Operative Neurosurgical Techniques

Indications, Methods and Results

Second Edition

Operative Neurosurgical Techniques

Indications, Methods and Results

Second Edition

Volume I

Edited by

Henry H. Schmidek, M.D., F.A.C.S.
Division of Neurosurgery
Department of Surgery
New England Deaconess Hospital
Harvard Medical School
Boston, Massachusetts

and

William H. Sweet, M.D., D.Sc.
Department of Neurosurgery
Massachusetts General Hospital
Harvard Medical School
Boston, Massachusetts

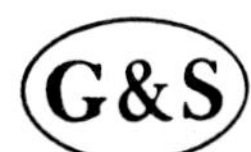

GRUNE & STRATTON, INC.

Harcourt Brace Jovanovich, Publishers
Orlando   New York   San Diego   London
San Francisco   Tokyo   Sydney   Toronto

Grune & Stratton, Inc.
Orlando, Florida   32887

Distributed in the United Kingdom by
Grune & Stratton, Ltd.
24/28 Oval Road, London NW 1

Library of Congress Catalog Number 87-082817
International Standard Book Number 0-8089-1862-1
Printed in the United States of America
87 88 89 90   10 9 8 7 6 5 4 3 2 1

Contents

1. **Surgery of the Scalp**
Peter C. Linton and David W. Leitner   1

2. **Repair of Defects of the Skull**
Michael S. Olin   11

3. **Surgical Management of Acute Head Injuries**
George F. Gade and Donald P. Becker   19

4. **Surgical Management of Acute and Chronic Subdural Hematoma**
J. Douglas Miller   33

5. **Surgical Management of Gunshot Wounds of the Head**
Maurice I. Saba   37

6. **Penetrating Missile Injuries of the Head**
Eugene D. George and T. Forcht Dagi   49

7. **The Management of Cerebrospinal Fluid Leaks**
T. Forcht Dagi and Eugene D. George   57

8. **Surgical Management of Intracranial and Intraspinal Infections**
R. Lewis Wright   71

9. **A Surgical Management of Tuberculosis, Cysticerocis, and Fungal Infections of the Central Nervous System**
R. Bhatia and P. N. Tandon   79

10. **Neurosurgical Aspects of Neurocysticercosis**
Francisco Escobedo   93

11. **Anesthetic Considerations and Techniques in Pediatric Neurosurgical Patients**
Mounir N. Abou-Madi and Davy Trop   103

12. **Management of Neurosurgical Problems in the Neonate**
R. Michael Scott   117

13. **Surgical Management of Craniosynostosis and Craniofacial Abnormalities**
Steven L. Wald and Henry H. Schmidek   125

14. **Surgical Management of Hydrocephalus**
Mel. H. Epstein   141

15. **Surgical Management of Meningoceles and Myelomeningoceles**
A. Loren Amacher   151

16. **Occult Spinal Dysraphism: Recognition and Surgical Management**
Paul H. Chapman   163

17. **Spinal Cord Tumors in Children**
Fred J. Epstein and Jeffrey H. Wisoff   175

18. **Current Surgical Management of Scoliosis and Kyphosis**
Morey S. Moreland   187

19. **Intraoperative Ultrasonography in Neurosurgery**
Robert A. Kane, Daniel H. O'Leary, and Ernest S. Mathews   213

20. **The Laser and Ultrasonic Aspirator in Neurosurgery**
Steven L. Wald and Henry H. Schmidek   223

21. **The Differential Diagnosis and Investigation of Unilateral and Bilateral Exophthalmos**
Don C. Bienfang   229

22. **Intraorbital Tumors**
Edgar M. Housepian   235

23. **Anterior and Lateral Microsurgical Approaches to Orbital Pathology**
Melvin G. Alper and Phil A. Aitken   245

24. **Sphenoethmoid Approach to the Optic Nerve**
Robert A. Sofferman   269

25. **Gliomas of the Anterior Visual Pathways**
William H. Sweet, Shirley H. Wray, and Paul F. New 279

26. **Surgical Management of Seller and Parasellar Lesions**
Peter Black and Nicholas T. Zervas 299

27. **Transsphenoidal Approach to Lesions in and about the Sella Turcica**
Edward R. Laws, Jr. 309

28. **Techniques of Reconstruction of the Sella and Related Structures**
Renata Spanziante, Enrico de Divitiis, and Paolo Cappabianca 321

29. **Transethmoidal Approach to the Pituitary**
Charles W. Cummings and Jonas Johnson 339

30. **Stereotactic Thermal Hypophysectomy**
Nicholas T. Zervas 345

31. **Craniopharyngiomas (With a note of Rathke's Cleft or Epithelial Cysts and on Suprasellar Cysts)**
William H. Sweet 349

32. **Transcallosal Approach to Tumors of the Third Ventricle**
Bennett M. Stein 381

33. **Transcallosal Interiornicial Exposure of Lesions of the Third Ventricle**
Michael L. J. Apuzzo 389

34. **Considerations in the Management of Masses in the Pineal Region**
Henry H. Schmidek 397

35. **Supracerebellar Approach for Pineal Region Neoplasms**
Bennett M. Stein 401

36. **The Occipital Transtentorial Approach to the Pineal Region**
Kemp Clark 411

37. **Brain Biopsy: Indications, Methods, and Complications**
Anthony Salerni, Steven Wald, and Henry H. Schmidek 419

38. **Neurologic Endoscopy**
C. Hunter Shelden, Skip Jacques, and Harold R. Lutes 423

39. **Surgical Management of Intracranial Gliomas**
Carrie L. Walters and Henry H. Schmidek 431

40. **Surgical Management of Intracranial Metastasis**
Perry Black 451

41. **Localization and Biopsy of Intracranial Lesions with Computed Tomography and Magnetic Resonance Imaging**
Robert J. Coffey and L. Dade Lunsford 463

41C. **Commentary: Stereotactic Techniques Using the Brown-Roberts-Wells Stereotactic Frame**
Peter Black 475

42. **Computed Tomographic and Magnetic Resonance Imaging Based Stereotactic Resection of Deep-Seated Intracranial Tumors**
Patrick J. Kelly 481

43. **Stereotactic Biopsy and Implantation of Radionuclides Guided by Computed Tomographic and Magnetic Resonance Imaging for Therapy of Brain Tumors**
F. Mundinger 491

44. **Stereotactic Radiosurgery with the Cobalt 60 Gamma Unit in the Surgical Treatment of Intracranial Tumors and Arteriovenous Malformations**
Ladislau Steiner 515

45. **Surgical Management of Olfactory Groove, Suprasellar, and Medical Sphenoid Wing Meningiomas**
Robert G. Ojemann and Karl W. Swann 531

46. **Preoperative Evaluation and Management of Meningiomas**
Robert E. Maxwell and Shelly N. Chou 547

47. **Convexity Meningiomas and General Principles of Meningioma Surgery**
Robert E. Maxwell and Shelly N. Chou 555

48. **Parasagittal and Falx Maningiomas**
Robert E. Maxwell and Shelly N. Chou 563

49. **Posterior Fossa Meningiomas**
Robert E. Maxwell and Shelley N. Chou 571

50. **Surgical Management of Lateral Intraventricular Tumors**
Dennis D. Spencer, William Collins, and Kimberlee J. Sass 583

51. **Surgical Approaches to Intraventricular Meningiomas of the Trigone**
Cecil L. Jun and Stephen L. Nutik 597

52. **Surgical Management of Extensive Tumors Involving the Skull and the Scalp**
Howard A. Richter 601

53. **Craniofacial Resection**
Narayan Sundaresan   609

54. **The Transbasal Approach to Tumors Invading the Base of the Skull**
Patrick J. Dermone   619

55. **Surgical Treatment of Tumors of the Clivus and Basloccipital Region**
R. B. Snow and R. R. Patterson, Jr   635

56. **Surgical Management of Tumors of the Tentorium and Clivus**
Edward Tarlov   647

57. **Surgical Management of Posterior Fossa Tumors**
John Duckworth and Henry H. Schmidek   653

58. **Transtemporal Approaches to the Poster Cranial Fossa**
Gale Gardner, Jon H. Robertson, and W. Craig Clark   665

59. **Tumors of the Cerebellopontine Angle: Clinical Features and Surgical Management**
William A. Buchheit and Robert H. Rosenwasser   673

60. **The Translabyrinthine Operation for the Removal of Acoustic Nerve Tumors**
T. T. King and A. W. Morrison   685

61. **Surgical Correction of Facial Palsy**
David W. Leitner   705

62. **The Surgical Treatment of Primary Brain Stem Tumors**
A. Konovalov and J. Atieh   709

63. **Glomus Jugulare Tumors—Skull Base Surgery**
Gale Gardner, James T. Robertson, Jon H. Robertson, Edwin W. Cocke, Jr., and W. Craig Clark   739

64. **Surgical Therapy of Diseases of the Extracranial Carotid Artery**
Robert A. Ratcheson and Robert L. Grubb   753

65. **Exposure of the Distal Internal Carotid Artery**
Calvin B. Ernst   765

66. **Surgical Management of Extracranial Lesions of the Vetebral Artery**
Edward F. Downing   771

67. **Direct Brain Revascularization**
Robert M. Crowell and Jafar J. Jafar   783

68. **Moyamoya Disease**
Tsuneyoshi Eguchi and Kazuo Ugajin   797

69. **Posterior Fossa Revascularization**
James I. Ausman, Fernando G. Diaz, Dante F. Vacca, R. A. de los Reyes, Carl E. Shrontz, Jeffrey E. Pearce, and Randy Gehrig   807

70. **Treatment of Intracerebral Vascular Lesions with Balloon Catheters**
Gerard M. Debrun   819

VOLUME II

71. **Surgical Management of Internal Carotid Artery Aneurysms within the Cavernous Sinus**
Dwight Parkinson   837

72. **Techniques of Thrombosis of Carotid Cavernous Fistulae**
John F. Mullan   845

73. **Commentary on the Transvenous Treatment of Anterioinferior Duval Venous Fistulae**
Henry H. Schmidek and Joseph R. Madsen   849

74. **The Surgical Approach to Arteriovenous Malformations of the Lateral and Sigmoid Dural Sinuses**
Thoralf M. Sundt, Jr., David G. Piepgras, and Glenn S. Forbes   855

75. **Surgical Management of Lesions of the Dural Venous Sinuses**
R. M. Peardon Donaghy   863

76. **Surgical Management of Dural Sinus Lacerations**
John P. Kapp   875

77. **Surgical Management of Intracerebral Hemorrhage**
David G. Pieparas and Michael J. Redmond   881

78. **Stereotactic Evacuation of Intracerebral Hematomas**
Edward I. Kandel and Vjacheslav V. Peresedov   889

79. **Cranial Arteriovenous Malformations**
Alfred J. Luessenhop   899

80. **Surgical Management of Cranial Arteriovenous Malformations**
Francis W. Gannoche, Jr. and Russell H. Patterson, Jr   905

81. **Proton Beam Therapy for Aeteriovenous Malformations of the Brain**
Raymond N. Kjellberg   911

82. **Surgical Treatment of Carotid Ophthalmic Aneurysms**
Jafar J. Jafar, Robert M. Crowell, and Roberto Heros   917

83. **Surgical Management of Aneurysms of the Internal Carotid: Posterior Communicating, Anterior Choroidal, and Bifurcation Aneurysms**
Henry H. Schmidek   929

84. **Surgical Treatment of Anterior Communicating Artery Aneurysms**
Robert M. Crowell and Jafar J. Jafar   939

85. **Surgical Management Aneurysms of the Middle Cerebral Artery**
Lindsay Symon   957

86. **Surgical Techniques of Posterior Cerebral Aneurysms**
Sidney J. Peerless and Charles G. Drake   973

87. **Surgical Management of Traumatic Aneurysms**
Dwight Parkinson   991

88. **Surgical Management of Bacterial Intracranial Aneurysms**
Robert G. Ojemann   997

89. **Treatment of Multiple and Asymptomatic Aneurysms**
Ronald Brisman   1003

90. **Stereotactic Clipping of Arterial Aneurysms and Arteriovenous Malformations of the Brain**
Edward I. Kandel and Vyacheslav V. Peresedov   1009

91. **Management of Unclippable Aneurysms**
Roberto C. Heros   1023

92. **Functional Neurosurgery**
Philip L. Goldenberg   1035

93. **Treatment of Intractable Psychiatric Illness and Chronic Pain by Stereotactic Cingulotomy**
H. Thomas Ballantine and Ida E. Giriunas   1069

94. **Intraventricular Morphine in the Treatment of Pain Secondary to Cancer**
Alberto Lenzi, Giuseppe Galli, and Giovanni Marini   1077

95. **Analgesia Induced by Brain Stimulation with Chronically Implanted Electrodes**
Yoshio Hosobuchi   1089

96. **Surgical Management of Disorders of the Lower Cranial Nerves**
Ronald I. Apfelbaum   1097

97. **Percutaneous Rhizotomy in the Treatment of Intractable Facial Pain (Trigeminal, Glossopharyngeal, and Vagal Nerves)**
John Tew, Jr. and Harry van Loveren   1111

97C. **Commentary: Percutaneous Rhizotomy**
William H. Sweet   1125

98. **Tetrogasserian Glycerol Injection as Treatment for Trigeminal**
William H. Sweet   1129

99. **Complications of Percutaneous Rhizotomy and Microvascular Decompression Operations for Facial Pain**
William H. Sweet and Charles E. Poletti   1139

100. **Intraspinal and Intraventricular Implantable Systems and Agents for Long-Term Relief of Cancer Pain**
Charles E. Poletti, William H. Sweet, Henry H. Schmidek, and Robert N. Pilon   1145

101. **Open Cordotomy Medullary Tractomy**
Charles E. Poletti   1155

102. **Dorsal Root Entry Zone Thermocoagulation**
D. G. T. Thomas   1169

103. **Longitundinal (Bishof's) Myelotomy**
Leslie P. Ivan   1177

104. **Commisural Myelotomy**
John E. Adams, Robert Lippert, and Yoshio Hosobuchi   1185

105. **Percutaneous Cordotomy: The Lateral High Cervical Technique**
Ronald R. Tasker   1191

106. **Percutaneous Electrothermocoagulation of Spinal Nerve Trunk, Ganglion, and Rootlets**
Sumio Uematsu   1207

107. **Surgery of Epilepsy—Current Technique of Cortical Resection**
Robert R. Hansebout   1223

108. **Cerebral Hemispherectomy: Indications, Methods, and Results**
Theodore Rasmussen   1235

109. **Section of the Corpus Callosum for Epilepsy**
David W. Roberts   1243

110. **Selective Vestibular Nerve Transection in the Treatment of Meniere's Disease**
Richard R. Gacek   1251

111. **Surgical Management of Spasmodic Torticollis and Adult-Onset Dystonia with Emphasis on Selective Denervation**
Claude M. Bertrand   1261

Contributors

Mounir N. Abou-Madi, M.B., Ch.B., F.R.C.P.(C), Department of Anesthesiology, Montreal Neurological Hospital and Institute, and McGill University, Montreal, Quebec, Canada

John E. Adams, M.D., Department of Neurological Surgery, University of California, San Francisco, San Francisco, California

Phil A. Aitken, M.D., Division of Ophthalmology, University of Vermont College of Medicine, Burlington, Vermont

Melvin G. Alper, M.D., Departments of Ophthalmology and Neurological Surgery, The George Washington University School of Medicine and the Washington Hospital Center, Washington, D.C.

A. Loren Amacher, M.D., Department of Neurosurgery, University of Connecticut, Farmington, Connecticut

Ronald I. Apfelbaum, M.D., Division of Neurosurgery, University of Utah Health Sciences Center, Salt Lake City, Utah

Michael L. J. Apuzzo, M.D., Department of Neurological Surgery, University of Southern California School of Medicine, Los Angeles, California

J. Atieh, M.D., Burdenko Institute of Neurosurgery, Moscow, Union of Soviet Socialist Republics

James I. Ausman, M.D., Ph.D., Department of Neurological Surgery, Henry Ford Hospital, Detroit, Michigan

H. Thomas Ballantine, M.D., Department of Neurological Surgery, Massachusetts General Hospital, Boston, Massachusetts

Janet W. Bay, M.D., Department of Neurological Surgery, Cleveland Clinic Foundation, Cleveland, Ohio

Donald P. Becker, M.D., Division of Neurosurgery, School of Medicine, University of California at Los Angeles, Los Angeles, California

Claude M. Bertrand, M.D., Division of Neurosurgery, Hospital Notre Dame and University of Montreal, Montreal, Quebec, Canada

R. Bhatia, M.S. (Surg), M.Ch. (Neuro), Department of Neurosurgery, All India Institute of Medical Sciences, New Delhi, India

Don C. Bienfang, M.D., Department of Ophthalmology, Brigham and Women's Hospital, Boston, Massachusetts

Perry Black, M.D., Department of Neurosurgery, Hahnemann University, Philadelphia, Pennsylvania

Peter McL. Black, M.D., Neurosurgical Service, Brigham and Women's Hospital, Boston, Massachusetts

Ronald Brisman, M.D., Department of Neurological Surgery, College of Physicians and Surgeons of Columbia University, Neurological Institute of New York, New York, New York

William A. Buchheit, M.D., Department of Neurosurgery, Temple University Health Science Center, Philadelphia, Pennsylvania

Robert C. Cantu, M.D., Neurosurgical Service, Department of Surgery, Emerson Hospital, Concord, Massachusetts

Paolo Cappabianca, M.D., Department of Functional Neurosurgery, Institute of Neurosurgery, University of Naples, Naples, Italy

112. **Surgery of the Sympathetic Nervous System**
Russell W. Hardy, Jr. and Janet W.
Bay   1271

113. **Craniovertebral Abnormalities and their
Treatment**
John C. VanGilder and Arnold H.
Menezes   1281

114. **Surgical Treatment of Rheumatoid Arthritis,
Ankylosing Spondylitis, and Paget's Disease
with Neurologic Deficit**
Ghaus M. Malik and James L. Sanders,
Jr.   1295

115. **Microsurgery of Syringomyelia and
Syringomyelic Cord Syndrome**
Albert L. Rhoton, Jr.   1307

116. **Anterior Cervical Disc Excision in the Treatment
of Cervical Spondylosis**
Henry H. Schmidek and Donald A.
Smith   1327

117. **Cervical Discography, Discometry, Cervical Disc
Distention Test**
William H. Sweet and Henry H.
Schmidek   1343

118. **Posterior Operations for Cervical Disc
Herniation and Spondylotic Myelopathy**
James C. Collias and Melville P.
Roberts   1347

119. **The Transthoracic Approach to the
Thoracolumbar Spine for Decompression and
Spinal Stabilization**
Henry H. Schmidek   1359

120. **Transthoracic Disc Excision**
Frederic A. Simeone and Ralph
Rashbaum   1367

121. **Lumbar Disc Excision**
Bernard Finneson   1375

121C. **Commentary: Lumbar Disc Excision**
Edward Tarlov   1393

122. **Microsurgical Lumbar Disc Excision**
Robert E. Harbaugh   1395

122C. **Commentary: Microsurgical Lumbar
Discectomy**
Richard L. Saunders   1399

123. **Posterior Lumbar Interbody Fusion**
Paul M. Lin   1401

124. **Anterior Lumbar Discectomy and Interbody
Fusion: Indications and Technique**
J. Leonard Goldner, Kenneth E. Wood, and James
R. Urbaniak   1421

125. **Chemonucleolysis**
Walter William Whisler   1437

125C. **Commentary: Chymopapain**
Charles A. Fager   1443

126. **Surgical Management of Trauma to the Spine**
David Yashon   1449

127. **Techniques of Fusion in the Cervical, Thoracic,
and Lumbar Spine**
Robert C. Cantu   1471

128. **Surgical Management of Thoracolumbar
Fractures: Indications, Methods, Results**
Carrie L. Walters and Henry H.
Schmidek   1481

129. **Surgical Management of Spinal Cord Tumors
and Arteriovenous Malformations**
Kalmon D. Post and Bennett M. Stein   1487

130. **Spinal Deformities Following Neurosurgical
Procedures in Children**
Edwin G. Fischer and John E. Hall   1509

131. **Metastatic Tumors of the Spine**
Eugene A. Quindlen   1515

132. **Surgical Approaches to Primary and Metastatic
Tumors of the Spine**
Narayan Sundaresan, George V. DiGiacinto, and
James E. O. Hughes   1525

133. **The Management of Malignant Epidural Tumors
Compressing the Spinal Cord**
Tzony Siegal and Tali Siegel   1539

134. **Surgery of the Peripheral Nerves and Brachial
Plexus**
Robert D. Leffert   1563

135. **Surgical Management of Peripheral Entrapment
Neuropathy**
Henry A. Young   1583

136. **Peripheral Nerve Tumors**
Alan R. Hudson, Fred Gentili, and David
Kline   1599

**The complete index appears following chapters
70 and 136.**

CHAPTER 1
Surgery of the Scalp

Peter C. Linton   David W. Leitner

THE SCALP is a vascular barrier that protects the skull and its contents and is a tight, unyielding cover that often presents a challenge when it must be closed or when coverage is needed.

This chapter is directed toward the neurosurgeon faced with a scalp closure problem. We shall therefore deal specifically with those characteristics of the scalp that cause these problems, some aspects of the closure of the defect, and last, the closure of some specific defects. It should be noted, however, that the principles of wound closure are paramount; to paraphrase Gertrude Stein, ''A hole is a hole is a hole.'' The origin of the defect is often irrelevant to the method of closure.

HISTORICAL BACKGROUND

The Egyptians as early as 3000 BC recognized that the uncovered and unprotected skull threatened life. In the United States, Patrick Vance (1776) treated scalping injuries by boring holes less than 1 inch apart with an awl, expecting healing to occur by epithelialization within 2 years.[1] Free skin grafting (Reverdin, 1869; Lawson, 1870; Ollie, 1872; Thiersch, 1874) greatly shortened time, and the discovery of methods for local and distant tissue transfer allowed early closure of even larger defects. The more recent additions of microvascular revascularization of scalp avulsions, microvascular free flaps, and skin expansion techniques have given surgeons the technology to close even the largest defects with relative safety.

ANATOMY

The five layers of the scalp consist of a tightly adherent sandwich of three layers loosely fitted over the periosteum. The first three layers are the skin, the subcutaneous tissue through which the major blood vessels run, and the galea aponeurotica. The galea is the fascia of the paired occipitofrontalis muscles (epicranium), which originate on the occipital skull, and is continuous with the fascia of the occipital and frontal muscles. These three layers are densely bound together by fibrous sheets and septa. Separating this sandwich from the periosteum is a loose connective tissue space that is the usual plane of avulsion, hematoma, or pus accumulation (the subepicranial space).

CIRCULATION

The circulation in the scalp is so rich that large flaps on tiny pedicles will often survive on their random or axial circulation. Because of the possibilities of microvascular anastomosis of free flaps, however, a more precise knowledge of the location of major vascular pedicles has gained greater importance.

The major circulation comes from three branches of the external carotid artery that anastomose richly across the midline and with each other. The occipital artery, the superficial temporal artery, and the posterior auricular artery run superficial to the galea, perforating the fascia high in the neck. The supraorbital artery is a terminal branch of the internal carotid and may anastomose with the external carotid through the angular artery. It perforates the galea at the supraorbital ridge. It is rarely available for anastomoses in trauma but is useful in an axial midline forehead flap.

The most useful of these vesseis is the large superficial temporal artery, which bifurcates just anterior to the external auditory canal into the frontal and parietal branches.

SENSATION

The anterior scalp is innervated by the ophthalmic division of the fifth cranial nerve through the supraorbital and supratrochlear nerves. The innervation of the posterior scalp comes from the second cervical nerve through the greater occipital nerve, and the temporal area from the maxillary division of the fifth cranial nerve.

GENERAL PRINCIPLES of DEFECT MANAGEMENT

As in any surgical effort, the completeness of the initial evaluation of the defect is critical. Many times an apparently large traumatic scalp defect is capable of being closed primarily after debridement, irrigation, and blunt mobilization in the areolar plane beneath the galea.

ASSESSMENT

The assessment of the defect should include the following:

1. Actual measured size.
2. Vascularity of the local tissue.
3. Nature of the defect bed, i.e. pericranium versus cortical bone.
4. Character and abundance of local tissue.
5. Potential for simple camouflage.

OPERATIVE NEUROSURGICAL TECHNIQUES
ISBN 0-8089-1862-1

Size

Measurement should be done before excision of scalp lesions or, in defects that are already present, with the slack in the edges taken up by gentle pulling. The real defect may be much smaller than is at first apparent because the edges of the wound retract.

Local vascularity

The choice of reconstruction depends upon the blood supply available to the graft. If the supply in the area of the defect is adequate, free grafting may suffice. If local supply is inadequate either because of scarring, radiation effects, or exposed bone, the graft must carry its own circulation for a successful take.

Nature of Defect Bed

The nature of the bed of the defect relates both to the circulation available for the graft and to the need for protecting the underlying structures. Exposed diploic bone will easily support a simple skin graft, as will the dura; however, a skin graft on the dura would hardly suffice for long-term protection of the brain.

Local Tissue Availability

The easiest reconstruction usually is accomplished with local tissue, and this will often be the first consideration. If tissue can be mobilized by the flap techniques to be described with primary closure of the donor site, then the most efficient closure will be accomplished.

Potential for Camouflage

The need for complex flap closure may be obviated if the defect can be covered by a simple change of hair style or by a hair piece or a hat.

CHOICE OF AVAILABLE RECONSTRUCTIONS

The reconstructive techniques for soft tissue applicable to scalp defects include all of those available in the management of defects elsewhere. Listed in general order of decreasing indications, these are:

1. Split thickness grafts. These are partial thicknesses of skin containing epidermis and variable thicknesses of dermis.
2. Full-thickness skin grafts. These consist of a complete thickness of skin with epidermis and dermis but without subcutaneous fat.
3. Local attached flaps. These flaps contain skin and subcutaneous tissue and carry their own circulation during transfer.
4. Distant detached flaps. Skin and subcutaneous tissue from a distant noncontiguous area is used that carries its own circulation during the transfer process until circulation is established in the recipient area. The flap then is detached from the donor vessels.
5. Distant reattached flaps (free flaps). Tissue is harvested from a distant donor site with its vascular supply included; this tissue is revascularized by microsurgical anastomosis at the recipient site. Such flaps include skin and subcutaneous tissue, musculocutaneous flaps, muscle flaps with skin grafts and omentum with an overlying skin graft.
6. Scalp expansion. Gradual expansion of adjacent scalp with subsequent advancement into the defect.

FREE SKIN GRAFTS

Free grafts containing epidermis and more or less dermis represent the first line of reconstruction of scalp defects. Two general principles govern their selection: (1) the thicker the graft, the lower the percentage of take; and (2) the more dermis that is included, the less the contraction. In large defects, such as in a granulating burn wound, initial closure may be done best by covering the wound with a thin, meshed graft even though reconstruction with flaps may be planned at a later date. The general principle of initial conversion of an untidy wound into a clean, closed wound with a temporary thin split graft is still a cornerstone of plastic surgery in any area of the body and will often convert an urgent situation into an elective one and give the best chance of success for a complex reconstruction at a later date.

The thickness of dermis in the graft determines the eventual contracture of the recipient bed. This fact can be used in defect management by intentionally selecting a thin graft in those defects where contraction over a long period of time will tend to minimize the defect. A thin split graft may contract 60 to 70 percent in area over the period of a year, gradually pulling in the edges of the wound to a degree that would be impossible to achieve at the time of initial closure because of suture necrosis. If this biologic process is not accompanied by dysfunction or deformity, it can be used in scalp reconstruction.

DONOR SITES

Free grafts can be harvested from any site. Grafts retain the characteristics of the donor site, therefore color match and texture can sometimes be preselected. Because of the occasional hypertrophic or keloidal scar that results at the donor site, whenever feasible the graft should be taken from an area that can be easily hidden by ordinary clothing. The upper thigh-lateral buttock area is perhaps the best of these donor sites and can be covered by most types of clothing.

TECHNIQUES

A split graft can be taken by any standard method, i.e., free-hand knife or one of the various dermatomes. Because the free graft must regain circulation from the recipient bed, close coaption of the graft to the bed is essential. Failure of the graft to take inevitably arises from the interposition of pus, clot, or serum between the graft and the bed, and this must be prevented. Pressure on the graft is most easily achieved with a tied-over stent dressing using enough bulk so that the resulting force is downward (Figure 1-1).

The full-thickness graft is cut by standard scalpel excision and is clearly limited in size to those donor sites where primary suture closure is possible. These include the retroauricular area where a graft 3×5 cm can be taken, the hairless supraclavicular area, and the groin crease. Since these grafts include all of the dermis, hair follicles will be transferred; therefore care must be taken in selection of the donor site. The graft is meticulously sutured to the defect, and a tie-over stent is applied as in a split-thickness graft. Unless suggestions of infection occur, there is no need to dress free grafts for 5 or more days. Disruption

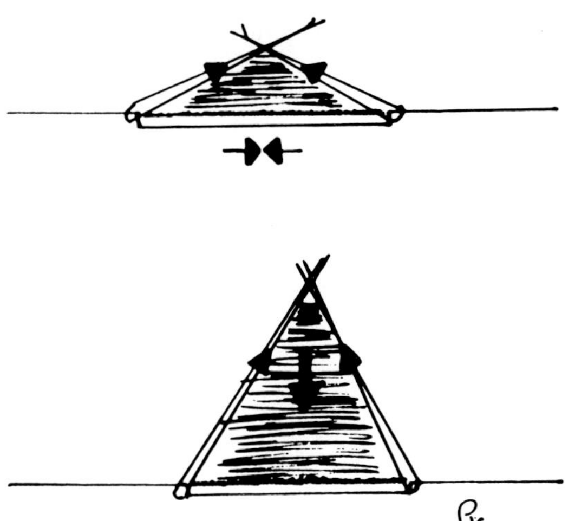

Fig. 1-1. (Top) Incorrect skin graft dressing. Inadequate bulk causes compressive distortion of the defect when the tie-over sutures are tied. (Bottom) Correct dressing. A large bulk of dressing converts the upward pull of the tie-over sutures into a downward force on the graft and the defect.

of the graft–defect interface can occur up to 7 to 10 days after grafting, and the fresh graft needs protection for that period.

FLAP THEORY

In order to successfully move a flap, knowledge of the skin circulation is essential. The end circulation to the skin (epidermis and dermis) lies in a random network of fine vessels in the subdermal plexus. This network is fed by different systems, depending upon the location. In some locations (e.g., head, groin, and finger) the subdermal plexus is the terminal branch of known arteries and veins running in the axis of the skin. In other areas (e.g., skin over the gastrocnemius muscle) the plexus is fed by perforating vessels from the underlying muscle.

This anatomic variance then defines the three types of available flaps; the random flap, the axial flap, and the musculocutaneous flap. In the scalp the circulation is primarily axial, with the intervening areas between large known vessels being of random circulation. Large flaps are therefore successful as long as the circulatory system between the galea and the skin is not violated either by poor flap design or by obstruction of venous

return by tight closure or by the accumulation of fluid between the galea and the pericranium.

LOCAL ATTACHED FLAPS

The basic concept of local flap transfer is to move available tissue with its circulation intact from an area of excess to an area of deficiency. In the scalp, the only areas of excess are laterally and posteriorly, since the movement of tissue from the anterior scalp causes distortion of the forehead and hairline. Although a profusion of complex local flaps have appeared in the literature, most are variants of the rotation flap and this will be dealt with in detail.

In any flap transfer, the surgeon must deal with the donor defect. On occasion, transfer of a local flap is essential to cover bare bone or exposed dura and the flap donor defect, over the pericranium, simply can be free grafted. The hairless free graft, however, is a noticeable deformity and should be avoided if possible.

ROTATION FLAPS

Planning a rotation flap requires an understanding of a simple geometric concept. Tissue is added to the defect by subtracting from the flap donor area, and the only way this can be effective is to change the defect shape from unclosable to closable. If the defect is a square 2 inches on a side, the total area is 4 in^2. Movement of a flap to fill a 4 in^2 defect creates a 4 in^2 donor defect. Primary closure will be impossible because of necrosis caused by excess suture tension. If a 10-inch-long circular incision could be made, the resulting flap would rotate into the defect, leaving an elliptical defect 10 inches long but still having a total area of 4 in^2. Because of the change in shape of the defect, primary closure might then be possible, since the maximum width of the defect would be 0.5 inch or less (Figure 1-2). In practice this requires that the flap be generous in size. Many problems arise from inexperienced surgeons because they use a flap that is too small. This results from a failure to grasp the geometry of design. The ideal defect should be triangular, suggesting the shape of a segment of pie, with the flap representing the remaining pie.

In some situations, single, long, large flaps are not possible and double or triple flaps can be planned on the same geometric principle (Figure 1-3).

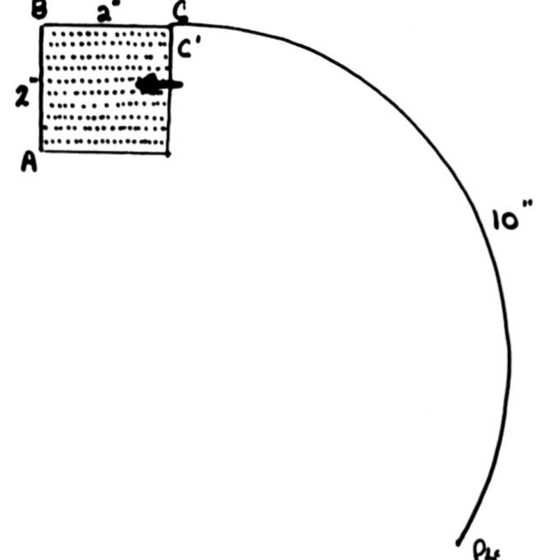

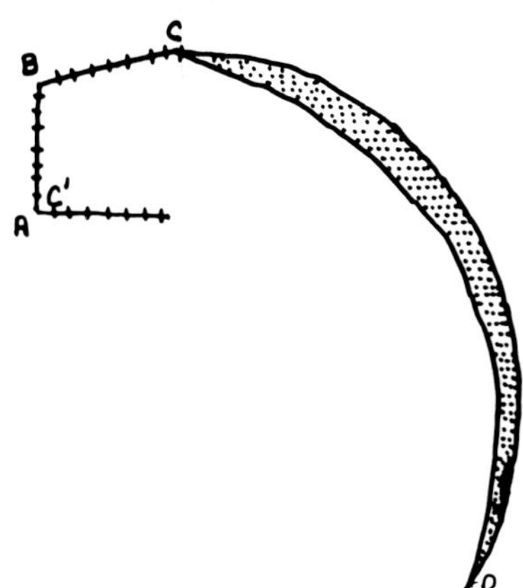

Fig. 1-2. The geometry of a standard rotation flap. The total area of the defect (stippled) remains the same even though the shape changes.

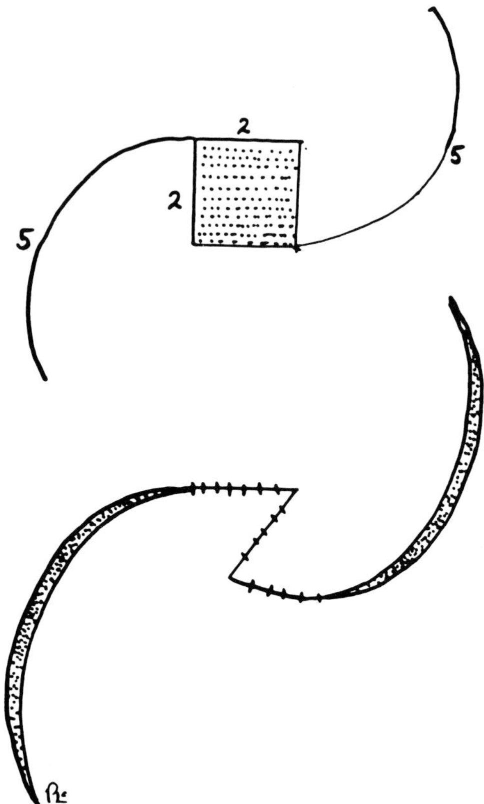

Fig. 1-3. A double-flap variation of a standard rotation flap. The geometry is unchanged but results in two elliptical donor defects rather than one.

TECHNIQUES

The defect as well as the location and quantity of available excess tissue should be evaluated, and a plan drawn on the scalp. The carpenter's adage "Measure twice, cut once" is of primary importance. A pattern of the flap then should be made with gauze dressing or a sterile towel and the flap pattern moved into the defect to assess the "fit." If easy rotation does not occur, the plan must be redone until it works, or another plan should be considered. Only when the pattern fits should the flap be incised, through the skin and galea but not through the pericranium. Elevation then can be done easily by blunt dissection to the base or beyond in the areolar plane found at this level. Minimal bleeding will be encountered except at the skin edges. If a bit of tension persists, the galea can be released by multiple shallow incisions from below with care taken to avoid

the vessels coursing to the flap that lie between the dermis and the galea. Rarely can more than a centimeter or so be gained by this maneuver, however, because the skin of the scalp itself is relatively stiff and inelastic. Suturing should commence at the original defect and usually consists of a simple layer of half-buried mattress sutures. The flap donor defect then can be closed or covered with skin grafts as required. At the point of flap rotation, a dog ear usually will occur. In general, this should be left for secondary adjustment after 3 to 4 weeks, since resection of this skin may interfere with flap circulation. Mild pressure dressings with or without drains usually are left undisturbed for 4 to 5 days unless trouble is suspected. The prevention of fluid accumulation beneath the flap is critical in preventing venous congestion in the flap. Virtually all flap failures are caused by venous obstruction rather than poor arterial flow and, if venous congestion is suspected, the prompt removal of tight sutures or a hematoma may restore circulation and save the flap.

BACK CUTTING

In any rotation flap, the axis of rotation is at A as depicted in Figure 1-4A. The movable length of the flap therefore is the line AB. If additional length is needed to reach point C as in Figure 1-4B (line CB), then an additional incision can be made at point A in the direction of line AB (dotted line) for the distance needed. This will result in advancement of the flap into the defect as well as rotation and will produce a donor defect as depicted in Figure 1-4C. The donor defect may well require skin grafting, but skin grafts usually do well on pericranium. The primary risk in back cutting is in narrowing the width of the flap base by the length of the back cut. This usually will not compromise circulation in the scalp, but it should be done with extreme care where the point of flap rotation and the back cut lie in an area known to contain major scalp vessels. In this situation, release of the galea from below and the skin from above may allow spreading dissection of the subcutaneous tissue with identification and preservation of visible vessels.

OTHER FLAPS

See the work of Juri,[2] Orticochea,[3] and others for details of other complex local flaps. Converse and Longacre[1] have reviewed this subject and the use of distant flaps in detail. It would be uncommon for the neurosurgeon to have to face these formidable challenges without the assistance of a plastic surgeon.

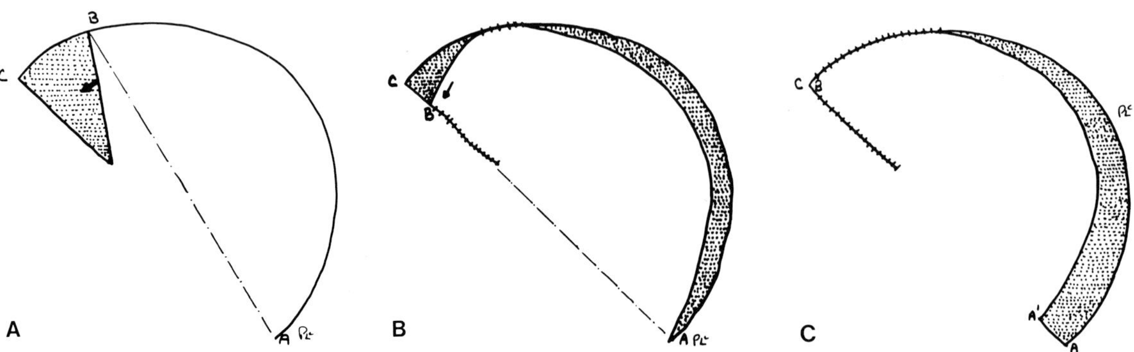

Fig. 1-4. The technique for back-cutting a rotation flap (see text for details).

Paul H. Chapman, M.D., Department of Neurological Surgery, Massachusetts General Hospital and the Harvard Medical School, Boston, Massachusetts

Shelly N. Chou, M.D., Ph.D., Department of Neurosurgery, University of Minnesota Hospitals, Minneapolis, Minnesota

Kemp Clark, M.D., Division of Neurological Surgery, Southwestern Medical School, The University of Texas Health Science Center at Dallas, Dallas, Texas

W. Craig Clark, M.D., Ph.D., Department of Neurosurgery, University of Tennessee-Memphis, Memphis, Tennessee

Edwin W. Cocke Jr., M.D., Department of Otolaryngology and Maxillofacial Surgery, University of Tennessee-Memphis, Memphis, Tennessee

Robert Coffey, M.D., Department of Neurological Surgery, University of Pittsburgh School of Medicine, Pittsburgh, Pennsylvania

James C. Collias, M.D., Department of Neurosurgery, Hartford Hospital, Hartford, Connecticut, and Division of Neurosurgery, University of Connecticut School of Medicine, Farmington, Connecticut

William F. Collins, M.D., Section of Neurological Surgery, Yale University School of Medicine, New Haven, Connecticut

Robert M. Crowell, M.D., Department of Neurological Surgery, University of Illinois College of Medicine, Chicago, Illinois

Charles W. Cummings, M.D., Department of Otolaryngology, University of Washington, Seattle, Washington

T. Forcht Dagi, M.D., Lt. Col. M.C., Neurosurgical Service, Walter Reed Army Medical Center, Washington, DC

Enrico De Divitiis, M.D., Department of Functional Neurosurgery, Institute of Neurosurgery, University of Naples, Naples, Italy

R. A. de los Reyes, M.D., Department of Neurological Surgery, Henry Ford Hospital, Detroit, Michigan

Gerard M. Debrun, M.D., Neuroradiology Section, The Johns Hopkins Hospital and the Johns Hopkins University School of Medicine, Baltimore, Maryland

P. J. Derome, M.D., Service de Neuro-Chirurgie, Centre Medico-Chirurgical Foch, Suresnes, France

Fernando G. Diaz, M.D., Ph.D., Department of Neurological Surgery, Henry Ford Hospital, Detroit, Michigan

George V. DiGiacinto, M.D., Division of Neurosurgery, St. Luke's-Roosevelt Hospital Center, and Department of Neurological Surgery, College of Physicians and Surgeons of Columbia University, New York, New York

R. M. Peardon Donaghy, M.D., Division of Neurosurgery, University of Vermont College of Medicine, Burlington, Vermont

Edward F. Downing, M.D., Neurological Institute of Savannah, Savannah, Georgia

Charles G. Drake, M.D., Division of Neurosurgery, University of Western Ontario University Hospital, London, Ontario, Canada

John W. Duckworth, M.D., Division of Neurosurgery, University of Vermont College of Medicine, Burlington, Vermont

Tsuneyoshi Eguchi, M.D., Division of Neurological Surgery, Kameda General Hospital, Kamogawa, Japan

Fred J. Epstein, M.D., Division of Pediatric Neurosurgery, Department of Neurosurgery, New York University Medical Center, New York, New York

Mel H. Epstein, M.D., Department of Clinical Neurosciences, Brown University, and the Department of Neurosurgery, Rhode Island Hospital, Providence, Rhode Island

Calvin B. Ernst, M.D., Division of Vascular Surgery, Henry Ford Hospital, University of Michigan Medical School, Detroit, Michigan

Francisco Escobedo, M.D., Instituto Nacional de Neurologia y Neurocirugia, Mexico City, Mexico

Charles A. Fager, M.D., Department of Neurosurgery, Lahey Clinic Medical Center, Burlington, Massachusetts

Bernard E. Finneson, M.D., Low Back Pain Clinic, Crozer-Chester Medical Center, Chester, Pennsylvania, and Department of Neurosurgery, Hahnemann University, Philadelphia, Pennsylvania

Edwin G. Fischer, M.D., Department of Neurosurgery, Children's Hospital and Department of Surgery, Harvard Medical School, Boston, Massachusetts

Glenn S. Forbes, M.D., Department of Radiology, Mayo Clinic, Rochester, Minnesota

Richard R. Gacek, M.D., Department of Otolaryngology and Communication Sciences, State University of New York Health Science Center at Syracuse, Syracuse, New York

George F. Gade, M.D., Division of Neurosurgery, School of Medicine, University of California at Los Angeles, Los Angeles, California

Giuseppe Galli, M.D., Department of Neurosurgery, University of Brescia and the Regional General Hospital, Brescia, Italy

Francis W. Gamache Jr., M.D., Division of Neurological Surgery, Cornell University Medical College, New York, New York

Gale Gardner, M.D., Department of Otolaryngology and Maxillofacial Surgery, University of Tennessee-Memphis, Memphis, Tennessee

Randy Gehring, M.D., Department of Neurological Surgery, Henry Ford Hospital, Detroit, Michigan

Fred Gentili, M.D., Division of Neurosurgery, University of Toronto, Toronto, Ontario, Canada

Eugene D. George, M.D., Col. M.C., Neurosurgical Service, Walter Reed Army Medical Center, Washington, D.C.

Philip L. Gildenberg, M.D., Ph. D., Division of Neurosurgery, University of Texas Mecical School, Houston, Texas

Ida E. Giriunas, R.N., Department of Neurological Surgery, Massachusetts General Hospital, Boston, Massachusetts

J. Leonard Goldner, M.D., Department of Orthopaedic Surgery, Duke University School of Medicine, Durham, North Carolina

Robert L. Grubb, M.D., Department of Neurology and Neurological Surgery, Washington University School of Medicine, St. Louis, Missouri

John E. Hall, M.D., Department of Orthopedics, Children's Hospital, and Department of Orthopedics, Harvard Medical School, Boston, Massachusetts

Robert R. Hansebout, M.D., F.R.C.S.(C), Department of Surgery, McMaster University, St. Joseph's Hospital, Hamilton, Ontario, Canada

Robert F. Harbaugh, M.D., Section of Neurosurgery, Dartmouth-Hitchcock Medical Center, Hanover, New Hampshire

Russell W. Hardy Jr., M.D., Department of Neurological Surgery, Cleveland Clinic Foundation, Cleveland, Ohio

Roberto C. Heros, M.D., Department of Neurological Surgery, Massachusetts General Hospital, Boston, Massachusetts

Yoshio Hosobuchi, M.D., Department of Neurological Surgery, University of California, San Francisco, San Francisco, California

Edgar M. Housepian, M.D., Department of Neurological Surgery, Neurological Institute of New York, College of Physicians and Surgeons of Columbia University, New York, New York

Alan R. Hudson, M.D., Division of Neurosurgery, University of Toronto, Toronto, Ontario, Canada

James E. O. Hughes, M.D., Division of Neurosurgery, St. Luke's-Roosevelt Hospital Center, and Department of Neurological Surgery, College of Physicians and Surgeons of Columbia University, New York, New York

Leslie P. Ivan, M.D., F.R.C.S.(C), Division of Neurosurgery, School of Medicine, Faculty of Health Sciences, University of Ottawa, Ottawa, Ontario, Canada

Skip Jacques, M.D., Advanced Neurosurgical Laboratory, Huntington Medical Research Institutes, California Institute of Technology, Pasadena, California

Jafar J. Jafar, M.D., Department of Neurological Surgery, University of Illinois College of Medicine, Chicago, Illinois

Jonas Johnson, M.D., Department of Otolaryngology, University of Pittsburgh, Pittsburgh, Pennsylvania

Cecil L. Jun, M.D., Department of Neurosurgery, Kaiser-Permanente Medical Center, Redwood City, California

Edward I. Kandel, M.D., D.Sc., Neurosurgery Clinic, Institute of Neurology, Moscow, Union of Soviet Socialist Republics

Robert A. Kane, M.D., Department of Radiology, New England Deaconess Hospital, Boston, Massachusetts

John P. Kapp, M.D., Department of Neurosurgery, State University of New York, Buffalo, New York

Patrick J. Kelly, M.D., Department of Neurological Surgery, Mayo Clinic, Rochester, Minnesota

T. T. King, F.R.C.S., Department of Neurosurgery, The London Hospital, Whitechapel, London, England

Raymond N. Kjellbeg, M.D., Department of Neurological Surgery, Massachusetts General Hospital, Boston, Massachusetts

David Kline, M.D., Division of Neurosurgery, Louisiana State University, Baton Rouge, Louisiana

A. Konovalov, M.D., Burdenko Institute of Neurosurgery, Moscow, Union of Soviet Socialist Republics

George Krol, M.D., Department of Radiology, Memorial Sloan-Kettering Cancer Center and Cornell University Medical Center, New York, New York

Edward R. Laws Jr., M.D., Department of Neurologic Surgery, Mayo Clinic, Rochester, Minnesota

Robert D. Leffert, M.D., Department of Orthopedic Surgery and Department of Rehabilitation Medicine, Massachusetts General Hospital, and Harvard Medical School, Boston, Massachusetts

David W. Leitner, M.D., Assistant Professor of Surgery, Division of Plastic Surgery, University of Vermont College of Medicine, Burlington, Vermont

Alberto Lenzi, M.D., Department of Neurosurgery, University of Brescia and the Regional General Hospital, Brescia, Italy

Paul M. Lin, M.D., Jenkintown, Pennsylvania

Peter C. Linton, M.D., Associate Professor of Surgery, Division of Plastic Surgery, University of Vermont College of Medicine, Burlington, Vermont

Robert Lippert, M.D., Department of Neurological Surgery, University of California, San Francisco, San Francisco, California

Alfred J. Luessenhop, M.D., Division of Neurosurgery, Georgetown University Hospital, Washington, D.C.

L. Dade Lunsford, M.D., Departments of Neurological Surgery and Radiology, University of Pittsburgh School of Medicine, Pittsburgh, Pennsylvania

Harold R. Lutes, O.D., Advanced Neurosurgical Laboratory, Huntington Medical Research Institutes, California Institute of Technology, Pasadena, California

Joseph R. Madsen, M.D., Department of Neurological Surgery, Massachusetts General Hospital, Boston, Massachusetts

Ghaus M. Malik, M.D., Department of Neurological Surgery, Henry Ford Hospital, Detroit, Michigan

Giovanni Marini, M.D., Department of Neurosurgery, University of Brescia and the Regional General Hospital, Brescia, Italy

Ernest S. Mathews, M.D., Department of Neurosurgery, New England Deaconess Hospital, Boston, Massachusetts

Robert E. Maxwell, M.D., Ph.D., Department of Neurosurgery, University of Minnesota Hospitals, Minneapolis, Minnesota

Arnold H. Menezes, M.D., Division of Neurosurgery, University of Iowa, Iowa City, Iowa

J. Douglas Miller, M.D., Ph.D., F.R.C.S., F.A.C.S., F.R.C.P.E., Department of Surgical Neurology, University of Edinburgh, Edinburgh, Scotland

Morey S. Moreland, M.D., Department of Orthopaedics and Rehabilitation, University of Vermont College of Medicine, Burlington, Vermont

A. W. Morrison, M.D., Department of Otolaryngology, The London Hospital, Whitechapel, London, England

John F. Mullan, M.D., Neurological Surgery, The University of Chicago Medical Center, Chicago, Illinois

F. Mundinger, M.D., Abteilung Stereotaxie and Neuronuklearmedizin, Neurochirurgische Universitätsklinik, Freiburg, Federal Republic of Germany

Paul F. New, M.D., Neuroradiology Section, Massachusetts General Hospital, Boston, Massachusetts

Stephen L. Nutik, M.D., Ph.D., Department of Neurosurgery, Kaiser-Permanente Medical Center, Redwood City, California

Daniel H. O'Leary, M.D., Department of Radiology, New England Deaconess Hospital, Boston, Massachusetts

Robert G. Ojemann, M.D., Department of Neurological Surgery, Massachusetts General Hospital and Department of Surgery, Harvard Medical School, Boston, Massachusetts

Michael S. Olin, M.D., Department of Neurosurgery, St. Joseph Hospital, Providence, Rhode Island

Dwight Parkinson, M.D., Department of Surgery, The University of Manitoba, Winnipeg, Manitoba, Canada

Russel H. Patterson Jr., M.D., Division of Neurosurgery, The New York Hospital-Cornell Mecical Center, New York, New York

Jeffrey E. Pearce, M.D., Department of Neurological Surgery, Henry Ford Hospital, Detroit, Michigan

Sidney J. Peerless, M.D., Division of Neurosurgery, University of Western Ontario University Hospital, London, Ontario, Canada

Vyacheslav V. Peresedov, M.D., Neurosurgery Clinic, Institute of Neurology, Moscow, Union of Soviet Socialist Republics

David G. Piepgras, M.D., Department of Neurosurgery, Mayo Clinic, Rochester, Minnesota

Robert N. Pilon, M.D., Department of Anesthesia, Athens General Hospital, Athens, Georgia

Charles E. Poletti, M.D., Department of Neurological Surgery, Massachusetts General Hospital, Boston, Massachusetts

Kalmon D. Post, M.D., Department of Neurological Surgery, College of Physicians and Surgeons of Columbia University, New York, New York

Eugene A. Quindlen, M.D., Department of Neurological Surgery, University of South Alabama College of Medicine, Mobile, Alabama

Ralph Rashbaum, M.D., Division of Neurosurgery, University of Pennsylvania School Medicine, and Pennsylvania Hospital, Philadelphia, Pennsylvania

Theodore Rasmussen, M.D., Montreal Neurological Institute and Hospital, Montreal, Quebec, Canada

Robert A. Ratcheson, M.D., Division of Neurological Surgery, Case-Western Reserve University, University Hospitals of Cleveland, Cleveland, Ohio

Michael J. Redmond, M.D., Department of Neurological Surgery, Mayo Clinic, Rochester, Minnesota

Albert L. Rhoton Jr., M.D., Department of Neurological Surgery, University of Florida College of Medicine, Gainesville, Florida

Howard A. Richter, M.D., Division of Neurosurgery, Lankenau Hospital and the Thomas Jefferson Medical College, Philadelphia, Pennsylvania

David W. Roberts, M.D., Section of Neurosurgery, Dartmouth-Hitchcock Medical Center, Hanover, New Hampshire

Melville P. Roberts, M.D., Division of Neurosurgery, University of Connecticut School of Medicine, Farmington, Connecticut, and Hartford Hospital, Hartford, Connecticut

James T. Robertson, M.D., Department of Neurosurgery, University of Tennessee-Memphis, Memphis, Tennessee

Jon H. Robertson, M.D., Department of Neurosurgery, University of Tennessee-Memphis, Memphis, Tennessee

Robert H. Rosenwasser, M.D., Department of Neurosurgery and Physiology, Temple University Health Science Center, Philadelphia, Pennsylvania

Maurice I. Saba, M.D., Division of Neurosurgery, American University Hospital of Beirut, Beirut, Lebanon

Ved Sachdev, M.D., Department of Surgery, Mount Sinai Medical Center and Mount Sinai Medical School, New York, New York

Anthony Salerni, M.D., Division of Neurosurgery, University of Vermont College of Medicine, Burlington, Vermont

James L. Sanders Jr., M.D., Department of Neurological Surgery, Henry Ford Hospital, Detroit, Michigan

Kimberlee J. Sass, Ph.D., Section of Neurological Surgery, Yale University School of Medicine, New Haven, Connecticut

Richard L. Saunders, M.D., Section of Neurosurgery, Dartmouth-Hitchcock Medical Center, Hanover, New Hampshire

Henry H. Schmidek, M.D., Department of Surgery, New England Deaconess Hospital, and Harvard Medical School, Boston, Massachusetts

R. Michael Scott, M.D., F.A.C.S., Department of Neurosurgery, New England Medical Center Hospitals and Tufts University, Boston, Massachusetts

C. Hunter Shelden, M.D., Advanced Neurosurgical Laboratory, Huntington Medical Research Institutes, California Institute of Technology, Pasadena, California

Carl E. Shrontz, M.D., Department of Neurological Surgery, Henry Ford Hospital, Detroit, Michigan

Tali Siegal, M.D., Spinal Surgery Unit, Beilinson Medical Center, Petah Tivka, and the Department of Oncology and Neurology, Hadassah University Hospital, Jerusalem, Israel

Tzony Siegal, M.D., D.M.D., Spinal Surgery Unit, Beilinson Medical Center, Petah Tivka, and the Departments of Oncology and Neurology, Hadassah University Hospital, Jerusalem, Israel

Frederick A. Simeone, M.D., Division of Neurosurgery, University of Pennsylvania School of Medicine, and Pennsylvania Hospital, Philadelphia, Pennsylvania

Donald A. Smith, M.D., Division of Neurosurgery, University of Vermont College of Medicine, Burlington, Vermont

Robert B. Snow, M.D., Ph.D., Division of Neurosurgery, The New York Hospital-Cornell Medical Center, New York, New York

Robert A. Sofferman, M.D., Division of Otolaryngology, University of Vermont College of Medicine, Burlington, Vermont

Renato Spaziante, M.D., Department of Functional Neurosurgery, Institute of Neurosurgery, University of Naples, Naples, Italy

Dennis D. Spencer, M.D., Section of Neurological Surgery, Yale University School of Medicine, New Haven, Connecticut

Bennet M. Stein, M.D., Department of Neurosurgery, Neurological Institute of New York, Columbia-Presbyterian Medical Center, New York, New York

Ladislau Steiner, M.D., Stockholm, Sweden

Narayan Sundaresan, M.D., Division of Neurooncology, St. Luke's-Roosevelt Hospital Center and Department of Neurological Surgery, College of Physicians and Surgeons of Columbia University, New York, New York

Thoralf M. Sundt Jr., M.D., Department of Neurosurgery, Mayo Clinic, Rochester, Minnesota

Karl Swann, M.D., Department of Neurological Surgery, Massachusetts General Hospital, Boston, Massachusetts

William H. Sweet, M.D., D.Sc., D.H.C., Department of Neurological Surgery, Massachusetts General Hospital and the Department of Surgery, Harvard Medical School, Boston, Massachusetts

Lindsay Symon, T.D., F.R.C.S., F.R.C.S.E., Gough-Cooper Department of Neurological Surgery, Institute of Neurology, University of London, National Hospital, London, England

P. N. Tandon, M.S., F.R.C.S.(E), Department of Neurosurgery, All India Institute of Medical Sciences, New Delhi, India

Edward Tarlov, M.D., Department of Neurosurgery, Lahey Clinic Medical Center, Burlington, Massachusetts

Ronald R. Tasker, M.D., Division of Neurosurgery, Toronto General Hospital, and Department of Surgery, University of Toronto, Toronto, Ontario, Canada

John M. Tew Jr., M.D., Department of Neurosurgery, University of Cincinnati College of Medicine, Cincinnati, Ohio

D. G. T. Thomas, M.A., F.R.C.P.(Glas.), F.R.C.S.(Ed.), Department of Neurological Surgery, Institute of Neurology, The National Hospital, London, England

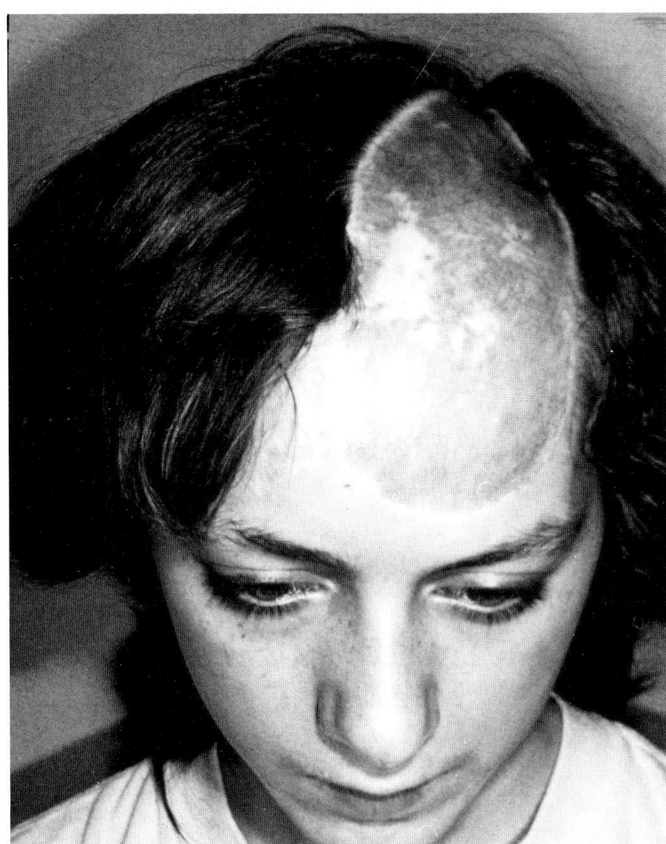

Fig. 1-5. The skin graft on the scalp after an avulsion injury suffered 10 years previously. (Reprinted from Argenta L: Controlled tissue expansion. Surgical Rounds 9:65, 1986. With permission.)

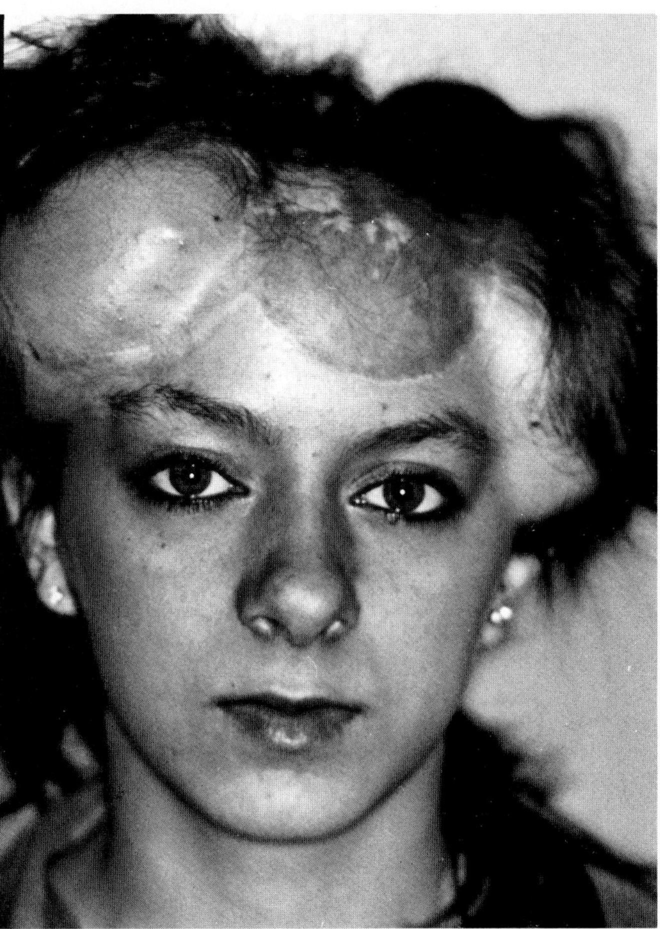

Fig. 1-6. The scalp was expanded 225 cc on each side. (Reprinted from Argenta L: Controlled tissue expansion. Surgical Rounds 9:65, 1986. With permission.)

TISSUE EXPANSION IN SCALP RECONSTRUCTION

The observation that skin expands to accomodate itself to gradual stretching was made in antiquity (i.e., the expansion of abdominal skin with pregnancy), but only recently has that observation been translated into a surgically useful principle. In 1978, Radovan[4] and, in 1982, Austed and Ross[5] published reports on the first clinically successful techniques of tissue expansion and demonstrated the prototypes of expanders clinically useful today. In essence, the expander is a silicone bag with a self-sealing fill valve that is placed beneath the tissue to be expanded. Expansion is then done percutaneously with incremental saline injections into the valve.

The morphology and pathophysiology of expanded tissue has been extensively studied.[6,7,8] In essence, the epidermis remains at its normal thickness; the dermis decreases in thickness but there is an increase in fibroblasts and myofibroblasts; the fat decreases in thickness as does muscle. A dense periprosthetic fibrous capsule develops with a marked increase in vascularity.

In the scalp, the expansion is planned in the normal scalp adjacent to the defect. The prosthesis is placed beneath the galea and expanded over a few months at 6- to 80-day intervals. With scalp expansion, the distance between hair follicles increases, but this should not be clinically noticeable.[9]

Following the desired expansion, the hairless scar is excised and primary closure accomplished by advancing the expanded scalp into the defect.[10] Disadvantages of scalp expansion include the need for two operations, the interim deformity, and an inability to apply the technique in situations of acute scalp loss. The latter disadvantage, however, can frequently be resolved by using a scalp flap to cover the cranial defect immediately with temporary skin grafts on pericranium to the flap donor site, then subsequent expansion of either the scalp flap or the unused scalp peripheral to the healed skin graft with removal of the hairless skin graft.

CASE REPORT

A 15-year-old girl had sustained a scalp avulsion at age 3 years, which had been treated with skin grafts (Figure 1-5). Two tissue expanders were expanded to 450 cc over 2 months (Figure 1-6). The graft was then excised and the expanded flaps closed primarily (Figures 1-7 and 1-8). (Case report courtesy of Dr. Louis C. Argenta, University of Michigan, and *Surgical Rounds.*)

SPECIFIC SCALP DEFECTS

CONGENITAL APLASIA OF THE SCALP

Congenital aplasia of the scalp (Aplasia cutis congenita) is a relatively rare deformity that usually appears as a scalp defect less than 2 cm in diameter in the midline over the posteriorfontanelle. The common course is for spontaneous healing to occur, resulting in a hairless scar. Skull defects occur in only 20 percent of cases. According to Lynch and Kahn,[11] associated anomalies can include hydrocephalus, myelomeningoceles, finger deformities, or clefts of the lip and palate. Thrombosis of the sagittal sinus has been reported. Management is the same as for any scalp defect and usually consists of rotation flaps.

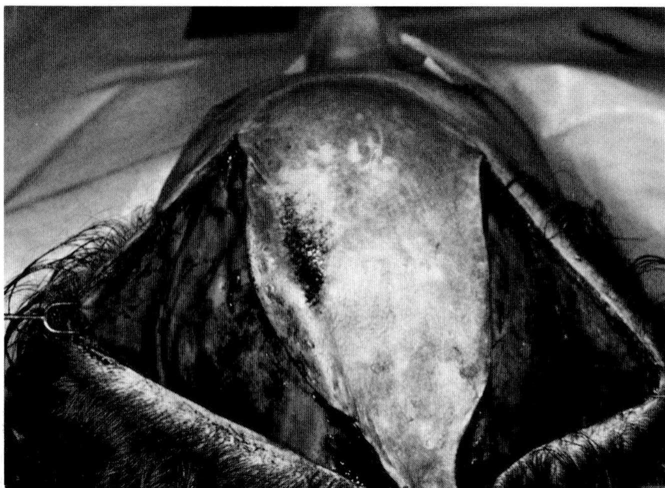

Fig. 1-7. At surgery, the skin graft was excised and the expanded scalp was used to close the wound. (Reprinted from Argenta L: Controlled tissue expansion. Surgical Rounds 9:65, 1986. With permission.)

INJURIES

Lacerations

Laceration injuries are primarily troublesome because of bleeding. Infection is extremely rare because of the rich blood supply. One-layer closure with continuous monofilament suture and locking of alternating sutures to prevent edge inversion usually is adequate. This suture technique helps control bleeding from the edge and permits rapid closure. Sutures are left in place for 10 to 14 days to allow maximal wound tensile strength to develop in order to prevent spreading of the scar, since a wide, hairless scar is more visible than any potential suture marks except in a bald scalp. Debridement of the edge of the wound should be parallel to the hair shafts rather than at right angles to the skin for the same reason.

Thermal Burns

The depth of a burn is a function of the burning temperature and the time of exposure as well as of the depth of the skin. In the scalp, with its thick skin and rich circulation, deep burns are less common. Because the hair follicles are in the subcutaneous space and are epidermal elements, re-epithelialization of even deep second-degree burns can be rapid in the absence of infection. Conservative treatment therefore is indicated where the depth of the burn is questionable.

Electrical Burns

Luce and Hoopes[12] showed that the noninfected burned skull can act as an in situ bone graft and regenerate if covered by tissue of good vascularity. The therapy for electrical burns therefore should consist of excision of the burned scalp and pericranium as soon as the margins of the burn are established and before infection occurs (1 to 3 days) and immediate coverage with vascularized flaps, either local or distant. The burned skull should be left intact unless it is infected or unless underlying damage to the dura or brain is suspected.

MICROVASCULAR REPLANTATION OF THE AVULSED SCALP

HISTORY

In 1960, Jacobson and Suarez[13] demonstrated that with the aid of an operating microscope blood vessels 1 mm in diameter could be anastomosed with a patency rate of at least 80 percent.

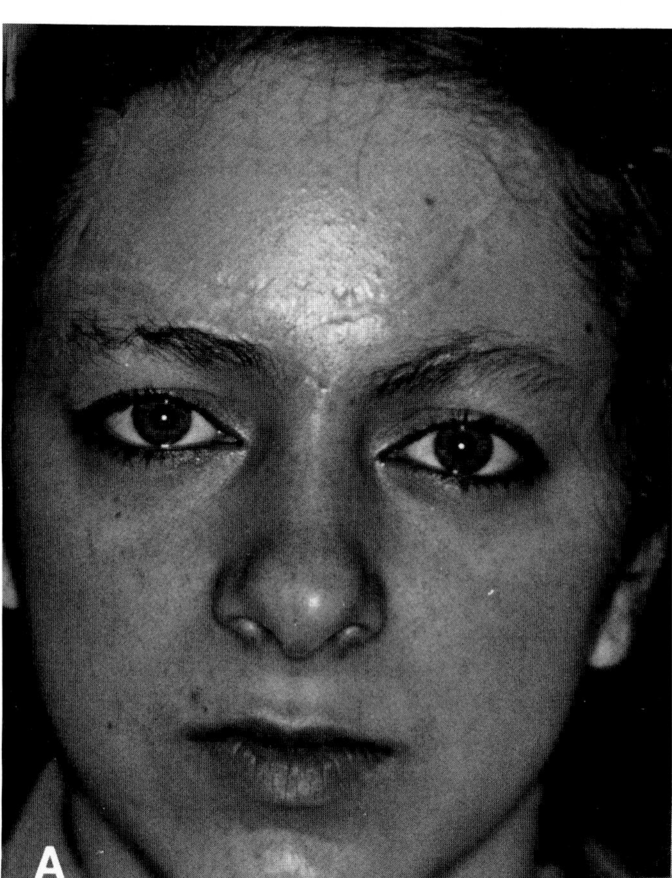

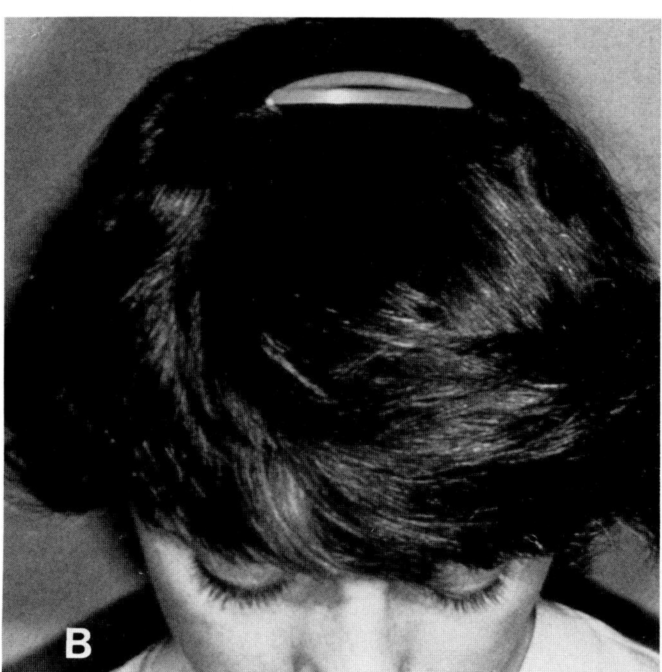

Fig. 1-8. The scalp 1 year postoperatively. (A) Note the elimination of the forehead graft, and (B) full hair coverage. (Reprinted from Argenta L: Controlled tissue expansion. Surgical Rounds 9:65, 1986. With permission.)

Davy Trop, M.D., F.R.C.P.(C), F.A.C.A., Department of Anesthesiology, Montreal Neurological Hospital and Institute and McGill University, Montreal, Quebec, Canada

Sumio Uematsu, M.D., Department of Neurosurgery, The Johns Hopkins University School of Medicine, Baltimore, Maryland

Kazuo Ugajin, M.D., Division of Neurological Surgery, Kameda General Hospital, Kamogawa, Japan

James R. Urbaniak, M.D., Department of Neurosurgery, Duke University School of Medicine, Durham, North Carolina

Dante F. Vacca, M.D., Department of Neurological Surgery, Henry Ford Hospital, Detroit, Michigan

Harry R. van Loveren, M.D., Department of Neurosurgery, University of Cincinnati College of Medicine, Cincinnati, Ohio

John C. VanGilder, M.D., Division of Neurosurgery, University of Iowa, Iowa City, Iowa

Steven L. Wald, M.D., Division of Neurosurgery, University of Vermont College of Medicine, Burlington, Vermont

Carrie L. Walters, M.D., Division of Neurosurgery, University of Vermont College of Medicine, Burlington, Vermont

Walter William Whisler, M.D., Ph.D., Department of Neurosurgery, Rush Medical College and Presbyterian-St. Luke's Hospital, Chicago, Illinois

Jeffrey H. Wisoff, M.D., Division of Pediatric Neurosurgery, Department of Neurosurgery, New York University Medical Center, New York, New York

Kenneth E. Wood, M.D., Department of Orthopaedic Surgery, Duke University School of Medicine, Durham, North Carolina

Shirley H. Wray, Neuroophthalmology Service, Massachusetts General Hospital, Boston, Massachusetts

R. Lewis Wright, M.D., Department of Neurosurgery, Stuart Circle Hospital and St. Mary's Hospital, Richmond, Virginia

David Yashon, M.D., Department of Neurosurgery, Ohio State University and St. Anthony's Hospital, Columbus, Ohio

Henry A. Young, M.D., Augusta, Georgia

Nicholas T. Zervas, M.D., Department of Neurological Surgery, Massachusetts General Hospital and the Department of Surgery, Harvard Medical School, Boston, Massachusetts

Subsequent to this report, clinical reconstructive microneurovascular surgery began to rapidly expand to include the replantation of amputated extremities and digits, one stage microneurovascular transplantation of a toe to the hand for reconstruction, and the coverage of large soft tissue or bone defects with microneurovascular free tissue transfers ("free flaps").[14]

Miller, Anstee, and Snell[15] were first to report a successful immediate scalp replantation by microvascular anastomosis in 1976. They described a patient who had his entire scalp avulsed at the subgaleal level. After a period of ischemia of 4 1/2 hours the circulation of the scalp was restored, and ultimately two arteries and three veins were anastomosed. The total operating time was 12 hours. The entire replanted scalp survived with subsequent normal hair growth and function of the frontalis muscle.[16,17]

ANATOMY OF THE AVULSED SCALP INJURY

Scalp avulsion requires a strong tearing or shearing force.[18,19] The scalp will detach from the skull along the path of least resistance, which is the loose areolar tissue layer between the galea aponeurotica and the pericranium. If the force is extensive enough the scalping will progress to the boundaries of the galea at the supraorbital ridges, and the zygomatic, mastoid, and occipital neucal line. At these points the muscular attachments of the galea (the paired occipitofrontalis muscles) do not offer much resistance, and the scalp tears away from the skull. The temporal scalp tear line is variable and can either be just craniad to the ear or include parts of the ear, because the galea inserts into the superior helix via the superior auricular muscle.

SCALP REPLANTATION PROCEDURE

When a scalp avulsion has occurred, the emergency facility receiving the patient should stabilize the patient's vital signs, determine the patient's tetanus prophlyaxis status, do whatever diagnostic procedures are necessary, administer a broad spectrum antibiotic and, if appropriate, administer analgesics. Preparation for blood transfusion should also be made. The exposed cranium should be covered with a saline-moistened gauze. The amputated scalp should be placed in a plastic bag and the bag placed in ice chips.

Ideally, two operating teams should be available for the replantation surgery. One team identifies and tags the vessels on the avulsed scalp and the other team works on the patient's head identifying vessels and debriding the wound.

Locating the vessels on an avulsed scalp can be time consuming and should be done with the aid of loupe magnification. The paired vessels that should be investigated are the supraorbital, temporal, postauricular and occipital. The diameters of the vessels in adults will range from 0.5 to 1.5 mm in diameter. The transected vessels are usually divided above (distal to) the level of the skin tear line. They also retract, and for this reason the galea will need to be incised radially in the respective locations of the vessels in order to expose them. As a result of stretching and retraction, the microanatomy of the vessels is often disrupted. Intimal cracking and separation must be identified by examining the transected vessel. If the intima is clearly separated from the media or if there are gossamerlike filaments in the lumen, the vessel must be transected until a point is reached at which the intima is smooth and adherent to the media. Such vessel evaluation must be done on both the proximal and distal vessels. In many cases vessel debridement will preclude direct anastomosis of the vessels. In such cases, an interposition vein graft with an autogenous vein must be done. This can be obtained from either the forearm or the dorsum of the foot.

Once the proximal and distal vessels have been identified and debrided and any cranial injuries repaired, the scalp is tacked into its appropriate position. An operating microscope is then used for the vascular repairs. Although it would be advantageous to anastomose the veins first and thus minimize blood loss once arterial continuity has been restored, this most often is not practical because of the scalp ischemia time. The arterial repairs thus should be done initially and microvascular clips placed on the major venous outflow vessels until such time as they are repaired. The smaller vessels can be allowed to bleed. When possible, it is best to repair multiple arteries and veins. However, there is no set ratio of veins to arteries that must be repaired. The vast interconnected network of arteries and veins in the scalp cross the midline, and major scalp replantations have been successful with only one arterial anastomosis and one venous anastomosis.[20] The most preferable artery for anastomosis is the one with the largest potential area of distribution—the superficial temporal artery. This should be repaired when possible.

There continues to be a great deal of variation between replantation centers over the treatment of the patient's vascular/coagulation status after flow in the replanted scalp has been restored. Low molecular weight dextran (20 ml/hour IV for 5 to 7 days), aspirin (300–600 mg orally), and heparin have been recommended,[21] but there is no control data to suggest that one regimen is better than the other. Another technique that has been employed in replantation surgery when venous congestion is a problem is medicinal leeches applied directly to the engorged replanted part.[22]

Once the vascular repairs have been completed, the scalp is sutured into place more precisely and dressed with a light bulky dressing. Several openings for observation of the scalp should be made in the dressing. The status of the replanted scalp can be monitored by such classical means as gross color, temperature to palpation, capillary refill, and the presence of bleeding when punctured with a needle. Other means of monitoring include Doppler assessment of the major vessels,[23] thermocouples,[24] fluorescein scanning,[25] transcutaneous oxygen measurement,[26] and various impedence techniques.[27] Indications of arterial or venous occlusion should be addressed by returning the patient to the operating room for exploration.

The patient should remain in the hospital for 5 to 10 days in most situations. Thereafter, the patient can be seen on an out-patient basis. Renewed hair growth may be seen within 2 weeks after the replantation.

CASE REPORT

A 27-year-old man avulsed greater than 50 percent of his scalp (20 × 22 cm) and had no underlying calvarial injuries. The scalp was replanted using the right superficial temporal artery and vein. The entire scalp survived (Figure 1-9).

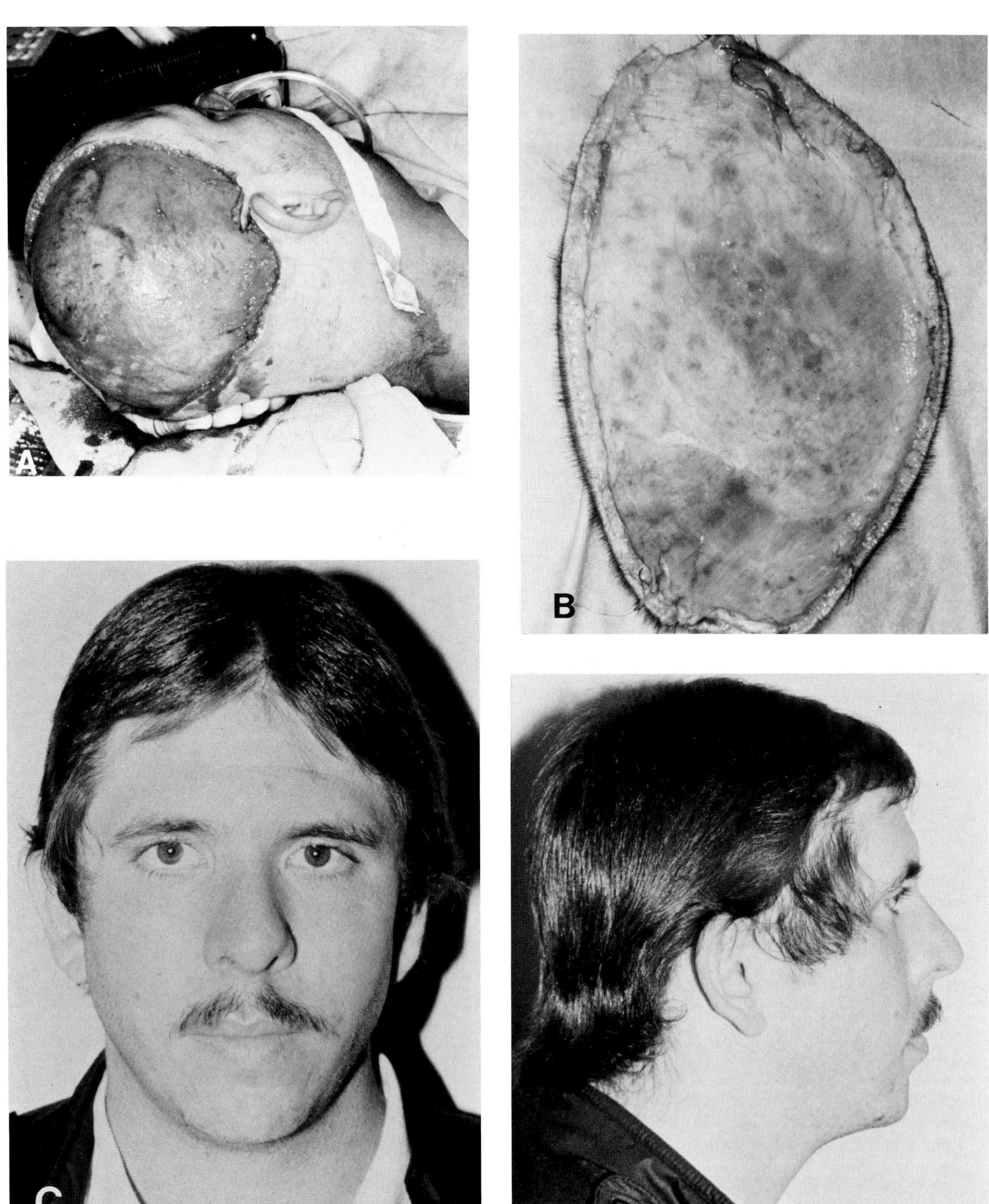

Fig. 1-9. (A) Exposed cranium. (B) Exposed scalp. (C,D) Frontal and lateral views of the patient 6 months after scalp avulsion and replantation. (Courtesy of J. Cassel, MD.)

REFERENCES

1. Longacre JJ, Converse JM: Deformities of the forehead, scalp and calvarium, in Converse JD (ed): Reconstructive Plastic Surgery, vol. 2. Philadelphia, WB Saunders, 1977, p 822

2. Juri J, Juri C, Arufe HN: Use of rotation scalp flaps for treatment of occipital baldness. Plast Reconstr Surg 61:23, 1978

3. Ortichchea M: New three flap reconstruction technique. Br J Plast Surg 24:184, 1971

4. Radovan C: Reconstruction of the breast after radical mastectomy using temporary expander. ASPRS Plast Surg Forum 1:41, 1978

5. Austed ED, Ross GL: A self-inflating tissue expander. Plast Reconstr Surg 70:588, 1982

6. Austad ED, Pasyk KA, McClatchey KD, et al: Histomorphologic evaluation of guinea pig skin and soft tissue after controlled tissue expansion. Plast Reconstr Surg 70:704, 1982

7. Pasyk KA, Austad ED, McClatchey KD, et al: Electron microscopic evaluation of guinea pig skin and soft tissue "expanded" with a self-inflating silicone implant. Plast Reconstr Surg 70:37, 1982

8. Sasaki GH, Pang GY: Pathophysiology of skin flaps raised on expanded pig skin. Plast Reconstr Surg 74:59, 1984

9. Nordstrom REA, Devine JW: Scalp stretching with a tissue expander for closure of scalp defects. Plast Reconstr Surg 75:578, 1985

10. Argenta LC, Watanabe MD, Graff WC: The use of tissue expansion in head and neck reconstruction. Ann Plast Surg 11:31, 1983

11. Lynch PJ, Kahn EA: Congenital defects of the scalp. A surgical approach to aplasia cutis congenita. J Neurosurg 33:198, 1970

12. Luce EA, Hoopes JE: Electrical burn of the scalp and skull. A case report. Plast Reconstr Surg 54:359, 1974

13. Jacobson J, Suarez E: Microsurgery in anastomosis of small vessels. Surg Forum 9:243, 1960

14. Daniel R, Taylor G: Distant transfer of an island flap by microvascular anastomosis. Plast Reconstr Surg 52:11, 1973

15. Miller G, Anstee E, Snell J: Successful replantation of an avulsed scalp by microvascular anastomoses. Plast Reconstr Surg 58:133, 1976

16. Lu M: Successful replacement of avulsed scalp. Plast Reconstr Surg 43:231, 1969

17. Osborne P: Complete scalp avulsion; Report of cases: Experimental basis for production of free, hairbearing grafts from avulsed scalp itself. Ann Surg 132:198, 1950

18. Koss N, Robson MC, Krizek TJ: Scalping injury. Plast Reconstr Surg 55:439, 1975

19. McGrath M: Scalping: The savage and the surgeon. Clin Plast Surg 10:679, 1983

20. Nahai F: Replantation of an entire scalp and ear by microvascular anastomoses of only one artery and vein. Br J Plast Surg 31:339, 1978

21. Buncke H, Rose E, Brownstein M, et al: Successful replantation of two avulsed scalps by microvascular anastomoses. Plast Reconstr Surg 61:666, 1978

22. Mutimer K, Banis J, Upton J: Microsurgical reattachment of totally amputated ears. Presented at the Second Annual Meeting of the American Society for Reconstructive Microsurgery, New Orleans, La., February 13–15, 1986

23. VanBeek A, Link W, Bennett J: Ultrasound evaluation of microanastomosis. Arch Surg 110:195, 1975

24. Stirrat C, Seaber A, Urbaniak J: Temperature monitoring in digital transplantation. J Hand Surg 3:342, 1978

25. Graham G, Gordon L, Alpert B, et al: Serial quantatative skin surface fluoresence: A new method for postoperative monitoring of vascular perfusion in revascularized digits. J Hand Surg l0A:218, 1985

26. Serafin D, Lesesne C, Mullen R: Transcutaneous PO monitoring for assessing viability and predicting survival of skin flaps: Experimental and clinical correlation. J Microsurg 2:165, 1981

27. Webster MH, Patterson J: The photoelectric plethysmograph as a monitor of microvascular anastomosis. Br J Plast Surg 29:2, 1976

CHAPTER 2

Repair of Defects of the Skull

Michael S. Olin

THE REPAIR OF SKULL DEFECTS is a problem endowed with a rich history that attests to the innovative abilities of the surgeon. Attempts at repair of skull defects date back to the ancients and have produced several isolated curiosities.[1] The late nineteenth century was marked by the successful adoption of autogenous, homogenous, and heterogenous bone grafting techniques. The major conflagrations of the twentieth century provided a high volume of cases and were associated with the testing and refining of new materials and surgical techniques, including the introduction of new alloplastic grafting materials and the eventual application of the single-stage repair.

Most defects of the skull are the result of trauma. Highway and industrial accidents and the shrapnel wounds of modern warfare have led to the increasing occurrence of skull defects. The support available for the patient's vital systems and intensive care now permit more patients to survive the initial injury. Improvements in the treatment of wound infections, osteomyelitis, congenital defects, and neoplastic diseases, along with the advent of decompressive craniectomy,[2] all have contributed to the increased caseload encountered by the neurosurgeon.

The list of materials in use for the repair of skull defects is impressive. Autogenous grafts have the advantage of being a biologically compatible material that causes minimal tissue reaction and donates a matrix allowing ingrowth of osteoblasts. The strength of the graft varies according to the site from which it is harvested. The tibia, ribs, iliac crest, scapula, sternum, and cartilage, as well as the adjacent outer table of the skull have been used.[3] Many of these early repair techniques remain popular. Split rib grafts, initially devised by Brown,[4] leave the inner lamina of the rib to protect the thoracic contents, while the strong graft material is used for large skull defects. Concave-convex grafts from the iliac crest, first used by Mauclaire,[5] permitted repair of the craniofacial contours; cartilage, although not as strong as bone, was used for the repair of small deformities of the supraorbital ridge. Homogenous grafting using pretreated cadaver bone has been advocated for use on the same basis as the frozen autogenous flap.[6–8] The advantage of this material is that in spite of a reduction in the bone thickness following chemical pretreatment, the graft can be frozen and stored indefinitely.[9] Perforation of the bone plate insertion also is possible and allows potential fluid collections to be drained. Heterogenous grafts are exemplified by the cranioplasties of sheep and ox bone used by Babcock.[10] The attractive features of metallic materials used in cranioplasty are their strength, malleability, and inertness. The early attempts involved the use of gold and silver, which is now precluded by their expense. Aluminum, platinum, Vitallium, titanium, tanta-

lum, and stainless steel also have been tried.[11–17] Lead also was used in one instance, resulting in lead intoxication.[18] Metals, for the first time, allowed satisfactory repair of even the largest defects. Tantalum mesh gained acceptance because of its strength and inertness. Malleability was less of a problem and no casting apparatus was necessary.

The experience with these different materials has produced a concept of the ideal material.[19] It should be inert, nontoxic, malleable, strong enough to protect the underlying brain, a poor thermal conductor, and radiolucent, allowing subsequent roentgenograms and computerized tomographic (CT) examinations to be made without disturbing the images.

After its introduction by Kleinschmidt in 1940,[20] the acrylic resin methyl methacrylate has fulfilled many of the criteria listed and now is widely used for the repair of skull defects. The ingredients for making this material are supplied in a kit form that contains a liquid monomer and the powdered polymer.* Methyl methacrylate is nonreactive, unaffected by temperature and electricity, has a tensile strength of greater than 4000 lb/in^2, and allows a one-stage implant that remains radiolucent to be formed rapidly.

GENERAL PRINCIPLES

The preoperative evaluation of patients with skull defects involves careful consideration of both the indications and the timing of surgery. A defect that results in a cosmetic aberration is one indication for repair, although the relationship between the size of the defect and the surgical indication is arbitrary. Since the frontal area is the most obvious cosmetically, a slight distortion of symmetry renders gross changes in appearance and is a significant handicap for the patient. Its complicated contours can make this area the most difficult to repair with satisfactory results. Defects of the calvarium in a bald patient might have the same disfiguring effect, but here much depends on the size of the defect and the self-consciousness of the patient. Generally, skull defects larger than 2 to 3 cm in diameter should be considered for repair, but this varies with location, since defects underlying a thick muscle mass, as in the temporal and occipital regions, are not normally operated upon.

The special circumstances of childhood deserve consideration.[21,22] In patients less than 3 years of age, the outer layer of the dura serves as periosteum and is capable of osseous regeneration. New bone formation molds well in respect to

---

*Cranioplastic kit, Codman & Shurtleff, Inc., Randolph, Massachusetts.

OPERATIVE NEUROSURGICAL TECHNIQUES
ISBN 0-8089-1862-1

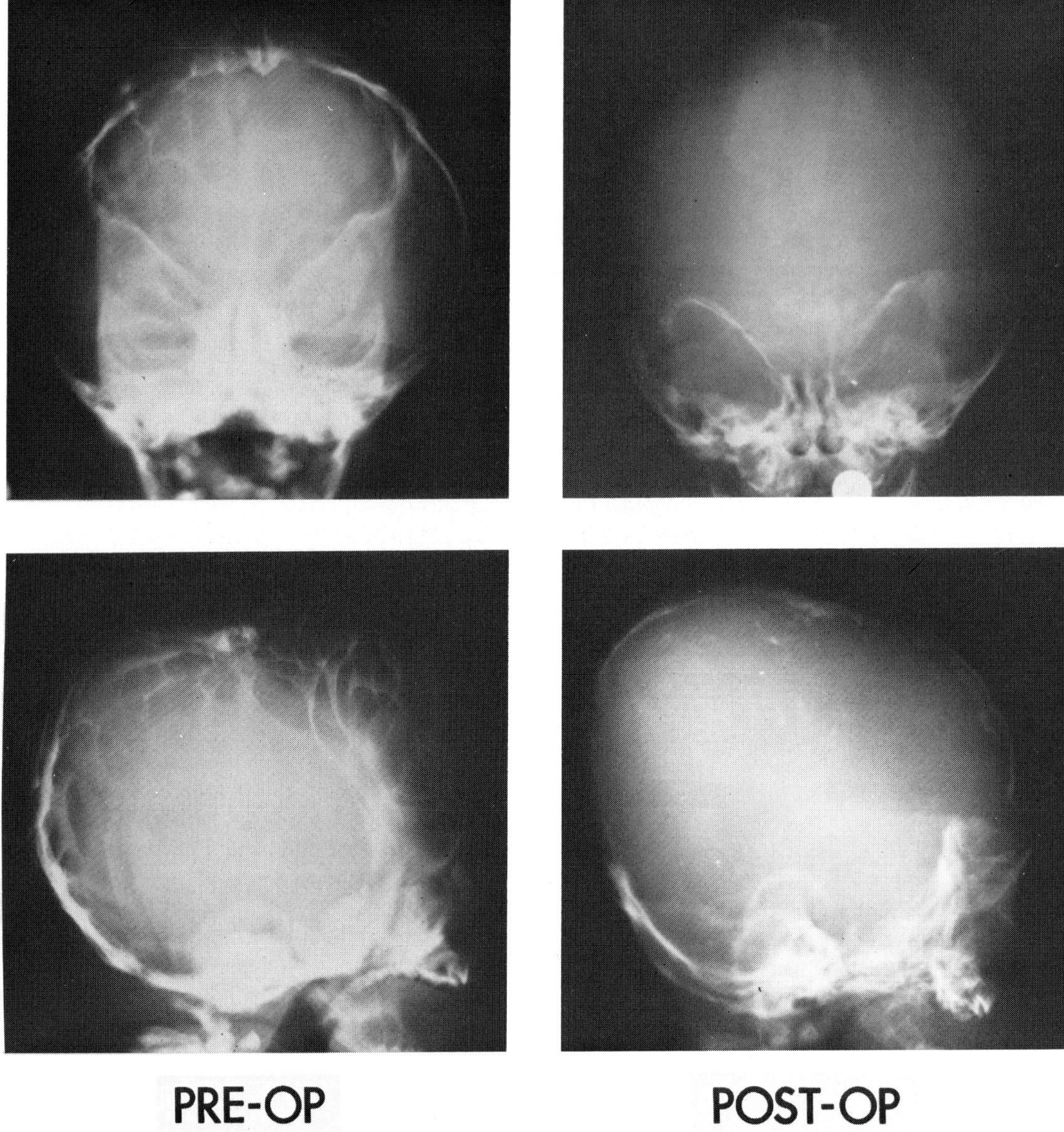

Fig. 2-1. Multisutural craniosynostosis. Preoperative films show total craniectomy. Corridors of bone are purposely left to protect the dural sinuses. New bone formation is expected in this patient.

brain growth, and total reossification occurs with 6 to 12 months. Thus, as long as dura is present, primary regeneration of even large defects can be anticipated. Total craniectomies have been accomplished for multisutural craniosynostosis (Figure 2-1), and protective headgear becomes essential until primary regeneration occurs. Another phenomenon of this age group is a tendency for the intracranial contents to herniate through a skull defect. The absence of bony countercompression results in asymmetry of brain growth with obvious ventricular disproportion, which has been termed *migration of the ventricle*. This is more apt to occur in cases with a coexistent dural defect, further loss of restriction to brain countercompression, and development of encephalocele (Figure 2-2). Other explanations for ventricular migration have been attributed to cerebral atrophy caused by the initial brain insult concomitant with the bony injury. The introduction of a rigid prosthesis offers countercompression but restricts brain growth and is not recommended for children under the age of 3 years.[23,24] The use of split rib grafts or assimilation of the older techniques involv-

ing osteoplastic flaps probably better serves this special situation.[22]

An intact cranium not only assumes a cosmetic significance, but also a protective role for brain growth and integrity. This concept of brain protection is an important indication for repair of a skull defect. Those patients exposed to occupational hazards are cautioned about the dangers of further injury. The true liability is readily appreciated in the patient with seizures, and here repair of the skull defect is performed as promptly as possible. The improvement or prevention of associated seizures does not appear to be related to cranioplastic repair. In a series of studies by Erculei and Walker consisting of 342 wartime injuries, the timing of defect repair did not seem to have an effect on the development or course of posttraumatic epilepsy.[25,26] They concluded that early cranioplasty may be desirable to shorten the convalescence of a patient, but probably has no influence on the development or relief of seizures. Previous reports of such improvement probably can be best explained by the simultaneous resection of a cortical cicatrix.

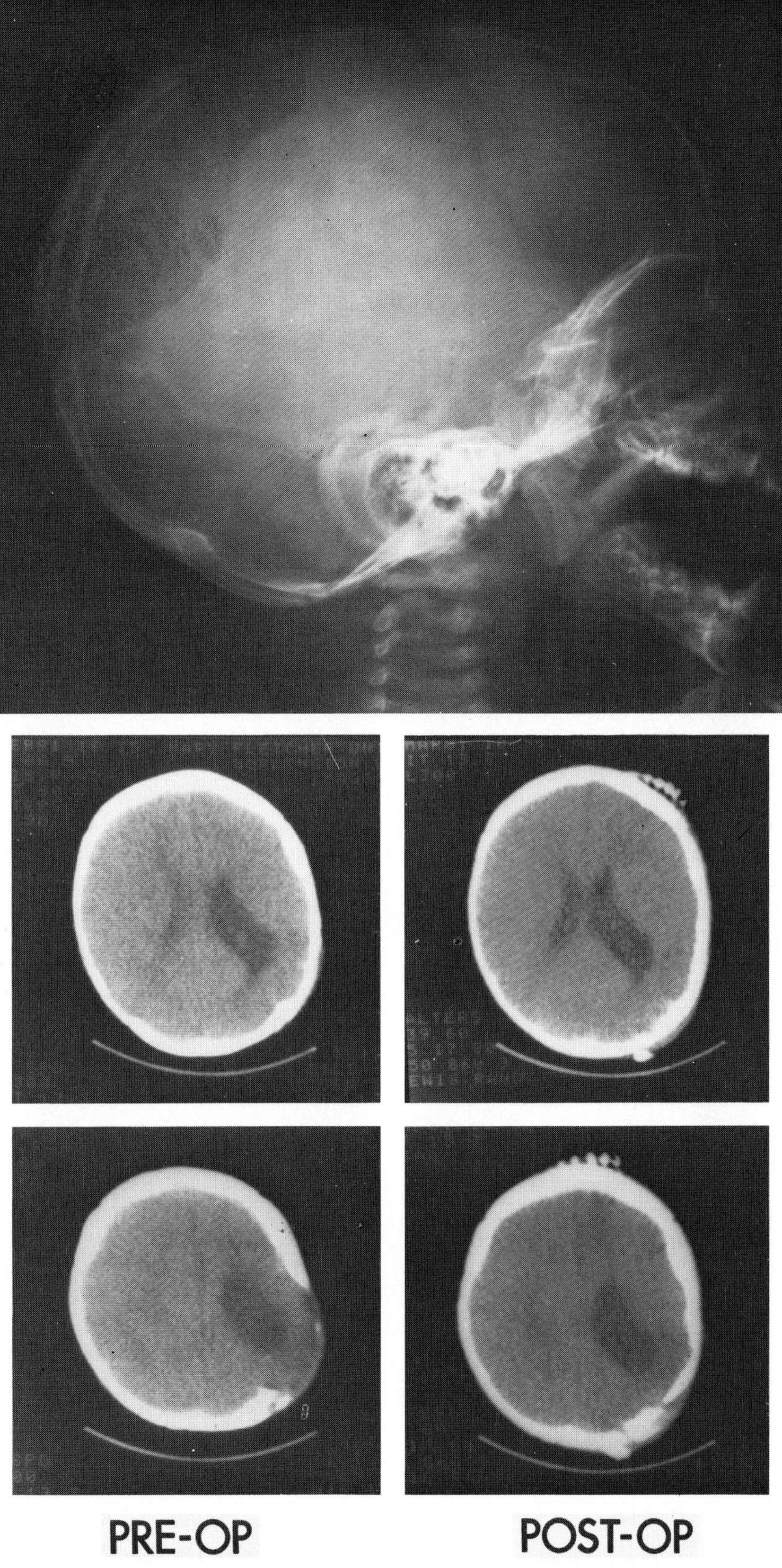

Fig. 2-2. A large traumatic parietal skull defect demonstrated on a lateral roentgenogram. Preoperative CT scans show the effects of loss of bony countercompression on brain growth with development of an encephalocele and ventricular disproportion, so-called ventricular migration. Postoperative CT scans show improvement of the disproportion and obliteration of the encephalocele through repair of the bony defect.

Routine electroencephalography has been suggested for preoperative and postoperative evaluation of patients undergoing cranioplasty.[27]

Other indications for cranioplasty include attempts to relieve local discomfort associated with a skull defect and the multiple somatic complaints sometimes observed in the posttraumatic period best described as neurasthenia.[28] Interestingly, some patients with even small defects are constantly aware of brain exposure and imaginatively seem to magnify their vulnerability. Grantham and Landis studied 100 cases of cranioplasty in patients with the "syndrome of the trephined."[29] They concluded that cranioplasty is indicated to eliminate a sense of insecurity caused by the presence of a skull defect, but warned that the success of cranioplasty in relieving headache and other associated symptoms is not universal. Silastic buttons to fill burr hole defects might be considered if one believes that this reassurance has an alleviating effect on the symptom complex mentioned above. Mount suggested tantalum discs to be fitted into disfiguring anterior burr holes,[30] while Ransohoff adapted stainless steel mesh for the same purpose.[31]

Operative timing addresses these indications plus the important complication of infection. Skull defects resulting from traumatic compound fracture have classically been managed by removal of contaminated bone fragments. Cranioplasty then is reserved for a later date. Replacement of flaps as primary repair of compound skull fractures was studied by Kriss et al.[32] in 79 patients with a follow-up period as long as 17 years. They reported an incidence of infection of 2.5 percent in patients treated by replacement of bone fragments. The use of live bone in these cases is preferred because it resists infection. In patients with heavily contaminated wounds or obvious infection, most neurosurgeons agree on a waiting period of 6 to 12 months to monitor the healing process. Preoperatively, all candidates are screened for possible sepsis, and if infection of the skin flap or bone edge is encountered, the procedure is abandoned. Kaslow and Ransohoff, however, utilized a primary wire mesh with cranioplasty in flap infections.[33] They reviewed the characteristics of cranioplastic materials, including negative effect on bacterial growth, and suggested that wire mesh might be utilized even in the presence of an infected wound. It is relatively inert and has a nonporous structure that prevents bacterial sequestration and allows fibrous tissue to grow through the interstices of the mesh. Reports also have appeared on the use of methyl methacrylate impregnated with antibiotic,[34,35] but further studies will be necessary to determine its advantage.

Other significant complications include the absorption of replaced bone flaps, especially after chemical or heat treatment. Ray and Parsons advocated free bone plates in routine craniotomies but noted the danger of resorption of treated bone if delayed replacement was anticipated.[36] Erosion of overlying soft tissue and skin, especially in the orbital region, is another possible complication of repair.[37]

TECHNIQUE

The most popular method of cranioplasty today is the use of the acrylic plastic methyl methacrylate. The method evolved from its introduction in 1940 by Kleinschmidt.[20] Initially, the procedure necessitated two stages and employed an impression technique.[38-40] The refinement of the polymerization process eliminated the need for heating and compression, and thus in 1948 Oliver and Blaine[41] introduced the single-stage cranioplasty using autopolymerization that terminated within 8 to 10 minutes at the relatively low temperatures of 70° to 80° F.

The three essential steps to single-stage methyl methacrylate cranioplasty are: (1) preparing the graft site, (2) forming and molding the methyl methacrylate, and (3) fitting and securing the plate. The steps are summarized in diagrammatic format, while the text provides a commentary on variations of the technique.

Adequate positioning of the patient facilitates the procedure by allowing the neurosurgeon to work in comfort and by giving him or her complete visual surveillance for appreciating symmetry while molding contours. Photographs showing the patient's previous features may aid in a successful cosmetic outcome and can be exhibited along with the x-ray portfolio. A skull should be available in the operating room at all times for ready reference to the contours, angulations, and landmarks. A draping technique that allows the upper half of the face to remain exposed is useful. This provides visual cues for repairing complex contours in the frontal region, where minor degrees of asymmetry have an undesirable cosmetic effect.

Intravenous administration of antibiotic is started at the time of the skin incision, and the previous scar is incised or resected. The skin flap is turned carefully to avoid damage to the dura underlying the skull defect. If the dura has been removed at a previous operation, the brain will be covered by dense fibrous tissue that will be adherent to the bone edge and underlying dura or brain and must be gently stripped away. Removal of this material allows the graft to be fitted snugly to the bone edge. It may be necessary to resect the bone edge to identify normal dura, at which point a tissue plane is initiated from which to begin stripping this fibrous material Figure 2-3). The dura, when exposed, should be carefully examined for tears and repaired by direct approximation or with appropriate grafting materials. The freed bone edge then is saucerized with rongeurs; this will form a beveled surface onto which the graft will rest, thus preventing slippage inward into the defect. The mold can eventually be formed to overlap this beveled edge by 5 to 10 mm, forming a lid-type covering.[37]

If methyl methacrylate is used, the kit contains a single dose consisting of 30 g of powdered polymer and 17 ml of liquid monomer. The mixing area should be well ventilated to avoid being overwhelmed by fumes, and the surgeon should use two pairs of gloves to keep the operating gloves clean and to avoid the unwanted introduction of material into the wound. The elements are placed in a stainless steel bowl and mixed with a spatula for approximately 30 seconds. Proper mixing promotes sterilization by the liquid monomer and has been shown to demonstrate bacteriostatic action.[42] The bowl then is covered to avoid evaporation of the monomer. The material becomes a doughlike mass that is ready to use after it no longer sticks to the surgeon's glove. Doughing time depends on temperature. Higher temperatures decrease doughing time. For example, at 82° F, doughing time is 4 minutes, while at 72° F, the time is 5 minutes. A quantity of the doughy mixture estimated to be sufficient for repair of the skull defect is then placed into a sterile plastic sleeve provided in the kit to prevent evaporation of the monomer.

Molding and fitting of the plastic graft proceeds until the final graft plate is secured. The initial shaping of plastic occurs while the material is still contained in the plastic sleeve. If exposed to air, the mixture will become crusty. The bag is

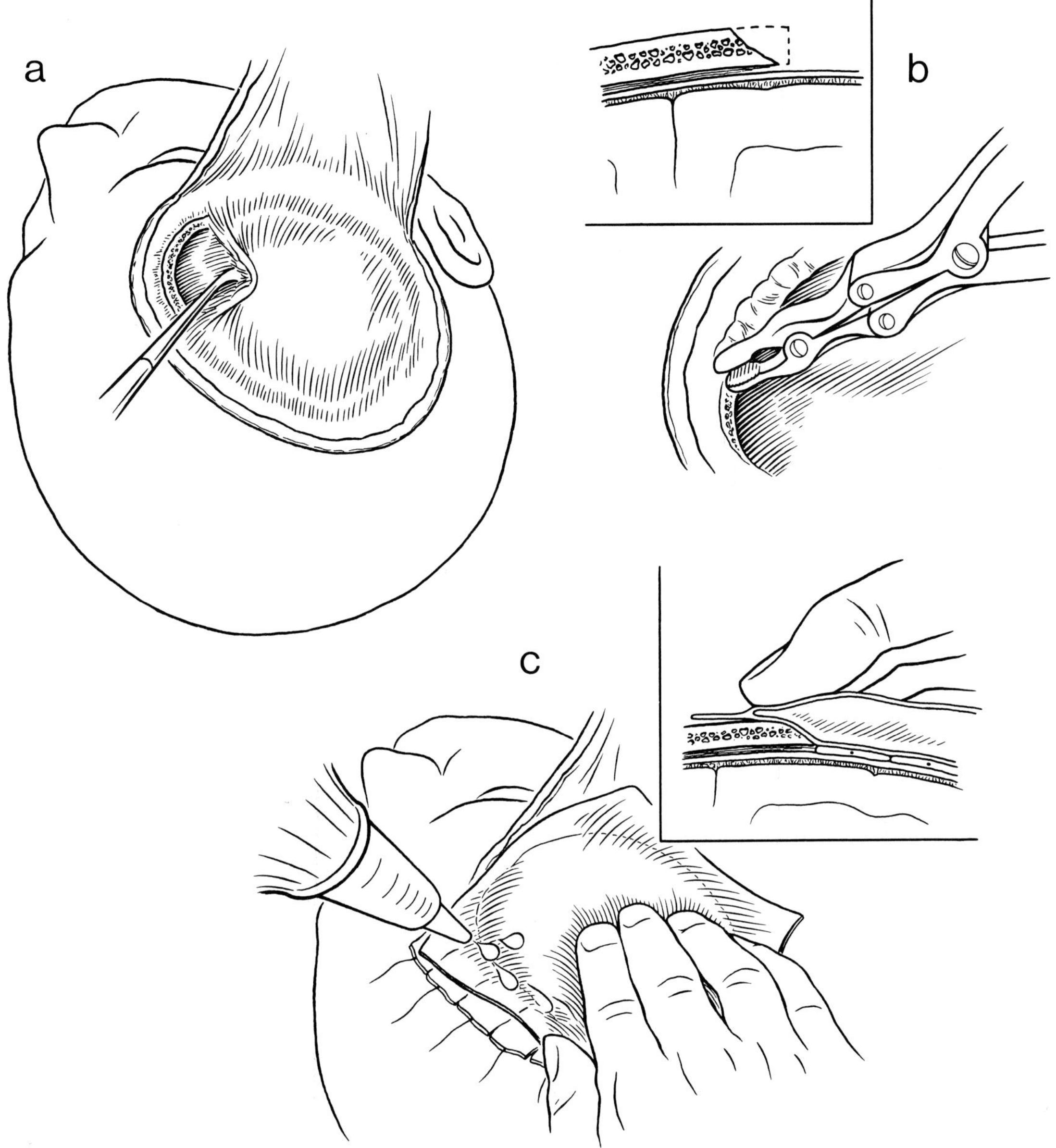

Fig. 2-3. The basic steps of single-stage methyl methacrylate cranioplasty showing (a) teasing of fibrous tissue from the bone edge to reveal the underlying dura; (b) saucerization of the edge of the defect to create a beveled edge on which the graft will rest; and (c) molding of the graft contours before the exothermic reaction occurs by gentle fingertip manipulation while the graft material is still in the plastic bag.

placed into the skull defect and digital compression is applied for flattening. This molds the plate into the defect and forms an overlapping beveled edge. The bag is stretched by the assistant while the surgeon lightly applies fingertip massage. Cool saline irrigation is used during this process to protect the dura from the heat of the chemical reaction within the bag (Figure 2-3). Further protection can be provided by covering the dura with cotton strips soaked in saline. This also provides definition of a space between the graft and the dura that prohibits the undersurface of the graft from resting directly on the dura and allows for possible brain expansion. A roller is used to flatten the material over the skull contour. A molding time of 6 to 8 minutes is normal; this is faster at higher temperatures. The essential process of polymerization takes place outside of the surgical field, thus avoiding the possibility of burning the brain

by the exothermic reaction that ensues. Preforming of sections of the graft may become necessary, especially to conform to areas of the frontal bone with its complicated contours. This can be accomplished by shaping the methyl methacrylate over a curved edge, such as the outside of a stirring basin, and then wiring this piece after it hardens to the larger piece of material (Figure 2-4). Visual cues from photographs, exposed facial features, and the skull specimen are essential here.[43]

A setting time of approximately 15 minutes is necessary. The graft then is secured with wire or other appropriate suture material. Rough edges are filed smooth. The pericranium and galea are approximated for snug adherence. A drain placed beneath the cranioplasty violates the tight fit unless a junction is purposely left open. Perforating the plate to promote ingrowth of connective tissue for fixation and drainage of underlying

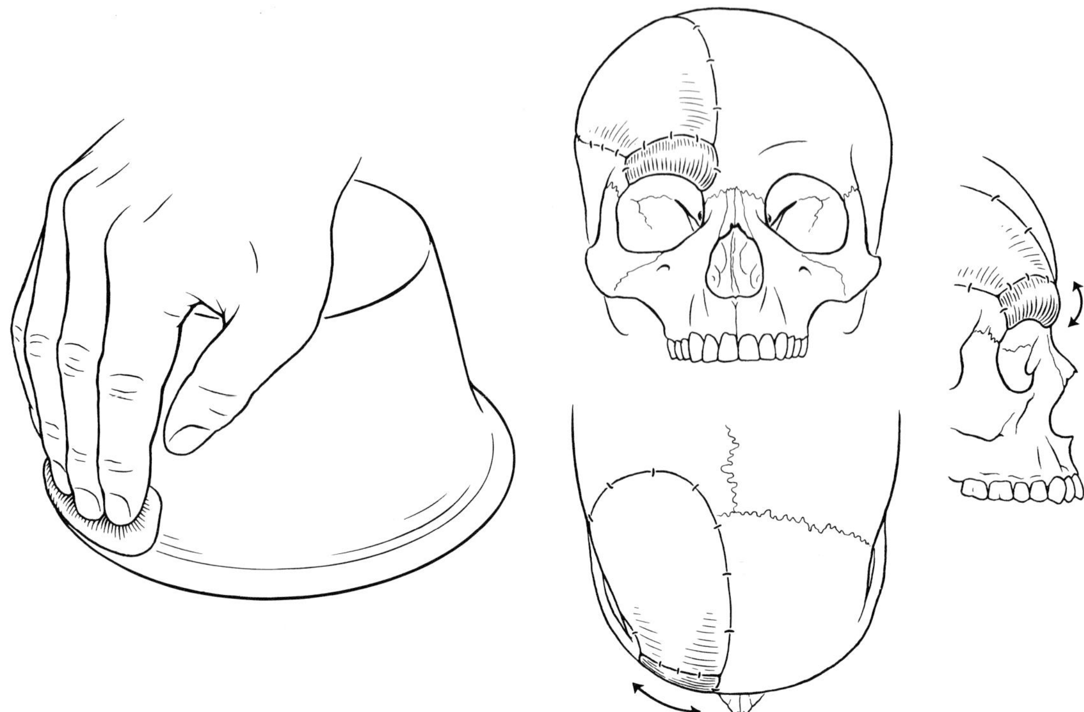

Fig. 2-4. Formation of a separate supraorbital ridge graft using a contoured surface for molding. This addition is subsequently attached to the larger graft.

collections also is advocated. Drains placed over the graft material can be used along with a compressive turban dressing and postoperative antibiotics for at least as long as the drain remains in place.

REFERENCES

1. Reeves DL: Cranioplasty. Springfield, IL, Charles C Thomas, 1950
2. Yamaura A, Sato M, Meguro K, et al: Cranioplasty following decompressive craniectomy—analysis of 300 cases. Neurol Med Chir (Tokyo) 5:345, 1977
3. Kyoshima K, Gibo H, Kobayashi S, et al: Cranioplasty with inner table of bone flap. Technical note. J Neurosurg 62:607, 1985
4. Brown RC: The repair of skull defects. Med J Aust 11:409, 1917
5. Mauclaire P: Autogreffe crânienne empruntée à la tubérosité iliaque, et homogreffe séreuse intermeningo-encephalique. Bull Soc Chir Paris 40:113, 1914
6. Bush LF: The use of homogenous bone grafts. Bone Joint Surg 29:620, 1947
7. Abbott KH: Use of frozen cranial bone flaps for autogenous and homogenous grafts in cranioplasty and spinal interbody fusion. J Neurosurg 10:380, 1953
8. Odom GL, Barnes W, Wrenn FR Jr: The use of refrigerated autogenous bone flaps for cranioplasty. J Neurosurg 9:606, 1952
9. Prolo DJ, Oklund SA: Composite autogeneic human cranioplasty: Frozen skull supplemented with fresh iliac corticocancellous bone. Neurosurgery 15:846, 1984
10. Babcock WW: "Soup bone" implant for the correction of defects of the skull and face. JAMA 69:352, 1917
11. Grekoff J: ü ber die deckung von sch ä deldefekten mit ausgegluhten knochen. Zentralbl Chir 25:969, 1898
12. Jaksch R: Zur frage der deckung von knochendefekten des sch ä dels nach der trepanation. Wein Med Wochenschr 39:1436, 1889
13. Weiford EC, Gardner WJ: Tantalum cranioplasty. Review of 106 cases in civilian practice. J Neurosurg 6:13, 1949
14. Bates JI, Reiners CR: The repair of cranial defects with zirconium. An experimental study. J Neurosurg 5:340, 1948
15. Simpson D: Titanium in cranioplast J Neurosurg 22:292, 1965
16. Scott M, Wycis MT, Murtagh F: Long term evaluation of stainless steel cranioplasty. Surg Gynecol Obstet 115:453, 1962
17. Black SPW, Kain CCM, Sights WP Jr. Aluminum cranioplasty. Technical note. Neurosurgery 29:562, 1968
18. Mauclaire P: Brèche crânienne restaurée par la prothèse mètal-lique. Bull Soc Chir Paris 34:232, 1908
19. Weisman S: Metals for implantation in the human body. Ann NY Acad Sci 146:80, 1968
20. Kleinschmidt O: Plexiglas zur deckung von schadellucken. Chirurgie 13:273, 1941
21. Shons AR, Press BH, Waite DE, et al: The use of methyl methacrylate in a two-stage correction of Crouzon's/Apert's defor-mity. Ann Plast Surg 10:147, 1983
22. Ventureyra EC, Da Silva VF: Reduction cranioplasty for neglected hydrocephalus. Surg Neurol 15:236, 1981
23. Timmons RL: Cranial defects and their repair, in Youmans JR (ed): Neurological Surgery, vol. 28 Philadelphia, WB Saunders, pp 903–1008
24. Matson DD: Neurosurgery of Infancy and Childhood. Springfield, IL, Charles C Thomas, 1969
25. Erculei F, Walker AE: Post traumatic epilepsy and early cranioplasty. J Neurosurg 20:1085, 1963
26. Walker AE, Erculei F: The late results of cranioplasty. Arch Neurol 9:105, 1963
27. Elkins CW, Cameron JE: Cranioplasty with acrylic plates. J Neurosurg 3:199, 1946
28. Jacobsen SA: The Post Traumatic Syndrome Following Head Injury. Springfield, IL, Charles C Thomas, 1969
29. Grantham EG, Landis MP: Cranioplasty and the post traumatic syndrome. J Neurosurg 5:19, 1948
30. Mount LA: Tantalum discs for covering trephine defects and tantalum clips for ligation of internal carotid artery intracranially. J Neurosurg 5:208, 1948
31. Ransohoff J: Stainless steel screen for covering trephine and other small cranial defects. J Neurosurg 7:589, 1950

32. Kriss FC, Taren JA, Kahn EA: Primary repair of compound skull fractures by replacement of bone fragments. J Neurosurg 30:698, 1969

33. Kaslow M, Ransohoff: Primary wire mesh cranioplasty in flap infections. Neurosurgery 4:290, 1979

34. Holm NJ, Vejlsgaard R: The in vitro elution of gentamicin sulfate from methyl methacrylate bone cement: A comparative study. Acta Orthop Scand 47:144, 1976

35. Marks KE, Nelson CL, Lautenschlager EP: Antibiotic impregnated acrylic bone cement. J Bone Joint Surg 58A:358, 1976

36. Ray BS, Parsons M: The replacement of free bone plates in routine craniotomies. J Neurosurg 4:299, 1947

37. Stula D: The problem of the "sinking skin flap syndrome" in cranioplasty. J Maxillofac Surg 10:142, 1982

38. Alesch F, Bauer R: Polyacryl prosthesis for cranioplasty—their production in silicon rubber casts. Acta Neurochir (Vienna) 77:68, 1985

39. Van Gool AV: Preformed polymethylmethacrylate cranioplasties: Report of 45 cases. J Maxillofac Surg 13:2, 1985

40. Seixas V, Dias MP, Resek J: Cranioplasty with pre-moulded and pre-sterilized methyl methacrylate plates. Neurochirurgia (Stuttg) 24:182, 1981

41. Oliver LC, Blaine G: A new one-staged method of cranioplasty with acrylic plastic. Med Press (London) 220:167, 1948

42. Axel Reitz K: The one-stage method of cranioplasty with acrylic plastic. With a follow-up study. J Neurosurg 15:176, 1958

43. Cabbabe EB, Shively RE, Malik P: Cranioplasty for traumatic deformities of the fronto-orbital area. Ann Plast Surg 13:175, 1984

CHAPTER 3
Surgical Management of Acute Head Injuries

George F. Gade   Donald P. Becker

PRIMARY HEAD INJURY occurs at the initial impact, which produces brain deformation and movement.[1] Cerebral contusion and laceration as well as diffuse shearing injury of the brain parenchyma are its major components. Injuries to the scalp and cranium also are part of the spectrum of primary head injury. Secondary brain injury is inflicted by subsequent hypoxia, hypotension, seizure, infection, brain swelling, and hematoma, which result in intracranial hypertension and brain shift. The focus of therapy is on preventing or rapidly treating any secondary injuries, while providing the victim with an optimal milieu for recovery from primary injuries. The major role of surgery is the evacuation of traumatic mass lesions, thereby relieving or preventing intracranial hypertension and brain shifts. The debridement and closure of wounds is important in preventing infection. To be effective, surgery must be undertaken before the patient deteriorates and suffers an irreversible secondary injury. In addition, surgery must not only be timely, it also must be extensive enough to deal adequately with the injury.

PREOPERATIVE CARE

Preoperative management of head injuries begins at the site of the accident; emergency personnel must stabilize the neck and assure the patient's airway, ventilation, and oxygenation levels. Fluid resuscitation, if required, should also be initiated at the scene of the accident. The injured brain does not tolerate hypoxia and ischemia well, and the best subsequent care may be futile if these are not prevented during the initial management.

In the emergency room the patient's neck should be protected until a lateral x-ray study of the entire cervical spine excludes the possibility of a cervical fracture. Airway patency, control of hemorrhage, and fluid resuscitation are attended to, appropriate blood studies obtained, and blood sent for crossmatch. A rapid but thorough general physical and neurologic examination should be performed pari passu with these initial therapeutic measures. If the patient is deteriorating rapidly, assessment of the level of consciousness, pupillary responses, extraocular eye movements, and motor function will allow the planning of further diagnostic studies and treatment.

After patients are stabilized and evaluated, they are triaged according to the severity of their brain injury (Table 3-1).[2] Grade I patients warrant a period of observation; evidence of significant cranial trauma necessitates skull x-ray films. Grade II patients have sustained a major brain injury and should undergo a CT scan on an urgent basis. Grade III patients require intubation and controlled ventilation. Many of these patients have hypoxia or intracranial hypertension, which are favorably affected by intubation.[3] It is important that the intubation be smooth. An emergency CT scan should be obtained after the patient is intubated. A patient who has or is developing signs of transtentorial herniation should be intubated immediately, hyperventilated, and given 1–2 g/kg mannitol intravenously as rapidly as possible. The use of steroids in the treatment of major head injury remains controversial.[4,5] We do not feel that the evidence convincingly supports their use; however, if used, massive, frequent doses beginning as soon as possible after the injury are indicated.[5] Grade II and grade III patients should receive prophylactic anticonvulsant medication. An initial dose of 18 mg/kg of diphenylhydantoin administered intravenously over 30 minutes while the ECG and blood pressure are monitored is usually sufficient.

Computed tomographic scanning is the diagnostic study of choice is assessing head injuries. In the majority of cases a study without contrast enhancement suffices. An adequate study frequently requires sedation or intubation and paralysis of the patient. A minimum of four cuts at the level of the parasagittal sulci, lateral ventricles, middle fossa, and posterior fossa should be obtained. In a patient whose neurologic condition is deteriorating, the use of mannitol will permit a limited preoperative CT scan to be carried out. This consists of a single cut through the cerebral hemispheres at the level of the lateral ventricles. This will reveal the majority of traumatic intracranial lesions, and is worth obtaining provided it does not delay surgery significantly. Even with major concomitant thoracic or abdominal injuries, a CT scan should have priority if the patient is hemodynamically stable. When studies are done on a machine that is capable of body imaging, limited scans of the chest and abdomen can also be obtained, thereby saving time in the evaluation of patients with multiple injuries. Should circumstances or the patient's condition preclude a CT scan, twist drill ventriculostomy and air ventriculography are an alternative form of assessment that can be performed in the emergency department. Such studies will demonstrate a ventricular shift indicative of a mass lesion. Emergency cerebral angiography remains another diagnostic option in identifying a surgical mass lesion and is the definitive study when vascular injuries are suspected.

OPERATIVE NEUROSURGICAL TECHNIQUES
ISBN 0-8089-1862-1

Table 3-1. Categorization of patients

Grade I: Transient loss of consciousness but alert, oriented, and without neurological deficit
Grade II: Impaired level of consciousness or focal deficit but able to follow at least some simple commands
Grade III: Unable to follow commands; speech if present inappropriate or incoherent. May localize to pain, posture, or may be flaccid.

Adapted from Youmans JR (ed): Neurological Surgery, ed 2. Philadelphia, WB Saunders, 1982, pp 2016.

INDICATIONS FOR SURGERY

If the condition of a patient with an intracranial hematoma begins to deteriorate, the hematoma must be evacuated. Likewise, a grade III patient with an intracranial hematoma that is causing ventricular compression or a midline shift of more than 5 mm, if bilateral clots are present, should undergo surgery. A cerebral contusion is an indication for surgery if it produces a significant mass effect associated with a deficit or deterioration. Involvement of a functionally important region of the brain should prompt close monitoring of the patient's clinical status and intracranial pressure, while medical therapy is used unless the patient's condition deteriorates. Deterioration is an indication for resection of the contused brain.

Scalp wounds less than 12 hours old should be closed. Older wounds should be treated by packing and secondary closure. Linear skull fractures of the vault, even if open, require no specific treatment. Care should be directed to the laceration. We do not recommend prophylactic antibiotic medications. Surgery for basilar fractures involves the treatment of CSF fistulas, cranial nerve injuries, and vascular injuries. Since the elevation of closed depressed skull fractures has little effect on subsequent resolution of neurologic deficits or the incidence of posttraumatic epilepsy, the indications for surgery in these cases is largely cosmetic.[6] The risk of infection in open depressed fractures mandates surgery.

Grade II and grade III patients in whom a surgically treatable lesion has been excluded can be admitted to the intensive care unit and watched closely. If indicated, their intracranial pressure is monitored.

SURGICAL TREATMENT OF SPECIFIC INJURIES

SCALP LACERATIONS

Sufficient hair must be removed from around the wound to allow its adequate visualization and handling. The scalp edges should be infiltrated with local anesthetic, after which the wound can be explored, thoroughly debrided, and copiously irrigated with sterile saline. Devitalized wound edges should be trimmed. Bleeding often is most easily controlled by upward traction on the galea rather than by attempts at direct clamping of individual vessels. A single-layer scalp closure with monofilament suture with approximation of the galea completes treatment. Tension free closure, if there is scalp loss, can be obtained by undermining or advancement flaps. Large or complex wounds often require specialized techniques (see Chapter 1).

DEPRESSED SKULL FRACTURES

Closed depressed fractures of the ''pond'' or ''ping-pong ball'' variety seen in very young children can be elevated by placing a burr hole at the edge of the depression and reducing the fracture by applying upward leverage on the depressed segment with a periosteal elevator inserted through the burr hole. These fractures can be extremely resistant to elevation; therefore, be prepared to proceed with the standard approach outlined below.

In the treatment of a closed depressed fracture the scalp incision should provide adequate exposure, since the fracture, particularly the involvement of the inner table, may be more extensive than apparent radiographically. Exposure can be obtained using either an S-shaped incision or a horseshoe flap. The curvilinear incision is the simplest and most rapid, can be enlarged readily, and interferes little with the scalp's blood supply. The horseshoe flap provides exposure without retraction and avoids the problem of placing a suture line over the fracture site. This incision requires more precise placement and takes longer to fashion and close. Enlarging it often means a T-shaped incision with its potential for poor healing. Compound fractures frequently require debridement of devitalized scalp, which may involve removal of an ellipse of tissue. Debridement should be carried down to the pericranium and extended back to viable tissue. Bone fragments are usually too firmly impacted to permit their direct extraction. Levering fragments free is dangerous to the underlying cortex; therefore a burr hole should be placed at the margin of the fracture to expose the normal dura; the fragments then can be removed with rongeurs.

Fractures crossing the dural venous sinuses are potentially treacherous. The injury may have lacerated the sinus and the depressed fragment may be tamponading the rent. Elevation of the fragment can provoke torrential bleeding. It is often better to leave a closed fracture crossing the dural venous sinuses undisturbed. If elevation is attempted, be prepared to deal with hemorrhage (see Chapter 75). The anesthetist is alerted to the possibility of sudden massive blood loss, and blood for transfusion should be available immediately. Burr holes are placed and sufficient bone removed to provide control of the sinus on either side of the depressed fracture before it is elevated. Should hemorrhage occur, it usually can be significantly slowed by raising the patient's head. Bone removal continues until all fragments are free and normal dura is exposed at the margins. Open fractures should be meticulously debrided of foreign material and copiously irrigated. Nasal sinuses that have been exposed are exenterated and filled with muscle or fat. If possible, a galeal flap can be pulled over the end of the violated sinus and tacked to the dura below to seal the opening. Intact, normal-appearing dura should be left unopened; however, if it appears tense or bluish in color, it is incised and the underlying brain examined. Intracranial hematoma or contused brain is removed. A dural laceration should be trimmed and extended to permit removal of foreign material, hematoma, and contused brain and to obtain hemostasis. The dura is closed in a watertight fashion with pericranium or a fascia lata graft if necessary. The bone fragments can be wired back into place with a low risk of infection, thereby saving the patient a further procedure.[7] This maneuver would be contraindicated if the wound is older than 24 hours or is grossly contaminated. The scalp can be closed in a single layer with monofilament suture and the galea approximated. The management of extensive scalp loss is discussed in Chapter 1.

Prophylactic coverage with a semisynthetic penicillin can be used in most cases of depressed skull fractures. Those patients who have sustained a dural laceration and a brain contusion should be started on anticonvulsants.

BASILAR SKULL FRACTURES

The surgical treatment of basilar skull fractures is directed at correcting CSF fistula, decompressing the optic and facial nerves, and repairing vascular injuries.

CSF FISTULAS

Most CSF leaks stop spontaneously, usually as a result of adhesions or herniation of brain into the fracture site. This type of closure is insecure and poses the risk of delayed meningitis. Accordingly, some neurosurgeons advocate an aggressive approach to this problem.[8] Because the magnitude of this risk is uncertain, we favor a trial of conservative treatment before resorting to surgery. This entails bed rest with the head elevated, and, if flow continues after 3 days, serial lumbar punctures. The use of prophylactic antibiotics in this situation is controversial, although some reports have shown an apparent benefit.[9] Other reports do not demonstrate a decrease in the incidence of meningitis[10,11,12] and suggest an increased risk of infection with resistant organisms.[13] We do not employ prophylactic antibiotics. A CSF leak that persists for over a week requires studies to localize the fistula.

Localization of the site of a CSF fistula requires a complete set of skull roentgenograms. These should be examined for fractures, air–fluid levels, or sinus opacification. Full delineation of fractures is aided by thin-section CT scans of the skull base, often supplemented by reconstructions in the coronal and sagittal planes. Radioisotope cisternography may be of help in localizing the site of a leak either by direct visualization with gamma camera imaging[14] or by nasopharyngeal pledgets placed at strategic locations to detect radioactivity. A variant of this technique involves the intrathecal instillation of fluorescein dye into the subarachnoid space rather than an isotope. This agent has been reported to cause status epilepticus and is no longer widely used.[15] Metrizamide cisternography with CT scanning is a relatively new technique capable of precisely defining the site of a fistula.[16]

The intracranial approach to correcting CSF fluid leaks in the anterior fossa is usually through a bifrontal craniotomy, although a localized fracture may be dealt with through a unilateral opening. Fractures of the petrous ridge can be exposed through a temporal or suboccipital craniectomy. The fistula can be visualized intradurally and closed primarily or with a pericranial or fascia lata graft. The intradural approach allows the brain to press against the graft, keeping it in place. The graft should be secured with sutures. In technically awkward situations, this can be most easily accomplished by first passing the sutures through the dura surrounding the defect and then through the edges of the graft while it is still outside of the wound. The graft then can be slid down the sutures into place and the sutures tied. Cyanoacrylic glue also can be used to secure and seal a repair.

Cerebrospinal fluid leaks involving the frontal sinus, ethmoid sinus, sphenoid sinus, and mastoid air cells can be repaired through extracranial approaches.[17] These approaches have less morbidity relative to the open procedures. Leaks arising in the parasellar area and involving the sphenoid sinus are particularly suited to a transsphenoidal repair. After the fistula is exposed, a fascial graft can be placed over the leak and reinforced with fat or muscle. Cyanoacrylic glue can be used to secure the graft and assure a seal.

CRANIAL NERVE INJURIES

Basilar fractures are often associated with trauma to the optic and facial nerves. The indications for decompression of the cranial nerves are controversial.[18] Trauma to the optic nerve in its passage through the optic canal is common with fractures of the skull base, but whether the injury to the nerve results from the fracture is uncertain. Surgical decompression is indicated if vision is present after the injury but subsequently deteriorates. In such situations prompt surgery has yielded good results.[19] Surgical decompression is unlikely to be of benefit in treating stable complete or partial visual deficits or partial visual deficits that are improving. If undertaken, the usual surgical approach is a frontal or pterional craniotomy. A high speed drill with a diamond bit under continuous irrigation is used to unroof the optic canal. Extracranial approaches that avoid retraction of contused or swollen frontal lobes have also been used for this purpose.[20,21,22] The value of steroids in treating optic nerve injuries remains unproved. Injury to the facial nerve within the temporal bone is common and the resultant paralysis can be immediate, delayed, or mixed in nature, reflecting the relative contribution of physical disruption and nerve swelling with compression to the loss of nerve function. Most patients undergo a good spontaneous recovery, which has led many surgeons to adopt a conservative approach to the issue of surgical decompression.[18] Although the timing and indications for surgery vary, the usual indication is that of immediate paralysis with electrophysiologic evidence of denervation or decreased conduction.[23] Delayed paralysis with axonal degeneration on electrical testing can also be an indication for exploration. Injuries distal to the geniculate ganglion can be exposed through standard mastoid and middle ear procedures, whereas those proximal to this point require an intracranial procedure. The nerve should be decompressed, and, if transected, sutured primarily or joined with a cable graft. Hypoglossal–facial nerve anastomosis and nerve grafts from the premeatal nerve stump to the nerve stump distal to the stylomastoid foramen[24] offer additional options. Steroids are frequently used in treating facial nerve injuries, although their value in this situation is unproved.

CAROTID-CAVERNOUS SINUS FISTULAS

Carotid-cavernous sinus fistulas are among the most common traumatic vascular lesions and often occur in the presence of a basilar fracture. Although life-threatening complications are rare with these lesions, a high proportion of patients with fistulas develop progressive monocular blindness, which justifies an aggressive approach. Surgical procedures employing proximal carotid ligation or trapping of the fistula carry the risk of ischemic complications. Embolization procedures combined with ligation of the ophthalmic artery were attempts to avoid this problem but they still presented the risk of stroke and were

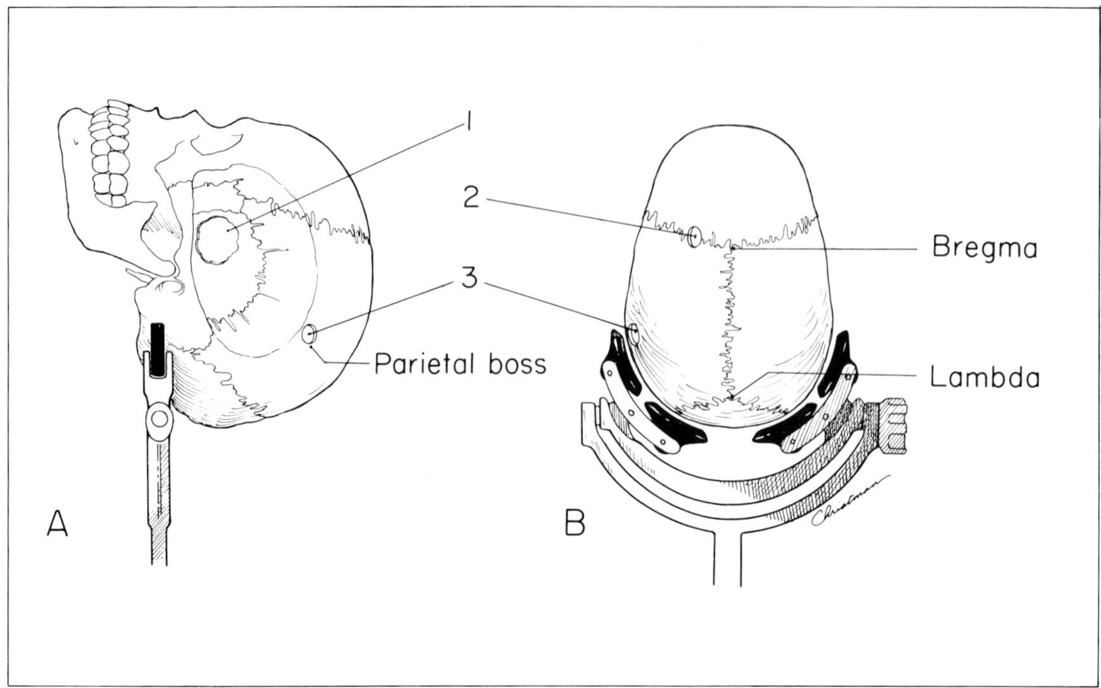

Fig. 3-1.   Positioning of exploratory burr holes. Placement begins in the temporal fossa ipsilateral to the suspected lesion.

not always successful in ablating the fistula.[25] The direct attack on the fistula used by Parkinson allows obliteration of the fistula with preservation of the carotid, but involves a major technical tour de force[26] with significant morbidity and mortality. Mullan developed an open surgical procedure in which the sinus is packed, blocking the fistula and preserving the carotid.[27] This has a high success rate with low morbidity and mortality. The therapy of carotid-cavernous sinus fistulas has been revolutionized by the advent of detachable balloon catheters.[28,29] These allow transcutaneous occlusion of most fistulas with preservation of the carotid lumen. Those fistulas that cannot be closed from the arterial side are often amenable to occlusion via the jugular vein.

TRAUMATIC MASS LESIONS

ANESTHESIA

Smooth intubation and induction of anesthesia in a patient with an intracranial mass and intracranial hypertension are critical. Mannitol is administered intravenously in a dose of 1–2 g/kg. Before intubation the patient should be paralyzed and given a bolus of thiopental. Lidocaine then should be instilled intratracheally. When the endotracheal tube is in place, the patient is hyperventilated to a $PaCO_2$ of 20–30 torr. Volatile anesthetic agents should be avoided because of their dilatory effect on cerebral vessels, which can adversely affect intracranial pressure.

EXPLORATORY BURR HOLES

There are situations in which a patient deteriorates so rapidly that diagnostic studies cannot be obtained. In such instances exploratory burr holes are placed. This procedure is of value only if the surgeon is prepared to proceed with a

craniotomy, since acute traumatic hematomas and contusions cannot be dealt with adequately through burr holes. The patient is placed in the brow-up position, which provides access to both sides of the head. The first burr hole should be made in the temporal region according to the following scheme (in order of localizing value): (1) ipsilateral to a dilated pupil; (2) contralateral to the most abnormal motor response, and (3) on the side of the fracture. Subsequent trephinations are undertaken in the parietal and frontal regions (Figure 3-1). The scalp incisions and burr holes should be placed to permit their incorporation into a formal craniotomy if a hematoma is encountered. When the procedure is completed on one side, it should be repeated on the other side.

BASIC TRAUMA CRANIOTOMY

Relatively small localized epidural hematomas or contusions of the temporal pole can at times be evacuated through a limited opening (Figure 3-2). However, the majority of traumatic injuries are best dealt through a generous frontotemporal craniotomy that provides access to the frontal and temporal poles and the area along the vertex (Figure 3-3). These are the most frequent sites of hematomas and contusions. Hemorrhage from bridging veins to the sagittal sinus can be controlled, and fractures, dural lacerations, and vascular injuries at the skull base visualized and treated.

The patient should be positioned with the head turned to the side, supported on a Richards headrest or donut, level, and elevated above the level of the heart. A bolster placed under the ipsilateral shoulder can help to prevent positional obstruction of cranial venous drainage. The scalp incision is begun a centimeter in front of the tragus and continued to several centimeters below the hairline. With a patient whose condition is deteriorating or who has a known temporal fossa lesion, the inferior end of the incision should be opened and a limited craniectomy performed immediately so that the dura can be opened,

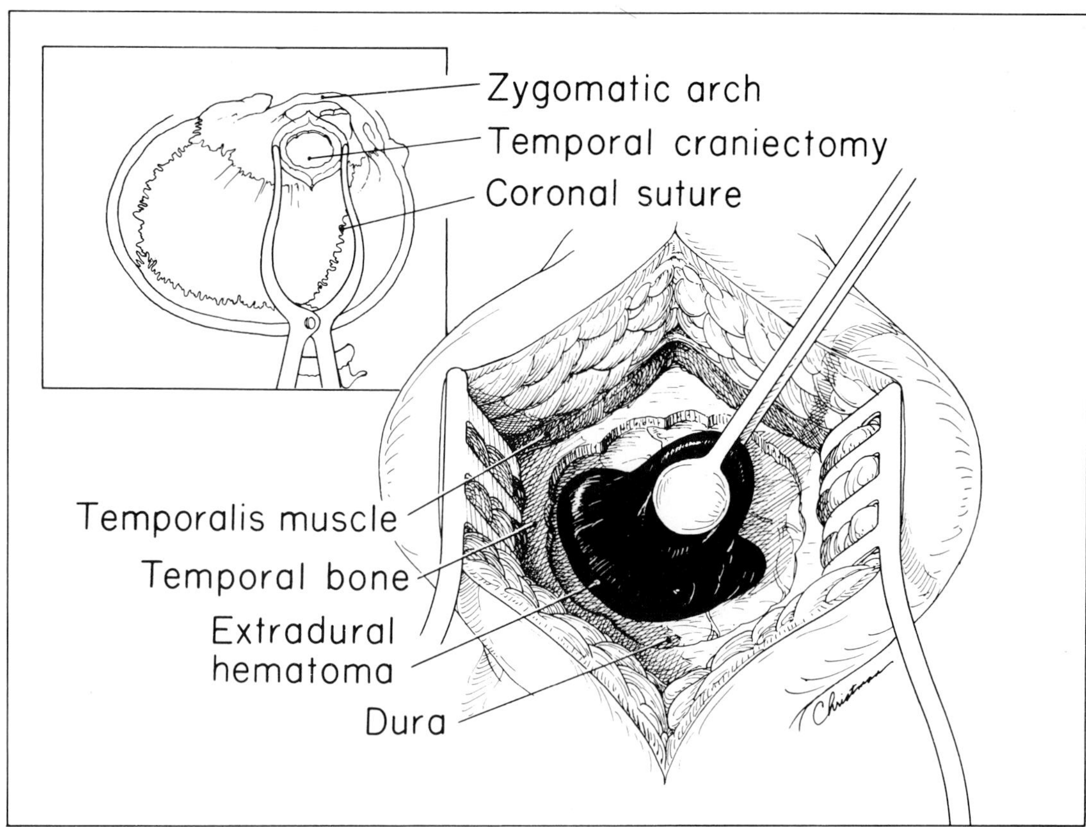

Fig. 3-2. A limited craniectomy for a small epidural hematoma. The same exposure provides access to localized contusion of the temporal pole.

hematoma evacuated, and contused brain decompressed, thereby affording immediate relief of the elevated intracranial pressure. The scalp incision then can be completed, and a large free or osteoplastic bone flap extending to within 2 or 3 cm of the midline and curving low over the frontal region elevated. Resection of the lateral sphenoid wing will further enlarge the exposure. If already begun, the temporal dural opening can be continued. Otherwise, the dural opening should be begun over the temporal region, since if brain herniates through the dural opening here, relatively silent cortex is affected. Often only contused temporal lobe will herniate, but if intact cortex begins to extrude, the intracranial pressure must be reduced. Hematomas and cerebral contusions are evacuated and the intracranial space explored. Gentle handling of the injured brain is critical during the procedure, since it cannot tolerate further mechanical trauma from rough instrumentation and forceful retraction. Meticulous hemostasis is vital in avoiding the disastrous third injury of a recurrent hematoma. After the procedure is completed, the dura should be closed with a pericranial or fascia lata graft, if necessary (Figure 3-4), and the bone flap secured with nonmetallic sutures. We use a subgaleal drain brought out through a separate incision and close the scalp in two layers. We do not recommend either leaving the dura open or the bone flap out for decompression.[30]

Sudden massive intraoperative brain swelling can develop during the surgery of a major head injury, particularly after evacuation of an intracerebral or subdural hematoma. A loss of cerebrovascular autoregulation with acute cerebral hyperemia is thought to account for this phenomenon. A brief period of arterial hypotension to a systolic pressure of 60–90 torr in combination with hyperventilation and additional mannitol of-

ten reverses this swelling, although these measures may need to be repeated several times. Brain swelling that is unrelieved by these means may respond to 500-mg boluses of thiopental to a total dose of 1–2 g. Only in the face of recalcitrant swelling should internal decompression by temporal or frontal lobectomy be used.

In the less common situations in which parietal, occipital, or posterior fossa lesions are present, the approach should be modified. Parietal lesions may be accessible by enlargement of the basic craniotomy flap. Otherwise, a reverse question mark or a Poppen type II scalp incision will provide the needed access. For posterior fossa masses a wide suboccipital craniectomy is used. The dural opening is begun on the side of the lesion.

EPIDURAL HEMATOMAS

Complete exposure of the hematoma out to normal dura is important. Although a more limited opening may suffice, the hematoma is usually best removed through the standard craniotomy described above (Figure 3-5). The clot should be removed and any bleeding controlled with bipolar coagulation. Fractures injuring the middle meningeal artery may require packing of the foramen spinosum with bone wax or bone wax mixed with cotton fiber to control hemorrhage. After hemostasis is achieved, the dura should be opened for several centimeters and the subdural space and brain inspected. The incision then can be closed and the dura tacked up to the craniotomy (Figure 3-6).

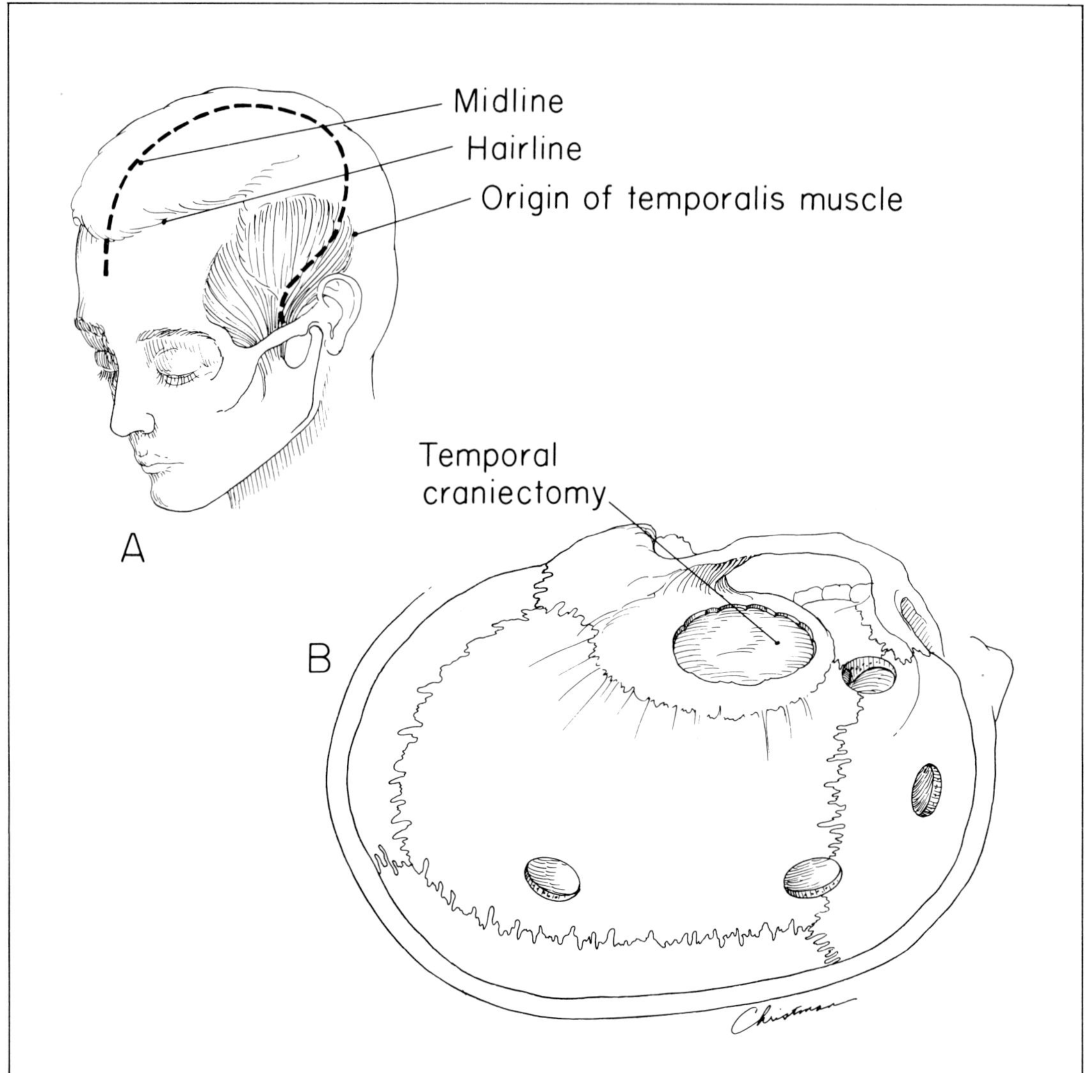

Fig. 3-3. Scalp incision and burr hole placement for a standard trauma craniotomy. Note the temporal craniectomy for initial decompression.

SUBDURAL HEMATOMA

After a generous opening has been made in the dura, the acute subdural hematoma can be removed by suction or gentle traction with cup forceps (Figure 3-7). Bleeding points on the brain surface should be coagulated. Hemorrhage from bridging veins arising from the sagittal sinus can be particularly troublesome. If coagulation is ineffective, tamponade with Gelfoam or Avitene-Surgicel packs will usually stop the bleeding. The subdural space and brain are then systematically inspected over the frontal, medial, occipital, and temporal surfaces for hematoma, contusion, or bleeding. Small amounts of clot that cannot be visualized adequately should be left undisturbed. Tentorial section and medial temporal lobectomy in an attempt to relieve a herniated medial temporal lobe are not recommended. After bleeding has been controlled, the dura can be closed in a watertight fashion and tacked up to the margins of the craniotomy.

CEREBRAL CONTUSION

Cerebral contusions are areas of irreparably damaged brain that serve as a nidus for brain swelling and further hemorrhage. As a general rule, contusions over the frontal and temporal regions larger than 1–2 cm should be removed. Judicious resection limited to purplish, mottled brain likewise is permissible in more eloquent areas (Figure 3-8).

INTRACEREBRAL HEMATOMAS

Intracerebral hematomas tend to occur in the frontal and temporal regions, but are generally more deeply situated than cerebral contusions. Computed tomographic scanning has made the diagnosis of these lesions common and their localization precise. Because they frequently are associated with the other traumatic lesions, in most instances the surgical approach should be the standard trauma craniotomy. Hematomas near the cortical surface and greater than 1–2 cm in diameter should be evacuated, whereas deeply placed hematomas are left undisturbed unless they produce significant shift and elevate intracranial pressure or are associated with a neurologic deficit.

POSTOPERATIVE MANAGEMENT

The goal of the medical management of patients with head injuries is to prevent secondary injury and to provide the ideal milieu in which the injured brain can recover. This requires that patients be closely monitored and that strict attention be paid to

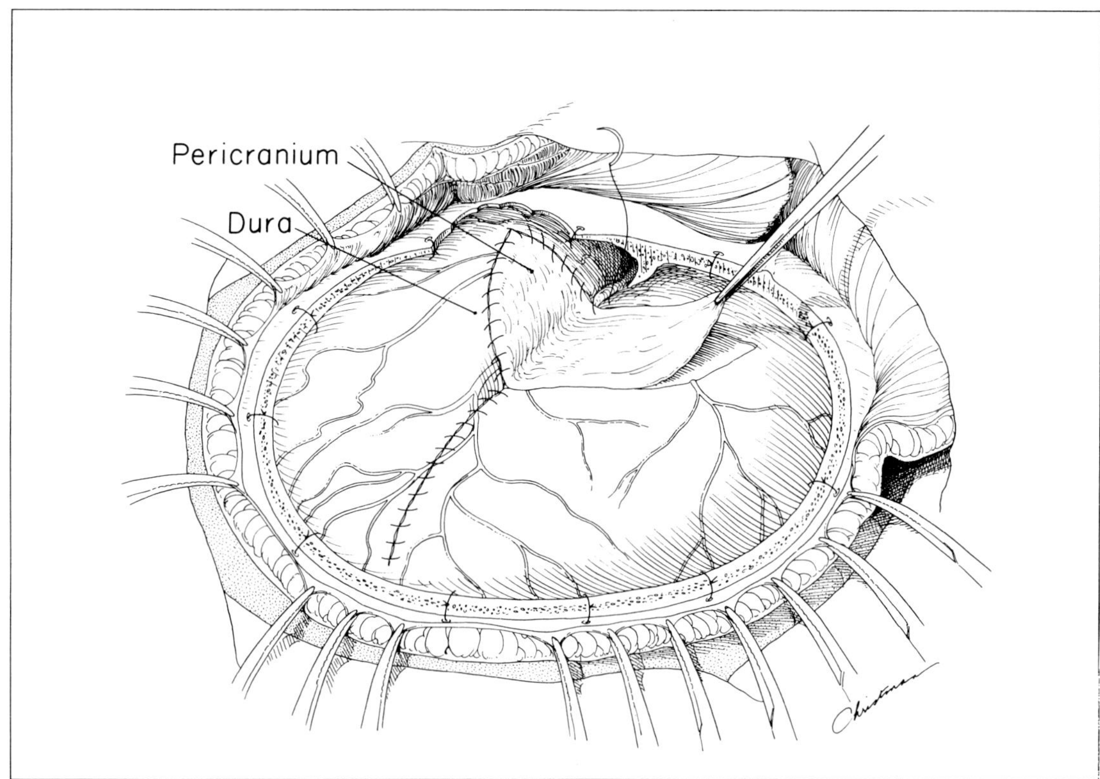

Fig. 3-4. Dural closure with a pericranium graft. Note the dural tacking sutures at the craniotomy edge.

maintaining the patient's normal physiologic and metabolic status. The patient's clinical condition should be re-evaluated and recorded at least hourly. In addition, many patients require invasive cardiovascular and intracranial pressure monitoring.

The injured brain tolerates hypoxia poorly, and supplementary oxygen and ventilatory support should be used to maintain the PaO_2 at 80 torr or above and the $PaCO_2$ between 25 and 30 torr. Sedation and paralysis may be necessary. Because cerebrovascular autoregulation is frequently impaired in head trauma, cardiovascular function must be strictly regulated.[31] Hypotension in conjunction with elevated intracranial pressure can result in cerebral ischemia, while hypertension promotes cerebral hyperemia and edema. Control of elevated blood pressure can usually be achieved with trimethephan camsylate. The effect of this agent is titratable and it does not have the cerebral vasodilator properties of nitroprusside. Fluid replacement should be aimed at maintenance levels with isotonic fluids. Strict fluid restriction is not recommended, since increased plasma volume in the absence of hypotonicity does not promote cerebral edema. Fluid restriction increases the risk of hypotension, electrolyte imbalance, and renal failure.[32] The monitoring of cardiovascular and fluid status in severe head injury requires an arterial line, a Foley catheter, and in many instances, a pulmonary artery catheter. The hematocrit, white blood cell count, electrolytes, and serum osmolality are checked at least daily. Head injury induces a hypermetabolic state similar to that seen in burn and multitrauma victims, and the early institution of enteral or parenteral feeding can favorably affect the outcome.[32]

COMPLICATIONS

We believe that the control of increased intracranial pressure is important, and intracranial pressure monitoring provides a rational means of guiding and gauging the effectiveness of

therapy. After a traumatic mass lesion is evacuated, 50 percent or more of patients develop an intracranial pressure of 20 torr or more.[33] We routinely monitor the ICP of these patients postoperatively. Grade II patients with mass lesions are also monitored, particularly if they require general anesthesia. Patients who are grade III and who have an abnormal CT scan are also monitored. Grade III patients with normal CT scans also are at a significant risk of developing intracranial hypertension and should be monitored if they have two or more of the following risk factors: an age greater than 40 years; a systolic blood pressure of less than 90 torr on admission, or abnormal posturing.[34]

Intracranial pressure can be lowered by elevation of the head, avoidance of jugular compression, and sedation or paralysis, especially if the patient is restless or posturing. Paralysis alone without sedation should be avoided since noxious stimuli can cause an elevation in intracranial pressure even in a comatose patient. Steroids traditionally have been given for their supposed effect on cerebral edema. If a ventricular catheter is in place, pressure can be reduced by venting CSF. Hyperventilation sufficient to lower the $PaCO_2$ to 25–30 torr is the mainstay of therapy. Mannitol can be given if the intracranial pressure remains elevated. With an ICP monitor to measure its effect, doses of 0.25–0.30 g/kg will often be adequate. Diuretics, particularly in combination with mannitol, are also effective in lowering elevated ICP. Elevated intracranial pressure that does not respond to these measures requires prompt re-evaluation of the patient for a surgically treatable lesion; if none is found, iatrogenic pentobarbital coma can be instituted. Since a recent randomized prospective trial of the prophylactic use of pentobarbital failed to show an effect on the development, severity, or outcome of elevated ICP, this drug should be considered as a last effort to treat an elevated ICP that is unresponsive to other measures.[35] A multicenter trial is

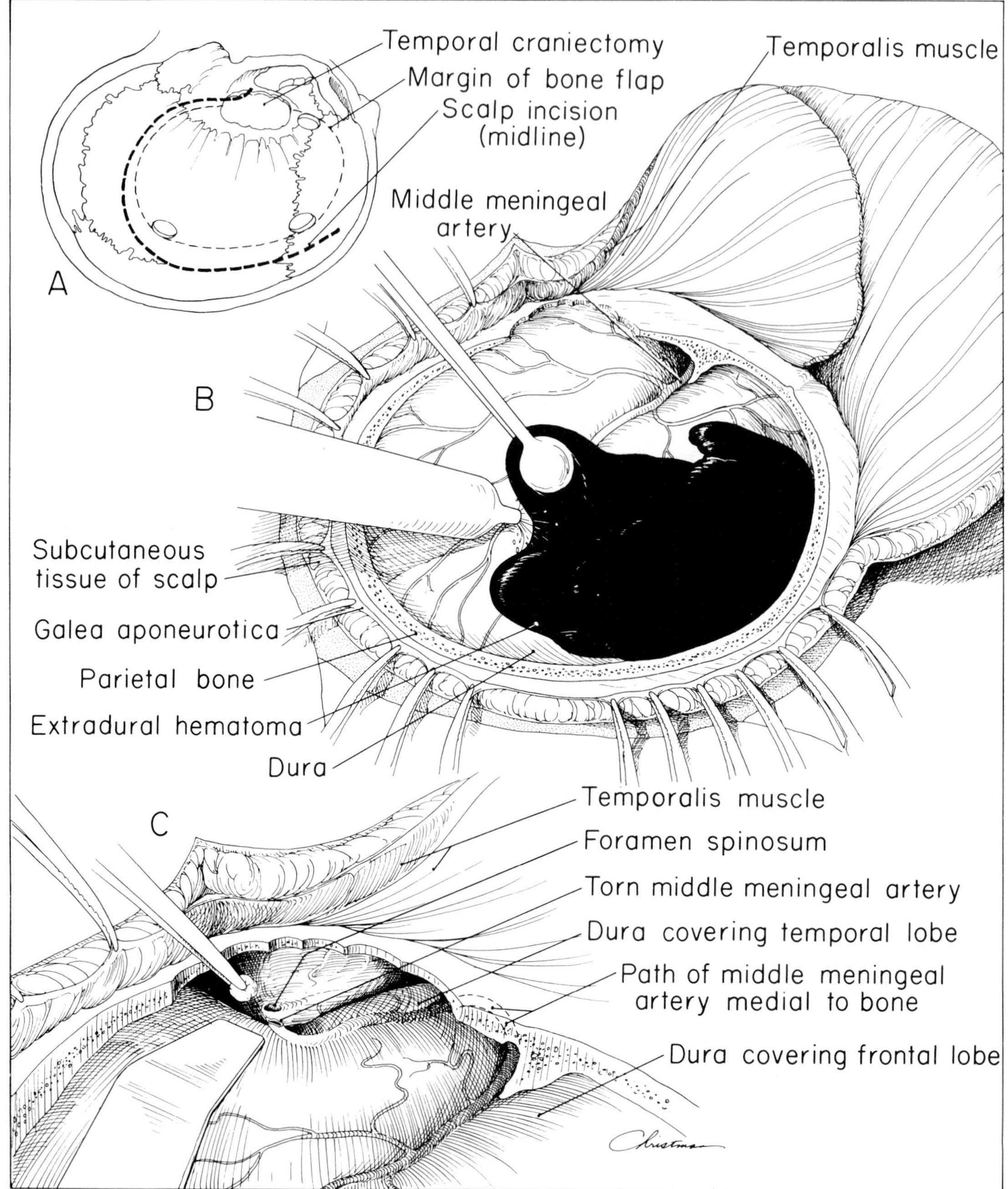

Fig. 3-5. (A) The scalp incision and bone flap for removal of a large extradural hematoma. (B) Removal of the clot. (C) Packing of the foramen spinosum.

now in progress that may better define the value of pentobarbital coma in the treatment of head injury. If used, 5–10 mg/kg of pentobarbital can be given as a loading dose and 1–3 mg/kg/hour administered by continuous infusion titrated to a burst suppression pattern on the EEG. Hypotension is a common problem and requires radial artery and pulmonary artery catheters to monitor blood pressure, cardiac output, and volume.

INFECTION

Postoperative infection in head injury may stem from contamination at the time of injury or it may be introduced at surgery. Meningitis, subdural empyema, and brain abscess, which are serious enough in otherwise normal patients, are often devastating complications in patients with head injuries. The brain tolerates the additional insult poorly, and the presence of intracranial infection may be masked by the traumatic deficit, leading to a delay in diagnosis. Local evidence of infection, fever, leukocytosis, seizure, and neurologic deterioration should call to mind this possibility and initiate aggressive evaluation and antibiotic treatment. Until culture results are known, large doses of a semisynthetic penicillin in combination with chloramphenicol should be administered. These provide wide ± spectrum coverage and good penetration into the central nervous system. Reviews on the use of antibiotics for central nervous system infections are available.[36] Third generation cephalosporins are playing an increasing role in their treat-

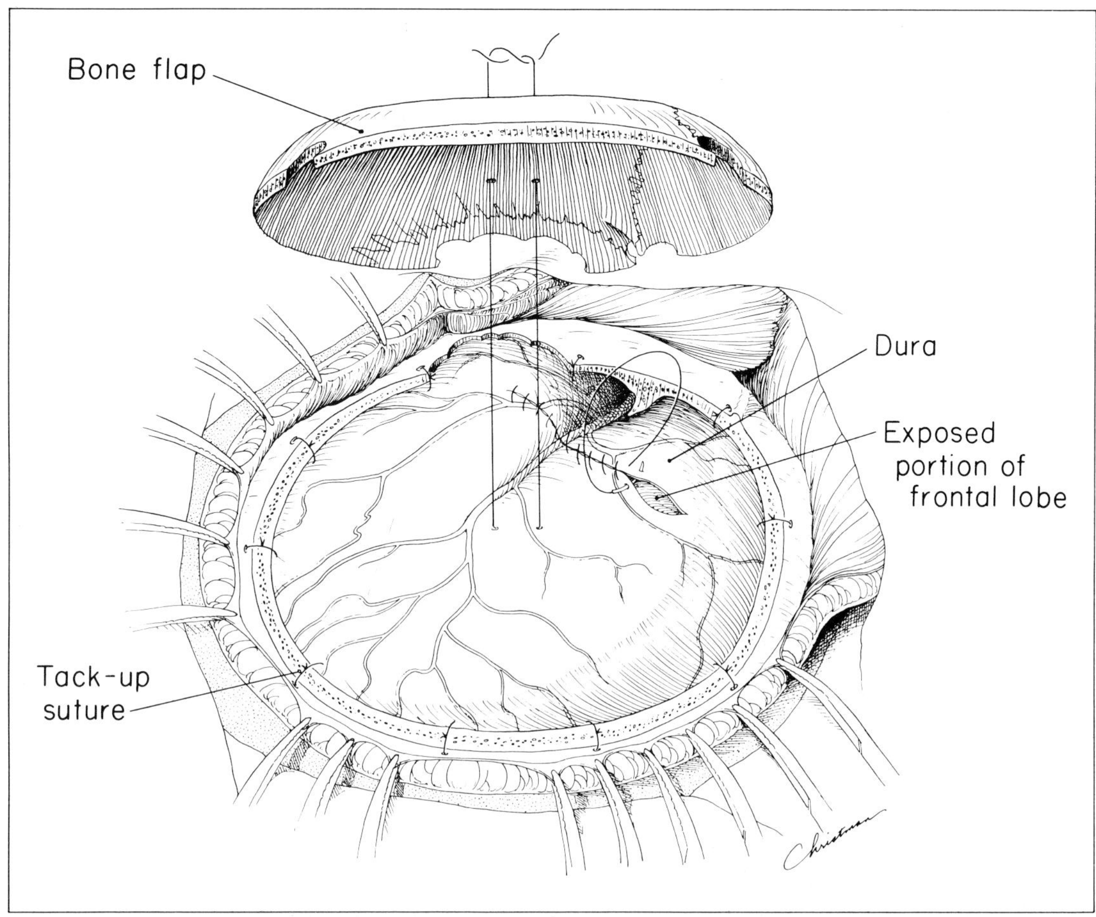

Fig. 3-6. Closure of an exploratory dural incision and tacking up of the dura to the bone flap and craniotomy edges.

ment.[37] Definitive therapy should be guided by the culture results and the infectious disease consultant.

An iatrogenic source of infection in head trauma warrants specific attention. An intracranial pressure monitoring device poses the risk of infection. This is particularly true with ventricular catheters. While meticulous technique during insertion and tunneling of the catheter and maintenance of a closed system may help reduce this risk, the most important factor is the length of time the catheter is left in place. In one series, the incidence of ventriculitis was 9 percent with catheters left in place for 5 days; this rose to 21 percent at 8 days and 37 percent at 10 days.[38] In over half of the cases the responsible organism was a Gram-negative bacterium. This study suggests that catheters should be removed quickly or relocated if they are left in place for more than 5 days. Although the incidence of infection is less with subarachnoid bolts and epidural devices, it is probably best to follow the same dictum and to remove them altogether as soon as possible.

RESPIRATORY COMPLICATIONS

Up to 65 percent of comatose head injured patients become hypoxic even with apparently adequate respirations or while hyperventilating.[39] The cause remains obscure, but disseminated miliary atelectasis with pulmonary shunting may underlie this phenomenon. The frequent occurrence of hypoxia in this group is a major indication for the routine intubation of grade III patients. Survival in head trauma has been shown to correlate with the degree of shunt.[39] Pulmonary edema is thought to occur as a direct result of severe head trauma[40,41] and is presumed to stem from a massive sympathetic discharge consequent to injury of the hypothalamus, which results in acute pulmonary hypertension. More often pulmonary edema in head injury is caused by fluid overload or the aspiration of gastric contents. Aspiration can also lead to bacterial pneumonia. Direct chest trauma with flail chest, pneumothorax or hemothorax, or pulmonary contusion can impair respiratory function in head injury. Concomitant long bone fractures that cause fat emboli can also occur. The patient with a head injury who is immobile is at risk of developing pulmonary emboli from deep venous thrombosis, particularly if injuries to the lower extremities or pelvis are present. These factors alone or in combination may trigger the development of adult respiratory distress syndrome (ARDS). Shock and disseminated intravascular coagulation (DIC) can also precipitate this condition. Once this syndrome develops, progressive respiratory failure and death ensues in a high proportion of patients.

In intubated, comatose patients many of the signs of respiratory insufficiency may be lacking, and the first indication is often a fall in the PaO_2. Radiographic changes usually lag behind the deterioration noted in arterial blood gases. Therapy should be aimed at supporting the level of oxygenation while reversing any underlying treatable lesion. The FIO_2 is increased to maintain the PaO_2 above 80 torr. If an FIO_2 of 100 percent fails to accomplish this, or an FIO_2 of 50 percent or more is required for a prolonged period, positive end-expiratory pres-

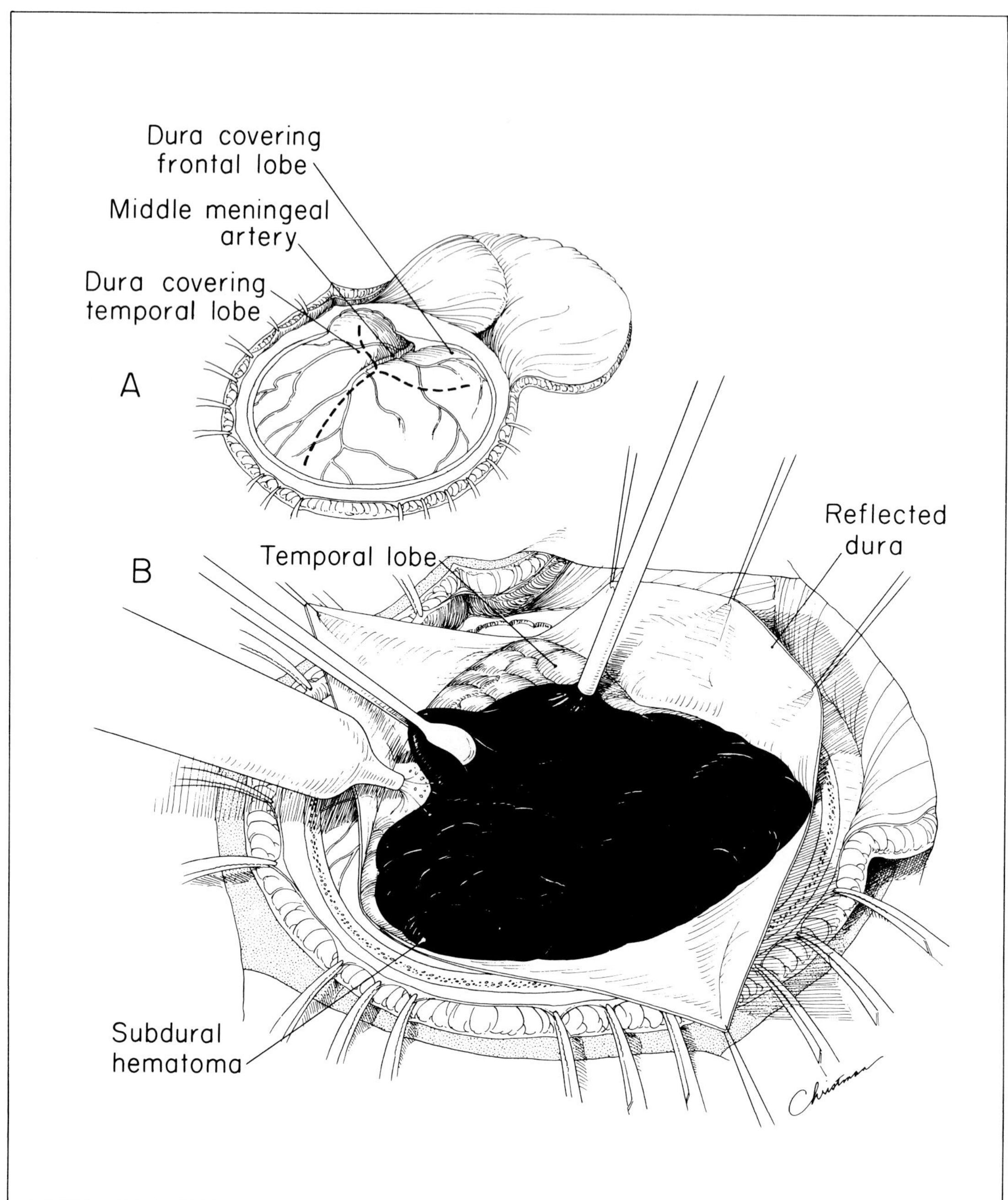

Fig. 3-7. (A) The dural opening for evacuation of a subdural hematoma. The incision begins over the temporal lobe. (B) Removal of clot.

sure (PEEP) should be instituted. Patients usually tolerate this to levels of 10 cm H_2O without an increase in the intracranial pressure when the head is elevated 30 degrees.[42] Intracranial pressure monitoring is required. Since PEEP can depress cardiac output, a pulmonary arterial catheter is useful as a guide to fluid management.

Oxygen therapy and positive pressure ventilation constitute the only treatment with demonstrated efficacy in treating ARDS. Steroids, fluid restriction, diuretics, and the use of colloid rather than crystalloid fluid replacement have been advocated, but whether they affect outcome has not been conclusively demonstrated. Central neurogenic pulmonary edema can also be treated with PEEP.[43] Pulmonary edema secondary to fluid overload responds to diuresis and fluid

restriction. Aspiration pneumonia can be treated with steroids, diuretics, and antibiotics. Suprainfections commonly complicate the other causes of respiratory failure, and frequent sputum cultures should be obtained for all such patients. Oxygen, positive pressure, and fluid resuscitation to treat concomitant shock are the most useful measures for treating fat emboli. Specific treatment designed to improve the microcirculation and to reduce serum lipid levels has produced inconsistent results.[44] Pulmonary emboli from deep vein thrombosis are best prevented with pulsatile stockings. Minidoses of heparin have been shown to be safe after craniotomy,[45] but hemorrhagic complications have been reported and this modality is best avoided in head injury. If a pulmonary embolus occurs and recent injury or surgery prevent

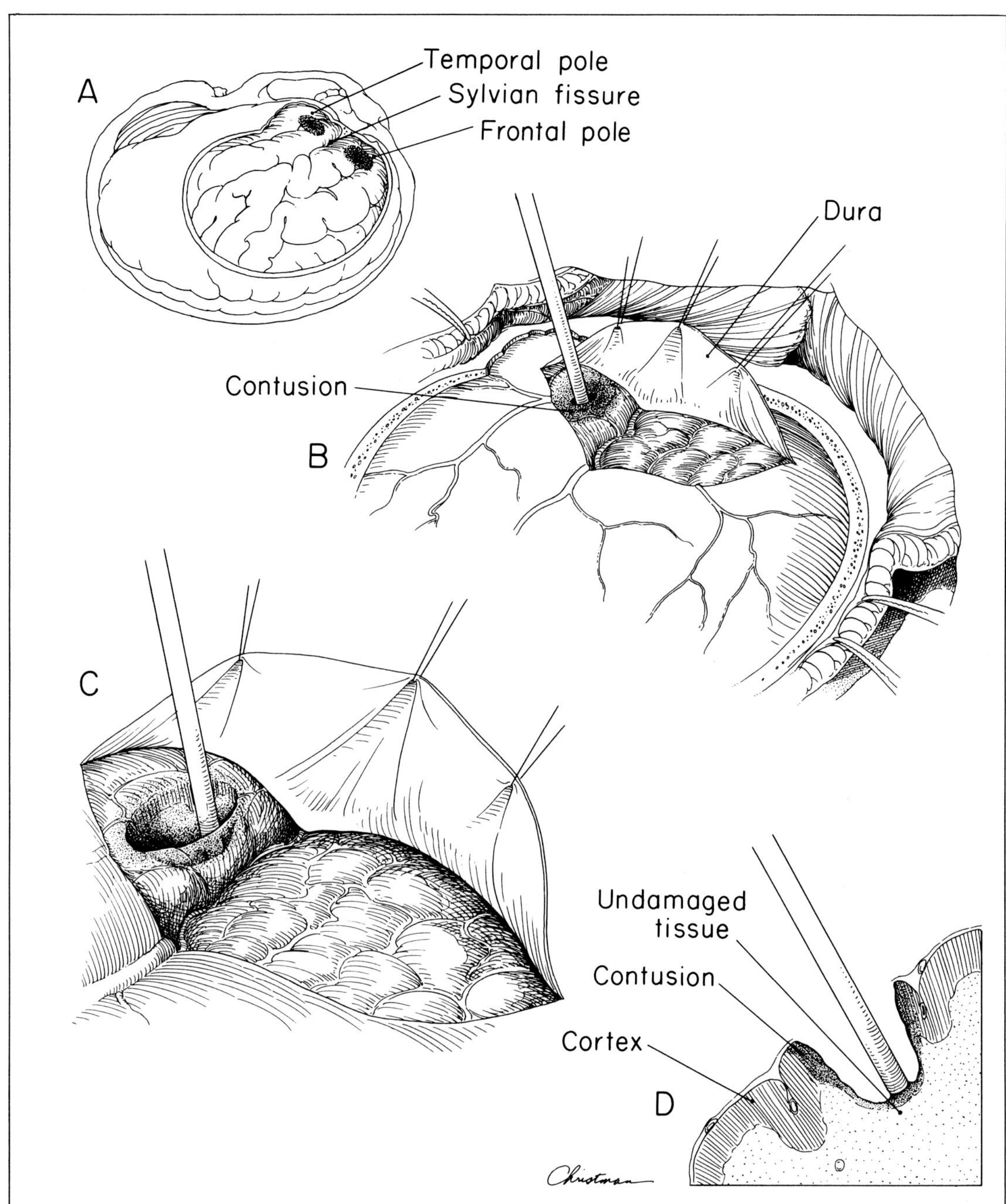

Fig. 3-8. (A) The usual location of contusions. (B) The dural opening for access to contusions. (C) Resection of contusion limited to damaged brain.

heparinization, ligation of the vena cava or placement of a caval umbrella should be considered.

FLUID AND ELECTROLYTES

Standard neurosurgical practice to date has been to maintain patients in a mild to moderate degree of hypernatremic hypovolemia by fluid restriction to combat cerebral edema. However, evidence suggests that plasma tonicity, not volume, is the significant factor that influences brain water.[46,47] It also appears that head injury induces a hyperdynamic cardiovascular state in which fluid restriction may be harmful and isovolemia will improve the overall outcome. This may be particularly true in the multitrauma patient in whom tissue

perfusion is vital.[32] Hypovolemia can also make the use of other measures to combat intracranial hypertension, such as controlled ventilation, osmotic diuresis, and pentobarbital, more difficult by predisposing the patient to hypotension. Fluid replacement at maintenance levels should be attempted with an isotonic fluid at a rate adjusted to avoid hypotonicity and in line with cardiovascular function and electrolyte balance. To this end, serum electrolytes and osmolality should be checked frequently and fluid intake and output monitored. A central venous or pulmonary artery catheter may be helpful in fluid management in more complex situations.

Most abnormalities involve sodium and water balance. However, serum potassium levels are frequently affected in head injury. Stress-induced aldosterone secretion, hyperventilation, therapeutic diuresis, and steroid administration can all result in hypokalemia. This can be corrected by potassium supplementation.

Hyponatremia is the most important electrolyte imbalance complicating head injury, since it promotes cerebral edema and, if severe enough or rapid in onset, seizures. It may be iatrogenic in origin as a result of inappropriate volume replacement with hypotonic fluid or a result of ADH secretion caused by the trauma, surgery, anesthesia, and mechanical ventilation. The syndrome of inappropriate antidiuretic hormone, SIADH, continues despite hypotonicity of the extracellular fluids. Expansion of the extracellular volume as a result of SIADH suppresses aldosterone secretion and increases glomerular blood flow and filtration, which leads to continued urine sodium loss despite plasma hyponatremia. Hyponatremia from SIADH results in hyponatremia, serum hypo-osmolality, increased urine sodium, and increased urine osmolality. Hyponatremia can occur in the absence of hypo-osmolality when another osmotically active substance accumulates in the serum. For example, serum sodium levels may be low when mannitol is being given. Plasma tonicity is increased and the hyponatremia in this case is not meaningful in terms of cerebral edema.

The treatment of hyponatremia depends on its severity. Mild degrees can be managed by restricting fluid intake 500 ml/day, whereas more severe symptomatic levels of hyponatremia may require 3 or 5 percent hypotonic saline in conjunction with furosemide.

Hypernatremia and hyperosmolality result from overzealous fluid restriction, treatment with osmotic agents, and diabetes insipidus, particularly in comatose patients. The iatrogenic forms respond to appropriate fluids. Diabetes insipidus can be treated with pitressin. This can be given in oil, which is more cumbersome to administer but lasts longer, or it can be given in aqueous form. The usual dose is 5–10 units, and this can be repeated until it has an effect. Pitressin in oil is administered subcutaneously, while aqueous pitressin is given either subcutaneously or intravenously. By the latter route it can cause hypertension. Fluid replacement should match urine output milliliter per milliliter on an hourly basis when pitressin is given.

Hypovolemia from the combined loss of sodium and water in head injury is usually caused by the use of diuretics and osmotic agents. Decreased skin turgor, dry mucous membranes, oliguria, and a low central venous or pulmonary wedge pressure are indications of hypovolemia. Serum creatinine and BUN levels are elevated. Serum sodium levels will vary with the relative losses of sodium and water. Treatment is volume expansion using a fluid appropriate to the serum sodium.

SEIZURES

Seizures occur in about 5 percent of patients with head injuries in the immediate postinjury period.[48] They can cause a disastrous increase in intracranial pressure even in a paralyzed patient because of an increase in cerebral blood flow.[49] If the blood flow cannot meet this metabolic demand because of intracranial hypertension, or if the seizure activity is prolonged, further ischemic injury may result.[50] Prophylactic antiseizure medication is therefore used. If seizures occur despite medication, an underlying cause such as hypoxia, electrolyte abnormality, or infection must be excluded. The serum diphenylhydantoin level should also be checked, and if at a subtherapeutic level, the dosage increased. If this is unsuccessful in preventing the seizures, phenobarbital can be added to the regimen. Acute control of seizures can be gained with intravenous diazepam or lorazepam (the latter has less of a cardiorespiratory depressant effect and a longer half-life). These agents can be used until the phenytoin or phenobarbital provides definitive control. Lorazepam is particularly effective in treating status epilepticus.[51] It is administered as an intravenous dose of 1–4 mg over 2 minutes and repeated to a total dose of 0.1 mg/kg if necessary.

GASTROINTESTINAL COMPLICATIONS

Gastrointestinal ulceration is common in conjunction with head injury. Its pathogenesis is unclear. Clinically significant hemorrhage is seen in about 10 percent of patients,[52] usually within 1 week of injury. Cimetidine (500 mg intravenously every 8 hours) is an effective and convenient prophylaxis against this eventuality.

COAGULOPATHY

A high percentage of patients with major head injuries develop clinical and laboratory signs of coagulopathy.[53] These tend to correlate with the severity of the head injury and may be initiated by the release of brain thromboplastin, injury to cerebral vascular endothelium, and neurohumoral alterations consequent to injury. Both hemorrhage and microvascular occlusion involving the brain and other organ systems result. Diagnosis rests on characteristic changes in the platelet count, PT, PTT, fibrinogen levels, and the level of fibrinogen split products. The ethanol gelatin and protamine sulfate paracoagulation tests are useful since positive results require both thrombosis and fibrinolysis to be occurring. When bleeding is a danger, therapy involves replacement of depleted clotting factor and platelets. The use of heparin to suppress ongoing clotting is questionable particularly with a major head injury.

REFERENCES

1. Miller JD, Becker DP: General principles and pathophysiology of head injury, in Youmans JR (ed): Neurological Surgery, ed Philadelphia, WB Saunders, 1982, pp 1896–1937
2. Becker DP, Miller JD, Young HF, et al: Diagnosis and treatment of head injury in adults, in Youmans JR (ed): Neurological Surgery, ed 2. Philadelphia, WB Saunders, 1982, pp 1938–2083
3. Gildenberg PL, Makela ME: The effect of early intubation and ventilation on outcome following head trauma, in Grossman R, Gildenberg PL (eds): Symposium of Neurological Trauma. New York, Raven Press, 1982
4. Gudeman SK, Miller JD, Becker DP: Failure of high dose steroid therapy to influence intracranial pressure in patients with severe head injury. J Neurosurg 51:301, 1979
5. Giannotta SL, Weiss MH, Apuzzo MLJ, et al: High dose glucocorticoids in the management of head injury. Neurosurgery 15:497, 1984
6. Jennett B: Epilepsy After Nonmissile Head Injuries, ed 2. London, Heinemann, 1975, p 179
7. Jennett B, Miller JD: Infection after depressed fracture of the skull: Implications for management of nonmissile injuries. J Neurosurg 36:333, 1972
8. Lewin W: Cerebrospinal fluid rhinorrhea in nonmissile head injuries. Clin Neurosurg 12:237, 1966
9. Leech P: Cerebrospinal fluid leakage, dural fistulae, and meningitis after basal skull fracture. Injury 6:141, 1974
10. MacGee EE, Cauthen JC, Brackett CE: Meningitis following acute traumatic cerebrospinal fistula. J Neurosurg 33:312, 1970

11. Klastersky J, Sadeghi M, Brihaye J: Antimicrobial prophylaxis in patients with rhinorrhea or otorrhea: A double blind study. Surg Neurol 6:111, 1976

12. Hoff JT, Brewin A, U HS: Antibiotics for basilar skull fractures. J Neurosurg 44:649, 1976

13. Raaf J: Posttraumatic cerebrospinal fluid leaks. Arch Surg 95:648, 1967

14. Mamo L, Cophignon J, Rey A, et al: A new radionucleotide method for the diagnosis of posttraumatic cerebrospinal fistula. J Neurosurg 57:92, 1982

15. Mahalay MS Jr, Odom GL: Complication following intrathecal injection of fluorescein: Case report. J Neurosurg 25:298, 1968

16. Calcaterra TC: Extracranial surgical repair of cerebrospinal rhinorrhea. Ann Otol Rhinol Laryngol 89:108, 1980

17. Ahmadi J, Weiss MH, Segall HD, et al: Evaluation of cerebrospinal fluid rhinorrhea by metrizamide computed tomographic cisternography. Neurosurgery 16:54, 1985

18. Rovit RL, Murali R: Injuries of the cranial nerves, in Cooper PR (ed): Head Injury. Baltimore, Williams & Wilkins, 1982, pp 99–114

19. Guyer DR, Miller MR, Long DM, et al: Visual function following optic canal decompression via craniotomy. J Neurosurg 62:631, 1983

20. Fukado Y: Diagnosis and surgical correction of optic canal fracture after head injury. Ophthalmologica Additanent ad. 158:307, 1969

21. Habal MB: Clinical observations on the isolated optic nerve injury. Ann Plast Surg 1:603, 1978

22. Niho S, Niho M, Niho K: Decompression of the optic canal by the transethmoidal route and decompression of the superior orbital fissure. Can J Ophthalmol 5:22, 1970

23. Boles R: Facial, auditory, and vestibular nerve injury associated with basilar skull fracture, in Youmans JR (ed): Neurological Surgery, ed 2. Philadelphia, WB Saunders, 1982, pp 2251–2260

24. Dott NM: Facial nerve reconstruction by graft bypassing the petrous bone. Arch Otolaryngol 78:426, 1963

25. Morley TP: Appraisal of various forms of management in 41 cases of carotid cavernous fistulas, in Morley TP (ed): Current Controversies in Neurosurgery. Philadelphia, WB Saunders, 1976, pp 223–236

26. Parkinson D, Downs AR, Whytehead LL, et al: Carotid cavernous fistula: Direct repair with preservation of carotid. Surgery 76:882, 1974

27. Mullan S: Treatment of carotid cavernous fistula by cavernous sinus occlusion. J Neurosurg 50:131, 1979

28. Mehringer CM, Hieshma GB, Grinnel V, et al: Therapeutic embolization for vascular trauma of the head and neck. AJNR 4:137, 1983

29. Debrun G, Lacour P, Vineula F, et al: Treatment of 54 traumatic carotid cavernous fistulas. J Neurosurg 55:678, 1981

30. Cooper PR, Rovit RL, Ransohoff J: Hemicraniectomy in the treatment of acute subdural hematoma: A reappraisal. Surg Neurol 5:25, 1976

31. Muizelaar JP, Obrist WD: Cerebral blood flow and brain metabolism with brain injury, in Becker DP, Povlishock JT (eds): Central Nervous System Trauma: Status Report 1985. Washington, DC, National Institute of Neurological and Communicative Disorders and Stroke, 1985, pp 123–138

32. Clifton GL, Robertson CS, Grossman RG: Management of the cardiovascular and metabolic response to severe head injury, in Becker DP, Povlishock JT (eds): Central Nervous System Trauma: Status Report 1985. Washington, DC, National Institute of Neurological and Communicative Disorders and Stroke, 1985, pp 139–160

33. Miller JD, Becker DP, Ward JD, et al: Significance of intracranial hypertension in severe head injury. J Neurosurg 47:503, 1977

34. Narayan RK, Kishore PRS, Becker DP, et al: Intracranial pressure: To monitor or not to monitor. J Neurosurg 56:650, 1982

35. Ward JD, Becker DP, Miller JD, et al: Failure of prophylactic barbiturate coma in the treatment of severe head injury. J Neurosurg 62:383, 1985

36. Everett ED, Strausburgh LS: Antimicrobial agents and the central nervous system. Neurosurgery 6:691, 1980

37. Nekson JD: Emerging role of cephalosporins in bacterial meningitis. Am J Med 79 (suppl 2A):47, 1985

38. Mayhall CG, Archer NH, Lamb VA, et al: Ventriculostomy related infection. N Engl J Med 310:553, 1984

39. Frost EAM, Arancibia CU, Shulman K: Pulmonary shunt as a prognostic indicator in head injury. J Neurosurg 50:768, 1979

40. Bean J, Beckman DL: Centrogenic pulmonary pathology in mechanical head injury. J Appl Physiol 27:897, 1969

41. Langfitt TW: Increased intracranial pressure and the cerebral circulation, in Youmans JR (ed): Neurological Surgery, ed 2. Philadelphia, WB Saunders, 1982, pp 864–866

42. Cooper KR, Boswell PA, Choi SC: Safe use of PEEP in patients with severe head injury. J Neurosurg 63:552, 1985

43. Shapiro HM: Intracranial hypertension. Therapeutic and anesthetic considerations. Anesthesiology 43:445, 1975

44. Kramer J, Klawans HL: Fat embolism, in Vinken PJ, Bruyn GW (eds): Handbook of Clinical Neurology, vol

24. Amsterdam, North Holland, 1975, pp 563–574

45. Barnett HG, Clifford JE, Llewllyn RC: Safety of minidose heparin administration for neurosurgical patients. J Neurosurg 47:27, 1977

46. Fishman RA: Effects of isotonic intravenous solutions on normal and increased intracranial pressure. Arch Neurol Psychiatr 70:350, 1953

47. Bakay L, Crawford JD, White JC: The effect of intravenous fluid on cerebrospinal fluid pressure. Surg Gynecol Obstet 99:48, 1954

48. Bricolo A: Electroencephalography in neurotraumatology. Clin Electroencephalogr 7:184, 1976

49. Lassen NA: Control of cerebral circulation in health and disease. Circ Res 34:749, 1974

50. Siesjo BK, Carlsson C, Hagerdal M, et al: Brain metabolism in the critically ill. Crit Care Med 4:283, 1976

51. Levy KJ, Krall RL: Treatment of status epilepticus with lorazepam. Arch Neurol 41:605, 1984

52. Swann K: Severe head injury, in Kennedy SK, Zervas NT (eds): Neurological and Neurosurgical Intensive Care. Baltimore, University Park Press, 1983, pp 207–230

53. Kaufman HH, Mattson JC: Coagulopathies in head injury, in Becker DP, Povlishock JT (eds): Central Nervous System Trauma: Status Report 1985. Washington, DC, National Institute of Neurological and Communicative Disorders and Stroke, 1985, pp 207–230

CHAPTER 4
Surgical Management of Acute and Chronic Subdural Hematoma

J. Douglas Miller

DEFINITIONS

The term *subdural hematoma* refers to all extracerebral collections of blood and serum, both clotted and liquid, that form under the dura mater but do not extend into the subarachnoid space or into the basal or other CSF cisterns. The term *acute subdural hematoma* refers to a collection that becomes evident soon, usually hours, after injury and that consists mainly of clotted blood. In a very fresh hematoma, however, there may be a zone of liquid blood within the clot. The term *chronic subdural hematoma* refers to a collection of almost always dark, altered liquid blood or serum of varying consistency that appears some considerable time, days or more often weeks, after a head injury that is almost always minor and may not even be recollected. A third term, *subacute subdural hematoma,* was coined by McKissock and his colleagues to refer to patients with neurologic deterioration 3 to 7 days after injury that was associated with a temporal mass consisting mainly of clotted subdural blood. With the advent of CT scanning early in the course of head injury of any degree of severity, this delayed presentation of an acute subdural hematoma has become much less common. This leads to the suspicion that most of these patients had an acute subdural collection, the effect of which was later amplified by contusion and vasogenic perifocal edema of the underlying brain, nearly always the temporal pole. Vasogenic edema reaches its peak on the third day after injury, which accounts the delay in presentation. In terms of surgical treatment, it is necessary only to distinguish between acute and chronic subdural hematoma.

PREOPERATIVE DIAGNOSIS AND MANAGEMENT

Acute subdural hematoma is more common in older patients in cases in which coma follows a fall rather than a road traffic accident; in the chronic abuser of alcohol, brain atrophy can permit major accumulation of hematoma before the intracranial pressure rises. In most cases, the diagnosis is made from CT scans after clinical examination has shown the patient to be in a high risk category. If the patient is comatose, scoring 8 or less points on the Glasgow Coma Scale with no eye opening, the risk of harboring a hematoma is 40 percent; if the patient scores less than 15 and has a skull fracture the risk is approximately 10 percent. Both acute and chronic hematomas can be isodense on CT scans, and both can be bilateral. These

are points worth remembering when there is a large visible hematoma on one side but little or no midline brain shift.

From time to time a patient's condition deteriorates at a rate that precludes CT scanning, and the surgeon must proceed immediately to surgical exploration if the patient's life is to be saved. Some simple guidelines may be of help here. If the patient develops a fixed and dilated pupil or the first of both pupils becomes dilated on one side and the patient has a skull fracture on that same side, the responsible lesion is most likely an extradural hematoma directly under the fracture; the burr hole should be made close to the fracture. If the dilated pupil is located on the side opposite the fracture, the lesion is most likely an acute subdural hematoma, almost always extending into the temporal fossa. The first burr hole therefore should be made just anterior to the ear on the same side as the dilated pupil. If the patient shows neurologic deterioration without any lateralizing signs, the possibility of a frontopolar, occipital, or posterior fossa hematoma (usually extradural) should be considered.

Steroids have no place in preoperative preparation of patients with subdural hematomas. In a comatose patient, intravenous mannitol is of considerable help when administered as soon as the hematoma is diagnosed to "buy" time until the surgical decompression can be started. Adequate intravenous hydration is most important, and arterial pressure must be carefully monitored, ideally from an indwelling arterial cannula in patients with acute subdural hematoma, in whom general anesthesia should be used. In selected cases of chronic subdural hematoma, where the surgical procedure is restricted to burr hole drainage, local anesthesia can be used.

SURGICAL TREATMENT OF ACUTE SUBDURAL HEMATOMA

The goals of the operative procedure are to decompress the brain at the earliest opportunity, especially in a patient who is already comatose; to evacuate all of the hematoma; to relieve tentorial herniation if this has already developed; to locate the source of the hemorrhage; and to secure hemostasis. To achieve these surgical objectives the operative exposure must provide access to the undersurface of the frontal lobe, the temporal lobe, and the floor of the middle fossa; both the venous drainage of the frontal lobe to the sagittal sinus and the

OPERATIVE NEUROSURGICAL TECHNIQUES
ISBN 0-8089-1862-1

vein of Labbé traversing the lateral surface of the temporal lobe some 5 or 6 cm from the pole should be accessible.

The skin incision can be of the question-mark type or the posterior limb can be taken behind the ear. If the patient is already in a coma, decompression must be started with minimum delay. In such cases the operative procedure begins with a 2-inch vertical incision starting at the zygomatic arch and extending up in front of the ear on the appropriate side. The temporal muscle is split, periosteum cleared, and a burr hole fashioned, which is quickly enlarged to 1 inch in diameter with rongeurs. The bulging blue dura mater is opened in a cruciate fashion and clotted blood is allowed to extrude; gentle pressure on the underlying brain with a periosteal elevator will often help much more clotted blood extrude from the relatively small opening. The surgical procedure to this point should not have taken more than 15 minutes. Surgical decompression has now been started, and the remainder of the operation can proceed at a less frantic pace.

As the large skin flap is opened, care should be taken to minimize blood loss. Patients with these injuries are often in a rather precarious hemodynamic state because of other injuries and because the blood pressure may have been pushed up or "propped up" by a vasopressor response related to the mass effect of the hematoma. In such cases hemorrhagic arterial hypotension will produce dangerous and damaging brain ischemia. It is important to alert the anesthetist to the fact that the dura is opened and decompression is achieved because there is often a drop in the arterial pressure at this point and the speed of the intravenous infusion may need to be increased.

When the bone flap is fashioned, the key openings are in the temporal bone at the level of the zygomatic arch, which is in line with the floor of the middle cranial fossa, and anteriorly at the edge of the temporalis muscle at the origin of the zygomatic arch. The flap is turned between these openings and should extend across the supraorbital part of the frontal bone close to the midline and backward above the ear, then upward toward the vertex, again close to the midline.

The dura mater should be opened with great care, especially if it is tense. Even if it appears uniformly blue, the underlying hematoma may be only a thin layer over the convexity of the cerebral hemisphere. If necessary several openings can be made to let clotted blood extrude and reduce dural tension before the wide dural opening, which is hinged on the sagittal sinus, is completed. Additional hyperventilation, increased head-up tilt, or intravenous mannitol may be required at this stage so that the dura can be safely opened.

All visible clotted blood should be irrigated, lifted, and gently sucked away and the underlying brain carefully inspected to determine the site of the hemorrhage. This may be a laceration of the brain with bleeding margins, usually extending from the temporal pole or from the frontal pole under the frontal lobe. It may arise from a torn vein linking the frontal lobe with the sagittal sinus, the temporal pole with the petrosal sinus, or the posterior temporal lobe with the sigmoid sinus (vein of Labbé). Sometimes the venous hemorrhage is from the sylvian veins. Finally, the source of the acute subdural hematoma may be from a ruptured cortical artery. This important subgroup, in which the bleeding vessel lies at the exact center of the clot, can be recognized on CT scans by a small area of radiolucency at the brain surface representing liquid blood in the center of the radiodense clot. It is important to realize that in these latter types of subdural hematoma there may be little or no damage to

the underlying brain and the ill effects on brain function have been produced entirely by compression.

When active bleeding from the brain surface has been controlled the next consideration is whether to excise contused, lacerated, or necrotic brain tissue. I favor a rather conservative approach, based on previous experience of an 88 percent incidence of intracranial hypertension following surgical excision of predominantly intracerebral hemorrhagic lesions. Brain that is obviously loose, pulped, necrotic, or mixed with clot should be gently aspirated. As tissue removal proceeds, hemostasis can be obtained by irrigation, bipolar coagulation, and application of hemostatic gauze in a single sheet with wet cotton wool packing, aided when necessary by dilute hydrogen peroxide. It is most important not to chase small bleeding vessels deep into the brain, and I no longer recommend opening and aspirating contused brain.

When the hematoma has been removed and hemostasis secured, the temporal lobe may remain impacted in the tentorial hiatus. In such cases, gentle elevation of the temporal lobe to expose the floor of the middle cranial fossa is recommended, proceeding until the free edge of the tentorium comes into view. As the medial part of the temporal lobe is slowly eased out of the hiatus, a flow of clear CSF will signal successful reduction of the tentorial hernia. On no account should attempts be made to disimpact the tentorial hernia by pressure injection in the lumbar subarachnoid space. This maneuver will be both unsuccessful and dangerous.

If severe brain swelling occurs during the operative procedure, the patency of the airway and the position of the head and neck must be checked and adequate muscle relaxation ensured. If no local or systemic cause can be found, the possibility of a contralateral hematoma should be considered. The anesthetist can administer mannitol or a bolus of barbiturate intravenously. Wound closure should proceed as rapidly as possible and a decision made whether to obtain an immediate postoperative CT scan or to make an exploratory temporal burr hole on the opposite side and, if there is a fracture, to make an additional burr hole close to it to look for an extradural hematoma. The dura should be closed as completely as possible, and the bone flap replaced but not wired into place. The skin is closed in the usual two layers with subgaleal suction drainage unless an emergency closure is being done as described above; in this event the skin can be closed in a single full-thickness layer, leaving the sutures in place for a longer period before removal.

If the patient was in a coma before removal of the hematoma, artificial ventilation should be continued after surgery and an intracranial pressure monitoring system should be installed. This is best located on the opposite side from the craniotomy through a separate burr hole made after the craniotomy has been completed (infection of the craniotomy and loss of the large bone flap is a complication to be avoided at all costs). The monitoring system can be a subdural catheter, bolt, or transducer or in some cases a ventricular catheter. If an ICP monitor is used, an arterial cannula should also be placed for continuous monitoring of arterial pressure and frequent measurement of blood gases and pH. Arterial ventilation is usually continued for at least 3 days, at which time the sedative and relaxant drugs are stopped and reversed so that an assessment of neurologic function can be obtained and a decision made to return to spontaneous respiration or to continue artificial ventilation for an additional 3-day period. Corticosteroids are not used, and antibiotics are given only for definite bacteriologic indications, not as prophylaxis.

Early postoperative problems include brain swelling and intracranial hypertension; this responds best to treatment with hyperventilation or infusions of hypnotic agents. At a later stage, after 48 to 72 hours, elevated intracranial pressure is more likely to be the result of brain edema; this is best treated by intravenous mannitol solution. Seizure activity can be difficult to detect when the patient is still under the influence of relaxant drugs, but should be suspected when the pupils become abruptly dilated and there is a sharp increase in arterial pressure. Monitoring of electrical activity in the brain using a compressed EEG display is helpful; unfortunately prophylactic anticonvulsant drugs are no guarantee that seizures will not occur in this critical early postoperative period.

SURGICAL TREATMENT OF CHRONIC SUBDURAL HEMATOMA

The goal of surgical treatment of chronic subdural hematoma is to evacuate as completely as possible and in a single procedure the liquid contents of the subdural collection. This can be achieved via two or more burr holes with a limited dural opening carried out under general or local anesthesia. The surgical procedure is simple but the penalty for operative inadequacy is severe for the patient. Close attention should be paid to details. Many of the affected patients are elderly and may have other significant medical problems.

With the patient in the supine position and lying very nearly flat, two burr holes should be made on the affected side. If there are bilateral hematomas, the larger should be evacuated first, but both sides should be done in a single operative session. The first (anterior) burr hole should be made in line with the coronal suture about 2 inches above the pterion. I prefer to make a large burr hole with a rose burr. The dura must be carefully inspected before it is opened to avoid cutting an underlying vein; this can mimic the blue color of underlying hematoma and is a mistake more easily made if the burr hole is small. The dura is opened in a cruciate manner and the corners coagulated. Sometimes troublesome dural bleeding occurs from just under the edge of the burr hole. This can be difficult to stop; a right-angled blunt hook can be used to compress the dura against the undersurface of the skull and the monopolar diathermy electrode applied. This simple maneuver nearly always stops the bleeding and avoids the need to enlarge the burr hole to a craniectomy.

Immediately after the dura is opened, dark brown liquid hematoma fluid may gush, spurt, or lap out according to its quantity and the level of the intracranial pressure. Sometimes, however, a thick brown, black, or even greenish membrane is encountered, and only when this has been opened is liquid hematoma encountered.

A second, posterior burr hole should now be made over the parietal eminence. When the dura has been opened and any residual fluid allowed to drain out, a soft rubber catheter is passed into the subdural space; great care is taken not to penetrate or injure the brain surface, since it is only too easy to provoke fresh bleeding. It is particularly important to direct the catheter posteriorly toward the inion, because it is here that the thickest and densest hematoma fluid will gravitate. Rather than aspirating fluid from here by suction, it is preferable to irrigate via the catheter then direct the proximal end of the catheter downward below the head to empty the subdural space by a siphon effect. This is a gentler technique and less likely to cause fresh bleeding in the subdural space. If the hematoma is thick and extensive, a third burr hole can be made in the anterior temporal region, as described in the section on acute subdural hematoma.

Once the subdural space yields only clear irrigating fluid, this phase of the procedure is complete; the depth of the subdural space must now be assessed. Attempts should be made to reduce this to less than 5 mm by tilting the table so that the patient is flat or even slightly head-down and by asking the anesthetist to gently compress the neck veins. If the brain comes up to the dural surface the burr holes are closed in two layers without drainage, but if a subdural space greater than 5 mm persists, a soft rubber drain is inserted into the posterior burr hole; this is connected to a bag but no suction is applied.

The patient is nursed flat for 48 hours, the drain is removed, and progress to the upright position and mobilization is taken slowly over the subsequent 48 or 72 hours. The temptation to obtain a postoperative CT scan should be resisted as long as the patient is making satisfactory clinical improvement. A CT scan nearly always shows some residual collection and an unnecessary reoperation may be carried out with the real risk of producing infection in the subdural space, which is a dangerous and devastating complication of chronic subdural hematoma. On the other hand, if the patient fails to improve rapidly or deteriorates again, a CT scan should be obtained without delay, remembering that a smaller isodense contralateral collection may have escaped notice on the preoperative CT scan. Other postoperative complications include infarction of the previously compressed brain, cortical thrombophlebitis, or severe focal epilepsy. As in the case of acute subdural hematoma, if the patient was in a coma before the evacuation of the hematoma, intensive neurologic care is likely to be required.

CHAPTER 5

Surgical Management of Gunshot Wounds of the Head

Maurice I. Saba

GUNSHOT WOUNDS OF THE HEAD are on the increase. The easy availability of handguns, revolvers, shotguns, and rifles and the continued and increasing armed struggle in various places in the world demand a renewed and serious interest in and a better understanding of both the ballistic characteristics of missiles and the surgical pathology of missile wounds. Suffice it to say that simple adherence to the general surgical principles of wound care leaves much to be desired when the neurosurgeon is confronted with a missile or gunshot wound of the brain. Gurdjian[1] has reviewed the stages through which the treatment of penetrating wounds of the brain sustained in warfare has come. An analysis of penetrating brain wounds from Vietnam by Hammon[2,3] has familiarized neurosurgeons with the difficult and multifaceted problems facing the surgeon who must deal with these types of wounds on a day-to-day basis. The high rate of complications,[4] bacterial contamination,[5] and the increased morbidity and mortality from reoperation will only be improved upon when the surgeon becomes familiar with certain specific surgical principles that are based upon vast experience in the care of such wounds. Meirowsky[6] has previously described some of the basic principles involved in the surgical care of such patients. It is recommended that both adherence to these basic surgical principles and a thorough understanding of ballistic characteristics and the mechanism of wounding and tissue damage be the prerequisite to a carefully executed and definitive surgical management. This management should begin as early as possible after wounding. This will ensure the saving of more lives and the preservation of more neurologic function.

BALLISTIC DATA

Most handguns and revolvers use heavy bullets weighing about 0.5 oz and have muzzle velocities ranging from 550 to 900 ft/sec. These are referred to as low-velocity missiles. In contrast, most rifles in use today use very light bullets of less than 10 g and have muzzle velocities averaging 3000 ft/sec with a range of 2300 to 6000 ft/sec. In our practice, in which an extraordinarily large number of patients have been seen since 1975, we have encountered and have become familiar with three basic types of missiles that cause penetrating wounds to the brain. These are:

1. The 7.62-mm bullet fired from the AK-47 assault rifle. This is an expanding type bullet that weighs 150 g and has a diameter of 0.311 inch and a length of 1.08 inch. It has a muzzle velocity of 2329 ft/sec[7] and is used for close range.
2. The 5.56-mm (.223) bullet fired from the M-16 rifle. This is a soft-point jacketed bullet weighing 55 g and has a muzzle velocity of 3250 ft/sec.[7] This is commonly used for sniping.
3. Fragments of high-explosive devices. These are of various shapes and sizes and can weigh as much as 100 g. These should be regarded as high-velocity missiles, since initially they travel at speeds of over 3000 ft/sec, although they rapidly lose speed because of their volume and irregular shape and become low-velocity missiles at distances of 10 m or more.

Although rifle and machine gun fire make up onlly 15 to 20 percent of such wounds in modern warfare, they will be encountered with greater frequency in civil strife and guerrilla warfare, where wounding usually occurs at very close range.

The ballistic analysis of shotgun and pellet injuries has been adequately discussed by Sights[8] and will not be discussed here.

SURGICAL PATHOLOGY

The behavior of a missile depends upon several variables, such as its size, shape, aerodynamic stability, and velocity. Tissue density and elasticity will greatly modify both the stability and the velocity of the missile. This, to a great degree, will limit the extent of tissue damage produced by the passage of the missile.

Because the center of velocity is behind the center of mass, bullets are aerodynamically unstable. This usually is overcome by the rifling of the barrel, which gives the bullet a spinning action and more stability. Stability is lost as the bullet hits the tissue, however, because the high density of the tissue retards the bullet as a result of the phenomenon of yaw. Human tissue on average is about 800 times denser than air.

The extent of tissue damage depends on the amount of energy expended by the missile at the point of tissue penetration. The physics of missile energy is beyond the scope of this discussion but in general tissue injury will exhibit itself in three different patterns:

1. Laceration and crushing of tissues. Here there is no significant energy transmitted to the tissues. This frequently occurs in low-velocity missile wounds. There is no cavitation except for the limited track produced by the passage of

the missile. A similar pathologic picture is produce by hand weapons and sharp objects. The wound is equal in size at the entry and exit points.

2. Shock waves. As the missile hits and enters the tissue, it compresses the tissue medium ahead of it, which momentarily spreads in the form of a spherical shock wave of very short duration but of considerable energy and produces damage distant to the missile track. According to Owen-Smith,[9] this energy can be in excess of 1000 lbs/in^2.

3. Temporary cavitation. Upon entry of a high velocity missile into tissue, the tissue moves both forward and sideways, producing what is referred to as temporary cavitation. The area affected may be as large as 30 times the diameter of the actual track of the missile. With the outward movement of the tissue, a sudden drop in pressure to subatmospheric levels occurs: this produces a sucking action that introduces debris, foreign material, and bacteria from the air into the cavity. This temporary cavitation is similar to a shock wave and of very short duration. It immediately collapses and forms the permanent cavity, which is invariably larger than the actual track of the missile. This mechanism of injury is exclusively produced by high-velocity missiles.

The extent of tissue damage in penetrating and perforating wounds of the head is modified by the existence of two distinct physical properties of the tissues involved. First, the brain is a semisolid medium (closer to a liquid system), and, second, it is encased in a rigid skull that has a physical property of being able to stretch. This ability of the skull to stretch perhaps accounts for the occurrence of limited cavitation in the brain. In contrast, because the skull is filled with the semisolid brain tissue, extensive fracturing of the skull occurs when the energy expended by the missile is great, such as occurs with high-velocity missiles. Owen-Smith[9] studied this phenomenon by firing bullets into empty skulls. The entry and exit wounds produced were small and neat. He then filled the skulls with gelatin medium and placed a pressure transducer in them. He noted extensive fracturing of the skull occurred with pressure recordings in excess of 400 lbs/in^2 when bullets were fired into these skulls. He therefore suggested that it is difficult to attain pressures high enough to extensively fracture an empty skull, while a gelatin-filled skull extensively fractured with much lower pressures. The brain therefore may actually aid in cracking the skull from within.

In summary, the surgeon should keep the following in mind:

1. High-velocity missiles traveling at speeds greater than 3000 ft/sec produce extensive tissue damage by shock waves and temporary cavitation.

2. The cavitary necrosis is much larger than the actual track of the missile.

3. The suction effect of temporary cavitation actively draws large volumes of bone, dirt, hair, skin fragments, clothing, and bacteria into the track, which also contains devitalized brain tissue.

4. Bacterial contamination of these wounds occurs as a result of the temporary cavitation and suction effect and is uniformly distributed throughout the wound.

5. Low-velocity missiles produce limited tissue damage consisting mainly of tissue laceration and crushing.

6. Larger wounds at exit sites are the result of the phenomenon of bullet deformation and yaw, occurring most commonly with high velocity bullets, and the degree of yaw angle is greatest at 10 cm or greater of tissue penetration.

Wound ballistics have been detailed by Weiner and Barrett.[10]

SURGICAL MANAGEMENT

Knowledge of the type of missile and the circumstances of injury will to some extent dictate the operative approach and the details of the technique. The presence of signs suggesting intracranial hypertension caused by an expanding hematoma or the presence of gross sepsis with meningitis may alter the timing and type of operative management.

PREOPERATIVE EVALUATION

If such information is available, a detailed history of the time, place, and circumstances of wounding is essential, as well as the type of weapon and the bullet used. A careful neurologic evaluation should be made in terms of any fixed neurologic deficit secondary either to the primary injury or to the effects of expanding intracranial hematomas. The picture of impending herniation and brain-stem compression must be immediately recognized. Plain roentgenograms of the skull in three projections (anteroposterior, lateral, and Towne) should be obtained to determine: (1) the entry and exit points of the missile, (2) the extent of bony fractures, (3) the volume of any bone that has been driven intracranially, (4) the presence of any metallic fragments, (5) the trajectory of the bullet, which may suggest the areas of penetration and bullet fragmentation and the extent of radial fragment scatter such as occurs with soft-point and copper-jacketed military bullets, to predict the expected neurologic deficit, (6) the type, caliber, shape, and size of the missile, and, (7) the location of the missile and its accessibility in terms of its removal at the time of the definitive surgery.

Computed tomography (CT) of the brain should be obtained in every case when feasible. The findings should be correlated with the plain roentgenograms (mainly for foreign material, bone, and metal) and the clinical picture. Computed tomographic scans can be obtained within 15 to 20 minutes and should be obtained even in patients with rapidly deteriorating clinical pictures. We have routinely used CT for gunshot wounds to the head at the American University of Beirut Medical Center since 1982. In addition to the information obtained from the plain roentgenograms, CT scans give added information in terms of (1) the extent of brain injury, (2) better assessment of hematomas along the track of injury, (3) the presence of subdural or epidural hematomas in close proximity or distant to the site of injury, (4) the extent of cerebral injury in tangential wounds, (5) the trajectory of the missile, predictive of outcome, such as in transventricular wounds, tracks through deep gray, or diagonal injury with crossover from one hemisphere to another, (6) the uncovering of cerebral injury distant from the surgical field, such as intracerebral hematoma or brain infarction secondary to vascular injury, and (7) the volume of in-driven bone as well as retained bone, which is best seen on CT scans.

Cerebral angiography is reserved for patients who are suspected of harboring a mass lesion and only when time permits. It is used only when CT is not available. Angiography is most helpful in cases in which there has been diagonal crossover of a bullet from one hemisphere into another, where the site of a hematoma is determined, and the operative procedure is planned. An incidental value of angiography has been the occasional discovery of a traumatic aneurysm on a postoperative angiogram. Our criteria for this has been the absence of such a lesion on a preoperative angiogram in the same patient. An analysis of 7 such cases, indicating the type of injury and the angiographic findings, has been reported.[11] These authors have additional cases totaling 17 to date. We believe that angiography should be performed postoperatively 2 to 3 weeks after injury in cases suspected of subarachnoid hemorrhage. Such aneurysms form more frequently after wounding by metallic shrapnel or fragmented bullets.

Preoperative osmotic diuretics have been used sparingly and only when an expanding intracranial lesion is suspected. In contrast, corticosteroids have been used routinely in a dosage range of 24 to 36 mg/day given in 6 divided doses. We have resorted to higher dosages when CT imaging revealed severe hemisphere swelling. All patients are started on anticonvulsants immediately, and Dilantin has been the drug most commonly used. Antibiotics are only started after all cultures are taken. We routinely take cultures from the entry and exit wounds, cerebral debris, bone fragments driven into the wound, and foreign matter. Since this is only feasible at the time of surgery, antibiotics are started either intraoperatively or immediately postoperatively. Specimens must be cultured in both aerobic and anaerobic media.

The entire scalp is shaved in the emergency ward and the wounds dressed with sterile gauze soaked with a solution of 1 percent Betadine, and a heavy sterile dressing is applied.

OPERATIVE TECHNIQUE

Accurate assessment of tissue loss can only be done in the operating room. The most crucial factor in successful closure of the wound is the amount of scalp loss. The primary aim of the surgical intervention is to save the patient's life and neurologic function. The most opportune time for cranial exploration after gunshot wounds of the head is early, preferably within the first 2 to 3 hours after injury. Every effort should be made to make this early exploration the definitive one, since reoperations carry a higher risk of mortality and morbidity from added neurologic insult.

The guidelines to follow for such operations are:

1. Adequate debridement or excision of the scalp wound.
2. Adequate debridement of all bone edges.
3. Exposure of the entire edge of the torn dura.
4. Thorough debridement of all necrotic brain tissue, hair, soil, skin fragments, blood clots, etc., from the cavity in the brain.
5. Hemostasis of the cerebral wound and torn dural venous sinuses.
6. Removal of all bone fragments driven into the wound. Bone fragments have the highest incidence of positive cultures and their retention in the depth of the cerebral wound predisposes the wound to the development of cerebritis, brain abscess, or both.
7. Watertight closure of the dura, preferably with a graft, and tight skin closure without tension.

We are in the habit of preparing the entire scalp and draping it to facilitate either the extension of scalp wounds across the midline or bilateral exploration of both the entry and exit wounds. Betadine solution is used for skin antisepsis. In the presence of entry and exit wounds, we prefer to debride the entry wound first because of the smaller amount of tissue damage. The entry wound, which is usually small, is excised and sent for culture. The wound is enlarged by Z extensions, and the bony defect is enlarged with ronguers to expose a clean and intact dural edge. The dura is opened with a cruciate incision and the cerebral wound is inspected. The cortical wound is usually much smaller than the track of the missile in the cerebral white matter. The track then is gently explored for debris and hematoma. For this maneuver we prefer to introduce the tip of an asepto syringe into the wound and wash the debris out by steadily and gently irrigating the track with saline under moderate constant pressure while the syringe tip is withdrawn slowly. Care is taken to avoid blocking the cerebral entry wound with the irrigating syringe since this allows water to dissect into brain with undesirable consequences instead of allowing back drainage with debris and necrotic hemorrhagic brain. This maneuver is repeated several times and effects a thorough debridement of the track. We avoid using the metal-tipped suction for fear of causing deep bleeding that could result in further neurologic deficit. Metal suction tips tend to suck up swollen brain from the wall of the track, brain that is not necessarily necrotic. We attempt to save as much viable brain tissue as possible and only debride necrotic brain in the center of the track. At times we have used diluted hydrogen peroxide solution, which remarkably stops all capillary oozing from the walls of the cerebral cavitary track. After this irrigation-debridement, attention is directed to removing all bone fragments embedded in the cerebral wound. Large fragments can be picked up easily with fine forceps; small lightweight chips float out with irrigation. We occasionally have encountered large buttons of bone driven deep into the center of a hemisphere as a bullet hit the skull and ricocheted tangentially after it had separated the bone button and drove it in as a secondary missile. In such cases the track created by the bone is small and not cavitary. Such fragments are easily found by sounding the track with a long brain needle, and the fragment can be picked up with a fine bayonet forceps. The track then is irrigated with saline. Hemostasis of the brain wound should be complete in order to avoid the use of Gelfoam or Oxycel. No attempt should be made to remove small metallic shrapnel fragments at the expense of further injury to brain tissue. These have a very low yield of positive cultures in comparison to bone fragments and it is doubtful whether such metallic fragments left in place form a nidus for brain abscess provided that all necrotic brain in their vicinity has been removed. The dural defect is patched with a piece of pericranium and sutured with fine monofilament nylon. The bone edge is waxed, and the skin edge is approximated with a continuous 2-0 nylon suture. There should be no tension on the skin edge. A rubber tissue drain is left in the subgaleal space within the craniectomy defect for 24 hours.

Attention then is directed to the exit wound, where a larger amount of tissue loss, particularly of the scalp, poses a challenge to closure. More skin exposure is necessary here, and extension of the skin is fashioned with easy closure in mind. The bone, which is usually extensively fractured, can be removed easily. Brisk and active bleeding may be encountered after fractured bone fragments are elevated, particularly over the high convexity or close to dural sinuses. Bleeding may occur from the torn surface of the dura or from lacerated brain where the bleeding points were tamponaded as the swollen brain pushed against the calvarium. The surgeon must alert the anesthesiologist to the possibility of brisk bleeding, especially

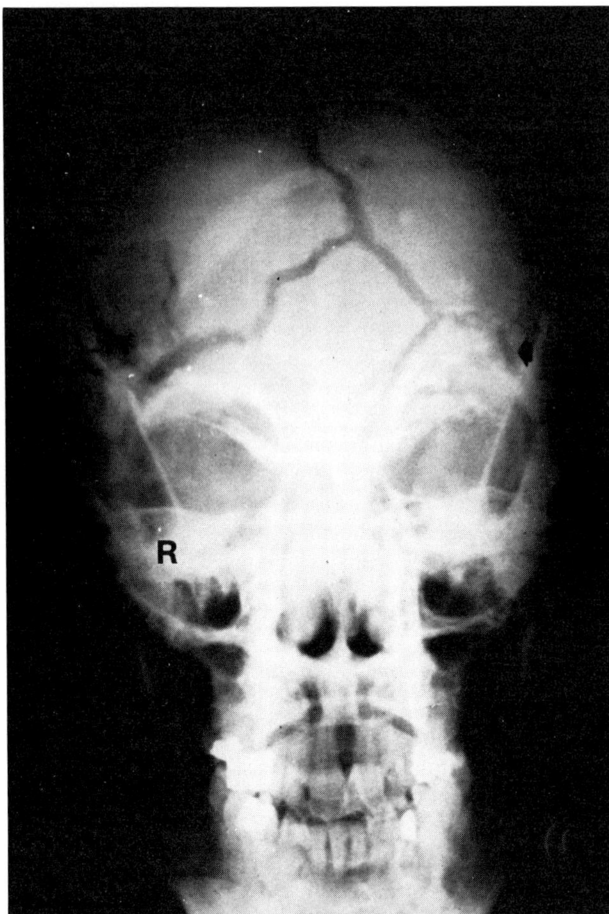

Fig. 5-1. Case 1. An anteroposterior x-ray film of the skull showing the entry wound (short arrow), the exit wound (curved arrow), and the blow-out and comminuted fracture of the entire frontal bone. Note the increased density medial to the entry wound representing the bone fragments that were driven into the brain and embedded deep in the left frontal lobe.

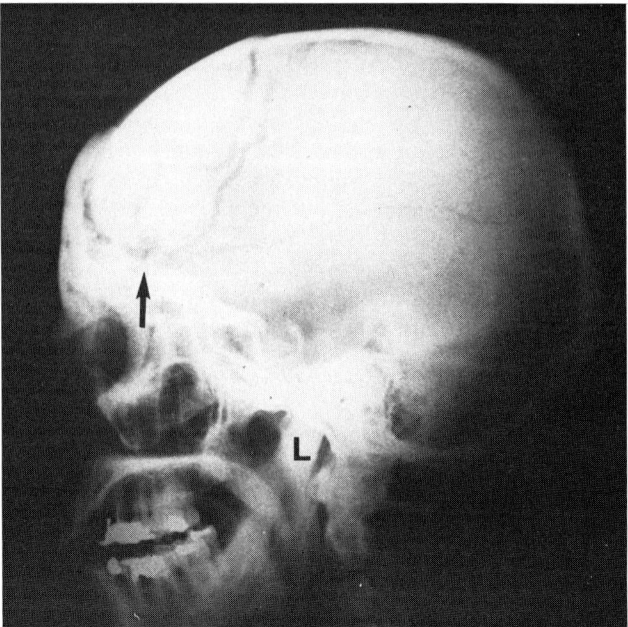

Fig. 5-2. Case 1. Lateral x-ray film of the skull showing the extensive frontal bone fractures. A frontoparietal linear fracture line is also visible. The bullet had entered just above the roof of the orbit (straight arrow).

when working close to the dural sinuses. He also must be readily equipped to control bleeding quickly with Gelfoam, Oxycel, and cottonoid patties. Sometimes several hundred milliliters of blood can be lost quickly from these sites. When torn sinuses are anticipated, it is important that a generous bone removal be done before removing the impacted bone fragment. After bone has been removed, the diploë are waxed; we do not hesitate to coagulate the dural surface for hemostasis since we rely on grafting for closure. Tears of the sinuses have at times been repaired with a patch of dura. More often, the tear is so irregular and extensive, with massive cerebral laceration in the vicinity, that packing with muscle and Gelfoam is necessary. The torn dural edge is excised completely and the dura is tacked up to the bone with interrupted 4-0 nylon sutures. The cerebral wound then is explored. Usually there is very little foreign material in the wound; in particular there are no bone fragments. The volume of necrotic brain tissue, however, is much larger than that in the entry wound. Both hemorrhagic brain and hematoma usually are found; this can be removed with saline irrigation. Care should be taken not to produce fresh bleeding from the adjacent swollen brain, since this may be difficult to control. Hemostasis of the edge of the lacerated cortex is secured by coagulation of the pia-arachnoid around the entire edge with bipolar coagulation. Again, we emphasize the

debridement of the necrotic brain tissue only; swollen brain should not be debrided, since this will function after the edema has subsided. Brain debridement should be thorough but gentle. Exploration of the bottom of the wound for hematoma is mandatory. If persistent brain swelling of a high degree is present, the surgeon should suspect a possible deep hematoma until it has been looked for and not found. Unless there is a deep hematoma, the bulk of brain will respond to a dose of mannitol with rapid decrease in size. In our experience, when brain swelling could not be satisfactorily explained, we have found a deep intracerebral hematoma in every instance. After evacuation of a hematoma, the cerebral wound is copiously irrigated with a solution of diluted hydrogen peroxide (half strength with saline, 1:1 v/v), and then with saline. This will ensure the removal of large amounts of devitalized brain. At times we have used a diluted solution of 1 percent Betadine (100 ml diluted in 1000 ml of saline). No untoward effects have been seen from the use of this solution.

Dural closure is routinely done with a graft. Pericranium or temporalis fascia usually suffice and are easy to handle. Pericranium is more accessible and has been used more frequently. We do not recommend fascia lata, since it withstands infection less than pericranium. Watertight closure of the dura is recommended and the patch is sutured with a running lock-stitch of 4-0 monofilament nylon. We share the opinion with many that dura is a good barrier to the intracranial extension of infection should the superficial wound become infected. The dural patch is not stretched and is left redundant to accommodate postoperative brain swelling. The devitalized edges of the scalp wound are excised, and with Z extensions, rotation flaps, or gridiron incisions into the galea, closure of the wound may be feasible. Tension on the edge produces necrosis and predisposes the wound to infection. After closure of the dura, the skin wound is irrigated with copious amounts of diluted Betadine solution and saline. Subgaleal rubber tissue

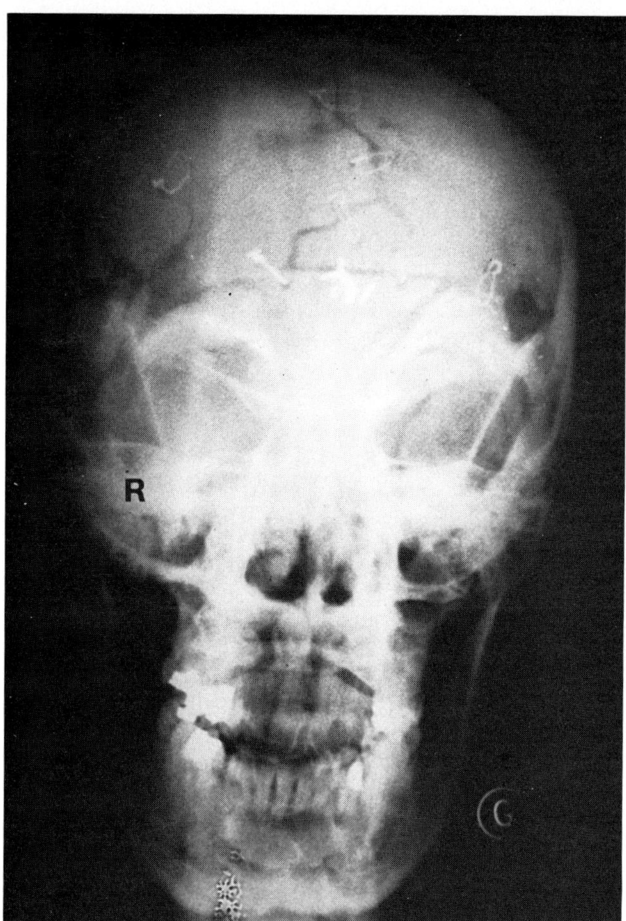

Fig. 5-3. Case 1. An anteroposterior x-ray film of the skull after debridement of the bone, dura, and brain. The bone fragments driven into the brain have been removed and the frontal fractures wired to reconstitute the normal contour of the forehead. The midline metallic clips were used to stop bleeding from a tear of the dural venous sinus.

drains are used routinely for 36 hours. The skin edge is approximated with 2-0 nylon sutures in one layer.

Unusual problems can occasionally be encountered that may require some modification of the recommended technique. The following case illustrations will demonstrate some of these unusual circumstances.

Case 1. A 35-year-old woman was hit with a sniper's high-velocity 5.56-mm bullet and was immediately rendered unconscious. She was brought to the hospital 1 hour after injury. She had a 0.8-cm entry wound in the left frontal area and a larger exit wound in the right frontal area, and extensive fractures of the frontal bone (Figures 5-1 and 5-2). She had no clinical evidence of expanding hematoma, but hemorrhagic necrotic brain was oozing out of both wounds. She underwent a large bifrontal craniotomy, debridement of brain, removal of all bone fragments, dural repair, and wiring of the extensive fractures of the frontal bone (Figures 5-3 and 5-4). Postoperatively, the wound healed without infection and within 3 weeks she was neurologically intact except for slight blunting of her affect and was discharged on anticonvulsants. Five years after injury this patient was doing well and was back to her job as a factory worker.

This case illustrates the extensive damage to the skull and the brain produced by high-velocity bullets, as has been previ-

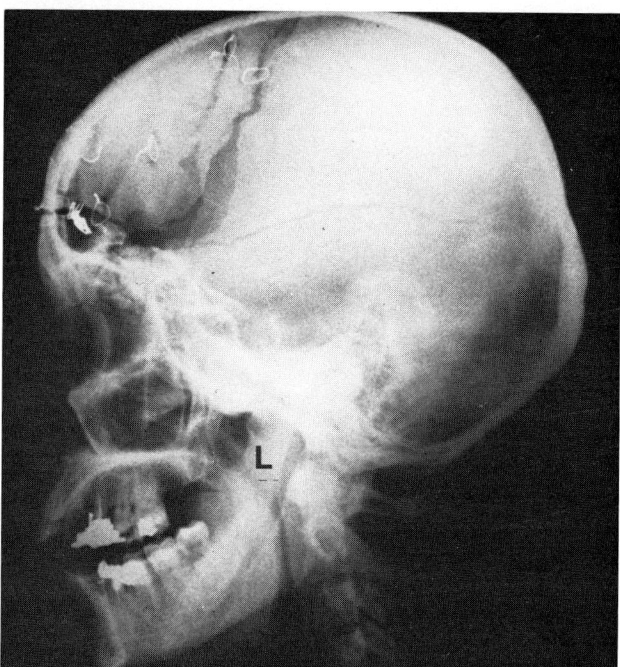

Fig. 5-4. Case 1. A postoperative lateral view of the skull with the fractured frontal bone wired in place. A bifrontal craniotomy had been done.

ously discussed in the section on surgical pathology. Meticulous operative technique as recommended above saved the life and neurologic function of this patient.

Case 2. A 20-year-old man was hit by a 7.62-mm bullet at close range. The injury produced a large scalp wound in the right frontal area with loss of skin, bone, and dura (Figure 5-5). When examined 48 hours after injury, the patient had necrotic and hemorrhagic brain coming out of his wound and producing a cerebral fungus. He had a fever of 104°F, a stiff neck, was

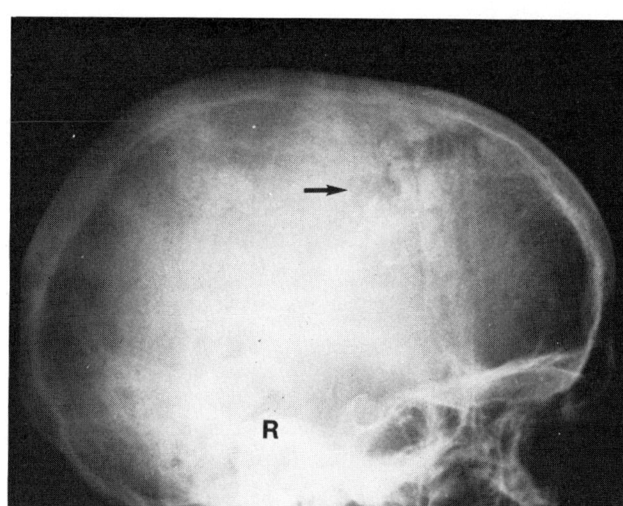

Fig. 5-5. Case 2. A lateral view of the skull demonstrating the bony defect produced by the entry of the bullet in the right frontal area. The bullet drove several large fragments of bone intracranially, ricocheted, and exited 5 cm posterolaterally at the level of the coronal suture (arrow).

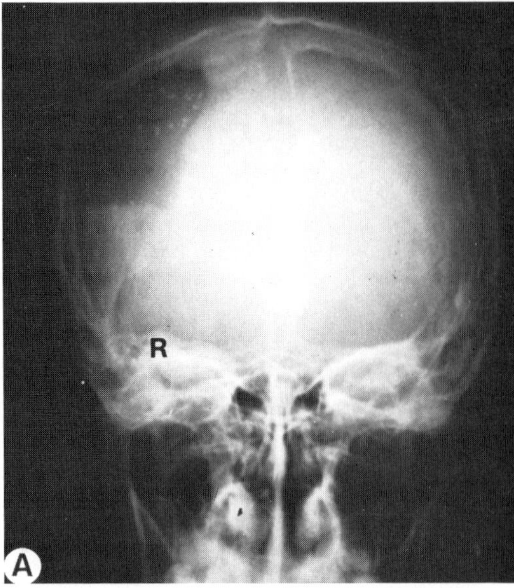

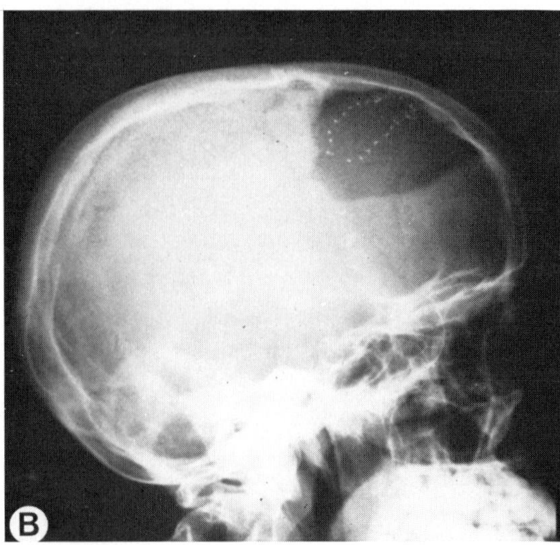

Fig. 5-6.   Case 2. Anteroposterior (A) and lateral (B) views of the skull demonstrating the extent of the craniectomy, the absence of any retained bone fragments, and the stainless steel wire suture outlining the pericranial dural patch.

somnolent, and had a left hemiplegia. A smear from the wound revealed Gram-negative rods, and the CSF as well as the wound subsequently grew *Proteus vulgaris,* which was sensitive to gentamicin. Because of his general condition, surgery was postponed. The head was shaved and the wound edge debrided, and the wound was packed with gauze soaked with 1 percent Betadine solution and an occlusive external dressing was applied. He was also given 80 mg of gentamicin intravenously every 8 hours and 5 mg of gentamicin intrathecally every other day along with 30 million units of crystalline penicillin G

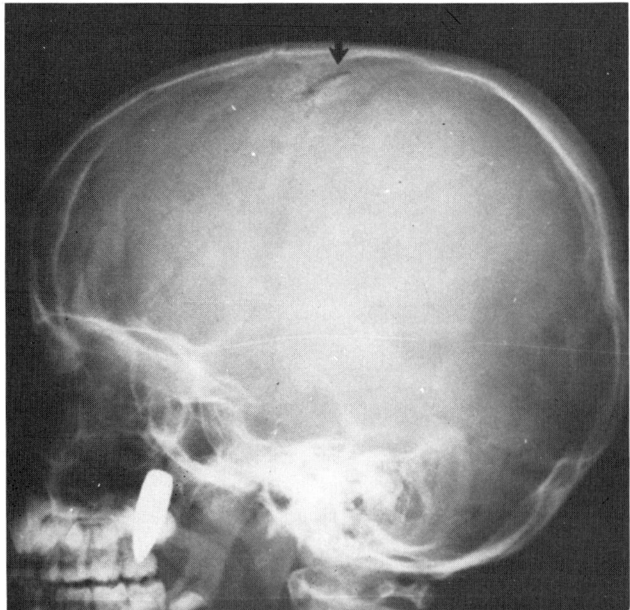

Fig. 5-7.   Case 3. The spent bullet, which was descending vertically, entered the skull just behind the coronal suture over the convexity (arrow), traveled through the white matter of the right hemisphere, and lodged in the facial bones just anterior and inferior to the zygoma. There were no bone fragments driven intracranially. The scalp wound was less than 1 cm in diameter.

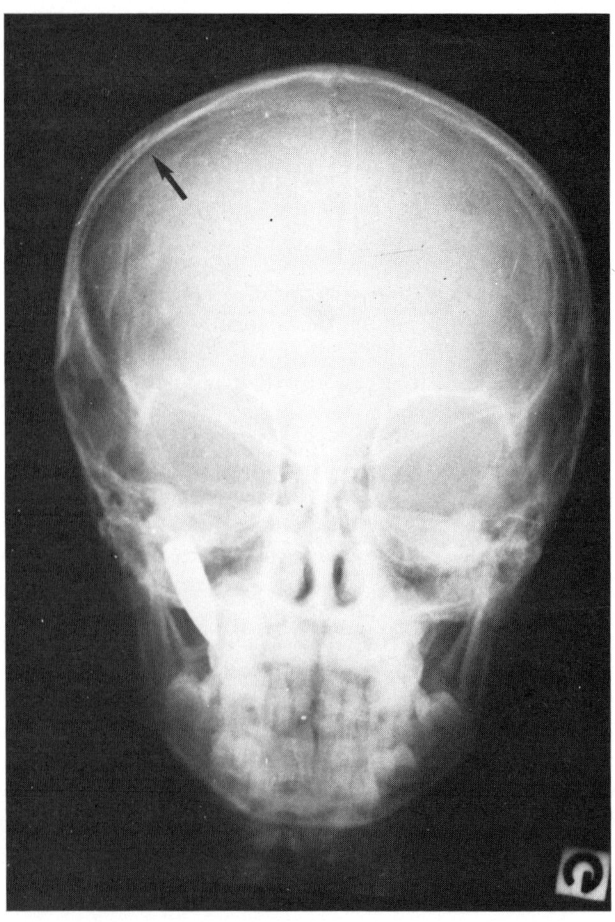

Fig. 5-8.   Case 3. An AP view of the skull showing the entry point of the bullet (arrow) and its position anterior to the zygoma.

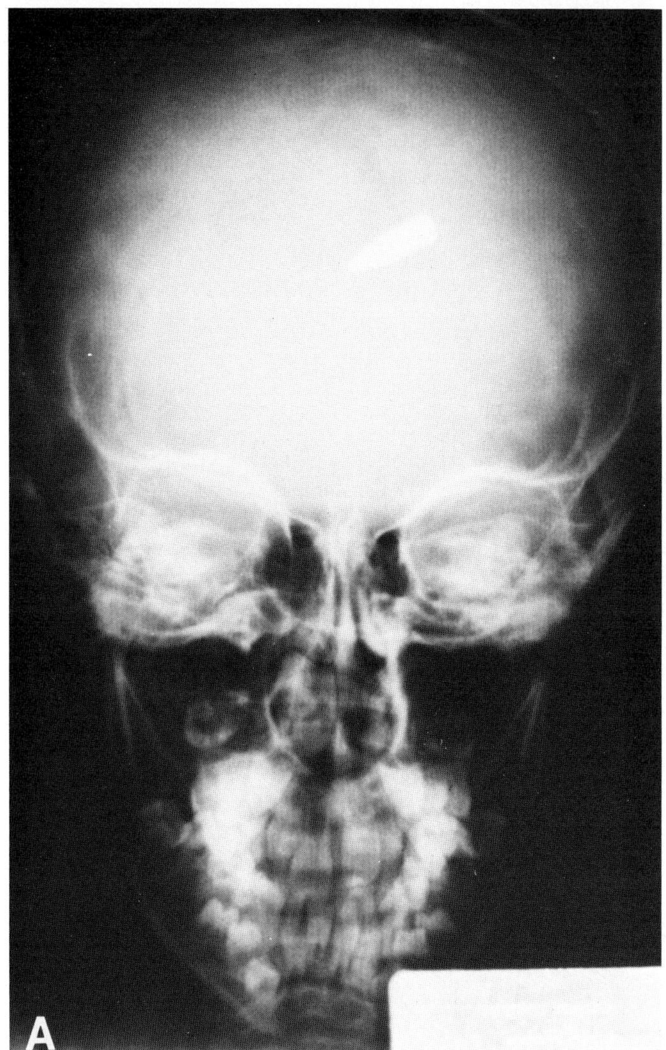

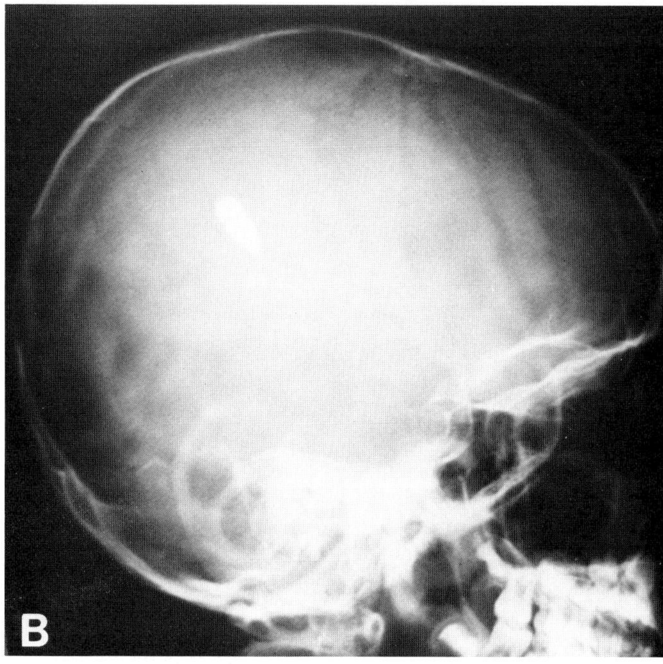

Fig. 5-9.   (A) Posteroanterior and (B) lateral projections showing a spent bullet in the center of the skull to the right of the midline. The injury occurred on May 20, 1985.

intravenously daily. On the sixth day after injury, the fever had reduced, the neck was less stiff, and the patient was more alert. Since admission, the head wound had been dressed with Betadine twice daily with some debridement of the brain wound with each dressing change, The wound looked clean on the sixth day. The previously swollen brain had shrunk back into the confines of the bony defect and was pulsating gently, and clear CSF welled up from around the brain wound. It appeared that the cerebral wound had been effectively debrided of necrotic brain with the daily dressings. On the seventh day, the patient was taken to the operating room, the wound was explored, and the basic principles of wound debridement as described in the section on operative technique were employed. All bone fragments were removed, the brain debrided with irrigation, the dura closed with a patch and stainless steel wire sutures (Figure 5-6), a clean craniectomy done, and excision of the skin wound and closure with relaxing incisions and gridiron galeal incisions. The skin was closed in one layer with 2-0 nylon over catheter drains that were used to irrigate the wound for 1 week with 2 mg of gentamicin diluted in 10 ml of saline. The wound healed without infection, and within 3 weeks after operative debridement, he was well, fully conscious, and his left hemiplegia had cleared completely. The patient was fol-

lowed up regularly and he showed no evidence of skull infection. Eighteen months later he had a cranioplasty. After 3 years he was still well and on anticonvulsants but without clinically apparent seizures.

Delayed definitive surgical debridement has been employed on several patients who came to the hospital 36 hours or longer from the time of injury. As this case illustrates, these patients have grossly infected wounds and the majority will have a Gram-negative rod as the infective organism. *Proteus* and *E. coli* have been the most common organisms cultured from these wounds. Treatment with aminoglycosides proved effective in controlling both the CSF and wound infections. Soaking with Betadine when dressing these wounds works both as a debriding agent for the necrotic brain and as an antiseptic for the wound. Continued use of the Betadine made delayed debridement an acceptable alternative to early surgical debridement of a cerebral fungus, where reoperation is often required for persistent infection. We have not encountered any deep persistent infections in a dozen such patients. In fact, we feel that delayed debridement of this kind of wound is an easy, less traumatic, and effective definitive surgical approach. The

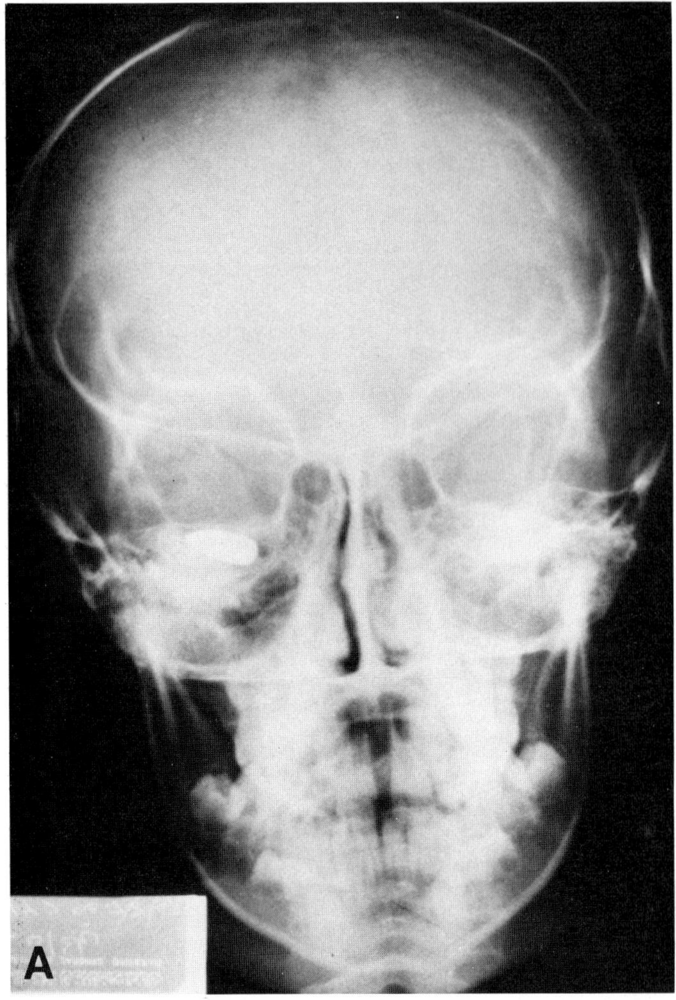

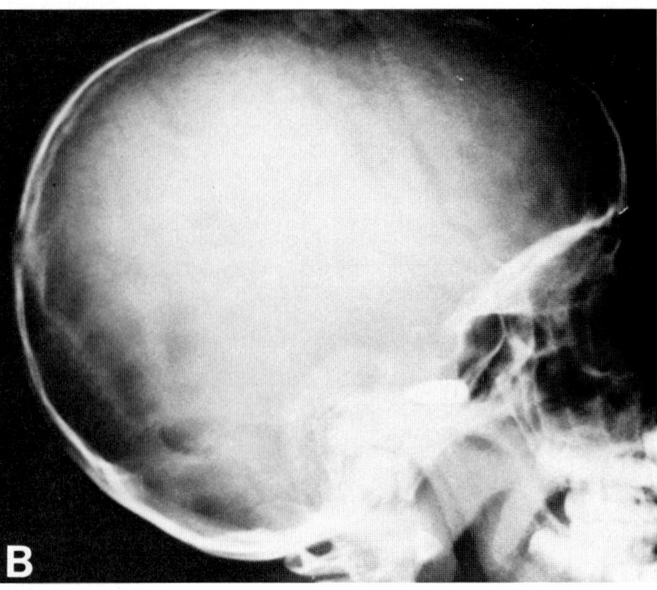

Fig. 5-10. (A) Posteroanterior and (B) lateral views of the skull of the same patient as in Figure 5-9 seven months after the initial injury illustrating the descent of the bullet through the brain substance to lie on the bone of the middle fossa. No clinical deficits occurred with the migration of the bullet.

postoperative result in terms of neurologic function has been satisfactory. This method is not to be recommended routinely, but can be a good alternative to early surgical intervention in a patient with a heavily infected wound with meningitis and cerebral fungus.

Case 3. A 7-year-old boy was struck by a bullet as it descended vertically. The bullet was 7.62-mm caliber and entered the head in the right frontoparietal area just posterior to the coronal suture (Figure 5-7) and 6 cm lateral to the midline. It made an 8-mm linear scalp wound, traversed the hemisphere after piercing the calvarium and produced a small depressed fracture (Figure 5-8) and lodged in the maxilla just anterior and inferior to the zygoma. The boy was dazed, fell to the ground, but soon got up and walked. Neurologic examination was normal except for a mild left facial weakness. There were no bone fragments driven into the wound on x-ray films of the skull. The scalp wound was excised and closed and the patient was treated conservatively with corticosteroids, an intravenous mannitol drip (15 ml hourly of 20 percent mannitol solution), anticonvulsants, and antibiotics. On the fourth day, his facial weakness had cleared and the patient was operated upon with a right frontoparietal craniotomy centered on the wound. The surface of the brain was hemorrhagic and the cortical wound

was covered with necrotic cerebral tissue. This was debrided with saline irrigation and the track was irrigated with the asepto syringe. All loose brain tissue separated easily with the water jet and there was no need for debridement with metal-tipped suction. There were no bone fragments and no foreign material. The dura was closed with a pericranial patch and sutured with fine nylon. The bone flap was anchored in place and the scalp flap closed in the usual fashion with 2-0 nylon. The bullet then was removed transorally through a mucosal incision above the last molar tooth. The postoperative course was smooth, and the patient was discharged on anticonvulsants on the sixth postoperative day, neurologically intact and without wound sepsis.

Patients who are injured by a spent bullet present a totally different pathologic picture from patients injured by a normal gunshot. These bullets descend vertically and are of sufficient energy to penetrate the calvarium and often go to the base of the skull, yet they produce only laceration of the brain and a small track during their passage. They do not produce cavitation nor do they drive bone fragments into the cerebral depths. Necrotic brain is limited to the passage track and bacterial contamination is very low. When the patient is neurologically intact at the time of admission, only the external wound is debrided, and a

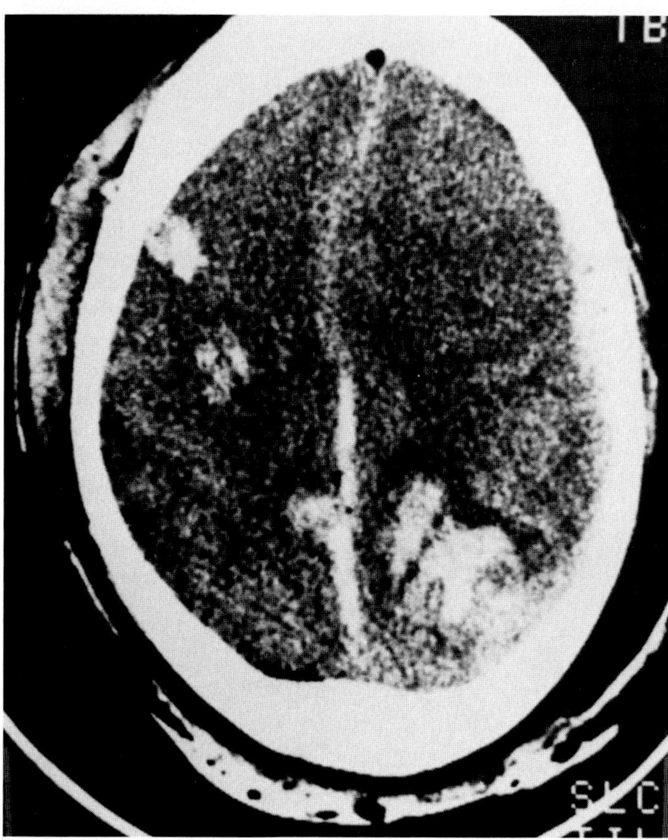

Fig. 5-11. A CT scan of a patient with a diagonal crossover of a bullet from the right hemisphere into the left. Note the larger hematoma toward the exit side.

delayed operation for brain debridement is done toward the end of the first week, when all brain edema has subsided and the necrotic brain tissue has separated. Under this setting, the operation is simple and bloodless, and effective cerebral debridement can be done without any risk of added neurologic deficit. We attempt to remove these bullets unless they are located in the depth of the brain. Our observation is that these bullets move with gravity within the brain substance because of their heavy weight, and, hence, it is important to obtain repeat x-ray films of the skull on the morning of the operation in order to locate their new position. The craniotomy is a routine one, and we prefer small flaps because of the limited cerebral pathologic process and the small passage track. Probing of the track with instruments often is not necessary, and irrigating the debris out of the wound with saline by introducing the tip of the asepto syringe into the depth of the track is sufficient. If the brain is unduly swollen 1 week after the injury, an intracerebral hematoma, usually in the depth of the track, must be sought. No foreign material such as Gelfoam is left in the wound.

Most of these injuries occur during the vertical descent of the bullet. The relative benignity of these injuries, unless penetration of deep structures with deep hemorrhage into the ventricles occurs, has been established from the large number of cases seen.[12] Although they behave like low-velocity missiles, they travel a distance into the skull and sometimes exit. Removal of these bullets may require a small additional craniotomy over the location of the bullet. Spent bullets in the depth of the cranium may change location and move with time to more accessible areas and can then be removed. This is

common in children with heavy smooth bullets as illustrated in Figures 5-9 and 5-10.

From the experience of 13 years of continued military operations and civil war in which over 2000 gunshot wounds to the head were treated at the American University of Beirut Medical Center, both civilian and military, we have come to recognize specific types of cerebral injury or unusual circumstances of ballistic wounds that carry with them a grim outlook and grave prognosis for both neurologic function and life. I have summarized these into the following categories:

1. Bullets penetrating areas of deep gray matter carry with them a fairly high mortality, over 50 percent. The explanation can be interpolated from the physiologic studies and experimental model of Gerber.[13]
2. Diagonal or crossover injuries from one hemisphere into another carry with them a bad prognosis in terms of residual cerebral function (usually devastating fixed neurologic deficit). The mortality here has been around 25 to 30 percent (Figures 5-11 and 5-12).
3. Transventricular penetrating wounds carry a high mortality, nearing 40 percent. These patients have a higher risk of developing meningitis or ventriculitis (Figure 5-13).
4. Tangential injuries. Although these look relatively benign to the inexperienced, frequently they are associated with large areas of local cerebral tissue damage and produce bad focal neurologic deficit. They occur with high-velocity bullets and the cerebral cavitary necrosis, with or without extensive skull fracturing, is substantial and involves the depth of the white matter down to the ventricular surface. The mortality is low but the neurologic deficit is profound. Figure 5-14 shows significant cerebral injury with minimal bony injury. Figure 5-15 illustrates a high convexity tangential wound with extensive fracturing, torn dura, sagittal sinus, and underlying cerebral injury. Figure 5-16 illustrates a large amount of in-driven bone.

A fairly common problem that one encounters is cerebrospinal fluid leak. This frequently occurs in gunshot wounds through the base of the skull, i.e., in the anterior cranial fossa with involvement of the paranasal sinus. In such instances, thorough debridement and closure of the craniofacial wound will allow the use of fascia lata for watertight closure of the dura. This has not been difficult nor fraught with a substantial increased risk of infection of the graft. Much greater difficulties, however, arise in gunshot wounds through the orbit with extensive damage to the globe and bony injury to the roof of the orbit or middle cranial fossa. Cerebrospinal fluid leaks are almost invariable after orbital exenteration or evisceration in such cases. Hence, the use of a fascia lata or pericranial patch over the cranial defect in the floor is mandatory at the time of the initial craniocerebral debridement procedure, despite the high risk of infection of the graft from an extension of orbital infection. Cerebrospinal fluid may not leak until after the globe has been exanthered. If the defect has not been patched at the initial operation and the globe exanthered later, that will certainly require a secondary cerebral operation for the leak. In general, the surgeon may be well advised to try to patch the defect of the cranial floor at the time of the first operation, provided that the injured and massively swollen brain will allow both good visualization and access. Although this may not be difficult in defects of the orbital roof, it may prove unattainable in the middle fossa and particularly below the sphenoid wing in

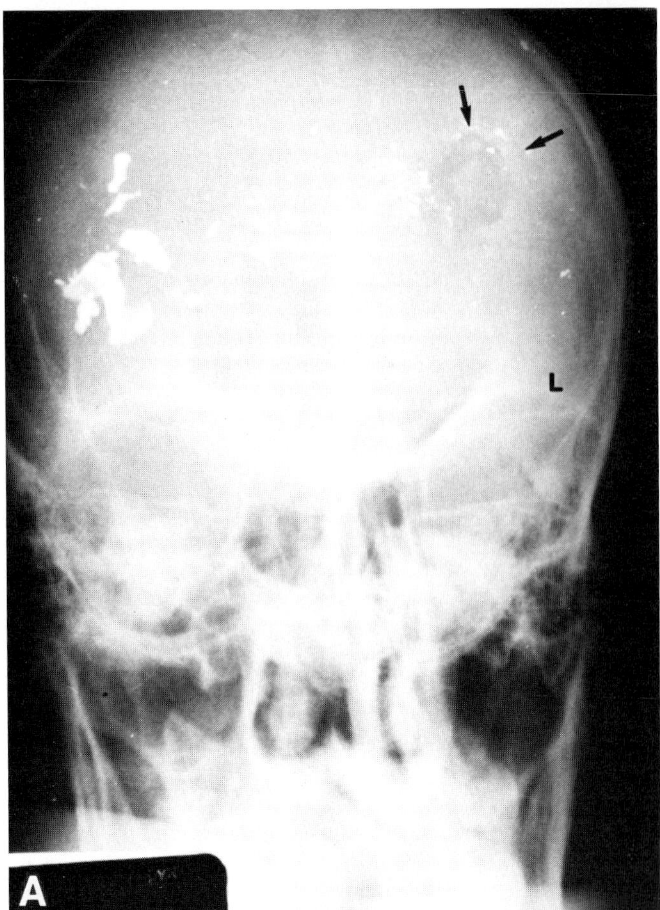
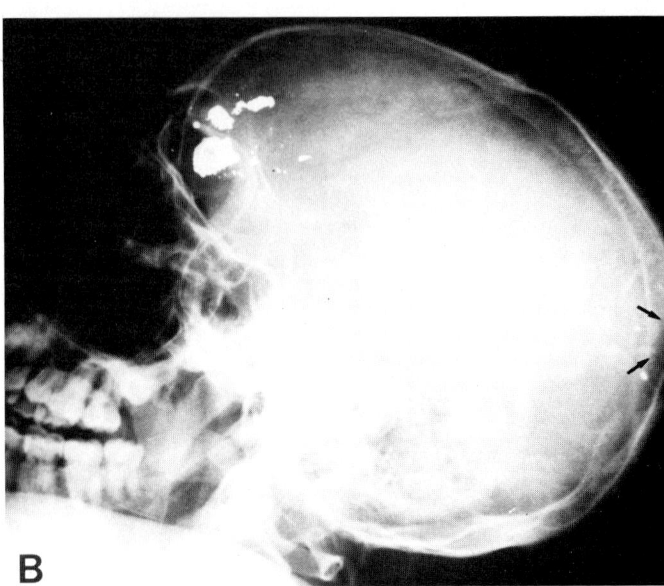

Fig. 5-12. (A) Anteroposterior and (B) lateral views of the skull of a patient with a diagonal injury from the right hemisphere into the left. Note the larger bony wound at the exit side in the left parietal area. The track of the bullet is clearly outlined by the fragmentation of the soft jacket of the bullet.

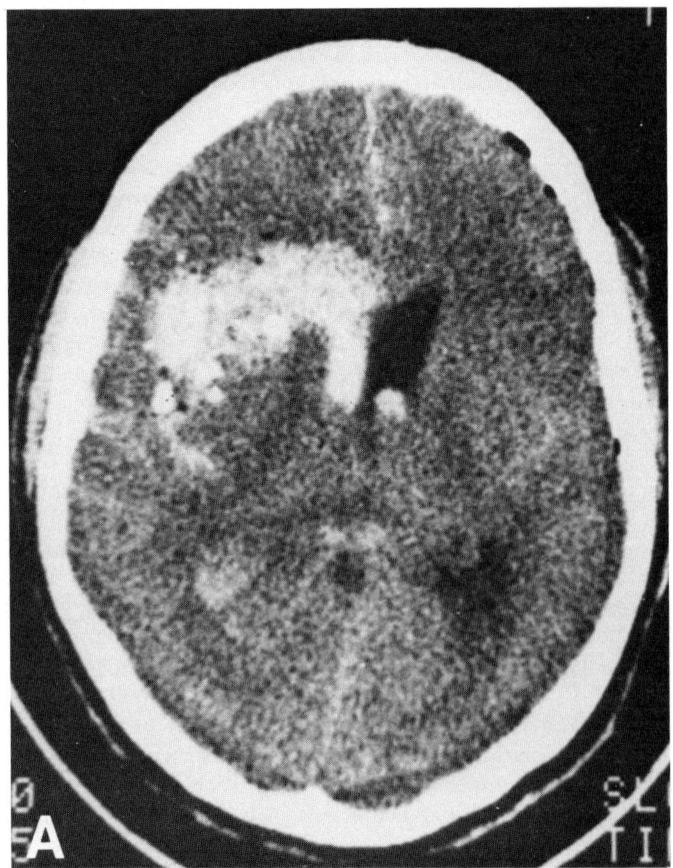
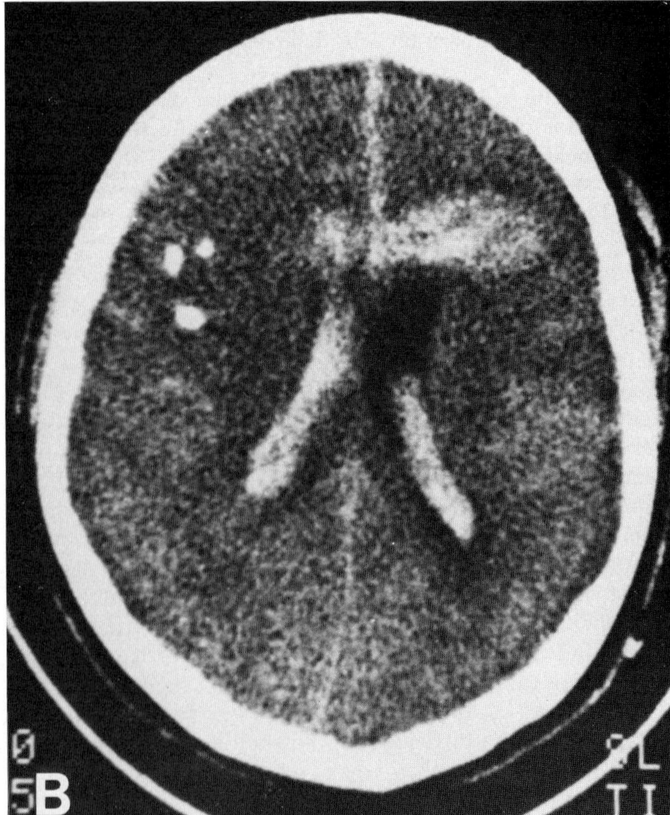

Fig. 5-13. Two CT scans in sequence illustrating a gunshot wound with a transventricular track. Note the in-driven bone in the right frontotemporal area at the entry and the track going through both frontal horns with a large hematoma along the track and intraventricular hemorrhage.

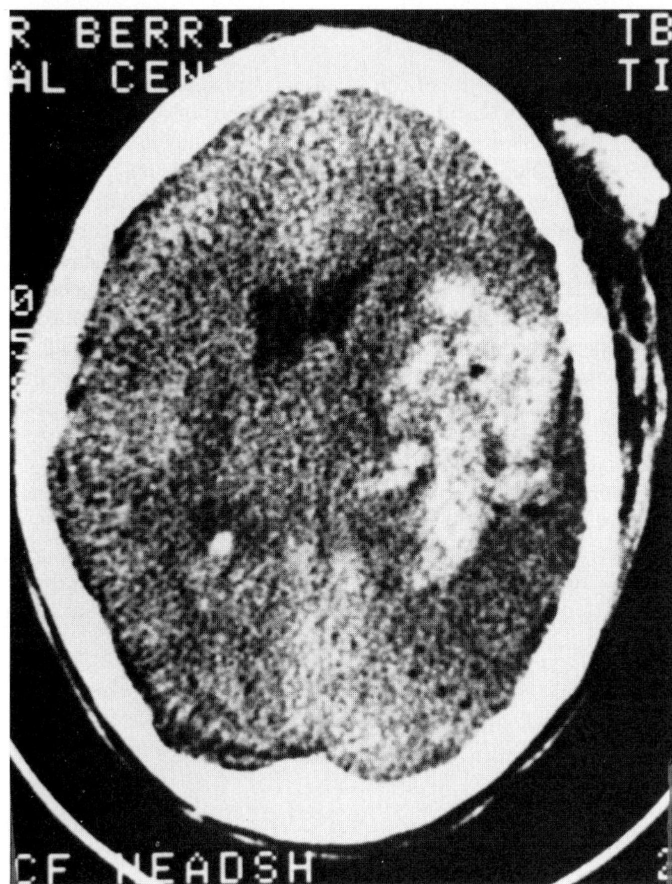

Fig. 5-14. A CT scan of a tangential gunshot wound to the left temporoparietal area with minimal bony injury and extensive cerebral injury with intracerebral hemorrhage and mass effect at the midline.

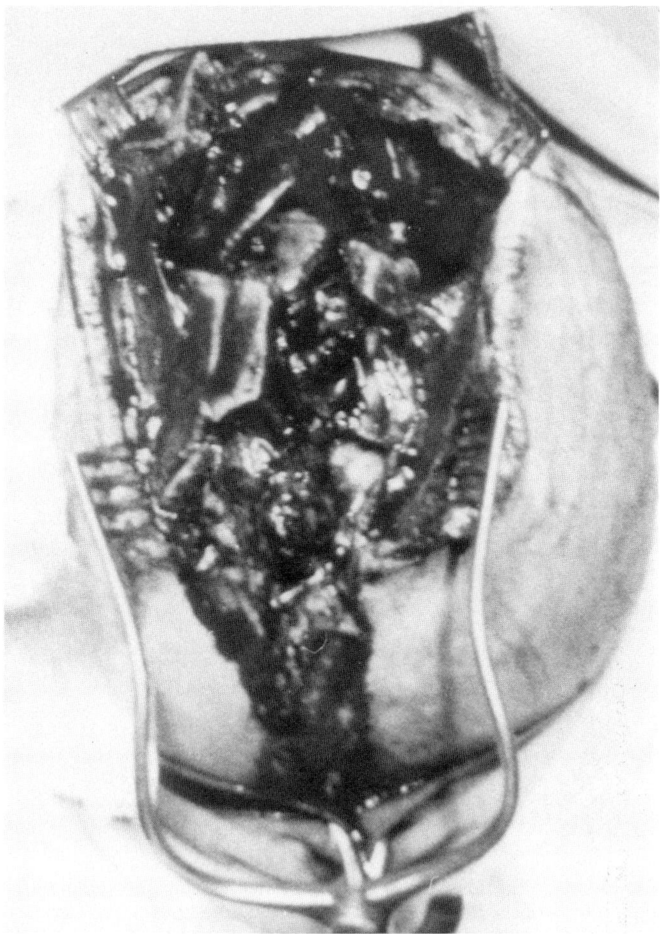

Fig. 5-15. The extent of a tangential gunshot wound to the left hemisphere convexity as seen at exploration. Note the extensive bony fracturing and the tearing of the dura to involve the sagittal sinus medially. Extensive cerebral injury in seen in the bottom of the wound into the depth of the white matter and hemorrhagic brain.

the posterior wall of the orbit. Leaks from these locations and into the orbit do not heal spontaneously.

The problem of retained intracranial bone remains of paramount importance to the surgeon in view of early reports of an increased risk of brain infection (abscess) associated with retained bone. Bone had a higher yield of positive cultures than metallic fragments.[5] Hence the long-standing dictum of the necessity to debride all bone driven into the brain. In principle, we concur with this dictum and we recommend strongly the removal of all accessible bone at the primary debridement operation. The issue becomes rather difficult when a substantial amount of bone is inaccessible or when a considerable volume of retained bone is discovered on a postoperative CT scan. It is our belief that small volumes, less than 1 cm^3, of retained bone do not pose an added hazard of infection after the necrotic brain has been thoroughly debrided, and the surgeon should not go after them at the risk of increased neurologic insult. However, larger volumes of bone located in or in proximity to infarcted or hemorrhagic necrotic brain may be a significant nidus for cerebral infection and another gentle debridement operation is in order. A total of 275 cases were reviewed with a mean follow-up of 3 years. These patients were grouped into three categories:

1. Those not debrided who had in-driven bone.
2. Those who were well debrided and had retained bone on follow-up CT scans.

3. Those who were well debrided and who did not have retained bone on follow-up CT scans.

Preliminary data[14] indicate that there is no significant statistical difference in the incidence of postinjury brain abscess related directly to retained bone among the three groups. Further detailed analysis with study of all the variables is necessary for final conclusions.

POSTOPERATIVE CARE

Postoperative care in most instances is indistinguishable from that for patients with severe closed head injury. These patients require an intensive care unit for general supportive therapy and specific therapy for their increased intracranial pressure. Postinjury or postoperative cerebral edema is combated with large doses of corticosteroids for 5 to 7 days. Repeated small boluses of osmotic diuretic or a continuous intravenous infusion of 20 percent mannitol solution for 3 to 5 days may be necessary to keep brain bulk down. Adequate monitoring of serum osmolarity is a must. Anticonvulsant therapy is maintained and patients are discharged on anticonvulsants for several years in view of the high incidence

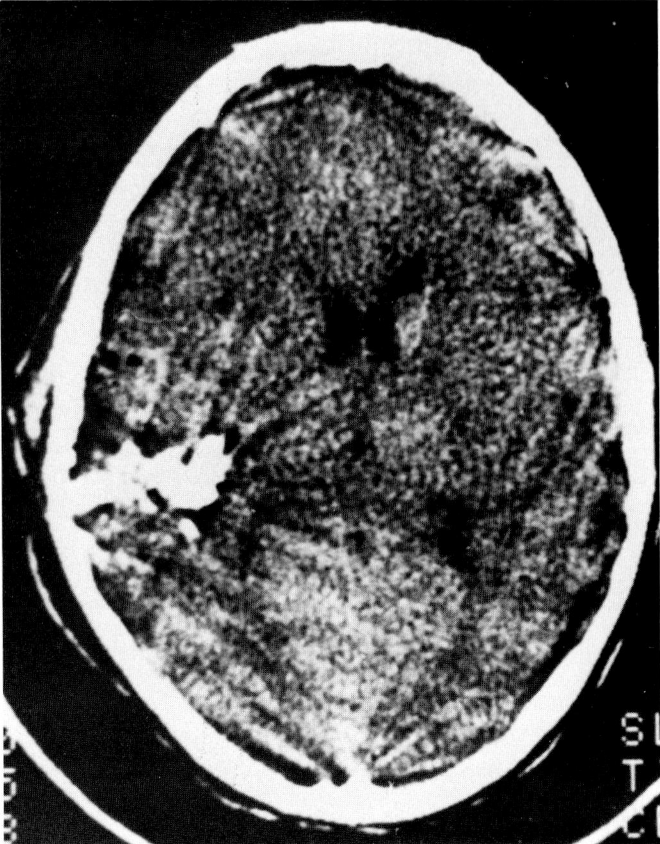

Fig. 5-16. A CT scan at the level of a tangential gunshot wound to the right temporoparietal area. Note the remarkable absence of significant cerebral injury and the large volume of in-driven bone in the hemisphere.

CONCLUSIONS

Gunshot wounds of the head can present different clinical pictures, largely based on the different types of damage inflicted on the brain. This is dependent on the size, shape, stability, and velocity of the missile. Low-velocity missiles may present a relatively benign clinical picture; high-velocity missiles, on the other hand, produce large areas of cavitary necrosis with extensive skull fracturing and are often incompatible with survival. A thorough knowledge of the pathology is essential in the execution of an early definitive operation, which basically consists of thoroughly debriding the cavitary track of all necrotic brain tissue, foreign bodies, and bone and metal fragments. This lessens the chances of deep cerebral wound infection with cerebritis or abscess. Closure of the dura is mandatory, and is easier with a graft. The scalp wound should be debrided well and excised if feasible, and closed without tension by relaxing incisions or rotation flaps. Unusual circumstances may present themselves, and the recommended operative technique may be slightly modified to suit the special case in an attempt to save more lives and preserve more neurologic function.

of posttraumatic epilepsy with penetrating brain wounds. Should a patient develop a CSF leak, this should be repaired soon as the patient's condition permits. The high yield of positive cultures from these wounds with both Gram-positive cocci and Gram-negative bacilli require prophylactic antibiotics. The use of antibiotics prophylactically is not to replace adequate wound debridement, since well-debrided wounds have a low incidence of infection. We have recently faced the problem of *Staphylococcus* species resistance to methicillin (nearly 50 percent) and resistant Gram-negative bacilli requiring the use of third generation cephalosporin for heavily contaminated wounds or when infection sets in. Postoperative CT scans are used routinely and as frequently as the patient's condition dictates. Postoperative CT scanning has been of great value in uncovering persistent brain swelling, retained foreign matter, areas of infarction, delayed hematomas, hydrocephalus, and, finally, abscess formation. We have not encountered increased bone flap infection and the majority of debrided cases had their bone flap replaced at the initial operation. Brain fungus has been seen in few cases, primarily those that were transferred to our facility longer than 3 or 4 days after wounding with no adequate treatment given in the peripheral hospitals.

REFERENCES

1. Gurdjian ES: The treatment of penetrating wounds of the brain sustained in warfare. A historical review. J Neurosurg 40:157, 1974
2. Hammon WM: Analysis of 2178 consecutive penetrating wounds of the brain from Vietnam. J Neurosurg 34:127, 1971
3. Hammon WM: Retained intracranial bone fragments: Analysis of 42 patients. J Neurosurg 34:142, 1971
4. Hagan RE: Early complications following penetrating wounds of the brain. J Neurosurg 34:132, 1971
5. Carey ME, Young H, Mathis JL, et al: A bacteriological study of craniocerebral missile wounds from Vietnam. J Neurosurg 34:145, 1971
6. Meirowsky AM: Neurological Surgery of Trauma. Washington, D.C, Office of the Surgeon General, Department of the Army, 1965
7. Smith WHB, Smith JE: The Book of Rifles, ed 4. Harrisburg, PA, Stackpole, 1972, pp 400, 434
8. Sights WP Jr: Ballistic analysis of shotgun injuries to the central nervous system. J Neurosurg 31:25, 1969
9. Owen-Smith Lt Col: Surgical Pathology of Missile Injuries. Graves Medical Audiovisual Library 77.38, Medical Recording Service Foundation, Chelmsford CMI 5HL
10. Weiner SL, Barrett J: Trauma Management. Philadelphia, WB Saunders, 1986, pp 1–12
11. Achram M, et al: Angiographic aspects of traumatic intracranial aneurysms following war injuries. Br J Radiol 53:1144, 1980
12. Hanieh A: Brain injury from a spent bullet descending vertically. J Neurosurg 34:222, 1971
13. Gerber A, Moody R: Craniocerebral missile injuries in the monkey: An experimental physiological model. J Neurosurg 36:43, 1972
14. Saba M, Taha J: The relationship of the volume of retained bone to cerebral infection in gunshot wounds of the head: Review of 275 cases. (in preparation)

CHAPTER 6

Penetrating Missile Injuries of the Head

Eugene D. George   T. Forcht Dagi

UNTIL THE TURN of the 20th century, penetrating missile injuries of the brain were almost universally fatal. During World War I, Cushing, Jefferson, and others demonstrated that the mortality could be reduced by early debridement and meticulous attention to neurosurgical technique. Since then, the focus of attention has shifted from survival to improvement of functional outcome.[1]

Historically, major conflicts have been separated by an interval sufficient to ensure that neurosurgeons who gained expertise in one war were not the ones to render front-line service in the next. Each war has different lessons to teach. World War I proved the efficacy of vigorous surgical intervention. The Spanish Civil War demonstrated that blast effect was a significant component of craniofacial injury after aerial bombardment. During World War II, the importance of initial dural repair and antibiotic medication was initially debated and finally universally accepted.[2–4] The Korean War confirmed the effectiveness of early evacuation and initial definitive surgery in improving survival and reducing infection.[2,5] The civil disturbances in Belfast took place so close to the neurosurgical center that the natural history of penetrating injury could be studied virtually from the moment of injury.[6] In the course of the Israeli expedition into Lebanon, all patients with head injuries were brought to a single institution, and for the first time the place of computed tomographic (CT) scanning in combat neurosurgery was evaluated. Finally, in the wake of the Vietnam conflict, the Vietnam Head Injury Study (VHIS), a unique cooperative effort funded by the Veteran's Administration and involving the U.S. Army, Navy, and Air Force, the American Red Cross, and the National Institutes of Health, was established to register and study outcome after penetrating head injury. For about 18 years, the VHIS has followed a large population of head injured patients using sophisticated epidemiologic, radiologic, and neuropsychologic techniques. Data that were often lost in the past, when injured veterans were not aggressively followed once they returned to their communities, have been successfully elicited.[7]

Regardless of the venue of the conflict, in every war a number of subjects come to be reconsidered:

1. The practical significance of distinguishing between high velocity and low velocity wounds.
2. The importance of early transport and treatment of the wounded.

3. The definition of what constitutes adequate surgical debridement.
4. Specific methods of dealing with complex wounds involving the orbit, the air sinuses, and major vascular structures.
5. The management of cerebrospinal fluid fistulas.
6. The prevention and diagnosis of acute infection and of delayed abscess and hematoma.
7. The epidemiology of posttraumatic seizure disorders.

Not surprisingly, these are the main questions that arise in the management of penetrating missile injuries. Dr. Maurice Saba, in his excellent chapter in this book, has provided a basic approach to the problem of penetrating missile injuries. Our companion chapter is directed at some specific areas of pathophysiology and treatment that draw heavily on lessons learned from military neurosurgery over the past 15 years from the Vietnam Head Injury Study, and, more recently, from evolving concepts in the treatment of open and closed head injury.

BALLISTICS AND THEIR CLINICAL SIGNIFICANCE

Injury to the brain is a function of energy release over time and of the volume and location of tissue disruption. The simplest useful classification divides penetrating missile injuries into high velocity and low velocity categories, relating the severity of the wound to the muzzle or initial velocity and energy content of the missile.[8,9] By convention, high velocity missiles exceed 2000 feet per second, a figure easily achieved by many bullets. Most modern high velocity rifle ammunition surpasses 2500 ft/sec. Most handgun ammunition has a velocity ranging between 800 and 1400 ft/sec. Penetrating fragments or shrapnel, however, typically have a velocity on the order of 600 ft/sec. The energy (E) released during the terminal ballistic events in tissue depends on the missile mass (M) and velocity (V). The greater the energy release, the greater the potential for damage, while the shorter the timespan over which release occurs, the more like an explosion it becomes. The relationship between E, M, and V can be construed in a number of ways, including momentum (MV), kinetic energy ($1/2\ MV^2$), and power (αMV^3). Each of these expressions places a different emphasis on velocity. At several important historical junctures, unavoidable compromises in ammunition design were defended by invoking a preference for momentum, kinetic energy, or power.

At the turn of the century, for example, the chamber pressures attainable in military weapons were limited by met-

---

The opinions expressed in this chapter are the personal views of the authors entirely and are not to be construed as reflecting the position of the Department of Defense or the Department of the Army.

OPERATIVE NEUROSURGICAL TECHNIQUES
ISBN 0-8089-1862-1

allurgical considerations, and ballistic design came to be focused on massive bullets with relatively low velocity, similar to those used for hunting big game. Modern ammunition is no longer limited in any practical sense by the design of the weapon, so that it can attain tremendous energy by emphasizing velocity at the expense of mass. This ballistic design tends to make weapons cycle more easily, and permits the foot soldier to carry a larger quantity of ammunition for the same weight. However, because light bullets are easily deflected and lose energy rapidly over distance, there is continued world-wide reliance on slower and more massive bullets. Thus, in most NATO and Warsaw Pact armies, low mass, small caliber, high velocity bullets such as the 55 grain .223 caliber fired in the American M-16 assault rifle or its Soviet equivalent are supplemented by slower more massive rounds, such as the 150 grain .308 caliber or 7.62 mm bullet for sniper use. This is not a trivial point, since sniper tactics emphasize aiming at the head, and terrorists who have been trained as snipers are taught to target prominent individuals in positions of leadership where disablement will be at least as demoralizing as death. Some sniper wounds will in fact be survivable, because most shots are taken at relatively great distance.

It is, unfortunately, increasingly likely that terrorist incidents will affect the innocent public throughout the world. The neurosurgeon may be called upon to deal with the consequences of terrorist acts that create injuries different from those he or she is accustomed to seeing. It is wise to shed any preconceived expectations regarding penetrating missile injuries. Experience with terrorist groups and organized crime has shown that many weapons and rounds can be modified to deposit more energy than one might predict: standard handgun ammunition, for example, can be hand-loaded to attain 1600 ft/sec; ''hot'' ammunition designed for submachine gun use can be discharged in most 9 mm pistols, and cast bronze or Teflon-clad bullets produce unusual cavitation. Moreover, blast effects from exploding bullets, grenades, plastic explosive, and incendiary devices in closed spaces create wounds that combine the worst characteristics of closed and penetrating head injury.[10]

A missile's energy is greatest at the moment at which it is launched and decays with time and distance. A .30/30 caliber, 170 grain bullet is discharged with a muzzle velocity of 2220 ft/sec, for example, but at 100 yards the velocity drops to 1350 ft/sec and at 200 yards to 1000 ft/sec, well within the range of handgun ammunition. Most survivable injuries occur at low impact velocity. From a practical standpoint, the terminal ballistic events—the striking velocity, the quantity of energy released, and the explosive force developed—are more important than muzzle velocity or bullet mass. What counts is the striking or impact energy rather than the muzzle velocity.

The degree of tissue injury is proportional to the quantity of energy delivered. The amount of energy imparted to tissue when a projectile strikes is limited by the energy at impact. As a rule, more energy is imparted by penetrating injuries than by perforating (through-and-through) injuries. Penetrating missiles release all their energy in the tissue, while in perforating injuries, the difference between the energy at impact and the residual energy at exit determines the energy delivered. The perfect bullet would release all of its energy instantaneously: dE/dt (t = time) would be infinite. Ballistic design therefore is calculated to create smooth, friction-free flight in air but infinite resistance to passage in tissue. This goal is achieved by physical changes that affect the shape or ballistic characteristics of the bullet by expansion, tumbling, yaw, or fragmentation. The

sudden loss of spin, for example, causes energy to be released in two ways: first, a significant quantity of angular energy is released; second, the bullet destabilizes, slows, tumbles, and sometimes fragments. Even a glancing, tangential injury can generate significant injury because of the energy transmitted to adjacent structures.[11,12]

Although many wartime injuries are sustained at a considerable distance from the weapons that inflict them, in civilian life, most injuries occur at less than 50 yards, and impact velocity is effectively equal to muzzle velocity. The distance at which a soldier in wartime is shot is usually the unknown variable that helps account for survival after ostensibly high energy bullet wounds.

PATHOPHYSIOLOGY

What happens when a missile strikes determines the limits of successful surgical intervention after a penetrating injury. Harvey[13] described the five events that accompany bullet penetration:

1. Shock waves develop at an angle to the bullet path.
2. A temporary cavity develops, lasting approximately 20 msec as energy is transferred to the tissue.
3. The temporary cavity pulsates before it collapses, sending pressure waves through adjacent tissue and causing remote injury and herniation.
4. The temporary cavity collapses, leaving a residual permanent cavity, the bullet track, and an area of surrounding tissue damage.
5. There is extravasation of blood around the missile track, occupying a space larger than but fairly concentric with the temporary cavity.

THE NATURE OF THE BULLET TRACK

At close ranges, the permanent cavity bears little relationship to the muzzle velocity of the missile. At greater distances, however, a high velocity bullet creates a beet-shaped cavity and a low velocity bullet creates a carrot-shaped cavity. With long range perforating injuries, the exit wound is always larger than the entrance wound; this rule does not hold true in short range injuries. The cavitary effect of low velocity missiles is inconsistent and determined both by the direction of travel and the extent of yaw. High velocity missiles, in general, create a more consistent cavity. When bullets fragment, specific cavitary characteristics cannot be projected because the configuration is a function of the complexities of energy transfer.[14]

BONE CHIPS

Bone chips invariably accompany penetration of the skull and may be thrown off by tangential injuries as well.[15] The path of a missile wound can often be determined on plain skull films by the track of bone chips. Bone chips occasionally form a secondary track different from that of the bullet, but the volume of this tract is usually small, and bone chips rarely act as secondary missiles of any significance. The volume of residual chips on plain skull films after surgery traditionally has been regarded as a measure of the adequacy of debridement (see below).[16]

ACUTE BURSTS OF INTRACRANIAL PRESSURE

Acute signs of intracranial pressure bursts are seen in over 90 percent of fatal head injuries. The significance of these pressure marks is controversial.[17–19] The degree of intracranial pressure does not correlate directly with missile velocity, cavity size, or duration of survival. Low velocity wounds observed in civilian practice have not been consistently associated with cerebral edema without direct brainstem injury.

CONTUSIONS AND HEMATOMAS

Cortical contusions are present at the site of entry in 50 percent of cases and elsewhere in another 50 percent. Irrespective of bullet path, subfrontal contusions occur in 25 percent. Other remote contusions are also commonly found.[17] Data obtained from CT scans in the VHIS substantiates the long-standing clinical impression that the degree of actual injury usually surpasses the surgeon's estimate.

During the Korean war, 46.2 percent of patients seen within 8 hours of injury had intracranial hematomas; this figure dropped to 27 percent after 12 to 35 hours, and to 7 percent after 48 to 72 hours.[20] In civilian practice, hematomas were found in 44 percent of patients seen within 5.5 hours of injury.[18] The decline in prevalence with time probably represents the early death of patients with significant mass effect or intracranial hematomas.

In a study of 316 cases seen within 8 hours of wounding, 3 percent had extradural clots, 21 percent had subdural clots, 23 percent had intracerebral clots, and 0.2 percent had intraventricular clots. Two or more hematomas were not uncommon.[20] It may be expected that the incidence of early and late hematomas will be recalculated when CT scans are obtained closer to the time of injury. In military practice, hematomas at the site of exit can be more significant than those elsewhere.[21]

FRACTURES AND FRACTURE LINES

Fracture lines that accompany gunshot wounds to the brain tend to pass from the point of impact to the opposite pole, shifting directions at and sparing buttress lines. Shock waves within the skull cause fractures of the orbital roofs and cribriform plate even when the missile proceeds elsewhere.[17] This helps to explain why CSF leaks after penetrating missile injuries are difficult to locate and treat; there are many widely separated areas where the leptomeninges could be lacerated by fracture lines.

TANGENTIAL INJURIES

Tangential injuries are common and carry the best prognosis of all types of missile injuries despite a significant morbidity. Before the advent of computed tomography, it was estimated that 75 percent of patients would have significant cortical contusions, subcortical hematomas, subdural hematomas, and venous sinus disruption. Comparable data have not been elicited using modern diagnostic techniques.

BLAST INJURIES

In urban battle, blast injuries complicate penetrating trauma with diffuse acceleration-deceleration forces akin to those encountered in closed head injury. This type of injury was characteristic in patients who were evacuated from the Lebanon conflict (M. Feinsod, Haifa: personal communication), and had as its major pathophysiologic component a rapid and diffuse increase in intracranial pressure.

OPERATIVE CONSIDERATIONS

GENERAL PRINCIPLES

The approach to penetrating missile injuries does not differ significantly between military and civilian practice, although specific concerns and limitations inherent to combat medicine in the military setting may affect certain details of operative management. The overall achievements of surgery are limited by the pathophysiologic events that accompany penetration of the brain by a missile. The goals of surgery thus are quite specific: to remove space-occupying lesions, to prevent infection, to produce hemostasis, and to repair and restore anatomic integrity to the injured structures.

The guiding principles of operative management were enunciated by Cushing and Jefferson and reiterated by Cairns, Lewin, Matson, and many others. In brief, vigorous operative debridement of the missile track is recommended to prevent abscess formation. The need for satisfactory dural closure and scalp reconstruction has become axiomatic. The dura should be closed in watertight fashion; a graft should be used when necessary to prevent tension. Dural grafts revascularize quickly, even though they are technically nonvital. In order of accessibility and preference, potential donor sites include temporalis fascia, pericranium, fascia lata, and transversalis fascia. Galea is usually needed to close the scalp; its use as a dural substitute is not recommended. All foreign materials should be avoided: artificial dural substitutes are contraindicated with the possible exception of lyophilized human dura, which seems to act like "true" autogenic dura despite having been irradiated and preserved.

Finally, a meticulous reconstruction and closure of the scalp is effected. Tension should be avoided in repair of the skin and subcutaneous tissues. Flaps can be rotated immediately, even over contaminated wounds, and may, in fact, facilitate healing of locally infected areas. If absolutely necessary, the dura can be left uncovered and a flap rotated once the dura has begun to granulate and heal by secondary intention. The older literature advocated this technique, but it is probably unnecessary when antibiotics are available. Absorbable suture material should be placed in the galea. Monofilament thread or stainless steel staples can be used for the skin. Single layer closures have been advocated for grossly contaminated wounds; the correct technique requires the use of interrupted vertically mattressed monofilament sutures spaced at 1–1.5-cm intervals. Because scalp closure is a major barrier to CSF leak, two-layer closure is always preferable. The use of drains does not seem to prejudice the development of wound infections.

Steroids and Alimentation

There is no evidence at this time to support the use of steroids in head injured patients. By the same token, aggressive dehydration has not been shown to be effective in controlling diffuse cerebral edema and cannot be recommended. Caloric intake, on the other hand, is highly correlated with improvements in outcome. The increased metabolic demands of head injured patients make hyperalimentation and careful nutritional support an integral part of the medical management.

Anticonvulsants

Anticonvulsant prophylaxis is routinely used. A number of factors influence the likelihood of seizure onset.[22,23] With long-term follow-up, it is becoming apparent that many patients who do not have seizures immediately after injury will do so within 5 to 15 years. There is no evidence, however, to suggest that the ultimate seizure history is affected by phenytoin, the anticonvulsant most commonly used for routine prophylaxis and treatment.[24] The correlation of hematomas with seizure disorders is well defined. Retained bone fragments do not seem to exert a deleterious effect on seizure prevalence, but whether the same holds true for retained metal fragments remains to be seen. Whenever the onset of seizures is other than immediately after injury, CT scans should be obtained to exclude hematoma and abscess formation, even as anticonvulsant treatment is begun.

Antibiotics

Antibiotics should be given prophylactically as soon as feasible. This is true regardless of whether or not proposed management includes surgery and has proved useful in both civilian and military experience. It will be necessary to determine in each situation which antibiotics are the most appropriate. To begin, skin flora should be covered. The use of antibiotics in this setting is therapeutic and not prophylactic; antibiotics should be prescribed in meningeal doses.[22,23,25,26]

Intracranial Pressure Monitoring

The role of intracranial pressure (ICP) monitoring is yet to be defined. It was rarely used in Vietnam. In Northern Ireland, other variables proved more useful in patient evaluation and management.[27] In contrast, ICP monitoring proved to be one of the cornerstones of therapy in Haifa between 1982 and 1985. This disparity can be accounted for by differences in the combat environment. Intracranial pressure monitoring can be especially useful where blast injury constitutes a significant component of the overall problem. In most patients who survive penetrating missile injuries, however, initial increases of intracranial pressure will be due to the mass effect of surrounding hematomas and collections of debris, and late increases will be the result of delayed hematoma formation[28] or abscess. These lesions can be visualized on CT scans and should be treated surgically, according to the usual indications for relief of mass lesions. Although angiography is not called for routinely, it should be considered as part of the evaluation and management of delayed or recurring hematoma to rule out the possibility of traumatic aneurysm or other vascular injury.

EVOLVING TECHNIQUES AND ONGOING CONTROVERSIES

Debridement and Management of Bone Fragments

With the advent of computed tomography, the existence of modern antibiotics, and the availability of intracranial pressure monitoring and neurosurgical intensive care, serious questions have been raised concerning the extent of necessary debridement: must all fragments of bone be removed to minimize the risk of abscess, even to the point of threatening relatively normal brain and performing secondary and tertiary operations, or can a more conservative approach be justified?

The reasons for pursuing this issue are several. First, from a number of sources, including the VHIS, the experience at Walter Reed Army Medical Center, and the follow-up experience with head trauma in a more general sense, it is becoming evident that there is no such thing as a truly "silent" area of brain and that there is a definable risk to reoperation in enthusiastic pursuit of retained fragments.[29] Second, several institutions have reported satisfactory outcomes with limited debridement under an antibiotic umbrella. Third, the extensive availability of CT scanning allows patients at risk of developing delayed abscess to be restudied serially.[30] Fourth, by using CT scanning rather than relying on plain skull films, the VHIS has demonstrated that "complete" debridement of all foreign material and bony fragments is achieved much less often than previously believed by the operating neurosurgeon.[31] Finally, recent experience in Israel suggests that many patients can be treated with relatively limited cerebral debridement, dural repair, and scalp closure without imperilling the eventual outcome, and then followed by intracranial pressure monitoring and serial CT scanning.[32]

This area is in flux, and dogmatic conclusions cannot be made on the basis of present levels of experience. At this time, it appears reasonable to withhold secondary surgery for retained fragments given three critical conditions: (1) adequate initial debridement was performed by qualified neurosurgeons; (2) serial CT scanning for long-term follow-up is available; and (3) satisfactory continuing neurosurgical care is readily obtainable. Should any of these conditions not be satisfied, a secondary operation may well be indicated.

As a practical matter, it is likely that the neurosurgeons primarily responsible for operative decisions in time of war will be required to tailor their approach to the situation. These points are by no means intended to inhibit or negate the importance of initial vigorous debridement of injured tissue. Rather, in our view, the practice of *uncritical* secondary or tertiary operation as a matter of policy is outdated so long as there is continued access to modern imaging techniques and satisfactory neurosurgical follow-up.

Metallic and Migrating Fragments

Although the possible epileptogenic effects of retained metal fragments—especially copper—have been mentioned,[33,34] there is at this time no definite indication to pursue metallic fragments beyond those that are readily accessible. An exception to this rule is the migrating metallic fragment.

There are two categories of migrating fragments: those in the ventricle, and those in the parenchyma of the brain. Intraventricular fragments have been implicated anecdotally in hydrocephalus, ventriculitis, and hypothalamic syndromes characterized by central disturbances of temperature control (central neurogenic hyperthermia) and obtundation. By judicious positioning, it is possible to position the fragment in the occipital horn of the lateral ventricle, where it can be reached relatively easily. Intraoperative x-ray films are necessary to confirm that the fragment is attainably lodged. Intraventricular metallic fragments associated with infection or obstructive hydrocephalus should also be removed, even if they do not appear migratory at the time. Ventriculoscopy and stereotactic techniques can be useful in retrieving intraventricular fragments.

Inaccessible fragments deep in the parenchyma of the brain

do not migrate as a rule, but when they do, the patient should be positioned in such a manner as to allow gravity to bring the fragment to the surface in an innocuous area. Fragments that spontaneously migrate to the cortex pose no particular technical difficulty and should be removed.

Exploding Bullets

Explosive bullets that detonate on impact or shortly thereafter are formally prohibited by the rules of war but have been available on the civilian market and are used by terrorist groups. When the bullet explodes, the surgeon will encounter a combination of blast effect and penetrating missile injury. When the bullet fails to detonate, the surgeon faces a certain risk of personal injury in removing or manipulating the missile. Some explosive bullets have a characteristic radiologic appearance: a central cavity filled with explosive, sometimes sealed with a ball bearing, a pellet, or a BB. Hollow-nosed and dum-dum (blunt tipped) bullets are not explosive. It is recommended that long handled instruments be used, that electrocautery not be applied in the vicinity of such missiles, that they be grasped gently from the base rather than the nose, and that, at all costs, the nose of the bullet not be crushed. The surgeon should wear goggles to protect the eyes. Although it has been suggested on theoretical grounds that ultrasound and microwaves could cause explosive bullets to detonate, we know of no published data on this point. (It may be of some small comfort to note that explosive bullets have a high failure rate.)

Dural Sinus Repair

Lacerations of the dural sinuses are common in wartime. Techniques for the repair of the dural sinuses have been well described.[35] In most respects, the classical approaches are not outdated. The application of modern microvascular techniques to trauma surgery, however, makes it possible to contemplate the functional repair of dural sinus injuries that in the past would have been treated by packing only.

A full complement of vascular instruments and clips should be available when undertaking sinus repair. The first step in repair involves hemostasis. Temporary hemostasis can usually be achieved by compressing the lacerated sinus with cottonoid over Gelfoam while elevating the head (reverse Trendelenburg position). Because of the risks of air embolus during sinus repair, the cottonoids covering the laceration and the wound edges should be soaking wet. A central line in the right atrium and Doppler echocardiography monitoring are mandatory. The use of positive end-expiratory pressure (PEEP) helps prevent air from entering the venous system but can be limited by cardiopulmonary constraints. Although PEEP can increase the amount of active bleeding, it is easier to contend with the bleeding than with massive air embolus.

Techniques for repair of the dural sinuses have been thoroughly described elsewhere in this book and will not be repeated here. The aim of sinus repair is to restore patency rather than simply staunch hemorrhage. For this reason, the surgery of penetrating missile injuries requires a familiarity with microvascular techniques, and a psychological preparedness to apply these techniques even under relatively primitive circumstances. For example, commercial shunts or Silastic T-tubes may not be available at all times. A workable alternative can be improvised from a floppy pediatric endotracheal tube to which a second balloon cuff has been affixed.

Cerebrospinal Fluid Leaks

At the time of initial debridement, a search should be made for potential sites of CSF fistulas, particularly when the air sinuses, skull base, and orbit have been violated. Complex craniofacial wounds are always treated more vigorously than other penetrating injuries; CSF fistulas are almost inevitable, and infection usually sets in if contaminated nasopharyngeal bone and mucosa is implanted within the brain. If a CSF leak has been detected, the entire frontal floor as far posteriorly as the optic foramina and the limbus sphenoidale must be inspected. The technique of repair is reviewed in Chapter 7.

Neither bone nor methylmethacrylate is needed to close a dural fistula leaking CSF from the skull base.* This can be done simply by patching or reinforcing the dura with pericranium, temporalis fascia, or an adjacent dural flap. The patch is tacked down with several 4–0 or 5–0 sutures intradurally. The pressure of the CSF and the brain holds the graft in place until it vascularizes and fuses to the dura. Sometimes fat must be used to plug a particularly large fistula and a dural graft or dural reflection used to hold the fat in place. Acrylic tissue adhesives for attaching the dural graft have been used with some initial success but are significantly toxic to neural elements. Furthermore, the seal produced by this type of tissue adhesive is not watertight; the cement separates the tissues, impeding contact, fibroblastic ingrowth, and eventual healing. Many of these problems may be solved by the fibrin glues, which are now undergoing clinical trials in the United States.

Cerebrospinal fluid fistulas can develop years after injury. They also can recur even after careful repair.

Hydrocephalus

There are a number of circumstances that predispose a patient to the development of hydrocephalus after a penetrating missile injury. The most obvious case is disruption or occlusion of the ventricular system by bone fragments (rarely) or metal. Where possible these should be removed (cf. "migrating fragments"). Ventriculitis and subarachnoid and intraventricular hemorrhage are known to cause both communicating and obstructive hydrocephalus. Lumbar puncture can be used as temporizing measure in communicating hydrocephalus.

Ventriculostomy (in contaminated or infected cases) and ventriculoperitoneal shunting can be used in both communicating and obstructive hydrocephalus. In diffuse intracerebral edema, the ventricles may be so small that they cannot be cannulated, but if a successful ventriculostomy can be placed, intracranial pressure should be measured at the same time. It is important to remember that the cause of any delayed rise in intracranial pressure as well as the onset of hydrocephalus needs to be understood before it is treated.

Replacement of Bone Fragments

Should bone fragments be replaced at time of initial debridement in order to achieve immediate reconstruction of the calvarium? In fresh injuries, large pieces of bone with aesthetically important functions, such as the forehead or the orbital ridge, can be replaced after they have been scrubbed and soaked with antibiotic solution or even sterilized. Moreover,

---

*Despite an initial enthusiasm for early repair of cosmetic and structural skull defects with methylmethacrylate, the infectious complications resulting from this practice make it inadvisable. Methylmethacrylate is also not a satisfactory substance for obtaining a watertight seal: it shrinks and can become porous over time.

most neurosurgeons have had reasonable success at treating smaller open skull fractures by immediate repositioning of bone fragments. Nonetheless, there is a risk of infection and osteomyelitis. Close neurosurgical observation must be available. If, because of a long evacuation path with multiple stations or because of other special circumstances, adequate neurosurgical follow-up cannot be assured, it is preferable to leave out the bone and perform a cranioplasty 9 to 12 months after injury. Obviously, delayed reconstruction is almost always preferable when an injury is not seen acutely. Under no circumstances should methylmethacrylate be incorporated into an initial bony repair. Infection is almost certain to supervene.

Strategic Considerations

In any future mass casualty situation, international conflict, terrorist incident, or natural disaster, improved transportation will reduce the interval between wounding and definitive care. In Vietnam, the interval between wounding and arrival at a treatment facility was frequently 1 hour or less, and rarely was it more than 6 hours.[36] In Israel during the Lebanon conflict, the average interval between wounding and CT scanning was less than 1 hour, with a physician-manned helicopter on the scene within 15 to 30 minutes. Resuscitation can be begun in the helicopter, and the neurosurgeon can expect to be close to the scene in time if not in actual distance. This should help minimize secondary hypoxic damage after injury and limit the number of untreated cases of acutely increased intracranial pressure; if the Vietnam experience holds true, most patients will be conscious when they arrive.

It can reasonably be anticipated that a CT scan will be available wherever the neurosurgeon operates. Ideally, a senior neurosurgeon would review the scan and be responsible for triage decisions in mass casualty situations. This arrangement proved quite satisfactory in Haifa, where the senior neurosurgeon was available to the emergency room and could accompany a patient to the CT scanner. Although it would be preferable to have at least two neurosurgeons at every location where neurosurgery is to be performed, a partially trained neurosurgeon or even a general surgeon could be called on to assist a single, fully qualified neurosurgeon working alone.

Patients can be moved as soon as they are stable according to the ordinary neurosurgical criteria. It may be necessary to relax these criteria under certain mass casualty conditions. If necessary, patients can be transferred intubated or under anesthesia.

SUMMARY

Compared with matched controls in the VHIS, patients with penetrating injuries have proved that there are no silent areas of the brain. Regardless of how well patients seem to recover, very complex psychobehavioral and cognitive functions are adversely affected, and community adjustment is never perfect. We would now emphasize the importance of preserving whatever brain tissue can be saved. With modern imaging techniques and dependable follow-up after an initially adequate debridement, multiple operations to achieve a ''perfect'' debridement of penetrating missile tracks are no longer routinely called for.

REFERENCES

1. Cushing H: A study of a series of wounds involving the brain and its enveloping structures. Br J Surg 6:558, 1918
2. Meirowsky AM (ed): Neurological Surgery of Trauma. Washington, DC, Office of the Surgeon General, 1964
3. Matson DD: The Treatment of Acute Craniocerebral Injuries due to Missiles. Springfield, Ill, Charles C. Thomas, 1948
4. British Journal of Surgery, 1947: War Surgery Supplement.
5. Lewin W, Gibon MR: Missile head wounds in the Korean campaign: A survey of British casualties. Br J Surg 43:628, 1956
6. Byrnes DP, Crockard HA, Gordon DS, et al: Penetrating craniocerebral missile injuries in the civil disturbances in Northern Ireland. Br J Surg 61:169, 1971
7. Meyers FW, Salazar AM: Vietnam Head Injury Study: Combat-caused penetrating head wounds—assessment 14 years after injury. Presented in part Sunday, April 27, 1986, Course No. 104, Annual Meeting the American Academy of Neurology (manuscript in preparation)
8. Demuth WE Jr: Bullet velocity as applied to military rifle wounding capacity. J Trauma 9:27, 1969
9. Demuth WE Jr: Bullet velocity and design as determinants of wounding capability. An experimental study. J Trauma 6:222, 1966
10. Dobbyn RC, Bruckly WL Jr, Shubin LD: An Evaluation of Police Handgun Ammunition: Summary report. Washington DC, U.S. Department of Justice, 1975
11. Dodge FR, Meirowsky AM: Tangential wounds of the scalp and skull. J Neurosurg 9:472, 1952
12. Adelola A, Odehu EL: A syndrome characteristic of tangential bullet wounds of the vertex of the skull. J Neurosurg 34:155, 1971
13. Harvey EW, Butler EG, McMillen JH, et al:. Mechanisms of wounding. War Med 8:91, 1945
14. Kirpatrick JB, DiMaio VD: Civilian gunshot wounds of the brain. J Neurosurg 49:185, 1978
15. Meirowsky AM: Secondary removal of retained bone fragments in missile wounds of the brain. J Neurosurg 57:617, 1982
16. Hammon WM: Retained intracranial bone fragments: Analysis of 42 patients. J Neurosurg 34:142, 1971
17. Freytag E: Autopsy findings in head injuries from firearms: Statistical evaluation of 254 cases. Arch Pathol 76:215, 1963
18. Raimondi AS, Samuelson GM: Craniocerebral gunshot wounds in civilian practice. J Neurosurg 32:647, 1970
19. Crockard HA: Bullet injuries of the brain. Ann R Coll Surg Engl 55:111, 1974
20. Barnett JC, Meirowsky AM: Intracranial hematoma associated with penetrating wounds of the brain. J Neurosurg 12:34, 1955
21. Matson DD, Wolkin J: Hematoma associated with penetrating wounds of the brain. J Neurosurg 3:46, 1946
22. Carey ME, Young H, Mathis JL, et al: A bacteriological study of craniocerebral missile wounds from Vietnam. J Neurosurg 34:145, 1971
23. Hagan RE: Early complications following penetrating wounds of the brain. J Neurosurg 34:127, 1971
24. Young B, Rapp R, Norton A: Failure of prophylactically administered phenytoin to prevent early posttraumatic seizures. J Neurosurg 58:231, 1983
25. Webster JE, Schneider RC, Loftram JE: Observations on early types of brain abscess following penetrating wounds of the brain. J Neurosurg 3:7, 1946
26. Ecker AD: A bacteriologic study of penetrating wounds of the brain from a surgical point of view. J Neurosurg 3:1, 1946
27. Crockard HA: Early intracranial pressure studies in gunshot wounds of the brain. J Trauma 15:339, 1975
28. Morin MA, Pitts FW: Delayed apoplexy following head injury (''traumatische Spaet-Apoplexie''). J Neurosurg 33:542, 1970
29. Carey ME, Tutton RM, Strub RL, et al: The correlation between surgical and CT estimates of brain damage following missile wounds. J Neurosurg 60:947, 1984
30. Rappaport ZH, Sahar A, Shaked I, et al: Computerized tomogra-

phy in combat-related craniocerebral penetrating missile injuries. Israel J Med Sci 20:668, 1984

31. Meyers FW, Salazar AM, Dillon JD, et al: The significance of retained intracranial bone fragments in penetrating combat head wounds. A preliminary report from the Vietnam Head Injury Study. Abstract presented at American Congress of Neurosurgeons, Chicago, November, 1983

32. Feinsod M: The Israeli experience with penetrating missile injuries in Lebanon. Presented to the Army-Navy Neurosurgical Conference, Walter Reed Army Medical Center, October, 1985

33. Caveness WF, Meirowsky AM, Rish BL, et al: The nature of posttraumatic epilepsy. J Neurosurg 50:545, 1979

34. Weiss GH, Feeney DM, Caveness WF, et al: Prognostic factors for the occurrence of posttraumatic epilepsy. Arch Neurol 40:7, 1983

35. Meirowsky AM: Wounds of the dural sinuses. J Neurosurg 10:496, 1953

36. Hammon WM: Missile wounds, in Vinken PJ, Bruyn GW, Braakman R (eds): Handbook of Clinical Neurology, vol

23. Part I: Injuries of the Brain and Skull. New York, American Elsevier, 1975, pp 505–526

The Management of Cerebrospinal Fluid Leaks

T. Forcht Dagi   Eugene D. George

CEREBROSPINAL FLUID FISTULA is a serious and potentially fatal condition, the successful management of which requires a fundamental understanding of the anatomy and pathophysiology of the problem. The evolution of the current operative approaches is best understood from an historical perspective.

HISTORICAL OVERVIEW

The correlation of posttraumatic rhinorrhea with leakage of cerebrospinal fluid (CSF) was initially suggested in the 17th century by a Dutch surgeon, Bidloo the Elder.[1,2] Cases in which nontraumatic CSF rhinorrhea resulted from increased intracranial pressure were then reported by Miller, in 1826,[3] and King, in 1834.[4] The full significance of CSF fistulas was not appreciated, however, until Chiari[5], in 1884, demonstrated a fistula connecting a pneumatocele in the frontal lobes with the ethmoid sinuses in a patient who died of meningitis following rhinorrhea. The introduction of roentgenography enabled the diagnosis of a fistula to be made in vivo through the detection of intracranial air,* ultimately leading to the development of pneumoencephalography as a diagnostic procedure,[7] and, less directly, to the refinement of surgical techniques for the repair of CSF fistulas.[8,9]

Despite a number of early attempts, successful repair was not consistently achieved until the mid 1930s. In 1937, Cairns published a report on a series of cases demonstrating that CSF leaks could be controlled by the extradural application of fascia lata.[10] The need for such intervention was not, however, universally acknowledged. World War II heightened interest in

this problem. By 1944, Dandy advocated surgical repair of any CSF leak within 2 weeks of onset in order to prevent meningitis.[11] Lewin's review of the British combat wound experience and of a large series of basilar skull fractures[12,13] strongly influenced the adoption of aggressive operative management as the standard of care. The cessation of a leak, he argued, did not eliminate the risk of meningitis. By the mid 1950s it became virtually axiomatic to operate on all CSF fistulas that did not close within several days.

There has never been a real consensus regarding what operative route is most successful. The extradural repair described by Cairns and Dandy was initially abandoned by neurosurgeons in favor of an intradural approach.[14] The extradural technique has recently enjoyed a resurgence of respect in both otolaryngologic and neurosurgical circles.[15–17]

Over the past 15 years the practice of early repair of all CSF fistulas without exception has come under increasing criticism. Three observations have been more or less responsible for this change:

1. Some fistulas seem to heal spontaneously with time, especially if external CSF drainage is used as an adjunctive maneuver.
2. A recurrence rate of 6 to 25 percent and operative morbidity and mortality of serious proportions have been recorded.
3. The incidence and severity of meningitis in otherwise uncomplicated CSF leaks can be diminished by treatment with antibiotics.[2,1826]

CONVENTIONS AND DEFINITIONS

The term *rhinorrhea* is used to describe fluid dripping from the nose, while the term *otorrhea* is used to describe fluid dripping from the ear. It must be understood that these terms reflect the site of the drip rather than the site of the leak. Cerebrospinal fluid leaking through a fracture in the temporal bone, for example, can easily reach the nasopharynx through the eustachian tube and mimic a leak through the cribriform plate. There is no specific term to describe leaks from the spinal subarachnoid space.

Transcranial CSF leaks fall into two major categories: *traumatic* leaks, and so-called *spontaneous* or *nontraumatic* leaks. The traumatic group has two subsets: acute or early leaks that appear within 1 week of injury, and delayed leaks that

---

The views presented in this chapter are the personal opinions of the authors alone, and must not be construed as representing the position of the Department of Defense or the Department of the Army.

*" . . . a middle-aged man was admitted with a head injury. . . . He was x-rayed by Dr. W. H. Stewart, who detected a fracture in the posterior wall of the frontal sinus. The patient was treated conservatively and discharged . . . but returned some three weeks later having suffered a relapse. On December 14, [1912], a further radiographic examination of the skull was undertaken. . . . These x-rays showed the ventricles enormously dilated by what was probably air or gas. As a result of these findings Dr. Luckett operated and during the course of the operation tapped one of the ventricles and noticed that air or gas was released. The patient died three days later and at autopsy the fracture in the posterior wall of the frontal sinus was confirmed and part of the bone was found to be depressed about one centimeter."[6]

OPERATIVE NEUROSURGICAL TECHNIQUES
ISBN 0-8089-1862-1

occur months and even years later. The nontraumatic group also contains several subsets, including those associated with intracranial mass lesions, with congenital defects of the skull base, with osteomyelitis and other causes of bony erosion, with focal cerebral atrophy,[4] and with an ill-defined group of acquired cerebral hernias, meningoceles, and myelomeningoceles perforating pneumatized bone in the anteromedial middle fossa.[27] Nontraumatic fistulas are further divided into high-pressure and low-pressure groups[4,28]; there is ample evidence to extrapolate this distinction to the traumatic group as well.[22] Iatrogenic or postoperative leaks are usually included in the category of traumatic fistulas.

In general, spinal CSF leaks are classified similarly. Most spinal CSF leaks are postoperative and therefore traumatic. A number of very rare congenital anomalies can give rise to meningopleural or meningoperitoneal fistulas. The distinction between high-pressure and low-pressure fistulas is particularly important in the management of spinal leaks. In children with spinal dysraphism or other anomalies, the leak may be the first expression of hydrocephalus.

ETIOLOGY AND EPIDEMIOLOGY

TRAUMATIC LEAKS

The most common cause of CSF leaks is head trauma, particularly basilar skull fracture.[29] In Lewin's series of 100 patients with head injury, 7 percent had basal skull fractures and 2 percent had CSF leaks.[12] A CSF leak was detected in 2.8 percent of 1250 head injuries and 11.5 percent of the basilar fractures studied by Brawley.[14] In another study of 1077 skull fractures, including a particularly large proportion of high-speed highway traffic accidents, 20.8 percent of 168 patients with basilar skull fractures had an acute CSF leak.[30] The incidence in cases of penetrating missile injuries is comparable: in 1133 cases, 101 (8.9 percent) developed a CSF fistula. The proportion was higher with transventricular penetration.[31] Thus, CSF leaks occur in approximately 3 percent of all head injuries, 9 percent of high energy penetrating injuries, and between 12 and 30 percent of basilar skull fractures, depending on the accelerative forces involved.

In children, however, CSF leaks are seen in 1 percent or less of closed head injuries.[32] This disparity may be the result of differences in fragility between adult and pediatric skulls, and also the lack of development of the air sinuses in children.*

SPONTANEOUS LEAKS

The term *spontaneous leak* is a 19th century misnomer, but remains in common use. Nontraumatic leaks have been reported in small series, but not in sufficient number or detail to allow any real estimate of incidence.[26] Anecdotally, pituitary tumors are the most common cause of CSF leaks accompanying intracranial mass lesions. Because of the structures eroded by

---

*As a rule, the frontal sinuses become visible between the 4th and 12th year, and are always detected by age 15 years. They are often assymetric until age 20 years. The ethmoids are present at birth, enlarge by age 3, and are fully formed by age 16 or 17. The cavity of the sphenoid sinus is usually recognizable by age 4, and fully developed by puberty. In the pediatric age range, the interpretation of sinus x-rays is often difficult because of small size, variations in development, and because of normal opacification and clouding.[32]

sellar masses, such leaks generally make their presence known as rhinorrhea.[28,33] Other presentations, including a serous otitis media, have been reported.[34]

POSTOPERATIVE LEAKS

Before the modern era of neurosurgery, subgaleal collections of CSF, representing altered preoperative CSF flow characteristics or unrecognized or untreated hydrocephalus, were common. These often leaked through the incision and represented one of the most common neurosurgical complications. Increased awareness of altered CSF dynamics and hydrocephalus as well as CT scanning have combined to diminish the magnitude of this problem in recent years. On the other hand, more radical approaches to surgery of the base of skull, including cerebellopontine angle lesions and tumors straddling the nasopharynx and anterior and middle fossa, have created problems of a different sort. The true incidence of incisional CSF leaks is difficult to estimate because the requisite figures are not published. After transfrontal surgery, the most common cause is failure to seal an opened frontal sinus. Rhinorrhea and otorrhea after cerebellopontine angle tumor resection are recorded in 2 to 22 percent of patients in large series.[35] The incidence has been reduced by waxing and plugging mastoid air cells as they are opened and placing a graft of adipose tissue in the opened porus acusticus.[36,37] Rhinorrhea in this setting is a false localizing sign. In the transsphenoidal approach to the pituitary, leaks occur in 1.4 to 6.4 percent of patients.[35,38,39]

PNEUMOCEPHALUS

The presence of intracranial air, a pathognomonic sign of CSF fistula after trauma or spontaneous rhinorrhea but not after surgery, is demonstrable in approximately 20 percent of patients with CSF leaks.[40] Pneumocephalus is posttraumatic in 75 percent and spontaneous or otherwise unexplained in 10 percent.[41]

MENINGITIS

Meningitis occurs in approximately 20 percent of acute posttraumatic leaks and 57 percent of delayed posttraumatic leaks.[29] These figures may vary somewhat in different series. Nevertheless, meningitis always appears more frequently in the delayed posttraumatic group. The incidence of meningitis in nontraumatic CSF leaks has not been well documented. Anecdotally, intermittent leakage is more likely to result in meningitis than copious continuous leakage of the high-pressure type.[28] The overall risk of meningitis from traumatic CSF leaks of all types is on the order of 25 percent.[13,42–45] In postoperative leaks, the incidence of meningitis has been calculated to be on the order of 20 percent, but the validity of this figure is diminished by the difficulty of distinguishing aseptic from bacterial meningitis as well as by factors that might precipitate both the leak and the meningitis through some common mechanism.

DEFINING AND LOCALIZING A FISTULA

The management of CSF leaks involves three steps: (1) proving that the fluid is really CSF; (2) delineating the site of the fistula; and (3) defining its mechanism.

CLINICAL EVIDENCE

Glucose

The presence of glucose has served historically to differentiate CSF from nasal secretions and serosanguinous drainage. The concentration of glucose in CSF equals or exceeds 50 percent of the serum concentration except during meningitis, after subarachnoid hemorrhage, or in other unusual circumstances. The glucose concentration in nasal secretions, in contrast, is 1O mg/100 ml or less.[46] Quantitative measurements of the glucose concentration are therefore differentially diagnostic. Qualitative spot tests (Clinistix, Dextrostix, Uristix, or Tes-Tape), in contrast, are *not* definitive for two reasons: (1) the glucose oxidase test on which they are based is too sensitive, turning positive at values under 2O mg/lOO ml of glucose; and (2) normal nasopharyngeal secretions will elicit falsely positive reactions even in the absence of glucose.[47,48] A negative glucose oxidase reaction effectively eliminates the possibility of CSF rhinorrhea.

Reservoir Sign

It is widely held that true CSF leaks will produce quantities of fluid sufficient for collection and quantitative analysis at some time in their course. The reservoir sign, that is, the abllity of a patient to voluntarily produce CSF at will by correct positioning of the head, is generally taken to be quite specific for a fistula with pooling in the sphenoid sinus.[27] Although Dandy[11] believed that this sign would differentiate leakage through the frontal sinus from ethmoidal and sphenoidal leaks, it is not reliably localizing.

Target Sign

The target sign refers to the differential, pseudochromatographic diffusion of CSF admixed with blood or other serosanguinous fluid on filter paper or bedclothes. Cerebrospinal fluid will migrate further, creating a bull's-eye stain with blood in the center. This is a convenient sign, but it can be deceiving, for whenever watery nasal secretions and blood are mixed, the same phenomenon is likely to occur.

Headache

Cerebrospinal fluid leaks can be accompanied by high-pressure or low-pressure headaches. Intermittent high-pressure leaks are characterized by *high* CSF pressure headaches that are relieved by the sudden discharge of fluid and build up again over time. Normal pressure leaks, in contrast, are characterized by postural *low* CSF pressure headaches, which are relieved by reclining or otherwise allowing pressure in the subarachnoid space to rise to normal levels.

Other Confirmatory Evidence

The finding of unusually *low opening pressure* in the lumbar subarachnoid space is corroborating evidence of a CSF leak. Unilateral or bilateral *anosmia* is associated with defects or leaks in the region of the cribriform plate and the fovea ethmoidalis. Olfaction may be preserved, however, in cases of spontaneous CSF rhinorrhea with congenital defects of the cribriform fossa.[28,42] *Optic nerve* lesions point to the tuberculum sella, the sphenoid sinus, and the posterior ethmoids. Impaired *vestibular function, facial nerve palsy,* and *cochlear damage* accompany fractures in the temporal bone.

IMAGING TECHNIQUES

Imaging techniques are used to detect intracranial air, fractures and defects in the skull base, mass lesions, and hydrocephalus, and to demonstrate flow through the fistula.[49] Plain films, multiplanar tomograms, computed tomographic (CT) scans, and magnetic resonance images (MRI) are obtained to delineate the anatomy and pathologic state of the skull base, sinuses, and calvarium. Stains, contrast agents, and radioactive tracers are injected into the ventricular or lumbar subarachnoid space to prove that leaking fluid is CSF and to show directly or by inference the location of the leak. Radiographic data must be interpreted in accordance with clinical information. As a general rule, *positive* data obtained from radiography studies is helpful, but *negative* data is often uninterpretable.

Plain Roentgenography and Computed Tomography

Plain films and CT scans are examined for evidence of fracture; air/fluid levels in the frontal, ethmoidal, and sphenoid sinuses; intracranial air; chronic increased intracranial pressure; erosion of bone by tumor or infection; congenital anomalies; and penetrating objects. Although multiplanar tomography provides exquisite detail of bony anatomy, it has been supplanted in most centers by high accuracy computed tompography with overlapping 2-mm cuts.[50] Contrast-enhanced cisternography in conjunction with CT scanning provides dynamic information about flow patterns of CSF.[51] Magnetic resonance imaging also provides superb detail of pathologic conditions of the soft tissue at the skull base and in the nasopharynx.

Tracers

The ultimate proof of a CSF fistula is the ability to retrieve extracranially a tracer substance injected into the CSF. Historically, the subtances injected into the CSF have included methylene blue, phenolsulfonphthalein, indigo carmine, and fluorescein.[52,53] Only *indigo carmine* and *fluorescein* remain in use; the others have proved toxic.[4]

In the presence of an active leak, cotton pledgets placed along the anterior roof of the nose, the posterior roof and the sphenoethmoid recess, the middle meatus, and below the posterior end of the inferior turbinate, can be used to confirm a leak and, when differentially stained or contaminated by radioactive isotopes, to infer the location.[26] The following procedure is used to trace with fluorescein:

1. A spinal tap is performed.
2. About 10 ml of spinal fluid is withdrawn after the opening pressure is measured.
3. The fluid is mixed with 0.5 ml of 5 percent fluorescein.
4. The mixture is slowly reinjected intrathecally.
5. The patient assumes a recumbent position for about 30 minutes, depending on the size of the leak.
6. The pledgets are removed and and examined under ultraviolet illumination. The interpretation of findings is given in Table 7-1.

In the presence of an active leak, tracer methods are sensitive and reasonably specific. With slow, low volume, or intermittent leaks, the test may produce falsely negative results. There is some controversy regarding the use of fluorescein intrathecally because transverse myelitis and other serious reactions have been reported.[54]

Indigo carmine is the tracer stain preferred by most

Table 7-1. Intrepretation of nasal pledget stains in locating cerebrospinal fluid fistulas

Location of Stain*	Probable Site of Fistula
Anterior nasal	Cribriform plate or anterior ethmoidal roof
Posterior nasal, Sphenoethmoidal	Posterior ethmoid or sphenoid sinus
Middle meatus	Frontal sinus
Below posterior end of inferior turbinate	Eustachian tube (middle fossa)

*Staining behind the tympanic membrane indicates a leak into the middle ear.

neurosurgeons. Indigo carmine is more visible than fluorescein to the unaided eye. This characteristic makes it useful in checking for the presence of CSF fistulas intraoperatively.[27]

Since it is easier to detect minute amounts of radioactivity than to distinguish faint color on plegets stained by bloody fluid or mucus, radioactive tracers are more sensitive than stains. Iodine 131 (RISA) was widely used for cisternography until quite recently; it has been replaced by Indium 111 DTPA, which is an isobaric tracer that combines improved physical properties, fewer adverse reactions, better imaging quality, and a shorter half life (2.8 days). Ytterbium (^{169}Yb DTPA) and Technetium (^{99m}Tc albumin) have also been approved for CSF imaging but suffer from inferior imaging characteristics and from excessively long (32 days) and short (6 hours) half-lives, respectively. Isotope cisternography is excellent for proving the existence of a CSF leak, but is inaccurate in localization; an active leak of any magnitude will quickly oversaturate the pledgets and surrounding tissues, making differential determination impossible.[29,55,56]

Active leaks will contaminate accurately placed pledgets within 30 minutes to 2 hours. Slow or intermittent leaks can be detected by leaving the pledgets in place or replacing them continuously over 6 to 48 hours. Careful interpretation is necessary over the extended time span: the isotope can be absorbed into the bloodstream from the CSF and undergo secondary secretion into the nasopharynx, resulting in a falsely positive test.[57] This alternate pathway for entry of the isotope into nasopharyngeal secretions was first recognized experimentally in normal dogs; whether this constitutes active transport from the CSF, passage via the olfactory nerves, or passive lymphatic drainage has yet to be fully understood.[58] In any event, the same phenomenon has been documented in normal human volunteers. Low level radioactivity in pledgets exposed to the nasal mucosa over many hours can therefore easily represent spurious contamination. The accuracy of faintly positive tests can be confirmed by calculating a radioactivity index ratio, a comparison of the radioactivity (RI) in counts per minute of an exposed pledget with that of 1 ml of blood:

$$\text{RI Ratio} = (^{RI}\text{pledget})/(^{RI}\text{1 ml blood})$$

A RI ratio of less than 0.3 is normal. Canine studies suggest that the ratio in the presence of a leak is at least five times greater.* The significance of tracer substances appearing in low concentrations more than 5 hours after injection thus should be very carefully evaluated.

It has been suggested that tracer injected into the cervical

subarachnoid cistern can be forced through a slow, intermittent, or low-pressure leak by raising the CSF pressure with saline or artificial CSF delivered via a constant infusion pump.[59] Delayed scans carried out 24 and 48 hours after injection of isotopes can help define the mechanism of a leak by detecting defects in CSF absorption and circulation.

Contrast

Early attempts at demonstrating CSF leaks by injecting air or Pantopaque into the subarachnoid space failed to produce consistently satisfactory images. The combination of CT and metrizamide cisternography, however, has yielded excellent visualization of *active* leaks. Smaller fistulas have been demonstrated by having the patient cough or perform a Valsalva's maneuver.[29] For maximal contrast, cisternal injections can be performed via punctures at C1-2. Overlapping views in both the coronal and axial planes are required.[50] Direct coronal studies are preferable to reconstructed images. The risk of provoking seizures and aseptic or chemical meningitis with metrizamide cisternography should be kept in mind.

Immunologic Methods

Irjala et al. described the use of an immunofixation technique for the identification of microaliquots (100 μ l) of CSF by demonstrating two electrophoretically characteristic bands of transferrin.[60] The β_1 fraction consists of normal transferrin and sometimes two variant fractions. The β_2 fraction characteristic of CSF contains smaller amounts of neuraminic acid. This method is not subject to contamination from other body fluids (tears, nasal secretions). The immunofixation method could theoretically be used for localization of the leak by differential suction techniques in the nasopharynx, but large scale clinical trials of this method have yet to be reported.

ANATOMIC CONSIDERATIONS: SITES OF LEAKAGE

TRAUMA

A CSF leak can occur wherever the dura is lacerated during an injury. It is more likely to persist or recur rather than close spontaneously where a meningeal hiatus is maintained by bony spicules, by dura entrapped in the edges of a fracture, or by herniating brain and leptomeninges. Avulsion of the olfactory fibrils can cause a dural fistula through the cribriform plate even without a fracture. Posttraumatic fistulas are frequently complex and multiple.

SPONTANEOUS LEAKS

Nontraumatic leaks are usually confined to one region where an anatomic defect is demonstrable. It is usually easier to demonstrate the defect than the leak. High-pressure leaks that

---

*In the canine model the RI ratio of nasal activity to CSF is 1:14 two to five hours after cisternal injection of radioisotope. The RI ratio of nasal activity to blood is 1:2–3, two to five hours after intravenous injection of radioisotope. The RI ratio of CSF to blood thus is 4.6–7.0.

act as "safety valves" for hydrocephalus occur where the skull is thinnest, usually the cribriform fossa and the sellar region. This is the case, for example, in Crouzon's disease and osteopetrosis (Albers-Schönberg disease).

The middle fossa can be the site of CSF leaks that are direct in the sense that they do not cross the inner ear. Such fistulas have been described mainly in conjunction with a pneumatized temporal fossa. Pulsatile CSF forces induce additional thinning of the bone and enlargement of pits and small bony defects that are normally present. The leptomeninges and brain herniate, thinning the dura and leading to rupture of the arachnoid. The leak can be constant or intermittent, depending on several factors including the underlying intracranial pressure; whether an arachnoid diverticulum is created; and whether brain tissue temporarily obliterates the leak. A similar sequence of events has been postulated to explain CSF leaks in the empty sella syndrome[27] and in focal atrophy.[28]

Indirect fistulas through the temporal bone are the most elusive. In *extralabyrinthine fistulas* the defect occurs in the middle fossa, in the region of the tegmen tympani. In *intralabyrinthine fistulas*, CSF escapes into the labyrinth through the subarachnoid space of the posterior fossa. In either case, the leak can appear as otorrhea, or, when the tympanic membrane is intact, as rhinorrhea.[40] The possibility of temporal bone dysplasia should be investigated whenever a patient with severe hearing loss develops unexplained or recurrent meningitis.[27,29,61] In the Mondini malformation, for example (unreactive ear with a shortened cochlear coil, dilated semicircular canal system, and widened inner ear vestibule), it is hypothesized that a widened, patent cochlear aqueduct allows CSF to pass from the subarachnoid space to the inner ear via a leak in the oval window. Other proposed routes include defects of the scala tympani, the footplate of the stapes, or the thin bony plate separating the internal auditory canal and the inner ear vestibule that is perforated by nerve fibers innervating the utricular and saccular macula.[61–64]

HIGH-PRESSURE VERSUS LOW-PRESSURE LEAKS

When a CSF leak is the expression of increased intracranial pressure from a mass effect or hydrocephalus, the underlying cause must be treated before the leak can be effectively repaired. The existence of increased intracranial pressure can be extrapolated from several sources. Skull films and CT scans disclose signs of pressure, mass effect, and tumors. Radiographic signs suggestive of defective circulation and absorption of CSF include periventricular lucencies, enlarged temporal horns, a disproportionately plump third ventricle narrowed at the massa intermedia, and an empty sella. Extracerebral collections of CSF can represent the so-called fifth ventricle phenomenon. Other concomitants of high-pressure leakage include papilledema and optic atrophy; pallor of the optic disc; enlarged central scotoma or subtle binasal visual field cuts; a history of headaches worse in the morning or while recumbent, and relieved by a gush of fluid; variable or intermittent diplopia; intermittent clonus or pyramidal tract signs that reverse spontaneously after leakage; and a history of granulomatous meningitis, subarachnoid hemorrhage, head trauma, or some other event that might adversely effect the circulation of CSF.

Infants with incisional leaks after fresh meningomyelocele repair can be assumed to have hydrocephalus, especially if there is an accompanying Arnold-Chiari malformation. In contrast to other cases of postoperative leak, where the temporizing maneuvers discussed below are frequently effective, CSF shunting will generally be required.

INITIAL MANAGEMENT

The initial management of CSF leaks is intended to slow or stop the leak and prevent meningitis. Usually, both these ends can be achieved simultaneously.

ANTIBIOTICS

Antibiotics have not proved effective in changing the incidence of meningitis in posttraumatic or postoperative CSF leaks. In traumatic leaks, they are no longer prescribed routinely.[14–16,18,30,65] For postoperative leaks, however, prophylactic antibiotics are commonly if not universally employed. There is some theoretical justification for distinguishing between the two situations. Whenever antibiotics are administered, several principles should be kept in mind.[66]

1. Patients should not be kept on antibiotics indefinitely in the hope that a leak will seal: a trial of conservative therapy is reasonable, but the endpoint should be decided a priori.
2. Wide-spectrum antibiotics are not desirable for prophylaxis: the most specific antibiotic capable of eliminating the potential pathogens should be used.
3. Patients of different ages and in different locations harbor different vulnerabilities because of changes in nasopharyngeal and environmental flora: thus *Hemophilus influenzae* is a very common cause of meningitis in children and in elderly persons, while *Diplococcus* is more common in healthy adults.
4. Patients can develop meningitis even while on prophylactic antibiotics: after the usual investigations are carried out, the antibiotics are changed to cover the appropriate organisms and sensitivities.
5. Bacteriocidal antibiotics are should be chosen whenever possible.

INTENSIVE CARE

The admission of patients with CSF leaks to intensive care was universally advocated in the older literature. This certainly may be warranted in some cases of trauma or spontaneous high-pressure leaks, but it is not always needed for recurrent or postoperative leaks. A great deal depends on the nursing and housestaff coverage in a given institution and other aspects of nursing policy. One consideration to keep in mind is that opportunistic infections arising in intensive care units are usually caused by resistant organisms and are often highly recalcitrant to treatment with the usual antibiotics.

POSITION

The head-up position reduces intracranial CSF pressure and raises the pressure in the spinal theca. For this reason, patients with cranial leaks should be nursed upright or at 45 degrees. Patients with a spinal leak should be kept flat.

EXTERNAL DRAINAGE OF CEREBROSPINAL FLUID

External drainage of CSF has been used in various forms for many years. External ventricular drainage[67,68] has been replaced in most centers by continuous lumbar drainage, which was first described in 1963.[23] Since then, lumbar drainage has proved useful in controlling and sometimes in curing CSF leaks of every etiology.[20–22] McCoy provided theoretical justification for the initial management of CSF fistulas with CSF diversion by demonstrating that granulation can seal the fistulas providing the leakage has stopped.[69] Lumbar drainage therefore should be considered whenever positioning alone does not eliminate or at least significantly diminish a leak within 24 hours.

TECHNIQUE

A 19-gauge Portex, Teflon, or polyethylene catheter is threaded percutaneously through a 17-gauge Touhy needle inserted into the lumbar subarachnoid space between L4-5 and L2-3. Aside from increased attention to sterile technique, there is no difference from a standard lumbar puncture procedure. After 10 to 20 cm of catheter has been threaded rostrally, the needle is removed over the catheter. If there is any significant resistance to passage, the needle and the catheter should be removed as a unit. Under no circumstances should the catheter be withdrawn through the needle once the tip has protruded: the needle tip may shear the catheter, leaving the tip irretrievably lost in the subarachnoid space or the subcutaneous tissue. The proximal end of the catheter is connected, via the appropriate adaptors, to a closed sterile drainage system. Prepackaged kits for epidural anesthesia generally provide all the necessary catheters, needles, and fittings. Several complete drainage systems have been marketed commercially. In their absence, a blood transfer pack connected to the catheter with intravenous tubing can be used for collection. Antibiotic ointment can be placed at the skin entry site. A waterproof occlusive dressing should be applied with the catheter coiled and taped to relieve strain and prevent disconnection.

PREVENTION OF INFECTION

The infection rate with indwelling catheters can be prohibitive, ranging in some series to 10 percent or more.[70] The risk is lower with lumbar catheters.[23] Infection can be controlled by prophylactic antibiotics, which are potentially capable of reducing infection by two thirds,[70] and by externalization of the catheter through an extended subcutaneous tunnel.[71] *Staphylococcus* species and other skin flora are the major threat: antibiotics should be chosen to reflect the sensitivities of local pathogens. Prophylaxis is continued for 8 to 24 hours after the catheter is withdrawn. Daily samples of CSF are obtained. The CSF is cultured and examined with Gram's stain. A separate sample is sent for cell count and differential and for sugar and protein analysis. The presence of a catheter does not of its own accord lower the CSF sugar level or evoke a major leukocytotic reaction; the cell count and sugar concentration remain quite stable in uninfected CSF over 4 to 9 days. Any persisting variation of 2 standard deviations or more from the cumulative average cell count and sugar concentration over several days is cause for concern and requires careful re-examination of the CSF for signs of opportunistic infection.[72]

External drainage has been maintained in large series for up to 10 days without infection. Longer periods have been reported in exceptional cases.[21] By analogy with central venous access lines, it may be wise to change catheters if drainage is continued beyond 7 days.

LENGTH OF DRAINAGE

Drainage should be continued for 3 to 5 days after the leak has stopped in order to allow healing. If the leak recurs, operative repair is indicated. If the underlying problem is increased intracranial pressure or hydrocephalus, implantation of a drain will act purely as a temporizing maneuver: no "cure" will be effected. Similarly, a patient whose leak is not controlled by external drainage should be considered for early operation. In Findler's series of 50 patients,[22] drainage of between 350 and 420 ml daily was continued for an average of 10 days, with a leak recurrence rate of 14 percent. There was an additional 8 percent incidence of delayed leak at the site of lumbar puncture.

As a rule, acute posttraumatic and postoperative normal pressure leaks will respond to external drainage. Transitory high-pressure leaks will also respond, so long as the pressure elevation recedes over the duration of the drainage. Delayed and recurring leaks cannot be definitively managed by drainage.

PHARMACOLOGIC ADJUVANTS

Pharmacologic agents such as Diamox (acetazolamide), which retards the production of CSF, can be helpful in reducing CSF pressure after the drain has been removed. They are not effective as a primary mode of therapy.

COMPLICATIONS

Very high CSF protein concentrations predispose a patient against a successful drainage. If for technical reasons patency of the drainage catheter cannot be maintained, the same effect can be achieved with repetitive lumbar punctures through a large needle.

Calcaterra recorded one case of fatal postoperative suboccipital hemorrhage in an elderly patient that was attributed to overdrainage of CSF.[17] Similar complications have followed spinal anesthesia.[73–75] Overdrainage of CSF can also cause life-threatening pneumocephalus.[42,76–78] The CSF pressure should be lowered substantially, but not reduced below zero. The acute reduction of CSF pressure can also precipitate headache, nausea and vomiting. This can be prevented, according to Findler, by gradually lowering the pressure and increasing the drainage incrementally over several days.[22] An accidental siphon effect can be avoided by adjusting the height of the drainage valve or the drainage bag to the level of the ventricular system rather than to the level of the bed. In this way, the pressure column remains constant as the bed is raised and lowered or as the patient is moved. Most commercial systems incorporate a micropore-filtered air port to prevent siphonage. Improvised systems are generally unable to include such a port, however, and positioning becomes critical.

There has been longstanding concern regarding the possibility of inducing meningitis by retrograde migration of bacteria into an open fistula under the influence of negative CSF pressure induced by an external drain.[4] This has not occurred in practice, however, and seems avoidable by maintaining a low but constant positive pressure in the CSF.

Catheters should not be forcibly removed. A catheter that

resists withdrawal should probably be removed in the operating room under direct vision. As the catheter is removed, the tip should be examined to ensure that no part of it has been left behind. An unused catheter should be available for comparison because the indwelling catheter can be distorted or elongated during withdrawal.

If the catheter is not intact, an effort should be made to locate and identify the retained segment. Although most catheters are intended to be radiopaque, they are easily missed on plain x-ray films and are better visualized on CT scans. There are two indications for retrieval of a broken catheter tip: infection, or radicular pain or paresis when the tubing can be shown to have lodged around the appropriate root. In the vast majority of cases, the retained fragment can be safely ignored.

Dural cutaneous fistulas can occur at the site of catheter insertion, particularly in the setting of a high-pressure leak. Most such fistulas will stop spontaneously or seal with a single stitch. Low-pressure or normal-pressure leaks can also be sealed by an injection of 10–20 ml of autologous blood as an epidural blood patch. This technique is favored by anesthetists and obstetricians for the treatment of low-pressure "spinal" headaches. It has been shown by a number of studies to improve the natural history of "spinal headaches"[79–83] with a success rate of 93 percent.[84] It should be noted, however, that epidural blood patching has resulted in symptomatic mass effect, hemorrhagic complications,[85] and infection. Surgical repair of the dura may still be needed. External lumbar drainage is obviously contraindicated in posterior fossa masses.

OPERATIVE MANAGEMENT

TIMING OF SURGERY

There is a continuing debate regarding the timing of surgery. The debate centers primarily on three considerations: (1) most CSF leaks stop spontaneously and do not recur; (2) surgery is neither universally successful nor without hazard; and (3) modern antibiotics have significantly reduced the morbidity from any infection that may develop while waiting for the leak to stop or that may ensue should the leak recur.

There are some leaks that should always be given the opportunity to stop spontaneously. Most acute posttraumatic leaks will stop within 10 days of injury: in Mincy's series of 54 cases of rhinorrhea in frontal fossa injury, 35 percent stopped within 24 hours, 68 percent within 48 hours, and 85 percent ceased within 1 week.[2] The use of lumbar drainage can further increase the rate of sealing.

In contrast, there are three classical criteria for surgical intervention: (1) a bout of meningitis, (2) pneumocephalus, or (3) an active leak (persistant or recurring). Lewin's insistence on surgery for virtually all leaks was based on a fear of meningitis rather than on accurate figures for recurrence. It has yet to be shown that surgery offers a real improvement over natural history in patients with acute posttramatic leaks that have stopped within the first week.

The great majority of leaks or dural tears associated with midface fractures will stop permanently when the facial fractures are reduced.[86] Oddly enough, meningitis is relatively uncommon in dural tears associated with facial fractures, despite the fact that the incidence of dural laceration in facial fractures (43 percent) is higher than in closed head injury (7 percent) and CSF leak occurs far more commonly (36 percent).[86]

Most postoperative incisional leaks will also stop spontaneously or with lumbar drainage, particularly if the incision is reinforced or oversewn and any underlying abnormality of intracranial pressure is properly treated. Postoperative rhinorrhea and otorrhea are less likely to seal. If positional adjustments and lumbar drainage do not stop the leak within 48 hours or if the leak stops and then recurs, most authors favor re-exploration of the wound and direct repair of the fistula. The air sinuses in these cases have usually been violated.

The data for transsphenoidal procedures are similar. In Spaziante's series of 140 cases, four of six leaks stopped with lumbar drainage alone.[38] Ciric estimates that 2 percent of transsphenoidal operations will require reoperation for CSF leak.[39]

Surgical intervention may be indicated without a waiting period in the following circumstances:

1. Acute traumatic or postoperative leaks that recur or persist after 10 to 13 days of conservative management, including external drainage.
2. Proven intermittent or delayed leaks.
3. High-pressure leaks acting as a "safety valve" for hydrocephalus.
4. Leaks associated with erosion, destruction, or severe comminution of the skull base or the paranasal sinuses.
5. Leaks associated with congenital dysplasias of the brain, skull base, orbit, or ear, particularly after a bout of meningitis.
6. Leaks caused by high-energy missile wounds.
7. Postoperative rhinorrhea and otorrhea that cannot be controlled by position and drainage, especially when the air sinuses have been violated as part of the operative route. High volume leaks through the petrous bone and the sella are particularly recalcitrant to conservative management.

OPERATIVE TECHNIQUE

There are three major operative approaches currently in use, both singly and in combination: (1) craniotomy, including intradural and extradural techniques; (2) extracranial extradural, with degrees of complexity ranging from simple packing to complicated mucoperiosteal grafts; (3) CSF shunting procedures.

Table 7-2 is a summary of current techniques and their applications.

Craniotomy

Anterior Fossa. Two techniques have been used in the anterior fossa: intracranial extradural, and intracranial intradural. The intracranial extradural approach has several substantial limitations: (1) dural tears are virtually inevitable in the course of dissection; (2) areas of cerebral tissue herniation into bony defects cannot be easily visualized; and (3) permanent dural repair is not reliably achieved. For these reasons, the intracranial intradural route is preferred when craniotomy is indicated.

Preoperatively, steroids, anticonvulsants, and antibiotics are given prophylactically. The patient is positioned in a Mayfield frame or on a cerebellar headrest, body flexed, knees bent, nose at the midline, head hyperextended with the malar eminences uppermost. A Doppler probe is used to monitor for air emboli during the procedure; arterial and central venous

Table 7-2. Operative procedures in the management of CSF leaks and their indications

Procedure	Indications
Intracranial intradural exploration	1. Acute or delayed traumatic leak from anterior or middle fossa. 2. Anterior fossa leak with extrasellar intracranial mass. 3. Congenital anomaly of brain. 4. Definable dysplasia of the anterior or middle fossa. 5. Postoperative leak after anterior or middle fossa surgery. 6. Complex penetrating or through-and-through injuries involving cerebral tissue as well as extracranial structures. 7. Whenever a craniotomy is indicated for other reasons. 8. Whenever a significant dural hiatus is demonstrable.
Extracranial extradural approach: transseptal, transsphenoidal, or transethmoidal with mucoperiosteal flap	1. Clearly defined ''spontaneous'' leaks from the anterior fossa, including the cribriform fossa and fovea ethmoidalis. 2. Postoperative leaks after treatment of sellar and parasellar lesions.
Extracranial extradual approach: dural repair and simple packing	1. Leaks associated with temporal bone dysplasia and ear anomalies. 2. Leaks through the mastoid air cells not originating in the middle fossa.
Primary repair of facial fractures: sinus repair and ablation as necessary	1. Le Fort type II or type III fracture with dural tear or CSF leak but without evidence of gross bony disruption of the skull base or significant cerebral contusion. 2. Complex facial fractures involving orbit or air sinuses in which the initial leak has spontaneously sealed without evidence of gross bony disruption of the skull base or significant cerebral contusion.
Osteoplastic sinusotomy: repair of posterior sinus wall or cranialization of sinus and packing	1. Leaks associated with simple fractures through the posterior wall of the frontal sinus without evidence of comminution of the skull base or significant cerebral contusion.
Ventricular or lumboperitoneal shunting	1. Carried out in conjunction with anatomic repair of a fistula or resection of a space-occupying mass in the fact of hydrocephalus. 2. Small leaks that cannot be identified.

access is obtained. A bicoronal scalp flap is turned. A bone flap is elevated ipsilateral to the leak for a unilateral exposure, bilaterally otherwise. Although in some situations satisfactory access can be obtained from a unilateral exposure, a full exploration of the anterior fossa generally requires a bifrontal flap. Should the frontal air sinus be entered, the mucosa is stripped from both the flap and the sinus, the sinus is packed with Bacitracin-soaked Gelfoam, and a pericranial flap reflected from the scalp is sutured over the open sinus to the dura. Instruments used to close the sinus are considered contaminated and replaced.

The intracranial intradural approach allows full exposure of the anterior fossa. A satisfactory exploration allows both sphenoid wings, both cribriform fossae, and both orbital roofs to be fully visualized. The middle fossa, however, is usually out of reach. The exposure should always extend as far posteriorly as possible to include the anterior clinoids. If the leak is to be repaired in conjunction with the definitive resection of an intracranial mass, other considerations may govern the exposure. Dehydrating agents and drainage of CSF facilitate retraction.

The fistula is often betrayed by a palpable or visible dural defect or by a contusion, adhesion, or herniation of cerebral tissue. An obvious fistula can be sealed by inserting a plug of abdominal fat and covering the defect with a free or reflected flap of dura. The dura is obtained from the adjacent bone or from the falx cerebri, depending on the location of the fistula. Alternatively, a free patch of pericranium, temporalis fascia, fascia lata, or lyophilized dura can be sutured to the surrounding dura, and, if needed, used to reinforce a plug of fat. Fat forms a more durable plug than muscle. Muscle fibroses and shrinks, whereas fat remains viable by recruiting a blood supply from adjacent tissues. It goes without saying that a simple dural laceration can be sutured primarily, with a dural patch graft inserted when necessary.

If no discrete fistula is visualized, the entire floor of the frontal fossa, including both cribriform plates and the limbus sphenoidale is invested with a large free pericranial graft. Sutures are placed to maintain approximation rather than to obtain a watertight seal. The vector of CSF pressure tends to approximate the graft to the dura and stop the leak. Although dural substitutes have been used to repair dural defects, there is usually enough pericranium available.

Middle Fossa. For leaks from the middle fossa, the temporal floor must be thoroughly inspected. This is most efficiently done with an intradural approach. An extradural dissection also runs the risk of damaging the facial nerve by traction on the geniculate ganglion.

The principles of repair are identical to those in the anterior fossa. Free pericranial grafts are easier to manipulate than dural flaps in the middle fossa. Additionally, because the middle fossa is bounded by venous sinuses, reflecting a flap of any substantial size is impossible. Because only a unilateral exposure can be obtained, it is particularly important to identify the site of the leak preoperatively. Craniotomy is the preferred route to the floor of middle fossa because of the anatomic consideration noted above. Leaks involving the petrous bone and the posterior margins of the temporal fossa are often better approached extradurally or in a combined fashion.

Air can be insufflated through specially designed tubes that seal the nares and occlude the posterior pharynx during surgery. By flooding the field with saline, it is sometimes possible to identify, by the bubbles, a fistula that would not otherwise be evident.[44] As a rule, it is simpler and more prudent to cover the entire anterior or middle fossa with a graft than to count on this technique.

Posterior Fossa. Cerebrospinal fluid does not leak from the posterior fossa except in fractures extending through the petrous bone and after surgery. Otorrhea from petrous fractures rarely presents a problem because it usually stops spontaneously or, at worst, with drainage. The same holds true for rhinorrhea emanating from the posterior fossa.

Cerebrospinal fluid leaks after surgery on the posterior fossa can also appear as rhinorrhea, as otorrhea, or as leaks through the incision. This is a recognized complication of cerebellopontine angle surgery, as previously noted. Postoperative leaks through the mastoid or through the temporal bone can be quite elusive and difficult to treat. For prevention as well as treatment, Montgomery, Ojemann, and others recommend that the porus acusticus be plugged with fat when it has been enlarged for tumor removal and that any opened mastoid air cells be sealed with bone wax if small and with a fat graft if large. These two sites are the most likely sources of leak. A water-tight dural closure is achieved with a dural graft.[35-37] Depending on the site of the leak, the clinical setting, and the surgeon's experience and preference, an extradural approach via a mastoidectomy may be a viable alternative, especially with recurrent leaks. When the ear is nonfunctional, this approach, combined with an obliteration of the inner and middle ear, has much to recommend it as the primary maneuver.

For "spontaneous" leaks such as those associated with the Mondini malformation, the extradural approach is generally adopted. Most incisional leaks after posterior fossa surgery can be repaired by oversewing the wound and draining CSF. As a rule, incisional leaks reflect increased intracranial pressure. If the leak recurs or if the wound bulges with subgaleal CSF after drainage is discontinued, permanent CSF diversion will probably be required.

Closure. A routine craniotomy closure is carried out. The patient is nursed in the upright position for 3 to 5 days postoperatively and treated with laxatives and stool softeners to prevent straining. All heavy labor and lifting is prohibited for 3 months.

Combined Craniotomy and Reduction of Facial Fractures

Most CSF leaks associated with fractures of the midface can be managed definitively by reducing the facial fracture. Complex fractures impacted into the skull base often require reduction via craniotomy before realignment of the facial fracture. No definitive rules can be given for these injuries: treatment must be carefully individualized and often requires a team approach that includes ENT, dental surgery, ophthalmology, plastic surgery, and neurosurgery.

Extracranial Approaches

Aside from the classic transsphenoidal operations, the extracranial approaches to the skull base are generally performed by or in conjunction with otolaryngologists. Only the broad principles of these techniques will be reviewed.

Indications. There are four situations to which the extracranial approach is particularly suited: (1) a discretely definable normal-pressure leak through the cribriform plate or adjacent ethmoid labyrinth; (2) fractures that abut upon an air sinus, particularly when the bony defect is limited to the cranial wall of that sinus; (3) postoperative leaks after transsphenoidal surgery; and (4) leaks through the oval window, petrous bone, or other parts of the ear.

Special Techniques. Intrathecal dye injected at the beginning of the procedure helps to visualize the leak intraoperatively. Indwelling catheters are often used: saline or artificial CSF can be injected intrathecally to distend the subarachnoid space and provoke an intermittent leak, and CSF can be drained postoperatively to encourage approximation of the flap and dural packing.

When CSF fistulas traverse an air sinus, the sinus is ablated with fat or muscle. The packing acts as a seal in its own right and serves to hold mucoperiosteal, periosteal, or free fascia lata grafts against the dura. To inhibit the formation of a mucocele, the mucosa of the sinus must be stripped before packing.

Transfrontal extradural procedures can be carried out either through a forehead incision or via a bicoronal incision. There is one important advantage to the bicoronal incision: should it be necessary to obtain a more generous view of the frontal fossa, a craniotomy can be carried out without difficulty. This eventuality should be considered and discussed with the patient before surgery. The anterior wall of the frontal sinus is removed with a Stryker saw or the Midas Rex with the C1 attachment following a template obtained from a 72-inch sinus film. The posterior wall is fully exposed; the mucosa is resected and enough bone is removed to display the dural defect. The dura can be patched or sutured primarily. Depending on the extent of damage, the fragments of the posterior wall can be replaced or totally removed, thereby cranializing the frontal sinus. In either case, the sinus is ablated with fat and the frontal wall is restored.

Depending on the angle required, the width of the desired window, the site of the leak, and the surgeon's preference, the sphenoid sinus and the sella can be approached transseptally via a sublabial or a transnasal route, or transethmoidally via an external rhinotomy incision. The first is more familiar to neurosurgeons, but the second is shorter, results in a wider exposure, and permits complete resection of the sphenoid septae. This is an important consideration in reoperation for CSF leak after transsphenoidal surgery and reconstruction of the sellar floor. The leak is sealed with a flap of mucoperiosteum elevated with or without the underlying cartilage and folded over the dural defect. Sometimes a free graft of fascia lata is interposed. The ethmoid or sphenoid sinus is packed to hold the graft in place. Lumbar drainage is carried out for 5 days.

The cribriform fossa and fovea ethmoidalis are best approached through a curved naso-orbital incision and a complete ethmoidectomy. A flap rotated from the middle turbinate or the septum is used to cover the cribriform plate and the ethmoid roof from below. The posterior ethmoidal artery is a landmark situated directly anterior to the optic nerve.

Extracranial techniques have a lower morbidity than craniotomy and do not produce anosmia. They are sometimes successful where multiple craniotomies have failed. On the other hand, they do not permit a wide visual inspection of the orbitofrontal cortex, nor of the floor of the anterior fossa.

Other Technical Considerations

Methylmethacrylate.   When methylmethacrylate first became available, it was hailed as the paean for CSF leaks.[40,87] Experience has not substantiated this initial enthusiasm. With time, methacrylate shrinks and the leak recurs. If infection sets in, the plug becomes a septic nidus. More importantly, it has become evident that the concept behind the use of methacrylate was faulty: it is the dura rather than the bone that requires repair. Leaks will seal when the dural fistula is closed. Except in rare instances the bony structures do not require reinforcement. When they do, however, autologous bone or cartilage is preferable to foreign material. Should the underlying problem be hydrocephalus or increased intracranial pressure, control of intracranial pressure should be carried out before or in conjunction with the exploration.

Lumbar Drainage.   Lumbar drainage is not generally carried out after craniotomy because it is hoped that the CSF pressure will compress the graft onto the dura surrounding the fistula and create a seal. In extracranial extradural approaches, on the other hand, drainage of CSF helps create a seal and promotes healing.

Tissue Adhesives.   The availability of cyanoacrylate tissue adhesive was also greeted with initial enthusiasm. Like methylmethacrylate, to which they are chemically related, cyanoacrylates seemed particularly suited to the management of CSF fistulas. It was hoped that adhesives might overcome some of the problems associated with obtaining a durable seal, especially in relatively inaccessible areas. Unfortunately, the first generation of acrylic tissue adhesives has proved disappointing. In addition to carrying a risk of meningitis and of neural toxicity, particularly to the optic apparatus, they form a barrier between layers of tissue, inhibiting granulation and preventing fibroblastic proliferation from fusing one layer to the next. With time, tissue adhesives become porous, and can result in recurring leaks.[88–91] More recently, the use of autogenous or prepackaged fibrin clot adhesives has prompted a reconsideration of the role of these agents. Initially encouraging results are now being subjected to large-scale clinical trials.

The Use of CSF Shunts

High-pressure leaks cannot be sealed without reducing the intracranial pressure. The primary pathologic condition must be treated first, either by resection of the space-occupying lesion, or by reduction of CSF volume and flow in hydrocephalus. Nonetheless, several types of recalcitrant fistulas have been successfully treated with lumboperitoneal shunts.[92,93]

Cerebrospinal fluid shunting can be attempted in normal pressure leaks when other means of repair have failed or when, after exhaustive investigation, the site of the leak cannot be located. Indeed, lumboperitoneal shunting has been advocated as the only treatment needed for small leaks that cannot be visualized.[59,94] This empirical approach assumes that the resistance to flow through the shunt will be less than the resistance to passage through the fistula. With shunt malfunction, the leak can recur. Moreover, tension pneumocephalus can occur when air is aspirated intracranially through an open fistula under negative pressure.[40,76,77] The treatment for this complication is ligation of the shunt initially and replacement of the valve with a higher pressure unit once the mass effect has been treated and the air resorbed.

THE TREATMENT OF SPINAL CSF LEAKS

Spontaneous spinal CSF leaks rarely occur outside the setting of spinal dysraphism or unusual spinal anomalies. Traumatic leaks occur after penetrating injury, after surgery, after lumbar puncture, and after spinal anesthesia. Prevention is far easier than cure in postoperative leaks. Dural defects should be closed in a watertight fashion whenever possible. The dura should not be closed under tension; a graft taken from the lumbodorsal fascia can be inserted. Dural flaps with the potential to become ball valves should be assiduously avoided. Closure of the fascial and superficial layers should not be left to inexperienced surgeons. Much has been said regarding the importance of intraoperative Valsalva's maneuvers in detecting small meningeal tears and proving the adequacy of dural repair. Although the emergence of CSF obviously implies that satisfactory repair has not been achieved, the absence of CSF with an increase in intrathoracic pressure does not eliminate the possibility of a delayed leak.

For patients undergoing elective repair of spinal anomalies such as spinal lipomas associated with dysraphism or in other situations where the skin or subcutaneous tissue is defective, consideration should be given to rotating a generous myocutaneous flap. This technique is also useful where there is a recurrence of CSF leak with breakdown of the wound edges, when difficulty with wound healing can be anticipated, and in the face of infection. Despite the dictum that infection should be cleared before a graft is applied, the myocutaneous flaps seem to survive rotation onto a clean but infected base and even to facilitate healing in chronically infected wounds.

Other principles of management are analogous to those already described for transcranial leaks. In meningomyeloceles and other dysraphic states, the repair of the leak becomes part of the repair of the anomaly. Increased ICP must be controlled before the leak will stop. Except in open injuries, transcutaneous leaks, and obvious anomalies, the site of the leak can be quite difficult to determine.[84] Isotope cisternography and contrast CT scanning are usually accurate in active leaks.[95] Most uncomplicated traumatic leaks will seal within several days so long as there is no ball valve dural defect to resist healing. Certain maneuvers may be helpful: incisional leaks should be initially repaired by resuturing the wound and applying an abdominal binder over a pressure pad to increase resistance to CSF flow. External CSF drainage from the cervical subarachnoid space via puncture at C1-2 has been used on several occasions to good effect at the Walter Reed Army Medical Center. The Touhy needle and drainage catheter must be inserted under fluoroscopic control. Although the cervical subarachnoid catheters are more likely to kink, no other major difficulties have been encountered. If the leak persists over 10 days and if the ICP is normal, re-exploration of the wound is generally indicated.

A number of other techniques have been reported. Three are mentioned as additions to the surgeon's armamentarium, although they cannot be recommended as a routine:

1. An infusion of 100 ml of 20 percent mannitol every 4 hours for 7 days and positioning the patient in a head-down attitude for 1 week.[96]
2. Insertion of a fat plug through a limited midline durotomy for small rents of the anterior and lateral thecal walls.[97]
3. The use of tissue adhesives to seal the dura.[98]

It is particularly important not to confuse an infected serous exudate with a delayed spinal CSF leak. We emphasize the need to re-explore a recalcitrant postoperative leak in order to determine what tissue layers need to be repaired for the leak to be contained.

CONCLUSIONS

The large number of solutions to the problem of CSF leak attests to the difficulty of the problem. Cerebrospinal fluid leaks can only be managed after the mechanism of causation, the anatomic origin, and the pathophysiology have been understood. Both extradural and intradural approaches are effective in the appropriate setting. Indeed, a team approach may well be desirable.

Leaks that act to decompress increased intracranial pressure will not stop until the pressure is reduced. The usefulness of CSF diversion should be kept in mind. A follow-up of long duration is necessary before the possibility of recurrence can be dismissed absolutely.

REFERENCES

1. Bidloo the Elder, quoted in Morgagni, De Sedibus et Causis Morborum, 1, 15, art 21. Cited in Lewin W: Cerebrospinal fluid rhinorrhea in nonmissile head injuries. Clin Neurosurg 12:237, 1966
2. Mincy JE: Post traumatic cerebrospinal fluid fistula of the frontal fossa. J Trauma 6:618, 1966
3. Miller C: Case of hydrocephalus chronicus with some unusual symptoms and appearances on dissection. Trans Med-Chir Soc Edinb 2:243, 1826
4. Ommaya AK: Spinal fluid fistulae. Clin Neurosurg 23:363, 1975
5. Chiari H: über einem Fall von Luftansammlung in den Ventrikeln des menschichen Gehirns. Z Heilkd 5:383, 1884
6. Luckett WH: Air in the ventricles of the brain, following a fracture of the skull. Report of a case. Surg Gynecol Obstet 17:237, 1913
7. Wilkins RH: Neurosurgical Classics. New York, Johnson Reprint Corporation, 1965, pp 242–256
8. Grant FC: Intracranial aerocele following fracture of the skull. Report of a case with review of the literature. Surg Gynecol Obstet 36:251, 1923
9. Dandy WE: Pneumocephalus (intracranial pneumatocele or aerocele). Arch Surg 12:949, 1926
10. Cairns H: Injuries of the frontal and ethmoidal sinuses with special reference to cerebrospinal fluid rhinorrhea and aeroceles. J Laryngol Otol 52:589, 1937
11. Dandy WE: Treatment of rhinorrhea and otorrhea. Arch Surg 49:75, 1944
12. Lewin W: Cerebrospinal fluid rhinorrhea in closed head injuries. Br J Surg 42:1, 1954
13. Lewin W: Cerebrospinal fluid rhinorrhea in nonmissile head injuries. Clin Neurosurg 12:237, 1966
14. Eden K: Traumatic cerbrospinal rhinorrhea. Repair of a fistula by a transfrontal intradural operation. Br J Surg 29:299, 1941
15. Dohlman G: Spontaneous cerebrospinal rhinorrhoea: Case operated by rhinologic methods. Acta Otolaryngol (Suppl) 67:2023, 1948
16. McCabe NF: The osteo-mucoperiosteal flap in repair of cerbrospinal fluid rhinorrhea. Laryngoscope 86:537, 1976
17. Calcaterra TC: Extracranial surgical repair of cerebrospinal rhinorrhea. Ann Otol 89:108, 1980
18. Appelbaum E: Meningitis following trauma to the head and face. JAMA 173:116, 1968
19. Brawley B, Kelly W: Treatment of skull fractures with and without cerebrospinal fluid fistula. J Neurosurg 26:57, 1967
20. Einhorn A, Mizrahia EM: Basilar skull fractures in children. Incidence of CNS infection and the use of antibiotics. Am J Dis Child 132:1121, 1978
21. Krayenbuhl HA: Questions and answers. Clin Neurosurg 14:23, 1967
22. Leech PJ, Patterson R: Conservative and operative management for cerebrospinal leakage after closed head injury. Lancet 1:1013, 1973
23. Vourc'h G: Continuous cerebrospinal fluid drainage by indwelling spinal catheter. Br J Anaesth 35:118, 1963
24. Aitken RR, Drake CG: Continuous spinal drainage in the treatment of postoperative cerebrospinal-fluid fistulae. J Neurosurg 21:275, 1964
25. McCallum J, Maroon JC, Janetta PJ: Treatment of postoperative cerebrospinal fluid fistulas by subarachnoid drainage. J Neurosurg 42:434, 1975
26. Findler G, Sahar A, Beller AJ: Continuous lumbar drainage of cerebrospinal fluid in neurosurgical patients. Surg Neurol 8:455, 1977
27. Kaufman B, Nulsen FE, Weiss MH, et al: Acquired spontaneous nontraumatic normal-pressure cerebrospinal fluid fistulas originating from the middle fossa. Radiology 122:379, 1977
28. Ommaya AK, di Chiro G, Baldwain M, et al: Nontraumatic cerebrospinal fluid rhinorrhoea. J Neurol Neurosurg Psychiatry 31:214, 1968
29. Park JI, Strelzow VV, Friedman WH: Current management of cerebrospinal fluid rhinorrhea. Laryngoscope 93:1294, 1983
30. Dagi TF, Meyer FB, Poletti CA: The incidence and prevention of meningitis after basilar skull fracture. Am J Emerg Med 3:295, 1983
31. Meirowsky AM, Caveness WF, Dillon JD, et al: Cerebrospinal fluid fistulas complicating missile wounds of the brain. J Neurosurg 54:44, 1981
32. Shulman K: Later complications of head injuries in children. Clin Neurosurg 19:371, 1971
33. Nutkiewicz A, DeFeo DR, Kohut RI, et al: Cerebrospinal fluid rhinorrhea as a presentation of pituitary adenoma. Neurosurgery 6:195, 1980
34. Piziak VK, Gilliland PF, Boyd G, et al: Pituitary tumor initially seen as serous otitis media. JAMA 251:3131, 1984
35. Horowitz NH, Rizzoli HV: Postoperative Complications of Intracranial Surgery. Baltimore, Williams & Wilkins, 1982, pp 76, 123–124
36. Montgomery WW: Surgery for acoustic neurinoma. Ann Otolaryngol 82:428, 1973
37. Ojemann RG: Microsurgical suboccipital approach to cerebellopontine angle tumors. Clin Neurosurg 25:461, 1978
38. Spaziante R, de Divitiis E, Cappabianca P: Reconstruction of the pituitary fossa in transsphenoidal surgery: An experience of 140 cases. Neurosurgery 17:453, 1985
39. Ciric I: Comment on Spaziante et al. Neurosurgery 17:458, 1985

40. Bakay L, Glasauer FE: Head Injury. Boston, Little Brown & Co., 1980, p 280

41. Markham JW: The clinical features of pneumocephalus based upon a survey of 284 cases with report of 11 additional cases. Acta Neurochir 16:1, 1967

42. Hubbard JL, Thomas JM, Pearson BW, et al: Spontaneous cerebrospinal fluid rhinorrhea: Evolving concepts in diagnosis and surgical management based on the Mayo Clinic experience from 1970 through 1981. Neurosurgery 16:312, 1985

43. Flanagan JC, McLachlan DL, Shannon GM: Orbital roof fractures. Neurologic and neurosurgical considerations. Ophthalmology 87:325, 1980

44. Ray BS, Bergland RM: Cerebrospinal fluid fistula: Clinical aspects, techniques of localization, and methods of closure. J Neurosurg 30:399, 1969

45. Jamieson KG, Yelland JDN: Surgical repair of the anterior fossa because of rhinorrhea, aerocele, or meningitis. J Neurosurg 39:328, 1973

46. Kosoy J, Trieff N, Winkelmann P, et al: Glucose in nasal secretions. Arch Otolaryngol 95:225, 1975

47. Healy CE: Significance of a positive reaction for glucose in rhinorrhea. Clin Pediatr 8:239, 1969

48. Kirsch AP: Diagnosis of cerebrospinal fluid rhinorrhea: Lack of specificity of the glucose oxidase Tes-Tape. J Pediatr 71:718, 1967

49. Ghoshhajra K: Radiologic techniques for identification and localization of cerebrospinal fluid fistulae. Semin Neurol 2:115, 1982

50. Levy JM, Christensen PK, Nykamp PW: Detection of a cerebrospinal fluid fistula by computed tomography. AJR 131: 344, 1978

51. Ahmadi J, Weiss MH, Segali HD, et al: Evaluation of cerebrospinal fluid rhinorrhea by metrizamide computed tomographic cisternography. Neurosurgery 16:54, 1985

52. Strauss H: Fluorescein als Indikator fur die Nierenfunktion. Berl Klin Wochenschr 50:2226, 1913

53. Fox N: Cure in a case of cerebrospinal rhinorrhea. Arch Otolarygol 17:85, 1933

54. Mahaley KS, Odom GL: Complications following intrathecal injections of fluorescein. J Neurosurg 25:298, 1966

55. Staab EV, Shirkhoda A: Cerebrospinal fluid scanning. Clin Nucl Med 6:103, 1981

56. Coletti PM, Siegel ME: Posttraumatic lumbar cerebrospinal fluid leak: Detection by retrograde In-111-DTPA myeloscintography. Clin Nucl Med 6:403, 1981

57. Hasegawa M, Watanabe I, Hiratsuka H, et al: Transfer of radioisotope from CSF to nasal secretion. Acta Otolaryngol 95:359, 1983

58. DiChiro G, Stein SC, Harrington T: Spontaneous cerebrospinal fluid rhinorrhea in normal dogs. Radioisotope studies of an alternate pathway of CSF drainage. J Neuropathol Exp Neurol 31:447, 1972

59. Spetzler RF, Wilson CB: Management of recurrent CSF rhinorrhea of the middle and posterior fossa. J Neurosurg 49:393, 1978

60. Irjala K, Suonpaa J, Laurent B: Identification of CSF leakage by immunofixation. Arch Otolaryngol 105:447, 1979

61. Parisier SC, Briken EA: Recurrent meningitis secondary to idiopathic oval window CSF leak. Laryngoscope 86:1503, 1976

62. Nenzelius C: On spontaneous cerebrospinal otorrhea due to congenital malformations. Acta Otolaryngol 39:314, 1951

63. Bottema T: Spontaneous cerebrospinal fluid otorrhea. Arch Otolaryngol 101:693, 1975

64. Rice WJ, Waggoner LG: Congenital cerebrospinal fluid otorrhea via defect in the stapes footplate. Laryngoscope 77:341, 1967

65. Ignelzi RJ, VanderArk GD: Analysis of the treatment of basilar skull fractures with and without antibiotics. J Neurosurg 43:75, 1975

66. Dagi TF, Ojemann RG, Zervas NT: Incidence and prevention of infection after neurosurgical operations, in Thompson RA, Green JR (eds): Infectious Diseases of the Central Nervous System. Jamaica, NY, Spectrum Publications, 1984, pp 155–173

67. Ingraham FD, Campbell JB: An apparatus for closed drainage of the ventricular system. Ann Surg 114:1096, 1941

68. White RJ, Dakters JG, Yashon D, et al: Temporary control of cerebrospinal fluid volume and pressure by means of an externalized valve-drainage system. J Neurosurg 30:264, 1969

69. McCoy G: Cerebrospinal rhinorrhea: A comprehensive review and a definition of the responsibility of the rhinologist in the diagnosis and treatment. Laryngoscope 73:1125, 1963

70. Wyler AR, Kelly WA: Use of antibiotics with external ventriculostomies. J Neurosurg 37:185, 1972

71. Friedman WA, Vries JK: Percutanous tunnel ventriculostomy. Summary of 100 procedures. J Neurosurg 53:662, 1980

72. Dagi TF, Ondra SL: The role of artificial intelligence systems in neurosurgical intensive care. Presented at the International Congress on Trends in Neurosurgery, Diagnostic and Surgical Perspectives: Vienna, Austria, 14–17 May, 1986 [manuscript in preparation]

73. Brownridge P: Spinal anesthesia revisited: An evaluation of subarachnoid block in obstetrics. Anaesth Intensive Care 12:334, 1984

74. Rudehill A, Cordon E, Rahn T: Subdural hematoma. A rare but life-threatening complication after spinal anaesthesia. Acta Anaesthesiol Scand 27:376, 1983

75. Benzon HT: Intracerebral hemorrhage after dural puncture and epidural blood patch: Nonpostural and noncontinuous headache. Anesthesiology 60:258, 1984

76. Ikeda K, Nakano M, Tani E: Tension pneumocephalus complicating ventriculoperitoneal shunt for cerebrospinal fluid rhinorrhea: Case report. J Neurol Neurosurg Psychiatry 41:319, 1978

77. Little JR, McCarty CS: Tension pneumocephalus after insertion of ventriculoperitoneal shunt for aqueductal stenosis. J Neurosurg 44:383, 1976

78. Jooma R, Grant DN: Cerebrospinal fluid rhinorrhea and intraventricular pneumocephalus due to intermittent shunt obstruction. Surg Neurol 20:231, 1983

79. Katz J: Treatment of a subarachnoid-cutaneous fistula with an epidural blood patch. Anesthesiology 60:603, 1984

80. Digiovanni AJ, Galbert MW, Wahle WM: Epidural injection of autologous blood for postlumbar-puncture headache. 1. Additional clinical experiences and laboratory investigation. Anesth Analg 51:226, 1972

81. Crawford JS: Experiences with epidural blood patch. Anaesthesia 35:513, 1980

82. Casement BA, Danielson DR: The epidural blood patch: Are more than two ever necessary? Anesthesia and Analgesia 63:1033, 1984

83. Rosenberg PH, Heavner JE: In vitro study of the effect of epidural blood patch on leakage through a dural puncture. Anesth Analg 64:501, 1985

84. Harrington H, Tyler HR, Welch K: Surgical treatment of postlumbar puncture dural CSF leak causing chronic headache. J Neurosurg 57:703, 1982

85. Reynolds AF, Hameroff SR, Blitt CD, et al: Spinal subdural epiarachnoid hematoma: A complication of a novel epidural blood patch technique. Anesth Analg 59:702, 1980

86. O'Brien MD, Reade PC: The management of dural tear resulting from mid-facial fracture. Head Neck Surg 6:810, 1984

87. Jakoby RK: The use of a methylmethacrylate seal in spinal fluid otorrhea and rhinorrhea. J Neurosurg 18:614, 1961

88. Lehman RAW, Hayes GJ, Martins AN: The use of adhesive and lyophilized dura in the treatment of cerebrospinal rhinorrhea. J Neurosurg 26:92, 1967

89. VanderArk GD, Pitkethly DT, Ducker TB, et al: Repair of cerebrospinal fluid fistulas using a tissue adhesive. J Neurosurg 33:151, 1970

90. Maxwell JA, Goldware SI: Use of tissue adhesive in the surgical treatment of cerebrospinal fluid leaks. Experience with isobutyl-2 cyanoacrylate in 12 cases. J Neurosurg 39:332, 1973

91. Mickey BE, Samson D: Neurosurgical applications of the cyanoacrylate adhesives. Clin Neurosurg 29:429, 1982

92. Greenblatt SH, Wilson DH: Persistant cerebrospinal fluid rhinorrhea treated by lumboperitoneal shunt: Technical note. J Neurosurg 38:524, 1973

93. Bret P, Hor F, Huppert J, et al: Treatment of cerebrospinal fluid rhinorrhea by percutaneous lumboperitoneal shunting: Review of 15 cases. Neurosurgery 16:44, 1985

94. Spetzler RF: Commentary on Bret P, et al. Neurosurgery 16:47, 1985

95. Gass H, Goldstein AS, Ruskin R, et al: Chronic postmyelogram headache. Isotopic demonstration of dural leak and surgical cure. Arch Neurol 25:108, 1971

96. Rosenthal JD, Hahn JF, Martinez GJ: A technique for closure of leak of spinal fluid. Surg Gynecol Obstet 140:948, 1975

97. Mayfield FH, Kurokawa K: Watertight closure of the spinal dura mater. Technical note. J Neurosurg 43:639, 1975

98. Papadakis N, Mark VH: Repair of spinal cerebrospinal fluid fistula with the use of a tissue adhesive: Technical note. Neurosurgery 6:63, 1980

CHAPTER 8
Surgical Management of Intracranial and Intraspinal Infections

R. Lewis Wright

IN THIS CHAPTER we consider bacterial infections of the nervous system that may require neurosurgical treatment for the control of infection or to relieve pressure on portions of the nervous system caused by the infection. These infections are mostly blood-borne, but they can at times occur by direct spread from nearby infections or as a result of a surgical procedure. They are of vital importance, however, because nowadays, as in the past, many cases are not diagnosed until irreparable damage to the nervous system or death has occurred (Figure 8-1). The chance of recovery is highly dependent upon the degree of damage to the nervous system that has taken place before diagnosis and treatment. Patients diagnosed early in the evolution of their disease and treated promptly have the best chance of recovery. A high index of suspicion on the part of the physician treating patients with possible intracranial and intraspinal infections remains of paramount importance.

OSTEOMYELITIS OF THE SKULL

Infection of the cranial bones occasionally can spread from infections in remote areas of the body via the bloodstream. More commonly, however, the infection develops from direct spread of bacteria to devitalized areas of bone. It is most often seen as an infectious complication after craniotomy or after the insertion of tongs for skeletal traction in the reduction of cervical fracture dislocations.[1,2] It also can originate from infections in the adjacent paranasal sinuses or in the middle ear or can follow penetrating injuries of the cranium. *Staphylococcus aureus* is the organism most often cultured from patients with osteomyelitis of the skull. Other bacteria, either alone or in mixture, can be causative organisms. Headache may vary considerably in patients with this condition, but swelling and local tenderness of the scalp usually are seen. Fever also may vary. Destruction of bone, as demonstrated on x-ray films, may not appear for up to 2 weeks after the clinical process begins. As the infection is visualized on x-ray films it spreads in an irregular fashion and follows no particular pattern or structure.

Once osteomyelitis is diagnosed, treatment usually consists of craniectomy for removal of the infected bone and eradication of any adjacent infections in the paranasal sinuses, the middle ear, or extensions into the extradural space. Antibiotics, effective as determined by laboratory testing for culture and sensitivity studies, should be continued for at least 3 to 4 weeks after all evidence of active infection has subsided. External drainage for several days postoperatively is recommended. Many of these patients will require subsequent cranioplasty for protection of the brain or for cosmetic purposes. This should be delayed several months to lessen the chance of recurrent infection around the implanted plastic or metal plates.

Theoretically, small areas of osteomyelitis of the skull can be treated medically with antibiotics, close clinical observation, and serial x-ray studies to document resolution and healing of the infectious process. To date, clinical experience with such cases is too scant for accurate evaluation of the effectiveness of medical treatment alone.

INTRACRANIAL EXTRADURAL ABSCESS

Intracranial extradural abscesses arise by direct spread from adjacent infections to the extradural space in patients with paranasal sinusitis, middle ear infections, and osteomyelitis of the skull.[1] These patients have fever and headache as initial complaints. As the lesion increases in size and intracranial pressure increases, lethargy occurs. In untreated patients the infectious process can result in intradural extension with meningitis, subdural abscess, brain abscess, or thrombosis of intracranial venous sinuses.

Clinical history and x-ray films of the skull and sinuses are important in the diagnostic evaluation of these patients. A computed tomographic (CT) scan will show the dura and brain displaced away from the skull at the site of abscess formation. This usually will be adjacent to the site of infection in the paranasal sinuses or the middle ear.

Treatment consists of craniectomy and removal of the infectious material from the dura. External drainage for several days is warranted, and, once again, antibiotics should be continued for 3 to 4 weeks after all clinical evidence of infection has cleared.

INTRACRANIAL SUBDURAL ABSCESS

Like extradural intracranial abscesses, those in the subdural space usually arise as complications of nearby infections in the paranasal sinuses and the middle ear.[3,4,5] Less often they follow penetrating wounds or operative procedures. Headache, fever, and neck stiffness occur early in these patients. Seizures, principally of the focal type, are common. Many patients

OPERATIVE NEUROSURGICAL TECHNIQUES
ISBN 0-8089-1862-1

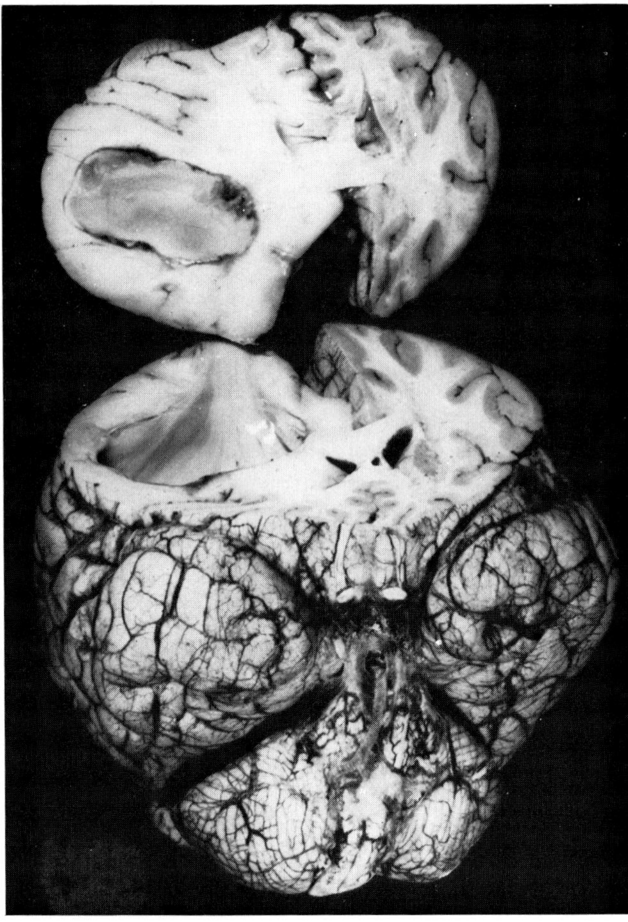

Fig. 8-1. A postmortem photograph showing a fatal undiagnosed frontal lobe abscess. Death was caused by temporal lobe herniation.

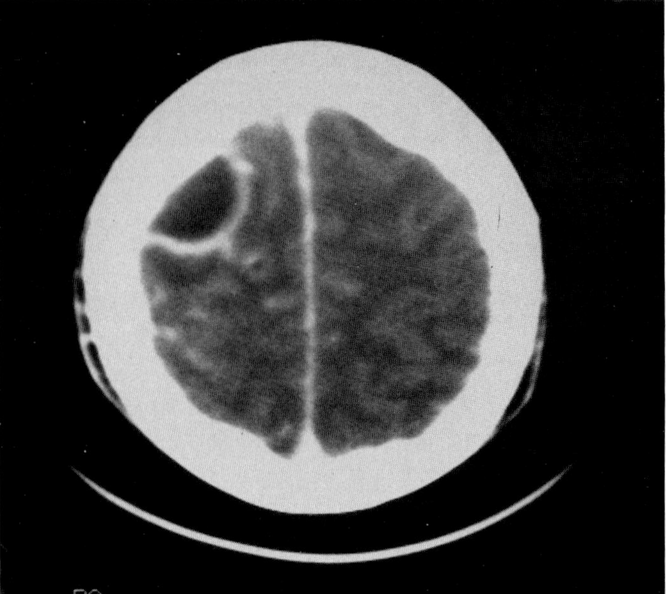

Fig. 8-2. A CT scan demonstrating a large subdural abscess that extended from frontal sinusitis.

with subdural abscesses deteriorate rapidly over a period of hours or a few days. Profound neurologic deficit and death can occur rapidly as the process evolves. Thrombosis of underlying cortical veins can occur, but meningitis rarely complicates this infection.

This lesion usually is easily visible on CT scans (Figure 8-2). Before the advent of CT scanning, nuclear scans were often accurate in diagnosing the lesion, and angiograms with oblique views, if necessary, would show the subdural abscess.

The only method of treating such lesions is craniectomy or craniotomy and removal of the contents of the abscess. Heavy encapsulation does not occur, and at times portions of the thin-walled capsule must be left adhering to vital areas of the cerebral cortex. Surgical removal of all infectious material, whether purulent or granulation tissue, should be done. Intracranial subdural abscesses are often multiloculated and at surgery care should be taken to make sure all pockets are drained. Serial CT scans every few days are of value in ensuring that this is the case. External drainage of the wound for a few days is wise. Once again, appropriate antibiotics should be continued systemically for 3 to 4 weeks.

ABSCESS OF THE BRAIN

Brain abscesses are less common now than formerly since infections throughout the body are commonly treated with antibiotics at an early stage. In approximately one fifth of

patients with brain abscesses, the parent infection will have been so mild that it escaped detection.

Healthy brain tissue has long been known to be resistant to the growth of bacteria. Experimental direct inoculation of the brain with pyogenic organisms has only rarely led to abscess formation. Necrotic tissue from infarction or trauma and dead spaces left after intracranial operations have seemed to favor abscess formation.

Clinically, brain abscesses have arisen most often from septic hematogenous emboli from distant infections (particularly pulmonary infections), from adjacent foci of infection in the paranasal sinuses and the middle ear, or as complications of intracranial surgery. Streptococci have been the organisms most often associated with brain abscess, although *Staphylococcus aureus,* coliform bacilli, diphtheroids, and mixed organisms are seen.

In most patients with brain abscess the early signs and symptoms are those of any lesion causing increased intracranial pressure: headache, somnolence, nausea, and vomiting. Seizures are common. With involvement of appropriate areas of the brain, hemiparesis, aphasia, or visual field defects may be encountered. Fever is usually absent. When the abscess arises from a septic hematogenous embolus, the abscess may develop in any one or a series of multiple sites, although these most often occur within the distribution of the middle cerebral artery and its branches. When the parent infection is otogenic or in the paranasal sinuses, the brain abscess is usually nearby, having spread by direct extension intracranially or by septic thrombophlebitis. Hence, infections of the middle ear or mastoid giving rise to a brain abscess usually will produce this lesion in the temporal lobe or occasionally in the cerebellum. Infections of the frontal, ethmoid, and sphenoid sinuses that produce brain abscesses usually do so in the adjacent portion of the frontal lobe.

In its early stages a brain abscess is characterized by cerebral softening, vascular congestion, and an adjacent margin of petechial hemorrhages. Within a few days the central portion undergoes a process of liquefaction and a capsule begins to

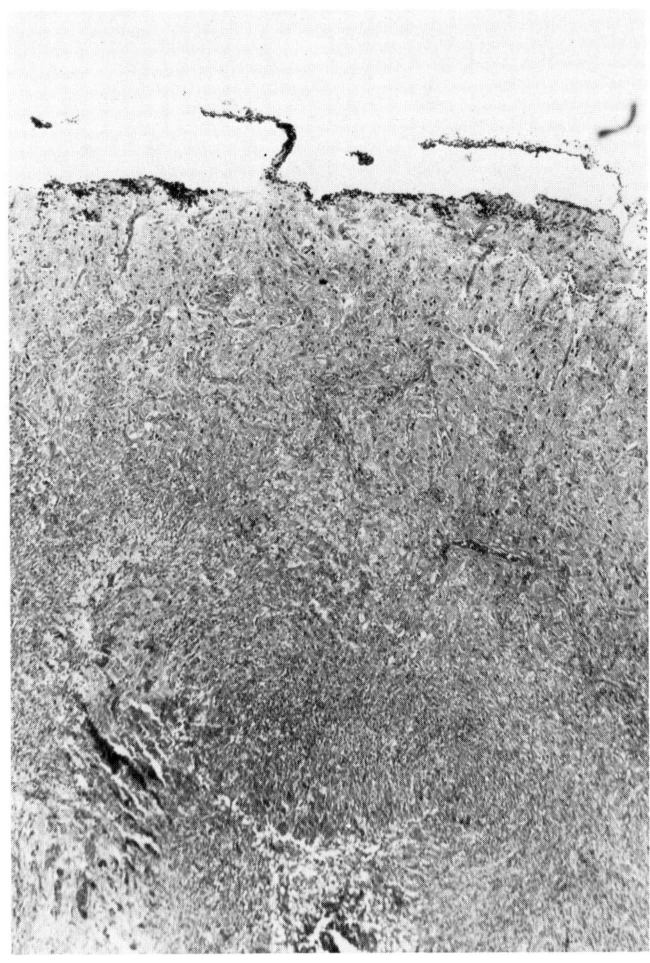

Fig. 8-3. A photomicrograph of the wall of a brain abscess. The central area of degenerating white blood cells is surrounded by a capsule consisting of reactive astrocytes and compressed brain tissue. (Magnification: × 50.)

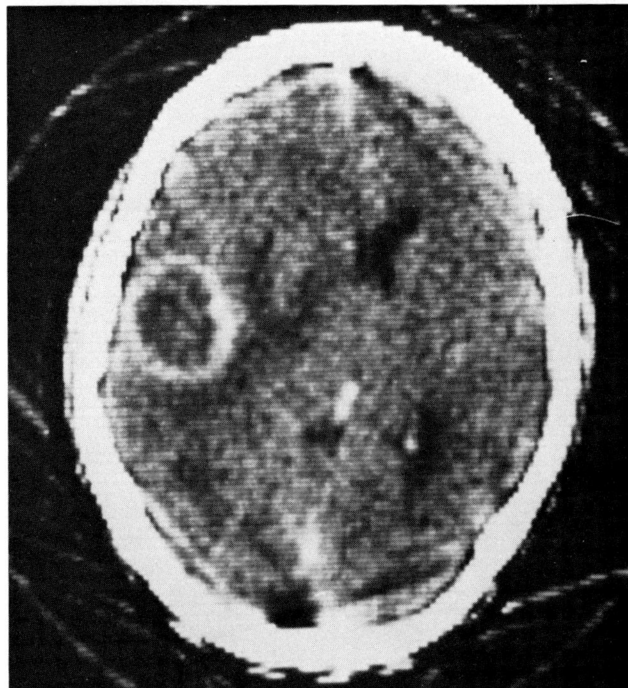

Fig. 8-4. A CT scan of a temporoparietal abscess showing the characteristic zone of ring-enhancement.

form. As additional time passes the capsule wall increases in thickness up to 4 to 5 mm. The inner layer of the abscess wall is composed of degenerating neutrophils, plasma cells, and lymphocytes enmeshed in fibrin. The outer layer is composed of compressed brain tissue and reactive astrocytes (Figure 8-3). Edema of the surrounding brain often is marked. If untreated, most patients with brain abscesses die of increased intracranial pressure with fatal herniation of the medial temporal lobe or the cerebellar tonsils; less commonly, death is caused by rupture of the abscess and fulminating meningitis.

Lumbar puncture is not indicated in the evaluation of a patient with a suspected brain abscess. In the past, when this was commonly done, findings were often normal. In others pressure was elevated to varying degrees, a leukocytosis was often present, and protein levels could be slightly elevated. Sugar content was normal unless rupture of the abscess had occurred.

A high index of suspicion on the part of the attending physician has long been emphasized as an important factor in the early diagnosis of brain abscesses. Routine x-ray films of the skull can be normal or at times can show a significant shift of a calcified pineal gland. Sinus infections can be visualized on x-ray films. An EEG usually shows a delta focus when the

abscess is superficial in location. In past years nuclear brain scans and angiograms have shown the mass lesion in most cases, but usually these have been indistinguishable from avascular tumors or hematomas.

The CT scan has become the single most valuable test in detecting brain abscesses.[6,7,8] In the early stages a mottled area of enhancement representing the area of cerebritis is seen. With subsequent liquefaction and formation of the capsule or wall the CT scan shows a ring-shaped lesion on enhancement with a central lucent area representing the area of liquefaction (Figure 8-4). Moreover, the CT scan provides data about the size, location, and age of the abscess and the presence of multiple abscesses.

In the past solely medical treatment of brain abscesses was condemned by many surgeons. With the use of the CT scan a few successful cures by medical treatment alone have been recorded.[6,7,8] This method should probably be limited to small, developing abscesses in which a wall has not formed and to those abscesses inaccessible to surgical treatment (abscesses located in basal ganglia, multiple small abscesses, etc.). Such patients should be followed closely with careful neurologic assessment and serial CT scans as appropriate drugs are administered. Antibiotics should be continued for at least 3 to 4 weeks in this group.

In a patient with a recent history of infection and findings on clinical examination and CT scans compatible with brain abscess, antibiotic therapy should be started promptly. Widespread antibiotic coverage with agents that cross the blood–brain barrier should be used. If the organism from the parent infection is known or when cultures taken at surgery for the abscess become available, this combination may need to be modified. Edema surrounding the abscess often is marked, and the use of steroids to control cerebral edema in these patients has been of great value. When appropriate antibiotic agents are

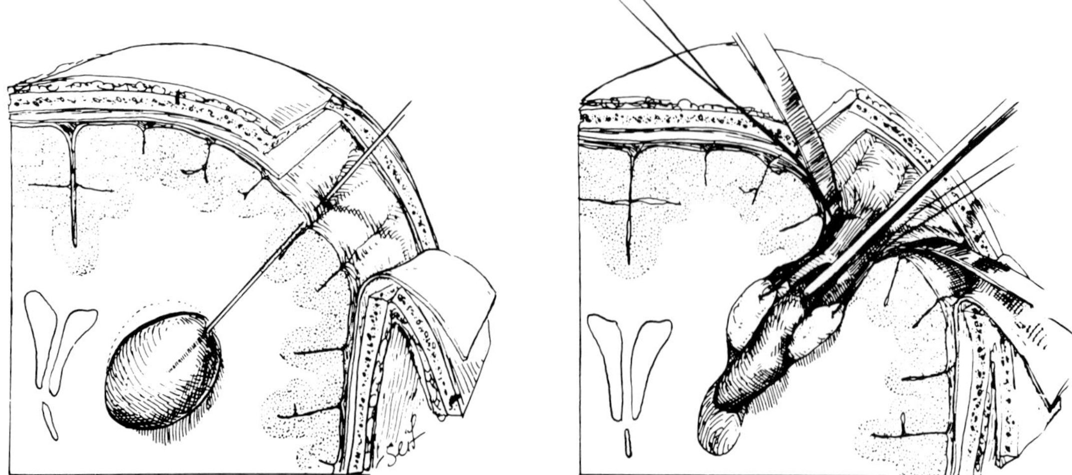

Fig. 8-5. Technique for removing a brain abscess. Total removal can often be done without resection of significant portions of the brain.

administered, the use of steroids in this situation has not led to spread of infection.

Although the relative merits of removal versus drainage of abscesses have been debated for decades, for large encapsulated brain abscesses surgical removal is the treatment of choice provided the lesion is in an area amenable to total removal.[4,9,10–13] Brain abscesses displace the brain tissue to a marked degree, but often little brain tissue is actually destroyed. Hence, many of the neurologic defects produced by an abscess are reversible.

At craniotomy the abscess is first aspirated as completely as possible. Large abscesses often must be opened as well to remove the contents and thereby decrease their size. The wall of the abscess then is gently dissected from adjacent white matter of the brain using small cottonoid patties to establish the plane between these two tissues. Gentle traction on the wall of the abscess facilitates its removal (Figure 8-5). In large abscesses removal of the wall is done in a piecemeal manner, but in smaller abscesses removal in toto may be possible. In certain situations, such as abscesses in the region of the basal ganglia and internal capsule and cases with multiple small abscesses, simple drainage may be better treatment, leaving the wall of the abscess intact. External drainage of brain abscesses that are operated upon is not necessary unless the abscess wall has been left in place. Replacement of the bone flap can be done in these patients unless intractable cerebral edema is present. Antibiotic coverage should continue for at least 3 to 4 weeks. In those patients in whom the wall or capsule of the abscess has been left intact and only simple drainage carried out, serial CT scans should be obtained.

SPINAL EXTRADURAL ABSCESS

Abscesses of the spinal extradural space can result from septic emboli to the extradural fat, by spread from paravertebral infections in the mediastinum or retroperitoneal space via an intervertebral foramen, or by direct extension from

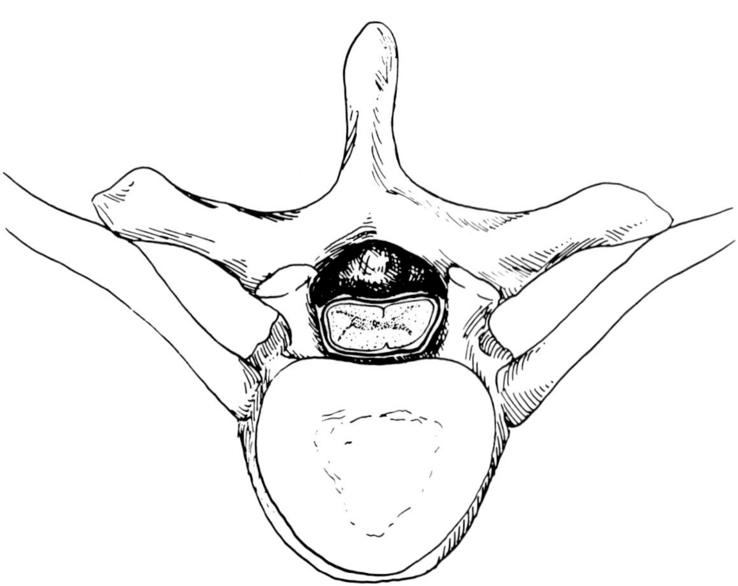

Fig. 8-6. Spinal extradural abscesses are characteristically located dorsal to the spinal cord.

osteomyelitis of the spine.[14–16] Rarely, they have arisen from penetrating injuries or as complications of surgery or lumbar puncture.

Initial symptoms are local backache near the infection and the presence of fever. Involvement of adjacent nerve roots may give rise to radicular pain. As compression of the spinal cord or cauda equina occurs, sensory and motor loss result distal to the site of compression and impairment of sphincter control develops. This process may extend over one or several vertebral segments. Rarely, the infection has extended through the entire length of the spine from the sacral to the upper cervical levels. The fact that extradural abscesses almost always occur dorsal to the spinal dura was first pointed out by Dandy (Figure 8-6).[16] Extradural fat and the extradural space are greater dorsally than either laterally or ventrally within the spinal canal.

Staphylococcus aureus is the organism most often responsible for these lesions, although *Streptococcus, Pseudomonas,* and typhoid bacilli may be the causative organisms. Fungus granulomas of the extradural space also can occur; in North America actinomycosis and blastomycosis are occasionally encountered.

In some patients deterioration occurs quickly, within a matter of hours or a few days. In others the disease has a prolonged course with the clinical picture extending over a period of days or weeks. The reason for such variability is not known. Fever and leukocytosis are often absent in this latter group. Whether progression is acute or prolonged, one fact is clear; the earlier surgical decompression is carried out, the better the outlook for neurologic recovery. The cauda equina withstands pressure from abscesses as well as other mass lesions better than the spinal cord itself.

Patients suspected of having spinal extradural abscesses should undergo a careful clinical evaluation with a detailed history and general and neurologic examinations. Spinal x-ray films are indicated but are often normal, unless paravertebral abscesses or adjacent osteomyelitic areas are demonstrated. At this time there is insufficient data to opine on the usefulness of the CT scan in this disease. Myelography should be done promptly via the lumbar route (unless the suspected abscess is thought to be lumbar in location, in which instance the cisternal route would be preferable). In most patients a total block will be demonstrated. The CSF usually shows an elevated protein content and increased white blood cells (both polymorphonuclear leukocytes and lymphocytes). If it is thought that the abscess extends well above the caudalmost extent outlined by the myelogram, cisternal myelography should be considered to outline its rostral extent.

Prompt decompressive laminectomy and removal of the abscess should be carried out. It is of vital importance that the laminectomy extend over the entire length of the abscess if good recovery is to be expected. In acute abscesses frankly purulent material will be encountered. In the chronic form only granulation tissue, which might be mistaken for a metastatic neoplasm, will be found. Radical removal of either of these is usually possible; bacterial smears and cultures should be obtained. If acute purulence is encountered, external drainage of the wound should be done for several days.

If an extradural abscess is suspected preoperatively, antibiotics should be begun before surgery. A choice is made on the basis of the antecedent infectious process. Some of the infectious chronic granulomas will show no growth on culture.

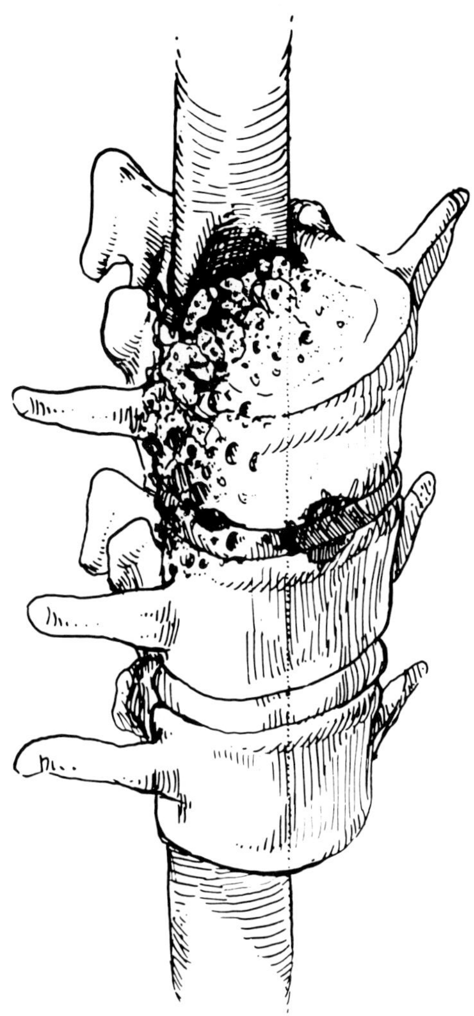

Fig. 8-7. Osteomyelitis of the spine characteristically involves several vertebral bodies and intervening discs.

SPINAL SUBDURAL ABSCESS

Abscesses of the spinal subdural space are uncommon. Most of these occur as extensions of infection in patients with midline congenital dermal sinuses;[15,17] rarely, blood-borne cases are encountered. Local back and radicular pain may be present or absent. As the lesion increases in size, symptoms and signs of compression of the cauda equina or spinal cord ensue. With leakage into the spinal subarachnoid space, meningitis may develop.

Myelography, prompt laminectomy, and drainage of the abscess are indicated. Laminectomy should extend over the length of the lesion, and external drainage should be employed for several days. The dura is probably best left open to ensure that maximal decompression is achieved. These abscesses probably never form a heavy wall or capsule. Appropriate antibiotic coverage should continue for a period of several weeks.

SPINAL INTRAMEDULLARY ABSCESS

Abscesses within the spinal cord itself are rare. These can arise via septic emboli or through penetrating injuries.[18] In the small number of cases reported, a variety of organisms have

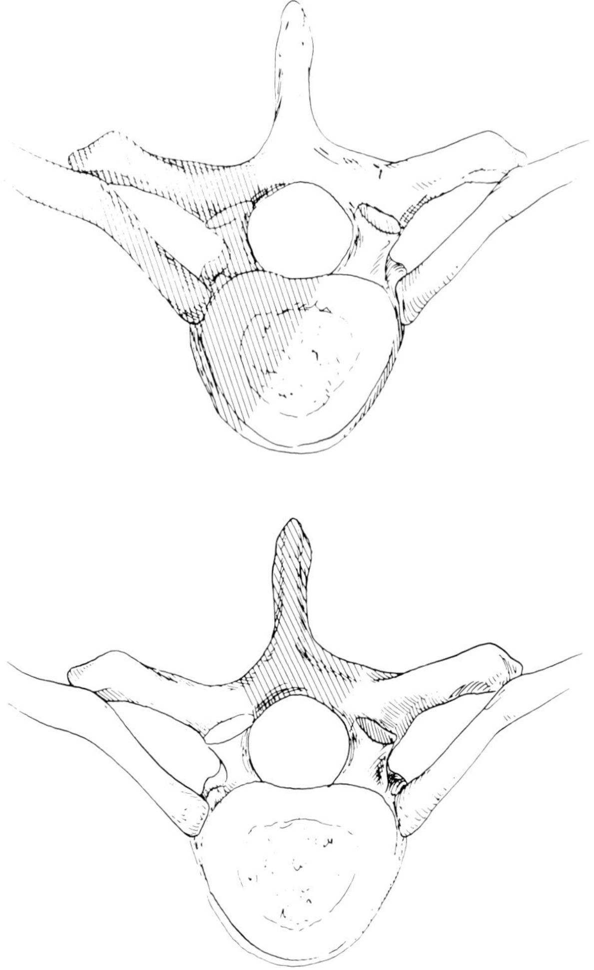

Fig. 8-8. Areas (shaded) of bone removal in costotransversectomy (above) and laminectomy (below).

been cultured. Progressive sensory and motor loss are the clinical picture, and pain is often absent. Systemic signs of sepsis, fever, and leukocytosis may be absent. Myelograms show a partial or complete block with evidence of widening of the spinal cord shadow. Decompression over the length of the process should be done promptly. Aspiration with a fine needle should be done for maximal decompression and to obtain cultures. It is unlikely that true encapsulation of these abscesses ever occurs. Once again, steroids to combat swelling and antibiotics for long periods are indicated.

OSTEOMYELITIS OF THE SPINE

Infections of the vertebral column can occur with pyogenic organisms, tuberculosis (Pott's disease), or fungi (especially actinomycosis and blastomycosis). These organisms most often reach this site via the hematogenous route. Among the pyogenic bacteria, *Staphylococcus aureus* and coliform bacilli are most common. Most cases of osteomyelitis do not concern the neurosurgeon. Compromise of the spinal cord can occur when an associated extradural abscess develops or when a bony deformity from a combined process of vertebral collapse with adjacent overgrown bone compromises the spinal canal (the

so-called gibbus formation). Rarely, operative procedures on the spine can result in osteomyelitis.

As a rule, the initial complaint is back pain, usually accompanied by local tenderness and muscle spasm. Fever and leukocytosis are common.

The earliest changes are seen on lateral x-ray films of the spine; tomograms may be helpful at times. The characteristic radiographic sign is erosion of several contiguous vertebral bodies with collapse and involvement of the associated discs (Figure 8-7). Characteristically, and for reasons unknown, metastatic tumors spare the intervertebral discs. Bone scans are usually positive at the site of infection, and the level alkaline phosphatase is elevated in most cases.

When compression of the spinal cord occurs, a clinical history, neurologic examination, and x-ray studies are all-important in determining the cause. Narrowing of the spinal canal by vertebral collapse or gibbus formation is assessed by tomography and by CT scanning. In the absence of spinal stenosis in patients with osteomyelitis of the spine, an extradural abscess or granuloma is the likely cause and should be treated by the aforementioned techniques. Myelography is indicated before surgery in all of the situations.

The thoracic area of the spine is most often the site of osteomyelitis. With progressive symptoms of cord compression here, costotransversectomy (removal of bone via an oblique posterior approach including the transverse processes, pedicles, and the involved portion of the diseased vertebral bodies) is the procedure of choice (Figure 8-8). Anterior operations are probably best for the rare cases in which the patient has progressive paralysis from osteomyelitis of the cervical spine, and retroperitoneal bone removal can be used for the rare cases in which the patient needs lumbar decompression for gibbus formation secondary to infection in this lower area of the spine. When spinal instability is present, long-term immobilization by casts, halo devices, or braces must be provided. Antibiotics in cases of osteomyelitis should be given intravenously for a period of 4 to 6 weeks.

Many patients with mild neurologic signs of spinal cord compression associated with tuberculosis of the spine will improve on a program of rest and antituberculous drugs and will not require surgery. It is essential that the neurologic findings in this group be followed carefully.

Spinal cord symptoms can occasionally occur in infectious diseases of the spine without compression of the cord itself. These cases are caused by vascular thrombosis secondary to the inflammatory process. It is of great importance to differentiate these patients from patients with compression of the cord by the tests previously mentioned, since surgical decompression of the spinal cord will not benefit this group of patients.

CONCLUSION

Although relatively uncommon now, infectious lesions causing dysfunction of the brain and spinal cord are neurologically devastating and sometimes fatal if they remain undetected and untreated. There is no substitute for prompt diagnosis and treatment. The CT scan has become invaluable in the diagnosis of intracranial abscesses and of deformities of the spinal canal caused by infectious diseases. Its utility in diagnosing intraspinal abscesses is as yet unproved.

In the surgery of all such lesions, adequate exposure and bony decompression over the extent of the abscess is mandatory. When the walls of brain abscesses are left in place and when frank purulence is present in abscesses at other sites, external drainage for several days is desirable. Surgical incisions usually can be closed primarily with absorbable sutures for the deep layers of the wound and nonabsorbable sutures, such as nylon or wire, for the skin. Some surgeons prefer to omit the deep sutures and use through-and-through wire sutures for the wound, leaving them in place for 2 to 3 weeks.

Proper postoperative care in all these patients may include the use of steroids when necessary to control swelling and appropriate antibiotic drugs for a prolonged period to ensure eradication of all bacteria. General supportive care, including physical therapy, is also of paramount importance.

REFERENCES

1. Woodhall B: Osteomyelitis and epi-, extra-, and subdural abscesses. Clin Neurosurg 14:239, 1966
2. Wright RL: Postoperative Craniotomy Infections. Springfield, Ill, Charles C Thomas, 1966
3. Bhandari Y, Sarkari NS: Subdural empyema: A review of 37 cases. J Neurosurg 32:35, 1970
4. LeBean J, Creissard P, Haripse L, et al: Surgical treatment of brain abscess and subdural empyema. J Neurosurg 38:198, 1973
5. Bannister G, Williams B, Smith S: Treatment of subdural empyema. J Neurosurg 55:82, 1981
6. Rosenblum ML, Hoff JT, Norman D, et al: Decreased mortality from brain abscess since advent of computerized tomography. J Neurosurg 49:658, 1978
7. Rotheram EB Jr, Kessler LA: Use of computerized tomography in nonsurgical management of brain abscess. Arch Neurol 36:25, 1979
8. Whelan MA, Hilal SK: Computed tomography as a guide in the diagnosis and follow-up of brain abscesses. Radiology 135: 663, 1980
9. Ballantine HT Jr, Shealy CN: The role of radical surgery in the treatment of abscess of the brain. Surg Gynecol Obstet 109:370, 1959
10. Lebeau J: Radical surgery and pencillin in brain abscess: A method of treatment in one state with special reference to the cure of three thoracogenic cases. J Neurosurg 3:359, 1946
11. Morgan H, Wood MR, Murphey F: Experience with 88 consecutive cases of brain abscess. J Neurosurg 38:698, 1973
12. Wright RL, Ballantine HT Jr: Management of brain abscesses in children and adolescents. Am J Dis Child 114:113, 1967
13. Choudbury AR, Taylor JC, Whitaker R: Primary excision of brain abscess. Br Med J 2:1119, 1977
14. Heusner AP: Nontuberculous spinal epidural infections. N Engl J Med 239:845, 1948
15. Wright RL: Infections of the spine and spinal cord, in Youmans (ed): Neurological Surgery. Philadelphia, WB Saunders, 1982, pp 3449–3458
16. Dandy WE: Abscesses and inflammatory tumors in the spine extradural space (so-called pachymeningitis externa). Arch Surg 13:447, 1926
17. Wright RL: Congenital dermal sinuses. Prog Neurol Surg 4:175, 1971
18. Wright RL: Intramedullary spinal cord abscess. J Neurosurg 23:208, 1965

A Surgical Management of Tuberculosis, Cysticercosis, and Fungal Infections of the Central Nervous System

R. Bhatia   P.N. Tandon

INFECTION OF THE CENTRAL NERVOUS SYSTEM (CNS) by *Mycobacterium tuberculosis* is invariably secondary to a primary focus elsewhere in the body. It occurs in several forms, including intracranial tuberculomas, tuberculous meningitis, spinal tuberculosis, and, uncommonly, tuberculous osteomyelitis of the skull. Spinal tuberculosis includes Potts' disease of the spine, which is a very common form of extradural compression in areas of the world in which tuberculosis is endemic; spinal arachnoiditis; and, rarely, intramedullary granulomas. This chapter deals only with tuberculomas and tuberculous meningitis.

Neurocysticercosis, which is caused by the pig tape worm, *Taenia solium,* is the most common worldwide parasitic infection of the nervous system. Although the disease is considered to be especially common in countries in which low socioeconomic conditions prevail, large numbers of cases also are reported in the more affluent countries.

Infections of the central nervous system by fungi are being recognized more frequently. This is partly because of better diagnostic facilities and partly because of their increased occurrence in immunosuppressed hosts and in patients with acquired immune deficiency syndrome (AIDS).

TUBERCULOSIS OF THE CENTRAL NERVOUS SYSTEM

With the advent of effective antituberculous drugs, the incidence of tuberculosis of the central nervous system has declined in both the developed countries and some of the less developed countries of the world. Indeed, in the western world this has resulted in tuberculosis being perceived by many as a rare disease of quaint historical interest.[1] In fact, even in the United States the decline has been slow; the number of cases among the elderly has actually increased.

In Britain, CNS tuberculosis has again become a problem in areas with large immigrant populations.[2] Immigration to the west, particularly an influx of refugees, coupled with the availability of more sophisticated diagnostic techniques contributes to the frequency with which CNS tuberculosis is encoun-tered and recognized. The incidence has declined in developing countries such as India, but its magnitude continues to be a serious medical problem.[3]

TUBERCULOMAS

Incidence

The incidence of tuberculoma in India ranges from 4.5 to 30 percent in different parts of the country.[3] Of 1487 space-occupying lesions studied in the series of Mathai and Chandy[4] from Vellore, South India, 10 percent were tuberculomas. In the neighboring city of Madras, only 82 miles away, Ramamurthi and Varadarajan[5] reported an incidence of tuberculomas of 24 percent. A high incidence has been reported from Chile (16 percent)[6] and from Rumania (7.3 percent).[7] It is interesting that although tuberculosis is widely prevalent in Nigeria, only 15 cases of tuberculomas were detected in a 5-year period. Misdiagnosis was ruled out, since a postmortem analysis of all patients dying of space-occupying lesions showed no cases of tuberculoma.[8] Similarly, in Taiwan, where CNS tuberculosis is common,[9] tuberculomas constituted only 1 percent of all intracranial mass lesions.[2] A combined series from several neurosurgical centers in Japan showed an incidence of only 2.6 percent.[10] Tuberculomas are certainly not rare even in industrial nations such as Great Britain[11–14] and the United States[15–19] and account for 1 to 2 percent of all intracranial mass lesions.

Location

Tuberculomas can occur at any site in the brain. In series of cases studied before the advent of computerized tomography, a a somewhat higher incidence in the posterior fossa was noted.[4,5,20] Of 50 tuberculomas evaluated with CT scans,[21] 82 percent were supratentorial, 8 percent were both supratentorial and infratentorial, and only 10 percent were located in the posterior fossa. Tuberculomas are rarely found in the thalamus, basal ganglia, ventricles, and the pituitary.

OPERATIVE NEUROSURGICAL TECHNIQUES
ISBN 0-8089-1862-1

Age and Sex

A preponderance for males was observed in earlier series. More recently, females with tuberculomas either just outnumber males or equal them in number.[4,20,21] This is a disease of the young; 60–70 percent of patients are below the age of 20 years. Tuberculomas are somewhat uncommon in children under the age of 4 years, although we treated a 9-month-old infant with multiple tuberculomas.

Clinical Features

The signs and symptoms of tuberculomas resemble those of other intracranial space-occupying lesions. Because they enlarge gradually, the clinical picture is one of a slowly progressive lesion although in at least 50 percent of patients the symptoms are less than 6 months in duration. Features that are of help in distinguishing tuberculomas from other brain tumors are constitutional symptoms, e.g., weight loss, fever or malaise, a history of active tuberculosis, a high frequency of seizures even in association with a cerebellar lesion, a positive Mantoux test, and a raised sedimentation rate. Infants and young children may have an enlarging head. At best, the clinical diagnosis is presumptive because even in endemic areas extracranial tuberculosis may coexist with a glioma. A review of several series shows that pyrexia is not invariable and may not be present in more that 20 to 25 percent of patients,[21] and that the Mantoux test may be negative.[4,7] The course may uncommonly show spontaneous remissions and relapses.[22] Clinical evidence of an active focus of tuberculosis, e.g., the lungs and lymph glands, may only be present in one third of patients[5,20] and in about 10 percent of close relatives. Rare signs include a scalp swelling, cerebrospinal fluid rhinorrhea, features of a pituitary tumor, unilateral proptosis, and trigeminal neuralgia.[20]

Pathologic Features

The typical tuberculoma is a solid, well-defined avascular mass with multiple nubbins extending to and compressing the surrounding brain. It is creamy white on the surface and has a pale yellow, often gritty caseating central core with a crenated margin. It has a firm collagenous capsule that at times has a pinkish appearance. This is usually referred to as the mature form of tuberculoma.[20] The immature form consists of multiple small tubercles, some with caseating or liquefied centers dispersed within an edematous brain. Severe edema, possibly caused by an allergic response,[20] may surround these tubercles. Tuberculomas vary in size from 1.5 to 8 cm and they vary in weight. Giant tuberculomas can occupy an entire cerebral hemisphere,[5] and a large number adhere to the dura. The dural attachment can be very tenuous or so firm that the tumor resembles a meningioma.

Microscopically the central zone of caseous necrosis is surrounded by tuberculous granulation tissue consisting of epithelioid cells, Langhans' giant cells, and some lymphocytes, polymorphonuclear leukocytes, and plasma cells (Figure 9-1). Acid-fast bacilli usually abound in both these layers. The brain surrounding a tubercle may show degenerated nerve fiber and nerve cells, thrombosed vessels, and, occasionally, swollen astrocytes and oligodendroglial cells. The changes in the small vessels can lead to microhemorrhages or microinfarcts, and these areas may coalesce.[23] Smaller satellite tuberculomas may surround the main mass.

Tuberculomas can take several unusual forms[24,25] representing the spectra of inflammatory reaction: (1) the incipient

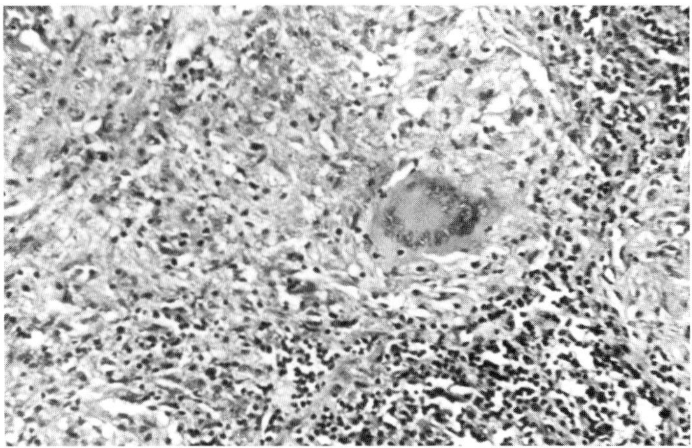

Fig. 9-1. A photomicrograph of a typical tuberculoma with Langhans giant cells, epithelioid cells, and lymphocytes. Hematoxylin and eosin stain: magnification X100.

tuberculoma, which may appear as an irregular, fleshy, gray cortical mass with associated meningeal tuberculomatosis or even grapelike clusters of tuberculoma along a cerebral vessel; (2) a subdural cyst overlying an intracerebral tuberculoma; (3) cystic tuberculoma; (4) tubercular abscess; (5) extensive edematous encephalopathy without a tuberculoma; (6) severe cerebral edema with a small "inconsequential" tuberculoma; and (7) rarely, tuberculoma that has spread transdurally to the calvarium. The factors that lead to a different type of tissue reaction associated with the presence of numerous live bacilli are not known. Tubercular abscesses were produced in BCG ±vaccinated and drug-protected monkeys by intracerebral injection of *Mycobacterium tuberculosis* var. *hominis*.[26] It is possible that previous antituberculous medication plays a role in the development of tubercular abscesses. The role of hydrolytic enzymes in liquefaction in tuberculous lesions at sites other than the brain has been extensively studied. Enzyme inhibitors from dead bacilli and necrotic tissue present in caseous material have been reported to prevent liquefaction in tuberculous lesions.[27] Brain tissue that is rich in hydrolytic enzymes may release large quantities of these enzymes and produce liquefaction, allowing tubercle bacilli to proliferate.

Radiologic Features

Tuberculomas cannot be differentiated from other CNS tumors on plain x-ray films of the skull. Calcification occurs in less than 6 percent of tuberculomas and is rarely extensive or dense.[5,6,7] Calcification is not indicative of an inactive lesion.[28] Cerebral angiography invariably reveals an avascular mass, although surface tuberculomas may show some peripheral vascularity.[5,28] An associated vascular spasm may be seen that is ascribed to tuberculous vasculitis.[29]

Before the advent of computed tomographic (CT) scanning, the diagnosis of an intracranial tuberculoma was established only by biopsy or excision. With CT scanning, it is possible to identify lesions as small as 3 or 4 mm in diameter and also to make an accurate diagnosis in a large percentage of cases.[11,13,18,21,22,30–34] These small lesions, existing without clinical evidence of elevated pressure, were excluded from earlier statistics based on surgical material.

The CT morphology[21,30,31] of tuberculomas can be classified in one of three categories:

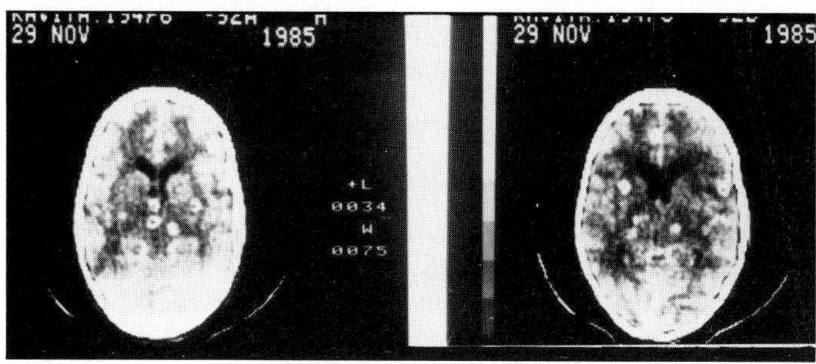

Fig. 9-2. A contrast-enhanced CT scan showing multiple rings and discs surrounded by areas of low attenuation indicating edema characteristic of tuberculosis. This 10-year-old patient had symptoms of elevated intracranial pressure and fever.

1. Small discs and rings measuring less than 1 cm in diameter with marked contrast enhancement and perilesional edema of low attenuation (Figure 9-2).
2. Large rings similar to an abscess but usually lacking the low central lucency of the latter (Figure 9-3). There may also be a central dense nidus within the ring lesion, the "target sign" of Welchman (Figure 9-4).[33]
3. Large nodular masses with an irregular outline, which may be the result of coalescence of multiple rings and discs (Figure 9-5).

A small discrete disclike lesion is the most common form of tuberculoma seen on CT scans. Such a lesion would be missed on conventional neuroradiologic studies. It also is the type that responds readily to antituberculous medication. These tuberculomas probably represent the early stage of parenchymal involvement ("immature tuberculoma").[20,23] The associated edema is disproportionately large compared with the size of the lesion. Tuberculoma should always be considered in the differential diagnosis of a mass lesion with intense ring enhancement, the center of which is approximately the same density as the normal brain substance.[33] The ring of a neoplasm tends to be variable in appearance and only uncommonly resembles a tuberculoma, but occasionally it may not be possible to distinguish between the two. A glioma ring tends to be more irregular and can often be seen on plain scans; with contrast enhancement it may have a beaded appearance.[31] The avascularity of tuberculomas on angiograms contrasts with the marked enhancement seen on CT scans.

Treatment

In 1961, Ramamurthi and Varadarajan[5] advocated an initial trial of medical treatment for selected tuberculomas in the early stages of the disease, this approach being followed by surgery if necessary. A year later, Roedenbeck[35] stated that medical treatment was effective even in the presence of raised intracranial pressure. Most older textbooks and papers espoused surgical excision of the lesion under the cover of antituberculous drugs. In recent years, the indications for surgical intervention have been greatly reduced[21,34] because medical treatment alone may be entirely effective.

Antituberculous Drugs. The drugs generally prescribed nearly always come from a group of six antibiotics known to be effective in treating extracranial tuberculosis (Table 9-1). The first line agents most commonly used are isoniazid and rifampicin (rifampin), which are bactericidal. Streptomycin and pyrazinamide, which also are bactericidal, are the drugs of second choice. Para-aminosalicylic acid (PAS) is seldom used today because of its poor penetrance into the CSF and because of its side effects. Ethambutol usually is used either in combination with isoniazid and rifampicin or as a second line drug. It is a bacteriostatic drug and usually cannot be given for periods longer than 3 or 4 months, whereas drug therapy is usually required for 16 to 18 months.[15,21,34] The optimal duration of treatment is unknown and there are no reports of controlled trials in the treatment of intracranial tuberculomas or tuberculous meningitis.[15] At present, three drugs are administered for the initial 3 or 4 months and two drugs for an additional 12 to 14 months. Usually the regimen involves a combination of rifampicin, isoniazid, and ethambutol or streptomycin for 3

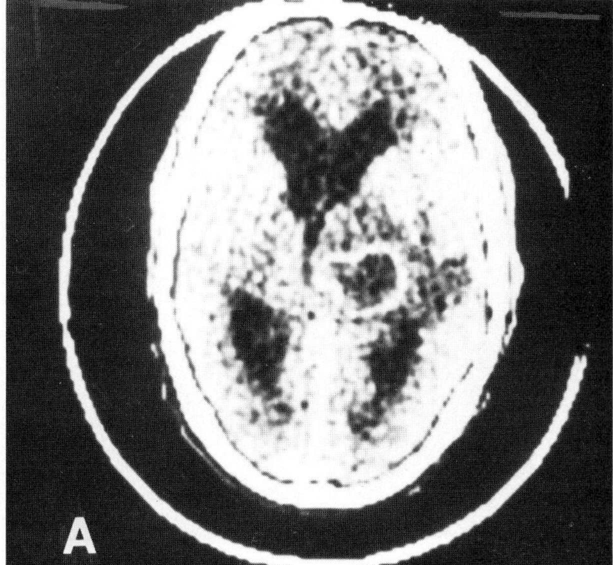

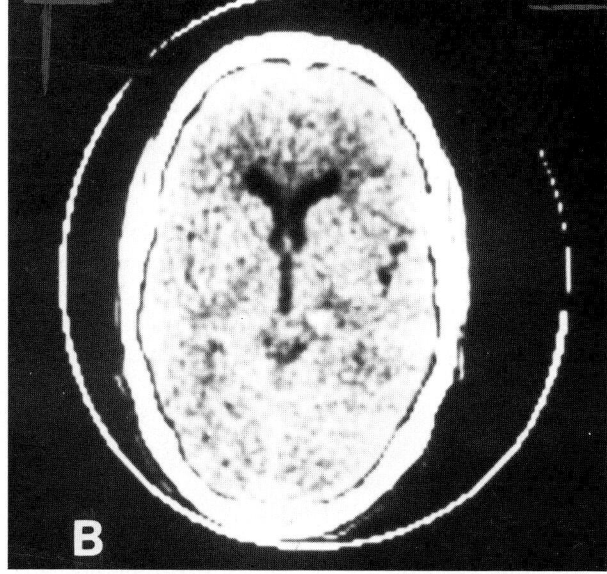

Fig. 9-3. This patient, who had undergone a kidney transplant 2 years earlier and was on regular immunosuppressants, developed hemiparesis over a 10-day period. (A) A contrast-enhanced scan shows a large ring-shaped lesion in the right thalamus. Stereotactic aspiration of pus revealed *Mycobacterium tuberculosis.* The patient improved rapidly on medical therapy. (B) A repeat scan shows almost complete resolution of the lesion.

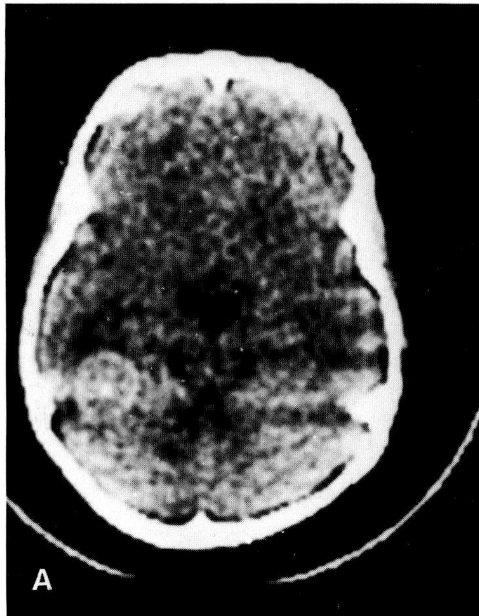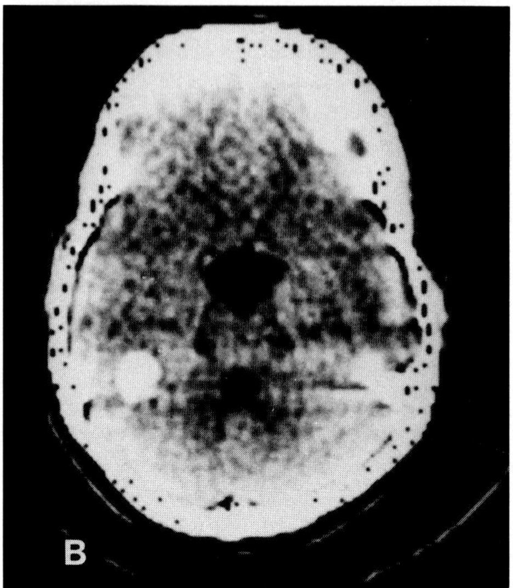

Fig. 9-4. (A) A contrast-enhanced scan of a 7-year-old girl with elevated intracranial pressure and cerebellar signs shows the target sign of a tuberculoma. She became asymptomatic after 6 weeks of medical therapy. (B) A scan made 4 1/2 years later shows only residual calcification.

months followed by isoniazid and rifampicin for an additional 12 to 14 months.

Intracranial tuberculomas may resolve with medical treatment alone (Figures 9-2 and 9-3).[15,21,32] The clinical and radiologic improvement is a result of the reduction of perilesional edema and actual regression of the tuberculoma. Lesions less than 1 cm in diameter on CT scans resolve partially within 4 to 6 weeks of the beginning of therapy with or without the addition of steroids; they often resolve completely within 10 weeks. Larger lesions may also respond readily to antituberculous medication and may resolve completely or nearly so within the same period. In about one third of cases residual evidence of the lesion is a speck of calcification or an area of low attenuation.[21] Medical treatment occasionally may result in liquefaction in the central part of the lesion without any reduction in its size.[36] In a remaining group of cases, the tuberculoma may either show no change or an increase in size.[13] Tuberculomas seem to enlarge and compress the surrounding brain without causing the destruction that is usually associated with a malignant tumor; as a result they can resolve with minimal residual deficits.

Cortiocosteroids. Corticosteroids are used in the presence of elevated intracranial pressure or severe cerebral edema as noted on CT scans. Treatment is seldom prolonged beyond 2 to 3 weeks, during which time corticosteroid therapy can produce dramatic improvement in the clinical state of the patient.

Anticonvulsant Medications. The high incidence of seizures with tuberculomas mandates the routine use of anticonvulsants. The drugs used are phenytoin, phenobarbitone, and carbamazepine, adjusted in dosage according to serum levels of the anticonvulsant. Patients on phenytoin and isoniazid may develop phenytoin toxicity because high levels of isoniazid in the serum can block the metabolism of the anticonvulsant.

Surgical Considerations

A tuberculoma that severely elevates intracranial pressure and threatens life or vision merits emergent surgical excision. With the exception of these lesions, most neurosurgeons familiar with tuberculomas restrict surgical intervention to (1) cases in which there is a lack of clinical or radiologic response to antituberculous drugs; (2) cases in which the diagnosis is in doubt, such as the case of an atypical CT image of the lesion; and (3) cases in which there is the presence of obstructive hydrocephalus.

Complete excision of tuberculomas is generally reserved for smaller lesions in noneloquent areas of the brain that have

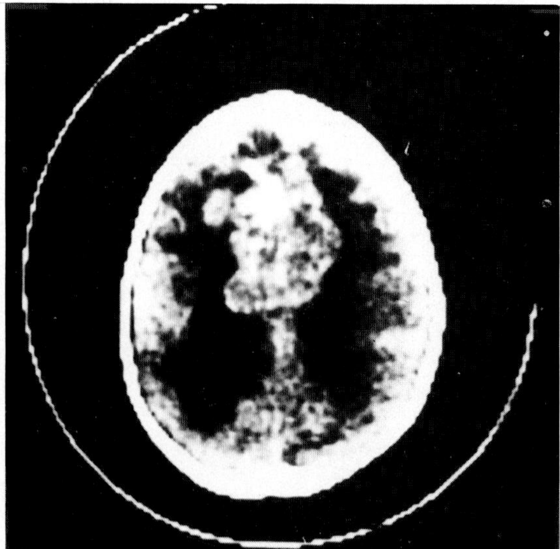

Fig. 9-5. A contrast-enhanced CT scan of a 6-year-old patient shows a large nodular tubercular mass in the corpus callosum. This was confirmed by stereotactic biopsy. The patient was originally diagnosed as having tubercular meningitis.

Table 9-1. Antituberculous Drugs

Drug	Dosage	Contraindications	Side Effects
Isoniazid	Oral or IM; 300 mg/day (adults: 3 mg/kg–10 mg/kg)	Drug-induced liver disease	Peripheral neuritis; convulsions, psychosis
Rifampicin	Oral 450–600 mg (10 mg/kg)	Jaundice, pregnancy	Liver, toxicity, GI symptoms. Rare: shock; Respiratory collapse
Ethambutol	Oral (15 mg/kg)	Optic neuritis	Optic neuritis, Color blindness, peripheral neuritis
Pyrazinamide	Oral (20–30 mg/kg)	Liver damage	
Streptomycin	1M. 1G/day in older patients and children 500–750 mg	Pregnancy	Ototoxicity; renal damage
Para-aminosalicylic acid	Oral 10–15 mg in divided doses	Peptic ulceration	GI disturbances; tinnitis; vertigo; blood dyscracias

been precisely localized on both coronal and sagittal reconstruction CT scans. Larger lesions require subtotal excision when they cause pressure-related symptoms; there is seldom a need for their complete removal. An insistence on total excision at the cost of an undesirable neurologic deficit is to be deprecated. In cases of multiple tuberculomas, only the largest mass need be removed.

An appropriate craniotomy or craniectomy is performed over the site of the lesion. Tuberculomas are generally avascular and readily separable from the surrounding edematous brain because of a clear plane of cleavage.[4,5,6,7,20,28] The edema is usually not as pronounced as that associated with metastatic deposits. Tuberculous lesions are often on the cortical surface and adherent to the overlying dura. Dural adhesions usually can be separated with ease, and the dura need not be excised. Surface tuberculomas attached to the dura at times can be extremely vascular, resembling meningiomas.[5] After the tumor's surface is identified, it is removed in piecemeal fashion, the procedure remaining within the confines of the granuloma. The Cavitron or ultrasonic aspirator is a useful aid to the decompression. En bloc removal is indicated only for small lesions. Where the center is liquefied or necrotic, aspiration of the contents is sufficient; no attempt should be made to excise the capsule.[36] Subcortical lesions are approached through a small corticectomy with preservation of as many vessels as possible. The incision is deepened until a tough gliotic layer is encountered. With the aid of the magnification and illumination provided by an operating microscope, the tuberculoma is decompressed. Parts of the tuberculoma adherent to any of the major venous sinuses are left in situ. The technique of frontal and temporal lobectomy and of ventricular punctures and instillation of streptomycin into the ventricles if they are opened is seldom indicated today.[37] Steroids have been advocated when the ventricles are entered during surgery.[4] Precise localization obviates preliminary needling of the brain, and the excision of edematous brain is seldom necessary to achieve decompression. After several months of antituberculous therapy, the lesion may be tough in consistency and resistant to curetting. If surgical exploration is undertaken for an atypical lesion and a tuberculoma is encountered, minimal surgical manipulation is advised.[36] After hemostasis is achieved, streptomycin powder is placed into the cavity.

Stereotactic biopsy and aspiration guided by CT scanning is the preferred mode of diagnosis and treatment for deep-seated lesions such as those in the thalamus or basal ganglia. Tubercular abscesses or tuberculomas with liquefied centers can be readily decompressed by this method. Atypical lesions may also merit a stereotactic biopsy instead of an open biopsy.[38] We prefer Backlund's biopsy kit for such procedures.

Results

Beginning with reports of a mortality ranging from 10 to 27 percent for intracranial tuberculomas, the results have improved dramatically in recent years. Harder et al.[32] reported no deaths in 20 cases, although 2 patients were lost to follow-up. In our experience,[31] of 50 consecutive cases in which the majority of patients were treated with drugs alone, one patient died in the hospital and one died 2 years after treatment, probably as a result of infection with a drug-resistant organism. Both of these patients had markedly elevated ICP and had multiple intracranial tuberculomas. Moreover, there have been numerous reports of patients with deep-seated inaccessible lesions and lesions in the brain stem who have enjoyed excellent recovery.

TUBERCULOUS MENINGITIS

Tuberculous meningitis, which is common in India and the far East, also remains an important cause of bacterial meningitis in the West.[39] Although considered predominately a disease of childhood, our own experience as well as that of others suggests that currently 50 percent of cases occur in adults. The major neurosurgical interest in tuberculous meningitis is the occurrence of hydrocephalus, which may be as high as 83 percent.[40] Hydrocephalus is almost invariable in children surviving for 4 to 6 weeks and is most often caused by blockage of the basal cisterns and the sylvian fissures by tubercular exudate in the acute phase of the disease. In more chronic phases hydrocephalus is caused by vascular adhesive arachnoiditis. In some cases this may be caused by obstruction at the outlet of the fourth ventricle; less commonly by obstruction at the level of the aqueduct either as a result of circumferential narrowing of the brain stem by exudates or as a result of an intraluminal

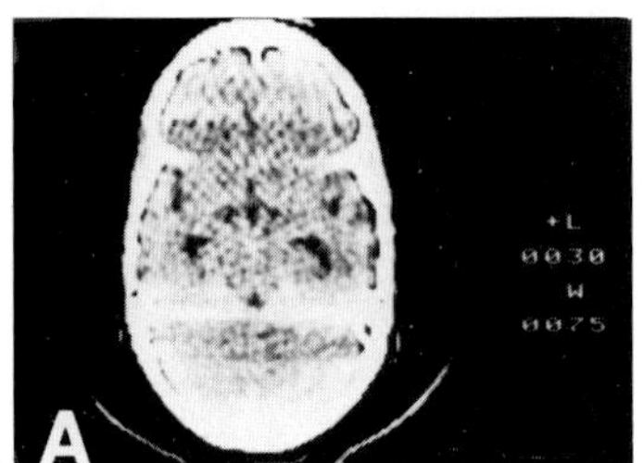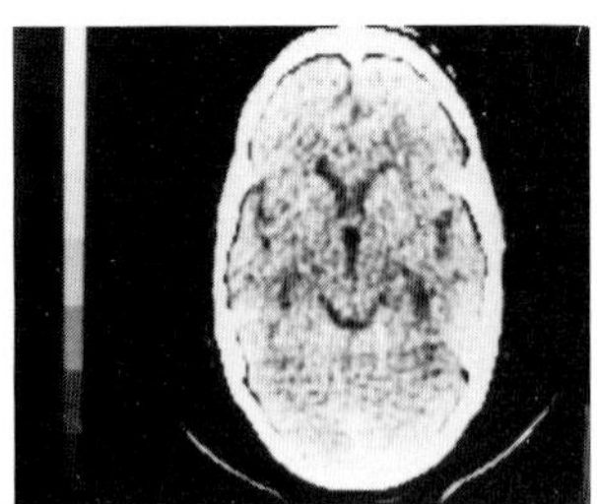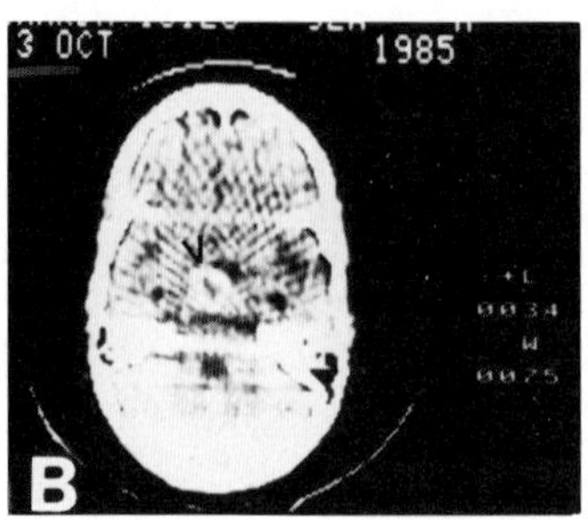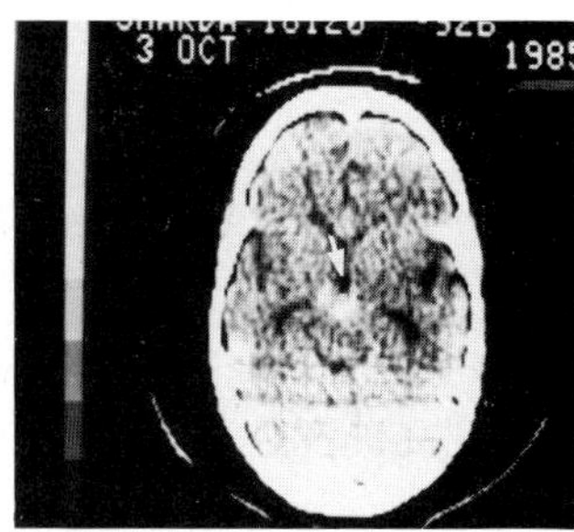

Fig. 9-6. The patient, a 20-year-old man, was treated for tuberculous meningitis. (A) A CT scan shows no definite abnormality. He was placed on medical therapy and improved. He then began to develop ataxia. (B) A repeat CT scan shows a highly attenuating lesion in the midbrain and third ventricle.

tuberculoma. The obstruction to the CSF circulation in tuberculous meningitis often occurs at multiple sites.[41]

Problems of Diagnosis

In a sizable number of patients the diagnosis of tuberculous meningitis still poses considerable difficulties. Examination of cerebrospinal fluid is often inconclusive, tubercle bacilli being found on direct smears in no more than 10 to 15 percent of initial samples. A notable exception was the report of Kennedy and Fallon,[39] who isolated *Mycobacterium tuberculosis* in 83 percent of 52 patients. Several tests have been devised to differentiate tuberculous meningitis from other forms of meningitis including the radioactive bromide partition test, measurement of adenosine deaminase activity in the CSF, and identification of mycobacterial antigen in the CSF by enzyme-linked immunoabsorbent assay (ELISA). Most of these, however, have not had widespread clinical application. More recently, a simpler method of detecting antigen by the later particle agglutination (LPA) test has been reported.[42]

The diagnosis of tuberculous meningitis is made on the presence of two or more of the following criteria: (1) clinical evidence; (2) evidence of CSF cellular and biochemical findings; (3) an associated tubercular focus elsewhere in the body; and (4) the clinical and CSF response of a suspected case to antituberculous treatment.

Computed Tomographic Scans

Computed tomographic scans of tuberculous meningitis demonstrate one or more of the following: (1) exudates in the basal cisterns; (2) hydrocephalus; (3) infarcts; (4) tuberculomas; and (5) edema in the white matter. Exudates that enhance with contrast infusion are characteristic of tuberculous meningitis. The most common sites are the suprasellar cisterns, the cisterna ambiens, and the sylvian fissures. Bhargava et al.[40] observed exudates in each of these regions in 81 percent of the cases. In general, severe grades of exudates are observed only in children. The degree of hydrocephalus correlates well with the duration of the illness; the longer the duration of the illness, the greater the incidence and severity of hydrocephalus. A periventricular lucency on a CT scan, which is usually indicative of transependymal CSF absorption caused by elevated ICP, is, in tuberculous meningitis, more likely to be a result of a spread of the inflammatory process.[43] The degree of hydrocephalus may not reflect the degree of elevation of the intraventricular pressure.

Antituberculous Therapy

The drug therapy for tuberculous meningitis and tuberculomas is similar (see Table 9-1). Controversy exists on the need for intrathecally administering streptomycin in the acute stage of the disease. A recent article concludes that the results are better if intrathecal streptomycin is used routinely.[44] The use of corticosteroids has also been controversial. It is generally accepted that steroids are a useful adjunct in treating (1) children under 1 year of age, (2) severely ill and toxic patients, and (3) those patients threatened with paraplegia. Intrathecal steroids have changed the course of tuberculous meningitis with associated spinal block and impending paraplegia in patients on adequate antituberculous therapy with or without oral corticosteroids.[41]

Surgery

Sir High Cairns first advocated ventricular decompression during the acute stage of meningitis. Since then a variety of procedures have been tried, and reports have conclusively documented the efficacy of ventriculoatrial (VA) or ventriculoperitoneal (VP) shunts for this condition.[26,41,43,45,46] The fear of spreading tubercle bacilli through the shunt is unfounded. Hydrocephalus may resolve under medical treatment alone; however, surgical diversion of CSF is indicated when hydrocephalus is associated with symptomatic elevated intracranial pressure. Surgery during the early acute stage of the disease to obviate the effects of a progressive increase of intraventricular pressure has been advocated.[43]

Ventriculoperitoneal shunts are generally preferred to VA shunts because of the numerous vascular complications associated with VA shunts. An unusual complication of VA shunts that we encountered was the development of chronic pulmonary hypertension. This occurred in 2 adults and 1 child 3 to 5 years after insertion of the shunt. The probable cause is either recurrent pulmonary thromboembolism from the shunt tube in the right atrium or an autoimmune reaction to the tubercular proteins. After insertion of a shunt, there is a progressive reduction in the size of the ventricles but the ventricles may not return to normal size. Uncommonly, while the lateral and third ventricles become smaller, the fourth ventricle remains enlarged and becomes isolated from the rest of the CSF pathways. This leads to pressure on the brain stem. This complication is treated either by deroofing the outlet of the fourth ventricle or inserting a second shunt from the fourth ventricular cavity. Rarely, optochiasmal arachnoiditis may be responsible for development of visual deterioration and may indicate a need for decompression of the optic nerves and chiasm. Cerebral tuberculomas can develop insidiously during treatment of tubercular meningitis (Figure 9-6),[34,47,48] and the patient may succumb as a result of elevated ICP. CT scans are helpful in recognizing and surgically removing these lesions. Infrequently, separate shunts are required from each lateral ventricle

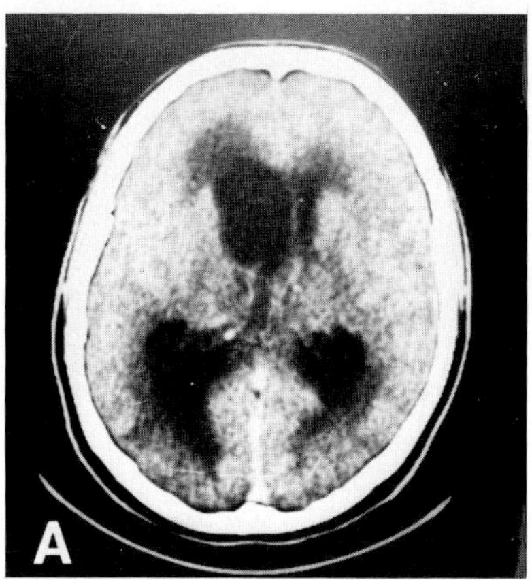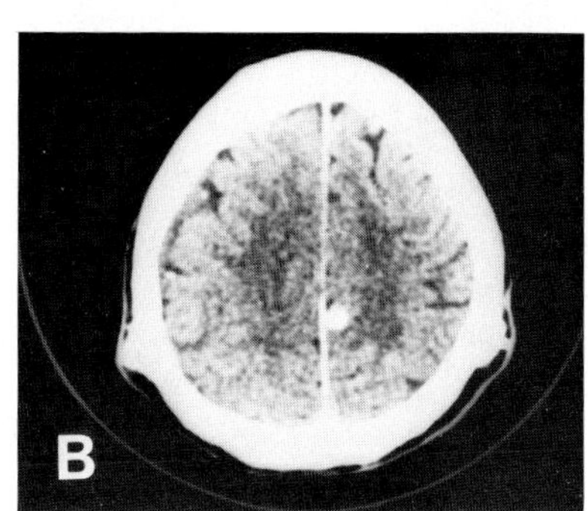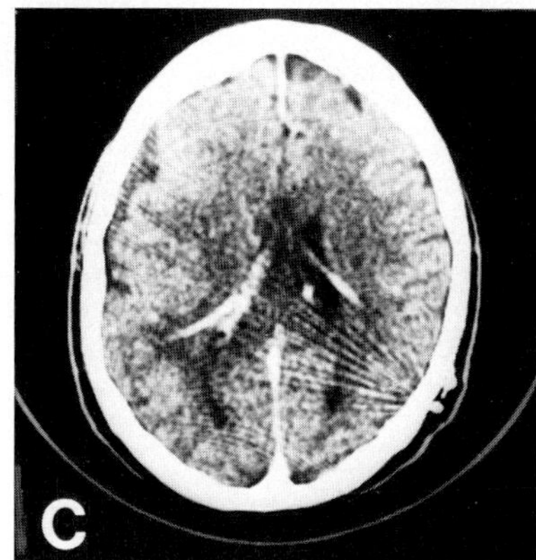

Fig. 9-7. This 52-year-old patient was being treated for tuberculosis and developed elevated intracranial pressure and neck stiffness. CT scans showed (A) hydrocephalus, and (B) a cortical tuberculoma. Noncommunication of the lateral ventricles was apparent on a ventriculogram. Bilateral ventriculoperitoneal shunts were placed and the symptoms rapidly disappeared. (C) A CT scan obtained 2 months later was nearly normal.

if there is a CSF block at the level of the third ventricle (Figure 9-7).

Results

The prognosis of tuberculous meningitis depends upon the patient's level of consciousness, the presence and degree of exudates, and the presence of hydrocephalus. The presence of cerebral infarcts often precludes a good recovery. Among 70 patients with tuberculous meningitis who underwent CSF diversion by a shunt,[46] 12 (17 percent) died; 6 of these patients died in the immediate postoperative period as a result of aspiration, hyperpyrexia, or herniation. The other 6 patients died 7 months to 6 years later of spontaneous intraventricular hemorrhage. Symptoms of raised pressure are relieved and remarkable improvements have been seen even in patients who were barely able to see or who were blind.

CYSTICEROSIS

The highest prevalence rate of cerebral cysticercosis has been reported from the developing countries, Latin America, and parts of Eastern Europe. In Mexico, 2.3 to 3.3 percent of all autopsies and 13 to 33 percent of all intracranial space-occupying lesions (ICSOLs) are caused by cysticercosis.[49] At the All India Institute, 2.5 percent of all verified ICSOLs and 2 percent

of all cases of focal epilepsy are caused by this disease. In a prospective study of 253 cases of late onset epilepsy from the All India Institute, 10.7 percent of the patients had space-occupying lesions and 5.1 percent had cerebral cysticercosis.[50] Infection results from eating the larval form of *Taenia solium* in uncooked or undercooked pork, by ingesting tapeworm eggs in water contaminated with raw sewage or vegetables fertilized with feces, through autoinfection from ano-oral contamination or reverse peristalsis (which allows the proglottides to travel up to the stomach), or direct contact with a tapeworm carrier, since the eggs can be found on clothing, under the fingernails, and on other parts of the body.[51]

PATHOLOGY

After the ova are ingested, the embryos are carried to all parts of the body. Their clinical importance lies in their invasion of the nervous system, muscles, and subcutaneous tissues. The incubation period between infection and development varies from less than 1 year to 30 years; the average interval being about 5 years.[52] Among 66 consecutive surgically verified cases, the following forms were encountered: (1) parenchymal—solitary in 16 percent and multiple in 56 percent; (2) meningeal or racemose—7.4 percent; intraventricular—16.4 percent; and (4) intraspinal or intraorbital—2.8 percent. The

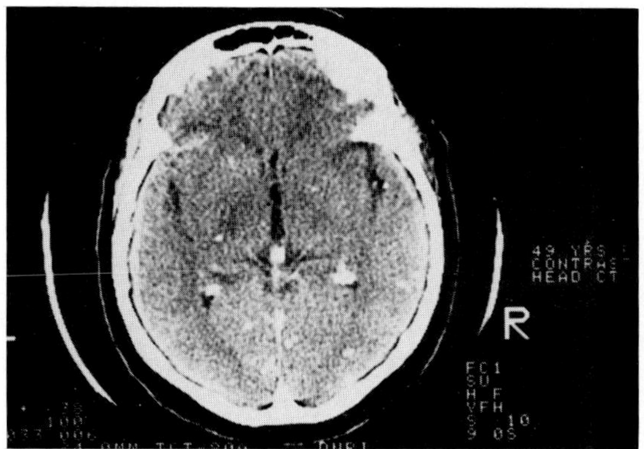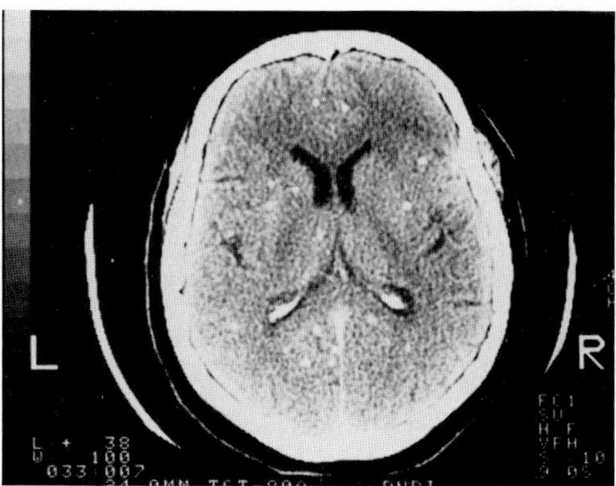

Fig. 9-8. This patient was diagnosed as having pseudotumor cerebri. Lateral subcutaneous nodules appeared. She remained well on regular anticonvulsant medication. A CT scan obtained 15 years after the initial diagnosis shows multiple grainlike calcific spots.

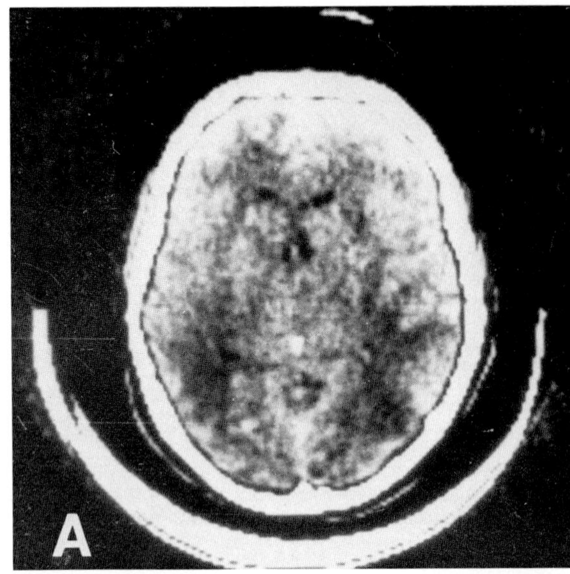

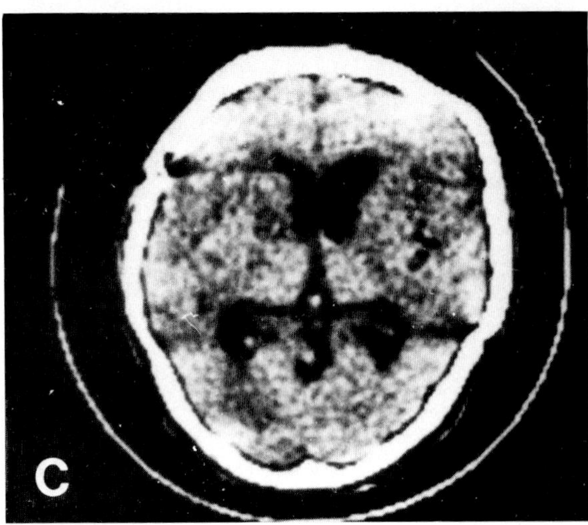

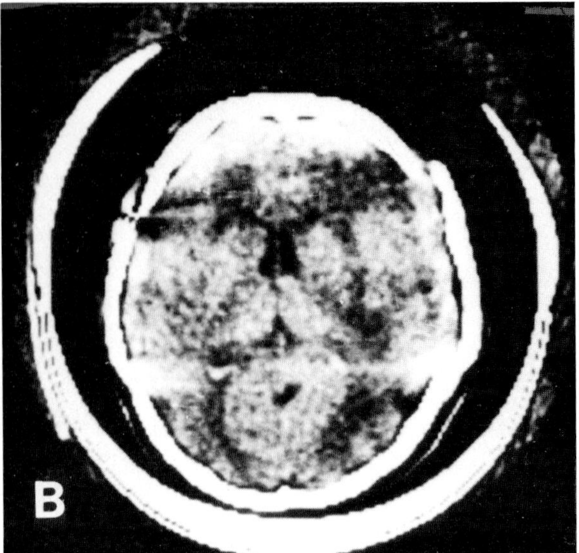

Fig. 9-9. A 19-year-old patient was admitted to the hospital with drowsiness and papilledema. (A) A contrast-enhanced scan shows bilateral edema with throttled ventricles. Bilateral decompression was performed and a biopsy confirmed cysticercosis. Successive scans (B, C) show "opening up" of the ventricles and a decrease in edema.

meningeal or racemose variety, which is the most common type of the disease reported from Mexico and Latin America, was surprisingly uncommon in reports from nearly all the neurosurgical centers in India.

CLINICAL FEATURES

Patients have (1) elevated intracranial pressure, which is a result of diffuse parenchymal involvement and is often labeled pseudotumor cerebri; or obstructive hydrocephalus, which results from an intraventricular cyst or racemose meningeal cysts; (2) focal, multifocal, or generalized seizures; (3) tumor syndrome; (4) meningoencephalitis, and (5) psychiatric disorders. The clinical features depend on the age of the patient, the location of the cysts, the severity of infestation, the duration of illness, and the severity of any allergic or immune response. There is a geographic variation in the relative incidence of the different clinical features. A characteristic aspect of the disease is the occurrence of unexplained spontaneous remissions and relapses.

DIAGNOSIS

Subcutaneous nodules are common, and cysts occasionally can be seen in an eye or in the tongue. The cysts often appear in crops. Eosinophilia in the blood and CSF is an infrequent

accompaniment. The current immunologic tests and specific radioimmunoassays are unreliable.[49,53]

The incidence of elevated ICP in plain x-ray films of the skull ranges from 9.8 to 50 percent in different series. Patients with epilepsy only have a low incidence of such findings compared with patients with the tumor syndrome. Calcification ranges from 2.8 to 39 percent, is nonspecific, and seldom exceeds 3 mm in diameter. However, multiple sago-grain calcifications occurring in a patient from an endemic area is a characteristic finding of cysticercosis (Figure 9-8).

Bhargava[54] has written an excellent account of the CT findings in cysticercosis. In the diffuse parenchymal variety, the CT scan is characterized by extensive bilateral areas of low attenuation in the white matter ranging in value from +5 to +10 Hounsfield units. The cortex stands out in contrast and the ventricles are invariably "throttled" by the surrounding edema. This picture is characteristic of neurocysticercosis and is seldom seen in any other condition (Figure 9-9). In some cases, single or multiple highly attenuating lesions 1 to 3 mm in size and occasionally small ring lesions are seen (Figure 9-10). Whether these lesions represent abnormal vascularity, an inflammatory response, or indeed, some other process is not known. Focal lesions in the parenchyma often appear as larger ring lesions or as highly attenuating nonspecific lesions that are indistinguishable from granulomas or abscesses. Intraventricular cysts do not enhance with contrast and cannot be distinguished from the CSF. A disproportionately large fourth ventricle with evidence of obstructive hydrocephalus would suggest the diagnosis in endemic areas. On positive contrast ventriculograms the entire smooth-lined cyst is outlined by the contrast material (Figure 9-11). It is usually difficult to visualize racemose cysts unless they are large and distort the basal cisterns. Ocular and orbital lesions appear as nonspecific cystic lesions and are invariably accompanied by intracerebral lesions. Spinal cysticerci are rare and appear as intramedullary lesions. Extradural cysticercus granulomas have also been reported.

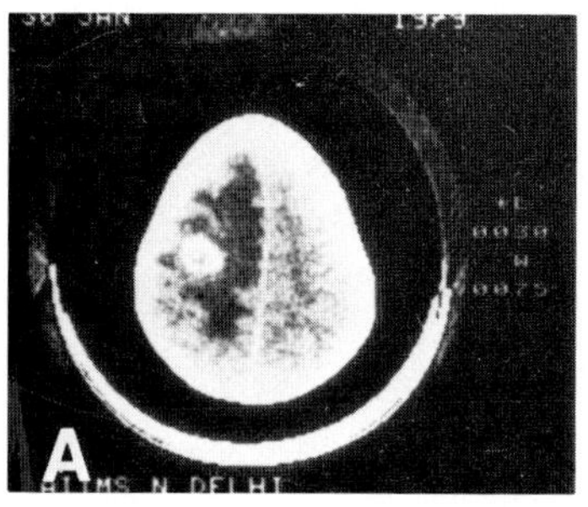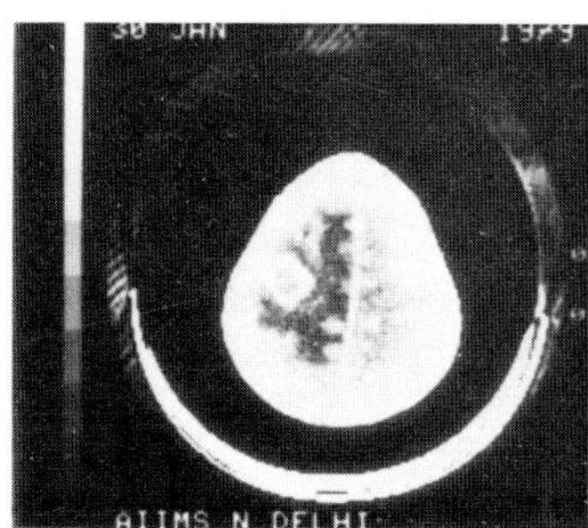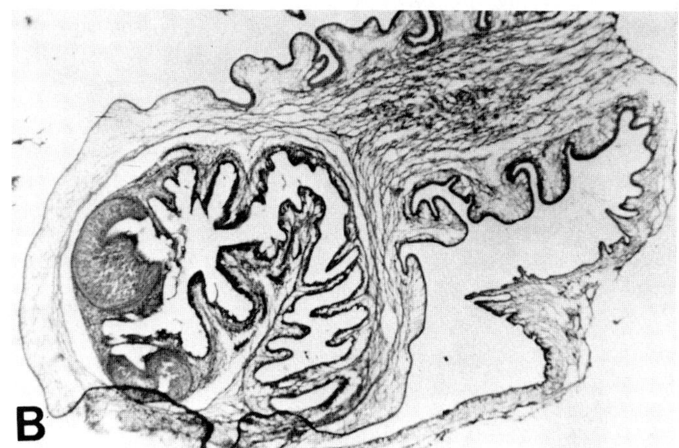

Fig. 9-10. This 22-year-old patient had a seizure disorder of recent onset. (A) A CT scan showed a single nodule with edema. (B) Surgical excision produced a typical cysticercus cyst.

MANAGEMENT

Drug Therapy

Until the introduction of praziquantel,[55] medical therapy was limited to control of the raised ICP and seizures. Praziquantel in doses of 50 mg/kg body weight for 10–15 days can markedly reduce the size of the brain cysts. Great caution needs to be exercised in administering this drug to patients with elevated ICP, since the intracranial pressure may rise alarmingly. One of our patients died after a single dose of praziquantel. This drug is of little value in the treatment of intraventricular cysts (and, in fact, may be hazardous because of cyst expansion), and calcified lesions without cerebral edema or elevated ICP. Other drugs that have been used in the treatment of cysticercosis include niclosamide and mebendazole. Niclosamide only effects the worm in the intestine; mebendazole may have therapeutic value in the treatment of CNS disease at a dosage of 400–600 mg daily for 4 weeks.

Surgery

The intraventricular lesions are mostly solitary cysts, which are often large in size, although multiple cysts also occur.[49,56]

Lateral ventricular cysts can be approached through a transcortical incision in the appropriate frontal lobe or through a transcallosal route.[56] Because the cysts are soft there is seldom need to decompress them, and they can be removed with ease. Cyst rupture does not pose a danger.[56] Occasionally they may be adherent to the choroid plexus. The septum pellucidum must be fenestrated to offer an alternative drainage pathway.

Cysts in the third ventricle are approached by a similar transventricular incision. The cyst appears to peep out of the foramen of Monro. The foramen does not need to be enlarged and because of the pressure differential, the cyst slips into the lateral ventricle. An alternative approach through the transcallosal interfornicial or the lamina terminalis can be used. Intraventricular cysts can migrate; this can lead to acute and lethal complications. Moreover, cyst migration is a potential surgical pitfall. Stereotactic endoscopic excision under CT guidance of a mobile cyst has been successful.[56] Ependymitis in association with a cyst in the third ventricle may necessitate bilateral VP shunts.

In treating cysts in the fourth ventricle, a preliminary VP shunt or external ventricular drainage is desirable. A limited

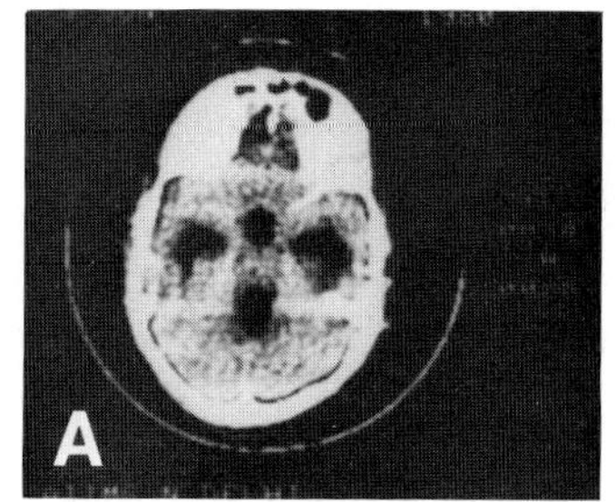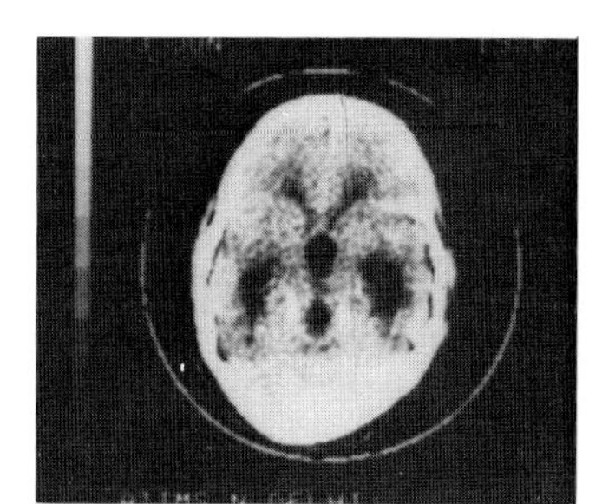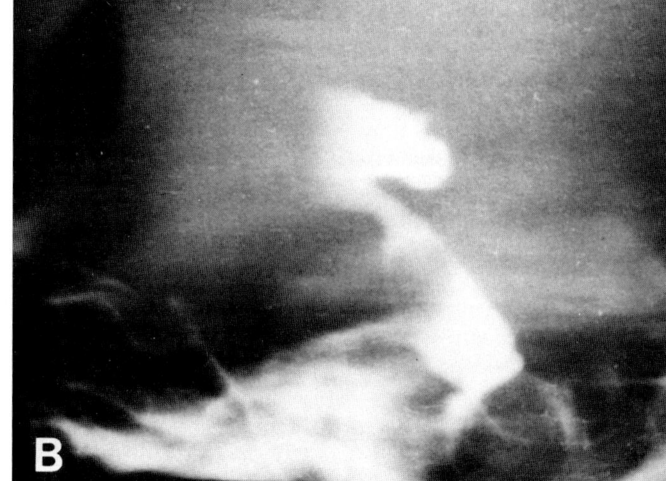

Fig. 9-11. Cysticercosis in the fourth ventricle. (A) A CT scan shows dilation of the fourth ventricle. (B) A ventriculogram shows a typical filling defect.

Table 9-2. Fungi identified in 27 consecutive patients in the Neurology and Neurosurgery services, All India Institute of Medical Sciences Hospital, 1965–1985

Fungi	Number of Patients
Aspergillus	14
Cryptococcus	7
Cladosporium	3
Mucor	2
Undentified	1

Table 9-3. Clinical features in 20 patients with intracranial fungal lesions, 1965–1985

Clinical Sign	Number of Patients
Elevated intracranial pressure	15
Drowsiness	10
Epilepsy	7
Impaired vision	5
Fever	5
Skin lesion	2
Proptosis	1
Nasal obstruction	1

suboccipital craniectomy subsequently is carried out with the patient in the sitting position. The arch of atlas is preserved. The tonsils are freed from the arachnoid, which may be adherent, and carefully separated. The lower part of the floor of the fourth ventricle is inspected; the cyst often will appear to bulge out. If the cyst is not visible initially, gentle retraction of the vermis and a slightly increased positive pressure in the expiratory phase will help to deliver the cyst. A small portion of the inferior vermis may need to be incised.

Localized parenchymal lesions, granulomas, or ring lesions require excisional or stereotactic biopsy, particularly when the diagnosis is in doubt. Intraventricular and meningeal cysticercosis may be associated with ventriculitis, which can result in double compartment hydrocephalus. This phenomenon is particularly observed in the fourth ventricle.[56] Extensive bilateral decompression rather than subtemporal decompression employing large bone flaps becomes necessary if symptoms of elevated pressure do not abate with drug therapy. The tense dura is incised, and the diagnosis usually becomes apparent. After biopsy of a cyst, a pericranial graft is used to bridge the dural gap. The bone flaps are replaced but not anchored. This allows the patient to survive the crisis and any subsequent relapses (Figure 9-9).

RESULTS

Patients with solitary intraventricular cysts and localized granulomas have a good prognosis, whereas patients with diffuse parenchymal disease and elevated ICP have a guarded prognosis. Patients with mature or calcified lesions who have epilepsy but do not have elevated ICP or brain edema are managed on long-term anticonvulsant therapy alone. Mortality ranges from 3 to 5.8 per thousand cases, deaths being caused by status epilepticus and intracranial hypertension.[52]

FUNGAL INFECTIONS

Until the advent of acquired immune deficiency syndrome (AIDS) and immunosuppressed hosts, fungal infections of the CNS were uncommon and therefore seldom considered in the differential diagnosis of space-occupying lesions of the brain or of chronic meningitis. In a large percentage of cases, the diagnosis is based on the morphology of the fungus in the tissues because by the time a histologic diagnosis is made, the formalin renders the tissue unsuitable for culture. It is also impossible to distinguish between different forms of fungi with certainty on the basis of the morphology of the lesion at surgery.

PATHOLOGIC FEATURES

Although more than 60 species of fungi have been identified as pathogenic to humans, those than come under the purview of the neurosurgeon are very few. These include *Cryptococcus neoformans, Cladosporium bantianum,* and species of *Aspergillus, Mucor,* and *Candida* (Table 9-2). The fungi usually enter the body through the respiratory system by inhalation of aerosolized fungi from the paranasal sinuses, the middle ear, or the skin. A primary focus of infection, which is often subclinical, is established in the lungs. The infection then spreads hematogenously.[57–60] Susceptibility to infection is facilitated by an altered immunity on the part of the host as a result of coexisting diseases such as a leukemia, diabetes, and lymphomas; immunosuppressive therapy, broad spectrum antibiotics, and cytotoxic drugs.[57,58]

Depending upon the tissue reaction and associated disease, fungal infections of the nervous system take three main forms. The first type of infection produces a chronic granulomatous reaction leading to a focal granuloma or abscess or, if in the basal meninges, obstructive hydrocephalus. Most of these patients have a long history of symptoms. The second type of infection produces diffuse cerebritis, often with areas of hemorrhagic infarction of the brain, microabscess formation, and intense cerebral edema. The history in these patients is usually short, often less than 7 to 10 days, and the clinical suspicion of a rapidly growing brain tumor or abscess is raised. The third type of infection produces signs similar to those of the second except that, in addition, the patients also usually have an underlying serious disease.

DIAGNOSTIC PROBLEMS

1. The illness is often a chronic one, often lasting several year and the mildness of the initial symptoms may be misleading. Among 20 cases at the All India Institute (Table 9-3), fever was present in only 5 patients and evidence of paranasal sinus infection or orbital and skin involvement in only 2 patients.
2. The CT findings in focal granulomas are not distinctive.[59,61,62] A clue may be provided by involvement of the paranasal sinuses, the orbit, and the frontal bone. The granulomas are indistinguishable from brain tumors and even tuberculomas.[61,63] Certainly there are no features by which to distinguish a fungal abscess from a pyogenic abscess (Figures 9-12, 9-13, and 9-14).
3. The diagnosis of a solitary fungal granuloma is seldom made with confidence preoperatively or even intraopera-

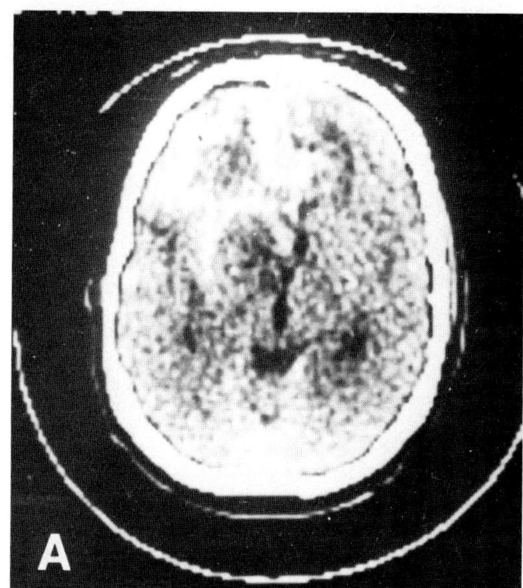 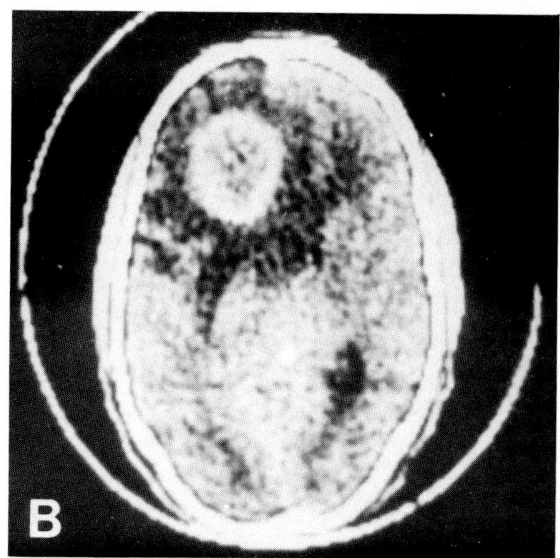

Fig. 9-12. Aspergillosis. (A) In this patient the aspergillosis appears as a diffuse frontal mass. (B) In this patient the aspergillosis appears as a well-defined enhancing lesion.

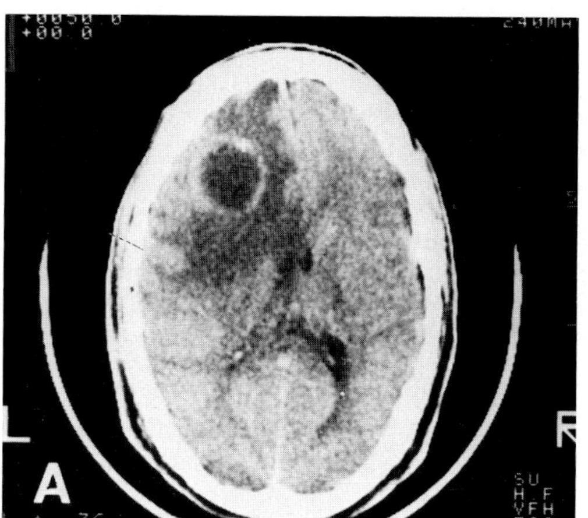 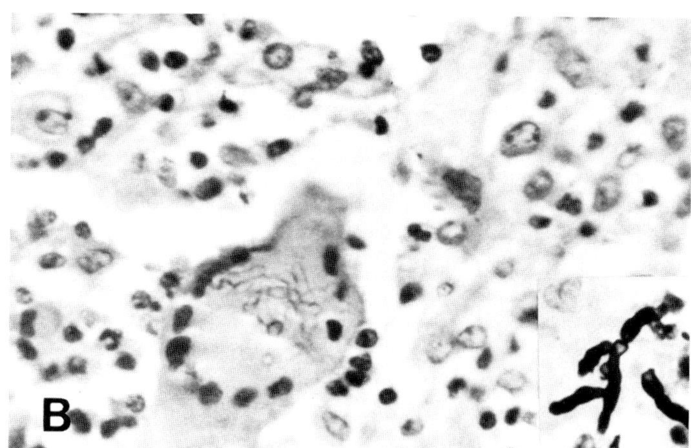

Fig. 9-13. Cladosporium abscess in a 40-year-old patient. (A) A CT scan shows a typical abscess. (B) A photomicrograph of the fungal abscess. Note the giant cells containing fungal hyphae. Inset: specimen stained with silver methiamine showing branching hyphae. Magnification: X240.

tively. There is both a macroscopic and microscopic resemblance to tuberculomas. The difficulty is compounded when the fungi in the tissue are few. The presence of numerous foreign body giant cells and fibrosis and the conspicuous absence of caseation necrosis may arouse a suspicion of a possible fungal etiology. Routine examination of pus from an abscess for fungi is useful even when a pyogenic organism has been isolated.

MANAGEMENT

Drugs

In the management of fungal infections of the CNS, amphotericin B and flucytosine remain the first line of drug therapy.[57,59,62] Amphotericin has a wider spectrum and is administered intravenously, intrathecally, or intraventricularly through an Ommaya reservoir.[57] The starting dose is 250 µg/kg/day; this dosage is gradually increased if tolerated to 1 mg/kg. The maximum dose in severely ill patients is 1.5 mg/kg daily or on alternate days dissolved in 500 ml 5-percent glucose in a very slow drip. These patients usually also receive steroids. Since the drug is nephrotoxic, frequent determinations of the levels of blood urea and serum creatinine are required. Toxicity is reduced by giving the patient an intravenous infusion of mannitol. Nausea, vomiting, fever, and hypokalemia are common side effects. Flucytosine has a narrower spectrum, is less toxic, and, unlike amphotericin B, can be absorbed orally. It is given at a dose of 150–200 mg/kg/day in divided doses. This drug is toxic to the liver and blood. The imidazole group of antifungal drugs, miconazole[64] and ketoconazole, have been used to treat CNS infections with anecdotal success.

SURGERY

Surgery (Table 9-4) is indicated for focal granulomas or abscesses and in cases of obstructive hydrocephalus. Fungal granulomas resemble tuberculomas except they tend to have a more fibrous consistency. They often need to be cut with a knife or scissors and resist curetting. The clear plane of cleavage seen

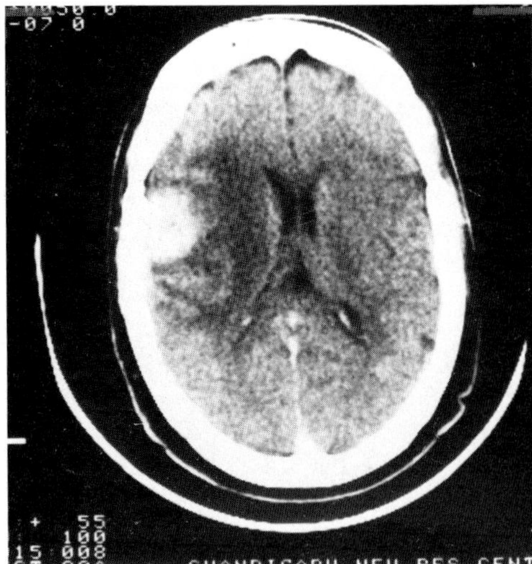

Fig. 9-14. Cryptococcal granuloma in a 56-year-old patient. The patient had been treated for a tuberculoma and the lack of response mandated excision.

Table 9-4. Surgical management of fungal lesions, 1965-1985

Procedure	Number of Patients
Excision of lesion:	
Granuloma	13
Abscess	4
Bilateral decompression	1
Ventriculoperitoneal shunt	3*
Decompression of sequestrated ventricle	1

*Two patients received shunts in addition to excision of the lesion.

with tuberculomas usually is not present, and adherence to the dura is firmer. Unlike tuberculomas, a fungal granuloma should be completely excised whenever possible. If pus aspirated from an abscess reveals evidence of a fungal infection, the abscess needs to be excised. Deep-seated lesions in the basal ganglia and thalamus are best stereotactically biopsied or aspirated. Ventriculoperitoneal shunts may be necessary to relieve symptoms of elevated ICP. Cryptococcal meningoencephalitis may appear as pseudotumor cerebri with narrowed ventricles requiring bilateral decompression. Antifungal drugs are complimentary to surgical therapy. However, we treated 4 patients with surgery alone. The results were good with follow-up ranging from 5 to 10 years.

ACKNOWLEDGMENTS

We are grateful to Professor S. Bhargava, Director of Radiology, All India Institute of Medical Sciences, for neuroradiologic assistance, and to Professor A. K. Banerji, who operated on many of these patients and was a constant source of new ideas on their management. Thank are due to Dr. V. S. Mehta and Dr. A. K. Mahapatra, who rendered help in many ways. The secretarial help of Miss Bimla Rani is gratefully acknowledged.

REFERENCES

1. Davidson PT: Tuberculosis—New views of an old issue. N Engl J Med 312:1514, 1985
2. Tang LM, Swash M: Tuberculosis of the nervous system, a modern problem. J R Soc Med 78:429, 1985
3. Lalitha VS, Dastur DK: Tuberculosis of the central nervous system. II. Brain tuberculomas vis-a-vis intracranial space-occupying lesions, 1953–1978. Neurol India 28:202, 1980
4. Mathai KV, Chandy J: Tuberculous infection of the nervous system. Clin Neurosurg 14:145, 1966
5. Ramamurthi B, Varadarajan MG: Diagnosis of tuberculomas of the brain. J Neurosurg 18:1, 1961
6. Asenjo A, Valladeres H, Fierro J: Tuberculoma of the brain. Arch Neurol 65:146, 1951
7. Arseni C: Two hundred and one cases of tuberculoma treated surgically. J Neurol Neurosurg Psychiatry 21:308, 1958
8. Ohaegbulam SC, Amuta J, Saddeqi N: Tuberculoma of the central nervous system in Eastern Nigeria. Tubercle 60:163, 1979
9. Tang LM, Chee CY, Cheng SY, et al: Neurological complications of tuberculous meningitis, in: 6th Asian and Occanian Congress of Neurology Abstracts. Amsterdam, Excerpta Medica, 1983, pp 93–94
10. Katsura S, Suzuki J, Wada T: A statistical study of brain tumors in the neurosurgical clinics of Japan. J Neurosurg 16:570, 1959
11. Peatfield RC, Shawdon HH: Five cases of intracranial tuberculoma followed by serial computerized tomography. J Neurol Neurosurg Psychiatry 42:373, 1979
12. Maurice-Williams RS: Tuberculomas of the brain in Britain. Postgrad Med J 48:678, 1972
13. Chambers ST, Hendrickse WA, Record C, et al: Paradoxical expansion of intracranial tuberculomas during chemotherapy. Lancet 1:181, 1984
14. Anderson JM, MacMillan JJ: Intracranial tuberculoma—an increasing problem in Britain. J Neurol Neurosurg Psychiatry 38:194, 1975
15. Mayers MM, Kaufman DM, Miller MH: Recent cases of intracranial tuberculomas. Neurology 28:256, 1978
16. Hirsch LF, Lee SH, Silberstein SD: Intracranial tuberculoma and the CAT scan. Acta Neurochir 45:155, 1978
17. Wilkinson HA, Ferris EJ, Muggia AL, et al: Central nervous system tuberculosis. A persistant disease. J Neurosurg 34:15, 1971
18. Leibrock L, Epstein MH, Rybock JD: Cerebral tuberculoma localized by EMI scan. Surg Neurol 5:305, 1976
19. Lehrer H, Venkatesh B, Girolamo R, et al: Tuberculoma of the brain (revisited). AJR 118:594, 1973
20. Dastur HM: Tuberculoma, in Vinken PJ, Bruyn GW (eds): Handbook of Clinical Neurology, vol 18. New York, Elsevier, 1975, pp 413–426
21. Tandon PN, Bhargava S: Effect of medical treatment on intracranial tuberculoma—a CT study. Tubercle 66:85, 1985
22. Mahanta A, Kalra L, Maheshwari MC, et al: Brain stem tuberculoma—an unusual presentation. J Neurol 227:249, 1982
23. Dastur DK: Neurosurgically relevant aspects of pathology and pathogenesis of intracranial and intraspinal tuberculosis. Neurosurg Rev 6:103, 1983
24. Sinh G, Pandya SK, Dastur DK: Pathogenesis of unusual intracranial tuberculomas and tuberculous space-occupying lesions. J Neurosurg 29:149, 1968
25. Sandhyamani S, Roy S, Bhatia R: Tuberculous brain abscess. Acta Neurochir 59:247, 1981
26. Tandon PN, Singh B, Mohapatra LN, et al: Experimental tubeculosis of the central nervous system. Neurol India 19:81, 1970
27. Dannenberg AM Jr, Sugimoto M: Liquefaction of caseous foci in tuberculosis. Am Rev Respir Dis 113:257, 1976
28. Tandon PN, Pathak SN: Tuberculosis of the central nervous system, in Spillane JD (ed): Tropical Neurology. London, Oxford University Press, 1973, pp 51–62
29. Dastur HM, Desai AD: A comparative study of brain tuberculomas

and gliomas based upon 107 case records of each. Brain 88:375, 1965

30. Bhargava S, Tandon PN: CNS tuberculosis—lessons learnt from CT studies. Neurol India 28:207, 1980

31. Bhargava S, Tandon PN: Intracranial tuberculomas—a CT study. Br J Radiol 53:935, 1980

32. Harder E, Al-Kawl MZ, Carney P: Intracranial tuberculomas—conservative management. Am J Med 74:570, 1983

33. Welchman JM: Computerized tomography of intracranial tuberculomata. Clin Radiol 30:567, 1979

34. Lees AJ, MacLeod AF, Marshall J: Cerebral tuberculomas developing during treatment of tuberculous meningitis. Lancet 1:1208, 1980

35. Roedenbeck SD: Tuberculomas of the nervous system in children. World Neurol 3:55, 1962

36. Pandya SK, Desai AD, Dastur HM: Caseative liquefaction within brain stem tuberculoma under drug therapy with simultaneous regression of cerebral tuberculomas. Neurol India 30:121, 1982

37. Descuns P, Garre H, Pheline C: Tuberculoma of the brain and cerebellum. J Neurosurg 11:243, 1954

38. Case Records of the Massachusetts General Hospital: Case 48-1984. N Engl J Med 311:1425, 1984

39. Kennedy DH, Fallon RJ: Tuberculous meningitis. JAMA 241:264, 1984

40. Bhargava S, Gupta AK, Tandon PN: Tuberculous meningitis—a CT study. Br J Radiol 55:189, 1982

41. Tandon PN: Tuberculous meningitis (cranial and spinal), in Vinken PJ, Bruyn GW (eds): Handbook of Clinical Neurology, vol 33. Amsterdam, North Holland, 1978, pp 195–262

42. Anonymous: A new diagnostic test for tuberculous meningitis. 66:157, 1985

43. Bullock MRR, Van Dellen JR: The role of cerebrospinal fluid shunting in tuberculous meningitis. Surg Neurol 18:274, 1982

44. Anonymous: Tuberculous meningitis in children. Br Med J 1:1, 1971

45. Bhagwati SN: Ventriculoatrial shunts in tuberculous meningitis with hydrocephalus. J Neurosurg 35:309, 1971

46. Upadhyaya P, Bhargava S, Sandaram KP, et al: Hydrocephalus caused by tuberculous meningitis—clinical picture, CT findings, and results of shunt surgery. Z Kinderchir 38:76, 1983

47. Borah NC, Maheshwari MC, Mishra NK, et al: Appearance of tuberculoma during the course of TB meningitis. J Neurol 231:269, 1984

48. Lebas J, Malkin JE, Coquin Y, et al: Cerebral tuberculomas developing during treatment of tuberculous meningitis. Lancet 2:84, 1980

49. Tandon PN: Cerebral cysticercosis. Neurosurg Rev 6:119, 1983

50. Ahuja GK, Mohanta A: Late onset epilepsy—a prospective study. Acta Neurol Scand 66:216, 1982

51. Richards F Jr, Schantz PM: Cysticercosis and taeniasis. N Engl J Med 312:787, 1985

52. Dixon HBF, Lipscomb FM: Cysticercosis, An Analysis and Follow-up of 450 Cases. Privy Council Medical Research Council Special Report Series No. 299. London, Her Majesty's Stationery Office, 1961, pp 1–58

53. McCormick GF, Zee CS, Heiden J: Cysticercosis cerebri, a review of 127 cases. Arch Neurol 39:534, 1982

54. Bhargava S: Radiology—including computed tompgraphy—of parasitic diseases of the central nervous system. Neurosurg Rev 6:129, 1983

55. Nash TE, Neva FA: Recent advances in the diagnosis and treatment of cerebral cysticercosis. N Engl J Med 311:1492, 1984

56. Apuzzo MC, Dobkin WR, Zee CS, et al: Surgical considerations in the treatment of intraventricular cysticercosis. An analysis of 45 cases. J Neurosurg 60:400, 1984

57. Utz JP: Fungal infections of the central nervous system. Clin Neurosurg 14:86: 1966

58. Mohandas S, Ahuja GK, Sood VP, et al: Aspergillosis of the central nervous system. J Neurol Sci 38:229, 1978

59. Mehta VS, Bhatia R, et al: Intracranial mycotic infection in nonimmunosuppressed individuals. J Ind Med Assoc 83:185, 1985

60. Deshpande DH, Desai AP, Dastur HM: Aspergillosis of the central nervous system. Neurol India 23:167, 1975

61. Tully RJ, Watts C: Computed tomography and intracranial aspergillosis. Neuroradiology 17:111, 1979

62. Sapico FL: Disappearance of focal cryptoccoccal brain lesion on chemotherapy alone. Lancet 1:560, 1979

63. Harper CG: Cryptococcal granuloma presenting as a mass lesion. Surg Neurol 11:425, 1979

64. Weinstein L, Jacoby L: Successful treatment of cerebral cryptococoma and meningitis with miconazole. Ann Intern Med 93:569, 1980

CHAPTER 10

Neurosurgical Aspects of Neurocysticercosis

Francisco Escobedo

MOST PARASITES THAT REACH NERVOUS TISSUE do so hematogenously. Considering the number of parasites that exist, it is surprising that so few cases of CNS invasion occur. This is probably the result of the protection afforded by the blood–brain barrier.[1]

The most important determinant affecting the incidence of parasitic diseases is the hygienic character of the environment. These diseases are seen more frequently in countries in which sanitary control of the water supply, agricultural systems, and food handling is poor. A tropical climate also favors the development of some parasites, and these disorders have often been considered tropical diseases. However, parasitic disorders are being seen increasingly in industrialized nations because of the migration of infected persons from endemic areas. Parasitic infections of the central nervous system have spread to groups and countries in which such diseases previously were rare.[2,3] Parasitic diseases affecting the CNS include amebiasis, malaria, coenurosis, echinococcosis, schistosomiasis, paragonimiasis, trichinosis, filariasis, angiostrongyliasis, *Toxocara canis* encephalitis, and gnathostomiasis. Most of these disorders are not subject to surgical treatment. The discussion in this chapter is restricted to cysticercosis, which is the most common of these disorders affecting the CNS.

CYSTICERCOSIS

Human cysticercosis results when a person serves as the intermediate host of *Taenia solium*, the porcine tapeworm; the larvae develop in various body tissues. The presence of the encysted larvae in the nervous tissue, its cavities, or its coverings constitutes the disease known as neurocysticercosis. The cysts are called *Cysticercus cellulosae*.[4]

Taenia solium infestation is endemic in parts of Asia (India, China), Africa, Eastern Europe, Indonesia, and Latin America. Cases occur sporadically in other parts of the world. The incidence varies according to the economic and social condition as reflected in the level of hygiene of a region, with the lower socioeconomic groups having a higher incidence of the disease.[1,2,3]

In Mexico, between 5 and 10 percent of all patients requiring surgery on the CNS are operated upon for cysticercosis. These patients constitute approximately 25 percent of all patients operated on for increased intracranial pressure.[5] In a study we conducted at the Institute of Neurology

and Neurosurgery in Mexico between 1964 and 1969, 206 cases were diagnosed; this corresponded to 3.1 percent of all patients undergoing neurologic surgery in those years. Fifty-three percent of these patients required surgical therapy. Of the 206 cases, 153 improved, 27 remained unchanged, and 26 died.[6] A second study conducted between 1977 and 1981 yielded 753 patients with neurocysticercosis confirmed by cerebrospinal fluid examination, computed tomography, surgery, or autopsy.[7] This chapter is based on our experience in the management of almost 1000 cases of neurocysticercosis.

THE PARASITE AND ACQUISITION OF INFECTION

In the usual cycle of transmission, only the pig harbors the larval stage of *T. solium*; human beings acquire the adult tapeworm by eating undercooked pork. The larval infection is acquired through the ingestion of food contaminated with *T. solium* eggs, each containing an active embryo or oncosphere. The oncospheres are liberated by digestive juices. They then penetrate the wall of the small intestine and burrow into the venules and lymphatics. From here they are carried to distant sites. The organisms lodge in various tissues, mainly muscle, skin, brain, and eye, and, once there, develop into larvae, the cysticerci, in 60 to 70 days. These cysticerci have an ovoid form and are about half an inch in diameter, consisting of a very fragile membrane, fluid, and a scolex with suckers and hooks. The cysts can live in tissue for long periods of time. Should they die and degenerate, a lipocalcareous infiltration will develop and become calcified. During this entire process, lasting months or years, the cysts can produce clinical manifestations in the host.[1,2,3]

PATHOPHYSIOLOGY

Cysticerci most commonly lodge in the brain and skeletal muscle. The larvae vary in size from about 5 mm up to 5 cm. Cysticerci can lodge in the parenchyma of the brain (around 60 percent), the subarachnoid space (meningobasal and cortical; around 40 percent), the ventricular system (around 10 percent), mixed areas (more than 50 percent), and the spine (near 1 percent). The location of these lesions determines the clinical manifestations.[1,5,8]

The clinical manifestations of this disease are the result of

OPERATIVE NEUROSURGICAL TECHNIQUES
ISBN 0-8089-1862-1

Table 10-1. Symptoms and signs
of neurocysticercosis*

Focal effect
Mass effect
Inflammatory response:
On nervous tissue
On meninges-arachnoid
On vessels
Hydrocephalus caused by obstruction:
Of foramina
Of aqueduct
Of cisterns
Of subarachnoid space

*All of these processes may coexist in the same patient.

the inflammatory response to the cysticerci in the nervous tissue, the meninges, or the vessels, the focal effect, the mass effect, and the effect of obstruction of the foramina, ventricular system, subarachnoid space, and cisterns of the brain. These processes can coexist in the same patient (Table 10-1). The combination of these factors and the distribution of the lesions makes neurocysticercosis a pleomorphic disease. Except when there is acute massive exposure, symptoms only appear after a latent period of a few years. This is because in most cases viable cysts incite little inflammatory response on the part of the host.[1,6,9]

The number of cysts, the duration of the illness, the location of cerebral cysticerci, their enlargement, and the local inflammatory response they provoke can lead to a clinical syndrome with focal neurologic manifestations, cranial nerve palsies, or a tumorlike presentation. When a cyst or a group of cysts (the ''racemose'' form) are located at the base of the brain in the subarachnoid space they incite chronic meningitis and arachnoiditis, after which a communicating or noncommunicating hydrocephalus frequently develops.

Cysts can lodge in the ventricular system and cause an obstructive hydrocephalus, either because of the cysts themselves or because of the inflammatory response they incite. Endothelial proliferation can occur in the cerebral arteries and arterioles as a result of a vasculitis, and the vessel may become occluded. Eventually, some of the older and nonviable cysts calcify, making them easier to diagnose.[4,8]

SIGNS AND SYMPTOMS

In almost every patient the disease has its own peculiarities depending upon the individual's immune response, the severity of infestation, the location of the cysts, and the size, site, and number of neurologic lesions. If the cysticerci are single or few in number and are lodged in a nonstrategic area of the brain, there may be no signs of disease. If there are large numbers of cysts or if they lodge in eloquent areas of the CNS, seizures, focal deficits, increased intracranial pressure secondary to mass effect or to communicating and noncommunicating hydrocephalus, and meningitis may develop. Not infrequently, the predominating signs or symptoms change during the course of infection. Focal, jacksonian, or generalized seizures occur in anywhere from 30 to 92 percent of patients, depending on the reported series. Headache is practically universal in patients with hydrocephalus. Nausea, vomiting, impaired vision, confu-

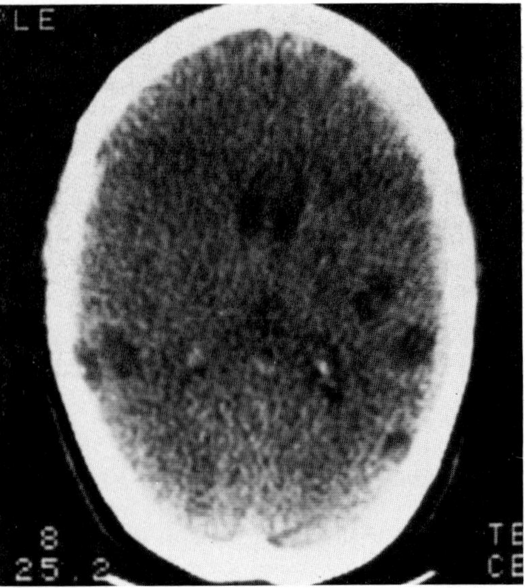

Fig. 10-1. A noncontrast CT scan showing multiple parenchymal cysts as hypodense round lesions.

sion, dizziness, and ataxia are also common manifestations of the disease. Papilledema and changes in mental status frequently occur in patients with hydrocephalus, and focal deficits are common in those with mass lesions.[6,7,10–12]

DIAGNOSIS

The diagnosis of neurocysticercosis is established by a combination of the clinical history and physical findings, signs, laboratory and serologic tests, and CT scans. A knowledge of the patient's country of origin and a history of exposure can be extremely helpful in making the diagnosis. The neurologic signs and symptoms are nonspecific, but the finding of multiple subcutaneous cysts strongly suggests the diagnosis. The cerebrospinal fluid is usually abnormal and suggests a chronic meningitis manifested as a lymphocytic pleocytosis and in some cases CSF eosinophilia, decreased glucose level, and elevated protein level.[7]

Computed tomography is the most useful study, and the findings are virtually diagnostic in most cases. The appearance of cerebral cysticercosis on CT scans varies and depends on the stage of the disease: a hyperdense nodular mass will be seen in the encephalitic phase; a hypodense round lesion of varying size sometimes surrounded by an enhanced ring will be seen when the lesion is cystic (Figures 10-1, 10-2, 10-3, and 10-4). In later stages of the disease the cysts may be calcified. Some lesions can be seen only on CT scans with contrast enhancement. The diagnosis is less certain when there are single lesions or nonspecific radiographic findings, such as hydrocephalus. Subarachnoid or intraventricular cysts are difficult to detect with CT scans and positive contrast medium (metrizamide) introduced into an obstructed lateral ventricle may be required to demonstrate them. In the case of suspected spinal neurocysticercosis, myelography and CT scans are the recommended studies.[13–17]

Serologic testing of the cerebrospinal fluid and the serum is useful in cysticercosis, but is neither highly sensitive nor specific. Although there are numerous tests, there are no standardized antigens or methods. *T. solium* antigen prepara-

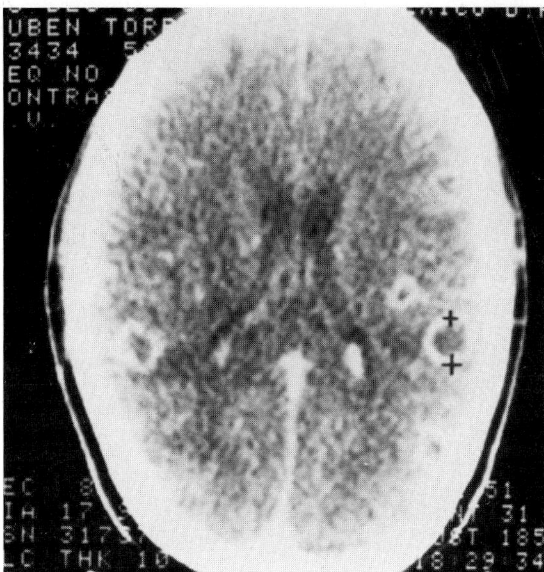

Fig. 10-2. A contrast-enhanced CT scan of the same patient as in Figure 10-1 showing the multiple parenchymal cysts as round lesions with a ring of enhancement.

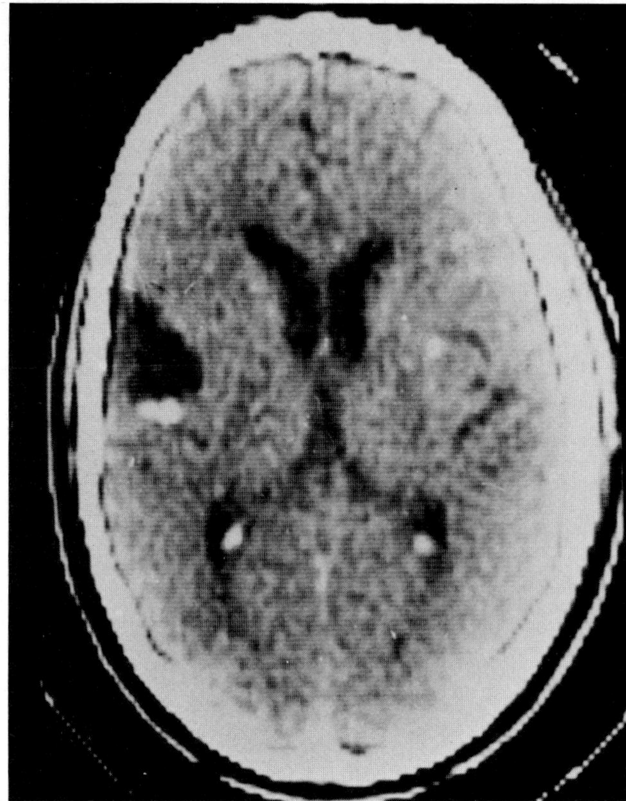

Fig. 10-3. A CT scan of a patient with a single large cyst and calcifications.

tions identify cross-reactive antibodies in some patients with echinococcosis, schistosomiasis, or occasionally other cestode infections. Despite these drawbacks, however, detection of antibodies in a patient with a typical clinical appearance and compatible CT findings generally establishes the diagnosis.[7]

PROGNOSIS

The prognosis of cysticercosis is variable and difficult to assess, and the course and tempo of the disease may change; this is caused in part by the individual's immunologic responses and by an increased inflammatory response in previously quiescent, viable cysts. Approximately one third of neurocysticercosis patients are asymptomatic; their disease is discovered incidentally on radiographic studies performed for other reasons; one third have minimal nonspecific complaints such as headache or dizziness and one third have major neurologic symptoms such as seizures, increased intracranial pressure, focal neurologic signs, mental deterioration, or involvement of the cranial nerves that requires immediate investigation.[18]

THERAPY

Supportive therapy includes anticonvulsant medications and steroids; the latter have been reported to cause short-term and sometimes long-term symptomatic improvement. Two specific antiparasitic drugs, praziquantel and albendazol, recently have been demonstrated to have a beneficial effect in parenchymal and cortical macroscopic viable cysts appearing on CT scans as hypodense images (Figure 10-5). These drugs interfere with the metabolism of the parasite but do not influence the calcified cysts, arachnoiditis, hydrocephalus, or subarachnoid, cisternal, or ventricular cysts associated with the disease.[19–25]

SURGICAL TREATMENT

The surgical approach in the treatment of neurocysticercosis depends on the number, size, and localization of the cysticerci and the anatomopathologic characteristics of the

infection. It is important to define the following aspects:

1. The number of cysts (single or multiple cysts).
2. The size of the cysts (more or less than 2 cm in diameter; mass effect?).
3. The location of the cysts (in the parenchyma of the brain or spinal cord; in the subarachnoid space of the base, cisterns, or convexity; in the ventricles; in the subarachnoid space of the spine; mixed types).
4. The biologic stage of the parasite (Figure 10-6) (encephalitic stage; viable cyst with clear fluid content; partially degenerated cyst with jellylike content; degenerated cyst that is calcified; racemose type of cyst).
5. The secondary pathologic conditions produced in the CNS by the presence of the cysts (Figure 10-7) (arachnoiditis-meningitis; ependymitis; vasculitis with or without ischemic sequelae; communicating or noncommunicating hydrocephalus).

The surgical approach varies depending on whether larvae are situated in brain or spinal cord parenchyma or are intraventricular in location, single or multiple; of the cellulosae or racemose variety, and whether they are located in the cortex or in the basal subarachnoid space or both, if there is a communicating or obstructive hydrocephalus, or if an adherent arachnoiditis or ependymitis is present. Most cases involve mixed types of the disease, calcified forms with parenchymatous cysts, cisternal cysts, basilar adhesive arachnoiditis and hydrocephalus.[5,18]

The surgical indications in a patient with neurocysticercosis include (1) viable cysts 2 cm or larger in diameter that produce focal neurologic symptoms and or a mass effect;

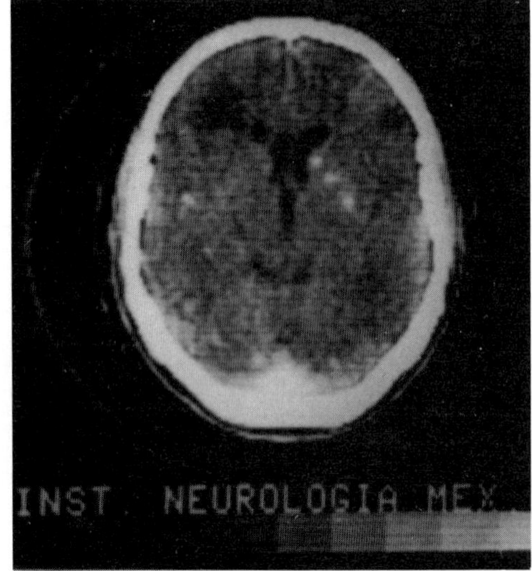
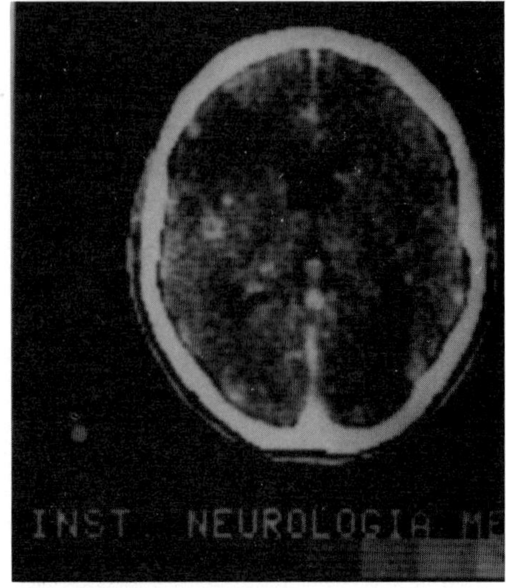
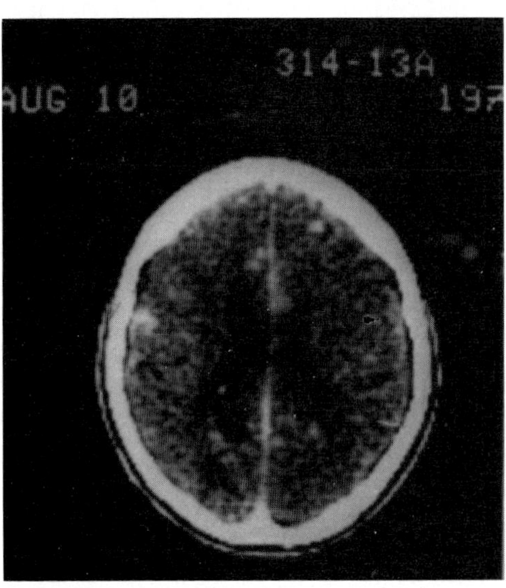
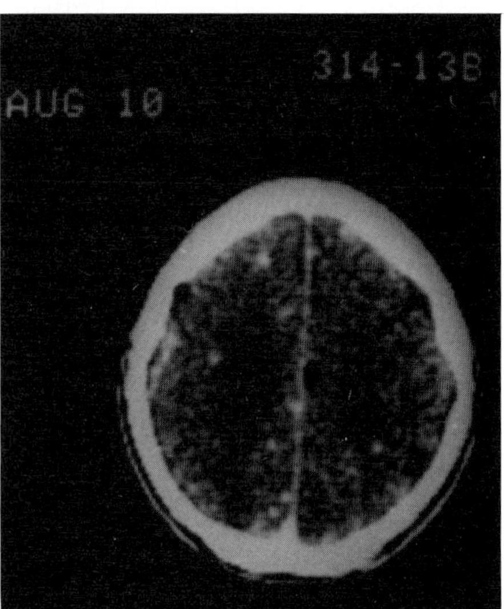

Fig. 10-4. A CT scan of a patient with the combined form of neurocysticerotic lesions: hydrocephalus, a large cyst, multiple small cysts, partially degenerated cysts, and calcifications (dead larvae).

(2) cysts obstructing ventricular pathways; (3) hydrocephalus; (4) spinal cord compression (Table 10-2).

Various clinical manifestations of neurocysticercosis and their surgical treatment are listed below (Figure 10-8):

1. A racemose lesion presenting as a tumorlike mass, predominantly localized in the parenchyma of the cerebral hemispheres or at a major cerebral sulcus such as the sylvian fissure. This mass has the appearance of an enhancing ringlike abscess or tumor up to 2 to 3 inches in diameter on CT scans. These lesions are treated by total excision. In cases of multiple cysts in which one large cyst appears to be primarily responsible for a focal neurologic symptom or deficit, its removal is also indicated. Microsurgical dissection attempts to separate the thin-walled cyst from the surrounding nervous tissue and vessels. We recently used a CO_2 laser, sharply focussed and at low power, to dissect and separate these structures and to extirpate as much as possible the inflammatory tissue that usually surrounds the cysts and is adjacent to vessels and adherent to nervous tissue (Color Plate 10-1). The cyst wall often is so thin and delicate there is always the danger that the cyst will tear during dissection and its fluid contents will spill into neighboring areas of the brain. Even though of concern, we have not found the spillage of the cyst contents to have subsequent deleterious consequences. In most cases steroid therapy is maintained throughout the perioperative period. If a cyst is firmly attached to surrounding structures and cannot be totally removed, the cavity is marsupialized, leaving it as open as possible so it has a connection with the subarachnoid space.

2. Patients with resistant partial seizures could be benefitted by the extirpation of the cysticercus or cysticerci (Color Plate 10-2).

3. Cysts that migrate within the ventricular system can obstruct the foramen of Monro, the aqueduct of Sylvius, the fourth ventricle, or the cisterna magna. The larvae, when accessible, are removed to re-establish CSF flow. Because of the possibility of future inflammatory reactions to the cysts, the removal of all accessible ventricular cysts is

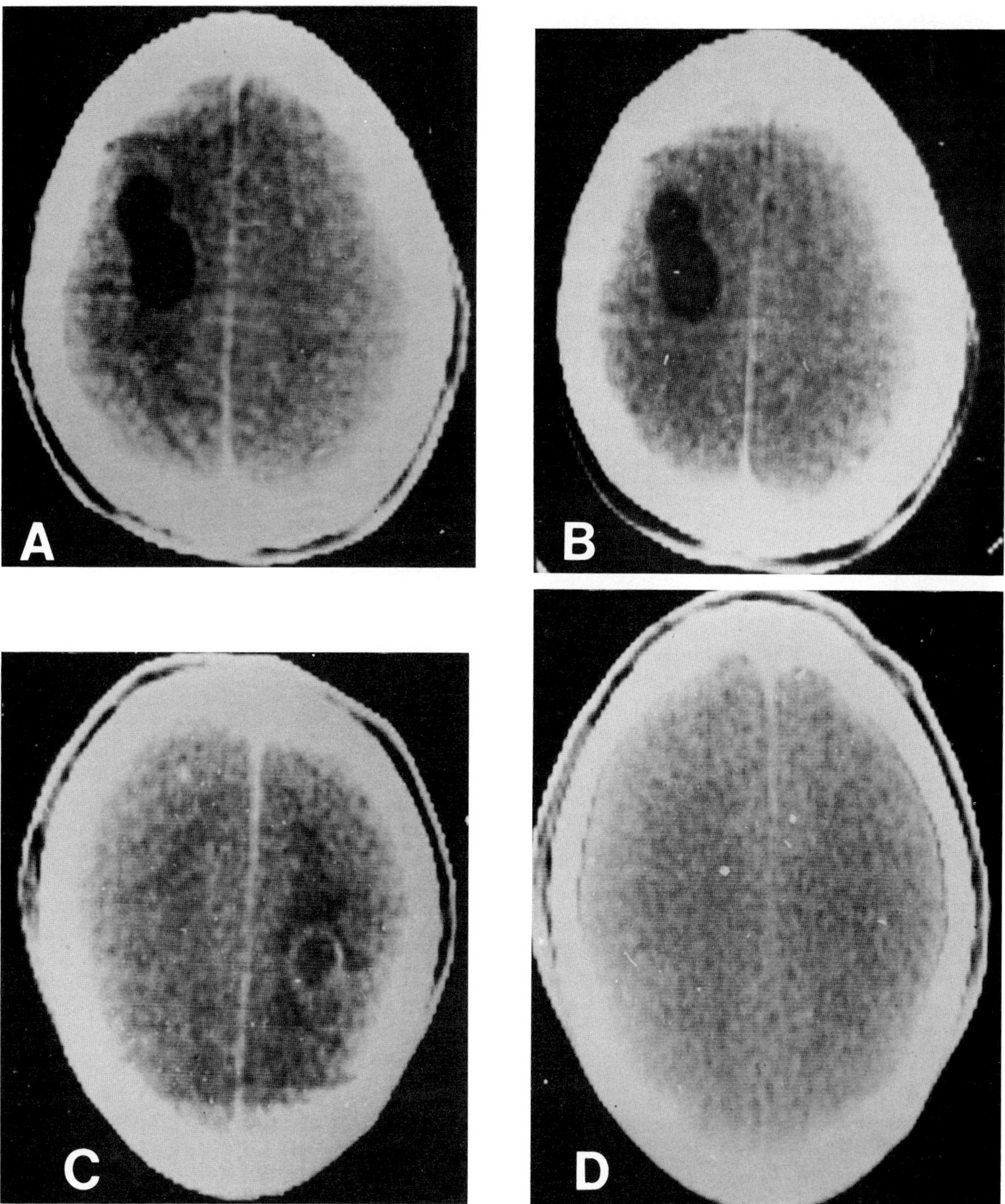

Fig. 10-5. Contrast-enhanced CT scans before and after praziquantel therapy. (A) A large cyst 2 months before treatment; (B) the same cyst immediately before treatment; (C) the cyst 3 weeks after treatment (note the intensely enhanced ring around the lesion as a result of the inflammatory process); (D) resolution of the lesion 3 months after treatment.

recommended. Although some of patients have multiple intraventricular cysts, a sufficient number of patients have solitary cysts, the removal of which may be curative. The tendency of intraventricular cysts to migrate may explain why so many tend to be found in the fourth ventricle. The radiographic studies in these cases demonstrate a large fourth ventricle, which is sometimes disproportionately large compared with the rest of the ventricular system. This finding in a patient with cysticercosis is highly suggestive of either an isolated ventricle or an intraventricular cyst.[11] A posterior fossa approach is performed using a suboccipital craniotomy with the patient in the sitting position. A midline exposure permits excision of a cyst or cluster of cysts if they are at the cisterna (Color Plates 10-3, 10-4, and 10-5). Cystic masses can also be found in the cerebellopontine angle, the lateral medullary recess, and even on the cerebellar hemispheres. When cysts are located within the fourth ventricle or the cerebral aqueduct, these areas are explored after the thickened tela choroidea is opened and both cerebellar tonsils are separated (Color Plate 10-6). In some cases it is necessary to divide the inferior vermis before the cysts can be extracted by gentle aspiration or

BIOLOGICAL STAGE

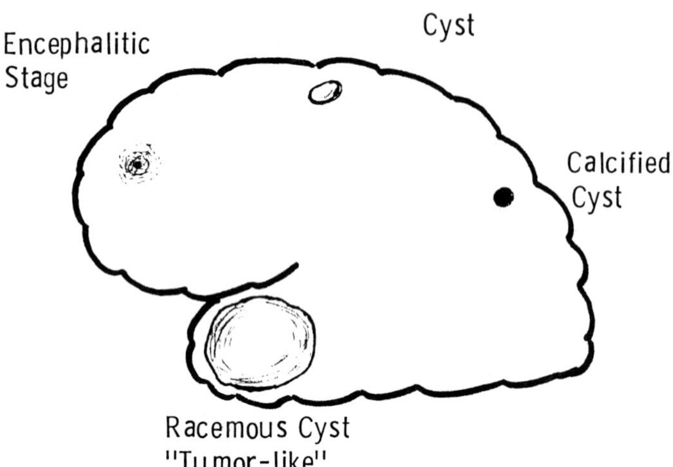

Fig. 10-6. The biological stage of neurocysticercosis.

traction with flat-bladed forceps on the walls of a smooth cyst. This can be supplemented by irrigation for hydraulic dissection and a Valsalva's maneuver, which assists in exposing and delivering lesions from deep recesses that may not have been previously suspected (Color Plate 10-7). These maneuvers often re-establish CSF flow. In some cases it is useful to inject 30 or 40 ml of saline into the lateral ventricle, which will push down cysts within the ventricular system and also confirm the free flow of CSF (Color Plate 10-8). If CSF flow is not re-established by these measures, a shunt should be performed immediately or within a short period of time. Cysts located in the lateral or third ventricle near the foramen of Monro are reached through a frontal craniotomy and either a transcortical or a transcallosal approach. In these cases the septum

SECONDARY PATHOLOGY

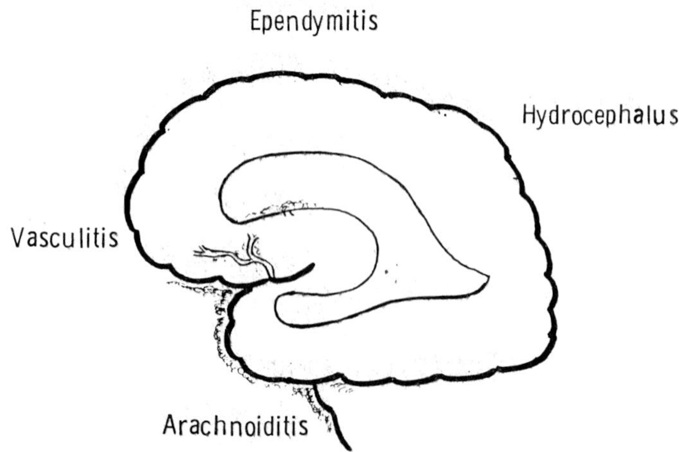

Fig. 10-7. The secondary pathologic conditions produced by neurocysticercosis.

Table 10-2. Indications for surgical treatment of neurocysticercosis

Cysts 2 cm or larger producing focal symptoms or a mass effect
Cysts obstructing ventricular channels
Hydrocephalus
Spinal cord compression

pellucidum should be fenestrated to ensure adequate bilateral ventricular drainage.

4. In cerebral cysticercosis the cysts are usually multiple and often in spite of these procedures the blockage of CSF circulation persists. Many of these intraventricular cysts are removable, however, hydrocephalus or increased intracranial pressure can persist as a result of ependymitis of the foramen of Monro or at the sylvian aqueduct or as a result of basilar adhesive arachnoiditis, which blocks the free circulation and absorption of CSF over the base or surface of the brain. In these cases shunting CSF into the blood stream or the peritoneal cavity is indicated. In most cases of neurocysticercosis the CSF protein content is high and the shunt system to be used must be selected carefully.

5. Cysticerci located in the chiasmatic region can produce an inflammatory reaction and adhesive arachnoiditis that affects the optic nerves and chiasm. These cases are very difficult surgical problems because the chronic basilar adhesive meningitis forms a thick membrane that surrounds all the structures on the ventral surface of the brain including the brain stem. Cysts are often blended into this mass of adhesions. These membranes are firmly attached to the optic nerves, the optic chiasm, and to the internal carotid arteries. Microsurgical dissection supplemented by bipolar coagulation and, in certain cases, a CO_2 laser is intended to decompress these structures and remove cysts.

6. Increased intracranial pressure without ventricular dilatation or hydrocephalus is often the result of diffuse parenchymatous disease without a focal mass effect. Current treatment methods for dealing with the increased intracranial pressure generally have been of little value, and surgical decompression by subtemporal craniotomy can be considered for persistently elevated ICP.

7. In the case of deep-seated cysts in the lateral ventricles, the posterior part of the third ventricle, or the lower areas of the hemispheres, the use of a stereotactic endoscopic system to introduce forceps, suction, or cannulas for the excision or draining of the cysts should be considered.[26,27]

8. Cysticerci located in the spine result in symptoms that indicate injury to the spinal cord or the nerve roots. Myelographic or CT studies show cysts or a block caused by arachnoiditis. In these cases laminectomy should be performed, the dura opened, the cyst or cysts removed, and adherent membranes removed or freed up in order to free the neural structures.

It must be recognized that surgery is not always indicated in all cases of neurocysticercosis and when performed is not necessarily curative, since multiple disseminated larvae cannot be treated surgically and the arachnoidal adhesions and cerebral arteritis and its sequelae may produce permanent neurologic complications. In selecting the surgical approach the surgeon

DIFFERENT SURGICAL APPROACHES

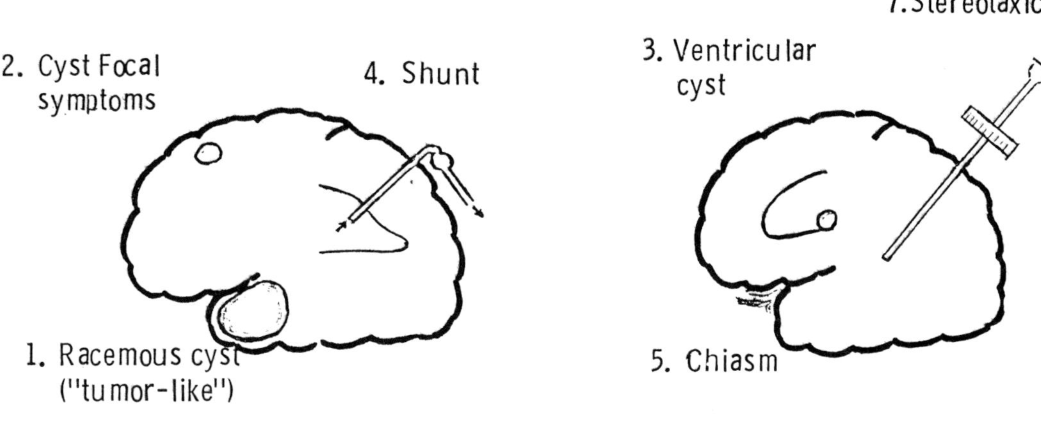

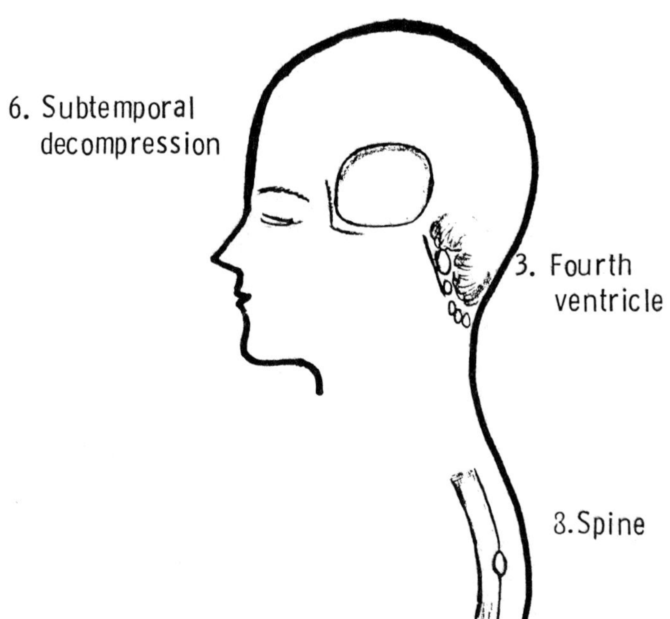

Fig. 10-8. The different surgical approaches to treating neurocysticercosis.

should be aware of the possibility of an associated ependymitis and the potential for current or eventual outlet obstruction in spite of the removal of a particular cysticercus. Direct surgical excision of simple cystic lesions, in the absence of radiographic evidence of arachnoiditis or ependymitis constitutes adequate primary therapy in the majority of these cases since the surgical approach is that of treating symptomatic manifestations. Most surgical procedures are palliative. Surgery can partially and temporarily relieve increased intracranial pressure and occasionally the focal symptoms caused by a cortical or subcortical cysticercus, even though this is not the rule.[18,28] Although improvement occurs, other evidence of disease precludes the idea of curing the underlying disorder surgically. Experience

with ventricular shunts indicates that although they are effective for alleviating CSF blockages, the catheter will eventually become occluded and require revision.

Unlike the complex problems and frustrations encountered with the mixed and disseminated forms of neurocysticercosis, removal of solitary intraventricular cysts is often followed by prompt improvement and excellent recovery. Such cysts are potentially curable.

Sometimes a patient will require staged surgical procedures. For instance, in some cases a shunt followed by the direct excision of cysts in the fourth ventricle or at the sylvian fissure is required; other cases require primary excision of cystic lesions and secondary shunting.

REFERENCES

1. Escobar A, Nieto D: Cysticercosis, in Minkler J (ed): Pathology of the Nervous System, vol 3. New York, McGraw-Hill, 1972, pp 2507–2515

2. Miller BL, Goldberg MA, Heiner D, et al: Cerebral cysticercosis: An overview. Bull Clin Neurosci 48:2, 1983

3. Gardner B, Goldberg M, Douglas H, et al: The natural history of parenchymal CNS cysticercosis. Neurology 34 (Suppl 1):90, 1984

4. Escobar A: The pathology of neurocysticercosis, in Palacios E, Rodríguez Carbajal J, Taveras J (eds): Cysticercosis of the Central Nervous System. Springfield, Ill, Charles C Thomas, 1983, pp 27–54

5. Escobedo F, González-Mariscal G, Revuelta R, et al: Surgical treatment of cerebral cysticercosis, in Cysticercosis. Present State of Knowledge and Perspectives. New York, Academic Press, 1982, pp 201–206

6. Escobedo F, García-Ramos G, Sotelo J: Parasitic disorders and epilepsy, in Nistico G, Di Perri R, Meinardi H (eds): Epilepsy. An Update on Research and Therapy. New York, Alan R. Liss, 1983, pp 227–233

7. Sotelo J, Guerrero V, Rubio F: Neurocysticercosis: A new classification based on active and inactive forms. A study of 753 cases. Arch Intern Med 145:442, 1985

8. Itabashi HH: Pathology of CNS cysticercosis. Bull Clin Neurosci 48:6, 1983

9. Gajdusek C: Introduction of Taenia solium into West New Guinea with a note on an epidemic of burns from cysticercus epilepsy in the Ekari people of the Wissel Lakes area. Papua New Guinea Med J 21:329, 1978

10. Feinberg W, Valdivia RF: Cysticercosis presenting as a subdural hematoma. Neurology 34:1112, 1984

11. Salazar A, Sotelo J, Martínez H, et al: Differential diagnosis between ventriculitis and cyst of fourth ventricle in neurocysticercosis. J Neurosurg 59:660, 1983

12. Wendy MG, Snodgrass RS: Intraparenchymal cerebral cysticercosis in children: A benign prognosis. Pediatr Neurol 1:151, 1985

13. Carbajal JR, Palacios E, Azar-Kia B, et al: Radiology of cysticercosis of the central nervous system including computed tomography. Radiology 125:127, 1977

14. Kerin D, Chi-Shing Zee, Tsai F, et al: Transventricular migration of a cysticercal cyst during pneumoencelography. Bull Clin Neurosci 48:61, 1983

15. Mehringer CM, Hieshima G, Grinnell VS, et al: Radiologic considerations in neurocysticercosis. Bull Clin Neurosci 48:24, 1983

16. Rodríguez Carbajal J, Salgado P, Gutiírrez R, et al: The acute encephalitic phase of neurocysticercosis: Computed tomographic manifestations. AJNR 4:51, 1985

17. Miller B: Spontaneous radiographic disappearance of cerebral cysticercosis: Three cases. Neurology 33:1377, 1983

18. Escobedo F: Surgical treatment of neurocysticercosis, in Palacios E, Rodrí guez Carbajal J, Taveras J (eds): Cysticercosis of the Central Nervous System. Springfield, Ill, Charles C Thomas, 1983, pp 114–148

19. Robles C, Chavarría M: Un caso de cisticercosis cerebral curado medicamente. Gac Med Mex 116:65, 1980

20. Botero D, Castaño S: Treatment of cysticercosis with praziquantel in Colombia. Am J Trop Med Hyg 31:811, 1982

21. Lawner PM: Medical management of neurocysticercosis with praziquantel. Bull Clin Neurosci 48:102, 1983

22. Kori SH, Olds R: PZQ therapy and NMR scans in cerebral cysticercosis. Neurology (Suppl 1):89, 1984

23. Sotelo J, Escobedo F, Rodríguez Carbajal J, et al: Therapy of parenchymal brain cysticercosis with praziquantel. N Engl J Med 310:1001, 1984

24. Sotelo J, Torres B, Rubio-Donnadieu F, et al: Praziquantel in the treatment of neurocysticercosis: Long-term follow-up. Neurology 35:752, 1985

25. Escobedo F, Penagos P, Rodríguez Carbajal J, et al: Albendazole therapy for neurocysticercosis. Arch Med (accepted for publication)

26. Seigel RS, Davis LE, Kaplan RJ, et al: CT-Guided aspiration of a cysticercotic thalamic cyst. Bull Clin Neurosci 48:48, 1983

27. Apuzzo MLJ, Dobkin WR, Chi-Shing Zee, et al: Surgical considerations in the treatment of intraventricular cysticercosis—an analysis of 45 cases. J Neurosurg 60:400, 1984

28. Stern EW: Neurosurgical considerations of cysticercosis of the central nervous system. J Neurosurg 55:382, 1981

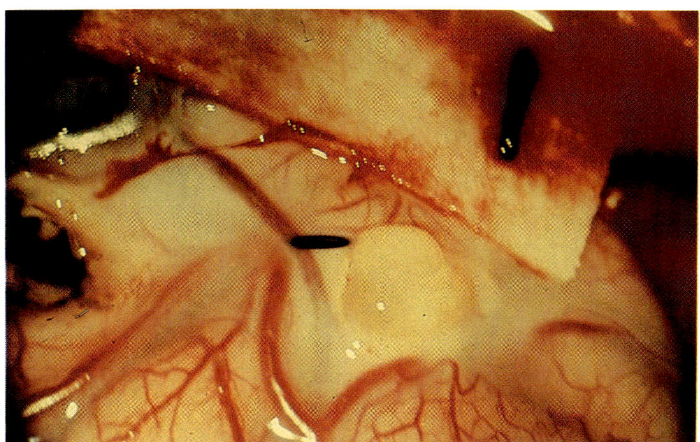

Color Plate 10-1. A cyst located in a brain fissure with associated inflammatory reaction. This is a milky white process over the cortex and around the vessels. A thrombosed vessel is also visible in the field.

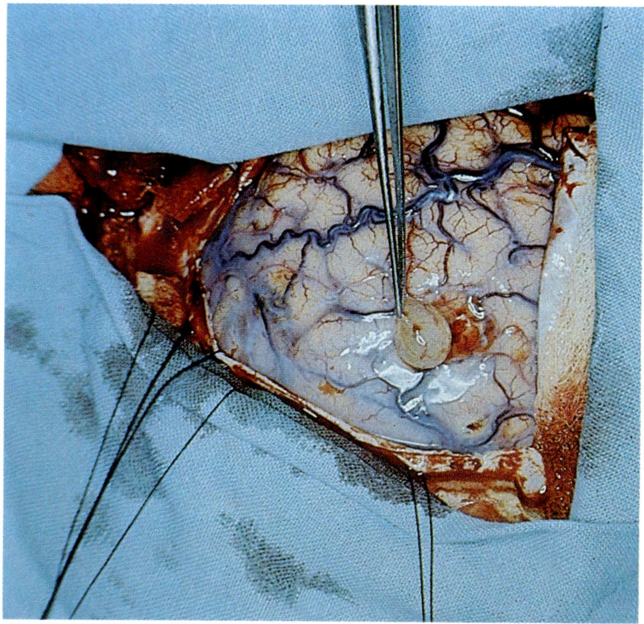

Color Plate 10-2. A cortical cyst dissected and ready for excision.

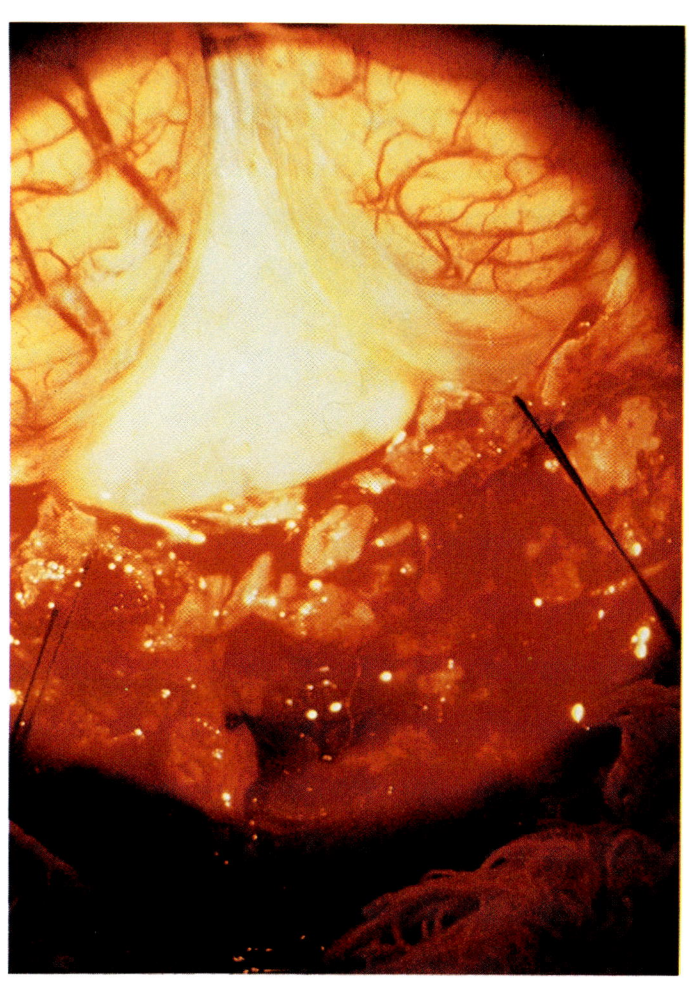

Color Plate 10-3. The suboccipital approach showing the thickened wall of the cisterna.

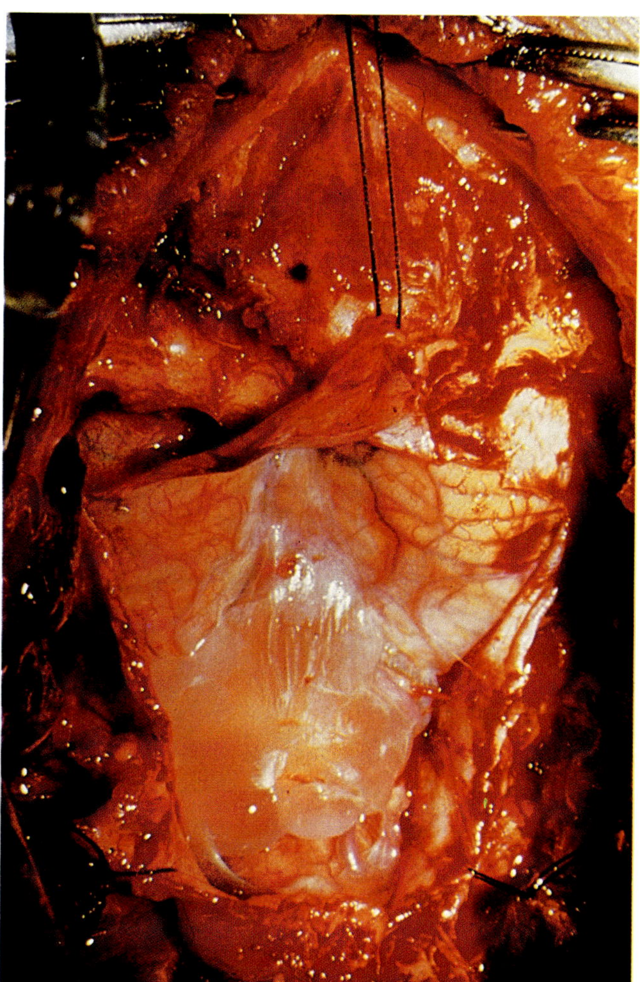

Color Plate 10-4. The suboccipital approach showing the cisterna containing several transparent cysts.

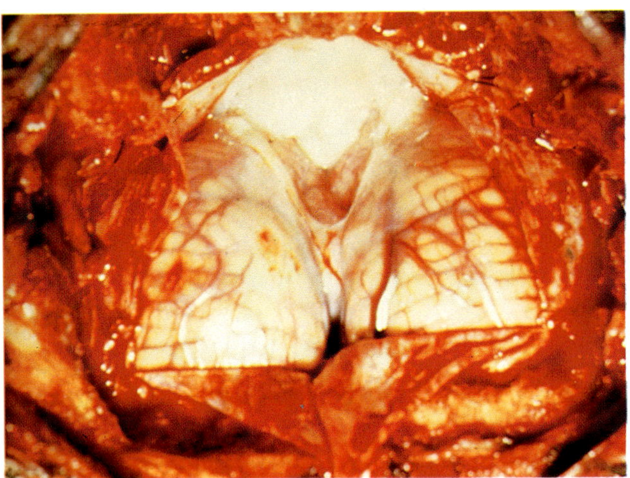

Color Plate 10-5. A cluster of cysts in the cisterna magna.

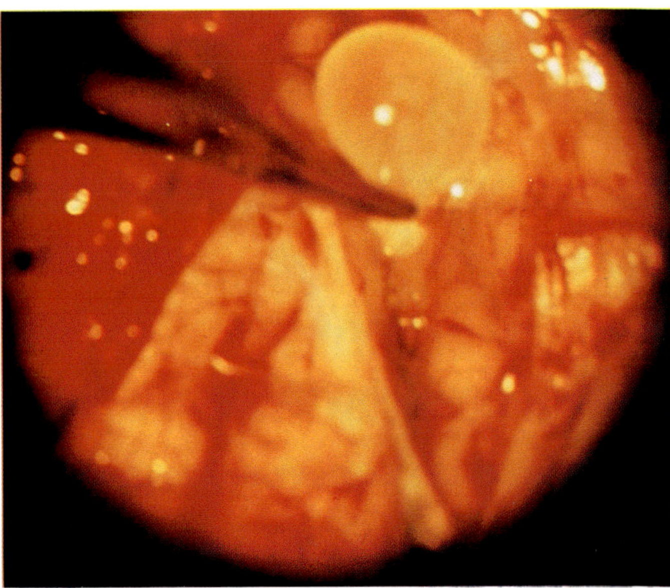

Color Plate 10-6. Extraction of a cyst from the lower part of the fourth ventricle.

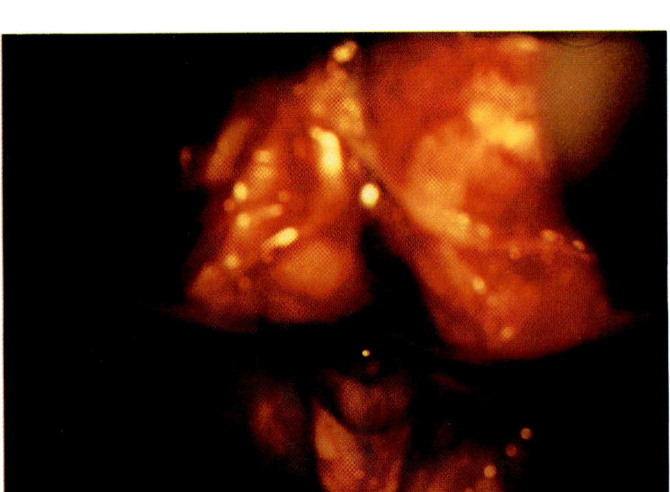

Color Plate 10-7. The suboccipital approach with separation of the cerebellar tonsils, exposure of the lower part of the fourth ventricle, and demonstration of part of a cyst.

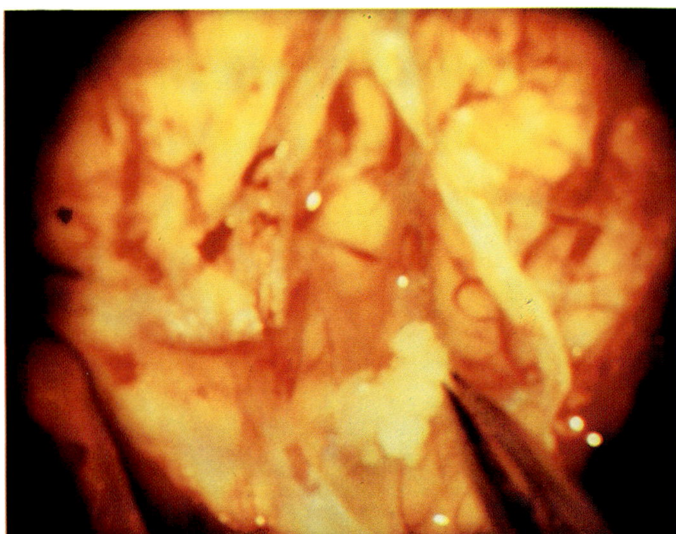

Color Plate 10-8. After the cyst has been removed from the cisterna and fourth ventricle, a creamy yellow inflammatory response (combined with dead parasites) is seen.

CHAPTER 11

Anesthetic Considerations and Techniques in Pediatric Neurosurgical Patients

Mounir N. Abou-Madi   Davy Trop

ALTHOUGH THE RECENT ADVANCES in contemporary anesthesia have paved the way for many of the rapid advances in neurologic surgery, pediatric neurosurgical patients have long been and continue to be a major challenge in the everyday practice of anesthesiology.

In a struggle to survive, newborn infants have to cope with six major obligations: lung expansion, circulatory conversion to an adult pattern, recovery from birth asphyxia, temperature regulation, establishment of renal function, and metabolic requirements.[1]

Pediatric anatomophysiologic features of significance to the anesthesiologist include:

- Problems related to intubation, ventilation and venipuncture.
- The immaturity of the central nervous system.
- The peculiar response of the cardiovascular system to stress, asphyxia, and hypovolemia.
- The overall relative immaturity of renal function in the neonatal period.
- Problems in maintaining core body temperature.
- Rapid depletion of body reserves of carbohydrates and fats in response to catecholamine release and fasting.
- The abnormal sensitivity or resistance to anesthetic agents, sedatives, analgesics, and muscle relaxants.
- Difficulties in calculating intraoperative blood and fluid requirements.
- The optimal time at which to undertake anesthesia and surgery for lesions requiring early correction.

BASIC NEUROPHYSIOLOGIC CONSIDERATIONS

The basic regulatory mechanisms of intracranial pressure, cerebral blood flow, and cerebrospinal fluid dynamics are the same in children and adults. The effects of changes in $PaCO_2$, PaO_2, and of abnormal blood pressure on the cerebral circulation and intracranial pressure are, however, less well understood in children and newborns than in adults. Two important features must be born in mind:

1. The intracranial pressure decreases during the early days after birth.[2] It usually parallels neonatal physiologic changes: dehydration, weight loss, redistribution of body fluids and increase in serum osmolarity. Under ordinary circumstances, loss of brain volume is compensated for by an increase in cerebrospinal fluid production. On the other hand, an incipient hydrocephalus may be progressive and severe with only a mild elevation of intracranial pressure.

2. Infants and small children can expand their intracranial volume while their fontanels and sutures are still open, and this affords them a greater margin of safety. Bulging of the fontanels accommodates some increase in intracranial volume and indicates that intracranial pressure is rising. Separation of the sutures occurs with chronically raised intracranial pressure.

Pathophysiologic factors causing derangement of normal brain function include hypoxia and ischemic insults, trauma to the central nervous system, cerebral compression by expanding space-occupying lesions, congenital neurologic malformations, and inflammatory diseases of the central nervous system. Derangement of normal brain function is manifested by tissue acidosis, loss of autoregulation, loss of regulation of intracranial pressure, loss of carbon dioxide reactivity, loss of central metabolic control, and brain edema.

ANESTHESIA FOR INTRACRANIAL SPACE-OCCUPYING LESIONS

The central nervous system is a common site for childhood tumors. Unlike those of adult life, they are most commonly situated in the posterior cranial fossa and in the region of the third ventricle and cause obstruction to cerebrospinal fluid flow and hydrocephalus. If a high intracranial pressure is suspected in these patients, preliminary shunting can be performed.

ANESTHETIC CONSIDERATIONS

There are a number of ways in which improper anesthetic techniques can adversely affect the intracranial pressure.[3] These include hypercarbia, hypoxia, disturbed cerebral autoregulation, increased cerebral venous pressure, the use of anesthetic agents known to be cerebral vasodilators, and improper intraoperative fluid therapy.

A proper approach to neurosurgical anesthesia should

OPERATIVE NEUROSURGICAL TECHNIQUES
ISBN 0-8089-1862-1

Table 11-1. Effects of anesthetics on cerebral blood flow and cerebral metabolic rate

	CBF	CMRO$_2$
Barbiturates	↓↓	↓↓
Etomidate	↓↓	↓↓
Althesin	↓↓	↓↓
Halothane	↑↑	↓
Enflurane	↑↑	↓↓
Isoflurane	↑	↓↓
Nitrous oxide	↑	↑
Narcotics	↓	↓
Droperidol	↓	↓
Ketamine	↑↑	↑↑

therefore involve the use of appropriate anesthetic agents, a smooth induction of anesthesia, prevention of reactions to laryngoscopy and intubation, maintenance of an unobstructed airway, maintenance of ventilatory pattern, maintenance of total neuromuscular blockade, proper positioning, adequate monitoring, maintenance of appropriate fluid therapy, maintenance of proper posture, control of intracranial pressure, and maintenance of temperature.

Appropriate Anesthetic Agents

Anesthetic agents that either reduce intracranial pressure or do not affect it adversely must be used. Of these, the most accepted is the nitrous-narcotic-relaxant-barbiturate technique (Table 11-1). Isoflurane often is used for neuroanesthesia because, of the currently available inhalation anesthetics, it has the least effect on cerebral blood flow and volume.[4] Its use, however, may not be benign in patients with increased intracranial pressure despite prior institution of modest hypocapnia.[5] The intermittent use of barbiturates throughout anesthesia reduces the cerebral oxygen consumption and, secondarily, the cerebral blood flow and intracranial pressure. Ketamine increases cerebral blood flow and oxygen consumption as well as intracranial pressure and therefore should be avoided.[6,7]

Smooth Induction of Anesthesia

One of the common problems facing the pediatric anesthesiologist is what method of induction to choose for the patient with mildly or questionably raised intracranial pressure. A rapid intravenous induction is mandatory for the patient who is genuinely compromised by a tight head or a full stomach. On the other hand, an inhalation induction may be indicated for the awake patient with no signs of intracranial hypertension. The intramuscular or rectal administration of a short-acting barbiturate (methohexital) before induction may be necessary for the frightened uncooperative patient.

Prevention of Untoward Reactions to Laryngoscopy and Endotracheal Intubation

Laryngoscopy and endotracheal intubation are done under deep general anesthesia, gently and rapidly and with full muscle relaxation. Depolarizing agents such as succinylcholine have a rapid onset of action and cause profound relaxation. However, the muscle fasciculation seen in children over the age of 5 years can transiently increase the intracranial pressure. Alternatively, a nondepolarizing muscle relaxant such as pancuronium bromide can provide rapid profound neuromuscular blockade without fasciculation if a sufficiently large dose is administered intravenously (0.15–0.2 mg/kg). D-Tubocurarine is less desirable than pancuronium because the resulting histamine release can simultaneously decrease blood pressure and increase intracranial pressure. The role of atracurium besylate in pediatric anesthesia has been well defined. Doses in the range of 0.5 to 0.6 mg/kg provide satisfactory conditions for intubation in all patients within 3 minutes.[8] The drug is safe to use in the presence of elevated intracranial pressure,[9] and its histamine-releasing action in children appears to be less than in adults and causes minimal cardiovascular changes.[10] Lidocaine (1.5 mg/kg) can be given intravenously a few minutes before endotracheal intubation to block cardiovascular responses[11] and the potential rise in intracranial pressure.[12]

Airway Maintenance

Meticulous attention to airway patency during bag-and-mask ventilation until the neuromuscular blocking agent has taken full effect is necessary. In certain instances, the head is flexed to an extreme degree on the body; this can cause the endotracheal tube to kink or to move caudad. After every change of position, careful auscultation of breath sounds is mandatory. The endotracheal tube should be securely fastened with waterproof tape after tincture of benzoin is applied to the face. Table 11-2 details the sizes of endotracheal tubes to be used.[13]

Maintenance of Proper Ventilatory Pattern

In patients with space-occupying lesions, hyperventilation has been clinically effective in lowering increased intracranial pressure and producing a relaxed brain. Hyperventilation is started as soon as the patient loses consciousness using the bag and mask; it is continued until full neuromuscular blockade is established and is immediately re-established after endotracheal intubation is carried out. Ventilation is controlled with a mechanical respirator aiming for a PaCO$_2$ of 25–30 mm Hg. This is usually accomplished with a tidal volume of 15 ml/kg. The frequency of the respirator is regulated as necessary. Positive end-expiratory pressure should not be used unless the patient's oxygenation is threatened. Inspired oxygen is adjusted to maintain a PaO$_2$ greater than 100 mm Hg.

Maintenance of Total Neuromuscular Blockade

In general, muscle relaxants have no significant effects on the central nervous system. Immobility, however, is preferably provided by pancuronium. Rapid administration of pancuro-

Table 11-2. Sizes of endotracheal tubes

Age of Patient	Internal Diameter (mm)
Premature	2.5–3.0
Full-term	3.0–3.5
6 months	4.0
12 months	4.0
18–24 months	4.5
4 years	5.0
6 years	5.5
8 years	6.0
10 years	7.0
12 years	7.0
14 years	8.0

Table 11-3. Preanesthetic fasting period

	Fasting Period (hours)	
Age of Patient	Milk & Solids	Clear Fluids
Neonate	4	2
1–6 months	4	4
6–36 months	6	6
36 months and older	8	8

Reprinted from Liu LMP: Pediatric blood and fluid therapy, in Hershey SG (ed): Refresher Courses in Anesthesiology, vol 12. Hagerstown, MD, J.B. Lippincott, 1984. With permission.

nium can result in tachycardia, but this is usually well tolerated by children. Curare is often avoided on theoretical grounds because histamine release can cause cerebrovasodilation. Intraoperative fluctuations of neuromuscular blockade are dangerous and must be avoided.

Positioning

In children most posterior fossa and upper cervical spine surgery is done with the child sitting. In children less than 2 years of age the prone position is recommended. Some authors advocate the use of the prone position for all children undergoing posterior fossa and upper cervical surgery.[14] They argue that in the sitting position, venous bleeding is frequently encountered from the superior surface of the cerebellum after a posterior fossa mass has been excised. This bleeding is usually caused by tearing of a communicating vein when the cerebellar hemispheres sag after the tension has been relieved. A further argument against the sitting position is that it will further diminish cerebral blood flow, which may already have been reduced by hyperventilation and hypotension. This is a critical situation that can be seriously aggravated by small amounts of blood loss in a pediatric neurosurgical patient. Also, while the threat of air embolism is not entirely removed with the patient positioned prone, it is considerably lessened.[14] The prone position also can present difficulties for the anesthesiologist; the endotracheal tube can be accidentally removed. To allow for free venous return and unimpeded respiratory movements, the patient should be supported on a special frame or blanket rolls to take the weight off the chest and abdomen.

Monitoring

Heart rate and rhythm are monitored continuously with a chest piece or esophageal catheter attached by a tube to the anesthesiologist's ear. An electrocardiogram is an important adjunct to cardiac monitoring to detect aberrantly conducted or ectopic ventricular beats, especially when surgical manipulation near the fourth ventricle is anticipated. The arterial pressure should be continuously measured with an arterial line. Twenty-two gauge catheters are usually appropriate for infants weighing less than 3 kg. Twenty-gauge catheters are appropriate for all other children. The arterial catheter is used for intermittent sampling of blood gases, electrolytes, osmolarity, and hematocrit. The central venous pressure of infants and children is normally 3–12 cm H_2O. Since small blood and fluid losses seriously decrease the atrial filling pressures of children, central venous pressure should be measured continuously, not intermittently. The catheter can be used to aspirate air that may

be entrained during a surgical procedure, especially one that is performed with the patient in the sitting position. Patients who are desperately ill may require pulmonary artery pressure monitoring. There is usually a 2–10 mm Hg difference between end-tidal and arterial PCO_2 during anesthesia. End-tidal CO_2 measurements are especially useful in patients undergoing sitting craniotomy where a sudden fall in end-tidal CO_2 is usually indicative of an air embolus. Early detection of air embolization can also be achieved with Doppler devices secured over the fourth or fifth intercostal space at the right sternal border. These devices are extremely sensitive and can detect as little as 0.05 ml/kg/min of air entering the circulation.[15] Intracranial pressure monitoring, although rapidly becoming routine in neurologic intensive care, is relatively uncommon in the operating room. The temperature of infants and children should be measured continuously (rectum, skin, esophagus, or tympanic membrane) and kept between 36° and 37°C. Urine output should be monitored during surgery if the blood loss or extracellular fluid shifts are expected to be large. This can usually be done in infants with either a straight catheter or a 5F or 8F feeding tube. Beyond the newborn period a Foley catheter can be used. Urine output should exceed 0.75 ml/kg/hr.

Maintenance of Proper Intraoperative Fluid Therapy

Children who are allowed to fast for prolonged periods can become severely dehydrated. The fasting period before anesthesia should be adjusted according to the age of the patient (Table 11-3). Numerous formulas have been used for calculating fluid requirements in children (Table 11-4). However, the administration of excessive free water to patients with intracranial masses can result in a potential increase in cerebral edema and intracranial pressure. In order to control brain water, balanced electrolyte solutions at about two thirds or three fourths the calculated maintenance requirements are administered. Intraoperatively, evidence of inadequate circulating volume such as hypotension, tachycardia, or excessive response to vasodilators is treated with 5 percent albumin, plasma, or blood. The

Table 11-4. Maintenance fluid requirements

Weight	Fluid Requirements
0–10 kg	4 ml/kg/hr
11–20 kg	40 ml + 2 ml/kg/hr for each kg over 10
over 20 kg	60 ml + 1 ml/kg/hr for each kg over 20

Reprinted from Graves SA: Pediatric blood and fluid therapy, in Hershey SG (ed): Refresher Courses in Anesthesiology, vol 11. Hagerstown, MD, J.B. Lippincott, 1983. With permission.

central venous pressure should be used to guide fluid therapy. The blood volume of an infant is roughly 85 ml/kg and decreases to 70–80 ml/kg for older children. Losses greater than 10 percent of the patient's total blood volume must be replaced. Glucose load should be controlled. Substantial experimental evidence suggests that the administration of glucose before an episode of hypoxia or ischemia exacerbates subsequent brain damage. This evidence has led some to recommend that patients at risk of intraoperative ischemia not be given glucose.[16] One problem with this recommendation in infants is the possibility that withholding glucose in a fasted patient may lead to intraoperative hypoglycemia, which in itself may cause brain damage.

Maintenance of Proper Posture

A frequently unrecognized problem, even in the supine position, is when the head is turned to allow a semilateral approach. One or both jugular veins may become obstructed, causing an increase in both cerebral venous pressure and intracerebral blood volume.

Control of Intracranial Pressure

Steps to lower intracranial pressure may be needed intraoperatively to avoid brain herniation. Mannitol (0.25–1.0 g/kg) is usually infused for this purpose. Additional doses of thiopental (1–4 mg/kg) are also helpful. Vigorous hyperventilation may be beneficial, even in the presence of an already low $PaCO_2$.

Normothermia

Attempts should be made to maintain normal body temperature. Anesthetized infants tend to become poikilothermic. It is therefore essential that core temperature be monitored continuously and prompt action taken to warm the patient if the temperature drifts below 32°–33°C. Aids in temperature control include room warming, limiting exposure during induction and surgical preparation, the use of warming blankets, and warmers for intravenous solutions.

ANESTHETIC MANAGEMENT

Preoperative Assessment of the Child

The child should be assessed for the presence of raised intracranial pressure that could become exacerbated during the administration of anesthesia. Some patients with intracranial space-occupying lesions may have delayed gastric emptying and their gastric fluid will have increased acid content. Full stomach precautions are necessary in these patients. Diabetes insipidus, volume depletion, excessive vomiting, and fluid restriction may render the child intolerant even to the lightest dose of cardiodepressant agents. Motor weakness may affect his or her ability to cough and to breathe adequately. Impaired gag and swallowing mechanisms may interfere with airway protection. Laboratory investigations should include urine analysis and hematocrit, BUN, serum and urine electrolytes, screening for clotting abnormalities, and cross-matched blood for transfusion.

Premedication

Premedication with respiratory depressant narcotics is avoided in the presence of signs and symptoms of raised intracranial pressure. Antisialagogues are usually used because

Table 11-5. Intravenous drug dosages commonly employed during anesthesia

Drug	Dosage
Atropine	0.01–0.02 mg/kg
Hyoscine	0.008 mg/kg
Thiopental	4–5 mg/kg
Althesin	0.05–0.07 ml/kg
Ketamine	1–2 mg/kg
Diazepam	0.2 mg/kg
Droperidol	0.15 mg/kg
Fentanyl	0.001–0.002 mg/kg
Morphine	0.1–0.2 mg/kg
Succinylcholine	1–2 mg/kg
D-Tubocurarine	0.3–0.6 mg/kg
Pancuronium	0.1 mg/kg
Atracurium	0.5–0.6 mg/kg
Neostigmine	0.05 mg/kg
Naloxone	0.005–0.01 mg/kg

the presence of secretions in the respiratory tract, especially in the narrow airways of infants, can cause partial respiratory obstruction. Atropine (0.02 mg/kg) is given intravenously at the time of induction.

Induction of Anesthesia

Extreme care is exercised in handling frightened patients. An intravenous infusion site is gently established using a plastic cannula. Monitoring includes an electrocardiogram, blood pressure with an appropriate sized cuff, and a precordial stethoscope. The patient is pre-oxygenated. Induction can be with intravenous (thiopental 4–6 mg/kg) or inhalation agents (nitrous oxide-oxygen-halothane or isoflurane). Thiopental induction is preferred. However, an inhalation induction might be necessary for uncooperative children and for very young infants. Intramuscular or rectal methohexital can be used in such circumstances. Succinylcholine (1 mg/kg) or pancuronium (0.15–0.2 mg/kg) is administered to facilitate endotracheal intubation.

The child is manually hyperventilated and adequate time is allowed for the relaxant to become fully effective before endotracheal intubation is attempted. Armored tubes are used to prevent tube kinking in extreme head positions.

MAINTENANCE OF ANESTHESIA

Anesthesia is either maintained with a nitrous oxide-narcotic-relaxant technique or with nitrous oxide-relaxant technique supplemented with intermittent thiopental (Table 11-5). Most anesthesiologists prefer to avoid using volatile anesthetic agents because of their vasodilatory effect on the cerebral vasculature. Adequate pulmonary ventilation must be ensured. Cerebral vasoconstriction and a slack brain can be achieved by subjecting the child to moderate hyperventilation ($PaCO_2$ 25–30 mm Hg). Apart from monitoring clinical signs, heart sounds, arterial blood pressure, central venous pressure, arterial blood gases, the electrocardiogram, temperature, and urine output, other specific monitors are considered:

1. A pulmonary artery catheter to monitor left heart function and for cardiac output measurements. However, it must be remembered that repeated determinations of cardiac output

can cause overhydration of small children, because 3–10 ml of fluid is required for each cardiac output estimation.
2. A capnograph to monitor expired CO_2.
3. A precordial Doppler to detect air embolism.
4. An intracranial pressure monitor.
5. A spectral compressed EEG display.
6. An evoked potential recorder.

Positioning the child will depend on the site of the operation and the surgeon's preferred approach. Meticulous attention is necessary to protect the eyes and other sensitive parts of the body. Measures are taken to keep the child normothermic. Blood loss can be difficult to estimate because of frequent wound irrigations and has to be assessed and replaced based on clinical judgment. Sponge weights can be misleading because of losses absorbed by the drapes. Intraoperative fluid management is an important aspect in the maintenance of anesthesia. Lactated Ringer's solution is chosen for fluid replacement because hypo-osmolar solutions increase brain edema. Both osmotic (mannitol 0.25–1.0 g/kg) and potent loop diuretics (furosemide 0.5–1.0 mg/kg) can be used to dehydrate the brain acutely to make more room for the surgeon to operate. Continuous cerebrospinal fluid drainage, deliberate hypotension, and induced hypothermia are specific intraoperative measures that may be required in particular situations.

Emergence

Drugs that cause respiratory depression or affect the pupillary reflexes should be wearing off at the end of the operation. At the conclusion of anesthesia, the pharynx is suctioned, the relaxant reversed with atropine (0.02 mg/kg) followed by neostigmine (0.05 mg/kg), and the endotracheal tube removed before the child starts coughing.

POSTOPERATIVE CARE

Complete monitoring is carried out to the recovery room, fluids are restricted, and the child is nursed in a head-up tilt. Pain is not a prominent feature following craniotomy. Steroids are usually continued in the early postoperative period and convulsions are stopped with diazepam and their recurrence prevented with diphenylhydantoin and phenobarbital.

ADJUNCT TECHNIQUES

Two specific techniques, not infrequently used in pediatric neurosurgical care, are controlled hypotension and induced hypothermia.

Controlled Hypotension

The use of hypotensive anesthesia in pediatric neurosurgery remains controversial. The success and safety of the technique is largely dependent on the skill, experience, and care of the individual anesthesiologist. The main hazard of hypotensive anesthesia is uncontrolled hypotension leading to inadequate cerebral perfusion and permanent brain damage.

Differences in response to induced hypotension between children and adults must be taken into consideration:

- Children are known to be more resistant than adults to hypotensive drugs[17,18] and are much less likely to have catastrophic falls in blood pressure if large doses of vasodilators are accidentally used.
- Because of their smaller size, the use of tilting in children

does not produce as great a pressure gradient and peripheral pooling of blood as in adults.
- Alveolar dead space does not increase during hypotension in infants and children.[19]
- The administration of 100 percent oxygen has been recommended to ensure a higher oxygen delivery to the brain during the period of hypotension.[20]

Indications for controlled hypotension

- Surgical correction of central nervous system arteriovenous malformations is greatly facilitated by deliberate hypotension.
- Clipping of cerebral aneurysms.
- To decrease operative blood loss and therefore reduce the need for blood transfusions.
- To reduce the blood pressure when it rises acutely to dangerously high levels.

Methods and drugs used. Ganglion blockade with trimethaphan in pediatric patients appears to be frequently associated with tachycardia, which may result in failure of the technique. The judicious use of a beta-adrenergic blocking agent (propranolol) before or after ganglionic blockade has proved effective in controlling the rise in heart rate.

The most commonly used vasodilator is sodium nitroprusside. This is a vascular smooth muscle relaxant that causes vasodilatation and a fall in blood pressure. In infants, the systolic blood pressure rarely falls below 50 mm Hg, whereas in adults similar doses can have a much greater hypotensive effect. Sodium nitroprusside is usually given by infusion in concentrations varying from 0.01 to 0.1 mg/ml. Its administration is best controlled by an infusion pump.

Apart from cases showing a normal response to sodium nitroprusside at total doses below 3 mg/kg, Davies et al.[21] have been able to recognize and define three abnormal responses to sodium nitroprusside in children:

1. A constant response to high doses (more than 3 mg/kg) with associated metabolic disturbances.
2. A tachyphylactic response needing increasing doses of the drug to maintain safe minimal levels of systolic blood pressure and therefore a potentially lethal situation.
3. Resistance to sodium nitroprusside exhibited very rapidly, soon after administration. Should the initial response show resistance to sodium nitroprusside, then the drug should be immediately stopped, for to continue will most likely kill the patient of cyanide poisoning. Patients resistant to sodium nitroprusside have shown high blood levels of cyanide and inappropriately low levels of thiocyanate, which is indicative of a gross disturbance of the cyanide-thiocyanate pathway. This may be the result of an inadequate supply of endogenous thiosulfate, a deficiency or abnormality of tissue rhodanase, an inhibition of tissue rhodanase by other drugs, or a combination of these.

Greiss et al.[22] suggest the following as mandatory disciplines to which to adhere when using sodium nitroprusside:

- Absolute contraindications to its use exist in patients who have (1) resistance to sodium nitroprusside; (2) Leber's hereditary optic atrophy; (3) severe liver disease; (4) severe renal disease; (5) malnutrition; (6) vitamin B = 1 = 2 deficiency; or (7) hypothyroidism.

- The use of solutions of not more than 0.02 percent sodium nitroprusside suitably protected from light and heat.
- The administration of infusions of sodium nitroprusside by a separate intravenous infusion by a microdrip or infusion pump.
- Direct and continuous intra-arterial pressure monitoring.
- Frequent (half-hourly) arterial acid-base determinations.
- Constant attention to the patient's dose-response characteristics, particularly in the first 30 minutes.
- If infusion rates are in excess of 10 μg/kg/min, determine the nature of the response: constant, tachyphylactic, or resistant.
- If the patient is tachyphylactic or resistant, discontinue the sodium nitroprusside and administer another hypotensive agent.
- Maintain normothermia throughout.
- Cyanide antidote therapy readily available[23]; this includes: (1) inhalation of amyl nitrite; (2) intravenous infusion of sodium nitrite, 5 mg/kg in 20 ml H_2O given over 3 to 4 minutes; (3) intravenous infusion of sodium thiosulfate (150 mg/kg in 50 ml H_2O over 15 minutes); (4) hydroxocobalamin, if available, can be given (0.1 mg/kg).

Because of the ability of sodium nitroprusside to dilate cerebral blood vessels and therefore to increase intracranial pressure, it has been suggested that its use be avoided in patients with raised intracranial pressure unless previous measures have been taken to improve intracranial compliance.[24]

Isoflurane recently has been recommended for deliberate hypotension because of its rapid onset of action, ease of control, and rapid reversal upon discontinuance. However, some investigators have demonstrated loss of autoregulation for 60 minutes after discontinuance of isoflurane and increases in cerebral blood flow, which could worsen edema, ischemia, and increase neurologic deficits.[25]

Monitoring During Controlled Hypotension

- The pulse becomes softer and more difficult to palpate.
- A delay in capillary refill indicates excessive hypotension.
- Intra-arterial pressure monitoring is mandatory when hypotensive anesthesia is employed.
- The electrocardiogram should be used to detect arrhythmias and possible myocardial ischemia.
- Temperature should be monitored because peripheral vasodilatation will increase heat loss unless steps are taken to prevent it.
- Arterial blood gases are regularly checked: low $PaCO_2$ levels may be not tolerated, causing cerebral vasoconstriction when cerebral perfusion pressure is low.
- Urine output measurement may be useful to monitor kidney function. Urine output normally should exceed 0.75 ml/kg/hr.
- Coagulogram for possible platelet-induced inhibition caused by sodium nitroprusside.[26]

In conclusion, induced hypotension is relatively safe in infants and children but is not devoid of complications. Monitoring during hypotension must be continuous and thorough if accidents are to be avoided.

Hypothermia

Induced hypothermia is used to reduce the metabolic rate and hence oxygen consumption, thereby increasing the duration of hypoxia that tissues will tolerate without developing irreversible damage. The fall in oxygen consumption with the reduction in temperature is not a linear process. Oxygen consumption will be reduced to 50 percent at 30°C, to 25 percent at 25°C, to 15 percent at 20°C, and to 10 percent at 15°C. Hypothermia causes a reduction in brain volume and cerebrospinal fluid pressure, changes much appreciated by the neurosurgeons. Surgical indications for hypothermia include intracranial aneurysms, cerebral vascular anomalies, and cerebral edema of surgical or traumatic origin. It makes hypotension safer and allows the circulation to be interrupted during resection of aneurysms and other vascular malformations. It also reduces the risk of cerebral ischemia caused by pressure on brain tissue. Cerebral vessels tend to show vasoconstriction and increased irritability down to 30°C. Below 30°C, vasodilatation becomes more apparent. Cooling below 30°C therefore should provide the best results.[27] Because hypocapnia increases cerebral vasoconstriction, some anesthesiologists prefer to maintain normocarbia during the progress of hypothermia. The tendency to develop arrhythmias, including ventricular fibrillation, is less in infants and occurs at lower temperatures compared with adults (26° to 27°C). Moderate hypothermia, achieved by surface cooling methods, is used most frequently in neurosurgical cases. The anesthetic management of patients undergoing hypothermia includes the use of muscle relaxants and controlled ventilation. Muscle relaxants abolish shivering, which would considerably increase oxygen consumption as the body temperature is lowered. Although anesthesia is usually induced and concluded at normothermia, it is relevant to understand the general principles of drug action at lowered temperatures, so that overdosage is avoided. At temperatures around 24°–26°C, cold narcosis occurs and EEG activity ceases. This depression of cerebral function means that lower concentrations of anesthetics are needed. Less D-tubocurarine is required at low temperature and recovery is also more gradual. Drugs that are inactivated by the liver or excreted by the kidneys will have a longer action at low temperature because of depression of hepatic and renal function.

Changing the patient's position can be particularly dangerous, because the sudden raising of the lower limbs can return a large quantity of very cold blood into the main circulation. Since the heart muscle is very sensitive to sudden changes in temperature, this sudden transfusion may be sufficient to provoke ventricular fibrillation. If the patient is placed upon the operating table in the correct position for surgery before cooling is commenced, this risk is obviated. The most likely cause of trouble is when immersion cooling is used for infants, because when the child is lifted out of the bath extra cold blood may enter the main circulation.

Monitoring. Continuous measurement of the temperature in the ear, nasopharynx, esophagus, rectum, and muscles gives guidance to the gradients achieved and to the brain temperature. Excessive rates of cooling leave some tissues rather warm and hence increase the risk of acidosis during circulatory arrest. The electrocardiogram and the venous and arterial pressures are monitored, the latter by electromanometry. Biochemical control and the control of blood clotting is essential, as is correct blood replacement using venous and arterial pressures as valuable guides. Hypothermia should be reversed before the patient is transferred to the recovery room. Hypothermic infants are slow to recover, remain acidotic, are more prone to vomit, and develop apnea.

ANESTHESIA FOR SPECIFIC NEUROSURGICAL PROCEDURES

POSTERIOR FOSSA TUMORS

Preoperative shunting is usually reserved for children who remain acutely ill because of intracranial hypertension. Even if intracranial pressure is normal, it must be assumed that intracranial compliance is reduced and that procedures which can increase intracranial pressure will be poorly tolerated. These patients may have motor weakness, impaired gag and swallowing mechanisms, pulmonary dysfunction from repeated aspirations, and inadequate hydration secondary to prolonged vomiting, poor appetite, diabetes insipidus, fluid restriction, and osmotherapy.

Issues of premedication, induction, and maintenance of anesthesia are similar to those discussed for patients with intracranial space-occupying lesion. If the sitting position is utilized a precordial Doppler, an end-tidal PCO_2 monitor, and a central venous line are mandatory. The sitting position will cause blood to pool in dependent limbs. Wrapping the legs and thighs can overcome this problem. Electrocardiographic monitoring is especially important in posterior fossa surgery, since irregular and ectopic beats are frequent during surgical manipulation of the floor of the fourth ventricle. The most serious intraoperative complication of the sitting position is air embolism.

If air embolization is detected, treatment must be prompt. Nitrous oxide is discontinued to prevent expansion of air bubbles. The patient is ventilated with 100 percent oxygen. The surgeon must be notified to cover the wound with saline. The jugular veins can be compressed, if accessible, to prevent further air entrainment. This maneuver, however, can lead to troublesome cerebral venous congestion. Attempts can be made to aspirate air from the central venous catheter. The addition of positive end-expiratory pressure can increase venous pressure but will aggravate an already decreasing arterial blood pressure and can predispose patients with a probe-patent foramen ovale to the risk of paradoxical air embolism.[28] Pressor support and full resuscitative measures may be needed in extreme cases.

CRANIOPHARYNGIOMAS

The preanesthetic assessment of patients with craniopharyngiomas must include complete neurologic and endocrine evaluations. The presence of headache, projectile vomiting, papilledema, or a decreased level of consciousness can indicate a significant increase in intracranial pressure. The presence of diabetes insipidus is suspected if the child is hypernatremic, hyperosmolar, has a negative fluid balance, and has very dilute urine (specific gravity less than 0.005). This should be corrected with a short-acting form of vasopressin, such as aqueous pitressin in a dose of 0.05–0.1 unit/kg. Cortisone administration is continued perioperatively. Anesthesia is induced with thiopental, succinylcholine, or pancuronium. The intracranial pressure may increase because of light anesthesia, coughing and straining, or the development of hypoxia or hypercarbia during the process of intubation, and these should be avoided. Anesthesia is maintained with nitrous oxide and oxygen, supplemented by the intravenous administration of narcotics and muscle relaxants. The patient is moderately hyperventilated ($PaCO_2$ 25–30 mm Hg). Manipulation of the hypothalamus may lead to loss of temperature regulation as well as to marked changes in heart rate and blood pressure. Visual evoked potentials, if available, can be used to monitor the optic pathways during the surgical procedure. The central venous pressure can be very helpful in determining the volume status of the patient. The quantity and quality of the urinary output must also be monitored. Postoperatively, major fluid and electrolyte imbalances are carefully corrected, the patient is extubated early and steroid coverage is continued.[29]

VASCULAR DISORDERS

Vascular disorders occur far less frequently in childhood than in adult life and constitute less than 1 percent of pediatric neurosurgical cases. They include intracranial aneurysms, arteriovenous malformations, and aneurysms of the vein of Galen.

Arteriovenous malformations constitute the most common cerebrovascular disorder of childhood to come to the attention of the neurosurgeon. The majority of hemispheric arteriovenous malformations remain clinically silent until they bleed. Convulsive seizures are an initial complaint in only 20 percent of cases, and a history of migraine-like headache is sometimes obtained in older children. Large arteriovenous shunts occasionally produce cardiomegaly and congestive heart failure, but such problems are much less common than in aneurysms of the vein of Galen. A common result of subarachnoid hemorrhage from arteriovenous malformations is the development of communicating hydrocephalus, which requires early intervention to relieve the obstruction.

Aneurysms of the great vein of Galen are a particular type of arteriovenous malformation in which hypertrophied cerebral arteries communicate either directly with the vein of Galen or through a mass of abnormal vessels. The vein enlarges considerably, as do the straight and lateral sinuses. As a result, a low resistance pathway is created that markedly increases cardiac output. In newborn infants, the symptoms are those of congestive heart failure.[30] Seizures are also common and hydrocephalus is present in almost every case. In older infants and young children, the symptoms are usually related to hydrocephalus. Spontaneous intracranial hemorrhage, so common with hemispheric arteriovenous malformations, is an exceptional complication of aneurysms of the vein of Galen.

In addition to the role of administering a stable and safe anesthetic to prevent rerupture of the vascular malformation, the anesthesiologist faces the particular challenge of maintaining adequate oxygen transport to the brain in the presence of cerebral vasospasm and deliberate hypotension. Premedication should be tailored to the child's state of consciousness. Patients who are obtunded because of heavy sedation or neurologic causes should not be given additional premedication. Children who are alert and asymptomatic can be given light oral premedication (diazepam 0.1 mg/kg). Full invasive vascular monitoring is deferred until the child becomes unconscious. Relatively deep levels of anesthesia must be reached before laryngoscopy and endotracheal intubation are attempted. Hypocarbia must be avoided, especially in the presence of vasospasm and deliberate hypotension, because it can further aggravate an already compromised cerebrovascular circulation; it can also increase steal to arteriovenous malformations. Mannitol and cerebral vasodilating drugs should be used only after the skull has been opened. Maintenance of anesthesia should aim at avoidance of abrupt changes in arterial blood pressure. Deliberate hypotension should be judiciously used in the pediatric age group. No data are available on the upper and lower limit of autoregulation, and the effects of abnormal blood pressures on cerebral blood flow and intracranial pressure are less well understood in children than in adults. Surface-induced profound hypothermia with circulatory arrest and low-flow extracorporeal circulation has allowed the safe excision of massive aneurysms of the great vein of Galen in infants.[31] Postoperatively, prompt endotracheal extubation should be possible in patients previously in grades I and II.

SURGERY FOR EPILEPSY

In children, the surgical treatment of epilepsy, except for that caused by an obvious structural lesion such as a brain tumor, should be undertaken reluctantly and only after all reasonable attempts at medical management have failed. Operative techniques for relieving intractable seizures include: (1) excising the epileptogenic area, (2) interrupting the pathways of seizure spread, and (3) altering the seizure threshold by neurostimulation. Of these, the most reliable by far is cortical excision of a discrete epileptogenic focus that has been precisely localized by EEG and electrocorticography.

In order to allow for intraoperative electrocorticography, surgery of temporal lobe epilepsy is usually performed under field block of the scalp and cranium supplemented by a form of neuroleptanalgesia in which no drugs that can depress or alter the cerebral cortical activity are utilized. Fentanyl and droperidol administered intermittently during the procedure are devoid of this effect and cause no respiratory depression. An alternative technique of anesthetic management is required for uncooperative patients and very young children.

An endotracheal nitrous oxide-oxygen-narcotic-relaxant technique is selected. Prior to electrocorticography, nitrous oxide is discontinued, and the dose and timing of neuromuscular blocking agents are so regulated that the residual neuromuscular blockade at the time of cortical stimulation is only minimal. The technique allows observation of motor phenomena only; testing of speech, memory, and sensory phenomena are not possible.

REPAIR OF DURAL TEARS

Continuous cerebrospinal fluid leak may persist following head trauma or previous neurosurgical operations. Recurrent pneumococcal meningitis can complicate dural tears if the dural leak communicates with the airway.

The major anesthetic problem involves the use of positive airway pressure during the induction of anesthesia. If positive pressure is used before the trachea is intubated, airway secretions may be forced through the dural defect into the central nervous system.

PEDIATRIC HYDROCEPHALUS

Hydrocephalic children may have their cerebrospinal fluid draining in a sealed system for some days before surgery. Fluid and electrolytes are therefore depleted and have to be adequately replaced before surgery. Children with obstructed shunts and elevated intracranial pressure frequently have apparent upper respiratory tract infections. Revision of the shunt should not be delayed; rhinorrhea and chest rales will improve as the raised intracranial pressure is corrected.[32] Babies with

hydrocephalus have very large heads, and special posturing may be necessary in order to intubate them. Ventilation is controlled to avoid hypercapnia and hypoxia, especially if a high intracranial pressure is suspected. Ketamine can cause acute rises of ventricular fluid pressure and therefore offers no advantages to these patients.[6] For ventriculoatrial shunts, the distal tip of the vascular end of the shunt catheter must be in the midatrium for maximal mechanical efficiency. Its correct placement can easily be verified by the use of a unipolar electrocardiogram, the chest lead of which is suitably connected to an electrolyte solution (3 percent sodium chloride) in the distal portion of the shunt tube. Between the sinoauricular node and the tricuspid valve, the P waves have a completely biphasic pattern. Pressure changes as the shunt tip descends down the jugular vein into the superior vena cava and into the right heart can also be used to check the position of the catheter tip inside the right atrium.[33] A final verification of the distal end of the shunt can be made by x-ray films of the chest. The introduction of the catheter into the heart can occasionally provoke cardiac arrhythmias, especially if the tube enters the right ventricle. Ventricular atrial shunts require that the distal end of the shunt be inserted into the jugular vein and hence require that the neck region be dissected. The neurosurgeon and anesthesiologist must pay particular attention to the possibility of air embolism. Multiple procedures are frequently required to relieve blockage, to treat shunt infections, and for elective lengthening of shunt tubes. If ventricular drainage is blocked, the child is lethargic and vomits frequently. There is a build up of cerebrospinal fluid and the intracranial pressure is elevated. Anesthesia for decompression is induced by establishing an intravenous line and doing a rapid sequence induction with a nondepolarizing muscle relaxant and a rapid-acting barbiturate while hyperventilating the child with a bag and mask and maintaining cricoid pressure to prevent regurgitation of stomach contents. Postoperatively, the patient is nursed in a slight head-up position and is kept on the left side to ensure proper functioning of the valve. Ventriculopleural shunts can cause postoperative respiratory failure if a large volume of cerebrospinal fluid accumulates in the pleural cavity and causes hydrothorax. Occasionally, a ventriculoperitoneal tube perforates a loop of bowel and causes abdominal distention and obstruction or intracranial infection by the cephalad migration of enteric organisms through the shunt tubing. Finally, care must be taken in patients with patent ventriculoatrial shunts who need postoperative pneumoencephalographic studies to avoid air embolism.[34] The decision to ligate or clamp the shunt before the injection of air should be contemplated and the use of another contrast medium instead of air should be considered. Extreme care is used in positioning the patient and in removing cerebrospinal fluid. Continuous electrocardiographic monitoring and the placement of a Doppler flow probe over the tricuspid area are strongly recommended.

ANESTHESIA FOR CONGENITAL MALFORMATIONS

Occipital Encephalocele

Anesthesia for correction of occipital encephalocele is often complicated by the presence of hydrocephalus, Klippel-Feil deformity, and a cleft palate. Other associated abnormalities can include micrognathia, a common cerebral ventricle with agenesis of the corpus callosum and septum pellucidum, subglottic stenosis, ventricular septal defect, patent ductus arteriosus, diastematomyelia, lumbar meningocele, and spina bifida occulta.[35]

Intubation. An armored endotracheal tube of suitable size should be used to prevent tube kinking when the patient is placed in the prone position. Intubation is performed with the patient lying on the left side. Although it is possible to support the patient supine on bolsters without damage to the encephalocele, the risk is minimized by using the lateral position. Intubation is performed with the patient awake. An assistant is instructed to press the shoulders back while supporting the head in the optimum position for laryngoscopy.

Temperature control. The maintenance of body temperature is a serious problem in these patients. The effect of any defect in the temperature regulating mechanism usually is compounded by the operating room environment. Using an overhead infra-red heating lamp during the preparatory stages and heating blankets during the operation might help to maintain temperature homeostasis.

Ventilation and posture. Ventilation is controlled and the prone position is preferred. Meticulous attention must be given to the positioning of the patient. Transverse bolsters under the chest and pelvic girdle ensure that the abdomen remains free from external pressure, permitting unimpeded movement and unobstructed venous flow.

Fluid therapy. In infants, the suboccipital bone is richly vascularized and the dural sinuses are extensive and undefined. Surgical blood loss is a problem and is estimated by careful observation and by changes in the patient's vital signs. Blood loss should be replaced in an amount sufficient to maintain a systolic blood pressure of 60 mm Hg during surgery.

Myelomeningocele

Myelomeningocele is a condition resulting from disturbance of the neural tube. The bony covering of the spinal canal is missing and the neural elements are usually on the surface. Hydrocephalus and Chiari malformation often complicate the initial defect. Surgery is usually undertaken within hours after birth to reduce the risk of infection and further neurologic damage. Respiratory obstruction causing stridor may also be seen in babies with hydrocephalus and myelomeningocele and may be caused by distortion and traction effects on the lower brain stem and cranial nerves. Therapy is operative neurosurgery.[36]

Adequate preoperative fluid replacement is required to compensate for the evaporative fluid loss from the meningocele. To eliminate the difficulty of positioning, the patient is intubated while awake in the lateral or semilateral position. The operation is performed in the face-down position. Positioning should allow free movement of the chest and abdomen. Controlled ventilation is likely to be required as spontaneous respirations, mainly diaphragmatic, are embarrassed in this position. These children tend to lose body heat during the surgical procedure and adequate means of warming the child are necessary. The significance of the blood loss depends on the size of the defect. Postoperatively the child is nursed in the prone position.

Posterior Fossa Decompression for Arnold-Chiari Malformation

The Arnold-Chiari malformation comprises a group of congenital hindbrain anomalies in which there is downward displacement of the vermis of the cerebellum into the cervical canal with caudal displacement and elongation of the lower pons and medulla. Usually the symptoms appear in the first 4 months of life, with hydrocephalus that results from narrowing of the aqueduct. A meningomyelocele is also commonly present. Children with Arnold-Chiari malformation may have laryngeal stridor. In these cases the vocal cords may be paretic or paralyzed. Respiratory arrest and loss of consciousness can follow flexion of the neck, a complication that can be missed if the patient is unconscious under general anesthesia.

During the preoperative assessment of these patients, particular attention must be paid to ensure that the airway is adequate. Whenever possible, endotracheal intubation with the patient awake to avoid undue positional changes of the neck is recommended. This will also provide a clear airway while anesthesia is being induced. If a pre-existing obstructive hydrocephalus has been decompressed, no special precautions for intracranial hypertension need to be taken.

Craniosynostosis

Craniosynostosis is a congenital deformity associated with premature closure of the cranial fissures. Surgery is required at an early age to relieve raised intracranial pressure, to avoid further neurologic damage, and for cosmetic purposes. The operation consists of removal of strips of bones alongside the fused sutures. To prevent refusion, polyethylene film strips are placed around the cut bone edges.

Various positions are employed according to the sutures involved and the surgeon's preference. Associated congenital abnormalities affecting the airway may render ventilation difficult to maintain. During removal of bone from the skull blood pours freely from the marrow space and may cause life-threatening hypovolemia. The anesthesiologist must prepare in advance to transfuse blood rapidly. Large-bore peripheral venous lines are required and blood loss should be estimated as accurately as possible and replaced milliliter for milliliter as it is lost. Inhalation induction can be performed satisfactorily in most cases. If difficulty with the airway is encountered during inhalation induction, intubation or tracheostomy with the patient awake should be considered. An armored tube should be used if extremes of head position are anticipated. If the surgery is performed in the prone position, the patient is supported on a U-shaped bolster. This will permit full diaphragmatic excursion and an unimpeded vena caval blood flow. Anesthesia is maintained with halothane, nitrous oxide, and oxygen, and ventilation is controlled. Blood pressure, fluid and electrolyte balance, and blood gases are monitored with intra-arterial and central venous catheters. A urinary catheter is placed in all patients to monitor urine output. Extubation is performed when the infant is warm and fully awake. Postoperatively, close observation for any sign of hypovolemia is especially important and the possibility of cerebral edema during the first 48 hours is carefully monitored.

Craniofacial Repairs

The operative procedure for craniofacial repairs consists of multiple craniectomies of fused sutures, forehead advancement, and reshaping of the cranial vault. Usually no intracranial pathologic condition is present, but an intracranial approach is necessary to provide access to the facial structures from within.

The major areas of concern for the anesthesiologist are airway establishment and maintenance, preservation of brain function, blood loss and fluid replacement, and temperature homeostasis. Frequently these children have abnormal airways that are very difficult to intubate. The obstructed nasal passages make inhalation induction difficult until the child is deep enough to tolerate an oropharyngeal airway. The endotracheal tube should be of an armored type and taped securely or stitched in position. The posterior pharynx is packed to prevent blood aspiration around the tube. Manipulation and retraction of the brain are unavoidable during the surgery and may lead to postoperative cerebral edema. Controlled hyperventilation, continuous CSF drainage, dexamethasone (0.2 mg/kg), and osmotic or potent loop diuretics are used to avoid retractor anemia and to reduce brain bulk. Considerable blood loss can occur from the highly vascular facial structures. Direct arterial pressure, central venous pressure, and urine output are continuously monitored to assess hypovolemia. Because of the danger of retractor anemia, deliberate hypotension should not be used for this operation. Bradycardia secondary to retraction of the frontal lobe can be eliminated with intravenous atropine (0.01–0.02 mg/kg). A further complication of this procedure manifests itself in the postoperative period as either excessive ADH secretion or diabetes insipidus and is caused by hypothalamic dysfunction.

ANESTHESIA FOR NEURORADIOGRAPHIC PROCEDURES

GENERAL CONSIDERATIONS

The diagnosis and localization of central nervous system lesions often necessitate the use of one or more invasive radiographic procedures. In infants and children, neuroradiographic procedures may be required in the investigation of congenital abnormalities, depressed fractures and intracranial hematomas, epilepsy, cerebral abscesses, and nervous system space-occupying lesions. Pediatric neuroradiographic anesthesia presents challenging problems for the anesthesiologist. Procedures are usually carried out far away from the familiar surroundings of the operating room. The child is frightened and apprehensive. Heavy premedication is always contraindicated, especially in the poor risk patient with intracranial hypertension. Postural changes are common during certain procedures: vomiting, aspiration, airway obstruction, hypoventilation, and hypotension are all known complications of sudden postural changes. The anesthesiologist should aim at a smooth induction; the avoidance of factors that increase cerebral blood flow and intracranial pressure; the use of unkinkable or cuffed armored endotracheal tubes; controlled ventilation; minimal depression of cardiovascular reflexes; and adequate monitoring. Rapid recovery is desirable, since these patients may receive more than one anesthetic within the course of a few days. Also the combination of fluid restriction, compounded by nausea and vomiting, may lead to inadequate hydration and hypovolemia in susceptible patients.

SPECIFIC PROCEDURES

Cerebral Angiography

In children, cerebral angiography is frequently performed through a catheter passed percutaneously via the femoral artery to demonstrate the displacement or compression of cerebral blood vessels by space-occupying lesions. It will also display intracranial aneurysms, vascular malformations, and occlusive vascular diseases.

Cerebral angiography is usually performed under general endotracheal anesthesia with controlled ventilation and adequate monitoring of the respiratory and cardiovascular systems. General anesthesia will provide complete immobility, adequate oxygenation, and avoid hypercarbia. Anesthesia is maintained with nitrous oxide, fentanyl, and relaxants. Potent inhalation agents (halothane-isoflurane) are less satisfactory because they dilate the cerebral blood vessels, cause more rapid transit of the dye through the cerebral circulation, and predispose the patient to hypotension, making arterial puncture more difficult to perform. Moderate hyperventilation will slow transit time of contrast medium and therefore allow for more films to be taken. Furthermore, the resulting inverse steal phenomenon will lead to a higher concentration of the contrast medium in the nonreactive and maximally dilated abnormal tumor and cerebral blood vessels. A $PaCO_2$ of 30 to 35 mm Hg is sufficient to provide good quality angiograms and to prevent any rise in intracranial pressure.[37] The anesthesiologist needs to be aware of the current limitations on dye dosages. At the end of the procedure, pressure should be applied over the artery until there is no evidence of hematoma formation. Adequate arterial pulsation in the foot is confirmed and the injection site is rechecked when the patient is returned to the ward. Serious neurologic problems sometimes follow angiography caused by arterial thrombosis, embolism, an increase in intracranial vascular spasm, or from systemic hypotension. Spasm of the artery at the site of insertion of the catheter can lead to reduced blood flow to the limb. Injection of procaine or papaverine around the artery can reduce the spasm. Carotid angiography can lead to massive hematoma and respiratory distress, necessitating urgent reintubation.

Myelography

With the patient in the prone position, a lumbar puncture is performed and a hyperbaric radiopaque contrast medium is injected in the subarachnoid space. The patient is then tilted head down, head up, supine, and prone while x-ray films are taken to visualize defects within the spinal canal. At the termination of the study, the contrast medium is aspirated back from the subarachnoid space as completely as possible. Air myelography has recently been introduced. Air is injected through a cisternal puncture and x-ray films are taken with the patient in the erect, supine, and prone positions. Like pneumoencephalography, it causes severe headache.

Myelography is usually performed under general anesthesia, and assisted spontaneous ventilation with nitrous oxide, oxygen, and halothane is often satisfactory. Care should be taken during posturing to avoid injury, disconnection from the anesthetic machine, displacement of the endotracheal tube and hypoventilation. Accidental puncturing of dural venous channels during cisternal air myelography can occasionally result in air embolism.[38] Children are particularly prone to this complication and the safety of the procedure can be increased by using nitrous oxide instead of air as the contrast medium.

Ventriculography

Ventriculography is the radiographic study of contrast medium within the ventricular system. The medium is injected into one or both lateral ventricles with a needle passing through the brain substance. Ventriculography is indicated to investigate the following conditions: (1) raised intracranial pressure and obstructive hydrocephalus; (2) Arnold-Chiari malformation in infants with spinal dysraphia; (3) intraventricular tumors in the presence of raised intracranial pressure; (4) congenital malformations accompanied by raised intracranial pressure. In infants with open coronal sutures a styletted needle is passed through the right coronal suture into the anterior half of the right lateral ventricle.

Infants weighing less than 10 kg are not anesthetized; a pacifier dipped in a sweet sedative syrup is often the best form of anesthesia. In older children without split sutures, a posterior frontal twist-drill hole is made through which a needle is inserted. The procedure usually necessitates a general anesthetic.

Computed Tomography (CT Scans)

Computed tomography is the procedure of choice for identifying the size and geography of the ventricles and the possible lesions obstructing the ventricular cerebrospinal fluid pathway. It is also best suited for determining the alteration of ventricular size in post-shunt hydrocephalic children.

The anesthesiologist's role is to keep the child still for the procedure. In older children some form of sedation is all that is needed, but in infants it may be necessary to intubate and ventilate the patient. In very sick or unconscious patients, no sedation may be needed, but the airway and ventilation must be carefully monitored.

Magnetic Resonance Imaging

Magnetic resonance imaging is a recently developed diagnostic technique that employs a strong magnetic field and radiofrequency pulses to generate images. It has specific advantages over CT scanning because there is an absence of bone artifact, which makes visualization of the posterior fossa and subdural and subarachnoid hemorrhage more precise. It can also clearly distinguish between white and gray matter.

Monitoring patients undergoing magnetic resonance imaging poses various problems. The ferrous metal contained in most monitoring equipment can distort the magnetic field and hence degrade the image. A monitoring system made up of commercially available components, permitting monitoring of blood pressure, heart rate, ECG, and chest-wall motion, and free of disturbances to magnetic resonance imaging function is now available.[39] The patient within the scanner is usually inaccessible for resuscitation. Defibrillators, pacemakers, and perfusion pumps may malfunction if needed. The anesthesia machine is at least 3 m away from the scanner's magnetic field and from the patient. Extension tubes on a Rees-type[40] modification of the Ayers T-system connect the patient to the anesthesia machine. In the neonate, in the very young, in those with involuntary muscular motion, and in children in whom sedation has been inadequate, a general anesthetic must be employed. Endotracheal intubation is mandatory if a general anesthetic is required. If the child has associated intracranial hypertension the anesthesiologist must be prepared to lower the intracranial pressure actively.

HEAD INJURIES

Pediatric head injury constitutes a very significant proportion of all childhood injuries. Distinguishing features from adult brain injury include (1) the special circumstances of birth trauma; (2) the amazing resiliency of the young brain; (3) the relatively low incidence of mass lesions; and (4) the high incidence of diffuse cerebral swelling. These differences have favored a different pathophysiologic response of the child's brain to injury, with an improved outcome and a better prognosis.[41,42] Early in the injury, however, evidence suggests that increased blood volume rather than edema is the cause of the brain swelling.[43] At that stage hyperventilation and not mannitol should be used to actively lower the intracranial pressure.

Pediatric head trauma is conveniently subdivided into three periods: (1) at birth, (2) during infancy, and (3) later childhood. The vast majority are blunt injuries resulting from bicycle or car accidents or from falls. A closed head injury can cause damage to the brain from direct contusion, intracranial bleeding, concussion injury with cerebral hyperemia and edema, or massively increased intracranial pressure.

In the management of acute head injuries, primary attention is given to maintain a free airway. The possibility of an unstable cervical spine injury must always be considered in any case of significant head injury. Vomiting and pulmonary aspiration are common. Injury can delay gastric emptying in children for more than 8 hours after the accident, and swallowed blood can result in a stomach distended with blood clots. Endotracheal intubation may be needed with more serious injuries or for respiratory dysfunction. The second consideration is hypovolemic shock. This is usually caused by bleeding from extensive scalp lacerations, from an expanding extradural hematoma, or from other associated injuries. Diagnostic studies required for a severe head injury include skull x-ray films, a lateral x-ray study of the neck, a CT scan, an arteriogram, and an echoencephalogram.

Emergency surgery is sometimes needed to evacuate an extradural hematoma or to explore compound injuries. Massive decompression may be considered in refractory brain swelling. Subdural hematoma of infancy, a relatively common problem, is usually tapped repeatedly and this may be the only treatment required.

Patients brought to the operating room require the most complete monitoring available. To prevent aspiration and an excessive increase in intracranial pressure, endotracheal intubation should be performed with minimal manipulations of the head and cervical spine, using the "full stomach" thiopental-relaxant technique. Radial artery cannulation is instituted for continuous monitoring of blood pressure and for frequent blood gas measurements. A central venous pressure line is inserted both to facilitate assessment of blood volume and to permit rapid transfusion of blood and fluid. Warming devices are used in the infusion line to prevent undue cooling of the infant. Temperature is monitored carefully to evaluate hypothalamic dysfunction. The bladder is catheterized to measure urinary output. The effect of drugs and anesthesia on the intracranial pressure must be carefully considered. It is believed that all inhalation anesthetic agents contribute to the increase in intracranial pressure and the use of such agents should be avoided whenever possible. Agents typically used are muscle relaxants, oxygen, and narcotics. Anesthesia techniques are conducted to prevent any sudden change in arterial and venous blood pressures. Ventilation is controlled to achieve moderate hyperventilation ($PaCO_2$ 25–30 mm Hg). During the course of anesthesia, it may be necessary to attempt to lower the intracranial pressure actively by the following techniques: (1) hyperventilation to a $PaCO_2$ of 20–25 mm Hg; (2) the use of osmotic diuretics (mannitol 0.25–1.0 g/kg); (3) the administration of dexamethasone (1 mg/kg); and the use of barbiturates (thiopental 1–4 mg/kg).

NONOPERATIVE MANAGEMENT OF SEVERE HEAD TRAUMA

Nonoperative management of severe head trauma is usually based on the principles of intensive neurologic and respiratory supportive cares. The main aspects are:

- Correction and avoidance of factors known potentially to increase the intracranial pressure. These include: hypercarbia; hypoxia; increased central venous pressure (coughing, straining, jugular vein compression, fluid overload, excessive PEEP, or mean airway pressure); hypertension, especially in response to painful or noxious stimuli; and cerebral edema (fluid overload, hyponatremia).
- Heavy sedation to reduce cerebral metabolic rate and somatic and autonomic reflexes.
- Total muscle paralysis to prevent gagging, straining, coughing, and shivering.
- Control of blood pressure to secure a within-normal cerebral perfusion pressure.
- Intracranial pressure monitoring. In children three methods of intracranial pressure monitoring are in use; the subarachnoid bolt, the intraventricular catheter, and the implantable epidural pressure transducer.[44–49] Continuous monitoring of intracranial pressure should be included in the management of all children suffering from severe head injuries.[50]
- Controlled hyperventilation to lower intracranial pressure and improve cerebral blood flow to damaged areas of the brain. Central causes of respiratory dysfunction following head injury include Cheyne-Stokes respiration, central neurogenic hyperventilation, apneustic breathing, and ataxic respiration. $PaCO_2$ values held in the range of 25 to 30 mm Hg will produce cerebral vasoconstriction; below 20 mm Hg cerebral oxygenation may be impaired.
- Maintenance of a PaO_2 slightly higher than normal. It has been observed that despite apparently adequate respiratory exchange, hypoxia occurs in approximately 70 percent of patients who are comatose following head injuries.[51] Intracranial pressure may be decreased by reversing hypoxic states.[52] In order to avoid toxic concentrations of oxygen, positive end-expiratory pressure has been used (5–10 cm H_2O) to normalize PaO_2. Intracranial pressure may not be affected if the patient is maintained in a 30-degree head-up position; however, intracranial pressure should be continuously monitored.[53,54]
- Neurogenic pulmonary edema can result from a centrally mediated massive sympathetic discharge.[55] Furosemide and positive end-expiratory pressure may improve alveolar ventilation. However, treatment aiming at supporting left ventricular performance and at reducing afterload has also been suggested.[56]
- Steroids are given commonly for severe head injuries. Dexamethasone is the drug of choice (0.5–1.5 mg/kg/day). Its use, however, remains controversial.[57,58]
- Mild hypothermia. Patients are placed on cooling blankets; the rectal temperature is lowered to approximately 33°–34°C. This decreases the cerebral metabolic rate and probably decreases cerebral blood flow as well[59];
- Five percent of trauma patients manifest seizure activity initially. Diazepam is the drug of choice and should be given intravenously when needed. The incidence of convulsions increases rapidly in the days and weeks following injury and the prophylactic use of diphenylhydantoin should be considered when there is gross brain damage.
- Fluids are restricted during the first few days to initiate cerebral dehydration. Only half the calculated fluid volume is infused. Euvolemic dehydration represents a state in which the central volume compartment is maintained euvolemic by the administration of colloid and blood products while the amount of free water that is administered is restricted to replacement of insensible losses.
- Osmotic and loop diuretics may be needed in severe trauma in addition to steroids and hyperventilation. Mannitol 20 percent is rapidly infused in a dose of 1 g/kg whenever brainstem compression is suspected. Furosemide 0.3–0.6 mg/kg causes no initial burden on the circulation.[60]
- Barbiturates. Indications for barbiturate coma include cerebral ischemia, raised intracranial pressure, and encephalopathy. An adequate depth of coma is achieved when the intracranial pressure is less than 20 mm Hg and the serum barbiturate level is 3 mg/100 ml. The use of high dose barbiturates in head injury rests on two uncertain propositions: that scrupulous control of intracranial pressure improves outcome and that barbiturates are effective in the long-term control of intracranial hypertension when other agents have failed.[61] The risks of this therapy are predictable and the complications are preventable and treatable.
- General Care. Fluid and electrolyte balance, respiratory care, adequate nutrition, and management of sepsis are routinely followed for all patients.

SPINAL CORD INJURIES

Spinal cord injuries are extremely rare in infants and children. They occur most commonly after breech extractions and in older children from falls and diving accidents. Most of the injuries in both groups involve the cervical region.

Respiratory insufficiency following high cervical injuries will lead to hypoxemia, hypoventilation, ineffective coughing, and pulmonary aspiration of gastric contents. Although the establishment of the airway is of paramount importance, this maneuver is frequently difficult and can result in extension of the cord injury. Tracheal intubation is performed with the neck maintained in a neutral position under topical anesthesia. In the absence of concomitant head injuries and raised intracranial pressure muscle relaxants and laryngoscopy are best avoided. Tracheal suctioning, intermittent ventilatory assistance, and tracheal intubation may result in reflex bradycardia or even cardiac arrest as a result of a vagovagal reflex in a sympathectomized child. This complication can be avoided by the prior intravenous administration of atropine. These patients develop muscle atrophy and are susceptible to severe hyperkalemia, leading to arrhythmias and cardiac arrest following succinylcholine injections.[62] Intravascular volume replacement is commonly used to treat hypotension in these patients. However, care must be taken with fluid administration in order to avoid overload leading to pulmonary edema. Gastric distension is common after spinal cord injury. Loss or diminution of protective pharyngeal reflexes makes aspiration an ever-present hazard. Temperature regulation is disturbed and the autonomic response to temperature changes is abolished. These patients are particularly susceptible to central depressant drugs such as thiopental, which can lead to severe hypotension. With spinal cord lesions at the C4-6 level followed by spinal fusion, respiration may initially appear adequate, but ascending edema of the cord can result in ventilatory difficulties after a few hours postoperatively. As laryngeal and pharyngeal reflexes are usually obtunded, intubation is relatively well tolerated with moderate sedation and assisted ventilation. Quadriplegics may develop autonomic hyperreflexia and may need anesthesia to control its signs and symptoms during surgery, even though the operative site is insensitive. Other common problems include pressure sores, urinary tract infections, anemia and other nutritional deficiencies, paralytic ileus and abdominal distension, and pulmonary embolism as a result of prolonged immobility.

THE REYE-JOHNSON SYNDROME

The Reye-Johnson syndrome is an acute neurologic disorder in children characterized by acute encephalopathy and brain swelling; fatty degeneration of viscera, especially the liver; and hyperammonemia. The illness is almost always preceded by a minor respiratory infection or, occasionally, chickenpox. The hepatic dysfunction that is manifested as hyperammonemia, hypoglycemia, and coagulopathy is transient and self-limiting. Intracranial hypertension, however, is intractable and results in death in a small number of children in spite of optimal care.[63]

Early diagnosis and rapid control of intracranial hypertension are mandatory to ensure full neurologic recovery. Control of the cerebral vascular volume and brain tissue water, while maintaining normal systemic circulation and cerebral perfusion pressure, are the main goals of therapy. Fluid overload, hypoxia, hypercarbia, vasodilating drugs, and obstruction of cerebral venous drainage must be avoided. The patient is cautiously sedated with diazepam, morphine, and phenobarbital and stimulated as little as possible. The head is elevated 30 degrees and kept in a midline position to help venous drainage. Attempts are made to keep the child normothermic. Fluids are restricted (1200 ml/m^2/day) to maintain serum osmolarity at 310–320 mOsm. Hypertonic glucose and vitamin K (2–5 mg IV) are given to treat hypoglycemia and coagulopathy, respectively, as they appear. Steroids, because they can induce protein catabolism, are avoided; evidence of their efficacy is scant. Exchange transfusions and peritoneal dialysis to treat hyperammonemia are now less frequently performed. Ventilation is mechanically controlled and muscular paralysis is maintained with pancuronium bromide (0.01–0.1 mg/kg). Nasotracheal intubation is contraindicated if a coagulopathy is present; the oral route is selected. The PaCO$_2$ is maintained between 20 and 25 mm Hg. If coma exceeds neurologic grade II[64] (disorientation, combativeness, and hyperventilation), intracranial hypertension is probable. Intraventricular monitoring of intracranial pressure and ventriculostomy are needed in neurologic grade III (decorticate) and grade IV (decerebrate) patients.[64,65] Acute elevations of intracranial pressure are managed with vigorous manual hyperventilation with 100 percent oxygen, cerebrospinal fluid drainage, and osmotic diuretics (mannitol 0.5–1.0 g/kg IV). High dose barbiturates to minimize

intracranial pressure rises have been advocated by many authors,[61,66] but currently their use is controversial.[61] Hypothermia, conducted according to a careful clinical protocol, can be effective in reducing intracranial pressure. Decompression craniectomy is indicated in individual cases where other methods have failed. The procedure, however, must be performed before severe brainstem compression has occurred. Treatment is terminated when the intracranial pressure remains below 15 mm Hg for 36 hours without therapy.

REFERENCES

1. Pang LM, Mellins RB: Neonatal cardiorespiratory physiology. Anesthesiology 43:171, 1975
2. Welch K: The intracranial pressure in infants. J Neurosurg 52:693, 1980
3. Michenfelder JD: Anesthesia for intracranial surgery. Refresher courses in anesthesiology, vol 3, chapter 12, 1975
4. Campkin TV: Isoflurane and cranial extradural pressure. Br J Anaesth 56:1083, 1984
5. Grosslight K, Foster R. Colohan AR, et al: Isoflurane for neuroanesthesia: Risk factors for increases in intracranial pressure. Anesthesiology 63:533, 1985
6. Crumrine RS, Nulsen FE, Weiss MH: Alterations in ventricular fluid pressure during ketamine anesthesia in hydrocephalic children. Anesthesiology 42:758, 1975
7. Dawson B, Michenfelder JD, Theye RA: Effects of ketamine on canine cerebral blood flow and metabolism: Modification by prior administration of thiopental. Anesth Analg 50:443, 1971
8. Goudsouzian NG, Liu LMP, Gionfriddo M, et al: Neuromuscular effects of atracurium in infants and children. Anesthesiology 62:75, 1985
9. Rosa G, Orfei P, Sanfilippo M, et al: The effects of atracurium besylate on intracranial pressure and cerebral perfusion pressure. Anesth Analg 65:381, 1986
10. Goudsouzian NG, Liu LMP, Cote CJ, et al: Safety and efficacy of atracurium in adolescents and children anesthetized with halothane. Anesthesiology 59:459, 1983
11. Abou-Madi MN, Keszler H, Yacoub J: Cardiovascular reactions to laryngoscopy and tracheal intubation following small and large intravenous doses of lidocaine. Canad Anaesth Soc J 24:12, 1977
12. Hamill JF, Bedford RF, Weaver DC, et al: Lidocaine before endotracheal intubation: Intravenous or laryngotracheal? Anesthesiology 55:578, 1981
13. Lee KW, Dougal RN, Templeton JJ, et al: Selection of endotracheal tubes in infants and children. Abstracts of the Meeting Section on Pediatric Anesthesia, Las Vegas, April 1980
14. Meridy HW, Creighton RE, Humphreys RP: Complications during neurosurgery in the prone position in children. Canad Anaesth Soc J 21:445, 1974
15. Frost EA: Anesthesia for elective intracranial procedures. Anesth Rev 7:13, 1980
16. Newberg LA: Use of intravenous glucose solutions in surgical patients. Anesth Analg 64:558, 1985
17. Anderson SM: Controlled hypotension with arfonad in paediatric surgery. Br Med J 2:103, 1955
18. Larson AG: Deliberate hypotension, review. Anesthesiology 25:682, 1964
19. Salem MR, Wong AY, Bennett EJ: Deliberate hypotension in infants and children. Anesth Analg 53:975, 1974
20. Salem MR, Kim Y, Shaker MH: Effect of alterations of inspired oxygen concentration on jugular bulb oxygen tension during deliberate hypotension. Anesthesiology 33:358, 1970
21. Davies DW, Greiss L, Kadar D, et al: Sodium nitroprusside in children: Observations on metabolism during normal and abnormal responses. Canad Anaesth Soc J 22:553, 1975

22. Greiss L, Tremblay NAG, Davies DW: The toxicity of sodium nitroprusside. Canad Anaesth Soc J 23:480, 1976

23. Jack RD: Toxicity of sodium nitroprusside. Br J Anaesth 46:952, 1974

24. Cottrell JE, Patel K, Turndorf H, et al: Intracranial pressure changes induced by sodium nitroprusside in patients with intracranial mass lesions. J Neurosurg 48:329, 1978

25. Van Aken H, Fitch W, Brussel T, et al: The influence of isoflurane induced hypotension on cerebral blood flow and cerebral autoregulation in baboons. Anesthesiology 63:A364, 1985

26. Saxon A: Inhibition of platelet function by nitroprusside. N Engl J Med 295:281, 1976

27. Benazon D: Hypothermia, in Scurr C, Feldman S: Scientific Foundations of Anaesthesia, ed 2. Chicago, Yearbook Medical Publishers, 1974, pp 344–357

28. Perkins NAK, Bedford RF: Hemodynamic consequences of peep in seated neurological patients. Implication for paradoxical air embolism. Anesth Analg 63:429, 1984

29. Roosen WA, Clar HE: Pre- and postoperative evaluation of hypothalamo-pituitary function in children with craniopharyngiomas. Acta Neurochir 45:287, 1979

30. Long DM, Seljeskog EL, Chou SN, et al: Giant arteriovenous malformations of infancy and childhood. J Neurosurg 40:304, 1974

31. Hood JB, Wallace CT, Mahaffey JC: Anesthetic management of an intracranial arteriovenous malformation in infancy. Anesth Analg 56:236, 1977

32. Frost EAM: The physiology of respiration in neurosurgical patients. J Neurosurg 50:699, 1979

33. Cantu RC, Mark VH, Austen WG: Accurate placement of the distal and of a ventriculo-atrial shunt catheter using vascular pressure changes. J Neurosurg 27:584, 1967

34. Youngberg JA, Kaplan JA, Miller ED: Air embolism through a ventriculo-atrial shunt during pneumoencephalography. Anesthesiology 42:487, 1975

35. Creighton RE, Relton JES, Meridy HW: Anaesthesia for occipital encephalocoele. Canad Anaesth Soc J 21:403, 1974

36. Bell WE, McCormach WF: Increased Intracranial Pressure in Children. Major Problems in Clinical Pediatrics, vol 8. Philadelphia, WB Saunders, 1972, p 70

37. Dallas SH, Moxon CP: Controlled ventilation for cerebral angiography. Br J Anaesth 42:597, 1969

38. Gardner LG: Air embolism during cisternal air myelography. Br J Anaesth 43:807, 1971

39. Roth JL, Nugent M, Gray JE, et al: Patient monitoring during magnetic resonance imaging. Anesthesiology 62:80, 1985

40. Rees GJ: Paediatric anaesthesia. Br J Anaesth 32:132, 1960

41. Berger MS, Pitts LH, Lovely M, et al: Outcome from severe injury in children and adolescents. J Neurosurg 62:194, 1985

42. Bruce DA, Schut L, Brunol A, et al: Outcome following severe head injuries in children. J Neurosurg 48:679, 1978

43. Obrist WD, Thompson HK, Wang HS, et al: Regional cerebral blood flow estimated by Xenon)133 inhalation. Stroke 6:245, 1975

44. Bruce DA, Berman WA, Schut L: Cerebrospinal fluid pressure monitoring in children: Physiology, pathology and clinical usefulness. Adv Pediatr 24:133, 1977

45. Gucer G, Vierstein LJ, Chubbock, et al: Clinical evaluation of longterm epidural monitoring of ICP. Surg Neurol 12:373, 1979

46. James H, Bruno L, Schut L, et al: Intracranial subarachnoid pressure monitoring in children. Surg Neurol 3:313, 1975

47. Mickell JJ, Reigel DH, Cooke DR, et al: Intracranial pressure: Monitoring and normalization therapy in children. Pediatrics 59:606, 1977

48. Ream AK, Silverberg GD, Corbin SD, et al: Epidural measurement of intracranial pressure. Neurosurgery 5:36, 1979

49. Vries J, Becker D, Young H: A subarachnoid screw for monitoring intracranial pressure. J Neurosurg 39:416, 1973

50. Miller JD, Becker DP, Ward JD, et al: Significance of intracranial hypertension in severe head injury. J Neurosurg 47:503, 1977

51. Frost EAM, Arancibia CU, Shulman K: Pulmonary shunt as a prognostic indicator in head injury. J Neurosurg 50:768, 1979

52. Frost EAM: Respiratory problems associated with head trauma. Neurosurgery 1:300, 1977

53. Frost EAM: Effects of positive end-expiratory pressure on intracranial pressure and compliance in brain-injured patients. J Neurosurg 47:195, 1977

54. Miller JD, Sullivan HG: Severe intracranial hypertension. Int Anesthesiol Clin 17:19, 1979

55. Graf CJ, Rossi NP: Catecholamine response to intracranial hypertension. J Neurosurg 49:862, 1978

56. Cohn JN, Franciosa JA: Vasodilator therapy of cardiac failure. N Engl J Med 297:254, 1977

57. Cooper PR, Moody S, Clark WK, et al: Dexamethasone and severe head injury. J Neurosurg 51:307, 1979

58. Miller JD, Leech P: Effects of mannitol and steroid therapy on intracranial volume-pressure relationships in patients. J Neurosurg 42:274, 1975

59. Lafferty JJ, Keykhah MM, Shapiro HM, et al: Cerebral hypometabolism obtained with deep pentobarbital anesthesia and hypothermia (30 C). Anesthesiology 49:159, 1978

60. Cottrell JE, Robustelli A, Post K, et al: Furosemide and mannitol induced changes in intracranial pressure and serum osmolarity and electrolytes. Anesthesiology 47:28, 1977

61. Piatt JH, Schiff SJ: High dose barbiturate therapy in neurosurgery and intensive care. Neurosurgery 15:427, 1984

62. John DA, Tobey RE, Homer LD, et al: Onset of succinylcholine induced hyperkalemia following denervation. Anesthesiology 45:294, 1976

63. Nelson DB, Hurwitz ES, Sullivan-Bolyai JZ: Reye's syndrome in the U.S. in 1977–1978. J Infect Dis 140:436, 1979

64. Lovejoy FH, Smith AL, Brenan MJ, et al: Clinical staging in Reye's syndrome. Am J Dis Child 128:36, 1974

65. Venes JL, Shaywitz BA, Spencer DD: Management of severe cerebral edema in the metabolic encephalopathy of Reye-Johnson syndrome. J Neurosurg 48:903, 1978

66. Marshall LF, Shapiro HM, Rasscher A, et al: Pentobarbital therapy for intracranial hypertension in metabolic coma: Reye's syndrome. Crit Care Med 6:1, 1978

CHAPTER 12
Management of Neurosurgical Problems in the Neonate

R. Michael Scott

IN PLANNING a neurosurgical procedure for a premature or newborn baby, the neurosurgeon must be concerned not only with technical considerations related to the child's size, but also with alterations in the routine neurosurgical protocol that must be made to protect the baby's fragile homeostatic mechanisms.

Hypothermia, because of its grave metabolic consequences in this age group, is an immediate risk when the child enters the operating room. Most neurosurgical cases require a relatively long period of preparation, and during this time significant heat can be lost by the baby into the environment, particularly if the operative field involves a large surface area. To prevent this problem, the child must be transported to the operating room in an Isolette, and the operating room temperature should be elevated before the child arrives. The baby must be kept covered during induction of anesthesia, and a rectal temperature probe should be positioned immediately upon the child's entry into the operating room. A heating blanket should be in place on the operating table; it is unwise, however, to rely on the blanket alone to maintain the child's temperature, and the room temperature should remain elevated until the child can be draped at the completion of the preparation. An overhead radiant heating device is often of help during the time the intravenous lines are being placed and the child is being anesthetized, since it permits observation of the child during these maneuvers and warms its extremities, making insertion of the intravenous lines easier. Other aids in maintaining thermal regulation are the use of warmed humidified anesthetic gases and warmed blood, intravenous fluids, and irrigation and skin preparation solutions. Antiseptic solutions such as alcohol that evaporate rapidly and result in skin cooling should be avoided.

Although one expects minimal blood loss in most of the common neurosurgical procedures in the neonate, there are enough exceptions in even the most routine procedures that a venous access route must be available to the anesthesiologist. One of the most frustrating preoperative delays in pediatric neurosurgery occurs when it is difficult to establish an intravenous line, and it is a good policy to limit this process to an agreed-upon time limit. Practical venipuncture sites in this age group include scalp veins (visualized with the aid of a circumferential rubber band tourniquet), an external jugular vein, and an almost constant but frequently nonvisible vein on the dorsum of the hand running parallel with the ring finger. Mild Trendelenburg positioning with fingertip pressure over the clavicle is a help in cannulating the external jugular vein. If a venous line cannot be placed rapidly, it is probably wise to proceed directly to a cut-down over the greater saphenous vein rather than delay surgery longer, although with most experienced pediatric operating room teams, a venous cut-down is rarely necessary.

As the child is positioned, care must be taken that all pressure points are completely padded and that the limbs are not so tightly restrained that traction is placed on the brachial or lumbar plexus. This caveat applies particularly to a neonate being prepared for shunt surgery in whom the head is typically turned fully to the side for an occipital burr hole, the neck extended over a roll to aid in passing the shunt subcutaneously (Figure 12-1); pulling the arm firmly down and to the side and anchoring it to the tablesheet can lead to traction palsies if care is not taken to avoid undue force. Pressure points can be protected with adhesive-backed foam cut to an appropriate size and fixed to the area of concern. In the neonate undergoing a posterior fossa procedure in the prone position, the foam can be placed over the entire face with apertures cut for the esophageal stethoscope and endotracheal tube (Figure 12-2).

INTRAOPERATIVE CONSIDERATIONS

Craniotomy techniques are modified when applied to the neonate. The skin is infiltrated with saline or a dilute solution of epinephrine (1:1 million) to aid in hemostasis when the skin flap is turned. In some children with relatively thick skin, the spring-loaded "Children's Hospital" or Cologne clips can be used on the skin edges hemostasis, but usually the limited bleeding that is encountered in younger children can be managed with bipolar cautery rather than skin clips. The Shaw scalpel, which uses a heated blade to effect hemostasis, dramatically reduces blood loss from the incision and eliminates the need for skin clips of any type. If monopolar cautery is used to incise the pericranium, care must be taken not to penetrate the thin skull with the cautery tip. Venous bleeding from the bone can be extensive in the neonate, and meticulous hemostasis should be maintained with bone wax and the flat blade of the cautery. The skin flap is secured with a 3-0 suture placed through the base of the flap and retracted with rubber bands to the drapes. The bone flap can be elevated, often without burr holes, by curetting near the fontanelle or a suture, identifying the epidural plane, and using a heavy scissors to cut a free flap. If necessary, a burr hole can be drilled in the pliable skull by rotating the perforator bit alone between the fingers while

OPERATIVE NEUROSURGICAL TECHNIQUES
ISBN 0-8089-1862-1

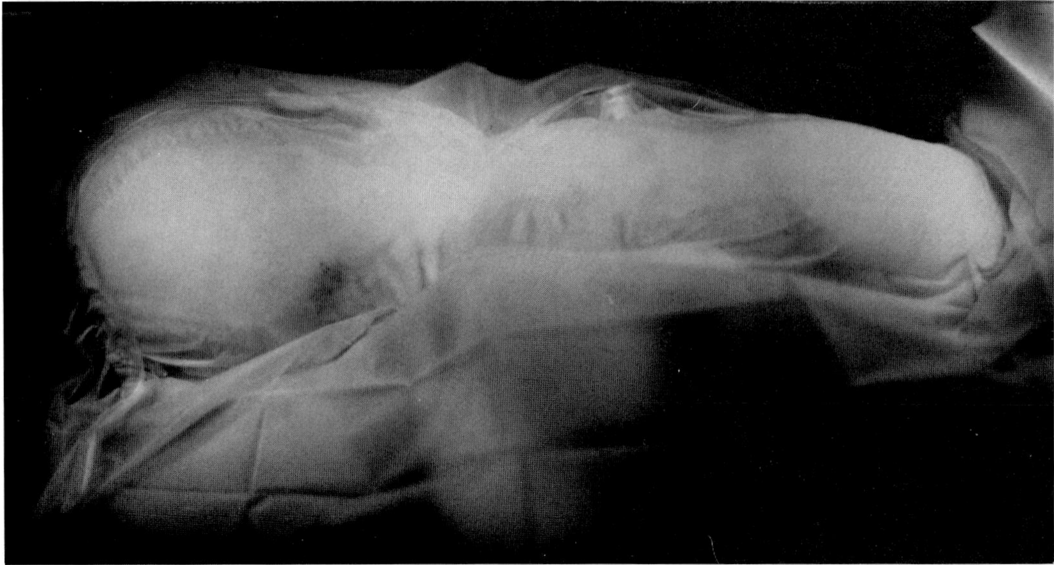

Fig. 12-1. Positioning of a baby for a ventriculoperitoneal shunt using a right parieto-occipital burr hole. The head is turned fully to the left, a roll is placed under the shoulder to elevate the chest and extend the neck, and the entire field is draped with plastic drapes before skin preparation. The burr hole should be made just anterior to the lambdoid suture, medial to a point midway between the ear and the sagittal suture, and the catheter directed toward the midline of the forehead several centimeters above the glabella. A more lateral burr hole will "migrate" laterally on the skull as the child grows, making re-entry into the ventricle difficult if revision is subsequently necessary.

exerting gentle pressure. Care must be taken to replace blood as it is lost, particularly in operations in the posterior fossa. In this location the dura can be laced with venous channels that can cause considerable rapid bleeding if opened inadvertently. Consideration of the child's limited blood volume must remain of foremost importance throughout every pediatric neurosur-

gical case. If bleeding is extensive, the surgeon should stop to allow the anesthesiologist to catch up on the blood replacement if necessary. Sponges must be weighed and irrigation and suction fluids measured to aid the anesthesiologist in the assessment of blood loss.

At the close of the procedure, the bone flap can be secured

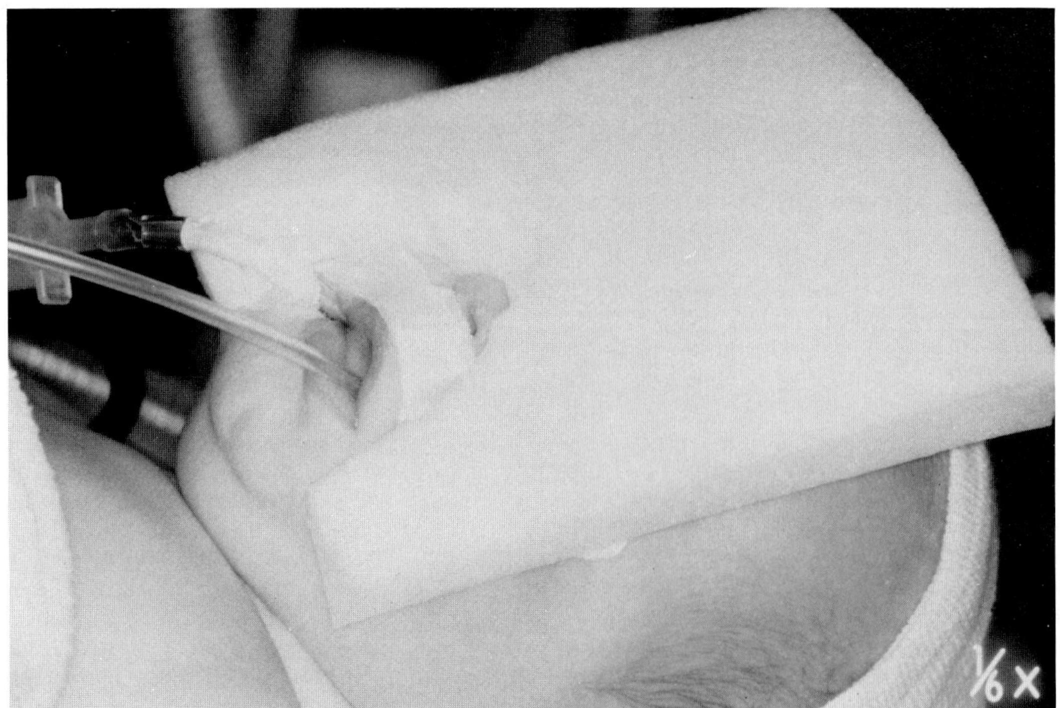

Fig. 12-2. A baby prepared for prone positioning on the horseshoe headrest. An esophageal stethoscope is in place, the baby's eyes taped closed, and the entire face covered with adhesive-backed foam.

with 3-0 nonabsorbable suture material. A baby's skull is sufficiently thin that it is not usually necessary to drill holes to secure the flap; the suture needle itself can be passed directly through the bone for this purpose.

Closure of the skin incision in the neonate can often be accomplished in two layers if desired. We presently use undyed Dexon or Vicryl for the galea, since black silk or braided nylon sutures are often visible through the thin skin of the neonate and can spontaneously extrude from the wound weeks or months after closure. Many pediatric neurosurgeons use single-layered closures for their neonatal patients, and we have noted no problems with wound healing with this technique.

The application of the dressing represents a final challenge to the healing process in neonates, since firm head wraps, which would be acceptable in a larger child, can cause skin and ear necrosis in a neonate. Dressings must be carefully applied, and pressure on the forehead and ears frequently checked, both during application of the dressing and subsequently.

HYDROCEPHALUS IN THE NEONATE

The ventricular shunt procedure is one of the most frequent neurosurgical operations performed on neonates. The major surgical hazards of this operation in this population are related to poor wound healing and cerebrospinal fluid (CSF) leak through skin that has been thinned by distension over a bulky shunt apparatus. In a premature child with hydrocephalus requiring a shunt, the apparatus should have the lowest possible profile and minimum size. All incisions should be designed so that the tubing does not cross or run directly beneath them. Since the premature infant with hydrocephalus is relatively immobile and usually kept recumbent because of the use of a ventilator or other medical concerns, frontal burr hole catheter placement is preferable to avoid pressure necrosis over the shunt catheter. In small premature babies with extremely thin and delicate skin, the valve and reservoir can be omitted, or only a low pressure distal slit valve utilized. The intracranial pressure can be adjusted by raising and lowering the child's head relative to the abdomen, depending on the fontanelle tension. When the child is older, the shunt can be revised to include the valve and reservoir. A single layer of running locked 5-0 nylon is the usual closure technique for the scalp incisions in these children, since CSF can easily leak through the most minute needle holes if an interrupted closure technique is used.

INTRAVENTRICULAR HEMORRHAGE IN THE PREMATURE INFANT

In premature infants with intraventricular hemorrhage, the major neurosurgical problem is the management of increased intracranial pressure and progressive hydrocephalus in a child who is a serious operative risk. Moreover, even if easily performed, standard ventricular shunting in this setting has a high likelihood of malfunction. In these babies we prefer to deal with the increased pressure nonoperatively, including daily lumbar punctures and the use of medications such as Diamox to reduce CSF production. An ultrasound study after lumbar puncture that demonstrates reduction in ventricular size suggests that the hydrocephalus is of a communicating type and that further lumbar punctures will be helpful. If these techniques are not successful, the ventricles can be decompressed

by placement, under local anesthesia, of a ventricular catheter with an attached subcutaneous reservoir. Percutaneous aspiration of the ventricular catheter reservoir using a small-gauge needle can then be carried out at the bedside to control intracranial pressure and remove CSF. Attempts can be made to gradually reduce the frequency of the aspiration in hopes of promoting the re-establishment of the child's own CSF absorptive mechanisms. External ventricular drainage can be instituted in this situation, although the risks of infection and subsequent ventriculitis are higher in these premature babies than in older children similarly treated, perhaps because of the extensive instrumentation and manipulation required as part of their daily care in the neonatal intensive care unit. A simple technique for the placement of external ventricular drainage in these babies is puncture of the skin and dura over the frontal or occipital bone with a 19-gauge needle-catheter assembly, threading the catheter into the ventricle, and connecting the opposite end to a standard external drainage system. A larger bore needle and catheter may be necessary if the CSF protein level is high. Before the skin puncture, the skin over the needle entry site is displaced laterally and the skin is entered at a slight angle so that the leaking of CSF through the needle puncture site will be minimized when the needle is withdrawn. The catheter should be fixed to the skin of the child with a suture and covered by an occlusive-type dressing, which should be changed as needed with meticulous technique by the neurosurgical staff. When these drains are eventually removed, it is often necessary to place a 5-0 nylon suture at the puncture site to stop a transient CSF leak. Frequent ultrasound scans should be carried out during all phases of treatment to assess ventricular size.

HYDROCEPHALUS AND MYELOMENINGOCELE

Once the decision to operate on a newborn with a myelomeningocele has been made, an important early surgical decision is the management of associated hydrocephalus. If the baby has been born with a large head and full fontanelle and CT scanning or ultrasound have confirmed the presence of significant ventriculomegaly, uncomplicated healing of the myelomeningocele dural closure will be facilitated by immediate CSF diversion. We previously used closed ventricular drainage in this situation, maintaining this system until back healing had progressed to the point where it was felt "safe" to proceed with ventriculoperitoneal shunting; however, simultaneous shunting following myelomeningocele repair has reduced hospitalization time and has not resulted in increased morbidity or infection. If indicated, therefore, we have usually placed the shunt after repair of the myelomeningocele if the repair has proceeded uneventfully, dural closure was secure, and the subarachnoid space was relatively uncontaminated. Since the infant will remain prone for several days after repair in this situation, the shunt is usually placed through an occipital burr hole.

NEONATAL TRAUMA

Most neonatal head trauma is related to either birth trauma or child abuse, and very little "operative" intervention has been necessary since CT and ultrasound scanning of neonates came into regular use. Acute epidural and subdural hematomas are rare and are dealt with by craniotomy or craniectomy, as in older children. Epidural hematomas are often quite focal, being sharply delimited by the dural attachments at the cranial sutures. The posterior fossa is a common site of neonatal intracranial hematoma. Characteristically this involves the area both above and below the tentorium. In neonates, the tentorium and dura of the posterior fossa are laced with large venous sinuses; lateral shear stress across the tentorium during delivery may rupture some of these sinuses or tear bridging veins from the cerebellum, leading to hematomas within the tentorium that can rupture through it and bleed into adjacent structures, causing subdural or cerebellar hematomas. It is difficult to be certain of the best neurosurgical treatment for these lesions, since when recognized, the child may be in extremis and die regardless of therapy. With the more frequent use of CT and ultrasound scanning of neonates, these lesions are being seen in neurologically stable children with greater frequency. If the mass effect from the hematoma is negligible and the child is neurologically stable or improving, the clot is best left alone. Bleeding from the tentorium is difficult to control, and if there is no appreciable mass effect, careful observation with follow-up scanning is probably the safest method of treatment. If surgery is necessary, the child should be operated upon in the prone position with head flexion to provide good visualization of the tentorium. Thorough preparation should be made for clip ligation of the venous sinuses, and blood replaced meticulously as surgery is carried out.

VEIN OF GALEN MALFORMATION

Vein of Galen malformations are detected in neonates when an intracranial bruit is heard in a newborn with intractable heart failure. Very rarely, subarachnoid hemorrhage or hydrocephalus secondary to mass effect is the initial symptom. Surgical management of children in heart failure is extremely difficult and is directed toward correcting the cardiac failure by decreasing the blood flow through the lesion. In neonates, the arterial feeders to the vein of Galen are usually numerous and originate at least partly from the medial and posterior choroidal arteries and the anterior and posterior cerebral arteries. Careful, complete selective preoperative cerebral angiography is essential and must be performed at a facility with specific expertise in pediatric neuroradiology.

Surgical positioning and approach depend on the number and location of the arterial feeders. A bilateral exposure is commonly necessary in neonates, and this is best carried out with the child in a supine, semi-sitting position, using a transcallosal approach to the area of the fistulae. Deliberate hypotension should be avoided since any hypoperfusion of an already compromised coronary circulation may lead to irreversible myocardial ischemia. Those centers in which intraoperative cardiac arrest with hypothermia is used as a surgical adjunct in neonates with these lesions almost universally report dismal results.[1] The procedure is best managed by an anesthetic team totally familiar with pediatric cardiac surgery, and cardiopulmonary bypass or other circulatory augmentation procedures available as necessary. Because of their symptomatology, these "aneurysms" in the neonate would be ideally treated by embolization techniques to reduce circulatory steal through the lesion and improve the baby's cardiac status; the selective techniques for catheterizing the numerous deep feeders to these lesions are becoming more widely available, and if the child can

be stabilized, referral to a facility capable of carrying out such techniques should be considered.

OCCIPITAL ENCEPHALOCELE

The variable size and complexity of occipital encephaloceles make generalizations regarding their surgical repair difficult. The initial question posed to the neurosurgeon inevitably is whether this often grotesque lesion should be repaired at all. This decision should be influenced by the extent of other congenital anomalies, the relative size of the encephalocele versus that of the remaining normal cranium, and the configuration of the "normal" cranium. Over the past decades, additional studies such as air ventriculography and arteriography have been used to elucidate how much of the normal brain has been involved in the encephalocele; certainly the most graphic test currently in use is magnetic resonance scan (MRI) which enables the cerebral deformity to be assessed and other associated brain anomalies to be clearly identified. Vascular anatomy of the lesion can often be inferred from the MRI, making formal arteriography unnecessary. Virtually all children with large encephaloceles will be retarded to varying degrees and a large percentage will develop hydrocephalus that will require treatment during the first several months of life—facts that must also be taken into consideration before initiating treatment.

Our policy is to repair the majority of these lesions unless the associated brain and somatic anomalies are severe or the lesion is so large that its repair would involve sacrifice of a major portion of cerebral tissue. An issue that may lend urgency to making the decision to operate is related to the quality of epithelialization of the sac and whether there is a CSF leak. If the skin over the distal sac is thin or eroded or if a CSF leak is present, repair must be carried out within the first 24 hours of life in order to avoid meningitis. Because ventricular shunting is so often required subsequently, avoiding meningitis at this stage of the child's treatment is of utmost importance.

Repair is almost always carried out with the child in the prone position, using the precautions in positioning outlined previously (Figure 12-3). Occasionally, a small lesion can be operated on with the child in the lateral position and the surgeon seated behind the patient. Since this position is often preferred by the anesthesiologist because of easy access to the airway, we make every effort to use it if the size of the lesion permits. As with an adult patient in the lateral position, a baby's brachial plexus must not be stretched by excessive downward traction on the uppermost shoulder, and the axillary nerve should be protected by placing a large roll in the axilla to prevent excessive pressure from being placed on the lateral aspect of the humerus. The child's head can be elevated 10 to 15 degrees, but not so high that an air embolus might occur. An intravenous line must always be established before surgery is begun in these children. In these midline lesions, the potential for rapid bleeding from large venous sinuses always exists, and the patient's blood must be cross-matched and replacement blood available before surgery begins.

A vertical elliptical incision around the base of the lesion is outlined high enough on the sac to provide enough residual scalp for easy closure without tension. It is carried cephalad and caudad to the lesion to provide room for additional supratentorial or infratentorial exposure should it be necessary. The bony and pericranial defect at the uppermost portion of the encephalocele is identified initially, the plane between the dural sac and the underlying skull and pericranium bluntly dissected, and the skin and dura sharply incised high on the sac around its circumference. If the lesion is small, it may be possible to preserve the arachnoid membrane surrounding the herniated brain and to reduce the entire contents of the sac into the cranial cavity. Cerebrospinal fluid cultures should be taken during the repair, particularly if there has been CSF leak prior to surgery. If the brain hernia cannot be reduced or if it is too large for this maneuver to be considered, the arachnoid is opened and the extracranial tissue amputated, using suction and bipolar cautery. Large venous and arterial channels are often encountered in this gliotic tissue, and every attempt should be made to preserve them, although it is often difficult to do so. When hemostasis has been obtained, the dura is trimmed and closed in a watertight fashion with a running suture of 4-0 braided monofilament nylon or Vicryl (polyglycolic acid suture). A Valsalva maneuver is performed to check for leaks in the dural closure, and pericranium flaps can be fashioned and closed over the dura if desired. The scalp is sutured in two layers if possible with Vicryl in the galea and nylon in the skin. No attempt is made to repair the bony defect at this time, since it often becomes less significant in size as the child grows. A head-wrap dressing is applied and changed daily to check for the presence of subcutaneous accumulation of CSF or CSF leaks through the incision, the presence of either of which may indicate developing hydrocephalus, which requires treatment. The child's head circumference should be monitored daily and a follow-up

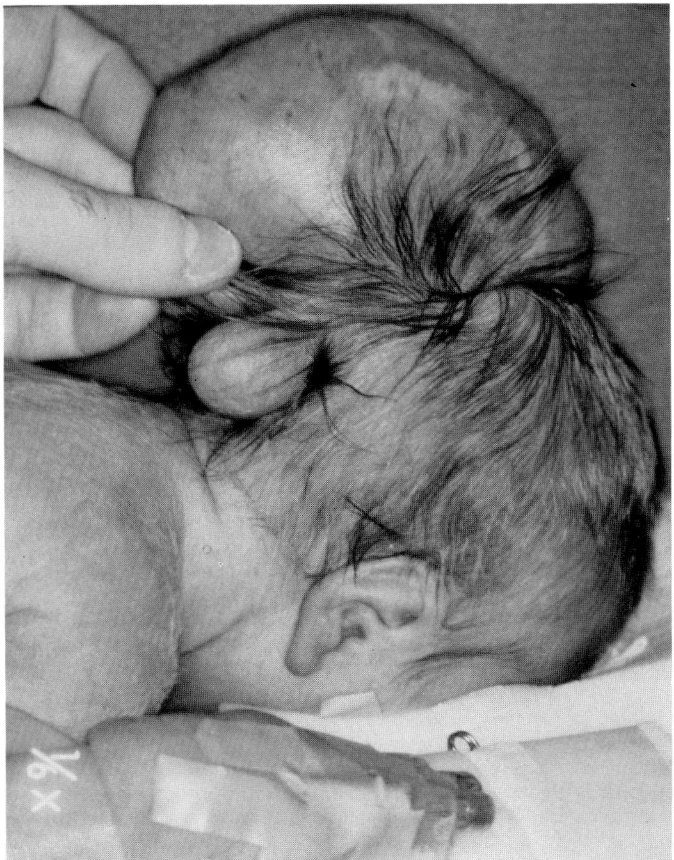

Fig. 12-3. A baby with an occipital encephalocele in the prone position for surgery. Note padding of the face with adhesive foam. It is difficult to shave the area around the encephalocele without injuring the delicate skin on its base and sides. This hair need only be trimmed with a clipper or scissors before the preparation begins.

ultrasound, CT scan, or MRI scan obtained before the child's discharge from the hospital to serve as a baseline for further observation.

FRONTONASAL ENCEPHALOCELE

Frontonasal encephaloceles should be treated as early as possible consistent with the child's general medical condition. Children with basal frontal encephaloceles in the pharynx or nares are at risk of developing meningitis because of direct inoculation of the meninges with nasal flora. The mass of the encephalocele can be large enough to obstruct the airway, and attempts to pass airways or endotracheal tubes through the nares or pharynx may rupture the encephaloceles with potentially dire consequences. Prophylactic tracheostomy should be considered in such situations. In certain patients it may be extremely difficult to be certain if the pharyngeal or nasal masses are encephaloceles, since tomograms and CT scans of this area of children are often quite difficult to interpret. The most helpful preoperative test is a CT scan enhanced with intrathecal metrizamide, since the presence of dye in the spaces around and adjacent to the mass is diagnostic of an encephalocele.

Sincipital encephaloceles at the root of the nose or projecting into the orbit are less of an emergency in a neonate, and surgical correction can be postponed for several weeks until anesthetic risks are somewhat reduced. The earlier these lesions are repaired, however, the less influence the lesion will have on subsequent orbital and nasal disfigurement, and repair should not be unduly delayed. A craniofacial team approach with plastic, otolaryngologic, and ophthalmologic surgeons represents optimal management of this problem in the majority of these patients.

The surgical approach to both the basal and sincipital lesions is similar. A bicoronal skin incision is used and the scalp reflected forward; bilateral frontal craniotomies are performed and the dura opened across the supraorbital margin bilaterally. The anterior sagittal sinus is ligated with 2-0 suture material, and an intradural exploration is carried out. Care must be taken to identify and preserve an intact olfactory tract and bulb when the frontal lobes are elevated. The brain herniation through the bony defects is usually readily identified, and the brain hernia amputated, hemostasis secured, and a dural flap or pericranial graft sutured in place over the bone defect. It is advisable to use care in attempting aspiration or removal of the nasal herniated tissue, lest the sac rupture and the intracranial contents become contaminated with nasal flora.

DANDY-WALKER MALFORMATION

The Dandy-Walker malformation is one of the causes of hydrocephalus apparent in the first several weeks of life. In neonates the resultant hydrocephalus is clinically similar to hydrocephalus resulting from other causes; the major surgical consideration in these patients is in the choice of the appropriate method for treating the hydrocephalus.

The CT diagnosis is based on a finding of lateral ventricular dilatation and a large posterior fossa containing a small anterior and superiorly displaced cerebellum with an ''open'' fourth ventricle extending into a large retrocerebellar CSF collection. Supratentorial anomalies, such as agenesis of the corpus cal-

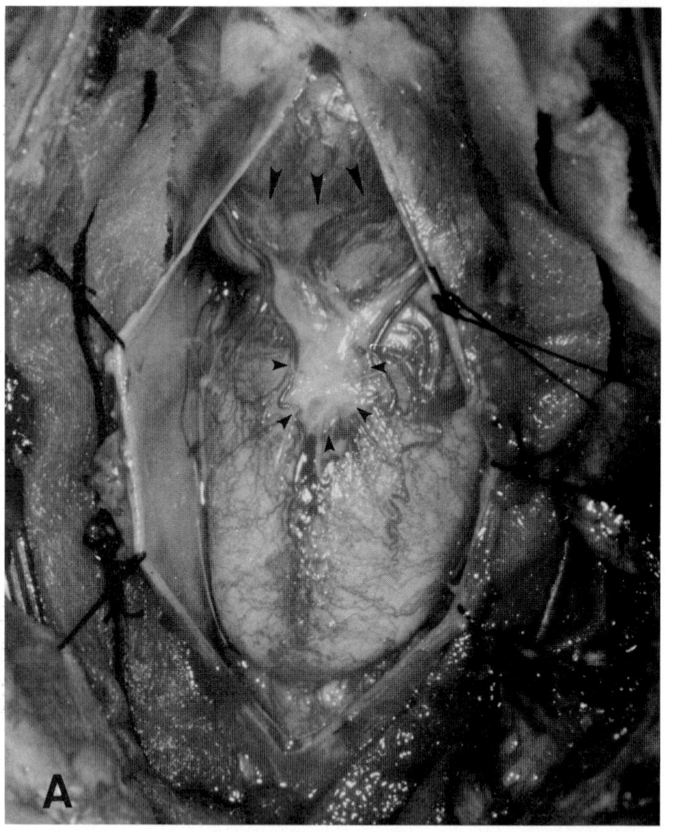
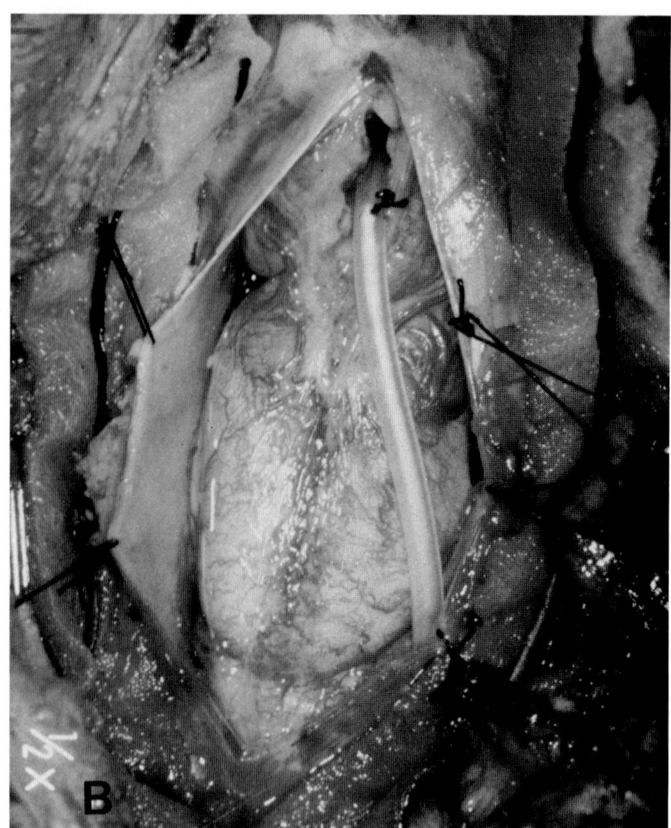
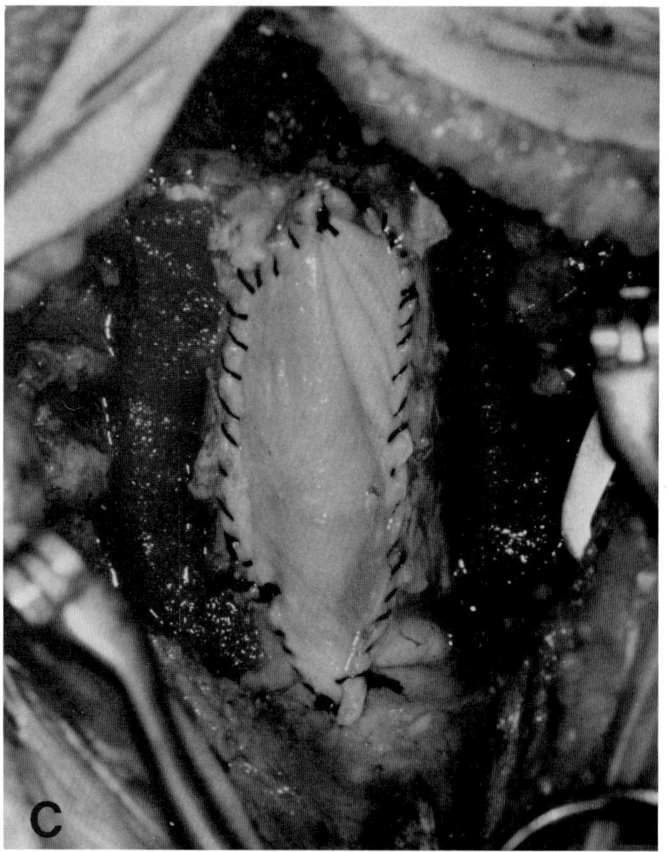

Fig. 12-4. (A) Appearance of a Chiari II malformation after cervical laminectomy and opening of the dura. The midline cerebellar peg is relatively short in this patient, extending to C1 only. The downwardly displaced medulla is swollen and cystic, probably from hydromyelia. The edge of the medullary kink is noted at the inferior portion of the exposure. The impression made on the herniated cerebellar tissue by the fibrous ligaments and dura at the cervicomedullary junction is easily visible (large arrowheads), as is the scarred and occluded foramen of Magendie (small arrowheads). (B) A midline opening has been made in the pia of the vermis peg, and, under magnification, dissection carried through dysgenetic cerebellum into the fourth ventricle. Care must be taken that this opening is made through the cerebellum above the foramen of Magendie and not through the medulla below. A Silastic catheter is placed into the fourth ventricle, threaded cephalad into the aqueduct, led out into the cervical subarachnoid space inferiorly, and secured with a 6-0 suture through its wall into the coagulated pia of the cerebellum. The obex was not visualized in this patient. (C) A graft of lyophilized dura has been sewn into the opening in the dura.

losum, may also be seen. The differential diagnosis between a retrocerebellar arachnoid cyst and the Dandy-Walker malformation occasionally can be difficult, but the visualization of a "covered" fourth ventricle that is normal in size and position relative to the cerebellar hemispheres tends to rule out Dandy-Walker malformation.

Regardless of the precise anatomic configuration, the surgical approach in these children is best determined by metrizamide ventriculography with CT scanning. Direct surgical removal of the cyst has been advocated in the past, but the majority of these patients will eventually require shunting despite cyst surgery, since wide fenestration of the cyst or removal of its walls fails to deal with the malabsorption of CSF over the cerebral hemispheres that is part of this syndrome.[2] The metrizamide CT study will indicate if shunting of both the cyst and the lateral ventricles is required, if the posterior fossa is isolated by a block at the aqueduct, or whether only one compartment need be shunted. In the latter situation, shunts placed directly into the cyst in the posterior fossa via a lateral suboccipital burr hole seem to have a longer revision-free life, perhaps because of the capacious area free of choroid plexus in which the shunt tip is placed. These children tend to tolerate shunt malfunction poorly, and questionable shunt function therefore should be evaluated promptly and the metrizamide study repeated if there is a question regarding communication between the cyst and the lateral ventricles.

CHIARI II MALFORMATION

The treatment of symptomatic Chiari II malformation in a neonate with a myelomeningocele remains highly controversial. There is general agreement regarding symptomatology. These babies, having undergone repair of their myelomeningocele and often with a shunt in place, will develop laryngeal stridor, difficulty in feeding, and occasionally opisthotonos. Laryngoscopy will reveal vocal cord weakness or paralysis. Brain stem auditory-evoked potential recordings (BAERs) are often abnormal or show sequential deterioration. It is rarely necessary to carry out myelography given this clinical presentation, since virtually all these children will have a type II Chiari malformation. Magnetic resonance imaging will vividly depict the typical caudal displacement of the fourth ventricle with or without generalized or terminal cystic enlargement, the downward prolongation of cerebellar vermian tissue, and medullary kinking.[3] A CT scan will demonstrate the well-recognized abnormalities associated with the Chiari malformation, and ultrasound study of the foramen magnum can demonstrate impaction of cerebellar tissue and cystic enlargement of the fourth ventricle. In a child symptomatic from the Chiari malformation, ventricular shunt function must be investigated by any appropriate method, since the symptoms of the Chiari II malformation can be exacerbated by hydrocephalus that is not adequately treated. If shunt malfunction has been ruled out, surgery for the Chiari malformation itself is performed with the baby in the prone position. It is usually not necessary to remove

any of the suboccipital bone at the time of surgery. Cervical laminectomy is carried out to a level required to decompress the herniated cerebellar tissue and brain stem angulation based on the preoperative radiographic studies and intraoperative ultrasound as a guide to the extent of bone removal. The dura must be opened to decompress the brain stem and spinal cord, since compression of the brain stem may be caused by a dural band at the junction of the posterior fossa and cervical dura (Figure 12-4A). This portion of the surgery is the most hazardous, since venous channels in the dura will bleed vigorously when opened. When encountered, these venous channels can be clipped with temporary metallic clips, which can be removed one at a time when hemostasis has been secured, while the venous channels are oversewn with nonabsorbable suture. We remove the metallic clips so that subsequent CT scans or magnetic resonance studies will not be degraded by clip artifact. In addition to the bony and dural decompression, it is important to reestablish normal CSF circulation in this area by opening the occluded foramen of Magendie. This structure can usually be identified at the base of the dysmorphic midline cerebellar peg (Figure 12-4A). Tufts of choroid plexus can frequently be seen in this area as well. If the region of the foramen cannot be identified with certainty, a midline opening is made in the lower portion of the "herniated" cerebellar tissue directed slightly cephalad under magnified vision. The elongated, low-lying fourth ventricle can then be entered; preoperative MRI studies or intraoperative ultrasound are helpful guides during this maneuver. Because hydromyelia can be a prominent part of the clinical syndrome, the obex should be identified and the opening of the central canal occluded with a plug of muscle tissue. To keep the foramen of Magendie open and to permit circulation of CSF outside the ventricular system rather than down into the central canal, we place a Silastic catheter into the fourth ventricle, threading it cephalad into the aqueduct as far as it will pass without resistance and placing the distal end in the cervical subarachnoid space. The catheter is anchored by placing a 6-0 suture through its walls into cauterized pia on the cerebellar peg adjacent to the opened "foramen." A dural graft of lyophilized dura is positioned to maintain wide decompression of the area (Figure 12-4B,C).

Postoperatively, these babies need continued monitoring in the intensive care unit. Their respiratory and feeding status remains fragile and tracheostomy may still be necessary despite successful surgery. The long-term results of this surgical procedure remain unclear.

REFERENCES

1. Hoffman HJ, Chuang S, Hendrick EB, et al: Aneurysms of the vein of Galen. Concepts in Pediatric Neurosurgery 3:52, 1983
2. Sawaya R, McLaurin RL: Dandy-Walker Syndrome. Clinical analysis of 23 cases. J Neurosurg 55:89, 1981
3. Venes JL, Black KL, Latack JT: Preoperative evaluation and surgical management of the Arnold-Chiari II malformation. J Neurosurg 64:363, 1986

CHAPTER 13
Surgical Management of Craniosynostosis and Craniofacial Abnormalities

Steven L. Wald

CRANIOSYNOSTOSIS, the premature fusion of the cranial sutures, was initially described and labeled as craniostenosis by Virchow in 1851.[1] The first attempted surgical correction occurred in 1890 and involved excision of the abnormal suture, an approach that is employed in many of today's surgical procedures.[2,3] It is estimated that synostosis in all its forms occurs with a frequency of 1 in every 4000 live births.[4,5]

ANATOMY AND PATHOPHYSIOLOGY

Two types of sutures are present in the infant skull. Structures of the skull base are joined together by a cartilaginous matrix termed a *synchondrosis,* while bones of the cranial vault are joined by a fibrous union termed a *syndesmosis.* Closure of the anterior fontanelle begins at 12 months and is complete by 18 months. The posterior fontanelle is closed by 3 months. The cranial sutures will functionally close during the early teenage years and ossify during the fourth and fifth decades of life. The maximum rate of cranial growth occurs during the first year of life, during which time brain volume doubles. The rapid growth of brain volume is the primary determinant of head size and shape. Many of today's operative procedures rely on this process to achieve normalization of the head shape.

Pritchard et al.[6] described a five-layer model of the vault sutures and proposed a five-stage maturation process. The development of synostosis is believed to occur in the middle layers with disruption of the normal architecture by a streaming proliferation of osteoblasts (Figure 13-1). Bone is then laid down and ossification is completed. Although this pathophysiologic concept of craniosynostosis has been confirmed in many cases, Hinton et al.[7] studied specimens from patients with lambdoid synostosis and found a different pathologic process than that seen in sagittal or coronal synostosis.

Although initial attention focused on the characteristic abnormalities associated with synostosis of the cranial vault sutures, Moss[8,9] proposed that cranial and facial development is best explained in terms of a "functional matrix," in which genetic information is encoded and all supporting structures develop secondarily in response to the needs of the matrix. He suggested that the dura of the skull base is an important intermediary in this process, with fixed points such as the

petrous ridges, sphenoid wings, and crista galli transmitting forces that influence growth of the membranous skull and distant calvarial suture lines. That this may be a reciprocal process has been shown by the experiments of Persson et al.,[10] who modified facial development in baby rabbits by early artificial fusion of cranial vault sutures. Park and Powers[11] suggested that an early insult to the mesenchymal blastema could lead to synostosis of both the cranial vault and base sutures. Graham and others have described an association of fetal constraint in the uterus with synostosis.[12–14] When there is crowding because of multiple births or a bicornuate uterus, premature fusion of the sutures has been shown to follow in those parts of infant's head that have not been permitted to expand. Graham also noted that 71 percent of cases of unilateral coronal synostosis occur on the right side, while 67 percent of all vertex presentations are in the left transverse or anterior occiput. This would presumably produce a restrictive force on the right side of the baby's forehead. The implication of various environmental factors such as birth trauma and infection as well as the association with endocrine and bone metabolism abnormalities suggests that the pathophysiology of craniosynostosis is diverse.[15–17] In most instances, the exact etiology cannot be determined.

Children with single suture craniosynostosis have a greater than average incidence of associated cerebral and systemic malformations. The incidence of these associated malformations will, however, vary depending on the involved suture. Cardiac malformations, syndactyly, hydrocephalus, convulsive seizures, and mental retardation constitute the major associated anomalies. A causal relationship is, however, difficult to establish. In one large series of patients with sagittal synostosis, 8.9 percent were ultimately diagnosed as mentally retarded, although over half of the patients were found to have unrelated but clearly identifiable reasons for the retardation.[4] The majority of children with a single suture synostosis, however, are likely to have appropriate cognitive function.

Preoperative investigation of a child with craniosynostosis requires evaluation for evidence of increased intracranial pressure. Computed tomographic (CT) scans may demonstrate alterations in ventricular contour, effacement of sulcal patterns, and obliteration of basal cisterns. This does not in itself indicate that the intracranial pressure is elevated. If there are any open

OPERATIVE NEUROSURGICAL TECHNIQUES
ISBN 0-8089-1862-1

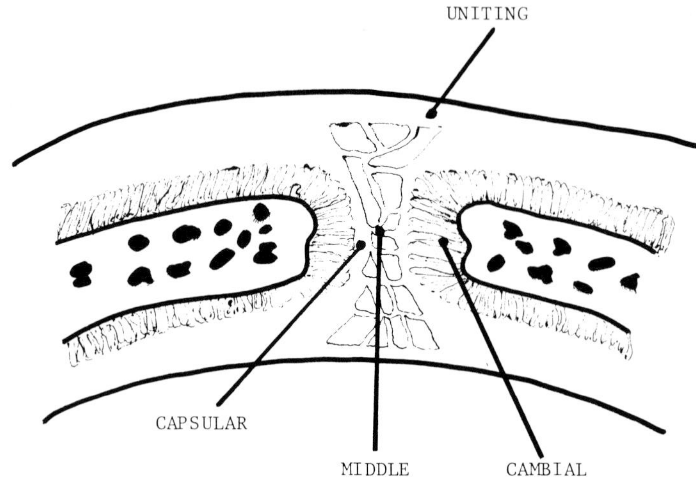

Fig. 13-1. The histologic structure of a cranial suture according to Pritchard.

sutures, the head will expand as a result of the growth of the brain, and intracranial pressure will only be moderately elevated. The relationship of chronic mild intracranial hypertension and functional outcome has not been established. Renier et al.[18] measured ICP using an epidural sensor in 75 children with various types of synostosis. Although normal intracranial pressure variables have not been established in neonates and infants, they found ICP to be evenly distributed between normal, mildly elevated, and elevated. The greatest proportion of cases with intracranial hypertension occurred in children with multiple sutural involvement. Gobiet et al.[19] confirmed the diversity of ICP measurement in children with single suture synostosis. Other studies, however, have generated conflicting data.[20,21]

Over 50 different syndromes have been described in which synostosis plays a part.[5,15] Many of these include severe deformities of the cranium and facial structures. The etiology of many of these syndromes is genetic. Input from neurosurgeons, plastic surgeons, geneticists, and other health professionals is required before undertaking surgical reconstruction. Such procedures should be done in centers where sufficient numbers of patients are concentrated in order to justify the facilities and expertise required.

Although there may be reluctance on the part of a neurosurgeon to advise surgery on a healthy infant for primarily cosmetic reasons, the decision should be made early and the operation undertaken by the time the patient is 6 weeks of age. At the initial meeting with the parents, we explain the nature of the pathologic process, its natural history, and the surgical options and risks. Photographs of children at various ages with and without treatment have proved helpful. We tell parents that the operation is limited to the superficial structures, that the brain is not disturbed, and that mental impairment is unlikely. The purpose of the operation is to improve the child's appearance, but, depending upon the surgical procedure, they should not expect the deformity to be immediately overcome. Cohen[22] recommended careful genetic study of each patient so that new, previously undescribed syndromes can be identified and the scientific implications better understood. We do not routinely suggest genetic referral except for cases of coronal synostosis.

SAGITTAL SYNOSTOSIS

DIAGNOSIS

Sagittal synostosis is the most common isolated suture synostosis.[23,24] Boys predominate in most series.[4] Nearly 20 percent of children will have associated systemic malformations, many of which are mild. Cerebral abnormalities are infrequent. Familial cases have been reported.[25]

Patients with sagittal synostosis have elongated, narrow skulls. There is a striking biparietal narrowing. Brain growth will cause either compensatory frontal or occipital bulging or both. These secondary changes can be quite prominent and are presumed to be caused by differences in growth at the coronal or lambdoid suture or may reflect the site of origin of the synostosis within the sagittal suture. A midline ridge is usually palpable and the anterior fontanelle is often obliterated. The finding of a patent anterior fontanelle, however, does not negate the diagnosis. The head circumference is usually above the mean percentile for age and may exceed two standard deviations from it. This does not mean that the infant has hydrocephalus, since the more a head deviates in shape from a sphere, the higher the circumference will be in relation to volume. The most useful and simple objective measurement is the cephalic index: width/length × 100. Values between 75 and 80 are normal. Children with sagittal synostosis will have values between 65 and 68. This value is not absolutely diagnostic but is especially useful during evaluation after surgery. Facial structures are normal except for a high, prominent forehead. The neurologic examination in uncomplicated cases is normal. The incidence of associated mental retardation ranges from 2.4 to 12.5 percent of patients.[26,27]

Lateral skull roentgenograms demonstrate a long, narrow skull with varying degrees of frontal or occipital bulge. Anteroposterior roentgenograms reveal biparietal narrowing and may demonstrate the fused sagittal ridge (Figure 13-2A,B). Isotope bone scanning is an imaging technique that attempts to display the metabolic status of the sutures. Fused sutures will have no osteoblastic activity and no isotope uptake. Although not routinely required, this procedure may be of value in patients with multiple sutural fusion or in equivocal cases. A false-positive isotope scan rate of 10 to 18 percent has been reported.[28,29] Computed tomographic scanning should be under-

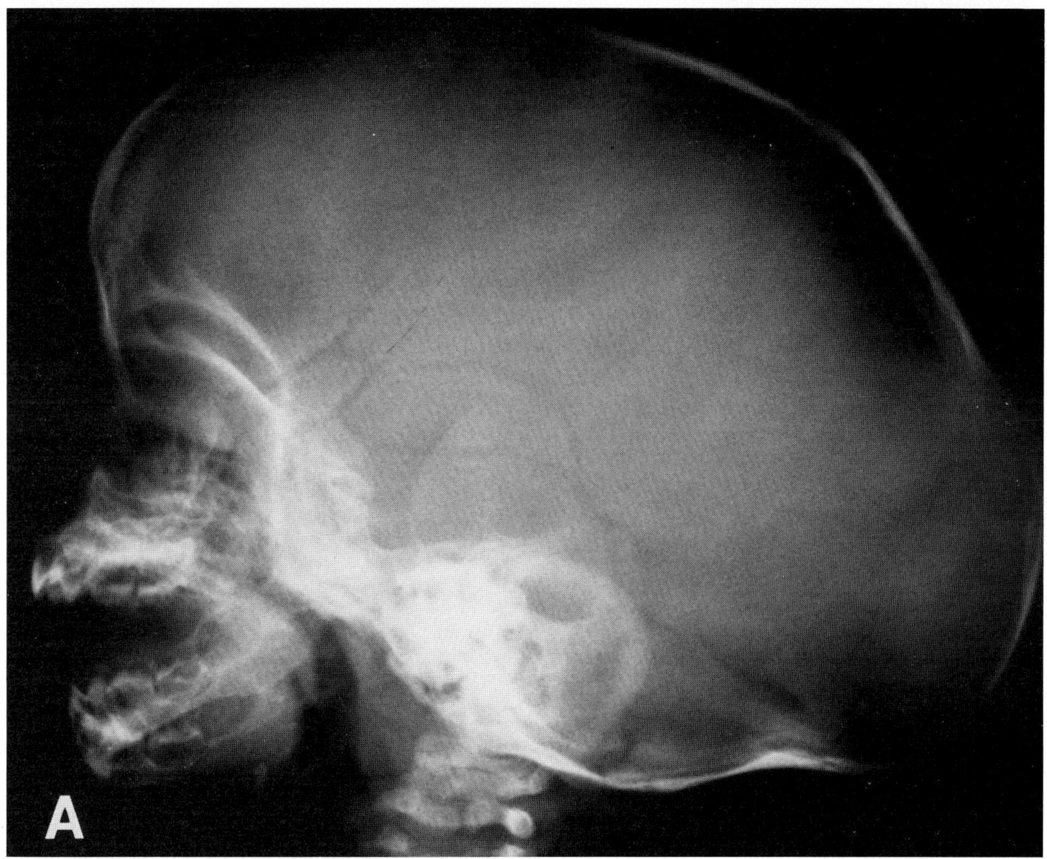

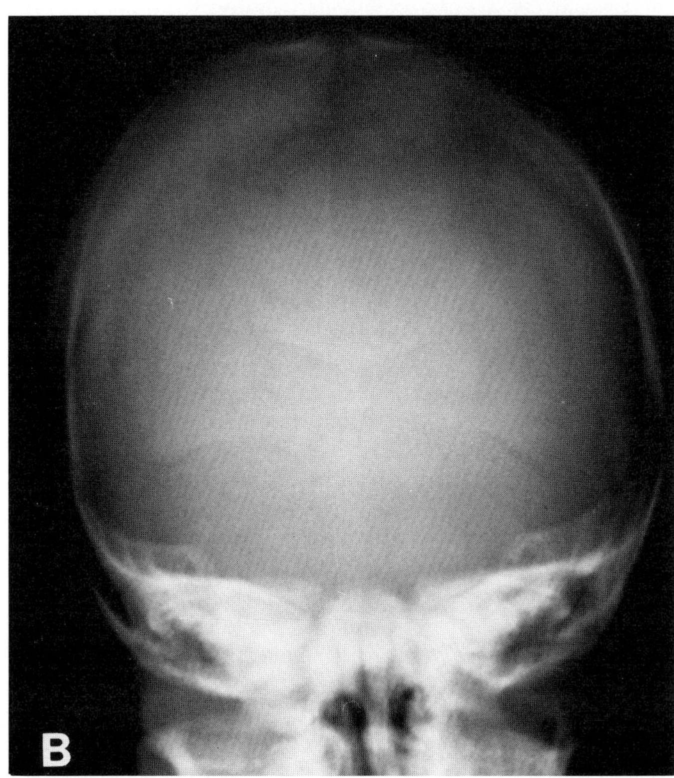

Fig. 13-2. (A) A lateral roentgenogram of an infant with sagittal synostosis demonstrates marked scaphocephaly and a prominent compensatory occipital bulge. (B) A Towne view demonstrates the lack of parietal prominences and a midline ridge with thickening of the perisagittal bone.

taken if there is suspicion of hydrocephalus or the neurologic examination is abnormal. Elongation of the calvarium is quite evident on CT scans (Figure 13-3). The fused suture may be well demonstrated when bone settings are used, a helpful finding in patients with partial or incomplete sutural synostosis.

Carmel et al.[30] reported attenuation of the basal cisterns, absence of the convexity sulcal patterns, and enlarged CSF spaces anteriorly and posteriorly. A prominent interhemispheric fissure may be evident.

In discussing options with the family, we explain that the

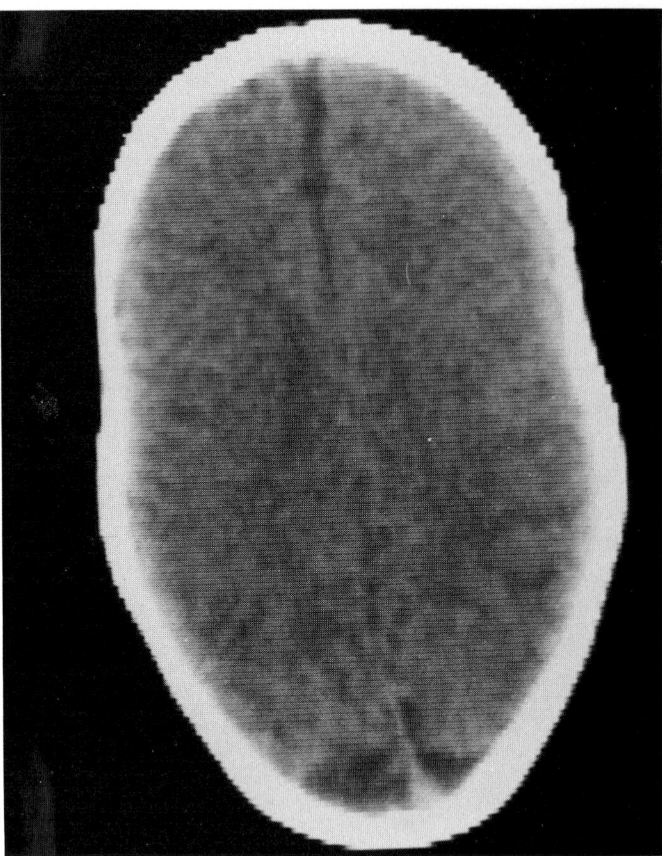

Fig. 13-3. A CT scan of an infant with sagittal synostosis demonstrates the elongation of the skull, prominence of the interhemispheric fissure, and an enlarged occipital CSF collection. The sulcal pattern is lost but the ventricles are normal.

deformity is unlikely to significantly worsen but the synostosis will not open without surgical intervention. Although Barritt et al.[26] found significant social and educational problems in some untreated children, we have rarely needed to discuss this with the parents.

OPERATIVE MANAGEMENT

The goal of surgery is to produce an aesthetically pleasing skull shape. Historically, the surgical options have included either midline sagittal craniectomy (synostectomy) or parasagittal craniectomies. Both these procedures create a ''suture,'' with normalization of the skull shape dependent on further cerebral growth. The importance of early surgery for the correction of sagittal synostosis has been stressed by many authors.[31-35] Variants of sagittal synostosis are not uncommon, and no single operation can always accomplish the desired result. Each patient must be individually evaluated and the operation tailored to that patient's specific deformity.

In common with all operations for synostosis is the need for careful and expeditious anesthetic management. Since these operations are performed on very young children, attention must be directed to careful control of blood volume, temperature, and airway. A major concern for the neurosurgeon is minimizing blood loss. Although the routine administration of transfusions at the time of skin incision has been advocated, we do not use this technique since nearly half of our patients do not require blood replacement. The following operative procedures have been used at our institution in the management of these patients.

Surgical Technique—Midline Sagittal Craniectomy

The infant can be placed in a supine, prone, or lateral decubitus position at the head of the operating table. With the prone or supine position, one must ensure access to both the coronal and lambdoid ends of the sagittal suture since the craniectomy must extend past each of these sutures. In the supine position, the head must be flexed and obstruction of the airway can occur. In infants it is prudent to avoid pin fixation devices to secure the head. We prefer a padded foam headrest. Park et al.[36] described a prone, hyperextended position for these operations. This position allows exposure from the supraorbital ridges to the foramen magnum. All extremities are padded. In young children, heat loss is a concern and blankets and heat lamps are required. A Foley catheter is rarely inserted.

A midline skin incision is drawn with a marking pen to extend 1 to 2 cm beyond the anterior fontanelle or medial coronal suture and the same distance beyond the posterior fontanelle or medial lambdoid suture. Draping should allow for additional extension of the skin incision. A sterile adhesive drape is used. Penetrating skin clips are avoided. Bupivacaine hydrochloride 0.5 percent with epinephrine is injected intradermally along the incision. The skin is incised in 3–5-cm segments down to the periosteum, and pediatric Raney clips are applied to the skin edges. Bipolar coagulation of small scalp bleeders is required. The scalp flaps are elevated and retracted laterally and the coronal and lambdoid sutures identified.

The periosteum is incised with cautery. Bleeding from the skull is controlled by cauterization or bone wax. Stripping of the periosteum is kept to a minimum to avoid bleeding. Depending on the patient's age and skull thickness, two to three burr holes are placed on each side of the midline 3 cm apart. The dura is stripped from the inner table of the skull. The craniotome is then used to create an island of bone 6 cm wide. If an anterior fontanelle is present, it can be opened first and used as the site of insertion of the footplate of the craniotome. The dura is not usually densely adherent to the inner table of the skull except at the suture lines. In very young infants the thin bone can be initially perforated by rotating a scalpel blade between the fingers.

Following the creation of the parallel cuts on each side of the midline, bone is ronguered at the coronal and lambdoid ends to create a completely free-floating island of bone. The island is elevated and the dura is stripped from the inner table. Adherence of the dura to bone over the sagittal sinus is common and care must be taken to avoid injuring it. Bleeding from the dura is controlled with bipolar coagulation or a hemostatic agent. The bone edges are waxed. It may be necessary to remove additional bone at the coronal and lambdoid sutures to ensure that the parietal bones are freely movable.

After creation of the craniectomy, pre-shaped Silastic material is sutured to the bone edges to prevent rapid reapproximation. The scalp then is approximated in two layers after irrigation with an antibiotic solution. Sterile adhesive strips are applied for skin closure. A non-bulky gauze head dressing is used to cover the incision. Drains are not used.

A one-day course of perioperative antibiotics is used. The child is returned to the ward and is allowed to eat or nurse as desired. The head dressing is removed at 48 hours so the skin incision can be inspected. Accumulation of subgaleal fluid is

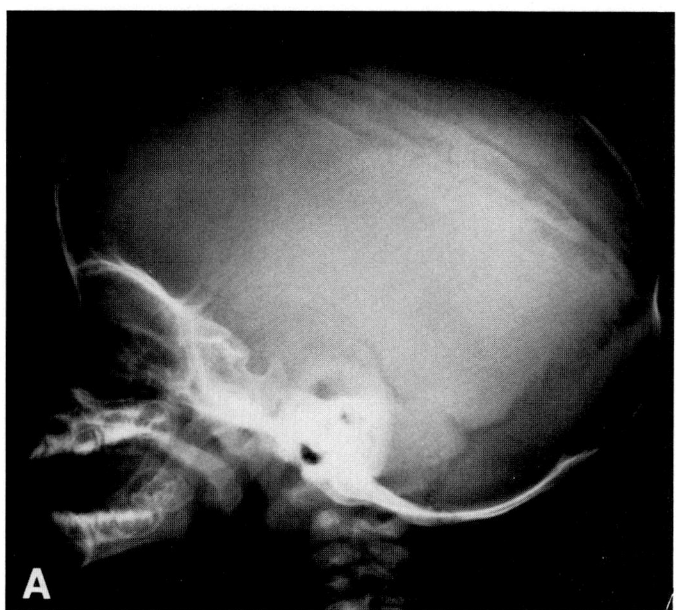

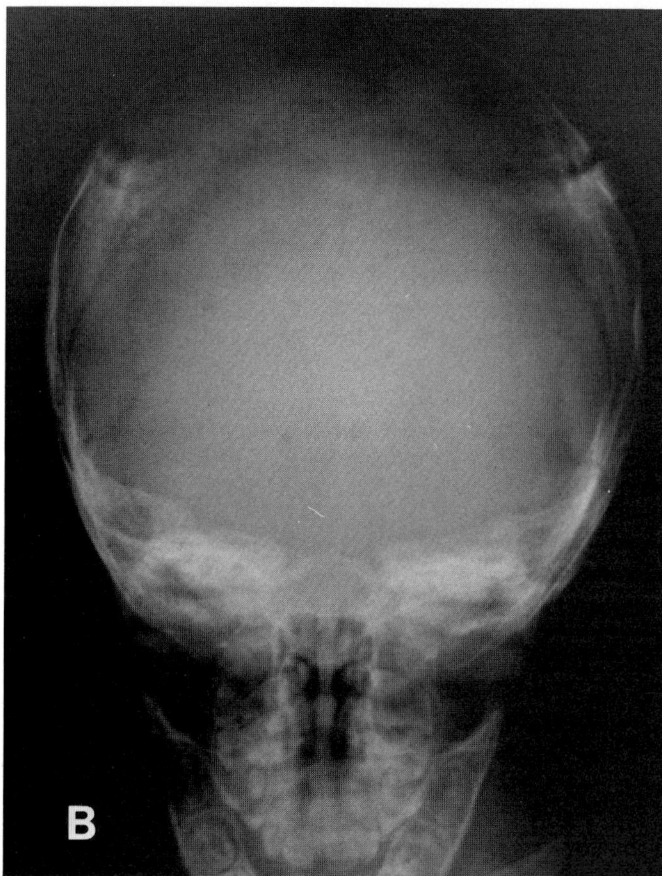

Fig. 13-4. (A) A lateral roentgenogram of the same patient in Figure 13-2 six months after midline sagittal synostectomy demonstrates less scaphocephaly, improvement in the occipital bulge and patency of both created suture lines. The synostectomy extends from the coronal to the lambdoid sutures. (B) A Towne roentgenogram reveals considerable improvement in the shape of the head, especially the biparietal region.

rarely a significant problem and tapping or aspiration of this fluid is avoided unless the suture line is under tension or there is clinical evidence of intracranial hypertension. The patient is discharged by the fifth postoperative day after routine skull roentgenograms demonstrate satisfactory craniectomy boundaries. No protective headgear is required for these infants. The adhesive strips are removed in 10 to 14 days.

Three to six months after surgery, regeneration of bone will have filled the craniectomy. Skull roentgenograms can be obtained to demonstrate that the craniectomy persists.

Surgical Technique—Midline Sagittal Craniectomy with Modifications

In many infants with sagittal synostosis, the compensatory occipital prominence is quite pronounced. Venes and Sayers[37] therefore advocated extending the craniectomy to include removal of the bony occipital prominence as well as additional lateral bone removal at the anterior and posterior extent of the sagittal suture. Immediate improvement in the lateral appearance of the head is evident, although the improvement in the biparietal diameter is still dependent on normal cerebral growth. Albright[38] added further modifications by creating bilateral wedge parietal craniectomies immediately anterior to the lambdoid suture. The base of the wedge is narrowed with sutures, which immediately and effectively improves the biparietal diameter. This method of immediate correction of head shape can also help prevent the problems of early refusion.

Surgical Technique—The Pi Procedure

In 1978, Jane et al.[39] described a new technique for immediate correction of sagittal synostosis. This operation involves creating a pi-shaped craniectomy and reducing the AP diameter of the skull by bringing together the sagittal strip and the frontal bone. Follow-up studies have indicated a lack of refusion of the sutures even though no artificial material is inserted to impede growth of the skull edges. This is thought to be a result of the changes in dural tension and stresses produced by the AP shortening at the time of operation.

In older children, more complex procedures are required to achieve correction of the deformity since the necessary growth of the brain and skull is limited. Vollmer et al.[40] reviewed the treatment of a group of patients with variations of sagittal synostosis. These individuals had been treated by modifying the pi craniectomy to alter the areas of compensatory bulging.

Surgical Technique—Vault Remodeling

In older children, significant growth of the brain does not occur and reshaping of the head can only be accomplished at the time of surgery. In addition, morphologic and radiographic studies may demonstrate the need for reconstruction of the supraorbital ridge. Vault remodeling can be accomplished by using the techniques of craniectomy, elevation of large bone flaps, and transposition of the bone flaps. The techniques of Rougerie et al.[41] or Marchac and Renier[42] are applicable in these situations. Creation of a plastic cast of the skull made by

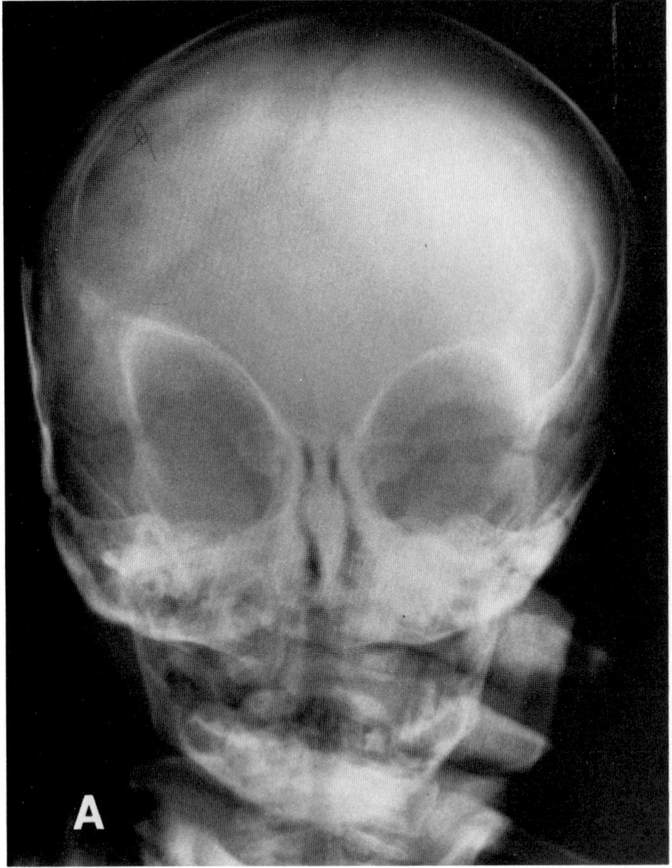
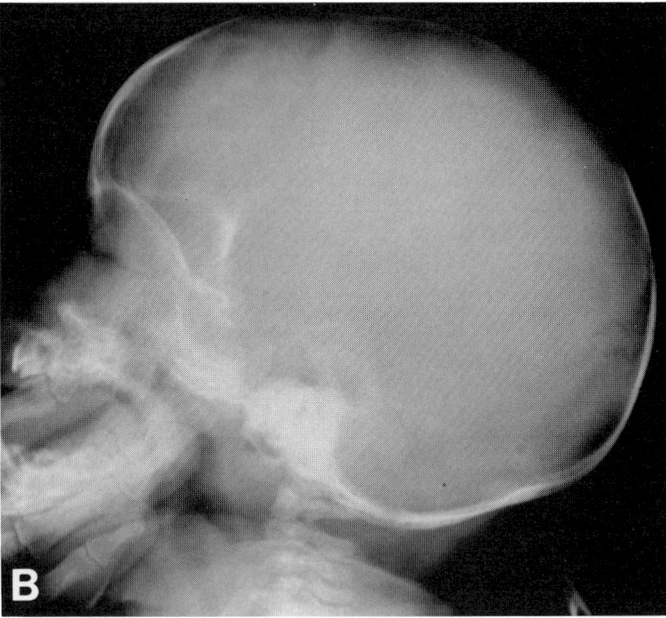

Fig. 13-5.   (A) Characteristic changes of coronal synostosis include the "harlequin" eye sign with elevation and obliquity of the lateral orbital wall. The sagittal and lambdoid sutures are clearly visible. (B) Elevation of the greater wing of the sphenoid, foreshortening of the anterior fossa and orbit, and absence of the coronal suture are apparent on this lateral roentgenogram.

a mold technique and modified according to data from x-ray studies is very useful in planning surgery. The surgeon can cut the model into various shapes and arrange the pieces to attain a satisfactory contour. The pieces of the model can serve as a template during the actual surgical procedure.

The carbon dioxide laser was used by James for skin incisions, subcutaneous tissue dissection, and creation of osteotomies in 5 patients with various types of synostosis.[43] The additional hemostasis obtained with the laser may make this a useful adjunct in the treatment of synostosis, although higher wattages are needed to expeditiously cut bone and it is necessary to protect the underlying dura from the laser energy. The water content of bone in older children is less than in neonates and infants, thereby diminishing the applicability of the laser in this group of patients.

COMPLICATIONS AND RESULTS

The list of potential complications includes those related to anesthesia and those related to the actual surgical procedure. Careful monitoring of respiratory and metabolic function and attention to hemodynamics and blood loss has resulted in a rate of significant complications of less than 1 percent.[44] Injury to the sagittal sinus is rare. Infection is unlikely, although the insertion of an interpositional material would seem to increase this relative risk. Wound closure problems are infrequent. Persistent bony defects have occasionally been reported.[45]

The results of any cosmetic procedure are subjective.

Midline sagittal synostectomy when performed at an early age is met with uniformly good results as judged by the family and the neurosurgeon (Figure 13-4A and B). Results of surgery in older patients and those with variants of sagittal synostosis are also good and appear to be improving as more radical procedures are employed.

CORONAL SYNOSTOSIS

DIAGNOSIS

Unilateral coronal synostosis accounts for about 15 percent of cases of craniosynostosis and is significantly more frequent in girls.[27,46,47] Bilateral coronal synostosis is frequently associated with craniofacial dysmorphic syndromes.

Patients with unilateral coronal synostosis demonstrate ipsilateral flattening of the frontal bone and lateral superior orbital ridge. Compensatory deformities of the contralateral frontal and ipsilateral temporal bones also occur. The nose may deviate toward the affected side, the globe may appear proptotic, and the eye on the involved side will be higher than the eye on the opposite side. Midface hypoplasia and flattening may be detected.

Skull roentgenograms demonstrate elevation of the greater wing of the sphenoid and foreshortening of the orbit (Figure 13-5). The anterior fossa is shallow and the ipsilateral frontal bone is flat. Bulging of the contralateral frontal and ipsilateral

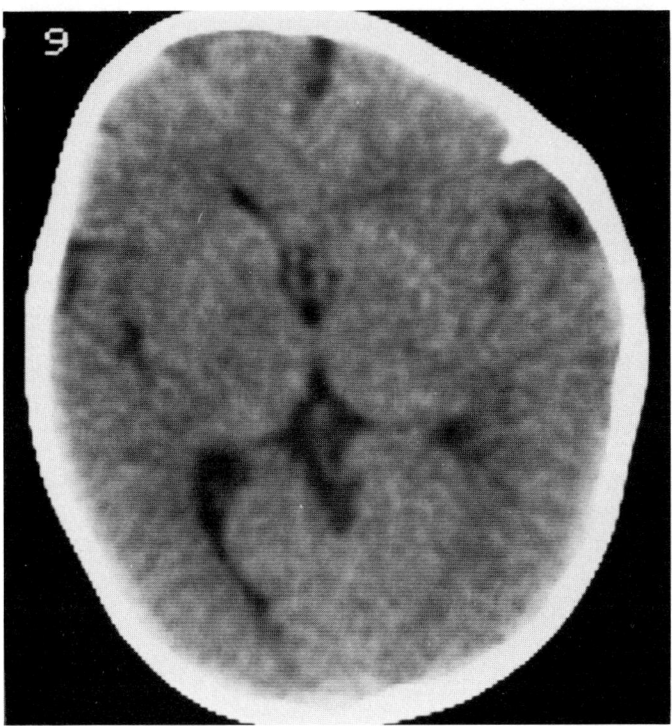

Fig. 13-6. A CT scan of an infant with coronal synostosis reveals anterior displacement of the sphenoid bone, effacement of the ipsilateral ventricular system, ipsilateral temporal bulging, and slight enlargement of the sylvian fissure CSF space. There is moderate bulging of the contralateral frontal bone.

temporal bone may be evident. The fused suture may not be visible, although thickening and perisutural sclerosis may be seen. The roentgenograms must be carefully reviewed for evidence of other sutural synostosis. Bilateral coronal synostosis will produce flattening of both sides of the forehead and of the supraorbital ridges. Computed tomographic scans demonstrate anterior displacement of the sphenoid wing with marked thickening of the pterion (Figure 13-6). The sphenoid-petrosal angle, which is normally 90 degrees, is reduced. Ipsilateral effacement of the cerebral sulci and frontal horn of the ventricle has been reported.[30]

SURGICAL TECHNIQUE-LATERAL CANTHAL ADVANCEMENT

Unilateral coronal synostosis, because of the asymmetry it creates, is more deforming than the bilateral version of this disorder. A unilateral lateral canthal advancement is currently the preferred method of treatment.[48,49] The major limitation of this procedure is that the contralateral deformity is not corrected. If this is a significant cosmetic problem, bilateral supraorbital and forehead remodeling should be considered. The operative procedure is carried out with the same precautions mentioned previously regarding surgery in young children. A bicoronal skin incision is used, and dissection of the skin flap over the forehead and frontal bone and into the orbit is accomplished in the subperiosteal plane. A unilateral bone flap is created, with the coronal suture serving as the posterior landmark and the sagittal suture as the medial boundary. The osteotomy is carried laterally to the pterion, which is thickened and elevated. The frontal bone flap is elevated and stored in an

antibiotic solution until it is replaced. A 10–12-mm supraorbital bar remains to be freed and advanced. If the compensatory contralateral bulge is prominent, bifrontal bone flaps should be elevated.

The frontal lobe is retracted epidurally to expose the orbital roof. To facilitate exposure and reduce retraction of the brain, hyperventilation is used and occasionally supplemented with osmotic agents. Careful attention must be directed to maintain serum electrolyte concentrations and balance the fluid intake and output in very young children. Lumbar drainage is not used.

After removal of the pterion, the surgeon proceeds across the orbital roof. The osteotomy across the orbital roof can be accomplished using a small angled Kerrison punch or craniotome. The periorbital fascia is thin and inadvertent tears must be repaired. We protect the fascia with a thin brain retractor, which is inserted from the external side. The osteotomy is carried to the edge of the crista galli. The frontozygomatic process is cut, leaving the supraorbital ridge hinged medially.

At this time it may be possible to bend the supraorbital bar to affect a curved lateral surface. Because the supraorbital bar is straight, the lateral edge may form a sharp corner when advanced to its final position. Bending the bar alleviates this sharp corner. This technique should not be tried in older children, since the bar is nonmalleable and will fracture.

A bone strut is created from the free frontal bone fragment. To ensure adequate room for frontal lobe expansion, the lateral canthus is advanced 1–2 cm. Although one tends to advance the supraorbital rim to achieve symmetry, it is better to overcompensate by a few millimeters in the amount of lateral canthal advancement.

The anterior aspect of the parietal bone is ensheathed with Silastic, which is sutured to the bone with 4–0 nylon. The strut is then sutured to the lateral canthus anteriorly and ensheathed parietal bone posteriorly.

The residual ipsilateral frontal bone flap is either loosely approximated to the supraorbital ridge or allowed to lie free on the dura, held in place by the periosteum and skin. The contralateral bone flap is positioned to achieve the best cosmetic effect.

The wound is closed in layers and sterile adhesive strips are used on the skin. A sterile, nonbulky head dressing is applied. Periorbital swelling is invariable but resolves within 48 to 72 hours. Postoperative skull roentgenograms are routinely obtained and the child is usually ready for discharge by day 5.

Modifications of the lateral canthal advancement procedure have addressed the problems of forehead ridging, which can occur after surgery in unilateral cases, and the failure to correct recession of the lower lateral orbital wall, which can produce a irregular step-off.[49] If the compensatory forehead bulging is prominent, bifrontal bone flaps should be elevated. Dural plication is then followed by positioning the bone plates to achieve the best cranial contour.[50]

COMPLICATIONS AND RESULTS

Operative procedures for correction of coronal synostosis share a similar list of complications as those for other forms of synostosis. The results of lateral canthal advancement are generally satisfactory if the procedure is done early. Long-term results are not yet available. Further surgery may still be required at a later date to correct serious midface hypoplasia and malocclusion.

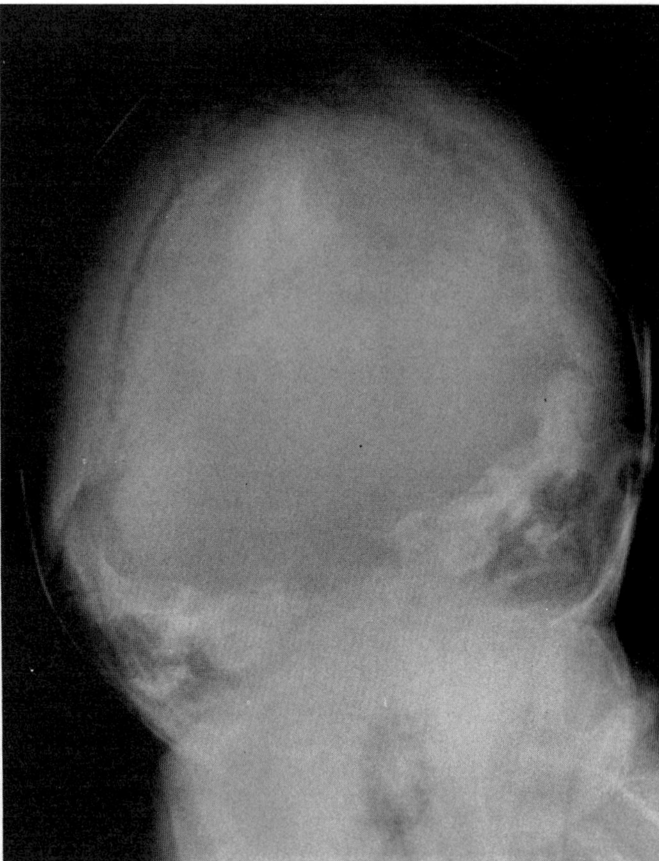

Fig. 13-7. A roentgenogram of an infant with lambdoid synostosis reveals assymetry of the petrous bones and a lucent line that could be mistaken for a patent suture.

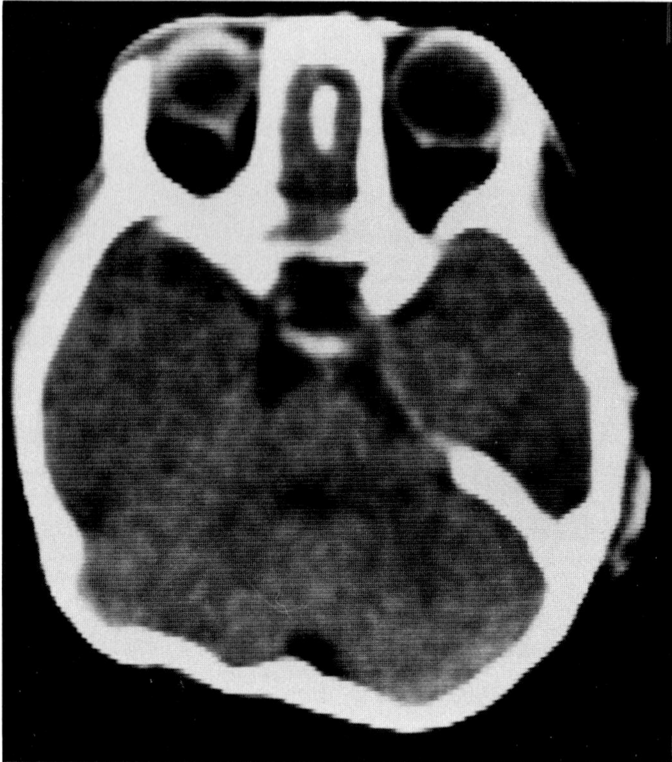

Fig. 13-8. A CT scan of a child with lambdoid synostosis demonstrates anterior displacement of the petrous bones, ipsilateral occipital flattening, and compensatory bulging of the contralateral occipital bone.

LAMBDOID SYNOSTOSIS

DIAGNOSIS

Isolated, unilateral lambdoid synostosis occurs with a frequency of 1 to 15 percent.[51,52] Boys predominate in most series. Associated systemic anomalies occur in 10 percent of children.

Occipital flattening and ipsilateral prominence of the forehead is characteristic of lambdoid synostosis. The ear on the involved side is located forward and downward. The ipsilateral occipital flattening and contralateral frontal flattening produce significant asymmetry. Head circumference measurements are enlarged for the age of the patient. Children with lambdoid synostosis tend to be referred to a neurosurgeon at a later age than children with other forms of synostosis. Many are initially thought to have positional molding and parents are told that the deformity will correct itself with time.

Skull roentgenograms may demonstrate a fused or united suture or may show only perisutural sclerosis (Figure 13-7). Hinton et al.[7] reported that the synostosis of the lambdoid suture is unlike that of the sagittal suture in that actual bone union was rare, occurring in less than 10 percent of cases examined pathologically. Lambdoid sutures without bone union demonstrated accelerated but normal histologic structure, often with cartilage in the intersutural space. These findings explain the lack of a palpable ridge over the involved suture and the absence of classical synostotic changes on plain roentgeno-grams. Occipital flattening is evident in all cases, and the forward migration of the petrous ridge can be identified. Muakkassa studied 57 patients using ^{99m}Tc bone scans, finding 50 abnormal sutures with this technique.[7] Proper evaluation of sutural bone scans requires experience in dosage, scanning time, and knowledge of normal suture activity at various stages of growth.[53] The characteristic findings on CT scans include ipsilateral occipital flattening and thinning of the occipital bone adjacent to the involved suture (Figure 13-8). The suture line itself may appear normal or thickened. Compression of the occipital horn of the ventricle can be seen, and the sphenoid-petrosal angle may be altered.

SURGICAL TECHNIQUE-LAMBDOID SYNOSTECTOMY

The therapeutic goals in the treatment of children with lambdoid synostosis are the achievement of a rounded, symmetric occiput and the normalization of ear position. Since the auditory canals cannot be directly mobilized, it is imperative that treatment be initiated early enough to allow migration and realignment of the ears. In older patients, one can expect to achieve a symmetric occiput but ear position will remain askew.

The child is placed in a prone position under general anesthesia. The weight of the head should rest on the frontal prominences with the orbits protected so no pressure is placed on the eyes. A linear skin incision over the lambdoid suture is made to expose it from the sagittal suture medially to the asterion laterally. The skin and subcutaneous tissues are opened down to the periosteum. The cutting current is em-

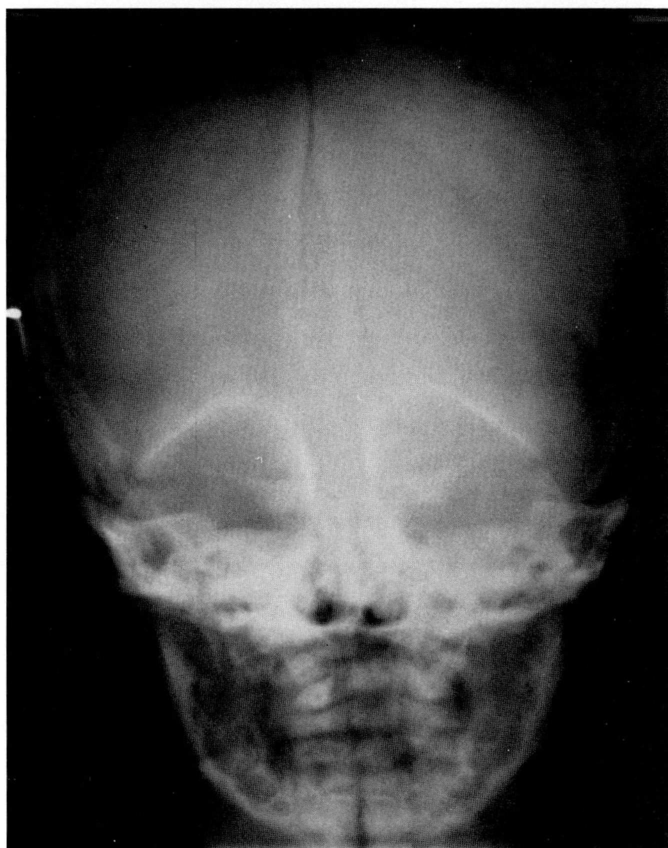

Fig. 13-9.　Metopic synostosis is demontrated by the vertical orientation of the medial aspects of the orbital walls, the "sad-sack" sign, and the double lucency in the midline that represents the fused suture.

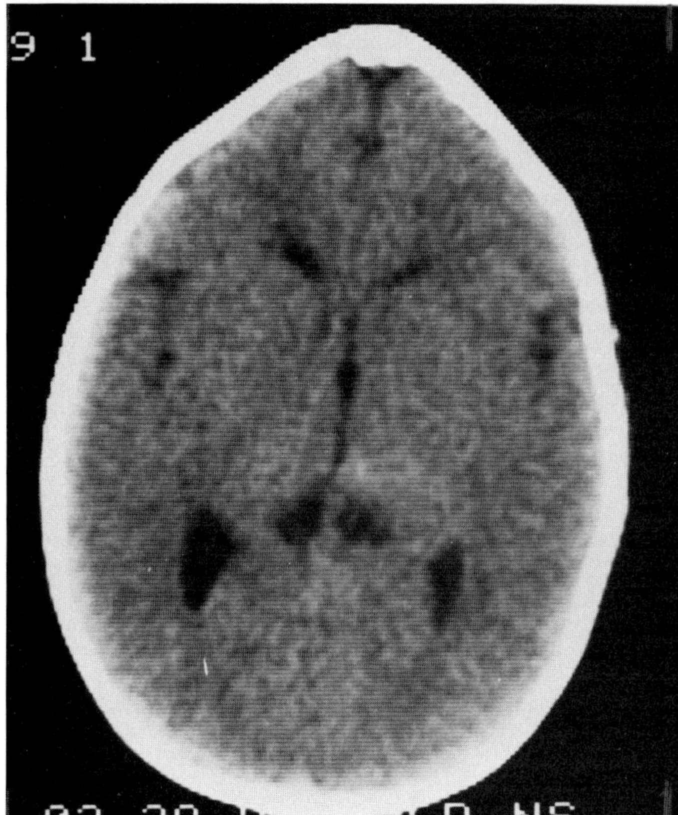

Fig. 13-10.　A CT scan of a child with metopic synostosis discloses the prominent pointed forehead. The ventricles and CSF spaces are normal.

ployed to open the periosteum, which is stripped only to the extent necessary to place the initial burr holes.

The craniotome is used to excise the suture extending from the sagittal to the squamosal suture. Although Rekate and Kaufman[54] suggested that it may be necessary to resect the lateral 2–3 mm of petrous bone, we have not found this to be necessary. It may be very difficult to accomplish this because of the dense adherence of the dura and the presence of the transverse or sigmoid sinus in this region. Dural plication may be required to achieve a rounded appearance of the occiput. Silastic is applied to both bone edges. The wound is closed in layers without drains.

COMPLICATIONS AND RESULTS

Complications are infrequent but similar to those previously cited. Injury to the transverse sinus is rare.

Gradual improvement and rounding of the occipital prominence can be expected in nearly all cases. The location of the ears, however, will depend to a great degree on the timing of surgery.

METOPIC SYNOSTOSIS

DIAGNOSIS

Premature closure of the metopic suture accounts for less than 5 percent of all synostoses.[5,27] A preponderance in boys is reported, and the synostosis is usually an isolated event.[55]

The forehead is narrow and shortened with absence of the normal frontal prominences. A midline ridge extending from the root of the nose to the anterior fontanelle is palpable. Hypotelorism is characteristic and epicanthal folds may be seen.

Skull x-ray films reveal a foreshortened frontal bone that may be convex in shape. The medial walls of the orbit are vertical, giving a typical appearance on plain roentgenograms (Figure 13-9). A midline bony prominence may be evident. A CT scan confirms the changes of the forehead and the associated hypotelorism (Figure 13-10). The suture usually appears thickened. The ventricular system and CSF pathways are not affected.

OPERATIVE THERAPY

Surgical procedures for the correction of metopic synostosis have evolved from Matson's limited strip craniectomy to more complex procedures that deal with the associated deformity of the supraorbital ridge.[27,56] As has become apparent with virtually all of the forms of craniosynostosis, the surgical procedure must be adapted to the degree of deformity. Conservative management has been advocated in cases with minimal forehead ridging and clinically inapparent hypotelorism on the basis of long-term clinical and roentgenographic results.[57] Neurosurgeons have advocated a procedure that involves excision of the involved suture and reapposition of the frontal bone.[44,58] However, this technique does not deal with the associated abnormality of the supraorbital rim as defined and characterized by Marchac and Renier.[59] Their technique creates a supraorbital bar, which is molded and

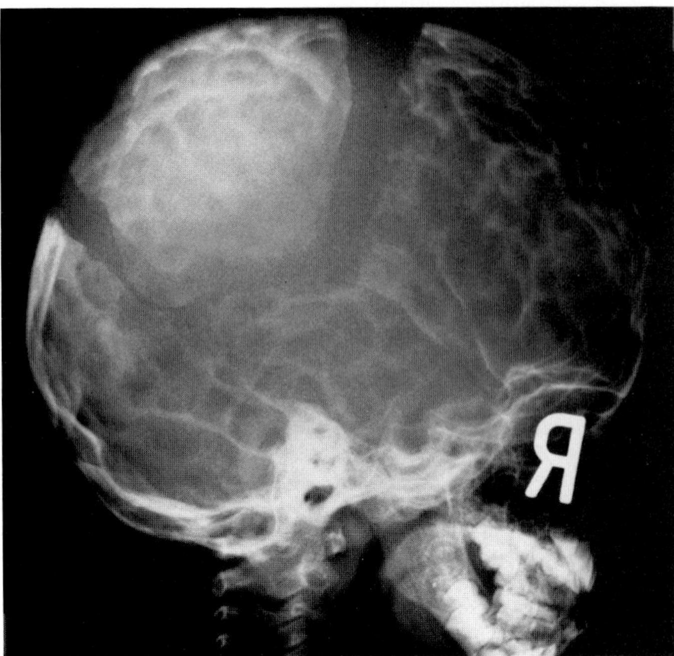

Fig. 13-11. A marked "beaten silver" appearance is evident. Bilateral parietal bone flaps have separated an additional 1 cm compared with an earlier postoperative roentgenogram.

shaped before replacement. Most neurosurgeons are not comfortable with attempting this procedure and an experienced team may be necessary.

Surgical Technique—Metopic Syntectomy

Following endotracheal intubation, the child is placed on a padded headrest in the supine position. A bicoronal skin incision is created and the forehead skin flap is developed. Burr holes are placed anterior to the coronal suture, and the craniotome is used to create bifrontal bone flaps. The metopic ridge must be removed down to the nasal root. A high-speed drill is used for this purpose.

The metopic ridge of the bifrontal bone flap is removed, creating two equal but separate frontal bone flaps. These are sutured together and reattached to the supraorbital rims. The wound is closed in the fashion previously described.

Surgical Technique—"The Floating Forehead"

A bicoronal skin incision is made and the frontal skin flaps are mobilized. The flap must extend to below the frontozygomatic suture. A bifrontal bone flap is removed and temporarily stored in a sterile antibiotic solution. The bone flap is designed to leave a supraorbital bar of 10–15 mm in height. The brain is elevated off the orbital roofs and in the area anterior to the crista galli. Tears in the dura should be immediately repaired. It is usually necessary to retract the dura of the anterior temporal fossa to facilitate placement of the osteotomies. The bone is cut across the orbital roofs and just anterior to the midline crista galli. The bone may be quite thick in the midline, requiring the use of a high-speed drill. The frontozygomatic suture is cut, freeing the entire supraorbital bar. The bar is then straightened by either fracturing the midline and suturing the two pieces back together or by actual removal of the thickened midline. The pterion are removed bilaterally.

Options are available for replacement of the supraorbital

bar. Marchac and Renier[59] advocated a single medial fixation point, which allows the entire bar to advance. Reported complications with this method are rare. Others prefer a more stable fixation by creating strut grafts between the supraorbital bar and the lateral wall of the orbit or posterior frontal bone, like that for a lateral canthal advancement.[60]

The frontal bone is reshaped by first excising the prominent midline ridge. The two halves are reapproximated and sutured to the supraorbital bar or left floating, being held in place by the periosteum and skin. The surgeon should attempt to achieve the best cosmetic shape possible, which may require rotating the bone flaps. We suture the frontal bone to the bar.

Salkind et al.[61] treated 13 patients by elevation of bilateral frontal bone flaps save for the midline medial metopic ridge, which was reduced with a drill.

COMPLICATIONS AND RESULTS

The list of complications for these procedures is similar to those previously cited. Excellent results have been reported with all of these procedures.

PAN SYNOSTOSIS

As suggested earlier in this chapter, there are instances of multiple suture involvement with actual or incipient intracranial hypertension that require decompression, not only for cosmetic effect but also to protect the growing brain. In these cases, a decision must be made regarding the urgency of decompression, whether the face or other body systems are involved, and whether correction of these deformities requires an integrated team approach.

The cloverleaf-skull deformity or kleeblattsch ä del is often associated with altered development in other areas of the body and most of these children die. Restriction of the growing brain may be an immediate life-threatening problem, and if the outlook is otherwise favorable, surgical treatment of this condition is indicated.[62]

In 1938, King[63] introduced "morcellation" of the skull: the cutting of the calvarium into multiple sections as in a jigsaw puzzle but leaving the fragments in place. This remains the essence of current treatment, although rather than leaving the pieces in place, these are now discarded and the dura and other connective tissues are relied on to reconstitute the skull as the child grows.[64] This approach should probably be limited to babies. Powiertowski[65] reported a series of children up to age 14 years in whom the increased intracranial pressure subsided after such extensive bone removal.

Patients with pansynostosis may be seen after the neonatal period. For example, a 5-year-old boy with congenital arthrogryposis, severe headaches, emesis, and papilledema underwent ICP monitoring that demonstrated a baseline pressure of 30 torr with one to three plateau waves daily. Clinical sequelae were not observed during these periods. Simple biparietal bone flaps resulted in resolution of the papilledema and headaches (Figure 13-11).

CRANIOFACIAL SYNDROMES

The management of the complex problems of children with craniofacial abnormalities requires a multidisciplinary team approach. The nature of these deformities often spans several surgical specialties with input from various team members affecting the timing and type of surgical procedure. The application of new concepts and surgical techniques has made cranio-orbital-facial surgery a safe and rewarding therapeutic modality.

It is not possible within this chapter to review all of the procedures available for the correction of craniofacial abnormalities. A review of several of the major problems and the applicable surgical procedures will be presented so that neurosurgeons will better understand the concepts and objectives employed in the evaluation and treatment of children and adults with facial anomalies.

CLASSIFICATION

The categorization of diverse craniofacial syndromes is difficult.[15,22,66] Attempts to arrange this group of diseases by a single clinical feature are misleading. Hydrocephalus, seizures, or mental retardation may be characteristic of a specific genetic entity, but because of multifactorial influences, expression of these specific characteristics may be varied or absent. Neurosurgeons must be aware that variable expression within a single genetic syndrome may present with a different synostotic suture than dictated by the classical condition. Detailed clinical, genetic, and roentgenographic evaluation is required.

There are approximately 40 genetic syndromes associated with craniosynostosis.[4,15,22,66–109] In addition, teratogenic syndromes and the multiple diseases that characterize the median cleft face syndrome may require neurosurgical evaluation and treatment.[110–113] Although the list of genetic syndromes will undoubtedly expand as new entities are described, Munro[114] reported that nearly 25 percent of the craniofacial deformities in children could not be properly labeled or classified.

DIAGNOSTIC EVALUATION

Neurologic, ophthalmologic, and neuroradiologic evaluation form the foundation for treatment (Table 13-1). Standard skull and facial roentgenograms and tomograms are especially valuable for precise cephalometric analysis. Computed tomography, including careful study of the cranial base, is carried out to identify associated cerebral anomalies. Subtle abnormalities of the involved suture and of remote sutures are enhanced by the CT bone window settings. Three-dimensional CT reconstruction can be most helpful in establishing a diagnosis and planning treatment.[115,116] An essential element of the pretreatment evaluation is clinical photography. This allows three-dimensional models to be constructed as well as comparisons to be made after the procedure.

TREATMENT

Clinical and experimental evidence suggest that early treatment during the neonatal period is preferable to a delayed approach and may abrogate the need for a more radical procedure in later years.[117,118] Attention is directed to the basal structures and their role in progressive facial growth.[8] Premature closure of the frontosphenoidal, frontoethmoidal, frontozygomatic, and sphenozygomatic sutures, accompanied by coronal synostosis, prevents the normal expansion of the frontal and temporal lobes.[119] Because the midface is attached to the

Table 13-1. Diagnostic evaluation of craniofacial abnormalities

Department	Diagnostic Evaluation
Radiology	Complete skull series
	Basal skull views
	Towne view
	Facial bones—Caldwell, Stereo Waters
	Orbital tomography
	Radionuclide bone scan
Neurosurgery	Neurologic assessment
	Radiologic evaluation and interpretation
Plastic surgery	Clinical orofacial-cranial evaluation
	Radiologic assessment
	Photographic analysis
Dental	Models, splints, occlusion studies
	Roentgenographic analysis
Anesthesiology	Airway evaluation
	Cardiopulmonary assessment
Neuro-ophthalmology	Visual acuity
	Visual fields
	Color vision
	Extraocular muscle function
	Funduscopic examination
	Prism testing
	Roentgenographic analysis
Psychology	Social history
	Psychologic evaluation
	Cognitive testing
	Counseling
Geneticist	Family history
	Syndrome labeling
	Counseling
	Chromosome evaluation

frontal bone, premature synostosis of these sutures results in retarded growth of the face, exorbitism, and proptosis. The anterior cranial fossa is foreshortened and its alignment with other bony landmarks abnormal. Creation of artificial sutures at an early stage can permit subsequent normal development of the midface structures.[120]

The neurosurgeon is responsible for the diagnosis and treatment of associated hydrocephalus. Standard cerebrospinal fluid shunting may be required. The shunt apparatus is placed in a parieto-occipital location so as not to compromise later frontal craniectomy.

The initial treatment of many craniofacial syndromes is directed toward correcting the problem of craniosynostosis. Bilateral coronal synostosis, which is a part of many of these syndromes, requires bilateral lateral canthal advancements at an early stage. Often, no further surgery is required until the child is older. Midface recession will ultimately require a LeFort III midface advancement. Ideally, it would be preferable to wait until the child reaches early adolescence, when mandibular growth has been completed, so as to avoid malocclusion, which will develop as growth continues. Many surgeons nevertheless feel that the midface advancement should be performed 5 to 6 years before the patient starts school.

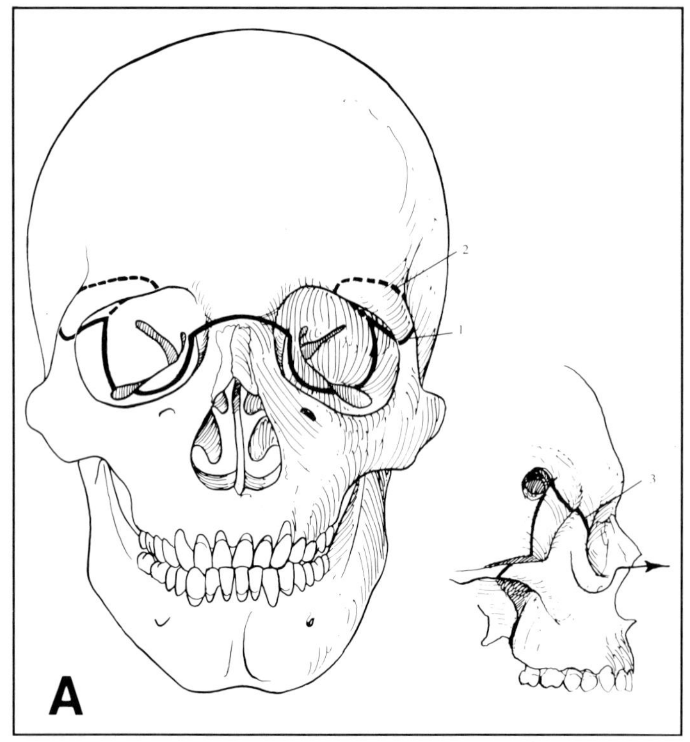
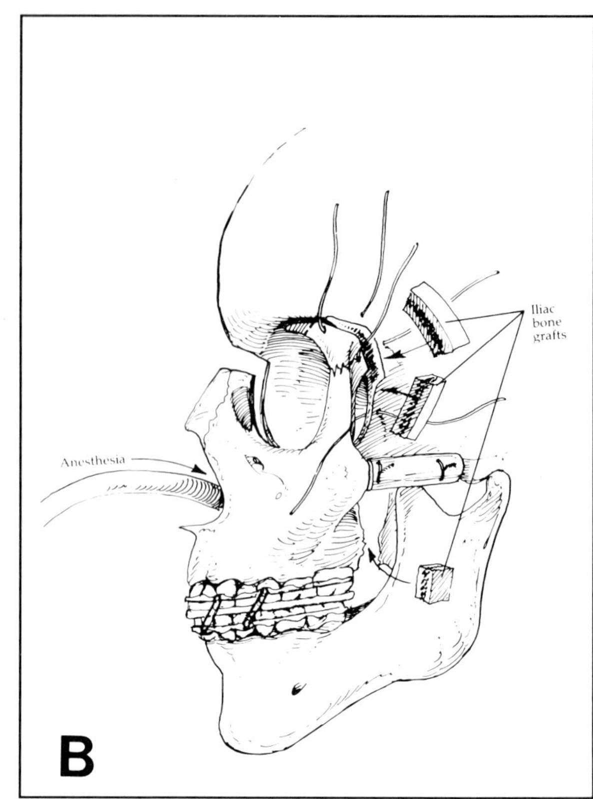

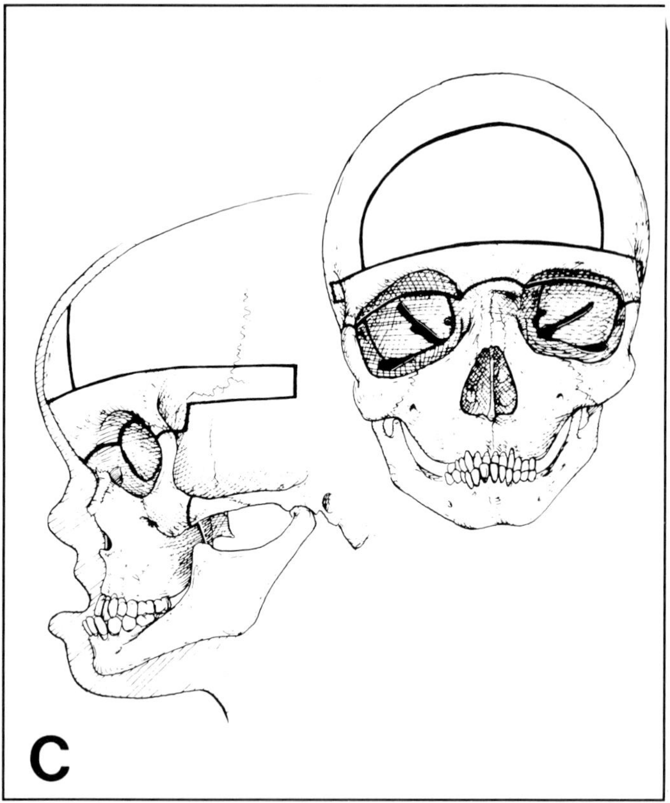
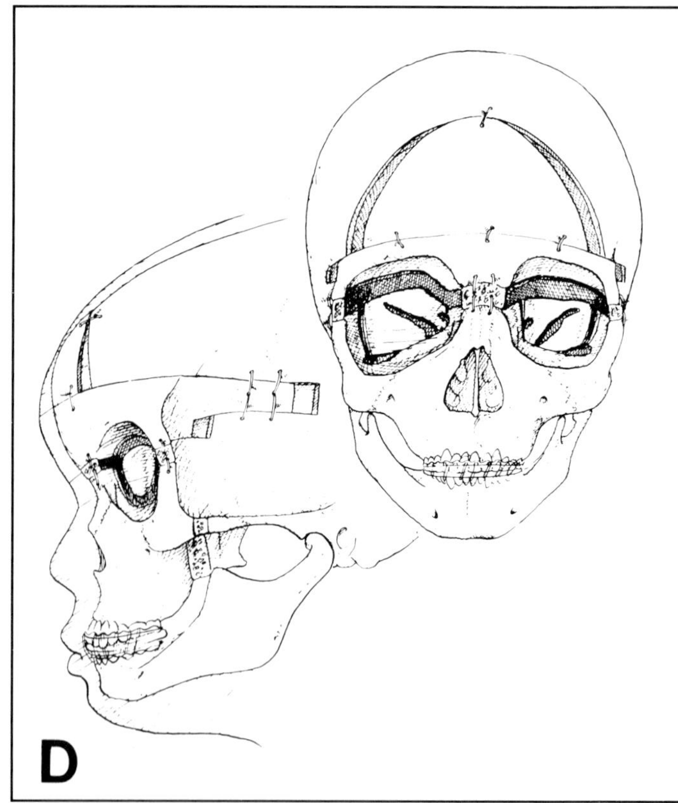

Fig. 13-12. (A) The three types of LeFort III osteotomies include (1) Tessier I, subcranial; (2) Tessier II, extended intracranial/entracranial; and (3) Tessier III, self-stabilizing. (B) Bone grafts are used after repositioning. (C) LeFort III osteotomy can be combined with forehead advancement. Osteotomy sites are demonstrated by bold lines. (D) Advancement of the forehead and midface is completed by bone grafting. (Reprinted from Jackson IT, et al: Atlas of Craniomaxillofacial Surgery. St. Louis, CV Mosby, 1982, pp 198, 206. With permission.)

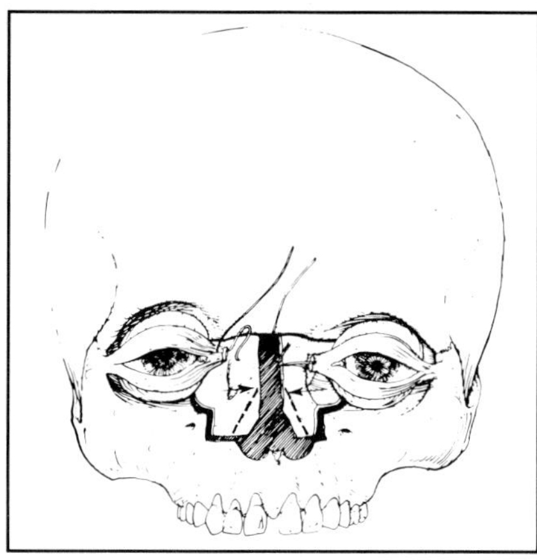

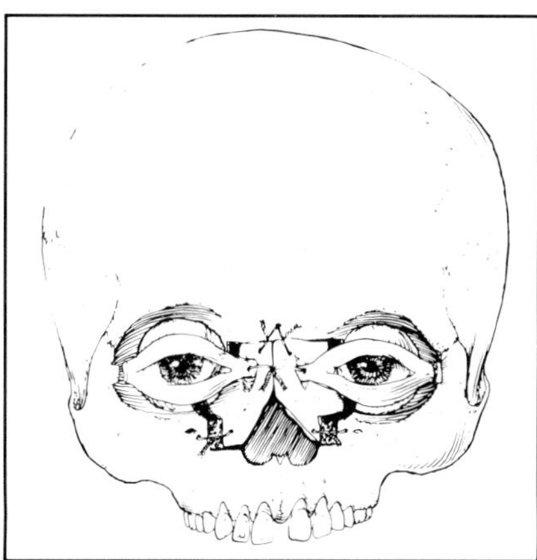

Fig. 13-13. Correction of orbital hypertelorism by a medial orbital wall osteotomy. (Reprinted from Jackson IT, et al: Atlas of Craniomaxillofacial Surgery. St. Louis, CV Mosby, 1982, pp 356, 357. With permission.)

LEFORT III MIDFACE ADVANCEMENT

Craniofacial reconstruction in older children and adults with craniofacial dysostosis requires creation of a LeFort III osteotomy and advancement of the frontal bone and supraorbital rims. Many surgeons feel that the LeFort III advancement should be performed in children with craniofacial syndromes at the preschool age, recognizing that this will necessitate correction of malocclusion at a later date. A bicoronal skin incision is used and a free bifrontal bone flap created. The dura is stripped from the floor of the anterior cranial fossa. The LeFort III osteotomies allow forward and downward displacement of the midface (Figure 13-12). This procedure produces an immediate increase in the orbital volume, relieving the apparent exophthalmos, and corrects the maxillary hypoplasia. The flattened nasal dorsum is advanced and the nose lengthened. Normal dental occlusion is restored. Corrective rhinoplasty and mandibular alterations may be required later. To stabilize the midface, it is necessary to wire the teeth together. A tracheostomy is usually required during the postoperative phase.

HYPERTELORISM

Correction of hypertelorism involves removal of a segment of nasofrontal bone, apposition of the bony margins, and bone grafts to the lateral orbital walls.[121] Correction can be accom-

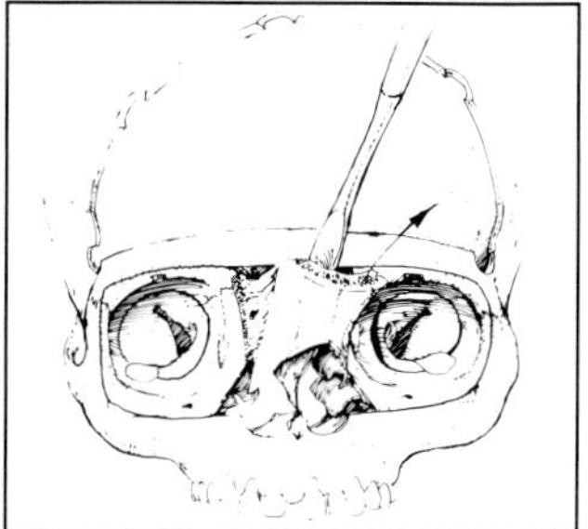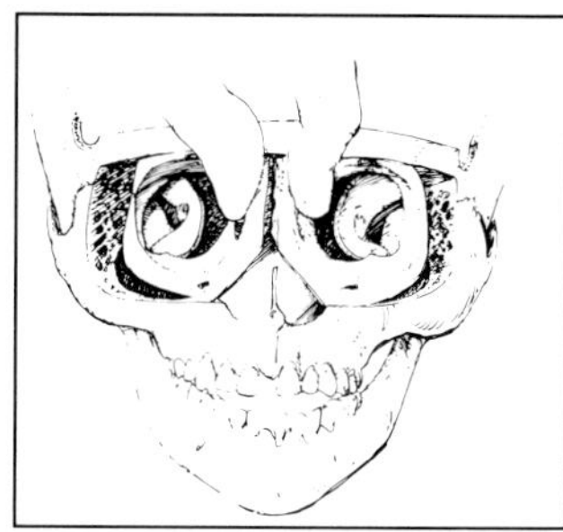

Fig. 13-14. An intracranial approach for correction of more severe orbital hypertelorism. (Reprinted from Jackson IT, et al: Atlas of Craniomaxillofacial Surgery. St. Louis, CV Mosby, 1982, pp 356, 357. With permission.)

plished when the patient is as young as 2 years of age. Cases requiring less than 1 cm of correction can be treated by medial orbital wall osteotomy (Figure 13-13). An intracranial procedure is best performed for more severe cases (Figure 13-14). The floor of the anterior fossa is exposed by the neurosurgeon using a bifrontal craniotomy. Retraction back to the crista galli necessitates occlusion of the anterior sagittal sinus at the foramen cecum. The cribriform plate is allowed to remain intact by placing the osteotomy lateral to this structure.[122] The entire orbit is freed and moved medially. Olfaction is thus uncompromised. Anterior encephaloceles, if present, are excised and the dura is closed.

Frequent postoperative monitoring of neurologic and ophthalmologic function in an intensive care unit is required. Parents should be forewarned of the inevitable lid edema and fluid accumulation.

COMPLICATIONS

The major complications related to radical craniofacial procedures include injury to the brain, blindness, cerebrospinal fluid leakage, and infection. Whitaker et al.[123] summarized the experience from six craniofacial centers noting a mortality of 1.6 percent, blindness in less than 1 percent, and an overall complication rate of 16.5 percent. Infection occurred in 4.4 percent of cases. Munro[124] reviewed his experience of over 2000 procedures, finding a mortality of 0.64 percent and major but often transient complications in 14.3 percent of cases.

RESULTS

Pyschosocial development and intellectual function are followed using standardized serial testing. Early surgical intervention can enhance the opportunity for normalization of cognitive and psychosocial development.[125-127]

The cosmetic effect is determined from interviews with the patient and family and the comparison of preoperative and postoperative photographs. Cephalometric measurements are compared from standard roentgenograms.[128] Preliminary data support the concept of early definitive surgical treatment.

REFERENCES

1. Virchow R: ü Uber den Cretinismus, namentlich in Franken, und über pathologische Schadelformen. Verh Phys Med Gesamte Wurzburg 2:230, 1851

2. Lane LC: Pioneer craniectomy for relief of mental imbecility due to premature sutural closure and microcephalus. JAMA 18:49, 1892

3. Lannelongue OM: De la craniectomie dans la microcephalie. Compt Rend Acad Sci 110:1382, 1890

4. Hunter AGW, Rudd NL: Craniosynostosis. I. Sagittal synostosis: Its genetics and associated clinical findings in 214 patients who lacked involvement of the coronal suture(s). Teratology 14:185, 1976

5. Hunter AGW, Rudd NL: Craniosynostosis. Teratology 15:301, 1977

6. Pritchard JJ, Scott JH, Girgis FG: The structure and development of cranial and facial sutures. J Anat 90:73, 1956

7. Hinton DR, Becker LE, Muakkassa KF, et al: Lamdoid synostosis. Part I: The lambdoid suture: Normal development and pathology of "synostosis." J Neurosurg 61:333, 1984

8. Moss ML: Functional anatomy of cranial synostosis. Childs Brain 1:22, 1975

9. Moss ML: New studies of cranial growth. Birth Defects 117:283, 1975

10. Persson KM, Roy WA, Persing JA, et al: Craniofacial growth following experimental craniosynostosis and craniectomy in rabbits. J Neurosurg 50:187, 1979

11. Park EA, Powers GF: Acrocephaly and scaphocephaly with symmetrical distributed malformations of the extremities. A study of so-called "acrocephalosyndactylism". Am J Dis Child 20:235, 1920

12. Graham JM, Badura RJ, Smith DW: Coronal craniosynostosis: Fetal head constraint as one possible cause. Pediatrics 65:995, 1980

13. Graham JM, Smith DW: Metopic craniosynostosis as a consequence of fetal head constraint. Pediatrics 65:1000, 1980

14. Higginbottom MC, Jones KL, James HE: Intrauterine constraint and craniosynostosis. Neurosurgery 6:39, 1980

15. Cohen MM: Craniosynostosis and syndromes with synostosis: Incidence, genetics, penetrance, variability, and new syndrome updating. Birth Defects 15:13, 1979

16. Clarren SK: Plagiocephaly and torticollis: Etiology, natural history, and helmet treatment. J Pediatr 98:92, 1981

17. Roy WA, Iorio RJ, Meyer GA: Craniosynostosis in vitamin D-resistant rickets. J Neurosurg 55:265, 1981

18. Renier D, Sainte-Rose C, Marchac D, et al: Intracranial pressure in craniostenosis. J Neurosurg 57:370, 1982

19. Gobiet W, Strahl EW, Bock WJ, et al: Direct measurement of ICP in cases of craniosynostosis as a diagnostic aid for operation, in Beks JWF, Bosch DA, Brock M (eds): Intracranial Pressure III. Berlin, Springer-Verlag, 1976, pp 336–339

20. DiRocco C, Iannelli A, Velardi F: Early diagnosis and surgical indication in craniosynostosis. Childs Brain 6:175, 1980

21. Scarfo GB, Tomaccini D, Gambacorta D, et al: Contribution to the study of craniostenosis: Disturbance of the cerebrospinal fluid flow in oxycephaly. Helv Paediatr Acta 34:235, 1979

22. Cohen MM: Genetic perspectives in craniosynostosis. J Neurosurg 47:886, 1977

23. Anderson FM, Geiger L: Craniosynostosis. A survey of 204 cases. J Neurosurg 22:229, 1965

24. Shillito J, Matson DD: Craniosynostosis: A review of 519 surgical patients. Pediatrics 41:829, 1968

25. Bell HS, Clare FB, Wentworth AF: Familial scaphocephaly. J Neurosurg 18:239, 1962

26. Barritt J, Brooksbank M, Simpson D: Scaphocephaly: Aesthetic and psychosocial considerations. Dev Med Child Neurol 23:183, 1981

27. Matson DD: Craniosynostosis in Neurosurgery of Infancy and Childhood. Springfield, Ill, Charles C Thomas, 1969, pp 122–167

28. Humphreys RP, Gilday DL, Ash JM, et al: Radiopharmaceutical bone scanning in pediatric neurosurgery. Childs Brain 5:249, 1979

29. Robinson WL, Gellad FE, Haney PJ, et al: Craniosynostosis. A clinical, radiological and pathological evaluation of 50 cases, in Humphreys RP (ed): Concepts in Pediatric Neurosurgery 5. Basel, S. Karger, 1985, pp 118–125

30. Carmel PW, Luken MG III, Ascherl GF Jr: Craniosynostosis: Computed tomographic evaluation of skull base and calvarial deformities and associated intracranial changes. Neurosurgery 9:366, 1981

31. Babler WJ, Persing JA, Winn HR: Compensatory growth following premature closure of the coronal suture in rabbits. J Neurosurg 57:535, 1982

32. Epstein N, Epstein F, Newman G: Total vertex craniectomy for the treatment of scaphocephaly. Childs Brain 9:309, 1982

33. Foltz EL, Loeser JD: Craniosynostosis. J Neurosurg 43:48, 1975

34. McLaurin RL, Matson DD: Importance of early surgical treatment of craniosynostosis. Review of 36 cases treated during the first six months of life. Pediatrics 10:637, 1952

35. Persing J, Babler W, Winn HR, et al: Age as a critical factor in the success of surgical correction of craniosynostosis. J Neurosurg 54:601, 1981

36. Park TS, Haworth CS, Jane JA, et al: Modified prone position for cranial remodeling procedures in children with craniofacial dysmorphism: A technical note. Neurosurgery 16:212, 1985

37. Venes JL, Sayers MP: Sagittal synostectomy. Technical note. J Neurosurg 44:390, 1976

38. Albright AL: Operative normalization of skull shape in sagittal synostosis. Neurosurgery 17:329, 1985

39. Jane JA, Edgerton MT, Futrell JW, et al: Immediate correction of sagittal synostosis. J Neurosurg 49:705, 1978

40. Vollmer DG, Jane JA, Park TS, et al: Variants of sagittal synostosis: Strategies for surgical correction. J Neurosurg 61:557, 1984

41. Rougerie J, Derome P, Anquez L: Craniostenoses et dysmorphies craniofaciales. Neurochirurgie 18:429, 1972

42. Marchac D, Renier D (eds): Scaphocephaly in Craniofacial Surgery for Craniosynostosis. Boston, Little, Brown & Co, 1982, pp 88–92

43. James HE: The role of the carbon dioxide laser in craniosynostosis and craniofacial dysostosis, in Raimondi AJ (ed): Concepts in Pediatric Neurosurgery 3. Basel, S. Karger, 1983, pp 202–206

44. O'Brien MS, Kee DB Jr: Surgical management of craniosynostosis. Part II: Surgical technique and results. Contemp Neurosurg 7:1, 1985

45. Olds MV, Storrs B, Walker ML: Surgical treatment of sagittal synostosis. Neurosurgery 18:345, 1986

46. Hoffman HJ, Hendrick EB, Munro IR: Craniosynostosis and Craniofacial surgery in Pediatric Neurosurgery. Surgery of the Developing Nervous System. New York, Grune & Stratton, 1982, pp 130

47. Tulasne JF, Tessier P: Analysis and late treatment of plagiocephaly. Scand J Plast Reconstr Surg 15:257, 1981

48. Hoffman HJ, Mohr G: Lateral canthal advancement of the supraorbital margin. A new corrective technique in the treatment of coronal synostosis. J Neurosurg 45:376, 1976

49. Marsh JL, Schwartz HG: The surgical correction of coronal and metopic craniosynostoses. J Neurosurg 59:245, 1983

50. Jane JA, Park TS, Zide BM, et al: Alternative techniques in the treatment of unilateral coronal synostosis. J Neurosurg 61:550, 1984

51. Matson DD: Neurosurgery of Infancy and Childhood, ed 2. Springfield, Ill, Charles C. Thomas, 1969, pp 122–167

52. Muakkassa KF, Hoffman HJ, Hinton DR, et al: Lambdoid synostosis. Part 2: Review of cases managed at The Hospital for Sick Children, 1972–1982. J Neurosurg 61:340, 1984

53. Gates GF, Dore EK: Detection of craniosynostosis by bone scanning. Radiology 115:665, 1975

54. Rekate HL, Kaufman B: Craniosynostosis of the lambdoidal suture: Surgical modification of migration of the external auditory canals, in Scientific Manuscripts of the 50th Anniversary Meeting of the American Association of Neurological Surgeons, Boston, 1981, Paper 25, pp 50–51

55. David DJ, Poswillo D, Simpson DA: The Craniosynostoses: Causes, Natural History, and Management. Berlin, Springer-Verlag, 1982

56. Marchac D: Radical forehead remodeling for craniostenosis. Plast Reconstr Surg 61:823, 1978

57. Dominguez R, Sang K, Bender T, et al: Uncomplicated trigonocephaly: A radiographic affirmation of conservative therapy. Radiology 140:681, 1981

58. Anderson FM: Treatment of coronal and metopic synostosis: 107 cases. Neurosurgery 8:143, 1981

59. Marchac D, Renier D: Trigonocephaly in Craniofacial Surgery for Craniosynostosis, ed 1. Boston, Little, Brown & Co, 1982, pp 94–105

60. Albin RE, Hendee RW, O'Donnell RS, et al: Trigonocephaly: Refinements in reconstruction. Experience with 33 patients. Plast Reconstr Surg 76:202, 1985

61. Salkind G, Sutton LN, Bruce DA, et al: Management of trigonocephaly. Surg Neurol 25:159, 1986

62. Muller PJ, Hoffman HJ: Cloverleaf skull syndrome. J Neurosurg 43:86, 1975

63. King JEJ: Oxycephaly, a new operation and its results. Arch Neurol Psychiatr 40:1205, 1938

64. Hanson JW, Sayers MP, Knopp LM, et al: Subtotal neonatal calvariectomy for severe craniosynostosis. J Pediatr 91:257, 1977

65. Powiertowski H: Surgery of craniostenosis in advanced cases, in Krayenbuhl H (ed): Advances and Technical Standards in Neurosurgery, vol. 1. Vienna, Springer-Verlag, 1974, pp 93–119

66. Cohen MM Jr: An etiologic and nosologic overview of craniosynostosis syndromes. Birth Defects 11:137, 1975

67. Anderson TH, Pindborg JJ: Et tilfaelde af total "pseudoanodonti"; forbingelse me Kraniedeformiter draergvaekst og e Ktodermal dysplasi. Odont T 55:472, 1947

68. Antley R, Bixler D: A-Trapezoidocephaly, midfacial hypoplasia and cartilage abnormalities with multiple synostoses and skeletal fractures. Birth Defects 11:397, 1975

69. Armendares S, Antillon F, Del Castillo V, et al: A newly recognized inherited syndrome of dwarfism, craniosynostosis, retinitis pigmentosa, and multiple congenital malformations. J Pediatr 85:872, 1974

70. Baller F: Radiusaplasie und Inzucht. Z Menschl Vererb Konstit-Lehre 29:782, 1950

71. Bell HS, Clare FB, Wentworth AF: Familial scaphocephaly. Case reports and technical notes. J Neurosurg 18:239, 1961

72. Berant M, Berant N: Radioulnar synostosis and craniosynostosis in one family. J Pediatr 83:88, 1973

73. Blank CE: Apert's syndrome (a type of acrocephalosyndactyly): Observations on a British series of thirty-nine cases. Hum Genet 24:151, 1960

74. Brown A, Harper RK: Craniofacial dysostosis: The significance of ocular hypertelorism. J Med 59:171, 1946

75. Christian JC, Andrews PA, Conneally PM, et al: The adducted thumbs syndrome. An autosomal recessive disease with arthrogryposis, dysmyelination, craniostenosis, and cleft palate. Clin Genet 2:95, 1971

76. Dodge HW, Wood MW, Kennedy RJL: Craniofacial dysostosis: Crouzon's disease. Pediatrics 23:98, 1959

77. Elejalde BR, Giraldo C, Jimenez R, et al: Acrocephalopolydactylous dysplasia. Birth Defects 13:53, 1977

78. Gerold M: Frakturheilung bei einen seltenen Fall kongenitaler Anomalie der oberen Gliedmassen. Zentralbl Chir 84:831, 1959

79. Gorlin RJ, Chaudhry AP, Moss ML: Craniofacial dysostosis patent ductus arteriosus, hypertrichosis, hypoplasia of labia majora, dental and eye anomalies. J Pediatr 56:778, 1960

80. Hall BD, Smith DW, Shiller JG: Kleeblatsch ä del (cloverleaf) syndrome: Severe form of Crouzon's disease? J Pediatr 80:526, 1972

81. Herrmann J, Opitz JM: An unusual form of acrocephalosyndactyly. Birth Defects 5:39, 1969

82. Herrmann J, Pallister PD, Opitz JM: Craniosynostosis and craniosynostosis syndromes. Rocky Mt Med J 66:45, 1969

83. Hootnick D, Holmes LB: Familial polysyndactyly and craniofacial anomalies. Clin Genet 3:128, 1972

84. Jabbour JT, Taybi H: Craniotelencephalic dysplasia. Am J Dis Child 108:627, 1964

85. Kushner J, Alexander E Jr, Davis CH, et al: Crouzon's disease (craniofacial dysostosis). Modern diagnosis and treatment. J Neurosurg 37:434, 1972

86. Levin LS, Perrin JCS, Ose L, et al: A heritable syndrome of craniosynostosis, short thin hair, dental abnormalities, and short limbs: Cranioectodermal dysplasia. J Pediatr 90:55, 1977

87. Lowry RB: Congenital absence of the fibula and craniosynostosis in sibs. J Med Genet 9:227, 1972

88. Marshall RE, Smith DW: Frontodigital syndrome: A dominantly inherited disorder with normal intelligence. J Pediatr 77:129, 1970

89. Martsolf JT, Cracco JB, Carpenter GG, et al: Pfeiffer syndrome. Am J Dis Child 121:257, 1971

90. McPherson E, Hall JG, Hickman R: Chromosome 7 short arm deletion and craniosynostosis. A 7p) syndrome. Hum Genet 35:117, 1976

91. Muller PJ, Hoffman HJ: Cloverleaf skull syndrome. J Neurosurg 43:86, 1975

92. Murphy JW: Familial scaphocephaly in father and son. US Armed Forces Med J 4:1496, 1953

93. Neuhauser G, Kaveggia EG, Opitz JM: Studies of malformation syndromes of man. XXXIX: A craniosynostosis-craniofacial dysostosis syndrome with mental retardation and other malformations: "Craniofacial dyssynostosis." Eur J Pediatr 123:15, 1976

94. Opitz JM, Kaveggia EG: Studies of malformation syndromes of man. 33: The FG syndrome. An X-linked recessive syndrome of multiple congenital anomalies and mental retardation. Z Kinderheilkd 117:1, 1974

95. Opitz JM, Patau K: A partial trisomy 5p syndrome. Birth Defects 11:191, 1975

96. Orbeli DJ, Lurie IW, Goroshenko JL: The syndrome associated with the partial D-monosomy. Case report and review. Humangenetik 13:296, 1971

97. Pantke OA, Cohen MM Jr, Witkop LJ, et al: The Saethre-Chotzen syndrome. Birth Defects 11:190, 1975

98. Partington MW, Gonzales-Crussi F, Khakee SG, et al: Cloverleaf skull and thanatophoric dwarfism. Report of four cases, two in the same sibship. Arch Dis Child 46:656, 1971

99. Sakati N, Nyhan WL, Tisdale WK: A new syndrome with acrocephalopolysyndactyly, cardiac disease, and distinctive defects of the ear, skin and lower limbs. J Pediatr 79:104, 1971

100. Saldino RM, Steinbach HL, Epstein CJ: Familial acrocephalosyndactyly (Pfeiffer syndrome). AJR 116:609, 1972 101. Say B, Meyer J: Familial trigonocephaly associated with short stature and developmental delay. Am J Dis Child 135:711, 1981

102. Schuch A, Pesch HJ: Beitrag rum Kleeblattsch ä del-Syndrome. Z Kinderheilkd 109:187, 1971

103. Simmons DR, Peyton WT: Premature closure of the cranial sutures. J Pediatr 31:528, 1947

104. Summitt RL: Recessive acrocephalosyndactyly with normal intelligence. Birth Defects 5:35, 1969

105. Temtamy SA: Carpenter's syndrome: Acrocephalopolysyndactyly. An autosomal recessive syndrome. J Pediatr 69:111, 1966

106. Temtamy S, McKusick VA: Synopsis of hand malformations with particular emphasis on genetic factors. Birth Defects 5:125, 1969

107. Terrafranca R, Zellis A: Congenital hereditary cranium bifidum occultum frontalis. Radiology 61:60, 1953

108. Ventruto V, DiGirolamo R, Festa B, et al: Familial study of inherited syndrome with multiple congenital deformities: Symphalangism, carpal and tarsal fusion, brachydactyly, craniosynostosis, strabismus, hip osteochondritis. J Med Genet 13:394, 1976

109. Waardenburg PJ: Eine merkwurdige Kombination van angeborenen Missbildungen: Doppelseitiger Hydrophthalamus verbunden mit Akrokephalosyndaktylie, Herzfehler, Pseudohermaphroditismus und anderen abweichungen. Klin Monatsbl Augenheilkd 92:29, 1934

110. Shaw EB, Steinbach HL: Aminopterin-induced fetal malformation. Survival of an infant after attempted abortion. Am J Dis Child 115:477, 1968

111. DeMyer W: The median cleft face syndrome. Neurology 17:961, 1967

112. Dodge H, Love J, Kernohan J: Intranasal encephalomeningoceles associated with cranium bifidum. Arch Surg 79:75, 1959

113. Walker EA, Resler DR: Nasal glioma. Laryngoscope 73:93, 1963

114. Munro IR: Orbito-cranio-facial surgery: The team approach. Plast Reconstr Surg 55:170, 1975

115. Hemmy DC, David DJ, Herman GT, et al: Three-dimensional reconstruction of craniofacial deformity using computed tomography. Neurosurgery 13:534, 1983

116. Marsh JL, Vannier MW: The "third" dimension in craniofacial surgery. Plast Reconstr Surg 71:759, 1983

117. Persing JA, Babler WJ, Persson M, et al: The effect of the timing of surgery in experimental craniosynostosis. Presented at the meeting of the American Association of Neurological Surgeons, 1980, pp 63–65

118. Persson KM, Roy WA, Persing JA, et al: Craniofacial growth following experimental craniosynostosis and craniectomy in rabbits. J Neurosurg 50:187, 1979

119. Seeger JF, Gabrielsen TO: Premature closure of the frontosphenoidal suture in synostosis of the coronal suture. Radiology 101:631, 1971

120. Menezes AH: Midface recession and exorbitism in anterior cranial base synostosis: Observations and surgical results in craniofacial dysmorphism in infancy. Presented at the meeting of the American Association Neurological Surgeons, Boston, 1981, pp 48–49

121. Converse JM, Ransohoff J, Mathews ES, et al: Ocular hypertelorism and pseudohypertelorism. Advances in surgical treatment. Plast Reconstr Surg 45:1, 1970

122. Epstein F, Ransohoff J, Wood-Smith D, et al: Correction of ocular hypertelorism. Childs Brain 1:228, 1975

123. Whitaker LA, Munro IR, Salyer KE, et al: Combined report of problems and complications in 793 craniofacial operations. Plast Reconstr Surg 64:198, 1979

124. Munro IR, Sabatier RE: An analysis of 12 years of craniomaxillofacial surgery in Toronto. Plast Reconstr Surg 76:29, 1985

125. Edgerton MT, Jane JA, Berry FA, et al: New surgical concepts resulting from cranio-orbital-facial surgery. Ann Surg 182:228, 1975

126. Murray JE, Swanson LT, Strand RD, et al: Evaluation of craniofacial surgery in the treatment of facial deformities. Am Surg 182:240, 1975

127. Powazek M, Billmeier GJ Jr: Assessment of intellectual development after surgery for craniofacial dysostosis. Am J Dis Child 133:151, 1979

128. Firmin F, Coccardo PJ, Converse JM: Cephalometric analysis in diagnosis and treatment planning of craniofacial dysostoses. Plast Reconstr Surg 54:300, 1974

CHAPTER 14
Surgical Management of Hydrocephalus

Mel H. Epstein

HYDROCEPHALUS is a term used to describe an excessive accumulation of cerebrospinal fluid (CSF) in the intracranial space. The term frequently is used by clinicians to characterize the state of ventricles enlarged under pressure. In point of fact, fluid accumulations resulting from porencephalic cysts, low-pressure ventricular dilatation, cerebral agenesis, and cerebral atrophy should be included under the term hydrocephalus. It is of considerable importance to differentiate between these conditions since the indications for surgical shunting vary.

PATHOPHYSIOLOGY

Hippocrates (460–377 BC)[1] was the first to recognize that water accumulating in the head could result in its abnormal enlargement. It was Vesalius, however, who first described internal hydrocephalus in a child. Internal hydrocephalus can result from either increased fluid production or decreased fluid absorption. Except for cases of choroid plexus adenoma, increased fluid production is not a documented cause of hydrocephalus. Most cases of internal hydrocephalus result from impeded fluid absorption, either at the level of the arachnoid villi, the basal cisterns, or the ventricles. Etiologic conditions take many forms. They include aqueductal stenosis; aqueductal atresia; Dandy-Walker syndrome;[2] Arnold-Chiari malformation;[3,4] arachnoidal cysts; porencephalic cysts; tumors (especially those located in the region of the pineal gland and the foramen of Monroe); viral, bacterial, yeast, or fungal infections; vascular malformations; and trauma.

INDICATIONS FOR SURGERY

The indications for surgical shunting are such that a careful analysis of each case on an individualized basis is required. Since a shunt may represent a lifelong commitment for the patient, the initial placement should not be taken lightly. In children, indications such as ventricles that appear enlarged on CT scans in the presence of a head that is crossing percentile growth lines constitute proper grounds for surgical shunting. If a child has enlarged ventricles, a stable head circumference, and is doing well clinically, however, continued observation may be the better part of valor. The use of ultrasound scanning offers a simple way to follow children with dilated ventricles.

Increased intracranial pressure occasionally forces the surgeon to perform a shunt before the usual criteria are met. Any patient with dilated ventricles, increased intracranial pressure, and alterations of vital signs, cranial nerve function, or state of consciousness should be treated promptly with a shunt. Children in particular can unexpectedly decompensate when intracranial pressure rises too high, usually resulting in respiratory arrest.

Porencephalic cysts will occasionally require shunting. This usually is indicated when there is a progressive neurologic deficit, seizures that elude control by medication, and when the skull progressively is being deformed by the enlarging cyst.

A complete discussion of low-pressure hydrocephalus is beyond the scope of this chapter. The indications for shunting are not clear-cut, and the complication rate in these patients can be high. Subdural hemorrhages and infections in particular can be most troublesome. Suffice it to say that a patient with the triad of gait disturbance, incontinence, and mental abberations of recent onset who has hydrocephalus with low pressure is a candidate for a shunt. If a patient has little visible cortical atrophy on CT scans together with ventricular stasis on cisternal isotope scans, the surgeon has sufficient grounds for offering a surgical shunt as treatment.

CLINICAL FINDINGS

In young children the hallmark of hydrocephalus is an enlarging head. In particular, the enlargement of the head continues beyond the normal growth percentiles.[5] Although hydrocephalus in utero now can be diagnosed with ultrasound scanning, it fortunately is not common. Most patients with hydrocephalus in utero are mentally retarded even with prompt surgical therapy. On the other hand, most cases of hydrocephalus develop insidiously some time after delivery. If detected early and treated properly with surgical shunting, normal mental development is the rule. It must be emphasized that a single measurement of head size is not as useful as repeated measurements, which indicate the growth rate of the head.

Transillumination with a halogen light should be done routinely in the examination of infants. Hydrocephalus causes the cranium to enlarge at a rate disproportionate to that of the face. The fontanelle can become full and dilated veins can be seen on a thin scalp. Macewen's sign is a tympanitic sound obtained on percussing the vault of the skull. Although it is extremely rare to see papilledema in young infants, sixth nerve

OPERATIVE NEUROSURGICAL TECHNIQUES
ISBN 0-8089-1862-1

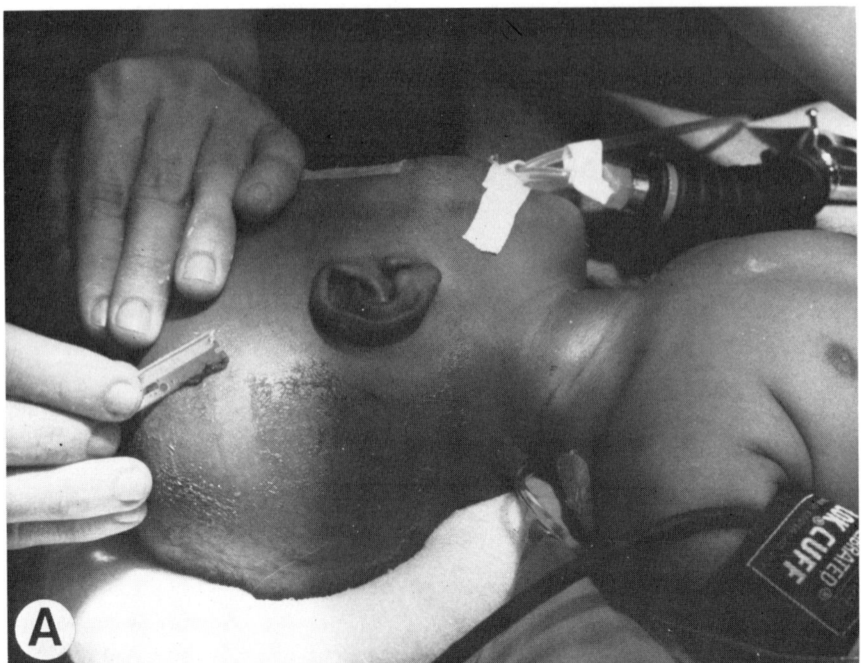

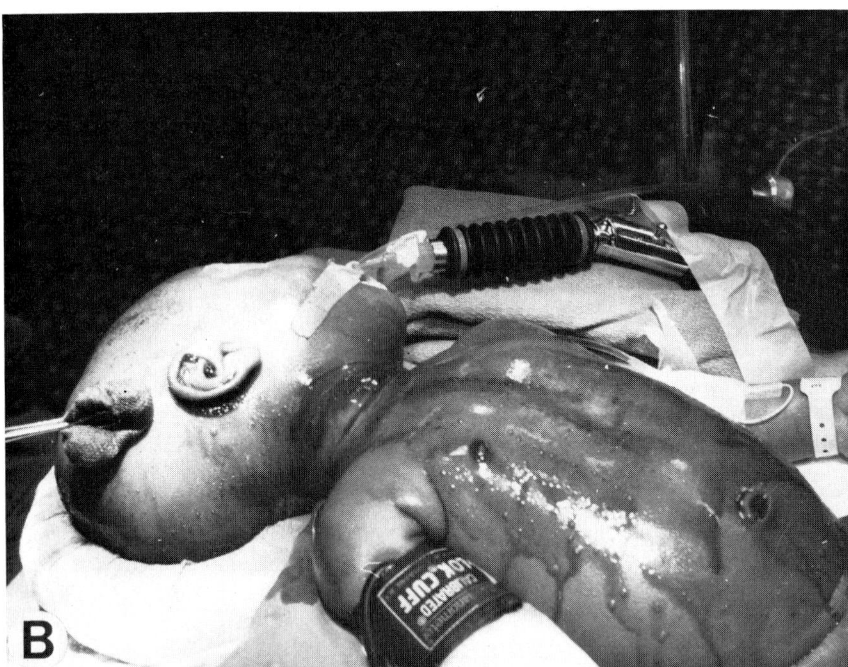

Fig. 14-1. (A) The hair should never be clipped or shaved until immediately before the operation. (B) The preparation of the surgical field is an important aspect of a shunt operation.

palsies are common. The sixth nerve is easily stretched as the progressing hydrocephalus causes the brainstem to descend down the clivus. Paralysis of upward gaze results in the "setting-sun sign," where the sclera is visible above the cornea. Hydrocephalus in infancy, if untreated, results in irritability, decreased appetite with vomiting, poor head control, retarded development, hyperactive deep tendon reflexes, periodic respirations, apneic spells, and, finally, respiratory arrest. In older children the rigid skull results in papilledema, headaches, nausea and vomiting, and gait disturbances. If, however, the ventricular dilatation occurs slowly, the patient can be symptom-free.[6]

OPERATIVE TREATMENT

Many surgical techniques have been tried in attempts to control progressive hydrocephalus. Lespinasse, Hildebrand, and Scarff[7] described attempts at coagulating or removing the choroid plexus. Complete removal of the plexus in the lateral, third, and fourth ventricles is difficult to achieve. In addition, it is now known that a considerable amount of fluid is produced at extrachoroidal sites. Dandy, Stookey, and Scarff described ventriculostomy of the third ventricle and incision of the lamina terminalis.[8] This has not become a popular procedure since shunting still is frequently required.

Shunting CSF via tubes from the ventricles to another part of the body has preoccupied neurosurgeons for a good part of this century. Attempts have been made to divert fluid to the distal ureter,[9,10] the fallopian tube, the pleural cavity,[11,12] the gallbladder and stomach,[13,14,15] the sagittal sinus, the cisterna magna, the right atrium,[16] and the peritoneal cavity.[17,18,19] Only the latter two sites have withstood the test of time. Since the development of the slit-valve catheter, the ventricular peritoneal (VP) shunt has become the procedure of choice for children. The VP shunt will lengthen with the growth of the child and has fewer long-term sequelae. The slit valve serves to control the opening pressure of the shunt and diminishes the probability that the tube will be blocked by omentum or scar tissue. Although the atrial shunt may still be used on special occasions (i.e., where the peritoneal cavity is unavailable, in children who have completed most of their growth, or where siphoning is a dangerous problem), 95 percent of the shunts carried out in our clinic are VP shunts. Lumbar peritoneal shunts have a place when the ventricles are small, but the laminectomy can lead to scoliosis in children. Recent work has suggested that lumboperitoneal shunts can be placed percutaneously.[20,21] The long-term complication rate, however, has not been demonstrated in the growing child. In addition, the small spine in neonates and infants makes this an impractical approach in young children. Because of the importance of peritoneal shunting, the remainder of this discussion will concern the VP shunt, including the operative technique and postoperative management.

HARDWARE

It should be emphasized at the outset that this discussion is not meant to endorse any manufacturer's product. There is a broad spectrum of implantable shunts on the market and most of them are quite good. It is more important that the surgeon become familiar with using one system than with using whatever is available at the time. This is one operation where repetition and good surgical technique lead to fewer complications.[22] Although we will describe the operation using the hardware we use in our medical center, it is to serve only as a model that demonstrates the general principles that apply to the insertion of most shunt products.

PREOPERATIVE PREPARATION

Unless the operation is an emergency, the preparation of the patient begins on the night before surgery. At least two sequential scrubs of the abdomen and scalp are performed using a slow-release, iodine-soap solution. The hair is not shaved until just before surgery. These preparations are important since the majority of shunt infections are caused by *Staphylococcus epidermidis,* which is commonly found on the skin.

THE OPERATION

Positioning the patient for a shunt operation is an important step. Because many of the patients undergoing this surgery have large heads, passing the peritoneal tubing through the neck can be quite awkward. This problem is mitigated by extending the neck. This is achieved by building up the sheets under the neck with linen rolls or by dropping the headpiece of the table. Ideally, the line from the cranial incision to the abdominal incision should be straight.

The skin is meticulously prepared with a slow-release iodine solution (Figure 14-1). A contact plastic drape is applied after the solution is thoroughly dry (Figure 14-2). This is to help decrease the loss of body heat in young babies and to diminish the possibility of skin contamination. Before the skin incision is made, the shunt is checked out carefully and any connections that are required are performed. If it is necessary to tie ligatures around any of the tubes, it is done at this time. Care must be taken not to make them too tight or the silicone rubber tubing

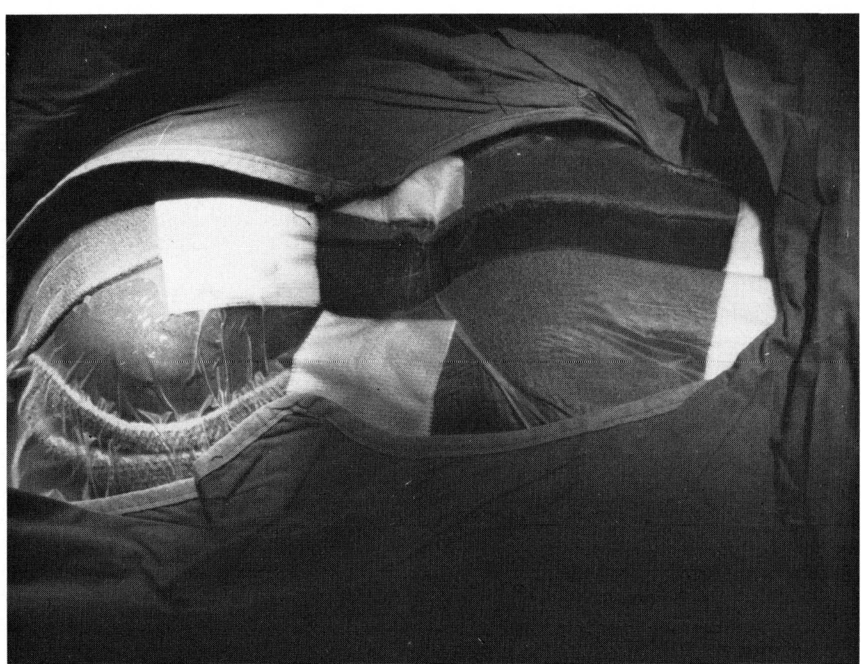

Fig. 14-2. A plastic drape not only decreases skin contact, but also helps to maintain the body temperature of small children.

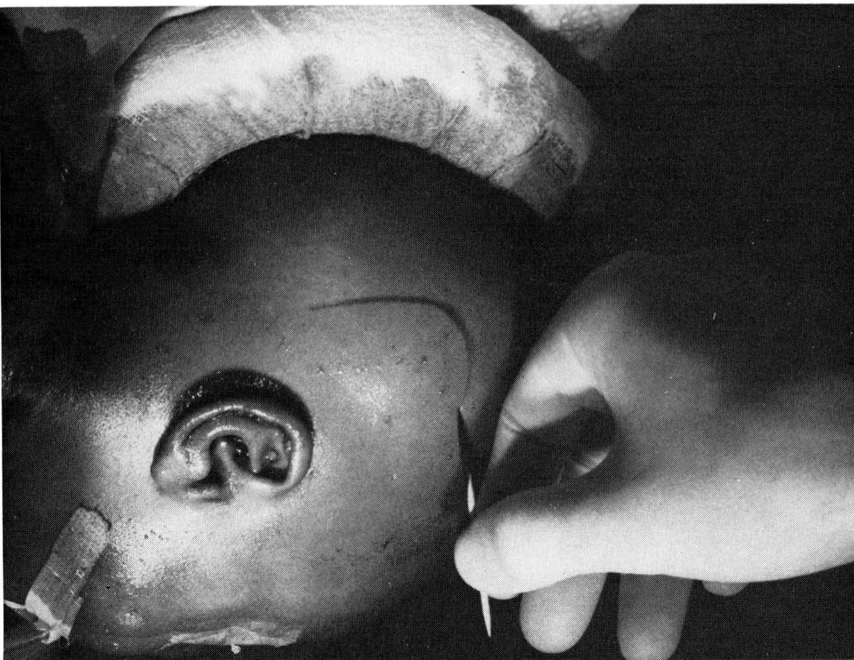

Fig. 14-3. A parietotemporal incision is outlined.

can be lacerated; if the knots are too loose, the tubing can slip off the connectors. The function of the shunt also is checked to make certain the opening pressure of the slit valve is per the manufacturer's specifications.

INCISION

An incision is made in the parietotemporal region (Figure 14-3). It is basically a half-moon flap with a broad base. If the patient is young and has a thin scalp, the incision must have a broader base to ensure a good blood supply. In premature infants the scalp will slough over the flushing device unless the shunt has a very low profile. In these individuals it is frequently necessary to eliminate the flushing device completely. If the child has severe hydrocephalus and has poor head movement, the shunt should be placed frontally (Figure 14-4). Babies with poor head control will frequently lie on the flushing device for prolonged periods of time and develop a decubitus ulcer. A decubitus ulcer invariably results in an infected shunt.

In a parietotemporal flap the burr hole is located one half the distance from the internal auditory meatus to the vertex. In the second dimension it is located one third the distance from

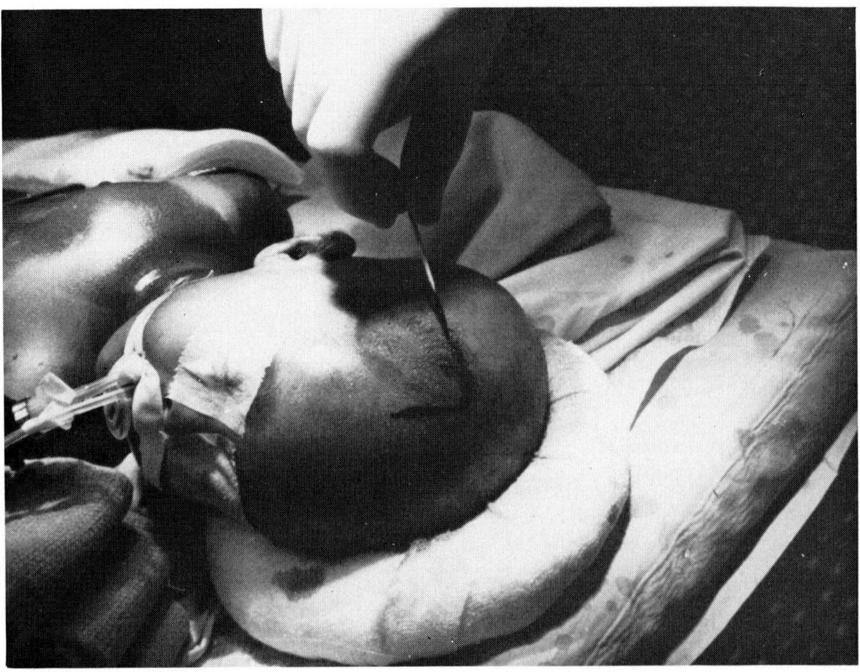

Fig. 14-4. A shunt occasionally must placed in a frontal location in cases of severe hydrocephalus, where decubitus ulceration over the shunt tubing and the flushing device might be a problem.

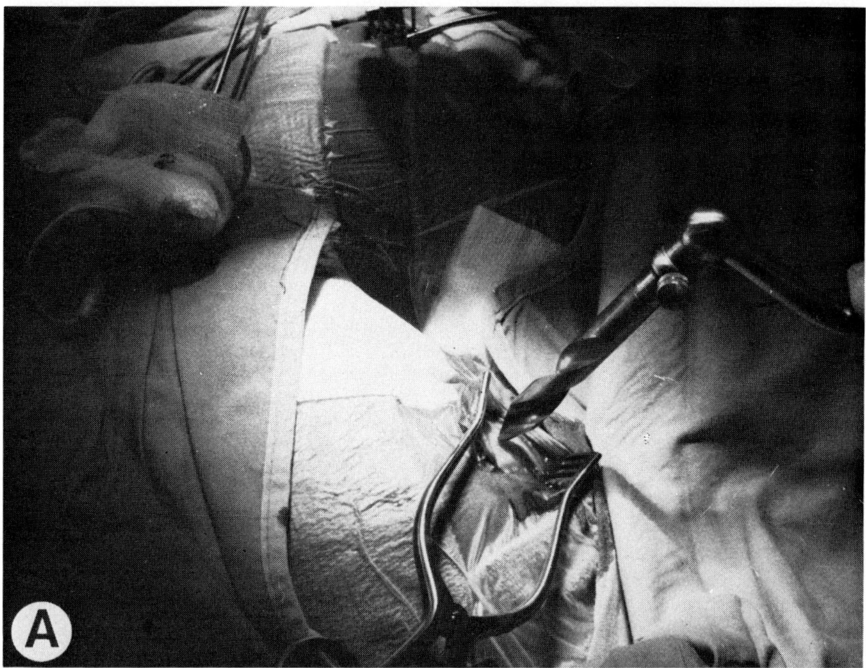

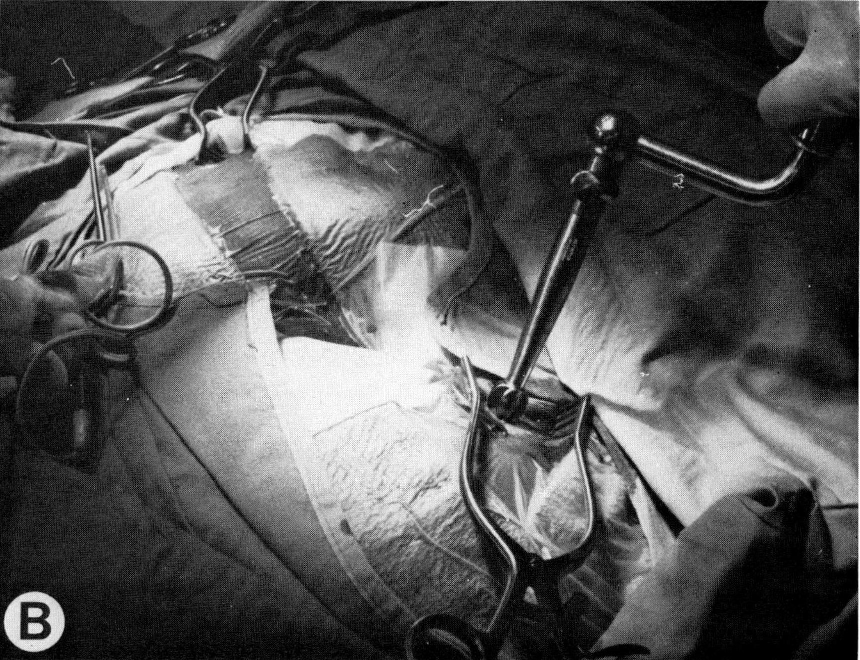

Fig. 14-5. (A) The burr hole for the flushing device must be made carefully since the bit will not lock in the normal fashion within the skull of young children. (B) It is important that the burr hole be large enough to accommodate the flushing device if it is the type that is seated in the burr hole. This lowers the profile and decreases the risk of decubitus ulcer.

the internal auditory meatus to the inion. In a frontal flap the burr hole is located just in front of the coronal suture in line with the pupils. Care must be taken to make the burr hole large enough to accommodate the shunt device (Figure 14-5). If the shunt sits too high on the skull, necrosis of the scalp can occur.

The abdominal incision generally is made two to three fingerbreadths below the costal margin. The incision usually is parallel to the costal margin and 3 to 4 cm in length. With standard muscle-splitting techniques, the peritoneum is identified and carefully clamped. It then is tented up so that a 3- to 4–mm incision can be made. It is essential to identify the bowel,

the liver, and the omentum at this time. There frequently is a small amount of free fluid in the peritoneal cavity, which easily can be identified. Occasionally it appears that the peritoneum has been incised when the preperitoneal space has been entered. Shunt catheters placed in this space will not work properly. After the peritoneum is properly identified, a purse-string suture is placed carefully around the peritoneal opening. The bowel in infants has a thin wall and care should be taken not to puncture or lacerate it. The previously tested distal peritoneal catheter then is inserted into the peritoneal cavity. We generally insert at least 25 cm of tubing to allow for growth.

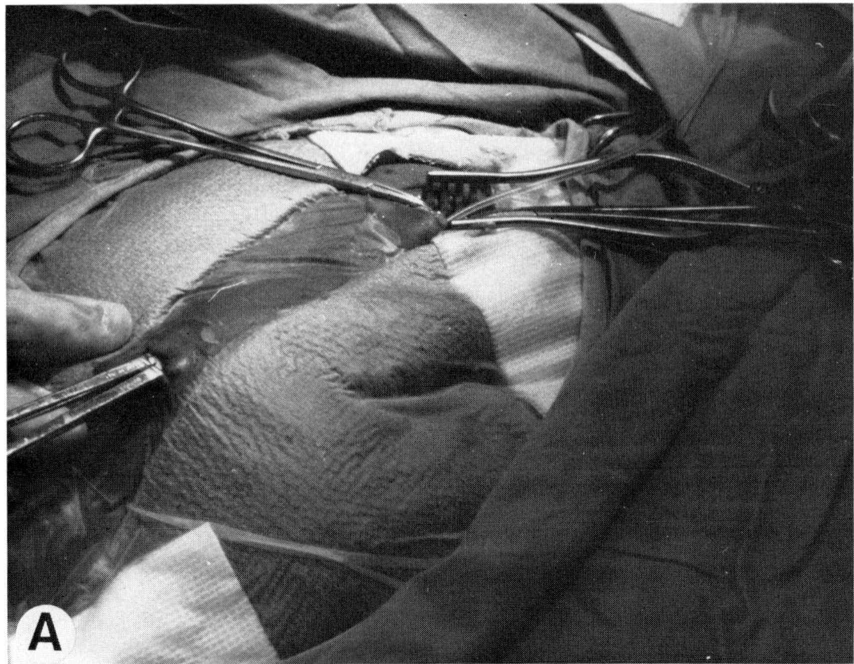

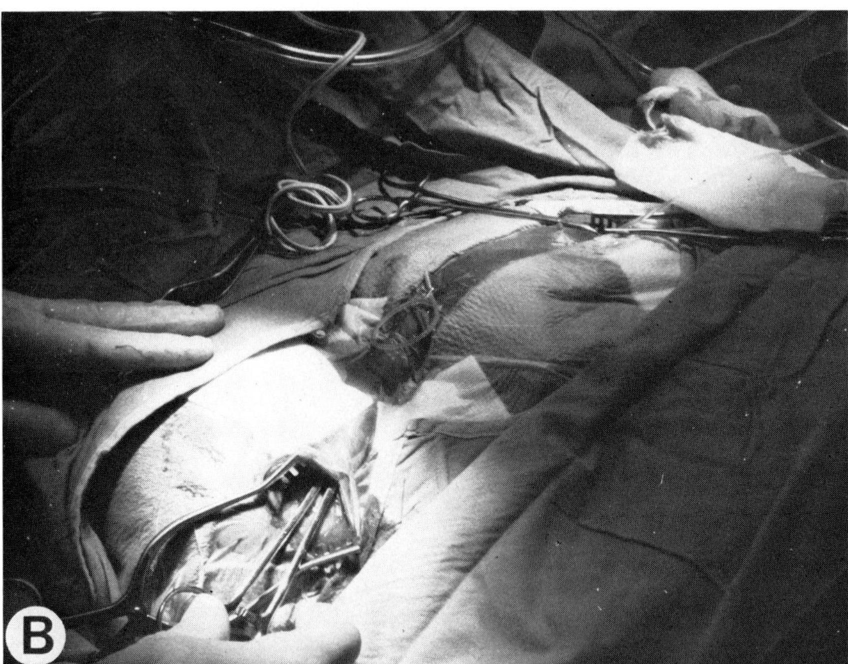

Fig. 14-6.   (A,B) The catheter is inserted into the peritoneum and then passed from the peritoneal incision up to the subclavicular stab wound.

The purse string then is snugged down to prevent bowel herniation but to allow the catheter to slide out of the abdominal cavity with growth. It is a good idea at this point to test the opening pressure of the distal tube by observing the descent of a column of water from the proximal end of the tube. If the water column stops above 20 cm, the shunt will not function properly.

The proximal end of the peritoneal catheter now must be passed under the skin to the cranial incision. In neonates it is usually possible to complete this pass without additional incisions. In most patients, however, an additional stab wound is necessary just below the clavicle (Figure 14-6). Through this chest incision a vaginal-packing forceps or similar passing instrument is inserted subcutaneously to the abdominal incision. The proximal peritoneal catheter is secured to the end of the instrument and passed to the stab wound in the chest. The passing instrument then is inserted from the cranial incision to the stab wound. The end of the catheter then is drawn up to the cranial incision.

INSERTION OF THE VENTRICULAR END

The dura over the exposed burr hole is coagulated with bipolar cautery (Figure 14-7). A small cruciate incision is made and the ventricle is tapped with a brain needle that is at least 14 gauge. If the parietotemporal approach is used, a burr hole is

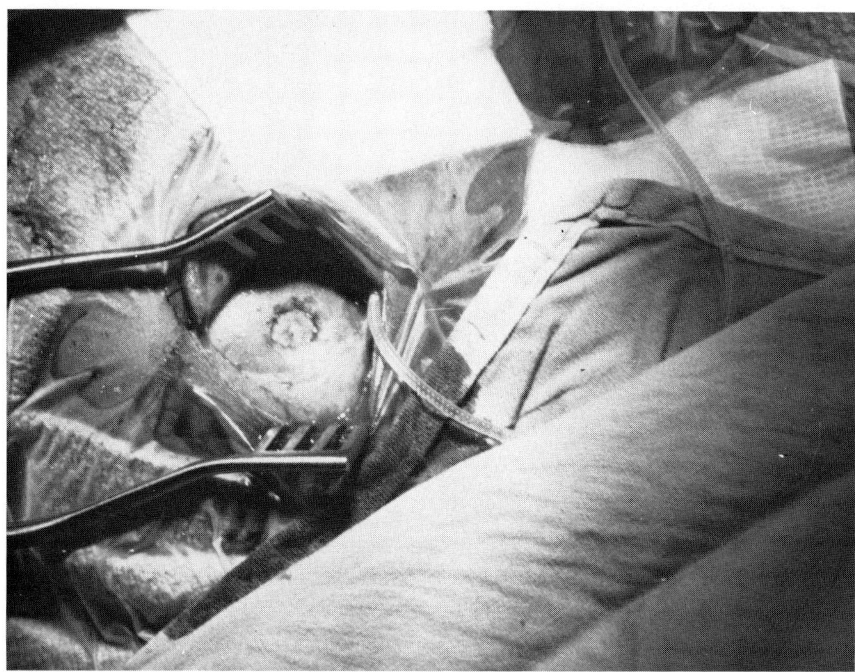

Fig. 14-7. The dura is coagulated with bipolar cautery and opened in a stellate fashion.

made at Keene's point. Because the size of the skull varies from person to person, it is best to approximate Keene's point based on a percentage of distances. To arrive at Keene's point, measure the distance between the external auditory meatus and the vertex of the skull in the lateral plane. Then measure 25 percent of that distance and mark it off superior to the external auditory meatus. From that point, measure the total distance in the lateral projection of the skull to the posterior aspect of the occiput along a line at right angles to the vertical line previously marked. From the vertical line, measure off two thirds of the total horizontal distance. In most patients, Keene's point will be 2.5 to 3 cm above the pinna and 2.5 to 3 cm directly posterior

from the external auditory canal. The needle is introduced into the ventricle through the burr hole at Keene's point angled 30 degrees forward and 10 degrees superiorly to encourage the catheter to enter the body of the lateral ventricle and work its way toward the frontal horn as opposed to entering the temporal horn (Figure 14-8). If the ventricle is approached from a frontal burr hole, this burr hole is made 1 cm anterior to the coronal suture and 2 to 3 cm from the midline, usually over the nondominant hemisphere. Using a CT scan, a premeasured catheter is introduced in a plane parallel to the falx cerebri and at a right angle to the plane bisecting the inferior orbits with the inion. When the ependymal wall is perforated, the needle will

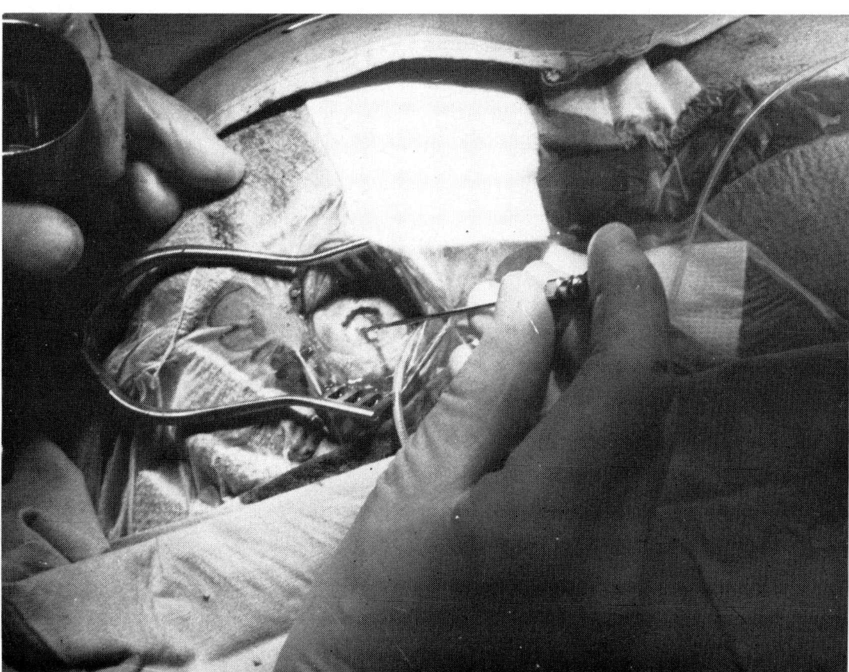

Fig. 14-8. The needle is passed carefully using a CT scan as a guide for placement in the ventricle.

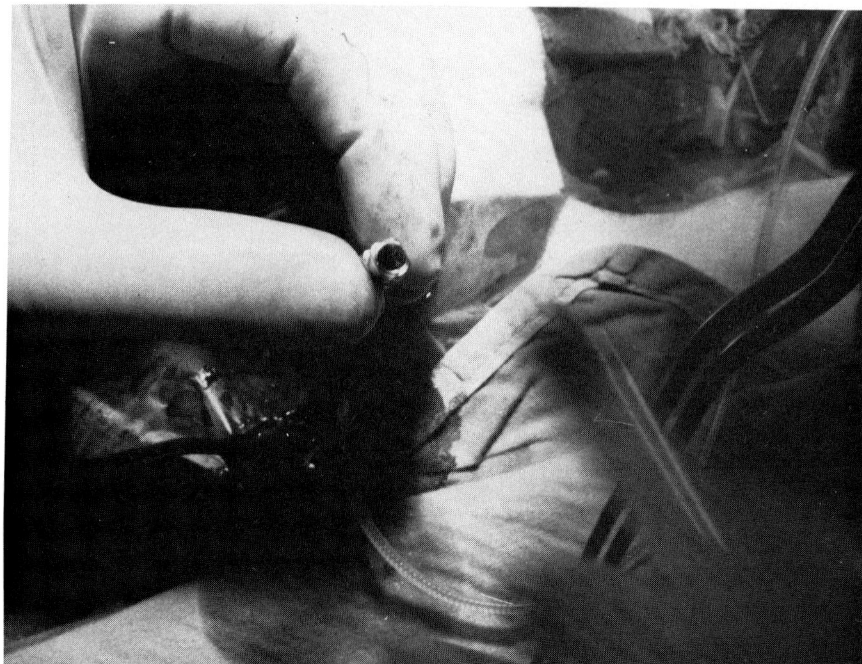

Fig. 14-9.   After the ventricle is entered, a small amount of fluid is allowed to escape from the needle to confirm that the needle is in the proper position.

give slightly. A small amount of ventricular fluid is allowed to escape by briefly withdrawing the stylet (Figure 14-9). After it has been confirmed that the needle is in the ventricle, it is withdrawn. The ventricular catheter connected to the flushing device is inserted into the needle track with a forceps until the flushing device is seated in the burr hole and CSF is seen flowing out of the outflow tube (Figure 14-10). The length of the ventricular catheter is determined by the size of the head and the amount of hydrocephalus. Generally from 5 to 9 cm will be adequate for most patients. The goal in the placement of a ventricular shunt is to have the tip of the catheter just anterior to the foramen of Monroe, thereby avoiding the choroid plexus.

After the catheter is properly placed, all connections are made between the flushing device and the peritoneal catheter. The tubing is held in place with a 0 silk tie. The extra tubing now is pulled down to the abdominal incision and slipped into the peritoneal opening. It is important to check that the outflow catheter from the flushing device has not kinked or twisted after this maneuver.

SKIN CLOSURE

Careful closure of the skin is important. It is our practice to place a subcutaneous suture line using slowly absorbable material (Figure 14-11). This allows the skin sutures to be removed earlier and gives the wound added strength if fluid collects under it postoperatively. The absorbable suture material also makes the long-term complication of suture abscess less likely. Because of the presence of a foreign body, suture abscess can have serious consequences.

POSTOPERATIVE CARE

The most common complication of shunt operations is infection. Even with the most meticulous care infection will occur between 3 and 20 percent of the time. There is some evidence that experience in doing repeated shunt operations leads to a reduction in the infection rate.[22] The use of prophylactic antibiotics has been demonstrated to greatly diminish surgically induced shunt infections.[23] A typical protocol involves giving the patient 40 mg/kg cephalothin intravenously 1 hour before surgery. A bath of cephalothin consisting of 500 mg in 100 ml of saline is used to soak all shunting devices. Cephalothin is administered to the patient intravenously, 160 mg/kg/day up to 2 g/day for a total of 3 days postoperatively. A protocol such as this has been shown to diminish the incidence of infection several hundred percent and appears to be a requirement for implantation of silicone rubber shunting devices. Our criteria for infection require satisfying one of the following three points:

1. Recovery of a bacterial isolate from two or more cultures of blood, CSF, shunt tubing, the flushing device, or a combination of two of these.
2. Recovery of a bacterial isolate from one of the above in addition to a clinically evident wound infection.
3. The presence of three of the following conditions: (a) bacteria on Gram's stain of CSF; (b) greater than 1000 WBC/cm^2 of CSF; (c) a temperature greater than 39°C; or (d) deteriorating consciousness.

If at any time in the postoperative period there is any evidence of infection, a shunt tap is indicated. This is frequently the only way to detect infection before gross ventriculitis occurs.

Shunt obstruction also is a common problem postoperatively. It usually is manifested by continued head growth, recurrence of symptoms, or fluid tracking down the wound. Sometimes shunt pumping can improve the situation, but most of the time a revision is necessary. Occasionally in small babies with large heads the peritoneum will not handle the fluid load. Time usually will resolve the problem as the abdominal distension abates.

Hemorrhage can occur in the ventricles, intracerebrally, or in the subdural space. Ventricular hemorrhage usually is a

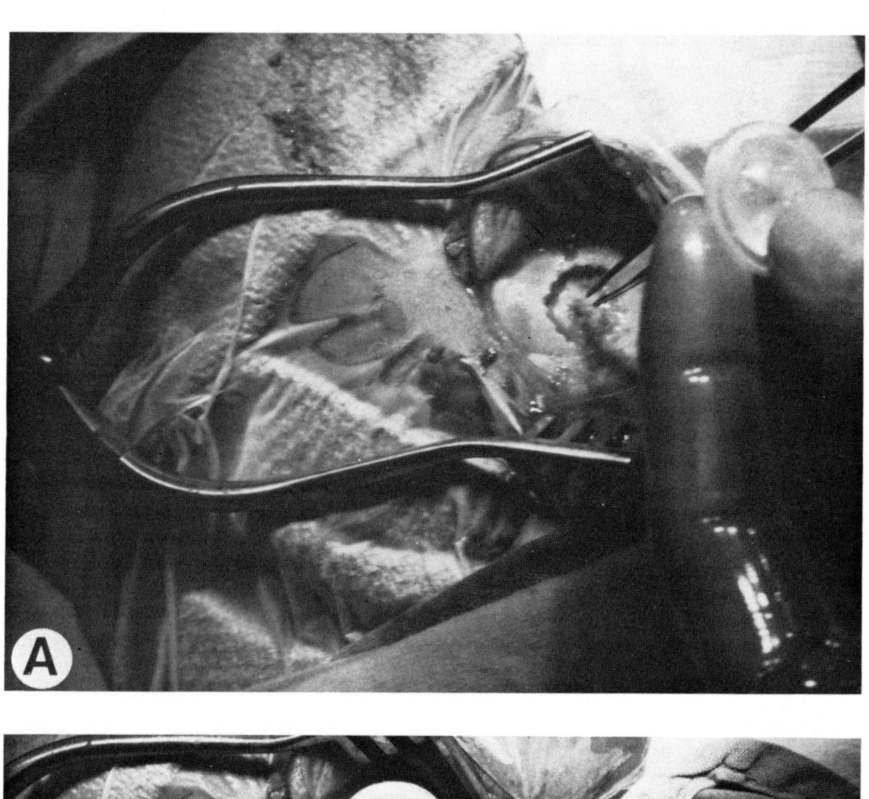

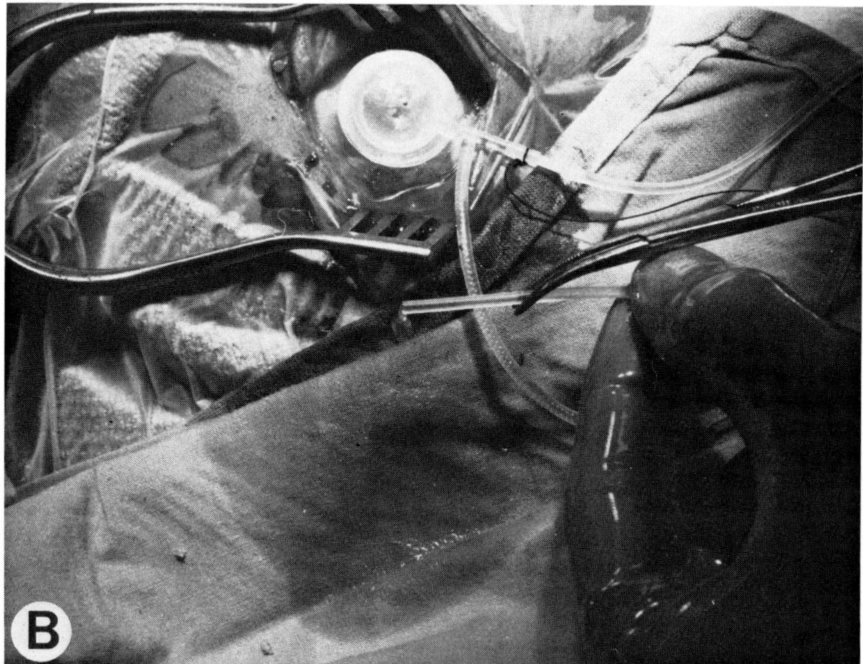

Fig. 14-10. (A) Immediately after the needle is withdrawn, the shunt tube is inserted along the needle track into the ventricular system. (B) If the needle enters the ventricular system properly, a free flow of fluid will be seen from the distal outflow catheter of the shunt device.

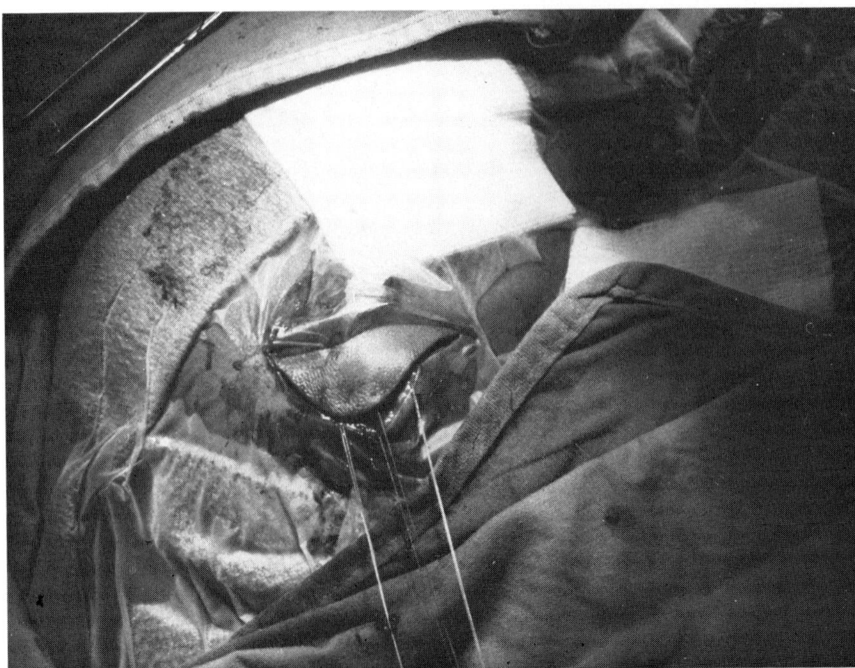

Fig. 14-11. Subcutaneous sutures are desirable in case there is a fluid leak around a malfunctioning catheter. They also allow earlier removal of the skin sutures. Absorbable sutures reduce the risk of suture rejection and suture abscess.

result of the choroid being caught in the ventricular catheter when it is removed for a revision. If a catheter is difficult to remove, it is sometimes wiser to abandon it and insert a new one. Subdural hemorrhage is not common in young children. It is most likely to occur in patients with fused sutures and large heads in the presence of significant hydrocephalus. If the patient is kept in bed postoperatively, the siphoning effect will be lessened and the risk of subdural hemorrhage diminished. We will occasionally keep high-risk patients in bed for 1 week postoperatively.

In summary, the VP shunt operation is one in which attention to detail is important. Repetition of the same operation with the same or similar hardware is necessary in developing rapid and consistent execution of the procedure.

REFERENCES

1. Walker AE: A History of Neurological Surgery. Baltimore, Williams & Wilkins, 1951
2. Taggart JK Jr, Walker AE: Congenital stenosis of the foramina of Luschka and Magendie. Arch Neurol Psychiatr 48:583, 1942
3. Bensman A, et al: Myelomeningocele birth defect: Habilitation of the child. Minn Med 54:599, 1971
4. Heile B: Zur chirurgischen Behandlung der Spina Bifida mit Hydrocephalus. Berl Klin Wochenschr 47:2298, 1910
5. Marburg A: Hydrocephalus, Its Symptomatology, Pathology, Pathogenesis and Treatment. New York, Oskar Piest, 1940
6. Yashon D, et al: The course of severe untreated infantile hydrocephalus: Prognostic significance of the cerebral mantle. J Neurosurg 23:509, 1965
7. Scarff JE: Nonobstructive hydrocephalus: Treatment by endoscopic cauterization of the choroid plexus. J Neurosurg 9:164, 1952
8. Stookey B, Scarff JE: Occlusion of the aqueduct of Sylvius by neoplastic and nonneoplastic processes with a rational surgical treatment for relief of the resultant obstructive hydrocephalus. Bull Neurol Inst 5:348,1936
9. Biddle A: Lumbar arachnoid-ureterostomy combining the Matson technique and the Pudenz-Heyer valve: Report of a case. J Neurosurg 24:760, 1966
10. Nashold BS Jr, Mannarino E: Treatment of hydrocephalus by ureteral-subarachnoid shunt: 14 year follow-up. South Med J 57:270, 1964
11. Heile B: Zur chirurgischen Behandlung des Hydrocephalus Internus durch Ableitung der cerebrospinal Flüssigkeit nach der Bauchhohle und nach der Pleurakuppe. Arch Klin Chir 105:501, 1914
12. Ransohoff J: Ventriculopleural anastomosis in treatment of midline obstructional neoplasms. J Neurosurg 11:295, 1954
13. Alther E: Die ventriculo-ventriculare liquor drainage in der Behandlung des Hydrocephalus. Acta Neurochir 12:26, 1964
14. Ferguson AH: Intraperitoneal diversion of the cerebrospinal fluid in cases of hydrocephalus. NY Med J 67:902, 1898
15. Neumann CG, Hoen TI, Davis DA: The adaptation of ileoentectrophy to the control of congenital communicating hydrocephalus. Plast Reconstr Surg 23:159, 1959
16. McClure RD: Hydrocephalus treated by drainage into a vein in the neck. Bull Johns Hopkins Hosp 20:110, 1909
17. Jackson IJ, Snodgrass W: Peritoneal shunts in the treatment of hydrocephalus: 4-year study of 62 patients. J Neurosurg 12:216, 1955
18. Picaza JA: Posterior-peritoneal shunt technique for treatment of internal hydrocephalus. J Neurosurg 13:289, 1956
19. Ransohoff J, Hiatt R: Ventriculoperitoneal anastomosis in the treatment of hydrocephalus: Utilization of the suprahepatic space: A preliminary report. Trans Am Neurol Assoc 77:147, 1952
20. Spetzler R, Wilson CB, Schulte R: Simplified percutaneous lumboperitoneal shunting, Surg Neurol 7:25, 1977
21. James HE, Tibbs PA: Diverse clinical application of Percutaneous Lumboperitoneal shunts. Neurosurgery 8:39, 1981
22. George R, Leibrock L, Epstein MH: Long-term analysis of cerebrospinal fluid shunt infections. J Neurosurg 51:804, 1979
23. Epstein M, Leitmen P, Hughes P, et al: A double blind prospective study of shunt infections. Abstract presented at the Meeting of the American Association of Neurological Surgeons, Honolulu, Hawaii, 1984

CHAPTER 15
Surgical Management of Meningoceles and Myelomeningoceles

A. Loren Amacher

FEW TOPICS RAISE MORE CONTROVERSY and distress among pediatric neurosurgeons than the timing of and the benefits to be expected from the closure of myelomeningoceles. Opinions, strongly held, range from nihilism, i.e., only exceptionally should the afflicted child be treated, to evangelistic enthusiasm, i.e., all must be treated at all costs.

We cannot explore such issues in all their complexities, but certain features of the condition are pertinent.

DEMOGRAPHIC AND GENETIC FACTORS

Across North America the incidence of myelomeningocele approximates 2 per 1000 live births. Regional differences are well known, reflecting a genetic pool high in Celtic ancestry. In southwestern Ontario, for instance, the incidence exceeds 3 per 1000 live births. On the other hand, the incidence is very low among such ethnic groups as Scandinavians, North American Indians, and blacks. In recent years, most pediatric neurosurgeons have noticed a decline in the number of newborns with myelomeningoceles. The reason for this welcome trend is unknown, although better nutrition, a generally more healthy populace, genetic screening, and counseling services all have been mentioned.

Geneticists suggest a ''multifactorial'' hereditary influence at work. Outbreaks of myelomeningocele in communities point to an environmental trigger as well. Once a woman has had a child with a myelomeningocele, her risk of producing another similarly afflicted baby is about 5 percent. If there is a family history of babies with spina bifida produced by a woman's first- or second-degree female relatives, the risk of recurrence may approach 10 percent. Any of the spinal or cranial dysraphic conditions increases the risk of recurrence for later siblings or offspring. Amniocentesis for α-fetoprotein (AFP) levels is useful in detecting recurrences in susceptible women, but its usefulness as a general screening procedure is offset by a risk of inducing abortion that exceeds the potential discovery rate. Serum AFP tests are not yet totally reliable.

CONCURRENT CARE

Over the past decade substantial improvements have been made in the ability to correct and prevent significant disease of the upper and lower renal tract, the relentless progression of which until recently was a major cause of late morbidity and mortality. Urodynamic evaluation of newborns with myelodysplasia and other spinal dysraphic states has a predictive value for the risk of upper tract deterioration; dyssynergia of detrusor-external sphincter coordination is an early warning signal of later trouble.[1] When indicated, early institution of an intermittent catheterization protocol usually is effective in preserving renal function.

Continuing developments in corrective orthopedics and in orthopedic appliances are making it feasible for more afflicted children to become and remain ambulatory. McLone reported that 47 percent of an unselected series were ambulatory within the community (not wheelchair-bound) 3.5 to 7 years after closure of the lesion.[2]

Early and long-term control of hydrocephalus, which becomes symptomatic in at least 80 percent of survivors, has contributed to the educability and eventual self-sufficiency of children with myelomeningocele.

Of major importance has been the development of well-equipped and well-staffed centers for the rehabilitation of handicapped children. Educational opportunities frequently are provided at such centers, but the trend is to establish as many such children as possible in normal schools. Public awareness of the problems and potentials of handicapped children is increasing, as is the quality of life for the growing number of such children reaching adolescence and young adult life.

There is no question that first-class care, in all of its aspects, for the victims of myelomeningocele is very expensive. One must not minimize the fact that the financial burden placed upon personal or public resources by adequately caring for and rearing a handicapped myelomeningocele child is heavy. It is estimated that the cost of caring for a myelomeningocele patient with a shunt, with renal tract problems, and with orthopedic requirements will reach $400,000 to $500,000 throughout childhood and adolescence.

SURVIVAL DATA

The Sheffield group has performed a valuable service by following and reporting upon their patients over a number of years. Of 200 unselected cases operated upon by the end of 1969, they found a 5-year survival rate of 58.5 percent and a 10-year rate of 56 percent. Among the survivors, 68.4 percent

OPERATIVE NEUROSURGICAL TECHNIQUES
ISBN 0-8089-1862-1

had normal intelligence, 27.4 percent were mobile without appliances, and 20.5 percent had normal renal tracts and urinary control.[3]

Naglo et al.[4] had an 81.4 percent survival rate over a 2- to 11-year follow-up, with 84 percent of the survivors normal mentally, 50 percent ambulatory with or without calipers, and 73 percent with normal renal function, with or without urinary diversions.

Of 163 consecutive cases evaluated by Stein et al.[5] using a selection procedure, 93 percent were alive at follow-up (mean: 7.5 years). Of the survivors, 72 percent were ambulatory, 75 percent were shunt-dependent, 72 percent had normal upper renal tracts, 65 percent had normal intelligence, and 64 percent had minimal or minor handicaps.

Evans et al., reporting upon a selected series from Wales, found that 75 percent of patients whose lesions were closed early were alive at follow-up. Sixteen percent of the unoperated patients were alive, even though patients with the most severe neurologic deficits or in poor medical condition generally were selected for nonsurgical treatment. They noted that of the treated survivors, 35 percent were continent, whereas none of the untreated survivors were. Early surgery had no effect upon the risk of development of hydrocephalus; it was correlated with better mobility and more likelihood of normal intelligence. One fifth of the patients selected for no early closure of their myelomeningoceles had normal intelligence; this finding is interesting and important, in that the selection process would create a bias against the latter group.[6]

McLone's report chronicles the outcome in 100 unselected infants (early closure in all) followed for 3.5 years to 7 years.[2] Fourteen percent were dead at follow-up. Of the survivors, 73 percent had normal mental development (IQ >80), and 87 percent of children were continent after 4.5 years. Thirty-two percent developed symptomatic hindbrain compression; of these, one in eight required posterior fossa and cervical decompression. McLone stated that 70 to 80 percent of survivors were independent and competitive in the community.

Such remarkably encouraging statistics from children treated some years ago may surprise the cynics but will seem neither unusual nor unattainable to those intimately associated with the care of these patients.

THE SELECTION CONTROVERSY

Between the extremes of opinion relating to the moral and ethical issues raised in the treatment of children with myelomeningocele, a large number of pediatric neurosurgeons employ some system of selection criteria in determining whether or not to initiate therapy. From the Sheffield experience, initial findings associated with an adverse physical or mental outcome or both include associated major congenital anomalies such as congenital heart disease or renal tract defects; megalencephaly present at birth; severe orthopedic problems such as pronounced gibbus at the site of the rachischisis, dislocated hips and ankles; and total paraplegia.

In their retrospective analysis of predictors of outcome, Stein et al.[5] found that poor outcome was predicted most reliably by the presence of lückenschädel and at least two more of the above adverse findings. The problem is that some infants with severe lückenschädel end up normal mentally, as do a few with any combination of adverse criteria.

The group at the Children's Hospital of Philadelphia made valuable observations in reporting upon their selected series.[7]

They emphasized that there was no difference for such criteria as the development of ventriculitis, developmental delay, or paresis between children whose myelomeningoceles were closed within 48 hours and those operated upon between 2 and 7 days or even later. No untreated child lived for more than 10 months. Their point was that if selection criteria are to be used, there is time in which to consider all of the factors.

Recent enactment of "Baby Doe" legislation has been accepted by some as justification for jettisoning any decision-making in these situations. Such attitudes are not in the best interest of the patient or the family, to say nothing of being a surrender of professional standards and responsibility in response to legislation, an action for which dangerous precedents exist.

Suggestions abound that special selection committees should be established for the triage of congenitally handicapped infants. A report of such a process and a severe critique of the committee and its actions have appeared in the literature.[8,9] Apart from the potential hazards of allowing such committees (which would be made up of various assortments of "socially conscious" people) to assume a triage role in any field of medicine, the person best equipped to assess the potential and the treatment requirements for such children is the one on whom falls the responsibility for the initial decision regarding therapy. In this difficult area, the conscientious, self-searching, and compassionate surgeon who will spend the next several years caring for the child is the best guarantee the public can have against irresponsibility.

EARLY CARE OF CHILDREN WITH MYELOMENINGOCELES

POSTNATAL CARE

There is no evidence that immediate or urgent closure of a myelomeningocele improves neurologic function or reduces the risk of infection.[7] Parents approached within minutes or hours after the birth of an afflicted child can be stampeded into signing uninformed consents by such statements as: "If we don't close it right away, the baby may end up paralyzed." Such attitudes are mischievous, as is a prolonged delay once a treatment plan has been reached. Forrest defined the issue precisely when he said: " . . . initial action or delay need in no way prejudice later decisions about management, and is not the most important factor determining survival." [10]

It is a common observation that lower extremity function or rectal tone increases during the first few postnatal days, whether or not the lesion is closed. It is as though delivery induces a state of spinal shock that begins to recede rather quickly.

A delay of a few days in closing the rachischisis allows proper initial evaluation of the child and proper briefing of the parents as well as of the total-care team and is perfectly safe if certain precautions are taken.

The infant should be nursed on his or her belly with soft rolls placed beneath the hips and ankles. The sac, even if leaking, can be maintained in a sterile state by using changes of saline and antibiotic dressings twice daily. Contamination of the site by stool and urine is easily avoided.

Duckworth et al.[11] used cortical evoked potentials in an attempt to predict later leg function. They found the results useful only for sensory levels in two thirds of the cases.

When the parents and the surgeon agree upon the desir-

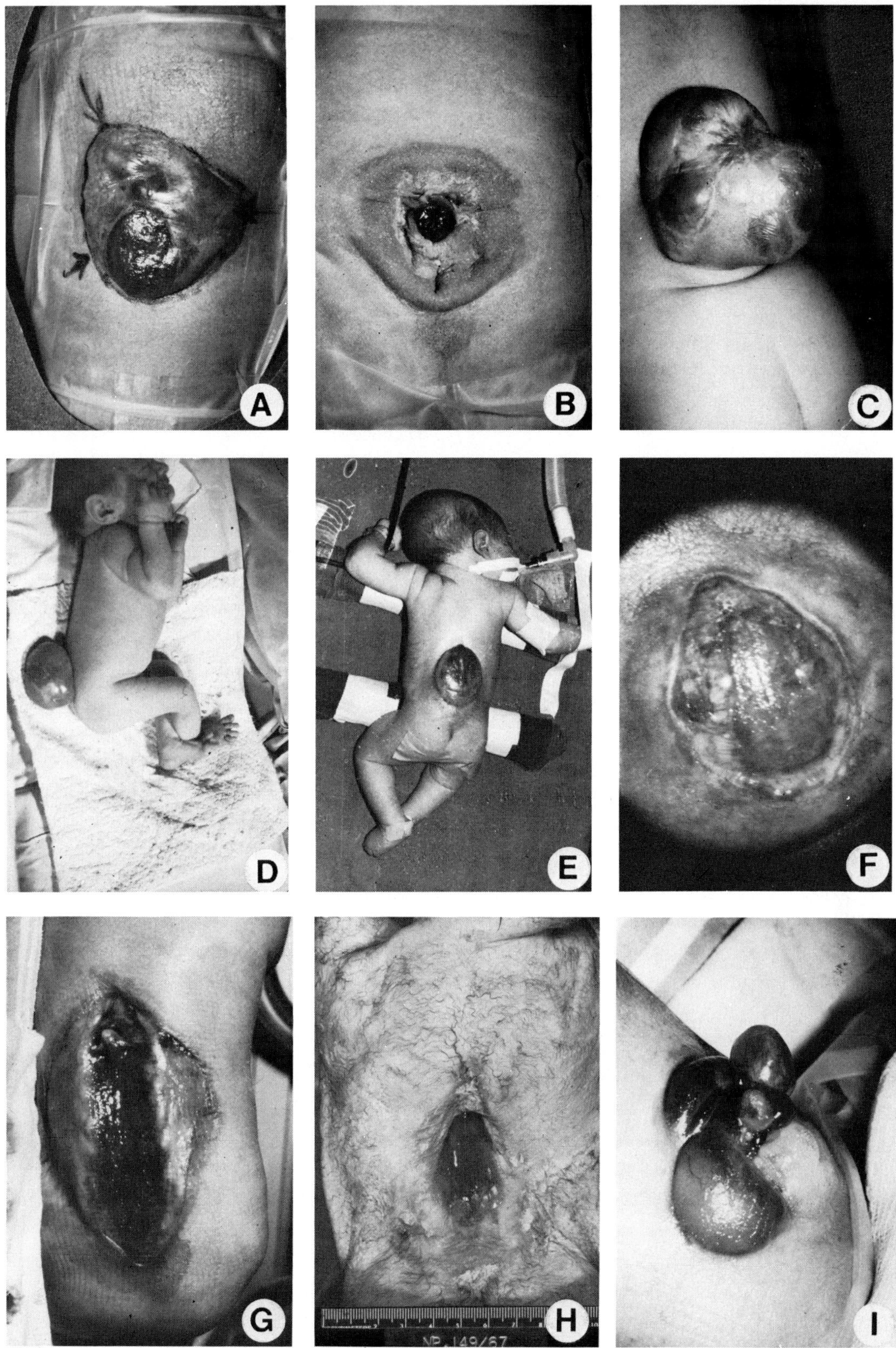

Fig. 15-1.   Examples of configurations of myelomeningoceles preoperatively.

ability of operative treatment, the child should be operated upon at the next convenient time. Parents should be made to realize that they have played a part in the decision-making, but only rarely can the final decision be theirs entirely. Whatever the initial decision, continuing support for the parents and their realization that early treatment decisions may be reversed or modified by later events are essential aspects of the overall approach to the child and the family.

An untreated infant with an open rachischisis is unlikely to survive for more than a few weeks, but some will live for several years. One cannot ask nurses or parents to provide suboptimal care for the infant in order to promote his or her demise. Under such circumstances, the situation must be reassessed and, often, initial decisions reversed.

TECHNICAL ASPECTS

Positioning

The lesion should be protected against pressure during intubation. Frequently a baby with a myelomeningocele requires a smaller endotracheal tube than may be apparent from the weight of the child.

Once the baby is in the prone position, soft rolls should be placed under the shoulders, hips, and ankles. The dressing should remain in place until one is ready to prepare the skin. A mild aqueous preparation is satisfactory and safe. If extensive skin undermining or preparation of rotation flaps is anticipated, a wide preparation of the skin and field is necessary.

Dissection

Figure 15-1 is a montage of commonly seen myelomeningocele defects. It is almost always possible to anticipate the type of skin closure that can be achieved, and using skin along the edge of a tense sac as closure material becomes much more likely once sac tension is released.

The dissection is begun at a site covered by the thinned leptomeninges. Only bipolar coagulation is permissible, and nothing less than 4.5-power loupes should be used. It is essential to remove all epidermal elements from the placode: I have had one epidermoid tumor arise within a retubulated spinal cord when a scrap of skin was left on the placode. Martinez-Lage et al.[12] described the finding of a dermoid tumor upon the surface of a neural placode at a delayed closure.

Extreme care must be taken at the upper end of the placode, especially when the placode abuts directly against the skin. The cord lies directly beneath the placode at this point. It is safe to remove the very outer edge of the placode with the skin in order to avoid leaving skin behind. The large, tortuous veins in the leptomeninges can be sacrificed, but rootlet arterioles must be preserved.

Once the placode is circumcised from its tetherings (Figure 15-2), the closure may be planned. Figure 15-3 indicates the potential layers available for closure. It is quite possible to retubulate the placode with a fine running suture,[13] but I have abandoned this maneuver because it is unnecessary. A leptomeningeal layer can be raised from off the deep fascia; the mobilization is begun just medial to the facet bulges. Almost always, a watertight closure can be obtained and a tubulated cord produced in the process (Figure 15-4).

Before the dura is closed, a gentle lifting of the placode will demonstrate the sensory (lateral) and motor (medial) rootlets (Figure 15-5). Undue lifting and jerking of the placode must be avoided at all stages of the dissection. In some of the large saccular types of myelomeningoceles, with redundant skin and elongated rootlets, the placode and some of the roots will be adherent to skin and scar tissue. A nerve stimulator is useful here in order to avoid damage to functional neural tissue. Damage to functioning lower sacral rootlets can be avoided by a combination of nerve stimulation and placement of an indwelling catheter attached to a water manometer (an operative cystometrogram).

A good fascial layer frequently can be raised from off the paraspinal muscles and closed over the spinal cord. A larger fascial flap can be raised from the thoracic wall, simply rotated down on its inferior pedicle.[14] I have never regretted eschewing the muscle-bone covering of the canal as advocated by Mustarde.[15] If this technique is used, considerable blood loss should be anticipated.

Skin Closure

Figure 15-6 outlines some strategies for skin closure. With experience, the surgeon will find it possible to close an increasing percentage of lesions by direct suture. The figure of 25 percent as stated by Paterson and Till as being uncloseable by direct suture is much higher than my current experience.[16] In 1985, a report appeared in a widely read journal advocating myelomeningocele closure by use of temporary porcine or split-thickness autologous grafts. The authors had experienced a 41 percent necrosis rate with primary closure of lesions the

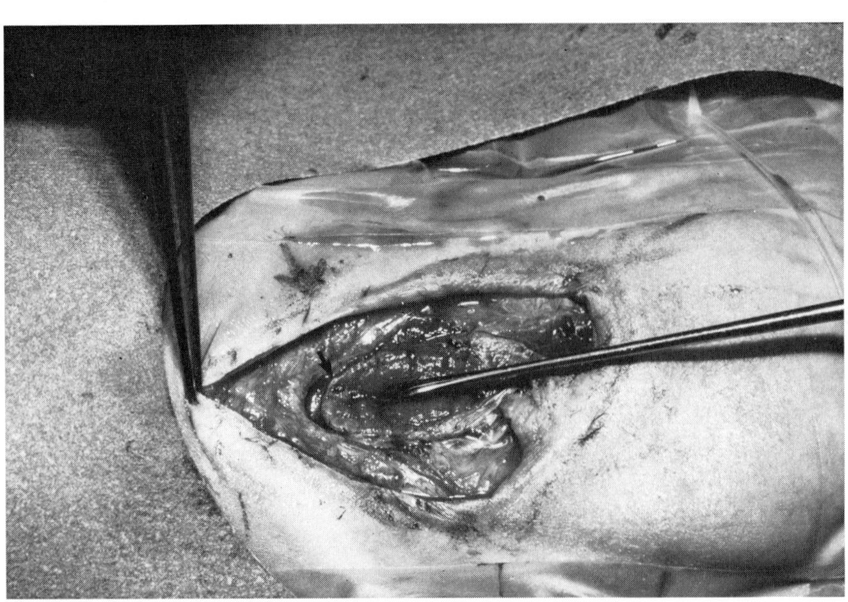

Fig. 15-2.   The neural placode is trimmed (the arrow marks the edge).

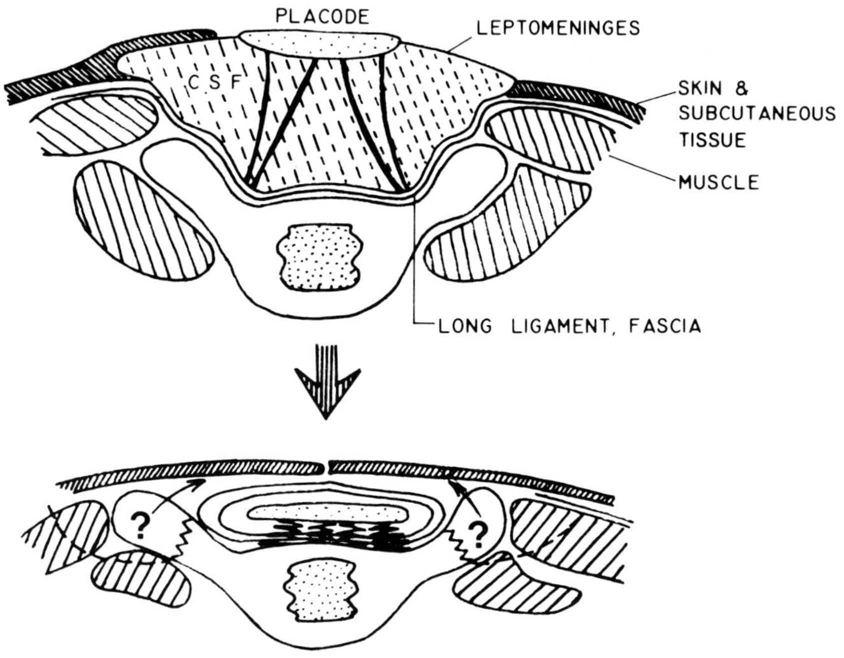

Fig. 15-3. Layers available for closure of myelomeningoceles.

mean area of which was 22.7 cm^2. This astounding failure rate prompted them to state: "the use of primary closure has no role in the treatment of myelomeningocele."[17] To such an arrogant and inane assertion one can reply emphatically: the great majority of myelomeningocele defects are closeable by primary suture with minimal to moderate undermining of dermal edges, and *all* are closeable by full-thickness coverage, which affords much greater protection to the neural placode than does split-thickness grafting.

In the case of large defects, surgeons unfamiliar with the techniques of raising viable rotation flaps should enlist the assistance of a plastic surgeon. It is quite safe to shave down the bony excrescences of a gibbus in order to allow easier and looser approximation of skin edges. When undermining the skin

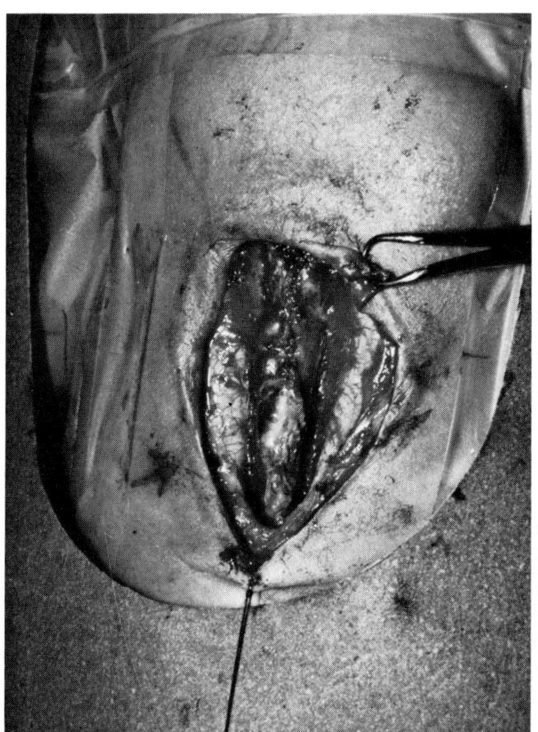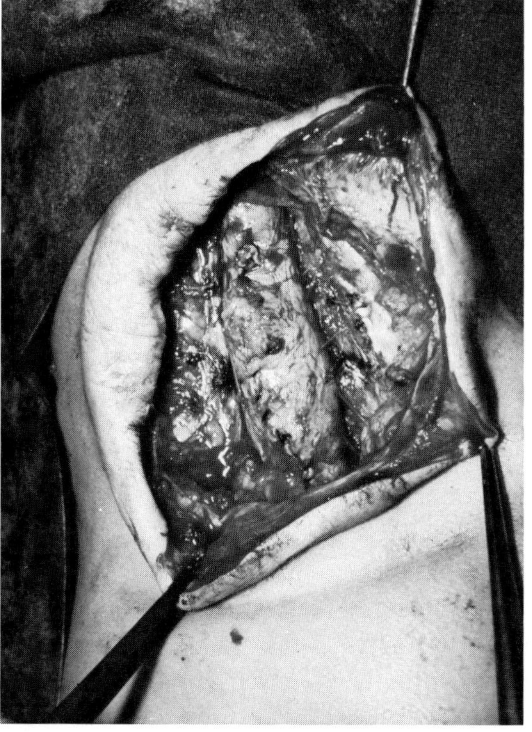

Fig. 15-4. Examples of dural tubes after closure.

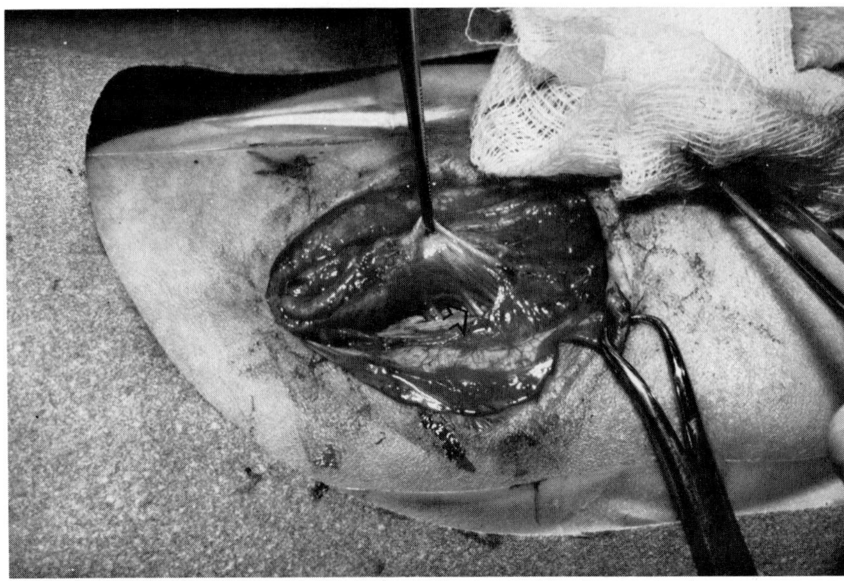

Fig. 15-5. Motor and sensory roots exiting from the placode (arrow).

edges, as much subcutaneous tissue as possible should be left with the skin, and buttonholing of the flap must be avoided.

In general, a rotation flap should have a length-to-base ratio of 1:1. As pointed out by Davies and Adendorff,[18] however, the infant usually will support a flap, even one that crosses the midline, that has a ratio of 1.5:1. Venes[19] has described a method of assessing skin edge vascularity with systemic fluorescein injection that may be most helpful in assessing flap viability. A recent suggestion that nitroglycerin paste rubbed onto a suture line may salvage dubious closures remains to be evaluated in a standard model.[20]

Bipedicle flaps may be useful in some situations, with the resulting elliptical defects closed by further undermining of the donor edges or by split thickness skin grafts.[21,22]

Double-Z rhomboid flaps[23] and latissimus dorsi or gluteus maximus myocutaneous flaps[24,25] may be necessary for some large defects. Marcias and Tena pointed out that triangular isolated skin flaps preserving a deep vascular pedicle may be advantageous at times.[26] When split-thickness grafts are used, they should be cut with sufficient thickness (0.011 of an inch or more) to ensure durable coverage. I have occasionally used secondary split-thickness grafting on small areas of flap necrosis with good success.

"Dog-ears" frequently occur at the distal corners of incisions following direct suture or flap rotation. Only the larger redundant ones need be trimmed; the smaller ones will mold out with time.

Skin edges that are white and strained at the end of closure will not survive; those that are blue probably will. The subcutaneous closure layer is the most important and should be done with interrupted sutures. Skin-edge approximation must be done loosely, with as few sutures as possible. Skin-edge approximation strips are excellent in this situation.

Figure 15-7 illustrates some direct suture closures corresponding to defects A, B, and C of Figure 15-1. Even round defects 6 to 7 cm in diameter are amenable to closure by direct suture if careful undermining techniques are used.

Aftercare

The baby must be kept off of his or her back until wound healing is secure. Newborns tolerate the prone position very well, and if soft rolls are kept beneath the hips and ankles and a small sheepskin mat beneath the child, skin irritation will be minimized. Collections of serous exudate or CSF beneath the closure should be evacuated if tension of the suture line is produced. I have not found it necessary to suspend the baby's abdomen in a soft sling, although this maneuver may help reduce lateral suture-line tension. Once it is obvious that the incision is stable and healthy, the baby can be nursed on its sides as well. Of recent years I have encouraged the picking up and cuddling of these children as soon as possible.

Any required physiotherapy or corrective casting of the lower extremities can begin immediately. Dressings should be changed frequently, and the viability of the closure assessed. A necrotic closure should be revised quickly in order to forestall serious infection of the closure site.

Progressive hydrocephalus or persistent CSF collection at the closure site should be dealt with by shunting. Whether or not myelomeningocele closure increases the likelihood of progressive hydrocephalus is moot,[27] but in that a small percentage of children with myelomeningocele will not require shunting, preclosure or concurrent insertion of a shunt should be done only for rigid indications. Mapstone et al.[28] presented evidence that myelomeningocele children who do not require a shunt exhibit higher mean IQs later on than do their shunted cohorts.

About 10 percent of infants with myelomeningocele will go on to develop laryngeal stridor of sufficient severity to require decompression of the posterior fossa and upper cervical cord within several days to several weeks of birth.

Later Major Closure-Site Procedures

For proper seating and bracing, it may be necessary to remove a prominent lumbar gibbus. The technique has been described by Hall and Poitras,[29] and can be done with safety by

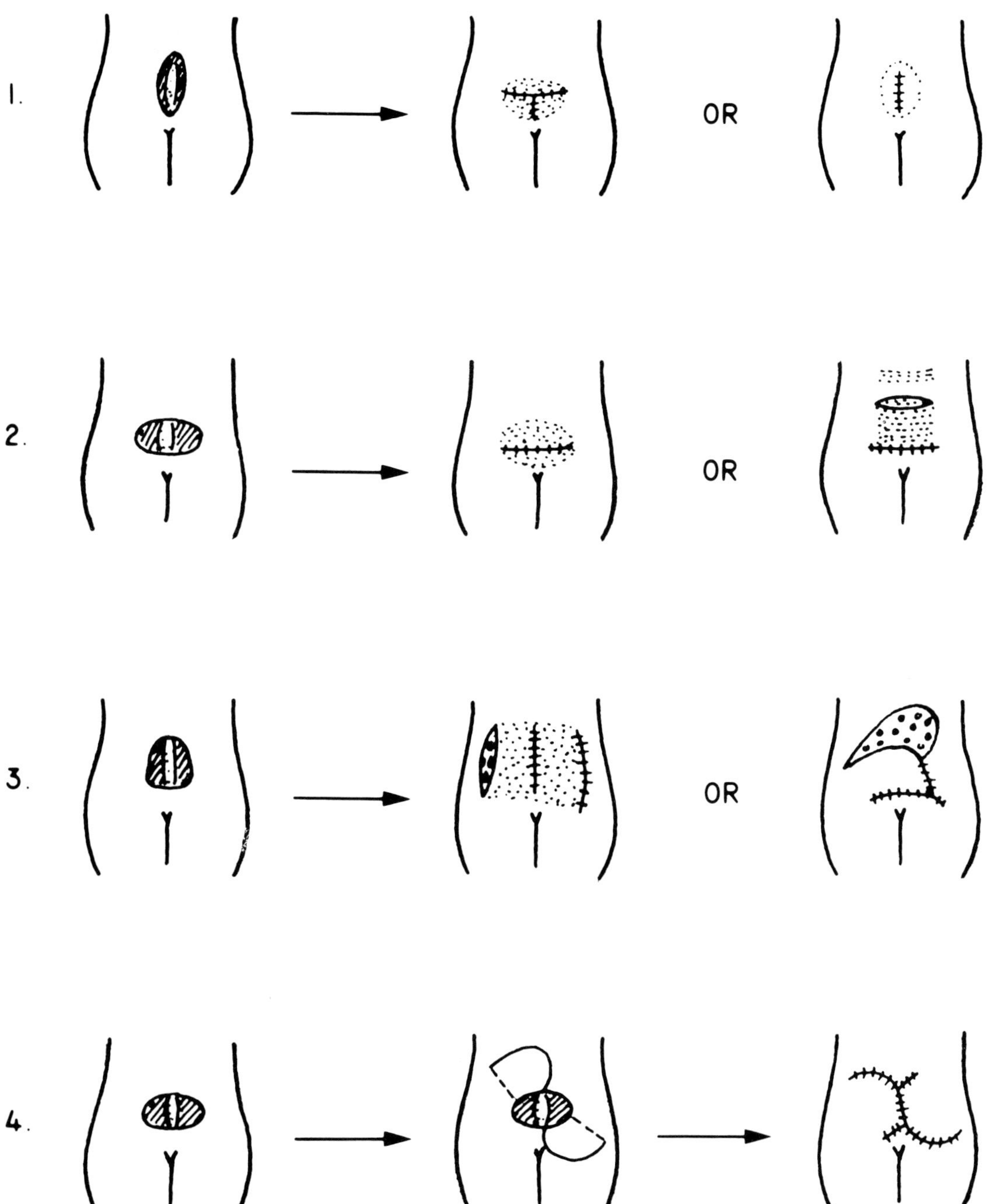

Fig. 15-6. Strategies for skin closure.

early to mid-childhood. Epstein et al.[30] recently described an exciting technique for reconstruction of the cauda equina, although long-term results are unknown as yet.

SUMMARY

Precise closure techniques for myelomeningocele will provide the maximum potential for rehabilitation of the little victims of this disorder. Only those surgeons who are willing to participate fully in the continuing care of such children should presume to expertise in this field.

POSTERIOR SPINAL MININGOCELES

Cystic lesions anywhere along the spinal axis and not containing neural elements usually are straightforward insofar as closure is concerned. Often there is an associated spinal anomaly such as spina bifida occulta, segmentation defect, or hemivertebra. Dissection along the neck of the sac with dural closure usually is accomplished easily, as is skin closure. There is a significant caveat, however: the likelihood of an intradural anomaly (cyst, diastematomyelia, bone spur, extradural or intradural lipoma, dermoid tumor, or short and thick filum) is very high.[31] These children deserve magnetic resonance imag-

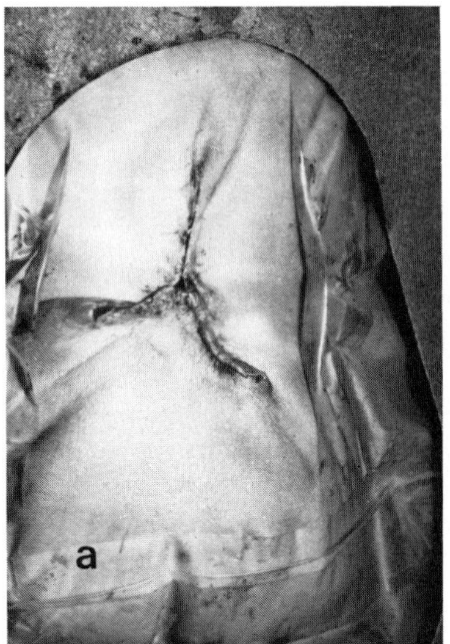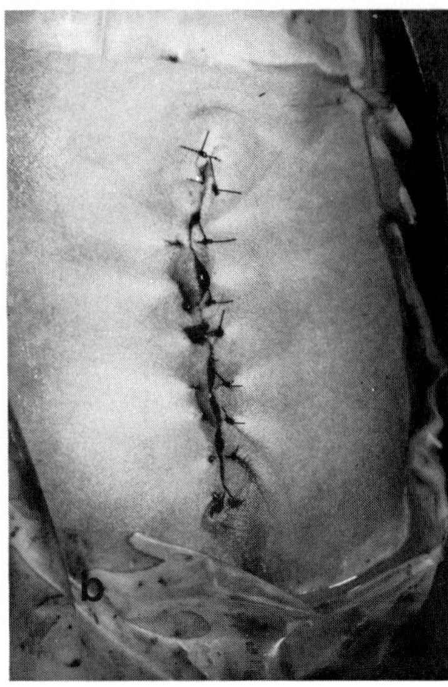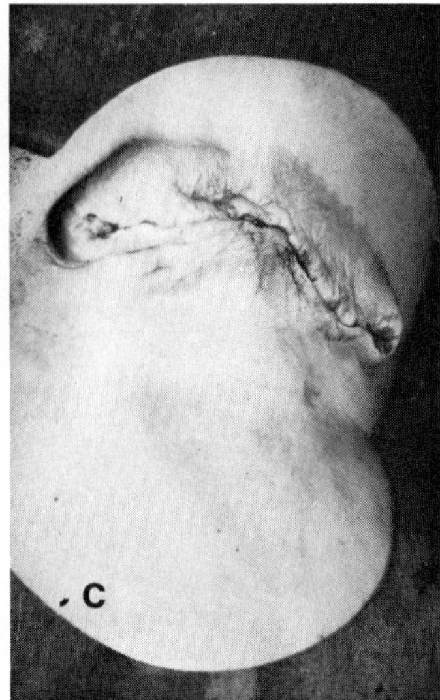

Fig. 15-7.   Completed incisions corresponding to the myelomeningoceles in Figure 15-1. a = Figure 7-1A; b = Figure 15-1B; c = Figure 15-1C.

ing (MRI) or metrizamide myelography at 12 to 18 months of age to rule out residual tethering of the spinal cord.

McLone and Naidich have drawn attention to the entity labelled terminal myelocystocele.[32] An intrasacral or retrosacral cyst representing an expanded central canal is associated with cloacal extrophy and sacral spina bifida occulta. There usually is a meningocele present as well. The extrasacral cyst may present very low, in my experience, as a bizarre overhang to the perineal area.

ANTEROLATERAL SPINAL MENINGOCELES

Meningoceles that emerge from the spinal column to lie anteriorly or laterally are very rare. Of Matson's total series of 1381 meningoceles and myelomeningoceles, only 0.43 percent were anterior or lateral.[33] Many anterolateral sacs, however, remain asymptomatic well into adult life; thus, the known prevalence of such meningoceles increases with age.

The review of the topic by Wilkins and Odom contains the pertinent literature up to the years 1974–1975.[34] This chapter supplies the pertinent English literature from 1975 through 1985.[35–68] It is apparent that both thoracic and sacral anterior meningoceles have been discussed with increasing frequency over the past 5 to 10 years. A fairly definitive description now can be given of the manifestations and treatment of such lesions.

CERVICAL MENINGOCELES

Only recently has the occurrence of these lesions been recognized. If present at birth as a swelling in the posterior cervical triangle, a diagnosis of cystic hygroma may be attached.[35] Multiple cervical meningoceles have been seen in association with neurofibromatosis.[36] Lastly, an example of a cervical meningocele above the clavicle following nerve root avulsion was reported by Jacobsen et al.[37]

THORACIC AND LUMBAR MENINGOCELES

Symptomatology

Probably the majority of thoracic and lumbar meningoceles are "occult," that is, asymptomatic until they are stumbled upon in the course of routine or other examinations. A rounded soft tissue density in the superior or posterior mediastinum on a routine chest x-ray film frequently heralds the meningocele. Occasionally, radicular pain in the thorax or abdomen or aching of the arm has been noted. Very occasionally, a myelopathy has been described, but such cord compression usually is ascribable to an associated spinal pathologic condition.

Headache of a paroxysmal nature, frequently associated with exercise or with prolonged upright posture, may occur because of pooling of CSF in large sacs.

Increasingly, an association of thoracic meningoceles with von Recklinghausen's disease (neurofibromatosis) is being reported.[38–44] Heselson and Goldberg found a 70 percent association in the literature to 1976.[41] A posterior or superior mediastinal mass in a patient with neurofibromatosis is likely to be either a dumbbell neurofibroma or a meningocele. Sometimes both are found. In addition, such patients may have multiple lesions.[45] These patients in particular may have kyphoscoliosis or gibbus formation of a degree sufficient to cause chronic cord compression. Intrathoracic meningoceles may exert sufficient chronic pressure to erode both bodies and lateral elements, rendering the spine unstable.[38]

Galzio has reported a unique case in which a giant lumbosacral meningocele opened into the abdominal cavity from a tiny neck that perforated the L5-S1 disc. The patient also had multiple congenital anomalies of the urogenital system and intracranial meningiomas.[46]

The very rare lumbar anterior meningocele usually is discovered incidentally as an abdominal or loin mass in children or adolescents. It occasionally produces back or loin pain,[34] and neurofibromatosis is associated commonly.

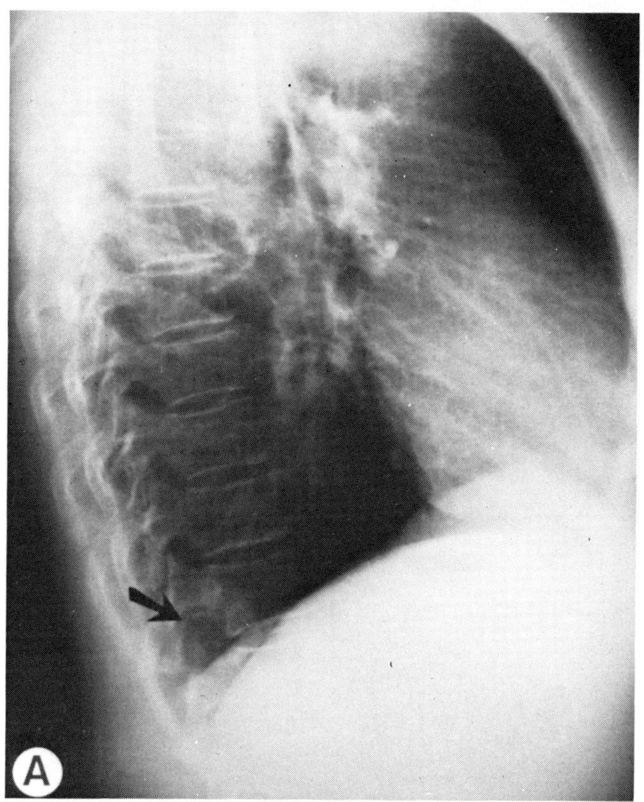

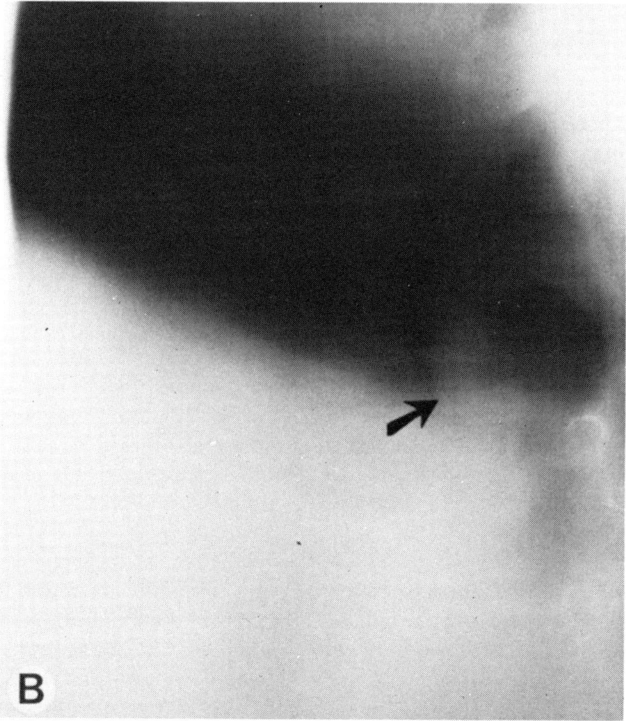

Fig. 15-8. (A) A lateral chest x-ray film showing an enlarged intervertebral foramen (arrow). (B) A lateral tomogram of the thoracic spine showing an enlarged intervertebral foramen and the shadow of a lateral thoracic meningocele.

Pathologic Anatomy

Usually the sac emerges from an enlarged intervertebral foramen (Figure 15-8), but rarely it may come straight forward through a disc or a vertebral body. When a kyphoscoliosis is present, the sac is seen most frequently on the convex side of the deformity.[34]

The capsule is made up of an amalgam of parietal pleura, retropleural connective and fibrous tissue, and dura. It is tough and resilient, and holds sutures well. They may enlarge with time.

The sac seems to originate from the root sleeve in front of the motor rootlet, emerging as a narrow stalk that balloons out into its sac. The segmental nerves and small vessels occasionally are stretched over the sac, as well as splayed out epidural veins. A neurofibroma rarely may be seen in the wall of the sac.[34] Almost always, the communication of CSF between the sac and the subarachnoid space is unimpeded, but not invariably.[47]

Radiology and Definitive Diagnosis

As with dumbbell neurofibromas, the hallmark of an anterolateral thoracic or lumbar meningocele is the finding of an enlargement of the intervertebral foramen on plain x-ray films (Figure 15-8). In addition, fused or hemivertebrae, posterior body scalloping, fused foramina, and kyphoscoliosis may be seen.

Myelography has been the most common method for defining the nature of the mass. At present, ultrasonography, magnetic resonance imaging (MRI), and CT scanning should be done first, as these may provide a reliable answer without resorting to invasive methods. When contrast-enhanced CT scanning is done, delayed images may be required to demonstrate the communication of the cyst and the subarachnoid space.

Treatment

There seems to be little purpose in attacking an asymptomatic anterolateral cervical, thoracic, or lumbar meningocele unless it is known to be enlarging. If pain or proven expansion are present, a posterior or posterolateral approach is advisable, with simple transfixation of the neck. The sac should be collapsed, but it need not be removed. Near the thoracolumbar junction, preoperative angiography is essential in locating the notoriously nomadic artery of Adamkiewicz. If this vessel is involved with the neck of the sac, it must be preserved at all costs. Hemilaminectomy may facilitate neck exposure, but pediculectomy or facetectomy are unnecessary.

INTRASACRAL AND ANTERIOR SACRAL MENINGOCELES

Since our report and search of the literature of 1968,[48] several accounts of anterior (ASM) and intrasacral (ISM) meningoceles have appeared.[34,47,68] The spectrum of presentations has been confirmed and widened, and a consensus for treatment has emerged.

Symptomatology

The incidence of ASMs and ISMs is unknown. Most seem to come to attention in adult women; since the discovery of ASMs in children appears to be likely equally in boys and girls,

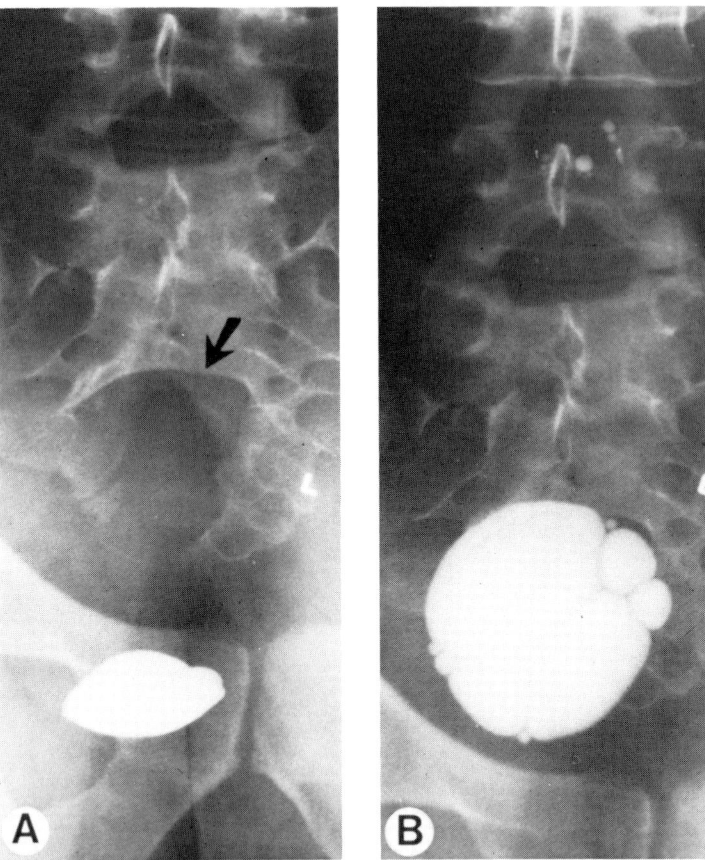

Fig. 15-9. (A) A posteroanterior sacral myelogram showing a "scimitar sacrum" (arrow). (B) A posteroanterior sacral myelogram with contrast falling to the anterior aspect of the sac.

it is improbable that there is a real sex preponderance at any age.

Among the commonly reported symptoms are headache, either because of excessive CSF pooling in the sac or reflux of CSF into the subarachnoid space; enuresis and encopresis, particularly in children; abdominal masses, usually discovered incidentally with or without vague abdominal complaints; pelvic masses discovered during labor or during routine rectal examinations; pain in the low back or pelvis, occasionally in a sacral nerve distribution; constipation and difficult defecation. Occasionally, lax sphincters and reduced perineal sensation may be discovered. Recently, an ASM presenting as a groin mass has been reported.[51]

Acute flexion injury to a sacrum ballooned out by an ISM may produce a transverse fracture of the sacrum, perhaps with neurologic findings.[52]

Of greater import is the potential for infection in the subarachnoid space in the presence of a rectomeningeal fistula, with either ASMs or ISMs. Such fistulas may occur spontaneously, following childbirth, or subsequent to attempted aspiration or needle biopsy of a presacral mass.[34,48,50,60] In the report of Brihaye et al.,[50] a fistulous, presumably congenital, tract was discovered between the rectum and an ISM in two cases.

Anterior sacral meningoceles have been reported in association with presacral teratoma,[55,56,58,68] intrasacral and presacral neurofibroma,[53] von Recklinghausen's disease,[40,53] intrasacral lipoma,[65] as well as with bony evidence of spinal dysraphism, particularly in the lumbar spine.[34] Quigley et al.

reported the case of a young woman who suffered repeated bouts of aseptic meningitis because of a dermoid tumor associated with an ASM.[61] Very rarely, a family incidence has been noted, as have anomalies in other organ systems.[34] Yates et al.[68] chronicled the remarkable occurrence of 11 members of one family pedigree with sacral bony defects, ASMs, and presacral teratomas. They suggested that these lesions may be transmitted as an autosomal dominant trait.

The Currarino triad consists of a complex of anal-rectal anomalies, sacral bony abnormality (scimitar sacrum), and presacral ASM, teratoma, or enteric cyst. The anorectal anomalies range from stenosis or ectopia to imperforation. Transmission is autosomal dominant of variable expression. There is a high risk of gastrointestinal-CSF fistulous connections.[57]

Pathologic Anatomy

Because of the associated bony abnormalities found in full measure in children as well as adults, it is likely that both ASMs and ISMs represent a congenital anomaly of the bone and the meninges. The sacs are thick-walled and contain elements of dura, leptomeninges, connective and fibrous tissue, epidural veins, and, occasionally, incorporated nerve fibers. They probably enlarge with time, perhaps because of hydrostatic forces.

Radiology and Definitive Diagnosis

The ISM produces a distinctive "ballooning" of the intrasacral canal, with thinning of posterior elements, scalloping of the posterior vertebral body, and expansion of the sagittal

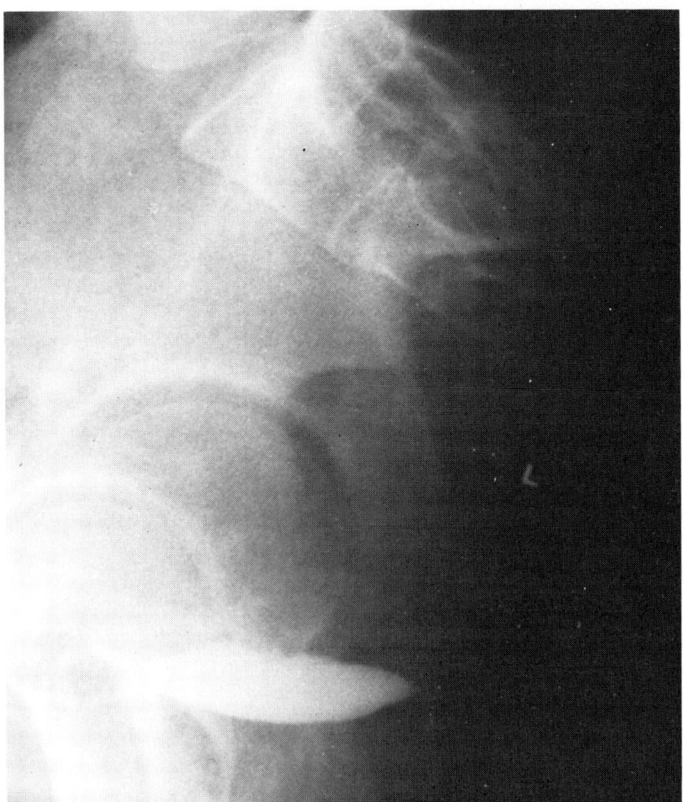

Fig. 15-10. The true size of an ASM is revealed by this lateral x-ray film. The patient is in the erect position.

diameter of the sacrum. Intervertebral foramina may be enlarged, but usually only to a moderate degree.

The ASM may be associated with complete agenesis of the lower sacrum and with marked enlargement or fusion of one or more intravertebral foramina. The most characteristic finding, however, is the so-called "scimitar sacrum". (Figure 15-9A).

The sac itself can be delineated by contrast myelography,[62] sonography,[59] computed tomography,[67] and, of course, MRI. Unless such measures have been used to rule out the presence of an ASM, needle aspiration of a presacral mass via a transrectal or perineal approach must never be done, since introduction of infection into an ASM is extremely serious.

The sac may be huge, filling the pelvis and extending into the abdomen (Figures 15-9B and 15-10).

Treatment

There is little that can be done for an ISM. If sacral pain or ingravescent or paroxysmal neurologic deficits occur, a cystoperitoneal shunt is advisable.

There are two approaches to treating ASMs. The vast majority should be approached by sacral laminectomy with plication of the neck, due care being taken to avoid damage to nerves in the wall of the sac. The neck of the meningocele may be much larger than anticipated from a myelogram or it may extend through more than one foramen.

The anterior approach to ASMs has a very bad reputation,[34,60] but it is a safe and useful approach when huge abdominal sacs are encountered.[48,58] With the sac in direct view, a great deal of operating space can be developed by sac aspiration and blunt dissection along the sac wall and in the

retrorectal space. Before the neck is ligated, the sac must be opened and any neural elements in the wall preserved.

SUMMARY

More frequent recognition of anterolateral spinal meningoceles has clarified the spectrum of symptomatology, the means of diagnosis, and the indications for and methods of treatment.

REFERENCES

1. Bauer SB, Hallett M, Khoshbin S, et al: Predictive value of urodynamic evaluation in newborns with myelodysplasia. JAMA 252:650, 1984
2. McLone DG: Results of treatment of children born with a myelomeningocele. Clin Neurosurg 30:407, 1983
3. Lister I, Zachary RB, Brereton R: Open myelomeningocele—a ten year review of 200 consecutive closures. Prog Pediatr Surg 10:161, 1977
4. Naglo AS, Heustrom B.:Results of treatment in myelomeningocele. Acta Paediatr Scand 65:565, 1976
5. Stein SC, Schut L, Ames ML: Selection of early treatment of myelomeningocele: A retrospective analysis of selection procedures. Dev Med Child Neurol 17:311, 1975
6. Evans RC, Tew B, Thomas MD, et al: Selective management of neural tube malformations. Arch Dis Child 60:415, 1985
7. Charney EB, Weller SC, Sutton LN, et al: Management of the newborn with myelomeningocele: Time for a decision-making process. Pediatrics 75:58, 1985
8. Gross RH, Cox A, Tatyrek R, et al: Early management and decision-making for the treatment of myelomeningocele. Pediatrics 72:450, 1983
9. Freeman JM: Early management and decision making for the treatment of myelomeningocele: A critique. Pediatrics 73:564, 1984
10. Forrest DM: Spina bifida: Some problems in management. Proc R Soc Med 70:233, 1977
11. Duckworth T, Yamashita T, Franks CL, et al: Somatosensory evoked cortical responses in children with spina bifida. Dev Med Child Neurol 18:19, 1976
12. Martinez-Lage JF, Masegosa J, Sola J, et al: Epidermoid cyst occurring within a lumbosacral myelomeningocele. J Neurosurg 59:1095, 1983
13. McLone DG: Technique for closure of myelomeningocele. Childs Brain 6:65, 1980
14. Voorhies RM, Fraser RAR: Fascial closure in low myelomeningocele repairs. J Neurosurg 58:144, 1983
15. Mustarde JC: Reconstruction of the spinal canal in severe spina bifida. Plast Reconstr Surg 42:109, 1968
16. Paterson TJS, Till K: The use of rotation flaps following excision of lumbar myelomeningoceles. An aid to the closure of large defects. Br J Surg 46:606, 1959
17. Luce EA, Walsh J: Wound closure of the myelomeningocele defect. Plast Reconstr Surg 75:389, 1985
18. Davies D, Adendorff DJ: A large rotation flap raised across the midline to close lumbo-sacral meningomyeloceles. Br J Plast Surg 30:166, 1977
19. Venes JL: The use of intravenous fluorescein in the repair of large myelomeningoceles. Technical note. J Neurosurg 47:126, 1977
20. Lehman RAW, Page RB, Saggers GC, et al: Technical note: The use of nitroglycerin ointment after precarious neurosurgical wound closure. Neurosurgery 16:701, 1985
21. Habal MB, Vries JK: Tension-free closure of large meningomyelocele defects. Surg Neurol 8:177, 1977
22. Moore TS, Dreyer TM, Bevin AG: Closure of large spina bifida cystica defects with bilateral bipedicled musculocutaneous flaps. Plast Reconstr Surg 73:288, 1984

23. Cruz NI, Ariyan S, Duncan CC, et al: Repair of lumbosacral myelomeningoceles with double Z-rhomboid flaps. J Neurosurg 59:714, 1983

24. Munro IR, Neu BR, Humphreys RP: Limberg-latissimus dorsi myocutaneous flap for closure of myelomeningocele. Childs Brain 10:381, 1983

25. Lehrman A, Owen MP: Surgical repair of large meningomyeloceles. Ann Plast Surg 12:501, 1984

26. Macias R, Tena L: Myelomeningocele: New technique for skin repair. Childs Brain 10:73, 1983

27. Linder M, Nichols J, Sklar F: Effect of myelomeningocele closure on the intracranial pulse pressure. Childs Brain 11:176, 1984

28. Mapstone TB, Rekate HL, Nulsen FE, et al: Relationship of CSF shunting and IQ in children with myelomeningocele. A retrospective analysis. Childs Brain 11:112, 1984

29. Hall JE, Poitras B: The management of kyphosis in patients with myelomeningocele. Clin Orthop 128:33, 1977

30. Epstein F, Spielholz N, McCarthy J, et al: Delayed cauda equina reconstruction in meningomyelocele. Childs Brain 7:31, 1980

31. Chaseling RW, Johnson IH, Besser M: Meningoceles and the tethered cord syndrome. Childs Nerv Syst 1:105, 1985

32. McLone DG, Naidich TP: Terminal myelocystocele. Neurosurgery 16:36, 1985

33. Matson DD: Neurosurgery of Infancy and Childhood, ed 2. Springfield, Ill, Charles C Thomas, 1969

34. Wilkins RH, Odom GL: Anterior and lateral spinal meningoceles, in Vinken PJ, Bruyn GW (eds): Handbook of Clinical Neurology, vol. 32. New York, North Holland, 1978, pp 198–230

35. Shore RM, Chun RWM, Strother CM: Lateral cervical meningocele. Clin Pediatr 21:430, 1982

36. O'Neill P, Whatmore WJ, Booth AE: Spinal meningoceles in association with neurofibromatosis. Neurosurgery 13:82, 1983

37. Jakobsen H, Røder OC, Bojsen-Møller: Large paracervical meningocele due to lesion of cervical spinal nerve roots. Acta Chir Scand 149:537, 1983

38. Kornberg M, Rechtine GR, Dupuy TE: Thoracic vertebral erosion secondary to an intrathoracic meningocele in a patient with neurofibromatosis. Spine 9:821, 1985

39. Brandt M, Altenburg H, Rode J: Occult thoracic and sacral meningocele. Neurochirurgia 20:118, 1977

40. Erkulvrawatr S, El Gammal T, Hawkins J, et al: Intrathoracic meningoceles and neurofibromatosis. Arch Neurol 36:557, 1979

41. Heselson NG, Goldberg S: Intrathoracic meningocele. A report of two cases. S Afr Med J 50:2108, 1976

42. Leech RW, Olafson RA, Gilbertson RL, et al: Intrathoracic meningocele and vertebral anomalies in a case of neurofibromatosis. Surg Neurol 9:55, 1978

43. Schechter FG, Carey ME, Bryant LR: Bilateral apical intrathoracic masses associated with von Recklinghausen's disease. Chest 75:367, 1979

44. Yagoobian J: Intrathoracic mass in a young woman with skin lesions. JAMA 242:2007, 1979

45. Weinreb JC, Arger PH, Grossman R, et al: CT Metrizamide myelography in multiple bilateral intrathoracic meningoceles. J Comput Assist Tomogr 8:324, 1984

46. Galzio RJ: Giant anterior lumbosacral meningocele associated with intracranial meningiomas and multiple congenital malformations. Surg Neurol 18:419, 1982

47. Roosen N, Van Vyve M, DeMoor J: Intrasacral meningeal cyst demonstrated by sacral epidurography. Neuroradiology 27:123, 1985

48. Amacher AL, Drake CG, McLachlin AD: Anterior sacral meningocele. Surg Gynecol Obstet 126:986, 1968

49. Anderson FM, Burke BL: Anterior sacral meningocele. A presentation of three cases. JAMA 237:39, 1977

50. Brihaye J, Gerard A, Kiekens R, et al: Rectomeningeal fistulae in dysraphic states. Surg Neurol 10:93, 1978

51. Dyck P, Wilson CB: Anterior sacral meningocele. Case report. J Neurosurg 53:548, 1980

52. Fardon DF: Intrasacral meningocele complicated by transverse fracture. J Bone Joint Surg 62A:839, 1980

53. Florez G, Ucar S: The occult intrasacral meningocele. Neurochirurgia 19:46, 1976

54. Frank JL: Pelvic mass in a 12-year-old girl. JAMA 237:1255, 1977

55. Head HD, Gerstein JD, Muir RW: Presacral teratoma in the adult. Am Surg 41:240, 1975

56. Jabre A, Ball JB, Tew JM: Anterior sacral meningocele. Current diagnosis. Surg Neurol 23:9, 1985

57. Kirks DR, Merten DF, Filston HC, Oakes WJ: The Currarino triad: Complex of anorectal malformation, sacral bony abnormality, and presacral mass. Pediatr Radiol 14:220, 1984

58. Leibowitz E, Barton W, Sadighi P, et al: Anterior sacral meningocele contiguous with a pelvic hamartoma. J Neurosurg 61:188, 1984

59. McCreath GT, MacPherson P: Sonography in the diagnosis and management of anterior sacral meningocele. J Clin Ultrasound 8:133, 1980

60. Oren M, Lorber B, Lee SH, et al: Anterior sacral meningocele: Report of five cases and review of the literature. Dis Colon Rectum 20:492, 1977

61. Quigley MR, Schinco F, Brown JT: Anterior sacral meningocele with an unusual presentation. J Neurosurg 61:790, 1984

62. Resjo IM, Harwood-Nash DC, Fitz CR, et al: Computed tomographic metrizamide myelography in spinal dysraphism in infants and children. J Comput Assist Tomogr 2:549, 1978

63. Skinner DW, Jacobson I: Anterior sacral meningoceles. J R Coll Surg Edinb 28:229, 1983

64. Smith HP, Davis CH: Anterior sacral meningocele. Two case reports and discussion of surgical approach. Neurosurgery 7:61, 1980

65. Sumner TE, Crowe JE, Phelps CR, et al: Occult anterior sacral meningocele. Am J Dis Child 134:385, 1980

66. Villarejo F, Scavone C, Blaquez MG, et al: Anterior sacral meningocele: Review of the literature. Surg Neurol 19:57, 1983

67. Wolpert SM, Scott RM, Carter BL: Computed tomography in spinal dysraphism. Surg Neurol 8:199, 1977

68. Yates VD, Wilroy RS, Whitington GL, et al: Anterior sacral defects: An autosomal dominantly inherited condition. J Pediatr 102:239, 1983

CHAPTER 16

Occult Spinal Dysraphism: Recognition and Surgical Management

Paul H. Chapman

THE TERM SPINA BIFIDA generally is understood to connote a wide variety of congenital pathologic conditions of the spine. Such dissimilar entities as myelomeningocele, dermal sinus with or without tumor, spinal lipoma, tethered filum terminale, and diastematomyelia have been variously included under the heading of spina bifida.[1] The common denominator is, as implied, a congenital defect in the posterior elements of one or more vertebral segments. Such a grouping on the basis of a single pathologic feature, however, has led to confusion regarding the relationship between these various conditions with regard to clinical presentation, course, and treatment. The major difficulty results from a juxtaposition of myelomeningocele (or meningocele, spina bifida cystica, spina bifida aperta, myeloschisis, etc.) with so-called spina bifida occulta and its associated conditions. Myelomeningocele, with its attendant problems, is a common and widely recognized entity (see Chapter 15). In such cases there is characteristically a dorsal protrusion of more or less severely malformed spinal cord elements and their coverings between the bifid bony elements on the surface of the back. Neurologic deficits in the lower extremities are often severe, with associated loss of bladder or bowel control. These deficits are present at birth and usually are unchanging. The Arnold-Chiari malformation of the cerebellum and brainstem is usually present, as are lesser deformities of the forebrain. Progressive hydrocephalus is common.

There is, on the other hand, a group of congenital lesions of the caudal spinal canal and its overlying tissues that involve the spinal cord to produce progressive neurologic deficits. Because spinal bifida is associated with these lesions, they are often discussed under the designation spina bifida occulta. Use of the term *spinal dysraphism* to designate them as a group is also common.[25] Pathologically, these lesions are not consistently associated with Arnold-Chiari malformation, hydrocephalus, or other cerebral anomalies and there is no clear pattern of heritability. The degree of spinal cord dysplasia is relatively minor compared with that found in the typical case of myelomeningocele. Likewise, the dysplasia of overlying tissues, in particular the skin, is usually of a minor sort, although it is extremely valuable in suggesting the presence of underlying difficulty. Occult spinal dysraphism typically causes progressive neurologic deterioration, whether of bladder, bowel, or lower extremity sensorimotor function. The deficits initially are often minor and may or may not occur in the context of pre-existing fixed deformities of the lower extremities, such as talipes or unequal size of the feet or legs. Finally, approximately two thirds of the patients are female, whereas in the case of myelomeningocele there is no clear sex predilection.

PATHOLOGY

The intraspinal pathologic features of spinal dysraphism are quite diverse. Certain common features, however, underlie this diversity. In most cases, the congenital abnormality, whatever it might be, exerts an immobilizing influence on the spinal cord, usually at its distal extremity. The use of the term *tethered spinal cord* reflects this feature. Occasionally, expanding lesions, such as intraspinal dermoid tumors or lipomas, produce neurologic symptomatology by direct compression of the adjacent spinal cord or nerve roots. Even in these cases, however, the presence of an ancillary immobilizing influence must be considered. In conjunction with tethering, the conus medullaris is found to lie at an abnormally low level within the spinal canal. This is demonstrable either during surgery or by myelography and constitutes an important feature in diagnosis. During fetal development, there is gradual relative ascent of the conus within the spinal canal because of the disparate rate of longitudinal growth of the spinal cord and spine.[6,7] At 17 weeks' gestation, the spinal cord ends opposite the L4 vertebral level. At term, the mean level of termination is at the lower border of L2. Several months postnatally it has reached the level of the L1-L2 interspace. There is no further ascent. As a general rule, therefore, if the conus terminates at the level of L3 or below after 5 to 6 months of age, it can be considered to be abnormally low.

In spinal dysraphism, the conus is not only low but also tends to be situated posteriorly within the spinal canal (see Figure 16-4). With caudal fixation of the conus, the lumbosacral lordosis tends to bring it into a posterior position. Another factor, which will be discussed below, may be actual fixation of the conus to the posterior dura by a thickened filum, lipomatous mass, or fibrous bands.

Aside from these general considerations, the spinal pathology usually assumes one of several forms. An understanding of the pathologic anatomy of these lesions is necessary for their proper recognition and surgical management. Intraspinal lipoma is a common pathologic entity (Figure 16-1A). Emery and Lendon[8] have studied its various forms in detail. A term that is synonymous in the literature is *lipomyelomeningocele*. The lipomatous mass usually is situated in the caudal extremity

OPERATIVE NEUROSURGICAL TECHNIQUES
ISBN 0-8089-1862-1

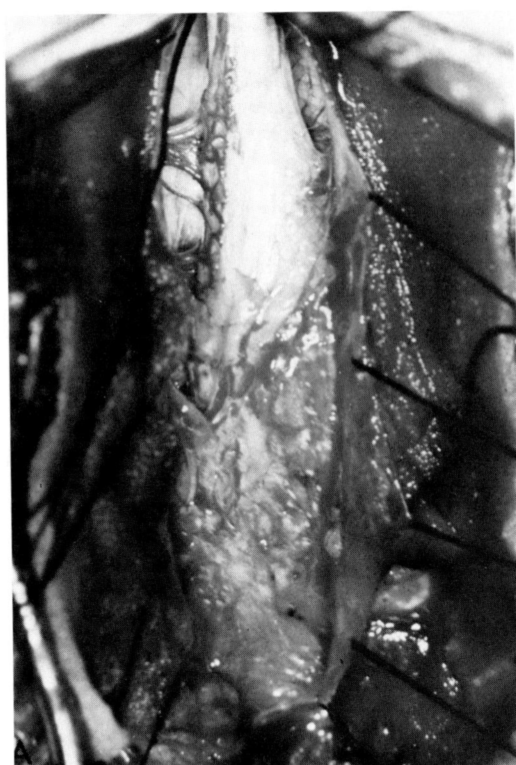

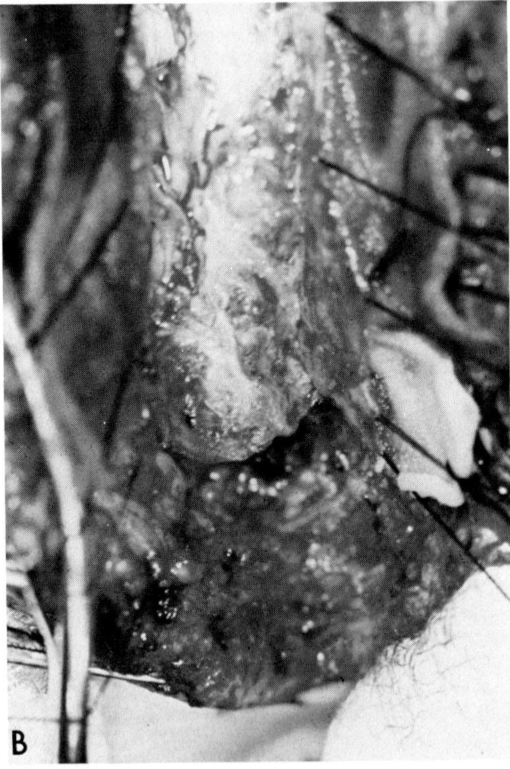

Fig. 16-1. (A) An intradural lipoma confluent with the conus medullaris. Note the horizontal direction of the exiting nerve roots. (B) A closer view of the lipoma shown in Figure 16-1A after subtotal resection. Surgery resulted in improved bladder function.

of the spinal canal and is coextensive with the conus medullaris. The connection with the conus may be a stalklike fibrolipomatous structure or the lipoma may gradually merge with the conus in such a way that there is extensive intermingling of fatty and

neural tissues at a rather indistinct interface. Careful histologic examination of the lipoma may, in fact, reveal a wide variety of mesodermal and ectodermal tissue elements including, on rare occasions, epithelium-lined cysts.[9] This finding does not have any special significance with respect to management or prognosis.

The site of fixation of the lipoma to the conus is of some importance surgically and serves to separate these lesions into two general categories.[10] On the one hand, the fatty mass may insert into the dorsal aspect of the conus. In this circumstance the lesion typically extends from the subcutaneous space into the spinal canal through widely bifid bony elements and a congenital posterior dural defect. This has been designated a leptomyelolipoma by Emery and Lendon.[8] The interface between the lipoma and the conus usually lies just posterior to the point of emergence of sensory rootlets so that neither these nor the more anteriorly situated motor rootlets are within the substance of the lipoma. On the other hand, the lipoma may insert into the distal extremity of the conus, in which case the fatty mass may be entirely intraspinal or, more commonly, may extend through a dural defect caudally to present as a subcutaneous mass. In this second type of lesion nerve roots are encountered running to their foramina of exit within the substance of the lipoma. These features are obviously of importance surgically and will be dealt with further in the discussion of operative technique.

A simpler type of abnormality is the short, thickened filum terminale (Figure 16-2A). The filum terminale is normally a threadlike structure. It represents a nonneural continuation of the conus medullaris. The filum inserts at the distal end of the dural sac and generally contains a microscopic continuation of the central canal of the spinal cord. In its abnormal state the filum is thickened to a diameter of 3 to 5 mm. It is shorter than normal by virtue of the low position of the conus and lies posteriorly within the dural sac, often in contact with the posterior dura. A lipoma in continuity with it may be present, particularly at the point of distal insertion of the filum. The thickened filum may insert posteriorly in the dura, proximal to the termination of the dural sac. Microscopically the abnormal filum is collagenous, with a centrally placed core of ependymal cells representing the remnant of the central canal. There may be small islands of fatty tissue within the collagenous substrate.

Occasionally fibrous bands may be found. These arise from the conus and insert on the dura posteriorly, laterally, or even anteriorly. Such bands may continue through the dura to end in relation to overlying bony elements or within subcutaneous tissue. At times these have the appearance of aberrant nerve roots with dorsal root ganglia present. Stimulation typically reveals no motor function. Lassman and James[11] have devised the term *meningocele manqué* for cases with adhesions of the conus, filum, or cauda equina rootlets to the inner aspect of the posterior dura, usually in the lumbosacral area.

Diastematomyelia is a less common form of spinal dysraphism. The pathologic features consist of a bony or fibrocartilaginous spur that traverses the spinal canal in an anteroposterior direction in the midline (see Figure 16-6).[12–14] It is attached anteriorly to the vertebral body and posteriorly to the arch of bone constituting the back of the spinal canal. The spur may incompletely span the canal, in which case it might be based either anteriorly or posteriorly. Abnormalities such as small or hemivertebrae, disc-space narrowing, fusion of anterior or posterior elements, or transverse widening of the canal generally occur at that level. The spur characteristically divides the

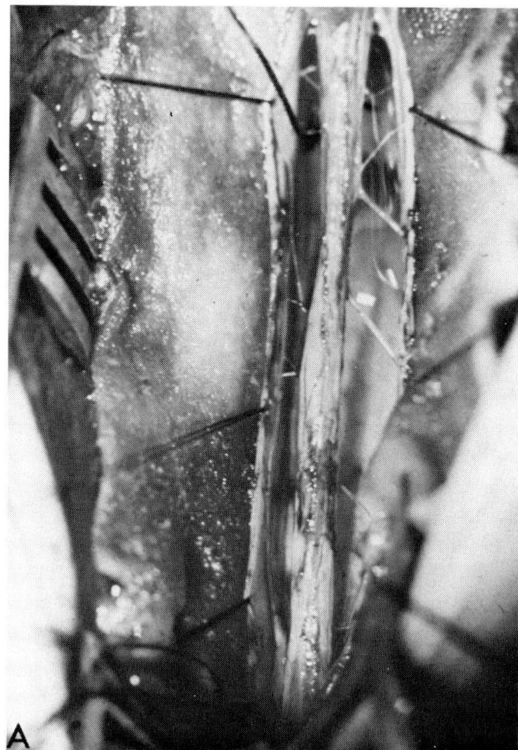

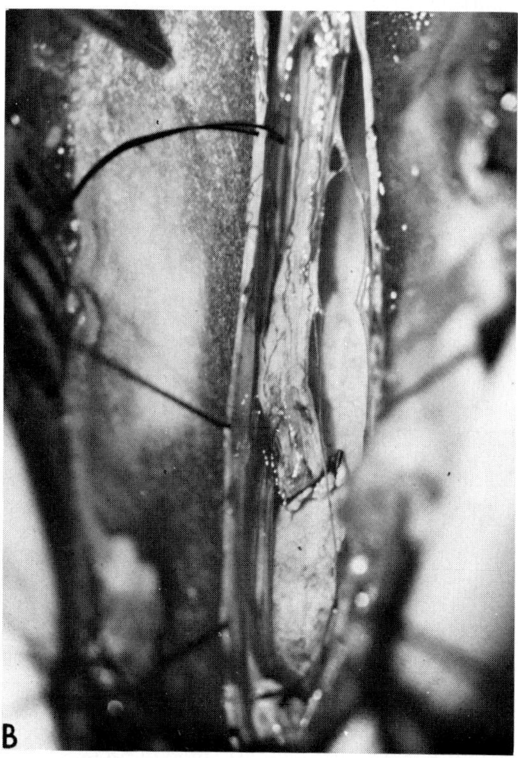

Fig. 16-2. (A) A thick filum with a low conus medullaris (top). (B) The filum shown in Figure 16-2A after division. Note the distance between the divided ends of the filum and the more vertical direction of the nerve roots, indicating upward migration of the conus and proximal filum after division of the filum.

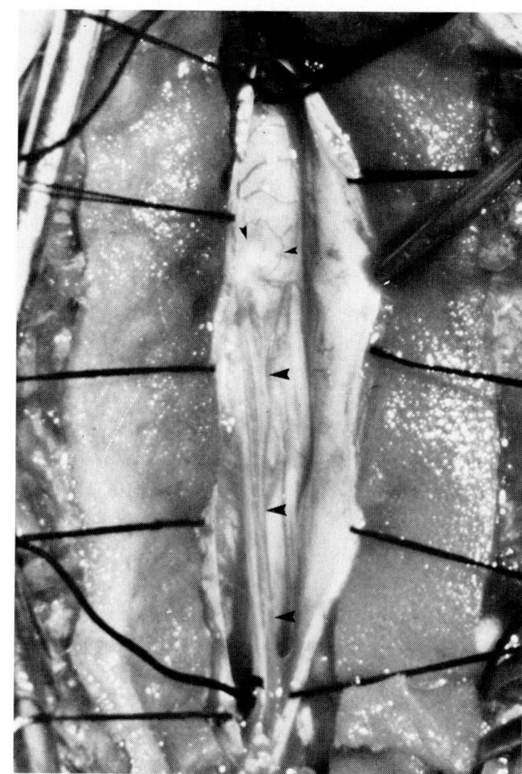

Fig. 16-3. Fibrous bands (large arrows, lower) attaching to the conus posteriorly in the region of an associated small intramedullary dermoid tumor (small arrows, upper). No sinus tract was demonstrated pathologically.

a peak incidence at L2.[15] The term *diastematomyelia* implies a division of the spinal cord into two halves. Uncommonly, one may in fact be dealing with actual duplication of the spinal cord or *diplomyelia*. Because these two conditions are indistinguishable clinically, the term diastematomyelia has been adopted by convention. Finally, diastematomyelia may occur without an associated spur or septum.

Dermal sinus, with or without a related intraspinal dermoid tumor, is found in association with occult spina bifida. The tumor is often situated partially within the substance of the spinal cord, particularly in the region of the conus. In such cases, it cannot be totally extirpated. Microscopically, these tumors consist of dermal elements, including appendages such as hair follicles with hair, sweat, and apocrine glands. Epidermoid tumors occur as well.

Although these various lesions have been described as discrete entities, the pathologic state often is more complex than such a description would indicate. There is a tendency for more than one type of lesion to occur in a single case (Figure 16-3). Thus, one occasionally finds a short, thick filum, fibrous bands, or intraspinal lipoma in the presence of diastematomyelia. Alternately, lipoma, tethering bands, and a thickened filum may occur in varying combinations. Finally, the lesions encountered are not strictly limited to those just described. Lesions such as occult meningocele and hydromyelia also have been observed either singly or in combination with the more common lesions, especially lipomas or diastematomyelia.[16] Despite the occasional lesion associated with Arnold-Chiari malformation, this hindbrain deformity generally has not been

spinal canal in a midsagittal direction, thus effectively skewering the divided cord, the halves of which rejoin above and below the spur. The spur may occur at any point along the spine but is most common in the lower thoracic and lumbar area with

found in cases of spinal dysraphism, where it has been specifically sought.[17]

The mechanism by which these diverse pathologic conditions produce neurologic impairment is unclear. Except when a mass lesion or fibrous bands exert obvious pressure on neural elements, the common denominator appears to be the immobilizing effect of the lesion on the distal spinal cord and, possibly, the nerve roots (see Figure 16-2B). It has been suggested that this prevents normal ascent of the conus with growth of the spinal cord in the canal, and that the traction thus exerted results in progressive neurologic deficits. Although the conus remains at the same vertebral level after several months of age, subsequent to that age there is relatively greater longitudinal growth of the vertebral column than of the spinal cord. In cases of caudal spinal-cord tethering, this has the effect of subjecting the cord to increasing tension, particularly during growth spurts of childhood and adolescence. In addition, a degree of mobility of distal spinal-cord elements in response to changes in position may be important. Some mobility can be demonstrated at myelography, although this alone has not provided a clear differentiation between normal and pathologic conditions. It is possible that immobilization of neural elements prevents normal protective accommodative movements in response to changes in position during activity. The possibility of vascular insult, as a result of cord immobility, also has been considered.[18,19] In this regard, Yamada et al.[20] have demonstrated reversibly impaired oxidative metabolism in the tethered cord, both experimentally and clinically.

SPINE ABNORMALITIES

The presence of spina bifida occulta is, as the name implies, an important feature in the diagnosis of this condition. Some confusion may arise in that a substantial proportion of the normal population harbors an occult spina bifida without intraspinal pathologic features. When spina bifida is a normal variant, the split element is generally at S1 and occasionally at L5. This degree of bifida has its highest incidence in early life and is more common in males. The incidence appears to vary with different racial groups.[21–24] In symptomatic spina bifida occulta associated with spinal dysraphism, spinal segments other than L5 and S1 usually are involved, often multiply, and the degree of diastasis is more pronounced. Although spina bifida may be the only demonstrable bony abnormality, other defects do occur. Examples of these were enumerated briefly in the discussion of diastematomyelia. Pang and Hoffman[25] have called attention to the possible existence of spinal-cord tethering in cases of sacral agenesis. Although uncommon, this is of particular significance since the sensorimotor and sphincter disturbances associated with this condition generally have not been considered amenable to surgery.

Although there is a general geographic relationship between the site of bony abnormality and the underlying intraspinal lesion, this is not exact. The two lesions may be separated by several segmental levels. This fact assumes importance in properly recognizing the site of an intraspinal pathologic condition at surgical exploration. It also emphasizes the need for careful preoperative radiographic evaluation.

SKIN ABNORMALITY

Cutaneous stigmata are often present and may provide a valuable clue to the problem. These abnormalities usually occur in the middle or lower back in the midline and, like the bony deformity, may not correspond to the segmental level of the intraspinal lesion. The nature of the skin lesion varies. It may consist of a circumscribed area of hyperpigmentation or capillary hemangioma. The latter is quite common as a normal variant over the inferior occipital area and is of no concern there. If such a lesion is found in the thoracic or lumbar midline region, unseen difficulties should be anticipated. There may be a hairy patch of skin, either with or without associated abnormal skin pigmentation. Hair growth can be extremely luxuriant, constituting what is aptly called a *fawn's tail*. A subcutaneous lipoma may be present. As indicated previously, such fatty masses are usually coextensive with intraspinal lipomas or other dysraphic anomalies. Other lesions associated with a subcutaneous lumbosacral mass that can be confused with lipoma include meningocele, myelocystocele, and sacrococcygeal teratoma. Myelocystocele represents a combined meningocele and focal hydromyelia. It tends to occur in association with omphalocele, bladder exstrophy, and imperforate anus.

A midline skin pore is common in association with intraspinal dermoid tumors. It represents the opening of a sinus tract that extends inward and attaches to the tumor. This tract is directed rostrally so that the skin pore lies caudal to the level of the tumor. It is important to distinguish between a true dermal sinus pore and a simple pilonidal dimple. The latter, which lies more inferiorly, usually at the tip of the coccyx, is of no consequence in the present context.

CLINICAL PRESENTATION

About two thirds of patients with spinal dysraphism are females. Although symptoms may arise at any age, most occur initially in the pediatric group. In most cases the presenting problem reflects neurologic impairment of the lower extremities or of bladder function. Gait disturbance is common and may represent simple weakness or postural deformity of one or both lower extremities, particularly distally. Equinus deformities are also common. In addition there may be shortening or wasting of the involved foot or leg. Orthopedic deformities are present at birth in some instances. Further neurologic impairment then may be superimposed on this pre-existing disability. In this context it may be difficult to detect progressive functional impairment at an early stage, especially in younger children. The problem might manifest itself, for instance, only as repeated failure of orthopedic corrections. A significant percentage of patients initially have urinary incontinence, which can be minor or severe. This problem may only become apparent when the child is well past the usual age of training, despite its presence from infancy. In infancy, patients often come to medical attention because of concern regarding the skin lesion alone. This is especially true for subcutaneous lipomas and hairy patches. At this time there is no neurologic abnormality. If the skin lesion is disregarded, the child may return later as a deficit appears, as sphincter disturbance is unmasked, or as he or she verbalizes discomfort. This shifting pattern of presenting features is well described for spinal lipomas[26] and diastematomyelia.[15] In most cases of tethered cord, the bladder dysfunction reflects partial denervation with hypotonicity and preserved sensation, although an atonic bladder can also occur.[27,28]

Although the foregoing covers the principal modes of presentation, occasionally other problems prompt initial con-

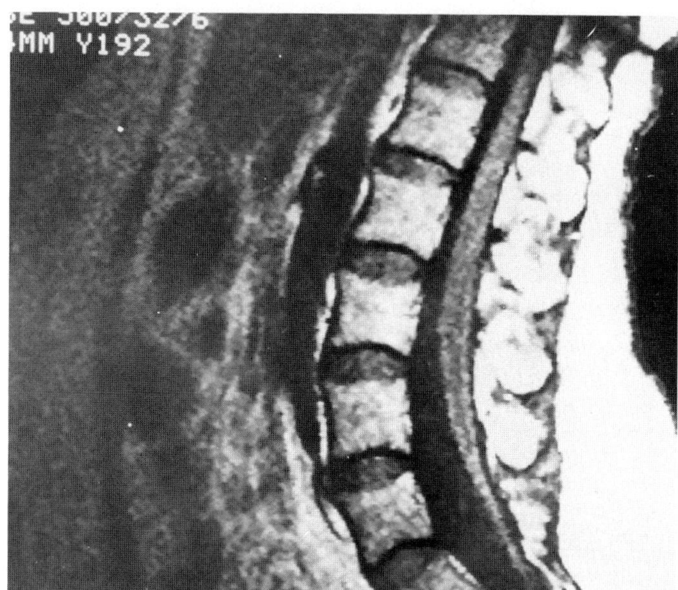

Fig. 16-4. A magnetic resonance scan of a 60-year-old woman with a thick filum terminale and recent onset of back pain, motor disturbance, and bladder dysfunction. The symptoms were relieved by surgical untethering.

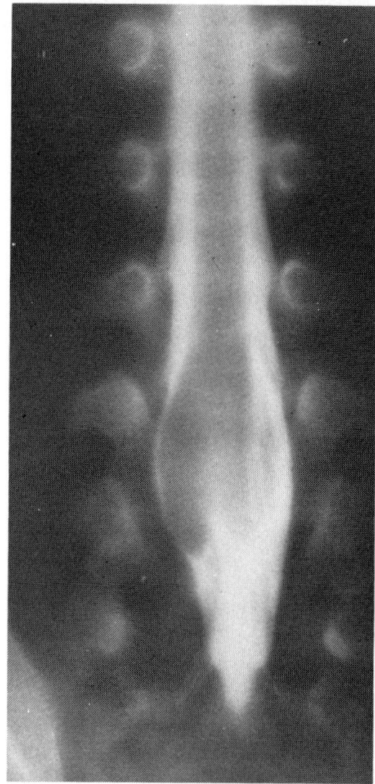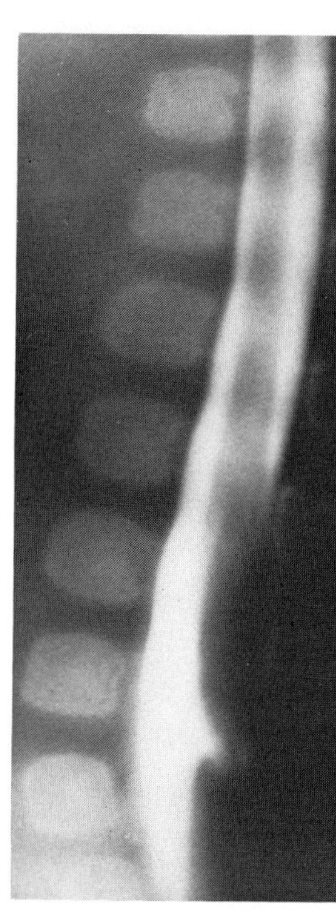

Fig. 16-5. An intraspinal lipoma with dorsal attachment to the conus medullaris.

cern. Impaired sensation in the lower extremities can result in trophic ulceration of the involved part. Septic meningitis, especially if recurrent or caused by an unusual organism, should elicit careful examination for the presence of a dermal sinus tract. Back pain may be the chief concern. This pain is characteristically exacerbated by movement or exercise and the child limits his or her activity, even though there may not be complaints about it specifically.[29] At one time it was felt that symptomatic dysraphism was exclusively a problem of childhood and adolescence. It is now recognized that symptoms may first appear in adulthood and even late life.[35] Figure 16-4 shows the MRI scan of a woman with a thick filum who initially presented at the age of 60 years with recent onset of urinary incontinence, leg weakness, and low back pain.

DIAGNOSTIC ASSESSMENT AND INDICATIONS FOR SURGERY

The initial assessment of these children requires a careful history and examination designed to detect what might be minor degrees of neurologic impairment. Any suspected case should be studied further. Also, a child with dermal sinus should be handled similarly, regardless of neurologic status. In the latter instance the high incidence of associated intraspinal tumor or potential communication with the subarachnoid space, with its attendant risk of meningitis, demands surgical intervention. An element of controversy arises regarding the proper management of patients with clinical and radiologic stigmata of spinal dysraphism but without evidence of deterioration or neurologic deficit. In cases of spinal lipoma, delayed neurologic deterioration is well documented, both in childhood[26,30–33] and in adult life.[34,35] This common phenomenon reflects our own experience. Because of such cases, we feel that the presence of a lumbosacral lipoma per se is an indication for further investigation and surgery. This opinion is shared by others,[26,36]

including Till,[4] who further felt that any child with clinical and radiologic stigmata of spinal dysraphism should undergo myelography, regardless of neurologic status. If the radiographic studies show either a specific lesion or a low conus, then surgical exploration is warranted. This view represents an extension of the concept of prophylactic surgery for all patients with spinal dysraphism. It is based on the observation that neurologic deficits that occur, even under close follow-up, cannot predictably be reversed by subsequent surgery. Implied is the fact that surgery, when properly executed, has a sufficiently low risk to warrant such action. Till[37] reviewed his own extensive experience with regard to the question of prophylactic surgery. In a detailed review of 65 cases of diastematomyelia, Kennedy[15] reached similar conclusions with respect to that condition. These considerations regarding preventative surgery do not apply to adults in whom surgery should be considered only on indication of progressive symptomatology.

SPECIAL RADIOGRAPHIC STUCIES

Because of the diverse and often complex intraspinal pathologic features associated with spinal dysraphism, it is important to gain maximum information from radiographic studies before surgical exploration. To do so requires a technique that clearly defines the structures within the caudal spinal canal. Iophendylate (Pantopaque, Lafayette Pharmaceutical, Inc.), introduced by the lumbar route, frequently has been used[17,36] but has several disadvantages. Because it is a dense contrast medium, structures, such as fibrous bands, tracts, or a thickened filum may be poorly visualized. The level of termination of the conus may not be apparent. The position of the conus is important. A low lying conus represents a more or less constant pathologic concomitant of spinal dysraphism and may

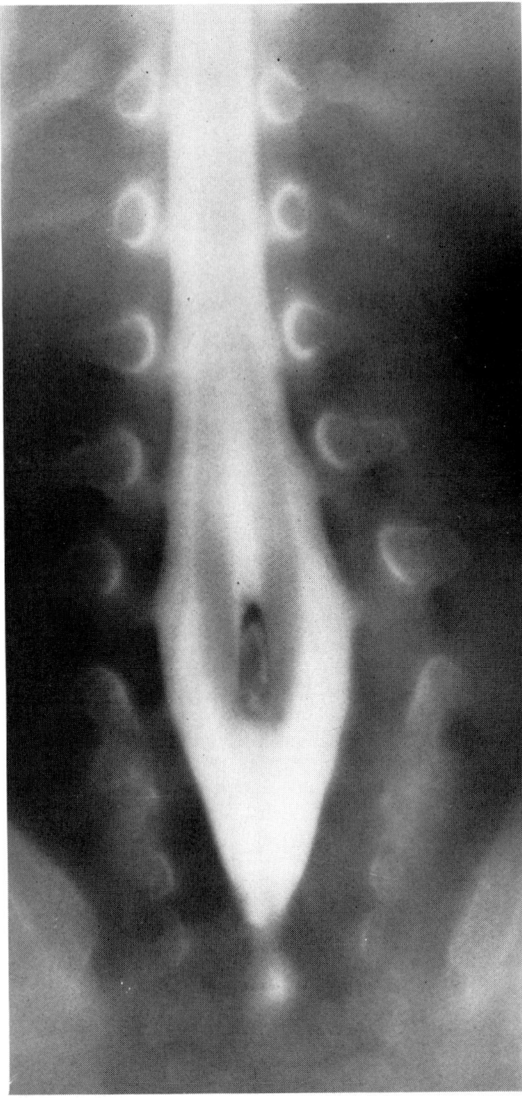

Fig. 16-6. Diastematomyelia of the lower lumbar region demonstrated by metrizamide-enhanced myelography.

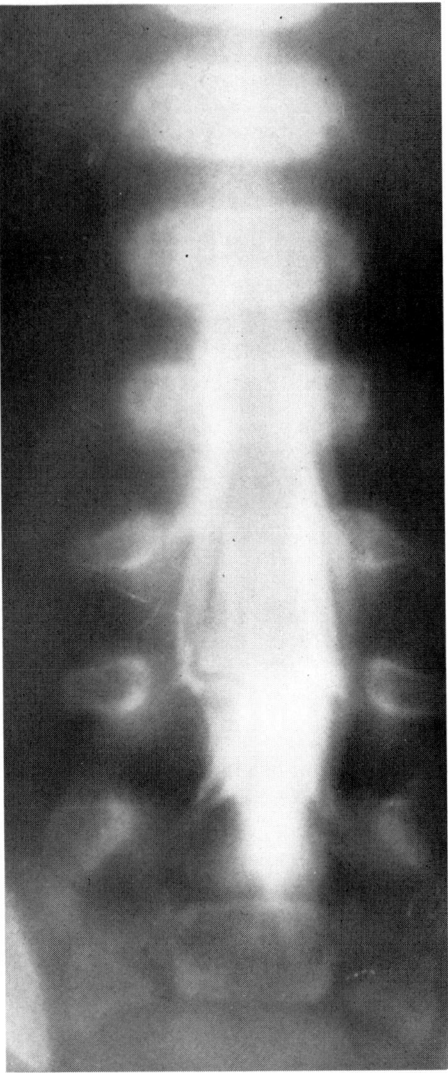

Fig. 16-7. An intraspinal lipoma with a major artery to the conus medullaris demonstrated by myelography. The vascular nature of the structure was confirmed at surgery.

be the only abnormality found on a myelogram. Puncturing the spinal canal in an area where displaced neural tissue may be situated logically presents the risk of injury to these structures. Finally, it may be difficult to enter the subarachnoid space, especially if a lipoma is present. Introducing the contrast by cisternal tap[17] presents problems in retrieving the substance.

Air myelography[4] represented a partial solution to these problems but has been superceded by computed tomographic scanning with intrathecal water-soluble contrast agents and, most recently, by magnetic resonance imaging (MRI). Conventional myelography with water-soluble contrast agents can also be performed but gives less anatomic detail, which may be important in the surgical approach to complex cases (Figures 16-5 through 16-7). Computed tomography and magnetic resonance imaging techniques also have the advantage of providing axial as well as sagittal and coronal projections (Figure 16-8).[38,39] High resolution MRI scanning is noninvasive and gives detailed three-dimensional information. With improved availability it will undoubtedly supplant other types of radiographic studies.

SURGICAL TECHNIQUE

Successful surgery of spinal dysraphism depends upon a detailed knowledge of the pathologic anatomy that will be encountered, especially when lesions are complex or multiple. In spite of preoperative studies, however, one often must rely on surgical observation to clarify the anatomic details. Intraoperative nerve stimulation is an important adjunct in this regard. It is of considerable help in identifying and avoiding injury to important neural structures, particularly in cases where anatomic relationships are seriously distorted. The patient is draped to allow examination of the feet and legs during stimulation. Electronic twitch monitors can also be placed on the toes to detect slight movement in response to stimulation. Manometric monitoring of bladder tone in response to stimulation may be helpful. At present, we also monitor bladder and rectal sphincter EMG responses using a ring electrode catheter and surface needle electrodes, respectively. The anesthetic technique should avoid the use of muscle relaxants, which might mask motor responses. In addition to nerve stimulation, we

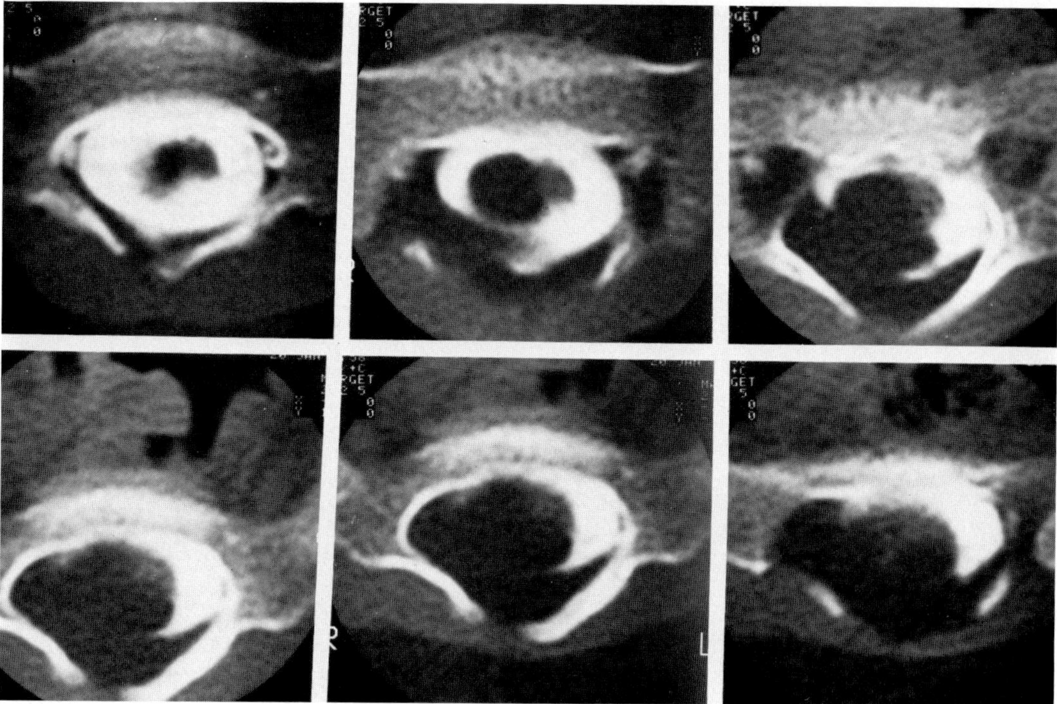

Fig. 16-8. Axial CT scans with intrathecal contrast showing the complex anatomic relationships of an intraspinal lipoma. (Reprinted from Raimondi AJ (ed): Concepts in Pediatric Neurosurgery, Volume 3. Basel: S. Karger AG, 1983, p 187. With permission.)

have occasionally used intraoperative recording of either cortical or spinal epidural evoked potentials. Such recording is useful principally to assess the effects of surgical manipulations rather than to identify neural elements. In view of the importance of accurate operative observations, we feel that microsurgical techniques should be used routinely.

The principle of surgery is usually to relieve the mechanical constraint exerted by the intraspinal lesion on the conus or nerve roots. In its simplest form this involves merely dividing a thickened filum or the tethering bands (see Figure 16-2). The filum should be sectioned well caudal to the point of emergence of the lowermost nerve roots. If the attenuated conus extends far distally, it may be necessary to divide the stalk virtually at its point of insertion into the dural cul-de-sac. There is often a small lipoma in continuity with the stalk at this point. The tethering bands of a *meningocele manqué* may be divided quite easily, or they may represent substantial displaced neural elements attached to the posterior dura, in which case it is advisable to free them by actually sectioning the dura itself. Occasionally one finds the conus and filum adherent to the inner aspect of the posterior dura over a considerable distance. Freeing neural elements in this circumstance represents a formidable and tedious surgical task. It is probably wisest, if possible, to excise the dura circumferentially about the point of attachment in order to free the conus. Dural closure then will require a watertight graft.

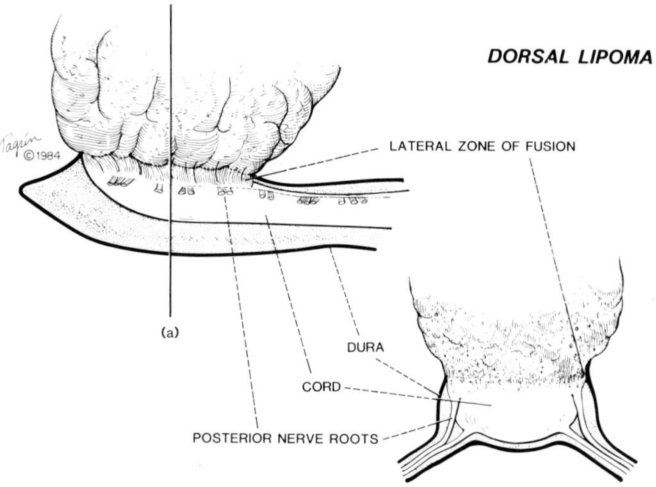

Fig. 16-9. Diagram of a dorsal lipoma.

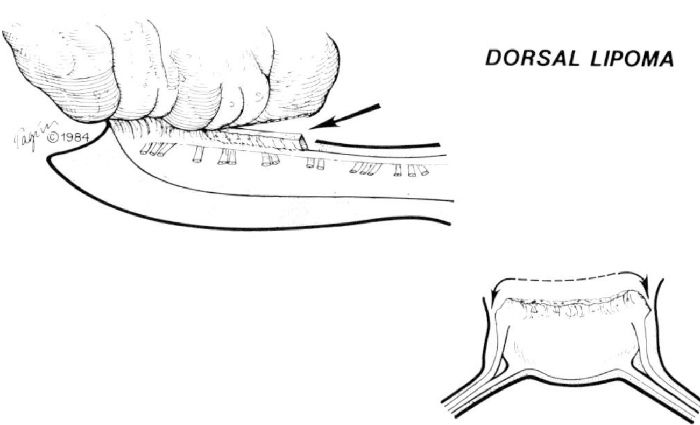

Fig. 16-10. Surgical steps in untethering a dorsal lipoma. Detaching the subcutaneous mass and releasing the circumferential zone of fusion at the edges of the dorsal defect.

CAUDAL LIPOMA

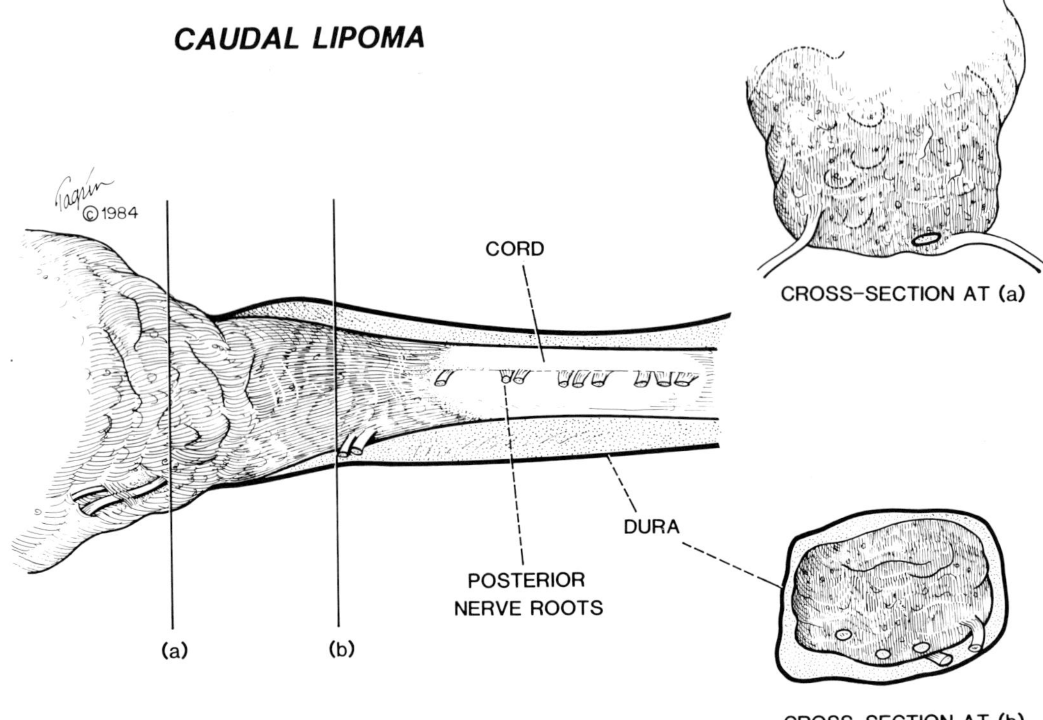

Fig. 16-11.   Diagram of a caudal lipoma.

In cases of diastematomyelia, the bony or fibrocartilaginous septum at the midline is excised along with the dural sleeve. It is not necessary to close the anterior dural defect. With spurs in the lumbar area one may find small, aberrant nerve roots, occasionally with dorsal root ganglia, entering the dural sleeve at the midline from the medial aspect of each hemicord. These nerve roots may end blindly or may re-enter the dura distally. It is generally necessary to sacrifice these structures in order to eliminate the midline septum. Finally, one must be alert to the fact that diastematomyelia at any point along the spine may be associated with caudal tethering of the conus because of a thickened filum or a lipoma in continuity with the conus. This should be detected on preoperative myelograms. If overlooked, it can cause functional deterioration at a later date, even though the bony spur has been dealt with successfully. Depending upon the level of the diastematomyelia, it may be necessary to correct the caudal tethering in a second operation.

Dermoid tumors, along with their associated dermal sinus tracts, should be excised in toto where possible in view of their propensity to recur. They may, however, be intimately associated with the conus (see Figure 16-3), making attempts at total excision inadvisable. Intraspinal lipoma represent a special problem.[10] The interface of the lipoma with neural tissue is often complex and indistinct, and nerve roots of the cauda equina may traverse its substance. The goal of surgery remains, however, to relieve the restraining influence the lipoma exerts on the distal spinal cord. This requires freeing the conus from the mass of the lipoma by dividing its fibrofatty attachment within the spinal canal (see Figure 16-1). In doing this, it is not necessary to completely eliminate the lipoma from the cord substance; in fact, attempts to do so are unnecessarily hazardous. Merely excising the extradural mass without freeing the conus intradurally does not relieve the problem and leaves the patient with a risk of subsequent neurologic deterioration. As previously described, the lipoma may insert into the posterior aspect of conus via a dural defect (Figure 16-9). This attachment usually is quite fibrous in its central portion and may contain substantial blood vessels. The edge of the dural defect is fused circumferentially to the conus–lipoma interface and the posterior rootlets lie just ventral to the line of fusion. Initially one opens the dura just rostral to the lipoma and identifies the conus. The dural opening is then continued caudally on either side of the point of entrance of the lipoma stalk so that the lipoma–conus interface can be identified. This attachment then is divided rostrocaudally. As this is done, the posterolateral line of attachment is progressively divided as well, first on one side, then on the other. The posterior rootlets provide a useful orientating landmark when doing this. Care must be taken to completely transect the caudal point of fixation of the conus in order to achieve a satisfactory result (Figure 16-10A,B).

CAUDAL LIPOMA

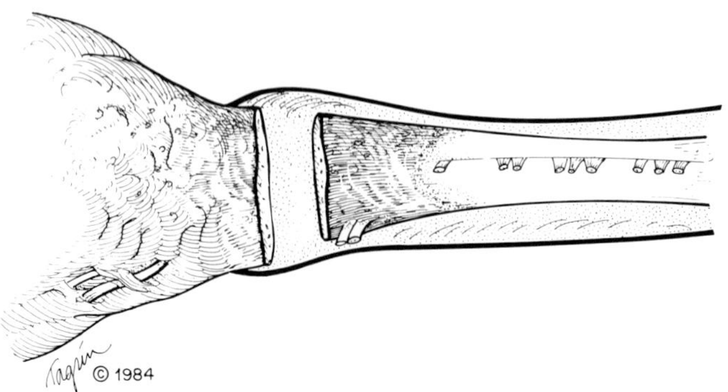

Fig. 16-12.   Surgical detachment of a caudal lipoma.

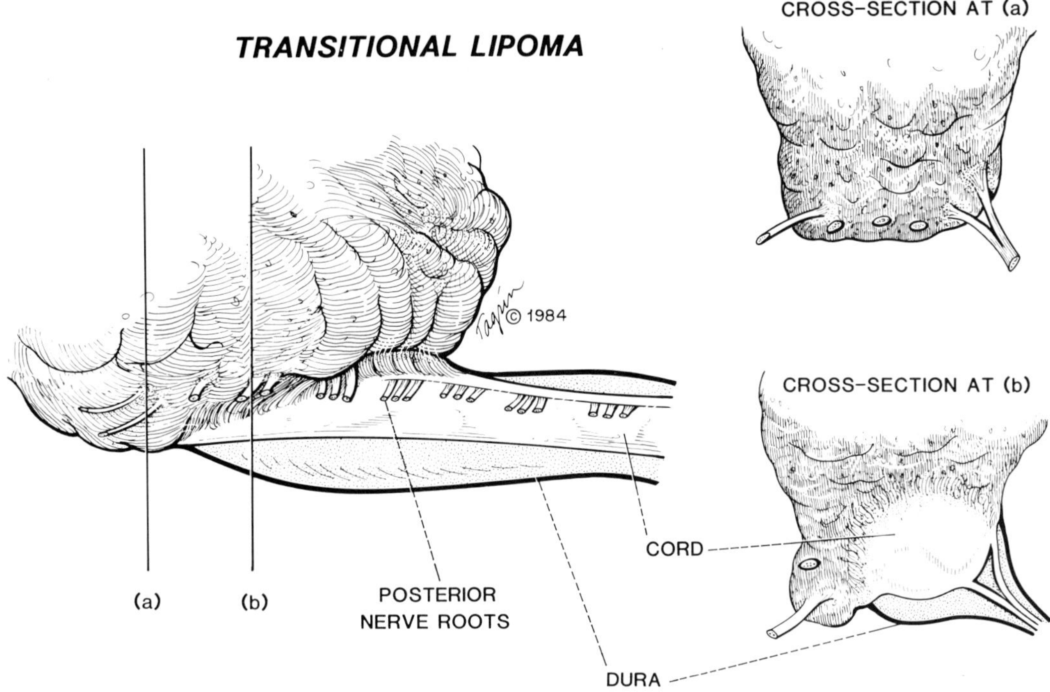

Fig. 16-13. Diagram of a transitional form of lipoma with features of both the dorsal and caudal varieties. Note the axial asymmetry of this lesion.

If a lipoma attaches to the distal extremity of the conus (Figure 16-11) and emerges from the dura caudally in the cul-de-sac or laterally to either side, one can expect nerve roots to traverse its substance. This circumstance presents a more serious surgical challenge and requires sparing all but the most caudal, rudimentary rootlets while progressively transecting the lipoma. Substantial arteries that might be critical to the blood supply of the conus should be sought and spared (see Figure 16-7). The conus should be circumferentially freed of all fibrous attachments to the lipoma as well as the adjacent dura before transecting the mass as far caudal as possible (Figure 16-12). Often one finds an admixture of the two lipoma types. Rostrally, the lipoma attaches to the posterior aspect of the conus so that the emerging rootlets are outside of its substance. As one proceeds caudally, however, elements of the fatty mass are found to insert into the distal or lateral dura in the region of the

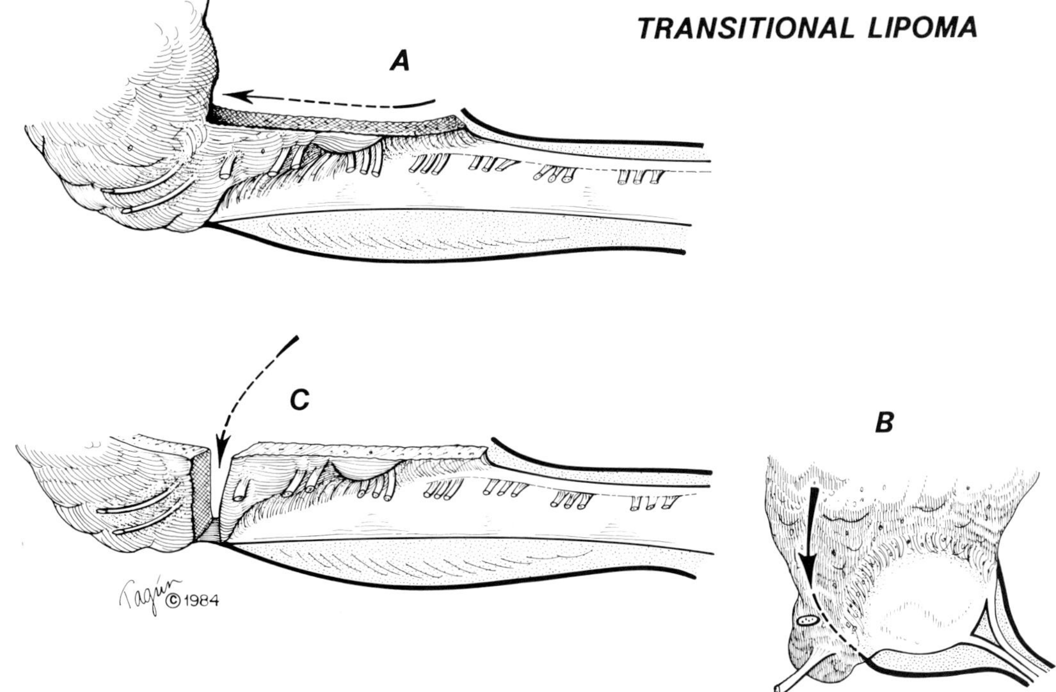

Fig. 16-14. Surgical steps in the release of a transitional lipoma.

neural foramina, with nerve roots traversing the mass accordingly (Figure 16-13). This situation can be anticipated by a careful study of the preoperative radiographs, with attention given to the relationship of the lipoma to the conus within the spinal canal. Surgically, such a lesion is approached as described above by adapting technique to the circumstances (Figure 16-14). Once the conus has been successfully untethered, it will relax anteriorly in the spinal canal and usually will migrate upward somewhat as well. During the dissection, any bulk of fatty tissue that is contiguous with the conus can be removed if necessary. The CO_2 laser and ultrasonic aspirator are quite useful for this. Cerebrospinal fluid leak is the most common complication of surgery. This is facilitated by the congenital absence of dura, particularly in cases of spinal lipoma. Careful attention must be given to obtaining a relaxed watertight dural closure using a dural graft if necessary. It is useful, during the initial exposure, to spare tissues that later can serve to buttress a tight wound closure.

RESULTS AND FOLLOW-UP

Most authors report some cases of improved sphincter or sensorimotor function after surgery. As a rule, however, surgery should not be undertaken in anticipation of achieving neurologic improvement. Rather it should be performed to prevent further deterioration. As stated previously, the rationale for prophylactic surgery rests, in part, upon this fact. It also implies that surgery should not be delayed once any degree of progressive impairment of sphincter or limb function is recognized in patients chosen for follow-up without initial studies. Finally, occasional instances of delayed postoperative deterioration in function have been reported. The deterioration may be the result of a previously undetected lesion, such as a thickened filum accompanying a treated diastematomyelia. Such cases warrant reinvestigation. In isolated instances of intraspinal lipoma one may find further worsening of a pes cavus foot deformity, which had been progressive pre-operatively. This can occur after seemingly satisfactory cord untethering. Despite one's best surgical efforts, retethering can occur, especially in the case of extensive lipomas of the transitional variety. In such circumstances, reoperation may be required to relieve progressive symptoms.

CONCLUSION

In summary, successful management of the patient with spinal dysraphism demands proper regard for the underlying problem. This requires, in the first instance, recognition of the true nature of the difficulties, which, at first glance, may appear to be orthopedic, urologic, or cosmetic. Early attention to lesions that will cause progressive deficits is vital. Finally, the surgeon dealing with these lesions must respect their often complex nature and the technical difficulties implicit in surgery. In such cases a thorough understanding of the pathologic anatomy, aided by appropriate preoperative studies, is necessary.

REFERENCES

1. Ingraham FD: Spina Bifida and Cranium Bifidum. Cambridge, Harvard University Press, 1944
2. James CCM, Lassman LP: Spinal dysraphism. An orthopedic syndrome in children accompanying occult forms. Arch Dis Child 35:315, 1960
3. James CCM, Lassman LP: Spinal Dysraphism. Spina Bifida Occulta. London, Butterworths, 1972
4. Till K: Spinal dysraphism. A study of congenital malformations of the lower back. J Bone Joint Surg 51B:415, 1969
5. Anderson FM: Occult spinal dysraphism: A series of 73 cases. Pediatrics 55:826, 1975
6. Reimann AF, Anson BJ: Vertebral level of termination of the spinal cord with report of a case of sacral cord. Anat Rec 88:127, 1944
7. Barson AJ: Vertebral level of termination of spinal cord during normal and abnormal development. J Anat 106:489, 1969
8. Emery JL, Lendon RG: Lipoma of the cauda equina and other fatty tumors related to neurospina dysraphism. Dev Med Child Neurol (Suppl) 20:62, 1969
9. Walsh JW, Markesbery WR: Histological features of congenital lipomas of the lower spina canal. J Neurosurg 52:564, 1980
10. Chapman PH: Congenital intraspinal lipomas. Anatomic considerations and surgical treatment. Childs Brain 9:37, 1982
11. Lassman LP, James CCM: Meningocoele manqué . Childs Brain 3:1, 1977
12. Naidich TP, Harwood-Nash DC: Diastematomyelia: Hemicord and meningeal sheaths; single and double arachnoid and dural tubes. AJNR 4:633, 1983
13. Houd RW, Riseborough EJ, Nehme AM, et al: Diastematomyelia and structural spine deformities. J Bone Joint Surg 62A:520, 1980
14. Guthkelch AN: Diastematomyelia with median septum. Brain 97:729, 1974
15. Kennedy PR: New data on diastematomyelia. J Neurosurg 51:355, 1979
16. Linder M, Rosenstein J, Sklar FH: Functional improvement after spinal surgery for the dysraphic malformation. Neurosurgery 11:622, 1982
17. Gryspeerdt GL: Myelographic assessment of occult forms of spinal dysraphism. Acta Radiol (Diagn) 1:702, 1963
18. Fitz CR, Harwood-Nash DC: The tethered conus. Am J Roentgenol Rad Ther Nucl Med 125:515, 1975
19. Beyerl B, Ojemann R, Davis KR, et al: Adult cervical diastematomyelia. Case report. J Neurosurg 62:449, 1985
20. Yamada S, Zinke DE, Sanders D: Pathophysiology of "tethered cord syndrome." J Neurosurg 54:494, 1981
21. Fawcitt J: Some radiological aspects of congenital anomalies of the spine in childhood and infancy. Proc R Soc Med 52:331, 1959
22. Lorber J, Levick K: Spina bifida cystica. Incidence of spina bifida occulta in parents and in controls. Arch Dis Child 42:171, 1967
23. Manley CB, Frech RS: Urinary tract infections in girls: Prevalence of spina bifida occulta. J Urol 103:348, 1970
24. Sutow WW, Pryde AW: Incidence of spina bifida occulta in relation to age. Am J Dis Child 91:211, 1956
25. Pang D, Hoffman HJ: Sacral agenesis with progressive neurologic deficit. Neurosurgery 7:118, 1980
26. Bruce DA, Schut L: Spinal lipomas in infancy and chiidhood. Childs Brain 5:192, 1979
27. Pavlakis AJ, Siroky MG, Goldstein I, et al: Neurologic findings in conus medullaris and cauda equina injury. Arch Neurol 40:570, 1983
28. Borzyskowski M, Neville BGR: Neuropathic bladder and spinal dysraphism. Arch Dis Child 56:176, 1981
29. Hoffman HJ, Hendrick EB, Humphrey RP: The tethered spinal cord. Its protean manifestations, diagnosis, and surgical correction. Childs Brain 2:145, 1976
30. Swanson HS, Barnett JC Jr: Intradural lipomas in children. Pediatrics 29:911, 1962
31. Dubowitz V, Lorber J, Zachary RB: Lipoma of the cauda equina. Arch Dis Child 40:207, 1965
32. Yashon D, Beatty RA: Tethering of the conus medullaris within the sacrum. J Neurol Neurosurg Psychiatry 29:244, 1966
33. Hoffman HJ, Taecholarn C, Hendrick EB, et al: The management

of lipomyelomeningoceles: Experience at the Hospital for Sick Children, Toronto. J Neurosurg 62:1, 1985

34. Loeser JD, Lewin RJ: Lumbosacral lipoma in the adult. Case report. J Neurosurg 29:405, 1968

35. Pang D, Wilberger JE: Tethered cord syndrome in adults. J Neurosurg 57:32, 1982

36. Villarejo FJ, Blazquez MG, Gutierrez-Diaz JA: Intraspinal lipomas in children. Childs Brain 2:361, 1976

37. Till K: Occult spinal dysraphism. The value of prophylactic surgical treatment, in Recent Progress in Neurological Surgery. Amsterdam, Excerpta Medica, 1973, pp 61–66

38. Naidach TP, Harwood-Nash DC, McClone DG: Radiology of spinal dysraphism. Clin Neurosurg 30:341, 1982

39. Naidach TP, McClone DG, Mutluer J: A new understanding of dorsal dysraphism with lipoma (lipomyeloschisis). Radiologic evaluation and surgical correction. AJNR 4:103, 1983

CHAPTER 17

Spinal Cord Tumors in Children

Fred J. Epstein   Jeffrey H. Wisoff

INTRAMEDULLARY SPINAL CORD ASTROCYTOMAS are uncommon neoplasms, accounting for 4 percent of all central nervous system tumors in children[16] and less than 10 percent of all CNS tumors in adults.[7,8] Patients frequently have minor clinical signs and symptoms and a radiographic picture of a diffusely widened spinal cord. The "traditional" approach to neurosurgical management is based on the assumption that it is not feasible to carry out extensive removal of the tumor within the centrum of the spinal cord without the great likelihood of inflicting additional neurologic injury. Faced with the clinical dilemma of an extensive tumor in a functional or nearly functional patient, a temporizing approach has been advocated, consisting of a laminectomy, dural decompression, and biopsy and the use of radiation therapy to control tumor growth.

The natural history of these tumors after radiation therapy unfortunately is one of progressive neurologic disability or death. This clinical course must be regarded as particularly tragic since most of these neoplasms are low grade gliomas and are microscopically identical to their "sister" tumors in the cerebellum, which are surgically curable. It was this perspective that encouraged the senior author to explore the technical feasibility of gross total excision of spinal cord astrocytomas. In this endeavor, 120 children underwent gross total excision of intramedullary astrocytomas over the past 6 years (1980–1986). This unusual series has provided a unique opportunity to use recent innovations in surgical technology and neurodiagnostic imaging to develop a radical surgical approach to intramedullary spinal cord tumors.

CLINICAL PRESENTATION

Clinical symptoms were often present from months to years before neurosurgical consultation.[1,2,9,10] In some cases the course was punctuated by exacerbations and remissions, possibly related to varying degrees of peritumoral edema.[1,2] Spinal pain caused by distention of the dura by a spinal cord expanded by tumor was the most common pain syndrome.[10] It was of a dull aching quality and was localized to the bony segments adjacent to the tumor. In some infants and young children pain from a distended dural tube with secondary rigidity and paravertebral spasm may be the initial symptom complex.[1,2,11,12,13]

Radiculopathy was present 10 percent of the time, was usually limited to one or two cervical dermatomes, and was similar to root pain from a variety of disease processes.[10] A sharp sensory level occurred less frequently with intramedullary tumors than with extramedullary lesions. Painful

dysesthesias occurred in 5 percent of the cases and were generally described as painful hot or cold sensations in one or more extremities. In rare circumstances, this was the primary symptom complex and was not associated with any signs of neurologic dysfunction. Paresthesias were occasionally associated with dysesthetic pain, and both of these symptoms were more common with neoplasms in the cervical spinal cord than with those in the thoracic spinal cord.

CERVICAL TUMORS

The most common early symptoms were nuchal pain and head tilt with torticollis. Mild upper extremity monoparesis was the next most common symptom and was often extremely subtle during the early stages of the illness. In young children, the first manifestation of weakness very often was a switching "handedness" in right-handed or left-handed patients. Neoplasms in the caudal cervical spinal cord commonly caused weakness and atrophy of the intrinsic muscles of the hand in contradistinction to tumors rostral to C5, which were less likely to cause significant weakness until relatively late in the clinical course. Interestingly, weakness of the lower extremities only evolved months or, rarely, 2 to 3 years after the first symptoms, and bowel and bladder dysfunction was rarely present at the time of primary diagnosis.

Sensory abnormalities were generally limited to one upper extremity, and a discrete sensory level was only noted very late in the course of the disease and then only in association with severe neurologic disability. In most patients, there was increased reflex activity in the lower extremities with or without extensor plantar signs and clonus.

THORACIC TUMORS

Mild scoliosis was the most common early sign of an intramedullary thoracic cord neoplasm. Pain and paraspinal muscle spasm commonly occurred before there were objective signs of neurologic dysfunction and were commonly assumed to be secondary to the evolving scoliosis. Insidious progressive motor weakness in the lower extremities was first manifest by "awkwardness" and only later by frequent falls and an obvious limp. Early sensory abnormalities were uncommon, although dysesthesias and paresthesias were occasionally present. Increased reflexes and extensor plantar signs, with or without clonus, occurred relatively early in the neurologic course.

An initial complaint of bowel and bladder dysfunction was most unusual and was diagnostic of a neoplasm extending into

OPERATIVE NEUROSURGICAL TECHNIQUES
ISBN 0-8089-1862-1

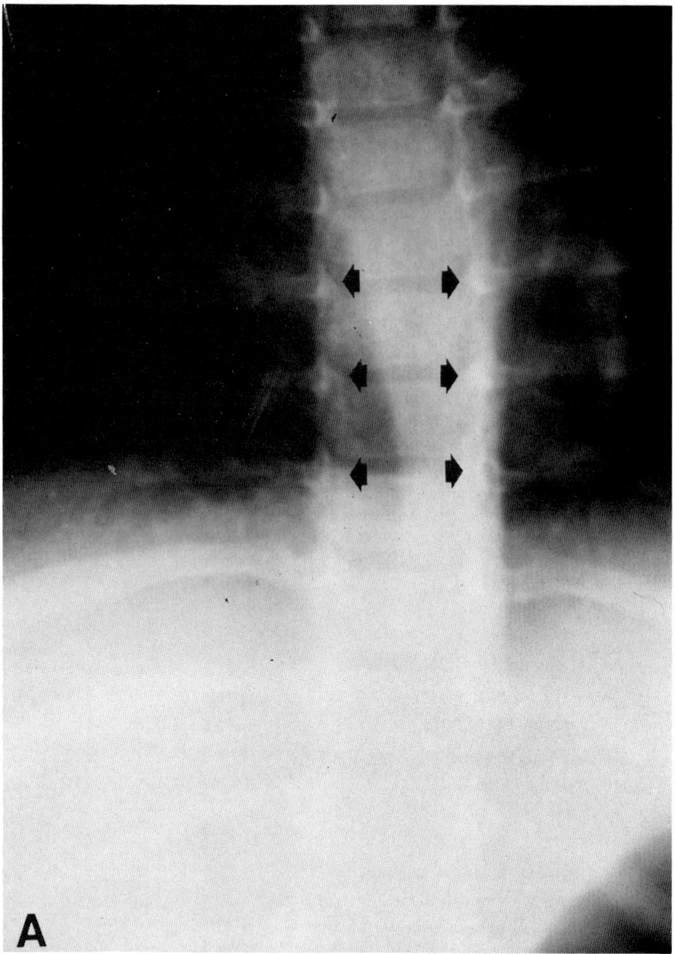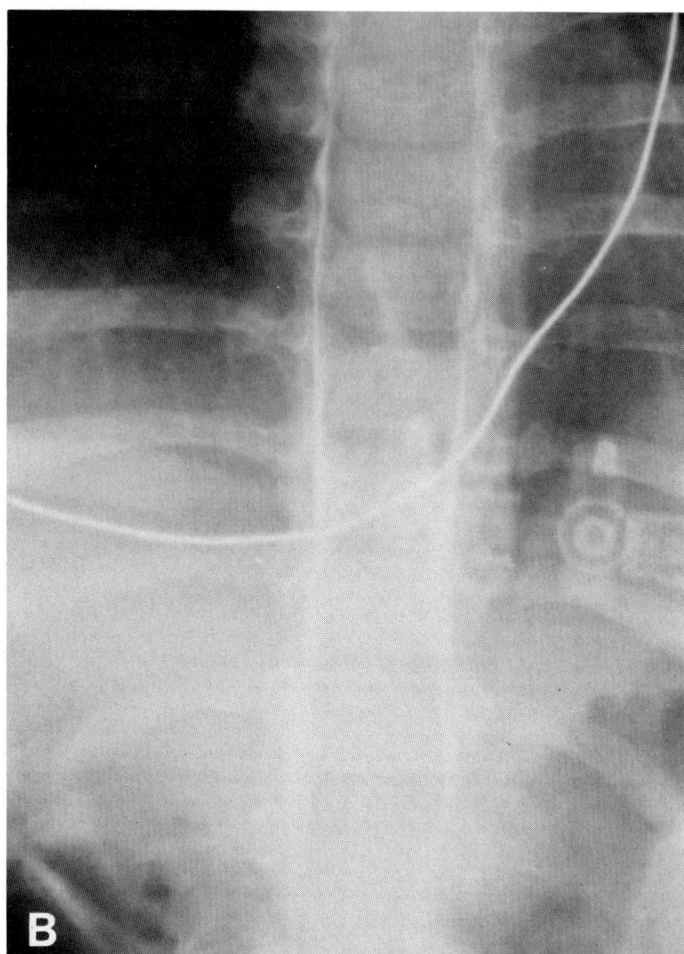

Fig. 17-1. (A) An AP x-ray film of the thoracic spine. (B) A metrizamide-enhanced myelogram. Note the diffusely widened canal with flattened pedicles (arrows) over the three to four segments corresponding to the solid tumor.

the conus. In general, these symptoms evolved only late in the clinical course if the tumor was rostral to the conus medullaris.

NEURODIAGNOSTIC EVALUATION

Spinal cord astrocytomas can be divided into two general categories, holocord and focal. Holocord widening occurred in approximately 60 percent of the pediatric spinal cord astrocytomas in this series.[11,14]

The first patients that had surgery for a presumed holocord neoplasm underwent a total laminectomy from C2 to L1.[15] It was subsequently recognized that much of the cord widening was secondary to rostral and caudal cysts, the walls of which were nonneoplastic. It therefore was subsequently recognized that it was only necessary to perform a limited laminectomy over the solid component of the neoplasm as documented by preoperative neurodiagnostic studies.[8,11]

Holocord Astrocytoma

Holocord astrocytomas were invariably cystic astrocytomas in which the solid component of the neoplasm spanned a variable length of the cord and was associated with huge nonneoplastic rostral and caudal cysts, which expanded the central canal above and below the tumor.

Plain spine x-ray films commonly disclosed a diffusely widened spinal canal, scoliosis, and relatively localized erosion or flattening of the pedicles.[1,2,10,16] Whereas widening of the spinal canal was secondary to long-standing expansion of the entire spinal cord, erosion or flattening of the pedicles occurred only adjacent to the solid component of the neoplasm (Figure 17-1).[4,11,12,14,15,17]

Although there were occasional early case reports of holocord widening, its relative frequency was probably not recognized because of the tendency to terminate neurodiagnostic studies when a lumbar myelogram disclosed a complete block secondary to an intramedullary neoplasm.[2,16] In the first patients in this series a cervical puncture was employed to identify the rostral extent of cord widening. It was subsequently recognized that although not apparent on myelograms, a small amount of metrizamide almost invariably "trickled" past the block and was obvious on the immediate or delayed spinal CT scan, which therefore defined the rostral extent of the expanded cord. A 12- to 24-hour delayed spinal CT scan may be helpful, since rostral and caudal as well as occasional intratumor cysts were identified as the water-soluble contrast medium diffused into them (Figure 17-2). It is for this reason that the availability of computed tomography (CT) of the spine is an invaluable adjunct to the neurodiagnostic evaluation of spinal cord tumors.

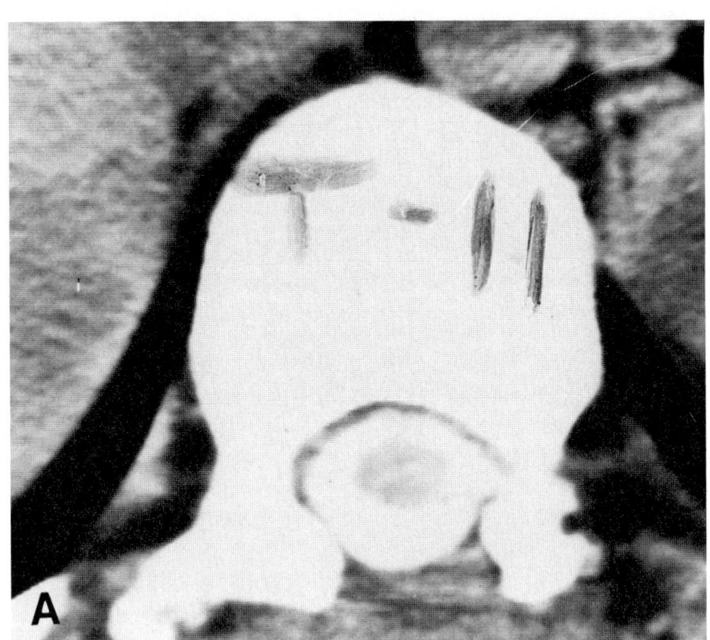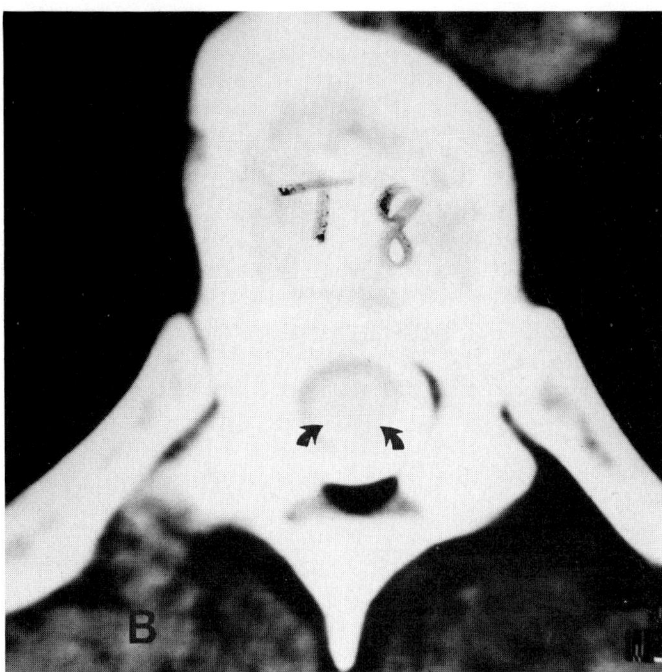

Fig. 17-2. (A) A CT scan obtained immediately after a myelogram, and (B) a CT scan obtained 12 hours later demonstrating an intramedullary cyst (arrows).

Focal Astrocytoma

Focal spinal cord astrocytomas were generally four to eight segments in length and commonly associated with flattening of the pedicles immediately adjacent to the neoplasm. In some cases, changes noted on plain films were as helpful in tumor localization as those noted on myleograms (although obviously never a substitute).

Focal astrocytomas were associated with a total subarachnoid block in 90 percent of cases and for this reason immediate and delayed CT scans were necessary to define the rostral extent of cord expansion. Intratumor cysts were rarely present in the previously unoperated and nonirradiated patient.

When available, MRI scanning with surface coils provides excellent definition of intramedullary neoplasms, and complete neuroradiologic evaluation can be performed with a MRI scan alone (Figure 17-3). It is essential to obtain a midsagittal view; this will occasionally be impossible in the presence of significant scoliosis or kyphosis.

Transcutaneous Ultrasonography

With patients who have had previous laminectomy, transcutaneous real time ultrasonography can be used to visualize the spinal cord and the neoplasm.[18] Ultrasonography may be more informative than conventional myelography, metrizamide CT scanning, or MRI scanning because it gives a direct view of the interior of the spinal cord. Real-time ultrasonography is performed utilizing 5.0 and 7.5 MHz transducers in both the sagittal and transverse projections. In occasional cases the tumor may be echogenic, affording a dramatic view of the neoplasm and its relationship to the spinal cord. The presence of cysts either within the tumor or at the rostral and caudal poles of the neoplasm is readily demonstrated (Figure 17-4A). Eighteen months or longer after radiation therapy there commonly appear multiple intratumoral cysts, which produce a "Swiss cheese" appearance (Figure 17-4A,B). The limitation of the technique is the length of the laminectomy, making it impossible to visualize the spinal cord rostral or caudal to the previous operative exposure.

OPERATIVE PROCEDURE

Intraoperative somatosensory evoked potentials are routinely used in our institution. However, this information is only valuable if it is immediately available and utilized by the surgeon to modify the operative dissection. Monitoring instruments that utilize optimized digital filtering for averaging the evoked potentials have the advantage of providing information updates every 5 to 10 seconds and of detecting evoked potentials less than 0.10 microvolts (e.g., Cordis Brain State Analyzer). The more common systems used in clinical practice update information every 2 or more minutes and require evoked potentials with amplitudes greater than 0.25 microvolts. These systems are unsatisfactory for intramedullary tumor surgery.

After the laminectomy is performed, the wound is filled with saline to allow intraoperative ultrasonography to confirm that the exposure encompasses the entire length of solid tumor. With a 5 MHz transducer probe the spinal cord is imaged in both the sagittal and transverse planes. The rostral and caudal ends of the tumor and the presence of rostral, caudal, and intratumoral cysts are immediately obvious. If the laminectomy is not long enough to expose the entire length of the solid neoplasm, additional laminae are removed with serial ultrasound guidance to limit excessive removal of bone (Figure 17-5A).

The dura is opened over the entire length of solid tumor as documented by the ultrasound. The spinal cord is commonly swollen, rotated, and distorted and it is essential to identify normal landmarks before placing the myelotomy. Since the posterior median raphe is generally obliterated it is important to

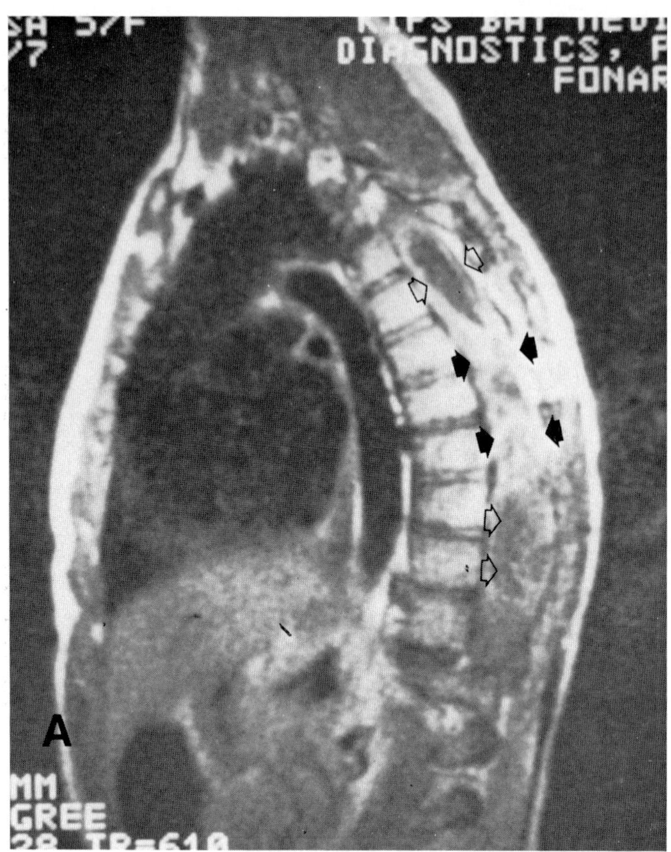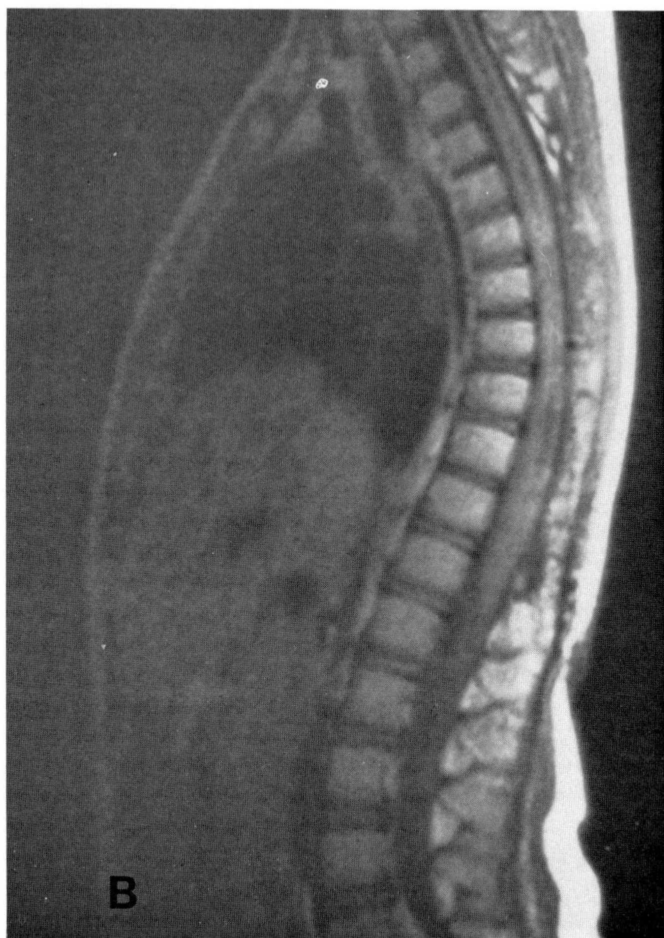

Fig. 17-3. (A) A preoperative MRI scan. Note the solid tumor (arrows) as well as the rostral and caudal cysts (open arrows). The subarachnoid space is obliterated. (B) A postoperative MRI scan. The subarachnoid space is expanded and there is an intramedullary cavity in the tumor bed.

identify the dorsal root entry zones to allow an approximation of the anatomic midline (Figure 17–5B).

In the presence of holocord widening associated with rostral and caudal cysts, the ultrasound will clearly define the juncture of the cyst and the neoplasm over both poles of the tumor (Figure 17-6A). It is in these "junctional" regions that the midline myelotomy is initiated utilizing an operating microscope and a carbon dioxide laser at 4–6 W of power. Although one is loath to interrupt blood vessels on the surface of the spinal cord, it is tedious and time consuming to preserve these vascular channels and not at all essential to the preservation of neurologic functions.

In our experience the rostral and caudal margins of the tumor were often demarcated by smooth, white-walled cysts containing xanthochromic fluid. Over the body of the tumor there was usually 1 to 2 mm of white matter, which was removed with laser or bipolar cautery with a small suction device. The astrocytomas were gray or pink in color and quite easily distinguished from white matter (Figure 17-6B).

Fine pial traction sutures were used to open the myelotomy incision, obviating the need for manual retraction of normal spinal cord (Figure 17-7). During the placement of pial traction sutures there was often a transient decrement in the amplitude of the evoked potentials, probably as a result of movement of the posterior columns. In most situations the normal potentials recovered within 1 to 2 minutes. If this did not occur, the sutures were removed and placed in an alternate location. In the patients without associated cysts, if the myelotomy was inadvertently extended beyond the limits of the tumor, there was a significant decrease in amplitude and an increase in the latency of the evoked potentials. This was apparently a result of manipulation of the posterior columns, which were in the normal anatomic position, not having been displaced by the tumor.

In cystic neoplasms, tumor removal was initiated at either the rostral or caudal pole of the solid component. Utilizing the Cavitron ultrasonic surgical aspirator (CUSA), the excision proceeded from within the center of the tumor laterally and anteriorly until the glial-tumor interface was identified (Figure 17-8). It is important to emphasize that no attempt must be made to define a plane of cleavage around the tumor, since this will result in unnecessary retraction and manipulation of normal functional neural tissue with the possibility of producing postoperative neurologic deficits.

After the central core of tumor was removed, the remaining wall of tumor was vaporized using the laser. If the instrument was used for bursts greater than 10 seconds the evoked potentials commonly decreased in amplitude and increased in la-

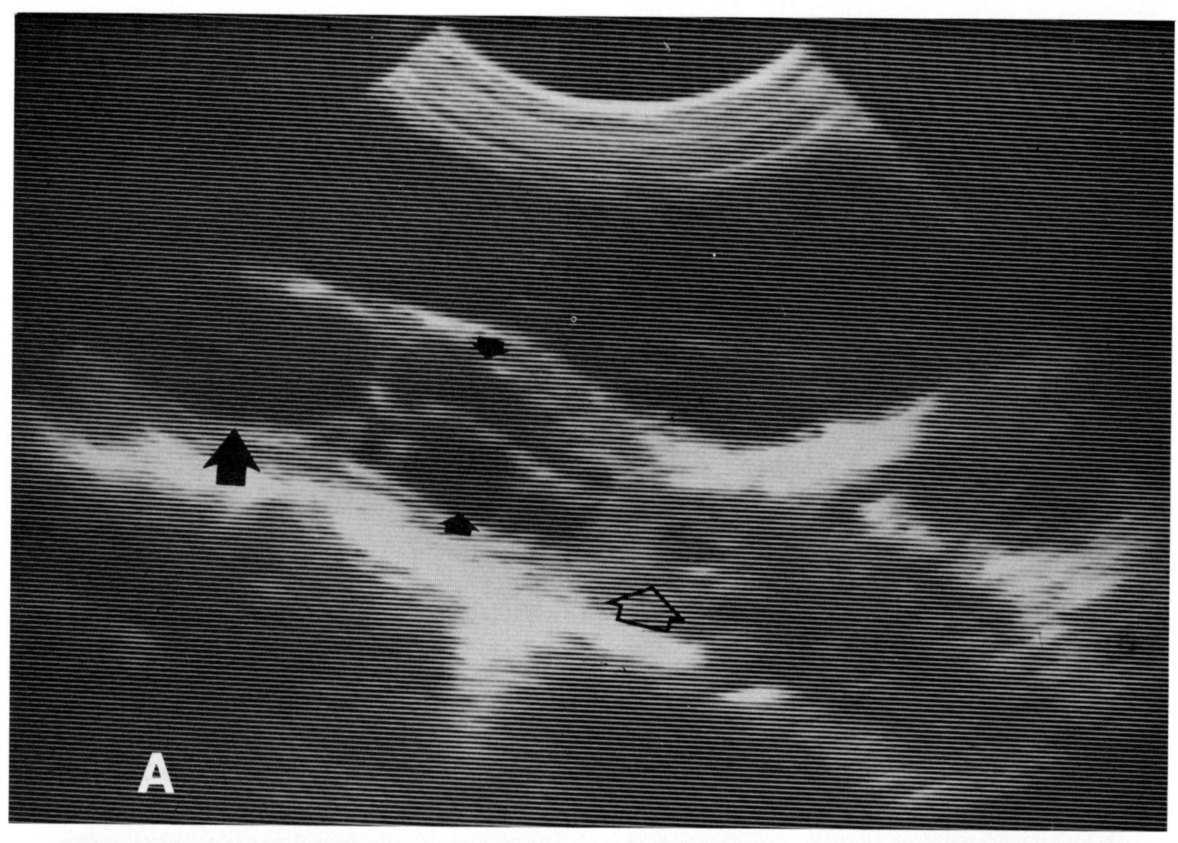

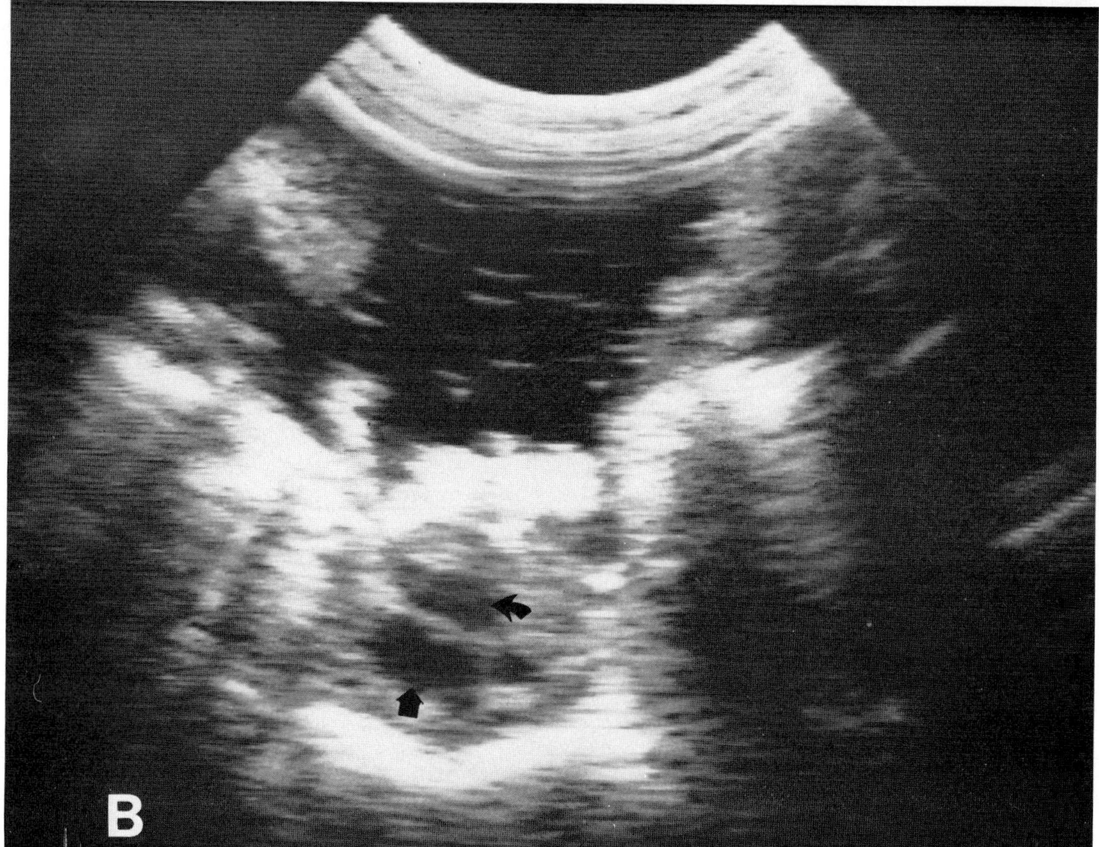

Fig. 17-4. (A) A sagittal ultrasound image demonstrating a rostral cyst (small arrows), an intratumoral cyst (small arrow), and solid tumor (open arrow). (B) A transverse ultrasound image showing intratumoral cysts (arrows).

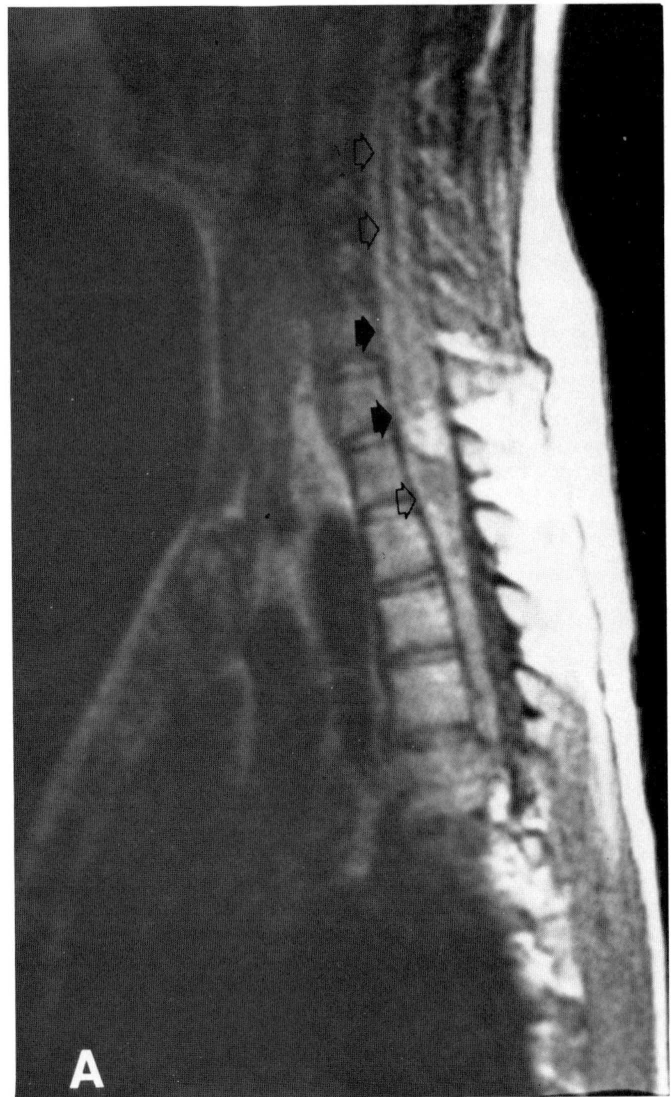

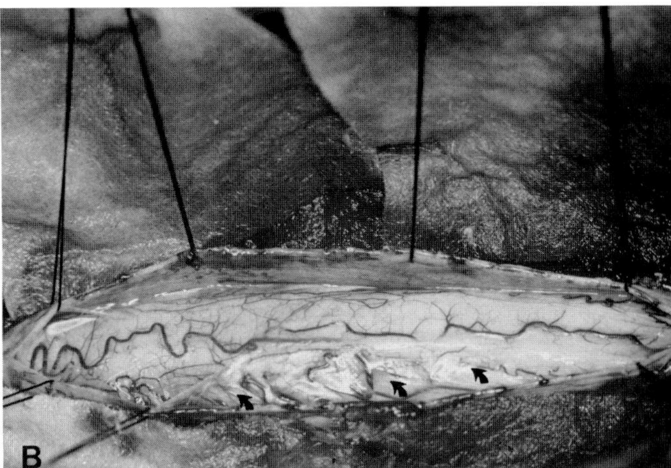

Fig. 17-5. (A) A preoperative MRI scan showing cysts (open arrows) and solid tumor (arrows). (B) The corresponding photograph of the surgical field. Note the expanded spinal cord that is rotated to expose left dorsal roots (arrows).

tency. This was probably an adverse thermal effect that was directly related to time and wattage. In these cases the dissection was temporarily suspended and the cord irrigated with cool Ringer's solution; electrical activity usually returned to normal within 30 to 90 seconds.

As tumor excision continues it is helpful to recognize that the anterior margins of the neoplasm rarely extend ventral to the anterior wall of the rostral and caudal cysts. The bulk of the tumor most often lies in the posterior two thirds of the spinal cord. The general dimensions of the tumor may be roughly conceptualized after inspection of the cysts.

Excision of a noncystic astrocytoma is initiated in the mid portion rather than the rostral or caudal poles of the neoplasm. Since there is no clear demarcation of the superior and inferior limit of the tumor, dissection of the final fragments must proceed slowly and cautiously with attention being paid to the evoked potentials as well as the appearance of the tissues. The "poles" of the neoplasm are the least voluminous part and the most hazardous since normal neural tissue can be easily disrupted.

Following gross total removal of the tumor the dura is closed in a water-tight fashion without the interposition of any dural graft. There is always ample decompression to allow for this closure (Figure 17-9).

Patients who have had radiation therapy are at risk of poor wound healing manifested by pseudomeningocele, CSF fistulae, and meningitis. In 26 previously irradiated patients, 12 developed a CSF leak and 8 of these meningitis. On the basis of this early experience, we use plastic surgical expertise for closing all "high risk" wounds. The technique of wound closure is based on the mobilization of healthy muscle and fascial layers from outside the radiation field.[19] Protruding spinous processes are removed to facilitate "water-tight" closure of the appropriate tissue planes. The competence of the "waterseal" is confirmed by the injection of saline through a catheter just beneath the suture line.

Skin closure must be hypereverted, leaving a "caterpillar" on the back. Interrupted and inverted 3-0 absorbable sutures are placed at 2-cm intervals. This will greatly evert the wound edge, making the incision look unusually humped. These deep sutures maximize dermis-to-dermis contact. The skin is then closed with interrupted or continuous 3-0 nylon sutures. Following suture removal the I-beam effect of the hypereverted skin closure will flatten out rapidly.

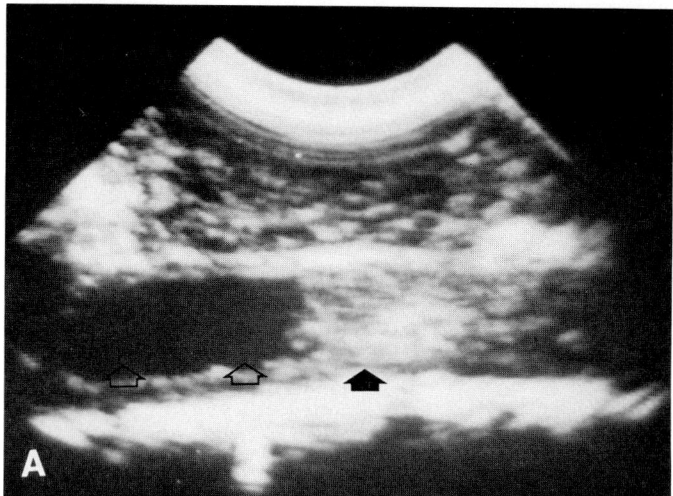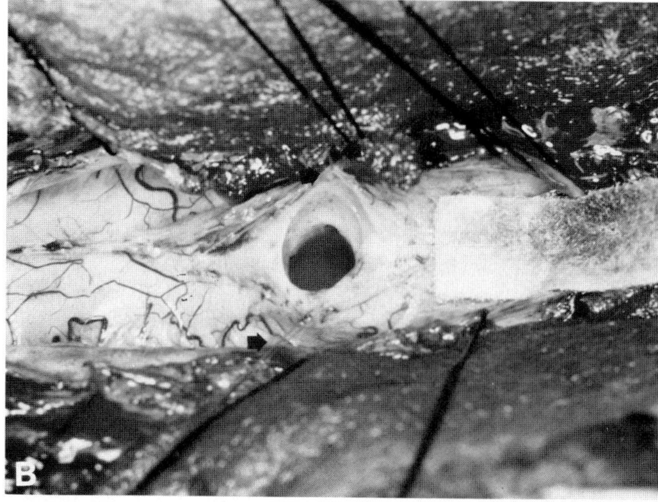

Fig. 17-6. (A) An intraoperative ultrasonogram (obtained before dural incision) demonstrates the tumor (solid arrow) and a cyst (open arrows). (B) Myelotomy is started over the rostral pole of the tumor exposing the cyst. Note the pial traction sutures (arrows).

SURGICAL COMPLICATIONS

MISSING ROSTRAL OR CAUDAL TUMOR FRAGMENT

In cases in which the entire spinal cord was expanded ("holocord astrocytomas"), it was a consistent finding that the neoplasm was associated with a rostral and caudal cyst that extended up and down the central canal but did not contain neoplasia. In three cases, a large intratumor cyst was confused with a rostral cyst, and the tumor removal was prematurely terminated on the assumption that the superior part of the tumor had been removed. In these cases, the symptoms re-curred 3 months, 6 months, and 18 months postoperatively as the cysts re-formed. The symptoms were rapidly evolving scoliosis in two patients and paraspinal and cervical pain in one. In all of these cases, re-exploration disclosed only residual tumor, which had been neglected as a direct result of misinterpreting a large tumor cyst for a rostral or caudal cyst. It is essential that when cysts are identified over the poles of the tumor they be opened up widely enough to be certain that it is a cyst extending above or below the tumor and not a cyst within the tumor. The former are lined by white matter, whereas cysts that occur within the neoplasm are lined by tumor tissue.

Intraoperative ultrasound may also be helpful in differentiating rostral and caudal cysts from intratumor cysts. The

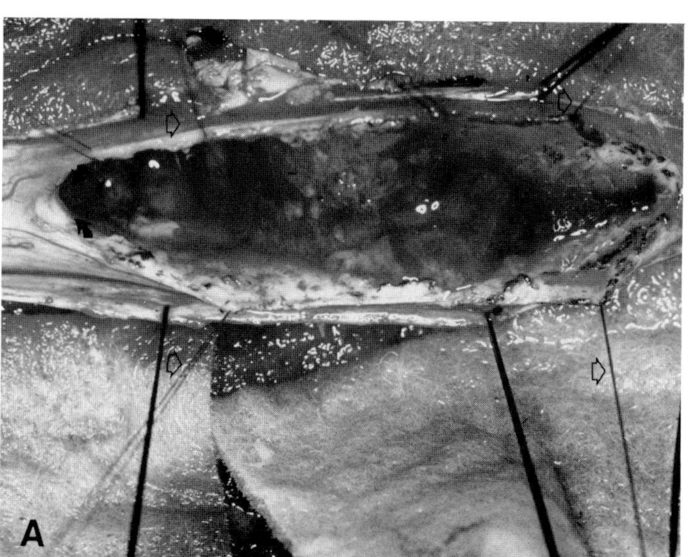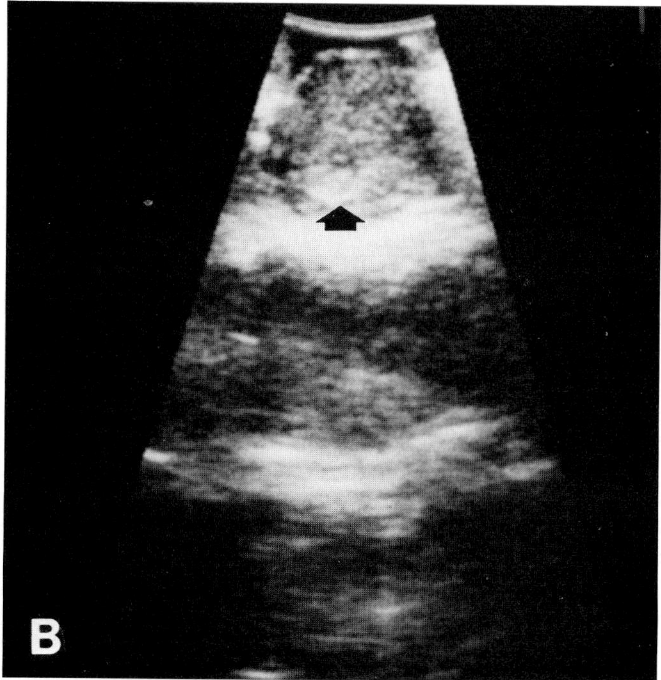

Fig. 17-7. (A) Myelotomy is completed by exposing solid tumor and the rostral cysts (arrows). The pial traction sutures (open arrows) obviate the need for manual retraction. (B) A transverse ultrasound image shows solid tumor (arrow).

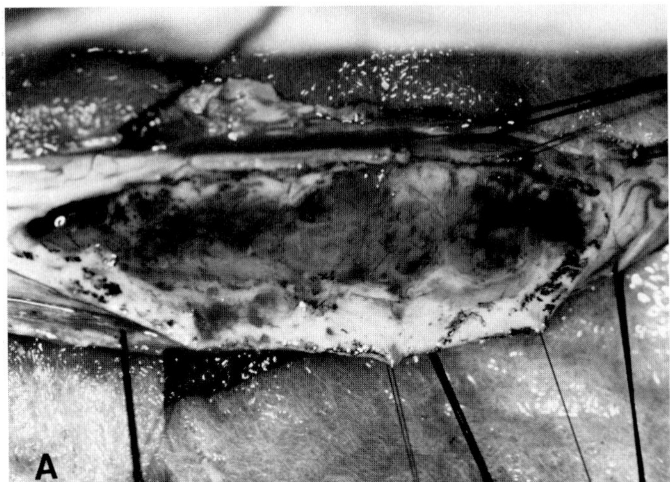

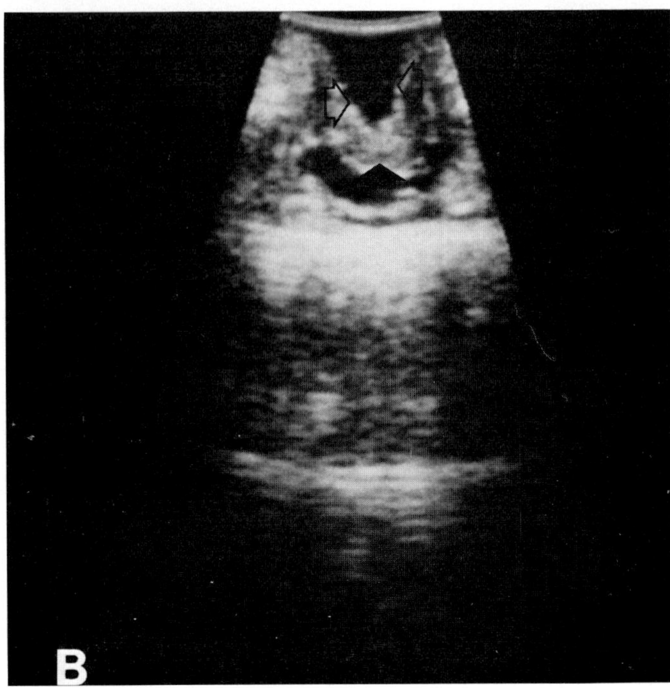

Fig. 17-8.   (A) Tumor resection is completed. (B) A transverse ultrasound image. Note the spinal cord (solid arrow) and the cavity (open arrows) remaining after tumor resection.

former symmetrically expand the cord, occupy two thirds of the diameter, and are smooth-walled. Intratumor cysts are eccentric and asymmetric, of varying volume, and often have irregular walls.

ANTERIOR SUBARACHNOID SPINAL FLUID LOCULATION

In six patients there was dramatic posterior extrusion of the spinal cord through the dural opening at some time during the tumor dissection. This was associated with a deterioration of somatosensory evoked potentials, and we initially misinterpreted this as acute spinal cord swelling. We now recognize that it is not uncommon for spinal fluid to become loculated anterior to the spinal cord and result in its posterior displacement. It is effectively dealt with by retraction of the lateral margin of the spinal cord and puncturing the cyst. It has been a consistent finding that this intraoperative problem only occurred in patients who had had previous surgery and in whom there were dense adhesions between the lateral spinal cord and the dural tube. It seems that the anterior subarachnoid space did not communicate freely with the posterior subarachnoid space, and this was responsible for the hydrodynamics that promoted this occurrence.

One patient in this series had a huge tumor in the lower thoracic cord, and although immediately neurologically stable, became paraplegic 1 week after surgery. A CT scan disclosed that the spinal cord had extruded from the spinal canal and at surgery there was a huge anterior loculation of spinal fluid, which had displaced the spinal cord posteriorly through the dural decompression, and the cord had become incarcerated in the rostral and caudal dura with secondary infarction.

Retrospectively, it was apparent that the dura had been excised at the time of the first operation and that it had not been closed at the time of the tumor resection. This permitted the trapped anterior subarachnoid compartment to displace the cord from the spinal canal with subsequent infarction. As a result of this experience, we no longer leave the dura open under any circumstances, and if it has been previously excised, a suitable dural substitute is used.

MALIGNANT ASTROCYTOMAS

Fourteen patients had grade III or grade IV astrocytomas. In each case there was rapidly progressive neurologic dysfunction, and all of the patients were moderately or severely disabled at the time of the primary surgery. Although it was technically possible to remove the bulk of the neoplasm, no patient was significantly improved by the surgery and all developed widespread neuraxis dissemination within 6 months of the procedure, 13 dying within 12 months. We now regard malignant spinal cord tumors as uniformly virulent and all patients receive neuraxis radiation and adjunctive chemotherapy.

HYDROCEPHALUS

Twelve patients developed symptomatic hydrocephalus within 36 months of definitive diagnosis and primary surgery. In each case there was involvement of the cervical cord, either by the neoplasm or a rostral cyst. Although the cause of the hydrocephalus remains unclear, it was probably related to mechanical obstruction of the outlet foramina of the fourth ventricle. Interestingly, the spinal fluid protein was not significantly elevated and therefore not etiologically related to the CSF obstruction.

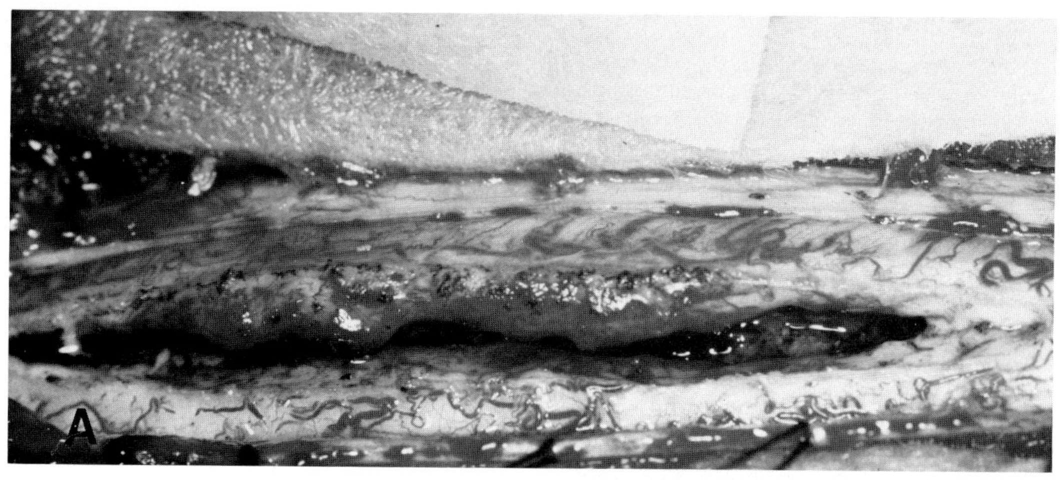

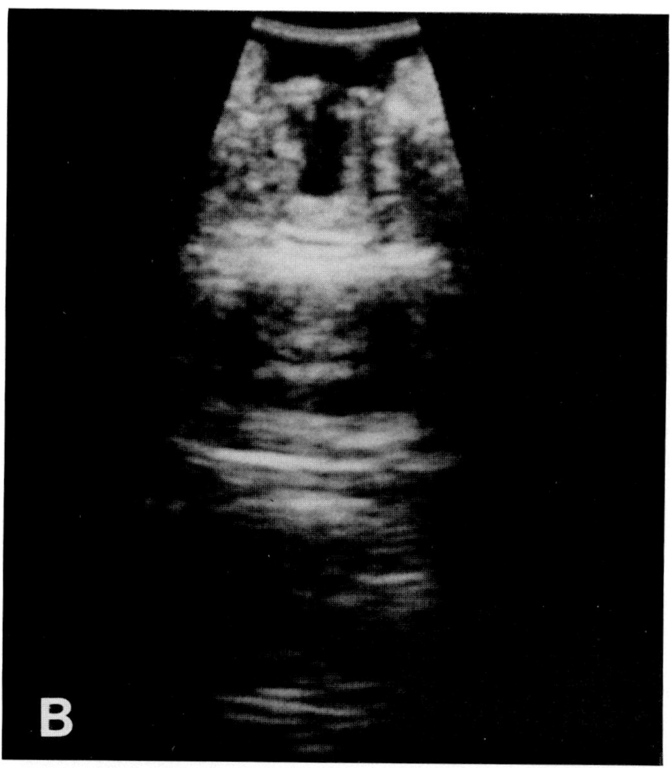

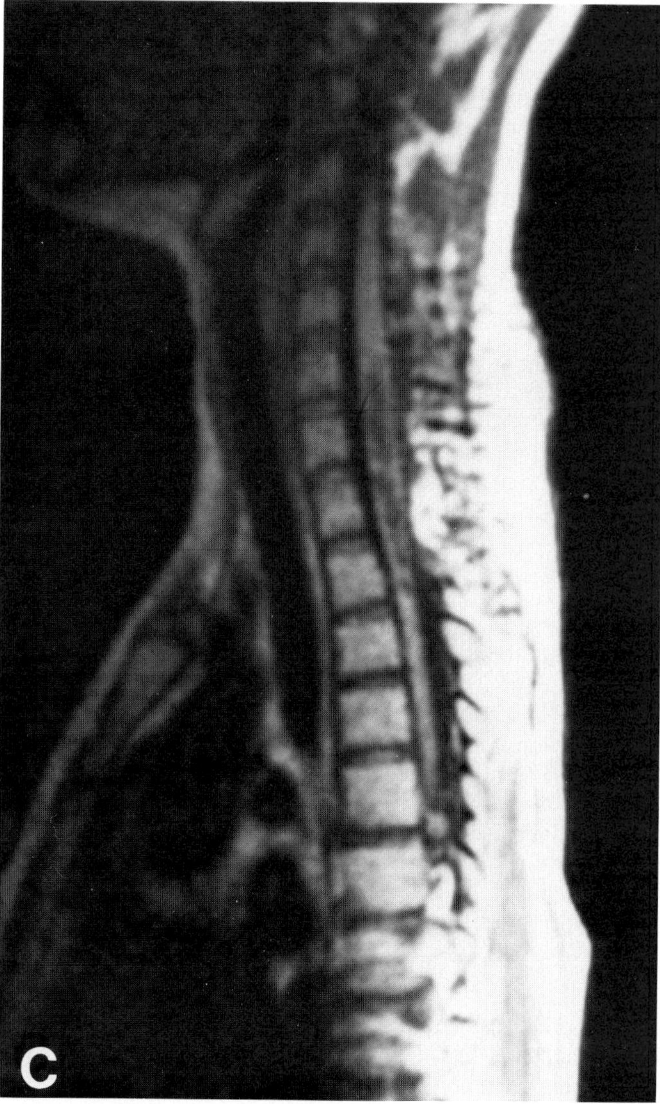

Fig. 17-9. (A) The pial sutures are removed before dural closure. (B) A transverse ultrasound image after removal of the pial sutures. (C) A postoperative MRI scan. Note the intramedullary cavity in the tumor bed and expansion of the subarachnoid space.

POSTOPERATIVE NEUROLOGIC MORBIDITY RELATED TO SEGMENTAL LOCATION OF THE NEOPLASM

Postoperative neurologic morbidity may be correlated with segments of spinal cord that are involved with the neoplasm. Whereas an extensive dissection can be carried out with little risk in those segments of spinal cord that are largely composed of white matter, this does not seem to be the case in the lowest segments, where gray matter is most abundant.

Dissections within the cervical spinal cord are associated with little morbidity, although it is not uncommon to note some anterior horn cell dysfunction as manifested by atrophy of one or more muscle groups of an upper extremity. When this occurred, it was permanent.

Dissection extending from the junction of the cervical and thoracic regions to T9 was associated with remarkably little neurologic morbidity. Tumors located in the lower spinal cord segments from T9 to T12 produced the greatest incidence of significant postoperative neurologic morbidity. This is because neoplasms in the conus or just above it compress or infiltrate gray matter, while tumors that occur in more rostral regions of the spinal cord compress white matter tracts and therefore the resultant signs and symptoms are based on pathologic anatomy and pathophysiology that is specific to the segmental location of the neoplasm.

Whereas an extensive intramedullary dissection may be carried out with relative impunity in white matter in the rostral cord, this is not the case in the gray matter in the region of the conus, and the surgeon must be aware of these technical limitations.

Significant preoperative sphincteric dysfunction suggests that the tumor extends into the conus, since such dysfunction rarely occurs if the tumor is rostral to T12. Conversely, the absence of bowel and bladder problems suggests that the tumor does not extend into the conus, although it may be asymptomatically expanded by a caudal cyst.

If there is no preoperative bowel and bladder dysfunction, it will occur postoperatively if the conus is disrupted. It is therefore essential that the myelotomy not be extended over the conus, since this will invariably result in sphincter dysfunction; such dysfunction may be permanent.

Intraoperative ultrasound is invaluable because it clearly discloses the location of the conus, which may not be obvious to the surgeon because of distortion and rotation as well as superimposed neural elements.

It is important that the patient be advised that at least a temporary increase in neurologic dysfunction is to be expected with surgery in this area, and we assume that the long-term or permanent morbidity will also be significant.

DISCUSSION

Holocord astrocytomas form a large subgroup (60 percent) of the spinal cord astrocytomas,[2,11,14] and in our series were a more common occurrence than the more limited neoplasms.[11,12,14] Although this has been described in occasional case reports, the prevalence has not been previously recognized because of the earlier tendency not to carry out complete neurodiagnostic studies when a complete intramedullary block was observed on myelograms.

There are a number of important observations that are clearly relevant in terms of understanding the biology of this group of neoplasms as well as in recommending proper surgical management. It has been a consistent observation that the solid component of the astrocytoma is often not as extensive as the myelograms alone suggest and, indeed, the actual location of the neoplasm will be in those segments of the spinal cord that correspond to neurologic dysfunction. Demonstration of the rostral and caudal cysts by delayed metrizamide-enhanced CT scanning, ultrasonography, and MRI is helpful. The lack of significant neurologic dysfunction relating to the spinal segments that are distended with fluid is probably directly related to the anatomic location of the cyst within the center of the cord as compared with the solid component of the neoplasm, which was relatively more diffuse. It was only necessary to expose and extirpate the solid portion of the neoplasm and drain the rostral and caudal cysts in order to obtain a satisfactory surgical result. A limited laminectomy over the solid portion of the neoplasm therefore was sufficient. The extent of the laminectomy was defined by the combination of neurologic deficit, eroded pedicles, and the area of maximal spinal cord widening on plain films and myelograms and confirmed intraoperatively with ultrasound.

The presence of cysts that were similar in appearance to those associated with the cystic astrocytomas of the cerebellum suggests that these neoplasms are congenital tumors that had their inception sometime during gestation. The fluid produced by the tumor extends up and down the spinal cord in the region of least resistance, that is, the central canal. It is our perspective that the presence of a widened spinal cord from the cervicomedullary junction to the conus that is associated with a relatively slowly evolving neurologic deficit is indicative of a very slowly growing and perhaps even hamartomatous type of lesion, which has a good long-term prognosis and should be treated aggressively. The rare malignant astrocytoma in this population has a different clinical picture: neurologic deficits develop rapidly, and the prognosis parallels that of glioblastomas elsewhere in the central nervous system.

Benign astrocytomas are often firm, contain calcium deposits, and have no obvious cleavage plane to delineate them from normal neural tissue. Traditional surgical techniques of suction and blunt dissection are relatively inefficient and may cause considerable traction on adjacent normal structures, which may account for the high incidence of neurologic deficit in older series. The CUSA and the surgical laser have been indispensable surgical adjuncts in the radical resection of these tumors.[11,12] The CUSA and the surgical laser permit fragmentation, emulsification, vaporization, and aspiration of the firmest tissue without any movement of adjacent normal spinal cord.

The outcome after radical resection of these tumors was directly related to the preoperative neurologic status. Although a transient increase in weakness or sensory loss was sometimes seen in the immediate postoperative period, only one patient had a significant permanent increase in neurologic deficit following surgery. Patients with paraparesis or quadriparesis, who were ambulatory before surgery, usually had neurologic and functional improvement over several weeks. The group with severe deficits preoperatively rarely made any significant improvement, although their downhill course often abated. There was no operative mortality and the 5-year survival for patients with grade I and grade II tumors was 90 percent. Malignant astrocytomas follow the same course as cerebral glioblastomas: 75 percent of the patients die within 1 year, often with widespread metastasis.

There is no evidence that radiation will cure benign astrocytomas of the spinal cord, and there is abundant evidence that it has a deleterious effect on the immature, developing nervous and skeletal system.[1,5,16,17,20] Spinal cord astrocytomas should be recognized as excisable lesions, and radiation therapy should be reserved for possible adjunctive use if there is a recurrence. At that time, it might be used after a second radical surgical resection.

Children who have undergone extensive laminectomy and, in addition, have denervation of the paravertebral muscles from tumor as well as operative muscle retraction are at risk of developing severe spinal deformities as they pass through periods of rapid growth.[21,22,23] They may need to be treated with body braces for several years after surgery. Close collaboration with a pediatric orthopedic surgeon experienced with kyphoscoliosis is helpful in managing these patients.

SUMMARY

This chapter summarized the authors' experience with radical surgery for spinal cord astrocytomas of childhood. The following conclusions were made:

1. Ninety percent of spinal cord tumors are "benign" gliomas.
2. In 60 percent of patients there is expansion of the entire spinal cord from the cervicomedullary junction to the conus ("holocord" tumor).
3. All holocord tumors are cystic astrocytomas and are similar or identical to cystic astrocytomas of the cerebellum.
4. Radical surgical excision of "benign" gliomas is compatible with neurologic recovery. The duration of remission or the likelihood of cure has not been established because the follow-up period is still too short.
5. Malignant gliomas have an extremely poor prognosis as a result of neuraxis dissemination.

REFERENCES

1. Anderson RM, Carson JJ: Spinal cord tumors in children: A review of the subject and presentation of 21 cases. J Pediatr 43:190, 1953
2. Aresnil C, Horvath L, Iliescu D: Intraspinal tumors in children. Psychiatr Neurol Neurochir 70:123, 1977
3. De Sousa AL, Kalsbech JE, Mealy J Jr, et al: Intraspinal tumors in children: A review of 31 cases. J Neurosurg 51:437, 1979
4. Garrigo E, Stein BM: Microsurgical removal of intramedullary spinal cord tumors. Surg Neurol 7:214, 1977
5. Ingraham FD: Intraspinal tumors in infancy and childhood. Am J Surg 39:342, 1938
6. Reimer R, Onogrio BM: Astrocytomas of the spinal cord in children and adolescents. J Neurosurg 63:669, 1985
7. Kopelson G, Lingood RM, Kleinman GM, et al: Management of intramedullary spinal cord tumors. Radiology 135:473, 1980
8. Cooper PR, Epstein F: Radical resection of intramedullary spinal cord tumors in adults. Recent experience in 29 patients. J Neurosurg 63:492, 1985
9. Elsberg CA, Beer R: The operability of intramedullary tumors of the spinal cord. A report of two operations with remarks upon the entrusion of intraspinal tumors. Am J Med Sci 142:636, 1911
10. Shenkin HA, Alpers BJ: Clinical and pathological features of glioma of the spinal cord. Arch Neurol Psychiatr 52:87, 1944
11. Epstein F: Spinal cord astrocytomas of childhood, in Symon L (ed): Advances and Technical Standards in Neurosurgery, vol 13. Berlin, Springer Verlag, 1986
12. Epstein F, Raghavendra N, John R, et al: Spinal cord astrocytomas of childhood, surgical adjuncts and pitfalls, in Humphreys RP (ed): Concepts in Pediatric Neurosurgery 5. Basel, S. Karger, 1985, pp 224–237
13. Richardson FL: A report of 16 tumors of the spinal cord in children: The importance of spinal rigidity as an early sign of disease. J Pediatr 57:42, 1960
14. Epstein F, Epstein N: Surgical treatment of spinal cord astrocytomas of childhood: A series of 19 patients. J Neurosurg 75:685, 1982
15. Epstein F, Epstein N: Surgical management of "holo-cord" intramedullary spinal cord astrocytomas in children. J Neurosurg 54:829, 1981
16. Coxe WS: Tumors of the spinal canal in children. Am Surg 27:62, 1961
17. Greenwood J: Surgical removal of intramedullary tumors. J Neurosurg 26:276, 1967
18. Raghavendra BN, Epstein FJ, McCLeary L: The use of intraoperative ultrasound in the localization of intramedullary spinal cord tumors of chldhood. AJNR 5:395, 1984
19. Zide B, Wisoff JH, Epstein F: Closure of extensive and complicated laminectomy wounds. J Neurosurg (in press)
20. Guidetti B: Intramedullary tumors of the spinal cord. Acta Neurochir 17:7, 1967
21. Catell HS, Clark GL Jr: Cervical kyphosis and instability following multiple laminectomies in children. J Bone Joint Surg 49:713, 1967
22. Sim FH, Svien HJ, Bickel WH, et al: Swan neck deformity following extensive cervical laminectomy. J Bone Joint Surg 49:564, 1967
23. Tachdjian MO, Matson DD: Orthopedic aspects of intraspinal tumors in infants and children. J Bone Joint Surg 47:223, 1965

CHAPTER 18

Current Surgical Management of Scoliosis and Kyphosis

Morey S. Moreland

THE TERM *scoliosis* is derived from the Greek word meaning "curvature." Scoliosis as it is currently applied to the description of deformities of the back means a lateral curvature or bend occurring in the coronal plane of the spine. Abnormal curvatures can also occur in the sagittal plane, i.e., abnormal kyphosis or increased degrees of lordosis. Combinations of deformities in both planes commonly occur.

In a broad sense, spinal deformities can be classified according to their origin, i.e., congenital or acquired. The Scoliosis Research Society has further classified both scoliotic and kyphotic deformities by etiology based on the disease state accompanying the deformity (Table 18-1).[1] Since there are 27 articulating elements in the spine (the skull, 24 presacral segments, and 2 fused vertebral segments, the sacrum and coccyx), abnormal curvatures are further classified by the location of the apex of the curvature: cervical (apex between C1 and C6); cervicothoracic (apex at C7 or T1); thoracic (apex between T2 and T11); thoracolumbar (apex at T12 or L1); lumbar (apex between L2 and L4); and lumbosacral (apex at L5 or S1). By adding the side on which the apex occurs (right or left), a complete anatomic description of the curve can be given.

In terms of classification, a word also must be said about the definition of structural curves and nonstructural curves. It has long been thought that true scoliosis produces physical changes within the skeletal elements of the spine itself. These structural changes consist of wedging of the disc spaces and vertebrae in the coronal or sagittal plane or a combination thereof; rotation of the vertebral bodies with respect to normal alignment in the transverse plane; distortion of the shape of the pedicles, laminae, or spinous processes; and anatomic remodeling of the facet joints. Nonstructural changes of scoliosis are those that are seen within the normal flexible accommodation of the spine and do not involve frank physical changes in the vertebral bodies themselves. For purposes of discussion in this chapter, consideration will be given only to those deformities that result in structural changes.

ETIOLOGY

In studying the classification of scoliosis, it becomes apparent that the vast majority of abnormal curvatures occurring in the spinal column are acquired. Notable exceptions are congenital curvatures, which represent a failure in the embryologic segmentation process, and, possibly, idiopathic scolio-

sis, for which an exact underlying mechanism of abnormal growth and development is not known. In other categories, the cause of the curvature is somewhat more evident. For example, in abnormal curves resulting from neuromuscular disease, there is clearly an unbalanced force relationship in the supporting elements of the long, thin spinal column. Persistent asymmetric forces on the spine lead to permanent structural changes, with abnormal curvatures being the resultant expression. The amount of asymmetric force applied over a specific length of time and the location of the applied forces combined with other antigravity activities may all play a role in the development of an abnormal curvature. However, the exact mechanism still remains an enigma, since not all patients with neuromuscular disease develop a scoliosis.[2] For example, in the case of cerebral palsy, only 30 to 60 percent of the patients will develop a curve[3–5]; in part, this depends on the severity of the disease. On the other hand, it appears that 85 to 92 percent of those children sustaining a traumatic paraplegia in childhood or preadolescence will develop a scoliotic deformity.[6–10]

One of the biggest problems in treating patients with scoliosis at the present time is our lack of understanding of the etiology of the idiopathic scoliotic curves. In these individuals, the scoliotic deformity usually appears in the preadolescent stage and may progress to a significant degree in a small minority of patients. In these individuals, there is no other obvious measurable associated abnormalities. Studies have failed to show an inherent bony abnormality suggestive of a vertebral growth disturbance that is primary.[11,12] There are some studies[13,14] suggesting that abnormal muscle functions specifically with reference to calcium transport, and, more recently, there is work suggesting that vestibular postural righting mechanisms may play a role.[15,16] The endpoint of the effect of these muscle abnormalities might be focused at the vertebral growth mechanism much as it is implicated in neuromuscular disease. The most obvious interruption of the growth mechanism occurs in trauma, either surgical or nonsurgical. Traumatic wedging of the vertebra or damage of the endplate growth mechanisms of the vertebral body could cause a curvature, although rarely this alone produces scoliosis, since only one or two levels are effected in this manner. Traumatic injuries, however, may have long-term effects if such injury occurs in a younger child. Surgical removal of all or a portion of the supporting elements of the spine can likewise effect the development of abnormal curvatures through destabilization of the ligamentous support, asymmetry of loading

OPERATIVE NEUROSURGICAL TECHNIQUES
ISBN 0-8089-1862-1

Table 18-1. Classification of scoliotic and kyphotic deformities

Scoliosis:

Idiopathic
  Infantile—0–3 years
    Resolving
    Progressive
  Juvenile—4 years to onset of puberty
  Adolescent—onset of puberty to epiphyseal closure
  Adult—epiphyses closed
Neuromuscular
  Neuropathic
    Upper motor neuron lesion
      Cerebral palsy
      Spinocerebellar degeneration
        Friedreich's
        Charcot-Marie-Tooth
        Roussy-Lévy
      Syringomyelia
      Spinal cord tumor
      Spinal cord trauma
      Other
    Lower motor neuron lesion
      Poliomyelitis
      Traumatic
      Spinal muscular atrophy
      Myelomeningocele (paralytic)
    Dysautonomia (Riley-Day)
    Other
  Myopathic
    Arthrogryposis
    Muscular dystrophy
      Duchenne (pseudohypertrophic)
      Limb-girdle
      Facio-scapulohumeral
    Congenital hypotonia
    Myotonia dystrophica
    Other
Congenital
  Congenital scoliosis
  Failure of formation
    Wedge vertebra
    Hemivertebra
    Failure of segmentation
      Unilateral bar
      Bilateral ("fusion")
    Mixed
  Associated with neural tissue defect
    Myelomeningocele
    Meningocele
    Spinal dysraphism
      Diastematomyelia
      Other
Neurofibromatosis
Mesenchymal
  Marfan's
  Homocystinuria
  Ehlers-Danlos
  Other
Traumatic
  Fracture or dislocation (nonparalytic)
  Postirradiation
  Other

Soft tissue contractures
  Postempyema
  Burns
  Other
Osteochondrodystrophies
  Achondroplasia
  Spondyloepiphyseal dysplasia
  Diastrophic dwarfism
  Mucopolysaccharidoses
  Other
Tumor
  Benign
  Malignant
Rheumatoid disease
Metabolic
  Rickets
  Juvenile osteoporosis
  Osteogenesis imperfecta
Related to lumbosacral area
  Spondylosis
  Spondylolisthesis
  Other
Thoracogenic
  Post-thoracoplasty
  Post-thoracotomy
  Other
Hysterical
Functional
  Postural
  Secondary to short leg
  Due to muscle spasm
  Other

Kyphosis:

Postural
Scheuermann's disease
Congenital
  Defect of segmentation
  Defect of formation
  Mixed
Paralytic
  Polio
  Anterior horn cell
  Upper motor neuron
Myelomeningocele
Posttraumatic
  Acute
  Chronic
Inflammatory
  Tuberculosis
  Other infections
  Ankylosing spondylitis
Postsurgical
  Postlaminectomy
  Post body excision (e.g., tumor)
Postirradiation
Metabolic
  Osteoporosis
    Senile
    Juvenile
  Osteogenesis imperfecta
  Other

Table 18-1. *(continued)*

Developmental
  Achondroplasia
  Mucopolysaccharidoses
  Other
Tumor
  Benign
  Malignant
    Primary
    Metastatic
Postural
Congenital
Paralytic
  Neuropathic
  Myopathic
Contracture of hip flexors
Secondary to shunts

Reprinted from Winter RB: Spinal problems in pediatric orthopaedics, in Lovell WW, Winter RB (eds): Pediatrics Orthopaedics. Philadelphia, JB Lippincott, 1986. With permission.

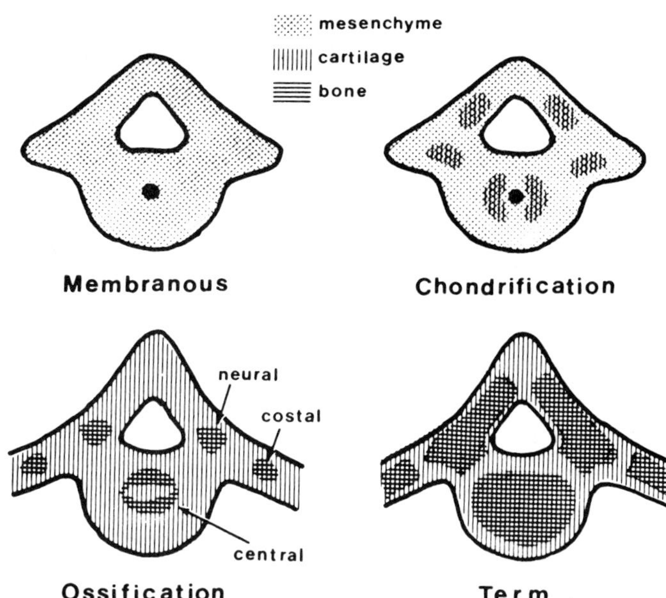

Fig. 18-1. The phases of vertebral column development: membranous development, chondrification, and ossification. (Reprinted from Parke WW: Development of the spine, in Rothman RH, Simone FA (eds): The Spine. Philadelphia, WB Saunders, 1975. With permission.)

across the spine, or interruption of the growth mechanism. A combination of all of these mechanisms may play a role in the case of wide excision of the posterior lateral elements of the spinal column for tumor excision, with likely production of a kyphosis or a scoliosis.

GROWTH AND DEVELOPMENT OF THE SPINE

An understanding of the development of the spinal cord and vertebral column is essential in understanding the development of spinal deformities occurring in children. Embryologically, the vertebral column begins as mesenchymal somite formation in close approximation to the ectodermal and endodermal plates. This formation occurs from a thickening along the paraxial regions adjacent to the notochord and neurotube. Segmentation begins at approximately the 12th day of gestation and is complete by the end of the 5th week. Excellent reviews of this process can be found in works by Lemire et al.,[17] Parke,[18] and Moe et al.[19] The formation of the vertebral column occurs through three separate phases, beginning with the initial formation of somites and sclerotomes. In the first phase membranous vertebral bodies form from mesenchymal cells, which migrate dorsally to form neural arches and ventrolaterally to form ribs. This segmental membranous cell structure then divides or resegments into two cell masses, a cranial mass and a more cellular caudal mass. The cranial portion of one somite condenses with the caudal portion of the somite above, incorporating the sclerotomic fissure, which contains the vascular supply for the newly formed somite. With this recombination, the spinal nerve root is located at the intersegmental level, while the vascular supply lies at the mid-vertebral body level. With condensation of the mesochyme, the membranous portion of the vertebral body surrounds the centrum of the somite, which in the region between the newly formed vertebral body becomes the intervertebral disc and nucleus pulposus. At approximately the 20th day of gestation, the second phase begins, with chondrification occurring in the mesenchymal membranous vertebral column (Figure 18-1). Chondrification begins around the lateral portion of the centrum, at the level of the transverse processes, and also in the neural arches lateral to the neurotube. This stage of chondrification overlaps that of the third phase, ossification, which begins at the 20th or 24th week. Primary centers of ossification occur at the centrum, at the level of the transverse process, and at the pedicles. Secondary centers of ossification develop much later, often not being seen radiographically until the 15th to 17th year. These include the ring hypothesis to which the annulus fibrosus attaches and the tips of the transverse and spinous processes. These secondary centers of ossification tend to be apophyses, that is, sites at which ligamentous structures attach and are not true epiphyseal structures.

Since the majority of spine deformities occur after birth and are acquired, it is important to understand the growth rate of the spine. The spine grows at a variable rate. This rate is more rapid from birth to age 3 year and again during the adolescent growth spurt[20,21] (Figure 18-2). The periods of rapid growth of the spine seem to correlate with similar periods of increase in curvature during the developmental sequences of scoliosis. The exact reason that idiopathic scoliosis particularly seems to have a propensity for increasing during this period of increased growth velocity is unknown. The possible role of growth hormones, somatomedin, and size of the vertebral bodies have been investigated but no definitive relationship was found.[22–25] Another implication of the rapidly growing spine during the adolescent period is the effect of spine fusion on the scoliotic segment during subsequent growth.[26] There is clear evidence that the fused portion of the spine does not grow significantly longitudinally.[27–29] There are rare instances in which the fusion mass may remodel, presumably under the forces of rapid growth in other areas, such as the anterior portion of the vertebral bodies. From standard growth tables the rate of growth of each vertebral segment per year in terms of height has been calculated as 0.07 cm.[19] Therefore, by calculating the number of segments of spine fused and the number of years with growth remaining one can estimate the

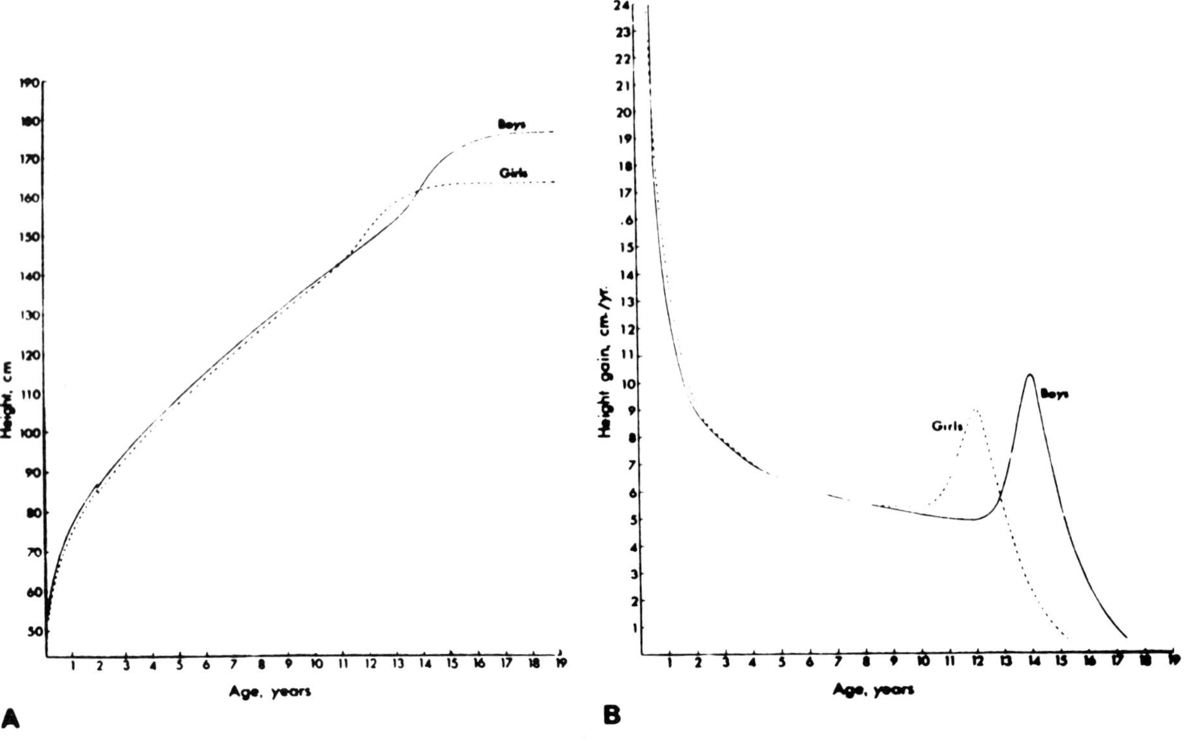

Fig. 18-2.   Growth rates of the spine. (A) Height achieved for boys and girls is plotted against years. (B) Growth plotted as growth gain (centimeters per year) against age. (Reprinted from Zorab PA (ED): Scoliosis and Growth. Proceedings of a Third Symposium held at the Institute of Diseases of the Chest, Brompton Hospital, London, November 13, 1970. London, Churchill-Livingstone, 1971. With permission.)

effect of shortening of the fusion mass on a spine. In most cases, the amount of shortening that occurs is less than that which would be anticipated has the curve continued to develop.[30]

NATURAL HISTORY AND PROGRESSION OF THE DEFORMITY

In order to have a proper prospective of the treatment options in scoliosis and kyphosis, it is appropriate to consider the natural history of the deformities. Described below are the currently understood patterns of development of deformities occurring for the more common forms of spinal curvatures.

IDIOPATHIC SCOLIOSIS

The vast majority of patients with scoliosis seen in North America are those with idiopathic scoliosis. For mild curves the actual incidence of this disease is about equal for boys and girls, while for curves greater than 15 to 20 degrees, girls predominate approximately 2 to 1. Actual prevalence for mild curves has been reported to be as little as 0.2 to 5.5 percent to as high as 13.6 percent of the population.[31–33] Most of the information on prevalence is based on physical findings of a positive rib hump with a forward bend test.[34,35] This has become the standard screening test for scoliosis, and is currently legislated to be a part of the screening examination in children from the fifth through the eighth grades in 23 states.[36] Of 14,900 students screened in Montreal, Canada, Rogala et al.[37] determined that 1252 merited further evaluation. Further screening clarified that 821 were believed to have scoliosis definitely, and x-ray films of this group revealed 610 with structural scoliosis of 5 degrees or more with rotational deformity. Idiopathic scoliosis was found

to be present in 603 of these, and 5 patients were felt to have Scheuermann's kyphosis. The overall instance of spine deformity was 4.6 percent and that of scoliosis was 4.1 percent. However, only 54 patients had curves greater than 20 degrees, with a male-to-female ratio of 1:6. Given the presence of scoliosis in a growing child, Lonstein has shown that the most accurate predictors of the likelihood of progression was the patient's age at initial examination, the magnitude of the curve, the degree of skeletal maturity, and the patient's menarche status.[36] In most studies of untreated idiopathic scoliosis, it has been determined that thoracic curves are more likely to increase over lumbar curves.[39,40] While the specific factors related to the likelihood of progression are not totally understood, it can be said that the younger the child and the greater the curve, the more likelihood for progression. A vast number of children with a small curvature, that is less than 10 degrees, remained unchanged or not significantly changed clinically. Because of the concern of increased spinal growth during the adolescent period, the most likely time for progression is during the adolescent growth spurt. For minor curves, there usually appears to be no significant progression after skeletal maturity is reached. It has long been thought that curves existing in adults were stable. However, in 102 patients examined by Weinstein and Ponseti and who had been followed for an average of 40.5 years, 68 percent progressed after skeletal maturity.[39] Again, this was felt to occur more often in thoracic curves, with increased rotation of the apical vertebra and with increased angulation of the ribs associated with scoliosis. Curves that measured between 50 and 75 degrees at skeletal maturity appeared to progress to the greatest degree. For minor and moderate curves, there appears to be no significant increase in mortality. For curves greater than 50 or 60 degrees, there appears to be significant increased morbidity with associated decreased pulmonary function and increased mortality, increased work disability, and a reduced chance of marriage.[41]

The degree of back pain occurring in adult scoliosis has been variably reported, although it continues to be a problem facing the orthopedist who treats individuals with severe idiopathic scoliosis.[42–44]

NEUROMUSCULAR DEVELOPMENT

Patients with neuropathic and myopathic types of scoliosis tend to have a somewhat different curve pattern. Their curves tend to be long sweeping curves, spanning several regions of the spine. At times they can be quite severe. Between vertebral segments, the rotation tends to be less but the total rotation occurring over the length of the curve segment can be considerable. The prevalence of scoliosis in these situations varies with the specific condition. It is remarkable that the incidence runs in the 30 to 50 percent range throughout all of the classified abnormalities. In the case of cerebral palsy, the incidence has been reported to be from 23 to 50 percent of those patients seen in cerebral palsy clinics.[3,4,45] Since the curves in these disorders usually develop as a result of muscle imbalance, there is a tendency for a curve to increase progressively over time. The contribution of a sitting imbalance, pelvic fixation, pelvic obliquity, and kyphosis make these curvatures more prominent when sitting, although they tend to maintain a relatively high degree of flexibility. Steady progression of the spinal curvatures occurs in spinal cerebellar degenerative diseases and is frequently seen with Friedrich's ataxia and Charcot-Marie-Tooth disease.[46] The incidence of scoliosis in patients with syringomyelia has been reported to be as high as 30 percent,[49] although in one report by Huebert[47] the incidence of severe curves is around 20 percent.

Poliomyelitis, while not frequently seen in this country, has been known to produce rather severe curves. These are long, C-shaped curves, which, depending upon the degree of muscle imbalance and the severity, may produce a significant cardiopulmonary decompensation with cor pulmonale. The late development of these myopathic curves depends upon the severity of the disease and the growth of the spine that remains at the onset of the disease. For example, in patients with spinal muscle atrophy, particularly those with Kugelberg-Welander disease, there is evidence of a persistently increasing severity of scoliosis with increasing age of the child.[50] In Duchenne muscular dystrophy, scoliosis occurring in the late phases of the disease is almost a universal finding. Scoliosis is rarely seen while patients are still ambulatory but it usually begins at the point at which the child ceases to ambulate and progresses invariably.[51] It is interesting to note that in a study by Wilkins and Gibson they found the least progression of scoliosis in those patients with diminished kyphosis or with thoracic frank lordosis.[52]

SPINE FRACTURES AND PARAPLEGIA, TUMORS

In children with acquired spinal cord injury with or without associated fracture, there is a high propensity for the development of scoliosis; this seems to be age related.[6,7,8,53,54] Bonnett analyzed 123 patients under the age of 18 with acquired spinal cord injury. Of 57 children who had progressive spinal deformity at the onset of injury the average age was 6.8 years, and of the 66 patients without significant deformity, the average onset of their spinal injury was age 16.[19] Finally, children with spinal cord tumors or tumors of the vertebral column may have a scoliosis or may have a scoliosis as a consequence of treatment.[55,56] In those cases in which tumors require wide excision, either for decompression or surgical resection, the growth plate mechanisms either in the posterior or anterior columns of the spine may be damaged. These growth centers may have been damaged by the tumor itself.[57–62] In those tumors requiring radiation therapy, selective growth inhibition may occur as a consequence of radiation, particularly, if it is applied in an asymmetric nature.[63,64]

NONOPERATIVE TREATMENT

OBSERVATION

Since the vast majority of scoliosis curves, particularly with respect to idiopathic scoliosis, are not progressive and are not of a sufficient degree to cause potential morbidity, a large number of these children are followed by observation.

In those patients with idiopathic scoliosis, no studies to date have shown that the use of physical therapy such as strengthening and stretching have had an effect in any way on the natural progression of scoliosis. The problem facing physicians treating scoliosis today is primarily an inability to predict which curves are going to progress and which curves are going to be static. At this time there is no specific diagnostic test that will differentiate those 9- or 10-year-old children who will progress from those who will not; by necessity, multiple observations over the course of time become the preferred management scheme. Most scoliosis patients are referred to an orthopedist from a primary care physician or school nurse who may have noticed an elevated rib hump on a physical examination. The children with idiopathic scoliosis have no other notable abnormalities, and the orthopedist is faced with a necessity of determining the best method and frequency for multiple observations. In the past, x-ray analysis was performed on a routine basis every 4 to 6 months, but there is now increasing concern over the potential adverse effects of multiple x-ray exposures, particularly of the abdomen and thorax, in scoliosis follow-up.[38,65] In those children with significant spinal deformity, truncal imbalance, and a positive rib hump, x-ray examination is usually warranted at least on a first-time basis. A single standing posteroanterior film is the preferred routine screening x-ray study, since this minimizes the x-ray dose to breast and ovarian tissue (Figure 18-3). Other x-ray studies such as lateral views would be indicated for those individuals who have back pain, increased kyphosis, or in whom there is a suspicion of other ongoing pathologic processes. X-ray studies to test the flexibility of the spine, such as bending films or traction films, would not be useful in otherwise asymptomatic mild idiopathic scoliosis. In children with congenital scoliosis or in those suspected of having intraspinal pathologic conditions, e.g., diastematomyelia or tumors, anteroposterior or lateral tomograms or computed axial tomograms may be helpful in delineating the lesion and defining the osseous pathologic condition.[66–69] Myelography, sonographic studies, and magnetic resonance imaging (MRI) may be helpful in the differentiation of intraspinal pathologic processes.[66–79] Follow-up examinations are scheduled for every 6 to 8 months during periods of very slow growth, but as often as 4 to 6 months during periods of more rapid growth. Recently, back surface shape analysis

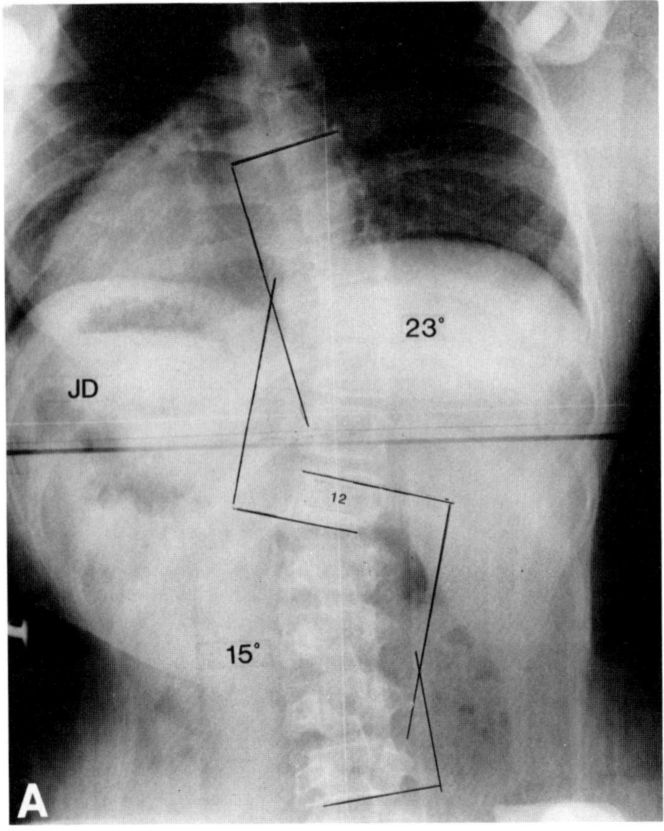

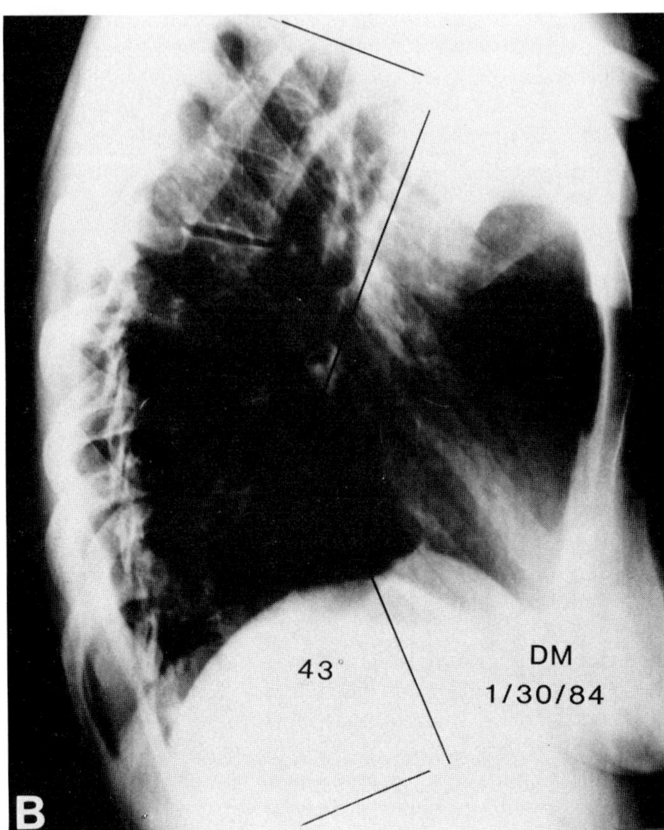

Fig. 18-3. (A) Posteroanterior roentgenogram of the entire spine of an 11-year-old girl with a 23-degree idiopathic right thoracic, 15-degree left lumbar double scoliosis. The standard Cobb measurement is made from the angle formed by perpendiculars to the end plates of the upper portion of the uppermost vertebral body and the lower portion of the lowermost vertebral body. (B) Lateral roentgenogram of the spine showing normal kyphosis (20–45 degrees) of the thoracic spine.

techniques to measure asymmetry from one side to the other, such as Moire fringe (Figure 18-4), or spirit levels, such as the scoliometer,[80,81] have been developed to measure more accurately the back surface deformity. In the case of those children with significant kyphosis, lateral x-ray films of the patient standing or in hyperextension may be helpful in terms of assessing the deformity in the sagittal plane. As long as the curvature does not exceed 20 to 25 degrees as measured by the Cobb technique of comparing the endplate angulation of the upper and lowermost vertebra (Figure 18-3), then observations could continue until spinal growth is complete or at least the patient has completed his of her adolescent growth spurt. If clear progression of the curve above 25 degrees is occurring and growth still remains, then more active treatment should be undertaken.

Follow-up for those patients with neuromuscular or paralytic types of curves is best done by comparing equivalent x-ray films from one visit to the next. If the patient is only capable of sitting, then follow-up anteroposterior films should be obtained with the patient sitting. Objective assessments of the back surface shape in neuromuscular and paralytic curves are less effective.

As long as the curve is mild at the beginning, that is, less than 25 degrees, observation is continued. As mentioned, physical therapy may not change the natural history of the disease, although in those children who tend to be rather sedentary, general recommendations are made for participation in some physical education programs on a routine basis to maintain general muscle tone. Although there is no specific indication for an exercise program, neither is there an indication that sports activities or any other specific activities, such as playing of musical instruments, carrying a book bag, or performing household chores, be avoided.

Once the skeleton has matured, the likelihood of mild curves progressing is so small that very little follow-up is required. If extenuating circumstances occur, such as an additional underlying disease process, significant truncal imbalance, or marked back surface rotation for the degree of curvature, then follow-up into early adult years may be warranted. Curves are considered mild if they are under 30 degrees and other than a mild cosmetic disturbance of back surface shape occasionally evidenced by an elevated shoulder or slight elevation of the hip, little to no functional impairment will occur.

BRACING AND ELECTRICAL STIMULATION

A group of patients exists in all classified categories of scoliosis in which the curvature and truncal imbalance has reached a degree that a more active means of intervention appears necessary. Those children with idiopathic scoliosis whose curves have reached at least 25 degrees, whose curves appear to be increasing, and who have growth remaining, are candidates for therapeutic intervention. In most recent years, bracing has been the standard of treatment in the group of patients having a moderate curve (25–45 degrees) with growth remaining. Historically, some type of bandaging or bracing has been attempted in scoliosis since the time of Hippocrates. Various metal plates, bandages, wooden splints, and leather

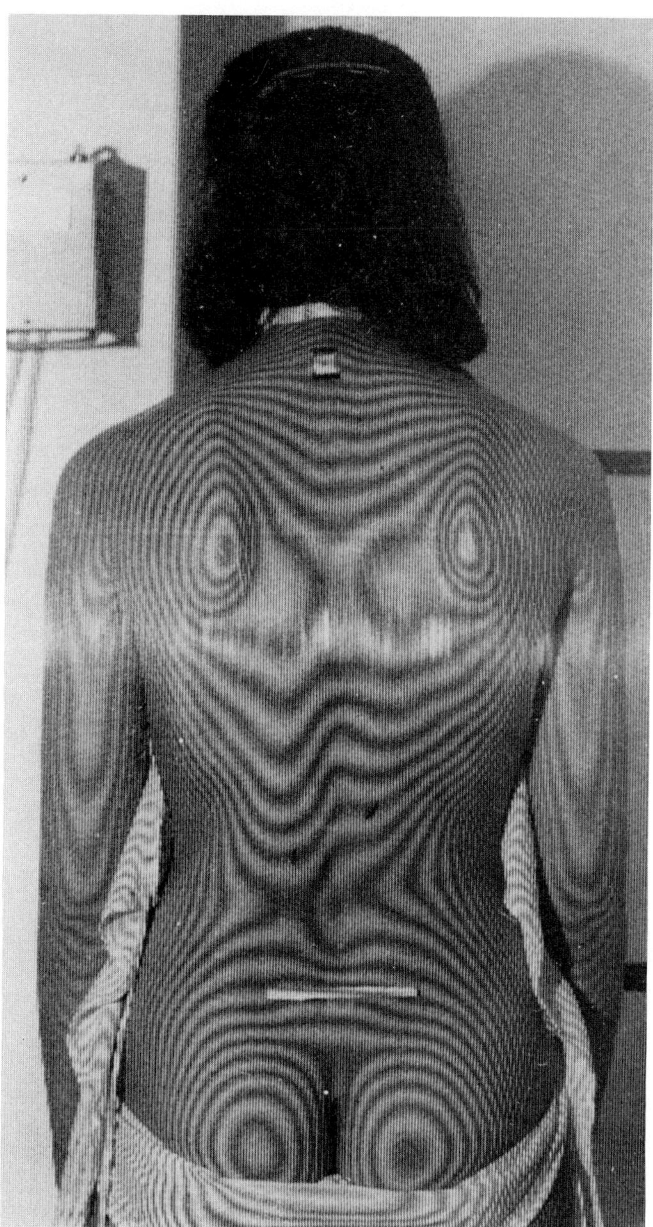

Fig. 18-4. Moire fringe of back surface. This effect, which is optically generated by projecting light through a grid and observing the projected lines through a second grid, gives a light pattern on the surface analogous to a contour map, where each dark line is 0.5 cm higher or lower in the anteroposterior plane. Such three-dimensional information allows comparison of the asymmetry of the back surface, reflecting the underlying rotation and lateral deviation of the spine. This patient has a right thoracic and left lumbar idiopathic scoliosis. Distortions can be seen in the pattern over the scapula and left lumbar paravertebral region.

braces have been used over the years. These early versions were not effective at controlling the curves, although this may have been in part a result of the failure to recognize curves until they had reached such a large degree that bracing could no longer be effective. The current effective means of brace therapy was developed by Blount and Schmidt in the early 1950s.[82] This brace consists of a molded leather pelvic girdle with fixed upright metal supports joining a ring placed about the neck. This brace, known as the Milwaukee Brace, was used to control the progression of curves that had reached the 20- to

30-degree level. It utilized a combination of static and dynamic forces to produce truncal alignment, elongation, and derotation and was worn 23 out of 24 hours a day. The brace was not used and not recommended for use in those patients who clearly qualified for a spine fusion, that is, patients whose curve had reached 45 to 50 degrees or more. Long-term follow-up results for patients treated with the Milwaukee Brace showed that the brace could be effective at controlling the curve, that is, preventing progression approximately 80 to 85 percent of the time.[83] The end results at 2 years after the discontinuance of bracing showed that the average curvature remained the same as at the time the brace was started plus or minus 5 degrees.[84] With the advent of thermal plastics and the nearly universal dislike on the part of patients of the upper neck ring of the Milwaukee brace,[19] low profile, primarily passive braces were designed. A typical example of this TLSO (thoracolumbosacral orthosis) is the Boston Brace (Figure 18-5), which fits more comfortably under clothes and provides a broader distribution of the external forces.[85,86] The indications for their application are similar to those of the Milwaukee brace, although recently some have advocated wearing the brace part-time.[87,88] The mechanism by which such braces prevent progression of the curve is at present unknown. In paralytic curves and in scoliosis curves occurring as a secondary phenomenon to other disease processes, bracing has also been effective. However, it is important to identify the presence of a curve while it is still within a moderate range, and while the curve remains flexible. In patients with congenital scoliosis caused by an unsegmented unilateral congenital bar in which progression is inevitable, with congenital kyphosis or kyphosis occurring in a myelodysplasia, and in idiopathic scoliosis in which thoracic lordosis is present, the use of the brace is contraindicated, since the brace can increase the lordosis.

The ability to mold the brace to the specific patient has allowed its application in those patients who have insensate skin, and their use has been extended to help control the trunk for improved sitting balance in both the adolescents and adults. In some spinal cerebellar diseases and myopathies, the rate of progression with bracing has been such as to lead some authors to recommend surgical intervention directly once the scoliosis has been clearly established.[46]

The length of application of the brace in the case of idiopathic scoliosis depends on the time that the child reaches skeletal maturity. At that point, there is generally a weaning process to wearing the brace part-time over the course of a year or more. In the case of neuromuscular diseases, there may not be a clear end point because most paralytic curves will continue to need some kind of support even after skeletal maturity. An exception would be if the degree of curvature increased significantly in the brace, truncal balance was not improved, or there was difficulty wearing the brace. Surgical intervention then would be necessary. An important consideration in the successful use of brace therapy is the presence of an adequately trained and competent orthotist.

In attempting to produce experimental scoliosis, Bobechko was able to successfully produce scoliosis in growing pigs with single-side paravertebral electrical stimulation. He extended that concept to the use of paraspinal electrical stimulation to improve the scoliosis previously created in these experimental animals and went on to test this clinically in patients.[89] His initial studies were based on the intraoperative insertion of paraspinal platinum electrodes. He was able to show some correction in scoliosis patients using this technique. In order to

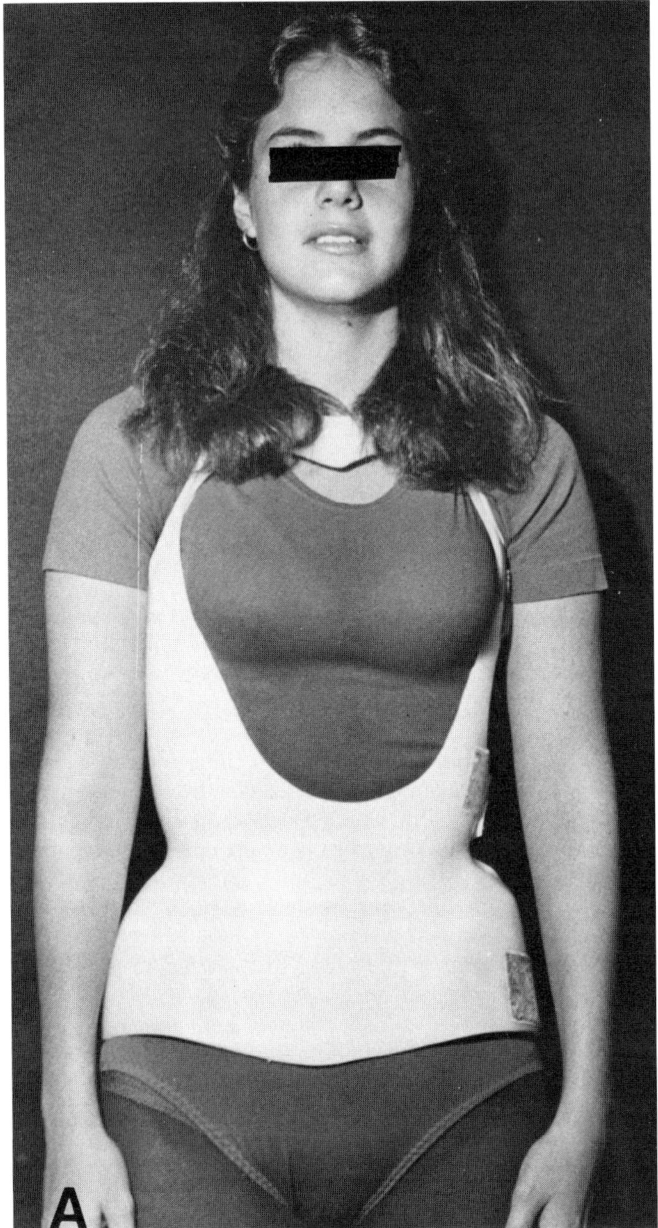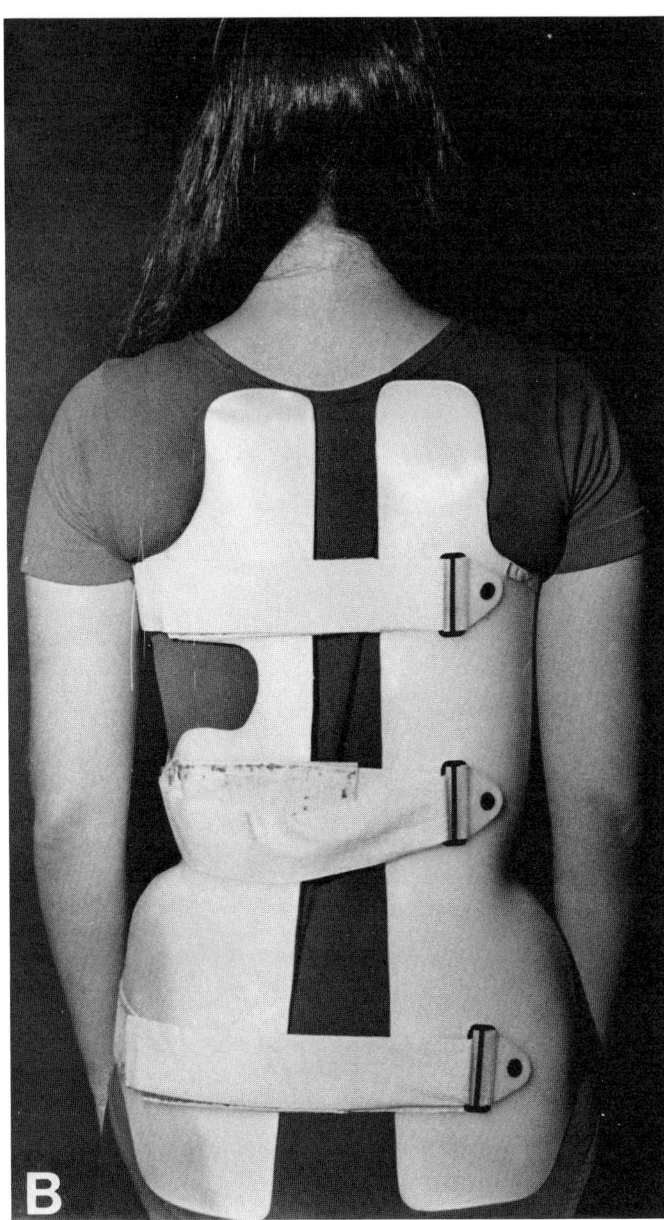

Fig. 18-5.   Boston brace. Modified from a modular molded thermoplastic, the custom fitted brace provides control for moderate curves. (A) The anterior is cut out for the chest. (B) The thoracic extension helps prevent thoracic lordosis.

avoid the operative aspect of this technique, transcutaneous stimulation of paraspinous muscles was investigated in the late 1970s and has subsequently been offered as an alternative method of treatment of moderate scoliosis.[90,91] The current criteria for the application of electrical stimulation are the same as those used for bracing, although many of the initial studies were limited to patients with single curves. Electrical stimulation is applied at night only, thereby avoiding the psychologic and physiologic discomforts that come from wearing a rigid plaster orthosis. Electrodes are positioned over the lateral-most portion of the paravertebral muscle mass. The optimum position is determined by that position that gives the best correction of the curve as measured on x-ray films taken during stimulation. Intermittent muscle stimulation seems generally well tolerated by patients, although there have been a significant number of difficulties with skin sensitivity at the sites of the electrode attachment. Results thus far would appear to indicate that surface electrical stimulation is effective in approximately 70 percent of those patients selected for treatment.[90,91,92] The mechanism of how electrical stimulation works to control progression of scoliosis is unknown, and further studies are needed to prove the effectiveness of the method.

SURGICAL TREATMENT

SURGICAL INDICATIONS

The primary goal of most surgical procedures for scoliosis deformities is to provide for the development of a bone fusion mass, usually to prevent further progression. There are also secondary benefits, such as, improvement of the curvature, elimination of pain, and decompression of the spinal cord and nerve roots. The specific indications for surgical intervention vary according to the underlying disease process. For example, in adolescent idiopathic scoliosis, general guidelines for surgery should include those immature curves that have reached 45 to 50 degrees and are showing signs of progression. In this instance, one is attempting to stop the progression of the scoliosis with the fusion and prevent further deformity. In most patients with scoliotic curvatures greater than 60 to 65 degrees, it may be anticipated that significant although slow progression will occur over the course of time even in adulthood and consideration may be given to surgical intervention in these patients to prevent a further increase, with continued trunk decompensation, back pain, and decreased pulmonary function. In adult scoliosis considerations for surgical intervention would include evidence of progressing curve or back pain. While pulmonary decompensation is clearly a problem in curvatures greater than 60 degrees, there is little improvement expected, at least in the first year postoperatively, although if one compares the eventual expected pulmonary function in the untreated patient with progressive scoliosis, then it is clear that a better state of pulmonary function would occur if the progression of chest deformity is controlled. Adult scoliosis with lateral translation of one vertebra on the other, often occurring in the junctional region between two curves, and frequently associated with back pain and degenerative arthritis, may be an indication for considering surgical intervention.[43,44]

Surgical fusion would be indicated in those neuromuscular or paralytic curves that cannot be managed successfully with a brace or that have reached a degree of curvature (usually 45 to 50 degrees) in which the mechanical distortion of the spine cannot be held satisfactorily with a brace. Early surgical intervention, even for curves in the 25–30-degree range are beneficial in muscle dystrophies and progressive spinal cerebellar disease in order to facilitate sitting without bracing. Surgical exploration and decompression of vertebral column tumors, and spinal cord tumors, usually require surgical fusion for stabilization. This is particularly true in the younger child who is undergoing a wide laminectomy and posterior lateral decompression in which a significant portion of the bone growth centers of the vertebral body have been removed. Because of the propensity for the development of a significant spinal deformity, providing for a fusion over the involved segments at the time of the decompression is most important.

HISTORY

Although scoliosis has been recognized and nonsurgical approaches to correction of the spinal deformity have been known since antiquity, the first actual fusion operation for a spinal deformity was first described by Hibbs in 1911,[93] although Albee,[94] in the same year, also described using a transplanted tibia in the spine for tuberculosis. While these first spine fusions were not intended for scoliosis, they suggested their possible use for spinal deformities. In 1931, Hibbs[95] published the results of 360 fusions for scoliosis. In many of these patients, corrections were accomplished preoperatively by a turnbuckle-type of corrective cast. However, there were a great number of failures of fusions and complications in the reported group in part related to the minimal immobilization that was used postoperatively. Complications associated with spine fusion and failure of fusion to occur continued to be prevalent through the next two decades. A report of the

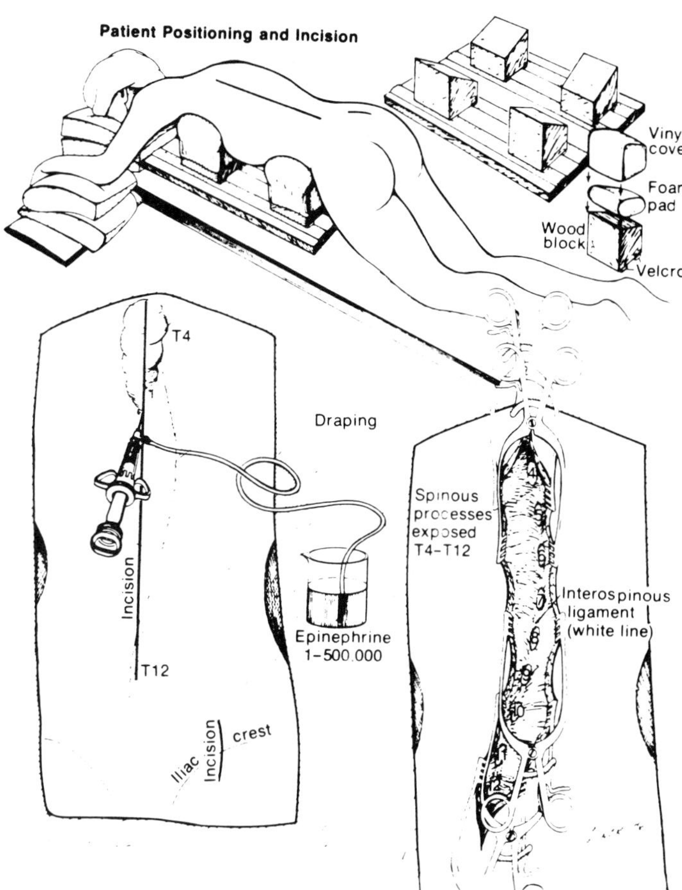

Fig. 18-6.   The patient is positioned on a well-padded four-poster frame, allowing the abdomen to remain completely free. Following skin preparation, a midline skin incision is made over the area of the spine to be fused. The incision is made just into the dermis, and the dermal and subcutaneous tissues are infiltrated with a 1:500,000 solution of epinephrine. The skin incision is then deepened down to the linea alba, dissection being facilitated by the use of Weitlaner self-retaining retractors. (Reprinted from Moe JH, Winter RB, Bradford DS, et al: Scoliosis and Other Spinal Deformities. Philadelphia, WB Saunders, 1978. With permission.)

American Orthopaedic Association[96] showed that of 180 cases reported, approximately 30 percent showed evidence of failure of union of the fusion mass, and 30 percent lost all of the correction. In the late 1950s, scoliosis procedures were being accomplished after corrective casts had been applied. This improved the nonunion rate and also improved the end results for curve correction. The use of autogenous iliac bone grafts also improved the rate of fusion. In the early 1960s, Harrington described a method of adding internal fixation to the spine for further stabilization during the fusion process.[97] This also had the secondary advantage of maintaining some of the correction. Both the fusion rates and the correction were markedly improved and this method became the mainstay of orthopedic corrections for spine deformities. More recent improvements on the technique have involved the use of segmental fixation to the posterior elements by passing wires beneath the lamina and incorporating the rod, thus gaining better fixation at multiple levels.[98,99]

Hodgson[100] first described the anterior approach to the spine for treatment of tuberculous spondylitis. He subsequently used this same approach for straightening a congenitally kyphotic spine and later went on to use this for releases for

Exposure of T4–T12

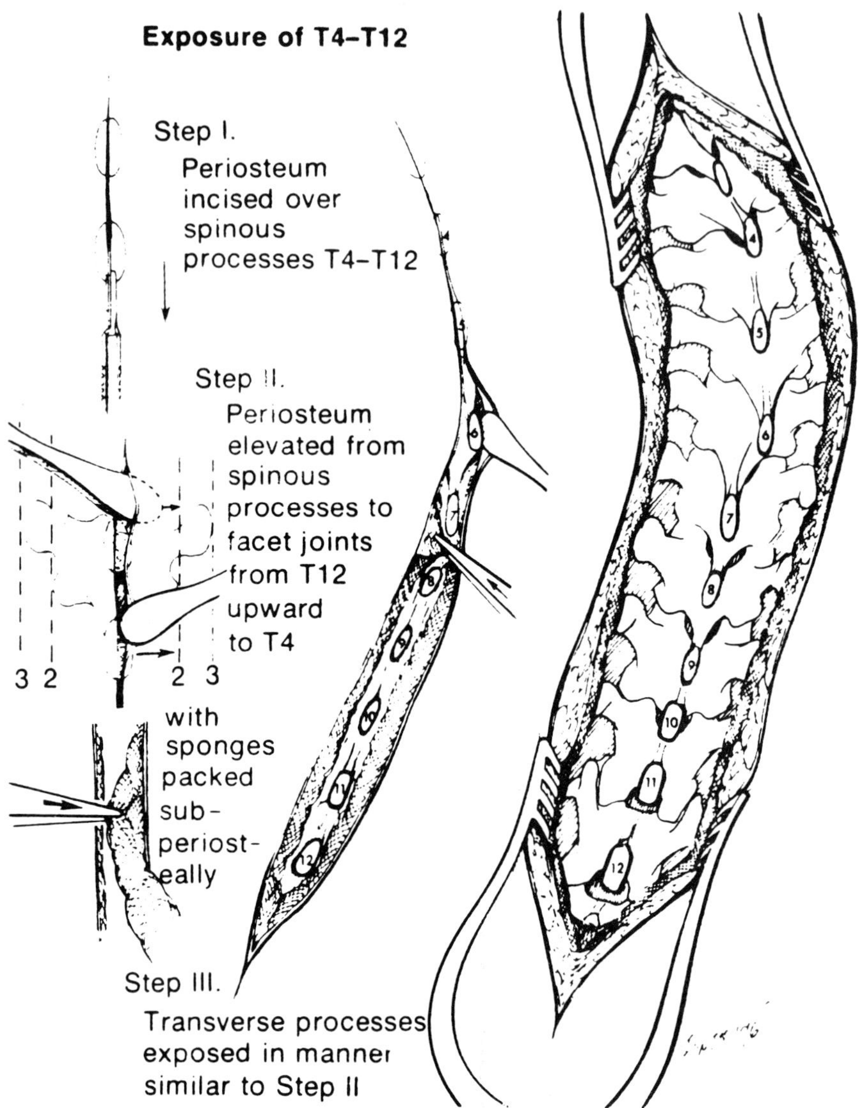

Fig. 18-7.   After the spinous processes have been identified, their centers are incised with a sharp scalpel through the cartilage cap and down into the bony tip. A careful sharp subperiosteal dissection is then carried out, beginning at T12 and working proximally to the upper vertebra to be exposed. Hemostasis is facilitated by subperiosteal sponge packing. A sharp incision is made into the superior facet and the pars interarticularis, allowing the soft tissue with periosteum to then be dissected laterally out to the transverse process. (Reprinted from Moe JH, Winter RB, Bradford DS, et al: Scoliosis and Other Spinal Deformities. Philadelphia, WB Saunders, 1978. With permission.)

other types of spinal deformities. With the introduction of skeletal fixation to the skull with the "halo" device, significant longitudinal and corrective tensions could be applied to the deformed spine.[101] This also improved postoperative management of severe spine deformities. In 1969, Dwyer introduced anterior instrumentation for correction of scoliosis deformity and ushered in yet another dimension in attempts to both correct the deformity and maintain the fusion of the spine.[102]

As previously emphasized, the primary goal of operative procedures for curvatures of the spine is to encourage formation of a bony fusion mass to prevent further progression. This singular proposition underlines the importance of obtaining an osseous fusion regardless of the technique used with or without instrumentation. There are a variety of approaches and techniques in current use, and modifications and refinements are constantly being added to improve the outcome. The selection

of a specific procedure depends on the location, severity, and underlying pathologic state of the deformity and the knowledge and experience of the surgeon. In general, approaches fall into two general categories, those done from the posterior aspect of the spine and those accomplished from the anterior aspect. Excellent descriptions of these techniques can be found in standard operative textbooks.[19,103]

POSTERIOR APPROACHES

In order to create an environment that is safe for the patient and produces relaxed intra-abdominal pressure to minimize bleeding, a prone position, usually on some type of truncal support, is preferred. Rolls placed on either side of the thorax while the patient is in prone position will allow the intra-abdominal contents to fall between the rolls as the abdomen

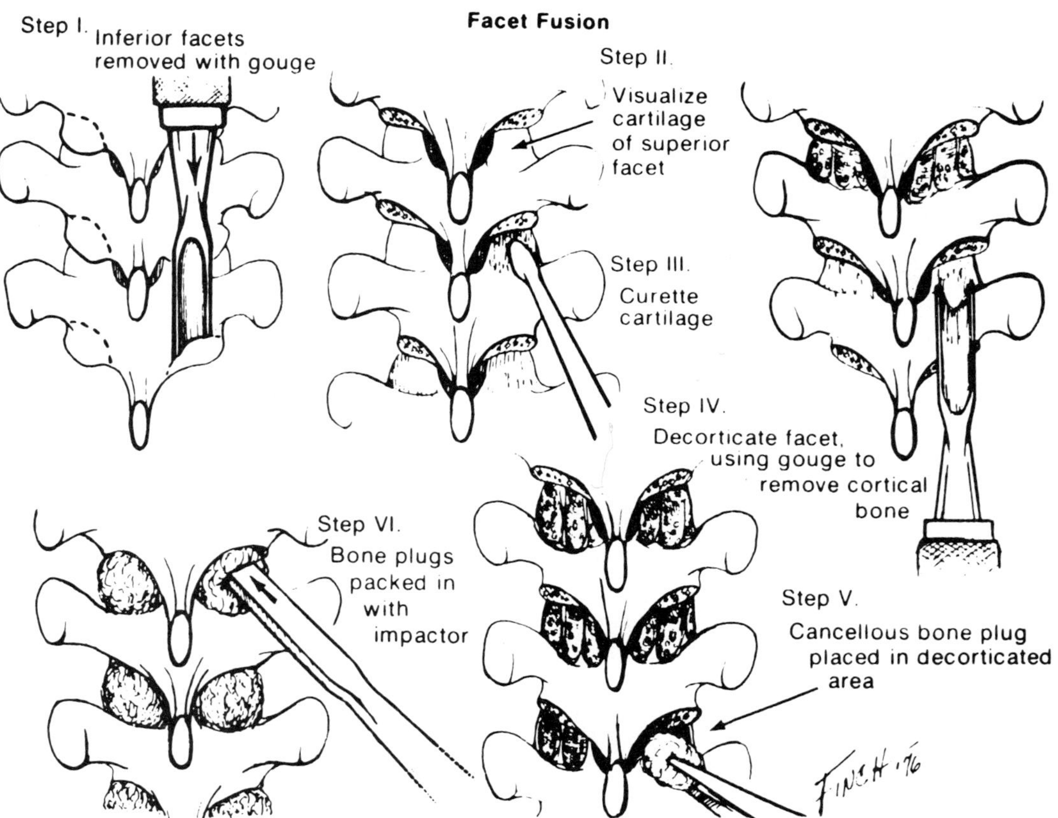

Fig. 18-8. An excellent facet joint fusion can be achieved by the methods described by Hall. In the first step, the inferior facet joint is sharply cut with a semicircular gouge in the manner outlined. The bone fragment with underlying articular cartilage is removed in one piece. The superior facet cartilage is then easily visualized and removed with a sharp curette. A trough is created by removing the outer cortex of the superior facet. Cancellous bone is then taken from the outer table of the ilium and snugly packed into the decorticated area previously created. (Reprinted from Moe JH, Winter RB, Bradford DS, et al: Scoliosis and Other Spinal Deformities. Philadelphia, WB Saunders, 1978. With permission.)

distends towards the table with gravity. The arms must be free, and care needs to be taken to prevent hyperextension of the shoulders and hyperabduction. Bony prominences need to be padded carefully. The Relton-Hall operating frame provides very adequate patient positioning with good control of the truncal position. This four-poster technique involves pads anterior over the clavicles and pectoralis region, and pads placed at the inguinal region. By adjusting the separation between the caudal and cephalad regions of the frame and by adjusting the width, adequate patient positioning can be obtained. Standard preparation with an iodine and soap scrub and meticulous attention to draping are important to ensure a minimal postoperative infection rate.

The following description gives the operative steps for posterior spine fusion in situ. This can be done alone without instrumentation, for example, in congenital scoliosis, but usually is combined with one or more forms of instrumentation.

Adequate visualization of the spine is created posteriorly through a straight incision made from the spinous process above the upper level of the anticipated fusion to the spinous process below the anticipated lowermost portion of the fusion (Figure 18-6). Epinephrine (1:500,000) can be infused into the subcutaneous tissues and into the muscle mass to minimize bleeding. The spinous processes are identified and, in the case of a child, the apophysis can be split and subperiosteal dissection carried over the lamina to the tips of the transverse process throughout the length of the spine to be fused (Figure 18-7). A

meticulous cleaning of the osseous structures to ensure a minimal amount of fibrous tissue will help to encourage a more vigorous osteoblastic response. Facet fusions are accomplished by osteotomizing the inferior articular process of the vertebral body above and isolating and removing the facet cartilage (Figure 18-8). The superior articular facet of the inferior vertebra can be curetted to expose cancellous bone. Facet fusions should be carried out at a minimum on the concave side and may also add beneficially to the fusion if carried out on the convex side of the curvature. Bone graft can be added at this stage.

The use of an autogenous bone graft significantly improves the fusion rate. Cancellous strips of bone obtained from the outer table of the posterior aspect of the iliac crest are harvested either through a separate lateral skin incision over the posterior crest or through the lower portion of the spinal incision. One or both iliac crests can be used. For this exposure, the posterior paravertebral muscles that attach to the superior portion of the iliac crest and the superior-most attachment of the gluteus maximus fibers are sharply dissected over the apophysis of the ilium. In children, sharp dissection is again carried down to bone, splitting the apophysis, which then leads to the subperiosteum over the lateral portion of the iliac wing. For the most part, the posterior one third of the ilium should be exposed and long cancellous strips harvested with either an osteotome or a curved gouge. Cancellous strips can be harvested following decortication.

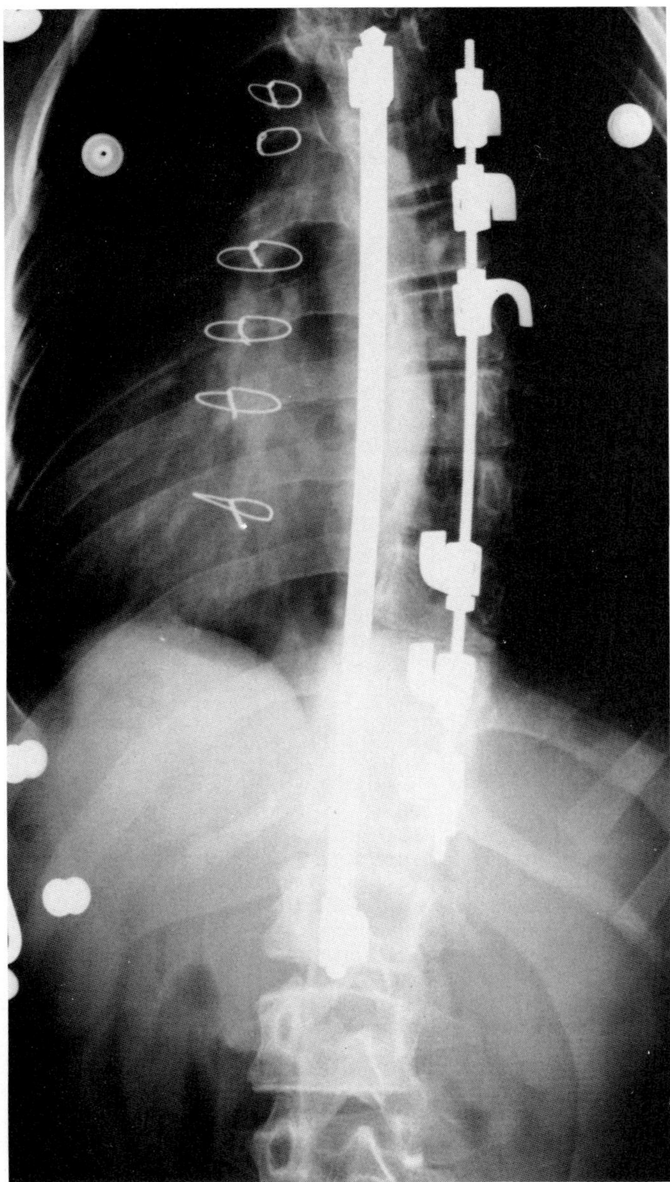

Fig. 18-9. Postoperative PA roentgenogram of a 15-year-old patient with a right thoracic scoliosis demonstrating a Harrington distraction rod on the concave side of the curve and a compression rod on the convex side. In most patients with reduced kyphosis or hypokyphosis, a single distraction rod is adequate.

Following this, the posterior elements of the spine, the laminae, transverse processes, and the spinous processes can be decorticated with a curved gouge. Some of the decorticated bone serves as a bone graft. This is supplemented with the autogenous iliac graft, which should be placed from the tip of the transverse process in the thoracic region all the way to the base of the spinous process. In the lumbar region it is important to obtain dissection beyond the facets to the level of the posterior lateral gutter and out on to the posterior aspect of the tips of the transverse processes. Decortication of the posterior aspects of these structures then allows the development of a posterior lateral fusion mass with bone grafting laid from transverse process to transverse process. Lumbar facets, which were previously debrided of cartilage, should have bone graft packed in between the surfaces. The bone grafts are allowed to

rest passively in place and the paraspinous muscles are closed to the midline over the top of them carefully. A Hemovac drain is placed and the facia and subcutaneous tissues are closed with interrupted absorbable sutures. The skin is closed subcutaneously with a running absorbable suture.

If a significant rib deformity is present with a considerable posterior rotation of the back surface and rib cage, transverse osteotomies across the thoracic transverse processes can be accomplished. This leaves a single rib attachment onto the lateral aspect of the vertebral body and produces increased flexibility of the rib cage, which may allow reduction in the rib hump with appropriate postoperative molding in a brace. More radical techniques of thoracoplasty have been advocated. The primary goal of an in situ fusion oftentimes is to prevent further curvature, particularly one related to congenital spine fusion. In this particular instance, there may be a fused mass along the concave side of the curve with open lamina and transverse processes on the convex side. By fusing the convex side further progression can be prevented.

Spine fusion after a laminectomy for decompression of the spine creates special problems.[104–106] Hopefully, in a child the laminectomy will be done in as conservative manner as possible in order not to disturb the inherent stability of the spine.[107] When stabilization needs to be accomplished, the fusion mass should bridge the laminectomy site, and specific attention should be directed to getting the bone mass lateral to the tips of transverse process in addition to across the laminotomy site if at all possible. If the laminotomy has taken place over several levels, it may not be possible to fuse over the large expanse of dura. If there is no satisfactory bone stock in the remaining transverse process, it may be necessary to consider an anterior interbody fusion for improved stability.

HARRINGTON ROD INSTRUMENTATION

The complete Harrington instrumentation applies two different forces to the spine. One is a distraction force distributed along a ¼-inch rod with hooks at either end. The second is a compression system distributed along a more flexible threaded rod with multiple compression hooks at either end[108] (Figure 18-9). The standard Harrington instrumentation for most idiopathic curves has been the distraction rod. A large majority of the patients with idiopathic scoliosis tend to have a hypokyphosis associated with their curvature. This lends itself ideally to distraction, which is usually carried out from a neutrally rotated vertebra above to a neutrally rotated vertebra below. Selection of the fusion area is important for two reasons. First, it is important to fuse and correct all of those vertebrae participating in the curve. This may be a difficult choice in a juvenile patient in whom progression of the curve can occur above or below the level of the curve present at the fusion by adding vertebrae onto the curve. In this instance, it may be necessary to anticipate the adding-on problem and fuse a level above and below the apparent neutral vertebrae. In those patients with two structural curves with equal degrees of stiffness, fusion should extend across both curves. Second, Cochran[109] has shown that the incidence of low back pain occurring in previously fused spines of patients with scoliosis tends to be higher the lower the fusion has been extended. Therefore, every attempt should be made, if possible, to select the caudal vertebra at a level that leaves as many interspaces from the L5–S1 junction as is possible and still incorporates the majority of the curve.

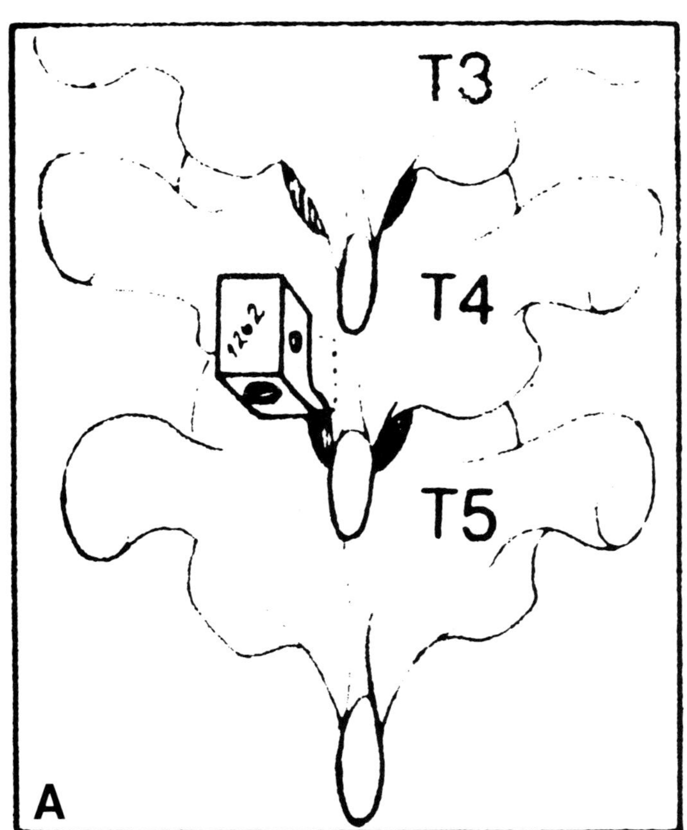

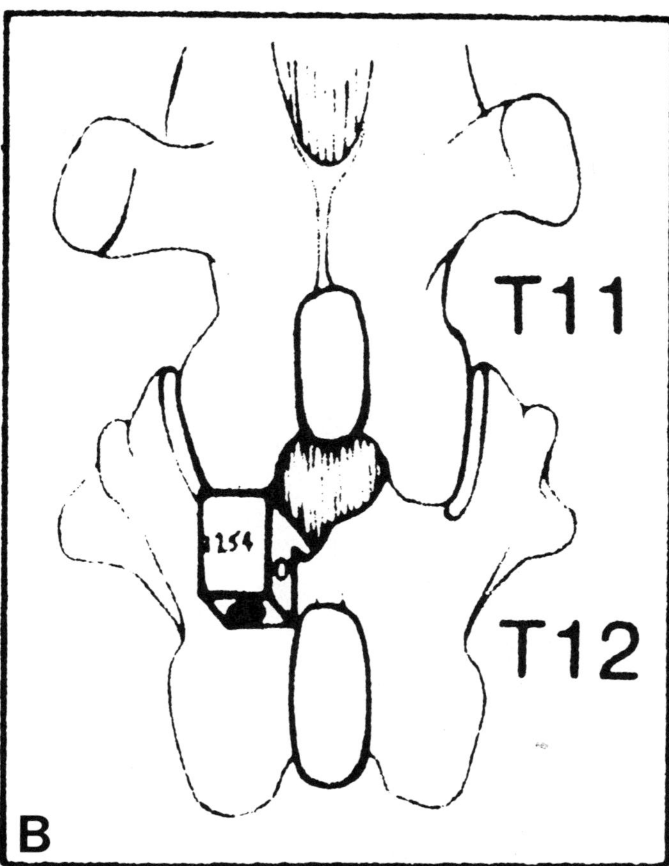

Fig. 18-10. Hook locations for the Harrington rod system. (A) The upper hook is seated against the caudal aspect of the thoracic lamina. (B) The lower hook seated over the cephalad portion of the inferior vertebra. (Reprinted from Moe JH, Winter RB, Bradford DS, et al: Scoliosis and Other Spinal Deformities. Philadelphia, WB Saunders, 1978. With permission.)

The hook sites inferiorly are usually placed in the lumbar vertebrae, occasionally in the thoracolumbar vertebrae (Figure 18-10). The inferior hook site is prepared by defining the superior edge of the lamina on the concave side of the inferior-most vertebra selected. The superior edge of this vertebra is freed of its ligamentum flavum attachments and a dull inferior hook is inserted over the edge of the lamina. It may be necessary to remove a small portion of the inferior articular facet or lamina from the vertebra above in order to allow the hooks to seat satisfactorily. It is important not to weaken the lamina with significant dissection of the superior border of the lamina onto which the hook sits.

The upper hook site is selected by defining the superior-most vertebra. The upper hook is seated under the inferior edge of the lamina on the concave side of the vertebra by again stripping the ligamentum flava from under the inferior surface of the lamina. This can be done by the insertion of a sharp upper hook followed by a dull hook. Adequate seating onto this lamina is exceedingly important and the position of the foot of the hook medial to the pedicle is an important factor in maintaining upper hook fixation. After satisfactory hook placement, the rod is engaged by advancing the rod through the ratchet system, the self-locking mechanism of the upper hook holds the distraction. The distraction is carried out to a single hand tightness, with care being taken not to overly distract so as to cause laminal fracture or hook cut out. A locking wire or washer is applied in the upper portion of the ratchet to prevent

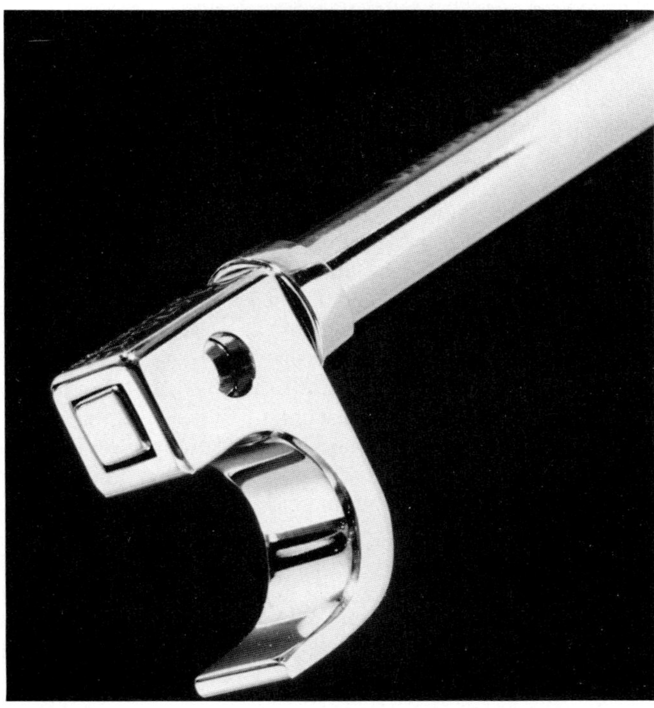

Fig. 18-11. Square-ended hook for the inferior or caudal hook site. The design of this hook prevents rotation of the rod and allows contouring to accommodate the normal lordosis in those patients who require instrumentation into the lumbar region.

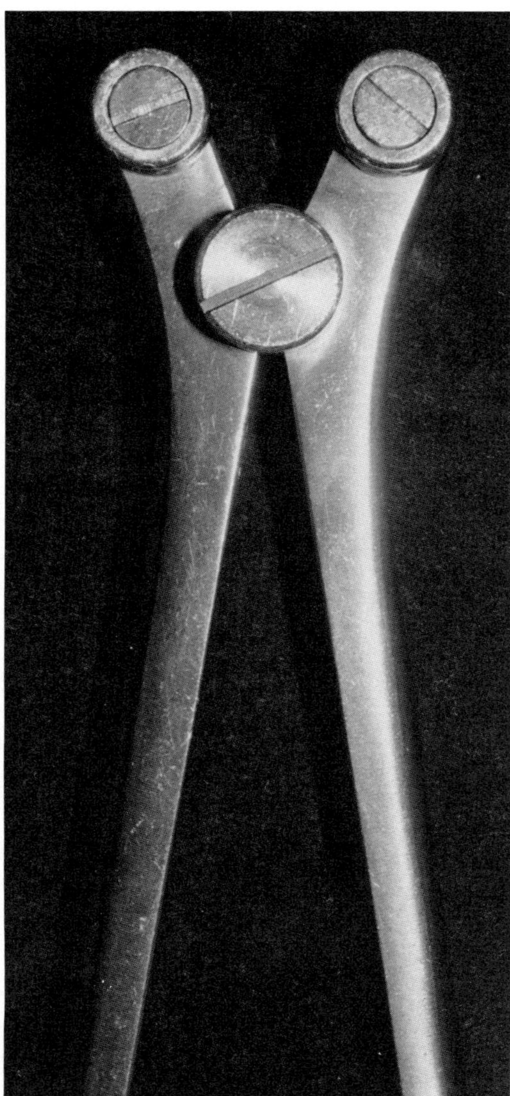

Fig. 18-12. Rod bender (DePuy, Inc., Warsaw, Indiana) for contouring Harrington rods into the appropriate kyphotic or lordotic curves.

the hook from backing and any excessive upper portion of the rod is removed with large bolt cutters.

Modifications of the original Harrington system have occurred over the course of time. The most significant of these is the addition of a square-ended rod for the inferior hook attachment in a square-ended hook assembly (Figure 18-11). Since many fusions extend past the thoracolumbar junction into the lumbar area, it is important to contour the Harrington rod to both the kyphosis superiorly and lordosis inferiorly. Failure to do so tends to produce a very straight segment through the normal lordotic portion of the spine and gives the patient a very flat back.

Maintaining the placement of a contoured rod is facilitated through the use of a square-ended hook. This prevents the rod from rotating and twisting when a significant portion of the rod is in a lordotic curved configuration. Contouring of the Harrington rod is facilitated with a special rod benders (Figure 18-12).

The compression device of the Harrington rod system is useful in those patients who also have a kyphosis deformity, particularly in the thoracic or thoracolumbar region. It is contraindicated in those patients who have a hypokyphosis, since the addition of compression on the convex side can accentuate the tendency for lordosis in the thoracic region. Hook sites for upper thoracic vertebra are prepared by clearing the superior edge of the transverse process. The hook is introduced over the superior edge of the transverse process onto the undersurface of the transverse process. At least three hook sites are prepared superiorly and inferiorly, the hook sites are selected at the inferior edge of the lamina. It occasionally is necessary to make a small cut in the inferior aspect of the lamina to be instrumented by using a small osteotome to cut a seat for the hook. The hooks are compressed by advancing the nuts on the threaded rod. When adequate compression has been obtained, the threads are crushed to prevent loosening of the nut.

SEGMENTAL INSTRUMENTATION

The concept of segmental instrumentation in posterior spine fusions was introduced by Luque in the late 1970s.[99] Although originally designed to provide an internal splint for nonfused spines, this rodding technique gained popularity because of the increased rigidity of fixation it provided. This allowed, for the first time, an opportunity to treat patients postoperatively without casts or braces because of the degree of security the instrumentation provides.[110] This technique has gained wide popularity, particularly in the treatment of neuromuscular patients for whom postoperative bracing presents a problem because of skin sensitivity and intolerance of unusual forces placed against the spine and rib cage. In addition, many of these patients are not as demanding of their back in terms of daily activities and therefore produce less stress on the instrumentation. The instrumentation consists of stainless steel L-shaped rods $\frac{3}{16}$ or $\frac{1}{4}$ inch in diameter. The selection of the fusion levels is based on criteria previously mentioned.[19,108,111] At each segmental level, the ligamentum flavum is incised in the midline and dissected laterally both on the convex and concave side. A doubled No. 16 or 18 stainless steel wire is bent into a loop with a radius of curvature of approximately $1\frac{1}{2}$ times that of the lamina and is carefully passed from the inferior edge of the lamina beneath the lamina to the interlaminar space of the next superior segment. Care is taken to keep the tip of the wire against the anterior surface of the lamina at all times. Segmental wires are passed at each level, care being taken to avoid anterior displacement of the wires during the procedure. Two L-shaped rods are cut to the appropriate length for the curvature and bent to accommodate for kyphosis and lordosis less any amount of correction to be obtained. In a similar manner, a degree of scoliosis less than that occurring in the noncorrected state is bent into each rod and approaching what is needed to achieve with correction. After the bends have been made the rods are placed against the posterior lamina.

The segmental wires are divided and one single strand wire is brought over the rod at each segmental level and tightened with a twisting instrument. By incrementally first tightening the ends of the rods on the concave side and working towards the center and, conversely, tightening the center wires on the convex side and working progressively towards either end of the deformity correction of the curvature will occur. The L rods are overlapped on either end (Figure 18-13).

For this procedure less extensive decortication is desired since this tends to weaken the lamina. However, some decortication may be desirable. Bone grafts are applied as for all fusions.

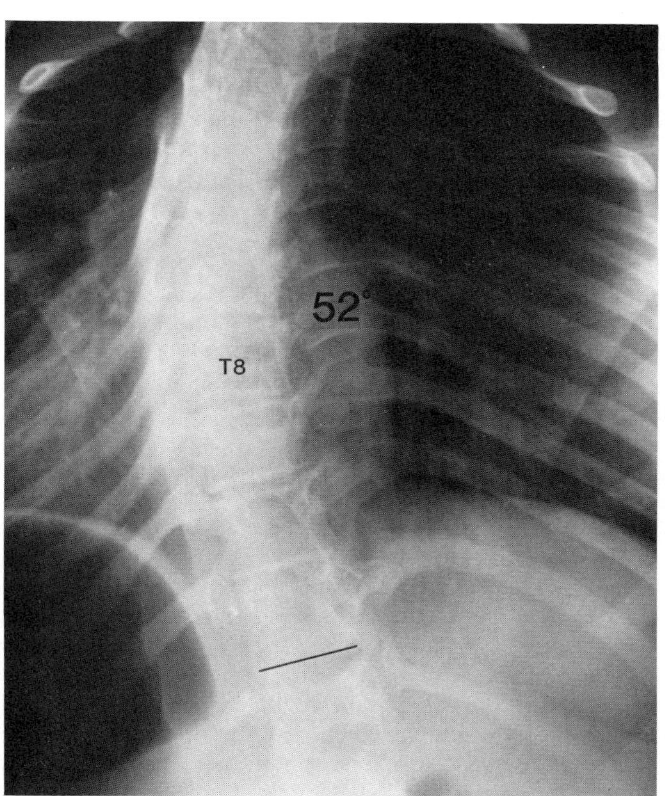
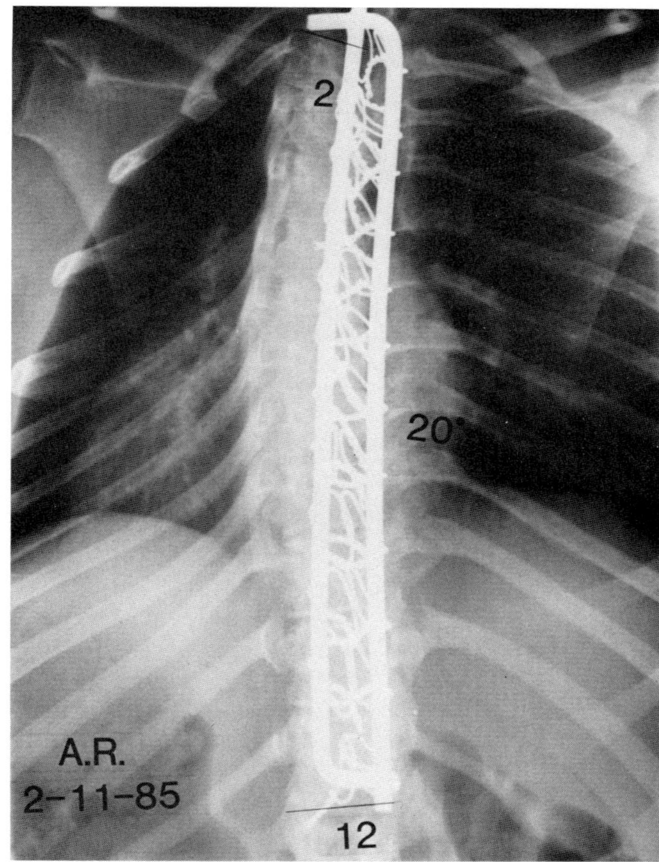

Fig. 18-13. Segmental wiring with Luque rods. (A) Anteroposterior sitting roentgenogram of a 14-year-old mentally retarded patient with neuromuscular scoliosis and a flexible left thoracic scoliosis. (B) Luque instrumentation in place with segmental wires for each rod. Stable fixation reduces demands for postoperative casting and bracing.

THE WISCONSIN SYSTEM

Because of the inherent dangers of inserting the segmental wires into the spinal canal, and the even greater potential dangers of removing these wires should this be necessary at a later time, Drummond has designed a segmental fixation system that does not require entrance into the spinal canal.[112,113] In this system, the base of the spinous process is used for fixation. Small holes are gouged through the cortical portion of the base of the spinous process above the cortex of the spinal canal from right to left and left to right. Wires are passed through these openings. They are secured around the rod in a twisted fashion. Small buttons prevent wire cut out through the base of the spinous process (Figure 18-14).

Combinations of Harrington instrumentation and Luque rod or a Harrington rod with segmental wiring have been used.[114] The instrumentation steps for this proceed according to the usual instrumentation technique for each type of instrumentation. If the Harrington rod is segmentally wired, care must be taken to make sure that the rod is sitting against a lamina in such a manner as to prevent hook protrusion into the spinal canal when the wires are tightened.

COTREL-DUBOUSSET FIXATION

A variation of the form of segmental fixation has been developed in Paris by Cotrel and Dubousset.[115] This system, not unlike the Harrington rod system, utilizes a combination of distraction and compression but allows application of the point of these forces in a more controlled manner onto several laminae of the involved vertebrae. In addition, the system allows transverse loading to be applied between the rods by cross-connecting pieces cephalad and caudad to turn the system into essentially a rigid four-part frame (Figure 18-15). Preparation for instrumentation proceeds in a standard fashion for fusion. The solid rod is bent for the concave side to fit the curvature that is present intraoperatively and in roughly the same proportion as the desired kyphosis after instrumentation. The proximal and distal hooks are engaged with the rod as are two intermediate open hooks on the concave side. Maintaining a slight distraction, the rod is rotated through 90 degrees to change the curve from a coronal plane deformity to a sagittal plane correction. Since the hooks are fitted under the lamina, this tends to bring the central portion of the curve into more of a kyphotic configuration. The convex side is reinforced by application of superior and inferior compression hooks and a central compression hook. The entire system is pulled together by transverse loaders. The rods have a irregular cut surface that allows each hook to be secured to the rod with individual set screws. This allows application of force at each specified level, which aids in correction and also improves the security of the fixation. In this particular instance, bone grafts should be applied before application of the rod, since the amount of instrumentation makes it difficult to accurately place the grafts after instrumentation. This system appears to have considerable advantages in maintaining increased rigidity in both the sagittal and coronal planes. A major advantage of this system is

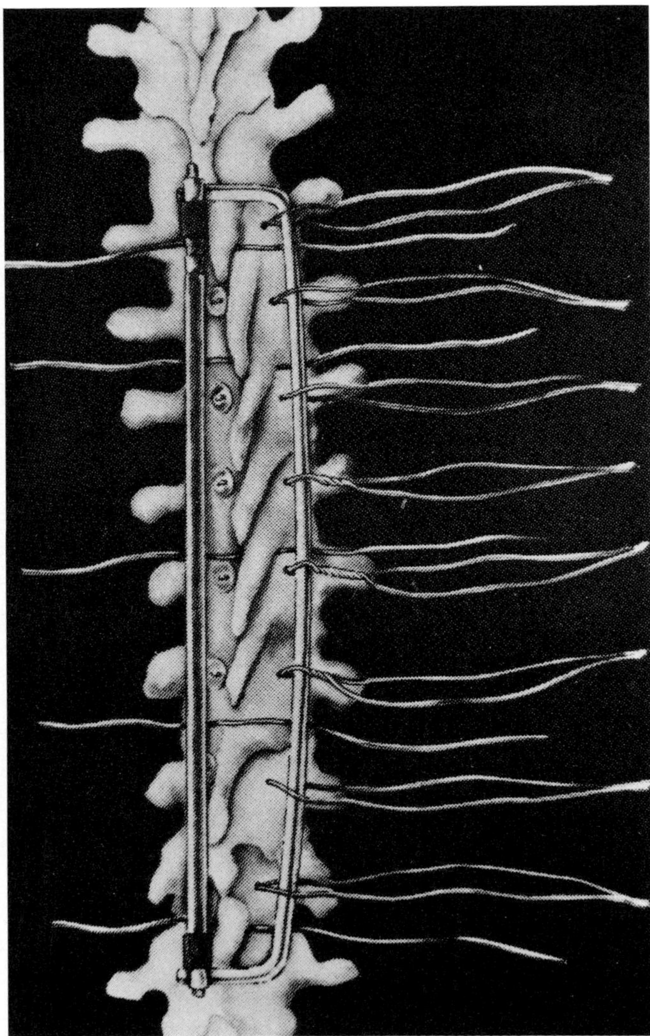

Fig. 18-14. Interspinous segmental spinal instrumentation. Wires are passed through the bone at the base of the spinous processes and then placed around the Luque rod. Note the additional wires to tie the Harrington and Luque rods together. (Reprinted from Drummond D, Guadagni J, Keene JS, et al: Interspinous process segmental spinal instrumentation. J Pediatr Orthop 4:399, 1984. With permission.)

its ability to correct a sagittal plane deformity as well as the underlying scoliosis curvature. However, as with all instrumentation systems, complete correction is rarely possible.

TRANSPEDICLE FIXATEURS

For a number of years, vertebral pedicles have held the interest of investigators as a site of fixation for instrumentation. Their lateral placement, bony configuration, location near the midpoint of flexion-extension stresses, and their ability to form a conduit to the anterior vertebral body from the posterior direction have led to interest in the development of multiple screw-type fixateurs.[116,117] The use of pedicles is attractive for spinal fusion, particularly where the lamina and spinous processes are deficient. Cancellous screws, inserted from posterior to anterior, are placed down the pedicle and into the anterior position vertebral body. These screws are angulated from the sagittal plane by 10 to 25 degrees and are fastened onto a rod (Vermont fixateur)[118] (Figure 18-16) or plate system.[117] Their

current use with or without plate attachments appears to be best suited for short segment fixation rather than the longer segment fixation required for scoliotic deformity. Subsequent design modifications may improve the desirability of this instrumentation for scoliosis fixation. Careful directional insertion of both the guide and the screw are necessary to avoid misplacement of the screw and to allow cancellous fixation into the anterior body. Following fixation, bone grafting is carried out in the usual manner.

ANTERIOR SPINE APPROACH

Spine deformities of long duration and great severity produce significant structural remodeling of the vertebral bodies in the anterior portion of the vertebral column. Significant wedging, fibrosis, and osteophyte formation occur around the vertebral bodies. In addition, spinal deformities caused by vertebral body infection, congenital abnormalities, such as, hemivertebra and congenital fusions, and tumors may have the greatest degree of structural changes and abnormalities in the anterior portion of the vertebral column. The most direct approach to correction of these deformities is to approach the vertebral column from an anterior direction. This can be done through transthoracic, transthoracolumbar, and either transperitoneal or retroperitoneal anterior lumbar approaches. Excellent descriptions of these procedures are available in the literature.[119–125] The type of incision will be dictated by the level of the deformity to be explored. The transthoracic operative procedures allow accessibility to the upper thoracic region, although for the cervical thoracic region. a combined cervical thoracic approach may be necessary. For deformities extending to the lower thoracic (T11, T12) and the upper lumbar (L1, L2) levels, a combined thoracoabdominal approach, dividing the diaphragm near its peripheral attachment, is necessary. The lumbar spine can be approached through a lateral lumbar sympathectomy type of incision retroperitoneally for exposure of L2 through L4. Either a transperitoneal approach or a retroperitoneal approach can be used for exposing the lumbosacral region at the L5-S1 interspace.

In those deformities occurring in the chest region, the approach involves rib removal. The incision is made over that rib extending from the vertebral margin posteriorly to the costal margin anteriorly. The rib selected is usually the rib at the most superior portion of the deformity, which because of the sloping nature of the ribs, will give adequate exposure to the deformity occurring below that level. The side of the incision should correspond to the convexity of the curve in most cases (Figure 18-17). Once the pleural cavity has been entered, the parietal pleura overlying the spine is divided, the great vessels are identified, and the segmental vessels are isolated and ligated anteriorly so as not to interfere with the longitudinal posterior lateral vessel anastomosis. The disc is incised sharply. Once this material is removed, the endplates are removed to facilitate fusion. The removed rib can be morcelled and used for graft. Additional autogenous grafts can be obtained from an iliac crest if necessary, for example, in kyphotic deformities. The anterior longitudinal ligament can be released. Decompression posteriorly to the posterior longitudinal ligament can be accomplished under direct vision (Figure 18-18). In those cases of significant kyphosis or hemivertebra, decompression of the anterior portion of the spinal canal should be accomplished over a wide area, with vertebrectomy of the hemivertebra. In addition to packing bone chips into the excised disc spaces, anterior strut

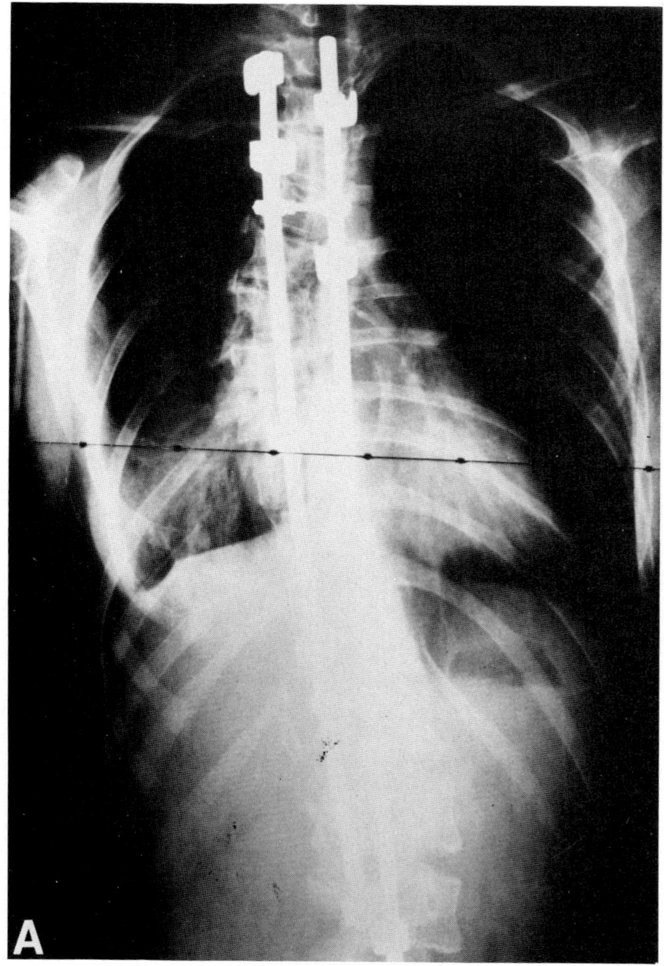

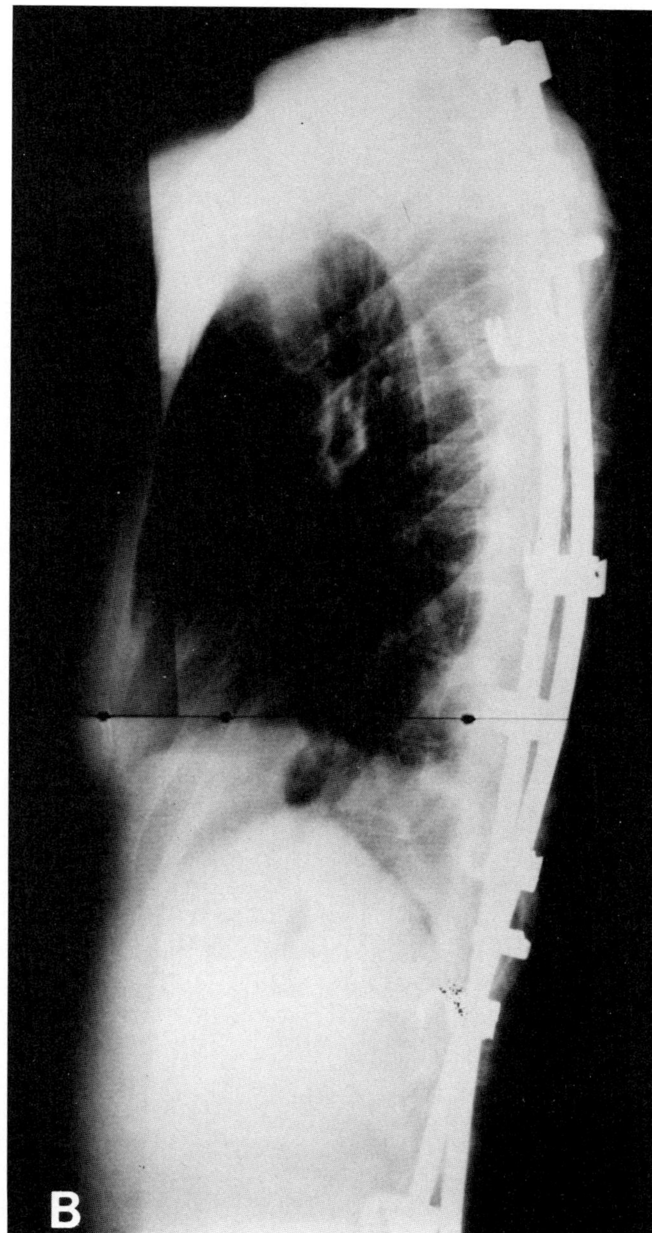

Fig. 18-15. (A) Posteroanterior roentgenogram of an 18-year-old patient after Coutrel-Dubousset instrumentation and fusion. Note the distraction rod with several fixation points, the compression rod on the convex side of the curve, and the transverse loading devices to decrease rotation. (B) Lateral roentgenogram showing a normal kyphosis pattern. (Courtesy of Dr. Richard Holt, Louisville, Kentucky.)

grafts of iliac crest, either fibula, or rib may be used. Recently, a vascularized pedicled rib graft was used successfully.[126]

Thoracolumbar approaches are usually made through the tenth rib, extending the incision onto the abdominal wall down to the level of the rectus abdominus. The junction of the diaphragm and anterior abdominal muscles allows retroperitoneal entrance to the abdominal cavity, and the lumbar region is exposed in a retroperitoneal manner. The diaphragm is incised, leaving a rim for repair, and the thoracolumbar disc spaces are approached in the same manner as for the thoracic region. Care must be taken to protect the great vessels, and segmental vessels should be ligated if any extensive dissection is necessary. It is important to obtain complete disc excision and to expose adequate cancellous bone at each vertebral level before grafting (Figure 18-19).

In 1969 Dwyer introduced an instrumentation system designed to correct scoliosis by direct application of controlled intervertebral force.[125] This is accomplished through a screw placed transversely through each vertebral body. A braided cable is then used to connect the screws from one vertebral level to the other, and by applying tension on the cable, the vertebral bodies can be drawn together on one side (convex), thereby correcting the scoliosis (Figure 18-20). Considerable gains in correction of the scoliosis can be obtained through the use of the Dwyer instrumentation. Large biomechanical forces can be applied to the spine. Care must be taken with the Dwyer instrumentation not to produce or increase a kyphosis deformity, particularly at the thoracolumbar junction.[125] To give better control of the rotational fixation and to maintain lordosis, Zielke developed a solid rod anterior system that works in a

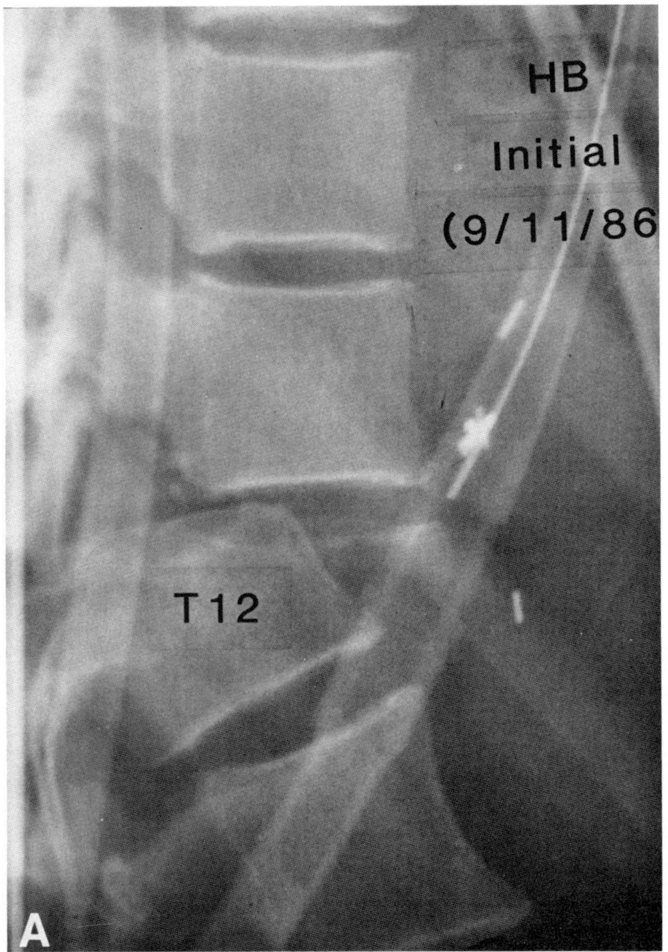

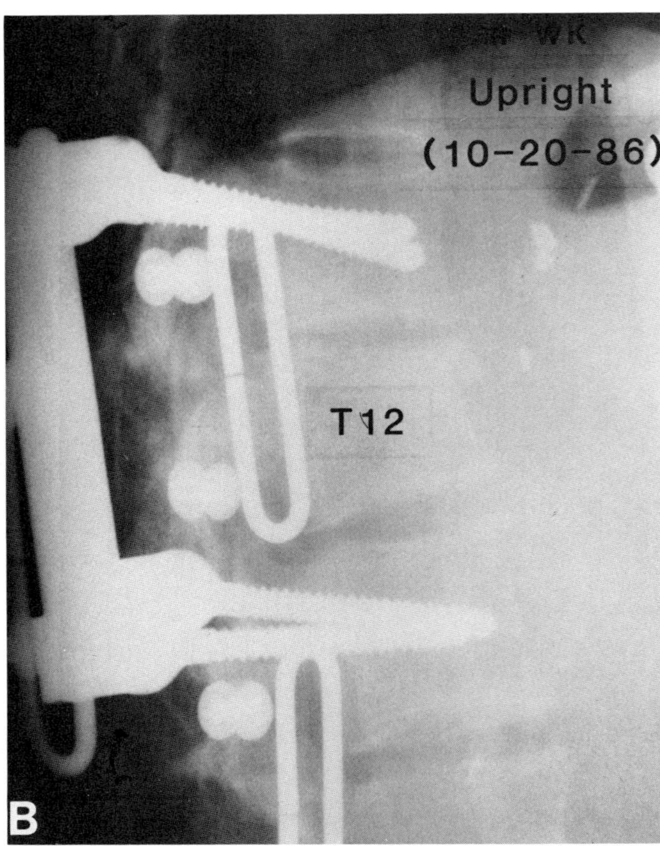

Fig. 18-16. The Vermont fixateur is a transpedicle fixation device that achieves fixation through pedicle screws placed from posterior to anterior with stabilization on adjustable attachments to rods. (A) Preoperative x-ray film showing a fracture dislocation of T11 on T12. (B) A lateral roentgenogram of the spine showing the Vermont fixateur in place 4 weeks after insertion. These devices currently seem best suited to short segment fixation. (Courtesy of Dr. M. Krag, University of Vermont.)

similar manner to the Dwyer system with transvertebral body screws.[127,128,129] The advantage of this system is that the entire fixation can be rotated into a position of lordosis at the completion of instrumentation.

The advantage of anterior spinal instrumentation is that a large degree of correction can be obtained per vertebral level, therefore, less vertebral levels may need to be fused. This has the advantage of leaving more mobile segments and thus not putting as much stress on the lumbosacral junction. In those patients with a thoracolumbar scoliosis, the lower extent of the required fusion may have to be no further than L3. Instrumentation of the thoracic spine anteriorly is rarely used today because of a decreased rate of fusion, the likelihood of producing increased kyphosis, and improved posterior instrumentation.

Combined anterior and posterior instrumentation has been used to increase stability and further correct the deformity particularly in those patients with very severe curves or curves occurring over a large number of segments.[130] With the development of improved posterior fixation techniques, often only anterior release and bone grafting are necessary. It occasionally is necessary to perform an anterior and posterior fusion in the same setting, although combined procedures generally are separated by a 10-day to 2-week interval to allow initial healing of the graft site anteriorly. Anterior release may give consider-

able flexibility and may make posterior fusion much more effective in a severe and well-established deformity.

POSTOPERATIVE MANAGEMENT

The amount of postoperative immobilization necessary to achieve a spinal fusion varies with the surgical technique. For example, in situ fusions particularly across multiple segments will require rather rigid fixation. While casts are rarely used today, bivalve polypropylene underarm bracing is usually employed.[131] Most commonly, the patients who are candidates for postoperative bracing are initially managed in a recumbent position. A Roto-kinetic bed has been used for the first few days postoperatively until fluid balances have readjusted and any postoperative abdominal distention has abated. With adequate adjustment of the brace, ambulation is begun on the fourth or fifth postoperative day. Postoperative bracing is maintained at least through 4 to 6 months on a full-time basis. Depending on the age of the patient, the degree of fixation of the spine, and the level of the spine fusion, the patient may use the brace for more vigorous activities such as sports for the next 6 months. Ambulation is usually undertaken in a progressive manner, and children can return to school within a period of 1 to 2 weeks

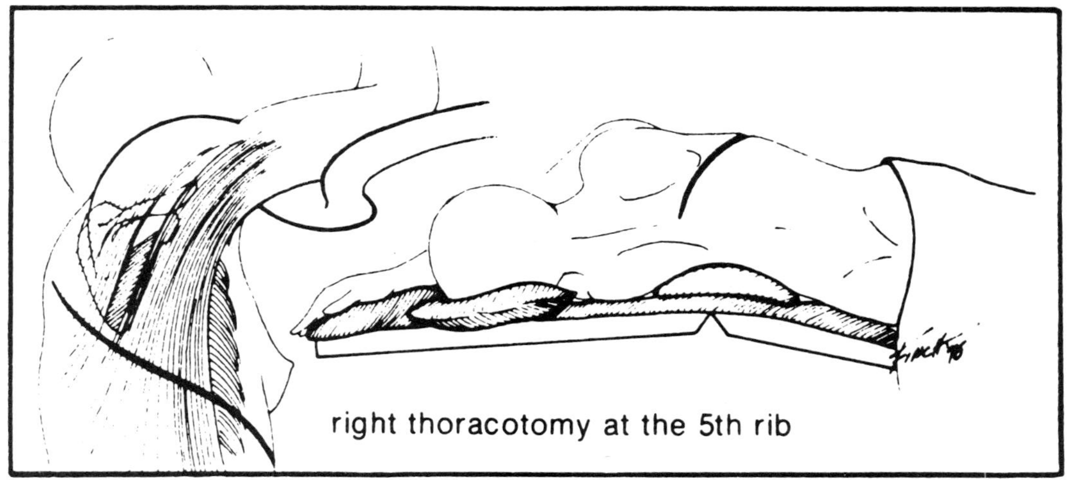

Fig. 18-17. The correct positioning for a patient undergoing a thoracotomy for exposure of the anterior spine at T5. (Reprinted from Moe JH, Winter RB, Bradford DS, et al: Scoliosis and Other Spinal Deformities. Philadelphia, WB Saunders, 1978. With permission.)

after discharge. In instances in which more rigid spinal fixation has been used, such as Luque or Cotrel-Duboussett, postoperative bracing may not be necessary, although patients still have a modified activity schedule and initially are allowed to ambulate only if lifting and sports are avoided. Once an adequate fusion mass is detected radiographically, usually at 4 to 6 months, increased activities can be undertaken.

COMPLICATIONS OF THERAPY

Operations on patients with scoliosis and kyphosis for spinal fusion, for correction of spinal deformities, and for spinal cord decompression are difficult and lengthy procedures. As a consequence, numerous complications have been encountered.[132] These are best considered under several categories.

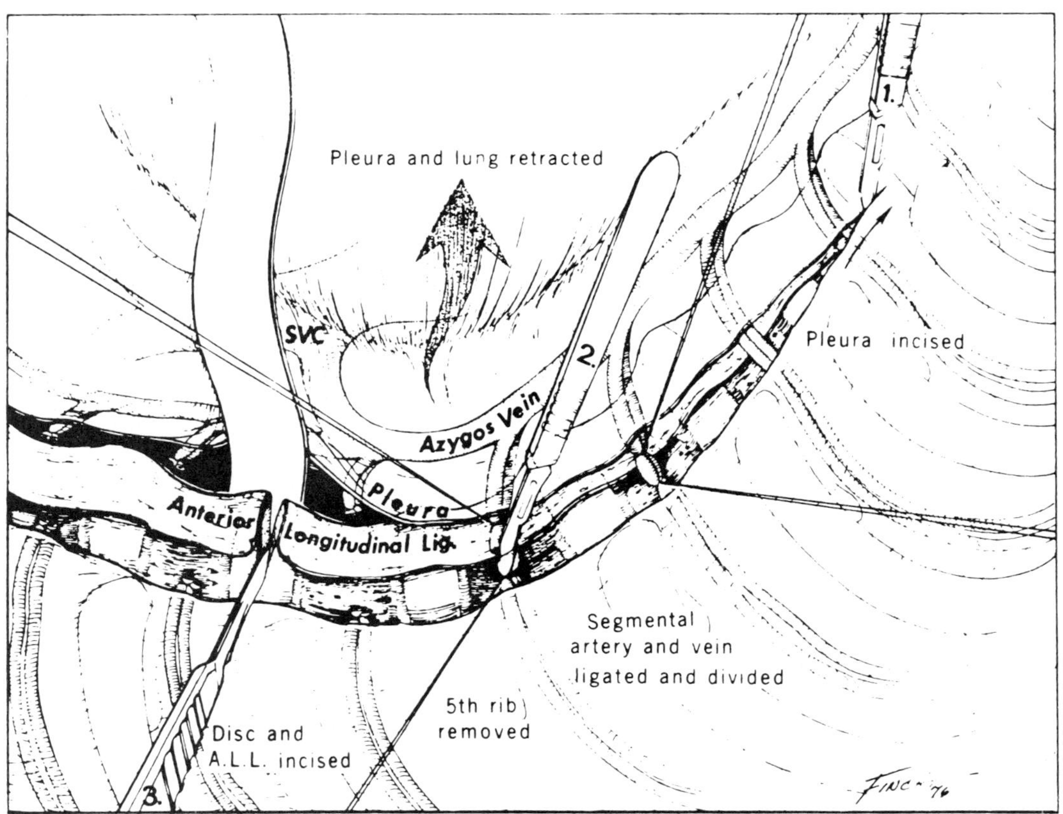

Fig. 18-18. The exposure of the spine following removal of the fifth rib. First, the parietal pleura is incised along the length of the spine to be exposed. The segmental vessels are identified overlying each vertebral body and are ligated and divided anterolaterally at least 1 cm away from the intervertebral foramen. By staying outside the periosteum, the areolar tissue with the divided vessels is pushed off the vertebral bodies and the anterior longitudinal ligament around to the opposite side and into the angle between the vertebral body and the transverse process. A malleable retractor provides excellent exposure. The disc and anterior longitudinal ligament can be incised and completely removed as necessary. (Reprinted from Moe JH, Winter RB, Bradford DS, et al: Scoliosis and Other Spinal Deformities. Philadelphia, WB Saunders, 1978. With permission.)

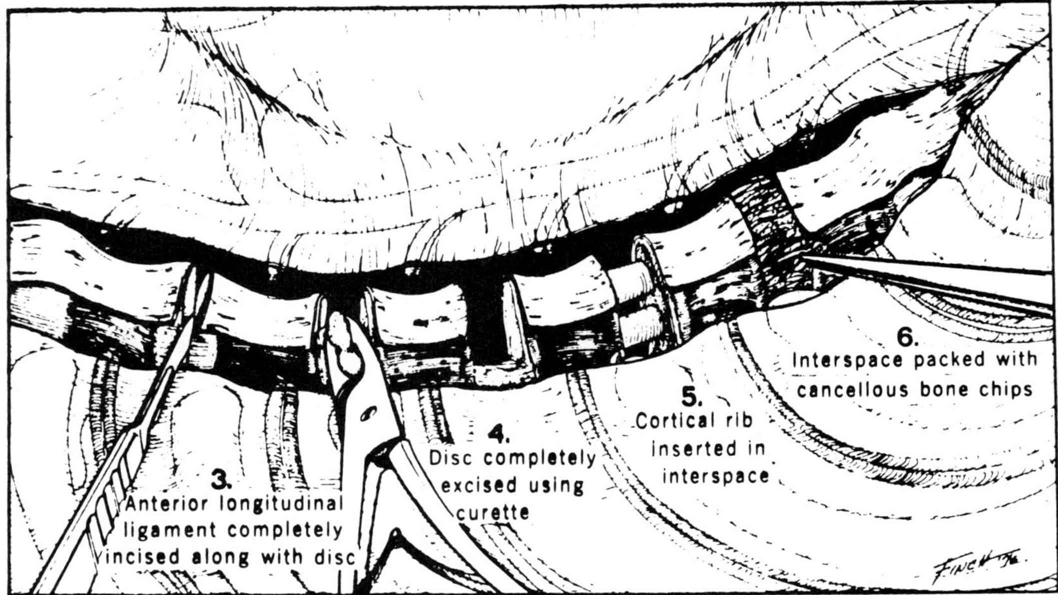

Fig. 18-19. Anterior interbody fusion is accomplished by complete excision of the anterior longitudinal ligament along with removal of the disc. The disc is removed to the posterior annulus and the intervening cartilage is removed to the bony end plate. If correction of the kyphosis is necessary, one should remove the posterior annulus along with the end plates up to the posterior longitudinal ligament. Generally, however, this will not be necessary, since removal of the disc material up to the posterior annulus will make it possible to hinge open the kyphosis and significantly correct the angular deformity. The rib bone that has been removed during the thoracotomy is cut into small pieces and wedged into each intervertebral space, hinging the vertebral bodies open and correcting the kyphosis. Remaining rib strips are then placed into the interspace or, if desirable, cancellous bone from the iliac crest is used to supplement the fusion mass. (Reprinted from Moe JH, Winter RB, Bradford DS, et al: Scoliosis and Other Spinal Deformities. Philadelphia, WB Saunders, 1978. With permission.)

MECHANICAL COMPLICATIONS

With instrumentation of the scoliotic spine, several mechanical problems can occur. Hook cut-out can occur with posterior Harrington instrumentation, particularly in cases of osteoporosis or when excessive attempts at correction have been made. This usually involves the upper hook, which may cut through or break the lamina. Hook dislodgement can occur following inadequate hook placement or inadequate hook site preparation. Screw cut-out with the Dwyer instrumentation occurs perhaps more frequently in the upper vertebral segments than the lower. In most instances, postoperative or brace management will provide for satisfactory fusion if the hook cut-out is noted late. If hook cut-out or dislodgement occurs intraoperatively, another level should be selected for the placement. Breakage of the Harrington rod will occasionally occur and is usually a result of metal fatigue and failure secondary to motion at a pseudoarthrosis. A common site for mechanical disruption is at the junction of the ratchet area and the smooth section of the rod.[133] If such a failure occurs, the presumption of pseudoarthrosis should be made and if the failure is accompanied by a change in the curvature or by pain, then re-exploration and re-instrumentation will be necessary. In some cases, the rod will fatigue and break late, the fusion will progress at that point and there will be no further pain, rod movement, or change of the curve.

In the early attempts at fusing the spine for scoliosis, pseudoarthrosis occurred in as many as 50 or 60 percent of patients. With better instrumentation, better postoperative immobilization, and more careful attention to the fusion techniques with adequate bone grafts, the current pseudoarthrosis rate is probably less than 2 percent.[19] Oblique x-ray films of the spine may be helpful in determining areas of failed fusion; examination for a complete obliteration of facet joints is also helpful. Bone scan techniques may be helpful in establishing areas of increased bone activity especially in those spine fusions in the late stages of maturing 1 to 2 years after fusion. Patients with neuromuscular curves, those with kyphoscoliosis, and adults can be expected to have a higher rate of pseudoarthrosis. If the presence of a pseudoarthrosis has been detected, re-fusion of the area with autogenous bone grafts obtained from the fusion mass or iliac crest and immobilization for up to a year may be necessary.[134]

Other mechanical problems that can occasionally occur include the prominence of a rod or hook, particularly in the upper region. This is more likely to occur if there is a lack of subcutaneous fat or muscles in this region. This can also be a problem if the upper end of instrumentation has been determined to be at the apex of a kyphosis. In these instances, it is important to select the upper hook site beyond the kyphosis so that it is not at the most prominent portion of the back. Presence of the square ended modification of the Harrington rod has allowed more complete contouring of the rod. This is particularly helpful in those cases where instrumentation is carried into the lumbar region. Maintaining lumbar lordosis is important in the overall sagittal plane and in maintenance of the center of gravity. If an uncontoured rod bridges the lumbar region, lumbar straightening and forward tilt of the trunk will occur.

NEUROLOGIC COMPLICATIONS

The possible occurrence of spinal cord injury accompanying spine fusion and instrumentation is a constant worry. Data collected from the Scoliosis Research Society for 1965 to 1971

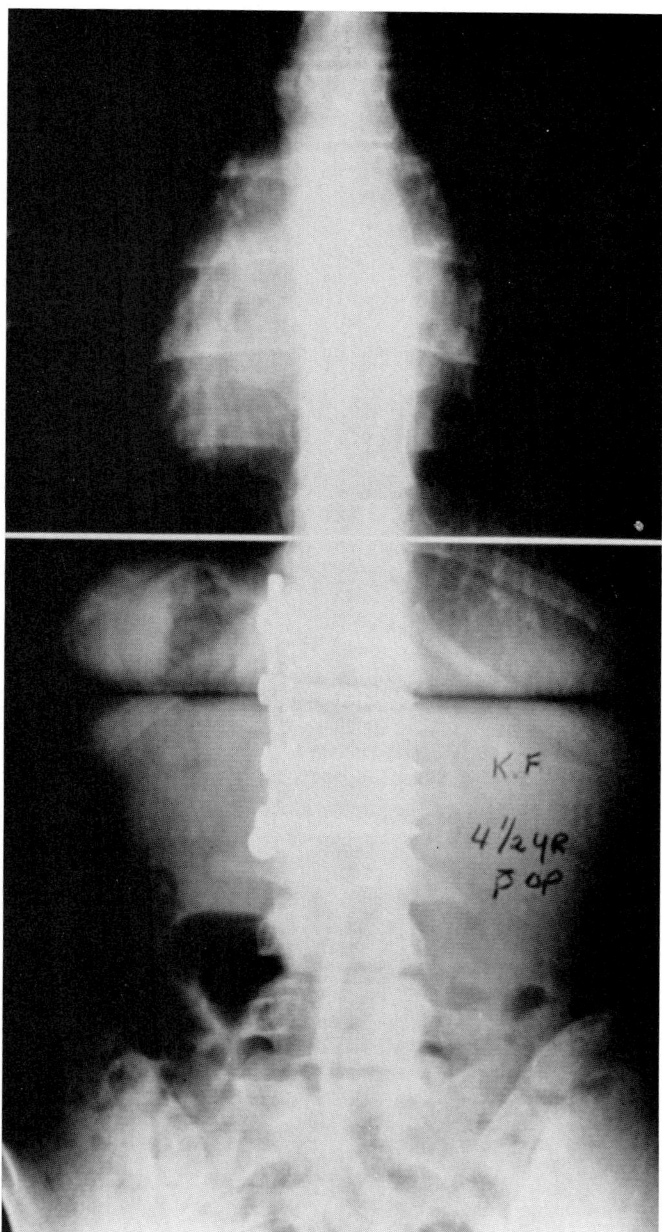

Fig. 18-20. Anterior spine fusion for an upper left lumbar idiopathic scoliosis 4½ years postoperatively showing anterior interbody fusion with instrumentation in place.

indicated that the overall incidence of acute neurologic complications resulting from the treatment of scoliosis was 0.72 percent.[135] This represented 57 major neurologic complications occurring out of 7885 patients. Of the reported spinal cord injuries, half were complete paraplegia and half were partial paraplegia; 36 percent of the patients recovered completely and 32 percent had no return of function.

The complication rate was considerably higher in those patients with congenital scoliosis, many of whom had occult interspinal abnormalities. As has been pointed out recently,[136] occult congenital interspinal anomalies were present in approximately 18.3 percent of patients with congenital scoliosis surveyed. These lesions included diastematomyelia, neurenteric epidermoid and dermoid cysts, teratoma, lipofibroma, fibrous bands, and tight phylum terminale. Oftentimes only one lower extremity had evidence of neurologic changes. Other factors associated with neurologic injury were the degree of severity of curve, presence of severe kyphosis, and neurologic deficit prior to the onset treatment. It was noted that in 6 out of 74 patients, paralysis occurred at the time of skeletal traction. During rapid application of skeletal traction, development of cranial nerve palsy has been reported. In a later survey by the Scoliosis Research Society, Kostiuk[137] reported that neurologic problems had occurred in 1.2 percent of the patients. Most of these patients had undergone Harrington rod instrumentation or wire instrumentation. Recent studies have shown increased risks for neurologic complications following segmental spinal instrumentation.[138,139] The main risk factor appeared to be the passage of the sublaminar wire, particularly in the thoracic and thoracolumbar regions. Because of the concern in congenital scoliosis curve, preoperative myelographic or tomographic evaluation should be done of the spinal cord to rule out dysraphism and underlying structural deformity of the spinal cord. Instrumentation in these individuals should be used only to support the fusion mass rather than to gain correction. In most cases in which paralysis, paraplegia, or quadriplegia have occurred as a result of traction related to halopelvic distraction,[140] kyphosis was the primary deformity. This may be particularly true when traction is used postoperatively and is also related to the severity of the deformity.

Because of the underlying concerns, Vauzelle and Stagnera[141] in France developed a technique of partially awakening patients during the operative procedure and asking them to move their extremities. By comparing the relative movement of upper extremities to the lower ones and the right side to the left side, a relative estimate of both sensory and motor neurologic function can be obtained. The patient is then reanesthetized.[142]

In the last decade, intraoperative monitoring of evoked potentials of spinal cord function has been advocated.[143–148] This technique is used to measure the spinal cord activity by monitoring conduction by the spinal cord of peripheral stimuli and monitoring these either from the epidural space, vertebral bone, or from the scalp. Previous work has shown that complete attenuation of spinal somatosensory evoked potentials (SSEP) can occur from traction, and recovery of these potentials may occur with release of traction. This is consistent with previous studies[135,137] in which at least half of those patients developing paraplegia have recovered following removal of instrumentation and release of traction. The sensitivity of the various elements within the cord to traction is yet to be determined. Dommisse[149] showed that a critical zone for the blood supply to the spinal cord extends from the fourth thoracic vertebra to the ninth thoracic vertebra. This region seems to correspond to those described in previous vascular studies, which show that the blood supply to this region tends to occur through single artery sources.[149]

The use of hypotensive anesthesia to help control blood loss during spinal fusion has been thought to play a contributing role to decreased blood supply to the cord. Studies by Hardy[50] and Kling[150] have shown that in most cases neurologic changes resulting from decreased blood flow are reversible with increasing blood pressure. Long-term significant neurologic consequences have not been documented to date in which hypotensive anesthesia has been used.[150,151,152]

Obviously, the role of spinal cord monitoring during surgery is most effective if intraoperative changes in the somatosensory evoked potentials can be detected.[153] Regardless of the site of recording, the sensitivity must be great enough to appreciate sudden changes that can occur with either instrumentation, traction, and other intraoperative events. It would appear that the current techniques of monitoring somatosensory potentials have applicability clinically, however, the possibility of multiple conduction pathways, the limitation of measuring only sensory conduction, and variability of the output depending on the monitoring sites requires that any changes in the SSEP be correlated carefully with other interoperative and postoperative neurologic findings.[154] Instrument removal, either intraoperatively or immediately postoperatively, depending on the time of discovery of the neurologic deficit, is correlated with the best chance of recovery. Avoidance of intraoperative complications through the careful positioning of instrumentation, avoidance of excessive force in traction particularly with regards to congenital abnormalities, and continuous appreciation of the potential for neurologic disturbance is essential.

OTHER COMPLICATIONS

A variety of other intraoperative complications can occur.[155–159] Hemothorax can occur as a result of penetration of an instrument during osteotomy of the transverse process or during decortication of the transverse process. Compression of the duodenum by the superior mesenteric artery as it passes anterior to the duodenum can occur with the duodenum laying between it and the aorta. This problem is related to elongation of the spine and tightening of the ligament of Treitz, and pulling the duodenum up under the superior mesenteric artery as elongation occurs. This can occur either with distraction at the time of surgery or with preoperative or postoperative traction. Symptoms of high intestinal obstruction with nausea and vomiting are usually noted and appear to be related to increased gastric intake. Positioning the patient with the left side down may be helpful. This complication seems to be more common in thin, asthenic individuals in whom there may not be as much mesenteric fat for protection of the duodenum. Postoperative hyperalimentation has been reported to be effective. Occasionally, operative release of the ligament of Treitz or gastrogastrostomy have been prescribed. Intraoperative cardiac arrest, acute renal failure, acute and chronic respiratory distress syndromes, and wound infections have also been reported.

All of these complications help emphasize that spinal fusions, by whatever approach, represent a large and stressful operative procedure for patients, especially those suffering from complications of other disease processes and especially those with attenuated cardiopulmonary function. Knowledge, experience, and circumspection should assist the surgeon in the selection and performance of spine fusion for spinal deformities.

REFERENCES

1. Winter RB: Spinal problems in pediatric orthopedics, in Lovell WW, Winter RB (eds): Pediatric Orthopaedics. Philadelphia, JB Lippincott, 1986
2. Duval-Beaupere G, Lespargot A, Grossiord A: Scoliosis and trunk muscles. J Pediatr Orthop 4:195, 1984
3. Rosenthal RK, Levine DB, McCarver CL: The occurrence of scoliosis in cerebral palsy. Dev Med Child Neurol 16:664, 1974
4. Samilson R, Bechard R: Scoliosis in cerebral palsy: Incidence, distribution of curve patterns, natural history, and thoughts on etiology. Curr Pract Orthop Surg 5:183, 1973
5. Madigan RR, Wallace SL: Scoliosis in the institutionalized cerebral palsy population. Spine 6:583, 1981
6. Kilfoyle RM, Foley JJ, Norton PL: Spine and pelvic deformity in childhood and adolescent paraplegia. J Bone Joint Surg 47A:659, 1965
7. Burke DC: Traumatic spinal paralysis in children. Paraplegia 11:268, 1974
8. Brown JC, Swank SM, Matta J, et al: Late spinal deformity in quadriplegic children and adolescents. J Pediatr Orthop 4:456, 1984
9. Mayfield JK, Erkkila JC, Winter RB: Spine deformity subsequent to acquired childhood spinal cord injury. J Bone Joint Surg 63A:1401, 1981
10. Lancourt JE, Dickson JH, Carter RE: Paralytic spinal deformity following spinal cord injury in children and adolescents. J Bone Joint Surg 63A:47, 1981
11. Roaf R: Spinal Deformities. Phildelphia, J.B. Lippincott Co., 1977
12. Langenskiold A, Michelsson JE: The pathogenesis of experimental progressive scoliosis. Acta Orthop Scand Suppl 59:26, 1962
13. Yarom R, Wolf E, Robin GC: Deltoid pathology in idiopathic scoliosis. Spine 7:463, 1982
14. Yarom R, Wolf E, Muhlrad A, et al: Neuromuscular causes of idiopathic scoliosis, in Jacobs R (ed): Pathogenesis of Idiopathic Scoliosis. Chicago, Scoliosis Research Society, 1982
15. Sahlstrand T, Petruson B: Study of labyrinthine function in patients with adolescent idiopathic scoliosis. Acta Orthop Scand 50:759, 1979
16. Herman RM: Postural and ocular motor control in patients with idiopathic scoliosis, in Jacobs R (ed): Pathogenesis of Idiopathic Scoliosis. Chicago, Scoliosis Research Society, 1982
17. Lemire RJ, Loeser JD, Leech RW, et al: Normal and Abnormal Development of the Human Nervous System. Hagerstown, Harper and Row, 1976
18. Parke WW: Development of the Spine, in Rothman RH, Simeone FA (eds): The Spine. Philadelphia, W.B. Saunders, 1975
19. Moe JH, Winter RB, Bradford DS, et al: Scoliosis and Other Deformities. Philadelphia, W.B. Saunders, 1978
20. Tanner JM, Whitehouse RH, Takaisni M: Standards from birth to maturity for height, weight, height velocity, and weight velocity. British children, 1965. Arch Dis Child 41:454, 1966
21. Zorab PA (ed): Scoliosis and Growth. London, Churchill Livingstone, 1971
22. Willner S, Nilsson KO, Kastrup K, et al: Growth hormone and somatomedin A in girls with idiopathic adolescent scoliosis. Acta Pediatr Scand 65:547, 1976
23. Nordwall A, Wilner S: A study of skeletal age and height in girls with idiopathic scoliosis. Clin Orthop 110:6, 1975
24. Misol S, Ponseti IV, Samaan N, et al: Growth hormone blood levels in patients with idiopathic scoliosis. Clin Orthop 81:122, 1971
25. Schultz AB, Ciszewski DJ, DeQald RL: Spine morphology as a determinant of progression tendency in idiopathic scoliosis. Presented at the meeting of the Scoliosis Research Society, Boston, 1978
26. Hallock H, Francis KC, Jones JB: Spine fusion in young children. A long term end-result study with particular reference to growth effects. J Bone Joint Surg 39A:481, 1957
27. Moe JH, Sundberg B, Gustilo R: A clinical study of spine fusion in the growing child. J Bone Joint Surg 46B:784, 1964
28. Winter RB, Moe JH, Wang JF: Congenital kyphosis. J Bone Joint Surg 55A:223, 1973
29. Johnson JTH, Southwick WO: Bone growth after spine fusion. A clinical survey. J Bone Joint Surg 42A:1396, 1960
30. Letts RM, Bobechko WP: Fusion of the scoliotic spine in young children. Clin Orthop Rel Res 101:136, 1974
31. Brooks HL, Azen SP, Gerber E, et al: Scoliosis: A prospective epidemiological study. J Bone Joint Surg 57A:968, 1975

32. Lonstein JE: Screening for spinal deformities in Minnesota schools. Clin Orthop 126:33, 1977

33. Kane WJ: Scoliosis prevalence: A call for a statement of terms. Clin Orthop 126:43, 1977

34. Sells CJ, May EA: Scoliosis screening in public schools. Am J Nurs 74:60, 1974

35. Willner S: A comparative study of the efficiency of different types of school screening for scoliosis. Acta Orthop Scand 53:769, 1982

36. Lonstein JE, Carlson JM: Prediction of curve progression in untreated idiopathic scoliosis during growth. J Bone Joint Surg 66A:1061, 1984

37. Rogala EJ, Drummond DS, Garr J: Scoliosis: Evidence and natural history; a prospective epidemiological study. J Bone Joint Surg 60:173, 1978

38. Drummond D, Ranallo F, Lonstein J, et al: Radiation hazards in scoliosis management. Spine 8:741, 1983

39. Weinstein SL, Ponseti JV: Curve progression in idiopathic scoliosis. J Bone Joint Surg 65A:447, 1983

40. Ponseti IV, Friedman B: Prognosis in idiopathic scoliosis. J Bone Joint Surg 32A:381, 1950

41. Bjure L, Nachemson A: Non treated scoliosis. Clin Orthop 93:44, 1973

42. Kostiuk JP: Recent advances in the treatment of painful adult scoliosis. Clin Orthop 147:238, 1980

43. Nachemson ALF: Adult scoliosis and back pain. Spine 4:513, 1979

44. Jackson RP, Simmons EH, Stripinis D: Incidence and severity of back pain in adult idiopathic scoliosis. Spine 8:749, 1983

45. MacEwen GD: Cerebral palsy and scoliosis, in Hardy JH (ed): Spinal Deformity in Neurological and Muscular Disorders. St. Louis, C.V. Mosby, 1974

46. Cady RB, Bobechko WP: Scoliosis in Freidrich Ataxia. J Pediatr Orthop 4:673, 1984

47. Huebert HT, MacKinnon WB: Syringomyelia and scoliosis. J Bone Joint Surg 51B:338, 1969

48. Simmons EH, Sue-A)Quan EA, Weber FA: An analysis of the indications for and results of Dwyer instrumentation of the spine. J Bone Joint Surg 56B:590, 1974

49. Fischer EG, Welch K, Shillito J Jr: Syringomyelia following lumboureteral shunting for communicating hydrocephalus. J Neurosurg 47:96, 1977

50. Hardy J: Neuromuscular scoliosis. J Bone Joint Surg 52A:407, 1970

51. Hsu JD: The natural history of spine curvature programs in the nonambulatory Duchenne muscular dystrophy patient. Spine 8:771, 1983

52. Wilkins KE, Gibson DA: The patterns of spinal deformity in Duchenne muscular dystrophy. J Bone Joint Surg 58A:24, 1976

53. Bazan UK, Paeslack V: Scoliotic growth in children with acquired paraplegia. Paraplegia 15:65, 1977–78

54. Audic B, Maury M: Secondary vertebral deformities in childhood and adolescence. Proceedings of the Scientific Meeting of the International Medical Society of Paraplegia, Jerusalem, November 6, 1968, pp 10–17

55. Tachdjian MO, Matson DD: Orthopaedic aspects of intraspinal tumors in infants and children. J Bone Joint Surg 47A:223, 1965

56. Haft H, Ransohoff J, Carter S: Spinal cord tumors in children. Pediatrics 23:1152, 1959

57. Raimondi AJ, Gutierrez FA, DiRocco C: Laminotomy and total reconstruction of the posterior spinal arch for spinal canal surgery in childhood. J Neurosurg 45:555, 1976

58. Pouliquen JC, Rigaoult P, Canevet M, et al: Les complications medullaires de la chirurgie des deviations rachidiennes. Chir Pediatr 21:215, 1980

59. Guidetti B, Mercuri S, Vagnozzi R: Long-term results of the surgical treatment of 129 intramedullary spinal gliomas. J Neurosurg 54:323, 1981

60. Fraser RD, Paterson DC, Simpson DA: Orthopaedic aspects of spinal tumors in children. J Bone Joint Surg 59B:143, 1977

61. Desousa AL, Kalsbeck JE, Mealey J Jr, et al: Intraspinal tumors in children. J Neurosurg 51:437, 1979

62. Citron N, Edgar MA, Sheehy J, et al: Intramedullary spinal cord tumours presenting as scoliosis. J Bone Joint Surg 66B:513, 1984

63. Arkin AM, Simon N: Radiation scoliosis. J Bone Joint Surg 32A:396, 1950

64. Neuhauser EBD, Wittenborg MH, Berman CZ, et al: Irradiation effects of roentgen therapy on the growing spine. Radiology 59:637, 1952

65. Nash CL, Gregg EC, Brown RH, et al: Risks of exposure to x-rays in patients undergoing long-term treatment for scoliosis. J Bone Joint Surg 61A:371, 1979

66. Humphreys RP, Hendrick EB, Hoffman HJ: Diastematomyelia. Clin Neurosurg 30:165, 1983

67. Frerebeau P, Dimeglio A, Gras M, et al: Diastematomyelia: Report of 21 cases surgically treated by a neurosurgical and orthopaedic team. Childs Brain 10:328, 1983

68. Galloway NT, Tainsh J: Minor defects of the sacrum and neurosenic bladder dysfunction. Br J Urol 57:154, 1985

69. Birkenfeld R, Kasdon DL: Congenital lumbar ridge causing spinal claudication in adolescents. Report of two cases. J Neurosurg 49:441, 1978

70. Naidich TP, Fernbach SK, McLone DG, et al: John Caffey Award, Sonography of the caudal spine and back congenital anomalies in children. AJR 142:1229, 1984

71. Modic MT, Handy RW, Weinstein MA: Nuclear magnetic resonance of the spine: Clinical potential and limitations. Neurosurgery 15:583, 1984

72. Agnoli AL, Schonmayr R, Popovic M, et al: The value of neuroradiological investigations in intraspinal malformations of the lumbosacral spine in childhood. Neuroradiology 16:91, 1978

73. Angelini L, Broggi G, Nardocci N, et al: Subacute cervical myelopathy in a child with cerebral palsy. Childs Brain 9:354, 1982

74. Gold LHA, Leach CG, Kieffer SA, et al: Large-volume myelography. Radiology 97:531, 1970

75. Harwood-Nash DCF, Fitz CR, Resjo IM, et al: Congenital spinal and cord lesions in children and computed tomographic metrizamide myelography. Neuroradiology 16:69, 1978

76. Levine RS, Geremia GK, McNeill TW: CT demonstration of cervical diastematomyelia. J Comput Assist Tomogr 9:592, 1985

77. Pettersson H, Harwood-Nash DCF, Fitz CR, et al: Conventional metrizamide myelography (MM) and computed tomographic metrizamide myelography (CTMM) in scoliosis. A comparative study. Radiology 142:111, 1982

78. Altman N, Harwood-Nash DC, Fitz Cr, et al: Evaluation of the infant spine by direct sagittal computed topography. AJNR 6:65, 1985

79. Raghavendra BN, Epstein FJ, Pinto RS, et al: The tethered spinal cord: Diagnosis by high-resolution real-time ultrasound. Radiology 149:123, 1983

80. Bunnell WP: An objective criterion for scoliosis screening. J Bone Joint Surg 66A:1381, 1984

81. Moreland M, Barce C, Pope MH: Moire topography in scoliosis: Pattern recognition and analysis, in Moreland MS, Pope MH, Armstrong GW (eds): Moire Fringe Topography and Spinal Deformity. New York, Pergamon Press, 1981, pp 171–185

82. Blount WP: Scoliosis and the Milwaukee Brace. Bull Hosp Joint Disease 19:152, 1958

83. Mellencamp DD, Blount WP, Anderson AJ: Milwaukee Brace treatment of idiopathic scoliosis. Clin Orthop Rel Res 126:47, 1977

84. Moe JH, Kettleson DN: Idiopathic scoliosis: Analysis of curve patterns and preliminary results of Milwaukee brace treatment in 169 patients. J Bone Joint Surg 52A:1509, 1970

85. Watts HG, Hall JE, Stanish W: The Boston brace system for the

treatment of low thoracic and lumbar scoliosis by use of a girdle without superstructure. Clin Orthop 126:87, 1977

86. Willner S: Effect of the Boston thoracic brace on the frontal and sagittal curves of the spine. Acta Orthop Scand 55:457, 1984

87. Green NE: Part time bracing of adolescent idiopathic scoliosis. J Bone Joint Surg 68A:738, 1986

88. Kahanovitz N, Levine DB, Lardone J: The part-time Milwaukee Brace treatment of juvenile idiopathic scoliosis: Long term follow-up. Clin Orthop 167:145, 1982

89. Bobechko WP, Herbert MA, Friedman HG: Electrospinal instrumentation for scoliosis. Current status. Orthop Clin North Am 10:927, 1979

90. Brown JC, Axelgaard J, Howson DC: Multicenter trial of a noninvasive stimulation method for idiopathic scoliosis. Spine 9:382, 1984

91. Bradford DS, Tanguy A, Vanselow J: Surface electrical stimulation in the treatment of idiopathic scolioses: Preliminary results in 30 patients. Spine 8:757, 1983

92. McCollough NC, Friedman H, Bracale R: Surface electrical stimulation of the paraspinal muscles in the treatment of idiopathic scoliosis. Orthop Trans 4:29, 1980

93. Hibbs RA: On operation for progressive spinal deformities. NY Med J 93:1013, 1911

94. Albee FH: Transplantation of a portion of the tibia into the spine for Pott's disease. JAMA 57:885, 1911

95. Hibbs RA, Risser JC, Ferguson AB: Scoliosis treated by the fusion operation. An end result study of three hundred sixty cases. J Bone Joint Surg 13:91, 1931

96. American Orthopaedic Association Research Committee: End result study of the treatment of idiopathic scoliosis. J Bone Joint Surg 23:963, 1941

97. Harrington PR: Treatment of scoliosis. Correction and internal fixation by spine instrumentation. J Bone Joint Surg 44A:591, 1962

98. Allen BL, Ferguson RL: The Galveston Technique for L-rod instrumentation of the scoliotic spine. Spine 7:276, 1982

99. Luque ER: The anatomic basis and development of segmental spinal instrumentation. Spine 7:256, 1982

100. Hodgson AR, Stock FE: Anterior spinal fusion. Br J Surg 44:266, 1956–57

101. Nickel VL, Perry J, Garrett A, et al: The halo: A spinal traction fixation device. J Bone Joint Surg 50A:1400, 1968

102. Dwyer AF: An anterior approach in scoliosis. A preliminary report. Clin Orthop 62:192, 1969

103. Goldstein LA, Dickerson RC: Atlas of Orthopaedic Surgery, vol 2. St. Louis, C.V. Mosby Co., 1974

104. Sim FH, Hendrik JS, Bickel WH, et al: Swan-neck deformity following extensive cervical laminectomy. J Bone Joint Surg 56A:565, 1974

105. McWhorter JM, Alexander E, Davis CH Jr, et al: Posterior cervical fusion in children. J Neurosurg 45:211, 1976

106. Holmes JC, Hall JE: Fusion for instability and potential instability of the cervical spine in children and adolescents. Symposium on the Upper Cervical Spine. Orthop Clin North Am 9:923, 1978

107. Cattell HS, Clark GL Jr: Cervical kyphosis and instability following multiple laminectomies in children. J Bone Joint Surg 49A:713, 1967

108. Dickson JH, Harrington PR: The evolution of the Harrington instrumentation technique in scoliosis. J Bone Joint Surg 55A:993, 1973

109. Cochran T, Irstam L, Nachemson A: Long-term anatomic and functional changes in patients with adolescent idiopathic scoliosis treated by Harrington rod fusion. Spine 8:576, 1983

110. Thompson GH, Wilber G, Shaffer JW, et al: Segmental spinal instrumentation in idiopathic scolioses, a preliminary report. Spine 10:623, 1985

111. King HA, Moe JH, Bradford DS, et al: The selection of fusion levels in thoracic idiopathic scoliosis. J Bone Joint Surg 65A:1302, 1983

112. Drummond D, Guadagni J, Keene JS, et al: Interspinous process segmental spinal instrumentation. J Pediatr Orthop 4:397, 1984

113. Guadagni J, Drummond D, Breed A: Improved postoperative course following modified segmental instrumentation and posterior spinal fusion for idiopathic scoliosis. J Pediatr Orthop 4:405, 1984

114. Herring JA, Wenger DR, et al: Segmental spinal instrumentation: A preliminary report of 40 consecutive cases. Spine 7:285, 1982

115. Cotrell Y, Dubousset J: A new technic for segmental spinal osteosynthesis using the posterior approach. Rev Clin Orthop 70:489, 1984

116. Roy-Camille RR, Saillant G, Mazel C: Internal fixateur of the lumbar spine with pedicle screw plating. Clin Orthop 203:7, 1986

117. Steffee AD, Biscup RS, Sitkowski DJ: Segmental spine plates with pedicle screw fixation. Clin Orthop 203:45, 1986

118. Krag MH, Beynnon BD, Pope MH, et al: An internal fixator for posterior application to short segments of the thoracic, lumbar, or lumbosacral spine. Design and testing. Clin Orthop 203:75, 1986

119. Burrington JD, Brown C, Wayne ER, et al: Anterior approach to the thoracolumbar spine. Arch Surg 111:456, 1976

120. Cook WA: Transthoracic vertebral surgery. Ann Thorac Surg 12:54, 1971

121. Hall JE: The anterior approach to spinal deformities. Orthop Clin North Am 3:81, 1972

122. Leatherman KD: Resection of vertebral bodies. J Bone Joint Surg 51A:206, 1969

123. Riseborough EJ: The anterior approach to the spine for correction of deformities of the axial skeleton. Clin Orthop 93:207, 1973

124. Bradford DA: Anterior spinal surgery in the management of scoliosis. Orthop Clin North Am 10:801, 1979

125. Dwyer AF: Experience of anterior correction of scoliosis. Clin Orthop 93:191, 1973

126. McBride GG, Bradford DS: Vertebral body replacement with femoral neck allograft and vascularized rib strut graft. A technique for treating posttraumatic kyphosis with neurologic deficit. Spine 8:406, 1983

127. Zielke K, Stunkat R, Beaujeau F: Ventrale Derotations - Spondylodese. Arch Orthop Unfallchir 85:257, 1976

128. Ogiela DM, Chan DPK: Ventral derotation spondylodesis. A review of 22 cases. Spine 11:18, 1986

129. Moe JH, Purcell GA, Bradford DS: Zielke instrumentation (VDS) for correction of spinal curvature. Analysis of results in 66 patients. Clin Orthop 180:133, 1983

130. Leatherman KD, Dickson RA: Two-stage corrective surgery for congenital deformities of the spine. J Bone Joint Surg 61B:324, 1979

131. Roberts RS, Price CT, Riddick MF: Use of a bivalved polypropylene orthosis in the postoperative management of idiopathic scoliosis. Clin Orthop 185:25, 1984

132. Moe JH: Complications of scoliosis treatment. Clin Orthop 53:21, 1967

133. Sturz H, Hinterberger J, Marzen K, et al: Damage analysis of the Harrington rod fracture after scoliosis operation. Arch Orthop Trauma Surg 95:113, 1979

134. Roy DR, Huntington CF, MacEwen GD: Pseudoarthrosis resulting in complete paraplegia fifteen years after spinal fusion. Arch Orthop Trauma Surg 102:213, 1984

135. MacEwen W, Bunnell WP, Sriram K: Acute neurological complications in the treatment of scoliosis. J Bone Joint Surg 57A:404, 1975

136. McMaster MJ: Occult intraspinal anomalies and congenital scoliosis. J Bone Joint Surg 66A:588, 1984

137. Kostuik JP: Morbidity and scoliosis surgery. J Bone Joint Surg 61B:11, 1979

138. Allen B, Ferguson RL: Neurologic injuries with the Galveston technique of L-rod instrumentation for scoliosis. Spine 11:14, 1986

139. Wilber RG, Thompson GH, Shaffer JW, et al: Postoperative

neurological defects in segmental spinal. Instrumentation J Bone Joint Surg 66A:1178, 1984

140. O'Brien JP, Yau ACMC, Smith TK, et al: Halo pelvic traction. J Bone Joint Surg 53B:217, 1971

141. Vauzelle C, Stagnara P, Jouvinroux P: Functional monitoring of spinal cord activity during spinal surgery. Clin Orthop 93:173, 1973

142. Hall JE, Levine CR, Sudhir KG: Intraoperative awakening to monitor spinal cord function during Harrington instrumentation and spinal fusion. Description of procedure and report of three cases. J Bone Joint Surg 60A:533, 1978

143. Dimitrijevic MR, Kehmkuhl LD, Dedgwick EM, et al: Characteristics of spinal cord evoked responses in man. Appl Neurophysiol 43:118, 1980

144. Engler GL, Spielholtz NI, Bernhard WN, et al: Somatosensory evolved potentials during Harrington instrumentation for scoliosis. J Bone Joint Surg 60A:528, 1978

145. Jones SJ, Edgar MA, Ransford AO, et al: Spinal cord monitoring during scoliosis surgery. J Bone Joint Surg 63B:631, 1981

146. Nash CL, Lorig RA, Schatzinger LA, et al: Spinal cord monitoring during operative treatment of the spine. Clin Orthop 126:100, 1977

147. Nuwer MR, Dawson EC: Intraoperative evoked potential monitoring of the spinal cord. Clin Orthop 183:42, 1984

148. Tamaki TH, Inue DI, Kobayashi H: The prevention of introgenic spinal cord injury utilizing the evoked spinal cord potential. Int Orthop 4:313, 1981

149. Dommisse GF: The blood supply of the spinal cord. J Bone Joint Surg 56B:225, 1974

150. Kling TF, Wilton N, Hensinger RN, et al: The influence of trimethaphan (Arfonad)-induced hypotension with and without spine distraction on canine spinal cord blood flow. Spine 11:219, 1986

151. Malcolm-Smith NA, McMaster MJ: The use of induced hypotension to control bleeding during posterior fusion for scoliosis. J Bone Joint Surg 65B:255, 1983

152. Grundy BL, Nash CL, Brown RH: Deliberate hypotension for scoliosis fusion (abstr). Anesthesiology 51:S78, 1979

153. Szaley EA, Carollo JJ, Ronch JW: Sensitivity of spinal cord monitoring to intraoperative events. J Pediatr Orthop 6:437, 1986

154. Bradshaw K, Webb JK, Fraser AM: Clinical evaluation of spinal cord monitoring in scoliosis surgery. Spine 9:636, 1984

155. Grimer RJ, Mulligan PJ, Thompson AG: Thoracic outlet syndrome following correction of scoliosis in a patient with cervical ribs. A case report. J Bone Joint Surg 65B:1172, 1983

156. Eismont FJ, Simeone FA: Bone overgrowth (hypertrophy) as a cause of late paraparesis after scoliosis fusion. J Bone Joint Surg 63A:1016, 1981

157. Pinto WC: Complications of surgical treatment of scoliosis. Israel J Med Sci 9:837, 1973

158. Bowen JR, Ferrer J: Spinal stenosis caused by a Harrington hook in neuromuscular disease. Clin Orthop 180:179, 1983

159. Court-Brown CM, McMaster MJ: Pseudarthrosis: A late cause of paraparesis after scoliosis surgery. J Bone Joint Surg 64A:1246, 1982

CHAPTER 19

Intraoperative Ultrasonography in Neurosurgery

Robert A. Kane   Daniel H. O'Leary   Ernest S. Mathews

INTRAOPERATIVE ULTRASONOGRAPHY (IUS) with portable real-time sonographic imaging equipment is widely used in a variety of operative settings. One of the most successful applications for IUS clearly has been in the realm of neurosurgery, initially in the brain and subsequently in the spinal cord as well. The clear and relatively straightforward depiction of normal and pathologic anatomy make IUS an extremely useful technique that can be used in academic centers and community hospitals, since the necessary ultrasound equipment is widely available. The only extra requirement is the acquisition of special purpose intraoperative probes, which can be operated through general purpose ultrasonography units.

Intraoperative ultrasonography can provide the neurosurgeon with a clearer and more complete depiction of diseases affecting the brain and spinal cord. It is particularly useful in accurate localization of disease processes, characterization of the solid and cystic components of lesions, and definition of the extent of disease. This information can be helpful in reducing operative time, minimizing tissue dissection or resection, and assessing the completeness of the surgical therapy. The site and type of surgical interventional procedure can be better planned by virtue of the ultrasonographic examination, which often provides information that is more complete than can be obtained by preoperative imaging procedures.

The rapid development of real-time ultrasonographic equipment, in particular the specially designed probes suitable for imaging through small surgical windows such as burr holes or laminectomy defects, has increased the quality of the information obtained and the ease of performing intraoperative ultrasonography. The relatively simple and straightforward techniques, the dynamic depiction of pathologic anatomy in real time, and the fairly straightforward interpretation of the imaging data make this a genuine growth area in imaging. Acceptance has been somewhat slow, perhaps in part because of the unfamiliarity of surgeons with the interpretation of ultrasound images. For this reason, it is often desirable that a partnership between the radiologist and the neurosurgeon be developed in order to utilize the radiologist's expertise in cross-sectional imaging and ultrasonography and in optimizing the quality of the images obtained. This partnership can reduce the learning curve time for interpretation of unfamiliar ultrasound images.

HISTORY

As with many other new imaging procedures, intraoperative ultrasonography of the brain is not really a new technique. There are several reported series utilizing ultrasonography for localization of brain lesions some 15 to 20 years ago.[13] These techniques used A-mode ultrasound (known as echoencephalography), a technique that does not produce anatomic images but merely demonstrates reflective surfaces along a single line from the ultrasound probe to the edge of the lesion. The returning echoes are displayed on an oscilloscope as an amplitude-modulated signal arising from the reflecting surface. The depth of this reflector can be calculated and calibrated on the oscilloscope by computing the speed of sound in the insonated tissues. While some success was had with this method of localization, its lack of anatomic imaging prevented its widespread application.

It was not until 1980 that the first report of real-time intraoperative ultrasonography of the brain was published.[4] In this preliminary report, a 3.5-MHz general purpose abdominal ultrasound transducer was utilized, resulting in a rather crude but nonetheless accurate depiction of cerebral anatomy. It was predicted that ultrasonography would prove useful in stereotactic localization of lesions as well as in guidance of biopsy procedures using specially designed biopsy probes. It rapidly became apparent that higher frequency probes (5 MHz and 7.5 MHz) resulted in a better depiction of normal and pathologic anatomy because of the greater axial resolution that results from a higher frequency transducer with shorter wave lengths.[5] However, the higher frequency transducers had less depth penetration because of greater attenuation of the sound beam. It was found that superficial lesions within a few centimeters of the brain surface were best imaged with the 7.5-MHz crystal, whereas deeper lesions were better seen with the 5-MHz probe.

Specially designed in-line transducers allowed for imaging through ever smaller craniotomy sites (Figure 19-1), with probes ultimately being developed that were small enough to be used through operative burr holes (Figure 19-2). Various guidance systems for biopsy under real-time observation utilizing a stereotactic system have also been developed, allowing for accurate needle and probe placement with minimum disruption of normal adjacent tissues.

Intraoperative ultrasonography of the spine and spinal cord was first described in 1983 and has developed rapidly since that

OPERATIVE NEUROSURGICAL TECHNIQUES
ISBN 0-8089-1862-1

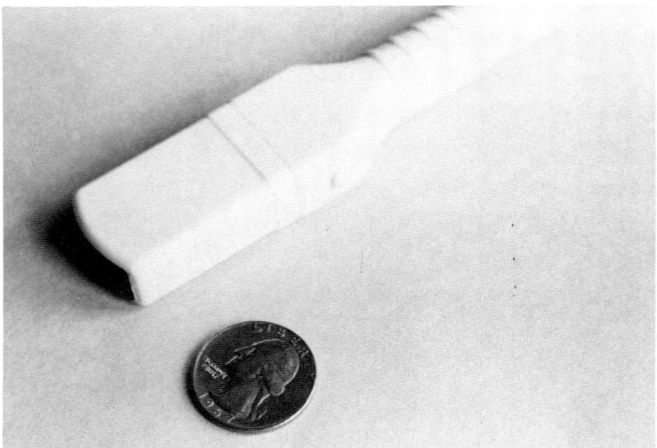

Fig. 19-1. A curved linear array ultrasound probe (7.5 MHz) suitable for imaging the brain and spinal cord through surgical bony defects.

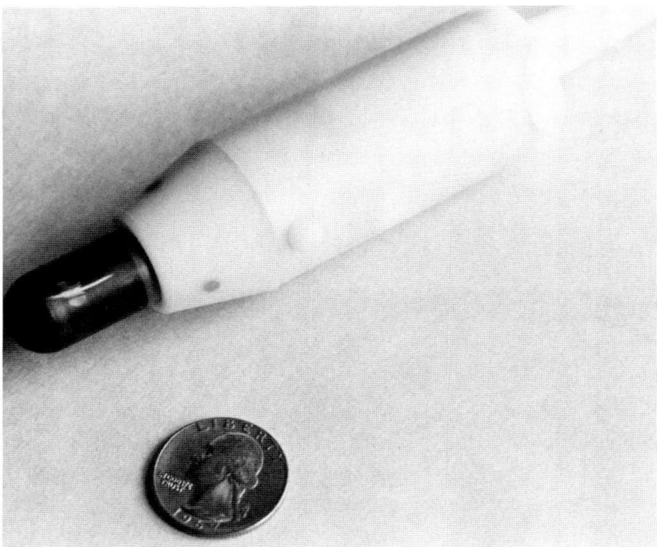

Fig. 19-2. A mechanical sector scanner (5 MHz) for intracranial imaging through surgical burr holes.

time.[6] A 7.5-MHz transducer was preferred because of its ability to depict normal intramedullary anatomy, which could not be well appreciated at lower frequencies because of the diminished spatial resolution. Ultrasound guidance for biopsy and drainage procedures in the spinal cord and for monitoring the extent of mass lesions and the completeness of surgical excisions has proved equally efficacious as IUS in intracranial imaging.

EQUIPMENT AND TECHNIQUES

Most, if not all, of the major manufacturers of ultrasound equipment now offer intraoperative probes. These are all real-time systems, ranging in frequency from 3.0 to 10.0 MHz. Mechanically driven sector scanners are most commonly employed, but electronic phased array systems and linear array systems are also available. The size of the scan head dictates the approach to intracranial imaging, since most transducers are larger than the standard burr hole and hence necessitate a craniotomy in order to be applied to the dural surface. Smaller mechanical sector probes are available that can be applied through a burr hole, but the small size of the crystal results in a much smaller field of view, which can make orientation to the surrounding anatomy somewhat difficult.

It is clear that one imaging frequency is not entirely adequate for all intraoperative neurosurgical purposes. A 7.5-MHz probe is ideal for imaging superficial lesions in the brain because of its short focal length. Similarly, the increased spatial resolution of a 7.5-MHz probe is necessary to demonstrate the fine anatomic detail of spinal cord and intramedullary lesions. However, the price paid for this increased resolution is a lack of penetration as a result of increased absorption of the sound waves. This results in inadequate depiction of deep structures beyond the usual 4–6-cm focal length of a 7.5-MHz transducer. A 5-MHz probe therefore is also necessary, particularly for imaging deep lesions in the brain as well as the normal deep anatomic structures such as the ventricles, choroid plexus, falx, and tentorium cerebelli. The 5-MHz probe will not adequately demonstrate very superficial lesions, however, because of reverberations in the near field and a focal zone that typically ranges from 2 to 10 cm. There is one mechanical sector probe available in which three separate crystals of 3.0, 5.0, and

7.5 MHz frequencies can be selected from the console without having to change probes (Figure 19-3).

Sterilization of the ultrasound probe and cord is essential. The temperatures of autoclaving are much too high for the ultrasound equipment, but some of the electronic transducers can be gas sterilized with ethylene oxide. Many probes, however, cannot undergo gas sterilization; this should be specifically determined from with the manufacturer in order to avoid damaging the transducers. Gas sterilization also requires a significant amount of time, primarily because of the prolonged aeration requirements following exposure of the probes to ethylene oxide. A minimum time of 12 to 16 hours is required, and this results in a 24-hour turn-around time.

Sterilization can be adequately achieved by enveloping the probe in a sterile sheath, usually made of latex or some other synthetic rubberlike compound. These frequently are available from the manufacturer and are designed specifically to fit the probe. Alternatively, a sterile surgical glove can be used. Scanning gel is placed on the surface of the probe, which is then enveloped in the sterile sheath. The sheath is fixed in place by means of sterile rubber bands or surgical sutures. A sterile sleeve, which can be of plastic, rubber, or surgical stockinette material, is then positioned over the probe and extended up along the cord. This preparation is sufficient for maintaining surgical sterility, although some users favor a double glove technique over the surface of the probe. It is important to provide an acoustic coupling agent (scanning gel) between the probe and the sterile covering and between each layer of sheathing if double layers are used. It is also important to press all entrapped air bubbles from the gel overlying the scanning surface of the transducer, since air in this position will seriously degrade the image quality.

Acoustic coupling is also necessary between the transducer and the target organ. Sterile saline is perfectly adequate for this and can be dripped directly on the dural surface of the brain with the ensheathed probe subsequently placed on the dura. Periodic replenishment of the saline helps to maintain optimal image quality. For spinal sonography, the laminectomy defect is filled with sterile saline and the transducer is placed within the fluid but not touching the surface of the dura mater. This helps to avoid a near-field reverberation effect and also avoids any inadvertent pressure upon the spinal cord. Microbubbles in the saline bath will degrade the image and can be minimized by slowly filling the laminectomy site with the fluid. If there is a considerable amount of blood or tissue debris within the surgical defect, suctioning before instillation of saline will help improve image quality.[7]

Scanning through the dural surface results in an image with a quality that is just as good as one produced by scanning directly on the brain surface, and hence scans are usually obtained before incision of the dura.[5] This pertains as well to spinal sonography, where, again, scanning through the dura does not in any significant way degrade image quality. If there is difficulty in satisfactorily imaging extremely superficial cortical or subcortical lesions in the brain, this is usually a result of near field reverberation artifacts. A water standoff can be made by filling the finger of a sterile surgical glove with saline, resting this on the dural surface and scanning through the fluid-filled glove, thereby moving the transducer 1 to 2 cm from the brain surface and improving resolution of superficial structures.

If a biopsy guide is to be used, the guide should be attached to the probe with great care in order to avoid any tearing of the sterile sheaths and consequent contamination of the operative field. The real-time images are presented on a monitor for immediate viewing, and images can be frozen for hard copy (on x-ray or Polaroid film). Alternatively, a videotape recording of the real-time examination can be made and a hard copy obtained subsequently from the videotape, although this results in somewhat degraded resolution.

Once the surgeon and radiologist are familiar with operation of the ultrasound equipment in the operating suite, the total time required for IUS, including the time of set-up and draping as well as the actual imaging, should add no more than 10 or 15 minutes to the surgical procedure and may in fact save much more time by quickly and precisely defining the appearance and location of the pathologic lesion. More time is required if biopsies are performed or sonographic assessment of the completeness of a surgical excision is to be utilized.

INTRACRANIAL SONOGRAPHY

PREOPERATIVE LOCALIZATION

There are two problems that confront the neurosurgeon: one is the accurate location of the burr hole, craniotomy flap, or laminectomy; the second involves precise localization of the lesion after bone removal and exposure of the operative field. Visual inspection is notoriously unreliable in defining the location and extent of lesions, even those that are quite superficial in location. Palpation is obviously quite limited and other means of exploration with needles, probes, and other devices can result in damage to normal brain or spinal cord structures.

Most focal lesions are now defined preoperatively by CT scanning, angiography, and magnetic resonance imaging. For intracranial lesions, it is helpful to plan the craniotomy or burr hole site using the CT scout image with slice localization markers to select the best point of entry. A metallic marker then can be placed on the scalp and repeat CT scans made to confirm the correct position of the marker. When satisfactory positioning of the marker is obtained, the skin of the scalp at that site is colored with an indelible ink marker. Once this is done, there is no danger of displacement of the marker and the indelible ink will remain visible after the scalp is shaved.

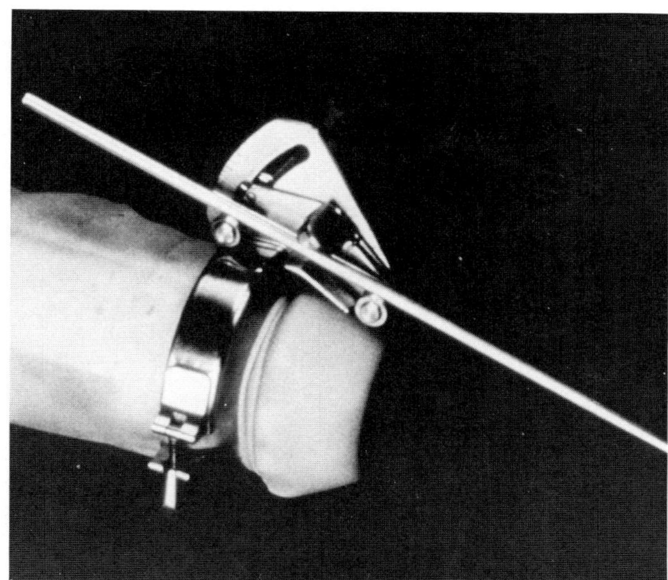

Fig. 19-3. A multiple frequency transducer (3, 5, and 7.5 MHz) suitable for imaging the brain and spinal cord. Note the attached guidance system with the needle in place for use in guiding biopsies and drainage procedures in real-time.

Skin marking guided by CT scanning can also be done for localization of the laminectomy sites for spinal surgery; alternatively, fluoroscopic guidance can be used during myelography. If this type of marking procedure is not performed, it is mandatory to know the precise number of cervical, thoracic, or lumbar vertebral bodies in order to correctly place the surgical incision and laminectomy.

Several CT-guided stereotactic biopsy systems are available and are quite accurate in guiding needle placement. However, this requires that a stereotactic frame to be attached to the calvarium and remain fixed in position after the CT scan until the surgery is performed. If there is any motion of the frame, the stereotactic calculations are no longer accurate. The stereotactic equipment is cumbersome and expensive and does not allow direct visualization of the target lesion during the actual surgical procedure. Real-time IUS is a much more satisfactory method of lesion localization, giving real-time information to the surgeon and thus ensuring accurate placement of probes and needles. An ultrasound-guided stereotactic biopsy device is available through which biopsies can be made via a burr hole.[8] With this system, a ringlike device is screwed into a specially modified burr hole (Figure 19-4A,B). The device contains a swiveling pivot into which the ultrasound probe is placed. When the lesion is localized and the optimal pathway selected, the pivot is stabilized by tightening a clamp plate, and the transducer is removed and replaced with a similar sized needle guide. The depth is calculated from the tip of the guide to the lesion and the biopsy needle then is passed directly to the target. This device has been used successfully with patients under general anesthesia and with conscious patients under local anesthesia only.

NORMAL ANATOMY

With proper setting of the time gain compensation controls on the ultrasound console, normal brain tissue has a homogeneous, hypoechoic appearance, while fluid-filled structures

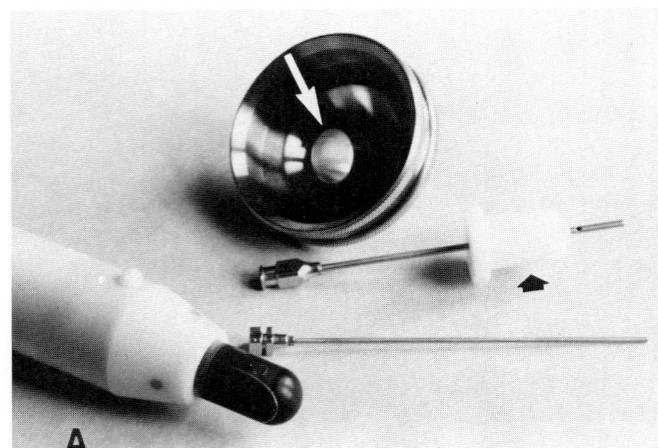

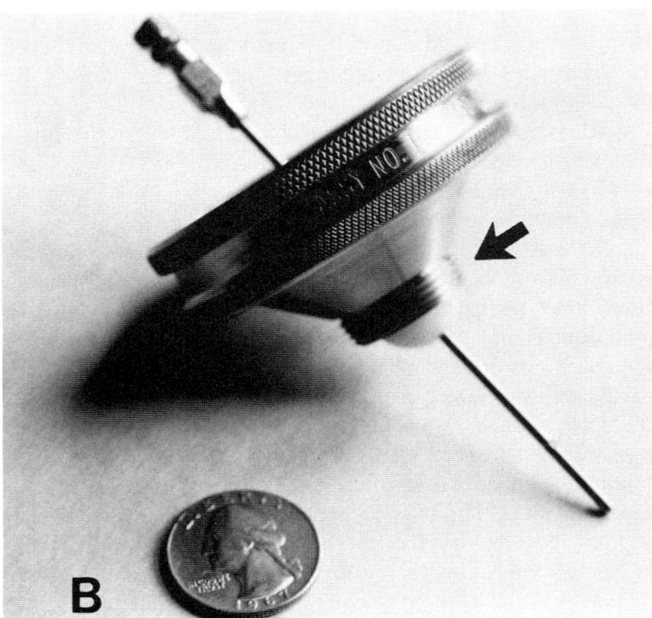

Fig. 19-4.   A Berger Neurobiopsy Device for stereotactic burr hole biopsies. (A) Note the ring with a central pivot (arrow) through which the burr hole probe and biopsy guide (arrowhead) fit. (B) The guide in place with a biopsy needle passing through the guide. Note the threaded portion of the ring (arrow), which screws into the burr hole for stability.

such as the lateral ventricles are anechoic (Figure 19-5). The lateral ventricles can usually be successfully imaged if there is sufficient penetration and the field of view is large enough. At times imaging through a small burr hole provides an insufficient acoustic window for complete definition of normal anatomy.[9] The walls of the lateral ventricles appear as thin hyperechoic linear structures. Similarly, the falx and tentorium cerebelli appear as linear hyperechoic structures.

The choroid plexus is hyperechoic relative to surrounding brain tissue and appears as a crescentic or arclike area of increased echogenicity in the temporal horns and trigone of the lateral ventricles. Sulcal grooves of the cerebral cortex can also appear moderately echogenic along the gyral surfaces (Figure 19-6) and in the region of the sylvian fissure. Major blood vessels can at times be visualized and have linear echogenic walls and anechoic lumens. Arteries are most easily recognized by virtue of their pulsatile expansion on real-time observation. Veins are much less consistently visualized.

PATHOLOGIC ANATOMY

Virtually all solid lesions in the brain are hyperechoic relative to surrounding normal or edematous brain tissue (Figure 19-6).[10] The increase in echogenicity is present whether there is calcification within the lesion or not, although calcified tumors are even more striking in their hyperechogenicity. Brain edema surrounding focal lesions is hypoechoic relative to normal brain tissue, but focal lesions are readily identified regardless of the presence or absence of edema. Hypoechoic or anechoic areas within solid tumors may represent areas of cyst formation, necrosis with cystic degeneration, or hemorrhage within the lesion (Figures 19-7 and 19-8).

Some lesions have zones of intermediate echogenicity between the focal hyperechoic mass and the surrounding hypoechoic brain tissue. This may represent locally invasive areas of tumor resulting in blurred, poorly defined boundaries. This invasive appearance is frequently seen with more aggressive higher grade astrocytomas, which also frequently contain hypoechoic areas secondary to necrosis.[11] Sonography, however, is not sufficiently characteristic to allow grading of astrocytomas, since similar appearances can occasionally be seen in lower grade lesions. Ultrasound is useful in evaluating low density areas on CT scans of lower grade astrocytomas (Figure 19-7A,B), which can represent areas of cyst formation, necrosis, or edema on the CT scan. Intraoperative sonography has been consistently successful in accurately defining the solid

Fig. 19-5.   An axial view showing normal homogeneous brain tissue and slightly dilated anechoic lateral ventricles (V).

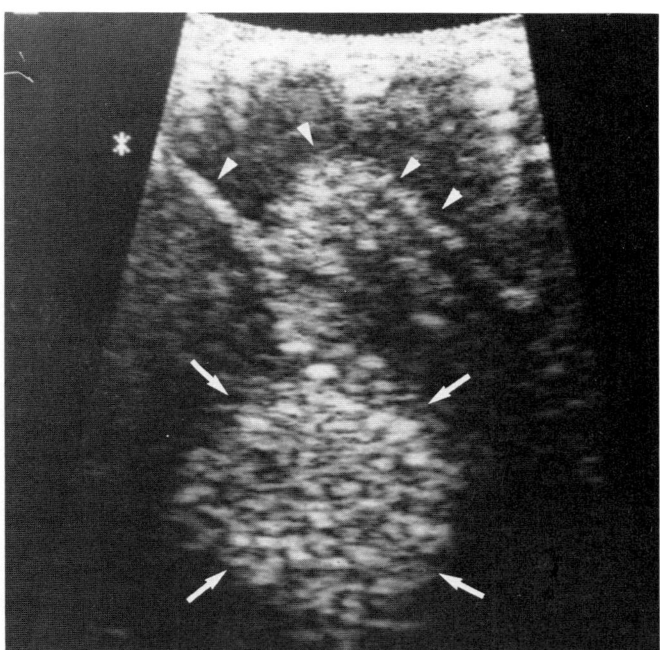

Fig. 19-6. A hyperechoic, sharply circumscribed brain metastasis (arrows) from a primary lung carcinoma. Note how well the lesion stands out from surrounding edematous brain tissue. Note also the undulating echogenic gyral folds (arrowheads).

component of tumors, thereby defining the most appropriate site for diagnostic biopsy.[12] Similarly, ring-enhancing lesions on CT scans with a central low density do not necessarily equate with areas of necrosis or cystic degeneration and are more completely evaluated by ultrasound (Figure 19-8A,B). In one series, three of four ring-enhancing lesions were nearly completely solid and echogenic on IUS images with no significant areas of cyst formation or fluid demonstrated.[13] In this series it was also noted that in 37 percent of a series of 22 cases, the extent of primary gliomas was greater on IUS images than had been predicted by preoperative CT scans. In 4 of 22 cases with nonenhancing astrocytomas on CT scans, the margins of the tumor were well delineated by ultrasonography despite being poorly visualized on the CT scans.

All metastatic brain tumors are hyperechoic and typically have a sharply marginated border and spherical shape (Figure 19-6).[11,13] They are typically subcortical in location and frequently difficult if not impossible to palpate. There are no characteristic ultrasound appearances to predict the nature of the metastatic lesion, be it carcinoma, melanoma, sarcoma, or lymphoma. For that matter, a well-circumscribed primary glioma will have an appearance identical to that of a metastatic lesion. Meningiomas are also sharply circumscribed and markedly hyperechoic. Some of the increased echogenicity may be related to tumoral calcification.

Nonneoplastic focal brain lesions also have a predominantly hyperechoic appearance. Brain abscesses are typically hyperechoic peripherally with a somewhat echo-poor central area. Even arteriovenous malformations appear as diffusely hyperechoic lesions.[13] If the shape of the echogenic lesion is nonspherical on the IUS image, this appearance is suggestive of a nonneoplastic lesion such as an AVM or an infarct.[14] Large feeding or draining vessels may suggest an AVM but can also be seen in hypervascular tumors.

Aneurysms are echo free or may contain some low level echogenicity if thrombus is present. A choroid plexus papilloma

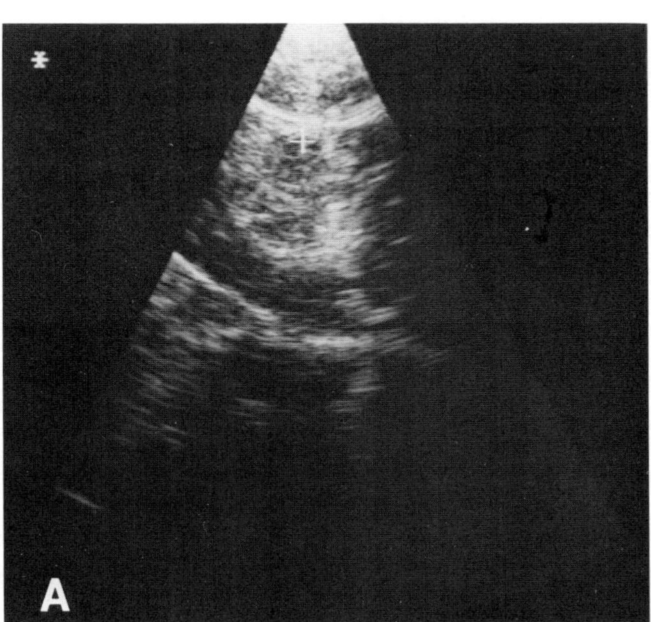

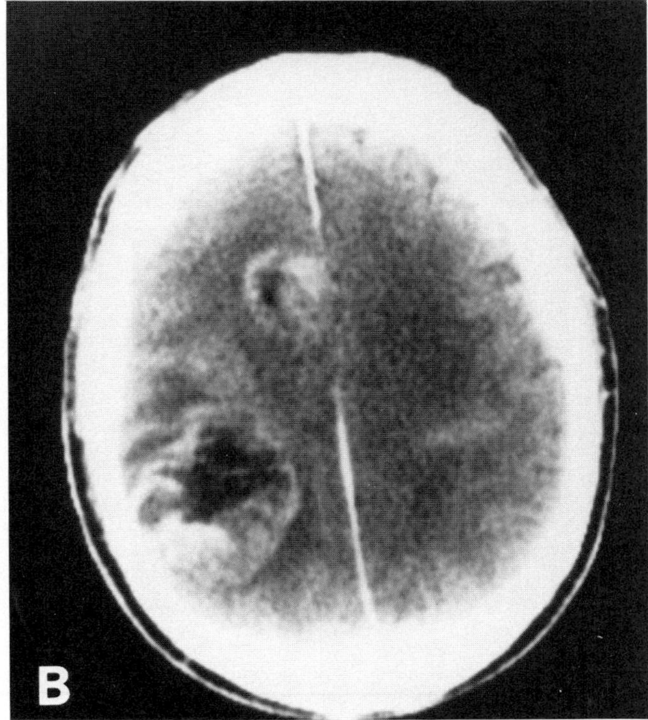

Fig. 19-7. A multifocal glioblastoma. (A) A hyperechoic lesion with a central area of lesser echogenicity caused by necrosis. The lesion is completely solid, however, with no cystic component. The caliper is measuring the distance from the transducer on the brain surface to the lesion. (B) A CT scan showing two focal enhancing lesions with low densities centrally suggesting fluid. The larger lesion corresponds to the ultrasound image in Figure 19-7A and was completely solid on IUS studies and at biopsy.

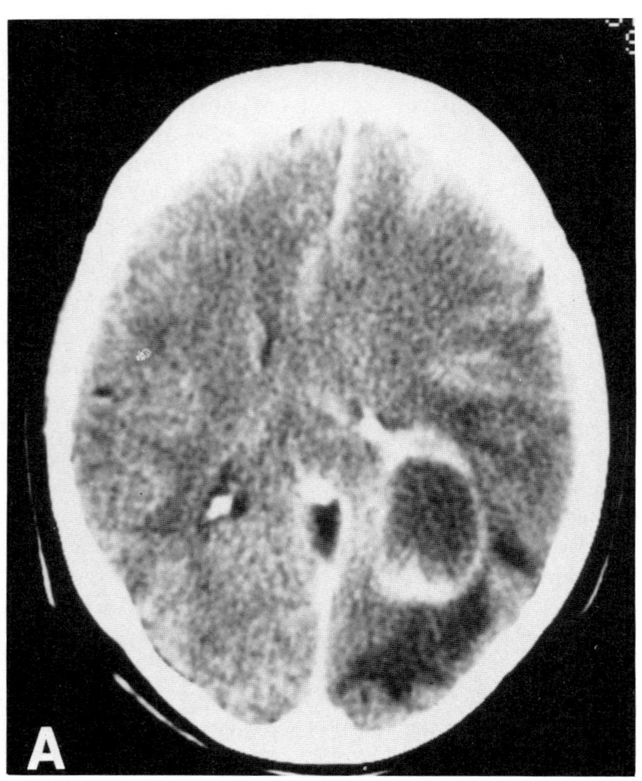

Fig. 19-8. Cystic astrocytoma. (A) A ring-enhancing lesion in left parietal lobe with surrounding edema. The lesion appears unilocular. (B) IUS reveals a multiseptated cystic mass with some solid components (arrows) and a much more complex consistency than suggested on the CT scan. Note also the similarity to the CT appearance of the lesion in Figure 19-7, which was totally solid.

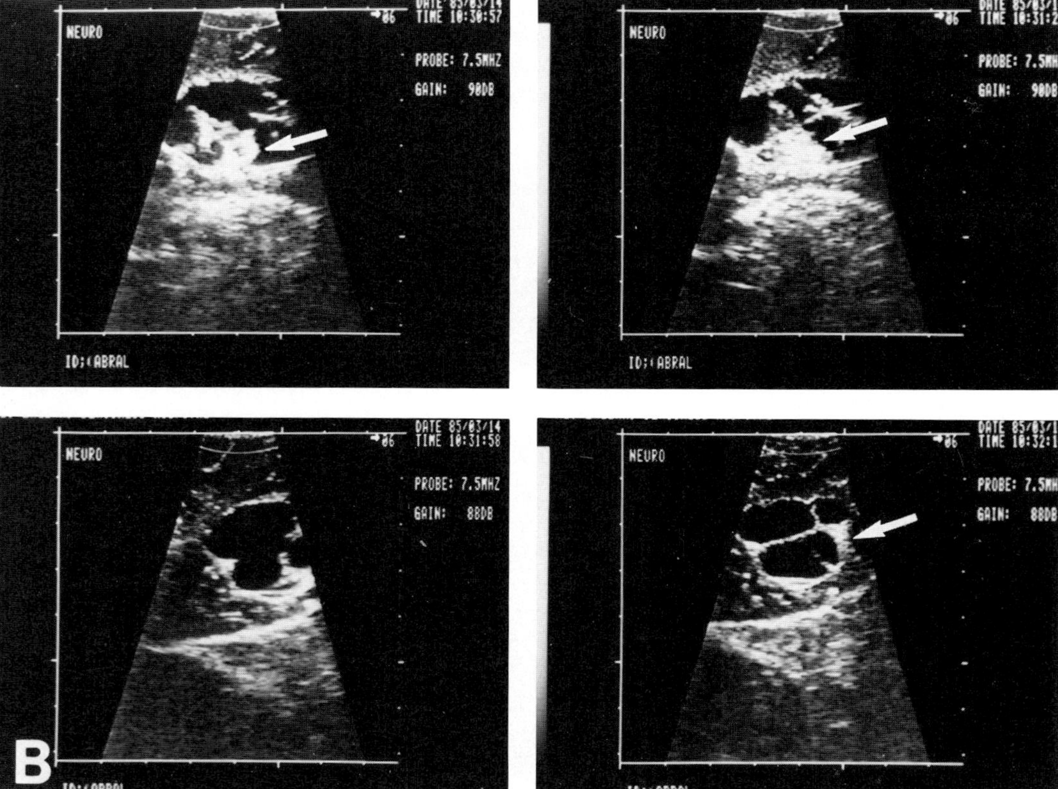

has been described as a highly echogenic lobulated mass arising from the atrium of the lateral ventricle and associated with hydrocephalus.[15] Colloid cysts of the third ventricle are one of the few nonechogenic brain lesions. These tumors usually originate in the roof of the third ventricle in the region of the foramen of Munro, just between the lateral ventricles. The cysts have an echogenic rim and an anechoic or hypoechoic central cavity. These lesions are usually associated with dilatation of one or both of the lateral ventricles, but occasionally a lesion causes only intermittent or partial obstruction and there is no significant hydrocephalus. In this setting, IUS is extremely helpful in localization of the colloid cyst, thereby minimizing

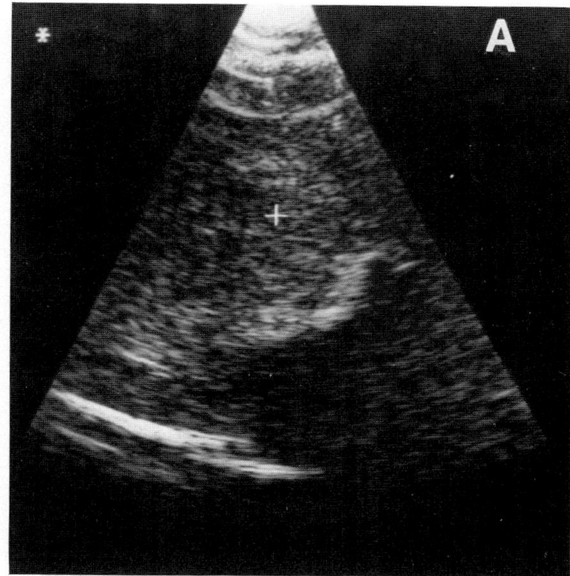

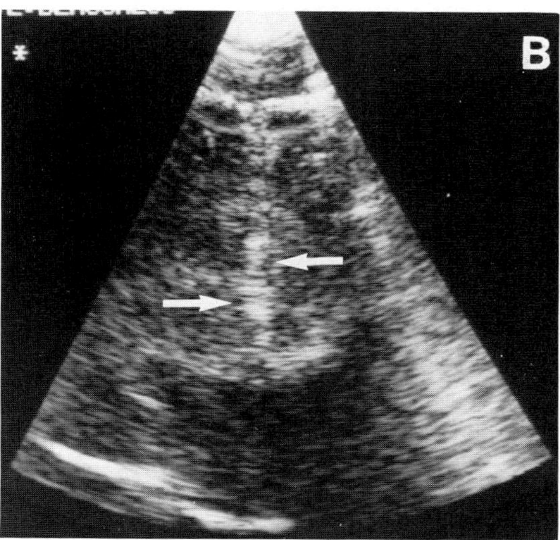

Fig. 19-9. (A) A moderately echogenic glioma. The calipers indicate depth and needle path. (B) A linear hyperechoic area centrally within the mass (arrows) indicating correct positioning of the biopsy needle.

the amount of exploration and brain manipulation required to successfully resect the lesion.[16]

BIOPSY AND OTHER INTERVENTIONAL PROCEDURES

It was recognized very early that IUS provided an ideal method for guidance of biopsy procedures, whether it was an excisional biopsy or merely a guided needle aspiration biopsy. In the former instance, the most direct path to the lesion can be selected, thereby avoiding unnecessary dissection and trauma to normal brain tissue. Needle aspiration biopsies result in even less disruption of normal tissue, and IUS provides extremely accurate guidance for needle placement.

Biopsies initially were performed freehand while being observed in real time, but direct visualization of the needle is difficult unless the path of the needle is directly within the imaging plane.[11] Needle guides consequently were developed

that were designed and calibrated for specific probe configurations. The guides fit over the sterile sheathing encasing the transducer (Figure 19-3) and typically provide a variety of different angled approaches to needle placement. Most of these systems have electronic representation of the needle pathway on a TV monitor, so that the target lesion is positioned within these electronic cursors. The transducer and guidance system are fixed in position, either manually or via clamps, and the needle is then passed through the brain into the lesion under direct real-time observation (Figure 19-9). In addition to needle biopsies, other aspiration procedures can also be performed in a similar fashion, including evacuation of brain abscesses, cysts, and cystic components of tumors. Intraoperative ultrasound biopsy guidance systems have also been proposed for stereotactic guidance in the placement of periventricular stimulating electrodes for control of intractable pain. This was successfully used in a series of experiments in dogs, in which electrodes were placed in the periventricular gray matter with a high degree of accuracy.[17]

Intraoperative ultrasonography has also been useful in guiding the placement of ventricular shunt catheters and for placement of Ommaya reservoirs.[5,10] The shunt catheters are readily visualized and can be manipulated under real-time observation. In infants, the catheter placement can be monitored via scanning over the anterior fontanelle, allowing for placement of the catheter via a small burr hole and manipulation of the catheter into the anterior horn. The effective life span of ventricular shunts has been shown to be increased in those infants who have had ultrasound-guided shunt placement.[18] In addition, any complications as a result of hemorrhage, perforation of the septum pellucidum, or entrapment of the catheter within the choroid plexus can be immediately detected.

It is useful to scan the patient for several minutes after any interventional procedure. Acute hemorrhage can be recognized by virtue of a change in echo texture. Acutely, the area of hemorrhage appears hypoechoic or echo free but rapidly undergoes transformation to a hyperechoic appearance (Figure 19-10A,B), presumably as a result of red cell aggregation and organization of the clot.[11] This has been shown to occur within a few minutes after hemorrhage. If the hematoma expands and threatens vital structures, evacuation can be undertaken under ultrasound guidance.

Intraoperative ultrasonography is also helpful in assessing the completeness of surgical resection. It was initially recommended that saline soaked surgical sponges be used to determine the progression of surgical resection.[19] The saline soaked sponges have a hyperechoic appearance and show some posterior enhancement. However, Gelfoam pledgets within the surgical field can actually obscure tumor margins because of their highly echogenic appearance and occasional reverberation or comet-tail artifact.[14] If this is a problem, the Gelfoam should be removed and the surgical cavity filled with sterile saline in order to better assess the resection margins.

INTRASPINAL SONOGRAPHY

NORMAL ANATOMY

The spinal cord is relatively hypoechoic and homogeneous in texture, although the anterior and posterior surfaces of the cord have a curvilinear hyperechoic appearance because of the

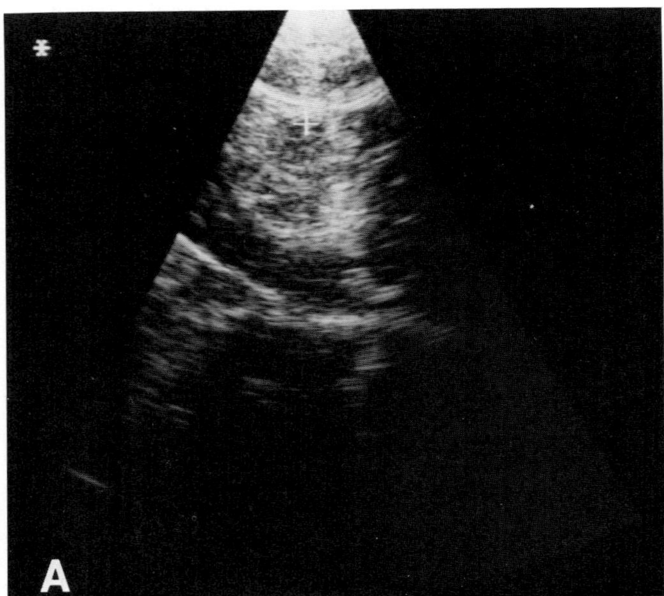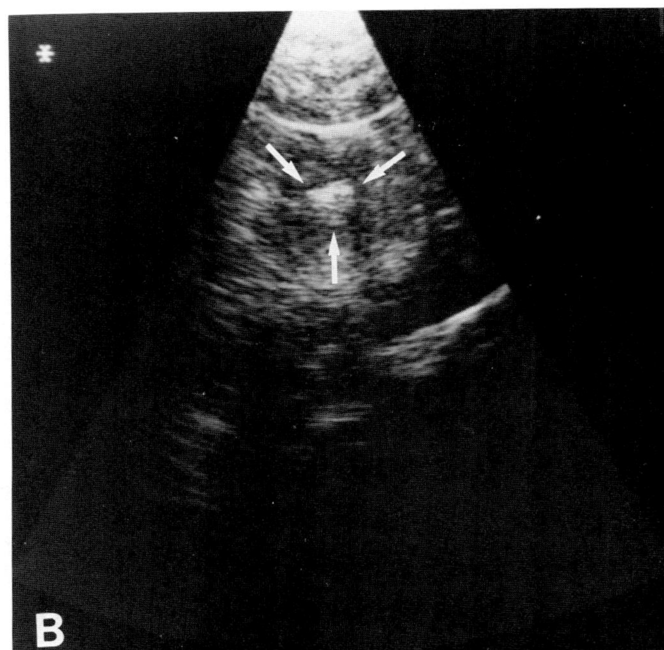

Fig. 19-10. (A) Calipers indicating the depth and path of needle biopsy to be performed. (B) An ultrasound image made 2 minutes following biopsy, demonstrating a focal hyperechoic area within the tumor (arrows) that was not seen before the biopsy. This represents a focal hematoma.

major change in reflectivity between the subarachnoid fluid and the soft tissue of the cord and its membranes. The only interruption of the homogeneous texture of the cord is the central canal, which appears as a linear hyperechoic area running up and down the length of the cord in its midportion (Figure 19-11). The central canal is an important anatomic landmark that should be sought after and identified on all scans. By scanning through the intact dura, fluid in the subarachnoid space can be visualized as crescentic or linear anechoic areas both anterior and posterior to the cord. The anterior spinal arteries can often be seen pulsating along the ventral surface of the cord.

In transverse section, the dentate ligaments are seen as

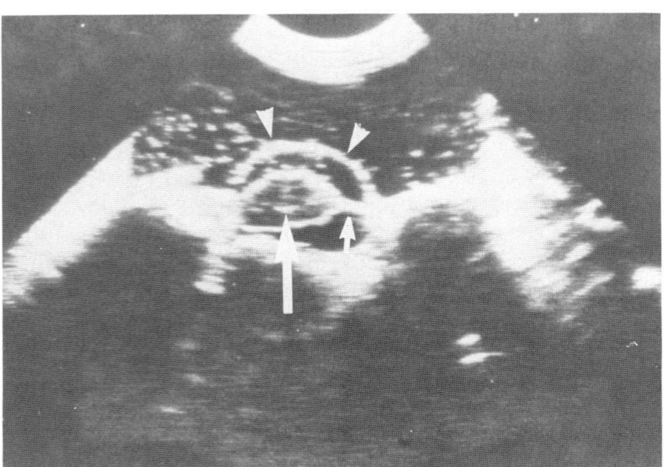

Fig. 19-11. A transverse ultrasound section of a normal spinal cord. Scans are obtained through a fluid-filled laminectomy defect, demonstrating the cord with its central canal (large arrow) surrounded by anechoic fluid in the subarachnoid space. Note the echogenic dentate ligament (small arrow) as well as the hyperreflective posterior dural surface (arrowheads).

linear hyperechoic structures extending from the lateral margins of the cord to the dura. Nerve roots can also be seen exiting from the cord along the ventrolateral surface, as well as distally below the cord at the level of the cauda equina. The nerve root bundles also have a linear hyperechoic appearance. In real time, a slight undulation of the thecal sac is observed as a result of respiratory activity.[11] The anatomic detail described above requires a 7.5-MHz frequency transducer for optimal demonstration.

PATHOLOGIC ANATOMY

Extramedullary Pathologic Conditions

Extramedullary tumors have a uniform hyperechoic appearance unless there are cystic components to the tumor or areas of hemorrhage or cystic necrosis.[11] The tumor margins are well defined and discrete, with an abrupt zone of transition between the spinal cord and the mass (Figure 19-12A,B). The cord is displaced to a variable extent by the mass and may be compressed and attenuated, but the central canal remains identifiable, which helps to distinguish an extramedullary mass from an intramedullary tumor.

It was previously thought that oscillations of the spinal cord in synchrony with the cardiac rate were an indication that the cord was free in the subarachnoid space without significant compression. This has been refuted by real-time IUS studies. In one series, 8 of 11 patients with lesions causing cord compression had these typical rhythmic oscillations despite the presence of a compressing lesion.[20] The oscillations were seen to be greatest near the site of compression, although they were diminished at the exact site of maximal compression. The oscillations appear to be caused by transmitted pulsations from the compressed anterior spinal arteries.

Intraoperative ultrasonography is particularly valuable in assessing the full extent of both neoplastic and nonneoplastic

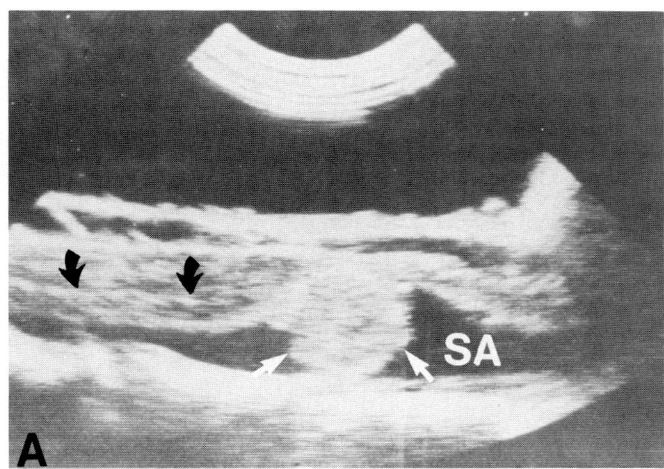
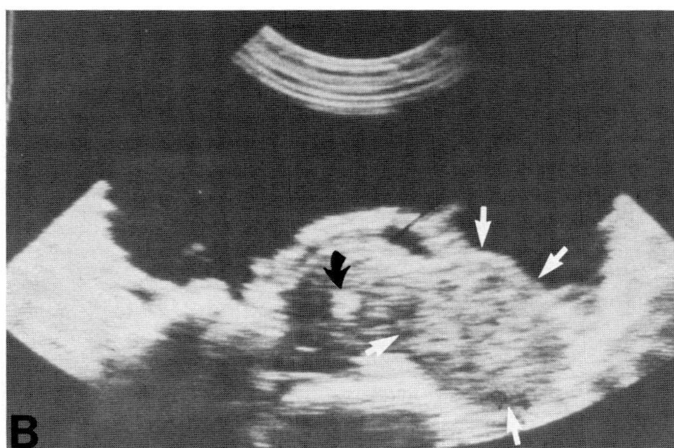

Fig. 19-12. Neurofibroma. (A) A sagittal image demonstrating a highly echogenic extramedullary tumor (arrows) causing compression and upward deflection of the cord with expansion of the subarachnoid space (SA). Note also the linear hyperechoic central canal (curved black arrows). (B) A transverse image demonstrating the intradural and extradural extent of the tumor (arrows). (Reprinted from Rubin JM, Dohrmann GJ: Work in progress: Intraoperative ultrasonography of the spine. Radiology 146:173, 1983. With permission.)

anterior extramedullary lesions. This is a relatively blind area for the neurosurgeon, but can be well assessed sonographically without resorting to retraction of the spinal cord, which carries some risk of damage to the cord.[21] Thus, the full extent of tumors can be defined, the surgical resection planned, and the completeness of resection assessed.

Nonneoplastic lesions such as protruding or herniated discs, hypertrophic bony bars (Figure 19-13), and posttraumatic lesions such as bone fragments, bullets, and other foreign bodies can also be readily assessed by IUS. A herniated disc is relatively echo-poor, especially in relation to extramedullary tumors. It appears as a homogeneous, relatively hypoechoic mass with a smooth convex margin arising from the ventral extradural plane and obliterating the ventral subarachnoid space, and to a varying degree indenting or compressing the cord.[7]

Intramedullary Pathologic Conditions

Unlike extramedullary spinal cord tumors and intra-axial brain neoplasms, intramedullary tumors of the spinal cord are relatively isoechoic to the cord itself.[11] Tumors within the cord consequently are difficult to recognize, and the boundary be-

tween neoplastic tissue and normal tissue is often impossible to determine. The presence of an intramedullary tumor is inferred by visualizing a localized bulging or swelling of the cord and by the lack of an identifiable central canal, which is usually obliterated by the tumor. However, absence of a definable central canal has also been reported in diffuse inflammatory swelling of the cord,[7] acute swelling of the cord following trauma,[11] and in posttraumatic myelomalacia with resultant cord atrophy.[22]

Intraoperative ultrasonography is clearly superior in demonstrating the cystic components of various cord lesions (Figure 19-14). In four of five cases reported by Rubin,[21] IUS produced considerably more information than either preoperative CT or myelography in demonstrating the presence of cystic degeneration within tumor and in completely demonstrating various loculations and outpouchings in two cases of

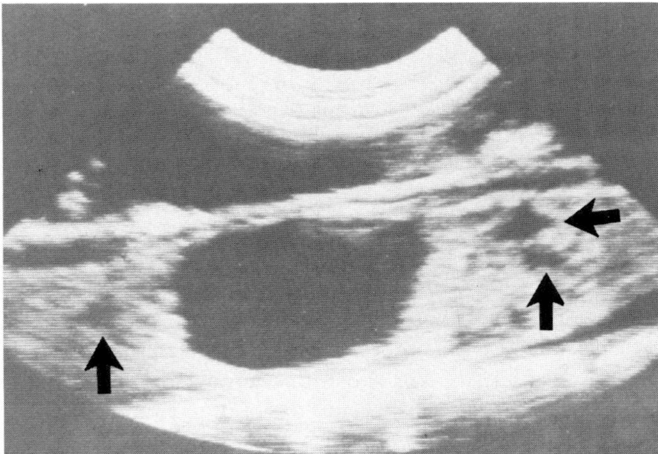

Fig. 19-14. A cystic intramedullary mass. A sagittal scan demonstrating a large anechoic cyst with several smaller cystic loculations (arrows). Note the fusiform expansion of the cord and the obliteration of the normal central canal. (Reprinted by permission of the publisher from Dohrmann GJ, Rubin JM: Intraoperative ultrasound imaging of the spinal cord: Syringomyelia, cysts, and tumors—a preliminary report. Surg Neurol 18:395. Copyright 1982 by Elsevier Science Publishing Co., Inc.)

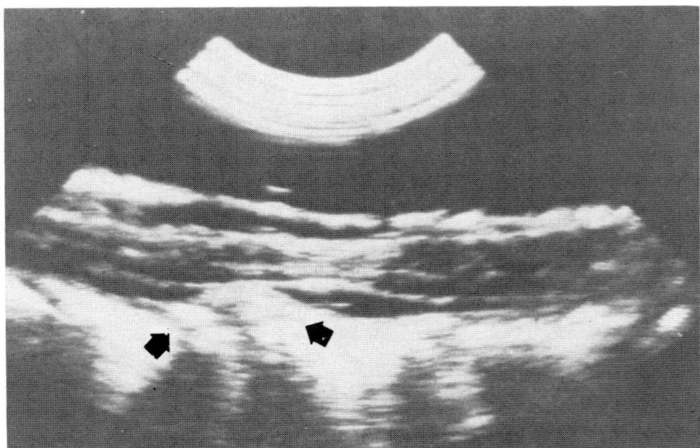

Fig. 19-13. A sagittal scan demonstrating elevation and flattening of the spinal cord by a hyperechoic bony bar (arrows).

syringomyelia in which even with metrizamide, the CT scan only demonstrated what appeared to be a single syrinx cavity. Intraoperative ultrasonography showed multiple loculations or outpouchings off of the main cavity. Small areas of cystic degeneration can also be seen in cases of myelomalacia, resulting in an inhomogeneous texture to the cord.[11] Intraoperative ultrasonography may also be of some value in surgery for spinal dysraphism, in particular for precise localization of the conus medullaris and filum terminale during surgery for tethered cord.[23]

In some instances it is impossible to distinguish intratumoral cysts from cystic dilatation of the central canal, although most often the central canal is obliterated by the tumor.[23] Postoperative imaging of the spine following tumor resections may provide useful information on the development of tumor recurrence, cyst formation, arachnoiditis, and cord atrophy. Raghavendra reported that in 70 percent of patients, postoperative scanning through the site of the previous laminectomy provided sufficiently detailed information that preoperative myelography or CT was judged unnecessary before reoperation.[23]

INTERVENTIONAL PROCEDURES

As in the brain, biopsies can be readily performed using ultrasound biopsy guidance systems. Similarly, ultrasound is quite useful in guiding the drainage of cysts or syrinx cavities. In particular, the presence of loculations or multiple separate cavities in syringomyelia can be determined and the effectiveness of the shunt catheter can be assessed. If residual fluid cavities are present after the initial drainage procedure, these are readily demonstrated and can be effectively dealt with by manipulation of the catheter or placement of further shunts.[7]

CONCLUSION

Intraoperative ultrasonography has been a major advance in diagnostic imaging of the brain and spinal cord, providing clearly superior information that cannot be obtained by preoperative imaging techniques or by direct visual inspection during surgery. It allows accurate depiction of normal anatomy and rapid identification of focal pathologic lesions; it provides an accurate means of guidance for biopsy procedures through burr holes or craniotomy flaps; it provides excellent guidance for placement of shunt catheters and drainage procedures; it allows for instantaneous assessment of the completeness of surgical excisions of tumors and the effects of various interventional procedures. The utilization of IUS results in a better planned surgical procedure, allowing for preservation of more normal CNS tissue and with consequently less adverse side effects of the surgical procedures. Intraoperative ultrasonography will continue to grow as more neurosurgeons become familiar with the uses and applications of this technique.

REFERENCES

1. Tanaka K, Ito K, Wagai T: The localization of brain tumors by ultrasonic techniques. A clinical review of 111 cases. J Neurosurg 23:135, 1965
2. Muller HR, Levy A: A simple method of two-dimensional intraoperative sonencephalography, employing the A-scan technique. Eur Neurol 1:31, 1968
3. Glasauer FE, Schlagenhauff RE: The use of intraoperative echoencephalography. Neurology 20:1103, 1970
4. Rubin JM, Mirfakbraee M, Duda EE, et al: Intraoperative ultrasound examination of the brain. Radiology 137:831, 1980
5. Rubin JM, Dohrmann GJ: Use of ultrasonically guided probes and catheters in neurosurgery. Surg Neurol 18:143, 1982
6. Rubin JM, Dohrmann GJ: Work in progress: Intraoperative ultrasonography of the spine. Radiology 146:173, 1983
7. Knake JE, Gabrielsen TO, Chandler WF, et al: Real-time sonography during spinal surgery. Radiology 151:461, 1984
8. Berger MS: Ultrasound guided stereotactic biopsy using the diasonics neuro-biopsy device for deep seated intracranial lesions. Presented at the Annual Meeting of the American Association of Neurological Surgeons, Atlanta, GA, April 21–25, 1985
9. Gooding GAW, Boggan JE, Powers SK, et al: Neurosurgical sonography: Intraoperative and postoperative imaging of the brain. AJNR 5:521, 1984
10. Chandler WF, Knake JE, McGillicuddy JE, et al: Intraoperative use of real-time ultrasonography in neurosurgery. J Neurosurg 57:157, 1982
11. Knake JE, Bowerman RA, Silver TM, McCracken S: Neurosurgical applications of intraoperative ultrasound. Radiol Clin North Am 23:73, 1985
12. Knake JE, Chandler WF, Gabrielsen TO, et al: Intraoperative sonographic delineation of low-grade brain neoplasms defined poorly by computed tomography. Radiology 151:735, 1984
13. Enzmann DR, Wheat R, Marshall WH, et al.: Tumors of the central nervous system studied by computed tomography and ultrasound. Radiology 154:393, 1985
14. Pasto ME, Rifkin MD: Intraoperative ultrasound examination of the brain: Possible pitfalls in diagnosis and biopsy guidance. J Ultrasound Med 3:245, 1984
15. Cappe IP, Lam AH: Ultrasound in the diagnosis of choroid plexus papilloma. J Clin Ultrasound 12:121, 1985
16. Rezvani L, Rubin J, Dohrmann GJ: Colloid cysts with and without ventriculomegaly: Role of intraoperative real-time ultrasound. Surg Neurol 22:515, 1984
17. Brown FD, Rachlin JR, Rubin JM, et al: Ultrasound-guided periventricular stereotaxis. Neurosurgery 15:162, 1984
18. Merritt CRB, Coulon R, Connolly E: Intraoperative neurosurgical ultrasound: Transdural and transfontanelle applications. Radiology 148:513, 1983
19. Gooding GAW, Edwards MSB, Rabkin AE, et al: Intraoperative real-time ultrasound in the localization of intracranial neoplasms. Radiology 146:459, 1983
20. Jokich PM, Rubin JM, Dohrmann GJ: Intraoperative ultrasonic evaluation of spinal cord motion. J Neurosurg 60:707, 1984
21. Rubin JM, Dohrmann GJ: The spine and spinal cord during neurosurgical operations: Real-time ultrasonography. Radiology 155:197, 1985
22. St Amour TE, Rubin JM, Dohrmann GJ: The central canal of the spinal cord: Ultrasonic identification. Radiology 152:767, 1984
23. Raghavendra BN, Epstein FJ: Sonography of the spine and spinal cord. Radiol Clin North Am 23:91, 1985

CHAPTER 20

The Laser and Ultrasonic Aspirator in Neurosurgery

Steven L. Wald   Henry H. Schmidek

THE INTRODUCTION of new neurosurgical instrumentation, including the laser, ultrasonic aspirator, and high-speed drills, provides the neurosurgeon with a range of tools with which to perform delicate and intricate craniospinal procedures. Although any of these instruments can prove quite useful for a particular operation, the use of these unique devices does not abrogate the requirement for meticulous neurosurgical technique. Specific training and experience are often required before the instrument can be applied to any specific clinical neurosurgical procedure.

THE LASER

OVERVIEW

The application of laser technology to neurosurgical procedures has enjoyed increasing popularity since Maiman constructed the first laser from a ruby crystal source in 1959.[1] The unique characteristics of laser energy have produced considerable excitement within the neurosurgical community, paralleling the rapid advances in diagnostic imaging and localization. Most experience has been gained with the carbon dioxide laser because of its ability to both vaporize and coagulate solid tissue.

The potential advantages of the laser are easily understood when the standard operative techniques for the total removal of a central nervous system neoplasm are considered. Adequate cerebral exposure; a defined line of demarcation between the tumor and normal brain; clear visibility, supplied in part by suction devices; and the ability to coagulate vascular structures are the minimum requirements for a successful procedure. It is frequently necessary to retract adjacent brain tissue, which can, in spite of gentle manipulation facilitated by hyperosmolar agents and cerebrospinal fluid drainage, produce serious neurologic sequelae. Dissection of tumor tissue near vital neural or vascular structures is potentially dangerous and can result in incomplete resection. Acute blood loss is a major consideration during any attempted tumor excision. The laser provides the neurosurgeon with the means to resect tumor tissue while potentially minimizing both retraction and blood loss.

LASER PHYSICS

The principle of quantum mechanics as elucidated by Bohr and Einstein maintains that atomic systems can exist at different states of energy. At the ground or stable state an atom or molecule can only absorb energy. In Figure 20-1, an atom, which has a characteristic nucleus and a unique arrangement of electrons in surrounding shells, has absorbed energy. The absorption of energy causes an electron to shift to a higher shell or orbit around the nucleus. When the electron spontaneously returns to its stable configuration, energy is emitted as a photon. An atom or molecule in the stable state can thus be excited by adding energy to it, and it can then spontaneously emit energy as it returns to its ground or steady state. Energy is always conserved. If an already excited atom is struck by another photon, it will stimulate the emission of two identical photons. The laser, an acronym for Light Amplification by the Stimulated Emission of Radiation, is a form of radiant energy generated by the emission of photons. A high voltage electric current is added to the active element or compound within the laser chamber (e.g., carbon dioxide) to raise it to an excited state. At a given time, more atoms are in the excited state than are in the stable state. Photons released during the process of decay may strike other electrons, producing a cascade or chain reaction effect. Within the laser chamber, parallel photons are captured and released to a delivery system. Non-parallel photons release their energy as heat within the chamber.

The emitted radiation of the laser is unique because the generated light waves are of a single length (monochromatic), parallel to each other (collimated), and in phase (coherent). The specific wavelength generated by any laser system is dependent on the activated medium. Carbon dioxide laser light, for example, has a wavelength of 10.6 μm, while the wavelength for a neodymium:ytterium argon garnet (Nd:YAG) laser is 1.06 μm. Different tissues will preferentially absorb a given wavelength. It is this characteristic that allows for a selective effect of the laser on various tissue components.

The available delivery systems generate a light beam with a spot size that can be altered by the operating surgeon. The spot size affects both the target surface area subjected to the laser and the amount of energy, termed power density, that the tissue will receive. Conventional laser systems can supply power densities from 100 to nearly 1,000,000 W/cm^2.

BIOLOGIC EFFECTS OF THE LASER

As a form of light, the laser beam can be absorbed, reflected, or transmitted by the tissue it strikes. Tissue absorption by any given laser is dependent on the wavelength generated by the active element or compound. The argon laser

OPERATIVE NEUROSURGICAL TECHNIQUES
ISBN 0-8089-1862-1

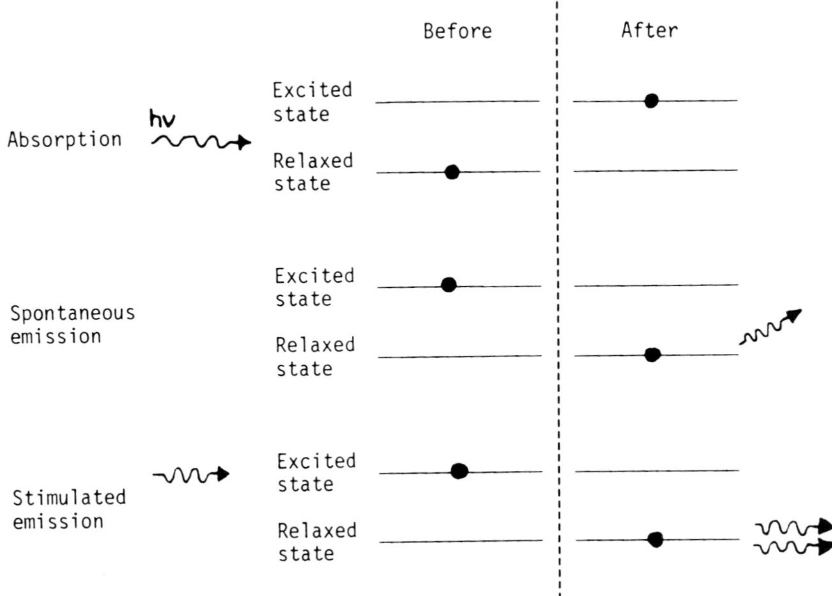

Fig. 20-1. The absorption of energy (photon) raises an atom in the ground state to an excited state. The photon can be spontaneously emitted. When an atom in the excited state is struck, two identical photons are emitted.

produces a visible green light and is selectively absorbed by red pigmented tissues and melanin. The energy produced by the carbon dioxide laser is invisible light and is absorbed primarily by water within tissue and converted to heat. Flash boiling of intracellular and extracellular water results in tissue vaporization and carbonization. A useful comparison is shown in Table 20-1. Since most cellular elements of the brain have a very high water content, nearly complete absorption of carbon dioxide laser energy is achieved at surface levels. The extinction coefficient, which is a measurement of energy absorption, indicates that 90 percent of the energy from a carbon dioxide laser will be absorbed by water molecules at a depth of 0.03 mm. The penetration of Nd:YAG laser energy is up to 60 mm in nonpigmented tissues.

Thermal injury to brain tissue is characterized by three concentric zones of change extending from the point of application.[2,3] A layer of charred debris covers a second deeper layer of destroyed, pyknotic, shrunken cells and empty spaces. A third or outer layer, partially destroyed by coagulation necrosis, consists of swollen neurons and glia. Large, swollen intracellular spaces are consistent with cerebral edema. Histologic studies on human brain tumor tissue have demonstrated viable cells below this third layer with little edema seen in normal tissue adjacent to tumor. The entire depth of these changes ranges from 3 to 8 cells in thickness or less than 1 mm of penetration. The characteristic lack of heat conduction and destruction by the carbon dioxide laser distant from the point of impact ensures the creation of a precise lesion with minimal thermal injury to adjacent structures.

Two studies compared lesions in the brains of cats produced by a carbon dioxide laser to similar lesions made with microbipolar coagulation and a scalpel.[4,5] In both studies, the hemisphere with lesions created with the laser demonstrated less cerebral edema than did the opposite hemisphere subjected to bipolar coagulation and sharp incision despite histopathologic similarities. Takizawa emphasized the more precise, localized demarcation produced by the laser in comparison with that created by electrosurgical units.[4] Normal healing of skin

and subcutaneous and fascial layers has been demonstrated when the laser is used as a cutting tool.

Dynamic studies of intracranial pressure, EEG patterns, and systemic arterial and venous pressures have shown that laser thermal injuries delivered through an intact dura produce changes similar to those seen in the classic cold or cryogenic injury.[6,7] Unlike the cold lesion, the stimulus can be accurately quantified and graded. Studies related to the treatment of this form of cerebral edema may prove useful in clinical situations. Studies of the cerebral microcirculation using the carbon dioxide laser have shown dilated and congested vessels adjacent to a wedge-shaped coagulated layer. Kuroiwa found focal bleeding in 28 percent of animals subjected to 4 or 8 W of laser energy for 2 seconds.[8] However, Toya found that the disturbances of the microcirculation were confined to an area within 3 mm of the center of the lesion.[9] Miller et al.[10] reviewed the long-term effects of intraocular photocoagulation in albino rabbits. Major retinal vessels were occluded without involvement of the underlying orbital structures. Lesions adjacent to the optic nerve exhibited no detectable involvement of the nerve on histologic review. The hemostatic effects of the carbon dioxide laser can be very helpful but are limited by the size of the vascular structure. Small vessels in the range of 0.5 to 1.0 mm are coagulated and sealed, while larger vessels are incised, requiring other methods for hemostasis.

LASER SYSTEMS

Commercially available laser units consist of a generating unit and a delivery system. The generating unit is composed of a portable console and a laser tube; the delivery system includes an articulated arm and either a free handpiece or an adapter for use with the operating microscope. The console houses the laser medium, the control functions, the gas cylinders, and the electrical circuits. A laser tube extends from the console and incorporates the series of mirrors necessary to transmit laser energy. Two lasers are actually generated; a helium-neon laser beam is used to guide or track the operational high-energy carbon dioxide laser. The laser is turned on and off

Table 20–1. Characteristics of lasers

Type	Wavelength (microns)	Spectrum Location	Absorption* (mm)	Power Output (watts)
Ruby	0.694	Visible	300	4
Argon	0.488–0.515	Visible	300	20
Nd:YAG	1.06	Infrared-near	60–100	Up to 50
Carbon dioxide	10.6	Infrared-far	0.3	Up to 100

* Absorption: Depth in water of 90 percent of radiant energy.

with a foot pedal. Mode structure refers to the characteristics of beam divergence and power distribution within the laser spot. The fundamental mode, designated TEM for Transverse Electromagnetic Mode, has a gaussian profile. Power is maximum at the center and decays at the edges. Higher order modes have multiple peaks and cold spots within the spot diameter. The mode is predetermined by the manufacturer and cannot be changed by the surgeon.

The carbon dioxide laser is a relatively efficient source of energy. The argon laser requires nearly 10,000 W of power to generate 1 W of laser power, while the carbon dioxide laser can produce 1 W of laser power with only 10 W of power input.

LASER TECHNIQUES

The manipulation of four variables determines the effect of laser energy on tissue. Power output, expressed in watts, is altered by an adjustment on the control panel. Current specifications allow a power range of 1 to 100 W depending on the laser model being used. The actual power delivered to the tissue will decay from 5 to 10 W because of conduction through the articulating arm. Twenty watts of power is required to vaporize 10 mm^3 of tissue with an 80 percent water content.[11] Spot size is limited by manufactured standards and ranges from 0.1 to 2 mm for carbon dioxide lasers. At comparable power outputs, a smaller spot size will produce more energy at the point of impact. The extent of laser injury and penetration is also dependent on the length of time tissue is exposed to the radiant energy. Commercially available laser systems are programmed to emit laser light either continuously or at intermittent, predetermined time intervals, called pulse mode. Finally, by adjusting the available lens systems or by moving the free handpiece, the surgeon can focus or defocus the laser light. A defocused beam will vaporize larger areas of tissue, while a focused beam will act as a laser scalpel. The goal of laser neurosurgery is to achieve an optimal thermal effect by manipulation of these variables with a minimal amount of laser energy.

When laser energy strikes a tissue, producing vaporization, a plume of smoke is emitted. The plume is composed of vaporized water, carbon, and cellular debris but is free of viable tumor cells.[12,13] Continuous suction is necessary to remove the smoke and provide an unobstructed view. The laser lenses are kept clean by a continuous wash of nitrogen across their surfaces. Carbonization on the surface of the tissue or on either side of an incision will be seen but is harmless and can be left in place.

A commonly cited disadvantage of the laser is its precise layer-by-layer vaporization. Debulking of large tumors is prohibitively time consuming. Using a defocused mode, we have employed a technique of outlining a block of tumor and undercutting the base. This allows for rapid bulk removal but still provides a degree of hemostasis in the tumor bed. Vessels larger than 0.5 to 1.0 mm continue to require conventional coagulation techniques. Surface bleeding from vessels must be evacuated or the energy from the laser will be absorbed by the pooled blood rather than the tumor tissue.

Certain safety precautions are required when using the laser. Signs are posted at each entrance to the operating room. Direct impact or reflected light can cause serious eye injuries and inflict third-degree burns. These injuries are less likely to occur when the laser is coupled to the operating microscope. Eye protection for operating room personnel is provided by wrap-around glasses of either plastic or glass. The surgeon and assistants are protected by the various lenses of the operating microscope. The laser is capable of igniting flammable gases or liquids, such as ether, alcohol, and acetone. Metal retractors should be covered with moist cottonoid strips, which will absorb the energy before it can strike the reflective surface. Additional wet cottonoids should be placed over any exposed brain tissue to prevent injury from stray or accidental laser discharge.

CLINICAL APPLICATION

The carbon dioxide laser is presently the most useful laser system for removing central nervous system neoplasms.[14–26] Any tumor is potentially amenable to laser excision. Lesions near vascular or neural structures can be removed "layer by layer" with fine adjustment of power and spot size to dissect tumor tissue off these structures. Intraventricular lesions can be excised after cerebrospinal fluid has been evacuated. Tumors of the brainstem and posterior fossa can be excised by laser vaporization without manipulating the tumor, which is a potential cause of seeding of neoplastic cells via the cerebrospinal fluid. While the long-term outcome for tumors treated with a laser has yet to be compared with conventionally treated tumors, the decreased mechanical trauma and increased precision of the laser appear to afford a potentially faster and smoother postoperative period. It is premature to suggest that outcome will be significantly improved in patients treated with the laser. If the extent of surgical resection of a malignant tumor plays a significant role in determining outcome, then the laser will be a valuable adjunct to the neurosurgeon. However, multiple factors usually influence outcome, and the role of the laser must be kept in perspective.[25] Although there was initial concern regarding the use of the laser in pediatric patients, no evidence has been forthcoming to support this concern.[24,27] Tumor masses adjacent to or within peripheral nerves can be excised or vaporized with the laser and peripheral nerves can be sectioned using this tool.

THE ARGON LASER

Hemostasis is an important factor in any neurosurgical procedure. Although the carbon dioxide laser is capable of coagulating small vessels, its wavelength is not optimal for this task. The argon laser, with a wavelength of 0.488 to 0.514 μm, produces a visible blue-green light that is highly transmissible through water and selectively absorbed by pigmented tissues such as blood vessels, melanin, and cytochromes. Although comparison of two different laser sources is difficult, Boggan et al.[3] found no significant differences in lesions created with the carbon dioxide laser versus the argon system. Theoretical advantages of argon lasers include the ability to deliver the energy through fiberoptic systems; improved precision, since a guiding or target light is not required; a smaller spot size; and greater hemostatic effects. The experience of Edwards et al.[28] indicates that the argon laser may be particularly helpful in areas where manipulation of neural structures must be minimized and in eradicating pigmented lesions. Large fibrous lesions require greater power densities than can normally be generated by argon systems.

THE ND:YAG LASER

Because of the inherent limitations of the argon and carbon dioxide lasers, attention has been directed to lasers with wavelengths that are preferentially absorbed by pigmented tissues but with higher potential power outputs. The invisible monochromatic light produced by the Nd:YAG laser is preferentially absorbed by hemoglobin pigments and can generate up to 100 W of power. In vivo and in vitro studies demonstrate rapid absorption of the thermal energy in tissue with histologic lesions resembling those found in animals treated with carbon dioxide lasers.[29–32] However, caution must be exercised in attempting to extrapolate this type of data. Jain presented an important series of clinical complications in a review of 32 patients treated with a Nd:YAG laser that serves to underscore the potential hazards of using this instrument.[33] Further experimental studies and clinical trials will be necessary before the Nd:YAG laser system can be appropriately adapted for neurosurgical use.

FUTURE DEVELOPMENTS

Techniques now exist that combine the benefits of laser surgery with data derived by computed tomography (CT) and magnetic resonance imaging (MRI) to perform stereotactic laser microsurgery.[34] This has been particularly useful in debulking lesions otherwise deemed inaccessible. While the ultimate goal is complete removal, the limiting factor appears to be the ability to precisely detect tumor margins.

Photoradiation therapy for malignant tumors has been reported by Laws et al.[35] Following intravenous administration of a hematoporphyrin derivative, which concentrates within tumor tissue, a stereotactic probe is placed within the tumor and is coupled to an argon laser. Empirically, the goal of the therapy is to administer red light at a wavelength of 630 nm for 45 minutes. Experimental studies have shown that hematoporphyrins accumulate in the cytoplasm and on membranes of tumor cells and that exposure to red light with a wavelength of 630 nm will kill cultured tumor cells.[36] Although the results must be considered preliminary, clinical improvement and CT evidence of tumor regression were seen in 3 of 5 patients.

Progressive occlusion of experimentally induced aneurysms without compromising the parent vessel was reported by Maira using an argon laser.[37] Jain and Gorisch employed a Nd:YAG laser to seal experimental arteriotomies and venotomies without producing mechanical or thermoelectric damage to the vessel.[38] Fasano et al.,[39] in a preliminary report, found the Nd:YAG laser useful in completely obliterating various types of arteriovenous malformations. Blood loss was substantially reduced and manipulation of surrounding structures was minimal. The potential application of these lasers for treatment of primary cerebrovascular abnormalities awaits further clinical reports.

Wet-field carbon dioxide laser surgery, which allows tissue vaporization through a fluid-filled compartment, is a neurosurgical application yet to be explored.[40,41]

The coupling of endoscopic techniques and laser technology is presently limited to the use of nonflexible systems.[42] An important advance will be the development of fiberoptic systems for the transmission of carbon dioxide laser beams.[43] These devices may result in even further reductions in tissue manipulation and exposure and allow the neurosurgeon to reach areas of the brain more easily.

Levy et al.[44] has demonstrated the ability of a laser to produce consistent and reproducible dorsal root entry zone lesions in cats. In comparison to the standard radiofrequency lesion, the laser injury was smaller, less variable in its size, and less time consuming. Clinical application of the carbon dioxide laser in the areas of functional and ablative pain surgery have yet to be fully explored.

Although the destructive characteristics of laser energy are well known, attention has now been directed to a reparative approach. Several investigators have reported favorable experiences using the carbon dioxide laser to weld or bond tissues.[45-51] Application of these techniques to vascular and neural anastomosis may simplify and expedite these procedures. Tissue bonding is apparently the result of local protein coagulation produced by the intense heat of the laser. Neural regeneration in severed rat sciatic nerves is not hindered by the imparted thermal injury, and morphologic studies indicate that there is less reactive scarring than is seen with standard epineural suture techniques.[45,51] Although it appears that tissue bonding can be accomplished using available standard laser systems, adapted systems employing milliwatt power outputs are preferable.

THE ULTRASONIC SURGICAL ASPIRATOR

OVERVIEW

Ultrasonic energy can be used to fragment and emulsify tissue. The success of this technique in ophthalmologic surgery prompted neurosurgeons to investigate its usefulness within the central nervous system. With the addition of suction and irrigation to a hand-held, self-contained unit, it is possible to fragment and evacuate tumor tissue simultaneously.

THE SYSTEM

The surgical aspirator consists of a portable control and a power console connected to a handpiece. The tip of the device vibrates at a frequency of 23 kHz through a range of 100 μm or 0.004 inches. The vibration is virtually imperceptible to the surgeon. Fragmentation and aspiration of tissue occurs within 1 to 2 mm of the vibrating tip. The flow rate of the irrigating solution, the magnitude of the vacuum or suction, and the intensity of the vibration are adjustable. As currently designed, the vibrating tip must make contact with the tissue, precluding direct integration with the operating microscope.

BIOLOGIC EFFECTS

The histologic characteristics of cortical and white matter resections performed with the ultrasonic aspirator have been studied by Flamm using the brains and spinal cords of cats.[52] Microscopic sections were compared with those obtained by the techniques of standard suction and cautery, cutting loop cautery, and rongeur removal. Characteristic areas of hemorrhage and necrosis were seen in the areas of resection surrounded by edema and swelling of axonal sheaths in all experimental preparations. No quantitative differences could be detected in the lesions created by the ultrasonic aspirator and those created by other standard techniques. Prolonged ultrasonic exposure of the spinal cord without actual tissue resection produced significant alterations of the evoked potentials. White matter edema, petechial hemorrhages, and cavitation were seen in microscopic sections of these spinal cords. The spinal cord exposure experiment, as the authors commented, does not, however, mimic the clinical application of this instrument.

Young et al.[53] studied blood flow and evoked potentials in the spinal cords of animals subjected to an ultrasonically created dorsal column lesion. Blood flow and action potential conduction were not significantly altered in the adjacent white matter regions despite characteristic histologic changes. Electrical studies of peripheral nerve demonstrated intact conduction even when the shank of the aspirator was placed in direct contact with the nerve. Only direct contact of the aspirator probe with the nerve produced abolition of action potentials.

CLINICAL APPLICATIONS AND TECHNIQUES

The primary advantages of ultrasonic emulsification and aspiration are the lack of mechanical manipulation of normal tissue, the preservation of tissue planes, the lack of thermal effects, and the ability to simultaneously aspirate and irrigate. After exposure of the tumor, the aspirator handle is applied to the tumor, producing a gradual removal of tissue with simultaneous irrigation and aspiration. Spread of vibration is negligible, and tumor can be removed near vital neural structures. We have found that at lower vibratory settings, the probe will not tend to fragment larger vascular structures but will aspirate them into the barrel at which time they can be coagulated by standard means. It must be emphasized that no hemostasis is provided with the ultrasonic aspirator. A useful technique is the ability to hold the aspirator in one hand and the bipolar forceps in the other hand. Gradual debulking of the tumor is carried out until the inside of the capsule is encountered, at which point other means should be used to complete the removal.

The emulsified and fragmented tissues are collected by the CUSA system and should be submitted for histologic review. Blackie found only minimal deterioration of specimens compared with material from conventional biopsies.[54] Diagnostic tissue was obtained in all cases.

The use of continuous irrigation and concern over tumor spillage prompted Oosterhuis to assess the viability of cells found in the irrigation fluid.[55] These studies demonstrated intact tumor cells that proved viable both in vitro and in vivo. The clinical relevance of this finding has yet to be fully explored.

Virtually all types of tumors are potentially amenable to ultrasonic fragmentation.[56–59] The usefulness of the ultrasonic aspirator in any given case is unpredictable. While it is extremely effective for extirpation of soft tumors, difficulty may be encountered when trying to aspirate firm, fibrous tumors or

tumors with a significant calcific component. We have found the ultrasonic aspirator to be useful in several unusual situations. Extensive removal of infected bone was expedited in a case of spinal osteomyelitis. Normal bony elements were spared since the device is not capable of aspirating rigid calcified structures. Caution must always be exercised when aspirating near a peripheral or cranial nerve. If the structure is not touched by the aspirator tip, however, function should be preserved.

The laser and ultrasonic aspirator are valuable adjuncts with unique characteristics that further improve our ability to effectively extirpate central nervous system neoplasms.

REFERENCES

1. Maiman TH: Stimulated optical radiation in ruby. Nature 187:493, 1960
2. Stellar S, Polanyi TG, Bredemeier HC: Experimental studies with the carbon dioxide laser as a neurosurgical instrument. Med Biol Eng Comput 8:549, 1970
3. Boggan JE, Edwards MSB, Davis RL, et al: Comparison of the brain tissue response in rats to injury by argon and carbon dioxide lasers. Neurosurgery 11:609, 1982
4. Takizawa T: Comparison between the laser surgical unit and the electrosurgical unit. Neurol Med Chir 17:95, 1977
5. Cozzens JW, Cerullo LJ: Comparison of the effect of the carbon dioxide laser and the bipolar coagulator on the cat brain. Neurosurgery 16:449, 1985
6. Tiznado EG, James HE, Kemper C: Experimental carbon dioxide laser brain lesions and intracranial dynamics: Part I. Effect on intracranial pressure, systemic arterial pressure, central venous pressure, electroencephalography, and gross pathology. Neurosurgery 16:5, 1985
7. Tiznado EG, James HE, Moore S: Experimental carbon dioxide laser brain lesions and intracranial dynamics: Part II. Effect on brain water content and its response to acute therapy. Neurosurgery 16:454, 1985
8. Kuroiwa T, Tsuyumu M, Takei H, et al: Effects of Nd:YAG and CO_2 lasers on cerebral microvasculature. Study in normal rabbit brain. J Neurosurg 64:128, 1986
9. Toya S, Kawase T, Iisaka Y, et al: Acute effect of the carbon dioxide laser on the epicerebral microcirculation. Experimental study by fluorescein angiography. J Neurosurg 53:193, 1980
10. Miller JB, Smith MR, Pincus F, et al: Intraocular carbon dioxide laser photocautery. Part I. Animal experimentation. Arch Ophthalmol 97:2157, 1979
11. Verschueren R: The CO_2 Laser in Tumor Surgery. Assen, The Netherlands, Van Gorcum, 1976
12. Voorhies RM, Lavyne MH, Strait TA, et al: Does the CO_2 laser spread viable brain-tumor cells outside the surgical field? J Neurosurg 60:819, 1984
13. Oosterhuis JW, Verschueren RCJ, Eibergen R, et al: The viability of cells in the waste products of CO_2 laser evaporation of Cloudman mouse melanomas. Cancer 49:61, 1982
14. Ascher PW: The use of the CO_2 laser in neurosurgery, in Kaplan I (ed): Laser Surgery II. Jerusalem, Israel, Jerusalem Academic Press, 1978, pp 76–78
15. Ascher PW, Ingolitsch E, Walter G, et al: Ultrastructural findings in CNS tissue with CO_2 laser, in Kaplan I (ed): Laser Surgery II. Jerusalem, Israel, Jerusalem Academic Press, 1978, pp 81–90
16. Hara M, Okada J, Takeuchi K, et al: Evaluation of laser surgery to treat brain tumor. Neurol Surg 8:363, 1980
17. Hudgins R, Moody J, Sanders M, et al: Microsurgical laser vaporization of inaccessible tumors of the central nervous system. Dallas Med J 76:245, 1981
18. Kelly PJ, Alker GJ Jr, Goerss S: Computer-assisted stereotactic laser microsurgery for the treatment of intracranial neoplasms. Neurosurgery 10:324, 1982

19. Kosary IZ, Shacked I, Farine I: Use of surgical laser in the removal of an osteoma of the skull. Surg Neurol 8:151, 1977

20. Salcman M, Kaplan RS, Ducker TB, et al: Effects of age and reoperation on survival in the combined modality treatment of malignant astrocytoma. Neurosurgery 10:454, 1982

21. Strait TA, Robertson JH, Clark WC: Use of the carbon dioxide laser in the operative management of intracranial meningiomas: A report of twenty cases. Neurosurgery 10:464, 1982

22. Takizawa T, Yamazaki T, Miura N, et al: Laser surgery of basal, orbital, and ventricular meningiomas which are difficult to extripate by conventional means. Neurol Med Chir 20:719, 1980

23. Gongbai C, Qiwu X: Carbon dioxide laser vaporization of brain tumors. Neurosurgery 12:123, 1983

24. James HE, Williams J, Brock W, et al: Radical removal of lipomas of the conus and cauda equina with laser microneurosurgery. Neurosurgery 15:340, 1984

25. Edwards MSB, Boggan JE, Bolger CA, et al: Effect of microsurgical and carbon dioxide and argon laser resection on recurrence of the intracerebral 9L rat gliosarcoma. Neurosurgery 14:52, 1984

26. Robertson JH, Clark WC, Robertson JT, et al: Use of the carbon dioxide laser for acoustic tumor surgery. Neurosurgery 12:286, 1983

27. Henderson BM, Goldman L, Martin LW, et al: The laser in pediatric surgery. J Pediatr Surg 3:263, 1968

28. Powers SK, Edwards MSB, Boggan JE, et al: Use of the argon surgical laser in neurosurgery. J Neurosurg 60:523, 1984

29. Wharen RE Jr, Anderson RE, Scheithauer B, et al: The Nd:YAG laser in neurosurgery. J Neurosurg 60:531, 1984

30. Eggert HR, Kiessling M, Kleihues P: Time course and spatial distribution of neodymium:yttrium-aluminum-garnet (Nd:YAG) laser induced lesions in the rat brain. Neurosurgery 16:443, 1985

31. Yamagami T, Handa H, Takeuchi J, et al: Histological study of normal rat brain tissue after neodymium-yttrium aluminum garnet laser irradiation. I. Cerebral hemisphere. Surg Neurol 23:475, 1985

32. Yamagami T, Handa H, Takeuchi J, et al: Histological changes in rat brain tissue cuased by neodymium-yttrium aluminum garnet laser irradiation. II. Cerebellum. Surg Neurol 24:421, 1985

33. Jain KK: Complications of use of the neodymium: yttrium-aluminum-garnet laser in neurosurgery. Neurosurgery 16:759, 1985

34. Kelly PJ, Alker GJ Jr: A stereotactic approach to deep-seated central nervous system neoplasms using the carbon dioxide laser. Surg Neurol 5:331, 1981

35. Laws ER, Cortese DA, Kinsey JH, et al: Photoradiation therapy in the treatment of malignant brain tumors: A phase I (feasibility) study. Neurosurgery 9:672, 1981

36. Dougherty TJ, Kaufman JE, Goldfarb A, et al: Photoradiation therapy for the treatment of malignant tumors. Cancer Res 38:2628, 1978

37. Maira G, Mohr G, Panisset A, et al: Laser photocoagulation for treatment of experimental aneurysms. J Microsurg 1:137, 1979

38. Jain KK, Gorisch W: Repair of small blood vessels with the neodymium-YAG laser. A preliminary report. Surgery 85:684, 1979

39. Fasano VA, Urciuoli R, Ponzio RM: Photocoagulation of cerebral arteriovenous malformations and arterial aneurysms with the neodymium:yttrium-aluminum-garnet or argon laser: Preliminary results in twelve patients. Neurosurgery 11:754, 1982

40. Miller JB, Smith MR, Pincus F, et al: Transvitreal carbon dioxide laser photocautery and vitrectomy. Ophthalmology 85:1195, 1978

41. Smith MR, Miller JB: New trends in carbon dioxide laser microsurgery. J Microsurg 1:354, 1980

42. Strong MS, Jako GJ: Laser surgery in the larynx. Early clinical experience with continuous CO_2 laser. Ann Otol Rhinol Laryngol 81:791, 1972

43. Pinnow DA, Gentile AL, Standlee AG, et al: Polycrystalline fiber optical wave guides for infrared transmission. Appl Phys Lett 33:28, 1978

44. Levy WJ, Gallo C, Watts C: Comparison of laser and radiofrequency dorsal root entry zone lesions in cats. Neurosurgery 16:327, 1985

45. Fischer DW, Beggs JL, Kenshalo DL, et al: Comparative study of microepineurial anastomoses with the use of CO_2 laser and technique, nerve action potentials, and morphological studies. Neurosurgery 17:300, 1985

46. Dew DK: Laser microsurgical repair of soft tissue: An update and review. Laser Surg Med 3:134, 1983

47. Harty RS, LoCicero J, McCarthy WJ: Microvascular applications of very low power CO_2 laser. Presented at the Congress on Laser Neurosurgery III, Chicago, Illinois, May 8, 1984

48. Jain KK: Sutureless microvascular anastamosis using a neodymium-YAG laser. J Microsurg 1:436, 1980

49. Mkrdichian EH: Nonvascular welding application in neurosurgery: Bone, dura, and others. Presented at the Congress on Laser Neurosurgery III, Chicago, Illinois, May 7, 1984

50. Neblett CR: History and future of tissue welding. Presented at the Congress on Laser Neurosurgery III, Chicago, Illinois, May 7, 1984

51. Fischer DW, Beggs JL, Shetter AG, et al: Comparative study of neuroma formation in the rat sciatic nerve after CO_2 laser and scalpel neurectomy. Neurosurgery 13:287, 1983

52. Flamm ES, Ransohoff J, Wuchinich D, et al: Preliminary experience with ultrasonic aspiration in neurosurgery. Neurosurgery 2:240, 1978

53. Young W, Cohen AR, Hunt CD, et al: Acute physiological effects of ultrasonic vibrations on nervous tissue. Neurosurgery 8:689, 1981

54. Blackie RAS, Gordon A: Histological appearances of intracranial biopsies obtained using the Cavitron ultrasonic surgical aspirator. J Clin Pathol 37:1101, 1984

55. Oosterhuis JW, Lung PFL, Verschueren RCJ, et al: Viability of tumor cells in the irrigation fluid of the Cavitron ultrasonic surgical aspirator (CUSA) after tumor fragmentation. Cancer 56:368, 1985

56. Boggan JE, Edwards MSB: The resection of central nervous system tumors using the CUSA TM and surgical lasers, in Surgical Update. Mountain View, California, Cooper Medical Devices Corp, 1982, pp 2–4

57. Wisoff JH: Surgical management of spinal cord astrocytomas, in Surgical Update. Mountain View, California, Cooper Medical Devices Corp, 1982, pp 8–9

58. Albright AL, Sclabassi RJ: Cavitron ultrasonic surgical aspirator and visual evoked potential monitoring for chiasmal gliomas in children. Report of two cases. J Neurosurg 63:138, 1985

59. Fasano VA, Zeme S, Fergo L, et al: Ultrasonic aspiration in the surgical treatment of intracranial tumors. J Neurosurg Sci 25:35, 1981

The Differential Diagnosis and Investigation of Unilateral and Bilateral Exophthalmos

Don C. Bienfang

THIS CHAPTER provides a framework for analyzing unilateral or bilateral exophthalmos and correctly diagnosing its cause in a particular patient. Twelve pathologic entities of children and twelve of adults are considered in this context. These pathologic entities constitute about 75 percent of the diagnostic possibilities related to the problem of exophthalmos. Not included are those entities that either are not diagnostic problems or are rare conditions.

The approach used in diagnosis involves obtaining answers to historical questions, detecting signs at physical examination, and selecting the appropriate array of diagnostic studies.

Historical questions include:

1. How old is the patient?
2. What is the tempo of the illness?
3. Is there pain?

Questions to be answered at physical examination include:

4. Is the exophthalmos unilateral or bilateral?
5. Is there a palpable mass?

Questions to be answered by special studies include:

6. What is the orbital location of the mass on CT scan?
7. What is the shape of the mass on CT scan?
8. Is there intracranial extension of the mass on CT scan?
9. Are the sinuses involved on CT scan?
10. What is the echogenicity of the mass on orbital ultrasound testing?
11. Are special laboratory studies required?
12. What is the response of the exophthalmos to systemic corticosteroids?

In many cases these twelve diagnostic questions will be redundant and a diagnosis may well be reached before they all have been applied.[1–5]

A list reduction algorithm can be used to arrive at the most likely diagnosis. First, decide if the patient is an adult or a child by determining if the patient has stopped developing physically or not. This is an area with fuzzy boundaries. Then determine if the onset of the exophthalmos was rapid or gradual. Whichever you decide, you will have to include the diverse entities in the variable onset group. Then apply the pain question, again including the "less frequently painful" diseases with whichever group the patient falls into. Note that some pathologic entities fall into two different groups. Proceed in the same way through orbital location, shape, character of B-scan echo, laterality, palpability of the mass, intracranial extension, sinus involvement, special laboratory tests, and, finally, steroid responsiveness. Questions for which there are no answers can be eliminated; stop as soon as there is only one possibility left. This approach is summarized in Tables 21-1 and 21-2.

   I. Age
      A. Childhood
          Dermoid
          Orbital cellulitis
          Thyroid eye disease
          Capillary hemangioma
          Lymphangioma
          Optic nerve glioma
          Neurofibroma
          Inflammatory pseudotumor
          Meningioma
          Metastasis
          Normal variant
          Rhabdomyosarcoma
      B. Adult
          Mucocele
          Orbital cellulitis
          Thyroid eye disease
          Vascular tumor other than cavernous hemangioma
          Cavernous hemangioma
          AV shunt
          Neurofibroma
          Inflammatory pseudotumor
          Lacrimal gland tumor
          Meningioma
          Metastasis
          Normal
  II. Tempo
      A. Rapid onset
          Orbital cellulitis
          Orbital pseudotumor
          Rhabdomyosarcoma
          Neuroblastoma

OPERATIVE NEUROSURGICAL TECHNIQUES
ISBN 0-8089-1862-1

Table 21-1. Orbital Diseases of Children

Disease Entity	Onset		Pain		Location in Orbit	Shape		B-Scan Echo		Laterality		Palpability		Intracranial as Well		Sinus Involved		Chemical Test	Steroid Response	
	Rapid	Gradual	Yes	No		Round	Irregular	High	Low	Unilateral	Bilateral	Yes	No	Maybe	Not usual	Maybe	No		Yes	No
Dermoid		X		X	Extra Conal	X			X	X		X			X		X			X
Orbital Cellulitis	X		X		Diffuse Mass		X	X		X		X	X		X	X				X
Thyroid Eye Disease	X	X		X	Enlarged Muscles		X	X		X	X		X		X		X	Thyroid Function Tests	X	
Capillary Hemangioma	X	X		X	Discrete Located Anywhere	X		X		X		X	X		X		X		X	
Lymphangioma	X	X		X	Diffuse Mass	X		X		X			X		X		X			X
Optic Nerve Glioma		X		X	Thickened Optic Nerve Outline	X		X		X			X	X			X			X
Neurofibroma		X		X	Discrete Mass Located Anywhere	X		X		X	X	X	X	X			X			X
Inflammatory Pseudotumor	X		X		Diffuse Mass		X	X		X		X	X		X		X		X	
Meningioma		X		X	Thickened Optic Nerve Outline	X		X		X			X	X		X				X
Metastasis	X		X	X	Discrete Located Anywhere		X	X		X	X	X	X	X		X		Urinary Catecholamines in Neuroblastoma	X	
Normal		X		X						X	X		X		X		X			X
Rhabdomyosarcoma	X			X	Discrete Located Anywhere		X	X		X			X		X	X				X

Table 21-2. Orbital Diseases of Adults

Disease Entity	Onset		Pain		Location in Orbit	Shape		B-Scan Echo		Laterality		Palpability		Intracranial Also		Sinus Involved		Chemical	Steroid Responsive	
	Rapid	Gradual	Yes	No		Round	Irregular	High	Low	Unilateral	Bilateral	Yes	No	Maybe	Not Usual	Maybe	No	Test	Yes	No
Mucocoele	X	X		X	Extraconal	X			X	X		X	X	X		X		None		X
Orbital Cellulitis	X		X		Diffuse mass		X	X		X		X	X		X	X		None		X
Thyroid Eye Disease	X	X		X	Enlarged node		X	X		X	X		X		X		X	X	X	
Vascular Tumor	X	X	X	X	Intraconal = Varix Discrete mass = Capillary hemangioma	X		X		X		X	X		X		X	None	Capillary Hemangioma	
Cavernous Hemangioma		X		X	Intraconal	X		X		X			X		X		X	None		X
A-V Shunt	X	X	X		Enlarged node	X			X	X			X	X			X	None		X
Neurofibroma		X		X	Discrete mass anywhere	X		X		X	X	X	X	X			X	None		X
Inflammatory Pseudotumor	X		X		Diffuse mass Enlarged muscle Thickened nerve outline		X	X		X	X	X	X		X		X	None	X	
Lacrimal Gland Tumor	X Malignant	X Benign	X Inflammatory Malignant	X Benign	Extraconal anterior	X		X		X		X			X		X	None	Inflammatory Swelling	
Meningioma		X		X	Thickened nerve outline	X		X		X			X	X		X		None		X
Metastasis	X	X	X	X	Discrete, located anywhere		X	X		X		X	X	X		X		None	Hematologic Tumors	
Normal		X		X	Normal orbit					X	X		X		X		X	None		X

231

B. Variable onset
    Any metastasis, lymphoma, or leukemia
    Mucocele
    Arteriovenous malformations and varices
    Thyroid eye disease
    Lacrimal gland tumor—malignant
    Capillary hemangioma
    Lymphangioma
C. Gradual onset
    Dermoid
    Lacrimal gland tumor—benign
    Glioma
    Meningioma
    Neurofibroma
    Cavernous hemangioma
    Normal
III. Pain
  A. Painful
    Orbital cellulitis
    Orbital inflammatory pseudotumor
    Malignant tumor of lacrimal gland—bone
      destruction
    Inflamed lacrimal gland—bone intact
  B. Less frequently painful
    Metastasis to orbit
    Arteriovenous malformation
    Neuroblastoma
  C. Rarely painful
    Thyroid eye disease
    Hemangioma
    Benign lacrimal gland tumor—bone intact
    Dermoid
    Rhabdomyosarcoma
    Lymphoma
    Meningioma
    Glioma of the optic nerve
    Lymphangioma
    Neurofibroma
    Normal
    Cavernous hemangioma
    Mucocele
    Capillary hemangioma
IV. Laterality
  A. Unilateral
    Dermoid
    Rhabdomyosarcoma
    Thyroid eye disease
    Normal
    Hemangioma
    Lymphangioma
    Pseudotumor
    Neurofibroma
    Optic nerve glioma
    Meningioma
    Cavernous hemangioma
    Mucocele
    Metastasis
    Orbital cellulitis
    Vascular tumors
    AV shunt
    Lacrimal gland tumor
    Capillary hemangioma
  B. Bilateral

    Thyroid eye disease
    Inflammatory orbital pseudotumor
    Neuroblastoma
    Normal
    Neurofibroma
V. Palpability
  A. Palpable mass
    Dermoid
    Lacrimal gland tumor
  B. May be palpable
    Metastasis
    Neurofibroma
    Capillary hemangioma
    Lymphoma
    Inflammatory pseudotumor
    Mucocele
    Orbital cellulitis
  C. Nonpalpable
    Rhabdomyosarcoma
    Thyroid eye disease
    Cavernous hemangioma
    Lymphangioma
    Glioma
    Meningioma
    Inflammatory pseudotumor
    AV shunts and orbital varices
    Normal
    Mucocele
VI. Location of the mass in the orbit based on computed
tomography
  A. Enlarged muscles
    Orbital myositis
    Thyroid eye disease
    AV Shunts
  B. Thickened optic nerve outline
    Meningioma (of the sheath)
    Glioma of the optic nerve
    Inflammatory pseudotumor
  C. Intraconal mass
    Cavernous hemangioma
    Lymphangioma
    Orbital varix
  D. Diffuse mass
    Lymphangioma
    Orbital cellulitis
    Inflammatory pseudotumor
  E. Discrete mass located anywhere
    Metastasis
    Neurofibroma
    Capillary hemangioma
    Rhabdomyosarcoma
  F. Always extraconal
    Dermoid
    Mucocele
    Lacrimal gland tumor
VII. Shape (usually by computed tomography)
  A. Smooth perimeter
    Dermoid
    Cavernous hemangioma
    Capillary hemangioma
    Lymphangioma
    Glioma of the optic nerve
    Neurofibroma

Meningioma
Neuroblastoma
Mucocele
Lacrimal gland tumor—benign
Lacrimal gland inflammation
B. Irregular perimeter
Rhabdomyosarcoma
Orbital cellulitis
Thyroid eye disease
Inflammatory pseudotumor
Metastasis
Lacrimal gland tumor—malignant
VIII. Can be intracranial as well
Meningioma
Glioma
Metastasis
Mucocele
Neurofibroma
IX. Can involve the sinuses
Mucocele
Orbital cellulitis
Any malignant tumor by invasion
Meningioma
X. Echogenicity on ultrasound testing
A. High (many acoustic interfaces internally)
Orbital cellulitis
Cavernous hemangioma
Lymphangioma
Neuroblastoma
Metastatic lesions
Thyroid eye disease
Vascular tumor
Neurofibroma
Inflammatory pseudotumor
Lacrimal gland tumor
Meningioma
Capillary hemangioma
Rhabdomyosarcoma

B. Low (more homogeneous interior)
Dermoid
AV Shunts
Mucocele
XI. Special laboratory tests
Tests of thyroid function in thyroid eye disease
Urinary catecholamines in neuroblastoma
XII. Response to systemic corticosteroids
May respond by reduction in size
Thyroid eye disease
Capillary hemangioma
Inflammatory pseudotumor
Neuroblastoma
Inflammatory lacrimal gland swelling
Certain tumors of hematologic origin

CONCLUSION

This chapter presents an approach to the differential diagnosis of exophthalmos and deals with the usual case rather than the exceptions and is therefore not encyclopedic. It should prove useful as a first step in the analysis of this problem.

REFERENCES

1. Hammerschlag SB, Hesselink JR, Weber AL: Computed tomography of the Eye and Orbit. Norwalk, CT, Appleton-Century-Crofts, 1983
2. Henderson JW: Orbital Tumors, ed 2. Stuttgart, Georg Thieme Verlag, 1980
3. Jakobiec FA: Ocular and Adnexal Tumors. Birmingham, AL, Aesculapius Publishing Co, 1978
4. Krohel GB, Stewart WB, Chavis RM: Orbital Disease: A Practical Approach. Orlando, FL, Grune & Stratton, 1981
5. Shammas HJ: Atlas of Ophthalmic Ultrasonography and Biometry. St. Louis, CV Mosby, 1984

CHAPTER 22

Intraorbital Tumors

Edgar M. Housepian

TO APPRECIATE THE DETAILS of a surgical technique, the objectives of the operation must be clearly understood. In turn, these objectives are derived from a clear understanding of the nature of the pathologic process and the detailed regional anatomy. Once achieved, the objectives, advantages, and limitations of a given surgical approach can be understood and a rational choice of technique made. The advantage of the transcranial neurosurgical approach to the orbit is apparent when dealing with disease processes that arise in or extend to the intracranial cavity; it also affords superior access to the apical portion of the optic nerve and to the medial and lateral superior quadrants of the orbit.

The great variety of tumors and other mass lesions that occur behind the eye and cause proptosis has been of interest to several surgical disciplines. Ophthalmologic surgeons can deal with many of these problems by one of a number of direct orbital approaches. The otolaryngologist can gain access to pathologic conditions arising within sinuses bordering the superior, medial, and inferior margins of the orbit. The neurologic surgeon has access to those tumors that involve both the intracranial and the intraorbital space. With the advent of modern neurosurgery, which allows safe access to the orbit by the cranial route, the neurosurgical literature began to reflect an increasing application of transcranial orbital exploration to a large number of orbital problems.[1–5] As one might expect, this encroachment on a traditionally ophthalmologic field led to a period of justifiable controversy regarding the proper approach to orbital problems.[6–10] Fortunately, the rapid development of diagnostic radiologic procedures has provided a means of more precisely defining the nature and extent of a problem and has brought some order to the chaos of orbital surgery.

SURGICAL ANATOMY

The purpose of surgical anatomy is to describe and define significant anatomic interrelationships and to correlate the anatomy with clinical and surgical considerations.[11–14]

THE ORBIT

The surgeon must be oriented to the medial obliquity of the apex of the orbit (Figure 22-1). The 5- to 10-mm-long optic canal enters the intracranial cavity medial to the anterior clinoid process, beneath which lies one of the two roots of the lesser wing of the sphenoid bone. This root forms the lateral wall of the optic canal and the medial margin of the superior orbital fissure. The lateral margin of the superior orbital fissure is bordered by the greater wing of the sphenoid bone, and together with the frontosphenoid process of the zygomatic bone forms the lateral wall of the orbit. The roof of the orbit and the floor of the anterior cranial fossa are, of course, one and the same, and the orbital plate of the maxillary bone forms both the floor of the orbit and the roof of the maxillary sinus. The medial wall of the orbit is formed by the lacrimal bone and the fragile lamina papyracea, which covers the ethmoid sinuses, and closer to the apex, the sphenoid sinus. The frontal sinus, to a variable extent, fills that portion of the frontal bone forming the supraorbital rim.

OPTIC NERVE

Starting at the chiasmal end, the optic nerve has a flattened horizontal oval shape and measures approximately 4 × 6 mm (Figure 22-2). After it enters the cranial end of the optic canal, it is circular and 5 mm in diameter, and continues to the globe as a 6 × 4-mm vertically oval structure. A pial membrane, carrying the blood supply, accompanies the nerve from the chiasm throughout its entire course to the sclera. The intracranial arachnoid, in like fashion, continues as a discrete structure through the optic canal and fuses with the pia at the globe. There are loose trabeculations in the subarachnoid space. At the apical orbital portion of the nerve, however, the pia and arachnoid are fused dorsomedially and ventrally with the dura and the fibrous annulus of Zinn, tethering the optic nerve and partially occluding the subarachnoid space but not obliterating its continuity. Normally, the intraocular pressure is slightly higher than the intracranial pressure; it is conceivable, therefore, that the papilledema found in conditions producing increased intracranial pressure is directly related to this continuity of the subarachnoid space from the cranial cavity to its termination at the lamina cribrosa.

PERIORBITA

The intracranial dura extends into and lines the optic canal, and at the orbital exit of the canal it splits into an outer periosteal (or periorbital) layer and an inner layer that accompanies the optic nerve to the globe, where it fuses with the arachnoid, pia, and sclera (Figure 22-3). To remove the optic nerve from the globe to the chiasm, as in cases of optic nerve glioma and meningioma, it is therefore necessary to section the annulus of Zinn and its fibrous attachment to the nerve. The periorbital dura also is continuous with the intracranial dura at the superior orbital fissure and, of course, lines the inferior orbital fissure as well as the other foramina, becoming contin-

OPERATIVE NEUROSURGICAL TECHNIQUES
ISBN 0-8089-1862-1

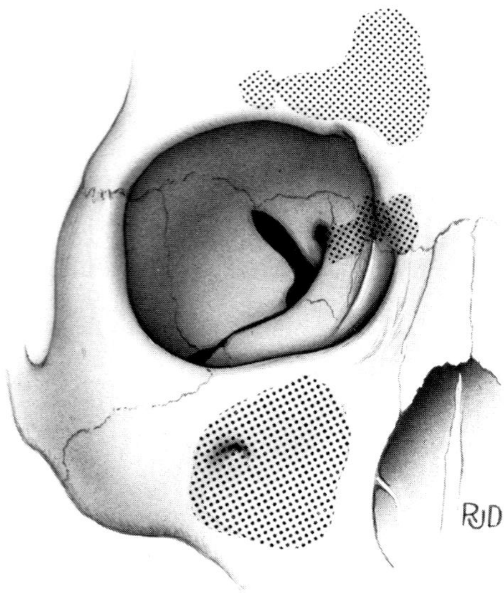

Fig. 22-1. The integrity of the bony orbit and the size and shape of its fissures and foramina can be defined by polytomography. The frontal, ethmoidal, and maxillary sinuses are shown in diagrammatic fashion. Attention is directed to one of the two roots of the lesser wing of the sphenoid, which lies beneath the anterior clinoid and forms the lateral margin of the optic canal in the medial margin of the superior orbital fissure.

uous with the periosteum of the skull at these sites. Anteriorly, the periorbita is continuous with the periosteum at the orbital margin; structural modifications in the periorbita enclose the lacrimal gland and fix the pulley of the superior oblique tendon.

This confluence of the periorbita with the intracranial dura at the superior orbital fissure may serve as a route of entry of en plaque meningioma. Arachnoidal rests at this border zone may be the source of intraorbital meningiomas that appear to arise from the periorbita. Resection of a meningioma invading the superior fissure cannot, of course, be achieved without injuring the important nerves passing therein. Primary optic nerve sheath meningiomas can be defined preoperatively and safely removed by the transcranial approach. When these tumors occur at the extreme apex, where the dural sheath of the optic nerve is fused with the origins of the extraocular muscles at the annulus of Zinn, total excision can be achieved without injury to these structures if they have not been invaded by the tumor.

Meningiomas may have a propensity for more rapid growth in children; exenteration therefore may be advisable in children if there is microscopic residual tissue at the annulus of Zinn or the superior orbital fissure. In older patients microscopic residual tissue within the muscle cone may be acceptable because the tumors grow more slowly. The annulus of Zinn provides no barrier against extension of a tumor through the optic nerve (Figure 22-4), and routine monitoring of the canal for hyperostosis, together with computed tomographic (CT) or magnetic resonance imaging (MRI) scans, will not always detect the presence of intracanalicular tumors.

MUSCLE CONE AND ANNULUS ON ZINN

The fibrous annulus tendineus (annulus of Zinn), previously described, serves as the origin of six of the seven extraocular muscles (Figure 22-4). Superiorly, the superior rectus muscle arises from the annulus, which, at this point, is fused with the leptomeninges and dura of the optic nerve. The origin of the levator palpebrae is medial and superior to that of the superior rectus muscle. More medial and inferior to this are the origins of the medial rectus and superior oblique muscles. Although firmly fused to the optic nerve dorsally, the annulus of Zinn loops widely around the nerve, laterally and inferiorly, giving rise to the lateral rectus muscle, which has its origin from two heads: the inferior rectus derives its origin from the inferior head; the space between the two heads of the lateral rectus muscle is known as the oculomotor foramen. It is thus evident that this arrangement separates the portal of entry of the nerves, arteries, and veins into essentially three spaces: the optic foramen, the superior orbital fissure, and the oculomotor foramen.

ARTERIAL SUPPLY AND VENOUS DRAINAGE

The ophthalmic artery arises from the internal carotid artery at its emergence from the cavernous sinus, passes on the medial side of the anterior clinoid, and runs in a split layer of dura beneath the optic nerves as it enters the orbital cavity through the optic foramen. Upon entering the orbit, it curves over the lateral margin of the optic nerve, gives off the central retinal branch, which perforates the dural sheath approximately 10 mm from the optic foramen, and then, within several millimeters, enters the nerve obliquely about 1.0 cm behind the globe. After giving off the central retinal branch, the ophthalmic artery crosses medially forward, giving off two long posterior

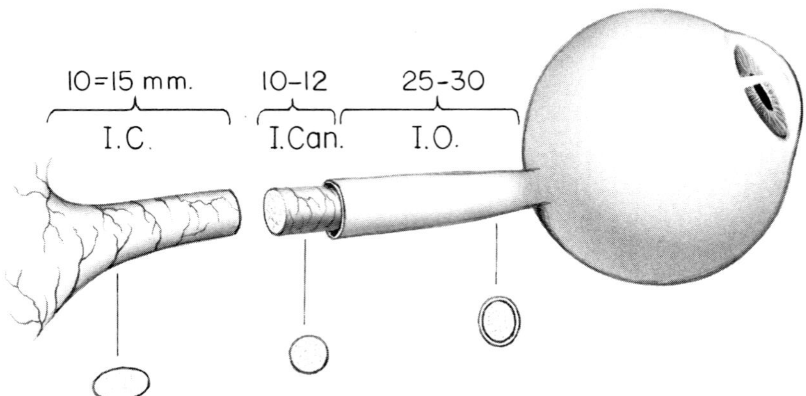

Fig. 22-2. The dimensions and contours of the intracranial, intracanalicular, and intraorbital portions of the optic nerve.

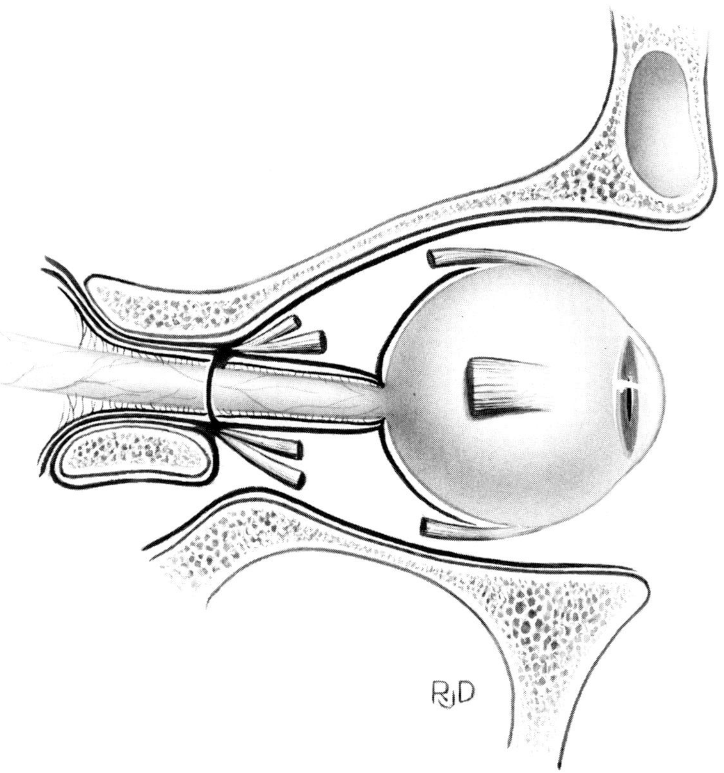

Fig. 22-3. The membranes investing the optic nerve and lining the intracranial cavity, optic canal, and orbit. A double-layered intracranial dura is seen extending through the optic canal and superior orbital fissure. The inner layer continues in the orbit as the dural sheath of Schwann. The outer layer forms the periorbita beyond the annulus of Zinn. There is a continuous subarachnoid space that extends from the intracranial space to the junction of the pia, arachnoid, and dura at the scleral margin. This space is partially obliterated at the annulus of Zinn.

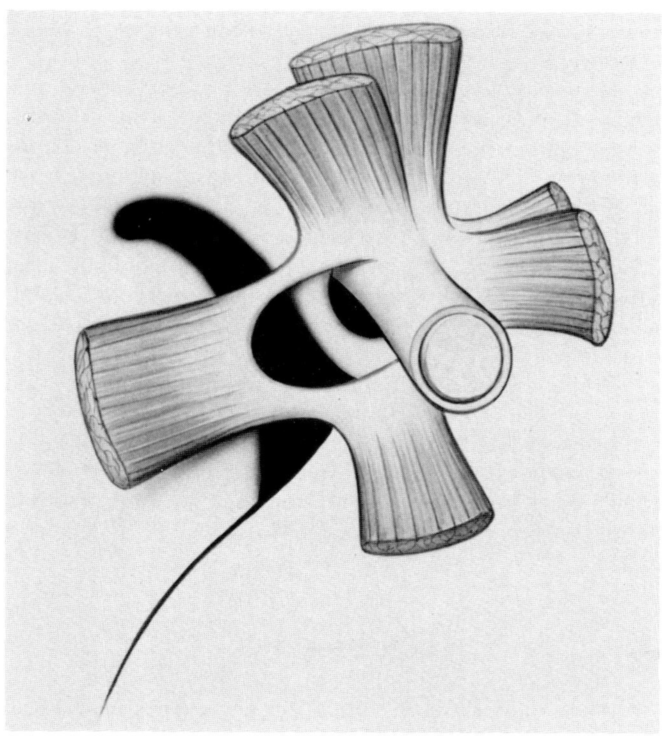

Fig. 22-4. The annulus of Zinn is a fibrous band giving rise to the origins of six of the seven extraocular muscles. This fibrous tissue is in continuity with the dural sheath of the optic nerve. The two heads of the lateral rectus loop around that portion of the superior orbital fissure known as the oculomotor foramen.

ciliary arteries, six or eight short posterior ciliary arteries, and then anastomoses freely with the external carotid circulation. Two small branches of the ophthalmic artery supply the ocular muscles at their origin near the annulus.[15,16]

Although obstruction of the central retinal artery results in a severe loss of visual acuity, obstruction of the ophthalmic artery may not if the arterial anastomoses are sufficient to preserve blood flow to the retina.

The orbital cavity is drained principally by the superior and inferior ophthalmic veins. Both of these valveless channels have extensive anastomoses with each other as well as with external tributaries. The superior ophthalmic vein passes above the lateral rectus muscle through the superior orbital fissure to drain into the cavernous sinus. The inferior ophthalmic vein, which primarily drains a network of channels on the medial wall and floor of the orbit, divides; one branch drains the pterygoid plexus through the inferior orbital fissure, the other joins the superior ophthalmic vein before it enters the superior orbital fissure. These extensive communications between the pterygoid plexus and the angular and deep facial veins accommodate minor alterations in venous drainage; however, occlusion of the superior ophthalmic vein may result in severe orbital venous congestion, chemosis, and proptosis.

ORBITAL NERVES

When the orbit is unroofed from above, the frontalis nerve is usually visible through the thin periorbita. Once the periorbita is opened, the surgeon will find the frontalis nerve

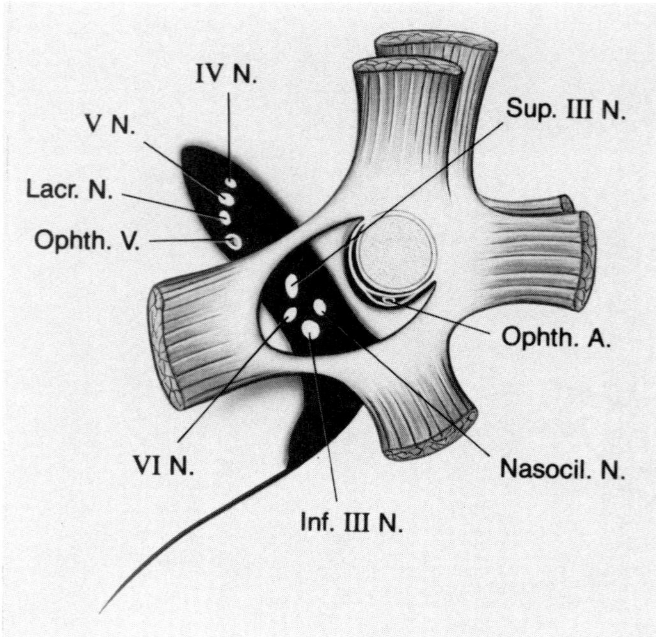

Fig. 22-5. Although partial obliteration of the subarachnoid space of the optic nerve at the annulus of Zinn is shown, the medial origin of the levator muscle is evident. The ophthalmic artery enters the orbit through the optic canal, whereas the superior division of the oculomotor nerve, the abducens nerve, nasociliary nerve, and the inferior division of the oculomotor nerve enter the muscle cone through the oculomotor foramen. The trochlear, frontalis, and lacrimal nerves and the ophthalmic vein enter through the superior orbital fissure and thus lie within the periorbita but outside the muscle cone.

overlying the levator and superior rectus muscles. In the same plane but closer to the apex lies the fine trochlear nerve. The trochlear nerve, the frontalis branch of the fifth nerve, and its lacrimal branch pass through the superior orbital fissure in that order and lie within the periorbita but over the extraocular muscles (Figure 22-5). The remaining nerves traversing the superior orbital fissure enter the orbit and the muscle cone through the so-called "oculomotor foramen" between the two heads of the lateral rectus muscle in the following order: the superior division of the oculomotor nerve, which supplies the superior rectus and levator muscles; the nasociliary branch of the ophthalmic nerve; the sixth nerve; and the inferior division of the third nerve. The nasociliary nerve crosses over the optic nerve to reach the medial wall of the orbit. The ciliary ganglion lies lateral to the optic nerve. The inferior division of the oculomotor nerve crosses beneath the optic nerve to reach the medial and inferior rectus muscles.

Because of this arrangement, it is clear that the optic nerve can be approached directly through the medial compartment, between the medial rectus and the levator muscles, without fear of injury to the nerve supply of any extraocular muscle (Figure 22-6). The trochlear nerve rarely can be spared. When optic nerve resection is the objective, however, there is little functional or cosmetic consequence of fourth-nerve section.

Careful dissection through the lateral compartment, between the lateral and superior rectus and levator muscles, allows access to solitary neurofibromas, which most frequently arise from branches of the long ciliary nerves lying lateral to the optic nerve.

Tumors or mass lesions that arise external to the muscle cone are most likely to cause proptosis without limitation of extraocular movements or loss of vision. Some tumors within the muscle cone cause proptosis without causing neurologic or ophthalmologic deficits; however, tumors that crowd the apex are most likely to lead to dysfunction of one or more of the extraocular muscles or their nerve supply, causing specific deficits.

A clear understanding of orbital apical anatomy should help the surgeon to approach the apical region safely and provides a basis for understanding the surgical limitations imposed by specific pathologic conditions.

DIAGNOSIS

When an orbital pathologic entity is suspected and, in particular, when unilateral exophthalmos exists, a logical sequential work-up should follow the clinical examination.[1519] This should begin with good quality roentgenograms of the skull, orbits, and optic canals. Calcified, hyperostosing, and grossly destructive lesions can be identified, and sinus disease also can be seen.

The recent availability of computed tomography has proved extremely useful in defining orbital pathologic processes. A well-performed study will show normal orbital anatomy, including the size and position of the globe, optic nerve, and extraocular muscles. The size and extent of a meningioma, optic glioma, or neurofibroma can be defined preoperatively. Most of these tumors enhance with contrast.

Magnetic resonance imaging (MRI) techniques are becoming widely available. The ability to define masses within the orbit without accompanying exposure of the lens to radiation is desireable, particularly when serial imaging is necessary. Although tumors of the orbit can be visualized in this way, the fat density contrast provided by CT may offer better definition except for the recognition of vascular lesions, for which MRI is superior.

Pleuridirectional tomography is also a critical radiographic diagnostic procedure for defining the integrity of the orbit. Polytomograms provide precise definition of the bony margins of the orbit. The precise extent of a hyperostosing process can be defined, perhaps more readily than on CT scans. Polytomograms also provide sagittal views, which CT cannot. Areas of dehiscence, dissolution, or destruction of bony structures can be shown that give clues to the presence of encephalocele, pathologic entities in the sinus, or destructive and invasive processes.

Orbital angiography and venography have a place in defining vascular lesions in the orbit. Nevertheless they are required with less frequency now that a combination of noninvasive studies is available, which together with a clinical evaluation allows the nature and extent of intraorbital pathologic processes to be defined with a high degree of accuracy.

CASE SELECTION

When a thoughtful sequential diagnostic work-up has been completed, the location and extent of the pathologic process can be defined. Is a tumor present at all? If so, is it confined within the muscle cone? Does it arise from, medial to, or lateral to the optic nerve? Is the optic canal enlarged or hyperostotic? Is the bony integrity of the orbit violated? Are the fissures normal? Is the process erosive or destructive? Does the pathologic process extend to or from a sinus or arise from or enter the cranial cavity?

The clinical diagnosis of optic nerve glioma can be made with a high degree of accuracy. In these cases primary treatment should be the transcranial approach when clinical evidence limits the tumor to a single optic nerve. There is no disagreement that surgical excision is the treatment of choice for a patient with a glioma of a single optic nerve who has proptosis and poor vision in the involved eye. The rationale for the transcranial orbital approach is based on the conclusion that a wide excision, from the globe to the chiasm, is necessary to ensure total removal. A simple orbital resection too often will leave residual tumor in the apical stump of the transected, tumor-bearing nerve.

Surgical resection would not be considered when there is multicentric optic glioma or chiasmal involvement. The place of radiotherapy is not as generally agreed upon; however, there is good evidence from our own large series of cases that astrocytoma of the optic nerve is a benign but often progressive process, similar to pilocytic astrocytoma of childhood in other locations. Our experience suggests that in many cases radiotherapy effectively arrests the course and improves proptosis and vision.

When a meningioma of the optic nerve or orbit is suspected, transcranial exploration is the preferred approach. These tumors frequently arise between the optic nerve and carotid artery and involve both the cranial and orbital cavities. The transcranial approach also allows direct and safe access to the apical part of the optic nerve. Tumors occurring distal to the orbital apex and close to the globe on CT scans can be explored by a direct approach.[20] Tumors arising in the lateral periorbita from arachnoidal rests near the superior orbital fissure are frequently associated with multicentric or en plaque lesions on the cranial side of the superior orbital fissure.

A microsurgical technique is essential for the successful removal of solitary neurofibromas, which usually are found lateral to the optic nerve. Although the transcranial approach provides good access to these lesions, they also can be accessible to lateral canthotomy (Krönlein operation). In view of the relative difficulty in making this diagnosis clinically, the latter approach may be advantageous.

Osteomas arising from the posterior ethmoid region can be defined and a transcranial approach selected for primary removal because of their medial epiperiorbital location. A two-stage procedure may be considered for very large lesions extending into intracranial spaces.

Obviously, encephaloceles must be treated by a neurosurgical approach, and some dermoid cysts and hemangiomas of the orbit also can be treated neurosurgically. Lesions such as ossifying fibromas and aneurysmal bone cysts that border both the orbit and the cranial cavity can be dealt with best by the transcranial approach.

Nevertheless, a vast majority of problems arising in the orbit can be dealt with more simply by a direct approach, including mucoceles, most hemangiomas, lymphangiomas, and others. Similarly, malignant processes of the orbit must *not* be exposed by the cranial route for fear of seeding. Finally, the surgeon dealing with proptosis must be aware of the very common nonsurgical causes, such as pseudotumor and thyrotoxicosis.

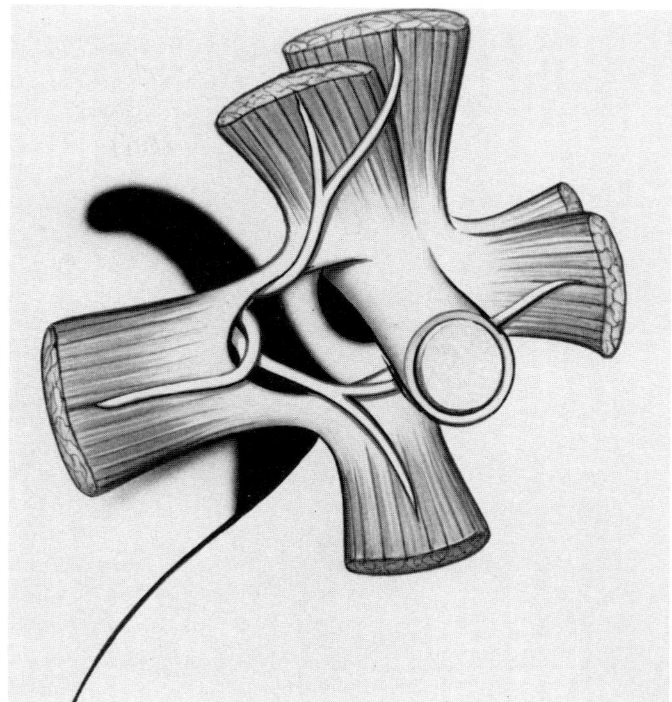

Fig. 22-6. The nerve supply to the extraocular muscles shown entering through the oculomotor foramen. A medial superior approach to the optic nerve between the lateral and medial rectus muscles provides direct access, with minimal chance of injury to this nerve supply to the extraocular muscles.

PREOPERATIVE MANAGEMENT AND ANESTHESIA

General anesthesia is used in all cases of transcranial orbital exploration. The principles of neuroanesthesia are adhered to and there are no special anesthesia requirements for exploring the orbit. Dexamethasone is used as an intraoperative and postoperative adjunct to reduce postoperative edema. Mannitol is used intraoperatively to reduce intraocular as well as intracranial tension so that a suitable surgical field is obtained without extensive retraction of the frontal lobe.

AIDS TO SURGERY

Besides deserving credit for systematizing the preoperative work-up in patients with orbital tumors, neurosurgery also can claim contributions to improved instrumentation and techniques for operating within the orbit. Thus, Maroon and Kennerdell[21] recently described the advantages of neurosurgical techniques in an ophthalmologic lateral approach to the orbit. Magnification with loupes or a microscope is mandatory when operating on the fine and attenuated structures within the orbit. Similarly, cottonoids and controlled suction are indispensable, as is the use of malleable retractors. Bipolar coagulation has materially added to the safety of operating within the orbit by either the cranial or the direct orbital approach. There may be a role for the laser in the surgical extirpation of certain orbital tumors.

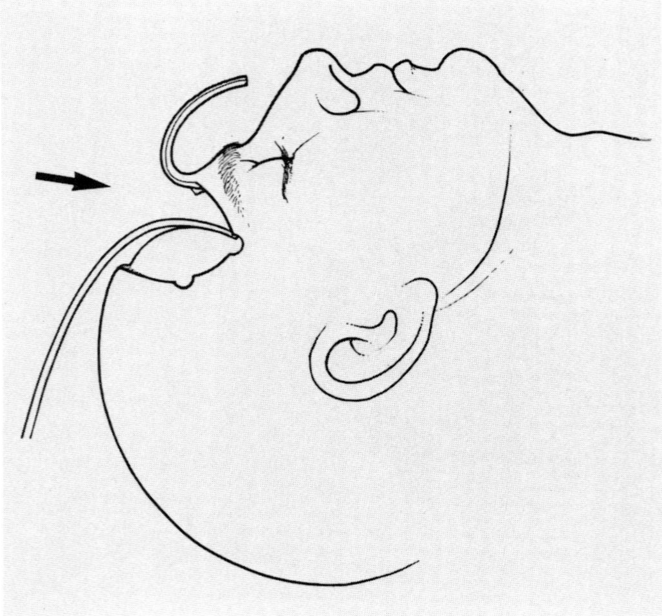

Fig. 22-7. The coronal incision and low frontal osteoplastic craniotomy flap used in exposing the floor of the anterior fossa. Osmotic diuretics and malleable retractors are used to gently retract the frontal lobe in this epidural approach.

OPERATIVE PROCEDURE[22–26]

It is not necessary to resect and replace the orbital rim to gain access to the apex of the orbit. It is most important, however, to plan a flap quite medial in order to allow a medial orbital approach to the optic nerve when dealing with primary tumors of the optic nerve. The frontotemporal approach, which is so useful for most invasive tumors of the lateral orbit, such as sphenoid wing meningiomas, thus is not adequate for surgery of optic nerve tumors.

After induction of anesthesia, intubation, and insertion of a Foley catheter, the patient is placed in the recumbent supine position on the operating table, with the knees flexed, the back slightly elevated, and the head slightly extended. A four-hole osteoplastic craniotomy is planned (Figure 22-7). An anteromedial trephination is located low in the midline, just above the glabella. A posteromedial trephination is marked off the midline but covering the sagittal sinus. An anterolateral trephination is marked at the temporal side of the temporal ridge, above the lateral margin of the orbit, and a posterolateral trephination is marked at the frontal convexity, beneath the insertion of the temporalis muscle.

A coronal incision is then planned, with the lower limb toward the side of the orbit to be explored. The incision should be placed approximately 1.0 cm behind the marked trephination sites.

After the patient is prepared and draped, the scalp and galea are incised and turned as one layer. Care is taken to keep from attenuating the periosteum. Hemostasis is achieved with Michelle clips or clamps. The reflected scalp and galea should be brought to within 1.0 cm of the glabella but *no lower;* if the galeal dissection extends to the orbital rim, there will be considerable postoperative ecchymosis and swelling; in addition there may be injury to the supraorbital vessel and nerve.

The periosteum is incised approximately 1.0 cm above the

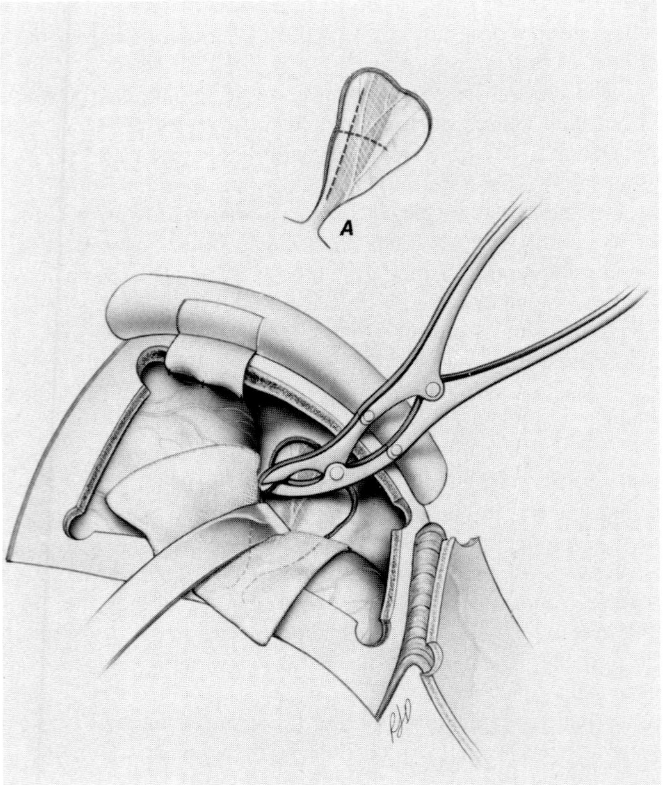

Fig. 22-8. The thin orbital roof is entered with a chisel or burr. The extent of orbital unroofing is outlined. The unroofing is completed with fine double action and Leksell rongeurs. When necessary, the optic canal is opened as illustrated. The frontalis nerve can be seen through the thin periosteum and is a landmark indicating the course of the levator and superior rectus muscles, which are often seen with difficulty. The dura is incised medial or lateral to these structures as indicated.

glabella in a horizontal direction tending from approximately 1.5 cm across the midline toward the side of the exposure and through the insertion of the temporalis fascia and muscle at the temporal ridge. Cutting current is frequently helpful for this portion of the procedure. The periosteum then is incised paramedially and along the posterior limb of the flap. It is preferable to make the periosteal exposure broader than the planned craniotomy to allow periosteal covering of the trephinations and bone cuts at the time of closure. A Gigli saw then is passed between the trephinations, and the bone is cut and notched. The medial posterior and lateral saw cuts are made on a bevel for reseating. The anterior limb is cut straight to prevent slippage.

If a large frontal sinus is exposed, it is recommended that this be repaired before the dura is opened. If the mucosa is intact, Gelfoam is simply placed over this. If the mucosa is lacerated, however, the entire sinus is exenterated, and the mucosa is rolled and impacted into the region of the ostium. Instruments used to handle the mucosa are not reused for the cranial procedure. A piece of temporalis muscle then is placed over the rolled mucosa, and the exenterated sinus is filled with Gelfoam dipped in an antibiotic solution. A rectangular flap of pericranium then is separated from the forward edge and sutured to the dura to prevent extrusion of the muscle and Gelfoam. After all bone margins are waxed and tenting sutures are placed at the posterior and lateral periphery of the dura and after the bone flap and its pedicle of temporalis muscle and fascia are covered with moist gauze, the wound is thoroughly irrigated. Fresh towels then are placed at the margins, and all exposed surfaces, except the area of dura to be incised, are covered with gauze or cottonoids.

If the orbit is being explored for optic glioma,[27] it is advisable to incise the dura and inspect the intracranial optic nerve before proceeding with the orbital unroofing. In so doing, the removal of cerebrospinal fluid from the chiasmatic cistern results in the development of an adequate operative exposure without the need for spinal drainage or excessive retraction. If the tumor is found to extend into the chiasm, indicating that gross total resection cannot be achieved, the procedure can be discontinued after a biopsy specimen is obtained. Once the tumor is identified within the nerve but not extending to the chiasm, the optic nerve is cut perpendicular to its direction at the chiasm. Hemostasis of the fine pial circulation is achieved with Gelfoam. If the tumor is not identified in the intracranial space, the optic nerve should not be sectioned until the glioma is identified intraorbitally.

Orbital exploration demands an epidural approach. This protects the underlying brain, which may require gentle retraction. In addition, it protects the olfactory nerve and bulb from avulsion. Since the dura inserts at the cribriform fossa lateral to the olfactory nerve, epidural retraction avoids injury in this location. Malleable self-retaining retractors are shaped and curved to expose the entire anterior fossa up to the clinoid. Moist cottonoids are placed at the lateral margins of the exposure to advance the epidural dissection, allow irrigation, and facilitate suctioning.

The orbital unroofing is begun with a chisel or a high-speed burr. Once a small opening is made in the midportion of the floor of the anterior fossa, the remainder of the resection is facilitated by the use of fine double-action mastoid or infant Leksell ronguers (Figure 22-8). The canal can be unroofed, if required, with orbital micropunches. The orbital unroofing does not need to come closer than 1.0 cm to the orbital rim anteriorly; it should extend approximately 1.5 cm from the medial margin and should be extended laterally to within 0.5 cm of the lateral orbital margin.

The periorbita is usually thin and transparent. When there is a significant orbital mass, the intraorbital structures are attenuated and blanched and may be difficult to see. The periorbita is incised in a cruciate fashion with a No. 11 blade. The vertical limb is placed lateral or medial to the levator and superior rectus muscles, depending upon whether a lateral or medial approach to the orbit is planned. The frontalis nerve is usually visible through the periorbita, as it lies over these muscles. It serves to approximate their location. The trochlear nerve, which lies beneath the periorbita but outside of the muscle cone, is only rarely visualized. It lies close to the apex, is extremely fine, and can rarely be spared if an apical pathologic process is encountered.

APPROACH TO THE MEDIAL ORBIT

A medial approach to the optic nerve is preferred when dealing with a meningioma or an optic glioma (Figure 22-9). The primary advantage of this approach relates to the nerve supply to extraocular muscles. We now are aware that the third nerve, after it enters the orbit through the superior orbital fissure and oculomotor foramen lateral to the optic nerve, sends branches over the nerve to supply the underbelly of the levator and superior rectus muscles and beneath the nerve to the inferior

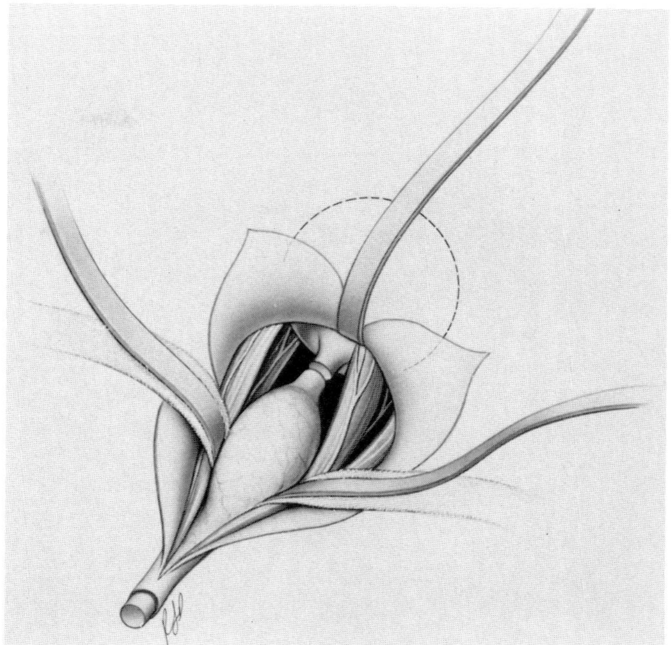

Fig. 22-9. Narrow malleable retractors and cottonoid pledgets are used to retract gently the orbital structures. The preferred approach to the optic nerve is shown.

and medial rectus muscles. A medial approach to the optic nerve thus can be made without traversing the course of these nerves to the extraocular muscles. Small malleable retractors are individually bent to retract the levator and superior rectus complex laterally and anteriorly. The tumor is approached by blunt dissection through residual orbital fat. Magnification and gentle handling of tissues are essential to this portion of the procedures. Both optic gliomas and primary optic nerve sheath meningiomas are fairly firm encapsulated tumors, and a plane of dissection is started directly on the tumor capsule. Gentle retraction and the placement of moist cottonoids allow the development of a plane entirely around the tumor capsule, which is not adherent to the surrounding residual areolar tissue. This tissue separates and protects the normal neurovascular structures, which can thus be spared during tumor removal. It is important *not* to dissect out structures protected in the periorbital fat.

The junction of the tumor and the posterior margin of the globe is readily found. At this point the nerve is transected between two fine mosquito forceps, which are used to clamp the tumor-bearing optic nerve. This technique will avoid injury to the posterior margin of the globe and the sclera. After the nerve is sectioned, the distal clamp is removed and any bleeding from the cut margin is carefully electrocoagulated with bipolar cautery. The proximal clamp can be used as a handle for further tumor dissection toward the apex.

In optic nerve glioma, in order to remove the tumor in one piece from the globe to the chiasm (Figure 22-10), the origin of the levator muscle, which inserts at the annulus of Zinn medial to the superior rectus, must be sectioned. Only in this way can the annulus of Zinn be opened from above to remove the canalicular portion of the optic nerve tethered at the orbital end of the canal. The origin of the levator muscle then can be resutured after the tumor is removed. This maneuver is difficult, and in young infants the structures are small and the exposure

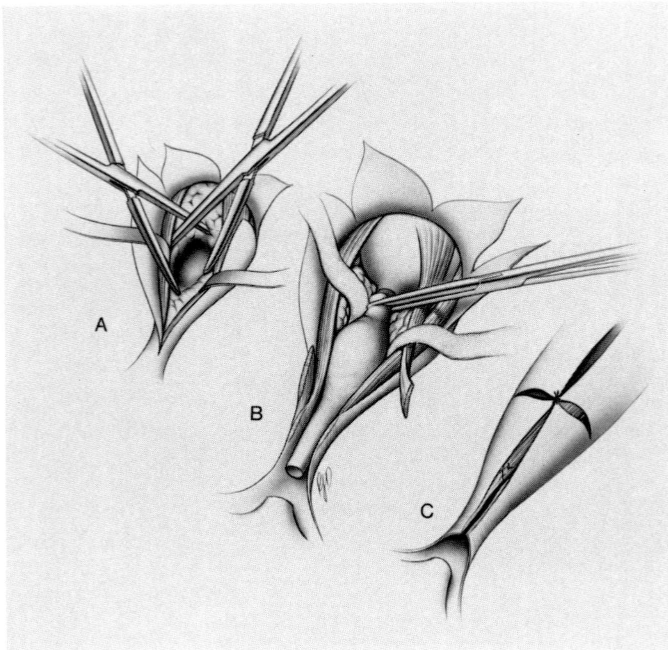

Fig. 22-10.　The technique of sectioning the levator. The annulus of Zinn cannot be opened without performing this maneuver. After resecting a tumor-bearing optic nerve from the globe to the chiasm, the origin of the levator muscle is resutured. This maneuver is useful in some cases of optic glioma and meningioma. (Reprinted from Housepian EM, Marquardt MD, Behrens M: Orbital tumors, in Wilkins RH, Renganchary SS (eds): Neurosurgery, vol 1. New York, McGraw-Hill, 1985. With permission.)

limited, making the procedure more difficult. The optic nerve can be sectioned with curved scissors at the extreme apex and the orbital specimen removed. At this juncture the ophthalmic artery is sometimes severed, but the bleeding can be controlled with bipolar electrocautery. The intracranial portion of the nerve then can be removed as a second specimen. In order to accomplish this, the epidural retractors must be removed and placed intradurally, re-exposing the intracranial optic nerve so that it can be pulled through the canal. If the surgeon feels that there may be a small amount of residual glioma at the canalicular face of the annulus, brief electrocoagulation on an angled nerve hook can be used safely without fear of recurrence. In any event, a small pledget of temporalis muscle placed within the canal will prevent the flow of cerebrospinal fluid into the orbital space in the immediate postoperative period.

When dealing with a primary optic nerve sheath meningioma, it is *mandatory* to unroof the optic canal, open the intracanalicular dura, section the origin of the levator at the annulus of Zinn, and open the annulus. This will permit inspection at high magnification and gross total removal of the intracanalicular tumor and optic nerve from the orbit close to the globe, back to the cranial end of the optic nerve near the chiasm. The annulus and levator origin should then be resutured with fine atraumatic silk or synthetic suture. Unlike the situation with optic nerve gliomas, electrocoagulation of residual meningioma at the orbital apex or in the canal is *not* an acceptable technique and *will lead to recurrence.*

There is ample histopathologic evidence for the primary intraorbital origin of optic nerve meningiomas. Cushing[1] described a psammotomatous meningioma arising at the sheath of Schwann and growing into the optic nerve. Although not clearly defined, it may represent the origin of some nerve sheath meningiomas. These tumors have been shown to traverse the optic canal by microscopic spread along the subarachnoid space without producing enlargement or hyperostosis of the optic canal.

The rare optic nerve sheath meningioma arising distal to the apex and encircling the optic nerve can be removed with

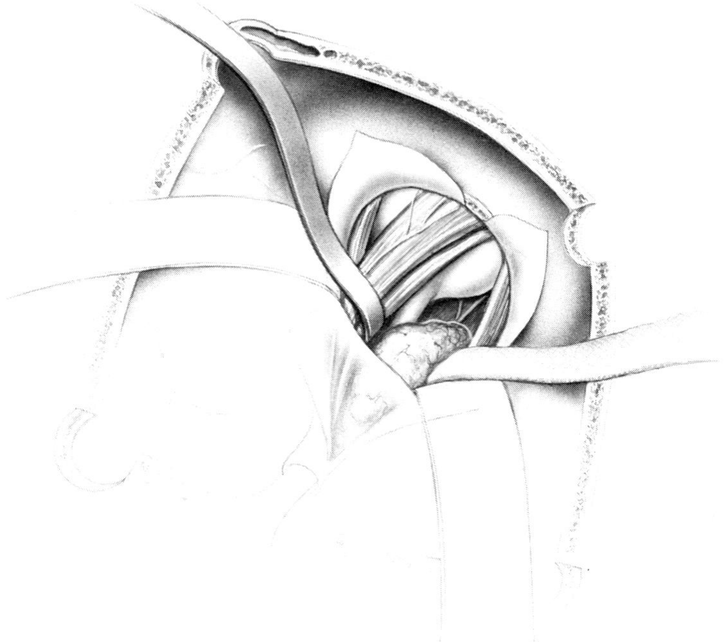

Fig. 22-11.　The lateral trancranial orbital approach to an apical neurofibroma. Dissection in the areolar tissue is avoided and cottonoid pledgets and narrow, shaped, malleable retractors are used to define a plane directly on the tumor capsule. Injury to the extraocular nerve supply is avoided in this way.

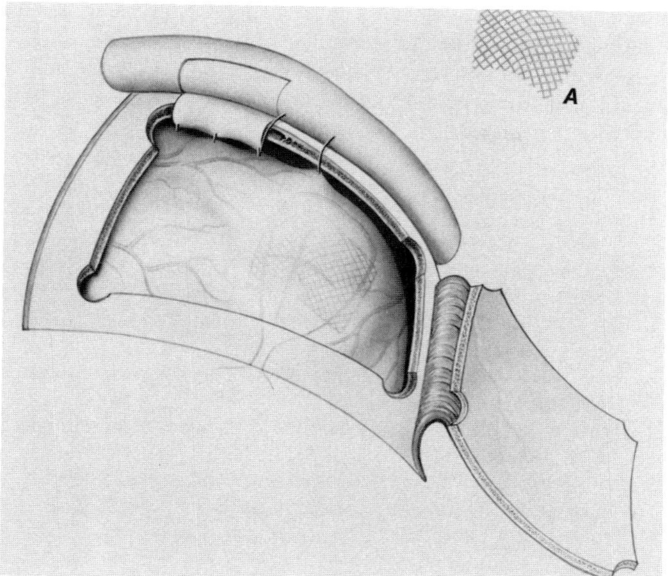

Fig. 22-12. Upon completion of tumor removal, the periorbita is closed with one or several fine atraumatic sutures; Gelfoam is placed over the periorbita; a wire mesh bridge is formed and placed at the orbital roof defect to avoid postoperative pulsation of the globe. Dural tenting sutures are then placed and any defect in the frontal sinus repaired and a flap of pericranium sutured to the dura to cover the bony defect.

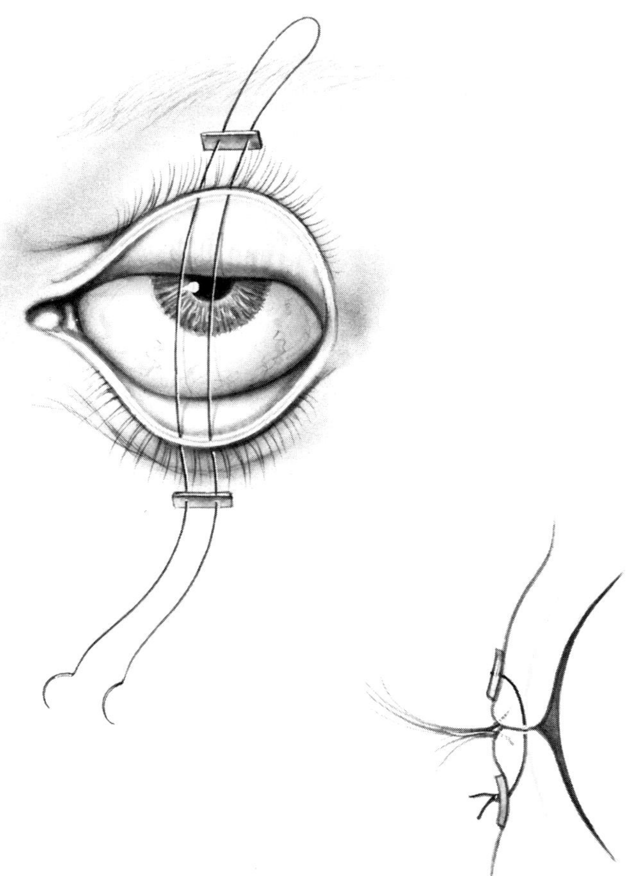

Fig. 22-13. The technique for temporary tarsorrhaphy. A fine double-ended atraumatic suture is placed though the tarsal plate of each lid. Small rubber bumpers prevent maceration of the thin skin of the lid.

preservation of the nerve and, in some cases, sparing of vision.[25]

LATERAL ORBITAL APPROACH

The transcranial orbital approach to the lateral superior quadrant of the orbit can be used for some cases of suspected solitary neurofibroma believed to arise from the long ciliary nerves. They are thus found in a position lateral to the optic nerve. In these cases the periorbital opening is made lateral to the superior rectus insertion (Figure 22-11), and, using the techniques described for orbital exploration with malleable retractors and cottonoids, a plane is developed directly on the tumor capsule. Efforts are made to separate the loose areolar tissue from the tumor itself and minimize dissection within this tissue. To achieve exposure of the lateral quadrant, the superior rectus is retracted medially. If the tumor is large, it can be broken into several pieces for removal. Efforts should be made to avoid the extreme apex in the lateral approach in order to minimize the chance of injury to the sixth nerve.

CLOSURE

Once removal of the tumor is complete and before retraction is released, cottonoids are carefully removed and the apical bed is inspected for hemostasis. Bipolar electrocoagulation should be used sparingly to achieve this. Extensive electrocauterization behind the globe should be avoided, since it can injure the retinal blood supply as well as the autonomic nerves and result in pupillary dilatation and corneal anesthesia. When the field is dry, all retractors and cottonoids are removed, the origin of the levator resutured, if sectioned, and the periorbita closed loosely by approximating the four corners.

Gelfoam then should be placed over the periorbita and a piece of stainless steel screen fashioned to bridge the defect in the orbital roof to avoid pulsation of the globe (Figure 22-12). This has not interfered with postoperative CT or MRI scanning. No attempt should be made to close the entire defect completely. The midportion is simply bridged and the prosthesis curved to approximate the normal curve of the orbital roof. Gelfoam then is placed on the outer surface of the screen, and the dura is allowed to fall back after retraction is removed. The cranial dura is sutured to the pericranium; this alone holds the screen in place, and no other effort need be made to secure it to the orbital roof. If the intracranial dura has been opened, it is sutured in a watertight fashion.

Closure of the craniotomy defect should follow standard practice. Epidural and subgaleal drains are recommended; however, if the sinus has been entered, suction drainage should be avoided. Thorough irrigation during all stages of closure is recommended to remove bits of bone dust or bone wax and dried blood.

The Berke modification of the Krönlein operation[6] may provide good access to pathologic processes in the lateral quadrant of the orbit. The application of neurosurgical techniques, as described by Maroon and Kennerdell,[21] and adherence to strict microsurgical technique should allow safe access to the lateral apex and minimize the possibility of injury to the sixth nerve. A direct approach is not recommended for primary optic nerve tumors, however, because of the anatomic configuration of the nerve supply to the extraocular muscles, as described previously.

TARSORRHAPHY

Before extubation and after the head dressing has been applied, tarsorrhaphy should be performed in all cases of orbital exploration, regardless of the route. The procedure is simple and atraumatic (Figure 22-13). The lids are washed with a cotton ball and pHisohex solution, and the cornea and conjunctiva are irrigated with saline. Sterile towels are placed to keep the sutures sterile. A double-ended 6-0 suture is used to place a horizontal mattress with two rubberband bumper guards. The thin skin of the lid is protected with the bumpers and makes removal of the tarsorrhaphy simple. In principle, the suture should be placed directly over the cornea, and should pass through the tarsal plate (gray line) of both lids. Care should be taken to see that there are no inverted lashes before the suture is tied. When the tarsorrhaphy is completed, an ophthalmic ointment is used to lubricate the cornea and conjunctiva. A pledget of Adaptic gauze is placed over the eye; fluffy cotton balls then are used to provide gentle pressure when taped to the head dressing. It is important for the surgeon to remove the tarsorrhaphy dressing daily to inspect the eye for signs of irritation and to reapply ophthalmic ointment. The tarsorrhaphy is left in place until the peak edema period has passed. It is advisable to remove the pressure dressing 1 day before the tarsorrhaphy suture is removed. In this way, if pressure has been removed prematurely and the eye begins to bulge, the cornea will be protected.

POSTOPERATIVE CARE

Intraoperative antibiotics are used routinely and dexamethasone is administered in high doses through the fourth postoperative day and then tapered over the ensuing week. With some care in hemostasis, blood transfusion usually is not required. Anticonvulsant therapy can be used, although there is usually little retraction injury to the orbital brain surface.

COMPLICATIONS

Transcranial exploration should be a relatively benign procedure. There is, however, transient palsy of the levator and superior rectus muscles in all cases. This may be complete or partial. Improvement usually is seen from within several days to 3 to 6 weeks and recovery is complete by 3 months. Ptosis and limitation of extraocular movement can, however, be a permanent accompaniment to the removal of orbital tumors by any approach. Postoperative keratitis is an infrequent but recognized complication. Seizures are rarely seen during the postoperative period. Recurrence of glioma within the orbit occurred in only one case. In this instance tumor was seeded by earlier Krönlein exploration.

CONCLUSIONS

The diagnostic techniques that are currently available have vastly improved our ability to predict the nature, precise location, and extent of tumors of the orbit. Familiarity with the variety of diseases that occur in the orbit and that can produce proptosis is essential for the neurosurgeon involved in the management of patients with orbital disease. A clear understanding of the regional anatomy will allow the surgeon to plan his or her surgical approach based on rational surgical objectives. It is not only good to know when and how to operate, but also when not to operate.

REFERENCES

1. Cushing H, Eisenhardt L: Meningiomas. Springfield, Ill, Charles C Thomas, 1938
2. Dandy WE: Results following transcranial attack on orbital tumors. Arch Ophthalmol 25:191, 1941
3. Love JG, Benedict WL: Transcranial removal of intraorbital tumors. JAMA 121:777, 1945
4. Matson DD: Unilateral exophthalmos in childhood. Clin Neurosurg 5:116, 1958
5. Van Buren JM, Poppen JL, Horax G: Unilateral exophthalmos: A consideration of symptom pathogenesis. Brain 80:139, 1957
6. Berke RN: A modified Kronlein operation. Trans Am Ophthalmol Soc 51:193, 1953
7. Davis FA: Primary tumors of the optic nerves. Arch Ophthalmol 23:735, 957, 1940
8. Jackson H: Orbital tumors. Proc Soc Med 38:587, 1945
9. Reese AB: Expanding lesions of the orbit. Trans Ophthalmol Soc UK 91:85, 1971
10. Spencer WH: Primary neoplasms of the optic nerve and its sheaths: Clinical features and current concepted pathogenetic mechanisms. J Am Ophthalmol Soc 70:490, 1972
11. Brash JP (ed): Cunningham's Manual of Practical Anatomy. London, Oxford University Press, 1948
12. Duke-Elder S, Wybar KC: The anatomy of the visual system, in System of Ophthalmology, vol 2. St. Louis, CV Mosby, 1961
13. Last RJ: Wolff's Anatomy of the Eye and Orbit, ed 6. Philadelphia, WB Saunders, 1968
14. Pernkopf E: Atlas of Topographical and Applied Human Anatomy, vol 1. Philadelphia, WB Saunders, 1963
15. Hanafee WN, Shiu PS, Dayton GO: Orbital venography. AJR 104:29, 1968
16. Lombardi G: Radiology in Neuroophthalmology. Baltimore, Williams & Wilkins, 1967
17. Potter GD, Trokel S: Tomography of the optic canal. Am J Roentgenol Radiother 106:530, 1969
18. Jakobiec FA, Depot MJ, Kennerdell JS, et al: Combined clinical and computed tomographic diagnosis of orbital glioma and meningioma. Ophthalmology 91:137, 1984
19. Bilaniuk LT, Schenck JF, Zimmerman RA, et al: Ocular and orbital lesions: Surface cell MR imaging. Radiology 156:669, 1985
20. Mark LE, Kennerdell JS, Maroon JC, et al: Microsurgical removal of a primary intraorbital meningioma. Am J Ophthalmol 86:704, 1978
21. Maroon JC, Kennerdell JS: Lateral microsurgical approach to intraorbital tumors. J Neurosurg 44:556, 1976
22. Housepian EM: Microsurgical anatomy of the orbital apex and principles of transcranial orbital exploration, in Keener EB (ed): Clinical Neurosurgery, vol 25. Baltimore, Williams & Wilkins, 1978, pp 556–573
23. Housepian EM: The surgical treatment of optic nerve sheath meningiomas, in Ransohoff JR (ed): Modern Techniques in Surgery: Neurosurgery. Mt Kisco, NY, Futura, 1981, pp 1–4
24. Housepian EM: Current concepts in the diagnosis and treatment of optic glioma, in Tindall G, Long D (eds): Contemporary Neurosurgery, vol 3. Baltimore, Williams & Wilkins, 1981, pp 1–5
25. Maroon JC, Kennerdell JS: Surgical approaches to the orbit. J Neurosurg 60:1226, 1984
26. Jane JA, Park TS, Doberskin LH, et al: The supraorbital approach: Technical note. Neurosurgery 11:537, 1982
27. Housepian EM: Surgical treatment of unilateral optic nerve gliomas. J Neurosurg 31:604, 1969

CHAPTER 23

Anterior and Lateral Microsurgical Approaches to Orbital Pathologic Processes

Melvin G. Alper   Phil A. Aitken

THE SURGICAL REMOVAL OF RETROBULBAR TU-MORS with retention of the globe was first devised by Krönlein in 1888.[1] Utilizing a lateral approach with a curvilinear incision parallel to the orbital rim and at right angles to Langer's lines in the skin, the procedure frequently resulted in cosmetic defects.

A review of the literature reveals that relatively few such operations were performed by ophthalmic surgeons in the decades before World War II. During this period, most orbital surgery in fact was performed by neurologic surgeons through a transcranial approach. Dandy[2] believed that 75 percent of orbital tumors arose within the cranial cavity and that the only proper surgical approach to them was by a transcranial route. He published a classical monograph, "Orbital Tumors: Results Following the Transcranial Attack," describing his experiences. Naffziger[3,4] advocated simultaneous bilateral orbital decompression for Graves' orbitopathy by removal of the orbital roof lateral to the frontal sinus through a bifrontal craniotomy.

In 1957, Iliff[5] restudied the Dandy series and added a group of orbital tumors from the Wilmer Eye Institute. He concluded that 75 percent of orbital tumors arose within the orbit and that orbital surgery properly lay within the province of the ophthalmic surgeon.

At about the same time, Reese[6,7] and Berke[8] modified the classical Krönlein lateral orbotomy and devised a better technique for orbital surgery through the lateral approach. Reese reported in his Bowman lecture[7] in 1970 that only 8 percent of 504 consecutive patients of expanding orbital masses qualified as candidates for the neurosurgical approach.

Benedict[9] and his colleagues at the Mayo Clinic accumulated a large experience with orbital surgery and advocated an anterior approach by a Killian or Lynch-type incision beneath the brow. Davis[10] recommended an anterior inferior approach to optic nerve gliomas by an incision through the skin at the inferior orbital rim.

From this cumulative experience, it is apparent that in the United States, at least, ophthalmic surgeons were performing most of the orbital surgery. In Europe, however, neurosurgeons continued to dominate the field.

John Foster[11] was thus prompted to report in 1948 in a symposium on orbital diseases that an accepted technique for treatment of orbital tumors was to "iodize and temporize—irradiate and exenterate."

Despite the admonitions of such authors as Long and Ellis[12] who, in 1971, reported that total unilateral visual loss was a common complication of exploratory orbitotomy, the past decade has witnessed a momentous change in orbital surgery. The advent of pleuridirectional polytomography and ultrasonography refined the diagnostic approach to orbital disease, making exploratory operations a rare experience. The use of computed tomography (CT) has further refined these diagnostic techniques so that the modern orbital surgeon can plan a surgical approach with confidence that there will be few surprises when the orbit is entered.[13] Utilizing modern fiberoptics,[14] magnification, and the innovative operative techniques of Wright[5] and Kennerdell,[6] orbital surgery today should produce few complications.

Adverse outcomes occur as a result of unfamiliarity with surgical anatomy and the operative techniques referred to above. Orbital surgery is performed for a variety of reasons—to biopsy and excise a tumor, to repair a congenital or traumatic defect, or to decompress the orbit for Graves' orbitopathy. To ensure a successful outcome, it is often necessary to use a team of specialists.

During the diagnostic period, neuroradiologists and endocrinologists as well as nuclear medical specialists are consulted. Frequently, the surgical team includes neurosurgeons, ENT specialists, and plastic surgeons working in cooperation with the ophthalmologist.

Before embarking on any of the above-described operations, however, the surgeon should be familiar with the diagnostic procedures available, the indications for surgery, the surgical anatomy, and the operative techniques at hand.

SURGICAL ANATOMY

The bony orbital cavity (Figure 23-1) is a four-walled, cone-shaped structure bounded medially by the lacrimal and ethmoid bones and laterally by the zygomatic bone and the greater wing of the sphenoid bone. The floor is slightly arched and composed by the zygoma, the maxillary, and the palatine bones (Figures 23-2 and 23-3). The roof arcs slightly upward and

OPERATIVE NEUROSURGICAL TECHNIQUES
ISBN 0-8089-1862-1

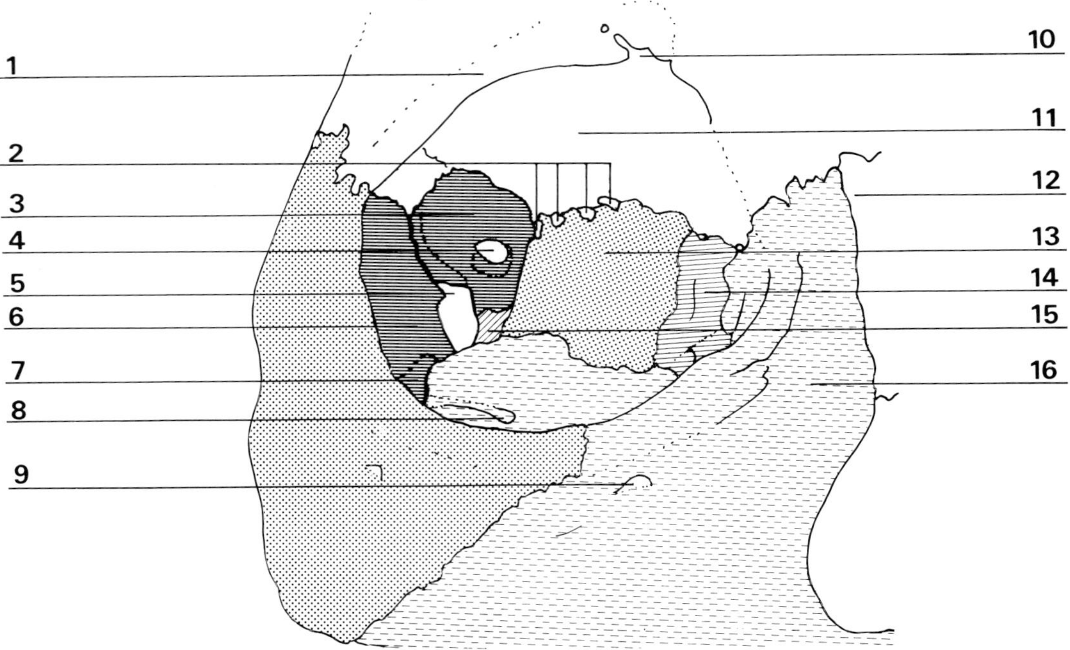

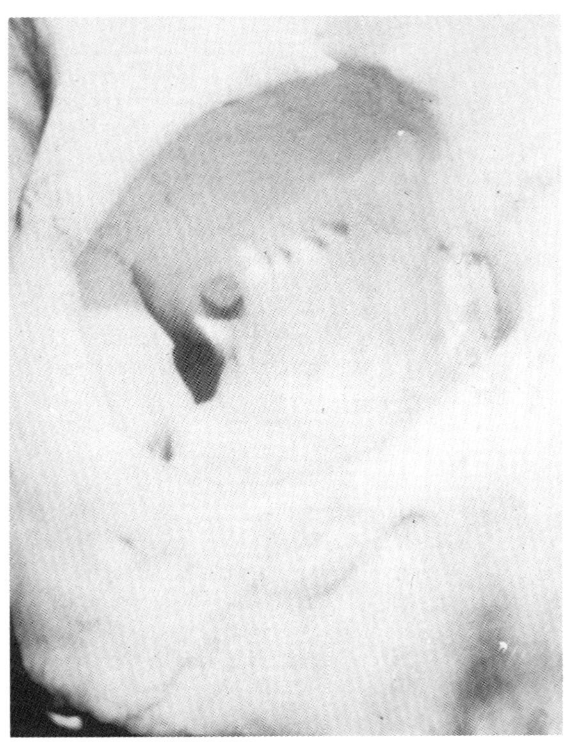

Fig. 23-1. A frontal view of the orbit with the optic foramen, the medial orbital wall, and the roof visible. 1 = supraorbital ridge; 2 = ethmoid foramina; 3 = lesser wing of the sphenoid bone; 4 = optic foramen; 5 = superior orbital fissure; 6 = greater wing of the sphenoid bone; 7 = inferior orbital fissure; 8 = infraorbital groove; 9 = infraorbital foramen; 10 = supraorbital notch; 11 = orbital roof(frontal); 12 = nasal bone; 13 = orbital plate of the ethmoid bone; 14 = lacrimal bone; 15 = orbital process of the palatine bone; 16 = maxilla. (Reprinted from Waddington MA: Atlas of the Human Skull, ed 1. With permission of Academy Books.)

is formed by the frontal bone. The anterior orbital rims form the base of the cone that encloses an opening that measures an average of 34 mm in height by 42 mm in width in an adult. The apex (Figure 23-4) is an enclosed bony structure penetrated by the superior orbital fissure, which is separated from the optic foramen by a bony portion of the lesser sphenoid wing called the "strut." The average depth of the lateral wall (Figure 23-5) in an adult measures 47 mm, and the medial wall measures 45 mm. The floor is 53 mm in length and the roof 52 mm in length. The volume of the orbit is 30 cc, with the globe making up an average of 6.5 cc.

The bony orbital cavity is lined by the periorbita or periosteum, which is an extension of the dural sheath from the anterior cranial cavity. The dura further extends forward with the optic nerve and encases it to form its leptomeningeal sheath.

There are four surgical spaces in which various lesions can be found:

1. The subperiosteal space.
2. The peripheral surgical space.
3. The central surgical space.
4. Tenon's space.

The subperiosteal space lies between the bone and the periosteum and harbors bony tumors and dermoid cysts. The

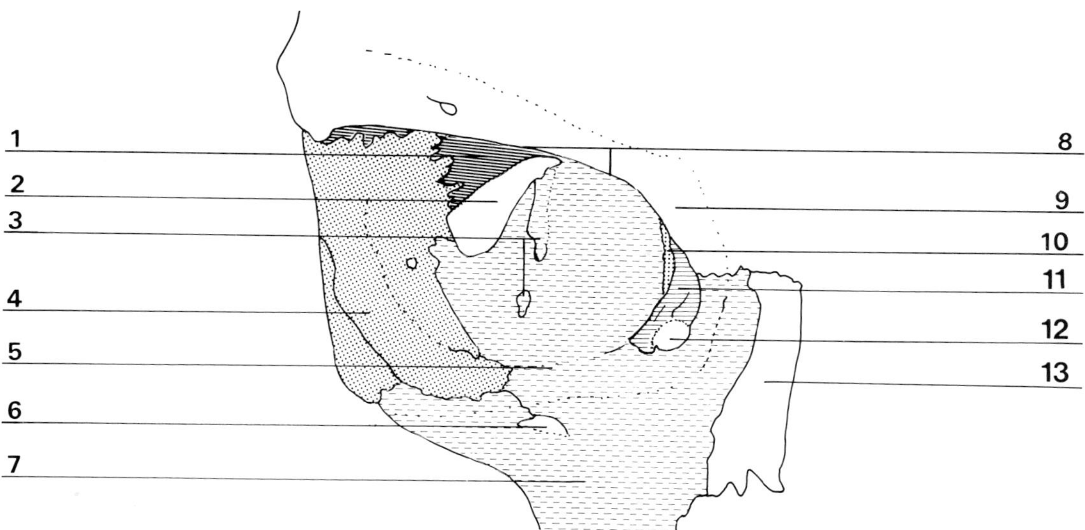

Fig. 23-2. A view of the inferior orbital surface and the medial wall of the orbit. 1 = greater wing of the sphenoid bone; 2 = inferior orbital fissure; 3 = infraorbital groove; 4 = zygomatic bone; 5 = inferior orbital margin; 6 = infraorbital foramen; 7 = maxilla; 8 = superior orbital margin; 9 = frontal bone; 10 = ethmoid bone; 11 = lacrimal gland; 12 = lacrimal canal; 13 = nasal bone. (Reprinted from Waddington MA: Atlas of the Human Skull, ed 1. With permission of Academy Books.)

peripheral surgical space or extraconal space lies between the periosteum and the extraocular muscles. Cavernous hemangiomas, fibrous histiocytomas, and lacrimal gland tumors as well as dermoid cysts commonly can be found here. The central surgical space or intraconal space lies within the muscle cone and contains the optic nerve with its vital blood supply. Here, one finds optic nerve tumors, cavernous hemangiomas, and neurilemomas. Inflammatory pseudotumors and rhabdomyosarcomas can be found in any of the above spaces as well as in Tenon's space, which surrounds the globe posteriorly. Tenon's space also can harbor intraocular tumors that have grown through the coats of the globe.

The most popular surgical approach to the orbit is a lateral approach. In this approach, few important or vital structures are encountered until the central surgical space is entered (see Figure 23-9). The lateral canthal ligament should be identified and preserved. The zygomatic artery and nerve are noted as they penetrate the zygoma at the malar eminence anteriorly. Posteriorly along the lateral wall, a small branch of the lacrimal artery—the meningeal branch—may be encountered coursing in the subperiosteal space.

The orbital roof may be quite thin and may have eroded into the anterior cranial cavity, especially if it is expanded by orbital tumors. The supraorbital nerve and vessels exit through the supraorbital notch or foramen at the juncture of the inner and middle one third of the superior orbital rim. As the

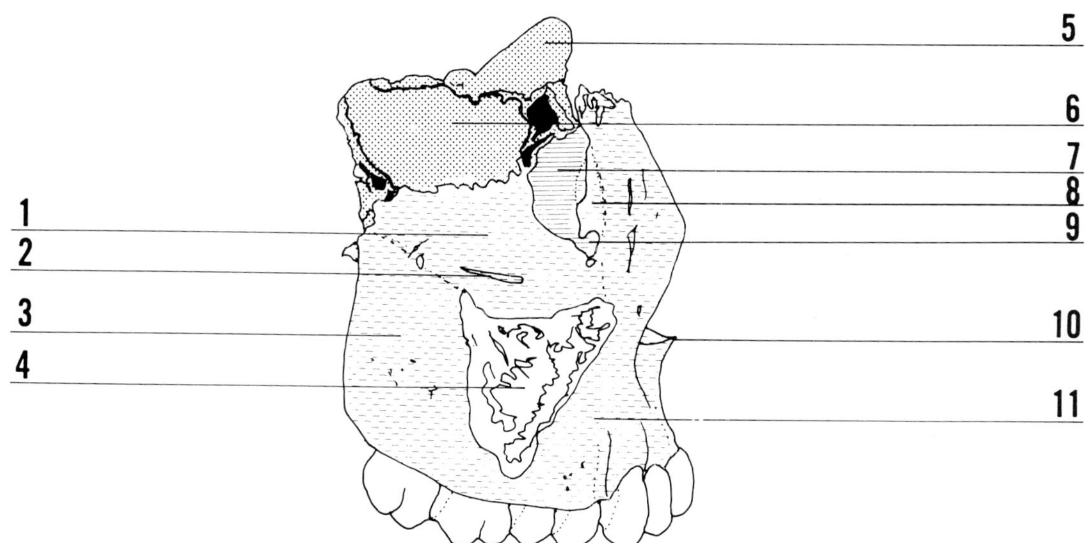

Fig. 23-3. A composite view of the floor of the orbit with the maxillary sinus exposed. 1 = orbital floor of the maxilla; 2 = infraorbital groove; 3 = infraorbital surface of the maxilla; 4 = articular surface for zygomatic bone; 5 = crista galli; 6 = orbital plate of the ethmoid bone; 7 = lacrimal gland; 8 = lacrimal fossa; 9 = lacrimal hamulus; 10 = anterior nasal spine; 11 = maxilla. (Reprinted from Waddington MA: Atlas of the Human Skull, ed 1. With permission of Academy Books.)

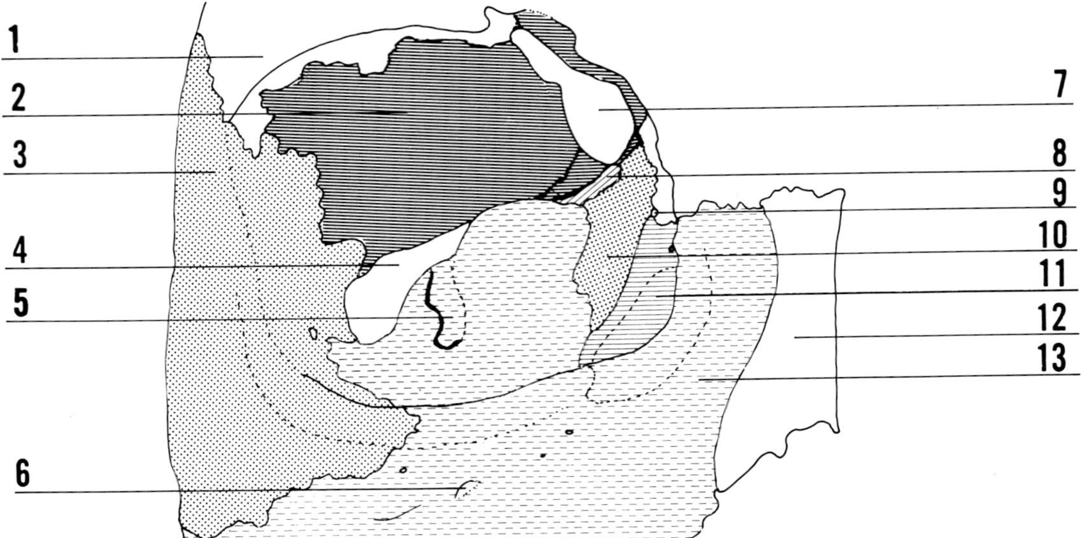

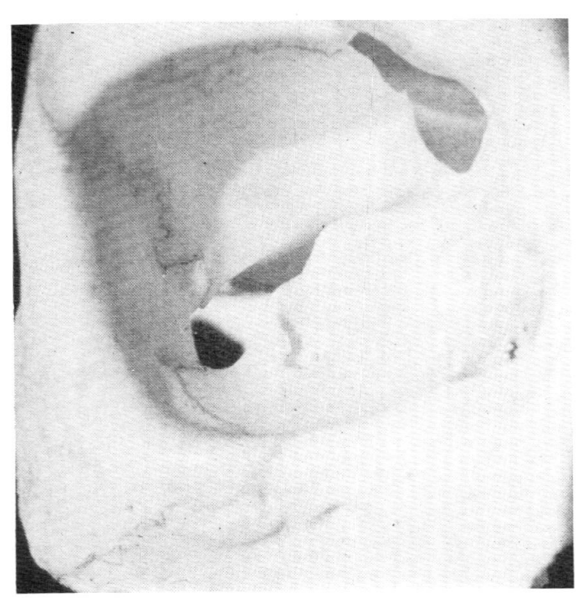

Fig. 23-4. View of the orbital floor and the orbital fissures near the apex. 1 = frontal bone; 2 = greater wing of the sphenoid bone; 3 = zygomatic bone; 4 = inferior orbital fissure; 5 = infraorbital groove; 6 = infraorbital foramen; 7 = superior orbital fissure; 8 = orbital process of the palatine bone; 9 = anterior ethmoid foramen; 10 = orbital plate of the ethmoid bone; 11 = lacrimal fossa; 12 = maxilla. (Reprinted from Waddington MA: Atlas of the Human Skull, ed 1. With permission of Academy Books.)

periosteum is reflected from the frontal bone in the anterior approach, the frontal nerve may be encountered in the subperiosteal space continuous with its two branches, the supratrochlear and the supraorbital, described above. Medially and superiorly, well behind the orbital rim, one encounters the trochlea and superior oblique tendon. Laterally, the lacrimal nerve and gland are encountered behind the orbital rim, Following the arched roof posteriorly in the subperiosteal space, the anterior part of the superior orbital fissure are encountered laterally.

The anterior inferior approach sometimes is used to approach tumors and is used most commonly for decompression of the orbital floor into the antrum for Graves' orbitopathy. Lying in the infraorbital groove at the junction of the inner and middle one third of the orbital floor is the infraorbital neurovascular bundle. This structure exits onto the face through a foramen or notch, the infraorbital foramen.

The medial orbital wall contains the attachment of the medial canthal ligament into the periosteum. By severing this ligament with its periosteal attachment and reflecting it laterally, the tear sac is carried off of the lacrimal bone and the medial wall is exposed (see Figure 23-1). Posteriorly along the medial wall, one encounters the anterior and posterior ethmoid artery in the subperiosteal space. Most posterior along the medial wall is the optic foramen at the apex of the orbital cavity. Here, one encounters the optic nerve if the subperiosteal dissection is carried out in too vigorous a fashion.

The ethmoid sinus lies medial to the ethmoid bone. This bone is quite thin, as is the lacrimal bone. Dissection that is too vigorous or pressure on these structures can result in entrance into the nasal cavity anteriorly beneath the lacrimal bone or into the ethmoid sinus beneath the ethmoid bone.

The medial walls of both orbits lie parallel while the lateral walls are at 90 to each other. The posterolateral aspect of each bony orbit abuts the temporal bone at its junction with the greater wing of the sphenoid. The temporalis muscle inserts along this juncture and is quite vascular with the subpterygoid plexus of veins quite apparent at this point.

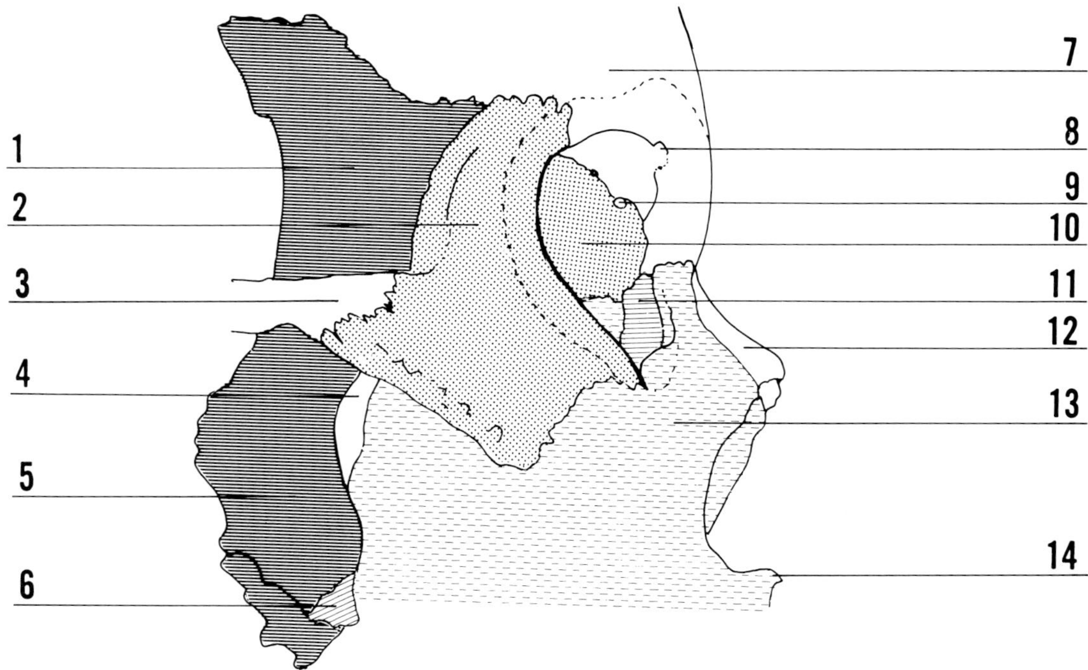

Fig. 23-5. Lateral external view of the orbital wall. 1 = greater wing of the sphenoid bone; 2 = zygomatic bone; 3 = temporal bone (zygomatic arch); 4 = pterygopalatine fissure; 5 = lateral pterygoid process of the sphenoid bone; 6 = pyramidal process of the palatine bone; 7 = frontal bone; 8 = supraorbital notch; 9 = ethmoid foramen; 10 = orbital process of the ethmoid bone; 11 = lacrimal gland; 12 = nasal bone; 13 = maxilla; 14 = anterior nasal spine. (Reprinted from Waddington MA: Atlas of the Human Skull, ed 1. With permission of Academy Books.)

The muscle cone is encased by an outer layer of Tenon's fascia, the integrity of which must be maintained separate from the overlying periorbita. These two layers are normally separated by a thin layer of fat located in the peripheral surgical space. After the muscle cone is entered from any surgical approach (lateral, anterior, or superior), an effort should be made to close the fascial layer separately from the periorbital layer. This is especially important when using the lateral approach, since the lateral rectus muscle can become encased in scar tissue and adhere to the periosteum, creating either limited motion in the field of action of this muscle or restriction in its antagonist's field of action (see below).

COMPLICATIONS DURING DIAGNOSIS

A successful outcome after orbital surgery begins with proper diagnostic procedures.[17] Unlike diagnosis in other fields of ophthalmology where the condition usually is apparent at first glance, in orbital disease, considerable thought must be given to the problem at hand. We must learn from our neurosurgical colleagues how to mount a proper diagnostic campaign.

The introduction of computed tomography (CT) has simplified our task to a great degree, but pitfalls in this relatively new technique still exist that may lead to surgical complications. In the era before CT scanning became available, certain diagnostic procedures themselves caused complications.

The criteria for use of any procedure in the diagnostic evaluation of orbital disease should include the following. The diagnostic procedure should (1) separate orbital from periorbital or intracranial disease; (2) delineate the surgical route of choice; (3) help in selecting the surgical team; (4) proceed in a logical sequence with little or no risk to the patient.

With these principles in mind, we have devised the following step-by-step schema for evaluating diseases of the orbit:

A. NONINVASIVE STUDIES

1. Establish presence of exophthalmos.
2. Rule out Graves' disease.
3. Roentgenographic studies of the skull, orbits, optic foramina and canals, sphenoid ridges, and paranasal sinuses by (a) plain x-ray films; (b) pleuridirectional polytomography, and (c) CT scanning without contrast.
4. Ultrasonography (A and B mode).
5. Radionuclide scanning.

B. INVASIVE STUDIES

1. CT scanning with contrast.
2. Orbital venography (including subtraction studies).
3. Cerebral angiography (including subtraction studies).
4. Trial of corticosteroids.
5. Orbital explora.

USE OF CONTRAST DYES

In any study involving the injection of iodinated dyes, it is important to take a careful history for allergy. Intolerance to seafood or other substances that may contain iodine should be queried. If there is a suspicion of Graves' disease, studies for this should be concluded before using any contrast material since the iodine contained in the dyes will vitiate any investigations for thyroid function. Anaphylactic reactions and even death from contrast dyes have been reported.

If there is a history of allergy to iodine, the test still can be carried out if the patient is properly prepared with antihistamines or corticosteroids or both. In the event that there has been a previous severe reaction to contrast dyes, any test with these substances can best be carried out with the patient hospitalized and the study performed with an anesthetist in attendance.

In many instances, CT scanning machines have been added to radiology departments without any planning for adequate facilities for resuscitation equipment and room for additional personnel in the event of an adverse reaction to contrast dyes. Since scanning with contrast is such an important part of most CT studies, the referring physician should be aware of the conditions under which the patient will be examined. If safe conditions do not exist, it may be well to defer contrast studies or to refer the patient to a clinic that has satisfactory facilities. By following these safeguards, reactions to iodine will be minimized but not completely eliminated.

CONVENTIONAL X-RAY EXAMINATION

In the years before CT scanning was available, we depended on conventional and special x-ray studies for diagnosis. Lloyd[8] has pointed out that in a series of 1070 patients, 33 percent showed an abnormality on plain x-ray films and that in 21 percent the features on the plain films were totally diagnostic without the necessity for further investigation. When hypocycloidal or pleuridirectional polytomography was added, the positive diagnostic yield approached 50 percent in Lloyd's broad experience.

Special x-ray studies include the use of orbital venography and contrast orbitography with water-soluble contrast medium to outline expanding masses in the orbit. We have encountered some complications with use of these two procedures, which should be familiar to the orbital surgeon.

ORBITAL VENOGRAPHY

Orbital venography is the visualization of orbital veins with radiopaque materials. The superior ophthalmic vein is of primary interest. The orbital veins are more constant in their course than the arteries and a mass lesion in the orbit often will produce displacement of the veins, especially if the lesion is posterior to the globe either inside or outside of the muscle cone. This procedure is of special use in investigating and differentiating orbital inflammatory disease processes from orbital tumors. Except for varices, venograms usually will not give clues to histology. We still use venography to outline orbital varices and to investigate orbital phlebitis or to rule out the Tolosa-Hunt syndrome in painful ophthalmoplegia.

The orbital veins can be demonstrated by injection of the angular, facial, or frontal vein. The easiest method by far is injection of the frontal vein. Injection through the facial vein at the mandibular angle sometimes necessitated open cut-down, which added to the difficulty of the technique. Hannafee[9] advocated filling the ophthalmic veins by a catheter study via the internal jugular-inferior petrosal sinus route. In one instance, we experienced an infarct of the pons, with partial recovery, using this latter route. Others have reported pontine stroke and hemorrhage from rupture of prepontine veins or the vasculature of malignancies because of excessive injection pressure in using the catheter study. In performing the cut-down technique at the mandibular angle, phlebitis and infection have been reported. Percutaneous injections have been associated with local hematomas, extravasation of dye, slough of tissue, and phlebitis.

Because of these complications, we use only the frontal vein as an injection site. It is necessary to wrap the forehead above the injection site with either an Ace bandage or a tourniquet to prevent the escape of the dye into the scalp veins, which form a negative pressure plexus into which the dye pours. By this technique we have had almost universal success without complications in demonstrating the veins of the orbit. We customarily perform this examination on an out-patient basis.

Few false-positives have been experienced with this technique, although false-negatives are not uncommon. Deviation of the superior ophthalmic vein from its normal course in an outward fashion implied a lesion within the muscle cone, while deviation inward indicated an extraconal mass. Obliteration of the final segment into the cavernous sinus indicated either thrombophlebitis, excessive orbital pressure, or the Tolosa-Hunt syndrome.

CONTRAST ORBITOGRAPHY

Contrast orbitography is the visualization of the muscle cone by retrobulbar injection of a water-soluble medium. Space-occupying lesions within the orbit deform the normal contour of the cone. Orbitography demonstrates the size, shape, and location of expanding masses in relation to the muscle cone, but gives no indication of their histopathology.

We customarily used 2 ml of Renografin 60 percent or Conray 60 percent diluted by 2 ml of 2-percent Xylocaine and 1 ml of hyaluronidase (150 u) to a 24 percent solution for retrobulbar injection. Initially, the bolus of material measured 5 ml, as recommended by Lombardi.[20] Because this resulted in increased retrobulbar pressure with chemosis in many cases, we reduced the volume to 2 ml and combined it with hypocycloidal polytomography to visualize the muscle cone. This proved quite satisfactory and reduced the danger to the ophthalmic artery and central retinal vessels from excessive retrobulbar pressure.

In a large series of cases, which we reported to the American Academy of Ophthalmology and Otolaryngology in a scientific exhibit in 1969,[21] we experienced a number of complications. These included retrobulbar hematomas in a few patients and chemosis with lid edema in the majority. This latter finding usually promptly resolved within 4 hours of the examination and was directly related to the volume of material injected. There frequently was extravasation of dye through the hernial orifices of the orbital septum into the lid. This complication was common and rarely interfered with the examination. If the retrobulbar bolus wase not properly placed into the muscle cone, however, the dye extravasated in such enormous quantity that the test had to be abandoned for another day.

In one of our patients, there was escape of the dye into the intracranial subdural space and into the terminal sac. Fortunately, it was absorbed without systemic reaction.

There were no false-negatives or false-positives in this series of contrast orbitographies. In several instances, however, findings were misinterpreted. Apical masses were misinterpreted as orbital or neurogenic tumors, but at surgery proved to be enlarged inferior rectus muscles associated with euthyroid Graves' disease in patients with monocular exophthalmos.

Others have reported temporary loss of vision and tissue slough[22] as well as optic atrophy.[23,24] Because of these complications, contrast orbitography has been abandoned in our hands. From these studies, however, we gained a great deal of experience in interpreting orbital masses in relation to surrounding vital structures. Clinicopathologic correlation of apical masses that were shown at surgery to be the inferior rectus muscle in euthyroid Graves' disease proved to be a most valuable lesson in our early experience with CT scanning.

COMPUTED TOMOGRAPHY

Computed tomographic scanning of orbital masses has revolutionized orbital surgery. By means of this new technique, the location of a tumor and its size and shape can be delineated in three dimensions. Evaluation of the density of the expanding lesion in comparison with surrounding structures should theoretically give an indication of the disease process. With use of fourth-generation scanners, which, in the most recent models, have the ability to make submillimeter sections, differences in tissue density have become more apparent. As Jakobiec and Henkind[25] have recently noted, the goal of making a specific tissue diagnosis preoperatively may be approaching.

In the early days of CT scanning, misinterpretation of findings and false-negatives were encountered. Thus, Susac and Smith[26] reported a case in their paper "The Impossible Meningioma" in which a meningioma of the orbital apex was missed on scans made by a first-generation EMI head scanner. The scans of this patient were restudied after exploratory surgery revealed the true diagnosis. By changing the window width on the scanner, the tumor was readily demonstrated. The reason for failure to perform this maneuver in the first instance resulted from a breakdown in communication between the referring physician and the neuroradiologist. Zimmerman[27] has recently emphasized the importance of close collaboration between clinicians responsible for the preoperative evaluation and the radiologist who must interpret the CT scan. Although it is not always possible, the referring physician should speak directly with the radiologist to offer pertinent clinical findings. After surgery, we advocate a multidiscipline conference between the orbital surgeon, the radiologist, and the pathologist so that clinicopathologic correlation can be made. Only through this type of learning experience will there emerge more accurate preoperative diagnosis and successful surgery.

In their early experience with CT orbital scans, misinterpretations were reported by radiologists. Most notable among these was the error that we made in our experience with contrast orbitography, namely, mistaking an inferior rectus muscle enlarged from Graves' orbitopathy for neurogenic or primary tumor of the orbital apex.[28] Extraocular muscle enlargement from Graves' orbitopathy may be interpreted as a variety of other conditions including inflammatory "pseudotumor," metastatic tumors, and even optic nerve tumors. Unfortunately, some of these misdiagnosed conditions were operated upon by both orbital and neurologic surgeons in other clinics.

Other frequent errors have arisen from malpositioning the patient for orbital CT scanning. This causes normal structures to appear abnormal and may result in missing lesions that are present. This error has arisen in some instances, in our observation, from lack of supervision of CT technicians who have only been trained in the more common examination of the brain. This is especially true when a new CT unit is installed in an existing radiology department where the radiologists must divide their time between conventional x-ray diagnosis and this new modality. Evaluation of the orbit must be carried out with the x-ray beam at an angle of 0 to 10 degrees to the canthomeatal (Reid's) line, whereas examination for intracranial disease is performed with the x-ray beam at an angle of 20 to 25 degrees to the canthomeatal line.

The examples of errors in CT diagnosis noted above have been cited to alert the uninitiated to the fact that CT scanning, like other diagnostic tests, is not without its own built-in limitations. Although it is better than most, it is not a "deus et machina," as Jakobiec and Henkind[25] expressed it. In our own experience, most of these errors have been obviated by close collaboration between the surgeon, the radiologist, and the pathologist. This re-emphasizes the need for a multidisciplinary approach to orbital tumors.

USE OF CORTICOSTEROIDS

A trial of therapy with corticosteroids in presumed inflammatory diseases of the orbit may be very helpful in ruling out acute inflammatory conditions. When combined with pre- and posttherapy CT scans that objectively reveal a resolution of the orbital condition, one can assume that the pathologic process is inflammatory in nature.

There are some who disagree with this approach and recommend biopsy of all orbital masses in order to be certain of the histopathology. Although we have witnessed impressive resolution of changes from both primary and metastatic tumors following the use of corticosteroids in some instances, we nevertheless still advocate its use as a trial of therapy in ruling out inflammatory disease. If the condition is neoplastic, the true nature of the process will be revealed by the clinical course in a short period of time despite the use of corticosteroids. By using this technique, fewer exploratory operations for orbital inflammatory masses with the attendant danger of exacerbation have been performed in our clinic in recent years.

SURGICAL APPROACHES TO THE ORBIT

As outlined in the introductory remarks, there are, in general, three surgical approaches to the orbit: (1) the superior approach; (2) the anterior approach; and (3) the lateral approach.

The superior approach, which was devised and popularized by Dandy, is transcranial and includes unroofing the orbit and optic canal. It is indicated for lesions arising in the orbital apex with or without extension into the optic canal or intracranial cavity or for those tumors that arise intracranially and extend into the orbit.

The anterior approach involves an incision either beneath the superior orbital rim or above the inferior rim. It affords entrance into the subperiosteal space either beneath the roof or above the floor of the orbit. From the subperiosteal space, one can enter the extraconal peripheral surgical space by an anteroposterior incision of the periorbita. The intraconal central

Table 23-1. Routes of Choice for Surgery
of Orbital Tumors

Location of orbital tumor	Surgical route
Intracranial extension	superior
Apex and canal	superior
Apex only	lateral
Superior extracoonal	anterior
Superonasal	anterior and lateral
Superotemporal	lateral and anterior
Inferior	lateral and anterior
Medial	anterior and medial
All others	lateral

surgical space then can be explored by merely retracting one of the rectus muscles. Its use is indicated for lesions lying in the anterior two thirds of the orbit superior or inferior to the optic nerve, inside or outside the muscle cone. This approach was devised by Knapp[29,30] in 1874 and popularized in more recent times by Benedict.[9]

The lateral approach is the most popular approach in use today. It reaches the retrobulbar spaces by removing the lateral bony wall or greater wing of the sphenoid bone to its junction with the temporal bone. It includes the classic Krönlein procedure as modified by Reese, Berke, and Wright. Its use is indicated for all intraconal lesions, and it can be used in combination with either the superior or anterior approach. It affords the best exposure by orbitotomy.

Combinations of the above approaches can be performed depending upon the location of an orbital tumor. As outlined under the discussion of CT scanning, by use of transaxial and coronal views, a preoperative three-dimensional analysis of orbital tumors can be made so that the orbital surgeon can tailor the surgical attack in the best fashion. Not only the surgical attack but also the surgical team can be selected preoperatively based on this analysis.

SURGICAL APPROACHES IN RELATION TO SURGICAL ANATOMY

Through the superior approach, the middle and posterior aspects of the orbital contents are readily visible (see Figure 23-23). By means of the lateral approach, one can see the anterior two thirds of the orbital contents. By removing the (greater wing of the sphenoid) posterolateral bony wall of the orbit to its junction with the temporal bone, the anterior two thirds of the orbit plus a portion of the posterior one third can be seen.

SURGICAL ROUTES OF CHOICE

From the foregoing discussion of surgical approaches influenced by preoperative CT analysis and related to the surgical anatomy, it is readily apparent that a team of surgeons is sometimes necessary for an attack on an orbital mass that may be in an inaccessible or contiguous area. Working with a seasoned team of ENT and neurologic surgeons, we have developed the routes of choice listed in Table 23-1 when performing surgery for orbital tumors.

The surgical approach chosen should (1) afford adequate exposure, (2) allow excision of the tumor at one sitting, (3) not cause a functional defect, and (4) not cause a cosmetic defect.

INDICATIONS AND CONTRAINDICATIONS

Before embarking upon orbital surgery, the surgeon should bear in mind the admonitions of Benedict,[9] who noted that "after dealing with more than 700 surgical cases of orbital tumors and cysts, one should be prepared to complete the necessary surgical treatment involved and to refrain from meddlesome interference to satisfy curiosity in indeterminate cases."

Orbital surgery is indicated for the following reasons: (1) when an orbital mass is demonstrated; (2) when vision of an exophthalmic eye is threatened; and, (3) for cosmesis.

In general, orbital surgery is contraindicated for the following reasons: (1) when the tumor is confined to an area anterior to the globe; (2) when an extraorbital tumor extends into the retrobulbar space; (3) when the tumor is metastatic; (4) when exophthalmos is caused by systemic disease; and (5) when inflammatory pseudotumor is present.

In some instances there are exceptions to these general rules. For example, it may be necessary to debulk a metastatic or inflammatory lesion surgically in order to be rid of the mass effect on vital structures before medical therapy has had time to act. It also may be necessary to operate upon a tumor extending from an adjacent structure; this can be done in league with a neurosurgeon or ENT surgeon to complete the excision of the lesion. In general, however, the contraindications listed above are good rules to follow to avoid trouble.

INSTRUMENTATION

Proper instrumentation should be available to ensure a successful conclusion to a surgical attack on the orbit. In addition to the usual instruments available for orbital surgery and neurosurgery, the following should be included: (1) adequate lighting and magnification; (2) self-retaining instruments for exposure; (3) bipolar electrocoagulation forceps for hemostasis; (4) hemostatic agents such as thrombin-soaked gelatin, oxidized cellulose (Surgicel), Avitene, and bone wax; (5) adequate suction; and (6) neurosurgical microscopic instruments.

Illumination can be provided by a fiberoptic headlight, which affords coaxial illumination. This can be combined with surgical telescopes (Designs for Vision) that afford up to $8\times$ magnification while providing a wide-angle view of the operative field. This combination allows the surgeon greater physical mobility than the use of a fixed-mount microscope. When using the operating microscope, we favor the Zeiss Microscope System with binocular eyepieces of $12.5\times$ magnification and a 300–mm objective zoom lens. The usual microscope in ophthalmic operating rooms uses either a 150-mm or 200-mm objective lens, which does not allow enough room to accommodate the long-handled instruments necessary for deep orbital surgery.

In order to free both hands for dissection, a self-retaining retractor is necessary. We prefer the self-retaining retractor designed by Kennerdell and Maroon. Use of this instrument, combined with neurosurgical cottonoid sponges to pack off the orbital fat that plagues the surgeon and obliterates the view when the muscle cone is entered, provides a clear field for dissection of vital structures.

Ophthalmic instruments are improper for use in orbital surgery. For orbital surgery we prefer the long spring-handled instruments designed by Jannetta and Yasargil for use in neurosurgery.

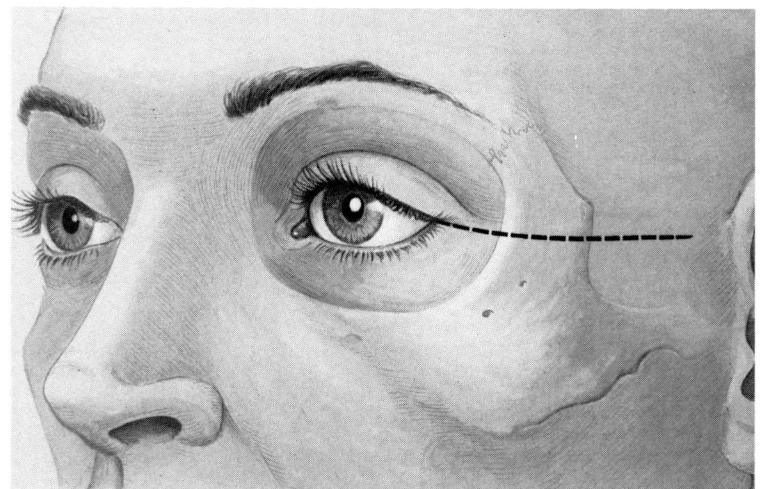

19-6

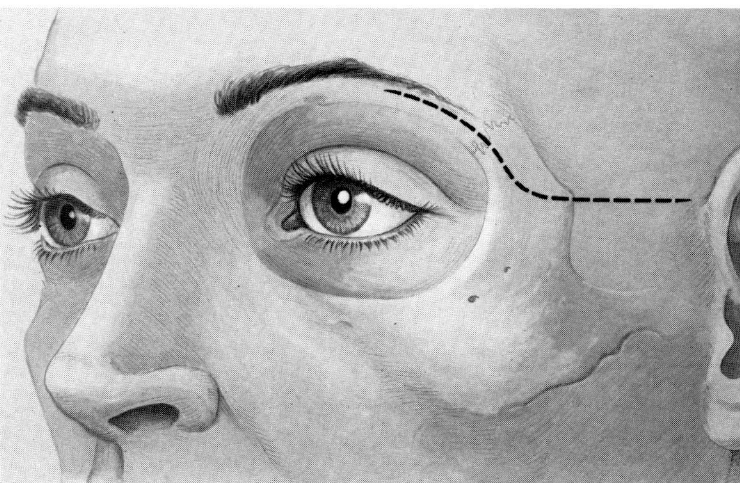

19-7

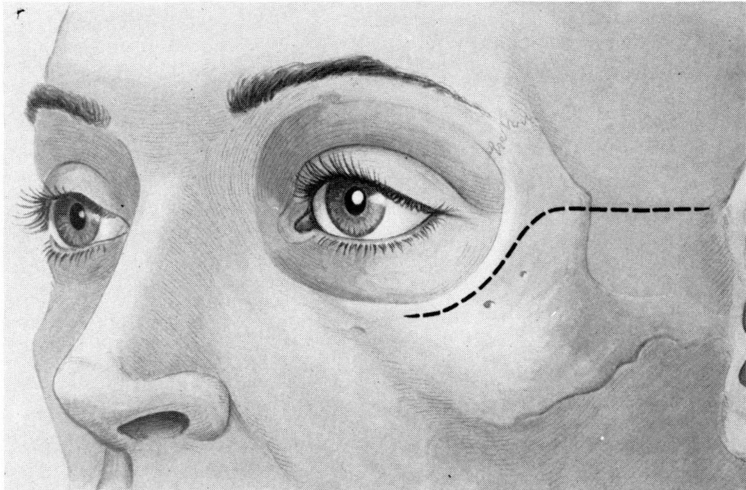

19-8

Figs. 23-6, 23-7, and 23-8. The lateral surgical approach may offer several options depending on the area of needed exposure and anatomic variations.

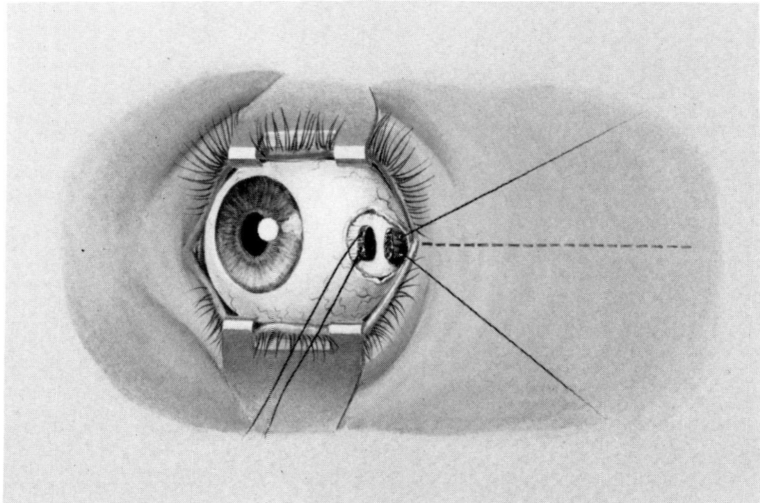

Fig. 23-9. Exposure is enhanced if the lateral rectus muscle is identified and separated. The globe can be held in place with sutures in the tendinous insertion.

LATERAL ORBITAL APPROACH

The lateral orbital approach (Figures 23-6 through 23-8) is the most popular one in use today for removal of orbital tumors. Its indications have been listed above. We use it in combination with the anterior approach or even with a medially situated incision to facilitate exposure by displacing the globe and orbital contents laterally. It is the sine qua non approach for intraconal tumors.

We advocate the use of general anesthesia for this and all deep orbital surgery, although we have performed orbital surgery under local anesthesia.

LATERAL CANTHOTOMY

Before the advent of CT scanning, when we did not know the exact location of a tumor, it was our custom first to perform a lateral canthotomy, disinsert the lateral canthal ligament, and explore the orbit by palpation before proceeding with the operation. The success of this procedure depends upon com-pletely disengaging the lateral canthal ligament, not only from the orbital tubercle but also from its extensive insertion up and down the lateral wall. Once this has been accomplished, an opening in the lateral fornix of the conjunctiva is made and finger exploration from the peripheral surgical space can proceed.

Finger exploration can allow palpation of the muscle cone and its contents. One must proceed cautiously, however, since heavy-handedness at this stage can damage vital structures. This is especially true when palpating the optic nerve or the apical area. The pupil should be monitored during this procedure and if dilatation occurs the pressure should be removed immediately.

We still use this operation for lesions that are laterally placed in the anterior one third of the orbit and for children in whom we may wish to avoid removing bone. In general, however, when we have localized a tumor by CT scanning and ultrasound as outlined above, we proceed immediately with the lateral orbitotomy.

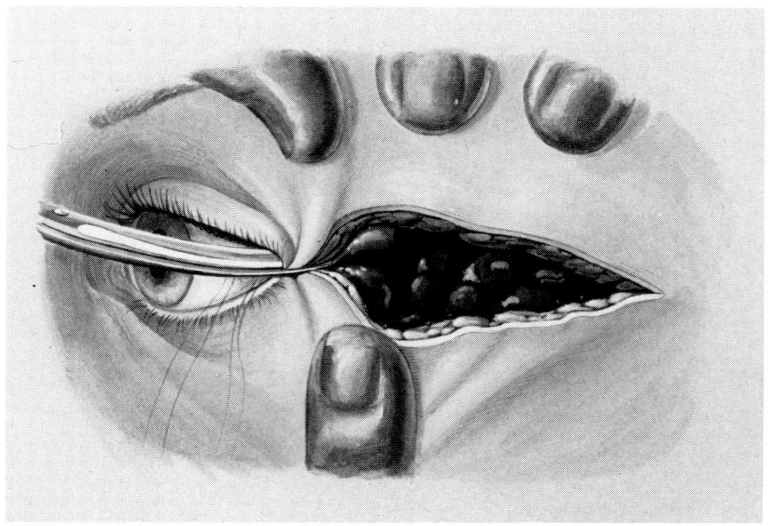

Fig. 23-10. The lateral approach to the orbit requires that the soft tissue be divided before exposing the zygomatic bone.

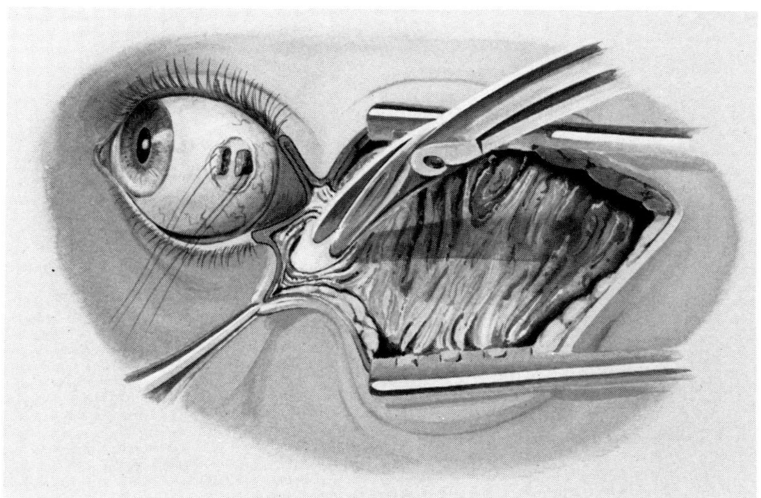

Fig. 23-11. The zygomatic bone is approached as the soft tissue is divided, exposing the periosteum of the orbital wall. A lateral canthotomy has been carried out with respect for the lateral canthal ligament.

LATERAL ORBITOTOMY

In the past, the lateral canthotomy was converted into a lateral orbitotomy (see Figure 23-6). Now, having practically abandoned lateral canthotomy, we proceed with an anterolateral skin incision similar to that advocated by Wright.[31]

We initially disinsert the lateral rectus muscle from its insertion and place "stay" sutures on the muscle as well as on the insertion site. These will serve for traction on the globe and the lateral rectus muscle to aid in dissection when the muscle cone is opened (Figure 23-9).

For lesions in the upper orbit, a running S-type skin incision beginning in the outer one third of the lateral supraorbital area is made extending along Langer's skin lines into the preauricular area for a distance of 30 to 40 mm (see Figure 23-7). Alternatively, if the tumor is located in the lower part of the orbit, we perform an inverted S-type skin incision beginning in the outer one third of the lateral infraorbital area and extending along Langer's skin lines into the preauricular area (see Figure 23-8).

Dissection then is rapidly carried down to the periorbita of the lateral orbital rim. With the combined anterolateral inci-

sions described above, it is unnecessary to remove the lateral canthal ligament from the periorbita. The orbicularis muscle insertions are then freed from the lateral orbital rim to an area above the zygomaticofrontal suture line and below the zygomaticomaxillary suture line (Figure 23-10). The temporalis muscle can be dissected off of the bone now exposed if the deep posterior one third of the orbit is to be explored, or it can be left intact on the posterior aspect of the lateral bony wall if more adequate exposure is not necessary (Figure 23-11). It is our custom to perform all cutting maneuvers on the muscle with electrocautery instruments. This obtains hemostasis at the same time and is a much faster technique than cutting and clamping bleeders. An incision now is made into the periorbita parallel to the lateral orbital rim (Figure 23-12) 4 mm behind the margin. It is then extended up and down the zygomatic arch using the suture lines described above to delimit the superior and inferior aspects of this incision. The periosteum then is stripped forward to the orbital rim and into the orbital cavity (Figure 23-13). It then is easily separated from the bony lateral wall posteriorly toward the apex of the orbit. "Bleeders" are usually encountered in the subperiosteal space and one can

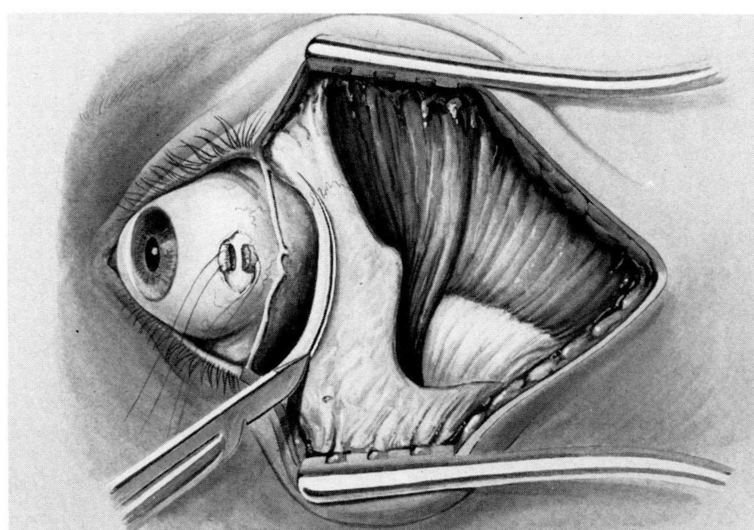

Fig. 23-12. After the lateral bony structures of the orbit have been exposed, the periosteum is incised on the surface. The divided lateral rectus is identified.

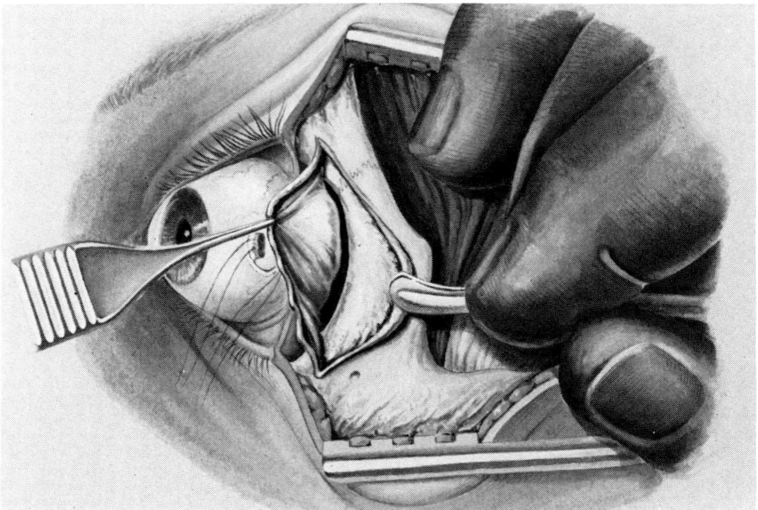

Fig. 23-13. The periosteum is divided and elevated using a periosteal elevator. Multiple orbital retractors developed by Kennerdell and Maroon are very helpful for surgery in this area.

identify the zygomatic artery anteriorly and the meningeal branch of the lacrimal artery posteriorly. These are usually coagulated by either electrocautery or bipolar coagulation and cause no bleeding problems. Attention is once again turned to the temporalis muscle, which is reflected posteriorly by blunt dissection to expose the posterolateral aspect of the orbital wall and free the muscle from the temporal fossa. Much bleeding may be encountered in this maneuver from the pterygoid plexus but is readily contained by electrocoagulation. Alternatively, the temporalis may be left adherent to the posterolateral bony wall and not cleared from the temporalis fossa until the bony wall is broken posteriorly.

Marks are now made with the Stryker saw in the bony lateral wall just above the zygomaticofrontal suture line and below the zygomaticomaxillary suture line. The orbital contents must be protected during this maneuver by means of a malleable ribbon retractor placed in the subperiosteal space (Figure 23-14). If the temporalis muscle has been disinserted, two drill holes are made at the upper and lower ends of the deep bone cuts so that the bone can be wired back into place after the operation is concluded. If the muscle is left intact, it acts as a

hinge for the later bony wall, which can be reflected posteriorly to expose the temporal fossa. Once the bone cuts have been made above the zygomaticofrontal suture and below the zygomaticomaxillary suture, the lateral bony wall can be removed. If the temporalis muscle is left intact, one can merely break back the bone with a Coker clamp. Alternatively, if the muscle has been disinserted, the Stryker saw can be used to join the upper and lower bone cuts by incising bone at the junction of the zygoma with the greater wing of the sphenoid. The bone becomes very thin at the sphenozygomatic suture, and in some patients it has been noted to be almost membranous in character, so that great care must be taken in joining the superior and inferior bone cuts with the Stryker saw. It is actually safer to break back the bone at this point as described above. More bone can be removed from the greater wing of the sphenoid with a rongeur until the temporal bone is exposed. By this technique, adequate exposure of the middle and posterior one third of the orbit can be obtained (Figure 23-15).

Hemostasis is very important in avoiding the postoperative problems that will be discussed below. Bleeding from soft tissue is contained by electrodissection, electrocoagulation, or by use

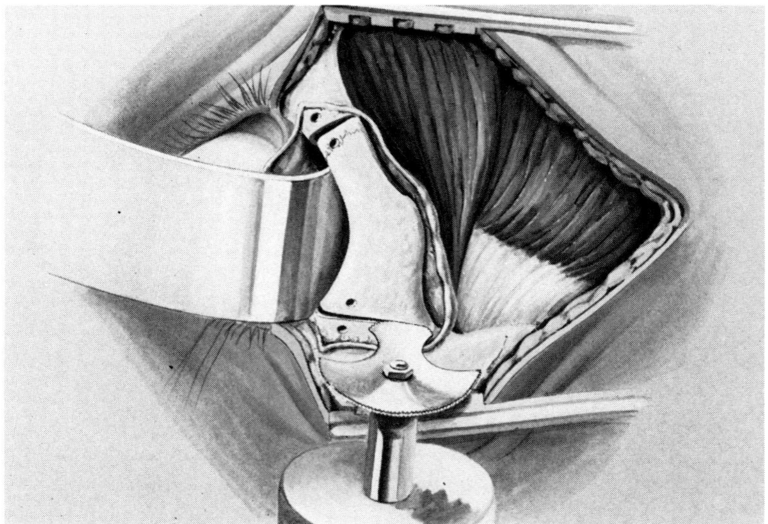

Fig. 23-14. The zygomatic bone is divided using a bone saw, being careful to protect the globe. Holes for wiring at the completion of surgery are prepared before sawing for better placement.

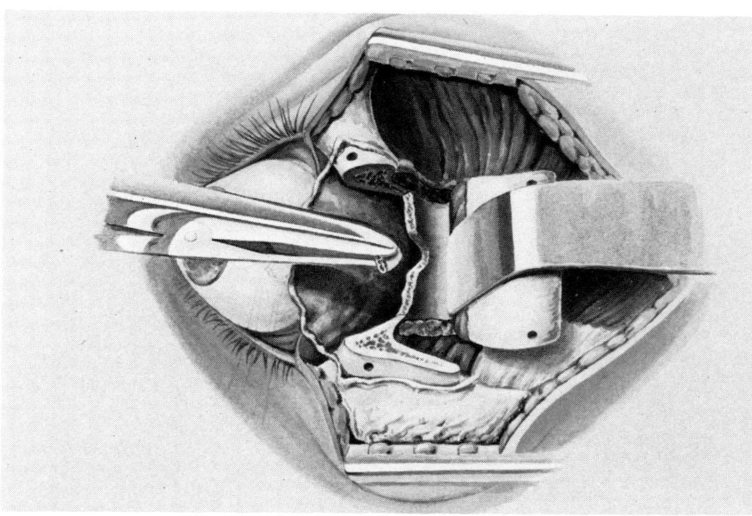

Fig. 23-15. Additional exposure is obtained by removing the lateral wall of the orbit using the rongeur.

of bipolar coagulation as the operation proceeds. Bleeding from bone is contained with bone wax or Avitene. Bone wax has been used successfully for many years without complications, but recently Trokel[32] reported a case of osteomyelitis in the sectioned bone that he attributed to bone wax. An alternative method of stopping bleeding from bone is by applying the electrocoagulator to the suction tip while the suction tip is in contact with the bone. Whatever method one chooses, complications are avoided by obtaining hemostasis as one proceeds with the operative dissection.

Once the bone has been removed, the retrobulbar contents are now visible from the subperiosteal space. Gentle palpation for the tumor now can be carried out and the surgical situation appraised. Careful observation of the pupil for dilation must be made when palpating the optic nerve; pressure should be immediately removed if this occurs. Some authors[33] have reported the use of continuous monitoring of visual evoked response (VER) during intraorbital surgery for more sensitive observation of adverse effects.

Tugging on the suture applied to the disinserted lateral rectus muscle aids in orientation before incising the periorbita (Figure 23-16). If the lesion has been localized above the plane

of the lateral rectus muscle, the incision through the periorbita into the peripheral surgical space is made above the superior edge of the muscle. If the tumor lies below the plane of the lateral rectus muscle, the incision through the periorbita into the peripheral surgical space is made below the inferior edge of the muscle.

Many lesions lie in the peripheral surgical space, and further dissection is carried out at this time to either biopsy or totally excise the mass. Surgery in the peripheral space is not as hazardous as that in the central surgical space, but use of an operating microscope with coaxial illumination is very helpful at this stage to avoid cutting vital structures.

Very little orbital fat is encountered in the peripheral surgical space, so that visibility usually is easily obtained by packing off the fat that does prolapse with neurosurgical cottonoid "patties." One must remember that orbital fat is laced with fine septae in which run vascular bundles, so that rough handling can precipitate additional bleeding that will have to be contained.

An incision next is made into the outer layer of Tenon's fascia just above or below the lateral rectus muscle. It is advisable not to strip the fascia from the muscle because this

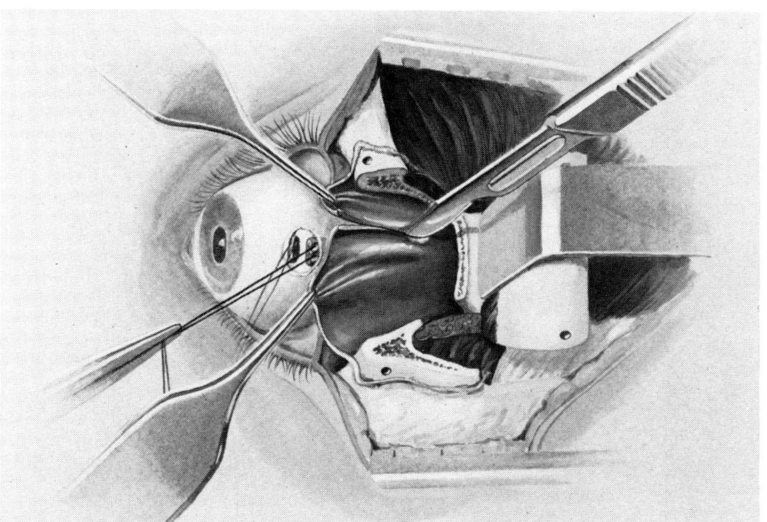

Fig. 23-16. The bony lateral wall has been removed and the periorbita is divided to provide exposure to the orbital contents.

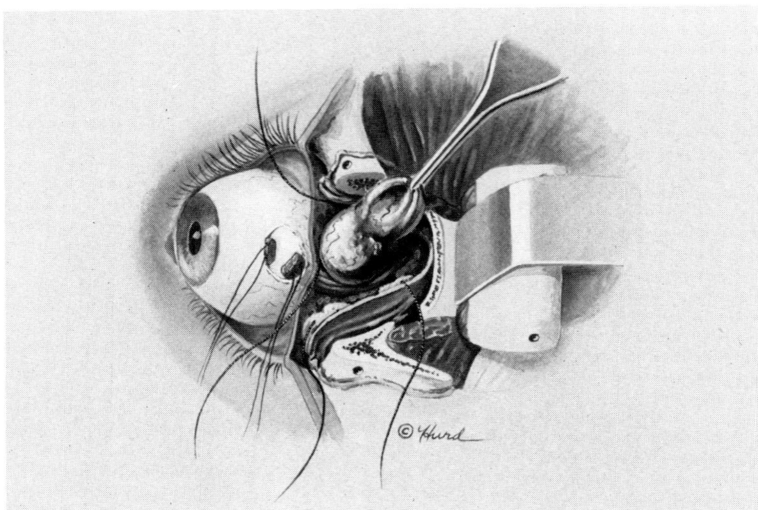

Fig. 23-17.   A tumor can be removed via the exposed site in the lateral orbital wall and the periorbita.

will promote scarring of the muscle itself or adhesions of the muscle to the canthotomy scar. Orientation by tugging on the sutures applied to the disinserted end of the muscle is helpful at this stage. The central surgical or intraconal space is now available for surgical intervention (Figure 23-17).

Exploration of the intraconal space must be done with uninhibited visibility. Magnification is essential at this stage to avoid vital structures. The lateral rectus muscle is retracted upward or downward depending upon the location of the mass within the muscle cone. Retraction of the muscle should be performed with a blunt instrument such as a malleable ribbon retractor or one of the "paddles" attached to the knobs on the self-retaining retractor designed by Maroon and Kennerdell. This avoids tearing or hemorrhage into the muscle from a traction suture. Avulsion of the lateral rectus muscle from its site of origin can occur if the assistant is too vigorous at this stage. By disinserting the muscle, however, this complication is readily avoided.

Blunt dissection within the muscle cone is dangerous but is quite helpful in delivering smooth encapsulated tumors from surrounding soft tissue when visibility is unobstructed. Instruments such as periosteal elevators or those designed by Penfield for neurosurgical use or by Freer for dissection in the nasopharynx are useful in stripping the encapsulated mass from the adjacent tissue. Vascular lesions such as cavernous hemangiomas are difficult to grasp with forceps. Traction can be obtained by engaging such masses with a cryoprobe or a Babcock hemorrhoid clamp. Other more solid masses can be grasped with an Allis forceps to help with delivery. By exerting traction with these methods with one hand and stripping the capsule with an instrument held in the other, the tumor is readily removed from its bed. Any vascular pedicle can be electrocoagulated and cut by scissors before delivery of the mass. Bulky cavernous hemangiomas or other vascular lesions can be reduced in size by squeezing out the bloody contents before applying the cryoprobe or Babcock clamp.

Cystic lesions can be removed intact with the aid of a cryoprobe, but if the mass is large it is safer to open the cyst wall and aspirate the contents before removing the capsule to avoid inadvertent rupture. Dermoid cysts contain sebaceous material that is quite toxic to the orbital soft tissue. Marked inflammation can result when the cyst wall leaks spontaneously into surrounding tissue. If rupture occurs inadvertently during surgery, copious irrigation must be performed to wash out as much of the material as possible and the patient given parenteral corticosteroids to suppress any ensuing inflammatory

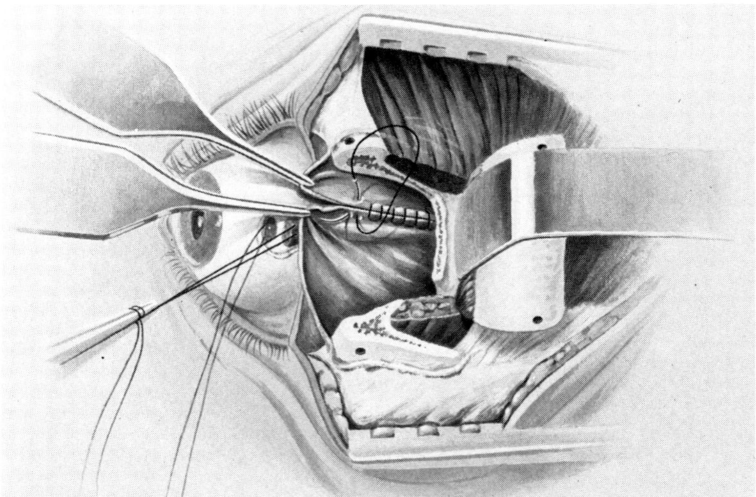

Fig. 23-18.   The periorbita is closed with 3-0 chromic gut as the first step in the repair of the lateral orbitotomy.

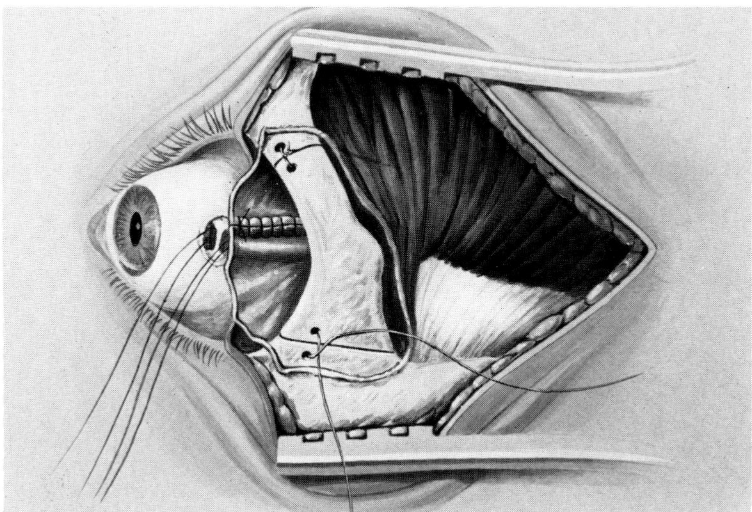

Fig. 23-19. Wire (No. 26 stainless steel) is used to fix the bone segment of the zygoma in place using the predrilled holes. The periosteum, soft tissue, and skin are closed in layers. This approach allows exposure to at least two thirds of the lateral orbit.

reaction. By using the above technique, postoperative inflammation with its attendant danger to vision is avoided.

Infiltrative lesions sometimes are difficult to separate from the surrounding structures without doing serious damage. It is in such situations that surgical judgment is important.

If, on clinical grounds, the surgeon feels that intraorbital surgery may not be the definitive treatment, then an adequate biopsy that debulks the orbit will suffice. Lesions such as sclerosing inflammatory pseudotumors, lymphomas, metastatic tumors, or rhabdomyosarcomas fall into this category. Frozen sections have been very helpful in such situations in our clinic, but these vary from institution to institution and depend upon the experience of the surgical pathologist. Before performing any radical surgery, it certainly is prudent to await permanent sections with review and consultation by pathologists who are familiar with orbital pathologic conditions.

We have found debulking, with incomplete surgical removal, to be useful in dealing with a host of incurable tumors that have invaded from adjacent structures. Lesions such as inverting papillomas from the nasal and paranasal cavities, chondrosarcomas, and sphenoid ridge meningiomas have been treated in this fashion. In some instances, vision has been restored or binocularity regained by debulking.

If the pathologic study is indeterminate at the time of the operation, even with frozen section, it is far better to terminate the surgical procedure than to proceed with total extirpation that may destroy vision unnecessarily. One can always return another day with a more certain plan.

In evaluating the central surgical space, gentle traction can be exerted on the suture placed into the stump of the scleral insertion of the lateral rectus muscle. This maneuver pulls the optic nerve into view without direct pressure by the surgeon. The short posterior ciliary arteries are readily seen and should not be torn. It is important to remember that the central retinal artery enters the optic nerve inferiorly about 10 to 15 mm behind the globe. If the dural sheath is to be opened, it is well to incise it on its anterolateral surface, well away from its vasculature.

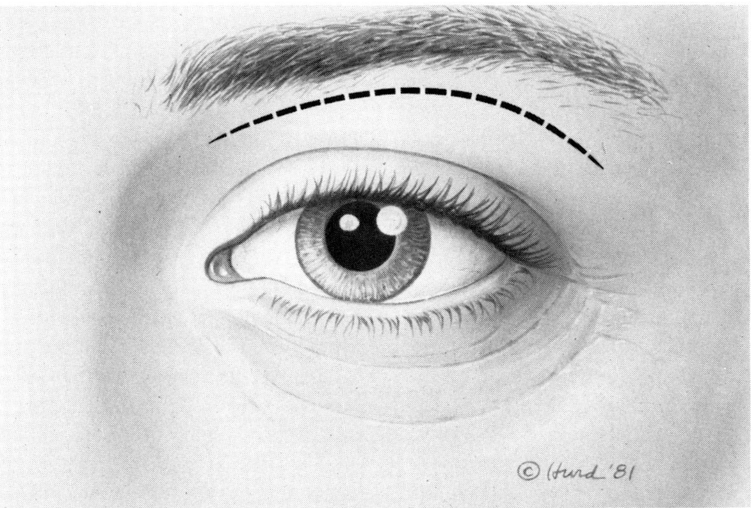

Fig. 23-20. The approach to the superior aspect of the orbit requires selection of folds in the lid or an initial incision above the brow. The area of the orbit to be approached determines the exact placement of the initial incision.

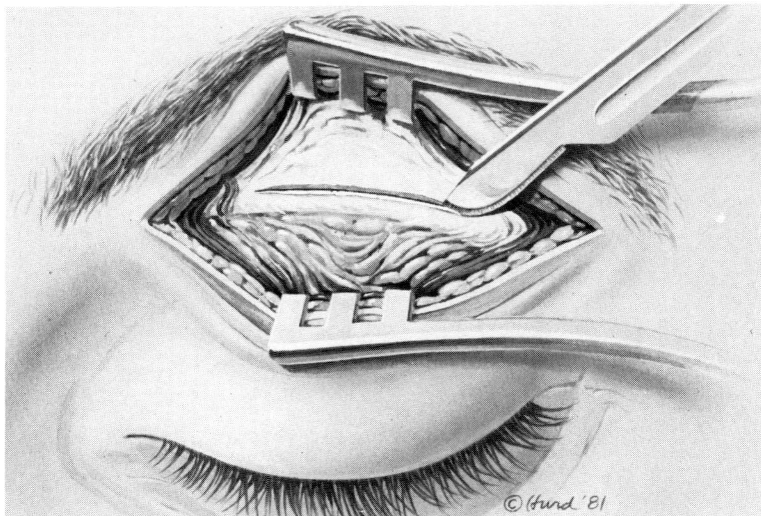

Fig. 23-21. The orbital rim and periosteum are exposed after separating the soft tissue and muscle. The periosteum is cleanly divided and the periosteal elevator is used to follow the roof of the orbit to the area of interest.

In dealing with a perioptic meningioma, the dural sheath should be opened as noted above. Gentle suction then should be applied to the subdural space to suck out the exuding tumor. It is easy to strip the blood supply of the optic nerve in operating on this kind of tumor, since it tends to invade the pial vessels in its natural course. Mark et al.[34] has recently reported successful removal of such tumors with restoration of good vision.

In the event that one decides to excise an optic nerve glioma for cosmetic reasons, care should be taken not to damage the nerve supply to the extraocular muscles. It is not our philosophy to remove these tumors, which we consider hamartomas. We do, however, recommend their biopsy to rule out meningioma or their removal for cosmetic reasons, but we advise retention of the globe.

Wright et al.[31] have recently reported the use of continuous monitoring of the visual evoked response (VER) during orbital surgery. Although we are not equipped for this procedure and have no experience with its use, it definitely would seem to be indicated in dealing with optic nerve tumors. This would be of special importance in those institutions using hypotensive anesthesia,[34] where hypoxia of the optic nerve is enhanced by the anesthetic.

We have adequately handled lesions in the nasal part of the orbit by an anteronasal type of approach modified from the classical Lynch incision for ethmoidectomy. In some instances it has been necessary to combine this with a lateral orbitotomy. This combination allows the globe and retrobulbar contents to be displaced laterally, making room for an adequate exposure of the medial portion of the orbit by a direct attack. The medial canthal ligament is disinserted in some cases by an incision through the periosteum high on the nasal bone. By tagging this with a 4-0 black silk suture and bluntly reflecting it laterally, the tear sac is displaced with the orbital contents to expose the medial subperiosteal space. By bluntly pushing the tissue off the medial wall, the entire ethmoid bone can be visualized almost to the apex. Care must be taken not to disinsert the trochlea, which lies approximately 4 mm behind the orbital rim in the nasal portion of the roof. The anterior and posterior ethmoid arteries may be encountered as well as branches of the ophthalmic artery but can be electrocoagulated as the dissection progresses since visibility by this approach is excellent.

Dermoids, mucoceles from the frontoethmoid group of sinus air cells, and ethmoid sinus tumors that have broken into the orbit have been encountered here.

Tumors lying in the nasal peripheral surgical space or the nasal portion of the central surgical space, nasal to the optic nerve, have been removed by us using this technique.

It must be remembered that the optic nerve lies nasally, so dissection in the intraconal space at this point should be performed with adequate exposure and not done in a "blind" fashion. It is most helpful in these instances to tug on the stay suture attached to the globe to move the eye laterally into the lateral orbitotomy for better exposure and orientation. It sometimes helps to further mobilize the globe by passing sutures under the other recti muscles for lateral traction.

After the mass is removed, a Penrose drain is placed in its bed to aid in the escape of blood or fluid that may collect in the dead space. The drain is brought out through the lateralmost edge of the incision, where it is anchored with 6-0 black silk to the skin after the wound is closed.

Closure is accomplished by suturing the outer layer of Tenon's fascia superior or inferior to the lateral rectus muscle with 4-0 chromic gut. The periorbita is closed as a separate layer with 3-0 chromic gut. Special care is given to a layer-by-layer closure to avoid incorporating the lateral rectus muscle in the wound (Figure 23-18).

If the bone has been left hinged to the temporalis muscle, there is no need to wire it back into place, since merely suturing the overlying periosteum accomplishes the repositioning of the bone flap. In the event that the muscle has been disinserted from the bone, however, wiring is necessary. This is accomplished with No. 26 stainless steel wire inserted through the previously prepared drill holes. Twisting the wire will firmly position the bone in its original location (Figure 23-19). The Penrose drain now lies behind the bone in the temporal fossa with its tip in the bed of the excised tumor and its other end in the lateral edge of the skin incision. The lateral canthal ligament is sutured to periorbita with 3-0 chromic gut. Subcutaneous tissue is closed in layers, using 4-0 chromic gut for the fascia of the temporalis and orbicularis muscles, and 5-0 plain gut for the superficial tissue. The skin is closed with a continuous running suture of either 6-0 silk or 6-0 nylon.

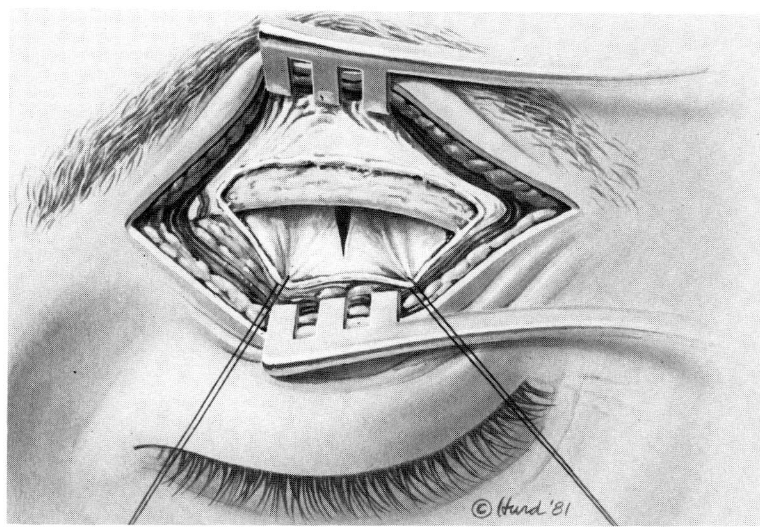

Fig. 23-22. The periorbita is divided and the orbital contents are exposed. Closure layer by layer is required.

Closure of the medial canthotomy is accomplished in a similar fashion. It is most important to resuture the medial canthal ligament with 4-0 chromic gut to the previously prepared area in the periosteum of the nasal bone. Failure to perform this step results in a marked cosmetic defect and tearing because of eversion of the lower punctum.

ANTERIOR ORBITAL APPROACH

For lesions lying in the superior anterior two thirds of the orbit outside of the central surgical space, the anterior orbital approach is an excellent approach and one that we prefer to the lateral orbitotomy (Figures 23-20 through 23-23).

An incision is made superiorly along the inferior margin of the eyebrow from the medial to the lateral canthus. If it is necessary to explore the superonasal quadrant as well, the skin incision is carried downward halfway between the medial canthus and the anterior aspect of the nasal bone, well down onto the lateral aspect of the nose.

The nasal aspect of the incision usually is quite vascular, and hemostasis should be obtained as the operation proceeds. The supraorbital notch is first encountered with its neurovascular bundle. This is usually sacrificed during the procedure so that anesthesia in the appropriate dermatome is expected. The patient should have been warned preoperatively to anticipate numbness in the forehead and scalp after surgery. The supratrochlear and dorsal nasal arteries also pierce the septum and must be coagulated at this time.

An incision is made into the periosteum along the entire length of the incision (see Figure 23-21). The subperiosteal space now is entered as the periosteum is elevated from the underlying bone (see Figure 23-22). Medially (Figures 23-24, 23-25; see also Figure 23-23), the anterior and posterior ethmoid arteries are encountered at the frontoethmoid suture line. Bleeding from these can be quite annoying but can be readily controlled by cautery and packing for a short period.

The periorbita is reflected downward with a malleable ribbon retractor. We have encountered dermoids, hematomas, metastatic tumors, mucoceles, and myelocytomas in this space (Figure 23-26).

It should be remembered that the levator muscle runs below the orbital roof and is separated from it by the periorbita, a thin layer of fat, and the frontal nerve. The levator is loosely suspended from the periorbita by connective tissue but is

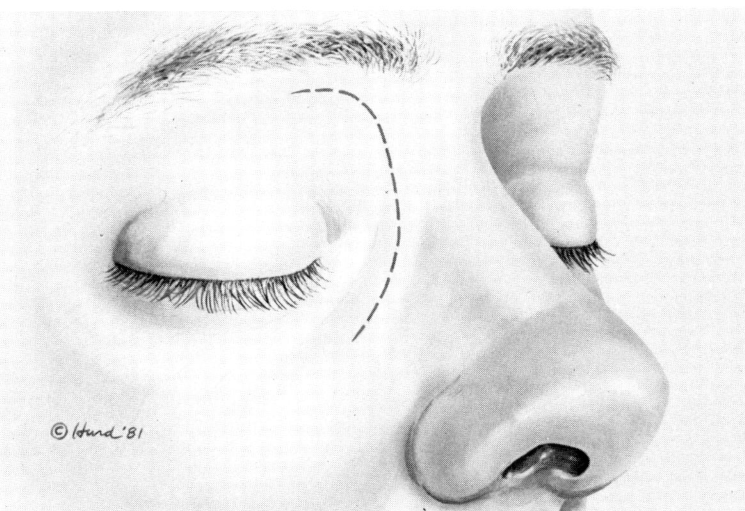

Fig. 23-23. The approach to the medial side of the orbit and the lacrimal fossa. The angular artery and vein may be encountered.

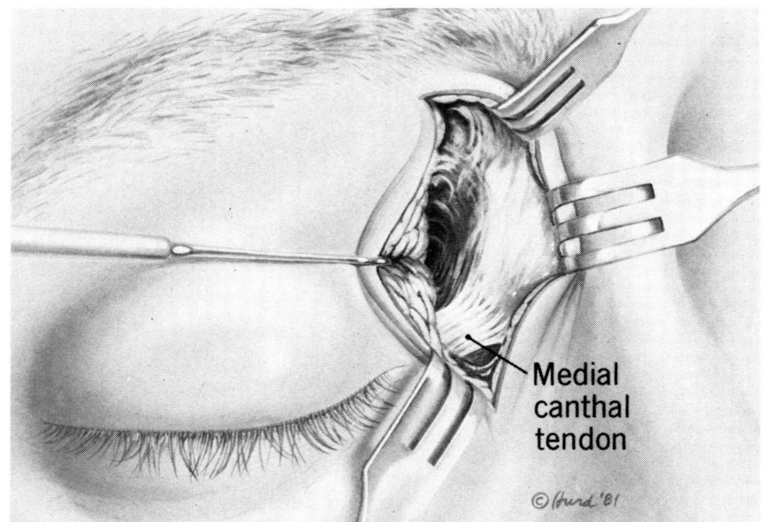

Fig. 23-24. The tissue is reflected until the medial canthal ligament is identified.

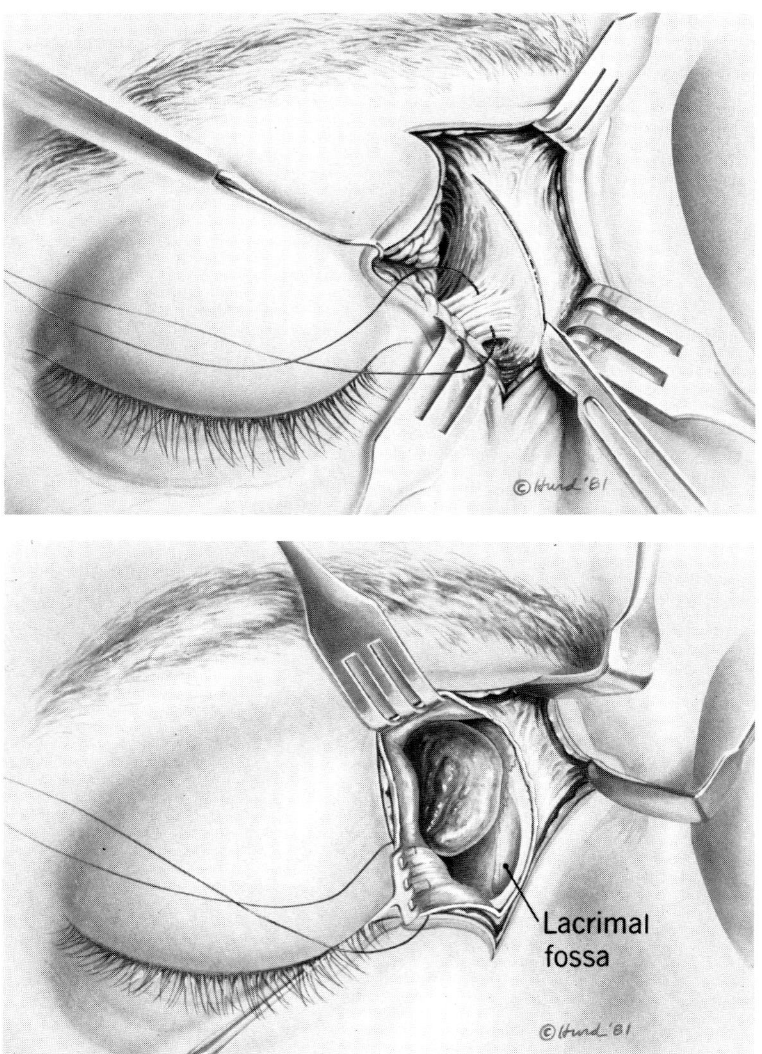

Figs. 23-25 and 23-26. The periosteum is divided anterior to the medial canthal ligament, and the ligament and tissue are reflected laterally to expose the lacrimal sac and fossa. Further exploration can be made with periosteal elevation. The ethmoidal vessels should be observed and recognized. See Figure 23-1, which shows the medial wall of the orbit as seen when the periosteum is reflected.

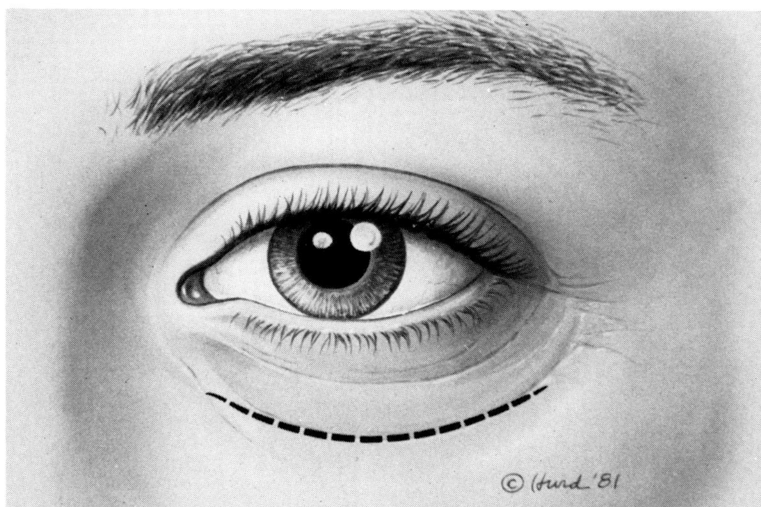

Fig. 23-27. The inferior approach to the orbit requires selection of an incision line along normal skin folds. Cosmetic closure and function can be improved if this is done.

continuous with the septum anteriorly as the levator aponeurosis approaches the tarsus. Injury to these anatomic relationships can result in a permanent ptosis. The patient should be warned about this preoperatively. In any event, there usually is some degree of postoperative ptosis that resolves after 2 to 3 weeks in most cases.

As exploration of the superior subperiosteal space continues, care must be taken in palpating the roof or in passing a periosteal elevator in this area. In many cases the bone is quite thin and becomes nonexistent from pressure of orbital expanding masses. Penetration at this point may tear the dura underlying the anterior cranial cavity and unnecessarily complicate the operation.

Exploration of the medial aspect may result in contact with the trochlea. Damage to this structure will result in postoperative diplopia from malfunction of the superior oblique muscle. If the tumor involves this area, the trochlea can be removed, but it should be replaced to avoid the above complication. Further dissection medially has already been described above.

The periorbita now should be opened in an anteroposterior vertical fashion to avoid damage to the structures described above that run at right angles to this plane. Evaluation of the superior peripheral surgical space may now proceed. We have encountered cavernous hemangiomas, inflammatory pseudotumors, and metastatic tumors most commonly in this space. Dissection should follow the techniques and caveats outlined under the discussion of lateral orbitotomy.

Closure is accomplished by suturing the periorbita with 3–0 chromic gut. It is most important to carefully reattach the periosteum to the orbital rim in order to support the upper lid. Drains are not usually inserted, but if drainage is deemed necessary, the Penrose drain can be brought out through the skin incision and anchored laterally or passed through the ethmoid air cells into the nasal cavity medially.

Incisions at the inferior rim are less common than those at the superior margin. Davis[10] used this approach to tumors of the optic nerve, but masses are encountered less commonly in the lower part of the orbit than in the upper in our experience. We have used this surgical approach most commonly to decompress the orbit into the antrum in cases of Graves' orbitopathy. We have encountered dermoids, rhabdomyosarcomas, and cavernous hemangiomas under the optic nerve

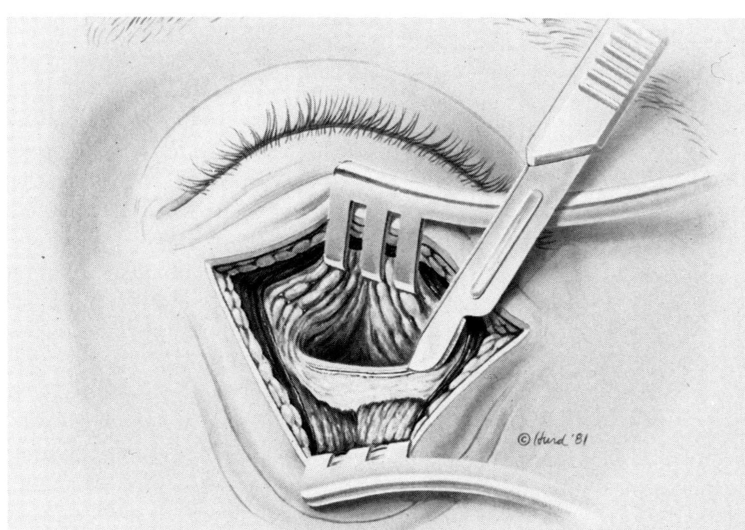

Fig. 23-28. The orbital rim is identified and the muscle and soft tissue divided so that they are directed toward the anterior surface of the rim.

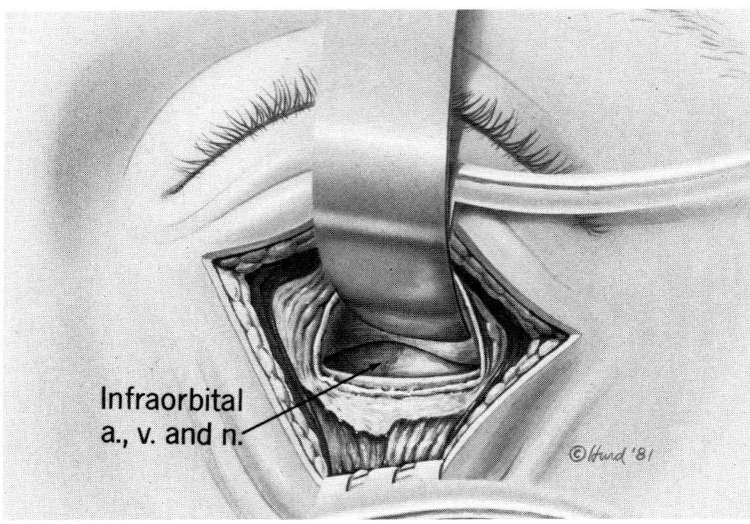

Fig. 23-29.   The periosteum is divided using a sharp blade. The periosteal elevator allows exposure back along the inferior aspect of the orbit. Upon completion of the operation the incisions are closed layer by layer and the periosteum is closed. The infraorbital artery, nerve, and vein are visible as the floor is exposed.

and extension from antral malignancies in the inferior part of the orbit.

The incision is made through the skin at the inferior orbital rim and is carried down to the periosteum (Figures 23-27 through 23-29). The septum should be avoided as the periosteum is incised below the rim. The periorbita is elevated and the subperiosteal space invaded. The infraorbital nerve and vessels are visible lying in the infraorbital canal and can usually be avoided. The patient should be warned of postoperative anesthesia of the lip, however. The periosteum is stripped from the floor up toward the apex and then is opened vertically in an anteroposterior direction to gain access to the peripheral surgical space. The origins of the inferior oblique muscle and tear sac lie medially and should be avoided. The optic nerve also lies medially and can be damaged if dissection is too vigorous after the central space is entered. It should also be remembered that the central retinal artery enters the nerve on its undersurface 10 to 15 mm behind the globe. Based on our experience, it is quite dangerous to approach lesions in this space in the deep orbit unless combined with a lateral orbitotomy that allows displacement of the globe and retrobulbar contents upward and laterally.

Closure is accomplished with interrupted sutures of 3-0 chromic gut to reattach the periosteum to the orbital rim. Drains can be brought out at the temporal aspect of the wound or through a separate stab wound, especially if the interior incision is combined with a lateral approach.

SURGERY OF LACRIMAL GLAND TUMORS

Special consideration should be given to tumors of the lacrimal gland. Wright and his co-workers,[36,37] Stewart and his fellow workers,[38] Henderson and Neult,[39] Henderson and Farrow,[40] and Font and Gamel[41,42] have published excellent papers on this subject.

As pointed out by Wright et al.,[36] if there is a history of a mass in the lacrimal fossa with a duration of less than 6 months, the lesion should be regarded as malignant until proved otherwise by an adequate biopsy. Adenoid cystic carcinoma of the lacrimal gland carries such a poor prognosis that very radical surgery is necessary to cure the patient.[36–42] The decision for

such a procedure should not be made on the basis of frozen sections but should await permanent sections for histopathologic diagnosis. Death usually results from intracranial extension with bony invasion, although lymph node metastases can occur.

It is important to obtain a satisfactory amount of representative lacrimal gland tissue for histopathologic examination. The surgical approach for biopsy must be adequate to achieve this goal. Rees and Jones[43] have stressed the importance of making a lateral approach without removal of bone for this purpose. This approach uses a modified anterolateral skin incision. The upper part of the lateral canthal ligament is disinserted from the bone and the skin undermined upward over the brow. This exposes the lateral portion of the superior orbital rim. The fossa of the lacrimal gland lies just behind the orbital rim in the lateral aspect of the roof. The lateral horn of the levator aponeurosis crosses the gland but is reflected upward with the detached lateral canthal ligament when the tumor of the lacrimal gland is exposed.

If the biopsy specimen proves to be adenoid cystic carcinoma of the lacrimal gland, exenteration with radical removal of bone must be accomplished. Wright et al.[36] advocated a radical combined neurosurgical and orbital procedure that removes the bony lateral wall and roof of the orbit together with exenteration of the orbital contents. Craniotomy is performed to remove the roof. Closure is by means of mobilization of scalp skin flaps to close the dead space. Henderson and Neult[39] designed a less radical procedure. We have used exenteration combined with removal of the bony lateral wall and roof without craniotomy. Closure is accomplished with split thickness skin grafts. Survival is rare from this most malignant of tumors, so that such radical methods of treatment are considered worthwhile to save life.

If the biopsy proves the tumor to be a lymphoma or an inflammation, treatment of the former condition by irradiation and the latter by corticosteroids is usually successful.

If the history of the mass is longer than 1 year, we have followed Wright's advice in removing the entire mass in the initial procedure. Benign mixed (pleomorphic) adenoma of the lacrimal gland is the most likely diagnosis. The gland should be removed with its overlying periorbita to prevent rupture of the capsule.

The best surgical approach for mixed tumor of the lacrimal gland is the anterolateral orbitotomy with removal of the bony lateral wall as described previously. The entire gland should be removed with its overlying periorbita to prevent rupture of the capsule with possible seeding and recurrence. If the bone appears to be involved, this should be removed also, together with the adjacent healthy bone.

The dura can be exposed during these procedures but can be covered with orbital soft tissue when closure is performed. If the dura is penetrated, it must be repaired to prevent cerebrospinal fluid leak and possible meningitis. The technique for dealing with this complication is discussed below.

COMPLICATIONS

Despite the many admonitions noted above in discussion of the various techniques, complications still occur from orbital surgery. With some experience, however, these are rare occurrences today.

COMPLICATIONS DURING SURGERY
INCISIONS IN SKIN

Improper incisions lead to poor exposure and compound the problems during the operation. Skin incisions should be made in Langer's skin lines to avoid cosmetic defects. They should be adequate and extend into the preauricular area for approximately 30 mm from the lateral canthus.

Incisions at a right angle to the skin lines can also result in severance of the facial nerve with ensuing paralysis of the orbicularis muscle. This can occur at the termination of the procedure if a stab wound is made at right angles to Langer's skin lines to bring out the Penrose drain from the wound at a separate site from the skin incision.

Incisions in the Bone

Bony cuts with the Stryker saw must be made judiciously, protecting the soft tissue with a malleable ribbon retractor to prevent damage to the retrobulbar tissues. In addition, if the cut is made too high above the zygomaticofrontal suture line, the anterior cranial cavity may be entered and the dura may be damaged. The dura also can be damaged if too vigorous a dissection is made along the roof where the bone is thin. In medial incisions, the lacrimal bone and ethmoid bone must be treated with similar respect since they are also thin and liable to be penetrated with ease. Penetration of the ethmoid bone exposes the orbit to infection from the paranasal sinuses.

Lacrimal Apparatus

Damage to the lacrimal gland can occur as the superotemporal quadrant is explored. Care must be taken to note the position of the normal lacrimal gland and to dissect posterior to it. The normal gland frequently prolapses into the wound, especially if there is an expanding mass behind it. Biopsy should exclude the normal gland since scarring can occur, which produces lack of tearing and subsequent keratitis from a dry-eye syndrome.

When operating in the nasal quadrant, damage to the tear sac can occur if it is not pushed away from the medial wall as described above.

Vascular Damage

Most problems from orbital surgery result from a failure to obtain hemostasis as the operation proceeds or from occlusion of the central retinal artery or short posterior ciliary arteries. Failure to assure proper hemostasis leads to postoperative oozing with increase of intraorbital pressure and occlusion of vital arteries. Insertion of a Penrose drain affords an escape path for a collection of blood and fluid postoperatively.

Overenthusiastic palpation and traction during surgery in the central (intraconal) space can lead to optic nerve ischemia, infarction of the retina, or vitreous hemorrhage. Retinal detachments also have occurred from rough handling of tumors adjacent to the posterior aspect of the globe.

It is our custom to give intravenous corticosteroids during surgery to prevent inadvertent edema of the optic nerve with its attendant complications.

Damage to Muscles and Nerves

Postoperative anesthesia is the rule in the area supplied by the supraorbital or infraorbital nerves when the anterior approach is used. The patient should be merely warned about this, since avulsion of these structures is practically a necessary part of the operation in obtaining proper exposure. The nerves usually regenerate, but we have seen a neuroma develop in the supraorbital scar following an anterior approach.

Ptosis is a common finding after the anterior superior approach. This usually subsides after a few weeks, but severe damage to the levator or nerve supply or to the levator aponeurosis can result in permanent ptosis. This can be prevented by maintaining the integrity of the orbital septum and ligamentous attachments of the levator to the medial and lateral aspects of the superior orbital rim. If ptosis persists for longer than 6 months, repair may be considered.

Damage to motor nerves that supply the extraocular muscles should be avoided when operating in the intraconal space to prevent palsy after surgery. Overzealous traction on the extraocular muscles in general and the lateral rectus muscle in particular should be avoided to prevent avulsion of the muscle or fracture of the muscle fibers with intramuscular hemorrhage. We have witnessed avulsion of the lateral rectus muscle from its origin. Disinsertion of the muscle before surgery has become routine in our hands to prevent this complication. As noted above under the description of technique of lateral orbitotomy, the muscle is tagged with a locked suture, and a traction suture is placed through the stump of the insertion on the globe. This serves the dual purpose of locating the lateral rectus muscle for orientation before entering the central surgical space during surgery and of mobilizing the optic nerve by traction on the globe.

Damage to the ciliary ganglion can result in permanent iridoplegia. Interruption of the ophthalmic branch of the trigeminal nerve in deep orbital surgery in the posterior or apical department results in corneal anesthesia. If this occurs, tarsorrhaphy must be performed as soon as possible to prevent corneal ulceration. Neuroparalytic keratitis is especially dangerous if associated with akinesia or paralysis of the orbicularis oculi muscle. If there is accompanying damage to the lacrimal gland that causes dryness of the eye, the outlook for corneal decompensation is almost certain.

Incarceration of the lateral rectus muscle into the scar of the lateral orbitotomy is a common complication that can be prevented during surgery. Care must be taken to close the outer layer of Tenon's fascia to prevent adhesions. The overlying periorbita must also be closed as a separate layer to further protect the integrity of the lateral rectus muscle. Pseudo-Duane's syndrome sometimes occurs when the muscle is incarcerated in the wound. Proof of mechanical restriction to differentiate it from paralysis of the muscle can be readily determined by a forced duction test. Computed tomographic scanning can also show this. It is difficult to correct this defect, even by careful lysis of the adhesions and encasing the muscle in a Supramid sleeve.

Dural Defects

In performing extensive orbital surgery for lesions near the orbital roof or in rough handling of the periorbita in stripping it from the roof during the superior anterior approach, the bone may be penetrated and the overlying dura torn. This is especially apt to happen in those cases of long-standing orbital tumor in which the bone has become quite thin from expansion of the orbital mass. If this occurs, it is most important to recognize the accident and deal with it at the time. Subsequent cerebrospinal fluid leak with the danger of meningitis can result if duraplastic repair is not performed.

We have encountered this complication and have been successful in repairing the torn dura with "postage stamp" grafts of fascia lata held in place by autopolymerizing glue. We have most recently used Histoacryl Blue tissue adhesive (butyl 2-cyanoacrylate) for this purpose.

A large specimen of fascia lata is taken and cut into small postage-stamp-sized grafts. A very thin film of Histoacryl is applied to the graft. The torn dura is dried adequately and the graft is applied to the defect. Overlapping grafts can be applied until the defect is completely covered and made watertight. Instruments or cottonoid swabs will stick to the tissue adhesive if they come in contact, so care must be taken in performing the repair to avoid this complication. Polymerization occurs within 10 seconds.

Some heat is given off during the process, therefore an excess use of the material should be avoided. Consultation with and the aid of neurosurgical colleagues can be helpful in this situation.

POSTOPERATIVE COMPLICATIONS VASCULAR DAMAGE AND TISSUE REACTION

In the early postoperative period, use of constrictive pressure dressings can elevate intraorbital pressure and occlude the central retinal artery. This is especially liable to occur if there is no Penrose drain in the deep orbital area to afford escape of slow bleeding or exudation. It is our custom to keep the drain in place for 48 to 72 hours postoperatively to obviate this difficulty, even after adequate hemostasis has been obtained at surgery.

Massive orbital edema with release of prostaglandins can complicate the postoperative period. We have already stated above that we begin intravenous corticosteroids during surgery to avoid inadvertent swelling of the optic nerve or orbital soft tissue. This is continued during the postoperative period for a varying duration depending upon the pathologic picture, the operative trauma, and the patient's response.

If the orbital soft tissue has been contaminated by the sebaceous material of a dermoid cyst, the tissue reaction may continue for a long period. Inflammatory pseudotumors or the myopathy of Graves' disease can be made worse by orbital surgery. In these events, corticosteroids will, of necessity, be used for a longer period of time than in less severe cases.

Infection and Foreign Body Reaction

Postoperative infection is a remote risk that accompanies any surgical procedure. Because orbital surgery usually takes several hours to complete with exposure of the orbital soft tissue to repeated irrigation and other surgical trauma, it is our custom to routinely use prophylactic broad-spectrum antibiotics during and after the procedure. Antibiotics are continued for 72 hours in the postoperative period.

In our experience with more than 200 orbitotomies, we have had one case of infection using this technique. The prophylactic use of an orbital drain and continuous use of systemic antibiotics prevented serious complication in this case.

Trokel[30] recently reported the occurrence of osteomyelitis in the bone flap. He attributed this to the use of bone wax.

We have experienced the occurrence of a postoperative orbital foreign body granuloma that resembled a tumor recurrence in the case of an optic nerve meningioma that was initially removed by craniotomy. Although tumor recurrence was present in this case, on histopathologic examination, organic fibers were identified in the granuloma.

Visual Loss

As indicated above, the most common cause of visual loss is optic nerve ischemia or infarction and occlusion of the short posterior ciliary arteries or of the central retinal artery. Optic atrophy, disorganization, and gliosis of the posterior pole become apparent several weeks after these episodes.

Another cause of visual loss in the postoperative period is persistence of choroidal and retinal folds that cross the macula. Even after removal of the tumor, these macular folds persist with failure of recovery of vision.

Tumor Recurrence

It is our custom to perform postoperative CT scanning 6 months after surgery to examine the anatomic state of the orbit and for tumor recurrence.

If reoperation becomes necessary in the event of a recurrence of an orbital tumor, it has been our experience that vascular embarrassment is more apt to occur than when the orbitotomy is initially performed.

Enophthalmos

After any surgical attack on the orbit, atrophy of the orbital fat can occur. Fat lobules are compartmentalized by connective tissue septae in which run a fine network of small and larger blood vessels. Disruption of these structures leads to bleeding, fibrosis, and ultimate atrophy of the adipose tissue. Enophthalmos then occurs. If this presents a cosmetic problem, there are oculoplastic procedures designed to correct it.

REFERENCES

1. Krönlein RU: Zur pathologie und operativen behandlung der dermoidcysten der orbita. Beitr Klin Chir 4:149, 1888
2. Dandy WE: Results following transcranial operative attack on orbital tumors. Arch Ophthalmol 25:191, 1941
3. Naffziger HC, Jones OW: The surgical treatment of progressive exophthalmos following thyroidectomy. JAMA 99:638, 1932

4. Naffziger HC: Pathologic changes in orbit in progressive exophthalmos with special reference to alterations in extra-ocular muscles and optic disks. Arch Ophthalmol 9:1, 1933

5. Iliff CE: Tumors of the orbit. Trans Am Ophthalmol Soc 55:505, 1957

6. Reese AB: Tumors of the Eye, ed 2. Hagerstown, MD: Harper & Row, 1963

7. Reese AB: Expanding lesions of the orbit (Bowman Lecture). Trans Ophthalmol Soc UK 91:85, 1971

8. Berke RN: A modified Kroenlein operation. Trans Am Ophthalmol Soc 51:193, 1953

9. Benedict WL: Surgical treatment of tumors and cysts of the orbit. Am J Ophthalmol 32:763, 1949

10. Davis FA: Primary tumors of the optic nerve. Arch Ophthalmol 23:735; 957, 1940

11. Foster J: The diagnosis and treatment of orbital tumors. Ann R Coll Surg Engl 17:114, 1955

12. Long JC, Ellis PP: Total unilateral visual loss following orbital surgery. Am J Ophthalmol 14:457, 1975

13. Alper MG: Computed tomography in planning and evaluating orbital surgery. Ophthalmology 87:418, 1980

14. Alper MG, Citrin CM: Computed Tomography of the Orbit, in Smith, Byron C (eds): Ophthalmic Plastic and Reconstructive Surgery, vol. 2. St. Louis, CV Mosby Co., 1987.

15. Wright JE: Surgery in the orbit, in Miller S (ed): Operative Surgery, ed 3. London, Butterworths, 1976

16. Kennerdell JS, Maroon JC: Lateral microsurgical approach to intraorbital tumors. J Neurosurg 44:556 1976

17. Kennerdell, JS: Orbital diagnosis, in Smith, Byron C (eds): Ophthalmic Plastic and Reconstructive Surgery, vol 2. St. Louis, CV Mosby Co, 1987

18. Lloyd GAS: CT scanning in diagnosis of orbital disease. Comput Tomogr 3:227, 1979

19. Hannafee WN: Orbital venography. Radiol Clin North Am 10:63, 1972

20. Lombardi G: Radiology in Neuro-ophthalmology. Baltimore, Williams & Wilkins, 1967

21. Alper MG, Rizzoli HV, Cowden J, et al: Value of x-ray and ultrasonography in evaluation of unilateral exophthalmos. Scientific Exhibit First Prize. Presented at the annual meeting of the American Academy of Ophthalmology and Otology, 1969

22. Manchester PT, Bonmati J: Iodopyracet (Diodrast) injection for orbital tumors. Arch Ophthalmol 54:591, 1955

23. Hansen E: Amaurose nach kontrastmittelfulung der kieferkohle. HNO 6:17, 1956–58

24. Sachsenweger R: Die roentgenologische darstellung des orbitalen optikus durch wasserlosische kontrastmitttel. Klin Monatsbl Augenheilkd 133:195, 1958

25. Jakobiec FA, Henkind P: Editorial. Ophthalmic CT scanning: The quest for precision and specificity. Ophthalmology 87:13A, 1980

26. Susac JO, Smith JL: The impossible meningioma. Arch Neurol 34:36, 1977

27. Zimmerman LE: Pathology and computed tomography. Ophthalmology 87:602, 1980

28. Hilal SK, Trokel SL: Computerized tomography of the orbit using thin sections. Semin Radiol 12:137, 1977

29. Knapp H: Exstirpation einer schnerven geschwulst mit erhaltung des augapfels. Klin Monatsbl Augenheilkd 12:439, 1874

30. Knapp H: A case of carcinoma of the outer sheath of the optic nerve, removed with preservation of the eyeball. Arch Ophthalmol 4:323, 1874

31. Wright JE: The role of surgery in the management of orbital tumors. Mod Probl Ophthalmol 14:553, 1975

32. Trokel SL: Case report to meeting of the Society of Orbital Surgeons, Bermuda, May, 1980

33. Wright JE, Arden G, Jones BR: Continuous monitoring of the visually evoked response during intraorbital surgery. Trans Ophthalmol Soc UK 93:311, 1973

34. Mark LE, Kennerdell JS, Maroon JC: Microsurgical removal of a primary intraorbital meningioma. Am J Ophthalmol 86:700, 1978

35. Smith GB: Anesthesia for orbital surgery: Observed changes in the visually evoked response at low blood pressures. Mod Probl Ophthalmol 14:457, 1975

36. Wright JE, Stewart WB, Krohel GB: Clinical presentation and management of lacrimal gland tumors. Br J Ophthalmol 63:600, 1979

37. Wright, JE: Factors affecting the survival of patients with lacrimal gland tumors. Can J Ophthalmol 17:3–9, 1982.

38. Stewart, WB, Krohel G., Wright JE: Lacrimal gland and fossa lesions,: An approach to diagnosis and management. Ophthalmology 86:886-895, 1979.

39. Henderson JW, Neult RW: En bloc removal of intrinsic neoplasms of the lacrimal gland. Am J Ophthalmol 82:905, 1976

40. Henderson JW, Farrow GM: Primary malignant mixed tumors of the lacrimal gland. Ophthalmology 87:466, 1980

41. Font RL, Gamel JW: Epithelial tumors of the lacrimal gland: An analysis of 265 cases, in Jakobiec FA (ed): Ocular and Adnexal Tumors. Birmingham, AL, Aesculapius Publishing Co., 1978

42. Font RL, Gamel JW: Adenoid cystic carcinoma of the lacrimal gland: A clinicopathologic study of 79 cases. In Nicholson DH (ed): Ocular Pathology Update. New York, Masson Publishing USA, 1980.

43. Reese AB, Jones IS: Bone resection in the excision of epithelial tumors of the lacrimal gland. Arch Ophthalmol 71:382, 1964

CHAPTER 24

Sphenoethmoid Approach to the Optic Nerve

Robert A. Sofferman

WITH CLOSED HEAD TRAUMA, visual impairment may develop as a complicating feature in nearly 5 percent of the cases.[1-4] In most instances the lesion can be localized to the canalicular segment of the optic nerve. Compressive edema or interruption of the proximal microvascular supply to the nerve are the most likely pathophysiologic mechanisms of injury.[2,4,5] Fractures of the optic canal can be missed with conventional canal views or polytomography, only to become apparent at surgery or postmortem analysis.[5]

The injury can be compared to traumatic facial nerve paralysis in temporal bone fractures. Both facial and optic nerves travel within a lengthy osseous canal and are covered by a noncompliant dural sheath. Both nerves receive their blood supply through a coaxial, subdural vascular network that enters at the open ends of the canal.[6,7] Although there are major differences in regeneration between these two "cranial nerves," it is likely that the potential for complete or partial recovery from ischemia depends in each system on osseous and sheath decompression. Most neurophthalmologists and neurosurgeons have learned through clinical experience that decompression in cases of total immediate traumatic blindness is unsuccessful.[1,2] This has been challenged somewhat in the Japanese literature.[8,9] The occasional successes cited in the American literature may have been a result of expedient decompression after the injury. Nevertheless, most neurosurgeons conservatively manage patients with immediate total traumatic amaurosis with the assumption that the optic nerve is avulsed at the proximal canalicular end or irreversibly infarcted.

The management of delayed traumatic peripheral facial paralysis can be compared with that of progressive visual deficits after head trauma. The facial nerve can be monitored by topognostic and electrophysiologic means with a relatively standard end point dictating surgical intervention. Most patients with traumatic canalicular visual loss are obtunded from the associated cerebral contusion, which complicates the monitoring of residual visual function or evidence of progressive impairment. Careful sequential neurophthalmologic examination to determine the development or progression of the Marcus-Gunn pupil may be the key to surgical preservation of vision. Perhaps the visual evoked response (VER) will play an important role in identifying residual vision in unconscious patients with a complete afferent pupillary defect. Most surgical

successes evolve from patients with delayed or partial visual loss,[1,2] analogous to the good result when decompression for facial nerve paralysis is undertaken early. These comments serve as an introduction to a new extracranial surgical approach to problems involving the canalicular segment of the optic nerve. The more comprehensive topic of optic nerve trauma and the precise timing of surgical intervention are beyond the intent of this chapter.

SURGICAL REQUIREMENTS FOR OPTIC NERVE DECOMPRESSION

As with facial nerve decompression, complete optic nerve decompression should include the following: (1) removal of at least half the circumference of the osseous canal; (2) removal of bone along the entire length of the optic canal, which measures between 5.5 and 11.5 mm;[10] and (3) total longitudinal incision of the dural sheath including the annulus of Zinn. These guidelines for adequate decompression allow for comprehensive surgical management of any lesion that might compress the optic nerve within the osseous canal. Depressed bone fragments or edema of the nerve in trauma, osseous proliferation states, and intracanalicular mass lesions are all conditions that might require optic nerve decompression. Since the canal is nearly circular, decompression can be successfully accomplished from a superior, inferior, medial, or lateral direction. Selection of one approach over another is determined by a few basic issues. For instance, if a frontal craniotomy is required for other neurosurgical problems, it would seem appropriate to approach the optic canal from a superior direction. A depressed medially or inferiorly located segment of a fractured canal might dictate an inferior or medial approach. In cases of traumatic edema of the nerve, an adequate decompression can in fact be accomplished by removing the bone and incising the sheath from any direction. Although otologic surgeons are conversant with the need to incise the confining dural sheath in mastoid and middle ear facial nerve decompression, the details of transcanalicular optic nerve decompression are vague regarding dural sheath incision.[1,2] Uemura[11] recently emphasized the specific importance of sheath incision in a representative clinical series.

HISTORICAL BACKGROUND

The transfrontal craniotomy is the standard surgical technique upon which virtually all reported series of optic nerve decompression are based.[1,2,12,13] This surgical approach

OPERATIVE NEUROSURGICAL TECHNIQUES
ISBN 0-8089-1862-1

to the junction of the anterior and middle cranial fossa is familiar to all neurosurgeons. Numerous disease entities such as anterior basal meningiomas, cerebral aneurysms, and suprasellar pituitary tumors demand consideration of optic nerve relationships.

The Krönlein procedure[14] approaches the orbit and anterior optic nerve from a lateral direction but is of limited usefulness. The procedure is unsuitable for total decompression of the optic canal since critical neurovascular structures in and about the superior orbital fissure and the cavernous sinus would be vulnerable to injury.

In 1926, Sewall conceived of the external ethmoidectomy as a medial approach to the optic canal.[15] Japanese surgeons Fukado[8] and Niho[9] reported large clinical series of optic canal decompressions with allegedly striking results. Conceptually, the technique is useful in approaching compression fractures of the orbital end of the canal. There are limitations to this technique, however, in that visibility is reduced even with the operating microscope. Bimanual instrumentation is virtually impossible posterior to the annulus. The most limiting feature is the narrow angle of surgical approach on the canal that is required. The operative direction is nearly parallel to the course of the optic nerve, severely limiting visibility in this confined area. The development of extremely narrow-shafted drills designed for use in stapes middle ear surgery may allow some surgeons to decompress the optic canal through an external ethmoidectomy incision with reasonable exposure and potential for manipulation.

In 1914, Cushing outlined his experiences with a transsphenoidal hypophysectomy and emphasized the advantages of using the approach to relieve chiasmal compression caused by expanding pituitary tumors.[16] Of 68 patients with visual impairment, 46 demonstrated stabilization or improved vision after surgery. Of greater relevance to this discussion, 2 of 5 patients who were totally blind before surgery had partial recovery of their visual acuity. The patterns of visual recovery after relief of compression in a variety of clinical situations have been well documented.[3] Cushing recognized the advantages of an extracranial approach to problems related to optic nerve compression, even with the limited technology of his day.[16] Coaxial illumination, magnification, and sophisticated intraoperative radiographic monitoring have allowed an expansion of the capabilities of this extracranial surgery.

In 1961, Hamberger reported a series of 163 hypophysectomies in which the sella turcica was exposed through the maxillary sinus.[17] The proposed advantage of this technique was improved exposure and thus added safety. The merits of this approach and the remarkably low incidence of complications were emphasized in a second series by Tollefsen.[18] These procedures were principally total hypophysectomies for carcinoma of the breast, performed before the common application of the operating microscope.

In 1976, Kennerdell et al. applied the transantral ethmoidal approach of Hamberger to a case of optic canal fracture.[19] A compressive canal fracture was apparently removed with total recovery of vision. The dramatic success in this case underscores the need for expedient surgery and represents an excellent alternative to the external ethmoidectomy for approaching the medial orbital apex and adjacent optic canal at the annulus level.

TECHNIQUE OF SPHENOETHMOID OPTIC NERVE DECOMPRESSION

Sphenoethmoid optic nerve decompression is the result of careful anatomic studies of cadaver dissections and actual model procedures on primates and cats.[20] Several surgical procedures on humans performed at the University of Vermont provide the clinical application for the technique. Although the procedure is in many ways a modification of the transantral-sphenoidal hypophysectomy of Hamberger, the introduction of drill technology and the concept of total decompression of the canal place new demands on surgical comprehension. The province of the operative procedure is the lateral wall of the sphenoid sinus, which is generally regarded as a site to be strictly avoided during hypophysectomy. Although the carotid artery and the cavernous sinus are vulnerable to injury by unplanned blind manipulation, understanding the anatomic relationships of the sphenoid and selective exposure will reward the surgeon with an exciting and logical extracranial approach to the optic nerves.

The preoperative assessment requires careful ophthalmologic consultation, as illustrated by the multiple concerns in case 5. Conventional views of the optic canal often are useful and should be obtained as part of an orderly work-up; they may be unremarkable, however, even in cases where the canal is fractured. Computed tomographic (CT) scans with specific views of the optic canal will be the most fruitful radiographic study. Carotid angiography is not usually required for strict optic canal fractures unless there has been an inordinately profuse epistaxis or concern about a carotid-cavernous sinus fistula. In the unconscious or noncommunicative patient with an afferent pupillary defect (Marcus-Gunn pupil), residual optic nerve function can be assessed via visual evoked responses (VERs). Once it has been established that a potentially reversible optic nerve injury exists, success probably depends on the expediency of surgical intervention.

The semi-Fowler position is used following orotracheal intubation and administration of general anesthesia. The image intensifier is positioned routinely as for transsphenoidal hypophysectomy, and electrodes can be placed for monitoring VERs intraoperatively.[21] The nose is inspected for septal deformity, cocainized, and the ipsilateral sublabial sulcus infiltrated with a 1:200,000 adrenaline solution. A Caldwell-Luc procedure is performed, and as a helpful option, the branches of the internal maxillary artery are clipped in the pterygomaxillary fossa. This maneuver reduces blood loss at the sphenoethmoid recess and thus enhances visualization. As depicted in Figure 24-1, the antrostomy bone cuts are extended and the anterior half of the inferior turbinate is resected. A complete ethmoidectomy is then performed with subsequent removal of the middle turbinate for better access to the sphenoid. An alternative and near equally effective exposure can be accomplished by disarticulating the nasal septum from the maxillary crest and displacing the septum into the opposite nasal vault (Figures 24-2, 24-3). This requires incising the mucoperiosteum along the entire ipsilateral floor and carefully elevating and preserving the mucoperiosteum of the contralateral floor. This modification allows similar access to the posterior ethmoids and sphenoid while eliminating the need for osteotomies along the upper maxilla and orbit. An inferiorly based septal mucosal flap, as described by Montgomery,[22] is fashioned and the ipsilateral sphenoid rostrum removed. For further visualization, the posterior osseous septum can be removed. A self-retaining

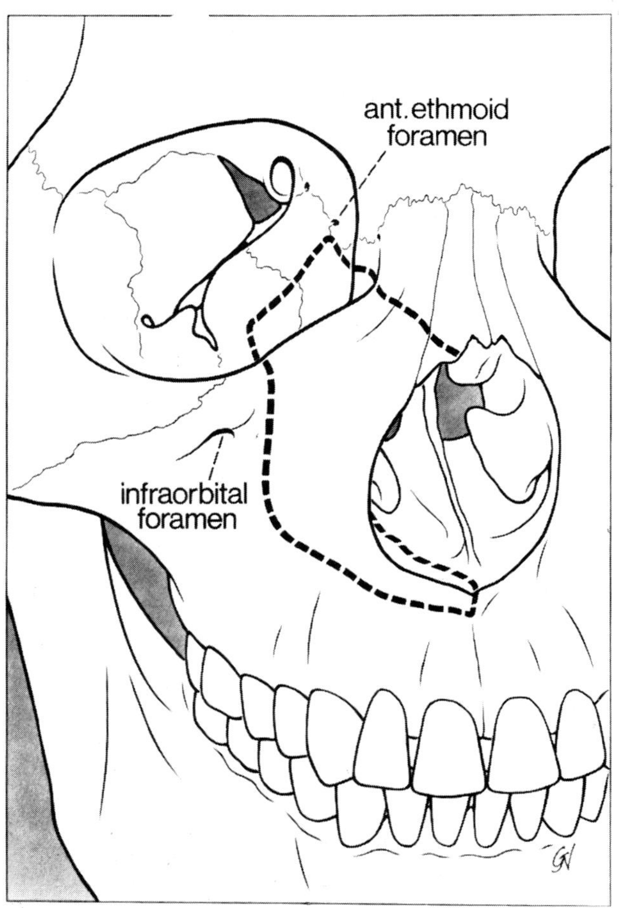

Fig. 24-1. The doted lines depict sublabial osteotomies. The infraorbital canal marks the lateral limit of the bone cut.

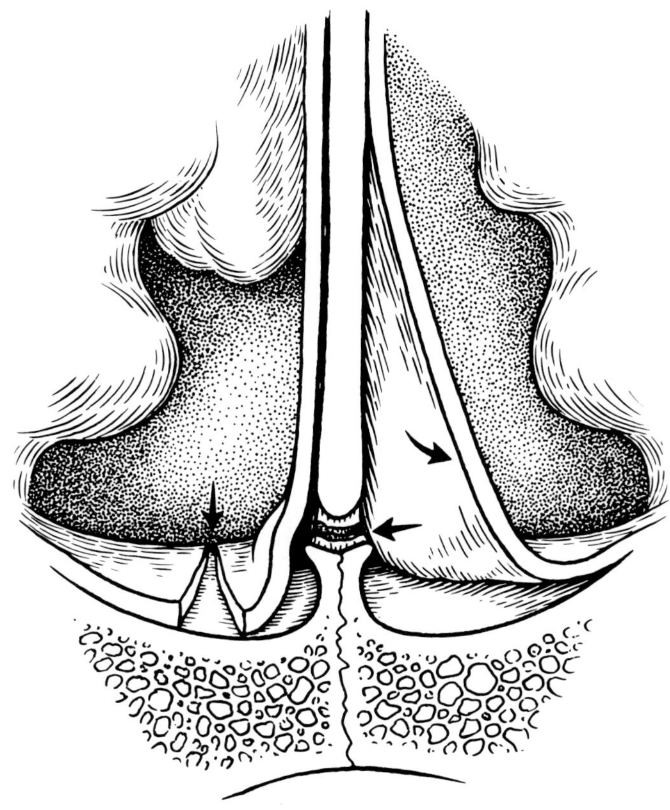

Fig. 24-2. A longitudinal mucosal incision along the nasal floor ipsilateral to the side of injury and elevation of the entire contralateral mucoperichondrium set the foundation for septal translocation.

hypophysectomy retractor is positioned on either side of the remnant of the lateral nasal wall (Figure 24-4), principally to retract the upper lip and allow unobstructed medioinferior to superolateral operative access within the nasal vaults. The operating microscope, with a 300-mm lens, is used at this point, which allows for careful removal of the sphenoid sinus mucosa under direct vision. Bleeding can be controlled with a dilute topical solution of adrenaline. The lateral sphenoid sinus is examined for fractures or rotated bone fragments, and the location of the carotid prominence is carefully identified. The carotid generally produces a bulge in the midportion of the lateral sphenoid and there is often an oblique bony septum extending from the sphenoid floor laterally toward the carotid imprint. The optic canal lies anterosuperior to the carotid bulge, but in cases where the carotid is not identified, the most anterosuperior aspect of the sphenoid will yield the optic canal. At this point, the posterior ethmoid cell and sphenoid sinus are separated by a heavy osseous partition. This bone segment also approximates the annulus tendineus. The image intensifier is most useful at this point in the procedure. Using a long hypophysectomy drill (OtoOsteotome 13, Stryker Corp., Kalamazoo, Michigan), diamond burrs, and continuous suction irrigation, the inferomedial optic canal is thinned. Figure 24-5 depicts the buttress of the bone, which should be preserved between the carotid artery and the optic canal. When the bone has been sufficiently thinned, it is removed in an "eggshell" fashion with microinstruments, exposing the dural sheath. The dural cover, including the thickened annulus tendineus, then is

incised with otologic hooks and a fine sickle knife (Figure 24-6). A cerebrospinal fluid leak occurs at this point and thin pia-arachnoid can be seen adhering to the nerve. These filaments should be left undisturbed to limit potential vascular interruption of the nerve. The ophthalmic artery usually enters laterally, but occasionally can be directly inferior in location (Figure 24-7). Care therefore must be observed when incising the inferomedial sheath to avoid this important vessel. Localized oozing can be controlled with Avitene. The entire sphenoid sinus is then obliterated by harvested abdominal, subcutaneous, adipose-free graft, and the septal mucosal flap is rotated against the obliterated sinus. A layer of Gelfoam is placed between the flap and antibiotic-impregnated gauze packing. Finger-cot packs are placed along the nasal floor. Postoperative care requires bed rest, with the head elevated, for 4 to 5 days and continuation of the prophylactic antibiotics begun during the preoperative period. Corticosteroids will usually have been instituted to cover the contusive cranial injury. The finger cots can be advanced in 5 to 6 days and the remainder of the packing gradually removed.

INDICATIONS FOR SPHENOETHMOID OPTIC NERVE DECOMPRESSION

Because of the relative infrequency of optic nerve problems, clinical experience with this surgical approach is still limited; however, laboratory experience with the technique and relatively consistent anatomic landmarks allow for reasonable

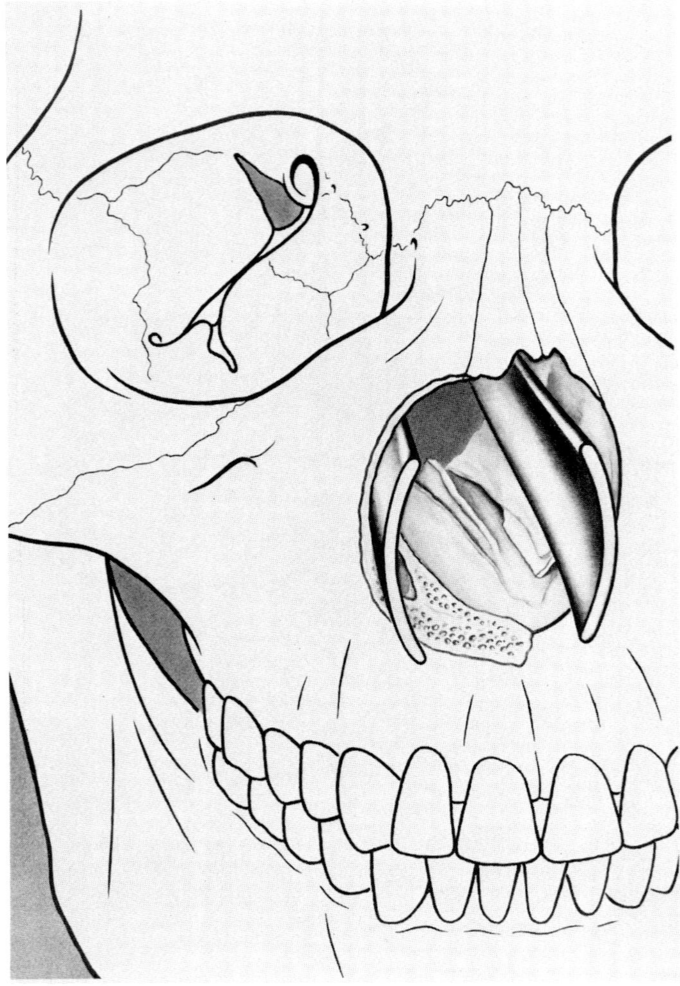

Fig. 24-3. The cartilaginous nasal septum is disarticulated from the perpendicular ethmoid plate and maxillary crest, allowing it to be transposed into the opposite nasal vault for excellent exposure of the ipsilateral sphenoid sinus and optic canal.

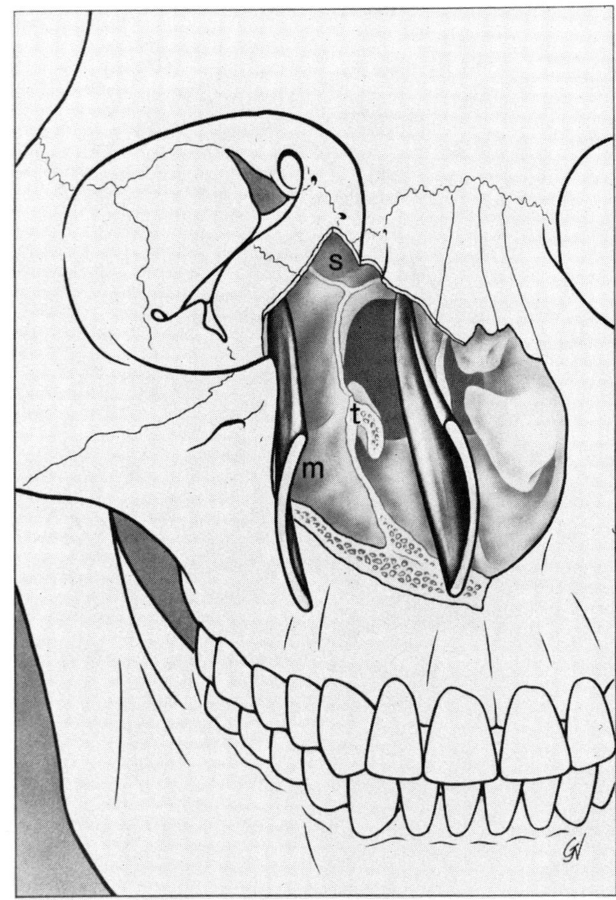

Fig. 24-4. The self-retaining hypophysectomy retractor is positioned with one blade against the nasal septum and the other within the maxillary sinus. The upper lip is elevated out of the visual field. m = maxillary sinus; t = remnant of the inferior turbinate; s = sphenoid sinus.

projection of its use for conditions other than optic canal trauma.

Osseous proliferation states can produce encroachment on the optic nerve through narrowing of the osseous foramina. Examples of successful surgical osseous decompression for Paget's disease, Albers-Schönberg disease, and fibrous dysplasia have been documented.[23–25]

Optic nerve glioma and meningioma[14,26] are examples of neoplasms that can arise within the osseous canal. The transsphenoidal approach could have some advantages for patients with optic nerve glioma since a common field would be produced for removal of both canalicular and orbital elements. Examples of other mass lesions that could be similarly addressed are sarcoidosis, canalicular arachnoid cysts, sheath hyperplasia in von Recklinghausen's disease, and metastatic malignant disease.[1,27]

Hypothetically, there may be some future uses for the approach for difficult cerebrovascular conditions. Aneurysms of the ophthalmic artery are relatively inaccessible through conventional craniotomy approaches; perhaps a transsphenoidal technique will provide the potential for an alternate direct attack.[28] Clipping the ophthalmic artery in carotid-cavernous sinus fistula via the sphenoid may provide a way to preserve retinal flow if embolization and "trapping" are used. Since good collateral flow via the anterior and posterior ethmoidal arteries (external carotid system) can enter the ophthalmic arterial systems, occlusion of the proximal ophthalmic artery may prevent embolization of the distal arterial network.

CASE REPORTS

Case 1. In 1977, a 23-year-old man was admitted with extremity and cranial facial trauma from a bicycle accident, objective findings included loss of light perception and a left Marcus-Gunn pupil. Radiographic analysis, including polytomography, confirmed a Le Fort II fracture, a nondisplaced frontal and multiple sphenoid fracture, and an optic canal fracture. The transsphenoethmoid decompression of the entire optic canal was accomplished 30 hours after admission, but in this early case the dura was not incised. Vision never returned in spite of the surgical procedure. Radiography confirmed adequate osseous canalicular decompression as depicted in Figure 24-8.

Case 2. A motor vehicle accident in 1978 left this patient with midfacial fractures, a left Marcus-Gunn pupil, and abducens paralysis. Ophthalmologic consultation revealed fin-

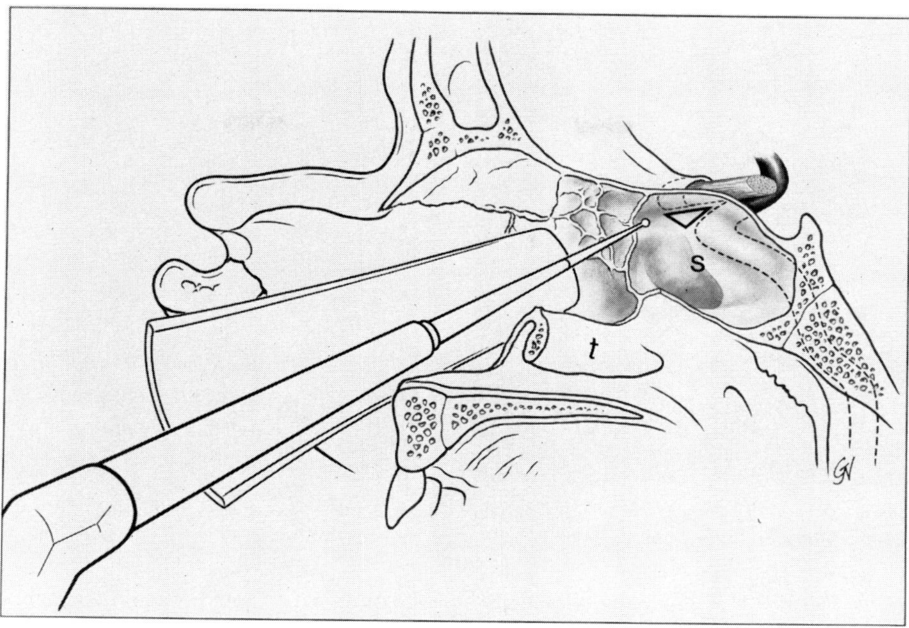

Fig. 24-5.   A sagittal view demonstrating the direction of the microdrill. The dark triangle indicates the osseous butress preserved between the carotid artery and the optic nerve.

ger counting only at 4 feet and a sluggish but reactive pupil. On the fifth day after injury, the patient contracted *Hemophilus influenzae* meningitis and was treated with a 10–day course of parenteral ampicillin. Although the meningitis resolved clinically, vision remained severely impaired and polytomography revealed fractures of the optic canal and the sphenoethmoid sinuses, and a "blow-in" component at the orbital apex. Two weeks after the injury, the procedure outlined in this chapter was accomplished. A 1.5 × 1.5-cm rotated bone fragment was removed from the floor of the apex and a totally unsuspected mucopyocele was identified upon opening the sphenoid sinus. Conventional views of the optic canal, obtained on admission,

did not demonstrate fractures, but polytomography done later clearly illustrated fractures of the sphenoid roof and canal. The sequence and evidence of adequate osseous decompression are demonstrated in Figure 24-9. The patient reported subjective visual improvement immediately after surgery and the objective measurement of the patient's acuity was 4/200 4 days after surgery.

Case 3.   In 1979, a 35-year-old woman sustained a severe frontal head injury while bicycling. Upon admission to the hospital, the patient was in a coma, had a dilated fixed right pupil, and absence of consensual left pupillary constriction with

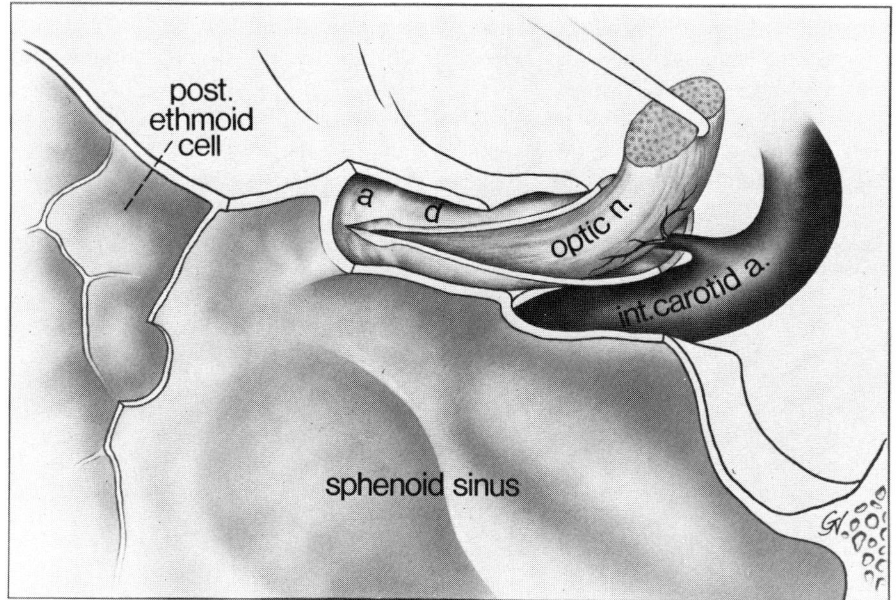

Fig. 24-6.   Canalicular decompression has been completed and the dural sheath incised. Note the inferolateral location of the ophthalmic artery internal to the dura. a = annulus tendineus; d = dural sheath.

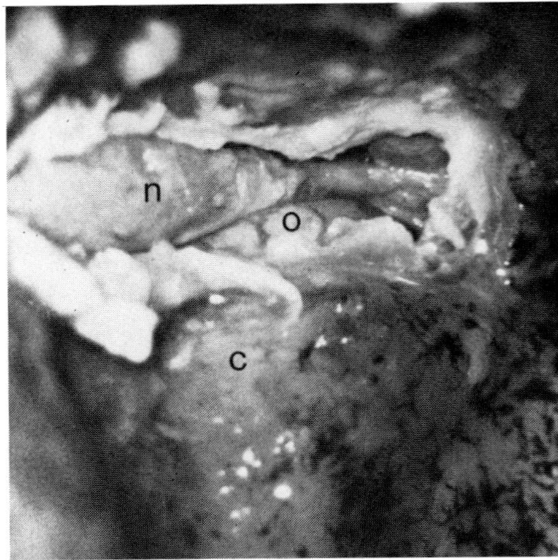
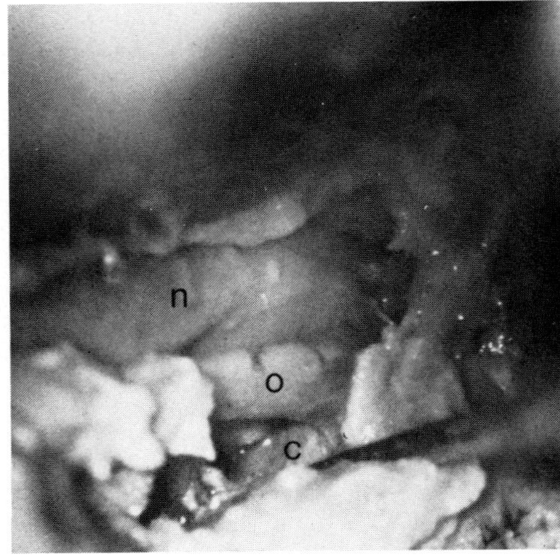

Fig. 24-7. A cadaver dissection of a lateral sphenoid showing the relationship of the carotid artery and the ophthalmic artery to the optic nerve. o = ophthalmic artery; c = carotid artery; n = optic nerve.

light stimulus in the right eye. Oculomotor and abducens paralysis also were noted. Fractures of the frontotemporal cranium, the posterior orbit, and the sphenoid were found, and a CT scan confirmed significant cerebral edema. The optic canal was moderately compressed by a lateral depressed fracture. Four hours after admission, a frontal craniotomy was performed for placement of a pressure monitor. Fractures of the posterior orbit, sphenoid, and optic canal were determined and free fragments were removed by the neurosurgical team. The entire thickened osseous roof of the optic canal was removed by the author toward the thickened anterior clinoid with the aid of a microdrill and suction irrigation. We were then able to incise the nerve sheath, revealing a contusion of the proximal canalicular segment of the optic nerve. Upon recovery from coma, the patient was able to read large print with the affected eye. A follow-up visual acuity of 20/30 with correction and some residual optic atrophy were confirmed by the consulting ophthalmologist. Although the lack of subjective responsiveness on admission precluded an assessment of her actual visual acuity, the lack of a consensual light pupillary response in the face of a compressive optic canal fracture led us to believe there was substantial nerve injury. Expedient decompression may have been the key to the successful visual result.

Case 4. In 1966, a 6-year-old girl was injured by an automobile and had complete bilateral blindness. Sphenoid fractures were noted, but no specific views of the optic canal were obtained. During preparation for craniotomy, the patient was able to count fingers with the right eye and the pupil became light-reactive. Surgery was canceled and the patient returned to the ward for observation. Two days after admission, her vision again deteriorated and there was residual function only in the temporal field. By the following day, she was totally blind again. She was given high-dosage parenteral corticosteroids. A frontal craniotomy performed 2 days later detected bilateral fractures of the roof of each optic canal with a groove across the right optic nerve at the fracture locus. Unfortunately, visual function never returned after this delayed decompression.

Case 5. In 1980, a 21-year-old man sustained craniofacial trauma in a motor vehicle accident. He experienced transient unconsciousness and retrograde amnesia. Physical examination revealed a dilated fixed right pupil, absence of light perception in the affected eye, and complete ophthalmoplegia. Central retinal artery occlusion was confirmed by ophthalmologic consultation (Figure 24-10). A CT scan identified right parasellar which resolved with appropriate antibiotic therapy.

Case 6. In 1986, a 12-year-old boy sustained a crush injury to the skull base in a bicycle-truck accident. He complained of complete bilateral loss of vision from the time of

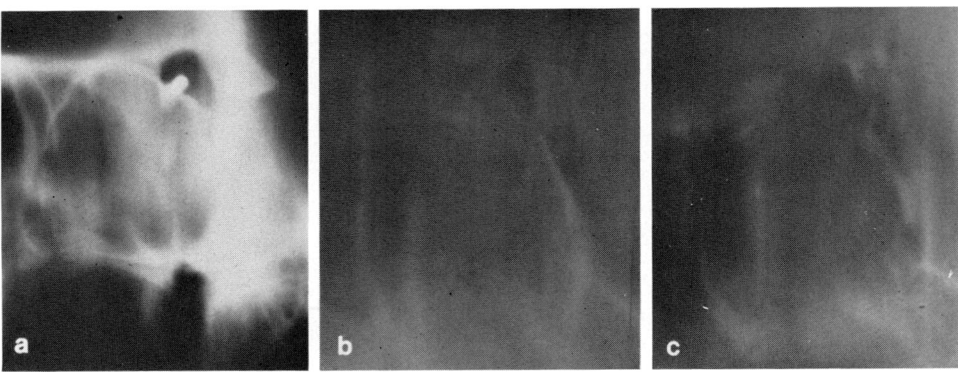

Fig. 24-8. Reverse Rhese polytomograms of the optic canal fracture in Case 1. (A) A radiograph of the dried skull in Figure 24-11 defining the location of the medial optic canal. (B) Preoperative x-ray film illustrating comminution and compression of the medial optic canal. (C) Postdecompression radiograph demonstrating complete removal of the medial canal.

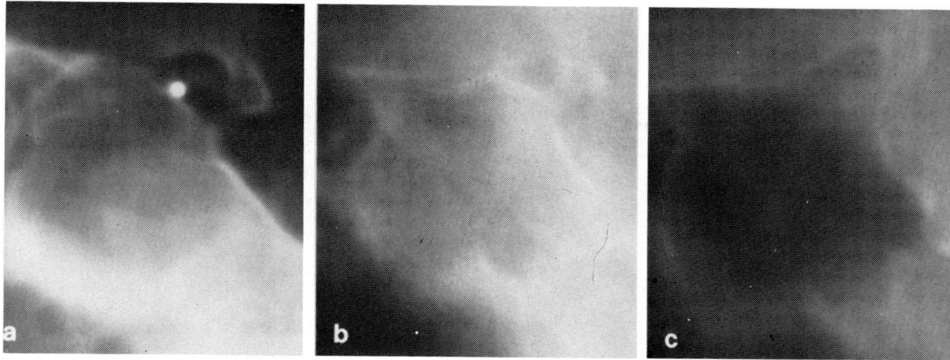

Fig. 24-9. A series of images for Case 2 similar to those in Figure 24-8. (A) dried skull, (B) Preoperative, and (C) postoperative decompression radiographs.

injury, and CT scans demonstrated bilateral optic canal, frontal sinus, sphenoid, and temporal bone fractures. The left retina displayed changes consistent with a central retinal artery occlusion and neither pupil reacted to direct or consensual light stimulus. A bilateral optic canal decompression through the sublabial sphenoethmoid route was performed 8 hours from the time of injury, with gradual recovery of vision. He has been able to return to school, reading large print with one eye, and functions independently.

DISCUSSION

The aim of this chapter is to introduce an alternate extracranial approach to the optic nerve. Since the transsphenoidal approach to the pituitary has achieved wide acceptance because of its low morbidity rate, this analogous surgical access to the optic canal may seem preferable to an intracranial procedure in several instances.

The potential advantages of an extracranial approach are many. In trauma, frontal lobe edema may preclude adequate exposure of the optic nerves from above; the inferomedial approach would, of course, obviate the need for frontal lobe elevation. Olfaction is preserved and rapid postoperative recovery approximates the course of transsphenoidal hypophysectomy. No external facial or cranial incisions are required. The medial and inferior aspects of the orbit and the entire sinus complex ipsilateral to the surgical field are readily accessible. This could have advantages for cases of expanding orbital hematomas with optic canal trauma, adjacent sinus infections as in case 2, combined orbital-canalicular tumors, and certain situations involving foreign bodies, such as gunshot wounds. The unfortunate complication of blindness following intranasal ethmoidectomy[29] can be addressed with this procedure since the surgical exenteration of the ethmoid is completed during the original procedure, allowing rapid canalicular exposure and sheath incision.

Some of the possible disadvantages should be outlined. As with transsphenoidal hypophysectomy, the field is nonsterile. Since the incidence of meningitis after hypophysectomy is remarkably low,[30] even when there is a cerebrospinal fluid leak through the diaphragma sella, this disadvantage may be only theoretical. In addition, pre-, intra-, and postoperative broad spectrum antibiotics are administered. Although there is a real danger of CSF rhinorrhea, the short sheath incision and obliteration technique minimize the likelihood of a leak. The carotid

artery and the cavernous sinus are adjacent to the operative site and require maximum care and surgical skill. Fujii et al., in a comprehensive cadaver analysis of sphenoid anatomy, demonstrated that 8 percent of carotid arteries and 4 percent of optic nerves are not entirely covered by an osseous plate in the lateral sphenoid.[31] The same study confirms the accessibility of the optic nerve through the sphenoid since 78 percent of the nerves were covered by 0.5 mm of bone or less. Reference to a horizontal section of the superior aspect of the sphenoid will make these relationships readily understood (Figure 24-11). Special microinstruments are required for this procedure and considerable cadaver practice must precede clinical surgery. Even the otolaryngologic surgeon, who is highly familiar with drill techniques, initially will find the longer hypophysectomy drill cumbersome to manipulate.

The case reports in which actual sphenoethmoid decompression was accomplished document the clinical application of the technique, and the radiographic sequences demonstrate the actual postoperative osseous surgical defect. The coaxial polytomographic views of the canal (reverse Rhese position)

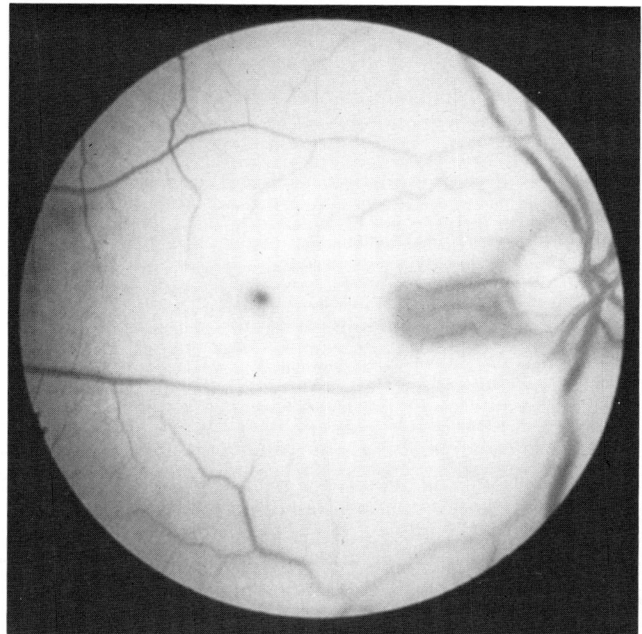

Fig. 24-10. A fundus photograph of the patient in Case 5 demonstrating central retinal artery ischemia with temporal sparing.

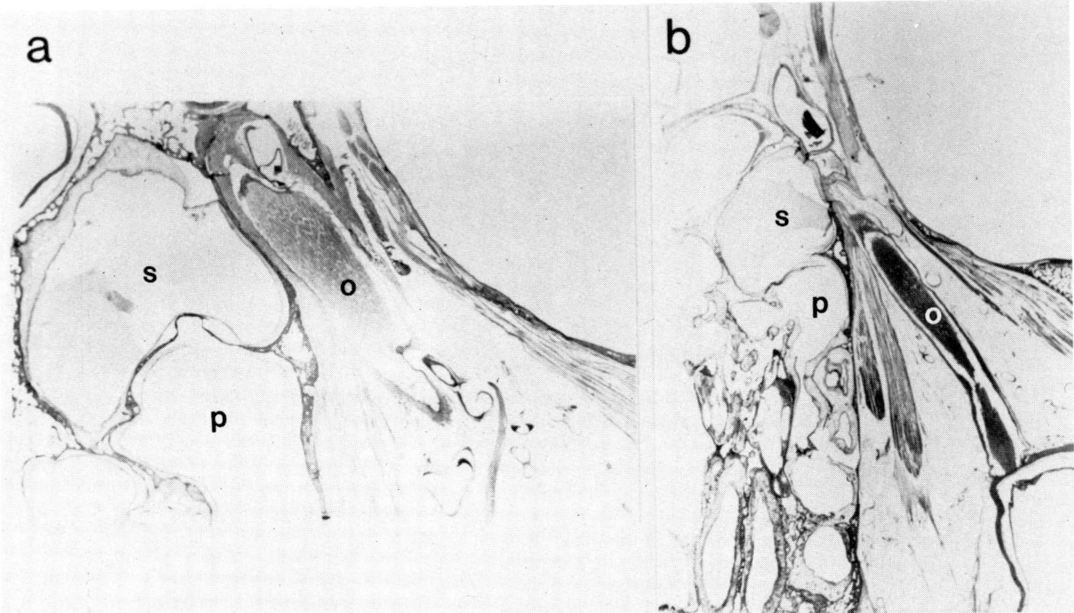

Fig. 24-11. Horizontal sections through the prepared head demonstrating the relationships of the optic nerve (o) to the sphenoid (s) and posterior ethmoid sinuses (p). (Reprinted from Bridges MWM, van Nostrand AWP: The nose and paranasal sinuses—applied surgical anatomy. J Otolaryngol 7:28, 1978. With permission.)

require special orientation for the reader. A wire brad affixed to the medial optic canal in a dried skull (Figures 24-8A, 24-9A) provides a point of reference for the sequential roentgenograms. Both patients have been free of complications subsequent to the procedure, with up to a 10-year follow-up. Specifically, neither patient has manifested nasal crusting, rhinitis, or CSF rhinorrhea.

The third case has been included to emphasize the flexibility of a team approach to optic nerve trauma. When the neurosurgical staff has determined that no concurrent intracranial injury exists, a mutual consideration to sphenoethmoid decompression will evolve. If a frontal craniotomy is required, decompression of the superior optic canal would be entertained. This case illustrates further that there may be a role for the otolaryngologist in transfrontal decompression. The optic canal in its superior aspect becomes thickened near the anterior clinoid, and the use of diamond burrs with suction irrigation is preferable to rongeur techniques. The otolaryngologist employs drills on a regular basis for otologic surgery in confined areas adjacent to important neurovascular structures. If a sound mutual relationship exists with the neurosurgical staff, the otolaryngologist can be as helpful in this procedure as in joint suboccipital surgery for acoustic neuroma. This particular case also emphasizes the benefits of expedient recognition of the problem and surgical decompression.

A review of 14 patients with traumatic amaurosis, evaluated at the University of Vermont from 1955 to 1975, raised some interesting questions regarding early recognition and treatment. Of the 14 patients who developed irreversible blindness, 7 were noted, either on admission to the emergency room or early in their hospitalization, to have ''pupils equally round and reactive to light.'' It is obvious that a retrospective interpretation cannot determine the validity of these observations, especially when they were not rendered uniformly by neurologists, neurosurgeons, or ophthalmologists. It is possible, however, that up to half of the patients who eventually became blind

might have had a rapidly progressive visual impairment. Perhaps these patients would have been the very individuals suitable for optic nerve decompression.

The fourth case represents a clear example of a progressive posttraumatic visual amaurosis with an unfortunate outcome. In fact, this is the very situation for which decompression would have been suitable. In retrospect, steroids were ineffective in restoring useful vision for this patient and probably should not be relied upon as the sole treatment modality in an evolving visual deficit.

The fifth case demonstrates that a very careful analysis of the entire visual system must develop before decompression is considered. One could argue that a rapid attempt at decompression might have somehow reversed the central retinal artery occlusion, but this would certainly have been unconventional in the face of the few hours of retinal ischemia. This case emphasizes that even though canalicular fractures may be identified radiographically, there may be other overriding clinical considerations precluding achievement of a successful result with decompression.

The sixth case emphasizes that an expedient and aggressive approach can have the hopeful favorable outcome. Although the eye with central retinal artery occlusion seemed beyond salvage, the surgical decompression may have been responsible for its strong recovery. Perhaps the presence of acute central retinal artery occlusion in the setting of trauma should demand optic canal decompression, but only future analysis of similar case problems will determine whether this proves to be a accurate consideration.

In conclusion, this discussion has focused on an alternate extracranial microsurgical approach to the optic canal. As described, the procedure has certain advantages and can present a safe alternative to existing intracranial techniques. The surgical methodology is quite specialized, however, and requires careful laboratory practice and thorough anatomic understanding before clinical surgery is undertaken. The optic canal injury is an emergency and there should be a sense of expediency in getting the patient to surgery. Adequate preliminary study and procurement of all necessary instruments will allow the surgeon to apply this technique properly.

REFERENCES

1. Gjerris F: Traumatic lesions of the visual pathways, in Vincen PJ, Bruyn CW (eds): Handbook of Clinical Neurology, vol 24. Amsterdam, North Holland, 1976, pp 27–57
2. Hughes B: Indirect injury of the optic nerves and chiasma. Johns Hopkins Med J 111:98, 1962
3. Kayan A, Earl CJ: Compressive lesions of the optic nerves and chiasm, pattern of recovery of vision following surgical treatment. Brain 98:13, 1975
4. Obenchain TG, Killeffer FA, Stern WE: Indirect injury of the optic nerves and chiasm with closed head injury. Bull Los Angeles Neurol Soc 38:13, 1973
5. Ramsey JH: Optic nerve injury in fracture of the canal. Br J Ophthalmol 63:607, 1979
6. Francois J: Vascularization of the optic nerve. Arch Ophthalmol 95:520, 1977
7. Hollinshead WH: Anatomy for Surgeons, vol 1. New York, Harper & Row, 1968, p 215
8. Fukado Y: Results in 350 cases of surgical decompression of the optic nerve. Translation of the Fourth Asia-Pacific Congress of Ophthalmology, 1972, pp 96–99
9. Niho S, Murakami I, Sato T: Decompression of the fractured optic canal by the transethmoidal route. Pac Med Surg 73:237, 1965
10. Maniscalco JE, Habal MB: Microanatomy of the optic canal. J Neurosurg 48:402, 1978
11. Uemura T, et al: Optic canal decompression—the significance of simultaneous optic canal sheath incision. Neurol Med Chir (Tokyo) 18:151, 1978
12. Keltner JL, et al: Optic nerve decompression. Arch Ophthalmol 95:97, 1977
13. Wennerstrand J, Galera R, del Corral-Gutierrez JF: A method for decompression and mobilization of the optic chiasm. Acta Soc Med Uppsala 72:272–276
14. Richards RD, Lynn JR: The surgical management of gliomas of the optic nerve. Am J Ophthalmol 62:60, 1966
15. Sewall EC: External operation in the ethmosphenoid-frontal group of sinuses under local anesthesia. Technic for removal of part of foramen wall for relief of pressure on optic nerve. Arch Otolaryngol 4:377–411
16. Cushing H: Surgical experiences with pituitary disorders. JAMA 63:1515, 1914
17. Hamberger CA, et al: Transantrosphenoidal hypophysectomy. Arch Otolaryngol 74:22, 1961
18. Tollefsen RH, Miller TR, Gerold FP: Transantral-sphenoidal hypophysectomy. Am J Surg 112:569, 1966
19. Kennerdell JS, Amsbaugh GA, Myers EN: A transantral-ethmoidal decompression of optic canal fracture. Arch Ophthalmol 94:1040, 1976
20. Sofferman RA: An extracranial microsurgical approach to the optic nerve. J Microsurg 1:195, 1979
21. Feinsod M, et al: Monitoring optic nerve function during craniotomy. J Neurosurg 44:29, 1976
22. Montgomery WW: Surgery of the Upper Respiratory System, vol 1. Philadelphia, Lea & Febiger, 1971, p 152
23. Liakos GM, Walker CB, Carruth JAS: Ocular complications in craniofacial fibrous dysplasia. Br J Ophthalmol 63:611, 1979
24. Caldron M, Brady HR: Fibrous dysplasia of bone. Am J Ophthalmol 68:513, 1969
25. Ellis PP, Jackson WE: Osteopetrosis. Am J Ophthalmol 53:943, 1962
26. Spencer WH: Primary neoplasms of the optic nerve and its sheaths; clinical features and current concepts of pathogenic mechanisms. Trans Am Ophthalmol Soc 70:490, 1972
27. Spencer WH, Borit A: Diffuse hyperplasia of the optic nerve. Am J Ophthalmol 64:638, 1967
28. Yasargil MG, et al: Carotid-ophthalmic aneurysms: Direct microsurgical approach. Surg Neurol 8:155, 1977
29. Griffin JF, Momose J, Wray SH: Optic canal fractures after rhinologic surgery. Am J Ophthalmol 87:526, 1979
30. McDonald TJ, et al: Surgical approaches to the pituitary gland, with emphasis on the transseptal route. Head Neck Surg 1:498, 1979
31. Fujii K, Chambers SM, Rhoton AL: Neurovascular relationships of the sphenoid sinus. J Neurosurg 50:31, 1979

CHAPTER 25
Gliomas of the Anterior Visual Pathways

William H. Sweet   Shirley H. Wray   Paul F. New

THE OPERATIVE TECHNIQUES for removal of gliomas of the anterior visual pathways are reasonably well worked out and require relatively brief description here. Highly controversial, however, are the indications for conservative management or for surgery, either alone or in combination with conventional radiation therapy. The major emphasis in this chapter will be on the precise documentation of clinical and neuroradiologic features that should prompt a physician to refer a patient for consideration of various types of surgery or radiation therapy or both.

Gliomas of the anterior visual pathways from the optic nerve back through the chiasm and optic tract exhibit extreme variation in their growth behavior from case to case. Correspondingly, extreme variations in recommendations for treating them have arisen with the sole exception of tumors that produce hydrocephalus. In these cases at least, all agree that the use of a shunt is advisable.

Gliomas of the anterior visual pathways are relatively rare, occurring in 1:10,000 to 1:100,000 ophthalmic patients[1]; they constitute 3.6 percent of intracranial tumors in children[2] and 1 percent of all of Cushing's brain tumors.[3] A massive amount of literature on optic gliomas has developed that reflects the difficulty of predicting the course of this disorder and of generalizing from small numbers of cases. There are, however, special diagnostic points of which a physician can and should take advantage.

SPECIAL DIAGNOSTIC POINTS

CALCIFICATION

Although the parasellar tumors most commonly showing calcification are craniopharyngiomas, calcification can also occur in optic gliomas. Schuster and Westberg[4] noted this in 5 of their 25 operatively verified cases; Fletcher et al.[5] in 3 of their 22 cases (11 histologically verified); Bynke et al.[6] in 1 of their 10 histologically proven cases; Myles and Murphy[7] in 2 of their 20 cases; and Kahn et al.[8] in 1 case. It was present in 9 of 21 of our verified cases and was often identifiable only with scans. A common misdiagnosis was craniopharyngioma. More surprising to us was perineoplastic calcification in extracerebral intradural fibrous tissue in 2 patients (Case 4 and Case 7 to be discussed later). Its presence was not associated with a recurrence of tumor. Of 16 patients irradiated by Fletcher et al.,[5] 2 developed progressive calcification of the lenticular nuclei and thalamus.

The clinical significance of this postirradiation calcification in the basal ganglia and elsewhere is uncertain. It was noted also in one of our patients and in one of 3 children treated by Beyer et al.[9] Hypothalamic and frontal lobe calcification accompanied by a progressive memory and learning deficit developed in a 4-year-old child with a craniopharyngioma after exposure to more than 5000 rads.[10]

COMPUTED TOMOGRAPHY AND MAGNETIC RESONANCE IMAGING

Computed Tomography

The development of computed tomography eliminated the need for cerebral pneumography. Technical advances in recent years have produced the capability of very high spatial resolution. Thin-section computed tomography allows reformating of coronal and sagittal images, albeit with some resultant loss of resolution in the process. Such high-resolution computed tomography has largely obviated the need for complex motion tomography and cisternography using water-soluble contrast agents. The position of the major cranial vessels can be determined from high-resolution contrast-enhanced computed tomographic (CT) scans, but dynamic contrast-enhanced CT scans with bolus intravenous injections are required for demonstration of the internal carotid arteries within the cavernous sinuses. Contrast-enhanced CT scans usually reveal enhancement of gliomas involving the optic pathways, e.g., in 6 of 10 cases reported by Byrd et al.,[11] and 18 of 22 cases reported by Fletcher et al.[5] In 3 of Byrd's 10 patients, clinically unsuspected bilateral lesions were found. Holman et al.[12] found that CT scans delineated orbital relationships better, whereas magnetic resonance imaging (MRI) was superior for identification of the optic nerves, chiasm, and optic tracts.

Magnetic Resonance Imaging

Magnetic resonance imaging (MRI) technology has advanced even more rapidly than that of computed tomography. It was very rapidly determined that contrast resolution of normal and pathologic tissues was generally higher in MRI scans than in CT scans provided that suitable radiofrequency pulse sequences were utilized. More recently, improvements in MRI have permitted high contrast resolution to be maintained as spatial resolution was improved, although the spatial resolution of MRI still does not quite match the best resolution that can be

OPERATIVE NEUROSURGICAL TECHNIQUES
ISBN 0-8089-1862-1

obtained with computed tomography. It is now becoming clear that MRI offers major advantages over computed tomography in the demonstration of anatomic and pathologic features in the optic pathways and adjacent structures. Superb anatomic detail within the orbits can be obtained with MRI using surface coils. Aron et al.[13] described one patient in whom MRI revealed involvement of the optic tract and optic radiation not seen on the CT scan. Daniels et al.[14] noted in particular that MRI was better in demonstrating the intracanalicular portion of the optic nerve. The comprehensive appraisal of suprasellar lesions by both MRI and CT scanning in 55 cases of Karnaze et al.[15] included 9 optic or hypothalamic gliomas. In the entire group of cases they found MRI superior in 14 cases and computed tomography better in 3 cases. In one of these 3 cases, the CT scans demonstrated a lesion that was not apparent on the MRI scans. In 11 cases, however, the extent of the lesion was better defined on the MRI scans. It should be noted that MRI is generally distinctly less effective in the demonstration of calcifications. The direct multiplanar capability of MRI precludes awkward posturing of the patient and the degradation of detail routinely produced by the need for reformating of axial images. The absence of ionizing radiation (indeed of any apparent biologic hazard) is of particular importance in the examination of children; this is especially noteworthy when multiple studies are desirable in long-term follow-up. Additional advantages of MRI include the lack of a need for contrast enhancement and its capacity to demonstrate the intracavernous portions of the carotid arteries and the other major basal arteries in any desired plane without injection of contrast into the vascular system.

Clinical testing of a MRI paramagnetic contrast agent has been completed, and it is expected that this agent will be cleared for routine clinical use in the near future. This agent, Gd-DTPA, is an effective agent for most of the purposes for which iodinated contrast agents have been used for computed tomography. Its pharmacokinetics are very similar to those of such agents, but it is extremely effective in very small doses and no neurotoxic or anaphylactoid complications have been observed.[16,17,18]

VISUAL EVOKED POTENTIALS

Only a few pattern visual evoked potential (PVEP) studies of gliomas of the optic nerve or chiasm have been done, but they have provided arresting data.[19-21] That is to say, abnormal PVEPs were recorded from the opposite "normal" eye in 6 patients with a tumor apparently confined to one optic nerve. Involvement of fibers from the opposite eye crossing at the chiasm was the only finding intimating involvement of the other eye. Whether such a finding should preclude removal of the obviously affected optic nerve is unclear, the more so since serial recording showed a remarkable spontaneous improvement in the pattern responses in 2 patients. In chiasmal gliomas the response to the usual checkerboard pattern stimulus may be almost eliminated despite good visual acuity.[20] These studies should be pursued further and correlated with color vision and other data in order to define their clinical significance.

CONTROVERSIAL DIAGNOSTIC POINTS

Combining our own experience with our appraisal of the literature we shall attempt a balanced judgment on three further disputed points: Are optic gliomas neoplasms or hamartomas?

Should gliomas of the optic chiasm and/or adjoining brain or optic nerves be exposed surgically? Which optic gliomas if any should be treated by radiation? Optic Gliomas—Neoplasms or Hamartomas?

Do optic gliomas, which often start in early childhood, continue to grow slowly or at times rapidly, or do they "tend to enlarge, cause symptoms early in life and remain static thereafter" so that "Excision of the tumor is justified only for the relief of severe proptosis of a blind eye" because "The tumor is non-neoplastic, self-limiting, and has a good prognosis for life."? The quotations are from Hoyt and Baghdassarian on the basis of 36 patients with chiasmal or optic nerve tumors (biopsy proven in only 58 percent).[22] The bases for this latter view have been augmented by Glaser et al.[23] Miller et al.[24] from the Wilmer Eye Institute of Johns Hopkins, studied 40 biopsy proven optic gliomas, 11 of an optic nerve and 29 of the chiasm. They "agree that this type of tumor probably represents a congenital hamartoma of low potential morbidity." Borit and Richardson of the Massachusetts General Hospital also said with respect to all gliomas of the optic pathways, "our findings . . . are in general agreement . . . that the mortality and morbidity are much the same regardless of whether the patients have been treated surgically or by irradiation, or have received no treatment directed against the tumors."[25] Wong and Lubow reached similar conclusions after follow-up of their 42 cases for 1 to 20 years.[26] The documentation and prestige of these groups have given their views widespread credence.

Three of our cases, with some of the longest follow-ups on record, present divergent answers about the self-limiting nature of these lesions.

Case Report

Case 1. The patient, a 3-year-old girl, underwent enucleation of her left eye and excision of some "glioma optic nerve." Fifteen months later further growth of the tumor extruded the glass eyeball implant. She underwent orbital exenteration of a "glioma of optic nerve." Despite requests, the patient and her mother did not return until 22 years later. She came to her ophthalmic surgeon with a mass "slightly smaller than a tennis ball" protruding from the left orbit. Donahue[27] reported she was a patient leading a comparatively normal life 22 years after orbitotomy. She had gone through high school and secretarial school and was working in an office. She declined surgery. Sweet first saw her when at age 32 she inquired about a cosmetic procedure for her extruding orbital mass, mentioning as symptoms only occasional dizziness and loss of taste of food for 2 years. She declined study, but returned at age 35 describing brief temporal lobe seizures, only about one per month for the previous 5 years, and consenting to hospitalization. Examination showed a visual acuity of 20/40 OD with relative temporal hemianopia to dim light but full field to bright light. Calcification in skull films and a pneumoencephalogram (PEG) outlined an additional subfrontal intracranial tumor the size of a grapefruit, 9 cm in transverse diameter. Sweet removed the intracranial tumor in one stage on September 3, 1965, the posterior segment of the intraorbital mass 1½ months later, and placed a ventriculoatrial shunt on January 19, 1966. An ophthalmic surgeon, Dr. Casten, removed the remaining 5 × 6 × 6.5-cm glioma on May 25, 1966. Removal of the intracranial tumor left her with a temporal hemianopia precisely splitting the macula and a corrected visual acuity of 20/30. Six years after these operations she was no longer experiencing seizures and

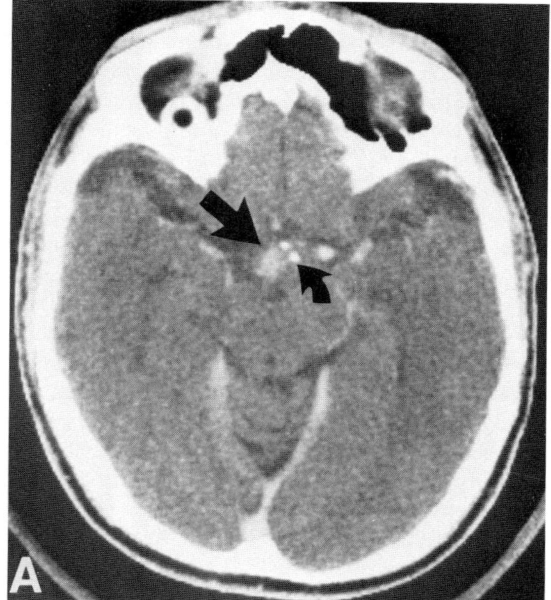

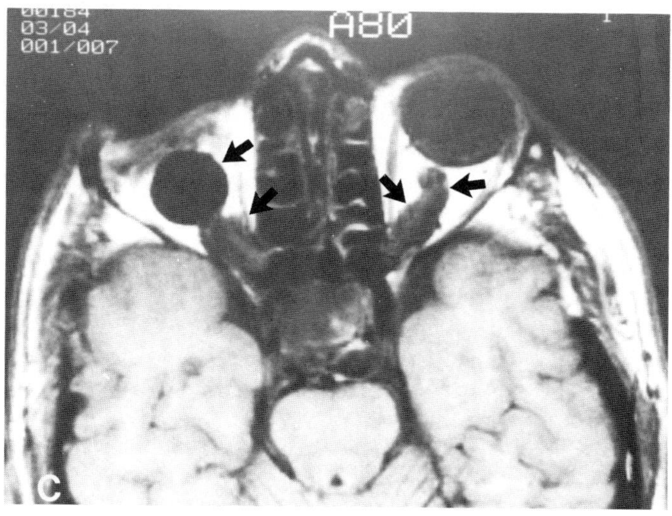

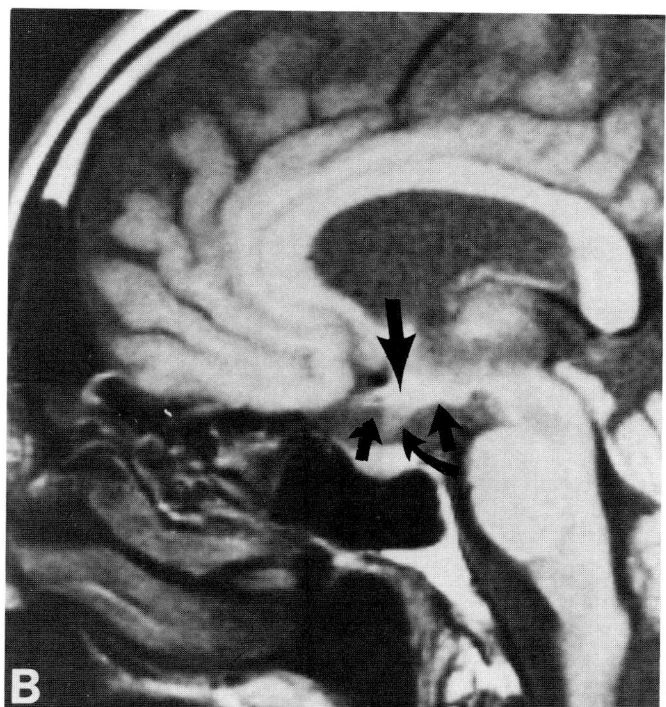

Fig. 25-1. Case 2. (A) A CT scan obtained February 21, 1982 showing an enhancing tumor of the chiasm (large straight arrow) with two calcified globules (small curved arrow). (B) A negative image of gliomas of each optic nerve enclosed by dense images of periorbital fat. (C) A MRI scan obtained on March 31, 1986 shows a dense chiasmal tumor (three large arrows) and the less dense enlarged pituitary stalk. Note the much less dense neighboring CSF.

was functioning well supported by cortisone, Synthroid, and Dilantin. She was lost to follow-up and it was later learned she had died with an infected shunt and ventriculitis on June 20, 1980 at age 50.

Summary: A glioma initially of one optic nerve apparently grew steadily for 32 years until totally removed.

Case 2. A 6-month-old boy was explored by Jason Mixter assisted by Sweet on February 18, 1941. We found a reddened right optic nerve, the pencil-sized enlargement of which extended back into the right side of the chiasm and optic tract. Examination of the biopsy specimen revealed a low grade glioma. He was seen again 6 years later, having gradually lost vision in the right eye with a sudden increase of the proptosis to an extreme degree for the previous 6 to 8 months. The ophthalmic surgeon removed the right eyeball and the orbital portion of the tumor on July 9, 1947. At that time his visual acuity was 20/200 (OS) with optic atrophy. He was followed assiduously every few years by his ophthalmologist. The visual field and acuity remained stable for 34 years until 1981. A new superior altitudinal defect and a decline in visual acuity to 20/400 were then found, but these were not accompanied by any

certain changes on CT scans obtained in February, 1982 and September, 1983 or on the MRI scan obtained in February, 1986. However, greater resolution of the involved structures was provided by the MRI studies. There was an enlargement of the intraorbital parts of both optic nerves and of the slightly calcified chiasm (Figure 25-1). He continued to work full time and, with an almost stable intracranial status for 37 years, without treatment. Slight further tumor growth may have occurred in the last 5 years.

Summary: A glioma initially of one optic nerve grew sporadically for 6 years, then remained virtually stationary for 37 years with, however, a visual acuity of only 20/200 in the remaining eye.

Case 3. The patient, reported in detail elsewhere, had her glioma of one optic nerve slightly invading the chiasm almost totally removed from in front of the chiasm to and including the globe and was given 4000 rad of radiation at age 4 years. Six years later the tumor, now a grade II astrocytoma, completely refilled the orbit and extended as a gray carpet from the tuberculum sellae to the hypothalamus. Only the intraorbital portion was removed. Further radiation therapy was thought useless. In the 33 years since then she has remained nearly normal, including a normal visual field and acuity in the remaining eye. Her menses, sleep patterns, and fluid intake and output were normal, but she had always had a problem of obesity, now weighing 245 pounds, as her only evidence of a hypothalamopituitary disorder. Closely spaced CT scans showed no intracranial tumor. Its previous site, the suprasellar fossa and most of the intrasellar fossas and the left subfrontal area were filled with CSF. The left posterior orbital and intraorbital canalicular spaces contained a mass, either residual tumor or fibrous tissue.

Summary: A glioma initially of one optic nerve and slightly involving the chiasm recurred massively despite removal of the nerve and 4000 rad of radiation at age 4. Extensive intracranial tumor seen at operation 6 years later then spontaneously disappeared almost completely in the next 33 years.

At the other end of the spectrum of growth rate are the relatively few malignant gliomas of the anterior visual pathways. As reported by Hoyt et al.,[28] their 5 cases and 10 they cited from the literature were adults. They were from 23 to 59 years of age at onset with an average age of 42 years. Since then there have been at least 19 other articles published describing malignant astrocytomas of the anterior visual pathways. While the majority have appeared in adults, Reese[29] described a grade IV and Brand and Hoover[30] a grade III optic glioma in infants. Helcl and Petrásková had one anaplastic glioma in their 18 otherwise pilocytic optic astrocytomas in children.[31] There are two Japanese reports of an aggressively growing type of optic glioma in infants.[32,33] Thus, of Kanamori's 6 patients aged 3 years or less at onset, 3 soon died and a fourth was bedridden. These four tumors were histologically malignant and gave rise to severe hypothalamic dysfunction. Hoyt also described two anaplastic astrocytomas as giant tumors in infants and five more "moderately anaplastic" gliomas in 12 children with chiasmal gliomas.[22] Borit and Richardson[25] described a 9-month-old infant with neurofibromatosis whose bilateral tumor of both optic nerves and chiasm at surgery was hypercellular with many mitoses, killing the patient 2 years later. Heiskanen et al.[34] reported on 2 children whose initially benign optic gliomas underwent malignant transformation with extensive invasion of the frontal lobes. One had had early hypothalamic signs; the first troubles in the other were visual. Wilson reported the case of a 7-year-old girl given 5670 rad in 6 weeks for her tumor, who died at age 27 with benign gliomatous areas in her visual pathways that became anaplastic in the massive basal spread of the lesion.[35] At post mortem no features of radiation effect were identified. These reports emphasize further the potential for erratic and dangerous growth of these lesions at all ages.

Hoyt and Baghdassarian[22] consider these mass lesions to have features of congenital hamartomas, citing as an example the events after partial excisions in 3 of their 7 patients with tumors of one optic nerve. Tumor, known to be present in the chiasm in these 3 patient, had not caused visual loss in the remaining eye thereafter (duration of follow-up not stated).

A "hamartoma" as defined in *Stedman's Medical Dictionary* (21st edition) is a "malformation resembling a neoplasm but developing and growing at virtually the same rate as normal components and not likely to result in compression of adjacent tissue." Similar definitions are given in other dictionaries. This definition simply does not fit the tumors in question, which nearly all grow faster than the child, like true neoplasms, for a long or a short time compressing or invading the optic pathways. As noted in Table 25-6, there were five publications by 1902 describing the recurrence of a glioma of one optic nerve

after intraorbital excision.[36–40] We see no justification then or thereafter for referring to them as hamartomas, a term that lulls the physician into a false sense of security with regard to the growth potential of the lesion. Indeed, Hoyt's colleagues, Andersen and Spencer, described three "mechanisms for enlargement of the tumor": (1) proliferation of tumor cells, (2) hyperplasia of surrounding tissues, and (3) accumulation of mucin within the tumor.[41]

With respect to excessive glial nonneoplastic growth in the anterior visual pathways, there are a few reported cases of neurofibromatosis in which one or both optic nerves became diffusely thickened as a consequence of proliferation of astrocytic, arachnoidal, and other connective tissue elements.[42] Such an unusual patient typically has neurofibromatosis, enlarged optic canals, pallor of the optic discs, but no visual complaints or visual field loss.[43] The 2 patients described in these two papers were 44 and 40 years of age, so the disorder had presumably been present for decades. Pfeiffer and Reese each described enlarged optic foramina without loss of vision in the presence of neurofibromatosis.[44,45]

Through the kindness of Robert Martuza, we describe here the case of an additional patient in whom the diagnosis of probable tumor rather than hyperplasia in the visual pathways was made even though she had no visual complaints.

Case Report.

The patient, aged 14, with the cutaneous stigmata of neurofibromatosis, had a similarly afflicted mother from whom a glioma of one optic nerve had been removed 10 years previously. The patient's visual fields showed the scotomas illustrated in Figure 25-2A, of which the asymptomatic patient was unaware. Her CT scan (Figure 25-2B,C) demonstrated a tumor in the chiasm and at least one optic nerve. By August, 1986, the scotoma in the left eye was larger and denser than in July, 1985. Radiation therapy was being considered at that time.

Careful follow-up was the course of action chosen by Horwich and Bloom for a similar patient with von Recklinghausen's disease and a tumor in one optic nerve with no evidence of progression of disease.[46] Even more dramatic surprises developed in one of our patients with neurofibromatosis, who at age 2 in 1971 had his right optic nerve containing a glioma removed from the chiasm to the globe. The visual field and acuity of his left eye were normal in 1975. Although he was totally asymptomatic and free of all neurologic deficits save those in his visual system, his follow-up studies at age 17 in 1986 revealed a quadrantic temporal field defect in his left eye, and the CT and MRI scans showed three large tumors in the third ventricle and right and left cerebellar hemispheres (Figures 25-3A and B). In addition the MRI scans revealed at least seven tiny nodules of indeterminate (astroglial?) nature scattered bilaterally in the frontal lobe white matter (Figure 25-3C shows two of these). The large left cerebellar astrocytoma was removed and radiation therapy given to the chiasmal region. Horwich and Bloom describe another patient with von Recklinghausen's disease whose bilateral optic nerve gliomas were treated by radiation. Thirty-one years later she had developed four other intracranial tumors, including a large grade III astrocytoma of the thalamus.[46] Lewis et al.,[47] in radiologic studies including CT scans on 207 patients diagnosed as having von Recklinghausen's neurofibromatosis, found tumors of the anterior visual pathways in 15 percent. In two thirds, such lesions were not suspected either from the patient's history or ophthalmologic examination. Aron et al.[13] recently

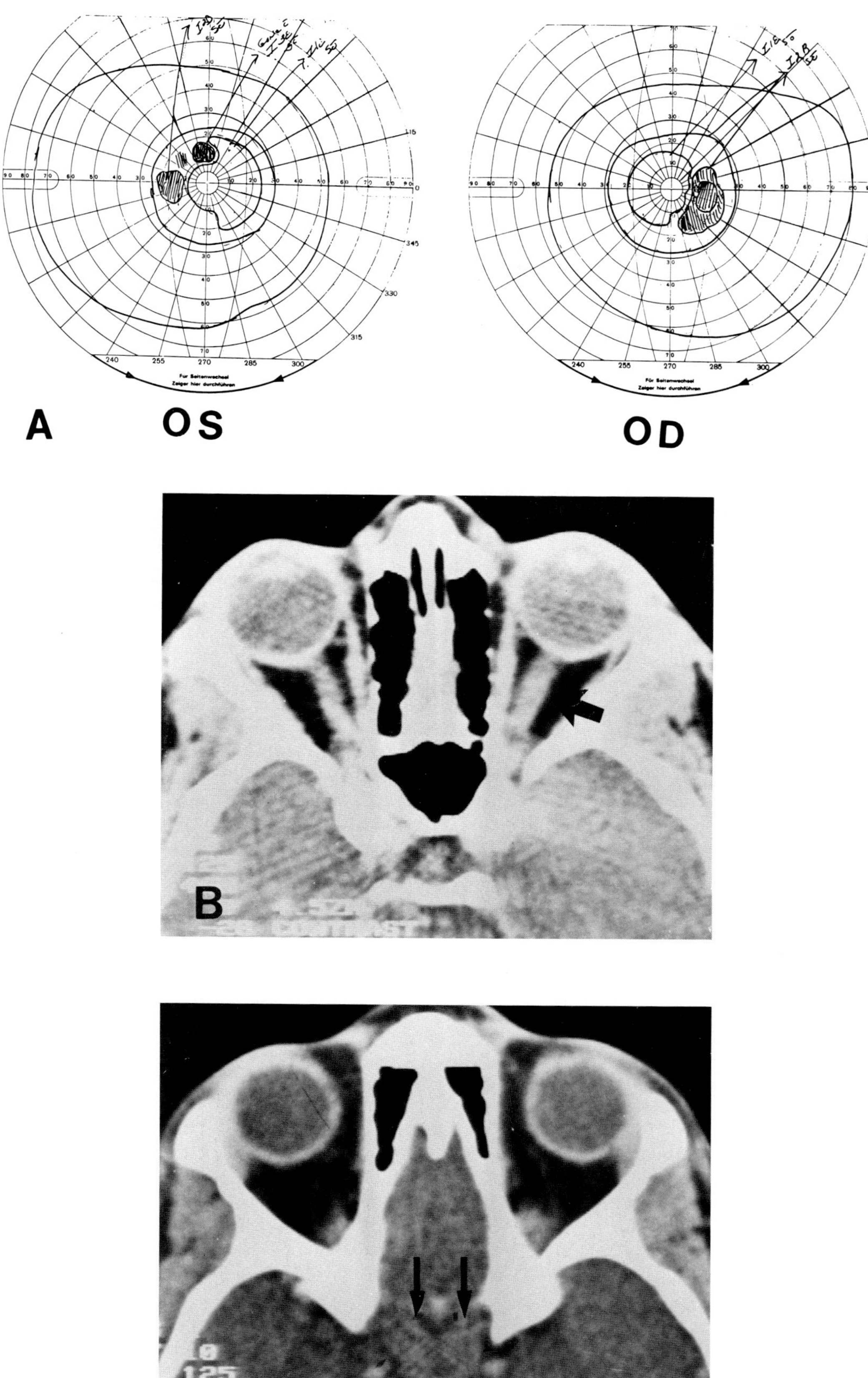

Fig. 25-2. This 14-year-old patient was asymptomatic, including subjectively normal vision. (A) The visual fields showed these scotomas. Those of the left eye worsened 13 months later. (B) A CT scan through the orbit shows a greatly enlarged left optic nerve (black arrow). (C) A CT scan through the chiasm shows substantial enlargement; estimated diameter, 1.5 cm (arrows).

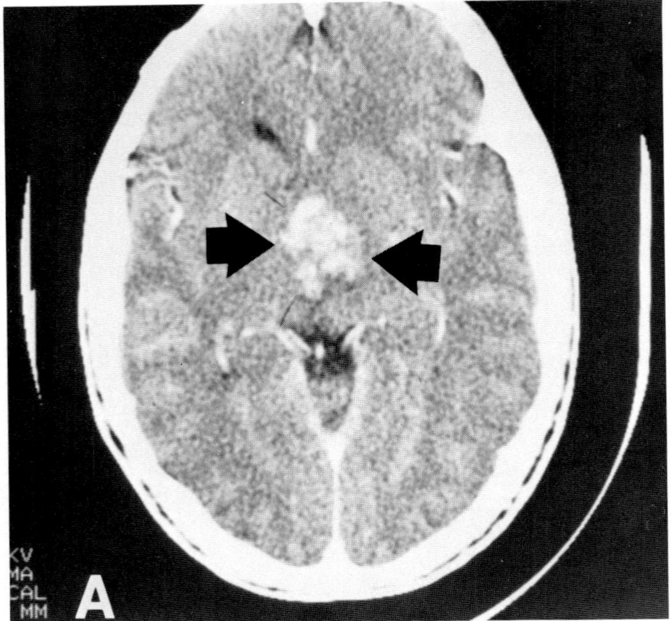

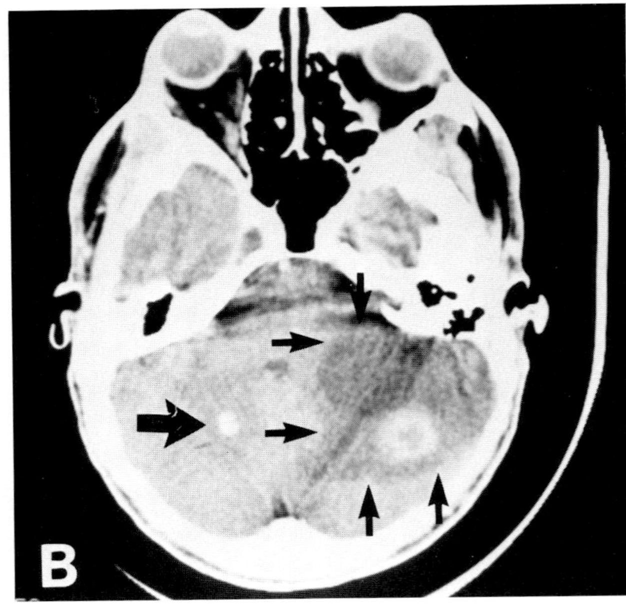

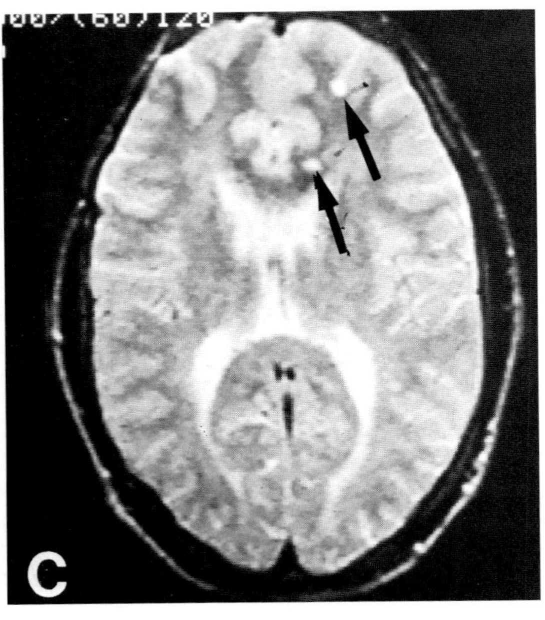

Fig. 25-3. Case 4. CT scans obtained on August 1, 1986. (A) Contrast-enhanced tumor in the region of the upper third ventricle. (B) The small arrows outline the huge cyst with a contrast-enhanced solid component near the surface of this left cerebellar cystic astrocytoma. (Large arrow: small tumor nodule in the center of the right cerebellar hemisphere). (C) One of a series of MRI scans showing a total of 7 small nodules of *f* indeterminate nature. The two in this image are indicated by the arrows.

reported on two more unsuspected chiasmal lesions detected on CT scans in such patients.

All patients with neurofibromatosis with or without pallor of an optic disc probably should be studied for optic and other gliomas and for smaller lesions, so that early diagnosis can be made and the natural history more fully documented. This group is favorable for conservative follow-up, with subsequent surgery or radiation therapy as and when advisable.

SPONTANEOUS REGRESSION OF OPTIC GLIOMAS

We have identified six other papers reporting significant although often modest spontaneous improvement in symptoms or findings in patients with operatively proven diagnoses. The report of Hoyt and Baghdassarian describes spontaneous improvement in 4 of 23 eyes in untreated patients—nearly all without surgical verification of the diagnosis.[22] The largest series of patients with verified diagnoses and protracted station-

ary status (3 cases), or actual regression (2 cases) is that of Tym.[48] It includes a patient followed 39 years whose chiasmal tumor had reduced visual acuity to less than J20 in each eye after 25 years of worsening. Vision then recovered to J6 and J18 over the next 14 years (case 3). In a 2-year-old child the optic nerves at transfrontal exploration "were swollen like spring onions in contact with each other"; the massively proptotic eyeball and the nerve on one side were removed. Eight years later she was developing normally with J2 vision in the remaining eye (case 6). In cases 1, 4, and 7 despite a swollen chiasm, one eye had conserved normal visual acuity and field for 16, 8, and 6 years, respectively. Other convincing reports include cases 9 and 21 of Borit and Richardson,[25] with residual tumor remaining at surgery but none found at autopsy in each case 13½ years later with no radiation therapy. In the first case, a 14-year-old girl, the eyeball and entire orbital and intracranial optic nerve had been resected, leaving only microscopic remnants in the chiasm, but in the second case, a 3-month-old boy, only a biopsy specimen had been taken. The case of Kahn et al.[8]

with a biopsy-proven glioma of the nerves and chiasm showed no progression of symptoms over a 9-year period; 20/20 vision remained in both eyes. With the advent of high-resolution CT scanning there is at least one case report of a marked spontaneous decrease in tumor size. A large suprasellar astrocytoma (grade II) of which only the exophytic component was surgically removed was far smaller in scans made 10 months after surgery compared with those made 3 months postoperatively; there also was some recovery of visual acuity.[47] As already noted, the visual evoked responses to pattern stimulation improved spontaneously in 2 patients with gliomas of an optic nerve.[20] Berke reported 2 patients in whom bilaterally enlarged optic canals both decreased in size after unilateral removal of a tumor via one-sided lateral orbitotomy.[50] Hird's patient had a blind right eye with no pupillary reaction to light plus blurred vision on the left at the time of a biopsy of the swollen right optic nerve and chiasm.[51] Bilateral papilledema subsided and vision and fields on the left recovered fully to the astonishment of her physicians. In one of the 17 patients of Wright et al. with presumed glioma of one optic nerve (no biopsy) the "proptosis resolved during a 3-year period."[52]

This extraordinary although infrequent tendency to spontaneous regression or even disappearance, which is also seen with a few other intracranial tumors, serves to differentiate them from hamartomas, which have not been shown to behave in this way.

The majority of patients suffer from significant enlargement of their neoplasm at some stage in the course of the disease. These cases will be analyzed in two groups: those with a tumor confined at least initially to one optic nerve, and patients with more extensive tumors.

GLIOMAS INITIALLY OF ONE OPTIC NERVE

One of the first comprehensive discussions of collations of gliomas of the optic nerve, that of Hudson in 1912,[53] includes 118 cases. His conclusion was that about 80 percent of optic nerve tumors were gliomas and 20 percent were "endothelial tumors," meningiomas of the nerve sheath. Widely quoted is his statement, "in no single instance has a recurrence of new growth in the orbit after removal of one of these tumors been recorded." The tumors were known to have been incompletely removed in 51 cases; yet freedom from recurrence was noted in 13 cases from 3 to 24 years later. This behavior led Hudson to suggest that the process is a "degenerative gliomatosis" rather than a true neoplasm. Not so widely quoted but picked up by Dandy[54] were the findings in 23 autopsies reported by Byers[38] between 1901 and 1903 and by Hudson on patients with intraorbital optic nerve gliomas.[53] *In only one instance did the cranial cavity contain no tumor.* Fourteen of them had died of meningitis a few days after removal of the orbital tumor; 3 died later of increased intracranial pressure, and 5 died of intercurrent disease. In Hudson's 15 autopsied cases the intracranial growth affected one or both optic nerves with or without the chiasm and including neighboring brain in 5. Recurrence of tumor caused death in 6; there was probable recurrence in 5 others. Although 34 had a 1 year "cure," there were follow-up reports at 6 years in only 6 patients. Fifty-seven of the patients had been followed less than 1 year. Hudson stated "The large size attained by the cerebral new formations without the production of severe symptoms has in several cases been very remarkable, and is to be attributed to the very slow rate of increase."

Stable defects in visual acuity and fields do not prove the tumor is not enlarging. For example, Aarabi, Long, and Miller reported that a patient had had pale optic discs and stable visual acuity from age 9 months to 13½ years, but only after 2 weeks of headache were studies and a craniotomy performed.[55] Her optic glioma had fanned out over the inferior surfaces of both frontal lobes and extended into the third ventricle, right basal ganglia, and temporal lobe. Fletcher et al.[5] also reported on 2 patients with CT evidence of slow growth of tumor but no change of visual function for several years. Follow-up by scans is clearly imperative.

A fairly complete survey of the literature of gliomas confined to one optic nerve and including our own cases is given in Tables 25-1 through 25-6.[2,7,20,24–26,31,34,36–40,52,56–85]

A remarkable patient illustrating the value of prompt surgery is the one reported by Goodman et al.[86] A 6½-year-old boy with normal visual findings in all respects except for papilledema, an enlarged blind spot, and minimal proptosis proved to have a huge glioma throughout one optic nerve, which when resected just in front of the chiasm showed a 1-mm cuff of normal nerve.

Two other unusual cases have recently been reported.[87] Each had von Recklinghausen's neurofibromatosis with a unilateral intraorbital optic glioma but without enlargement of the optic foramen or intracanalicular portion of the optic nerve. Exclusively intraorbital removal in one at age 2 and in the other at age 4 revealed no tumor in the posterior cut edge of the excised optic nerve, so no radiation was given. Proptosis recurred in 2 months and 2 years, respectively, but reoperation in each revealed only an intensely fibrotic mass without tumor cells. Neither of these masses increased in size during the follow-up period, which was 5 years in the younger patient.

The case reports cited make clear the erratic growth potential. Yet there is almost unanimous agreement that juvenile pilocytic astrocytomas (also called polar spongioblastomas) that continue to grow cannot be distinguished from those that do not by light microscopy. Indeed, Borit and Richardson in their detailed analysis of 30 patients noted that some tumors with well localized and apparently quiescent growth also had small areas of unusually dense cellularity.[25] It is obviously highly desirable to determine, if possible, which tumors are not going to grow in order to spare these patients unnecessary surgery or radiation treatment. There are very few reports of electron microscopically evaluated ultrastructure in these cases, and we found none correlating subsequent growth patterns with any aspect of such structure.

Wright et al.[52] thought that in their 17 patients with gliomas of one optic nerve they could distinguish two groups: a group of 9 patients in whom the tumors followed a "slow indolent course," justifying follow-up for 1 to 8 years without immediate therapy; and a group of 8 patients in whom growth progressed more rapidly, and whom they referred at once to the neurosurgeon. They have, however, lost to follow-up 3 of the 9 patients in the first group, illustrating one hazard of this tactic. Our summary of patients with continuing growth of these tumors on the one hand along with the minimal morbidity and mortality of the neurosurgical techniques of the last 15 years leads to our unequivocal recommendation for surgery in nearly all cases of tumors of one optic nerve. The tiny streamer of tumor that can gradually spread backward within the nerve to the chiasm will not be seen by the best scans now available. Indeed, Fog et al.[88] had one case of an intraorbital glioma in which the optic foramen and the intracranial portion of the optic nerve appeared normal. However, the poste-

Table 25-1. Glioma of one optic nerve; grossly complete excision from variable distances in front of chiasm to globe

Reference	Number of Cases	Outcome
Cuneo and Rand, 1952	1	OK 13 years later
Jain, 1961	1	Removal in front of chiasm in two stages OD; (No microscopy cut poterior end of nerve) followed by radiation treatment. Dose not stated. 17 1/2 months after right optic nerve cut, new enlargement left optic foramen, OS nearly blind from recurrence
Bane and Long, 1964	1	No recurrence at 22 months
Richards, 1966	4	No tumor in posterior cut end of nerve; no recurrence
Matson, 1969	7	Six certainly and 1 possibly totally removed. No recurrence; 5 followed 4–18 years
Wong and Lubow, 1972	10	No recurrence in 3–14 years
Lloyd, 1973	8	No recurrence 1–14 years
Myles and Murphy, 1973	4	One postoperative death before 1932; 3 OK at 14 months, 17 and 19 years
Miller 1974	11	Two died postoperatively—1 seizures, 1 cardiac arrest; 1 meningitis. All "complete resections"—no mention of microscopy at cut end of nerves
Heiskanen, 1978	5	"Total excisions"—3 of 5 irradiated; other eye normal 4–18 years later
DeSousa, 1979	3	Two alive; 1 dead of malignant trigeminal schwannoma years later
Karaguisov, 1979	10	No recurrences 3–23 years
Marejeva, 1979	0	Fifty-seven optic nerves (cut just in front of chiasm posterior to area of grossly visible tumor) microscopic tumor in posterior cut end in 44 of 57. Recurrence in 4 of 44 at 1 to 12 years
Visot, 1980	4	No recurrence, all more than 10 years; 1 with normal CT scan at 12 years; in all 4 histologic invasions of posterior cut end of nerve given radiotherapy
Wright, 1980	1	Case 1—intraorbital biopsy with spillage much mucinous material; later removed from chiasm to "behind the globe"; in 9 months *orbital recurrence*; partial exenteration
Tenny, 1982	29	(Nine with irradiation also)—all alive
Helcl, 1985	4	Aged 6–13 years; no recurrence
Sweet, 1986	14	Aged 5 months–10 years at 1st symptom, average 5 years; 1 recurrence at 15 years postoperatively; follow-up 6–34 years, average 21 years; 1 recurrence chiasm
		Posterior cut end of nerve: 8 inadequate data or uncertain data; follow-up 12–30 years—average 21 years; 3 clearly free of tumor; follow-up 6–13 years—average 9½ years; no recurrences, 2 clearly contained tumor; follow-up 10–34 years; average 22 years

Summary: 117 grossly total removal; 3 recurrences, 2 into chiasm, 1 into orbit; 3 died after operation in earlier decades.

rior end of the nerve cut at the chiasm showed microscopic evidence of tumor. It therefore appears to us to be advisable to resect nearly all gliomas that appear to be confined to one optic nerve before such backward spread has occurred. Exceptions to this are the early cases of neurofibromatosis. In such patients independent tiny foci of tumor can be present elsewhere in the anterior visual pathway, as in Martuza's case reported earlier and the cases of Lewis et al.[47] In such cases, frequent follow-ups are required to determine when, where, and how to intervene. In particular, the advisability of a course of immediate radiation therapy once minor microscopic tumor strands are seen in the posterior cut end of the nerve is uncertain. Richardson pointed out that the distinction between neoplastic astrocytes grade I and "reactive" astrocytes is difficult.

SURGERY FOR GLIOMAS OF ONE OPTIC NERVE

Once it is determined that surgery is necessary, the subfrontal transcranial approach to the intracranial, intracanalicular, and intraorbital portions of the optic nerve is the procedure of choice.

Housepian's account of refinements of the original Dandy approach emphasizes diagonal division of the origin of the levator palpebrae superioris muscle just anterior to the annulus of Zinn and medial to the superior rectus, with resuture of the annulus and muscle after the removal.[89,90] (See the excellent series of figures in his chapter on Intraorbital Tumors in this text.) We recommend preliminary verification by histologic examination of a biopsy specimen. Luccarelli described 2 patients in whom the gross appearance was of swelling confined to the anterior optic pathways.[91] In one 39-year-old woman only the full extent of one optic nerve was involved. In the other, a 32-year-old woman, the swelling involved both optic nerves and the chiasm. Histologic examinations revealed a highly radiosensitive ectopic pinealoma, more properly termed a dysgerminoma, unfortunately only after the optic nerve had been resected in one of the patients. Excision of an optic glioma, usually in one stage, should be from globe to chiasm.

In view of reported recurrences when the intracanalicular portion of the nerve has been left behind, we disagree with Housepian's statement that it is not essential to remove this part of the nerve in the treatment of these gliomas.[90] Frank

Table 25-2. Glioma of one optic nerve; incomplete excision in front of chiasm to globe—recurrence

Reference	Number of cases	Outcome
Hanbery, 1956	1	Chiasm looked normal; death 8 months later with huge glioma arising in chiasm spreading to hypothalamus
Suarez, 1971	0	Four patients with microscopic or macroscopic infiltration of chiasm or even tract by tumor; all irradiated: all without recurrence 15, 14, 2, and 1 year later
Spencer, 1972	1	Removal of tumor in front of chiasm to just behind entrance of central retinal artery. Tumor still in oculobulbar part of nerve: 4 recurrences of intraorbital tumor in this patient 7, 2, 3, and 1 year later—all "benign astrocytoma"
Wong and Lubow, 1972	0	No progression; follow-up 1 to 20 years 11 patients
Visot, 1980	0	Three microscopic tumors posterior cut end of optic nerve; 0 sine such tumor; all 3 irradiated; all had normal CT scans 10 years later
Wright, 1980	0	Cases 4 and 5 had microscopic tumors in posterior end of cut optic nerve—only 6 months follow-up
Kalifa, 1981	0	Three microscopic tumors in posterior end of optic nerve; 0 sine such tumor; 1 irradiated 5000–5300rad; no recurrence 10, 10, or 4 years
Gaini, 1982	1	Five patients with microscopic tumors in posterior cut end of optic nerve; all irradiated: no recurrence in less than 5 to 20 years. In 1 patient tumor left in optic canal—regrew in both directions 11 years later
Tenny, 1982	3	Deaths from intracranial tumor at 3 months, 3, and 4 years—no follow-up data re recurrence without death
Groswasser, 1985	0	Four microscopic tumors in posterior cut end of optic nerve—follow-up not stated
Sweet, 1986	2	One globe invaded by tumor recurrence at 15 months; 1 chiasm invaded by tumor recurrence at 6 years

Summary: Histologic examination of posterior end of cut optic nerve is important. In 8 cases there was known recurrence following incomplete removal. (Inadequate follow-up in most.) Data do not permit evaluation of radiation for microscopic infiltration of posterior cut end of nerve.

Walsh concluded in 1947, "The fact that a glioma (of an optic nerve), incompletely removed, may occasionally cease to grow does not seem sufficient reason for doing an incomplete operation."[92] The long follow-ups of the ensuing 39 years support the wisdom of that advice. How to treat the patient when the eye is minimally involved remains a matter of uncertainty and will depend to some extent on the accuracy with which the latest generations of CT and MRI scanners can detect growth of these tumors once they are discovered. Maisongrosse's solution was to give radiotherapy to a child whose acuity was $7/10$ or less in the affected eye.[93]

GLIOMAS OF THE CHIASM AND/OR OPTIC NERVES AND/OR ADJOINING BRAIN

Most optic gliomas involve some combination of the chiasm, optic nerves, and adjoining brain. Whether they should be operated on is a question to be carefully weighed in each individual case. The decision as to open operation and its extent should be guided by the following considerations.

SURGERY—ITS RATIONALE AND PITFALLS

Because of the hazards and "little likelihood of a good result," many critics favor no surgical attack on these tumors. Opponents of surgery point out that Martin and Cushing[3] had 3 deaths within 48 hours of operation and no useful results in the 4 other patients treated in this way. Dandy's 4 patients[54] all succumbed soon after surgery. Such results are irrelevant, since they occurred many years before the controllability of hypothalamo-pituitary deficits, infection, and cerebral edema and the use of the operating microscope. Housepian and his colleagues at the New York Neurological Institute recommend an attempt to reach a presumptive diagnosis of such tumors without surgery so that one can proceed forthwith to radiation therapy. Wright et al. usually advise against surgery when the chiasm is involved,[52] as did Throuvalas et al.[94] and Jefferson.[70] Robertson and Brewin stated that in chiasmal gliomas "the effect of surgery (on vision) will almost inevitably be to make it immediately and permanently worse."[95] They conclude that survival "is probably not affected by surgery or by radiotherapy."

However, a number of writers think that the clinical and radiographic features of pituitary tumors, Hodgkin's disease, reticulum cell sarcomas, suprasellar ganglioneuromas, and ectopic pinealomas (dysgerminomas), cannot be distinguished with certainty from optic gliomas unless the patient has neurofibromatosis.[1,24,63] A tongue projecting from a craniopharyngioma has enlarged an optic canal simulating a glioma.[96] The preoperative diagnosis of "chiasmatic hypophyseal glioma" in a case reported by Giuffrè et al.[97] proved to be radionecrosis of this region caused by ^{60}Co therapy to the pituitary gland many

Table 25-3. Glioma of one optic nerve; no excision

Reference	Outcome
Jefferson, 1940	First eye symptoms 18 months; blind OD age 5; always at top of class until age 12—then rapid downhill course to death. Autopsy: glioma of right optic nerve, chiasm, brain stem
Smith, 1977	2-year-old boy with neurofibromatosis; OD 2 mm proptosis 20/25 vision with central field depression. 10 months later vision 20/30 or 20/40. CT scan showed optic glioma OD. At surgery tumor into chiasm—"radiation with little response"
Wright, 1980	Case 3—5½-year-old girl. No neurofibromatosis. Blind OD with 3 mm proptosis; OS vision and VEP normal. 1 year later VEP-nasal fibers OD involved. Age 8½ tumor at surgery in both optic nerves, chiasm, and hypothalamus. Radiation: no progression 4 years later
Borit, 1982	Intraorbital tumor—operation refused—5 years later operation accepted but chiasm involved
Summary: Tumor spread in visual pathways in all 4 cases 2–15 years without operation or radiation.	

Table 25-4. Glioma of one optic nerve; intraorbital excision thought complete

Reference	Number of Cases	Outcome
Lloyd, 1973	1	Normal optic foramen; normal nerve at each end of intraorbital glioma
Klug, 1977	3	OK 14 months, 17 and 19 years
Wright, 1980	1	20-year-old woman with glioma in orbit only; transfrontal operation; no tumor
Gaini, 1982	3	Glioma in orbit only; no recurrence less than 5 to more than 20 years
Sweet, 1986	4	Aged 1½ to 14 years at first symptom, average 6.1 years; intracranial optic nerve looked normal; removed behind optic canal; No recurrence at 7–28 years—average 19½ years
Summary: A few tumors are confined to orbit and canal		

months before (Giuffré R: Personal communication, September 15, 1986). For all of these reasons many favor operative exposure. Pitfalls include one described by Miller of two cases in which the neurosurgeon's biopsy specimens of enlarged intracranial optic pathways were misdiagnosed by the operator and the first pathologist as glioma.[24] More extensive tumor material revealed Hodgkin's sarcoma in one case and reticulum cell sarcoma in the other. The need for caution in the face of unexpectedly normal neural appearances was pointed out by Wright.[52] In one patient with an enlarged optic foramen the intracanalicular and intracranial portions of the optic nerve were excised but contained neither glial hyperplasia nor glioma. The need for caution even in the face of the expected gliomatous appearance has already been mentioned in two cases in which the tumor proved to be a dysgerminoma.

When only a small biopsy specimen is taken one must attempt to remove it from a portion of the visual pathway related to a blind area of the visual field to avoid the experience reported by Montgomery et al. in which 75 percent of their 15 patients undergoing biopsy suffered a surgically related increase in the visual field deficit.[98]

By using a Cavitron ultrasonic surgical aspirator while monitoring visual evoked potentials, Albright and Sclabasse removed 60 to 85 percent of 2 chiasmal gliomas without worsening of already severely impaired vision.[99]

FEATURES FAVORABLE FOR PARTIAL OR MORE COMGLETE RESECTION

Some optic gliomas clearly have surgically remediable aspects.

Edema without Neoplastic Invasion

The first of these is the situation seen by Walsh.[100] At intradural exposure the left optic nerve was the size of his middle finger and the ipsilateral two thirds of the chiasm was greatly swollen. The affected nerve was excised from the chiasm forward into normal nerve. On histologic examination the tumor proved to have been completely removed; the

Table 25-5. Glioma of one optic nerve; incomplete (?) intraorbital excision: No recurrence

Reference	Number of Cases	Outcome
Knapp, 1926	3	Large optic canals but only intraorbital operation well with good vision other eye 15–18 years later
Bane and Long, 1964	1	4-year-old girl—followed 37 years
Chutorian, 1964	16	Followed up to 24 years; normal vision other eye
Spencer, 1972	1	Case 1—proptosis 4–11 mm in 18 months; no recurrence 5 years after orbitotomy
Wong and Lubow, 1973	4	Followed for "years"
Wright, 1980	1	Followed 4 years
Sweet, 1986	2	Intraorbital excision known incomplete; no recurrence at 4 years
Summary: 27 patients (7 articles): No recurrence		

Table 25-6. Glioma of one optic nerve; Incomplete (?) Intraorbital Excision—Recurrence

Reference	Outcome
Szokalski, 1861	Five years later intraorbital recurrence size of small apple—removed; meningitis; Death—Autopsy: walnut-sized tumor on chiasm
Goldzieher, 1873	Case 3, orbital recurrence
Byers, 1901	Orbital recurrence at 1 year; exenteration; death in 8 years of huge intracranial glioma
Barraquer, 1902	Intracranial extension 9 years after operation
Pagenstecher, 1902	Orbital recurrence 25 years later; death from meningitis after 2nd removal. Autopsy: tumor did not reach chiasm
Seefelder, 1931	Intraorbital recurrence at 2 years, again 1 year later
Davis, 1940	Case 3, distal half of right optic nerve removed; slow progression, enlargement of optic foramen, tumor into intracranial optic nerve, chiasm 4½ years later. Autopsy: "Independent" large tumor anterior and medial right temporal lobe
Levitt, 1940	Case 2, 9-year-old girl, 4½ years later semicoma, atrophy other optic disc; diagnosis: extension of tumor to chiasm and hypothalamus
Christensen, 1952	Two of 11 with glioma of nerve or nerve plus chiasm: reoperation 1 and 2 times, respectively. Intraorbital as well as intracranial recurrences
Zülch 1960	Age 3 intraorbital removal; chiasmal growth operated on age 28
Yanoff, 1978	Five-year-old boy; enucleation; intraorbital removal 4 times in 1 year; death at 6½ years huge chiasmal glioma spreading to anterior and middle fossas. All orbital tumors "juvenile pilocytic astrocytomas"; 1 specimen this patient only rare mitoses and more cells than usual
Rougier, 1973	Thirty-year-old woman 3½ years after excision loss in contralateral eye of inferior temporal quadrant with arc central scotoma other 3 quadrants; optic foramen much larger ipsilateral eye
Mullaney, 1976	Four-year-old boy, 48 years later gross proptosis "for many years." Intraorbital re-operation only; histology: malignant features
Chang and Wood, 1977	Three patients—"recurred in orbit or extended intracranially" several years later. "Grossly total tumor removal" originally
Nicole, 1980	6 children: 4 good results 15, 14, 13, and 2 years; 1 died 6 months (?) cause; 1 intracranial spread at 8 years
Iraci, 1981	Six-year-old girl, normal optic foramen—intraorbital removal—3 years later optic foramen enlarged, suprasellar mass, vision decreased other eye
Borit, 1982	Fourteen children: *4 orbital recurrences*; 1 patient 3 such recurrences with intracranial spread.

Summary: 23 patients (17 articles) with recurrence

chiasmal swelling was not neoplastic. After 7 years the vision in the other eye was still normal (p 2087). Walsh wrote "Resection of the nerve is indicated whether or not the chiasm is swollen and appears to be affected and whether or not the patient is a child." (p 2092).

Cystic or Hemorrhagic Component

Another favorable but likewise infrequent finding is of cystic fluid compressing the optic pathways. Kahn described a 9-year-old girl who in 1961 had advanced primary optic atrophy of her left eye with a visual acuity of only 20/400 OS, 20/50 OD and a right homonymous hemianopia in each eye.[8] There was a semilunar calcification 15 mm above and slightly behind the sella turcica. At surgery the posterior part of the left optic nerve, the left half of the chiasm, and the left optic tract were grossly swollen with a "blue domed" cyst bulging inferolateral to these structures. He aspirated 4 ml of yellow fluid, whereupon the swelling in the nerve, chiasm, and tract collapsed. The biopsy specimen from the tract revealed glioma. The findings after examination of her eyes in March, 1981, were the same except her visual acuity improved (20/30 OD). Her general health was excellent. Computed tomographic scans showed no abnormality except multiple tiny calcifications and a normal-sized optic chiasm, left optic tract, and medial left temporal lobe. Myles and Murphy evacuated a cyst involving the chiasm and one optic nerve with a good result that remained 10 years later.[7] Pellet et al.[101] and Visot et al.[63] also recommended surgical attack on a major cyst. Uihlein removed a blood clot caused by a "telangiectatic" astrocytoma that had ballooned out much of the right chiasm and the right optic nerve.[102] The visual acuity OS and much of the temporal field in that eye, previously lost, recovered. The right eye remained blind. These are infrequent occurrences.

Exophytic Growth of Tumor

Much more common but not widely enough recognized is the tendency of optic gliomas to break through their pial sheath and grow more readily in the subarachnoid space, as noted in 1940 by Wolff.[103] In the same symposium at the Royal Society of Medicine this growth pattern was confirmed in a specimen from a 1½-year-old-child shown by Neame.[104] Cogan stated "the glioma itself may invade the subarachnoid space and extend a considerable distance forward or backward about a portion of the nerve which itself shows minimal neoplasia."[105]

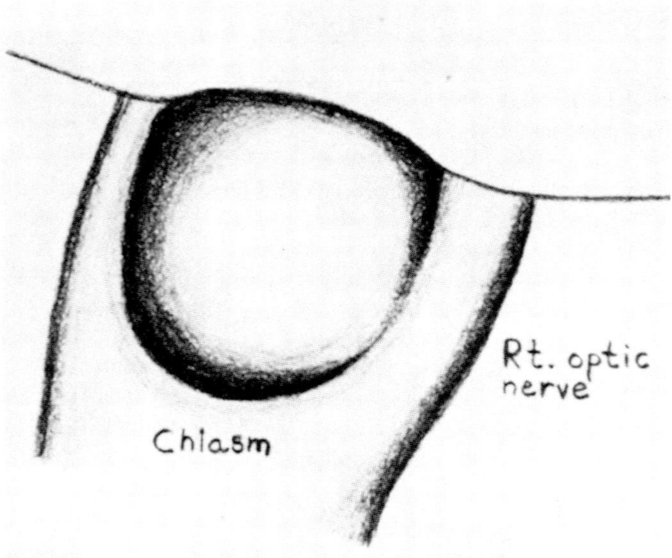

Fig. 25-4. Bynke's diagram of his patient with a completely exophytic glioma attached to the right optic nerve. (Reprinted from Bynke H, Kagström E, Tjernströom K: Aspects on the treatment of gliomas of the anterior visual pathways. Acta Ophthalmol 55:276, 1977. With permission.)

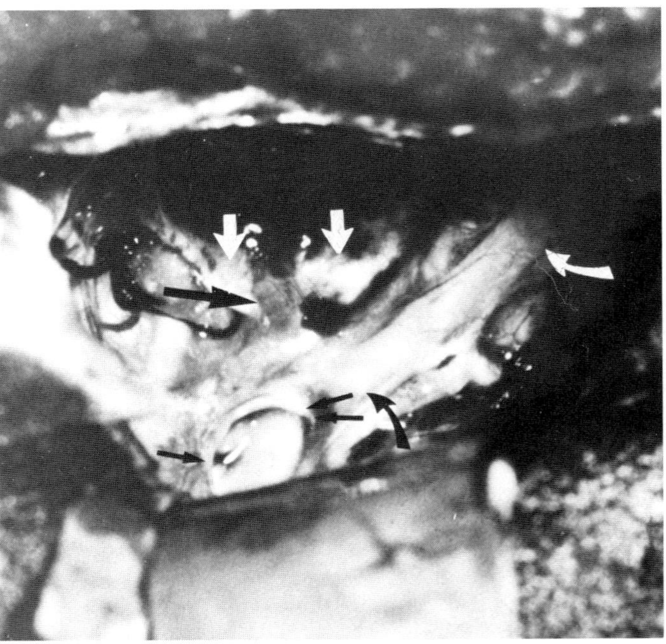

Fig. 25-5. This intraoperative photograph shows the parasellar field after removal of the tumor in Case 1. An ovoid erosion in the lamina terminalis disclosing the interior of the third ventricle lies just posterior to the narrow strip of chiasm, the left side of which was virtually compressed out of existence and not attached to the tumor. All these structures are displaced markedly backward. White arrows: dorsum sellae; large black arrrow: pituitary stalk; small straight arrows: inferior rim of the hole in the lamina terminalis; curved black arrow: junction of the right optic nerve and chiasm; curved white arrow: anterior end of the intracranial portion of the right optic nerve. Intact arachnoid covers the posterior communicating, posterior cerebral, and basilar arteries.

Walter[106] and Stern et al.[107] made essentially the same statement. In the latter paper the contention was that the "tumor eruption and proliferation in the subarachnoid space correlated with the presence of neurofibromatosis." However, this was not the diagnosis of our 6 cases with this growth pattern. Borit and Richardson commented, "in the chiasmatic group the tumor always extended into the chiasmatic cistern and frequently involved the interpeduncular fossa and the lumen of the third ventricle. In most cases . . . with minimal evidence of invasion of brain tissue."[25]

Neurosurgeons should take advantage of these possibilities. Northfield observed that the intracranial portion of an optic nerve glioma can compress and displace the chiasm without invading it.[108] Bynke et al.[6] (Figure 25-4) recorded a most favorable example of this. In a patient with severe impairment of the fields and acuity in both eyes an exophytic glioma arose by a mere 3×3-mm attachment to the medial caudal aspect of the right optic nerve. It pushed apart both nerves and the chiasm, was attached nowhere else, and its removal restored visual acuity and fields to normal on the left and nearly to normal on the right. There was further improvement 5 years later. Heiskanen described a similar case arising from the front of the chiasm.[34] In case 4 of Löhlein and Tönnis a mushroomlike cap of tumor overlay the chiasm but arose from one optic nerve more than 5 mm in front of its junction with the chiasm and was successfully removed.[109]

CASE REPORTS

One of the authors (Sweet) has sought to utilize this phenomenon in 6 patients in whom it was not so well developed. The most striking was in the patient described in Case 1 mentioned earlier. She illustrates another attractive feature of this growth pattern which can occur, namely that as the exophytic mass expands it may compress the adjacent optic pathway even to the point of slowly separating itself from the neural bundle rather than infiltrating into it.

Case Report.

The patient's gigantic intracranial tumor (9 cm in diameter) burgeoned out of the left optic canal and in the course of its 3 decades of growth appears to have completely cut off its connections with the chiasm and left optic tract (Figures 25-5A and B). After much of the interior of this tough avascular mass with multiple small cysts had been cored out it proved simple to separate the capsule from all of the normal structures including, to our amazement, the chiasm, the left side of which was compressed almost to disappearance. The left optic tract was never identified but the capsule separated with the greatest of ease from all the numerous identifiable structures in this region, and with no visible vascular ooze. The slow although extreme displacement of all the normal anterior basal structures had produced mild preoperative symptoms yet it took 4 months for her mental and endocrine systems to regain reasonably normal levels after operation.

Case 4. The patient, aged 4 at the time of surgery on April 4, 1970, was another child with a large intracranial glioma to show this growth behavior. He had a proptotic blind right eye and a temporal defect in the left eye. His right intracranial optic nerve expanded into a circular tangerine-sized mass 5 cm in largest diameter. This engulfed the chiasm but had severed its connection with the right optic tract, which was not visible. Figure 25-6A is a diagram of the two remarkably similar tumors,

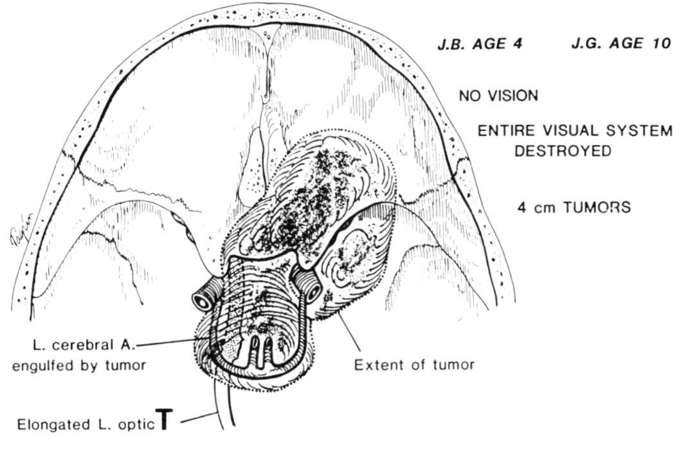

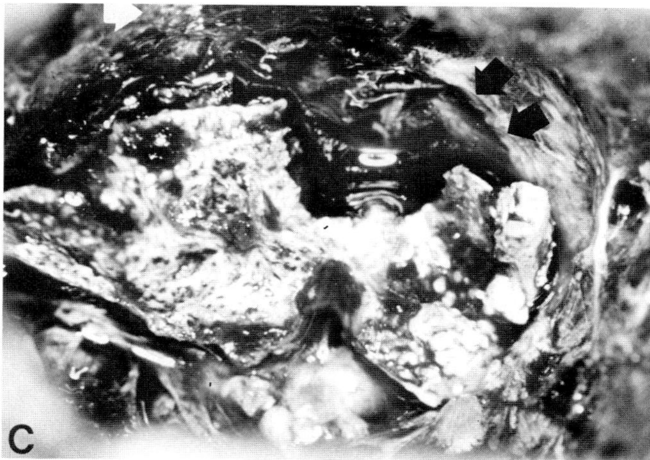

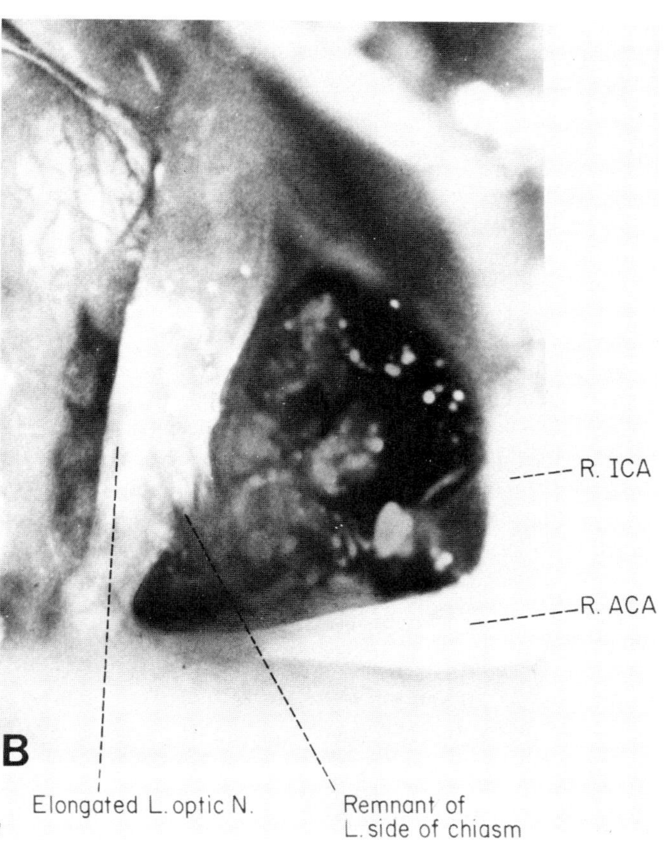

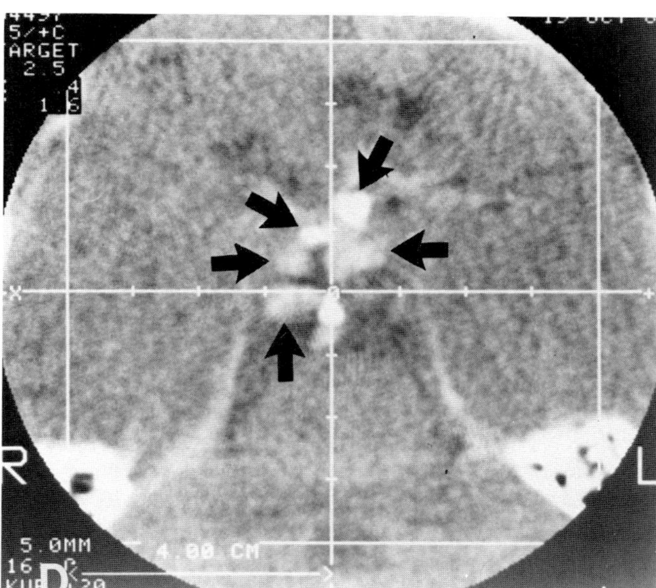

Fig. 25-6. (A) Diagram of the remarkably similar tumors in cases 4 and 5. (B) Case 4. An intraoperative photograph obtained April 8, 1970 after removal of the main tumor. Note the ragged area on the medial aspect of the left optic nerve, which was the site of attachment of the grossly swollen chiasm to the somewhat swollen nerve, compared with the optic tract. (C) Case 4. Intraoperative photograph obtained November 1, 1976. The suprasellar region is exposed during this subfrontal operation; almost no normal structures are visible. The glistening irregular jagged features are calcific masses embedded in fibrous tissue. Black arrow: posterior edge of the lesser wing of the right sphenoid bone. White arrows: planum sphenoidale. (D) Case 4. A contrast-enhanced CT scan obtained October 19, 1983. Arrows point to five separate islands of suprasellar calcification and soft tissue nodules (these were unchanged in CT and MRI scans obtained 3 years later).

one in this patient and the other in the patient in Case 5. Figure 25-6B shows the bed after tumor removal in this case. The extremely elongated left optic nerve had a rough gray area for a few millimeters on its medial aspect where the neoplastic chiasm had not separated itself totally from the nerve. After surgery the lateral fibers of this optic nerve did not function and an uncertain reduction in the field and acuity of the left eye preoperatively was converted to blindness. We waited in vain for 7 months for some recovery of vision before removing the intraorbital and intracanalicular portions of the right optic nerve

and tumor as well as the now infiltrated left optic nerve intracranially. We saw him again 6 years later because he had had retro-orbital headaches of increasing severity for 6 weeks. A broad irregularly calcified suprasellar mass diagnosed as recurrent tumor was accompanied by massive enlargement of all four ventricles in the PEG but with no subarachnoid air passing above the prepontine cistern. A ventriculoatrial shunt restored the ventricles to normal size but did not help the headaches. Figure 25-6C shows how the rectangular fibrous mass with rough calcified inclusions looked at subfrontal oper-

J.C. AGE 9

PRESERVED NASAL FIELD   LEFT EYE

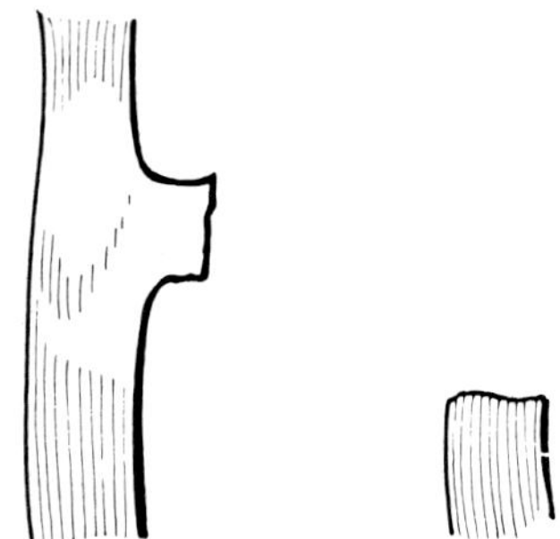

Fig. 25-7.   Case 6. Diagram of the appearance of the left lateral chiasm and right optic tract after nearly complete amputation of those portions invaded by tumor.

C.H. AGE 18

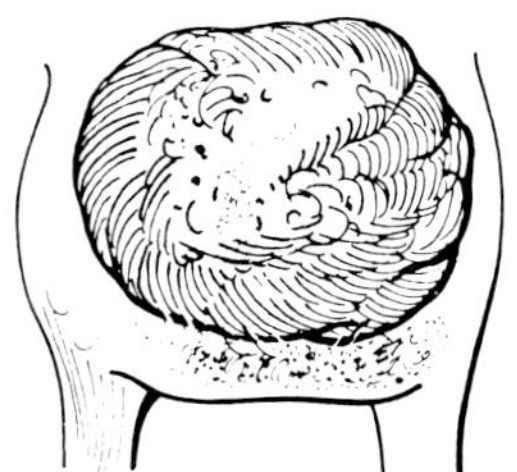

PRESERVED NASAL FIELD

LEFT EYE

Fig. 25-8.   Case 7. Diagram of the appearance of the tumor at surgery.

ation on November 1, 1976. When this relatively circumscribed fibrocalcific mass had been removed there was a smooth bed remaining on the floor of the sellar and parasellar area. No neoplastic elements were identified histologically in the specimen. The headaches were greatly reduced. We cannot find any similar reports in the literature. Ten years after this operation and 16 after the tumor removals he was leading a dramatically effective life. He had recently won in a statewide competition one of a few scholarships for gifted students and did A minus work in his first year of university. Computed tomographic scans with and without contrast in October, 1983 with improved resolution and including direct coronal scans discriminated five small separate islands of suprasellar calcification and small soft tissue nodules (Figure 25-6D). These remained unchanged on CT and MRI scans obtained in August, 1986.

Case 5.   The patient, aged 10 at his first operation on January 3, 1970, had a clinical picture and sequence with an initial two-stage operation that was remarkably similar to the patient in Case 4. His tumor, somewhat larger than the one in Case 4, had rendered him bilaterally blind before surgery and he did not recover any vision in the left eye even though the left optic nerve looked fairly normal with only tiny nubbins of obvious tumor at the left chiasmal remnant. He made a good adjustment to his blindness and has excellent general health. A CT scan obtained in July, 1983 was normal. At age 25 he had completed a college degree and was training with the US Internal Revenue Service.

Case 6.   The patient, a 9-year-old boy, had been completely blind in his right eye for at least 3 years. He was found to have low normal intelligence after he failed a year in school. A PEG outlined a large mass in the region of the right optic nerve from which 3 ml of light yellow fluid were aspirated during surgery on July 29, 1960. The tumor, which covered all of the optic structures and extended above and beyond them in all directions, was removed piecemeal until we could demonstrate that it was expanding only the right optic nerve, the right

side of the chiasm, and the anterior end of the right tract. The large tumor nubbin seemed to separate cleanly from the normal-sized portions of the chiasm and the tract. Figure 25-7 diagrams the intracranial visual pathways that remained after the tumor was removed. The full visual field of the left eye before surgery was reduced by a temporal hemianopia. Acuity and general performance remained satisfactory in the 23 years since but we do not yet have detailed follow-up data.

Case 7.   A 17-year-old girl had steadily lost vision in both eyes for 10 years to an acuity of 20/100 OD and 20/200 OS, with only small seeing fields in the nasal quadrants of each eye. Numerous small suprasellar calcified areas had led to the diagnosis of craniopharyngioma. At surgery July 5, 1966, the frontal lobes were eased readily off of a fluctuant, encapsulated tumor mass that bulged upward between the laterally displaced optic nerves. Aspiration yielded only 1.8 ml of yellow fluid. After a reddish gray neoplasm was gently sucked out of the interior, continuous attachments to both optic nerves and to the chiasm were seen with the operating microscope. The normal looking portions of the chiasm and both optic nerves were preserved (Figure 25-8). Although postoperatively she had no vision in the right eye, the nasal field of the left eye remained larger and the visual acuity was still 20/200 17 years later. Almost none of the suprasellar calcification was removed at surgery. The concern that this calcium might represent residual tumor seemed untenable to us in the light of the operative findings. She returned to work 2 months after surgery and 18 years later was working a 65-hour week. A CT scan obtained in June, 1984 showed no tumor.

Case 8.   The patient, aged 18 with a visual acuity of 20/60 OD and a right nasal field defect, had a huge right optic foramen and her intraorbital mass extended to the chiasmal region according to findings on PEG. At surgery on January 15, 1973, a 2.2-cm dark red mass covered the visual structures and both internal carotid arteries (Figure 25-9A). It could be separated easily from all of these normal structures with the exception of its expansion into the right optic nerve. Posteriorly there was a large overhang superior to the right optic tract but there was only a small attachment of tumor to the lateral aspect of the tract and chiasm. Most of these two structures looked normal. Removal was facilitated by transection of the intracranial mass just behind the optic foramen and at the junction of the optic nerve and chiasm. The main intracranial portion of the tumor (Figure 25-9B) having been lifted out, the critical final dissection

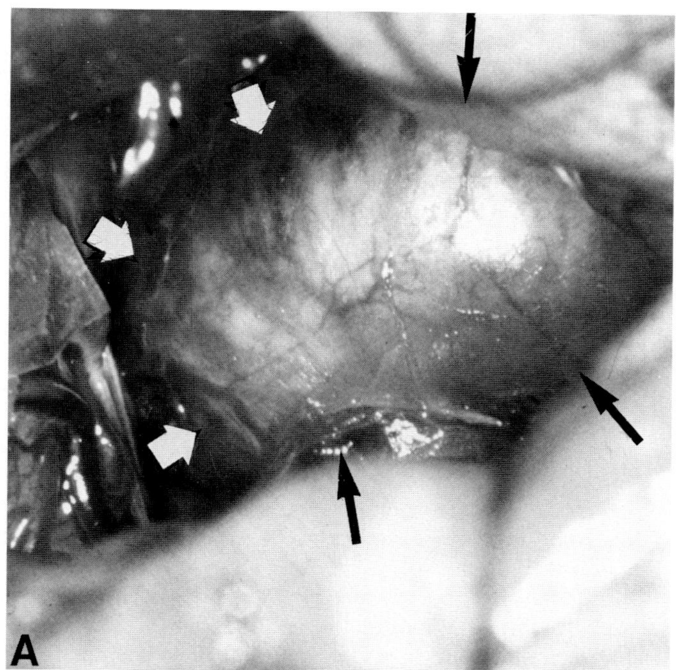

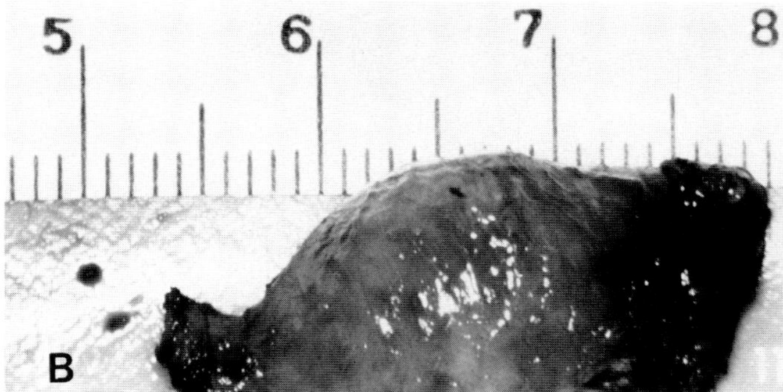

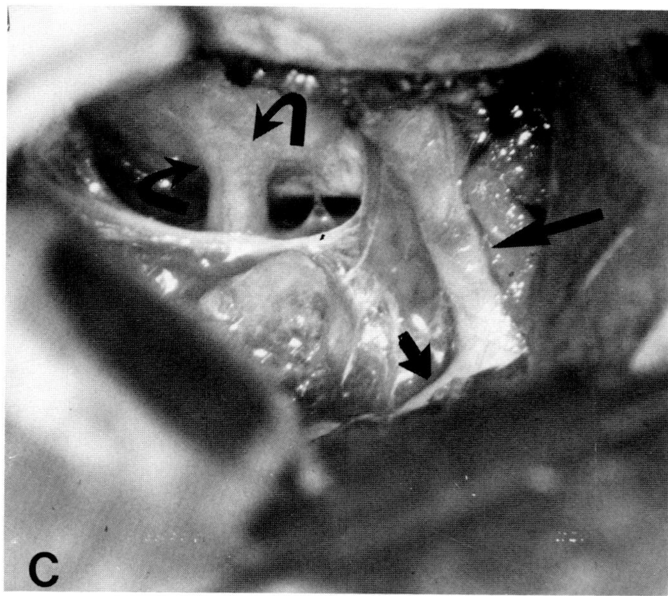

Fig. 25–9.   Case 8. (A) Subfrontal exposure of tumor (bounded by white and black arrows) covering the normal parasellar structures. (B) The excised intracranial portion of the tumor expanding the right optic nerve; the huge optic foraminal end of tumor is to right. (C) Following tumor removal, the normal structures can be seen in glistening intact arachnoid. Long straight arrow: right internal carotic artery. Short straight arrow: right anterior cerebral artery. Curved arrow: pituitary stalk. The left optic nerve, chiasm, and right optic tract were so grossly displaced by the tumor that they are covered by brain in this view. (D) Diagram of the relationship of the intracranial portion of the tumor to the visual pathways.

of tumor from the posterior visual pathways was more precise (Figure 25-9D). The roof of the optic canal and the orbit were then removed and the anterior end of the tumor to behind the globe was dissected out as a separate specimen. The full visual field and acuity of the left eye were normal and the patient has maintained an excellent work record since the operation. Her CT scans with and without contrast obtained on January 11, 1984 showed no tissue suggestive of neoplasm in the suprasellar cistern. A single low suprasellar clip interferes with the resolution in its vicinity both in the CT and MRI scans. We should not use metal clips for hemostasis in these patients now.

Hypothalamic Invasion

All of the foregoing patients had no intimation of a hypothalamic or other cerebral invasion by tumor. Only in the case of a Chinese male, aged 21 when first diagnosed, have we had a fruitful result from a partial removal of a tumor invading the hypothalamus.

Case 9.   Unlike the tumors whose primary origin in the visual pathways leads to initial symptoms of visual disturbance, this patient had had increasing polydipsia and polyuria for 2 years with visual impairment for only 6 months when we saw

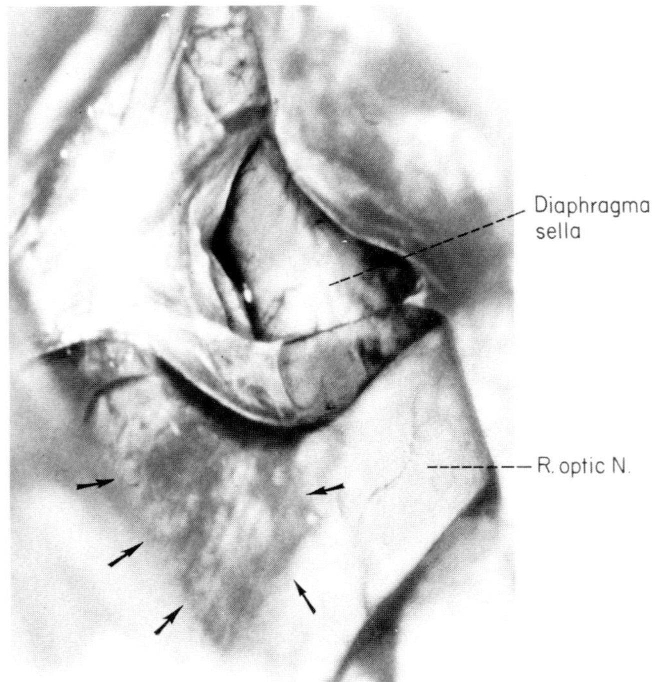

Fig. 25-10. Case 9. Subfrontal exposure. Before removal the gray tumor can be seen invading the lamina terminalis and much of the chiasm. The small black arrows mark the tumor boundaries. The chiasm is markedly postfixed.

him. Although his irregular field defects were largely confined to the inferior temporal quadrants, his visual acuity was down to 20/200 in each eye. A PEG showed an anteriorly situated mass in the third ventricle about 2.5 cm in diameter. His optic nerves and anterior chiasm looked normal on February 3, 1967, but the lamina terminalis and the posterior chiasm were covered with a gray mass, which as seen from the right side largely spared the optic tract (Figure 25-10). Accordingly, the gray tissue within the anterior third ventricle was removed to and including a 7-mm hole in the hypothalamic floor through which the arachnoid covering the pons could be seen. The pathologic diagnosis was astrocytoma grade I. Four weeks postoperatively he was reading J2 slowly with the right eye and J4 with the left; the field defects were about the same. Kjellberg gave the patient 1500 rad of proton radiation at the Bragg peak at a single sitting—roughly equivalent to 3000 rad of gamma rays. His visual acuity worsened slowly down to 20/50 each eye and by August 1967 was 20/200 OD and less than 20/400 OS with a nearly complete right homonymous hemianopia. No increase in tumor size was apparent on PEG. No more radiation was given. The visual acuity improved to J1 on the right and J3 on the left by February 1977. His field defects still precluded his driving a car. In the ensuing 19 postoperative years he became an energetic, effective business man, travelling extensively.

Other aggressive removals of the anterior portions of huge tumors invading nerves, chiasm, and hypothalamus in patients blind or virtually so have failed to achieve a useful result. One patient died postoperatively; another, although living 17 years later, were better dead. He is incontinent, unable to feed himself, and has limited speech. Two of our colleagues have had similar experiences with one case each. Sweet's third case seemed at first similar to Cases 4 and 5. A 15-cc cyst out in the right sylvian fissure continued into solid glioma of the right optic nerve and chiasm, but then also invaded the left optic tract

and hypothalamus, which were left behind. The boy had a disappointing course to death 12 years later. In 18 other chiasmal or hypothalamic gliomas of our colleagues and in 2 more of Sweet's cases we thought the situation called for no more than a biopsy. The 6 more favorable cases add to the evidence that operative exploration is the most certain means of determining operability of a tumor. These operations, all performed before 1974, were usually without the benefit of the operating microscope.

EXPERIENCES OF OTHERS

There are many other accounts of one or more good results of major removals of gliomas invading the chiasm. Ray reported the case of a boy 13 years old when Cushing resected his tumorous right half of the chiasm and adjacent segments of the right nerve and tract in 1929.[110] Vision was preserved in the nasal field of the left eye until he died of another cause 32 years later. A postmortem examination revealed a tiny nodule of tumor at the chiasm.

Gaini did "a macroscopically complete removal" of a tumor invading one optic nerve and the chiasm on the same side. The child, blind in the left eye with a hemianopia in the other had no evidence of recurrence 4 years later.[69] Comparison of the postoperative with the preoperative CT scans documented a major removal here and in one case of Helcl and Petrásková.[31]

Myles and Murphy[7] (9 cases) and Helcl Petrásková[31] (11 cases) did partial or subtotal removal of tumors where there was considerable extension of tumor outside the visual pathways. Baram et al.[111] used acute or subacute visual deterioration as the basis for a partial surgical removal in 3 children with improvement of vision in 1 eye in 2 of them. Full details are not given in these three accounts.

Other reports given in sufficient detail to make it clear that a worthwhile result ensued after nearly total removal are provided by Posner and Horrax[112] (3 cases), Löhlein and Tönnis[109] (3 cases), Matson[2] (2 cases), and Boudet et al,[113] Francois,[114] Karagiusov,[62] MacCarty,[115] and Helcl and Petrásková[31] with 1 case each. If it can be determined that a portion of the tumor lies outside of visual and hypothalamic tissues or fails to enlarge some of the chiasm or opposite nerve, we see no good reason for leaving it in. It is usually avascular and readily removable. Chang and Wood[83] pointed out that small optic gliomas respond better to radiation than large ones, which is an additional reason for partial extirpation rather than no removal.

A most encouraging report is that of Koos et al.[116] They stated that under the operating microscope they can distinguish both tumor tissue and vessels from intact optic neural elements and normal vessels upon longitudinal opening of the tight nerve sheath. Under high magnification "tumor was differentiated from compressed neural tissue and resected safely." By selective coagulation of tumor vessels they stated they provoked degeneration of unresectable tumor remnants. They reported that in 10 children 3 to 5 years of age such operations for spongioblastomas of the optic system yielded "unexpected and rapid improvement of vision as a persistent finding." In 2 other children aged 3 to 5 years extensive hypothalamic spongioblastomas were similarly resected "with rapid improvement in level of consciousness and endocrine disturbances." The improvement in vision of one eye remained constant in one of the two 3 years after surgery. Their figure showed that in one patient an intrinsic rather than an exophytic tumor of right optic nerve and chiasm was attacked. Four years after partial removal of this "optic spongioblastoma" the 6-year-old lad continues to have improved acuity in the right eye and normal vision in the left.

We agree with Matson's 1969 dictum to which many other authorities subscribe that it is of primary importance to establish the degree of operability by surgical exploration of the optic chiasm in every case.[2]

SUMMARY OF DATA ON RADIATION THERAPY

We summarize here the data concerning the advisability of radiation therapy.

There are 16 publications (including ours) that describe 64 cases in which a significant decrease in tumor size following radiation therapy was ascertained by air studies or CT measurements. In all but 3 of these publications the documentation consists of CT scans "before and after." The total number of cases studied in this way is given in only 8 publications[5,6,61,63,117,118,119,12020] and in this chapter. In this group of 105 irradiated patients, 50 were described as showing a significant reduction in tumor size, in 15 of which virtual disappearance of tumor was recorded. An additional 7 articles describe a significant radiographically proven reduction in tumor size in 16 patients without indicating the total number of patients studied.[13,46,74,121–124] Other than the patient described in Case 3, we found only one report of a measured spontaneous decrease in size.[49]

A comparison between the outcomes with and without radiation is given in 10 publications (including this chapter) in reasonably similar groups of patients.[2,24,26,34,64,85,118,125,126] In 7 of the publications describing a total of 203 cases the irradiated group fared significantly better. In three reports, however, describing 42 cases, there was no clearcut difference in outcome.[2,26,34]

Of 96 patients with assessable vision reported in 7 articles, 29 or 30 percent showed improvement after radiotherapy.[46]

Major radiation injury was described in at least 7 reports of 9 children receiving 4200 to 5500 rad to this part of the brain.[34,63,68,97,125,127,128] Less disabling but serious are disorders of learning and intellect, especially at doses in the 5000-rad range.[63,122,129]

The relevant facts are: (1) the risks of such therapy are substantially greater in children; (2) the disorder is subject to spontaneous stabilization or improvement, and (3) innocuous CT and MRI scans permit critical appraisal of status in addition to neurologic studies. These lead us to recommend initial radiation doses for children in the first decade of 4000 rad in fractions no greater than 180 rad for significant residual tumor following operative verification of tumor type in most cases. Initial doses of 5000 rad are appropriate for adults. Assiduous follow-up is needed and a second course of radiation is in order if the tumor continues to grow or clinical worsening occurs. The major sequelae of radiation therapy should be clearly presented to the patient or a responsible relative. We have documented much more fully the basis for these recommendations elsewhere.[130]

ADDENDUM

Through the courtesy of Mr. C. B. T. Adams of Oxford University we add the report of another hypothalamic grade I astrocytoma in a 9-month-old boy successfully treated by surgery plus radiation. Beginning at age 3 months, the baby failed to gain weight and lost subcutaneous fat to an alarming degree despite normal growth in length and head circumference and normal electrolyte and growth hormone levels (6 mg/ml). The diagnosis of wasting as a result of a diencephalic syndrome was confirmed by a CT scan, which revealed an enhancing hypothalamic mass. A left temporal field defect and a hemoglobin of 8 g were the only other abnormal findings. At right frontotemporal craniotomy the soft, gray, avascular hypothalamic tumor, although adherent to both internal carotid arteries, was partially removed, decompressing the chiasm and pituitary stalk. The smooth postoperative course included a brief period of diabetes insipidus; the visual field defect recovered. Cobalt 60 radiotherapy, 3000 rad in 20 fractions, was given to the tumor bed and adjacent areas via a parallel pair technique. At the end of a month, the patient had gained 0.5 kg in weight and regained some of the subcutaneous fat.

CONCLUSIONS

1. A mass in the anterior visual pathways is nearly always a neoplasm, not a hamartoma or arachnoidal hyperplasia. Even though it may remain quiescent for decades, its potential for unpredictable growth remains. If a watch and wait course is pursued, follow-up examinations including scans at appropriate levels are needed.

2. Calcification may develop not only within but outside the tumor. The latter locus should be identified to avoid the mistaken assumption of recurrence of tumor.

3. Computed tomographic scans, inclusive of coronal views, and MRI scans all at close spatial intervals provide essential critical diagnostic and postoperative follow-up information. The procedures complement each other and both are helpful. Visual evoked potentials especially those with a checkerboard pattern stimulus are in an early stage of evaluation and are advisable.

4. A glioma confined to one optic nerve should be treated by neurectomy from the chiasm to the globe via a subfrontal approach as soon as it is diagnosed in the great majority of symptomatic cases. Exceptions to this rule are mainly patients with neurofibromatosis.

5. More extensive probable gliomas should be explored transfrontally to confirm the diagnosis and to remove some or nearly all of the tumor in the minority of patients favorable for such attack. Happily, some large tumors partially amputate their connections with the normal visual pathways rather than infiltrate them. Metal clips for hemostasis at surgery should be avoided because they disturb interpretation of both CT and MRI scans.

6. Cautious radiation therapy of residual gross tumor is clearly indicated. Careful clinical and neuroradiologic follow-ups will determine optimal dosage schedules. More comprehensive data are required to determine variables associated with a significant risk of radiation injury, but doses of approximately 4000 rad in fractions no greater than 180 rad are probably advisable as initial treatment for children to age 10, including those with only grade I or grade II gliomas.

ACKNOWLEDGMENT

Dr. Sweet wishes to express his gratitude to the Neuro-Research Foundation for its support during the preparation of this manuscript.

REFERENCES

1. Lloyd LA: Gliomas of the optic nerve and chiasm in childhood, in Smith JL (ed): Neuro-Ophthalmology Update. New York, Masson Publishing, 1977, pp 185–197

2. Matson DD: Neurosurgery of Infancy and Childhood. Springfield, Ill, Charles C Thomas, 1969, pp 533–536

3. Martin P, Cushing H: Primary gliomas of the chiasm and optic nerves in their intracranial portion. Arch Ophthalmol 52:209, 1923

4. Schuster G, Westberg G: Gliomas of the optic nerve and chiasm. Acta Radiol 6:221, 1967

5. Fletcher WA, Imes RK, Hoyt WF: Chiasmal gliomas: Appearance and long-term changes demonstrated by computerized tomography. J Neurosurg 65:154, 1986

6. Bynke H, Kagström E, Tjernström K: Aspects on the treatment of gliomas of the anterior visual pathways. Acta Ophthalmol 55:269, 1977

7. Myles ST, Murphy SB: Gliomas of the optic nerve and chiasm. Can J Ophthal 8:508, 1973

8. Kahn EA, Crosby EC, Schneider RC, et al: Correlative Neurosurgery. Springfield, Ill, Charles C Thomas, 1969, pp 111–113

9. Beyer RA, Paden P, Sobel DF, et al: Moyamoya pattern of vascular occlusion after radiotherapy for glioma of the optic chiasm. Neurology 36:1173, 1986

10. Cavazzuti V, Fischer EG, Welch K, et al: Neurological and psychophysiological sequelae following different treatments of craniopharyngioma in children. J Neurosurg 59:409, 1983

11. Byrd SE, Harwood-Nash DC, Fitz CR, et al: Computed tomography of intraorbital optic nerve gliomas in children. Radiology 129:73, 1978

12. Holman RE, Grimson BS, Drayer BP, et al: Magnetic resonance imaging of optic gliomas. Am J Ophthalmol 100:596, 1985

13. Aron AM, Taff I, Wallace SA, et al: Neurofibromatosis and chiasmal glioma: Reappraisal for future management. Ann Neurol 20:399, 1986

14. Daniels DL, Herfkins R, Gager WE, et al: Magnetic resonance imaging of the optic nerves and chiasm. Radiology 152:79, 1984

15. Karnaze MG, Sartor K, Winthrop JD, et al: Suprasellar lesions: Evaluation with MR imaging. Radiology 161:77, 1986

16. Brant-Zawadski M, Berry I, Osaki L, et al: Gd-DTPA in clinical MR of the brain. 1. Intraaxial lesions. AJR 147:1223, 1986

17. Berry I, Brant-Zawadzki N, Osaki L, et al: Gd-DTPA in clinical MR of the brain. 2. Extraaxial lesions and normal structures. AJR 147:1231, 1986

18. Schörner W, Laniado M, Niendorf HP, et al: Time-dependent changes in image contrast in brain tumors after gadolinium-DTPA. AJNR 7:1013, 1986

19. Kupersmith MJ, Siegel IM, Carr RE, et al: Visual evoked potentials in chiasmal gliomas in four adults. Arch Neurol 38:362, 1981

20. Groswasser Z, Kriss A, Halliday AM, et al: Pattern and flash-evoked potentials in the assessment and management of optic nerve gliomas. J Neurol Neurosurg Psychiatry 48:1125, 1985

21. Cohen ME, Duffner PK: Visual evoked responses in children with optic gliomas, with and without neurofibromatosis. Childs Brain 10:99, 1983

22. Hoyt WF, Baghdassarian SA: Optic glioma of childhood. Natural history and rationale for conservative management. Br J Ophthalmol 53:793, 1969

23. Glaser JS, Hoyt WF, Corbett J: Visual morbidity with chiasmal glioma. Long-term studies of visual fields in untreated and irradiated cases. Arch Ophthalmol 85:3, 1971

24. Miller NR, Iliff WJ, Green WR: Evaluation and management of gliomas of the anterior visual pathways. Brain 97:743, 1974

25. Borit A, Richardson EP: The biological and clinical behaviour of pilocytic astrocytomas of the optic pathways. Brain 105:161, 1982

26. Wong IG, Lubow M: Management of optic glioma of childhood: A review of 42 cases, in Smith JL (ed): Neuroophthalmology, vol 6. St. Louis, CV Mosby, 1972, pp 51–60

27. Donahue HC: An exceptional lesion of the orbit. Arch Ophthalmol 54:259, 1955

28. Hoyt WF, Meshel LG, Lessell S, et al: Malignant optic glioma of adulthood. Brain 96:121, 1973

29. Reese AB: Tumors of the Eye, ed 3. Hagerstown, Harper and Row, 1976, pp 134–145

30. Brand WN, Hoover SV: Optic glioma in children. Review of 16 cases given megavoltage radiation therapy. Childs Brain 5:459, 1979

31. Helcl F, Petrásková H: Gliomas of visual pathways and hypothalamus in children—a preliminary report. Acta Neurochir Suppl 35:106, 1985

32. Sugita K, Kageyama N: Treatment and follow up studies of the optic gliomas. Infant and child types. Shoni no Noshikei 2:97, 1977

33. Kanamori M, Shibuya M, Yoshida J, et al: Long-term follow-up of patients with optic glioma. Childs Nerv Syst 1:272, 1985

34. Heiskanen O, Raitta C, Torsti R: The management and prognosis of gliomas of the optic pathways in children. Acta Neurorchir 43:193, 1978

35. Wilson WB, Feinsod M, Hoy WF: Malignant evolution of childhood chiasmal pilocytic astrocytoma. Neurology 26:322, 1976

36. Szokalski V: Tumeur squorho-cancé reuse du nerf optique. Ann d'Oculistique 46:43, 1861

37. Goldzieher W: Die Geschw ̈u lste des Sehnerven. Graefes Arch Ophthalmol 19:119, 1873

38. Byers WGM: Primary intradural tumours of the optic nerve: Fibromatosis nervi optici, in Studies from the Royal Victoria Hospital Montreal. Toronto, J.A. Carveth & Co, 1901, pp 3–82

39. Barraquer J: Mixoma quístico del nervioó ptico de la papila y retina derechas y de la cavidad craneal y órbita izquierda. Arch Oftal Hispanoam 2:132, 1902

40. Pagenstecher AH: Ueber Opticustumoren. Graefes Arch Ophthalmol 54:300, 1902

41. Anderson DR, Spencer WH: Ultrastructural and histochemical observations of optic nerve gliomas. Arch Ophthal 83:324, 1970

42. Spencer WH, Borit A: Diffuse hyperplasia of the optic nerve in von Recklinghausen's disease. Am J Ophthalmol 64:120, 1967

43. Spencer WH: Primary neoplasms of the optic nerve and its sheaths: Clinical features and current concepts of pathogenetic mechanisms. Trans Am Ophthalmol Soc 70:490, 1972

44. Pfeiffer RL: Personal communication to Taveras, Mount & Wood. Radiology 66:518, 1956

45. Reese AB: Tumors of the Eye, ed 2. New York, Harper and Row, 1963, pp 171,191,192

46. Horwich A, Bloom HJG: Optic gliomas: Radiation therapy and prognosis. Int J Radiat Oncol Biol Phys 11:1067, 1985

47. Lewis RA, Gerson LP, Axelson KA, et al: von Recklinghausen neurofibromatosis. II. Incidence of optic gliomata. Ophthalmology 91:929, 1984

48. Tym R: Piloid gliomas of the anterior optic pathways. Br J Surg 49:322, 1961

49. Venes JL, Latack J, Kandt RS: Postoperative regression of opticochiasmatic astrocytoma: A case for expectant therapy. Neurosurgery 15:421, 1984

50. Berke RN: A modified Krönlein operation. Arch Ophthalmol 51:609, 1954

51. Hird B: Discussion on tumours of the optic nerve. Proc R Soc Med 33:690–692, 1940

52. Wright JE, McDonald WI, Call NB: Management of optic nerve gliomas. Br J Ophthalmol 64:545, 1980

53. Hudson AC: Primary tumors of the optic nerve. R London Ophthalmol Hosp Reps 18:317, 1912

54. Dandy WE: Prechiasmal intracranial tumors of the optic nerves. Am J Ophthalmol 5:169, 1922

55. Aarabi B, Long DM, Miller NR: Enlarging optic chiasm glioma with stable visual acuity. Surg Neurol 10:175, 1978

56. Cuneo HM, Rand CW: Brain Tumors in Childhood. Springfield, Ill, Charles C Thomas, 1952, pp 126–143

57. Jain NS: Two-stage intracranial and orbital operation for glioma of the optic nerve. Br J Ophthalmol 45:54, 1961

58. Bane WM, Long JC: Glioma of the optic nerve. Am J Ophthalmol 57:649, 1964

59. Richards RD, Lynn JR: The surgical management of gliomas of the optic nerve. Am J Ophthalmol 62:60, 1966

60. Lloyd LA: Gliomas of the optic nerve and chiasm in childhood. Trans Am Ophthalmol Soc 71:488, 1973

61. De Sousa AL, Kalsbeck JE, Mealey J Jr, et al: Optic chiasmatic glioma in children. Am J Ophthalmol 87:376, 1979

62. Karaguiosov L: Surgical treatment of gliomas of the optic nerve and chiasma. Acta Neurochir Suppl 28:411, 1979

63. Visot A, Rougerie J, Derome PJ, et al: Gliomes opto-chiasmatiques. Neurochirurgie 26:181, 1980

64. Tenny RT, Laws ER, Jr, Younge BR, et al: The neurosurgical management of optic glioma. Results in 104 patients. J Neurosurg 57:452, 1982

65. Hanbery JW: Gliomas of the optic nerve. Stanford Med Bull 14:34, 1956

66. Suárez J, Garzón F, Schuster G, et al: Gliomas del nervio y quiasma óptico en la infancia. Acta Neurol Latinoam 17:46, 1971

67. Marejeva TG, Rostotskaya VI, Sokolova ON, et al: Tumours of the optic nerve and chiasm in children. Diagnosis and surgical treatment. Acta Neurochir (Suppl 28):409, 1979

68. Kalifa C, Ernest C, Rodary C, et al: Les gliomes du chiasma optique chez l'enfant. étude rétrospective de 57 cas traités par irradiation. Mémoires Originaux. Arch Fr Pediatr 38:309, 1981

69. Gaini SM, Tomei G, Arienta C, et al: Optic nerve and chiasm gliomas in children. J Neurosurg Sci 26:33, 1982

70. Jefferson G: Discussion on tumours of the optic nerve. Proc R Soc Med 33:688, 692, 1940

71. Smith JL (ed): Neuro-ophthalmology Update. New York, Masson Publishing, 1977, pp 396

72. Klug GL: Gliomas of the optic nerve and chiasm in children. Aust NZ J Surg 47:596, 1977

73. Knapp A: On the intracranial extension of optic nerve tumors, in: Contributions to Ophthalmic Science. Menasha, Wisconsin, George Banta Publishing Company, 1926, pp 69–73

74. Chutorian AM, Schwartz JF, Evans RA, et al: Optic gliomas in children. Neurology 14:83, 1964

75. Seefelder R: Beiträge zu den Gliomen des Sehnerven. Wien Klin Wochenschr 44:838, 1931

76. Davis FA: Primary tumors of the optic nerve. Arch Ophthalmol 23:735, 1940

77. Levitt JM: Discussion of Davis: Primary tumors of the optic nerve. Arch Ophthalmol 23:1019, 1940

78. Christensen E, Andersen SR: Primary tumors of the optic nerve and chiasm. Acta Psychiatr Neurol Scand 27:5, 1952

79. Zülch KJ, Nover A: Die Spongioblastome des Sehnerven. Graefes Arch Ophthalmol 161:405, 1960

80. Yanoff M, Davis RL, Zimmerman LE: Juvenile pilocytic astrocytoma ("glioma") of optic nerve: Clinicopathologic study of sixty-three cases, in Jakobiec FA (ed): Ocular and Adnexal Tumors. Birmingham, Ala, Aesculapius, 1978, pp 685–707

81. Rougier J, Rambaud G, Joyeux O: Spongioblastome du nerf optique. A propagation chiasmatique. Oto-Neurol-Ophthalmol 45:53, 1973

82. Mullaney J, Walsh J, Lee WR, et al: Recurrence of astrocytoma of optic nerve after 48 years. Br J Ophthalmol 60:539, 1976

83. Chang CH, Wood EH: The value of radiation therapy for gliomas of the anterior visual pathway, in Brockhurst RJ, Boruchoff SA, Hutchinson BT, et al (eds): Controversy in Ophthalmology. Philadelphia, WB Saunders, 1977, pp 878–886

84. Nicole S, Palma L, Giuffrè R, et al: 31 primary orbital lesions in infancy and childhood. Childs Brain 6:255, 1980

85. Iraci G, Gerosa M, Tomazzoli L, et al: Gliomas of the optic nerve and chiasm. A clinical review. Childs Brain 8:326, 1981

86. Goodman SJ, Rosenbaum AL, Hasso A, et al: Large optic nerve glioma with normal vision. Arch Ophthalmol 93:991, 1975

87. Abellan P, George J-L, Lesure P, et al: Tumeurs orbitaires apres exerese d'un gliome du nerf optique. A propos de deux cas. Bull Soc Ophtamol Fr 85:113, 1985

88. Fog J, Seedorff HH, Vaernet K: Optic glioma. Clinical features and treatment. Acta Ophthalmol 48:644, 1970

89. Housepian EM: Intraorbital tumors, in Schmidek HH, Sweet WH (eds): Operative Neurosurgical Techniques: Indications, Methods, and Results. New York, Grune & Stratton, 1982, pp 227–244

90. Housepian EM: The surgical treatment of optic nerve sheath meningiomas. Mod Tech Surg Neurosurg 21:1, 1981

91. Luccarelli G: Ectopic pinealomas of the optic nerves and chiasma. Report of two personal cases. Acta Neurochir 27:205, 1972

92. Walsh FB: Tumors ocular and intracranial and related conditions, in: Clinical Neuro-Ophthalmology. Baltimore, Williams & Wilkins, 1947, p 1140

93. Maisongrosse G, Blanchard M, Antiphon R, et al: Gliomes du nerf optique et du chiasma. A propos de 10 cas. Bull Soc Ophtalmol Fr 82:207, 1982

94. Throuvalas N, Bataini P, Ennuyer A: Les gliomes du chiasma et du nerf optique. Bull Cancer 56:231, 1969

95. Robertson AG, Brewin TB: Optic nerve glioma. Clin Radiol 31:471, 1980

96. Block MA, Goree JA, Jimenez JP: Craniopharyngioma with optic canal enlargement simulating glioma of the optic chiasm. J Neurosurg 39:523, 1973

97. Giuffrè R, Bardelli AM, Taverniti L, et al: Anterior optic pathways gliomas. J Neurosurg Sci 26:61, 1982

98. Montgomery AB, Griffin T, Parker RG, et al: Optic nerve glioma: The role of radiation therapy. Cancer 40:2079, 1977

99. Albright AL, Sclabassi RJ: Cavitron ultrasonic surgical aspirator and visual evoked potential monitoring for chiasmal gliomas in children. J Neurosurg 63:138, 1985

100. Walsh FB, Hoyt WF: Clinical Neuro-Ophthalmology. Baltimore, Williams & Wilkins, 1969, pp 2076–2094

101. Pellet W, Rakotobe A, Paillas JE: Evolution tardive des gliomes du chiasma traités par opération et irradiation. Rev Otoneuro-ophtalmol 43:241, 1971

102. Uihlein A, Rucker CW: The neurosurgeon's role in acute visual failure. Arch Ophthalmol 60:223, 1958

103. Wolff E: Discussion on tumours of the optic nerve. Proc R Soc Med 33:687, 1940

104. Neame H: Discussion on tumours of the optic nerve. Proc R Soc Med 33:692, 1940

105. Cogan DG: Tumors of the optic nerve. Handbook Clin Neurol 17:350, 1974

106. Walter GF: Kleinhirnastrocytome und Opticusgliome—eine vergleichende feinstrukturelle Untersuchung. Virchows Arch (A Pathol Anat Histol) 380:59, 1978

107. Stern J, DiGiacinto GV, Housepian EM: Neurofibromatosis and optic glioma: Clinical and morphological correlations. Neurosurgery 4:524, 1979

108. Northfield DWC: The Surgery of the Central Nervous System. Oxford, Blackwell Scientific, 1973, pp 183–185

109. Löhlein W, Tönnis W: Die operative Behandlung der das Foramen opticum überschreitenden Sehnervengeschwülste. Graefes Archiv Ophthalmol 149:318, 1949

110. Ray BS: Surgical lesions of optic nerves and chiasm in infants and children, in Smith JL (ed): Neuro-ophthalmology, vol 3. St. Louis, CV Mosby, 1967, pp 77–99

111. Baram TZ, Moser RP, van Eys J: Surgical management of progressive visual loss in optic gliomas of childhood. Ann Neurol 20:398, 1986

112. Posner M, Horrax G: Tumors of the optic nerve. Long survival in three cases of intracranial tumor. Arch Ophthalmol 40:56, 1948

113. Boudet A, Arnaud, Bullier, et al: Gliome du chiasma optique. A propos de quartre cas. Bull Soc Ophtalmol Fr 75:1045, 1975

114. Francois J: Gliome du chiasma. J Fr Ophtalmol 1:125, 1978

115. MacCarty CS, Boyd AS, Childs DS: Tumors of the optic nerve and optic chiasm. J Neurosurg 33:439, 1970

116. Koos WT, Böck FW, Salah S, et al: Microsurgery of gliomas of the optic nerves, the optic chiasm, and the hypothalamus, in Koos WT, Böck FW, Spetzler RF (eds): Clinical Microneurosurgery. Stuttgart, Georg Thieme, 1976, pp 58–63

117. Danoff BF, Kramer S, Thompson N: The radiotherapeutic management of optic nerve gliomas in children. Int J Radiat Oncol Biol Phys 6:45, 1980

118. Gould RJ, Hilal SK, Chutorian AM: Efficacy of radiotherapy in optic gliomas. Ann Neurol 10:285, 1981 119. McFadzean RM, Brewin TB, Doyle D, et al: Glioma of the optic chiasm and its management. Trans Ophthal Soc UK 103:199, 1983

120. Marks JE, Gado M: Serial computed tomography of primary brain tumors following surgery, irradiation, and chemotherapy. Radiology 125:119, 1977

121. Harter DJ, Caderao JB, Leavens ME, et al: Radiotherapy in the management of primary gliomas involving the intracranial optic nerves and chiasm. Int J Radiat Oncol Biol Phys 4:681, 1978

122. Packer RJ, Savino PJ, Bilaniuk LT, et al: Chiasmatic gliomas of childhood. A reappraisal of natural history and effectiveness of cranial irradiation. Childs Brain 10:393, 1983

123. Redfern RM, Scholtz CL: Long-term survival with optic nerve glioma. Surg Neurol 14:371, 1980

124. Taveras JM, Mount LA, Wood EH: The value of radiation therapy in the management of glioma of the optic nerves and chiasm. Radiology 66:518, 1956

125. Gauthier N: Gliomes du chiasma et des nerfs optiques chez l'enfant: 65 observations. Paris, Thèse Médecine, 1973

126. Oxenhandler DC, Sayers MP: The dilemma of childhood optic gliomas. J Neurosurg 48:34, 1978

127. Bignami A, Giuffrè R, Riccio A: Radionecrosi tardiva del chiasma, dei nervi ottici, e dell'ipotalamo conseguente a cobaltoterapia dell'ipofisi e simulante un processo espansivo. Riv Neurol 33:709, 1963

128. Bojsen-Moller M, Knudsen V: Radiation induced meningeal sarcoma. Acta Neurochir 37:147, 1977

129. Bamford FN, Jones PM, Pearson D, et al: Residual disabilities in children treated for intracranial space-occupying lesions. Cancer 37:1149, 1976

130. Sweet WH, Linggood R, Seymour MA: Radiation therapy of glioma of anterior visual pathways. Submitted to Brain

CHAPTER 26

Surgical Management of Sellar and Parasellar Lesions

Peter McL. Black   Nicholas T. Zervas

THE REVIVAL of transsphenoidal surgery and the improvement in intracranial microsurgical techniques for approaching tumors at the base of the brain have made the management of lesions around the sella turcica a rapidly evolving area in neurosurgery. This chapter is based on our experience with approximately 400 sellar and parasellar lesions over a 5-year period. It begins with a brief overview of the variety of lesions found around the sella turcica; moves briefly to preoperative evaluation, including endocrinologic, radiologic, and visual testing; discusses surgical aspects including techniques of resection; and concludes with surgical results for various lesions including pituitary and other tumors.

LESIONS IN AND AROUND THE SELLA TURCICA

Although pituitary tumors are the most common abnormality in the sellar region, a multitude of other processes can be found there. Table 26-1 lists the lesions other than pituitary tumors encountered in 100 sequential transsphenoidal procedures done by the authors. Among neoplasms, craniopharyngiomas were the most common, followed by meningiomas and metastatic tumors. Primary tumors of the clivus including chordomas were virtually always diagnosed successfully as such before surgery. Inflammatory disorders including hypophysitis or sarcoidosis were thought to be neoplasms preoperatively. Both the surgeon and pathologist should be prepared for unusual histologic findings in approaching sellar and parasellar lesions.

PREOPERATIVE EVALUATION OF SELLAR AND PARASELLAR LESIONS

Sellar lesions commonly produce endocrine dysfunction, visual loss, headache, or abnormal x-ray findings without apparent symptoms.[1] Most patients with *endocrine dysfunction* will have had a complete evaluation by an endocrinologist before referral to the neurosurgery service; visual field testing is indicated if the mass is suprasellar on CT scans. Patients with *visual loss* usually are seen initially by a neurologist or ophthalmologist; basic endocrine testing including determinations of growth hormone, prolactin, and cortisol levels should be done before surgery in these cases. *Headache* is a common concomitant of pituitary tumors, but one particular form is especially important for the neurosurgeon to recognize. This is pituitary apoplexy, a condition with severe sudden headache and obtundation resembling subarachnoid hemorrhage. Visual loss may occur several hours after the initial event or may not occur at all. It is crucial to evaluate the sella in cases of acute headache by obtaining a CT scan with representative sections through the sella. Finally, in the list of possible presentations, some patients only have an *enlarged sella* on skull x-rays or CT scans. If endocrine testing for elevated growth hormone, cortisol, or prolactin levels is negative and a tumor is not apparent on a CT scan with thin section cuts through the sella, these patients can be considered to have "empty sella syndrome" and can be followed regularly with CT scans. If there is doubt, cisternography with omnipaque or another contrast medium will establish whether there is an empty sella.

The major preoperative considerations for sellar and parasellar lesions are endocrinologic, radiologic, and visual.

ENDOCRINE CONSIDERATIONS

Four endocrine syndromes relevant to pituitary tumors are well-described; these are summarized in Table 26-2. Prolactin hypersecretion is the most common, occurring in about 30 percent of all patients with pituitary tumors and resulting in amenorrhea/galactorrhea in women and subtle loss of libido in men. Hypersecretion is best diagnosed by a single serum prolactin determination; dynamic testing does not appear to add accuracy. A prolactin level above 20 ng/ml is abnormal. Between 20 and 200 ng/ml, elevated levels can either be from a tumor or from a nonspecific drug or stalk effect. A level above 200 ng/ml is generally accepted as indicating a prolactinoma.

Elevated growth hormone levels produce gigantism in children or acromegaly in adults (Figure 26-1). Hypersecretion of growth hormone is diagnosed by a basal growth hormone level above 10 ng/ml or a growth hormone level that on glucose tolerance testing fails to fall below 5 ng/ml (Figure 26-2). Somatomedin C, a peptide whose release from the liver is a reflection of growth hormone activity, is another substance whose measurement can establish the diagnosis of acromegaly. Normal values are 0.34 to 2.0 IU/ml in men and 0.45 to 2.2 IU/ml in women.

Cushing's disease is usually clinically evident (Figure 26-3); its endocrine diagnosis is the most problematic of the pituitary endocrine syndromes (Figure 26-4). The diagnosis has two steps: establishing hypercortisolism, and establishing that

OPERATIVE NEUROSURGICAL TECHNIQUES
ISBN 0-8089-1862-1

Table 26-1. Lesions other than pituitary adenomas in 100 consecutive transsphenoidal procedures at the Massachusetts General Hospital

Lesion	Number of Patients
Craniopharyngioma	4
Meningioma	3
Malignant tumors (metastatic, dysgerminoma, myoblastoma, chordoma)	4
Arachnoid cyst	1
Inflammatory disorders (granuloma, lymphocytic hypophysitis)	2
Mucocele	1

hypercortisolism is from a pituitary tumor and not from an adrenal or ectopic source of ACTH. Plasma ACTH assays, if they are reliable at a specific institution, may help to separate pituitary from adrenal sources. The dexamethasone suppression test is usually employed to separate pituitary from ectopic sources. An oral dose of 2 mg dexamethasone should not suppress an elevated cortisol level if it is the result of a pituitary adenoma, but 5 mg should do so. Neither the larger nor the smaller dosage of dexamethasone usually suppresses a high cortisol level from an ectopic source. Recently, catheterization of the petrosal sinuses to establish a differential in ACTH levels between right and left sinuses, or one between the sinuses and the vena cava, has been very useful in making the distinction between pituitary-dependent Cushing's disease and adrenal or ectopic forms.[2]

The fourth well-established endocrine syndrome of pituitary adenomas is that of pan-hypopituitarism. All tested hormones may be low or only one or two may be deficient in partial states.

Diabetes insipidus, an inability to secrete the posterior pituitary hormone arginine vasopressin into plasma and therefore to concentrate urine, is a very rare symptom of anterior pituitary tumors. Its occurrence should raise the possibility of a metastatic lesion or other malignant process in the sella.

RADIOLOGIC CONSIDERATIONS

In our experience, one aspect of the radiologic appearance is crucial in determining whether a lesion should be approached transsphenoidally; this is the size and shape of the sella. For lesions that extend into the suprasellar space, an enlarged sella

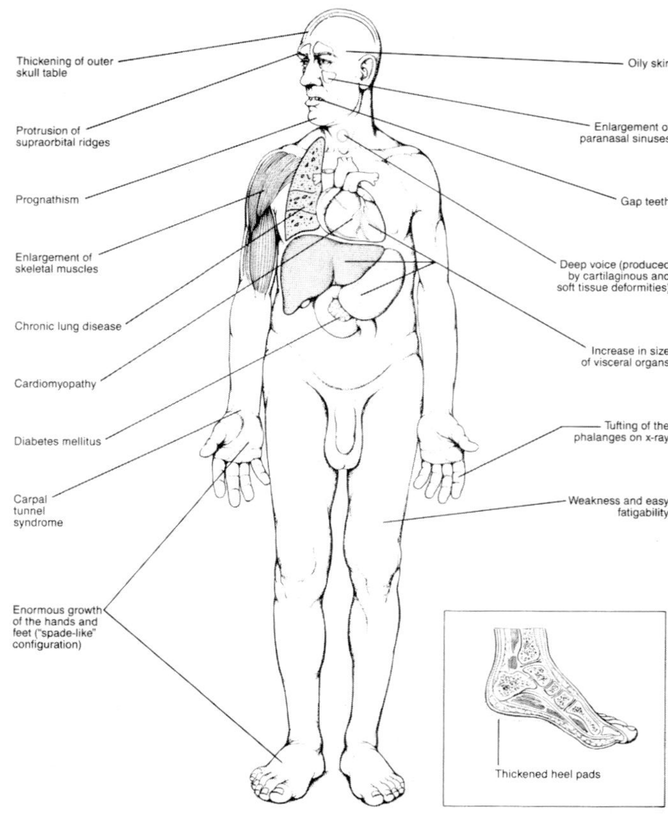

Fig. 26-1. Typical clinical findings in a patient with acromegaly. (Reprinted from Black PMcL: Diagnosis: Pituitary tumor. Hosp Med 21:43, 1985. With permission.)

is necessary for the transsphenoidal approach. Plain skull films, sellar polytomograms, or CT scans may provide the required information. For intrasellar lesions and those with only modest enlargement of the sella, we still find hypocycloidal polytomography a useful adjunct.

Computed tomography is by far the most useful technique for diagnosing sellar and intrasellar lesions. For tumors extending outside the sella, virtually any scanner is satisfactory: care must be taken to look carefully at the base of the skull, however. For definitive diagnosis two modifications of the

Table 26-2. Clinical syndromes of pituitary tumors

Tumor Product	Clinical Syndrome	Laboratory Diagnosis
Prolactin	Amenorrhea/glactorrhea (women); loss of libido (men)	Elevated prolactin level
Growth hormone	Gigantism (children); acromegaly (adults)	Elevated fasting growth hormone level and somatomedin-C; Failure to suppress on glucose tolerance testing
Adrenocorticotropic hormone	Cushing's disease	Elevated plasma and urinary cortisol levels and failure to supress cortisol level after high dose dexamethasone administration
Unknown (? glycoprotein hormones)	Panhypopituitarism; visual field defect	Low FSH, LH, testosterone, cortisol, T4

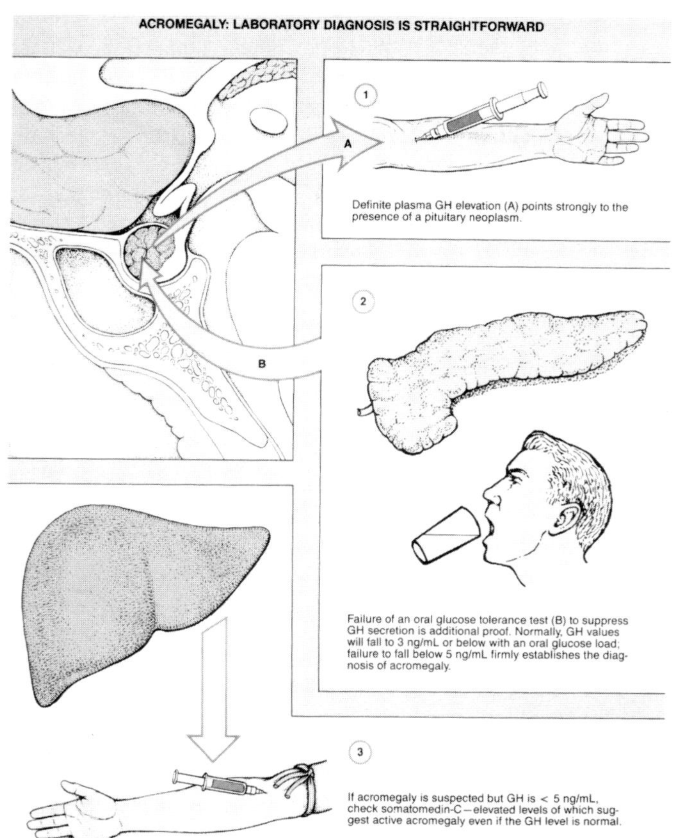

Fig. 26-2. Laboratory diagnosis of acromegaly. (Reprinted from Black PMcL: Diagnosis: Pituitary tumor. Hosp Med 21:43, 1985. With permission.)

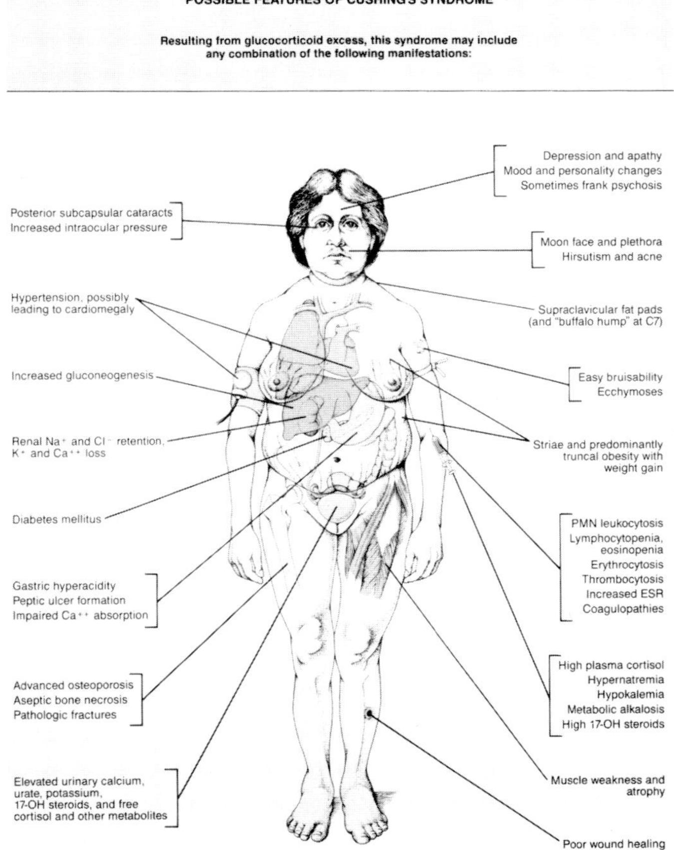

Fig. 26-3. Typical clinical findings in a patient with Cushing's disease. (Reprinted from Black PMcL: Diagnosis: Pituitary tumor. Hosp Med 21:43, 1985. With permission.)

standard scan are helpful: thin (3 mm) sections with overlap through the region of the sella; this is possible on all third generation scanners such as the GE 9800; and coronal sections either directly (the preferred method) or by reconstruction using special computer software. With these, some attempt at least can be made at visualizing the extent of suprasellar extension and of lateral outgrowth. A scan without contrast enhancement can demonstrate tumor and exclude recent hemorrhage as well. Enhancement with contrast material should also be carried out routinely.

When tumor is suspected, fast CT scanning during administration of a bolus of contrast material may help to establish vascularity of the lesion and specifically exclude an aneurysm. We obtain digital or conventional angiograms in cases where the configuration of the lesion is roughly globular or the apparent tumor is brightly enhancing on contrast CT scans.

Even more useful than the CT scanner in imaging sellar lesions is magnetic resonance imaging (MRI). Its advantages are sagittal and coronal as well as transaxial views (Figure 26-5); insensitivity to bony artifact around the sella; and potentially greater information about the nature of the lesion, especially whether it is vascular and possibly whether it is fibrous. Snow et al. suggested that a tumor appearing isointense with brain on spin echo sequences 30 and 90 is likely to be fibrous.[3] As MRI becomes more widely available, it may become the single radiologic study required to assess sellar and parasellar lesions.

VISUAL TESTING

Formal neuro-ophthalmologic testing should be done on any patient whose CT scan shows suprasellar extension and is an important part of the follow-up of such patients. Especially important are visual fields, funduscopic examination, and extraocular movements.[4] Table 26-3 summarizes the field defects in 113 patients with extrasellar extension at our institution.

SURGICAL CONSIDERATIONS

SURGICAL TECHNIQUES

There are a variety of approaches to the sellar and parasellar region; these are presented diagrammatically in Figure 26-6. In another chapter of this text, Laws presents the surgical technique for transsphenoidal approaches to the sella; the technique we use for transsphenoidal surgery will therefore be described only briefly. At our institutions, the neurosurgeon carries out the entire procedure. The patient is positioned with the upper trunk horizontal or slightly elevated, the head turned 30 degrees to the right and flexed 15 to 30 degrees, with the arms of a C-arm fluoroscope cradling the head. We do not usually use a lumbar drain. The nostrils are packed with cottonoid pledgets soaked with 3 percent cocaine. The oropharynx is packed around the orotracheal tube. Prophylactic oxacillin (1 g) and gentamicin (80) mg are given intravenously; an alternative is

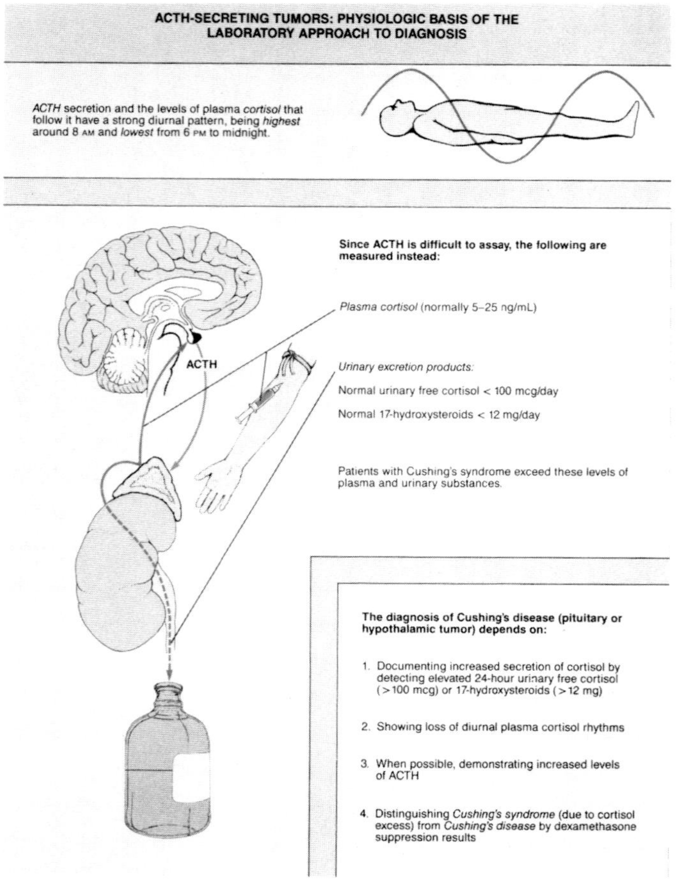

Fig. 26-4. Laboratory diagnosis of Cushing's disease. (Reprinted from Black PMcL: Diagnosis: Pituitary tumor. Hosp Med 21:43, 1985. With permission.)

vancomycin (500 mg); the nasal mucosa is infiltrated with 1:400,000 epinephrine. Either a sublabial or a transnasal approach is used. The transnasal approach is used more often: it is simple, direct, and effective. The microscope is brought in at the beginning of the operation. An incision is made in the septal mucosa of the left nostril 2 mm behind the mucocutaneous junction, and the mucosa is dissected from the septum with a periosteal elevator. The septum is cracked from left to right, and submucosal dissection is contained bilaterally. The C-arm is used to confirm that the trajectory is appropriate for the sella. A Hardy speculum is placed, usually with the superior aspect of the blades just below the sphenoid ostia. The sphenoid prow is removed, leaving enough bony rim to allow later packing if necessary; the sella is entered with a diamond drill. The dura is focally coagulated and punctured with a 20-gauge spinal needle to be certain there is no unusual vascularity; it is then opened in an H pattern. Curettes of varying size are used to remove tumor, beginning inferiorly and laterally. The principle of resection is to allow capsule to fall into the center of the sella and remove it as it does so. If the tumor is fibrous, a microscope-guided laser may be helpful. Complete resection is indicated by prolapse of the diaphragm into the field.

We have recently found that a radiofrequency electrode is a useful adjunct in assuring complete resection of a functional microadenoma producing known hormone products. After complete apparent tumor resection, a radiofrequency ball electrode is used to produce small lesions on the surface at 60

degrees; these do not injure deeper structures. After tumor resection the sella is packed, unless the tumor is a microadenoma, using fat harvested from a small incision in the right lower quadrant: the fat is held in place by a bone stent.

For transcranial surgery we generally use a pterional approach from the right side. The patient's head is turned 45 degrees to the left with the zygoma uppermost. A lumbar drain is often used and mannitol (100 g) and furosemide (20 mg) are given with induction of anesthesia. A standard pterional craniotomy proceeds. The frontal lobe is retracted until the junction of the olfactory tract and optic nerve is identified; CSF is released from the chiasmatic cisterns. The tumor can be removed from the prechiasmatic recess if the chiasm is postfixed, from the space between carotid artery and optic nerve, or through the lamina terminalis. The principle of resection is again internal decompression with an attempt to avoid traction or devascularization of the optic apparatus or hypothalamus. The dura is closed as watertight as possible and the bone is replaced with wire sutures. No attempt is made to remove tumor completely from the optic nerves.

SPECIFIC SURGICAL ISSUES

1. Deciding whether to approach a lesion transsphenoidally or transcranially (Figure 26-6).

The transsphenoidal approach increasingly has been advocated in approaching sellar lesions even when such lesions have significant extrasellar extension. Its morbidity is less than that of transcranial surgery, it can be repeated readily, and its results are as good as transcranial surgery in terms of visual improvement and resection of the sellar lesion (Black PMcL, Zervas NT, Candia GL: unpublished observations).[5-9] The following considerations have been useful in our experience in deciding whether to approach a lesion transsphenoidally.

A. For microadenomas (lesions with a diameter less than 10 mm on a CT scan or endocrine active lesions not seen on the CT scan), the transsphenoidal approach is preferred.
B. For lesions above the sella turcica with a normal configuration of the sella, a transcranial approach is best.
C. For all other lesions with suprasellar or parasellar extension, the transsphenoidal approach is preferred initially unless: (1) The lesion has a significant hourglass configuration suggesting a small diaphragmatic opening; (2) there is significant extension into the anterior or middle cranial fossa, which can be expected to be removed by a transcranial approach; or (3) there is reason to believe the lesion will be fibrous enough to prevent collapse into the sella with resection from below. In our experience, approximately 1 percent of pituitary tumors will require transcranial surgery with this set of guidelines.

2. Deciding whether to proceed transsphenoidally or transethmoidally.

The transethmoid approach, which begins with an incision medial to the medial canthus and dissects medial to the globe, is known to otolaryngologists as an expeditious route to the sella turcica. The exposure is best performed by an otolaryngologist. It is helpful in children in whom the sphenoid is not pneumatized and in patients with recurrent tumors who have had previous transsphenoidal procedures. It has a less capacious view than transsphenoidal surgery and has the potential danger of injury to the globe.

3. Deciding which transcranial approach to use. Three

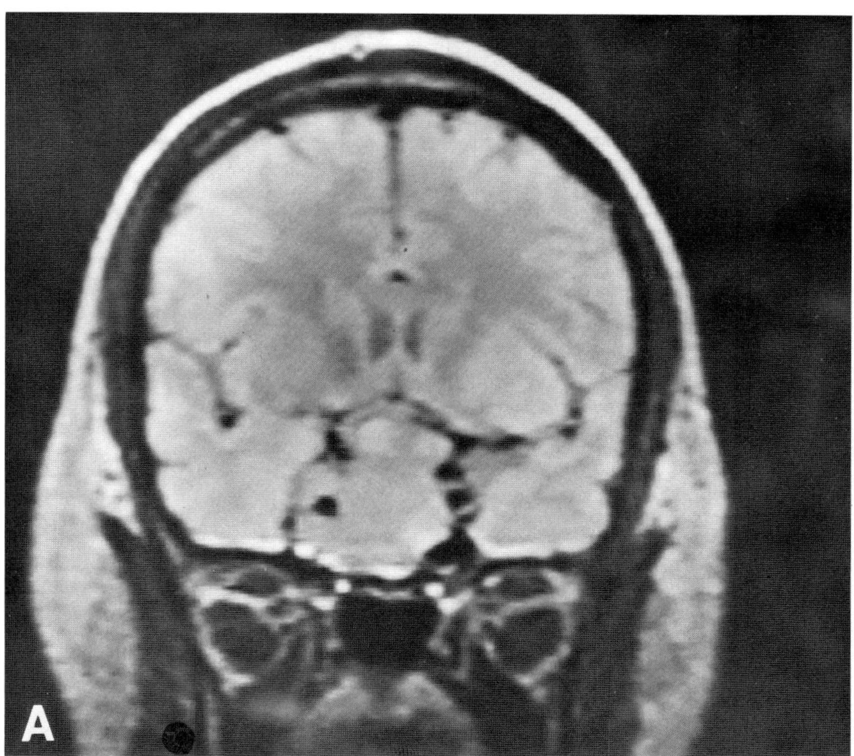

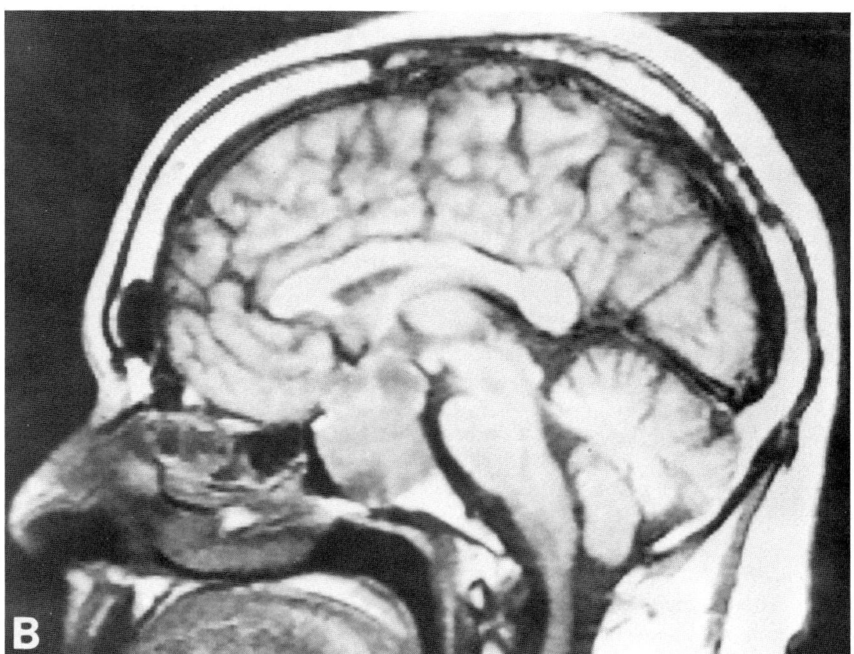

Fig. 26-5. A MRI scan of a patient with a large prolactinoma. (A) Sagittal view. The relationship of the tumor and surrounding structures can be readily appreciated. The clivus has been eroded superiorly. (B) Coronal view. Again, the extent of parasellar extension can be readily assessed. The carotid arteries are seen as black "flow voids."

approaches can be used in gaining access to tumors of the sellar region; subfrontal, pterional, or subtemporal. All should be done with microsurgical technique. The subfrontal approach uses a bifrontal bone flap with the patient's head extended and often a lumbar drain to increase access to the infrachiasmatic region. It has the advantage of bifrontal direct-on exposure but is difficult with a prefixed chiasm, requires substantial retraction of both frontal lobes, and may result in anosmia because of tension on both olfactory tracts.

The pterional approach is now familiar to most neurosurgeons in its exposure of the circle of Willis for aneurysms: it is satisfactory for tumors that can be removed through

Table 26-3. Visual defects in patients with sellar lesions

Defect	Percentage
Bitemporal hemianopia or quadrantopia	75
Unilateral hemianopia	15
Homonymous hemianopia	3
Extraocular movement palsy	4

the triangle between the optic nerve, tubercular sella, and chiasm. Tumors lying more posteriorly must be approached from the subtemporal direction. The subtemporal approach, however, limits access to the suprasellar space and has the potential complication of temporal lobe herniation from edema postoperatively.

4. Deciding whether to begin a transsphenoidal approach sublabially or transnasally.

Two approaches to the sphenoid can be used routinely in neurosurgery: a transseptal incision, which leads to unilateral submucosal dissection, cracking of the septum from left to right, and wide satisfactory exposure of the sella for most purposes, and a sublabial approach, which is that described by Hardy and others. The transnasal approach is quick and straightforward: in acromegalic patients the speculum may not be long enough to get to the sphenoid prow, however, and in all patients the view is not as wide. The sublabial approach gives a slightly wider view and provides better visualization of the superior aspect of the sella; it has the disadvantage of leaving the upper teeth numb posteriorly and in patients with dentures may change the fit of their plate.

5. Deciding how widely to open the sella. Generally speaking, the wider the sellar opening the better. However, if the goal is decompression of a cyst or if there is a strong possibility of a CSF leak, a small initial bone opening may be enough. After the initial bone opening, we use dural coagulation locally and gentle insertion of a needle to establish that there is no vessel behind the sellar floor. It is important to leave enough sellar rim to allow packing at the end of the case.

6. Deciding how vigorous to be with the attempted resection. Experience in transsphenoidal surgery is required in deciding how vigorous to be in attempting removal of a lesion. In general, complete resection should be the goal of the case. Points to consider are the following:

A. Gentle curetting is the usual technique, whenever possible done under direct vision.
B. Many lesions are encapsulated and by getting outside the lesion's capsule with the curette and peeling it forward it is possible to obtain a visibly complete removal.
C. Pulling on fragments still adherent to sellar walls or diaphragm with pituitary rongeurs is a dangerous move.
D. The resection is best approached in an orderly fashion: the central soft portion first, the inferior portion next, then the firmer sides, which may act as pillars holding up the tumor; finally the portion adherent to diaphragm.
E. When the diaphragm prolapses into the field the resection is complete. Some surgeons use suprasellar air placed via a lumbar drain to confirm that the diaphragm has descended, but we have not found this routinely helpful.

7. Deciding whether to pack the sella and how to do so. With microadenomas with pituitary tissue left between the surgeon and the diaphragm sellae, it is usually unnecessary to

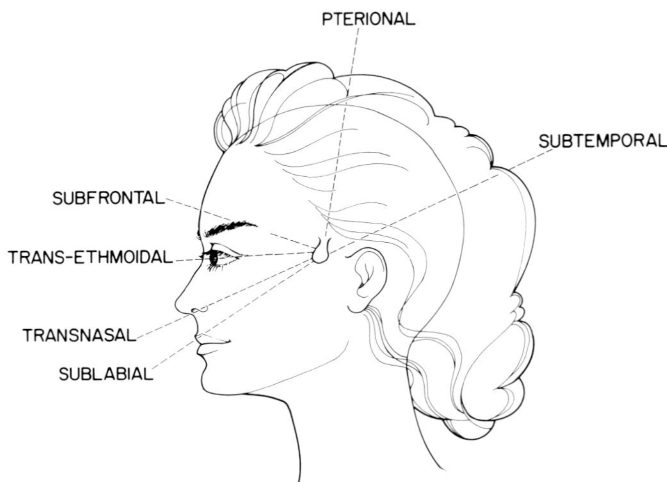

Fig. 26-6. Approaches to the sella turcica. With craniotomy, subfrontal, pterional, or subtemporal approaches can be used depending on tumor configuration or extension. Transsphenoidally, either a sublabial or transnasal route is possible. The transethmoidal route provides an alternative to transsphenoidal access.

pack the sella unless CSF is seen at surgery. With macroadenomas that abut the diaphragm, sellar packing has routinely been carried out by the authors since our early experience had a higher incidence of CSF leak in these patients than in others. In adenomas that have grossly expanded the diaphragm, sellar packing is also done routinely. We use fat harvested from the right lower quadrant of the patient.

It has been our practice to pack the sphenoid sinus as well using fat and Oxycel if a significant CSF leak is seen at surgery. In evaluating a CSF leak, it is important to remember that with the patient's head elevated, air may be sucked in instead of CSF being lost. The C-arm fluoroscope allows an assessment of intracranial air at surgery.

MANAGEMENT OF INTRAOPERATIVE PROBLEMS

BLEEDING

Sinus bleeding from the circular or other dural sinuses around the sellar capsule can usually be packed with oxidized cellulose. An alternative is bipolar cautery on either side of the sinus, but this is usually unhelpful; packing is more satisfactory. As more dura is opened away from the sinus, the sinus margins may retract, and there is often autohemostasis. Attempting to apply clips is not usually helpful. Substantial bleeding from the lateral recesses suggests carotid injury: the best course is to pack the sella firmly and stop. A postoperative arteriogram should be done, since a carotid cavernous fistula or pseudoaneurysm may form.

CEREBROSPINAL FLUID LEAK

A cerebrospinal fluid leak may vary from a small amount of clear liquid seen mixed with blood in the sella to an obvious gush of CSF that fills the field. If any CSF leak is suspected at surgery, it has been our policy to pack the sella with fat harvested from the patient's abdomen: others have suggested fascia lata along with fat taken from the lateral thigh. Bone or cartilage from the nasal septum or sphenoid prow is modelled to fit the sellar opening and the sella is sealed with tissue adhesive.

If there is a copious leak, enough to see CSF empty into the sella with each respiration, our recent policy has been to exenterate and pack the sphenoid sinus as well as the sella. The sphenoid mucosa is stripped and oxidized cellulose in cotton form is placed in the recesses of the sphenoid. Fat is then placed centrally and buttressed with further sheets of Oxycel.

FAILURE TO IDENTIFY ADENOMA

For small tumors secreting prolactin, growth hormone, or adrenocorticotropic hormone, initial evaluation of the pituitary may not reveal tumor. The first step is widening the sellar opening, then fileting the gland left to right in equal thirds. High power magnification is a helpful adjunct. The posterior lobe should be examined as a potential site of tumor.

It is important in Cushing's disease and any other endocrinopathy in which the radiographic findings are uncertain to have discussed the course of action to be taken if no tumor is readily found at surgery. We do not operate on patients with an entirely normal CT scan and elevated prolactin levels unless the prolactin level is greater than 200 ng/ml.

The major problem is the patient with Cushing's disease in whom no adenoma is found. We remove a wedge of the central portion of the anterior pituitary. If that fails to produce a cure, the options vary depending on the patient's age and wishes. In postmenopausal patients, complete hypophysectomy is suggested; in younger patients, the choice is adrenalectomy or radiation therapy.

POSTOPERATIVE CONSIDERATIONS

THE FIRST WEEK

Immediately after surgery, primary attention is directed at visual field examination as part of postoperative nursing care; early hematomas can be detected by such examination. Close measurement of fluid balance is a second important feature. Diabetes insipidus will not usually appear before 12 to 24 hours: it is sometimes hard to distinguish from an appropriate postoperative diuresis in this period. We use Pitressin only if the diagnosis of diabetes insipidus is clear (urine outputs over 200 ml/hour with a specific gravity of 1000). Pitressin in oil, well mixed, is the usual short-term agent. If the condition continues, intramuscular ddAVP is the material of choice; it is long-acting and effective. Levels are checked 3 or 4 days postoperatively for prolactin and growth hormone; cortisol usually takes longer to return to normal. A prolactin level less than 25 ng/ml, a growth hormone level less than 5 ng/ml, and a plasma cortisol level less than 25 ng/ml are hopeful signs of long-term remission if not cure. Dexamethasone (1–2 mg po q6h) is rapidly tapered in the first few days.

The packs are removed on the third postoperative day. Rarely a pack will slip into the oropharynx: it should be removed promptly from the back of the throat and the nostril should be repacked with gauze covered with petroleum jelly. The patient is watched for 1 to 2 days after removal of the packs to be certain there is no CSF leak and discharged with instructions not to blow his or her nose. The typical patient goes home on the fifth postoperative day, usually on Prednisone (5 mg/day)

Table 26-4. Criteria for remission in pituitary adenomas

Tumor Product	Current Criteria for "Remission"
Prolactin	<25 ng/ml
Growth hormone	<5 ng/ml
Adrenocorticotropic hormone	cortisol <5 ng/dl dexamethasone suppressibility

until there is documentation of satisfactory pituitary dynamics. Follow-up examination is performed at 1 to 3 weeks.

For transcranial surgery the patient is kept in an intensive care unit overnight with careful monitoring of arterial pressure and visual fields. A Foley catheter is left in for 24 hours. He or she is encouraged to be up the next day. Sutures are removed on the seventh postoperative day. The patient is kept on Dilantin or some other anticonvulsant.

SUBSEQUENT EVALUATION

The surgeon should remember that a surgical procedure is only the first step in treatment for many tumors. By 1 month after the surgery the hormone levels are usually at their minimal level: at this time decisions need to be made about subsequent care. Possible situations include:

1. For endocrine active tumors: (A) Apparent complete remission. In most cases annual endocrinologic evaluation is adequate. One caution is that some tumors may produce hormones but not be primarily endocrine active; it is important to follow the patient with CT or MR scans as well as determinations of hormone levels, especially if the tumor was large at the time of initial resection. (B) Incomplete endocrine remission. For prolactinomas, bromocriptine is the treatment of choice; for acromegaly and Cushing's disease, radiation therapy, either proton beam or conventional, is preferred.
2. If there is evidence of major residual tumor, either transcranial surgery or radiation therapy should be considered. In general, surgery is preferred if there is a reasonable possibility of improvement.

LONG-TERM RESULTS

Endocrinologic Results

Endocrinologic results in pituitary adenoma resection depend on the criteria for remission, the surgeon, and the size of the lesion. Criteria for remission and surgical results from various series are presented in Tables 26-4 through 26-7.[10–20] Rough estimates are a remission rate of 70 to 90 percent for microadenomas and of 30 percent for macroadenomas.

Table 26-5. Endocrine "cure" rates by transsphenoidal surgery for prolactinomas in representative series

Series	Microadenomas	Macroadenomas
Zervas[16]	74%	30%
Faria and Tindall[12]	76%	46%
Hardy[17]	78%	29%

Table 26-6. Endocrine "cure" rates by transsphenoidal surgery for growth hormone producing adenomas

Series	Microadenomas	Macroadenomas
Zervas[16]	78%	33%
Baskin et al[11]	78%	na
Laws et al[18]	65%	55%

Visual Results

In a series of 113 adenomas with extrasellar extension of the tumor, we found that postoperative visual improvement was produced in 81 percent of patients and worsening occurred in none (Black PMcL, Zervas NT, Candia GH: unpublished observations). In general, the improvement rate varies from 80 to 90 percent in most transsphenoidal series.[6–8] Using longer-term follow-up after radiation therapy was completed, Symon and Jakubowski[9] showed improvement in 90 percent of patients; other craniotomy series have an 70 to 80 percent improvement rate, but there also is a significant incidence of visual worsening with transcranial surgery. The major argument for transsphenoidal surgery as the procedure of choice is that it has less potential morbidity and mortality than transcranial surgery and has results at least as good as craniotomy.[10,13–15]

COMPLICATIONS

There is a long list of potential complications in transsphenoidal surgery for pituitary adenomas.[13] Table 26-8 outlines many of them; most are not serious. Management of the most common will be briefly discussed here.

CSF LEAK

Establishing that nasal fluid is CSF is best done by assessing its chloride content—it should be higher than serum chloride levels. The best test to confirm that a leak is present is to provoke it by positional change. A leak that is primarily evident in the morning and does not result in visible dripping of clear fluid from the nostril on lowering the head may be treated expectantly for 10 days. A lumbar drain for 5 days or repeat lumbar punctures may keep the pressure low and allow closure. Be wary of pneumocephalus in this period; it is worse than a CSF leak and should be watched for on regular lateral skull films.

A leak that visibly drips or does not resolve in 10 days requires repeat surgery. This can be done transsphenoidally if

Table 26-7. Endocrine "cure" rates by transsphenoidal surgery for ACTH producing adenomas

Series	Microadenomas	Macroadenomas
Zervas[16]	91%	61%
Boggan et al[19]	87%	48%
Laws et al[20]	79%	

Table 26-8. Possible complications in transsphenoidal surgery

Nasal or Oral
  Septal perforation
  Septal deviation
  Tearing of the nares
  Persistent nasal discharge
  Recurrent nosebleeds
  Tooth analgesia
  Asymmetry of mucosal contour
  Dentalization of pulp of anterior teeth
  Aspiration of blood postoperatively
Sphenoid Sinus
  Sinusitis
  Mucocele
  Fracture, possibly with optic nerve injury
Sellar Region
  CSF leak
  Hemorrhage into sella
  Carotid artery damage
  Extraocular nerve damage
  Basilar artery damage
Brain Injury
  Optic nerve, chiasm, or tract
  Hypothalamus
  Ventral pons
  Medial frontal lobe
  Anterior cerebral artery

the surgeon feels there is further packing to do: transethmoid exposure is another possibility.

SINUSITIS

Sinusitis should be treated vigorously, including the use of intravenous antibiotics and sinus drainage if it does not resolve.

Table 26-9. Possible complications of craniotomy

Associated with Bone Flap and Incision
  Wound infection
  Dehiscence
  CSF leak
  Frontalis palsy
  Cosmetic deformity
  Subdural abscess
Associated with Brain Manipulation
  Seizure disorder
  Intellectual slowing
  Frontal lobe edema
  Subdural or epidural hematoma
  Frontal lobe contusion
Associated with Parasellar Region
  Visual loss
  Hypothalmic injury
  Carotid injury
  Panhypopituitarism
  Anosmia
  Vegetative state
  Autonomic disturbances
  CSF leak

DIABETES INSIPIDUS

Diabetes insipidus can be handled very well with ddAVP snuff, 0.1 cc given nasally every 2 days or as needed.

The potential complications of transfrontal surgery are even longer and more serious than transsphenoidal surgery (Table 26-9). Most of them are those anticipated in any craniotomy. A particularly upsetting problem is failure of the patient to awaken immediately, a condition that should lead to CT scanning and then close observation if the CT scan shows no hematoma or other cause. Damage to the hypothalamus, either directly or indirectly through vascular compromise, is the usual cause: recovery is variable. Memory loss, disorientation, and agitation or stupor are components of this syndrome as it resolves.

REFERENCES

1. Black PMcL: Diagnosis: Pituitary tumor. Hosp Med 21:43, 1985
2. Doppman JL, Oldfield EH, Cruddy AG, et al: Petrosal sampling for Cushing's syndrome: Anatomical and technical considerations. Radiology 150:99, 1984
3. Snow RB, Lavyne MH, Lee BCP, et al: Craniotomy versus transsphenoidal excision of large pituitary tumors: The usefulness of magnetic resonance imaging in guiding the operative approach. Neurosurgery 19:59, 1986
4. Trautman JC, Laws EG Jr: Visual status after transsphenoidal surgery at the Mayo Clinic. Am J Ophthalmol 96:200, 1983
5. Ciric I, Mikhael M, Stafford M, et al: Transsphenoidal management of pituitary macroadenomas with long-term followup results. J Neurosurg 59:395, 1982
6. Cohen AR, Cooper PR, Kupersmith MJ, et al: Visual recovery after transsphenoidal removal of pituitary adenomas. Neurosurgery 17:446, 1985
7. Nicola G: Transsphenoidal surgery for pituitary tumors with extrasellar extension. Prog Neurol Surg 6:149, 1975
8. Symon L, Jakubowski J: Transcranial management of pituitary tumors with extrasellar extension. J Neurol Neurosurg Psychiatry 42:123, 1979
9. Wilson CB: Neurosurgical management of large and invasive pituitary tumors, in Tindall GT, Collins (eds): Clinical Management of Pituitary Disorders. New York, Raven Press, 1979, pp 335–342
10. Black PMcL, Zervas NT, Candia G: The incidence and management of complications in transsphenoidal operation for pituitary adenomas. Neurosurgery (in press)
11. Baskin DS, Boggan JE, Wilson CB: Transsphenoidal microsurgical removal of growth hormone-secreting pituitary adenomas: A review of 137 cases. J Neurosurg 56:634, 1982
12. Faria MA, Tindall GT: Transsphenoidal microsurgery for prolactin-secreting pituitary adenomas. J Neurosurg 56:33, 1982
13. Laws ER Jr, Kern EB: Complications of transsphenoidal surgery. Clin Neurosurg 23:401, 1976
14. Nakane T, Kuwayama A, Watanabe M, et al: Transsphenoidal approach to pituitary adenomas with suprasellar extension. Surg Neurol 16:225, 1981
15. Wilson CB, Dempsey LC: Transsphenoidal microsurgical removal of 250 pituitary adenomas. J Neurosurg 48:13, 1978
16. Zervas NT: Surgical results in pituitary adenomas: Results of an international survey, in Black PMcL, Zervas NT, Ridgway EC Jr, Martin JB (eds): Secretory Tumors of the Pituitary Gland. New York, Raven Press, 1984, pp 377–385
17. Hardy J: Transsphenoidal microsurgery of prolactinomas, in Black PMcL, Zervas NT, Ridgway EC Jr, et al (eds): Secretory Tumors of the Pituitary Gland. New York, Raven Press, 1984, pp 73–82
18. Laws ER, Randall RV, Abboud CF: Surgical treatment of acromegaly: Results in 140 patients, in Givens J (ed): Hormone-Secreting Pituitary Tumors. Chicago, Year Book, 1982, pp 225–228
19. Boggan JE, Tyrrell JB, Wilson CB: Transsphenoidal microsurgical management of Cushing's disease. Report of 100 cases. J Neurosurg 59:195, 1983
20. Laws ER Jr, Ebersold MJ, Piepgras DG, et al: The results of transsphenoidal surgery in specific clinical entities, in Laws ER Jr, Randall RV, Kern EB, et al (eds): Management of Pituitary Adenomas and Related Lesions. New York, Appleton-Century-Crofts, 1982, pp 277–305

CHAPTER 27

Transsphenoidal Approach to Lesions In and About the Sella Turcica

Edward R. Laws, Jr.

THE TRANSSPHENOIDAL APPROACH is commonly used for the operative treatment of pituitary adenomas. It is also highly suitable for ablative hypophysectomy and for the management of certain other tumors of the area such as craniopharyngiomas, tumors of the clivus such as chordomas or cholesteatomas, and for the management of disease involving the sphenoid sinus, such as mucoceles, carcinomas, or cysts.

The technique employed is essentially that used by Cushing,[1] Hirsch,[2] and Dott,[3] with the technical advances introduced by Guiot[4] and by Hardy.[5]

The patient is placed in a semirecumbent position on an operating table, using a Mayfield headrest with horseshoe (Figure 27-1). Although some surgeons fix the head in a pinion headrest, we prefer the horseshoe support so that small lateral movements of the head can be used to improve visualization of the cavernous sinus area. The patient is positioned so that the left ear is cocked downward toward the left shoulder, allowing the surgeon a more comfortable midline approach to the nose and head. If a suprasellar extension of a pituitary tumor is anticipated, an intraoperative pneumoencephalogram can be performed through a malleable needle or catheter placed into the lumbar subarachnoid space. A special split mattress is used so that the needle remains undisturbed. Once the endotracheal tube is in place, the oropharynx is carefully packed with cotton gauze to prevent the accumulation of blood in the throat and eventually in the stomach. Details of anesthetic management have been described.[6]

At our institution the rhinologist usually performs the initial portion of the procedure, up to and occasionally including the entrance into the sphenoid sinus. The rhinologic aspects of this procedure have been described in detail;[4–13] however, the steps used when the neurosurgical service performs the entire operative procedures will be repeated.[14,15]

OPERATIVE PROCEDURE

After the skin of the face is prepared with an aqueous antiseptic solution, the nostrils are packed with pledgets of cotton gauze soaked in 5 percent cocaine and inserted with a nasal speculum and bayonet forceps. The pledgets are allowed to remain in contact with the nasal mucosa for 5 to 10 minutes, while draping of the patient is completed. A solution of 0.5 percent Xylocaine in 1:200,000 epinephrine is injected submucosally. Using a 25-gauge needle, 10 to 20 ml of the solution is infiltrated, first along the upper gingiva, then along the inferior portion of the nasal septum, and finally along the lateral aspects of the nasal septum. A conscious effort is made to dissect the nasal mucosa away from the cartilaginous septum with the injection solution. This is done under direct vision with the aid of a nasal speculum and a headlight.

We have adopted the initial approach of the rhinologist, i.e., a right-sided hemitransfixion incision in the nostril (Figure 27-2), since this greatly simplifies dissecting the left anterior nasal mucosal tunnel away from the septum. This incision is made along the inferior border of the nasal septum as the columnella is retracted laterally to the patient's left. The inferior border of the cartilaginous septum is exposed with sharp dissection and the left side of the septum is exposed submucosally with a combination of sharp and blunt dissection, thereby creating the left anterior tunnel. The premaxillary region then is undermined with blunt dissection using small scissors. In many patients, the entire procedure can be performed through the nostril, and this route is routinely used by Zervas[16] and Ludecke.[17]

In most cases, the sublabial approach permits a wider exposure. The upper lip then is retracted, and an incision is made in the buccogingival junction from one canine tooth to the other (Figure 27-3). Mucosa is elevated from the maxillary ridge and the anterior nasal spine until the inferior border of the pyriform aperture is exposed. Using curved dissectors and working from the lateral border medially, the two inferior nasal tunnels are created by dissecting the mucosa away from the superior surface of the hard palate (Figure 27-4). With sharp dissection, the left anterior tunnel and the left inferior tunnel are connected (Figure 27-5), and the entire left side of the nasal septum is exposed back to the perpendicular plate of the ethmoid (the bony portion of the nasal septum). Using firm blunt dissection along the left side of the base of the nasal septum, the cartilaginous portion of the nasal septum is dislocated and reflected to the right, and a right posterior mucosal tunnel is developed along the right side of the bony septum. At this point it should be possible to insert the transsphenoidal retractor. It should be spread gently, and care should be taken to place all tears in the nasal mucosa lateral to the retractor blades. As the retractor is opened, the turbinates will fracture; it is unwise to apply a great deal of force in opening the retractor. Once the retractor is in place, the vomer should be visualized and submucous dissection then carried up to the face

OPERATIVE NEUROSURGICAL TECHNIQUES
ISBN 0-8089-1862-1

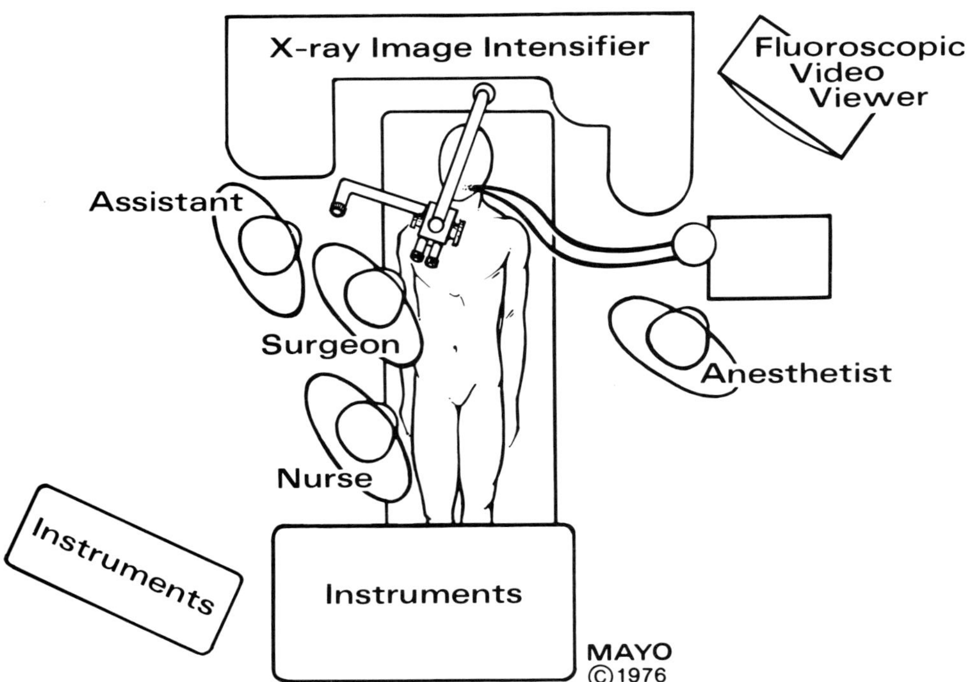

Fig. 27-1. Diagram of the arrangement of the operating room for transsphenoidal surgery.

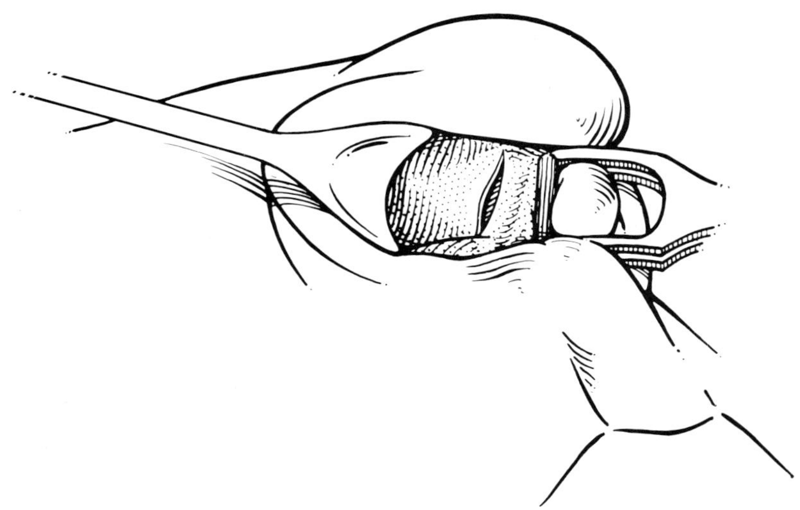

Fig. 27-2. The right-sided hemitransfixion incision exposing the caudal end of the nasal septum.

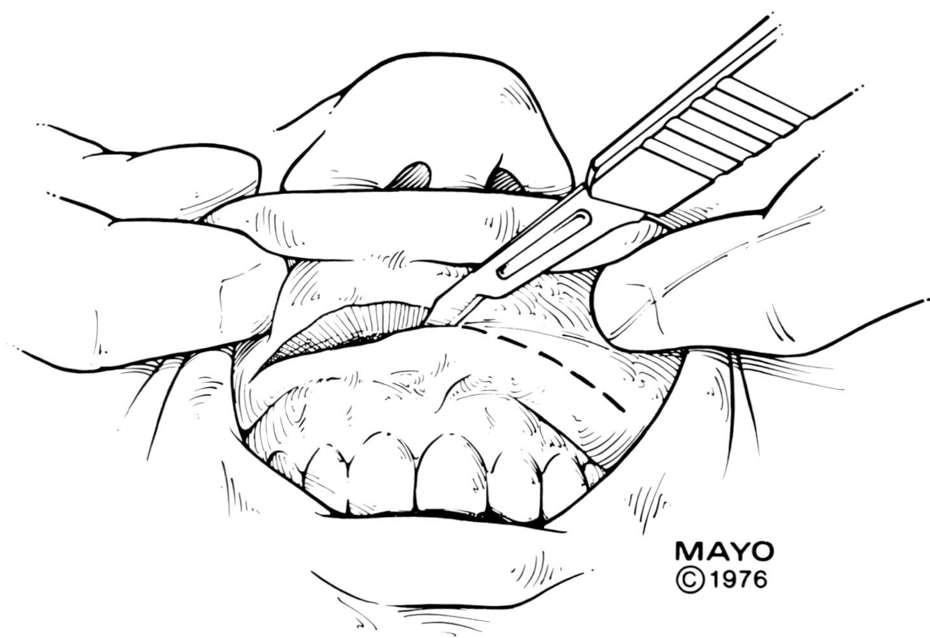

Fig. 27-3. The sublabial incision.

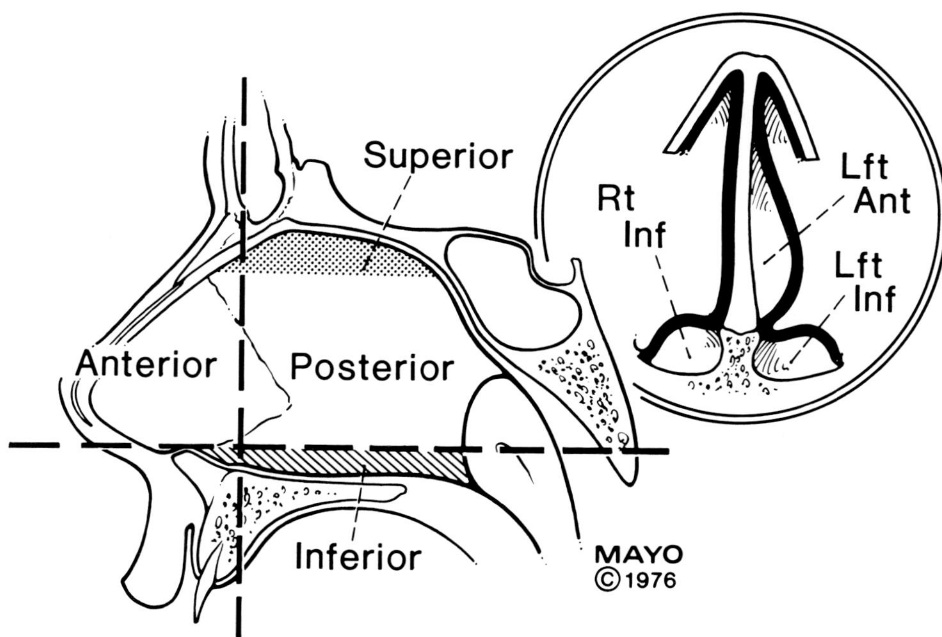

Fig. 27-4. Diagram of the tunnels created by elevating the nasal mucosa.

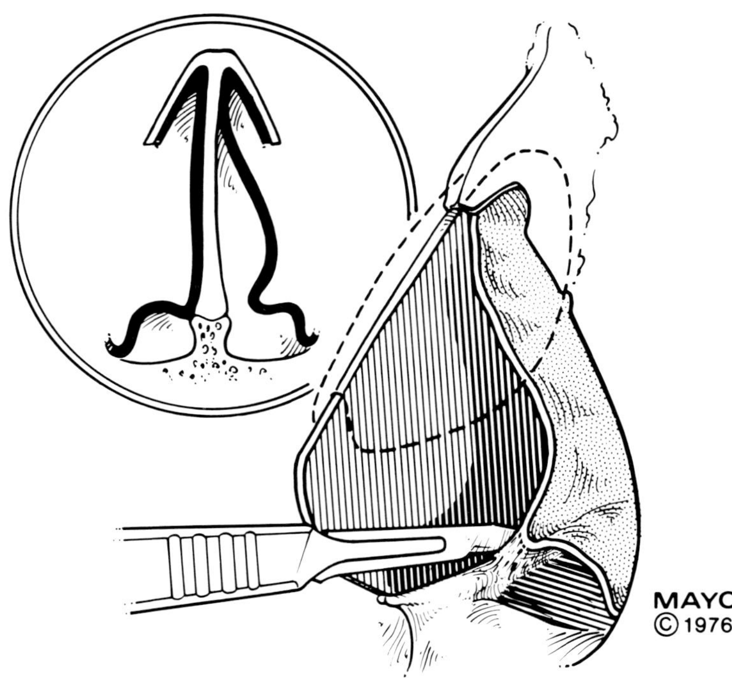

Fig. 27-5. Sharp dissection is used to connect the anterior tunnels of the nasal mucosa with the inferior tunnels.

of the sphenoid sinus. The transsphenoidal retractor then can be repositioned and secured in place.

The bony nasal septum in the operative field should be resected, using a Lillie-Koffler tool or a Ferris-Smith punch (Figure 27-6). This cartilage and bone is saved so that it can be used during the closure. With experience, the nasal spine anteriorly does not represent a major obstacle, and it is preferable, from a cosmetic standpoint, to preserve this structure rather than chisel it away.

With the transsphenoidal retractor properly positioned, the keel of the vomer and the face of the sphenoid sinus will be seen (Figure 27-7). On either side of the central ridge the ostia of the sphenoid sinus can be identified.

At this point, either a lateral skull x-ray film is obtained or the portable image intensifier is used so that bony landmarks and the relationship of the transsphenoidal retractor to the eventual pathway of operative approach can be determined. Any corrections, either mental or physical, are then made and the operating microscope is introduced.

It usually is possible to fracture into the sphenoid sinus by grasping the vomer with a Lillie-Koffler tool or Ferris-Smith punch. A chisel can be used, if necessary. Detailed CT images or tomograms of the sphenoid sinus are helpful in determining the anatomy and internal landmarks to be visualized, and the operative approach may need to be adjusted if anomalies of sinus formation are present. Once the sphenoid sinus is entered, a right-angled sphenoid punch can be used to complete the exposure. The mucosa within the sphenoid sinus is resected with a cup forceps. Resection of the mucosa aids in reducing bleeding and probably decreases the risk of postoperative mucocele formation.

The floor of the sella should now be clearly visible, and the bony landmarks should be confirmed with x-ray films or with the portable image intensifier. With some tumors, the face of the sella will have been eroded or will be extraordinarily thin, so that it can be fractured with a blunt nerve hook. Occasionally a midline septum within the sphenoid sinus can be used to gain entry into the sella simply by grasping the base of the septum where it joins the face of the sella and twisting as this bone is removed. If the floor of the sella is thick, a small chisel can be used to remove a triangle or square of bone, fracturing it from the face of the sella. Exposure of the dura of the pituitary region is completed with a miniature right-angle Kerrison-type punch. In certain cases in which the floor of the sella is thick or the sphenoid bone poorly pneumatized, a high-speed air drill can be used to provide exposure. A poorly pneumatized sphenoid can usually be hollowed out with a curette to remove medullary bone, exposing the inner cortical surface, which is the sellar floor.

Exposure of the sella proper is carried out using the operating microscope with a 300-mm objective lens and 12.5 × oculars. In most cases the magnification is set at 6 or 10 ×, but it is advisable to alter the magnification so that the sella fills the entire field of vision once the intrasellar portion of the operation is begun.

An invasive pituitary tumor may erode through the anterior dura of the sella, but in most cases the dura will be intact. It is exposed as widely as feasible, and careful attention is paid to its appearance. Transverse, blue, intercavernous sinuses crossing the sella at the top and bottom of the operative exposure of the anterior dura are common, particularly in microadenomas. On rare occasions the entire anterior dura is laced with venous structures, appearing as one huge sinuous intercavernous sinus.

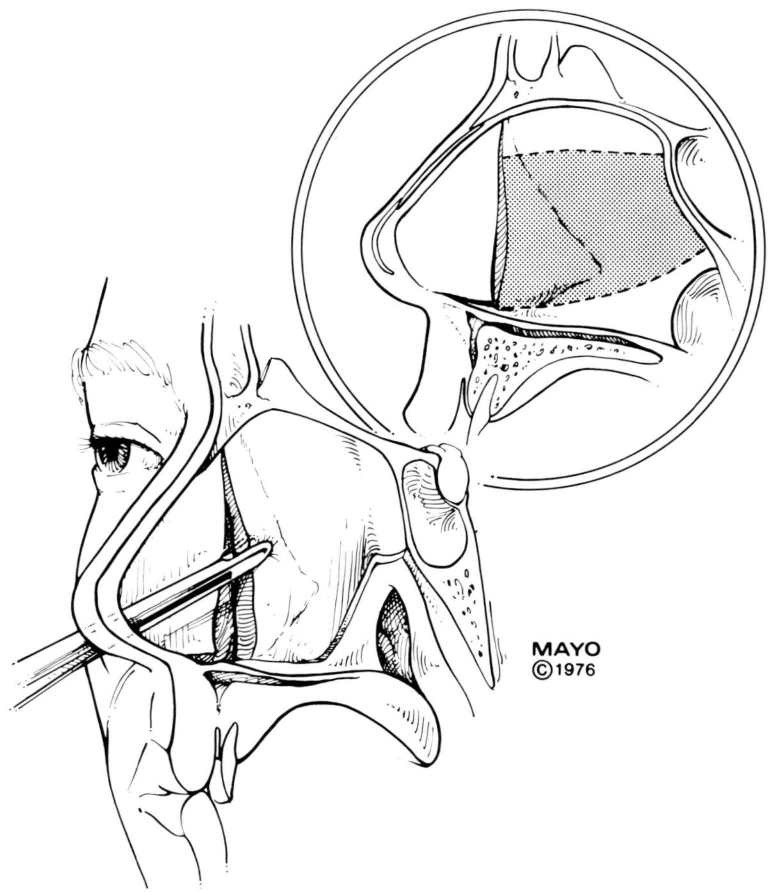

Fig. 27-6. Removal of the inferoposterior aspect of the nasal septum.

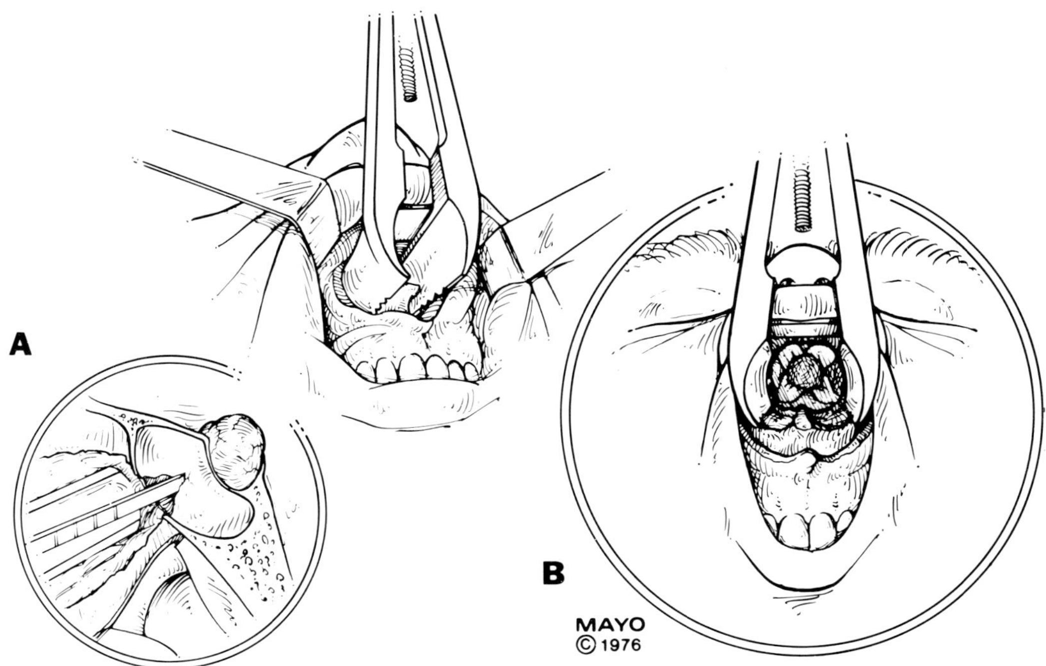

Fig. 27-7. (A) Insertion of the transsphenoidal retractor; (B) entrance into the sphenoid sinus; (C) exposure of the sellar floor.

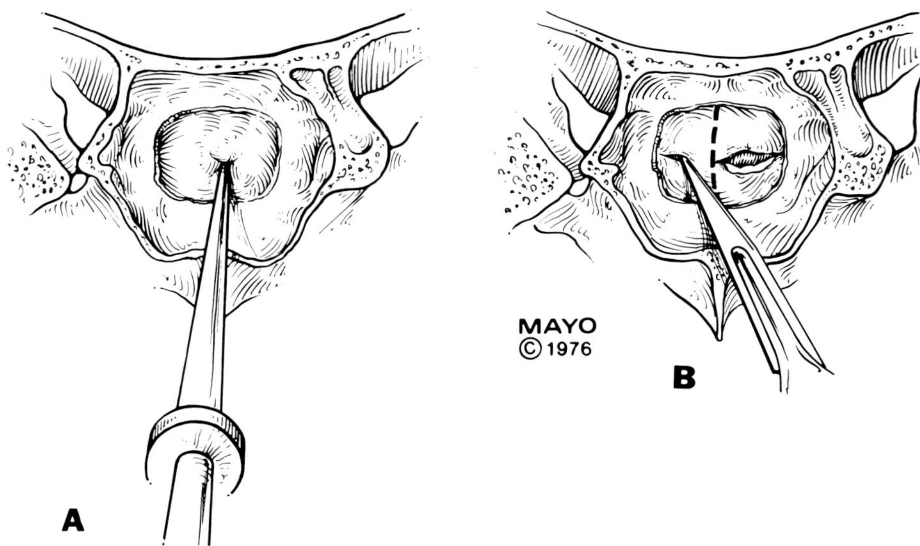

Fig. 27-8. (A) Aspiration of the sella, and (B) incision of the dura.

The anterior dura may appear totally blue and very thin; this may indicate the presence of an empty sella. Once the dura is exposed completely, it is cauterized with a suction-cautery device, usually around the periphery where the dural incision will be made. Before the dura is opened, the sella is aspirated with a long, 19–gauge needle (Figure 27-8). This procedure is monitored with the x-ray image intensifier. The goals are (1) to be certain there is no aneurysm within the sella, and (2) to detect either a cystic tumor or an empty sella. After needle aspiration, the dura is opened. A horizontal incision is made between the intercavernous sinuses with a bayonet-handled knife. In most cases, a central vertical incision then is made to complete a cruciate opening of the dura. Alternatively, the incision can be performed as an ''X'', or an ellipse of anterior dura can be excised.[18] Current practice favors excision of a rectangular dural window. If possible, a blunt hook then is used to establish a definite subdural cleavage plane between the pituitary gland or tumor and the dura. A plane of dissection between the two layers of the dura should be carefully avoided, as this will allow entrance into the cavernous sinus and produce a great deal of venous bleeding. Once the dura has been reflected, the suction-cautery is used to cauterize and shrink the leaves of dura to provide an unobstructed view into the sella. Bipolar cautery can be useful in controlling bleeding from venous channels within the dural margins.

In the case of the typical diffuse pituitary adenoma, the tumor is entered, using a ring curette, and the tumor tissue is carefully loosened and removed (Figure 27-9). This is accomplished with a relatively blunt ring curette, first cleaning tumor away from the inferior dura of the sella. Once the inferior aspect is free of tumor, dissection is continued laterally, from inferior to superior on both sides, against the medial wall of the cavernous sinus. During this portion of dissection, the carotid arteries can be seen, and injury to them must be avoided. Tissue is never pulled away from the lateral aspect of the sella, since doing so could avulse a vascular structure. It is preferable to use a ring curette to loosen tissue and to remove only loosened tissue with a cup forceps and very little traction. With the floor of the sella and both sides cleaned of tumor, the next step is to work from the lateral walls to the superior aspect of the tumor, starting anteriorly within the sella. Here a special effort must be made not to tear the diaphragm and thus create a cerebrospinal fluid leak. Decompression of the intrasellar portion of the tumor frequently allows a suprasellar extension to herniate directly into view within the sella. The diaphragma sellae or the capsule of the tumor will subsequently prolapse. If this does not occur, air injected through the malleable lumbar needle will outline the suprasellar extension of the tumor and produce a pressure differential favoring herniation of tumor into the sella. Ordinarily 15 to 25 ml of air is adequate both for x-ray visualization and to alter pressure relationships. If prolapse of the capsule does not occur, a ring curette can be used cautiously in the intracranial space, under x-ray control with the image intensifier. The capsule can be re-expanded, if necessary, by withdrawing cerebrospinal fluid through the lumbar needle. The fact that no residual tumor is present can be confirmed by visual inspection, with the help of a dental mirror, a nasopharyngoscope, or a small flexible-tipped fiberoptic endoscope.

In most cases it is worthwhile to attempt to save normal pituitary tissue. In a large diffuse adenoma, this usually appears as a thin, superolaterally placed membrane. A biopsy specimen can be taken for confirmation, but usually the appearance is typical and this tissue can be left behind with some confidence.

If a pituitary microadenoma is not visible immediately when the dura is opened, a transverse incision is made into the pituitary gland proper. Once this incision is made, subdural dissection of the lateral wings of the pituitary gland is started, first on one side and then on the other, with the Hardy dissectors. If the incision into the gland has been made deeply enough, lateral pressure with the Hardy dissector usually causes the microadenoma to herniate into the operative field. Its location therefore can be delineated, its cavity entered, and

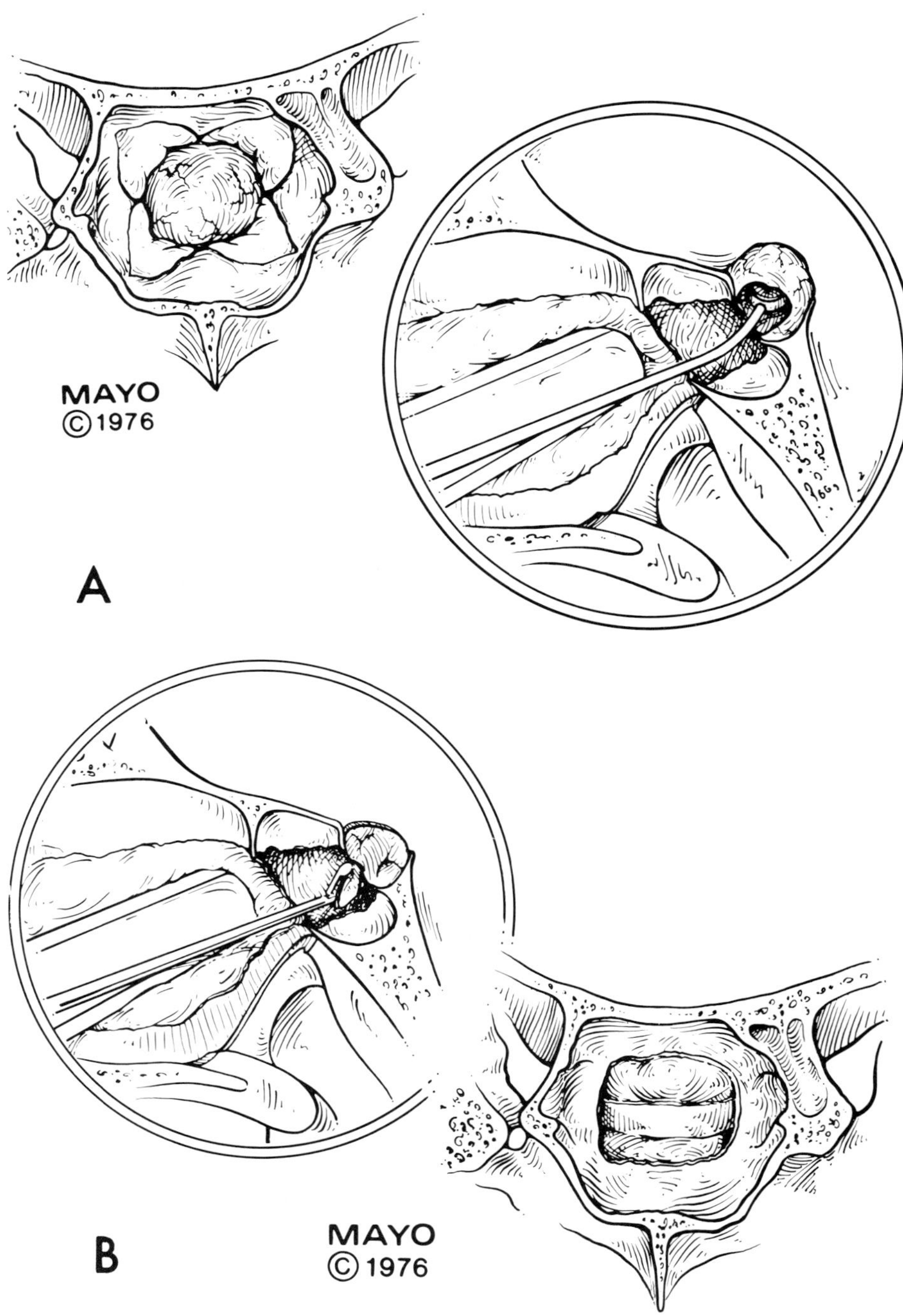

Fig. 27-9. (A) Removal of adenoma with a ring curette; (B) packing of the sella with muscle and a stent of nasal cartilage.

its removal completed, using a small ring curette and cup forceps. All tissue that appears suspicious is removed and the residual, presumed normal, pituitary gland is occasionally biopsied. The tumor cavity can be treated with applications of absolute alcohol or Zenker's solution, but there is no evidence that this step improves either the immediate result or the risk of recurrence.

The technique of hypophysectomy for metastatic carcinoma or diabetic retinopathy is similar to that described for microadenomas. The pituitary gland is dissected subdurally; the lateral wings are dissected first and then the inferior aspect of the gland. The subdural plane of dissection is maintained, and considerable pressure is used to strip the lateral aspects of the

gland, from anterior to posterior, away from the walls of the cavernous sinus. This is done cautiously and little by little, working first on one side then the other and then on the inferior aspect of the gland, repeating this sequence many times. The gland will, in effect, shrink, and once some mobility has been achieved, the superior aspect of the gland can be dissected and then depressed, permitting the pituitary stalk to come into view. The stalk is then transsected with an alligator scissors or a No. 11 blade knife. Once this has been accomplished, a Hardy dissector is placed along the floor of the sella and used to dissect behind and then over the superior surface of the gland to free it completely. In some cases the dissection does not go smoothly and the gland may have to be removed piecemeal, in which case

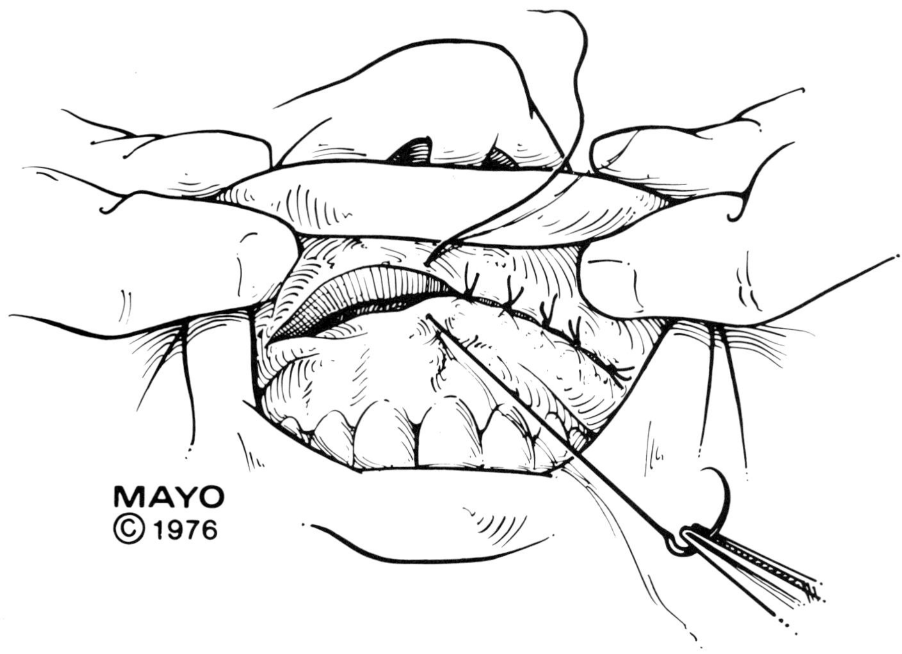

Fig. 27-10. Closure of the sublabial incision.

the sella must be searched thoroughly for retained fragments of the gland. Total hypophysectomy must be achieved for optimum results.

After the tumor has been removed, or after hypophysectomy, the sella is packed, as is the tumor cavity of a microadenoma once the lesion has been removed. Most often, homograft fat or muscle taken from the right lower quadrant of the abdomen is used. A piece of fat that has been soaked in chloramphenicol solution is trimmed to approximate the size of the operative defect and is placed within the sella, using the sucker and cup forceps. Once it is in place, it is secured with a piece of nasal bone or cartilage cut in the shape of a narrow rectangle or rhomboid and placed in a subdural position as a wedge to hold the muscle securely (Figure 27-9). On occasion, more than one piece of fat or muscle or more than one piece of cartilage or bone is employed.

If a cerebrospinal fluid leak has developed during surgery, the roof of the sella can be reconstructed with a piece of homologous dural graft material or fascia lata. This step probably adds little to the security of the seal, and autograft muscle or fat usually is satisfactory. Sellar closure with a relatively large epidural plate of nasal bone also adds security to the seal.

When a cerebrospinal fluid leak has been present, usually the sphenoid sinus is also packed with muscle or fat, but in the absence of a cerebrospinal fluid leak, it is left free of packing or foreign material.

Assuming that adequate hemostasis has been achieved and the sella has been suitably packed, the nasal phase of the procedure is completed by packing the nostrils with gauze impregnated with petroleum jelly and closing the gingival and nasal incision with loose interrupted 4-0 catgut sutures (Figure 27-10).

A compression dressing is applied in the form of a gauze pad placed beneath the nostrils and over the upper lip as a drip pad, and the nose is taped to ensure a satisfactory cosmetic result.

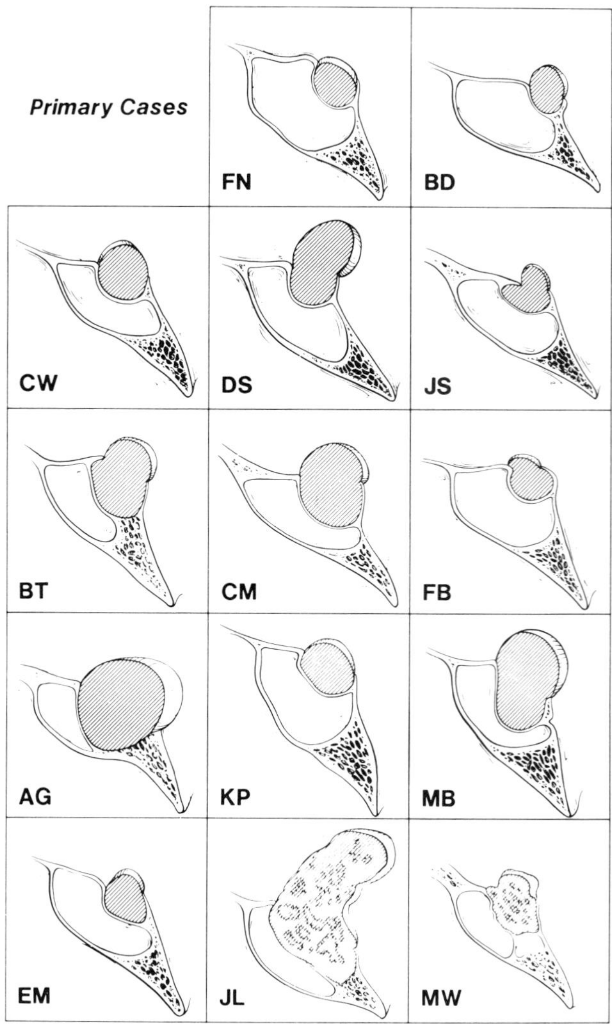

Fig. 27-11. Diagrammatic representation of types of craniopharyngiomas treated primarily by transsphenoidal excision.

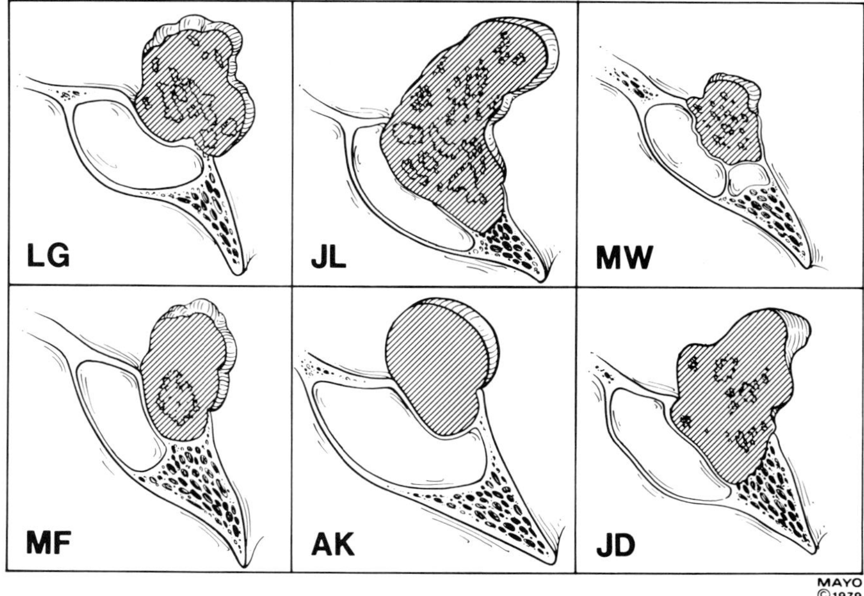

Fig. 27-12. Diagrammatic representation of previously treated craniopharyngiomas operated upon transsphenoidally.

Prophylactic antibiotics are continued until the nasal packing is removed, usually on the fourth postoperative day. In uncomplicated cases, the patient can be dismissed from the hospital on the sixth postoperative day.

The transsphenoidal approach has been used successfully to treat 66 patients with craniopharyngiomas. Although some of these patients had been diagnosed preoperatively as having pituitary adenomas, the majority had been diagnosed correctly.[19] If a craniopharyngioma produces enlargement of the sella, its origin is likely to be intrasellar and below the diaphragm, and it is therefore amenable to a transsphenoidal approach.

There are two general categories of craniopharyngioma patients: those whose primary treatment is transsphenoidal, where a "total" removal is attempted, and those with recurrent tumors previously treated by craniotomy, where palliation is the goal. Examples of the tumors treated are shown in Figures 27-11 and 27-12.

Important aspects of the surgical technique include the following points. Complete exposure of the floor of the enlarged sella is desirable, and wide bony excision to the margins of the cavernous sinuses laterally and to the dural reflection at the tuberculum superiorly is recommended. After the dura is opened widely, a subdural dissection is begun. The normal anterior pituitary gland is usually seen as a membranous structure that occasionally can be preserved. Within the sella, an extracapsular plane of dissection is established around the capsule of the craniopharyngioma. Adhesions of the tumor capsule to the walls of the cavernous sinus and the floor of the sella usually will yield to cautious use of the Hardy dissectors. This is not true of the diaphragm, however, and sharp dissection with removal of the diaphragm is necessary for total removal of the lesion. The diaphragm is detached from the tuberculum initially with a No. 11 scalpel blade working laterally to medially. This creates a large CSF leak that must be ignored until closure. The fused superior tumor capsule and diaphragm then are depressed and the stalk is visualized. With microscissors or scalpel blade hugging the superior capsule, the stalk is divided as close to the capsule as possible. It then is usually possible to complete the intrasellar dissection and remove the lesion (Figure 27-13). Closure in these cases is accomplished as outlined earlier, with intrasellar muscle held in place by a plate of nasal bone placed epidurally to reconstruct the floor of the sella.

Transsphenoidal decompression of a recurrent craniopharyngioma can be an effective palliative procedure. If no CSF leak has occurred, an attempt can be made to provide continuing drainage of the lesion by placing a Silastic tube into the tumor cavity and leading it out into the posterior septal space where it can drain into the nasopharynx (Figure 27-14). An alternative to tubing is a piece of thin Silastic sheeting rolled into a cylinder. In either case, it is prudent to mark the internal

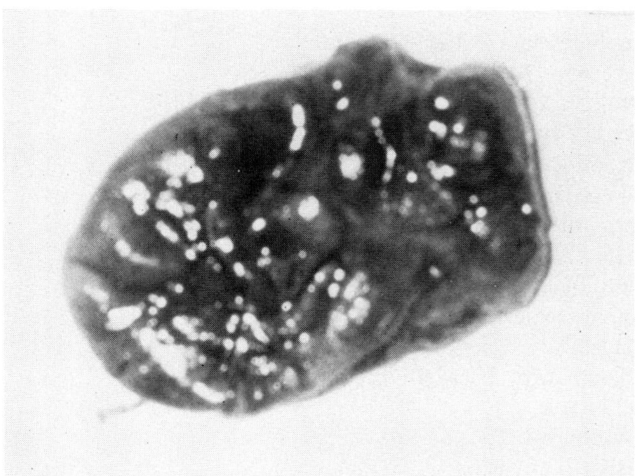

Fig. 27-13. A craniopharyngioma 2 cm in diameter. Gross total removal was accomplished using the transsphenoidal approach.

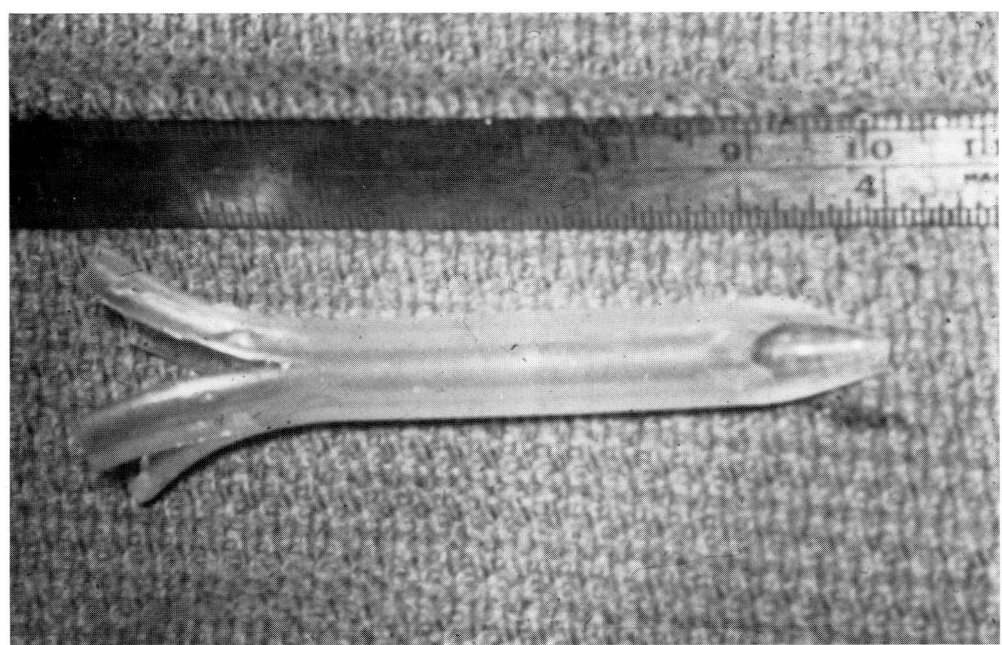

Fig. 27-14. Silastic tube used to provide drainage of cystic craniopharyngiomas.

end of the tube with a clip, since the tubes can become displaced or work their way out.

These techniques have been most satisfactory for the management of selected craniopharyngiomas. It should be emphasized again that the transsphenoidal route generally is only suitable for those patients with an enlarged sella.

Table 27-1. Clinical entities treated by transsphenoidal microsurgery, Mayo Clinic, 1972–1986

Clinical Entity	Number of Patients
Pituitary adenoma	1598
Craniopharyngioma	66
Metastatic carcinoma (hypophysectomy)	18
Diabetic retinopathy (hypophysectomy)	4
Empty sella/arachnoid cyst	37
CSF rhinorrhea	38
Clivus chordoma	18
Miscellaneous lesions	41

Table 27-2. Pituitary adenomas treated by transsphenoidal microsurgery

Clinical Entity	Cases Number	Cases Total
Functioning adenomas		1157
Acromegaly	284	
Prolactin-secreting adenomas	622	
Nelson-Salassa syndrome (postadrenalectomy ACTH)	44	
Primary Cushing's disease	207	
Nonfunctioning adenomas (includes FSH/LH, Null, etc.)		441
Total pituitary adenomas		1598

The clinical entities treated in a 12-year period,[20–23] along with the complications observed,[24–26] and the results of treatment are presented in Tables 27-1 through 27-5.

The transsphenoidal approach has proved to be safe and effective in the management of a variety of problems associated with the sella turcica.[20,21,22,27–30] Not only have the results been as satisfactory or better than those achieved with more traditional approaches, but a new group of pathologic lesions, i.e., microadenomas, has become amenable to surgical correction.

Table 27-3. Miscellaneous lesions treated by transsphenoidal microsurgery

Clinical Entity	Number of Patients
Mucocele/pyocele	5
Nasal glioma	3
Meningioma	3
Sphenoid sinus carcinoma/sarcoma	5
Sphenoid sinus cyst	2
Ganglioglioma of the sphenoid sinus	1
Cavernous hemangioma (parasellar)	1
Myeloma (sellar)	2
Fibrous dysplasia (parasellar)	1
Carotid-cavernous fistula	1
Tolosa-Hunt syndrome (granuloma)	1
Germinoma/teratoma	2
Hypothalamic hamartoma	1
Schwannoma	1
Hemangioblastoma	1
Metastatic carcinoma	12
Inflammatory disease/hypophysitis	3
Melanoma	1
Colloid cyst	3
Basilar impression	1
Total	49

Table 27-4. Complications of transsphenoidal surgery, Mayo Clinic, 1972 to 1985 (1696 cases)[24–27]

Complication	Number of Patients
Operative mortality (30-day)	
Hypothalamic injury/hemorrhage	3
Meningitis	2
Vascular injury/occlusion	3
CSF leak, pneumocephalus, MI	1
Postoperative MI	1
Total	10 (0.6%)
Major morbidity*	
Vascular occlusion/spasm/subarachnoid hemorrhage (stroke)	5
Visual loss	10
Vascular injury	8
Meningitis (nonfatal)	2
Sellar abscess	1
Sellar pneumatocele	1
Sixth nerve paralysis	2
Third nerve paralysis	1
CSF rhinorrhea	29
Total	59 (3.5%)
Lesser morbidity	
Hemorrhage, intraoperative or postoperative	5
Postoperative psychosis	5
Nasal septal perforation, webbing	5
Sinusitis, lip infection, postoperative	2
Transient third or sixth nerve palsy	3
Diabetis insipidus (usually transient)	22
Cribriform plate fracture	2
Maxillary fracture	2
Hepatitis	1
Total	49 (3.0%)

Table 27-5. Results of transsphenoidal surgery in patients with preoperative visual field defects[28,29]

Postoperative Vision	Patients (%)
Improved	81
Unchanged	13
Worse	6

REFERENCES

1. Cushing H: The Weir Mitchell Lecture: Surgical experience with pituitary disorders. JAMA 63:1515, 1914
2. Hirsch 0: Ueber Hypophysentumoren und deren Behandlung. Klin Monatsbl Augenheilkd 85:609, 1930
3. Dott NM, Bailey P: A consideration of the hypophyseal adenomata. Br J Surg 13:314, 1925
4. Guiot G: Transsphenoidal approach in surgical treatment of pituitary adenomas: General principles and indications in non-functioning adenomas. Excerpta Medica International Congress Series. No. 303, 1973, pp 159–178
5. Hardy J: Transsphenoidal microsurgery of the normal and pathological pituitary. Clin Neurosurg 16:185, 1969
6. Messick JM, Laws ER Jr, Abboud CF: Anesthesia for transsphenoidal surgery of the hypophyseal region. Anesth Analg 57:206, 1978
7. Kern EB, Laws ER Jr, Randall RV, et al: A transseptal, transsphenoidal approach to the pituitary. An old approach—a new technique in the management of pituitary tumors and related disorders. Trans Am Acad Ophthalmol Otolaryngol 84:997, 1977
8. Kern EB, Laws ER Jr, Randall RV, et al: A transseptal, transsphenoidal approach to the pituitary. Postgrad Med 63:97, 1978
9. Kern EB, Laws ER Jr: The transseptal approach to the pituitary gland. Rhinology 16:59, 1978
10. Kern EB, Pearson BW, McDonald TJ, et al: The transseptal approach to lesions of the pituitary and parasellar regions. Laryngoscope 89:1, 1979
11. Kern EB, Laws ER Jr, Randall RV: Transseptal, transsphenoidal pituitary surgery. Min Endocrinol 3:187, 1978
12. McDonald TJ, Kern EB, Laws ER Jr, Pearson BW: Surgical approaches to the pituitary gland with emphasis on the transseptal route. Head Neck Surg 1:498, 1979
13. Pearson BW, Kern EB, McDonald TJ, et al: Anatomical aspects of the transseptal approach to the sphenoid sinus, in Post KD, Jackson IMD, Reichlin S (eds): The Pituitary Adenoma. New York, Plenum Press, 1980, pp 365–377
14. Laws ER Jr: Transsphenoidal tumor surgery, for intrasellar pathology. Clin Neurosurg 26:391, 1979
15. Laws ER Jr, Randall RV, Kern EB, et al CF (eds): Management of Pituitary Adenomas and Related Lesions with Emphasis on Transsphenoidal Microsurgery. New York, Appleton-Century-Crofts, 1982
16. Zervas NT, Martin JB: Management of hormone-secreting pituitary adenomas. N Engl J Med 302:210, 1980
17. Ludecke DK, Saeger W, William T: Effectiveness of microsurgery in acromegaly. Study of 210 cases. Period Biol 85:59, 1983
18. Wilson CB: A decade of pituitary microsurgery. The Herebert Olivecrona Lecture. J Neurosurg 61:814, 1984
19. Laws ER Jr: Transsphenoidal microsurgery in the management of craniopharyngioma. J Neurosurg 52:661, 1980
20. Laws ER Jr, Piepgras DG, Randall RV, et al: Neurosurgical management of acromegaly—results in 82 patients treated between 1972 and 1977. J Neurosurg 50:454, 1979
21. Laws ER Jr: Transsphenoidal microsurgery in the management of acromegaly, in Smith JL (ed): Smith's Neuro-ophthalmology Focus. New York, Masson, 1980
22. Laws ER Jr, Randall RV, Abboud CF: Surgical treatment of acromegaly: Results in 140 patients, in Givens J (ed): Hormone-Secreting Pituitary Tumors. Chicago, Year Book, 1982, pp 225–228
23. Laws ER Jr, Onofrio BM, Pearson BW, et al: Successful management of bilateral carotid-cavernous sinus fistulae with a transsphenoidal approach. Neurosurgery 4:162, 1979
24. Laws ER Jr, Kern EB: Complications of transsphenoidal surgery. Clin Neurosurg 23:401, 1976
25. Laws ER Jr, Kern EB: Complications of transsphenoidal surgery, in Tindall GT, Collins WF (eds): Clinical Management of Pituitary Disorders. New York, Raven Press, 1979, pp 435–445
26. Laws ER Jr: Complications of transsphenoidal microsurgery for pituitary adenoma, in Brock M (ed): Modern Neurosurgery 1. Berlin, Springer-Verlag, 1982, pp 181–186
27. Laws ER Jr, Fode NC, Redmond MJ: Transsphenoidal surgery following unsuccessful prior therapy. J Neurosurg 63:823, 1985
28. Laws ER Jr, Trautmann JC, Hollenhorst RW Jr: Transsphenoidal decompression of the optic nerve and chiasm. J Neurosurg 46:717, 1977
29. Trautmann JC, Laws ER Jr: Visual status after transsphenoidal surgery at the Mayo Clinic, 1971–1982. Am J Ophthalmol 96:200, 1983

CHAPTER 28

Techniques of Reconstruction of the Sella and Related Structures

Renato Spaziante   Enrico de Divitiis   Paolo Cappabianca

THE TRANSSPHENOIDAL APPROACH to the sella turcica is influenced at each step of its execution by the specific regional anatomy through which it is carried out. Specifically, to rebuild the pituitary fossa and nasal and paranasal structures, traditional neurosurgical methods—obtaining hemostasis by coagulation of the operative site under direct visual control, suspending and suturing the dura mater, and fusing the bone flap—cannot be used. Alternative methods have been devised to deal with the transsphenoidal approach and will be discussed in this chapter.

GENERAL PRINCIPLES

The fundamental goals of reconstruction of the region of the sella are:

1. Hemostasis.
2. Reduction of intrasellar dead space.
3. Support for suprasellar structures (the diaphragma sellae, chiasmal cistern, optic structures, and third ventricle).
4. Prevention or arrest of cerebrospinal (CSF) leakage.
5. Reconstitution of the integrity of the sellar floor.

To satisfy these aims the sellar cavity must be adequately packed and the breech in the bone and dura in its floor sealed.

PACKING OF THE PITUITARY FOSSA

An intrasellar tumor often causes an increase in the size of the sella turcica. This can be barely perceptible in the case of a microadenoma or it can be huge in the case of some types of giant adenomas. During its development an intrasellar lesion first stretches and then causes atrophy or even the disappearance of the diaphragma sellae. This structure normally forms the roof of the pituitary fossa, dividing it from the cranial fossa, the chiasmal cistern, and the optic structures.

After a sellar tumor (or the normal pituitary in cases of hypophysectomy) is removed, a free space is formed within the sellar cavity (Figure 28-1). Because the walls of this space are potentially hemorrhagic unless obliterated, the space will tend to fill with blood. There is therefore the danger of intrasellar hematoma formation with a mass effect or of meningitis or an intrasellar abscess because of the communication of the sellar space with the sphenoidal sinus. When the pituitary fossa is not properly separated from the intracranial contents either because of congenital incompetence of the diaphragma sella or,

more commonly, because of its secondary atrophy, the pulsatile action of the brain can force the arachnoid of the chiasmal cistern downward toward the sellar floor; it then can involve the optic nerves and cause their downward displacement. In the most serious cases the third ventricle may herniate into the sellar cavity. The onset or worsening of a CSF fistula is markedly favored.[1]

To avoid these problems the free intrasellar space is obliterated by packing it with substances that will ensure hemostasis, provide both immediate and future support for the suprasellar structures, and create a barrier between the inside and the outside of the pituitary fossa (Figure 28-2). The substances that best fulfill these requirements are subcutaneous fat, fascia, or muscle, usually harvested from the thigh or the abdomen[2,3]; fragments of cartilage and bone from the nasal septum or the sphenoid[2]; reabsorbable materials such as fibrin sponge, oxidized cellulose hemostat, Gelfoam, or collagen[4,5]; and lyophilized dura mater.[3,6] These various substances can be used alone or in combination. Because they are commercially available, the prepared reabsorbable substances and lyophilized dura mater are the easiest to use and most frequently used, with bone-cartilage fragments being added where necessary. When the surgical situation requires the packing to be particularly effective, the best materials are muscle or subcutaneous fat, even though it takes time to procure them and they may be a source of contamination.[7] Fat is preferable to muscle because it undergoes less necrosis and less scar retraction that would result in a reduction in the volume of the packing. This could be a problem when the packing is insufficient or if an excessive amount of material needs to be inserted to compensate for later loss in volume.[8,9]

CLOSURE OF THE SELLAR FLOOR

Classically,[2] the pituitary fossa is reached by removing a 1 cm^2 segment of the floor of the sella, opening the dura in a cruciate fashion, and coagulating its edges for hemostasis and to provide wider access to the sella. The resulting defect, which now forms the floor of the sella, needs to be repaired, since it must support the materials that eventually will be used to fill the pituitary fossa and because it is the most effective barrier between the intrasellar and extrasellar spaces. Only rarely should the sellar floor be left open.

The simplest and most effective method of restoring the integrity of the sellar floor is to use a disc of cartilage or bone

OPERATIVE NEUROSURGICAL TECHNIQUES
ISBN 0-8089-1862-1

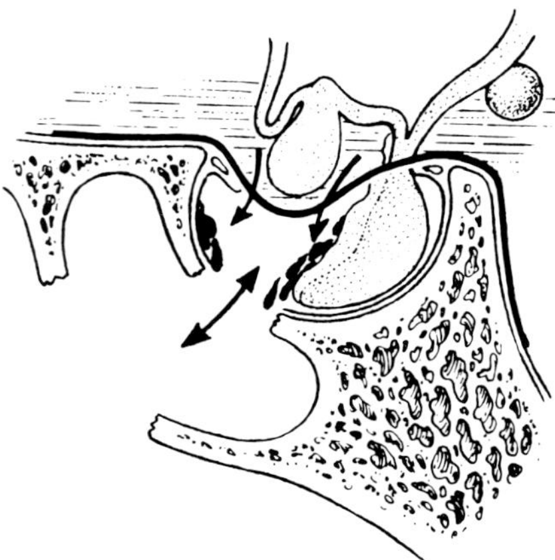

Fig. 28-1.　The conditions that frequently need to be corrected after removal of pituitary fossa lesions. The surgical site is bloody because of many small hemorrhages arising from the cut surface of the hypophysis and the dura mater covering the sellar floor and the cavernous sinuses. The suprasellar structures tend to be pushed toward the sellar floor because of the ineffectiveness of the sellar diaphragma. Preoperative adhesions, surgical damage, or downward distension of the chiasmal cistern favor the development of CSF leaks (upper arrows). Communication with the septic sphenoidal sinus may lead to contamination of the sellar cavity (double-faced arrow).

harvested from the nasal septum or paranasal structures during the initial stages of the surgical exposure.[2] This material is cut to the correct shape and size and inserted below the edges of the opening in the bone, in the epidural space, so that pressure from the dura mater will help maintain its position until healing provides a true union (Figure 28-3). Analogous results can be obtained with discs of lyophilized dura mater or fascia lata.[10] Prostheses of synthetic histoacrylic resin, ceramic, and lyophilized bone have also been used.[11–13] Furthermore, for fusion of the plug, whatever its nature, histoacrylic biologic glues or natural derivatives have been used.[3,14–16]

In cases in which the floor of the sella is paper thin, it can be opened by cutting two small lateral bone flaps, which can be

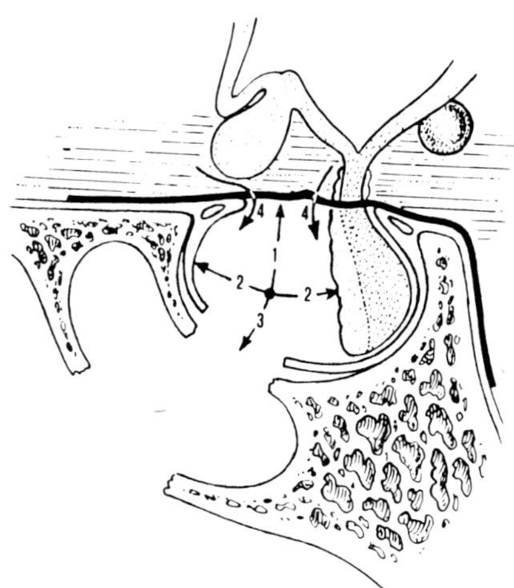

Fig. 28-2.　The basic problems at which packing of the pituitary fossa is aimed (in addition to reducing the amount of intrasellar dead space): (1) to support the diaphragma sellae, the chiasmal cistern, and the suprasellar structures; (2) to ensure hemostasis of the surgical bed by contact and light compression; (3) to seal the intrasellar space against external (sphenoidal) agents; and (4) to prevent or arrest CSF leaks.

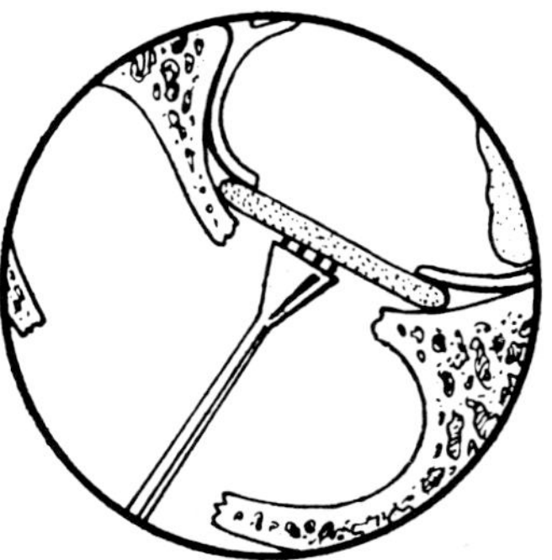

Fig. 28-3.　The sellar floor is usually easily closed by slipping a disc of cartilage or bone (or lyophilized dura mater or synthetic materials) into the extradural space. This disc generously overlaps the breech in the bone and in the dura on all sides.

turned to the side (Figure 28-4); when the floor is reconstructed the bone flaps are returned to their natural position and secured either by fixing them to each other and to the edges of the breech in the bone or by threading a strip of cartilage beneath the upper and lower margins of the hole in the bone, bridging the medial edge of the two juxtaposed bone flaps (Figure 28-5). Because the bone edges fit together perfectly and the periosteum has been preserved, the chances for physiologic union of the sella floor are improved.[17]

PACKING AND CLOSURE OF THE SPHENOIDAL SINUS

Packing is not universally accepted to be mechanically useful in closing the sphenoidal sinus,[18,19] but we use this technique to support the sellar floor when it is particularly stretched and inconsistent (''ghost'' sella) and to create a less septic postoperative environment by using reabsorbable substances soaked in an antibacterial solution.

The same materials are used as for packing the pituitary fossa. The simplest method is to use a fibrin or gelatin sponge soaked in antibiotic solution together with residual bone-cartilage fragments. The largest fragment can be used to approximately reconstruct the anterior wall of the sphenoidal sinus and separate it from the nasal fossa. Hermetic closure of the sphenoidal sinus by synthetic materials, bone cements, or resins does not prevent the mechanical complications mentioned above nor CSF leakage and adds the risks of foreign body reaction and chemical osteitis.[18,20] Moreover, it prohibits or greatly impedes reoperation by the transsphenoidal route, which may be necessary if, in spite of careful rebuilding of the sellar region, mechanical complications arise.

There are some conditions in which it may be useful to avoid any filling of the sphenoidal sinus. This is the case when hemostasis at the operative site is not adequate; a permeable sphenoidal sinus is an excellent way of draining blood that may collect in the pituitary fossa during the first hours after surgery. Likewise, not packing the pituitary fossa facilitates the spontaneous delivery of residual intrasellar and suprasellar tumor, e.g., hourglass adenoma or cystic craniopharyngioma in which only an intracapsular removal has been performed. In these cases a free sphenoidal sinus is absolutely necessary to allow further emptying of the sellar tumor.[10,21]

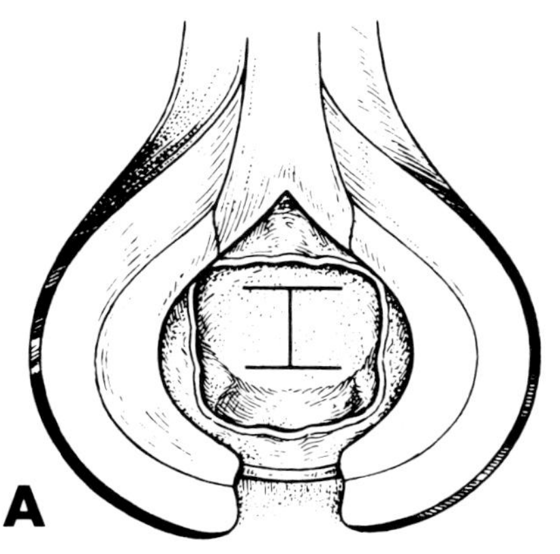

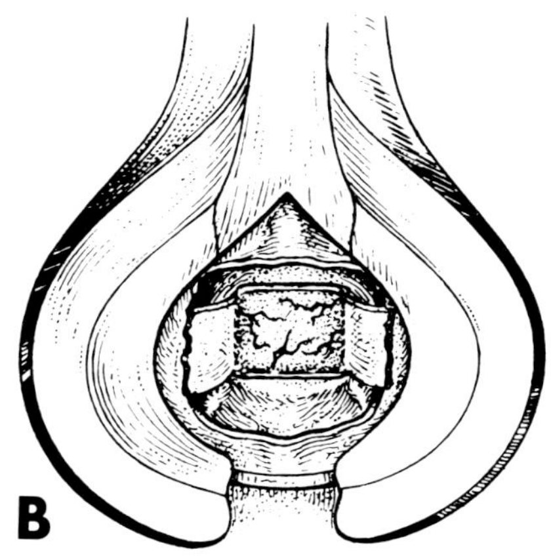

Fig. 28-4. (A) Lines along which the sellar floor can be cut if it has a paperlike consistency. (B) Two small flaps are reflected to the sides, parallel to the carotid artery grooves.

RECONSTRUCTION OF NASAL STRUCTURES

Reconstruction of nasal structures is usually limited to (nonobligatory) reapposition of the cartilage of the nasal septum where this has been removed or to returning the nasal septum to the midline in the case of a unilateral transseptal approach.[22] The two nostrils are filled with medicated, nonadhesive gauze. In the transnasal approach the columella is held by 3 or 4 sutures, of which one transfixes deeply. In the transoral route the gingival mucosa can be reapposed with a few stitches or can even be left open.

METHODS FOR RECONSTRUCTING THE PITUITARY FOSSA

The underlying lesion and conditions encountered during surgery will determine the manner in which the sellar region is reconstructed. Although the needs of the patient in each case at surgery will be the main guide, general criteria can be formulated for the principal methods possible.

SIMPLE INTRADURAL PACKING

Simple intradural packing is the fundamental method suggested in most classical descriptions of transsphenoidal surgery.[2] Materials for packing the sellar cavity are introduced into the intradural space and the plug that closes the floor is fixed into the epidural space (Figure 28-6). This is easily and rapidly performed and is the ideal solution when the empty space left at the end of the operation is no larger in size than the sella turcica.

This approach has two main limitations: the packing cannot be very tight, even when this is needed, because the pressure developing within the sella is transmitted to suprasellar and parasellar structures; and the packing material is not solidly adherent to the walls of the fossa and can move about.

ANCHORED INTRADURAL PACKING

To avoid the limitations of simple intradural packing, the packing material can be fixed to the floor of the sella so that it is more stable and offers a more complete closure.

There are two slightly different methods by which this can be accomplished; both are based on the same principles. The first consists of interposing the disc of cartilage used to close the sella between two muscle fragments that are larger in size than the hole in the sella.[23] One is placed intradurally, the other in the sphenoidal sinus (Figure 28-7A). A suture, which previously has been passed through the entire packet, is then tied, consolidating the mass and fixing it to the sellar floor so that it cannot move either into the sella nor outward. A later variant consists of interposing a large muscle fragment between two cartilage discs, one intradural and the other intrasphenoidal (Figure 28-7B).[24] A suture that previously has been passed through all the components is tightened and tied. As well as securely

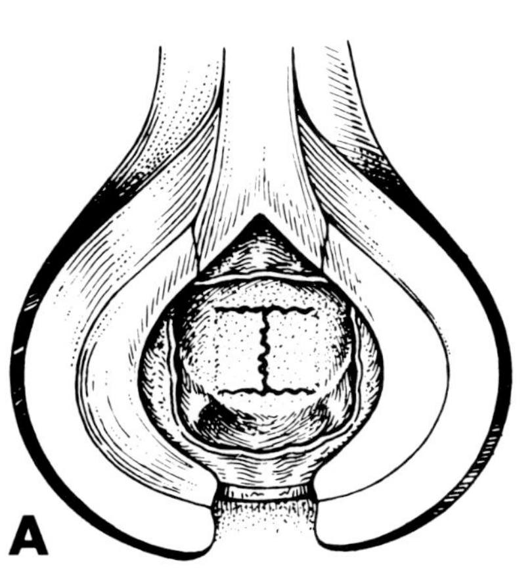

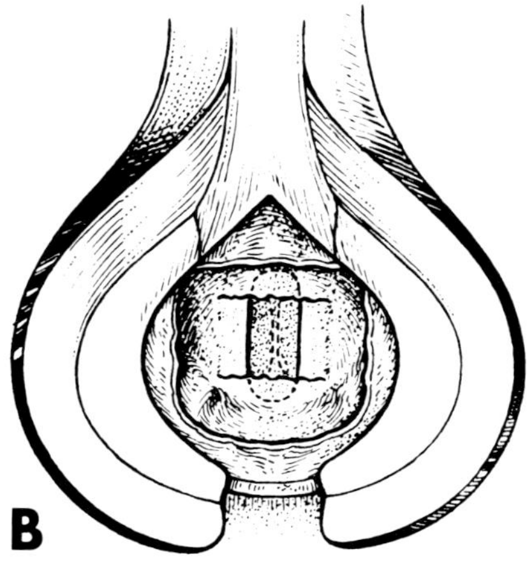

Fig. 28-5. To reconstruct the sellar floor after it is opened at noted in Figure 28-4, the bone flaps are returned to their natural position. They can be secured by fitting in them to each other and to the edges of the sellar opening (A). When this proves unreliable a strip of cartilage can be threaded beneath the edges of the hole in the bone bridging the medial edge of the two juxtaposed bone flaps (B).

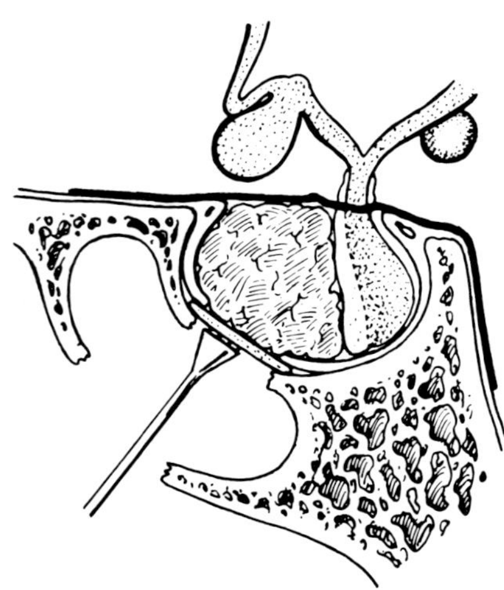

Fig. 28-6. Simple intradural packing. The packing materials are inserted intradurally, completely filling the intrasellar space. A disc of cartilage or similar material is fitted extradurally to close the sellar floor. (Reprinted from Spaziante R, De Divitiis E, Cappabianca P: Reconstruction of the pituitary fossa in transsphenoidal surgery: An experience of 140 cases. Neurosurgery 17:453, 1985. With permission.)

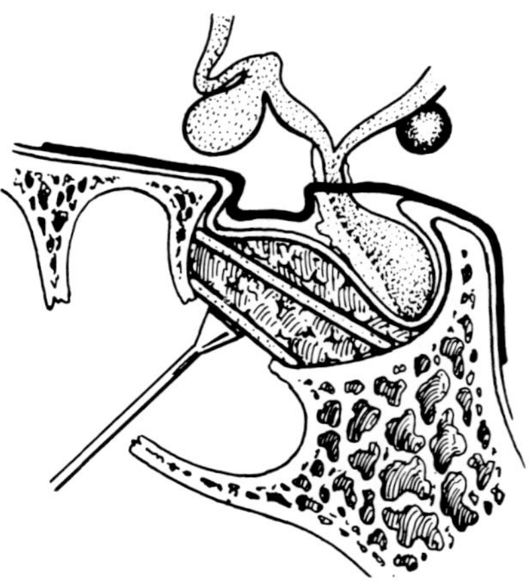

Fig. 28-8. Extradural packing. Intradural free-space is markedly reduced by detaching the dura mater from the sellar floor. The extradural space is filled with the usual materials interposed between the two cartilage discs, the larger one in contact with the dura mater, the other closing the hole in the sella. (Reprinted from Spaziante R, De Divitiis E, Cappabianca P: Reconstruction of the pituitary fossa in transsphenoidal surgery: An experience of 140 cases. Neurosurgery 17:453, 1985. With permission.)

anchoring the packing to the sellar floor, the ligature pushes the muscle centrifugally, thus filling the lateral recesses of the pituitary fossa and providing better hemostasis of the wall of the cavernous sinus.

EXTRADURAL PACKING

The dura covering the sellar floor can easily be detached from the floor and elevated as far as the insertion to the cavernous sinus, of which it forms the medial wall, prevents further elevation. The wide space thus obtained then can be packed with the same materials as mentioned above (Figure 28-8), which are interposed between two large bone-cartilage discs, one corresponding to the dural hole, the other to the breech in the bone.[25,26,27]

This type of packing can be particularly tight and hermetic because the elastic forces produced by distending the dura mater make it more compact and stable. Furthermore, there is no risk of introducing an excessive amount of packing material because the dura cannot be interrupted nor elevated beyond the limits imposed by its own elasticity (unless exceptionally violent

maneuvers are used). There thus is no risk of excessive pressure being transmitted to perisellar structures (Figure 28-9).

COMBINED EXTRADURAL-INTRADURAL PACKING

Extradural packing is advantageous from many points of view; it does not allow a particularly large residual cavity to be packed completely, however, because there is a limit to the degree of dural movement at the sellar floor. In this situation the ideal solution is to make part of the packing intradural (producing volume) and part extradural (providing stability, solidity, and watertight closure) (Figure 28-10).

PACKING IN THE CASE OF CSF LEAKAGE

The method of sellar reconstruction for repair of a CSF leak must be meticulous because such a leak can create serious postoperative problems.[28–30] A strip of fascia lata or lyophilized dura is placed to protect the arachnoid and the diaphragma sellae; the sellar cavity is then partially filled with muscle or subcutaneous fat inserted into the intradural space. A second

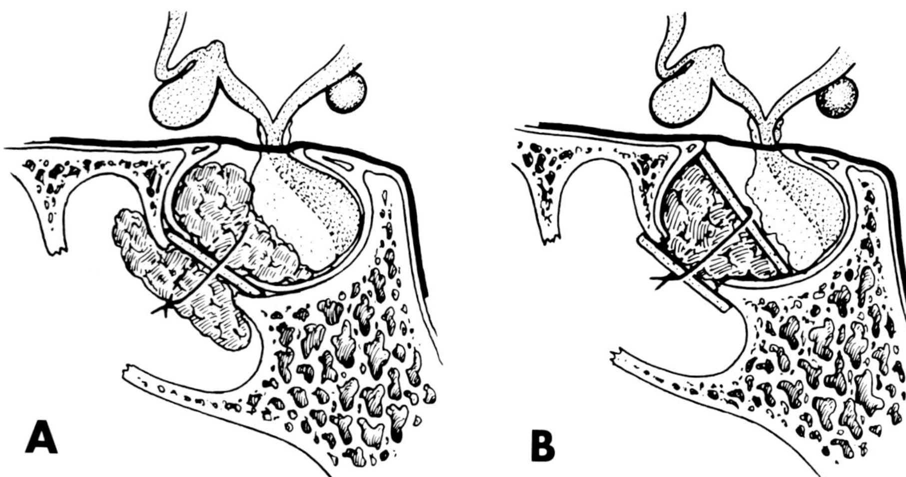

Fig. 28-7. Anchored intradural packing. (A) The disc of cartilage closing the sellar floor is interposed between two large muscle fragments, one inside and the other outside the sella. By tying a suture previously passed through them, the mass is consolidated and firmly fastened to the sella. (B) Two cartilage discs, one intradural and the other intrasphenoidal, sandwich a large muscle fragment and close the breech in the sella. The packet is solidly anchored by tightening a suture previously passed through the discs and muscles; in addition, the muscle splits laterally, filling the lateral recesses of the sellar cavity. (Reprinted from Spaziante R, de Divitiis E, Cappabianca P: Reconstruction of the pituitary fossa in transsphenoidal surgery: An experience of 140 cases. Neurosurgery 17:453, 1985. With permission.)

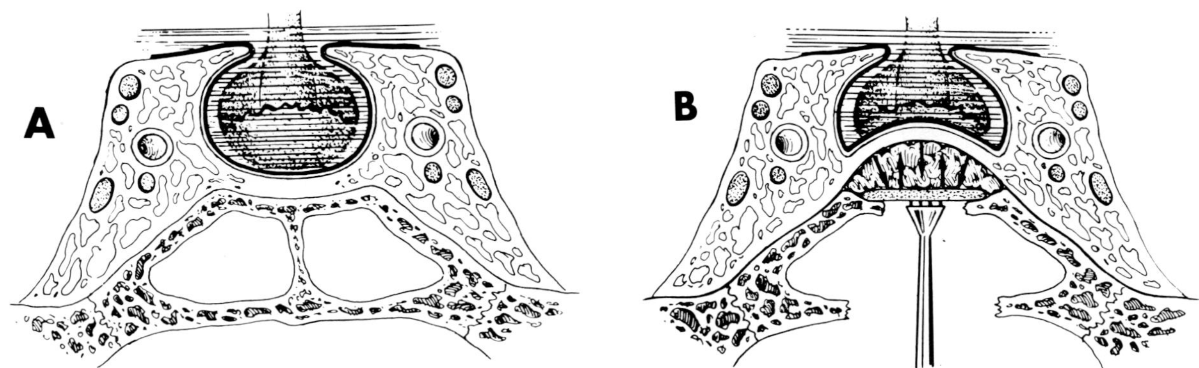

Fig. 28-9. Crossection of the pituitary fossa along a coronal plane (A) before and (B) after extradural packing. The dura mater of the sellar floor is joined to the walls of the cavernous sinuses. When it is detached from the floor and pushed upward, its distension creates elastic forces that compress the packing materials. The risk of overpacking is avoided because the dura cannot be elevated to an unlimited degree; increased pressure inside the packed space is not transmitted to suprasellar and perisellar structures. (Reprinted from Spaziante R, De Divitiis E, Cappabianca P: Reconstruction of the pituitary fossa in transsphenoidal surgery: An experience of 140 cases. Neurosurgery 17:453, 1985. With permission.)

strip of fascia or lyophilized dura is used on the inner surface of the dura mater to close it.[2,3,5,20,26,31] A particularly precise extradural packing then is performed (Figures 28-11 and 28-12).

INDICATIONS IN RELATION TO THE MOST FREQUENT SELLAR DISEASES

There are a number of factors that determine the technique used to reconstruct the pituitary fossa. The possibilities range from situations in which no packing or reconstruction of the sellar walls is necessary to those in which they must be performed with obsessive precision. Although it is extremely difficult to indicate absolute rules for every case, we will indicate those approaches we have found to be most frequently useful and adaptable to a variety of situations.

PITUITARY MICROADENOMA

The size and topographic relationships of pituitary microadenomas mean that there is hardly ever any need to pack the residual cavity after their removal. Hemostasis usually occurs

within a few minutes of the removal of the lesion. Suprasellar structures are not involved by the adenoma and are supported naturally (Figure 28-13). Reconstruction of the sellar floor with a cartilaginous plug fixed in the epidural space is useful in separating the pituitary fossa from the sphenoidal sinus (Figure 28-14). Two situations, however, may require effective packing: (1) extension of the microadenoma toward the cavernous sinus with persistent hemorrhage after its removal[32]; and (2) a co-existing spontaneous or intraoperatively formed intrasellar arachnoidocele, which rarely occurs. In the infrequent event of CSF leakage the provisions already outlined would have to be implemented.

INTRASELLAR ADENOMAS

In cases of intrasellar adenomas (adenomas confined to the sella or slightly indenting the chiasmal cistern), the sellar cavity is wider than normal and can be very large (e.g., in the case of giant adenomas developing downward). The diaphragma sellae is usually atrophied as a result of pressure from the adenoma; nonetheless, suprasellar structures (the cisterns and optic pathways) are virtually unaffected by the growth of the adenoma. Packing the cavity is useful both in ensuring hemostasis of the

Fig. 28-10. Combined extradural-intradural packing. The free space within the pituitary fossa is partly filled intradurally; extradural packing, as mentioned above, is performed afterward. (Reprinted from Spaziante R, De Divitiis E, Cappabianca P: Reconstruction of the pituitary fossa in transsphenoidal surgery: An experience of 140 cases. Neurosurgery 17:453, 1985. With permission.)

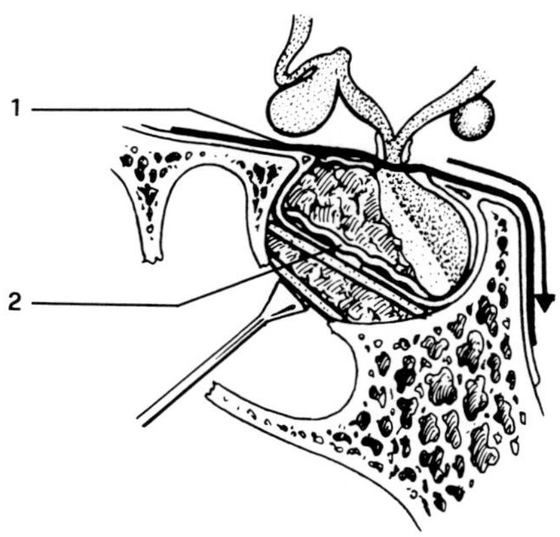

Fig. 28-11. General rules for packing to treat CSF leakage. The first strip of fascia lata or lyophilized dura mater reinforces the diaphragma sellae and arachnoid of the chiasmal cistern (1). Partial intradural packing is performed and the dura mater of the sellar floor is closed and reinforced with a second strip of fascia or lyophilized dura (2). Reconstruction of the sella is completed by extradural packing. The arrow running along the dorsum sellae demonstrates the usefulness of continuous spinal lumbar drainage during the operation and for the first few postoperative days.

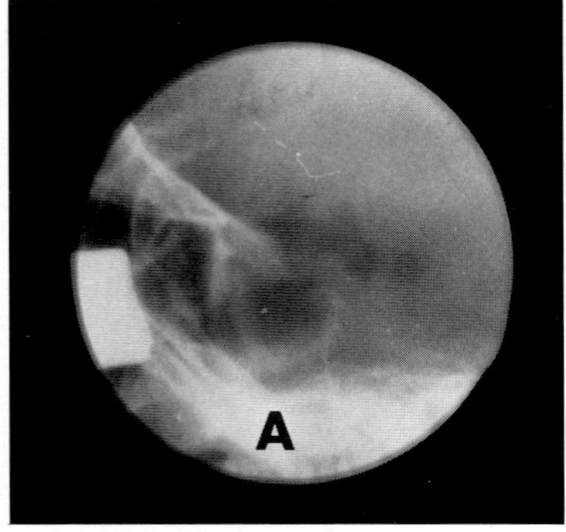
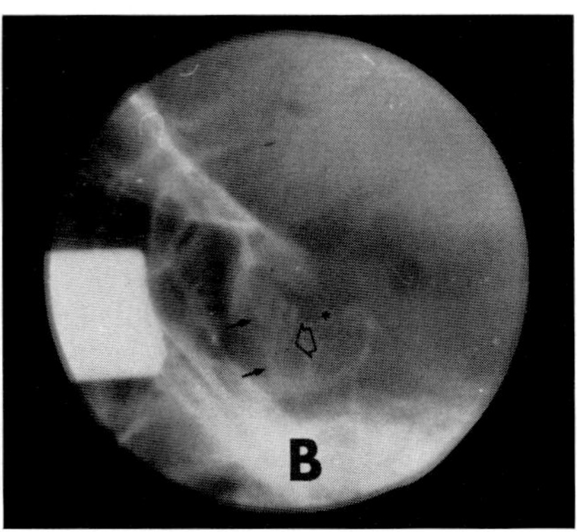

Fig. 28-12. Intraoperative fluoroscopic image. (A) Intraoperative CSF leakage after complete removal of a pituitary tumor with intrasellar and suprasellar extensions is clearly demonstrated by spontaneous entrance of air into the suprasellar cistern. (B) Combined extradural-intradural packing of the sellar cavity. The first strip of lyophilized dura (not visible and indicated by the asterisk) reinforces the arachnoid. A second strip of lyophilized dura marked with iodinated contrast medium reinforces the dura mater of the sellar floor (open arrow). The packing is completed extradurally (arrows).

large cavity and in supporting the suprasellar structures, which could otherwise herniate downward and cause immediate or delayed onset of the empty sella syndrome. Since there is much downward distension of the dura of the sella (Figure 28-15), extradural packing can be very easy and efficacious and does not carry the risk of overpacking (Figure 28-16). If intradural packing is used, its upward extent must be checked fluoroscopically (Figure 28-17) to ensure that the packing does not extend above the interclinoid plane.[3,5]

ADENOMA WITH LARGE SUPRASELLAR EXTENSION

After a large tumor with suprasellar extension is removed, the residual cavity is very large and most of it is not beyond direct visual examination. The diaphragma sellae is incompetent and there is compression, stretching, and adherence of the dome of the adenoma to suprasellar and cerebral structures; in some places adenomatous tissue may reach beyond the capsule. The sella turcica is larger than normal although its volume is not always proportionate to the overall volume of the adenoma. In these situations mechanical complications can arise because of hemorrhage and hematoma formation in relation to the size and

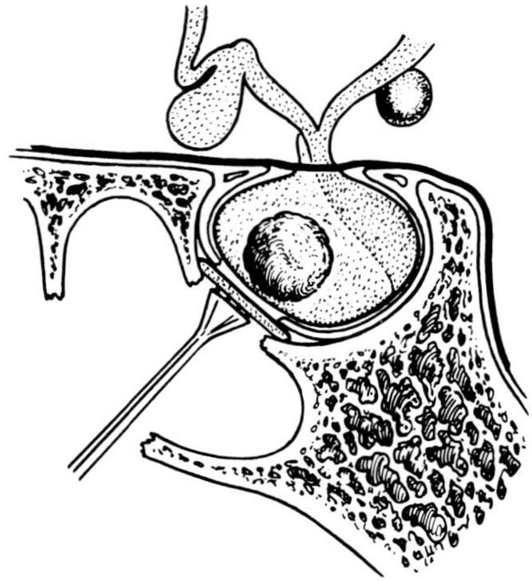

Fig. 28-13. After removal of a microadenoma there is usually no need to fill the sellar cavity because of the relationships between the residual cavity and the surrounding anatomic structures. However, plugging the sellar floor with a cartilage disc fitted extradurally may be advisable to restore the sellar wall.

vascularity of the incised surface; an empty sella can develop because of descent of the previously stretched chiasmal cistern into a large residual sellar cavity, which also pulls with it the optic nerves and, in the most severe cases, the anterior part of the third ventricle; or CSF leakage can develop because of accidental rupture of the chiasmatic cistern during surgery as a result of excessive stretching postoperatively or interruption of its continuity by the adenoma.

Adequately packing this space can be a difficult problem. To fill the cavity completely (Figure 28-18) would create the same conditions as those caused by the adenoma.[10,15,33] To prevent overpacking, it must be strictly limited to the intrasellar space and beneath the interclinoid plane. Such packing, which is disproportionate to the volume of the residual cavity, risks being mobile and thus ineffective. These difficulties can be greatly reduced after the adenoma has been removed by returning the chiasmal cistern to its natural position. This can be spontaneous (58 percent of cases according to Nakane et al.[34]) or it can be effected (20 percent of cases[34]) by introducing either a small amount of air or Ringer's solution into the subarachnoid space via a lumbar catheter (peroperative pneumoencephalography (PEG) or by compressing the jugular vein in the neck for a few seconds (Figure 28-19). The capsule of the adenoma then returns to the sellar cavity. Adhesions to structures above it usually are modest and not tenacious and the situation becomes analogous to that of an intrasellar adenoma, although it must be remembered that the diaphragma sellae is completely incompetent. If the capsule remains raised, however (Figure 28-20), packing will be necessary, both to correct this situation and also to prevent the probability that at some point in time the dome of the adenoma will invert its curve and descend into the sellar cavity.[15,25,35] It is then best to perform anchored intradural packing or mixed intradural-extradural packing (Figure 28-21).[36] In the same way one must check during the operation to see if the capsule spontaneously descends into the sellar cavity (Figures 28-22 and 28-23). Special consideration must be given to cases of hourglass adenoma in which removal of the suprasellar portion is inevitably incomplete. To encourage descent into the sellar cavity of the residual suprasellar portion with a view to further surgery or radiotherapy or to obtain better optic decompression, it may be useful not to do any packing nor to close the floor, but simply to sterilize the sphenoidal sinus.[10,21] Although there are risks attached to it, this approach may prove to be the most advantageous.

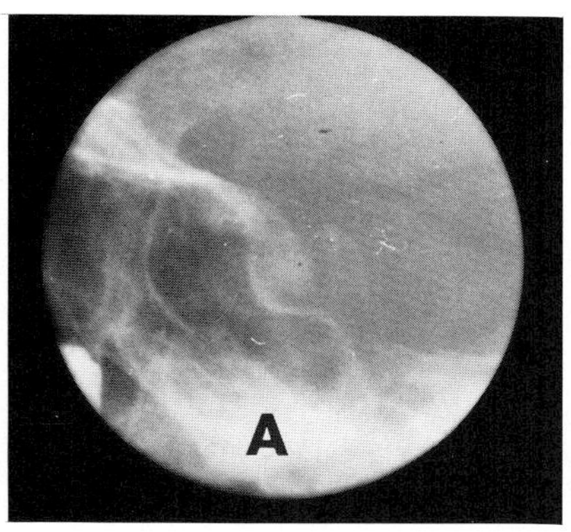 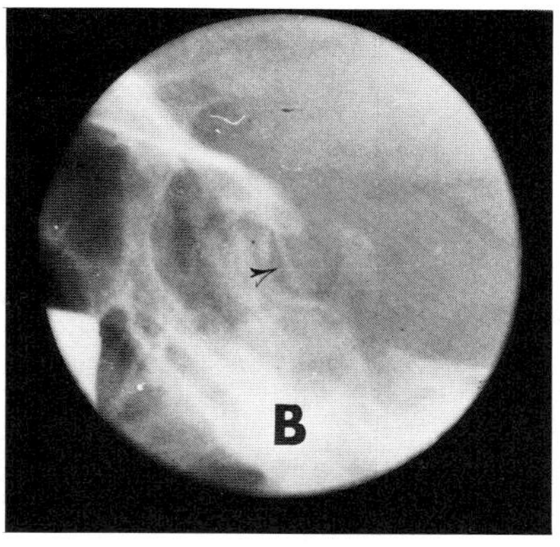

Fig. 28-14. Intraoperative fluoroscopic image. (A) The residual cavity filled with a sponge soaked in iodinated contrast medium after removal of a microadenoma. (B) An extradural cartilage disc (arrowhead) closes the sellar floor and reduces the intradural free space.

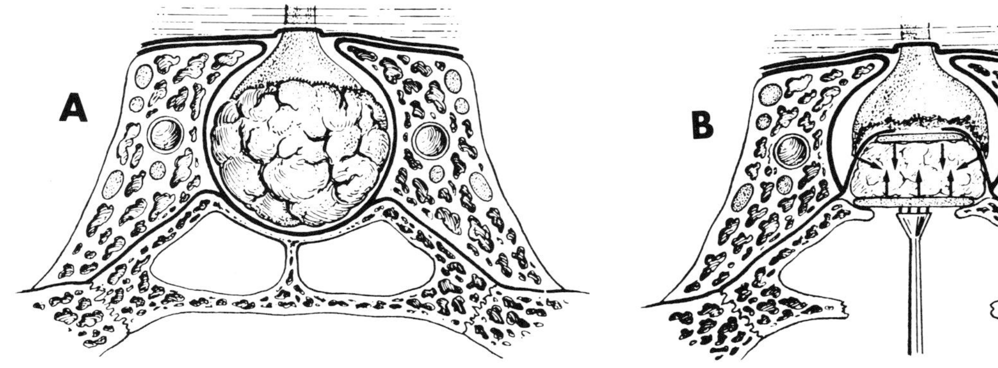

Fig. 28-15. Crossection of the pituitary fossa along a coronal plane (A) before and (B) after removal of a large intrasellar adenoma followed by extradural packing of the residual cavity. Because the dura mater of the sellar floor has been markedly distended it can be detached very easily and extensively raised before the walls of the cavernous sinus are tightened. Almost the entire intrasellar residual cavity can be filled in this way.

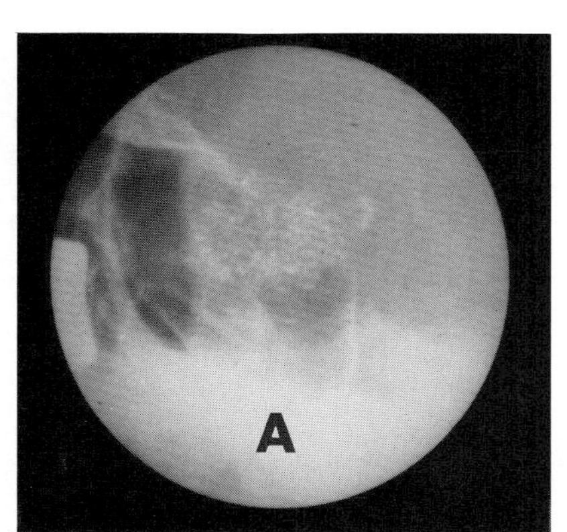 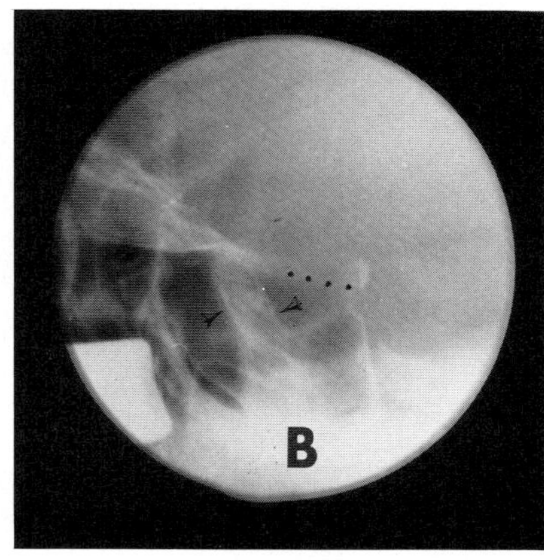

Fig. 28-16. Intraoperative fluoroscopic image. (A) The residual cavity after removal of a large intrasellar adenoma is visualized by a radiopaque cottonoid. (B) The outside and inside limits of extradural packing (open arrowheads). The correct position of the diaphragma sellae is outlined by the air bubble remaining within the pituitary fossa (dotted line).

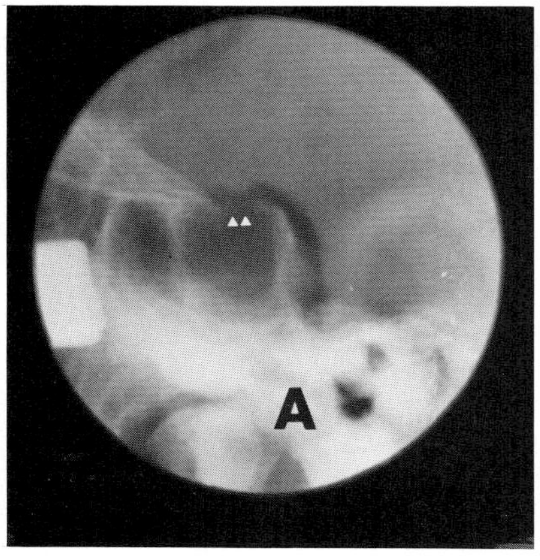 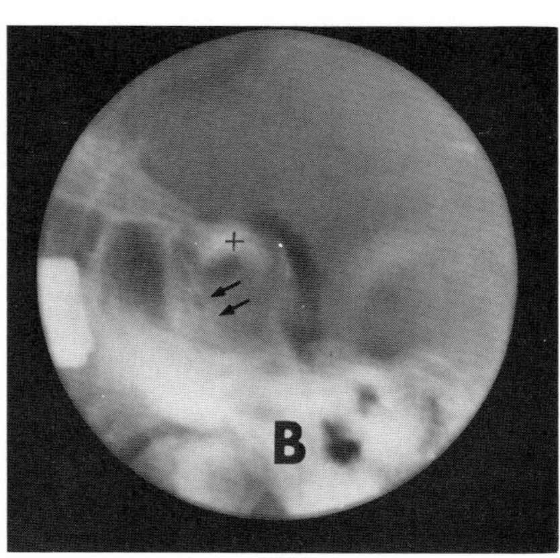

Fig. 28-17. Intraoperative fluoroscopic image of the removal of a large intrasellar adenoma. (A) The diaphragma sellae (white arrowheads) is outlined by an air bubble within the pituitary fossa, while the chiasmal cistern is visualized by means of peroperative pneumoencephalography (PEG). (B) Intradural filling of the defect with reabsorbable materials, the upper limit of which is marked with a sponge soaked in iodinated contrast medium (cross). The sellar floor is closed with numerous bone and cartilage fragments that have been inserted extradurally (arrows).

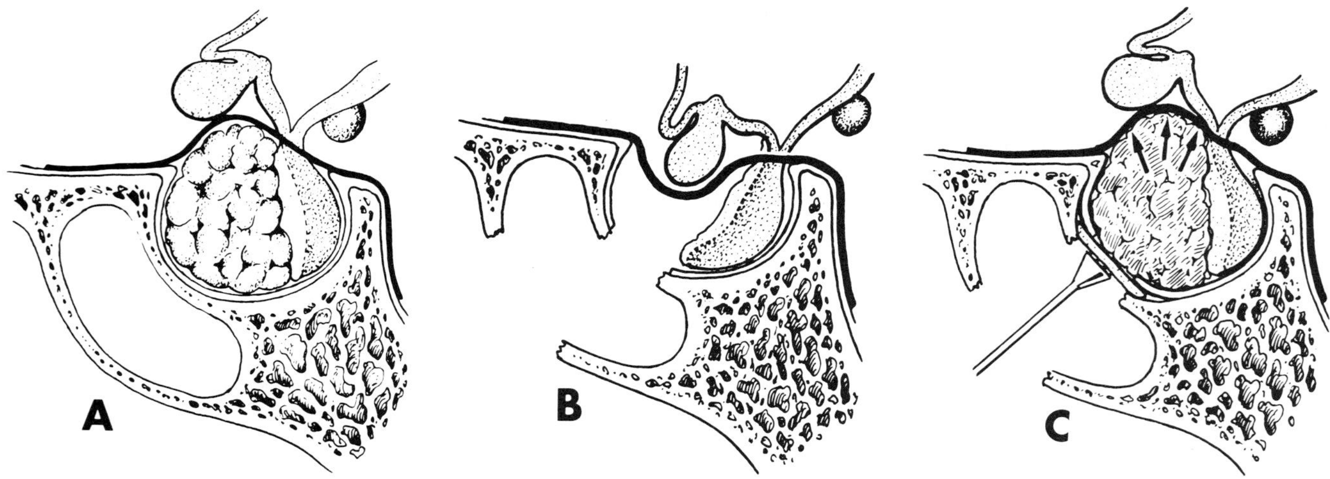

Fig. 28-18. After removal of an adenoma with suprasellar extension (A) there are many features that predispose the patient to postoperative mechanical complications such as empty sella syndrome, CSF rhinorrhea, and hemorrhage. (B) An effective intradural tamponade carries the risk of being too tight, causing compression of the suprasellar structures similar to that produced by the growth of the adenoma (C). (Reprinted from Spaziante R, De Divitiis E, Cappabianca P: Reconstruction of the pituitary fossa in transsphenoidal surgery: An experience of 140 cases. Neurosurgery 17:453, 1985. With permission.)

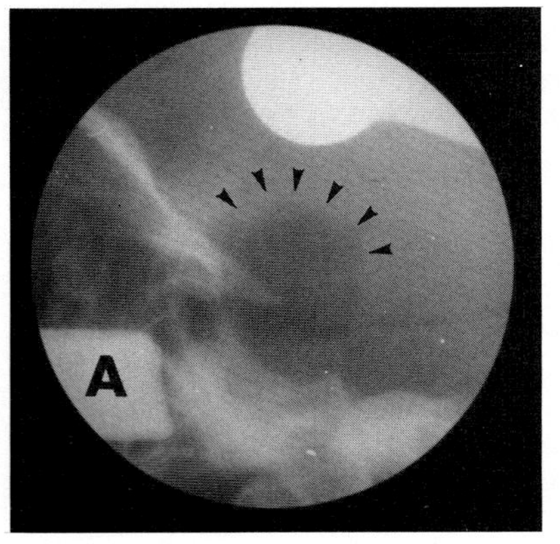

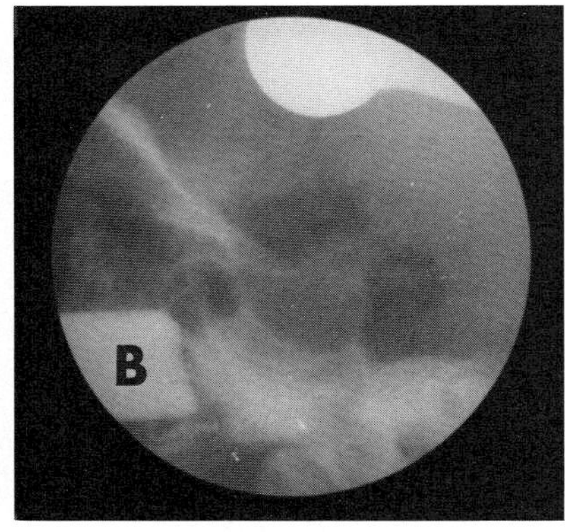

Fig. 28-19. Intraoperative fluoroscopic image. (A) Following removal of an adenoma with an extensive suprasellar extension the dome of the tumor remains raised (arrowheads). (B) Injection of fractionated amounts of air through a lumbar spinal catheter pushed it downward, refilling the chiasmal cistern and dissecting the loose adhesions from surrounding structures.

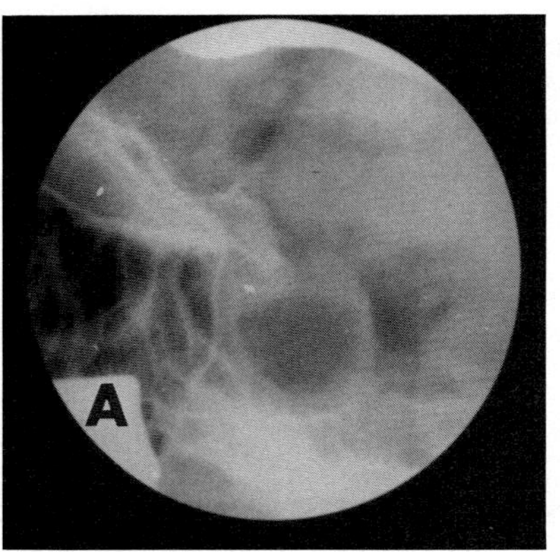

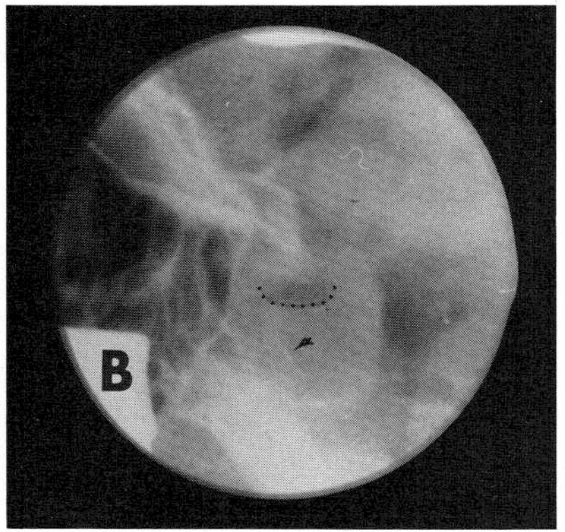

Fig. 28-20. Intraoperative fluoroscopic image. (A) After complete removal of an adenoma with suprasellar extension its dome collapsed as demonstrated by peroperative PEG. (B) Combined intradural-extradural packing. The upper limit beneath the interclinoid plane is outlined by an air bubble remaining inside the pituitary fossa (dotted line). The arrowhead points out the bone disc that constitutes the inner surface of the extradural packing.

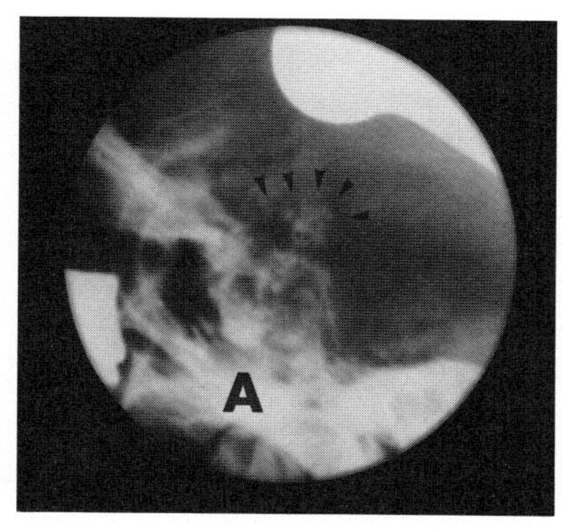
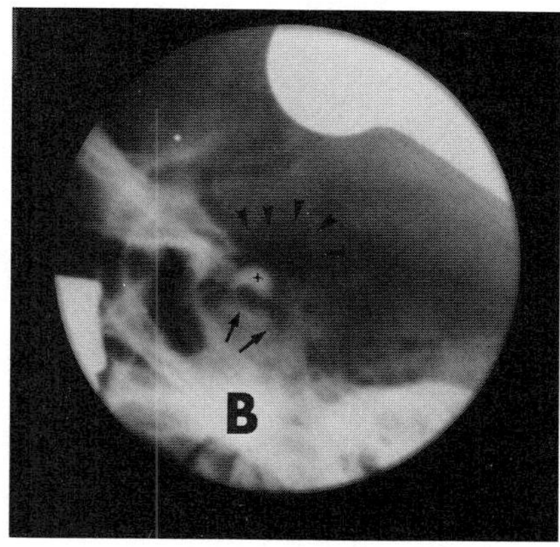

Fig. 28-21. Intraoperative fluoroscopic image. (A) Adenoma with suprasellar extension (arrowheads) visualized by diluted water-soluble nonionic contrast medium that was injected into it before the dura mater was opened. (B) The dome of the tumor (arrowheads) failed to descend despite repeated maneuvers to collapse it. A proper tamponade was achieved by combined intradural (the upper limit is marked with a sponge soaked in iodinated contrast medium +) and for the most part extradural packing (arrows).

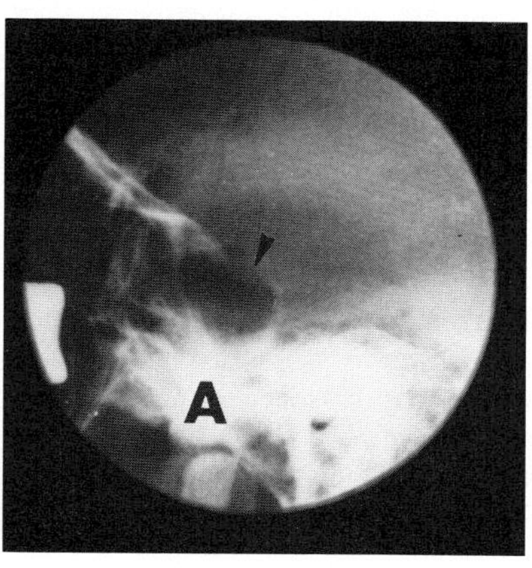
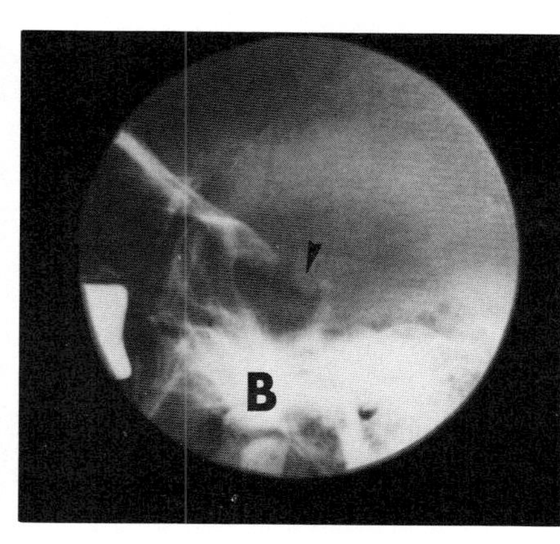
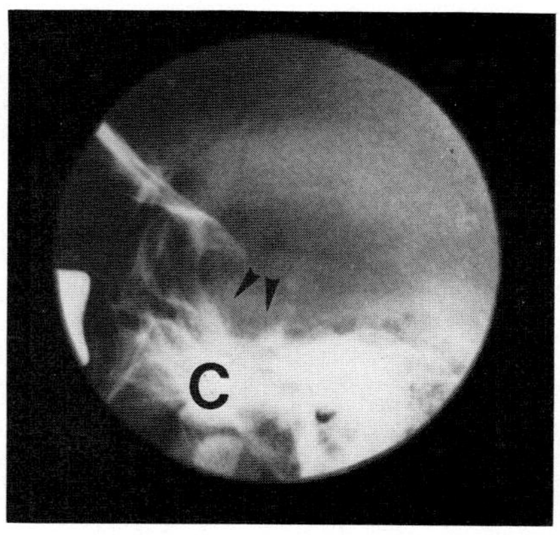

Fig. 28-22. Intraoperative fluoroscopic image. After complete removal of a pituitary cystic tumor with extensive suprasellar extension, the dome of the tumor (arrowhead) spontaneously returned to the interclinoid plane (A). Afterward it appeared in the sellar cavity (B) and soon after it descended deep toward the sellar floor (C).

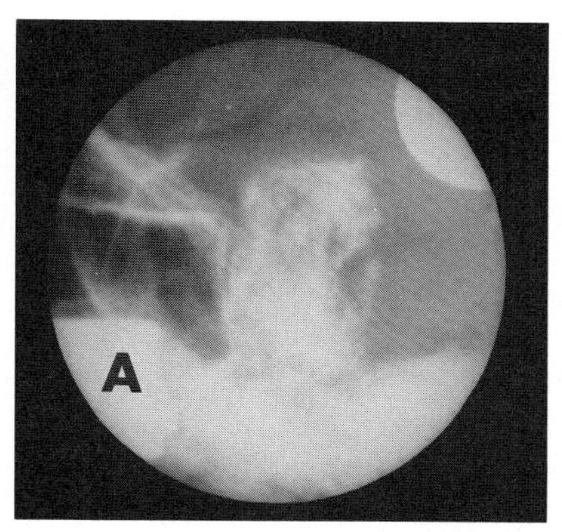
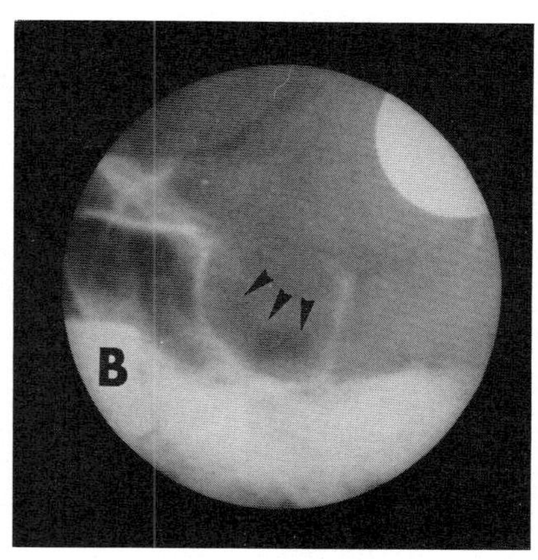

Fig. 28-23. Intraoperative fluoroscopic image. (A) A pituitary adenoma with suprasellar extension visualized by diluted water-soluble nonionic contrast medium that was injected into it before the dura mater was opened. (B) After removal of the adenoma, the diaphragma sellae spontaneously descended deep into the sellar cavity (arrowheads). (Reprinted from Spaziante R, De Divitiis E, Cappabianca P: Reconstruction of the pituitary fossa in transsphenoidal surgery: An experience of 140 cases. Neurosurgery 17:453, 1985. With permission.)

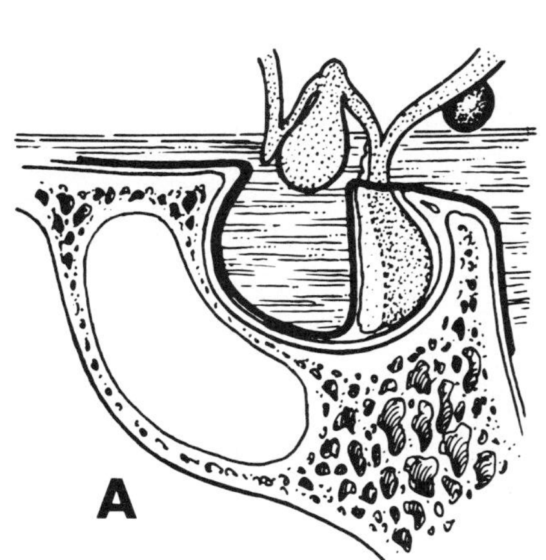
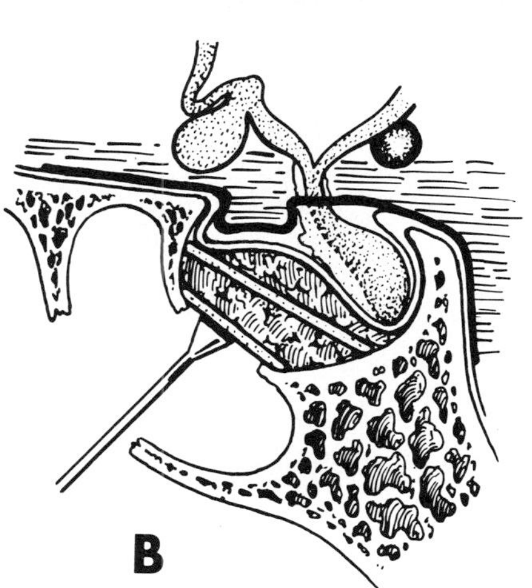

Fig. 28-24. (A) The most suitable method for achieving the primary goals of the surgical treatment of a pure empty sella (reduction of arachnoidocele, chiasmapexy, protection of the pituitary gland and sellar floor against pulsatile action of CSF, and prevention of CSF leakage) is extradural packing (B). Besides being very stable and well proportioned, it does not carry the risk of intrasellar and suprasellar structures being damaged by the surgical maneuvers.

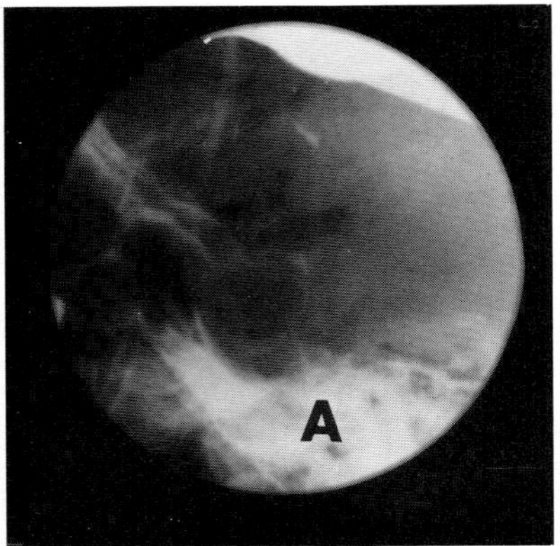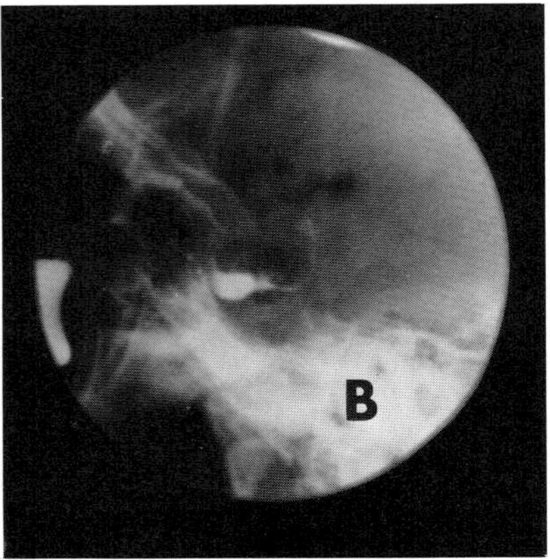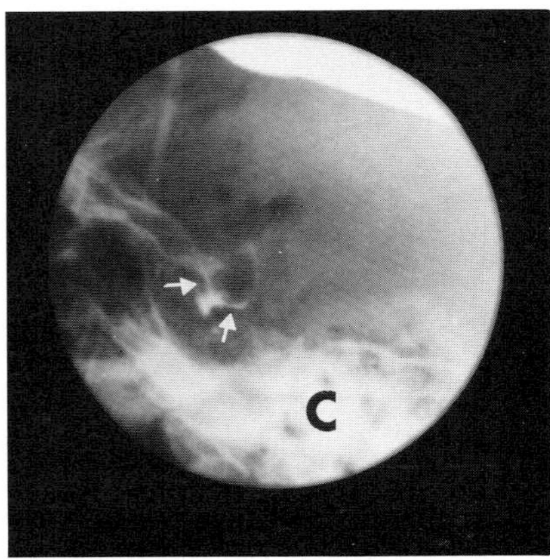

Fig. 28-25.   Intraoperative fluoroscopic image. (A) An empty sella visualized by peroperative PEG. (B) A small amount of nonionic water-soluble contrast medium was injected through a thin needle into the dura mater within the arachnoid pouch to mark its bottom. (C) The sellar cavity was packed extradurally, raising the arachnoid diverticulum and delineating the pituitary gland (white arrows).

EMPTY SELLA

A pituitary adenoma often may be accompanied by an intrasellar arachnoidocele as a consequence of spontaneous necrosis or previous treatment.[1] During removal of the adenomatous tissue the arachnoid must be protected and elevated and put back in its natural position,[2,5] to avoid risk of CSF leakage and to prevent the serious complications that an empty sella can provoke with time.[26,37] Packing must be of sufficient volume, consistency, and stability to avoid recurrence of an empty sella. Extradural mixed packing is probably the best type of repair in this situation since the arachnoid is protected with a strip of lyophilized dura before being very carefully elevated.[36]

Correction of a pure empty sella presents different problems. The aims of such an operation are to elevate the chiasmatic cistern and optic structures; to prevent progressive stretching and erosion of the sellar floor (involving dura and bone) as a result of transmission by the CSF of the pulsatile action of the brain; to prevent compression and distortion of the pituitary and its stalk, repositioning them in an anatomic position; to prevent (or arrest) CSF leakage; and to prevent late recurrence.[1,30,38] The packing in this situation must be well-proportioned, carried out with minimal trauma, and very stable. The ideal is an extradural repair (Figure 28-24).[27,38] Elevation of the dura mater will markedly reduce the space within the sella; intrasellar and suprasellar structures are lifted without being damaged by the surgical maneuvers since the arachnoid pocket protects them; the sellar floor is protected against cerebral pulsation. The best packing material for this purpose is either subcutaneous fat or bone-cartilage fragments, which will not undergo much necrosis or retraction with time so that the initial volume will not excessively decrease later. Peroperative PEG fluoroscopic visualization of the chiasmal cistern and of the intrasellar diverticulum during the entire procedure (Figure 28-25) is almost indispensible.[8]

GHOST SELLA

Ghost sella is a special problem because the large size of the sella and the flimsiness of the floor may prevent efficient performance of any of the methods of repair described.[36] This occurs very rarely, but when it is encountered it may be necessary to resort to intradural packing (Figure 28-26), com-

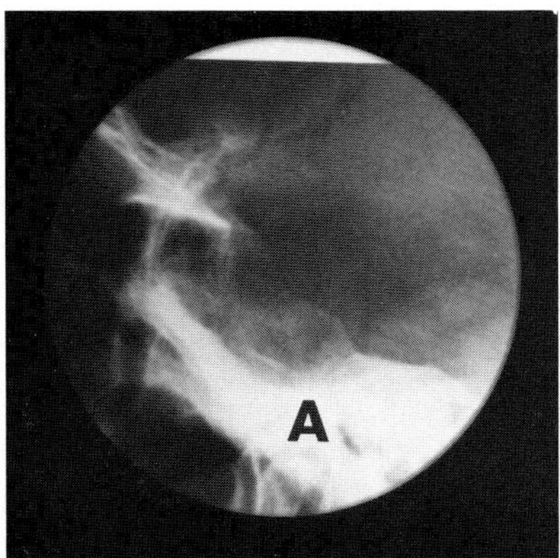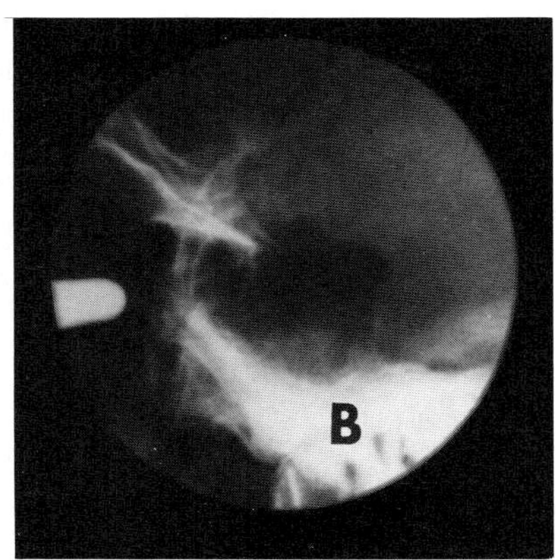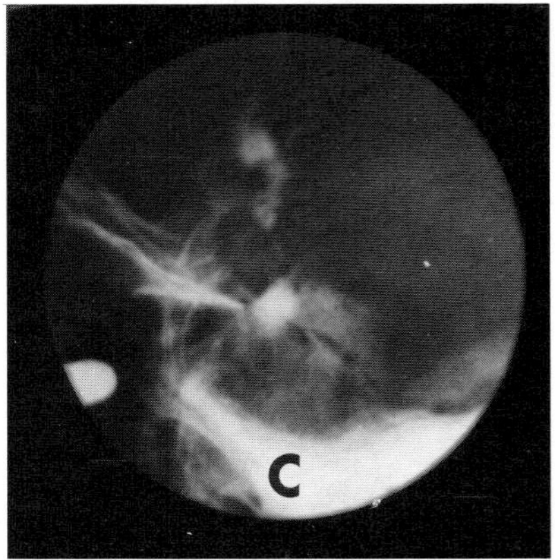

Fig. 28-26.   Intraoperative fluoroscopic image. (A) A giant pituitary adenoma with extensive suprasellar extension. The sella turcica has completely disappeared. (B) The residual cavity after removal of the tumor spontaneously filled with air. (C) Widespread intradural packing with fat lightly soaked in water-soluble nonionic iodinated contrast medium to avoid the risk of overpacking. Some contrast has escaped into the cisternal spaces through an apparently spontaneous disruption of the subarachnoid layer. (Preoperatively the patient complained of a spontaneous intratumoral hemorrhage).

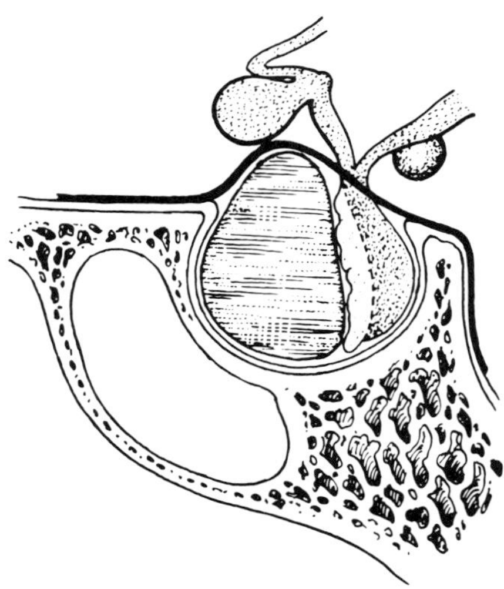

Fig. 28-27. An intrasellar and suprasellar arachnoid cyst. The anatomic conditions are similar to those of an adenoma with suprasellar extension (see also Figure 28–18). Even if emptying is surgically more favorable, the structural characteristics of the cyst wall and its relationship with CSF pathways may favor the development of postoperative mechanical complications.

bined with packing of the sphenoidal sinus with muscle, fat, and bone-cartilage fragments.[26,31]

OTHER SELLAR LESIONS

Other lesions more rarely approached by the transsphenoidal route (craniopharyngiomas, arachnoid cysts, dermoid cysts, chondromas, metastases) involve similar intraoperative factors to those of the more common conditions and can be treated in an analogous manner.

Arachnoidal cysts have both intrasellar and suprasellar

growth and features similar to those of pituitary adenomas with suprasellar extension (Figure 28-27); however, their walls do not readily heal solidly postoperatively and they can communicate through a unidirectional valve mechanism with the subarachnoid space, favoring the entry and accumulation of CSF under pressure and the subsequent development of CSF rhinorrhea.[39] Postoperative mechanical complications are therefore more frequent.[40]

In the case of removal of a cystic craniopharyngioma that is restricted to emptying the tumor cyst without completely removing the capsule (provided there is no evident communication with the cerebral space nor passage of CSF across the tumor wall), it may prove useful not to attempt a hermetic closure of the sellar floor. Instead, the cyst cavity should be allowed to communicate with the sphenoidal sinus to improve drainage of the contents of the cyst and avoid its recurrence (Figure 28-28).[41]

FUNCTIONAL HYPOPHYSECTOMY

The residual cavity is small after functional hypophysectomy and its reconstruction may be unnecessary. There are two exceptions to this rule: when there is diffuse hemorrhage caused by the wide dissection surface of the gland or when there is CSF leakage caused by section of the pituitary stalk in total hypophysectomy (Figure 28-29). This problem arises in about 11 percent of cases.[42] In view of the satisfactory condition of the diaphragma sellae, intradural packing and closure of the sellar floor constitute an adequate repair.[2,26]

CSF RHONORRHEA

Frequently but not exclusively a nontraumatic CSF rhinorrhea occurs as the consequence of the development of an empty sella or a pituitary adenoma. This is perhaps the most difficult condition to be treated by the transsphenoidal approach.[28,29] It

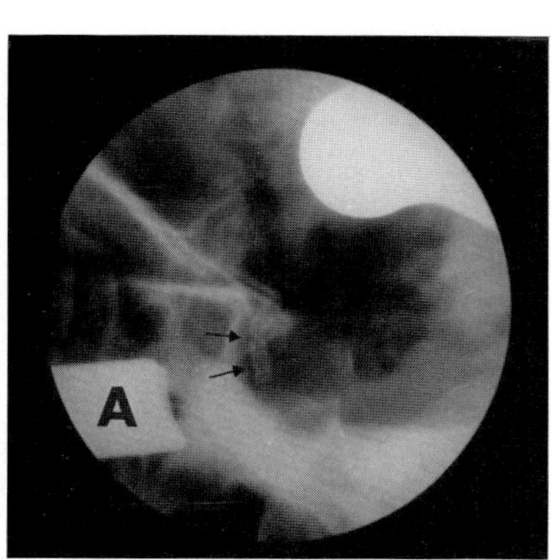
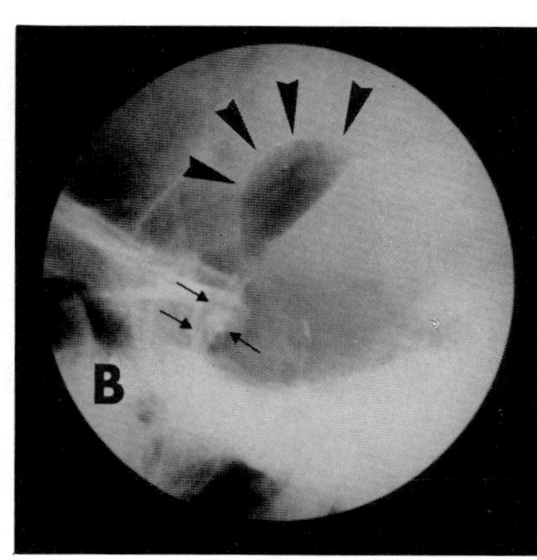
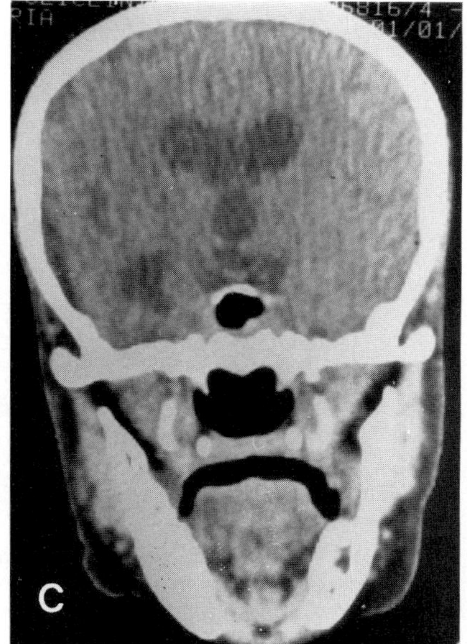

Fig. 28-28. (A) The dome of this cystic craniopharyngioma with suprasellar extension collapsed when it was completely emptied as demonstrated by peroperative PEG. A short Silastic tube was used to establish a permanent communication between the cyst and the sphenoid sinus (arrows). (B) Two days later the cyst cavity was empty but its dome retained it suprasellar extension (arrowheads). (C) One month after surgery the tumor cavity was empty as evident on this CT scan and occupied only the intrasellar region.

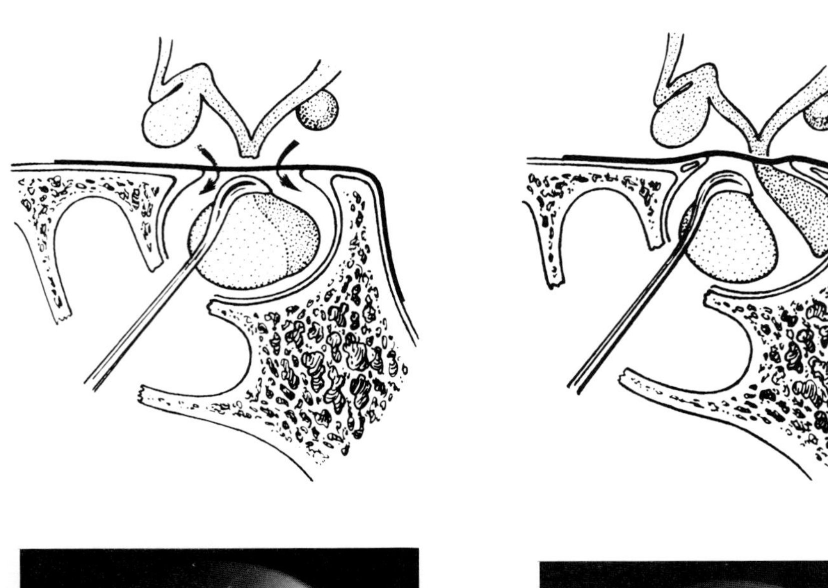

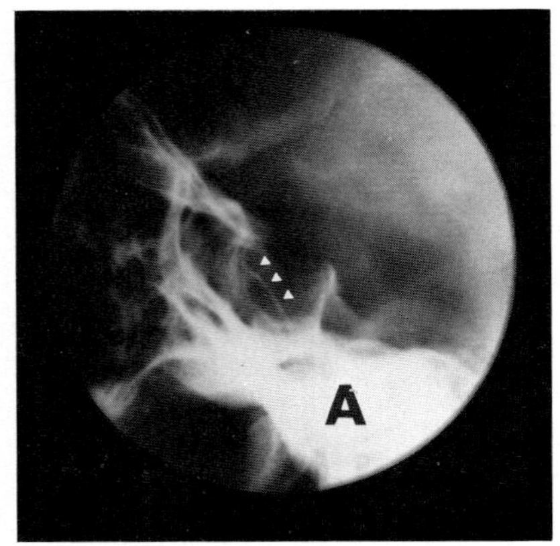

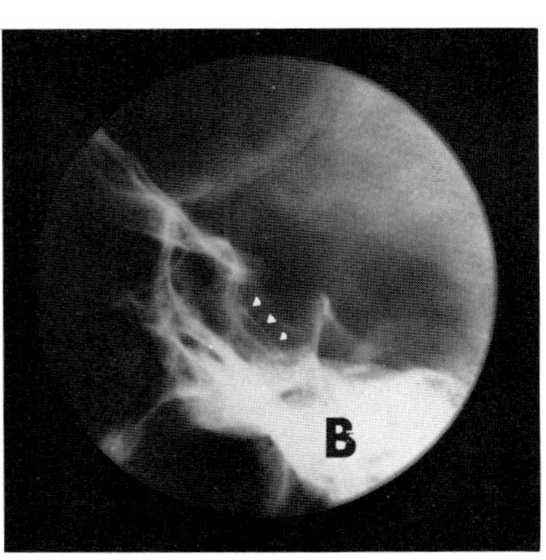

Fig. 28-29. (A) Total and (B) anterior selective functional hypophysectomy. In (A) section of the pituitary stalk is a factor predisposing the patient to CSF leakage (arrows) and requires proper treatment.

Fig. 28-30. A roentgenogram of the sella turcica (lateral view) (A) 5 days and (B) 3 months after a transsphenoidal operation. The bone fragment limiting the extradural packing (arrowheads) is lowered because of scarring and retraction of the packing material.

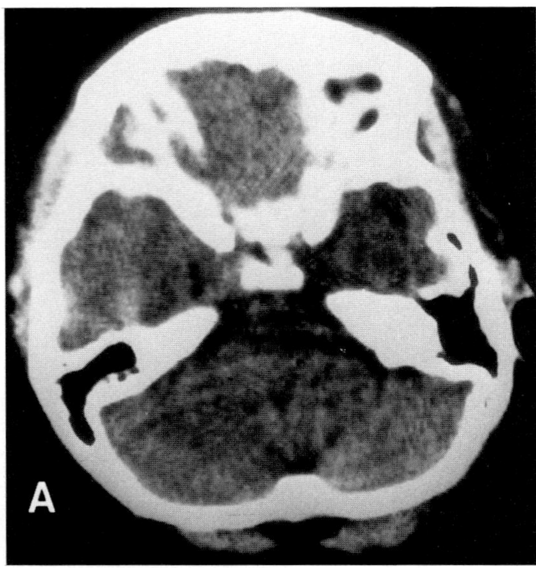

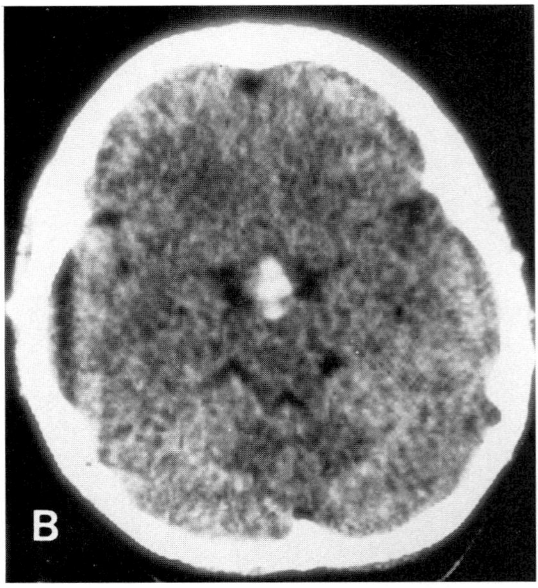

Fig. 28-31. A CT scan obtained 24 hours after a transsphenoidal operation for an ACTH-secreting intrasellar and suprasellar adenoma demonstrating a bloody hyperdensity simulating a hematoma within the tumor bed that appears to be both intrasellar (A) and suprasellar (B). Because the patient was complaining of worsening vision, she was operated on again. A hemostatic sponge was found.

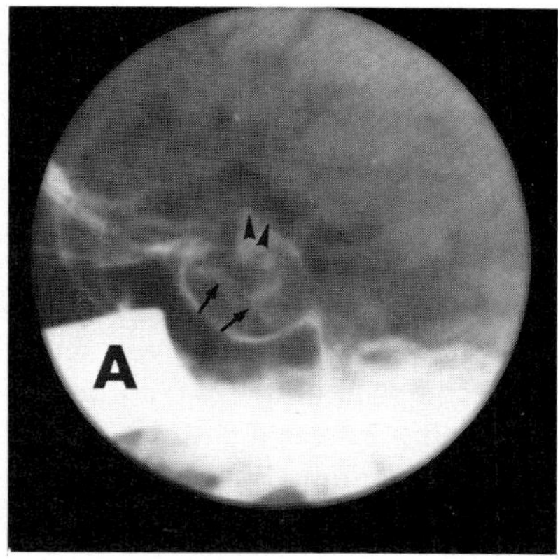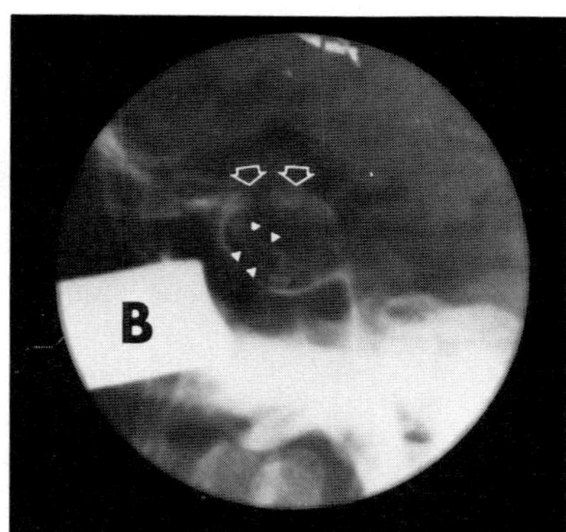

Fig. 28-32. Intraoperative fluoroscopic image. (A) An intrasellar adenoma bulging into the chiasmal cistern. Combined extradural (arrows) and intradural packing. There is so much intradural packing material (lightly soaked in iodinated contrast medium) that its upper limit (arrowheads) indents the suprasellar cistern demonstrated by means of peroperative PEG. (B) The amount of packing was reduced, freeing the chiasmal cistern. Its upper limit (open white arrows) is at the interclinoid plane. The white arrowheads outline the extradural packing.

can occur as an intraoperative complication in 6 to 20 percent of cases depending on the characteristics of the sellar lesion.[43,44] Furthermore, it can occur as an immediate or delayed postoperative complication in 3 to 6.4 percent of cases,[31,45,46] requiring reoperation in 1.5 to 2 percent of cases,[26,30,40] although the frequency is decreasing in recent clinical series. The success of an operation or reoperation for CSF rhinorrhea remains disappointing, with cure rates of approximately 80 percent even after multiple operations.[19,29]

Table 28-1. Synopsis of 165 transsphenoidal surgical procedures performed from 1978 through 1985

Cause	Number of Cases
Pituitary tumors	
Microadenoma	30
Intrasellar adenoma	33
Intrasellar adenoma indenting the chiasmal cistern	13
Suprasellar adenoma	50
Invasive adenoma	7
Total	133
Other sellar tumors	
Craniopharyngioma	5
Metastasis	2
Epidermoid tumor	1
Neurohypophyseal tumor	1
Chondrosarcoma	1
Total	10
Empty sella	8
Benign (arachnoidal) cyst	4
Reoperation for recurrence	
Pituitary adenoma (suprasellar)	5
Epidermoid tumor	1
Total	6
Reoperation for postoperative complications	
CSF rhinorrhea	2
Empty sella syndrome	1
Suspected hematoma	1
Total	4

ERRORS AND COMMON COMPLICATIONS

Reconstruction of the pituitary fossa may be ineffective either because a nonsuitable method was chosen or because the volume of packing material inserted was inadequate (or excessive), either from the outset or because of its subsequent retraction or necrosis (Figure 28-30).[8,12] The consequences can be (1) an intrasellar hematoma, (2) contamination of the cavity, (3) postoperative empty sella, or (4) CSF leakage. Care must be taken not to interpret a hyperdense lesion seen on an early postoperative CT scan as a true postoperative hematoma (the actual frequency of which is less than 1 percent of cases[44]) (Figure 28-31), since materials such as oxidized cellulose, Avitene, and fibrin sponge absorb blood and have an appearance on CT scans similar to a true blood clot.[12,44,47] Also, a certain degree of intrasellar arachnoidocele is a common finding on postoperative radiographic studies and is not a complication unless there are symptoms of an empty sella syndrome,[12] but this is a very rare occurrence.[33]

Cerebrospinal fluid rhinorrhea can be transitory or prolonged. Prolonged CSF rhinorrhea persists for days after surgery and when it does not improve despite suitable provisions requires surgical intervention (using the transsphenoidal, transethmoidal or transcranial routes or even a CSF shunting procedure).[29,30] Transitory CSF leakage is frequently seen in

Table 28-2. Factors influencing the surgical procedure.

Factor	Number of Cases
Intrasellar arachnoidocele associated with pituitary tumor	14
Pre- or intraoperative CSF leakage	20
Previous treatment	
Transsphenoidal surgery	7
Transcranial surgery	3
External radiotherapy	3
External radiotherapy plus transsphenoidal surgery	3
External radiotherapy plus transcranial surgery	2
Total	18

Table 28-3. Postoperative mechanical complications.

Complication	Number of Cases
Requiring reoperation	
CSF rhinorrhea	2
Empty sella syndrome	1
False hematoma	1
Total	4
Not requiring reoperation	
CSF rhinorrhea	5
Visual field defect	2
Diplopia	3
Total	10

the early postoperative period but usually stops within a few hours or days, either spontaneously or after continuous CSF drainage. We believe this measure should be used whenever a CSF leak occurs, whether it is before, during, or immediately after surgery.[48,49] We routinely insert a lumbar spinal subarachnoid catheter at the outset of the operation in all patients operated upon for tumors with suprasellar extension or in those in whom problems related to CSF leakage are anticipated.

Excessive packing of the sella is a less frequent event; its most serious and perhaps most common consequence is extension into the suprasellar cistern (Figure 28-32), which recreates de novo chiasmal compression and alteration in the visual fields.[32,33,47] Besides the case of unperceived introduction of overabundant filling materials, overpacking is usually consequent to the efforts of curing intraoperative CSF leakage, a diffuse hemorrhage from a cut surface, or a severe hemorrhage originating from a cavernous sinus. If moderate in amount it may regress because of the expected reduction in the volume of packing materials, otherwise it is best to reoperate and remove this material rather than risk a useless and probably damaging wait. Excessive intrasellar compression, excessive traction, or distortion of the dura mater of the sellar floor and of the wall of the cavernous sinus may cause paresis of the oculomotor nerves,[44,50] postoperative trigeminal syndrome,[5] or intense and persistent postoperative headaches. More exceptional complications caused by overpacking of the sella include compression or spasm of the carotid artery in its intracavernous segment.[46,50]

CONCLUSIONS

Although the transsphenoidal approach to the pituitary fossa and removal of the lesion are carried out by all workers in a virtually identical fashion, there is little agreement concerning reconstruction of the surgical site. In part this is because insufficient emphasis is placed on its importance and in part because there are conflicting ideas about the usefulness and the timing of careful reconstruction and hermetic closure of the sella, which for some authors is advisable only in cases with elements of risk.[10,21,51]

The relative rarity of mechanical complications with this type of surgery demonstrates the validity of the different methods used, largely suggested by personal experience, which

has led to little consideration being given to this aspect. It should not be underestimated, however, for although such complications are rare, they are very difficult to treat and may be more incapacitating and more severe than the original lesion. Preventing them with such sophisticated surgery is therefore imperative.[26,38]

Our experience is based on the 165 transsphenoidal operations summarized in Table 28-1. Tables 28-2, 28-3, and 28-4 show the procedure used, the risk factors that influenced surgery, and the postoperative complications observed, respectively. These findings have convinced us that the sellar region must routinely be reconstructed in the most careful and opportune way unless there are very specific reasons for a different approach.[52] The greater frequency of complications we encountered in our first 15 patients (one case of secondary empty sella the reappearance in one patient (Figure 28-33) of visual problems because of overpacking[39]) is certainly a result, in part, of the standard method of intradural packing. In the following 150 cases, in which we used the repair techniques described in this chapter, there were no serious mechanical complications even though the conditions in many of the cases were particularly unfavorable (invasive giant adenoma, associated empty sella, spontaneous preoperative CSF rhinorrhea). Only one patient had to undergo repeat surgery and even that proved to have been unnecessary; following a slight subjective deterioration of vision a postoperative CT scan suggested the presence of an intrasellar hematoma which on reoperation turned out to be a blood-soaked hemostatic sponge, while visual function recovered spontaneously (see also Figure 28-31).

Of the most feared complications of transsphenoidal surgery, intrasellar hemorrhage with hematoma formation is extremely infrequent[46,51] and intrasellar abscess is even more rare.[53] The possibility of a CSF leak with related dangers of septic meningitis, on the other hand, should be considered more frequently as well. So too should a secondary empty sella, which only exceptionally causes involvement of suprasellar structures.[26]

Multiple risk factors favor postoperative complications; reconstruction of the region therefore should be performed meticulously and with extra special care. The most important risk factors are:

1. Preoperative or intraoperative CSF leakage.
2. A large residual cavity.[33,38]
3. Marked suprasellar extension of the lesion.[25,38,45,51]
4. Anomalous positioning of the dome of the adenoma after removal of neoplastic tissue.[20,38]

Table 28-4. Summary of the techniques of sellar packing performed in 165 transsphenoidal procedures.

Technique	Number of Cases
No packing	29
Intradural packing	41
Intradural-extradural packing	46
Extradural packing	36
Intradural with sphenoidal sinus packing	13

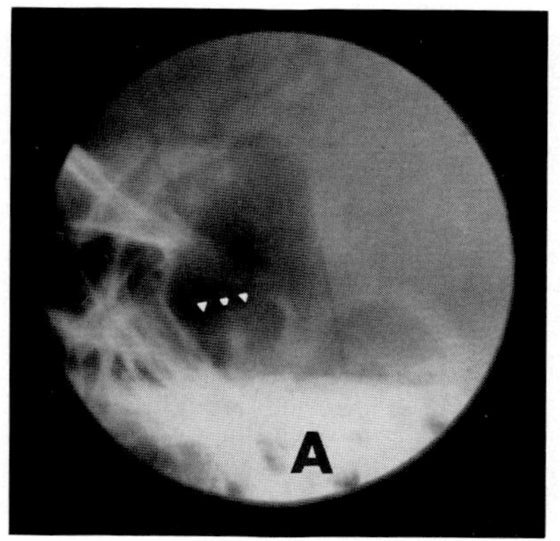 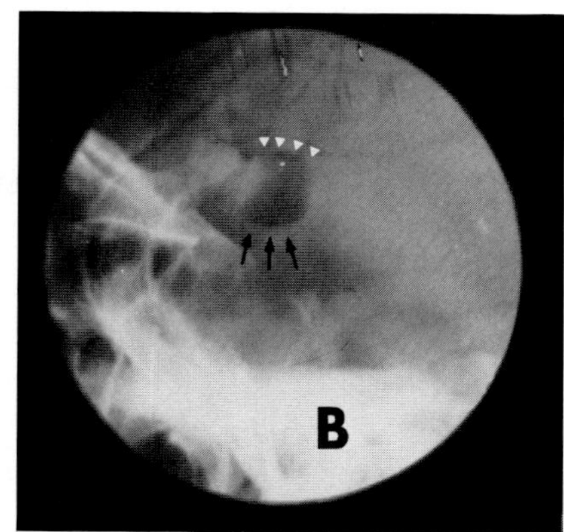 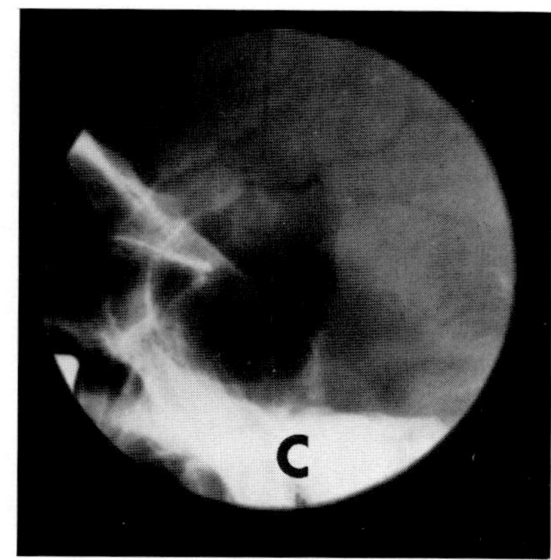

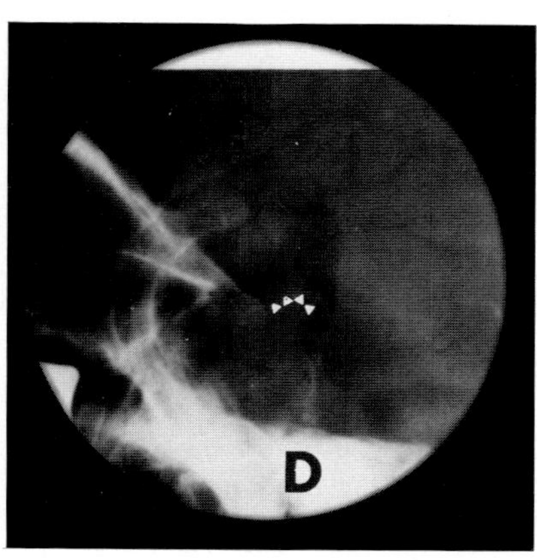

Fig. 28-33. Intraoperative fluoroscopic image. (A) An intrasellar and suprasellar arachnoid cyst emptied through a transsphenoidal approach. The dome of the cyst failed to descend. The intrasellar portion of the cavity was partly filled with muscle (arrowheads). (B) An x-ray film of the skull performed 5 days later because the patient developed CSF rhinorrhea, fever, and mild meningeal reactions. The unmodified upper limit of the cyst was spontaneously outlined by an air bubble (arrowheads) while a fluid level can be seen within it (arrows). (C) At reoperation a unidirectional valvelike mechanism through the capsule was recognized that supplied the cyst with CSF. (D) Intradural packing of the cyst cavity (more tight than the first time) the upper limit of which (arrowheads) went above the interclinoid plane. Patient recovered but because of such overpacking the bitemporal hemianopia and diplopia of which she originally complained transiently reappeared.

5. A co-existing preoperative or intraoperative empty sella.
6. Persistent bleeding after removal of an adenoma, even after prolonged compression and irrigation.
7. Precarious preoperative visual function because of involvement of the chiasm. 8. Previous surgery or radiotherapy.[5,7,30,54]
9. "Ghost" sella.[26,31,36,51]

Natural biologic substances obtained during surgery or common reabsorbable materials used in neurosurgery will fulfill the packing requirements in almost any situation.[26] Extradural packing used on its own or together with intradural packing constitutes the best method for producing a solid, stable closure of the sella, both immediately and with the passage of time. The consolidation is so effective that cases are often seen in which all the extradural packing undergoes pronounced ossification

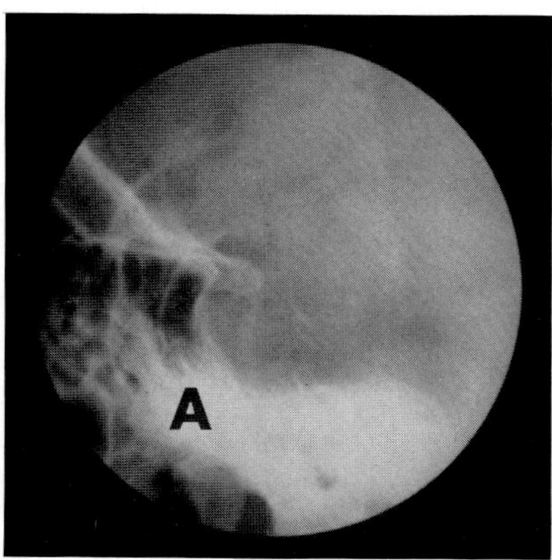 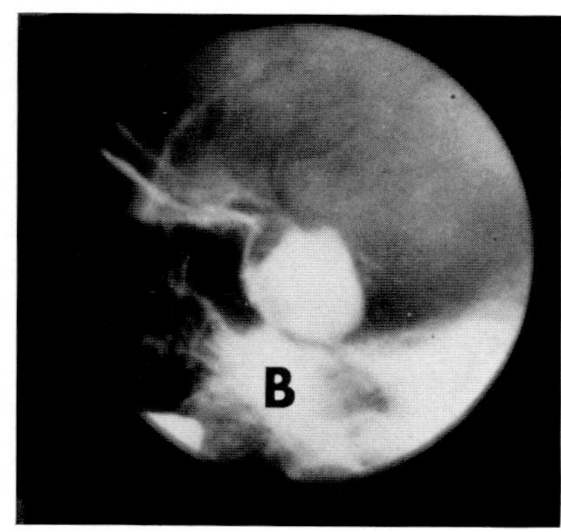 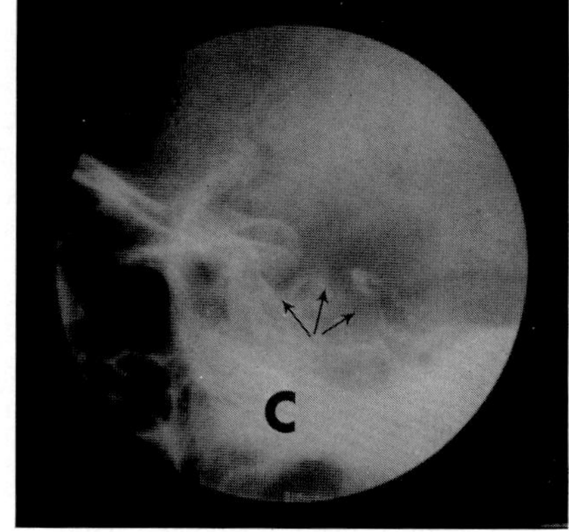

Fig. 28-34. (A) A preoperative x-ray film of the skull showing an enlarged and eroded sella turcica with disappearance of the dorsum in a case of a GH-secreting intrasellar adenoma. (B) Intraoperative fluoroscopic image. The dimensions of the adenoma are shown by a sponge soaked in iodinated contrast medium introduced into the residual cavity. (C) An x-ray film of the skull obtained 3 years later. The sellar boundaries and the dorsum sellae are recalcified. The materials used for intradural and extradural packing (arrows) are thinly calcified and ossified as are the bone fragments lying in the sphenoidal sinus.

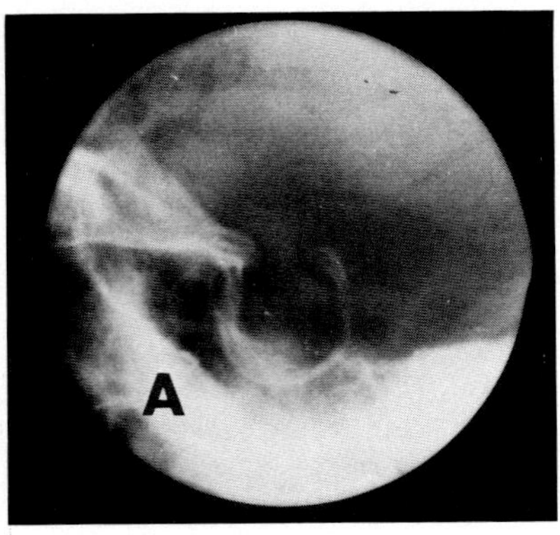
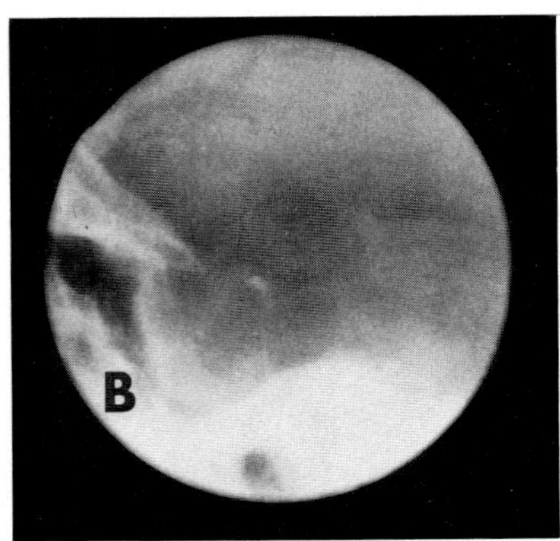
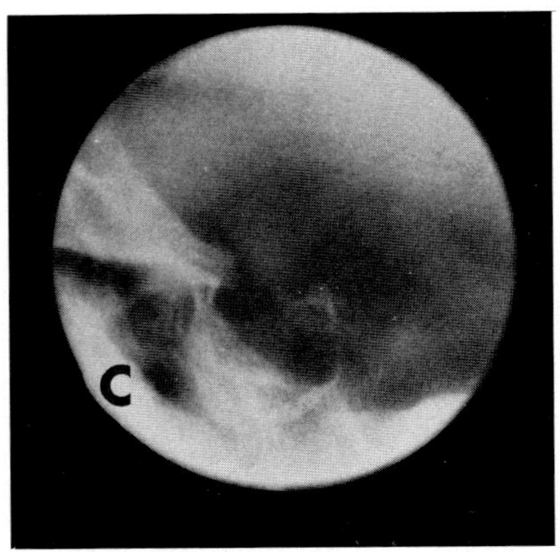

Fig. 28-35. A roentgenogram of the skull (A) before, (B) 1 year after, and (C) 3 years after a transsphenoidal operation for empty sella with CSF rhinorrhea that was cured with extradural packing. Progressive ossification of the packing material is clearly visible.

(Figures 28-34 and 28-35). It would be extremely difficult to conceive of a better result than this.

ACKNOWLEDGMENTS

The authors wish to thank Mr. Antonio D'Agostino, who lovingly and patiently prepared the drawings, Mr. Ciro Varchetta, who carefully prepared the photographs, and Mr. Fabrizio Naselli, whose agency prepared the English translation with swiftness and efficiency.

REFERENCES

1. de Divitiis E, Spaziante R, Stella L: Empty sella and benign intrasellar cysts, in Krayenb ̈u hl H (ed): Advances and Technical Standards in Neurosurgery, vol 8. Berlin, Springer Verlag, 1981, pp 3–74
2. Hardy J: Transsphenoidal microsurgery of the normal and pathological pituitary. Clin Neurosurg 16:185, 1969
3. Laws ER Jr: Transsphenoidal approach to lesions in and about the sella turcica, in Schmidek HH, Sweet WH (eds): Current Techniques in Operative Neurosurgery. New York, Grune & Stratton, 1977, pp 161–172
4. Ciric IS, Tarkington J: Transsphenoidal microsurgery. Surg Neurol 2:207, 1974
5. Wilson CB, Dempsey LC: Transsphenoidal microsurgical removal of 250 pituitary adenomas. J Neurosurg 48:13, 1978
6. Ludecke D, Kautzky R, Saeger W, et al: Selective removal of hypersecreting pituitary adenomas? Acta Neurochir 35:27, 1976
7. Faria MA Jr, Tindall GT: Transsphenoidal microsurgery for prolactinomas, in Givens JR (ed): Hormone-Secreting Pituitary Tumors. Chicago, Year Book Medical Publishers, 1982, pp 275–297
8. Hudgins WR, Raney LA, Young SW, et al: Failure of intrasellar muscle implants to prevent recurrent downward migration of the optic chiasm. Neurosurgery 8:231, 1981
9. Peer LA: The neglected "free fat graft". Its behavior and clinical use. Am J Surg 92:40, 1956
10. Griffith HB: Transsphenoidal pituitary surgery, in Symon L (ed): Operative Surgery. London, Butterworths, 1979, pp 187–194
11. Afshar F, Thomas A: Bromocriptine-induced cerebrospinal fluid rhinorrhea. Surg Neurol 18:61, 1982
12. Kaplan HC, Baker HL Jr, Houser OW, et al: CT of the sella turcica after transsphenoidal resection of pituitary adenomas. AJNR 6:723, 1985
13. Kobayashi S, Sugita K, Matsuo K, et al: Reconstruction of the sellar floor during transsphenoidal operations using alumina ceramic. Surg Neurol 15:196, 1980
14. Armenise B, Montinaro A: The prevention of nasal liquorrhea caused by transsphenoidal surgery for pituitary adenomas. J Neurosurg Sci 29:57, 1985
15. Nicola G: Transsphenoidal surgery for pituitary adenomas with, extrasellar extension, in Krayenbuhl H, Maspes PE, Sweet WH (eds): Progress in Neurological Surgery. Basel, S. Karger, 1975, pp 142–199
16. Young WC, Gates GA: The use of cyanoacrylate in transsphenoidal hypophysectomy. Laryngoscope 88:1784, 1978
17. de Divitiis E, Spaziante R: Osteoplastic opening of the sellar floor in transsphenoidal surgery. Technical note. Neurosurgery (in press)
18. Mickey BE, Samson D: Neurosurgical applications of the cyanoacrylate adhesives. Clin Neurosurg 28:429, 1981
19. Ommaya AK: Spinal fluid fistulae. Clin Neurosurg 23:363, 1976
20. Landolt AM, Strebel P: Technique of transsphenoidal operation for pituitary adenomas, in Krayenb ̈u hl H (ed): Advances and Technical Standards in Neurosurgery, vol 7. Berlin, Springer Verlag, 1980, pp 119–177
21. Rand RW: Fifteen years experience with transnasal transsphenoidal operation for pituitary tumours, in Brock M (ed): Modern Neurosurgery 1. Berlin, Springer Verlag, 1982, pp 173–180
22. Tindall GT, Collins WF Jr, Kirchner JA: Unilateral septal technique for transsphenoidal microsurgical approach to the sella turcica. J Neurosurg 49:138, 1978
23. Weiss MH, Kaufman B, Richards DE: Cerebrospinal fluid rhinorrhea from an empty sella. Transsphenoidal obliteration of the fistula. J Neurosurg 39:674, 1973
24. Landolt AM: Therapeutic aspects of the empty sella syndrome, in Glaser JS (ed): Neuro-ophthalmology, vol 9. St. Louis, CV Mosby, 1977, pp 229–235
25. Guiot G, Derome P, Demailly P, et al: Complications inattendue de l'exérèse compléte de volumineux adénomes hypophysaires. Rev Neurol 118:164, 1968
26. Derome PJ, Visot AM, Delalande O, et al: Mechanical complications after the transsphenoidal removal of pituitary adenomas, in Derome PJ, Jedinak CP, Peillon F (eds): Pituitary Adenomas. Paris, Asclepios, 1980, pp 233–235
27. Olson DR, Guiot G, Derome P: The symptomatic empty sella. Prevention and correction via the transsphenoidal approach. J Neurosurg 37:533, 1972
28. Garcia-Uria J, Carrillo R, Serrano P, et al: Empty sella and rhinorrhea. A report of eight treated cases. J Neurosurg 50:466, 1979

29. Hubbard JL, Mc Donald TJ, Pearson BW, et al: Spontaneous cerebrospinal fluid rhinorrhea: Evolving concepts in diagnosis and surgical management based on the Mayo Clinic experience from 1970 through 1981. Neurosurgery 16:314, 1985

30. Laws ER Jr, Fode NC, Redmond MJ: Transsphenoidal surgery following unsuccessful prior therapy. An assessment of benefits and risks in 158 patients. J Neurosurg 63:823, 1985

31. Landolt AM: Cerebrospinal fluid rhinorrhea: A complication of therapy for invasive prolactinomas. Neurosurgery 11:395, 1982

32. Hardy J, Beauregard H, Robert F: Prolactin-secreting pituitary adenomas: Transsphenoidal microsurgical treatment. Clin Neurosurg 27:38, 1980

33. Laws ER Jr, Kern EB: Complications of transsphenoidal surgery, in Tindall GT, Collins WF (eds): Clinical Management of Pituitary Disorders. New York, Raven Press, 1979, pp 435–445

34. Nakane T, Kuwayama A, Watanabe M, et al: Transsphenoidal approach to pituitary adenomas with suprasellar extension. Surg Neurol 16:225, 1981

35. Goldman JA, Hedges TR III, Shucart W, et al: Delayed chiasmal decompression after transsphenoidal operation for a pituitary adenoma. Neurosurgery 17:962, 1985

36. Wilson CB: Neurosurgical management of large and invasive pituitary tumors, in Tindall GT, Collins WF (eds): Clinical Management of Pituitary Disorders. New York, Raven Press, 1979, pp 335–342

37. Spaziante R, de Divitiis E, Stella L, et al: The empty sella. Surg Neurol 16:418, 1981

38. Guiot G, Derome P: Surgical problems of pituitary adenomas, in Krayenbühl H (ed): Advances and Technical Standards in Neurosurgery, vol 3. Berlin, Springer Verlag, 1976, pp 3–33

39. Spaziante R, de Divitiis E, Stella L, et al: Benign intrasellar cysts. Surg Neurol 15:274, 1981

40. Baskin DS, Wilson C8: Transsphenoidal treatment of non-neoplastic intrasellar cysts. A report of 38 cases. J Neurosurg 60:8, 1984

41. Laws ER Jr: Transsphenoidal microsurgery in the management of craniopharyngioma. J Neurosurg 52:661, 1980

42. Tindall GT, Payne NS, Nixon DW: Transsphenoidal hypophysectomy for disseminated carcinoma of the prostate gland. Results in 53 patients. J Neurosurg 50:275, 1979

43. Balagura S, Derome P, Guiot G: Acromegaly: Analysis of 132 cases treated surgically. Neurosurgery 8:413, 1981

44. Hardy J, Mohr G: Le prolactinomes. Aspects chirurgicaux. Neurochirurgie 27(Suppl 1):41, 1981

45. Ciric I, Mikhael M, Stafford T, et al: Transsphenoidal microsurgery of pituitary macroadenomas with long-term follow-up results. J Neurosurg 59:395, 1983

46. Horwitz NH, Rizzoli HV: Postoperative Complications of Intracranial Neurological Surgery. Baltimore, Williams & Wilkins, 1982, pp 472

47. Dolinskas CA, Simeone FA: Transsphenoidal hypophysectomy: Postsurgical CT findings. AJNR 6:45, 1985

48. Findler G, Sahar A, Beller AJ: Continuous lumbar drainage of cerebrospinal fluid in neurosurgical patients. Surg Neurol 8:455, 1977

49. Loew F, Pertuiset B, Chaumier EE, et al: Traumatic, spontaneous and post-operative CSF rhinorrhea, in Symon L (ed): Advances and Technical Standards in Neurosurgery, vol 11. Berlin, Springer Verlag, 1984, pp 171–207

50. Laws ER Jr: Complications of transsphenoidal microsurgery for pituitary adenoma, in Brock M (ed): Modern Neurosurgery 1. Berlin, Springer Verlag, 1982, pp 181–186

51. Nicola GC, Tonnarelli GP, Griner AC: Complications of transsphenoidal surgery in pituitary adenomas, in Derome PJ, Jedinak CP, Peillon F (eds): Pituitary Adenomas. Paris, Asclepios, 1980, pp 237–240

52. Spaziante R, de Divitiis E, Cappabianca P: Reconstruction of the pituitary fossa in transsphenoidal surgery: An experience of 140 cases. Neurosurgery 17:453, 1985

53. Robinson B: Intrasellar abscess after transsphenoidal pituitary adenomectomy. Neurosurgery 12:684, 1983

54. Baskin DS, Boggan JE, Wilson CB: Transsphenoidal microsurgical removal of growth hormone-secreting pituitary adenomas. A review of 137 cases. J Neurosurg 56:634, 1982

CHAPTER 29
Transethmoidal Approach to the Pituitary

Charles W. Cummings   Jonas Johnson

THE INTENT OF THIS CHAPTER is to present the advantages and disadvantages as well as a procedural description of the transethmoidal sphenoidotomy approach to the pituitary gland. This procedure, in conjunction with the transseptal sphenoidotomy approach, represents one distinct anatomic pathway to the pituitary region. The ease of approach and the relatively benign postoperative course merit consideration of the procedure when an approach to the pituitary is warranted.

INDICATIONS

The indications for surgical approach to the pituitary gland have previously been discussed. Hyperprolactinemia, acromegaly, Cushing's disease, and metastatic carcinoma of the breast and prostate are paramount among these indications.

CONTRAINDICATIONS

1. This procedure should not be used in cases of extensive suprasellar displacement of the tumor.
2. An underpneumatized sphenoid sinus, which occurs 3 percent of the time, is a distinct contraindication to the surgical approach because the sella is difficult to identify.
3. An overpneumatized sphenoid sinus is a relative contraindication in that the optic canal can be completely surrounded by sphenoid air cells, thus making identification exceedingly difficult and injury more likely.
4. Chronic ethmoid sinusitis or sphenoid sinusitis or both impair surgical access because of mucosal edema, hyperemia, and the potential for introducing an infection.
5. Acute sinusitis or nasal sepsis presents a high risk of contamination or infection.
6. Abnormal development of the cavernous sinus or medial displacement of the carotid arteries into the sphenoid make this surgical approach hazardous.

ADVANTAGES

The advantages of the transethmoid approach to the sphenoid, and thus to the pituitary, over other procedures are:

1. A shorter anatomic distance is traversed to enter the sphenoid sinus.
2. The procedure allows for two-plane instrumentation, i.e., transnasal as well as transethmoid.
3. The operative procedure can be performed on a plane parallel to the floor of the anterior fossa.
4. There is minimal postoperative discomfort.
5. The risk of septomucosal perforation is avoided by this procedure.
6. Contamination from the oral cavity is avoided.
7. Devitalization of the teeth is avoided.

DISADVANTAGES

1. An external scar is necessary.
2. Procedure is not a midline approach.

COMPLICATIONS

Although these complications do not represent problems specific for this surgical approach, they should be mentioned. Diabetes insipidus is by far the most frequent complication, occurring in 15 percent of cases, according to Collins.[1] Usually this problem can be managed by replacement therapy without difficulty.

Cerebrospinal fluid leaks occur in 4 to 9 percent of cases.[2,3] If the sinus has been obliterated with fat or a fascia lata and a nasal-mucosal pedicle flap, a permanent leak is unusual.

Meningitis, either alone or in concert with a cerebrospinal fluid leak, is the most significant postoperative complication, and occurs less than 2 percent of the time.

Immediate surgical complications are:

1. Injury to the optic nerve by dissection of the superolateral aspect of the posterior ethmoidal cell or sphenoid sinus.
2. Injury to the carotid artery as it traverses the lateral wall of the sphenoid sinus. Kirchner[3] has recommended needle aspiration of the uncapped area if there is any suspicion that the region may not be the sella.

WORK-UP

Several special studies are necessary to obviate procedural difficulties. These should be obtained in addition to necessary diagnostic procedures.

1. Routine sinus films.
2. Tomograms of the sphenoid and sella region, both from a lateral and basilar projection.

OPERATIVE NEUROSURGICAL TECHNIQUES
ISBN 0-8089-1862-1

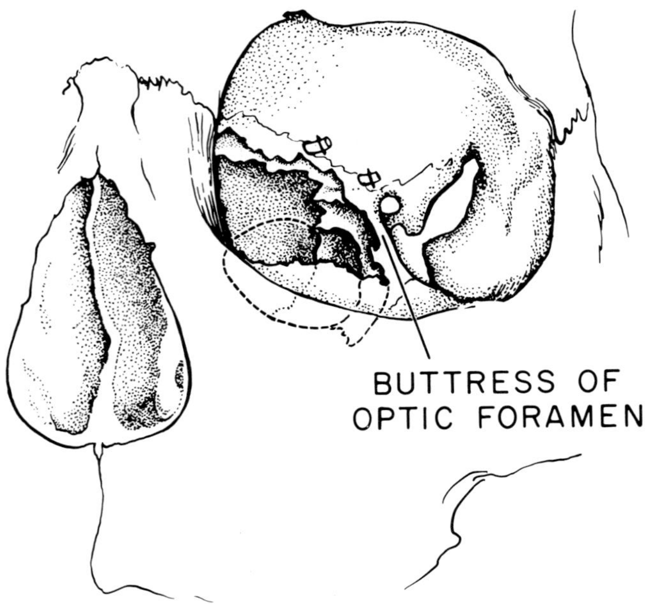

Fig. 29-1. The middle turbinate, ethmoid labyrinth, and anterior wall of the sphenoid are removed. The medial buttress of the optic foramen is identified.

3. Diagnostic measures to eliminate the possibility of suprasellar extension of disease (computerized axial tomography, air-contrast tomography, magnetic resonance imaging). Optional: Carotid arteriograms to ascertain adequate intercarotid space within the sphenoid.

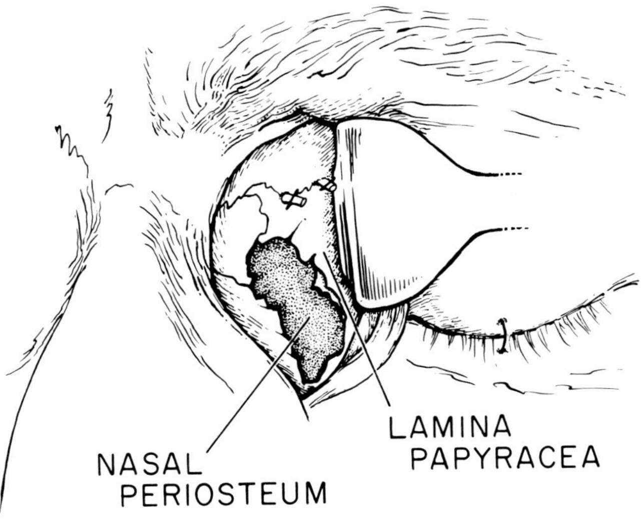

Fig. 29-3. The lamina papyracea is partially removed.

TECHNIQUE

The surgical technique for this procedure will be outlined in stepwise fashion. There are several anatomic landmarks, however, that must be kept in mind when performing the operation.

1. The middle turbinate. Medial to the insertion of the middle turbinate lies the cribriform plate area. This area must be avoided to eliminate trauma to the cribriform and the potential for a cerebrospinal fluid leak. The ethmoid air cells lie lateral

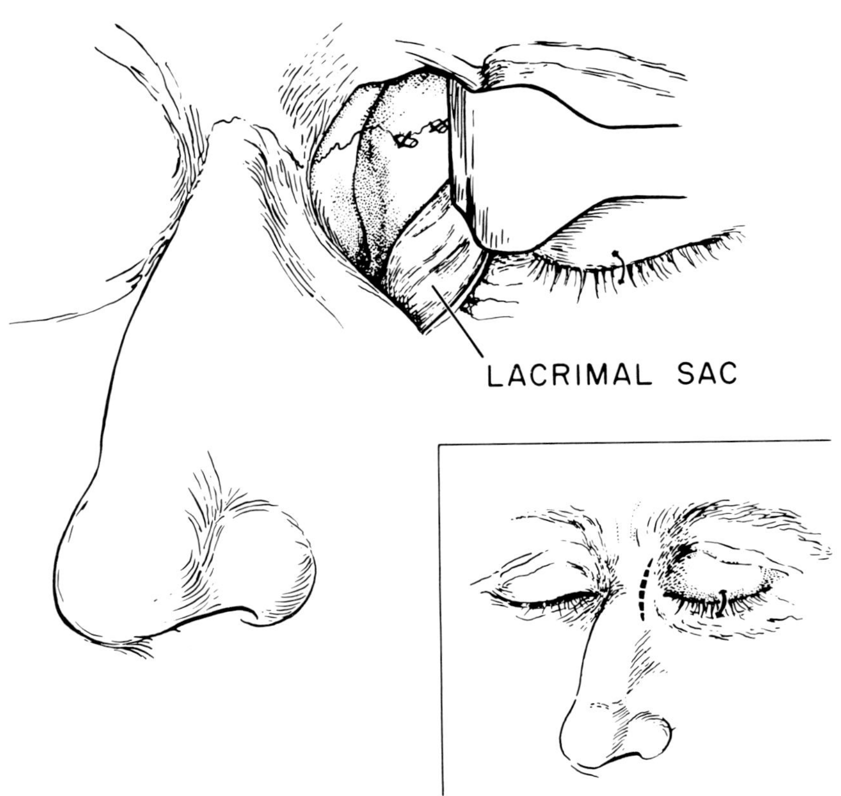

Fig. 29-2. A curvilinear incision is made one half the distance between the dorsum of the nose and the medial canthus. The periorbitum is reflected laterally and the anterior and posterior ethmoid arteries are divided.

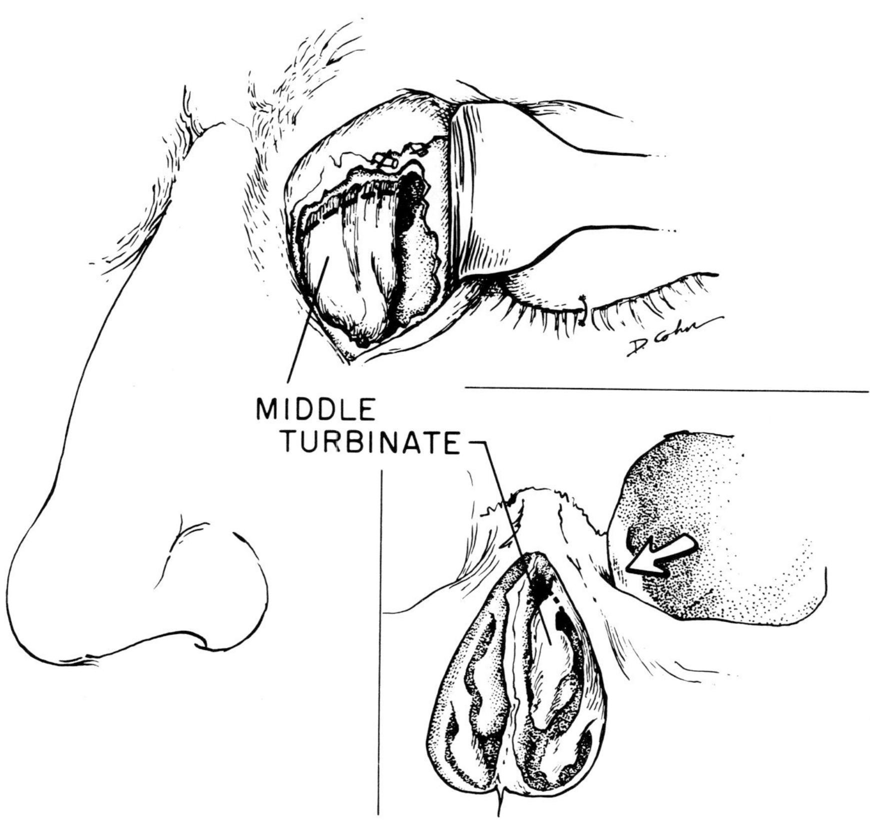

Fig. 29-4. The lateral nasal mucosa is removed and the middle turbinate identified.

to the insertion of the middle turbinate. These represent an area of relative safety if the roof of the ethmoid is not violated.

2. The cribriform area offers superior plane orientation and is directly parallel with the floor of the anterior fossa.

3. The anterior and posterior ethmoid arteries form a plane at the level of the cribriform plate area and therefore represent the superior limits of surgical dissection.

4. The posterior ethmoid artery is the posterior limit of ethmoidal dissection. The optic foramen is 4 to 7 mm posterior to the posterior ethmoid artery and is protected by a medial rim of bone (Figure 29-1). This artery also traverses the roof of the posterior ethmoid cell, enabling its identification. The posterior wall of this cell represents the anterior wall of the sphenoid sinus. The canal of the optic

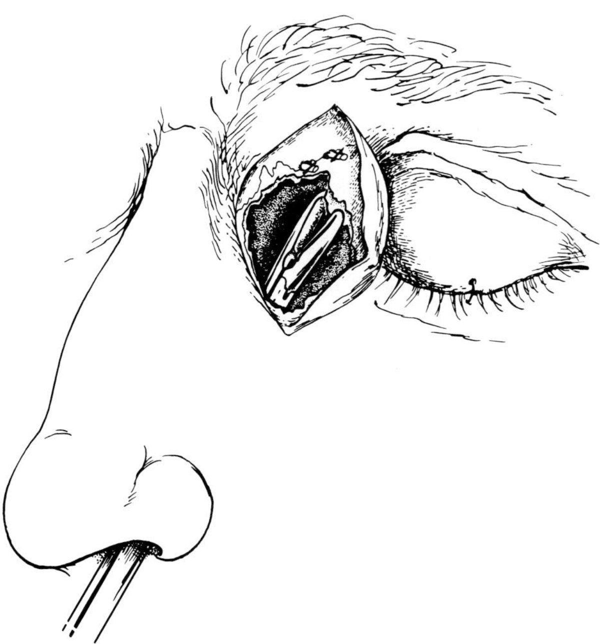

Fig. 29-5. The ethmoid air cell mucosa is removed transnasally under direct vision via the external ethmoidectomy exposure.

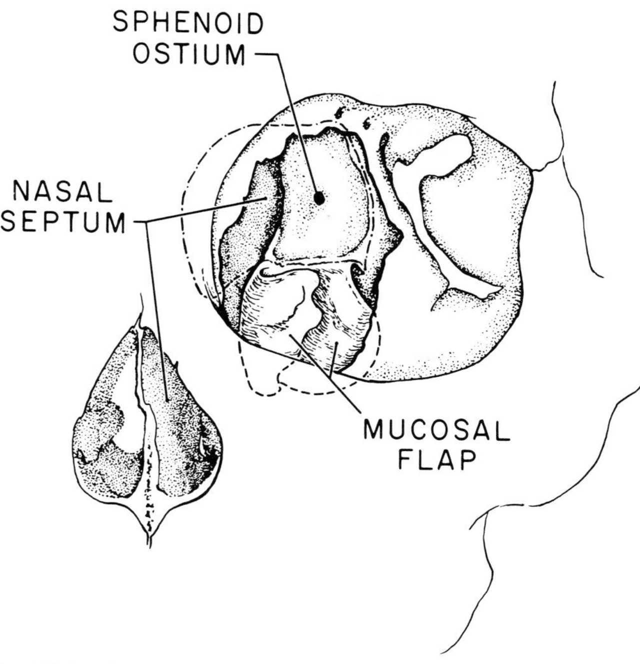

Fig. 29-6. A nasal septal mucosal flap based posteroinferiorly is developed. The sphenoid ostium is well visualized.

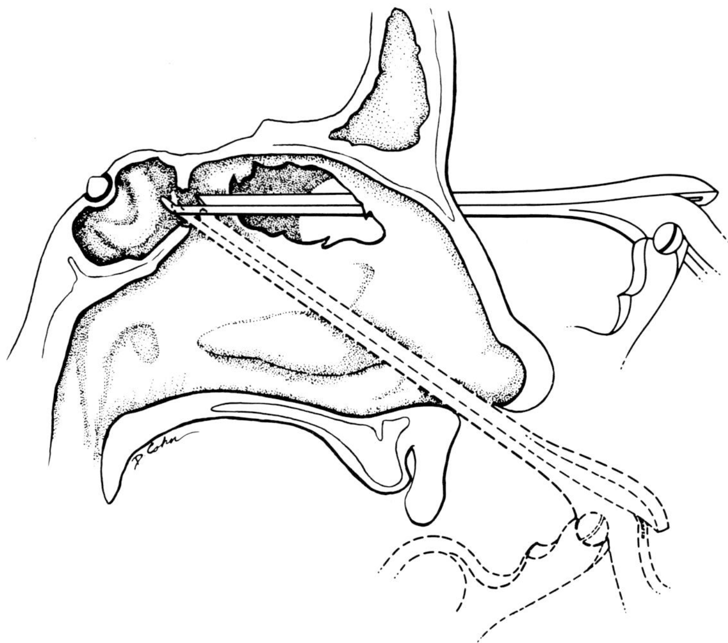

Fig. 29-7. The entrance into the sphenoid is made anteriorly adjacent to the ostium. A Cloward biting forceps can be used either transnasally or transethmoidally.

nerve intrudes upon the superolateral aspect of the posterior ethmoid cell.

5. The rostrum of the sphenoid allows for location of the inferior aspect of the sphenoid sinus.

6. The sphenoid septum does not necessarily reside in the midline and is of no value for orientation other than by comparison to the sinus laminograms.

7. The medial projection of the carotid canal can be visualized within the sphenoid sinus and must not be interpreted as a sphenoid septum or the sella. As this bone is unroofed,

aspiration with a thin needle is advocated to rule out the contralateral carotid artery.[3] This artery will be exposed (if at all) because of the slightly off-midline approach through the ethmoid.

8. Localization of the midline can be performed by passing a flat instrument along the superior aspect of the nasal septum into the sphenoid sinus. This will identify the midline and the region of the sella.

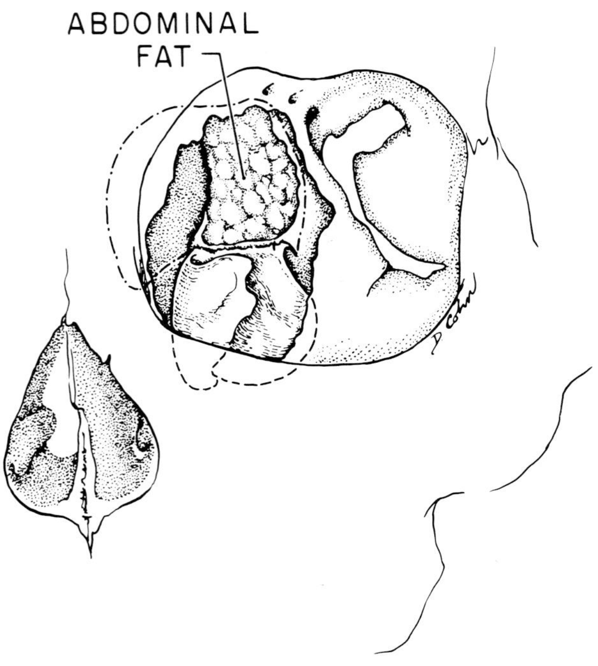

PROCEDURE

1. The head is elevated 20 degrees.
2. The eyes are protected with either lid sutures or plastic eye shields.
3. An incision is made at a point one half the distance from the dorsum of the nose to the canthus, approximately 3 cm in length (Figure 29-2).
4. The inner canthal ligament and lacrimal sac are retracted laterally.
5. The anterior ethmoid artery is identified, clipped or ligated, and divided.
6. The posterior ethmoid artery is identified.
7. The lamina papyraceous portion of the lacrimal fossa is taken down (Figure 29-3).
8. An incision is made through the lateral nasal mucosa, and the middle turbinate is identified (Figure 29-4).
9. The middle turbinate is removed and its insertion is preserved as a landmark.
10. The ethmoid mucosa is removed and the posterior ethmoid cell is uncapped (Figure 29-5).
11. An inferiorly based nasal mucosal flap is created.
12. The sphenoid ostium is identified (Figure 29-6).
13. The position is corroborated with image intensifying fluoroscope with a C-arm.

Fig. 29-8. Abdominal fat is used to obliterate the sphenoid sinus.

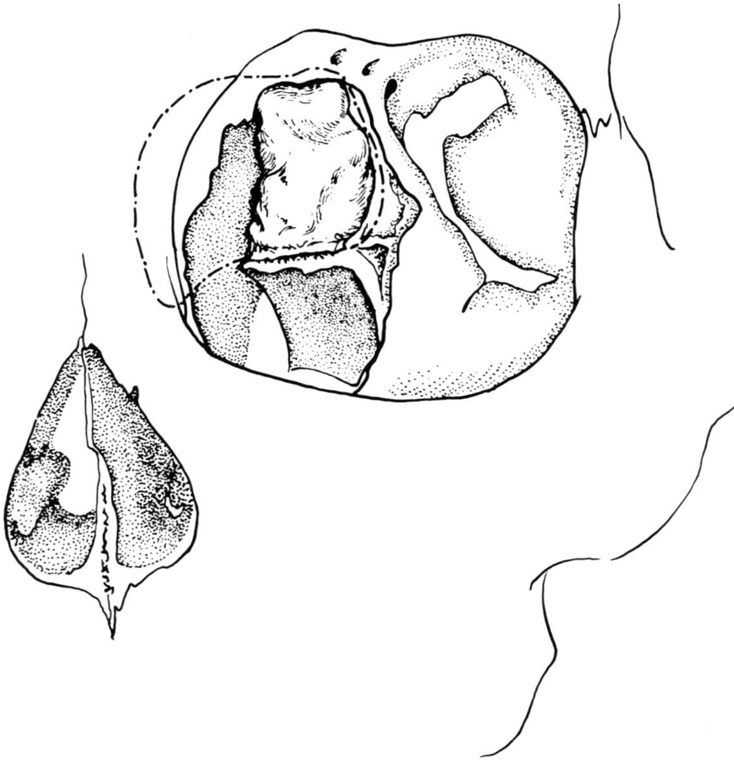

Fig. 29-9. The nasal septal mucosal flap is placed over the fat graft.

14. An entrance into the sphenoid is made by taking down the anterior wall (Figure 29-7).
15. The sphenoid sinus mucosa is removed. An operating microscope with a 300-mm objective lens is used to aid visualization.
16. The region of the sella is uncapped from bone. The uncapped area can be aspirated with a long needle to rule out the presence of the carotid artery.
17. A cruciate incision is made in the capsule and the gland is exposed.
18. The pituitary fenestration is obliterated with fat (abdominal) or fascia lata (Figure 29-8).
19. The sphenoid is obliterated with fat and the nasal mucosal flap is placed over the defect (Figure 29-9). Gelfoam is placed over the flap.
20. The inner canthal incision is closed in two layers.

REFERENCES

1. Collins WF: Hypophysectomy: Historical and personal perspective. Clin Neurosurg 21:68, 1974
2. Richards SH, Thomas JP, Kilby D: Transethmoidal hypophysectomy for pituitary tumors. Proc R Soc Med 67:889, 1974
3. Kirchner JA, Van Gilder JD: Transethmoidal hypophysectomy: Some surgical landmarks. Trans Am Acad Ophthalmol Otolaryngol 80:391, 1975

CHAPTER 30

Stereotactic Thermal Hypophysectomy

Nicholas T. Zervas

THE INDICATIONS FOR STEREOTACTIC THERMAL HYPOPHYSECTOMY have diminished markedly in the past decade. The procedure is now indicated rarely for patients with diabetic retinopathy who might benefit from total hypophysectomy without undergoing the slightly greater rigors of an open transsphenoidal procedure. Operations for the relief of pain and breast and prostatic cancer are now rare in my experience. Nonetheless, there are times when this procedure may be utilized in these instances or in cases where previous transsphenoidal removal of a pituitary gland has not been successful. The technique as described below has not been altered in the past few years.

Stereotactic hypophysectomy was introduced into the neurosurgical armamentarium by Jean Talairach. He first employed radioactive gold to induce ablation of the pituitary gland. Since that time, radioactive yttrium, radioactive strontium, heat, cold, and ultrasound have been used as alternate methods to induce destruction. Since 1964, we have produced heat lesions in the pituitary gland using radiofrequency current. This has proved to be a satisfactory way to bring about total destruction of the gland in most cases without the risk of damage to surrounding vascular or cranial nerve structures. Perhaps the major objection to stereotactic transnasal procedures was the high incidence of cerebrospinal fluid rhinorrhea. This virtually has been eliminated by the tactic of packing the sella turcica with fascia lata at the end of the operation and occluding the defect in the anterior wall of the sella turcica with a silicone plug. The need for this procedure has been reduced by pharmacologic methods to treat metastatic cancer and laser therapy for diabetic retinopathy.

METHODS

PREPARATION OF THE PATIENT

No special precautions are required before surgery. A nasal culture may be indicated in patients with a previous history of sinus infections. It is essential, however, that all patients receive antibiotics before, during, and after the operation. Accordingly, patients are given 1 g of oxacillin intravenously, beginning at 6 AM on the morning of the operation. Also, patients are given 50 mg of hydrocortisone intramuscularly before the operation. No other special measures are required. When the patient enters the operating room, the nasal cavity can be sprayed on either side with a vasoconstrictive agent such as Neo-Synephrine.

ANESTHESIA

Radiofrequency thermal lesions can be produced in patients while they are under anesthesia because damage to visual structures has been a very rare event. In the few instances in which injury did occur, it was first manifested as anisocoria, and the production of the lesion was quickly terminated. To perform the procedure under local anesthesia is very trying for both the patient and the professional staff and is not necessary.

OPERATION

Following the induction of general anesthesia, the oral pharynx is packed with a 1.0-inch moistened gauze roll. The patient's head is fixed securely in a stereotactic frame. We use the Todd-Wells frame (Figure 30-1). The electrode holder then should be centered on the anterior wall of the sella turcica as close to the midline as possible. Quite obviously, it is very necessary to ensure that the electrode enters the pituitary gland directly and does not go above or lateral to it. There is little security in the bony landmarks of plain films. The surgeon never can be certain where the diaphragma sellae is, nor of where the lateral margins of the pituitary gland lie in an individual patient. We have not found angiography and pneumoencephalography necessary. As long as the surgeon is careful to be as close to the midline as possible and no more than 4 mm above the sellar floor when entering the pituitary gland, poor placement of the electrode can be minimized. Perhaps the most variable location is the position of the diaphragma sellae. Although this should run horizontally from the tuberculum sellae to below the dorsum sellae, we have repeatedly found that it often lies quite low in the sella turcica and, of course, may be deficient in the midline. Accordingly, the target point on the anterior wall of the sella turcica must be kept rather low to avoid penetrating above the diaphragma sellae. We never enter the sella turcica more than 4 mm above the floor, regardless of its apparent configuration. If the sella turcica has a peculiar shape, one is best advised to obtain a pneumoencephalogram to be certain of the position of the diaphragma. Once the target point has been set, a nasal cannula can be advanced into the nasal cavity on either side, whichever side appears to be more expedient from the standpoint of easy advancement of the instruments. A 4-mm drill hole then is made in the anterior wall of the sphenoid sinus, and a cannula is inserted just short of the anterior wall of the sella turcica. The sphenoid sinus then is washed copiously with a solution of bacitracin (50,000 units/500 ml N saline). A 2.2-mm drill hole is made in the anterior wall of the sella turcica. Care must be taken so that the head of the drill does not extend more than 1.0 or 2.0 mm into the sella turcica.

OPERATIVE NEUROSURGICAL TECHNIQUES
ISBN 0-8089-1862-1

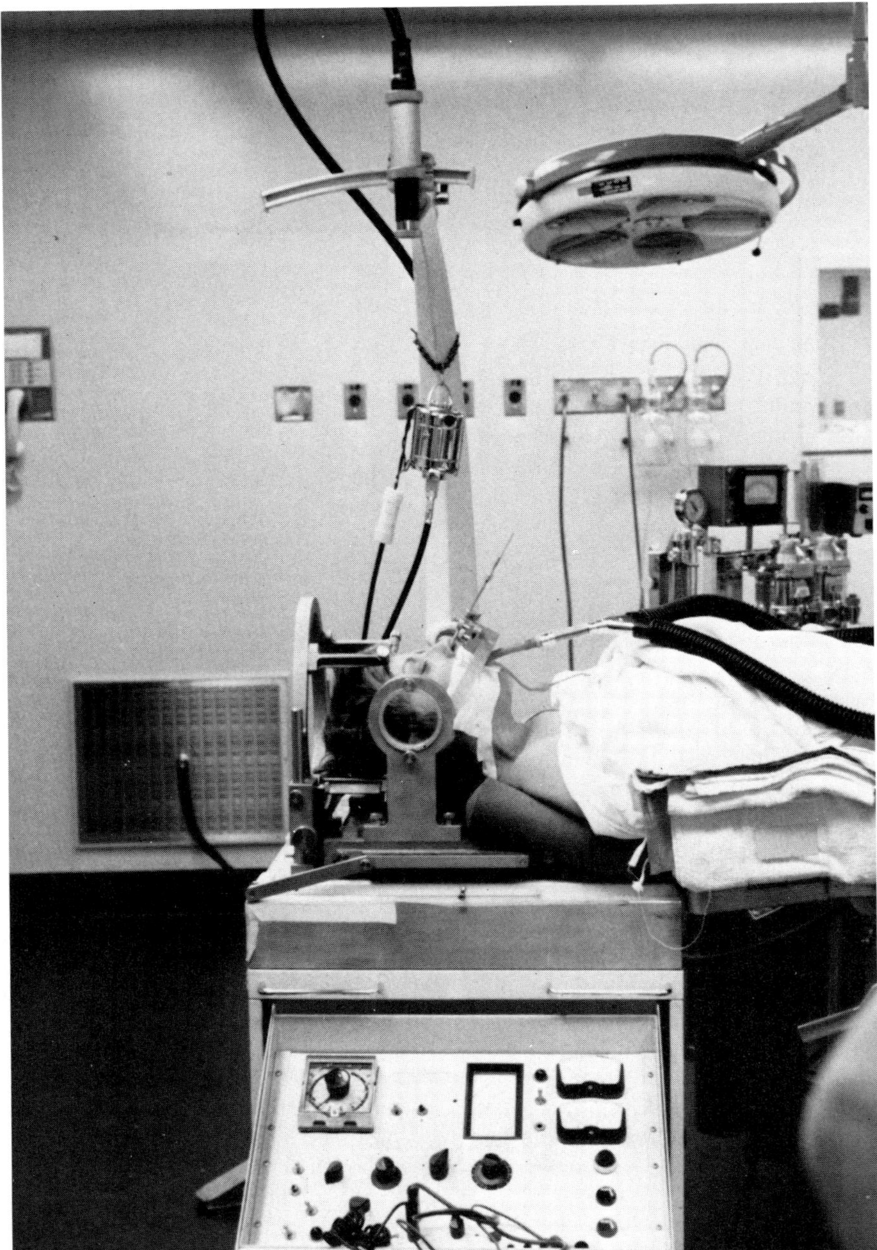

Fig. 30-1. Operative scene: the patient's head is fixed in the stereotactic frame. The electrode is in place. The miniature x-ray tubes are aligned orthogonally with the frame. The radiofrequency generator is in the foreground.

This is done to prevent stripping the dura away from the bone. The dura then is punctured with a series of double-ended instruments, each one larger than the one before, so that the length of the opening in the dura finally is larger than the diameter of the electrode tip.

The radiofrequency electrode then is inserted into the sella turcica. The electrode we employ is a totally insulated, hollow stainless steel cannula. The end is closed, but there is a side hole 1 mm short of the tip (Figures 30-2 and 30-3). A stainless steel, coiled wire electrode with a preformed curve can be projected through the side hole. As this is forced through the side hole it becomes a semicircular stylet. It is quite malleable and not likely to puncture surrounding structures, such as dura or the carotid artery. There is a thermocouple within the spring that is used to monitor the temperature at the tip. In the past we used thermistor tips, but these were easily broken. Thermocou-

ples have a much longer life. The electrode is mounted on the stereotactic frame and then advanced into the sella turcica. It is possible to easily palpate the anterior dorsum sellae with the electrode tip. At this point the electrode is withdrawn 1 or 2 mm. The lateral stylet then is advanced through the side hole until resistance can be felt as it encounters either the diaphragma sellae or the floor or the lateral dura surrounding the pituitary gland, depending on the angle of rotation of the outer cannula. Thus, the surgeon can estimate the actual size of the gland. Passage through the gland is unimpeded, since it is rather soft. The dura or the diaphragma sellae however, offers resistance.

In order to bring about total destruction of the gland, we usually place the electrode tip in the posterior and then anterior sectors of the gland. In each position, a series of lesions is made in various quadrants by alternately retracting and extending the

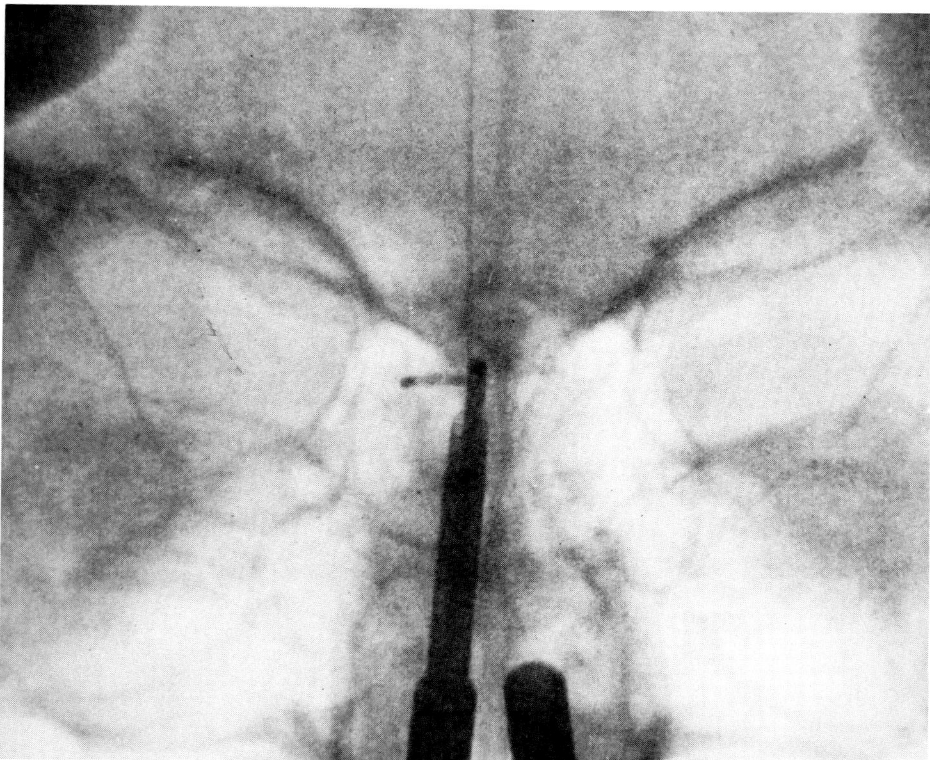

Fig. 30-2. A frontal roentgenogram showing the electrode in position and the sidearm projecting to the right.

side arm after the electrode has been turned to a new angle. It is very important to confirm the actual position of the electrode tip with a plain roentgenogram, since very often the malleable spring will be diverted from its true radiant as it bumps obliquely against the diaphragma sellae or the floor of the sella. Also, if the electrode inadvertently is placed above the diaphragma sellae, the latter may catch the lateral stylet and prevent it from being directed downward into the gland. These problems can be detected easily if films are taken at each projection.

Before a lesion is made, stimulation is carried out at each lateral position of the spring electrode to detect any possible eye movements. If ocular motion is not observed at voltages less than 2 V, the lesion can then be produced. The stimulating current is 60 Hz, 2 msec.

The lesion is made with a radiofrequency generator. The ground is a 3.5-inch, 18-gauge spinal needle implanted in either deltoid. Each lesion is produced by bringing the temperature around the electrode tip as monitored by the thermocouples to 80°–90°C. The lesion duration is 120 seconds. As mentioned above, a series of lesions is made in anterior and posterior positions. This usually requires turning the outer cannula 22 degrees after each lesion. It is important, however, to be certain that the electrode tip is not above the line joining the dorsum sellae to the tuberculum sellae. In most instances the diaphragma sellae can be palpated, but it should not be taken for granted that it is intact. Lesions in the midline made with the electrode are to be carefully considered and avoided if possible. We have produced bitemporal hemianopsia in 2 patients, probably related to a positioning of the lateral spring that was excessively superior so that it apparently came into contact with the optic chiasm a few millimeters above the sella turcica. Such a high placement of the electrode is to be strenuously avoided.

Once the series of lesions has been completed, the electrode can be removed. To prevent cerebrospinal fluid rhinorrhea, fascia lata should be packed into the sella turcica using a double-pointed stylet with a tip 1 mm in cross section. Using the double-pronged instrument, small squares of tissue can easily be carried along the cannula directly through the anterior wall of the sella into the electrode tract. As these are advanced, the surgeon can feel the tract becoming filled. In order to avoid having to remove tissue from the patient, bovine fascia lata (Ethicon) can be used. This is very satisfactory material and has caused neither infection nor rejection. Once the tract appears to be filled, a dumbbell-shaped silicone plug can be impacted into the bone opening with the proper instrument. The plug we use contains silver particles so that its proper positioning can be confirmed radiographically. The cannula in the sphenoid sinus then is removed partially, and the sinus is again washed copiously with bacitracin solution. The cannula then is totally removed and a Vaseline gauze pack is placed in the appropriate nostril. This can be removed 8 hours later.

Following the operation the patient usually is in very good condition and has few restrictions.

POSTOPERATIVE MANAGEMENT

REPLACEMENT THERAPY

Hydrocortisone is given in the postoperative period, beginning with 200 mg/day, and is gradually reduced over a 6-day period to 30 mg/day in divided doses. Thyroid replacement can begin at any time in the postoperative period; usually 60 mg of thyroid extract will suffice.

It is very important that antibiotics be continued in the postoperative period for 5 days. Intravenous oxacillin, 1 g every

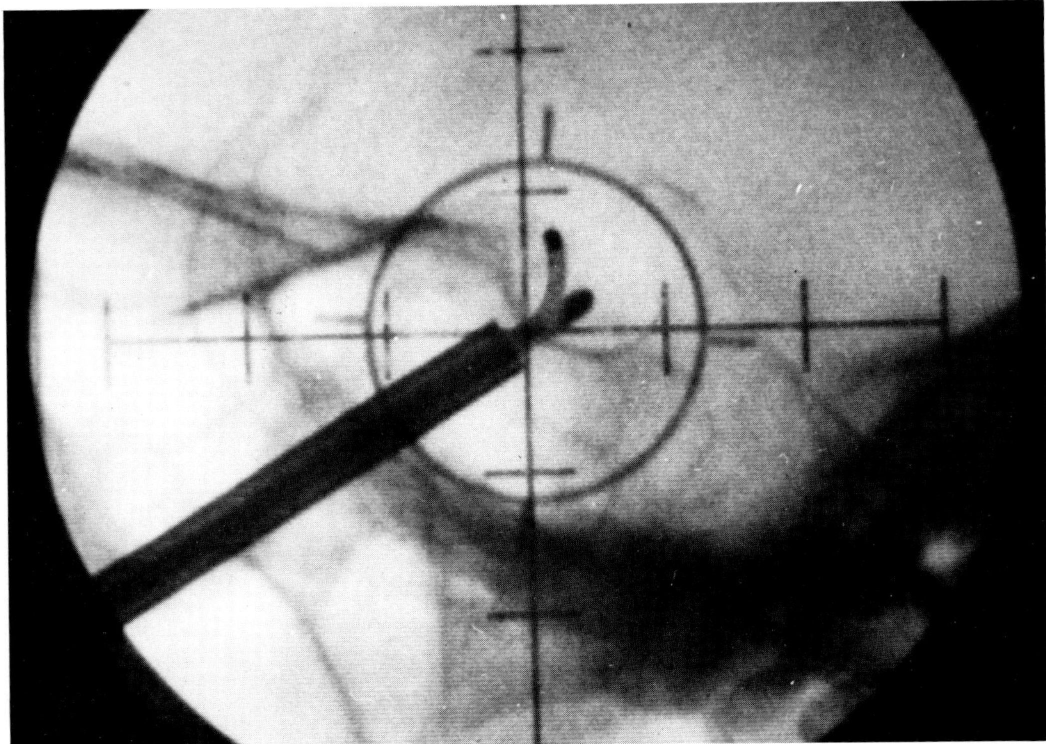

Fig. 30-3. A lateral roentgenogram showing the sidearm projecting up.

6 hours, is used for the first 2 days and then oral dicloxacillin, 1 g every 6 hours, for the final 3 days.

Diabetes insipidus occurs in almost every patient within 2 or 3 days after operation. It generally subsides within 1 to 2 weeks. If excessive in the beginning, it can be controlled with Pitressin Tannate in oil. Thereafter, it can be minimized by giving the patient chlorpropamide in a dose of 125 to 250 mg/day. If this is not adequate, desmopressin acetate (DDAVP) can be given as a nasal spray twice a day. The latter virtually eliminates diabetes insipidus in all patients who require long-term therapy. In our hands 1 patient in 20 will require treatment beyond 1 month after surgery. Desmopressin acetate appears to be the most satisfactory agent in controlling diabetes insipidus in the long term.

COMPLICATIONS

CEREBROSPINAL FLUID RHINORRHEA

Cerebrospinal fluid rhinorrhea is very rare when the sella has been packed and the anterior wall defect occluded. If it does occur, it should be repaired surgically, using the open transsphenoidal method to inspect the defect quickly. Some patients complain of wetness in the nose, particularly after eating spicy foods. Others worry excessively that a wet nose may mean that they have a cerebrospinal fluid leak. The surgeon should not be hastened into an unnecessary operation by concluding that wetness itself indicates rhinorrhea. The diagnosis should be confirmed by the actual collection of fluid from the nose that contains glucose and has a higher potassium level than serum. When in doubt, the diagnosis should be confirmed by radioactive isotope scanning after the intrathecal introduction of labeled isotope.

LOCAL INFECTION

We have not encountered an instance of infection in the sphenoid sinus or nasal cavities in over 600 cases with the exception of 1 patient who continuously complained of a greenish discharge from the nostril. However, 2 patients did develop intrasellar abscesses. The prodromal symptoms and signs were periorbital pain and fever in these 2 cases. As the processes developed rapidly, higher fever and stiff neck with pleocytosis of the cerebrospinal fluid developed. There was no evidence of cerebrospinal fluid rhinorrhea. In both instances, the sella turcica was opened stereotactically to permit drainage. This tactic, together with the administration of very large doses of antibiotics, resulted in total recovery in both instances. In both cases, these unfortunate complications developed in patients with diabetic retinopathy, and it is probable that the diabetic state was partially responsible for the development of the abscess. In addition, 1 patient inadvertently was not given antibiotics after operation.

HEMORRHAGE

Intraoperative hemorrhage from the sella turcica has not been encountered in any of the patients we operated upon. Two patients did develop epistaxis at the very beginning of the procedure, necessitating termination of the operation. Both of these hemorrhages were the result of thrombocytopenia, caused by chemotherapy for breast cancer.

CHAPTER 31

Craniopharyngiomas (With a Note on Rathke's Cleft or Epithelial Cysts and on Suprasellar Cysts)

William H. Sweet

SINCE ERDHEIM'S 1904 ACCOUNT, many have thought that slow-growing craniopharyngiomas arise from squamous epithelial rests persisting after most of the cells of the embryonic evagination from the stomodeum (Rathke's pouch) have differentiated into the pars anterior and intermedia of the pituitary gland.[1] These rests lie anywhere from the thin pars tuberalis, which encloses much of the upper end of the pituitary stalk and its junction with the hypothalamus, to down along the stalk and less often to the main adenohypophysis itself. Carmichael[2] found masses of cells resembling squamous epithelium in 33 percent of 55 postmortem specimens upon serial section of the human infundibulohypophyseal region, confirming earlier studies of Kiyono.[3] Other names for these tumors are adamantinoma, ameloblastoma, epithelioma, hypophyseal duct tumor, Rathke's pouch tumor or cyst, interpeduncular cyst, and suprasellar cyst. The terms *Rathke's cleft cyst* and *suprasellar cyst* are now applied properly to two other types of lesion that will be described separately.

In most countries of the world craniopharyngiomas constitute only about 3 percent of all intracranial tumors.[4] An exception is Japan, where the figure rises to 8 percent.[5] The incidence of craniopharyngioma is higher in childhood the world over, constituting 9 percent of 750 tumors in the report by Matson.[6] At the Mayo Clinic, Love and Marshall[7] noted that about half of the patients with craniopharyngioma were over 20 years old when they were treated, an age distribution also reported from several other clinics, including ours, treating both children and adults.

GROWTH CHARACTERISTICS

RATE OF GROWTH

Matson summarized one view on the growth rate of craniopharyngiomas, namely that "growth of this lesion is not neoplastic, but by desquamation of epithelial debris into closed spaces and by simple cellular proliferation of the epithelium" (p 544).[6] He therefore concluded that radiation had no place in the therapeutic regimen. However, a substantial group of distin-

Radiographic studies prepared in collaboration with Paul F. J. New

guished investigators proposed that these tumors arise by metaplasia of anterior pituitary cells into the squamous epithelium, which usually constitutes much of the solid part of the tumor (see Pertuiset[8] for relevant literature). There is an abundance of evidence to support Shillito's statement that "Recurrence of a large mass from a microscopic fragment left behind is almost certain." (p 198).[9] As an example, I left a tiny tumor fragment firmly attached to the chiasm in a 61-year-old patient (A.B.) because I presumed this congenital rest would give him no more trouble for the rest of his life. He returned 3½ years later with a massive, almost entirely cellular, solid tumor that had destroyed his chiasm and his left optic nerve. This sequence of events plus symptomatic recurrences in every major series after radical or presumed total removals has made a convincing case that these lesions are nearly always true tumors. The radiosensitivity of most of these masses is also consonant with their classification as neoplasms.

SITE AND DIRECTION OF GROWTH

Despite the relatively limited suprasellar area in which most of these tumors arise, they can grow in any of the possible directions therefrom or can exist in unusual sites. Where they come to lie is a major determinant of the route by which they should be attacked.

The most common sites for craniopharyngioma are immediately suprasellar, either (1) anterior to the chiasm, pushing it backward and rising up between and separating the optic nerves; (2) beneath the chiasm, pushing it upward and appearing to the surgeon in the prechiasmal area and perhaps behind the chiasm in the third ventricle after the lamina terminalis is opened, or (3) posterior to the chiasm, pushing it forward and the hypothalamus to either side, so that the tumor also lies within the third ventricle. Indeed, the craniopharyngioma was located here in 23 of the 40 patients in whom my initial operation was a radical resection. In this posterior position a modest-sized tumor can seem nonexistent at initial subfrontal inspection. Figure 31-1A shows the normal appearance of the suprasellar area upon easy exposure of virtually the entire lamina terminalis. The tumor was 2 cm in diameter and lay completely within the third ventricle. Figure 31-1B shows the

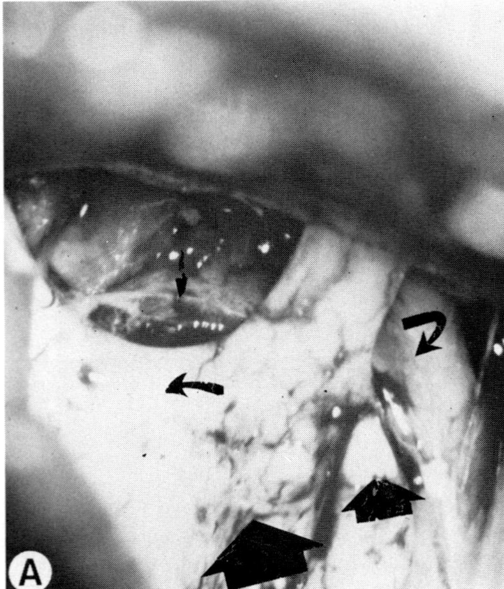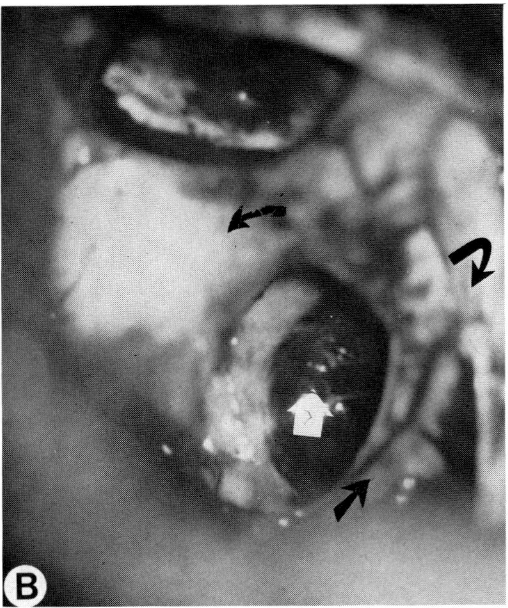

Fig. 31-1. Patient G.J. Right subfrontal approach to the suprasellar area. The CT scan showed a 2-cm mass filling the anterior end of the third ventricle. (A) Although the mass also indented the posteroinferior aspect of the frontal horns, at the initial exposure no mass was obvious and the lamina terminalis (large arrowhead pointing upward) looked normal, as did all the other structures. The small curved arrow pointing downward indicates the dorsum sellae with empty space behind it; the curved arrow overlies the chiasm; the recurring arrow lies on the right internal carotid artery; the medium-sized arrowhead lies on the right optic tract. (B) After removal of the thinned-out lamina terminalis and the entire tumor, the deep-lying intact floor of the hypothalamus became evident (white arrowhead). The more superficial structures of Figure 31-1A are out of focus. The curved black arrow is on the chiasm; the straight black arrow is on the right anterior cerebral artery, the medial part of which has eased downward and forward into view after removal of the tumor; the recurving black arrow on the right internal carotid artery points to the origin of the right anterior cerebral artery from the internal carotid.

appearance of the suprasellar area after the tumor presumably had been totally removed.

Autopsies of 30 Czech and Russian patients, 11 of whom did not undergo surgery and 19 in whom the tumor was only partially removed, permitted Steno to analyze the precise microsurgical topographic relationship of these lesions.[10] Four were intrasuprasellar, and of the 26 suprasellar tumors 4 were extraventricular, 14 intra-extraventricular, and 8 intraventricular.

A small percentage of these tumors are exclusively intrasellar. This was the site in 3 of Northfield's 37 patients.[11] Although the early account of Love and Marshall stated that in 33 of 100 cases "the principal part of the tumor was in the sella, deepening it in all directions,"[7] improved diagnostic methods have shown that the great majority of craniopharyngiomas are largely extrasellar. There are seven recent reports of largely intrasellar craniopharyngiomas with a clinical picture of a prolactin-secreting adenoma, i.e., amenorrhea, galactorrhea, and hyperprolactinemia. No calcification was present in one of the tumors. All three abnormalities disappeared soon after transsphenoidal operations.[12,13] Neoplastic compression of the hypothalamus or the region of the stalk presumably prevented the portal system from delivering the prolactin-inhibiting factor. These authors cite 4 previous cases. There is a report of a single case of a tumor wholly within the chiasm, which was diagnosed by biopsy and treated by radiation.[14]

In case 1 of Hamberger et al.,[15] the craniopharyngiomatous cyst filled the sphenoid sinus and completely eroded away the bony sellar floor but did not invade the capsule of the hypophysis and was radically removed by a transsphenoidal

approach. The tumor also arose in the sphenoid bone in a patient described by Cooper and Ransohoff.[16] They cited three other cases from the literature. In their patient the tumor had eroded the base of the skull as seen on roentgenograms obtained in 1933. By the time of the patient's death in 1970, the tumor had replaced the sphenoid body, its left greater wing, and both left pterygoid processes, plus the medial temporal bone and had extended upward as a large intradural mass invaginating the left temporal lobe. The pituitary gland and diaphragma sellae looked normal! A happier sequence ensued in a similar case reported by Pheline et al.[17] The typical intrasellar calcification of this tumor in a 12-year-old girl was accompanied by a downward growth that wiped out the body of the sphenoid and filled the nasopharynx down to the palate. The basilar artery was displaced posteriorly and the right carotid laterally. The tumor recurred after an attempt at removal through a nasoseptal approach but was apparently completely removed through an antroethmoidal route. The authors cited seven other such cases since 1970 from four centers; these should be consulted if one has such a problem. Fitz et al.[18] described still another patient with a tumor 76 mm in greatest dimension with a calcified high suprasellar shell extending straight downward and nearly filling the patient's nasopharynx. It was when it reached this site that it caused the first symptom, a change of voice. Mukada et al.[19] described another similarly placed tumor, largely infrasellar and nasopharyngeal, that destroyed the central part of the sphenoid bone but with a major suprasellar calcified portion. A sublabial, rhinoseptal approach revealed the cheerful fact that the tumor originated extradurally and was therefore largely removable by the route used. In a unique autobiographical account, Maier[20]

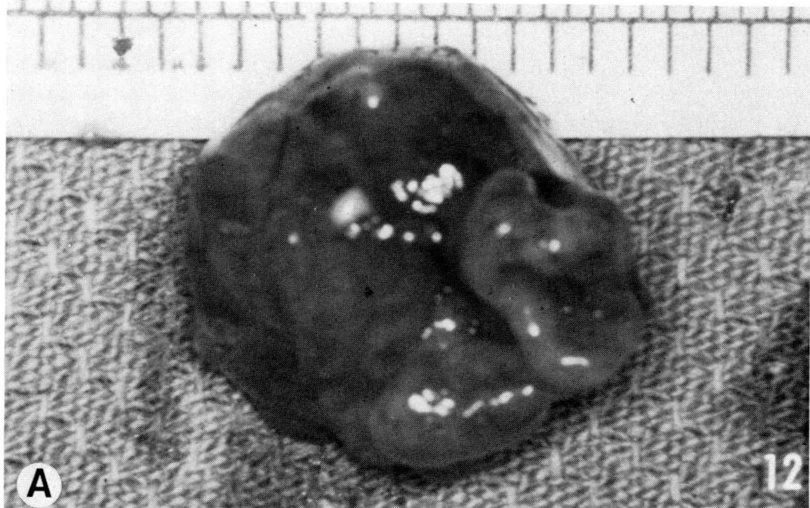

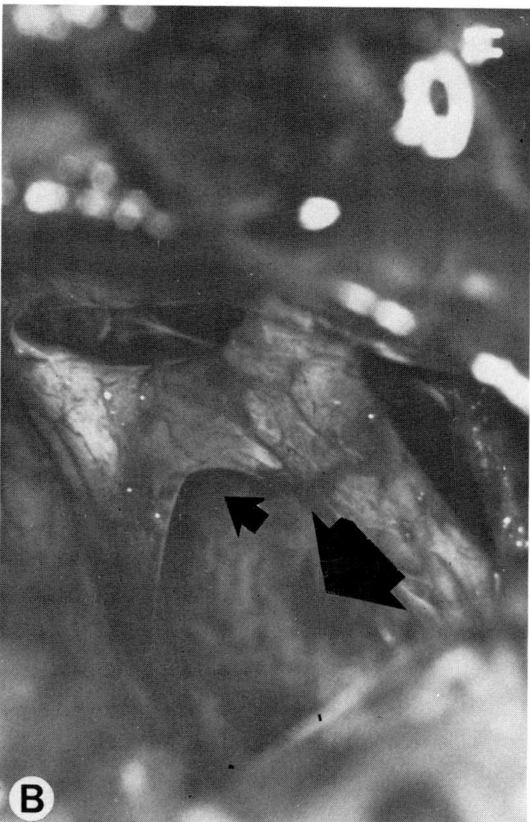

Fig. 31-2. Patient S.S. (A) A relatively intact tumor capsule after removal of its entirely solid content. The specimen is 19 mm at its longest point and without gaps, suggesting removal may have been complete. (The scale at the top is in millimeters.) The capsule was maintained during removal to avoid loss of any of it. (B) The chiasm and retrochiasmal area after radical removal via the lamina terminalis of the craniopharyngioma of Figure 31–2A, which was mostly within the third ventricle. At the base of the large black arrowhead on the right is the optic tract; the arrowhead is pointing at thin hemorrhage in the hypothalamic floor. The small arrow on the hypothalamic floor points toward the posterior edge of the middle of the chiasm. Beneath the chiasm and not visible except with a mirror is a hole in the anteroinferior wall of the third ventricle. A small amount of tumor anterior and inferior to the chiasm is more readily removed by pushing it behind into the third ventricle through this hole than by withdrawing it from in front of the anteriorly displaced chiasm.

described the 65-year history of his intrasellar and intrasphenoid tumor that treated itself by intermittent drainings of its cystic content into the nasopharynx for 30 years, supplemented by two courses of radiation, the first of 2400 rad and, 25 years later in 1963, of 4100 rad. The second case of Halves[21] demonstrated another odd type of growth. Having removed the tumor in two stages using a subfrontal approach right down to emptying the sella, he completed via a transsphenoidal third stage the removal of both a solid and cystic tumor that lay below a thin layer of bone thought to have been the intact sellar floor at the previous operation.

Several of us have seen the cyst extend backward and downward the full length of the posterior fossa to the foramen magnum.[22,23] Petito et al.,[24] studying 245 cases of craniopharyngioma in the files of the Armed Forces Institute of Pathology, found that 12 percent of the tumors extended into the posterior fossa. Altinörs et al.[25] described a lad in whom the predominant location of the mass in one cerebellopontine angle produced localizing deficits only in the ipsilateral fifth, seventh, and eighth cranial nerves.

Despite its customary origin from cells lying on the outer surface of the infundibulum or hypothalamus, a craniopharyngioma can unquestionably arise from above the intact hypothalamic floor and lateral walls, filling some or all of the third ventricle. This important possibility precludes an approach inferolaterally via the middle fossa unless the tumor erodes through the hypothalamic floor. Figure 31-2A shows a craniopharyngioma after it was removed from the third ventricle via a window in the lamina terminalis, and Figure 31-2B shows the

intact inferoposterior hypothalamic floor after the tumor had been removed. Figure 31-3A illustrates another similar disposition of tumor causing constriction of the right anterior cerebral artery. After the tumor, which was entirely within the third ventricle, was removed, the artery became much larger. Cashion and Young[26] found such a locus in 2 cases they studied critically at post mortem. Long and Chou,[27] Fitz et al.,[18] King,[28] Papo et al.,[29] Rush et al.,[30] and Al-Mefty et al.[31] also reported such cases. Solarski et al.,[32] in a postmortem study, described an asymptomatic, partially cystic craniopharyngioma that replaced the pineal gland; there was no tumor in the third ventricle or hypothalamus. A significant posterior extension from the third ventricle into the region of the pineal gland led Wilson to use a suboccipital approach in 2 patients.[33]

A common direction of growth is upward and forward, displacing one or both frontal ventricular horns upward as illustrated by my case 2 (p 55).[22] Still another growth quirk of these tumors is illustrated by the computed tomographic (CT) scan shown in Figure 31-4. The largest component of this dumbbell-shaped tumor, which greatly dilated the sella, extended into the anterior part of the interhemispheric fissure and expanded on the right side in a configuration somewhat simulating the right frontal horn. This radiographic series obtained with the next-to-last generation of CT scanner demonstrates less detail than can now be seen with the latest devices. Craniopharyngiomas may follow along any or many of the basal arteries laterally into the medial sylvian fissure with the middle cerebral artery, posteriorly along the posterior communicating

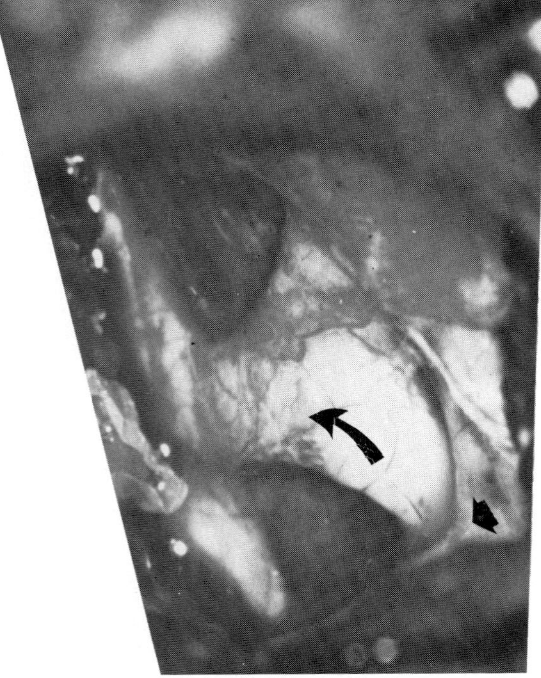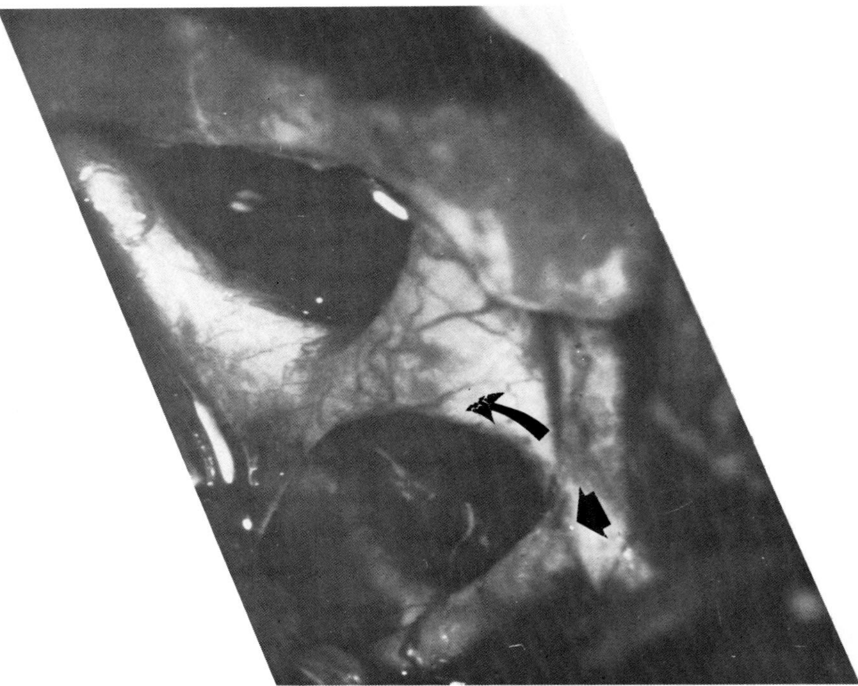

Fig. 31-3.   Patient C.N. (A) A craniopharyngioma after partial removal from behind the chiasm. The curved arrow points to the still-bulging chiasm. The arrowhead lying on the right internal carotid artery points to a still tiny right anterior cerebral artery. (B) The craniopharyngioma after radical removal from behind the chiasm. Arrows as in Figure 31-3A. The chiasm is now flat. The anterior cerebral artery is now dilated after removal of neoplastic pressure from deep to it. Note the much larger working space behind the chiasm and between the optic tracts as tumor has been withdrawn forward; this permits backward displacement of the anterior cerebral arteries toward the empty third ventricle.

artery, and around the brainstem with the posterior cerebral artery.

In children, craniopharyngiomas rarely may compress enough of one or both cerebral arteries to produce the abnormal local small vessel network characteristic of moyamoya or "puff of smoke" disease.[34,35]

MICROSCOPIC FEATURES

Numerous authors have described a dense gliotic covering to craniopharyngiomas which intervenes between the epithelial neoplastic cells and the normal brain tissue. Such articles were cited in my 1976 paper beginning with the graphic accounts in the book of Bailey, Buchanan, and Bucy[36] and including those of Van den Bergh and Brucher.[37] The gliosis often includes an abundance of the eosinophilic tadpole-shaped Rosenthal fibers.

Pertuiset[8] is a recent exponent of the view that the "layer of gliosis surrounding the small papillary tumor extensions and separating them from the nerve cells" makes it "obvious that any dissection can damage the normal tissue." Landolt[38] studied biopsy specimens of five of these tumors under an electron microscope. In three of the specimens he found extensive glial tissue on that aspect of the retrochiasmatic portion of the tumor in contact with the brain. In these sections there was not only a gliotic boundary zone, but also penetration of glia well into the tumor. In the biopsy specimen of one tumor entirely within the third ventricle, however, he identified no glial tissue. In general he noted that the basal membranes of the epithelial tumor cells were separated from the basal membranes of the glia by a few collagen fibers. This may possibly be the plane of cleavage that helps the surgeon draw frankly neoplastic epithelial cells away

Fig. 31-4.   Patient S.A. Craniopharyngioma. (A,B,C, and D) CT scans with contrast enhancement (horizontal slices) obtained preoperatively (December 19, 1980). (A) At the level of the upper sella. The arrow indicates the intrasellar cyst with its thick wall enhanced by contrast. (B) At the suprasellar level through the lowest parts of the frontal lobes. The arrow indicates the neck of the tumor with only a tiny cystic component. (C) At a level through the full length of the third ventricle and the lowest part of the frontal horn of the left lateral ventricle. The right frontal horn is compressed to invisibility by an upward extension of the cyst into the interhemispheric fissure. In the lateral wall of the cyst is an obvious plaque of calcification. The recurving arrow points to an interval between the two small forward-projecting horns of the cyst. The posterior arrow is pointing forward and to the right to a less obvious calcified plaque at the posteromedial surface of this cyst. (D) A higher horizontal level (the right side of the head is on the left in this scan from a later-generation scanner). The configuration suggesting a dilated right anterior horn is in fact an expansion of the cyst. The anterior arrow points to its irregular anterior wall; the middle arrow points to the calcification in its medial wall; the posterior arrow points to the posterior wall. (E) Coronal reconstruction obtained preoperatively (December 19, 1980). (The right side of the patient is on the right.) The arrows with curved shafts point to the medial and lateral bits of calcification in the cyst wall. The straight-shafted arrow points to the bulbous lateral expansion of the cyst. (F) (The right side of the head is on the right. We have deliberately presented the illustrations in this way to draw attention to the confusion caused by the convention in early generation scanners of showing the right side of the patient on the right—a convention that has been reversed in the later models.) That the interpretation of neoplastic cyst replacing the anterior part of the right lateral ventricle is correct is shown further by this scan obtained 4 months later with metrizamide in the ventricles and subarachnoid space. The head has been tilted to the left to show that a small amount of metrizamide is filling the posterior part of the cyst, forming a horizontal fluid level corresponding to the angle of tilt. The short straight-shafted arrow points to the small dense metrizamide shadow. The curved arrows point to the main cyst, which is communicating only slightly with the ventricles.

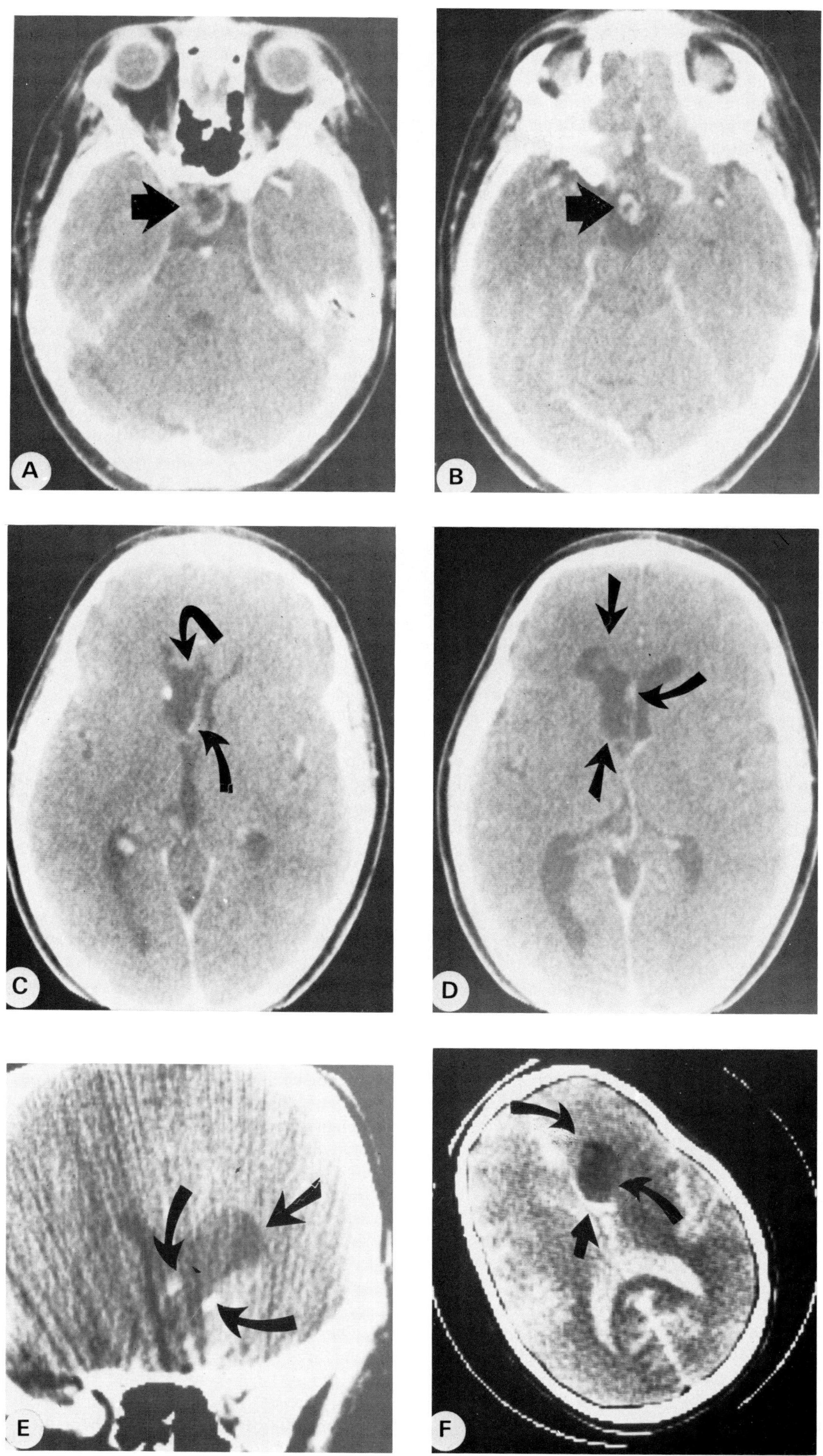

from the glia, decreasing the injury to the brain beyond. The gliosis surrounding and penetrating well into the main mass of tumor has been and continues to be regarded by some as a feature that precludes total removal of that portion of a craniopharyngioma impinging on brain tissue. Shillito stated that "the layer of gliosis around the tumor may be either too dense and adherent to the brain or too non-existent to be of value."[23] I should add that both problems can be present in the same tumor. Kobayashi et al.[39] studied at autopsy 7 patients from three different centers who had had "no major surgery on these tumors." They examined particularly the relationship between the tumor and adjacent neural tissue. In the cystic parts of the tumors they found a layer of Rosenthal fibers and fibrillary astrocytes, from several hundred microns to a few millimeters in thickness, between the cyst wall and viable ganglion cells in the thalamus or hypothalamus.

Bartlett[40] also studied the relationships of craniopharyngioma to surrounding brain in 12 cases. He found the gliotic or collagenous reaction to be a feature of "the fast-growing tumors." Although he concluded that in these it was only in the exceptional case that one could remove the tumor totally, his illustration showed *"gliotic reaction which separates the tumor from normal brain."* (italics are mine). In the slow-growing type of craniopharyngioma it "usually fell out of its bed at the autopsy," because there was so little reaction to it or tissue invasion by it—which is surely an encouraging finding from the surgeon's standpoint. Hoffman et al.[41] also saw bits of tumor so intimately invading the wall of the internal carotid artery as to be irremovable.

From the standpoint of what is feasible surgically, I point out that of 43 patients on whom my first operation was the first attempt at radical removal, I decided against continuing the attempt in only three. The operative specimen of only one of them (J.D.) showed histologically hypothalamic tissue firmly adherent to the dense astroglia, and hence the cleavage plane lay within the hypothalamus. This patient died postoperatively from both wound infection and hypothalamic injury. The second extensive removal transfrontally in this patient followed 14 years after my first such effort on him, at which time I had left tumor behind attached to the internal carotid artery. The second effort was 9 years after symptomatic tumor recurrence, by which time he was desperately ill. Another patient (A.M.) was treated with 3000 rads of radiation to her presumed third ventricular pinealoma in 1949. By 1973 the center of her brain was a solid mass of tumor. The central part was cored out readily via the lamina terminalis, but separation of the periphery from the brain was clearly impossible. In another patient (W.W.), a partial removal elsewhere in 1970 was followed 18 months later by a ventriculoatrial shunt, 4500 rad of radiation delivered during 6 weeks, and 2 months later by aspiration of a cyst at another craniotomy. At our operation in October, 1979, Poletti and I concluded with only a partial removal; as we sought to separate the tumor from the main arteries, the bleeding we encountered was in contrast to the usual absence of this problem when radiation has not been given years earlier. The patient remains disabled.

These 3 patients are the only ones in my series of initial radical operations in whom continuing gentle traction and dissection applied to the mixture of gliotic, fibrous, and epithelial cells in contact with brain did not bring forth a specimen free of neurons yet rid the patient of all or nearly all the tissue suggestive of tumor. The peripheral portions of some surgically removed specimens, however, have looked frighteningly like normal brain upon inspection at the operating table. In 10 such cases I called this worrisome gross appearance to the attention of our neuropathologist, but he saw no neurons or nerve fibers, only gliosis with occasional epithelial pearls.

In summary, my experience has been that in the great majority of patients the actual cleavage plane, either through glia or beyond a capsule, did not include neuronal nuclei or visual fiber tracts. The only three exceptions to this had their tumors growing for 9 to 24 years; two of these had had radiation therapy to the region 7 and 24 years before operation, presumably furthering a fibrotic reaction. It is reasonable to conclude that the histologic appearance, which has been interpreted by some as a tenacious, glial, insurmountable barrier to total or nearly total removal, may in fact be the reverse. The functionless glia may provide a significant margin of safety between the growing epithelial cells to be excised and the vitally important thalamohypothalamic and visual structures that should be preserved intact. I venture to regard this concept as my principal contribution to the subject.

Once that gliotic barrier has been removed during a presumed total excision, but recurrence nevertheless takes place, the glial cells probably do not regrow. This may be the reason that secondary efforts after an initial radical excision are more dangerous.

Shillito's other point that portions of the capsule may be extremely fragile is well taken.[23] This feature has led me to preserve the capsule so that, after intracapsular removal, intact sheets of it remain even if the boundary tissues are torn at a number of points. One can thus stay oriented to the plane for final dissection and avoid leaving behind torn-off bits of thin capsule. The islands of tumor cells remaining within functioning thalamus and hypothalamus described by Kobayashi et al.[39] cause clinical recurrences when a "total removal" was thought to have been achieved in markedly varying percentages of patients, depending on the surgeon.

Kahn et al.[42] described histologically a childhood type of tumor in 48 of their 60 cases with a tendency for more rapid growth and recurrence, and an "adult type" with nonkeratinizing squamous epithelium similar to that of the oropharyngeal mucosa in the remaining 12 patients, 11 of whom were adults. In this smaller group "some tumor was knowingly left in the majority; yet none of these has required reoperation for recurrence." Exactly the reverse position was taken by Cogen and Carmel[43] after their study of 109 craniopharyngioma patients (66 adults and 44 children) operated on between 1952 and 1977 at the New York Neurological Institute. Although they found no histologic differences in the two age groups, the children did much better than the adults. This was especially convincing in the relapse-free survival rates after "total" removal. In the children 77 percent had no recurrence after 5 years and 47 percent had no recurrence after 10 years, whereas in the adults far fewer were free of recurrence—36 percent at 5 years and 16 percent at 10 years. Bloom[44] also found that children do much better than adults. Studying material from our service under the electron microscope, Liszczak et al.[45] defined an "atypical" "aggressive" morphology in 3 of 13 cases. Only one of the three tumors has in fact grown rapidly clinically, and none of the other 10 "typical" types has recurred either. In a study of the 125 operative survivors who underwent less than a "total" tumor removal between 1950 and 1979 at the University of Tokyo, Manaka et al.[46] in 1985 found slightly better survival times for adults than children both in the groups with and without postoperative irradiation. The difference in survival

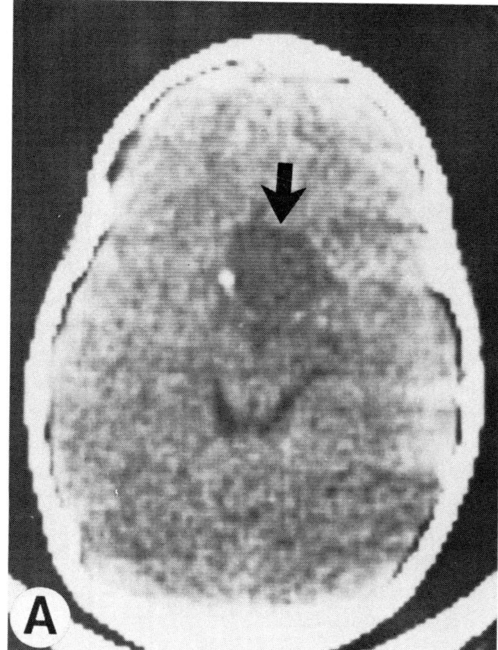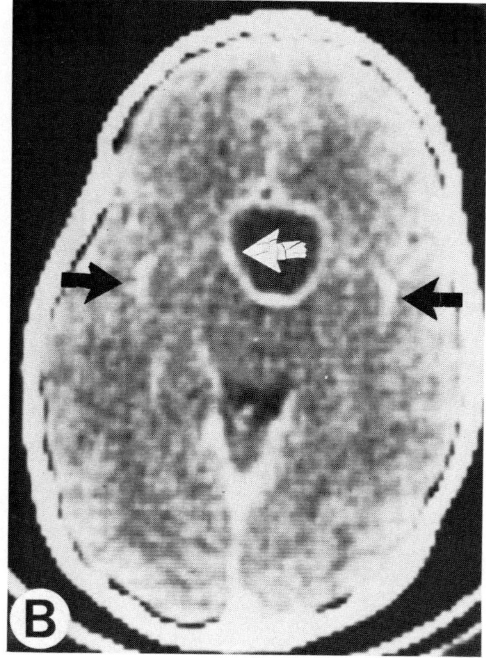

Fig. 31-5. Patient A.B. Craniopharyngiomatous cyst. Comparison of scans with and without contrast at a horizontal level about 1 cm above the floor of the anterior cranial fossa. (A) Area of decreased photon density (black arrow) with a fleck of calcification at one point in the wall. (B) Striking demonstration of the neoplastic wall after injection of Renografin IV; the white arrow points to calcification still visible in the wall. The black arrows point to the middle cerebral arteries.

times between the two cell types, squamous versus adamantinomatous, was "minimal."

CLINICAL PRESENTATION

The multiplicity of possible directions of growth of craniopharyngiomas is mirrored by a corresponding variation in the clinical pictures they may present. The first mechanisms to be involved are usually visual or hypothalamo-hypophyseal or both. Frontal, temporal, or posterior fossa symptoms will develop later or may be the initial features if the growth is in those directions, along with manifestations of blockage of cerebrospinal fluid pathways. Because moderate visual disturbances are so often missed, especially in children, the symptoms that finally bring these patients to the physician may be those of increased intracranial pressure. Six of our patients (four children, two adults) were nearly blind when we first saw them. A number of articles plead for a high index of suspicion vis-à-vis such a locus of lesion upon any intimation of visual trouble. Special techniques may be necessary to discover field defects in young children, such as fixed and moving balls, observation of play, of other behavior and specifically the use of toys.[47] The neurosurgeon would do well to make sure the ophthalmologic consultant is using these methods of examination. There is a single case report in which the only visual deficit was an internal ophthalmoplegia—a paralysis of accommodation and dilated sluggish pupils.[48]

In another group of patients, often adults, a symptom wrongly attributed to psychiatric or diffuse mental disorder dominates the clinical picture. The patient of Klotz et al.[49] thus was treated for 8 years for anorexia nervosa and "secondary amenorrhea," despite an initial episode of polydipsia, until loss of vision led to the correct diagnosis. Three of Kahn's adult patients had Korsakoff's syndrome.[42] He found only one such report of a child.

Now that CT and MRI scanning achieve such high resolution and are being used so much we shall be seeing more patients in whom the diagnosis is made incidental to studies for other reasons. The pediatrician of our most astutely diagnosed patient suspected an endocrine growth problem when the patient at age 16 was only 5 feet 4 inches (163 cm) tall and weighed only 115 pounds (52 kg). He entertained this suspicion even though the father did not reach his full height of 5 feet 11 inches until age 19 and a maternal uncle "matured slowly." Despite this minimal symptom and normal neurologic and visual examination the CT scan revealed a tumor 2 cm in diameter. Rather than observe the patient with serial scans we removed the tumor radically, and 7 years later having completed his university degree "with flying colors," he is a computer expert.

RADIOGRAPHIC STUDIES (WITH THE COLLABORATION OF PAUL F. NEW)

Cranial computed tomography (CT) and magnetic resonance imaging (MRI) scans have added dramatically to our preoperative and postoperative knowledge in these patients. In the CT scans without contrast the solid portions of the tumor have a radiographic density equal to or a little higher than normal brain. Contrast enhancement occurs in the majority of the cases (in 29 of 32 reported by Cabezudo et al.[50] and in 27 of 40 reported by Gardeur et al.[51]). This is seen in various portions of the solid tumor or in the wall of the cysts (Figure 31-5). The cystic fluid rarely contains enough cholesterol-like material to

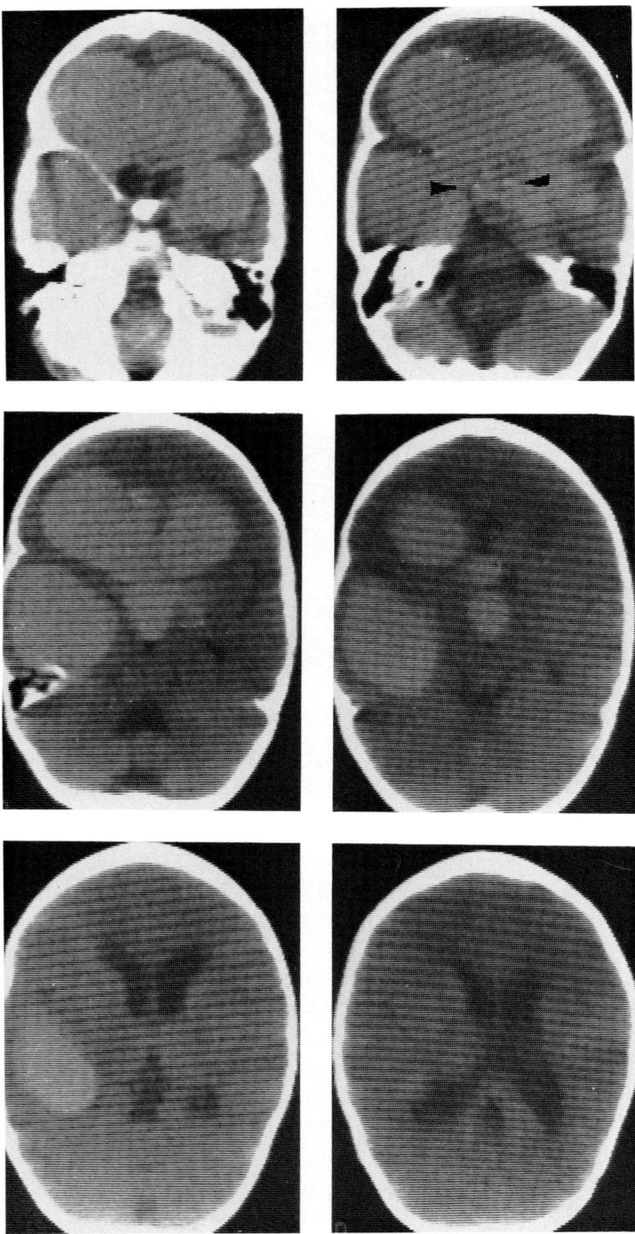

Fig. 31-6. An extraordinary craniopharyngioma reported by Maurice Lipper. Enormous high-density lesions are present bilaterally in the frontal and temporal regions; the left is larger than the right. A clue to the diagnosis were the low-density zones in the suprasellar regions containing calcification (arrows in upper right-hand scan).

give it a density as low as −80 Hounsfield units (reference level 0 = absorption of water). The cystic fluid nearly always has a density less than the 28 to 35 Hounsfield units (HU) characteristic of normal white matter but may have a similar or even greater density on occasion. (Normal gray matter is 36 to 48 HU). The cyst range usually is from 2 to 19 HU.[52,53] As New and Aronow[54] have shown, however, protein in fluid, such as the globin fraction of hemoglobin, can greatly increase the density on CT scans. Craniopharyngiomas may extend in all possible directions from their usual immediately suprasellar locus, even into the cerebellopontine angle cistern, and these extensions may be graphically portrayed in the scan. For example, one extraordinary lesion reported by Lipper et al.[55] not only obliterated the third ventricle but extended as huge,

lobulated, high-density cysts into the lower frontal and temporal regions on both sides! It originally was thought to be a solid tumor because of its high density of 46–54 HU (Figure 31-6). In another case an isodense, nonenhancing, noncalcified left temporal mass proved to be a huge cystic craniopharyngioma with a protein content of 9.2 g/100 ml.[56]

Even minute bits of calcification are also more clearly brought out in CT scans than in ordinary skull films, and their characteristic calcific density of greater than 100 HU is measured precisely on the plain scan as the numerical absorption value at which the suspicious point changes from white to black (on measure mode). Thus, Cabezudo et al.[53] found calcification on CT scans in 82 percent of 33 patients but on plain films in only 57 percent. In Symon's 20 cases the figures for the presence of calcification were 45 percent on CT scans compared with 25 percent on plain films.[57] Histologic examinations show calcification in even more of the patients, e.g., in 91 percent of 43 cases at the Columbia Medical Center.[58] It was also seen on CT scans in all but 1 of the 20 "giant" tumors reported by Al-Mefty.[31] Postradiation calcification in the basal ganglia has been reported by Danoff et al.[59] and Fischer et al.[60] Fischer and his colleagues described "brain mineralization in 12 of 23 children, in the basal ganglia in 10 and in the hypothalamus and frontal lobes in 1 case." In this last case it was accompanied by a progressive learning and memory defect.

Converting the data to coronal and sagittal or other projections than the standard horizontal plane is fruitful since successive scans at 1-mm intervals can now be made. These are especially valuable in studying the sellar and parasellar region in the case of craniopharyngiomas to detect tumor remnants in order to guide either a further prompt removal, radiation therapy, or a follow-up of any further growth. The series in Figure 31-4 shows another unusual configuration, portrayed conclusively in the scans, in which a large intrasellar cyst is connected by a narrow midportion to an expanded cyst extending up between the frontal lobes.

We compare the relative merits of CT and MRI scans for parasellar tumors in Chapter 25 "Gliomas of the Anterior Visual Pathways."

PNEUMOGRAPHY AND TOMOGRAPHY OF THE SELLAR AREA

The progressively increasing resolution of the scanners and facile means of data analysis that have been developed in the last few years have eliminated the need for pneumography and tomography. Until recently, when greater detail was required to elucidate any questionable points, a small dose of isotonic metrizamide introduced into the subarachnoid space was likely to give the same or more information with less risk and discomfort than the use of air or oxygen. Figure 31-4F illustrates this point. Patterson and Danylevich[61] reported the case of a patient in whom two CT scans 16 months apart were normal on an older type scanner, but in whom a pneumoencephalogram revealed a suprasellar mass.

ANGIOGRAPHY

The use of rapid intravenous injections of boluses of contrast medium in conjunction with rapid, high-resolution CT scanning usually permits satisfactory evaluation of the relationship of a tumor to the cavernous sinuses and major basal arteries. As Hoffman recently pointed out, the largely intrasellar tumors displace neither the A1 segments of the anterior

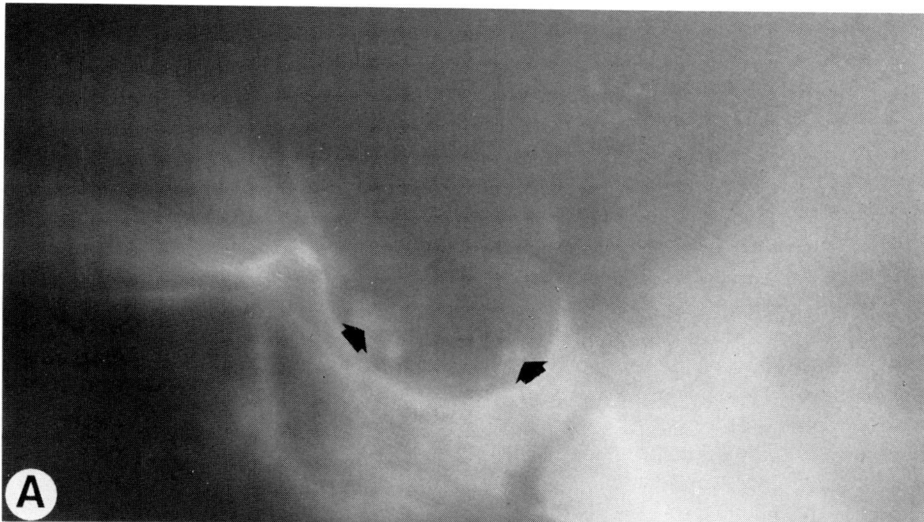

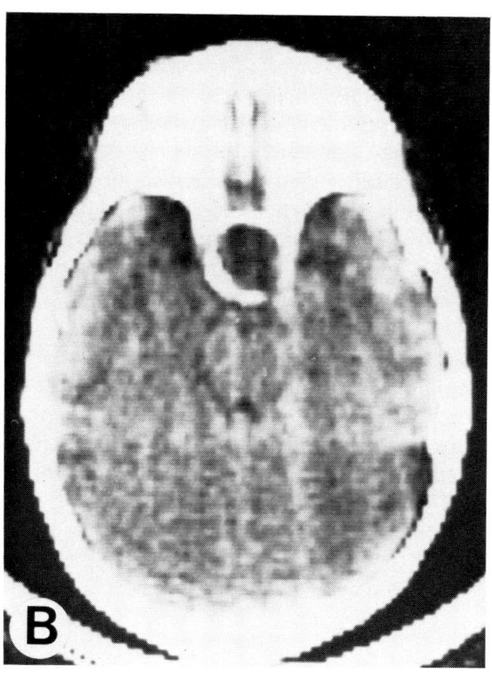

Fig. 31-7. Patient R.L. (A) A pneumoencephalogram. The large craniopharyngioma is almost obliterating the third ventricle with suprasellar and retrosellar calcification. Black arrow: wisps of air in the posterosuperior aspect of the third ventricle. (B) Vertebral arteriogram. The anterior thalamo-perforating arteries are displaced markedly backward in an arc that is concave forward (curved black arrows). This suggests that the tumor could be approached laterally after elevation of the temporal lobe or removal of the temporal tip as advocated by Symon and Logue. Straight black arrow: calcification in the tumor.

cerebral arteries nor the basilar artery, whereas tumors bulging up between the two optic nerves elevate the former vessels, and those pushing the basilar artery backward also push the chiasm forward into a "prefixed" position.[62] The anterior and posterior thalamo-perforating arteries cannot be demonstrated consistently without direct arteriography (Figure 31-7). If a lateral approach to a lesion invading the third ventricle is considered, knowledge of the locus of these vessels is helpful. Otherwise, angiography may be unnecessary because craniopharyngiomas have an insignificant arterial supply, especially if appropriately configured and placed calcification supports the diagnosis. We know of only a single case report of this type of tumor staining at angiography.[63] A sizeable suprasellar aneurysm, however, may have a deceptively thin calcified shell and contain a large amount of lamellar thrombus, which may be misconstrued as a craniopharyngioma unless the high density of the contrast-enhanced fluid blood in a portion of the aneurysm is recognized. This density should be compared with that in the larger cerebral vessels displayed at the same time. Jakubowski and Kendall[64]

described aneurysms coincidental with intrasellar or suprasellar tumors. They found only one aneurysm among the angiograms of their 33 craniopharyngiomas; it extended medial to the intracavernous carotid and was not seen during surgery.

Other lesions that can occasionally appear on CT scans as craniopharyngiomas and for which angiography may be helpful in the differential diagnosis and the planning of the operation include suprasellar meningiomas and pituitary adenomas with cystic extensions. Cavernous angiomas, suprasellar teratomas, and hypothalamic gliomas or hamartomas are all rare but possibly can be mistaken for a craniopharyngioma. Chiasmal or chiasmohypothalamic gliomas may have calcification in or near them and are often misdiagnosed as craniopharyngiomas.

TREATMENT: RADICAL SURGERY

The relatively benign growth characteristics of craniopharyngiomas have made their aggressive surgical management seem logical to neurosurgeons since the first decades of neurosurgery. However, their villous prolongations into the surrounding brain and the protean metabolic derangements consequent upon dissections in and about the hypothalamus led to disillusionment, especially after attempts at total removal. Northfield[11] concluded that the treatment of these patients "is fraught with difficulty and disappointment to a degree probably not offered by any other intracranial tumor with the exception of the glioblastoma." The report of Svolos on 106 patients operated upon by Olivecrona from 1924 to 1958 and who were followed for up to 31 years typifies other data on which such pessimism was founded.[65] Although only 25 patients, presumably the most favorable, underwent radical extirpation of their tumors, 40 percent of them died. Of the 50 patients who did not die until later, only "15 could be classified as useful survivals." There were only 30 alive at the time of the report.

Kahn's earlier experience with craniopharyngiomas led him to recommend a radical approach,[66] but he later withdrew from this stance with respect to these tumors in children. Rapid recurrence in this age group "where we were quite certain the tumor had been totally removed," and greater difficulty in controlling the endocrine deficits of children than those of adults led him to settle for less than a total removal "unless the tumor can be readily mobilized." These conclusions were based upon his experience with 28 children upon whom he had operated between 1947 and 1970. Nine of his 12 adults were in good or excellent shape and "led a relatively normal life," whereas this was achieved in only 21 percent of the children. Even three adults who preoperatively had marked confusion and memory loss "due to compression of the mammillary bodies" made a complete recovery.

The first neurosurgeon to maintain a record that he felt justified a radical operation as the initial procedure was Matson. His last report of 34 patients in this category, who had been operated on between 1950 and 1968, the last 18 years of Matson's operative career, revealed 22 still living without recurrence. He had achieved the spectacular record of no postoperative mortality in this group. On the other hand, there were six postoperative deaths in 24 patients on whom he reoperated—9 of his original 34 patients because of recurrence and 15 patients whose first operation was performed by another surgeon. The quality of survival was classified by Katz as follows: "Excellent"—normal independent functioning; "good"—functioning well despite deficiency; "fair"—functional but dependent; and "poor"—nonfunctional. Of the 22 survivors of the initial radical operation, 9 had "excellent" results and 6 had "good" results.[67]

On the basis of an independent appraisal of the facts and concurrently with Matson, I too began a program of radical removal. I was stimulated to do this in the first instance by a distinguished neurologist who referred to me for operation a much-loved close relative with the proviso that I would totally remove her tumor even if my impression at surgery was that persistence toward this goal would cause a greater than 95 percent chance of mortality. He said he took this remarkable attitude because of his conclusion that the life of a patient undergoing repeated partial removals and cyst aspirations became progressively less worth living. The total extirpation of her solid craniopharyngioma in 1953 went surprisingly well and provided a strong impetus to continue the series. The late results of my radical removals were similar to those of Matson and will be presented after a discussion of operative methods. My loneliness in 1975 in advocating an aggressive attack on these lesions was dissipated by the publications of Hoffman et al.,[41,62,68] Patterson and Danylevich,[61] Symon et al.,[57,69] Till,[70] Al-Mefty et al.,[31] and Sorva and Heiskanen.[71]

TECHNIQUE FOR RADICAL REMOVAL VIA TRANSFRONTAL ROUTE

Initial Phase

Matson and I have confined our approaches almost exclusively to the transfrontal route, a view shared by Hoffman[41] and by Patterson and Danylevich.[61] Despite the many directions in which a craniopharyngioma can grow, we all found that any firm attachments of tumor have been to the pituitary stalk, the thalamohypothalamus, the visual pathways, or nearby arteries of the anterior part of the circle of Willis. The transfrontal route gives good exposure of these critical areas—as does the pterional route recommended by Symon.[69]

I have used a unilateral frontal flap in all cases, operating from the side of the worse vision, where the larger mass of tumor nearly always lies. Some distinguished neurosurgeons prefer to work from the patient's right side so that they can hold a retractor in their left hand and have more effective use of the right hand from this angle. I prefer to use a self-retaining retractor in order to have both of my hands and occasionally an assistant's hand available to work on the tumor. Infrequently a tumor is lateral to the left optic nerve and is virtually unapproachable from the right side, as shown in Figure 31-8. Another reason for operating on the side of the worse vision is to provide maximal protection to the better optic nerve and tract by drawing the tumor away from that side as soon as possible.

The scalp incision usually can be made entirely behind the frontal hairline, extending a few centimeters to the contralateral side of the midline and down to the zygoma on the side of the flap. The frontal scalp flap must be pushed far enough forward to permit the supraorbital saw cut to lie just above the roof of the orbit. The inferomedial burr hole should be at the midline. This cut usually enters the frontal sinus. I still prefer the narrow kerf of a Gigli saw to the wider chasm made by a craniotome, especially for a bone flap in the frontal region. The pericranium is incised in the horizontal plane about 1 cm above where the saw cut will lie, so that this flap of pericranium can be turned backward over the hole into the frontal sinus and sewn to the dura, sealing the sinus and discouraging the spread of bacteria from there. The dura is opened only with a linear incision 8 to 10 mm above the saw cut. Intravenous urea, mannitol, or Lasix or combinations thereof are given as the bone flap is being cut in order to decrease cerebral volume. If there is significant ventricular enlargement, tapping the anterior part of the ipsilateral lateral ventricle may aid in decompression so that the frontal lobe can be slowly and gently be elevated. As this is done more cerebrospinal fluid will slowly ooze into the field; this increases when the carotid cistern is reached (if it is not filled with tumor). I have not needed to withdraw CSF with a lumbar needle for over a decade, nor have I removed a small 1–2-cm strip of inferomedial frontal lobe from the frontal pole to the chiasm as recommended "in most cases" by Patterson and Danylevich.[61] Magnifying loupes were used in the earlier years, the operating microscope more recently.

As soon as the craniopharyngioma or the lamina terminalis with tumor beyond it in the third ventricle is exposed, the entire intradural area is lined with cottonoid or Telfa strips to prevent spread of the irritating crystalline content of the cyst or solid

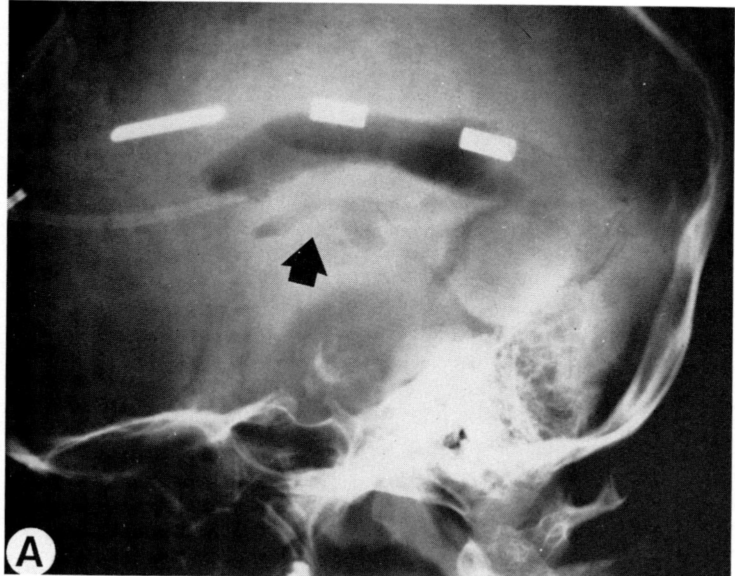
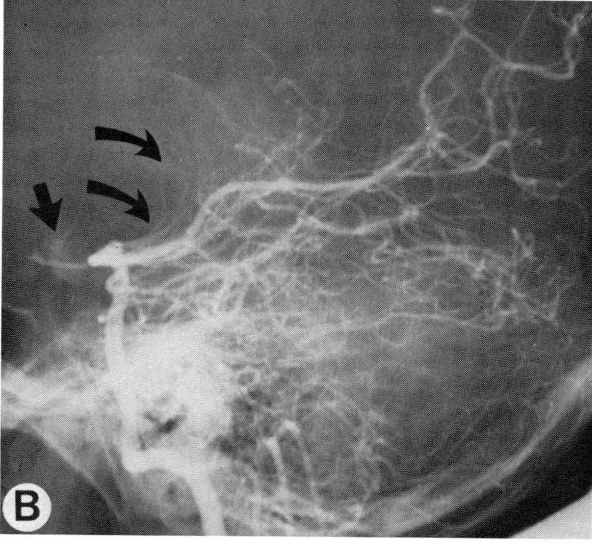

Fig. 31-8. Patient C.W. After removal of the tumor from lateral to the left optic nerve and from between the two optic nerves. The tumor had extended inferoposteriorly into the left cerebellopontine angle (straight black arrow on the left optic nerve points to the black void of the empty angle). Proceeding clockwise, the black arrowhead to the right of the left optic nerve points to the intact pituitary stalk; the black recurving arrow on the right optic nerve points to the origins of the right posterior communicating artery and anterior choroidal artery from the right internal carotid. The closed triangles lie on the zigzag left optic tract, which was sharply displaced by the tumor to lie lateral to the chiasm for about 1 cm then angled sharply backward. The right closed triangle lies between the perforating branches running backward from the anterior and middle cerebral arteries. The large white arrow at the top left points to the anterior end of the left internal carotid artery. The black arrow just below and to the right of this points to the largest artery feeding the capsule, which was electrocoagulated and divided several millimeters from its origin from a large anomalous artery running inferomedial and parallel to the anterior end of the left internal carotid. The shaft of the arrow lies on that anomalous artery.

tumor onto the brain or away from the field into the CSF. These mica-like cholesterin crystals can lead to a major and at times dangerous aseptic meningeal reaction postoperatively if any escape removal. They float to the surface of the irrigating fluid, and we try to get all loose debris from inside the cyst wall out of the patient by generous irrigation before attacking the solid part of the tumor. The patient of Patrick and his colleagues[72] in whom such a cyst ruptured spontaneously developed an intracranial pressure greater than 300 mm H_2O, a total protein of 7.5 g/ml, and a white count of 23,700/mm^3 in the CSF at the peak of the reaction. Horoupian et al.[73] reported aqueduct gliosis caused by keratin and cholesterol in one patient. Possibly a failure to preclude contamination of the CSF with such cyst contents led to the necessity for a CSF shunt after 5 of my 62 operations. Although multilocular cysts are less frequent, entry into a new pocket of fluid should be handled in the same thorough way. A single self-retaining retractor usually suffices to maintain just enough exposure. The ipsilateral olfactory tract will be sacrificed, but one can usually avoid lifting the opposite olfactory bulb off the cribriform plate. Not all of these cyst fluids are irritants, as demonstrated by another case of spontaneous rupture in which the only clinical change was an abrupt cessation of headache accompanied by a disappearance on the CT scan of the large hypodense cyst. Cholesterin crystals were seen in the CSF and the diagnosis of craniopharyngioma was confirmed at operation.[74]

EXTRACEREBRAL REMOVAL

Often the surface of a craniopharyngioma is readily identified between the two optic nerves or lateral to one of them. Aspiration of any cyst is the first step. In agreement with

Hoffman,[68] I find it useful to work with the patient's head looking straight upward or extended a little to help the brain fall backward. Craniopharyngiomas tend to roam, however, e.g., posterolaterally into a cerebellopontine angle or laterally into the sylvian fissure, and rotation of the head may be required for a better view of these pseudopodia. The dislocation of the normal structures and unusual directions of tumor growth make frequent checks on one's orientation advisable. Figure 31-8 illustrates how the normal structures can be grossly distorted. There is a zigzag course to the left optic tract with the first section going straight laterally from the chiasm, then turning posteriorly at a right angle. The intracranial portions of the optic nerves are fully 2 cm long; there is a large anomalous artery running parallel to and below the anterior end of the left internal carotid artery. As viewed obliquely from the left side, the pituitary stalk appears to arise from beneath the right internal carotid artery. The right posterior communicating and anterior choroidal branches are parallel to and adjoining the stalk, which is displaced to the right.

When working on extracerebral portions of the tumor, not only the sizeable named arteries but the smaller ones as well should be preserved insofar as possible and separated from the capsule. Anomalies are not uncommon. I have seen a branch from an anterior cerebral artery go forward to an optic foramen. Since the main arterial supply of the intracranial portions of the optic nerves enters from below, a planned search for the little vessels is important. The capsule must then be teased away from them. The tiny feeding arteries to the tumor should be gently coagulated as they enter the capsule as far as possible from their trunk vessel of origin to avoid thrombosis in that vessel. Removal can be especially tedious from solid tumors, since they must be cored out from within, tiny bits at a time, as one nears the numerous critical structures at their periphery.

It is better to initiate no intradural arterial bleeding at all—not because the bleeding cannot be readily stopped by gentle application of Oxycel or another hemostatic agent to small holes, even in the side walls of the larger vessels, but, again, because of thrombosis spreading from these sites into the lumina of one or more main channels. In one patient (I.Z. in 1961), for example, I placed divergent retractors on the frontal and temporal lobes in a way that caused a slight tear at the angle of origin of the anterior cerebral artery from the internal carotid artery. Since then I have sought to make a single self-retaining retractor suffice. Radiation treatment 1 year earlier may have decreased the elasticity of the vessel in this patient. Wisps of Oxycel into the angle stopped the bleeding at once, so I proceeded with the extirpation. The same sequence was followed in another patient (M.Z.), in whom numerous tiny holes were made in one anterior cerebral artery and the opposite internal carotid artery as the tumor capsule was separated from them. My pleasure at the smoothness of the early postoperative recovery in both was abruptly dashed when they died 25 and 5 days later, respectively, from thrombosis gradually spreading from the affected arteries. Since these two experiences, once I have made one or a few little holes in a significant artery I stop the operation after achieving complete hemostasis, wait some weeks for an endothelial covering to form at the site of the clot in the arterial wall, and then complete the operation at a second stage. Hakuba et al.[75] followed a similar tactic in their second case, soaking their Oxycel in "Biobond," which is an EDH adhesive, and waiting a month before resuming tumor removal.

In another patient, recurrent tumor, after an extensive partial removal at another center 16 months earlier, was so adherent to the orbital surface of both frontal lobes, one temporal tip, and the middle cerebral artery that I stopped after removing this portion, covered the suprasellar stump of remaining tumor with gutta percha to prevent it from adhering to the brain above, and returned to complete the removal in 4 weeks. Ten years later he is working and has had no recurrence.

I agree with Symon[76] and with Hoffman[68] that tenacious adhesions of tumor to essential arteries are the usual obstacle to achieving a presumed total removal. As Symon pointed out, it is especially densely calcified material which may adhere to a major artery and preclude development of a plane of cleavage. My last postoperative death occurred in 1969 and was described above (M.Z.). It was caused by my obstinate conviction that I ought to be able with impunity to free tumor from the medial wall of an internal carotid artery just below the anterior clinoid process. One of the only two postoperative deaths of Wilson[33] was caused by an intraoperative tear in a carotid artery. In another patient of mine (C.N.), tumor adhering to the medial wall of each cavernous sinus was apparently not cleanly removed; the tumor recurred 10 years later.

The arachnoid often intervenes between the arteries and the tumor, however, and its capsule is likely to fall away from many of the vessels. After a craniopharyngioma is removed from in front of and below the chiasm, the basilar and proximal posterior cerebral and superior cerebellar arteries may be seen through the intact prepontine arachnoid membrane. The same view is obtained after removal behind the chiasm from the third ventricle if the tumor has pushed the ventral hypothalamic structures to each side, which leaves a gaping hole in the floor of the third ventricle. I have only once seen a craniopharyngioma invade the arachnoid of the posterior fossa and adhere to

the vessels beyond. Hoffman's exposition at the 50th anniversary meeting of the American Association of Neurological Surgery made many of the points already mentioned.[77] Although his exposure is almost always subfrontal, of 21 cases on whom he operated in the previous 6 years, he used a pterional approach on one and a subtemporal approach on another.

REMOVAL OF BONE ANTERIOR TO THE SELLA

Earlier in my series I thought I could remove the anterior intrasellar portions of a craniopharyngioma beneath the tuberculum sellae by vigorously scraping it away with a curette after electrocoagulation and division of the anterior limb of the circular sinus. The curette clearly cannot be used with impunity anterolaterally in the neighborhood of the intracavernous carotid arteries. More recently I have reflected dura from the tuberculum sellae and planum sphenoidale and, using a diamond-tipped air drill followed by antrostomy forceps, have taken away the tuberculum, some of the planum, and the anterior wall of the sella turcica and in one patient part of the roof of one optic canal. Slight elevation of the optic nerve permitted a clean dissection of the tumor from its adherence to the intracavernous carotid artery beneath. One can usually keep the sphenoid sinus mucosa intact, pushing it forward into the ostium of the sinus, and after the tumor is removed, fill the sinus with fat. I close any dural opening over the sinus with a pericranial graft if necessary and start prophylactic antibiotics as soon as any of the sphenoid sinus (or the frontal sinus earlier in the operation) is entered.

Patterson and Danylevich[61] have recently emphasized the value of routine removal of the tuberculum sellae and anterior wall of the sella with division of the dura beyond that wall after coagulation of the circular sinus. They do this even when the optic nerves are long and the tumor is being removed from behind as well as in front of the chiasm. They note the safety to the optic nerves provided by pushing bits of tumor downward and forward away from the optic chiasm and hypothalamus and removing them from the exposed sphenoid sinus. Although I do not think this approach is helpful if the tumor is within the third ventricle and the anterior wall of the ventricle is intact, it may well represent a major technical step forward in many cases, as is strongly intimated by their encouraging results with 11 patients. My impression is that the surgeon's best tactic is to remove the tumor from those gaps between normal structures which the tumor itself has made the widest. Figure 31-8 shows a situation in which the logical main access to the tumor was lateral to the left optic nerve and tract and to a lesser extent between the two optic nerves.

RETROCHIASMAL REMOVAL

In 25 of my 43 patients the tumor had grown up from below, first indenting and then breaking into the third ventricle, or had arisen from within that ventricle. The tumor is then covered by a normal looking or somewhat bulging lamina terminalis (see Figure 31-1). This extends from side to side between the optic tracts, often with no clear boundary indicating the medial border of the tract on either side. In this situation the longitudinal incision into this structure should be halfway between the lateral borders of the two optic tracts. Usually the tumor is obvious just deep to the ultra-thin white lamina terminalis. In two of my patients, however, the tissue behind

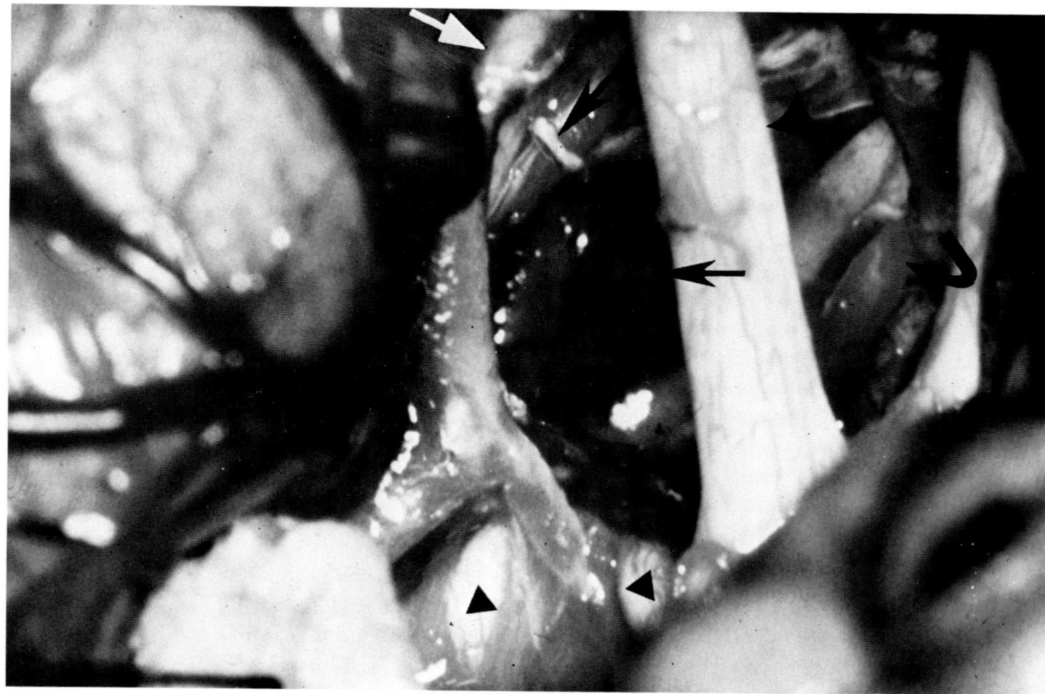

Fig. 31–9.   Special instruments needed at times in the removal of craniopharyngiomas. (A) Long, ultra-delicate alligator forceps with or without terminal mouse teeth and a tiny mirror with a flexible silver shaft. (B) Up-biting and down-biting rongeurs with cups only 2 mm in outside diameter may be needed to remove calcification.

the chiasm had the whitish gray firmness of a glioma of the visual pathways and I could find no cleavage plane between a possibly swollen chiasm and optic tract and the frank tumor. In one of these patients, whose roentgenograms had shown no intracranial calcification, I could aspirate no cyst fluid. My biopsy specimens from midway between the lateral borders of the optic tracts were reported as glial tissue, so I assumed the diagnosis was glioma of the visual pathways and closed the wound. The neuropathologist continued to study the slides, however, and, as I was placing the last scalp stitches, notified me that he had found one epithelial cluster characteristic of craniopharyngioma. Upon at once re-exposing the operative field, I decided the best place to find a surface tumor would be on its superior aspect where the air study had shown it to be in contact with CSF. Once this clear-cut boundary was felt, the central part of the tumor was removed and a cleavage plane readily followed as the wall of the tumor was teased toward the empty center all the way around. A complete homonymous hemianopia and visual acuity of 20/65 in each eye improved 1 week after surgery to an inferior temporal defect in the right eye only. The patient later recovered an acuity of 20/20 in each eye. Twenty-three years later she has no evidence of recurrence. In my second patient in whom the tumor looked to me like a glioma, the pathologist promptly diagnosed craniopharyngioma amid the glial cells. I then found the cleavage plane and did a radical removal in the same way as in the first case.

In another of my patients who underwent biopsy elsewhere 3 years earlier, the specimen had been identified as fibrous tissue with chronic inflammation, and the wound closed by that surgeon.

In one patient (G.W.) there was only an 8-mm interval between the posterior edge of the chiasm in front and the anterior cerebral artery behind. It seemed at first impossible to think of a radical removal of this entirely solid tumor. As bits of

the interior were removed, however, more tumor from behind descended into the narrow interval, making it possible to displace the anterior cerebral vessels a little farther posteriorly. In the end we had a satisfactory view of an empty third ventricle and the patient has had no recurrence in her 17½ years since. Another patient had such obviously widened optic tracts that the lamina terminalis was only a narrow band between them. The pressure of the tumor from behind was responsible for this distortion, and again as enough minute bits of tumor were removed, a similar phenomenon occurred. The optic tracts gradually resumed their normal oval contour with over a centimeter between them. This patient also has had no recurrence in the 23 years since surgery.

Although at first I was very concerned about blindly pulling a craniopharyngioma forward into the field of view from its more posterior loci, experience has shown that its tenacious attachments are happily only anterior, as already described. The capsule does, however, tend to draw back into the third ventricle and I have found it valuable to have an assistant maintain a grasp on one point of the visible capsule while I hold another part of it with one of my hands, using my other hand to ease more tumor into view. For this tactic the double-headed binocular microscope is indispensable. Only with the microscope can both surgeons see into the tiny field. Very thin-shafted, alligator-type, mouse-toothed forceps (Figure 31-9) are helpful instruments for this task. This blind, hand-over-hand hauling out of tumor has never caused any bleeding or yielded a trophy containing neurons.

At times I find that tumor already in the field can be conveniently pushed forward out of the third ventricle via a hole in the hypothalamus below the chiasm; at other times removal has gone more easily by pressing beneath an optic tract laterally. This displaces the lateral hypothalamus medially and thereby facilitates a dissection of the tumor from the third ventricular wall under direct vision. Carmel and I found that a small mirror with a flexible silver shaft may be needed to see tumor beneath the chiasm or in other obscure spots (Figure 31-9).

Suzuki et al.[78] described a modification of this approach via a bifrontal craniotomy and separation of the two frontal lobes after dividing the anterior end of the superior sagittal sinus and the falx.

This certainly provides a broad access to the lamina terminalis, which has permitted him to save both olfactory tracts in 80 percent of his cases. He also thinks that one can divide "a sufficiently long" anterior communicating artery with impunity to improve the exposure. He had no postoperative mortality in 13 cases of craniopharyngioma in the third ventricle. In 9 of these cases the craniopharyngiomas were thought to be totally removed; however, 3 of these 9 patients have since died at 4 months, 9 months, and 7½ years, as has one of the patients at 16 months in whom the removal was subtotal, illustrating that careful CT or MRI follow-up and additional treatment are often needed.

RADICAL REMOVAL VIA THE LATERAL ROUTE—PTERIONAL OR SUBTEMPORAL

Symon at the National Hospital for Nervous Diseases has developed a "radical temporal approach," that he has used in his last 20 cases of radical removal, all of which showed a large third ventricular filling defect.[57] He found that the posteroinferior portion of such tumors, lying free in the interpeduncular cistern, is best attacked from laterally along the sphenoid wing with a small resection of the anterior 2 cm of the temporal lobe. He opens the inner end of the sylvian fissure, if necessary removing also the uncus by suction to improve access to the interpeduncular fossa. The internal carotid artery and its anterior choroidal and posterior communicating branches with the thalamo-perforating branches of the latter, invested in their own arachnoid, intervene between the surgeon and the tumor. Behind them, the posterior cerebral and basilar arteries can be identified. He gently dissects the third nerve clear and protects it so well that only transient third nerve palsies have occurred—partial in 4 patients and complete in 1 patient. He recommends not dividing any of the small arteries including the small thalamic perforators. He commonly mobilizes the posterior communicating artery forward, working in the space between that and the most anterior thalamo-perforating branch (see Figure 31-7). After internal decompression of the tumor, he then enters the third ventricle just in front of the mammillary bodies. We both agree that one can commonly dissect in the glial tissue reactive to the tumor "without actual transgression of the nuclear masses in the walls of the third ventricle." We both found that after the interior of the tumor is removed, the capsule can be brought down out of the upper third ventricle with gentle traction. Probably less of the procedure is blind by this approach than in mine via the lamina terminalis. He succeeds in protecting the optic tract while retracting it under cottonoid, emphasizing protection of the perforating arteries supplying it. We further agree that the tumor is almost always densely adherent to the anterior third ventricle in the region of the posterior part of the optic chiasm. He stated that, "the preservation of a line of the top of the capsule, and the excellent exposure of the ipsilateral optic nerve and optic tract, enables calculation of the line of the chiasm and under reasonable magnification, sharp dissection of the tumor from the posterior aspect of the chiasm." I am at times uncertain where the posterior edge of the chiasm lies vis-à-vis the lamina terminalis, but his selection of a line for sharp dissection may protect the chiasm in a way I have not done. His description is worth detailed study.

I have not shared King's reluctance to dissect small definite tumor remnants away from the third ventricular floor behind the chiasm, as he felt inadvisable in three of four intraventricular tumors of this type.[28] Guiot and Namin[79] were among the first to advocate the subtemporal approach for retrochiasmatic tumors, stating that it is usually useless to resect a part of the temporal lobe and that it suffices to tap the dilated ventricle. They had no mortality in 6 patients, three of whom had craniopharyngiomas, but they were not able to remove the entire capsule in any of these 3 patients. Malis[80] and Hunt and Miller[81] also recommended this approach for these tumors in this position. While I have not used either of these routes, the excellent results of Symon et al.[57] make it important to present a summary of his lucid description.

RADICAL REMOVAL VIA THE LATEROPOSTERIOR TRANSPETROSAL-TRANSTENTORIAL ROUTE

Still another approach to retrochiasmatically placed craniopharyngiomas was developed by Hakuba et al.[75] They gave an excellent detailed description of their extraordinary tactic of removing much of the petrous portion of the temporal bone and incising the tentorium to expose the lateral ambient cistern on the way to the third ventricle. Of seven radical removals by this route, two were disasters but five produced excellent results on all scores. I think one should await further reports from this group before attempting this approach.

INFLUENCE OF SIZE AND CYSTIC CONTENT ON THE TYPE OF OPERATION

Although Petito et al.[24] stated that 60 percent of craniopharyngiomas are exclusively cystic, most of them are in fact a mixture of cystic and solid portions. Only 8 of the 43 tumors in my series were essentially all solid, and only 4 were almost all cystic, with from 20 to 56 ml of fluid in them. In Backlund's recent series, only one of nine craniopharyngiomas was predominantly cystic.[82] If even a few milliliters of fluid are available for aspiration, this helps in that it permits prompt withdrawal of the capsule away from the better optic nerve and tract. Shapiro et al.[83] achieved a grossly total removal in almost all of their eight predominantly cystic lesions, regardless of size; whereas in their 27 mixed types the likelihood of radical removal varied inversely with the size of the lesion. This was accomplished in only 20 percent of their tumors over 3 cm in diameter.

Size played a major role in Kobayashi's operative results with 15 patients.[39] Of his 7 patients who had tumors with volumes greater than 25 ml, 5 were dead within 1 year. The other 2 patients who had cystic tumors of 30 and 45 ml had excellent results, however. Of my 8 patients who had recurrences, 6 had tumors over 3 cm in diameter. On the other hand, Hoffman found that tumor size had no influence on the success rate of radical removal,[41,62] and, indeed, there have been no recurrences of the largest tumors in my series, examples of which I have cited elsewhere.[22] Al-Mefty, working in Saudi

Arabia, recently achieved total removal as determined from CT scans of eight of ten giant craniopharyngiomas, i.e., 5 to 11 cm in diameter.[31] Two late postoperative deaths occurred from septicemia, but none of the survivors had mental deficits or behavioral problems. A bilateral subfrontal approach was used for eight of the ten tumors.

Symon et al.[69] stated that "a craniopharyngioma which is almost completely cystic is unsatisfactory for radical excision by any route, since every movement of dissection of the wall is accompanied by considerable disturbances of the third ventricular structures." At the other extreme stands Bartlett,[40] who found that slow-growing cystic-type craniopharyngiomas tend to fall out of their brain beds at post mortem. In Belgrade, cystic craniopharyngiomas are the favorites of Djordjevic et al.[84] They totally remove only those with thin, noncalcified, nonfibrous capsules; large size is no contraindication to such an attack. The cystic contents of three of their subfrontal, interhemispheric lesions came to 100, 150, and 200 ml! They stated "craniopharyngiomas of this type can be removed in one operation and there is no recurrence." Gelabert et al.[85] removed a craniopharyngioma from the bilateral frontal area of a patient containing 620 ml of cystic fluid. Total removal was achieved as demonstrated by examinations early after the operation and again at 1 year. The precaution of draining the fluid at the rate of 100 ml/hour was their initial gesture.

THE PITUITARY STALK

Hoffman stated that "the very nature of the tumor necessitates sacrifice of the pituitary stalk."[77] In eight of my patients I thought I had either dissected the tumor cleanly from the entire length of the stalk or found no tumor in its vicinity and preserved it intact. In three of these patients, however, the tumor recurred. In a ninth patient (K.A.), I divided the long stalk a few millimeters above the pituitary gland but kept it intact on up to the hypothalamus. At the end of the operation, it was lying on the diaphragma sellae. This patient rarely requires antidiuretic hormone 18 years later; possibly the stalk reattached. In another patient, having with effort preserved the stalk, I thought its 3–4-mm diameter excessive, cut into it, and found a central core of tumor running the length of the stalk, so I sacrificed the entire structure. Often I have not succeeded in identifying the stalk and found after removal of the tumor only an empty space between the diaphragma or sellar cavity and the brain above. Al-Mefty preserved the stalk in three of his ten radical removals of giant tumors.[31]

When a wholly intraventricular tumor has pushed the chiasm forward against the tuberculum sellae but has left the anterior wall and floor of the third ventricle intact, the stalk almost surely remains intact, although never seen. Unless the craniopharyngioma separates from the stalk with essentially no dissection, it may be better to eliminate this entire potential source of recurrence; DDAVP can provide adequate replacement.

HANDLING A MAJOR CALCIFIED SECTOR OF THE TUMOR

Infrequently a large irregular, almost cauliflowerlike mass, often with sharp flanges on it, nestles around the visual pathways, the arteries, and/or the dorsum sellae. Comments on these masses are sparse in the literature, probably because their removal has seemed neither technically feasible nor necessary.

I have left in two such masses. One of the patients came to post mortem from other causes 9 months after the last removal of the soft-tissue tumor attached to the mass, and there was no evidence of soft tissue recurrence after that rather short interval. In a more recent case 9 years ago, I could free the jagged mass nearly completely from its position half embracing one optic tract from below, but had no instrument small enough and powerful enough to break it up without trauma to the tract. The patient's condition has gradually worsened until he no longer does productive work. Since then I have found that the tiny antrostomy-type rongeur (see Figure 31-9) enabled me to fragment a smaller calcified mass in a subsequent case so that I could remove it. Talalla[86] reported the successful use of a high-speed drill to bisect a rock-hard solid mass totally intrasellar. He was apparently able to push the mass against the sellar floor and drill against it, having first removed all of the soft tissue tumor. Alvarez-Garijo et al.[87] described a remarkable case of a 2-year-old girl whose large, dense calcification was 6 cm in diameter and above the sella. Using "sharp rongeurs" they brought forth an operative specimen that included 20 microscopically identified teeth, three of them complete with crown and root. Although some of the capsule was left behind, follow-up roentgenograms 3 years later showed no change in the size of her residual tumor.

The Cavitron ultrasonic surgical aspirator may increase the safety of removal of hard or calcified portions of the tumor. It is not clear, however, from the meager available reports just how safely one can remove these large residual calcified masses with ultrasonic or laser methods.

TRANSSPHENOIDAL APPROACH

Shortly after the turn of the century Hirsch's use of the transsphenoidal route included tapping some craniopharyngiomatous cysts.[88] This maneuver had only limited value with two large cysts thus treated by my colleague Hamlin. Since microscopy and Guiot's[89] introduction of televised radiofluoroscopic control have both been called into play to aid this approach, substantial suprasellar components of pituitary adenomas burgeoning upward have often been successfully removed by this low-risk route. Even Guiot, however, with his tremendous experience and skill, thought that only those craniopharyngiomas that are "essentially intrasellar" are suitable for this approach.[90] Of 57 such tumors on his service that were operated on after 1957, only four were attacked exclusively by this route; approaches both from above and below were used for four more patients in whom tumor removal was incomplete by the first approach, whether from above or below. These figures are representative of the percentage of these tumors seen by others as suitable for removal by the nasal route. Thus, transsphenoidal operations were done in 3 of 37 patients of Lichter et al.[91] and in 2 of 50 patients by McMurry et al.[92] An intrasellar locus was described by Northfield in 3 of 37 patients at operation or necropsy,[11] and by Cabezudo et al.[53] in 4 of 33 patients from CT scans. Kobayashi performed radical removals in 5 patients and subtotal removals in 2 more treated primarily by this approach.[39,93]

At the Mayo Clinic, Laws used the transsphenoidal route on 26 of 50 patients in a recent 7-year period.[94] In 14 patients this was the first definitive surgical procedure, and in 9 of the 14 he described a "total" removal; there was one operative death. His excellent diagrams of each tumor indicate an essentially intrasellar position in only 5 of the 14. In a subsequent report covering the previous 12 years he increased dramatically the number of patients to 60, achieving "total" removal in 36 with three recurrences and still only one operative death.[95] I remain surprised that a significantly suprasellar craniopharyngioma, with its frequent intimate attachments to arteries and brain, can be safely dissected out via this route.

Wilson used the transsphenoidal approach for 39 percent of the 74 craniopharyngiomas he removed, selecting intrasellar and slightly suprasellar tumors for removal by this route. Excision was total, however, in only 7 of the 74, the rest being subtotal removals.[33] A comparison of the results and problems with this approach and the subfrontal approach, which was used in 47 percent of the patients, is not given.

TRANSCALLOSAL, TRANSCORTICOVENTRICULAR, OR SUBOCCIPITAL APPROACH

The ease of reaching large craniopharyngiomas within the third ventricle via the dilated lateral ventricle or through the corpus callosum has for decades tempted neurosurgeons to use this route. I read the results as indicating that this temptation should usually be resisted. All five of Northfield's attempted extirpations via the transventricular route and 5 of the 12 biopsies via this route failed, resulting in the death of the patient—a "forbidding mortality" in his opinion.[11] Kahn commented that he and the experienced Parisian Rougerie "have given up any attempt to remove a craniopharyngioma through the foramen of Munro as the mortality and morbidity are too great."[42] Pertuiset described the transventricular and transcallosal approaches as "dangerous."[8] Katz mentioned that all three of Matson's patients in whom the transventricular approach was used died.[67] Asari's patient, who underwent transcallosal subtotal removal, died in 4 months.[96] Shucart and Stein[97] attempted "subtotal" removals in 2 patients and noted "the complete boundaries of the craniopharyngiomas were not defined despite enlarging the foramen of Munro, and the completeness of tumor removal was uncertain." One of the 2 patients had the serious complication of mutism. Patterson was able to do only a partial removal by a transcallosal approach, and had to do his subfrontal procedure (q.v.) (see above) 11 months later, then achieving a "presumed total removal."[61] A major problem in the exposure by the translateroventricular route is that one should not increase the access to the third ventricle by cutting the second anterior column of the fornix. Although in the 1 patient on whom I have used this approach the exposure was delightful for the simple removal of a colloid cyst, she has had an undesirable memory deficit for the 25 years since.[98] Milner described the same type of deficit of lesser degree in a patient who was treated similarly.[98]

In all four of Long and Chou's cases, two in which a transcallosal approach was used and two in which a transcorticoventricular approach was used, a grossly total removal was achieved, but three of the patients died with massive gastrointestinal hemorrhage during the first postoperative week.[27] The fourth patient, after a less serious hemorrhage, survived without neurologic deficit. Transcallosal removal was also undertaken in two children whose tumors had recurred largely within the third ventricle after subfrontal operations but had also herniated into both lateral ventricles. A "grossly total removal" was followed again by recurrence in both patients. Long and Leibrock[99] added four more transcallosal operations on these tumors.

Recurrent neoplasm was thus attacked in three, and the fourth patient had a second-stage operation on the intraventricular portion of the tumor. This patient and one with a recurrence were "unchanged by surgery." The other two were rendered "normal." Baskin and Wilson[33] used a transcallosal approach in 4 cases and a suboccipital route on 2 of their 74 patients. Tumor location in the first group in the middle portion of the third ventricle and significant extension into the pineal region in the latter group were the bases for these approaches. The results in these specific cases were not described. However, Bose et al.[100] reported full details on two totally intraventricular tumors that were completely removed with resultant neurologic normality and no recurrence as determined from CT scans at 18 and 12 months. In one of them a vascular pedicle arising from the floor of the third ventricle was identified and divided. Hoffman saw in the postoperative scan after his initial radical subfrontal operation that there was still "considerable tumor in the third ventricle."[62] This he promptly removed by the transcallosal route.

Although as Northfield pointed out these approaches are intrinsically safe as demonstrated by their successful use in the treatment of colloid cysts, they may not provide an adequate view of the main sites of tumor adherences at the base of the brain.[11] Whereas the subfrontal, pterional, or subtemporal approach can apparently be used with impunity to draw the almost certainly unattached tumor from the upper third ventricle down into the field of view, the reverse is not true in the approach from above.

TREATMENT VIA RESERVOIR DRAINAGE SYSTEM

Gutin et al.[101] reported on 4 patients, each of whom had a ventricular catheter placed in the cavity of a predominantly cystic tumor and connected to a subcutaneous reservoir for aspiration as needed. They cited in support of this method the examples of Oh[102] and of Miles,[103] who used drainage to a reservoir, and of Muller et al.,[104] who used a T-tube with its superficial end in the subcutaneous tissues. Gutin et al. recommended this "in grossly cystic craniopharyngiomas whenever it becomes apparent that complete resection is impossible."[101] Symon's procedure in these cases is to "insert a large Silastic tube (5 mm internal diameter) with several side holes, anchored to the dura along the sphenoidal wing, its free end lying within the cavity of the cyst, and the tube brought out along the sphenoid wing to a Rickham reservoir in the temporal muscle."[69] It is evident that some of us are finding the essentially cystic tumors the most favorable for removal, while others heartily disagree and prefer the drainage tactic.

SHUNTING PROCEDURES

Not only hydrocephalus associated with increased intracranial pressure, but also dilated ventricles of modest degree associated with normal pressures may contribute to a lethargic or unsatisfactory mental state and require a shunt of cerebrospinal fluid out of the ventricles. This was needed in five of my patients. One should be especially alert to such a need if an aseptic cellular meningitis occurs after operation.

METABOLIC AND ENDOCRINE STUDIES AND MANAGEMENT

Knowledge in the metabolic and endocrine world continues to increase at a pace that makes it advisable for a neurosurgeon to work with a consultant in this field from the time he suspects that there may be a sellar or parasellar lesion and throughout the follow-up in the years after the operation. Kliman's newest chapter on the subject merits intensive study, especially if the neurosurgeon plans on handling this role.[105]

One of the most vulnerable deficits in patients with craniopharyngioma may be their failure to increase their secretion of cortisone with stress such as infection. This has been emphasized especially by Till.[70] Among the late deaths in his group of 23 children undergoing total removal of their craniopharyngiomas, four occurred from 3 to 9 years after operation and were the result of inadequate treatment of the patients' suprarenal insufficiency "at the time of an otherwise straightforward infection." (Autopsies in all 4 patients showed no residual tumor.) Happily, emergency life-saving treatment ensued in 9 other of his other 51 postoperative craniopharyngioma patients. We are aware of a similar fatality in one of our patients. Instruction of patients and responsible relatives and the doubling or tripling of the maintenance dose of steroid during any infection or other illness is essential. Clinical studies on these patients require awareness of their vulnerability. A patient of Hoffman et al.[41] thus died of unrecognized hypoglycemia during a metapyrone test in another hospital.

Some endocrinologists prefer to treat the almost inevitable diabetes insipidus early in the postoperative period by replacing fluid as fast as urine pours out, relying on antidiuretic hormone only modestly. Others are more liberal in replacing this deficient substance. The endocrinologic and neurosurgical staffs must agree on the tactic to avoid confusion.

Once the patient goes home, desmopressin acetate (DDAVP) can be used. With its prompt but long-lasting action it is an example of the improvements in endocrine therapy. The irregular action of Pitressin Tannate keeps some patients either a little depleted or enough overloaded with water that their initiative and energy are reduced. One patient told me that with these peaks and valleys of hydration smoothed out by the DDAVP she works "an order of magnitude" better in the past 7 years. While on the Pitressin Tannate she also had incessant hyperphagia; no sense of satiety ever developed. She had to stop eating as an exercise in self-discipline. She now feels satisfied at the end of a normal meal, and the constant fight against weight gain is going better.

In general, the use of average doses in endocrine replacement therapy fails to take advantage of the fine tuning as to type, timing, and dosage of the many supplemental agents now available, or the need to update the regimen as new knowledge and substances appear. A point I learned only a few years ago is that the rate of metabolism of adrenal glucocorticoids is dependent on the level of thyroid hormone. The steroids burn in a thyroid flame, just as fats require the carbohydrate flame for their metabolism. If the thyroxin level is too low, the steroids accumulate, causing Cushing's syndrome to appear. This occurred in one of my patients (N.D.). Although only 1 in 20 patients requires 0.3 mg thyroxin per day, this man was found by Dr. John Crawford, endocrinologist, to need that dose. By reducing the dosage of prednisone to 4 mg/day (from 25 mg hydrocortisone per day), and adding 5 mg of dexedrine per day and DDAVP instead of Pitressin Tannate, alertness, weight loss, even visual fields, and acuity improved to nearly normal. The symptoms I was attributing to recurrence vanished.

Formerly, some physicians urged deferral of radical surgery in small children in the hope that further somatic growth would take place. Presumed total removal of these tumors, however, has frequently been followed by normal or even accelerated growth.[106] This occurred in all eight of our patients who underwent radical removal and who were critically studied in an attempt to find out why they grew three times as fast in the year after surgery as in the year before despite subnormal levels of growth hormone. Postoperative growth without somatotropin treatment also took place in 12 of Carmel's 34 children, including 5 with radical removals.[43]

In general, the assiduous management of the multiple endocrine deficiencies has been so successful that these problems no longer plague the neurosurgeon and have not received detailed attention here.

COAGULOPATHIES IN PARASELLAR TUMORS

An increased incidence of thromboembolic complications in the presence of parasellar tumors was reported by Brisman et al.[107] The literature has been augmented by Sawaya et al.[108] with a report of a case of massive preoperative fatal pulmonary embolism and by Hoogenhout et al.[109] with two adults dying of postoperative pulmonary embolism among 17 patients who underwent subtotal removal of craniopharyngiomas. Special alertness to this complication seems in order.

TWO UNUSUAL SEQUELAE

A complication related to intracranial tumors causing hypopituitarism and chiasmal compression has been described by Heatley et al.,[110] namely, slipped upper femoral epiphyses. They found this bilaterally in each of 4 patients: 2 with craniopharyngiomas, 1 with an optic nerve glioma, and 1 with an ectopic pinealoma. This lesion might be milder and asymptomatic on one side. In 2 patients the diagnosis was made at the initial admission for the tumor, in one 3 years later, and in 1 (with a craniopharyngioma) not until 9 years after such admission. All 4 patients had hypogonadism, and 3 also had low gonadotropin and sex hormone levels. Three earlier papers reporting such cases are mentioned. A patient of Klotz[49] developed a more serious problem—major necrosis of the heads of both femurs and of the right humerus. One of our patients (G.J.) developed a unilateral slipped epiphysis 2 years after his tumor was removed.

Another rare development is that of a pyogenic abscess within a craniopharyngioma. Obrador and Blazquez[111] described five earlier cases in addition to their own. An outpouring of pus when the tumor capsule is first incised is the rude, surprising first indication of this problem, and is another reason why cottonoid pledgets should line the entire intradural area before the capsule is entered. Vigorously energetic treatment of the infection is required; 3 of the 6 patients died.

RESULTS OF RADICAL REMOVAL

Personal Record

In the 43 patients with craniopharyngioma on whom I have operated since 1950, my objective at my first operation was to do a radical removal if this seemed at all feasible as the operation evolved. At the time of that operation, 21 patients, 16 males and 5 females, were under 17 years of age and 22 patients, 12 males and 10 females, were 17 years or older. Only with the three cases described earlier did it seem unreasonable to carry forward to a removal that was total or nearly so. In the

Table 31-1. Results of radical excision (19 children, 21 adults)*

Years Since First Radical Operation	Number Operated On Who Might Have Lived for Stated Interval (Number "At Risk")	Number Alive for Stated Interval	Death Caused by Surgery and/or Recurrent Tumor	Death from Unrelated Disease
3	40	32 (80%)	0–3 years 4 (13%)	4
5	32	31 (97%)	3–5 years 1 (3%)	0
10	31	27 (87%)	5–10 years 2 (3%)	2
10–15	24	22 (92%)	10–15 years 0 (0%)	2
15–38	15	14 (93%)	15–38 years 0 (0%)	1

* Note: Of the 24 patients surviving from 10 to 38 years, none of the three deaths in this period were related to tumor—a record not equalled by any reports regarding radiation therapy at these late dates.

remaining 40 patients my first operation was with one exception the first radical removal the patient had undergone.

Matson[6] and Katz[67] and I[22] each described separately the results of radical surgery at the initial operation and at a secondary craniotomy, since the operative mortality in the latter group was much greater. In reviewing my cases I find that if the operation that preceded my aggressive effort was only a partial or subtotal removal the operative mortality was not very discouraging. Thus, of my 32 patients on whom my radical operation was their first craniotomy, 2 died, and of 8 patients who had had a less extensive resection before my radical effort, 1 died. As already described, this patient (I.Z.) died 20 years ago of a technical error at operation that is easily avoidable. This patient had had a course of radiation therapy (dose not stated) 1 year before my operation, as had the following 2 patients: In a 14-year-old child 5050 rads of ^{60}Co photons was administered over 36 days, finishing 11 months before my radical operation. In a 38-year-old woman a partial removal was followed by a course of 4000 rad given through 4.5 × 4.5) cm fields by rotation at the Massachusetts General Hospital during 29 days. Because of failing vision the radiation was stopped and I performed a radical removal, encountering no major technical problems. The result in the child was hard to assess because he also had Huntington's chorea, from which he died 8 years later. The woman's good postoperative result was followed by death from unrelated causes at 1 year. On the basis of these eight cases I had earlier concluded that a radical attempt may reasonably follow a subtotal operation, radiation, or both, performed in the previous year or two. However, an appraisal of my 12 radical removals in my last decade of such operations reveals that the worst result, initially graded "fair," was in a patient who had undergone a "grossly total removal" by another surgeon followed a few months later by a cyst aspiration in the year prior to my operation. Although the patient has had no recurrence in the 14 years since my operation, he remains a useless creature; I should not have attempted a second radical removal.

Death ensued within a maximum of 6 months in every one of the 5 patients in whom I carried out a second radical removal following a recurrence after my own first radical procedure. Consequently, of the other 2 patients who had a recurrence in this situation, I did only a subtotal removal at the second operation (without mortality but with continuing deterioration).

Behavioral problems have grossly marred the quality of the survival in another 5 of my 24 still-living patients. The principal problem seems to be a lack of mental and physical capacity and/or motivation to do productive work. Two have held nondemanding jobs intermittently; the other three, as one relative put it, are "about as useful as a household pet," doing little more than feeding and dressing themselves. Gradual deterioration to this level occurred in the 2 patients who underwent only subtotal removals at my second craniotomy. Of the other 19 survivors, 5 are in the "good" category and 14 in the "excellent" category as described by Katz,[67] and 10 of 14 who died were in one of these categories after recovery from surgery. The classification anent quality of survival of Katz and of the radiotherapists Bloom[44,112] and Danoff et al.[59] will be used insofar as possible for comparison of results. Katz's "excellent" (group 1) consists of those patients who are "independent, functioning normally"; "good" (group 2) are those patients who are "functioning well with some deficiency"; "fair" (group 3) are those patients who are "functioning but dependent"; "poor" (group 4) are those patients who are "non-functional." Similarly the radiotherapist's group 1 equals excellent, no disability; group 2 equals good, mild handicap; group 3 equals fair, major disability, capable of self care; group 4 equals poor, incapable of self care.

The problems that may be associated with leaving behind a large calcified mass are illustrated by the case of one of my patients (P.B.), a top-ranked student in his first 2 years of high school. He had the gigantic frustration 5 years after operation of barely making a "C" average in university; he has gradually worsened to loafing around his apartment refusing to support himself with the "menial kinds of work" of which he is capable.

A possible symptom patients and relatives need to be warned about is verbally explosive, unreasonable attacks of ill-temper or rage. Five of the young men we have treated have or have had this problem, which has not progressed to physical assaultiveness or destructiveness in any of them, perhaps because they are deficient in androgenic hormones. This can be a disabling symptom, however, from the standpoint of employability. Both relatives and employers need to learn that this is an unequivocal symptom of the brain disorder and not just innate surliness. Shillito has stated that an overaggressive surgeon dealing with these tumors may produce an overaggressive patient.[9]

Table 31-1 gives the mortality data on my 40 radical removals. In the 5 years since these were last published none of the 24 patients then surviving has died, and only one has developed an asymptomatic soft tissue recurrence (shown on CT scan). Very long follow-ups may be required to determine how the "total removal" cases compare with those treated by lesser surgery plus radiation.

Patients Operated on in the 1970s

There have been no postoperative deaths in any of the 12 patients on whom I performed radical surgery in the 1970s; my last such operation was in July, 1979. One of these patients, who was asymptomatic at 13 months, nevertheless showed a small probable recurrence on both a routine CT scan and a subsequent pneumogram. A linear accelerator was then used to deliver 5520 rad in 46 elapsed days (the dose recommended by Kramer after presumed total removal).[113] Massive radiation necrosis developed, which killed him by 5 1/2 months later. The case has already been fully described.[114] Of the remaining 11 patients, 7 are in the "excellent" category, 1 in the "good" category, and 1 in the "fair" category. Unrelated causes have killed one who was also in the "excellent" class until her terminal illness. The 12th patient (P.B.), for 5 years in the "good" category, has at 10 years dropped to "fair." An asymptomatic recurrence developed in one; this small lesion, which appeared 3 years postoperatively, has not increased in size on CT scans for 5 years. The patient has received no radiation therapy. In a second asymptomatic patient a recent high-resolution scan disclosed a small nodule of intrasellar calcification with no contrast-enhancing tissue. The extraordinary resolution of the latest scans makes it reasonable to follow patients, subjecting them to radiation only when its need is clear-cut. In summary, of 12 patients operated on in the decade of the 1970s only two had results as bad as the "fair" category, one on whom a "grossly total removal" was done prior to my radical operation and one in whom a major calcified mass was not removed. There have been asymptomatic recurrences in 2 of the 11 patients who underwent total removal.

Results of Others

Hoffman's most recent of his steady contributions to the field described the results of 29 primary microsurgical excisions of craniopharyngioma from 1976 through mid)1985.[62] He achieved the handsome record of presumed total removal in 25 patients with, to date, no clinical recurrence in 21 and no operative mortality. The CT scans of these patients showed contrast-enhancing residual lesions in 4 of the 25. One patient with a considerable tumor in the third ventricle was treated promptly by transcallosal total excision. The other 3 patients had clinical recurrences at 8 months, 2 years, and 3 years. These 3 patients and the 4 who underwent known subtotal removal all had a subsequent operation followed by radiotherapy. These 7 patients have IQ levels of 63, 73, 86, 90, and 91 with two "normal." The IQs in the 21 patients who underwent total resection range from 84 to 128. All but one of the 29 patients is being treated for diabetes insipidus and all but 1 require cortisone replacement. Weight gain occurred in 5 of the 21 patients who underwent total resection; this was excessive in 4 of the 8 who underwent reoperation and radiotherapy for recurrence. The CT scans in 15 of the 21 patients who underwent total resection showed either no lesion or small bits of calcification with no recurrence to date.

Although Hoff and Patterson,[115] reporting the earlier New York Hospital experience, described only four presumed total excisions of craniopharyngioma in 51 operative cases, Patterson and Danylevich[61] gave detailed accounts of 11 patients in whom a total removal was the goal, which was achieved in 8 of the 11. In one patient "only a small scrap densely adherent to the hypothalamus" was left behind; in another the postoperative CT scan showed residual tumor, which had given no sign of growth in the 3 years of follow-up. Only in a patient treated 14 months earlier by partial excision and 5750 rad of radiation were the yellow optic nerves and hypothalamus so densely adherent to the tumor that only a partial removal was feasible, and the patient still required custodial care. There were no postoperative deaths; the only patient to receive supplemental radiation was the one with "a scrap of tumor" remaining. Patterson succeeded in carrying out his total removals with a satisfactory result in 5 patients who had undergone a previous partial removal from less than 1 year to 14 years earlier. The patient whose first operation had been 14 years earlier had also received 3000 rad to the tumor after that operation. Even in this especially difficult situation, Patterson succeeded in removing all but a tiny remnant of tumor. These are encouraging achievements.

One of the first neurosurgeons to follow Matson's lead and remove the craniopharyngioma when this seemed safely advisable was Till.[70] He had in the 20 years before 1982 accomplished an apparently complete removal in 23 patients and a less complete removal in the remaining 28 of his 51 patients. His operative mortality, only two deaths, one in each of the two groups, was achieved entirely without the operating microscope. Recurrence has been recognized in only 3 of the 23 patients undergoing radical removal at 2, 4, and 4 years. Only the patients undergoing partial removal were treated by radiation. Till favors total excision, but "not at the risk of disabling morbidity."

Symon[57] reported results on 20 primary microsurgical radical excisions since 1977, his preferred treatment since that date. His only exceptions were a recurrent tumor in a patient whose first operation was performed elsewhere and massive cystic lesions inaccessible by a single approach. He had only one surgically related death in the first postoperative month. One patient died at 15 months as a result of hypothalamic damage and a third patient died because of a malfunction of a ventriculoperitoneal shunt that was improperly treated in another country. Follow-up CT scans of all patients revealed one recurrent cyst at 8 months; drainage of this was followed by radiation therapy. Continuing but decreasing loss of memory was noted in 2 patients at 3 months after operation. Gross weight gain was a problem in 2 patients. Decreasing doses of DDAVP sufficed and less than half the cases still required this at the end of 2 years. Symon's likewise noteworthy earlier results were described in our second edition.

The good results of Al-Mefty after his total removal of eight of ten giant craniopharyngiomas have already been noted.[31]

However, some neurosurgeons whose records include earlier operations had much less attractive results after attempted total resections of craniopharyngiomas. Thus, on one university service, of 30 patients treated primarily by surgery in the 16 years beginning in 1965, "total" removal was thought to have been attained in 14; 2 patients died postoperatively and 4 had recurrences.[116] Three of these 4 patients died 1, 2, and 8 years after surgery. Of the 8 patients surviving for an average of 10.2 years, only 3 were in the group 1–2 category, i.e., a good result.

MANAGEMENT OF SMALL TUMORS

Tumors that Produce Minimal or No Symptoms

Hoffman's last series included 2 patients whose craniopharyngiomas were found incidental to skull films taken for other symptoms.[77] Both of his patients and one of mine (G.J.) in a

Table 31-2. Bloom's survival rates (%) for patients treated with radiation therapy for craniopharyngioma—"new cases"

Interval (years)	Children (46)	Adults (66)
3	86	80
5	85	74
10	74	60

similar state had presumed total extirpations with excellent results.

The danger of merely observing such a patient is exemplified by the report of Fitz et al.[18] A diagnosis of craniopharyngioma was made from a CT scan of a 17-year-old girl with minimal signs and symptoms. No treatment was given. One year later a rapid loss of visual field, tinnitus, ataxia, and nystagmus were associated with a large, nonenhancing dense mass in the posterior fossa on another CT scan. The preoperative diagnosis of clot because of the sudden onset of symptoms and the lack of calcification was controverted by the operative finding of a large subpeduncular extension of calcified tumor.

Small Soft Tissue Remnants of Tumor

In four of my patients in whom I thought I had left behind a bit of tumor no clinical recurrence has taken place to date. Three (E.B., A.P. and D.W.) are still living 19, 21, and 22 years after surgery, and the fourth (J.G.) died 11 years after surgery from a myocardial infarct. In two other patients I was uncertain about some of the residual tissue and they too have had no recurrence after 20 and 29 years. Of the 7 patients with clinical recurrences, I knew I had left some tumor in three but thought I had totally removed the tumor in four. In a patient treated recently (C.W.), a CT scan and PEG obtained 1 year after my presumed total removal showed a small nonsymptomatic recurrence. I opted to act on the cheering reports regarding radiation therapy. This killed him. Patterson[61] carried out no further treatment in his case 1, in which residual tumor was noted on the postoperative CT scan. Hoffman[78] explicitly counsels against prophylactic radiotherapy for asymptomatic residual tumors.

However, Till commented that on several occasions reoperation was easier than at the first attempt and there are several examples of apparently total removal being achieved months or years after a subtotal removal.[70] When the sole recurrence took place in the seven radical removals of Wilson he removed it and the patient has had no recurrence after 7 years.[33] With the superb CT and MRI scanning now available, it may be possible to determine more precisely the best choice for each patient.

RADIATION THERAPY

The value of radiotherapy has been unequivocally demonstrated by the sustained efforts of Kramer et al.,[117] first reported in 1961, and by Bloom and Harmer.[118] They proved this by combining radiotherapy with the minimal surgery of biopsy and cyst aspiration followed by "radical radiotherapy."[113,114,118] Bloom's latest reported survival figures as computed by Life Table methods are given in Table 31-2. He judges the quality of survival after his treatment by the results at 2 years. At that point "90 percent of his cases had no significant neurological or mental disability and vision was good or useful in 83 percent."[118] Since these figures do not indicate the degree of deficit caused by radiation, it is difficult to assess the value of treatment in terms of the percentage of patients who had vision restored, e.g., two of my patients were legally blind before surgery and remained so. All but two of the remainder recovered or maintained useful vision. Kramer's comprehensive 1976 report of his total experience with 43 patients since 1952 ascribes death in only 5 cases to the failure of radiation therapy to control the disease or to the production of damage.[113] He noted that "16 of 19 children have survived and are either in school or leading normal adult lives without major deficits." His 1983 report is on 19 patients under 20 years of age irradiated between 1961 and 1978. The doses were 3500 to 5900 rad in 12 children and 6000 to 6500 rad in 7 adolescents. The preceding surgery was subtotal removal in 10 patients, minimal operation in 6, and "total excision" in 3, who were irradiated only after clinical recurrence. Nine of 13 patients (69 percent) survived 5 years; 8 of 12 (66 percent) survived 10 years. The Katz-Kramer performance ratings were: group 1, 36 percent; group 2, 43 percent; and group 3, 21 percent. In 10 patients the mean full scale IQ was 90; 4 of 5 were employed at nonprofessional work.

The ground swell of proof of the value of radiation therapy in these cases has now approached the proportions of a major wave. It has become abundantly clear in a score of reports that when surgical removal is short of total the addition of radiotherapy (RT) greatly improves both the recurrence and survival rates. The data supporting this conclusion are overwhelming. The uncertainty is related to a comparison between minimal up to subtotal removals plus RT on the one hand and total removals and no radiation on the other hand.

There are several reports in which the value of minimal surgery plus radiation is compared with that of other treatment. Thus, Fischer et al.[60] compared a group of 23 children having minimal surgery with a group of 14 in whom total excision was the tentative goal; this was thought to have been accomplished in eight. Radiation treatment was given to the 2 of these 8 patients with recurrence and to 9 other of the 14 patients in the second category as well as to all 23 of those patients undergoing

Table 31-3. Results of radiation therapy correlated with extent of operative tumor removal— University of Tokyo*

Extent of Removal	Radiation Therapy	Number of Cases	5-Year Survival (%)	10-Year Survival (%)
Minimal	−	20	35	24
	+	13	85	59
Partial	−	28	29	25
	+	14	79	79
Subtotal	−	11	45	36
	+	18	100	87
Total	−	21	81	81

* Adapted from Manaka S, Teramoto A, Takakura K: The efficacy of radiotherapy for craniopharyngioma. J Neurosurg 62:648, 1985.

Table 31-4. Radiation therapy at Columbia-Presbyterian Medical Center

	Number of Cases	Group 1 (%)	Group 2 (%)	Group 3 (%)	Group 4 (%)
All Ages Sung et al.[122]					
Total resection	27	26	30	18	26
Subtotal resection and RT	14	64	14	22	0
Minimal operation and RT	11	27	46	9	18
Sung et al.[123]					
Surgery plus RT	33	51		21	27
Children Carmel et al.[58]					
Total resection	14	29	29	13	29
Subtotal resection and RT	13	23	31	31	15

minimal surgery. The dose was 5000 to 5700 rad in 180) to 200-rad fractions, usually in a radiation field of 36 cm^2 over an average of 45 days. The CT scans showed similar reductions in maximum tumor diameter in the two groups; by 48 percent in the first group and by 55 percent in the second. At follow-up no tumor was seen in 3 of the 11 patients in the second group (major operation-radiation) and in 2 of the 23 patients in the first group. Follow-ups were from 1 to 9 years and 10 years. Diabetes insipidus required treatment in only 2 patients in the first group and in all of the patients in the second group.

A massive study emanated from Tokyo University, where Manaka et al.[46] selected 125 well-documented cases treated in the 30-year period beginning in 1950. Only 45 of these patients were irradiated at doses of 4500 to 6000 rad, average 5000 rad. They divided the patients into four categories vis-à-vis extent of removal as shown in Table 31-3. Regardless of the extent of subtotal removal, the irradiated patients did dramatically better in each group. As this fact became steadily more evident the percentage of patients referred for radiation increased during the three decades from 10 percent to 54 percent to 73 percent, respectively. The best survival figures were found in the group of subtotal removal plus radiation. It is noteworthy that the 10-year and 5-year survival rates are the same after total removal, which corresponds with other data that a presumably totally removed tumor is less likely to recur after 5 years than an irradiated one.

In the small group of 8 children of Richmond et al.[119] from the University of California, San Francisco, treated by minimal surgery plus radiation, all 8 survived 5 years and the 4 patients treated 10 or more years before were also living. Of the 8 patients treated by presumed total excision, 7 were alive at 5 years and 2 of 4 were alive at 10 years—not quite as good as the irradiated group, although all of these were in the "good" category regarding the quality of survival. Thomsett et al.[120] from the same institution also concluded from a comparison between 14 patients undergoing total excision and 11 patients receiving subtotal removal plus RT that the latter course yielded more survivors with a good outcome. Cabezudo et al.[50] added their voices to the chorus. Total excision in 16 cases was followed by three deaths and four recurrences, whereas subtotal removal plus 5000 to 6100 rad of radiation in 5 to 7 weeks yielded no deaths and one recurrence. Resch et al.[121] also treated residual tumor in 5 children with about 5000 rad, with regression of tumor size as determined from CT scans in all cases.

Some of the difficulty in assessing the data can be gleaned from a comparison (Table 31-4) of three different reports from the same institution. On the important issue of the quality of survival the radiation oncologist Sung found nearly twice as many patients in the two worse groups after total excision as after either of two lesser extents of surgery plus radiation.[122] The next year, however, he found the percentage of fair and poor results to be about the same in the group undergoing total excision as in the group treated with radiation[123]—a finding that Carmel the neurosurgeon corroborated in the same year with respect to children.

The excellent results of Wilson deserve special mention.[33] Although his objective "in all cases" was total removal of the tumor, he thought he could do this "without unacceptable morbidity" in only 7 of his 74 patients operated on between 1969 and 1985. Recurrence has taken place in 1 of the 7 patients, who underwent reoperation with, again, presumed total removal. The remainder have been treated by "*radical subtotal removal*" followed by radiation therapy. The operation led to only two deaths early in the series. Multiple procedures to "provide significant relief of compressive symptoms" were required in 15 percent of the patients. A transsphenoidal approach was used in 39 percent of the patients; no statement

Table 31-5. Recurrence-free survival rates (%) (R); Comparison of radical operation with nonradical operation plus radiotherapy*

	Number of patients	5 years	Number of Patients	10 years
Radical operation	27	72 ± 6	12	60 ± 8
Nonradical operation and radiotherapy	8	62 ± 12	2	25 ± 13
Nonradical operation without radiotherapy	7	36 ± 10	4	26 ± 9

* Adapted from Sorva R, Heiskanen O: Craniopharyngioma in Finland. Acta Neurochir 81:85, 1986. Sorva and Heiskanen state, "Radical operation is the best treatment."

Table 31-6. Comparison between Massachusetts General Hospital and Boston Children's Hospital series

	Sweet 1970–1979 Up to 9 of 10 patients tested; Followup 7–17 years	Cavazzuti-Fischer 1972–1981 Group I 18 of 21 patients tested; Radiation with or without biopsy confirmation; Followup 1–9 years	Sweet 1955–1979 18 of 24 patients tested; Followup 7–38 years
Psychological Testing			
Full scale IQ	(7)* 97.2	101.4	(9) 97.9
Frontal lobe function			
Thurstone word			
Fluency	(3) 56.0	40.5	(4) 50.2
Wisconsin Card			
Sorting			
Category Achieved			
> 4	(4) 100%	94%	(5) 80%
Learning and Memory			
Memory Quotient			
(Wechsler Memory Scale)	(7) 101.0	101.6	(7) 102.4
Rey-Osterrieth Test	(4) 26.8	19.3	(5) 18.9
(Reproduction complex figure)			
Manual Dexterity			
Thurstone tapping			
Normal R 104.0	(5) 86.0	86.0	(3) 84.7
Normal L 98.0	79.2	76.8	82.2
General Performance Category			
	12 pts	21 pts	
Excellent	76%	86%	
Good	16%	14%	
Fair	8%	0%	
Visual Status†			
Better	42%	33%	38%
Same	25%		33%
Worse	33% (1 eye only)		29%
Residual Tumor or Late Recurrence	25%	91%	

* Numbers in parentheses = number given specific test. In the WHS scores in column in the seventies group in column 1 the lone case in the "good" and one in the "fair" categories were tested, hence the excellent group is inadequately represented.
† Initial good vision always preserved in one eye. In both series normal vision preoperatively was maintained.

was made about whether or not a presumed total removal was attained in any of these. However, the total results are impressive. Further growth of tumor leading to death occurred in only 1 patient and only 1 patient was totally blinded by the operation. Significant improvement in visual field defects was achieved in 48 of 52 patients; in 17 the fields reverted to normal. The mean follow-up period was over 4 years. Diabetes insipidus, which was produced in only 23 percent of patients who did not have it, was attributed in most of them to the radiation therapy, since it usually developed 6 to 18 months after that therapy. Three died of unrelated causes. The state of remission of 67 of the patients is described as one of "stable ophthalmological and neurological disease" with a continued decrease or stable tumor size as assured radiologically. This full report did not include any statement about the mentation and general performance level of the group.

The aggressively oriented neurosurgeon will be happy to learn the experience at Finland's University Central Hospital in Helsinki. Sorva and Heiskanen reported on 123 histologically verified cases of craniopharyngioma in the 32 years between 1951 and 1982.[71] Their surgical mortality dropped as the case load increased: 29 percent of 24 patients in the 1950s, 25 percent of 28 in the 1960s, 7 percent of 54 in the 1970s, and none since 1979. They do more "radical" removals than lesser removals in a ratio of 61:48. Their recurrence-free survival rates: R ± SEM% are given in Table 31-5.

The most complete comparative data are perhaps those of Fischer[60] and Cavazzuti et al.[124] Their excellent record at the Boston Children's Hospital has already been cited. It was achieved in 23 children following either radiation alone or radiation plus conservative surgical measures. The diagnosis was not confirmed histologically in 10 cases. The treatment was given in the decade from 1972 to 1981; 21 of the 23 patients were followed. Reaspiration of cysts in 5 patients was helpful in maintaining the happy status shown in Table 31-6. Further asymptomatic tumor growth occurred in only 1 patient given a smaller than usual dose and radiation field. A shrunken calcified mass was the usual appearance of these lesions on CT scans in the 21 patients. Visual perceptual tests, visual acuity, and occulomotility improved in one third of the patients.

Clear-cut radiation injury from their relatively large dose to children occurred in only 2 patients. One was a 4-year-old who showed progressive impairment in memory and learning tests along with calcification in the frontal lobe and hypothalamus. The other child after the sequence of radical surgery and two courses of radiation to control tumor growth became deaf in both ears. They also had two disasters of delayed coma at 1 year after treatment in their group of patients treated by radical surgery plus radiation. At autopsy one of these had "severe gliosis and cavitation of the infundibulum and mammillary bodies." The other recovered only to a severely disabled, category "poor" level. Neither had a cyst or solid tumor as determined from CT scans. The time interval seems to me to be typical for radiation necrosis, and I suggest that these two sequelae were perhaps caused at least in part by radiation damage such as occurred more conclusively in one of my cases (C.W.). I have not seen this sequela in any of my nonirradiated patients.

These authors[124] and Galatzer et al.[125] have added an important further variable of detailed psychological testing to their appraisals. We have followed their lead and have had the benefit of some of the same psychologists under the aegis of Professor Suzanne Corkin for much of this work. Table 31-6 compares the test results after my radical removals in 18 patients with their group of 18 patients undergoing minimal surgery plus RT with a shorter follow-up. As these data stand, the slightly better level of frontal lobe function in my patients may not be significant because of the small number of studies and may not be worth the added hazard of a major operation. However, a longer follow-up might possibly reveal late radiation injury or late tumor regrowth after radiation. This was seen in a Parisian series of 52 children which provided a very long follow-up comparison on the same service between radical removal and subtotal removal with RT.[126] The recurrence rate in the former group, 24 percent at 10 years, remained the same at 15 years (as has been my experience), whereas the recurrence rate in the group with lesser removal plus radiation jumped from 20 percent at 9 years to 50 percent at 15 years. One of their irradiated patients also became deaf. Earlier diagnosis plus improved surgical skill and techniques may all make radical removal safer. At present it is something approaching a dead heat between the Massachusetts General Hospital and the Boston Children's Hospital for the shorter follow-ups at less than 10 years. The latter group did not publish data to compare with our group of 24 patients followed for 10 to 38 years.

SHARPLY CIRCUMSCRIBED RADIATION

The specialized procedure developed by Leksell and Backlund[127] involves use of the Leksell stereotactic system to inject colloidal β-emitting yttrium 90 in any cystic parts of the tumor carefully calculated to deliver 20,000 rad to the inside of the cyst wall. The solid portion receives primarily photons from cobalt 60 via many channels appropriately constructed in a heavy helmet. Thirty-five patients have been treated in the 10-year period ending in 1975. Only 2 patients were dead and 2 partially disabled. A definitive report on the series now totaling well over 100 patients has not appeared.

FOLLOW-UP PATHOLOGIC FINDINGS AFTER RADIATION THERAPY

Amacher[128] described an autopsy in which serial sections at 5-μ intervals showed complete radiation necrosis of the remaining tumor except for "a microscopic collection of viable epithelial cells in each hypothalamus." Because of a malfunctioning shunt this patient died 13 months after a 5000-rad dose to the tumor. Landolt also published reports on 2 children whose partial removals were followed by treatment of 4000 rad in 1 patient and 5000 rad in the other.[38,129] Exploratory operations after 4 and 3 years, respectively, revealed in each only cellular calcified "parakeratotic" masses embedded in collagenous scar without proliferating tumor. One of the patients was "stable" 2 years later.

In the same vein is the report of Weiss and Raskind.[130] Their 2 patients received 4860 rads in 37 days and 5400 rads in 55 days. At 1 and 5 years later, respectively, re-exploration disclosed no tumor, but pronounced radiation changes in the meninges, brain, and optic nerves were seen.

The magnitude of the problem is intimated by the 1983 review of the literature of Fukamachi et al.[131] on radiation necrosis after treatment of tumors in the sellar region of adults. They found 40 such cases in 23 articles dating back to 1951, 16 of which were after 1970. The dose was 5000 rads or less in 12 cases and from 5100 to 6100 rads in 12 more. The incidence of proven major radiation injury to vision in pituitary adenomas and craniopharyngiomas was 9 percent in 55 cases of Harris and Levene.[132] The destructive doses were 4500 rads in 3, 5000 rads in 1, and 7000 rads in the 5th, given in 250-rads fractions in all 5. The patients were all middle aged or older adults.

Another problem is the late development of a malignant glioma, usually in the radiation field of a more benign lesion. Although rare, Piatt et al.[133] and Maat-Schieman et al.[134] collected 21 cases of this complication after doses from 2400 to 6000 rads in 14 of them (much less in the other 7).

APPROPRIATE RADIATION DOSE LEVELS

Given the lead of Kramer and of Bloom that "radical" radiation therapy should involve high dose levels, others have followed suit after recurrences at lower initial doses. Onoyama et al.,[135] treating children experienced a worse survival rate with doses less than 5000 rads than with doses at that and higher levels. Sung et al.[122] described recurrence in 4 of 8 patients following treatment by minimal surgery plus 4000 to 5000 rads of radiation. They then jumped the dose to the 5500–6900-rad level in both children and adults and have had only three recurrences to date in the next 19 patients (followed for a shorter time). Similarly, Chin et al.[136] had a recurrence in 1 of 3 patients whose partial tumor removal was supplemented by less than 5600 rads of radiation before 1970. Thereupon they increased the dose to as high as 6500 rads with but one recurrence in 6 patients. Likewise, Vyramuthu and Benton[137] who treated 15 patients postsurgically with 1350 to 1600 CRE (rets*) noted recurrences only in the 7 of the 10 patients whose doses were less than 1520 rad. Follow-up was from 5 to 23 years.

---

*"Rets" refers to nominal standard dose (NSD), computed by the formula

$$NSD = (D)/(n^{0.24} \times t^{0.11})$$

where D is the total dose in rads, n is the number of fractions, and t is the time in days over which radiation given.

FINAL CONCLUSION

The decisions regarding increasing the dose of radiation or striving maximally for total excision were all reached before high resolution scanners became available to detect tumor regrowth before clinical recurrence. Now that the diagnosis of asymptomatic tumor growth is readily attainable, it is imperative to follow patients at reasonable intervals because some clinical recurrences are the universal experience whatever the treatment. A conservative course both in regard to radiation dose on the one hand and pushing for total excision on the other hand seems appropriate. In my professional lifetime the outlook for craniopharyngioma has gone from grim in most patients to excellent in the great majority.

RATHKE'S CLEFT OR EPITHELIAL CYSTS

Rathke's pouch, the superiorly directed evagination from the stomodeum of the 4-week-old human embryo, becomes obliterated at all but its cranial portion by the seventh week of gestation. The anterior wall of the remaining small cavity, "the pituitary pouch," develops into the anterior lobe of the pituitary gland and its posterior wall becomes the pars intermedia of the gland. A residual lumen between a portion of these two structures was found by Shanklin at autopsy to have persisted in 22 of 100 normal pituitary glands.[138] Small, asymptomatic, fluid-containing cysts were found in 13 of these 22 specimens. Rarely, these cysts enlarge enough to produce symptoms; by 1977, Yoshida et al.[139] had collected 35 such cases from the world literature and at least that many more have been reported since then. Cuboidal or columnar epithelial cells, often mucin-secreting goblet cells that stain positively by the periodic acid-Schiff (PAS) method and often ciliated, line these residual clefts of Rathke's pouch and fill them with a fluid that is usually white and "mucoid" or "colloid." In two cases it was clear and colorless; yellow, blue, or green fluid has been seen. A few have had an appearance more suggestive of craniopharyngioma with brown or machine-oil fluid and cholesterin crystals. In at least four of the cases in which the fluid looked like creamy white pus, the surgeon diagnosed an abscess, but an organism was grown in only one case. This will be discussed further.

In 26 of Yoshida's 35 cases the cyst was wholly or largely intrasellar, often with significant bony sellar enlargement or destruction or both. A suprasellar component may give some of the lesions a dumbbell shape. Ringel and Bailey[140] described the precise relationship in a patient who died preoperatively after a Conray ventriculogram. The $2.8 \times 2.5 \times 2.0$-cm histologically typical lesion emerged from the center of a normal pituitary gland, lying almost entirely above it. A totally suprasellar position has now been reported in 9 other cases, 7 collected by Barrow et al.[141] In four cases there was calcification in the cyst wall.[142] Of Yoshida's 35 patients, only 5 were under 25 years of age; 21 were female.

Fager and Carter,[143] with the earliest reported series of 5 living patients, found no solid abnormal tissue other than the thin wall in any of them. Visual fields and acuity, grossly abnormal in four of the patients preoperatively, improved markedly after the operation. Fager did not remove the cyst wall completely, but no symptoms recurred in any of the patients followed for as long as 9 years. He therefore regards total excision of the wall as unnecessary, concluding that a less radical approach suffices for these purely cystic intrapituitary or parapituitary lesions containing milky or mucoid fluid. Baskin

and Wilson[144] took the same position after their experience with 10 such cases; seven intrasellar and three intrasellar and suprasellar with visual field defects. Their operations, all by the transsphenoidal route, included histologic examination of a cyst wall biopsy specimen, with drainage only, if no neoplasm was found. These authors pointed out the need for establishing the clinical significance of hypodense intrasellar areas on CT scans in the 20 percent of persons who show them.[145] If, despite complaints of headache and symptoms of possible endocrine malfunction, detailed studies of the endocrine and visual systems are normal, they logically counsel against operation. Shuangshoti et al.[146] presented evidence that the intrasellar epithelial cysts are histologically and histochemically indistinguishable from the higher neuroepithelial or colloid cysts, which also tend to refill slowly after aspiration.

Totally benign behavior is far from invariable, however. One of Yoshida's patients had a small nodule on her cyst wall, which was scraped out with a curette.[139] Only part of the cyst wall was removed and a serious recurrence took place within 1 year. Raskind's patient, whose cyst contained a clear, colorless fluid, experienced a recurrence requiring reoperation 26 years later.[147] The patient reported by Berry and Schlezinger[148] had only a fragment of the cyst wall removed at the first craniotomy. At a major recurrence 37 months later the cyst was three times the original size, but contained the same clear, colorless mucoid fluid. The recurrences described by Yoshida et al.,[139] Iraci et al.,[149] and Matsushima et al.[150] were in patients with solid components to their lesions containing stratified epithelium. In Matsushima's case, although the cyst was filled with the typical mucinous, puslike material and some of its lining was ciliated columnar cells containing mucin, most of it consisted of stratified squamous epithelium. This latter component determined the outcome, namely death from recurrent tumor 20 months after its subtotal removal. Clearly, it is the solid portion of the tumor more than the appearance of the cystic fluid that determines the prognosis. Two patients of Marcincin and Gennarelli[151] experienced recurrences within 2 years after transsphenoidal evacuation of the cysts even though the cyst fluid and wall were typical of pure Rathke's cleft lesions. A permanent visual loss ensued in one of the patients. The lesion was approached intracranially upon recurrence in the second patient and the entire cyst wall removed.

As the reports have accumulated, it has become clear that many patients have transitional lesions. Russell and Rubinstein[4] were among the first to point this out, describing in 2 patients dumbbell cysts the intrasellar portion of which was lined by a single layer of ciliated epithelium that changed abruptly at the diaphragma sellae to the squamous epithelium characteristic of a craniopharyngioma for the suprasellar portion. In a case of Yoshida's there was a tumor nodule with an inner lining of columnar cells covering many layers of stratified squamous epithelium. Matsushima's case was just mentioned. Tajika et al.[152] found some areas of stratified epithelium in 2 of their 3 patients with Rathke's cleft cysts; in 1 of the 2 patients there were cholesterol crystals, calcification, and brown fluid. Conversely, some ciliated combined and columnar cell areas were found in 2 other patients with histologic findings otherwise typical of a craniopharyngioma. Goodrich et al.[153] described a suprasellar soft necrotic tumor rather than a fluid-containing tumor containing many ciliated cuboidal or columnar cells typical of the lesion under discussion, but other parts of the tumor included masses of squamous epithelium. Another Rathke's cleft cyst was reported with characteristics as well of an epidermoid cyst.[154] In another group of at least 7 patients the solid tumor of a chromophobe adenoma was associated with the typical histologic form of a Rathke's cleft cyst.[155–157] The more solid tissue there is associated with the cyst, the more likely it is to include a chronic inflammatory process, the stratified epithelium of a craniopharyngioma, or the glandular tissue of a pituitary adenoma. These tissues are likely to show enhancement in a scan, whereas the cyst fluid is low on the Hounsfield Unit scale.

The reports of recurrences upon mere evacuation of cysts have provided support for those who from the first included readily removable cyst walls as part of the surgical objective. One of the earlier reports of a patient with typical pathologic findings described piecemeal removal of the capsule, leaving small fragments attached to the hypothalamus.[158] More recently Nagasaka et al.[159] resected all of the cyst wall in one of their 2 cases and the suprasellar part of it in the other, leaving behind the portion occupying much of the intrasellar region. The first case was followed for 5 years without a recurrence. Subtotal or partial excision of the cyst wall was also elected by Rout et al.[160] in their 2 cases. In a 1984 publication (high resolution CT scanning available), Shimoji et al.[161] noted enhanced capsules around low density cysts in all three of their patients.

They therefore elected to remove "as much as possible of the capsule" in all three with good clinical results. Specimens from all 3 patients showed the typical histologic pattern of the Rathke's cleft cyst with the addition of squamous epithelium in the third case. They also gave 3000 rad of radiation therapy in two of these cases—a tactic described in no other report for a pure Rathke's cleft cyst. Yamamoto et al.[162] also elected to excise the capsule of the cysts in their 2 patients. A thick, faintly enhancing cyst wall was "radically" removed by Okamoto et al.[163] It proved to contain stratified squamous as well as ciliated columnar epithelium plus inflammatory cells. Only parts of the cyst wall were resected in their other 2 cases, one of which showed no contrast enhancement. Swanson et al.[155] also used the fact of capsular enhancement at CT scanning of an intrasellar mass to guide them to a transfrontal excision of the cyst wall. Nonfunctional pituitary adenomatous cells constituted a part of that wall, so they then gave the patient a course of radiation therapy.

Since then Dietemann et al.[164] also have drawn attention to the low attenuation of the cystic fluid in CT scans (15–17 HU in their 3 cases), leading them to approach the enlarged sella transsphenoidally and successfully. In the first 2 of 3 cases the entire cyst wall and in the third a part of the cyst wall was removed. Fluid similar to machine oil in the second case was not accompanied by any squamous epithelium in the cyst wall. In general the transsphenoidal route has been favored for many cases, especially when the suprasellar portion shows minimal enhancement. However, simple transsphenoidal aspiration of 7 ml of thick brown fluid in one case was followed by a prompt recurrence in 4 months. At subsequent transsphenoidal operation the cyst wall proved to be pure Rathke's cleft in type.[160]

BOUTS OF CHEMICAL MENINGITIS; THE SYNDROME OF THE TOXIN-LEAKING CNS CYST

An important point emerges from collating the data on scattered individual case reports of patients with curious repeated febrile episodes, often with CSF pleocytosis. In only one case was an organism cultured. Attacks of a recurrent chemical febrile meningitis in a craniopharyngioma, presumably from a leakage of keratin or cholesterol, is an extremely rare but well authenticated occurrence.[165]

In the first such case of Rathke's cleft cyst (reported as an abscess by Obenchain and Becker[166]), the patient had had five episodes in 3 years of severe headaches, nausea, vomiting, general malaise, and fever, all leading to hospital admissions but which resolved spontaneously in a few days. Finally, blurring of vision in her inferior temporal quadrants led to the diagnosis of her intrasellar and minimally suprasellar mass from which via a subfrontal route 2 ml of "purulent" fluid was aspirated. *Staphylococcus epidermidis* was cultured from this fluid, and the patient was given penicillin, INH, and ethambutol for 1 month. Then via the transsphenoidal route 3 ml of "pus" was aspirated and the capsule removed. Histologically the wall was fibrous and lined by columnar epithelium with chronic inflammatory cells. Recovery was excellent and sustained. The absence of acute inflammatory cells and the spontaneously subsiding brief attacks for 3 years cast doubt on the role of the staphylococci.

In the next case there were similar recurrent brief episodes, each lasting only 2 or 3 days, characterized by intense supraorbital pains, fever to 39° or 40°C plus about 50 clear-cut temporal lobe seizures a day, each lasting several seconds, mainly during the bouts of fever. These mysterious episodes continued for 10 years, during which the patient's weight went from 50 to 72 kg. Although she did not develop nuchal rigidity in the attacks, a lumbar puncture finally done in 1977 revealed a largely lymphocytic pleocytosis with a normal protein level. Demonstration of an infratemporal quadrantanopsia was followed by pneumography, which revealed a suprasellar mass. At a subfrontal exposure thick puslike fluid was removed from a subchiasmatic cyst, the capsule of which was also largely removed. The cyst wall was heavily vascularized and infiltrated with inflammatory cells but lined with the typical ciliated columnar and cuboidal epithelium. The patient gradually made a full recovery.[167]

The following year Verkijk and Bots[154] described a patient in whom meningeal reactions developed after surgery on a cyst; these resolved spontaneously in 9 months. In the case of Steinberg et al.[168] the initial symptoms pointed to the pituitary region, but then over the next 2 years the patient was in the hospital numerous times with bouts of severe headache, nausea, vomiting, confusion, stiff neck, decreased visual acuity, and ataxic gait. On different occasions the CSF showed pleocytosis and an increased protein level with elevated pressure. All manner of cultures were always negative. The episodes either resolved spontaneously or disappeared promptly with increases in the dexamethasone dosage. The sella was found to be enlarged, containing a mass without suprasellar extension; the sella was, however, partially empty, its anterior portion filling with air. These were apparently considered incidental findings. The lateral and third ventricles became increasingly dilated and there was delayed egress of contrast through the aqueduct and out of the fourth ventricle. The hydrocephalus was treated by ventriculoatrial shunt in 1972. Intracranial obstruction of the shunt required two revisions; each time the symptoms promptly resolved. The patient died a year later of pneumonia. At autopsy the Rathke's cleft cyst occupying the entire sella was filled with thick yellow-green fluid. The cyst epithelium was ciliated columnar in some cases and squamous in one area, keratinized in others. The

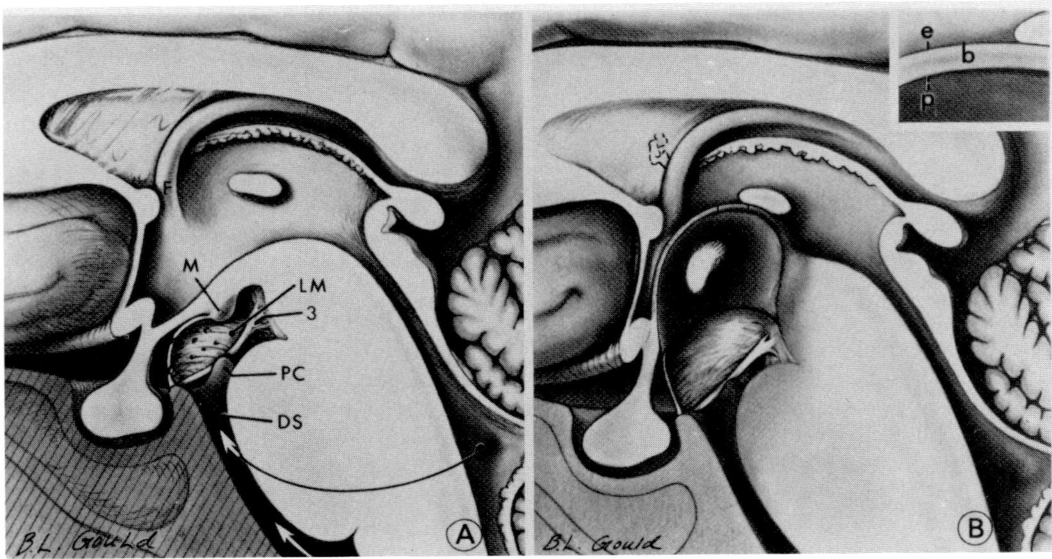

Fig. 31-10. Anatomy of a suprasellar cyst. (A) Artist's conception of the sagittal section of a normal brain and the sellar region, looking to the right. F, fornix; M, mammillary body; LM, Liliequist's membrane; 3, right oculomotor nerve; PC, right posterior clinoid process; DS, dorsum sellae; arrows, normal flow of cerebrospinal fluid through the prepontine and interpeduncular cisterns. (B), The membrane of Liliequist has ballooned forward and upward, compressing the floor of the third ventricle to the level of the massa intermedia. The left base of the semi-three dimensional "cyst" has been cut away to show the right oculomotor nerve. Inset: enlargement of the compressed cyst-ventricular floor junction; e, ependymal lining of the floor of the third ventricle; b, brain parenchyma of the compressed hypothalamus; p, pia. (Reprinted from Fox JL, Al-Mefty O: Suprasellar arachnoid cysts: An extension of the membrane of Liliequist. Neurosurgery 7:617, 1980. With permission.)

leptomeninges adjacent to the chiasm and third ventricle were "moderately fibrotic with mild chronic inflammation."

Episodes of severe meningeal symptoms and signs also with completely negative cultures characterized a patient of Gomez Perun.[169] When a suprasellar lesion was demonstrated and explored 1½ years later, the cyst contained a thick white fluid with an intense inflammatory reaction and numerous vessels in the cyst wall along with a lining of ciliated columnar epithelium. There was also an extensive frontal basal arachnoiditis not noted in the other cases. The "pus" was sterile and the patient made a prompt recovery but soon regressed, with similar episodes of aseptic meningitis. Despite three more operations he died; no organism was ever grown.

Sonntag's patient had only two episodes of a lymphocytic aseptic meningeal reaction before his intrasellar/suprasellar mass was subfrontally exposed.[170] Seven milliliters of "pus" was aspirated, and the cyst wall was subtotally removed. The aspirate was sterile, but rare Gram-negative rods were seen and chloramphenicol was administered for a week. The symptoms recurred in a month, leading to transsphenoidal drainage of 5 ml of "pus" and "extensive removal of its wall." Cultures from this fluid were also negative. Chloramphenicol was continued for a month and the patient has remained well for almost 2 years.

In Shimoji's second case, brief episodes of headache, nausea, vomiting, and fever were accompanied by enough eye signs to point to the sellar region and its cyst.[161] The "abscess-like viscous fluid" was sterile. As much cyst wall as possible was removed, with an excellent result that persisted 2 years later. The first suggestion of infection in their third case was an intermittent fever to 38°C on hospitalization. After pneumoencephalography this rose to 39°C; the patient had meningeal signs and a CSF pleocytosis of 456 neutrophiles and 74 lym-

phocytes. There was no growth on culture. A week of antibiotics brought no change, but 30 mg prednisone per day and other antibiotics dropped the temperature to normal the next day. The yellowish-white gelatinous cyst fluid and its capsule were removed. The PAS-positive stratified squamous epithelium was heavily infiltrated with inflammatory cells. The good recovery persisted at 28 months.

Thick yellow puslike material and a cyst wall accompanied by squamous epithelium and thick connective tissue infiltrated with inflammatory cells was described in two other reports (case 1[160]; case 1[163]).

CONCLUSIONS

1. There are at least 8 patients in less than a hundred with reported Rathke's cleft cysts demonstrating recurrent episodes of systemic or usually meningeal febrile illness. The suggestion is that some of these typically thin-walled cysts may contain a peculiar chemical irritant that can leak out enough to contaminate the blood stream or CSF at intervals and produce these dangerous responses. At surgery the area should be protected by cottonoid before aspiration with as complete a removal of the wall as is consistent with the avoidance of morbidity.

2. The features of CT contrast enhancement of the wall, dark cyst fluid containing cholesterin crystals or creamy "pus" content and/or the biopsy specimen at operation revealing evidence of craniopharyngioma or pituitary adenoma all call for a more serious effort to remove the cyst wall. Since most cases have been reported within a few years of operation, we do not have long-term pathologic data to correlate with recurrence rates.

SUPRASELLAR CYST

The term *suprasellar cyst,* formerly one of the synonyms for craniopharyngioma, designates a small group of lesions, usually congenital, with a thin, even transparent wall filled with a clear colorless or light yellow fluid with the same radiographic density in Hounsfield units as CSF. Constituting less than 1 percent of all intracranial mass lesions, the congenital defect was severe enough to cause symptoms in the first two decades in 46 of the 54 reports collated by Hoffman et al.[171] The lesion evolves as a consequence of prevention of continuing CSF circulation forward into the chiasmatic cistern or laterally from the interpeduncular cistern beneath the hypothalamus and behind the pituitary stalk and optic chiasm. The presence of CSF from below the pontine cistern then pushes the hypothalamic floor upward and thins it markedly so that above the arachnoid dome are only at most a few glial and ependymal cells, as described by Harrison[177] in 3 of his 4 cases. In many of the cases thin, even transparent connective tissue is the only lining to the cyst. By the time the diagnosis is made much or all of the third ventricle usually is filled by the intruder, causing obstruction of one or both foramina of Monro, lateral ventricular dilatation, and a huge head. Indeed, the dome of the cyst is usually much higher than shown in Figure 31-10, lying just beneath the corpus callosum. One possible mechanism for this block is excessive development of an arachnoidal curtain extending from the posterior hypothalamus above to the dorsum sellae below, originally described by Key and Retzius.[172] Its presence, confirmed by Liliequist[173] and by Fox[174] becomes a menace when it and the arachnoid lateral to it become imperforate. Another mechanism of pathogenesis proposed by Starkman et al.[175] is that intra-arachnoidal spaces in the embryo persist and expand exclusively within the arachnoid, as demonstrated in a careful dissection by Krawchenko and Collins[176] for an intact suprasellar cyst in a patient who came to post mortem with this as an incidental finding.

The clinical picture often includes, in addition to hydrocephalus with a big head and ataxia, disturbed visual acuity and fields because of forward and upward displacement of the chiasm and hypopituitarism because of pressure on the hypothalamus and pituitary stalk. A constant forward and backward nodding of the head and neck, the bobble-head syndrome, has been seen in 9 patients. A rotary shaking of the head and shaking arms occurred in one case.[177] The likewise unusual precocious puberty has been seen in 8 children.[171] Headache may occur in the older patients. On CT scans the cyst has the density of CSF; its wall shows neither enhancement nor calcification and it is often mistaken for a dilated third ventricle. The diagnosis is clarified by injection of metrizamide into a lateral ventricle, whereupon the cyst's shadow fails to intensify. Air injected from below often fills the cyst via prepontine and interpeduncular cisterns, but in advanced cases may not do so. The dynamic changes associated with pneumoencephalography or placement of a catheter for third ventriculography may rupture the cyst wall, connecting it with the ventricle, as occurred in all five of Segall's cases.[178]

Surgical treatment which would seem to involve the simple task of making a big opening between the cyst and a normal CSF compartment, proves to be surprisingly difficult to keep effective. Various combinations have been tried, including transfrontal removal of the lower anterior wall of the cyst beneath the chiasm, transcorticoventricular or transcallosal approach to remove much of the dome, catheters between the cyst and ventricle or chiasmatic cistern, and shunts from the lateral ventricles. Any one of these operations alone has a poor chance of sustained success. Agreement seems to be converging on a combination of shunts from the lateral ventricles to the peritoneal cavity with either a transcallosal route to remove the cystic dome as done with sustained success by Hoffman in 5 cases, or subfrontal removal of the anterior cyst wall. This latter tactic was successful in 2 cases of Gonzalez et al.,[179] 3 cases of Raimondi,[180] and 2 cases of Murali and Epstein.[181] However, the lower opening closed with recurrence of symptoms in 1 case of each of the last two groups and in one of Hoffman's cases. That shunts from the ventricles alone may not suffice was demonstrated by a case of Murali and Epstein in a child in whom a neonatal shunt kept the ventricles small but who also 9 years later required opening of a suprasellar cyst to control bilateral visual loss. Ventriculoperitoneal shunting alone was satisfactory in Raimondi's fourth case.

Although nearly all of the cysts represent developmental abnormalities, there are exceptions on a posttraumatic or postinflammatory basis. Thus, Sansregret et al.[182] had one patient whose cyst they presumed had formed in relation to a small typical sarcoid lesion found in the floor of the third ventricle as a postmortem surprise. Many of the patients are severely impaired by the time of initial diagnosis so that prompt aggressive effort and close follow-ups are required.

ACKNOWLEDGMENT

Dr. Sweet wishes to express his gratitude to the Neuro-Research Foundation for its support in the preparation of this manuscript.

REFERENCES

1. Erdheim J: über Hypophysenganggeschwülste und Hirncholesteatome. Sitzber Akad Wiss (Vienna) 113:537, 1904
2. Carmichael HT: Squamous epithelial rests in the hypophysis cerebri. Arch Neurol Psychiat 26:966, 1931
3. Kiyono H:über das Vorkommen von Plattenepithelherden in der Hypophyse. Zugleich ein Beitrag zur Kenntnis der Hypophysenganggewächse. Virchows Arch Pathol Anat 252:118, 1924
4. Russell DS, Rubinstein LJ: Pathology of Tumours of the Nervous System, ed 3. Baltimore, Williams & Wilkins, 1971
5. Araki C, Matsumoto S: Statistical reevaluation of pinealoma and related tumors in Japan. J Neurosurg 30:146, 1969
6. Matson DD: Neurosurgery of Infancy and Childhood. Springfield, Charles C Thomas, 1969
7. Love JG, Marshall TM: Craniopharyngiomas. (Pituitary adamantinomas). Surg Gynecol Obstet 90:591, 1950
8. Pertuiset B: Craniopharyngiomas, in Vinken PJ, Bruyn GW (eds): Handbook of Clinical Neurology, vol 18, 1975, pp 531–572
9. Shillito J: Craniopharyngiomas. Special Lecture. American Association of Neurological Surgeons, New Orleans, April 26, 1978
10. Steno J: G. sella. Microsurgical topography of craniopharyngiomas. Acta Neurochir (Suppl) 35:94–100, 1985
11. Northfield DWC: Rathke-pouch tumours. Brain 80:293, 1957
12. Arem R, Zoghbi W, Chan L: Amenorrhea-galactorrhea and craniopharyngioma. Surg Neurol 20:109, 1983
13. Gamblin GT, James LP, Thomas J, et al: Simulation of a prolactin-secreting adenoma by an intrasellar craniopharyngioma. Neurosurgery 16:689, 1985

14. Duff TA, Levine R: Intrachiasmatic craniopharyngioma. J Neurosurg 59:176, 1983
15. Hamberger C-A, Hammer G, Norlén G, et al: Surgical treatment of craniopharyngioma. Radical removal by the transantrosphenoidal approach. Acta Otolaryngol 52:285, 1960
16. Cooper PR, Ransohoff J: Craniopharyngioma originating in the sphenoid bone. Case report. J Neurosurg 36:102, 1972
17. Pheline C, Jamois Y, Engel Ph, et al: Craniopharyngiome extopique basi-sphénoïdal. Abord par voie basse, naso-septale, puis antro-ethmoïdale. Neurochirurgie 27:221, 1981
18. Fitz CR, Wortzman G, Harwood-Nash DC, et al: Computed tomography in craniopharyngiomas. Radiology 127:687, 1978
19. Mukada K, Mori S, Matsumura S, et al: Infrasellar craniopharyngioma. Surg Neurol 21:565, 1984
20. Maier HC: Craniopharyngioma with erosion and drainage into the nasopharynx. J Neurosurg 62:132, 1985
21. Halves E: Die ergänzende transsphenoidale Operation bei Kraniopharyngiomen im Kindes- und Jugendalter. Neurochirurgia 23:71, 1980
22. Sweet WH: Radical surgical treatment of craniopharyngioma. Clin Neurosurg 23:52, 1976
23. Shillito J: The treatment of craniopharyngiomas of childhood, in Morley TP (ed): Current Controversies in Neurosurgery. Philadelphia, WB Saunders, 1976, pp 332–335
24. Petito CK, DeGirolami U, Earle K: Craniopharyngiomas. A clinical and pathological review. Cancer 37:1944, 1976
25. Altinörs N, Senveli E, Erdogan A, et al: Craniopharyngioma of the cerebellopontine angle. Case report. J Neurosurg 60:842, 1984
26. Cashion EL, Young JM: Intraventricular craniopharyngioma. Report of 2 cases. J Neurosurg 34:84, 1971
27. Long DM, Chou SN: Transcallosal removal of craniopharyngiomas within the third ventricle. J Neurosurg 39:563, 1973
28. King TT: Removal of intraventricular craniopharyngiomas through the lamina terminalis. Acta Neurochir (Wien) 45:277, 1979
29. Papo I, Scarpelli M, Caruselli G: Intrinsic third ventricle craniopharyngiomas with normal pressure hydrocephalus. Neurochirurgia 23:80, 1980
30. Rush JL, Kusske JA, DeFeo DR, et al: Intraventricular craniopharyngioma. Neurology 25:1094, 1975
31. Al-Mefty O, Hassounah M, Weaver P, et al: Microsurgery for giant craniopharyngiomas in children. Neurosurgery 17:585, 1985
32. Solarski A: Craniopharyngioma in the pineal gland. Arch Pathol Lab Med 102:490, 1978
33. Baskin DS, Wilson CB: Surgical management of craniopharyngiomas. J Neurosurg 65:22, 1986
34. Tsuji N, Kuriyama T, Iwamoto M, et al: Moyamoya disease associated with craniopharyngioma. Surg Neurol 21:588, 1984
35. Lau YL, Milligan DWA: Atypical presentation of craniopharyngioma associated with Moyamoya disease. J R Soc Med 79:236, 1986
36. Bailey P, Buchanan DN, Bucy PC: Intracranial Tumors of Infancy and Childhood. Chicago, University of Chicago Press, 1939, pp 349–375
37. Van den Bergh R, Brucher JM: L'abord transventriculaire dans les cranio-pharyngiomes du troisième ventricule. Aspects neurochirurgicaux et neuro-pathologiques. Neurochirurgie 16:51, 1970
38. Landolt A: 8. Die Ultrastruktur des Kraniopharyngeoms. Schweiz Archiv Neurol Neurochir Psychiat 111:313, 1972
39. Kobayashi T, Kageyama N, Yoshida J, et al: Pathological and clinical basis of the indications for treatment of craniopharyngiomas. Neurol Med Chir (Tokyo) 21:39, 1981
40. Bartlett JR: Craniopharyngiomas. An analysis of some aspects of symptomatology, radiology and histology. Brain 94:725, 1971
41. Hoffman HJ, Hendrick EB, Humphreys RP, et al: Management of craniopharyngioma in children. J Neurosurg 47:218, 1977
42. Kahn EA, Gosch HH, Seeger JF, et al: Forty-five years experience with the craniopharyngiomas. Surg Neurol 1:5, 1973
43. Cogen PH, Carmel PW: Craniopharyngioma growth potential: Therapy response of children vs. adults (abstr). Neurosurgery 9:469, 1981
44. Bloom HJG: Recent concepts in the conservative treatment of intracranial tumours in children. Acta Neurochir 50:103, 1979
45. Liszczak T, Richardson EP, Phillips JP, et al: Morphological, biochemical, ultrastructural, tissue culture and clinical observations of typical and aggressive craniopharyngiomas. Acta Neuropathol 43:191, 1978
46. Manaka S, Teramoto A, Takakura K: The efficacy of radiotherapy for craniopharyngioma. J Neurosurg 62:648, 1985
47. Duchen LW, Schurr H: The pathology of the pituitary gland in old age, in Everitt AV, Burgess JA (eds): Hypothalamus, Pituitary and Aging. Springfield, Charles C Thomas, 1976, pp 137–156
48. Freeman JW, Cox TA, Batnitzky S, et al: Craniopharyngioma simulating bilateral internal ophthalmoplegia. Arch Neurol 37:176, 1980
49. Klotz HP, Raymond JP, Beaufils F, et al: Adipsie et syndrome de Korsakoff après intervention hypothalamohypophysaire pour craniopharyngiome. Obésité et ostéonécrose fémorale postopératoires. Ann Endocrinol (Paris) 34:158, 1973
50. Cabezudo JM, Vaquero J, Areitio E, et al: Craniopharyngiomas: A critical approach to treatment. J Neurosurg 55:371, 1981
51. Gardeur D, Nachanakian A, van Effenterre R, et al: Analyse tomodensitométrique des craniopharyngiomes. Incidences thérapeutiques. J Radiol 60:51, 1979
52. Naidich TP, Pinto RS, Kushner MJ, et al: Evaluation of sellar and parasellar masses by computed tomography. Radiology 120:91, 1976
53. Cabezudo JM, Vaquero J, Garcia-de-Sola R, et al: Computed tomography with craniopharyngiomas: A review. Surg Neurol 15:422, 1981
54. New PFJ, Aronow S: Attenuation measurements of whole blood and blood fractions in computed tomography. Radiology 121:635, 1976
55. Lipper MH, Kishore PRS, Ward JD: Craniopharyngioma: Unusual computed tomographic presentation. Neurosurgery 9:76, 1981
56. Nagasawa S, Handa H, Yamashita J, et al: Dense cystic craniopharyngioma with unusual extensions. Surg Neurol 19:299, 1983
57. Symon L, Sprich W: Radical excision of craniopharyngioma. Results in 20 patients. J Neurosurg 62:174, 1985
58. Carmel PW, Autunes JL, Chang CH: Craniopharyngiomas in children. Neurosurgery 11:382, 1982
59. Danoff BF, Cowchock FS, Kramer S: Childhood craniopharyngioma: Survival, local control, endocrine and neurologic function following radiotherapy. Int J Radiat Oncol Biol Phys 9:171, 1983
60. Fischer EG, Welch K, Belli JA, et al: Treatment of craniopharyngiomas in children: 1972–1981. J Neurosurg 62:496, 1985
61. Patterson RH, Danylevich A: Surgical removal of craniopharyngiomas by a transcranial approach through the lamina terminalis and sphenoid sinus. Neurosurgery 7:111, 1980
62. Hoffman HJ: Craniopharyngiomas. Canad J Neurol Sci 12:348, 1985
63. George AE, Lin JP, Kricheff II: Craniopharyngioma with abnormal vasculature. Radiology 95:93, 1970
64. Jakubowski J, Kendall B: Coincidental aneurysms with tumours of pituitary origin. J Neurol Neurosurg Psychiatry 41:972, 1978
65. Svolos DG: Craniopharyngiomas. A study based on 108 verified cases. Acta Chir Scand [Suppl] 403:1, 1969
66. Kahn EA: Some physiologic implications of craniopharyngiomas. Neurology 9:82, 1959
67. Katz EL: Late results of radical excision of craniopharyngiomas in children. J Neurosurg 42:86, 1975
68. Hoffman HJ: Craniopharyngioma: The continuing controversy on management, in Concepts in Pediatric Neurosurgery II. Basel, S. Karger, 1982, pp 14–28
69. Symon L, Jakubowski J, Logue V: The surgical treatment of craniopharyngioma (abstr). Neurochirurgia [Suppl]:262, 1981

70. Till K: Craniopharyngioma. Child's Brain 9:179, 1982

71. Sorva R, Heiskanen O: Craniopharyngioma in Finland. Acta Neurochir 81:85, 1986

72. Patrick BS, Smith RR, Bailey TO: Aseptic meningitis due to spontaneous rupture of craniopharyngioma cyst. Case report. J Neurosurg 41:387, 1974

73. Horoupian DS, Wisniewski HM, Gamble R, et al: Aqueduct gliosis caused by keratin and cholesterol in a case of craniopharyngioma. Can J Neurol Sci 1:185, 1974

74. Okamoto H, Harada K, Uozomi T, et al: Spontaneous rupture of a craniopharyngiomatous cyst. Surg Neurol 24:507, 1985

75. Hakuba A, Nishimura S, Inoue Y: Transpetrosal-transtentorial approach and its application in the therapy of retrochiasmatic craniopharyngiomas. Surg Neurol 24:405, 1985

76. Symon L: Microsurgery of the hypothalamus with special reference to craniopharyngioma. Neurosurg Rev 6:43, 1983

77. Hoffman HJ: Craniopharyngioma—the continuing controversy on management. Presented at the American Association of Neurological Surgeons, Boston, April 6–9, 1981

78. Suzuki J, Katakura R, Mori T: Interhemispheric approach through the lamina terminalis to tumors of the anterior part of the third ventricle. Surg Neurol 22:157, 1984

79. Guiot G, Namin P: L'abord des tumeurs rétrochiasmatique par voie sous-temporale. Neurochirurgie 1:226, 1955

80. Malis L: Craniopharyngiomas. Presented at the Congress of Neurological Surgeons, Atlanta, October 20–24, 1975

81. Hunt WE, Miller CA: Parasellar tumors: Variations on a theme. Clin Neurosurg 25:425, 1978

82. Backlund EO: Solid craniopharyngiomas treated by stereotactic radiosurgery, in Szikla G (ed): Stereotactic Cerebral Irradiation. Amsterdam, Elsevier, 1979, pp 271–281

83. Shapiro K, Till K, Grant DN: Craniopharyngiomas in childhood. A rational approach to treatment. J Neurosurg 50:617, 1979

84. Djordjevic M, Djordjevic Z, Janicijevic M, et al: Surgical treatment of craniopharyngiomas in children. Acta Neurochir [Suppl] 28:344–347, 1979

85. Gelabert M, Reyes F, Bollar A, et al: Successful treatment of a giant cystic craniopharyngioma. J Neurosurg Sci 29:263, 1985

86. Talalla A: Total removal of a craniopharyngioma. Technical note. Acta Neurochir 32:297, 1975

87. Alvarez-Garijo JA, Froufé A, Taboada D, et al: Successful surgical treatment of an odontogenic ossified craniopharyngioma. Case report. J Neurosurg 55:832, 1981

88. Hirsch O: Hypophysentumoren ein Grenzgebiet. Acta Neurochir 5:1, 1957

89. Guiot G: Adénomes Hypophysaires. Paris, Masson, 1958

90. Guiot G: Par ou faut-il aborder l'hypophyse? Presse Med 78:209, 1970

91. Lichter AS, Wara WM, Sheline GE, et al: The treatment of craniopharyngiomas. Int J Radiat Oncol Biol Phys 2:675, 1977

92. McMurry FG, Hardy RW, Dohn DF, et al: Long term results in the management of craniopharyngiomas. Neurosurgery 1:238, 1977

93. Kobayashi T, Kageyama N: Combined transsphenoidal and intracranial surgery of craniopharyngioma (abstr). Neurosurgery 19:326, 1986

94. Laws ER: Transsphenoidal microsurgery in the management of craniopharyngioma. J Neurosurg 52:661, 1980

95. Laws ER: Craniopharyngioma (abstr). Neurosurgery 19:326, 1986

96. Asari S, Sakurai M, Suzuki K, et al: Craniopharyngioma in the third ventricle. Neurol Med Chir (Tokyo) 20:1039, 1980

97. Shucart WA, Stein BM: Transcallosal approach to the anterior ventricular system. Neurosurgery 3:339, 1978

98. Sweet WH, Talland GA, Ervin FR: Loss of recent memory following section of fornix. Trans Am Neurol Assoc 84:76, 1959

99. Long DM, Leibrock L: The transcallosal approach to the anterior ventricular system and its application in the therapy of craniopharyngioma. Clin Neurosurg 27:160, 1980

100. Bose B, Huang P, Myers D, et al: Intrinsic third ventricular craniopharyngioma: Two case reports with review of the literature. Del Med J 57:389, 1985

101. Gutin PH, Klemme WM, Lagger RL, et al: Management of the unresectable cystic craniopharyngioma by aspiration through an Ommaya reservoir drainage system. J Neurosurg 52:36, 1980

102. Oh S: Rickhamklappen-drainage bei rezidivierendem zystischem Kraniopharingeom. Schweiz Arch Neurol Neurochir Psychiat 113:57, 1973

103. Miles J: Sump drainage: A palliative manoeuvre for the treatment of craniopharyngioma. J Neurol Neurosurg Psychiatry 40:120, 1977

104. Muller PJ, Russell NA, Morley TP: Craniopharyngioma: Results of surgical treatment without radiotherapy, in Morley TP (ed): Current Controversies in Neurosurgery. Philadelphia, WB Saunders, 1976, pp 344–350

105. Kliman B: Metabolic derangements, in Ropper AH, Kennedy S, Zervas NT, et al (eds): Neurological and Neurosurgical Intensive Care, ed 2. Rockville, Aspen, Inc., (in press)

106. Holmes LB, Frantz AG, Rabkin MT, et al: Normal growth with subnormal growth-hormone levels. N Engl J Med 279:559, 1968

107. Brisman R, Mendell J: Thromboembolism and brain tumors. J Neurosurg 38:337, 1973

108. Sawaya R, Decourteen-Meyers G, Copeland B: Massive preoperative pulmonary embolism and suprasellar brain tumor: Case report and review of the literature. Neurosurgery 15:566, 1984

109. Hoogenhout J, Otten BJ, Kazem I, et al: Surgery and radiation therapy in the management of craniopharyngiomas. Int J Radiat Oncol Biol Phys 10:2293, 1984

110. Heatley FW, Greenwood RH, Boase DL: Slipping of the upper femoral epiphyses in patients with intracranial tumours causing hypopituitarism and chiasmal compression. J Bone Joint Surg 58:169, 1976

111. Obrador S, Blazquez MG: Pituitary abscess in a craniopharyngioma. Case report. J Neurosurg 36:785, 1972

112. Bloom HJG: The role of radiotherapy in the management of chiasmal compression. Proc R Soc Med 70:319, 1977

113. Kramer S: Craniopharyngioma: The best treatment is conservative surgery and postoperative radiation therapy, in Morley TP (ed): Current Controversies in Neurosurgery. Philadelphia, WB Saunders, 1976, pp 336–343

114. Sweet WH: Recurrent craniopharyngiomas: Therapeutic alternatives. Clin Neurosurg 27:206, 1980

115. Hoff JT, Patterson RH: Craniopharyngiomas in children and adults. J Neurosurg 36:299, 1972

116. Amendola BE, Gebarski SS, Bermudez AG: Analysis of treatment results in craniopharyngioma. J Clin Oncol 3:252, 1985

117. Kramer S, McKissock W, Concannon JP: Craniopharyngiomas: Treatment by combined surgery and radiation therapy. J Neurosurg 18:217, 1961

118. Bloom HJG, Harmer CL: Craniopharyngioma: General aspects and treatment, in Bucalossi P, Veronesi V, Emanuelli H, et al (eds): I Tumori Infantili. Milano, Casa Editrice Ambrosiana, 1976, pp 119–128

119. Richmond IL, Wara WM, Wilson CB: Role of radiation therapy in the management of craniopharyngiomas in children. Neurosurgery 6:513, 1980

120. Thomsett MJ, Conte FA, Kaplan SL, et al: Endocrine and neurologic outcome in childhood craniopharyngioma: Review of effect of treatment in 42 patients. J Pediatrics 97:728, 1980

121. Resch R, Haas H, Schwarz S, et al: Kraniopharyngeom. Dtsch Med Wochenschr 106:1502, 1981

122. Sung DI, Chang CH, Harisiadis L, et al: Treatment results of craniopharyngiomas. Cancer 47:847, 1981

123. Sung DI: Suprasellar tumors in children. A review of clinical manifestations and managements. Cancer 50:1420, 1982

124. Cavazzuti V, Fischer EG, Welch K, et al: Neurological and

psychophysiological sequelae following different treatments of craniopharyngioma in children. J Neurosurg 59:409, 1983

125. Galatzer A, Nofar E, Beit-Halachmi N, et al: Intellectual and psychosocial functions of children, adolescents and young adults before and after operation for craniopharyngioma. Child Care Health Dev 7:307, 1981

126. Pierre-Kahn A, Hirsch JF, Renier D, et al: Craniopharyngiome de l'enfant—indication therapeutique et devenir a long terme. Analyse retrospective de 52 observations. Abstract for the meeting of the Société de Neurochirurgie de Langue Francaise, December 8–11, 1986, Paris, France

127. Backlund EO: Stereotactic treatment of craniopharyngiomas—a ten years material (1966–1975). Presented at the 6th International Congress of Neurological Surgery, Sao Paulo, June 19–25, 1977

128. Amacher AL: Craniopharyngioma: The controversy regarding radiotherapy. Childs Brain 6:57, 1980

129. Landolt AM: Can craniopharyngiomas be treated by radiotherapy (histologic and ultrastructural considerations)?, in Bushe KA, Spoerri O, Shaw J (eds): Progress in Paediatric Neurosurgery. Stuttgart, Hippokrates-Verlag, 1974, pp 232–236

130. Weiss SR, Raskind R: Non-neoplastic intrasellar cysts. Int Surg 51:282, 1969

131. Fukamachi A, Wakao T, Akai J: Brain stem necrosis after irradiation of pituitary adenoma. Surg Neurol 18:343, 1982

132. Harris JR, Levene MB: Visual complications following irradiation for pituitary adenomas and craniopharyngiomas. Radiology 120:167, 1976

133. Piatt JH, Blue JM, Schold SC, et al: Glioblastoma multiforme after radiotherapy for acromegaly. Neurosurgery 13:85, 1983

134. Maat-Schieman MLC, Bots GTAM, Thomeer RTWM, et al: Malignant astrocytoma following radiotherapy for craniopharyngioma. Br J Radiol 58:480, 1985

135. Onoyama Y, Ono K, Yabumoto Y, et al: Radiation therapy of craniopharyngioma. Radiology 125:799, 1977

136. Chin HW, Maruyama Y, Young B: The role of radiation treatment in craniopharyngioma. Strahlentherapie 159:741, 1983

137. Vyramuthu N, Benton TF: The management of craniopharyngioma. Clin Radiol 34:629, 1983

138. Shanklin WM: The incidence and distribution of cilia in the human pituitary with a description of microfollicular cysts derived from Rathke's cleft. Acta Anat (Basel) 11:361, 1951

139. Yoshida J, Kobayashi T, Kageyama N, et al: Symptomatic Rathke's cleft cyst. Morphological study with light and electron microscopy and tissue culture. J Neurosurg 47:451, 1977

140. Ringel SP, Bailey OT: Rathke's cleft cyst. J Neurol Neurosurg Psychiatry 35:693, 1972

141. Barrow DL, Spector RH, Takei Y, et al: Symptomatic Rathke's cleft cysts located entirely in the suprasellar region: Review of diagnosis, management, and pathogenesis. Neurosurgery 16:766, 1985

142. Adelman LS, Post KD: Calcification in Rathke's cleft cyst. J Neurosurg 47:641, 1977

143. Fager CA, Carter H: Intrasellar epithelial cysts. J Neurosurg 24:77, 1966

144. Baskin DS, Wilson CB: Transsphenoidal treatment of non-neoplastic intrasellar cysts. A report of 38 cases. J Neurosurg 60:8, 1984

145. Chambers EF, Turski PA, LaMasters D, et al: Regions of low density in the contrast-enhanced pituitary gland: Normal and pathologic processes. Radiology 144:109, 1982

146. Shuangshoti S, Netsky M, Nashold BS Jr: Epithelial cysts related to the sella turcica. Proposed origin from neuroepithelium. Arch Pathol 90:444, 1970

147. Raskind R, Brown HA, Mathis J: Recurrent cyst of the pituitary: 26-year follow-up from first decompression. J Neurosurg 28:595, 1968

148. Berry RG, Schlezinger NS: Rathke cleft cysts. Arch Neurol 1:48, 1959

149. Iraci G, Giordano R, Gerosa M, et al: Ocular involvement in recurrent cyst of Rathke's cleft: Case report. Ann Ophthalmol 11:94, 1979

150. Matsushima T, Fukui M, Ohta M, et al: Ciliated and goblet cells in craniopharyngioma light and electron microscopic studies at surgery and autopsy. Acta Neuropathol 50:199, 1980

151. Marcincin RP, Gennarelli TA: Recurrence of symptomatic pituitary cysts following transsphenoidal drainage. Surg Neurol 18:448, 1982

152. Tajika Y, Kubo 0, Kamiya M, et al: Clinico-pathological features of 5 cases of pituitary cyst including Rathke's cleft cyst. Neurological Surgery (Tokyo) 10:1055, 1982

153. Goodrich JT, Post KD, Duffy P: Ciliated craniopharyngioma. Surg Neurol 24:105, 1985

154. Verkijk A, Bots GthAM: An intrasellar cyst with both Rathke's cleft and epidermoid characteristics. Acta Neurochir 51:203, 1980

155. Swanson SE, Chandler WF, Latack J, et al: Symptomatic Rathke's cleft cyst with pituitary adenoma: Case report. Neurosurgery 17:657, 1985

156. Matsumori K, Okuda T, Nakayama K, et al: A case of calcified prolactinoma combined with Rathke's cleft cysts. Neurological Surgery (Tokyo) 12:833, 1984

157. Hiyama H, Kubo O, Yato S, et al: A case of pituitary adenoma combined with Rathke's cleft cyst. Neurological Surgery (Tokyo) 14:435, 1986

158. Eisenberg HM, Sarwar M, Schochet S: Symptomatic Rathke's cleft cyst. Case report. J Neurosurg 45:585, 1976

159. Nagasaka S, Kuromatsu C, Wakisaka S, et al: Rathke's cleft cyst. Surg Neurol 15:402, 1981

160. Rout DL, Das L, Rao VRK, et al: Symptomatic Rathke's cleft cysts. Surg Neurol 19:42, 1983

161. Shimoji T, Shinohara A, Shimizu A, et al: Rathke cleft cysts. Surg Neurol 21:295, 1984

162. Yamamoto M, Takara E, Imanaga H, et al: Rathke's cleft cyst. Report of two cases. Neurological Surgery (Tokyo) 12:609, 1984

163. Okamoto S, Handa H, Yamashita J, et al: Computed tomography in intra- and suprasellar epithelial cysts. (Symptomatic Rathke Cleft Cysts). AJNR 6:515, 1985

164. Dietemann JL, Bonneville JF, Buchheit F, et al: CT findings in symptomatic Rathke's cleft cysts of the pituitary gland. Report of three cases. Neuroradiology 24:263, 1983

165. Martin JB: Case records of the Massachusetts General Hospital. Case 17-1980. N Engl J Med 302:1015, 1980

166. Obenchain TG, Becker DP: Head bobbing associated with a cyst of the third ventricle. J Neurosurg 37:457, 1972

167. Menault F, Sabouraud 0, Javalet A, et al: Kyste de la fente de Rathke. Rev Otoneuroophtamol 51:383, 1979

168. Steinberg GK, Koenig GH, Golden JB: Symptomatic Rathke's cleft cysts. J Neurosurg 56:290, 1982

169. Gomez Perun J, Eiras J, Carcavilla LI: Abcès intrasellaire au sein d'un kyste de la poche de Rathke. Neurochirurgie 27:201, 1981

170. Sonntag VKH, Plenge KL, Balis MS, et al: Surgical treatment of an abscess in a Rathke's cleft cyst. Surg Neurol 20:152, 1983

171. Hoffman HJ, Hendrick EB, Humphreys RP, et al: Investigation and management of suprasellar arachnoid cysts. J Neurosurg 57:597, 1982

172. Key A, Retzius G: Studien in der Anatomie des Nervensystems und des Bindegewebes, vol 1, plate III. Stockholm, P.A. Norsted and Soner, 1875

173. Liliequist B: The anatomy of the subarachnoid cisterns. Acta Radiol 46:61, 1956

174. Fox JL, Al-Mefty O: Suprasellar arachnoid cysts: An extension of the membrane of Liliequist. Neurosurgery 7:615, 1980

175. Starkman SP, Brown TC, Linell EA: Cerebral arachnoid cysts. J Neuropathol Exp Neurol 17:484, 1958

176. Krawchenko J, Collins GH: Pathology of an arachnoid cyst. Case report. J Neurosurg 50:224, 1979

177. Harrison MJG: Cerebral arachnoid cysts in children. J Neurol Neurosurg Psychiatry 34:316, 1971

178. Segall HD, Hassan G, Ling SM, et al: Suprasellar cysts associated with isosexual precocious puberty. Neuroradiology 111:607, 1974

179. Gonzalez CA, Villarejo FJ, Blazquez MG, et al: Suprasellar arachnoid cysts in children. Report of three cases. Acta Neurochir 60:281, 1982

180. Raimondi AJ, Shimoji T, Gutierrez FA: Suprasellar cysts: Surgical treatment and results. Childs Brain 7:57, 1980

181. Murali R, Epstein F: Diagnosis and treatment of suprasellar arachnoid cyst. J Neurosurg 50:515, 1979

182. Sansregret A, Ledoux R, Duplantis F, et al: Suprasellar subarachnoid cysts: Radioclinical features. AJR 105:291, 1969

CHAPTER 32

Transcallosal Approach to Tumors of the Third Ventricle

Bennett M. Stein

TUMORS WITHIN THE THIRD VENTRICLE are strategically located and of a nature that makes them difficult to expose and remove.[1-3] Although they can be reached by a number of routes, it is difficult to expose the region widely. At the very least such surgery requires an operating microscope and microsurgical instruments.

The tumors arise from structures surrounding the third ventricle, including the hypothalamus and thalamus, or from within the third ventricle, originating from the ependyma or the paraphysis. Craniopharyngiomas, when they arise from the median eminence, may grow almost entirely within the third ventricle.[4] Tumor histology varies greatly and the region of the third ventricle rivals the pineal region for a gamut of pathologic entities.[5-9] The more common lesions encountered include astrocytomas of all grades, ependymomas, craniopharyngiomas, colloid and ependymal cysts, choroid plexus papillomas, and other rare lesions. It is important to realize that a wide variety of tumors occur in this region and attempts should be made to diagnose the type of tumor accurately before operative intervention. The dorsal part of the tumor is related to the velum interpositum, which contains folds of arachnoid, the internal cerebral veins, and the choroid plexus. The tumors often reach the foramen of Monro and may enlarge it or grow through it into the lateral ventricles. They are related to the lamina terminalis anteriorly, to portions of the hypothalamus inferiorly, and to the thalamus laterally.

The anatomic location, size, and possible nature of the tumor have a bearing on the choice of approach to be used to expose the third ventricle. Lesions that impinge upon or enlarge the foramen of Monro can be approached most easily from a transcallosal route. It appears that even though the tumor may arise in the chiasmatic or suprasellar area, if it is large enough to reach the foramen of Monro, it will have so thinned out the hypothalamic region that it can be approached directly by a transventricular route.

SURGICAL APPROACHES TO THE THIRD VENTRICULAR REGION

A number of surgical approaches have been used for tumors that fill the third ventricle and encroach upon the lateral ventricles. A transfrontal route requires a frontal craniotomy, usually on the right side, with incision into cortical and subcortical tissue, until the ependymal surface of the right lateral ventricle is reached.[10] At this point an enlarged foramen of Monro usually permits access to the third ventricle. Rhoton et al. recommended this approach for certain tumors of the third ventricle, believing that the angulation and exposure is superior to that obtained by a transcallosal exposure.[11] Furthermore, access to the middle and posterior third ventricle appears to be easier via this route. The interhemispheric, parafalx, or transcallosal approach was used by Dandy[9] and others.[12-16] The advantages of the transcallosal approach to the third ventricle are numerous. Retraction rather than incision into the right hemisphere provides an easy route and brain tissue is not sacrificed. Sacrifice of an occasional cortical vein as it enters the sagittal sinus has not resulted in significant neurologic deficit; arteries on the surface of the corpus callosum can be easily mobilized and spared, while small veins that run directly on the corpus callosum are of no significance and can be sectioned. The amount of corpus callosum that is removed is not enough to result in neurologic deficit.[17,18] Unlike the transfrontal exposure, which is carried out through amorphous gray and white matter, the transcallosal exposure is quick and is facilitated by an excellent view of the normal anatomy in the interhemispheric fissure. The transcallosal approach can also be used when the ventricles are not enlarged or slightly enlarged. In this circumstance a transfrontal approach is contraindicated.

The greatest advantage of the transcallosal exposure is that it permits entry into either or both lateral ventricles and provides direct access to deep regions of the third ventricle through the foramen of Monro. The surgeon is not encumbered by entering the lateral ventricle at an angle that limits the view of the deep recesses of the third ventricle, especially the optic recesses. In a dilated ventricular system, the exposure is virtually bloodless.

Once the lateral ventricles are reached, there are various approaches to the third ventricle. The classic one is via the enlarged foramen of Monro without any additional enlargement. If enlargement is required, it has been previously recommended that the fornix on one side, preferably the nondominant hemisphere side, be opened anteriorly into the fibers of the corpus callosum and the adjacent septal region. However, this violates functional brain tissue. A better approach, which appears to be safe, is to section the thalamostriate vein and proceed posteriorly. A variation on this latter approach is the subfornicial approach, which is direct through the choroid fissure, posterior to the formen of Monro, entering the third ventricle through its roof under the velum interpositum. This

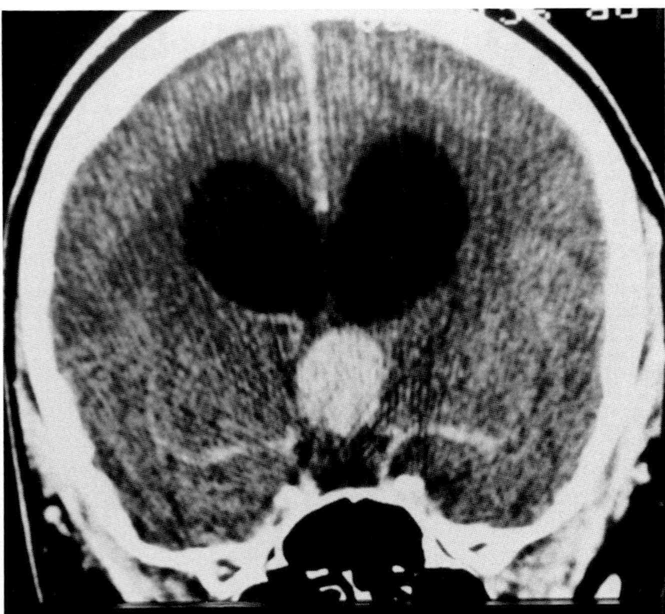

Fig. 32-1. A coronal CT scan with contrast showing a large contrast-enhanced tumor producing marked hydrocephalus. The dorsal surface of the tumor reaches to the foramina of Monro and is easily approached through a transcallosal exposure.

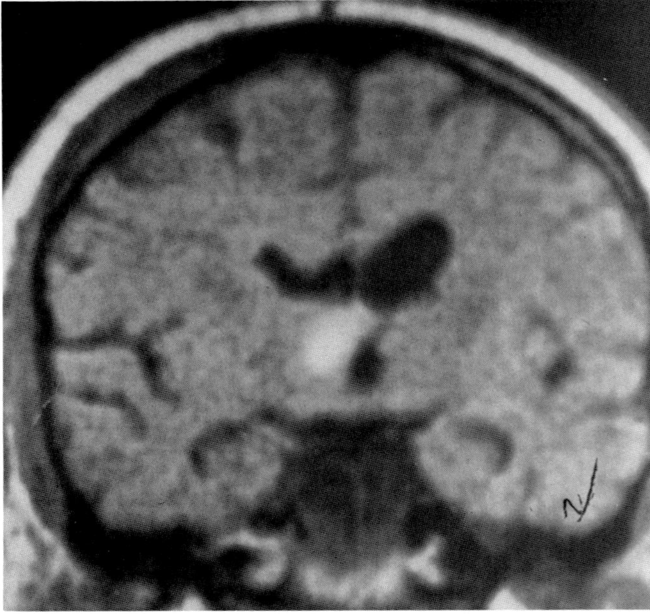

Fig. 32-2. A coronal MRI scan showing a craniopharyngioma eccentric in the third ventricle extending to the region of both foramina of Monro. This tumor was totally removed through a transcallosal approach.

requires cautery of the choroid plexus, section of the thalamostriate vein, and manipulation of the medial posterior choroidal arteries. It does provide excellent exposure of the entire third ventricle. In association with large tumors that originate from the velum interpositum and separate the columns of the fornix, an interfornicial approach can be used. This is directly through the septum with a small incision exactly in the midline and a careful separation of the fornices. The advantage of this approach is its central midline nature directed at the attachment of most of the tumors. The disadvantage is injury to one or both of the fornices.

PREOPERATIVE EVALUATION

The most informative radiographic procedures are those that outline the extent of the tumor. These include contrast ventriculography with either air or Pantopaque, computed tomographic (CT) scans, and magnetic resonance imaging (MRI). Although arteriography may be valuable for demonstrating the vascularity of a tumor, giving some indication of its pathologic structure, it rarely outlines the tumor sufficiently to disclose its exact relationship to the foramen of Monro and other structures of the third ventricle. Because the surgical approach depends upon the size and exact position of the tumor, it is important to outline the extent of the tumor, and, particularly, its relationship to the foramen of Monro. If the tumor lies deep within the third ventricle or is basically a suprasellar tumor indenting the third ventricle and not large enough to reach the foramen of Monro, it is better approached from a subfrontal or trans-lamina terminalis route. If the surgeon can be certain that the tumor impinges upon the foramen of Monro or goes through it, then a transventricular approach, especially the transcallosal, is appropriate (Figure 32-1). The CT or MRI scan (Figure 32-2) supplants ventriculography,

which is rarely used, thereby shortening the operative procedure and the morbidity of the diagnostic work-up and operation.

DETAILS OF THE OPERATIVE APPROACH TO THE THIRD VENTRICLE

The patient is positioned in the recumbent supine position, with the head flexed. Care is taken so that an air embolism can be diagnosed and treated appropriately. This requires placement of a central venous catheter and Doppler and end-tidal PCO_2 monitoring. The patient's head generally is best held by a pin-type head holder so that there will be no change in position during the operative procedure. The angle of the head in the flexed position should be memorized by the surgeon. Also, it is essential that the head not be tilted so that a direct perpendicular approach can be carried out. If the patient's position varies, and the operating surgeon is not aware of the changes, entry into the lateral ventricular system may be rostral or caudal to the foramen of Monro, or the ventricle opposite to the intended one may be entered.

Either a horseshoe[3] or a question-mark incision[12] (anterior to posterior along the midline then curving inferior toward the zygoma) is used. A free bone flap is elevated, with the superior margin just to the left of the midline so that the sagittal sinus is exposed. The anteroposterior position of the flap is situated so that two thirds will be anterior to the coronal suture and one third posterior. Mannitol, spinal drainage, or aspiration of the ventricle can be used for brain relaxation, depending on the degree of obstruction within the ventricular system. The dura is then opened in a U-shaped fashion with its base along the sagittal sinus. It is important to make the cuts directly to the edge of the sinus so that the dural flap can be reflected firmly to the left side and the falx visualized. A number of cortical veins entering the sagittal sinus are generally encountered. Some of these can be dissected from the sagittal sinus a considerable

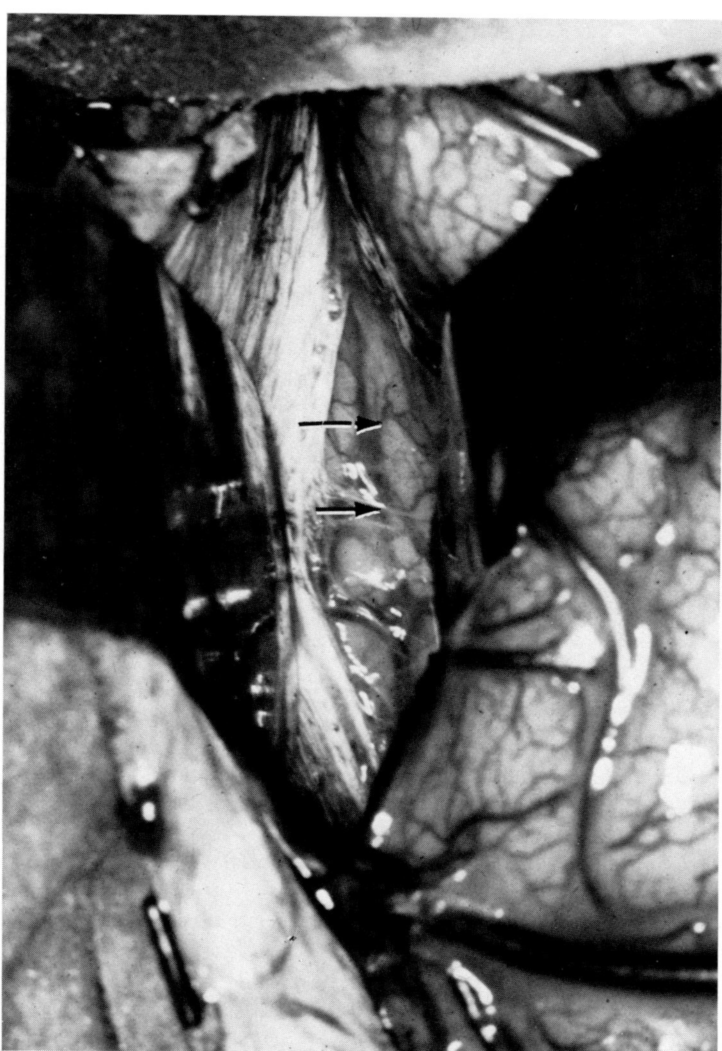

Fig. 32-3. Exposure of the cingulate gyrus (arrows). Compare the texture with that of the corpus callosum (Figure 32-4).

distance so that they can be displaced out of the operative area. Others can be sacrificed; this should not result in neurologic deficit. When the medial margin of the hemisphere is free, gentle retraction is applied to separate it from the falx. If tension exists, the right lateral ventricle can be tapped with a ventricular needle and cerebrospinal fluid evacuated to facilitate retraction of the hemisphere. When the interhemispheric fissure is entered, the cingulate gyrus may be confused with the corpus callosum (Figure 32-3). The cingulate gyri are often adherent to each other and may be displaced to the left or right of the midline, making a direct approach to the corpus callosum somewhat difficult. This situation should be recognized immediately, otherwise a great deal of difficulty will be encountered and the brain injured. The cingulate gyrus is more vascular than the dorsal surface of the corpus callosum, which is very white and relatively avascular. At this point the operating microscope with a 250-mm or 275-mm objective is used. The dissection is carried to the corpus callosum, where the main trunks of the anterior cerebral artery or the pericallosal arteries will be encountered. A brief appraisal of the situation will indicate that both arteries can be displaced either to the left or right without sacrificing all but one or two small branches to the cingulate gyrus, or, more commonly, the exposure can be made between these two arteries. Having displaced the arteries appropriately, the dorsal surface of the corpus callosum, upon which a number of small veins run, is encountered (Figure 32-4). These veins are cauterized to facilitate section of the corpus callosum. The falx is held sharply toward the left by a self-retaining retractor, whereas the brain is held in position, covered by Telfa, by two self-retaining retractors. An anteroposterior oval-shaped resection of the corpus callosum, amounting to approximately 2 to 3 cm, is sufficient exposure. The measurement, of course, depends upon the age of the patient and the relative size of the corpus callosum.

The pial margin of the corpus callosum is cauterized and an incision made with cautery, suction, and a blunt dissector. The thickness of the corpus callosum varies according to the degree of ventricular expansion and the age of the patient. When the ependymal margin is reached, the color of the tissue changes and veins will be encountered on the ependymal surface. Additional corpus callosum can be resected in order to afford adequate exposure of either the left or right lateral ventricle.

It is often difficult, at first, to determine whether the exposure has been made into the left or right lateral ventricle. The surgeon should immediately look for landmarks, which include the septal vein of the septum pellucidum; the choroid

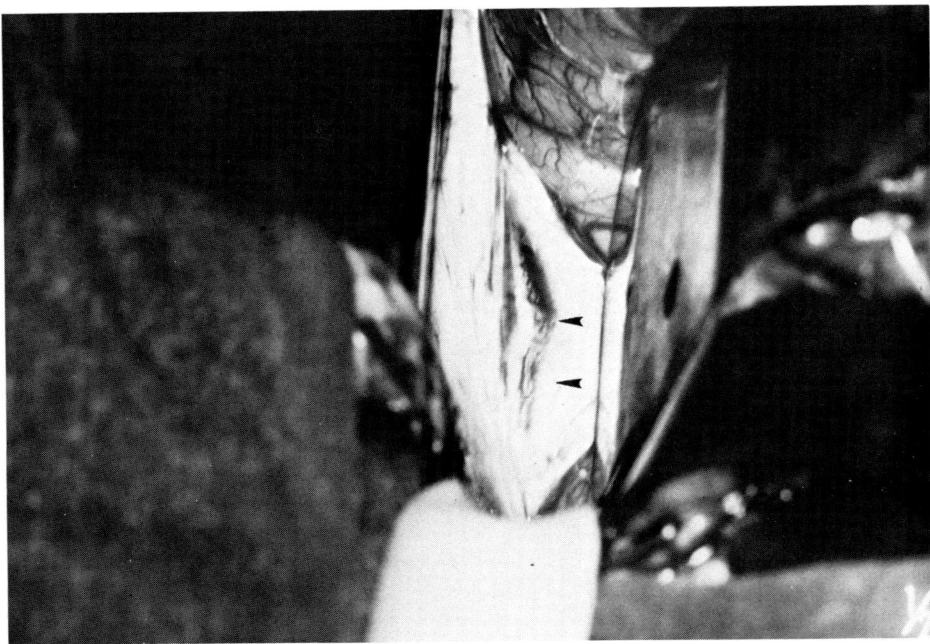

Fig. 32-4.   Exposure of the corpus callosum (arrows).

plexus, which terminates in the region of the foramen of Monro; and the thalamostriate vein.[19] With a small amount of effort, these landmarks can be identified and at this point one can be certain which ventricle has been opened. The self-retaining retractors are then extended deeper to retract the sectioned corpus callosum, affording an excellent view of the lateral ventricle and the region of the foramen of Monro (Figure 32-5). If the preoperative diagnosis was accurate, the foramen of Monro will be dilated and the tumor easily visible, either within or just below the foramen of Monro (Figure 32-6). If the exposure is directly in the midline and the septum thin, exposure of both foramina of Monro will be advantageous (Figures 32-7 and 32-8).

To facilitate removal of tumor or surgery within the third ventricle, it may be necessary to retract or open the foramen of Monro. To do so, an incision can be made anteriorly through one of the fornices. The anterior opening of the foramen of Monro is relatively avascular and section of one fornix will not produce a neurologic deficit. Because of hemisphere dominance, it appears preferable to section the nondominant fornix. Care should be taken, however, not to section both fornices or to damage the septal region. Additional experience with exposures to the third ventricle indicates that the foramen of Monro can be opened safely in a posterior direction.[20] This avoids section of the fornix. The thalamostriate vein must be sacrificed and the choroid pelxus mobilized from the choroidal fissure.[21]

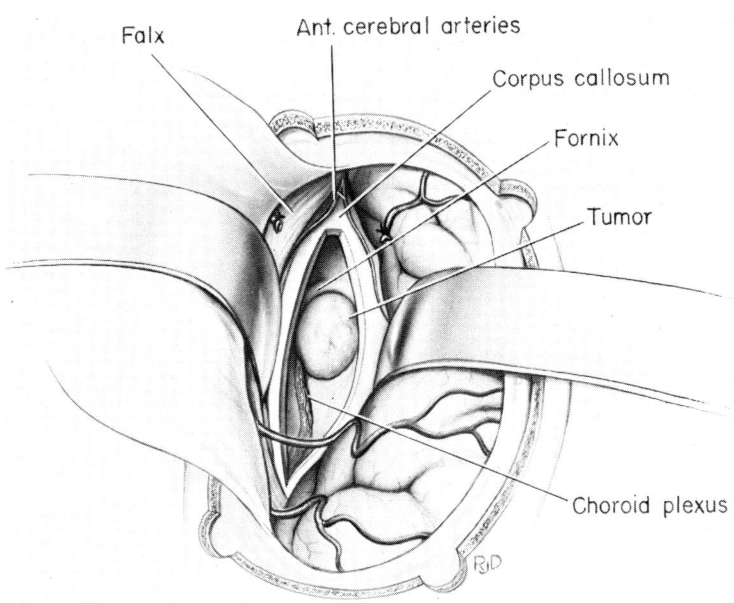

Fig. 32-5.   Intraventricular exposure.

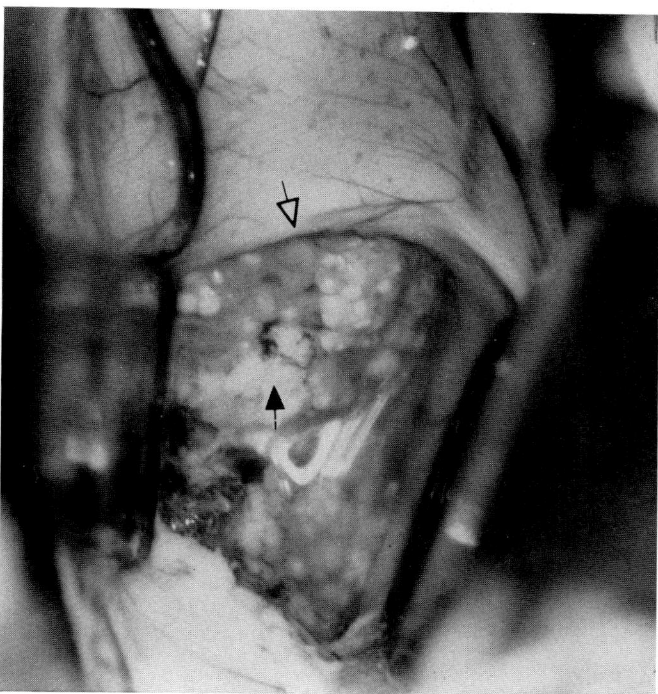

Fig. 32-6. Operative exposure of the right lateral ventricle demonstrating the fornix (open arrow) and a large craniopharyngioma (solid arrow) dilating the foramen of Monro.

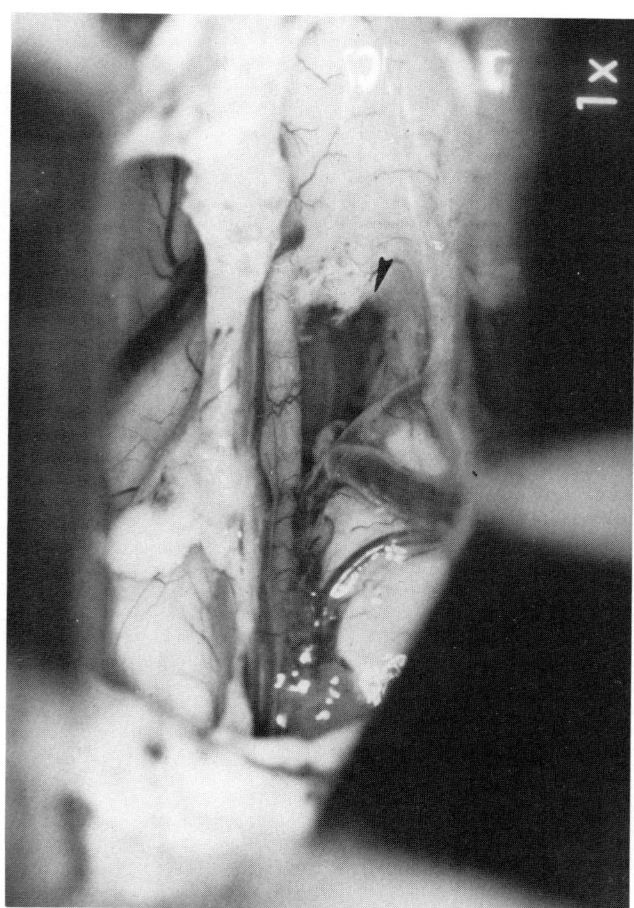

Fig. 32-8. The same patient as in Figure 32-7 after removal of the colloid cyst through a somewhat tattered but intact right foramen of Monro (arrow).

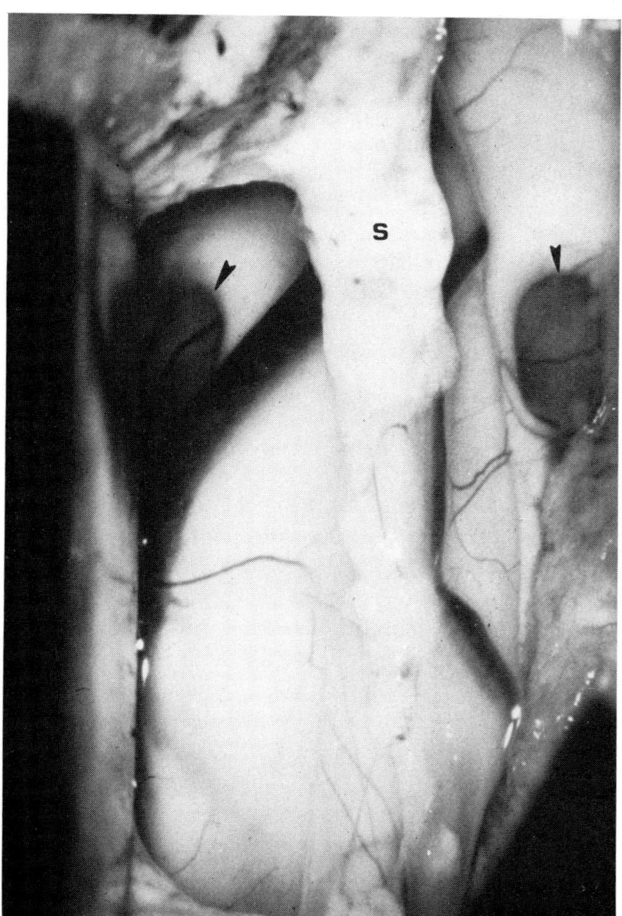

Fig. 32-7. Transcallosal exposure directly into the septum pellucidum (S) providing an exposure of both foramina of Monro (arrows) through which a colloid cyst is visualized.

This requires cautery of the choroid plexus and mobilization of the branches of the medial posterior choroidal arteries. However, the opening in the posterior direction is almost limitless and gives excellent exposure to the attachment of most tumors in the region of the tela choroidea or roof of the third ventricle posterior to the foramina of Monro. The latter extension is termed a subfornicial approach to the third ventircle.[22] It is carried out through the choroidal fissure below the tela choroidea and over the superomedial surface of the thalamus. An interfornicial approach has also been advocated.[14,15] This should only be carried out if preoperative testing with CT and MRI indicates a separation of the septum and thereby the fornices by a large tumor extending upward (Figure 32-9). The route is directly along the septum with careful separation of the columns of the fornices. Situations in which it is possible to accomplish this are recognized when one observes both lateral ventricles and a wide separation of the foramina of Monro by the underlying tumor (Figure 32-10).

A cavum pellucidum represents a confusing anatomic variation of the midline transcallosal approach. There are, of course, none of the usual ventricular landmarks and it becomes obvious after exploration that this is the situation. The first case I encountered was not recognized as a cavum on the CT scan and this resulted in a brief period of confusion until we were able to direct the exposure to the lateral ventricle and discover the error.

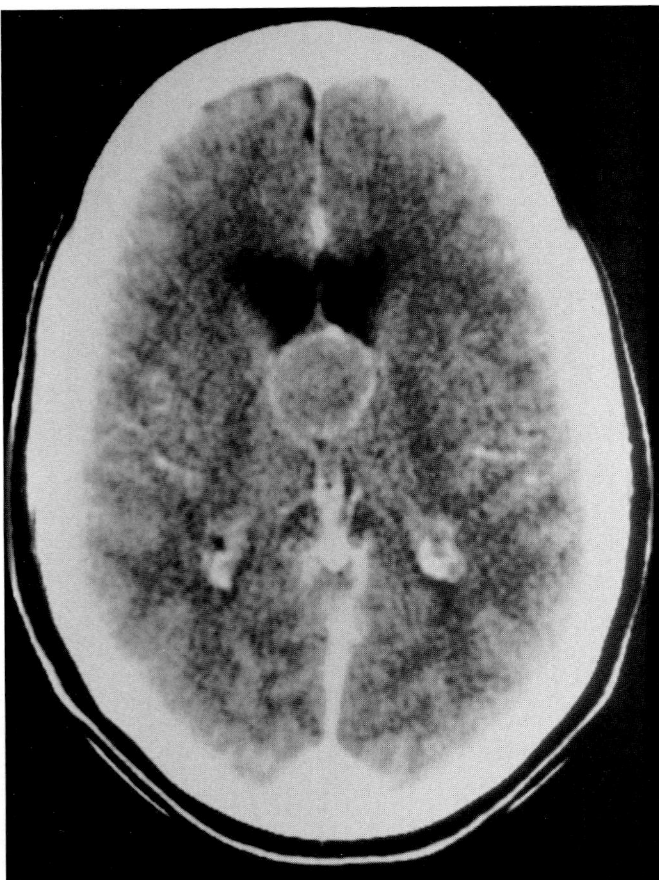

Fig. 32-9. A horizontal CT scan with contrast showing a large anterior tumor of the third ventricle separating the two foramina of Monro. An interfornicial approach might be anticipated.

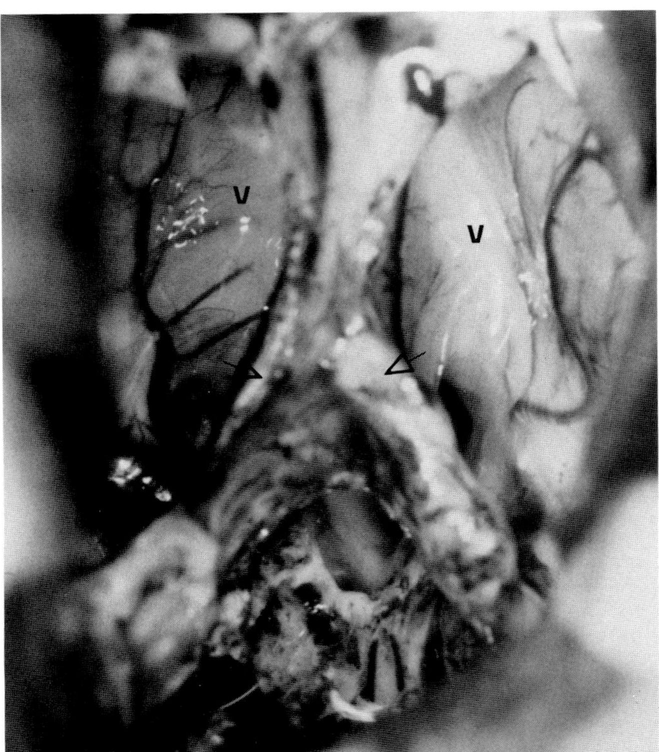

Fig. 32-10. Operative photograph of the same patient as in Figure 32-9 showing a midline interfornicial approach via the septum. Both lateral ventricles are marked by a V. The fornices are separated and shown by arrows. The tumor, a colloid cyst, has been totally removed. There was no memory deficit.

With the exposure enlarged, biopsy specimens of the tumor can be taken or the tumor can be removed by microsurgical techniques.[23] Care must be taken not to injure any of the ependymal surfaces and to keep bleeding to a minimum, since blood could permeate the ventricular system and perhaps cause secondary obstruction where there otherwise would be an open ventricular system following operative resection of the tumor. The long curved tip of the Cavitron has been useful in decompressing the interior of some tumors. Certain colloid cysts have firm irregular grumous material within them and the Cavitron is particularly useful in these circumstances. Otherwise, tumors can be removed by the usual techniques of suction, cautery, tumor forceps, and dissectors. When work on the tumor is complete, hemostasis must be accurate and no bleeding left within the ventricular system. Hemostatic agents such as Gelfoam are not used, since they can dislodge and occlude the aqueduct or other portions of the ventricular system.

Tumors that are located in the posterior third ventricle or the posterior thalamic region extending into the lateral ventricle can be approached through a para posterior parietal lobule route so as to section the posterior corpus callosum and enter the trigone of the lateral ventricle and thus through the choroidal fissure into the posterior region of the third ventricle. This is similar to the subfornicial approach but is carried out through a distinctly posterior route.

The major problem encountered in closure is collapse of the lateral ventricular system after the hydrocephalus has been relieved. There appears to be no way to satisfactorily close the corpus callosum, so postoperatively cerebrospinal fluid will undoubtedly leak into the interhemispheric region and then subdurally. Attempts have been made to inflate the ventricular system by placing a small Foley catheter into the opening in the corpus callosum, the balloon occluding it and the catheter being removed when dural closure has been completed. This is temporary at best, however, and had not been very satisfactory. Generally, collapse of the ventricular system, especially on the operative side, is ignored. Since hydrocephalus has been controlled, either by decompression or secondary shunt, the hemisphere, after a period of time, appears to assume a more normal configuration and position. Difficulty has occasionally been encountered because of subdural hygromas. The closure of the craniotomy is routine.

If a shunt is to be employed because of residual tumor or persistent obstruction of the ventricular system, the ventricular end of the shunt tubing may be placed, at the primary operative procedure, into the appropriate lateral ventricle. If the obstruction remains in the region of the foramen of Monro, an opening is made through the septum pellucidum so that shunting one ventricle will decompress both. This maneuver ensures that both lateral ventricles will be decompressed and that the tubing will be accurately located within the ventricular system. The shunt tubing is then brought out through the opening in the corpus callosum, via the interhemispheric fissure, then subcutaneously, exiting through a stab wound in the posterior scalp for external drainage. If needed, it subsequently can be connected into a shunt system by removing some of the subcutaneous portion and attaching it to appropriate distal tubing, or, if not required, it can be abandoned in the subgaleal space.

SUMMARY

In this series, 50 transcallosal approaches have been used for lesions within the third ventricle, both in children and in adults. Many of the tumors were infiltrating noncystic astrocytomas, presumably of the thalamic region. Therefore, the tumor usually could not be radically removed. In 50 percent of the cases, however, benign pathologic entities, including craniopharyngiomas, colloid cysts, and a cystic teratomatous tumor of the third ventricle, were encountered and could be largely or totally removed. In cases in which only a biopsy or subtotal resection was done, important data about tumor type helped in the planning of subsequent therapy. There was 1 operative death in this series. The procedure is deemed reasonably safe and allows the best visualization of the third ventricle for lesions that arise primarily within that region and extend to the level of the foramen of Monro, no matter what their nature.

REFERENCES

1. Antunes JL, Muraszko K, Quest DO, et al: Surgical strategies in the management of tumours of the anterior third ventricle, in Brock EM (ed): Modern Neurosurgery 1. Berlin, Springer-Verlag, 1982, pp 215–224

2. Matson DD: Neurosurgery of Infancy and Childhood. Springfield, Ill, Charles C Thomas, 1969

3. Stein BM, Fraser RAR, Tenner MS: Tumors of the third ventricle in children. J Neurol Neurosurg Psychiatry 35:776, 1972

4. Van den Bergh R, Brucher JM: L'abord transventriculaire dans les cranio-pharyngiomes du troisieme ventricule. Aspects neurochirurgicaux et neuro-pathologiques. Neurochirurgie 16:51, 1970

5. Buchsbaum HW, Colton RP: Anterior third ventricular cysts in infancy. Case report. J Neurosurg 26:264, 1925

6. Cassinari V, Bernasconi V: Tumori della parte anteriore del terzo ventricolo. Acta Neurochir 11:236, 1963

7. Lakke JPWF: Report on 16 intraventricular brain tumors: A clinical study. Eur Neurol 2:158, 1969 8. Pecker J, Ferrand B, Javalet A: Tumeurs du troisieme ventricule. Neurochirurgie 12:7, 1966

9. Dandy WE: Benign Tumors in the Third Ventricle of the Brain. Diagnosis and Treatment. Springfield, Ill, Charles C Thomas, 1933

10. Geffen G, Walsh A, Simpson D, et al: Comparison of the effects of transcortical and transcallosal removal of intraventricular tumors. Brain 103:773, 1980

11. Rhoton AL, Yamamoto I, Peace DA: Microsurgery of the third ventricle: Part 2. Operative approaches. Neurosurgery 8:357, 1981

12. Shucart WA, Stein BM: Transcallosal approach to the anterior ventricular system. Neurosurgery 3:339, 1978

13. Long DM, Chou SN: Transcallosal removal of craniopharyngiomas within the third ventricle. J Neurosurg 39:563, 1973

14. Apuzzo MLV: Transcallosal interfornicial exposure of lesions of the third ventricle, in Schmidek HH, Sweet WH (eds): Operative Neurosurgical Techniques, vol 1. New York, Grune & Stratton, 1982, pp 585–594

15. Apuzzo MLV, Chikovani O, Gott P: Transcallosal, interfornicial approaches for lesions affecting the third ventricle. Surgical considerations and consequences. Neurosurgery 10:547, 1982

16. Koos WT, Pendl G (eds): Lesions of the Cerebral Midline. Acta Neurochir 35:1, 1985

17. Jeeves MA, Simpson DA, Geffen G: Functional consequences of the transcallosal removal of intraventricular tumors. J Neurol Neurosurg Psychiatry 42:134, 1979

18. Winston KR, Cavazzuti, V, Arkius T: Absence of neurological and behavorial abnormalities after anterior transcallosal operation for third ventricular lesions. Neurosurgery 4:386, 1979

19. Yamamoto I, Rhoton AL, Peace DA: Microsurgery of the third ventricle: Part 1. Microsurgical anatomy. Neurosurgery 8:334, 1981

20. Ciric I, Zivin I: Neuroepithelial (colloid) cysts of the septum pellucidum. J Neurosurg 43:69, 1975

21. Hirsch JF, Zouaoui A, Renier D, et al: A new surgical approach to the third ventricle with interruption of striothalamic vein. Acta Neurochir 47:135, 1979

22. Viale GL, Turtas S: The subchoroid approach to the third ventricle. Surg Neurol 14:71, 1980

23. Little JR, MacCarty CS: Colloid cysts of the third ventricle. J Neurosurg 40:230, 1974

24. Apuzzo MLJ (ed): Surgery of the Third Ventricle. Baltimore, Williams and Wilkins, 1987

CHAPTER 33

Transcallosal Interfornicial Exposure of Lesions of the Third Ventricle

Michael L.J. Apuzzo

MASS LESIONS OF THE THIRD VENTRICLE provide the neurosurgeon with a major technical challenge. In spite of the advent of the microsurgical era, improvements in anesthetic methods, high potency glucocorticoids, and increased sophistication in roentgenologic techniques that provide strict three-dimensional definition of lesions and the deformation they cause of normal anatomic elements, surgery of the diencephalic region continues to require the utmost in preoperative and intraoperative planning and precision.

Following lateral ventricular entry, the neurosurgeon has a variety of alternatives for exposing the region of the third ventricle. These include: (1) transforaminal entry, either unilaterally or bilaterally; (2) section of one or both of the fornicial columns with appropriate exposure of the anterior region of the third ventricle; (3) incision of the lamina affixa with lateral to medial mobilization of the choroid plexus and fornicial columns and body; or (4) development of the interfornicial plane at the levels of the columns and body with entry through the roof of the third ventricle into that region (Figure 33-1). It is apparent that with the exception of the strict foraminal approach, all options for entry of the third ventricle via the translateral ventricular avenue incorporate some element of fornicial manipulation. This chapter will describe the technique of midline interhemispheric exposure directly via the corpus callosum and fornicial component of the roof of the third ventricle.

In consideration of any operative corridor, and particularly one that deals with deep cerebral lesions, the surgeon must be cognizant of the advantages afforded in terms of the *exposure* of a given lesion and the *physiologic consequences* that are attendant to the elements of the exposure itself. In this regard, we have found the transcallosal interfornicial approach to neoplasms of the third ventricle most advantageous. The interfornicial maneuver was originally described by Busch[1] in 1944, and in 1963 Baldwin et al.[2] suggested a midline approach for entry into the third ventricle via an incision of the corpus callosum and interfornicial space in the laboratory setting. We have had the opportunity to use this technique in the treatment of a variety of mass and vascular lesions occurring in the region of the third ventricle and feel that it is an important surgical alternative in approaching this area, particularly in the absence of ventriculomegaly or sufficient access via the foramen of Monro.[3]

CASE MATERIAL, OUTCOME, AND ANALYSIS

Of our first 25 cases treated by the midline interfornicial technique, there were 5 colloid cysts, 7 craniopharyngiomas, 3 intrinsic gliomas, 8 cysticercosis cysts, an arteriovenous malformation, and a 22-caliber bullet (Table 33-1). These lesions ranged in size from 1 to 4 cm, and in texture from cystic with a filmy capsule to dense and fibrous-type masses. Five of the lesions involved not only the third ventricular region, but also the sellar and parasellar regions as well.

RESULTS

Total excision was accomplished in 19 of the 22 potentially excisable lesions. This included 4 of the 7 craniopharyngiomas, where no evidence of tumor was apparent on postoperative imaging studies. Small to moderate tumor remnants were apparent in 3 cases in which subfrontal parasellar extension of tumor existed, and this argues for consideration of a *combined subfrontal* and *midline* exposure in the event that parasellar extension of a mass is extensive.

Exposure was found to be adequate in all compartments of the chamber, especially in the anterior and middle thirds, with posterior-third lesions accessible with minor manipulations of head and microscope position. On a number of occasions the basilar artery and prepontine cisterns or the sellar contents were visualized upon completion of mass excision.

COMPLICATIONS

There were no deaths and no incidences of gastrointestinal hemorrhage. There was no incidence of hemiparesis, nor alteration in endocrine status, preoperative visual status, or level of consciousness.

The major adverse observation was the development of a transient amnesic syndrome in 8 of 25 patients. This was characterized by an inability to retain recent events. The manifestation of the complaint was evident from 3 to 22 days postoperatively, with 6 of the 8 patients being normal or returned to preoperative baselines of mental status evaluation in 7 days. At 3 months postoperatively no detectable amnesia or

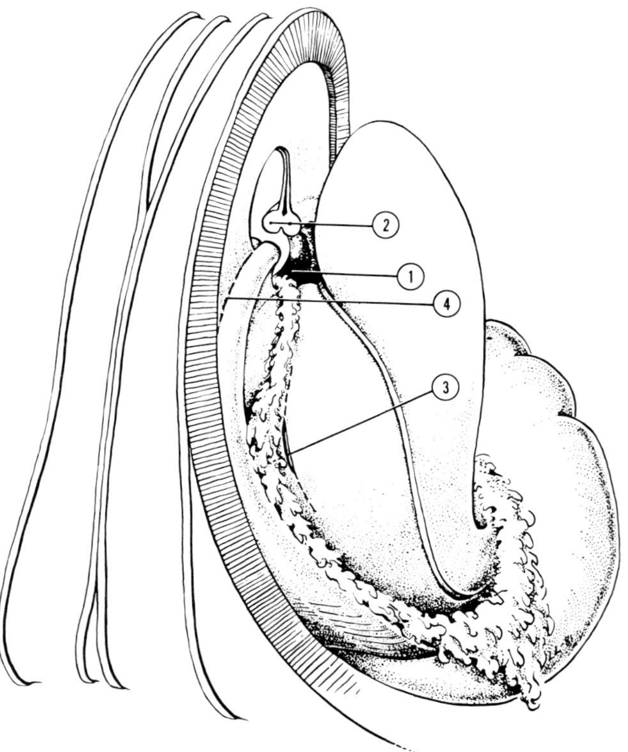

Fig. 33-1. Dorsolateral view of the right lateral ventricle with the corpus callosum to the left. The options for access to the third ventricle include: (1) the foramen of Monro; (2) incision of one or both fornicial columns; (3) mobilization of the lamina affixa with development of the subchoroidal plane; and (4) development of the interfornicial raphe.

alteration in memory patterns was appreciated by the patients, their families, or examining physicians.

Although this corridor does not alter fornicial structures by section, but rather employs division of the natural raphe separation in order to enhance exposure, transient amnesic syndromes have been observed in approximately one third of the cases. It should be stressed that these are temporary phenomena and did not last more than 3 weeks in any of our 25 cases. Moreover, no alteration of mentation was observed on clinical assessment nor indicated in statements of patients or relatives at 3 months postoperatively. None of 6 patients who underwent formal neuropsychiatric assessment at 3 months manifested abnormal profiles. The cause for this observation in the strictly physiologic sense is arguable, but probably is related to transmission of pressure to regions adjacent to the third ventricle during manipulation of the local pathologic process. Examination of these data would appear to imply that lesions of progressively firmer texture require greater manipulation and thus increased local trauma. This would appear to be evident from our data, with only 2 of 8 pliable cysticercosis cysts but 4 of 7 dense craniopharyngiomas manifesting postoperative memory dysfunction. No clear relation of the size of the lesion to observed incidence appears to exist.

In addition to the benefit of providing the surgeon with a corridor of minimum physiologic cost, this midline exposure offers the capability for simultaneous manipulation of the lesion, not only through the 2-cm fornicial exposure, but also simultaneously via both foramina of Monro, thereby adding the technical opportunities for manipulation and lesion excision.

ANATOMIC AND PHYSIOLOGIC CONSIDERATIONS

It is essential in preparing for any surgical endeavor to have strict comprehension of the normal anatomic elements constituting the surgical avenue and of those that may have potential influence on the procedure. Of particular importance are the major landmarks in the midline approach.[4,5] These include all topographic elements of the interhemispheric fissure, the sagittal sinus, the parasagittal veins, the falx cerebri, the cingulate gyrus, the anterior cerebral arteries (pericallosal arteries), the corpus callosum, the fornix, the tela choroidea, the medial posterior choroidal arteries, and the internal cerebral veins. In consideration of each one of these anatomic elements, one can envision certain risks inherent in the manipulation and techniques of the approach.

At the level of the cerebral cortex in the parasagittal region, direct cortical injury[6,7] or potential injury secondary to sacrifice or manipulation of parasagittal draining veins poses an important problem, but one that is easily resolved with proper planning. It has been our experience that appropriate placement of the bone flap can be enhanced by a study of the venous pattern of parasagittal drainage in the individual patient. We have had the opportunity to study 100 normal angiograms in consideration of this topic.[3] Optimal entry for this approach is at the level of the coronal suture. Forty-two percent of patients, however, demonstrate significant parasagittal veins which have tributaries that provide venous drainage from the middle and posterior frontal lobe within 2 cm anterior or posterior to the coronal suture. Seventy percent of these are within 2 cm posterior to the coronal suture, while 30 percent are in the anterior 2-cm sector. This is an important consideration in interhemispheric entry and retraction in the region, and we therefore have planned our craniotomies in view of these elements of venous anatomy (Figure 33-2). In addition, appropriate placement of the bone flap in the midline or slightly to the left of the midline obviates the need for excessive retractor pressure.

A second possible risk is related to the incision of the corpus callosum.[6,8–10] This approach requires an incision of 2.5 cm or less in the callosal body. There has been some indication that such an incision could cause impairment of interhemispheric transfer of tactile information.[6] Data derived from the study of our patients and from others, however, tend to refute this concept and would imply that the physiologic impact of such an incision is minimal.[3]

A third area of concern is the possible implications of fornicial manipulation.[11–21] Considerable controversy has existed in this regard. A review of the literature indicates a somewhat nebulous risk in fornicial manipulation, with a number of authors considering that this is attended by significant memory loss and others contending that no significant physiologic consequence is related to isolated fornicial injury. Our studies and observations on a group of patients who underwent bilateral fornicial manipulation as required in this approach indicate that a short-term memory loss of a transient nature may be observed in the early postoperative period. With extended follow-up, however, no significant memory loss has been apparent.[3]

A fourth consideration is the handling and the possible occlusion of the internal cerebral, the thalamostriate, and the septal veins in the region.[22,23] A review of the literature does not provide ample evidence for hard conclusions in this regard. Our experience, however, has not indicated any adverse effects related to manipulation of the internal cerebral veins as was necessary for excision of mass lesions via this approach.

Table 33-1. Interfornicial exposure

Case Number	Location	Pathologic Process
1	Anterior third ventricle	Colloid cyst (1.5 cm); ventriculomegaly; transient memory loss; total excision
2	Anterior third ventricle	Colloid cyst (2.0 cm); ventriculomegaly; total excision
3	Anterior third ventricle	Colloid cyst (1.0 cm); total excision
4	Anterior third ventricle	Colloid cyst (1.5 cm); total excision
5	Third ventricle	Colloid cyst (2.5 cm); ventriculomegaly; transient memory loss; total excision
6	Third ventricle	Craniopharyngioma (3.0 cm); ventriculomegaly
7	Third ventricle	Craniopharyngioma (2.5 cm); ventriculomegaly; total excision
8	Third ventricle	Craniopharyngioma (2.0 cm); ventriculomegaly, transient memory loss; total excision
9	Third ventricle	Craniopharyngioma (2.5 cm); ventriculomegaly; total excision
10	Third ventricle	Craniopharyngioma (4.0 cm); ventriculomegaly; transient memory loss
11	Third ventricle	Craniopharyngioma (3.0 cm); ventriculomegaly; transient memory loss; total excision
12	Third ventricle	Craniopharyngioma (2.5 cm); ventriculomegaly; transient memory loss
13	Foramen of Monro, anterior third ventricle	Cysticercosis (1.7 cm); ventriculomegaly; total excision
14	Foramen of Monro, anterior third ventricle	Cysticercosis (2 cm); ventriculomegaly; total excision
15	Foramen of Monro, anterior third ventricle	Cysticercosis (2.0 cm); ventriculomegaly; total excision
16	Foramen of Monro, anterior third ventricle	Cysticercosis (2.0 cm); ventriculomegaly; total excision
17	Anterior third ventricle	Cysticercosis (2.0 cm); ventriculomegaly; transient memory loss; total excision
18	Third ventricle	Cysticercosis (2.5 cm); ventriculomegaly; total excision
19	Third ventricle	Cysticercosis (2.0 cm); ventriculomegaly; total excision
20	Posterior third ventricle	Cysticercosis (1.5 cm); transient memory loss; total excision
21	Third ventricle	Glioma; ventriculomegaly
22	Third ventricle	Glioma; ventriculomegaly
23	Third ventricle	Glioma; ventriculomegaly
24	Foramen of Monro, third ventricle	AVM; transient memory loss; total excision
25	Posterior third ventricle	Bullet (.22 caliber)

A final consideration addresses the potential for diencephalic injury. Many factors bear on this risk in an individual patient. Important variables among these are related to the exposure that an individual approach affords, as well as the nature of the pathologic process to be managed. Soft and cystic lesions provide a more favorable substrate for excision than do denser solid masses where the possibility for transmission of pressure is greater.

ADVANTAGES OF THE APPROACH

The transcallosal interfornicial approach to the third ventricle offers rapid, safe, and extensive anterior and superior exposure of mass lesions of the third ventricle. Its advantage is that it is a technique that provides visualization of the entire region of the third ventricle without depending upon hydrocephalus or an extra-axial mass to enhance the exposure. With proper planning and technique, it can be accomplished with a minimum of physiologic consequence.

PREOPERATIVE PLANNING

Major enterprises in the preoperative period include obtaining appropriate computed tomographic (CT) scans, magnetic resonance imaging (MRI) scans, and cerebral angiograms. As previously noted, angiography is of value not only for the definition of vascular components in the region of the pathologic process and attendant to the lesion itself, but also for

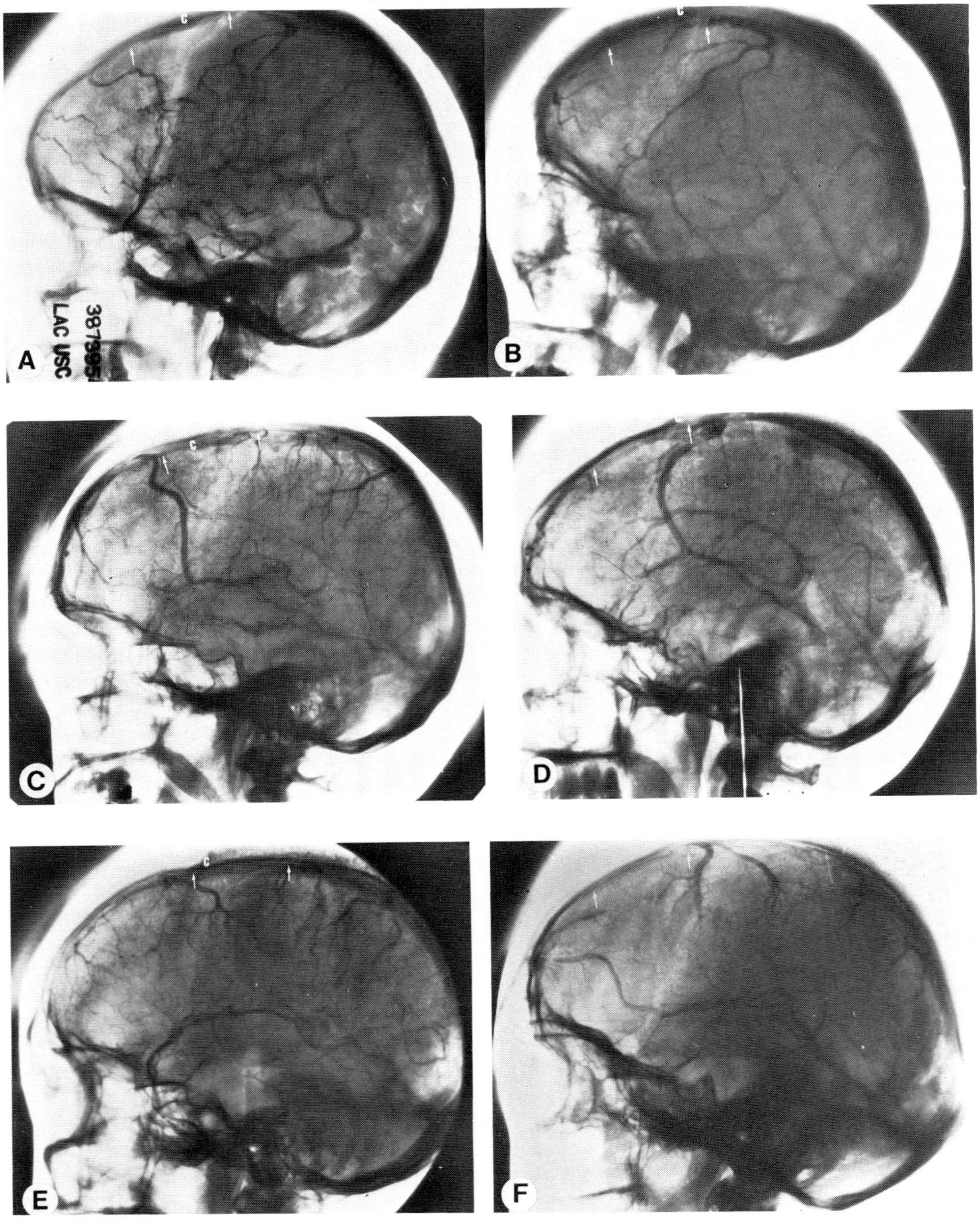

Fig. 33-2. Right lateral cerebral angiograms during the venous phase in 6 patients, demonstrating placement of the bone flap (arrows) as dictated by the situation of parasagittal venous tributaries. C indicates the coronal suture.

strict definition of the parasagittal venous anatomy in the area of the proposed entry. Of critical importance for optimal surgical planning and intraoperative manipulation is the development of an *absolute three-dimensional concept,* not only of the lesion in question, but also of the deformities the lesion has created in normal anatomic elements in the region. This is best obtained by multiple-view CT or MRI scans. These should include not only axial views, but also, from the standpoint of this approach, coronal cuts through the region of the lesion as well as sagittal views in midline and paramedian areas. Having made such appropriate anatomic definitions, the surgeon should be ready to undertake the approach and the management of the lesion within the region of the third ventricle with a minimum of risk to the patient.

ESSENTIAL FEATURES OF OPERATIVE TECHNIQUE

The surgery is performed with the patient in the supine position, with the head elevated 20 degrees and supported in a Mayfield pin-fixation headrest. In patients with hydrocephalus, a left frontal ventriculostomy is placed. This serves not only as a potential landmark during the course of surgery, but also as a method for postoperative assessment and control of intracranial pressure.

A right-sided 5 × 4-cm trapezoidal free *bone flap* is used for transcalvarial entry. The flap is placed in relationship to the parasagittal venous anatomy at the level of the coronal suture. The suture either can bisect the central point of the flap or the

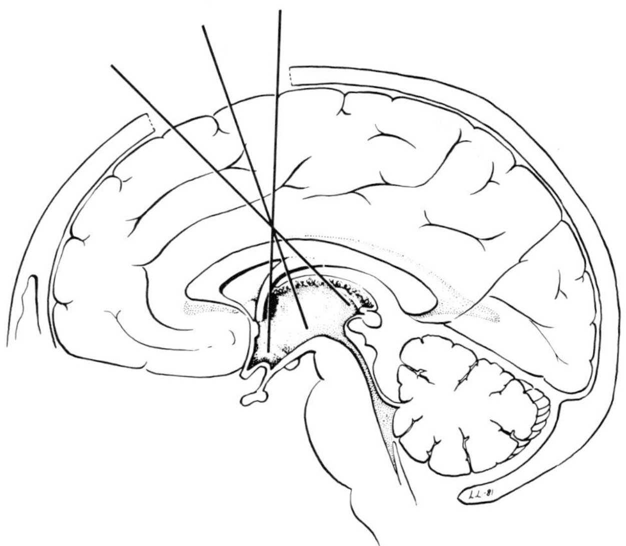

Fig. 33-3. Sagittal representations of anatomic elements at the level of the interhemispheric fissure. A bone flap is removed. Lines indicate planes of visual access that can be achieved by retractor angle variations in the midline.

flap can be moved posteriorly or slightly anteriorly according to the venous anatomic substrate. Depending on calvarial thickness, the flap is usually placed in the midline or slightly to the left of midline. This is essential, not only because of the superficial entry in relation to the interhemispheric fissure, but also because retraction is minimized from the medial to the lateral plane by appropriate flap placement. With regard to the midline extent of flap placement, it is important to appreciate that the midline approach to the third ventricle requires an absolute sagittal plane in the line of the falx, and, therefore, if this plane can be initiated at a superficial level, retraction can be minimized. We have found that all retraction and deformation of the parasagittal brain parenchyma can be localized to a 5 cm anterior-to-posterior plane. Having used a triangular craniotomy in the past, we have found that the trapezoidal shape is most appropriate for the retraction that is necessary for proper exposure.

With regard to the bone flap, we have used a two-limbed, curvilinear *scalp flap.* This flap is fashioned in the midline or slightly to the left of the midline, depending on the thickness of scalp tissue. Once we have initiated a scalp incision, we generally administer mannitol or Lasix to reduce cerebral tissue mass, with the idea of facilitating the interhemispheric exposure and minimizing retractor pressure.

A trapezoidal *dural incision* is then made with the broad base of the form positioned medially. Traction sutures are arranged so that the dural flap is turned over the sagittal sinus with some element of compression of this structure and absolute exposure of the midline plane at the level of the falx. A Budde self-retaining ring retractor system is prepared with a 14- or 19-mm blade to enter from the right side of the operative field. Dissection commences in the sagittal plane, employing a Penfield No. 1 instrument initially, followed by the self-retaining Budde blade. A secondary retractor can be placed on the falx from left to right, but in our experience this is not usually required for adequate exposure and may carry a risk of mutism secondary to bilateral cingulate manipulation. Protection of the parasagittal cortical tissue is provided by the application of

collagen sponge.[24] Once the inferior edge of the falx is appreciated, the operating microscope with a 275-mm objective lens is brought into the field, and, employing a combination of blunt- and broad-tipped instruments, the *cingulate gyri* are separated in the interhemispheric plane. As has been stressed,[9] the cingulate gyrus can occasionally be confused with the corpus callosum. With experience, however, it is apparent that this structure bears a strict resemblance to other cortical tissue, whereas the corpus has a striking white hue that is, in general, unmistakable as a cortical pial surface.

With identification of the *corpus callosum,* the pericallosal arteries are visible bilaterally, usually without difficulty. At this point it should be remembered that the transcallosal incision measuring 2–2.5 cm will generally be extensive enough to provide adequate exposure for biopsy, mobilization, and excision of most third ventricular lesions. The disposition of the anterior cerebral arteries will, in effect, dictate their management during the course of the transcallosal portion of the incision. Of critical importance is maintaining the midline exposure in reference to the falx, and this should be considered in the management of the anterior cerebral artery component of entry. Callosal incision can be made in the interarterial space or after retraction of the arteries laterally. Incision of the corpus callosum is initiated with a 5F irrigating suction apparatus and fine-tipped (0.3 mm) bipolar coagulating forceps. The thickness of the corpus will vary according to the degree of hydrocephalus and will be delineated on the coronal-view CT or MRI scan. In the event that a *strict midline transition* of the corpus is effected, it will be possible to identify a plane between the inferior margin of the corpus callosum and the *dorsal fornicial body.* Incision of this tissue in the sagittal plane with a Sheehy canal knife and fine-tipped bipolar forceps will provide entry through the diencephalic roof.

It is important to note that the surgeon should be constantly aware of entry angles related to head position, flap placement, and general ventricular anatomy as it is related to the particular case. Minimal changes in entry angles may make the site of ventricular visualization and access confusing. We have found that in the event a significant mass is present within the third ventricle, further medial-to-lateral retraction of fornicial tissue is not necessary. A secondary 9-mm retractor blade, however, can be introduced during the course of dissection and decompression of the mass from within the third ventricular cavity. In the event that the mass is small or significant hydrocephalus does not exist, identification of fornicial body tissues and the raphe is done without difficulty. A Sheehy canal knife is introduced, with excellent exposure through the roof of the third ventricle being attained rapidly. The internal cerebral veins come into view and can be retracted in the midline from right to left using a 9-mm retractor or a blunt microinstrument. Exploration of the area then can be undertaken.

Our development of the interfornicial plane has not exceeded 2 cm in any case. Of importance in considering this incision is its relationship to the hippocampal commissure in the posterior component of the fornicial structure. There is suggestive evidence in the literature that compromise of this area may lead to permanent memory loss,[16,21] so we have been reluctant to include the posterior portion of the fornicial structure in our line of incision. We therefore have limited incision in the fornicial elements to the region of the interface of the body and anterior column at the level of the anterior commissure.

In general, in the event that further exposure of the third

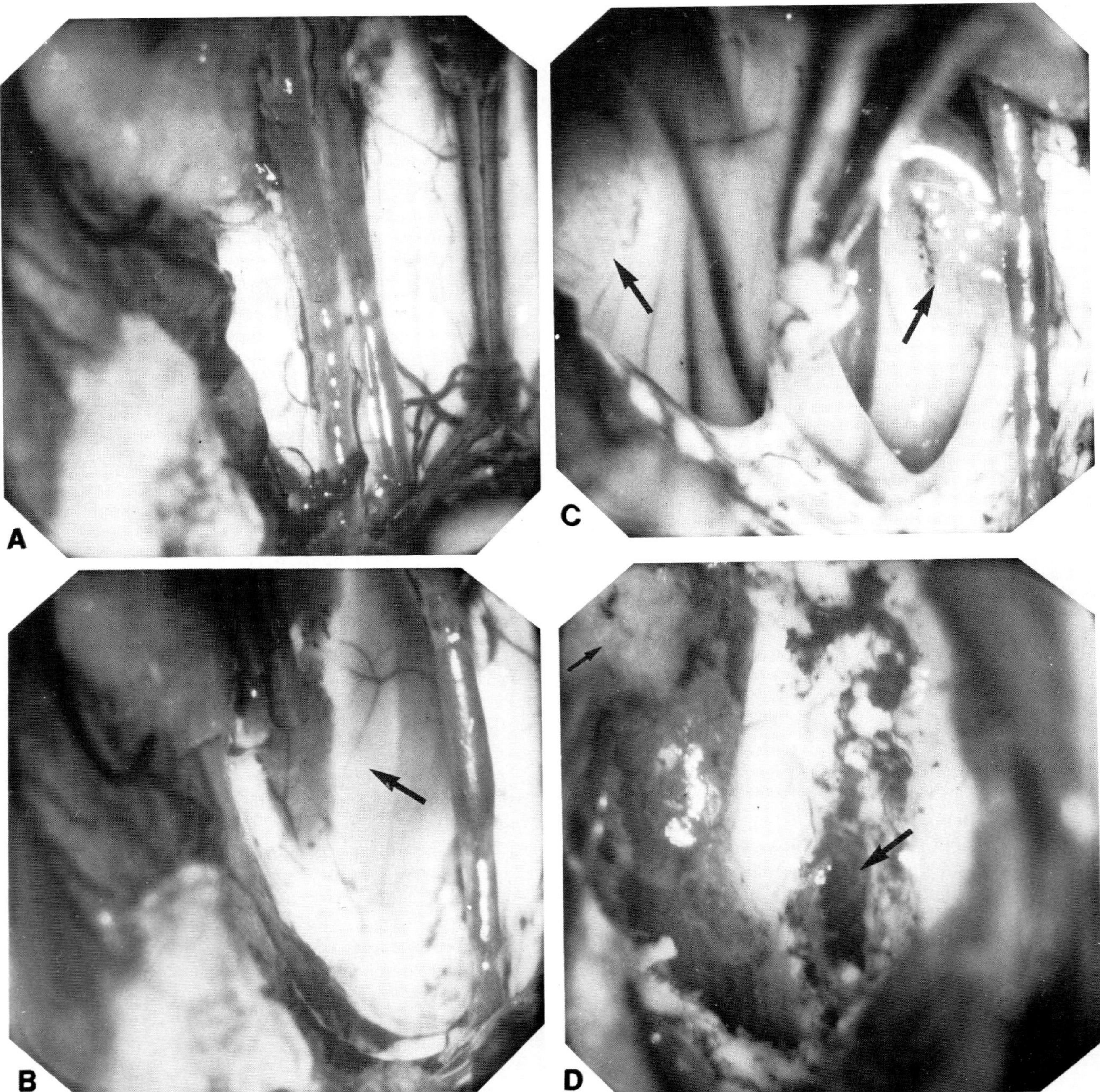

Fig. 33-4. Midline entry to the third ventricle in a case of ependymoma of the third ventricle. The series of intraoperative micrographs illustrates a common variable in the midline approach with initial identification of the septum pellucidum–callosal junction. (A) White callosal bed with pericallosal arteries. Note the cingulate surface with cottonoids to the left and the retractor blade to the right. (B) The corpus callosum is incised, and the pericallosal arteries are displaced laterally (right artery well visualized). The point of junction of the septum pellucidum and the corpus callosum is evident as the defined white line to the left of the arrow. The septum is bowed to the right frontal horn. A 5F irrigating suction tip is visible over the left lateral ventricle. The ependyma is intact. (C) Midline bilateral entry of the lateral ventricle has been accomplished. The bipolar forceps in the center of the field grasp the septum pellucidum as it is resected to the fornix. Note tumor tissue (arrows) emerging from the foramina of Monro bilaterally. (D) The fornicial raphe is partially incised (large arrow), with tumor tissue apparent in the third ventricle. There is a remnant of the base of the septum pellucidum superiorly. The small arrow indicates tumor emerging from the left foramen of Monro. The choroid plexus of the left lateral ventricle is evident in the left of the field as it approaches the foramen. The midline fornicial plane will be developed further to enhance exposure.

ventricle, either anterior or posterior, is desired, minimal alteration of the retractor angle will allow visualization of the appropriate area (Figure 33-3). We have not found manipulation of the internal cerebral veins when necessary during the course of this dissection to have been attended by significant operative morbidity.

In some cases entry of the *lateral ventricle* is effected during the course of transcallosal incision. This can result from either a failure to adhere to the strict midline plane during the course of callosal incision or some element of shift of the midline related to the placement of the ventriculostomy. Entry of the lateral ventricle is recognized by the identification of the ependyma, which initially appears as a dark plane when the inferior surface of the corpus callosum is transgressed. The *ependyma* is carefully entered with bipolar coagulating forceps and microscissors. The presence of cerebrospinal fluid (CSF) is readily identified in the ventricular cavity. Once the ventricular space is identified, the retractor blade is introduced to further enhance exposure. At this point it is necessary to gain orientation in relation to the plane of entry, and this is accomplished by identifying the anatomic elements in the region. We have found that the *choroid plexus* is the most striking and reliable element for orientation following entry of the lateral ventricle, and orienting the structure from a posterior-to-anterior direction aids in identification of the intraventricular foramen of Monro. In addition, one can identify the thalamostriate vein, the septal vein, and the septum pellucidum. Once these structures are identified, the fornicial column is readily appreciated.

With entry of the lateral ventricle, it is possible to effect a fenestration of the *septum pellucidum,* and with midline exposure bilateral identification of the foramen of Monro is realized. This maneuver is important because unilateral shunting will effect complete ventricular drainage in the event that a subtotal excision of a third ventricular mass is accomplished. Following fenestration of the septum pellucidum in cases where masses of the third ventricle are significant, it is possible to identify the mass bilaterally and effect manipulation of the lesion via the transforaminal route. Once anatomic orientation is realized, a Sheehy canal knife or Krayenbuhl hook can be used in the interfornicial raphe, at the level of either the columns or the body, to develop this plane and provide access through the roof of the third ventricle to the lesion in question. In many cases we have found that transforaminal as well as interfornicial manipulation of lesions is advantageous during the course of their excision (Figure 33-4).

Occasionally the presence of a cavum septum pellucidum as defined on CT or MRI scans will offer another variable in midline entry. Cavum access will provide a well-defined corridor to the midline fornix.

Having gained proper exposure, the lesions then are managed by standard microsurgical techniques. Management of the offending pathologic process having been completed, copious irrigation of the region with body-temperature Ringer's lactate solution then is undertaken, with care being taken to remove from the system all elements of blood and debris that could block CSF circulation. This is particularly important within the cavity of the third ventricle.

The patient is taken to the intensive care unit, where intracranial pressure monitoring is maintained for a 48- to 72-hour period. In the event that there are no abnormal excursions of intracranial pressure during this period, a small amount of indigo-carmine dye is placed through the ventriculostomy and a lumbar puncture performed 1 hour later to assess the status of flow dynamics. In the event that the patient is asymptomatic and the course uneventful, a CT scan is performed at the end of the first postoperative week.

SUMMARY AND CONCLUSIONS

The midline corridor, which transgresses the corpus callosum and interfornicial space at the level of the coronal suture, provides rapid, safe, and extensive anterior and superior exposure of mass lesions of the third ventricle. With appropriate roentgenologic evaluation and meticulous attention to preoperative and intraoperative planning and technique, the approach can be accomplished with a minimum of physiologic consequence and offers a valuable adjunct that merits consideration in the management of tumors of the third ventricle.

REFERENCES

1. Busch E: A new approach for the removal of tumors of the third ventricle. Acta Psychiatr 19:57, 1944
2. Baldwin M, Ommaya AK, Farrier R, et al: Mesial cerebral incision. J Neurosurg 20:679, 1963
3. Apuzzo MLJ, Chikovani O, Gott P, et al: Transcallosal, interfornicial approaches for lesions affecting the third ventricle: Surgical considerations and consequences. Neurosurgery 10:547, 1982
4. Seeger W: Atlas of Topographical Anatomy of the Brain and Surrounding Structures. Vienna, Springer-Verlag, 1978
5. Yamamoto I, Rhoton AL Jr, Peace DA: Microsurgery of the third ventricle: Part 1. Microsurgical anatomy. Neurosurgery 8:334,1981
6. Jeeves MA, Simpson DA, Geffen G: Functional consequences of the transcallosal removal of intraventricular tumours. J Neurol Neurosurg Psychiatry 42:134, 1970
7. Shucart WA, Stein BM: Transcallosal approach to the anterior ventricular system. Neurosurgery 3:339, 1978
8. Dimond SJ, Scammell RE, Brouwers EYM, et al: Functions of the centre section (trunk) of the corpus callosum in man. Brain 100:543, 1977
9. Stein BM: Transcallosal approach to third ventricular tumors, in Schmidek HH, Sweet HW (eds): Current Techniques in Operative Neurosurgery. New York, Grune & Stratton, 1977, pp 247–256
10. Winston KR, Cavazzuti V, Arkins T: Absence of neurological and behavioral abnormalities after anterior transcallosal operation for third ventricular lesions. Neurosurgery 4:386, 1979
11. Bengochea FG, De La Torre O, Esquivel O, et al: The section of the fornix in the surgical treatment of certain epilepsies. Trans Am Neurol Assoc 79:176, 1959
12. Cairns H, Mosberg WH Jr: Colloid cyst of the third ventricle. Surg Gynecol Obstet 92:545, 1951
13. Ciric I, Zivin I: Neuroepithelial (colloid) cysts of the septum pellucidum. J Neurosurg 43:69, 1975
14. Dott NM: Surgical aspects of the hypothalamus, in Clark WEL, Beattie J, Riddoch GG, et al. (eds): The Hypothalamus: Morphological, Functional, Clinical and Surgical Aspects. Edinburgh, Oliver and Boyd, 1958, pp 131–185
15. Hassler R, Riechert T: Uber einen Fall von doppelseitiger Fornicotomie bei sogenannter temporaler Epilepsie. Acta Neurochir 5:330, 1957
16. Heilman KM, Sypert GW: Korsakoff's syndrome resulting from bilateral fornix lesions. Neurology 27:490, 1977
17. Horel JA: The neuroanatomy of amnesia. A critique of the hippocampal memory hypothesis. Brain 101:403, 1978
18. Little JR, MacCarty CS: Colloid cysts of the third ventricle. J Neurosurg 39:230, 1974
19. Sweet WH, Talland GA, Ervin FR: Loss of recent memory following section of fornix. Trans Am Neurol Assoc 84:76, 1959
20. Woolsey RM, Nelson JS: Asymptomatic destruction of the fornix in man. Arch Neurol 32:566, 1975
21. Zaidel D, Sperry KW: Memory impairment after commissurotomy in man. Brain 97:263, 1974
22. Caron JP, Debrun G, Sichez JP, et al: Ligature des veines cerebrales internes et survivantes: A propos de deux pinealomectomies. Neurochirurgie 20:81, 1973
23. Hirsch JF, Zouasui A, Reiner D, et al: A new surgical approach to the third ventricle with interruption of the striothalamic vein. Acta Neurochir 47:135, 1979
24. Kurze T, Apuzzo MLJ, Weiss MH, et al: Collagen sponge for surface brain protection. J Neurosurg 43:637, 1975

CHAPTER 34

Considerations in the Management of Masses in the Pineal Region

Henry H. Schmidek

ALTHOUGH OFTEN the discussion regarding the treatment of pineal region mass lesions evolves around which is the most suitable surgical approach, one should realize that subjecting all these patients to surgery is a rather simplistic way of dealing with a complex problem.

Pineal tumors are a heterogeneous group of mass lesions originating in or located adjacent to the pineal gland. Neoplasms in this region cause symptoms when they compress or invade local structures or are disseminated beyond the confines of the tumor. When these tumors occlude the cerebral aqueduct, obstructive hydrocephalus with intracranial hypertension occurs; if the superior colliculus and pretectal area are involved, characteristic eye signs develop, which may include impairment of upward gaze and abnormalities of the pupil, paralysis or spasm of convergence, and nystagmus retractorius. This sylvian aqueduct syndrome is indicative of a periaqueductal lesion. Parinaud's syndrome, the paralysis of upward gaze alone, is often and incorrectly used as a synonym for sylvian aqueduct syndrome. The anatomic substrate underlying these functions is located just anterior to the aqueduct and below the posterior part of the third ventricle. Downward gaze, which can also be impaired in these patients, has its localization caudal to that of upward gaze in the brain stem. Compression or invasion of the cerebellum results in dysmetria, hypotonia, and intention tremor. There may be altered consciousness as a result of intracranial hypertension or direct invasion of the brain stem by tumor. Some of these tumors metastasize to the spinal cord or cauda equina or to structures outside the nervous system. These metastases may pass through the shunts inserted to treat intracranial hypertension. Less common symptoms, occurring in less than 10 percent of male patients with pineal tumors, are precocious puberty or delayed onset of sexual maturation. Even less common is the occurrence of pineal apoplexy, in which a patient undergoes sudden neurologic deterioration secondary to intratumoral hemorrhage and sudden expansion in the size of the posterior third ventricular tumor.

The lesions in the posterior third ventricle represent a diverse group of tumors; however, the crucial differentiation prognostically is between those lesions that are benign and those that are malignant. Approximately 10 percent of lesions in this area are truly benign, including cysts, lipomas, arteriovenous malformations and aneurysms, pineocytomas, and meningiomas. Another 5 to 10 percent of tumors are relatively benign, including the low-grade gliomas and dermoid cysts. The remaining 80 to 85 percent of pineal region neoplasms are highly malignant lesions. These include the germ cell tumors typified by the atypical teratoma (pineal germinoma), also teratocarcinoma, choriocarcinoma, endodermal sinus tumor, pineoblastoma, glioblastoma, metastatic tumor, sarcoma, and mixed tumors with two or more of these components.

The suprasellar germinomas are included in this family of neoplasms. These tumors, which are histologically identical to pineal germinomas, arise in or beneath the anterior part of the third ventricle.

Many suprasellar germinomas represent anterior extension of a pineal germinoma; however, suprasellar germinomas have been shown to exist free of pineal involvement. Kageyama and Belsky[1] categorized these suprasellar tumors. The type 1 suprasellar germinoma is a metastatic tumor from the pineal which invades the floor of the third ventricle, hypophysis, and optic pathways. The symptoms are those of pineal tumor and of hypothalamic and chiasmatic involvement. There is commonly an admixture of these signs and symptoms indicating involvement of both anterior and posterior third ventricular structures. Type 2 germinomas are those which arise within the third ventricle and produce an obstructive hydrocephalus early in the disease; later findings are indicative of invasion of the hypothalamus, pituitary, and optic pathways. Type 3 germinomas are those which originate in the region of the optic chiasmal region, grow outside the ventricular system, and only late in the disease invade the third ventricle and hypothalamus.

When there is suprasellar involvement, the patient may have a triad including diabetes insipidus, visual defects, and other evidence of endocrine dysfunction. Diabetes insipidus is the most common manifestation of these tumors and may precede the development of other findings by years. The abnormalities of the visual system encountered include reduction in visual acuity, often in conjunction with optic atrophy. There are isolated reports of extraocular paralysis or severe exophthalmos caused by infiltration of the tumor into the optic chiasm, nerves, and orbit. Papilledema may not be evident, even in the presence of severe intracranial hypertension, because of the associated optic atrophy. Visual field studies may demonstrate bitemporal inferior scotomas, indicating a lesion

---

Portions of this chapter are reprinted from Schmidek HH (ed): Pineal Tumors. New York, Masson, 1977, ch 5, and Schmidek HH, Waters A: Pineal masses: Clinical features and management, in Wilkins RH (ed): Neurosurgery. New York, McGraw-Hill, 1984, pp 688–693. With permission.

OPERATIVE NEUROSURGICAL TECHNIQUES
ISBN 0-8089-1862-1

on the dorsum of the chiasm. Macular fiber involvement by tumor growing into the posterior and superior part of the chiasm, associated with a bitemporal inferior scotomatous defect, is particularly characteristic of this tumor. Hypopituitarism is the third most common finding, after diabetes insipidus and visual abnormalities, and is often associated with growth arrest when the tumor occurs before puberty or with hypogonadism and amenorrhea when it occurs in older patients. Pathologic obesity, neurogenic hypernatremia, abnormalities in temperature regulation, and excessive somnolence are uncommon manifestations reported in conjunction with these lesions. Elevated intracranial pressure is seen in tumors arising by extension from pineal region neoplasms. Suprasellar germinomas can also metastasize throughout the neuraxis.

The skull roentgenograms are abnormal in approximately 50 percent of patients with pineal region tumors, indicating changes secondary to chronic intracranial hypertension, and there may be abnormalities in the amount and configuration of calcification in the pineal region aneurysm, dermoid cyst, meningioma, low-grade glioma, or germinoma. Chest radiography is part of the investigation to exclude a primary malignant disease of the lung or a tumor that may have metastasized to both lung and brain.

Computed tomography of the head with enhancement indicates the size and position of the lesion; whether there is a calcific, cystic, or hemorrhagic component; the degree of hydrocephalus; and whether there is evidence of subependymal extension or extension into the lateral ventricles or the suprasellar region. The suprasellar extension from a posterior third ventricular mass can be quite subtle and may require serial thin sections for detection, especially of the subependymal enhancement. The suprasellar germinomas may show obliteration of the suprasellar cistern, irregular margins, moderate enhancement by contrast material, and tumor infiltration of the wall of the third ventricle and both lateral ventricles. There may also be extension into the orbit and expansion of the optic nerves or chiasm as a result of tumor infiltration.

Cytologic examination of the cerebrospinal fluid is important, since the presence of malignant cells may establish the nature and extent of the lesion. Seeding of the cerebrospinal fluid is a particularly characteristic feature of the germinomas, although this property is exhibited by an occasional pineoblastoma. The incidence of this phenomenon in patients with malignant pineal tumors is not known. There are reports of this occurrence in up to 60 percent of cases, especially when the sensitivity of the cerebrospinal fluid examination is improved by the use of millipore-filtered CSF + tissue culture techniques.

Angiographic examination of both the carotid and the vertebral systems should allow identification of aneurysms of the posterior cerebral artery, arteriovenous malformations, abnormalities of the vein of Galen, and meningiomas, allowing these lesions to be appropriately treated. Although germinomas are vascular, it is unusual for them to contain neovascularity demonstrable by angiography, whereas embryonal carcinoma and teratocarcinoma show tumor vessels, and the presence of such tumor vascularity is suggestive of these malignant tumors. In addition, angiography provides important preoperative information about the relationships of the internal cerebral veins, the vein of Galen, the basal veins of Rosenthal, and the precentral cerebellar vein to the lesion.

Whether a myelographic examination of the spinal axis should be performed in patients with a posterior third ventricular neoplasm of undefined character is problematic. It is my policy to undertake this examination as part of the investigation both during the initial set of diagnostic studies and often serially in the patient with a malignant tumor in order to identify asymptomatic spinal metastases or assess the response of these to therapy. The presence of such lesions is of major diagnostic and therapeutic importance, particularly since one cannot determine with a high degree of accuracy the nature of an isolated posterior third ventricular mass on the basis of radiographic studies alone. Currently, benign and malignant posterior third ventricular tumors cannot be distinguished on the basis of tumor enhancement, size, and tumor margination alone.

The patient with a posterior third ventricular tumor requires as part of the investigation a careful assessment of endocrine function.[2] Diabetes insipidus is the most common endocrine abnormality associated with pineal tumors; when present, it is probably caused by anterior third ventricular extension of the neoplasm. Such cases are often overlooked. The physician should be suspicious and should undertake appropriate provocative tests. Tests of anterior pituitary function are also part of the investigation, to exclude ACTH deficiency and secondary, possibly life-threatening, adrenocortical insufficiency. Abnormalities of sexual maturation require that the levels of LH, FSH, testosterone, prolactin, and growth hormone and the melatonin-forming activity of the cerebrospinal fluid and serum be surveyed.

Neuro-ophthalmologic examination is mandatory in search of the defects seen in conjunction with these lesions and to provide evidence of the extent of the tumor involvement, which may not be apparent from the other studies, as well as a baseline for comparison after treatment.

Immunoassay for alpha fetoprotein (AFP) and the beta chain of human chorionic gonadotropin (hCG) may allow the diagnosis of an intracranial germ cell tumor (i.e., germinoma, teratocarcinoma, choriocarcinoma, or embryonal carcinoma). Forty to 50 percent of germinomas and embryonal carcinomas are hCG-producing tumors, and the embryonal carcinoma can also produce AFP. Cases have been reported in which the tumor produces both AFP and hCG, although no tumor has been reported as producing AFP alone.[3] In addition, the plasma level of these tumor markers correlates with tumor growth and regression and may be used to assess the response to therapy.[4] Plasma melatonin has also been used as a marker of pineal tumors, although there may be extrapineal sources of melatonin, so that even when a pineal tumor and raised melatonin levels exist, the value of this test has been questioned.[5]

Since pineal region tumors are dangerous intracranial masses to excise, there has been an ongoing debate for at least the half-century concerning their surgical management. The debate centers on whether it is in the patient's best interest to explore these lesions at the time of their diagnosis, or whether the obstructive hydrocephalus should be treated with a shunt and the posterior third ventricular tumor irradiated without a tissue diagnosis—maneuvers that can be carried out with a mortality of under 5 percent. Until the last decade the high morbidity and mortality associated with attempts to biopsy or excise tumors in this location provided ample reason for this debate. In response to the challenge, the last decade has seen increasingly frequent reports of exploration of these tumors with standard microsurgical techniques, with an ever lessening mortality and morbidity. These reports by Jamieson,[6] Neuwelt et al.,[7] Chapman and Linggood,[8] Sano and Matsutani,[9] Ventureyra,[10] and Stein[11] represent an aggregate of 128 cases of posterior third ventricular tumor subjected to direct exploration. In this combined series there were two operative deaths, one from hemorrhage into a glioblastoma occurring 1 week after surgery, the other related to a large infiltrating tumor of the midbrain which had been previously irradiated.[11]

Even though it is now feasible for highly experienced surgeons to operate on lesions in the posterior third ventricle with an acceptable risk, patients in whom cytologic examination of the cerebrospinal fluid shows malignant cells, patients with evidence of either spinal or extraneural metastases, and patients in whom both an anterior and a posterior third ventricular tumor are demonstrable (particularly if one of the tumor marker assays is abnormally high) are harboring a germinoma or other malignant germ cell tumor and may not require direct intervention. In contrast to these cases, there is a strong indication for surgical intervention in those tumors which, on the basis of the investigations, have a particularly high likelihood of being benign, e.g., the cyst or dermoid; those cases in which investigations do not allow characterization of the tumor; and those patients previously treated with shunt and radiation without a tissue diagnosis who have progressive neurologic problems in the presence of a functioning shunt. Patients in this latter group have often survived for a period of years, and benign or relatively benign tumors are particularly frequent among this select group of cases, whereas the danger of radionecrosis from further radiotherapy is high. A significant percentage of cases in surgical series with a favorable outcome include cases of this type.

There is controversy whether, in treating malignant pineal tumors, radiation should be confined to the head or extended to include the entire neuraxis. The exquisite responsiveness of the germinoma to radiation, as assessed by serial CT scans performed during treatment in five cases of presumed (i.e., not histologically confirmed) germinoma, has been described by Takaki et al.[12] It was possible to detect evidence of clinical improvement when the patient had received 1200 rad, with a change in the clinical effects preceding the changes to be seen on CT scanning. At 1500 rad a marked decrease in tumor size was detectable, coincident with a decrease in the tumor's contrast enhancement. With further radiation there was gradual normalization of the ventricular system and cisterns, and by 5000 rad the tumor had disappeared entirely. The concern is whether the prophylactic irradiation of the entire neuraxis is necessary in tumors such as the germinoma and pineoblastoma, which have a propensity to seed throughout the nervous system, since bone marrow suppression, growth arrest of the spine, and radiation effects on the ovaries or testes attend this approach. The other reason for controversy is that reliable figures are not available on the incidence of spinal metastases, although there are estimates of 15 to 57 percent.[13] Symptomatic spinal metastases occur in approximately 15 percent of cases.

On my service, neuraxis radiation is currently reserved for patients with histologically proven germinomas and for patients with a posterior third ventricular neoplasm and cerebrospinal fluid cytology positive for malignant cells or in whom spinal implants are revealed on myelography. The remaining patients are treated on an individualized basis in consultation with the radiotherapist.

The absence of the blood–brain barrier in the pineal gland suggests that lesions located there may have an increased vulnerability to systemic chemotherapy. Objective remission has been reported in a pineal tumor with pulmonary metastases treated with chlorambucil, methotrexate, and dactinomycin. In addition, testicular germinomas, which are histologically identical to pineal germinomas, have shown an 82 percent remission rate when treated with bleomycin, Vinblastine, and cis-platinum.[7] These forms of chemotherapy are currently reserved for patients with systemic, extraneural metastases or those with recurrent disease within the neuraxis following full courses of radiation therapy in whom further radiation is not an option.

REFERENCES

1. Kageyama N, Belsky R: Ectopic pineloma in the chiasma region. Neurology 11:318, 1961
2. Schmidek HH (ed): Pineal Tumors. New York, Masson, 1977
3. Haase J, Nielsen K: Value of tumor markers in the treatment of endodermal sinus tumors and choriocarcinomas in the pineal region. Neurosurgery 5:484, 1979
4. Gindhart TD, Tsukahara YC: Cytologic diagnosis of pineal germinoma in cerebrospinal fluid and sputum. Acta Cytol 23:341, 1979
5. Barber SG, Smith JA, Hughes RC: Melatonin as a tumour marker in a patient with pineal tumour. Br Med J 2:328, 1978
6. Jamieson KG: Excision of pineal tumors. J Neurosurg 35:550, 1971
7. Neuwelt EA, Glasberg M, Frenkel E, et al: Malignant pineal region tumors: A clinico-pathological study. J Neurosurg 51:597, 1979
8. Chapman PH, Linggood, RM: The management of pineal area tumors: A recent reappraisal. Cancer 46:1253, 1980
9. Sano K, Matsutani M: Pineloma (germinoma) treated by direct surgery and postoperative irradiation: A long-term follow-up. Childs Brain 8:81, 1981
10. Ventureyra ECG: Pineal region: Surgical management of tumors and vascular malformations. Surg Neurol 16:77, 1981
11. Stein BM: Supracerebellar approach for pineal region neoplasms, in Schmidek HH, Sweet WH (eds): Operative Neurosurgical Techniques: Indications and Methods. New York, Grune & Stratton, 1982, pp 599–607
12. Takaki S, Hikita T, Ishii C, et al: Serial computed tomographic studies of pineal region tumor treated by irradiation. Kurume Med J 26:163, 1979
13. Sung DI, Harisiadis L, Chang CH: Midline pineal tumors and suprasellar germinomas: Highly curable by irradiation. Radiology 128:745, 1978

CHAPTER 35

Supracerebellar Approach for Pineal Region Neoplasms

Bennett M. Stein

PINEAL TUMORS can arise from the pineal gland including the pineal cells and supporting cells. In addition, tumors are included in this group that arise from the medial walls of the thalamus and midbrain. We therefore have tumors of the pineal region.[1–4] These tumors lie in a central position that is equidistant from various cranial points traditionally used as routes of exposure. The deep central location places such tumors in intimate contact with the important deep venous system, including the vein of Galen, the precentral cerebellar vein, and the internal cerebral veins.[5] In almost all instances, including malignant and benign tumors, the bulk of the tumor, if not all of the tumor, lies below the internal cerebral veins and the vein of Galen. In some instances there may be a dense attachment to these structures, including the tela choroidea. The arteries that are concerned with these tumors are small caliber branches of the posterior choroidal arteries and branches of the quadrigeminal arteries. In most cases they are destined strictly for the tumor and supply no areas of the brain beyond the tumor. In a highly vascular tumor, these arteries may be a problem in terms of intraoperative and postoperative hemorrhage.

Although the number of patients who have tumors in this region is relatively small, the fact that the tumors represent a wide variation in histology and have been a challenge to expose surgically has led to a comparatively voluminous literature on them. Cushing[6] indicated the difficulty with surgical treatment of pineal tumors by stating "Personally, I have never succeeded in exposing a pineal tumor sufficiently well to justify an attempt to remove it." Others[7,8,9] also emphasized the high mortality following operation on pineal tumors. Dandy,[10] however, despite the high operative mortality, continued to advocate surgical exposure and removal of these tumors. Later, Suzuki[11] reported a large series of pineal tumors in which total or near total removals were effected without overwhelming morbidity or mortality. This history of attempts to treat pineal tumors underscores the evolving surgical attitude toward these tumors. Initially, there was an aggressive attitude that bore no fruit. Based on these early disasters, a more conservative approach subsequently advocated control of the hydrocephalus and "blind" radiation to the tumor.[7,8,9] With the advent of the operating microscope, a better understanding of the anatomy, and sophistication of surgical techniques, many neurosurgeons advocated an aggressive surgical approach to these lesions, with removal of benign tumors and decompression and identification of malignant tumors.[11–16] The mortality and morbidity

from the surgical approaches has been dropping steadily. As will subsequently be detailed, there are a number of surgical approaches to this region.

The well-recognized fact that a wide variety of tumors can occur in this region and that approximately 25 percent of them are encapsulated and benign lends further justification to attempts to remove those that are encapsulated and can be dissected free of surrounding brain tissue (Table 35-1). With more invasive tumors, exact histologic identification results in enlightened therapeutic management, since the germinoma type of tumor has a tendency to spread widely throughout the central nervous system. In such instances radiation of the entire neuraxis and chemotherapy may be indicated. On the other hand, astrocytomas and ependymomas tend to invade locally and may best be treated by high-dose local radiation and supplemental chemotherapy. We have recently encountered mixed tumors of the pineal region. These are generally large and for the most part benign teratomas with small components of malignancy. The malignancy is represented by germinomas, embryonal carcinomas, and choriocarcinomas. This finding that tumors may show a small malignant component while for the most part being benign demands surgical exploration with removal of as much tumor as possible so that the malignant features can be identified by a pathologist. Furthermore, even with malignant tumors, oncologists now feel that debulking procedures can be done safely and are of benefit in reducing the tumor burden in view of subsequent therapy, whether it be radiation or chemotherapy.

CLASSIC SURGICAL TECHNIQUES

Dandy[10] was a master at approaching deep-seated brain tumors and was particularly interested in pineal region tumors. He advocated an interhemispheral approach with section of the posterior portion of the corpus callosum to gain access to the pineal region. This required sacrificing a number of parietal cortical veins and retracting a large portion of the parietal hemisphere, usually the right. In the region of the pineal gland, difficulties were encountered in dissecting through or around the deep venous system, and many of the fatalities appeared to arise from uncontrolled deep-vein thrombosis and edema of the diencephalic region. VanWagenen[17] advocated an approach through the right lateral ventricle, which is almost always dilated when tumors compromise or obstruct the aqueductal

OPERATIVE NEUROSURGICAL TECHNIQUES
ISBN 0-8089-1862-1

Table 35-1. Fifty consecutive pineal region tumors

Type of Tumor	Benign		Malignant	
	Number	Percent	Number	Percent
Germ cell origin	4	8	12	24
Pineal cell origin	0	0	8	16
Glial origin	6	12	12	24
Meningiomas	5	10	0	0
Others	2	4	1	2
Total	17	34	33	66

region. Exposure of the tumor still involved dissection of the deep venous system, since the approach was primarily dorsal to the tumor. In addition it had the disadvantage of a transcortical incision and possible hemispheral collapse when the ventricle was opened. Poppen[18] advocated an approach under the occipital lobe, in which bridging veins were sacrificed, a large portion of the hemisphere retracted, and the free edge of the tentorium sectioned to expose the deep venous plexus in a more favorable attitude relative to the underlying tumor. Reid and Clark have reviewed the merits of this approach.[13] Krause,[19] in 1926, reported 3 cases, each a different variety of tumor in the pineal or quadrigeminal region, which he approached through the posterior fossa, over the cerebellar hemispheres, and under the tentorium. Since most of these tumors are central, the posterior fossa approach with the patient in the sitting position allows an excellent midline, central exposure to these tumors. In addition, (with those tumors lying primarily beneath the deep venous system) injury is avoided to this important group of veins. This exposure gives room commensurate to supratento-

rial approaches and avoids injury to the parietal or occipital lobes and subsequent defects in sensation or peripheral vision. The disadvantages to the posterior fossa approach are realized when the tumor extends dorsally above the incisura and when the tumor extends laterally to the trigone of the lateral ventricles. The tentorium may be cut, but it is still difficult to reach these extremes of the tumor (Figure 35-1). This approach provides excellent access to these tumors and is the one that I use.[15,16]

DIAGNOSIS

CLINICAL FEATURES

The classic symptomatology of Parinaud's syndrome is not always encountered in cases of pineal tumor or, at best, variations of this syndrome may be encountered. More likely are signs of raised intracranial pressure and ataxia caused by compromise of the aqueduct and compression of the superior cerebellar peduncle in the midbrain. Precocious puberty occurs primarily in a select group of boys and in less than 10 percent of patients. A similar incidence of diabetes insipidus is encountered, in which case seeding of the tumor into the hypothalamic region may be suspected.

With the prevalent use of computed tomographic (CT) scans after head injuries or to evaluate individuals with headaches, we are now encountering a few pineal tumors that appear to be asymptomatic. It is therefore apparent that tumors can reach a significant size, certainly large enough to be visualized with modern-day imaging systems, and not produce symptoms. The evolution of symptoms appears to be primarily on the basis of hydrocephalus caused by compression or infiltration of the aqueductal region. This can occur late in some tumors.

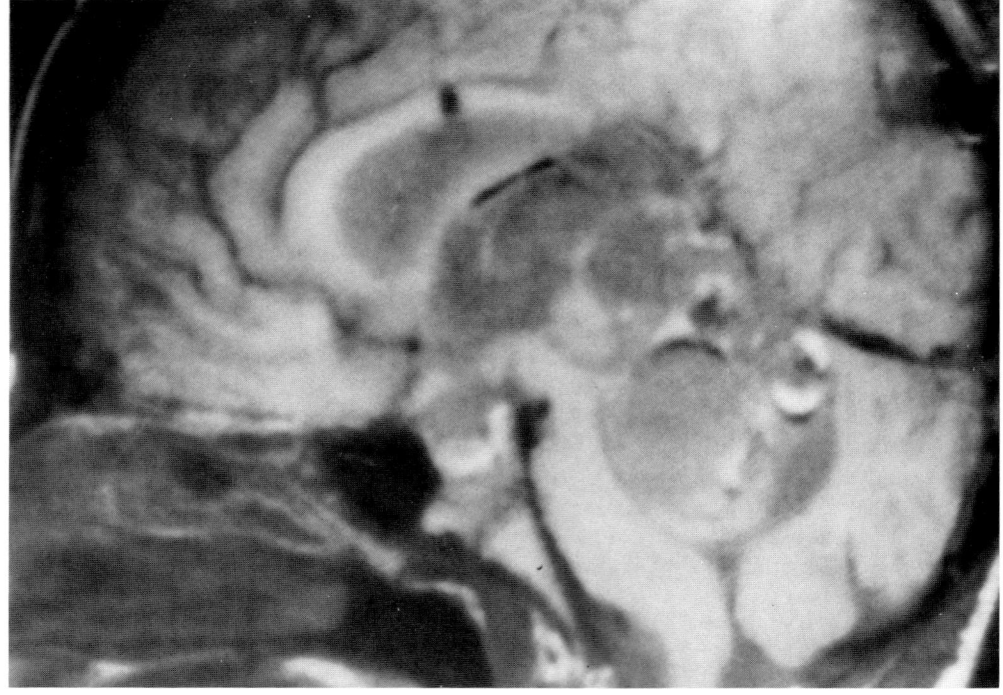

Fig. 35-1.   A sagittal MRI scan showing a huge tumor of the teratoma type extending well above the level of the incisura.

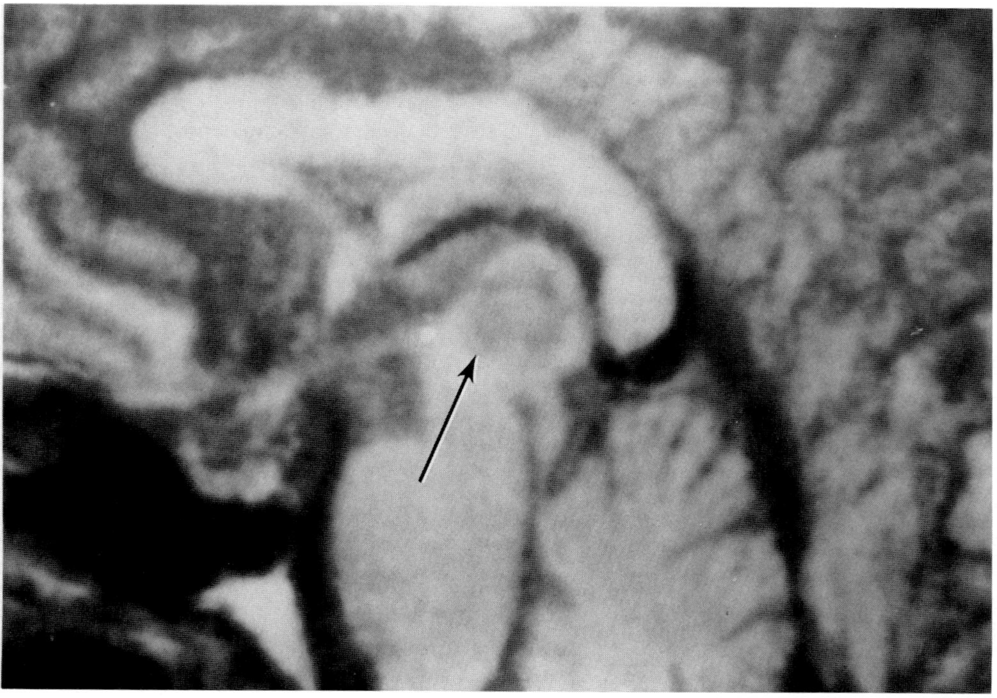

Fig. 35-2. A sagittal MRI scan showing a large, variegated tumor compressing the aqueductal region (arrow).

DIAGNOSTIC TESTS

Air- or positive-contrast ventriculography was once the backbone of diagnosis in cases of tumor of the pineal region. These techniques have been surpassed by the use of computed tomographic (CT) scanning, which is now the foundation for diagnosis. The scan must be done both with and without contrast. The scan not only precisely defines the limit of the tumor, its relationship to the third ventricle, midbrain, and quadrigeminal cisterns, but has also in some instances indicated cysts within the tumor and the characteristic findings of a benign teratoma with the presence of fat, calcium, and a variegated type of tissue. Radiologists also believe that the CT characteristics may lead to a closer understanding and diagnosis of these tumors.[20] The CT scan, of course, will also indicate the degree and presence of hydrocephalus, which is an important feature in determining the need for preoperative ventricular decompression.

Magnetic resonance imaging (MRI), as it gains increased use, is replacing the CT scan in the diagnosis of pineal region tumors. The ability to obtain sagittal, horizontal, and coronal views with precision in MRI scanning has greatly increased our knowledge of the anatomic relationships of these tumors, and in many instances, it may be possible to visualize displacement or occlusion of the aqueduct (Figure 35-2). Rarely is the tumor shown better by CT scan than it is by sophisticated MRI. The disadvantage, of course, it the long time required for imaging and the impracticality of using MRI on children.

Arteriography is now of little help in defining the location of pineal tumors. If, however, a vascular abnormality such as an AVM or vein of Galen anomaly is suspected as a result of prior CT or MRI studies, then arteriography is mandatory.

The use of the biologic markers, alpha fetoprotein, and human chorionic gonadotropin has been of value in gauging the effectiveness of therapy.[21] In our hands, it has not been infallible in predicting the histologic type of tumor, even when both CSF and serum samples are obtained.[22] We have no experience in the use of melatonin assay in these tumors.[23]

The selection of patients for surgery must be considered on the basis of clinical features and radiographic findings, especially CT and MRI. In most instances surgery for these tumors is advocated, since the exact nature of the pathologic process must await surgical verification. In certain instances, when the tumor is eccentric or grows laterally to the region of the trigone or superiorly through the corpus callosum, we have selected the

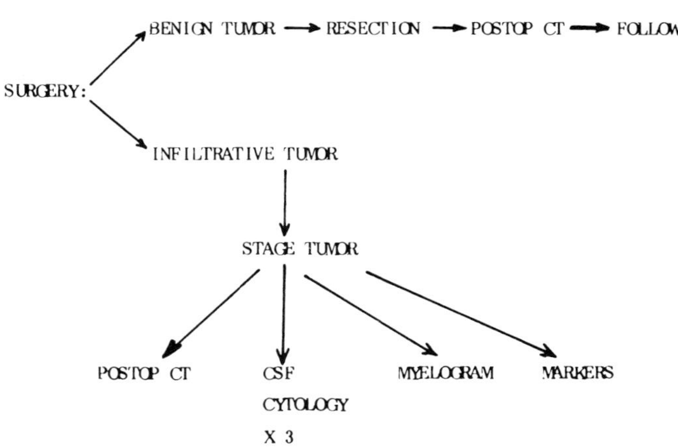

Fig. 35-3. Modes of treating

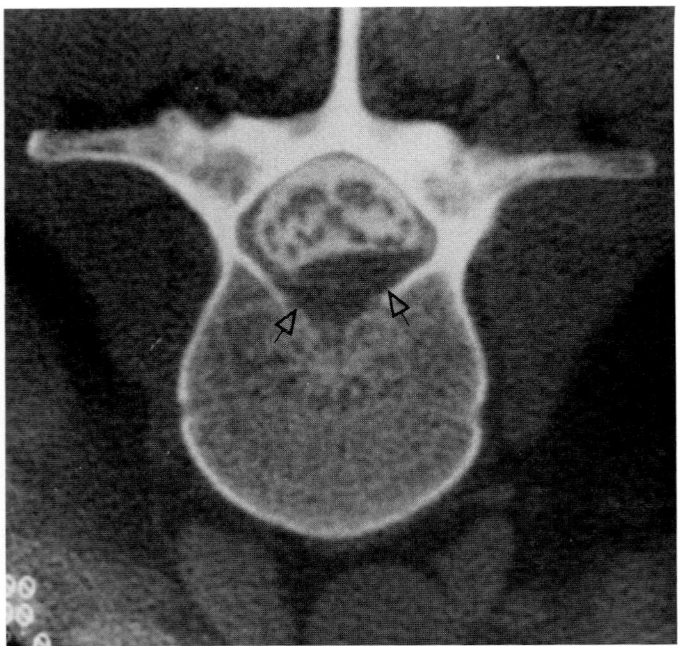

Fig. 35-4 A metrizamide-enhanced CT myelogram showing subarachnoid metastases (arrows) from a pineocytoma.

more effectively. With the supratentorial approach, however, one has difficulty in reaching the opposite side of the approach or into the posterior fossa. It may be necessary to widely cut the tentorium on the opposite side. Even so, a portion of the tumor in the posterior fossa opposite the exposure is difficult to reach and dissect. In some cases, it may be necessary to use a supratentorial and infratentorial approach to remove all of a large benign tumor. If there is evidence of seeding when the areas adjacent to the tumor are exposed, then conservative management with a shunt and radiotherapy might be considered.

COMPREHENSIVE THERAPY FOR PINEAL REGION TUMORS

Surgery, although representing a major aspect of pineal tumor therapy, is only one of the modes that is used (Figure 35-3). One must consider in malignant tumors the addition of chemotherapy and radiation therapy after the operative procedure.[2,9,21,24,25] If there is no direct evidence of seeding at the time of surgery, then the patient is subjected to three cytologic analyses of the spinal fluid to determine whether or not malignant cells are present and a lumbosacral, thoracic myelogram in the first week after surgery (Figure 35-4).

Pineal tumors fall into three main categories:

interhemispheric, posterior parietal, parafalx approach (Figure 35-1). This requires section of a portion of the thinned out corpus callosum by which these large tumors can be reached

1. Germ cell tumors, including malignant and benign varieties. In this group of tumors are germinomas, embryonal carcinomas, choriocarcinomas, yolk sac tumors, benign teratomas, and dermoid and epidermoid cysts.

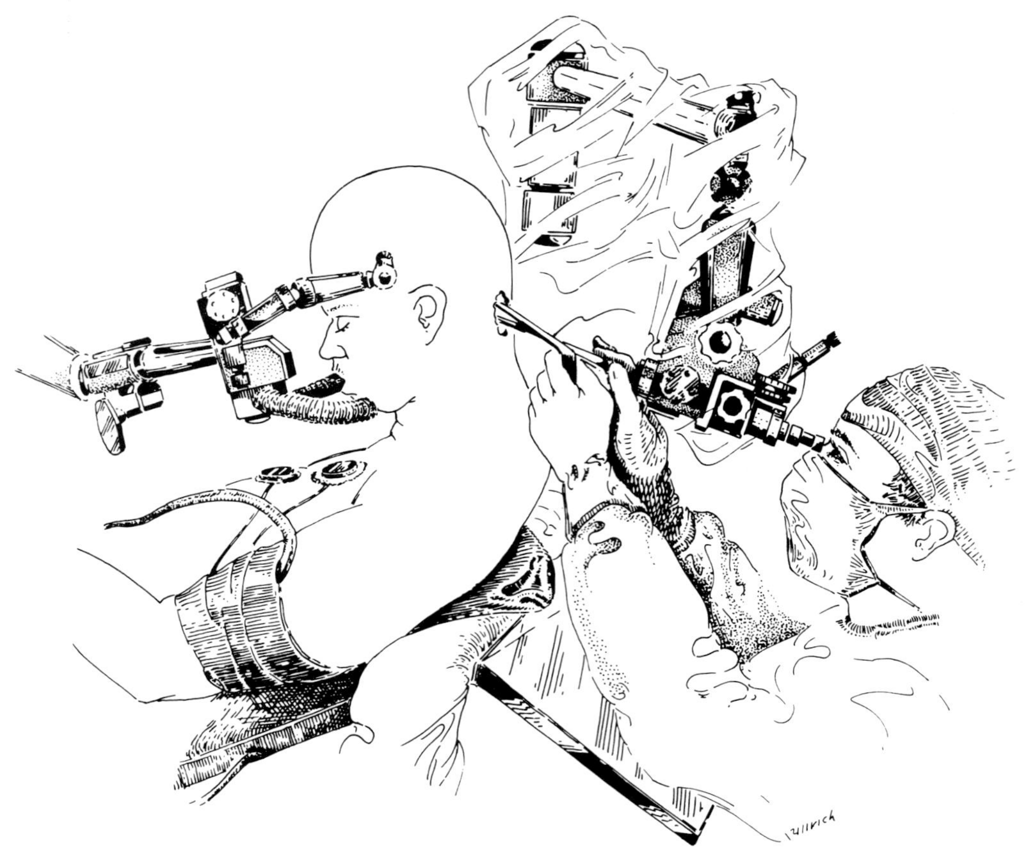

Fig. 35-5 Diagram of the position for craniotomy and the microscope.

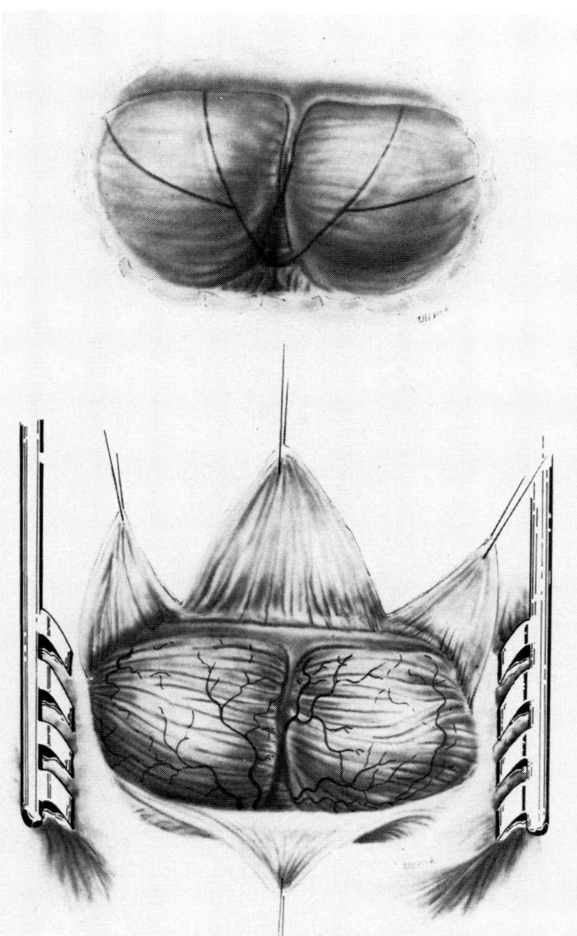

Fig. 35-6 Drawing showing the dural opening.

2. Pineal cell tumors, including benign and malignant varieties. Tumors in this group are pineocytomas (benign and malignant) and pineoblastomas, which are always malignant.
3. Tumors of supporting elements (both benign and malignant). In this group are astrocytomas of all grades, meningiomas, other glial tumors, and a miscellaneous group of tumors.

Reviewing all three categories, approximately 25 to 30 percent of the tumors are benign and encapsulated (Table 35-1). These are removed with low morbidity by radical surgery. The more malignant tumors are treated on the basis of histologic identification and the presence or absence of seeding. Radiotherapy is specific for the germinomas, astrocytomas (malignant variety), other glial tumors, the pineocytomas, and pineoblastomas. Chemotherapy of the Einhorn[25] method is reserved for germ cell tumors of high malignancy, such as the choriocarcinomas, yolk sac tumors, and embryonal carcinomas or malignant tumors that have previously received a full course of radiotherapy.

OPERATIVE TECHNIQUE—POSTERIOR FOSSA APPROACH

Most patients have raised intracranial pressure and hydrocephalus as a result of obstruction or compromise of the aqueduct. In such cases, the hydrocephalus must be relieved before a direct attack is made on the tumor. This can be carried out by an extracranial shunt performed a week or two before the primary operative procedure or by ventricular drainage at the time of the craniotomy. The disadvantages of performing ventricular drainage at the time of craniotomy in the face of a markedly enlarged ventricular system is the distinct probability of cortical collapse following release of the obstruction in the aqueductal region. Unless the patient is under 2 years of age and suffering from a severe degree of hydrocephalus, the sitting position is preferred.

The patient is positioned on the operating table in a "C" shaped configuration. This necessitates placing a pillow under the shoulders and positioning the patient low on the operating table. The head, neck, and shoulders are brought forward by a pin vise head-holder fixation. This is termed the "sittingouch" position. The patient's head must be strongly flexed so that the best exposure of the tentorial notch can be achieved with the greatest comfort to the surgeon. In addition to strong flexion of the neck, the patient is tilted somewhat forward once he or she is positioned on the operating table, so that the surgeon actually works over the back of the patient's shoulders to the posterior fossa (Figure 35-5). Care is taken to avoid or to recognize an air embolism, using a Doppler probe, central venous catheter, end-tidal PCO_2 evaluation, and modest positive-pressure ventilation during the opening or when large venous sinuses are exposed.

A self-retaining retractor of the Greenberg type is used. This is fixed via a bar to the operating table on the left side. The bars are then arranged in a U shaped configuration with the open end ventral. Two retractors are used, one in the superior direction to elevate by millimeters the tentorium and one in the inferior position to depress the cerebellum. A cottonoid tray is affixed to the self-retaining retractor system and an irrigator consisting of a bent 18-gauge needle is directed toward the surgical wound and held by one of the retractor arms.

A long midline incision is used, extending from C2 high up into the occipital region, so that the pericranium and muscle attachments can be elevated to either side without disrupting their continuity. This greatly facilitates closure, since all muscle attachment must be elevated. A wide craniectomy generally is performed, which includes the lateral sinuses and torcular in all instances. In recent cases we have been doing a limited craniectomy, which involves the superior region of the posterior fossa but does not extend to the foramen magnum. Adjuvants, such as mannitol or ventricular drainage, can be used to reduce volume and to facilitate retraction of the cerebellum. The opening of the dura is important, for it must be opened bilaterally to the region of the lateral sinus. These incisions should not be carried too far laterally, however, since in doing so one is unable to retract the flap of dura adequately in the region of the torcular (Figure 35-6). Once this is accomplished, the tentorium can be elevated with a self-retaining retractor. The weight of cottonoids and a copper retractor is sufficient to depress the cerebellum (Figure 35-7). When the patient is in the sitting position, gravity helps in this latter maneuver. The operating microscope with a 250- or 275–mm objective has been used in all instances. If a greater focal distance is used, the surgeon is too far from the incisura region and, even with an armrest, the focal length results in fatigue. Therefore, the microscope and surgeon must be relatively close to the field. An armrest is recommended.

After the dura is opened, all bridging veins over the dorsal surface of the cerebellum, including the hemispheres and

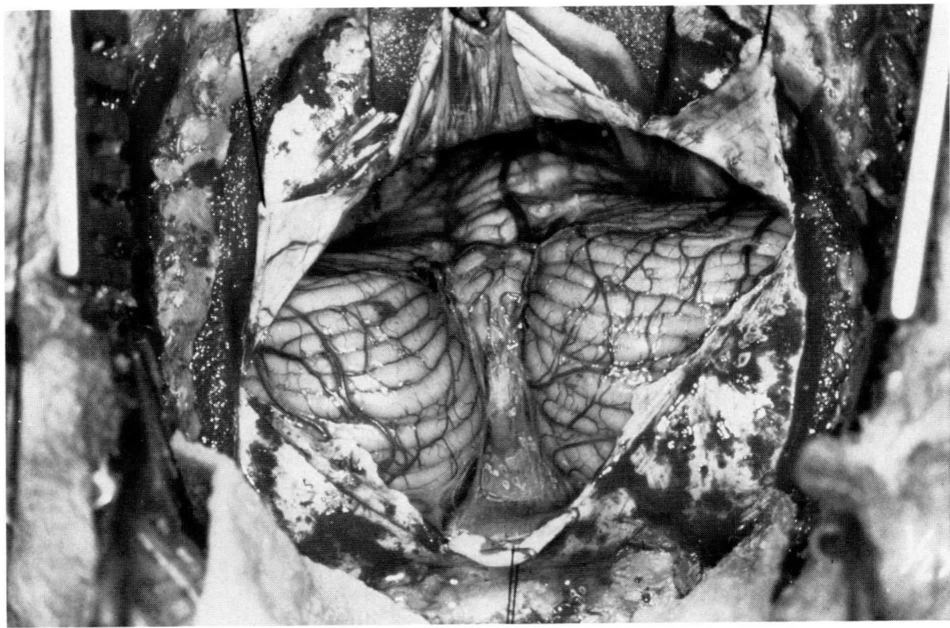

Fig. 35-7 Full dural opening and the cerebellum, which is sagging because of gravity after the bridging veins have been divided.

vermis, can be sacrificed in order to open the quadrigeminal region and the incisura. The arachnoid in this region is almost always thickened and opaque in the presence of tumors and must be opened by microdissection techniques to expose the surface of the tumor. The great vein of Galen and the internal cerebral veins generally are well above the tumor and are not encountered in these initial maneuvers.[5] Laterally, the medial aspect of the temporal lobe and the veins of Rosenthal can be seen as they course upward toward the confluence of veins in this region. The thickened arachnoid over most of these tumors can obscure the underlying anatomy. The arachnoid should be opened by sharp dissection and the opening kept close to the anterior surface of the vermis and cerebellar hemisphere so as not to injure the deep venous system, remembering that the initial trajectory is toward the vein of Galen. Upon opening either lateral side, the precentral cerebellar vein is cauterized and divided. The anterior portion of the cerebellum is then retracted by the inferior self-retaining retractor, exposing a

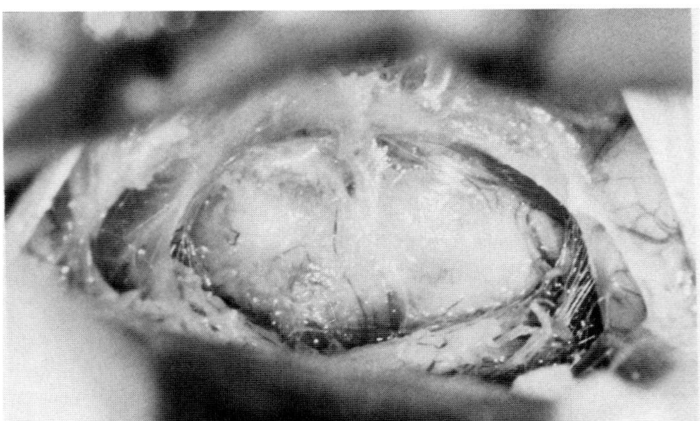

Fig. 35-8 Operative view showing exposure of the posterior surface of a large meningioma, without dural attachment, in the pineal region.

large posterior surface of the tumor (Figure 35-8). This tumor surface may be invested by small or large branches of the choroidal arteries, which nourish the tumor. The tumor capsule is then cauterized and opened by sharp dissection. The tumor, depending on its consistency, is removed with tumor forceps, small curettes, suction, and cautery. Since many of these tumors extend well into the third ventricle, some to the region of the foramen of Monro (Figure 35-9), long instruments are required to reach the posterior third ventricular region and beyond. With tumors of firm consistency, we have been using the long curved tip of the Cavitron for debulking. The instrument is large and it is difficult to insert it into the operative field, especially if an objective lens less than 275 mm is used on the microscope.

In general terms, the trajectory of the operation is toward the velum interpositum (Figure 35-10). This must be considered when attempts are made to remove portions of the tumor in the inferior position of the third ventricle or directly over the quadrigeminal plate in relationship to the anterior lobe of the cerebellum. This is the most difficult aspect to be dealt with; small dental mirrors and angled instruments may be required to remove tumor in this region. The lateral extent of the tumor can be pursued through this particular exposure.

Even with nonresectable tumors, benefit may be accrued through internal decompression of or an opening through the tumor adequate to expose the posterior third ventricle. This will allow placement of an internal shunt tube from directly within the third ventricle, through the interior of the tumor, and over the cerebellar hemisphere to the region of the cisterna magna. Even in instances in which this tubing occludes, a passageway has been established for cerebrospinal fluid. If the tumor cannot be removed completely or an internal shunt placed, ventricular drainage with subsequent conversion to a shunt may be necessary in the postoperative period.

With adequate decompression of the tumor, especially unblocking of the obstructed ventricular system, the dura can be closed in a loose fashion in order to support the cerebellum.

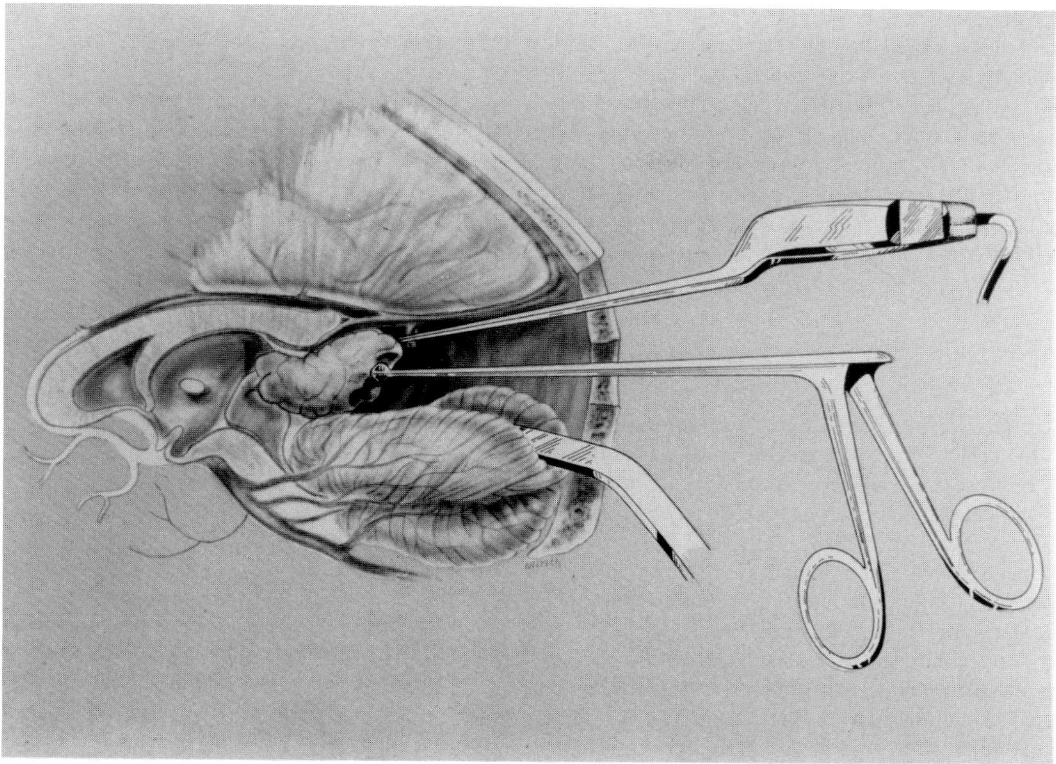

Fig. 35-9 Drawing in the sagittal view showing the position of the pineal tumor and the extra long instruments used in the posterior fossa approach.

This would appear to make the postoperative course smoother and may limit the degree of postoperative aseptic meningitis. A 12-hour drain is used in the layers of muscle and fascia.

When the tumor is large and one can anticipate a total removal, such as in the case of a benign teratoma that extends dorsally as well as to the trigonal region, a different approach must be used. The working area through the posterior fossa exposure is too limited to allow removal of such tumors. In these instances, we switch to a supratentorial approach, generally between the falx and the medial posterior parietal lobule. This brings us to the region of the incisura and the posterior corpus callosum. The latter structure must be opened for a small distance. The internal cerebral veins are generally compressed and displaced laterally in such large tumors and have not been a problem in removal of the tumor from this route. The difficulties encountered are visualizing the opposite side and the portion that extends into the posterior fossa, especially the opposite side. On the same side, the tentorium can be cut from the incisura posteriorly to gain improved exposure of the posterior fossa component.

COMPLICATIONS

Complications related to the posterior fossa approach are in general those related to operations on hydrocephalic patients in the sitting position. These include collapse of the ventricular system and entry of air into the ventricular system and into the subdural space. The general complications of air embolism have been previously commented upon. A unique complication of this position has been the occurrence of temporary sciatic nerve palsy in two patients out of a large series of operations done with the patient in the sitting position. The ease with which the tumors can be exposed through the posterior fossa demands a sitting position and therefore these complications must be watched for, accepted, and treated as they occur. Cortical collapse or entry of air into the ventricular or subdural space generally improves with time and nothing special has to be done to correct this. Unrelieved hydrocephalus should be corrected by an appropriate shunting procedure.

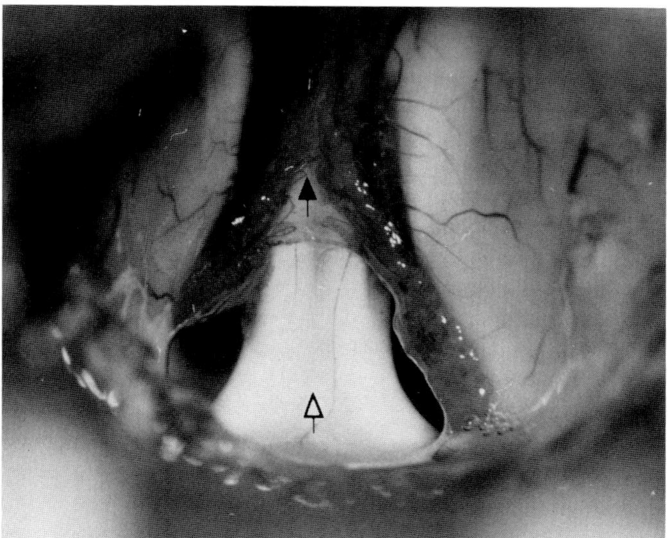

Fig. 35-10 View of the interior of the third ventricle showing the columns of the fornix (open arrow) and relachoroidea (closed arrow) after removal of a pineal region tumor.

Specific complications related to tumor removal are generally those related to injury of the quadrigeminal region. This results in deranged eye movements, which in almost all cases is a temporary condition. There is often an increase in paralysis of upward gaze, convergence and pupillary accommodative responses. This happens most frequently with those tumors that are benign and encapsulated and must be dissected off the delicate tectal region, with interruption of the blood supply that is common to both the tumor and the tectum.

SUMMARY

To date, 100 pineal region tumors have been operated on. Experience with this series of cases has led to a two-part plan applicable to all pineal region tumors (Figure 35–3). First and most essential is control of hydrocephalus; second is operation on the tumor. In the case of benign tumors, the tumor is removed and no further treatment is necessary. In the case of malignant tumors, it is possible to identify the exact nature of the tumor. In those tumors that are mixed, even though the malignant component is small, this essential part of the diagnosis will be realized. This is necessary because contemporary treatment modalities, which include various forms of radiation and chemotherapy, demand a firm histologic diagnosis. The variability within tumors often will preclude a stereotactic biopsy where there is a high chance of sampling error. Furthermore, many oncologists believe that debulking of a malignant tumor may be useful in itself. There is obviously less tumor to treat and the result of effective additional therapy should be improved. For example, in two tumors with large cysts, germinoma was a surprise finding. These tumors are not generally cystic and, accordingly, the preoperative diagnosis in these cases was cystic astrocytoma. The difference in longevity of these two types of tumors is obvious and bears upon subsequent therapy. Even in the germinoma-type tumor radiation appears to be more effective after a thorough debulking of the tumor.

There have been three operative deaths for a mortality of 3 percent. This is a relatively good figure, indicating the safety of an operation that was once associated with a 50 to 75 percent mortality. The three deaths were the result of postoperative hemorrhage; two in cases of malignant pineocytomas in which death occurred within 24 hours and one in a case of a glioblastoma in which hemorrhage was delayed by 1 week postoperatively. It should be kept in mind that all three deaths were related to malignant tumors;—tumors known to respond erratically to radiation therapy.

In almost all cases where radical resection of the tumor was carried out, especially benign tumors, disturbances in extraocular movements ensued and gradually improved over months postoperatively. Eventually, there was excellent return of functional vision in all of these individuals. A multitude of problems associated with cortical collapse and entry of air into the ventricular or subdural spaces has been short lived. In 3 percent of the patients, there has been a permanent morbidity taking the form of an akinetic state. These have been in cases of infiltrating tumors, and I suspect that they are related to involvement of the periaqueductal region by the tumor, which was manipulated at the time of surgery. These cases have not responded well to radiation therapy.

Exposure of all tumors in the pineal region is therefore advocated. Confirmation of the histology; removal if feasible, and, in malignant tumors, an internal decompression or debulking of the tumor should be accomplished. In those cases in which hydrocephalus has not been relieved, a preoperative or postoperative shunt is necessary. In a few cases an internal shunt has been placed from the third ventricle through the decompressed tumor into the cisterna magna. This functions satisfactorily if the incisura is not blocked and provided that there is no infection in the CSF, which would necessitate removal of this shunt through reoperation.

REFERENCES

1. DeGirolami U, Schmidek H: Clinicopathological study of 53 tumors of the pineal region. J Neurosurg 39:455, 1973
2. Neuwelt EA: The challenge of pineal region tumors, in Neuwelt EA (ed): The Diagnosis and Treatment of Pineal Region Tumors. Baltimore, Williams & Wilkins, 1984, pp 130
3. Sano K: Pinealoma in children. Childs Brain 2:67, 1976
4. Schmidek HH: Pineal Tumors. New York, Masson, 1977
5. Quest DO, Kleriga E: Microsurgical anatomy of the pineal region. Neurosurgery 6:385, 1979
6. Cushing H: Intracranial Tumors: Notes Upon a Series of Two-Thousand Verified Cases with Surgical Mortality Pertaining Thereto. Springfield, Ill, Charles C Thomas, 1932
7. Camins MB, Schlesinger EB: Treatment of tumors of the posterior part of the third ventricle and the pineal region: A long-term follow-up. Acta Neurochir 40:131, 1978
8. Cummins FM, Taveras J M, Schlesinger EB: Treatment of gliomas of the third ventricle and pinealomas: With special reference to the value of radiotherapy. Neurology 10:1031, 1960
9. Horrax G, Daniels JT: The conservative treatment of pineal tumors. Surg Clin North Am 22:649, 1942
10. Dandy WE: Operative experience in cases of pineal tumors. Arch Surg 33:19, 1936
11. Suzuki J, Iwabuchi T: Surgical removal of pineal tumors (pinealomas and teratomas): Experience in a series of 19 cases. J Neurosurg 23:565, 1965
12. Page LK: The infratentorial supracerebellar exposure of tumors in the pineal area. Neurosurgery 1:36, 1977
13. Reid WS, Clark K: Comparison of the infratentorial and transtentorial approaches to the pineal region. Neurosurgery 3:1, 1978
14. Sano K: Pineal region tumors: Problems in pathology and treatment. Clin Neurosurg 30:59, 1982
15. Stein BM: The infratentorial supracerebellar approach to pineal lesions. J Neurosurg 35:197, 1971
16. Stein BM: Surgical treatment of pineal tumors, in Carmel PFW (ed): Clinical Neurosurgery. Baltimore, Williams & Wilkins, 1979, pp 490–510
17. VanWagenen WP: A surgical approach for the removal of certain pineal tumors: Report of a case. Surg Gynecol Obstet 53:216, 1931
18. Poppen JL: The right occipital approach to a pinealoma. J Neurosurg 25:706, 1966
19. Krause F: Operative Freilegung der Vierhugel, nebst Beobachtungen uber Hirndruck und Dekompression. Zentralb Chir 53:2812, 1926
20. Ganti SR, Hilal SK, Stein BM, et al: CT of pineal region tumors. AJNR 7:97, 1986
21. Allen JC, Nisselbaum J, Epstein F, et al: Alphafetoprotein and human chorionic gonadotropin determination in cerebrospinal fluid, An aid to the diagnosis and management of intracranial germ-cell tumors. J Neurosurg 51:368, 1979

22. Fetell MR, Stein BM: Therapy of pineal region tumors. Neurology 34 (Suppl 1):184, 1984

23. Neuwelt EA, Glasberg M, Frenkel E, et al: Malignant pineal region tumors. A clinico-pathological study. J Neurosurg 51:597, 1979

24. Abav EO, Laws ER, Grado GL, et al: Pineal tumors in children and adolescents. Treatment by CSF shunting and radiotherapy. J Neurosurg 55:889, 1981

25. Einhorn LH, Donohue J: Cis-diamine dichloroplatinum, Vinblastine, and bleomycin combination chemotherapy in disseminated testicular cancer. Ann Intern Med 87:293, 1977

CHAPTER 36
The Occipital Transtentorial Approach to the Pineal Region

Kemp Clark

NEUROLOGICAL SURGEONS recently have recognized the importance of obtaining histologic confirmation of the nature of masses lying in the pineal region.[1] Several series have reported that as many as 40 percent of these lesions are benign and surgically resectable.[2-4] Further emphasis on the direct surgical treatment of these tumors has been generated by evidence that radiation of the brain, particularly in young children, may produce long-term deleterious effects.

Clearly, the major advance that made surgery possible for tumors of the pineal region was the development of the operating microscope, which provided an improved view of the area.[5,6] Development of appropriate tools for dissection of the deep cerebral plexus in this region is the other significant technical advance.

Attempts to operate on the pineal region were made early in the development of neurosurgery. The original approaches were either transcallosal, as proposed by Dandy,[7] or along the falx medial to the occipital lobe. This was introduced by Poppen[6] and expanded by Jamieson.[1] It was Jamieson who began the renaissance of pineal surgery with his report in 1971.

Exposure of this region by a parietal flap and transection of the splenium of the corpus callosum were advocated by Dandy.[7] The difficulty with this approach is that it is extremely deep. The surgeon approaches the pineal region with the internal cerebral vein, the vein of Galen, and the vein of Rosenthal lowermost in the surgical field. Injury to any of these vessels can occur before the surgeon can successfully deal with the neoplasm. It is unclear from the literature what effect ligating components of the deep venous plexus would have.[8]

There are three possible positions on the operating table for the patient undergoing this particular surgical approach. The first is the prone position, which is the one we prefer in the treatment of vein of Galen aneurysms; because of the small size of an infant, this makes it somewhat easier to accomplish than other positions. However, the surgeon is standing at the head of the patient, which inverts the usual perspective of the anatomy. The second useful position is the semi-sitting one. If this is used, a central venous catheter should be inserted in the right atrium and a Doppler monitor should be placed over the precordium in order to reduce the possibility of air embolus or to ensure its early detection. The patient is positioned in the semi-sitting position with the neck and knees flexed and at the same level. The likelihood of air embolization is markedly reduced. This position allows for a comfortable arrangement for the surgeon. The operative field is directly in front of and

slightly below the surgeon at all stages. This allows the surgeon to work in a comfortable, relaxed position. The final position is the park-bench position. With this position, we have found that placing the patient on his or her right side and turning a right occipital bone flap enables gravity to let the occipital pole fall away from the falx. This eliminates the necessity of a retractor on the occipital pole. This has, in turn, eliminated any danger to the visual cortex, which was one of the concerns regarding this approach (Figure 36-1).

The approach preferred on the neurosurgical service at the University of Texas Health Science Center at Dallas is a supratentorial, transtentorial approach. The rationale for this approach over others was set forth in the paper by Reid and Clark in 1978.[3] A right occipital craniotomy extends slightly across the midline and then turns. The bone flap should extend to the transverse sinus. This will ensure that the exposure is low enough and right to the midline. It may be safer to do the medial and inferior part of the craniotomy with a rongeur to reduce the chance of damage to the posterior superior sagittal and transverse dural sinuses (Figure 36-2).

The bone flap should be generous in size, but not so large as to allow the occipital lobe to herniate. If this happens, the lobe may infarct as the result of interference with the venous drainage to the calcarine cortex, and a visual field cut will result (Figure 36-3).

Once the bone flap has been turned, the dura is opened along the superior sagittal sinus and the transverse sinus, producing a triangularly shaped flap that is reflected laterally. Enough margin should be left for a dural closure. The small margin is turned out of the operative field with retention sutures. The striking thing about this approach is that no bridging veins enter the superior sagittal sinus from the occipital lobe. It is this fact that makes the approach possible. Drainage of the occipital lobe is by way of the great cerebral vein, which is quite lateral. It occasionally can be seen at the lateral inferior edge of the craniotomy. This vein must not be coagulated or ligated; infarction of the occipital lobe will result (Figure 36-4A).

A self-retaining retractor should be used to elevate the occipital lobe in an upward and outward direction. The tentorium then is incised along the straight sinus, exposing the superior part of the cerebellar hemisphere. The opened tentorium is retracted with sutures. At this point, the microscope should be brought into the operating field.

What is done at this point depends on the patient's

OPERATIVE NEUROSURGICAL TECHNIQUES
ISBN 0-8089-1862-1

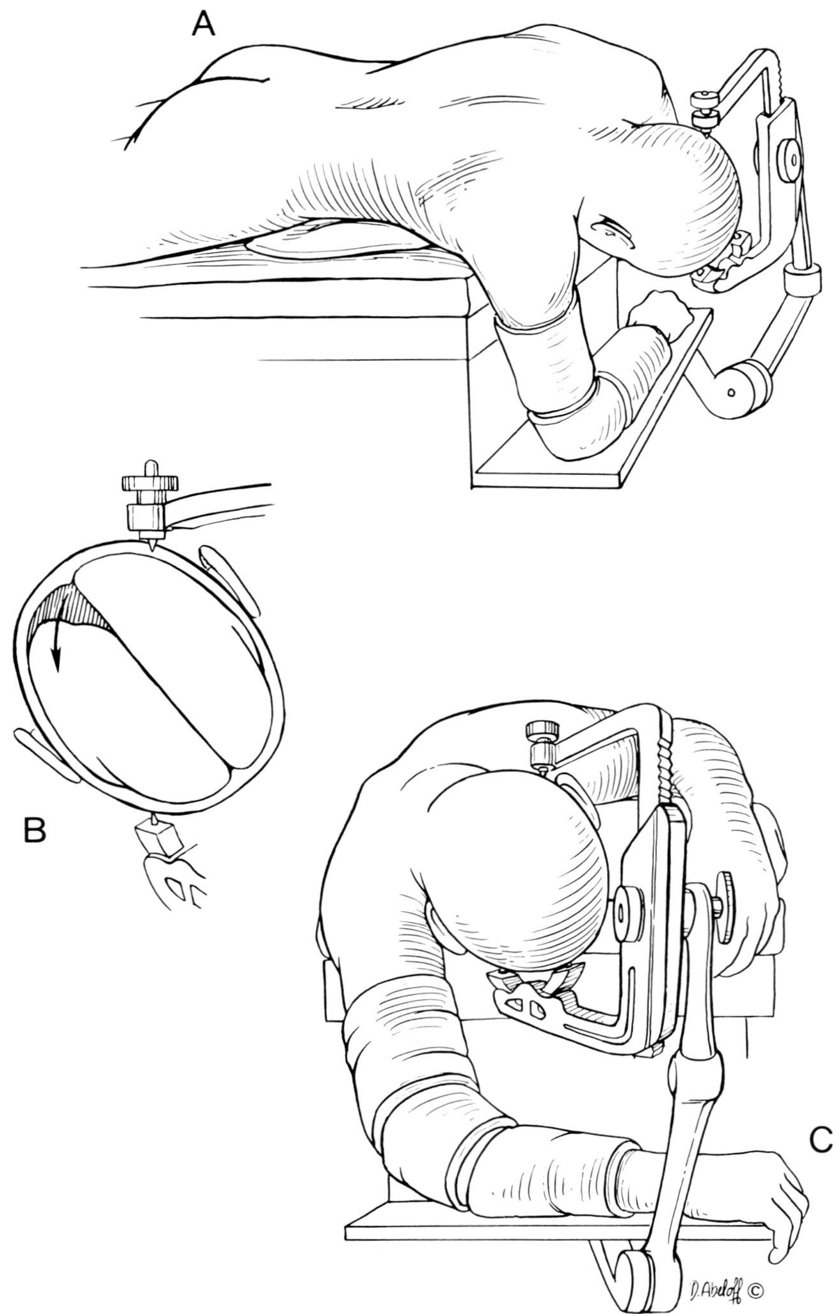

Fig. 36-1. The semiprone position. (From Clark WK: Occipital transtentorial approach, in Puzzo A (ed): Surgery of the Third Ventricle. Baltimore, Williams & Wilkins, 1987, p. 593. With permission.)

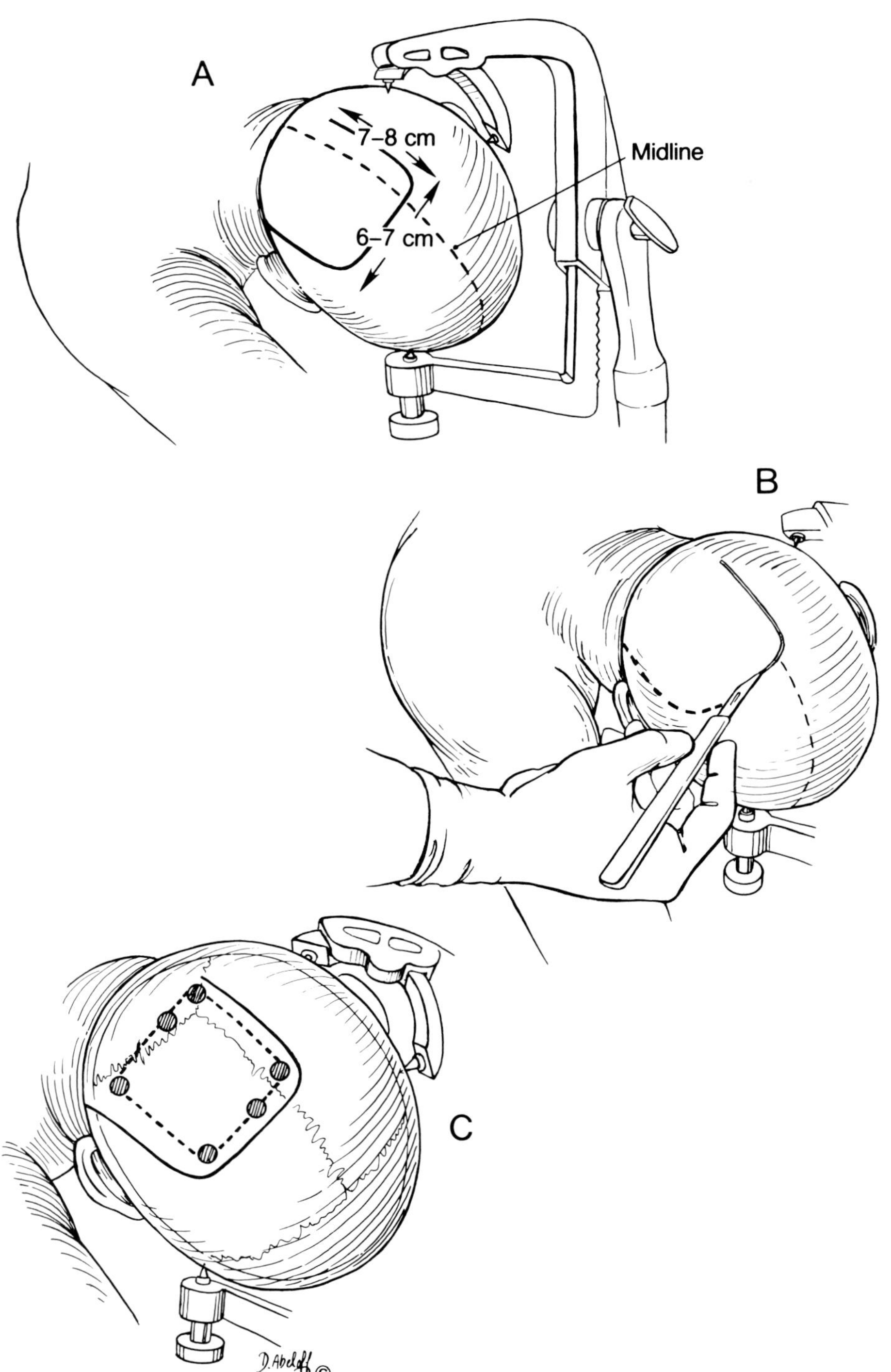

Fig. 36-2. The skin incision. (From Clark WK: Occipital transtentorial approach, in Puzzo A (ed): Surgery of the Third Ventricle. Baltimore, Williams & Wilkins, 1987, p. 595. With permission.)

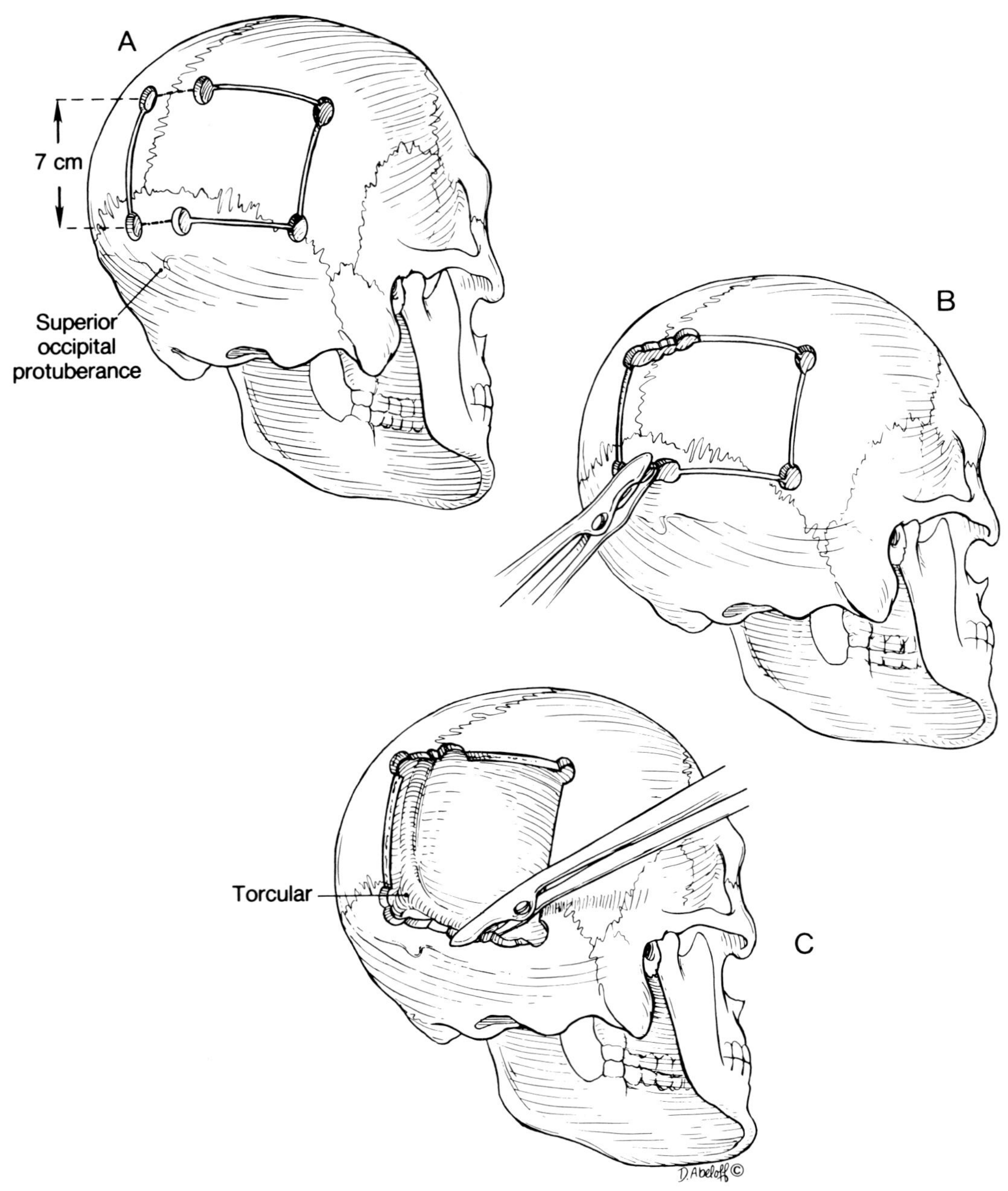

Fig. 36-3. The bone flap showing removal of bone over the sagittal and transverse sinuses. (From Clark WK: Occipital transtentorial approach, in Puzzo A (ed): Surgery of the Third Ventricle. Baltimore, Williams & Wilkins, 1987, p. 596. With permission.)

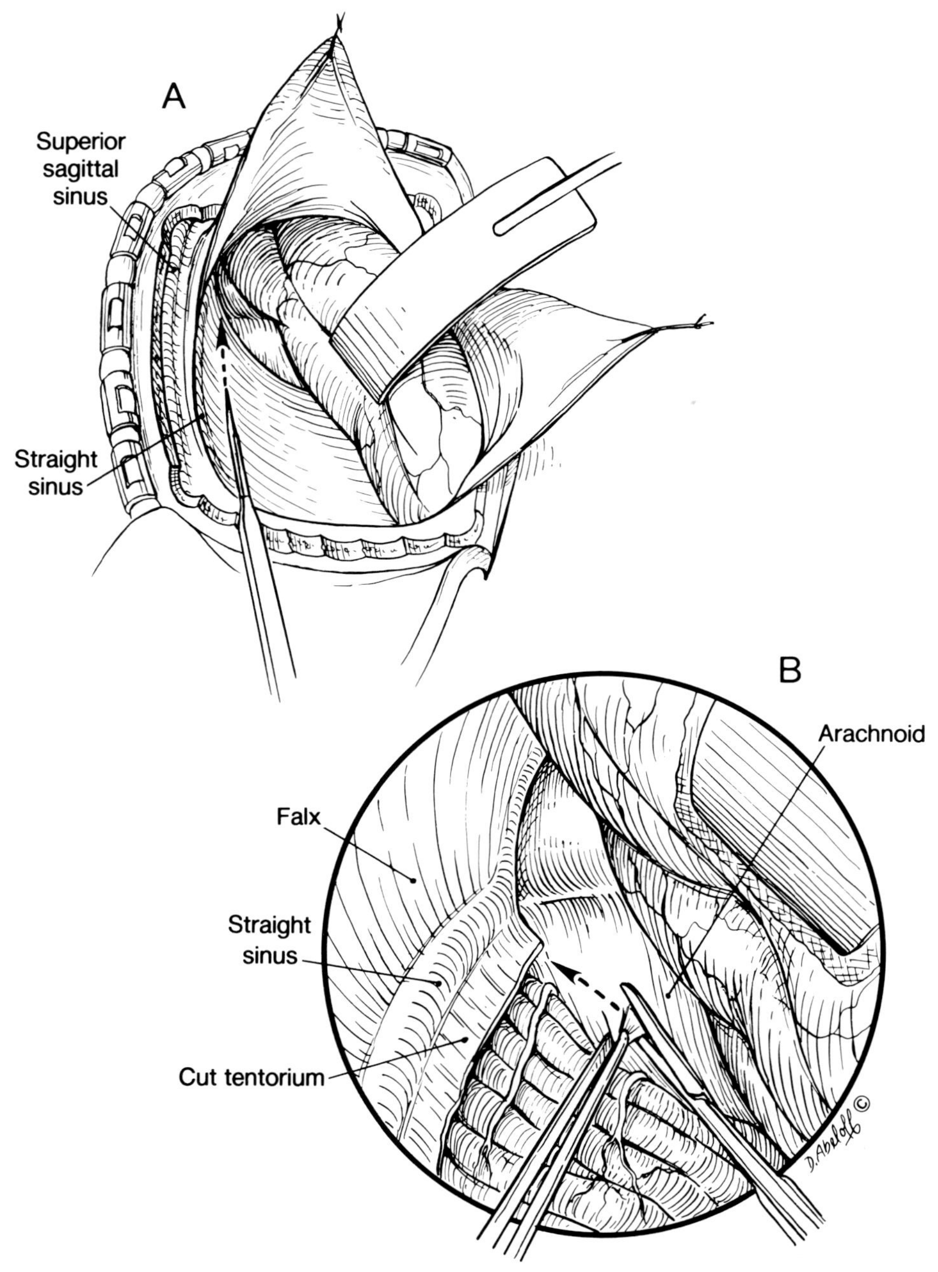

Fig. 36-4. (A) Opening of the tentorium. (B) Opening of the arachnoid of the quadrigeminal cistern. (From Clark WK: Occipital transtentorial approach, in Puzzo A (ed): Surgery of the Third Ventricle. Baltimore, Williams & Wilkins, 1987, p. 599. With permission.)

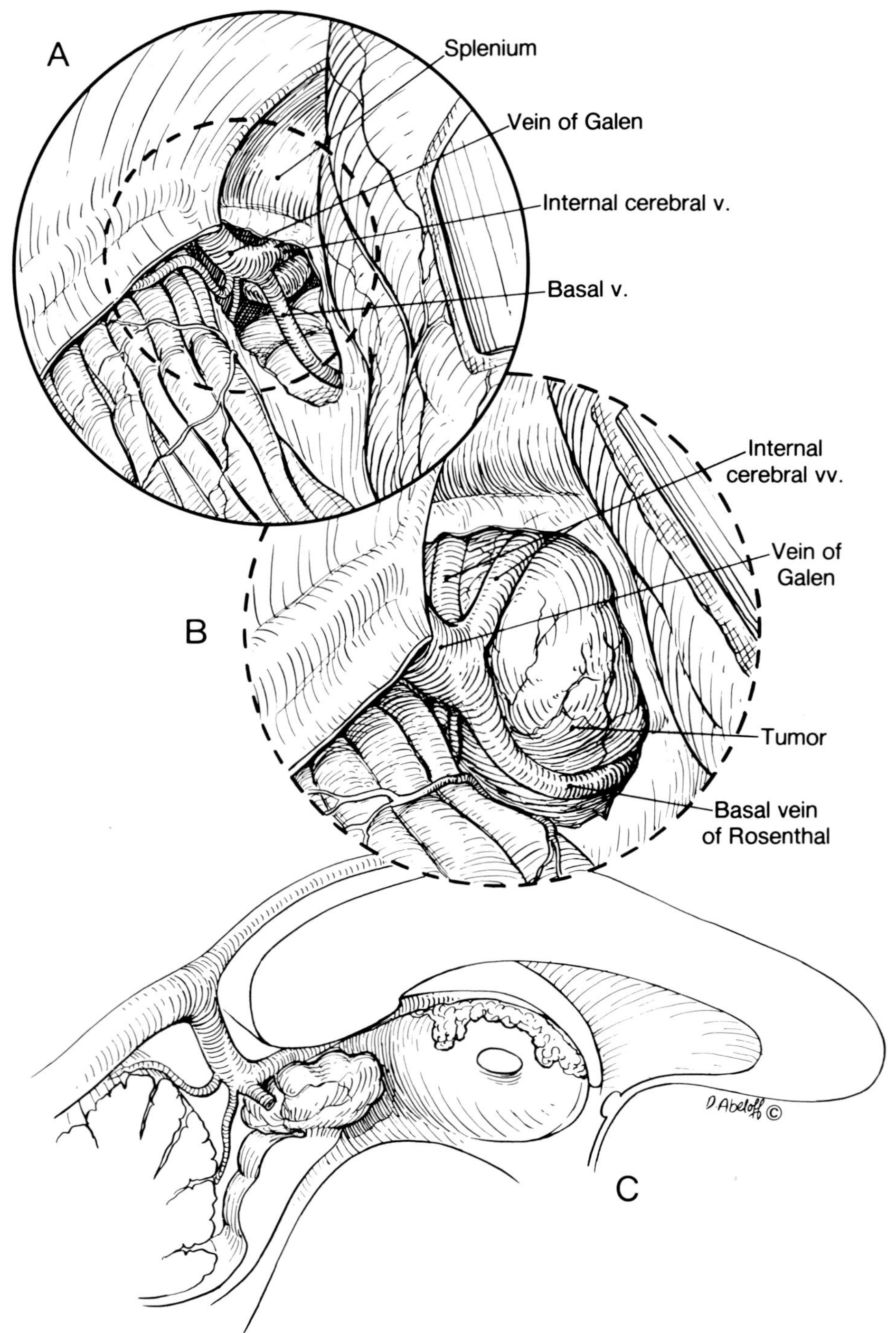

Fig. 36-5. The usual relation of the deep venous structures to a pineal tumor. (From Clark WK: Occipital transtentorial approach, in Puzzo A (ed): Surgery of the Third Ventricle. Baltimore, Williams & Wilkins, 1987, p. 602. With permission.)

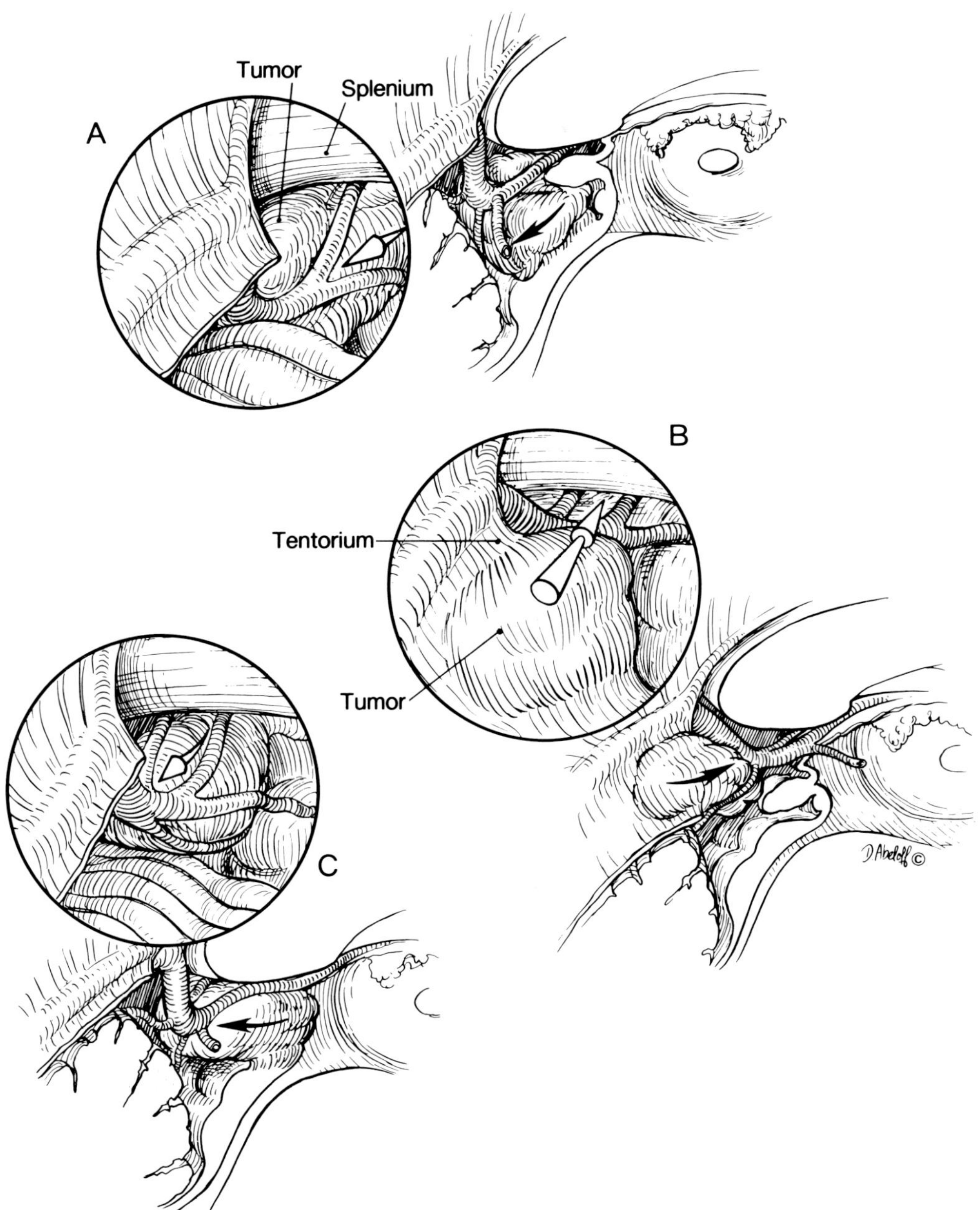

Fig. 36-6. The location of the deep venous structures when the tumor arises from the tectum (A), tentorium (B), or pineal structure (C). (From Clark WK: Occipital transtentorial approach, in Puzzo A (ed): Surgery of the Third Ventricle. Baltimore, Williams & Wilkins, p. 603. With permission.)

pathologic entity. An arteriogram, which should have been done as part of the preoperative work-up, will reveal the relationship of the internal cerebral veins, the great vein of Galen, the basilar veins of Rosenthal, and the precentral vein to the mass. If a meningioma is arising at the junction of the tentorium and the falx, for instance, these vessels will be displaced anteriorly and will lie on the anterior surface of the tumor. If there is a glioma arising from the quadrigeminal plate, these vessels will be displaced superiorly and posteriorly and will lie draped over the mass. A similar arrangement will be found if the tumor arises from the pineal gland itself. If the tumor arises from the splenium of the corpus callosum, the veins usually are displaced inferiorly.

The arachnoid overlying the deep cerebral vein always is opaque and very tough. It must be divided sharply with a knife and scissors. No attempt should be made to tear it. To do so invariably will damage one of the major venous structures (Figure 36-4B).

Once the arachnoid is dissected off the veins, the relationship of the tumor can be identified. If the tumor is a glioma, a biopsy specimen should be obtained and a modest decompression done. If it is a benign pineal tumor, total extirpation is the goal. If the tumor proves to be of embryonal origin, such as a teratoma or dermoid, piecemeal or en bloc resection is carried out. The surgeon should attempt complete tumor removal. If the tumor is a germinoma, as much tumor as possible is carried out, one goal of surgery being to visualize the interior of the third ventricle thereby ensuring that there is no block of the CSF pathways at this level (Figures 36-5 and 36-6).

Through this approach, one can reach the fourth ventricle by going through the superior vermis. One can adequately deal with tumors of the superior part of the cerebellar vermis. Tumors lying in the posterior part of the third ventricle also can be reached. In fact, it is possible to reach as far forward as the foramen of Monro in the third ventricle by opening the suprapineal recess.

Following hemostasis, the retractors are removed from the wound, and the wound is closed in layers in an appropriate manner.

Our experience indicates that the occipital transtentorial approach is the preferred approach to the pineal region. Complications have been few in the postoperative period. One patient suffering from metastatic adenocarcinoma died. Two patients had homonymous hemianopsia, and one pediatric patient suffered a small infarct in the right posterior thalamus. Our total experience now includes 17 patients on whom we have used this approach. From this experience, we can state our satisfaction with it.

REFERENCES

1. Jamieson KG: Excision of pineal tumors. J Neurosurg 35:550, 1971
2. Araki C, Matsuroto S: Statistical re-evaluation of pinealoma and related tumor in Japan. J Neurosurg 30:146, 1969
3. Reid WS, Clark WK: Comparison of the infratentorial and transtentorial approaches to the pineal region. Neurosurgery 3:1, 1978
4. Stein BM: The infratentorial supracerebellar approach to pineal lesions. J Neurosurg 35:197, 1971
5. Lazar ML, Clark K: Direct surgical management of masses in the region of the vein of Galen. Surg Neurol 2:17, 1974
6. Poppen JL: The right occipital approach to a pinealoma. J Neurosurg 25:706, 1966
7. Dandy NE: Operative experience in cases of pineal tumor. Arch Surg 33:19, 1936
8. Suzuki J, Iwabuchi T: Surgical removal of pineal tumors. J Neurosurg 23:565, 1965

CHAPTER 37

Brain Biopsy: Indications, Methods, and Complications

Anthony Salerni   Steven Wald
Henry H. Schmidek

BIOPSY OF THE HUMAN BRAIN is performed for a variety of neurologic conditions. In general, the techniques used for this procedure are safe and technically straightforward. A few of these techniques as well as the risks, benefits, and complications of cerebral biopsy are discussed in this chapter. Since brain biopsy in some illnesses is of no direct benefit to the patient, moral and ethical considerations are also examined.

INDICATIONS

The conditions that require brain biopsy for definitive diagnosis, that is, those that cannot be diagnosed by histologic and biochemical examination of tissue or by enzymatic assays of body fluids, white blood cells, and cultured skin fibroblasts, are few (Table 37-1). However, virtually all neurologic diseases can be accurately identified by the examination of cerebral tissue. The processes requiring brain biopsy form a pathologic spectrum, from entities that require prompt and specific therapy to disorders with no known effective treatment. Diseases for which there are specific treatments provide the clearest indications for brain biopsy. Patients in this group often have an acute, rapidly progressive neurologic illness. Herpes simplex encephalitis and acquired immune deficiency syndrome (AIDS) are two clinical situations in which the benefit of identifying a potentially treatable illness outweighs the risks of biopsy.[1–11] In these patients, brain biopsy is a highly sensitive and reliable diagnostic technique. Positive results have been reported in 60 to 100 percent of cases.[3,5,6,8–10] In addition, previously unsuspected diseases for which there are specific therapies have been discovered in 60 to 70 percent of such patients.[3,5,10]

The other extreme of illnesses considered for brain biopsy are the chronic, progressive disorders for which there is no known specific therapy. Although the information obtained by biopsy for diseases in this category may be useful for prognostic purposes, genetic counseling, or research purposes, it is rarely of any direct benefit to the patient.[12,13] The establishment of indications for biopsy in this group therefore represents an ethical as well as a surgical problem.

Between these two extremes are those conditions for which there is either innocuous or questionably effective treatment. In the former category there is frequently a propensity to treat the patient without obtaining a definitive diagnosis. This practice can allow unsuspected disease processes to progress unchecked.

LEGAL, MORAL, AND ETHICAL CONSIDERATIONS

In contrast to brain biopsy performed in patients with acute diseases, biopsies for those patients with chronic neurologic illnesses have only a 35 to 45 percent chance of yielding a diagnosis in adults and a 13 percent chance in children[12,14–18] (Table 37-2). Moreover, if a diagnosis is obtained, the chance that it will lead to effective therapy is remote. Nevertheless, the diagnosis may be useful. In the diagnosis of individuals with dementia, a normal biopsy suggests an indolent process and a longer life span, which is information that may be important to the family in making plans for the patient's care.[18–20]

Informed consent requires a rational mind capable of understanding the issues surrounding brain biopsy and possessing the judgment necessary to give consent for an operation. Most conditions for which brain biopsy is considered result in a loss of insight, intellect, and judgment, so that the permission for this procedure must be obtained from others responsible for the patient's care. Cerebral biopsy for chronic neurologic disease is appropriate when the following criteria have been satisfied[19]:

1. There is a chronic progressive cerebral disorder of diffuse character accompanied by dementia.
2. All other possible diagnostic methods have been tried and have failed to provide a diagnosis.
3. Consulting specialists are in agreement regarding the indications.
4. The general condition of the patient permits performance of the procedure.
5. Permission from parents or relatives can be obtained after the aim of the procedure has been fully explained.

OPERATIVE TECHNIQUES

The operative approaches for obtaining cerebral tissue for analysis include open craniectomy, stereotactic CT-guided procedures, and biopsy with intraoperative ultrasound. The surgery can be performed under local or general anesthesia.

Since certain disorders show predilections for different areas of the brain, a knowledge of the topography of pathologic lesions is helpful in selecting the area of brain for biopsy (Table

OPERATIVE NEUROSURGICAL TECHNIQUES
ISBN 0-8089-1862-1

Table 37-1. Diagnoses that can only be established by brain biopsy

Patient Group	Disease
Children	Alexander's disease
	Canavan's spongy degeneration
	Progressive myoclonic epilepsy*
Adults†	Alzheimer's disease
	Jakob-Creutzfeldt disease
	Pick's disease
	Kuf's disease

*Progressive myoclonic epilepsy (Lafora body type) in principle can be diagnosed from skeletal muscle biopsy.

†Alper's disease and sudanophilic leukodystrophy (Pelizaeuspathologically ill-defined.

37-3). This information is supplemented by electrophysiologic and neuroradiologic studies.[11]

Prophylactic antibiotic coverage starting preoperatively is not recommended in cases with a potentially infectious cause, since this will reduce the chances of in vitro growth of the organism. If desired, antibiotics can be administered during surgery, immediately after the specimen is obtained. Anticonvulsants are routinely administered preoperatively and postoperatively in selected cases.

After burr-hole, trephine, or standard craniotomy, the dura is opened in a cruciate fashion to provide the greatest exposure of the underlying cortical surface. A meningeal biopsy is usually not required, although its value in certain instances must be kept in mind. Cauterization is avoided on the cortical surface until after the specimen has been removed. The amount of tissue necessary is based on the sum of the tissue required for the individual studies to be performed. As a rule a 1.0 to 1.5 cc tissue sample is needed.[12,17,21–23] It is paramount that the specimen contain both gray and white matter and, when possible, a sulcus. In the vast majority of cases in which a diagnosis cannot be established, the reason is that an inadequate amount of tissue was taken for examination.

The cortical area to be sampled is sharply incised with a No. 15 scalpel blade. The incision is then carried 1.0 to 1.5 cm through the cortex and into the white matter. The procedure involves taking a core sample using four separate stab incisions

Table 37-3. Preferred site of biopsy according to suspected disease

Disease	Location
Neurodegenerative	
Alzheimer's disease	Frontal
Pick's disease	Frontal, temporal
Hallervorden-Spatz disease	Globus pallidus
Alper's disease	Frontal, parietal
Metabolic	
Metachromatic leukodystrophy	Frontal, parietal
Krabbe's disease	Frontal, parietal
Hurler's disease	Frontal
Tay-Sachs disease	Frontal
Infectious/parainfectious	
Herpes simplex encephalitis	Frontal, temporal
Other encephalitides	Frontal
Jakob-Creutzfeldt disease	Frontal, parietal
Subacute sclerosing panencephalitis	Frontal
Unknown	
Sudanophilic leukodystrophy	Frontal, parietal
Canavan's spongy degeneration	Frontal, parietal
Progressive myoclonic epilepsy (Lafora type)	Frontal, cerebellum

along the base of a tetrahedron; the base being at the pia (Figure 37-1).

The biopsy specimen should immediately be given to those persons directly responsible for its further handling. A pathologist should be present in the operating room. Tissue for culture and biochemical studies is obtained from the perimeter of the block or by incising the block parallel to the crest of a gyrus 3 mm from the edge. Diagnoses that require microbiologic analysis usually will not require biochemical analysis and vice versa.[23] Virtually all of the remaining neuropathologic studies require 2–3-mm slabs from the remaining block of tissue (Figure 37-2). These slices should be made across the depth of the sulcus. The center slabs should be reserved for studies that are most dependent on preserved cytoarchitecture. These sections consequently are sent for electron microscopic and histologic examination. To ensure adequate fixation, the piece of tissue

Table 37-2. Bibliographic summary of brain biopsy results and complications

Study	Type	Number of Patients	Biopsy Results (%) Positive	Biopsy Results (%) Negative	New Deficit (%)*	Complications (%) Deficit	Complications (%) Clot	Complications (%) Seizure	Complications (%) Dead
Boltshauser[14]	Pediatric chronic	45	13	87	?	2	0	7	0
Kaufman[24†]	Adult chronic	50	37	73	2	0	0	2	2
Groves[15]	Adult chronic	127	35	65	?	0.8	?	?	0
Moosy[17]	Adult chronic	31	39	61	3	3	?	?	0
Kohl[5]	HSE‡ acute	12	58	42	58	?	?	?	0
Whitely[11§]	HSE acute	132	83	17	65	1	1	?	0
DiSclafani[3]	HSE acute	10	100	0	70	?	?	?	0

*Unsuspected treatable conditions

†One death secondary to postoperative aspiration pneumonia.

‡Herpes simplex encephalitis.

§Complication from a group of 182 patients.

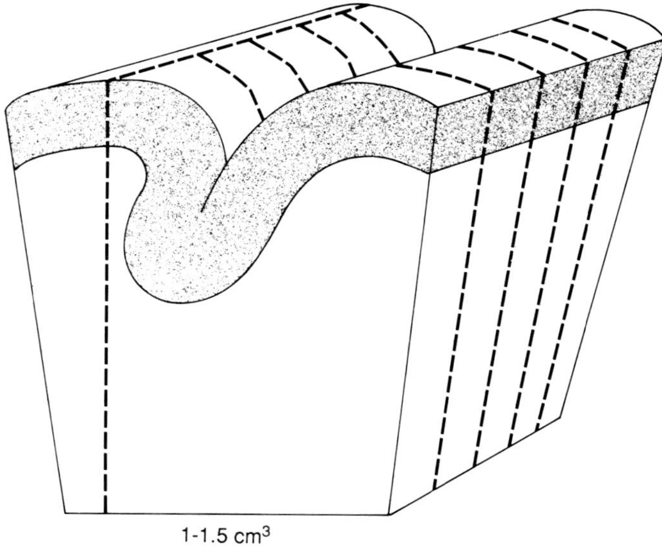

Fig. 37-1. The tetrahedral-shaped, 1- to 1.5-cc brain biopsy specimen must include both gray and white matter. It is recommended that the specimen also include a sulcus. The proposed manner of tissue division is depicted by the dashed lines.

Table 37-4. Possible complications with open biopsy and needle biopsy of the brain

Complication	Incidence (%)	Reference
Seizure	10(?)	14, 16, 17, 19, 23, 27
Neurologic deficit	1–3	10, 15–17, 23–25
Intracerebral hematoma	~1	10, 16, 17, 24–26
Subdural fluid	?	23, 24
Stroke	?	23, 24
Fever	?	19, 23, 24
Death	0–2	3, 5, 10, 14–17, 24–26
CSF leak	?	23, 24
Wound infection	1–2	17, 23, 24, 34
Porencephaly	?	23, 24
Herniation of brain tissue	1	10
Transmission of slow virus	?	23, 24, 30, 31

for electron microscopy is divided into 1–2-mm blocks and immediately immersed in Karnovsky's solution or its equivalent. The remaining tissue may be rapidly frozen should assays of biogenic amines or oxidative enzymes be needed.

To use the tissue optimally requires a combination of meticulous organization, gentle tissue handling, and immersion of the sections into their proper fixatives as expeditiously as possible. This must be done in conjunction with pathologists, virologists, and other specialists present in the operating room who are prepared to receive and process the specimen.[17,22,24] Any handling of tissue in a less formal way is unacceptable.

COMPLICATIONS

The complications of brain biopsy occur with a frequency of 1 to 3 percent and are usually transient[7,14–18,22–28] (Tables 37-22 and 37-4). Complications, however, can affect persons other than the patient. In general, it has been shown that surgeons run a 28 percent risk of being seropositive for hepatitis B.[29] In the case of brain biopsy, it is the potential for transmission of slow virus disease by contact with the infected tissue that concerns the neurosurgeon, his or her staff, and any patient subsequently treated with the same surgical instruments. Although transmission of slow virus disease to other patients via contaminated electrodes has been documented, infection of health care and laboratory workers remains only a theoretical

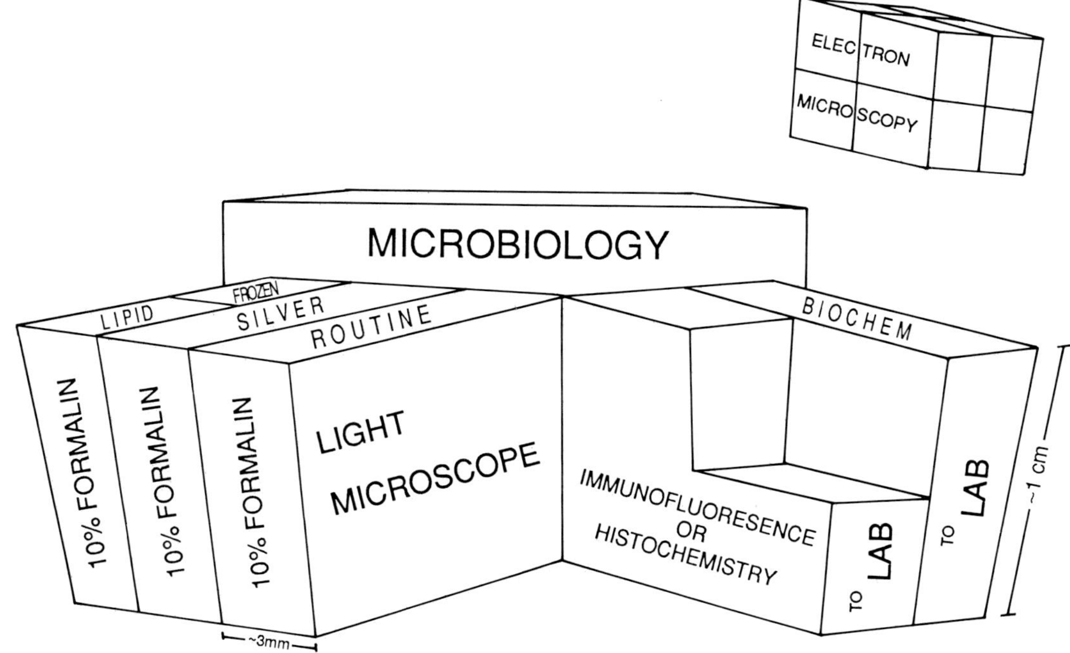

Fig. 37-2. The proposed schema for the proper handling of a biopsy specimen. Dividing the brain tissue into aliquots such as these will ensure its optimal utilization.

danger.[30,31] Current recommendations call for careful handling of the tissue and sterilization of equipment along specific guidelines.

Although the mechanism of transmission of the human T-lymphocyte (AIDS) virus in the community and its spread to recipients of contaminated blood products is well recognized, its transmission to health care workers is felt to be an extremely rare event.[32,33] Nevertheless, the virus can be spread to health care workers either by extensive unprotected exposure to a patient's blood secretions, or excretions or via inadvertent percutaneous innoculation with contaminated instruments.[37] The nature of these injuries, which are usually needle sticks, may, in fact, be quite trivial.[37] The nonspecific transmission of the HTL virus through casual contact with infected individuals is thought not to occur.[38] Although the risk to health care workers is felt to be small, caution must be exercised when in contact with a potential carrier, given the serious nature of becoming HTLV-positive. The measures taken to keep the possibility of inadvertent transmission of the virus to an acceptable minimum follow the same rationale as the isolation procedures for patients with hepatitis.[33]

REFERENCES

1. Barza M, Pauker SG: The decision to biopsy, treat, or wait in suspected herpes encephalitis. Ann Intern Med 92:641, 1980
2. Baumann RJ, Walsh JW, Gilmore RL, et al: Brain biopsies in cases of neonatal herpes simplex encephalitis. Neurosurgery 16:619, 1985
3. DiSclafani A, Kohl S, Ostrow PT: The importance of brain biopsy in suspected herpes simplex encephalitis. Surg Neurol 17:101, 1982
4. Griffith JF, Ch'ien LT: Herpes simplex virus encephalitis. Med Clin North Am 67:991, 1983
5. Kohl S, James AR: Herpes simplex virus encephalitis during childhood: Importance of brain biopsy diagnosis. J Pediatr 107:212, 1985
6. Levy RM, Pons VG, Rosenblum ML: Central nervous system mass lesions in the acquired immunodeficiency syndrome (AIDS). J Neurosurg 61:9, 1984
7. Morawetz RB, Whitely RJ, Murphy DM: Experience with brain biopsy for suspected herpes encephalitis: A review of forty consecutive cases. Neurosurgery 12:654, 1983
8. Moskowitz LB, Hensley GT, Chan JC, et al: Brain biopsies with acquired immune deficiency syndrome. Arch Pathol Lab Med 108:368, 1984
9. Snow RB, Lauyne MH: Intracranial space-occupying lesions in acquired immune deficiency syndrome patients. Neurosurgery 16:148, 1985
10. Whitely RJ, Soong SJ, Hirch MS, et al: Herpes simplex encephalitis: Vidarabine therapy and diagnostic problems. N Engl J Med 304:313, 1981
11. Whitely RJ, Soong SJ, Linneman C, et al: Herpes simplex encephalitis: Clinical assessment. JAMA 247:317, 1982
12. Brett EM, Berry CL: Brain biopsy in infancy and childhood. Dev Med Child Neurol 10:263, 1968
13. Mahendra B: Some ethical issues in dementia research. J Med Ethics 1:29, 1984
14. Boltshauser E, Wilson J: Value of brain biopsy in neurodegenerative disease of childhood. Arch Dis Child 51:264, 1976
15. Groves R, Moller J: The value of cerebral cortical biopsy. Acta Neurol Scand 42:477, 1966
16. Kaufman HH, Catalano LW: Diagnostic brain biopsy: A series of 50 cases and a review. Neurosurgery 4:129, 1979
17. Moosy J: Diagnostic cerebral biopsy, in Toole JE (ed): Special Techniques for Neurological Diagnosis. Contemporary Neurology Series No. 3. Philadelphia, F.A. Davis Co., 1969, pp 184–194
18. Sevush S, Turkewitz LJ: Brain biopsy: Risks, benefits, and indications. Mt Sinai J Med 52:380, 1985
19. Biemond A: Indications, legal and moral aspects of cerebral biopsies, in Proceedings of the Fifth International Congress of Neuropathology, Zurich, August 31–September 3, 1965. Amsterdam, Excerpta Medica, 1966, pp 362–375
20. Torack RM: Adult dementia: History, biopsy, pathology. Neurosurgery 4:434, 1979
21. Kovarsky J, Schochet SS, McCormick WF: Modern use of the biopsy in the diagnosis of neurological disease. J Iowa Med Soc 62:424, 1972
22. Wagner JA, Wisotzkey H: Cerebral cortical biopsy: A new vista for the pathologist. South Med J 56:415, 1963
23. Ellis WG, Youmans JR, Dreyfus PM: Diagnostic biopsy for neurological disease, in Youmans JR (ed): Neurological Surgery, ed 2. Philadelphia, WB Saunders, 1982, pp 382–422
24. Kaufman HH, Ostrow PT, Butler IJ: Diagnostic brain biopsy, in Wilkins RH, Rengachary SS (eds): Neurosurgery. New York, McGraw-Hill, 1985, pp 289–293
25. Barnwell S, Barboro N, Gutin P: Results, complications and factors affecting CT directed stereotaxic biopsies in 47 consecutive patients. Poster Session, No. 97, AANS Annual Meeting, Denver, Colorado, 1986
26. Crevier PH: Post-stereotaxic intracranial hematomas. Acta Neurochir 21:71, 1974
27. Elian M: Late effects of brain biopsy. J Neurol 211:95, 1975
28. Guthkelch AN: Brain biopsy in infancy and childhood. Dev Med Child Neurol 10:107, 1968
29. Denes AE, Smith JL, et al: Hepatitis B infection in physicians: Results of a nationwide seroepidemiological survey. JAMA 239:120, 1978
30. Bernoulli C, Regli F, Gajdusek DC, et al: Danger of accidental person-to-person transmission of Creutzfeldt-Jakob disease by surgery. Lancet 1:478, 1977
31. Gajdusek DC, Gibbs CJ, Asher DM: Precautions in medical care of, and in handling materials from patients with transmissible virus dementia (Creutzfeldt-Jakob disease). N Engl J Med 297:1253, 1977
32. Centers for Disease Control: HTLV-III/LAV: Agent summary statement. Morbidity and Mortality Weekly Report 35:540, 1986
33. Francis DP, Chin J: The prevention of acquired immunodeficiency syndrome in the United States. JAMA 257:1357, 1987
34. Centers for Disease Control: Apparent transmission of human T-lymphocyte virus type III/lymphadenopathy-associated virus from a child to a mother providing health care. Morbidity and Mortality Weekly Report 35:76, 1986
35. Anonymous: Needlestick transmission of HTLV-III from a patient infected in Africa. Lancet 2:1376, 1984
36. Stricof RL, Morse DL: HTLV-III/LAV seroconversion following deep intramuscular needlestick injury. N Engl J Med 314:1115, 1986
37. Okenhendler E, Harzic M, Le Roux JM, et al: HIV infection with seroconversion after a superficial needle stick injury to the finger. N Engl J Med 315:582, 1986
38. Centers for Disease Control: Acquired immunodeficiency syndrome. United States. Morbidity and Mortality Weekly Report 35:757, 1986

CHAPTER 38
Neurologic Endoscopy

C. Hunter Shelden   Skip Jacques   Harold R. Lutes

ENDOSCOPY ORIGINALLY WAS CONCEIVED as a method that would permit the direct inspection of the interior of a hollow organ. Over the years, a large number of excellent endoscopic instruments have been developed that allow inspection of the bladder, the intestine, the bronchus, and almost every other air- or fluid-filled cavity in the body. Numerous historical and descriptive reviews have been published,[1] particularly in recent years.

General endoscopy probably began with biopsy and removal of pedunculated polyps from the rectosigmoid portion of the colon. The first large-scale success in surgical endoscopy resulted from the development of instruments to inspect the interior of the urinary bladder. During the past 20 years, a resectoscope such as that developed by Braasch and Thompson provided the technology for a transurethral approach to the bladder and prostate that supplanted open surgery on those organs. During this same period, endoscopy assumed a vital role in the investigation and management of many problems affecting the gut, bronchus, bladder, and even the synovial spaces of large joints.

The recent widespread interest in endoscopy stems from technological advances that have afforded flexibility, illumination, and optical qualities all markedly improved over those previously available. These technical developments have led to the remarkable expansion and worldwide acceptance of endoscopy as a diagnostic and surgical tool. Although many people have played some role in this development, it is apparent that Harold Hopkins, professor of applied optical physics at the University of Reading in England, deserves the major credit (Hopkins H: personal communication). He developed a solid-rod lens system that has been adopted as the basic design for all present-day nonflexible endoscopes. This rigid segmental design created an instrument in which maximum target illumination is achieved by elimination of most of the transmission loss. This breakthrough, plus recently developed high-intensity light sources such as xenon, affords ample light even for microsurgical procedures. A further asset of the Hopkins system is the increase in image resolution and elimination of chromatic aberration and ghost images.

Professor Hopkins also developed a fore-oblique lens, which consists of triple prisms with mirrored surfaces that afford a 30-degree-wide angle of visibility; this added a new technical ingredient vital to stereotactic tumor removal. The K prism was redesigned by Hopkins, and his improvements led to correction of the inverted image without chromatic aberration.

In addition to his interest in rigid endoscopes, Hopkins made valuable contributions to the flexible variety; the most significant of these was his improved method for producing the fiberoptic bundle. Hopkins described a simple but effective method for producing a ''coherent'' bundle of fibers. Coherency basically requires a bundle of fibers that are identical in length and that match in size at each end. Hopkins proposed wrapping a long, continuous fiber around the circumference of a drum as many times as the size of the optical bundle required. All of the fibers then were cut at one linear marker across the drum surface. This produced as many fibers as there were turns of the original fiber on the drum. These fibers are termed ''coherent'' because they are identical in length, and at each end the bundles of the fibers exactly match. This is a key factor in flexible (fiberoptic) endoscopy. Unmatched quartz fibers will transmit light and will produce illumination at the distal end, but they will have the capability of transmitting an image only if they form a coherent bundle.

NEUROLOGIC ENDOSCOPY

Neurologic endoscopy began with the earliest efforts to control primary hydrocephalus in children.[2] The enlarged lateral ventricle that was filled with clear fluid afforded an inviting target for the endoscope.[3] Initial success in visualizing the ventricular surfaces naturally led to attempts at control of cerebrospinal fluid volume either by third ventriculoscopy or by coagulation or resection of the choroid plexus.[46] Although the rationale was logical, and endoscopic procedures were well executed for that period, the long-term results were disappointing. A variety of endoscopic techniques were developed, but no satisfactory animal model for hydrocephalus was available for study. An experimental obstructive hydrocephalus could be produced, but all too often the animal would die from a rapid increase in intracranial pressure before a stabilized form of internal hydrocephalus could develop. Interest in endoscopy of the lateral ventricles declined rapidly following the outstanding investigation of hydrocephalus by Pudenz. Although his shunt system received international acclaim, a lesser-known observation may have had the most lasting impact. He realized that for half a century neurosurgeons had been attempting to reproduce an infantile disease in an adult animal. The substitution of kittens for cats allowed researchers to produce marked chronic hydrocephalus in animals.

In recent years there has been little interest in the endoscopic visualization of the lateral ventricles. Computed tomography (CT) has replaced all but very special studies in evaluating the nature and degree of internal hydrocephalus. Shunting procedures have supplanted surgical endoscopic technique.

OPERATIVE NEUROSURGICAL TECHNIQUES
ISBN 0-8089-1862-1

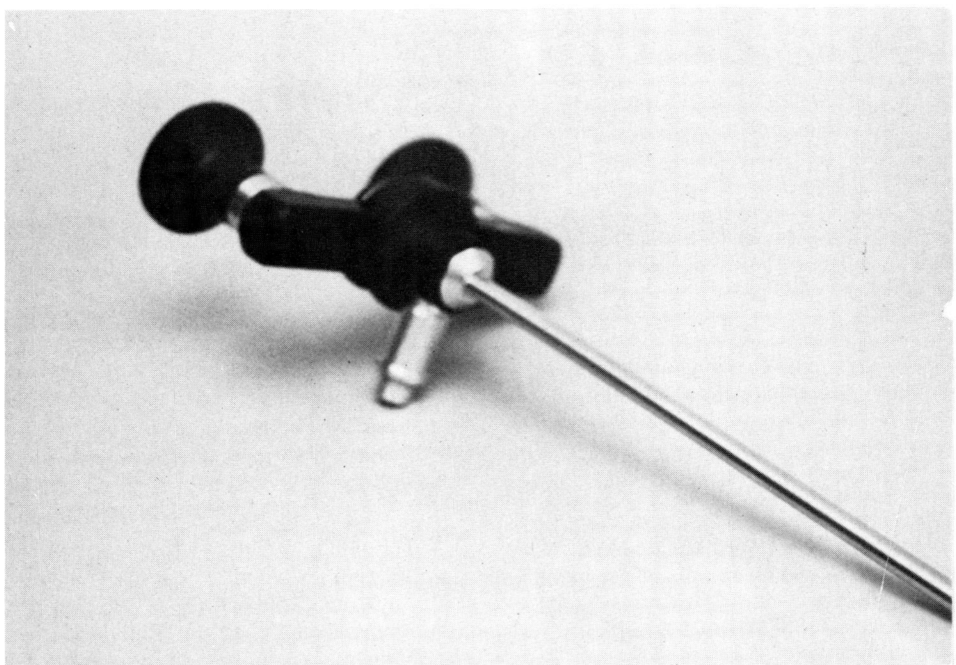

Fig. 38-1. The optical system of an endoscope showing the binocular eyepieces and a long double barrel. Each barrel contains two Hopkins fiberoptic units. The threaded attachment is for xenon illumination.

Neurosurgeons, however, continue to have sporadic interest in visualizing other cerebrospinal fluid-filled cavities. Crue developed a unique fiberoptic needlescope (1.7 mm in diameter) that he used successfully to visualize the cisterna magna.[7] It was designed to visually enhance the accuracy of electrode placement in the medulla during percutaneous tractotomy.

Meckel's cave, the cisterna magna, and the cerebellopontine angle have been explored clinically by Fukushima through a very small (1.45 mm) endoscope equipped with a Selfoc lens that had a 54-degree-wide angle of view.[8] Prott initiated specific endoscopic studies of the cerebellopontine angle.[9] Burham,[10] Olinger and Ohlgaber,[11] Pool,[12] and Stern[13] inspected intraspinal structures by myeloscopy. Historically, endoscopy has been an interesting, innovative, yet rather unproductive aspect of the developments in neurosurgery.[14] It commanded justifiable attention during the period of neurologic diagnosis based on indirect evidence, i.e., the era of diagnosis based on ventricular shift, intraventricular obstruction, local distortion or asymmetry of specific portions of the ventricular system, and displacement of intracranial vascular structures. Often the nature of the offending lesion could not be determined, and one quick look through any type of endoscope was better than exploratory craniotomy.

The CT scanner, however, has made endoscopy almost obsolete in neurosurgery. Even a two-dimensional Polaroid picture is so clear that visualization by an invasive technique is not justified. It would seem that endoscopy is about to follow encephalography, ventriculography, and arteriography (other than for aneurysm) into history—the victim of computed tomography.

We believe, on the contrary, that with a few major changes, endoscopy can occupy a very prominent role in the future of neurosurgery. To accomplish this:

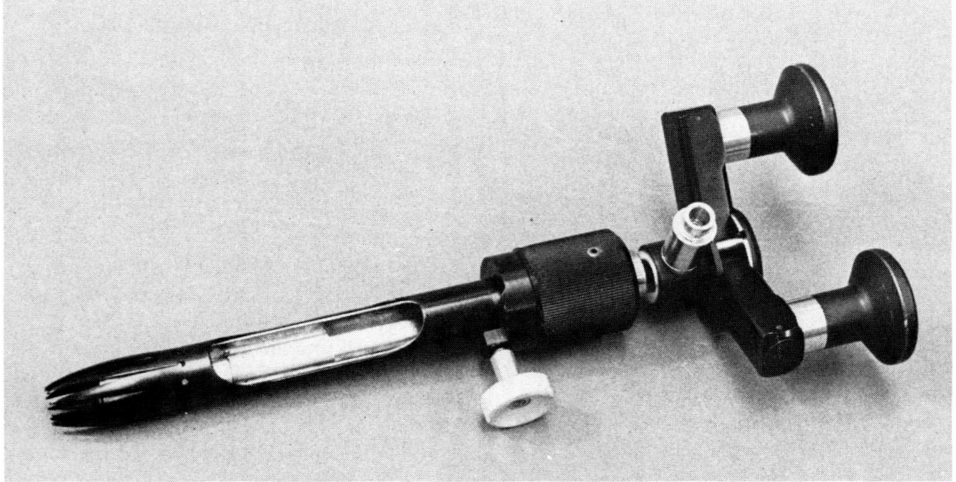

Fig. 38-2. A tumorscope assembly with the tulip blades in the open position. The side port is for the introduction of special surgical instruments. The binocular optic system is shown.

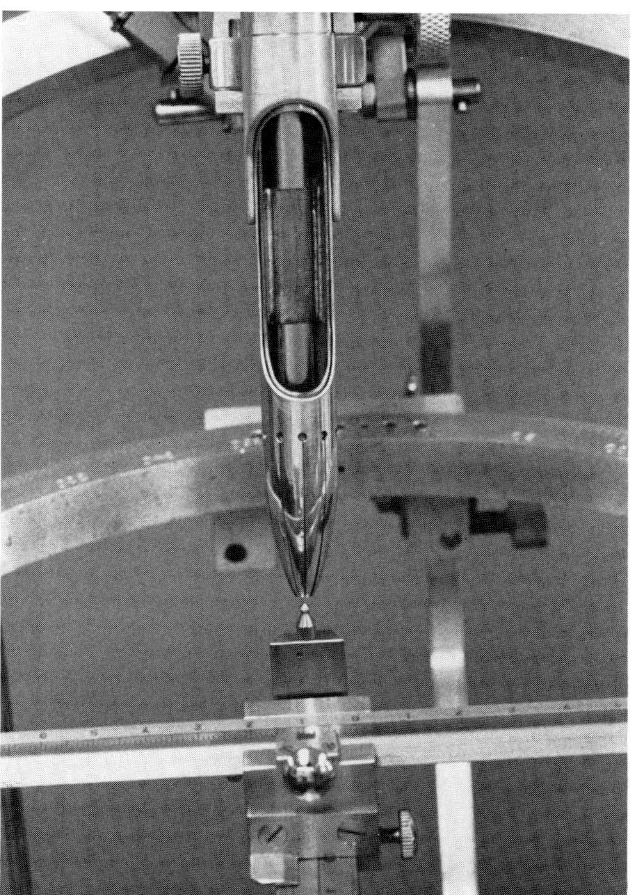

Fig. 38-3. The tumorscope exactly at the target point on the phantom. The target is pre-set in three planes representing the X, Y, and Z axes. The barrel of the optical unit can be seen through the side port intended for instruments.

1. The brain itself, rather than fluid-filled cavities, must become the principal target of the endoscope.
2. The endoscope must be computer-directed and mated to CT or MRI digital data.
3. The endoscope must provide its own air-filled cavity for visualization of tumors or, in the future, for areas suitable for brain transplant.
4. Illumination must be full-spectrum, of high intensity, and provided by an adjustable external source. The optic system must be binocular and stereoscopic.

Table 38-1. Preoperative procedures

Routine CT data is transferred to tape then disc
Lesion Enhancement
  1. Subtraction algorithms, digital printout
  2. Color coding
  3. Magnification
  4. Three-dimensional reconstruction
Lesion Inspection
  1. Surface detail, depth, density
  2. Boundaries, contours
  3. Outline of the edema
  4. Base of the tumor (mathematical removal)
Determination of the X, Y, and Z coordinates
  1. Position ring and vertical pins
  2. Define circle—X and Y axes
  3. Perform algorithms
  4. Determine the Z axis

5. The endoscope must incorporate a tumor-identifying system, a method of tumor removal, and capabilities for in situ adjuvant therapy.

Binocular stereoscopic vision is essential for intracranial procedures. Although it should be adopted for all endoscopic techniques, this would require redesign to afford 360 degrees of rotary capability in order for it to be useful in most areas of nonneurosurgical endoscopy.

OPTICAL SYSTEM

The optical design requirements for a surgical endoscope are much more demanding than for instruments developed purely for inspection purposes. Our futile attempts to utilize a monocular system demonstrated to us the need for greater depth perception under high-intensity illumination in a surgical field with minimal landmarks or other monocular clues. Lutes, who developed our optical system, is an authority on stereoscopic vision, photography, and imaging. He believes that a three-dimensional capability is essential if surgical endoscopy is to occupy a prominent role in treatment. In his evaluation of our visual requirements, he emphasized the need for a new design. The instrument must be of a small size; it must be capable of clear definition; it must have a short focal length; and it must possess a wide-angle field with universal focus.

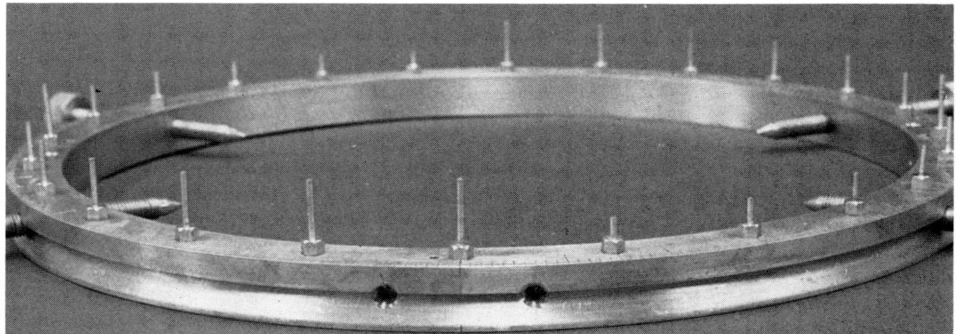

Fig. 38-4. A close-up of the stereotactic ring. Four identical long pins are at quadrants. There are two sets of graduated pins, varying by 1 mm in length. One set begins with the shortest pin, near the 180-degree marker. The pins are critical in the determination of the Z axis.

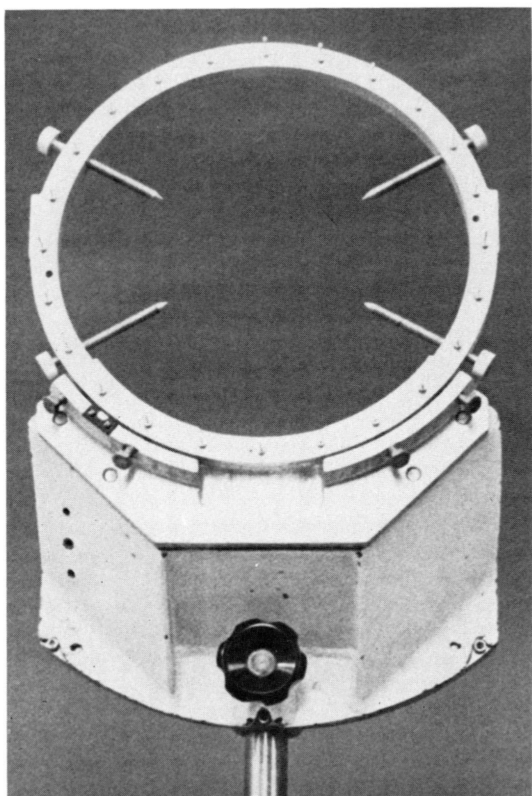

Fig. 38-5. The operating ring with four pins for skeletal fixation. The ring is held in a constant fixed position by the attachment that fits both the scanner and the operating table.

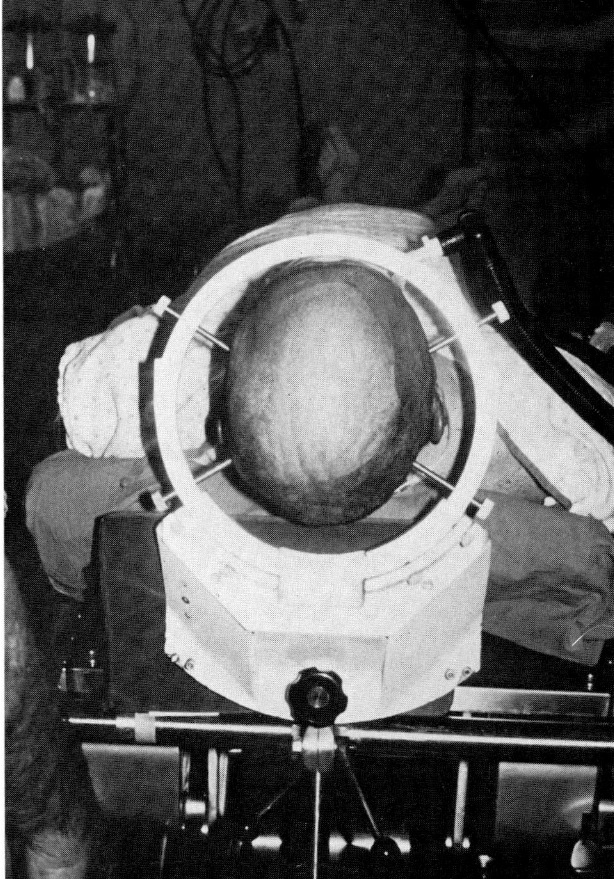

Fig. 38-6. The ring attached to a patient, demonstrating the ring holder attached to the operating table. The ring serves as an excellent head holder during the operation.

Table 38-2. Operative procedures

Patient Selection
Enhancement and inspection of the preoperative lesion, positioning of the ring placement, and localization of the lesion
  1. CT scan with ring in place and a table mount
  2. Coordinate calculation by computer
  3. Prepare operating table mount
  4. Transfer coordinates to phantom
Lesion Removal
  1. Determine ANGLE OF APPROACH by computer
  2. Coordinate transfer to patient ring
  3. Prepare instruments
    a. Stereotactic system
    b. Micromanipulators
    c. Tulip "RESECTOSCOPE"
    d. Binocular optics
    e. Dilators
    f. Roto-sucker-dissector
    g. Laser, cryoprobes, heat
    h. Adjuvant therapy reservoir
Adjuvant therapy
  1. Immediate—holds cells "in limbo"
  2. Prolonged—localized immunotherapy, chemotherapy
    a. Photolysis
    b. THORACIC DUCT STUDIES

The Storz pediatric-type Hopkins endoscope is a monocular device that has a focal length of 10 mm, has a nearly universal focus, and contains a fiberoptic bundle that allows illumination at the operating site. Experiments soon revealed that the monocular image presented by the instrument was inadequate for the specialized requirements of neurologic endoscopy.

The neurosurgeon needs to work, if possible, through a burr hole approximately 15 mm in diameter. He or she must look at objects of unknown color, size, shape, and texture. It is imperative that as near normal a visual experience as possible be achieved in order to perform the task at its highest level. Such normality of vision requires a single simultaneous binocular stereoscopic vision.

It is often stated that experienced surgeons can acquire so-called "stereotactic" vision using a monocular device. Such a surgeon is really using some of the monocular clues to depth, which are (1) texture, (2) overlapping contours, (3) known size and distance, (4) parallax, (5) perspective (convergence of parallel lines), (6) apparent position on a horizontal surface, (7) density gradient, and (8) aerial perspective. Obviously, many of these clues are not available in a body cavity as they are in real life, as utilized by an individual with only monocular vision. This ability varies greatly with surgeons, and at best represents a substandard visual picture of the objects viewed.

In addition, the factor of object size is one of the greatest

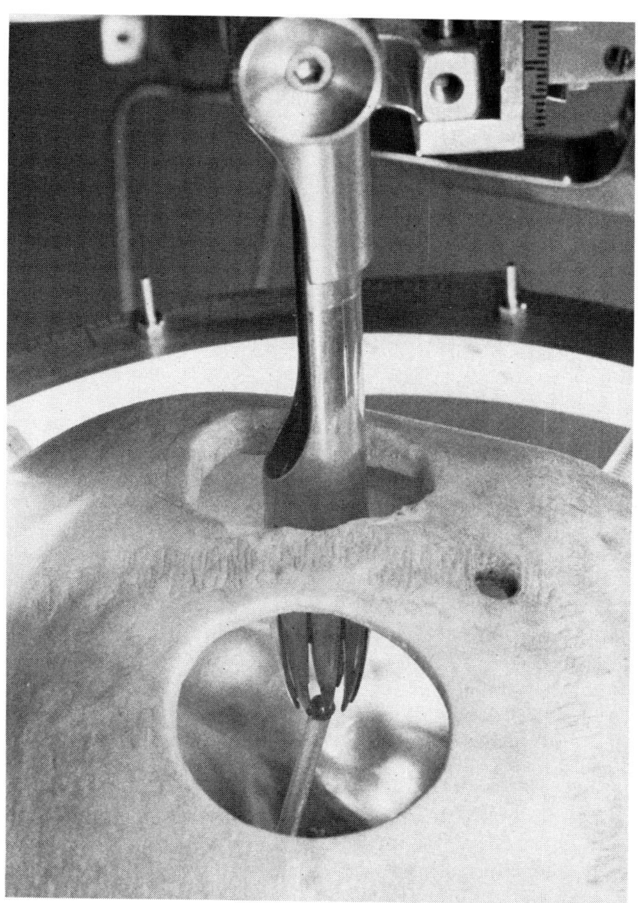

Fig. 38-7. The tulip blades of the tumorscope open to enclose a target point within a test skull. The ring with pins is visible in the background.

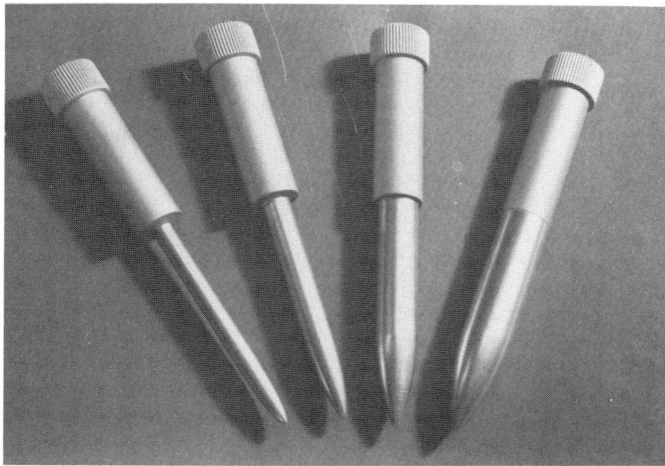

Fig. 38-8. A set of cerebral dilators that allow gradual separation of cerebral fibers before introduction of the tumorscope. Each dilator is maintained on the exact axis in order to ensure atraumatic insertion.

variables. Using a very short focal length lens, such as that found in all endoscopes, perspective is forced and objects at greater distances appear much smaller than they really are. Since size and distance are interrelated, one factor must be known if the other is to be correctly judged. In a monocular view down a restricted tube, a view of unfamiliar objects of unknown size, there is no basis for judgment except the experience of repeated operations in a restricted anatomic area.

Further limitations of monocular endoscopy arise from the nature of the illumination. Light of high intensity is emitted from the instrument adjacent to the optics and parallel to the optic axis, causing very "flat" lighting, which is the poorest way to illuminate surface texture. It is a well-established principle of photography that oblique or side lighting is essential in order to create a true image of texture. Furthermore, stereoscopic vision is required in order to see texture properly.

When it was determined that a binocular, dual-channel endoscope was essential, it was found that no such stereoscopic instrument was available. We therefore designed a system using two endoscopes mounted in a position of convergence at their focal distance on the usual axis; this provided a stereoscopic image. This instrument proved to be bulky and was redesigned with parallel tubes and a Hopkins-rod-lens system (Figure 38-1). With the lens objectives 3.5 mm apart and at a working distance of 20 mm, the convergence required to fuse the two images is equal to viewing an object 16 inches (41 cm) from the observer. At this point the object appears at life size. When the

object is moved to a working distance of 10 mm, it appears twice life size, and if moved to a working distance of 40 mm, it appears half-size, which means that the linear perspective changes rapidly at a very high angle. A 4:1 change in size ratio takes place with an associated convergence change that is equal to an object being moved from 8 to 32 inches. This does not fit the average background of visual experience or the geometry of learned perspective and thus may be rejected, with resultant blurring, diplopia, or subjective visual discomfort. The use of any endoscope requires practice if it is to be used effectively over extended periods. The viewing of close-up stereo pictures in a hand viewer can provide such practice.

The use of the stereo endoscope in the Shelden tumorscope with the "tulip" tissue-dilating expandable tube provides an additional advantage. A plane of reference is created by the blades of the tulip, such that the tumor appears to be seen through a window. In viewing stereo pictures, the window aperture serves as a plane of reference and objects appear to be in front of, in line with, or behind the window plane. In our experience, if the object appears even with the tulip blade tips, it serves as a true size control: the object appears twice normal size.

The correct perception of size, texture, perspective, stereopsis, and so forth, enhances the ability of the surgeon to place dissecting instruments in precise position with binocular accuracy. The ability to align two objects in a common plane (stereopsis) is one of the highest orders of precision and should serve to reduce errors of visual judgment.

Presently we are using three tumorscope sizes:

1. Standard (15.5 mm diameter—Figures 38-2 and 38-11)
2. Large (25 mm diameter—Figures 38-11 and 38-12)
3. Small (10.2 mm diameter—Figure 38-13)

Sizes 1 and 2 have been modified for use with the carbon dioxide laser (Figure 38-11). A neurosurgical endoscope should have:

1. A tubular shaft, 14 mm or less in diameter, containing a binocular scope.
2. Tulip-like blades at the distal end that can be opened when the target is reached along the Z axis. Proper tension of the blades on brain tissue stretches tiny vessels and prevents

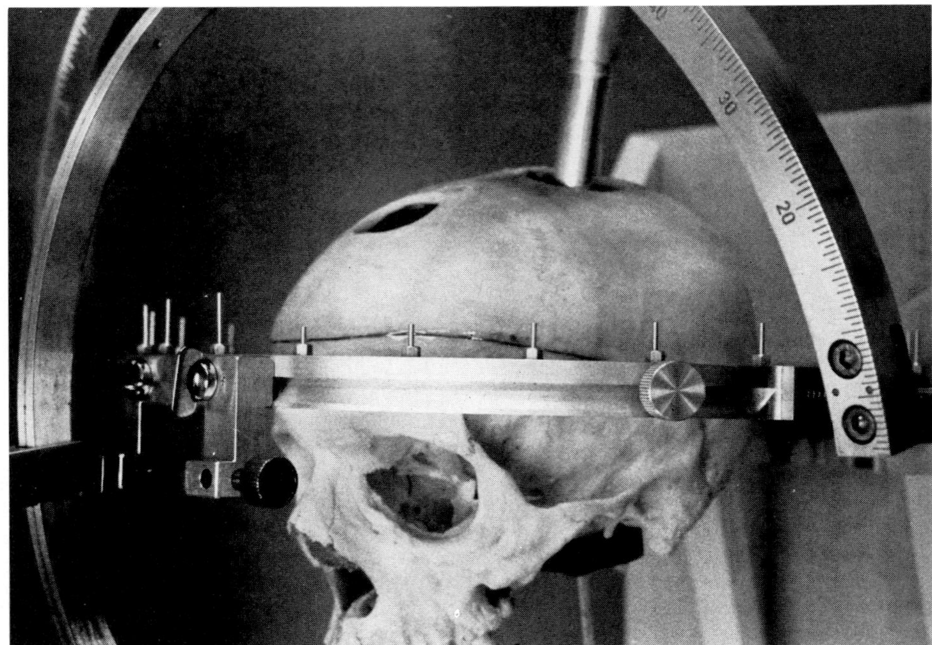

Fig. 38-9. A test skull showing the attached rings and pins. Arched structures support the tumorscope assembly.

bleeding from the brain area exposed between the open blades (Figures 38-2 and 38-13). The working distance between tips is 10 mm.

3. An air-filled cavity between the end of the optical system and the tumor.

4. A side port for introducing instruments, suction, and the carbon dioxide laser for tumor removal (Figures 38-3, 38-11, 38-12, and 38-14). The addition of a carbon dioxide laser greatly enhances the precision of tumor removal. In the future, when specialized markers are available, a minute area of tumor tissue will be identified by hema-

toporphyrin derivatives excited by ultraviolet light and seen at surgery by the emitted red light.

5. A fiberoptic system consisting of 6 Hopkins units in each parallel unit, which provides adequate distance from the skull to allow freedom of movement for the surgeon. An additional set of quartz fibers for excitation of porphyrin derivatives will provide for tumor identification or for excitation of other substances for photoradiation and lysis of the lesion.

STEREOTACTIC PROTOCOL

The stereotactic protocol designed for patients with a small brain tumor can be detailed in the following steps that are used at the Huntington Memorial Hospital.

All patients selected for this type of neurosurgical endoscopy have had evidence of a small intracerebral lesion based on CT data from a General Electric 9800 Scanner (CT/T 9800 Scanner manufactured by General Electric Medical Systems Division, Milwaukee, Wisconsin). Unless the original scan has been done in our laboratory, the scan is repeated because of slight variations in digital output, and the information is transferred from the General Electric tape to a floppy disk on a PDP 1145 computer for further treatment. Scanning enhancement techniques, subtraction, color coding, magnification, and other algorithm manipulations are performed (Table 38-1). All lesions are reconstructed three-dimensionally in order to better define the exact volume, size, density, and shape of the lesion before stereotactic surgery.[15–19]

On the day before the operation, the patient is admitted to the hospital for routine preoperative work-up. On the morning of surgery, the patient is taken to the CT scanning suite, where the modified stereotactic ring with localizing pins is placed on the head, and skeletal fixation is obtained by the placement of four long screws after local infiltration of the scalp (Figure

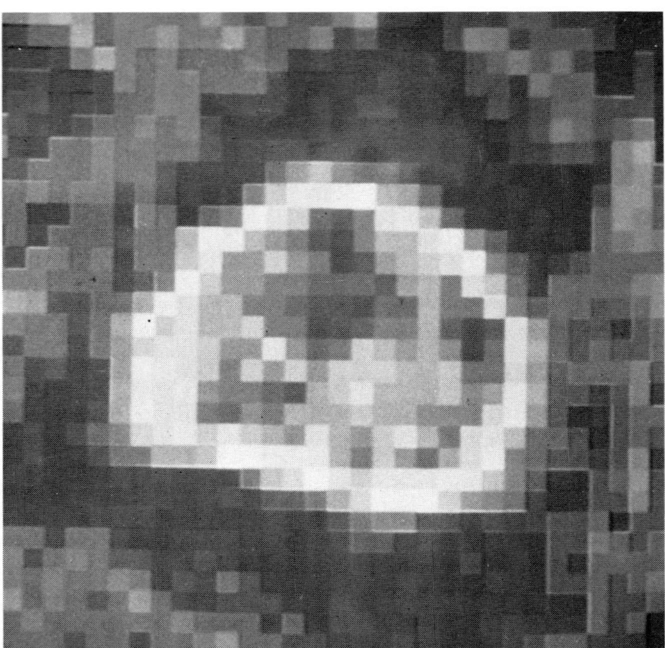

Fig. 38-10. An enhanced and enlarged digital printout of a small tumor. Variations in outline and density are apparent.

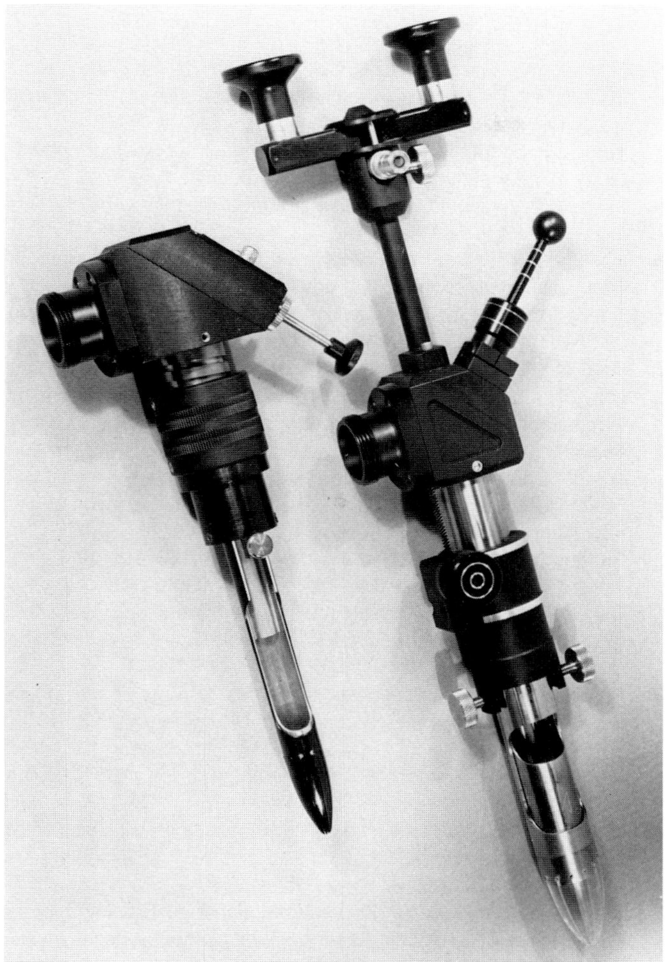

Fig. 38-11. Standard and large-size tumorscopes for carbon dioxide laser adaptation.

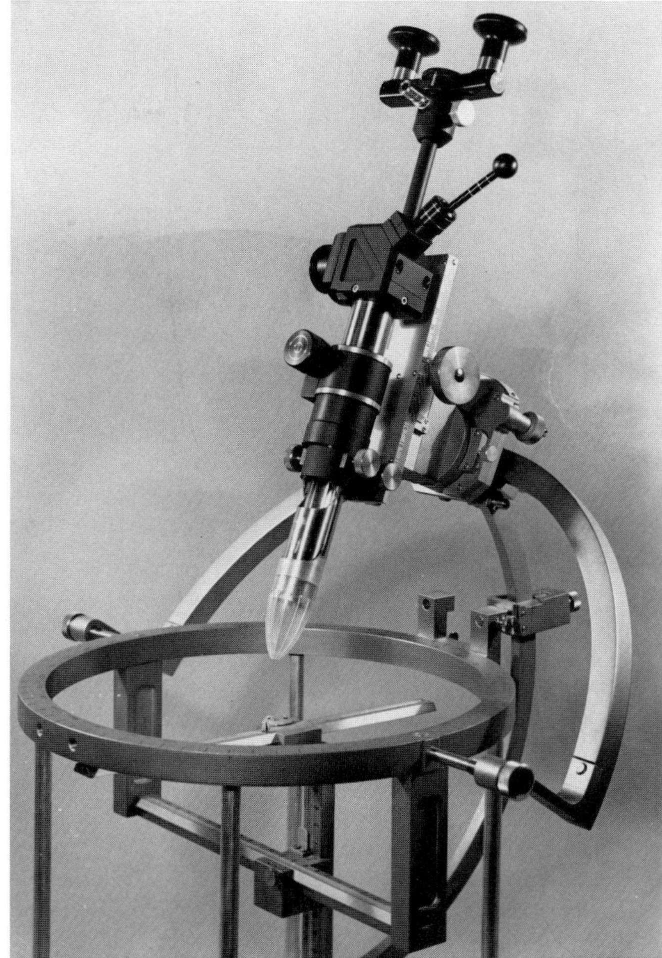

Fig. 38-12. A large tumorscope for laser surgery. A stereo endoscope in place. The unit is mounted on a phantom ring.

38-4). The hair is clipped and routine scalp preparation is carried out.

The patient is placed on the CT scan table, and the ring is secured to the base-mounting system (Figure 38-5; Table 38-2). A repeat scan through the lesion area and the ring is carried out, and the information is transferred to magnetic tape. The tape is then taken to the computer for XYZ-coordinate calculation. Meanwhile, the patient and ring are removed from the base-mounting system and transferred to the operating room.

In the operating room, the patient is intubated and the head-ring is attached to the operating table fixation mount (Figure 38-6). Final preparations for surgery are made and the patient is draped.

During this time, the exact XYZ coordinates have been processed by the computer and returned to the operating room. The "phantom," which had been sterilized, is placed on a draped table and the adjustable target is set in accordance with the coordinates derived from the computer. The halo bearing the tumorscope assembly is attached to the phantom and the desired angle of entry is determined. While still on the phantom, the micromanipulator is advanced to the depth of the lesion, and the readings from the micromanipulator and the halo-stabilizing bar are recorded (Figure 38-7). The halo is removed from the patient ring so that a routine scalp incision and a small trephination can be made coincident with the desired angle of entry. After the dura is opened and the pia incised transversely over a length of approximately 4 mm, the halo is reapplied to the patient ring. A series of dilators (Figure 38-8) are then used to approach the appropriate depth along the Z axis.[20] Finally, the tulip is mounted on the micromanipulator, introduced into the brain after the pia mater is incised, and opened at the appropriate coordinate setting to expose the lesion (Figure 38-9).

The actual surgical removal of the lesion is performed using a series of biopsy forceps, small dissectors, and a CO_2 laser plus a roto-sucker-dissector designed specifically for use within the

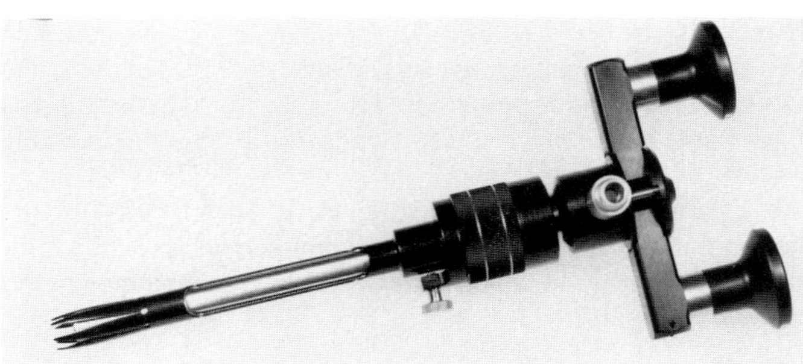

Fig. 38-13. A small tumorscope with a stereo endoscope. The tulip open in operating position.

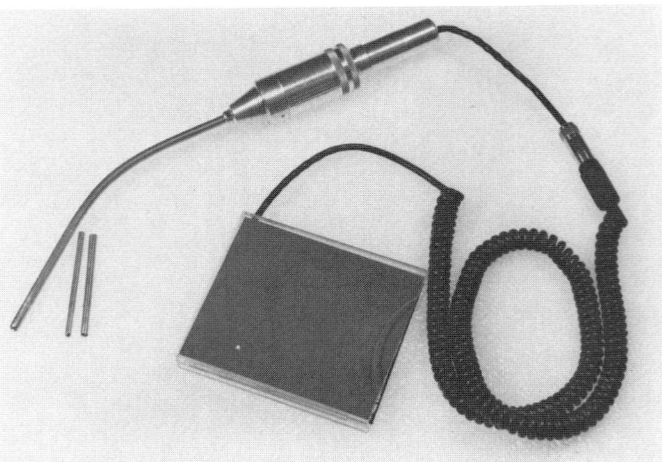

Fig. 38-14. A Roto-resector used with the Shelden-Jacques tumorscope.

tulip.[21] Lesion removal is simplified by preoperative inspection of the three-dimensional reconstruction of the tumor (Figure 38-10), as well as by excellent depth perception afforded by the stereoscopic optical system designed for use with the tulip. After the lesion is removed, routine neurosurgical closure is performed. The patient and ring are removed from the base-mounting system, the ring is removed, and the patient is sent to the recovery room for routine (3-day) postoperative care.

CONCLUSIONS

Historically, endoscopy has had a powerful and beneficial effect on many disciplines in medicine. Artificial barriers that have developed between the medical and surgical groups in gastroenterology have been eliminated largely because of endoscopy. Those groups interested in the urinary tract and the respiratory system have become more closely linked as the result of the interdisciplinary aspect of endoscopy. It will be interesting to observe the effect of endoscopy on neurology and neurosurgery. It is our hope that it will bring these two disciplines much closer together at a time when many disturbing influences are apparent. In particular, the diagnosis of intracranial lesions is frequently made solely on the basis of CT data before the patient has seen either a neurologist or a neurosurgeon. As a result, the subsequent referral or even the entire program for treating a patient is determined by someone unqualified to make such decisions. Too often patients are referred to someone who will perform a simple biopsy followed by irradiation, or even to someone who will advise radiation as the sole treatment. Although the condemnation of such a practice is justified theoretically, the fact must also be accepted that the previous policy of orderly diagnosis, investigation, and primary open surgical treatment has not led to statistical results that would make neurologists enthusiastic about continuing with that program.

On the other hand, the past failure to "cure" brain tumors does not justify abandoning a competent surgical program, but, rather, demands the development of new, potentially better clinical methods.

REFERENCES

1. Mitchel J: Endoscopy. Ann R Coll Surg Engl 62:106, 1980
2. Pudenz RH: The surgical treatment of hydrocephalus. An historical review. Surg Neurol 15:15, 1980
3. Temple F, Grant FC: Ventriculoscope and intraventricular photography in internal hydrocephalus. JAMA 80:461, 1923
4. Mixter WJ: Ventriculoscopy and puncture of the third ventricle. Bos Med Surg J 188:277, 1923
5. Scarff JE: Third ventriculoscopy as the rational treatment of obstructive hydrocephalus. J Pediatr 6:870, 1935
6. Dandy WE: Cerebral ventriculoscopy. Bull Johns Hopkins Hosp 33:189, 1922
7. Crue BL: Needle scope attached to stereotactic frame for inspection of cisterna magna during percutaneous radiofrequency trigeminal tractotomy. Appl Neurophysiol 39:58, 1977
8. Fukushima T: Endoscopy of Meckels' cave, cisterna magna and cerebello-pontine angle. J Neurosurg 48:302, 1978
9. Prott W: Cisternoscopy-endoscopy of the cerebellopontine angle. Acta Neurochirurg 31:105, 1974
10. Burham MS: Myeloscopy or the direct visualization of the spinal canal and its contents. J Bone Joint Surg 13:695, 1931
11. Olinger CP, Ohlgaber RL: Eighteen-gauge microscopic-telescopic needle endoscope and electrode channel. Potential clinical and research application. Surg Neurol 2:151, 1974
12. Pool JL: Direct visualization of dorsal nerve roots of the cauda equina by means of a myeloscope. Arch Neurol Psychiatr 39:1308, 1938
13. Stern EL: The spinascope: A new instrument for visualizing the spinal canal and its contents. Med Rec 143:31, 1936
14. Guiot G, Rougrie J, Fouristier M, et al: Une nouvelle technique endoscopique explorations endoscopiques intracraniennes. Presse Med 1:225, 1963
15. Shelden CH, McCann GD, Jacques S, et al: Bio-information systems. Basic research on brain tumors. Computer based investigation of minute tumors (5 mm); composition, development, and early detection. Localization and determination of base-line for Z-axis calibration. Annual Engineering Report, California Institute of Technology, 1978
16. Jacques S, Shelden CH, McGann GD, et al: A microstereotactic approach to small CNS lesions. Part 1: Development of CT localization and 3-D reconstruction techniques. Neurol Med Chir (Tokyo) 8:527, 1980
17. Shelden CH, McCann GD, Jacques S, et al: Development of a computerized microstereotactic method for the localization and removal of minute CNS lesions under direct 3-D vision. Technical report. J Neurosurg 52:21, 1980
18. Jacques S, Shelden CH, Clayton C: A microstereotactic approach to small CNS lesions. Part 2: Adjuvant therapy. Clinical potential and toxicity of intraventricular lymph infusion. Neurol Med Chir (Tokyo) 8:615, 1980
19. Jacques S, Shelden CH, Pudenz RH, et al: Micro-surgical cannulation of the thoracic duct in cats. Technical note. J Immunol Meth 21:383, 1978
20. Jacques S, Shelden CH, McCann GD, et al: Recognition of minute (5 mm) cerebral gliomas by advanced computer technology, in Marguth F, et al (eds): Neurovascular Surgery—Specialized Neurosurgical Techniques. Berlin, Springer-Verlag, 1979, pp 365-370
21. Jacques S, Shelden CH, McCann GD, et al: Computerized 3-dimensional microstereotactic removal of small central nervous system lesions in patients. Case reports. J Neurosurg 53:816, 1980

CHAPTER 39

Surgical Management of Intracranial Gliomas

Carrie L. Walters   Henry H. Schmidek

DESPITE ADVANCES in detection; surgical techniques; and radiation therapy, chemotherapy, and immunotherapy, the outlook for patients suffering with gliomas remains bleak. Over 50 years ago, Foster Kennedy[1] observed:

> He who cares for the patients suffering from brain tumors must bring to his problem much thought and stout action. There is need also for formidable optimism, for the dice of the Gods are loaded!

Few would argue that surgery will ever be the answer to the cure of gliomas, just as few would deny that the skills of the surgeon have much to offer in the diagnosis and treatment of these lesions. At present, most gliomas are not curable, but they are treatable. Our present-day task is to offer the patient the best surgical and biologic therapy available; our present-day challenge is to unravel the cellular mysteries that constitute the basis of glioma formation.

ASTROCYTOMA GRADES 3 AND 4 (GLIOBLASTOMA MULTIFORME)

Approximately 50 percent of all intracranial neoplasms are gliomas.[4] Of any 100 tumors in this group, 55 are glioblastomas, 20 to 30 grade 1 and 2 astrocytomas, and 5 are oligodendrogliomas.[3–5] Glioblastomas are most common in men aged 50 to 60 years.[6] Rubenstein suggested that glioblastoma multiforme may in fact represent the end stage in the progression of anaplasia in a pre-existing astrocytoma.[3] This tumor grows rapidly, and patients usually seek medical attention within 6 months of the onset of symptoms. If untreated, they have a life expectancy of 2 months from the time of diagnosis.[7,8] The frontal lobe is involved in 36.7 percent of these tumors, the temporal lobe in 33.9 percent, the parietal lobe in 25 percent, and the occipital lobe in 2.2 percent.[6] These tumors characteristically extend along the commissures and fiber tracts within the white matter; conversely, the cortex appears to constitute a relative barrier to spread the tumor. Glioblastomas are multiple in 2.5 to 4.9 percent of cases,[3,9] and bilateral in 11 to 47 percent.[7] Tumors originating above the level of the corpus callosum tend to spread to the opposite hemisphere, resulting in the ''butterfly glioma''; whereas those originating below the level of the corpus callosum spread to involve the basal ganglia.[10] Tumors in the temporal lobe are least likely to spread and theoretically are therefore the most suitable to radical resection. These tumors may invade the cerebral ventricles, but distant metastases are rare without previous surgical intervention.[11–14]

Although these tumors appear encapsulated, their margins are ill defined and infiltrate adjacent gliotic brain tissue.[15,16] These tumors are usually gray or pinkish with firm outer margins, and a softer necrotic center. Cysts may be present and are occasionally multiple. Foci of recent and old hemorrhage also may be seen. A subclass of encapsulated glioblastomas, usually 3 to 5 cm in diameter, grossly circumscribed with a gray-red surface, frequently adherent to the dura, with a propensity to occur in the temporal lobe has been described.[17,18] Bucy found both the quality and duration of survival better in this subgroup of cases than among the infiltrative glioblastomas,[18] a finding that was not confirmed by Davidoff and Feiring.[17]

SUPRATENTORIAL GRADE 1-2 ASTROCYTOMAS

Supratentorially located grade 1-2 astrocytomas comprise approximately 30 percent of intracranial tumors. The onset of symptoms is at age 30 to 40 years in adults[5] and age 6 to 12 years in children, with a male preponderance.[6] Symptoms usually are present for an average of 2 years before diagnosis.[3,19] They are present in the frontal lobe (40 to 50 percent), temporal lobe (31 to 35 percent), parietal lobe (14 to 16 percent), and the occipital lobe (0 to 1.2 percent).[6] Their appearance at the time of surgery is that of ill-defined, firm, sometimes white to pinkish-gray lesions that merge imperceptibly into surrounding brain tissue and obliterate the distinction between cortex and white matter.

CYSTIC PILOCYTIC ASTROCYTOMA OF THE CEREBRAL HEMISPHERES

Cystic pilocystic astrocytoma constitute about 3 percent of hemispheric gliomas and usually presents as a large cyst contiguous with the lateral ventricle and containing a small mural nodule, which enhances on CT scans.[20] The mean age of patients is 18 years and the average clinical history is 14 months. These patients present with seizures (68 percent), headache (63 percent), and vomiting (51 percent). The temporal lobe is involved in 49 percent of the cases, the parieto-occipital lobe in 35 percent, and the frontal lobe in 16 percent. Unlike astrocytomas grades III and IV,[21] neither the patient's age nor radiation therapy are relevant prognostic factors. The important

OPERATIVE NEUROSURGICAL TECHNIQUES
ISBN 0-8089-1862-1

favorable prognostic variable is the total excision of the tumor nodule.[20]

OLIGODENDROGLIOMAS

Oligodendrogliomas represent about 5 percent of intracerebral gliomas,[4,5] particularly in men 30 to 50 years of age.[22,23] Oligodendrogliomas occur most frequently in the frontal lobes (50 percent), often extending to the opposite side, followed by parietal lobes (30.6 percent); and the temporal lobes (19.4 percent of cases)[6] and are frequently in close proximity to the ventricular wall. Occasionally these tumors seed through the CSF to other parts of the nervous system.[22,24,25] Spontaneous intratumoral hemorrhage occurs in approximately 41 percent of cases. Gross calcification is present in 50 percent and histologic calcification is present in 75 percent of cases.

At surgery the tumor appears as a well-defined, globular, occasionally gelatinous mass that often is cystic and hemorrhagic.

Approximately 50 percent of oligodendrogliomas are actually mixed gliomas containing both astrocytic[3] and oligodendrocytic elements.

PREOPERATIVE ASSESSMENT

Cerebral gliomas often present either with mental deterioration, personality change, grand mal seizures, or headache; raised intracranial pressure; or a seizure or focal neurologic deficit. The initial complaint among patients with low-grade astrocytomas in one large series was headache in 32 to 35 percent of the cases, mental changes is 13 to 15 percent, visual failure in 3 to 15 percent, and vomiting in 6 to 8 percent.[6] Forty percent of the patients with glioblastomas had headache, 21 percent had mental changes, 12 percent had dysphasia, 12 percent had hemiparesis, 10 percent experienced vomiting, and 5 percent had miscellaneous symptoms. Headache and mental changes were the initial symptoms in 17 percent of patients with oligodendrogliomas, and hemiparesis was an initial finding in 14 percent. The Brain Tumor Study Group found that in patients with glioblastomas, 31 percent had headaches as an initial symptom, 18 percent had seizures, 16 percent had personality changes, 13 percent motor symptoms, and 7 percent sensory symptoms.[26] Among patients with all grades of gliomas, 38 percent of the National Hospital series had seizures, 35 percent had headache, 16 percent had mental changes, 10 percent had hemiparesis, and 8 percent experienced vomiting.

RADIOGRAPHIC ASSESSMENT

Computed tomographic scans with contrast enhancement involve administering 25.2 g of iodine, which produces an immediate blood iodine level in the adult of 1.5 to 2.5 mg/ml. Since the cerebral volume varies between 2 and 5 percent, the increased attenuation of brain tissue with contrast ranges up to 2 EMI units; however, with disruptions of the blood/brain barrier or increased tumor vascularity, contrast medium seeps into the interstitial spaces resulting in the tumor's enhancement.[27] The horizontal resolution with current CT scanners is 0.5 mm, and the depth resolution is 1.5 mm. Imaging can be performed in coronal, oblique, sagittal, and horizontal planes.

In a recent NCI multicenter study of 1071 brain tumors and the radiographic studies that best detected them, it was found that plain roentgenograms failed to reveal 65 percent of the tumors, radionuclide studies 25 percent of the tumors, plain CT scan (using an EMI Mark I Head Scanner) 7 percent, cerebral angiograms 4 percent, and contrast-enhanced CT scans 3 percent.[28] Considering only gliomas, among centrally placed tumors plain radiographic studies are negative in 63 percent of patients as were 62 percent of the radionuclide studies, 6 percent of the CT scans, 14 percent of the angiograms, and 5 percent of the enhanced CT scans. In the subgroup of supratentorial tumors, 77 percent of the plain roentgenograms were negative, 16 percent of the radionuclide studies were negative, 2 percent of the CT scans were negative, 2 percent of the angiograms were negative, and 2 percent of the enhanced CT scans were negative. Of the infratentorial tumors, 67 percent had negative skull roentgenograms, 40 percent negative radionuclide studies, and none had negative CT scans, enhanced CT scans, or cerebral angiograms. Tumor-specific diagnosis was subsequently confirmed in 85 to 90 percent of the cases based on CT scans and angiograms compared with a histologically accurate diagnosis in 30 to 40 percent of tumors diagnosed from radionuclide studies. False-positive diagnosis occurred in 2.8 percent of 464 cases. Most of these false-positive results were based on CT scans. In all but two of the 13 patients in whom this occurred, the diagnosis was subsequently changed after further nonsurgical evaluation; the remaining two patients underwent surgical exploration and were found to have an infarct in one case and in area of necrotic inflammation in the second case.

Certain CT characteristics provide clues to the nature of the tumor.[29] Calcification and homogeneous enhancement were more frequent in cases of oligodendrogliomas, and cerebral edema less likely than in other gliomas, whereas calcification and hydrocephalus were more frequent in low-grade gliomas, and irregular CT enhancement was more frequent in high-grade astrocytomas (Table 39-1).

The CT scan distinction between an area of cerebral infarct and a brain tumor can be very difficult in that as many as 60 percent of recent cerebral infarcts (1–4 weeks) will show contrast enhancement.[30] In most cases this enhancement will decrease or disappear in an area of infarction, whereas it will either persist or increase in amount in a tumor. The xenon inhalation study performed by having the patient inhale the readily diffusible gas xenon while a CT scan is performed can help clarify whether a tumor or an infarct is present since an infarct will barely increase in density whereas a neoplasm will demonstrate considerable enhancement.[31,32]

In the immediate postoperative period, CT scanning is a routine form of patient assessment. In Saloman's comparing the results of 70 postoperative CT scans with the patient's clinical status, 46 scans were improved or unchanged from preoperatively and these findings paralleled the patient's clinical course. Of 24 scans which had worsened, 62 percent of the patients deteriorated clinically.[33] These studies allow one to detect both the positive effect of surgical treatment in stable postoperative patients as well as alerting the surgeon to CT demonstrated abnormalities mandating reoperation or therapy. Twenty percent of studies showed asymptomatic ventricular enlargement.

In the later postoperative period, incidence of tumor recurrence is diagnosed by the presence of new areas of contrast enhancement and/or an increase in peritumoral edema. Biopsy of the enhancing ring in 7 patients with glioblastoma subjected to surgery and radiation revealed that the enhancing ring

Table 39-1. Gliomas: Incidence of manifestations in each type and grade of tumor

	Astrocytoma (%)		Oligodendroglioma (%)		Total (%)
	Grades 1-2	Grades 3-4	Grades 1-2	Grades 3-4	
Calcification	11 (31)	9 (8)	7 (70)	5 (45)	32 (18)
Edema	30 (83)	106 (90)	5 (50)	10 (91)	151 (84)
Midline shift	31 (86)	95 (81)	8 (80)	9 (82)	143 (80)
Obliteration of ventricle	34 (94)	109 (92)	8 (80)	11 (100)	163 (91)
Hydrocephalus	22 (61)	37 (31)	6 (60)	3 (27)	68 (38)
High attenuation	7 (19)	18 (15)	2 (20)	1 (9)	28 (17)
Total	135	374	36	39	585

Reprinted from Claveria LE, Kendall BE, DuBoulay GH: Computerized axial tomography in supratentorial gliomas and metasteses, in *First European Seminar on Computerized Axial Tomography in Clinical Practice*. Berlin, Springer-Verlag, 1977. With permission of the authors and publisher.

represented viable tumor, whereas a tumor's hypodense center is often cellular necrosis or radiation change.[34] Distinguishing radiation necrosis from recurrent tumor can be difficult. One series, for example, included 3 cases of partial enhancement of a mass lesion indistinguishable from that occurring in previously treated gliomas. A nonspecific avascular mass was seen on the angiograms and this study was not helpful in arriving at a specific diagnosis.[35,36,37] The CT scan appearance of viral encephalitis, AVMs, metastatic brain tumor, cerebral abscess, resolving intracerebral hematoma, and demyelinating disease[32,38] can all present as a mass lesion difficult to distinguish from gliomas.

Computed tomographic scanning after intrathecal administration of metrizamide[38,39] outlines structures encroaching on the basal cisterns. In conjunction with coronal sections this technique is particularly useful in studying the area around the pituitary and parasellar structures.

The Wada intra-arterial sodium amytal test is occasionally used preoperatively in planning surgery in patients in whom resection are planned which could interfere with the patient's language ability.[40] From 150 to 200 mg sodium amytal is injected over 1 to 2 seconds into the internal carotid artery while the patient's speech and motor power are examined repeatedly. If speech arrest occurs at the same time as a transient contralateral hemiplegia speech is localized on the side of the injection. If speech becomes garbled after the onset of the contralateral hemiplegia and the patient is able to resume counting and naming objects within 15 to 20 seconds while the contralateral hemiplegia is still present, speech probably is localized on the opposite side. The same procedure then is performed on the opposite side for verification.

Lee et al. compared MRI and CT scanning with regard to their ability to detect glial tumors and to distinguish between the various histologic grades. In 20 of 28 low grade gliomas, the CT scans showed low attenuation and in 11 of these cases no enhancement after intravenous administration of contrast agent. The MRI studies were abnormal in all 28 cases with the signal abnormality, especially in the T2 weighted scan, often considerably larger than the altered attenuation and contrast enhancement seen on the CT scan.[41] Lee compared the MRI studies of the eight patients with biopsy proven grade III and IV gliomas with those of 28 patients with low grade gliomas/gangliogliomas. The MRI appearances of the two groups were similar, whereas the CT scans of malignant gliomas on the other hand are more likely to show contract enhancement than the lower-grade gliomas. The MRI scan is better at detecting the presence of a glial tumor than the enhanced CT scan, but does not help in

determining its degree of malignancy. At present MRI scanning does not allow one to differentiate edema from tumor infiltration, nor is it possible to distinguish tumor from surgical changes.[41,42] The MRI scan presently is particularly useful in cases in which the CT scans are either normal or equivocal, especially if a lesion is adjacent to where calvarial artifacts are present on the CT scan.

Patronas et al. reported on an experience with 45 patients with histologically proven high-grade astrocytomas studied using positron emission tomography with fluorine)18 (18F))2-deoxyglucose (FDG).[43] This study showed that the mean survival time of patients with tumors exhibiting high glucose utilization was 5 months, whereas patients with lower glucose utilization had a mean survival of 19 months. Enhanced CT scans performed on these patients revealed no consistent features that could be used to distinguish the very aggressive tumors from the less aggressive ones. Lilja et al. reported improved delineation of gliomas from surrounding edema using PET with L-methyl-C-methionine (C-L-methionine) compared with computed tomography, angiography, and in some instances, PET with 68 Ga-EPTA.[44]

High resolution real time intraoperative sonography is a useful modality in localizing tumors; determining their size and boundaries; and distance from the cortical surface, and differentiating cystic from solid neoplasms.[45,46] In addition, this tool can be used postoperatively if an adequate surgical cranial window exists.[46]

OPHTHALMOLOGIC ASSESSMENT

Visual fields should be performed on any patient in whom the tumor or the surgical approach might endanger the optic radiations. The optic radiations carrying visual information from the ipsilateral half of each retina begin in the lateral geniculate body and terminate in the striate cortex on the medial aspect of the occipital cortex. The geniculocalcarine tract leaves the lateral geniculate body and passes through the retrolenticular portion of the internal capsule. The more dorsal fibers subserving the superior retina (inferior visual field) pass directly laterally and posteriorly to enter the portion of the visual cortex that is superior to the calcarine fissure. The ventral fibers (superior visual field), on the other hand, follow a less distinct route and turn forward and inferiorly into the temporal lobe, where they spread out over the tip of the inferior horn of the lateral ventricle before looping backward to run close to the outer wall of the ventricle until reaching the inferior striate cortex. Thus, the more ventral the fiber, the longer is the loop and the greater the chance that it will be damaged either by tumor or by the operative approach. Temporal lobe tumor, except for those located at the temporal tip, frequently produce a complete or partial homonymous superior quadrantanopsia. Occipital tumors usually produce a partial or complete homonymous hemianopsia; however, a superiorly placed tumor can present with an inferior quadrantanopsia just as inferiorly placed tumors can produce a superior quadrantanopsia. Parietal tumors are less likely to produce a discrete field deficit, although large parietal lobe tumors may produce an inferior homonymous quadrantanopsia.

NEUROPSYCHOLOGIC TESTING

Patients undergoing resection of intracranial gliomas should be evaluated by neuropsychologic testing pre- and postoperatively. This is of help in counseling the patient and his or her family and can alert the surgeon to subtle deficits that are difficult to delineate fully on routine neurologic examination.

The complexity of human abilities subserved by the cerebral hemispheres requires that a battery of test should measure (1) sensory perceptual functions (vision, hearing, touch); (2) speed and strength of motor function; (3) complex tests of psychomotor functions (i.e., patients ability to organize an integrate sensory information with the motor output necessary to solve relatively complex problems); (4) language and communications skills; (5) visuospatial abilities of various kinds; (6) areas of abstraction, analytical reasoning, and concept formation; and (7) memory. Since cerebral organization in humans more closely resembles a complex of integrations rather than a set of specific and independent locations of a function, a well-localized disease process can have far-reaching effects on total brain function. When treatments such as radiation and chemotherapy, which are known to effect the total brain, are added, the need for qualitative as well as quantitative assessment of higher brain function is clear. Specifically, one needs to know if there is impairment of cognitive function, to what degree it exists, and how this is going to alter the patient's ability to function in his or her environment. IQ testing alone does not adequately answer these questions. The full-scale IQ tends to return to premorbid or near premorbid levels shortly after insult to the brain; this may occur even when damage is severe and obvious impairment remains.

At our institution, a neuropsychologic evaluation consists of administration of either the Wechsler Adult Intelligence Scale (WAIS) or the Wechsler Intelligence Scale for Children (WISC-R), the Halstead-Reitan neuropsychologic test battery, and the Minnesota Multiphasic Personality Inventory (MMPI).

The Wechsler Adult Intelligence Scale includes a verbal and a performance section and is reported as a verbal IQ, a performance IQ, and a full-scale IQ. The verbal score reflects language function and is indicative of left hemisphere function in a left-brain dominant patient. The performance score reflects the ability to deal with visual spatial relationships, and is thought to be indicative of right hemisphere function. The verbal IQ taps material that is familiar to the patient, some of it falling into the category of overlearned information, whereas the performance subtests are largely unfamiliar or novel tasks.

Verbal IQ test are subdivided into tests of (1) the patient's general fund of information; (2) social judgement and abstractions; (3) mathematical problems presented orally; (4) digit span, which test the recall of a series of digits both forward and backward; (5) similarities between words or objects; and (6) vocabulary, which requires appropriate definition of words.

The performance IQ is divided into five subtests: (1) picture arrangement, which requires the subject to arrange pictures in a proper sequence in order to tell a meaningful story; (2) picture completion, which requires the patient to identify missing parts in a series of pictures; (3) block design, which requires the subject to duplicate spatial configurations shown on cards using a set of colored blocks; (4) object assembly, which requires the subject to put together parts of a puzzle to complete a picture; and (5) digit symbol, which requires the subject to substitute symbols for numbers, using a code that is presented with the test.

In evaluating the WAIS one looks at not only the absolute scores but inconsistencies between the two IQ scores. A difference between the verbal and performance score of 15 to 20 points is considered significant. Verbal IQ is affected primarily by rapidly developing lesions in the left hemisphere or in the acute stages of trauma. Performance IQ, since it entails performing new and unfamiliar tasks, is easily lowered by either right hemisphere lesions or diffuse brain pathology.

While useful in the total evaluation, it should be noted that the WAIS was not developed to assess psychologic consequences of cerebral lesions and that the other tests are more sensitive to the presence of cerebral damage. One of the most noted of these is the Halstead-Reitan neuropsychologic test battery, which looks at the general performance of the individual and categorizes him or her as either impaired or not impaired; is able to detect specific pathognomonic findings such as constructional apraxia; and compares right hemisphere function with left hemisphere function. This comparison of right-versus-left-hemisphere function in a given patient helps control for individual variation in the level of cognitive function; information on age, educational level, and occupation also is considered in the final determination of impairment and degree of deficit. The test battery takes approximately 5.25 hours to administer, and can be done in sections. The battery ranges from procedures that measure an isolated function, such as the Finger Oscillation Test, to highly complex tests, such as the Category Test that judges abstract conceptualization, problem solving, and new learning.

In the Finger Tapping Test the patient depresses as rapidly as possible for a 10-second period a key attached to a counting apparatus. The score is the average of five consecutive trials for each hand.

The Seashore Rhythm Test consists of 30 pairs of rhythmic beats that are presented by a taped recording. The patient must indicate which pairs of beats are the same and which are different. This task requires sustained attention and auditory nonverbal skill. While the latter is primarily a right temporal lobe function, Seashore Rhythm does not consistently lateralize lesions, since decreasing attention span can override the lateralization effects of the test.

The Speech Sound Perception Test utilizes a tape to present 60 spoken nonsense words (the middle phoneme is constant, while the beginning and the ending sounds change, i.e., "theeg" or "zeets"). The patients must identify the "word" spoken by selecting it from four "words" on a written form. Receptive auditory ability, visual recognition of spoken words, and a sustained attention and concentration, which are primarily a left temporal lobe function, are measured by this test.

In the Tactile Performance Test the patient is blindfolded

and at no time is allowed to see the board or the blocks. The task is to place the blocks into the board as quickly as possible. This is done once with the dominant hand, once with the nondominant hand, and finally with both hands. Once the test has been completed and the blocks and boards have been removed, the patient is asked to draw a outline of the board and to draw in as many blocks as he or she can in their appropriate positions. The test requires tactile and kinesthetic feedback, motor movement, some degree of learning, and efficacy in the face of a new problem, and the ability to remember without specifically having been directed to do so. This test is particularly sensitive to parietal lobe function.

The most complex of the tests in the Halstead battery, the Category Test, uses a slide projector to present a number of stimulus situations on screen. An answer panel contains four levers, numbered 1 to 4, and the patient is told that something about the stimulus will suggest a number from 1 to 4. If the patient depresses the correct level, a bell sounds. If the choice is incorrect, a buzzer sounds. The task is to determine through hypothesis testing and trial-and-error learning the underlying principle that determines the correct response. The test is divided into several subtests, each of which has only one principle or solution. The Category Test requires considerable learning efficiency, mental flexibility, abstractive skills, and the ability to identify critical from noncritical aspects of new and unfamiliar situations.

These five tests provide the data for the Halstead Impairment Index and allows one to decide whether or not a patient is brain damaged.

Several other tests and measures complete the Halstead-Reitan battery and are used in the final judgment or determination of impairment, although their scores are not specifically included in the Impairment Index. In the Trailmaking Test the patient's task is to connect circles distributed on a sheet of paper. In part A of this test, the circles are numbered 1 to 25, and are to be connected in order. In part B, there are 25 circles numbered 1 through 13 and lettered A through L. The patient is to connect the circles, alternating between numbers and letters (i.e., 1A2B3C, etc.). This test requires number and letter recognition, visual scanning, motor speed, mental flexibility, and the ability to deal with two separate requirements of a situation simultaneously.

As part of the Lateral Dominance Examination grip strength is measured in kilograms in each hand using dynamometer. An aphasia screening test covers all language functions, and the Sensory-Perceptual Examination tests response to unilateral and bilateral simultaneous stimulation via the tactile, auditory, and visual modalities, and tests for graphesthesia, stereognosis, and finger agnosia.

To evaluate the emotional status of a patient, the Minnesota Multiphasic Personality Inventory provides quantitative scores for individual subjects on the basis of answers to a large number of questions. The test can be scored with respect to normative data on a series of scales that include hypochondriasis, depression, hysteria, psychopathic deviance, paranoia, psychoasthenia, schizophrenia, and hypomania. In addition to these scores, the test also includes validational scales that provide some assistance in judging whether the answers of the subjects are consistent and reasonable and therefore open to valid interpretation.

PREOPERATIVE MANAGEMENT

STEROIDS

Once a glioma is suspected, the patient is placed on anticonvulsants and steroids. The appropriate dose of steroids is determined by trial and error, and must be re-evaluated from time to time as the stage and activity of the disease changes. The conventional dose of steroid to be given for cerebral edema and raised intracranial pressure is 100 mg prednisone or its equivalent per day in divided doses.[47] Dexamethasone has no sodium-retaining properties and a biologic half-life of 2 to 4 days so that if one or two doses are missed, there is less likelihood of adrenal crisis. Neurologic improvement may occur within 4 hours of the administration of the first dose of dexamethasone.[47] The side effects of short-term steroid administration (less than 4 weeks duration) including psychic effects, increased appetite, leukopenia, and hyperglycemia. Long-term administration can lead to hypothalamus-pituitary-adrenal axis suppression, cushinoid appearance, hypertension, psychologic disturbances, growth retardation, osteoporosis, myopathy, infection, poor wound healing, glaucoma, and cataracts. The most immediate effect of steroid therapy is the reduction of cerebral edema. Recently, however, there has been some evidence that particularly high-dose steroid therapy might in and of itself result in tumor inhibition.[26,48,49]

High-dose steroids have been used when conventional dosages have failed. Liberman reported neurologic improvement in 8 out of 11 patients with inoperable brain tumors treated with methylprednisone (200 to 2000 mg/day). The patients had previously been on conventional doses of methylprednisone (80 to 120 mg/day). In 2 of these patients, it was possible to discontinue the steroids after high-dose therapy.

Patients on steroids are maintained on either antacids or cimetidine (Tagamet). There has been concern about confusional states in the elderly with the use of cimetidine.[50] Its advantage is that it can be given intravenously in the perioperative period.

ANTICONVULSANT THERAPY

The average patient who is in no neurologic distress is given a loading dose of diphenylhydantoin (Dilantin), which consists of 600 to 1000 mg in divided doses over 8 to 12 hours. This will provide effective plasma concentrations within 24 hours in most patients.[47] Maintenance therapy is, in most adults, 300 to 400 mg/day. Blood levels are determined periodically and plasma concentrations adjusted to 10 to 20 mg/ml.[51] Chloramphenicol, dicumarol, disulfiram, and isoniazid, and sulthiame can inhibit the inactivation of Dilantin and thus lead to an increase in plasma levels. Conversely, carbamazepine (Tegretol) may lower Dilantin levels. The interaction of phenobarbital and ethanol with Dilantin is variable. Because two of the side effects of Dilantin are gingival hyperplasia and hirsutism, young adults frequently are started on phenobarbital in lieu of Dilantin. The initial daily dose for children is 2 to 3 mg/kg in 2 divided doses, which then can be adjusted as needed for seizure control and as plasma levels indicate. If the seizures persist despite adequate blood levels of either the diphenylhydantoin or the phenobarbital the two then are used concurrently. In cases of temporal lobe seizure, Tegretol frequently is used.

INTRAOPERATIVE MANAGEMENT

Craniotomies for intracranial glioma are performed under general endotracheal anesthesia. All patients are monitored using a Foley catheter, arterial line, ECG, and central venous line. At the beginning of the operation the patient receives intravenous dexamethasone and cefazolin (Kefzol). If the dura is tense when it is exposed, 500 ml of a 20 percent solution of mannitol is administered rapidly. This agent may be supplemented by lasix (30–40 mg IV) given concurrently. The dura is not incised until it is seen to pulsate well, indicate a lowering of the intracranial pressure.

SURGICAL ALTERNATIVES

There are four alternatives in the surgical management of gliomas: (1) External decompression, mentioned as an historical curiosity, involves removing portions of the skull over the site of the tumor and allowing the intracranial contents to herniate through the defect providing temporary decompression.[52] This technique was employed until the 1940s, when more aggressive attempts at tumor removal became feasible; (2) biopsy, (3) craniotomy and internal decompression of the tumor mass until either normal brain tissue is encountered or further dissection encroaches on vital brain tissue; and (4) lobectomy, consisting of the removal of tumor and a margin of adjacent brain.

SURGICAL BIOPSY

The surgical biopsy of intracerebral gliomas allows one to establish the nature of the tumor, drain its cystic components, and instill therapeutic agents into a tumor cavity when that is deemed appropriate. The morbidity of brain biopsies of gliomas has been reduced with the advent of stereotactic biopsy, CT-guided biopsy, and stereotactic biopsy with CT control.[53,54,55] Morbidity has been associated with multiple needle insertions into brain with resultant cerebral edema and hemorrhage. In more recent years, with use of stereotactic guided biopsies and steroids the mortality of biopsy has been reduced to 1 or 2 percent, and morbidity to between 2 and 4 percent.[56–61] Even in stereotactically guided biopsies, however, the histologic diagnosis cannot be made in 12 to 20 percent of patients.[62] Shetter reported on 34 patients biopsied using a stereotactic apparatus and 20 patients biopsied using "freehand" procedures. A positive diagnosis was obtained in 95 percent of the freehand cases and 82 percent in the stereotactic group. The 1 death in the series followed a stereotactic biopsy. No permanent neurologic defects were seen in patients in the stereotactic biopsy group and only 9 percent experienced temporary worsening. This contrasts with a permanent complication rate of 10 percent and transient deterioration of 20 percent in patients undergoing freehand biopsy. Marshall and Langfitt, in their series of 29 patients in whom high-dose steroids (dexamethasone; 40 mg/day or greater) were used in combination with needle biopsy of the glioma and 6000 rad of radiation, reported a median survival of 29 weeks with a mean of 34 weeks and no surgical mortality. Stereotactic biopsy is usually reserved for masses that lie deep within cortical structures (thalamus, basal ganglia); are in the vicinity of the third ventricle or medial temporal lobe; and for situations in which bulk removal would be dangerous and of little significant therapeutic benefit.[63–65]

A major problem of biopsy—either freehand or stereotactic—is that of tissue sampling. It is well known that the more malignant forms of gliomas have less malignant sections within them, frequently at the periphery. With the use of CT scanning in conjunction with stereotactic biopsy, this problem has been all but solved.[66] Using CT imaging with its computer analysis, a trajectory can be planned that allows multiple biopsies to be taken throughout the various densities of the tumor without actually having to remove the needle. Gleason et al. combined stereotactic localization with radiofrequency treatment of brain lesion.[67] Others have used CT scanning in conjunction with the implantation of interstitial radiation such as iridium 192 or iodine 125.[68–70]

INTERNAL DECOMPRESSION

The extent of internal decompression and survival rates in the management of patients with glioblastomas has been compared in several series. These studies have tended to indicate that the more extensive the removal of tissue, the longer the survival in the first 1 to 2 years after surgery; however, by 3 to 5 years groups undergoing radical and less radical surgery have the same survival rates.[8,71] Roth and Elvidge, analyzing their results in 163 patients with glioblastomas undergoing partial removal, achieved a mean survival time of 8.4 months, whereas the 236 patients with "complete" removal survived an average of 11.5 months.[8] The difference in survival in the two groups became progressively less after 6 months, and at 5 years they were the same.

These studies are not supported by those of Weir, who concluded that while the extent of tumor removal in glioblastomas is associated with an increased postoperative survival, this factor is of negligible importance compared with the patient's age and whether the patient received radiation therapy.[21] Hitchcock and Sato also found no difference in survival between patients with glioblastomas who underwent partial removal followed by radiation therapy compared with those who underwent "complete" removal followed by radiation therapy.[7]

The extent of surgical removal compared with survival in astrocytoma grades I and II has been reviewed by Laws et al. In this series of 461 cases of low grade glioma, 356 treated with biopsy, 48 with radical but subtotal removal, and 57 treated by "total" removal, survival at 5 years was 32 percent, 44 percent, and 61 percent, respectively ($P <0.0001$).[72] In this study, age of the patient at the time of surgery was the most important variable in predicting the length of survival.

LOBECTOMY IN THE MANAGEMENT OF CEREBRAL GLIOMAS

FRONTAL LOBECTOMY

When feasible, a formal lobectomy represents the most complete form of surgical removal of cerebral glioma. In the following discussion, the surgical management of a dominant hemisphere glioma will be considered.

Surgical Positioning and Exposure

The patient is positioned on the back with the left shoulder elevated by a sponge wedge, allowing the head to be turned toward the right 20 to 40 degrees (Figure 39-1). A transcoronal skin incision is made behind the hairline, extending the left limb

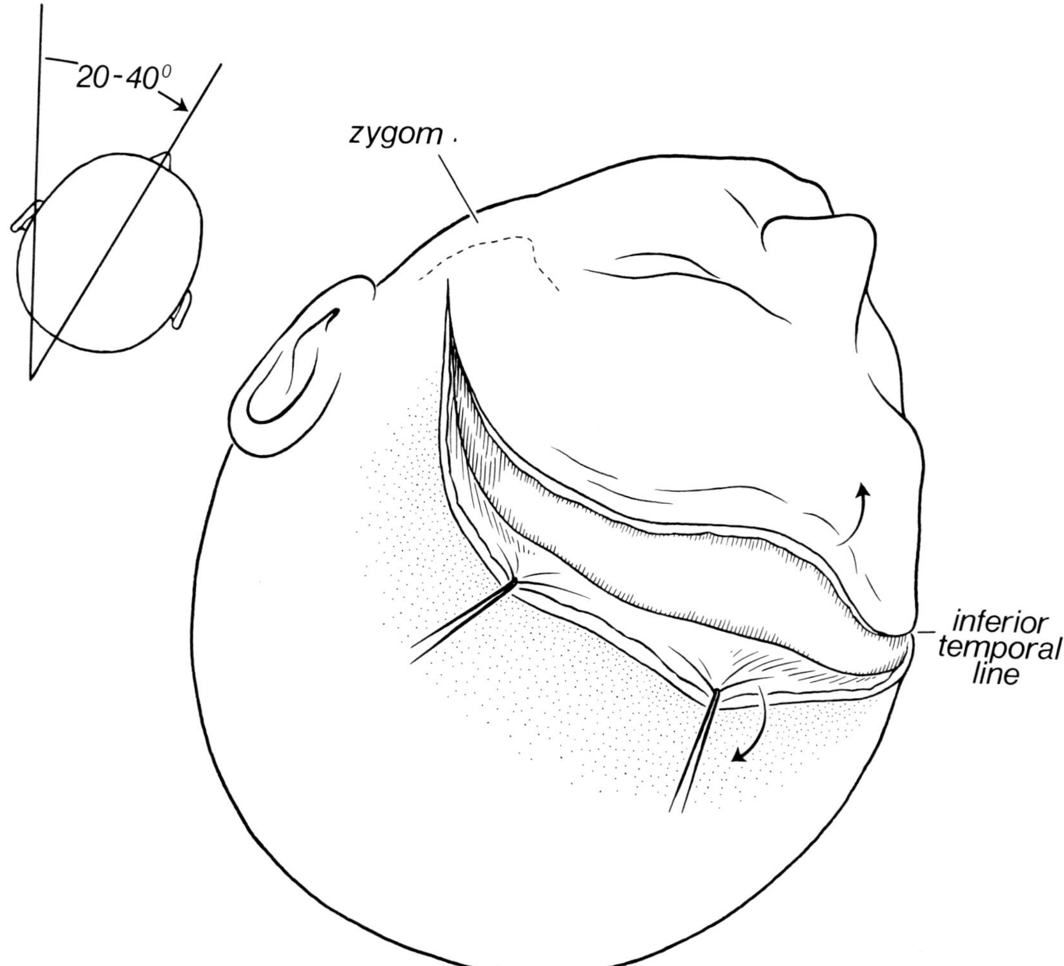

Fig. 39-1. Transcoronal skin incision extending from just above the zygoma on the left to the inferior temporal line on the right. Inset: Patient's position with respect to the surgeon.

of the incision to the zygoma and the right limb to the inferior temporal line (Figure 39-1). The facial nerve courses below the zygoma and is to be avoided (see Figure 39-6). The skin flap is reflected anteriorly over a roll of sponges and is held in place by fishhooks on elastic bands (Figure 39-2). The temporalis muscle is incised with the cautery leaving its insertion into the frontoparietal bone intact (Figure 39-2). It is reflected laterally and covered with a moist sponge. The bone flap is fashioned to allow exposure of the frontal pole and the anterior portion of the sylvian fissure. Burr holes are placed as shown in Figure 39-2. Medially, the bone flap extends to 1 to 1.5 cm lateral to the midline to avoid the superior sagittal sinus and its large draining veins. The posterior medial burr hold (No. 3) is placed immediately behind the coronal suture; the posterior lateral burr hold (No. 4) 1 to 2 cm behind the suture. The inferior burr hole (No. 5) is placed immediately posterior to the pterion. The anterior lateral burr hold (No. 6) is placed medial to the insertion of temporalis muscle with care being taken to avoid entering the orbit. The anterior medial burr hold is placed 1.0 to 1.5 cm lateral to the superior sagittal sinus sand as low on the frontal bone as possible without entering the frontal sinus. The burr holes are connected using a craniotome. At the pterion it may be necessary to use a Kerrison rongeur to negotiate the lateral aspects of its sphenoid wing (Figure 39-3). The bone is removed and the dura is inspected and if it is tense despite preoperative

steroids and intraoperative hyperventilation to a PCO_2 of 25, 500 ml of 20 percent mannitol and 20 to 40 mg of Lasix IV is given as rapidly as possible. If the tumor has a cystic component a small area of the dura over lying the cyst is cauterized and the cyst tapped with a ventricular needle. Once the dura is no longer tension it is opened in a "U" shape medially to protect the sagittal sinus and any draining veins (Figure 39-3). The temporal tip, the sphenoid wing, the inferior frontal gyrus, and Broadmann's area[73] localized in the posterior half of the inferior frontal gyrus are identified. The cortical incision starts 7 to 8 cm from the frontal pole and extends laterally to the level of the lesser wing of the sphenoid. The pia-arachnoid is coagulated with the bipolar forceps and cut with fine scissors. Large cortical vessels are isolated and coagulated. (Figure 39-4). The gray and white matter then are sectioned with a metal suction tip. It is important to keep the plane of dissection at the same depth throughout the length of the incision. Lining the posterior wall of the resection plane with moist cotton strips, the portion of the frontal lobe to be removed is retracted with a broad brain retractor. When the medial veins draining into the superior sagittal sinus are coagulated and sectioned, care should be taken to divide them close to the brain and not the sinus. As the incision is carried toward the base of the frontal lobe, the lateral ventricle will be entered. To prevent bleeding into the ventricle a cotton ball should be placed over gently over the ventricle.

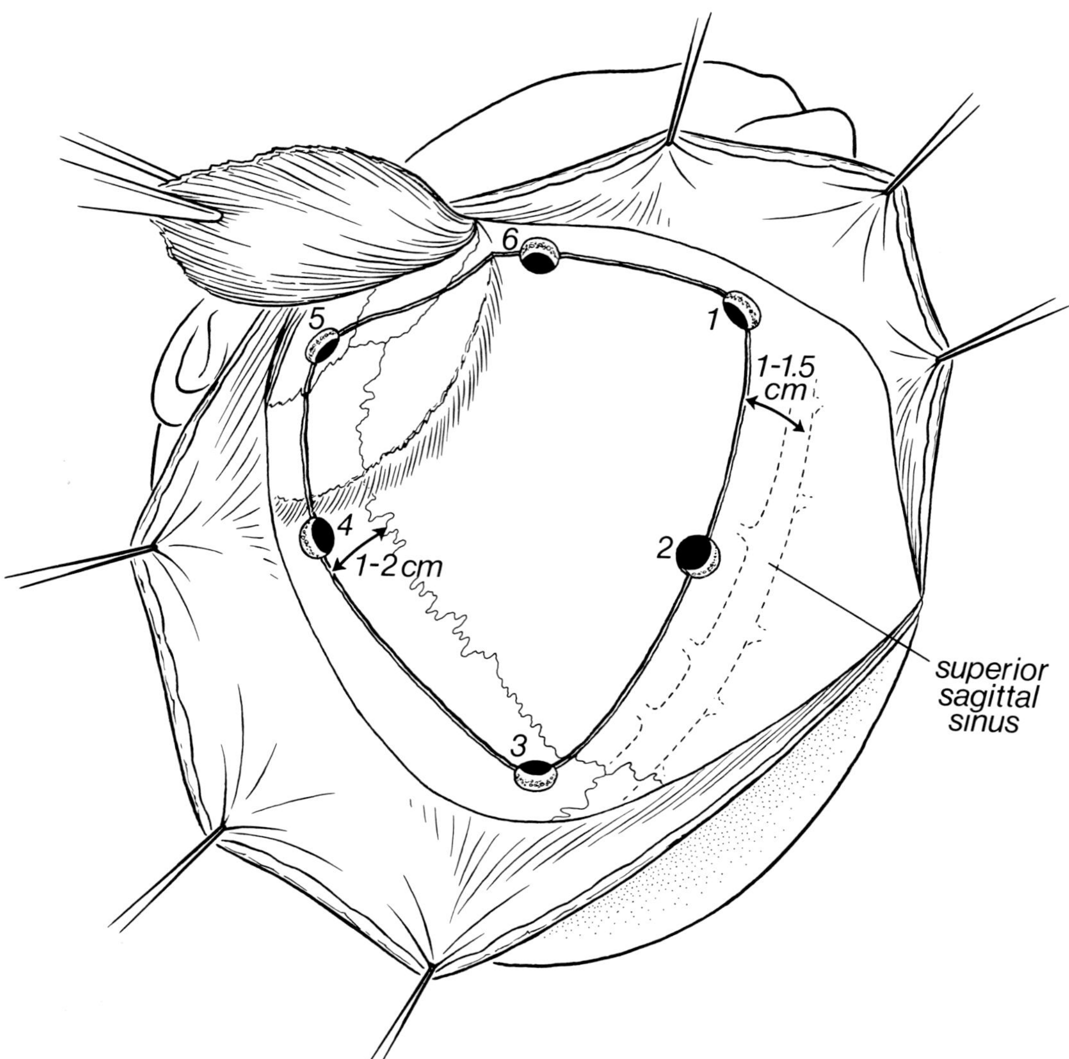

Fig. 39-2. Placement of the burr holes for a frontal bone flap after the temporalis muscle has been reflected laterally. Medial extent 1 to 1.5 cm lateral to the superior sagittal sinus.

Should it not be desirable to open the ventricle, the medial aspect of the cortical incision is made at the level where the two hemispheres are clearly separate. This approach is anterior to the corpus callosum, the ventricle, and the anterior cerebral artery. To carry out a more complete lobectomy, for low-grade or high-grade tumors whose margins can be circumvented by such a resection, the anterior cerebral arteries from both sides must be identified. The ipsilateral frontopolar artery on the medial surface of the frontal lobe is then divided near the cortical surface. The contralateral frontopolar artery must be avoided. This artery is near the midline and easily can be mistaken for its opposite counterpart (Figure 39-5). As the floor of the frontal fossa is approached, the olfactory tract lying in the olfactory groove is encountered. To avoid bleeding and the possibility of opening the cribriform plate and a CSF leak, this structure should be left in place. The frontal tip is now held only by the draining veins over the medial orbital surface and the tip of the frontal lobe. These vessels are coagulated and divided. If the tumor extends caudal to the line of resection, additional tumor is removed by suction, leaving the more infiltrating margins alone to prevent further injury to functioning brain. Following removal of the resected tissue the entire cavity is filled with wet cotton balls, to which suction is applied. These are left in place several minutes. Just before removal, they are irrigated with saline to prevent small vessels from adhering to the cotton. After removal, obvious remaining bleeding points are coagulated. The raw surface of the frontal lobe may be covered with Avitene. The fluffy cotton is removed from the ventricle. The dura is closed in a watertight fashion. Before the last several stitches are placed the cavity is filled with saline to prevent air from remaining in the ventricle. An epidural Jackson-Pratt drain is left in place in the epidural space and the bone flap replaced. The reflected temporalis muscle is sutured to the muscle left on the bone flap. A separate linear skin incision and burr hold are placed adjacent to the craniotomy for placement of an epidural Ladd pressure switch (Ladd Instrument Co., Burlington, Vermont). This allows for monitoring of the intracranial pressure in the postoperative period.

Potential Postoperative Deficits

The frontal lobectomy described above is designed to avoid the motor strip and Broca's speech area. Patients undergoing frontal lobectomy usually have no noticeable postoperative deficits. It is possible however, for such a patient to show some

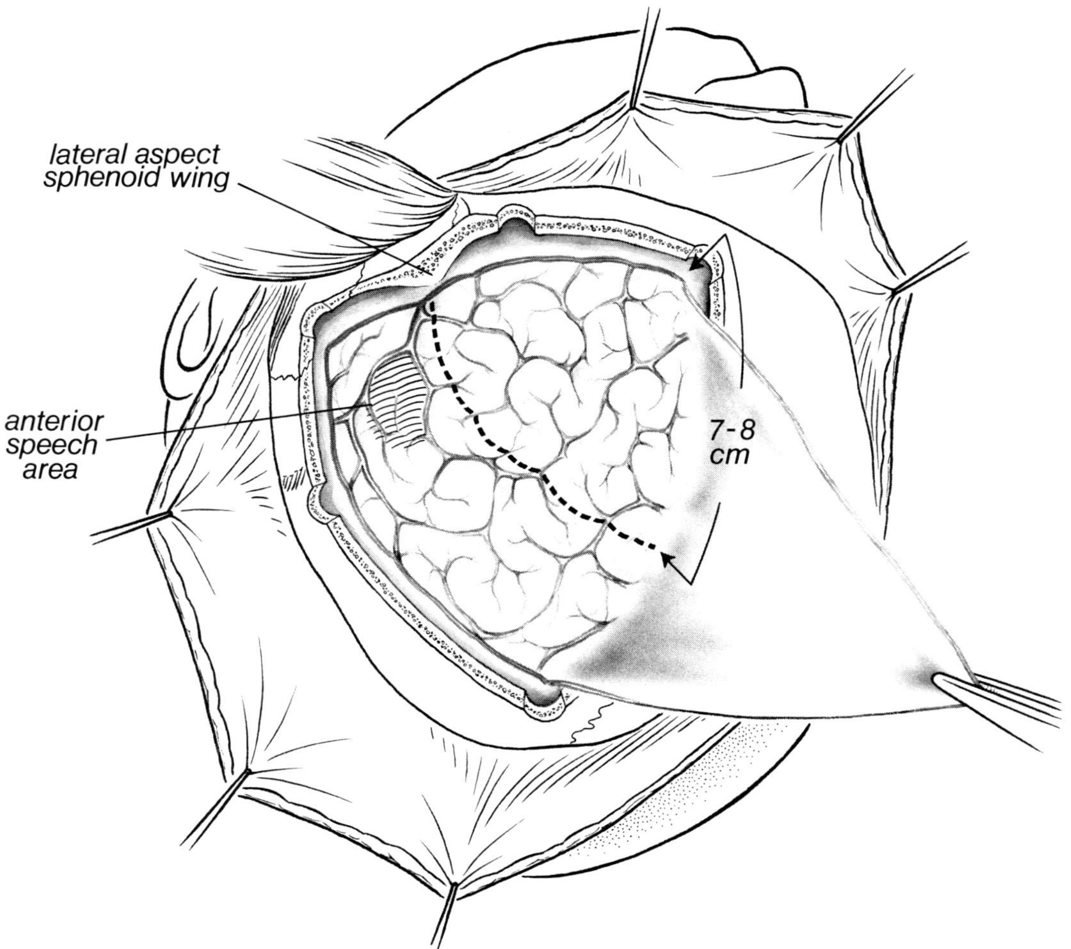

Fig. 39-3. Line of incision showing the relationship of the anterior speech area to the lateral aspect of the sphenoid wing.

signs of apathy and general slowing of the intellect, especially if the lobectomy has been done on the dominant hemisphere. Occasionally, impairment of recent memory and of voluntary and serial memorization can occur.[74] While lesions limited to the frontal pole region do not result in motor paresis or paralysis, voluntary and more complex control can be impaired. The "high motor deficit" usually presents itself with difficulty with serial, alternate, or novel tasks.[74]

TEMPORAL LOBECTOMY

A temporal lobectomy is usually performed with the patient's body in either full lateral or three-quarters lateral position, using a wedge-shaped sponge and blanket under the axilla. These positions allow the head to be at full lateral (Figure 39-6). Care must be taken to protect the brachial plexus. The question-mark skin incision is used, starting above the zygoma, passing along the anterior margin of the pinna, and curving posteriorly so the incision is 3.5 cm behind the external auditory meatus (Figure 39-6). This incision spares the branch of the facial nerve to the frontalis muscle and the superficial temporal artery. The scalp flap is reflected anteroinferiorly over a roll of gauze and is held in place by fishhooks. The temporalis muscle may be dealt with either as a separate flap or as part of an osteoplastic flap. If the former is chosen, electrocautery is used to incise the muscle approximately 0.5 cm from its line of insertion. It then is reflected laterally and placed under the same

fishhooks as the skin. The burr holes are placed as with the osteoplastic flap and connected by craniotome. The free flap is removed and set aside until the end of the craniotomy. If an osteoplastic flap is chosen, three incisions are made in the temporalis muscle, allowing burr holes to be placed beneath it (Figure 39-6). Two additional burr holes are placed above the muscle (Figure 39-6). The anteroinferior burr hole is placed just posterior to the outer canthus of the eye and anterior to the pterion, allowing exposure of the anterior tip of the temporal lobe. The inferior-most burr hole is placed above the zygoma. Burr holes are connected when necessary by rongeuring bone beneath the temporalis muscle (Figure 39-7A). The remaining bone is fractured and the bone flap reflected while hinged on the temporalis muscle (Figure 39-7B). The bone flap is reflected inferiorly and the remaining temporal bone is removed to the floor of the middle fossa (Figure 39-7B). The middle meningeal vessels are coagulated. The dura is opened several millimeters from the bony edge and reflected anteroinferiorly over the temporalis muscle (Figure 39-8A). A moist sponge is placed over the dura and anchored in place behind the skin flap. The cortical resection can involve removal of the anterior 5 to 6 cm of the temporal lobe; or alternatively, the vein of Labbé may be used as a landmark for the posterior extent of the resection. Both, however, can be misleading because of the variability of the position of the vein of Labbé and the size of the temporal lobe. More consistent landmarks therefore are recommended. The junction of the rolandic and sylvian fissures is the most

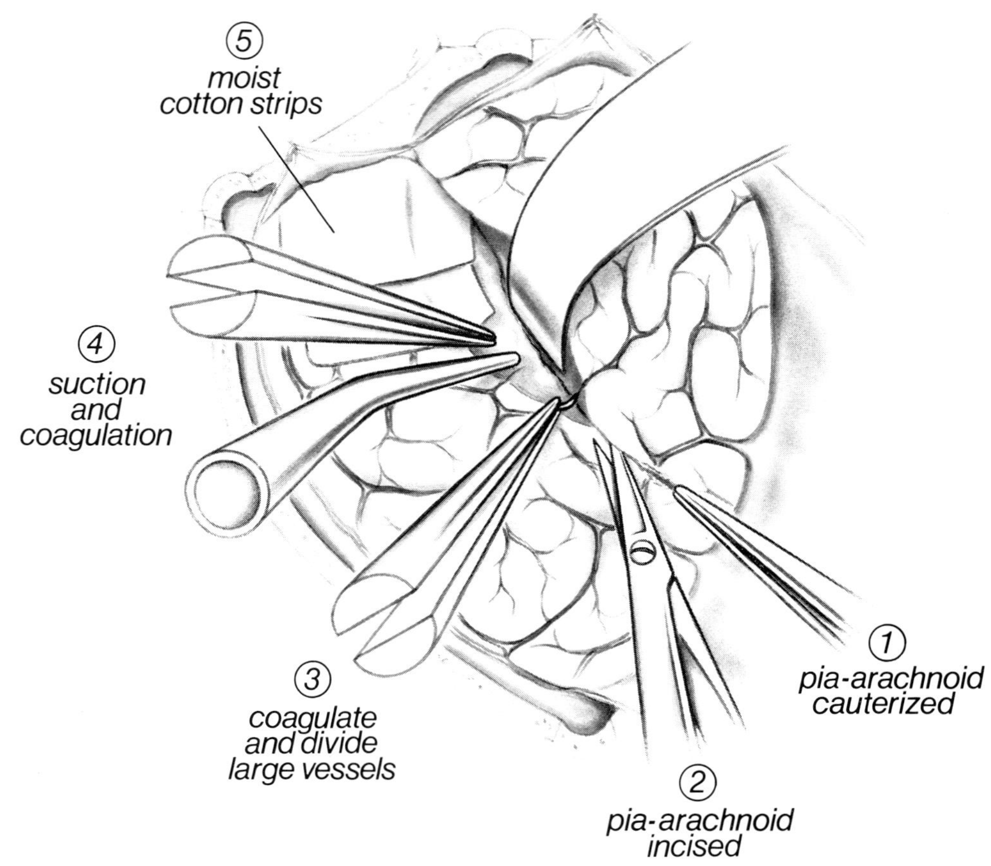

Fig. 39-4. Steps in performing a cortical resection; see text for details. Note moist cotton strips protecting area of brain to be left.

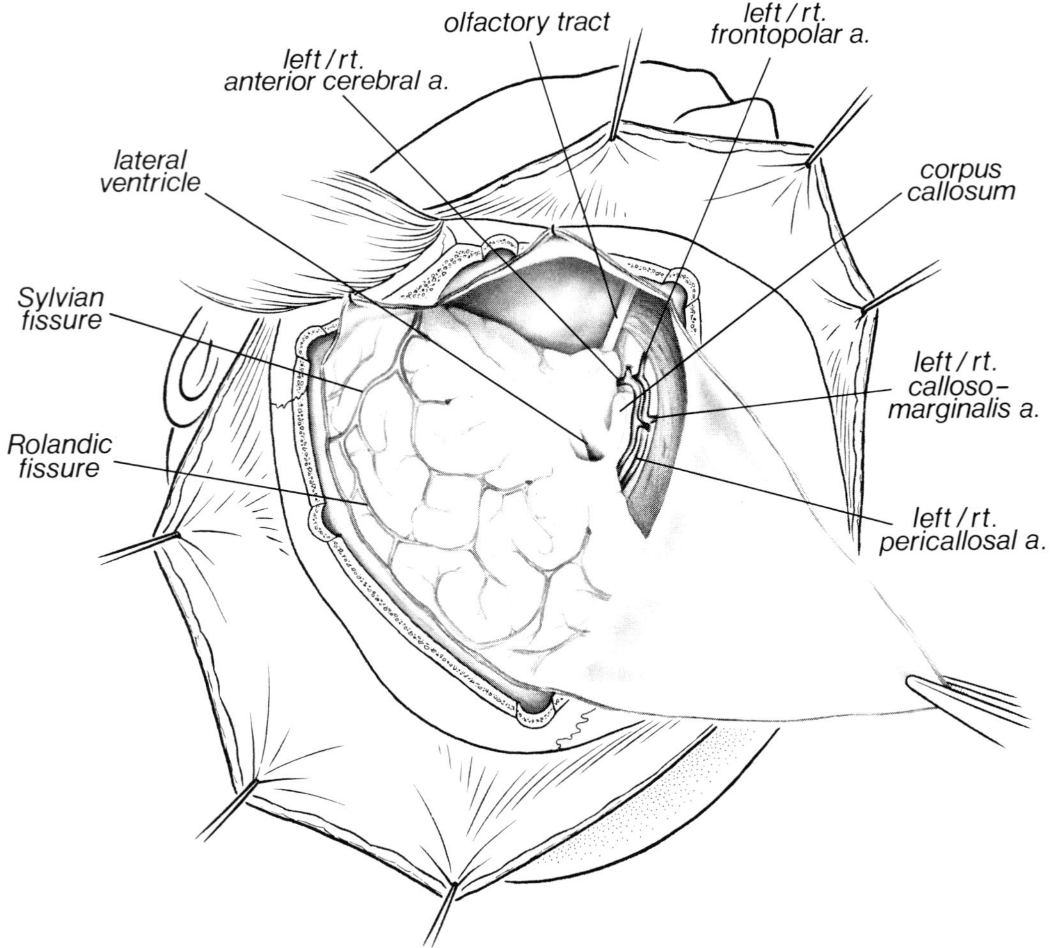

Fig. 39-5. Structural relationships at the base and medial aspect of the frontal fossa after removal of the frontal tip.

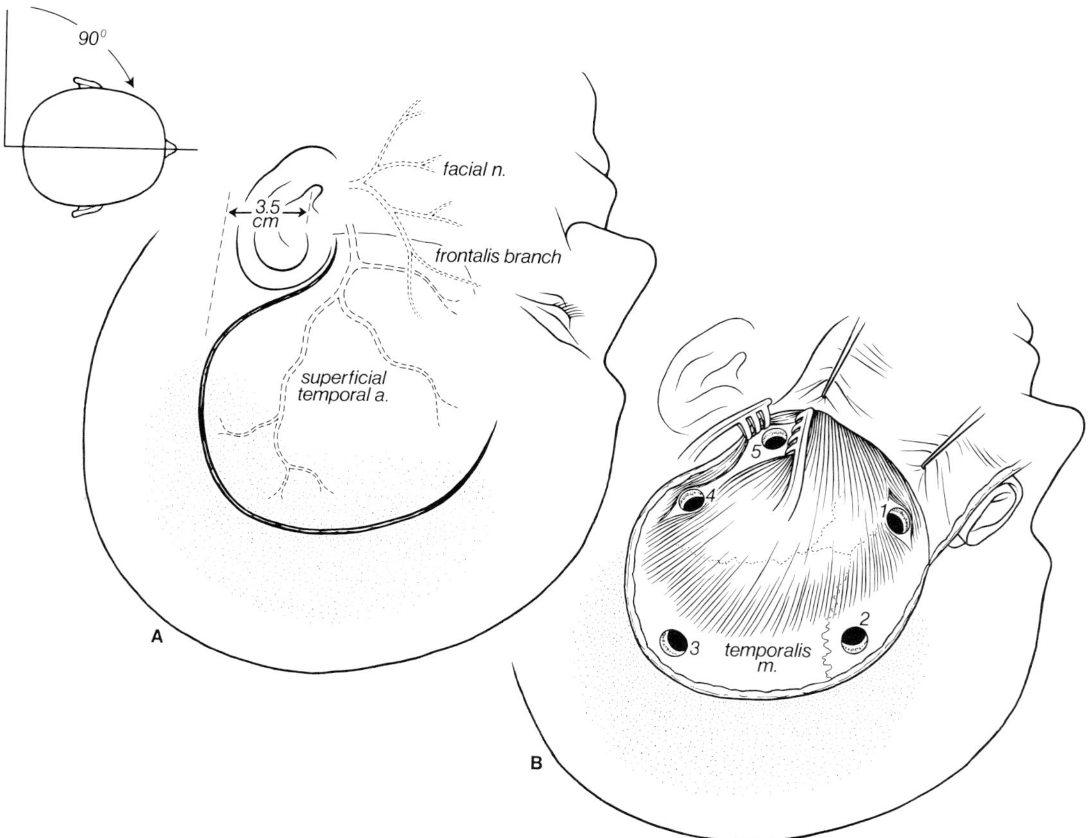

Fig. 39-6. (A) Skin incision for a left temporal lobectomy. Note position of zygoma, superficial temporal artery, and facial nerve. (B) Placement of burr holes for an osteoplastic flap. Inset: position of the patient relative to the surgeon.

reliable. The first and second temporal convolutions posterior to that intersection are to be avoided. When starting the cortical dissection along the superior temporal gyrus it is best to leave a thin layer of the superior temporal gyrus cortex to protect the middle cerebral vessels (Figure 39-8A).

The dissection is started at the anterior edge of the first temporal gyrus and carried posteriorly to the junction of the rolandic and sylvian fissures, where the line of incision turns inferiorly and across the middle and inferior temporal gyri. As the dissection is carried medially through the superior temporal gyrus one incises the pia-arachnoid, gray matter, minimal white matter, and the pia-arachnoid overlying the insula. The dissection proceeds so as not to cross the deep pia-arachnoid barrier protecting the insula and the middle cerebral vessels (Figure 39-9). Failure to do so can lead to postoperative hemiparesis. After the insula has been exposed, the dissection is carried into the white matter of the temporal stem. Once into the temporal stem the incision is directed downward through the uncus to the floor of the middle fossa. Attention is then directed to the posterior portion of the incision, which is extended from the superior temporal gyrus on the inferior aspect of the temporal lobe (Figure 39-9). The temporal horn is entered and dealt with as described above. As these two incisions meet on the inferior surface of the temporal lobe, the resection is complete; the draining veins, however, are still in place.

To allow maximum venous drainage and to prevent edema secondary to venous stasis, it is preferable to leave as many draining veins as possible until this stage of the procedure. At this time the bridging veins over the anterior part of the

temporal lobe are coagulated and out near the brain as are the medial and inferior veins which drain into the cavernous sinus on the undersurface of the temporal lobe. Once the lobe is excised, the resultant cavity is dealt with as previously described. If the tumor extends toward the uncus, it is possible to remove the parahippocampal gyrus and the lateral aspect of the uncus. The medial aspect of the uncus is left in place to protect the optic tract. If the dissection is carried this far medially care must be taken to preserve the third nerve, the posterior cerebral artery, and the cerebral peduncle (Figure 39-9). The transverse temporal gyrus of Herschl on the superior surface of the temporal lobe also is left intact. On nondominant temporal lobe resections, the posterior extent of the cortical incision can be carried out to the supramarginal and angular gyri. Closure of the wound is carried out as previously described.

OCCIPITAL LOBECTOMY

Surgical Positioning and Exposure

The three-quarters prone position or a semi-sitting may be used for easy access to the midline (Figure 39-10). With the face down, care must be taken to protect the patient's eyes. The skin incision starts in the midline at the superior nuchal line, is carried forward on the midline, and swings laterally to end just below the squamosal suture (Figure 39-10). The skin flap is reflected inferiorly to preserve the occipital artery and the greater and lesser occipital nerves. Burr holds for the bone flap are made 1 cm lateral to the midline, 1 cm above the transverse

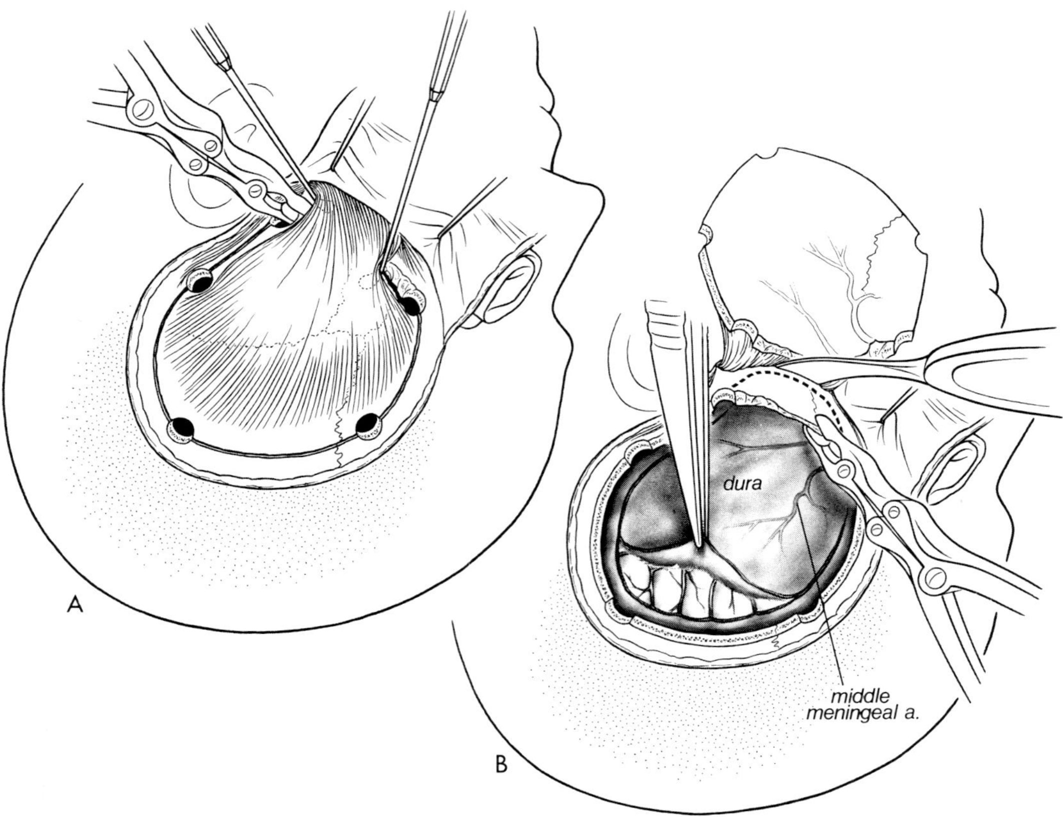

Fig. 39-7.   (A) Connecting burr holes No. 1 and No. 5 beneath the temporalis muscles to allow muscle to remain intact. (B) Removal of remaining temporal bone to expose inferior to lateral aspect of temporal bone. Dura reflected laterally after coagulation of middle meningeal artery.

sinus inferiorly and in the posterior superior portion of the temporal bone (Figure 39-10). A free bone flap is removed. The dura is opened in a "T" fashion to allow reflection toward both the superior sagittal sinus and the transverse sinus (Figure 39-11). In the dominant hemisphere the cortical incision is started 3.5 cm from the occipital tip on the superior cortical margin to avoid damage to the angular gyrus. On the nondominant side, it is started 7 cm from the occipital tip (Figure 39-11). The cortical incision and subpial dissection is performed as previously described (section on frontal lobectomy). The occipital horn of the lateral ventricle may or may not be entered. It is covered with cotton fluffs. As the calcarine fissure is approached, the posterior cerebral artery can be seen in its depths (Figure 39-12). This is coagulated and divided. Before removing the occipital lobe, the draining veins that enter the torcular must be coagulated and sectioned near the cortex. Following removal of the occipital lobe the cavity is filled with saline and the dura closed. The remainder of the operation follows general neurosurgical practices. Following occipital lobectomy the patient will have a contralateral homonymous hemianopsia. In the dominant hemisphere, damage to the cerebral hemisphere in the area of the junction of the parietal, occipital, and temporal lobes can produce dyslexia, dysgraphia, and acalculia. Van Buren has mapped the cortical areas in which electrical stimulation causes interference with speech and has shown that these extend into the angular and supramarginal gyri.[75] The position of the angular gyrus then was measured in 10 cadavers. The distance from the angular gyrus to the occipital pole is 3.5 cm and from the angular gyrus to the parietal-occipital midline is 2.4 cm

(Figure 39-11).[75] In the dominant hemisphere, damage to the angular gyrus, Wernicke's area, and the surrounding parietal temporal cortex (Figure 39-13) leads to deficits in recognition of complex visual and auditory symbols, including those of written and spoken language, defects in the visual-spatial-body image, and severe communication abnormalities. The general deficit is a profound asymbolia.

DECOMPRESSION WITHOUT LOBECTOMY

Although not amenable to lobectomy, a glioma that occurs in areas of important neurologic function should be considered for radical removal. This position is adopted for several reasons: first the tumor mass may displace vital areas without actually infiltrating them,[19] so that dysphasia and hemiparesis caused by local compression and edema can be improved. Second, if the tumor has infiltrated vital areas and rendered them nonfunctional their surgical removal, if one stays within the limits of grossly evident tumor, should not increase the patient's neurologic deficit.

EXPOSURE

When operating on tumors of the dominant temporal lobe, Broca's area, or the motor strip, the exact location of the tumor will determine the specific placement of the craniotomy. For example, in the case of a posterior temporal parietal tumor, a modification of the approach used for either temporal

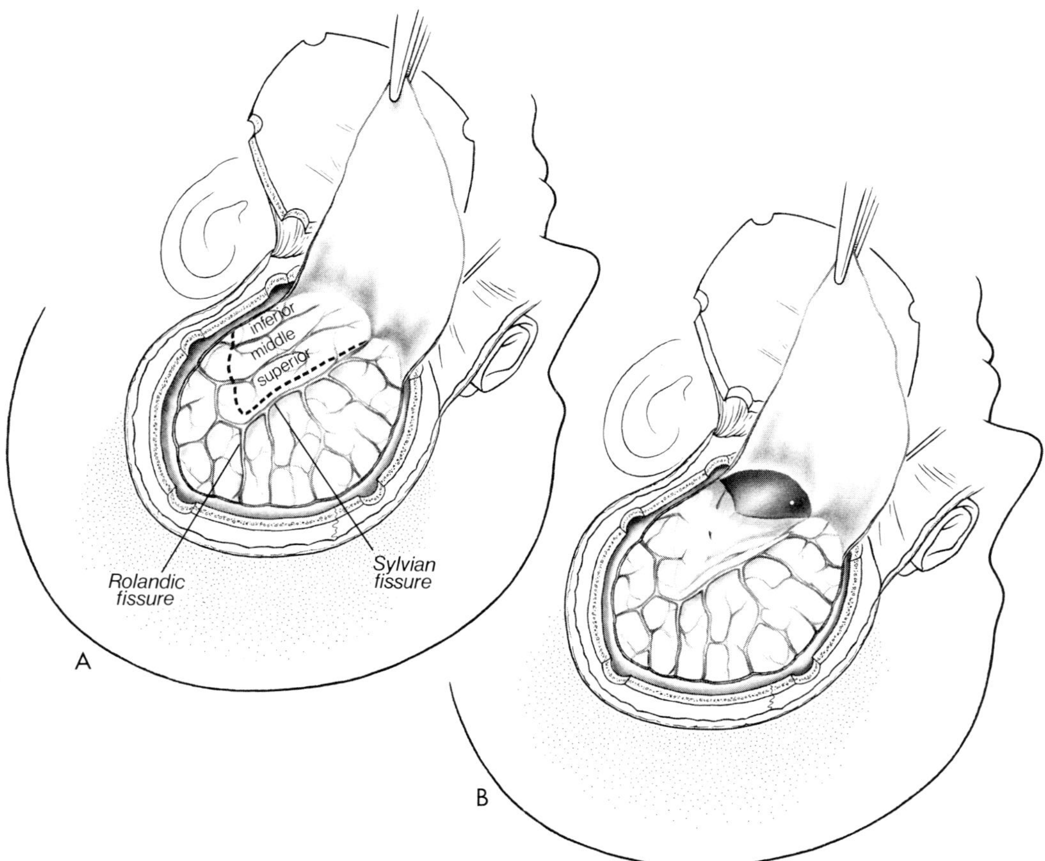

Fig. 39-8. Left temporal lobectomy. (A) Cortical incision, sparing posterior speech area and middle cerebral vessels (see text). (B) Operative site after removal of tissue.

lobectomy or occipital lobectomy may be used. Tumors located in Broca's area can be approached either through a modification of the craniotomy used for frontal or temporal lobectomy. For tumors beneath the motor strip, a rectangular skin and free bone flap craniotomy centered over the tumor is preferred. After the skull is opened, the dura is reflected superiorly to protect the sagittal sinus. Upon opening the dura, the cortex is inspected. Rarely, a tumor nodule will be present on the surface, or in the case of a subcortically located tumor, which is more common, gyri may be widened over the tumor. Equally frequent, however, are broadened gyri secondary to edema in the cortex adjacent to the tumor. Gentle palpation of the cortex with a moistened, gloved finger is occasionally helpful, but often edema is mistaken for solid tumor. Using the CT scan, angiography, MRI or intraoperative sonography, the tumor usually can be located to within 1 to 2 cm. After the tumor is located, a small cortical incision is made either anterior or posterior to the motor cortex (or other vital cortical area), and a blunt brain cannula is inserted searching for areas of increased or decreased consistency. Once the tumor is located, the cortical excision is expanded. Biopsies then are taken and sent for frozen section analysis of both the peripheral and central portions of the tumor. If the tumor is destructive and necrotic, the resection may extend directly into motor and speech areas if the surgeon remains within the tumor mass. The necrotic and softened portions of the tumor are best removed by routine suction, or the ultrasonic aspirator. If the tumor is infiltrative and firm with the anatomy of the brain preserved, resection should not be undertaken. In this instance an adequate decom-

pression can usually be obtained by removal of the tumor up to but not within the vital area. If the infiltrative nature of the tumor precludes removing most of it, removal of adjacent frontal, temporal, or occipital tissue may provide necessary internal decompression.

If the tumor is cystic upon initial insertion of the cannula, enough fluid is drained through the cannula to decompress the brain. Once the cyst is opened through the cortical incision, retractors are gently inserted into the interior of the cyst, which is inspected for tumor nodules. If these are present the nodule and the surrounding cyst wall is excised, hemostasis is established, and the dura closed. For patients in whom an adequate internal decompression is not possible, monitoring intracranial pressure for several days is essential. In these patients an epidural pressure switch is inserted prior to closure of the craniotomy.

POSTOPERATIVE CARE

Following craniotomy, patients are routinely nursed in a surgical intensive care unit for 1 to 3 days depending on their condition. This allows for constant monitoring of the patients' general and neurologic condition and of their ICP. Epidural and subdural drains are routinely removed on the first postoperative day unless there has been considerable drainage, in which case they remain for 14 to hours. All patients remain on dexamethasone at a dose of 4 to 10 mg every 6 hours for the first 3 days and then are tapered as tolerated down to a level of 2 mg

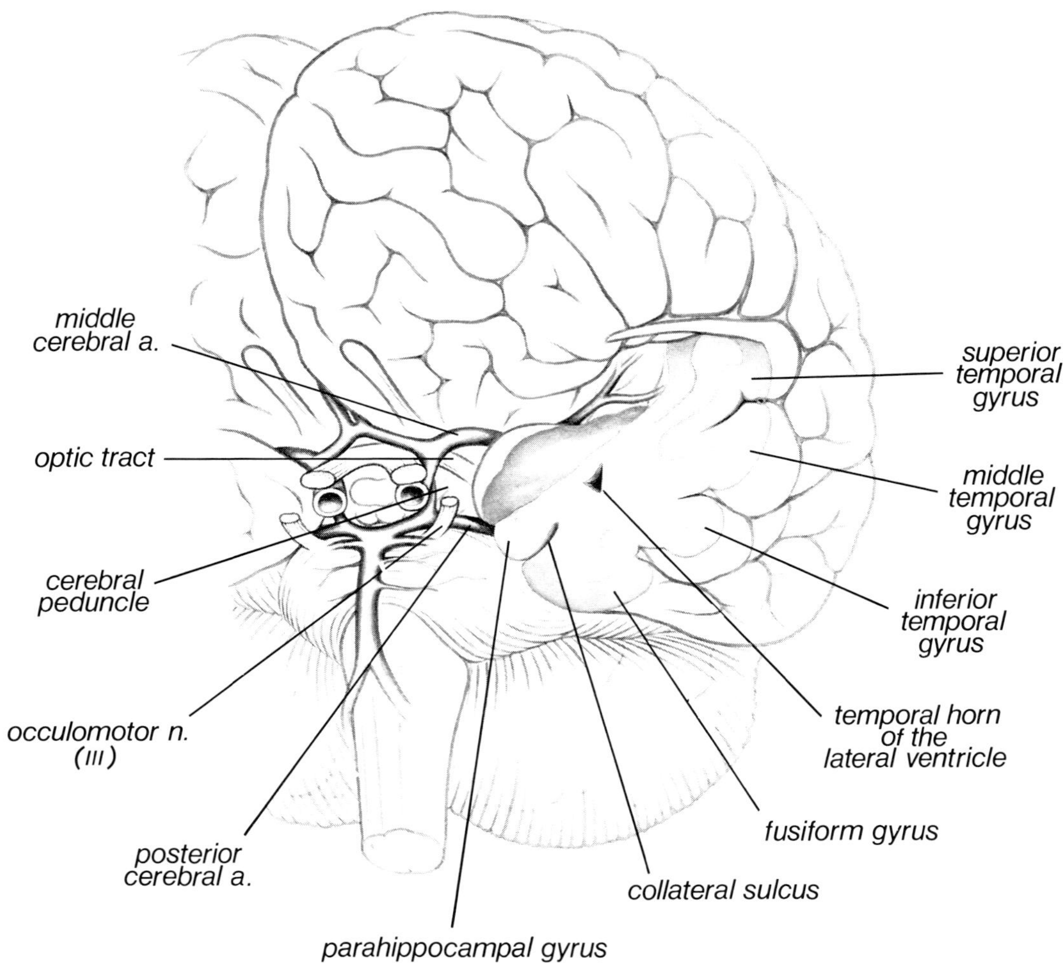

Fig. 39-9. Basal to lateral view of the left side of the brain with partial temporal lobectomy. Note proximity of the middle cerebral artery, optic tract, oculomotor nerve, posterior cerebral artery, and cerebral peduncle to medial extent of the incision.

q.i.d. They remain on this dosage through radiation therapy unless the neurologic signs and symptoms increase, at which time the dosage may be increased. In the usual case the ICP switch is removed when the values registered are consistently under 20 mm Hg. An elevated intracranial pressure or a worsening in the patient's neurologic status mandates an immediate CT scan to exclude a postoperative hematoma, acute hydrocephalus, or massive cerebral edema. Given a major elevation of ICP or neurologic deterioration while investigative procedures are being undertaken, one should consider among the treatment options reintubation and hyperventilation, intravenous lasix (20 to 40 mg) intravenous mannitol (0.25 to 2 g/kg) and increasing the dexamethasone (25 to 100 mg IV). If a surgical lesion is identified, it is dealt with; if no surgical lesion is found the patient continues on the treatment as outlined above. If the ICP is not responsive to medical management, removal of the bone flap, particularly in low-grade gliomas, is considered.

A CT scan is routine performed within the first postoperative week even in the case of an uneventful recovery. This serves as a baseline before beginning other forms of therapy. Sutures in most instances are removed at 1 week, and radiation therapy is started. Neuropsychologic testing is often repeated before the patient is discharged.

REOPERATION FOR CEREBRAL GLIOMAS

The concept of reoperation for cerebral gliomas originated with Cushing.[76,77] He described patients who had a tumor removed and then subsequently underwent a second operation for removal of a recurrence. One such patient had 6 operations.

Since the advent of the CT scan several series have addressed the issue of reoperation in management of patients with anaplastic gliomas. Young reported on 24 reoperated patients with astrocytoma grades III or IV whose median survival time after reoperation was 14 weeks.[78] The most important prognostic factor was the Karnofsky rating (KR) at the time of the second operation.[79] Patients with a score of 60 or greater had a median survival time after the second surgery of 22 weeks. Patients with a KR of less than 60 had a median survival time of 9 weeks. Age, sex, and location of tumor were not significantly correlated to the duration of survival. This is in contradistinction to Soloman, who reported on 40 reoperated patients with glioblastoma.[80] Median survival after the second operation was 37 weeks; neither the patient's KR, tumor grade, interoperative interval, nor age significantly effected the outcome. The influence of age on total survival was also reflected in the patients undergoing reoperation, median survival after the second operation was 36 weeks for the 23 patients over 40 and approximately 55 to 60 weeks for the 17 patients under 40;

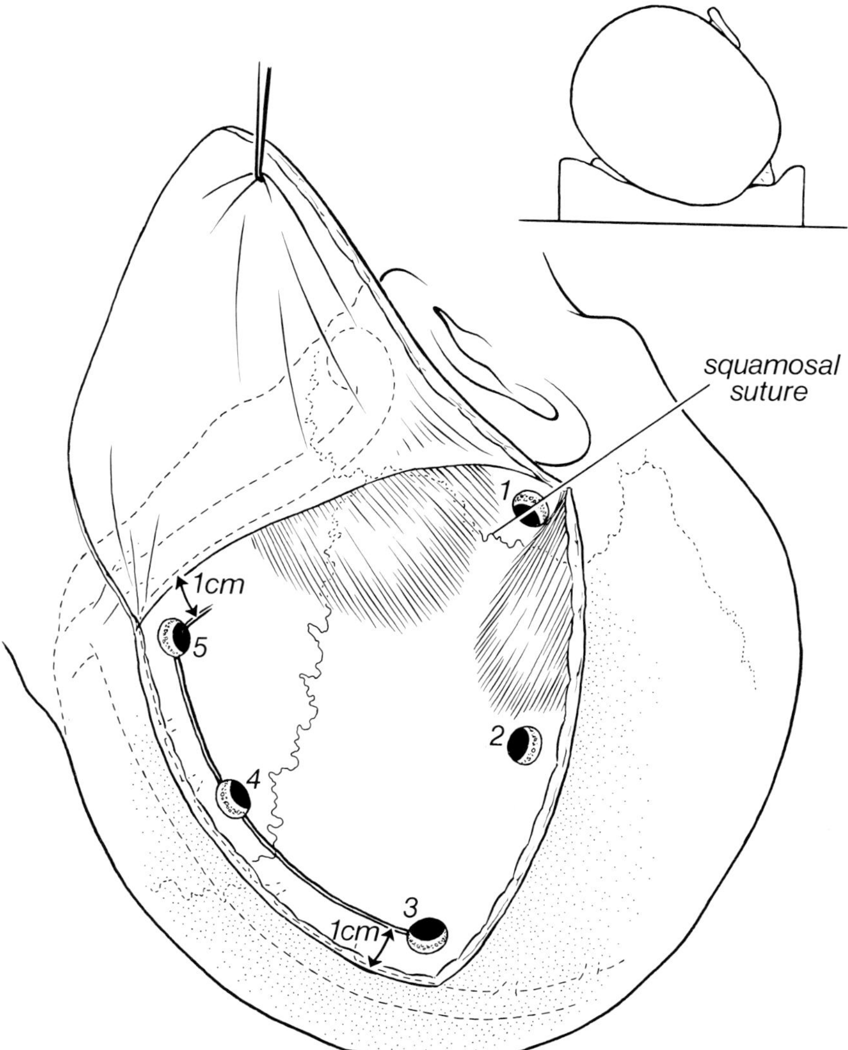

Fig. 39-10. Occipital lobectomy skin incision and burr hole placement. Inset: Patient's posotion with respect ot the surgeon.

however, survival after the second operation was not significantly different in young and old patients. Harsh reported a series including 39 patients with glioblastoma and 31 patients with anaplastic astrocytomas. Median survival for patients with glioblastoma was 35 weeks, 11 of the patients had a KR or 70 or greater, and 84 weeks for patients with anaplastic astrocytomas. For patients with glioblastomas, both age and preoperative KR had a statistically significant effect on the duration of postoperative high quality survival but not on postoperative survival independent of quality; for anaplastic astrocytomas only age was significant.[81]

Reoperation can improve severe neurologic deficits if the recurrent tumor is compressing and not infiltrating vital structures. Starting the patient on high-dose steroids for several days frequently can help to distinguish between neurologic deficits secondary to edema and compression and deficits caused by structural damage from the infiltrating tumor. Curable lesions such as cyst, abscesses, and, less frequently, resolving hematoma can be mistaken for tumor recurrence even with today's sophisticated radiologic techniques and should enter into the decision of whether or not to reoperate. Delayed radiation necrosis of the brain can also be mistaken for recurrent tumor.[35–37,82] Diagnostic studies are rarely helpful in distinguishing between the two since they both may elevate CSF protein, appear on a radionuclide brain scan as an area of increased uptake, produce focal delta slowing of the EEG, present angiographically as an avascular mass, and appear as a hypodense area on the CT scan. Patients with delayed radiation necrosis often respond to steroid therapy as do those with recurrent gliomas. Unfortunately, it is not possible at the present time to distinguish between the two without a biopsy, and if the radiation necrosis has resulted in a swollen, necrotic brain, surgical excision of part of the brain may be necessary to save the patient's life. If, however, the mass is small and the patient is not in danger of herniation, a trial of dexamethasone may carry the patient over the period of maximum swelling and make surgery unnecessary. There have been reports of even large masses secondary to radiation necrosis resolving without surgery, while some patients continue to deteriorate despite surgery and steroids.[36] The history of the standard brain tumor dose of 5000 to 7000 rad being fractioned at greater than 200 rad per day should alert one to the possibility of radiation necrosis.[36]

Some technical points regarding the surgical technique in a second surgical approach deserve consideration. If possible, the same skin flap as that used for the initial surgery should be

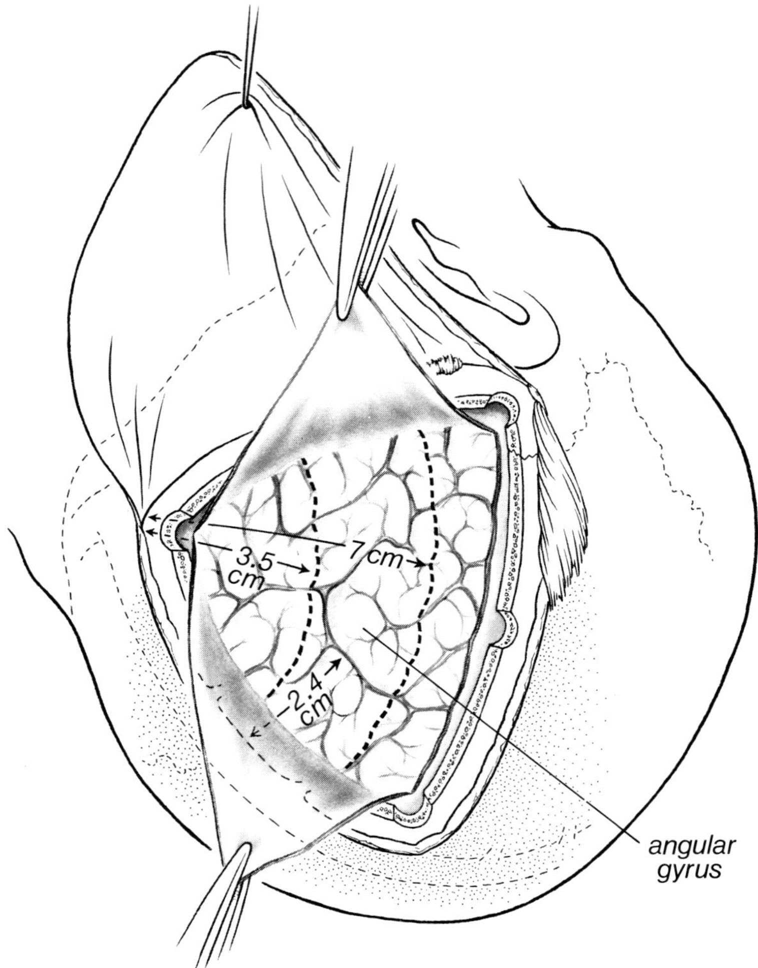

Fig. 39-11.   Reflection of dura in a "T" shape to protect both the superior sagittal and transverse sinus. Cortical incisions for both dominant (3.5 cm) and nondominant (7 cm) hemispheres are shown. Note proximity to midline of angular gyrus (see text).

used, if not, it must be extended in such a manner as not to compromise a major blood supply to the already radiation damaged scalp. The dura and the fibrous tissue growing from the dura are frequently adherent to the bone flap at its margins and at the burr hole sites and need to be separated gently. If there is any question of adequate exposure, extension of the bone flap is to be encouraged. The dura usually is adherent to the cortex at the line of previous dural incision, and the two must be carefully separated. Sometimes this is best accomplished by creating a second dural opening in the same shape, but slightly larger than the initial one, allowing the surgeon to develop a plane of dissection between unscarred cortex and the dura. This is particularly important if the line of incision is close to the motor or speech area. If the surgery is in the vicinity of the rolandic fissure, inoperative electrical stimulation for identification of the motor strip may be useful since normal anatomic landmarks are frequently distorted or absent. Pool[83] points out that recurrent tumor close to the motor strip may make it relatively insensitive to electrical stimulation and cites 1 case requiring 30 V at reoperation to elicit motor responses, when 2 years earlier at the initial surgery, under the same type of anesthesia, 5 V was sufficient.[83] Identification of the recurrent tumor is not usually a problem, since it is nearly always adjacent to the area of previous surgery. As in the case of the

first operation the recurrent tumor should be removed as radically as possible without damaging vital structures. In cases where a large cystic cavity is found with a mural nodule, the nodule and the surrounding cyst wall are removed, the cystic fluid drained, and the cyst irrigated.

Meticulous hemostasis is a general rule. Closure and insertion of a pressure switch for immediate postoperative monitoring are done as described above.

In general, reoperation should be reserved for patients harboring lower grade gliomas and mixed tumors in a surgically accessible area, whereas the reoperation of patients with glioblastoma should be carefully tailored to the patient's neurologic state and the likelihood of a functionally useful result being achieved which is likely to provide the patient with a better quality of survival than would have been accomplished without further operation.

CONCLUSION

Even the most enthusiastic proponents of surgical therapy do not suggest that surgery alone is the answer for gliomas. To date, the only adjuvant treatment that has consistently added to mean survival of the patient is radiation therapy. Comparison of

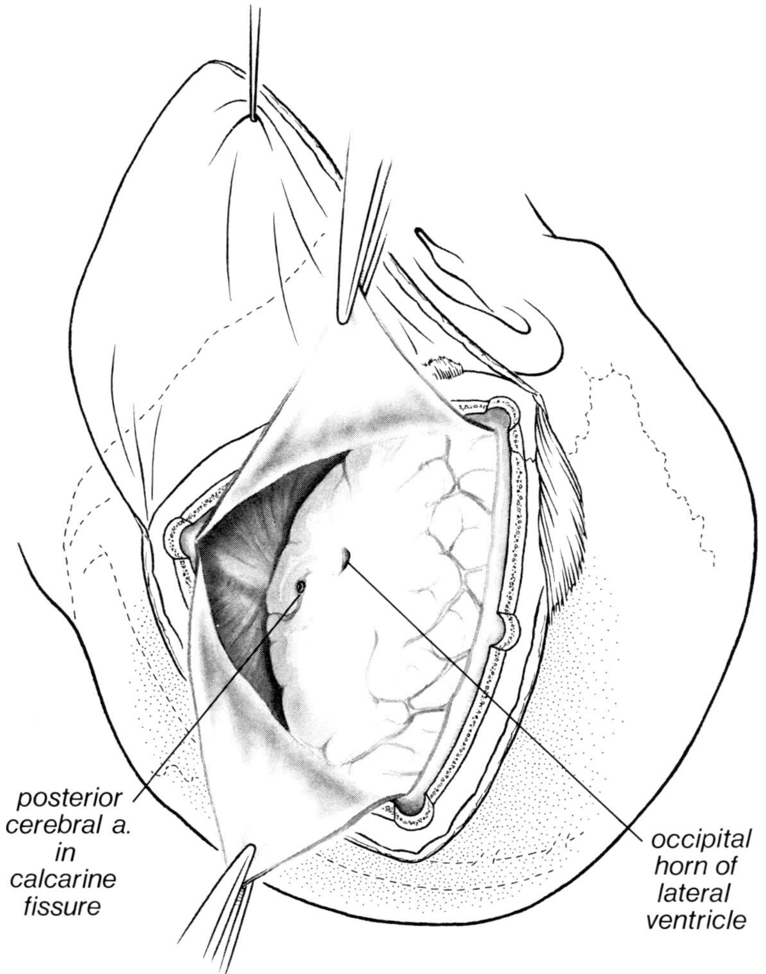

Fig. 39-12. Posterior cerebral artery as seen in the depths of the calcarine fissure after removal of the occipital pole.

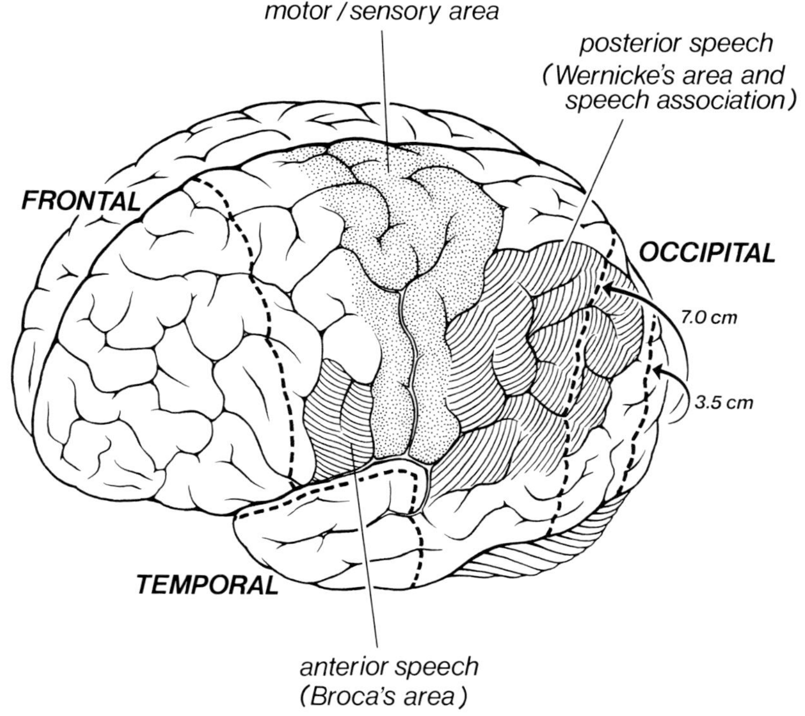

Fig. 39-13. Cortical incisions for dominant hemisphere lobectomies (occipital lobe nondominant hemisphere lobectomy also shown) and their relationships to pre) and postcentral gyri and speech areas.

the efficacy of the other modes of therapy such as chemotherapy, immunotherapy, and interstitial radiation for gliomas is difficult. In most reported series patients have undergone multiple treatment protocols either with various chemotherapy agents (frequently administered via differing routes) or chemotherapy agents combined with other forms of therapy such as interstitial radiation or immunotherapy. To isolate the benefit of any one form of therapy is difficult. Chemotherapy, both systemic and intrathecal, is under active investigation, but to date the results are less than encouraging, although earlier reports from the Brain Tumor Study Group suggested that 1,3-bis (2-chloroethyl)-1-nitrossourea (BCNU) might be of some value.[84,85] BCNU is currently being investigated both systemically and intra-arterially as well as in combination with other agents such as vincristine, procarbazine, cisplatin, 2-deoxy-5-fluorouridine (FUDR) and dichloromethotrexate (DCMTX).[86–89]

Radiosensitizers such as misonidazole and bromouridine are being studied but preliminary work is not encouraging.[90,91] Interstitial radiation therapy and laser extraction treatments are being developed at several centers and may well be important tools in the next decade.[65,69,92–96] Experimental work with immunotherapy is still in its infancy and while theoretical consideration make an enhanced immune response an attractive alternative to conventional therapy, more clinical data is needed.[97–101]

REFERENCES

1. Baily P (ed): Intracranial Tumor. Springfield, Ill, Charles C Thomas, 1933
2. Kernohan JW, Saye GP: Tumors of the central nervous system. Fascicle 35, Atlas of Tumor Pathology. Washington, Armed Forces Institute of Pathology, 1952
3. Rubenstein LJ: Tumors of the central nervous system. Second series, Fascicle 6, Atlas of Tumor Pathology. Washington, Armed Forces Institute of Pathology, 1972, pp 55–56
4. Gartner J: Statistische untersuchungen an 654 intrakranielles raumfordernden prozessen. Beitrag zur biologie der hirngescheviilste. Zentralbl Neurochir 15:333, 1955
5. Penman J, Smith MC: Intracranial gliomata: some clinical, radiological and therapeutic aspects of 298 cases. London, Medical Research Council, Publ. 616-006:384, 1954, pp 1–70, 284
6. McKeran RC, Thomas DGT: The clinical study of gliomas, in Thomas PGT, Graham DI (eds): Brain Tumours, Scientific Basis, Clinical Investigation and Current Therapy. London, Butterworths, 1980, pp 194–230
7. Hitchcock E, Sato F: Treatment of malignant gliomata. J Neurosurg 21:497, 1964
8. Roth JG, Elvidge AR: Glioblastoma multiforme: A clinical survey. J Neurosurg 17:736, 1960
9. Chadduck WM, Roycroft D, Brown MW: Multicentric glioma as a cause of multiple cerebral lesions. Neurosurgery 13:170, 1983
10. Maxwell HP: The incidence of interhemispheric extension of glioblastoma multiforme through the corpus callosum. J Neurosurg 3:54, 1946
11. Rubenstein LJ: Development of extracranial metastases from a malignant astrocytoma in the absence of previous craniotomy. J Neurosurg 26:542, 1967
12. Anzil AP: Glioblastoma multiforme with extracranial metastases in the absence of previous craniotomy. J Neurosurg 33:88, 1970
13. Sodek AR, Port R, Garfienkel B, et al: Extracranial metastasis of cerebral glioblastoma multiforme: Case report. Neurosurgery 15:549, 1984
14. Pang D, Ashmead JW: Extraneural metastasis of cerebellar glioblastoma multiforme. Neurosurgery 10:252, 1982
15. Scherer HJ: The forms of growth in gliomas and their practical significance. Brain 63:1, 1940
16. Hockberg FHI, Pruitt A: Assumptions in the radiotherapy of glioblastoma. Neurology 30:907, 1980
17. Davidoff LM, Feiring EH: Circumscribed glioblastoma multiforme. J Neuropathol Clin Neurol 1:161, 1951
18. Jelsma R, Bucy P: Glioblastoma multiforme—its treatment and some factors effecting survival. Arch Neurol 20:161, 1969
19. Pool JL, Kamrin RP: The treatment of intracranial gliomas by surgery and radiation. Prog Neurol Surg 1:258, 1966
20. Palma L, Guidette B: Cystic pilocystic astrocytomas of the cerebral hemispheres. J Neurosurg 62:811, 1985
21. Weir B: The relative significance of factors affecting postoperative survival in astrocytomas grades 3 and 4. J Neurosurg 38:448, 1973
22. Shenkin HS, Grant EC, Drew JH: Postoperative period of survival of patients with oligodendroglioma of the brain. Reports of 125 cases. Arch Neurol Psychiatry 58:710, 1947
23. Horrax G, Wu WQ: Postoperative survival of patients with intracranial oligodendroglioma with special reference to radical tumor removal. A study of 26 patients. J Neurosurg 8:473, 1951
24. Beck PK, Russell DS: Oligodendrometosis of the cerebrospinal pathway. Brain 65:352, 1941
25. Strang RR, Nordenstan H: Intracerebral oligodendrogliomas with metastatic involvement of the cauda equina. J Neurosurg 18:683, 1961
26. Walker M, Alexander E, Hunt W, et al: Evaluation of BCNU and/or radiotherapy in the treatment of anaplastic gliomas. J Neurosurg 49:333, 1978
27. Neuwelt EA, Maravilla K, Frankel E, et al: The use of enhanced computerized tomography to evaluate osmotic blood brain barrier disruption. Neurosurgery 6:49, 1980
28. Baker HL Jr, Houser OW, Campbell JK: The National Cancer Institute Study: Evaluation of computerized tomography in the diagnosis of intracranial neoplasms. Neuroradiology 136:91, 1980
29. Claveria LE, Kendall BE, DuBoulay GH: Computerized axial tomography in supratentorial gliomas and metastases, in DuBoulay GH, Moseley IF(eds): First European Seminar on Computerized Axial Tomography in Clinical Practice. Berlin, Springer-Verlag, 1977
30. Wing SW, Norman D, Pollack J, et al: Contrast enhancement of cerebral infarcts in computed tomography. Radiology 121:89, 1976
31. Drayer BP, Wolfson SK, Boehnke M, et al: Physiologic changes in regional cerebral blood flow defined by Xenon-enhanced CT scanning. Neuroradiology 16:220, 1978
32. Radue EW, Kendall BE: Xenon enhancement in tumors and infarcts. Neuroradiology 16:224, 1978
33. Saloman M, Levine H, Rao K: Value of sequential computed tomography in the multimodality treatment of glioblastoma multiforme. Neurosurgery 8:15, 1981
34. Selker RG, Mendolow H, Wilker M, et al: Pathological correlations of CT ring in recurrent, previously treated gliomas. Surg Neurol 17:251, 1982
35. Pennybacke J, Russell DS: Necrosis of the brain due to radiation therapy: Clinical and pathological observations. J Neurol Neurosurg Psychiatry 11:183, 1948
36. Martins AN, Johnson JS, et al: Delayed radiation neurosis of the brain. J Neurosurg 47:336, 1977
37. Mikhail M: Radiation necrosis of the brain: Correlation between computerized tomography, pathology and dose distribution. J Comput Assist Tomogr 2:71, 1978
38. Spetzler RF, Norman D, Selman WR, et al: Computerized tomographic diagnosis: Pitfalls for neurosurgeons. Neurosurgery 5:231, 1979
39. Scarabin JM, Pecker J, et al: Stereotaxic exploration in 200

supratentorial brain tumors: Its value in addition to computerized tomography. Neuroradiology 16:591, 1968

40. Wada J, Rasmussen T: Intracranial injection of sodium amytal for the lateralization of cerebral speech dominance. J Neurosurg 17:266, 1960

41. Lee BCP, Kneeland JB, Cahill PT, et al: MR recognition of supratentorial tumors. Am J Neuroradiol 6:871, 1985

42. Brant-Zawadzki M, Davis PL, Crooks LE: NMR demonstration of cerebral abnormalities: Comparison with CT. Am J Neuroradiol 4:117, 1983

43. Patronas NJ, DiChina G, Kufta C, et al: Prediction of survival in glioma patients by means of positron emission tomography. J Neurosurg 62:816, 1985

44. Lilja A, Bergstron K, Hartvig P, et al: Dynamic study of supratentorial gliomas with L-methyl-^{11}C-methionic and positron emission tomography. Am J Neuroradiol 6:505, 1985

45. Grode ML, Komaiko MS: The role of intraoperative ultrasound in neurosurgery. Neurosurgery 12:624, 1983

46. Godding GAW, Boggan JE, Powers SK: Neurosurgical sonography: Intraoperative and postoperative imaging of the brain. Am J Neuroradiol 5:521, 1984

47. Goodman LS, Gilman A: Steroids for Raised ICP. The Pharmacological Basis of Therapeutics, ed 5. New York, Macmillan, 1975, pp 1472–1506

48. Gercay O, Wilson CB, Barker M: Corticosteroid effect of transplantable rat glioma. Arch Neurol 24:266, 1971

49. Garfield JS: Neurosurgical aspects of supratentorial malignant gliomas. Proc Roy Soc Med 69:53, 1976

50. Priebe H, Skillman, Bushnell, et al: Antacid versus cimetidine in preventing acute gastrointestinal bleeding. N Engl J Med 302:426,

51. WIlson CB, Baker M, Hoshimo T: Steroid induced inhibition of growth in glial tumors—a kinetic dialysis, in Neulan HJ, Schurmann K (eds): Steroids and Brain Edema. Berlin, Springer-Verlag, 1972, pp 99—100

52. Horsley V: Discussion on the treatment of cerebral tumors. Br Med J 2:1365, 1893

53. Heilbrun MP, Roberts TS, Apuzzo MLJ: Preliminary experience with Brown-Roberts-Wells (BRW) computerized tomography stereotaxic guidance system. J Neurosurg 59:217, 1983

54. Apuzzo MLJ, Sabskin JK: Computed tomographic guidance stereotaxis in management of intracranial mass lesions. Neurosurgery 12:272, 1983

55. Yeates A, Emzmann DR, Britt RH, et al: Simplified and accurate CT-guided needle biopsy of central nervous system lesions. J Neurosurg 57:390, 1982

56. Edner G: Stereotaxic brain tumor biopsy—5 years experience. Acta Neurochir 31:261, 1975

57. Heath RG, John S, Foss O: Stereotactic biopsy: A method for the study of discrete brain regions of animals and man. Arch Neurol 4:291, 1961

58. Marshall LF, Jennnett B, Langfitt TW: Needle biopsy for the diagnosis of malignant glioma. JAMA 228:1417, 1974

59. Marshall LF, Langfitt TW: Needle biopsy, high dose corticosteroids, and radiotherapy in the treatment of malignant gliomas. Presented at the 44th annual meeting of the American Association of Neurological Surgeons, San Francisco, April 7, 1976

60. Shetter AG, Bertuccini TV, Pittman HW: Closed needle biopsy in the diagnosis of intracranial mass lesions. Surg Neurol 8:341, 1977

61. Spence JW, Richards GE, Nulsen FE: Indication for brain tumor biopsy by trephine and needle: Review of results. Presented at the 42nd annual meeting of the American Association of Neurological Surgeons, St. Louis, April 24, 1974

62. Hahn JF, Levy WJ, Weinstein MJ: Needle biopsy of intracranial lesions guided by computerized tomography. Neurosurgery 5:11, 1979

63. Maroon JC, Bank WO, Drayer BP, et al: Intracranial biopsy assisted by computerized tomography. J Neurosurg 46:740, 1977

64. Conway L: Stereotactic diagnosis and treatemnt of intracranial tumors including an initial experience with cryosurgery for pinealomas. J Neurosurg 38:453, 1973

65. Mundinger F, Birg W, Ostertag CB: Treatment of small cerebral gliomas with CT-aided stereotactic curietherapy. Neuroradiology 16:564, 1978

66. Soloman M, Levine H, Rao K: Value of sequential computed tomography in the multimodiality treatment of glioblastoma multiforme. Neurosurgery 8:15, 1981

67. Gleason C, Wise B, Feinstein B: Stereotactic localization (with computerized tomographic scanning), biopsy, and radiofrequency treatment of brain lesions. Neurosurgery 2:217, 1978

68. Mundinger F: Rationale and methods: Interstitial iridium 192 brachycurie therapy and iridium 192 or iodine 125 protracted long-term irradiation, in Zilka GS (ed): Stereotactic Cerebral Irradiation, No. 12. Amsterdam, Elsevier, 1979, pp 101–115

69. Birg W, Schneider J, Bauer S, et al: An interactive program system for the stereotactic interstitial implantation of radionuclides in brain tumors, in Zilka GS (ed): Stereotactic Cerebral Irradiation, No. 12. Amsterdam, Elsevier, 1979

70. Jelsma R, Bucy P: The treatment of glioblastoma multiforme of the brain. J Neurosurg 27:388, 1967

71. Frankel SA, German WJ: Glioblastoma multiforme: Review of 219 cases with regard to natural history, pathology, diagnostic methods, and treatment. J Neurosurg 15:489, 1958

72. Laws ER, Taylor WF, Clifton MB, et al: Neurosurgical management of low-grade astrocytomas of the cerebral hemispheres. J Neurosurg 61:665, 1984

73. Gol A: The relatively benign astrocytomas of the cerebrum. A clinical study of 194 verified cases. J Neurosurg 18:501, 1961

74. Needham CWL Neurosurgical Syndromes of the Brain—Frontopolar Syndromes. Springfield, Ill, Charles C Thomas, 1973

75. Van Buren JM, Fedio P, Frederick GC: Mechanisms and localization of speech in the parietal temporal cortex. Neurosurgery 2:233, 1978

76. Cushing H: The surgical mortality percentages pertaining to a series of two thousand verified tumors. J Neurosurg 22:191, 1965

77. Cushing H, Bovie WT: Electrosurgery as an aid to the removal of intracranial tumors. J Neurosurg 23:85, 1965

78. Young B, Oldfield EH, Markesbery WR, et al: Reoperation for glioblastoma. J Neurosurg 55:917, 1981

79. Karnofsky DA, Abdmann WH, Carver LF, et al: The use of the nitrogen mustards in the palliative treatment of carcinoma with particular reference to bronchogenic carcinoma. Cancer 1:634, 1948

80. Soloman MJ, Kaplan RS, Duchen TB, et al: Effect of age and reoperation on survival in the combined modality treatment of malignant astrocytomas. Neurosurgery 10:454, 1982

81. Harsh IV, Levin GR, Gutin VA, et al: Reoperation for recurrent glioblastoma and anaplastic astrocytomas. Presented at the Amercan Association of Neurological Surgeons, Atlanta, 1985

82. Diengdoh JV, Booth AE: Post-irradiation necrosis of the temporal lobe presenting as a glioma. Case report. J Neurosurg 44:732, 1976

83. Pool JL: The management of recurrent gliomas. Clin Neurosurg 15:265, 1967

84. Walker MD: Treatment of brain tumors. Med Clin North Am 61:1045, 1977

85. Walker MP, Alexander E, Hunt WE, et al: Evaluation of BCNU and/or radiotherapy in the Treatment of Anaplastic Gliomas J Neurosurg 49:333, 1978

86. Phillips TW, Chandler WF, Kindt GW, et al: New implantable continuous administration and bolus dose intracarotid drug delivery system for the treatment of malignant gliomas. Neurosurgery 11:213, 1982

87. West CR, Avellanosa AM, Barva NR, et al: Intraarterial 1,3-bis(2-chloroethyl)-1-nitrosourea (BCNU) and systemic chemotherapy

for malignant gliomas: A follow-up study. Neurosurgery 13:420, 1983

88. Kapp JP, Parker JL, Tucker EM: Supraophthalmic carotid infusion for brain chemotherapy. J Neurosurg 62:823, 1985

89. Oldfield EH, Dedrick RL, Yeager RL, et al: Reduced systemic drug exposure by combining intra-arterial chemotherapy with hemoperfusion of regional venous drainage. J Neurosurg 726, 1985

90. Bleehan NM: The Cambridge glioma trial of misonidazole and radiation therapy with associated pharmacokinetic studies. Cancer Clin Trials 3:267, 1980

91. EORTC Brain Tumor Group: Misonidazole in radiotherapy of supratentorial malignant brain gliomas in adult patients: A randomized double-blind study. Eur J Cancer Oncol 19:39, 1983

92. Kelley PJ, Olsen MH, Wright AE, et al: CT localization and stereotactic implantation of Ir-192 into CNS neoplasms, in Szilka G (ed): Stereotactic Cerebral Irradiation. INSERM Symposium No. 12. Amsterdam, Elsevier, 1979

93. Mundinger F: Rationale and methods of interstitial iridium 192 brachycurie therapy and iridium 192 or iodine 125 protracted long-term irradiation, in Szilka G (ed): Stereotactic Cerebral Irradiation. INSERM Symposium No. 12. Amsterdam, Elsevier, 1979

94. Kelley PJ, Elker GJ Jr: A stereotactic approach to deep seated central nervous system neoplasms using the carbon dioxide laser. Surg Neurol 15:331, 1981

95. Gutin PH, Phillips TL, Wara WM, et al: Brachytherapy of recurrent malignant brain tumors with removal high-activity iodine 125 sources. J Neurosurg 60:61, 1984

96. Dyck P: Stereotactic Biopsy and Brachytherapy of Brain Tumors. Baltimore, University Park Press, 1984

97. Gerosa MA, Olivi A, Rosenblum ML, et al: Impaired immunocompetence in patients with malignant gliomas: The possible role of T-lymphocyte subpopulations. Neurosurgery 10:571, 1982

98. Mahaley MS, Urso MB, Whaley RA, et al: Interferon as adjuvant therapy with initial radiotherapy of patients with anaplastic gliomas. Neurosurgery 61:1069, 1984

99. Bullard DE, Bigen DD: Applications of monoclonal antibodies in the diagnosis and treatment of primary brain tumors. J Neurosurg 63:2, 1985

100. Mahaley MS, Urso MB, Whaley PS: Immunobiology of primary intracranial tumors. J Neurosurg 63:719, 1985

101. Jacobs SK, Wilson DJ, Kornblith PL, et al: In vitro killing of human glioblastoma by Interleukin-2-activated autologous lymphocytes. J Neurosurg 64:114, 1986

CHAPTER 40

Surgical Management of Intracranial Metastasis

Perry Black

ALTHOUGH IT HAS BEEN ESTIMATED that 18 percent of cancer patients develop intracranial metastases at some stage of their disease,[1] only a small proportion come to the attention of the neurosurgeon. In different neurosurgical series reported during the past 2 decades, metastatic tumors constituted 7 to 17 percent of all brain tumors seen clinically[2]; this variation probably reflects differences in selection of clinical material. Leptomeningeal metastases (meningeal carcinomatosis) are found in approximately 4 percent of cancer patients at autopsy[3]; in about half of these patients, there is no other metastatic involvement of the central nervous system (CNS).

PATHOLOGIC ASPECTS

ORIGIN OF METASTASES

The most common sources of metastases to the brain are tumors of the lung, breast, and kidney, and malignant melanomas.[4] Other sources are relatively infrequent, including tumors of the gastrointestinal tract, the thyroid, the uterus, the ovary, the pancreas, the prostate, and sarcomas.[5–11] Although melanoma is not the most common tumor metastasizing to the brain, it ranks highest in its proclivity to spread to the brain,[12] with a greater tendency for metastasis to the brain to occur in males than in females.[13] In some series, about 50 percent of the patients have neurologic symptoms or signs as the first manifestation of malignant disease.[2,9,11,14] The primary origin in these cases is usually discovered later (Figures 40-1 and 40-2), but occasionally the primary tumor cannot be identified, even at autopsy. In patients in whom the primary tumor is unknown initially, more than half are subsequently found to have bronchogenic carcinoma.[2]

DISTRIBUTION IN BRAIN

About two thirds of intracranial metastases are located within the brain parenchyma (intracerebral); the remaining one third are situated in the subdural or extradural space and may compress but not necessarily invade the brain. In some series, a predominance of parenchymal metastases has been observed in the distribution of the middle cerebral artery,[7,11] which has been explained on the basis of laminar arterial flow.[15] The cerebellum has also been reported as a site of predilection[3,5]; this may be related, however, to the fact that mass lesions in the cerebellum tend to manifest themselves clinically earlier than those in relatively "silent" areas, such as the frontal lobes. In general, reports in the literature indicate wide variability in the location of brain metastases. It seems that tumor emboli may settle in any part of the brain and that the distribution probably reflects the relative mass of the different areas of the brain.[16,17]

SOLITARY VERSUS MULTIPLE BRAIN METASTASES

Brain metastases from solid tumors are solitary (Figure 40-1) in about 50 to 65 percent of the cases when the diagnosis is made while the patient is alive.[12,17] The advent of computed tomographic (CT) scanning has increased the likelihood of detecting multiple lesions (Figure 40-3). Although CT scanning may reveal multiple metastases, high-resolution scans may detect solitary metastases earlier than in the past.

CHARACTERISTICS OF LESIONS

Intracerebral metastases generally are soft, nodular, circumscribed masses, often with central necrosis (Figure 40-1). They vary in size from minute (requiring a microscope for identification) to centimeters in diameter (Figures 40-1 through 40-4). Even small metastases are characteristically associated with enormous surrounding reactive edema, which further compresses the brain tissue and increases the neurologic symptoms and signs.

LEPTOMENINGEAL METASTASES

Apart from the solid metastatic lesions, leukemias and lymphomas constitute another major category of CNS metastases. They generally invade the leptomeninges in a diffuse or multifocal manner,[18] usually with widespread seeding of tumor cells in the CSF rather than as solid tumor deposits (Figure 40-5). Although hematologic malignancies contribute the largest proportion of cases of leptomeningeal metastases, an increasing number of solid tumors—especially carcinoma of the breast—are being found as a source of this form of CNS metastasis.

LATENT INTERVAL

There is wide variability in the interval between the clinical appearance of the primary cancer and that of the cerebral metastasis. It is not uncommon for the cerebral metastasis to represent the first manifestation of a malignant neoplasm. For

OPERATIVE NEUROSURGICAL TECHNIQUES
ISBN 0-8089-1862-1

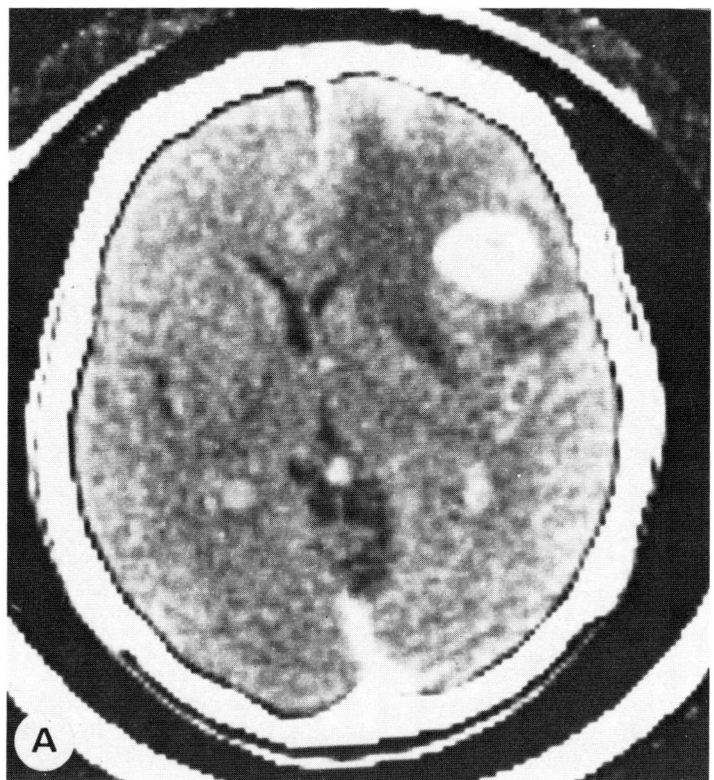

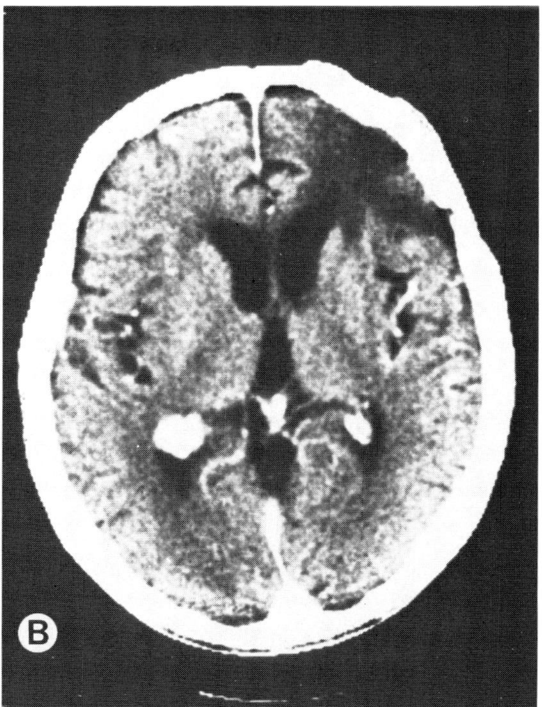

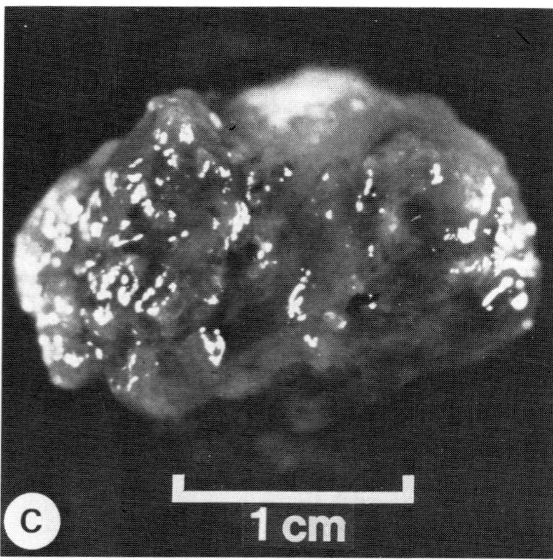

Fig. 40-1. A solitary brain metastasis in a patient whose initial presentation was related only to cerebral symptoms. Despite a search for a possible primary source, the bronchogenic site of origin did not declare itself until 8 months after surgical excision of the brain metastasis, when the patient began to complain of chest pain. (A) A CT scan with contrast showing a solitary frontal mass that was surgically excised and proved to be metastatic. (B) A CT scan of the same patient 1 year later; there is no evidence of recurrence of brain metastasis, but patient's general condition was declining secondary to the bronchogenic carcinoma. (C) A gross photograph of the solitary mass removed from the frontal region. (D) Histopathologic study of lesion showing well to moderately differentiated adenocarcinoma infiltrating the brain tissue, narrow bands of which are visible between the epithelial elements; original magnification: 420×. (Pathologic interpretation courtesy of Dr. Jeffrey Stead, Hahnemann University Hospital, Philadelphia.)

example, in one series, 14 of 35 patients with brain metastasis from lung cancer had an intracranial lesion as the first manifestation of malignancy.[14] The symptoms of cerebral metastasis, however, may appear anywhere from months to as long as 15 years after the diagnosis of the primary tumor.[2,17] How long that interval is tends to be a function of the tissue of origin on the metastatic tumor; the average interval between the diagnosis of lung carcinoma and the development of brain metastases is 4 to 10 months,[14] whereas the average interval between the diagnosis of breast cancer and the development of brain metastasis is 3 years.[2] The reverse can also occur—a cerebral metastasis may be excised, followed by a delay of months or years before the primary cancer (usually bronchogenic) manifests itself.[8] Although metastases are generally regarded as rapidly growing lesions, they can rarely grow so slowly that calcification may occur.[19]

MANAGEMENT

EVALUATION OF TREATMENT MODALITIES

Management of metastasis to the brain is almost always palliative, with cure the rare exception. Because the results of therapy (in terms of restoration or maintenance of neurologic function) are usually limited, there is considerable controversy regarding the appropriate mode of therapy and, indeed, regarding whether any therapy is warranted at all. Evaluation of

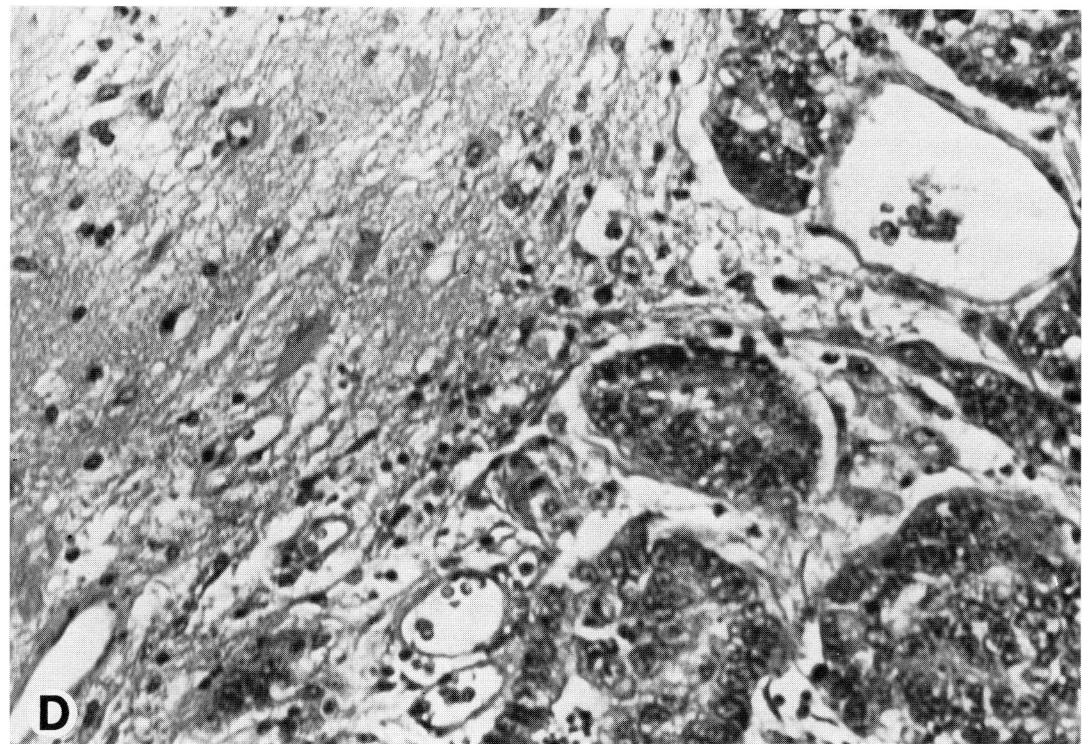

various therapeutic modalities—radiation, chemotherapy, or surgery—has been confounded by a lack of controlled, randomized studies whereby the relative benefit of the respective modalities could be assessed objectively. Almost all of the numerous published studies on the management of cerebral metastasis are limited by the failure to control for critical variables such as the stage of the systemic disease, the degree of neurologic deficit, the number or location of metastatic lesions, or the cell type or radiosensitivity of the primary lesion; the studies are also confounded by the use of a combination of treatment modalities.

Despite these limitations, some progress is being made in the identification of those patients for whom therapy is likely to be of benefit. Such benefit should be measured in terms of both quality (remission of symptoms) and duration of survival. In one surgical series, excision of a solitary brain metastasis was considered beneficial if the patient's condition was not made worse and if the patient survived for at least 6 months.[16] In another series, craniotomy was thought worthwhile if the patient could lead a functional home life, did not require continuous nursing care, and was appreciative of normal daily living.[20] For purposes of rough comparison, the respective therapeutic modalities may be viewed in relation to a baseline of "no treatment," in which case the median survival is approximately 1 month (Table 40-1).

STEROID THERAPY

Administration of adrenocorticosteroid hormones may be expected to ameliorate neurologic symptoms and signs in about two thirds of patients with intracranial metastasis. The benefits often are evident within 24 hours (Figure 40-6). Steroids are believed to exert their beneficial effect primarily by reducing cerebral edema surrounding the tumor; to a lesser extent, there may be a direct oncolytic effect on the tumor itself.[21]

RADIATION THERAPY

Aside from the use of steroids to control cerebral edema, radiotherapy is currently the most commonly used therapeutic modality for cerebral metastases. It also plays an important role in the postoperative management of those patients with intracranial metastasis who are selected for surgical excision. The ideal dose of radiation and fractionation have not been established, but in general 2500 to 5000 rad is given over a variable course ranging in different series from 1 to 5 weeks.[22–24] The major portion of the therapy is delivered to the whole head because of the presence of multiple metastases in about half of the cases, with a smaller proportion of the radiation cone to the

Table 40-1. Brain metastasis: Results of treatment

Therapeutic Modality	Survival Time		
	Median (months)	1 Year (%)	>2 Years (%)
No treatment[3]	1		
Steroids alone[3]	2		
Radiation alone[3,24]	3–6	3–20	4–8
Surgery alone[5,7,24]	5–6	22–31	3–7
Surgery* plus radiation and/or chemotherapy[6,14,30]	6–12	38–53	25
Chemotherapy[3]		Benefit not established	
Immunotherapy[3]		Benefit not established	

* Solitary metastasis.

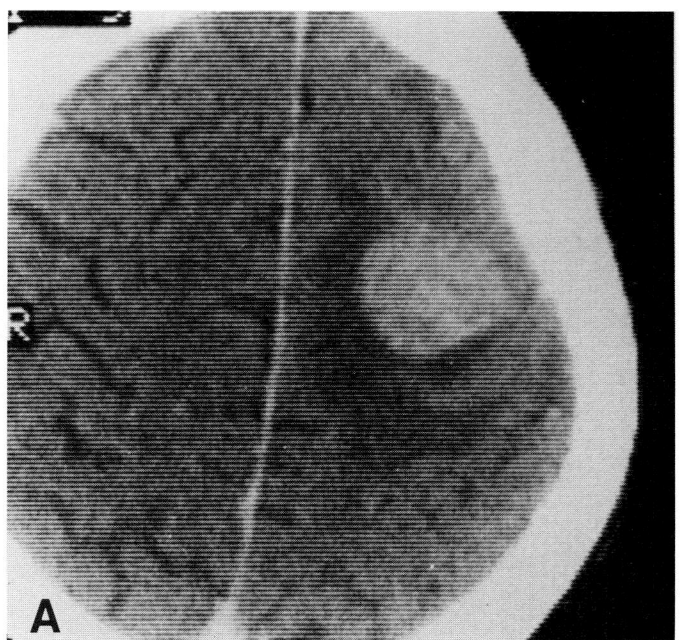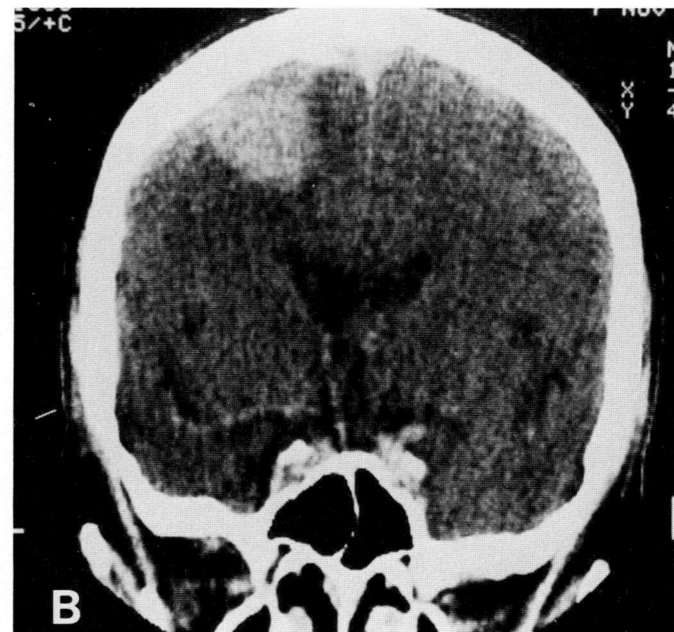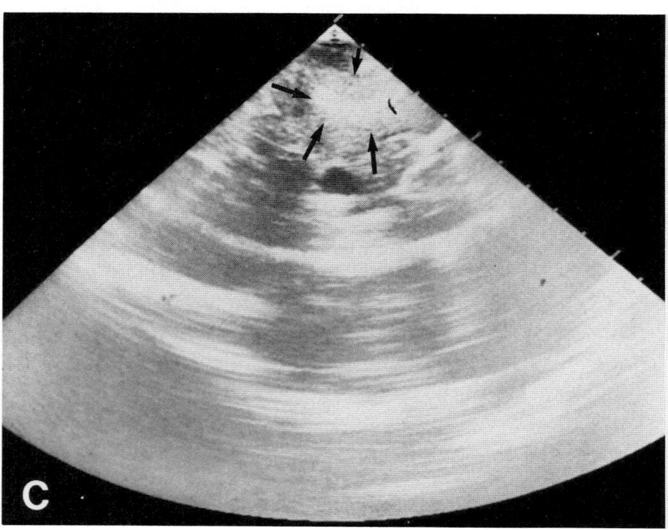

Fig. 40-2. A 50-year-old man with mild neurologic symptoms but without any evidence of neoplasm elsewhere in the body. (A) A CT scan showing a lesion in the left frontoparietal area, suspicious for metastasis; note the lesion is relatively circumscribed and surrounded by moderate edema. (B) Because the lesion appeared to be surgically accessible, excisional biopsy was undertaken (rather than CT-guided biopsy). In view of the fact that lesion appeared subcortical, a coronal CT scan was carried out in order to obtain further imaging of the geometry of the lesion. (C) When the bone flap was turned, the cortex appeared normal, and intraoperative ultrasound was used to precisely localize the lesion (arrows) and thereby aid in placement of the cortical incision.

site of the known cerebral metastasis. A rapid fractionation technique, consisting of a course of radiation of 1000 rad given as a single dose or distributed over 1 week, has been recommended for convenience and economy.[25] Radiation therapy to the brain is not believed to cause further neurologic deterioration or death except when it is given in high doses to patients already showing signs of cerebral herniation.[24]

Radiotherapy affords temporary improvement of neurologic symptoms in about 60 percent of patients.[3,23] Those who show initial improvement may show temporary benefit after undergoing irradiation again. Steroids generally are given during each course of radiation and are sometimes given in low doses for indefinite periods. In a different series, as shown in Table 40-1, median survival after radiation therapy has varied from 3 to 6 months, with 1-year survival ranging from 3 to 20 percent; the overall 1-year survival is about 15 percent.[3,23] Finally, the effectiveness of radiotherapy depends in part on the cell type of the tumor; radiosensitive tumors such as small-cell carcinomas of the lung, lymphoma, and breast cancer respond best, whereas non-small-cell carcinomas of the lung, hyper-

nephromas, and malignant melanomas are less responsive. Progression of the systemic disease also plays a role in the survival time.

SURGERY

The consensus among neurosurgeons concerning cerebral metastatic disease is that surgical excision should be restricted to patients with a solitary intracerebral metastasis whose general medical status is satisfactory. French and Ausman extend this concept to include excision of an incapacitating metastasis even when it is known that the tumor is not solitary; they also advocate the excision of multiple metastases if the lesions are surgically accessible.[26] This approach has been advocated by Fernandez et al.[27] in a case of malignant melanoma, which is generally viewed as carrying a poor prognosis for surgical intervention; they reported, in one case, repeated surgical excision of metastatic malignant melanoma with relatively long survival of good quality.

The radiosensitivity of the tumor may play a role in the

decision regarding surgery; patients with radioresistant tumors such as renal carcinomas or melanomas are more likely than other patients to be offered surgical excision with or without postoperative radiotherapy. Surgery may also be favored in patients with slow-growing tumors, as suggested by the natural history of the disease or by a long latency period after diagnosis of the primary malignancy.[20] It has been suggested that a long latency period signifies good host defense mechanisms against the primary tumor and that the outcome of surgical excision of the cerebral metastasis is therefore likely to be favorable.[6] Surgical intervention is also often recommended for patients who are presumed to have metastatic disease when the nature of the primary extracranial tumor is unknown or where none can be found (Figures 40-1 and 40-2). The need to establish a tissue diagnosis is most imperative if the intracranial lesion is solitary, so that the possibility of a benign, curable lesion, such as a meningioma, a hematoma, or an abscess, can be ruled out.[5–8] In the case of a patient with a confirmed primary malignancy elsewhere in the body, a single intracranial lesion is probably metastatic, but excisional biopsy (when surgically feasible) is desirable.

Surgical Excision Alone

The median survival time after excision of a solitary metastasis (in most cases without radiotherapy) is 5 to 6 months. This figure is based on three surgical series reported since 1970[5,7,24]; the benefits of improved anesthesia, surgical technique, and control of cerebral edema are thus more uniformly applicable than in those series reported before 1970 (Table 40-1). The 1-year survival rate after surgery varied from 22 to 31 percent of patients; this represents some improvement in surgical results over the 14–21-percent survival for 1 year in three surgical series reported during the previous decade (1960–1970).[8,11,16] The median and 1-year surgical survival statistics (surgery alone) seem approximately the same as or slightly better than those for radiation alone. Strictly speaking, however, it is not appropriate to make a direct comparison between these two modalities of therapy, because patients selected for surgery are likely to have only a solitary metastasis and are more likely to be in better general condition. Aside from other considerations, an appealing aspect of surgical intervention is the possibility, although rare, of achieving a cure or long-term survival.[28]

Combined Therapy: Surgery plus Radiotherapy

Ransohoff has reported a series of 100 patients on whom combined modalities were used.[6] Surgical excision of a single cerebral metastasis (various tumor types) was followed by radiotherapy, chemotherapy, or both. This resulted in a median survival time of 6 to 12 months; 38 percent of the patients survived 1 year, and 13 percent survived beyond 2 years (Table 40-1). The operative mortality (death during the first postoperative month) was 10 percent. These results seem to be superior to those obtained with any single therapeutic modality.

In another combined-therapy study reported by Magilligan et al.,[29] 22 patients with solitary cerebral metastases from bronchogenic carcinoma had a median survival of about 6 months and an average survival of 14 months. Forty-five percent of the patients survived longer than 1 year (Table 40-1); 32 percent of these patients remained free of symptoms, indicating that the quality of survival was reasonable. The operative mortality was 4 percent. The patients in this series underwent resection of the pulmonary lesion before removal of the brain

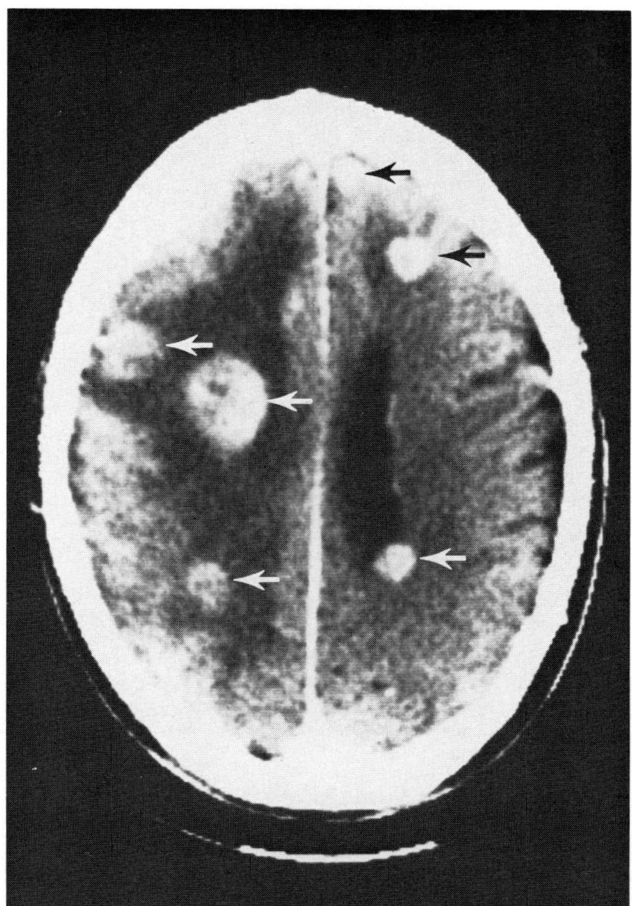

Fig. 40-3. A CT scan showing multiple intracranial metastases (black and white arrows).

metastasis, and most had whole-brain radiotherapy after craniotomy. The authors concluded that the following factors had a favorable bearing on the outcome: a history of prior pulmonary resection of stage 1 lung cancer (no nodal metastases and no tumor at the bronchial margins) and a long interval between the pulmonary resection and the onset of the cerebral metastasis. The use of whole-brain radiation therapy in these patients was also thought to contribute to a relatively favorable outcome. In another series (1983), Sundaresan et al.[14] reported surgical resection of brain metastases in 35 patients with non-small (oat) cell lung cancer. The histologic make-up of the primary tumor was predominantly adenocarcinoma, the remainder being squamous cell or bronchiolar carcinoma. The overall median survival time was 14 months; the 1-year survival rate was 53 percent, and the 2-year survival rate was 25 percent (Table 40-1). Favorable prognostic variables included: (1) absence of local or systemic disease at time of craniotomy (median 23 months survival); (2) aggressive treatment of the primary tumor (median 18 months survival); and (3) metachronous (brain metastases occurring at varying periods following treatment of the primary tumor) onset of brain metastases (median 15 months survival). The results of these studies are encouraging, particularly in view of the historical median 6-months survival for patients with pulmonary metastasis.[30]

Comparison of the 1-year survival rates for surgical excision of a brain metastasis from lung before and after 1970 (0 percent in 1954, increasing to 45 percent in 1976,[29] and 53

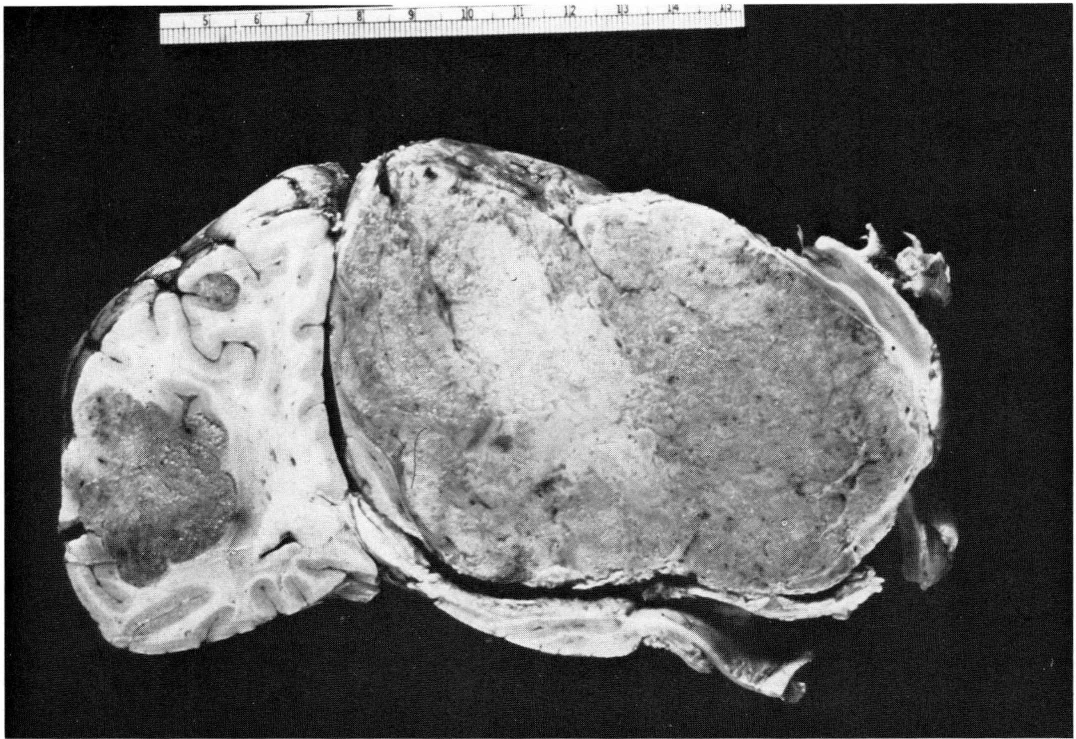

Fig. 40-4. Coronal section of an autopsy specimen of brain showing an enormous metastasis in one cerebral hemisphere and a smaller nodule in the other.

percent in 1983[14]) suggests a trend toward an improved prognosis.[4,14,29] The better prognosis reflects more aggressive treatment of the primary lung cancer, earlier detection of the brain metastasis by CT scanning, and post-craniotomy radiotherapy, as well as improvements in surgical technique and postoperative care. In the past, brain metastasis from lung cancer had been viewed as having a worse prognosis than did metastasis from some other major categories (breast, kidney). The apparently improved results of the combined surgical-radiotherapeutic approach for lung metastases should provide an impetus for even more aggressive application of this approach to the other types of metastasis.

Another histologic tumor type with a traditionally dismal outlook is malignant melanoma. In a series of 125 patients with brain metastasis from malignant melanoma, median survival of untreated patients was 3 weeks; 6 weeks for patients given steroids only; 9 weeks for those given radiotherapy; 11 weeks with intra-arterial chemotherapy; and 26 weeks for those patients who underwent successful surgical excision of a solitary lesion.[13]

In a series of 36 patients with brain metastasis from choriocarcinoma,[31] 5 of 10 patients with surgical excision of the intracranial lesion survived more than 6 months; these authors recommend the following management for intracranial metastasis of choriocarcinoma: (1) in the presence of increased intracranial pressure, removal of the intracranial tumor or at least decompression followed by multi-drug chemotherapy and whole-brain irradiation; and (2) in patients without severe neurologic symptoms, chemotherapy combined with irradiation as the primary mode of therapy.

Clonogenic Assay

A further consideration in surgical excision of metastatic lesions is the possibility that the tumor tissue may be grown in tissue culture for the purpose of identifying chemotherapeutic agents that can be used postoperatively for treatment of the systemic disease. This is comparable to antibiotic sensitivity testing for bacteria. The technique, known as clonogenic assay,[32] consists of placing small samples of the tumor tissue in different dishes containing growth medium; different chemotherapeutic agents, or combinations of agents, are added to each of the tissue culture dishes. The growth of tumor cells is monitored under the microscope at intervals over the course of several weeks, in order to determine which of the chemotherapeutic agents suppresses growth of the tumor cells. This process can be facilitated by the use of an automatic image analyzer. Based upon this information, the patient may then be offered chemotherapy specific for the tumor involved.

Surgical Mortality and Morbidity

Yet another factor that enters into the decision regarding selection of patients for surgical intervention is that of the operative mortality from the surgical procedure itself. The mortality within 30 days after surgery has ranged from 11 to 21 percent in various series reported from 1971 to 1976, with an average mortality of 11 percent.[30] The mortality in a series reported in 1983 was 3 percent.[14]

In a study reported in 1978, postoperative complications (morbidity) occurred in approximately 24 percent of patients after craniotomy for excision of a solitary cerebral metastasis.[33] Re-operation was required in approximately one third of those patients with complications, which included worsening of neu-

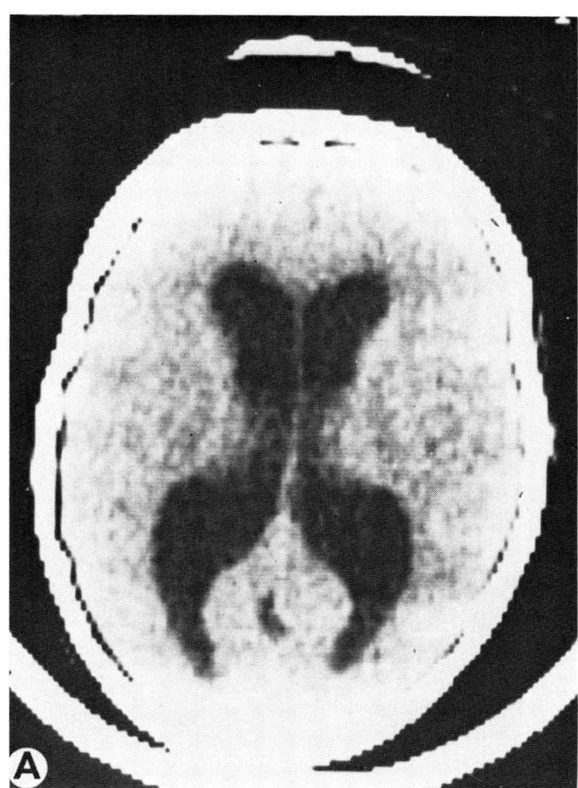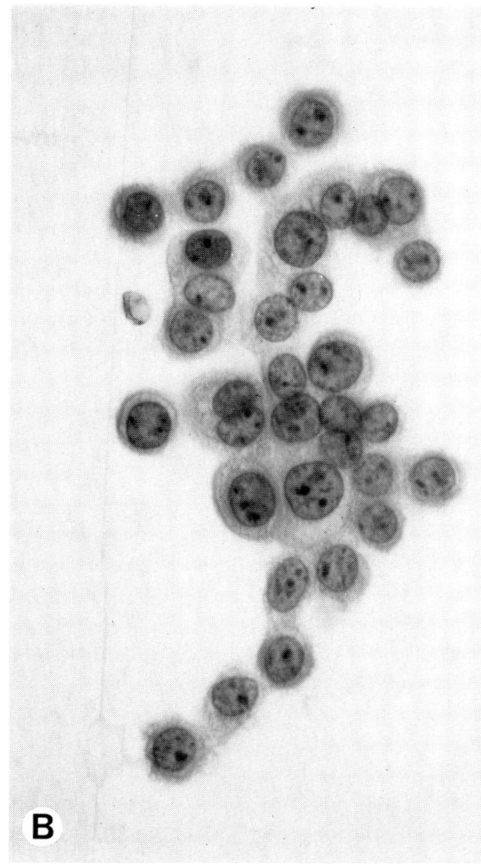

Fig. 40-5. A. CT scan of a 47-year-old woman with history of breast carcinoma, treated 2 years earlier with a mastectomy and chemotherapy. She then had a 3-month history of headaches, confusion, and lethargy. Aside from papilledema, the neurologic examination was normal. The CT scan showed symmetric hydrocephalus with no evidence of a mass lesion. Meningeal carcinomatosis (carcinomatous meningitis) was suspected, so a lumbar puncture was performed. Precautions were taken to have available at the bedside a twist-drill set, to permit a ventricular puncture in the event of cerebral herniation. She tolerated the spinal tap without incident, although her cerebrospinal fluid pressure was elevated. (B) Cytopathologic examination of the cerebrospinal fluid revealed sheets of tumor cells compatible with metastasis from the patient's primary breast tumor. The patient was given a course of whole-head radiation therapy as well as a course of intraventricular methotrexate via an implanted ventricular (Ommaya) reservoir. She did not respond to this therapy and she continued to decline until her death 6 weeks later. Although this particular patient failed to respond to this mode of therapy, some others with meningeal carcinomatosis do show improvement.

rologic deficit, intracranial hematoma, and wound infection. More recently (1983), the morbidity following surgical excision has been reported as 14 percent, with re-operation required in only 6 percent.[14] In the future, further improvement in surgical technique and control of cerebral edema and infection might be expected to reduce the incidence of both postoperative mortality and morbidity.

Surgical Technique

Haar and Patterson have observed that the operative mortality for brain metastasis surgery is correlated with the extent of tumor removal; in their series, the mortality was 8 percent with total excision, 18 percent with partial excision, and 30 percent with biopsy.[5] A similar experience was reported in the series of Richards and McKissock.[8] This suggests that total excision is preferable, although the mortality probably also reflects the depth and accessibility of the lesion, which influences the extent of removal. Moreover, the extent of surgical intervention in patients in poor condition is more likely to be limited to biopsy or partial excision. The reported results therefore may not be entirely a function of the extent of tumor removal.

Metastatic lesions deep in the dominant hemisphere generally are not amenable to surgical excision.[6] This restriction is also said to apply to thalamic lesions in either hemisphere,[6] although the transcallosal approach is being used increasingly for biopsy or excision of various types of thalamic tumors.[33] An inoperable metastasis in the brainstem is shown in Figure 40-7. Needle biopsy may be used for diagnosis of deeply situated lesions not amenable to direct surgical attack; needle biopsy may also be used for a superficial lesion suspected of being an abscess. A biopsy needle with a sharp cutting edge but without a bevel, specifically designed for tissue biopsy, should be employed, rather than the more widely used regular brain or ventricular cannula; the biopsy needle, with its nonbeveled open end, enables a long, thin core of tissue to enter the needle lumen.

A major technical development has been the introduction of CT-guided stereotactic biopsy for deep lesions or when surgical excision of a relatively superficial lesion is not feasible. CT-guided biopsy offers a precise and reasonably safe approach to the lesion for biopsy. The CT-guided technique can also be used to target the lesion as part of an open craniotomy for precise localization and open excision of subcortical lesions. Figure 40-2 illustrates the case of a metastatic lesion that,

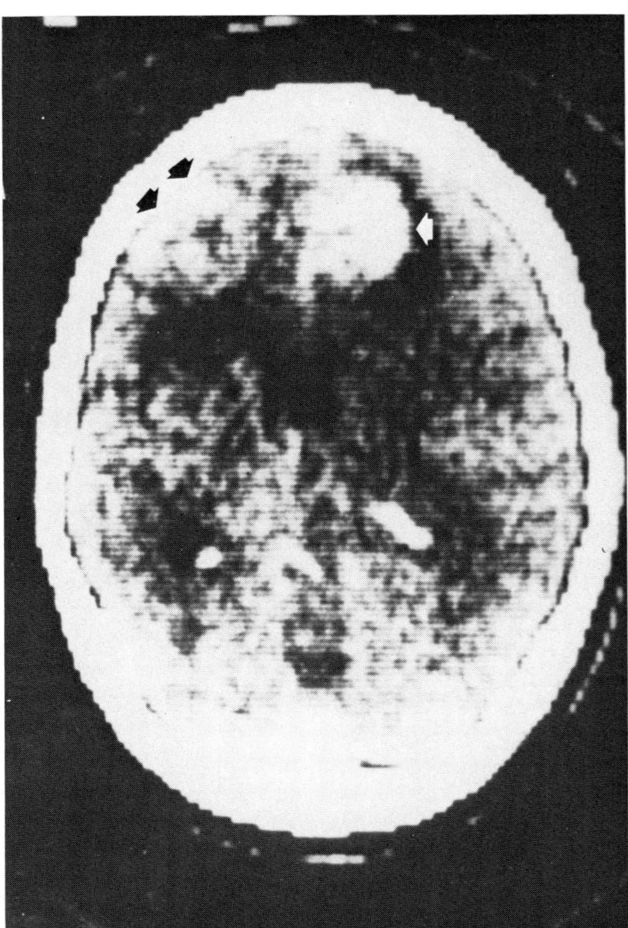

Fig. 40-6. A CT scan of a 42-year-old woman with a 1-week history of severe headaches, progressing to confusion and lethargy. On admission, she had papilledema and mild right hemiparesis. The CT scan, enhanced with contrast, showed multiple circumscribed mass lesions, two of which are shown in this tomographic cut. The lesion close to the lateral frontal cortex (two black arrows) had a ringlike appearance with a low-density center, suggesting necrosis or cyst. The multiple intracranial lesions strongly suggested metastasis, but complete investigation failed to reveal a primary malignancy. Under these circumstances, for establishment of a tissue diagnosis, an excisional biopsy of the accessible lesion in the left frontal area (black arrows) was made; this was done under local anesthesia. The circumscribed lesion, a reddish-black mass, was easily separated from the surrounding brain tissue and was totally excised. It was apparent there had been hemorrhage into the tumor, probably accounting for the rather rapid onset of symptoms and appearance of central necrosis on the CT scan. Pathologic examination revealed malignant melanoma. A subsequent search for melanotic lesions in the skin was unrevealing. The patient was given a course of whole-brain radiotherapy and was maintained on low-dose steroids. She did well for 6 weeks, at which time she was re-admitted with evidence of rapid neurologic deterioration; this was presumed, on the basis of repeat CT scan, to be related to hemorrhage around one of the other intracranial tumor metastases. She responded transiently to high-dose steroids and finally succumbed 1 month later.

although surgically accessible, was subcortical. This requires careful planning of the bone flap in order to ensure surgical access to the lesion. After the cortex is exposed, placement of the cortical incision (when the lesion does not appear on the cortical surface) can be guided either by use of the CT-stereotactic probe or by the use of intraoperative ultrasound (see Figure 40-2C).

Metastatic tumors are commonly circumscribed, although not encapsulated, and often can be totally separated macro-

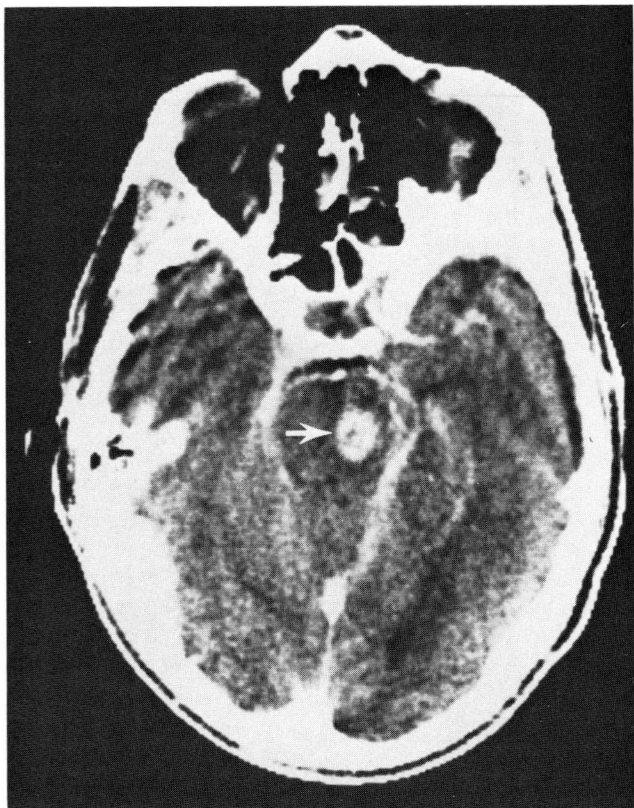

Fig. 40-7. A CT scan of a 51-year-old man with mild hemiparesis who had a history of bronchogenic carcinoma treated 2 years previously. The scan revealed an inoperable solitary enhancing lesion, presumably metastasis, in the midbrain (arrow).

scopically from brain tissue (Figures 40-1, 40-2, 40-6, and 40-8).[6,17] At autopsy, the completeness of the tumor resection has been confirmed in about 75 percent of the cases, the remainder of cases showing tumor infiltration in the surrounding brain parenchyma.[17] In another autopsy study, no residual tumor was found at the site of the previous surgical excision in 58 percent of the cases, although a number of these patients were found to have metastases elsewhere in the brain[16]; postoperative radiation was not used in either of the latter two series.[16,17] The 50–75 percent chance of eliminating the local metastasis by surgical excision is encouraging, and the addition of postoperative radiation might be expected to further improve these results (see Figure 40-1).

GUIDELINES FOR SELECTING PATIENTS FOR SURGICAL INTERVENTION

Although there are not yet any clear-cut criteria for the selection of patients for surgery, the following guidelines are suggested.

Solitary and Surgically Accessible Metastasis

Implicit in the decision regarding surgical accessibility of a lesion is the anticipation that its excision would not leave the patient with a severe neurologic deficit. In general, surgery is recommended only for patients with relatively superficial solitary lesions. It seems reasonable, however, as suggested by French and Ausman,[26] to consider the excision of a metastatic

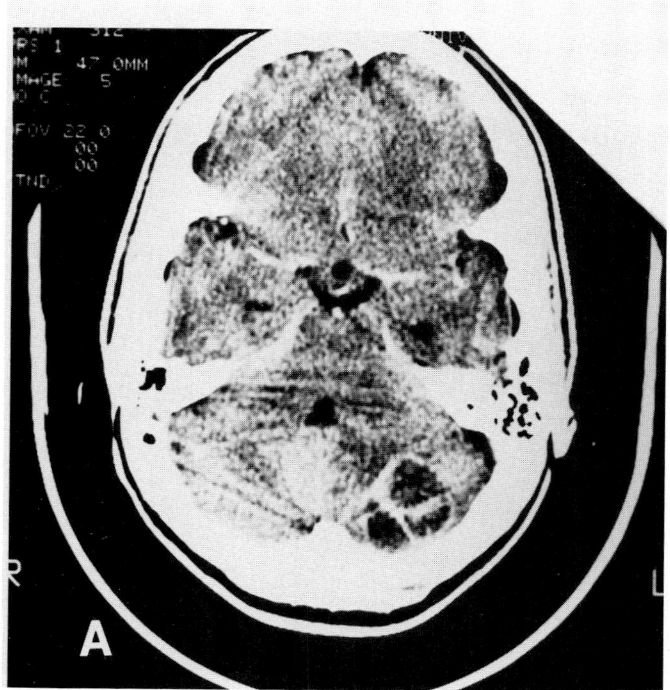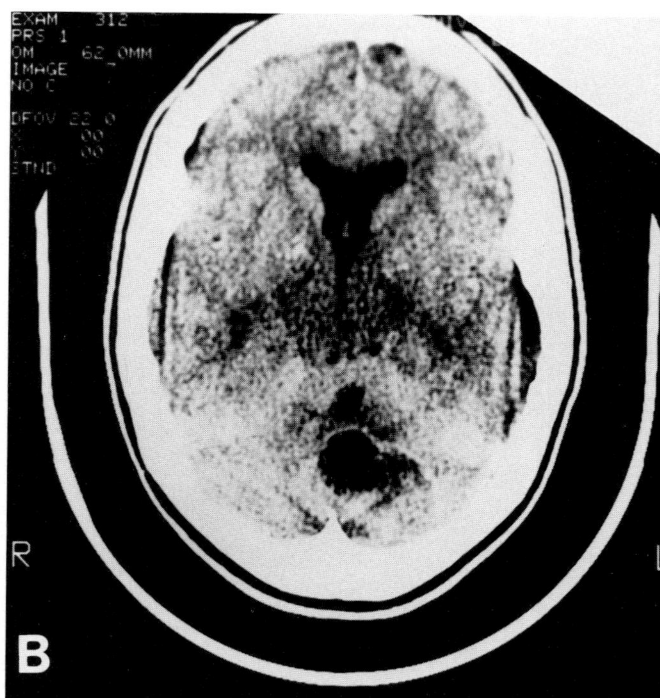

Fig. 40-8. Contrast-enhanced CT scan of 39-year-old woman with history of mastectomy for cancer 4 years earlier; 1 year earlier she had a right metastatic nodule removed from the lung. At the time of these studies she had a several-week history of headaches and ataxic gait. Chest x-ray films showed possible local recurrence of lung metastasis. (A) A contrast-enhanced CT scan showing a multiloculated lesion (left cerebellar hemisphere) causing shift of the fourth ventricle. (B) A CT scan slice through upper cerebellum and cerebral hemispheres showing the midline component of the cerebellar lesion with compression of the fourth ventricle and acute hydrocephalus. In view of the imminent danger of brain stem compression and despite the presence of other extracranial metastases (lung), incision of the cerebellar lesion appeared reasonable. She tolerated the surgery well; both the headache and ataxic gait were improved. She died 2 months later of further systemic spread of the cancer.

lesion that is immediately life-threatening or incapacitating, even in the presence of more than one metastatic brain lesion; this may be extended to the removal of multiple metastatic brain tumors if they are surgically accessible. Based on the improved results of combined therapy, it seems wise to follow the surgical excision of a metastatic lesion with a course of radiotherapy, chemotherapy, or both (see Figure 40-1).

Status of the Primary Tumor

The second consideration is whether the primary tumor can or has been treated, or if it will permit reasonably long survival. In many instances, the primary tumor may be symptomatically quiescent, and the immediate threat to life is the intracranial metastasis. Under such circumstances, management of the brain metastasis takes precedence over the management of the primary tumor.

Extracranial Metastases

The patient is a much better candidate for surgical intervention if there are no metastases elsewhere in the body. There are borderline situations in which the patient may not be a good surgical candidate in terms of there being evidence of unsatisfactory control of the primary lesion or systemic spread. When, however, the intracranial lesion is life-threatening but surgically accessible, it is reasonable to consider craniotomy for resection of the lesion, as illustrated by the case shown in Figure 40-8.

General Condition Satisfactory

The patient should be able to tolerate intracranial surgery. Needle or excisional biopsy of a small, superficial lesion can be carried out under local anesthesia (Figure 40-6).

Uncertain Diagnosis

Excisional or needle biopsy may be necessary in order to establish a tissue diagnosis, which is important in planning further management. For example, the patient may have a past history of a malignancy that had presumably been cured; the presence of a solitary intracerebral mass lesion does not necessarily indicate a metastasis. It also, of course, is conceivable that an intracranial lesion in a patient with known malignancy may prove to be an unrelated benign or treatable process, as illustrated by Figure 40-9. A third consideration is exemplified by the patient shown in Figure 40-6, in whom multiple intracranial lesions are demonstrated without evidence of a primary malignancy; in such cases, the differential diagnosis may include brain abscess, which can be by CT-guided stereotactic needle aspiration if the lesion is deep, or by excisional biopsy if it is near the surface of the brain.

Shunt for Hydrocephalus

Patients with hydrocephalus secondary to obstruction of the CSF pathway by tumor or edema can be offered a shunt procedure, which can provide significant temporary relief of symptoms. The shunt can be done in conjunction with excision of a metastatic tumor. Alternatively, the shunt can be used as an adjunct to radiation therapy. In either event, the incorporation of a Millipore filter (Millipore Corporation, Bedford, Massachusetts) within the shunt adds a measure of protection against further dissemination of the malignancy.[34] The placement of this filter within the shunt system prevents tumor cells from entering the bloodstream (for ventriculoatrial shunts) or from entering the peritoneal cavity.

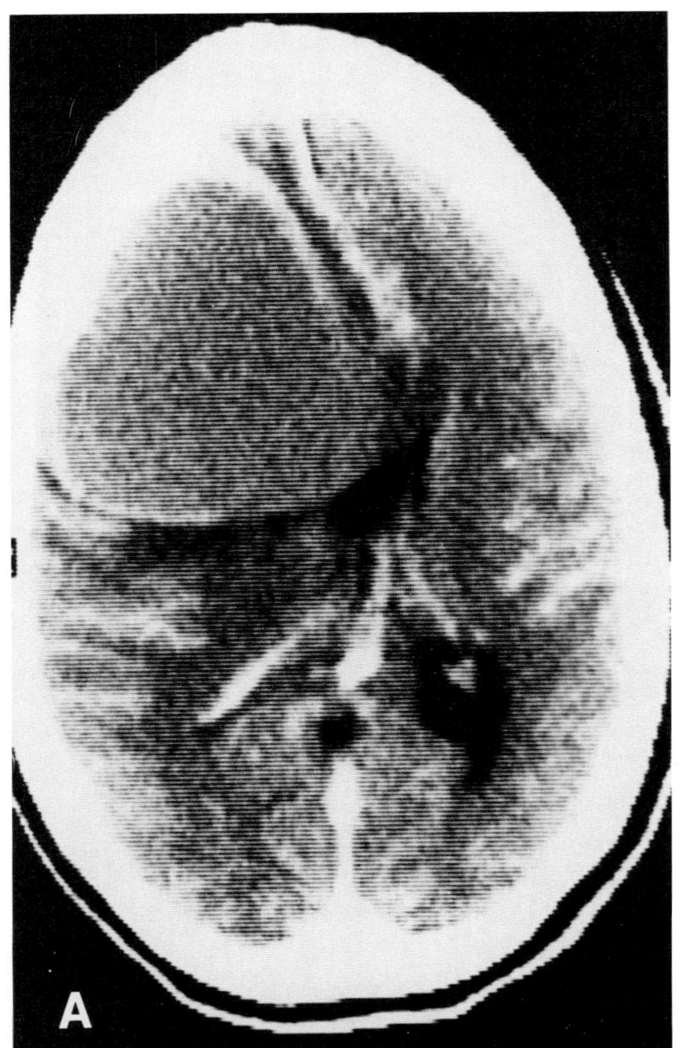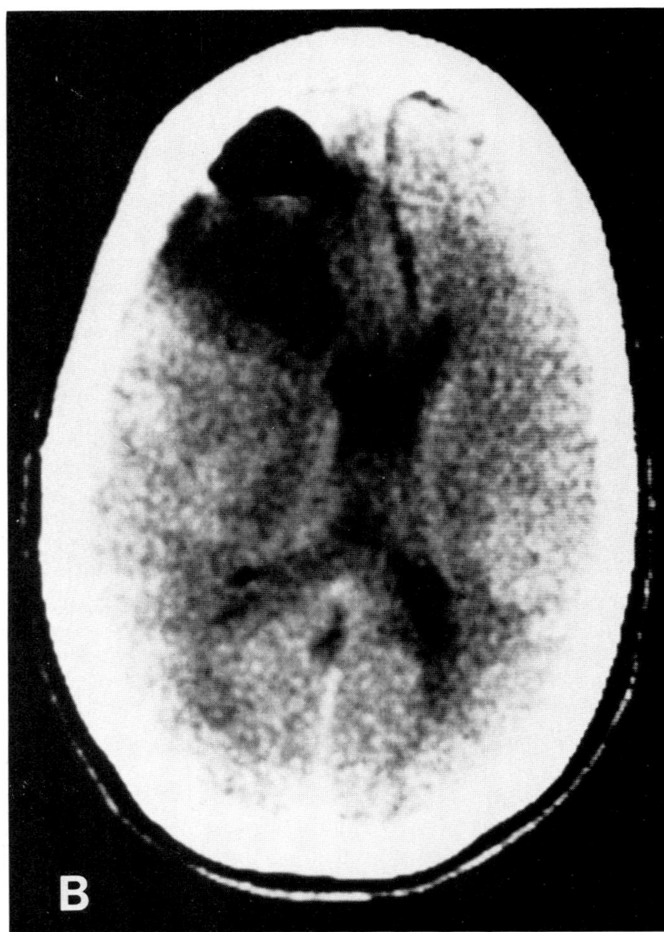

Fig. 40-9. A CT scan of a woman, age 55, with a history of squamous cell carcinoma of the lung, for which she had had a left lower lobectomy 1 month earlier. At the time of these studies she had a several-day history of progressive lethargy, frontal headache, and mild left hemiparesis, as well as nausea and vomiting. (A) Initial CT scan of head with contrast enhancement showing homogeneous, relatively isodense right frontal mass with a rim of enhancement. To rule out the possibility that the mass could be a hematoma, a right frontal twist-drill trephine was made, with needle evacuation of 100 ml dark blood. In an effort to reduce the chance of further bleeding, presumed to be from an adjacent tumor metastasis, thrombin (5000 units) was instilled into the hematoma cavity. A rubber catheter was left in the hematoma cavity for drainage overnight. Her neurologic condition improved considerably. (B) A follow-up CT scan 12 hours after aspiration of hematoma.

CHEMOTHERAPY AND IMMUNOTHERAPY

Neither chemotherapy nor immunotherapy has been shown to be of benefit in the management of cerebral metastasis. The failure of antitumor drugs has been attributed, in part, to the inability of most of these drugs to cross the blood-brain barrier.[35] The lipid-soluble nitrosoureas that cross this barrier are of some value in the management of primary brain tumors (gliomas), but these agents have not as yet been found to be useful for the management of brain metastases.[3] An exception is choriocarcinoma, which responds well to a combination of radiation therapy and chemotherapy.[21] Wilson and de la Garza also reported a favorable response to carmustine in a small series of patients with metastatic melanoma and a similar response to lomustine in some patients with metastatic bronchogenic carcinoma.[35] It has been suggested that prophylactic chemotherapy may reduce the incidence of brain metastases, particularly in breast carcinoma and melanoma.[36]

MENINGEAL CARCINOMATOSIS

Metastatic involvement of the leptomeninges implies that the entire neuraxis is exposed to the malignancy, as illustrated by the presence of tumor cells in the CSF (Figure 40-5). Without treatment, survival is usually limited to about 6 weeks.[3] This gloomy outlook can be improved by treatment combining radiotherapy and chemotherapy. Young et al. recommended delivering radiotherapy to the major site of the neurologic symptoms (the brain or spine), and treating the remainder of the neuraxis with intrathecal drugs (methotrexate and/or arabinosylcytosine).[37] The drugs are given in repeated doses by lumbar puncture or via an indwelling ventricular catheter with a subcutaneous reservoir under the scalp (Ommaya device; Heyer-Schulte Corporation, Goleta, California). The ventricular route is preferable because this entails simply puncturing the scalp for penetration of the subcutaneous reservoir, which the patient tolerates better than repeated lumbar punctures; the

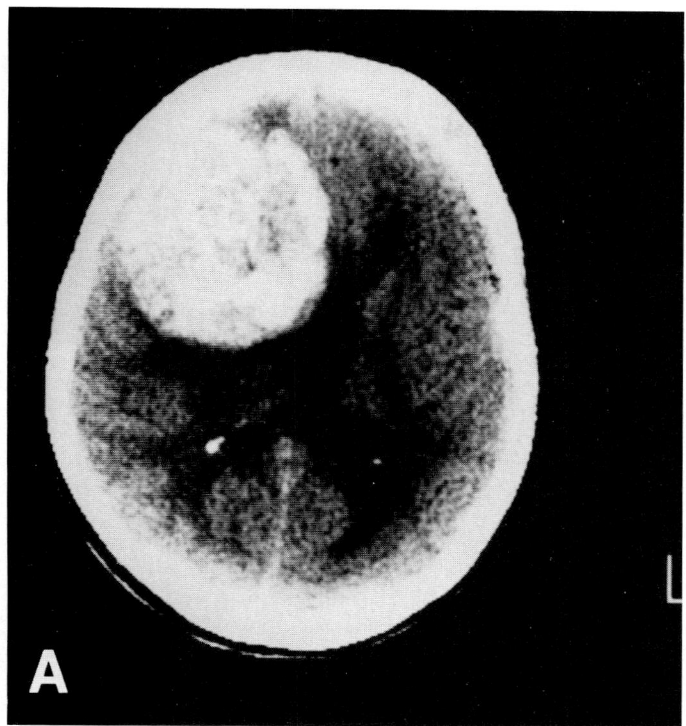
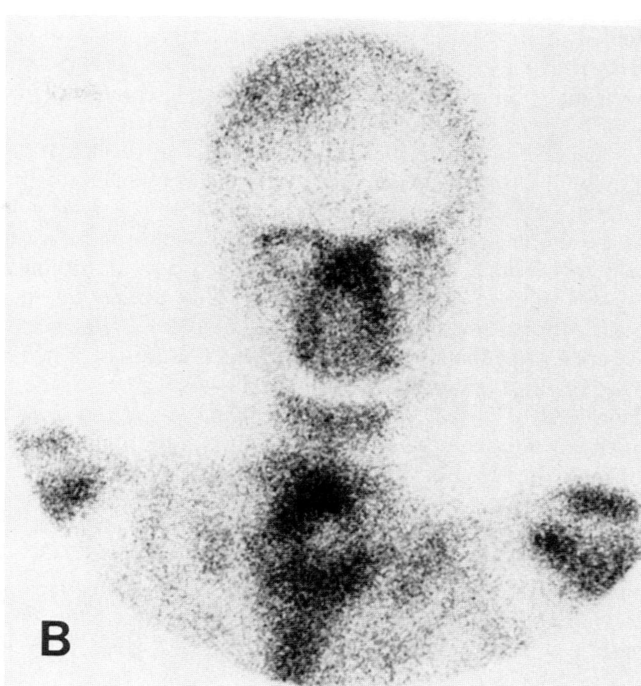

Fig. 40-10. A 42-year-old woman with a history of left upper lobectomy 16 months earlier for adenocarcinoma of lung. She received 6000 rad postoperatively for the lung lesion, and a high cervical cordotomy was performed for pain secondary to upper thoracic nerve root compression. She then experienced headache and recurrence of severe pain in upper posterior thorax. (A) A CT-scan of the head (nonenhanced) showing a large right frontotemporal mass, suspicious for metastatic tumor with irregular densities (thought to be hemorrhage) and considerable mass effect. (B) Isotope bone scan showing increased uptake (right side of head—corresponding to mass lesion seen on CT scan) and dense uptake in area of upper thoracic spine, corresponding to plain roentgenograms showing vertebral metastatic involvement. The patient refused biopsy or resection of right frontal lesion. Because the patient's primary concern was upper posterior chest wall pain, therapeutic efforts were directed to pain relief with intercostal phenol denervations.

ventricular route also has the advantage of better CSF dispersion of the antitumor agent. In the series treated by Young et al., patients with lymphoma and, to a lesser degree, those with breast carcinoma, responded well to this combined therapy, with the median survival time extended to about 5 months.[37] The response of bronchogenic carcinoma, melanoma, and other malignancies is less predictable.

THERAPEUTICALLY HOPELESS SITUATIONS

There are circumstances when it is reasonable to withhold active therapy of any kind. This applies to cases in which the patient seems terminally ill, with the expected survival time limited to a matter of days or weeks. The decision is readily made to withhold treatment in a terminally ill patient with widespread metastases outside the nervous system. Figure 40-10 illustrates the case of a patient with a presumed brain metastasis from a lung primary but in whom there was extensive metastatic involvement of the thoracic spine; in this situation, the primary goal became one of management of pain rather than tumor control. A more difficult decision arises with patients with severe neurologic deficit secondary to one or more intracranial metastases. Surgical intervention does not seem warranted in the presence of profound deficit, except for the purpose of biopsy when the diagnosis is in doubt. This is especially true when there are multiple brain or extracranial metastases in critical locations. In such situations, the chance of reversing profound neurologic deficit with either surgery or

radiotherapy is remote. Although there are borderline situations in which a course of radiotherapy and steroids might be considered, such patients are probably best treated symptomatically with medication for the relief of specific symptoms such as pain, rather than treated with the aim of prolonging life with little hope of recovery of neurologic function.

CONCLUSION

Advances in the radiotherapeutic and neurosurgical approaches to brain metastasis gradually are improving the outlook for such patients and are extending the duration of palliation. Although chemotherapy in the management of brain metastasis has not seemed promising thus far, this adjunct may contribute by helping to control the systemic component of the cancer. It seems clear that controlled prospective studies are now needed to compare the various available therapeutic modalities, as well as to investigate their combined use. Such objective evidence would place management on a more rational basis. Carefully planned protocols might be developed, with the collaboration of multiple hospitals in order to enlarge the patient population and thereby maximize the validity of the results.

It is important to assess the outcome of a given treatment modality without setting unrealistic objectives. Any advance in management is likely to come slowly, with further extension in the duration of palliation and, it is to be hoped, improvement in the quality of survival. It would be unreasonable at this stage to set goals for complete cure, because this would serve only to obscure other positive gains. Within the framework of these limited objectives, an improved outlook for patients with brain metastasis may emerge. Statistical analysis of controlled studies using various treatment modalities may eventually point to criteria for selecting treatment for a given patient.

Despite an overall slight improvement in results, for the present it should be kept in mind that a percentage of these patients may not be helped, and some may even be made worse as a result of therapeutic intervention. A philosophical as well as practical public health decision must be made concerning the relative value of short-term salvage weighed against the therapeutic effort, financial cost, and potential for prolonging the suffering of patients who are treatment failures. The history of progress in other spheres of medicine—for example, the advances made in the treatment of leukemia—suggests that the price will probably be worthwhile in the long run. Using the currently inadequate criteria for selection of treatment, the clinician must decide with the individual patient and family whether to invest in aggressive therapy with its high cost and risk. A number of disciplines—medical oncology, radiation oncology, neurosurgery—should participate in the decision-making process, because the management of these patients can best be achieved through a team effort.

ACKNOWLEDGMENTS

The assistance of Carol Lynn Daly, MA in the preparation of the manuscript is gratefully acknowledged.

Portions of this chapter are reprinted from previous publications by the author: "Metastatic tumors of the central nervous system: Cerebral metastases," in Abeloff M (ed): Complications of Cancer: Diagnosis and Management, Baltimore, Johns Hopkins University Press, 1980; and "Brain metastasis: Current status and recommended guidelines for management." Neurosurgery 5:617–631, 1979. Used with permission of the publishers.

REFERENCES

1. Aronson SM, Garcia JH, Aronson BE: Metastatic neoplasms of the brain: Their frequency in relation to age. Cancer 17:558, 1964
2. Van Eck JHM, Go KG, Ebels EJ: Metastatic tumours of the brain. Psychiatr Neurol Neurochir 68:443, 1965
3. Posner JB: Management of central nervous system metastases. Semin Oncol 4:81, 1977
4. Black P: Metastatic tumors of the central nervous system: Cerebral metastasis, in Abeloff MD (ed): Complications of Cancer: Diagnosis and Management. Baltimore, Johns Hopkins University Press, 1979, pp 283–312
5. Haar F, Patterson RH Jr: Surgery for metastatic intracranial neoplasm. Cancer 30:1241, 1972
6. Ransohoff J: Surgical management of metastatic tumors. Semin Oncol 2:21, 1975
7. Raskind R, Weiss SR, Manning JJ, et al: Survival after surgical excision of single metastatic brain tumors. AJR 111:323, 1971
8. Richards P, McKissock W: Intracranial metastases. Br Med J 1:15, 1963
9. Simionescu MD: Metastatic tumors of the brain: A follow-up study of 195 patients with neurosurgical considerations. J Neurosurg 17:361, 1960
10. Taylor HG, Lefkowitz M, Skokog SJ, et al: Intracranial metastases in prostate cancer. Cancer 53:2728, 1984
11. Veith RG, Odom GL: Intracranial metastases and their neurosurgical treatment. J Neurosurg 23:375, 1965
12. Walker MD: Brain and peripheral nervous system tumors, in Holland JF, Frei E (eds): Cancer Medicine, vol 3. Philadelphia, Lea & Febiger, 1973, pp 1385–1407
13. Madajewicz S, Karakousis C, West CR, et al: Malignant melanoma brain metastases: Review of Roswell Park Memorial institute experience. Cancer 53:2550, 1984
14. Sundaresan N, Galicich JH, Beattie EJ: Surgical treatment of brain metastases from lung cancer. J Neurosurg 58:666, 1983
15. Kindt GW: The pattern of location of cerebral metastatic tumors. J Neurosurg 21:54, 1964
16. Lang EF, Slater J: Metastatic brain tumors: Results of surgical and nonsurgical treatment. Surg Clin North Am 44:865, 1964
17. Stortebecker TP: Metastatic tumors of the brain from a neurosurgical point of view: A follow-up study of 158 cases. J Neurosurg 11:84, 1954
18. Olson ME, Chernik NL, Posner JB: Infiltration of the leptomeninges by systemic cancer: A clinical and pathologic study. Arch Neurol 30:122, 1974
19. Murray JJ, Houston MC: Calcified intracranial metastases from breast carcinoma with a therapeutic response to tamoxifen therapy. South Med J 79:253, 1986
20. MacGee EE: Surgical treatment of cerebral metastases from lung cancer. The effect on quality and duration of survival. J Neurosurg 3:416, 1971
21. Shapiro WR, Posner JB: Corticosteroid hormones: Effects in an experimental brain tumor. Arch Neurol 30:217, 1974
22. Deutsch M, Parson JA, Mercado R Jr: Radiotherapy for intracranial metastases. Cancer 34:1607, 1974
23. Order SE, Hellman S, von Essen CF, et al: Improvement in quality of survival following whole-brain irradiation for brain metastasis. Radiology 91:149, 1968
24. Posner JB: Diagnosis and treatment of metastases to the brain. Clin Bull 4:47, 1974
25. Shehata WM, Hendrickson FR, Hindo WA: Rapid fractionation technique and retreatment of cerebral metastases by irradiation. Cancer 34:257, 1974
26. French LA, Ausman JI: Metastatic neoplasms to the brain. Clin Neurosurg 24:41, 1977
27. Fernandez E, Maira G, Puca A, et al: Multiple intracranial metastases of malignant melanoma with long-term survival. J Neurosurg 60:621, 1984
28. McCann WP, Weir BKA, Elvidge AR: Long-term survival after removal of metastatic malignant melanoma of the brain: Report of two. J Neurosurg 28:483, 1968
29. Magilligan DJ Jr, Rogers JS, Knighton RS, et al: Pulmonary neoplasm with solitary cerebral metastasis: Results of combined excision. J Thorac Cardiovasc Surg 72:690, 1976
30. Black P: Brain metastasis: Current status and recommended guidelines for management. Neurosurg 5:617, 1979
31. Ishizuka T, Tomoda Y, Kaseki S, et al: Intracranial metastasis of choriocarcinoma: A clinicopathologic study. Cancer 52:1896, 1983
32. Salmon SE: Human tumor colony assay and chemosensitivity testing. Cancer Treat Rev 68:117, 1984
33. Shucart WA, Stein BM: Transcallosal approach to the anterior ventricular system. Neurosurg 3:339, 1978
34. Hoffman HJ, Hendrick EB, Humphreys RP: Metastasis via ventriculoperitoneal shunt in patients with medulloblastoma. J Neurosurg 44:562, 1976
35. Wilson WL, de la Garza JG: Systemic chemotherapy for CNS metastases of solid tumors. Arch Intern Med 115:710, 1965
36. Costanza ME, Nathanson L, Lenhard R, et al: Therapy of malignant melanoma with an imidazole carboxamide and bischloroethylnitrosourea. Cancer 30:1457, 1972
37. Young DF, Shapiro WR, Posner JB: Treatment of leptomeningeal cancer (abstr). Neurology 25:370, 1975

Localization and Biopsy of Intracranial Lesions with Computed Tomography and Magnetic Resonance Imaging

Robert J. Coffey   L. Dade Lunsford

THE INTRODUCTION of computed tomography (CT) in the mid 1970s radically altered the practice of both neuroradiology and stereotactic neurosurgery. Ten years later, the widening availability of magnetic resonance imaging (MRI) has again provided a greatly superior diagnostic tool for the evaluation of pathologic processes in the central nervous system. Computed tomography and now multiplanar MRI directly image various intracranial lesions and reveal their relationship to neighboring cerebral, osseous, vascular, or cerebrospinal fluid (CSF)-containing structures. Small lesions have been recognized earlier in the course of many diseases before significant neurologic deficits or mass effect have developed. These imaging modalities, combined with new surgical techniques capable of reaching the depths of the brain with millimeter precision, were of paramount importance.

Computed tomography and MRI have demonstrated the dimensions and contours of complex lesions, as well as the vascularity, the solid or cystic nature of the masses, or the presence of calcification or hemorrhage. Sophisticated image production using computer techniques permitted multiplanar and three-dimensional displays of the cranial contents. Both CT and MRI have proved to be safe, noninvasive, and easily repeatable, allowing the evolution of pathologic processes to be monitored with serial studies. Both CT and MRI images can be used to obtain coordinate information for localization of various intracranial targets free of the magnification, rotation, and parallax effects encountered when conventional radiography is used. Combinations of these imaging tools with precise guiding devices have evolved significantly in the past 10 years. Table 41-1 indicates the current uses of CT- and MRI-guided stereotactic surgery in the evaluation and treatment of lesions of the brain and for functional neurosurgery.

HISTORY OF CT GUIDED LOCALIZATION TECHNIQUES

While it may seem unusual to talk about a history of only 10-years duration, the field of imaging-directed neurosurgery has evolved rapidly. The initial techniques reported with early generation CT scanners have now been supplanted by the use of more sophisticated and precise surgical tools. Shortly after the introduction of CT, work began on a variety of methods to guide biopsy instruments to brain lesions demonstrated on CT scans. Several approaches of variable complexity and usefulness evolved simultaneously at various centers over the past decade. These techniques can be classified according to the following criteria:

1. Free-hand techniques guided by intraoperative imaging.
2. Transposition techniques (transfer of CT data to stereotactic roentgenographic plane films).
3. Modifications of traditional stereotactic frames for CT and MRI compatibility.
4. Simple and plane of target devices.
5. Development of new CT or MRI stereotactic systems.

THE DEVELOPMENT OF FREE-HAND TECHNIQUES

Biopsy of brain tumors monitored by CT was reported by Maroon et al. in 1977.[1] An early generation CT scanner was used in conjunction with a localization device fashioned from a rubber bathing cap that contained radiodense reference lines. These lines left marks at the periphery of each axial CT image and were used to guide the drawing of additional reference and trajectory lines directly on the patient's scalp. Burr hole placement and free-hand biopsy needle placement were carried out in the CT scanner and were interrupted frequently to obtain CT images from which the progress of the needle was monitored. Subsequent corrections of the trajectory were made as needed. Variations in this technique were widely used and occasionally were reported by others.[2] More elaborate external localization devices were employed using grids.[3] Although less sophisticated than the techniques currently available, those procedures were often successful in obtaining diagnostic tissue or draining fluid from relatively large lesions. More importantly, they served as the impetus to develop more sophisticated and precise techniques.

TRANSPOSITION OF CT DATA TO STEREOTACTIC ROENTGENOGRAMS (PLAIN X-RAY FILMS)

Various methods of augmenting conventional radiographic data by including CT data into established stereotactic systems were developed in several centers in the 1970s. Gildenberg

OPERATIVE NEUROSURGICAL TECHNIQUES
ISBN 0-8089-1862-1

Table 41-1. Indications and uses of CT and MRI stereotactic surgery

Type of Surgery	Diagnosis	Therapy
Morphologic	Mass lesions of the cerebrum and brain-stem	Tumor resection; cyst evacuation; shunt placement; abscess drainage; hematoma evacuation; interstitial irradiation; intracavitary irradiation; linear accelerator adaptations; stereotactic radiosurgery
Physiologic (functional)	Epilepsy; chronic pain; movement disorders	Thalamotomy; internal capsulotomy; pituitary ablation; deep brain electrodes

reported a method by which CT data could be transposed onto stereotactic anteroposterior (AP) and lateral plain roentgenograms taken with the patient's head fixed in a traditional stereotactic instrument.[4,5] The angle of the CT gantry and resulting axial images relative to the bony landmarks of the skull base were determined from the lateral CT electronic radiograph (scout film). A particular axial image was selected to represent the zero slice. The line representing this plane plus a second line perpendicular to its midpoint were transcribed onto the stereotactic roentgenograms. Using CT cursor-derived measurements, the target point could be plotted on these roentgenograms after which stereotactic frame coordinates for the targets were calculated. The CT slice thickness and distance between images determined the vertical coordinate. Thus, the accuracy of this technique depended upon the accuracy of the CT table movements. Kaufman and Gildenberg subsequently developed a head holder to allow repeatable nonoperative fixation of the patient's head in the CT table.[6] This device permitted serial CT scans with the head in exactly the same position. A standard stereotactic frame could then be applied in precise relation to the head holder, allowing immediate or delayed operations after an initial CT scan. This technique was reported to have an accuracy within 3 mm.[4,6] Unfortunately, patient motion during any portion of the scanning sequence destroyed the accuracy of the system, and errors could be

introduced as well by inaccuracy of table movement or slice thickness measurements.

SIMPLE DEVICES

A number of relatively simple and inexpensive CT-guided stereotactic biopsy systems have been developed.[2,7,8,9] Most represented the mechanical refinement of earlier free-hand techniques requiring the entry point to be in the same axial plane as the target. Trajectory selection with such devices has been limited, making large regions of the brain relatively inaccessible. For example, the risk of vascular entry during trans-sylvian "plane of target" approaches to "the basal ganglia" has remained a serious limitation. Patil has constructed a plane of target device that permits coordinates of various targets to be obtained from the CT image.[9] The Patil stereotactic coordinate frame is compatible with both CT and MRI imaging modalities and has been used both for functional as well as morphologic neurosurgery.

Carol developed a skull-mounted stereotactic system having a circular central aperture.[10] Convenient trajectories have been limited to frontal or parietal convexity entry points. A three) dimensional "phantom" apparatus, simulating the relationship between the skull-mounted disc, the entry point, the target point, and the CT table and gantry was employed. The "phantom" mechanically set the trajectory of the ball and socket probe guide as well as the depth of the biopsy probe. The device has relied upon the scanner table index to determine the vertical (depth) coordinate. A table calibration device available from the manufacturer helped to minimize errors in this calculation. One limitation of the system has been that the trajectory to the target was predetermined by application of the skull disc before imaging. Any change in trajectory would require removal and replacement of the disc followed by repeat CT imaging.

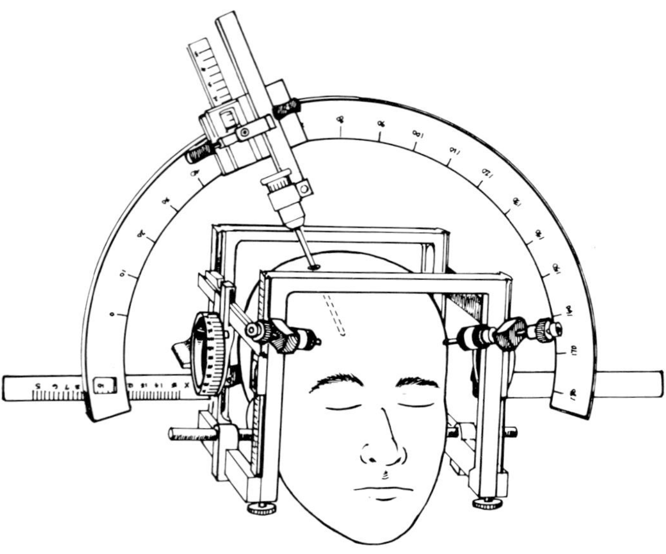

Fig. 41-1. The Leksell stereotactic system, arc-radius principle. The probe is equal in length to the radius of the arc and thus reaches the geometric center of the arc regardless of arc rotation around the supporting gimbals, or movement of the probe carrier along the arc circumference. The side bars and gimbal supports, which are adjustable in three dimensions, move the probe impact point (arc center) to coincide with the target coordinates.

MODIFICATION OF TRADITIONAL STEREOTACTIC FRAMES FOR CT AND MRI

Virtually all current stereotactic instruments employ rigid fixation of the device to the head during both the imaging and surgical phases of the procedure. Accuracy of probe placement to within 1 mm of the selected target is the accepted mechanical accuracy of any stereotactic device. Adaptations of traditional stereotactic devices for CT have been reported for the Leksell stereotactic system,[11] the Riechert-Mundinger system,[12–18] and the Todd-Wells stereotactic system.[19–22]

Using an early generation CT scanner, Bergstrom and Greitz in 1976[23] and subsequently Boethius et al. reported development of a large base ring with a localization device

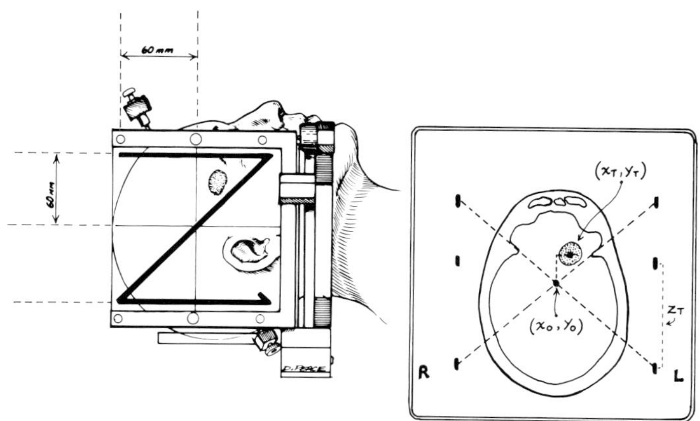

Fig. 41-2. Direct CT coordinate determination. The "N" shaped strips of the localizer devices (left) produce three marks in the lateral margins of each axial CT image (right). Connecting the marks at opposite corners with the CT cursor locates the center of the frame (X = O, Y = O). The cursor also gives CT coordinates for the target point (X = T, Y = T). The arithmetic difference between these two coordinate pairs (X = T − X = O, Y = T − Y = O) is the distance of the target in millimeters from the center of the frame in the AP and lateral planes. The vertical frame coordinate of the target is obtained by subtracting the distance Z = T from 60 mm, half the height of the stereotactic frame, (60 − Z = T). This value is the distance of the target above or below the center of the frame. Cursor position and distance functions are standard features of all current generation CT scanners.

attached to it for CT imaging.[24,25] The localization device could be replaced by a conventional Leksell frame, after which standard stereotactic procedures were performed.

The Leksell stereotactic device itself was subsequently redesigned for CT compatibility by Leksell and reported by Leksell and Jernberg in 1980.[11] By this time modifications in CT scanners had eliminated such encumbrances as the water bag. Enlargement of the CT scanner aperture allowed conventional stereotactic devices to be used with only minor modifications. The new Leksell instrument (Figure 41-1) was constructed entirely of aluminum. Head fixation was achieved by steel drills, which were replaced by carbon fiber pins after penetration of the outer table. Direct coordinate determination was obtained from fiducial markers located within removable side plates and producing index marks in the margins of the CT images. Coordinates could be determined by using standard CT scanner software or a grid scaled for standard CT film images. In 1984, further modification of the stereotactic device was performed for MRI.[26] The frame was magnetically isolated by a special anodization process. Fiducial markers in the new MRI side plates consisted of tubes filled with a dilute aqueous solution of copper sulfate, replacing the aluminum strips used during CT imaging. Stereotactic coordinates were obtained from both axial magnetic resonance and CT images, as well as from coronal and sagittal magnetic resonance images. The addition of a vertex fiducial plate allowed direct sagittal MRI localization according to the geometric principles described below.

With the Leksell CT system, target localization is performed from axial images. Each image contains along its margins the small fiducial markers created by the "N" shaped metal strips encased in the removable plastic side plates (Figure 41-2). Using the CT computer, cursors deposited at opposite corners of the image containing the targets are connected to form an "X" determining the center of the cubical stereotactic coordinate frame. The distance in millimeters along each axis between the center of the coordinate frame and the target point is measured by the cursor. This gives the stereotactic target coordinates in the anteroposterior (Y) and left-right (X) planes.

The vertical (superoinferior or Z) coordinate is derived

from the fiducial markers on the side plates as follows: the diagonal line of each "N" is at a 45-degree angle to each vertical line, thereby forming a set of isosceles right triangles. An imaginary line connecting the midpoints to the two diagonal fiducials passes through the geometric center of the frame. Axial imaging must be performed parallel to the base of the frame. The distance between the marks produced by the vertical and diagonal fiducials on the target slice is subtracted from half the distance between the two vertical fiducials (60 mm), thus giving the distance of the target in millimeters above or below the frame's center. Vertical coordinate determination by the use of "N" shaped localization devices has been a unifying theme in many successful CT-guided stereotactic instruments. The Leksell CT coordinate frame is attached by steel feet to a magnetic adapter on the CT table. For MRI, these are replaced by plastic feet, which snap into an adapter designed for the various MRI units.

In 1983, Bullard[12,13] in the United States and Gahbauer et al.[15] in Germany both described modifications of the Riechert-Mundinger stereotactic system to permit direct target coordinate determination from axial CT images. A localization attachment having either "N" or "V" shaped marker rods was attached to the base ring. As in the Leksell and other devices, the relative positions of the artifacts created by the fiducial markers allowed calculation of the vertical coordinate.

Birg and Mundinger in 1982 described the commercially produced CT adaptation of the Riechert-Mundinger system.[27] A detailed description of the operation and limitations of a similar system was published by Dyck.[14] No "N" or "V" localizer attachments were used in this modification. Instead, an adjustable calibrated adapter clamped the head ring to the CT table. By serial adjustments, the ring and gantry were made isocentric and coplanar. The origin of the head frame coordinate system (the center of the head ring) then coincided with the center of each actual CT image. Consequently, scanner coordinates were equivalent to anteroposterior (Y) and the left-right (X) frame coordinates. The vertical (Z coordinate) was obtained from CT cursor distance measurements on sagittal or coronal reformatted images or from the electronic sagittal radiograph. Entry point coordinates, necessary to establish a trajectory in the

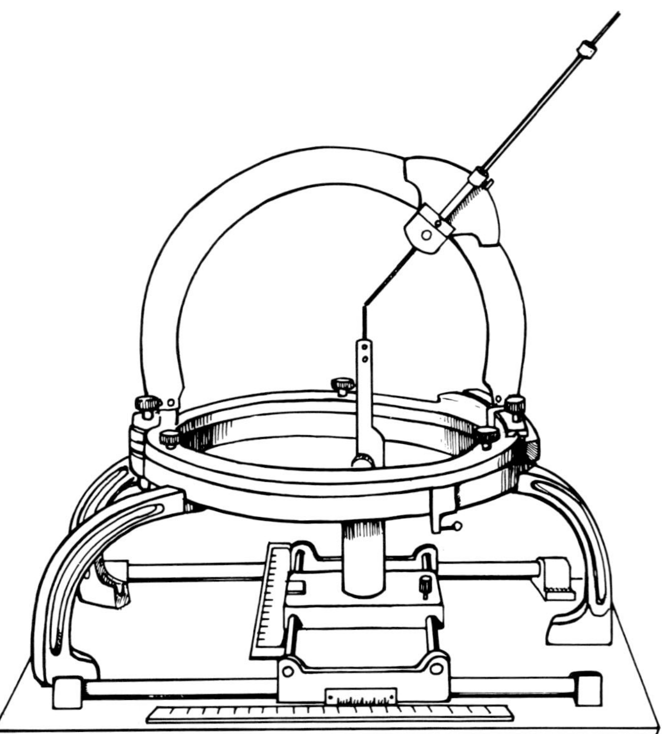

Fig. 41-3. The BRW stereotactic frame showing the arc-guidance system mounted on the phantom-target simulator. The latter, having adjustments in the AP, lateral, and vertical dimensions, places a pointer at the target or entry point as determined by the system's microcomputer. The arc-guidance system, with its polar (angular) coordinates and depth, also set according to the microcomputer, is placed on the phantom as a final visual/mechanical check before commencing the surgical phase of the operation.

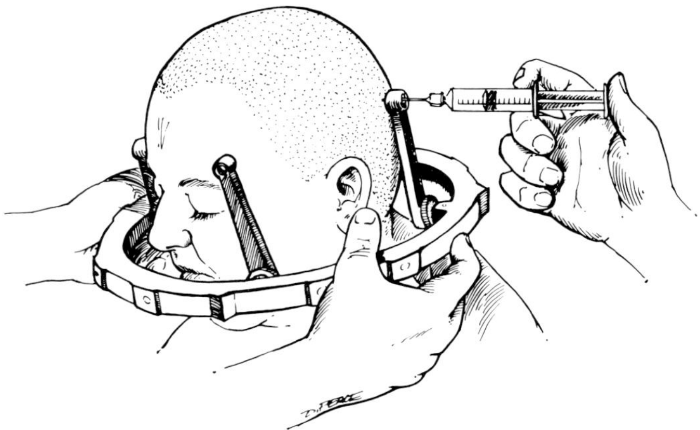

Fig. 41-4. Application of the BRW head ring. The support posts are adjusted such that the penetrating pins will be located at the supraorbital and parieto-occipital convexity regions of the skull. Local anesthetic is injected through the support post apertures, after which the sharpened pins are threaded in to penetrate the outer table of the skull.

Riechert-Mundinger system, were obtained from the anteroposterior and lateral electronic radiographs taken with strips of radiopaque markers attached to the patient's head. A phantom device set at the appropriate target point, entry site, and trajectory was used to check those variables before actually inserting the probe into the brain.

Kelly et al. developed a system that contained major modifications of an original Todd-Wells sterotactic device.[19–22] The original pin supports were replaced by imaging-compatible materials, and head fixation was obtained with carbon fiber pins. Low artifact CT imaging could be performed, as well as calculation of the target coordinates. The head ring was adjustable such that the target point was moved to the focal point of an arc-quadrant frame system. Later modifications of this device made it compatible with MRI, digital subtraction angiography, and ultrasonography. By greatly enlarging the radius of the original arc of the Todd-Wells stereotactic system, Kelly was able to incorporate an operating microscope and a carbon dioxide laser to perform stereotactic vaporization of brain lesions identified by various imaging modalities.[20,21] Imaging was performed in a separate radiology suite, after which surgery was carried out in a stereotactic operating room equipped with the computer and display consoles of the CT scanner. Magnetic resonance imaging, CT, and angiographic digitized information could be ''dumped'' into an independent computer in the operating room. This information was used to create three-dimensional images of the lesion and surrounding brain structures to be approached by stereotactic technique. Imaging

and surgery were often performed on different days, necessitating precise repositioning of the frame in the exact orientation as when imaging was performed. The safety and efficacy of this system were demonstrated in several reports.[19–21]

NEW STEREOTACTIC SYSTEMS

Brown et al., beginning in 1979, first detailed the development of a new stereotactic system subsequently referred to as the Brown-Roberts-Wells (BRW) stereotactic system.[28–34] Six major components constitute the currently marketed system: a head ring, a CT localizing system, an arc guidance system, a phantom simulator, a mini computer, and a floor stand (Figure 41-3). The detailed operation of the BRW system has been described elsewhere[31,32,34] but will be summarized here. The head ring is attached to the patient by pins penetrating the scalp (Figure 41-4). It serves as a base for the CT localization system during the imaging phase and for the arc-guidance system during the surgical portion of the procedure. The orientation in which the head ring is applied determines the position of the patient's head during surgery (Figure 41-5). The arc-guidance system, which resembles a surveyor's transit, has four separate angular adjustments in two orthogonal planes. Depth to target is the fifth and only linear setting in the polar coordinate system. The phantom simulator, which also accepts the arc-guidance system, has a base ring identical to the actual head ring. As with other similar devices, entry points and trajectories can be verified mechanically before surgery begins (Figure 41-3).

The localization system consists of a circular array of three ''N'' shaped carbon fiber figures. These produce nine fiducial marks around the circumference of the axial CT image. Using the CT scanner cursor, coordinates for each of these marks plus the intended target are compiled. Entering the ten coordinate (X,Y) pairs into the notebook-sized BRW computer gives the three-dimensional frame coordinates of the target. The mathematical transformation of CT data into three-dimensional target coordinates and polar frame settings is relatively complex and cannot be performed easily without the aid of a computer. The frame settings and probe depth are calculated by the computer

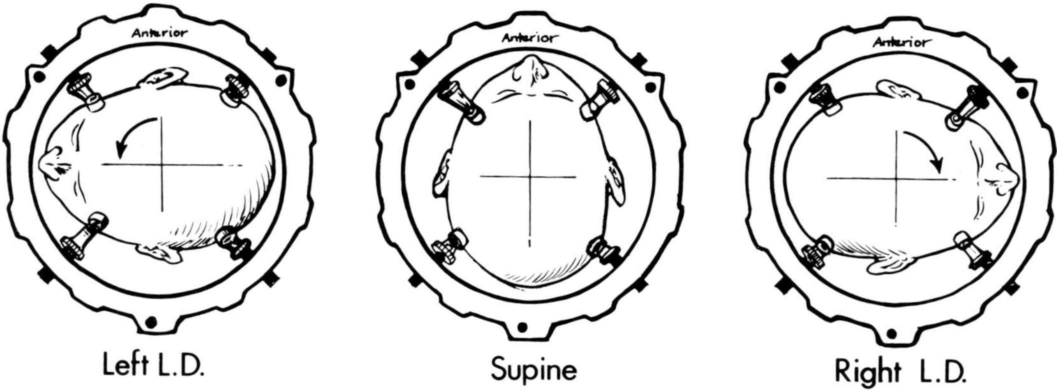

Fig. 41-5. Ring application is performed to position the patient's head with the entry point upward and the Mayfield adapter of the head ring downward. For frontal entry points the patient is supine (center); for right parietal or occipital entry points the patient lies in the left lateral decubitus position (left). The situation is reversed for left parietal or occipital entry (right). In each case, the "Anterior" mark engraved on the head ring faces upward, permitting use of the Mayfield adapter to firmly clamp the patient's head to the operating table.

after selection and input of an entry point. This point is determined in one of three alternate ways depending upon the nature of the operation being performed: visually, from the CT image as in target point selection; mechanically, by transfer of the arc-guidance system having the probe at the desired spot on the patient's scalp to the phantom simulator; or mathematically, by specifying a desired set of trajectory angles to the computer.

Brown's original computer software employed matrix algebra solutions to coordinate determination and allowed the processing of data from nonparallel CT images.[28–30] The current production model, with its micro-computer, employs vector analysis to convert linear CT data to polar frame coordinates. Complex operations involving reformatted CT images and tabulations of coordinate data from multiple CT slices are greatly facilitated by keeping the axial images, the head ring, and the CT gantry parallel. An adapter to clamp the head ring to the CT table accomplishes this at the present time. Transsphenoidal and suboccipital trajectories are usually not possible with the BRW instrument. The metal arc guidance system also does not permit artifact-free intraoperative CT imaging, although a limited number of low artifact plastic (Delrin) arcs have been fabricated.

Rhodes et al. in 1982 described a polar coordinate instrument constructed entirely of plastic, permitting surgery and intraoperative imaging in the CT scanner.[35] Similarities between this device and the BRW device are obvious. The Rhodes-Glenn instrument required access to a mainframe computer to operate its full range of advanced imaging software programs. Localizer coordinates from every CT image were entered in the computer by an automated visual search program. The computer could then display tentative probe trajectories in any one of several reformatted viewing planes. More recently, the localization components of the frame (having four "N" shaped rods) have been linked to a computer via a robot arm, thus eliminating the manually set stereotactic frame. The robot instrument has proved accurate and reliable in phantom tests and has been successfully used to a limited extent on patients.[36] The future role of robotics in stereotactic surgery remains to be defined.

Perry et al. in 1979 developed a CT-compatible stereotactic frame linked to the computer operating software of a Pfizer (Pfizer Medical Systems, Baltimore, MD) scanner.[37] A combination of linear and polar coordinates were employed. Target localization was again attained by means of "N" shaped markers followed by a computer vector analysis to determine the stereotactic coordinates. Those portions of the frame appearing in the CT image were fabricated of low artifact materials specifically designed to allow intraoperative imaging of the target with the probe in position. Limitations of this device included the relatively narrow range of artifact-free imaging as well as a limited number of trajectories (vertex) that were available. Lunsford et al. utilized this device at the University of Pittsburgh in a series of cases in 1979 and 1980.[37,38] We subsequently adopted the simpler and more versatile Leksell stereotactic instrument.

INDICATIONS FOR STEREOTACTIC SURGERY

Despite advances in neurodiagnostic imaging, accurate histologic diagnosis of brain lesions remains mandatory. In our initial series, in as many as 26 percent of cases a histologic diagnosis that differed from the preoperative diagnosis was obtained when stereotactic biopsy was performed.[38] Such findings always altered postoperative treatment. Stereotactic surgery has also provided 1-mm precision when accurate biopsy and precise therapies were planned. We advocate stereotactic surgery when lesions are small, deep, multiple, or not amenable to traditional neurosurgical approaches. When despite lesion size the patient's symptoms or signs are insignificant or likely to be exacerbated by conventional craniotomy or resection, stereotactic surgery is a good option. When lesions are multiple, adverse medical conditions exist, or the patient is of advanced age, stereotactic surgery is the treatment of choice. At the present time, lesions of the cerebrum, brain stem, and cerebellum are all amenable to stereotactic surgery. Bosch also has discussed the current role of stereotactic biopsy in brain tumors.[39]

Histologic definition is also dependent upon the type of biopsy instrumentation that is used. Various instruments currently used for stereotactic biopsy are shown in Figure 41-6. These instruments include varous modifications of suction or aspiration needles, a "cork-screw" spiral, and tissue biopsy forceps. At the University of Pittsburgh, we have chosen the Backlund biopsy instrument. It has proved to be relatively

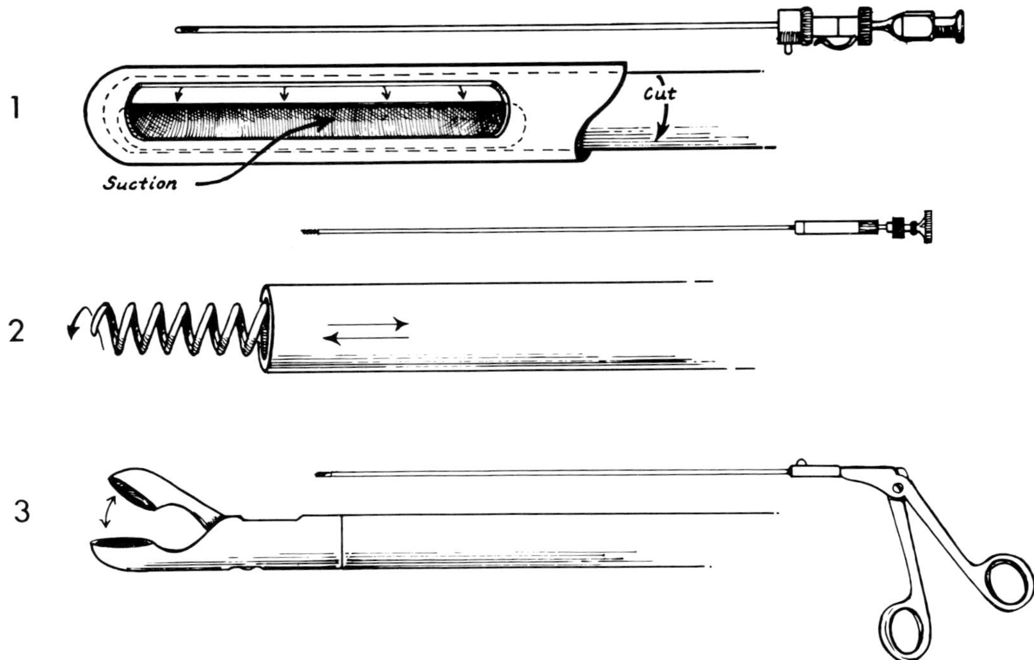

Fig. 41-6. Biopsy instruments used with CT-guided stereotaxis. (1) Nashold/Sedan biopsy needle (most suitable for soft, suckable tissue). Gentle syringe suction applied to the Luer-lok fitting draws tissue into the cannula through the side port. Rotation of the inner cannula 180 degrees severs the core of tissue, holding it within the instrument until removed with a small needle or forceps. (2) Backlund spiral (for firm, nonsuckable tissue). Once the probe has reached the target, the spiral-tipped instrument is screwed into the tissue. The outer cannula is then advanced over the spiral, after which the entire device is withdrawn. A core of tissue, held within the spiral, is removed by gently unscrewing the spiral held between moistened fingers. (3) Endoscopic forceps. Cup tipped biopsy forceps, of the type used during endoscopy, are available in sizes to fit through stereotactic probes. Substantial hemorrhage can result from the inadvertent grasping of a blood vessel with the instrument's jaws. (4) Aspiration cannulas (not shown). Cannulas varying in diameter and tip sharpness are available for the puncture and aspiration of cystic lesions. The sampling of liquid or soft, solid material for cytologic examination is also possible with these devices.

atraumatic, preserving the histologic nature of the tissue specimens. In most cases both aspiration as well as spiral biopsy specimens are obtained.

TECHNIQUE OF STEREOTACTIC SURGERY AT PRESBYTERIAN-UNIVERSITY HOSPITAL OF PITTSBURGH

We performed 333 stereotactic operations between 1981 and 1985. The usage of stereotactic surgery has increased from 26 cases in 1981 to an estimated 125 cases per year in 1985. Approximately 15 percent of all neurosurgical operations are now done with stereotactic technique at Presbyterian-University Hospital, and approximately 50 percent of all brain tumors are diagnosed or treated by stereotactic surgery.

Patients are referred for stereotactic surgery after review of the appropriate preoperative CT scan or MRI study. Cerebral angiography is not considered mandatory prior to surgical intervention unless the lesion is within the anterior third ventricle, the suprasellar space, or the pineal region. We have found no correlation between the angiographic appearance of brain neoplasms and the subsequent risk of post biopsy hemorrhage.

OPERATIVE TECHNIQUE

Patients are premedicated with an anticholinergic and an anxiolytic agent before entering the operating room. With the patient sitting on a chair, the head is prepared with isopropyl alcohol. The Leksell coordinate frame is attached to the head under local anesthesia supplemented by intravenous narcotic administered by the anesthesiologist in attendance. An intravenous contrast infusion is given to all patients prior to CT target identification. Serial axial CT scan images of the brain are performed in our operating room, which is equipped with a dedicated CT scanner.[38,40] Stereotactic coordinates of the target are obtained using either the standard CT computer software, a plastic grid overlay scaled to the filmed CT image, or a special computer software program created for the Leksell stereotactic frame (Lunsford LD, et al., in preparation, 1986). The target is chosen to allow serial sampling through the entire lesion along a single trajectory having the least risk to the brain.

The scalp is shaved in a limited area at the entry point after which the entire frame and head is again cleansed with alcohol. Skull entry in the majority of diagnostic-brain biopsy cases is performed percutaneously, using a twist drill held by the arc of the frame in the intended probe trajectory (Figure 41-7). For lesions approached laterally through the parietal lobe or sylvian fissure, we normally perform a burr hole followed by inspection of the pia before passing the probe to the target. This reduces the risk of laceration of a pial vessel. The biopsies are performed at the sites specified on the CT or MRI images. Spiral biopsies are performed throughout the lesion, including the area identified by both contrast-enhanced CT scan or MRI as well as the surrounding brain in an attempt to identify tumor margins[41] (Figure 41-8). Should bleeding occur from the tip of the needle, the probe is left in position until the egress of blood ceases.

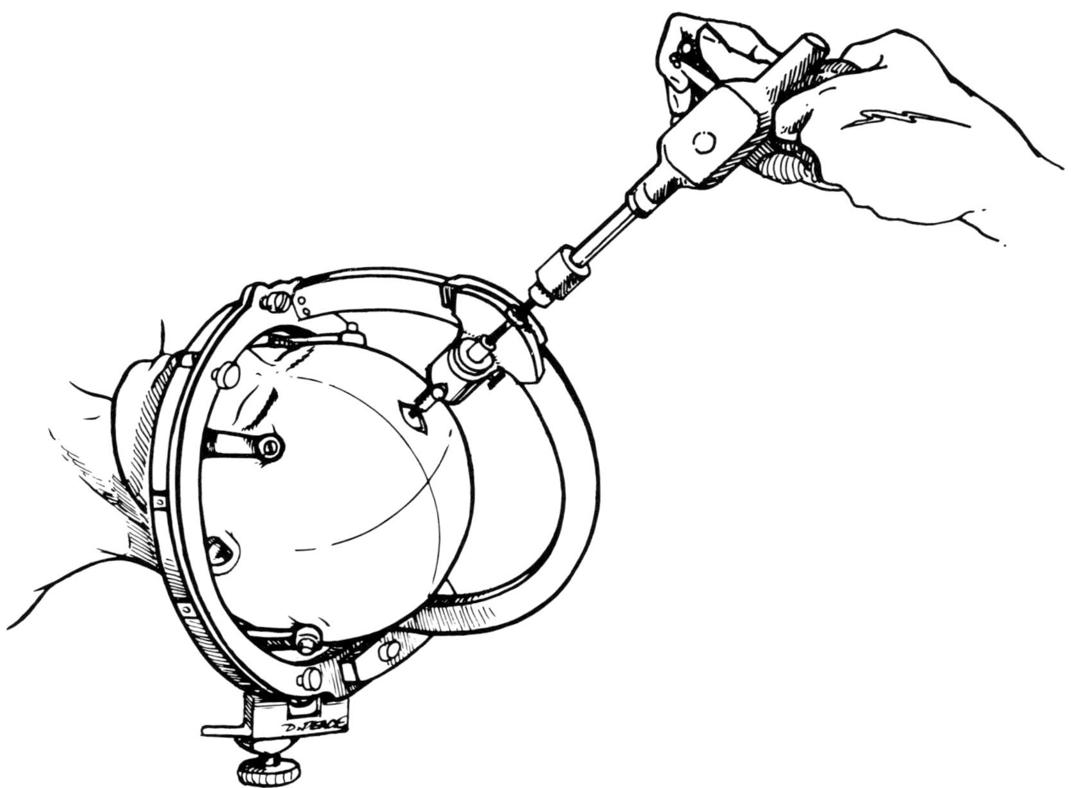

Fig. 41-7. Percutaneous twist drill skull entry. Stereotactic operations with most frames can be accomplished through a small twist drill hole (BRW system shown). After the frame has been set to the target coordinates, an appropriate drill bit and guide is used to perforate the skull along the same trajectory as the stereotactic probe.

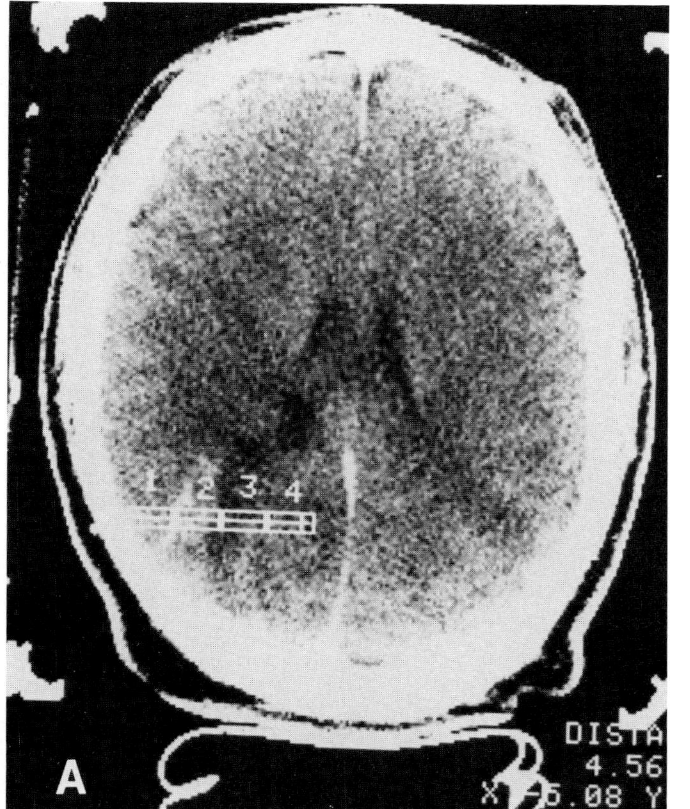
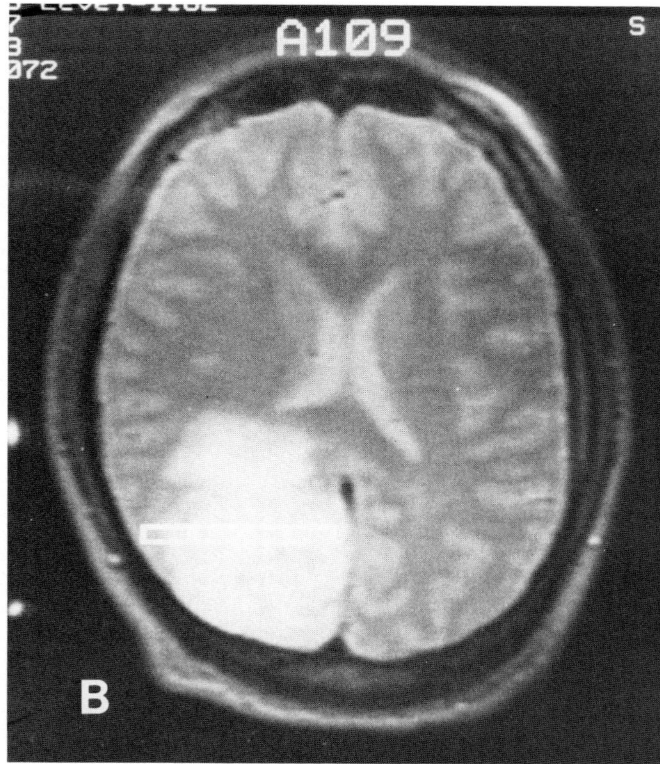

Fig. 41-8. (A) A stereotactic axial CT scan of a right occipital low attenuation mass in a 32-year-old man with seizures. (B) Stereotactic axial MRI of the same lesion. Biopsy of the areas shown disclosed a well-differentiated astrocytoma. The coordinates are the same using both MRI- and CT-derived techniques.

Table 41-2. CT-guided stereotactic surgery at Presbyterian-University Hospital, Pittsburgh, Pennsylvania (Diagnoses obtained in 240 cases)

Diagnosis	Number of Cases	Percent
Glioblastoma	70	29.1
Anaplastic astrocytoma	34	14.1
Well-differentiated astrocytoma	25	10.4
Metastatic tumor	22	9.1
Lymphoma	16	6.7
Brain abscess*	14	5.8
Hematoma	9	3.8
Encephalitis	7	2.9
Vascular malformation	6	2.5
Colloid cyst	5	2.1
Germinoma	4	1.7
Neuroepithelial cyst	4	1.7
Degenerative disease	4	1.7
Epidermoid tumor	3	1.3
Other†	7	2.9
Nondiagnostic	10	4.2
Total	240	100.0

*Eight patients had catheter drainage; 3 patients had acquired immune deficiency syndrome (AIDS).
†Includes one case each of infarct, porencephaly, leukoencephalopathy, neurosarcoid, vasculitis, granuloma, and PML.

Immediate postoperative CT images are obtained in our CT scanner-equipped operating room to assess potential complications.

Table 41-2 indicates the location of the various lesions in a series of 240 patients undergoing diagnostic stereotactic surgery between 1981 and 1985. The majority of patients had brain

Table 41-3. CT-guided stereotactic surgery, Presbyterian-University Hospital, Pittsburgh, Pennsylvania, 1981–1985 (diagnostic surgery in 240 cases)

Lesion Location	Number of Cases	Percentage
Cerebral hemisphere	149	62.0
Basal ganglia	27	11.0
Thalamus	12	5.0
Third ventricle	11	5.0
Corpus callosum	10	4.1
Pons	10	4.1
Pineal region	7	2.9
Cerebellum	5	2.1
Midbrain	4	1.7
Suprasellar	4	1.7
Intrasellar	1	0.4

lesions located in the subcortical cerebral hemisphere. Lesions of the basal ganglia, thalamus, third ventricle, pineal region, and cerebellum have all been biopsied or aspirated using stereotactic technique. The results of CT stereotactic surgery at Presbyterian-University Hospital are summarized in Table 41-3. Of our patients, 53.6 percent proved to have astrocytomas of the brain, including 29.1 percent who had glioblastomas. A follow-up study to determine the results of multimodality treatment after stereotactic biopsy for malignant gliomas (104 cases) has begun. Primary CNS lymphoma was diagnosed in 16 cases. In 14 cases stereotactic drainage of brain abscesses was accomplished. Eight patients had an indwelling catheter drainage system placed; six underwent a single aspiration. We now regard stereotactic drainage as the primary treatment for brain abscesses. Vascular malformations have been identified in six

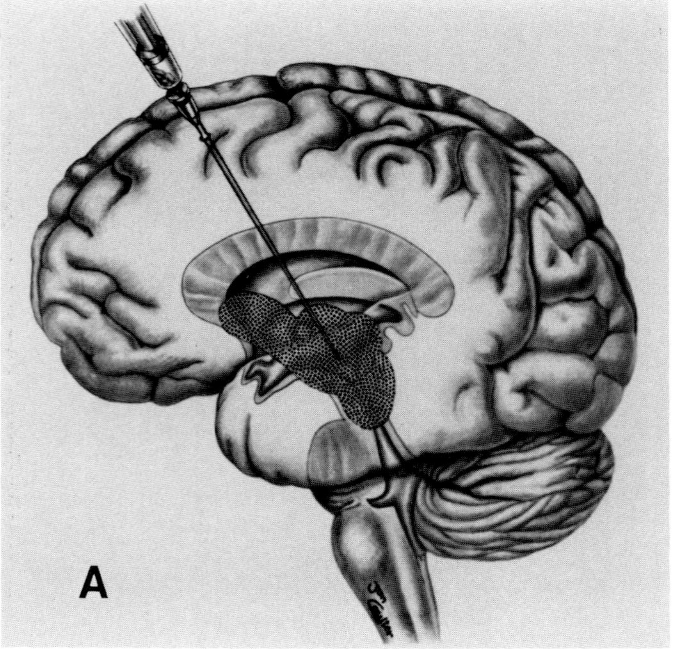

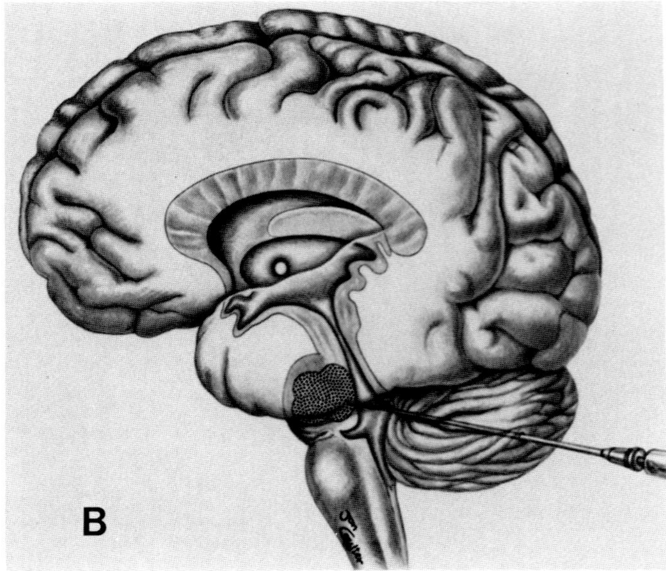

Fig. 41-9. (A) Transfrontal stereotactic approach to midbrain or pontine lesions above the level of the middle cerebellar peduncle. (B) Transcerebellar approach to lesions located at or below the middle cerebellar peduncle. (Reprinted from Coffey RJ, Lunsford LD: CT-guided stereotactic surgery for mass lesions of the midbrain and pons. Neurosurgery 17:12–18, 1985. With permission.)

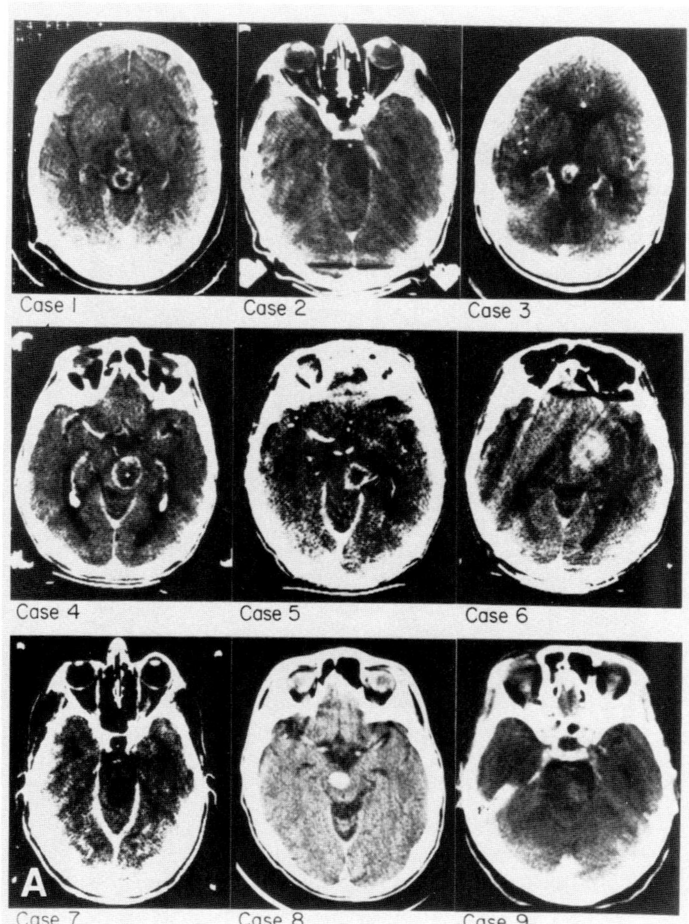

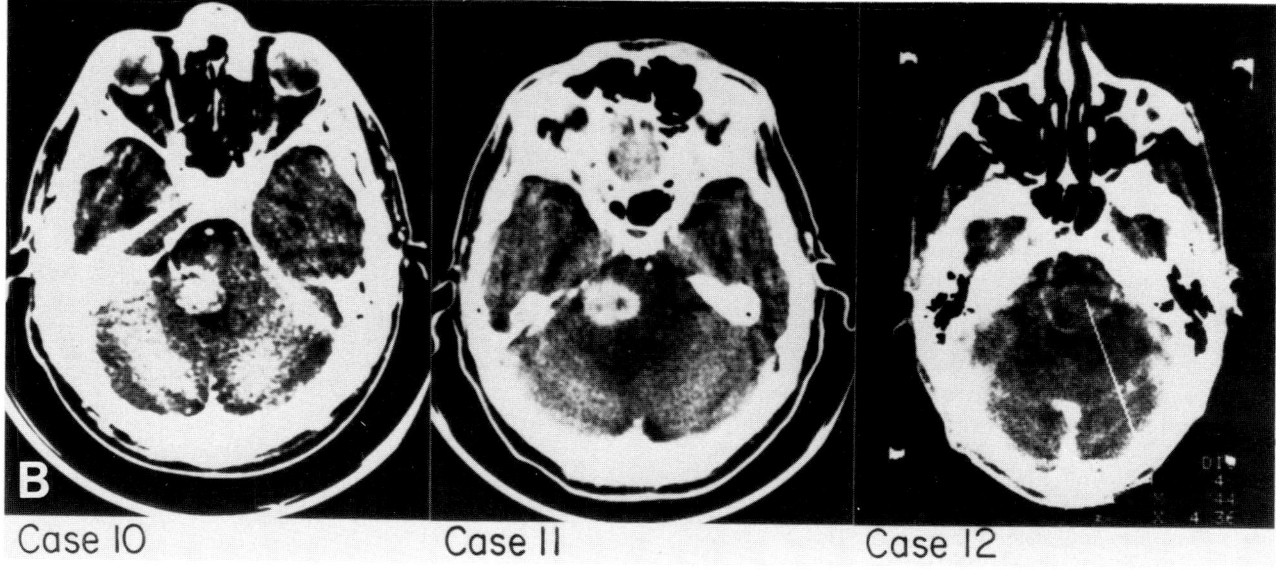

Fig. 41-10. (A) A composite photograph of the CT scans of nine patients with lesions of the midbrain or rostral pons. All nine patients underwent a transfrontal stereotactic biopsy or aspiration procedure. (B) Composite photograph of the CT scans of three patients with lesions of the caudal lateral pons or middle cerebellar peduncle. All three patients underwent a transcerebellar stereotactic biopsy (± aspiration) procedure. ((Reprinted from Coffey RJ, Lunsford LD: CT-guided stereotactic surgery for mass lesions of the midbrain and pons. Neurosurgery 17:12–18, 1985. With permission.)

patients, none of whom sustained postoperative hemorrhages following biopsy. Using the technique described by Bosch et al.[42] colloid cysts were aspirated in five cases. Because of persistent symptoms, three subsequently required craniotomy and removal of the cyst remnant.

Brain biopsy proved diagnostic in 95.8 percent of our cases. No patient died as a result of stereotactic surgery. Eight patients developed postoperative intracerebral hematomas; five had clinical symptomatology that required craniotomy and evacuation of the hemorrhage. Two patients had infections at the burr hole site, which in part has led us to abandon this technique whenever possible. One patient suffered a wound seroma. Thirty percent of patients improved immediately as a result of stereotactic surgery. This usually resulted from aspiration of necrotic masses or reduction in the volume of cystic lesions.

Our therapeutic uses for imaging-directed stereotactic surgery, now combining CT with MRI, include intracavity irradiation for cystic brain neoplasms, interstitial irradiation for solid tumors, catheter placements for cyst or ventricular decompres-

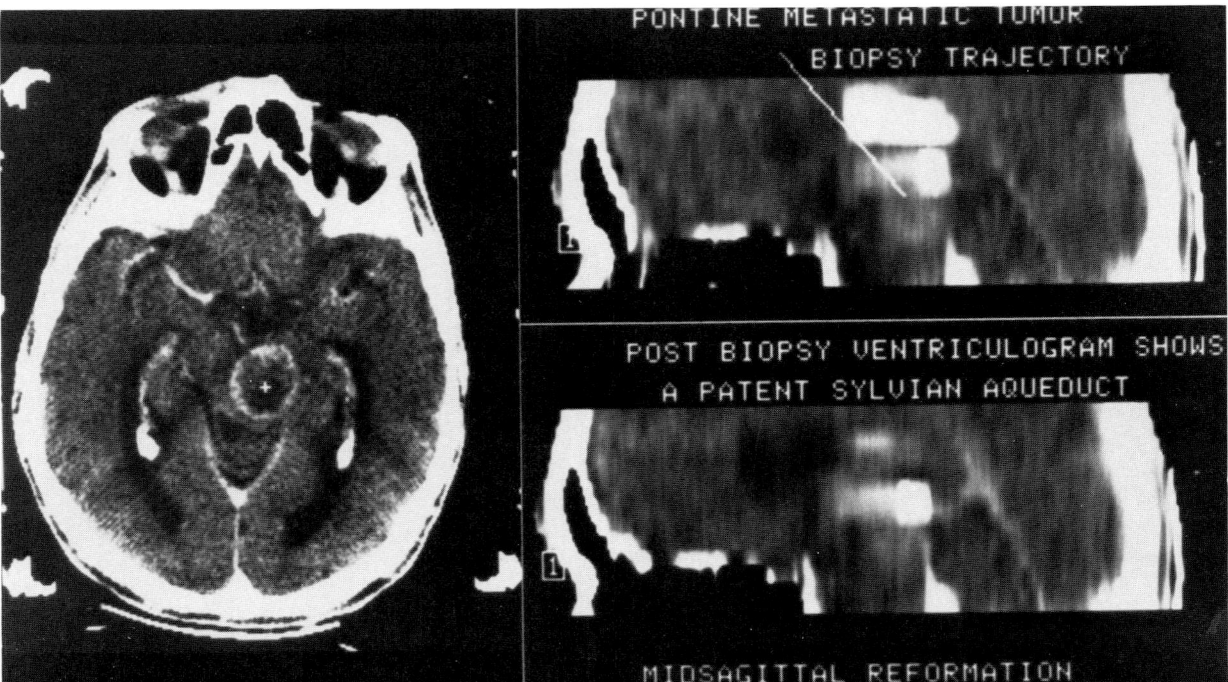

Fig. 41-11. Stereotactic CT scan (left) of a left pontomesencephalic mass prior to biopsy. The approach is demonstrated by a reformatted parasagittal image (right, upper). Post biopsy CT ventriculogram demonstrated a patent adqueduct of Sylvius (right, lower). (Reprinted from Coffey RJ, Lunsford LD: CT-guided stereotactic surgery for mass lesions of the midbrain and pons. Neurosurgery 17:12–18, 1985. With permission.)

sion, and accurate tumor volume assessments. Comparison of the imaging attributes of both CT and MRI are underway (Figure 41-8). We currently perform all functional neurosurgical intervention with stereotactic technique directed by computed tomography. Such procedures include thalamotomy and placement of depth electrodes for electrical recording as well as for pain treatment using deep brain stimulation.

STEREOTACTIC SURGERY OF THC MIDBRAIN AND PONS

Lesions of the midbrain and pons can be approached by stereotactic technique.[43–45] Fourteen such patients have been treated at our hospital since 1980. Two techniques have been described.[45] For lesions of the midbrain and pons above the middle cerebellar peduncle, a transfrontal approach through an entry point at the coronal suture has been selected (Figure 41-9, left). For lesions at the level of the middle cerebellar peduncle or below within the pons, a transcerebellar stereotactic approach has been selected (Figure 41-9, right). The neurologic examination localized the brain stem lesions in all 14 cases. Diagnostic CT scanning (Figure 41-10) was largely confirmatory. Despite accurate clinical and radiographic localization of these lesions, the preoperative diagnosis was in error in half of the patients. In all 14 patients a diagnosis was achieved by surgery, and no neurologic morbidity occurred as a result of the operations. Ten therapeutic interventions were carried out in nine patients including aspiration of cysts, hematomas, necrotic tumors, and stereotactic placement of ventriculostomies. Six of seven patients who underwent aspiration of cystic masses improved neurologically in the early postoperative period. This improvement was only temporary in three patients harboring cystic malignancies.

The vast majority of stereotactic operations were performed under local anesthesia. For those patients harboring lesions approached through the cerebellum in the prone position on the CT scanner table, we have elected to use general anesthesia. It is possible, however, to perform transcerebellar stereotactic surgery in cooperative adults with the patients awake in a semisitting position on a standard operating room table. The high diagnostic yield in an area where clinical diagnosis has often been in error, the relative lack of postoperative morbidity, and the lasting benefits of therapeutic intervention in selected cases has made imaging directed stereotaxis an attractive surgical option in patients harboring mass lesions of the brain stem. An example of such a case is demonstrated in Figure 41-11.

DISCUSSION

The value of and indications for stereotactic surgery have been radically altered by the development of sophisticated imaging modalities such as CT and MRI. With a few notable exceptions in Europe, until development of CT guidance techniques, stereotactic surgery was largely a tool of investigative and functional neurosurgeons.[46] Various reports by Bosch,[39] Edner,[49] Ostertag et al.,[17] and Pecker et al.,[47] among others, demonstrated that stereotactic biopsy guided by ventriculography or angiography reached a correct diagnosis in 55 to 90 percent of cases. The integration of data from early generation CT scanners (either mechanically or mathematically) into the stereotactic target calculations consistently improved the diagnostic rate to greater than 90 percent.[18] The introduction of CT-guided instruments has led to a dramatic increase in the number of patients undergoing stereotactic biopsies. In the recent series of Apuzzo et al.,[33,34] Bouvier et al.,[48] Bullard et al.,[12,13] Edner,[49] Heilbrun et al.,[31] Lunsford and Martinez,[38] and Mundingeret al.[16] the diagnostic biopsy rate has varied between 91 and 100 percent. The histologic diagnosis differed from the preoperative clinical radiographic diagnosis in 25 to 50 percent of cases.

A decision about whether to obtain diagnosis by conventional or microsurgical techniques through an open craniotomy or by stereotactic technique is dependent on several factors, including the location, size, multiplicity, vascularity, and solid or cystic nature of the lesion. Stereotactic surgery is most useful in approaching small lesions in relatively inaccessible regions of the brain. More superficial regions of the brain subserving critical neurologic functions such as language, movement, or higher cortical functions have also been biopsied by stereotactic technique without incurring additional neurologic deficit. Patients with multiple lesions, usually representing metastatic neoplasm or infection, have been the subject of stereotactic biopsy or drainage when appropriate.

The decision to employ stereotactic biopsy should not precede a thorough neurologic and radiographic assessment of the patient. When a list of possible clinical diagnoses in a patient harboring a brain lesion is excessively long, brain biopsy may not provide the answer. Errors in pathologic interpretation are most common in this situation, especially for very small lesions. This problem can be avoided in most cases by adequate serial sampling of the lesion and demonstration of the images to the neuropathologist at the time of histologic review. Proper interpretation is dependent upon an experienced neuropathologist who can evaluate small tissue samples. Of equal importance is proper care of the specimens themselves by a well-trained histologist. At the University of Pittsburgh, we do not perform frozen section diagnoses because of the inherent inaccuracies in interpreting such tissue and because rarely is treatment immediately affected by frozen section diagnosis. The mechanical accuracy of reaching a target is 1 mm, and there can be no question that sampling of the target site was performed. In addition, postoperative CT imaging, which frequently discloses a small air bubble at the site at which the biopsy specimens were taken, confirms target accuracy. We review our histologic specimens after permanent fixation within 18 to 24 hours after the biopsy was performed. Only in cases of suspected brain infection, where appropriate antimicrobial treatment can be life-sustaining, do we perform frozen section diagnosis.[50]

At the present time, there is virtually no reason for empiric therapy of brain lesions identified by CT or MRI. Despite the development of these advanced imaging tools, histologic diagnosis remains mandatory, even in lesions of the brain stem or cerebellum. The accuracy and safety of imaging-directed stereotactic surgery has been demonstrated many times. The current goals of stereotactic surgery rest in the introduction of new therapeutic techniques dependent upon the inherent accuracy of the available tools. The development of stereotactic microsurgical[19–21] or stereotactic endoscopic resection of lesions[51,52] and the introduction of robotics into the operating room[36] demonstrates the growing importance of image-guided neurosurgical techniques.

Stereotactic surgery has now become as well established in the practice of morphologic neurosurgery as it had been in the practice of functional neurosurgery. Advanced imaging modalities and precise guidance instrumentation are as essential to modern stereotactic surgery as the operating microscope is to microsurgery. The future rests in further development and application of these valuable tools.

REFERENCES

1. Maroon JC, Bank WO, Drayer BP, et al: Intracranial biopsy assisted by computerized tomography. J Neurosurg 46:740, 1977
2. Greenblatt SH, Rayport M, Savolaine ER, et al: Computed tomography-guided intracranial biopsy and cyst aspiration. Neurosurgery 11:589, 1982
3. Wester K, Sortland O, Haughlie-Hanssen E: A simple and inexpensive method for CT-stereotaxy. Neuroradiology 20:255, 1981
4. Gildenberg P: Stereotactic neurosurgery and computerized tomographic scanning. Appl Neurophysiol 46:170, 1983
5. Gildenberg PL, Kaufman HH, Murthy KSK: Calculation of stereotactic coordinates from the computed tomographic scan. Neurosurgery 10:580, 1982
6. Kaufman JJ, Gildenberg PL: New head-positioning system for use with computed tomographic scanning. Neurosurgery 7:147, 1980
7. Levy WJ: Simple plastic stereotactic unit for use in the computed tomographic scanner. Neurosurgery 13: 182–185, 1983.
8. Levy WJ, Oro JJ: Curved biopsy needle for stereotactic surgery: A technical note. Neurosurgery 15:82, 1984
9. Patil AA: Computed tomography-oriented stereotactic system. Neurosurgery 10:370, 1982
10. Carol M: A true burr-hole mounted stereotactic device. Presented at the IX Meeting of the World Society for Stereotactic and Functional Neurosurgery, Toronto, 1985 (Abstract)
11. Leksell L, Jernberg B: Stereotaxis and tomography. A technical note. Acta Neurochir 52:1, 1980
12. Bullard DE, Nashold BS, Osborne D, et al: CT-guided stereotactic biopsies using a modified frame and Gildenberg technique. J Neurol Neurosurg Psychiatry 47:590, 1984
13. Bullard DE, Nashold BS, Osborne D, et al: Experience using two CT-guided stereotactic biopsy methods. Appl Neurophysiol 46:188, 1983
14. Dyck P: Stereotactic Biopsy and Brachytherapy of Brain Tumors. Baltimore, University Park Press, 1984
15. Gahbauer H, Sturm V, Schlegel W, et al: Combined use of stereotaxic CT and angiography for brain biopsies and stereotaxic irradiation. AJNR 4:715, 1983
16. Mundinger F, Birg W, Klar M: Computer-assisted stereotactic brain operations by means including computerized axial tomography. Appl Neurophysiol 41:169, 1979
17. Ostertag CB, Mennel HD, Kiessling MK: Stereotactic biopsy of brain tumors. Surg Neurol 14:275, 1980
18. Sturm V, Pastyr O, Schlegel W, et al: Stereotactic computer tomography with a modified Reichert-Mundinger device as the basis for integrated stereotactic neuroradiological investigations. Acta Neurochir 68:11, 1983
19. Kelly PJ, Earnest F, Kall BA, et al: Surgical options for patients with deep seated brain tumors: Computer assisted stereotactic biopsy. Mayo Clin Proc 60:223, 1985
20. Kelly PJ, Kall BA, Goerss B, et al: Computer-assisted stereotaxic laser resection of intra-axial brain neoplasms. J Neurosurg 64:427, 1986
21. Kelly PJ, Kall BA, Goerss B: Results of computer-assisted stereotactic laser resection of deep-seated intracranial lesions. Mayo Clin Proc 61:20, 1985
22. Goerss S, Kelly PJ, Kall B, et al: A computed tomographic stereotactic adaptation system. Neurosurgery 10:375, 1982
23. Bergstrom M, Greitz T: Stereotaxic computed tomography. AJR 127:167, 1976
24. Boethius J, Bergstrom M, Greitz T: Stereotactic computerized tomography with a GE 8800 scanner. J Neurosurg 52:794, 1980
25. Boethius J, Collins VP, Edner G, et al: Stereotactic biopsies and computer tomography in gliomas. Acta Neurochir 40:223, 1978
26. Leksell L, Leksell D, Schwebel J: Stereotaxis and nuclear magnetic resonance. Neurol Neurosurg Psychiatry 48:14, 1985
27. Birg W, Mundinger F: Direct target point determination for stereotactic brain operations from CT data and calculation of

setting parameters for polar coordinate devices. Appl Neurophysiol 45:387, 1982

28. Brown RA: A computerized tomography-computer graphics approach to stereotaxic localization. J Neurosurg 50:715, 1979

29. Brown RA: A stereotactic head frame for use with CT body scanners. Invest Radiol 14:300, 1979

30. Brown RA, Roberts TS, Osborn AG: Stereotaxic frame and computer software for CT-directed neurosurgical localization. Invest Radiol 15:308, 1980

31. Heilbrun MP, Roberts TS, Apuzzo MLJ: Preliminary experience with Brown-Roberts-Wells (BRW) computerized tomography stereotaxic guidance system. J Neurosurg 59:217, 1983

32. Roberts TS, Brown R: Technical and clinical aspects of CT-directed stereotaxis. Appl Neurophysiol 43:170, 1980

33. Apuzzo MLJ, Chandrasoma PT, Zelman V, et al: Computed tomographic guidance stereotaxis in the management of lesions of the third ventricular region. Neurosurgery 15:502, 1984

34. Apuzzo MLJ, Sabshin JK: Computed tomographic guidance stereotaxis in the management of intracranial mass lesions. Neurosurgery 12:277, 1983

35. Rhodes ML, Glenn WV, Azzawi Y-M, et al: Stereotactic neurosurgery using 3–D image data from computed tomography. J Med Systems 6:105, 1982

36. Young RW: A robotic system for stereotactic neurosurgery, in Lunsford LD (ed): Modern Stereotactic Surgery. Boston, Martinus Nijhoff, 1987

37. Perry JH, Rosenbaum AE, Lunsford LD, et al: Computed tomography-guided stereotactic surgery: Conception and development of a new stereotactic methodology. Neurosurgery 7:376, 1980

38. Lunsford LD, Martinez AJ: Stereotactic exploration of the brain in the era of computed tomography. Surg Neurol 22:222, 1984

39. Bosch DA: Indications for stereotactic biopsy in brain tumors. Acta Neurochir 54:167, 1980

40. Lunsford LD, Leksell L, Jernberg B: Probe holder for stereotactic surgery in the CT scanner. A technical note. Acta Neurochir 69:297, 1983

41. Lunsford LD, Martinez AJ, Latchaw RE: Stereotaxic surgery with a magnetic resonance and computerized tomography compatible system. J Neurosurg 64:872, 1986

42. Bosch DA, Rahn D, Backlund EO: Treatment of colloid cysts of the third ventricle by stereotactic aspiration. Surg Neurol 9:15, 1978

43. Beatty RM, Zervas NT: Stereotactic aspiration of a brain stem hematoma. Neurosurgery 13:204, 1983

44. Bosch DA, Beute GN: Successful stereotaxic evacuation of an acute pontomedullary hematoma. Case report. J Neurosurg 62:153, 1985

45. Coffey RJ, Lunsford LD: CT-guided stereotactic surgery for mass lesions of the midbrain and pons. Neurosurgery 17:12, 1985

46. Hankinson J, Hudgson P, Pearce GW, et al: A simple method for obtaining stereotaxic biopsies from the human basal ganglia. A case of cerebral porphyria. Acta Neurochir (Suppl) 21:227, 1974

47. Pecker J, Scarabin JM, Brucher JM, et al: Stereotactic Approach to Diagnosis and Treatment of Cerebral Tumors. Paris, Laboratoires Pierre Fabre, 1979

48. Bouvier G, Couillard P, Leger SL, et al: Stereotactic biopsy of cerebral space-occupying lesions. Appl Neurophysiol 46:227, 1983

49. Edner G: Stereotactic biopsy of intracranial space occupying lesions. Acta Neurochir 57:213, 1981

50. Lunsford LD, Martinez AJ, Latchaw RE, et al: Rapid and accurate diagnosis of herpes simplex encephalitis by stereotaxic computed tomography. Surg Neurol 21:249, 1984

51. Jacques S, Shelden CH, McCann GD, et al: Computerized three-dimensional stereotaxic removal of small central nervous system lesions in patients. J Neurosurg 53:816, 1980

52. Shelden CH, McCann G, Jacques S: Development of computerized microstereotactic method for localization and removal of minute CNS lesions under direct 3-D vision. J Neurosurg 52:21, 1980

Commentary: Stereotactic Techniques Using the Brown-Roberts-Wells Stereotactic Frame

Peter McL. Black

THE CHAPTER BY Coffey and Lunsford has outlined the use of the Leksell frame for stereotactic biopsy. There are a number of other systems available[1] including those of Kelley et al.,[2,3] Gildenberg,[4,5] and Tailarach.[6] At the present time, however, the major alternative for the practicing neurosurgeon is the Brown-Roberts-Wells frame. This commentary describes the Brown-Roberts-Wells stereotactic system, which has four major components: the head ring, the localizer ring, the arc system, and the phantom base. Through the work of Roberts,[7] Brown,[8,9] Heilbrun,[10,11] Apuzzo,[12] and others it has become widely used in stereotactic tumor biopsy. This commentary will outline techniques for this frame and summarize the experience with it at Massachusetts General Hospital over a 3-year period.

TARGET LOCALIZATION AND SELECTION

Target localization is accomplished by applying a base ring to the scalp, adding a localizing carbon arc ring, and using the CT cursor system to establish coordinates. The base ring (Figure 41-12) can be applied at the bedside with local anesthesia; Renografin or another contrast agent can be administered intravenously during placement. Usually the anterior pins are positioned just above the superior temporal line and the posterior pins in the parieto-occipital region. If a temporal biopsy is planned, however, the pins will have to be placed in the supraorbital region to have the frame low enough to achieve temporal access. The ring should be placed as symmetrically as possible with the square ball socket in line with the inion. At least one pin should be short to allow easy placement and removal of superstructure components.

Four important points to note in pin placement are the following:

1. The computer trajectory cannot direct the probe up from horizontal; therefore the bone entry site has to be cephalad to the lesion. The ring has to be placed appropriately to allow this. Ring placement must also allow space for the nose when the arc system is added.
2. An estimate of the lesion location should be made before pin placement because the pins may produce an artifact that will obscure the target.

3. For superficial lesions the arc must be high enough to allow the probe apparatus to fit over the scalp.
4. The pins should be fixed firmly in place so as not to slip when the frame is held or lifted with some force.

The next steps are placement of the localizer ring assembly, CT scanning, and target localization. Third generation scanners such as the GE 9800 are much to be preferred in biopsies because of fast scan times and high resolution. Using the cursor system of the GE software, the locations of the nine carbon arc rods are now entered on a calculation sheet beginning with the large rod, which is at approximately 9 o'clock. The rod locations are entered clockwise as X and Y coordinates.

Selecting the target is a crucial part of judgment in performing a stereotactic biopsy. The CT scan sections are usually 5-mm thick, producing at least this much imprecision in selecting a target. If a lesion is homogeneous, aiming at the center will ensure that representative tissue is obtained. If, as is more often the case, there is an enhancing rim with a necrotic or low absorption center, it is important to choose sites that are on the rim and therefore allow selection of representative tissue of the growing tumor. If the central portion of the lesion is cystic, entering it on the initial pass may distort the anatomy of the surrounding lesion, and it is therefore important to biopsy the edge before trying to drain the cyst. Similarly, if the lesion is beside a ventricle, draining ventricular fluid initially may distort the anatomy for subsequent biopsy.

Targets that are in the path of major blood vessels should be avoided. This is especially true in the midline, in the subfrontal region, around the circle of Willis, and where the biopsy path might transgress the middle cerebral artery arcade. If a temporal lobe lesion is to be biopsied it is best approached from a temporal burr hole.

It is useful to choose at least two targets for each scan slice selected. It is also prudent to choose two different scan slices showing the lesion to be certain that there is adequate information to proceed if the first passes do not produce diagnostic material.

The calculation of the BRWT coordinates will not be discussed in detail; it is described in the Radionics instruction manual for the Brown-Roberts-Wells stereotactic system obtainable from Radionics Incorporated (P.O. Box 438, 76

OPERATIVE NEUROSURGICAL TECHNIQUES
ISBN 0-8089-1862-1

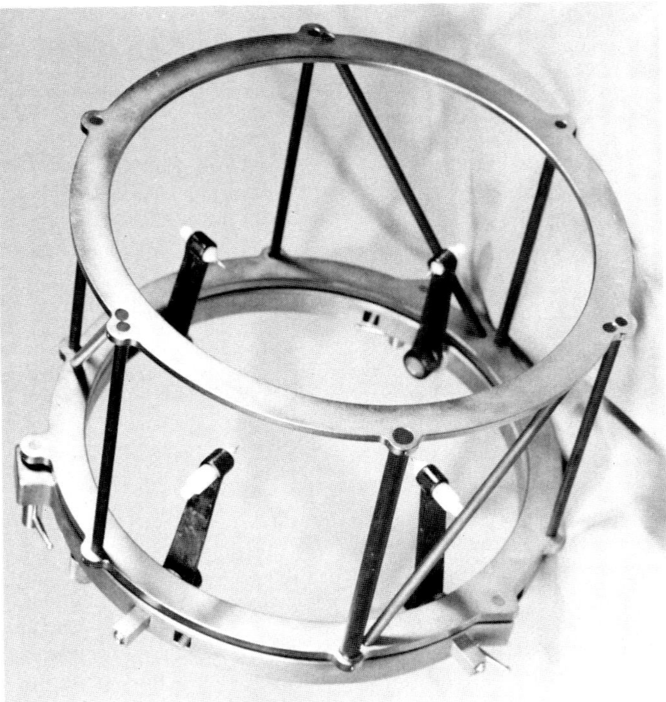

Fig. 41-12.   The base plate with localizing ring for the BRWT system. The metal-tipped plastic pins are screwed into the scalp under local anesthesia.

Cambridge St., Burlington, MA 01803). The sequences in this program are first to enter patient data and date, and then to enter the coordinates of the carbon arc rods and the target; the computer will provide target coordinates. The entry point is entered as described below and the computer will provide the angles and depth for biopsy.

BIOPSY

After the scan has been obtained, the biopsy itself can either be done in the operating room or the scanning area if there is adequate surgical equipment. At the Massachusetts General, a dedicated stereotactic suite associated with the scan room becomes an operating theater for the biopsy procedure. Appropriate equipment includes lighting, coagulation, and suctioning capacity. Virtually all biopsies can be done through one of three burr holes: a frontal hole at the coronal suture and 3 cm lateral to the sagittal suture, a parietal burr hole 7 cm above the inion and 3 cm lateral to the midline, or a temporal burr hole 2 to 3 cm above the zygoma. With these placements, important brain is not transgressed by the biopsy probe. Some surgeons feel that the probe can be safely directed through an entry site placed anywhere convenient to the lesion.

In preparing for skull entry, only enough hair to allow adequate sterility need be shaved. This greatly diminishes the psychologic impact of the biopsy. Sterile towels are placed around the margin of the shaved skin to keep hair out of the biopsy site.

The steps in the biopsy itself are as follows: (1) placement of the entry site in the skull and insertion of its coordinates into the BRWT calculator; (2) alignment of the target on the phan-tom and verification that the trajectory is correct; and (3) placement of the arc system and biopsy.

Two methods of entry site selection can be used. The first is to place the burr hole and then calculate its coordinates, inserting them into the BRWT computer program; the second is to select the entry site en route to doing the biopsy. The first system is somewhat more cumbersome, but more traditional in stereotactic surgery. For this the scalp is prepared with anti-septic solution and a vertical linear incision is made. Meticulous hemostasis is achieved to prevent later bleeding into the subdural space. Either a brace and bit perforator or an air-driven drill is used to make the burr hole; if the hand-held perforator is used the burr hole may need modification depending on the precise trajectory of the probe. The skin is temporarily closed with a single suture and the drapes are removed. A sterile drape is then placed over the entire scalp surface, covering the previously placed sterile towels but not covering the base ring. This provides a sterile scalp surface. The arc assembly is placed on the base plate and the probe is positioned to touch the dural surface. It should be placed so that its tip is in the center of the burr hole. The arc assembly is moved from the patient to the phantom and the phantom pointer tip is positioned at the opening of the probe. The AP, lateral, and vertical coordinates are entered into the BRWT program as the entry point, and the trajectory is calculated and confirmed as follows.

The target coordinates have been established by inserting the CT and localizer ring data into the BRWT computer program. The phantom pointer is set at these to represent the target and a mock-up of the biopsy is done by inserting the biopsy instrument in the probe and measuring its length (Figure 41-13). The length measurement on the computer is provided from the holder fixed to the arc; the inner sleeve and probe measurements must be added to this. The use of the phantom allows the surgeon to set the instruments that will be used for the biopsy directly at the target. With a side-biting aspirator the center of the side-biting hole is set on the target; for the pituitary forceps, the forceps itself is set on the target, which places the obturator approximately 1 cm short of the target.

An alternative to the method just described is to set the target on the phantom base, align the carbon arc system so that it appears to be at an appropriate angle to pass through prepared scalp, and place the burr hole to allow that trajectory using a twist drill included in the BRWT kit. The twist drill allows visualization of dura but requires only a 2-cm skin incision. This method saves the steps of draping and redraping and ensures that the orientation of the entry site is appropriate for the biopsy trajectory. It requires that some thought be given to the site of head preparation and the biopsy trajectory.

With the phantom assembly now set up to guide the probe to the target, the arc system is placed on the base ring. The biopsy device is inserted and appropriate biopsy specimens are taken. A variety of instruments can be used; I have found either a pituitary rongeur or a side-biting instrument to be most useful. The side-biting instrument is best for soft lesions and obtains a core 1 cm long and 3 to 4 mm wide. The pituitary forceps are useful for firm lesions such as low-grade astrocytomas, and although the biopsy is smaller, it is more precise in that the bite is taken exactly at the target site. Hemorrhage has not been a problem with the pituitary forceps. Angiograms are obtained routinely before biopsy if lesions look hypervascular on CT scans.

Several important points can be made about the selection

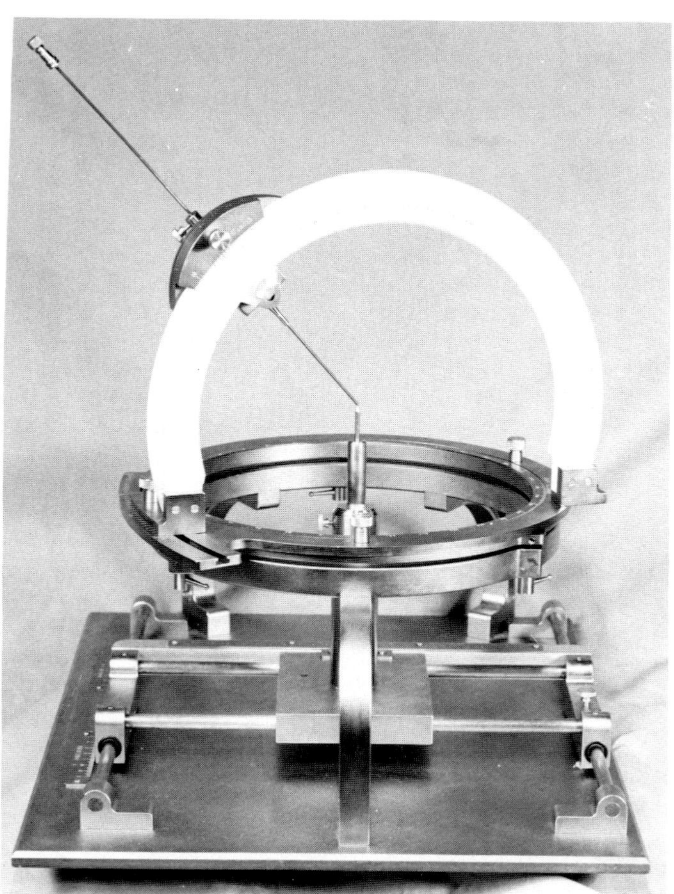

Fig. 41-13. The BRWT base and phantom. Here a CT-compatible arc is displayed with a side-biting biopsy instrument in place, demonstrating the way in which the target is localized and its position confirmed.

of targets and calculations. First, all measurements from the frame are in millimeters. Second, the computer will not allow the biopsy trajectory to be upward, so that the entry point, especially in the temporal fossa, has to be above the target. Third, there are some entry points that will not allow a satisfactory trajectory, especially in superficial lesions where the burr hole has to be almost directly above the lesion. Fourth, if the ring assembly is placed very low, the arc may not be large enough to fit around the head. Finally, on occasion the head may be too big to allow the ring to fit over it; if there is doubt, the carbon rod localizing ring which is not sterile can be placed over the head before the biopsy begins to be sure there is adequate room.

The usefulness of doing frozen sections or smears on biopsy specimens varies from institution to institution.[13] I have found that frozen sections are invaluable if an experienced pathologist examines them. It has not been possible to make definitive diagnoses from them in about 15 percent of cases.

INSTRUMENTATION

For CT scanning, an adapter for the base ring which slots into the CT headholder can be machined to hold the head in a stable position. In the operating theater the Mayfield headrest can position the head with an adapter especially made for this. Required in all biopsies are the assembly ring and pins,

Table 41-4. Location of 120 tumors diagnosed by stereotactic biopsy techniques (several neurosurgeons)

Location	Percent
Left frontal or temporal	25
Right frontal or temporal	9
Bifrontal	8
Parietal or occipital	25
Brainstem	3
Thalamic	15
Other	15

the localizing ring, the arc system, the phantom base, and the BRWT calculator and its energy pack. Optional accessories include a Del-Ran arc system for biopsies in the CT scanner, a set of endoscopic instruments, an MRI-compatible localizing ring and base ring assembly, and head ring post extenders and shorteners for pediatric patients or those with large heads. Stereotactic microdrives can be adapted to this system as well.

BIOPSY RESULTS AND ILLUSTRATIVE CASES

One of the important features of the BRW system is that it allows a number of surgeons to do stereotactic biopsy as part of their surgical management of particular lesions. Table 41-4 presents the location of lesions biopsied at this institution over the last 3 years by six different surgeons; Table 41-5 presents a summary of the diagnosis in these cases. Unexpected lesions include lymphomas (Figure 41-14); an area of gliosis that proved to be precisely that at autopsy 3 years later and that prevented radiation therapy; and demyelinating disease. Two cases are illustrative; a 21-year-old graduate student noted subtle changes in the dexterity of her right hand and slight occasional word-finding difficulties. With an EEG proving abnormal in the left hemisphere, CT and MRI scanning were done which showed a low absorption lesion several centimeters in diameter in the left centrum semiovale. Multimodality evoked potentials were all normal. A stereotactic biopsy demonstrated demyelinating disease and no evidence of neoplasm. In the second case, a woman with diabetes insipidus and memory loss had enhancement noted in the region of the hypothalamus. Under CT guidance and in the CT scanner itself it was possible to localize the biopsy precisely to the region of enhancing abnormality noted

Table 41-5. Pathologic diagnosis of 120 tumors

Tumor Type	Percentage
Astrocytoma	
Grade I-II	18.0
Grade III	27.0
Glioblastoma	30.0
Lymphoma	2.7
Abscess	2.7
Metastatic tumor	2.7
Parasitic infection	2.0
Insufficient tissue	1.7

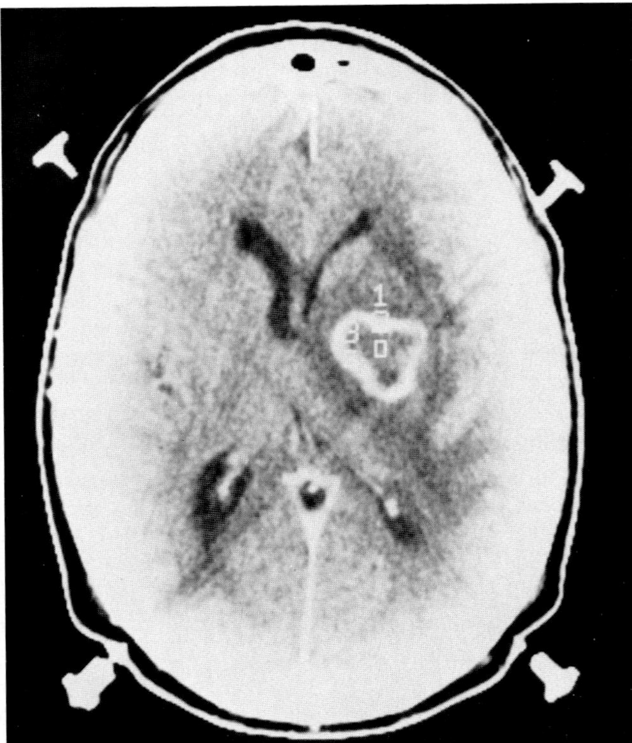

Fig. 41-14.   A CT scan of a patient in whom the distinction between abscess and neoplasm was impossible radiographically. This lesion proved to be a lymphoma.

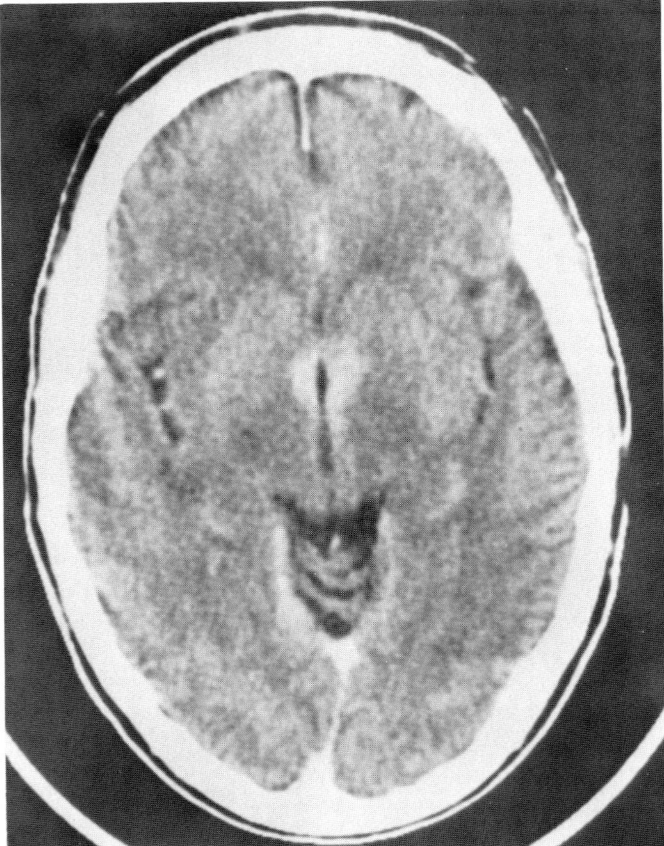

Fig. 41-15.   A hypothalamic glioma successfully biopsied without complication.

(Figure 41-15). This proved to be a grade II glioma. She had no postoperative hypothalamic deficits. These cases illustrate the power and precision of the biopsy technique. Definitive diagnosis is not possible in 5 percent of cases in the combined experience at this institution.

COMPLICATIONS

The complication rate for stereotactic biopsy is low but not negligible. Mortality at our institution is 0.8 percent. Clinically important hematomas occurred in 1.2 percent of cases. Superficial infections were found in 2 percent of patients.

POSTOPERATIVE CARE

The patient is sometimes observed in the recovery room for 1 to 2 hours, or more often allowed to return to the neurosurgical ward with careful postoperative clinical monitoring. Discharge is usually 24 to 48 hours after the biopsy. I routinely administer anticonvulsants and steroids at the time of biopsy and continue anticonvulsants for at least a year after the biopsy. Steroids are tapered over several days. At the time of suture removal approximately 1 week later the final pathology report is available, and at that time there is further discussion about treatment.

OTHER USES OF THE BRWT FRAME

The stereotactic techniques described here were adapted to improve tumor management. They have made lesions that were previously considered inaccessible capable of safe and accurate biopsy as well as lessening the morbidity of biopsy for such lesions as corpus callosum gliomas. Compatibility with MRI is possible using a nonmagnetic localizing system with mineral oil inserted into hollow carbon localizing rods: this provides very satisfactory localization without distortion.

It is clear that with increasing sophistication of target localization, especially with MRI scanning, the BRWT frame can be used for placement of lesions as well as for biopsy within the central nervous system. These applications have not been discussed here. It may be appropriate, however, to point out other important potential applications. It is possible to drain some cystic lesions for diagnosis and possibly therapy; Figure 41-16 presents a scan sequence from one of my patients demonstrating virtually complete evacuation of a colloid cyst. Ventricular or cyst catheters can also be positioned: a Silastic catheter made by Radionics is specifically designed for use with the system. This is invaluable in placement for tumor drainage and may also be useful in ventricular tumors or slit ventricles where the ventricles can be difficult to reach. Finally, interstitial radiation techniques can be applied to this system. These are of increasing importance in tumor surgery.[14] Mundinger reported in 1980 on interstitial brachytherapy using iridium 192 or iodine 125 long term in 251 malignant inoperable tumors, commenting that it produced 5-year survival in 43 to 68 percent of patients and had a mortality of 2.6 percent.[15] Short-term implantation of ^{32}P, ^{198}Au, or ^{90}Y colloid was accomplished in 247 patients. Applications of this frame to stereotactic diagnosis and therapy are increasing with time and

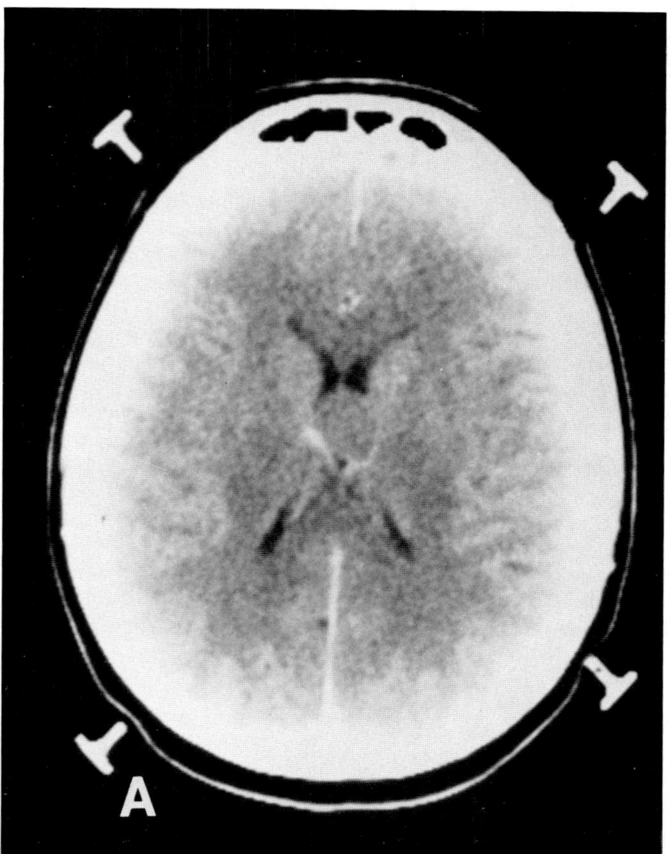
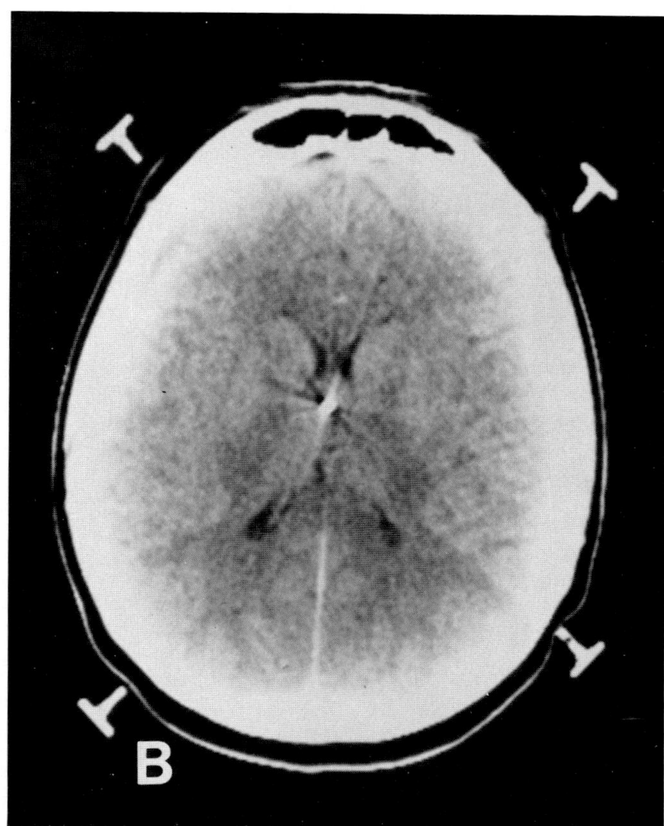
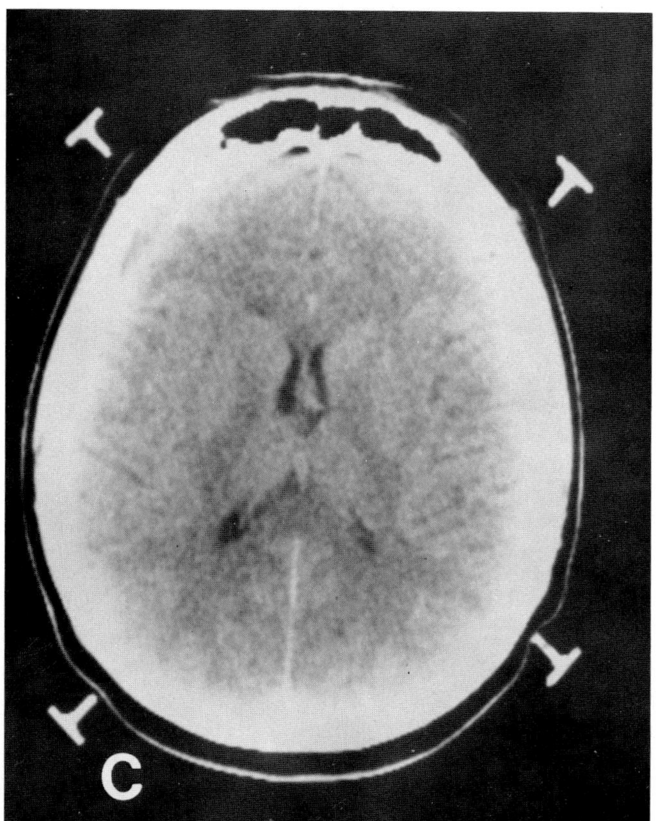

Fig. 41-16. Use of the BRWT technique for aspiration of a colloid cyst. (A) A preoperative scan; (B) scan obtained during aspiration with the open-ended biopsy instrument, which produced a scatter artifact; (C) a scan obtained postoperatively. There was no recurrence at 6 months.

make it and similar devices an important adjunct in contemporary neurosurgery.

REFERENCES

1. Horner NB, Potts DB: A comparison of CT-stereotactic brain biopsy techniques. Invest Radiol 19:361, 1984
2. Kelley PJ, Koll B, Goerss S: Stereotactic CT scanning for the biopsy of intracranial lesions and functional neurosurgery. Appl Neurophysiol 46:193, 1983
3. Kelley PJ, Earnest F, Koll BA, et al: Surgical options for patients with deep-seated brain tumors: Computer-assisted stereotactic biopsy. Mayo Clin Proc 60:223, 1985
4. Gildenberg PL, Kaufman HH, Krishnamurthy KD: Calculation of stereotactic coordinates for the computerized tomographic scan. Neurosurgery 10:580, 1982
5. Bullard DE, Nashold BS, Osborne D, et al: CT-guided stereotactic biopsies using a modified frame and Gildenberg techniques. J Neurol Neurosurg Psychiatry 47:590, 1984
6. Bouvier G, Couillard P, Leger SL, et al: Stereotactic biopsy of cerebral space-occupying lesions. Appl Neurophysiol 46:227, 1983
7. Roberts TS, Brown R: Technical and clinical aspects of CT-directed stereotaxis. Appl Neurophysiol 43:170, 1980
8. Brown RA: A computerized tomography-computer graphics approach to stereotactic localization. J Neurosurg 50:715, 1979
9. Brown RA, Roberts TS, Osborn AG: Simplified CT-guided stereotactic biopsy. AJNR 2:181, 1981
10. Heilbrun MP, Roberts TS, Apuzzo ML, et al: Preliminary experience with Brown-Roberts-Wells computerized tomography stereotactic guidance system. J Neurosurg 59:217, 1983
11. Heilbrun MP, Roberts TS, Wells TH, et al: Technical Manual: Brown-Roberts-Wells (BRW) CT Stereotactic Guidance System. Burlington, MA, Radionics, Inc., 1982
12. Apuzzo M, Sabshin JK: Computed tomographic guidance stereotaxis in the management of intracranial mass lesions. Neurosurgery 12:277, 1983
13. Willems JGMS, Alva-Willems JM: Accuracy of cytologic diagnosis of central nervous system neoplasms in stereotactic biopsies. Acta Cytol 28:243, 1984
14. Dyck P, Bongaglon A, Solit-Bohman L, et al: Computer-assisted CT guided biopsy and brachytherapy of brain tumors. Bull Clin Neurosci 48:122, 1983
15. Mundinger F, Ostertag CB, Birg W, et al: Stereotactic treatment of brain lesions: Biopsy, interstitial radiotherapy (iridium-192 and iodine-125) and drainage procedures. Appl Neurophysiol 43:1980

Computed Tomographic and Magnetic Resonance Imaging Based Stereotactic Resection of Deep-Seated Intracranial Tumors

Patrick J. Kelly

DEEP-SEATED PRIMARY OR METASTATIC intra-axial neoplasms can be difficult to locate during conventional craniotomy because a surgeon's three-dimensional orientation decreases as the procedure extends below the cortical surface, and the definition between primary glial neoplasm and surrounding brain tissue may not be apparent. In addition, maintaining spatial orientation within various extensions of geometrically complex neoplasms can also pose a significant problem. Since most deep-seated lesions lie within important brain tissue, neurosurgeons are reluctant to be too aggressive in the resection of these lesions. Nevertheless, some advocate conventional craniotomies to establish the tissue diagnosis and "decompress" the lesion.[1,2] Others prefer not to operate on deep-seated tumors, infer the diagnosis from neuroradiologic studies, and prescribe empirical therapy.[3,4] However, a significant number (17 percent) of deep-seated lesions are found to be nonneoplastic at stereotactic biopsy.[5]

Computed tomography and magnetic resonance imaging provide information on the three-dimensional extent of intra-axial tumors. Computer reconstructions of stereotactically gathered computed tomographic (CT) and magnetic resonance imaging (MRI) data can provide a three-dimensional model of the neoplasm in stereotactic space.[6–9] With proper interfacing an operating room computer system can monitor and display the position of stereotactically directed instruments in relationship to that three-dimensional model.[9,10]

We have performed these so-called computer-assisted stereotactic procedures since January, 1980[10–13] During this time, we have refined the methodology, increased the number of preoperative data bases, and developed new instrumentation for efficient operations.

This chapter will describe current methodology for computer-assisted stereotactic laser resection of intra-axial lesions, detailing the data acquisition, treatment planning, and interactive surgical phases of the procedure. In addition, we will outline our clinical experience to date with the procedure.

DATA ACQUISITION

The preoperative data base consists of stereotactically gathered computed tomographic (CT), magnetic resonance imaging (MRI), and digital angiographic (DA) data. These studies are performed in image-compatible stereotactic head holders applied to the sedated patient under local anesthesia. The head holder can be placed and replaced in precisely the same manner for data acquisition, surgery, and subsequent procedures.

STEREOTACTIC HEAD HOLDER

The head holder consists of a base ring, vertical supports, sleeves, fixation pins, and detachable micrometers (Figure 42-1). The base ring is constructed of aluminum for the CT-compatible unit and molybdinum disulfide for the magnetic-resonance-compatible head holder. Four molybdinum disulfide vertical supports extend from the base ring. Collett devices in each vertical support secure hollow sleeves that maintain the distance between the patient's scalp and the vertical support. Carbon fiber fixation pins (3 mm in diameter) are inserted through the hollow sleeves into holes drilled through the outer table of the patient's skull into the diploe. A flange located 4 mm from the tip of the fixation pin rests on the outer table of the patient's skull. The depth of each pin is measured by micrometer, and these micrometer readings are recorded for each pin location. This provides a mechanism for precise replacement of the head holder.

Data acquisition and surgery are rarely performed on the same day. Once the required data on a patient has been accumulated, the head frame is removed and replaced on the day of surgery.

For reapplication of the head holder, the surgeon taps the four fixation pins into the previously made drill holes, slides the sleeves over them, and secures the sleeves with the colletts after reproducing the micrometer measurements.

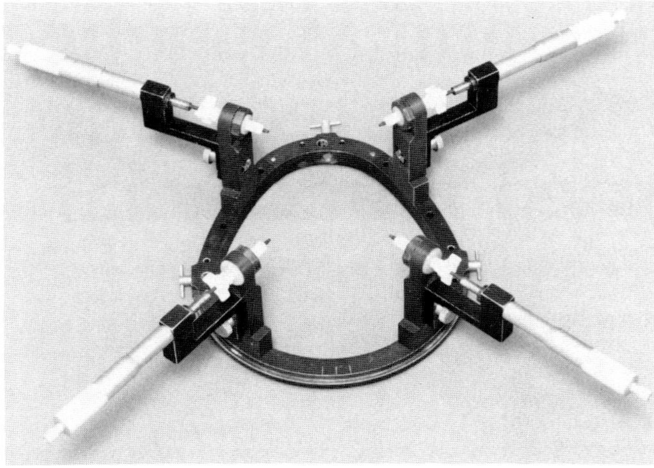

Fig. 42-1. A CT compatible stereotactic head holder. Note the detachable micrometers on the vertical supports.

Posterior fossa procedures are performed with the patient in the prone position. The stereotactic head holder is applied in the inverted position for data acquisition and surgery. This allows unobstructed access to the posterior fossa.[14]

STEREOTACTIC CT SCANS

Computed tomographic data is gathered on General Electric 8800 or 9800 standing units. A CT table adaptation plate attaches to the scanning table. The adaptation plate has a slot that receives the base ring of the stereotactic head holder, similar to the fixation system that exists on the stereotactic surgical frame.[6,8,9] Alignment of indexing marks on the adaptation plate and headholder baseline ensure that no rotational errors between CT scanning and surgery occur.

A CT localization system, applied to the base of the head holder, contains nine carbon fiber rods arranged in the shape of the letter N located on either side of the head and anteriorly (Figure 42-2). This creates nine reference marks on each CT slice from which the height and inclination of the slice above the base ring can be determined. The CT slices are gathered through the lesion for computer calculation of the entire lesional volume.

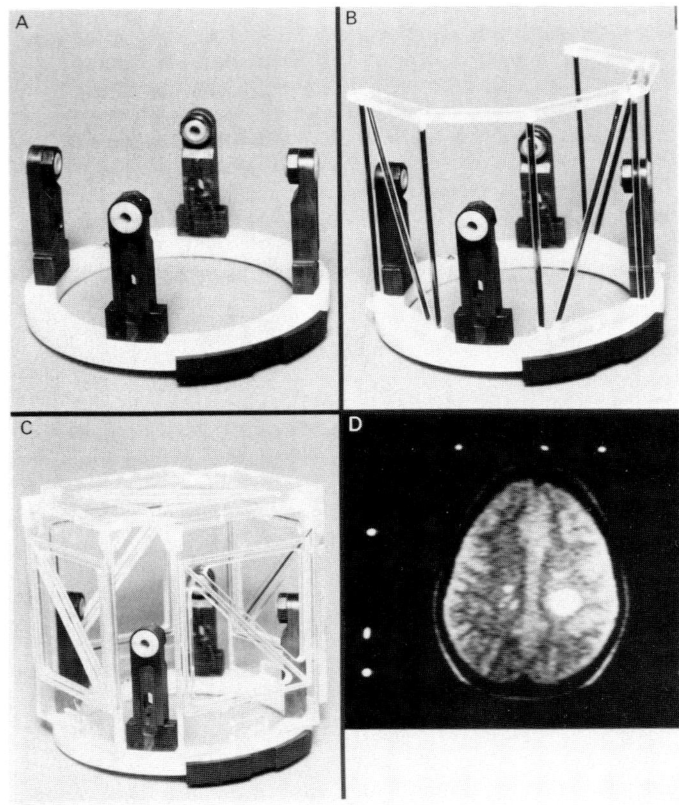

Fig. 42-3. (A) A MRI compatible head holder, (B) transverse, and (C) multiplanar localization systems. (D) The localization systems create nine reference marks on each MR image.

STEREOTACTIC MAGNETIC RESONANCE IMAGING

A table adaptation plate developed for a Picker 1.5 Tesla Resistive MRI Unit receives the MRI compatible stereotactic head holder. This holds the patient rigid during the MRI examination. A transverse localization system resembles that designed for CT scanning, having nine capillary tubes filled with copper sulfate ($CuSO_4$) solution (Figure 42-3B). This creates a series of nine reference marks around each MRI image from which stereotactic coordinates of any point or sets of points on each MRI slice can be calculated. A multiplanar localization

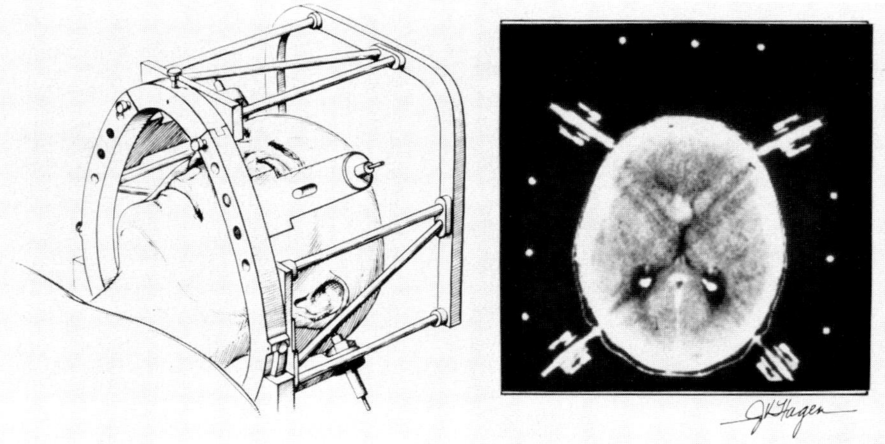

Fig. 42-2. The localization system attaches to the base ring of the stereotactic head holder. This creates reference marks on each CT slice.

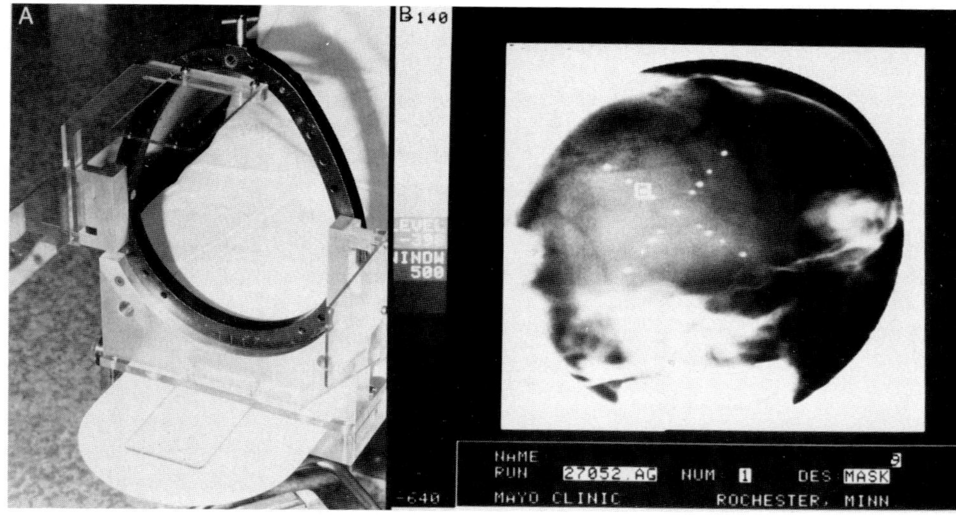

Fig. 42-4. (A) A stereotactic head holder mounted on a DF table adaptation plate. The angiographic reference system (ARS) attaches to the base ring. (B) A mask image demonstrates 18 reference marks created by the ARS.

system has also been developed to utilize coronal and sagittal as well as transverse images (Figure 42-3C).

STEREOTACTIC DIGITAL ANGIOGRAPHY

A table adaptation plate is also used to secure the stereotactic head holder during the angiographic examinations on General Electric DF 3000 or 5000 units (Figure 42-4A). An angiographic reference system (ARS), which consists of four radiolucent plates, each having nine radiopaque reference points, attaches to the base ring of the stereotactic head holder. The reference plates are positioned bilaterally, anteriorly and posteriorly. These create 18 reference marks on each AP and lateral DA image (Figure 42-4B).

The reference marks define coordinate axes for the ARS and provide grids for computer calculation of x-ray magnification at any three-dimensionally defined point in space. Orthogonal and 6-degree oblique series are obtained for AP and lateral images.

A computer program transforms the X-Y-Z points in space from stereotactic CT and MRI calculations as a function of the distances from the central beam defined by each reference plate and interpolates the magnification factor for the correct annotation of that point on DA images.

TUMOR VOLUME INTERPOLATION

The archived data tapes from the CT, MRI, and DA examinations are transferred to the operating room computer system (Data General Eclipse Sl40 with l28Kb RAM and 192 Mb disc storage). Each CT and MRI slice that displays the tumor is viewed on a raster display console. A tumor volume is then interpolated from CT and MRI data and registered in an image matrix as follows.

First, the computer automatically digitizes the nine reference marks produced by the localization systems on each CT and MRI slice utilizing an intensity detection algorithm. The surgeon then traces around the lesion on each sequential slice using a cursor and trackball subsystem and enters a series of points on the boundary of the lesion by the deposit key (Figure 42-5). The digitized points are then suspended into a three-dimensional image array at levels corresponding to the location of each CT or MRI slice defined by the reference fiducials. The surgeon also selects a target point at some location within the lesion from a CT or MRI slice for which stereotactic frame coordinates are calculated. The tumor volume is constructed around and surgical approach angles are based on this point.

The digitized boundary points are connected by computer into a closed contour within the matrix at each sequential level. The computer then interpolates intermediate slices at 1-mm intervals between the digitized slices. Finally, each of the digitized and interpolated slices is filled with 1-mm cubic voxels. This creates a three-dimensional solid volume within the image matrix for the CT-based tumor boundaries and for the MRI defined limits (Figure 42-6). A shaded graphic display,

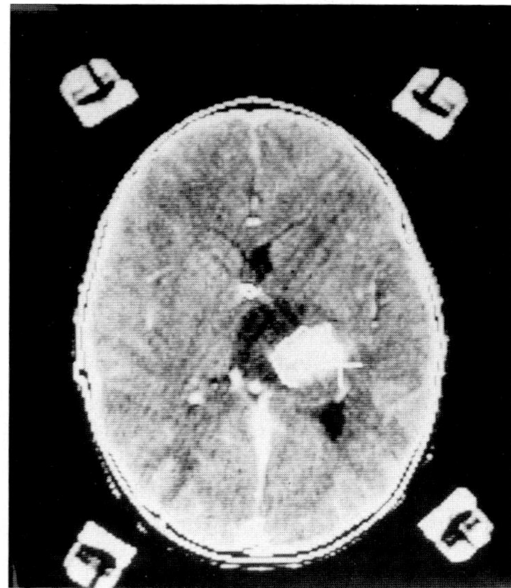

Fig. 42-5. Digitizing a CT slice using the cursor and trackball.

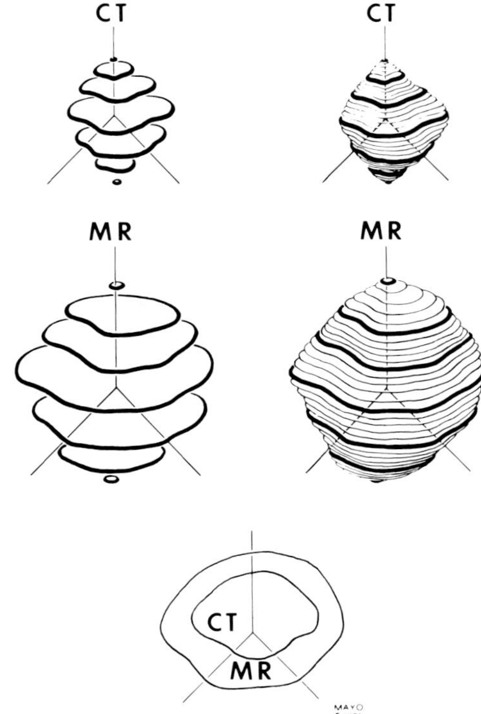

Fig. 42-6. Each CT and MRI slice is suspended in an image matrix; intermediate slices are interpolated at 1-mm intervals, volumes defined by CT and MRI are then created and reformatted along the line of view.

presented as a stereo pair, is useful for the surgeon to understand the geometric complexities of the tumor as a three-dimensional volume.

The CT and MRI defined tumor volumes can also be sliced perpendicular to a specified surgical viewline defined by arc and collar angle settings on the stereotactic instrument. The limits of the tumor defined by CT and those defined by MRI are designated by specific gray levels in the display (Figure 42-7). These slices are displayed on a monitor in the operating room during surgery. The computer also displays the position of the stereotactic retractors and the position of the carbon dioxide laser beam in relationship to each tumor slice. The stereotactic frame settings corresponding to the displayed tumor slice are also shown on the monitor. These include the X, Y, and Z frame adjustments and the patient rotation and arc and collar angles. The actual numbers for patient rotation and arc and collar angles are determined during the surgical planning procedure.

SURGICAL PLANNING

All intracranial lesions can be accurately localized and resected with computer-assisted stereotactic techniques. However, an opening through the brain of at least 2 cm in diameter will be required in order to expose the subcortical lesion. Several routes provide access to deep-seated tumors from the cortical surface. Cortical and subcortical incisions made in nonessential brain tissue in directions parallel to major white matter projections can be used to expose some tumors. Microsurgical splitting of deep sulci and gentle retraction of the opposing gyral banks provide another means of gaining access to tumors lying deep to them in important subcortical areas. An incision in the trough of the sulcus can then be used to expose

the tumor. We have used this approach in centrally located lesions by splitting the rolandic fissure or the pre- or post-central sulci depending on the precise location of the tumor in relationship to the overlying gyrus. In addition, subinsular lesions have been successfully removed by splitting the sylvian fissure and making an incision in the insular cortex.

The sylvian and rolandic fissures constitute important barriers that should not be traversed if neurologic deficit is to be avoided. Therefore, lesions located anterior to the rolandic fissure are approached anteriorly, those located posterior to the rolandic fissure are approached from behind, and those located below the sylvian fissure are exposed inferior to the plane of the fissure. The stereotactic relationships of the lesion to overlying sulci, fissures, and gyri are determined from their location on CT slices or MR images. In addition, the position of the major sulci and fissures can be established in stereotactic space by identification of the deep segments of cortical vessels visualized on stereotactic stereoscopic angiography.[15] The stereotactic coordinates of sulci are then determined from calculations based on the reference marks created by the arteriographic reference system.

Centrally located lesions deep to the mesial hemisphere are best approached through the interhemispheric fissure. The cortex overlying the lesion is localized stereotactically and incised. When using this approach, stainless steel reference balls are placed by stereotactic cannula before the trephine craniotomy is opened. Preliminary and subsequent stereotactic radiographic images are used to detect and correct for possible movements of the tumor caused by retraction of the hemisphere (see below).

Deep-seated lesions lying medially can also be approached transcortically, provided that the overlying brain tissue is expendable. This approach is appropriate for paraventricular posterior frontal lesions (approached from a cortical entry point anterior to the coronal suture) or parietal lesions located lateral to the trigone of the lateral ventricle (approached by incision into the superior parietal convolution).

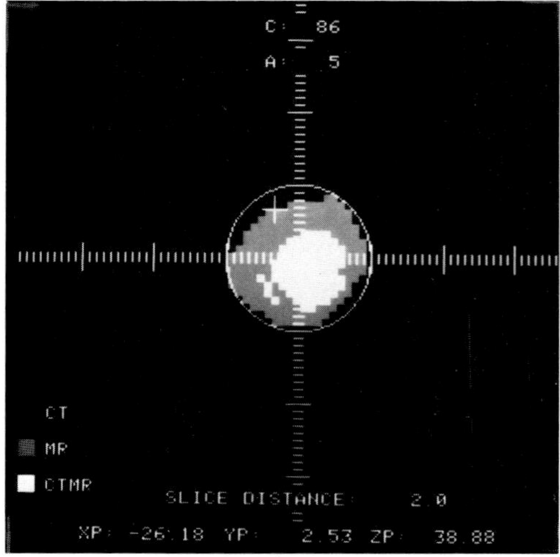

Fig. 42-7. A tumor sliced perpendicular to surgical viewing. The CT- and MRI-defined limits are designated by specific gray levels in the display. The position of the stereotactic retractors in reference to the tumor slice is shown (circle) against the millimeter scale grids. The position of the surgical laser is represented by the cursor. The stereotactic (X, Y, and Z) frame settings, the arc and collar approach angles, and the patient rotation are shown as in the slice distance in millimeters from the focal point of the stereotactic instrument.

In planning the surgical approach to thalamic lesions, the surgeon must define the location of the uninvolved regions of the thalamus in relationship to the tumor. These intact regions cannot be incised and retracted without risking substantial neurologic deficit. Tumors located in the anterior thalamus therefore are approached through the anterior limb of the internal capsule. Tumors in the dorsal thalamus are exposed through the lateral ventricle. Posterior thalamic tumors are approached posterolaterally from a temporo-occipital cortical and subcortical incision through the posterior aspect of the temporal horn of the lateral ventricle.

Midline posterior fossa lesions are exposed through the vermis; lateral lesions through cerebellar hemisphere. Midline pontine lesions that elevate and extend to the floor of the fourth ventricle are resected through a midline incision in the floor of the ventricle. Lateral pontine lesions are exposed through the middle cerebellar peduncle.

STEREOTACTIC DEFINITION OF THE SURGICAL APPROACH

A surgical approach is defined by three settings on our stereotactic frame: patient rotation, arc (angle from the vertical plane), and collar (angle from the horizontal plane) settings. Patient rotation is indicated by indexing marks on the base ring of the stereotactic head holder aligned with the index mark on the receiving yoke of the stereotactic three-dimensional slide apparatus.

PATIENT ROTATION

Three-hundred-sixty degrees of patient rotation are possible: 0 degree represents the supine position, 90 degrees corresponds to left lateral decubitus, 180 degrees indicates the prone position, and 270 degrees corresponds to the right lateral decubitus position. Intermediate settings are also possible and frequently employed. The major aim in patient rotation is to provide the surgeon with the most comfortable working situation. For instance, a left posterior temporal occipital approach would use a patient rotation of 150 degrees. Computer software rotates the stereotactic data base and calculates stereotactic coordinates based on the selected rotation.

Arc and collar approach angles are derived from the stereotactic coordinates of two points: target and entry. The selected reference point within the tumor target volume (see tumor volume interpolation) is the deep point. An entry point, digitized on a stereotactic CT or MRI slice, represents the optimal entry point on the cortical surface. This can be located on the superficial aspect of a deep sulcus or on an area of nonessential cortex. Alternatively, the stereotactic coordinates of the entry point can be calculated from the stereotactic angiogram.

The computer calculates arc and collar approach angles based on the following equations:

$$\text{Arc angle} = \text{TAN} - 1\ (X_2 - X_1)/Z_2 - Z_1)$$

$$\text{Collar angle} = \text{TAN} - 1\ (Y_2 - Y_1)/(Z_2 - Z_1)$$

where X_2, Y_2, and Z_2 are the coordinates of the entry point and X_1, Y_1, and Z_1 are the target point coordinates.

INSTRUMENTATION

STEREOTACTIC FRAME

The instrument presently used for computer-assisted stereotactic laser microsurgery consists of a servomotor-controlled three-dimensional slide system that positions an intracranial target point into the focal point of the arc quadrants attached to the instrument's base plate.[9,10] A 400-mm radius arc-quadrant indexes into position when stereotactic control during a craniotomy is required. Smaller arc quadrants (135-mm and 160-mm radii) are used to direct intracranial biopsy probes and hold the stereotactic retractors through which tumors are exposed and removed (Figure 42-8).

A microscope and laser manipulator apparatus (microslad) travels perpendicular to a tangent to the 400-mm arc quadrant and thus is directed to the focal point of the arc quadrant regardless of the arc or collar angles selected. The focal distance of the microscope and microslad from the focal point of the arc quadrant is controlled by a servomotorized drive system on the carriage. Optical encoders (Acu-Rite II, Bausch & Lomb, Rochester, NY) on the microscope/microslad carriage

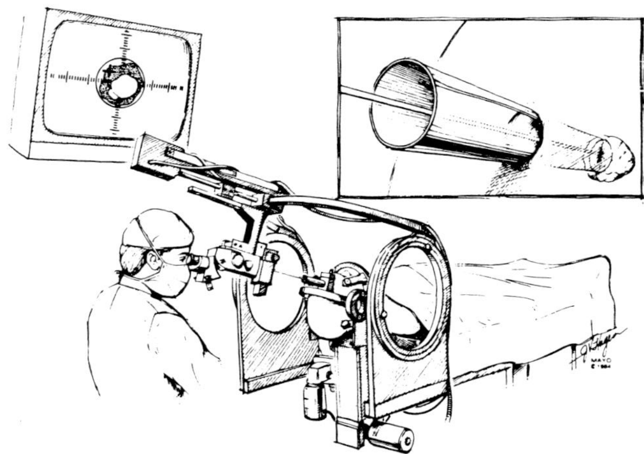

Fig. 42-8. The stereotactic instrumentation consists of a three-dimensional servomotor controlled slide system that positions the patient's head into the focal point of an internal arc quadrant, which directs a stereotactic retractor toward its focal point. A microscope and laser manipulator apparatus is suspended from a carriage that runs perpendicular to the tangent of the 400-mm arc quadrant. A video monitor displays the computer-generated information depicted in Figure 42-7.

and on the three-axis slide system record the distance of the
microscope and laser foci from the focal point of the arc
quadrant and the X, Y, and Z stereotactic coordinates, respectively, and relay this information to digital display units on the
control panel. The microscope/microslad drive system is controlled by foot pedal and the X, Y, and Z frame coordinates are
set by switches on the control panel operated by a technician.

MICROSLAD

The CO_2 laser and HE-NE aiming beam are delivered to
the microslad from a Sharplan 743 surgical laser (Sharplan 743,
Laser Industries, Tel-Aviv, Israel) by an articulated optical
arm. The beams pass through a variable focus lens system
(which changes the focal length and thus the spot size) and then
reflect off two mirrors that ultimately direct the laser beams into
the surgical field. These mirrors are mounted on the shafts of
galvanometers, the pitch of which is controlled by the voltage
output of the digital-to-analogue (DAC) board of the operating
room computer system. Specific voltages supplied by the DAC
to the galvanometers deflect the laser beam in a precise and
reproducible manner at a given focal length in the surgical field.

A joystick, controlled by the surgeon, transmits the desired
positions of the laser beam in the surgical field to the computer
system by optical encoders within the joystick assembly. The
digital pulses from the encoders are instantaneously converted
to voltages related to galvanometers in the microslad that
position the laser beam at the required location in the surgical
field. The computer also displays the position of the laser beam
as a cursor in relationship to an X,Y grid centered on the
surgical viewline on an operating room display monitor (Figure
42-7).

ACCESSORY INSTRUMENTS

STEREOTACTIC RETRACTORS

Cylindrically shaped retractors attach to the 135-mm or
160-mm arc quadrants and are secured by a collett. Extra long
bipolar forceps with a shaft length of 150 mm are required to
control bleeding in the surgical field when working through the
stereotactic retractors (Radionics Incorporated, Burlington,
MA). In addition, 150–160-mm long suctions, tips, dissectors,
and alligator scissors are also used.

SURGICAL PROCEDURE

The patient is placed under general anesthesia
endotracheally and the stereotactic headframe is replaced using
the same pin placements and micrometer settings used during
the data acquisition phase. The patient is positioned in the
stereotactic frame so that the index marks on the frame line up
with the marks on the head holder indicating the desired
rotation. The patient's head is moved in order to position the
desired target point into the focal point of the arc quadrant.
After the head is prepared and draped, the desired arc and
collar angles are set on the arc quadrant.

In order to monitor possible intracranial shifts in the tumor
after the skull and dura have been opened, the tumor is
traversed by a stereotactically directed biopsy cannula through
a ⅛-inch drill hole and a series of (0.5-mm diameter) stainless

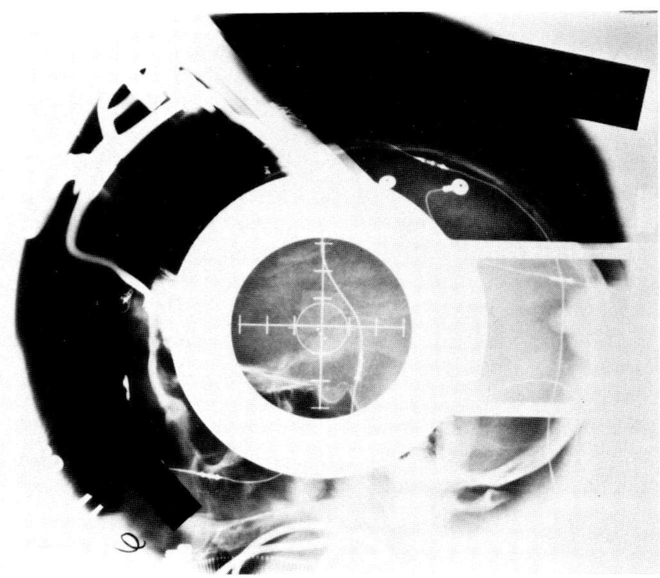

Fig. 42-9. Stainless steel reference balls stereotactically inserted at
5-mm intervals along the surgical line of view.

steel reference balls are deposited at 5-mm intervals along the
viewline (Figure 42-9). The position of these markers on anteroposterior and lateral stereotactic teleradiographs provides reference points so that any subsequent intracranial shifts can be
detected. If movement of the reference balls is detected (extremely uncommon in our experience), the position of the
tumor volume can be shifted in the computer image matrix in
order to take these spatial shifts into account in subsequent
image displays.

The patient's scalp is then opened with a linear incision and
the skull is opened with a 1½–2-inch cranial trephine centered
on the twist drill hole used to deposit the reference balls. The
dura is opened in a cruciate fashion.

In the removal of superficial lesions, the computer displays
the configuration of the trephine in relationship to the reformatted tumor outlines (Figure 42-9). This will keep the surgeon
oriented during removal of the tumor. A plane is created around
the tumor with bipolar cautery or the stereotactically directed
laser using the computer-generated images as a guide. In this
manner, even high grade gliomas can be removed as intact
specimens where a plane of dissection corresponds to the
contrast-enhanced margins on CT scans.

Deep-seated tumors are removed with a stereotactically
directed retractor that maintains the exposure. The position of
the cylindrical retractor is shown as a circle on the display
monitor in relationship to the tumor slice. The position of the
surgical laser is shown as a cursor. A ''Lookahead'' option also
displays deeper tumor slices along the viewline. This alerts the
surgeon to the configuration of the tumor to be encountered as
the procedure progresses. Using the computer display as a
guide, the surgeon creates a plane of dissection around the
lesion with the laser, advances the retractor, and deepens the
incision, circumscribing the tumor.

Tumor tissue within the retractor is removed with 65–85 W
of defocused laser power utilizing the manual or automatic
mode (in which the computer sweeps the laser beam according
to a specified programmed sequence based on the CT) or
MRI-defined tumor limits). In this manner the tumor is removed
slice by slice extending from the most superficial slices to the

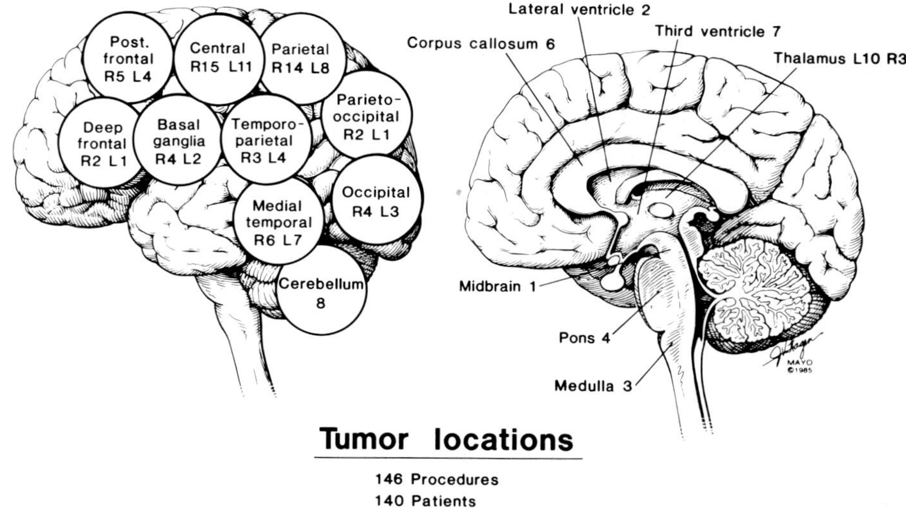

Tumor locations

146 Procedures
140 Patients

Fig. 42-10. Tumor locations in 140 patients.

deepest. The surgeon monitors not only the surgical field of view through the operating microscope but also the display monitor for information on the location of the laser and retractor in relationship to the CT- and MRI-defined tumor boundaries. Anteroposterior and lateral teleradiographs are obtained to document the progress of the procedure and record possible movements of the reference balls (which are removed as they are encountered during the procedure). Hemostasis is secured utilizing the extra long bipolar forceps.

CLINICAL EXPERIENCE

We have performed 146 computer-assisted stereotactic craniotomies on 140 patients since January, 1980. Five patients underwent repeat procedures (three for residual tumors and two for recurrent tumors). One patient underwent a third procedure for recurrent tumor. The age of the patients ranged from 2 to 78 years; the average age was 46.8 years. Lesion locations are illustrated in Figure 42-10; histologic results are listed in Table 42-1. Table 42-2 shows the results of neurologic examinations performed 1 week postoperatively: 67 patients improved, 59 patients were unchanged, and 17 patients were worse. Superior quadrant visual field deficits followed posterior temporal approaches to medial temporal or thalamic lesions in 7 patients; 1 patient had a complete homonymous hemianopsia following an occipital approach to a posterior thalamic lesion and 9 patients had worsening of neurologic deficits noted preoperatively.

Three deaths occurred within 1 month after surgery: one from massive brainstem edema following removal of a thalamic astrocytoma with brainstem infiltration apparent on the MRI, one from a ventricular infection after resection of a previously irradiated third ventricular teratoma, and one from massive pulmonary embolism 2 weeks after resection of a thalamic cavernous hemangioma.

Based on this overall experience, we have certain opinions on the appropriateness of computer-assisted stereotactic laser microsurgery in specific lesions. In addition, technical maneuvers useful in the stereotactic removal of various lesions depending on histologic findings and anatomic location have been developed.

Computer-assisted stereotactic resection can remove all

Table 42-1. Histologic findings in 140 patients undergoing computer-assisted stereotactic resection of tumors.

Tumor type	Number of Patients
Astrocytoma grade IV	32
Astrocytoma grade III	12
Astrocytoma grade II	23
Metastatic	38
Oligodendroglioma	9
Vascular	14
Miscellaneous:	
Lymphoma	2
Tuberous sclerosis	2
Meningioma	3
Abscess	1
Choroid plexis papilloma	1
Colloid cyst	1
Ganglioglioma	2
Total	140

Table 42-2. Postoperative results following 146 computer-assisted stereotactic laser resections

Result	Number of Patients
Improved	67
Unchanged	
Normal preoperatively	39
Deficit preoperatively	20
Worse	
Superior quadrantanopsia	7
Homonymous hemianopsia	1
Preoperative deficits worse	9
Dead	
Brainstem edema	1
Pulmonary embolism	1
Infection	1

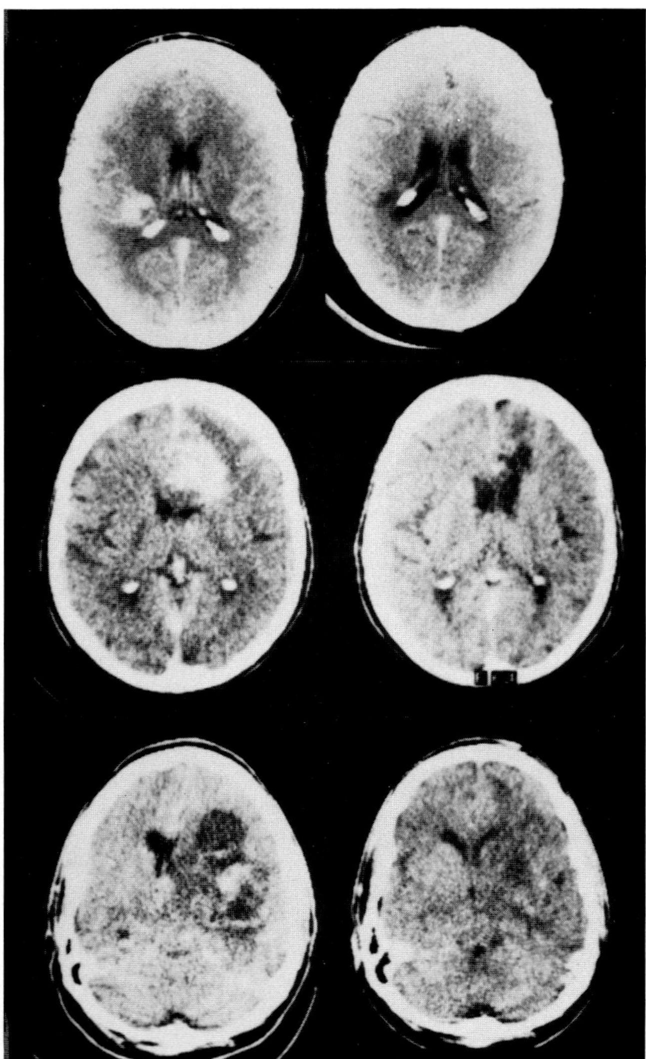

Fig. 42-11. Preoperative and postoperative CT scans of a deep parietal grade 4 astrocytoma (top), a grade 3 posterior fossa astrocytoma invading the corpus callosum (middle), and a basal ganglia grade 3 astrocytoma (bottom).

CT-defined, contrast-enhancing portions of glioblastomas from neurologically important subcortical areas with acceptable levels of mortality and morbidity (Figure 42-11). However, even though postoperative CT studies in our series demonstrated an absence of contrast enhancement around the surgical defect, new areas of contrast enhancement developed, within low density areas close to and remote from the surgical defect within 6 to 9 months after the procedure. Death in the majority of these cases was therefore a result of tumor ''recurrence'' and progression.

The average postoperative survival of our patients harboring grade 4 astrocytomas and treated with postoperative external beam radiation therapy was 38 weeks. It should be noted that all of these patients had lesions in central and deep-seated locations that have historically been associated with poor survival and high surgical morbidity and mortality.[4,8] Nevertheless, the survival of our patients is similar to survival times quoted in other series, where a high percentage of patients harbor lesions in the frontal and temporal lobes, which are more amenable to radical resection by lobectomy.[16–21]

Resection of the volume defined by the MRI abnormality would theoretically prolong postoperative survival.[22] Histologic examination of tissue specimens obtained from regions corresponding to hypodensity on CT scans and increased T2 on the MRI revealed intact edematous brain parenchyma infiltrated by aggressive, isolated tumor cells, which surrounds the mass of solid tumor tissue represented by CT contrast enhancement.[23–25] This edematous infiltrated parenchyma appears to extend as far as the area of signal prolongation abnormality on the T2-weighted MR image indicates.[25] However, unacceptable neurologic deficits would result from removal of the intact although infiltrated parenchyma. Isolated tumor cells also infiltrate intact and surrounding edematous parenchyma in patients having grade 3 astrocytomas and oligodendrogliomas. Computer-assisted stereotactic resection does not cure these patients either. Tumor recurrences are seen later in the patient's postoperative course than with glioblastomas but generally in the same spatial pattern. However, the procedure removes all of the solid tumor tissue component of the neoplasm defined by contrast enhancement on stereotactic CT scanning and permits a reduction in tumor border that is as aggressive as possible with preservation of neurologic function in the majority of patients.[10]

Low grade glial tumors in adults are usually manifested by an area of low density on CT scans and prolongation of signal on MRI. Stereotactic serial biopsies of the areas defined by the low density areas on CT scans and signal prolongation on MRI reveal infiltrated intact parenchyma with little tumor tissue proper.[24,25] Resection of this infiltrated parenchyma therefore results in postoperative neurologic deficits.[5,10]

On the other hand, pilocytic astrocytomas, which tend to occur in children, are histologically circumscribed. They can be completely resected by computer-assisted stereotactic technique with excellent postoperative results in spite of the fact that many are located in the thalamus (Figure 42-12).[10] The borders of these lesions are accurately defined by the contrast enhancement that these tumors exhibit on CT scans.[24,25]

Adults occasionally may harbor pilocytic or other circumscribed low grade glial tumors. However, this is so unusual that we now perform a preliminary stereotactic biopsy procedure to exclude the more common fibrillary astrocytoma or infiltrating oligodendroglioma before considering computer-assisted stereotactic laser resection of the lesion.

METASTATIC TUMORS

Metastatic tumors are histologically circumscribed and can be completely resected (Figure 42-13). In patients with stable disease, solitary metastases can be completely resected stereotactically with more favorable levels of postoperative morbidity than associated with conventional craniotomy for these lesions.[26,27]

Stereotactic resection is useful for superficial as well as deep-seated metastatic lesions. Stereotactic localization helps locate small cranial trephines directly over superficial lesions or over the sulcus that will be opened to provide access to more deeply seated lesions. The trephine need be no larger than the cross-sectional area of the neoplasm. The computer display provides the surgeon with useful information on the global configuration of the neoplasm when the margins between the neoplasm and brain tissue are not readily apparent. Thus, complete resection can always be achieved. Nevertheless, external beam radiation therapy has followed surgery in all of our patients in order to treat possible microscopic metastatic lesions not visible on CT scans.

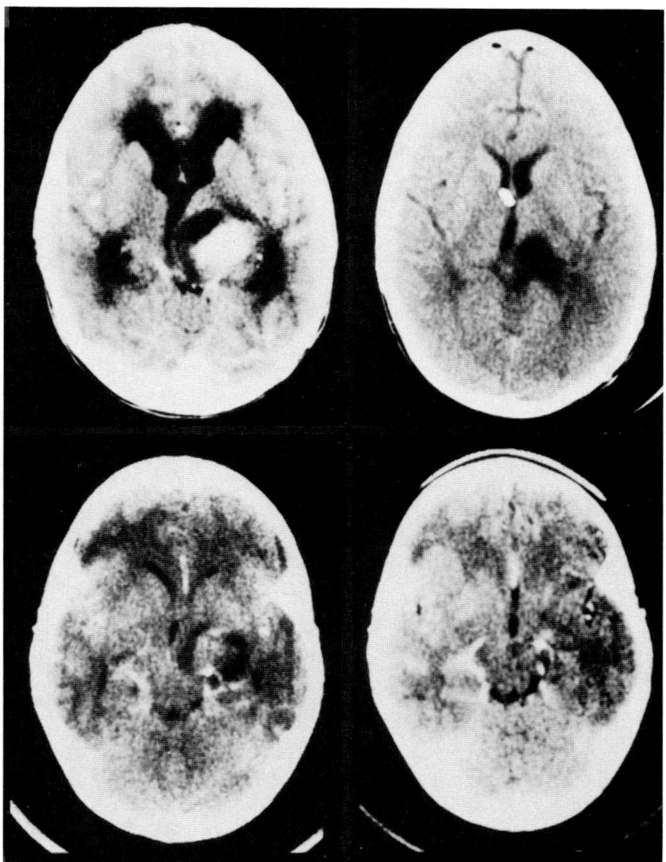

Fig. 42-12. Preoperative and postoperative CT scans of two patients with pilocytic astrocytomas in the thalamus.

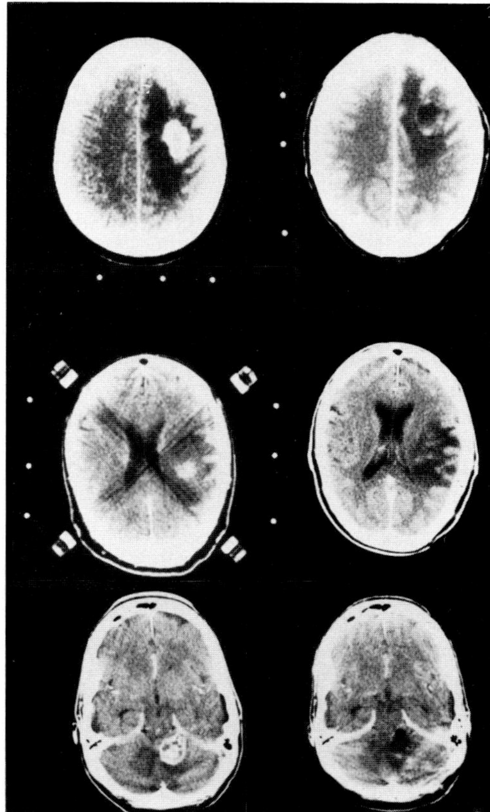

Fig. 42-13. Metastatic tumors. (Top) Precentral adenocarcinoma resected through the precentral sulcus. (Middle) Left subinsular lesion resected through the sylvian fissure. (Bottom) Adenocarcinoma of left middle cerebellar peduncle (transcerebellar approaches).

In a 6-year experience with computer-assisted stereotactic resection of intracranial metastases, we have yet to have a single local recurrence of the tumor. However, one patient with adenocarcinoma (lung) developed a second metastatic lesion in the left hemisphere 4 years after stereotactic resection of a right posterior frontal metastasis.

VASCULAR MALFORMATIONS

Surgeons should be reluctant to perform stereotactic biopsies on circumscribed lesions demonstrating intense contrast enhancement on CT scans. These could represent cryptic AVMs or cavernous hemangiomas, even though arteriography is negative. However, cryptic AVMs and cavernous hemangiomas are well circumscribed and can be completely removed stereotactically with relatively low risk. A by-product of establishing the histologic characteristics is that a cessation or significant reduction of seizures, when present, usually results.

Small, deep-seated, active arteriovenous malformations can also be resected with similar techniques.[28] The position of the feeding vessels is established in the three-dimensional surgical planning matrix and approached and clipped or coagulated first, before the remainder of the lesion is dissected away from the surrounding parenchyma.

INTRAVENTRICULAR LESIONS

Intraventricular landmarks can be used to maintain surgical orientation in the approach to and resection of interventricular lesions by conventional craniotomies. This is easier in patients having large lateral ventricles; more difficulty is encountered locating and staying oriented in small or normal-sized ventricles. A more limited but direct approach to intraventricular lesions can be made stereotactically. Brain and ventricular incisions need to be only large enough to remove the lesion. Thus, intraventricular lesions are removed through a 1.5-inch trephine and 1- or 2-cm cylindrical retractors.

Third ventricular lesions are approached through the right lateral ventricle. One fornix is incised in order to extend the stereotactic retractor into the third ventricular lesion. Here an internal decompression of the lesion is performed with the laser until only a thin rim of the capsule remains. The computer display of the cross sections of the digitized tumor volume is extremely useful in this step, since the surgeon can be quite aggressive within the tumor with no risk of extending through the capsule and damaging the walls of the third ventricle. Following this internal decompression, the retractor is withdrawn to the level of the roof of the third ventricle, and the capsule is carefully dissected from the walls of the third ventricle. The tumor capsule can be contracted with the defocused laser, which facilitates the dissection of the capsule from the wall of the third ventricle.

LARGE LESIONS

Deep-seated tumors 5 cm in diameter or even larger can be removed with the technique and instrumentation described even though the size of the largest retractor is only 3 cm in diameter. Here the surgeon gains access to and removes different parts of the tumor, which are sequentially positioned into the focal point of the stereotactic frame and therefore under the opening of the retractor. This is accomplished by first translating the cross-sectional image of the tumor on the display screen in order to place the desired portion of the tumor within the circle that designates the cylindrical retractor as viewed by the surgeon. The computer calculates new frame coordinates, which are then duplicated on the stereotactic frame by activating the switches that control the servomotors of the three-dimensional slide system.

In the resection of large lesions, a plane of dissection is first developed around the borders of the tumor in order to isolate it from surrounding brain tissue before any of the lesion is removed. This maneuver will prevent shifts of the neoplasm within the intracranial compartment as a result of tumor decompression, which could render the stereotactic coordinates no longer accurate. Extra large lesions can be resected at two or in some cases more successive operations. Repeat procedures are easily performed after acquisition of a new data base that represents the tumor volume (reduced in size after the first procedure) as a new target volume in space. The same skin and trephine cranial openings and white matter incision down to the lesion that were made during the initial procedure are used for the second procedure.

CONCLUSION

The computer-assisted stereotactic technique maintains a surgeon's three-dimensional orientation for precise and direct exposure of subcortical intracranial lesions. In addition, the location of surgical instruments (stereotactic retractor and $CO=2$ laser) are displayed in relationship to planar contours of the lesion displayed intraoperatively. With this method and instrumentation, aggressive resection of subcortical lesions is possible with minimal damage to surrounding brain tissue, and lesions can be resected from neurologically important areas with acceptable levels of morbidity and mortality.[5,10,13]

The benefits to patients with high grade glial neoplasms appear small with regard to long-term survival when stereotactic resection is compared with other more conventional surgical methods. However, a maximal reduction of tumor burden can be achieved with computer-assisted stereotactic resection with better postoperative neurologic results than would be associated with conventional procedures for lesions in central and deep-seated locations.

The procedure more clearly benefits patients with histologically circumscribed lesions such as pilocytic astrocytomas, metastatic tumors, intraventricular lesions, and vascular lesions.[10] In fact, the postoperative neurologic status seems more dependent on the degree of histologic circumscription than on the actual location of the lesions.

REFERENCES

1. Bernstein M, Hoffman HJ, Halliday WC, et al: Thalamic tumors in children. J Neurosurg 61:649, 1984
2. Greenwood J: Radical surgery of tumors of the thalamus, hypothalamus and third ventricular area. Surg Neurol 1:29, 1973
3. Cheek WR, Taveras JM: Thalamic tumors. J Neurosurg 24:505, 1966
4. Lee F: Radiation of infratentorial and supratentorial brain-stem tumors. J Neurol 43:65, 1975
5. Kelly PJ: Computer assisted stereotaxis: New approaches for the management of intracranial intra-axial tumors. Neurology 36:535, 1986
6. Goerss SJ, Kelly PJ, Kall BA, et al: A computed tomographic stereotactic adaptation system. Neurosurgery 10:375, 1982
7. Kelly PJ, Alker GJ Jr, Goerss SJ: Computer-assisted stereotactic laser microsusgery for the treatment of intracranial neoplasms. Neurosurgery 110:324, 1982
8. Kelly PJ, Kall BA, Goerss SJ: Transposition of volumetric information derived from computed tomography scanning into stereotactic space. Surg Neurol 21:465, 1984
9. Kall BA, Kelly PJ, Goerss SJ: Interactive stereotactic surgical system for the removal of intracranial tumors utilizing the CO_2 laser and CT derived data base. IEEE Trans Biomed Eng BME-32:112, 1985
10. Kelly PJ, Kall BA, Goerss SJ, et al: Computer-assisted stereotactic laser resection of intra-axial brain neoplasms. J Neurosurg 64:427, 1986
11. Kelly PJ, Alker GJ Jr: A method for stereotactic laser microsurgery in the treatment of deep-seated CNS neoplasms. Appl Neurophysiol 43:210, 1980
12. Kelly PJ, Alker GJ Jr: A stereotactic approach to deep-seated central nervous system neoplasms using the carbon dioxide laser. Surg Neurol 15:331, 1981
13. Kelly PJ, Kall BA, Goerss SJ, et al: Precision resection of intra-axial CNS lesions by CT-based stereotactic craniotomy and computer-monitored CO_2 laser. Acta Neurochirurg 68:1, 1983
14. Kelly PJ, Kall BA, Goerss SJ: Computer-assisted stereotactic resection of posterior fossa lesions. Surg Neurol 25:530, 1986
15. Szikla G, Bouvier G, Hori T, et al: Three-dimensional angiography for stereotactic localization of normal and pathological cortical structures. Presented at the meeting of the European Society of Stereotactic and Functional Neurosurgery, Paris, 1979
16. Gehan EA, Walker MD: Prognostic factors for patients with brain tumors. Natl Cancer Inst Monog 46:189, 1977
17. Hitchcock E, Sato F: Treatment of malignant gliomata. J Neurosurg 21:497, 1964
18. Jelsma R, Bucy PC: The treatment of glioblastoma multiforme of the brain. J Neurosurg 27:388, 1967
19. Jelsma R, Bucy PC: Glioblastoma multiforme: Its treatment and some factors effecting survival. Arch Neurol 20:161, 1969
20. Salcman M: Survival in glioblastoma: Historical Perspective. Neurosurgery 7:435, 1980
21. Walker M, Green SB, Byar DP, et al: Randomized comparisons of radiotherapy and nitrosoureas for the treatment of malignant glioma after surgery. N Engl J Med 303:1323, 1980
22. Hoshino T, Barker M, Wilson CB, et al: Cell kinetics of human gliomas. J Neurosurg 37:15, 1972
23. Burger PC, DuBois PJ, Schold SC, et al: Computerized tomographic and pathologic studies of the untreated, quiescent, and recurrent glioblastoma multiforme. J Neurosurg 58:159, 1983
24. Daumas-Duport C, Monsaingeon V, Szenthe L, et al: Serial stereotactic biopsies: A double histological code of gliomas according to malignancy and 3-D configuration, as an aid to therapeutic decision and assessment of results. Appl Neurophysiol 45:431, 1982
25. Kelly PJ, Daumas-Duport C, Kispert DB, et al: Imaging based stereotactic serial biopsies in untreated intracranial glial neoplasms. J Neurosurg (in press)
26. Haar F, Patterson RH Jr: Surgery for metastatic intracranial neoplasm. Cancer 30:1241, 1972
27. MacGee EE: Surgical treatment of cerebral metastases from lung cancer: The effect on quality and duration of survival. J Neurosurg 35:416, 1971
28. Kelly PJ, Alker GJ Jr, Zoll JG: A microstereotactic approach to deep-seated arteriovenous malformations. Surg Neurol 17:260, 1982

Stereotactic Biopsy and Implantation of Radionuclides Guided by Computed Tomography or Magnetic Resonance Imaging for Therapy of Brain Tumors

F. Mundinger

THE EFFECT of curietherapy or brachycurietherapy* of intracranial tumors by direct interstitial or intracavitary implantation of radioactive isotopes was first demonstrated in the early 1950s in tumors or cysts. In some cases the effect was found to be curative.[1–55]

This form of therapy requires a stereotactic operation in which the stereotactic device is attached to the patient's head, a biopsy specimen of the tumor is obtained, and, if indicated, a radioactive isotope is implanted into the tumor or cyst.

STEREOTACTIC INSTRUMENTS

When a stereotactic operative procedure is used on the central nervous system, the intention is to make small, sharply circumscribed lesions with sparing of the surrounding brain tissue in the subcortical structures, the nuclei of the brain stem, the basal ganglia, or the pain tracts.

The use of guided probes in subcortical structures dates back to the second half of the 19th century, when a guiding device was used in Ludwig's laboratory to reach the medulla oblongata.[56] In 1908, Horsley and Clarke[57] devised their stereotactic apparatus to study the deep cerebellar nuclei in experimental animals.

The types of apparatus used in humans are modeled after Clarke's[58] and are available in several forms:

1. The Horsley-Clarke apparatus[57] consists of two parts, a quadrangular or ring-shaped head-holder in which the head is fixed in a plane, and a frame on the head-holder on which a movable electrode or cannula holder can be mounted. In the first of these models movement of the electrode was possible in only one direction, whereas in later models modifications allowed inclination of the electrode in the sagittal plane. Most instruments for use in humans employ this basic principle.

2. The equatorial apparatus consists of a head-holder that is built in a ring. In the plane of the head-holder there is a second shallow disc, which is movable through 360 degrees. Fastened to this disc is a semicircular arc that moves over the head. The electrode-holder is attached to the semicircular arc and can be inclined in various angles independent of the position of the circular base. This principle is used in the Todd-Wells and Gianciulli-Mosso instruments and allows placement of a cannula at any angle anywhere within the dimensions of the enclosed space.

Spiegel and Wycis pioneered the use of stereotactic surgery in humans when they modified the Horsley-Clarke device and undertook a series of psychosurgical stereotactic procedures (1947 and 1949) (Figure 43-1). Spiegel and Wycis subsequently developed 17 models of this stereotactic device, three of which have been in use. In their third model (1951, 1952), the basal frame, a rectangular frame, is held to the head with four supports. A right-angled tubular frame is screwed to the basal frame and the electrode carrier can then be fastened above, behind, or to the side as desired.[59] Uchimura and Narabayashi[60] built and reported their use of a simplified Spiegel-Wycis apparatus.

Talairach and his coworkers[61] developed a stereotactic apparatus (Figure 43-2) in which the right-angled basal frame is fixed to the skull with four conical removable graduated cutting burrs. These are set into previously made corresponding trephine openings in the external table of the skull. The perforations in the skull permit the apparatus to be repeatedly replaced in the same position if necessary. The apparatus can also be firmly fixed to the operating table. The procedure using this device is carried out in two stages. In the first stage, roentgenographic studies are made in two planes using an attached frame from a distance of 4 m to reduce divergence to a minimum. The central x-ray beam is directed parallel to the horizontal plane and perpendicular onto the sagittal plane of the skull or the

---

*The term *brachytherapy* in the English literature means "therapy at short range." This is incorrect etymologic usage, since the ancient Greek adjective *brachy* in combination with a noun is used to characterize lapses of time, in the sense of "short-term therapy." We therefore proposed the alternative term *curietherapy* to define "low dose rate interstitial irradiation with radioisotopes" when the implant is permanent and the term *brachycurietherapy* for "interstitial afterloading techniques with high dose rates."

OPERATIVE NEUROSURGICAL TECHNIQUES
ISBN 0-8089-1862-1

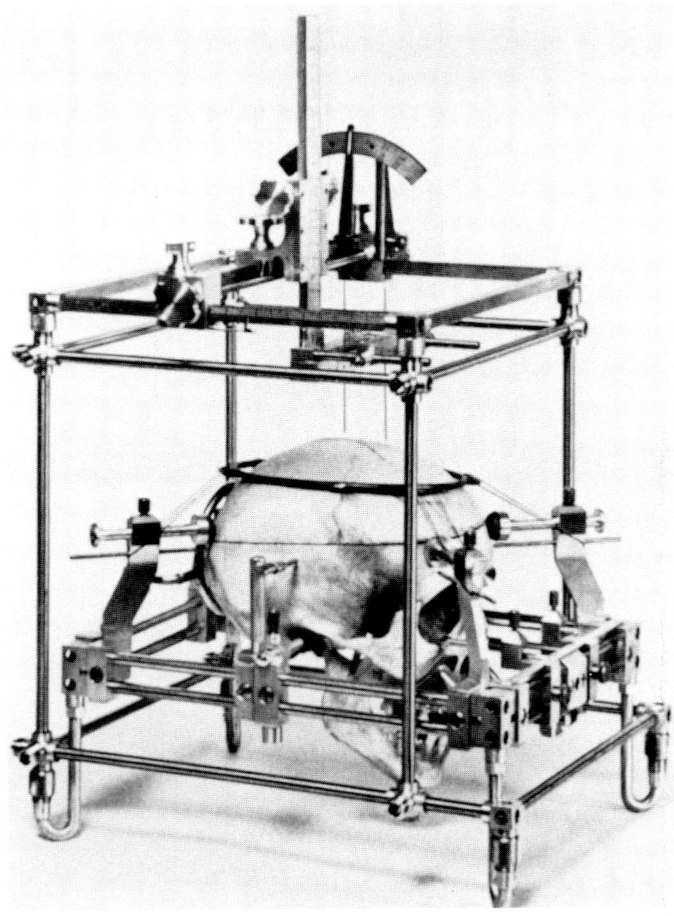

Fig. 43-1. A model 3 stereoencephalotome. (Reprinted from Spiegel EA, Wycis HT: Stereoencephalotomy, Part I. New York, Grune & Stratton, 1952. With permission.)

apparatus and the axis of the central radiation beam is focused on the center of the grid. These adjustments are obtained through a two-part sighting-system and transparent double-grid plates with perforations at 1-mm intervals, which must be superimposed. The double grids serve as an indicator of the exact centering and for carrying the electrodes and cannulas. The localization of the target results from visualization of specific landmarks, such as those associated with the ventricles.

In the second stage the electrodes or cannulas are introduced using the double grids photographed on the roentgenograms. One determines on the lateral film to which perforation of the sagittal grid the target coincides. The graduated electrode passing through the appropriate perforation must intersect the target, the depth at which it reaches the target being determined on the AP film. With a stereometer the actual placement of the electrode can be pretested on a phantom to roentgenologically ascertained points.

In Leksell's stereotactic apparatus,[62] the axis of a semicircular bow is brought into the axis of the roentgen beam, which runs through the target point (Figure 43-3). The middle point of the bow axis is adjusted to coincide with the target. A smaller inner frame is fastened to the head, the target is established, and a relationship between this point and the transverse and horizontal axes determined. A trephine opening is then made, and the outer semicircular bow is adjusted in the axis of the central radiation beam in such a way that the target point corresponds with the midpoint of the axis of the bow. The electrode, which is carried by a movable electrode holder in the circuit of the bow, is then advanced toward the target, which is in the midpoint of the axis of the bow.

Other types of stereotactic apparatuses are usually variations of the Horsley-Clarke device adapted for use on humans. For example, Lorimer, Segal, and Stein[63] described an apparatus of plastic material with a semicircular bow, the calibration of

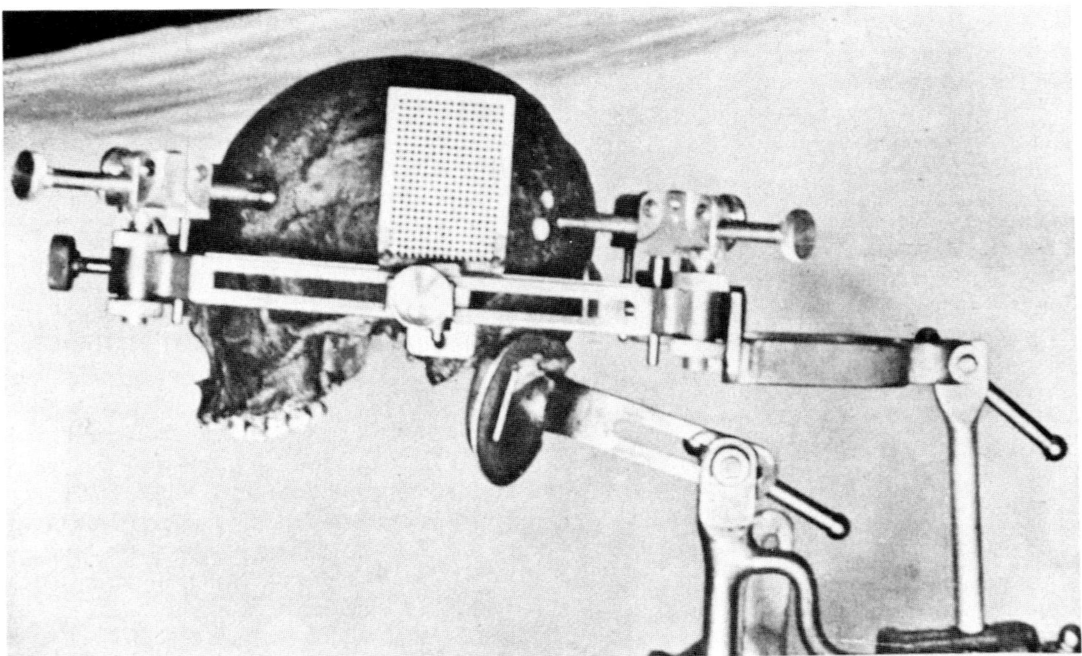

Fig. 43-2. The stereotactic apparatus of Talairach and collaborators. (Reprinted from Talairach J, Hecaen H, David A, et al: Recherces sur la coagulation therapeutique des structures soucorticales chez l'homme. J Rev Neurol 81:4-24, 1959. With permission.)

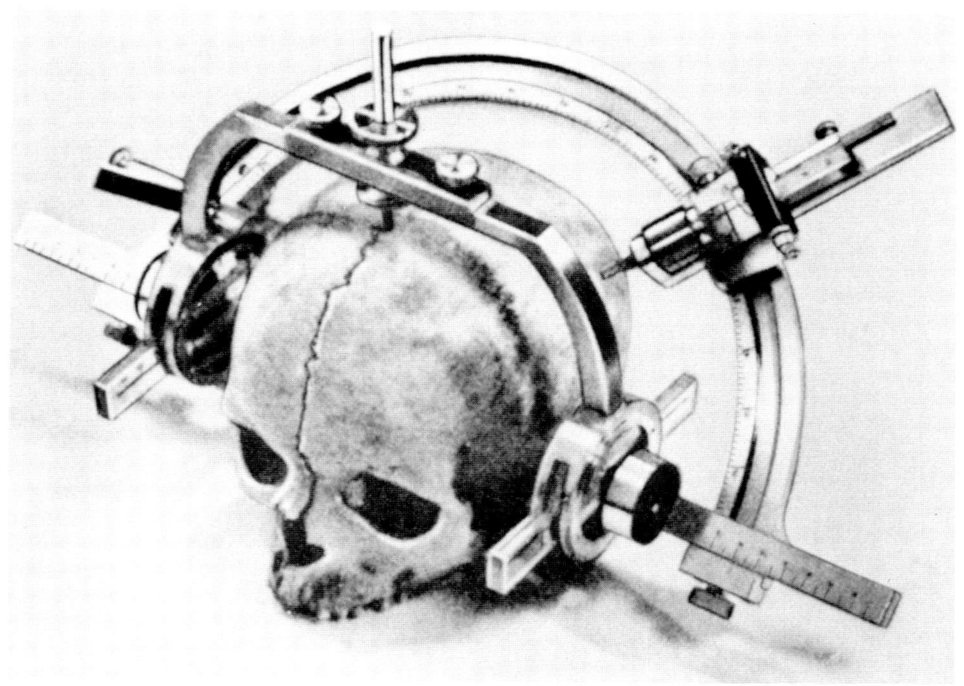

Fig. 43-3. The stereotactic apparatus of Leksell. (Reprinted from Leksell L: A stereotactic apparatus for intracerebral surgery. Acta Chir Scand 99:229-233, 1949. With permission.)

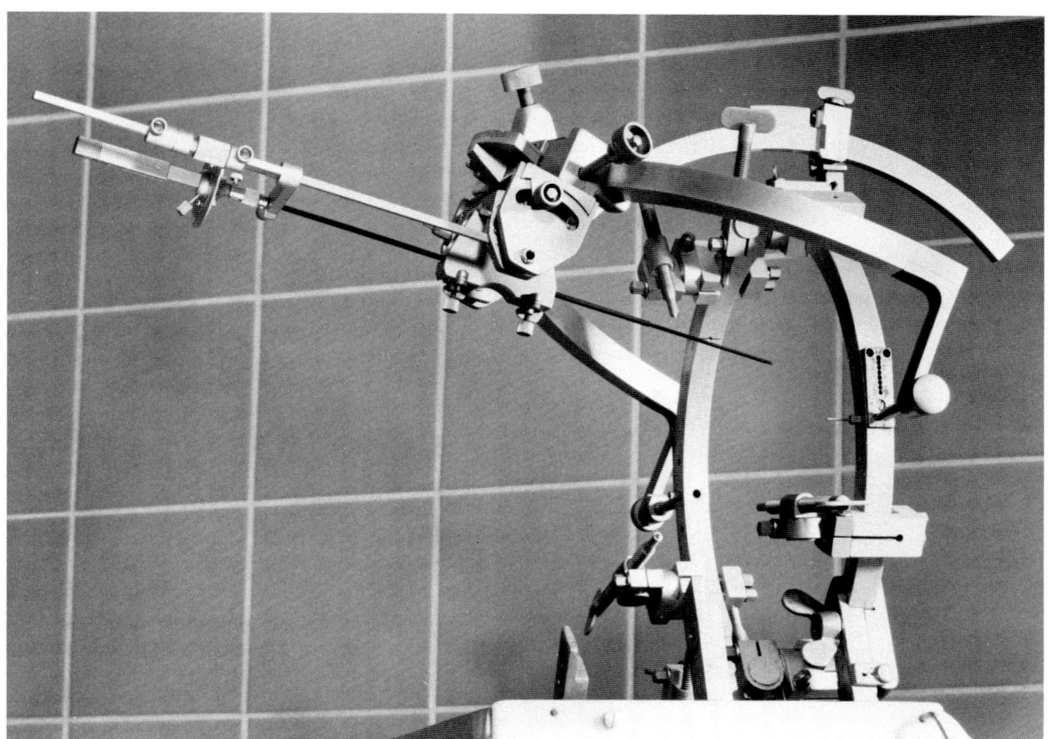

Fig. 43-4. With the Mundinger-Birg CT-, MRI-, and computer-compatible version of the stereotactic system of Riechert and Mundinger any target within the brain can be reached from any site on the face or skull. The mechanical accuracy is $\pm$ 0.1 mm. The base ring is fixed to the patient's skull and is unmovable. The ring is attached to a U-shaped holder, which can be fixed anywhere. The target arc with the electrode holder can be attached to the patient's skull in 16 different positions. The electrode or probe position can be checked radiographically since the brain and skull structures are not covered by any parts of the device. For x-ray control, long x-ray distances are desirable but not necessary since even an image converter can be used for the x-ray technique. The device does not need to be used in a special room; because of its flexibility it can be used in any operating room or x-ray suite.

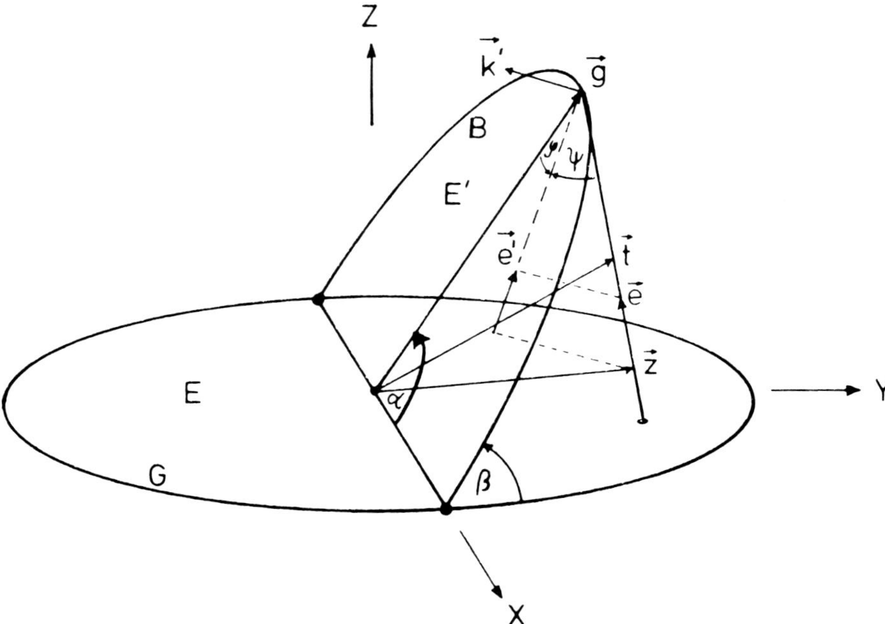

Fig. 43-5. This stereotactic system works according to the polar coordinate principle. Plane E is the plane of the base ring, plane E′ is the effective plane of the target arc. The trephination point is indicated by a t, the target by a z. The position of the target arc is determined by angle β, that of the electrode holder by angle α. The direction of the electrode is indicated by the two polar coordinate angles φ and σ. The needle depth corresponds to the distance g1 − Z, marked with NT (Nadeltiefe). The details of the mathematical deduction of the five seating parameters, α, β, φ, σ, and NT, will not be given here. They are described elsewhere. The final formulae for the determination of the parameters are as follows:

$$\alpha = \text{Arctan (W2/gx)}$$
$$\beta = \text{Arctan (gz/gy)}$$
$$\sigma = \text{Arctan (W1/sqr (w2-w2} - \text{w1-w1)}$$
$$\phi = \text{Arctan (sqr (1} - \text{w1-w1/w2-w2} - \text{ex-ex)/ex)} - \alpha \text{ (if ex = 0)}$$
$$\phi = \text{PI/2} - \text{Alpha (if ex = 0)}$$
$$\text{NT} = 312.5 - \text{L1}$$

The abbreviations are:

$$t = \text{(tx,ty,tz), the trephination point}$$
$$z = \text{(zx,zy,zz), the target point}$$
$$r = \text{radius of the target arc}$$
$$\text{L1} = \text{sqr ((t} - \text{z)*(t} - \text{z))}$$
$$\text{ex} = \text{(tx} - \text{zx)/l1}$$
$$\text{ey} = \text{(ty} - \text{zy)/l1}$$
$$\text{ez} = \text{(tz} - \text{zz)/l1}$$
$$1 = - \text{(z-e)} + \text{sqr ((z*e)*(z*e)} - \text{z*z} + \text{r:r)}$$
$$\text{gx} = \text{zx} + 1 * \text{ex}$$
$$\text{gy} = \text{zy} + 1 * \text{ey}$$
$$\text{gz} = \text{zz} + 1 * \text{ez}$$
$$\text{W1} = \text{ey*gz} - \text{ez*gy}$$
$$\text{W2} = \text{sqr (gy*gy} + \text{gz*gz)}$$

The advantage of the mathematical calculation is that sterility problems resulting from the transfer procedure can be avoided. Moreover, this method is not time-consuming. Above all, in cases in which it is only necessary to aim at one or a few targets, it is much more favorable to determine the new setting with the computer than with a phantom. Cases in which an exact predetermination of the trephination point is needed as well as cases of CT and MRI stereotaxy require computer calculation.

which was checked on cadaver specimens, although no data concerning its use on patients has been published. Mark, MacPherson, and Sweet[64] designed a ring-shaped frame as a base, to which the arrangements for holding and moving the operative instruments are attached. The correction for the roentgen deviations they take up with two scales and constant focus-plate distance. The target is localized graphically on an index card.

Hayne and Meyers[65] constructed an apparatus related to the midsagittal, interaural, and Reid basal line in the form of a rectangular "understructure" with an attached double rectangular bridge and a needle-holder. Hayne, Belinson, and Gibbs[66] used a modified Horsley-Clark apparatus. Wada[67] developed a very sturdy apparatus weighing 40 kg based on the Horsley-Clarke model.

There are other models, which are mostly modifications or combinations of the above two principle types of apparatus, including those of Hitchcock,[68] Laitinen,[69] Kelly,[70,71] and others. These and the previously described devices allow a target to be hit with a very high degree of accuracy, especially when used in conjunction with CT or MRI imaging.

The Riechert-Mundinger universal apparatus[33,72–75] is adapted for CT- and MRI-guided operations (Mundinger-Birg[76–84]) (Figures 43-4 through 43-13).* This stereotactic apparatus can be utilized for all known clinical situations in which this type of approach is required (Figure 43-7). Moreover, this device allows approaches through the facial part of the skull for biopsy or implantation of isotopes, for example, transnasally for hypophysectomy, transbuccally for clival disorders, and transorbitally for retro-orbital pathologic processes or for pathologic processes in the region of the facial part of the skull. In addition, using the transcerebellar approach, the cerebellum, cerebellopontine angle, and the brain stem can be reached (Figure 43-8). Using the ventral or dorsal and lateral-cervical approach, structures in the neck, the cervical vertebral column, and the cervical spinal cord can be reached (Table 43-1).

STEREOTACTIC BIOPSY OF INTRACRANIAL LESIONS

Every unverified, progressive intracranial lesion should be histologically studied to determine its pathologic nature. This rule applies irrespective of its location and whether or not the process is solitary or multiple, since this information is essential for planning rational treatment. A stereotactic approach is used except when an open exploratory operation is primarily indicated, during which an adequate biopsy can be performed. A biopsy of such CNS lesions must be carried out even when modern CT or MRI imaging offers improved diagnosis, since CT and MRI do not offer the accuracy of a histologically verified diagnosis.[85]

Stereotactic biopsy is the method of choice in many of these situations since it can be performed at low risk, tissue can be obtained with a precision of 1 mm from foci 3 mm in diameter, pathologic tissue can be histologically compared with surrounding tissue, and treatment can be decided upon immediately.[30] This means, for example, that in cases of inflammatory, hemorrhagic, or necrotic foci or systemic diseases appropriate medical treatment can be initiated, in cases such as localized low grade astrocytoma of the brain stem, pons, or basal ganglia, interstitial curietherapy can be initiated immediately, or, in cases in which there is a cyst, a catheter can be placed for drainage of the cyst or intracystic irradiation can be implanted. In the case of a nonresectable tumor, e.g., a malignant glioma, the tumor grade can be established intraoperatively and a decision made whether a combination of curietherapy or brachycurietherapy with percutaneous irradiation or percutaneous irradiation in combination with chemotherapy is indicated.

One of the advantages of the stereotactic method is that the focus to be punctured can be reached exactly, to the nearest millimeter, using a thin needle or a biopsy probe.[24,26,70,78,79,83,84,86–89] With our stereotactic device any intracranial, intracerebral, or intracerebellar point can be punctured from any point on the surface of the skull, thereby avoiding functionally important areas and larger vessels.

The biopsy specimens are taken beginning in healthy

---

*Manufacturer: F. L. Fischer MET D-78 Freiburg, West Germany.

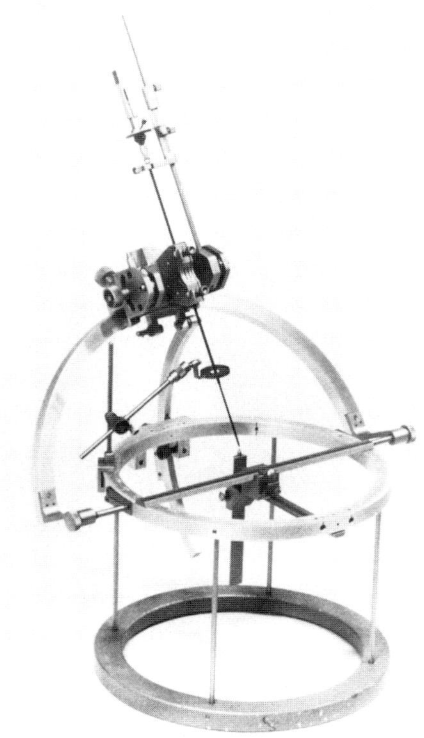

Fig. 43-6. Determination of parameters can also be carried out without mathematical calculations by means of the phantom device. A ring marking the burr hole is set to the planned trephination point on the patient's head, using a holder which is fixed to the base ring. In the same position, it is transferred to the base ring of the phantom device. Subsequently, the target marker of the phantom device is set to the target point by means of a holder that is movable in three axes. The target arc is then empirically adjusted in such a way that the introduced electrode precisely hits the predetermined target point via the phantom burr hole. The angles and needle depths thus obtained are documented and the target arc with preset target parameters is transferred to the base ring attached to the patient's head. The target point can thus be reached even without previous calculation.

tissue, then through the pathologic tissue and into reactively changed or healthy tissue on the other side of the lesion. A morphologic profile of the lesion can thus be provided. This procedure has a further advantage in that it includes the infiltration zone of tumors. Stereotactic biopsy, particularly of multiple foci, was made more simple and more reliable by computer stereotaxy as developed in the 1970s with Birg, using a modification of the stereotactic device of Riechert and Mundinger.[76–79,82–84] This technique has been further improved by its combination with computed tomography (CT) and magnetic resonance imaging (MRI).[3,4,43,70,71,89–93]

The stereotactic biopsy procedure is generally performed under local anesthesia. General anesthesia is used only in the transcerebellar approach and in children under 6 years of age. There are three possibilities of combining CT, MRI, and stereotaxy: the indirect method, the direct method, and the "ex-post" method.

In the indirect method, the position of the stereotactic device in relation to the CT sections is determined by means of wire or synthetic glass structures scanned simultaneously. This method is recommended if the size of the stereotactic device is larger than the gantry of the CT scanner or if the spatial

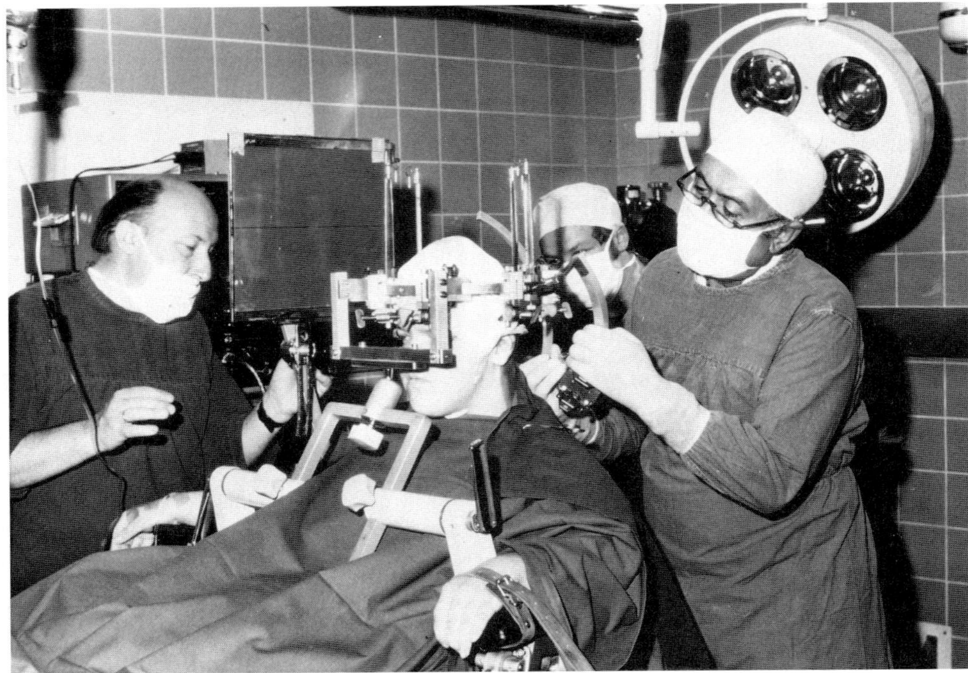

Fig. 43-7. A CT-guided stereotactic biopsy and nuclide implantation with a transcerebellar approach to a brain stem glioma. The patient is in a half-sitting position. The stereotactic ring is attached to the operating table by means of supports. The semicircular target bow with the holding device for the probes is being attached. (The intervention can also be carried out in a prone position).

synchronization of the two coordinate systems cannot be achieved for other reasons.

With the direct method, the CT or MRI scans are produced while the stereotactic device is attached to the patient's head. After the correct adjustment of both systems, the target coordinates can be measured directly.

With the "ex-post" method, the projected CT or MRI sections scaled according to their x-ray distortion are plotted onto a transparent sheet and the images are then transposed to the corresponding roentgenograms, either manually or by a computer program. Thus, the shape of the tumor, the ventricles, or other brain structures taken from the CT or MRI

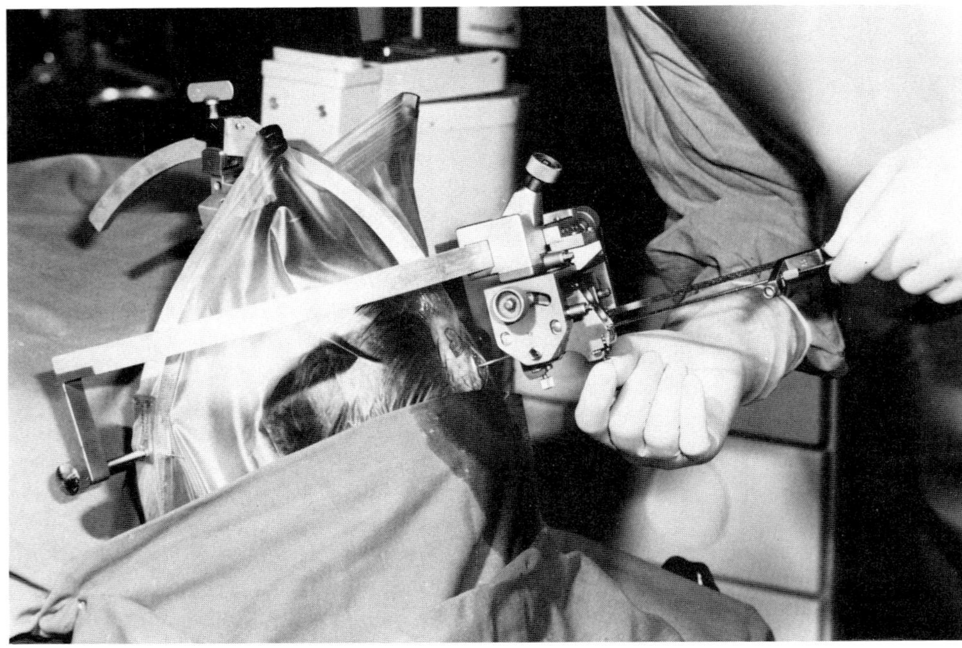

Fig. 43-8. Example of a transfrontal approach with the patient in the dorsal position. The semicircular target bow with the holder for the probes is attached to the base ring in the previously calculated position. The four angles are set. The combination cannula for the biopsy and nuclide implantation is being inserted into the encephalon.

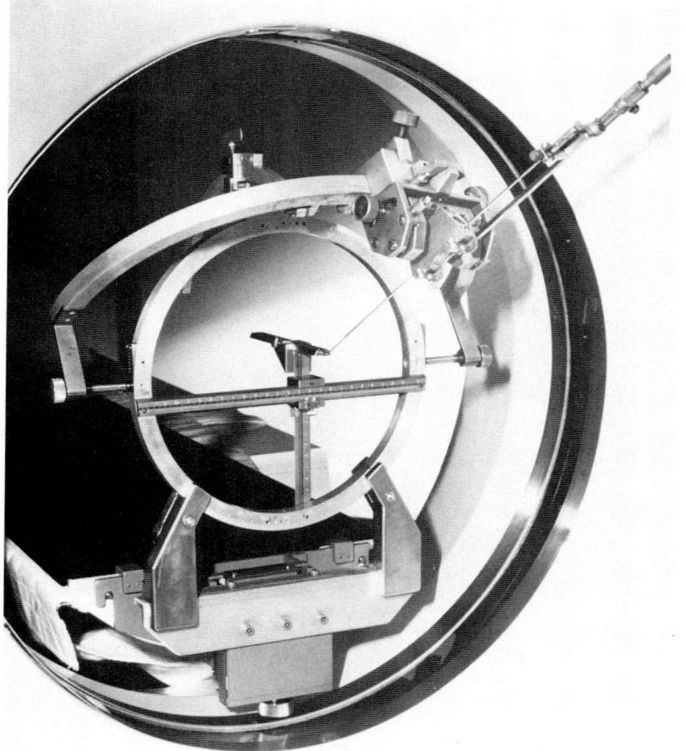

Fig. 43-9. For CT-guided stereotactic procedures a holder is attached to the bed of the CT scanner to fix the stereotactic device so that the base ring of the device, which is attached to the skull either in a high cranial or low basal position, can be adjusted in the center of the CT gantry in a precise orthograde way. For obtaining a CT scan with the device fixed as described above, the same x and y coordinates apply to both the stereotactic device and the CT scan. Biopsy or tumor implantation coordinates can thus be determined on the CT scans and calculated with the software of the CT device. The corresponding coordinates can subsequently be put in the computer in order to calculate the setting parameters. It is also possible to choose the trephination point and hence the approach angle for the probe directly on the CT monitor. All parameters required for the operation thus are determined immediately after the CT examination. For optimum documentation purposes and for the comparison with the surgical x-ray films, the target and trephination points taken from the CT scans are additionally transposed to the corresponding stereotactic x-ray films.

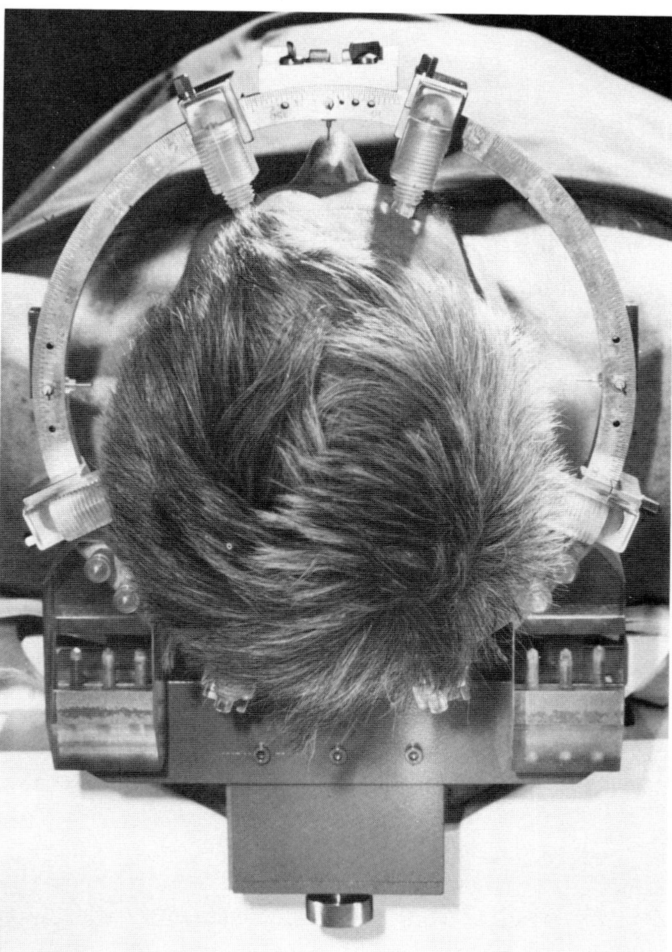

Fig. 43-10. For CT- or MRI-guided stereotactic procedures, the ring can be fixed to the examination devices in an orthograde position by means of an adapted holder, so that coordinate calculations are unnecessary. The stereotactic coordinates can be taken directly from the CT or MRI images.

sections coincide automatically with the corresponding structures shown on the x-ray films.

The direct method is the most exact but requires that the patient be scanned with the stereotactic base ring attached to his or her head. In this case, any stereotactic device can be used; however, the base ring or polygonal frame of the device must fit into the CT scanner or MRI gantry and it must be adjustable so that the origin of the device coincides exactly with the center of the CT scanner or the center of the magnetic field.

During the scanning process, none or only few artifacts can be allowed to originate from the surgical site and we therefore use a Riechert-Mundinger stereotactic device[33,73–75] in a computer compatible version of the Mundinger-Birg apparatus[25,26,76–84] (Figures 43-8 through 43-13). With this instrument the base ring is fixed to the patient's head by acrylic screws, which produce few artifacts on the x-ray films or magnetic field (Figure 43-10).

Metal holders and screws can be used in a CT scanner if the base ring is fixed to the skull at such a level that the area to be scanned is either above or below the ring. For MRI stereotaxy, nonmagnetic alloys or synthetic materials are obligatory for the base ring (Figure 43-14). The targeting procedure is shown in Figures 43-11 through 43-15.

The procedure is performed in the operating room using a 2.5-cm incision. A burr hole 6 mm in diameter is made in the direction of the first target point, the dura is coagulated, and the outer cannula of the biopsy probe or implantation probe is directed incrementally to the target point (Figures 43-16, 43-17, and 43-18).

The first biopsy specimens are taken before the tumor surface is reached, mainly from the zone of perifocal edema or reactive gliosis. The next biopsy specimens are taken at distances of 1 mm or 2 mm, sometimes through the target and to the opposite side of the lesion into the perifocal tissue. Anywhere from 5 to 20 samples are submitted to the neuropathologist for paraffin embedding and special staining.[68,86,94,95] Smear preparations of other specimens are prepared, stained with methylene blue, and examined immediately. In our series there is a 95 percent correlation between the results of the smear preparations and those of the permanent sections.[94,95]

The classification and grading of tumors can readily be established from the smear preparations. This makes it possible to decide immediately on further therapeutic procedures. The

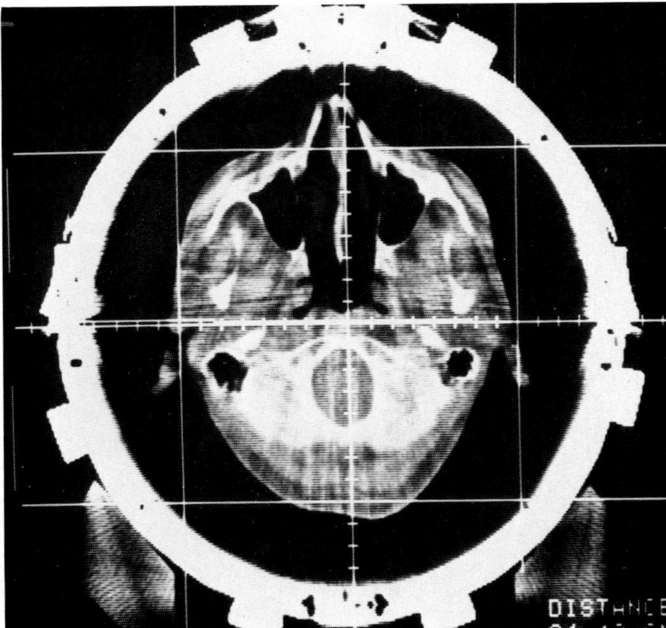

Fig. 43-11. A stereotactic operation showing the following: After the stereotactic ring is fixed to the patient's head, the patient is laid on the CT table and the stereotactic base ring is fixed to the adjustable holder (see Figure 43-10). The coordinates of the stereotactic base ring are adjusted to coincide with the coordinates of the CT gantry. The zero-plane of the base ring is thus in coincidence with the zero-plane of the CT gantry.

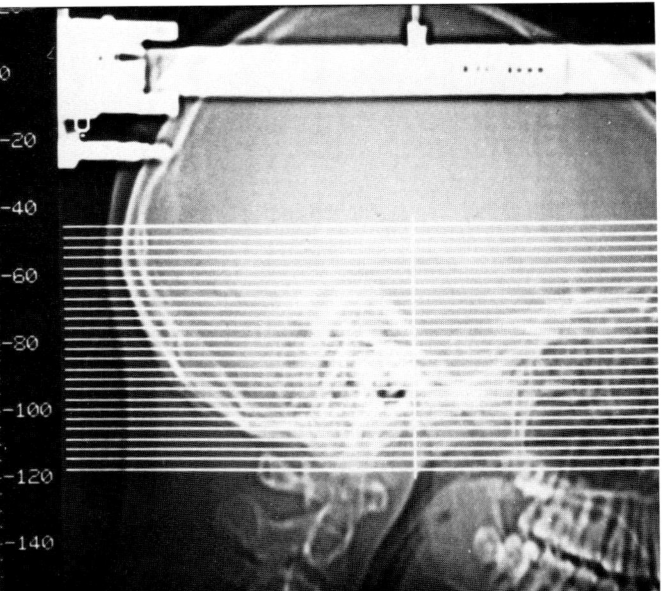

Fig. 43-12. CT-guided stereotaxy. By means of the scout-view feature of the CT scanner the levels of the CT cuts are selected. The zero point of the ring is in coincidence with that of the CT system and the scan planes must be parallel to the ring plane.

confirmation of the tumor's extent and infiltration enables us to correct the dosimetry if necessary.

Stereotactic biopsy is done in the peripheral areas of a lesion in the case of a recurrent tumor or where progressive growth of the focus has been established on the CT or MRI scans following a previous operation, interstitial radiotherapy, or percutaneous irradiation, in order to examine the residual tumor after operation or parts of a recurrent tumor, as well as to distinguish viable tumor and radiation necrosis. Multiple biopsy specimens can be obtained through a small burr hole (6 mm in diameter) using various approach angles calculated by computer. For lesions in both hemispheres, bilateral burr holes may be necessary.

CLINICAL RESULTS OF BIOPSY

Since 1952, our group has performed over 3238 stereotactic biopsies, 1407 of these between January, 1981, and April 30, 1987 being CT-guided stereotactic interventions (Table 43-2). In most cases, a CT-guided stereotactic biopsy was performed in order to categorize the nature of a tumor and to administer curietherapy or brachycurietherapy or to demarcate inflammations, abscesses, necroses, hemorrhage, or infarcts.

Review of the biopsy results obtained from 600 patients produced the following results.[94,95] Combined smear preparations and paraffin-embedded samples revealed the tumor type and grade in 492 (82 percent) cases; in 66 (11 percent) cases a clinically suspected neoplasm was ruled out; in 42 (7 percent) cases a tumor was confirmed but the samples did not allow its classification.

CONSECUTIVE PROCEDURES AFTER BIOPSY

Since the nature of the biopsied lesion can usually be established intraoperatively, one can decide whether curietherapy should be started immediately after the biopsy procedure during the same operation or whether the lesion should be resected by open operation. A stereotactic biopsy does not limit subsequent microsurgical resection of benign tumors such as intraventricular tumors, ependymomas, meningiomas, or teratomas, and possessing the histologic diagnosis is often of advantage in planning the open surgical procedure. The same rules apply to anaplastic gliomas, which, as a result of their size and localization, are not appropriate for either direct operative intervention or curietherapy. They also apply to patients in poor general condition or of advanced age who cannot be further burdened with an operation. In these cases, having the results of a biopsy facilitates the decision of whether further operative intervention is advisable. Percutaneous irradiation of malignant tumors is carried out after a diagnosis of benign cyst, necrosis, low-grade glioma, or inflammatory foci has been excluded.

Abscesses, cysts, and hemorrhages (Figures 43-19 and 43-20) are punctured immediately after the biopsy and, if necessary, drained through stereotactically implanted catheters[32,96] (Figure 43-21). Inflammatory diseases are diagnosed and then treated medically. Aneurysms and vascular lesions are an obvious contraindication to this procedure and are a reason why angiography is absolutely indispensable before a stereotactic biopsy is performed. In the case of cystic tumors such as astrocytomas, glioblastomas, and craniopharyngiomas, interstitial or intracavitary radiation intervention is used after drainage of the lesion through a catheter. In the case of cystic craniopharyngiomas the catheter is directed in such a way that it drains the contents of the cyst through the ventricular system. The catheter is connected to a Rickham reservoir, which is fixed into the trephination point so that the reservoir subsequently can be percutaneously aspirated and thus the cyst

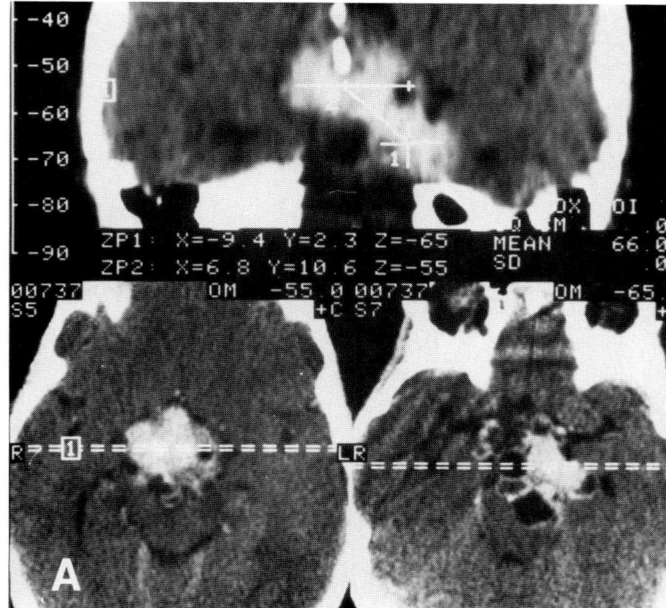

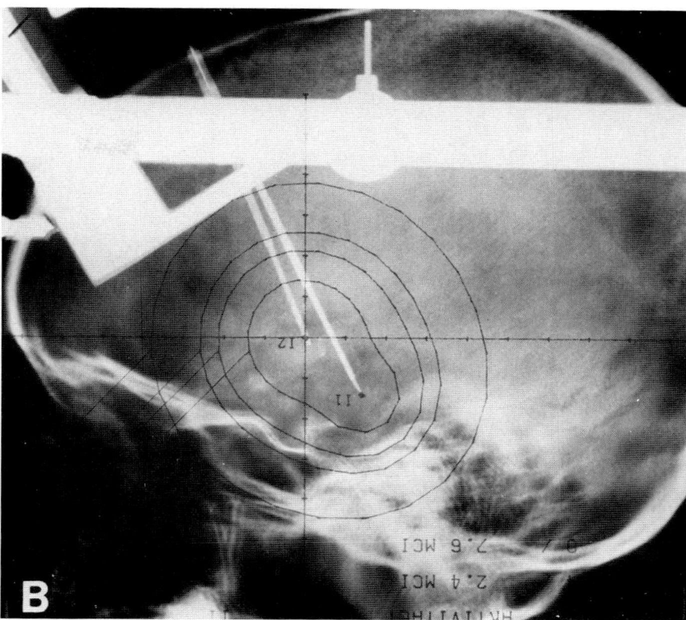

Fig. 43-13. A 13-year-old patient with a pilocytic astrocytoma (WHO I) of the diencephalon. CT-guided stereotactic biopsy and curietherapy with iodine 125. (A) An oblique CT section through the space-occupying diencephalic process, which with enhancement is clearly demarcated. Determination of target points 1 and 2 for implantation of ^{125}I seeds following volumetric determination of the suspected tumor. The coordinates for target points 1 and 2 have been plotted. (B) Implantation cannula in the corresponding target points. The ^{125}I seeds are implanted. The inner ring indicates the peripheral tumor dosage (= 100 Gy).

repeatedly emptied if necessary. If an obstructive hydrocephalus is present because of obstruction of the third ventricle or the sylvian aqueduct, an additional ventricular catheter is stereotactically introduced either unilaterally or bilaterally after the instillation of the isotope into the tumor cyst. The ventricular catheter can subsequently be converted into a ventriculoatrial or ventriculoperitoneal shunt.

CURIETHERAPY AND BRACHYCURIETHERAPY

The CT-guided stereotactic biopsy and interstitial or intracavitary curietherapy or brachycurietherapy for intracranial processes or skull base lesions are principally neurosurgical operations carried out in collaboration with a radiotherapist. There are two kinds of local irradiation (see Table 43-1):

Table 43-1. Stereotactic operations performed at University Hospital, Freiburg, West Germany, between 1950 and April 30, 1987

Indication	Number of Procedures
Parkinsonism	3932
Hyperkinesia	1380
Curietherapy	1831
Biopsy since 1965	1407
Intractable pain	437
Psychiatry	174
Epilepsy	111
Angioma	22
Combined stereotactic/open pituitary surgery	107
Miscellaneous	543
Total	9944

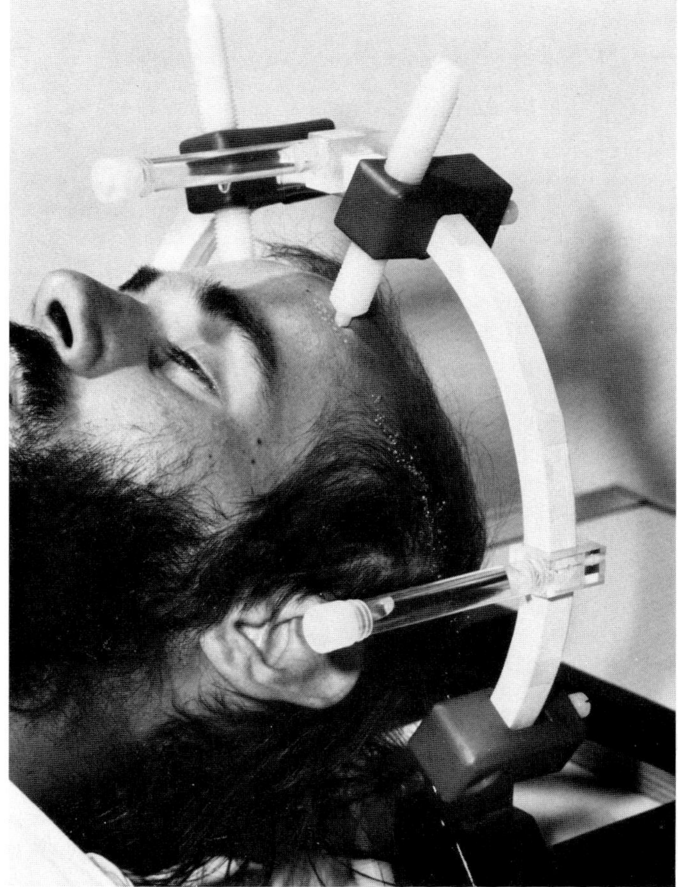

Fig. 43-14. For magnetic resonance imaging (MRI), the base ring must be modified. The metal alloy of the stereotactic apparatus is replaced by plastic, since any metal parts in the examination area of the MRI scanner produce strong artifacts. In order to precisely localize the plastic base ring, it is provided with a concentrically arranged reservoir on the inside filled with a paramagnetic liquid. This produces light projection spots on the sagittal and coronal images; their communication lines mark the corresponding coordinate axes.

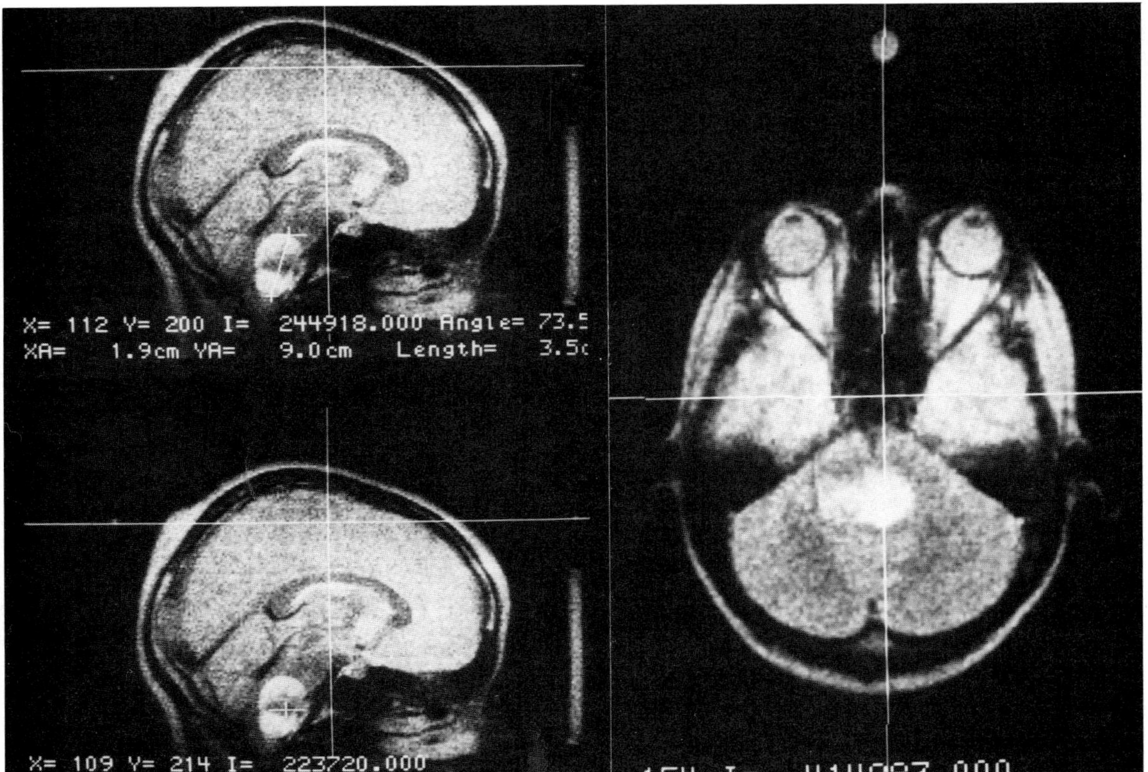

Fig. 43-15. As with CT scans, coordinates can be taken directly from the MRI scans which correspond to those of the stereotactic device. Any indirect determination of the coordinates is hence unnecessary. The operator takes the required target and trephination coordinates directly from the MRI monitor and can then calculate in the coordinate system of the stereotactic device the PE and implantation structures to be treated. The accuracy range is approximately ± 0.6 mm.

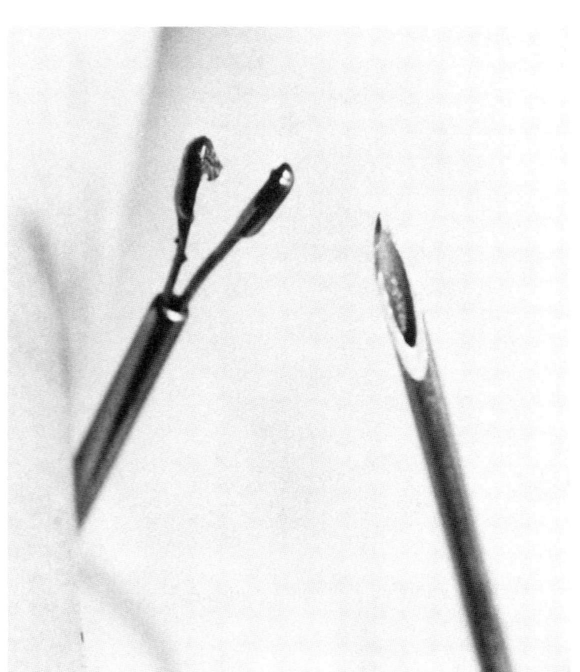

Fig. 43-16. The biopsy cannula has a diameter of 1 mm, the two clamps 0.4 mm each. The samples to be taken are 3 mm^3 in size.

1. Brachycurietherapy using an emitter with high curie activity inserted into the tumor for a short time, giving the tumor a dose of radiation within minutes or a few days.
2. Curietherapy, involving the permanent implantation of a radioactive emitter which irradiates the tumor over a period of a few days to months while it spontaneously decays.

The radiobiologic differences between high dose rate brachycurietherapy using an after-loading contact irradiation device with ^{192}Ir (GammaMed),[97] i.e., with the dose administered within minutes, and temporary implantation over a period of several days are only minor because the tumor necrosis is replaced by a glial scar or cyst.

With low-dose curietherapy, especially using ^{192}Ir, perifocal edema is minimal, which means this form of therapy is better tolerated than brachycurietherapy. However, curietherapy is indicated only for certain disorders. There is not enough time for protracted long-term irradiation in cases of anaplastic gliomas or other malignant tumors. In such cases, brachycurietherapy must be used, if necessary in combination with long-term irradiation or percutaneous irradiation (a combination we frequently employ).

The radiopharmaceuticals that are most commonly used are listed along with a description of their physical characteristics in Table 43-3. Because of the various radiation protection laws, some radionuclides are not available in spite of their very favorable physical characteristics and demonstrated clinical success.[17,72,98] I introduced the use of ^{192}Ir for brain tumor therapy in 1959 and the use of ^{125}I seeds in 1979 for very low dose rate long-term irradiation. Iodine 125 seeds can also be

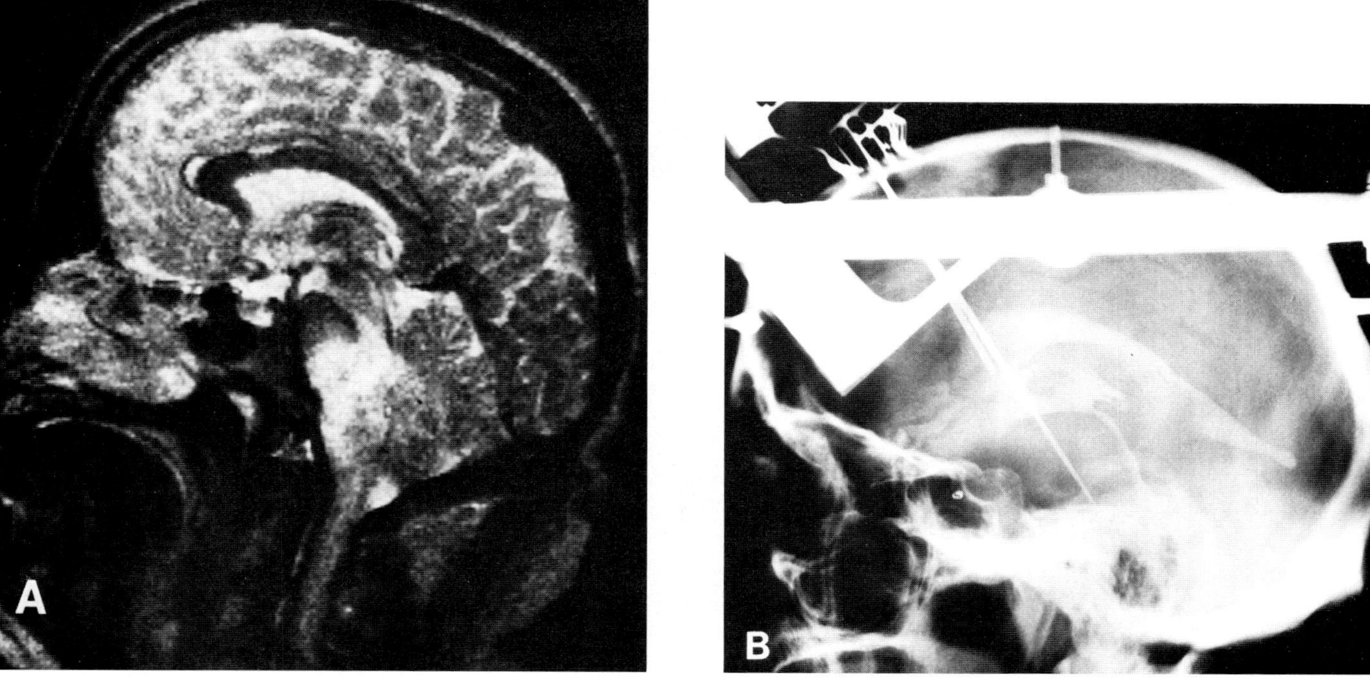

Fig. 43-17. This 48-year-old patient had a fibrillar astrocytoma (WHO II) as confirmed by CT-guided stereotactic biopsy of the brain stem. (A) MRI with a significant T2 weighted signal diffuse in the mid brain stem and pons area. (B) An x-ray film obtained after stereotactic ventriculography (note the cannula in the foramen of Monro). The biopsy cannula is situated in the center of the brain stem focus. For bioptic confirmation, 13 samples were taken at 1-mm intervals.

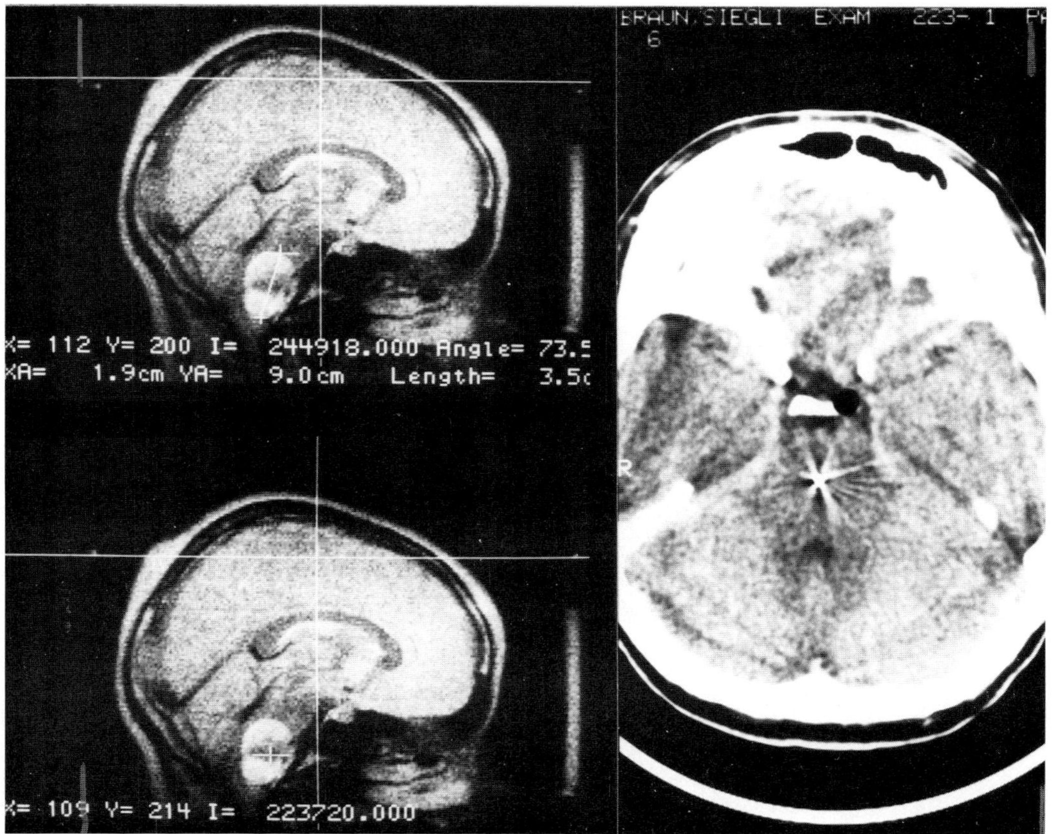

Fig. 43-18. MRI-guided stereotaxy. (Left) Fixation of the MRI ring in the high position. A pear-shaped focus 9 cm in orocaudal diameter is visible with decreased central signal intensity. Coordinate lines are determined by the markings of the ring. The coordinate values show the distance from the point of origin of the coordinate system that coincides with the center of the magnetic field. On the bottom left the target point has been marked with a cross. The biopsy, performed step by step, revealed an astrocytoma (WHO II) with a central cyst. (Right) Control CT scan. The silver wire (artifact) proves that the previously calculated MRI target point has been precisely reached.

Table 43-2. Diagnoses in 928 CT-guided stereotactic biopsies performed between January, 1981 and April 30, 1987

Histologic Finding	Number of Cases
Glial tumors	
Astrocytoma I	177
Astrocytoma II	393
Astrocytoma III	270
Glioblastoma IV	242
Oligodendroglioma	68
Total	1150
Nonglial tumors	
Ependymoma	19
Papilloma	8
Medulloblastoma	6
PNET	39
Meningioma	14
Germinoma	34
Teratoma	11
Epidermoid	6
Craniopharyngioma	55
Colloid cyst	24
Metastases	159
Unclassified tumors	23
Total	398
Nontumorous processes (appearing as tumors on CT and MRI scans)	
Hemorrhage	70
Glioses	111
Abscesses	34
Total	215

distributed in larger volume tumors without any conflict with the radiation protection laws. Restrictions, however, do exist for the use of ^{192}Ir in larger tumors. (In such cases, a combination of ^{192}Ir and ^{125}I or ^{192}Ir after-loading brachycurietherapy is the "way out.") Both ^{192}Ir and ^{125}I are indicated for permanent implantation, which is the method of choice in the treatment of low-grade astrocytomas, brain midline tumors, and tumors at the base of the skull. We have previously reported on the techniques and on our long-term results. In cases of malignant intracranial tumors, brachycurietherapy is indicated.

The decision of which isotopes to use is based on the tumor volume to be irradiated. The variation with which the dosage decreases from the emitter surface must also be taken into consideration. The tumor volume also determines whether one or more radiation sources is to be implanted and where these are to be placed geometrically, so that the dose distribution within the tumor is sufficiently high and as homogeneous as possible.

A first approximation is carried out with the CT or MRI software. Subsequently, the number and locations of the implants and their coordinates are defined, even for geometrically complicated tumor volumes, as well as the activity to be implanted in order to adapt the peripheral tumor isodose lines to the tumor surface. This is done with the help of our interactive dosimetry program system.[99] Other programs have been described by Dyck,[3] Dutreix,[100] Hilaris,[6] Pierquin,[101–103] and others.[104,105]

TECHNIQUES OF PERMANENT IMPLANTATION OF ISOTOPES (CURIETHERAPY)

Where interstitial curietherapy is to be used, the isotope, either ^{125}I or ^{192}Ir, is implanted into the precalculated target points directly after the biopsy procedure and using the same hollow cannula. The seeds are enclosed in a radiation-protected magazine. The magazine is then put into an intermediate piece,

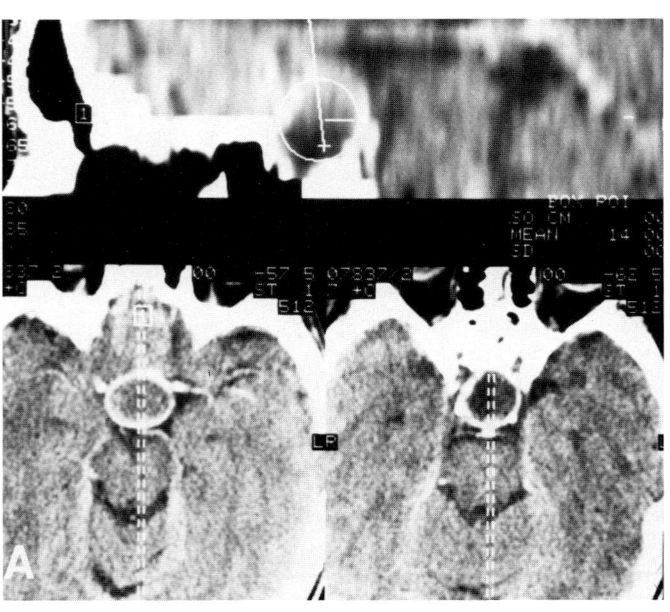
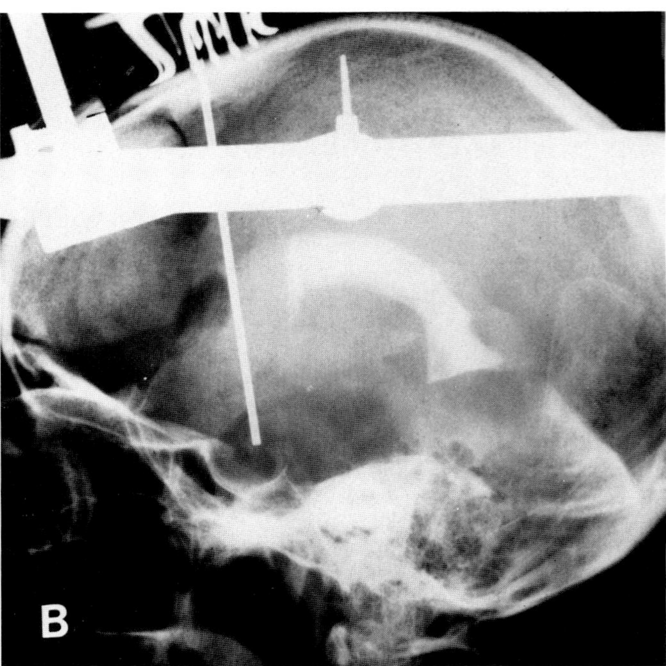

Fig. 43-19. A 31-year-old patient with a recurrence of a cystic craniopharyngioma 2 years after open exploration and resection. CT-guided stereotactic puncture of the craniopharyngioma cyst. (A) CT-guided determination of the target point and cannula approach to the cyst. (B) An x-ray film obtained after stereotactic ventriculography. The cannula is placed exactly in the center of the cyst. Discharge of 5 cm^3 of cyst liquid containing cholesterol crystals.

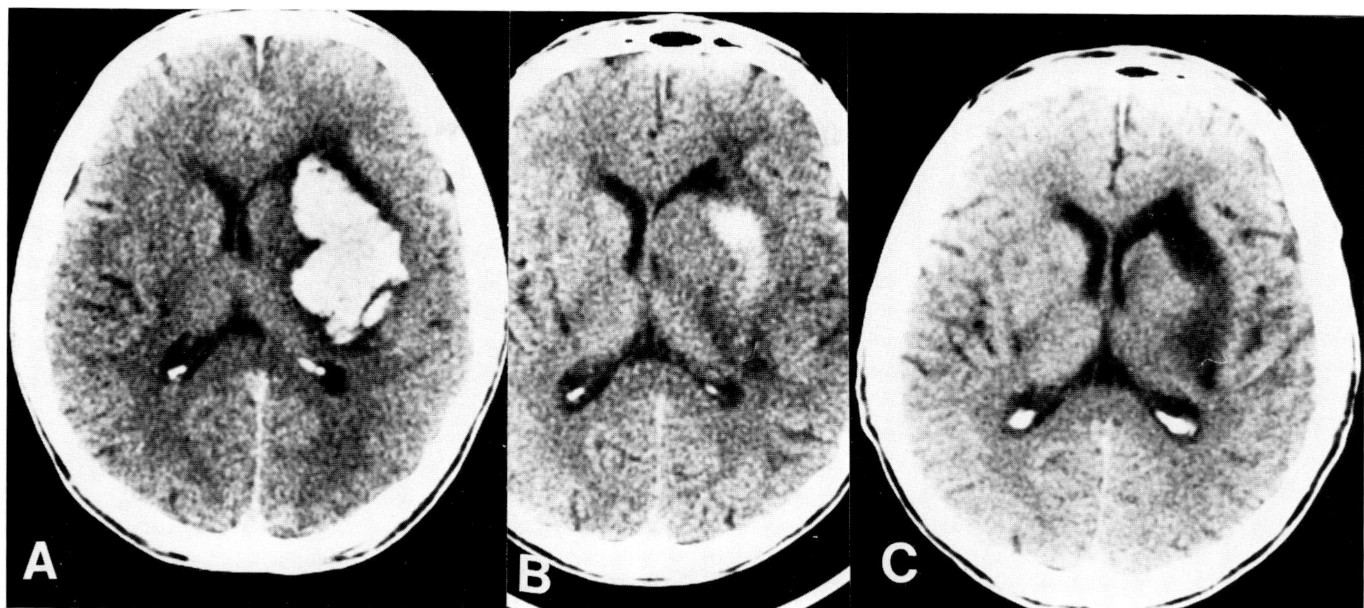

Fig. 43-20. A 49-year-old patient with apoplectic encephalorrhagia in the left hemisphere, typical localization. (A) CT scan obtained before stereotactic evacuation. (B) A CT scan obtained immediately after stereotactic evacuation. (C) A CT scan obtained 6 weeks later. The mass effect has completely disappeared. There is a hypodense tissue effect in the area of the circulation of the middle cerebral artery. Prior to evacuation, the patient was clinically comatose and hemiplegic on the left. Twelve hours after the evacuation he was fully conscious and his hemiparesis began to abate. Four weeks later, he was capable of working in his profession and was without neurologic symptoms.

which, in turn, is put into the cannular cone. The seeds are ejected from the magazine at the target site with the aid of a mandrin (Figure 43-22). If the isotope is to be distributed at several targets within the tumor, the probe is adjusted to the precalculated angles sequentially to bring the point of the cannula to these targets.

Smaller cortical or subcortical cerebral tumors or metastases are stereotactically resected as completely as possible through the small bony opening with a cortical incision of 10 mm; subsequently, intracavitary irradiation of the surgical site can be performed either intraoperatively by means of a contact radiation device, (e.g. [192]Ir GammaMed; Figure 43-23) or using ^{125}I in an after-loading catheter implantation. Cysts or cystic tumors are first drained and then irradiated intracavitarily. In the case of cystic craniopharyngiomas, intracavitary beta-radiation with ^{90}Y-glucose, [198]Au or [186]Re colloid is helpful.[1,33,38,44,46,49,55] In the case of inoperable solid craniopharyngiomas, we treat these with implanted ^{125}I seeds or after-loading catheter implantation (Figure 43-24).

TECHNIQUE OF TEMPORARY IMPLANTATION OF RADIOISOTOPES (BRACHYCURIETHERAPY)

At present we use ^{192}Ir or ^{125}I and after-loading techniques for temporary implantation in the following way: the isotope is encapsulated in hollow needles or threaded in synthetic catheters and administered to the tumor either for 4 to 10 days or for a period of minutes or hours.

In the first case, one or more implants are inserted, depending on the size of the tumor. Compared with the permanent implantation system, the dose rate of brachycurietherapy is higher, e.g., amounting to a peripheral tumor dose of 60 Gy in 6 days or 0.4 cGy/hour.[5,6,8,10,14,19,23,24] Brachycurietherapy with

[192]Ir applied over the course of several days requires considerable radiation protection for the nursing staff and we therefore abandoned this technique, giving preference to intraoperative brachycurietherapy using the [192]Ir GammaMed contact radiation device[67] or the after-loading ^{125}I catheter system.

In the case of the after-loading ^{125}I brachycurietherapy technique, a stiff silicone outer catheter is stereotactically

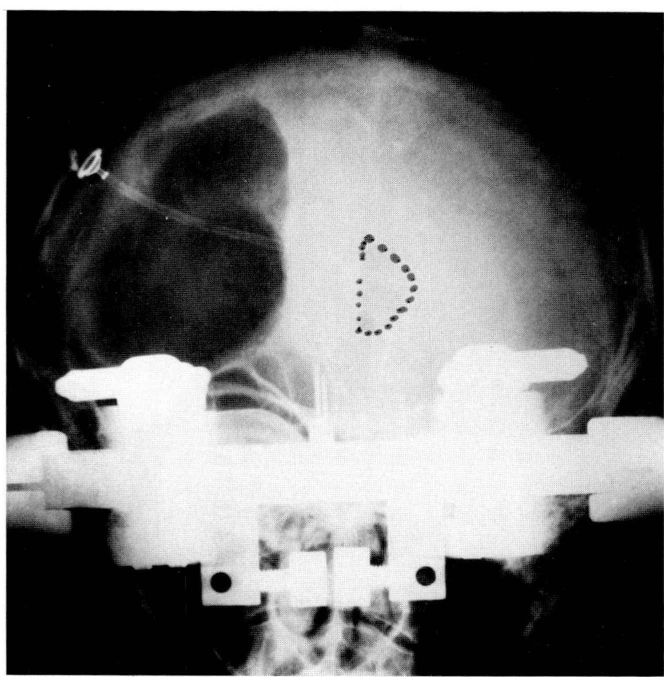

Fig. 43-21. This 74-year-old patient had a large right cerebral arachnoidal cyst and underwent CT-guided stereotactic implantation of a Rickham catheter with drainage into the ventricular system on the left.

Table 43-3. Principal physical properties of the nuclides used in interstitial radiation therapy of brain tumors

Nuclide	T½	E_γ	E_β	K	Legend	
$^{32}_{15}$P	14.3 days		1.71 (~100%)	—	$T_{1/2}$:	Physical half-life
$^{60}_{27}$Co	5.27 years	1.17 (100%) 1.13 (100%)	0.31 1.48 (0.15%)	13.2	E_γ:	maximum intensity of radiation in MeV
$^{90}_{39}$Y	2.7 days	1.75 (<0.005%)	2.27 (~100%)	—	E_β:	maximum intensity of β radiation in MeV
$^{109}_{46}$Pd	13.8 hours	0.31-0.77 (<0.005%)	1.02 (100%)	—	(%):	intensity of quants per 100 decays
$^{125}_{53}$I	60.2 days	0.0275 (73.8%) 0.0272 (37.8%) 0.031 (19.9%)		1.4		
$^{134}_{55}$S	2.15 days	0.61 (100†) 0.80 (72†)	0.66 (76%)	3.4	(†):	relative frequency of decays
$^{182}_{73}$Ta	115 days	1.12 (100†) 1.19 (60†)	0.51 (100†) 0.44 (60†)	6.1	K:	point source dose rate constant in (r · cm²)/(h · mCi)
$^{186}_{75}$Re	3.7 days	0.137 (100†)	1.07 (71%) 0.93 (21%)	0.062		in br · Cm²dh · mCie for gamma radiation
$^{192}_{77}$Ir	74.6 days	0.31 (100†) 0.47 (164†) 0.1-1.06	0.67 (44%) 0.54 (40%)	5.0		
$^{198}_{79}$Au	2.7 days	0.41 0.68 (0.5%) 1.09	0.96 (98.6%) 0.29 (1%)	2.3		

introduced. For radiation protection the inner catheter, filled with ^{125}I seeds, is inserted into the outer catheter and both catheters are clipped together with a Hemoclip. The catheters are cut off directly above the clip, having been secured subgaleally, and the incision is closed with a few sutures (Figure 43-25). No wound infections have occurred, even in cases where the catheter remained in situ over a period of 5 to 7 days. At the end of the radiation treatment, the catheter is removed and the wound is reclosed. In some cases we remove the inner catheter only and exchange it with a inner catheter filled with a fresh supply of ^{125}I. We have experienced no complications with this approach over a period of several years. The introduction of various catheters filled with ^{192}Ir seeds in a grid pattern[86,93] to obtain a more homogeneous dose distribution within a tumor is not necessary, since necrosis with possible cystic liquefaction is a desired reaction and inner decompression is obtained by puncture of the cyst.

CONTACT RADIATION DEVICES

Contact radiation devices are for use with high dose irradiation. A variety of different devices and application systems exist; we use an automated apparatus for irradiation with ^{192}Ir called "GammaMed"* (Figure 43-26). The design of this device is such that it fulfills all requirements for intraoperative or postoperative application. With the aid of the after-loading method it is possible to obtain doses of radiation capable of producing necrosis in a tumor within a few minutes.

The ^{192}Ir emitter of up to 120 Ci in strength is manufactured by Philips-Ouphar, Amsterdam, The Netherlands, in the form of a cylinder 1 mm in diameter and of variable length. It is contained in a Monel metal shell 1.8 mm in diameter and of appropriate length, usually of 10 mm. When not in use, the emitter is placed in a heavy metal container of ellipsoid shape, which eliminates all environmental radiation. This shielding device weighs 30 kg and has a shielding capacity for 150 Ci of ^{192}Ir. The shielding device is placed in a protective container, which hangs on a mobile stand or support and can be moved automatically.

The ^{192}Ir emitter is attached to a flexible cable or tube and

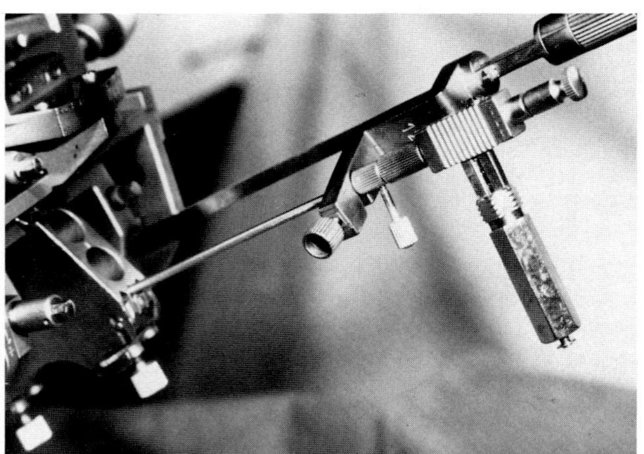

Fig. 43-22. A number of radiation-protected ^{192}Ir and ^{125}I seeds, the activity of which is calculated by means of a specialized program (developed together with Birg), are distributed within the tumor using this special applicator (modified "Mick" applicator).

*Manufacturer: Isotopen-Technik, Haan, West Germany.

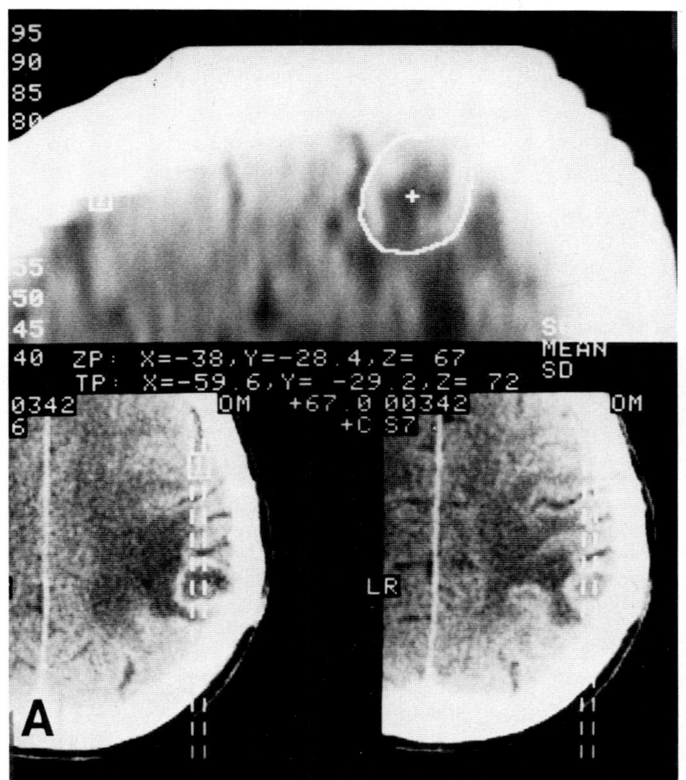

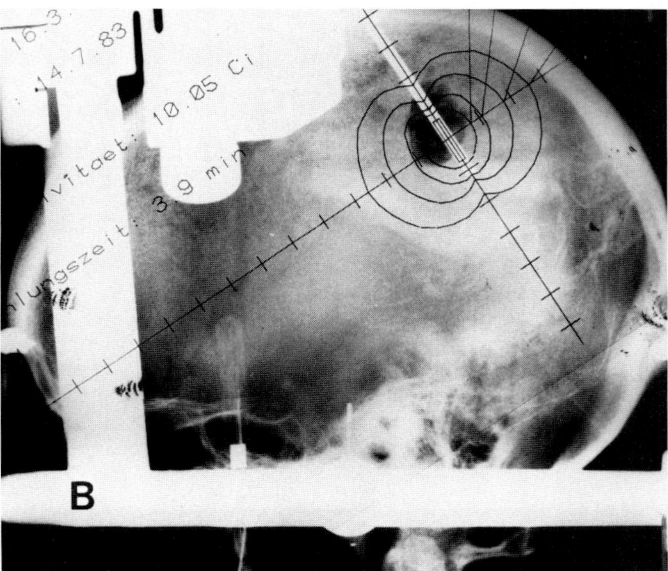

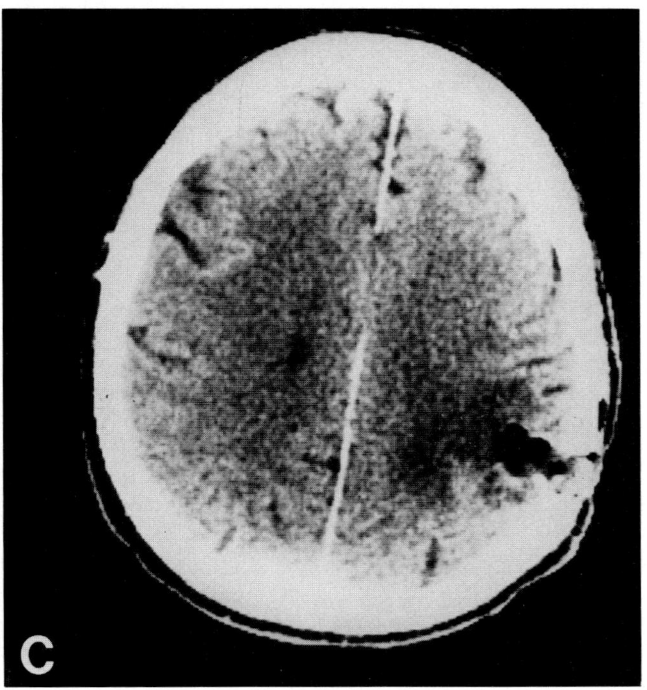

Fig. 43-23. This 63-year-old patient had a glioblastoma (WHO IV) and underwent combined CT-guided stereotactic open resection and intraoperative brachycurietherapy with the GammaMed ^{192}Ir contact radiation device. (A) Sagittal reconstruction depicting the subcortically located tumor, which is hypodense in the center. Determination of the target (cross) and approach. (B) The trephination hole is made directly above the tumor (diameter 11 mm). Intraoperative contact irradiation after resection of the tumor. The radiation cannula is placed in situ. The resection cavity has inflated with air. (C) Postoperative control CT scan. The tumor is completely resected. Following this combined treatment, the patient survived 22 months with the glioblastoma.

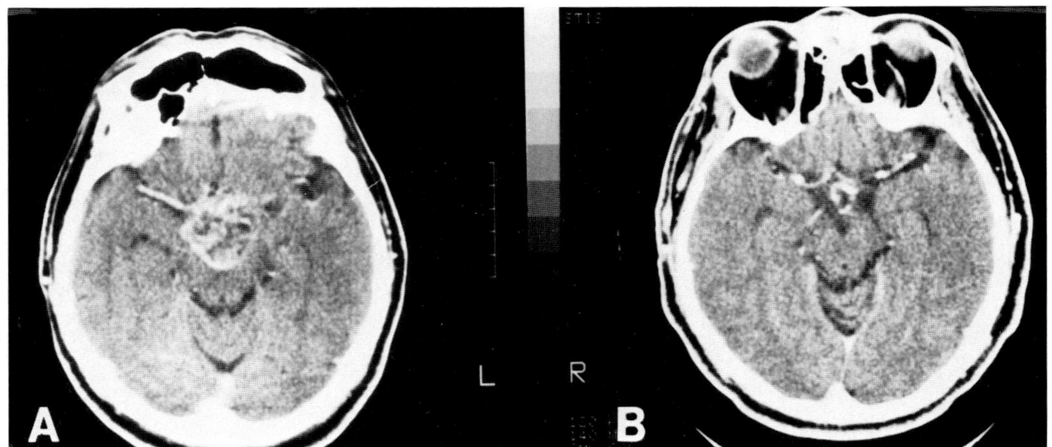

Fig. 43-24. Craniopharyngioma. This 56-year-old patient was in a poor general state of health and thus the craniopharyngioma was inoperable. Anesthesia and open resection were contraindicated. (A) The CT-stereotactically confirmed craniopharyngioma, 4 cm in diameter. (B) Ten months after ^{125}I curietherapy. The craniopharyngioma can no longer be identified. There was a dramatic improvement in the patient's general state of health with an almost normal endocrine state and without any narrowing of the visual field.

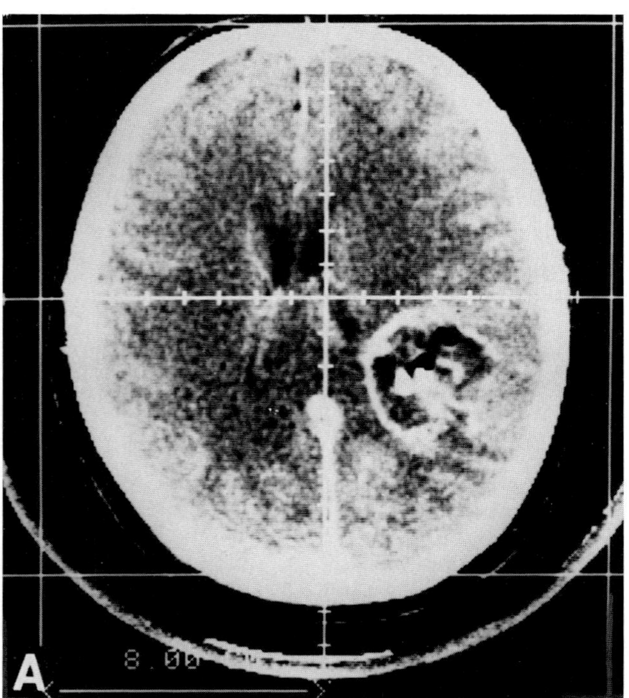

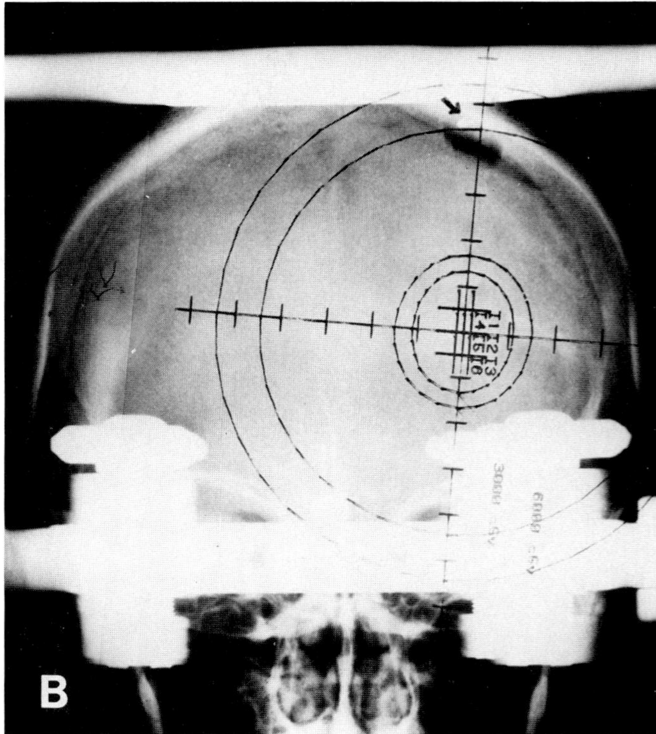

Fig. 43-25. The anaplastic glioma (WHO III) in this 53-year-old patient was treated by CT-guided stereotactic biopsy and after-loading brachycurietherapy with two catheters loaded with ^{125}I seeds. (A) This AP x-ray film shows the isodose distribution (peripheral tumor dosage 40 Gy). (B) A control CT scan shows the catheter positions in the anaplastic glioma. The dark circles correspond to air insufflation through the cannula caused by repeated insertion of the biopsy forceps.

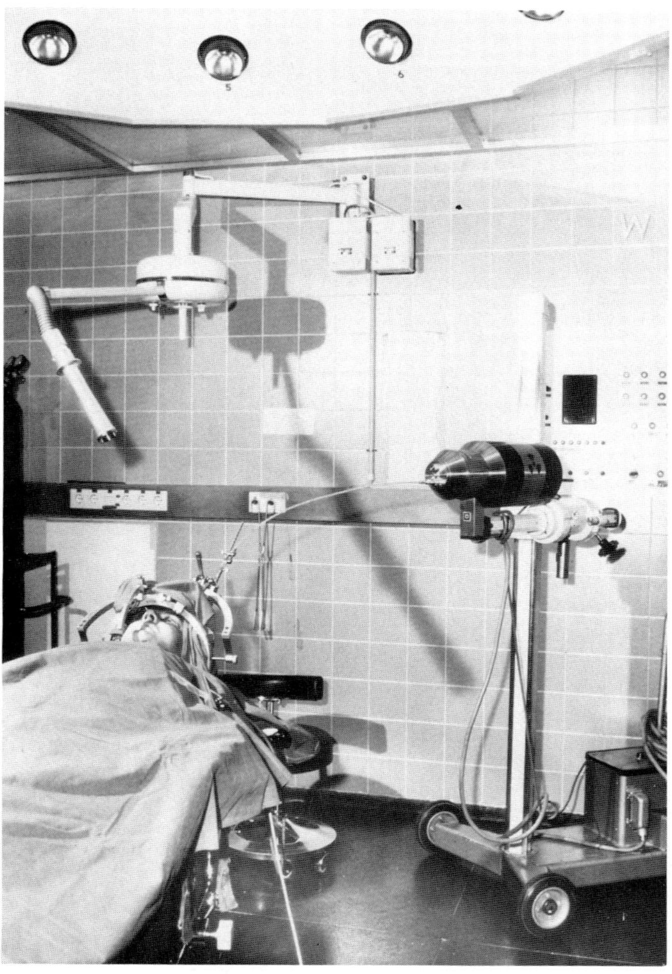

Fig. 43-26. The GammaMed iridium 192 contact radiation device developed by Mundinger and Sauerwein. The connecting tube is attached to the stereotactically introduced application cannula at one end and to the exit channel of the shielding container at the other. With the aid of the remote automatic control the emitter is introduced into the application cannula and is automatically withdrawn into the shielding container after the calculated exposure has been reached.

can be automatically moved from the shielding container through a channel equipped with a shutter and guided by a sterilizable extension of the cable or tube, which is attached to the cannula used for the radiation treatment. After delivery of the desired dose of radiation as determined by a time program, the emitter is automatically withdrawn to its original position within the device, which is, in turn, automatically closed by a shutter. A radiation detector incorporated into the protective container monitors and safeguards the correct placement of the emitter into the shielding device.

If primary stereotactic or postoperative ^{192}Ir brachycurietherapy is indicated after partial resection of a tumor, the cannula is stereotactically introduced to the target point for the intraoperative after-loading of the contact irradiation, which is carried out after the cannula position has been checked radiographically. Depending on the size and geometry of the volume to be irradiated, several cannulas may be introduced, through which the emitter is successively introduced (Figure 43-27). By shifting one cannula in the tumor axis to different positions, the peripheral tumor dose can be adapted to complicated tumor shapes.

The more recent GammaMed II device has an emitter drive that can be programmed. In addition, several different activity levels can be programmed so that optimal interstitial or intracavitary irradiation is carried out more easily on even complicated tumor forms. The dose for the tumor surface is, depending on the volume, 40 to 45 Gy in one sitting.

In cases where a fractionation into two, three, or more sessions is planned possibly in combination with fractionated external radiation, the single dose can be correspondingly reduced. The additional peripheral tumor dose should not exceed 100–120 Gy. One radiation session lasts, depending on the activity level, from a few minutes to about half an hour.

Radionecrosis takes place in about one third of cases, followed by cystic liquefaction. Two to 5 weeks after treatment, an increased perifocal edema occurs in many cases, requiring that the patient receive higher doses of dexamethasone. According to our experience, the application of the ^{192}Ir contact radiation of high dosage is limited to tumor volumes of under 125 cm^3 (5 cm in diameter). When the full dosage is applied, this "radiosection" is only tolerated in tumors of the cerebral and cerebellar hemispheres. For larger hemisphere malignant gliomas a combination of percutaneous irradiation and contact irradiation is advisable. In tumors that infiltrate into the gray substance (basal ganglia), the tumor surface dose should not exceed 20 Gy per session. In such cases, a combination with permanent implantation is indicated for tumors of smaller volume; combination with percutaneous irradiation is recommended for larger volumes. In cases of recurrences after percutaneous irradiation or insufficient regression of the tumor volume, additional brachycurietherapy is indicated for smaller lesions.

RESULTS OF BRACHYCURIETHERAPY

We have interstitially and stereotactically treated a total of 1707 patients. Tables 43-4 and 43-5 show the isotopes that were used and the tumor histology in these cases.[10,11,14,18,19,21,23,28]

INDICATIONS FOR CURIETHERAPY, BRACHYCURIETHERAPY, AND COMBINED RADIOTHERAPY

The decision on which method to use and which radioactive source to apply depends on the histologic diagnosis, the grade of the tumor, its location within the brain, the tumor volume, and the extent of infiltration (Table 43-6).

Local (focal) interstitial and intracavitary application of isotopes has in cases of intracranial tumors effectively expanded the therapy or has even become the treatment method of choice for nonresectable low-grade midline tumors (Figures 43-28 and 43-29). In cases of larger brain tumors of the hemispheres, open surgery with, if possible, total or subtotal removal of tumor should be the goal. Should, however, the removal or partial resection of a tumor prove impossible, then stereotactic curietherapy or brachycurietherapy is indicated (Table 43-7; Figure 43-30).

1. In the case of anaplastic tumors (grade III or IV) of the hemispheres, the combination of interstitial brachy curietherapy and percutaneous radiation therapy provides an effective increase in the local dosage, thus improving the palliative result. If the anaplastic tumor is detected at an

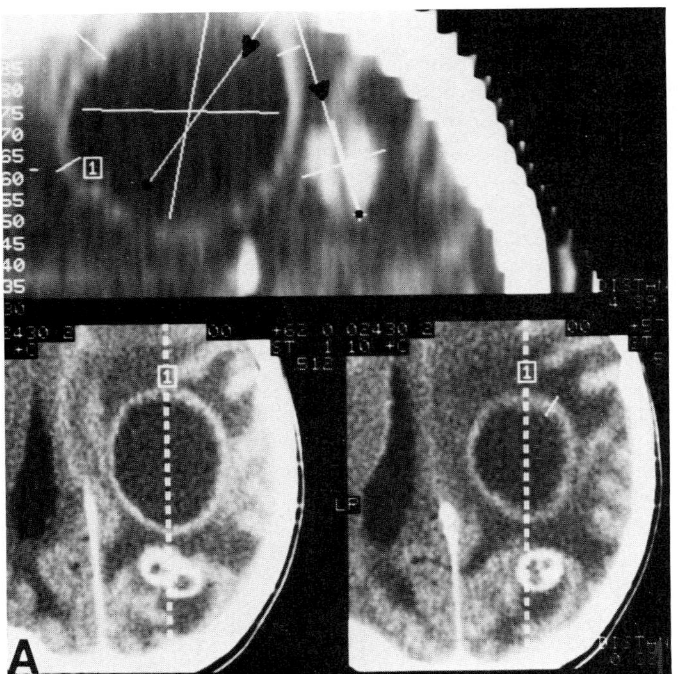
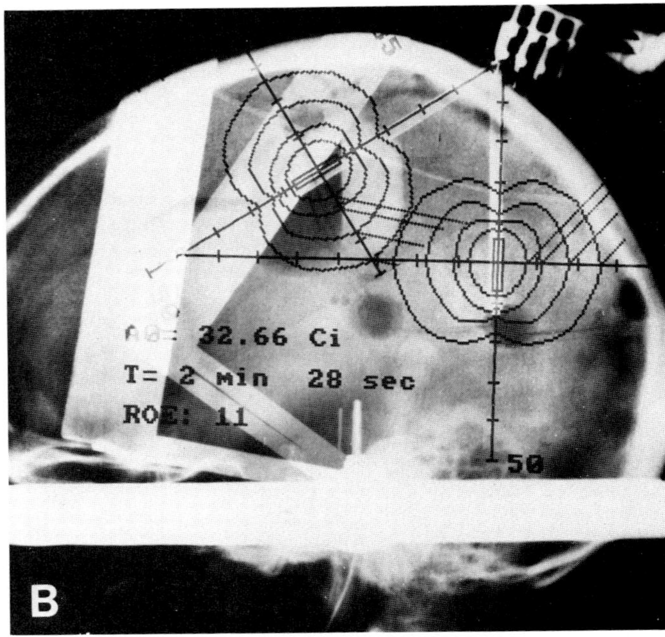

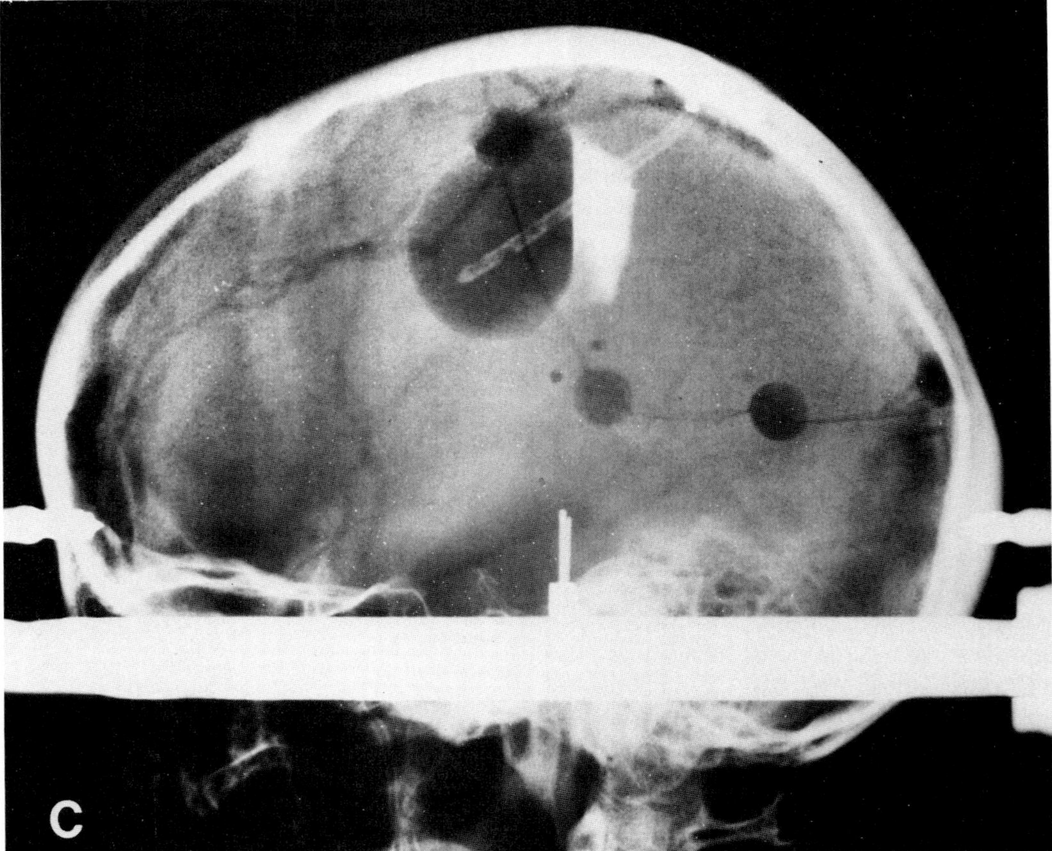

Fig. 43-27. This 43-year-old patient had a recurrent melanoma metastasis following open resection and external radiation. (A) Sagittal reconstruction. Centroparietally, the large tumor cyst with a hyperdense halo can be seen with enhancement. It continues parieto-occipitally as a mainly hyperdense metastatic tumor. (B) Intraoperative brachycurietherapy with the GammaMed ^{192}Ir contact radiation device. The lateral x-ray film shows the ^{192}Ir isodose distribution (peripheral tumor dosage = 40 Gy). (C) Following intracavitary intraoperative radiation, a Rickham catheter with enlarged perforations was also stereotactically inserted into the cyst cavity.

<table>
<tr><td valign="top">

Table 43-4. Radionuclides and number of interstitial irradiation procedures, 1952–1987

Radionuclide	Number of Procedures
^{32}P	6
^{60}Co	179
^{90}Y	44
^{182}Ta	21
^{198}Au	129
^{125}I	546
^{125}I (brachycurie)	40
^{192}Ir (GammaMed)	340
^{192}Ir	609
Total	1878

</td><td valign="top">

Table 43-5. Bioptically confirmed histology and number of interstitial irradiation procedures, 1952–1987

Tumor Type	Number of Procedures
Glioblastoma	455
Astrocytoma	907
Oligodendroglioma	141
Ependymoma	53
PNET	72
Meningioma	29
Metastases	116
Sarcoma	14
Pituitary adenoma	263
Craniopharyngioma	69
Other lesions	268
Hypophysectomy	57
Pallidotomy	21
Total	2425

</td></tr>
</table>

Table 43-6. Indications of CT-guided stereotactic low-dose-rate ^{192}Ir or ^{125}I curietherapy (permanent implantation)

	Biopsy Obligatory
Primary curietherapy	Nonresectable low-grade tumors (WHO I, II) around the cerebral/cerebellar midline
	Nonresectable tumors (WHO II-III, III) followed by external irradiation
Secondary curietherapy	Resting low-grade tumors (WHO I, II) after partial resection
	High-grade tumor recurrences after operation and external irradiation
	After external irradiation only
	Brachycurietherapy not indicated

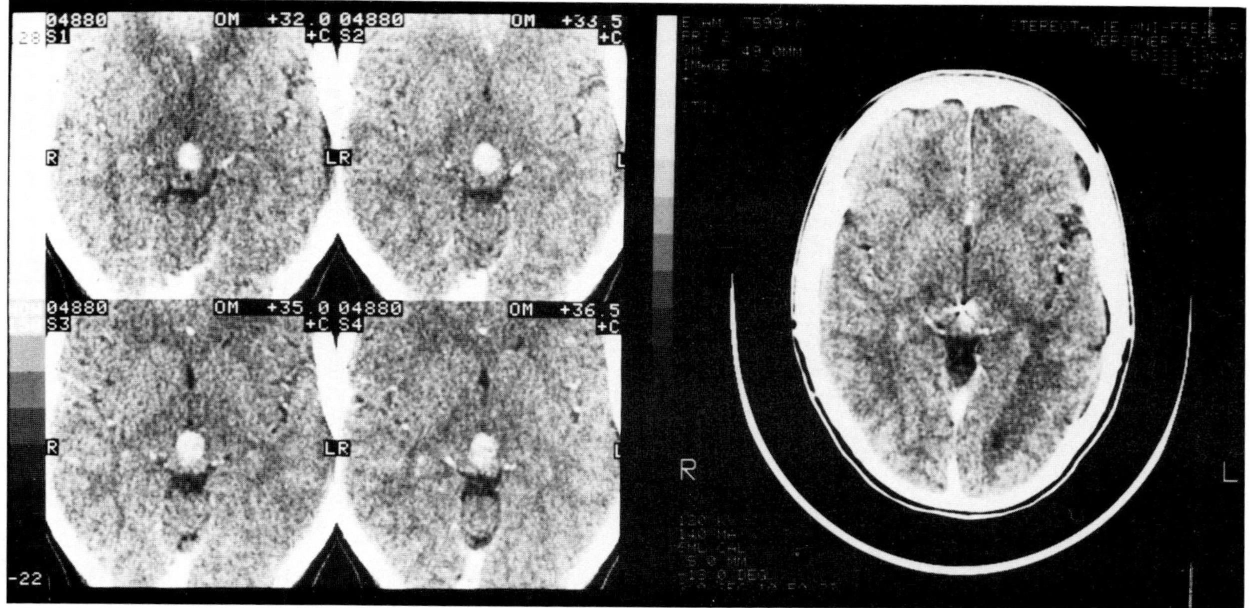

Fig. 43-28. (Left) This 18-year-old patient had an astrocytoma (WHO I) of the upper brain stem as confirmed by CT-guided stereotactic biopsy with a clinical picture of occlusive hydrocephalus and oculomotor disturbances. (Right) Three years after ^{192}Ir implantation and ventriculoatrial shunt there were no neurologic findings. The oculomotor disturbances had completely receded and there was no evidence of recurrence.

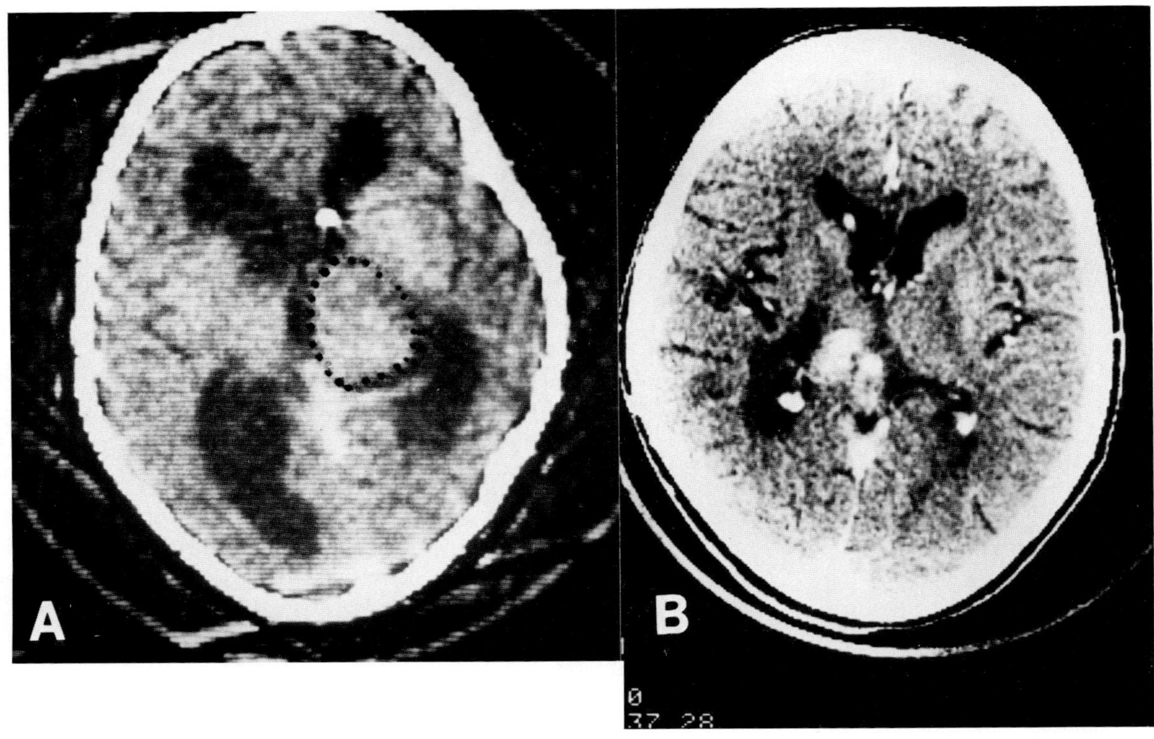

Fig. 43-29. (A) This 16-year-old patient had a large astrocytoma of the right thalamus with occlusive hydrocephalus as confirmed by CT-guided stereotactic biopsy. (B) Eight years after ^{192}Ir implantation and atrioventricular shunt, artifacts of the ^{192}Ir can be recognized surrounded by scarred areas that appear hyperdense with enhancement. The tumor can no longer be seen. The ventricular system has shifted back to the midline and there is no evidence of pathologic involvement of the peripheral subarachnoid space. The patient had neither psychologic nor neurologic symptoms.

Table 43-7. Indications for CT-guided stereotactic high-dose-rate ^{192}Ir or ^{125}I brachycurietherapy (temporary implantation) of intracranial malignant tumors

	Biopsy Obligatory
Primary brachycurietherapy	Small volume hemispheric tumors
	Tumors in functionally important regions (central, temporal, parietal)
	Nonresectable deep-seated tumors
Secondary brachycurietherapy	After operation and external irradiation
	Recurrences after external irradiation
	Not indicated in process around midline structures

Indications for nonresectable deep-seated malignant tumors around cerebral/cerebellar midline structures	
	Biopsy Obligatory
Grade III (WHO)	Iridium 192 or iodine 125 curietherapy (permanent implantation)
Grade IV (WHO)	External beam irradiation only
	Brachycurietherapy not indicated

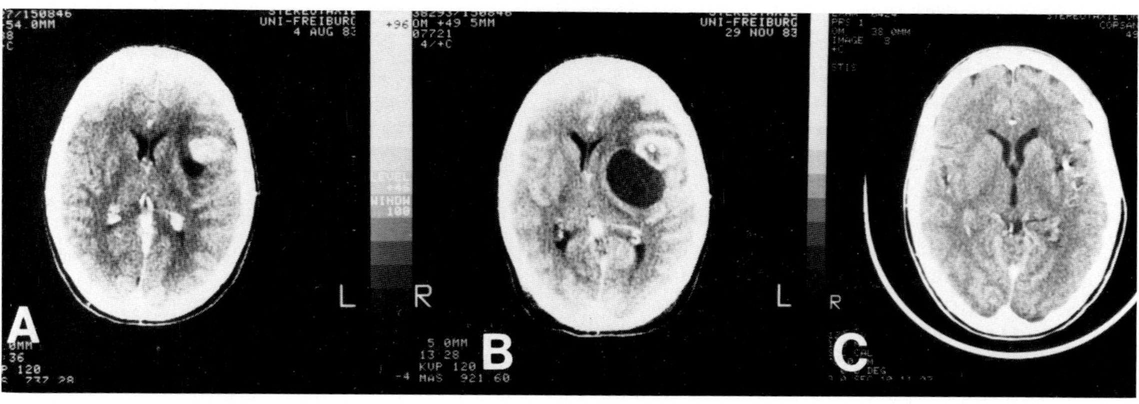

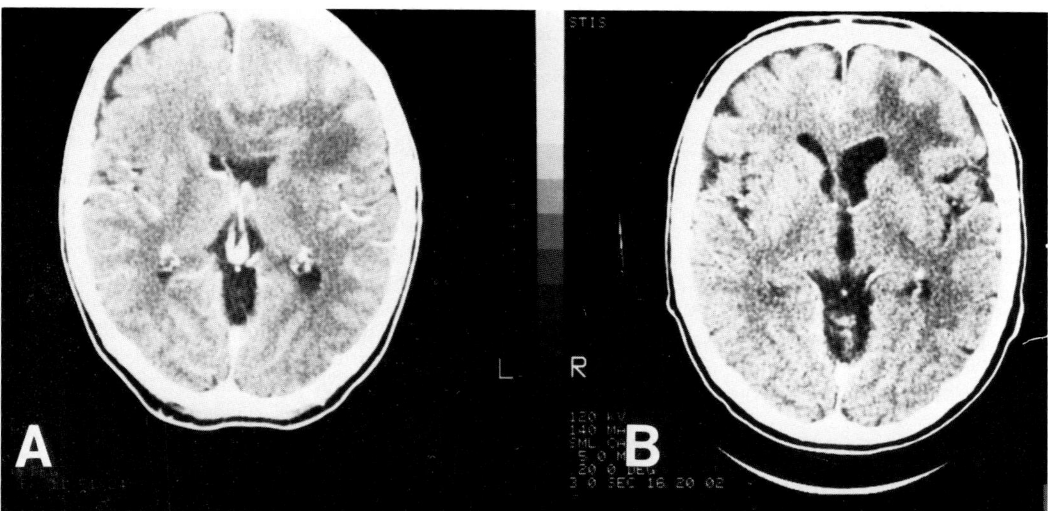

Fig. 43-31. CT-guided stereotactic biopsy was used to confirm the presence of an anaplastic glioma in this 54-year-old patient. The tumor was treated by stereotactic curietherapy with ^{125}I combined with external radiation. (A) Before treatment. The anaplastic glioma, located frontally on the left and infiltrating the entire corpus callosum, had compressed the ventricular system, shifting it caudally. (B) Five months after ^{125}I curietherapy and external radiation the ventricular system has shifted back to the midline. There is extension of the left anterior horn as a result of shrinking of the tumor and there is reactive gliosis in the area of the left frontal lobe. The tumor is no longer visible. The patient was fully capable of working in a responsible position. As of February, 1986, he had survived 13 months.

early stage and if it fulfills the conditions for small volume irradiation, brachycurietherapy alone is indicated.

2. Regular CT control is used to decide whether reimplantation or additional percutaneous irradiation is indicated. After combined treatment, recurrent tumors can again be treated with brachycurietherapy.

3. Experience has shown that tumors of grades I and II do not react satisfactorily to external irradiation. If the boundaries of the tumor can be demarcated, curietherapy combined with additional therapeutic measures such as cyst puncture, catheter systems, etc., is indicated, and long-term palliative and curative results can be achieved. For extended, nondelimited, nonresectable hemisphere gliomas of grades I and II, corticoid therapy alone should be applied. A surprisingly long palliative effect can sometimes be achieved with this treatment.

4. For the transition to anaplastic tumors (grade II and III), curietherapy is preferred in combination with percutaneous irradiation (Figure 43-31).

5. External radiation therapy may be indicated if necessary in combination with radiosensitizers and chemocytostatic agents whenever the anaplastic tumor (grades III or IV) has infiltrated extensively and when the patient's general condition and functional deficits, as well as any spread into the brain stem and basal ganglia do not any longer justify curietherapy or brachycurietherapy. In such cases, priority must be given to enabling the patient to live a worthwhile life rather than merely accomplishing long-term survival.

REFERENCES

1. Backlund EO: Studies on craniopharyngiomas. III. Stereotaxic treatment with intracystic yttrium 90. Acta Chir Scand 139:237, 1973

2. Bond WH, Richards D, Turner E: Experiences with radioactive gold in the treatment of craniopharyngioma. J Neurol Neurosurg Psychiatry 28:30, 1965

3. Dyck P: Stereotactic Biopsy and Brachytherapy of Brain Tumors. Baltimore, University Park Press, 1983

4. Gutin PH, Bernstein M: Stereotactic interstitial brachytherapy for malignant brain tumors. Prog Exp Tumor Res 28:166, 1984

5. Hilaris BS: Techniques for interstitial and intracavitary radiation. Cancer 22:745, 1968

6. Hilaris BS (ed): Handbook of Interstitial Brachytherapy. Acton, MA, Publishing Sciences Group, 1975

7. Mundinger F: Eine einfache Methode der lokalisierten Bestrahlung von Grosshirngeschwülsten mit radioaktivem Gold. MMW 98:23, 1956

8. Mundinger F: Beitrag zur Dosimetrie und Applikation von Radio-Tantal (Ta[182]) zur Langzeitbestrahlung von Hirngeschwülsten. Fortschr Roentgenstr 89:86, 1958

9. Mundinger F: Die interstitielle Radio-Isotopen-Bestrahlung von Hirntumoren mit vergleichenden Langzeitergebnissen zur Röntgentiefentherapie. Acta Neurochir 9:89, 1963

10. Mundinger F: Treatment of brain tumors with radioisotopes, in Krayenbühl H, Maspes M, Sweet C (eds): Progress in Neurological Surgery. Basel, S. Karger, 1966, pp 202–257

11. Mundinger F: Erfahrungen mit der stereotaktischen interstitiellen Brachytherapie mit Ir[192]-"GammaMed" bei infiltrierenden Hirntumoren. Fortschr Roentgenstr 110:254, 1969

12. Mundinger F: Die intrasell äre protrahierte Langzeitbestrahlung von Hypophysenadenomen mittels stereotaktischer Implantation von Iridium 192. Acta Radiol 8:55, 1969

13. Mundinger F: Intrasell äre Iridium 192—Permanent-Implantation bei Hypophysenadenomen, in Bushe KA (ed): Fortschritte auf dem Gebiet der Neurochirurgie. Stuttgart, Hippokrates, 1970, pp 83–87

14. Mundinger F: The treatment of brain tumors with interstitially applied radioactive isotopes, in Wang Y, Paoletti P (eds): Radionuclide Applications in Neurology and Neurosurgery. Springfield, Ill, Charles C Thomas, 1970, pp 199–265

15. Mundinger F: Interstitial radioisotope therapy of intractable diencephalic tumors by the stereotaxic permanent implantation of iridium 192, including bioptic control. Confin Neurol 32:195, 1970

16. Mundinger F: Combined treatment of experimental DS-tumors and infiltrating cerebral gliomas with interstitial curietherapy and radiosensitizing drugs, in Proceedings of the Fourth European Congress of Neurosurgery. Present Limits of Neurosurgery. Prague, Avicenum, 1972, pp 77

17. Mundinger F: Interstitial curietherapy in the treatment of pituitary adenomas and for hypophysectomy. Prog Neurol Surg 6:326, 1975

18. Mundinger F: Die stereotaktische interstitielle Therapie nicht resezierbarer intracranieller Tumoren mit Ir-192 und Jod-125, in Wannenmacher M, Schreiber HW, Gauwerky F (eds): Kombinierte chirurgische und radiologische Behandlung maligner Tumoren. Munich, Urban & Schwarzenberg, 1981, pp 90–112

19. Mundinger F: Implantation of radioisotopes (curietherapy), in Schaltenbrand G, Walker AE (eds): Textbook of Stereotaxy of the Human Brain. Stuttgart, Georg Thieme, 1982, pp 410–435

20. Mundinger F: Stereotactic interstitial therapy of nonresectable intracranial tumors with iridium 192 and iodine 125, in Kärcher KH et al (eds): Progress in Radio-Oncology II. New York, Raven Press, 1982, pp 371–380

21. Mundinger F: Stereotaktische intrakranielle Bestrahlung von Tumoren mit Radioisotopen (Curie-Therapie), in Dietz H, Umbach W, Wüllenweber R (eds): Klinische Neurochirurgie. Vol 2: Klinik und Therapie. Stuttgart, Georg Thieme, 1984, pp 519–565

22. Mundinger F: Langzeitbestrahlung nicht resezierbarer intracranieller Hirntumoren. Die CT-stereotaktische interstitielle Curie-Therapie mit Jod-125-Seeds. MMW 41:1176, 1984

23. Mundinger F: Technik und Ergebnisse der interstitiellen Hirntumorbestrahlung, in Heilmann HP (ed): Handbuch der medizinischen Radiologie. Vol XIX/4. Spezielle Strahlentherapie maligner Tumoren. Berlin, Springer Verlag, 1985, pp 179–214

24. Mundinger F: Stereotactic biopsy and technique of implantation (instillation) of radionuclei, in Jellinger K (ed): Therapy of Malignant Brain Tumors. New York, Springer Verlag, (in press)

25. Mundinger F: CT-Guided stereotactic implantation with iridium-192 and iodine-125 of nonresectable intracranial tumors, in Winkler C (ed): Nuclear Medicine in Clinical Oncology. Berlin, Springer Verlag, 1986, pp 378–380

26. Mundinger F: CT-Guided stereotactic biopsy and interstitial curietherapie with Ir-192 and I-125 of nonresectable midline and brain stem gliomas, in Samii M (ed): Surgery In and Around the Brain Stem and the Third Ventricle. Berlin, Springer Verlag, 1986, pp 509-517

27. Mundinger F, Birg W, Ostertag C: Treatment of small cerebral gliomas with CT-aided stereotactic curie-therapy. Neuroradiology 16:564, 1978

28. Mundinger F, Busam B, Birg W, et al: Results of interstitial iridium-192 brachy-curie therapy and iridium-192 protracted long term irradiation, in Szikla G (ed): Stereotactic Cerebral Irradiation. INSERM Symposium No. 12. Amsterdam, Elsevier/North Holland, 1979, pp 303-320

29. Mundinger F, Hoefer T: Protracted long-term irradiation of inoperable midbrain tumors by stereotactic curie-therapy using iridium-192. Acta Neurochir 21:93, 1974

30. Mundinger F, Metzel E: Interstitial radioisotope therapy of intractable diencephalic tumors by the stereotaxic permanent implantation of iridium-192, including bioptic control. Confin Neurol 32:195, 1970

31. Mundinger F, Noetzel H, Riechert T: Erfahrungen mit der

lokalisierten Bestrahlung von malignen Hirngeschwülsten mit Radio-Isotopen. Acta Neurochir Suppl 6:171, 1959

32. Mundinger F, Ostertag CB, Birg W, et al: Stereotactic treatment of brain lesions: Biopsy, interstitial radiotherapy (iridium-192 and iodine-125) and drainage procedures. Appl Neurophysiol 43:198, 1980

33. Mundinger F, Riechert T: Hypophysentumoren—Hypophysektomie. Klinik, Therapie, Ergebnisse. Stuttgart, Georg Thieme, 1967

34. Mundinger F, Vogt P, Jobski C, et al: Klinische und experimentelle Ergebnisse der interstitiellen Brachy-Curietherapie in Kombination mit Radiosensibilisatoren bei infiltrieren den Hirntumoren. Strahlentherapie 143:318, 1972

35. Mundinger F, Weigel K: Stereotactic curietherapy of thalamic tumors. J Neuro-Oncol 2:278, 1984

36. Mundinger F, Weigel K: CT-Stereotactic biopsy and interstitial radiotherapy of pineal region tumors. Presented at the 8th Mexican Congress of Neurological Surgery, Acapulco, July 26–30, 1983, in Bamberg M (ed): Aktüelle Onkologie. Munich, Fückschwendt Verlag, (in press)

37. Mundinger F, Weigel K: Indications and results of stereotactic curietherapy with iridium-192 and iodine-125 for nonresectable tumors of the hypothalamic region. Acta Neurochir Suppl 33 1984

38. Mundinger F, Weigel K: Long-term results of stereotactic interstitial curietherapy. Acta Neurochir Suppl 33:367, 1984

39. Mundinger F, Weigel K: Long-term results of stereotactic curietherapy (permanent implantation) with iridium-192 and iodine-125 in nonresectable cerebral gliomas or recurrent tumors. Presented at the International Congress of Radiology, Hawaii, July 8–12, 1985

40. Mundinger F, Weigel K: CT-Stereotactic interstitial irradiation therapy of nonresectable and recurrent intracranial tumors in children and adolescents, in Voth D, Krauseneck P (eds): Chemotherapy of Gliomas. Basic Research, Experiences, and Results. Berlin, Walter de Gruyter, 1985, pp 241–259

41. Mundinger F, Weigel K: Results of CT-guided stereotactic curietherapy of midline tumors of the brain. Presented at the 3rd International Meeting on Progress in Radio-Oncology, Vienna, March 27–30, 1985

42. Mundinger F, Weigel K, Mohadjer M: CT-Stereotaktische Biopsie und/oder interstielle-extern kombinierte Strahlenbehandlung von Hirnmetastasen. Aktuelle Onkologie 13:128, 1984

43. Murray KJ, Blumberg A, Strubler K, et al: Permanent radioactive iodine seed implants following radical resection in recurrent human malignant high grade astrocytomas. J Neuro-oncol 2:282, 1984

44. Musolino A, Munari C, Blond S, et al: Traitement stéréotaxique des kystes expansifs de craniopharyngiomes par irradiation endocavitaire beta (Re 186, Au 198, Y 90). Neurochirurgie 31:169, 1985

45. Rougier A, Pigneux J, Cohadon F: Combined interstitial and external irradiation of gliomas. Acta Neurochir Suppl 33:345, 1984

46. Schaub C, Bluet-Pajot MT, Videau-Lornet C, et al: Endocavitary beta irradiation of glioma cysts with colloidal 186-rhenium, in Szikla G (ed): Stereotactic Cerebral Irradiation. INSERM Symposium No. 12. Amsterdam, Elsevier/North Holland, 1979, pp 293–302

47. Szikla G et al: Interstitial and combined interstitial and external irradiation of supratentorial gliomas. Results in 61 cases treated between 1973 and 1981. Acta Neurochir Suppl 33:355, 1984

48. Szikla G, Betti O, Szenthe L, et al: L'expérience actuelle des irradiations stéréotaxique dans le traitement des gliomes hémisphériques. Neurochirurgie 27:295, 1981

49. Szikla G, Musolina A, Miyahara S, et al: Colloidal Rhenium-185 in endocavitary beta irradiation of cystic craniopharyngiomas and active glioma cysts. Long term results, side effects, and clinical dosimetry. Acta Neurochir Suppl 33:331, 1984

50. Szikla G, Peragut JC: Irradiation interstitielle des gliomes. Neurochirurgie 21 (suppl 2):187, 1975

51. Wara WM, Gutin PA, Leibel SA, et al: Treatment of malignant brain tumors with high-activity iodine-125. J Neuro-oncol 2:284, 1984

52. Weigel K, Mohadjer M, Mundinger F: CT-Stereotaxy for differential diagnosis and radiotherapy of intracranial metastases. Adv Neurosurg 12:87, 1984

53. Weigel K, Mundinger F: Permanent drainage of cysts—A simple therapy for cystic craniopharyngiomas. Presented at the 9th Scientific Meeting of the European Society for Paediatric Neurosurgery, Vienna, October 10–13, 1984

54. Weigel K, Ostertag CB, Mundinger F: Interstitial long-trem irradiation of tumors in the pineal region, in Szikla G (ed): Stereotactic Cerebral Irradiation. INSERM Symposium No. 12. Amsterdam, Elsevier/North Holland, 1979, pp 283–292

55. Wycis HT, Robbins R, Spiegel-Adolf M, et al: Studies in stereoencephalotomy. III. Treatment of a cystic craniopharyngioma by injection of radioactive P-32. Confin Neurol 14:193, 1954

56. Dittmar C: über die Lage des sogenannten Gehörzentrums in der Medulla Oblongata. Ber Sächs Ges Wiss Leipzig Math-Physik Klasse 25:449, 1873

57. Horsley V, Clarke RH: The structure and functions of the cerebellum examined by a new method. Brain 31:45, 1908

58. Clarke RH: I. Investigation of the central nervous system. Methods and instruments. Johns Hopkins Report, Special Volume, 1920

59. Spiegel EA: Guided Brain Operations. Basel, S. Karger, 1982

60. Uchimura Y, Narabayashi H: Stereoencephalotomy. Presented at the 47th Japanese Neuropsychiatry Conference, Kyoto, April 9, 1950

61. Talairach J, Hécaen H, David M, et al: Recherches sur la coagulation therapeutique des structures sous-corticales chez l'homme. Rev Neurol 41:4, 1949

62. Leksell L: A stereotactic apparatus for intracerebral surgery. Acta Chir Scand 99:229, 1949

63. Lorimer FM, Segal MM, Stein SN: Path of current distribution in brain during electro-convulsive therapy. EEG Clin Neurophysiol 1:343, 1949

64. Mark VH, McPherson PM, Sweet WH: A new method for correcting distortion in cranial roentgenograms. With special reference to a new human stereotaxic instrument. AJR 71:435, 1954

65. Hayne R, Meyers R: An improved model of a human stereotactic instrument. J Neurosurg 7:463, 1950

66. Hayne RA, Belinson L, Gibbs FA: Electrical activity of subcortical areas in epilepsy. EEG Clin Neurophysiol 1:437, 1949

67. Wada T: A modified stereotactic apparatus for brain surgery of deep portions. Tohoku J Exp Med 58:299, 1953

68. Hitchcock E, Morris CS, Sotelo MG, et al: Comparison of smear and imprint techniques for rapid diagnosis in neuro-oncology. Surg Neurol 26:176, 1986

69. Laitinen LV, Liliequist B, Fagerlund M, et al: An adapter for computed tomography guided stereotaxis. Surg Neurol 23:559, 1985

70. Kelly PJ, Kall BA, Goerss SG: Computer-assisted stereotactic biopsies utilizing CT and digitized arteriographic data. Acta Neurochir Suppl 33:233, 1984

71. Kelly PJ, Kall BA, Goerss S, et al: Computer-assisted stereotactic laser resection of intra-axial brain neoplasms. J Neurosurg 64:427, 1986

72. Mundinger F: Stereotaktische Operationen am Gehirn—Grundlagen, Indikationen, Resultate. Stuttgart, Hippokrates, 1975

73. Mundinger F, Uhl H: über die Genauigkeit der röntgenologischen Zielpunktbestimmung bei stereotaktischen Operationen. Fortschr Rontgenstr 103:419, 1965

74. Riechert T, Mundinger F: Beschreibung und Anwendung eines Zielgerätes für stereotaktische Hirnoperationen (2. Modell). Acta Neurochir 3:308, 1956

75. Riechert T, Mundinger F: Stereotaktische Geräte. in Schal-

tenbrand G, Bailey P (eds): Einführung in die stereotaktischen Operationen mit einem Atlas des menschlichen Gehirns. Stuttgart, Georg Thieme, 1959

76. Birg W, Mundinger F: Computer calculations of target parameters for a stereotactic apparatus. Acta Neurochir 29:123, 1973

77. Birg W, Mundinger F: Computer programmes for stereotactic neurosurgery. Confin Neurol 36:326, 1974

78. Birg W, Mundinger F: Direct target point determination for stereotactic brain operation from CT data and the calculation of setting parameters for polar-coordinate stereotactic devices. Appl Neurophysiol 45:387, 1982

79. Birg W, Mundinger F: CT-guided stereotaxy with the Riechert-Mundinger apparatus for biopsy and interstitial curietherapy of intracranial processes. J Neuro-oncol 2:280, 1984

80. Birg W, Mundinger F, Klar M: Computer assistance for stereotactic brain operations. Adv Neurosurg 4:287, 1977

81. Birg W, Mundinger F, Mohadjer M, et al: X-Ray and magnetic resonance stereotaxy for functional and nonfunctional neurosurgery. Appl Neurophysiol 48:22, 1985

82. Mundinger F, Birg W: CT-Aided stereotaxy for functional neurosurgery and deep brain implants. Acta Neurochir 56:245, 1981

83. Mundinger F, Birg W: CT-Stereotaxy in the clinical routine. Neurosurg Rev 7:219, 1984

84. Mundinger F, Birg W: Stereotactic biopsy of intracranial processes. Acta Neurochir Suppl 33:219, 1984

85. Mundinger F, Weigel K, Fürmaier R, et al: CT and MRI diagnosis of intracranial tumors compared with the results of stereotactic biopsy, in Poeck K, Freund HJ, Gänshirt H (eds): Neurology. Berlin, Springer Verlag, 1986, pp 469–476, 1986

86. Gruskin P, Saeger KL, Carberry JN: Neuropathology of stereotactic biopsies, in Dyck P (ed): Stereotactic Biopsy and Brachytherapy of Brain Tumors. Baltimore, University Park Press, 1983, pp 63–78

87. Mundinger F: CT-Stereotactic biopsy of brain tumors, in Voth D, Gutjahr P, Langmaid C (eds): Tumors of the Central Nervous System in Infancy and Childhood. Berlin, Springer Verlag, 1982, pp 234–246

88. Mundinger F: CT stereotactic biopsy for optimizing the therapy of intracranial processes. Acta Neurochir Suppl 35:70, 1985

89. Powell M, Olney J, Darling J, et al: Correlation of target site with histology and cell culture in CT-directed stereotactic biopsy. J Neuro-oncol 2:275, 1984

90. Apuzzo MLJ, Sabshin JK: Computed tomographic guidance stereotaxis in the management of intracranial mass lesions. Neurosurgery 12:277, 1983

91. Bergstroem M, Greitz T, Steiner I: An approach to stereotaxic radiography. Acta Neurochir 54:157, 1980

92. Hoefer T, Mundinger F, Birg W, et al: Computer calculations to localize subcortical targets in plane x-rays for stereotactic neurosurgery. Confin Neurol 36:334, 1974

93. Salcman M, Sewchand W, Amin P, et al: CT-Guided stereotactic surgery and interstitial irradiation for glial tumors. J Neuro-oncol 2:282, 1984

94. Kiessling M, Kleihues P, Gessaga E, et al: Morphology of intracranial tumors and adjacent brain structures following interstitial iodine-125 radiotherapy. Acta Neurochir Suppl 33:281, 1984

95. Kleihues P, Volk B, Anagnostopoulos J, et al: Morphologic evaluation of stereotactic brain tumor biopsies. Acta Neurochir Suppl 33:171, 1984

96. Mohadjer M, Ruh E, Hiltl DM, et al: CT-Stereotactic evacuation and fibrinolysis of hypertensive intracerebral hemorrhages. Presented at the 8th International Congress on Fibrinolysis, Vienna, August 25–29, 1986

97. Mundinger F, Sauerwein K: "GammaMed," ein neues Gerätzur interstitiellen, nur einige Minuten dauernden Bestrahlung von Hirngeschwülsten mit Radioisotopen, auch intraoperativ anwendbar. Acta Radiol 5:48, 1966

98. Mundinger F: Rationale and methods of interstitial iridium-192 brachy-curietherapy and iridium 192 or iodine 125 protracted long term irradiation, in Szikla G ((ed): Stereotactic Cerebral Irradiation. INSERM Symposium No. 12. Amsterdam, Elsevier/North Holland, 1079, pp 101–106

99. Birg W, Schneider J, Bauer S, et al: An interactive program system for the stereotactic interstitial implantation of radionuclides in brain tumors, in Szikla G (ed): Stereotactic Cerebral Irradiation. INSERM Symposium No. 12. Amsterdam, Elsevier/North Holland, 1979, pp 77–80

100. Dutreix A, Marinello G, Wambersie A: Dosimétrie en Curiethérapie. Paris, Masson, 1982

101. Pierquin B: Précis de Curiethérapie. Paris, Masson, 1964

102. Pierquin B: The destiny of brachytherapy in oncology. AJR 127:495, 1976 103. Pierquin B, et al: The Paris system in interstitial radiation therapy. Acta Radiol Oncol 17:33, 1978

104. Selker R, Eddy M, Anderson L: A method of dosimetry planning and implantation of interstitial irradiation in glioma patients utilizing I-125. J Neuro-oncol 2:281, 1984

105. Sommermeyer K, Mittermaier L: Untersuchungenüber die Dosisverteilung in der Umgebung reiner Gammapräparate mit dem Fluoreszenzdosimeter. Strahlentherapie 102:78, 1957

Stereotactic Radiosurgery with the Cobalt 60 Gamma Unit in the Surgical Treatment of Intracranial Tumors and Arteriovenous Malformations

Ladislau Steiner

STEREOTACTIC RADIOSURGERY was defined by Leksell[1,2] as a technique for the destruction of intracranial targets without opening the skull using single high doses of ionizing radiation in stereotactically directed narrow beams. The current definition is the use of a "single high dose of radiation to destroy an intracranial target or to induce in the target a certain biologic effect." Leksell deliberately used the term radiosurgery to stress that the method had little to do with conventional radiotherapy and that although beams of ionizing radiation replace the scalpel or diathermy, the technique is nonetheless surgery.

Radiosurgery employs accurate stereotactic localization of the target and steep dose gradients that match the periphery of the target tissue volume. This allows delivery of a single high dose to the target with minimal involvement of surrounding nontarget brain substance. Radiosurgery is a one-session procedure, and the dose given in a single sitting is biologically equivalent to a three-fold higher fractionated dose.

The concept of biologic radiosensitivity is much less important in radiosurgery than in radiotherapy. Instead, the physical factors that determine the sharp dose gradients in large measure define the magnitude of the allowed dosage.

After initial tests with x-rays, heavy particle beams from a synchro-cyclotron, and photons from a linear accelerator,[3,4] with the intent of devising a simple and practical tool, the Gamma Unit was developed 1968. The Gamma Unit is a stereotactic device with multiple ^{60}Co sources in which both the sources and the target are rigidly fixed to ensure high mechanical accuracy.

Soon after the Gamma Unit was introduced, its application, which initially consisted of functional brain surgery, was expanded to include the treatment of arteriovenous malformations (AVMs) and tumors. The small disk-shaped lesions produced by the first prototype were inadequate for the new applications, and subsequently, three generations of Gamma Units with cylindrical apertures and wider distribution were developed. The main characteristics for all these devices are the sharp boundaries of the irradiated field and a high degree of spatial accuracy.

The source of radiation in the Gamma Unit are ^{60}Co rods, each of which is 20 mm in length and 1 mm in diameter, distributed over a segment of hemisphere and heavily shielded in the core of the apparatus (Figures 44-1 and 44-2). The number of 60Co rods varies in the different prototypes of the Gamma Unit between 179 to 202. The second component of the Gamma Unit is a collimator system with an outer section enclosed in the central body of the unit and an inner section called the collimator helmet provided with an arrangement for the suspension of the head of the patient (Figure 44-2). The size and form of the apertures of the collimators determines the size and shape of the cross-sections of the beams. The isodose configurations obtained with three available collimators are illustrated in Figure 44-3. By using a number of interchangeable collimator helmets with different apertures, single or overlapping fields of radiation of required size and configuration can be tailored to match the target volume. The stereotactic frame is fixed on the head of the patient (Figure 44-4).

Following visualization of the target by one or several appropriate stereotactic imaging techniques, the x, y, and z coordinates of the target are computed and the head of the patient is positioned in the collimator helmet according to the coordinates (Figure 44-5). The target is always situated in the center of the collimator helmet where the beams converge. A remote control hydraulic system moves the table with the patient in and out of the unit.

For further details concerning the Gamma Unit, the radiosurgical procedure, and the pre-, peri- and posttreatment management of the patient, see previously published papers.[2,5–9] In this chapter experience with the radiosurgical treatment of intracranial tumors and AVMs is summarized.

INTRACRANIAL TUMORS

CRANIOPHARYNGIOMA

Stereotactic radiosurgery is an appealing alternative to conventional radiotherapy, permitting precise irradiation that is limited to the tumor. To date we have treated 36 craniopharyngiomas using radiosurgery.

OPERATIVE NEUROSURGICAL TECHNIQUES
ISBN 0-8089-1862-1

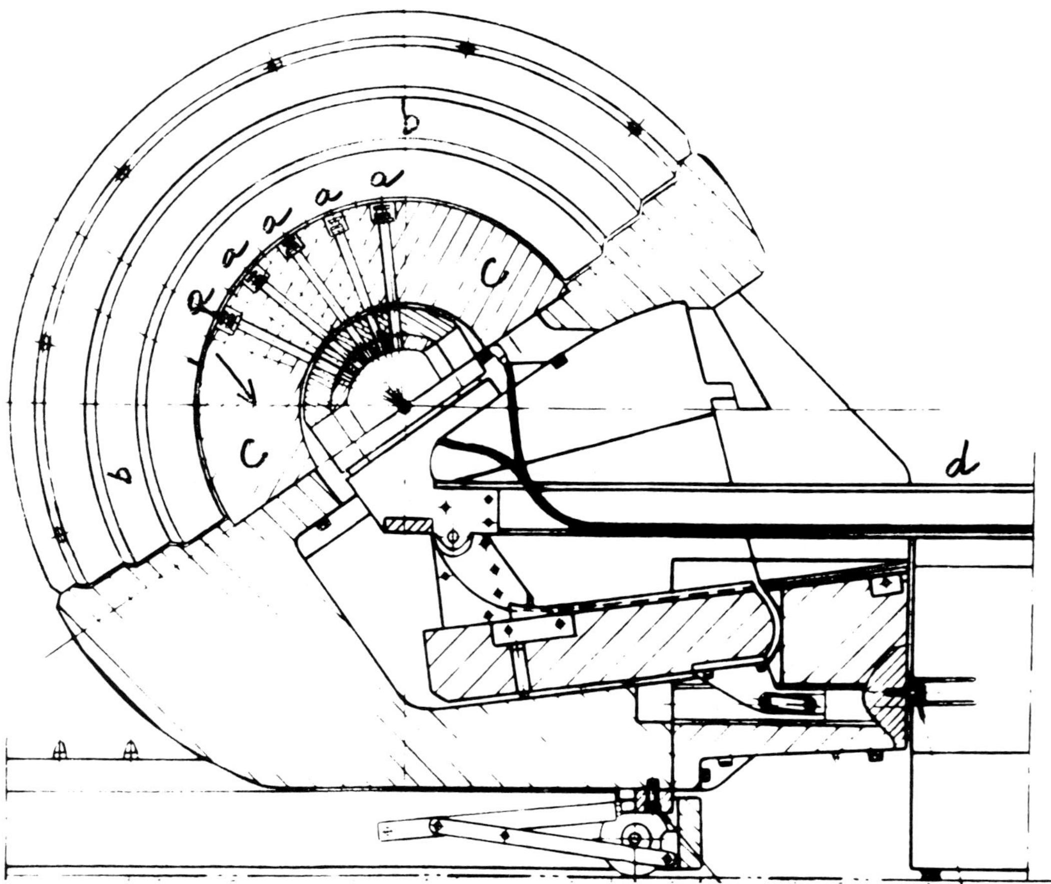

Fig. 44-1. Schematic drawing of the stereotactic ^{60}Co Gamma Unit. a = cobalt 60 sources; b = the hemispheric core made of shielding material and containing the outer segment of the collimator system; c = inner collimator or collimator helmet with a device for suspending the patient's head; d = moveable operating table; arrows = central beam.

Backlund[7] reported the results from combining intracystic radionuclide treatment with radiosurgery to solid tumor portions in 11 patients (approximately 15 percent of all craniopharyngiomas treated in the Department of Neurosurgery of Karolinska Hospital between 1968 and 1979). In 3 patients radiosurgery was the primary treatment. The diagnosis was verified by open or stereotactic biopsy.

In the cases of tumors with a cystic component, radiosurgery was applied only to the solid portion of tumor after shrinkage of the cyst by the intracystic injection of radiocolloid ^{90}Y.

The target dose varied between 20 and 50 Gy and the dose at the periphery of the tumor was limited to 10 Gy. In a few cases, however, it was no higher than 2 or 3 Gy. The average period of observation to date has been 4 years with some patients being followed for 10 years. The usual course after the irradiation is a progressive decrease in the size of the tumor and (Figure 44-6) regression of clinical symptoms associated with the decrease in the bulk of the tumor. The majority of the patients are in good condition and working.

It was difficult to establish a definite cause-effect relationship for symptoms that occurred after irradiation in a young girl who had had open surgery previously and had impaired sight in her right eye (finger counting). This improved following injection of radiocolloid into a large cyst and the visual acuity of her affected eye was 20/100 at the time of radiosurgery. One year later she became blind in the same eye and after another 6 months she developed a left-sided transitory oculomotor paresis as well as a transitory hypothalamic syndrome. Subsequently, a progressive recovery occurred and the patient is now well except for right-sided amaurosis. Backlund suspected that the pronounced shrinkage of the tumor may have induced untoward effects as a result of traction; however, a late radiation effect cannot be excluded as a cause of the patient's deterioration. At present we feel radiosurgery permits precision irradiation of the solid component of a craniophayngioma, although to date it has not been possible to determine the optimal single dose necessary to induce necrosis of a solid craniopharyngioma. It seems that a peripheral dose of 10 Gy is sufficient for satisfactory results. The steepest gradient of the radiation field should coincide with the periphery of the tumor.

HYPERSECRETING PITUITARY TUMORS

Pituitary Dependent Cushing's Disease

Since 1975 our neurosurgical unit has treated 90 patients with Cushing's disease using the Gamma Unit. Part of this experience has been reported by Rähn and by Degerblad.[10–12] In 76 percent of cases clinical remission was obtained using a single dose of radiation of 70 Gy in adults and of 60 Gy in children. The dexamethasone suppression test usually showed that a previously poor or absent suppressibility was more pronounced following treatment. When the suppression test

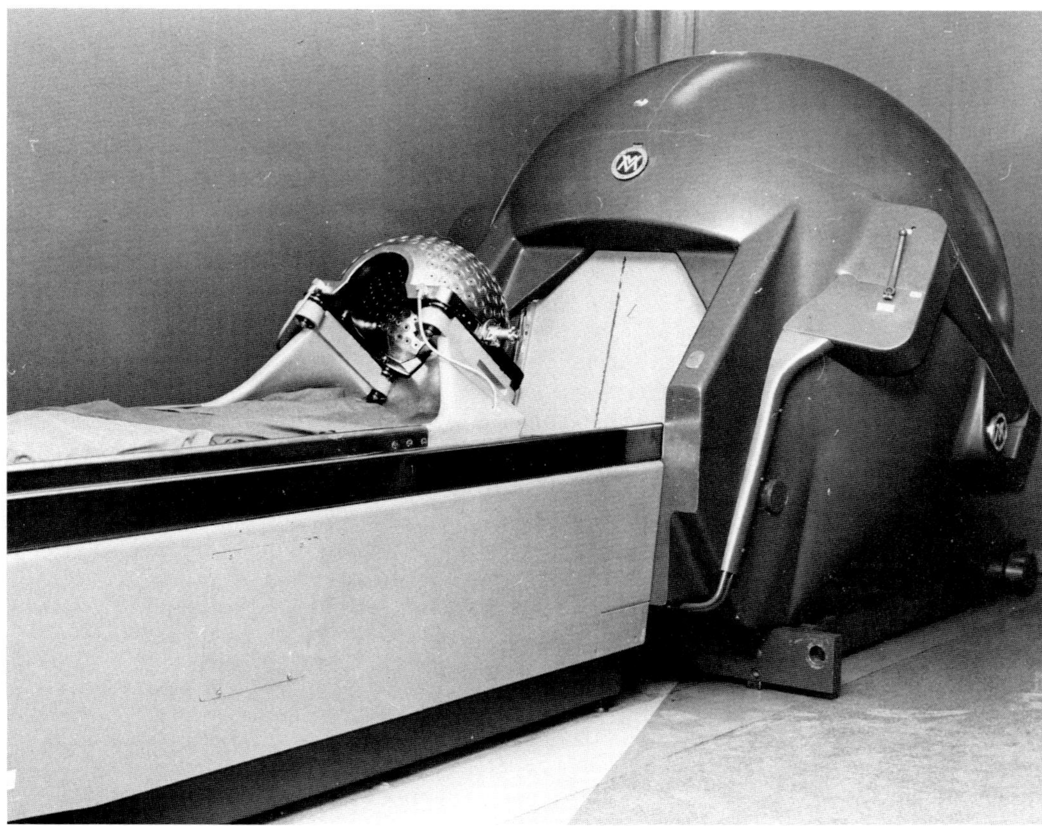

Fig. 44-2. The stereotactic ^{60}Co Gamma Unit.

was followed by ACTH-stimulation, a preoperative increased cortisol secretion level decreased to a normal rise in the plasma cortisol level after ACTH administration. The basal plasma cortisol levels were within the normal range after treatment.

In a long-term study[12] of 29 adult patients observed for 3 to 9 years after their irradiation, clinical remission with normal urinary cortisol levels occurred in 14 cases following the first treatment. Fourteen patients improved clinically with a decrease in the urinary cortisol level. One patient did not respond to the irradiation. Of the 14 patients who were somewhat improved, 11 were irradiated a second time 0.4 to 2.2 years after the first treatment. Two patients underwent adrenalectomy and one did not receive further treatment. Following the second irradiation, remission occurred in 4 patients, and 7 patients did not improve. Six of them received a third irradiation 0.4 to 2.4 years after the second treatment. Remission occurred in 2 and improvement in 1 case. Remission was obtained in 2 patients after a fourth irradiation. Remission after radiosurgery therefore occurred in this series in 22 of 29 (76 percent) of the patients and 2 of 29 patients improved.

In addition to these 29 patients, 6 patients with Cushing's disease treated by radiosurgery had an observation time of less than 3 years. Two of these underwent clinical remission after one irradiation. Four patients improved.

Recurrences were not observed in any of the 24 patients with clinical remission; however, in 12 patients pituitary deficiency developed 4 months to 7 years after irradiation. ACTH deficiency, which was noted in 9 cases, was usually the first symptom, with TSH deficiency in 2 cases and TSH and LH-FSH deficiency in 4 patients. One patient had a TSH deficiency only. This series did not include children, and growth hormone levels were not evaluated.

The parameters of the irradiation at the second, third, and fourth treatments were not given in the study and information was not provided concerning the relationship between the incidence of pituitary deficiency and the cumulative dose involved in repeat treatments. We presume that pituitary deficiency occurs because important parts of the sella contents are included in the irradiated field. Confronted with the difficulties in visualizing small pituitary tumors, Rähn based the localization of the tumor on the bone changes in the sella and found the predilection site of ACTH-producing adenomas to be the mid-anterior part of the adenohypophysis. Rähn did not trust the criteria for the localization and used fields of radiation that covered a larger part of the sella contents in order to treat a microadenoma. This lack in precision of the localization often led to failures and the need to repeat the radiation.

To decrease the risk of pituitary deficiency after radiosurgery, Bunge, Chinella and Guevara[13] in the Centro de Radiocirurgia, Clinica Del Sol, Buenos Aires, use stereotactic CT scans for the localization and the 4-mm-diameter collimator for the radiation of microadenomas, which produces a lesion measuring 60 mm^3. Two overlapping fields include a tissue volume of 100 mm^3 compared with a 520-mm^3 volume if the collimator with a diameter of 8 mm is used, as when Rähn irradiated patients with Cushing's disease.

Although a wealth of reports exist on the possibility of visualizing pituitary microadenomas by CT scan,[14,15,16] technical factors make the interpretation of these images ambiguous, a problem that the advent of magnetic resonance imaging may reverse, thereby allowing visualization of pituitary microade-

1.2

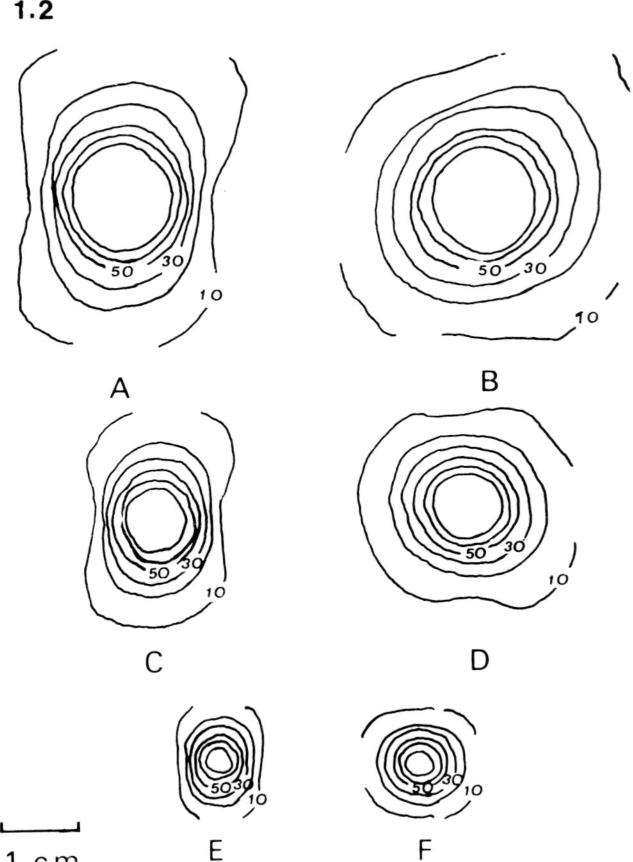

Fig. 44-3. Dose distributions obtained with the (A, B) 14 mm, (C, D) 8 mm, and (E, F) 4 mm collimators. (A, C, E) Frontal views; (B, D, F) transverse views.

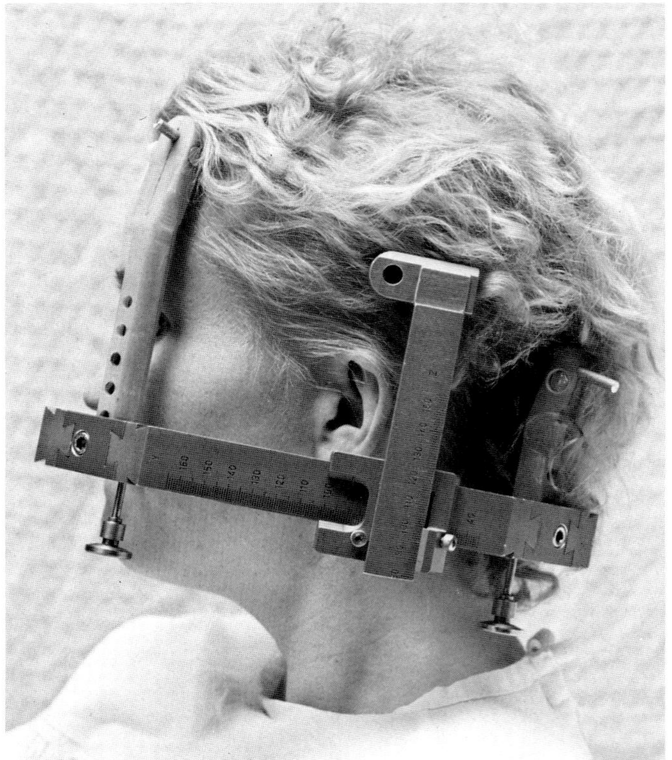

Fig. 44-4. A Patient with the stereotactic frame.

nomas and the use of the smallest collimator size in most cases to better match the geometry of the radiation field to the limits of the tumor. Until these technical problems have been resolved, radiosurgery of microadenomas should be restricted to cases in which the identification of the tumor is unequivocal and to high-risk surgical patients.

NELSON'S SYNDROME

Backlund reported on 3 cases of Nelson's syndrome treated by radiosurgery. In 2 cases 50 to 70 Gy was delivered to a target point at the center of the anterior lobe of the pituitary. In a third case, the maximum dose was placed in the right part of the anterior lobe. Twenty-five to 30 months later the hyperpigmentation seen in this disorder was markedly reduced in 2 patients and disappeared completely in 1 patient and the laboratory findings normalized. A small unilateral visual field defect occurred 1 year after the treatment in a patient who had received 70 Gy of irradiation. A follow-up encephalogram revealed that the volume of the sellar contents had decreased and that there had been an increase in the herniation of the suprasellar cisterns into the sella.

ACROMEGALY

Pituitary microadenoma resulting in acromegaly is a disorder treatable by radiosurgery. Our experience in the Department of Neurosurgery in Stockholm and the experience of the Clinica Del Sol, Buenos Aires[13] prove this disorder is curable if the tumor causing it is small, whereas the results of such treatment seem to be less favorable among larger tumors.

In most cases, an early transient improvement of the acromegalic symptoms occurs and in isolated cases the growth hormone values are lowered. Delayed improvement can occur after a hiatus of several years. In a number of cases, hypopituitarism was observed.

TUMORS IN THE PINEAL REGION

Tumors in the region of the pineal gland and the quadrigeminal plate, if of the appropriate size and shape, can be treated by radiosurgery, irrespective of their histologic character. Among these cases stereotactic biopsy should always precede treatment. Backlund[7,17] reported 3 pineocytomas, 2 ependymomas, 3 astrocytomas, and 1 medulloblastoma subjected to radiosurgery. The average tumor diameter among these cases varied between 1 and 3 cm and target doses of 20 to 75 Gy were delivered to the lesions. The average duration of follow-up was 5 years. In 3 pineocytomas and in 2 cases in which the biopsy had failed to provide the histologic diagnosis, the therapeutic results were excellent. In 1 ependymoma and in 2 astrocytomas, the results were also good 1 to 3 years after the treatment. One ependymoma and 1 astrocytoma increased in size following treatment. A patient with a medulloblastoma and a patient with a tumor erroneously classified as a pineocytoma died 2 and 3 years, respectively, after treatment.

Bunge's[14] results in Buenos Aires confirmed the results from our institution.

Benign tumors of the pineal region should be treated by radiosurgery whereas malignant tumors of the pineal region should be treated by conventional radiotherapy. However, if the size and the shape of the malignant tumor permits the use of

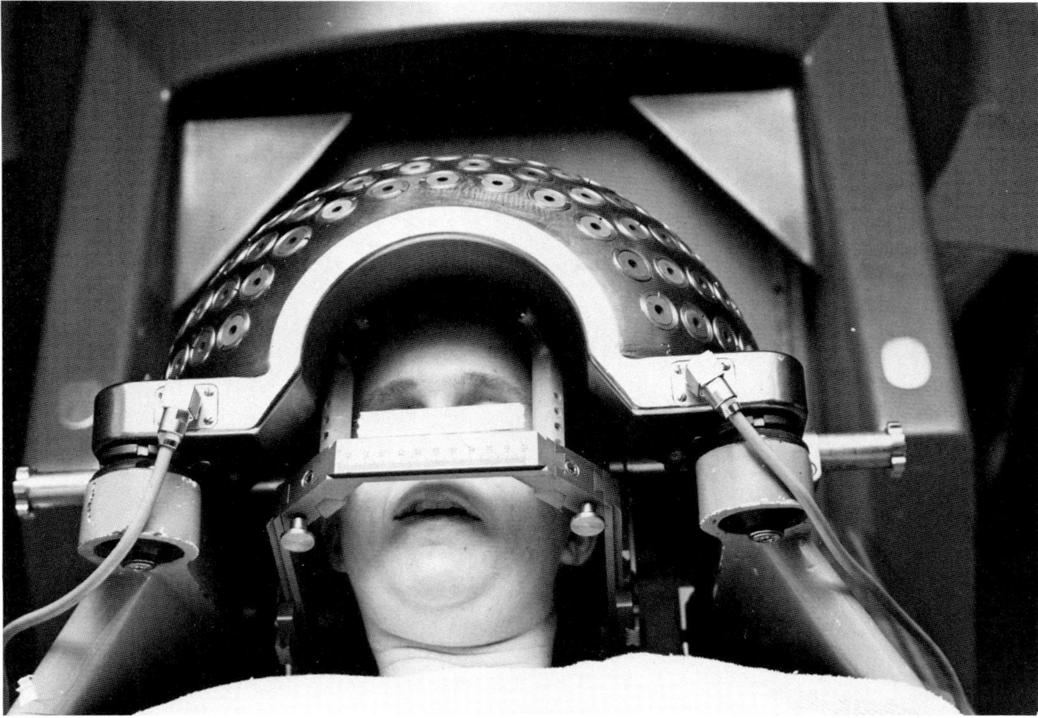

Fig. 44-5.　Patient's head positioned in the collimator helmet according to the x, y, and z coordinates.

radiosurgery this is probably advantageous because the results are comparable with those of radiotherapy without the side-effects of the latter. Radiosurgery has the additional advantage that treatment is completed in one day instead of several weeks.

INTRACRANIAL MENINGIOMAS

Over 40 intracranially situated meningiomas to date have been treated by radiosurgery in the departments of Neurosurgery, Karolinska Hospital, Stockholm, and Centro de Neurocirurgia, Clinica del Sol, Buenos Aires. Meningiomas ranging in diameter from 10 to 30 mm were treated using one or multiple overlapping fields of irradiation. The aim was to deliver 20 or 25 Gy to the periphery of the tumor, although in order to avoid damage of the adjacent cranial nerves this dosage was sometimes lowered. If possible, the arterial feeders of the tumor were included in the 90 percent of the isodose configuration. Both stereotactic CT scanning and stereotactic angiograms were performed in order to plan the radiosurgical lesions. Six to 12 months after treatment decreased contrast enhancement was observed in the center of a few of the tumors. Shrinkage ranging from a few millimeters to two thirds of the size of the tumor and improvement in the neurologic deficits occurred in a few patients within 1 to 2 years, but usually the size of the tumor did not increase. Only long-term follow-up will reveal whether the radiosurgery actually stopped the growth of the tumor.

A specific subcategory of meningiomas are those involving the cavernous sinus. These tumor should be managed by being explored by open operation, and the feasibility of their extirpation with low morbidity should be assessed. With the exception of a few cases, total extirpation with reasonable risks is not possible. Radiosurgery should be carried out on residual tumor tissue following maximal reduction of the bulk of the tumor without endangering the cranial nerves. In addition, high surgical risk patients harboring meningiomas can be treated by radiosurgery alone.

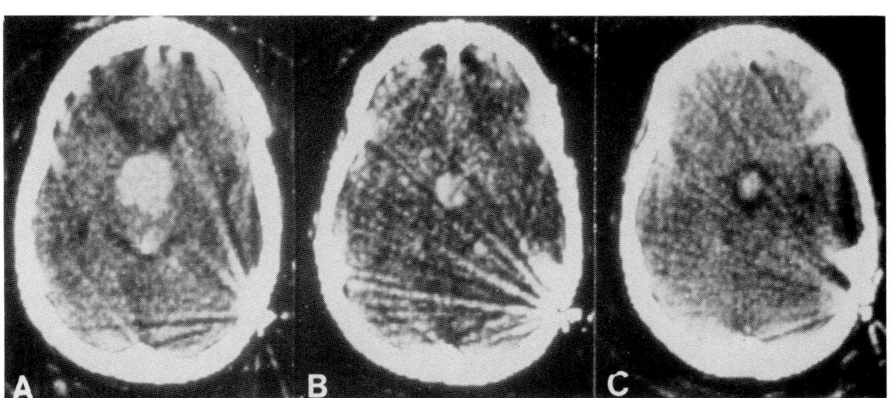

Fig. 44-6.　Craniopharyngioma. CT scans obtained before (A) and after (B, C) radiosurgery showing progressive decreases in the size of the tumor.

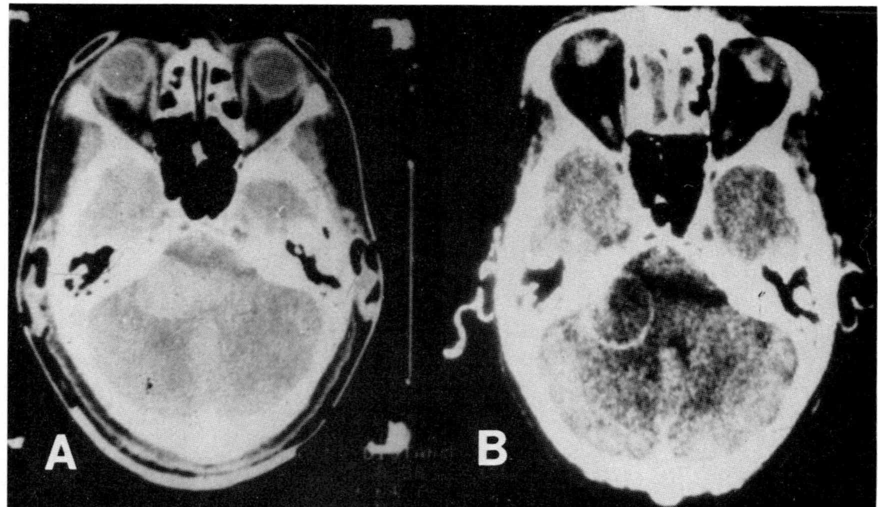

Fig. 44-7.   Acoustic neurinoma. CT scans obtained before (A) and after (B) treatment. Note the transitory loss of contrast enhancement in the tumor 6 months after treatment.

ACOUSTIC NEURINOMAS

In 1969, Leksell asked me to assist him in the treatment of a patient with acoustic neurinoma using radiosurgery for the first time in the treatment of such lesions. I participated in the procedure without enthusiasm, since I felt dubious about the potential value of this technique in the treatment of acoustic neurinoma. In a subsequent publication a short footnote acknowledged my help with this case. In the intervening 18 years Leksell, Noren, D. Leksell, Lindquist, and Arndt[8,9,18] refined the techniques for the visualization of these tumors, introduced CT and MRI scanning for the determination of stereotactic coordinates,[1,7] improved dose planning and stereotactic technique, and accumulated a wealth of knowledge concerning the response of the tumor and the adjacent tissues to single high dose radiation. The total experience based on the experience with 160 patients treated in Stockholm and of 17 cases treated by Bunge in Clinica Del Sol, Buenos Aires, is now available for analysis.

The data presented in this chapter are based on personal communications with Noren and summarize his experience in 110 patients with 115 acoustic neurinomas treated by radiosurgery who have also had recent detailed neurologic, radiologic, audiologic follow-up. The follow-up period ranged from 0.5 to 12.8 years (mean 4.0 years).

The tumors selected for treatment had a diameter of up to 30 mm. Beyond this size, the dose distribution may become inhomogeneous. Since the dose gradient is steepest at the 90-to*50 percent of isodose configuration, this gradient was made to coincide with the periphery of the tumor. The intracanalicular portion is also included in the radiation field.

Doses of 18 to 25 Gy to the periphery of the tumor are considered optimal. The maximum dose within the tumor usually ranges from 22 Gy to 50 Gy, which are dosages that seem to be tolerated by the critical structures surrounding the tumor.

Computed tomographic follow-up performed in the 6 to 24

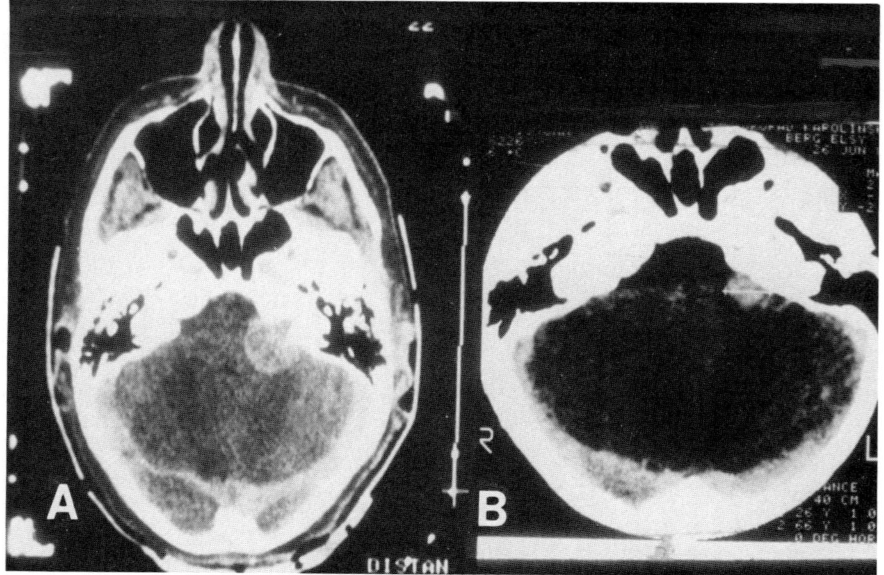

Fig. 44-8.   Acoustic neurinoma. CT scans obtained before (A) and 1 year after (B) radiosurgery. Note the significant decrease in the size of the tumor.

months following the treatment revealed in 60 percent of the cases a transitory loss of contrast enhancement in the center of the tumor (Figure 44-7). This did not seem to be related to the pattern of the subsequent radiologic findings. The tumor either remained unchanged or decreased or increased independently of the initial changes in contrast enhancement. Among unilateral tumors, progressive shrinkage occurred in 45 cases (49 percent) (Figure 44-8); an increase in size was noticed in 8 cases (9 percent), and no changes were observed in 38 cases (42 percent). Of the 24 tumors associated with neurofibromatosis, 6 (25 percent) decreased in size, 10 (42 percent) remained unchanged and 8 (33 percent) increased in size. There was no surgical mortality related to the treatment.

UNTOWARD EFFECTS FOLLOWING RADIOSURGERY OF ACOUSTIC NEURINOMA

Peritumoral Edema

Peritumoral edema developed in 5 percent of the cases of acoustic neuroma treated by radiosurgery and this caused varying degrees of cerebellar symptoms and trigeminal nerve dysfunction, which subsided 6 to 12 months after the onset.

Hydrocephalus

Communicating hydrocephalus, manifest either before treatment or developing within 1 to 2 years after irradiation occurred in 10 percent of these patients. Although not directly related to radiosurgery the hydrocephalus probable arose because the tumor bulk was not eradicated and a continued level of increased CSF protein persisted after radiosurgery which may contribute to the development of the hydrocephalus.

Cranial Nerve Abnormalities

Varying degrees of facial weakness occurred in 15 percent of patients within 4 to 15 months after radiosurgery, a problem which improved within 6 months of onset. In severe cases, synkinesias appeared during the process of reinnervation. There is close correlation between the incidence of facial palsy and the maximum dose of radiation. Palsy occured after doses of 40 Gy, occasionally (one case) after a dose below 30 Gy, and was not seen with a dose of less than 27 Gy.

Deterioration of Hearing

In most cases, there was a tendency toward slow deterioration of hearing after the radiosurgical treatment of acoustic neuroma. The cochlear impairment is presumably the result of vascular insufficiency. One year after treatment, 27 percent of the patients demonstrated a change in hearing equal to or less than 5 dB and a discriminiation score equal to the value before treatment.[18] Significant improvement of hearing was observed in 2 patients and deafness occurred in 20 percent. The remaining patients exhibited a deterioration of the hearing thresholds and/or lowering of the discrimination score. In one case with bilateral neurinomas, sudden and irreversible deafness occurred within 24 hours of the irradiation. A deterioration of hearing was also noted during follow-up in most cases. If we accept a limited hearing loss of 20 dB pure tone average or less compared with the preoperative value as "preserved hearing," 56, 54, and 28 percent were included in this group 1, 2, and 6 years after radiosurgery.

Damage to the Trigeminal Nerve

In 18 percent of the cases, hypesthesia was observed in the fifth nerve distribution 6 to 9 months after treatment. In 5 patients treated early in the series, the hypesthesia was severe, irreversible, and in some cases, was associated with deafferentation pain syndrome. These complications were related to the dosage; the worst side-effects occurred when doses of 50 to 100 Gy were given. Total or almost total regression of the symptoms occurred after 1 year in the mild cases.

It is currently premature to predict the future role of radiosurgery in the treatment of acoustic neurinomas. All the facts necessary to allow for such a prediction are not yet available. The significance of the lack in change of tumor size after radiosurgery is still unknown. It might not necessarily mean that the treatment arrested the growth. To establish whether or not it is the normal behavior of an acoustic neurinoma, the growth rate of the specific tumor before the treatment should be known. The observations of Newman et al.[19] and of Hirsch[20] suggest that in the long term, acoustic neurinomas show signs of growth. If it were proved that tumor growth is arrested following radiosurgery, the group of patients in whom tumor shrinkage occurred together with the group in whom there were no changes in the size of the neurinoma after radiosurgery would constitute 86 percent of the all the cases. Moreover, if the cases associated with neurofibromatosis are excluded, 91 percent of the neurinomas responded to radiosurgery. Should tumor growth occur in the long term, radiosurgery would appear to be a less attractive treatment alternative.

To have any significant share in the management of acoustic neurinoma, radiosurgery must match the results obtained by microsurgery. Preservation of the function of the facial nerve and preservation of hearing are the most important problems in the microsurgical treatment of acoustic neurinomas. While facial nerve function never constitutes a problem in radiosurgery, since the risk of weakness is currently only 3 percent and when it does occur is transitory, the preservation of hearing remains a challenge even though the results with this technique compare favorably with the results obtained by the microsurgical excision of these tumors. Improvements in radiologic imaging and the increasing experience in dosimetry will probably increase the number of cases in which hearing is preserved following radiosurgery for acoustic neuroma.

Intracranial tumors of small and moderate size, if accurately delimited, can be treated by single high dose irradiation. However, the traditional criteria for assessment of the results cannot be applied. Radiosurgery does not eradicate a meningioma or an acoustic tumor since it only causes them to shrink or arrests their growth. This can be obtained without mortality and with a low incidence of side-effects if the basic principle of radiosurgery—a steep dose gradient at the borderline between the tumor periphery and surrounding normal structures—is respected.

ARTERIOVENOUS MALFORMATIONS

Radiosurgery in the treatment arteriovenous malformations (AVMs) was initiated in 1970. Today, although the limits of the applicability of this technique to the problem of intracranial AVMs is still being defined, radiosurgery is an established therapeutic option to be used in selected cases.

Following Roentgen's discovery of x-rays there was intense interest in the application of this new modality in the treatment of AVMs. The enthusiasm waned as the results of surgery improved and because it was not possible to see results with radiotherapy. Since data concerning the treatment parameters are scarce in these case reports, one can only speculate about the dosimetric and localization factors used in the cases that resulted in failure. The reassessment of the potential value of irradiation in vascular malformations came about as a result of the increasing body of evidence that the cells constituting the vessel wall are responsive to ionizing radiation; their replicative or metabolic functions may be temporarily or definitively inhibited, and proliferation and formation of collagen may also occur. Perivascular or subendothelial edema, hemorrhages, thrombi, degeneration of endothelial cells, increased interstitial colloid deposits, and increased fibroblastic activity are followed by proliferation of endothelial cells and subendothelial connective tissue and the formation of collagen and hyaline in the subendothelial space. These progressive effects may culminate in the occlusion of the vascular lumen.

The second factor leading to the use of irradiation in the treatment of AVMs was the stereotactic Gamma Unit.

Based on a 17-year experience with over 600 cases, it is now possible to define the possibilities and limitations of radiosurgery in relation to the variables of the AVM and to the patients, and to the parameters of the procedure.[5,6,22–27]

PATIENT MATERIAL

Over 600 patients with intracranial AVMs have been treated by radiosurgery. These patients ranged in age from 4 to 70 years; their sex distribution was equal. Over 90 percent of these patients had intracranial hemorrhages: 4 percent of the patients had as their only symptom a seizure disorder. The remaining patients were hospitalized for headache, hydrocephalus, or exophthalmus. Included in this series are a number of high surgical risk patients, or cases with residual malformations following microsurgery or embolization referred for radiosurgery.

The AVMs were both supra- and infratentorial in location and a large number of them involved deep brain structures. In 8 cases, the malformation was situated in the brain stem, and in another group of cases the AVM surrounded a segment of the brain stem or involved only the tectum. Several dural AVMs and rare cases with cerebral-dural AVMs were also treated. A few patients had 2 AVMs or an AVM associated with a venous malformation. The volume of the AVMs treated ranged from 0.2 to 35 ml.

DECISION MAKING

Our treatment strategy for an AVM is based on the patient's clinical profile and initial symptoms, on the specific characteristics of the AVM, and what we now know about the natural history of this disease. The rate of rehemorrhage of an AVM is between 2 and 6 percent, while the risk of hemorrhage from an AVM that has not bled previously is 1.5 percent. The anticipated results of the therapeutic alternatives should be compared and should weigh heavily in the decision-making process. The neurosurgeon trained in both microsurgical and radiosurgical techniques can then select the most appropriate technique for each individual case.

Our strategy for treating AVMs is as follows. Standard microsurgical approaches and techniques are used to excise rupture AVMs situated in noneloquent areas of the brain if surgery is not contraindicated by the patient's general condition. Ruptured AVMs in eloquent areas and nonruptured AVMs in all parts of the brain that are of suitable size and configuration are treated by radiosurgery. Malformations that have not bled carry a relatively low risk for hemorrhage and have a high chance of being obliterated during the 1 to 2 years required for a total effect of radiosurgery to become apparent.

To date radiosurgery was usually carried out weeks to months after the hemorrhage; however, the idea of irradiating an AVM soon after it has bled and when it is surrounded by a hematoma is appealing because in this way less adjoining normal brain tissue is irradiated. Nevertheless, early cerebral angiography sometimes led to false-positive findings and the hematoma may influence the shape and size of the AVM and make the definition of the target volume difficult, although it is possible to avoid this pitfall by defining the target volume slightly beyond the visible boundaries of the malformation.

The most reliable way to cure an intracranial AVM is to eliminate the entire cluster of pathologic arteriovenous shunts: AVMs are permanently cured if all feeding vessels are occluded. Focused gamma beams can easily reach and obliterate feeding arteries anywhere within the skull. These ideas required modification when we came to realize that the feeding vessels of an AVM are often elusive and cannot always be visualized on the arterial angiograms. Furthermore, if visualized, their stereotactic coordinates must calculated from both the lateral and the anteroposterior views, but it is difficult to identify the same segment of a vessel on both angiographic projections, and a mistaken assessment will result in a therapeutic failure. If these technical difficulties can be solved, the logical targets for radiosurgery may prove to be both the cluster of pathologic shunting vessels and the feeding arteries. In this series, irradiation of the feeding vessels was carried out in a few cases only. More frequently the cluster of pathologic shunting vessels was partially covered while the feeding vessels together with part of the arteriovenous shunt were included in the radiation field.

TREATMENT PARAMETERS

Target doses ranging from 20 to 125 Gy in single or multiple overlapping fields have been tested. Since the periphery of the malformation is made to coincide with the steepest isodose gradient, i.e., at the 90–50 percent isodose configuration, the dose at the periphery was 10 to 62.5 Gy. It seems that a minimum dose of 20 to 25 Gy at the periphery gives the best chances for obliteration. The same dosage schedule is used in adults and children.

The interplay between dose and volume of the irradiated tissue is still not completely elucidated. Observations in cases with radiation-induced brain tissue changes indicate that the size of the tissue volume irradiated is more important for their occurrence than the dose factor. However, there is no clear-cut evidence that in large AVMs the desired obliterative effect can be obtained with a lower dose than that effective in smaller malformations.

In 20 cases in which the AVM did not respond to the first radiosurgical treatment, the procedure was repeated. The amount of radiation initially delivered was taken into account in planning the second treatment.

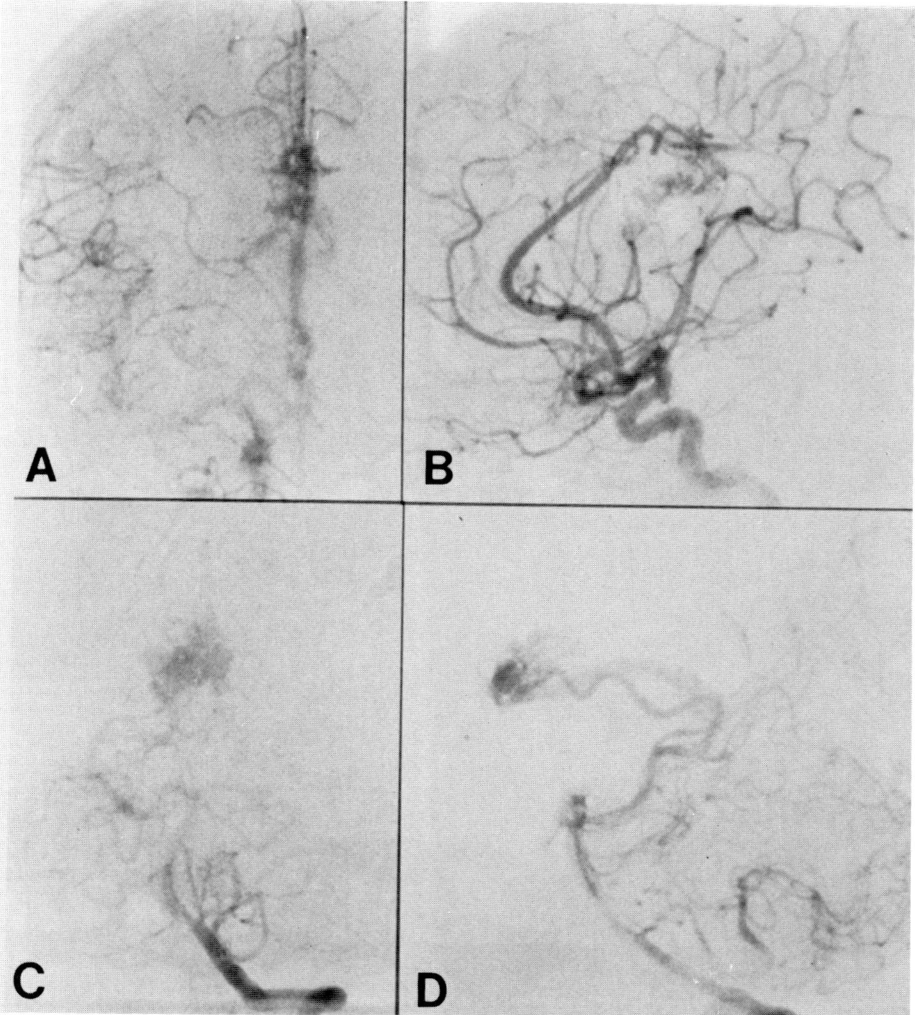

Fig. 44-9. An AVM in the septum pellucidum and in the wall of the lateral ventricle close to the right foramen of Monro fed by vessels from a wide right-sided pericallosal artery as well as from the posterior pericallosal artery and draining into the internal cerebral veins. The size of the malformation was 30 ml. (A, B) Carotid angiogram (frontal and lateral views) and (C, D) vertebral angiograms (frontal and lateral views) before treatment.

FOLLOW-UP

Starting 3 months after radiosurgery, repeated serial angiography is carried out. Our experience has led us to monitor the neuroradiologic changes in the early follow-up period by CT scan where the arteriovenous malformation is visible on the CT scan before radiosurgery. Computed tomographic scanning repeated every 6 months is also used to detect an asymptomatic radiation-induced brain injury, changes in the size and shape of the AVM, or development of hydrocephalus. Magnetic resonance imaging can also be used for follow-up. In those cases in which the AVM is not visualized by CT or MRI scanning before the treatment, annual digital subtraction angiography provides an alternative means of follow-up; however, even when the AVM is no longer revealed on CT or MRI scans or on digital substraction angiograms, serial arteriography is still performed to provide definitive proof of total obliteration of the AVM. Conventional angiography is important because the early filling of a tiny vein may be the sole indication of a persistent shunt and this can often be missed on digital angiograms.

Twenty patients were subjected to follow-up cerebral angiography 5 to 8 years after the obliteration of an intracranal arteriovenous malformation to assess the late effects of the irradiation on the cerebral vasculature.

In addition these follow-up studies included periodic neurologic examinations, reports from the patient and family concerning the patient's condition, social adjustment, working capacity and employment, repeated EEG studies, and psychological testing (especially in children).

Of the 600 patients treated by radiosurgery, over 100 did not have optimal treatment, i.e., only partial covering of the AVM, irradiation of all or part of the feeding vessels, or an inadequate dosage of radiation. Another 100 cases were treated less than 12 months ago. One-hundred-thirty-seven patients were treated more than 5 years ago and 332 patients more than 2 years ago.

FOLLOW-UP ANGIOGRAMS

An analysis of the angiograms performed subsequent to irradiation of the AVMs indicates that hemodynamic changes occur before changes are visible in the size or shape of the AVM. The flow-rate through the malformation and the size of the feeding arteries and outflow veins is decreased progressively and partial obliteration of the AVM can sometimes be

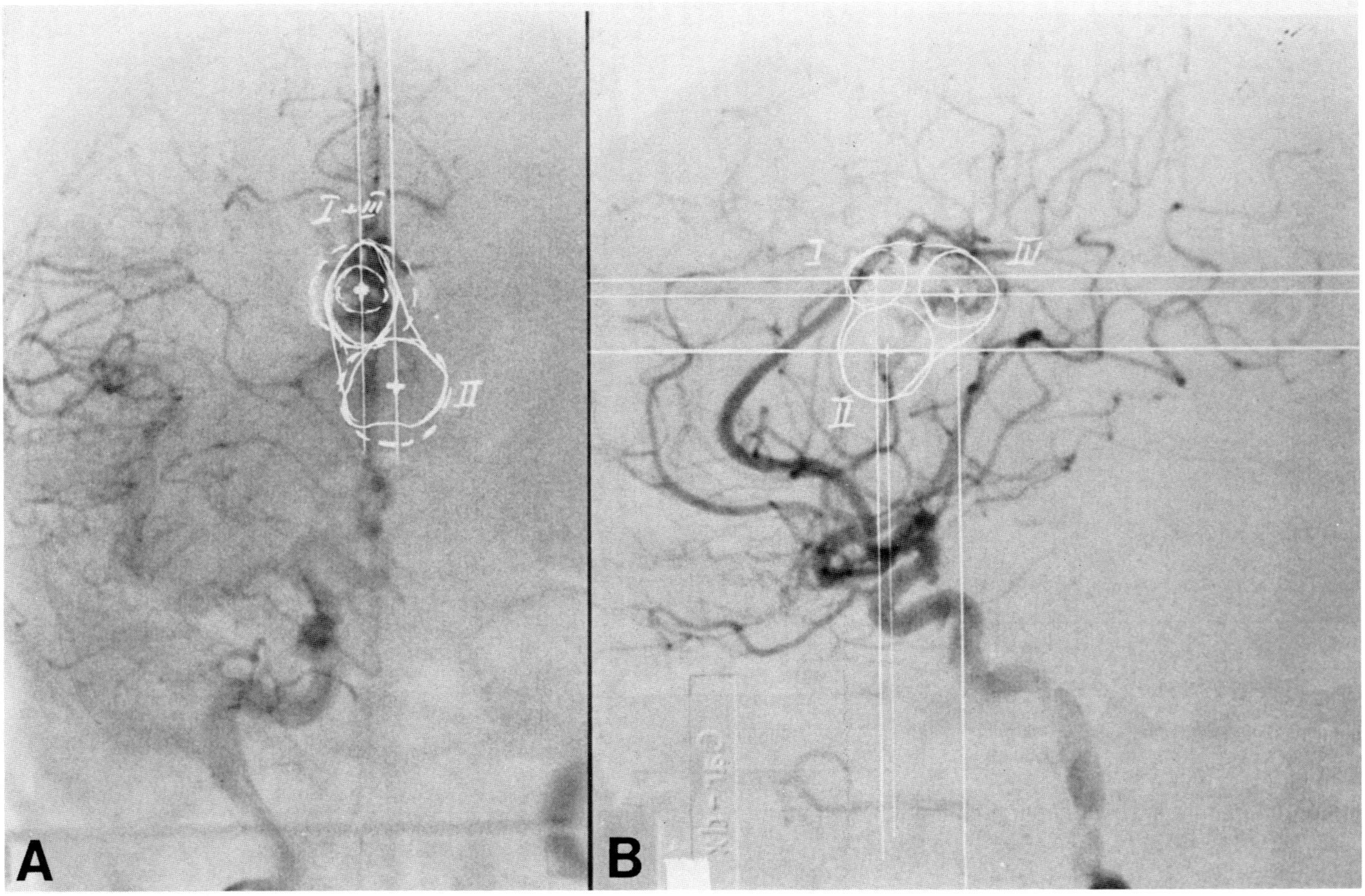

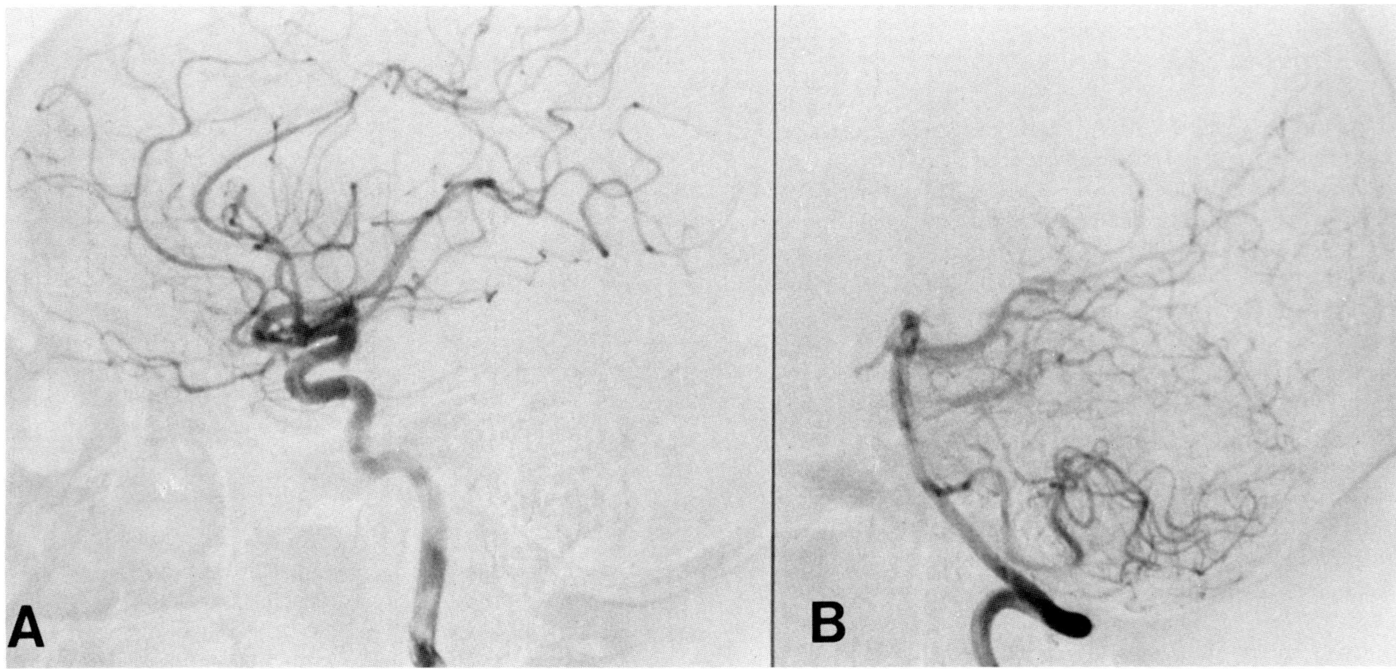

Fig. 44-10. The same AVM as in Figure 44-10. (A and B) Carotid angiograms (frontal and lateral views). During the radiosurgical treatment, the malformation was covered by 3 fields of radiation.

Fig. 44-11. The same AVM as in Figures 44-9 and 44-10. (A and B) Carotid and vertebral angiograms (lateral views). Three years after the treatment the malformation was totally obliterated.

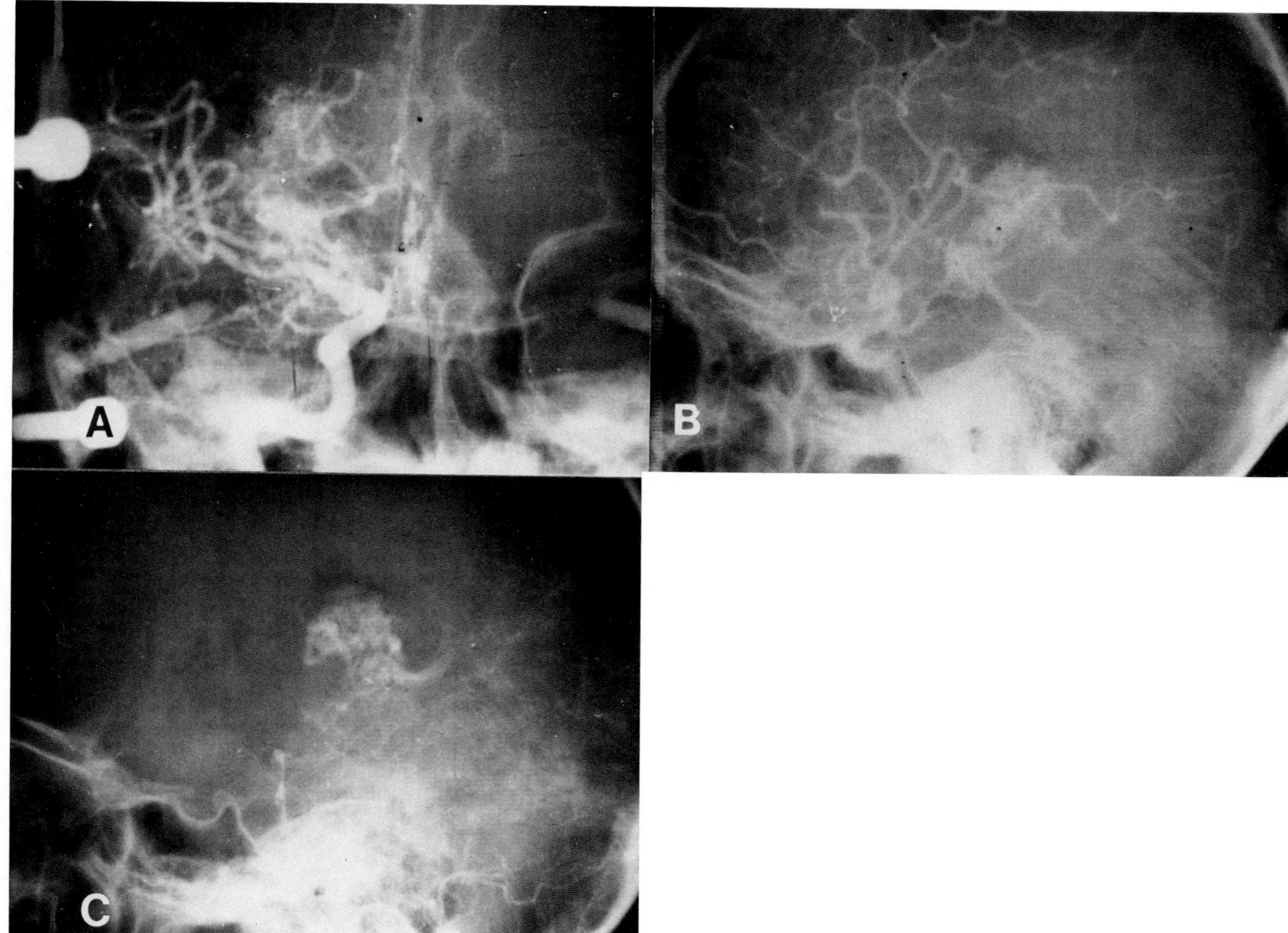

Fig. 44-12. (A and B) Carotid angiograms (frontal and lateral views) and (C) vertebral angiograms (lateral view) of an AVM in the right basal ganglia. The size of the malformation was 36 ml. (Courtesy of Dr. Hernan Bunge, Centro de Radiocirurgia, Clinica Del Sol, Buenos Aires.)

noticed a few months after treatment. The process continues over the subsequent months and at 2 years no filling of the malformation occurs in most cases responding to the radiation; although in a small group total obliteration of the AVM requires 3 to 5 years following radiosurgery.

Case Reports

Case 1. A 30-year-old woman had 3 hemorrhages from an AVM measuring about 30 ml in size located adjacent to the formation of Monro. This lesion was fed by arteries from the internal carotid and the vertebral arteries (Figure 44-9A, B, and C) treatment consisted of covering the malformation with 3 overlapping fields of irradiation and target doses of 40, 30, and 20 Gy (Figure 44-10A and B). The periphery of the malformation received approximately 20 Gy. The total time required for irradiation was 65 minutes. On follow-up angiograms obtained 1 year after the treatment, there was a marked decrease in the size of the malformation, by 2 years after the treatment there was a subtotal obliteration of the AVM, and on an angiogram 3

years after the treatment, the malformation was no longer visible (Figure 44-11A and B).

Case 2. The patient, a boy aged 13, had a history of seizures since the age of 8, and was initially seen for an intracerebral hemorrhage secondary to an AVM located in the right basal ganglia and fed by multiple arteries from the vertebral and the internal carotid artery territories (Figure 44-12A, B, and C). Radiosurgery was carried out using 3 overlapping fields (Figure 44-13A and B). The target dose was 50 Gy. The dose to the periphery of the AVM was 25 Gy. An angiogram obtained 2 years after the lesion's irradiation revealed total obliteration of the malformation (Figure 44-14A, B, C, and D).

The angiographic results following treatment of an AVM using optimal doses overlapping the lesion entirely has been consistent throughout the years (Table 44-1 summarizes the results in 159 and 165 cases with angiographic follow-up). Complete obliteration of the malformation occurred in 80 to 86 percent of the cases. Partial or subtotal obliteration occurred in 1 to 5 percent of the cases. Angiograms carried out 5 to 8 years

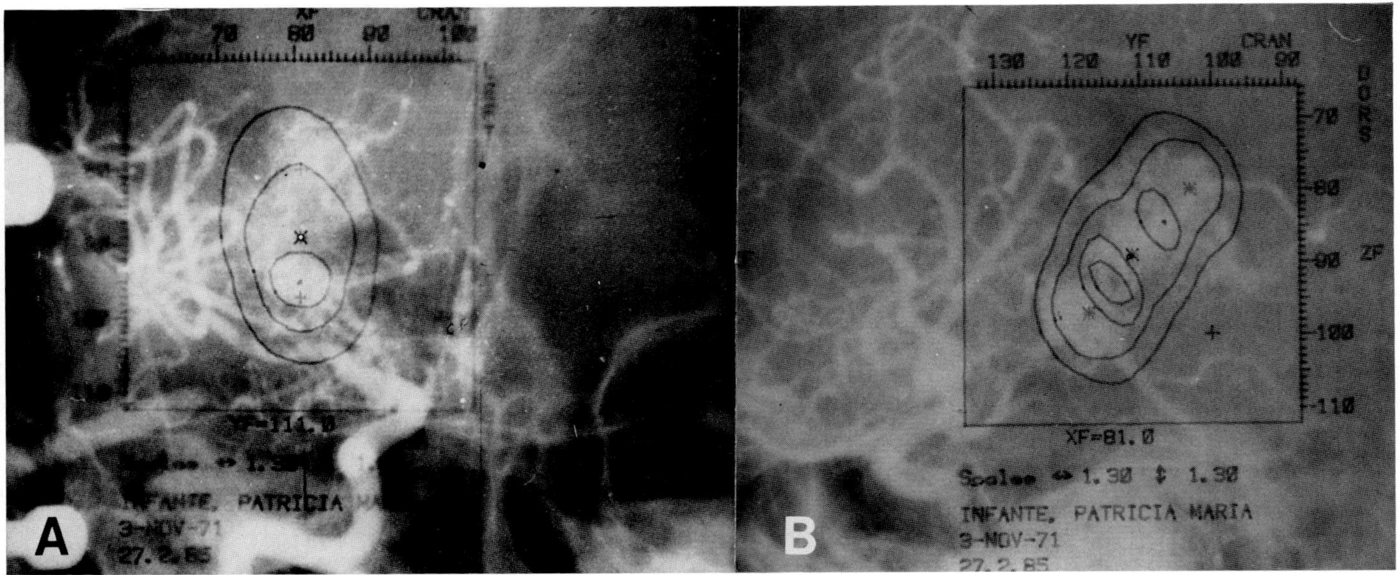

Fig. 44-13.　The same AVM as in Figure 44-12. (A and B) Stereotactic right carotid angiograms (frontal and lateral views). Three overlapping fields of radiation were used and the 50 percent isodose configuration (outer ring) corresponded to the periphery of the malformation. The target dose was 50 Gy, given over a period of 25 minutes. The inner ring represents the 90 percent isodose curve. The middle circle represents the 70 percent isodose curve. (Courtesy of Dr. Hernan Bunge, Centro de Radiocirurgia, Clinica Del Sol, Buenos Aires.)

after the total obliteration of the AVM proved that neither recanalization of the AVM nor progressive obliterative changes in the normal vessels occurred.

RADIATION-INDUCED CT SCAN CHANGES FOLLOWING IRRADIATION

In 20 cases, adverse effects of different degrees occurred after irradiation; the diagnosis of radiation-induced changes in the brain was usually made from CT scans. Computed tomographic investigation with and without contrast enhancement is routine in our follow-up scheme. The first follow-up CT scan is carried out 6 months after the treatment, although this is performed earlier if clinical symptoms appear.

The first clinical manifestations caused by the radiation usually occur after a latency of 3 to 8 months. In a few cases, the delay is up to 12 months and more. In these cases the patient suddenly develops increased intracranial pressure and simultaneously or within a few days, focal symptoms characteristic of the irradiated region. These symptoms can be severe or slight, progressive, stationary, or transitory. Occasionally, asymptomatic radiation damage is detected on the routine CT scan follow-up. Experimental observations based on animal studies regarding the basic mechanisms underlying delayed central nervous system destruction by ionizing radiation[28] explain the clinical CT findings. These consist of delayed tissue breakdown, small areas of focal necrosis, and larger areas of coalescing necrosis, plus pronounced vascular changes resulting in capillary permeability, and brain swelling distant from the region receiving the radiation. These adverse effects of irradiation can be local or diffuse, with or without an associated mass effect. Sometimes low-density, isodense, or high-density lesions can be seen. In some cases, enhancement after contrast injection is obtained. The enhancement has an irregular form, and is always present when a necrosis develops.

In Figure 44-15A, a severe radiation-induced lesion is presented. The patient was a 12-year-old child with a hemi-

plegia following a hemorrhage from a deep right-sided AVM. The lesion occurred 6 months after radiosurgery with 50 Gy as the target dose in the malformation with a volume of roughly 30 ml and a time of irradiation of 26 minutes. Treatment with steroids was started. A follow-up examination 6 months later showed that the slightly expansive high density lesion surrounded by a low density area had decreased in size (Figure 44-15B). The low density component, extending corticosubcortically, was still present. The lesion was no longer expansive. The left-sided hemiparesis improved progressively. The patient walked without help, but the paresis of the upper extremity was still marked. An angiogram obtained 2 years after the treatment no longer demonstrated the AVM.

The wide range of changes revealed by the CT scan, and the varied clinical pattern from cases without neurologic deficit to cases with slight transitory symptoms and others with marked and persistent neurologic symptoms presumably correspond to a gamut of morphologic changes. Adverse effects, occurring relatively early, usually appear as extensive low-density lesions in the white matter and are probably the result of diffuse demyelination or are of vascular origin.[29] These changes are reversible, while the changes caused by coagulation necrosis are irreversible.

Of our 20 patients with evidence of radiation-induced brain injury, 6 were asymptomatic, 6 had slight or moderate transitory or persistent neurologic deficits, while 8 had a moderate or marked neurologic syndrome. All patients were self sufficient and were able to return to their previous or to some other kind of work. However, some of these patients were not employable either because of their disability or because of personal or social factors.

THE CLINICAL OUTCOME

We recently evaluated the outcome of 239 of 247 patients (97 percent).[22] Although it is often difficult to differentiate improvements occurring in the natural course of the disease or

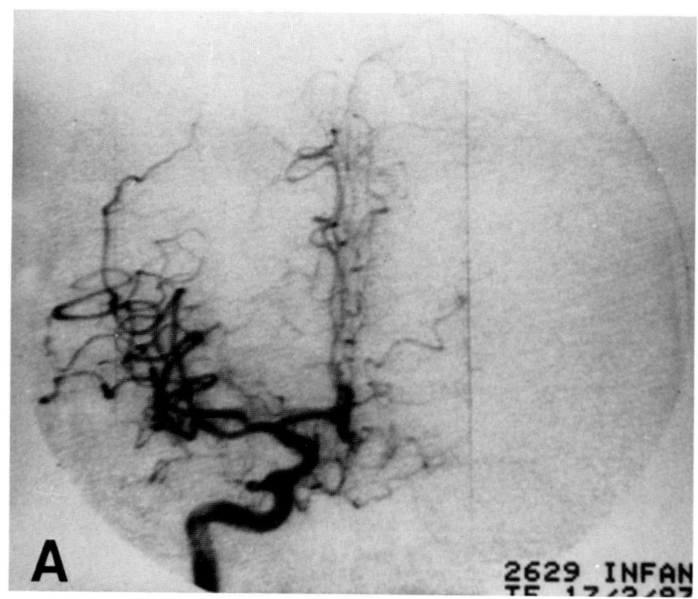
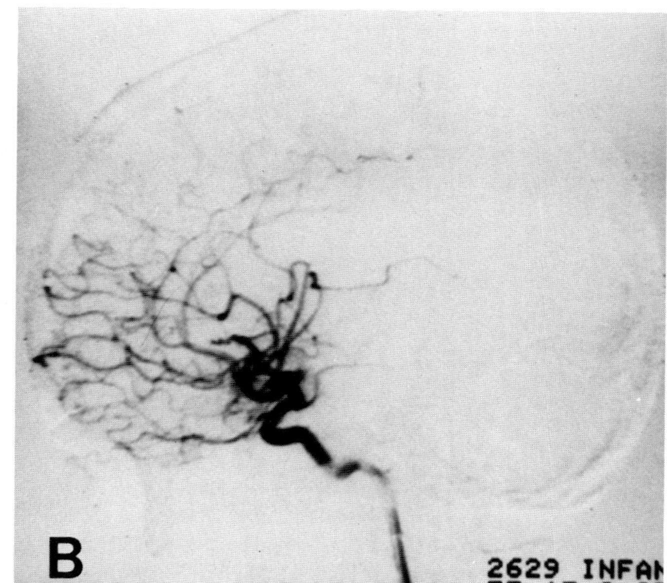
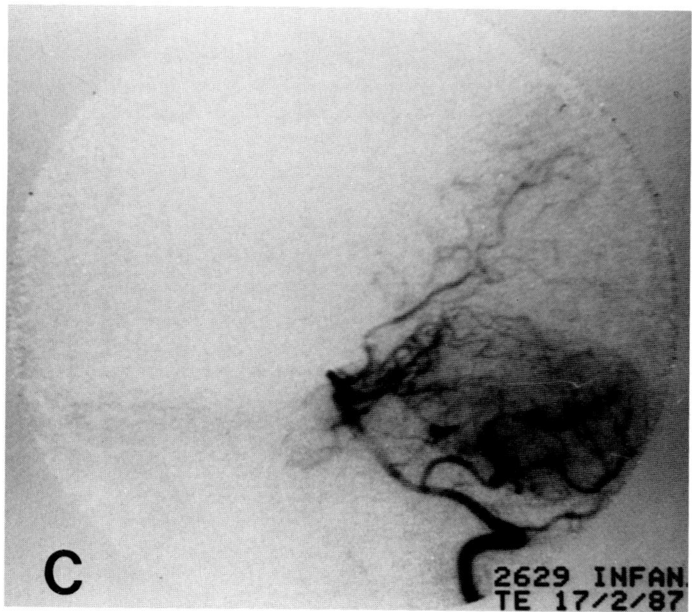
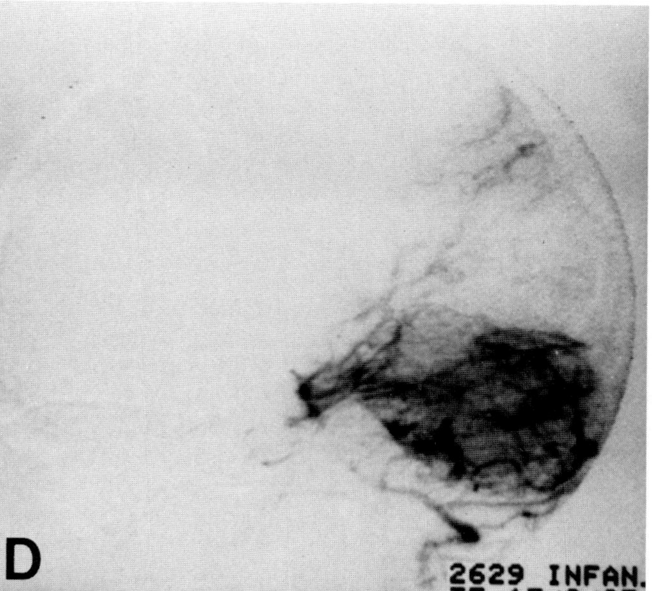

Fig. 44-14. The same AVM as in Figures 44-12 and 44-13, 2 years after the treatment. (A and B) Right carotid angiograms (frontal and lateral views) and (c and d) vertebral angiograms (lateral views in early and later arterial phase). The malformation no longer fills. (Courtesy of Dr. Hernan Bunge, Centro de Radiocirugia, Clinica Del Sol, Buenos Aires.)

caused by placebo-effects or by medication, the preliminary findings indicate that there is improvement in headache, decreases in the frequency in seizures (and in a number of cases the seizures stopped entirely). There were, however, cases in which seizures began after treatment. These patients had all had preoperative hemorrhage with severe intracerebral lesions.

The relationship between radiosurgery and the appearance of neurologic deficits following the treatment was easy to establish. These symptoms, hemihypoesthesia, hemiparesis, dysphasia, transitory or persistent, were caused by radiation-induced morphologic changes in the brain tissue. For example, a 52-year-old woman developed a contralateral homonymous quadrantanopsia after the treatment of an occipital AVM. The

Table 44-1. Incidence of obliteration of AVMs after radiosurgery assessed on follow-up angiograms during the years 1983 to 1987

Year	Number of Patients	No AVM Visible	Obliterated (%)
1983	63	53	84.1
1984	104	90	86.5
1987	166	126	79.2
1987	166	133	80.0

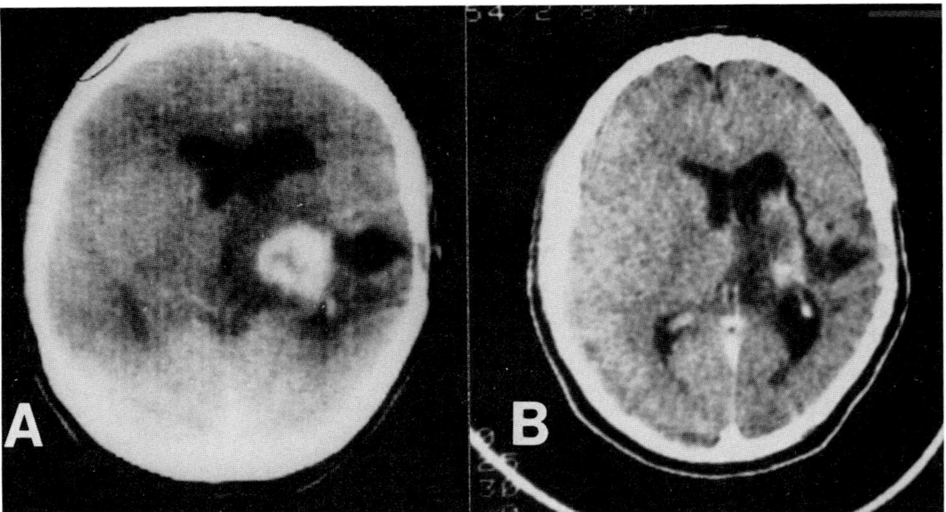

Fig. 44-15. A CT scan revealing radiation-induced delayed necrosis of the brain tissue occurring 6 months after radiosurgery. There is a slightly expansive high density area corresponding to the irradiated region. Low density changes extending up to the cortex surround the high density component of the lesion (A). Six months later (B) the central high density lesion decreased in size. The low density area did not change significantly. (Courtesy of Dr. Hernan Bunge, Centro de Radiocirurgia, Clinica Del Sol, Buenos Aires.)

malformation was occluded 7 months after the treatment. A few small vessels serving the calcarine cortex were filled in the follow-up angiogram.

In 57 children treated by radiosurgery between the ages of 4 and 13 years no psychological problems or endocrinologic deficits were noted following irradiation of their AVMs.

RECURRENT HEMORRHAGE

During the interval between the time of irradiation and before the lesion was completely obliterated there were 24 episodes of rehemorrhage in the entire series (a recurrent hemorrhage rate of 4 percent). Included among the cases analyzed are the cases with nonoptimal treatment. If one considers only the optimally treated cases there were 12 cases of rehemorrhage before the AVM was totally obliterated (an incidence of 2.2 percent). In a recent study,[22] our rebleed rate was estimated at between 2.0 and 4.9 percent, figures that are no higher than the rebleed rate of 2 to 3 percent reported for untreated AVMs. It appears that radiosurgery confers protection against rebleeding only after the malformation is completely occluded. Recurring hemorrhage may cause new deficits or death. In the group of optimally treated patients there was one fatal hemorrhage (less than 0.2 percent) before the AVM obliterated.

Since sterotactic angiography is part of the radiosurgical procedure in the treatment of AVMs, the risks of angiography as well as the risks due to the latency period preceding the total occlusion of the AVM must be included among the risks related directly to the single high dose of radiation.

With an optimal radiosurgical treatment in selected cases of AVM, a total obliteration of the lesion can occur in 80 percent of cases. A further 11 to 15 percent of the AVMs are partially obliterated within approximately 2 years of the treatment. The defining of the target and the accuracy of the stereotactic localization could be further improved and—with better knowledge of the doses needed for the occlusion of the AVM nidus—the present incidence of successfully treated cases could be increased. The incidence of untoward effects is

approximately 3 percent and the rate of rehemorrhage before the total obliteration of the AVM is comparable with the occurrence among untreated cases and resulted in a rebleed-related mortality of 0.2 percent.

FINAL CONSIDERATIONS

Radiosurgery is currently evolving into an established neurosurgical method. The problem is no longer that of not being accepted; on the contrary, there is a risk that if this method is not soon incorporated into neurosurgery, radiosurgery will be carried out under the aegis of departments of radiotherapy. Hence the involvement of the neurosurgeon in the selection of the patients will be restricted and the number of improperly biased decisions will increase.

To ensure sound development, research should go hand in hand with routine clinical work. There are a number of problems still waiting to be solved. The dose-volume-time relationships need further investigation. The minimum dose necessary to achieve the therapeutic effect and the maximum dose allowable to the cranial nerves, to the hypothalamus, and to the brain stem should be established. Secondary supported factors to be used in association with radiosurgery should be tested. These could increase the success rate and decrease the incidence of complications. The role of biologic factors to explain the different responses to similar treatment parameters should be studied.

Although no radiation-induced brain tumors were observed in our series of over 1300 cases treated in the past 19 years, the answer to this problem remains uncertain, since the latency for radiation-induced tumors is up to 26 years. In any event the incidence of tumors after radiation is so low that when it occurs, it is—in Deck's formulation—little more than a curiosity.

A number of technical problems, such as the improvement of imaging procedures (CT and MRI scanning) in the visualization of microadenomas and acoustic neurinomas, and arteriography for the identification of feeding vessels, could widen the limits of radiosurgery. The yield of continuous research will determine the final boundaries of radiosurgery and its relationship to other lines of development in neurosurgery.

REFERENCES

1. Leksell L: The stereotaxic method and radiosurgery of the brain. Acta Chir Scand 102:316, 1951

2. Leksell L: Stereotactic radiosurgery. J Neurol Neurosurg Psychiatry 46:797, 1983

3. Leksell L, Larsson B, Rexed B: The use of high-energy protons for cerebral surgery in man. Acta Chir Scand 125:1, 1963

4. Larsson B, Liden K, Sarby B: Irradiation of small structures through the skull. Acta Radiol Oncol Radiat Phys Biol 13:512, 1974

5. Steiner L: Radiosurgery in arterio-venous malformations in the brain, in Wilson C, Stein B, (eds): Intracranial Arteriovenous Malformations, Current Neurosurgical Practice, 1984

6. Radiosurgery in cerebral arteriovenous malformations, in Fein J, Flamm E (eds): Cerebrovascular Surgery, vol 4. New York, Springer-Verlag, 1985

7. Lindquist C, Steiner L: Radiosurgery in arteriovenous malformations, in Lundsford D (ed): Stereotactic Techniques. Orlando, Grune & Stratton, 1987

8. Noren G: Stereotactic radiosurgery in acoustic neurinomas. A new therapeutic approach. (Thesis) Sundt Offset, Stockholm, 1982

9. Noren G, Arndt J, Hindmarsh T, et al: Treatment of acoustic neurinomas, in Lundsford D (ed): Stereotactic Techniques. Orlando, Grune & Stratton, 1987

10. Backlund EO: Stereotactic radiosurgery in intracranial tumors and vascular malformations, in Krayenbuhl H (ed): Advances and Technical Standards in Neurosurgery, vol 6. New York, Springer-Verlag, 1979

11. Rähn T, Thorn N, Hall K, et al: Stereotactic radiosurgery in Cushing's syndrome: Acute radiation effects. Surg Neurol 2:85, 1980

12. Rähn T: Stereotactic radiosurgery in Cushing's disease. (Thesis) Sundt Offset, Stockholm, 1980

13. Degerblad M, Rähn T, Bergstrand G: Long term results of stereotactic radiosurgery to the pituitary gland in Cushing's disease. Acta Endocrinol 112:310, 1986

14. Bunge HG, Chinela AB, Guevara JA (personal communication).

15. Belloni G, Baciocco A, Borelli, P, et al: The value of CT for the diagnosis of pituitary microadenomas in children. Neuroradiology 15:179, 1978

16. Bonafe A, Sobel D, Saladine AM, et al: Diagnostic value of CT scanning in pituitary microadenomas. Neuroradiology 20:263, 1981

17. Hemminghytt S, Kalkhoff K, Daniels D, et al: Computed tomography study of hormone secreting microadenomas. Radiology 146:65, 1983

18. Hagerman B: Reliability in the determination of speech discrimination. Scand Audiol 5:219, 1976

19. Newman H, Sheline GE, Boldrey EB: Radiation therapy of tumors of the eighth nerve sheath. AJR 120:562, 1974

20. Hirsch A, Noren G, Andersson H: Audiologic findings after stereotactic radiosurgery in nine cases of acoustic neurinomas. Acta Otolaryngol 88:155, 1979

21. Forster DMC, Steiner L, Hakansson S: Arteriovenous malformations of the brain. A long term clinical study. J Neurosurg 37:562, 1972

22. Steiner L, Lindquist C, Adler J: Clinical outcome of radiosurgery for cerebral arteriovenous malformations. J Neurosurg (in press)

23. Steiner L: Radiosurgery in intracranial tumors and arteriovenous malformations in children, in Voth D, Gutjahr P, Langmaid (eds): Tumors of the Central Nervous System in Infancy and Childhood. Berlin, Springer-Verlag, 1982

24. Steiner L, Greitz T, Backlund EO, et al: Radiosurgery in arteriovenous malformations of the brain, in Szikla G (ed): Stereotactic Cerebral Irradiation. Amsterdam, Elsevier/North-Holland, 1979, pp 257–269

25. Steiner L, Greitz T, Leksell L, et al: Radiosurgery in intracranial arteriovenous malformations. II. A follow-up study. Proceedings of the 6th International Congress of Neurological Surgeons. Amsterdam, Excerpta Medica, 1977

26. Steiner L, Leksell L, Forster DMC, et al: Stereotactic radiosurgery in arteriovenous malformations. Acta Neurochir (Suppl) 21:195, 1974

27. Steiner L, Leksell L, Greitz T, et al: Stereotaxic radiosurgery for cerebral arteriovenous malformations. Report of a case. Acta Chir Scand 138:459, 1972

28. Caveness FE: Experimental observations: Delayed necrosis in normal monkey brain, in Gilbert HA, Kagan AR (eds): Radiation Damage to the Nervous System. New York, Raven Press, 1980

29. Groothuis DR, Vick NA: Radionecrosis of the central nervous system: The perspective of the clinical neurologist and neuroradiologist, in Gilbert HA, Kagan AR (eds): Radiation Damage to the Nervous System. New York, Raven Press, 1980

30. Graf I, Perret GE, Torner JC: Bleeding from cerebral arteriovenous malformations as part of their natural history. J Neurosurg 58:331, 1983

31. Leksell L: A note on the treatment of acoustic tumors. Acta Chir Scand 137:763, 1971

32. Backlund EO, Rähn T, Sarby B: Treatment of pinealomas by stereotaxic radiation surgery. Acta Radiol (Ther Phys Biol) 13:368, 1974

Surgical Management of Olfactory Groove, Suprasellar, and Medial Sphenoid Wing Meningiomas

Robert G. Ojemann   Karl W. Swann

IN 1938, CUSHING, in his classic two-volume work on meningiomas, included chapters on suprasellar meningiomas, meningiomas of the olfactory groove, and meningiomas of the sphenoidal ridge (those of the deep or clinoidal third).[1] This chapter is based on experience with the surgical management of 55 consecutive patients with meningiomas in these locations treated from 1968 to 1985: 23 of these patients had suprasellar meningiomas, 11 had olfactory groove meningiomas, and 21 had meningiomas of the medial sphenoid wing.

As expected, the majority of the patients were women (44 of 55). Their ages ranged from the early 30s to mid 70s. Age should not be a deterrent to surgery if the patient is losing vision or showing progressive signs of frontal lobe dysfunction and the general medical condition is satisfactory.

Good preoperative radiographic studies are essential. Computerized tomographic (CT) scan with contrast enhancement should include coronal views, which are particularly useful in defining the relationship of the tumor to the skull base.[2] Cerebral angiography with subtraction views define the vascular relationships and blood supply. We have not seen a patient in this group where preoperative embolization was needed and Al-Mefty et al. could not find any reports of its use in the management of suprasellar meningiomas.[3]

Careful preoperative medical evaluation is done. All patients are pretreated with steroids for several days before surgery. General anesthesia is used with controlled ventilation to keep the PCO_2 in the low 30 range. After intubation the patient is given 10–20 mg Lasix (Hoechst-Roussel Pharmaceutical, Somerville, New Jersey) and while the exposure is being made, 500 ml 20 percent Mannitol (Abbott Laboratories, North Chicago, Illinois) is administered.

Portions of this chapter are reproduced with permission from Ojemann RG: Meningiomas of the basal para-pituitary region; technical considerations. Clin Neurosurg 27:233–262, 1980, and Ojemann RG: Clinical features and surgical management of meningiomas, in Wilkins RH, Rengachary SS (eds): Neurosurgery. New York: McGraw-Hill Book Co, 1985, Vol 1, pp 635–654.

SUPRASELLAR MENINGIOMAS

PRESENTATION

Suprasellar meningiomas usually arise in the midline from the region of the tuberculum sellae and planum sphenoidale but they can arise from the diaphragm sellae or be located primarily to one side arising from the anterior clinoid region.[4–7] In this series 18 were midline, 2 extended more to one side, and 3 arose from the anterior clinoid region.

The most common initial symptom is an asymmetric loss of vision starting with unilateral decreased acuity or blurring in the visual field followed by progression to bilateral involvement. In Symon and Rosenstein's series of 101 patients with suprasellar meningiomas, symptoms recorded on admission were visual loss in 99 percent, headache in 45 percent, and mental changes in 10 percent.[8] Other symptoms included hyposomia, seizures, diplopia, eye pain, and endocrine dysfunction.

On examination there is almost always a reduction of visual acuity in at least one eye and a visual field defect.[2,8,9] Incongruity and asymmetry of the field defect is the common finding. Optic atrophy is frequently seen.[10]

RADIOGRAPHIC FINDINGS

The typical CT scan shows a densely enhancing round mass in the midline above the sellae and extending laterally and anteriorly (Figure 45-1). The tumor may arise in the region of the anterior clinoid as shown in Figure 45-2.

Lateral angiograms may show little abnormality or there may be slight displacement of the distal internal carotid artery inferiorly and posteriorly (Figure 45-3A). There may be a stain. In large lesions, the proximal pericallosal arteries can be elevated over the tumor (Figure 45-4A). On anteroposterior views, elevation of the A1 segments of the anterior cerebral arteries is seen (Figures 45-3B and 45-4B) and the distal internal carotid artery may be displaced laterally (Figure 45-4B). The blood supply to these tumors usually comes from small vessels passing through the area of the dural attachment, but these are not usually visible on angiograms.

OPERATIVE NEUROSURGICAL TECHNIQUES
ISBN 0-8089-1862-1

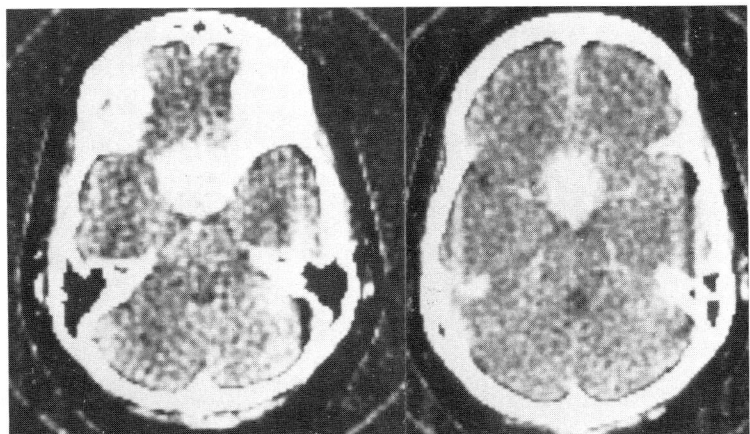

Fig. 45-1. Suprasellar meningioma. The CT scan shows an enhancing midline mass above the sella and extending over the region of the tuberculum.

OPERATIVE TECHNIQUE

Smaller suprasellar meningiomas compress the optic nerves laterally, the chiasm posteriorly, and do not involve the internal carotid or anterior cerebral arteries (Figure 45-5). Larger tumors may extend both above and below the optic nerves and chiasm, at times displacing the internal carotid arteries laterally or the anterior cerebral arteries away from the chiasm. In some patients the tumor may adhere to or encase the anterior cerebral artery or the anterior communicating artery complex (Figure 45-6).

The operative approach we prefer in most patients is a right frontal temporal craniotomy with a lateral subfrontal exposure just in front of the sphenoid wing unless the tumor arises from the left anterior clinoid region. A bifrontal exposure occasionally is indicated in large tumors. Kempe also approaches meningiomas in this region with a right lateral subfrontal exposure.[11] MacCarty et al.[12] use the subfrontal approach from the side of greatest visual loss; they also use a bifrontal craniotomy if the tumor is very large, as does Al-Mefty et al.[3] Morley[13] and Kadis et al.[2] prefer a bifrontal craniotomy. Logue[14] and Symon[6] use a unilateral right subfrontal exposure but approach the tumor along the midline. In large tumors, Symon resects a portion of the frontal lobe.

After the satisfactory induction of anesthesia, a lumbar puncture can be done to insert a catheter for CSF drainage if it is thought that drainage of CSF from the basal cisterns may not be adequate. This is done in addition to the use of Lasix and mannitol. The patient then is carefully placed in the supine position. The head is elevated and rotated 60 degrees to the left so that the anterior zygoma is uppermost and is held with a three-point Mayfield-Kees skeletal fixation headrest.

An incision is made beginning just above the zygoma a few millimeters anterior to the ear and then, staying behind the hairline, is extended medially to end in the midline of the forehead (Figure 45-7). The skin, underlying temporalis muscle, and pericranial tissue are turned down together exposing the inferior lateral frontal and anterior temporal bone (Figure 45-8). The most important burr hole is the one placed just below the anterior end of the superior temporal line at the level just behind the zygomatic process of the frontal bone (Figure 45-8). It is important that this hole be properly placed so that the exposure will be on the floor of the anterior fossa. Two or three other burr holes are placed and the free bone flap is cut.

The lateral portion of the sphenoid wing is removed, as is bone over the anterior superior temporal region. After dural sutures are placed to control epidural bleeding, the dura is opened over the inferior frontal and anterior temporal region (Figure 45-9). The draining veins from the anterior temporal lobe along the sphenoid wing are divided. The frontal lobe is carefully elevated along the sphenoid wing. The posterior part of the olfactory tract is seen and normally will lead the surgeon

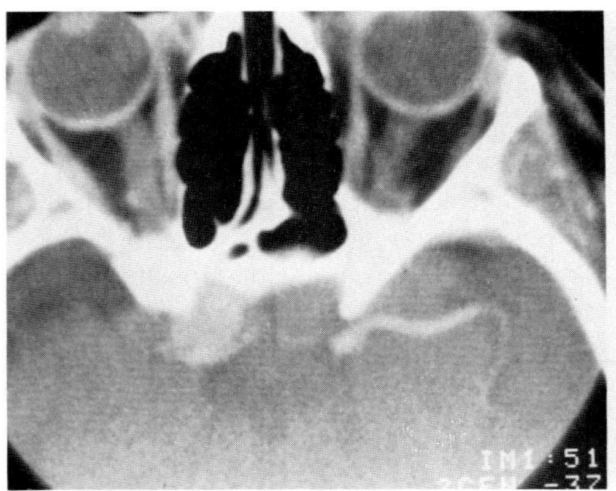
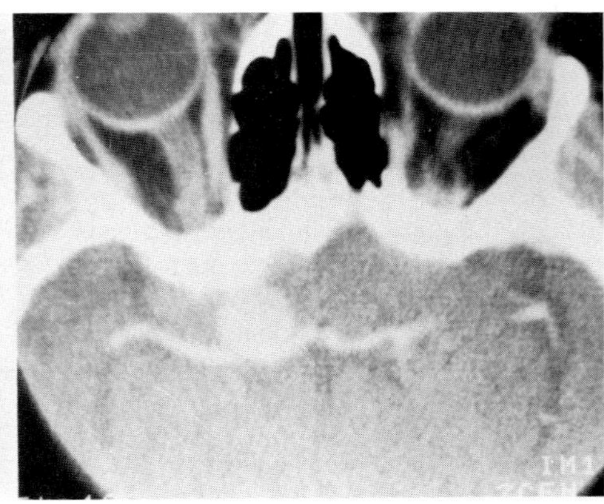

Fig. 45-2. Suprasellar meningioma. The tumor arises from the region of the left anterior clinoid process.

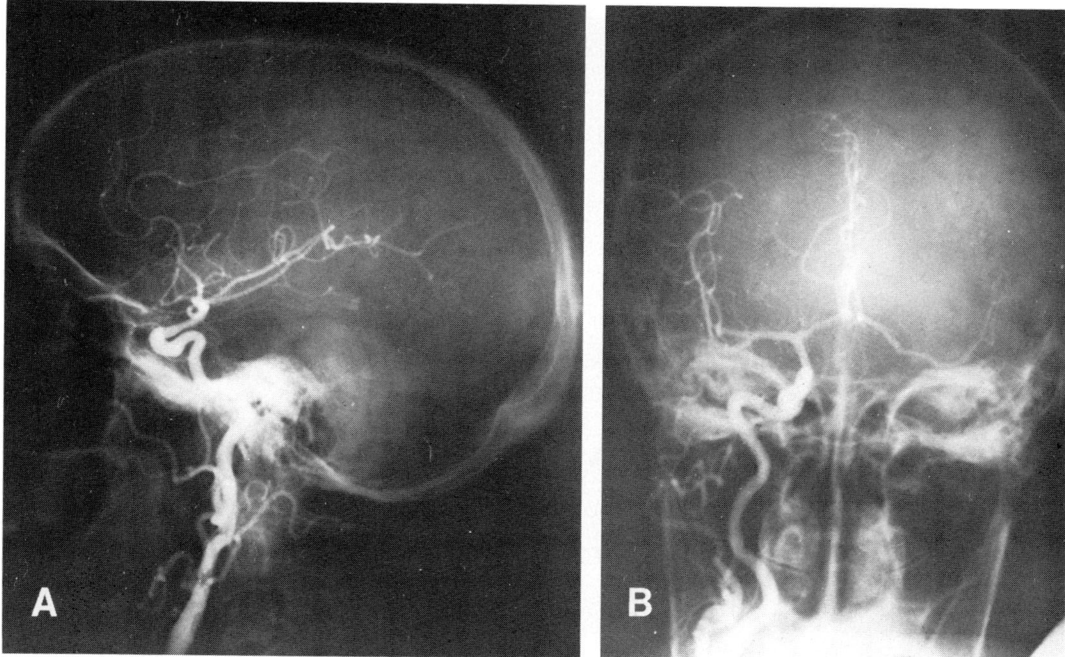

Fig. 45-3. Suprasellar meningioma. (A) A lateral angiogram shows slight compression of the distal internal carotid artery with displacement inferiorly and posteriorly. (B) An AP angiogram reveals elevation of the A1 segments of the anterior cerebral arteries.

to the optic nerve unless there is significant displacement (Figure 45-10).

Evidence of the tumor may be seen in the dura anterior to the optic nerve. The dura may be reddish and have increased vascularity. Slightly more exposure reveals the anterior clinoid process, the internal carotid artery, and a varying portion of the right optic nerve, depending on the size of the tumor (Figure 45-11). In patients with smaller tumors, the arachnoid over the lateral optic nerve and internal carotid artery is opened, and CSF is aspirated to provide further decompression. Large tumors may surround both optic nerves; grow beneath the optic nerves to involve the medial wall of the internal carotid artery and its branches; lift the A1 segments of the anterior cerebral arteries off the chiasm; and may be adherent to the A2 segments of these arteries (Figure 45-6). The frontal lobe tissue is carefully freed from the surface of the tumor, and self-retaining retractors are placed. Up to this point, the operation has been done with the aid of surgical loupes. The operating microscope is used for the remainder of the operation.

The tumor capsule is opened. The attachments of the tumor along the planum, tuberculum, and anterior clinoid are divided to interrupt the blood supply as it comes into this area. Internal decompression of the tumor is done using bipolar coagulation, the Cavitron, or laser.

In cases of large tumors where the tumor has projected beneath or surrounded the right optic nerve, it will often be possible to free the tumor from above and below the nerve, to remove it from its loose attachment to the carotid artery, and to roll it out from beneath the right optic nerve (Figure 45-12). In smaller tumors, the left optic nerve may be seen just proximal to the optic canal initially or, after decompression, along the tuberculum. In large tumors, it is sometimes best to identify the

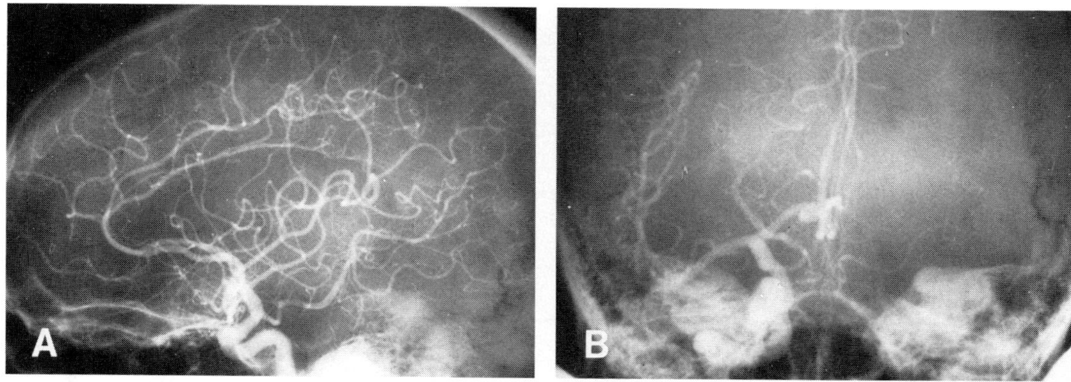

Fig. 45-4. Suprasellar meningioma. A larger tumor than that illustrated in Figure 45-3. (A) On this lateral angiogram, the anterior cerebral arteries are elevated and curved over the surface of the tumor. The distal internal carotid artery is straightened and displaced. (B) On the AP angiogram the A1 segment is elevated, and the distal internal carotid artery is displaced laterally.

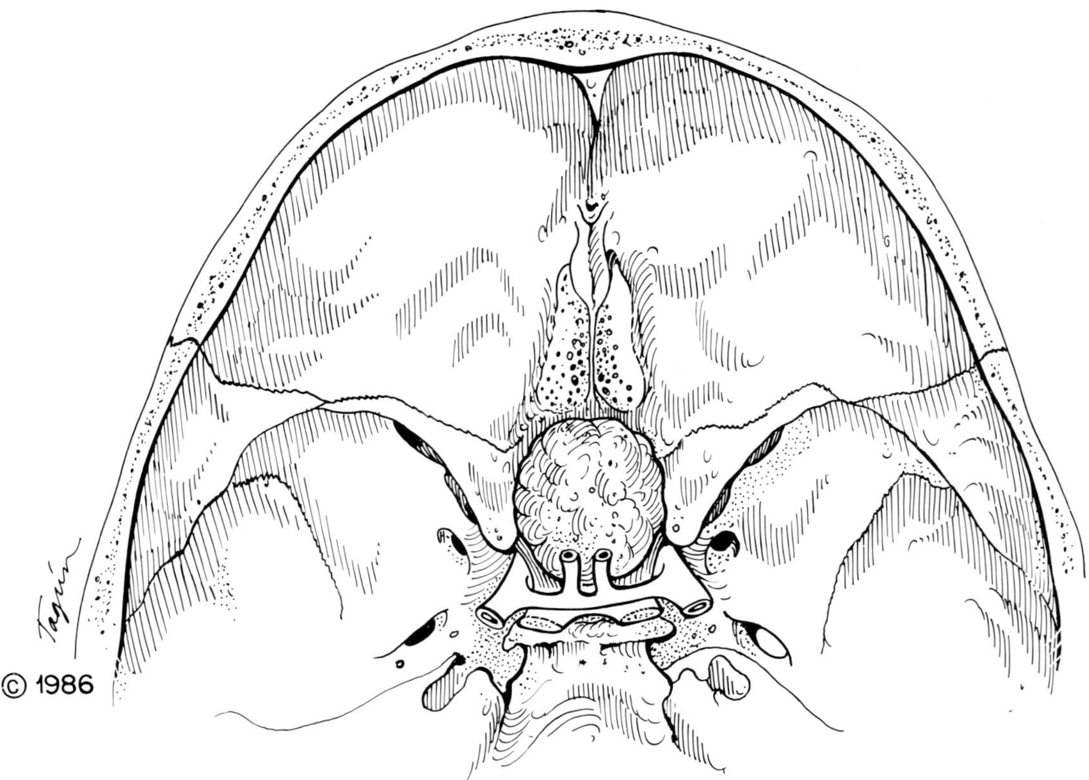

Fig. 45-5. Suprasellar meningioma. In this drawing the tumor arises from the dura over the tuberculum. The smaller tumor compresses the optic nerves and chiasm but does not involve the internal carotid and anterior cerebral arteries.

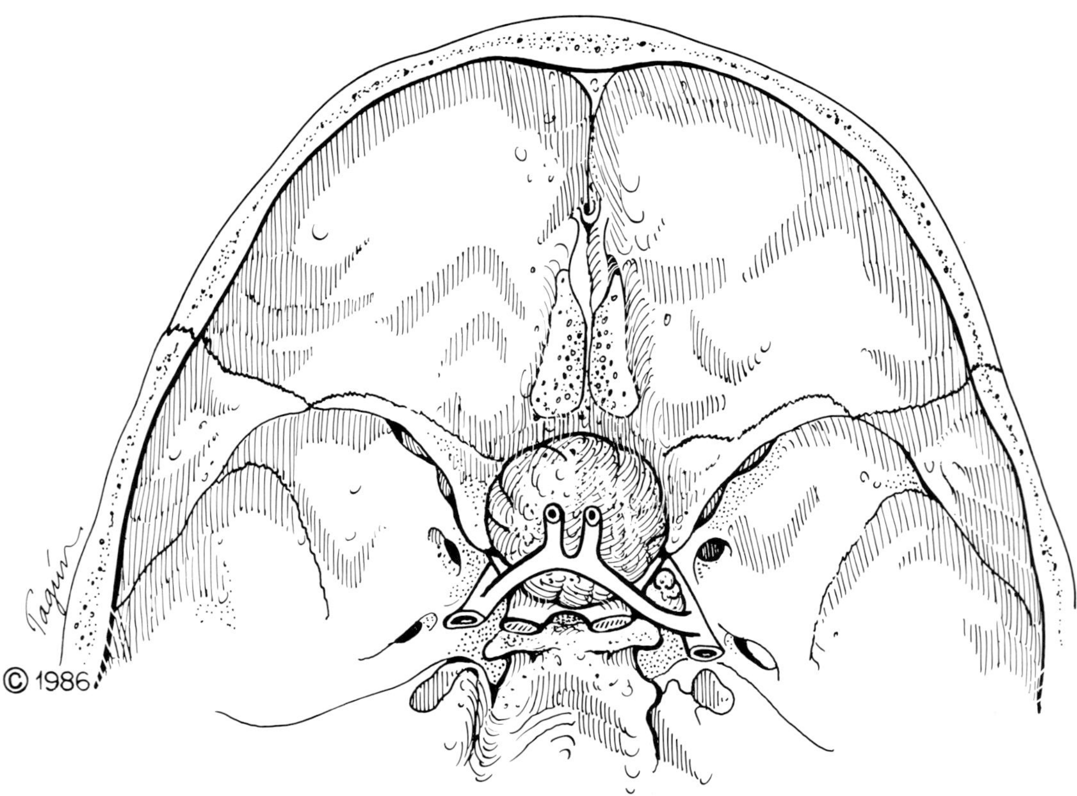

Fig. 45-6. Suprasellar meningioma. In this drawing a larger tumor (dashed lines) has displaced the anterior cerebral artery complex away from the optic chiasm and has grown beneath the right optic nerve to displace the distal internal carotid artery laterally.

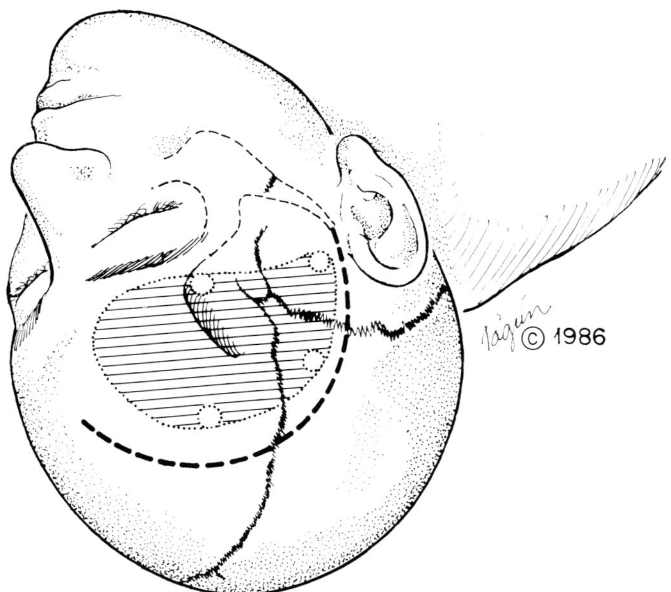

Fig. 45-7. Position of the head, skin incision, and bone flap for the frontotemporal approach to suprasellar and medial sphenoid wing meningiomas.

chiasm and the left optic nerve by dissection of the posterior capsule, taking great care to visualize directly any attachment to the anterior cerebral vessels (Figure 45-13), or to approach the tumor from a bilateral exposure so each optic nerve can be seen.

Occasionally the A1 segments of the anterior cerebral arteries and the anterior communicating artery complex are encased in tumor, and the tumor cannot be removed from the artery. A small portion of the tumor will need to be left on the artery in this circumstance.

As the tumor is removed from between the optic nerves and from in front of the chiasm, arachnoid may be encountered that is thickened. Just beneath this is the pituitary stalk, which may have been displaced by the tumor. This structure usually can be preserved. After removal of the tumor is completed, the dura over the tuberculum and adjacent area is removed. Usually this is all that is required, but on occasion there may be hyperostosis that needs to be removed with a diamond burr. In some patients the tumor may grow into the optic foramen or involve the dura under the optic nerve, and tumor may need to be left in this area. Surgicel (Surgikora, New Brunswick, New Jersey) is placed over the area where the tumor was removed from the frontal lobe. The dura is closed and the bone flap replaced and held with No. 28 wire to the adjacent skull.

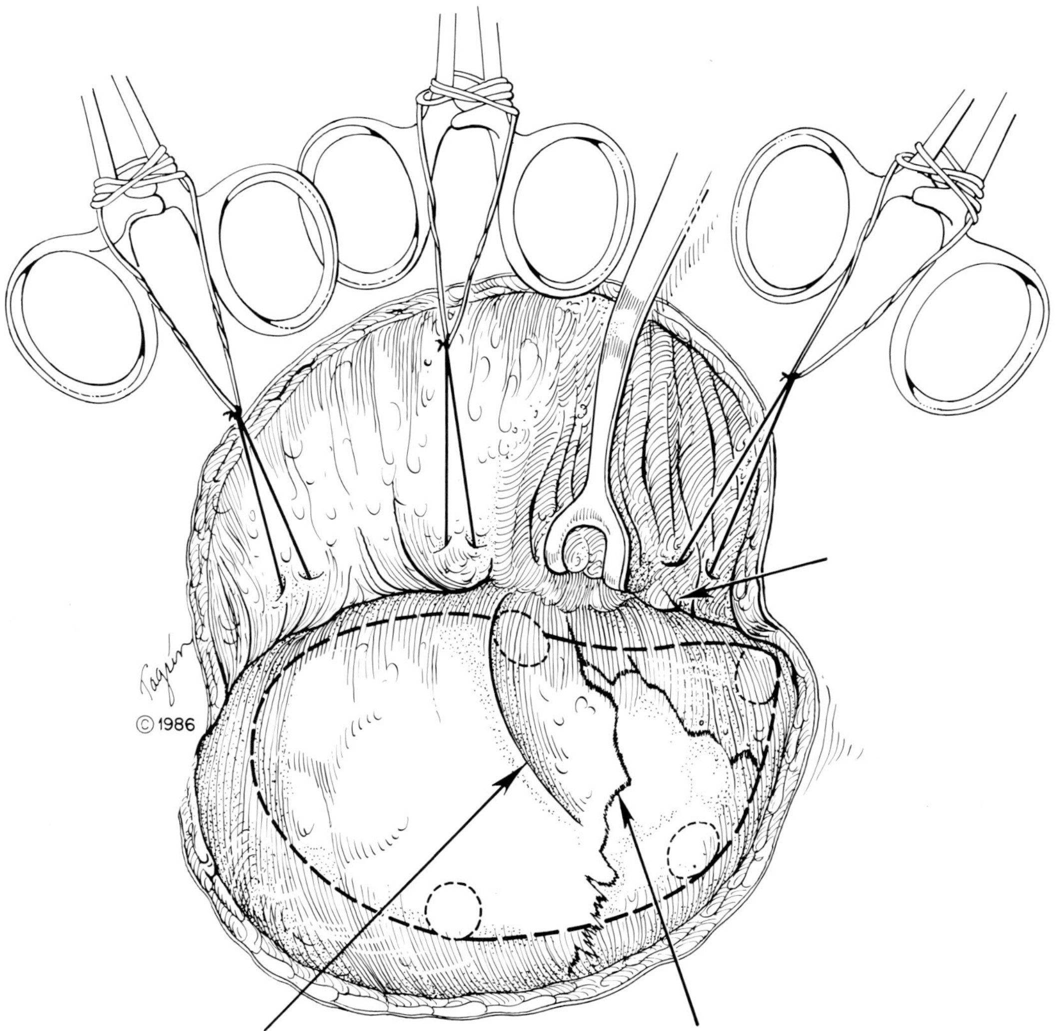

Fig. 45-8. The skin, temporalis muscle, and pericranial tissue have been turned down together. The bone flap is outlined (dashed line). It is very important that the burr hole just below the anterior end of the superior temporal line be properly placed so the exposure will be on the floor of the anterior fossa.

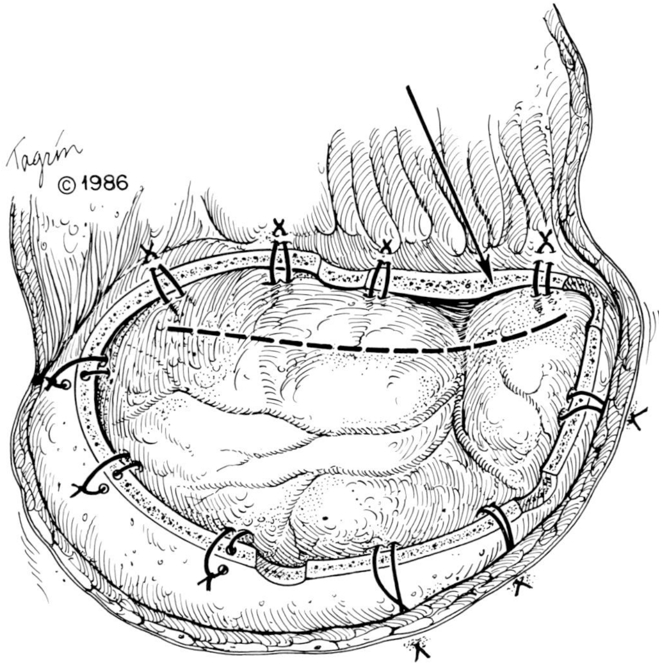

Fig. 45-9.   The bone flap has been elevated, and bone has been removed over the anterior temporal region and from the lateral sphenoid wing. Tenting dural sutures have been placed. The dural incision is shown (dashed line).

RESULTS

There was no operative mortality in the patients in this series and Symon and Rosenthal had only one death, due to aspiration, in the patients operated with microsurgical technique.[8] These authors also outlined the complications that may be associated with this operation and we have previously discussed the morbidity in these patients.[4,5,7,15] The most important morbidity outside the visual system has been the

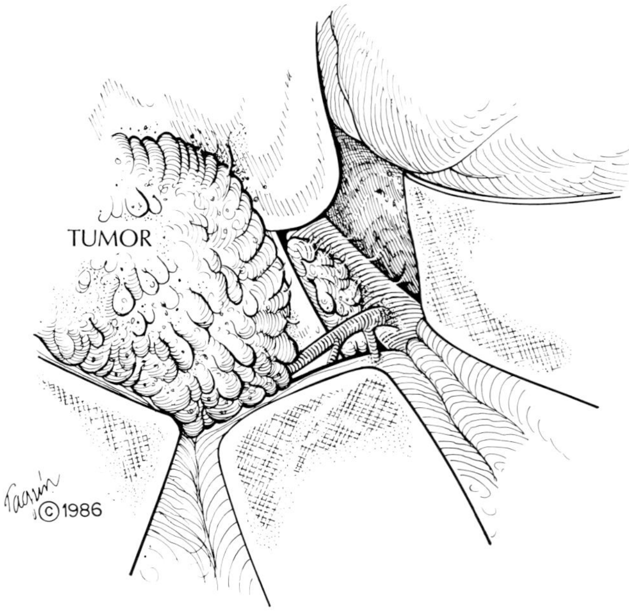

Fig. 45-11.   Suprasellar meningioma. Tumor surrounds a portion of the right optic nerve and right anterior cerebral artery and displaces the right internal carotid artery laterally.

small incidence of permanent frontal lobe syndrome, postoperative seizures, and diabetes insipidus. However, in our series and in Symons' the patients operated upon with microsurgical techniques had a very high percentage of good or excellent results, usually returning to their normal way of life.

Vision improved in many of our patients, but some patients with extensive growths, particularly recurrent tumors, could not be helped and were occasionally made worse.[4,5,15] Gregorius et al. found that a long history of decreased visual acuity or a severe visual field defect did not preclude postoperative recovery of vision.[10] They noted that improvement

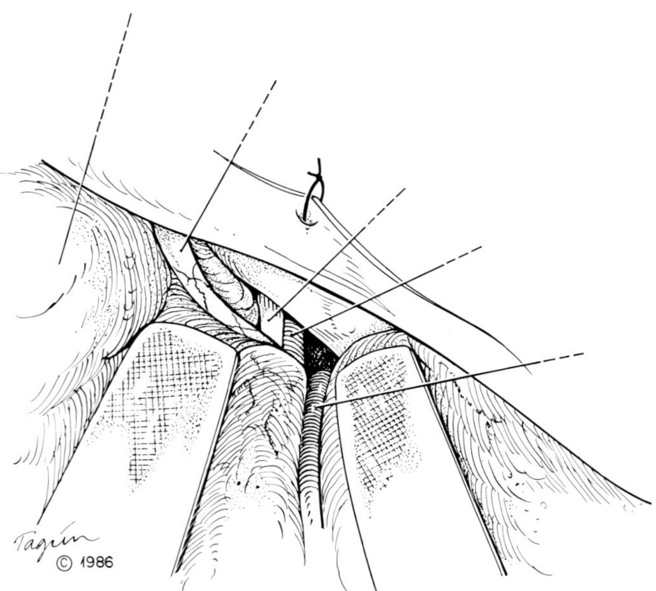

Fig. 45-10.   The normal anatomy in a frontotemporal craniotomy. The right frontal lobe has been elevated. The olfactory tract is seen first and then the right optic nerve and internal carotid artery come into view. A second retractor is on the anterior temporal lobe.

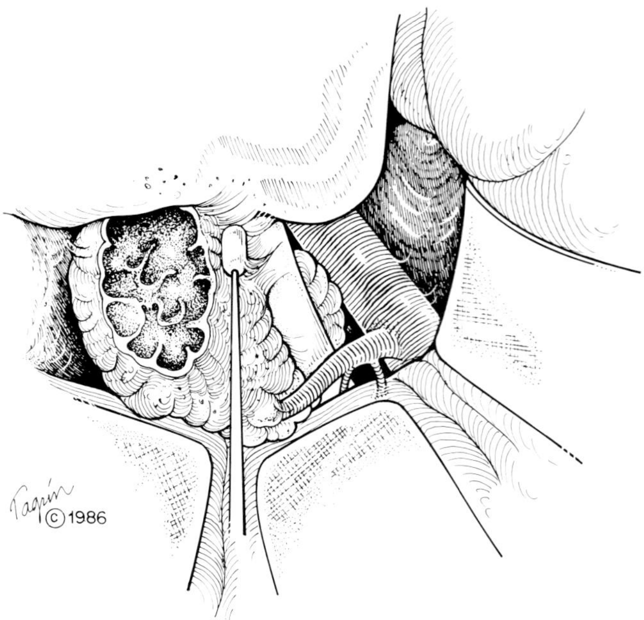

Fig. 45-12.   Suprasellar meningioma. Internal decompression of the tumor has been accomplished. The attachments to the right optic nerve are being separated.

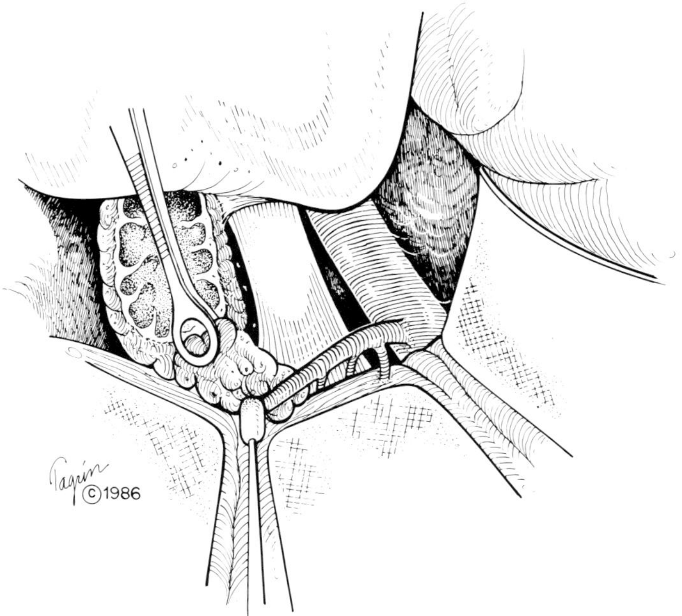

Fig. 45-13.   Suprasellar meningioma. The tumor surrounding the right anterior cerebral artery is being carefully separated and then the chiasm can be followed to the left optic nerve.

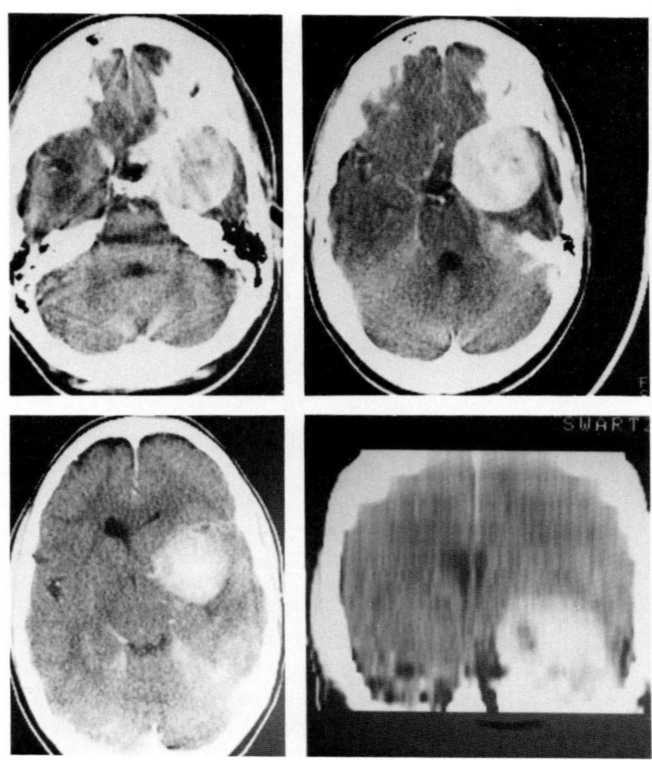

Fig. 45-15.   Medial sphenoid wing meningioma. The CT scan shows a large mass extending predominantly into the middle fossa.

occurred most frequently within the first several weeks after surgery and that further return of vision did not occur after a year. Rosenstein and Symon found that 74 percent of patients in whom preoperative visual symptoms had been present for 2 years or less were improved postoperatively, compared with only a 43 percent improvement rate for patients in whom symptoms had been present for more than 2 years.[9] Furthermore, there was a higher incidence of postoperative visual deterioration in patients in whom there had been a longer duration of symptoms (43 percent versus 15 percent). Other factors that favorably influenced the prognosis for visual function were a tumor size less than 3 cm and the presence of normal optic discs.

Residual tumor was left in some patients because of adherence to the visual pathways or vascular structures. This is almost always true when the patient has had previous surgery. Some of these patients received radiation therapy, with apparent arrest of tumor growth. This is usually done when the CT scan shows evidence of recurrence and further surgery is considered inadvisable. Benefits of radiation in this group of patients has also been reported by others.[16]

From our experience it is best to do as complete a removal of tumor as possible at the initial operation. The patient should then be carefully followed with regular CT scanning and visual field examination and reoperation or radiation therapy considered if there is evidence of recurrence.

MEDIAL SPHENOID WING MENINGIOMAS

PRESENTATION AND RADIOGRAPHIC FINDINGS

Patients with tumors in the region of the medial sphenoid wing can be divided into two general categories. In one, the tumors are predominantly masses arising from the medial sphenoid wing; involving the internal carotid and middle cerebral arteries to varying degrees; and compressing or surrounding the optic nerves, optic tract, or the adjacent frontal and temporal lobes (Figure 45-14). These patients usually have evidence of compression of the visual pathways, but a seizure disorder or progressive hemiparesis may also be the initial symptom. The CT scan will reveal a dense enhancing mass in the region of the medial sphenoid wing extending into the frontal or middle fossa (Figure 45-15). The angiogram will show elevation of the proximal middle cerebral artery and stretching of the distal internal carotid artery. At times, encasement of the internal carotid and middle cerebral arteries is indicated by

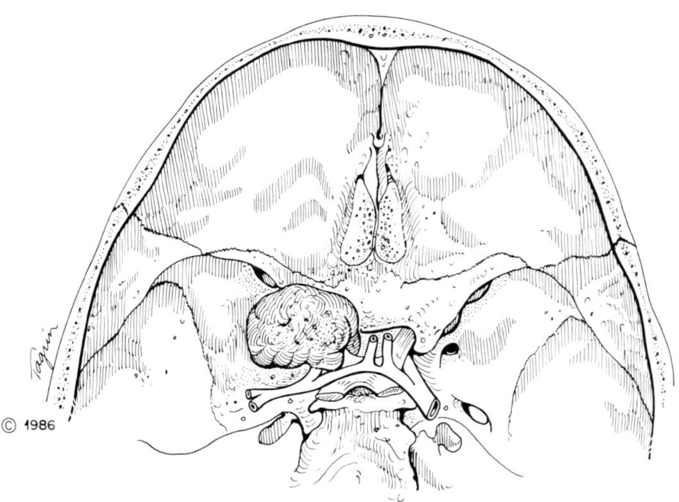

Fig. 45-14.   Medial sphenoid wing meningioma. Some tumors grow as a mass and may involve the optic nerve, internal carotid, and/or middle cerebral arteries and compress the frontal lobe, the temporal lobe, or both.

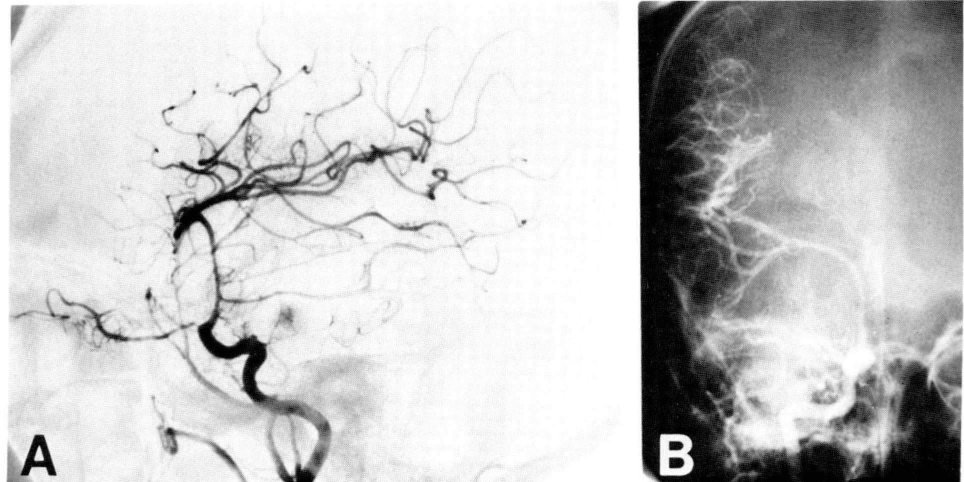

Fig. 45-16. Medial sphenoid wing meningioma (same patient as in Figure 45-15). (A) The lateral study shows marked elevation of the proximal middle cerebral artery complex and stretching and irregular narrowing (suggestive of tumor encasement) of the internal carotid artery. (B) The AP study reveals marked stretching and displacement of the internal carotid and proximal middle cerebral arteries.

segmental narrowing or irregularity of the vessel (Figures 45-16A and B). In the second category are those patients in whom the tumor grows diffusely in the region of the anterior clinoid, cavernous sinus, and adjacent medial sphenoid wing, often without significant intracranial mass (Figure 45-17). These patients may have evidence of optic nerve involvement, third nerve palsy, or sensory loss in trigeminal nerve distribution. The CT scan will show an enhancing parasellar lesion (Figure 45-18). Angiograms will reveal hypertrophied vessels and stain in the region of the cavernous sinus (Figure 45-19). This type of tumor may be best treated with radiation therapy.[5,16]

OPERATIVE TECHNIQUE

The operative approach is similar to the frontotemporal exposure outlined in the section on suprasellar meningiomas with more temporal exposure; the side is determined by the site of the tumor. A similar subfrontal approach is used by Kempe, MacCarty, and Bonnal et al.[11,12,17] Logue does an elective resection of the lateral inferior frontal lobe.[8] Morley may resect the temporal lobe tip.[13]

Great care must be taken in the approach to these lesions since the carotid and middle cerebral arteries may be embedded

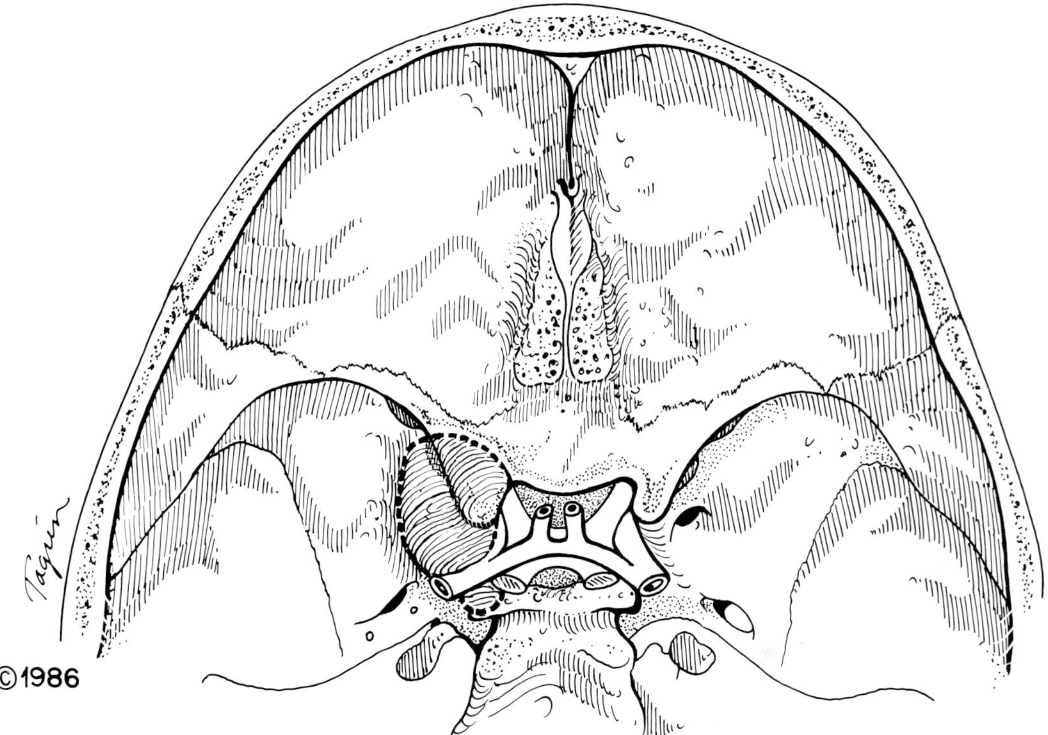

Fig. 45-17. Medial sphenoid wing meningioma. Some tumors grow as a plaque involving the anterior clinoid, the medial middle fossa, and the cavernous sinus.

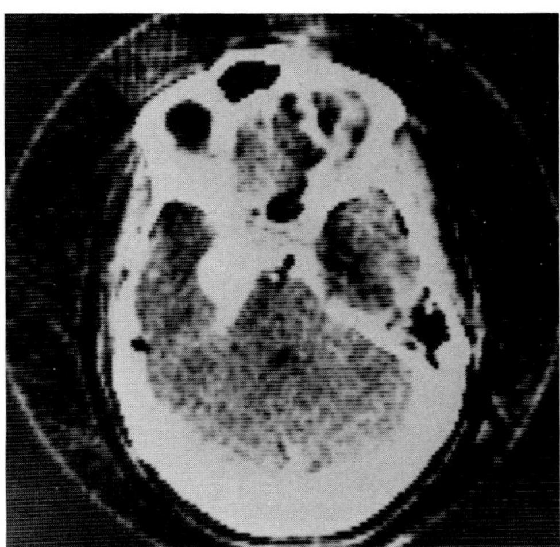

Fig. 45-18. Medial sphenoid wing meningioma. A CT scan of a tumor growing diffusely in the cavernous sinus and medial wall of the middle fossa.

the bone around the foramen and superior orbital fissure, the dura over this area is excised. The bone is removed using a diamond-burr with the air drill and a fine curette under the operating microscope. Even when it is possible to extensively remove the tumor with the involved bone and dura, it is difficult to totally excise these meningiomas; recurrent growth, however, usually is very slow.[17]

RESULTS

In none of the 21 patients in this series was it possible to be absolutely sure that a total removal had been done. Improvement in visual function with optic nerve decompression was the exception. There was no operative mortality, but two late deaths were caused by recurrent tumor. Five other patients have had to undergo reoperations for significant recurrence of a mass. Radiation therapy has been used in some patients when there was a recurrence and in those with a diffuse involvement in the cavernous sinus region with apparent arrest of growth in all but one with an atypical pathologic process.

in the tumor. On occasion, the tumor can be split and removed from around the artery using microsurgical techniques, but usually only a subtotal tumor removal is indicated to avoid arterial injury.

After the initial exposure, it may be necessary to open the medial aspect of the sylvian fissure. Internal decompression of the tumor is done and blood supply along the sphenoid wing, often a hypertrophied branch of the middle meningeal artery, is divided. As the dissection progresses on the lateral aspect of the tumor, it is important to look for the middle cerebral artery branches and to follow these medially to determine if they or the internal carotid artery are involved with tumor.

When the tumor grows into the optic foramen or involves

OLFACTORY GROOVE MENINGIOMAS

PRESENTATION

Olfactory groove meningiomas arise from the midline of the anterior fossa in the region of the cribriform plate and adjacent floor of the anterior fossa extending from the crista galli back to the planum sphenoidal. They are usually bilateral and often attain a large size before causing symptoms that lead to the diagnosis.[19] In Bakay's series of 36 patients the complaints that led to evaluation were failing vision in 12 cases; dementia in 8 cases; a combination of dementia and failing vision in 5 cases; seizures in 4 cases; seizures and dementia in 3 cases; headache in 3 cases; and urinary incontinence in 1

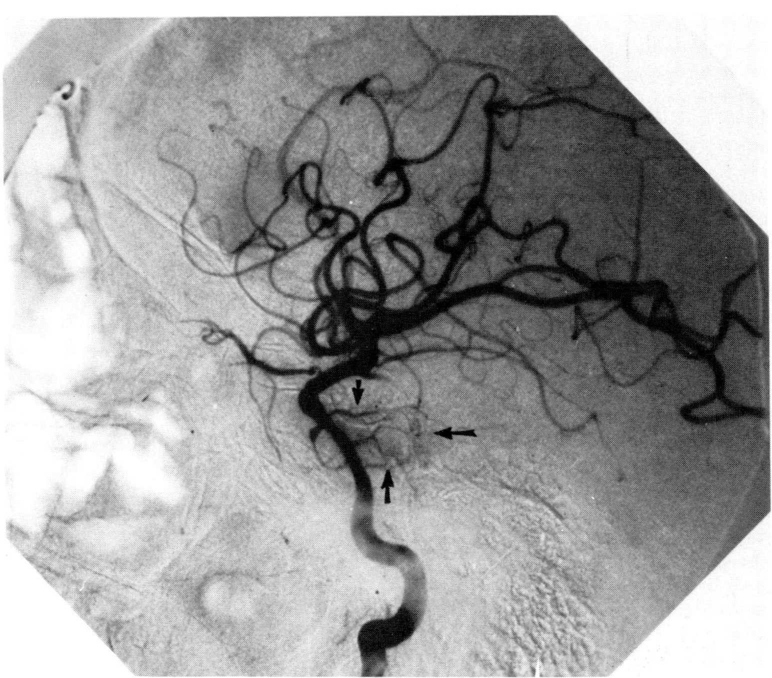

Fig. 45-19. Medial sphenoid wing meningioma. This angiogram shows a stain and abnormal hypertrophied arteries arising from the intracavernous portion of the internal carotid artery (arrows).

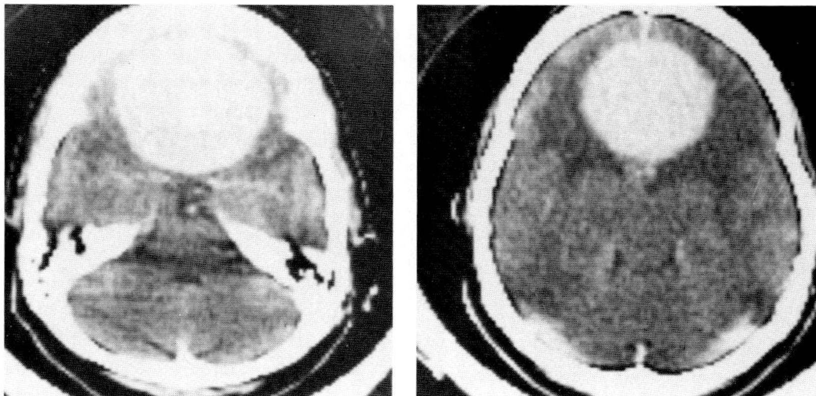

Fig. 45-20. Olfactory groove meningioma. Typical CT scan findings in a case of meningioma of the olfactory groove. A large, round, midline enhancing mass extends from the floor of the anterior fossa. There is edema in the adjacent frontal lobes.

case.[18] All patients except one had anosmia on examination but in none was it the initial symptom. Loss of a sense of smell was recorded "as possibly" the primary symptom in only three of 28 patients in Cushing's series, and he questioned the reliability of this finding.[1] In our series, the most common initial symptom was a subtle change in mental function or headache alone or in combination, but a disturbance in vision or seizure disorder was also the initial manifestation. None complained of impairment of the sense of smell, although it was found on examination.

RADIOGRAPHIC FINDINGS

The typical CT scan shows a large well-circumscribed mass in the low, midline frontal region with edema in the adjacent frontal lobes (Figure 45-20). Lateral cerebral angiograms show the typical stretched, curved course of the frontal polar artery over the superior surface of the tumor (Figure 45-21). The primary blood supply comes from branches of the ethmoidal, middle meningeal, and ophthalmic arteries, which enter through the midline of the base of the skull.

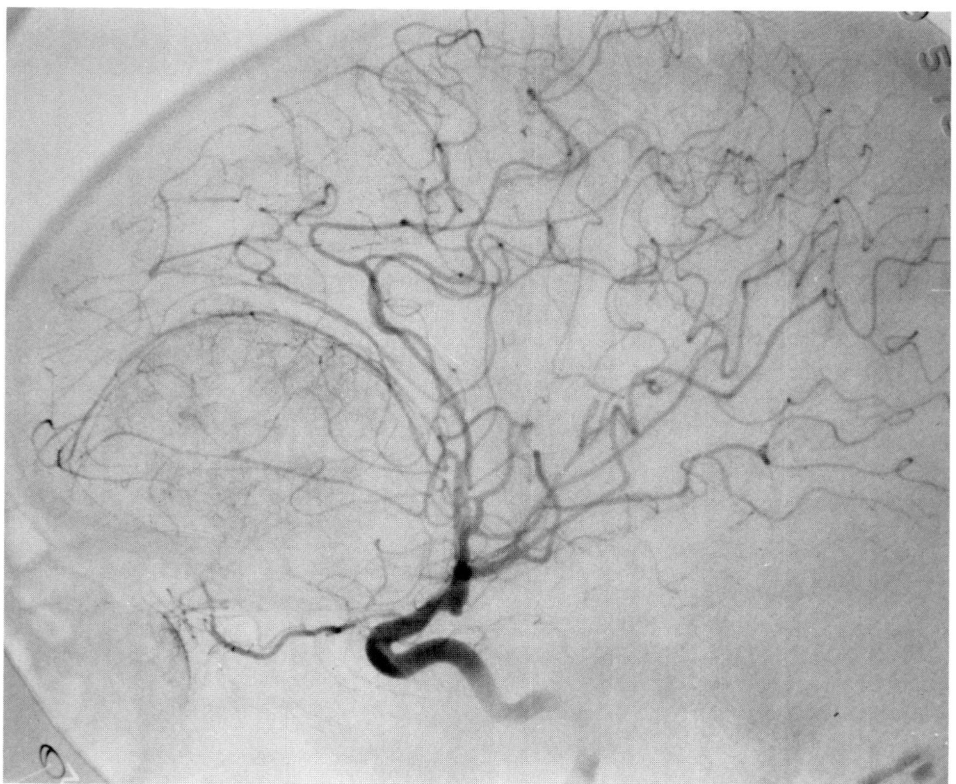

Fig. 45-21. A lateral angiogram shows the typical appearance of an olfactory groove meningioma. There is stretching and elevation of branches of the anterior cerebral artery over the superior surface of the tumor. The blood supply is coming into the base of the tumor from branches of the ethmoidal, middle meningeal, and ophthalmic arteries (arrows).

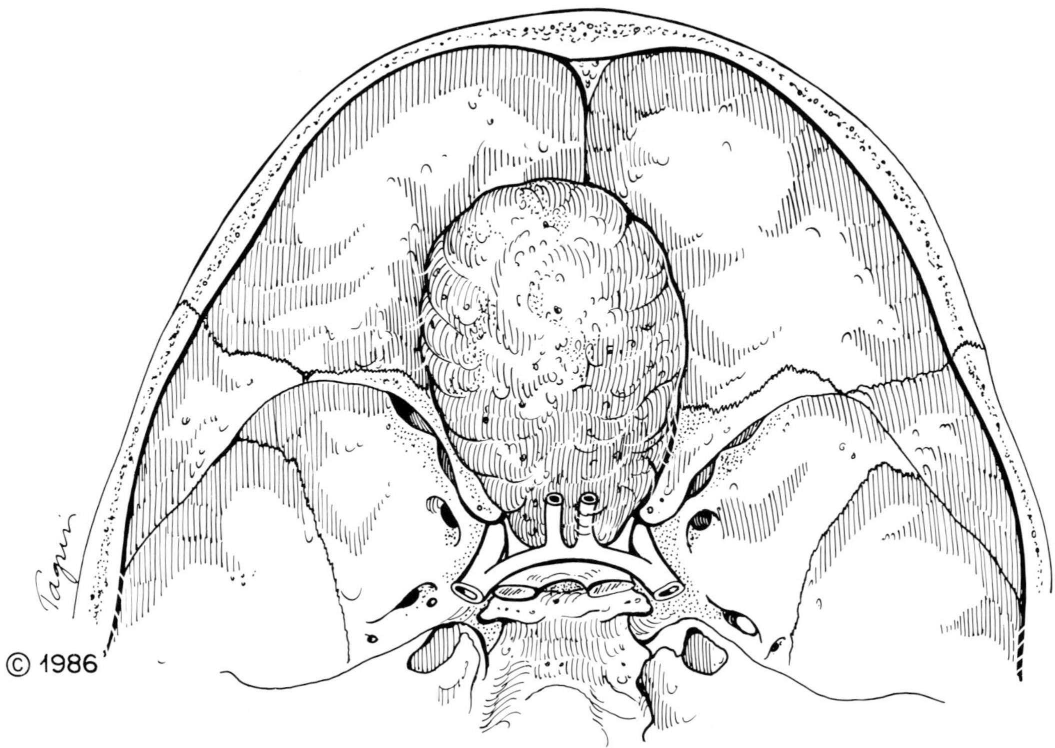

Fig. 45-22. The relationship of a large olfactory groove meningioma to the base of the skull, the optic nerves, the chiasm, and the anterior cerebral arteries.

OPERATIVE TECHNIQUE

In planning the operation, it is important to remember that the main blood supply comes into the tumor through the bone in the midline of the anterior fossa and the posterior capsule may be attached to the optic nerves, chiasm, and anterior cerebral arteries (Figure 45-22).

A bifrontal craniotomy for removal of these tumors is our usual approach. This allows the least amount of traction on the frontal lobes and gives direct access to both sides and the posterior surface of the tumor. MacCarty and Morley also prefer the bifrontal exposure.[12,13] Kempe described a unilateral right subfrontal approach.[11] Symon[6] and Logue[14] use either exposure and also resect part of the frontal lobe. Solero et al. use a right frontal craniotomy with frontal lobe resection.[19]

The patient is carefully placed in the supine position with the head elevated, slightly extended, and held with the Mayfield-Kees three-point skeletal fixation headrest. A coronal incision is made. The skin flap and underlying tissue, including the pericranial tissue, are turned down together. Burr holes are placed just below the end of the anterior temporal line and on each side of the sagittal sinus at the level of the skin incision (Figure 45-23). The bone cut just above the supraorbital ridge is made from each side as far medially as possible. Usually this leaves a centimeter or less of bone in the midline. Because of the irregular bone projecting from the inner table of the skull in this area, it usually is impossible to cut completely across the area. The outer table is cut with a small high-speed air drill; the inner table then can be broken and the free bone flap removed. The frontal sinuses are almost always entered. The mucosa is removed and the sinuses are packed with Bacitracin-soaked Gelfoam (Upjohn Co., Kalamazoo, Michigan). A flap of pericranial tissue from the back of the skin flap is turned down

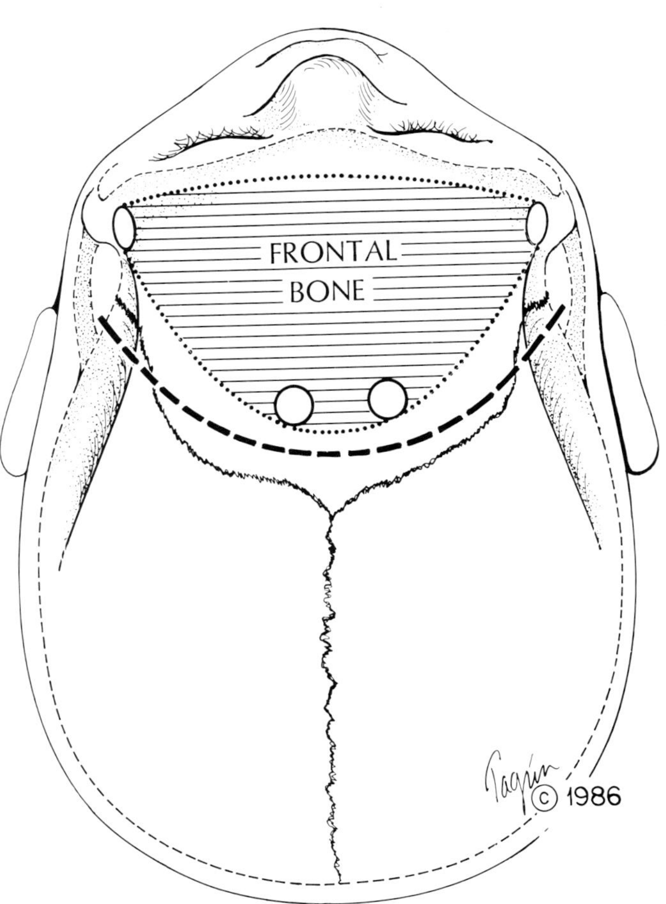

Fig. 45-23. Olfactory groove meningioma. The skin incision (dashed line) and free bone flap (dotted line) are outlined.

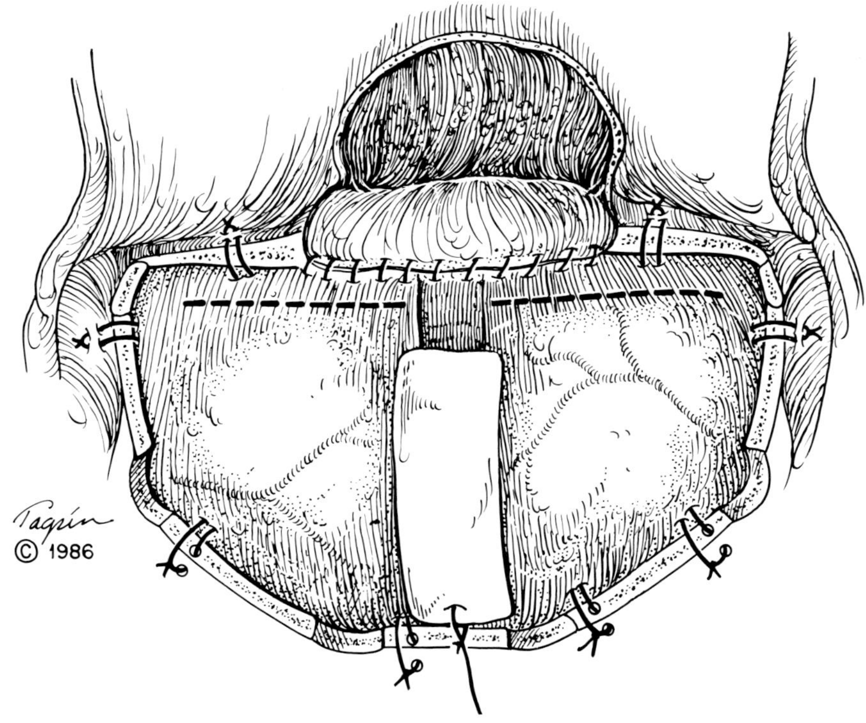

Fig. 45-24. Olfactory groove meningioma. The frontal sinuses are almost always entered. The mucosa is removed, the sinuses packed with bacitracin-soaked Gelfoam, and the opening covered with a flap of pericranial tissue.

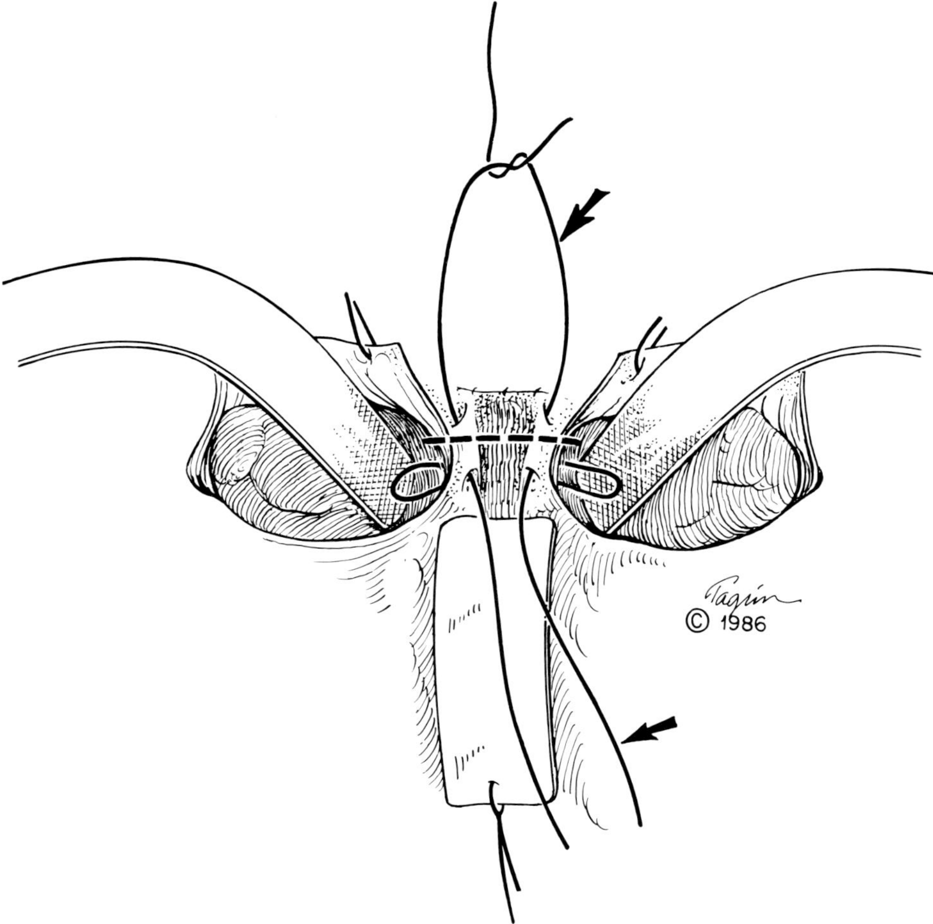

Fig. 45-25. Olfactory groove meningioma. The anterior sagittal sinus is being ligated.

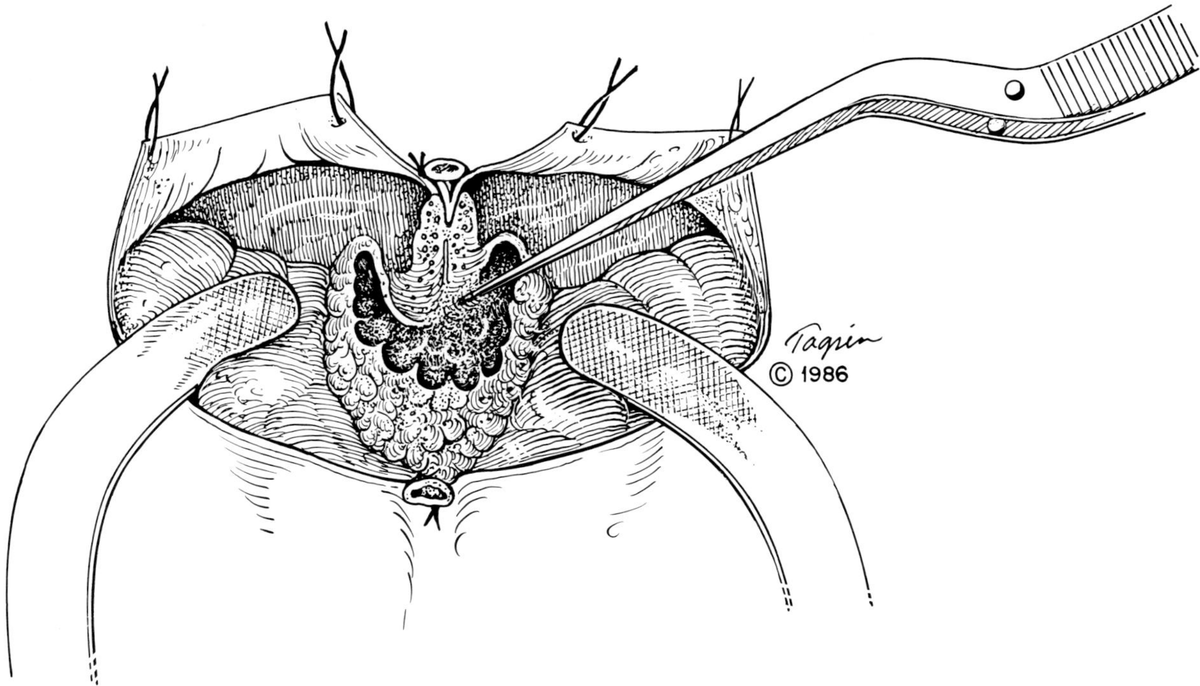

Fig. 45-26. Olfactory groove meningioma. Internal decompression of the tumor has been accomplished. The blood supply coming through the midline of the frontal fossa is being interrupted.

over the sinuses and sewn to the adjacent dura (Figure 45-24). Sutures are placed along the edge of the craniotomy to control epidural bleeding.

The dural incision is made over each medial inferior frontal lobe just above the edge of the craniotomy opening. The frontal lobes are carefully retracted, the sagittal sinus is divided between two silk sutures, and the falx is cut (Figure 45-25). The frontal lobes are then carefully retracted laterally and slightly posteriorly. The tumor will come into view in the midline and at times grow into the region of the crista galli and falx.

The anterior capsule of the tumor then is exposed; an extensive internal decompression is done using the Cavitron. The attachments of the tumor in the midline along the base of the frontal fossa are gradually divided, interrupting the blood supply which enters the tumor through numerous openings in the bone in this area (Figure 45-26). These feeding arteries are

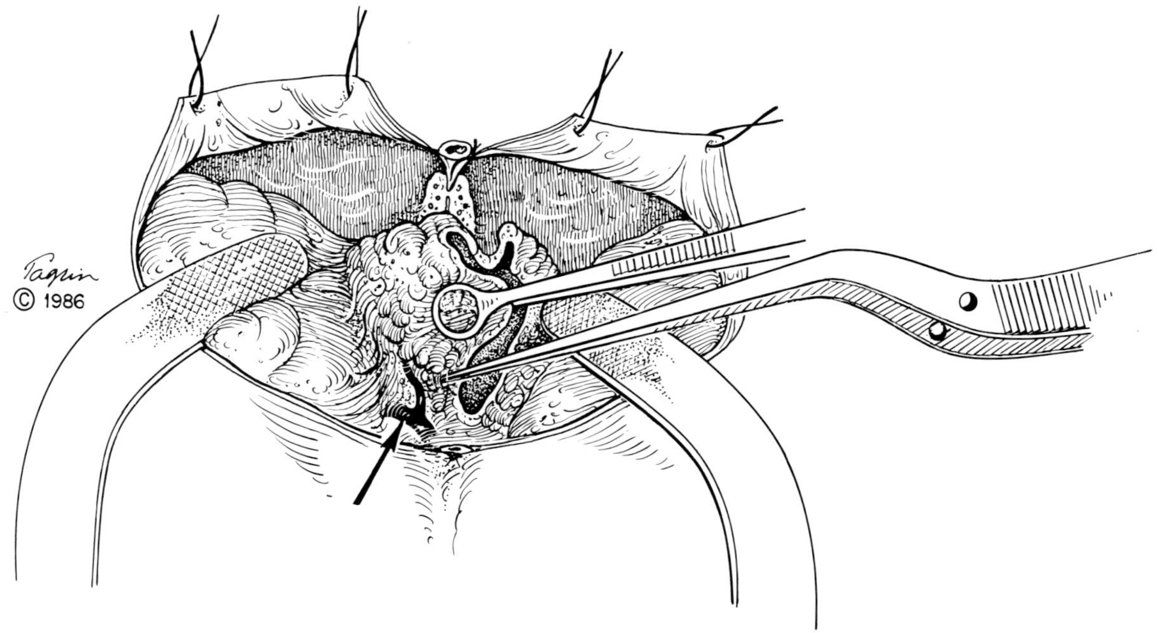

Fig. 45-27. Olfactory groove meningioma. The posterior capsule is being separated from the frontal lobe. The frontal polar artery is often adherent to the tumor and may need to be divided.

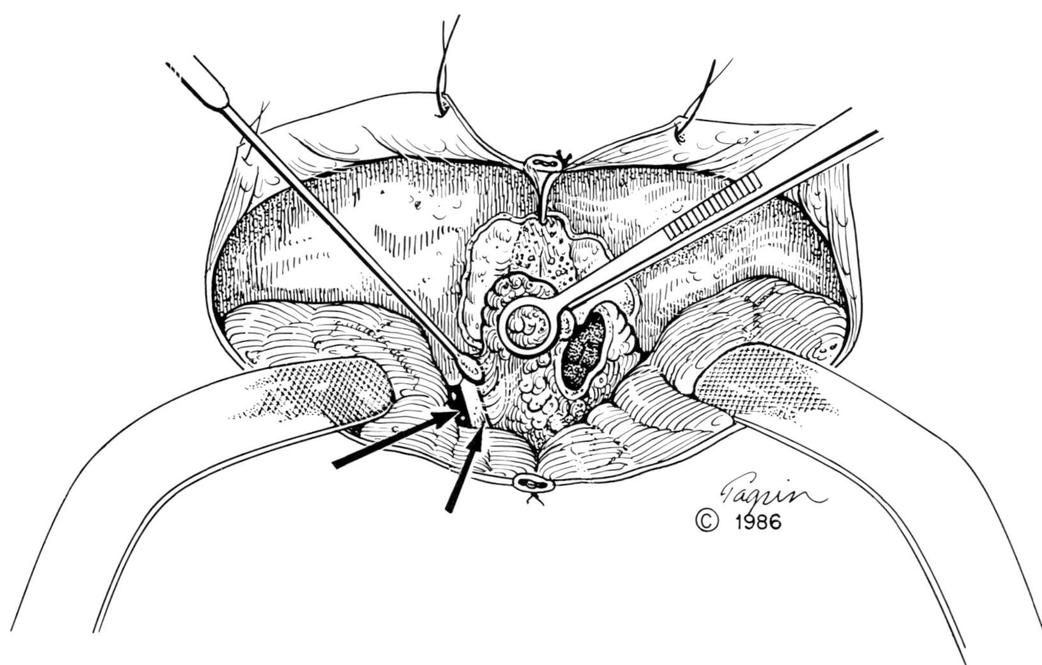

Fig. 45-28.   Olfactory groove meningioma. The left optic nerve and carotid artery (arrows) have been exposed. The tumor is being separated from the arachnoid over the nerve.

occluded with coagulation and bone wax. The capsule now can be reflected into the area of the decompression without undue pressure on the frontal lobes. Great care is taken during the dissection of the posterior portion of the capsule, reflecting it anteriorly and being careful to look for the pericallosal branch of the anterior cerebral artery complex, which may be embedded in the tumor. The frontal polar branch often will be adherent to the tumor and may need to be divided (Figure 45-27). It usually is possible to follow the capsule back to the

sphenoid wing, and then, working medially, to identify the anterior clinoid process and the optic nerve. At times it may be difficult to see the nerve because of the posterior and inferior compression and the reaction in the arachnoid. However, under magnification, the tumor can be reflected off the optic nerve (Figure 45-28).

Once the bulk of the tumor is removed, the dural attachment is totally excised, and any major bone enostosis is removed, with care being taken to avoid entering the ethmoid

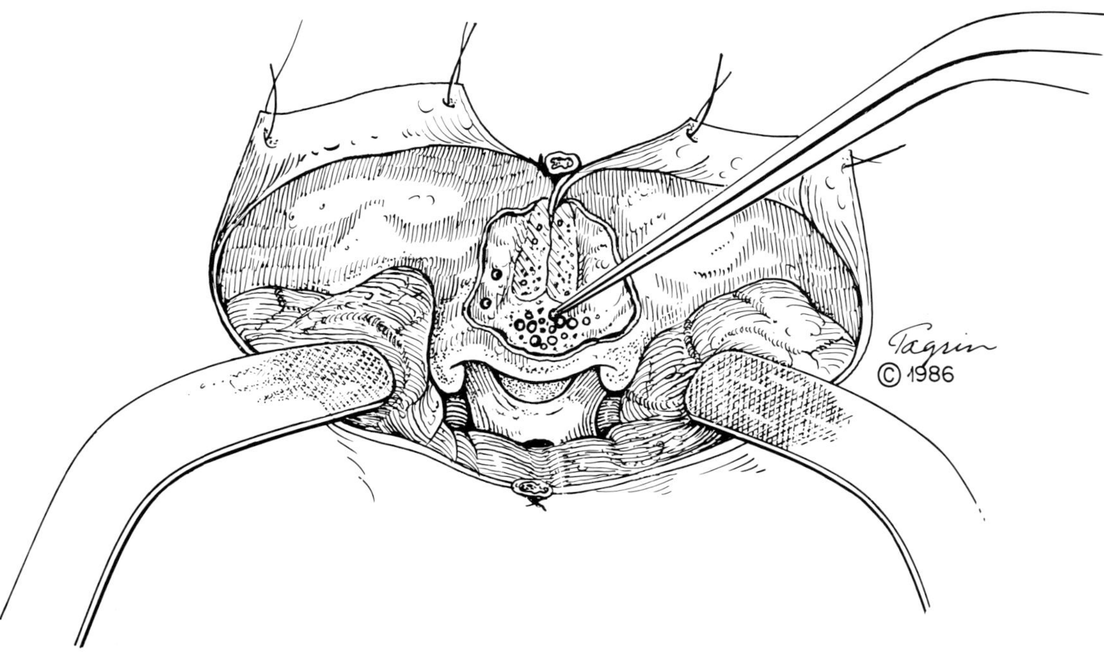

Fig. 45-29.   Olfactory groove meningioma. The tumor has been removed. Multiple holes are seen in the bone where the blood supply entered the tumor.

sinus (Figure 45-29). The region of the cribriform plate is covered with a graft of pericranial tissue and Gelfoam. Symon reported that the recurrence rate of these tumors is so low that there is no need to extensively treat the bone and one should avoid entering the ethmoid air cells if possible.[6]

RESULTS

In this series all 11 tumors were totally removed, with restoration of normal mental function and full activity in 10 patients. The postoperative course in 1 patient was complicated by a subdural hydroma that required a subdural peritoneal shunt. Another had a postoperative wound infection and a third had a CSF leak through the ethmoid sinus that required transethmoid repair. Bakay[18] reported one death in his last 11 patients, and MacCarty et al.[12] reported a very low mortality rate in their most recent series of meningiomas.

REFERENCES

1. Cushing H, Eisenhandt I: Meningiomas. Their Classification, Regional Behaviour, Life History and Surgical End Results. Part 1. Springfield, IL, Charles C Thomas, 1938
2. Kadis GN, Mount LA, Ganti SR: The importance of early diagnosis and treatment of the meningiomas of the planum sphenoidale and tuberculum sellae: A retrospective study of 105 cases. Surg Neurol 12:367, 1979
3. Al-Mefty O, Holoubi A, Rifai A, Fox JL: Microsurgical removal of suprasellar meningiomas. Neurosurgery 16:364, 1985
4. Ojemann RG: Meningiomas of the basal parapituitary region: Technical considerations. Clin Neurosurg 27:233, 1980
5. Ojemann RG: Clinical features and surgical management of meningiomas, in Wilkins RH, Rengachary SS (eds): Neurosurgery, vol 1. New York, McGraw-Hill, 1985, pp 638-684
6. Symon L: Olfactory groove and suprasellar meningiomas in Krayenbuhl H (ed): Advances and Technical Standards in Neurosurgery, vol 4. Berlin, Springer-Verlag, 1977, pp 67-91
7. Ojemann RG, Swann KW: Meningiomas of the anterior cranial base, in Sekhar L, Schram V (eds): Tumors of the Cranial Base: Diagnosis and Treatment. Futura (In press)
8. Symon L, Rosenstein J: Surgical management of suprasellar meningioma. Part 1: The influence of tumor size, duration of symptoms and microsurgery on surgical outcome in 101 consecutive cases. J Neurosurg 61:633, 1984
9. Rosenstein J, Symon L: Surgical management of suprasellar meningioma. Part 2: Prognosis for visual function following craniotomy. J Neurosurg 61:642, 1984
10. Gregorius FK, Hepler RS, Stern WE: Loss and recovery of vision with suprasellar meningiomas. J Neurosurg 42:69, 1975
11. Kempe LG: Operative Neurosurgery, vol 1. New York, Springer-Verlag, 1968
12. MacCarty CS, Piepgras DG, Ebersold NJ: Meningeal tumors of the brain, in Youmans J (ed): Neurological Surgery, ed 2. Philadelphia, WB Saunders, 1982, pp 2936-2966
13. Morley TP: Cranial meninges, in Youmans J (ed): Neurological Surgery. Philadelphia, WB Saunders, 1973, pp 1388-1411
14. Logue V: Surgery of meningiomas, in Symon L (ed): Operative Surgery: Neurosurgery. London, Butterworths, 1979, pp 128-173
15. Ojemann RG: Clinical features and surgical management of meningiomas, in Wilkins RH, Rengachary SS (eds): Neurosurgery, vol 1. New York, McGraw-Hill, 1985, pp 638-654
16. Carella RJ, Ransohoff J, Newall J: Role of radiation therapy in the management of meningiomas. Neurosurgery 10:332, 1982
17. Bonnal J, Thibaut A, Brotchi J, et al: Invading meningiomas of the sphenoid ridge. J Neurosurg 83:587, 1980
18. Bakay L: Olfactory meningiomas. The missed diagnosis. JAMA 251:53, 1984
19. Solero CL, Giombini S, Morello G: Suprasellar and olfactory meningiomas; Report on a series of 153 personal cases. Acta Neurochir 67:181, 1983

CHAPTER 46

Preoperative Evaluation and Management of Meningiomas

Robert E. Maxwell   Shelley N. Chou

HARVEY CUSHING coined the term *meningioma* in 1922 to define and distinguish a class of benign tumors arising from the meninges of the brain and spinal cord.[1] Meningiomas are the most common neoplasms of nonglial origin arising within the central nervous system and account for approximately 15 percent of all primary intracranial tumors.[2,3] Meningiomas are a neoplasm of adult life with a peak incidence in the fifth through seventh decades. A female preponderance is seen, especially for the spinal cord meningiomas.[4] Less than 2 percent of primary intracranial tumors in childhood and adolescence are meningiomas.[5] Bailey et al.[6] reported that when meningiomas occur in children, they tend to be large and are prone to sarcomatous elements. These tumors are less favorable for total resection than those occurring in adults.[6] Globus et al. also reported a higher incidence of meningiomas with sarcomatous features in children.[7] Distinctive features in childhood meningiomas are: (1) a relatively high incidence in the lateral ventricles (11.1 percent), (2) a high incidence of cyst formation in the tumor (16.7 percent), and (3) a predominance of male patients to female patients in contrast to the female predominance in adults.[8] One fourth of patients with meningiomas in childhood have neurofibromatosis.[9]

Ninety percent of intracranial meningiomas are supratentorial and 10 percent infratentorial. Approximately one third of supratentorial meningiomas arise along the superior sagittal sinus or falx, one third over the convexity of the hemispheres, and one third from basal regions such as the sphenoid ridge, the perisellar region, and the olfactory groove. Intraventricular meningiomas are rare and account for only 1 to 2 percent of all intracranial meningiomas. The intracranial site of origin determines the clinical presentation of the tumor, the size the tumor attains before symptoms occur, the operative approach, and, perhaps, the success of surgery. A clival meningioma encompassing the basilar artery presents technical problems not encountered with a small convexity meningioma. Tumor location, configuration, distribution, accessibility, histology, and vascularity compete with the surgeon's talent, experience, judgment, and applied state of the art directed toward achieving total tumor removal with preservation of function. Unfortunately, meningiomas recur.

Skullerud and Loken reported recurrence rates of 25 percent for suprasellar meningiomas and 33 percent for tentorial and posterior fossa meningiomas. This compares with a 9 percent recurrence rate for convexity meningiomas.[10] Meningiomas are benign tumors and the completeness of sur-

gical removal of the tumor is the single-most important prognostic factor.[2,11,12] Mirimanoff et al.[13] found that following a total resection, the recurrence-free rate at 5, 10, and 15 years was 93 percent, 80 percent, and 68 percent, respectively, at all sites. In contrast, after a subtotal resection, the progression free rate was only 63 percent, 45 percent, and 9 percent during the same period. The probability of having a second operation following a total excision after 5, 10, and 15 years was 6 percent, 15 percent, and 20 percent, whereas after a subtotal excision the probability was 25 percent, 44 percent, and 84 percent, respectively.[13] Borovich and Doron recently found, however, that solitary globular meningiomas represent only the most visible growth in the midst of a neoplastic field change spreading over a wide area of dura mater. The authors believed that this can explain some unexpected "recurrences," and that a wide resection of dura around globular meningiomas, whenever possible, could reduce the incidence of clinical growth after true total excision of the most visible lesion.[14]

The tumor recurrence rate is higher in children with meningiomas. Deen et al.[9] reported a 39 percent tumor recurrence rate in 51 patients under 21 years of age. The 15-year survival rate in patients with intracranial meningiomas was 68 percent. Factors adversely affecting survival were brain invasion, papillary histology, and location in the posterior fossa.

Meningiomas are of neuroectodermal origin and probably arise from arachnoid granulation tissue.[15] Their preferential sites correspond closely with the locations where arachnoid villi are most frequently encountered, namely, along the major venous sinuses and their contributory veins, at the foramina of exit of the cranial nerves, and where arachnoid cell clusters are found within the trunk of the perineurial sheaths of cranial nerves within or adjacent to the basal foramina.[16] Courville[17] and Russell and Rubinstein[18] have classified meningiomas into syncytial, transitional, fibroblastic, and angioblastic types based on the histologic appearance. Tumors without a predominating histologic pattern are classified as a mixed type. There are two subtypes of angioblastic meningiomas; one resembles the capillary hemangioblastoma found in the cerebellum (type IV, variant III of Cushing and Eisenhardt) and the other resembles the hemangiopericytoma (type IV, variant I of Cushing and Eisenhardt).[2]

The prognostic significance of tumor histology is controversial. Angioblastic meningiomas have been considered more aggressive and even potentially malignant.[18,19] Recent studies have shown a modest recurrence rate for angioblastic

OPERATIVE NEUROSURGICAL TECHNIQUES
ISBN 0-8089-1862-1

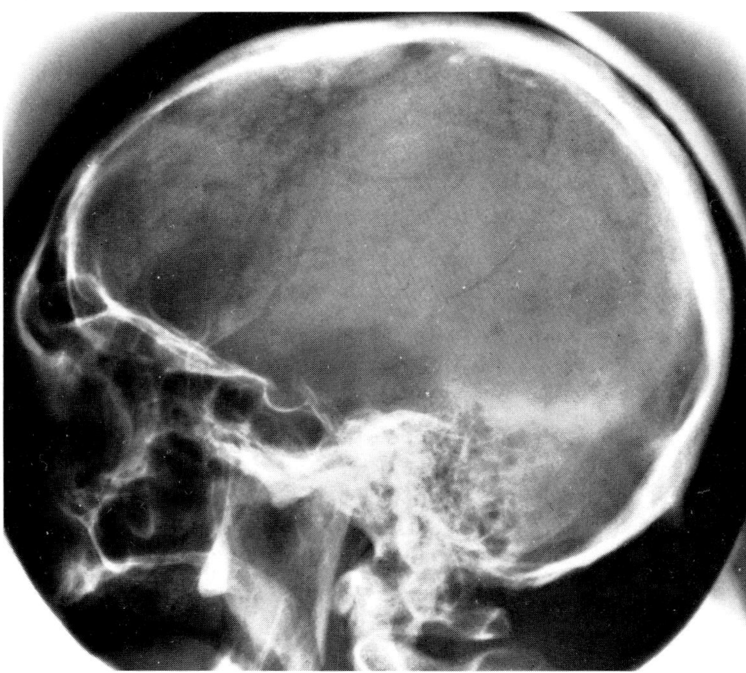

Fig. 46-1.   A plain x-ray film showing hyperostosis of the skull with a striated appearance overlying a meningioma.

meningiomas on the whole,[11,12] but the hemangiopericytoma subtype of the angioblastic meningioma has a higher recurrence rate than other meningiomas.[20–22]

Skullerud and Loken studied the prognostic significance of the histologic features of tumors in 161 patients with meningiomas in whom "total excision" was accomplished at the time of surgery.[10] The tumors were classified according to Courville.[17] Only the small subgroup of the angioblastic meningiomas resembling hemangiopericytomas recurred with significantly greater frequency. The prognostic significance of histologic and cytologic detail also was examined for 84 syncytial meningiomas. Only a high degree of cellularity could be statistically correlated with recurrence. There was also a predominance of high vascularity, mitoses, focal necrosis, and infiltration into bone and cortex among the recurrences, but these difference were not statistically significant.[10] Boker et al. found that the presence of mitoses, brain invasion and focal necrosis could be linked to a higher tumor recurrence rate, however, and tumors exhibiting all three of these characteristics recurred in every case in their series of 60 recurring meningiomas.[23]

Jellinger and Slowik[24] reviewed the incidence of the histologic subtypes of meningioma in 1238 patients using the classification of Courville. They found a recurrence rate of 14.2 percent for intracranial meningiomas among patients surviving 5 years. The symptomatic recurrence rate was twice as high after partial removal. Only the hemangiopericytoma type of angioblastic meningioma and atypical (malignant) meningiomas recurred more frequently or at shorter intervals after the initial surgery. In malignant meningiomas, the recurrence rate is high even in cases of total removal. The outcome for these patients is good with the papillary type meningioma, relatively good with the hemangiopericytic type, and poor with the anaplastic type.[25] The initial clinical course of malignant meningiomas tends to be short, but is otherwise indistinguishable from that of

benign meningiomas. The chances of recurrence and eventual death are high, however, and extracranial metastases are not rare. The tumors are most often hemangiopericytomas, but not exclusively so, and men are particularly at risk.[26]

Cystic meningiomas are rare but also have a tendency to recur.[27] These tumors have angioblastic components and display a histologic similarity to hemangioblastomas of the cerebellum, which are often cystic. Although the walls of large cysts associated with some meningiomas have been composed of reactive glia or collagen, neoplastic cells may be found in the distant cyst walls underscoring the need for resection and careful pathologic evaluation of the large cyst associated with meningiomas.[28]

Multiple meningiomas are being seen more frequently with the advent of CT scanning. The incidence of 8.9 percent reported by Lusins and Nakagawa is significantly higher than the 1 to 3 percent incidence reported previously.[29] Multiple meningiomas sometimes occur as forme fruste of Von Recklinghausen's disease, but this is not always the case.[30]

PREOPERATIVE ROENTGENOLOGIC STUDIES

The history and clinical examination vary according to the location, size, and configuration of the tumors and are best discussed in the context of specific meningiomas classified according to their sites of origin. Radiographic studies are necessary and are selected not only to confirm the presence of a tumor, but also to assess key anatomic and pathologic features that aid the surgeon in planning surgery.

PLAIN ROENTGENOGRAMS

Although computed tomographic (CT) scanning and angiography are the most useful radiographic studies for assessing meningiomas, anteroposterior (AP) and lateral chest and skull

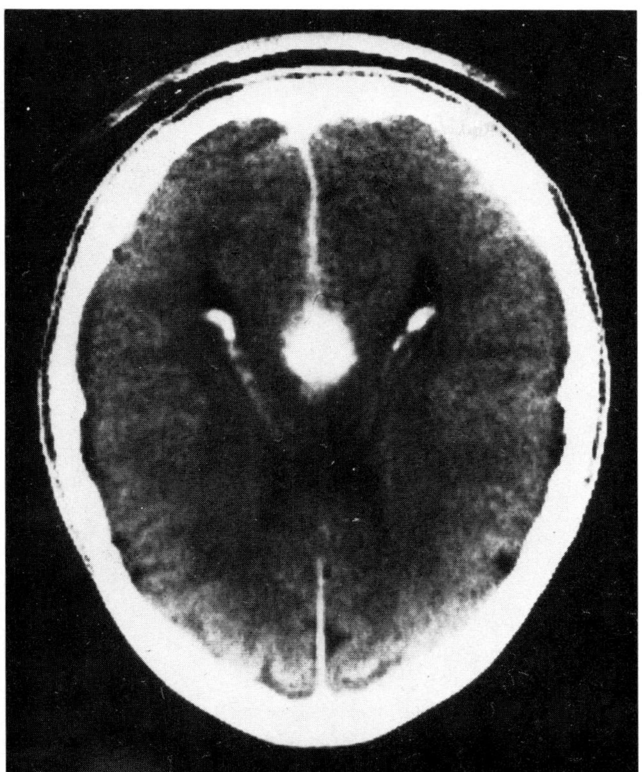

Fig. 46-2. A CT scan showing the bilateral configuration of a falx meningioma.

x-ray studies are not neglected. The chest reontgenograms may reveal pulmonary, cardiovascular, or metastatic disease.

Cushing reported that 14 of 65 meningiomas were associated with hyperostosis of the skull along the vertex and particularly in the region of the bregma.[2] The changes seen on plain skull x-ray films may take the form of diffuse, homogeneous bone-thickening, exostosis, or enostosis. The hyperostosis is often striated in appearance (Figure 46-1). The extent of hyperostosis is not indicative of the size of the associated soft tissue mass.[31] Bone erosion is not common, but occasionally a meningioma infiltrates the calvaria and produces bone destruction. Gilbertson and Good reported radiographic calcification in 18 percent of 154 meningiomas.[32] This is similar to the incidence reported by others.[33,34]

Hyperostosis of the skull associated with the en plaque form of meningioma may present a diagnostic challenge since the intracranial part of the tumor is not visualized by skull radiography, computed tomography, or other neuroradiologic methods. Kim et al. recently reported 4 cases of hyperostosing meningioma en plaque demonstrating the characteristic features of a subdural layer of ossification along the hyperostic bone with a dural lucent interface. Polytomography or high resolution CT scanning at bone window settings is necessary to identify the dural lucent line. The absence of this sign, however, does not exclude meningioma en plaque.[35]

Abnormal vascularity is difficult to recognize with certainty on plain skull x-ray films. A cluster of punctate radiolucencies may indicate the site where enlarged branches of the superficial temporal and middle meningeal arteries penetrate the skull to supply the meningioma. The vascular trunks leading to a meningioma usually are large. Distal enlargement and tortuosity of the middle meningeal arterial groove on the inner table of the skull near the convexity suggests the possibility of a parasagittal meningioma.

COMPUTED TOMOGRAPHIC SCANNING

The CT scan is the diagnostic screening procedure of choice for recognizing and accurately localizing meningiomas. The contrast-enhanced CT scan has been shown to detect over 96 percent of intracranial meningiomas and has been found to be significantly more accurate than radionuclide studies and plain radiography and slightly more accurate than angiography.[36] The tomographic cuts are taken at sufficiently close intervals so that the exact location, size, configuration, and area of dural attachment can be determined preoperatively. Biplane or triplane tomography is helpful in predicting the relationship of the tumor to important contiguous structures and in assessing

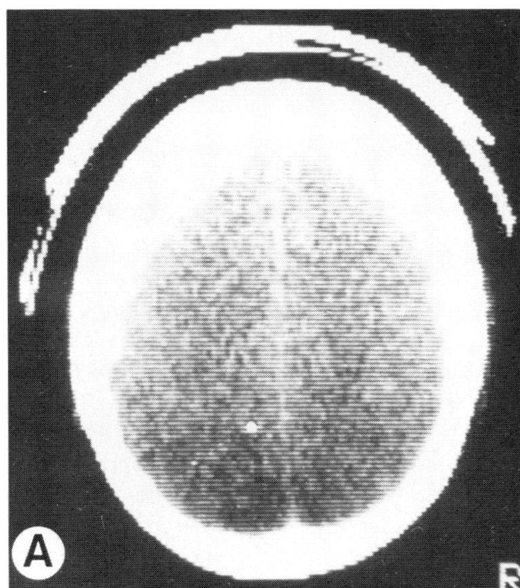
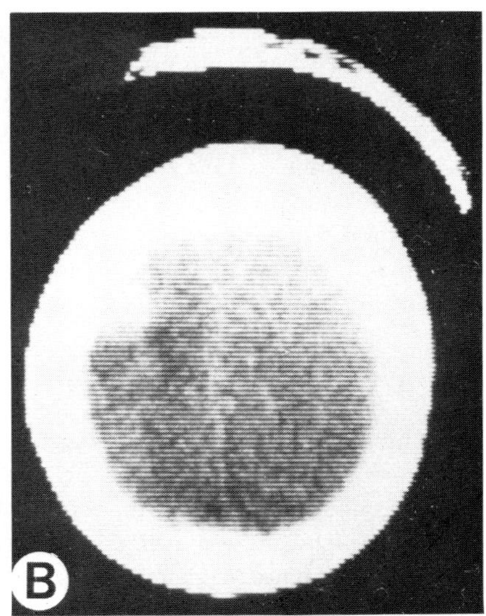

Fig. 46-3. (A) This CT scan failed to demonstrate a small meningioma adjacent to the vertex of the skull. (B) This subsequent CT scan with close tomographic cuts near the vertex shows a small meningioma.

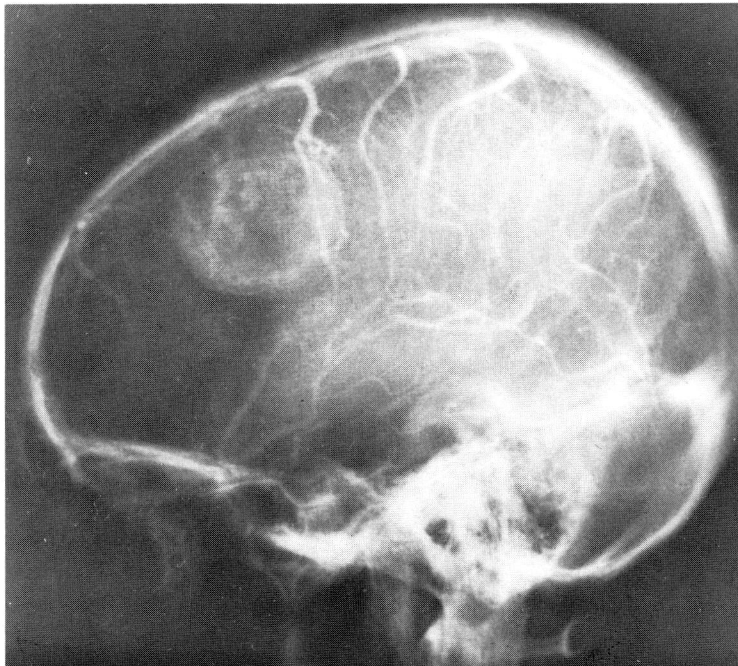

Fig. 46-4. An angiogram showing a meningioma tumor stain that is characteristiccally diffuse and persistent into the venous phase.

the amount of brain edema and the degree of brain distortion or shift. The procedure is particularly helpful for determining that the tumor is bilateral (Figure 46-2). Falsely negative scans are uncommon. They usually are associated with technical deficiencies such as the omission of contrast enhancement or failure to examine the vertex or high parietal region adequately with close tomographic cuts (Figures 46-3A and B).

Techniques are being developed to precisely localize tumors according to skull landmarks. This will assist the neurosurgeon in planning the operation. The CT scan is useful in the immediate postoperative period to detect the presence of a hematoma, brain edema, or brain shift. Serial CT scanning can be used along with the catamnesis to detect or follow recurrent tumors.

New et al. correlated histologic features associated with malignancy and a high rate of recurrence with radiologic features. On CT scans, most of the malignant meningiomas were moderately hyperdense before contrast enhancement, but showed no or minimal calcification. Marked perifocal edema was common. Indistinct tumor margins or, occasionally, deeply extending fringes of tumor interdigitating with brain substance, marked bone destruction, or prominent pannus or tumor extending well away from the globoid mass, termed "mushrooming," were correlated with histologic and clinical malignancy in meningiomas.[37]

MAGNETIC RESONANCE IMAGING

Meningiomas are often more clearly seen on CT scans than with magnetic resonance imaging (MRI) scans. This is a result of poor contrast between the tumor and the adjacent brain on all spin-echo and inversion-recovery pulse sequences. Those sequences that provide the greatest anatomic detail are best for identifying this low-contrast lesion. Inversion-recovery scans in particular demonstrate the tumor as a discrete hypointense mass (relative to nearby white matter) with excellent visualization of the dural base and white matter buckling indicative of extra cerebral

mass affect. Other characteristic features of meningiomas on the MRI scan include: a hypointense rim because of the venous capsule (66 percent); mottling due to hypervascularity; a well defined edema collar that demarcates the tumor from adjacent brain; and hyperostosis with thickening of the calvaria and obliteration of its normal landmarks. A MRI scan does not demonstrate tumor calcification but does demonstrate vascular encasement, displacement, and occlusion better than CT scans and as well as digital venous angiography.[38]

Preliminary work suggests that intravenous gadolinium-diethylenetriamine pentaacetic acid (Gd-DTPA) administration may enhance the display of meningiomas on MRI scans. Inversion-recovery has been shown to be the most useful sequence for demonstration of the tumor prior to administration of intravenous Gd-DTPA and also displayed the highest level of contrast enhancement after Gd-DTPA.[39]

ANGIOGRAPHY

Preoperative angiography is important in the assessment of intracranial meningiomas, not only for diagnostic purposes, but also for planning the management of the tumors. The amount and source of tumor vascularity are determined along with the involvement of adjacent vascular structures. The blood supply of meningiomas is primarily derived from dural vessels, but the tumor usually parasitizes pial vessels by the time it reaches 2 cm in diameter.[40]

Angiography demonstrates the primary blood supply to the tumor so that the surgical approach can be planned and preoperative embolization of the tumor performed if it is deemed advantageous. A tumor stain is often seen that is homogeneous and persistent into the venous phase (Figure 46-4). If important arteries are encased by tumor, this may be recognized in advance. The venous phase of the angiogram is important for assessing the patency of the major dural venous sinuses and the proximity of large draining cortical veins to the tumor. The presence of cortical venous collateral pathways is important in planning surgery so that venous occlusion, hemorrhagic infarction, and intraoperative and postoperative brain swelling are avoided.

Selective external carotid injection is combined with internal carotid angiography in the preoperative assessment of supratentorial meningiomas. The vertebrobasilar arterial system also is studied when a posterior fossa meningioma is suspected or demonstrated.

AIR OR POSITIVE CONTRAST ENCEPHALOGRAPHY

Very small meningiomas, particularly in the parasagittal or falcine area, may produce focal motor seizures when they are so small that angiographic studies are equivocal. Air pneumoencephalography or ventriculography (in the patient with symptoms or signs of increased intracranial pressure) was formerly necessary to detect a depression in the roof of one or both lateral ventricles. Water-soluble contrast ventriculography also can be used for this purpose. Computed tomographic scanning now circumvents the need for this invasive procedure provided that the tomographic cuts are obtained at sufficiently close intervals near the vertex and contrast enhancement is used.

Air encephalography also may aid the neurosurgeon in the preoperative assessment of parasellar and suprasellar meningiomas when three-dimensional CT tomography is not available. A small amount of air may help define more precisely the lateral, postchiasmal, and retroclival extent of these tumors.

INDICATIONS FOR SURGERY AND RADIATION THERAPY

Meningiomas as a class are benign tumors, potentially curable by total excision, and with few exceptions surgery is the sole treatment of choice. Even when total excision is deemed unlikely because of the location, configuration, or extent of the tumor, surgery is performed for the purpose of confirming the diagnosis and obtaining tissue so that alternative modes of therapy can be considered. An occasional patient is encountered for whom surgery is contraindicated because of advanced age, poor general condition, or an associated disease. Papo reported that since the advent of CT scanning the number of meningiomas operated upon and the average age of the patients diagnosed with meningiomas have increased. The mortality rate with surgery increased steeply for patients over 65 years of age and for this reason Papo recommended that the indications for surgery should be carefully evaluated in the geriatric age group.[41]

Many clinicians have reported that radiotherapy is not appreciably effective in the treatment of most meningiomas.[12,42–44] Recurrence of meningioma is uncommon when the surgeon is confident that the tumor has been totally excised. Wara et el.[45] reported 84 patients for whom the operating surgeon thought complete tumor removal was achieved and there were no recurrences among this group, with an average observation time longer than 6 years. The symptomatic recurrence rate approaches 75 percent, however, when only a subtotal resection is achieved. Several authors have suggested that postoperative irradiation is of value for meningiomas that are partially removed.[45–48] Wara and associates[45] found that postoperative irradiation of at least 5000 rad reduced the symptomatic recurrence rate to 22 percent and also delayed

recurrence. They were unable to correlate the tumor response to radiation therapy with the specific histologic subtype as defined by Courville.[17] Solan and Kramer could find no difference in ultimate outcome between patients with benign meningiomas irradiated in the immediate postoperative period as opposed to those irradiated at time of progression or recurrence.[49] Forbes and Goldberg reported data suggesting that moderate-dose radiation therapy can offer long-term symptom-free survival with few complications in patients having unresected or partially resected benign meningiomas. No patients, however, with malignant meningiomas were relapse-free 3 years after radiation therapy.[50] Carella et al. concluded on the basis of a review of 68 patients with meningiomas treated by radiation therapy that radiation therapy has an established role in the treatment of incompletely excised, recurrent, or malignant meningiomas and, in some cases, as the initial management of meningiomas.[51]

At the Cushing Society Meeting in 1965, Boldrey advocated preoperative radiation therapy to decrease the vascularity of the meningioma in selected cases.[45] The recommended tumor dose was 5000 to 5500 rad administered over a 6-week period approximately 6 months before the contemplated surgery. Wara et al. suggested the use of preoperative radiation for extremely vascular meningiomas where total removal is doubtful. They recommended that 5000 to 5500 rad be given over 5½ to 6 weeks with a 6-month delay between irradiation and surgery. This approach allowed the successful extirpation of 8 of 12 meningiomas for which surgery had not been considered feasible. Fukui et al.[52,53] concluded on the basis of their results and a review of the literature that preoperative irradiation may be helpful in the treatment of angioblastic meningiomas of the hemangiopericytoma type if the tumor is highly vascular and hardly accessible. Meningotheliomatous meningiomas and angioblastic meningiomas of the hemangioblastoma type were less radiosensitive.

PREOPERATIVE EMBOLIZATION OF MENINGIOMAS

Djindjian et al. demonstrated the effectiveness of embolizing branches of the external carotid artery feeding vascular tumors.[54] Presurgical embolization of meningiomas can be used to lessen operative hemorrhage, shorten the time in surgery, and make total tumor extirpation more feasible.

Hekster et al.[55] used pieces of Gelfoam (spongostan) and a transfemoral selective catheter technique to occlude feeder vessels originating off branches of the external carotid artery. Surgery was performed the following day with minimal blood loss. Gelfoam presents some difficulties when used for tumor embolization, however. Feeder vessels tend to recanalize, and it is difficult to see with fluoroscopy. There also is a danger of Gelfoam refluxing into the internal carotid artery distribution and occluding branches important for cerebral circulation unless retrograde flow is prevented. Rutka et al. carried out transfemoral Gelfoam embolization preoperatively in 8 patients with supratentorial meningiomas. In 7 of the cases, post-embolization, contrast-enhanced computed tomography was carried out. Areas of low-density tumor necrosis were identified in 5. In 3 of the 8 patients, post-embolization angiography demonstrated elimination of the tumor blush and in the other 5, the blush was reduced in intensity. Histologic evidence of tumor embolization was identified in each case to a varying degree. Preoperative embolization resulted in an identifiable

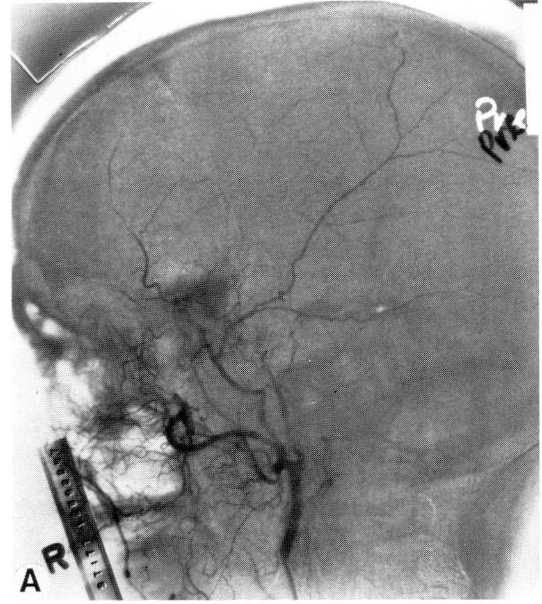

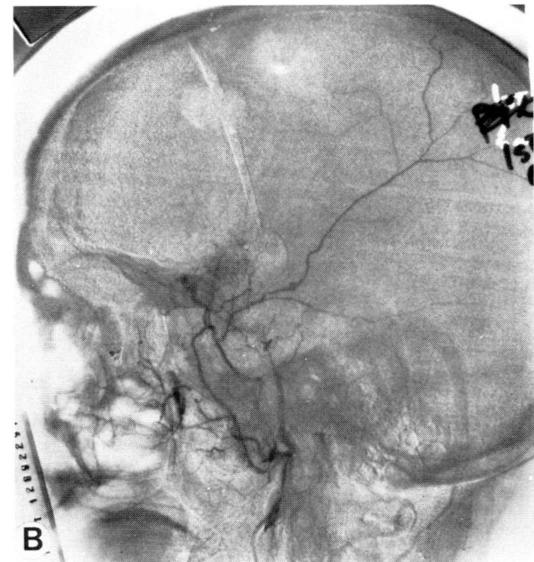

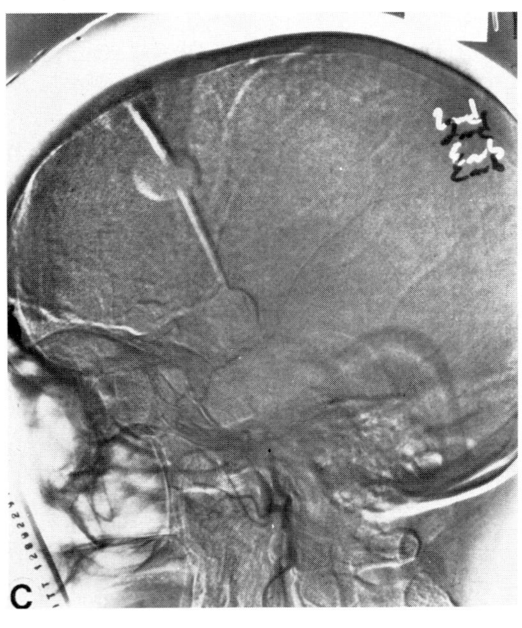

Fig. 46-5. (A) Following partial resection of a large right frontal meningioma, this right external carotid angiogram shows residual tumor stain in the distribution of the middle meningeal artery. (B) Partial embolization of the distal right external carotid artery with PAF obliterated the tumor stain by obstructing vessels within the tumor parenchyma. (C) Subsequent embolization obliterated the middle meningeal artery.

radiologic change in the majority of these tumors, but the authors could not determine whether intraoperative bleeding was reduced.

Hilal and Michelsen described the use of Silastic spheres and a low-viscosity Silastic elastomer to occlude vessels that fed a tumor originating from the branches of the external carotid artery.[57] A percutaneous puncture of the common carotid artery is performed, and the catheter is advanced into the lumen of the branches of the external carotid feeding the tumor. Double-lumen balloon catheters allow embolization and angiography without retrograde reflux of embolic particles. Radiographic control is essential throughout the procedure and Gelfoam or Silastic adhesives can be mixed with a radiopaque tantalum powder (1 μ particles) to permit detection of the emboli by fluoroscopy or radiography.

Polyvinyl alcohol foam (PAF) (Unipoint Laboratories, High Point, NC) is an effective material for embolizing vascular meningiomas.[58] PAF shavings occlude small vessels within the tumor as well as the major feeding vessels (Figure 46-5). Following PAF embolization, meningiomas unresectable because of excessive vascularity can be excised with far less bleeding. Multiple blanched areas are seen throughout the tumor at the time of surgery.

Teasdale et al.[59] cautioned that CT and dynamic radioisotope scan findings were unable to predict the degree of vascularity of the tumor or its suitability for embolization. Futhermore, these tests, repeated after embolization, were unreliable in detecting either the extent of necrosis or reduction in blood flow. They did find, however, that subselective embolization was simple, safe, and effective for producing tumor necrosis and intraoperative hemostasis in selected patients.

Arterial digital subtraction angiography has been reported to have some advantages over conventional angiography when monitoring the intravascular embolization of hypervascular tumors.[60] Arterial digital subtraction angiography may reduce the time of waiting for regular film development and subtraction. The smaller amount of contrast material used in arterial digital subtraction angiography minimizes the discomfort to the patient and may also prevent further renal damage in those patients with poor renal function.

PREPARATION OF PATIENT FOR SURGERY

The operative approach and contingency plans should be thought out in advance based on the clinical and radiographic information available to the surgeon. The objectives, priorities, risks, and indications of surgery are discussed thoroughly with the patient and family before consent for the operation is obtained.

Modern instrumentation, drugs, lighting, magnification, and anesthetic techniques make total resection feasible for meningiomas previously considered unresectable. An aggressive posture in pursuit of a "permanent cure" is always tempered, however, by surgical judgment born of the awareness that the first priority is to preserve and improve function. The surgical objectives are flexible and adapted to the age, condition, desires, social responsibilities, and specific tumor characteristics of each patient.

Corticosteroid (dexamethasone or methylprednisolone) therapy is initiated at least 24 hours before surgery in order to reduce brain edema and intracranial pressure. Diphenylhydantoin also is administered, and a serum drug level of 15–20 mg/ml is attained for seizure prophylaxis. The increase in metabolic activity, hypercarbia, and hypoxia associated with a major motor seizure can rapidly and profoundly elevate pressure within an intracranial compartment where compliance already may be exhausted from accommodating the mass effect of the tumor. In a study of a consecutive series of 127 surgically treated meningiomas, Ramamurthi et al.[61] found that 29 percent of the patients had reported convulsions as their initial symptom. In this group, surgical excision of the meningioma stopped the convulsions in about half of the patients, but the others continued to have seizures after their operations. Among those patients with meningiomas who did not have preoperative convulsions, about one sixth developed postoperative seizures. Patients in both groups required prolonged anticonvulsant medication. Factors predisposing a patient to the occurrence of postoperative seizures were the site of the tumor, faulty surgical technique, and preoperative history of seizures.

Cefoxitin sodium or a comparable antibiotic with broad spectrum and antistaphylococcal properties is administered parenterally in a dosage of 1 g/kg on call to surgery and in four divided doses during the first 24 hours following surgery. Cefoxitin is well tolerated after intramuscular or intravenous injection. It can be administered less frequently and in smaller doses than cephalothin because of its longer half-life.[62]

A smooth induction of general anesthesia and a nontraumatic intubation without straining or coughing in a well-paralyzed patient is crucial. Controlled hyperventilation then is used to maintain a well-oxygenated patient with a PCO_2 of 25–28 torr. An intra-arterial catheter is used to monitor blood gases and arterial pressure throughout the procedure. A catheter is placed in the right atrium of the heart with radiographic confirmation of location for monitoring central venous pressure and for aspiration of air should air embolism occur. The head is positioned higher than the heart and the neck is not flexed or rotated to such a degree that jugular venous drainage is impeded.

An indwelling Foley catheter is inserted following the induction of anesthesia so an osmotic dehydrating agent can be administered to reduce brain swelling. Urine output is measured throughout the procedure and during the postoperative recovery phase. A 20 percent solution of mannitol in a dosage of 1 g/kg is started intravenously after induction of anesthesia so that diuresis is achieved by the time dura mater is opened and the tumor is exposed. J Maxwell and Chou

REFERENCES

1. Cushing H: Meningiomas, Macewen Memorial Lecture, 1927. Glasgow, Jackson Wylie and Company, 1972
2. Cushing H, Eisenhardt L: Meningiomas. Their Classification, Regional Behavior, Life History and Surgical End Results. Springfield, Ill, Charles C Thomas, 1938, p 785
3. Zulch KJ: Brain Tumors: Their Biology and Pathology. New York, Springer, 1965
4. Challa VR, Markesbery WR: Meningiomas: Pathology, in Wilkins RH, Setti SR (eds): Neurosurgery. New York, McGraw-Hill, 1984, pp pp 613–622
5. Leibel SA, Wara WM, Sheline GE, et al: The treatment of meningiomas in childhood. Cancer 37:2709, 1976
6. Bailey O, Buchanan DN, Bucy PC: Intracranial Tumors in Infancy and Childhood. Chicago, University of Chicago Press, 1948, pp 441–500
7. Globus JH, Zucker JM, Rubinstein JM: Tumors of the brain in children and adolescents—a clinic and anatomic survey of ninety-two verified cases. Am J Dis Child 65:604, 1943
8. Sano K, Wakai S, Ochiai C, et al: Characteristics of intracranial meningiomas in childhood. Childs Brain 8:98, 1981
9. Deen HG Jr, Scheithauer BW, Ebersold MJ: Clinical and pathological study of meningiomas of the first two decades of life. Neurosurgery 56:317, 1982
10. Skullerud K, Loken AC: The prognosis in meningiomas. Acta Neuropathol 29:337, 1974
11. Crompton MR, Gautier-Smith PC: The prediction of recurrence in meningiomas. J Neurol Neurosurg Psychiatry 33:80, 1970
12. Simpson D: The recurrence of intracranial meningiomas after surgical treatment. J Neurol Neurosurg Psychiatry 20:22, 1957
13. Mirimanoff RO, Dosoretz DE, Lingood RM, et al: Meningioma: Analysis of recurrence and progression following neurosurgical resection. J Neurosurg 62:18, 1985
14. Borovich B, Doron Y: Recurrence of intracranial meningiomas: The role played by regional multicentricity. Neurosurgery 64:58, 1986
15. Wolman L: Role of the arachnoid granulation in the development of meningioma. Arch Pathol 53:70, 1952
16. Nager GT, Heroy J, Hoeplinger M: Meningiomas invading the temporal bone with extension to the neck. Am J Otolaryngol 4:297, 1983
17. Courville CB: Pathology of the Central Nervous System, ed 3. Mountain View, Ca, Pacific Press Publishing, 1950
18. Russell DS, Rubenstein LJ: Pathology of Tumors of the Nervous System, ed 3. London, Edward Arnold, 1971
19. Bailey R, Cushing H, Eisenhardt L: Angioblastic meningiomas. Arch Pathol 6:953, 1928
20. Kruse F: Hemangiopericytoma of the meninges. Neurology 11:771, 1961
21. Kernohan JW, Vihlein A, Gould SE (eds): Sarcomas of the Brain. Springfield, Ill, Charles C Thomas, 1962
22. Pitkethly DT, Hardman JM, Kempe LG, et al: Angioblastic meningiomas. J Neurosurg 32:539, 1970
23. Boker DK, Meurer H, Gullotta F: Recurring intracranial

meningiomas. Evaluation of some factors predisposing for tumor recurrence. J Neurosurg Sci 29:11, 1985

24. Jellinger K, Slowik F: Histological subtypes and prognostic problems in meningiomas. J Neurol 208:279, 1975

25. Inoue H, Tamura M, Koizumi H, et al: Clinical pathology of malignant meningiomas. Acta Neurochir 73:179, 1984

26. Thomas HG, Dolman CL, Berry K: Malignant meningioma: Clinical and pathological features. J Neurosurg 55:929, 1981

27. Lake P, Heiden JS, Minkler J: Cystic meningioma. Case report. J Neurosurg 38:638, 1973

28. Bowen JH, Burger PC, Odom GL, et al: Meningiomas associated with large cysts with neoplastic cells in the cysts' walls. Report of two cases. J Neurosurg 55:473, 1981

29. Lusins JO, Nakagawa H: Multiple meningiomas evaluated by computed tomography. Neurosurgery 9:137, 1981

30. Nahser HC, Grote W, Lohr E, Gerhard L: Multiple meningiomas. Clinical and computer tomographic observations. Neuroradiology 25:259, 1981

31. Peterson HO, Kieffer SA: Introduction to Neuroradiology. Hagerstown, Md, Harper & Row, 1972, p 267

32. Gilbertson EL, Good CA: Roentgenographic signs of tumor of the brain. AJR 76:226, 1956

33. Gold LHA, Kieffer SA, Peterson HO: Intracranial meningiomas: A retrospective analysis of the diagnostic value of plain skull films. Neurology 19:873, 1969

34. Traub SP: Roentgenology of Intracranial Meningiomas. Springfield, Ill, Charles C Thomas, 1961

35. Kim KS, Rogers LF, Lee C: The dural lucent line: Characteristic sign of hyperostosing meningioma en plaque. AJR 141:1217, 1983

36. New PF, Aronow S, Hesselink JR, National Cancer Institute study: Evaluation of computed tomography in the diagnosis of intracranial neoplasms. IV. Meningiomas. Radiology 136:665, 1980

37. New PF, Hesselink JR, OCarroll CP, Kleinman, GM: Malignant meningiomas: CT and histologic criteria, including a new CT sign. AJNR 3:267, 1982

38. Zimmerman RD, Fleming CA, Saint-Louis LA, et al: Magnetic resonance imaging of meningiomas. AJNR 6:149, 1985

39. Bydder GM, Kingsley DP, Brown J, et al: MR imaging of meningiomas including studies with and without gadolinium DTPA. J Comput Assist Tomogr 9:690, 1985

40. Tenner MS: The role of conventional neuroradiologic techniques in relation to computed tomography, in Sher JH, Ford DH (eds): Primary Intracranial Neoplasms. New York, SP Med and Sci, 1971, pp 71–85

41. Papo I: Intracranial meningiomas in the elderly in the CT scan era. Acta Neurochir 67:195, 1983

42. Dyke CG, Davidoff LM: Roentgen Treatment of Diseases of the Nervous System. Philadelphia, Lea and Febiger, 1942, p 113

43. Rubinstein LJ: Tumors of the central nervous system, in Atlas of Tumor Pathology. Washington, Armed Forces Institute of Pathology, 1972

44. Schulz MD, Wang CC, Zinniger GF, et al: Radiotherapy of intracranial neoplasms. With a special section on the radiotherapeutic management of central nervous system tumors in children. Progr Neurol Surg 2:318, 1968

45. Wara WM, Sheline GE, Newman H, et al: Radiation therapy of meningiomas. AJR 123:453, 1975

46. Bouchard J: Central nervous system, in Fletcher C (ed): Textbook of Radiotherapy, ed 2. Philadelphia, Lea and Febiger, 1973, pp 316–418

47. Cooper M, Dohn DF: Intracranial meningiomas in childhood. Cleve Clin Q 41:197, 1974

48. King DL, Chang CH, Pool JL: Radiotherapy in the management of meningiomas. Acta Radiol (Ther) 5:26, 1966

49. Solan MJ, Kramer S: The role of radiation therapy in the management of intracranial meningiomas. Int J Radiat Oncol Biol Phys 11:675, 1985

50. Forbes AR, Goldberg ID: Radiation therapy in the treatment of meningioma: The Joint Center for Radiation Therapy experience 1970 to 1982. J Clin Oncol 2:1139, 1984

51. Carella RJ, Ransohoff J, Newall J: Role of radiation therapy in the management of meningioma. Neurosurgery 10:332, 1982

52. Fukui M, Kitamura K, Ohgami S, et al: Radiosensitivity of meningiomas—analysis of five cases of highly vascular meningiomas treated by preoperative irradiation. Acta Neurochir 36:47, 1977

53. Fukui M, Kitamura K, Nakagaki H, et al: Irradiated meningiomas: A clinical evaluation. Acta Neurochir 54:33, 1980

54. Djindjian R, Cophignon J, Theron D, et al: Embolization by super selective arteriography from the femoral route in neuroradiology. Review of 60 cases. I. Technique, indications, complications. Neuroradiology 6:20, 1973

55. Hekster RE, Metricali B, Luyendijk W: Presurgical transfemoral catheter embolization to reduce operative blood loss. Technical note. J Neurosurg 41:396, 1974

56. Rutka J, Muller PJ, Chui M: Preoperative Gelfoam embolization of supratentorial meningiomas. Can J Surg 28:441, 1985

57. Hilal SK, Michelsen JW: Therapeutic percutaneous embolization for extra-axis vascular lesions of the head, neck and spine. J Neurosurg 43:275, 1975

58. Latchaw RE, Gold LHA: Polyvinyl foam embolization of vascular and neoplastic lesions of the head, neck and spine. Radiology 131:669, 1979

59. Teasdale E, Patterson J, McLellan D, et al: Subselective preoperative embolization for meningiomas. A radiological and pathological assessment. J Neurosurg 60:506, 1984

60. Tsai FY, Hieshima G, Mehringer CM, et al: Arterial digital subtraction angiography with particulate intravascular embolization and angioplasty. Surg Neurol 22:204, 1984

61. Ramamurthi B, Ravi B, Ramachandran V: Convulsions with meningiomas: Incidence and significance. Surg Neurol 14:415, 1980

62. Quintiliani R, Nightingale CH: Cefazolin-diagnosis and treatment. Ann Intern Med 89:650, 1978

CHAPTER 47

Convexity Meningiomas and General Principles of Meningioma Surgery

Robert E. Maxwell   Shelley N. Chou

CLASSIFICATION OF CONVEXITY MENINGIOMAS

Cushing separated the convexity meningiomas into seven groups based on surgical considerations relevant to their radiographic localization, neurologic presentation, and prognosis.[1] He first classified the convexity meningiomas according to location in 1922 as frontal, paracentral, parietal, occipital, and temporal.[2] This classification proved inadequate for precise localization of these tumors, however, since the frontal lobe includes the large region anterior to the rolandic fissure. Thirty eight (70 percent) of 54 convexity meningiomas reported in the monograph by Cushing and Eisenhardt (1938) were anterior to the rolandic fissure. Cushing therefore later reclassified the convexity meningiomas into seven categories by subdividing the frontal meningiomas into precoronal, coronal, and postcoronal groups.[1] This classification proved more relevant for surgical considerations based on the clinical and radiographic presentation.

SYMPTOMATOLOGY OF CONVEXITY MENINGIOMAS

PRECORONAL CONVEXITY MENINGIOMAS

Patients with frontal convexity meningiomas are notable for the absence of mental symptoms that are seen in patients with anterior parasagittal or olfactory groove meningiomas. Dementia, personality change, and incontinence are much less common with frontal convexity meningiomas away from the midline.

CORONAL CONVEXITY MENINGIOMAS

Cushing found in his series that one third of all convexity meningiomas were primarily attached along the coronal suture. Twenty nine of these tumors were pterional and 17 were between the pterion and bregma.[1] Compared with frontal convexity meningiomas located further posteriorly, the coronal tumor remains symptomatically silent for long periods. These tumors become quite large and cause pressure symptoms. Visual blurring, diplopia, and choked discs or secondary atrophy may occur. A contralateral paresis of the arm and face eventually occurs, but the leg remains relatively spared. Focal motor seizures start in the hand or face. Paraphasia may occur with tumors compressing the dominant hemisphere.

Cushing observed that there is a tendency for bregmatic and pterional meningiomas at either end of the coronal suture to cause hyperostosis, but hyperostosis is unusual with convexity tumors arising along the central portion of the suture. En plaque meningiomas midway along the coronal suture may produce hyperostosis, however.

POSTCORONAL CONVEXITY MENINGIOMAS

Convexity meningiomas overlying Brodmann's areas 6 and 8 of the cerebral cortex often produce simple partial motor seizures characterized by conjugate movement of the head and eyes with twitching of the contralateral face and arm. Some patients describe a sensory aura characterized by a sense of tingling or warmth in the contralateral face or arm. A contralateral, central-type facial and arm paresis eventually occurs.

PARAROLANDIC MENINGIOMAS

The pararolandic region includes the sensory postcentral gyrus (Brodmann's area 3,1,2) and the motor precentral gyrus (Brodmann's area 4). Jacksonian seizures involving the contralateral arm and face combined with dysarthria when the dominant hemisphere is compressed characterize meningiomas over the convexity in this region. Cushing noted that the seizures produced by pararolandic tumors usually have a motor rather than sensory aura initially.[1] The 9 cases he described were all on the dominant side and were prone to recurrence.

PARIETAL MENINGIOMAS

The majority of parietal meningiomas produce sensory seizures and compress or irritate the postcentral gyrus. Meningiomas located posteriorly nearer the lambdoid suture (posterior portions of areas 5 and 7) are less epileptogenic.[1] The sensory auras experienced with convexity meningiomas over the parietal lobe are restricted to the contralateral face and arm with sparing of the leg and foot initially. Receptive dysphasia is found with meningiomas over the dominant parietal cortex, but this is not always the case.

TEMPORAL MENINGIOMAS

Convexity meningiomas compressing the outer surface of the temporal lobe are relatively uncommon if the pterional meningiomas arising along the outer third of the sphenoid wing

OPERATIVE NEUROSURGICAL TECHNIQUES
ISBN 0-8089-1862-1

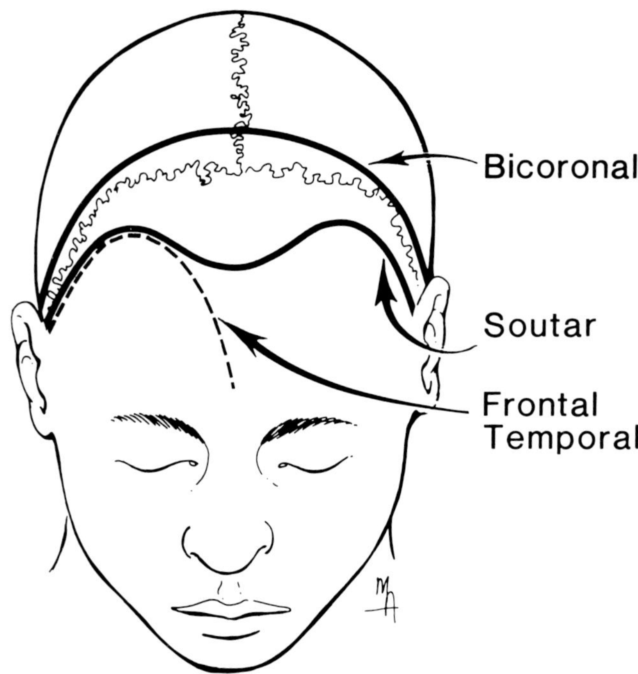

Fig. 47-1. A bicoronal or Soutar scalp incision positioned behind the hairline provides wider exposure and less cosmetic deformity than a frontotemporal incision with the anterior limb of the incision crossing the forehead.

are excluded. Patients with these meningiomas have contralateral seizures and weakness involving the face and upper extremity. Later, when signs and symptoms of increased intracranial pressure are apparent, an ipsilateral spastic weakness of the leg may occur associated with a contralateral shift of the brainstem and compression of the opposite cerebral peduncle against the edge of the tentorium cerebelli. Visual disturbance usually is associated with choked discs or secondary optic atrophy. An incongruous, homonymous visual field deficit may be detected if the patient can cooperate and concentrate sufficiently for testing.

OCCIPITAL MENINGIOMAS

Occipital convexity meningiomas are very uncommon. Cushing found no tumors in this location among 54 convexity meningiomas. Signs and symptoms of increased intracranial pressure are associated with a congruous, homonymous hemianopsia and visual hallucinations in patients with tumors in this location.

GENERAL PRINCIPLES OF MENINGIOMA SURGERY

Preoperative awareness of the precise location, size, configuration, and vascularity of each meningioma considered for surgery is essential. The general principles applicable to meningioma surgery are primarily determined by these tumor characteristics. The principles of meningioma surgery discussed in this chapter are applicable to all meningiomas whether convexity, parasagittal, falcine, posterior fossa, or basal in location. The feature of convexity meningiomas requir-

ing special consideration is involvement of the skull, which may hinder elevation of the bone flap. Special technical considerations regarding parasagittal, falx, posterior fossa, and basal parapituitary meningiomas are discussed in subsequent chapters.

The location and configuration of the tumor dictate the operative approach. The primary concern is the preservation of function by avoiding injury to important vessels, cranial nerves, and brain tissue. The size of the meningioma may work for or against the surgeon depending on other features such as tissue vascularity or firmness. A large tumor easily debulked by aspiration with little bleeding may be excised with very little additional tissue trauma. A very vascular, angioblastic meningioma in a poorly accessible location may preclude total extirpation.

The preferred operative approach is one that provides options for dealing with technical contingencies. It is best if problems are anticipated rather than reacted to after the fact. The experienced surgeon learns to never underestimate the potential problems inherent in meningioma surgery. In this regard, it seems appropriate to quote Cushing from his classic monograph on meningiomas, where he stated: "To other than beginners much of what follows may seem trifling, but it is on a multiplicity of trifles, carefully observed, that the success of one of these operations depends."[1]

POSITION

Meningioma surgery may take several hours and proper positioning is important. The head should be higher than the heart and excessive angulation or twisting of the neck should be avoided. The head also should be secured so there is no chance for motion or instability during the procedure that could reduce or distort the operative field and surgical perspective, result in contamination of the field, or disturb the patient's airway. Pressure points on vulnerable areas such as the eyes, brachial plexus, and peripheral nerves should be prevented by careful positioning and padding. Care should be exercised that scrub solutions do not run into the eyes or pool about the cautery plate, increasing the risk of burns. The relationship of the tumor to the brain and other contiguous structures should be considered in advance so gravity can be used to minimize the need for brain retraction. The head position and operative field are planned taking into consideration the handedness of the surgeon and the optimal location for instruments such as self-retaining retractors and the operating microscope. It is often helpful if the surgeon has a surface on which to rest and steady the forearms, particularly when working under the operating microscope in the sitting position.

SCALP INCISION

The first priority for the scalp incision is that it be appropriate for the site and size of the craniotomy or craniectomy that is required to adequately expose the tumor. A scalp flap need only be slightly larger than the proposed bone flap provided that the tumor location, size, and site of dural attachment are known in advance. If there is any doubt, it is better to err on the side of a scalp and bone flap that is too generous when exposing a meningioma.

The scalp is very vascular and rarely devascularized if good surgical principles are adhered to. Unfortunately, some meningiomas recur and scalp incisions are reopened, extended,

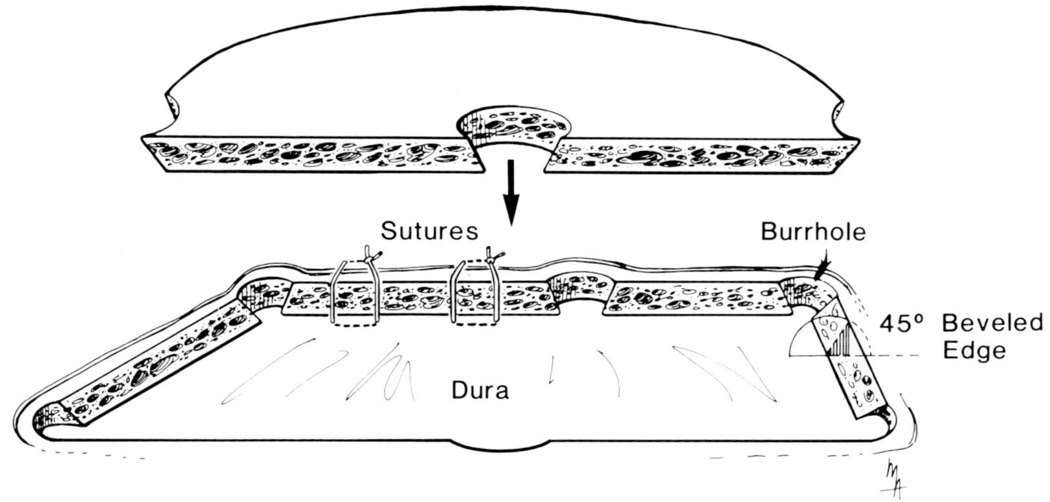

Fig. 47-2.   The bone edge is beveled when cut to prevent the bone flap from sinking when sutured in place. The craniotomy cuts join the outer tangent of the burr hole to increase dural exposure. The dura is tacked up to lessen epidural bleeding.

or revised. The blood supply to the scalp should be considered and flaps based on a vascular pedicle where practical. The length of a scalp flap ideally should not exceed the width by more than a 3:2 ratio, and a flap should be designed to be widest at its base.

The cosmetic result of an incisional scar also should be considered. A bicoronal or Soutar incision is preferable to a frontal or frontotemporal scalp flap where the anterior limb or the incision crosses the forehead and leaves a cosmetic deformity (Figure 47-1). The temporal branch of the facial nerve to the frontalis muscle can be spared if the scalp incision extends no lower than the top of the zygomatic arch and is barely in front of the external ear. Necrosis of the scalp edge can be avoided by using plastic Raney skin clips rather than the metallic clips, which have more tensile strength. They are effective for achieving hemostasis provided the galea aponeurotica is included in the clip. The galea is always closed at the end of the procedure whether a single- or two-layer suture technique is used. Approximation of the galea aponeurotica and subcutaneous tissue with an interrupted, inverted, absorbable suture and the dermis with stainless steel skin staples provides an efficient, cosmetic, scalp closure.

ELEVATION OF BONE FLAP

The true osteoplastic bone flap in which the scalp, muscle, and skull bone are turned as a unit is disadvantageous in meningioma surgery for two reasons. First, it preserves the excessive blood supply from the branches of the external carotid artery. Second, the flap also tends to be bulky, difficult to handle, and limits exposure if the tumor and dura mater are attached to the bone flap. The choice between a free bone flap and a flap hinged on periosteum and muscle is governed by the location and other peculiarities of the specific tumor and the preference of the surgeon. Free bone flaps more often are turned high on the convexity, near the vertex, and in the midfrontal region.

The edges of the bone flap are beveled to prevent a postoperative depression of the bone flap and a cosmetic

deformity (Figure 47-2). This problem is more likely to occur when the air osteotome is used rather than the Gigli saw. The Gigli saw and guide also lessen the risk of fenestrating the dura mater and tearing adherent venous channels. The air osteotome occludes diploic vascular channels with fine bone dust as it cuts, however, and thereby reduces bone bleeding. The skull bone is waxed only when necessary to control bleeding or seal mastoid air cells. Bone wax acts as a foreign body and should not be applied routinely or in excess. Burr holes are joined at

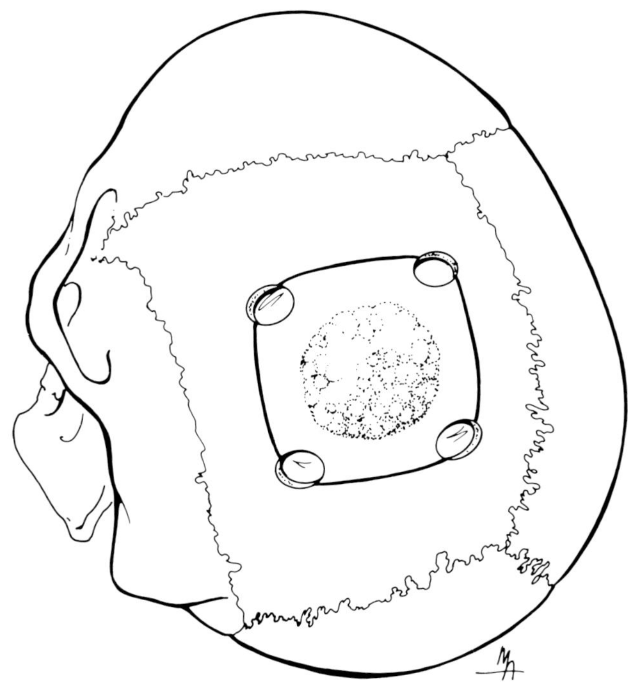

Fig. 47-3.   The bone flap over a convexity meningioma is wider than the tumor and is centered over the tumor. A free bone flap is turned high on the convexity or at the vertex. The saw cut is made last so the bone flap can be elevated quickly if sinus bleeding occurs.

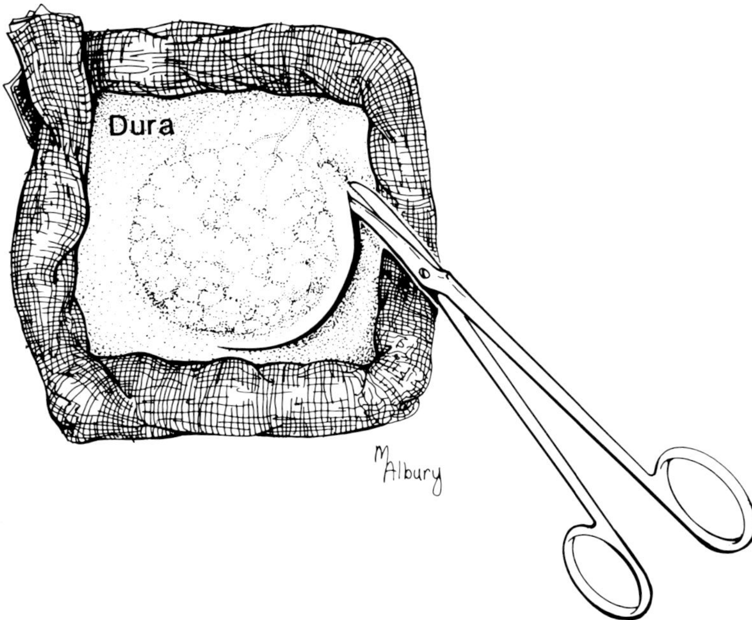

Fig. 47-4. The dural incision is extended circumferentially about the margin of the tumor with blunt-tipped scissors. Very little cortex need be exposed when excising convexity meningiomas.

their outer margins to ensure maximum exposure of the dura (Figure 47-2).

The bone flap must be large enough to ensure that the tumor is not attached to dura mater beyond the margins of the craniotomy. The bone flap is centered over the meningioma to lessen the likelihood of tumor crossing the margin of the craniotomy flap. The final bone cut is made on the side of the flap closest to a large dural venous sinus (Figure 47-3). If the dura and a venous channel are torn, the bone flap then can be more quickly turned and the bleeding more rapidly controlled.

DURAL HEMOSTASIS AND OPENING

The assistant waxes the bone edges and retracts the bone flap while the surgeon achieves dural and extradural hemostasis. Bipolar rather than diathermy coagulation is used to control bleeding vessels in order to reduce dural shrinkage. Troublesome ooze from arachnoid granulation tissue over dural sinuses or dura infiltrated by vascular tumor can be controlled by placing oxidized cellulose (Surgicel) or spongostan (Gelfoam) on the bleeding surface and applying gentle pressure with cottonoid strips. Bleeding from the epidural space beneath the margins of the skull can be controlled by placing pledgets of Gelfoam between the dura and skull and then tacking the dura to the inner table of the skull to obliterate the epidural space (see Figure 47-2). After hemostasis is achieved, the wound is irrigated, cottonoid pledgets are placed at the bone margins, and clean, dry skin towels are applied to the margins of the scalp wound before the dura is opened.

The dura mater is inspected and gently palpated to assess the location of the venous sinuses, the meningeal vessels, the attached tumor, and the relative tightness of the underlying brain. The dura mater is opened at the margin rather than over the center of the tumor. The dura is opened so the absolute minimum of brain is exposed. The dura should not be opened primarily over functionally important cortex until increased intracranial pressure is relieved. If all measures such as steroids, mannitol, head elevation, and hyperventilation are in effect and the patient is well anesthetized and paralyzed, lateral ventriculostomy and cerebrospinal fluid (CSF) decompression are another option for reducing intracranial pressure. The dura mater should not be opened widely over a tight brain until the precise position of the tumor is known.

The dura is incised and the dural incision is extended circumferentially about the margin of the tumor using blunt-tipped scissors (Figure 47-4). The dura mater is hinged toward the nearest venous sinus in order to avoid damage to bridging cortical veins. Dura mater involved by the tumor is isolated from surrounding dura and left attached to the neoplasm. Sutures can be passed through the dura and used for indirect gentle traction and manipulation of the meningioma, thereby reducing or eliminating the need for retraction applied directly to the tumor or the brain (Figure 47-5).

TUMOR EXPOSURE AND EXCISION

The priority in meningioma surgery is to preserve and restore function, and all technical principles and procedures are dedicated to this purpose. Injury to the brain and cranial nerves is avoided by preserving the blood supply while exposing and excising the tumor with minimal or no brain retraction. Every technical alternative to forceful brain retraction is explored as the situation dictates. Traction is applied to the tumor capsule or the dura attached to the tumor as previously described, rather than to the adjacent brain. Position of the head should be adjusted so that gravity works to the surgeon's advantage. The single-most useful technique for removing all but the smallest meningiomas is to exenterate the core of the tumor early in the resection. This creates a space into which the thinned tumor capsule can be retracted (Figure 47-6).

At this stage the magnification and cold light provided by the operating microscope are helpful adjuncts in the dissection and development of the arachnoidal plane between tumor and brain. The bipolar coagulator and miscroscissors can be used to take down fine arachnoidal adhesive bands and small tumor vessels parasitized from the pia mater (Figure 47-7). If brain

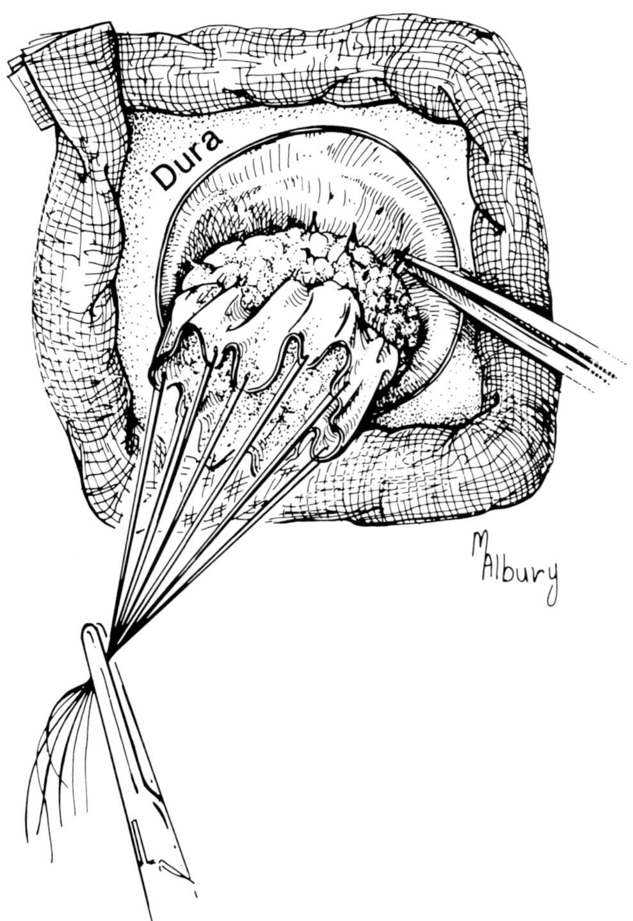

Fig. 47-5.   Dura mater left attached to a convexity meningioma provides a useful handle for retracting and manipulating the tumor.

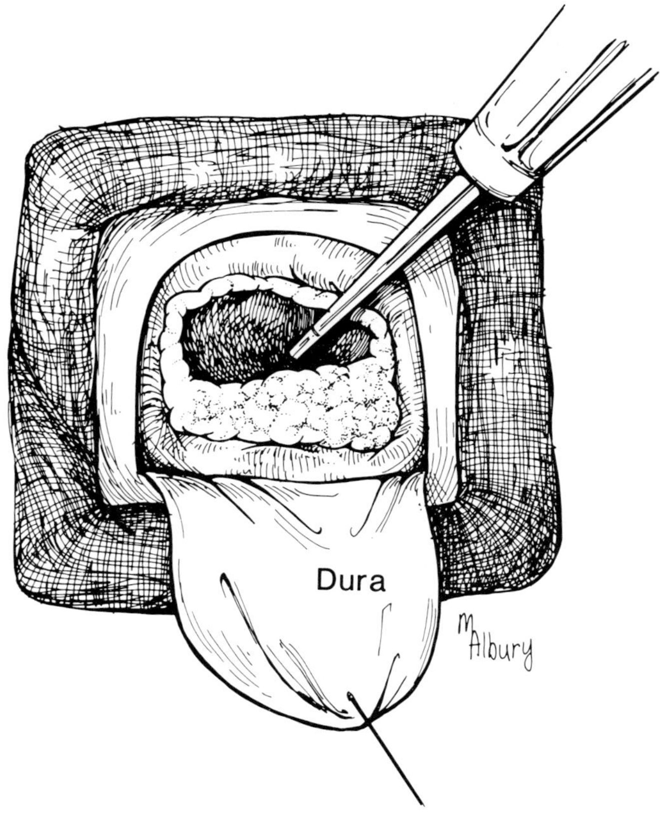

Fig. 47-6.   Intracapsular enucleation of tumor tissue permits invagination of the tumor capsule and development of the plane between the meningioma and the brain without forceful retraction.

retraction is necessary, moist cottonoid sponges are placed between the retractors and brain tissue. Self-retaining retractors produce less tissue damage than hand-held retractors provided they are not applied too forcefully for too long. The surgeon may, on rare occasions, judiciously elect to resect a small amount of brain tissue in order to expose the tumor, thereby obviating the need for forceful brain retraction.

Few technical difficulties are encountered during the tumor excision if the tissue is accessible, soft, and relatively avascular or necrotic so that suction and curettage can be used to reduce the tumor bulk before the tumor capsule is delivered. A large tumor with tough, tenacious tissue that cannot be aspirated can be excised piecemeal with a cutting loop cautery. This technique carries the risk of damage to important nerves or vessels encompassed by or adjacent to the tumor, however. The ultrasonic aspirator and CO_2 laser sometimes facilitate the excision of firm, gritty, or vascular tumors.[3,4]

The ultrasonic aspirator (Cavitron Corp., Stamford, CT) selectively fragments and aspirates tissue exposed at the tip of the instrument, which vibrates longitudinally at a frequency of 23,000 times per second. Fragmentation of tissue is dependent on the water content of the tissue; less power and exposure are required to fragment tissue with high water content, such as areolar tissue, than tissue with considerable collagen or elastic tissue, such as blood vessels.[3] This selective tissue removal permits the identification and elective preservation or coagulation of blood vessels. Visibility is improved because the tissue is shaved from the surface rather than by cutting beneath the surface with cautery loops, spoon curettes, or biopsy forceps. The simultaneous aspiration immediately removes blood from the tumor bed. Flamm and Ransohoff reported the advantage of ultrasonic aspiration in the surgical removal of 30 meningiomas.[5]

The CO_2 laser is also sometimes useful in brain tumor surgery.[4] Laser energy is converted to heat when it is absorbed by tumor tissue, and thermal coagulation occurs. If sufficient energy is absorbed the tissue vaporizes. The advantages of surgical lasers include: (1) the ability to operate with smaller exposures, (2) reduced brain retraction, (3) a reduced amount of mechanical manipulation by vaporizing the tumor mass, (4) vaporization of the dural attachment after removal of the tumor, (5) improved operative precision, and (6) thereby enhanced ability to remove meningiomas that might otherwise prove difficult to extirpate by conventional means.[6]

Beck has suggested that there is an advantage of combining the use of the CO_2 laser for cutting with that of the Nd-YAG laser for coagulation. He prefers the Nd-YAG laser for use on tumors with a rich vascular supply and reported a decreased need for blood transfusions in patients operated upon with this laser.[7] The Nd-YAG laser produces a homogeneous coagulation with an energy-dependent depth effect.[8] The penetration of the laser beam in tissues is controlled by the output wattage, the grade of coagulation is controlled by duration of radiation time and by the output wattage.[9] Tumor shrinkage and demarcation based on different absorbtion properties facilitates dissection, and allows the preservation of healthy tissue.[10]

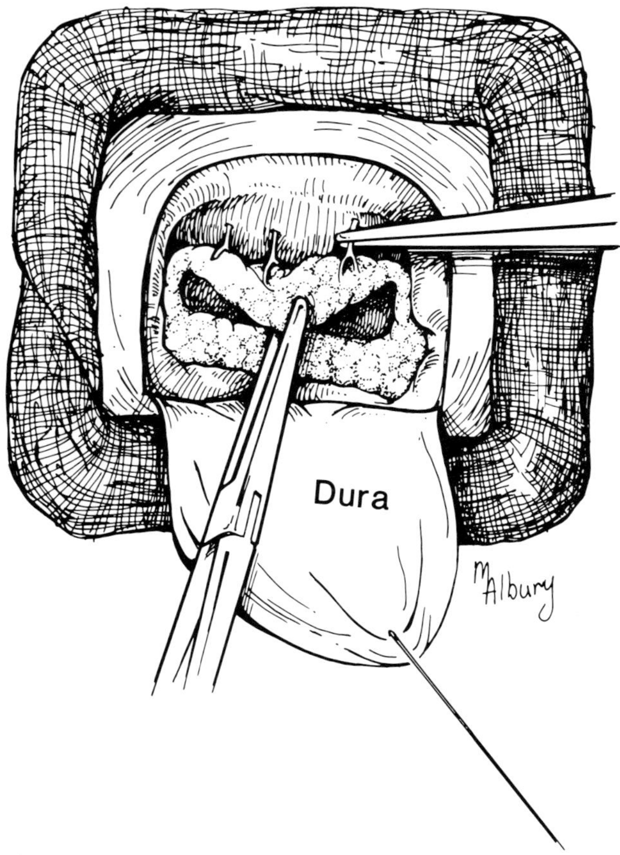

Fig. 47-7. The bipolar coagulator and microscissors are used to take down arachnoidal adhesive bands and tumor-feeding vessels as a plane is developed between the cortex and the thinned tumor capsule.

Hemostasis is a major problem when large, firm, extremely vascular meningiomas are encountered. Dandy stated: "Because of the great dural vascularity, dura endotheliomas offer the most difficult battles in cranial surgery."[11] Preoperative irradiation and embolization of feeding vessels from branches of the external carotid artery can reduce intraoperative bleeding of the tumor. Intraoperative arterial hypotension also can be induced with sodium nitroprusside to help control bleeding from the tumor and reduce turgor of the brain. Large feeding vessels to the tumor are coagulated when accessible before the tumor capsule is entered. If the site of attachment of the meningioma to the dura mater can be identified and exposed early in the resection, the major arterial feeders are coagulated and divided at this point.

Meningiomas not only tend toward greater vascularity but also have reduced hemostatic properties relative to other common brain tumors such as gliomas. In gliomas the local tissue factors favor the deposition of fibrin and the persistence of these deposits; in meningiomas the amount of fibrin deposited is smaller, and the fibrin products are broken down faster because of comparatively low thromboplastic activity and high fibrinolytic activity.[12] It is possible to depress the fibrinolytic activity of intracranial tumors by antiplasmin drugs in order to lessen bleeding from the tumor.[13]

The brisk intracapsular bleeding encountered during the resection of angioblastic meningiomas may not be controlled by simple pressure with cotton balls or cottonoid pledges. Thrombin-soaked Gelfoam, Surgicel, or Avitene can be applied with gentle pressure to control tumor bleeding. The surgeon must judge, based on the size and location of the tumor, the condition of the patient, and the rate of bleeding, whether it may be more expedient to tolerate moderate bleeding in order to rapidly enucleate the tumor and thereby shorten the operating time and perhaps reduce the overall blood loss and chance of morbidity.

The operating microscope and microinstrumentation are very helpful during the extracapsular tumor dissection but may be a hindrance during the intracapsular debulking of large tumors. The surgeon should not be distracted by insignificant ooze and anatomic trivia within the tumor stroma that is magnified out of proportion by the operating microscope. The microscope is essential, however, if important arteries, veins, or nerves are passing through crevices in the capsule of a multilobulated tumor. Although the operating microscope, bipolar coagulation, and microinstrumentation now make it possible to perform precise dissection around important vessels and nerves, the primary objectives of preserving and improving function are not sacrificed in a heroic attempt for a "cure."

Whenever possible, the dura and bone should be excised when involved by the tumor to reduce the possibility of recurrence. Wide resection of the dura around globular meningiomas has been recommended because of recent histologic evidence of regional multifocality.[14] Cauterization of bone and dura is less effective, and the recurrence rate is higher.

WOUND CLOSURE

The necessity of formally closing a dural defect by fashioning an autologous dural graft or inserting a dural substitute is open to question.[15] Experimental and clinical evidence shows that a neodural membrane forms in the absence of a graft. Many neurosurgeons prefer to close the dura and reconstitute the subdural space even when the surgery requires excision of dura because of involvement by the tumor. Abbott and Dupree recommend dural closure to prevent CSF leakage, brain herniation, wound infection, and cortical scarring and adhesions.[16] The use of pericranium, temporalis fascia, and fascia lata is widespread for closing dural defect. These autologous materials have the advantages of being readily available and pliable. It also has been shown that lyophilized dura mater can be used without complications and precludes the need for additional incisions at the time of surgery.[15]

There appears to be little advantage other than ready accessibility in repairing the dura mater with inorganic or synthetic dural substitutes. Banerjee et al.[17] reported delayed postoperative subdural hematomas associated with bleeding from neovascularized membranes provoked by Silastic dural substitutes. Implanted synthetic foreign materials also increase the risk of infection.

Following closure of the dura, the bone flap is sutured in place with a nonabsorbable, synthetic suture. An acrylic or wire mesh cranioplasty can be performed to repair a defect necessitated by the excision of bone involved by the meningioma. The cranioplasty occasionally is delayed and done as a second procedure. This approach may be indicated if there is severe swelling of the brain, suspected contamination, or if a patient in poor general health has had to endure a long period of anesthesia. Care should be taken to approximate the galea during the scalp closure.

POSTOPERATIVE CARE

The primary concern in the postoperative period is that a hematoma or brain edema will produce a focal or generalized increase in intracranial pressure, progressive neurologic dysfunction, and transtentorial herniation. The anesthesiologist strives for a smooth extubation without straining to avoid unnecessary elevation of blood pressure and intracranial pressure.

The patient is observed closely in the recovery room and the intensive care unit for deterioration in the level of consciousness, focal neurologic deficit, or seizure activity. Vital signs, pulmonary function, blood gases, and fluid and electrolyte balance are monitored. The head is elevated 20 to 30 degrees. Corticosteroid therapy should be continued at full dosage for 72 hours, or through the expected period of maximum brain swelling, before a steroid taper is started. Seizure prophylaxis with parenteral diphenylhydantoin is continued. A computed tomographic (CT) scan without contrast enhancement is advisable to distinguish brain swelling and postoperative hematoma in a patient with persistent or progressive lethargy or obtundation or progressive focal neurologic deficit.

REFERENCES

1. Cushing H: Meningiomas, Macewen Memorial Lecture, 1927. Glasgow, Jackson Wylie and Company, 1972

2. Cushing H, Eisenhardt L: Meningiomas. Their Classification, Regional Behavior, Life History and Surgical End Results. Springfield, Ill, Charles C Thomas, 1938, p 785

3. Zulch KJ: Brain Tumors: Their Biology and Pathology. New York, Springer, 1965

4. Challa VR, Markesbery WR: Meningiomas: Pathology, in Wilkins RH, Setti SR (eds): Neurosurgery. New York, McGraw-Hill, 1984, pp pp 613–622

5. Leibel SA, Wara WM, Sheline GE, et al: The treatment of meningiomas in childhood. Cancer 37:2709, 1976

6. Bailey O, Buchanan DN, Bucy PC: Intracranial Tumors in Infancy and Childhood. Chicago, University of Chicago Press, 1948, pp 441–500

7. Globus JH, Zucker JM, Rubinstein JM: Tumors of the brain in children and adolescents—a clinic and anatomic survey of ninety-two verified cases. Am J Dis Child 65:604, 1943

8. Sano K, Wakai S, Ochiai C, et al: Characteristics of intracranial meningiomas in childhood. Childs Brain 8:98, 1981

9. Deen HG Jr, Scheithauer BW, Ebersold MJ: Clinical and pathological study of meningiomas of the first two decades of life. Neurosurgery 56:317, 1982

10. Skullerud K, Loken AC: The prognosis in meningiomas. Acta Neuropathol 29:337, 1974

11. Crompton MR, Gautier-Smith PC: The prediction of recurrence in meningiomas. J Neurol Neurosurg Psychiatry 33:80, 1970

12. Simpson D: The recurrence of intracranial meningiomas after surgical treatment. J Neurol Neurosurg Psychiatry 20:22, 1957

13. Mirimanoff RO, Dosoretz DE, Lingood RM, et al: Meningioma: Analysis of recurrence and progression following neurosurgical resection. J Neurosurg 62:18, 1985

14. Borovich B, Doron Y: Recurrence of intracranial meningiomas: The role played by regional multicentricity. Neurosurgery 64:58, 1986

15. Wolman L: Role of the arachnoid granulation in the development of meningioma. Arch Pathol 53:70, 1952

16. Nager GT, Heroy J, Hoeplinger M: Meningiomas invading the temporal bone with extension to the neck. Am J Otolaryngol 4:297, 1983

17. Courville CB: Pathology of the Central Nervous System, ed 3. Mountain View, Ca, Pacific Press Publishing, 1950

18. Russell DS, Rubenstein LJ: Pathology of Tumors of the Nervous System, ed 3. London, Edward Arnold, 1971

19. Bailey R, Cushing H, Eisenhardt L: Angioblastic meningiomas. Arch Pathol 6:953, 1928

20. Kruse F: Hemangiopericytoma of the meninges. Neurology 11:771, 1961

21. Kernohan JW, Vihlein A, Gould SE (eds): Sarcomas of the Brain. Springfield, Ill, Charles C Thomas, 1962

22. Pitkethly DT, Hardman JM, Kempe LG, et al: Angioblastic meningiomas. J Neurosurg 32:539, 1970

23. Boker DK, Meurer H, Gullotta F: Recurring intracranial meningiomas. Evaluation of some factors predisposing for tumor recurrence. J Neurosurg Sci 29:11, 1985

24. Jellinger K, Slowik F: Histological subtypes and prognostic problems in meningiomas. J Neurol 208:279, 1975

25. Inoue H, Tamura M, Koizumi H, et al: Clinical pathology of malignant meningiomas. Acta Neurochir 73:179, 1984

26. Thomas HG, Dolman CL, Berry K: Malignant meningioma: Clinical and pathological features. J Neurosurg 55:929, 1981

27. Lake P, Heiden JS, Minkler J: Cystic meningioma. Case report. J Neurosurg 38:638, 1973

28. Bowen JH, Burger PC, Odom GL, et al: Meningiomas associated with large cysts with neoplastic cells in the cysts' walls. Report of two cases. J Neurosurg 55:473, 1981

29. Lusins JO, Nakagawa H: Multiple meningiomas evaluated by computed tomography. Neurosurgery 9:137, 1981

30. Nahser HC, Grote W, Lohr E, Gerhard L: Multiple meningiomas. Clinical and computer tomographic observations. Neuroradiology 25:259, 1981

31. Peterson HO, Kieffer SA: Introduction to Neuroradiology. Hagerstown, Md, Harper & Row, 1972, p 267

32. Gilbertson EL, Good CA: Roentgenographic signs of tumor of the brain. AJR 76:226, 1956

33. Gold LHA, Kieffer SA, Peterson HO: Intracranial meningiomas: A retrospective analysis of the diagnostic value of plain skull films. Neurology 19:873, 1969

34. Traub SP: Roentgenology of Intracranial Meningiomas. Springfield, Ill, Charles C Thomas, 1961

35. Kim KS, Rogers LF, Lee C: The dural lucent line: Characteristic sign of hyperostosing meningioma en plaque. AJR 141:1217, 1983

36. New PF, Aronow S, Hesselink JR, National Cancer Institute study: Evaluation of computed tomography in the diagnosis of intracranial neoplasms. IV. Meningiomas. Radiology 136:665, 1980

37. New PF, Hesselink JR, OCarroll CP, Kleinman, GM: Malignant meningiomas: CT and histologic criteria, including a new CT sign. AJNR 3:267, 1982

38. Zimmerman RD, Fleming CA, Saint-Louis LA, et al: Magnetic resonance imaging of meningiomas. AJNR 6:149, 1985

39. Bydder GM, Kingsley DP, Brown J, et al: MR imaging of meningiomas including studies with and without gadolinium DTPA. J Comput Assist Tomogr 9:690, 1985

40. Tenner MS: The role of conventional neuroradiologic techniques in relation to computed tomography, in Sher JH, Ford DH (eds): Primary Intracranial Neoplasms. New York, SP Med and Sci, 1971, pp 71–85

41. Papo I: Intracranial meningiomas in the elderly in the CT scan era. Acta Neurochir 67:195, 1983

42. Dyke CG, Davidoff LM: Roentgen Treatment of Diseases of the Nervous System. Philadelphia, Lea and Febiger, 1942, p 113

43. Rubinstein LJ: Tumors of the central nervous system, in Atlas of Tumor Pathology. Washington, Armed Forces Institute of Pathology, 1972

44. Schulz MD, Wang CC, Zinniger GF, et al: Radiotherapy of intracranial neoplasms. With a special section on the radiotherapeutic management of central nervous system tumors in children. Progr Neurol Surg 2:318, 1968

45. Wara WM, Sheline GE, Newman H, et al: Radiation therapy of meningiomas. AJR 123:453, 1975

46. Bouchard J: Central nervous system, in Fletcher C (ed): Textbook

of Radiotherapy, ed 2. Philadelphia, Lea and Febiger, 1973, pp 316–418

47. Cooper M, Dohn DF: Intracranial meningiomas in childhood. Cleve Clin Q 41:197, 1974

48. King DL, Chang CH, Pool JL: Radiotherapy in the management of meningiomas. Acta Radiol (Ther) 5:26, 1966

49. Solan MJ, Kramer S: The role of radiation therapy in the management of intracranial meningiomas. Int J Radiat Oncol Biol Phys 11:675, 1985

50. Forbes AR, Goldberg ID: Radiation therapy in the treatment of meningioma: The Joint Center for Radiation Therapy experience 1970 to 1982. J Clin Oncol 2:1139, 1984

51. Carella RJ, Ransohoff J, Newall J: Role of radiation therapy in the management of meningioma. Neurosurgery 10:332, 1982

52. Fukui M, Kitamura K, Ohgami S, et al: Radiosensitivity of meningiomas—analysis of five cases of highly vascular meningiomas treated by preoperative irradiation. Acta Neurochir 36:47, 1977

53. Fukui M, Kitamura K, Nakagaki H, et al: Irradiated meningiomas: A clinical evaluation. Acta Neurochir 54:33, 1980

54. Djindjian R, Cophighon J, Theron D, et al: Embolization by super selective arteriography from the femoral route in neuroradiology. Review of 60 cases. I. Technique, indications, complications. Neuroradiology 6:20, 1973

55. Hekster RE, Metricali B, Luyendijk W: Presurgical transfemoral catheter embolization to reduce operative blood loss. Technical note. J Neurosurg 41:396, 1974

56. Rutka J, Muller PJ, Chui M: Preoperative Gelfoam embolization of supratentorial meningiomas. Can J Surg 28:441, 1985

57. Hilal SK, Michelsen JW: Therapeutic percutaneous embolization for extra-axis vascular lesions of the head, neck and spine. J Neurosurg 43:275, 1975

58. Latchaw RE, Gold LHA: Polyvinyl foam embolization of vascular and neoplastic lesions of the head, neck and spine. Radiology 131:669, 1979

59. Teasdale E, Patterson J, McLellan D, et al: Subselective preoperative embolization for meningiomas. A radiological and pathological assessment. J Neurosurg 60:506, 1984

60. Tsai FY, Hieshima G, Mehringer CM, et al: Arterial digital subtraction angiography with particulate intravascular embolization and angioplasty. Surg Neurol 22:204, 1984

61. Ramamurthi B, Ravi B, Ramachandran V: Convulsions with meningiomas: Incidence and significance. Surg Neurol 14:415, 1980

62. Quintiliani R, Nightingale CH: Cefazolin-diagnosis and treatment. Ann Intern Med 89:650, 1978

CHAPTER 48

Parasagittal and Falx Meningiomas

Robert E. Maxwell   Shelley N. Chou

THE DESIGNATION "parasagittal" for meningiomas along the superior sagittal sinus was first suggested by Cushing in 1922.[1] The anatomic and surgical distinction between parasagittal and falx meningiomas is more critical than the clinical distinction based on symptomatology. The term *parasagittal* implies that a tumor arising from the dura mater high on the convexity of the hemisphere involves the wall and possibly the lumen of the sagittal sinus. The falcine meningioma arises from the falx cerebri and only gains a secondary attachment to the walls of the sagittal sinus if it is large or widely spread en plaque.[2] Although it is difficult to determine with certainty in all cases whether a large tumor is parasagittal or falcine, the former predominate consistent with the predilection of meningiomas to arise where arachnoidal granulation tissue is most abundant. The practical operative criterion proposed by Cushing for distinguishing a primary tumor of the falx cerebri rests on its complete concealment by overlying cerebral cortex. The parasagittal meningiomas were approximately seven times more frequent than the falcine tumors in Cushing's series Cushing found hyperostosis of the skull associated with one fourth of parasagittal meningiomas, but not with meningiomas limited to the falx. There is no appreciable difference in the clinical presentation or symptomatology of these two classes of meningiomas. They do, however, present different technical considerations for the surgeon.

Olivecrona was the first to distinguish parasagittal meningiomas according to their site of origin along the sagittal sinus.[4] He reported that 52 percent of parasagittal meningiomas involved the middle third of the sinus; 37 percent were attached to the anterior third of the sinus, and 11 percent to the posterior third of the sinus. Thirteen of Olivecrona's 27 cases of parasagittal meningiomas showed evidence of bilateral growth.

Cushing found at the time of surgery that the frontal and occipital tumors were all sizable, but many tumors along the middle third of the sinus were small. He ascribed this finding to the tendency of tumors adjacent to the paracentral lobule to produce earlier and more obvious symptoms than occipital tumors and tumors in more frontal locations. Both Olivecrona and Cushing emphasized the symptomatic differences between parasagittal meningiomas depending upon whether they were located along the anterior, middle, or posterior third of the sinus. The division of the sinus into thirds also proves useful because of technical considerations concerning the operative management of the sagittal sinus itself when it is involved by tumor.

The sagittal sinus extends from the crista galli to the torcular Herophili. The anterior one third of the sinus extends from the crista galli to the coronal suture; the middle third runs between the coronal and lambdoid sutures; the posterior third encompasses the length of sinus from the lambdoid suture to the torcular. The middle third of the sagittal sinus lies adjacent to the paracentral lobule and the motor and sensory cortex for the foot and lower leg, which borders the rolandic fissure. This area is drained by a cortical vein, or group of veins, that is important to preserve if it is still patent at the time of surgery.

SYMPTOMATOLOGY

One of the more publicized brain tumors was that of General Leonard Wood who came Cushing in 1910 with focal jacksonian seizures of the left foot and progressive numbness and spasticity of the left lower leg. Subsequent surgery revealed a parasagittal meningioma involving the middle third of the sagittal sinus in the region of the paracentral lobule. The seizures in a given patient may initially be either motor or sensory, but usually spread to involve the other modality. Sometimes loss of consciousness ensues and the patient has a residual Todd's paralysis. Signs and symptoms of increased intracranial pressure are not common because the patient usually is evaluated and the tumor diagnosed before it attains great bulk. If the seizures are controlled with anticonvulsant medication and the spastic weakness of the contralateral lower extremity is ignored, however, the tumor may grow and extend laterally to compromise fibers from the arm area of the pararolandic cortex.

Meningiomas adjacent to the anterior third of the sagittal sinus tend to attain greater size before diagnosis and surgery because of the more insidious onset and progression of symptoms (Figure 48-1). These tumors produce a "frontal lobe syndrome" with progressive dementia characterized by apathy and alterations of personality. Twenty-five percent of the patients with anterior third parasagittal meningiomas have seizures, but they are less frequent and nonfocal.[5] Symptoms and signs of increased intracranial pressure including headache and papilledema or optic atrophy accompany the dementia. Failing vision may prompt the patient to seek a medical opinion.

Patients with meningiomas involving the posterior third of the sagittal sinus usually have a chief complaint of headache. The characteristic localizing sign, however, is a hemianopsia, the pattern of which depends on the size and precise location of the tumor. The visual field deficit is often so slowly progressive it goes unnoticed by the patient, particularly if only the peripheral visual field is involved. Sometimes the patient is aware of visual hallucinations.

OPERATIVE NEUROSURGICAL TECHNIQUES
ISBN 0-8089-1862-1

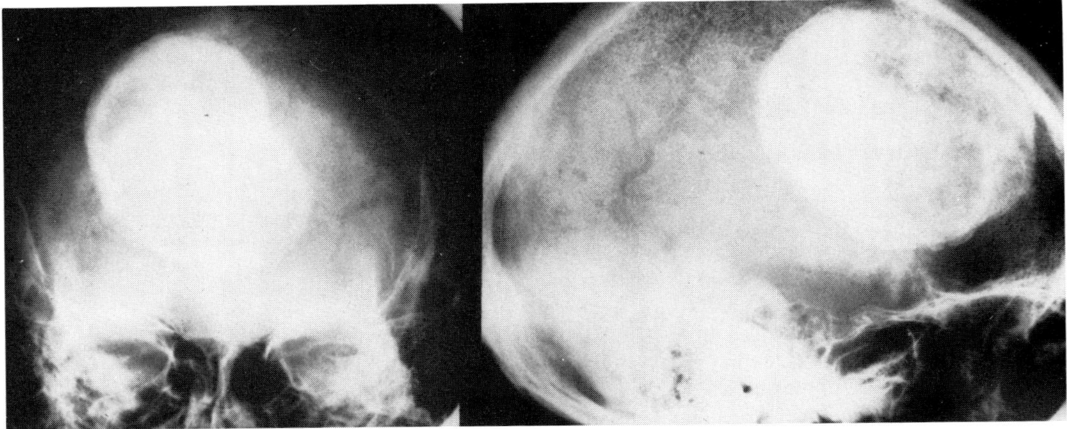

Fig. 48-1. Parasagittal and falx meningiomas adjacent to the anterior third of the sagittal sinus often attain a large size before they are diagnosed because of the insidious onset and progression of symptoms. This meningioma is unusual because of the dense calcification on plain skull x-ray films.

Patients with a long history of headaches are more likely to have a complete homonymous hemianopsia because the tumor is large. Smaller tumors located above the calcarine fissure may cause an inferior quadrant anopsia and tumors adjacent to the tentorium cerebelli may spare the upper banks of the calcarine fissure and produce a superior quadrant anopsia. Epilepsy, if visual hallucinations are not considered such, is uncommon with meningiomas involving the posterior third of the sagittal sinus.

RADIOGRAPHIC INVESTIGATION

Radiographic studies should be designed to answer specific questions about parasagittal and falcine meningiomas that are critical for the proper design and performance of surgery.

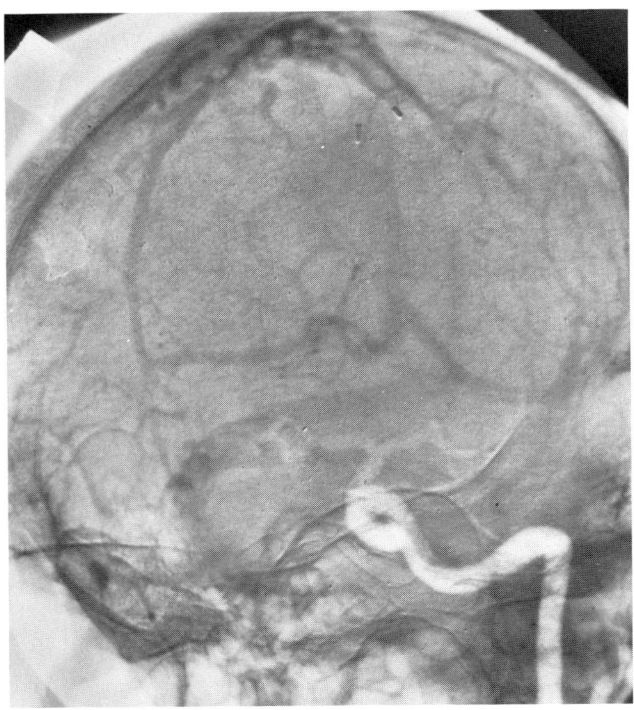

Fig. 48-2. Subtraction carotid angiography with contralateral carotid compression using the half-axial oblique view during the venous phase demonstrates occlusion of the superior sagittal sinus by a parasagittal meningioma.

PLAIN SKULL X-RAY FILMS AND COMPUTED TOMOGRAPHIC SCANS

Plain skull x-ray films should be examined for hyperostosis, enostosis, striations, and other evidence of tumor involving the skull. Vascular markings give information about skull vascularity in the vicinity of the tumor and the site of the craniotomy. The computed tomographic (CT) scan can provide information about the size, location, and configuration of the tumor. The scan also can show the site of dural attachment and is the most reliable means of determining if the tumors extends across the midline (Figure 48-2). Contrast enhancement and tomographic cuts near the vertex are necessary to avoid missing very small parasagittal and high convexity meningiomas (Figures 48-3A and B).

ANGIOGRAPHY

Preoperative angiography is important for answering the following questions:

1. How vascular is the tumor itself? The very vascular angioblastic meningioma is often more difficult to excise without significant blood loss unless en bloc dissection of a small tumor is feasible.
2. What is the relationship of the branches from the anterior cerebral artery to the tumor and where are the major arterial feeders of the tumor?
3. Is the sagittal venous sinus widely patent, partially occluded, or totally occluded by tumor involvement?
4. What is the relationship of major cortical draining veins, such as the anastomotic vein of Trolard, to the tumor?

It is critical that large draining cortical veins entering the sagittal sinus and the sinus itself, if still patent, be spared when exposing and excising parasagittal or falx meningiomas along the middle third or posterior third of the sinus. Attention therefore should be given to the location of these large draining veins and the surgery planned so these vessels are spared. The acute surgical occlusion of the middle third of the sagittal sinus may result in spastic diplegia. Occlusion of the posterior third of a widely patent sinus may be fatal. The technical decision to effect a "cure" by total extirpation of a parasagittal meningioma by excision or reconstruction of the sinus by duraplasty or vein grafting may depend on the preoperative angiographic assessment of the patency of the superior sagittal

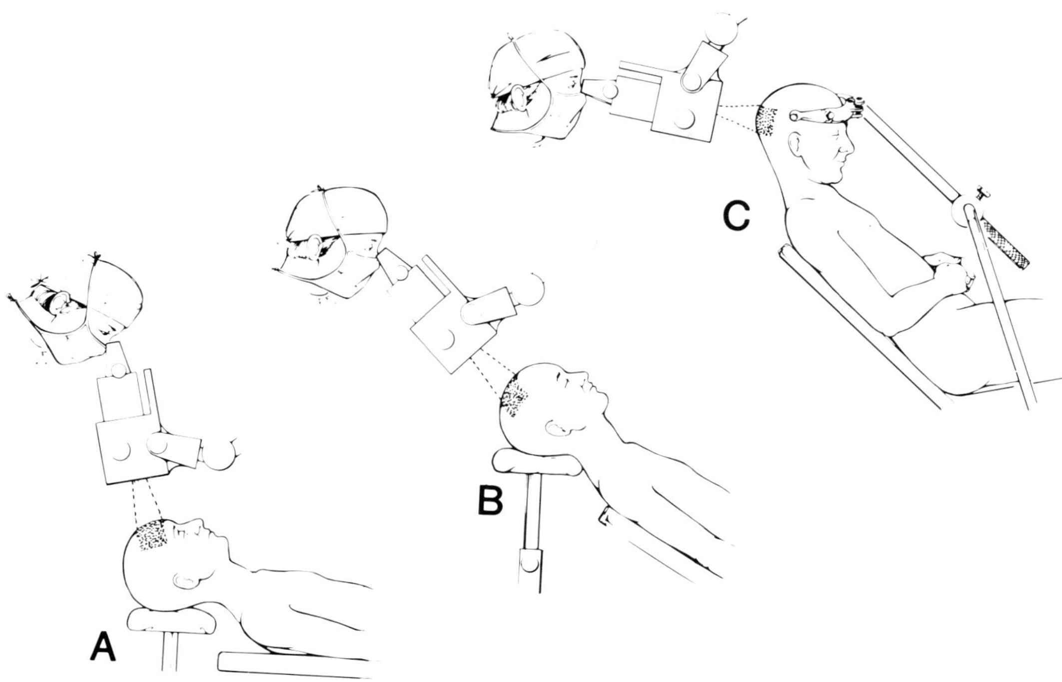

Fig. 48-3. Head position of the patient for approaching meningiomas involving (A) the anterior third, (B) the middle third, and (C) the posterior third of the sagittal sinus.

sinus and on the presence of collateral anastomotic channels to the sylvian veins.

Morris recommended an oblique half-axial view to show the entire sinus.[6] This view may be misleading if a segment of the sinus is not visualized, however. To overcome this problem, Yasargil and Damur recommended half-axial oblique phlebography obtained by simultaneous bilateral injection of the internal carotid artery.[7] Waga and Handa recommend an alternative technique of using contralateral carotid compression during the injection of 10 to 12 ml of contrast medium for half-axial oblique phlebography.[8] Subtraction angiography also is advised because the inner table of the skull can mimic an opacified superior sagittal sinus (Figure 48-2).[9]

Marc and Schechter believe that occlusion of the superior sagittal sinus by a slowly growing tumor can be predicted with reasonable accuracy from the lateral projection of the venous phase of a carotid angiogram providing the findings include:

1. Nonvisualization of a segment of the superior sagittal sinus.
2. Failure of cortical veins to reach the superior sagittal sinus.
3. Delay of venous drainage in the area of obstruction.
4. Reversal of the normal venous flow with large collaterals connecting the anterior superior sagittal sinus with the superior sagittal sinus distal to the obstruction, the transverse sinus, or the middle cerebral vein.[9]

Nonvisualization of a segment of the superior sagittal sinus without the other signs on the lateral view could be due to the sinus receiving a large volume of unopacified blood from the opposite cerebral hemisphere through a large cortical vein at that location.

Phlebography also may show collateral venous drainage through enlarged scalp veins.[8] These dilated scalp veins also are seen when the scalp is shaved and should be considered when planning the scalp incision and flap.

Walkenhorst reviewed 79 parasagittal meningiomas involving the dural sinus angle and 35 falx meningiomas to determine if angiography provided signs conclusive for differentiating the

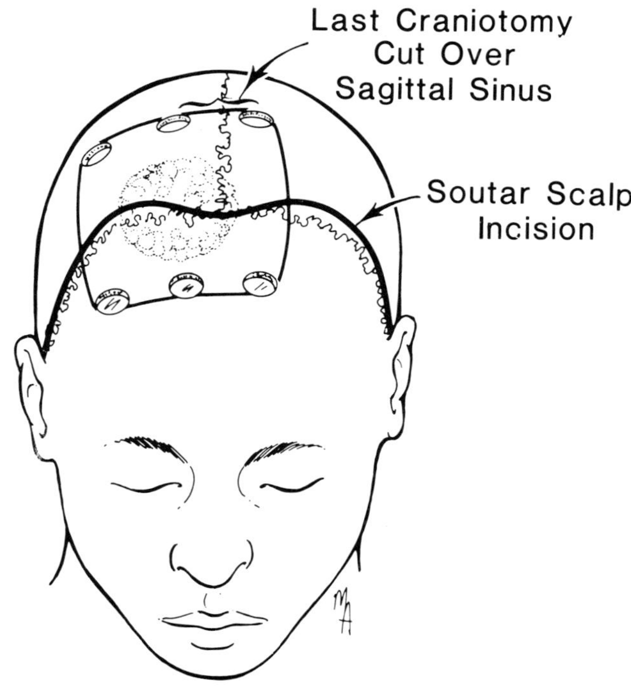

Fig. 48-4. The scalp incision bisects the anteroposterior plane of a parasagittal or falx meningioma. The free bone flap crosses the midline to the extent determined by the size and configuration of the tumor. Burr holes are placed on either side rather than directly over the sagittal sinus.

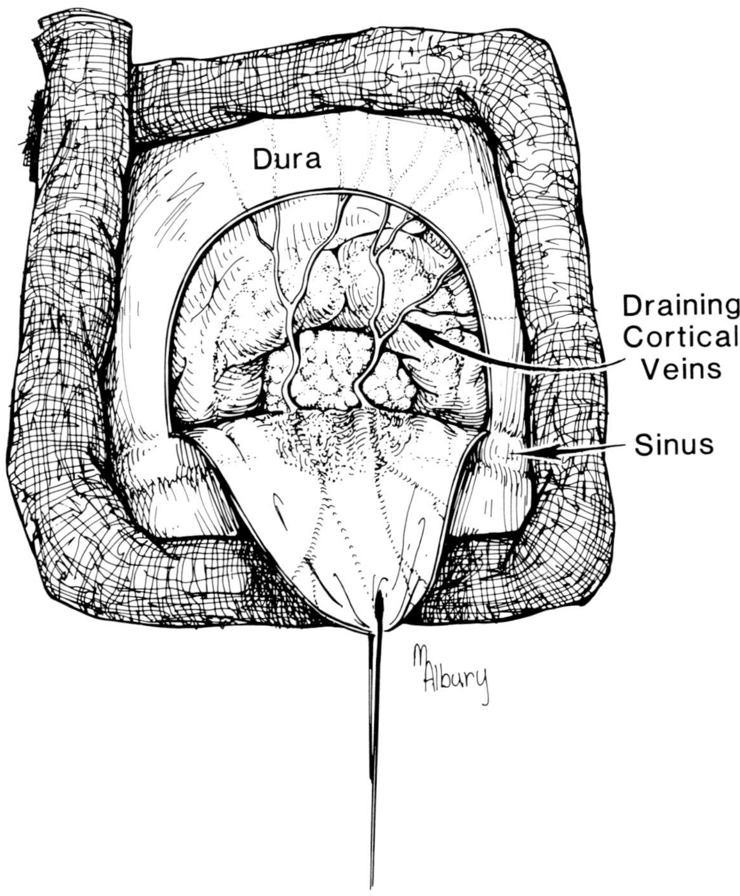

Fig. 48-5.   The dura mater is carefully peeled away from a parasagittal meningioma. Bridging veins that drain the cerebral cortex and enter the sagittal sinus are spared.

two tumor types preoperatively.[10] He reported that a falx meningioma is excluded angiographically when the blood supply is from branches of the middle cerebral artery or when the external carotid artery contributes to the tumor circulation. Marked basal convex meandering of the pericallosal artery on the lateral angiogram is evidence for a falx rather than a parasagittal meningioma.

Selective injection of the external carotid artery may be helpful in determining the site of tumor attachment at the convexity or along the falx cerebri. The tentorial branches from the internal carotid artery may delineate the site of dural attachment of posterior falx meningiomas. Subtraction studies, angiotomography, and magnification also may improve definition of tumor vascularity. Internal carotid artery injection of contrast agents with digital subtraction angiography is an effective method for demonstrating venous anatomy and patency of the sagittal sinus.

SAGITTAL SINOGRAPHY

Sagittal sinography is largely of historical interest and is considered only when angiography does not provide a satisfactory venous phase for determining sinus patency with middle and posterior third parasagittal tumors. A burr hole is placed in the exact midline 8 cm above the nasion. The sinus this far forward may be small and less blue than in the parietal region. The lateral margins of the sinus usually are delineated, how-

ever, by thickened white strands in the dura. A No. 11 scalpel blade is used to fenestrate the sinus wall and a fine catheter is inserted 3 cm into the sinus. Aspiration of venous blood confirms the catheter position before the contrast medium is injected.

Direct sagittal sinography has several disadvantages and often is not necessary when good angiograms are available. The procedure does not always provide complete information regarding collateral venous flow and the cerebral pattern of venous drainage is not seen at all. The procedure may be technically troublesome, time consuming, and is not without risk. Sinography may be thrombogenic, and Krayenbuhl cautioned that sinography may be dangerous in patients who have an acute thrombotic process or a thrombotic process in evolution.[11] There also is the potential for air embolism with direct sinography.[12]

MAGNETIC RESONANCE IMAGING

Magnetic resonance imaging (MRI) is often not as effective as CT scanning for demonstrating meningiomas. The MRI scan can, however, demonstrate evidence of vascular occlusion better than CT scans and can be an effective noninvasive way of demonstrating a sagittal sinus or transverse sinus occlusion. Sagittal sinus thrombosis has been demonstrated by means of a spin-echo technique with T1 and T2 weighted images and may prove to be an effective, noninvasive way of assessing the

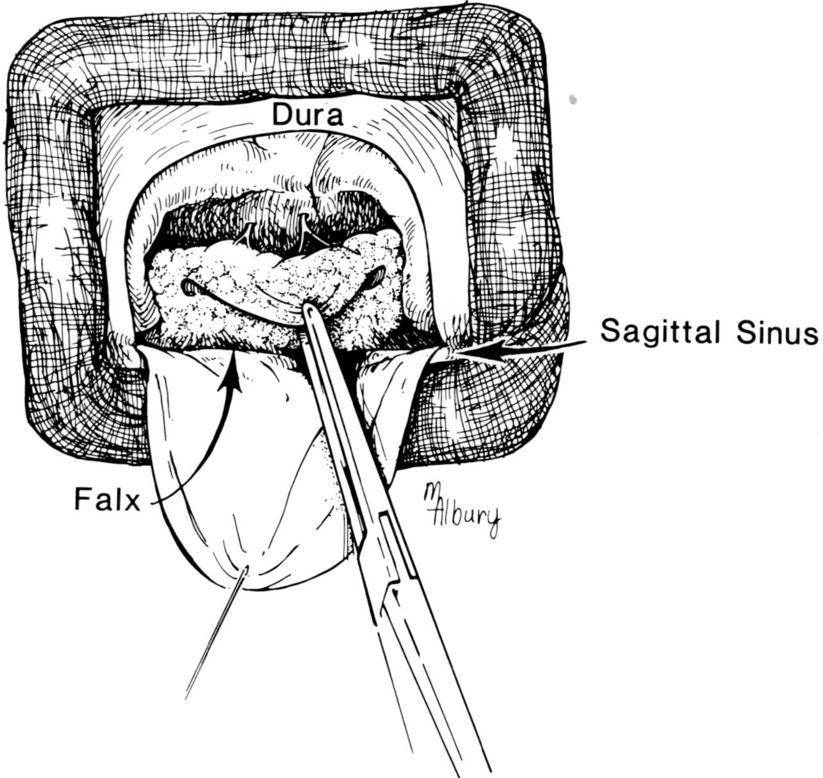

Fig. 48-6. A parasagittal meningioma is first debulked by intracapsular enucleation. The thin capsular wall is then delivered into the tumor cavity as arachnoidal adhesive bands and feeding vessels are divided. The capsule is removed piecemeal until only the attachment to the falx and the sagittal sinus remains.

patency of venous sinuses involved by meningiomas (Roll J, Elias D: Personal communication on work in progress). One advantage of MRI is the ease with which sagittal, coronal, and axial views can be obtained (Roll J, Elias D: Personal communication on work in progress).

OPERATIVE APPROACH AND TECHNIQUES

POSITION

The head is positioned with the sagittal plane of the head parallel to the walls and perpendicular to the ceiling. The patient is supine for tumors along the anterior third of the sagittal sinus with the head of the table flat or slightly elevated. The head is supported in a donut head holder or by three-point skeletal fixation. Tumors involving the middle third of the sinus are more easily approached if the head is elevated a few degrees and the neck slightly flexed so the surgeon is looking directly down on the vertex. Tumors between the lambdoidal suture and torcular Herophili can be approached with the patient in a three-quarter semisitting position with the neck flexed and the head secured by three-point skeletal fixation (Figure 48-3) or with the patient in the prone position in three-point skeletal fixation. It is important that it be possible to raise or lower the head quickly to control sagittal sinus venous pressure in the event of bleeding from the sinus or the occurrence of air emboli.

SCALP INCISION

The incision is outlined on the shaved and prepared scalp with a scratch or skin marking pencil before draping but after positioning, so there is no confusion about the relationship of the incision to key landmarks. The midline is identified with a cross-hatch mark that can be identified easily.

The curvilinear or sinusoidal transverse scalp incision offers several advantages over the more traditional scalp flap. The incision is quickly opened and closed. It is readily extended on either side of the midline if more exposure is needed. The blood supply to the scalp is not compromised. The incision is less restrictive and can easily be adapted to additional surgery at a later date, if necessary. The transverse incision is in the plane bisecting the anteroposterior diameter of the tumor and extends equidistant on either side of the tumor (Figure 48-4).

BONE FLAP

A free bone flap is preferred to an osteoplastic or periosteal hinged flap high on the convexity or across the midline at the vertex. The skull is thick in this region and not easily fractured. There is no muscle or fascia to remove from the bone or to secure the bone flap. Troublesome bleeding from the bone is easier to control and the flap can be manipulated more safely in the region of the sagittal sinus.

The bone flap is extended to or just across the midline for unilateral tumors. The bone flap is carried well across the midline to the extent dictated by the size and shape of the tumor when the CT scan shows a bilateral meningioma (Figure 48-4).

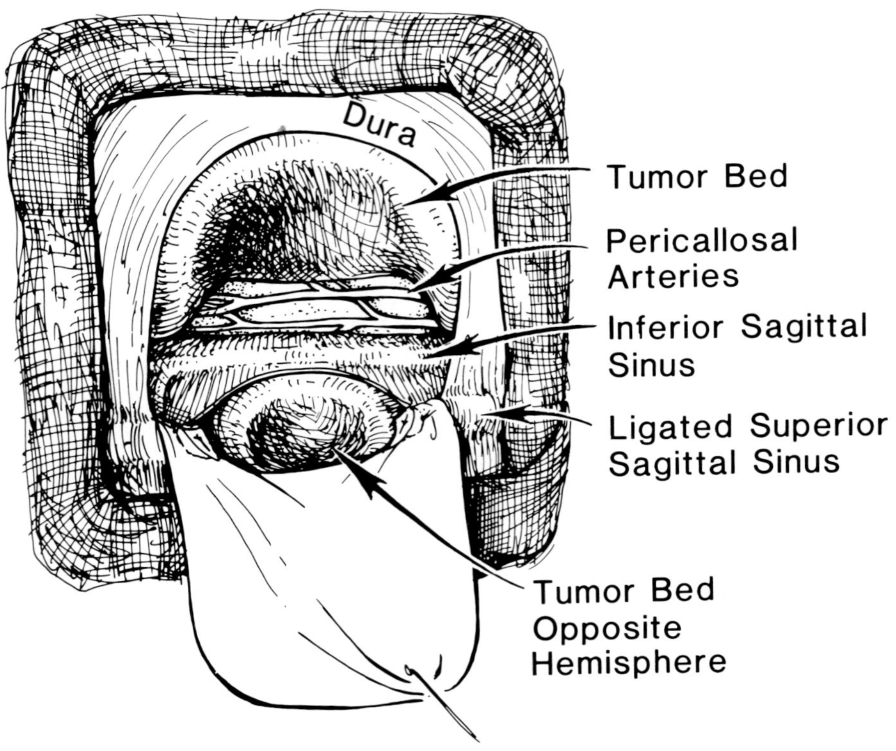

Fig. 48-7. A bilateral parasagittal meningioma has been excised along with a segment of the involved falx and occluded sagittal sinus, which was first ligated, then divided. A collateral vein from the sagittal sinus proximal to the occlusion is spared along with the patent inferior sagittal sinus. The pericallosal arteries that supplied feeding branches to the tumor are seen on the dorsal surface of the corpus callosum.

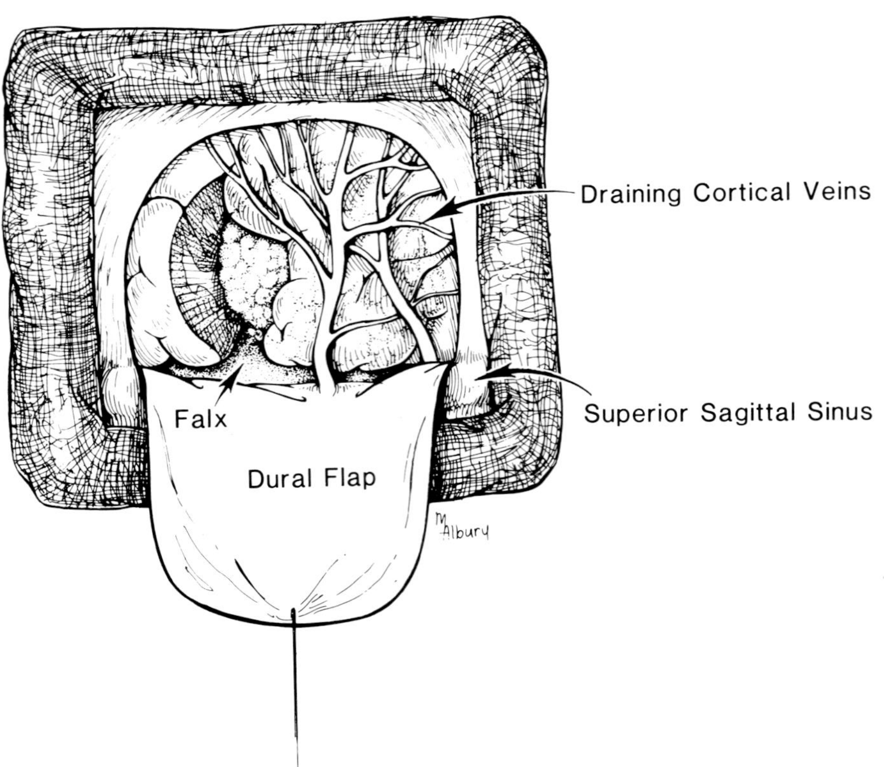

Fig. 48-8. A large falcine meningioma invaginates the paracentral lobule beneath large draining cortical veins. An anterior wedge resection of premotor cortex adjacent to the falx provides access to the tumor without forceful retraction on the motor cortex or injury to the important bridging veins.

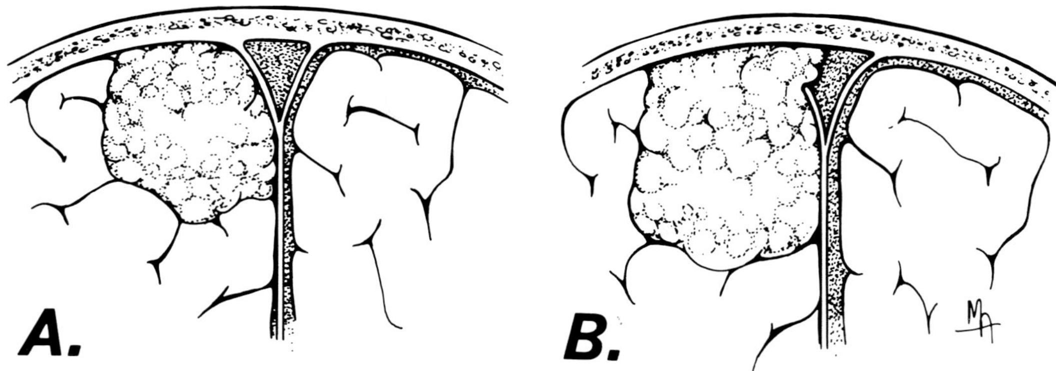

Fig. 48-9. (A) A coronal view of the superior sagittal sinus illustrates a meningioma involving one wall. A parasagittal meningioma usually infiltrates both layers of dura mater while a falx meningioma may be attached to the outer layer only. (B) A coronal view of the superior sagittal sinus illustrates a meningioma infiltrating the lateral wall and angle of the sinus and protruding into the lateral recess of the lumen.

The bone flap is centered over the tumor. Care is taken to make the bone flap extra generous when the meningioma is adjacent to the paracentral lobule so that functionally important sensory and motor cortex does not have to be removed or manipulated for exposure of the tumor.

Burr holes are placed immediately on both sides of the sagittal sinus at the anterior margins of the bone flap but not directly over either the sinus or the tumor (Figure 48–4). The dura mater and sinus are carefully separated from the inner table of the skull with a dural separator. Whether the Gigli saw or air osteotome is used, it is important to bevel the cuts. The bone cuts across the sinus are performed last, and the anterior cut is made before the posterior cut.

If the bone flap is attached to the dura mater or involved by tumor over or near the sagittal sinus, it is preferable to rongeur the bone away, rather than risk tearing the sagittal sinus by avulsing the tumor with the bone. If it is known or strongly suspected in advance that the tumor involves the skull over the sinus, the bone flap is not freed on all sides with the saw for fear the rocking action of the rongeur on the free bone flap that is tethered by tumor may tear the sagittal sinus or injure adjacent brain.

Brisk venous bleeding is sometimes encountered coming from the sagittal sinus and should be anticipated. Strips of Surgicel or thrombin-soaked Gelfoam that have been prepared previously are placed over the bleeding sinus immediately and gentle pressure is applied with cottonoid strips. The dura and epidural bleeding is otherwise handled as previously described with bipolar coagulation and dural tacking stitches.

DURAL OPENING, TUMOR EXPOSURE, AND EXCISION

The sagittal sinus is readily identified, but bridging cortical veins just beneath the dura mater can easily be torn if not anticipated and carefully dissected off the dural flap as it is turned. The flap is hinged on the sagittal sinus to avoid damaging these important draining veins, which can cause serious neurologic deficit if interrupted posterior to the coronal suture (Figure 48-5).

Parasagittal meningiomas often can be palpated through the dura mater and the dura opened accordingly so that unnecessary brain exposure is avoided. The dura mater is peeled away from the tumor immediately and is not used to retract the tumor, as suggested for convexity meningiomas, because of the risk of initiating bleeding from the sinus or bridging cortical veins (Figure 48-5).

The capsule is partially exposed using bipolar cautery to coagulate small vessels parasitized from the pia arachnoid over adjacent cortex that are feeding the tumor. This is done without excising any cortex and with very little retraction of surrounding brain. An intracapsular enucleation then is performed and the capsule delivered into the tumor cavity. If the tumor is not excessively vascular and aspirates well, it generally works best to then deliver the capsule invaginating the cortex (Figure 48-6). After the tumor mass is removed, the attachment to the falx and sagittal sinus is excised and coagulated.

Bilateral tumors infiltrating the falx and presenting on the medial side of both cerebral hemispheres require a resection of the falx along the anterior and posterior margins of the tumor. It is important to identify and preserve collateral venous channels passing through the falx to the inferior sagittal sinus, particularly when the superior sagittal sinus is occluded. The inferior sagittal sinus and pericallosal arteries are preserved as feeding vessels coming off the pericallosal branches are coagulated and divided (Figure 48-7).

If a large meningioma invaginates the medial surface of the hemisphere along the middle third of the falx in the vicinity of the paracentral lobule, it may on rare occasion be preferable to expose the tumor by performing a wedge cortical resection well anterior to the motor cortex, rather than to attempt to expose the tumor through forceful retraction of the brain and interruption of cortical draining veins passing to the sagittal sinus (Figure 48-8). Gentle retraction on the cortex is always attempted initially, however, to see if the tumor can be exposed and excised without brain resection.

Technical problems are fewer when the tumor is at or anterior to the coronal suture. Draining cortical veins can be coagulated and divided and a patent superior sagittal sinus ligated and divided if necessary. The falx then is excised with the infiltrating tumor attached.

Surgical judgment determines how the superior sagittal sinus infiltrated with tumor is best managed according to the peculiarities of the specific case. Factors to be considered include the age and condition of the patient, the amount of time the patient has been under anesthesia, the blood loss and tissue trauma associated with the exposure and excision of the main

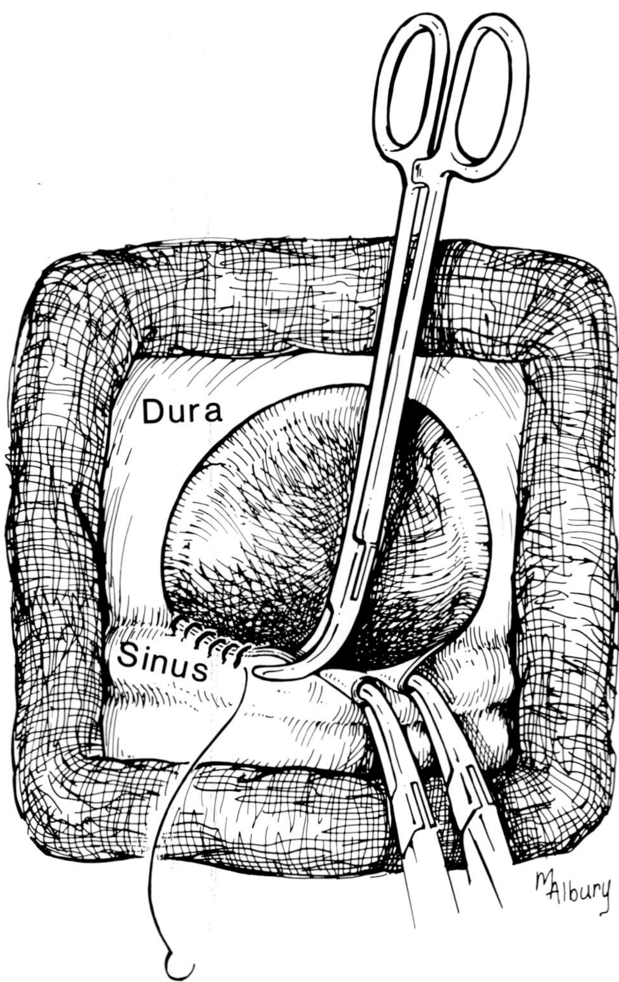

Fig. 48-10. The patent sagittal sinus with a meningioma involving the lateral recess is opened longitudinally along the inside curve of vascular clamps. The clamps are applied sequentially as the dural walls forming the lateral angle are partially excised along with the contained tumor. The clamps are then removed in reverse order as a sinorrhaphy is performed with a running vascular stitch.

tumor mass, and the location and extent of involvement of the sinus by the tumor. The sinus can be clipped or ligated and divided in order to accomplish total tumor removal when involved anterior to the coronal suture, whether patent or not. The sinus also can be sacrificed anywhere along its length when totally occluded by tumor. If a tumor involves the middle or posterior third of a patent sinus, one of several options can be exercised.

The tumor attached to one wall of the sinus without significant infiltration of the dura or lumen is best peeled off the sinus wall and the dura coagulated (Figure 48-9A). If the tumor has infiltrated the sinus lumen in the lateral angle but not obliterated the sinus, it usually is feasible to grasp the superior and lateral wall of the sinus with the contained nubbin of tumor with curved vascular clamps or hemostats (Figure 48-9B). The dural wall of the sinus then is excised by cutting along the inner curve of the clamps. The clamps then are rotated one-half turn and a running vascular suture is used to perform the

sinorrhaphy as the clamps are removed one at a time (Figure 48-10).

The sinus grossly invaded by tumor with involvement of all three dural walls but still carrying blood is often best left intact. Hartman and Klug reported enclosing the superior sagittal sinus still carrying blood despite invasion by tumor in a sleeve fashioned from the falx and convexity dura. This sleeve of dura contains and directs any possible future recurrent growth of tumor in such a way that it eventually obliterates the sinus. Collateral circulation gradually develops and the segment of sagittal sinus occluded by tumor then can be excised without risk.[13]

Simpson found that complete excision of a meningioma with its dural attachment is followed by fewer clinical recurrences (5–9 percent) than is complete removal of the tumor with coagulation of the dural attachment (17 percent), complete removal without treatment of the dural attachment (29 percent), or partial removal of the tumor (39 percent).[14]

Bonnal and Brotchi have demonstrated the technical feasibility of using partial or total autogenous vein grafts to repair the superior sagittal sinus when one, two, or all three sinus walls are infiltrated with tumor.[15] The procedure adds to the time and complexity of the operation, however, and the tumor still may recur.

REFERENCES

1. Cushing H: The meningiomas (dural endotheliomas): Their source and favored seats of origin (Cavendish Lecture). Brain 45:282, 1922
2. Northfield DWC: The Surgery of the Central Nervous System. Oxford, England, Blackwell, 1973, p 884
3. Cushing H, Eisenhardt L: Meningiomas. Their Classification, Regional Behavior, Life History and Surgical End Results. Springfield, Ill, Charles C Thomas, 1938, p 785
4. Olivecrona H: Die Parasagittalen Meningiome. Leipzig, Georg Thieme, 1934
5. Lund M: Epilepsy in association with intracranial tumours. Acta Psychiatr Scand (Suppl) 81:149, 1952
6. Morris L: Angiography of the superior sagittal and transverse sinuses. Br J Radiol 33:606, 1960
7. Yasargil MG, Damur M: Thrombosis of the cerebral veins and dural sinuses, in Newton TH, Potts DG (eds): Radiology of the Skull and Brain, vol 2. St. Louis, CV Mosby, 1974, pp 2375–2400
8. Waga S, Handa H: Scalp veins as collateral pathway with parasagittal meningiomas occluding superior sagittal sinus. Neuroradiology 11:119, 1976
9. Marc JA, Schechter MM: Cortical venous rerouting in parasagittal meningiomas. Radiology 112:85, 1974
10. Walkenhorst A: Angiographic aspects of parasagittal meningiomas. Acta Neurochir 31:288, 1974
11. Krayenbuhl H: Cerebral venous and sinus thrombosis. Clin Neurosurg 14:1, 1967
12. Askenasy HM, Kosary IZ, Braham J: Thrombosis of the longitudinal sinus diagnosis by carotid angiography. Neurology 12:288, 1962
13. Hartman K, Klug W: Recurrence and possible surgical procedures in meningiomas of the middle and posterior parts of the superior sagittal sinus. Acta Neurochir 31:283, 1975
14. Simpson D: The recurrence of intracranial meningiomas after surgical treatment. J Neurol Neurosurg Psychiatry 20:22, 1957
15. Bonnal J, Brotchi J: Surgery of the superior sagittal sinus in parasagittal meningiomas. J Neurosurg 48:935, 1978

CHAPTER 49

Posterior Fossa Meningiomas

Robert E. Maxwell   Shelley N. Chou

LESS THAN 9 PERCENT of intracranial meningiomas occur in the posterior fossa.[1,2] Castellano and Ruggiero reported on 68 posterior fossa meningiomas, including 20 of the tentorium cerebelli, among 803 intracranial meningiomas in Olivecrona's series of 4185 brain tumors.[3] Tumors of the posterior fossa can be difficult to excise totally and the recurrence rate for symptoms is relatively high. The clinical presentation varies with the size and location of the tumor and depends primarily on the degree of involvement of the lower cranial nerves, cerebellum, brainstem, and fourth ventricle with secondary obstructive hydrocephalus. Tumors of the posterior fossa are classified according to their site of attachment in the cerebellopontine angle (CPA), the posterior surface of the petrous ridge, the tentorium cerebelli, the clivus, the foramen magnum, the fourth ventricle, and the occipital squama over the cerebellar hemispheres.

Midline tumors arising along the basilic groove displace the brain stem and cause a stretching of the cranial nerves. The symptoms and signs are those associated with dysfunction of the long motor tract and the lower six cranial nerves. The extremely rare tumors arising from the tela choroidea in the fourth ventricle produce an early obstructive hydrocephalus. Meningiomas arising from the posterolateral petrous ridge, from the occipital squama over the posterior cerebellar convexity, and from the tentorium cerebelli produce symptoms of cerebellar dysfunction. These tumors often are well tolerated by the patient because of their slow growth until signs and symptoms of increased intracranial pressure associated with hydrocephalus develop.

Meningiomas arising adjacent to the porus acousticus in the cerebellopontine angle cause symptoms similar to those associated with acoustic neuromas and cannot be distinguished with assurance on clinical findings alone. Ten to 15 percent of CPA tumors are meningiomas.[4] There is a tendency for meningiomas to involve the fifth and seventh cranial nerves more frequently than acoustic neuromas do, and additional involvement of any of the lower four cranial nerves suggests either a meningioma or metastatic tumor. Meningiomas tend to produce less auditory and vestibular nerve dysfunction than acoustic neuromas.[5]

Meningiomas arising from the tentorium cerebelli account for 3 to 5 percent of all meningiomas and 18 percent of posterior fossa meningiomas.[6] These tumors present clinically in one of three ways. They may produce disturbances of gait with ataxia. There may be a long history of progressive facial numbness and eighth nerve dysfunction. Some patients have an obstructive hydrocephalus and increased intracranial pressure.[7]

Foramen magnum meningiomas account for about 3 percent of brain and spinal cord meningiomas.[8] Meningiomas occur more frequently than either neurilemomas or neurofibromas in this region and two thirds of foramen magnum tumors are meningiomas.[8,9]

Cushing classified foramen magnum meningiomas into "craniospinal" and "spinocranial" groups according to whether the site of origin was above or below the foramen magnum.[1] Cerebellar signs, increased intracranial pressure, and cranial nerve deficits are more characteristic of "craniospinal" meningiomas.

Foramen magnum meningiomas tend to go unrecognized and undiagnosed for long periods because of their ubiquitous symptoms and lack of good localizing signs. Foramen magnum meningiomas are sometimes misdiagnosed because incomplete myelographic studies fail to define the anatomy around the foramen magnum adequately. The diagnostic pitfalls associated with these tumors are emphasized in numerous reports.[9–11]

In the early stages of tumor growth the clinical picture may be mistaken for cervical spondylosis with a secondary radiculopathy. In advanced stages, an intramedullary, rather than extramedullary, lesion may be suspected. Elsberg and Strauss emphasized that the size of the upper spinal canal and the foramen magnum permits tumors in this region to attain large size and manifest radicular symptoms without myelopathy.[12]

The most frequent initial symptom of foramen magnum tumors is suboccipital or neck pain (49 percent) and dysesthesia in the extremities (37 percent).[7] By the time patients have surgery, often many months after their initial symptoms develop, 95 percent have dysesthesia in their hands and fingers and 75 percent have posterior cervical or suboccipital pain. About 50 percent of these patients have weakness in the upper extremities or gait disturbance, and one third complain of bladder disturbance. Almost one half of patients with foramen magnum tumors have a normal neurologic examination when first evaluated for their initial complaint. Hypalgesia in the C2 dermatomal distribution and spinal accessory nerve palsy are reliable localizing signs. Stereoanesthesia of the hands also occurs with foramen magnum tumors that compress or interfere with the blood supply to the posterior columns or their nuclei.[13,14]

RADIOGRAPHIC STUDIES

COMPUTED TOMOGRAPHIC SCANNING

The differential diagnosis of posterior fossa tumors is aided by radiographic studies. Moller et al.[15] analyzed CPA tumors with computed tomographic (CT) scanning and concluded that

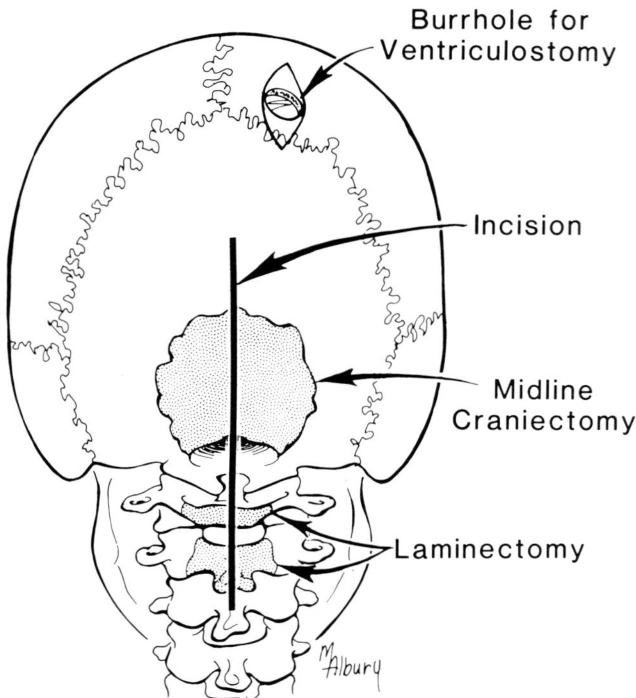

Fig. 49-1. A burr hole is placed 7 cm above the inion and 3 cm to the right of the midline for a lateral ventriculostomy when posterior fossa surgery is performed without previous ventricular drainage. Tumors in the region of the foramen magnum, the fourth ventricle, or the occipital squama overlying the medial posterior cerebellar hemisphere are approached by a midline suboccipital craniectomy.

there were features that differentiated CPA meningiomas from acoustic neuromas. They found that cerebellopontine angle meningiomas were often calcified and were more likely to be attenuated on unenhanced CT scans. The center of an acoustic neuroma rarely is anterior to the porus acusticus and the tumor rarely extends as high as the dorsum selli, both of which may occur with CPA meningiomas. Meningiomas of the CPA may also protrude into the suprasellar cistern. Porus changes are rare with CPA meningiomas, unlike acoustic neuromas. Meningiomas characteristically show a broad-based mass aligned with the petrous ridge rather than one centered over the internal auditory canal.[16] Valavanis et al.[17] carried out a detailed analysis of the CT findings in 16 surgically verified cases of meningioma of the posterior surface of the petrous bone. They concluded that a correct preoperative diagnosis is possible in almost every case. Frequently occurring specific CT criteria for meningioma of the posterior surface of the petrous bone include a hyperdense, homogeneously enhancing, extra-axial CPA mass; an inverse relationship between precontrast attenuation values and degree of contrast enhancement of the tumor; an oval shape; an obtuse angle between the lateral tumor border and the posterior surface of the petrous bone; and evidence of transcisternal, supratentorial tumor extension. Infrequently occurring specific CT criteria include tumor calcification; hyperostosis or exostosis of the posterior surface of the petrous bone; a comma-shape tumor configuration in cases with transcisternal tumor extension; and evidence of transtentorial tumor extension.

Computed tomography may miss small foramen magnum meningiomas unless contrast enhancement is used and cuts are obtained at close intervals through the region of the lower medulla and upper cervical spinal canal. Oxygen CT cisternography is a sensitive and reliable technique for detecting small tumors.

MAGNETIC RESONANCE IMAGING

Mikhael et al.[18] reported that magnetic resonance imaging (MRI) has shown interesting capabilities as a noninvasive study for the visualization of the internal auditory canal, the neural bundle entering the canal, the brain stem, and cerebellum. Magnetic resonance imaging was successful in detecting all cerebellopontine angle tumors in their series. They concluded that MRI can replace invasive air and metrizamide cisternography in the diagnosis of CPA lesions and can help in the differentiation between acoustic neuromas and meningiomas.[18] Recent experience suggests that nuclear magnetic resonance imaging will become a useful noninvasive means of evaluating the foramen magnum region as well and may supplant or provide an adjunct to metrizamide-enhanced CT scanning for assessing meningiomas in this region.[19]

ANGIOGRAPHY

The dura mater anterior to the foramen magnum is supplied by meningeal vessels from the carotid siphon, the ascending pharyngeal artery, and the middle meningeal artery. The dura mater posterior to the foramen magnum is supplied primarily by the occipital artery and also by the posterior meningeal branch of the vertebral artery.[20] Selective angiography of the internal carotid, the external carotid, and the vertebral arteries assist in the preoperative diagnosis of meningiomas of the posterior fossa. An abnormal meningeal artery, whether arising from the middle meningeal, the ascending pharyngeal, or the internal carotid artery, is strong evidence for a meningioma rather than an acoustic neuroma in the cerebellopontine angle.[20] Although meningiomas attached to the dura over the squamous part of the occipital bone are rare, they can be recognized when dilated meningeal vessels from the posterior meningeal branch of the vertebral artery or meningeal branches of the occipital artery are seen. Only 50 percent of posterior fossa meningiomas can be diagnosed with a tumor stain.[21]

Angiography of the vertebral and internal and external carotid arteries is important when a tentorial meningioma is a possible diagnosis. A tentorial meningioma may receive its blood supply from the terminal branches of the basilar, middle meningeal, occipital, and ascending pharyngeal arteries. The blood supply is mainly from meningeal branches off the internal carotid artery.[22-24] The most prominent of these branches was described by Bernasconi and Cassinari[25] and has been called the "artery of the free margin of the tentorium."[23] This artery normally is small and may not be visible on routine angiograms. The artery enlarges and may be prominent in the presence of a tentorial meningioma, however.

Angiography also is helpful in the assessment of foramen magnum meningiomas. A diffuse tumor stain suggests the tissue diagnosis. Preoperative awareness of the tumor's vascularity and the location of prominent feeding vessels suggest the optimum operative approach. It is especially helpful to understand the relationship of the tumor to the foramen magnum.

MYELOGRAPHY

Complete cervical myelography with contrast medium carried through the foramen magnum is necessary to exclude small meningiomas in this area.[26-28] Myelography is performed with

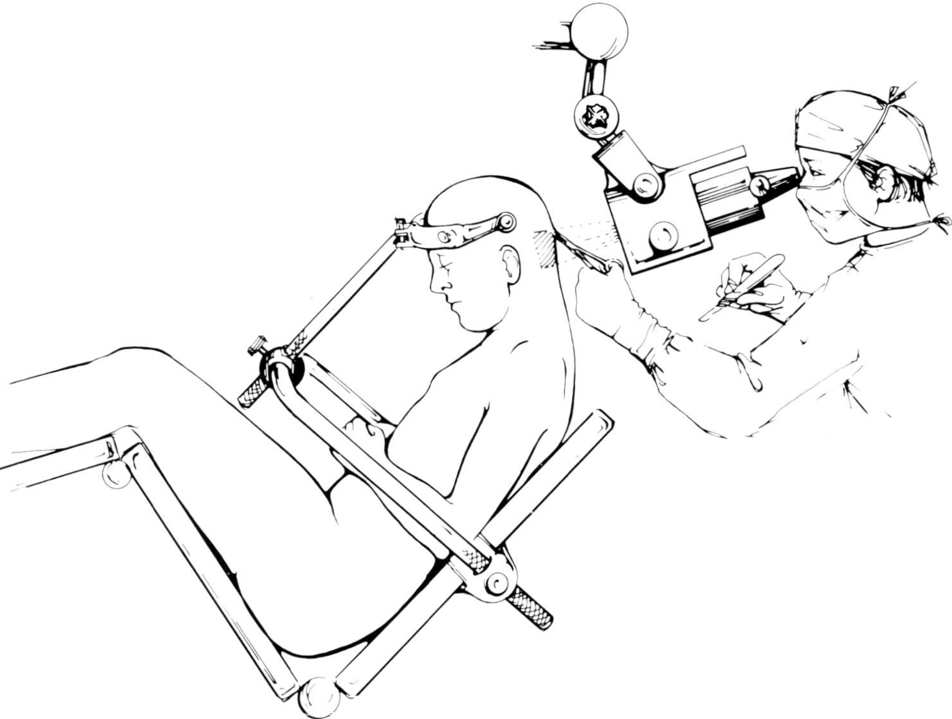

Fig. 49-2. The prone, three-quarter prone, or sitting position can be used to approach a posterior fossa meningioma. The head holder is attached to the back of the table so the head can be lowered quickly without disengaging the head holder.

the patient supine if a tumor is not defined with the patient in the standard prone position. Cerebrospinal fluid (CSF) examination is routine at the time of myelography. Approximately 90 percent of patients with foramen magnum tumors have elevated total protein levels in the CSF.[7] Clivography has been supplanted by CT scanning in the evaluation of cerebellopontine angle meningiomas. Brookler et al.[29] reported that computed axial tomography with contrast enhancement is of limited value in detecting small tumors adjacent to the temporal bone or within the internal auditory canal. If the CT scan is normal, they state that a positive contrast posterior fossa myelogram is indicated.

VENTRICULOGRAPHY

Ventriculography is not without risk in patients with posterior fossa meningiomas. Knupling and Fuchs reported 6 of 18 patients with posterior fossa meningiomas and secondary hydrocephalus suffering complications from upward transtentorial herniation after ventricular taps.[30] These patients had a disturbance of transtentorial CSF flow and developed brain stem dysfunction because of herniation with mesencephalic and bulbar dysfunction. The operative mortality was high for this group. Computed tomographic scanning now obviates the need for ventriculography in most cases.

VENTRICULAR DRAINAGE FOR OBSTRUCTIVE HYDROCEPHALUS

Control of increased intracranial pressure and hydrocephalus is urgent. Lumbar puncture and drainage is contraindicated because of the risk of transtentorial or foramen magnum hernia-

tion. If any delay in posterior fossa surgery is elected or necessary, the increased intracranial pressure associated with hydrocephalus is relieved by lateral ventriculostomy and ventricular drainage. Care should be taken to ensure that the CSF pressure is controlled and gradually, not suddenly, reduced, since upward transtentorial herniation or a subdural hematoma can be induced by sudden changes in pressure. The sterile ventricular drainage system is kept open, but the height of the tubing is adjusted so drainage occurs only at pressures exceeding 100 mm of water (7–8 torr). The CSF pulsations or pressure waves are continually observed to ensure that the drainage system is not obstructed. The patient's vital signs and neurologic status are closely monitored for evidence of brainstem compression or ischemia associated with transtentorial herniation. Ventricular drainage is preferred to ventricular shunting because the system is better monitored and a foreign body is not permanently left in place. If a prolonged delay in definitive surgery is anticipated, however, a ventriculoperitoneal or ventriculoatrial shunt is preferred to lessen the risk of ventriculitis and to make nursing care easier.

A preoperative ventriculostomy performed through a frontal twist drill or burr hole is preferred to one in the occipital or posterior parietal region. This lessens the potential for contamination of the posterior fossa craniectomy wound. The right frontal site is chosen for primary shunting or ventriculostomy drainage. If ventriculostomy is necessary but there is concern that subsequent shunting may become necessary or if it is a possibility, consideration should be given to placing the frontal ventriculostomy on the left side. If immediate posterior fossa surgery is carried out, an occipital burr hole is placed 7 cm above the inion and 3 cm to the right of the midline for lateral ventriculostomy (Figure 49-1).

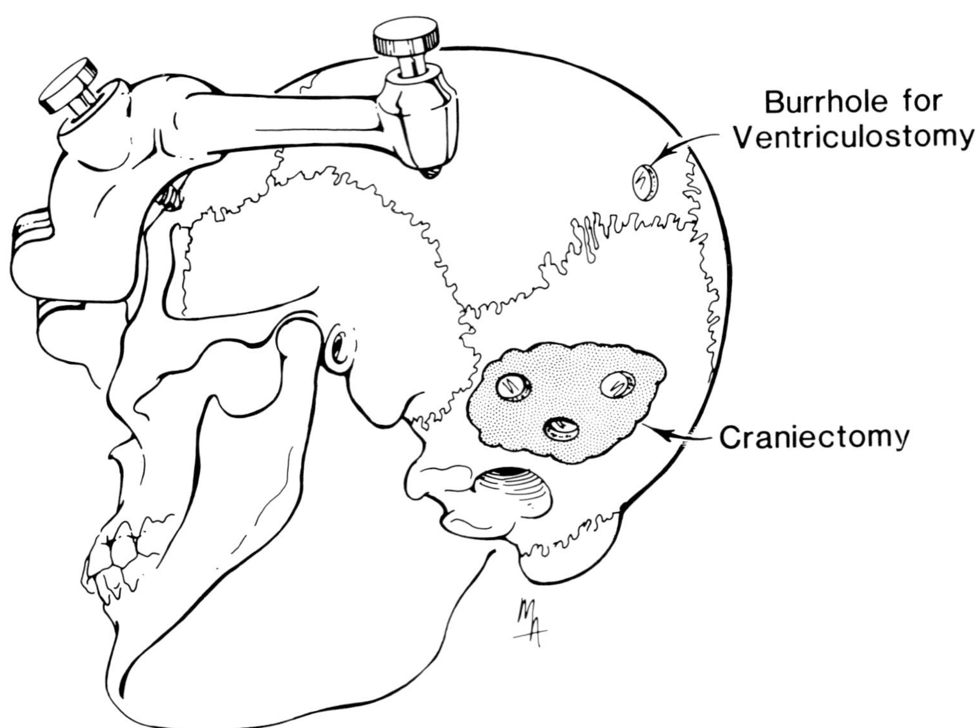

Fig. 49-3. Small meningiomas in the cerebellopontine angle are exposed by a unilateral craniectomy. The head is rotated toward the side of the lesion and the chin is flexed toward the ipsilateral shoulder.

ANESTHESIA

The general principles of anesthesia applicable for surgery on supratentorial meningiomas are even more critical when applied to posterior fossa surgery, where the implications of any complications are compounded. In addition, it is necessary to make adaptations imposed by the technical considerations and risks inherent with tumors of the posterior fossa.

Posterior fossa surgery for meningioma resection is performed under general anesthesia with nasotracheal intubation. There is an advantage to leaving the endotracheal tube in place several hours and preferably overnight following major posterior fossa procedures. Brain stem or cranial nerve dysfunction is heralded by respiratory distress and an inability to manage secretions. The cuffed nasotracheal tube is not removed until the patient is stable and alert with no evidence of posterior fossa swelling or hematoma. The patient is observed closely in the intensive care unit for several hours after the nasotracheal tube is removed. Patients tolerate a nasotracheal tube very well without undue coughing or straining, unlike an orotracheal tube, which is not tolerated once the patient is awake.

If the sitting position is used, a catheter is placed in the right atrium and the position of the catheter is confirmed by a chest roentgenogram and ECG. This permits the anesthesiologist to maintain the central venous pressure between 5 and 10 cm of water by blood, colloid, and crystalloid fluid replacement. The catheter also provides the means for aspirating air from the right atrium if air embolism occurs. A Doppler ultrasonic monitor, esophageal stethoscope, and ECG all facilitate the detection of an air embolism. If an air embolism occurs, the head is lowered quickly and the patient is rotated into the left lateral decubitus position. Air trapped in the right atrium is aspirated with the patient in this position. To lessen the risk of an air embolism in the sitting position, positive end-expiratory

pressure (PEEP) is applied to achieve an end-expiratory pressure of $+3$ to $+10$ cm of water. PEEP can be adjusted according to the degree of brain tightness and the tendency for venous bleeding.

The advantages of controlled respiration outweigh the single advantage of spontaneous respiration, namely, the ability to monitor spontaneous brainstem respiratory activity. The ECG should be monitored for extrasystoles and bradycardia during tumor manipulation in the posterior fossa. The ECG is a sensitive indicator of medullary dysfunction and it is not necessary to risk depending on spontaneous respirations for this purpose. Continuous CO_2 recording of expired air and blood gas analyses at regular intervals also is valuable for detecting respiratory and metabolic dysfunction, both during surgery and in the immediate postoperative period.

POSITION

The optimum position for posterior fossa surgery is still a controversial issue and is partly a matter of preference and experience. As the methodology has improved for controlling intracranial and cerebral venous pressure, providing better lighting and magnification and reducing blood loss through improved instrumentation, the prone and three-quarter prone positions have gained favor over the more traditional sitting position (Figure 49-2).

There are several disadvantages to having patients sit up for posterior fossa surgery. The positioning is time consuming and prolongs the time they will be anesthetized. The patient is vulnerable to sudden hypotension and cerebral ischemia. Air embolism is a constant threat. The surgeon is working with the arms elevated and tends to tire during a long procedure.

The disadvantage of the prone position is that blood, CSF,

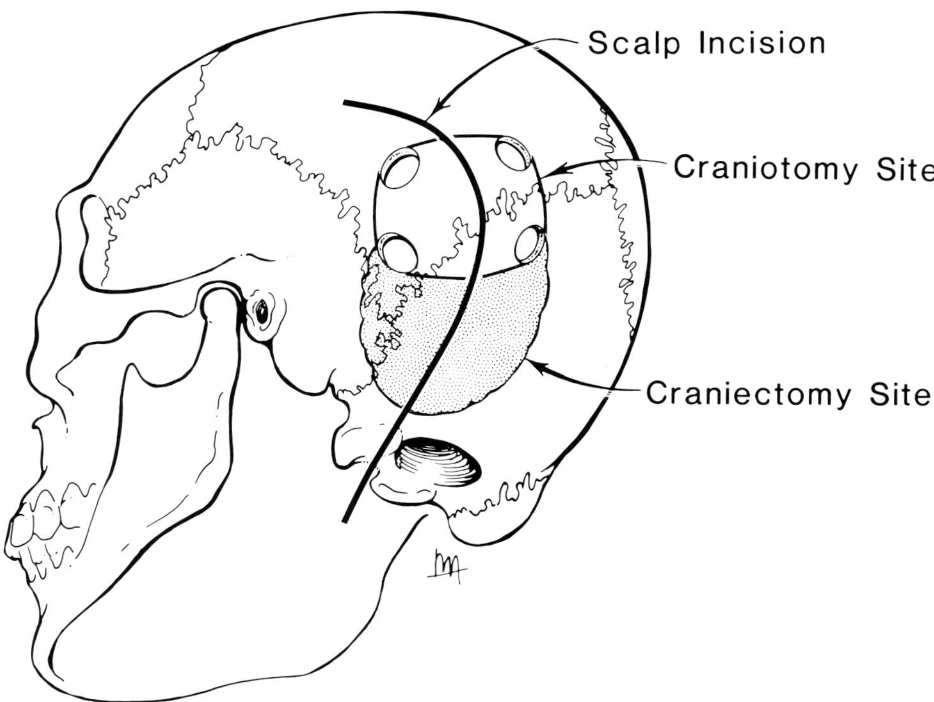

Fig. 49-4. A unilateral approach that combines a supratentorial craniotomy and an infratentorial craniectomy is used to expose large meningiomas of the posterior petrous ridge, the inferior surface of the tentorium cerebelli, or large CPA tumors extending upward through the incisura.

and irrigating fluid tend to collect in the wound and restrict vision, particularly under the operating microscope. When the patient is in the prone position, it is also important to keep pressure off the eyes and to prevent fluids from pooling about the face and eyes. This is especially important when a padded horseshoe headrest is used.

In either position, it is important to keep the patient's abdomen free and to avoid excessive flexion or rotation of the neck in order to prevent venous hypertension and poor pulmonary compliance. In the sitting position the legs and hips are flexed to avoid postoperative low-back pain and sciatica. The legs are raised and wrapped from the feet up to the thighs to prevent venous pooling in the lower extremities.

Three-point skeletal fixation generally is preferable in posterior fossa surgery whether the prone or sitting position is used. The head position is more secure. There is less risk of widespread skin irritation, necrosis, or burns from prolonged pressure on the face or from fluids collecting between the head holder and skin. The surface area of the scalp is not compromised by tape or padding. The head holder is always attached to the back of the frame of the operating table, rather than to the seat or foot of the table (Figure 49–2). The table can then be unflexed and the head quickly lowered without taking the patient's head out of the holder and contaminating the surgical field in the event of sudden vascular hypotension or air embolism.

OPERATIVE APPROACH AND TECHNIQUE

The surgical approach to meningiomas in the posterior fossa is determined primarily by the location of the tumor. Tumors in the region of the foramen magnum, the fourth ventricle, or the occipital squama overlying the posterior cere-

bellar hemisphere are approached by a midline suboccipital craniectomy. Usually the arch of the atlas and sometimes the lamina of the axis are also removed (Figure 49-1).

Small meningiomas in the cerebellopontine angle are exposed through a smaller, unilateral craniectomy (Figure 49-3). Large meningiomas in the CPA, tumors arising from the dura over the posterior petrous ridge, those growing downward from the tentorium cerebelli, or any of these tumors extending upward through the incisura often are best exposed by a unilateral combined supra) and infratentorial approach (Figure 49-4).

MENINGIOMAS OF THE TENTORIUM CEREBELLI AND POSTERIOR PETROUS RIDGE

Tentorial meningiomas present diagnostic and operative difficulties that have in previously reported series resulted in an operative mortality rate between 16 and 34 percent and a case mortality rate, partly due to recurrences, as high as 54 percent.[5] Castellano and Riggiero analyzed Olivecrona's patient material in 1953 and concluded that tentorial meningiomas are best removed from above whether they are on the superior or inferior surface of the tentorium.[5] Small tumors growing downward into the posterior fossa are approached by a subtemporal-occipital approach with tentorial splitting (Figure 49-5). Meningiomas with a large element in the posterior fossa or those involving the posterior petrous ridge are better approached by a combined supra) and infratentorial approach. This approach is also useful for large CPA tumors protruding through the incisura.

The patient is placed in a three-quarter prone position with the ipsilateral shoulder elevated to avoid unnecessary twisting of the neck and obstruction of venous return. The head is

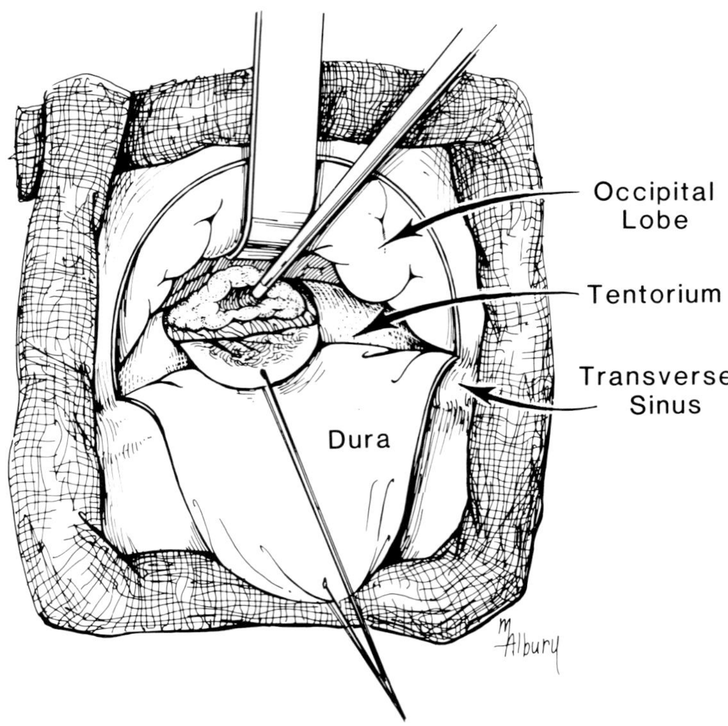

Fig. 49-5. Small tumors growing downward into the posterior fossa from the tentorium cerebelli are approached by a subtemporal-occipital approach with tentorial splitting.

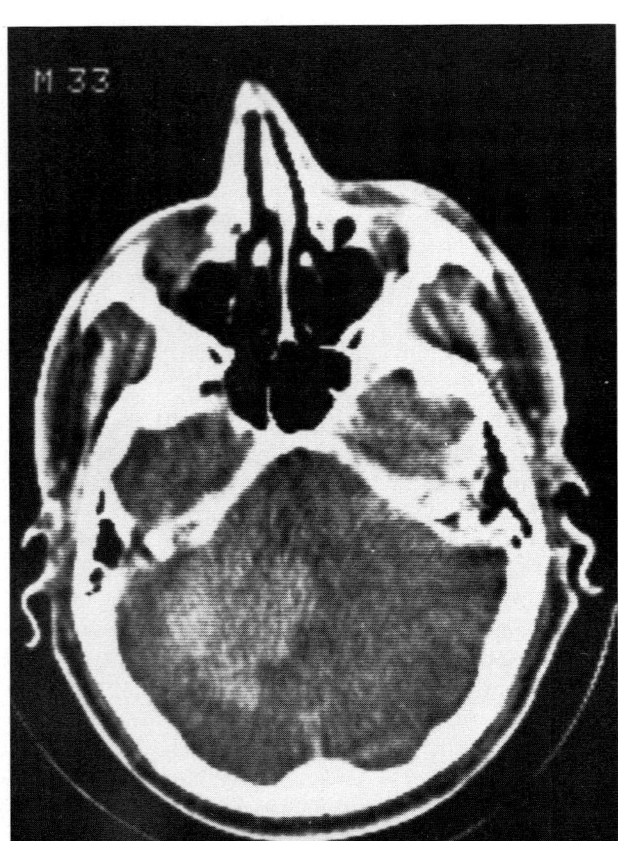

Fig. 49-6. This CT scan shows a large meningioma attached to the posterior surface of the left petrous ridge. This tumor was resected by a combined supra) and infratentorial approach.

slightly flexed and canted toward the opposite shoulder. The ipsilateral shoulder is pulled downward to provide better access to the suboccipital region, being careful to pad the shoulder and avoid compression of the cervical or brachial plexus.

A slightly curved or hockey stick-shaped incision is started 6 cm above the ear and is extended in a posteromedial direction, passing midway between the inion and the mastoid process. The neck in the suboccipital region is prepared and draped so the incision can be extended as far as necessary to expose large tumors displacing the ipsilateral cerebellar hemisphere. The incision is carried down to the skull so subperiosteal dissection with periosteal elevators and the scalpel permits adequate exposure.

After self-retaining retractors are inserted to maintain exposure, burr holes are placed in the temporal squama above the lateral sinus and in the posterior fossa below the lateral sinus and medial to the mastoid air cells. A small temporo-occipital free bone flap is elevated. If there is strong evidence of extensive posterior fossa involvement by the tumor, it is probably best to proceed immediately with a unilateral suboccipital craniectomy below and across the lateral sinus before opening the dura (Figure 49-4); thus the posterior temporal and occipital lobes of the brain are protected by dura while bone is being rongeured.

The dura mater is opened over the occipital lobe with the base of the dural flap at the lateral sinus. This promotes dural drainage and lessens the risk of tearing bridging cortical veins passing toward the sinus before they are well exposed. The occipital lobe is gently retracted to expose the superior surface of the tentorium. Occipital bridging veins can be coagulated electively under direct vision at this time, but care should be taken to cut the veins well away from the dura and lateral sinus.

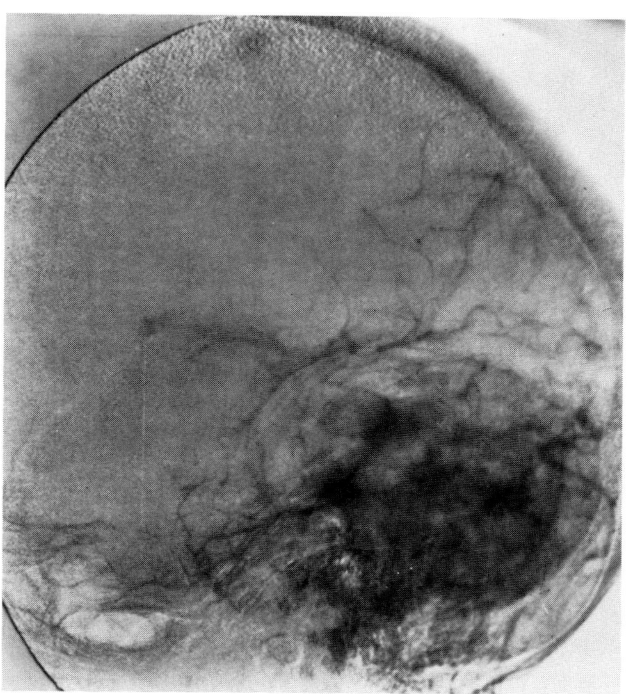

Fig. 49-7. An angiogram showing a very vascular tumor arising from the posterior petrous ridge, which proved to be a hemangiopericytic type of angioblastic meningioma.

The superior surface of the tentorium is inspected for tumor and the incisura is inspected for tumor growing upward along the brainstem.

The tentorium is elevated with a sharp hook and incised posteriorly but well away from tumor attachment and the lateral sinus. The incision is carried toward the incisura, care being taken to identify and preserve the trochlear nerve adjacent to the tentorial edge. Where possible, bipolar coagulation is used to control bleeding from the cut edge of the tentorium rather than metallic clips. Metallic clips may cause refractive distortion of the CT scan later and hinder follow-up examinations for tumor recurrence.

Opening the tentorium back to the transverse sinus exposes the region of the CPA from above, provided the tumor is not large. Although some tumors arise primarily from the underside of the tentorium, many tumors in this region arise from the posterior surface of the petrous ridge. These often grow to be large and may be quite vascular with angioblastic features of the hemangiopericytic type (Figures 49-6 and 49-7). It is best in this situation to elevate and incise the dura mater below the lateral sinus. Usually a thin rim of cerebellum is stretched over the tumor. It is preferable to excise this rim of nonfunctional tissue rather than retract and undermine it, which leaves devascularized, necrotic, swollen tissue behind.

If the tumor is huge and vascular, as meningiomas in this area are wont to be, a very useful technique is to temporarily cross-clamp the ipsilateral transverse sinus and observe the brain and cortical veins for 5 minutes. If there is no swelling of the brain or venous engorgement, the transverse sinus can be safely ligated and divided, since sufficient collateral venous drainage is available. This maneuver improves the exposure and obviates the need to work on the tumor resection alternately from above and below the lateral sinus (Figure 49-8).

The large, firm, vascular tumor arising from the posterior surface of the petrous ridge is technically challenging. Extracapsular dissection before enucleation of the tumor for the purpose of interrupting feeding vessels and devascularizing the tumor is precluded by the sensitivity of the brain stem and cranial nerves to compression or traction during tumor manipulation. Intracapsular debulking of the tumor is tedious if the tumor does not aspirate well. Troublesome bleeding is encountered when the cautery wire loop is used on very vascular tumors. Heat spread to the brain stem and cranial nerves also is a concern. The ultrasonic aspirator, the CO_2 laser, or both will perhaps expedite this phase of the procedure.

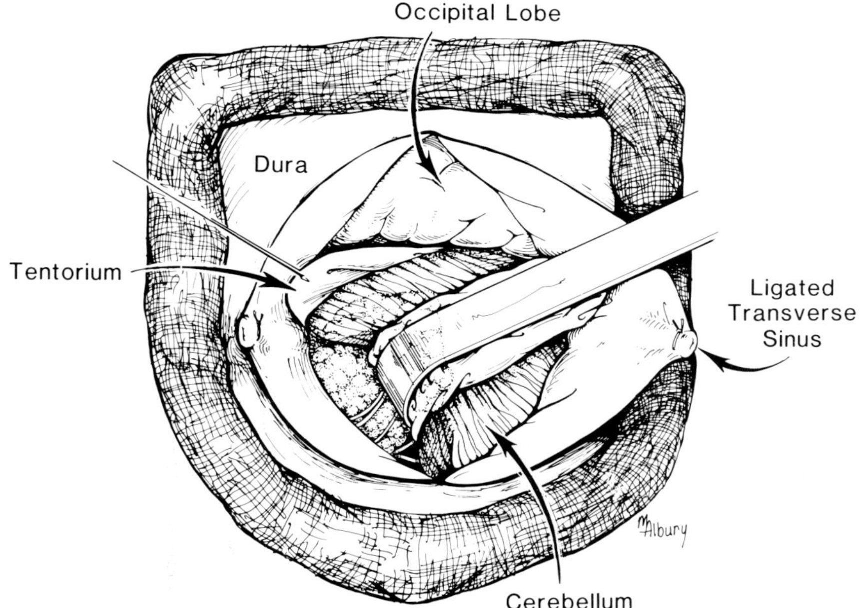

Fig. 49-8. The dura mater is opened above and below the transverse sinus, which was ligated and divided after cross-clamping for 5 minutes produced no swelling of the brain or venous engorgement. The tentorium cerebelli is divided to the incisura. A large meningioma arising from the posterior petrous ridge is exposed.

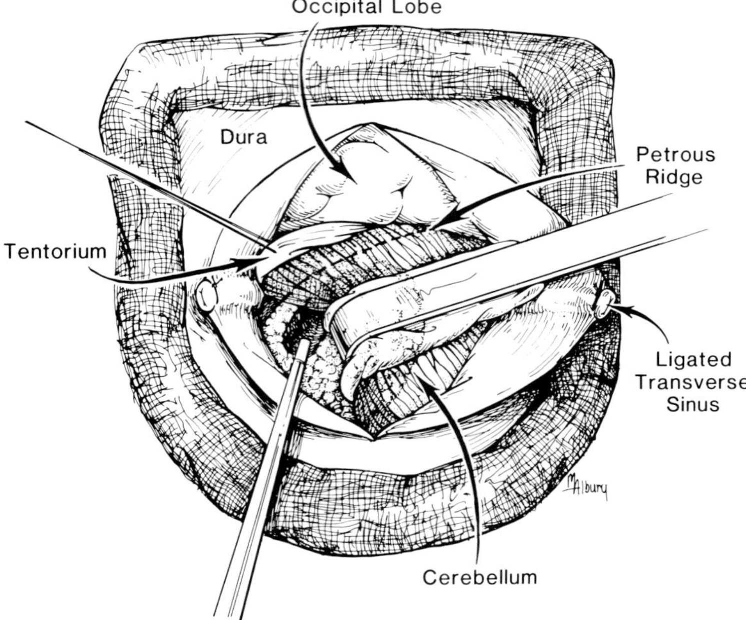

Fig. 49-9. A large, firm, vascular posterior petrous ridge meningioma is resected by first furrowing parallel to the ridge. The attachment to the dura and large feeding vessels from the middle meningeal artery can be coagulated. The remaining tumor is then debulked with less bleeding and the thinned capsule adjacent to the brain stem is excised.

An alternative approach to debulking the entire tumor is to furrow quickly across the interior of the tumor near the pole attached to the petrous ridge (Figure 49-9). Avitene followed by light pressure with dry cotton pledgets is applied to stem brisk bleeding. This allows selective invagination of the capsule wall along the petrous ridge and coagulation and interruption of the main feeding vessels from the middle meningeal and ascending pharyngeal arteries through the dura at this site. Once this detachment is accomplished, the tumor is less vascular and can be widely debulked much more quickly with far less bleeding. The capsule is never placed under forceful traction. Extracapsular dissection is performed with magnification and microinstrumentation in order to spare the cranial nerves, important blood vessels such as the perforating arteries to the brain stem coming off the basilar artery, and the brain stem tissue itself.

On occasion, a huge, vascular posterior fossa meningioma is encountered arising from the posterior petrous ridge, extending up along the clivus in front of the brainstem, and through the incisura alongside the brainstem. If the debulking is tedious, blood loss substantial, and brainstem function precarious as heralded by transient bradycardia and extrasystoles, consideration is given to performing the procedure in stages. The dura is left open, the bone flap is freeze-preserved and stored in a saline-antibiotic solution, and the scalp is meticulously closed by carefully approximating the galea and dermis. Within 10 to 14 days the second stage is carried out and the tumor excised much more expeditiously. During the interim, the partially devascularized tumor tends to herniate into the site of the decompressed craniotomy (-ectomy) and away from the brain stem, clivus, and incisura. Further debulking is accompanied by less blood loss and the tumor capsule is more easily dissected off the brain stem without evidence of medullary dysfunction.

Following tumor removal, CSF flows freely through the tentorial incisura, and the cranial nerves and carotid artery are well visualized. The surgeon often realizes or suspects that some tumor cells are left in the dura and bone of the petrous ridge. Postoperative irradiation is especially recommended if the tumor is the hemangiopericytic type of angioblastic meningioma.

After meticulous hemostasis is achieved, a "watertight" dural closure is attempted and attention is given to obliterating any exposed mastoid air cells with bone wax or muscle. This may prevent the occurrence of a CSF fistula in the immediate postoperative period before a dural neomembrane has a chance to form. The freeze-preserved bone flap is sutured in place and the scalp is closed as previously described.

CEREBELLOPONTINE ANGLE MENINGIOMAS

Meningiomas in the cerebellopontine angle can be approached through a paramedian incision and suboccipital craniectomy if the tumor is relatively small and confined to the posterior fossa (see Figure 49-3). The face is turned 45 degrees toward the side of the tumor and the neck is flexed. The head is held in three-point skeletal fixation. A separate paramedian incision is made 7 cm above and 3 cm lateral to the inion and a burr hole is placed for ventriculostomy in case CSF decompression is necessary either during or after surgery. The foot plate for the self-retaining retractor can be inserted at this site and is well out of the main operative field.

Subperiosteal dissection is performed and one or more burr holes are placed in the occipital squama. The craniectomy is enlarged using instruments such as the Leksell double-action rongeur and the large Kerrison bone punches. The limits of the exposure, at least initially, are the transverse sinus superiorly, the mastoid air cell laterally, and the foramen magnum inferiorly. Sufficient bone is removed medially to obtain good visualization of the tumor.

The dura mater is opened in a triradiate (Y) fashion and dural retention sutures applied (Figure 49-10). The cerebellum

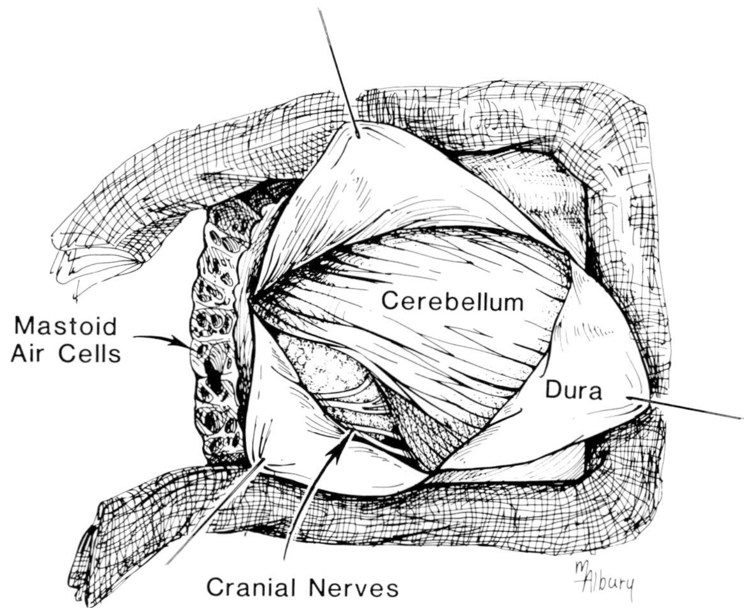

Fig. 49-10. A unilateral posterior fossa craniectomy is enlarged until the mastoid air cells are seen. The dura is opened in a triradiate (Y) fashion and dural retention sutures applied. The CPA meningioma is seen displacing the lower cranial nerves.

is gently retracted to expose the tumor, and a self-retaining retractor with the blade placed on cottonoid padding maintains exposure with minimal tissue trauma. The operating microscope and microinstrumentation are important adjuncts for dissecting the capsule away from cranial nerves, vessels, and the brain stem. An en plaque meningioma may be unresectable and surgery limited to tissue biopsy. A globoid tumor may be multilobulated, but usually it has a limited area of dural attachment and is accessible for operative excision.

After the lower cranial nerves are identified and carefully dissected off the capsule wall, they are protected with moist cottonoid strips. The tumor capsule is incised and the intracapsular debulking of the tumor is carried out using the techniques for tissue removal and hemostasis discussed for meningiomas in other locations. When only a thin, pliable capsule remains, the capsular wall is carefully involuted while contiguous structures are dissected off the capsule.

Cerebellopontine angle meningiomas have a propensity to extend further up the clivus toward the dorsum sellae than do acoustic neurinomas. They also are multilobulated, and important structures such as the anteroinferior cerebellar artery (AICA) and the facial nerve may be bound within the interstices of these lobules and surrounded by tumor, although technically still extracapsular. The seventh nerve may be displaced in almost any direction, or completely concealed by the tumor. The nerve may be displaced anteriorly by the capsular wall, but this is far more variable than with acoustic neurinomas. Even with the aid of electrical nerve stimulation it may not be possible to identify and save the nerve and still accomplish complete tumor removal. Seventh nerve palsy is an even more profound problem if the trigeminal nerve root or descending tract also is compromised by tumor or damaged during surgery. Tarsorrhaphy is then necessary to prevent corneal exposure keratitis, ulceration, and possible loss of ipsilateral vision. The corneal reflex and the ability to close the eye and blink should

be checked as soon as the patient is awake in the recovery room. An eye ointment, artificial tears, and an eye patch may be indicated in the immediate postoperative period. If the lower cranial nerves are damaged and the gag reflex and ability to handle secretions are lost, a feeding gastrostomy and tracheostomy may prove necessary until function improves.

The surgeon's technical judgment is sorely taxed by large meningiomas in this region. It is important for the patient and the patient's family to realize in advance the problems the surgeon may confront. Their understanding and philosophy regarding total or subtotal excision and possible functional loss complement the surgeon's judgment based on the patient's age and condition and the surgeon's previous experience with similar tumors.

Once the fifth nerve root and seventh nerve are successfully identified, it is usually possible to dissect them off the capsule. The tumor is gently delivered from above into the space created by the intracapsular debulking of tissue. Arterial feeders from the AICA, the internal carotid artery, and the ascending pharyngeal artery are visualized, coagulated with the bipolar cautery, and divided. Bridging veins passing from the tumor to the superior petrosal sinus are similarly coagulated and are divided close to the tumor, rather than the sinus.

Tumor attached to the brain stem or involving the basilar artery, its perforating branches, or the AICA is better left behind. The AICA can loop out to the region of the porus acusticus, give off an internal auditory branch, then return to supply the brain stem (Figure 49-11). It is important to spare this vessel even when it appears to be well away from the brain stem in the vicinity of the porus acusticus.

Hemostasis is readily achieved if the tumor is totally removed. Otherwise, oozing tumor tissue remains. This bleeding is stopped with light bipolar coagulation and saline irrigation. Avitene, Surgicel, or Gelfoam are applied directly to the oozing surface if necessary.

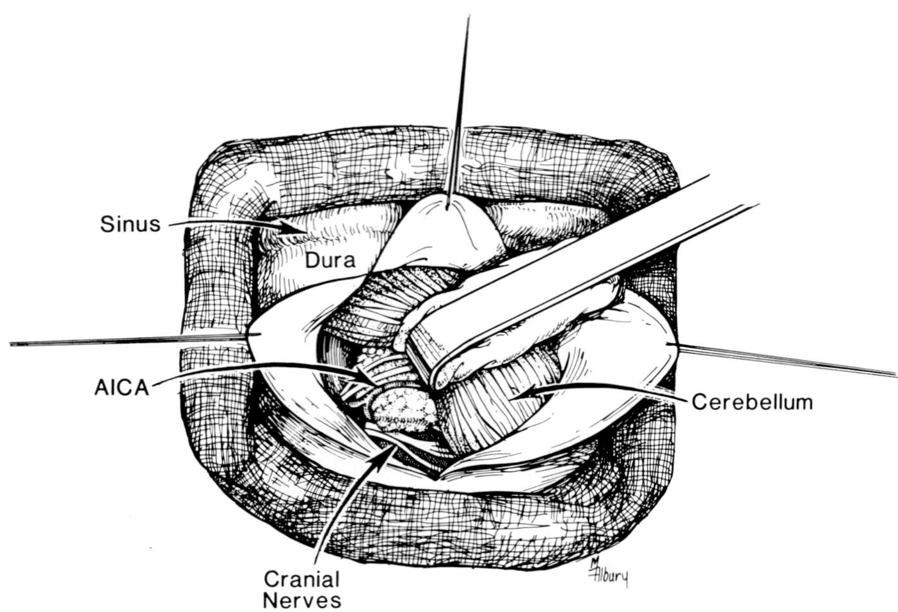

Fig. 49-11.   The meningioma capsule is exposed and the AICA is seen giving off an internal auditory branch before looping back to supply the brain stem. It is better in this situation to leave a small amount of tumor attached to the artery than to risk sacrificing the AICA.

FORAMEN MAGNUM MENINGIOMAS

Foramen magnum meningiomas usually are removed through the posterior approach by suboccipital craniectomy and upper cervical laminectomy (see Figure 49-1). This limited posterior exposure is not adequate for large tumors extending along the clivus. These tumors are exposed by an incision starting above the helix of the external ear, then angling across the occipital squama and down the posterior midline of the neck. This then combines the exposure outlined for posterior petrous ridge and cerebellopontine angle meningiomas with the approach for small tumors limited to the region of the foramen magnum. An anterior, transoral approach has also been reported for exposing and resecting clival meningiomas.[31]

Ascertaining the location, size, and probable site of dural attachment of the tumor is important in planning the operative approach. The majority of foramen magnum meningiomas are located ventrolateral to the upper cervical cord. Kempe stated that the anterior rim of the foramen magnum is the second-most frequent site of origin for meningiomas in the posterior fossa.[32] Tumors arising along the rim of the foramen magnum also tend to be attached to the vertebral artery where it enters the cranial cavity. The magnification and lighting provided by the operating microscope are important for exposing these anatomic relationships and safely excising the tumor.

With the patient seated, legs flexed and elevated, and vulnerable areas padded, the neck is flexed and the head stabilized by three-point skeletal fixation. Hyperflexion of the neck is contraindicated. This is checked by placing three fingers between the patient's chin and sternum before tightening the headrest. A posterior midline incision is used extending from above the inion to the level of the spinous process of C5. The head and neck are draped so this incision can be extended if necessary to improve exposure. A separate vertical incision is made and an occipital burr hole is placed 7 cm above the inion and 3 cm lateral to the midline in case intraoperative or postoperative ventriculostomy for CSF decompression is required (see Figure 49-1).

A subperiosteal dissection is carried out bilaterally over the occipital squama and an Adson self-retaining retractor inserted. The spinous processes and lamina of at least the upper three cervical vertebrae are exposed by sharp dissection. Care should be taken to avoid injuring the vertebral arteries where they pass over the posterior arch of the atlas in the lateral recess. Emissary veins opened during subperiosteal dissection should be waxed immediately. The condyloid veins in the vicinity of the foramen magnum may require bipolar coagulation if troublesome bleeding occurs.

Burr holes are drilled bilaterally in the occipital squama, being careful to stay well off the midline so a persistent occipital sinus is not perforated. The burr holes are placed well below the nuchal line and transverse sinus. The craniectomy is then enlarged by connecting the burr holes with double-action rongeurs (Leksell) and bone punches (Kerrison). The dura is carefully stripped away from the inner table of the skull with a dural separator. The craniectomy is enlarged until the edge of the transverse sinus is seen and the posterior rim of the foramen magnum is removed. Initially, the craniectomy may not have to be enlarged so far laterally that the mastoid air cells are opened. Once entered, the mastoid air cells are sealed with bone wax. The posterior arch of the atlas is removed and if there is preoperative evidence of pronounced tonsillar herniation or a significant intraspinal component to the tumor, the lamina and spinous process of C2 are also removed at this time.

Should the Doppler, ECG, or vital signs suggest air embolism, PEEP is increased, the wound is filled with saline and covered with saline-soaked cotton sponges, and the patient immediately lowered into the left lateral decubitus position. Air is aspirated through the catheter that was placed preoperatively in the right atrium. Meticulous attention to venous hemostasis with prompt bone waxing of open emissary veins will lessen the risk of this complication, but veins and sinuses may be open without bleeding in spite of PEEP.

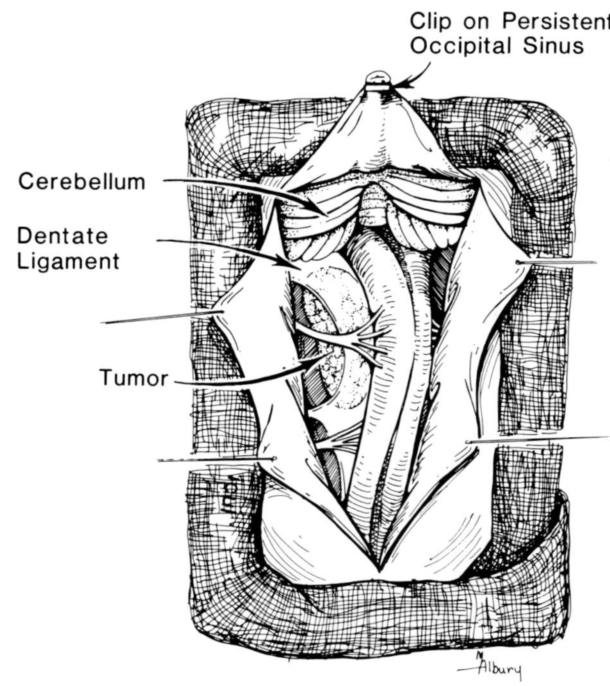

Fig. 49-12. The dura mater is opened by a Y incision and a persistent occipital sinus is clipped. The foramen magnum meningioma is more on the left side ventrolateral to the spinomedullary junction. The dorsal root of C2 is stretched over the tumor and will have to be sectioned. The upper dentate ligament serves as a landmark to where the displaced vertebral artery enters the intrathecal space.

If elevated intracranial pressure and hydrocephalus are apparent before surgery, a ventriculostomy usually is performed preoperatively as described previously (see section on ventricular drainage for obstructive hydrocephalus). The dura mater is always inspected and gently palpated, however, before it is opened widely in the posterior fossa or upper cervical spinal canal. If the dura is unexpectedly tight or not pulsating, it is necessary to pass a cannula into the atrium of the right lateral ventricle through the occipital burr hole that was drilled earlier in the procedure for this purpose. Sudden intraventricular decompression is avoided, however, lest subdural or intraventricular bleeding result.

The dura mater is opened with a Y-shaped incision. The cephalad leaf of dura is reflected cephalad and tacked up with dural sutures over a strip of cottonoid or Gelfoam to protect the transverse sinus. The inferior tail of the Y incision extends below the level of the C1 arch and is tacked laterally with dural sutures over cottonoid strips or Gelfoam pledgets. A persistent occipital sinus may be encountered at the junction of the Y limbs (Figure 49-12). Bleeding from the sinus is controlled with metallic surgical clips or bipolar coagulation. The dura is kept moist throughout the procedure and only bipolar coagulation is used on the dura. This reduces shrinkage and permits a tight dural closure without necessitating a dural substitute graft.

Foramen magnum meningiomas are most often ventrolateral to the spinomedullary junction and attached along the anterior rim of the foramen. The upper cervical spinal cord is displaced dorsally and is rotated away from the side on which the main tumor mass is located. The dorsal root of C2 may be stretched over the posterior surface of the tumor (Figure 49-12). It may be necessary to section this nerve root and accept some

ipsilateral scalp numbness. To the extent possible, it is important to ascertain the relationship of the tumor to the vertebral artery before surgery and at this stage of the operative exposure. If the artery is not seen, a helpful landmark is the highest dentate ligament that normally marks the level where the vertebral artery enters the intrathecal space. The dentate ligament is sectioned where it is stretched over the tumor capsule (Figure 49-12). The spinal accessory nerve is identified, preserved, and protected with cottonoid strips. It may be necessary to dissect the nerve off the tumor capsule. Before the tumor capsule is opened for internal debulking, the tumor is isolated from the intrathecal space with cottonoid strips in order to lessen the incidence and degree of postoperative aseptic meningitis associated with subarachnoid blood. The tumor then is enucleated using the techniques discussed previously.

As the capsule is collapsed inward, adhesions to the pia arachnoid over the cerebellum, spinal cord, and medulla are dissected using microinstrumentation and bipolar coagulation. The capsule is dissected off the vertebral artery if this is feasible. The site of dural attachment is cauterized with bipolar coagulation if the dura cannot be readily excised in this area.

After hemostasis is obtained, the cottonoid strips protecting the spinomedullary junction, spinal accessory nerve, and subarachnoid space are removed. A watertight closure of the dura mater is desirable to prevent an occipital pseudomeningocele. If necessary a dural graft is used to achieve a tight closure. Meticulous hemostasis and a multilayered muscle closure with interrupted, nonabsorbable sutures lessens the possibility that a postoperative serosa will form and cause a complication to result from the wound. Inverted, interrupted absorbable sutures are used subcutaneously and the skin is closed with an interrupted, nonabsorbable suture.

As with other posterior fossa procedures, it is wise to keep the nasotracheal tube in place until the patient's respiration is strong and spontaneous, his or her vital signs and blood gases are stable, and the patient's alertness indicates that an uncomplicated extubation can be done.

REFERENCES

1. Cushing H, Eisenhardt L: Meningiomas. Their Classification, Regional Behavior, Life History and Surgical End Results. Springfield, Ill, Charles C Thomas, 138, p 785

2. Morley LP: Tumors of the cranial meninges, in Youmans JR (ed): Neurological Surgery, vol 3, Philadelphia, WB Saunders, 1973, pp 1389–1411

3. Castellano F, Ruggiero G: Meningiomas of the posterior fossa. Acta Radiol (Suppl) 104:1, 1953

4. Laird F, Harner S, Laws E Jr, et al: Meningiomas of the cerebellopontine angle: Otolaryngol Head Neck Surg 93:161, 1985

5. Katinsky SE, Toglis JV: Audiologic and vestibular manifestations of meningiomas of the cerebellopontine angle. J Speech Hear Disord 33:351, 1968

6. Frowein RA: Meningiomas of the tentorium. Acta Neurochir 31:283, 1975

7. Barrows HS, Harter DH: Tentorial meningiomas. J Neurol Neurosurg Psychiatry 25:40, 1962

8. Yasuoka S, Okazaki H, Daube J, et al: Foramen magnum tumors: Analysis of 57 cases of benign extramedullary tumors. J Neurosurg 49:828, 1978

9. Dodge HW Jr, Love JG, Gottlieb CM: Benign tumors of the foramen magnum. Surgical considerations. J Neurosurg 13:603, 1956

10. Howe JR, Taren JA: Foramen magnum tumors. Pitfall in diagnosis. JAMA 225:1061, 1973

11. Krayenbuhl H: Special clinical features of tumors of the foramen magnum. Schweiz Arch Neurol Neurochir Psychiatr 112:205, 1973

12. Symonds CP, Meadows SP: Compression of the spinal cord in the neighborhood of the foramen magnum. Brain 60:52, 1937

13. Elsberg CA, Strauss I: Tumors of the spinal cord which project into the posterior cranial fossa-report of a case in which a growth was removed from the ventral and lateral aspects of the medulla oblongata and upper cervical cord. Arch Neurol Psychiatr 21:261, 1929

14. Boshes B, Padberg F: Studies on the cervical spinal cord of man. Sensory pattern after interruption of the posterior columns. Neurology 3:90, 1953

15. Rubenstein JE: Astereognosis associated with tumors in the region of the foramen magnum. Arch Neurol Psychiatr 39:1016, 1938

16. Moller A, Hatam A, Olivecrona H: The differential diagnosis of pontine angle meningioma and acoustic neuroma with computed topography. Neuroradiology 17:21, 1978

17. Valavanis A, Schubiger O, Hayik J, et al: CT of meningiomas on the posterior surface of the petrous bone. Neuroradiology 22:111, 1981

18. Mikhael MA, Ciric IS, Wolff AP: Differentiation of cerebellopontine angle neuromas and meningiomas with MR imaging. J Comput Assist Tomogr 9:852, 1985

19. Meyer FB, Ebersold MJ, Reese DF: Benign tumors of the foramen magnum. J Neurosurg 61:136, 1984

20. Salamon GM, Combalbert A, Raybaud C, et al: An angiographic study of meningiomas of the posterior fossa. J Neurosurg 35:731, 1971

21. Nadjmi M, Ratzka M, Moissi G: Angiographic aspects of meningiomas in the posterior fossa. Acta Neurochir 31:289, 1974

22. Berkmen YM: Angiographic demonstration of blood supply to the tentorium: Case report and review of the literature. J Neurosurg 25:90, 1966

23. Papo I, Salvolini V: Meningiomas of the free margin of the tentorium developing in the pineal region. Neuroradiology 7:237, 1974

24. Schechter MM, Zingesser LH, Rosenbaum A: Tentorial meningiomas. AJR 104:123, 1968

25. Bernasconi V, Cassinari V: Un segno carotidografico zipico di meningioma del tentorio. Chirurgia 11:586, 1956

26. Bakes HL Jr: Myelographic examination of the posterior fossa with positive contrast medium. Radiology 81:791, 1963

27. Malis LI: The myelographic examination of the foramen magnum. Radiology 70:196, 1958

28. Margolis MI: A simple myelographic maneuver for the detection of mass lesions at the foramen magnum. Radiology 119:482, 1976

29. Brookler KH, Hoffman RA, Camin M, et al: Trilobed meningioma: Ampulla of posterior semicircular canal, internal auditory canal and cerebellopontine angle. Am J Otol 1:171, 1980

30. Knupling R, Fuchs E: Meningiomas of the posterior fossa-disturbances in CSF circulation and brain stem function. Acta Neurochir 31:284, 1974

31. Mullan S, Naunton R, Hekmatpanah J, et al: The use of an anterior approach to ventrally placed tumors in the foramen magnum and vertebral column. J Neurosurg 24:536, 1966

32. Kempe LG: Posterior fossa, spinal cord and peripheral nerve disease; in Operative Neurosurgery, vol 2. New York, Springer Verlag, 1970, p 269

CHAPTER 50

Surgical Management of Lateral Intraventricular Tumors

Dennis D. Spencer   William Collins   Kimberlee J. Sass

TUMORS OF THE LATERAL VENTRICLES of the cerebral hemisphere are frequently benign or of low malignancy; thus, their removal often results in cure or a long period of palliation. Effective therapeutic intervention, however, is often difficult. The tumors are typically large and, because they have grown slowly within the ventricles, symptoms and signs are usually secondary to mass effect or ventriculomegaly. A low rate of replication and benign morphology leave them resistant to most forms of therapy other than surgical excision. Constituting less than 1 percent of all intracranial tumors, they are relatively rare and are outside the usual experience of most neurosurgeons. Problems that are unique to the excision of intraventricular tumors and that require modification of typical approaches for removal of hemispheric masses are not obvious. To illuminate the unique problems in removal of intraventricular tumors, we have evaluated our own experience and related it to relevant literature.

Although tumor location and patient variables will dictate which of the various surgical approaches to use, all approaches share several features. Functional areas should be identified and avoided if possible. Early visualization of feeding arteries by piecemeal removal of tumor, even at the expense of some blood loss, is important, particularly when evidence of unusual vascularity is present. Control of the main blood supply of the tumor is established as early as possible. The border of the tumor is visualized by tumor removal rather than by brain retraction to prevent retraction damage in the white matter, which may be partially demyelinated by chronic pressure. The use of a solute diuretic may aid exposure and stiffen the white matter, but does not allow retraction of the periventricular region for rapid en bloc removal of the tumor without unacceptable neurologic loss. Hemispheric retraction should be minimal and retractors released at 15- to 20-minute intervals. Under certain conditions, the intraoperative release of cerebrospinal fluid (CSF) by ventricular tap is helpful to increase the exposure utilizing an enlarged portion of the ventricle.

These techniques can result in blood loss and the anesthesiologist must be aware of this possibility, preparing for rapid blood replacement and using hypotension to control bleeding. Deep anesthesia and mild hypothermia can be helpful in protecting the brain against hypoperfusion during removal of the tumor. Preoperative steroids and the use of osmotic diuretics are helpful in controlling edema, protecting against ischemia, and gaining exposure.

The position, type, vascularity, and blood supply of the tumor, in addition to the function of adjacent nervous system tissue, are factors that must be considered when planning a surgical approach. Preoperative studies should include computed axial tomography (CT scanning) with sagittal and coronal reconstructions and direct coronal cuts, magnetic resonance imaging, and magnified subtraction angiography of the anterior and posterior circulation.[1] The identification of a trapped portion of one lateral ventricle or of the entire opposite lateral ventricle is easily determined by CT scanning. Preoperative neurologic findings, such as a homonymous hemianopsia, may make a parietal incision or occipital lobectomy exposure more acceptable. When confronting extremely large tumors, the loss of an occipital lobe or some optic radiations may constitute an acceptable neurologic loss in exchange for the function of the remaining hemisphere. However, when the hemianopsia originates in the dominant hemisphere, a transcallosal approach through the splenium is contraindicated. This would isolate the intact visual cortex in the nondominant hemisphere from the language areas of the dominant hemisphere. Similarly, a callosotomy is contraindicated in patients whose preoperative evaluation (which includes intracarotid amytal studies if patients are left-hand dominant or have a history of significant early onset left hemisphere trauma or disease) documents opposite hemisphere control of speech and the dominant hand. Most important, the surgeon should not feel confined to a single approach in treating these tumors.

In the sections that follow, the surgical approaches will be described separately for tumors at the trigone, body, frontal horn, and temporal horn, because each presents a unique surgical problem.

TUMORS IN THE TRIGONAL REGION

The trigonal region is the most common site of origin for lateral ventricular tumors. The frequency of intraventricular meningiomas in this location is striking. In Ladenheim's review of 100 intraventricular meningiomas, 68 were found in the trigone.[2] A predisposition for this region may be accounted for by the abundance of choroid plexus arachnoidea in the glomus from which arise choroid plexus papillomas and meningiomas. All other types of intraventricular tumors, including ependymomas, subependymomas, astrocytomas, angiomas, and epidermoid tumors, can also originate here.[3,4,5] Hydrocephalus is a common concomitant to these tumors. This may range from

OPERATIVE NEUROSURGICAL TECHNIQUES
ISBN 0-8089-1862-1

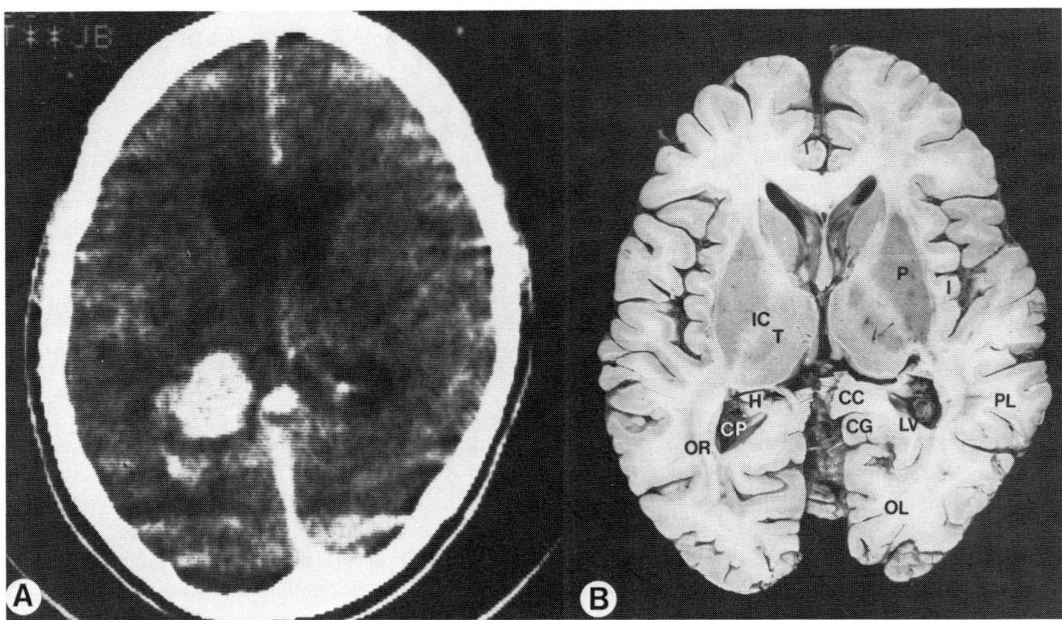

Fig. 50-1.   (A) A CT scan showing a tumor of the trigonal region. (B) Horizontal slice of a human brain at the level shown in A. Note the surrounding structures, especially the visual projections, thalamus, and corpus callosum. P = putamen; I = insula; IC = posterior limb of the internal capsule; T = thalamus; CC = splenum of the corpus callosum; H = hippocampal fimbria; CP = choroid plexus; OR = optic radiations; CG = cingulate gyrus; OL = occipital lobe; PL = parietal lobe.

a trapped temporal horn to ventriculomegaly associated with CSF overproduction produced by a choroid plexus papilloma.[6]

ANATOMY

Figure 50-1A depicts a CT scan of a tumor of the trigonal region. Figure 50-1B shows a cadaver brain sliced at the same angle, which is presented to identify the important anatomic structures adjacent to a trigonal tumor. Since many of the tumors in this region arise from the choroid plexus or its arachnoid, the base may be broad and adherent to the limbic projections, the tail of the caudate nucleus, visual projection fibers, and/or the pulvinar of the thalamus. When these tumors are vascular (e.g., meningiomas), they often are supplied by both the anterior and posterior choroidal arteries,[711] with displacement, tortuosity, and enlargement of these vessels on carotid and vertebral angiograms.

COMMON SURGICAL APPROACHES

Several surgical approaches to the trigone have been designed. These are portrayed schematically in Figure 50-2. None is completely satisfactory for circumventing all potential operative problems, such as adequate visualization of the tumor and early obliteration of feeding vessels, without unacceptable neurologic loss. However, each of the approaches has been advocated as a satisfactory compromise. The ability of each approach to obtain adequate visualization of the tumor and to avoid neurologic deficit is addressed in the following paragraphs.

Lateral Temporal Parietal Lobe Incision

Contrasted with other approaches, lateral temporal parietal cortical incision (Figure 50-2, LTP) transgresses less brain from the cortical surface to the tumor. This single advantage, however, is often outweighed by the frequent postoperative loss of neurologic function. Damage to the angular gyrus of the domi-

nant hemisphere may produce dyslexia,[12,13] agraphia,[14] acalculia,[15] or ideomotor apraxia[16] or combinations of all the above. Gerstmann's syndrome is generally believed to result from lesions in this area.[17,14] Damage to the submarginal gyrus has been associated with conduction difficulties (when the arcuate fasciculus is involved), agraphia,[14] and apraxia.[16] Cortical stimulation studies suggest that lesions to this area in the nondominant hemisphere may impair memory for visual information.[13] Lesion studies also identify neglect,[19] construction deficits,[20] and receptive aprosodia (i.e., the inability to discriminate enhanced inflection)[21] as potential deficits from surgery involving the nondominant temporal-parietal area. A homonymous field deficit is almost assured, since the visual projection fibers, which parallel the lateral aspect of the ventricle, must be transected. Highly vascular masses are particularly difficult to remove by this approach since they require both manipulation of the tumor and brain to visualize important vessels, and piecemeal resection before control of the feeding blood vessels can be obtained. This almost always results in blood loss.

Middle Temporal Gyrus Incision

The middle temporal gyrus approach (Figure 50-2, MTG) again brings the surgeon close to the tumor, but for trigonal tumors it also risks significant neurologic deficits. Language functioning may be compromised by lesions to the middle temporal gyrus of the dominant hemisphere. Cortical stimulation techniques indicate that capabilities for phoneme identification (i.e., Wernicke's area), reading, and naming are often impaired by lesions in this area.[13,22] This is consistent with clinical studies that show this area to be involved in anomic aphasia.[23] Geffen et al.[24] reported such a result following excision of a meningioma of the left lateral ventricle via left middle temporal gyrus approach. When the tumor involves the right lateral ventricle, this approach may be more acceptable. Although dysfunction of the nondominant middle temporal

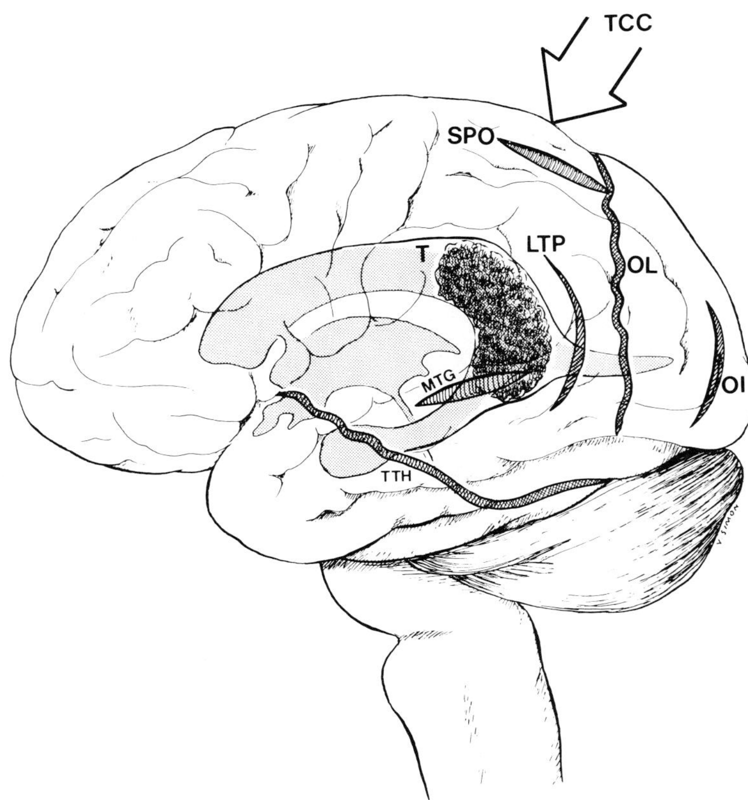

Fig. 50-2. A sketch illustrating the various approaches suggested for trigonal tumors. T = tumor; TCC = trans-corpus callosum approach; SPO = superior parietal occipital incision; LTP = lateral temporal parietal incision; OL = occipital lobectomy; OI = occipital lobe incision; MTG = middle temporal gyrus incision; TTH = transtemporal horn-occipital temporal gyrus incision.

gyrus is associated with impaired recognition of emotion, as evidenced in faces[3] or speech,[21] our experience indicates that patients with such impairments do not consider them important to their daily functioning. Postoperative homonymous visual field loss also is seen with this incision, although theoretically there should be less danger of this since the optic projections are parallel to the incision.

The anterior choroidal artery can be dealt with relatively early in vascular tumors supplied by this artery, but piecemeal resection may be required. In large tumors, a significant portion of the mass may be obscured by the posterior thalamus. If the tumor takes its blood supply from the posterior choroidal artery, the vessel will remain unattended until the entire tumor has been removed. The incision may have to be extended into the parietal lobe for proper visualization of the medial ventricular component.

Occipital Lobectomy or Incision

The two obvious disadvantages to occipital lobectomy are the resultant homonymous field defect and the surgeon's inability to deal with the blood supply early in the resection (Figure 50-2, OL). However, occipital lobectomy may obviate the need for prolonged cortical retraction with its concomitant complications. When a patient has a homonymous hemianoptic field cut from a relatively large avascular tumor, this approach may be an appropriate choice.[25]

Superior Parietal Occipital Incision

Superior parietal occipital incision (Figure 50-2, SPO) extends from the postcentral fissure to the parieto-occipital fissure, approximately 3 cm from the falx, and lies medial to the majority of visual fibers and parallels their projection. Fornari et al. found that this approach preserved vision in 2 of 18 patients undergoing surgery. Visual loss in their other patients was ascribed to damage caused by manipulation of the tumor at the border of the lateral ventricular ependyma.[11] These authors reported no lasting motor or speech deficits in their patients. Parietal lobe functioning was not addressed. Other neurologic deficits that may be associated with this approach within the dominant hemisphere include apraxia,[16] acalculia,[15] and deficits in visual-spatial processing. Associated impairments in the nondominant hemisphere are limited to those in visual-spatial information processing. With this approach a certain amount of blood loss from piecemeal resection again must be accepted until the tumor can be resected to the point that it can be gently displaced to allow control of the feeding blood vessels.

Transcallosal Approach

Kempe and Blaylock, using the transcallosal approach, reported no new neurologic deficits in 3 patients who underwent surgery for apparently small trigonal tumors. Indeed, a developing literature supports the benign nature of a corpus callosum section when used in carefully selected patients and limited to the anterior two thirds of the body and the genu. In their report

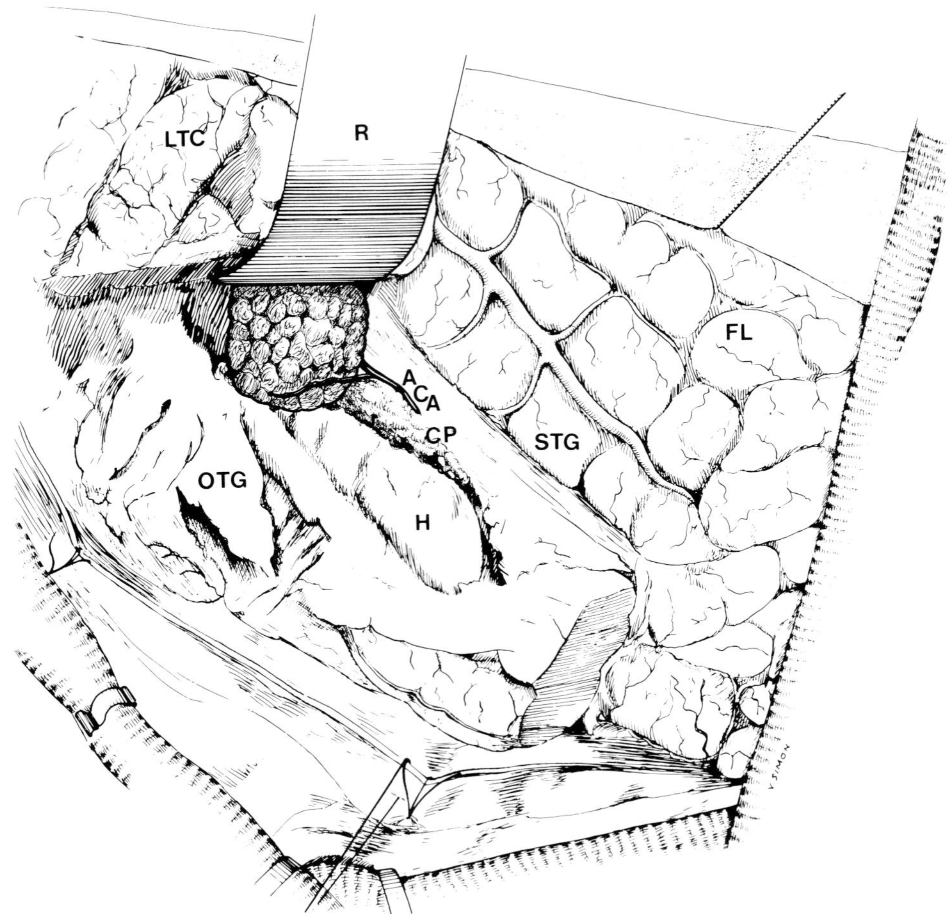

Fig. 50-3. In this sketch, the anterior 5 cm of the middle and inferior temporal lobe gyri have been excised and the occipital temporal fasciculus sectioned posteriorly along the temporal horn. The posterior lateral temporal cortex is shown gently retracted to expose the entire hippocampus, the choroid plexus, and the trigone tumor with its anterior choroidal blood supply. H = hippocampus; CP = choroid plexus; ACA = anterior choroidal artery; STG = superior temporal gyrus; LTC = lateral temporal cortex; OTG = occipital temporal gyrus; FL = frontal lobe; R = retractor.

of patients undergoing a transcallosal approach for excision of lateral or third ventricular lesions, Shugart and Stein[27] reported no significant postsurgical deficit that could be attributed to the disconnection procedure. Our experience with callosotomy for medically refractory epilepsy is similar; disconnection signs, when present, abate quickly.

Serious consequences may arise, however, if patient selection criteria are inadequate. As mentioned above, when the splenium of the corpus callosum is sectioned in the presence of a homonymous field cut resulting from damage to the dominant hemisphere, alexia without agraphia may result. Geschwind[28] described this, and Levin and Rose[29] reported such a disconnection syndrome in a patient operated upon for a lateral ventricular tumor of the dominant hemisphere. Speech and writing may be affected when the callosotomy is performed on a patient whose preferred hand for writing is ipsilateral to his or her hemispheric localization for speech, as can be demonstrated with the intracarotid amytal test.[30] These impairments are not lessened by sparing the splenium. Sass et al. also reported motor impairments in some patients with evidence of a preexisting cortical pathologic condition. Although studies occasionally report impaired memory following callosotomy,[24,31] this finding is less robust. In our patients, a mild but statistically significant loss in verbal memory accompanies anterior cal-

losotomy. However, patients and their families do not complain of significant changes in this regard.

Many tumors, especially meningiomas, can attain large proportions (50 to 400 g in one series),[2] inducing only minor symptoms. Given the limited exposure that results from a posterior callosal section, this large tumor bulk may prevent any effective lateral retraction of the involved hemisphere. The approach does provide for early exposure and obliteration of the feeding branches of the posterior choroidal artery. Thus, in a large, primarily trigonal, tumor, the presence of a preoperative homonymous field cut in the dominant hemisphere, or ipsilateral speech representation and handedness, are contraindications to this approach.

There are few reports of callosal sectioning for lateral ventricular tumor removal (Figure 50-2, TCC). We feel it should play an increasing role and, for this reason, an illustrative case is presented at the conclusion of this chapter.

Transtemporal Horn Occipital Temporal Gyrus Incision

The transtemporal horn occipital temporal gyrus approach had been developed for the resection of the posterior hippocampus in temporal lobe epilepsy. It affords an excellent

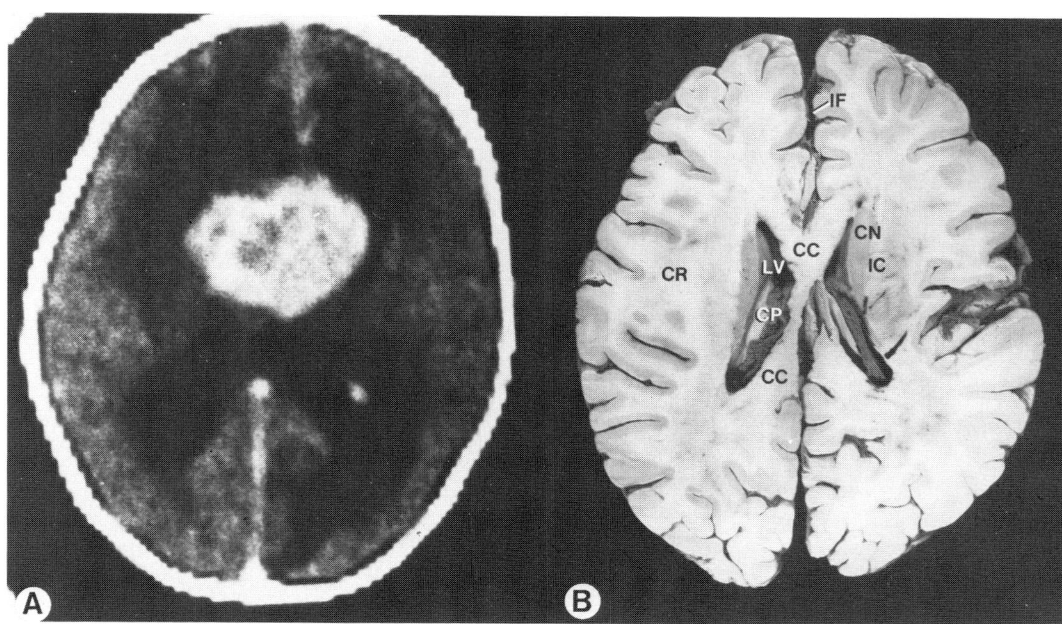

Fig. 50-4.   (A) A CT scan showing a midbody intraventricular tumor. (B) A horizontal brain slice at the level shown in A. Note the relationship of the surrounding structures, especially the corpus callosum and internal capsule. IF = interhemispheric fissure; CC = corpus callosum; CN = caudate nucleus; IC = internal capsule; CR = corona radiata; CP = choroid plexus.

view of the ventricular atrium and its use can be extended to the resection of tumors in this region. It also can be combined with other approaches for larger trigonal tumors extending into the temporal horn. There currently are no reports of this approach for intraventricular tumors.

As shown in Figure 50-3, the procedure involves a frontotemporal craniotomy with the temporal craniectomy rongeured even with the floor of the middle fossa for inferior exposure. Resection of the pterion is performed for anterior oblique visualization. A limited lateral temporal lobectomy of the middle and inferior temporal gyri is performed, 5 cm from the temporal tip on the nondominant side or 4 cm on the dominant side. The temporal horn is opened, exposing the hippocampus, and an incision along the occipital temporal fasciculus is extended from the ventricle through the occipital temporal gyrus, posterior to the petrous ridge of the temporal bone. A wide self-retaining retractor is used to elevate this temporal lobe neocortex, exposing the trigone region. This offers two advantages; it provides access to the choroidal fissure for ligation of the anterior choroidal artery, and it is useful in either the dominant or nondominant hemisphere with minimal neurologic complications. An upper-quadrant homonymous visual field defect is possible, and naming difficulties may follow surgery in the dominant hemisphere. Like the middle temporal gyrus and lateral temporal parietal incisions, it does not provide adequate visualization of tumors extending superior and medial to the thalamus that derive their blood supply from the posterior choroidal artery.

SELECTION OF THE BEST SURGICAL APPROACH

No single approach for excision of trigonal tumors is clearly superior to the other alternatives. Radiologic examination, including CT scanning, MRI, and stereoangiography, will provide the precise size, location, and vascularity of each tumor. Hemispheric dominance for language should be determined. With this information, the surgeon can adapt his or her approach to the presumptive pathologic entity and the hemisphere involved. For example, a small or medium-sized, medially positioned tumor that derives its major blood supply from the posterior choroidal artery might be most expeditiously removed transcallosally, provided there is not a preoperative hemianopia in the dominant hemisphere and speech representation is not ipsilateral to the dominant hand. Small or medium-sized lateral trigonal tumors irrigated primarily by the anterior choroidal artery can be most safely approached by the restricted anterior temporal lobectomy and occipital temporal fasciculus incision. Large, relatively avascular tumors that are not associated with a major field cut may be best removed piecemeal from the vertical parieto-occipital incision. This incision could be used in a patient with the same type of tumor but with a homonymous field cut, but an occipital incision or lobectomy are viable alternatives.

Very large and vascular tumors fed by both the anterior and the posterior choroidal arteries are the most hazardous when any single approach is utilized. The morbidity and mortality from the blood loss alone in children with piecemeal resection of these tumors is extremely high. Manipulation of the tumor or retraction of the hemisphere to secure the blood supply through either the temporal, parietal, or occipital incisions risks severe neurologic complications. Under these conditions, a combination of approaches should be considered. One can approach a large vascular trigone tumor beginning with the modified anterior temporal lobectomy (Figure 50-2, TTH) and occipital temporal fasciculus incision. The anterior choroidal artery can be controlled, thereby permitting piecemeal resection of that portion of the tumor directly visualized in the atrium. This is accomplished more easily when the temporal horn has been obstructed and is dilated. With the mass decompressed, a transcallosal or parieto-occipital incision would allow the posterior choroidal blood supply to be ligated and the

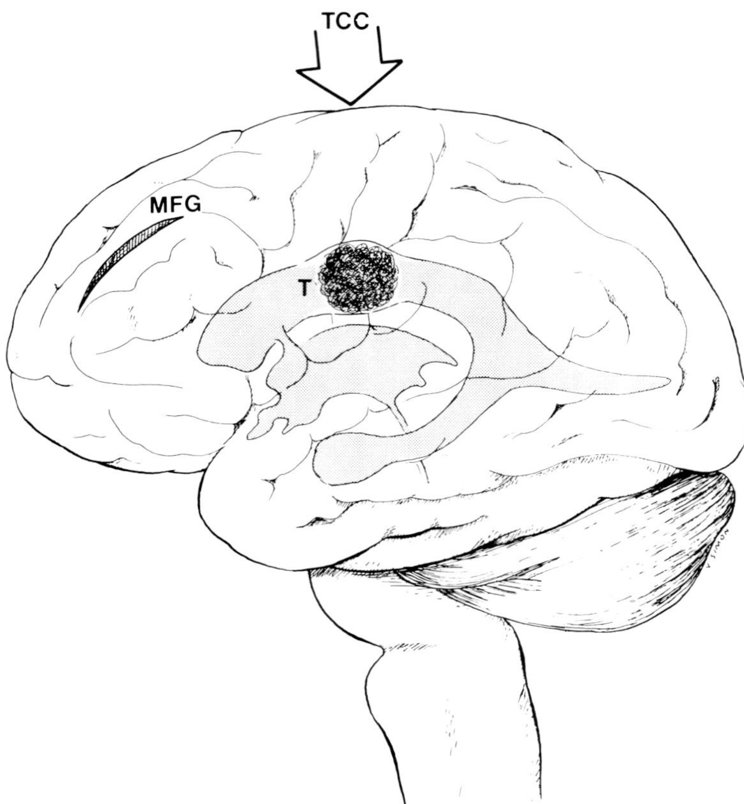

Fig. 50-5. The relationship of the transcallosal approach and the middle frontal gyrus incision to a midventricular body tumor. T = tumor; TCC = trans-corpus callosum approach; MFG = middle frontal gyrus incision.

remaining tumor to be resected piecemeal (Figure 50-2, SPO, TCC).

MIDVENTRICULAR BODY TUMORS

ANATOMY

A unique property of tumors arising in the midventricular body is their tendency to present in both lateral ventricles by compression of the thin septum pellucidum. The anatomic relationships of such a tumor are shown in Figure 50-4. They also deform the roof of the third ventricle. Vascular tumors, such as meningiomas, parasitize the choroidal blood supply of the posterior choroidal arteries. The internal capsule becomes compressed bilaterally. Both frontal horns and atrial regions may be trapped and dilated by the central position of this tumor in the narrowest portion of the lateral ventricles.

SURGICAL APPROACH

A lateral transcortical approach is contraindicated because midventricular body tumors lie beneath the primary motor and sensory gyri. The middle frontal gyrus may be chosen for some tumors (Figure 50-5, MFG), such as those that are purely unilateral, take their blood supply anteriorly, or are bulky, avascular, and situated forward in the body. This approach with tumors that have a posterior choroidal blood supply and are

positioned in the middle to posterior aspect of the body may cause inordinate blood loss during piecemeal resection.

The best approach to most tumors in this region is transcallosal, and several features of this need elucidation (Figure 50-5, TCC). Preoperatively, the angiographic venous phase must be examined to locate the veins draining into the superior sagittal sinus. The bone and dural flap then should be designed so that the major venous drainage is not interrupted by the exposure. One of two major neurologic complications in one series was a venous infarction that resulted from the division of two anterior draining cortical veins.[27] For tumors confined to one ventricle, the patient's head should be placed in a pin-fixation headrest and turned laterally with the involved ventricle in the superior position. As the tumor is resected piecemeal, it will then migrate into the field. Access to the contralateral ventricle in this position has been, in our experience, excellent, with partial callosotomy for excision of lateral intraventricular tumors and treatment of medically refractory epilepsy. The approach has also been reported in a case of intraventricular AVM.[32] With a large bilateral tumor such as that shown in Figure 50-4, the nondominant hemisphere should be placed in the inferior position and retracted, as required. This allows tumor to be delivered more easily from the opposite lateral ventricle.

In treating such tumors, the bone flap should extend across the sagittal sinus, permitting gentle retraction of the falx. Care must be taken, however, to avoid compression of the sagittal sinus, which can result in intraoperative swelling and postoperative thrombosis. Figure 50-6 shows a bone flap position for the midbody tumor. Note that there are no major draining veins

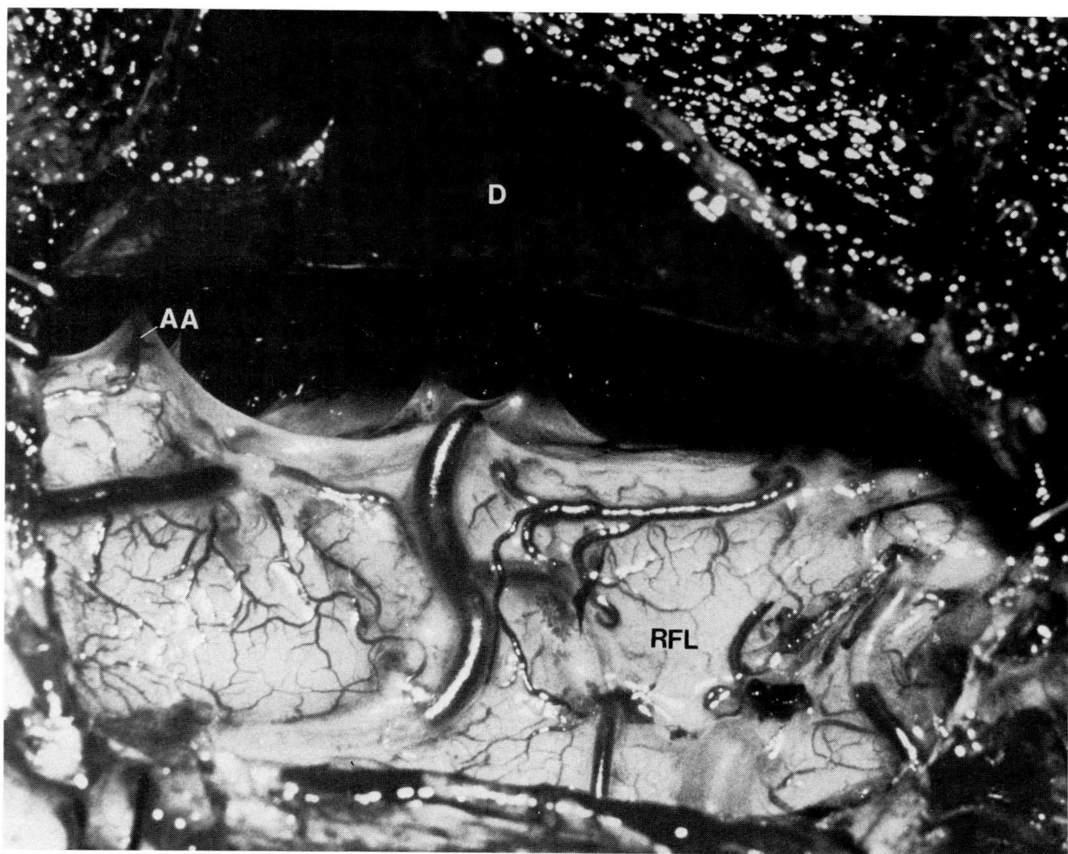

Fig. 50-6.   Intraoperative photograph showing the dural opening for the transcallosal approach to a midbody ventricular tumor. Note that the bony opening should be to the center of or on the opposite side of the sagittal sinus and the dura turned toward the sinus. Multiple arachnoid adhesions to the falx and opposite hemisphere as pictured here are common. RFL = right frontal lobe; D = dura; AA = arachnoidal adhesions.

in the field. Osmotic diuresis, hyperventilation, and less often, CSF drainage will allow the hemisphere to fall from the midline without mechanical retraction.

Arachnoidal adhesions are common between the medial hemisphere and the falx. Particular care must be taken to separate the often approximated cingulate gyri, especially when a large, bilaterally placed tumor or dilated contralateral ventricle shifts the opposite medial hemisphere under the falx. The pericallosal artery seen in Figure 50-7 must be carefully preserved when the callosum is sectioned between the medial and lateral longitudinal stria and preferentially between the two pericallosal arteries.

At the middle portion of the callosal body, the fornices are compact bundles running side by side. Both can be damaged by a cut at the absolute midline of the callosum. Instead, the callosum should be divided from 5 mm to 1 cm off the midline. It is becoming more clearly established that division of the neocortical commissure alone does not result in severe cognitive or memory disturbances,[33,34,30] but division of both fornices proximal to the foramen of Monro may cause short-term memory deficits.[24,35,36]

The callosal section should begin at the pole of the tumor that receives the major blood supply. The tumor again is resected piecemeal. Consideration must be given to a combined approach if any portion of the tumor is not visualized or easily delivered. This combined approach would require the remaining tumor to be removed via a midfrontal gyrus incision on the appropriate side.

TUMORS OF THE FRONTAL HORN

Tumors of the frontal horn are most often gliomas, either astrocytomas or ependymomas, but meningiomas occasionally are found in this area.[37] Early histopathologic identification of the type of tumor aids intraoperative decision making. The approach therefore should allow direct access for a biopsy. Tumors of the frontal horn may block the foramen of Monro, trapping spinal fluid within the same or the opposite ventricle. The release of such fluid will improve visualization and the control of bleeding.

ANATOMY

The frontal horn of the lateral ventricle is bordered medially by the septum pellucidum and laterally by the caudate nucleus. The floor is formed by the rostrum of the corpus callosum and the apex by the genu of the corpus callosum (Figure 50-8). The lateral ventricle communicates to the third and opposite lateral ventricles via the intraventricular foramen of Monro, which is bordered anteriorly and posteriorly by the columns of the fornix. With large tumors, the columns of the fornix can be compressed against each other. Bilateral fornicial damage can result if the anterior border of the foramen is not carefully identified. With an anterior oblique approach to the ventricle, unless the anatomy of the ventricular wall is clearly defined, the dissection can extend to the vascular ependyma overlying the thalamic nuclei, resulting in bleeding that is

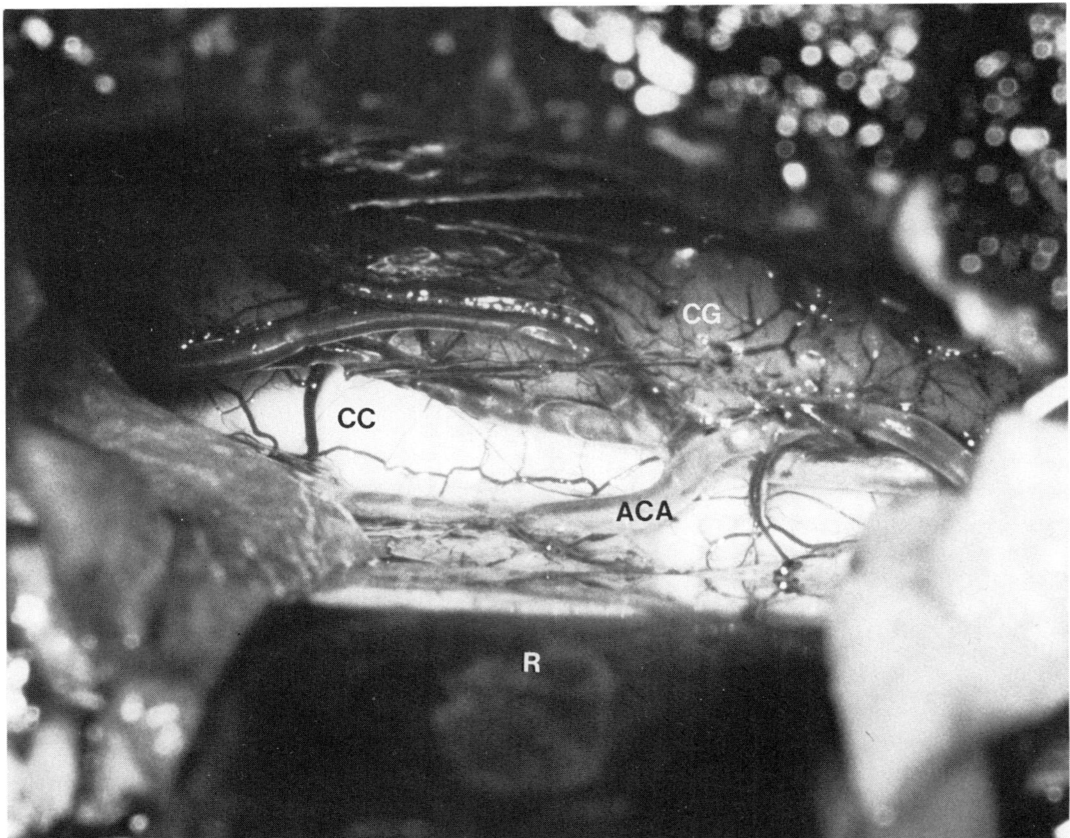

Fig. 50-7. The surface of the body of the corpus callosum is easily seen in this intraoperative photograph. Note the important relationship of the pericallosal segment of the anterior cerebral artery. These vessels must be preserved. The callosum is entered by bipolar coagulation of the fine vascular network on the surface. CC = corpus callosum; ACA = anterior cerebral artery; CG = cingulate gyrus; R = retractor.

difficult to control safely. The choroid plexus of the lateral ventricle often is contiguous along the roof of the third ventricle with the choroid plexus of the opposite lateral ventricle. Manipulation of either the roof of the third ventricle or the choroid plexus of the lateral ventricle can cause undetected bleeding at a distance from the operative field.

SURGICAL APPROACH

Tumors of the frontal horn are also often accessible via a transcallosal incision, which we generally prefer. This section will be used, however, to describe the middle frontal gyrus approach, with the understanding that the intraventricular anatomy and the resection technique are much the same, regardless of whether a transcallosal or transcortical incision is used.

An incision through the middle frontal gyrus allows direct access to the frontal horn and the tumor (Figures 50-8 and 50-9). We prefer an incision rather than a circular cortical resection. Either can be used. The patient's head is positioned supine in a pin-fixation headrest with the head turned 30 to 40 degrees to the opposite side. Some surgeons prefer the straight supine position, but rotation of the head simplifies the use of the operating microscope.

A bicoronal skin incision is made and a 4- or 5-hole osteoplastic flap is turned using the ipsilateral temporalis muscle. The margins of the bony opening extend 1 to 2 cm from the midline just above the frontal sinuses, to 2 to 3 cm behind the

coronal suture and laterally to the pterion. If the opposite ventricle contains trapped CSF, a burr hole is made on the opposite side just anterior to the coronal suture and about 3 cm off the midline. A ventriculostomy is performed, and the ventricle is decompressed before the dura is opened. A U-shaped dural incision is reflected medially. The middle frontal gyrus is identified, the pial surface coagulated, and the pia and cortex incised for a distance of 2 to 3 cm in front of the posterior extent of the gyrus.

Two hand-held, 1-cm flat brain retractors are used to "walk" through the cortex and white matter. The 1-cm square surface, which is exposed at the base of the retractors during the dissection allows identification of the various layers, including the ependymal surface of the ventricle. As an assistant holds one retractor, the ventricular wall is identified and opened with bayonet forceps. The surface of the tumor usually can be identified at this point. A biopsy specimen is taken for diagnosis of tumor type.

The anterior superior surface of the tumor is identified. If the tumor is large, the incision is extended in an anterior direction, and self-retaining retractors are fixed in place. The operating microscope is brought into the field. Low-power magnification usually is adequate for most of the dissection. The central portion of the tumor is gutted with suction dissection, ultrasonic aspiration, or the CO_2 laser, depending on its consistency. The dissection is planned to demarcate the borders of the tumor, the medial ventricular structures are noted and exposed. After identification of the fornix and the foramen of

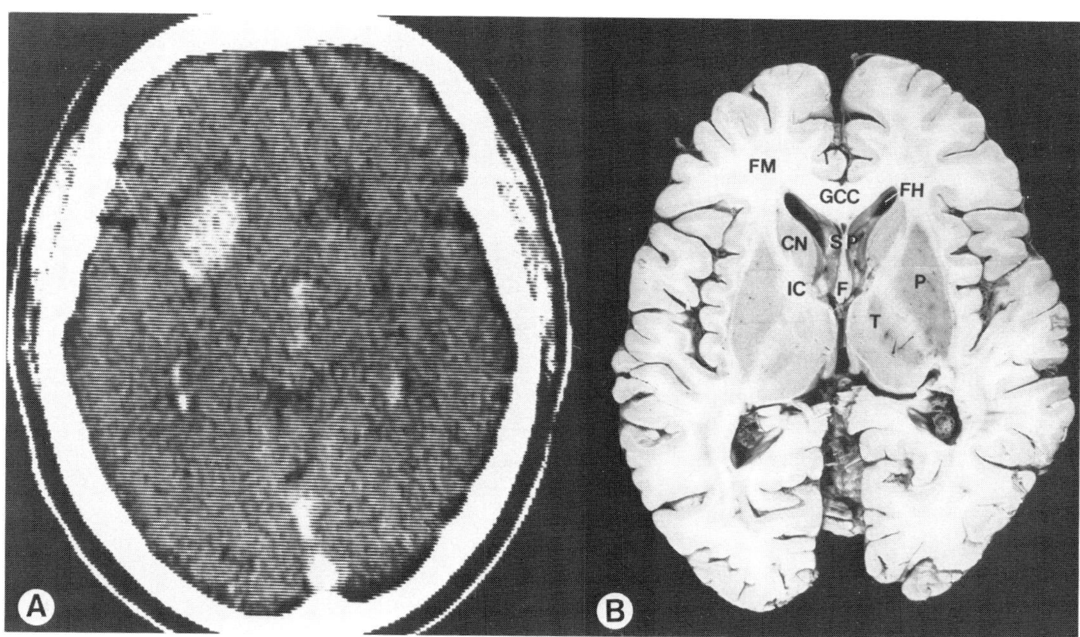

Fig. 50-8. (A) A CT scan showing a left frontal horn intraventricular tumor. (B) A horizontal section through a human brain at the same level and angle as shown in A to depict the relationship of important neural structures to the frontal horn. FM = forceps minor; GCC = genu of corpus callosum; FH = frontal horn of lateral ventricle; SP = septum pellucidum; CN = caudate nucleus; F = fornix; IC = internal capsule; P = putamen; T = thalamus.

Monro, a cottonoid is placed over this area to decrease the pooling of blood in the opposite lateral and third ventricles.

Preoperative determination of the tumor position, size, and areas of attachment and the planned central tumor resection allow the free ventricular wall to be used as a guide to the attached tumor border. Since the blood supply of these tumors is usually at a distance from the approach, attempts at early control of blood vessels are not possible, except on the surface of the resection area. In glial tumors, the excision is continued until the point of attachment is reached and the ventricular wall around the attachment is identified. Using higher magnification, the tumor, when possible, is removed from the underlying white matter. A primary intent is to restore communication of the ipsilateral and contralateral ventricles with the third ventricle, thus achieving interventricular communication. This determines the minimum necessary resection in tumors that are not confined to the ventricle.

Meningiomas usually adhere to the choroid plexus. As the piecemeal resection proceeds, the blood supply of the tumor can be identified and coagulated. The choroid plexus is resected with the specimen since removal of the tumor and its attachments may devascularize the remaining choroid, resulting in vascular stasis, infarction, and delayed postoperative intraventricular hemorrhage. The dura then is closed, and a ventricular catheter is inserted through the superior posterior burr hole and is exteriorized through a separate scalp incision.

Often following resection of tumors via the middle frontal gyrus, no neurologic deficit is detected. Lesion studies suggest, however, that damage to the prefrontal areas may impair attention, executive functions (e.g., self-monitoring and regulation), visual searching, speech (even with preservation of Broca's area), and new learning. Nondominant prefrontal lesions may produce attention deficits, visual searching difficulties, and unilateral inattention.

TUMORS CONFINED TO THE TEMPORAL HORN

The temporal horn is an unusual location for intraventricular tumors. It is shown schematically in Figure 50-10.

ANATOMY

Although any of the intraventricular tumors may be found in the temporal horn, meningiomas are most common. Anatomically, this tumor will be based on the choroid plexus and derive its blood supply from the anterior choroidal artery or from branches of the posterior cerebral artery. The important anatomic structures surrounding this tumor are the hippocampus and limbic projections medially and inferiorly; the choroidal fissure, posterior cerebral artery, and brain stem medially; the fibers of Meyer's loop, the arcuate fasciculus, and in the dominant hemisphere, portions of Wernicke's speech area laterally and superiorly.

SURGICAL APPROACH

Tumors confined to the temporal horn can be removed by either the middle temporal gyrus incision (Figure 50-10. MTG) or by the modified anterior temporal lobectomy and occipital temporal gyrus incision (Figures 50-3 and 50-10). The latter approach is probably best suited for this location since it allows early ligation of the anterior choroidal artery. It also should preserve the lower-quadrant visual fibers and Wernicke's area in the dominant hemisphere.

GENERAL COMPLICATIONS OF ALL SURGICAL APPROACHES

The complications associated with removal of intraventricular tumors include the neurologic deficits associated with the particular approach for each tumor; these have been detailed

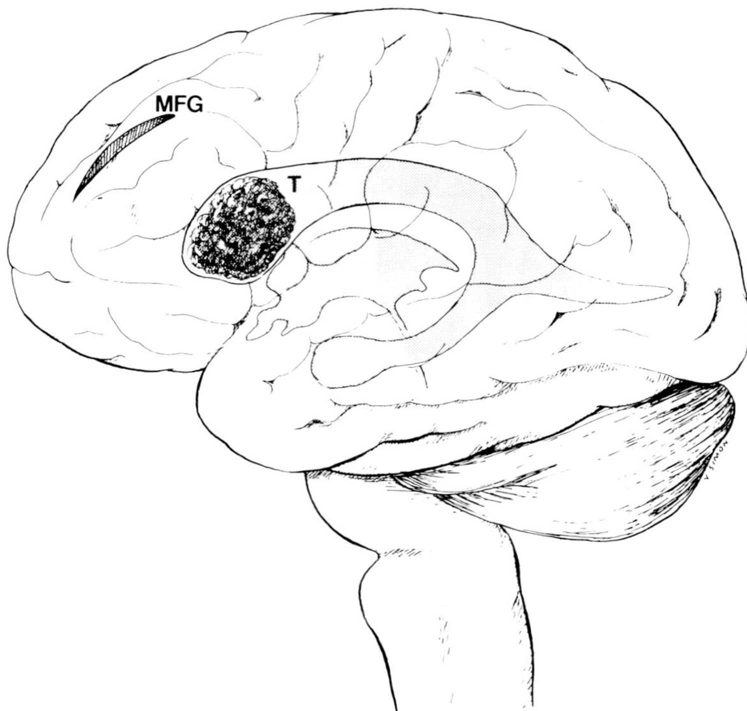

Fig. 50-9. A sketch showing the relationship of a middle frontal gyrus incision to a frontal horn tumor. MFG = middle frontal gyrus incision; T = tumor.

above. Other complications are those that may be encountered during or after removal of a tumor from any intraventricular location and include:

1. Intraoperative hemorrhage.
2. Delayed postoperative intraventricular hemorrhage.
3. Cortical collapse and subdural hematoma or hygroma following removal of a large tumor from a dilated ventricle.
4. Postoperative cerebral edema.
5. Postoperative hydrocephalus.

POSTOPERATIVE CARE

The basic tenets of good postoperative care in cases of intraventricular tumors are those that should be followed after any major craniotomy. They are:

1. An adequate blood volume is maintained without overhydration. This requires serial serum electrolytes and blood determination.
2. An airway with good oxygenation is essential.
3. Preoperative steroids are maintained and tapered during the first postoperative week.

There are, however, certain postoperative care requirements unique to the intraventricular tumor. They are:

1. A ventricular catheter should be placed in the involved ventricle at the conclusion of the operation. This is left for at least 48 hours to monitor rises in intracranial pressure and occurrence of intraventricular hemorrhage.
2. Before removing the catheter, indigo carmine may be injected and a lumbar puncture performed within thirty minutes to ensure adequate CSF circulation.
3. CT scans should be performed on the second and fifth postoperative days to check for ventricular size, intraventricular blood, and subdural hygroma or hematoma. Scans also should be obtained in case of any neurologic deterioration, unexplained rises in ICP, or fresh blood noted in the ventricular drainage.

ILLUSTRATIVE CASE

Since so few cases with a transcallosal approach to intraventricular tumors are reported in the literature, the following case is presented to illustrate that callosal sectioning can be safely accomplished and may provide the needed flexibility for total removal of very large lateral ventricular tumors without resorting to additional cortical incisions. It demonstrates that a major portion of the callosal body can be entirely divided without persistent disconnection signs or cognitive or neurologic loss. This patient returned to his premorbid level of function. Finally, the case demonstrates the need to remain attentive to postoperative complications, particularly the collapse of a decompressed attenuated hemisphere.

The patient was a 21-year-old, right-hand dominant, white male college student. His initial complaints included a mild bifrontal headache of several months duration, a more acute progressive bilateral loss in vision, and mild academic difficulties. Four days before admission, the patient underwent ophthalmologic examination, which revealed bilateral papilledema.

Neurologic examination was notable for a bilateral decrease in visual acuity, a mild bilateral sixth nerve palsy, and a left upper extremity drift. Bilateral Babinski reflexes were intermittently demonstrated. Admission laboratory studies were within normal limits. Endocrine function test results were within normal limits, except for mild hypothyroidism.

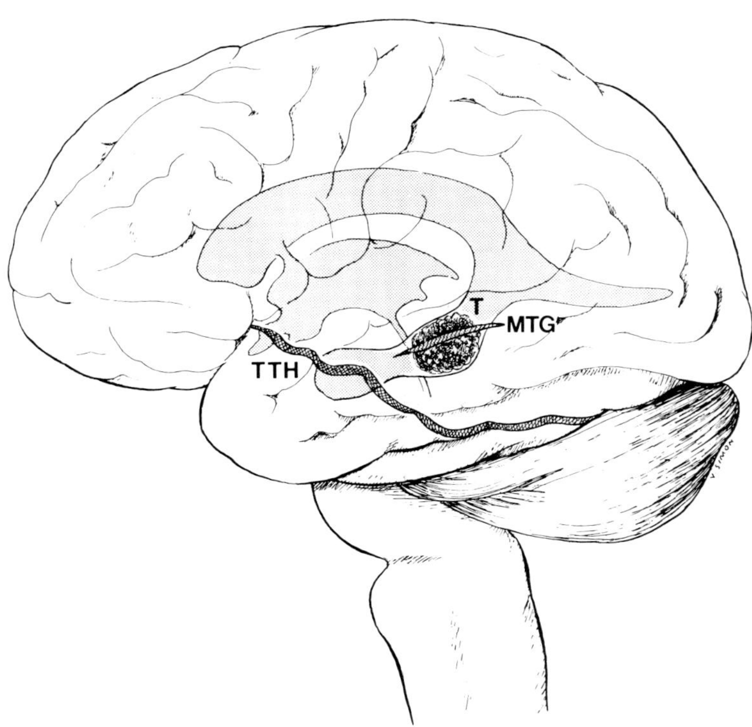

Fig. 50-10. A temporal horn tumor is shown in this sketch with two possible incisions for removal. T = tumor; MTG = middle temporal gyrus incision; TTH = trans-temporal horn occipital temporal gyrus incision.

Neuropsychologic examination revealed mild left upper extremity weakness, slowing, incoordination and deep tendon reflexes that were symmetrically brisk. Left upper extremity two-point discrimination, visual perception, visual searching, judgment of body position, and discrimination of nonspeech sounds (i.e., rhythm and prosody) were moderately impaired. New nonverbal learning and memory were moderately impaired and the performance IQ index was significantly below the verbal IQ index (VIQ = 109: PIQ = 72). The neuropsychologic findings were indicative of acute, diffuse right hemisphere dysfunction.

Computed tomography revealed an irregular cystic mass of mixed attenuation occupying the anterior horn of the right lateral ventricle (Figure 50-11). The mass appeared to be solely within the right ventricle, which was enlarged, and it displaced the midline and compressed the third ventricle. Angiography revealed lateral displacement of the sylvian triangle on the right with a questionable mild shift of the anterior cerebral artery. There was tumor blush from the middle anterior and posterior cerebral arteries. Major draining veins were identified.

The patient was taken to the operating room and placed on the table in the right lateral position, with the head fixed in the pin headrest. A horseshoe-shaped incision was made, extending from the hairline anteriorly across the midline approximately 2 cm medially and to the mastoid posteriorly. A parasagittal frontoparietal flap was turned, extending just across the midline.

The dura was open based medially on the sagittal sinus. Two small draining veins were sacrificed. When the interhemispheric fissure was visualized, the right hemisphere was gently retracted. Cingulate gyri adhesions were dissected, revealing the corpus callosum.

The corpus callosum was divided posteriorly from the genu

to include approximately 75 percent of the body. Both pericallosal arteries were preserved.

When the ependyma was opened, the tumor was immediately visible as a dark reddish-gray mass. Biopsy specimens

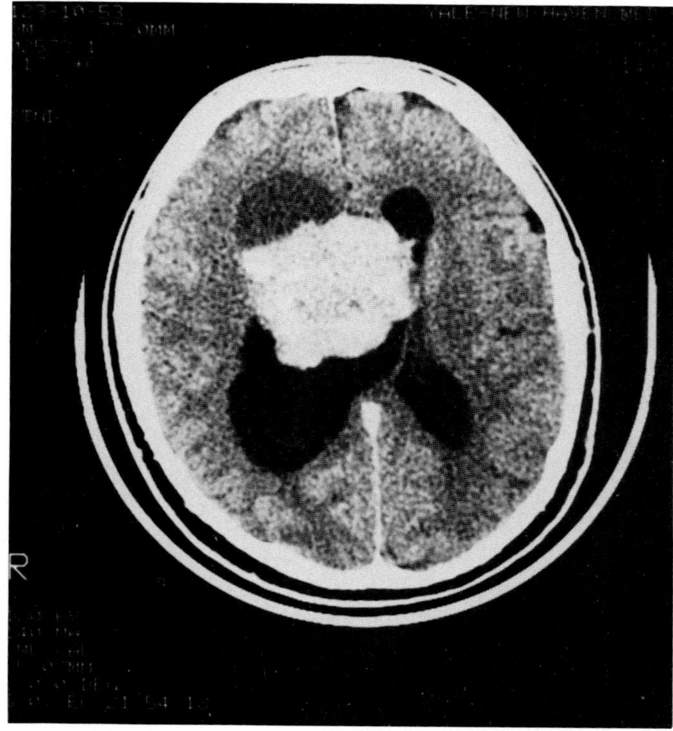

Fig. 50-11. A CT scan of the patient illustrating the striking enhancement of this tumor, the trapped right lateral ventricle from obstruction at the foramen of Monro, and the protrusion into the opposite ventricle with displacement of the septum pellucidum.

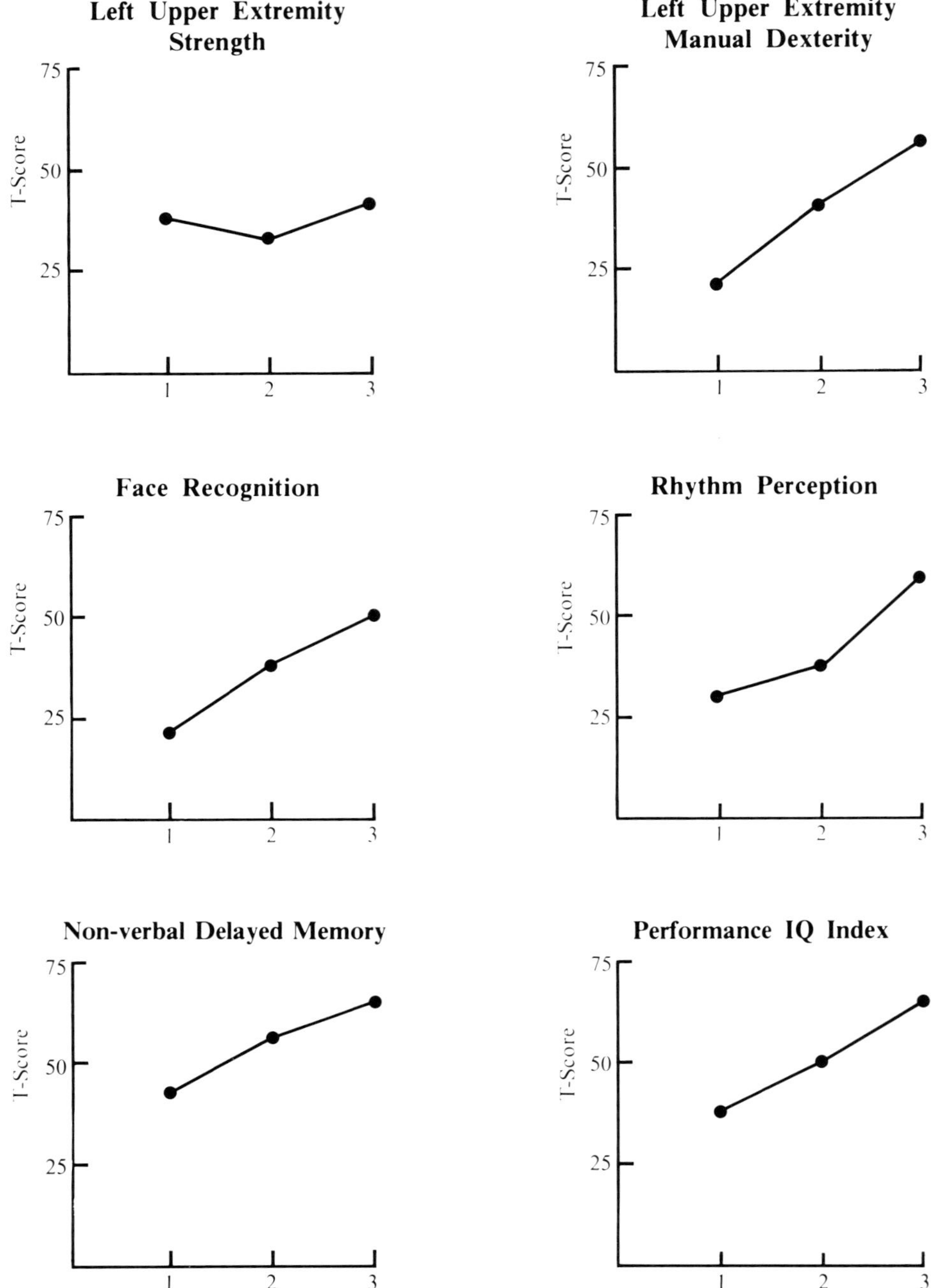

Fig. 50-12. Results for the patient of repeated neuropsychologic examinations conducted (1) before surgery, (2) 2 weeks after surgery, and (3) 3 months after surgery. The T-score transformations were computed using norms compiled for a comparable population of neurologically impaired patients.

were sent for frozen section, and were diagnosed as low grade ependymoma. The tumor was debulked in a piecemeal fashion, using suction and bipolar coagulation and ultrasonic aspiration. The anterior, posterior, and left lateral margins were established. After the left half of the tumor was removed, the septum pellucidum was opened and free communication was established between the lateral ventricles.

To remove the right portion of the tumor, the head of the bed was lowered. The foramen of Monro was identified and a small fingerlike projection of tumor was removed from the third ventricle. Tumor debulking continued with suction and ultrasonic aspiration. The tumor was eventually removed entirely, including the lateral portion, which was adherent to the ven-

tricular wall. A Silastic ventriculostomy catheter was placed in the ventricle, and brought out interhemispherically through the dural incision. Permanent histologic sections later were diagnosed as oligodendroglioma.

Postoperatively, the patient was alert and oriented. A mild right sixth and a central left seventh nerve paresis were observed in addition to left upper extremity pronation with drift. Acute disconnection phenomena were not present. On the seventh postoperative day, the ventriculostomy was removed. Lumbar punctures were intermittently used to control intracranial pressure. By 14 days postoperatively, the patient's left drift had resolved, and his left facial weakness was barely perceptible.

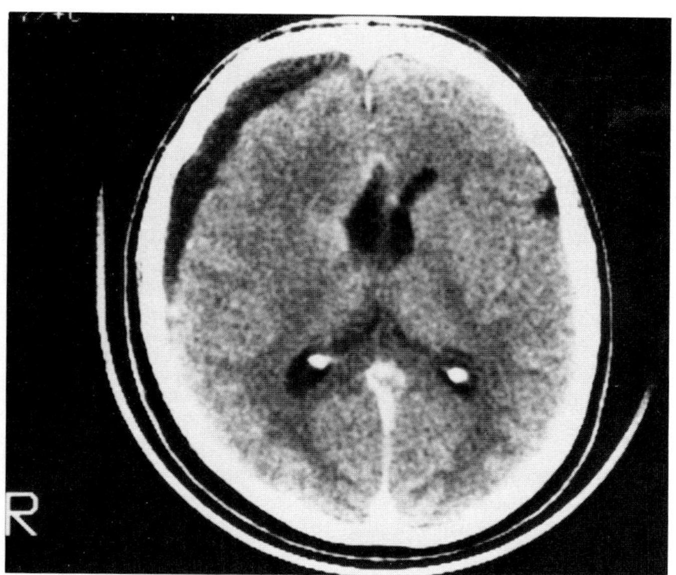

Fig. 50-13. A postoperative CT scan showing that the tumor has been resected with resultant collapse of the previously dilated right frontal horn and the accompanying subdural fluid collection.

Approximately 3 weeks after surgery, the patient was examined neuropsychologically. Improvements were noted in left upper extremity manual dexterity, left upper extremity two-point discrimination, visual searching, visual perception, position sense, discrimination of nonspeech sounds, nonverbal new learning, and performance IQ. His improvement in selected areas is portrayed graphically in Figure 50-12. Interhemispheric transfer of information was demonstrated in the three major modalities. Further improvement in neuropsychologic functioning was documented when the patient was re-examined 3 months after surgery. By this time the patient had returned to his premorbid level of functioning.

Four months after surgery, the patient returned to the emergency room with complaints of a 6-day history of right-sided headache. Neurologic examination revealed mild right papilledema on fundoscopic examination. A CT scan significant for a right frontal subdural fluid collection with near total effacement of the lateral ventricle and a 2–3-mm right to left shift (Figure 50-13). The patient was taken to the operating room where a right frontal burr hole was performed to drain a chronic subdural hematoma. No postoperative declines in neurologic functioning were detected. Neuropsychologic examination, performed 7 days after the patient's craniotomy, also revealed no increased neurologic deficit, relative to the findings obtained at 3 months after surgery.

The patient is now 1 year 4 months post-surgery. He has returned successfully to college. Following his graduation, he will pursue advanced study in veterinary science.

CONCLUSION

The rarity and relative seclusion of the lateral intraventricular tumor demands of the neurosurgeon a careful preoperative evaluation and thoughtful consideration of the peritumoral anatomy. The various surgical approaches to these challenging tumors provide a clear example of how one must consider the possible cognitive and neurologic consequences of removing or excising normal brain for proper exposure. A variety of approaches have been presented from which either a single or combination of approaches can be selected, depending upon tumor position, size, vascularity, feeding blood vessels, presumptive pathology, and residence in either the dominant or nondominant hemisphere. These factors are properly determined by CT scanning, MRI, angiography, and the intracarotid amytal procedure (under special circumstances). Then, after careful neurologic and neuropsychologic examinations, the surgeon should list the approaches in order of technical ease of tumor removal and ask "What are the behavioral and neurologic consequences of this approach?". The approach can then be logically selected. Today's intraoperative technology, using laser, ultrasonic aspiration, and minimal retraction through a hemisphere or callosal incision, should make the care of these patients one of the most satisfying challenges in neurosurgical practice.

REFERENCES

1. Silver AJ, Ganti SR, Hilal SK: Computed tomography of tumors involving the atria of the lateral ventricles. Radiology 145:71, 1982
2. Ladenheim JC: Chroid Plexus Meningiomas of the Lateral Ventricle. Springfield, Ill, Charles C Thomas, 1963
3. Eekhof JLA, Thomeer RTWM, Bots GThAM: Epidermoid tumor in the lateral ventricle. Surg Neurol 23:189, 1985
4. Lobato RD, Cabello A, Carmena JJ, et al: Subependymoma of the lateral ventricle. Surg Neurol 15:144, 1981
5. Afra D, Turoczy L, Deak G: Ependymomas extending into both lateral ventricles: CT-diagnosis and operability. Report of 2 cases. Zbl Neurochirugie 42:255, 1981
6. Turcotte JF, Copty M, Bedard F, et al: Lateral ventricle choroid plexus papilloma and communicating hydrocephalus. Surg Neurol 13:143, 1980
7. Bernasconi V, Cabrini GP: Radiological features of tumors of the lateral ventricles. Acta Neurochir 17:290, 1967
8. Falk B: Radiologic diagnosis of intraventricular meningiomas. Acta Radiol 46:171, 1956
9. De La Torre E, Alexander E Jr, Davis CH Jr, et al: Tumors of the lateral ventricles of the brain: Report of eight cases, with suggestions for clinical management. J Neurosurg 20:461, 1963
10. Mani RL, Hedgcock MW, Mass SI, et al: Radiographic diagnosis of meningioma of the lateral ventricle: Review of 22 cases. J Neurosurg 49:249, 1978
11. Fornari M, Savoiardo M, Morello G, et al: Meningiomas of the lateral ventricles: Neuroradiological and surgical considerations in 18 cases. J Neurosurg 54:64, 1981
12. Friedman RB, Albert M: Alexia, in Heilman KM, Valenstein E: Clinical Neuropsychology. New York, Oxford University Press, 1985
13. Mateer CA: Localization of language and visuospatial functions by electrical stimulation, in Localization in Neuropsychology. New York, Academic Press, 1983
14. Roeltgen D. Agraphia, in Heilman KM, Valenstein E: Clinical Neuropsychology. New York, Oxford University Press, 1985
15. Levin HS, Spiers PA: Acalculia, in Heilman KM, Valenstein E: Clinical Neuropsychology. New York, Oxford University Press, 1985
16. Heilman KM, Gonzales Rothi LJ: Apraxia, in Heilman KM, Valenstein E: Clinical Neuropsychology. New York, Oxford University Press, 1985
17. Gerstmann J: Zur Symptomatologie der Hirnlasionen in Uebergangsgebiet der unteren parietal- und mittleren. Occipitalwindung. Nervenarzt 3:691, 1930
18. Benton A: Visuoperceptual, visuospatial, and visuoconstructive disorders, in Heilman KM, Valenstein E: Clinical Neuropsychology. New York, Oxford University Press, 1985

19. Heilman KM, Watson RT, Valenstein E, et al: Localization of lesions in neglect, in Heilman KM, Valenstein E: Clinical Neuropsychology. New York, Oxford University Press, 1985

20. Kertesz A: Right-hemisphere lesions in constructional apraxia and visuospatial deficit, in Heilman KM, Valenstein E: Clinical Neuropsychology. New York, Oxford University Press, 1985

21. Ross ED: Right-hemisphere lesions in disorders of affective language, in Kertesz A: Localization in Neuropsychology. New York, Academic Press, 1983

22. Ojemann G: Individual variability in cortical localization of language. J Neurosurg 50:164, 1979

23. Mazzocchi R, Vignolo LA: Localization of lesions in aphasia: Clinical CT scan correlation in stroke patients. Cortex 15:627, 1979

24. Geffen G, Walsh A, Simpson D, et al: Comparison of the effects of transcortical and transcallosal removal of intraventricular tumors. Brain 103:773, 1980

25. Olivecrona H, Tonnis W: Handbuch der Neurochirurgie. Berlin, Springer-Verlag, 1967, pp 175–177

26. Kempe LG, Blaylock R: Lateral-trigonal intraventricular tumors: A new operative approach. Acta Neurochir 35:233, 1976

27. Shucart WA, Stein BM: Transcallosal approach to the anterior ventricular system. Neurosurgery 3:339, 1978

28. Geschwind N: Disconnexion syndromes in animals and man. Brain 88:237, 1965

29. Levin HS, Rose JE: Alexia without agraphia in a musician after transcallosal removal of a left intraventricular meningioma. Neurosurgery 4:168, 1979

30. Sass KJ, Novelly RA, Spencer DD, et al: Corpus callosotomy in treatment of epilepsy: Neuropsychological outcome. J Clin Exp Neuropsychol 7:618, 1985

31. Zaidel D, Sperry RW: Memory impairment after commissurotomy in man. Brain 97:263, 1974

32. Nehls DG, Marano SR, Spetzler RF: Transcallosal approach to the contralateral ventricle. Technical note. J Neurosurg 62:304, 1985

33. Ledoux JE, Risse GL, Springer SP, et al: Cognition and commissurotomy. Brain 100:87, 1977

34. Goldstein MN, Joynt RJ, Hartley RB: The long-term effects of callosal sectioning: Report of second case. Arch Neurol 32:52, 1975

35. Jeeves MA, Simpson DA, Geffen G: Functional consequences of the transcallosal removal of intraventricular tumors. J Neurol Neurosurg Psychiatry 42:134, 1979

36. Heilman KM, Sypert GW: Korsakoff's syndrome resulting from bilateral fornix lesions. Neurology 27:490, 1977

37. Busch E: Meningiomas of the lateral ventricles of the brain. Acta Chir Scand 82:282, 1930

CHAPTER 51
Surgical Approaches to Intraventricular Meningiomas of the Trigone

Cecil L. Jun   Stephen L. Nutik

INTRAVENTRICULAR MENINGIOMAS are relatively rare tumors; consequently, most neurosurgeons will not have an extensive experience with them. The widespread availability of computed tomographic scanning can expedite the diagnosis. However, because these tumors can remain silent for a long time, they may reach a large size before diagnosis.

Numerous surgical approaches have been devised for trigonal meningiomas, each with its proponents. All carry the risk of potentially serious morbidity. Since the description of the transcallosal approach was published by Kempe and Blaylock,[1] negative comments[2] and reports[3] have questioned the value of the procedure. This is unfortunate, because the Kempe-Blaylock approach deserves serious consideration, along with other approaches, when plans are made for removal of any intraventricular meningioma of the trigone.[4,5]

Meningiomas of the lateral ventricle constitute 0.5 to 4.5 percent of all meningiomas.[6,7] They occur mainly at the trigone of the ventricle, where they constitute from 20 to 50 percent of the tumors at that site.[8–10] As with other meningiomas, there is a female-to-male preponderance of about 2:1.[2,7,11,12] They occurred slightly more frequently in the left hemisphere in some series[1,2,6,13] but not in all series.[7,11,12] Intraventricular meningiomas are usually seen in adults. In children, meningiomas constitute only 1 to 2 percent of all intracranial tumors, although 17 percent of these meningiomas are intraventricular.[14]

There is no characteristic clinical syndrome associated with trigonal meningiomas. The first symptoms may be intermittent. The signs and symptoms frequently found include headaches, personality changes, motor and sensory abnormalities, seizures, visual field defects, ataxia, alexia, and dysphasia. Preoperative visual field defects, which are important in choosing among the various surgical approaches, have been seen in 40 to 70 percent of patients in the reported series.[2,6,7,15]

A correct preoperative diagnosis of trigonal and paratrigonal tumors can usually be made from the radiologic features. The most useful studies are cerebral angiograms and computed tomographic scans. Magnetic resonance imaging does not demonstrate these lesions as clearly as CT scanning. Tumors within the ventricle at the trigone usually arise from the choroid plexus, whereas paratrigonal tumors are mainly of ependymal or glial origin. A CT scan reveals the size of the tumor and aids in differentiating paratrigonal from intraventricular neoplasms. Silver et al.[16] noted that benign trigonal tumors are homogeneous, cause localized dilatation of the lateral

ventricle, engulf the choroid plexus, and result in enlarged choroidal arteries. The paratrigonal tumors compress the lateral ventricle, displace the choroid plexus, and shift the midline to the contralateral side. The most common tumors of the choroid plexus are meningiomas and papillomas, according to Zimmerman and Bilaniuk.[17] They noted that smooth margins distinguish the benign tumors from the malignant ones. Papillomas of the choroid plexus can usually be differentiated from meningiomas by the following features: their greatest incidence is in children; they are frequently associated with asymmetric hydrocephalus; and they blush more intensely on angiograms. On CT scans, meningiomas are usually of increased density; they enhance homogeneously; and calcification is evident in 47 percent of them on CT scans but rarely on plain x-ray films.[11] There may be peritumoral edema around meningiomas, which Kendall et al.[11] related to disruption of the ependyma by the tumor. In a series reported by Mani et al.,[18] carotid angiography showed enlargement of the anterior choroidal artery in nearly half and tumor blush in 30 percent of patients with trigonal meningiomas. They noted enlargement of the posterior choroidal artery in 7 of 9 patients studied with vertebral injection. Similar findings were noted in another series.[2] However, these findings can occur with other types of intraventricular and paraventricular tumors.

There are several factors to bear in mind when considering a surgical approach to a trigonal meningioma. The tumors are frequently large, requiring piecemeal removal, as stressed by Fornari et al.[2] Early control of the arterial supply to vascular tumors is desirable, especially in children.[9,19] No single approach, however, will allow access to both the anterior and posterior choroidal arteries as a preliminary step. Cortical incisions or excessive retraction can cause neurologic deficits. In the dominant hemisphere, the result may be dyslexia or dysphasia. In either hemisphere, visual field defects can occur from surgical damage to the optic radiations or visual cortex. A preoperative right hemianopsia is a relative contraindication to a transcallosal approach but may justify a temporal or parietal incision. Cortical incisions carry a risk of postoperative epilepsy, in contrast to the low risk theoretically expected from a purely transcallosal approach.

An inferior parietal incision directly over the tumor has been used by many surgeons.[6–8,15,20–22] It has the advantage of minimizing the depth of brain transgressed, especially in very large meningiomas. However, it results in homonymous hemianopsia, since the incision cuts across the optic radiations.

OPERATIVE NEUROSURGICAL TECHNIQUES
ISBN 0-8089-1862-1

Furthermore, there is a risk to language function in the dominant hemisphere and to spatial perception in the nondominant hemisphere. Finally, neither of the main feeding arteries can be controlled early in the procedure.

Occipital lobectomy has been used to approach some trigonal meningiomas.[23] This may reduce cerebral retraction, but it has several disadvantages. Again, the vascular pedicles are not accessible early. A homonymous hemianopsia results from the procedure. Also, if the lobectomy is carried too far forward, alexia can occur secondary to damage to the angular gyrus. This was seen in 7 cases of occipital lobectomy reported by Hécaen et al.[24] Although this improved slowly over a period of months, recovery was incomplete; reading facility and enjoyment were never regained. Van Buren[25] also described a patient who developed severe dyslexia, moderate dysgraphia, and dyscalculia following occipital lobectomy. He stressed the fact that the angular gyrus is only about 3.5 cm from the tip of the occipital lobe.

A high parietal paramedian incision has been used in order to avoid the optic radiations. Fornari et al.[2] spared a normal preoperative visual field in 1 case and noted recovery of a preoperative hemianopsia in another. However, 4 previously normal patients developed a visual field defect following the procedure, probably as a result of damage to the periventricular optic radiations during tumor dissection. With this approach, no permanent speech deficits were found, but mild motor weakness was present in 3 cases. Seizures occurred in 29 percent of the patients. Parietal sensory loss was not commented upon by these authors. Astereognosis does not usually follow an incision made 2 to 3 cm from the midline in this area.[26] However, deficits of higher cortical function not apparent on routine examination may be delineated by neuropsychologic testing as a result of a parasagittal approach in the dominant hemisphere.[27] These deficits arise from disturbance of kinesthetic feedback function and damage of the tertiary parieto-occipital zone of the dominant hemisphere. Visuomotor ataxia can occur after lesions in the posterior parietal lobe and is thought to be the result of interruption of occipital-frontal or cortical-cortical connections or damage of posterior parietal neurons with supramodal integrative function.[26,30] A parasagittal incision 4 to 5 cm in length will also damage a variable number of radiating commissural fibers of the corpus callosum, which can cause deficits evident on sophisticated testing.[31]

A surgical approach through the temporal horn allows preliminary occlusion of the anterior choroidal artery. This is facilitated if the temporal horn is dilated. An incision in the posterior middle temporal gyrus is usually used.[32] Although this incision passes through the fibers of the optic radiation, it is parallel to them, lessening the damage. However, in the dominant hemisphere there is a risk to language function. Ojemann[33] showed that the cortical sites of speech representation vary greatly when mapped with electrical stimulation in awake patients. Furthermore, de la Torre et al.[9] reported a transient dysphasia in 1 of 2 patients operated on by the middle temporal gyrus approach. Finally, auditory comprehension deficits can result from retraction damage to the posterior supratemporal or supramarginal areas.[34]

Spencer and Collins[35] gain exposure to the anterior temporal horn and trigone by utilizing a limited anterior temporal lobectomy, with continuation of the exposure posteriorly in the ventricle by a more inferior temporo-occipital incision. This lessens the risk to speech centers in the dominant hemisphere. It is, however, associated with a superior quadrant field defect postoperatively. It is also conceivable that a temporary subangular alexia could result from damage to fibers from the visual cortex coming together inferior to the occipital horn or trigone in the dominant hemisphere.[36]

Kempe and Blaylock[1] described a transcallosal approach to small trigonal meningiomas of the dominant hemisphere. They utilized an occipital craniotomy in the sitting position, retraction of the occipital lobe laterally, and complete division of the splenium and posterior body of the corpus callosum to reach the choroid fissure medial to the trigone. The fissure was then opened, and the choroid plexus was followed laterally to the tumor. The mobile meningioma could then be worked medially into the operative field and removed after the feeding vessels and choroid plexus were sectioned. Theoretical advantages of the procedure include a lower incidence of postoperative seizures, no risk to speech centers, no incision in the optic radiations or cortex, and early control of the posterior choroidal blood supply to the tumor. In fact, Kempe and Blaylock[1] reported excellent results in their 3 cases; the only postoperative deficit was the persistence of a preoperative "minimal right lower quadrantanopsia" in 1 patient.

Complete section of the splenium of the corpus callosum interrupts the transfer of cortical visual information from the nondominant hemisphere to the speech centers. The resulting hemialexia in the nondominant visual field is only noticeable with tachistoscopic examination and is not clinically significant.[37,38] Kempe and Blaylock[1] did not mention evaluating their patients for this postoperatively. However, some patients who have had careful postoperative testing after splenial section have not shown the expected disconnection syndrome.[39-41] These cases can best be explained by the presence of some ventrally placed splenial fibers that have escaped section. These fibers carry interhemispheric visual information. The fear of producing the disabling disconnection syndrome, alexia without agraphia, is a significant deterrent to the transcallosal approach. When a right homonymous hemianopsia is associated with a complete splenial section, alexia without agraphia occurs. Levin and Rose[3] described this complication after removal of a trigonal meningioma via the transcallosal route. Their patient not only had a preoperative right homonymous hemianopsia, but, at surgery, developed a left occipital lobe necrosis, which prevented any chance of recovery from the hemianopsia. A preoperative right hemianopsia is a relative contraindication to the transcallosal approach, since only a small number of patients recover the visual field after surgery. Recovery of the field was seen in 1 of 12 and 3 of 9 cases in 2 reported series.[2,42] This limits the use of the procedure, because preoperative field defects have been described in 40 to 70 percent of cases.[2,6,7,15] Partial visual field defect sparing the ventral optic radiations, as in the case described by Kempe and Blaylock, may not cause this complication.[43] In patients with normal preoperative visual fields, care must be taken to avoid causing a postoperative hemianopsia. This can result from prolonged occipital lobe retraction. Chronic occipital lobe ischemia, as a result of transtentorial herniation of the posterior cerebral artery seen in some cases of large tumors, may predispose the lobe to retractor damage.[3] Finally, damage to periventricular optic radiations during tumor mobilization may cause hemianopsia.[2] Large tumors can disrupt the ependyma and become adherent to gliotic periventricular white matter,[22] increasing the risk. Peritumoral edema seen on CT scan may indicate the ependymal disruption,[11] suggesting an increased risk to visual fibers.

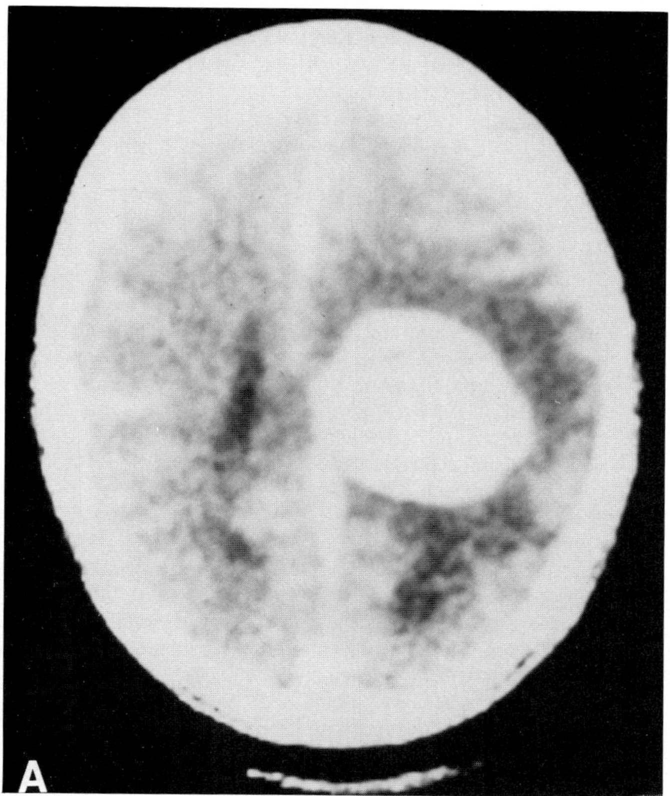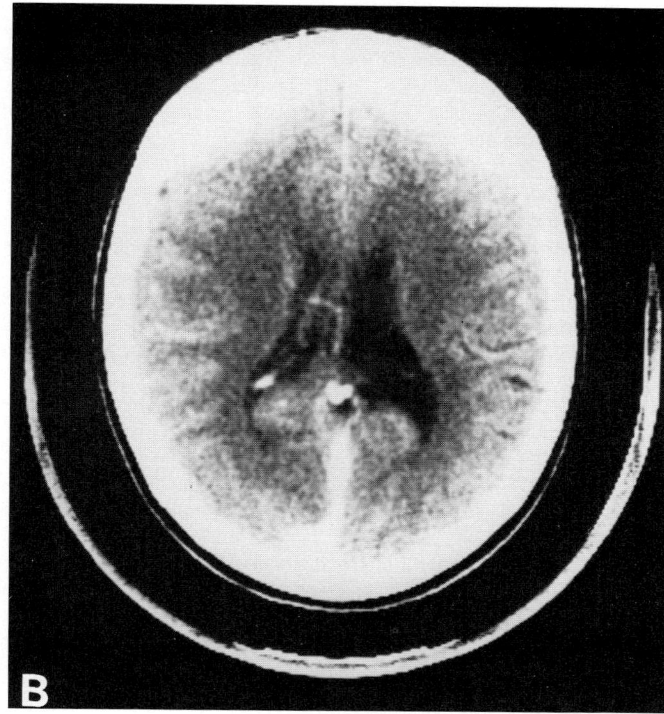

Fig. 51-1. Preoperative (A) and postoperative (B) CT scans of a 6-cm left trigonal meningioma removed via a transcallosal approach with no significant postoperative deficit.

Attention to technical details and some modifications can facilitate and lower the risks of the transcallosal approach to the trigone. Positioning the head of the patient with the tumor-containing ventricle down can minimize the retraction on the medial surface of the hemisphere.[44] The use of mannitol and hyperventilation widens the initially narrow exposure. Drainage of the cerebrospinal fluid from the posterior pericallosal, quadrigeminal, and superior cerebellar cisterns improves brain relaxation. Retraction becomes progressively easier as the tumor is debulked and cerebrospinal fluid is released from the ventricle. There is considerable variation in the length and width of the tentorial notch,[45] and it may be necessary to divide the tentorium if the tentorial notch is narrow. Large tumors may be evident under the thinned-out corpus callosum, obviating the need for tedious opening of the choroidal fissure and complete sectioning of the splenium.[4] Even a large tumor can be removed through a 2- to 3-cm incision (Figure 51-1). As the tumor is progressively gutted, it can be mobilized medially into the incision. Conceivably, meningiomas demonstrating peritumoral edema may be less mobile than other tumors. Minimizing the length of the callosal incision and saving some posteroventral fibers may prevent the development of both tactile and visual-verbal disconnection. To preserve part of the splenium, a parieto-occipital approach rather than a purely occipital one should be used, allowing the splenium to be exposed from a more vertical angle, as suggested by Greenblatt.[46] This also decreases the risk to visual cortex from retraction. The more anterior section of the corpus callosum may result in an auditory disconnection, since the auditory pathway crosses just anterior to the splenium.[4,8,46–48] However, this disconnection syndrome has no clinical importance. A parieto-occipital ap-proach may be prevented by important bridging veins, but this can be predicted from the angiogram.[44]

Meningiomas of the trigone can be successfully removed by a number of different routes. Careful consideration of the risks and demands of each approach and the nature of the preoperative deficit should lead to the correct choice. Only detailed neuropsychologic testing can give a comprehensive evaluation of the postoperative status of these patients.

REFERENCES

1. Kempe LG, Blaylock R: Lateral-trigonal intraventricular tumors: A new operative approach. Acta Neurochir 35:233, 1976
2. Fornari M, Savoiardo M, Morello G, et al: Meningiomas of the lateral ventricles: Neuroradiological and surgical considerations in 18 cases. J Neurosurg 54:64, 1981
3. Levin HS, Rose JE: Alexia without agraphia in a musician after transcallosal removal of a left intraventricular meningioma. Neurosurgery 4:168, 1979
4. Jun CL, Nutik SL: Surgical approaches to intraventricular meningiomas of the trigone. Neurosurgery, 416, 1985
5. Kempe LG: Meningiomas of the lateral ventricles (letter). J Neurosurg 54:848, 1981
6. Gassel MM, Davies H: Meningiomas in the lateral ventricles. Brain 84:605, 1961
7. Kobayashi S, Okasaki H, MacCarty CS: Intraventricular meningiomas, Mayo Clin Proc 46:735, 1971
8. Busch E: Meningiomas of the lateral ventricles of the brain. Acta Chir Scand 82:282, 1939
9. de la Torre E, Alexander E Jr, Davis CH Jr, et al: Tumors of the lateral ventricles of the brain: Report of eight cases, with suggestions for clinical management. J Neurosurg 20:461, 1963

10. Morrison G, Sobel D, Kelley W, et al: Intraventricular mass lesions. Radiology 153:435, 1984

11. Kendall B, Reider-Grosswasser I, Valentine A: Diagnosis of masses presenting within the ventricles on computed tomography. Neuroradiology 25:11, 1983

12. Ladenheim JC: Choroid Plexus Meningiomas of the Lateral Ventricles. Springfield, Ill, Charles C Thomas, 1963

13. Abbott KH, Courville CB: Intraventricular meningiomas: Review of the literature and report of two cases. Bull Los Angeles Neurol Soc 7:12, 1942

14. Merten DF, Gooding CA, Newton TH, et al: Mengiomas of childhood and adolescence. J Pediatr 84:696, 1974

15. Tukanowicz SA, Grant FC: The meningiomas of the lateral ventricles of the brain. J Neuropathol 17:367, 1958

16. Silver AJ, Ganti SR, Hilal SK: Computed tomography of tumors involving the atria of the lateral ventricles. Radiology 145:71, 1982

17. Zimmerman RA, Bilaniuk LT: Computed tomography of choroid plexus lesions. CT 3:93, 1979

18. Mani RL, Hedgcock MW, Mass SI, et al: Radiographic diagnosis of meningioma of the lateral ventricle: Review of 22 cases. J Neurosurg 49:249, 1978

19. Diehl PR, Symon LTD: Supratentorial intraventricular hemangioblastoma: Case report and review of literature. Surg Neurol 15:435, 1981

20. Cushing H, Eisenhardt L: Meningiomas: Their Classification, Regional Behavior, Life History, and Surgical End Results. Springfield, Ill, Charles C Thomas, 1938

21. Vassilouthis J, Ambrose JAE: Intraventricular meningioma in a child. Surg Neurol 10:105, 1978

22. Wall AE: Meningiomas within the lateral ventricle. J Neurol Neurosurg Psychiatry 17:91, 1954

23. Olivecrona H, Tonnis W (eds): Klinik und Behandlung der raumbeengenden intrakraniellen prozesse, in Handbuch der Neurochirurgie, ed 2, vol 4. Berlin, Springer-Verlag, 1967, pp 175–179

24. Hécaen H, de Ajuriaguerra J, David M: Les Déficits fonctionnels après lobectomie occipitale. Monatsschr Psychiatr Neurol 123:239, 1952

25. Van Buren JM: Anatomical study of a posterior cerebral lesion producing dyslexia. Neurosurgery 5:1, 1979

26. Lapras C, Deruty R, Bret P: Tumors of the lateral ventricles. Adv Tech Stand Neurosurg 11:103, 1984

27. Conley FK, Moses JA, Helle TL: Defects of higher cortical function in two patients with posterior parietal arteriovenous malformation. Neurosurgery 7:230, 1980

28. Castaigne P, Pertuiset B, Rondot P, et al: Ataxie optique dans le deux hémichamps visuels homonymes gauches après exèsrése chirurgicale d'un anevrysme artériel de la paroi du ventricule latéral. Rev Neurol I24:262, 1971

29. Castaigne P, Rondot P, Ribadeau-Dumas JL, et al: Ataxie optique localisée au côte gauche dans les deux hémichamps visuels homonymes gauches. Rev Neurol I31:23, 1975

30. Levine DN, Kaufman KJ, Mohr JP: Inaccurate reaching associated with a superior parietal lobe tumor. Neurology 28:556, 1978

31. Oepen G, Schulz-Weihing R, Zimmerman P: Long term effects of partial callosal lesions. Preliminary report. Acta Neurochir 77:22, 1985

32. Kempe LG: Lateral intraventricular tumors (choroid plexus papilloma of the lateral ventricle), in Operative Neurosurgery, vol 1. Berlin, Springer-Verlag, 1968, pp 196–202

33. Ojemann GA: Individual variability in cortical localization of language. J Neurosurg 50:164, 1979

34. Selnes OA, Knopman DS, Niccum, et al: Computed tomographic Iscan correlates of auditory comprehension deficits in aphasia: A prospective recovery study. Ann Neurol 13:558, 1983

35. Spencer DD, Collins WF: Surgical management of lateral intraventricular tumors, in Schmidek HH, Sweet WH (eds): Operative Neurosurgical Techniques: Indications, Methods, and Results, vol 1. New York, Grune & Stratton, 1982, pp 561–574

36. Greenblatt SH: Subangular alexia without agraphia or hemianopsia. Brain Lang 3:229, 1976

37. Gazzaniga MS, Freedman H: Observations on visual processes after posterior callosal section. Neurology 23:1126, 1973

38. Trescher JH, Ford FR: Colloid cyst of the third ventricle: Report of a case; operative removal with section of posterior half of corpus callosum. Arch Neurol Psychiatry 37:959, 1937

39. Ajax ET, Schenkenberg T, Kosteljanetz M: Alexia without agraphia and the inferior splenium. Neurology 27:685, 1977

40. Greenblatt SH, Saunders RL, Culver CM, et al: Normal interhemispheric visual transfer with incomplete section of the splenium. Arch Neurol 37:567, 1980

41. Vincent FM, Sadowsky, CH, Saunders RL, et al: Alexia without agraphia, heminaopsia, or color-naming defect: Disconnection syndrome. Neurology 27:689, 1977

42. Guidette B, Delfini R, Gagliardi FM: Meningiomas of the lateral ventricles. Surg Neurol 24:364, 1985

43. Greenblatt SH: Alexia without agraphia or heminaopsia: Anatomical analysis of an autopsied case. Brain 96:307, 1973

44. Collins, WF: Surgical approaches to intraventricular meningiomas of the trigone (Comment). Neurosurgery 16:419, 1985

45. Sunderland S: The tentorial notch and complications produced by herniations of the brain through that aperture. Br J Surg 45:422, 1958

46. Greenblatt SH: Neurosurgery and the anatomy of reading: A practical review. Neurosurgery 1:6, 1977

47. Damasio H, Damasio A: "Paradoxic" ear extinction in dichotic listening: Possible anatomic significance. Neurology 29:644, 1979

48. Pandya DN, Karol EA, Heilbronn D: The topographical distribution of interhemispheric projections in the corpus callosum of the rhesus monkey. Brain Res 32:31, 1971

CHAPTER 52

Surgical Management of Extensive Tumors Involving the Skull and the Scalp

Howard A. Richter

THE PURPOSE OF THIS CHAPTER is to outline a rational approach to the treatment of patients with large skull and scalp tumors excepting the skull base and face. The combined craniofacial approach to the paranasal sinuses, orbit and anterior skull base has been described by Ketchum et al.,[1] Schramm et al.,[2] and in this book by Derome.

The infratemporal approach to lesions of the temporal bone and base of the skull has been delineated by Fisch and Pillsbury[3] and glomus jugulare tumors are discussed by Gardner in this volume. The reader also is referred to chapters herein by Linton on surgery of the scalp and Olin on repair of skull defects.

Extensive tumors of the skull and scalp occur infrequently enough so that there are many scattered single-case or small series reports but no definitive review articles. Table 52-1 is a listing of tumor types, reported in a search of the literature from 1966 through 1980. It will be seen that there are benign and malignant, primary and metastatic tumors with a large variety of cell types.

It is rare that a tumor of the skull or scalp cannot be approached surgically. Although some of these lesions are formidable and initially appear to be inoperable, careful planning and use of a team approach when necessary can effect cosmetically acceptable and medically correct treatment.

Large scalp tumors often will be treated without neurosurgical consultation. Occasionally these skin tumors involve the skull and warrant neurosurgical involvement in the management. Extensive skull tumors are certainly subject to the neurosurgeon's scalpel, be it cold steel, plasma arc, ultrasonic aspirator, or laser.

Two cases are presented as specific examples. The general principles of management then will be outlined.

Case 1. A 35-year-old, right-handed woman was admitted with a "2-month" history of an enlarging mass on the right side of her head. She only came to the emergency room at the insistence of her employer, who noted the large mass on the right side of her head and overheard her complaining of double vision and headache. She also complained of right posterior neck pain. The patient claimed that the mass had increased rapidly in size over the 2 preceding months and reported a 10-pound weight loss.

Past medical history revealed that 10 years previously a mass in the left iliac region had been biopsied. She was told she had a tumor that was either a granulosa-cell tumor of the ovary or an undifferentiated sarcoma. She received x-ray treatment to the pelvic area following biopsy.

Her vital signs were normal upon admission. General physical examination revealed a grapefruit-sized, firm, nontender fixed mass in the right parietal region, extending out from the surface of the skull 12 cm (Figures 52-1 and 52-2). There was bilateral, one-diopter papilledema. There was a small well-healed scar over the left iliac crest. In all other respects her general physical examination was within normal limits. Neurologic examination was normal. Skull x-ray films showed an extensive destructive process involving the right parietal-occipital region with a large soft tissue component. Calcification in the base of the mass was seen and the mass was considered to be most likely of metastatic origin. There was an irregular bony defect in the left iliac wing on plain x-ray films. A bone scan was abnormal only with respect to the skull. A liver scan showed slight hepatomegaly without evident metastatic lesions. Bilateral carotid and vertebral arteriograms showed a very large vascular neoplasm with destruction of skull and extension to the meninges. The blood supply was predominantly through the right and left external carotid arteries.

Multiple needle biopsy specimens of this large mass were obtained in the operating room under local anesthesia. The pathologists were able to say only that the tumor was malignant and consisted of small cells. They felt the diagnosis was consistent with Ewing's sarcoma, but ovarian tumor could not be completely ruled out. Because of the extreme vascularity of this tumor, a preoperative course of radiotherapy was given. The patient was treated on the ^{60}Co Theratron 80 unit through right and left lateral parallel opposing fields with the right side being off-loaded 2 to 1. The tumor was exposed to 3600 rad in 27 lapsed days.

One week following radiation therapy, the patient was taken to the operating room and placed under general endotracheal anesthesia. The right external carotid artery was ligated at the carotid bifurcation in the neck. She was then turned to the prone position and the head was placed in a 3-point skull-fixation headrest. The tumor was positioned so that it was uppermost and pointing to the right side (Figures

Table 52-1. A survey of the extensive tumors of the scalp and skull reported in the literature

Type of Tumor	Location	Reference
Primary benign		
Aneurysmal bone cyst	skull	Chalapati et al[4]; Mufti[5]
Angioma	skull	Marchac & Cophignon[6]
Cavernous hemangioma	scalp & skull	Gupta et al[7]; Kawai et al[8]; deKlerk & Northover[9]; Wojtanowski et al[10]
Dermoid cyst	skull	Glasauer et al[11]; Ojikutu & Mordi[12]
Giant cell tumor	skull	Hlavacek & Jolma[13]
Hemangioendothelioma	scalp	Cantu[14]
Hemangiopericytoma	scalp	Tam'as et al[15]
Meningioma	skull	Galicich et al[16]; Ohaegbulam[19]; Rahoria & Gulati[20]
Osteoblastoma	skull	Doron et al[21]
Osteoma	skull	Betkowski[22]; Gorschkhov[23]; Resanovic & Stojanovic[24]
Peculiar congenital	skull & scalp	Yamada et al[25]
Plexiform neurofibroma	scalp	Garcia-Uria et al[26]
Teratoma	skull	Goretskii[27]
Turban tumor	scalp	Kupchik et al[28]
Primary malignant		
Angiosarcoma	scalp & skull	Didcott & Hammer[29]
Basal cell carcinoma	scalp & skull	Gormley & Hirsch[30]; Parkin & Steven[31]
Epidermoid carcinoma	scalp	Yamada et al[32]
Ewing's sarcoma	skull	Hara et al[33]
Fibrosarcoma	scalp	Chaudhari et al[34]
Hemangiosarcoma	scalp	Bennett et al[35]
Malignant melanoma	scalp	Close et al[36]; Simoes et al[37]; Zhang et al[38]
Osteogenic sarcoma	skull	Bito et al[39]; Caron et al[40]; Kosary et al[41]; Thompson et al[42]
Rhabdomyosarcoma	skull & scalp	Deutsch & Felder[43]
Malignant metastatic		
Breast carcinoma	scalp	Thiers et al[44]
Endometrial adenocarcinoma	scalp	Rasbach et al[45]
Hepatoma	scalp	Reingold & Smith[46]
Prostate carcinoma	skull & scalp	Peison[47]
Renal carcinoma	scalp	Livingston et al[48]
Retroperitoneal liposarcoma	scalp	Peison et al[49]
Thyroid carcinoma	skull	Hamer & Piotrowski[50]

52-3 and 52-4). An incision was drawn with methylene blue that allowed for the extensive scalp over the tumor to be excised. An exploratory incision was made over the galeal plane. Once the galeal plane was seen, an extensive scalp incision, starting in the right occipital region, extending over the temporoparietal region into the frontal region, was carried through the skin and galea, and Dandy clamps were applied to the galea on either side. The subgaleal plane was developed to expose the large, massive encapsulated tumor (Figure 52-5). The tumor was firmly attached to the skull; therefore, periosteal elevation was carried out around the tumor and multiple burr holes were placed circumferentially approximately 1½ inches apart (Figure 52-6). These were then connected with a craniotome circular saw. Once this was accomplished, the tumor mass was removed as part of a large frontoparietal, occipitotemporal craniectomy free-bone flap (Figure 52-7). The dura was carefully separated from the skull as this was accomplished. Hemostasis in the bone was secured with wax. A small tear in the lateral sinus was repaired with suture closure and a piece of Oxycel. The dura was covered with Gelfoam. The wound was vigorously irrigated. A cranioplasty (Figure 52-8) was fashioned of 20-gauge stainless steel wire mesh and methyl methacrylate and wired in place. An epidural Hemovac placed beneath the cranioplasty and another subgaleal Hemovac were left in place and brought out through separate stab wounds, and the wound was closed in two layers with 3-0 Vicryl sutures in the galea and 3-0 wire sutures in the scalp.

Postoperatively, the patient's papilledema receded rapidly. She had no neurologic deficit. She did develop a generalized macular rash with pruritus and fever. A discontinuation of the antibiotics and Dilantin led to defervescence of these symptoms. She was discharged from the hospital 18 days after surgery and was followed as an outpatient for 6 years. She had a recurrence of the malignant tumor in her hip, which has been treated by further biopsy and radiation. It is now the consensus that this was a metastatic Ewing's sarcoma. One pathologist, from the Armed Forces Institute of Pathology, still felt it might be an ovarian tumor. The patient has remained neurologically intact and has an excellent cosmetic result.

Case 2. A 73-year-old woman was admitted to the oncology service because of an 8-week history of a mass in the

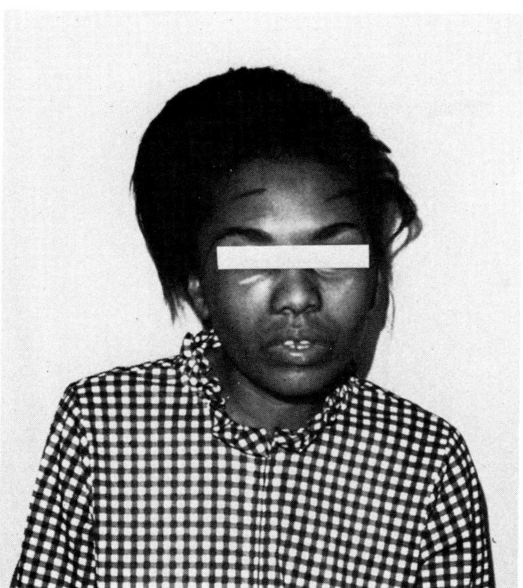

Fig. 52-1. Case 1. A frontal photograph of the patient while she was receiving radiation therapy. Note the marks on the forehead. The patient had fashioned her hair on the right side of her head to hide the large mass lesion.

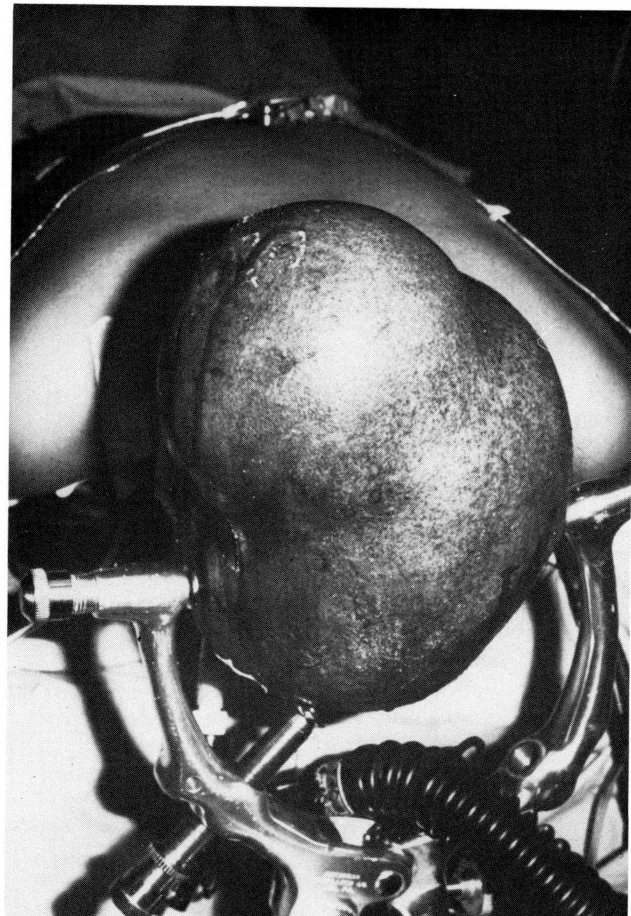

Fig. 52-3. Case 1. A photograph of the head of the patient showing the preoperative position in the skull-fixation headrest. Note the methylene-blue incision drawn over the mass.

left neck and suboccipital area. As the mass gradually enlarged she sought medical attention and was admitted to the hospital for further evaluation. No distant lesions were found on metastatic survey. A CT scan revealed a soft tissue mass in the left skull base and in the soft tissues of the suboccipital and upper cervical region.

Ten days after admission, the patient was taken to the operating room, placed under general endotracheal anesthesia, and placed in the prone position. A left paramedian cervical-occipital scalp incision was made in a routine fashion, as if to perform a suboccipital craniectomy. Immediately upon incising the galea in the occipital region, it was apparent there was a large tumor mass in the plane between the galea and skull that extended into the occipital muscles and posterior cervical muscles in the upper cervical region. The tumor was dissected to the skull and freed from the skull along the suboccipital bone.

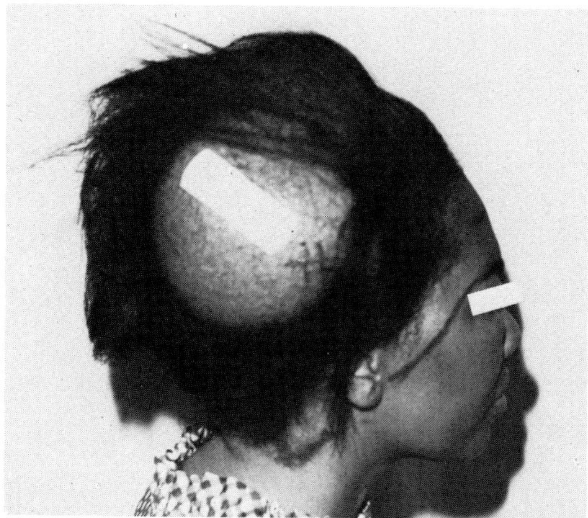

Fig. 52-2. Case 1. A lateral photograph showing the large right skull tumor. Hair has been removed over the tumor for biopsy and the patients was receiving preoperative radiation therapy.

It was attached firmly to the ligaments of the foramen magnum and the ligaments at C1, but it was possible to remove it in a subperiosteal fashion from these structures. It was then further dissected from the muscles in the cervical region and resected in a single en bloc fashion. Bleeding points were coagulated with bipolar cautery. The left occipital artery was both coagulated and ligated. The left occipital nerve had to be sectioned because it was involved in the tumor. The left vertebral artery was identified and preserved. Frozen section confirmed malignancy, and the final pathologic diagnosis was undifferentiated sarcoma. Closure of the wound was accomplished over a medium Hemovac in the large suboccipital space. The very thin scalp and neck muscle-skin combined tissue was closed with 3-0 wire. Postoperative radiation of 4000 rad was given to the entire region of the left occiput in the neck. The patient did well enough postoperatively to receive some of the radiotherapy treatments on an outpatient basis. She had no neurologic deficit following surgery. She survived in a useful fashion for 1 year and succumbed to metastatic disease.

PREOPERATIVE MANAGEMENT

Preoperative evaluation should include a careful description of the tumor, including photographs if indicated. Every patient should have a complete history, general physical and neurologic examinations, complete blood count, urinalysis, and

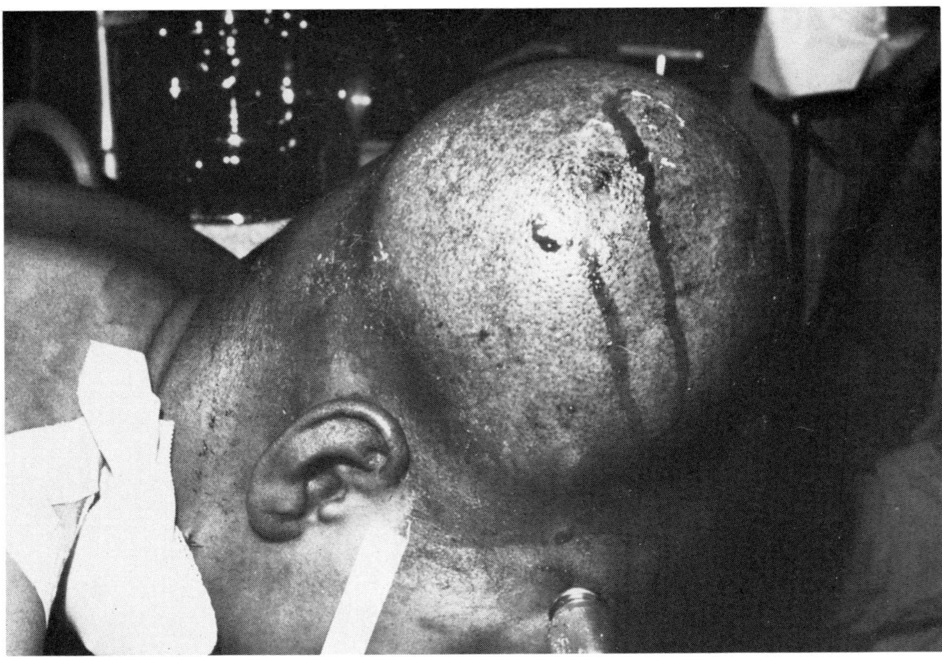

Fig. 52-4. Case 1. A lateral photograph taken from the patient's right side in the operative position. The extent of the mass clearly can be appreciated.

other routine laboratory studies as indicated by his or her age and condition and the tentative diagnosis. If the tumor appears primary in the skull or scalp and malignant, a search for metastases should be made. If the tumor appears metastatic, a search for the primary tumor and other metastases should be made. If the tumor involves the skull, x-ray films and CT scans should be obtained. Arteriography should be employed with selective external and internal carotid and vertebral injections if indicated. Consideration should be given to the desirability of preoperative needle biopsy, radiation, chemotherapy, and embolization. If extensive scalp removal is required, preoperative planning for scalp replacement is in order and may require consultations with a plastic surgeon. One of the many examples of reconstructive flap coverage for full-thickness removal of the scalp, skull, and dura is presented by Krupp.[51]

SURGICAL MANAGEMENT

The principles of tumor surgery must always be kept in mind. The tumor should be removed in its entirety and recurrence is ideally prevented by en bloc dissection whenever

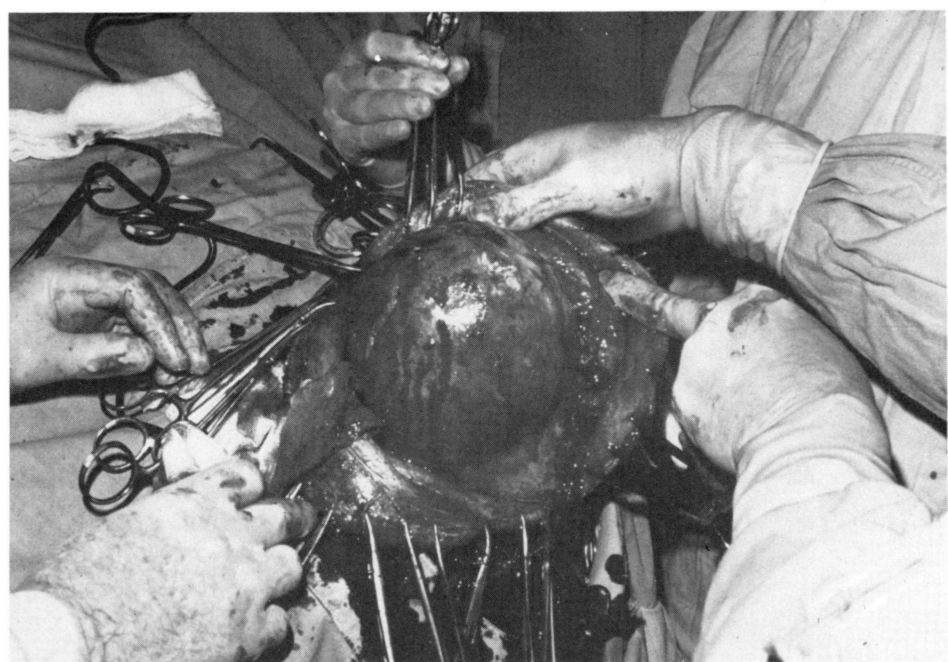

Fig. 52-5. Case 1. Subgaleal dissection of the tumor mass early in the operation. Note the hemostasis with Dandy clamps in the galeal layer.

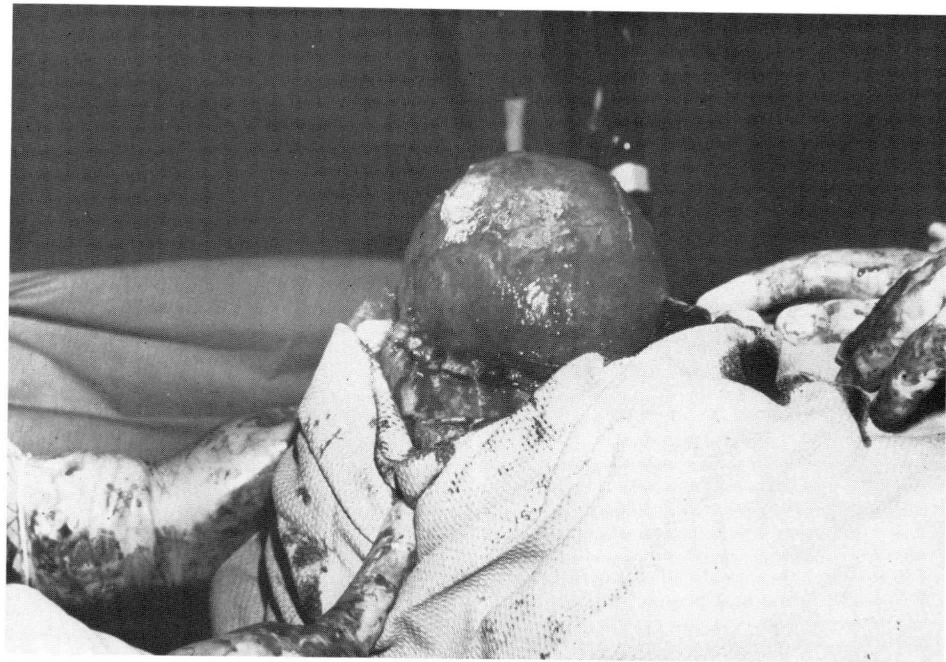

Fig. 52-6.   Case 1. The exposed tumor with burr holes and connecting cuts around the base of the tumor at its attachment to the skull.

possible. Meticulous hemostasis, adequate exposure, and careful sharp and blunt dissection are always in order. Incisions should be planned with the blood supply of the scalp, exposure of the lesion, and reconstruction after removal in mind. If scalp loss will be coincident with a large dural exposure, coverage with a full-thickness flap is desirable. It is often wise to repair the cranial defect at a later date. Split-thickness grafts take very well on pericrania or bleeding skulls, but rotated flaps may be more desirable for cosmetic reasons, particularly in the frontal or hair-bearing areas. Resection of redundant scalp after removal of a large skull lesion also must be planned.

If the tumor involves only the outer table of the skull, it can often be gouged and chiseled out without disturbing the integrity of the inner table. When full-thickness skull removal is necessary, burr holes and saw cuts should be made circumferentially outside the margin of the tumor. If the tumor compresses the underlying brain, it is important to use anti-edema measures, anticonvulsants, proper anesthesia, and care-

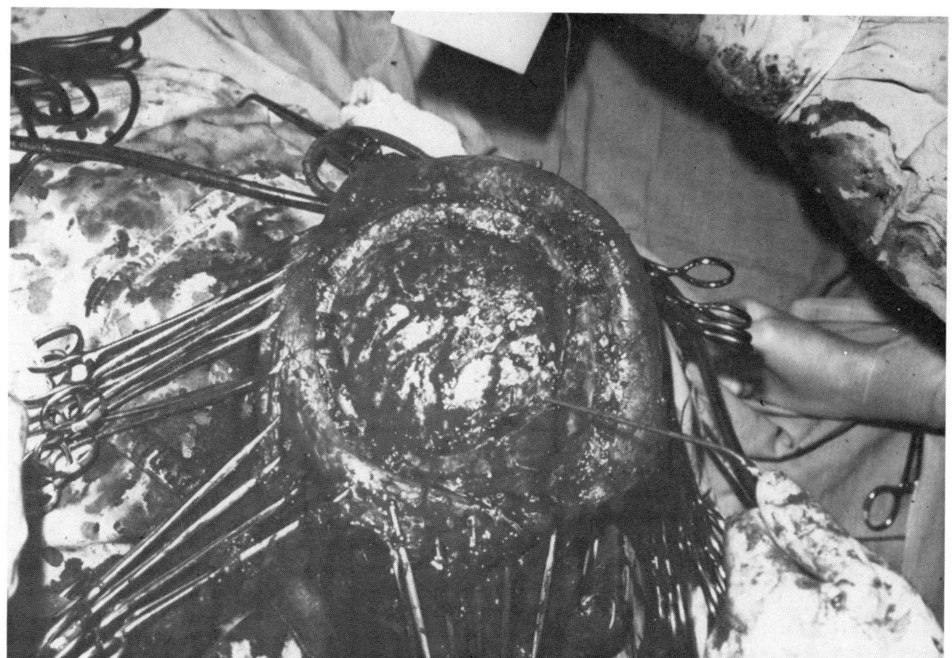

Fig. 52-7.   Case 1. A photograph of the site after complete removal of tumor with the dura exposed. The bony margins were negative for tumor circumferentially.

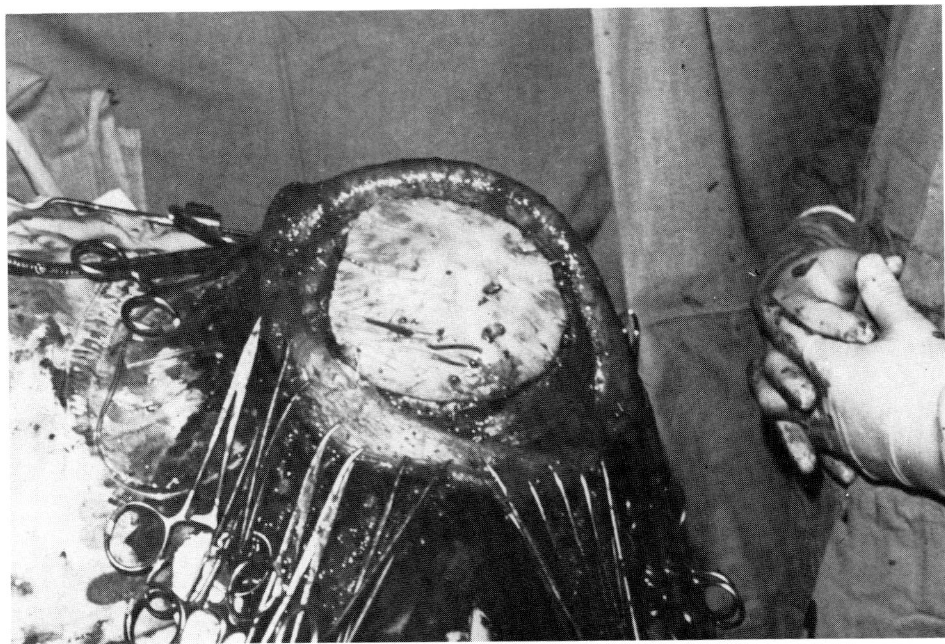

Fig. 52-8. Case 1. The cranioplasty, composed of 20-gauge stainless steel mesh and methyl methyacrylate, completed and in place.

ful positioning to prevent swelling of the brain and trauma during removal. Careful separation of the dura from the portion of the skull being removed must be accomplished. In this regard, liberal use of multiple burr holes is advised. If the tumor invades the dura, the involved dura should be excised. If the tumor invades the brain, meticulous dissection of the tumor from the brain is required using microsurgical and bipolar techniques as necessary. Tenting the dura to the pericranium to prevent epidural hematoma is advised when feasible. Dural repair can be performed with temporalis fascia, fascia lata, or lyophilized human cadaver dura. I prefer the latter. Dural suturing with 4-0 silk is customary, but if absorbable sutures are desired, 4-0 Vicryl may be used. When the scalp can be closed primarily, it is recommended that skull defects be repaired. I perform cranioplasty with 20-gauge stainless steel mesh coated with methyl methacrylate and secured with 2-0 wire. If there is any question about brain swelling, a subdural or epidural silicone rubber catheter can be placed, brought out through separate stab wound, and used to monitor intracranial pressure. I frequently place a medium Hemovac drain in the subgaleal space, which is also brought out through a separate stab wound. Scalp closure is preferable in two layers. Sutures of 3-0 Vicryl in the galea and 3-0 wire in the skin work very well. Routine use of intraoperative antibiotic prophylaxis is recommended. I use 1.0 g cephalosporin administered by IV push when the skin incision is made and 1.0 g administered by slow IV during the procedure. An additional 1.0 g by IV push is given every 4 hours while the scalp is open. Steroids are not recommended unless there is preoperative evidence of increased intracranial pressure or focal cerebral compression. If dural exposure is planned, phenytoin is used pre-, intra-, and postoperatively for 30 days. If a patient is allergic to phenytoin, appropriate substitute drugs are used. Intraoperative hemorrhage greater than 1000 ml should be replaced.

POSTOPERATIVE MANAGEMENT

Proper care after surgery must never be neglected. The cliche that "the operation was a success but the patient died" can be avoided by strict attention to detail in postoperative management. I treat patients who have had an extensive skull and scalp tumors removed as carefully as if they had just had a deep brain tumor removed. Monitoring in an intensive care unit is clearly in order with all that it implies. Monitoring the patient's airway, vital signs, neurologic status, blood gases, chemistries, and intake and output must be vigilant. If a subgaleal drain has been used, it is removed and the head re-dressed at 48 hours, unless the drainage is excessive. Catheters for monitoring ICP are removed when no longer needed; this depends directly on the neurologic examination and the ICP measurement. I do not hesitate to monitor arterial and venous pressures if warranted and have even used Swan-Ganz catheters in appropriate circumstances.

If a patient deteriorates neurologically in the postoperative period, a CT scan usually will differentiate between edema, subdural hematoma, and epidural hematoma. Prompt re-exploration and evacuation of the hematomas or removal of the cranioplasty plates may save the patient's life. If postoperative fever persists without explanation, it may be advisable to assume that the cranioplasty is the cause and remove it.

The sutures usually are removed on the seventh postoperative day, but in patients receiving x-ray treatment or chemotherapy, a delay may be indicated. Discharge from the hospital is dictated by the patient's condition.

SUMMARY

In this chapter an overview of the surgical management of extensive skull and scalp tumors has been presented. Specific references to all tumor types reported in the last 15 years may be found by consulting Table 52-1 and the reference list. Two cases from the author's experience were presented for illustration, and the general principles of pre-, intra-, and postoperative care have been summarized. It is hoped that a neurosurgeon facing his or her first tumor of this type would use this chapter as a guide and that the experienced colleague might find a reference to a fine point not previously considered.

REFERENCES

1. Ketcham AS, Wilkins RH, VanBuren JM: A combined intracranial facial approach to the paranasal sinuses. Am J Surg 106:698, 1963

2. Schramm VL Jr, Myers EN, Maroon JC: Anterior skull base surgery for benign and malignant disease. Laryngoscope 89:1077, 1979

3. Fisch U, Pillsbury HC: Intratemporal fossa approach to lesions of the temporal bone and base of skull. Arch Otolaryngol 105:99, 1979

4. Chalapati KV, Rao BS, Reddy CP, et al: Aneurysmal bone cyst of the skull. Case report. J Neurosurg 47:633, 1977

5. Mufti ST: Aneurysmal bone cyst of the skull. Case report. J Neurosurg 49:730, 1978

6. Marchac D, Cophignon J: [Angioma and fronto-orbital bone swelling: complete excision and immediate bone restoration]. (French) Ann Chir Plast 17:73, 1972

7. Gupta SD, Tiwari IN, Pasupathy NK: Cavernous hemangioma of the frontal bone. Case report. Br J Surg 62:330, 1975

8. Kawai K, Fukui M, Tanaka A, et al: Extracerebral cavernous hemangioma of the middle fossa. Surg Neurol 9:19, 1978

9. deKlerk DJ, Northover RC: Giant haemangiomas of the scalp. A report of 2 cases. S Afr Med J 55:59, 1979

10. Wojtanowski MH, Mandal MA: Seizures abolished by excision of a cavernous hemangioma of the scalp and skull. Plast Reconstr Surg 64:831, 1979

11. Glasauer FE, Levy LF, Auchterlonie WC: Congenital inclusion dermoid cyst of the anterior fontanelle. J Neurosurg 48:274, 1978

12. Ojikutu NA, Mordi VP: Congenital inclusion dermoid cyst located over the region of the anterior fontanelle in adult Nigerians: Report of two cases. J Neurosurg 52:724, 1980

13. Hlavacek V, Jolma VH: Giant cell tumors of bone in the ENT organs. Report of two cases in the frontal sinus. Acta Otolaryngol 77:374, 1974

14. Cantu RC: Successful excision of a giant scalp hemangioendothelioma in an infant. Int Surg 53:293, 1970

15. Tam'as A, Korom L, Csepregi E, et al: [Recurrent hemangiopericytoma of the scalp]. Orv Hetil 120:1637, 1979

16. Galicich JH, Robinson JS, Beattie EJ, et al: Extradural angioblastic meningioma presenting as a neck mass. 1CDB/80/67516, Clin Bull 10:21, 1980

17. Siegel GJ, Anderson PJ: Extracalvarial meningioma. Case Report. J Neurosurg 25:83, 1966

18. Smith AT, Selecki BR, Stening WA: Ectopic meningioma. Med J Aust 1:1100, 1973

19. Ohaegbulam SC: Ectopic epidural calvarial meningioma. Surg Neurol 12:33, 1979

20. Rahoria SK, Gulati DR: Intraosseous meningioma. A case report. Neurol India 26:79, 1978

21. Doron Y, Gruszkiewica J, Gelli B, et al: Benign osteoblastoma of vertebral column and skull. Surg Neurol 7:86, 1977

22. Betkowski A: Osteoma of temporal squama. Wiad Lek 28:137, 1975

23. Gorshkhov VM: [Osteoma of the frontal sinuses and the ethmoid labyrinth]. Vestn Otorinolaringol 35:86, 1973

24. Resanovic D, Stojanovic S: [Osteomas of the head]. Med Preg 125:163, 1972

25. Yamada H, Sakata K, Kashiki Y, et al: Peculiar congenital parieto-occipital head tumor: Report of 3 cases. Childs Brain 5:426, 1979

26. Garcia-Uria J, Sola RG, Carrillo R, et al: Epicranial plexiform neurofibroma. Surg Neurol 11:390, 1979

27. Goretski KG: [Case of mastoid teratoma]. Zh Ushn Nos Gorl Bolezn 2:105, 1977

28. Kupchik BM, Kozlov VG, Kripalski LN: [Treatment of an extensive turban tumor of the scalp (in a single observation)]. Vopr Onkol 12:77, 1973

29. Didcott C, Hammer A: Harare staff round: Angio-sarcoma of the scalp with penetration to involve brain. Cent Afr J Med 18:214, 1972

30. Gormley DE, Hirsch P: Aggressive basal cell carcinoma of the scalp. Arch Dermatol 114:782, 1978

31. Parkin JL, Stevens MH: Basal cell carcinoma of the temporal bone. Otolaryngol Head Neck Surg 87:645, 1979

32. Yamada S, Schuh FD, Harvin JS, et al: Enblock subtotal temporal bone resection for cancer of the external ear. J Neurosurg 39:370, 1973

33. Hara N, Kaneko H, Inoue K, et al: [Primary Ewing's sarcoma of the temporal bone—case report (author's transl)]. No Shinkei Geka 8:557, 1980

34. Chaudhari AB, Ladapo F, Duncan JT: Fibrosarcoma of the scalp. Case report. J Neurosurg 49:893, 1978

35. Bennett RG, Keller JW, Ditty JF Jr: Hemangiosarcoma subsequent to radiotherapy for hemangioma in infancy. J Dermatol Surg Oncol 4:881, 1978

36. Close LG, Goepfert H, Ballantyne AJ, et al: Malignant melanoma of the scalp. Laryngoscope 89:1189, 1979

37. Sim-oes JC, Abr-ao T, Gulin D, et al: [Epidermoid carcinoma of the scalp with disseminated bone metastases]. AMB 25:111, 1979

38. Zhang GY, Yan GH, Chen YT, et al: Experiences in surgical treatment of carcinoma of the scalp. Plast Reconstr Surg 64:622, 1979

39. Bito S, Sakaki S, Gohma T: Primary osteosarcoma of the skull—a case report (author's transl). Neurol Surg 4:191, 1976

40. Caron AS, Hajdu SL, Strong EW: Osteogenic sarcoma of the facial and cranial bones. A review of forty-three cases. Am J Surg 122:719, 1971

41. Kosary IZ, Braham J, Bubis JJ: Primary osteogenic sarcoma of the skull. Case report. J Neurosurg 25:87, 1966

42. Thompson JB, Patterson RH Jr, Parsons H: Sarcomas of the calvaria; surgical experience with 14 patients. J Neurosurg 32:534, 1970

43. Deutsch M, Felder H: Rhabodomyosarcoma of the ear-mastoid. Laryngoscope 84:586, 1974

44. Thiers H, Moulin G, Perrot H: [Cephalic cutaneous metastasis 20 years after cancer of the breast]. Lyon Med 217:1195, 1967

45. Rasbach D, Hendricks A, Stoltzner G: Endometrial adenocarcinoma metastatic to the scalp. Arch Dermatol 114:1708, 1978

46. Reingold IM, Smith BR: Cutaneous metastases from hepatomas. Arch Dermatol 114:1045, 1978

47. Peison B: Metastasis of carcinoma of the prostate to the scalp. Simulation of a large sebaceous cyst. Arch Dermatol 104:301, 1971

48. Livingston WD Jr, Becker DW Jr, Lentz CW III: Solitary scalp metastasis as the presenting feature of a renal carcinoma. J Plast Surg 30:319, 1977

49. Peison B, Benisch B, Williams MC: Retroperitoneal liposarcoma metastatic to scalp. Arch Dermatol 114:1358, 1978

50. Hamer J, Piotrowski W: [Tumor of the cranium in metastasizing thyroid adenoma]. Zentralbl Neurochir 34:139, 1974

51. Krupp S, Levy A: Coverage of large defects of skin, galea, periosteum, bone and dura with transposition flaps of skin and galea, in Chambers RG, et al (eds): Cancer of the Head and Neck. Amsterdam, Excerpta Medica, 1975, pp 357–361

CHAPTER 53

Craniofacial Resection for Anterior Skull Base Tumors

Narayan Sundaresan　　　Ved Sachdev　　　George Krol

THE COMBINED CRANIOFACIAL APPROACH for anterior skull base tumors is based on the concept of en bloc surgical resection of malignant and aggressive tumors involving the anterior cranial fossa. When successfully accomplished, it can be regarded as the best procedure that allows local control of the wide variety of neoplasms arising in this region.[1–15] Tumors involving the anterior skull base may be divided into three major groups: (1) primary tumors of the paranasal sinuses that involve the cribriform plate and extend intracranially; (2) other neoplasms arising from the skin or appendages (lacrimal gland) that may ultimately erode into the orbit and anterior cranial fossa; and (3) primary intracranial tumors arising from the basal meninges (meningioma) or metastases that originate within the cranium and extend extracranially into the sinuses.

Malignant tumors of the paranasal sinuses are rare,[16–21] with an annual estimated incidence of less than 1:100,000 population. These cancers account for less than 3 percent of all reported cancers in the United States. Compounding the rarity are the diverse histologic types that develop within this anatomic area, all with a significantly different biologic behavior.[22–25] Paranasal sinus tumors predominate in the fifth and sixth decades of life, with a general male preponderance by a ratio of 2:1. The ethmoid sinuses represent the primary site in 5 to 30 percent of such cancers, although frequently the site of origin may not always be obvious in locally advanced tumors (Figure 53-1). Carcinoma of the ethmoid sinuses also represents an occupational hazard in workers exposed to nickel, chromates, polyaromatic hydrocarbons, as well as organic dusts, especially from hardwoods.[26] The most common epithelial tumor is the epidermoid cancer, followed by undifferentiated and adenocarcinoma; less than one third are tumors of minor salivary gland origin.[22] A variety of sarcomas also arise within this region, as well as other tumors including lymphomas, melanoma, and ectopic meningiomas. Of particular interest is the esthesioneuroblastoma, which is encountered in a younger age group.[27–29] These tumors constitute a rare group of tumors of neural crest origin which arise from the olfactory neuroepithelium high in the nasal cavity in close proximity to the

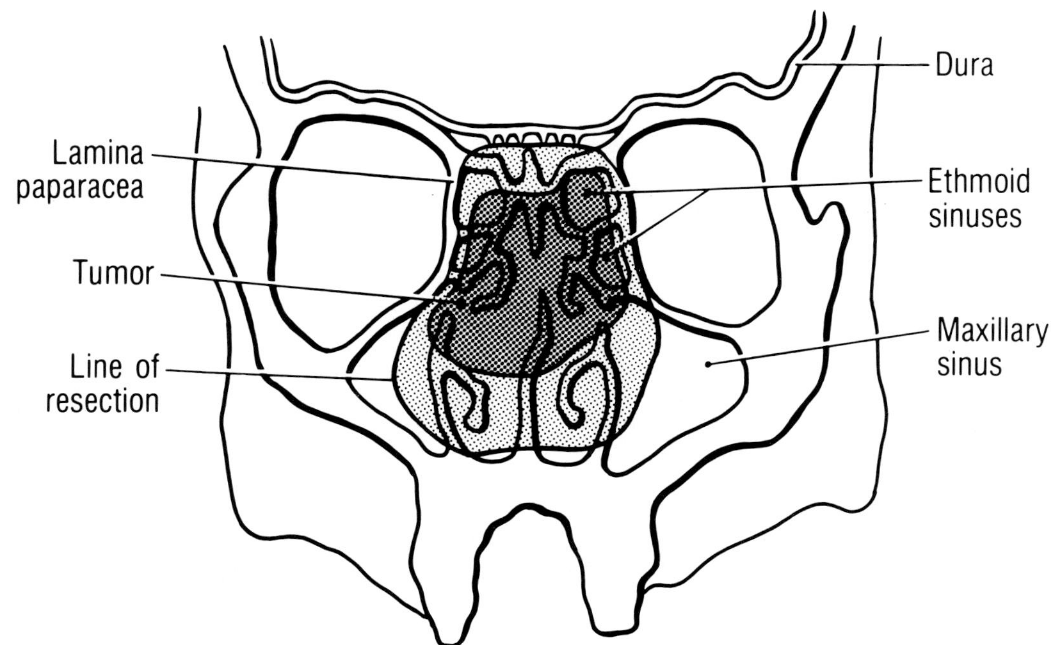

Fig. 53-1. Anatomic line drawing depicting sites of origin of paranasal tumors with anterior cranial fossa invasion.

OPERATIVE NEUROSURGICAL TECHNIQUES
ISBN 0-8089-1862-1

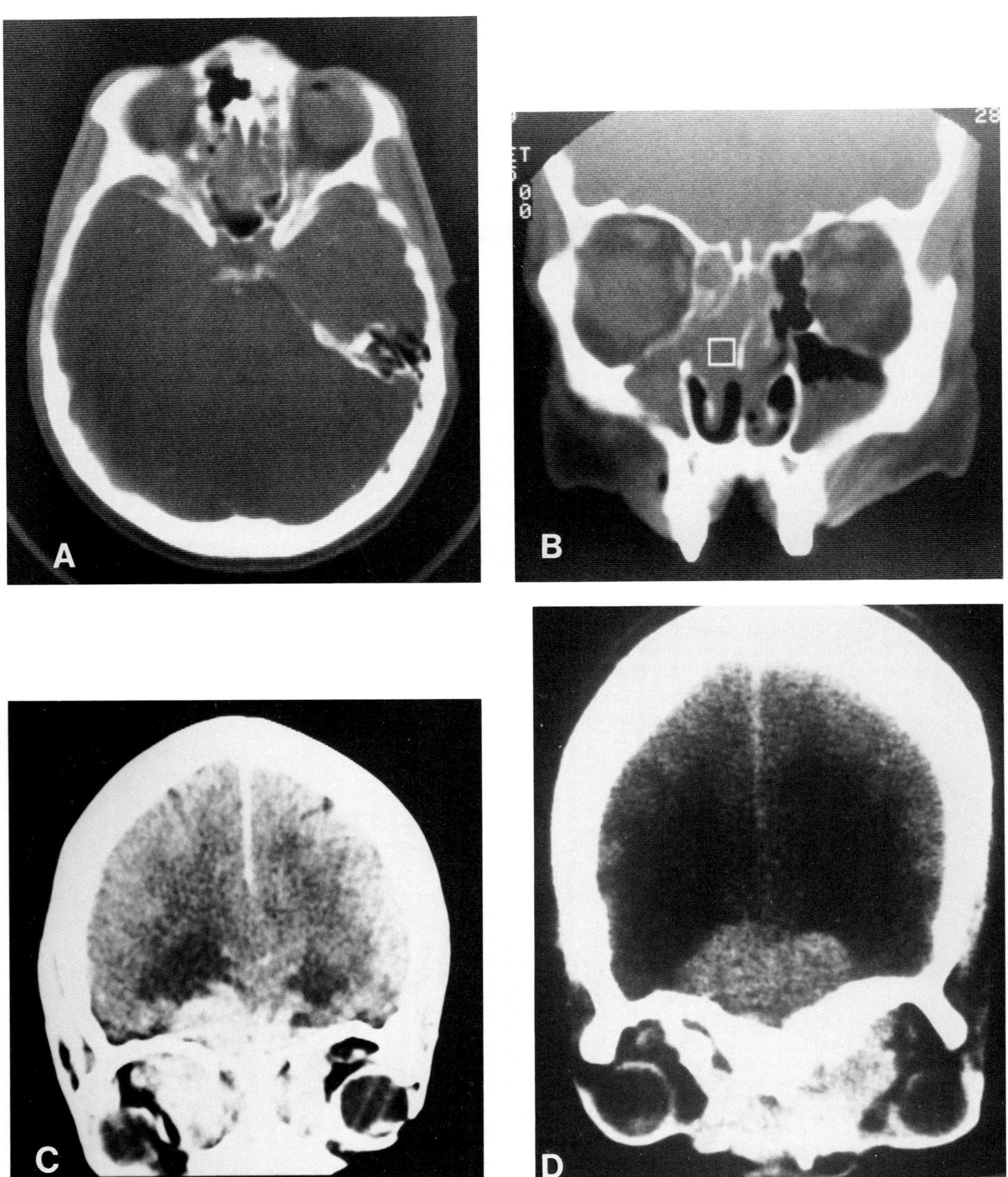

Fig. 53-2

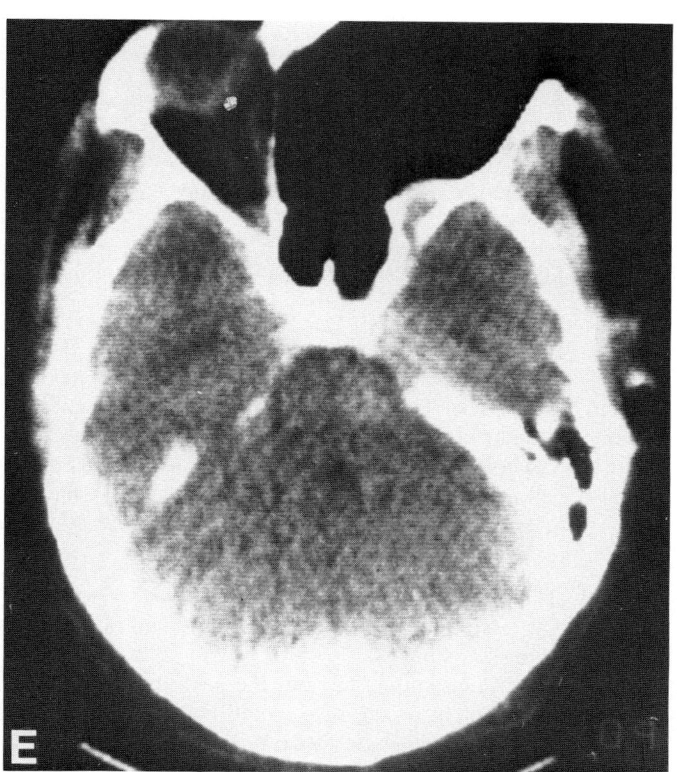

Fig. 53-2. Computed tomographic scans in the (A) axial and (B) coronal plane showing tumor configuration in two planes. (C) Coronal CT scan with contrast showing intracranial invasion by poorly differentiated ethmoid cancer. Despite intracranial invasion, craniofacial resection was successfully accomplished. (D) Coronal CT scan showing another example of intracranial and paranasal sinus involvement by meningioma. These patients require combined craniofacial approaches for tumor resection. (E) Postoperative CT scan showing completed resection. Follow-up CT scans should be obtained periodically to rule out tumor recurrence.

cribriform plate. The vast majority of reported cases in the literature have been diagnosed only within the past two decades, mainly because of an increased awareness of this neoplasm by clinicians and pathologists. We would agree with Newbill et al.[29] that any nasal tumor in which the biopsy report is read as "undifferentiated carcinoma" should be suspected of being an esthesioneuroblastoma until definitive electron-microscopic studies exclude squamous carcinoma or lymphoma. The diagnosis of esthesioneuroblastoma is based on light-microscopic findings of (1) plexiform intercellular neurofibrils; (2) poorly defined or nonexisting cytoplasm; (3) round to oval nuclei; (4) palisading sheets of neoplastic cells separated into lobules by slender vascular fibrous septa, and (5) true rosettes or pseudorosettes. The demonstration of argyrophilic reaction with the Gremelius or the fume-induced fluorescence technique may aid in identifying biogenic amines in this tumor by light microscopy. Under electron microscopy, the presence of neurosecretory granules, cytoplasmic fibrils, and microtubules can also be seen. The clinical presentation of all paranasal sinus tumors and nasal cavity tumors is relatively uniform; they consist of nonspecific sinus discharge or obstruction, nasal stuffiness, with occasional epistaxis. These symptoms may be attributed to "sinusitis" or "allergic rhinitis" and treated conservatively with antibiotic therapy until there is further progression of disease. Plain roentgenographic findings of this region are generally unrewarding in the early stages, with the result that median duration of symptoms is generally 6 months before establishment of the proper diagnosis (unless epistaxis is present). Symptoms suggesting extension of tumor *outside* the sinuses include anosmia (secondary to involvement of the olfactory nerves), visual symptoms resulting from orbital invasion, anesthesia or pain in the cheek from involvement of the maxillary nerve, and trismus secondary to invasion of the pterygoid fossa. Clinical assessment should therefore include a complete neurologic examination of the cranial nerves II–VI, as

well as endoscopic evaluation of the nasal cavity and posterior nasopharynx. Regional lymphadenopathy should be sought, although early lymphatic metastases are relatively uncommon in these tumors. Hematogenous dissemination is rare except in patients with embryonal rhabdomyosarcoma and lymphomas. Radiologic evaluation should include both plain x-ray films of the skull including sinus views, as well as computed tomographic (CT) scans obtained in the transverse and coronal planes.[30–33] With the advent of CT scans, most other studies for evaluation of tumors within this region are superfluous (Figure 53-2A and B). For axial studies, a series of transverse sections at 5–10-mm intervals are taken parallel to Reid's baseline, and coronal sections are taken at 60 to 80 degrees to Reid's baseline using the hanging-head technique to obtain an additional 15 percent angulation. In patients with paranasal sinus tumors, sinus opacification is common and may suggest a more extensive tumor than is actually present. A soft-tissue tumor mass extending beyond the bony confines of the sinuses is frequently seen in most patients. This soft-tissue extension should be carefully sought, both in the infra-temporal fossa and in the parapharyngeal space. In these regions, tumor can be recognized as a well-defined mass or simply as a loss of soft tissue planes between the muscles and the surrounding fat. Enhancement following contrast injection is rarely noted with tumors within the sinuses but may be seen when intracranial extension is present (Figure 53-2C). With the use of thin sections and bone windows, invasion of the skull base should be carefully evaluated together with the radiologist. The critical areas that determine operability include the pterygoid region, nasopharynx, sphenoid sinus, cribriform plate, and orbital apex. To determine early involvement of the cribriform plate, coronal scans are the most helpful in determining whether a craniofacial procedure is required, or whether the tumor can be successfully extirpated from below using a maxillectomy approach We now use cerebral

Table 53-1. TNM American Joint Committee staging system for carcinoma of the paranasal sinuses

T1: Tumor confined to the antral mucosa of the infrastructure* with no bone erosion or destruction.
T2: Tumor confined to the suprastructure† or mucosa without bone destruction or to the infrastructure with destruction of the medial or inferior walls only.
T3: More extensive tumor invading skin of cheek, orbit, anterior ethmoid sinuses, or pterygoid muscles.
T4: Massive tumor with invasion of the cribriform plate, posterior ethmoids, sphenoids, hypopharynx, pterygoid plate, or base of skull.

* Structures lying anteroinferior to Ohngren's line (an imaginary plane running between the angle of the mandible and the medial canthus).
† Structures lying posterosuperior to Ohngren's line.

angiography only when a hypervascular tumor is suspected, for presurgical embolization, or for intra-arterial therapy.

PREOPERATIVE EVALUATION AND PATIENT SELECTION

All patients should undergo an initial biopsy to determine the histologic nature of the tumor, which allows proper treatment planning. The American Joint Committee uses the TNM staging system for paranasal sinus cancer,[34] but this classification is applicable mainly to tumors arising in the maxillary antrum (Table 53-1). The severity of disease as represented by tumor extension into sinuses may elevate the T1 stage to T4 when the ethmoid, sphenoid, cribriform, or pterygoid areas are involved; all patients undergoing craniofacial surgery have T4 lesions. In patients with esthesioneuroblastoma, the staging system proposed by Kadish[27] is generally used:

Stage A: Tumor confined to the nasal cavity.
Stage B: Disease confined to the nasal cavity and one or more paranasal sinuses.
Stage C: Disease extending beyond the nasal cavity including involvement of the orbit, skull base, cervical lymph nodes, or metastatic disease.

Occasionally, the decision to perform a combined craniofacial procedure can only be made at the time of operation, pending biopsy evaluation of nonspecific involvement of the ethmoid and cribriform plate. We cannot overemphasize the value of close cooperation between the neurosurgeon and the surgical oncologist in careful patient selection for optimal management of these tumors.

Once the decision for craniofacial resection has been made, and accepted by the patient, we prefer to institute steroid coverage (dexamethasone 4 mg p.o. q6h) 48 hours before surgery. Antibiotics beginning 6 hours before surgery are routinely used and continued during the perioperative period after nasal cultures have been taken. It is also important to have the patient evaluated by a prosthodontist before surgery for the prefabrication of a temporary and permanent maxillary prosthesis.

OPERATIVE TECHNIQUE*

Our techniques of craniofacial surgery have been described in several previous reports[6,7,35] and are described specifically from the neurosurgeon's viewpoint. General anesthesia using oral endotracheal intubation is used in all patients, and the oral cavity packed with gauze. Because of the propensity for blood loss in some tumors, arterial lines and central venous pressure monitoring are routinely used. Although some authors have advocated a preliminary tracheostomy, we have rarely had to use it. As soon as the patient is anesthetized, the thigh is prepared and two split-thickness skin grafts are obtained and preserved in antibiotic and saline solution. The patient is then turned to his or her side, and a constant spinal drainage system instituted. We prefer to leave an indwelling catheter in place, which is inserted through a 14-gauge Touhy needle through the fourth or fifth lumbar interspace. Following these maneuvers,

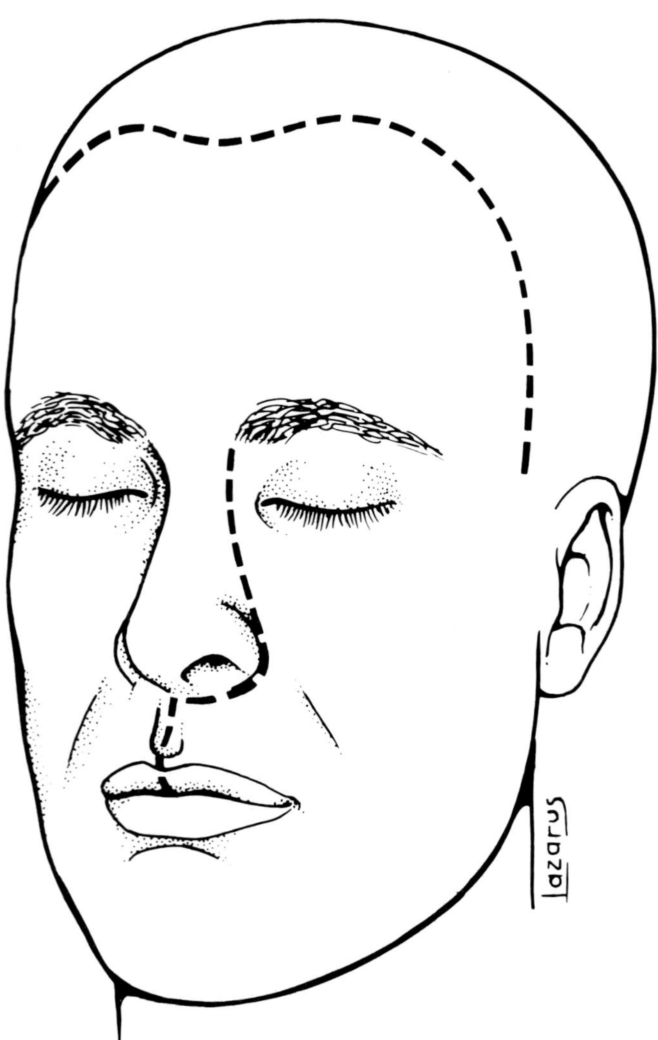

Fig. 53-3. Skin incisions include a bicoronal scalp incision for craniotomy and a Weber-Ferguson incision for the facial approach.

---

*The technical details of the operative procedure vary considerably, especially those used at Mount Sinai Hospital by one of the coauthors (V.S.) and H. Biller, MD.

the patient is positioned in the Mayfield headrest, and the head shaved and prepared. The decision to use the Mayfield skull clamps or the U-shaped rest is based on individual preference. It is important, however, to keep the head elevated 30 degrees and at the same time extended so that the base of the anterior cranial fossa can be visualized without retraction of the brain. Both the face and head are prepared with Betadine solution, and the skin incisions outlined with methylene blue. We prefer a bicoronal incision, which allows a bifrontal craniotomy, and a modified Weber-Ferguson incision for the facial approach (Figure 53-3). The skin is infiltrated with 1:200,000 epinephrine solution with Xylocaine ½ percent. After the skin incision is made, both galeal edges are held either with Dandy hemostats or scalp clips for additional hemostasis. We prefer to use the subgaleal plane for dissection because additional pericranium can be obtained by retracting the posterior edge of the flap as far back as possible to harvest the pericranium (Figure 53-4). The pericranium itself is dissected from the outer table of the skull with periosteal elevators, and the temporalis muscles on either side are stripped from the superior temporal lines using cautery. The subperiosteal dissection should proceed inferiorly to the supraorbital ridges and glabella. An oscillating saw (a trephine can also be substituted) is then used to remove the anterior wall of the frontal sinus (Figure 53-5). The mucosa of the frontal sinus is removed completely with pituitary rongeurs, and the sinus packed with Gelfoam. A formal bifrontal craniotomy is performed by making six other burr holes, which are then connected by means of a craniotome or Gigli saw (Figures

53-6A and B). The posterior wall of the frontal sinus can also be drilled out with a high-powered drill or removed piecemeal with rongeurs. The inferior cut of the craniotomy should be flush with the supraorbital ridges. The dura is carefully separated from the inner table with curved Penfield dissectors. In older female patients with hyperostosis frontalis interna, or others who have received prior radiotherapy, this dissection may result in tears of the cranial dura. Once the free bone flap is elevated, all dural tears should be repaired, and the superior sagittal sinus covered with Avitene (microfibrillar collagen) and Gelfoam.

The decision to perform an extradural or intradural dissection depends on whether the tumor has extended intracranially. For the more standard extradural dissection, self-retaining retractors of the Greenberg or Leyla variety are positioned. For extradural exposures, the posterior wall of the frontal sinus is removed with rongeurs or a high-speed drill, and the dura gently stripped from the floor of the anterior cranial fossa (Figures 53-7A and B). Using sharp microdissection, the dura should be freed on either side of the crista galli, which protrudes into the dura. The crista is removed with fine Leksell or needle-nosed rongeurs. The olfactory rootlets are cut sharply at this level, and the dissection proceeds posteriorly towards the planum sphenoidale. The dura is protected with cottonoids and stripped laterally from the orbital roofs. These maneuvers are facilitated

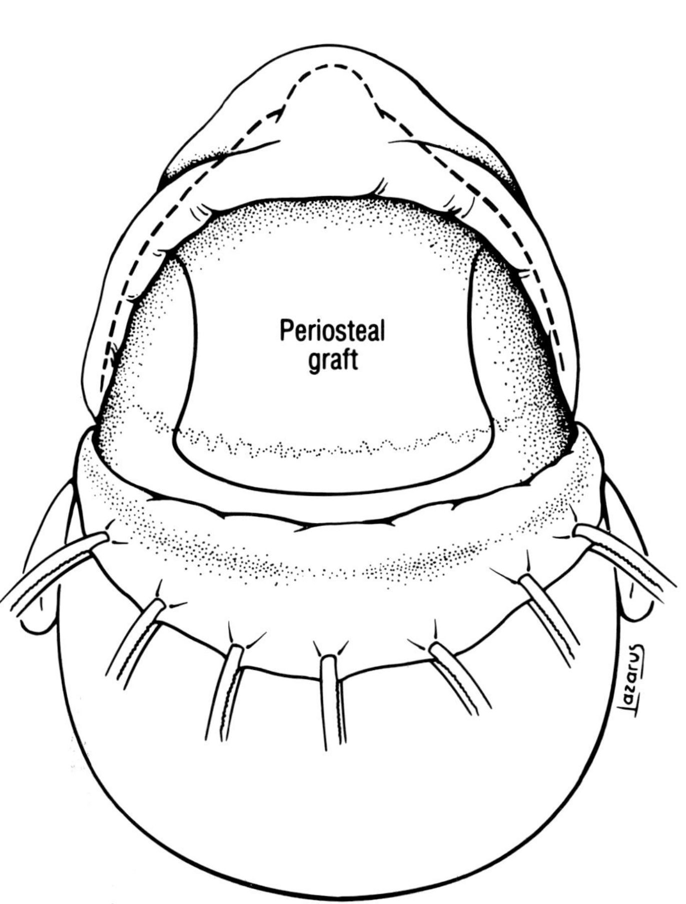

Fig. 53-4. Drawing showing reflection of the scalp flap posteriorly to harvest the periosteal (pericranium) graft.

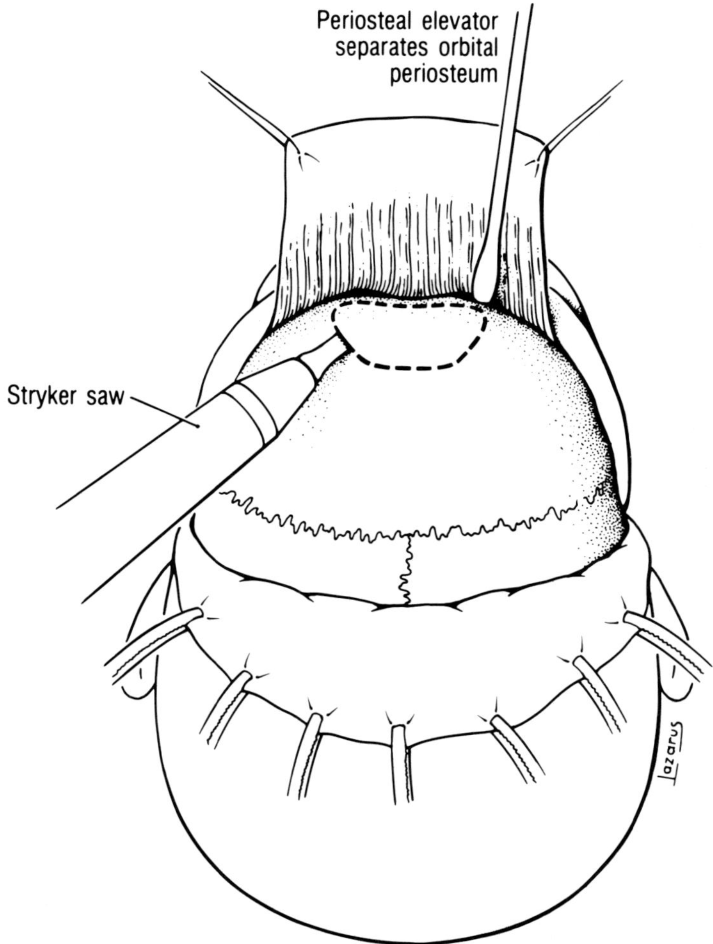

Fig. 53-5. Using a Stryker saw, the anterior wall of the frontal sinus is removed for cosmetic closure. The mucosa of the frontal sinus is removed completely and sinuses packed with Gelfoam.

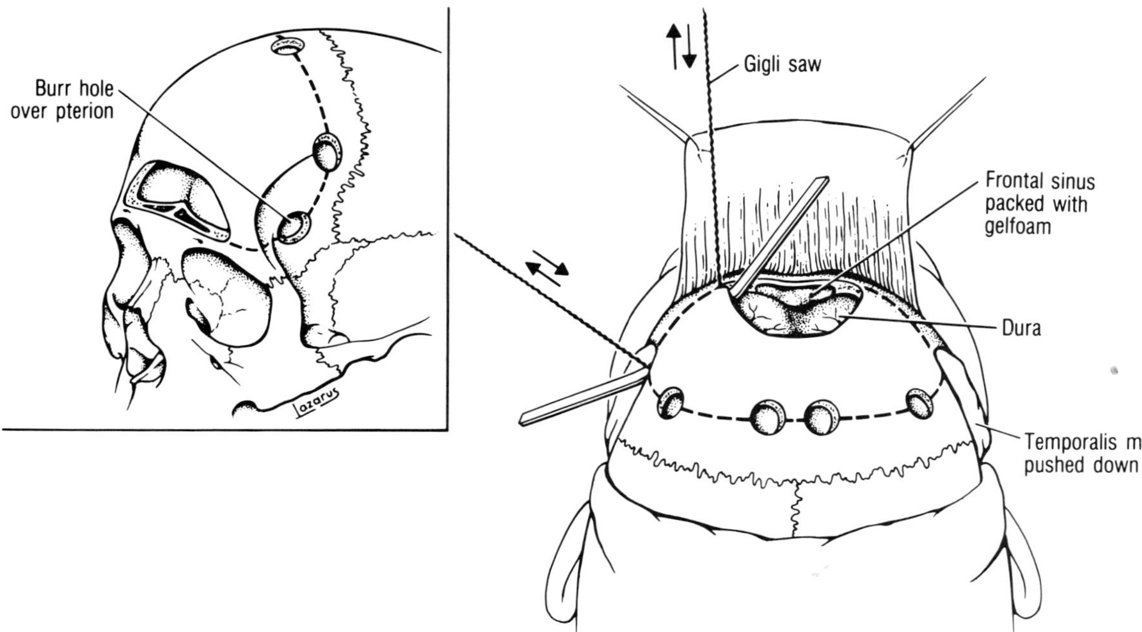

Fig. 53-6.   (A,B) Line drawings illustrating the position of burr holes. Key burr holes include those anterior to the pterion. A Gigli saw is used for the inferior cuts. Both osteoplastic and free bone flaps can be used.

by gentle removal of CSF in increments of 10–20 ml. Hemostasis is secured with the microtipped bipolar cautery. In more complicated cases with intracranial extension, the dura is opened along the floor of the anterior fossa anteriorly, and the falx cerebri sectioned between two sutures of 00 silk or Nurolon (Ethicon, New Jersey). Cortical draining veins anteriorly may be carefully coagulated and clipped, and the brain itself protected with cottonoid strips. By gentle retraction of the brain, the floor of the anterior cranial fossa involved by tumor can be displayed. Using microdissection, tumor involving the floor of the anterior cranial fossa and the brain is carefully dissected from the rest of the frontal lobes. We prefer to use the Cavitron ultrasonic tumor aspirator for removal of the intracranial tumor. Once the intracranial portion of the tumor has been removed, that portion of the frontal fossa dura that is involved by tumor should be included in the tumor specimen. The dura therefore is cut circumferentially around the tumor and the portion that has to be sacrificed dissected off the bone of the orbital roofs on

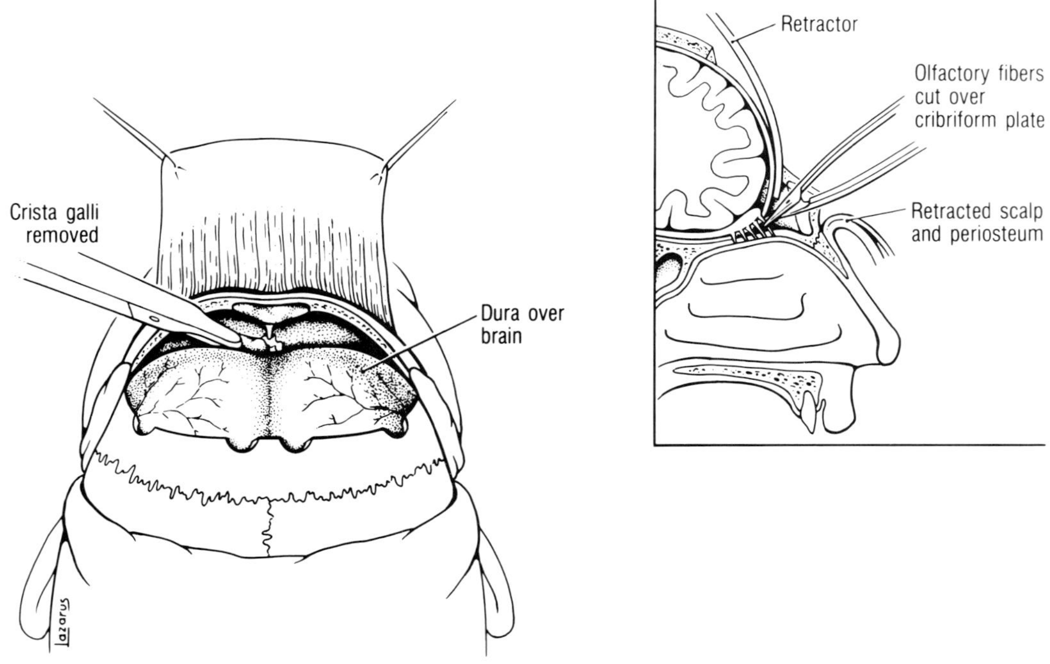

Fig. 53-7.   (A,B) With spinal drainage, an extradural dissection can be accomplished with minimal or no brain retraction. Olfactory rootlets are carefully clipped and cut.

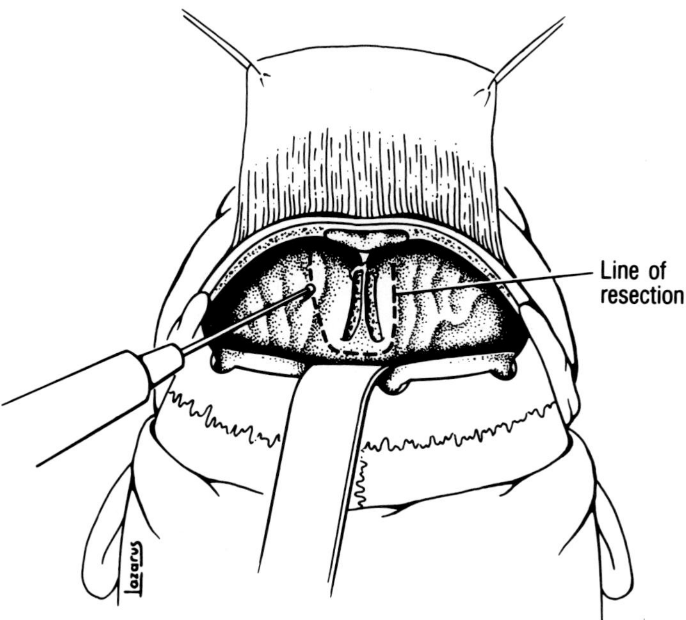

Fig. 53-8. Following exposure of the planum sphenoidale, the mid-portion of the anterior cranial fossa is mobilized by drilling through the ethmoid sinuses on either side. If orbital invasion is suspected, the lateral cut is made over the orbital roof as shown without injury to the orbital periosteum.

either side. The final phase of the intracranial operation is an osteotomy through the planum sphenoidale and the roof of the ethmoids on either side (Figure 53-8). This can be performed with fine chisels or a Hall microdrill. We also prefer to repair all dural defects primarily at this point. Following this, the bone flap is replaced and held loosely by 00 sutures to protect the

brain during the next phase of the operation. The facial portion begins with a standard or modified Weber-Ferguson incision for maxillectomy. After the skin is cut down to the dermis, we prefer to use the pencil-tip electrocautery to ensure hemostasis while the facial flap is cut down to the periosteum. The skin flaps are reflected laterally with skin hooks and dissected off the bone. At the upper end, the medial canthal ligament must be carefully identified with silk sutures so that it can be reapproximated at the end with silk sutures. Inferiorly, the infraorbital nerve is cut and the anterior wall of the maxilla exposed. The maxillary antrum is entered from the front and inspected (Figures 53-9A and B). If there is tumor extension into the antrum, a total maxillectomy is required. For tumors arising in the orbit or ethmoids, with little or no tumor in the maxillary antrum, the hard palate can be preserved and a partial maxillectomy performed on that side (Figure 53-10). Whenever possible, we prefer to preserve the hard palate, since palatal defects may predispose the patient to long-term eating and talking problems. However, a portion of the hard palate and nasal septum is frequently removed to provide access to the ethmoid sinuses. For tumors requiring palatal resection, a dissection is made through the alveolar ridge at or just off the midline so as to leave as many teeth as possible for fixation. The incision is carried through the midline of the hard palate and about the maxilla on that side. Laterally, the osteotomies go through the zygomatic arches. If the orbit is to be preserved, the medial orbital walls are carefully freed from the orbital periosteum. By reflecting the nose and the nasal septum laterally, it is possible to remove the entire specimen with the ethmoid sinuses of the opposite side. The most difficult portion of the mobilization is posteriorly, where the maxilla attaches to the pterygoid plates and has to be freed by blind dissection from the sphenopalatine fossa.

At this point, the neurosurgical team rejoins the operation

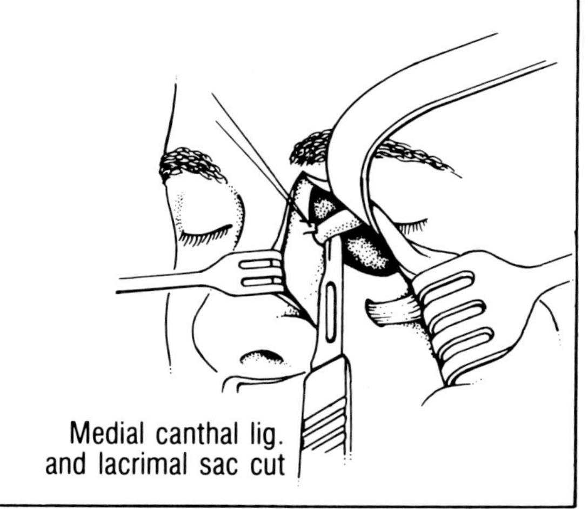

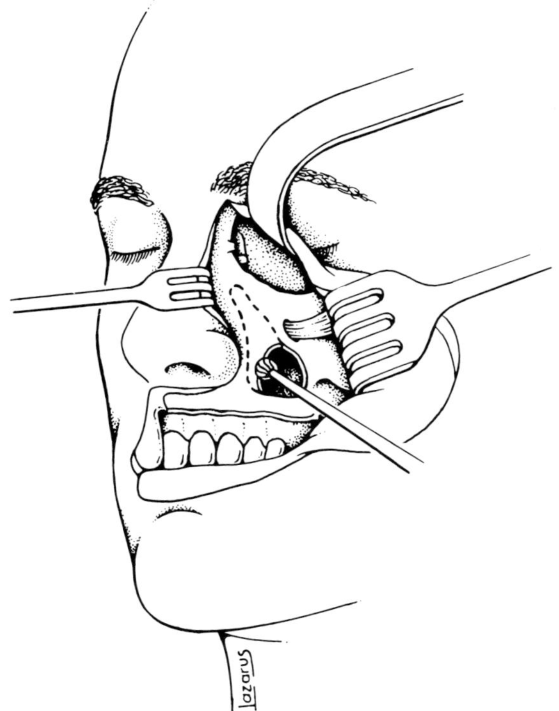

Fig. 53-9. (A,B) The facial portion of the operation begins with a modified Weber-Ferguson incision. The medial canthal ligament is carefully identified by sutures. The maxillary antrum is entered from in front to determine the extent of maxillectomy required.

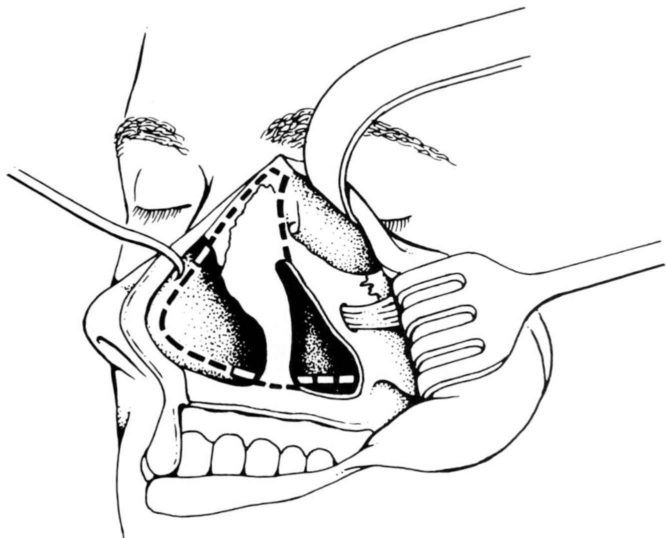

Fig. 53-10. Dotted lines indicate osteotomies to extend exposure by resection of the nasal septum and vomer. A portion of the palate can be removed for tumor access if additional exposure is required.

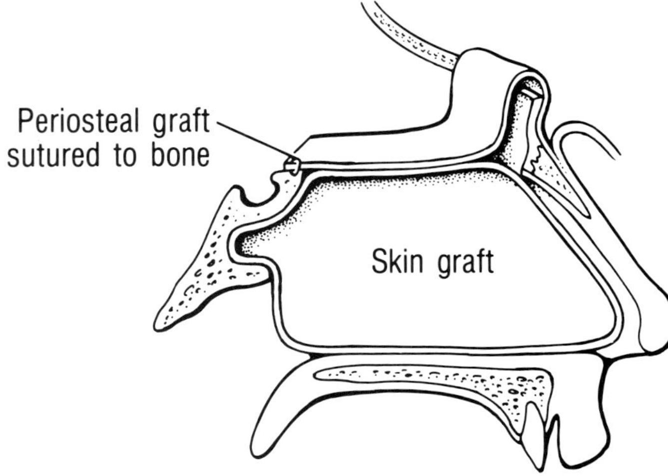

Fig. 53-11. Reconstruction of the anterior skull base is performed with a pedicled periosteal flap from above and a skin graft applied from below. In the occasional benign tumor, additional bone reconstruction can be accomplished by bone grafts obtained from the ribs or outer table.

for the final stage of tumor resection. By a combination of sharp dissection and traction from below and downward pressure from above, the entire specimen is removed en bloc. This dissection is more difficult when the orbital contents are preserved as opposed to when they have to be sacrificed. When an orbital exenteration is performed as part of the operation, the muscular attachments and the vascular pedicle at the apex of the optic foramina should be secured with a suture ligature applied under a long right-angled clamp. Once the main specimen is removed, hemostasis is secured and all irregular bone edges are rongeured off or drilled to provide a smooth surface for reconstruction. All redundant mucosa should be carefully trimmed and removed to prevent formation of postoperative polyps. The resected specimen should include the entire cribriform plate and the superior and middle turbinates on either side.

Reconstruction of the skull base is done as follows: initially, all dural defects are sutured primarily with 0000 silk or Nurolon sutures. Larger defects are closed with a free flap of temporalis fascia or cadaver dura. A viable pedicled flap of pericranium is then placed on the anterior cranial fossa, and secured to the basal dura and the bone of the skull base by 0000 sutures. Against this periosteal flap, a split-thickness skin graft is applied from below (Figure 53-11). The skin graft is painstakingly positioned into the bony and soft tissue surfaces in the large facial defect. It is important to obtain a good approximation of the graft against the pericranial flap. The graft is sutured peripherally to the skin edges while centrally a stent of Xerofoam gauze is used for packing. The packing is supported in place by a previously fabricated dental obturator that obliterates the defect in the hard palate. Closure of the craniotomy flap is performed in routine fashion. The bone flap is replaced and the epidural space lined with Avitene after the dura is tented to the bone edges. We generally leave an epidural suction drain and close the scalp routinely in two layers. Sterile dressings and antibiotic ointment are used to cover the skin wounds.

POSTOPERATIVE MANAGEMENT

Patients are monitored in the intensive care unit and placed on fluid restriction. Intravenous broad-spectrum antibiotics, Dilantin, and steroid therapy are used postoperatively in all patients. The spinal drain may be left in place for 2 to 3 days at the discretion of the surgeon. In patients who continue to require ventilation postoperatively, we obtain a noncontrast scan within 24 hours to document the absence of a postoperative clot.

The antral packing is kept in place for 5 to 10 days, during which time the patient remains on antibiotics. When it is removed, the defect is repacked or filled with a space-occupying prosthesis to maintain the contour of the facial skin. In our experience, there is rarely a complete "take" of the graft, but this does not represent a major problem. Sutures are kept in place for 10 days to 2 weeks. Patients are taught to irrigate the wound with saline solution twice a day to remove crusts and promote healing. Generous and frequent irrigations combined with localized debridement usually bring about rapid epithelialization of the exposed surfaces. Follow-up CT scans and further therapy are recommended depending on the histologic composition of the tumor (see Figure 53-2D).

COMPLICATIONS

Despite the extensive nature of the operative procedure, it is surprising how few complications are encountered when the surgery is performed by experienced teams. We divide complications into minor and major: minor complications include local seromas, sloughing of the graft, epidural or subdural infections requiring antibiotic therapy or removal of the bone plate, as well as serous otitis. Approximately 10 to 20 percent of patients in our series have developed localized infections requiring eventual removal of the frontal bone flap. More serious neurologic complications include cerebral edema, CSF leakage, cranial nerve dysfunction, and neurologic deficits, including pituitary insufficiency from frontal lobe retraction. It is our impression the major cause of morbidity at present is related directly or indirectly to infection in the parameningeal space. With experience, the major complication rate should vary from 5 to 15 percent in major centers. At present, the reported mortality rate in our hands, as well others, ranges from 3 to 5 percent.[5,35]

RESULTS

The current median survival of all patients following craniofacial resection is 5 years and varies according to the histologic composition and grade of the tumor. It is impossible to compare results from one surgical series to another, because selection criteria have varied widely. The value of this operation in the de novo treatment of paranasal sinus cancers is also difficult to assess because many centers often use radiation therapy for initial treatment, and offer craniofacial resection to palliate patients with recurrences following radiation.[17,36] In Ketcham's series, the median survival was 5 years but varied according to whether orbital contents were spared or not. Thus, the 5-year survival was 30 percent in those in whom the orbits were spared, compared with 50 percent in those in whom the orbital contents were sacrificed. He therefore advocated orbital exenteration whenever tumor invasion of the bony medial orbit was seen. In our experience, it is often possible to accomplish the same goal, i.e., gross total resection, while preserving the orbit without compromising the results unless invasion of the orbital fat is present. In Jackson's series of 79 patients, only 53 patients had malignant tumors; 3 deaths over 12 years are mentioned but no other details of survival are given.[12] In our recent series of 30 patients, followed for a minimum of 2 years, median survival was 5 years despite the fact that more than half the patients had failed prior treatment and one third had intracranial invasion at presentation.[35] We therefore believe that craniofacial resection is the procedure of choice for most patients with neoplasms involving the anterior skull base; the presence of limited intracranial invasion and involvement of pterygoid plates are not necessarily contraindications to surgery providing complete tumor resection can be accomplished. In patients with well-differentiated tumors, we advocate surgery prior to radiation therapy because this approach results in a higher proportion of local control. In patients with esthesioneuroblastoma, current evidence indicates that combined modality treatment including chemotherapy and radiation should be used along with surgery. Since the majority of such patients have microscopic intracranial invasion along the olfactory rootlets, we believe that the initial surgical procedure should be a craniofacial procedure even in the presence of a tumor limited radiologically to the sinuses. Following surgery, cyclic alternating combination chemotherapy including cytoxan, vincristine, VP-16, and cisplatin should be used along with local radiation therapy. In other epithelial neoplasms cisplatin-containing chemotherapy regimens may produce complete and partial responses in close to 50 percent of untreated patients, but their impact on survival is marginal to date. Nevertheless, current data suggests that both radiation and chemotherapy are more effective in the treatment of microscopic rather than gross bulk disease, and we have therefore offered craniofacial resection for palliation in good risk surgical patients, despite the presence of limited intracranial invasion. We believe that with more effective methods of sealing the basal dura,[37] the scope and indications for this procedure should increase.

REFERENCES

1. Cheesman AD, Lund VJ, Howard DJ: Craniofacial resection for tumors of the nasal cavity and paranasal sinuses. Head Neck Surg 8:429, 1985
2. Jackson IT, Marsh WR, Hide TA: Treatment of tumors involving the anterior cranial fossa. Head Neck Surg 6:901, 1984
3. Ketchum AS, Chretien PB, Van Buren JM, et al: The ethmoid sinus: A re-evaluation of surgical resection. Am J Surg 126:469, 1973
4. Ketchum AS, Wilkins RH, Van Buren JM, et al: A combined intracranial facial approach to the paranasal sinuses. Am J Surg 106:698, 1963
5. Ketchum AS, Van Buren JM: Tumors of the paranasal sinuses: A therapeutic challenge. Am J Surg 150:406,1985
6. Sundaresan N, Shah JP: Cranio-facial resection for paranasal sinus tumors. Indian J Cancer 16:74, 1979
7. Arbit E, Sundaresan N, Galicich JH, et al: Cranio-facial resection following chemotherapy. Surg Neurol 13:395, 1980
8. Tomita T, Sundaresan N, Huvos A, Shah J: Giant ossifying fibroma with intracranial extension. Acta Neurochir 56:65, 1981
9. Chapman P, Carter RL, Clifford P: The diagnosis and surgical management of olfactory neuroblastoma: The role of craniofacial resection. J Laryngol Otol 95:785, 1981
10. Sisson GA: Carcinoma of the paranasal sinuses and cranio-facial resection. J Laryngol Otolaryngol 90:59, 1976
11. Terz JJ, Young HF, Lawrence WE Jr: Combined craniofacial resection for locally advanced carcinoma of the head and neck. I. Tumors of the skin and soft tissue. Am J Surg 140:613, 1980
12. Terz JJ, Alksne JF, Lawrence W Jr: Craniofacial resection for tumors invading the pterygoid fossa. Am J Surg 118:782, 1969
13. Terz JJ, Young HP, Lawrence W JR: Combined craniofacial resection for locally advanced carcinoma of the head and neck. II. Carcinoma of the paranasal sinuses. Am J Surg 140:618, 1980
14. Westbury G, Wilson JSP, Richardson A: Combined craniofacial resection for malignant disease. Am J Surg 130:463, 1976
15. Bridger GP: Radical surgery for ethmoid cancer. Arch Otolaryngol 106:630, 1980 16. Cheng VST, Wang CC: Carcinomas of the paranasal sinuses. Cancer 40:3038, 1977
17. Ellingwood KE, Million RR: Cancer of the nasal cavity and ethmoid sinuses. Cancer 40:1517, 1979
18. Elner A, Koch H: Combined radiological and surgical therapy of cancer of the ethmoid. Acta Otolaryngol 78:270, 1974
19. Bush SE, Baghshaw MA: Carcinoma of the paranasal sinuses. Cancer 50:154, 1982
20. Frazell EL, Lewis JS: Cancer of the nasal cavity and accessory sinuses: A report of the management of 416 patients. Cancer 16:1293, 1963
21. Saunders SH, Ruff T: Adenocarcinoma of the paranasal sinuses. J Laryngol Otolaryngol 90:157, 1976
22. Weber AL, Stanton AC: Malignant tumors of the paranasal sinuses: Radiologic, clinical and histopathologic evaluation of 200 cases. Head Neck Surg 6:761, 1984
23. Robin PE, Powell DJ, Stansbie JM: Carcinoma of the nasal cavity and paranasal sinuses. Incidence and presentation of different histologic types. Clin Otolaryngol 4:431, 1979
24. Helliwell TR, Yeoh LH, Still PH: Anaplastic carcinoma of the nose and paranasal sinuses. Cancer 58:2030, 1986
25. Robbins KT, Fuller LM, Vlasak M, et al: Primary lymphomas of the nasal cavity and paranasal sinuses. Cancer 56:814, 1985
26. Klintenberg C, Olofsson J, Hellquist H, et al: Adenocarcinoma of the ethmoid sinuses: a review of 28 cases with special reference to wood dust exposure. Cancer 54:482, 1984
27. Kadish S, Goodman M, Wang CG: Olfactory neuroblastoma. Cancer 35:1571, 1976
28. Elkon D, Hightower SI, Mengi LL: Esthesioneuroblastoma. Cancer 44:1087, 1979
29. Newbill ET, Johns ME, Cantrell RW: Esthesioneuroblastoma: Diagnosis and management. South Med J 78:275, 1985
30. Kondo M, Horiuchi M, Shiga E: Computed tomography of malignant tumors of the nasal cavity and paranasal sinuses. Cancer 50:226, 1982
31. Parsons C, Hodson W: Computed tomography of paranasal sinus tumors. Radiology 132:641, 1979

32. Som PM: The role of CT in the diagnosis of carcinoma of the paranasal sinuses and nasopharynx. J Otolaryngol 11:340, 1982

33. Som PM, Lawson W, Biller HF, Langier DF, Sachdev VP, Rigamonti D: Ethmoid sinus disease:CT evaluation in 400 cases. Part III. Craniofacial resection. Radiology 159:605, 1986

34. American Joint Committee on Cancer: Manual for Staging of Cancer. Philadelphia, JB Lippincott, 1983, pp 23–48

36. Sundaresan N, Shah JP: Cranio-facial resection for anterior skull base tumors. Head Neck Surg (in press)

36. Harrison DFN: A critical evaluation of present day attitudes to the treatment of antro-ethmoidal cancer. J Otolaryngol 11:148, 1982

37. Rosen M, Simeone FA, Bruce DA: Single stage composite section and reconstruction of malignant anterior skull base tumors. Neurosurgery 18:7, 1986

CHAPTER 54
The Transbasal Approach to Tumors Invading the Base of the Skull

Patrick J. Derome

BECAUSE THEY ARE LOCATED IN A "FRONTIER AREA" between the skull and the face (a no-man's-land for the different specialties), lesions that invade the base of the skull, particularly the middle areas, have been treated by neurosurgeons, ENT surgeons, ophthalmologic surgeons, and plastic surgeons. It often was impossible to remove the mass completely. In addition, many patients were not offered further treatment after a single biopsy through a narrow anterior approach and gradually became blind before the base of the skull was massively invaded and all of the cranial nerves were involved by the lesion.

Although it is perfectly acceptable not to remove certain malignant tumors, a benign tumor should always be removed, and many of the tumors that invade the base of the skull are benign. Tumors in the region of the ethmoid, sphenoid, or clivus admittedly present many problems and are extremely difficult to remove. In the past, close collaboration between neurosurgeons and plastic surgeons was required. Today the entire procedure can be completed by a neurosurgeon alone using the transbasal approach.

Tessier[1] developed the transbasal approach in 1960 for craniofacial abnormalities and used it to reduce his first cases of hypertelorism and craniofacial dysostosis. It then was adapted for the surgical removal of basal tumors.[2]

GOALS WITH THE TRANSBASAL APPROACH

The first goal with the transbasal approach is the complete removal of the tumor. Some tumors are located at the midline, but most extend laterally toward the orbital walls, the lesser and greater sphenoid wings, and the middle fossa. The second goal is to free the cranial nerves and to open the optic foramina, the sphenoidal fissures, and even the foramen rotundum and foramen ovale, areas that cannot be reached through narrow anterior approaches. If the anterior and, possibly, the middle fossae are to be seen, an anterior subdural and extradural approach is required. Anosmia, which very often is present before the procedure, is the only side effect. An anterior approach that can be combined with the intracranial approach to remove certain tumors of the clivus will be discussed later.

HAZARDS OF THE TRANSBASAL APPROACH

The most important complication of the transbasal approach is the possibility of creating a communication between the subarachnoid spaces and the upper air-filled cavities of the face (Figure 54-1). Resection of a ethmoidosphenoidal mass widely opens the frontal and sphenoidal sinuses and the ethmoidal air cells. The floor of the nasal fossae and the pharyngeal or cavum mucosae can be reached through the cranial approach. Meningeal tears and dural defects occur frequently. Well-known possible complications are pneumatoceles or cerebrospinal fluid leaks, ascending infections, and meningitis.

The three structures superimposed between the intradural spaces and the air-filled cavities of the face are the dura, the bone involved by the tumor, and the rhinopharyngeal mucosal plane. These structures must be repaired carefully to prevent the above-mentioned complications. The dura must be closed tightly and strengthened with (depending on the size of the defect) a pericranial or dermal graft. The base of the skull must be reconstructed with bone autografts to eliminate a medial dead space, which can lead to meningoceles or encephaloceles and postoperative extradural hematomas or infections (Figure 54-2). The mucosal plane must be preserved as much as possible, since it sustains and feeds the lower aspect of bone grafts. When these dicta are rigidly applied, the transbasal approach is a benign procedure.

PREOPERATIVE ORGANIZATION

Prophylactic antibiotic therapy should be administered routinely for 2 days before the procedure, during the operation, and for 1 week postoperatively. The frontal lobe must be well retracted so that the base of the skull is readily exposed. All available methods can be used simultaneously, i.e., assisted ventilation with negative pressure, administration of mannitol, and continuous intraoperative lumbar drainage. Because the procedure is a very long one (10 to 12 hours and sometimes longer), the anesthesiologist must maintain the patient in a state of normothermia and strict biologic control and must prevent hyponatremia. Blood losses must be carefully replaced and strict hemostasis applied at each step. If the tumor has a tendency to bleed, special techniques, such as ligation of the

OPERATIVE NEUROSURGICAL TECHNIQUES
ISBN 0-8089-1862-1

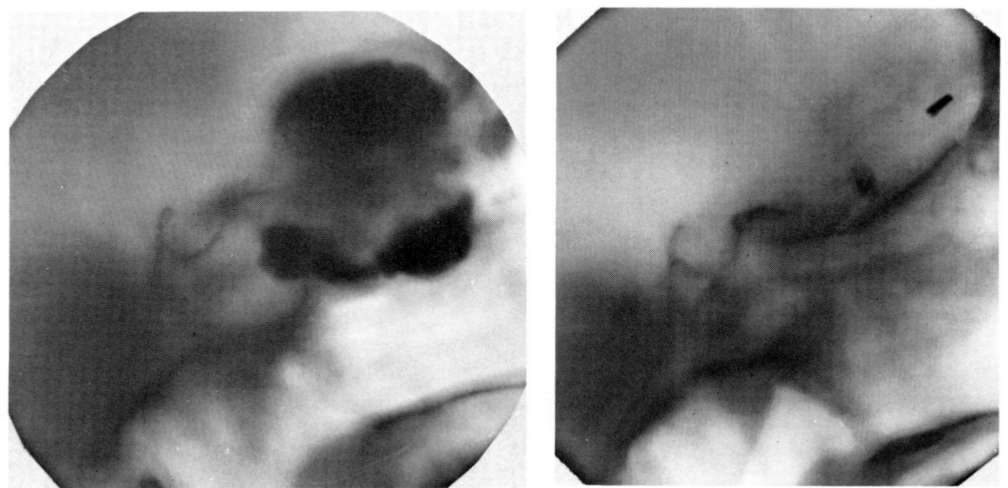

Fig. 54-1. (Left and Right). Resection of an ethmoidosphenoidal tumor (osteoma ?) opens the upper air cavities of the face widely.

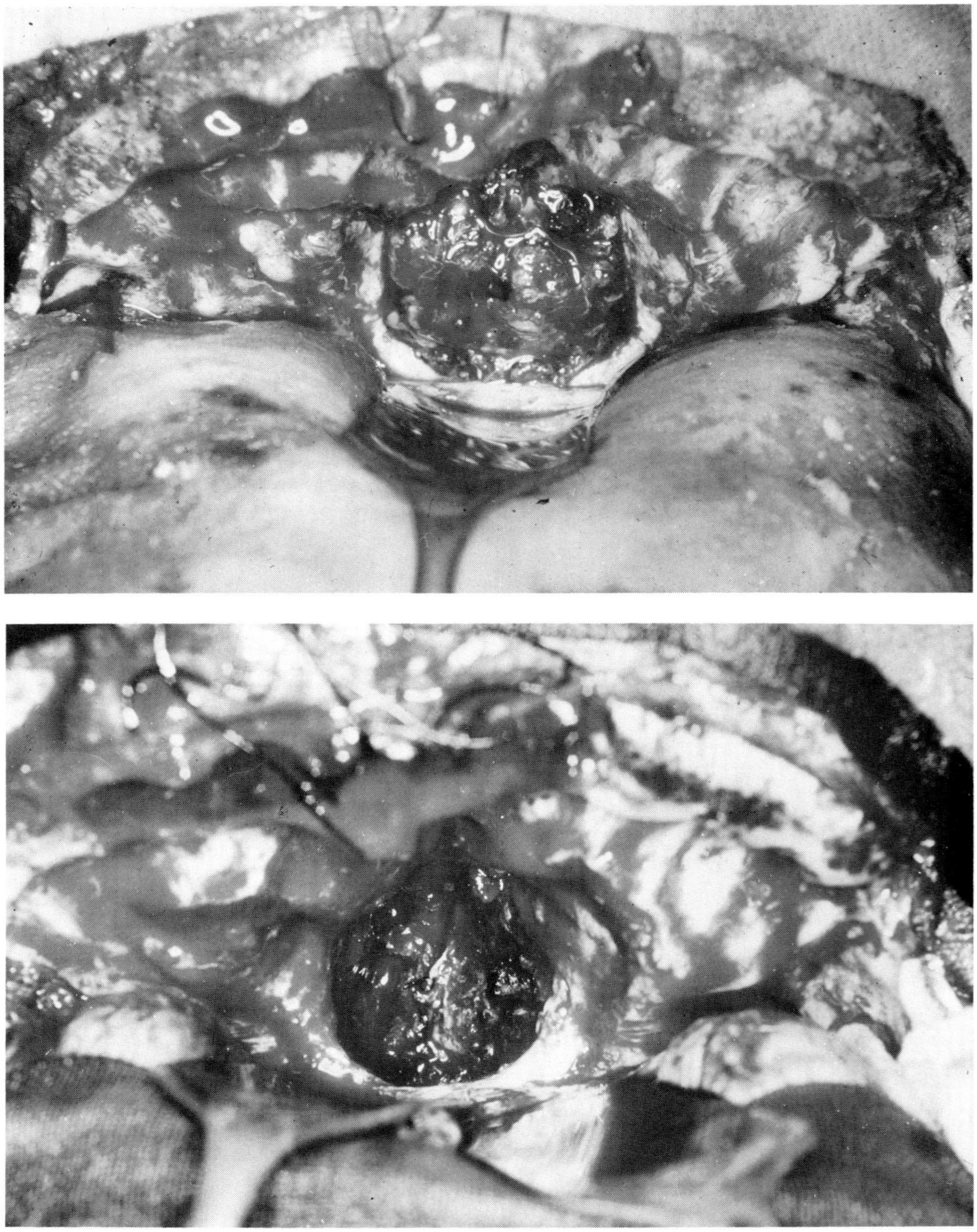

Fig. 54-2. (Left) Intraoperative view of an ethmoidosphenoidal chordoma responsible for extradural compression of both optic nerves. The orbital roofs are partially removed. (Right) After the tumor has been removed, a large dead space extends to the nasal fossae and the deeper aspects of the pharyngeal mucosae. Note the free optic nerves.

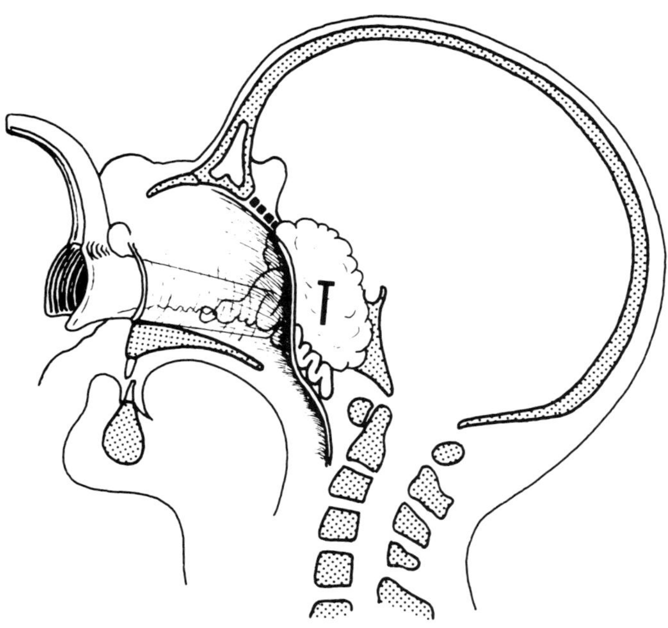

Fig. 54-3. A rhinoseptal approach permits the surgeon to preserve the rhinopharyngeal mucosae. A packing is introduced both for protection and to serve as a deep landmark.

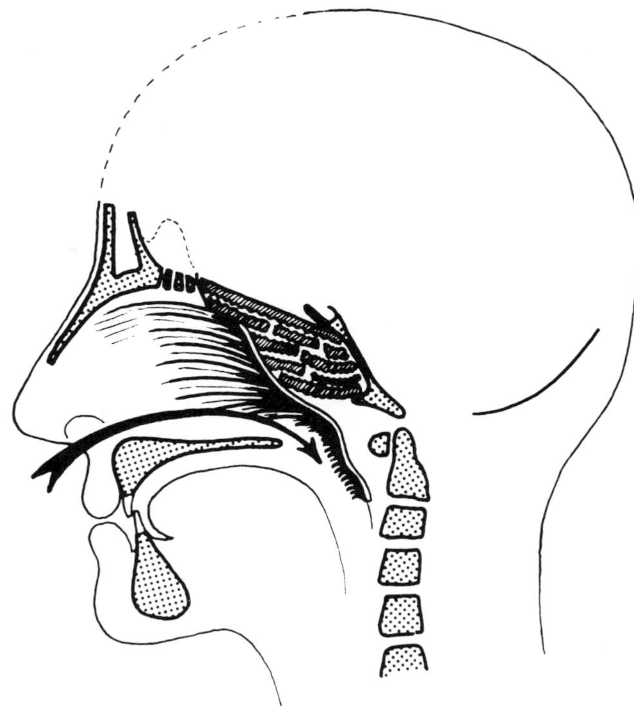

Fig. 54-4. The mucosae are reapplied close to the ethmoidosphenoidal mass, which was reconstructed with bone autografts.

external carotid artery or preoperative embolization, can be used.

The patient should be placed in the dorsal decubitus position without fixation of the head, so that all aspects of the positioning (rotation and declivity) can be modified intraoperatively.

PRESERVING THE MUCOSAL PLANE

To preserve the rhinopharyngeal mucosae, they should first be dissected through a rhinoseptal approach, as in the first steps of a classic transsphenoidal access to sellar tumors, i.e., an incision is made under the upper lip, the inferior nasal spine is resected and the mucosae are separated up to the rostrum; a dissector then is pushed backward and the mucosae of the choanae are separated as much as possible from the vomer and the inferior aspect of the body of the sphenoid. Two tents can be introduced, both for protection and as deep landmarks, before the tumor is attacked from above (Figure 54-3). At the end of the procedure, nasal packing can be used to position the mucosae against the cancellous bone grafts used to repair the base of the skull and the sphenoethmoid (Figure 54-4).

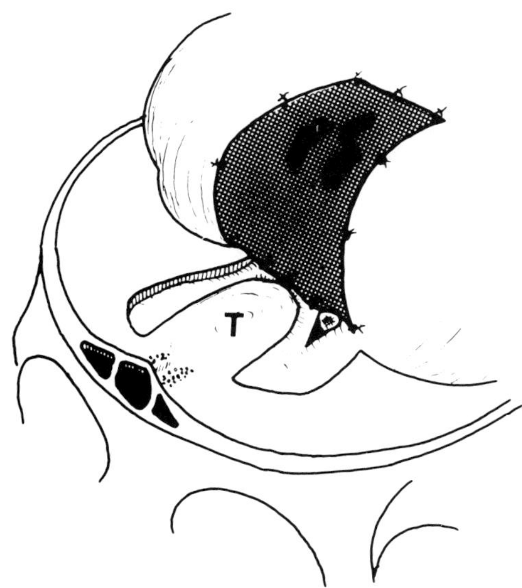

Fig. 54-5. Strengthening of the subfrontal dura at the midline with a pe ricranial graft. T = tumor.

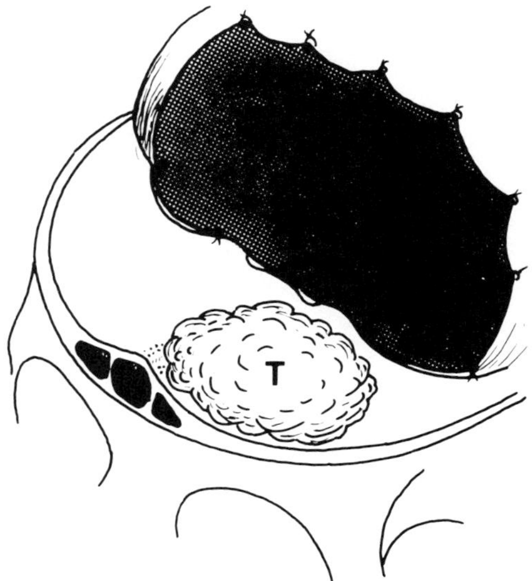

Fig. 54-6. A dural defect closed with a large graft. Note the suture at the remote edges of the anterior fossa. T = basal insertion of the tumor.

With sufficient surgical experience, this first operative step can be avoided and the mucosal plane dissected from above after the tumor is removed.

In the case of huge tumors involving the nasal fossa, the mucosal flap disappears. When such a case is expected, a large anterior pericranial flap is cut and preserved at the beginning of the operation, before the bifrontal free flap is turned. This pericranial flap will close the nasal fossae and its posterior edge will be sutured at the most remote limits of the subfrontal dura; the bone autografts will then be inserted between the subfrontal dura (or its repair) and this new ''mucosal plane.''[17]

EXPOSING THE BASE OF THE SKULL

We use a temporotemporal incision made just behind the hairline. The pericranial incision follows both temporal crests laterally to the coronal sutures and then is curved upward. If it is necessary to proceed more laterally, the entire temporal muscle is dissected from the temporal fossa and from the retromalar area to the zygomatic process.

The bone flap is usually a bifrontal free flap; its inferior margin is strictly supraorbital without regard for the frontal sinuses. If these sinuses are wide, their posterior walls and mucosae are removed and their ostia closed with bone grafts.

After the subfrontal dura is dissected, the anterior fossa is exposed. This dissection is fairly easy, except for the area of both olfactory grooves (sometimes it is possible to avoid meningeal tears by a primary resection of the crista galli apophysis and by cutting the olfactory nerves one by one). The dissection must reach the posterior limits of the anterior fossa: the posterior edge of the lesser sphenoid wings, the tuberculum sellae, and the base of the anterior clinoid processes. A partially invaded dura or a tumor growing through the meninges into the intradural spaces may cause some problems. The subfrontal and intracerebral parts of the tumor are removed through a

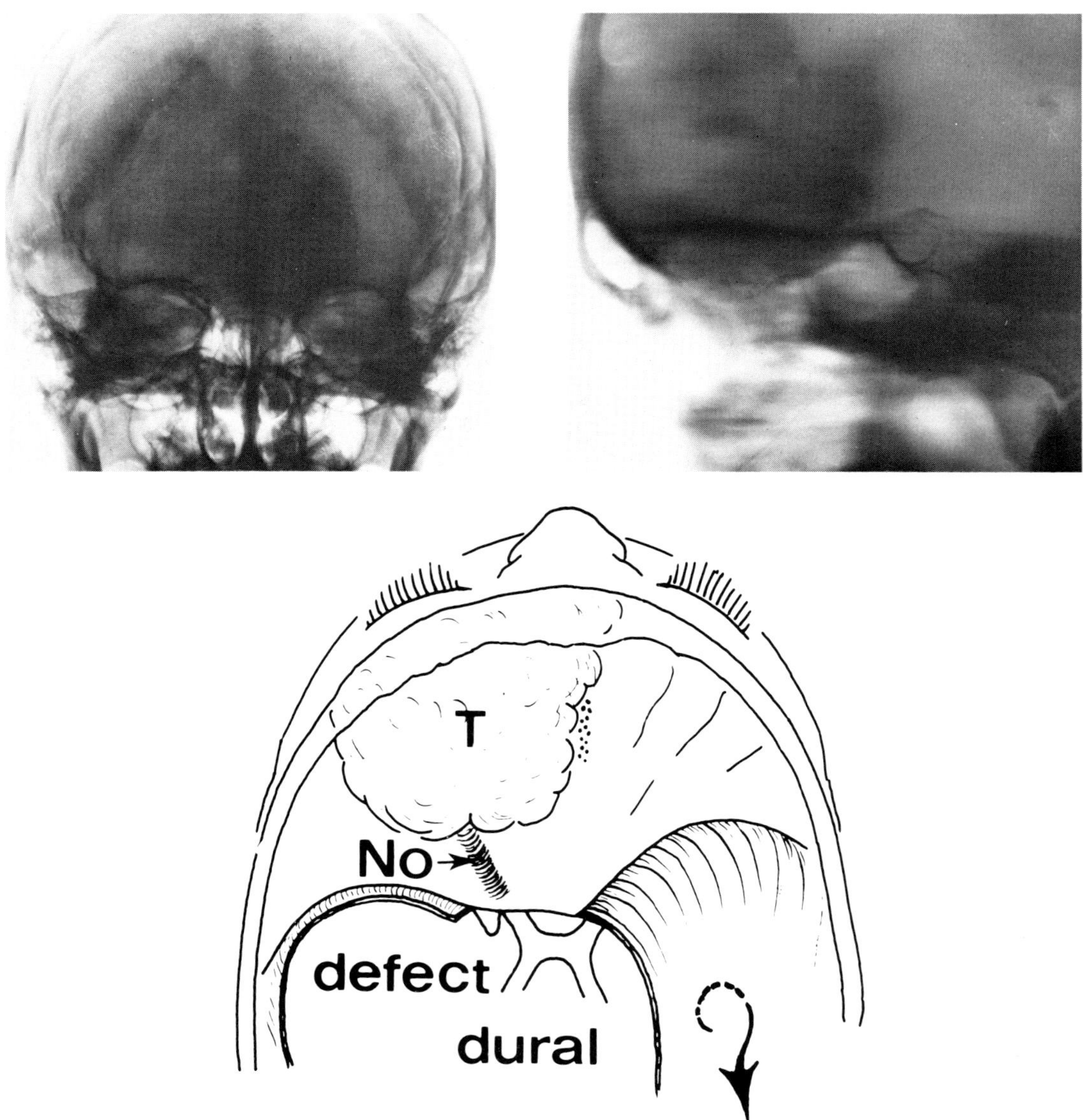

Fig. 54-7. An ossifying fibroma with a large intracranial extension. T = basal insertion of the tumor; No = extradural portion of the left optic nerve. After the intracranial portion of the tumor is removed, the optochiasmatic cistern is opened widely. In this case a dermal graft is necessary because it is more adhesive.

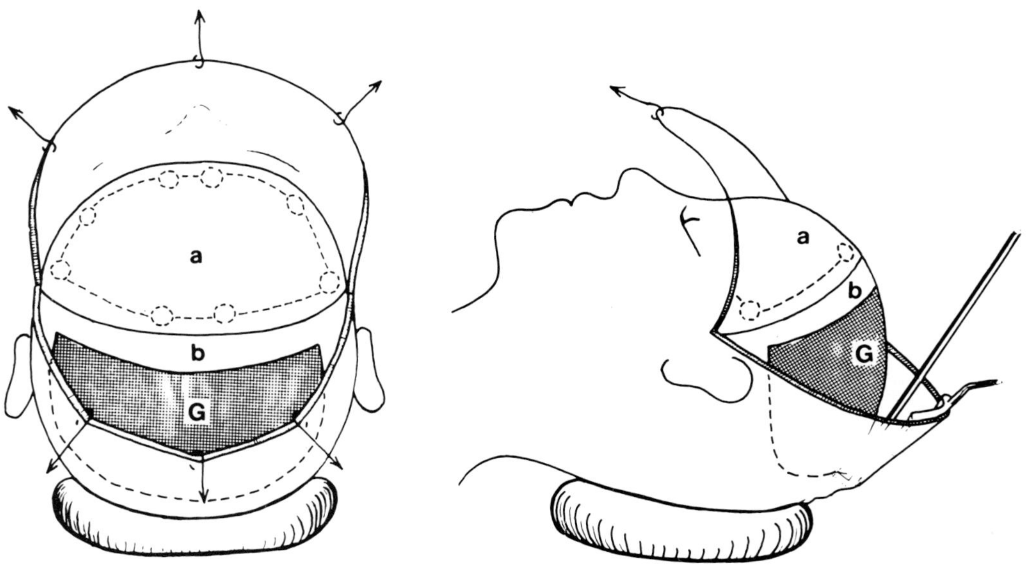

Fig. 54-8. Extracting a pericranial graft. a = anterior pericranium; G = graft; b = pericranial band preserved to allow sutures to be placed at the end of the procedure.

classic intradural approach before the subfrontal dura around the basal insertion of the tumor is dissected.

MENINGEAL REPAIR

The dura is closed before the base is resected and the upper air-filled cavities are opened. There are three possibilities:

1. The dura is preserved and there are only a few meningeal tears, generally located in the area of the olfactory grooves.

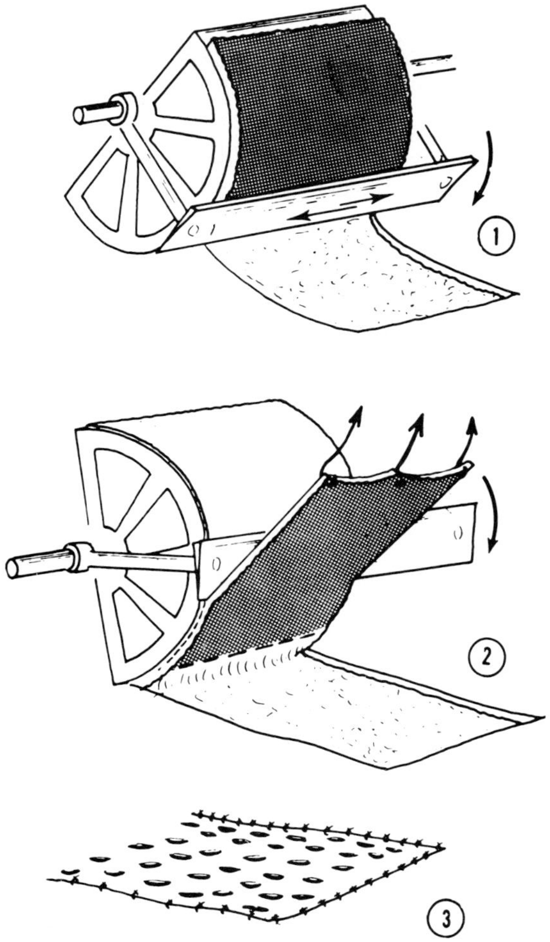

Fig. 54-9. Obtaining a dermal graft from the abdominal area.

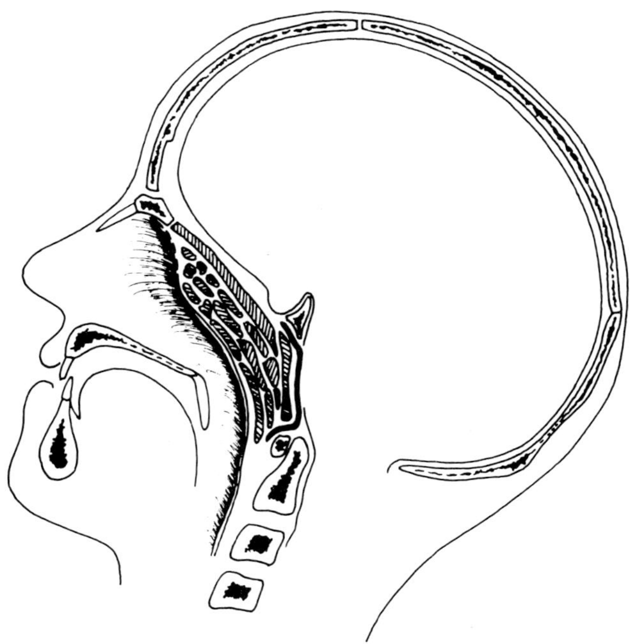

Fig. 54-10. Repair of a clival dural defect. The graft is applied to the bone reconstruction.

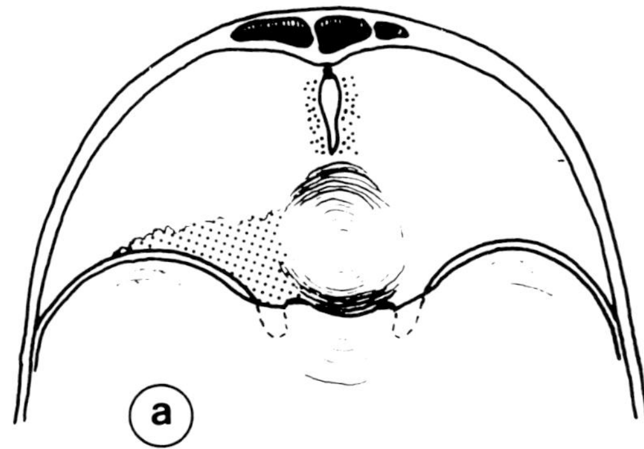

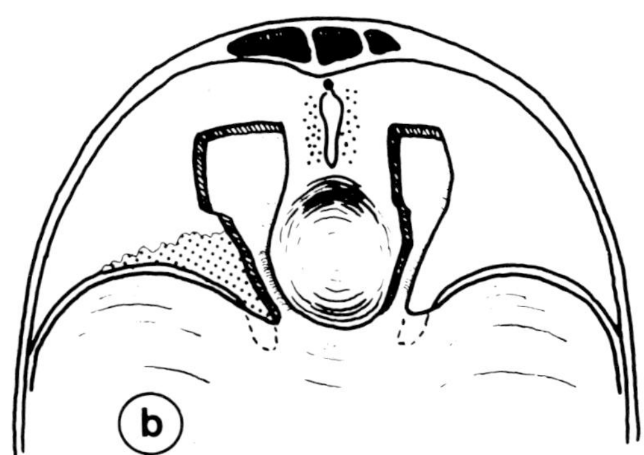

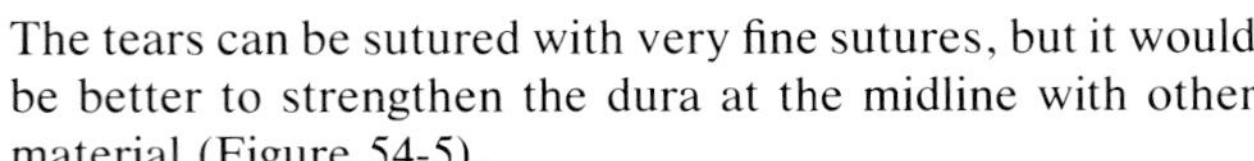

Fig. 54-11.   (a) Fibrous dysplasia involving the body and the left lesser wing of the sphenoid. (b) Opening of the optic canals.

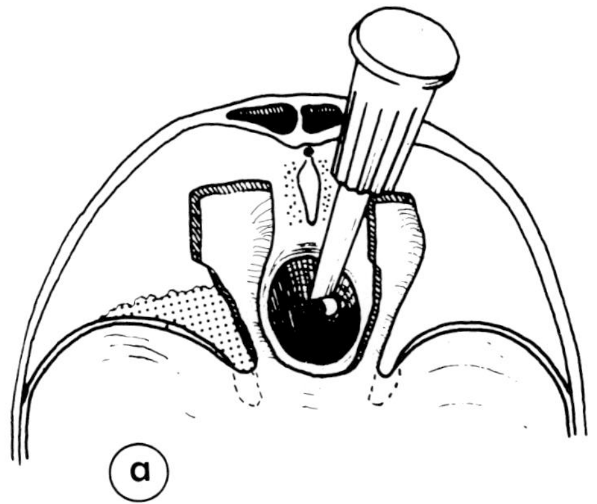

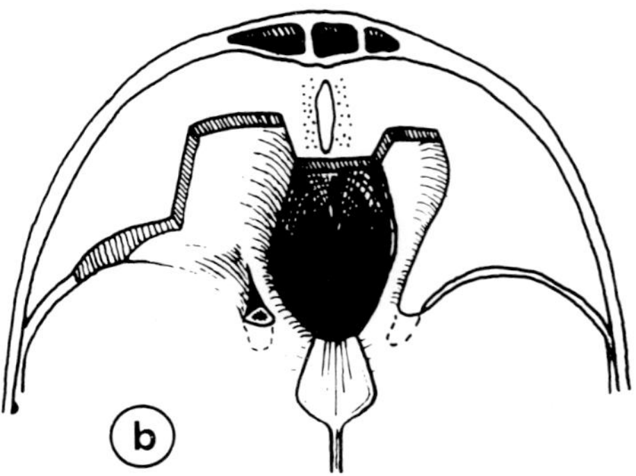

Fig. 54-12.   (a) Intratumoral resection between the optic nerves. (b) Total removal of the sphenoid body leading to the pharyngeal mucosae. Opening of the left sphenoidal fissure and resection of the left anterior clinoid process.

The tears can be sutured with very fine sutures, but it would be better to strengthen the dura at the midline with other material (Figure 54-5).

2. There is a true dural defect. This must be closed with a dural substitute more than twice the size of the defect. This substitute is sutured to the dura at the most remote margins of the anterior fossa (Figure 54-6).

3. The defect is exceptionally large and the posterior dura in front of the optochiasmatic cistern has disappeared (Figure 54-7A, B, and C). It is impossible to suture the dural substitute posteriorly, which is folded like a leaf in a book. When it is impossible to achieve an immediate tight closure, the basal part of the tumor is resected in a second stage 3 or 4 months after the meninges is repaired.

The choice of a dural substitute depends on many factors. The material must be thick enough and tight enough to prevent leaks and ascending infection, supple enough to permit brain re-expansion, and must revascularize rapidly for quick adherence and to feed the bone grafts used to reconstruct the base of the skull. In our experience, a pericranial or dermal autograft is preferable to prosthetic materials, lyophilized dura, or fascia lata.

A pericranial autograft has the same properties as periosteum. For a thicker material and to preserve the anterior pericranium (covering the bifrontal free flap at the end of the procedure), the graft should be taken from the biparietal area through the same scalp incision (Figure 54-8). If necessary, the size of the sample can be as large as the entire subfrontal dura. We use this type of pericranial graft in almost all cases. Its periostic face is placed toward the basal reconstruction.

A dermal autograft is excellent, provided epidermal implants are avoided. It can be obtained from the abdominal area with a Padgett's dermatome. A thick dermoepidermal graft (1 to 1.2 mm thick) is cut from the subumbilical area. The graft stuck on the dermatome is recut on the drum to obtain a purely dermal graft (0.5 to 0.6 mm thick). The epidermal part is folded backward and sutured (Figure 54-9). This substitute is used when the pericranial graft is not available. The epidermal face of the graft is placed on the skull base (the deeper face of the graft close to the frontal lobes).

It must be emphasized that subsequent steps in the procedure depend on the quality of dural repair. In contrast to the anterior approach, the transbasal approach makes this repair easier, even with a clival dural defect (Figure 54-10).

REMOVAL OF THE BASAL TUMOR

The difficulties encountered in removing a basal tumor vary according to the location, extension, and consistency of the tumor. All types of rongeurs and drills can be used to remove pathologically involved bone.

Tumors in the ethmoidal area can be removed easily because there are no structures in the vicinity that can be injured. The nasal fossae are quickly reached, where the turbinates, the septum, and septal mucosae are identified and preserved if they are not invaded by tumor.

In the sphenoidal area the first step is to locate both optic nerves (Figure 54-11A and B). Partial resection of the orbital roofs therefore is the first step after the periorbita has been separated through an orbital approach. For this reason, the frontal bone is scraped to the upper margin of the orbits. When the supraorbital fissures are closed, resection of their lower rim helps to preserve the supraorbital vessels and nerves. The optic canals then are opened and the extradural part of the optic nerves identified. The tumor is attacked between the nerves on the jugum plate (Figure 54-12A). After intratumoral resection, the margins of bone are progressively removed. The medial walls of both orbits and the entire body of the sphenoid then are resected to the packing introduced through the rhinoseptal approach to preserve the pharyngeal and cavum mucosae (Figure 54-12B). The medial rim of the sphenoidal fissure can be opened from the midline (Figure 54-13), and it is possible to reach the foramen rotundum and the vidian canal in the root of the pterygoid process.

Laterally, if the tumor involves the lesser and greater wings of the sphenoid, resection of the orbital roof is extended to the temporal dura so that the lesser wing and the upper margin of the sphenoidal fissure disappear. Working between the sphenoidal fissure and the optic foramen, the anterior clinoid process is progressively removed. This resection must be done very carefully, step by step, because of the proximity of the internal carotid artery and the insertion of the small circumference of the tentorium just below the dura. Resection of the greater wing, between the periorbita and the temporal dura, is now easy and opens the inferior margin of the sphenoidal fissure, leading toward the floor of the middle fossa, the foramen rotundum, and the foramen ovale (Figure 54-13). At the end of this procedure, all upper cranial nerves are free.

Posteriorly, it is now possible to reach the clivus after the tuberculum sellar area and the vertical part of the sellar floor have been removed. Some bleeding may occur in this area because the dura of the sella is extremely vascular. This bleeding, however, generally is not significant.

Proceeding downward, the clivus is removed and the clival dura dissected to the anterior margin of the foramen magnum, which is opened. If dissection of the pharyngeal mucosa follows, the precervical space, the anterior arch of the atlas, and even the bodies of C2 and C3 can be reached (Figure 54-14A and B). The base of the skull, after this wide dissection, looks much different than usual: the bony tissue has disappeared, the soft tissues of the orbits are attached only to the frontal and temporal dura by the optic nerves and sphenoidal fissures, and between them there is a large dead space bounded by the rhinopharyngeal mucosae.

REPAIR OF THE BASE OF THE SKULL

Reconstruction of the skull base is necessary for three reasons: (1) in the midline, it is necessary because of the dead space and risk of later meningoceles and encephaloceles; (2) laterally, in the orbital area it is necessary to avoid postoperative enophthalmos and pulsatility of the eyeball; and (3) in the frontal area it is necessary for cosmetic reasons, if the orbitofrontal band and supraorbital margins are involved and therefore removed.

Maxillofacial and plastic surgeons have taught us that the best material to use to close air-filled cavities of the face that have been opened widely and are generally septic is autogenous bone. Grafts can be taken from the iliac bone, where it is possible to get a large specimen in one procedure. The advantage of an iliac graft is that it provides cancellous rather than cortical bone. If the specimens are not sufficient, which is often the case in children, one, two, or even three rib grafts also can be used. Ribs must be split to get a cancellous face, which is applied close to the upper air-filled cavities and the rhinopharyngeal mucosae (Figure 54-15A, B, and C). After the medial walls and the roofs of the orbits have been repaired with two single grafts or one modeled graft, the dead space should be packed with cancellous bone. A final cortical graft can be used to close the ethmoidosphenoidal area. It should be implanted between the nasion and the clivus, beneath the horizontal portion of the sellar floor. If the clivus also has been removed, the graft should be applied close to a vertical graft, fitted between the floor of the sella and the anterior margin of the foramen magnum or the anterior arch of the atlas. The optic nerves must remain completely free. Last, bone dust should be packed intracranially to give a tight closure. (Figures 54-16 through 54-19 illustrate the principles of this reconstruction.) If necessary, the supraorbital margins can be reconstructed with an iliac graft or with one single-modeled split rib graft wired to both orbital processes of the malar bone. Removal of the greater sphenoid wing and anterior half of the middle fossa generally does not require repair.

CLOSURE

Clips should be placed medially on the subfrontal dura, which has been strengthened by the pericranial graft. These serve as landmarks that can be used to follow postoperative brain re-expansion radiographically. The bifrontal free flap should be replaced with dural suspensions. If the tumor also invaded a part of the flap, the pathologically involved bone must be resected and a cranioplasty performed at the same stage. Again, a bone autograft is preferred to prosthetic material. (The possible need for such reconstruction must be anticipated when grafts are being obtained.) The anterior pericranium should be turned down to cover the bifrontal free flap. Two drains should be placed before the scalp is sutured, one extradurally in the

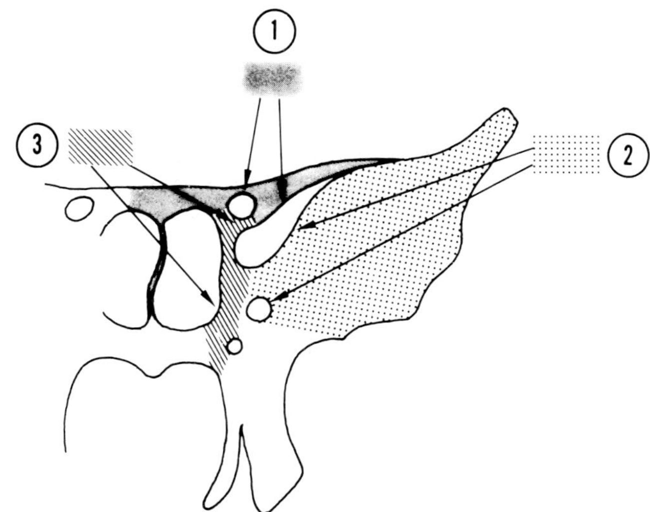

Fig. 54-13.   (1) Vertical attack; (2) medial attack; (3) lateral attack.

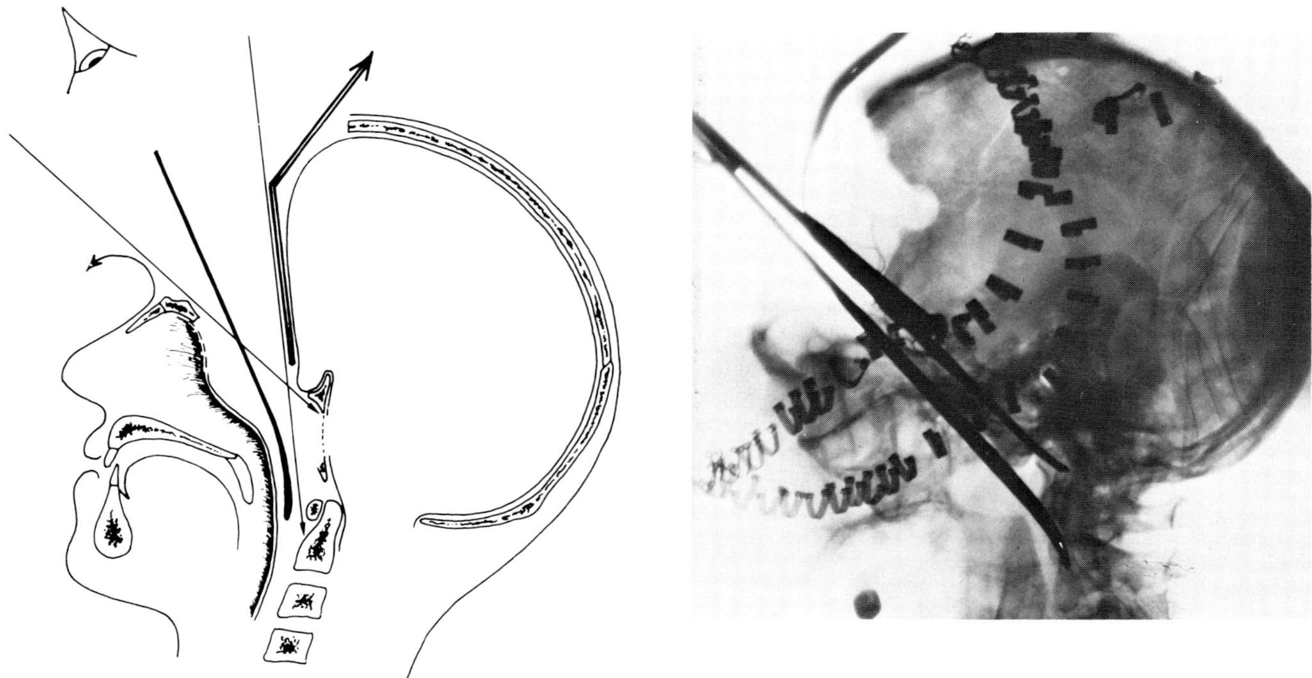

Fig. 54-14. (Left) Through the transbasal approach it is possible to reach the clivus, the anterior arch of the atlas, and the bodies of C1 and C2. Notice the preservation of the pharyngeal mucosae. (Right) An intraoperative radiogram. The tips of the instruments are located at the anterior margin of the foramen magnum and the body of C2.

subfrontal area and the other in the parietal area where the pericranial graft was extracted.

In the presence of preoperative exophthalmos, the eyelids can be closed temporarily with silk sutures and the eyes included in the dressing to avoid postoperative edema of soft orbital tissues. Lumbar drainage should be removed at the end of the procedure.

LIMITS OF THE TRANSBASAL APPROACH AND COMBINATION OF SEVERAL APPROACHES

Only the subfrontal approach provides the exposure required for extensive removal of tumors invading the base of the skull. The entire anterior fossa and the largest part of the middle fossa can be resected. It is possible to free the vessels and nerves that pass through the optic canals, the sphenoidal fissures, the foramen rotundum, and the foramen ovale (Figure 54-20). The posterior limit is the petrous bone, which can be reached through a posterolateral approach, but its removal is not consistent with conservative surgery because the seventh and eighth nerves are destroyed. Resection of a pathologically involved skull base in front of the petrous bone preserves all upper cranial nerves except the olfactory tracts.

Bone resection does not present problems; problems occur only when soft tissues are involved, as with meningiomas. In the orbital area it is often possible to overlap the limits of the tumor by careful intraorbital dissection under a surgical microscope. When the cavernous sinus is invaded, overlapping is generally impossible. Also, with the exception of rare encapsulated tumors such as chondromas, the usual invasive and adhesive characteristics of the lesion make its complete removal impossible.

Possibilities for removing the clivus through different anterior approaches are summarized in Figure 54-21. The transcervical[3] and transoral approaches provide access only to its lower half. The rhinoseptal route is convenient for gaining access to the sella, but it is narrow, lateral structures are not visible, and only the upper part of the clivus can be resected. Except for the subsellar area, which is hidden by the bulging sellar dura, the body of the clivus and sphenoid can be resected most extensively through the transbasal approach. A rhinoseptal approach can be used in the same procedure to preserve the rhinopharyngeal mucosae. Thus, both approaches can be combined, adding the advantages of each to remove the clivus completely (except for the dorsum sellae, which can be reached only intradurally).

The approach to a clival tumor depends on its nature, consistency, level of insertion, main expansion, and location relative to the dura of the clivus. Some tumors can be removed through a single anterior approach. In a few cases, however, the transbasal approach has certain advantages:

1. Tight closure of the dura is possible if there is any risk that the subarachnoidal spaces will have to be opened.
2. The procedure can be combined with a rhinoseptal or pseudotransoral approach (introducing a finger in the mouth to push an anteriorly bulging tumor backward) for tumor removal (Figure 54-22).
3. It is possible to add an intradural approach (subtemporal or through the posterior fossa) without risk of leaks, 2 to 3 months after the anterior part has been removed and the base of the skull reconstructed.

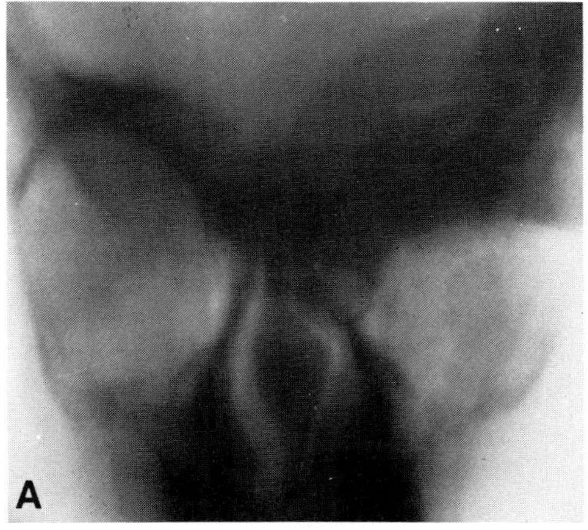

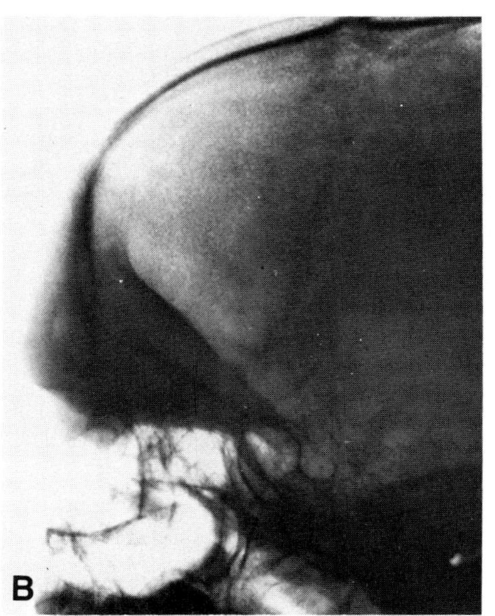

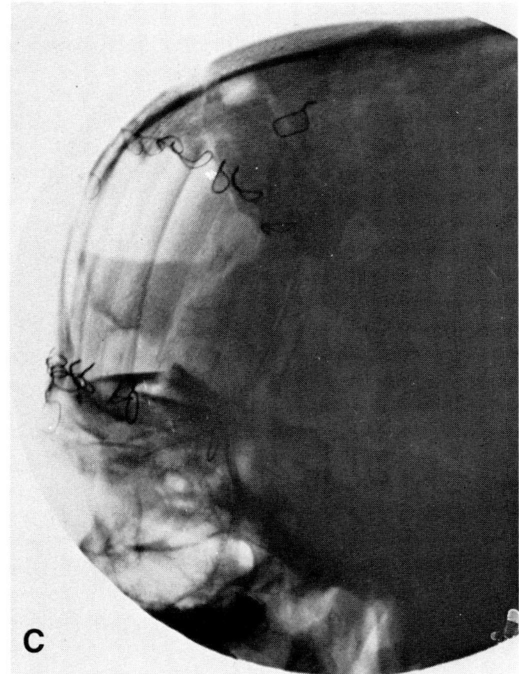

Fig. 54-15. (A and B) Fibrous dysplasia in an 8-year-old child. (C) Frontal, orbital, and basal reconstruction with split rib autografts.

INDICATIONS FOR THE TRANSBASAL APPROACH

A transbasal approach is not required to gain access to all tumors at the base of the skull. Its use depends on the exact anatomic location of the lesion. The transbasal approach, however, should be used each time it is likely to increase chances for total removal of a tumor. Table 54-1 summarizes those cases in which this approach seemed to be absolutely necessary.

Diagnosis of a tumor invading the base of the skull does not routinely lead to the same concept of treatment. The choice zbetween complete removal, decompression, or radiotherapy without surgery must be based on the histologic characteristics and extent of the lesion. For example, it is illogical to resect the base widely if an invasive malignant tumor involves the cavernous sinus. These factors must be assessed during the preoperative examination.

Arteriography, phlebography, and sometimes pneumoencephalography can detect upward extension toward the intradural spaces and cavernous sinus. Radiography, tomography, gammagraphy, and, more recently, computed tomography (CT) provide the most complete information about the nature and extent of bone invasion. The nature of the lesion may be very difficult to diagnose, however, in which case rhinoseptal

biopsy is suggested. Biopsy will prevent errors; some invasive adenomas and sphenoidal mucoceles are often confused, clinically and radiologically, with destructive chordomas.

Lesions involving the base of the skull can be divided into three groups: (1) tumors of intracranial origin, such as meningiomas; (2) true bone tumors; and (3) tumors of rhinopharyngeal origin, which generally are malignant.

MENINGIOMAS

Meningiomas invade the base of the skull in three different ways. (1) Sometimes the anterior fossa is ruptured at its weakest point, the ethmoidal area and cribriform plates, as with intranasal extension of olfactory meningiomas[2,4–9] in which there is no true bone invasion. (2) With an en plaque meningioma,[2,5,10] the dural tumor is less important than hyperostosis, which is not a single reaction but a true tumoral infiltration of bone. The hyperostosis is responsible for the entire clinical syndrome and compression of the optic nerve into the optic canal. The dural plaque as well as the bone must be removed to avoid recurrence. A pterional location is not an indication for the transbasal approach. This approach is necessary and useful, however, when the lesion overlaps the optic Zcanal and involves the sphenoidal area medially. (3) A bone reaction may be found close to the basal insertion of some en

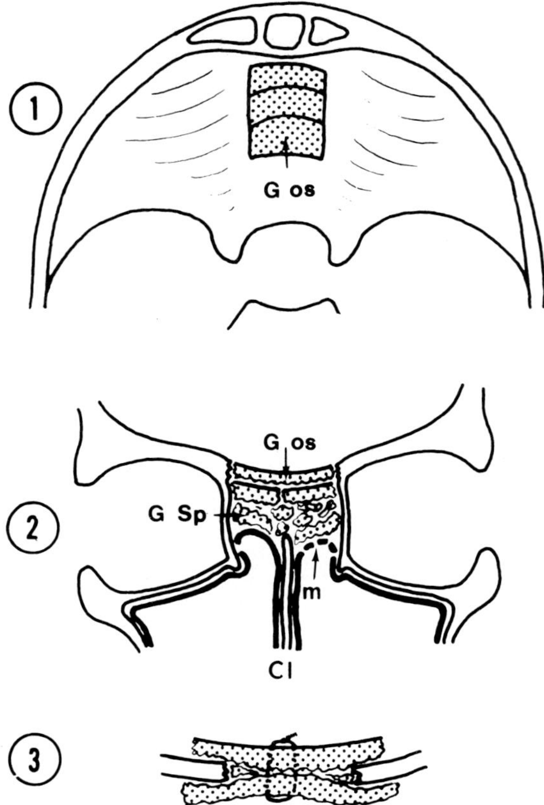

Fig. 54-16. Ethmoidal reconstruction. (1) Endocranial view of the anterior floor. G os = split rib grafts. (2) Frontal section. G sp = cancellous bone grafts; m = mucosae; Cl = nasal septum. (3) "Studlike" technique ensuring the closure of a defect when the bone is thin.

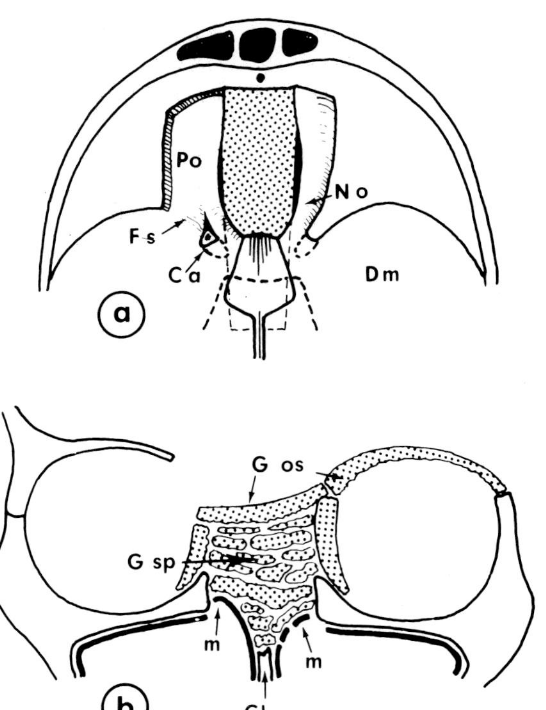

Fig. 54-17. Ethmoidosphenoidal reconstruction. (A) Endocranial view. Po = periorbita; No = optic nerve; Fs = sphenoidal fissure; Ca = anterior clinoid process; Dm = dura. (B) Frontal section. G os = cortical bone grafts; G sp = cancellous bone grafts; m = mucosae; Cl = nasal septum. Note the simultaneous repair of an orbit roof.

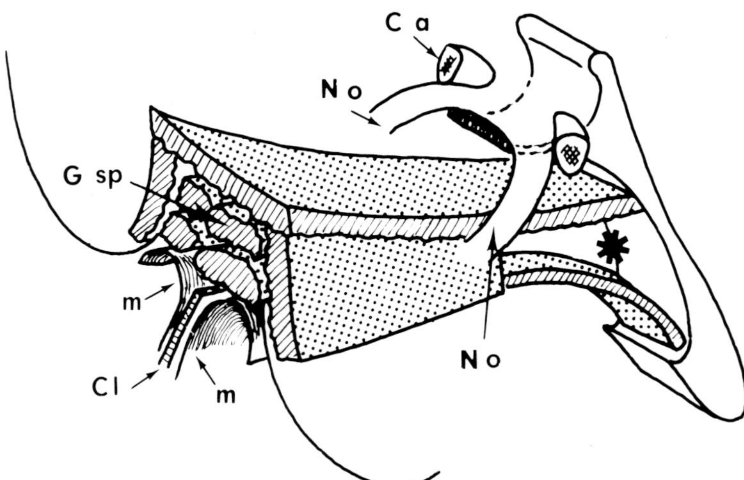

Fig. 54-18. Sphenoethmoidal reconstruction at the midline. The dead space is packed with cancellous bone grafts between the new orbital walls and the large upper graft packed below the sellar floor. Notice that both optic nerves are free. G sp = cancellous bone grafts; No = optic nerve; Ca = anterior clinoid process; m = mucosae; Cl = nasal septum.

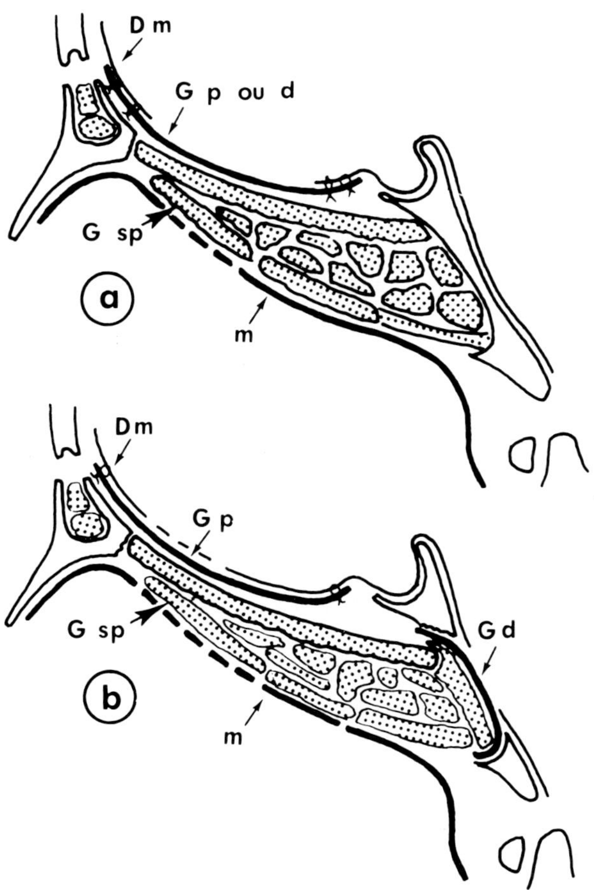

Fig. 54-19. Sagittal section of the reconstruction. (A) The upper graft is impacted between the nasion and the remnants of the clivus. (B) If the clivus is removed, the posterior edge of the upper graft is impacted close to a graft fitted between the floor of the sella and the anterior margin of the foramen magnum or the anterior arch of the atlas. Dm = dura; G p or d = pericranial or dermal graft; m = mucosae; G sp = cancellous bone grafts.

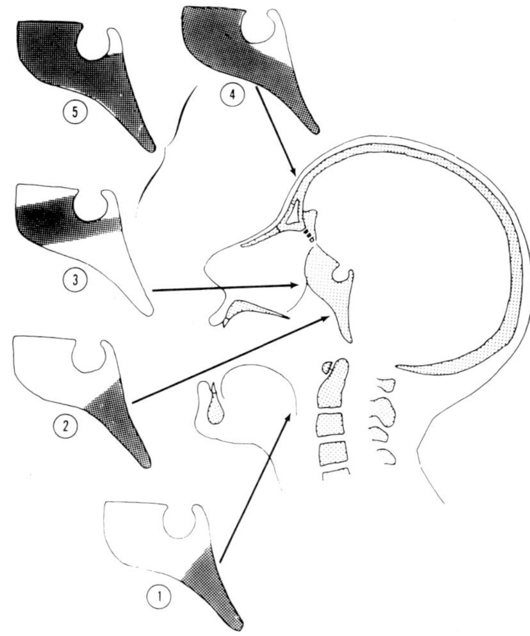

Fig. 54-21. Limits of sphenoidal and clival resection through anterior approaches. (1) transcervical approach; (2) transoral approach; (3) rhinoseptal approach; (4) transbasal approach; (5) combination of transbasal and rhinoseptal approaches.

masse meningiomas.[11] The pathologic features of such a reaction are difficult to confirm, but it may be a true invasion, causing the basal malignancy to recur several years after the intracranial part has been removed. The basal invasion of a meningioma must be removed along with the intradural mass in one or two stages, depending on the size of the dural defect and the duration of the intracranial procedure.

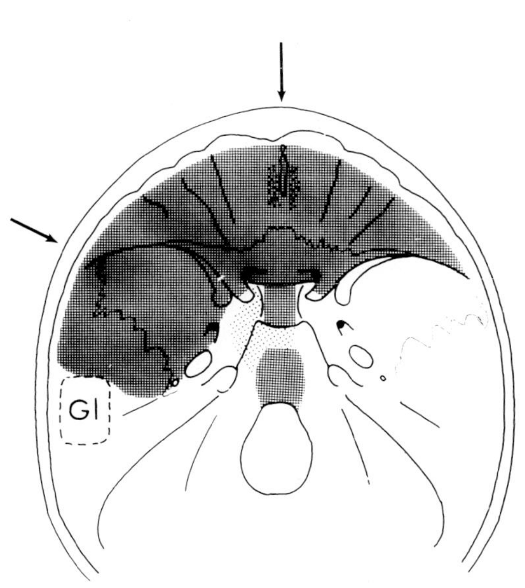

Fig. 54-20. Limits of basal resection through a bifrontal approach.

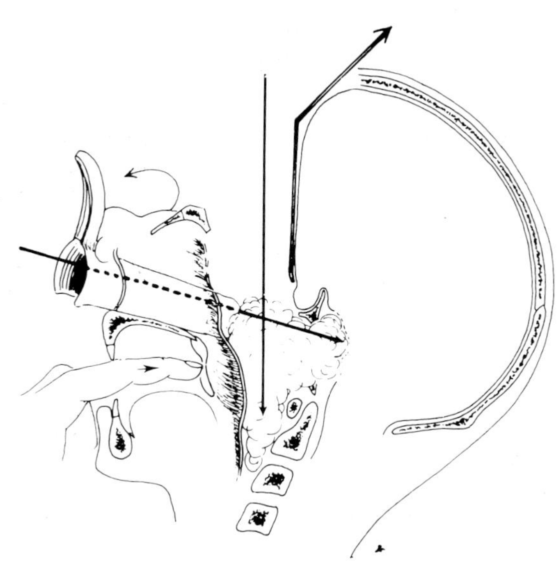

Fig. 54-22. Combination of several approaches during the same procedure (transbasal, rhinoseptal, and "pseudotransoral" approaches).

Table 54-1. Cases in which a transbasal approach was used (to December, 1985)

Tumor	Number of Patients
Fibrous dysplasia	42
Meningioma	28
Chordoma	11
Olfactory placode tumor	6
Chondroma	5
Osteoblastoma	4
Ossifying fibroma	4
Osteoma	2
Sarcoma	2
Cylindroma	1
Hemangiopericytoma	1
Nasopharyngeal fibroma	1
Total	107

TRUE BONE TUMORS

Bone tumors include many types of lesions.[11,12] Some are malignant and usually inoperable, such as sarcomas or metastases. Many are benign, such as osteomas, osteoblastomas, hemangiomas, ossifying fibromas,[2,13] or fibrous dysplasia.[2,8,14,17] Although fibrous dysplasia is not a tumor, it can be considered one clinically and is sometimes responsible for visual disturbances. It is very difficult to predict the evolution of this type of lesion, which is often found in young patients, but progressive fibrous dysplasias with rapid visual loss are not uncommon (Figure 54-23).

Our experience suggests that preventive surgery is required if the fibrous dysplasia is progressive or the area of the optic foramen is involved. Also, there are bone tumors that are difficult to classify because their pathologic potential is doubtful, even though some are malignant. Their malignancy, however, is localized, probably because it is impossible to remove them completely. Examples of these tumors are giant cell tumors,[4] chondromas,[6] and chordomas.[2,7] Surgery is certainly advised for chondromas because radiotherapy is ineffective. These tumors are more or less encapsulated and they probably can be removed almost completely, even when they develop within the cavernous sinus. With chordomas, the decision lies between surgery with or without radiotherapy, implantation of radioactive material, or radiotherapy alone. Because the transbasal approach increases the possibility that a tumor in the clival area can be removed, surgery, in my opinion, is warranted. Even if the tumor cannot be removed completely, the effectiveness of postoperative radiotherapy is improved when pathologic remnants have been reduced to a minimum. The combination of the most complete removal possible and radiotherapy gives the patient the best chance for long-term survival without recurrence.

TUMORS OF RHINOPHARYNGEAL ORIGIN

Among the rhinopharyngeal tumors that involve the base of the skull, very few are benign, i.e., benign olfactory placode tumors[11] (esthesioneurocytomas) or nasopharyngeal fibromas. These tumors generally are malignant carcinomas or epitheliomas, and the approach to each may vary. If the tumor extends toward the anterior fossa, the intracranial approach is suggested, but extensive resection of the base of the skull is only indicated when it is possible to widely overlap the area of the tumor, as in surgery for carcinoma.[1,3,13,16] Extensive removal in these cases is more important than reconstruction. Unfortunately, when a patient with this type of tumor is seen by the neurosurgeon, it is often too late to remove all tumorous

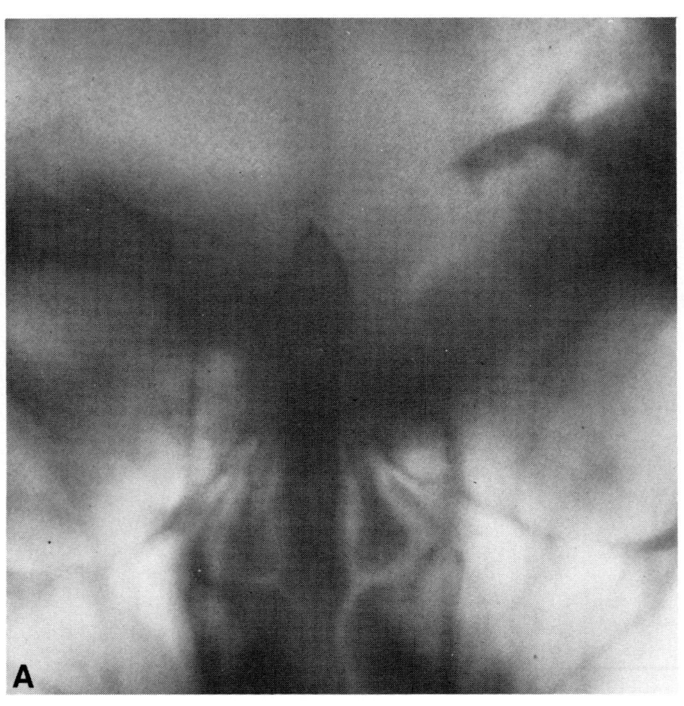

A

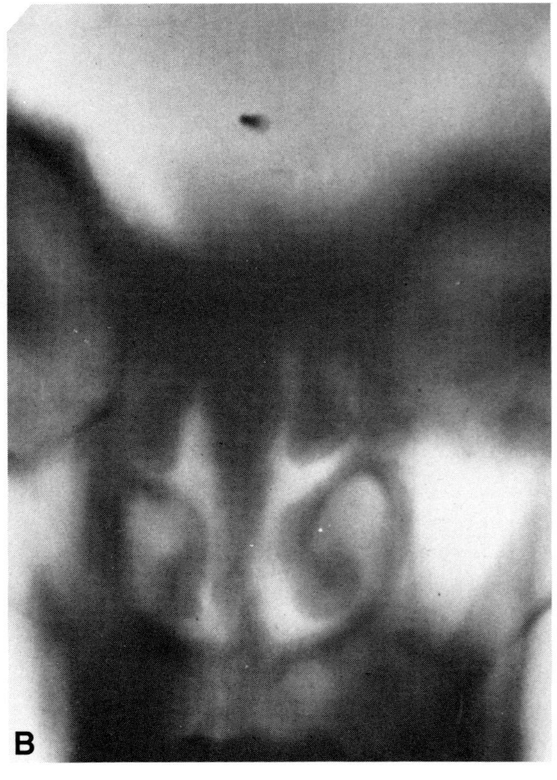

B

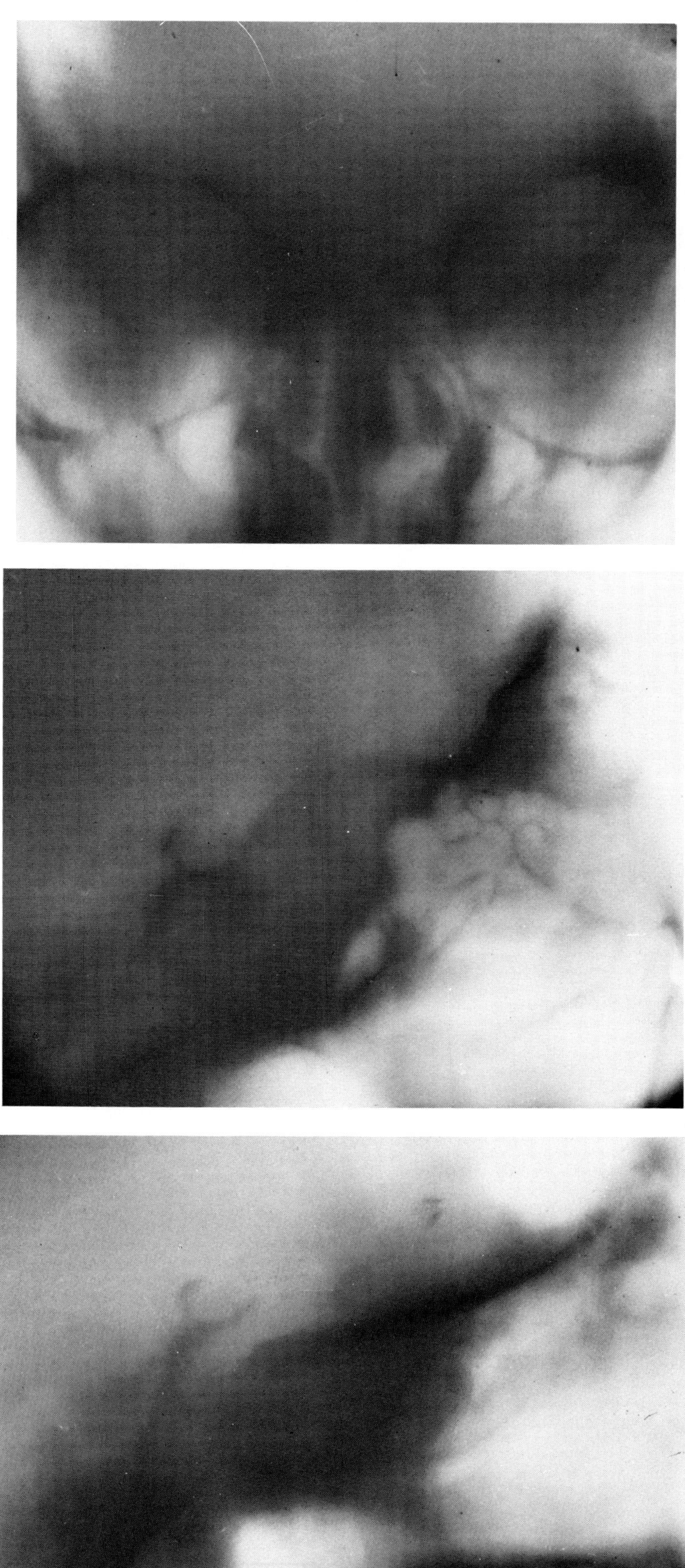

Fig. 54-23. Fibrous dysplasia responsible for visual loss. (A) Preoperative tomogram showing invasion of the entire anterior fossa. (B) Tomogram obtained 15 days after the procedure. Both orbits and the sphenoethmoidal mass have been reconstructed. (C) Tomography obtained 2 years after the procedure. Note the normal aspect of the skull base. (D) Preoperative sagittal tomogram. (E) Sagittal tomogram obtained 15 days after the procedure. Note the large upper graft covering the sphenoidal reconstruction.

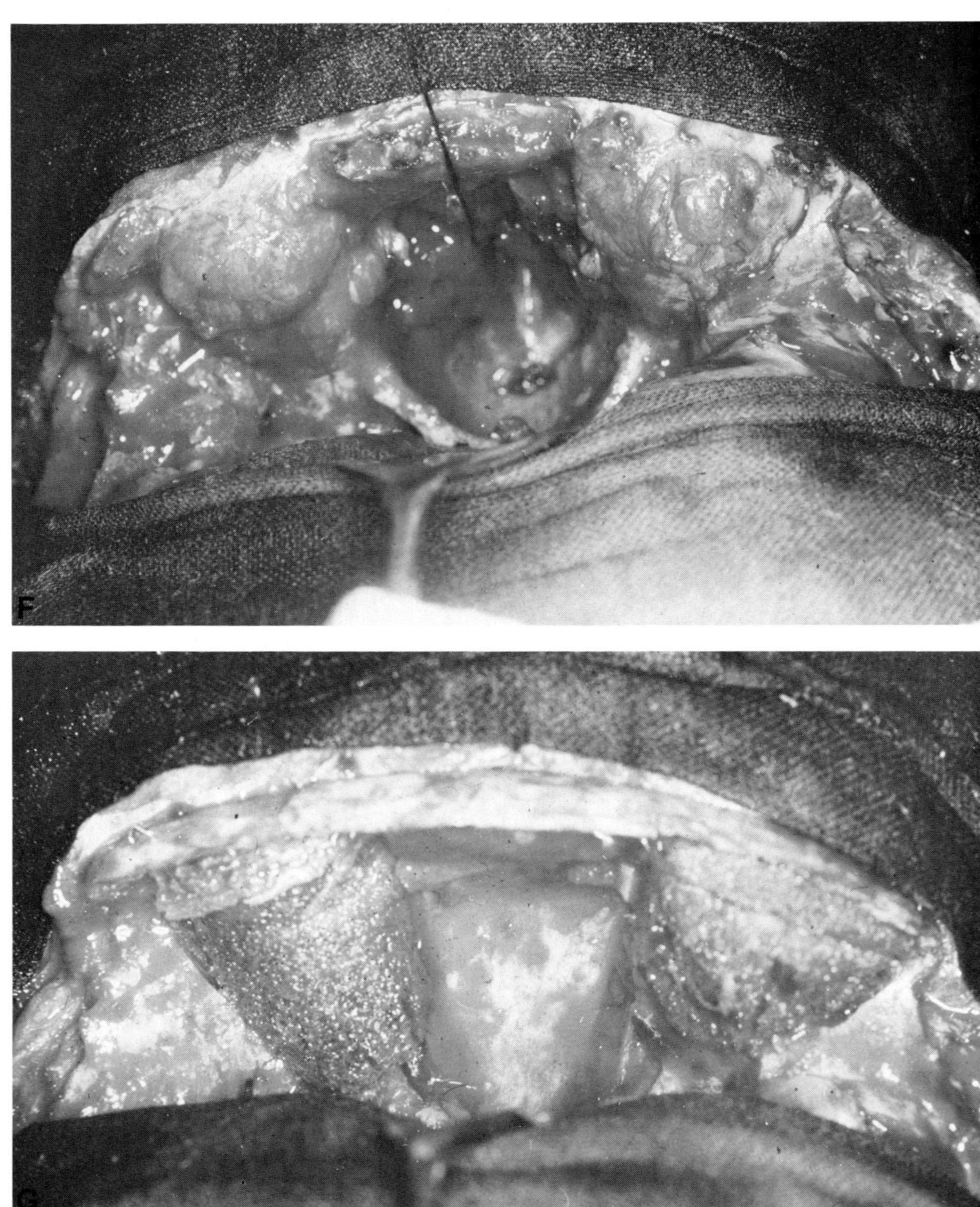

Fig. 54-23 (continued). (F) Intraoperative view of the removal of the entire anterior fossa. The upper orbital margins, roofs, and medial walls; the ethmoid; the body and lesser wings of the sphenoid; and the anterior clinoid processes have been resected. Medially this resection leads to the nasal fossae and pharyngeal mucosae. Both optic nerves are totally free and the sphenoidal fissures are opened. (G) Intraoperative view of the reconstruction. Both upper orbital margins have been repaired with a single wired split rib graft. Note the large medial graft between the reconstruction of both orbits. (H) The patient 15 days after surgery. The cosmetic result was good and she had normal vision.

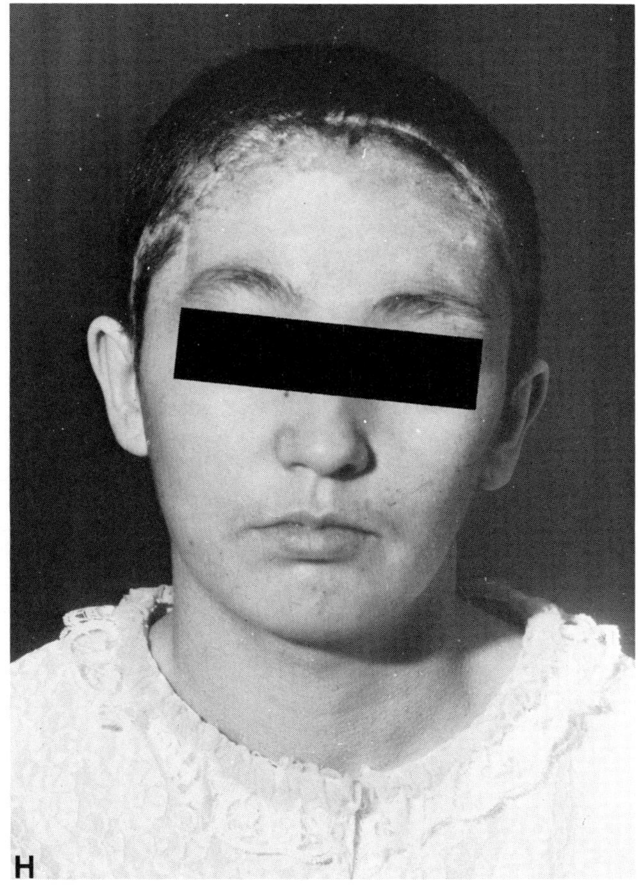

tissue completely. These patients must be seen very early in the course of tumor development, and to do so requires close cooperation between neurosurgical, ENT, and maxillofacial teams.

REFERENCES

1. Tessier P, Guiot G, Derome P: Orbital hypertelorism. II. Definite treatment of orbital hypertelorism by craniofacial or by extracranial osteotomies. Scand Plast Reconstr Surg 7:39, 1973
2. Derome P, Akerman M, Anquez L, et al: Les tumeurs spheno-ethmoidales, Possibilities d'exerese et reparation chirurgicales. Rapport de la Societe de Neurochirurgie de Langue Francaise. Neurochirurgie 15 (suppl 1):1, 1972
3. Stevenson GC, Stoney RJ, Perkins RK, et al: A transcervical, transclival approach to the ventral surface of the brainstem for removal of a clivus chordoma. J Neurosurg 24:544, 1966
4. Geissinger JD, Siqueira EB, Ross ER: Giant cell tumors of the sphenoid bone. J Neurosurg 32:665, 1970
5. Guiot G, Derome P: A propos des meningiomes en plaques du pterion. Le traitement chirurgical des meningiomes osseux hyperestosants. Ann Chir 20:C1109, 1966
6. Lehrer HZ: Ossifying fibroma of the orbital roof: Its distinction from blistering or intraosseus meningioma. Arch Neurol 20:536, 1969
7. Krayenbuhl H, Yasargil MG: Cranial chordomas. Prog Neurol 6:380, 1975
8. Liechtenstein L, Jaffe HL: Fibrous dysplasia of bone. A condition affecting one, several or many bones the graver of which may represent abnormal pigmentation of skin, premature sexual development, hyperthyroidism, or still other extraskeletal abnormalities. Arch Pathol 33:777, 1942
9. Pertuiset B, Beciric T: La voie intracranienne dans l'exerese du prolongement nasal des meningiomes olfactifs. Presse Med 63:1863, 1958
10. Castellano F, Guidetti B, Olivecrona H: Pterional meningiomas en plaques. J Neurosurg 9:188, 1952
11. Dahlin D: Bone Tumors. Springfield IL, Charles C Thomas, 1964
12. Reynaud J, Courson B: A propos des osteodysplasies et osteopathies fibreuses craniofaciales et de leur traitement. Ann Chir Plast 15:312, 1970
13. Scott M, Peale AR, Croissant PD: Intracranial midline anterior fossae ossifying fibroma invading orbits, paranasal sinuses, and right maxillary antrum. J Neurosurg 34:827, 1971
14. Plewes JL, Jacobson I: Familial frontonasal dermoid cysts. Report of four cases. J Neurosurg 34:683, 1971
15. Saunders WH, Miglets A: Surgical techniques for eradicating far advanced carcinoma of the orbital ethmoid and maxillary areas. Trans Am Acad Ophthalmol Otolaryngol 7:426, 1967
16. Van Buren JM, Ommaya AK, Ketcham AS: Ten years' experience with radical combined craniofacial resection of malignant tumors of the paranasal sinuses. J Neurosurg 28:341, 1968
17. Derome PJ, Visot A, et al: Fibrous dysplasia of the skull. Neurochirurgie 29 (suppl 1), 1983

CHAPTER 55

Surgical Treatment of Tumors of the Clivus and Basioccipital Region

R. B. Snow   R. R. Patterson, Jr.

THE REMOVAL of a tumor of the clivus or basioccipital region is a formidible surgical challenge. However, lesions that were previously regarded as inaccessible can now be removed using new surgical approaches to the skull base developed by neurosurgeons and otolaryngologists. Advances in imaging such as magnetic resonance imaging (MRI) have aided surgeons in precisely defining the margins of these lesions and in planning the optimal surgical approach.

The aim of this chapter is to briefly review the relevant surgical anatomy of the clivus region, discuss the most common tumors that develop here, discuss the neurodiagnostic evaluation of this area, and review some surgical approaches that have been developed to resect tumors in this region.

ANATOMY OF THE CLIVUS

GROSS ANATOMY

The boundaries of the clivus have not been consistently delineated. The term was used by von Sommering,[1] Blumenbachü,[2] and Virchow[3] to describe the region of the skull base between the dorsum sellae and the foramen magnum. Common neurosurgical and radiologic usage employs the entire thickness of the basioccipital bone and the body of the sphenoid bone as a definition (Figure 55-1).[4] The lateral extent of the clivus is demarcated superiorly by the petro-occipital fissure in which lies the inferior petrosal sinus, and inferiorly by the synchondrosis between the basioccipital and exoccipital bones (Figure 55-2).[4]

The posterior boundary of the clivus is formed by the slightly concave sloping surface from the base of the dorsum sellae to the anterior margin of the foramen magnum. The anterior margin is not well defined, since it blends with the sphenoid sinus. The inferior margin of the clivus consists of the nasopharyngeal surface of the lower portion of the sphenoid and basiocciput.[4]

The surfaces of the clivus are composed of cortical bone, while the central portion is composed of cancellous bone pneumatized to a variable degree by the sphenoid sinus.[4] The endocranial cortical surface is normally smooth. The inferior, or exocranial cortical surface, on the other hand, is typically irregular due to the attachments of the muscles of the nasopharynx and of the fibrous raphe of the pharynx.

The inferior petrosal sinuses drain into their respective jugular bulbs lateral to the jugular tubercles (Figure 55-2). The basilar venous plexus lies on the endocranial surface of the clivus covered by the dura.[4] Just posterior to the basilar venous plexus are the pontine and medullary cisterns that separate the pons and medulla from the clivus.

EMBRYOLOGY

The development of the clivus proceeds by the process of enchondral bone formation. The notochord begins to develop in the cephalic region of the fetus by the third week of gestation.[5] It is thought to be epithelial in origin beginning as a tubular structure, and later condensing to a solid cord of undifferentiated epitheloid cells. These undifferentiated epitheloid cells eventually undergo vacuolation and fibrillation and serve as a supporting structure for the bone formation of the base of the skull, vertebrae, and sacrum.[6]

The notochord runs a winding course through the clivus, projecting superiorly, ventrally, or dorsally.[4,7] The notochord is usually, but not exclusively, a midline structure. As originally described by Virchow in 1846, remnants of notochordal tissue may persist into adulthood.

TUMORS OF THE CLIVUS AND BASIOCCIPITAL REGION

Because of the large variety of specialized tissues present in the clivus and basioccipital region, a multitude of neoplasms and neoplasm-like lesions can occur.[8] A nonexhaustive, representative listing is given in Table 55-1. Of these lesions, chordomas, chondromas, and meningiomas are the ones most frequently seen by neurosurgeons.

CHORDOMA

Cranial chordomas are uncommon lesions representing from 0.15 to 0.2 percent of primary brain tumors. They occur more often in men than in women with a mean age at diagnosis of 38 years.[7,9] The tumor arises from notochord remnants, which explains the various sites of predilection along the clivus. Excrescences of cartilaginous tissue in the clivus found as incidental findings at postmortem examination were named *ecchondrosis spheno-occipitalis physalyphora* by Virchow in 1846. Tumors that arise from the most rostral aspect of the notochord, in the dorsum sellae, present as sellar or parasellar

OPERATIVE NEUROSURGICAL TECHNIQUES
ISBN 0-8089-1862-1

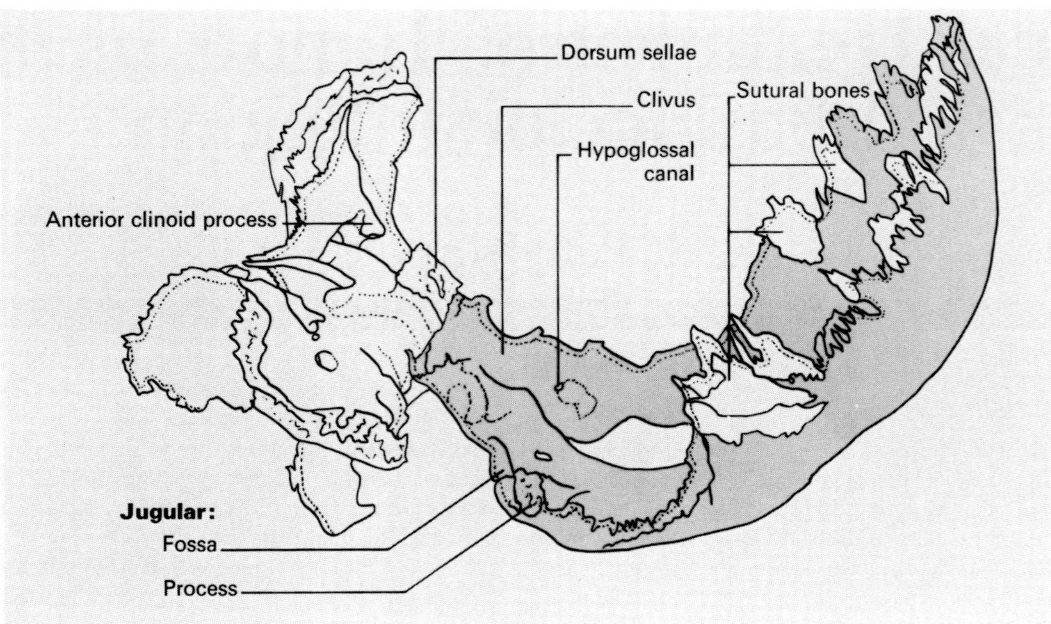

Fig. 55-1. Lateral view of the clivus.

masses. Tumors that originate in the body of the clivus ventrally present as nasopharyngeal masses, and dorsally lead to multiple cranial nerve palsies and obstructive hydrocephalus. Tumors that originate from the most caudal region of the clivus present clinically with either cerebellopontine angle syndromes or foramen magnum syndromes.

In reported series of tumors affecting the clivus, chordomas are the most common lesion.[10] The primary therapy of chordomas is surgical, but complete extirpation is rarely possible because of the location and extent of the lesion at the time of diagnosis. Radiation therapy in conjuction with surgery appears to be the best treatment plan at the present time.[11–13]

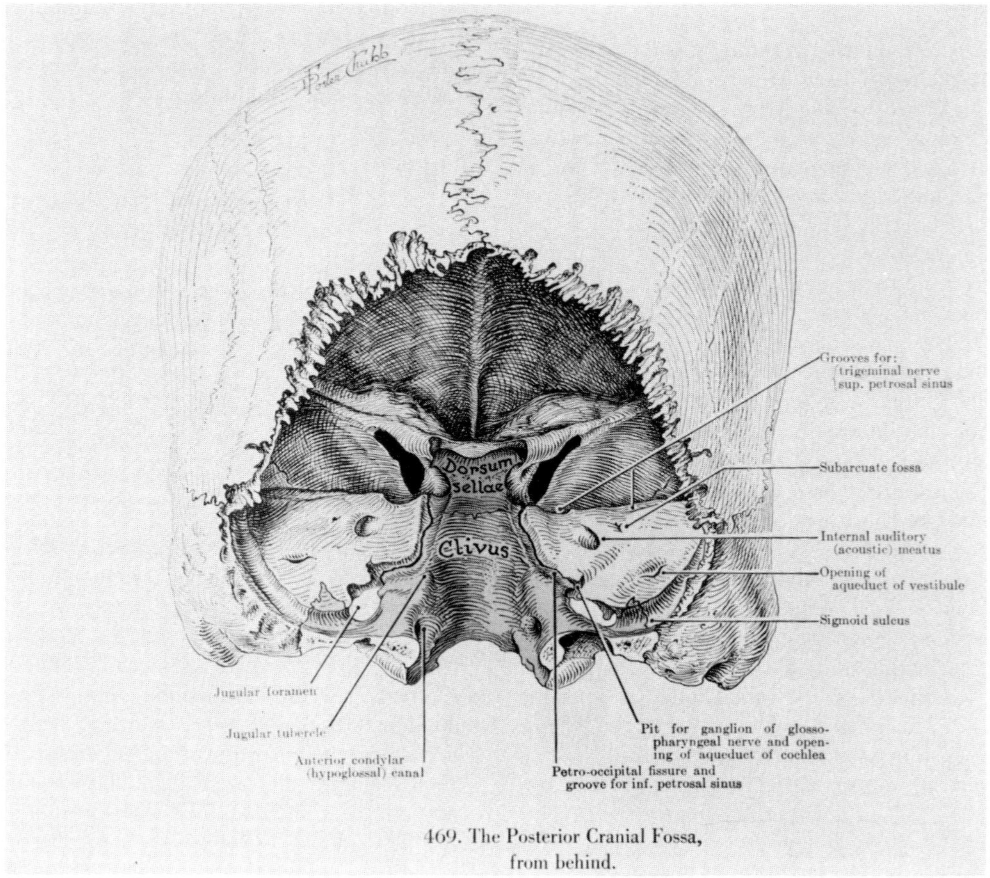

Fig. 55-2. Posterior view of the clivus.

Table 55-1. Tumors of the clivus and basioccipital region

Chordoma
Chondroma
Chondrosarcoma
Meningioma
Squamous cell carcinoma
Dermoid cyst
Arachnoid cyst
Teratogenic cyst
Giant cell tumor
Craniopharyngioma
Pituitary adenoma
Plasmacytoma
Acinic cell carcinoma
Adenoid cystic carcinoma
Metastatic carcinoma

CHONDROMAS

Chondromas are a subtype of chordoma which account for about 25 percent of the group.[11,14,15] Their significance is that the mean survival of patients with this subtype is substantially longer than in the nonchondroid type.[11] In a series of 155 chordomas seen at the Mayo Clinic reported by Heffelfinger et al.,[11] 19 of the 55 intracranial tumors were of the chondroid subtype. The average survival among patients with chondroid elements in the tumor was 15.8 years, compared with 4.1 years among those with the nonchondroid type of chordoma.

Meningiomas constitute roughly one sixth of primary intracranial tumors.[16] They occur more frequently in women (the female-to-male ratio for clivus meningiomas was 4:1 in Yasargil's series[17]) with a mean age in the 40s. Posterior fossa meningiomas constituted 1 to 1.7 percent of all brain tumors in the large series of Cushing and Olivecrona.[18,19] Clivus meningiomas made up 11 percent of the posterior fossa meningiomas in Olivercrona's series,[18] and 38 percent in Yasargil's series.[17] In the past 3 years we have operated on 193 cranial meningiomas at our institution. Approximately 708 of these patients are women. Twenty percent of these tumors originated in the posterior fossa. Four of these cases were clivus meningiomas.

Surgery is the primary therapeutic modality for clivus meningiomas, with radiation therapy of benefit in subtotally removed tumors.[20] The possibility of medical treatment through hormone modulation of these tumors has been suggested, but thus far there has been no proven clinical efficacy for this approach.[21,22,23] Nonetheless, as more in vitro evidence is accumulated, anti-estrogen drugs such as tomoxifen and progestational agents such as medroxyprogesterone acetate,[21,22,23] may play an adjuvant role in unresectable base of skull meningiomas. Total excision of these tumors is typically quite treacherous because of their proximity to multiple cranial nerves. Yasargil[17] was able to radically extirpate 7 of 20 clivus meningiomas. Five of these patients were judged in good condition postoperatively, and two were judged in fair condition.

CLINICAL PRESENTATION

The clinical presentation of clivus region tumors depends on the exact location of the tumor. The various lesions found in this area have different growth patterns and sites of precise origin and therefore produce a variety of clinical syndromes. For the purpose of this review we will only detail the clinical presentation of the more common lesions: clivus chordomas and meningiomas.

CHORDOMA

Chordomas that originate from the most rostral fingers of notochord remnants in the dorsum sellae produce symptoms and signs suggestive of optic chiasm and/or nerve damage, pituitary dysfunction, and/or a cavernous sinus syndrome. Commonly, these patients also have headaches.[7,12]

When tumors arise from the mid-clival region they may fungate ventrally and present as a nasopharyngeal mass, or grow dorsally and present with multiple cranial nerve palsies. The most common presenting symptom from these tumors is diplopia due to either unilateral or bilateral lateral rectus palsy.[12] The sixth cranial nerve is particularly susceptible to the effects of these tumors because of its relatively long course in the dura of the clivus. As midclival chordomas become larger they produce multiple cranial nerve palsies (fifth through twelfth), brain stem compression syndromes (ataxia, dysarthria, vertigo, pyramidal signs), syndromes of the cerebellopontine angle, and obstructive hydrocephalus.[7,12]

Chordomas that arise from notochordal remnants in the basion typically produce twelfth cranial nerve palsy and/or a foramen magnum syndrome. Headache and neck pain commonly occur with chordomas in this location as well.

MENINGIOMA

Meningiomas that originate from the mid and rostral clivus region typically produce multiple cranial nerve palsies, gait ataxia, and headaches. The cranial nerves most commonly affected are the fifth, eighth, and seventh, in that order.[17]

In Yasargil's series[17] over 70 percent of patients with clivus or cerebellopontine angle meningiomas produced gait ataxia. Headaches occur in roughly 25 percent of the patients.[17]

Meningiomas arising from the inferior clivus region around the foramen magnum produce occipital-nuchal pain and/or accessory nerve palsies.[17,24] These patients also may develop Brown-Sequard syndromes and dysfunction of cranial nerves 9, 10, and 12.[17]

Inexplicably, although clivus meningiomas often encase or displace cranial nerves III, IV, and VIII, patients seldom develop palsies of these cranial nerves.[17] This is in sharp contrast to clivus chordomas and may be a point of differential diagnosis based on clinical presentation.

NEURODIAGNOSTIC EVALUATION

PLAIN ROENTGENOGRAPHY

The clivus is not adequately visualized in roentgenograms of the skull in the standard projections. However, the bony anatomy of the clivus is demonstrated adequately by sagittal tomography in the lateral projection and by frontal tomography in which the plane of the cut is parallel to the slope of the clivus.[4]

Chordomas of the clivus typically demonstrate dense nodular calcification associated with bone erosion on tomography.[25] Clival meningiomas, on the other hand, rarely demonstrate bone erosion on plain roentgenograms.[17,25] Rather,

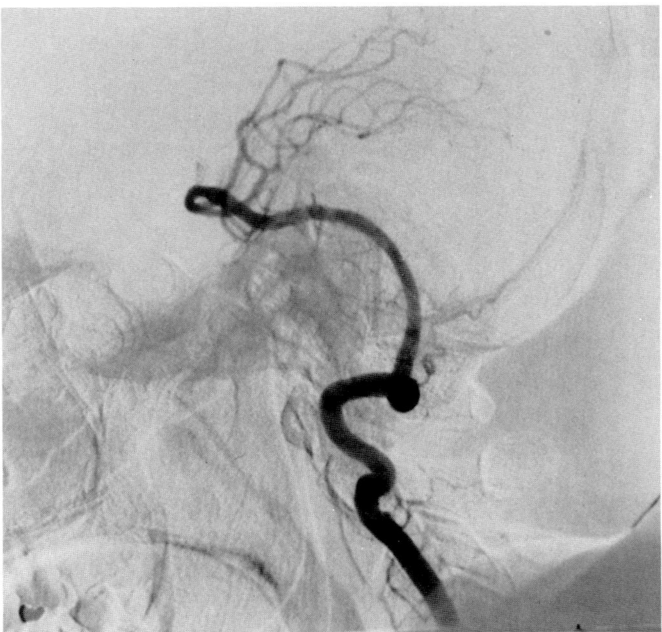

Fig. 55-3. Lateral angiogram of a clivus meningioma demonstrating posterior displacement of the basilar artery.

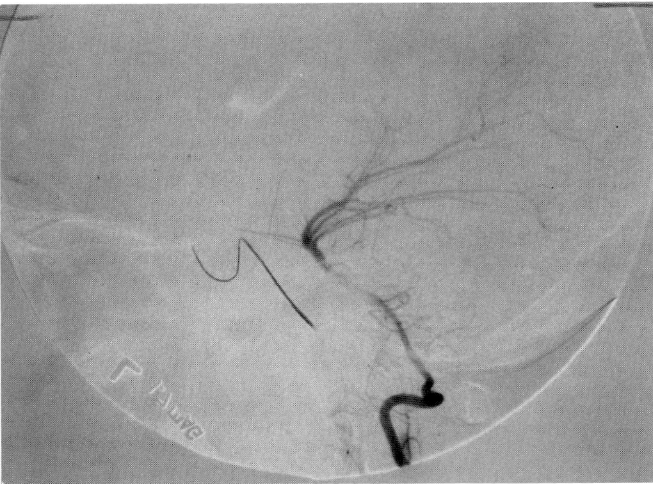

Fig. 55-5. Lateral angiogram of clivus chordoma with posterior displacement of basilar artery from clivus (highlighted).

hyperostosis consisting of a generalized increased bony density or irregularly sclerotic clival border is more characteristic.[4] In Yasargil's[17] series of 20 clivus meningiomas, the tomograms were entirely normal in six cases.

ANGIOGRAPHY

Vertebral and carotid (selective internal and external) angiograms are helpful in the preoperative evaluation of patients with clival tumors. Abnormal vessels or a tumor blush are sometimes seen with clival meningiomas[17] and chordomas.[26] The most characteristic finding in chordomas as well as

meningiomas is posterior displacement of the basilar artery (Figures 55-3, 55-4, and 55-5), although occasionally the artery may run along the anterior aspect of the tumor along its base.[17,18] Knowledge of the relation of major vessels to the tumor as well as the origin of the principal feeding vessels can be helpful in planning extirpation of the tumor. We therefore obtain an angiogram in most cases of clivus tumors.

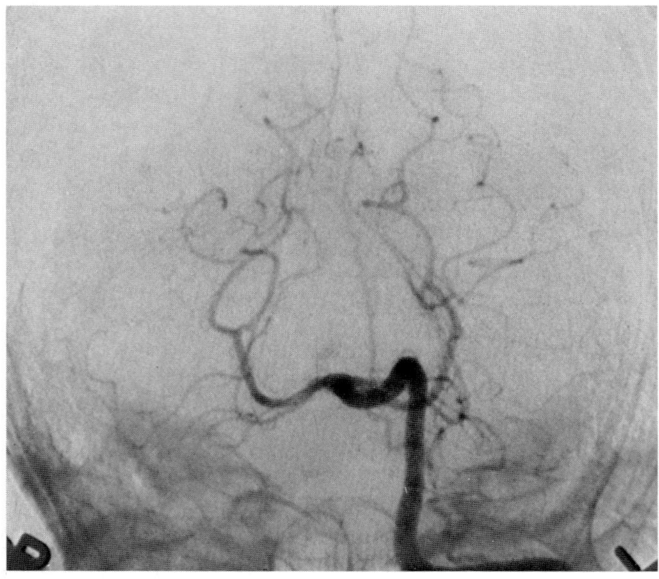

Fig. 55-4. An AP angiogram of the same patient as shown in Fig. 55-3 demonstrating displacement of the basilar artery.

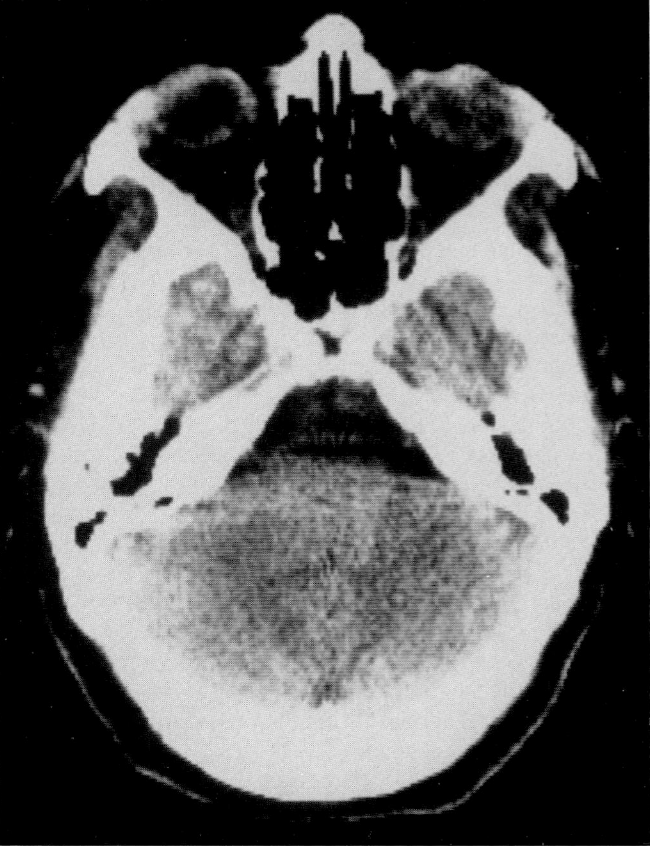

Fig. 55-6. Noncontrast CT scan of a patient with a clivus meningioma demonstrating the mass in the posterior fossa, which is isodense before contrast administration.

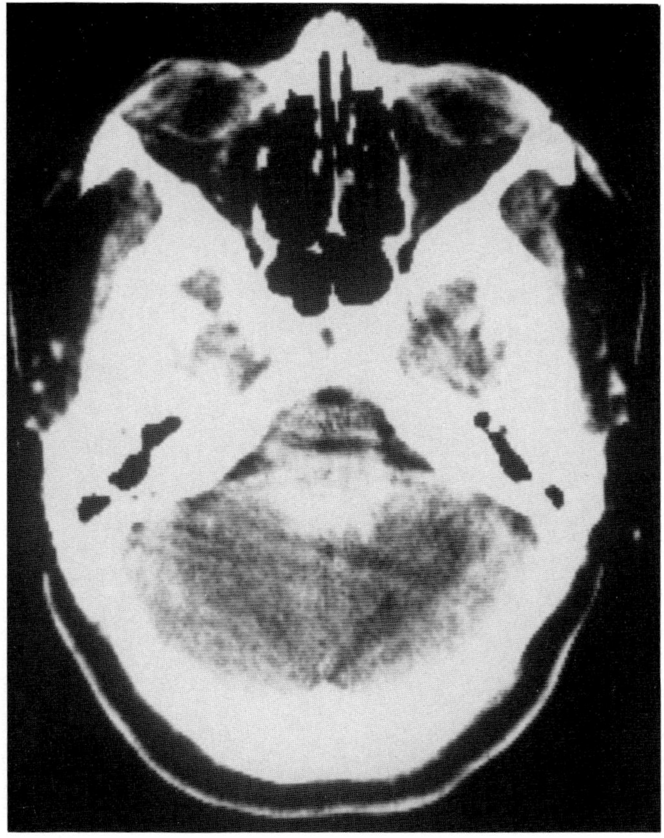

Fig. 55-7.   Contrast CT scan of same patient as shown in Fig. 55-6 demonstrating intense tumor enhancement which is typical for clivus meningiomas.

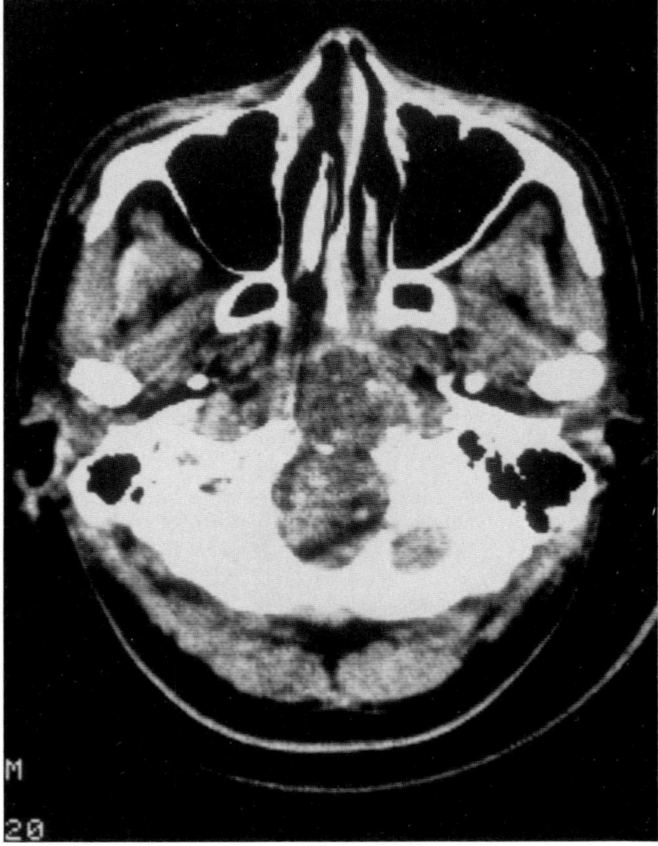

Fig. 55-8.   Noncontrast CT scan of a patient with a clivus chordoma. Apparent is bony destruction of the clivus and typical calcification within the tumor mass.

COMPUTED TOMOGRAPHY

High resolution computed tomography (CT) enables visualization of bony foramina, fissures, and canals as well as the juxtaposed soft tissues and thus is helpful in the neurodiagnostic evaluation of base of skull tumors.[27,28] Cranial chordomas commonly demonstrate bone erosion and occasionally calcification within the tumor.[26] Following administration of intravenous contrast, chordomas may or may not enhance, with the degree of enhancement generally less than is the case with meningiomas.[26] Clival meningiomas typically show marked enhancement following intravenous contrast. Hyperostosis is commonly seen, and rarely bone destruction.[17] Examples of the typical CT appearance of these tumors are shown in Figures 55-6 through 55-9.

MAGNETIC RESONANCE IMAGING

Because of the absence of bone artifacts, magnetic resonance imaging (MRI) demonstrates the exact relationship of clival tumors to the brain stem. Additionally, the relationship of large blood vessels to the tumor can be seen on MRI scans (Figure 55-10). Meningiomas tend to be isointense on MRI scans, while chordomas tend to be slightly hyperintense on T2-weighted images (Figure 55-11). We have found MRI in conjunction with CT invaluable in diagnosing and revealing the extent of clival region tumors (Figure 55-12). In the future, with improved resolution using magnets of greater strength, MRI

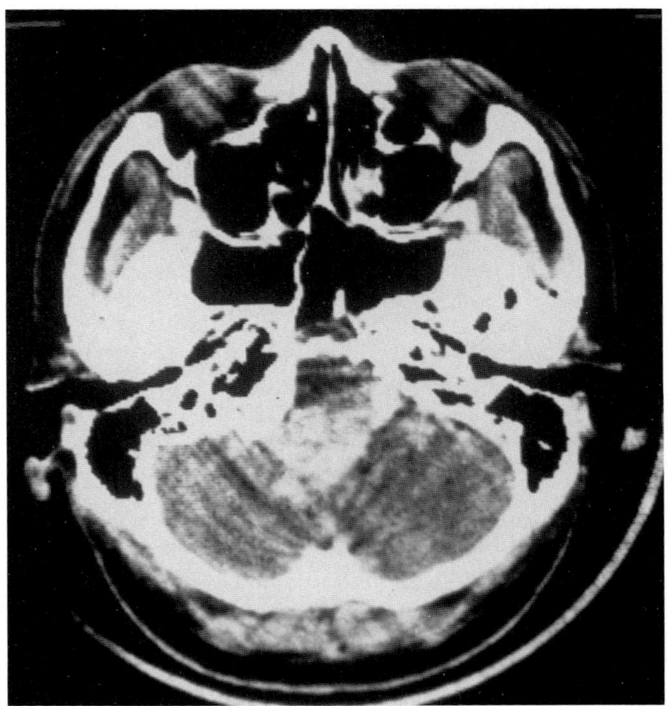

Fig. 55-9.   Contrast CT scan of same patient as shown in Fig. 55-8, which demonstrates enhancement of the chordoma.

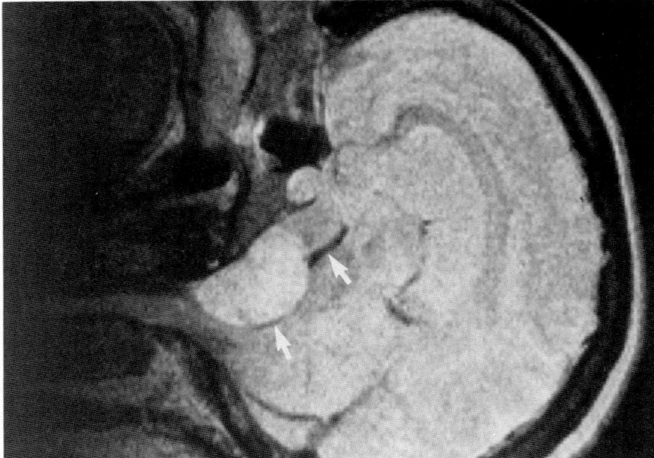

Fig. 55-10. Sagittal MRI scan of a patient with a clivus meningioma demonstrating posterior displacement of the basilar artery (arrows) and brain stem.

may eliminate the necessity of cerebral angiography in the preoperative evaluation of patients with these tumors.

SURGICAL APPROACHES TO THE CLIVUS

Multiple surgical approaches have been devised to explore the clivus area including primarily extradural anterior, extradural posterolateral, and intradural (frontotemporal, subtemporal and suboccipital) routes. All of these approaches have limitations and none provides completely satisfactory exposure in cases of particularly extensive tumors.[17] In this section, some of these approaches will be discussed including the advantages, limits, and complications of each.

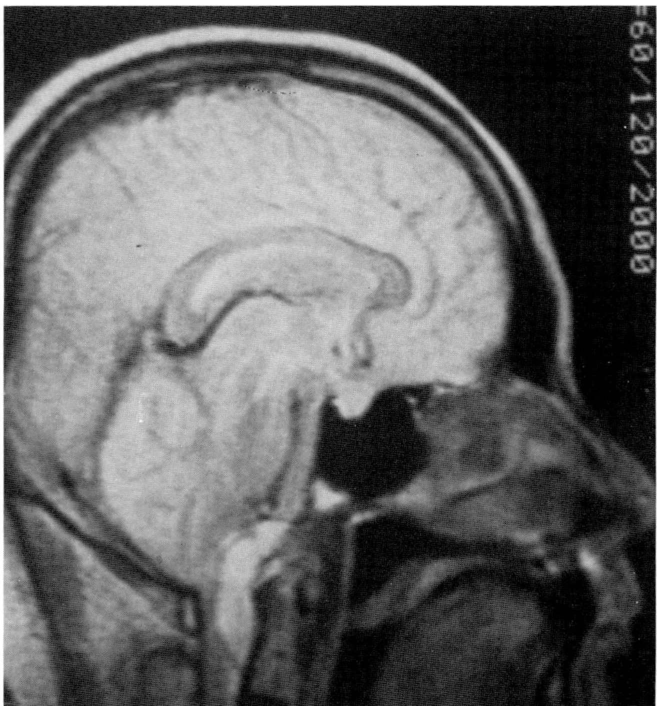

Fig. 55-11. A T2-weighted MRI scan of a clivus chordoma demonstrating the hyperintense tumor relative to adjacent brain stem.

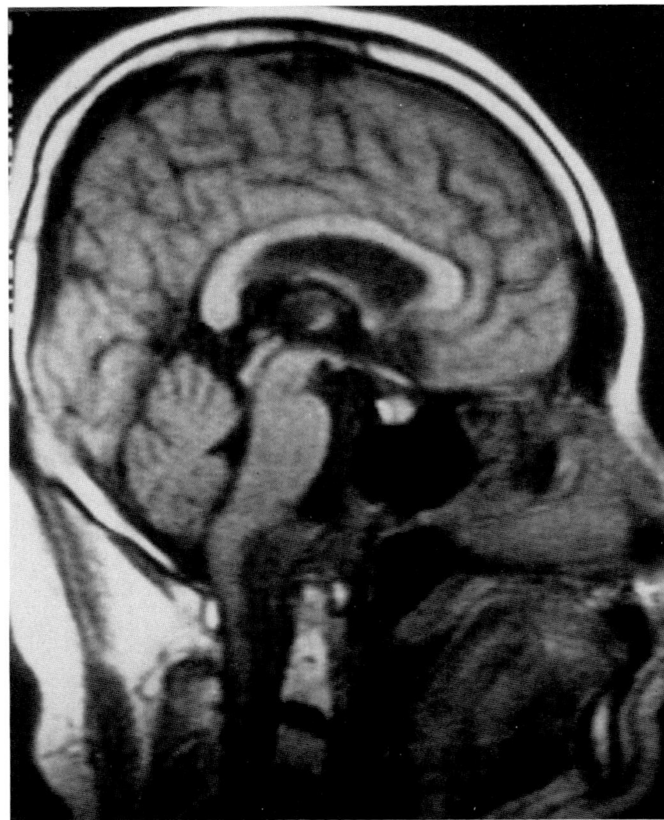

Fig. 55-12. Sagittal T1-weighted MRI scan of a clivus chordoma demonstrating the tumor compressing the medulla as well as a tumor mass in the retropharyngeal space.

INTRADURAL APPROACHES

Frontotemporal Approach

The frontotemporal (pterional) approach, as described by Yasargil[29] for internal carotid artery aneurysms, has been used in approaching rostral clivus tumors with extension laterally to the petrous bone and anteriorly to the anterior middle fossa and region of the optic nerves and internal carotid artery.[17] Clivus meningiomas at times grow extensively in these regions—filling the floor of the middle fossa and extending deep in the cerebellopontine angle. Yasargil[17] has discussed the removal of clivus meningiomas via this route in detail. The hazards are numerous and include damage to the internal carotid arteries, optic nerves, pituitary stalk, cranial nerves III, IV, V, and VI, and pontine perforating arteries when dissecting tumor from around the basilar artery. However, the major problem with the pterional approach is that the clivus below the posterior clinoids is impossible to visualize, and this by definition is the origin of clival meningiomas. Consequently, only a partial removal of tumor can be achieved through this approach.

Subtemporal Approach

The subtemporal approach is excellent for tumors of the upper clivus which compress the brainstem.[17,30] The patient is positioned supine with a roll under the ipsilateral shoulder and a question mark frontotemporal incision is made (Figure 55-13). Alternatively, a horseshoe-shaped incision over the ear can be utilized. We advocate employing spinal drainage since the dura

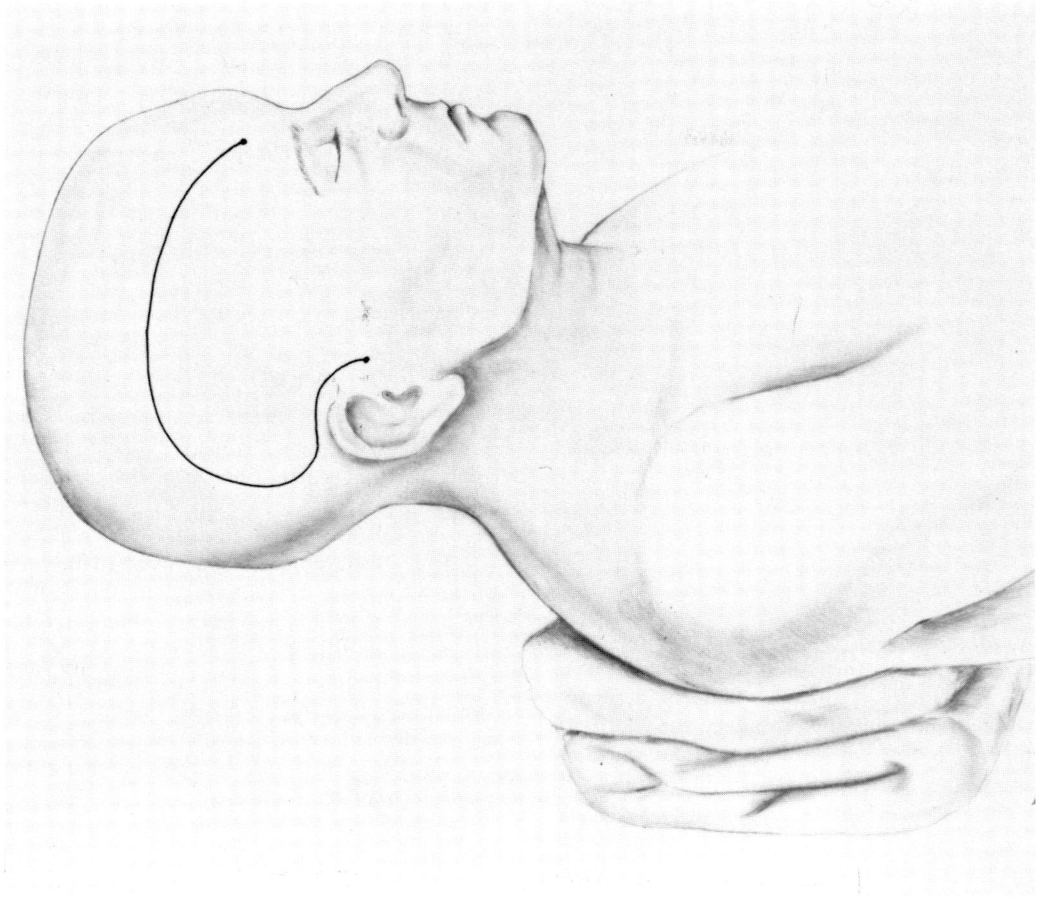

Fig. 55-13.   Skin incision for subtemporal approach to upper clivus tumors.

is often tense with large tumors, and removal of cerebrospinal fluid facilitates temporal lobe retraction.

Once the dura is opened, the middle fossa is explored by careful successive retraction of the temporal lobe from its posterior one third. The vein of Labbé needs to be preserved to avoid the risk of a venous infarction of the temporal lobe. Tumor is removed first from the middle fossa, then more anteriorly toward the chiasmatic area. Once tumor is removed from the middle fossa, the tentorium is incised parallel to the petrous ridge from the free edge to the lateral sinus, taking care to preserve the trochlear nerve. The cerebellopontine angle and prepontine regions are thus exposed and tumor is removed. During tumor removal, the surgeon must always be on the lookout for cranial nerves III, IV, V, and VI. Should these structures be seen to be passing through portions of the tumor, as particularly may occur with meningiomas, the operation should be terminated, for dissection places these nerves at great risk for permanent damage.

If necessary, a paramedian suboccipital posterior limb skin excision can be made, allowing a suboccipital craniectomy to increase exposure. In this regard, Malis[31] has developed a procedure to preserve the vein of Labbé that allows a wide petrosal approach.

The posterior fossa is exposed in similar fashion to removing an angle tumor. The mastoid process is removed with a high speed drill and rongeurs, and bone resection is carried out completely across the sigmoid and lateral sinuses. The dura is then opened in a curved fashion with its base medially in the posterior fossa just beneath the line of the lateral sinus. The dura in the temporal region is opened parallel to the base, extending backward over the first anterior centimeter of the lateral sinus.[31] The vein of Labbé enters the lateral sinus from the temporal lobe posterior to this point.

The next step in Malis's[31] approach is to ligate the lateral sinus distal to the vein of Labbé and proximal to the junction of the sigmoid sinus and petrosal sinus. Once the sinus is divided, the tentorium is divided along the petrosal apex taking care to preserve the petrosal sinus.

Once the tentorium is incised all the way to the free edge, a retractor is placed under the tentorium, and the tentorium, lateral sinus, temporal lobe, and vein of Labbé are lifted together. This serves to expose widely subtemporally in the anterior direction and all the way down the clivus toward the foramen magnum. Of importance, the vein of Labbé is able to drain through the medial portion of the lateral sinus, across the torcular, and then through the opposite lateral and sigmoid sinus into the opposite jugular vein.[31]

The subtemporal approach affords good exposure to the upper and mid-clival areas, but risks postoperative deficits such as aphasia and epilepsy due to temporal lobe retraction.[17,30] These deficits are often transient and can be minimized by limiting the retraction of the temporal lobe to less than 15 mm.

Other complications with this procedure include damage to cranial nerves III through VIII, as well as brain stem ischemia if perforators off the basilar artery are sacrificed with the tumor dissection.[17,31] These latter complications can be avoided if the

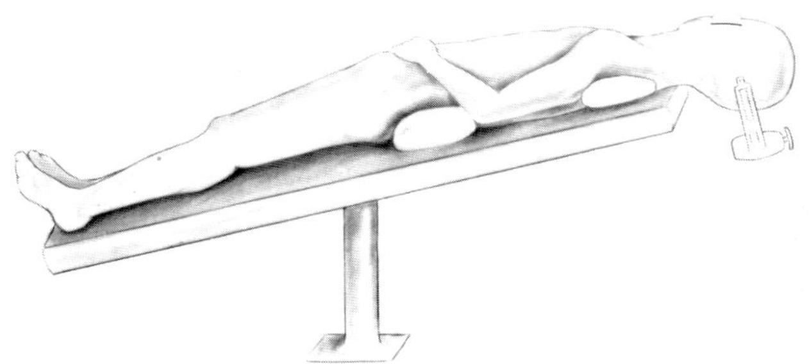

Fig. 55-14. Position and skin incision employed for suboccipital approach to lower clivus tumors.

surgeon recognizes that clival tumors that engulf multiple cranial nerves and the basilar artery are not amenable to total resection and terminates the operative procedure following tumor debulking.

Suboccipital Approach

The suboccipital approach affords exposure of the lower portion of the clivus down to the foramen magnum. The positioning and skin incision is similar to that for acoustic neuromas, except the skin incision may be carried superiorly to allow for an occipital craniotomy with splitting of the tentorium for greater exposure if necessary. We position the patient supine with a roll under the ipsilateral shoulder and hip. A lumbar spinal needle is employed for removal of CSF as necessary. The head is placed in Mayfield pins, moderately flexed, and rotated about 20 to 30 degrees away from the side of the approach (Figure 55-14). The posterior fossa is exposed widely from the transverse sinus-sigmoid sinus junction laterally, to the midline, and below to the posterior ridge of the foramen magnum.

If an occipital-temporal craniotomy is used in conjunction with the suboccipital approach, as described above, it is helpful to know preoperatively that the two lateral sinuses join through the torcular and that the jugular vein of the opposite side is open.[31] Therefore, good quality bilateral venous phase angiography is required preoperatively.

Tumor resection proceeds with surgical debulking once the dura is opened. Removal of large amounts of tumor is difficult with the suboccipital approach because the fifth through eleventh cranial nerves are likely to be interposed between the surgeon and the tumor.[30,31] When the tumor extends caudally to the foramen magnum and below, the vetebral arteries may be deflected backwards over the tumor surface as well.[30] Nonetheless, total tumor removal can at times be accomplished by intratumoral debulking using aids such as bipolar cutting cautery forceps, ultrasonic aspirator, or laser.

The principal problems with this operation for meningioma are postoperative cranial nerve palsies and ataxia. Most patients will sustain at least a partial facial palsy, deafness, and great difficulty swallowing leading to aspiration pneumonia. A cerebrospinal fluid shunting procedure may also be required. If a patient is debilitated before surgery it is reasonable to consider a prophylactic tracheostomy, a percutaneous gastrostomy, and a ventricular shunt. Fortunately, these complications are likely to be transient since it should be possible to preserve the cranial nerves. The alternatives, partial removal, shunting alone, or radiation therapy are not attractive because the tumor inevitably continues to grow with progressive disability and death the result.

An alternative to the one-staged procedure advocated by Malis is a two-staged procedure attacking the posterior fossa at one sitting and the tumor at or above the tentorial notch at a second. This plan has merit particularly if tumor removal is tedious and time consuming due to the small space available in which to operate between the nerves coupled with the likelihood that the tumor itself is tough, fibrous, and highly vascular.

EXTRADURAL ANTERIOR APPROACHES

Transcervical Approach

This approach, first described by Stevenson et al.,[32] is best suited for low clivus lesions. A curvilinear submandibular skin incision is made from the tip of the mastoid to the symphysis menti, with a "T" extension across the sternocleidomastoid to the level of C8. The axis and atlas are then exposed between the neck vessels and the trachea. Using high speed drills, as well as various rongeurs, the anterior arch of the atlas and the odontoid are removed. The microscope is then brought into the field and a window is drilled in the clivus from the anterior rim of the foramen magnum to just anterior to the sphenoccipital synchondrosis. Once exposed, tumor is removed with standard techniques and the aid of the microscope.

A drawback to this approach is that exposure is limited to the width of the odontoid process. However, it offers an advantage over other anterior approaches, such as a transoral approach, in that the surgeon is not operating through a contaminated field. Thus, should the dura be opened either voluntarily or accidently, the risk of a cerebrospinal fluid leak into a septic cavity is not present.

Complications of the procedure mainly relate to injury to structures encountered in the course of the exposure, and are similar to those inherent in removing cervical discs from the anterior approach.[33] These include perforation of the pharynx, esophagus, or trachea; recurrent laryngeal nerve palsy; injury to the vertebral artery, carotid artery, or jugular vein; a cerebrospinal fluid fistula; and, only if dissection extends lateral to the longus colli muscles, Horner's syndrome.

Transoral Approach

The transoral approach to the low clivus and upper cervical spine has been employed for a variety of problems including tuberculosis, atlantoaxial dislocation, and osteoma of the axis[34,35]; as well as for low clival neoplasms,[36] and the correction of choanal atresia.[37] After retraction or incision of the soft palate, a midline cut is made from the hard palate to the uvula, where the incision becomes paramedian.[30] The soft tissues are retracted laterally, and the exposure is extended by resecting the posterior edge of the hard palate. C1 and C2 are exposed by a midline vertical incision of the pharyngeal mucosa. After removal of the arch of the atlas, the odontoid and clivus can be visualized. The odontoid and inferior clivus can be resected using a high speed drill. By so doing, the anterior rim of the foramen magnum is opened, permitting extradural decompression of the brain stem.

Chordomas are usually extradural, and thus can be removed via this approach. However, tumors that invade the dura and require dural opening cannot be removed safely by this approach. This is because the dura is very adherent to the clivus and nearly impossible to suture closed. Instead, the surgeon

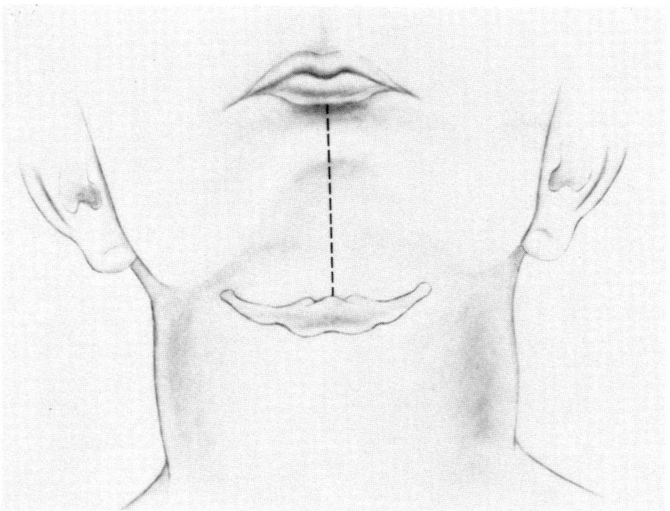

Fig. 55-15. Skin incision for transoral median labiomandibular approach to tumors of the clivus.

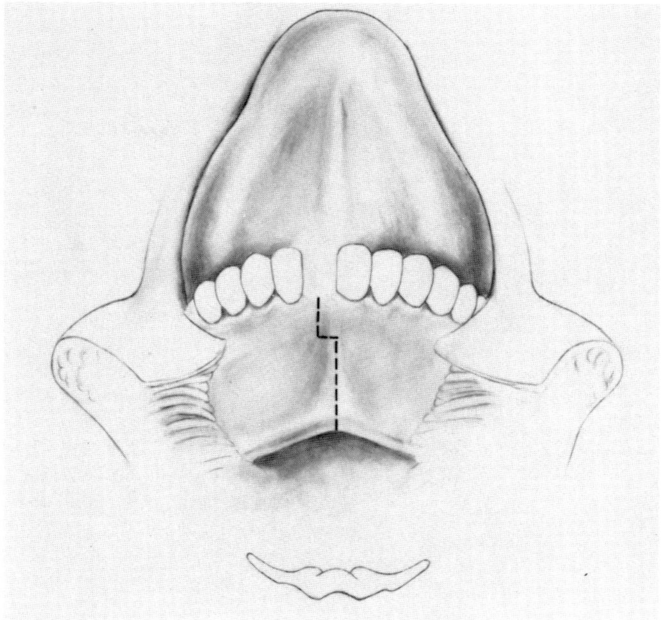

Fig. 55-16. Removal of one tooth and steplike mandibular incision.

must rely on packing with muscle, aponeurosis, or lyophylized dura, risking a cerebrospinal fluid leak and meningitis.[30]

A major disadvantage of this approach is meningitis from a persistent cerebrospinal fluid leak should the dura be opened. A further disadvantage is the rather limited exposure one can achieve via this route. Only the midline aspect of the bottom half of the retroclival area can be exposed and the opening in the clivus is less than 2 cm wide and 3 cm long.[17] Rare but potential complications of this approach are injury to the twelfth cranial nerves, or the structures entering the jugular foramen and foramen lacerum should the surgeon not remain medial to the atlantooccipital facet joints in removing the clivus.[38]

TRANSSPHENOIDAL APPROACH

The transsphenoidal technique is well known and used extensively in pituitary surgery.[39] Through this approach the upper half of the clivus can be reached. It is limited by the interposition of the sella turcica. It is facilitated by a large sphenoid sinus, especially a large posterior recess with a thin clival wall.[30]

Through this exposure one achieves a narrow midline surgical window, 10 to 12 mm, and it is difficult to remove a firm tumor.[40] Furthermore, controlling bleeding from a vascular tumor in such a deep space can be difficult. This approach is very well suited for biopsy of mid- and upper clival tumors.[7] Occasionally a soft chordoma can be removed via this approach.

TRANSORAL MEDIAN LABIOMANDIBULAR APPROACHES

The transoral operation allows exposure down to C2. Further exposure down to C4 can be achieved by splitting the tongue and mandible. This procedure, which seems at first to be excessive and mutilating, is suprisingly well tolerated by patients. Besides increasing the number of vertebrae in the field, medial labioglossotomy widens the approach and makes the back of the pharynx more superficial and accessible than is possible operating through the mouth.

The nasopharynx is cultured 72 hours preoperatively, and the appropriate antimicrobial agents are begun prior to starting the procedure. A tracheostomy is performed and the neck, oropharynx, mouth, and jaw are washed with Povidone iodine solution. The head is placed in a pin fixation headrest in slight extension.

The lower lip and chin are incised in the midline inferiorly to the hyoid bone (Figure 55-15). The mandible is then sawed through with a power saw in steplike fashion in order to prevent postoperative slippage (Figure 55-16). The tongue is incised in the median raphe with an electrocautery to the glossoepiglottal fold and sutures are used to retract the tongue superiorly and laterally.

The floor of the mouth is split between the submaxillary ducts to the hyoid bone. The mandibular-lingual halves are retracted laterally with self-retaining retractors. The uvula is then incised in the midline and retracted laterally by retention sutures, thereby exposing the posterior pharyngeal wall, which covers the upper cervical vertebrae (Figure 55-17).

In order to expose the clivus, the hard palate is removed to 1 cm off the midline on each side. The osteotomy is restricted to the horizontal part of the palatine bone and therefore does not run the risk of injuring the sphenopalatine artery and the nasopalatine nerve, which exit via the sphenopalatine foramen. Virtually the entire clivus is exposed via this approach (Figure 55-18).

After excision of the tumor using standard neurosurgical techniques with the microscope, the posterior pharyngeal wall is closed with 0 nonabsorbable retention sutures in addition to buried absorbable sutures and a buried mucosal closure with catgut.

The patient is continued on antibiotics for a week postoperatively. The tracheostomy is usually discontinued after a week as well.

The advantage of this approach to the clivus is the wide exposure in the vertical and sagittal planes. The major complication is meningitis from an oropharyngeal organism. Another

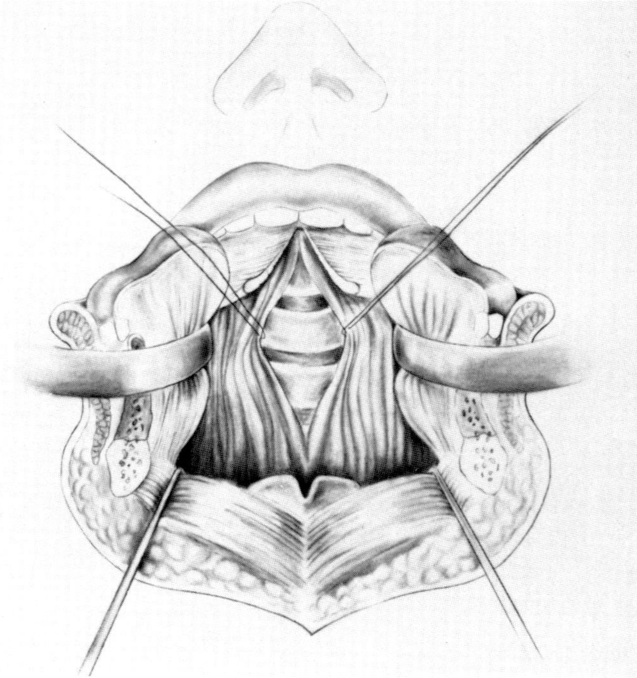

Fig. 55-17. Exposure of upper cervical vertebrae.

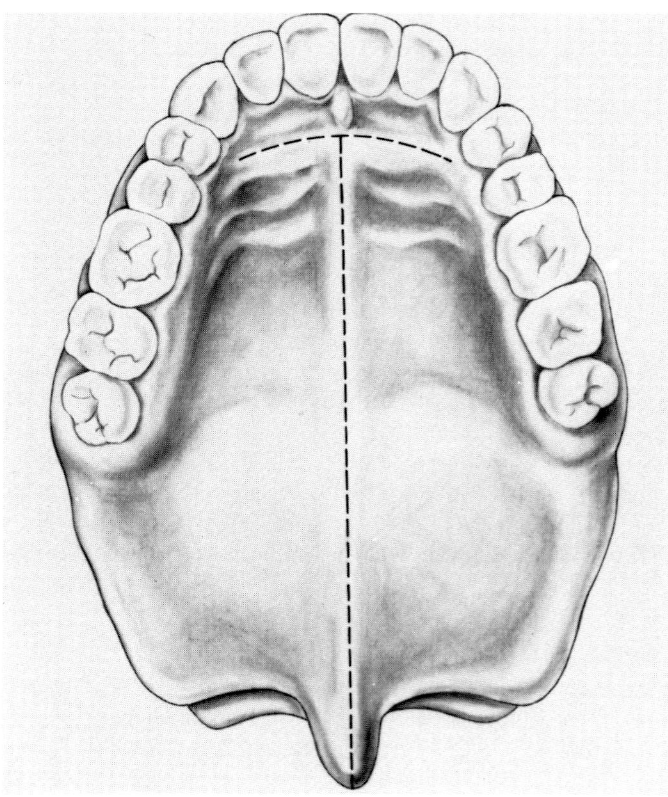

Fig. 55-18. Incision in hard palate, overlying soft tissue and uvula necessary to expose clivus.

drawback is the midline scar which is cosmetically displeasing to some patients.

TRANSBASAL APPROACH

The transbasal approach to the clivus and base of skull developed by Derome[30,41] allows resection of tumors extending from the upper clivus to C2. Only the most rostral aspect of the clivus cannot be resected due to obstruction by the sella dura.

A bicoronal, bifrontal opening is performed and the dura is dissected away from the base of the skull. The olfactory nerves are sacrificed at the level of the cribriform plate. With careful dissection, tumor is dissected from neurovascular structures which pass through the optic canal, sphenoid fissure, foramen rotundum, and foramen ovale.

A major hazard in this procedure is an unrecognized dural tear with subsequent cerebrospinal fluid leak and meningitis. Any dural tears must be primarily closed if possible and reinforced with pericranium. Furthermore, Derome[30,41] recommends that the base of the skull be reconstructed with bone autografts, thereby eliminating dead space that might encourage an extradural hematoma, abscess, or meningoencephaloceles. Additionally, in the initial exposure, the nasopharyngeal mucosal plane must be preserved because it provides physical support, as well as vascularization to bone grafts.

In our experience, bony reconstruction of the base of the skull can usually be omitted. The best way to prevent a CSF leak is to make the coronal scalp incision far back and dissect a large flap of pericranium from the under surface of the scalp flap just at the brow. The pericranial flap then is placed over the floor of the frontal fossa. The pericranial flap should be large enough to be redundant and cover the defect in the skull base with pericranium to spare.

EXTRADURAL POSTEROLATERAL APPROACHES

Infratemporal Fossa Approach

Fisch and colleagues have developed an infratemporal fossa approach to the skull base which has been utilized in removing chordomas and meningiomas of the clivus.[10,42,43] This approach is best suited for posterolateral clivus tumors involving the jugular foramen and temporal bone. Its scope is limited, therefore, and is best used in conjunction with an additional route such as the above discussed anterior approaches. A detailed presentation of this elegant approach is beyond the scope of this chapter, but can be found elsewhere.[10,42,43] It involves a subtemporal, extradural approach with mastoidectomy, ligation of the sigmoid sinus, and anterior transposition (or ligation with reanastomosis) of the facial nerve. If the clival tumor is parasellar in location, Fisch[43] divides the maxillary and mandibular divisions of the trigeminal nerve at the level of the foramina rotundum and ovale.

The main disadvantage of this approach, in addition to its limited lateral exposure to the clivus, is permanent conductive hearing loss due to obliteration of the middle ear cleft. Additionally, temporary paresis of facial function, and loss of facial sensitivity and ipsilateral masseter function may occur due to damage to cranial nerves seven and five respectively.

In a series of 121 patients treated with the infratemporal approach, 7 percent developed a cerebrospinal fluid leak, 3 percent developed an infection, and there was one death.[43]

CHOICE OF SURGICAL APPROACH

The choice of the surgical approach depends on multiple factors such as the intent of the operation (i.e., biopsy for diagnosis versus complete excision), the tumors relation to the dura, the consistency of the tumor, the histology of the tumor, and the localization and extent of the tumor. These factors will be discussed briefly below.

INTENT OF THE OPERATION

In some cases, despite extensive preoperative neuroradiologic evaluation, the preoperative diagnosis remains elusive and the surgeon and patient may elect to perform a simple biopsy procedure prior to contemplation of further treatment. A transsphenoidal approach can be employed for many of these tumors when a simple biopsy is the aim. Tumors solely located in the lower half of the clivus may need to be approached for a biopsy procedure via another route such as a transcervical or transoral approach.

TUMOR RELATION TO THE DURA

Tumors that are primarily intradural, such as a clival meningioma, are best approached via an intradural route. As discussed above, these tumors present a formidable risk of postoperative meningitis if a transsphenoidal or transoral approach is employed.

CONSISTENCY OF THE TUMOR

Soft, "suckable" tumors can often be removed in a narrow surgical field such as that offered by transsphenoidal surgery irrespective of their size.[7,30,40] On the other hand, hard, "fibrous" tumors need to be removed with laser, rongeurs, drills, and Cavitron, and necessitate a larger surgical field. MRI can often distinguish "hard" from "soft" tumors preoperatively.[40]

TUMOR HISTOLOGY

The choice of operative approach also depends on the histology of the tumor. Assuming a diagnosis has been made previously, further treatment might consist of radical surgical removal for some tumors (i.e., chordoma, schwannoma), or biopsy and debulking followed by radiation therapy or chemotherapy for others (e.g., metastasis).

LOCALIZATION AND EXTENT OF THE TUMOR

The most important factor influencing the surgical approach is the localization and extent of the clival tumor. Clival chordomas and meningiomas can grow in any direction and are often quite extensive at diagnosis.

When the tumor is purely extradural, transoral and transcervical approaches can be used in tumors limited to the lower half of the clivus. The infratemporal fossa approach of Fisch or the transbasal route are indicated for tumors in the upper and midclival regions.

Occasionally very large tumors are not amenable to complete resection by a single approach. In these cases, combined approaches can be performed in multiple stages. For example, a large chordoma that has invaded bone and dura extensively may be attached in this fashion. In this instance, the extradural component could be resected 2 or 3 months before an intradural route is employed for the remainder of the tumor. The 2 or 3 month interval between procedures allows for the mucosal planes to heal and therefore minimizes the risk of cerebrospinal fluid leak and meningitis.[30]

REFERENCES

1. von Sommering ST: Vom Bane des menschlichen Korpers, vols 1–5. Frankfurt, Varrentrapp & Wenner, 1791–1798
2. Blumenbachü JF: Geschichte und Bescheibung der Knochen des menschlichen Korpers. Gottingen, Dieterich, 1807
3. Virchow RLK: Untersuchungen uber die Entwicklung des Schadelgrundes im gesunden und krankhaften Zustande und uber den Einfluss derselben auf Schadelform, Gesichtsbildung und Gehirnbau. Berlin, Reimar, 1857
4. Coin CG, Malkasian DR: Clivus, in Newton TH, Potts DG (eds): Radiology of the Skull and Brain, vol 1. St. Louis, CV Mosby, 1971, pp 348–356
5. Arey LB: Developmental Anatomy: A Textbook and Laboratory Manual of Embryology. Philadelphia, WB Saunders, 1965
6. Gray H: Anatomy of the Human Body. CM Goss (ed). Philadelphia, Lea & Febiger, 1967
7. Laws ER: Cranial chordomas, in Wilkins RH, Rengachary SS (eds): Neurosurgery. New York, McGraw-Hill, 1985, pp 927–929
8. Bingas B: Tumors of the base of the skull, in Vinken PJ, Bruyn GW (eds) Handbook of Clinical Neurology, vol 17. New York, American Elsevier, 1974, pp 136–233
9. Sassin JF: Intracranial chordoma, in Vinken PJ, Bruyn GW (eds): Handbook of Clinical Neurology, vol 18. New York, American Elsevier, 1975, pp 151–164
10. Kumor A, Fisch U: The infratemporal fossa approach for lesions of the skull base. Adv Tech Stand Neurosurg 10:187, 1983
11. Heffelfinger MJ, Dahlim DC, MacCarty CS, et al: Chordomas and cartilaginous tumors at the skull base. Cancer 32:410, 1973
12. Raffel C, Wright DC, Gutin PH, Wilson CB: Cranial chordomas: Clinical presentation and results of operative and radiation therapy in twenty-six patients. Neurosurgery 17:703, 1985
13. Suit HD, Goitein M, Munzenrider J, et al: Definitive radiation therapy for chordoma and choadrosarcoma of base of skull and cervical spine. J Neurosurg 56:377, 1982
14. Ericksson B, Gunterberg B, Kindblom LG: Chordoma. A clinicopathologic and prognostic study of a Swedish national series. Acta Orthop Scand 52:49, 1981
15. Valderrama E, Kahn LB: Chondroid chordoma. Electron microscopic study of two cases. Am J Surg Pathol 7:625, 1983
16. Schoenberg BS, Christie BW, Whisnant JP: The resolution of discrepancies in the reported incidence of primary brain tumors. Neurology 28:817, 1978
17. Yasargil MG, Mortara RW, Curcic M: Meningiomas of basal posterior cranial fossa. Adv Tech Stand Neurosurg 7:3, 1980
18. Castellano F, Ruggiero G: Meningiomas of the posterior fossa. Acta Radiol (Suppl) 104:1, 1953
19. Cushing H, Eisenhardt L: Meningiomas. Springfield, Ill, Charles C Thomas, 1938
20. Wara WM, Sheline GE, Newman H, et al: Radiation therapy of meningiomas. Amer J Roentgenol Radium Ther Nucl Med 128:453, 1975
21. Jay JR, MacLaughlin DT, Riley KR, et al: Modulation of meningioma cell growth by sex steroid hormones in vitro. J Neurosurg 62:757, 1985
22. Markwalder TM, Zava DT, Goldhirsh A, et al: Estrogen and progesterone receptors in meningiomas in relation to clinical and pathologic features. Surg Neurol 20:42, 1983
23. Martuza RL, Miller DC, MacLaughlin DT: Estrogen and progestin

binding by cytosolic and nuclear fractions of human meningiomas. J Neurosurg 62:750, 1985

24. Krayenbuhl H: Special clinical features of tumors of the foramen Magnum. Schweiz Arch Neurol Neurochir Psychiat 112:205, 1973

25. DiChiro G, Anderson WB: Clivus. Clin Radiol 16:211, 1985

26. Kendall BE, Lee BCP: Cranial chordomas. Br J Radiol 50:687, 1977

27. Arbit E, Patterson RH: Combined transoral and median labio-mandibular glossotomy approach to the upper cervical spine. Neurosurgery 8:672, 1981

28. Nakagawa H, Wolf BS: Delineation of lesions of the base of the skull. Neuroradiology 17:1, 1978

29. Yasargil MG, Smith RD, Gosser JR: Microsurgery of the aneurysms of the internal carotid artery and its branches. Prog Neurol Surg 9:58, 1978

30. Derome PJ, Guiot G: Surgical approaches to the sphenoidal and clival areas. Adv Tech Stand Neurosurg 6:101, 1979

31. Malis LI: Surgical resection of tumors of the skull base. In Wilkins RH, Rengachary SS (eds): Neurosurgery. New York, McGraw-Hill, 1985, pp 1011–1021

32. Stevenson GC, Stoney RJ, Perkins RK, Adams JR: A transcervical, transclival approach to the ventral surface of the brainstem for removal of a clivus chordoma. J Neurosurg 24:544, 1966

33. Tew JM, Mayfield FH: Complications of surgery of the anterior cervical spine. Clin Neurosurg 23:424, 1978

34. Fang HSY, Ong GB: Direct anterior approach to the upper cervical spine. J Bone Joint Surg 44A:1588, 1962

35. Southwick WO, Robinson RA: Surgical approaches to the vertebral bodies in the cervical and lumbar regions. J Bone Joint Surg 39A:631, 1957

36. Mullan S, Naunton R, Helemot-Panah J, et al: The use of an anterior approach to ventrally placed tumors in the foramen magnum and vertebral column. J Neurosurg 24:538, 1966

37. Kennedy DW, Papel ID, Holliday M: Transpalatal approach to the skull base. Ear Nose Throat J 65:48, 1986

38. Decker RE, Malis LI: Surgical approaches to midline lesions at the base of the skull: A review. Mt Sinai J Med. 37:84, 1970

39. Landolt AM, Strebel P: Technique of transsphenoidal operation for pituitary adenomas. Adv Tech Stand Neurosurg 7:119, 1980

40. Snow RB, Lavyne MH, Lee BCP, et al: Craniotomy versus transsphenoidal excision of large pituitary tumors: The usefulness of magnetic resonance imaging in guiding the operative approach. Neurosurgery 19:59, 1986

41. Derome PJ: The transbasal approach to tumors invading the base of the skull, in Schmidek HH, Sweet WH (eds): Current Techniques in Operative Neurosurgery. New York, Grune & Stratton, 1977, pp 223–245

42. Fisch U: Infratemporal fossa approach to tumors of the temporal bone and base of the skull. J Laryngol Otolaryngol 92:949, 1978

43. Fisch U, Pillsbury HC, Sasaki CT: Infratemporal approach to the skull base, in Sasski CT, McCabe BF, Kirchner JA (eds): Surgery of the Skull Base. Philadelphia, JB Lippincott, 1984, pp 141–160

44. Biller HF, Shugar JMA, Krespi YP: A new technique for wide-field exposure of the base of the skull. Arch Otolaryngol 107:698, 1981

45. Ahn HS, Sexton CS, Zinreich SJ, et al: Neuroradiologic techniques in the evaluation of lesions of the skull base. Ear Nose Throat J 65:53, 1986

46. Krespi YP, Sisson GA: Transmandibular exposure of the skull base. Am J Surg 148:534, 1984

47. Delgado TE, Garrido E, Harwick RD: Labiomandibular, trans-oral approach to chordomas in the clivus and upper cervical spine. Neurosurgery 8:675, 1981

CHAPTER 56

Surgical Management of Tumors of the Tentorium and Clivus

Edward Tarlov

PRIMARY TUMORS OF THE TENTORIUM and clivus are occasionally encountered, perhaps with increasing frequency with computed tomographic (CT) scanning. The clinical presentation of tumors in these regions and the earlier experience with radiologic diagnosis and surgical management have been extensively reviewed elsewhere.[1–7] The impact of improved computed tomographic and microsurgical techniques, patient positioning, neurosurgical handling of the dural sinuses, methods of brain retraction, and the applicability of supratentorial, infratentorial, and other operative approaches will be reviewed in this chapter.

Surgical lesions on the tentorium are meningiomas; surgical lesions of the clivus itself are most frequently meningiomas but occasionally are chordomas. Metastatic lesions are excluded from this surgical discussion. In the Olivecrona series, meningiomas of the tentorium are less unusual.

TENTORIAL TUMORS

A review of the historical aspects of tentorial meningiomas is included in the analysis of the Olivecrona series by Castellano and Ruggiero.[1] In this large group of tumors, approximately an equal number arose from the upper and lower surfaces of the tentorium. The clinical features of the tumors in that earlier era were elevated intracranial pressure, seizures, and occasionally hemianopsia. Cranial nerve involvement was cited later. The tumors may involve the transverse and sigmoid sinuses, which they tend to infiltrate. The sinus rectus may be involved by the more medial lesions. Fortunately for the surgeon, their most frequent site of attachment is the posterior part of the tentorium. Earlier diagnosis should now be possible in most instances.

RADIOLOGIC DIAGNOSIS

Computed tomographic scanning has simplified the radiologic diagnosis of tentorial tumors and their differentiation from other lesions. With high-resolution CT scanning, preoperative differentiation of a tentorial meningioma from a glioma of the superior vermis or corpora quadrigemina, a pinealoma, or a metastatic lesion is possible in most instances. On CT scans, the findings indicating a meningioma usually are quite characteristic. The tumor borders typically are round or lobulated and the lesion usually is fairly homogeneous, although this is not always the case. Enhancement with contrast is the rule. Cal-

cium density may be detectable within the tumor mass. Rarely, the lesion may have a low CT absorption.[8] The improvements in CT resolution have been a very significant development, allowing the recognition of characteristics that indicate the presence of meningioma. Computed tomographic scanning technology now also permits, by patient positioning or reconstruction, the display of an image in the coronal plane in addition to the usual horizontal oblique CT plane. In some instances this may allow better judgment regarding the relationship of the lesion to the tentorium or the falx and thereby clearly indicate the relative volumes of supratentorial and infratentorial tumors (Figure 56-1).

Experience with MRI scanning is developing. This modality is, in general, less straightforward in its use and interpretation and even with an alert radiologist at the controls of the machine a large meningioma can be missed with present technology. As we become more familiar with MRI, it will no doubt become more and more useful.

Cerebral angiography may help in planning the operative approach so that important draining cerebral veins can be avoided, and, in special instances discussed below, may help the surgeon visualize the relationship between the lateral sinus and draining temporal anastomotic veins in large tumors of the clivus. It may also help the surgeon to judge the patency of the dural sinuses and the blood supply of the lesion, although tentorial meningiomas are not ordinarily highly vascular.

POSITIONING

Careful anesthetic technique can reduce the hazards of intraoperative hypotension, and careful surgical technique can reduce the risks of venous air embolism in the sitting position. Nevertheless, these risks must be calculated when the sitting position is used. For more and more patients, especially elderly patients, it is advantageous to place them in a horizontal position, either prone or supine with the head turned laterally, or in a full lateral or "park bench" position. Once the surgeon is accustomed to them, these horizontal positions do not greatly interfere with the exposure, and they somewhat reduce though do not abolish the risks of air embolism or arterial hypotension. The prevention of air embolism is the responsibility of both the surgeon and the anesthesiologist. The patient must have adequate intravascular volume. The surgical techniques for handling the bone edges, emissary veins, and dural sinuses are well known. High-speed drills such as those used for drilling out the

OPERATIVE NEUROSURGICAL TECHNIQUES
ISBN 0-8089-1862-1

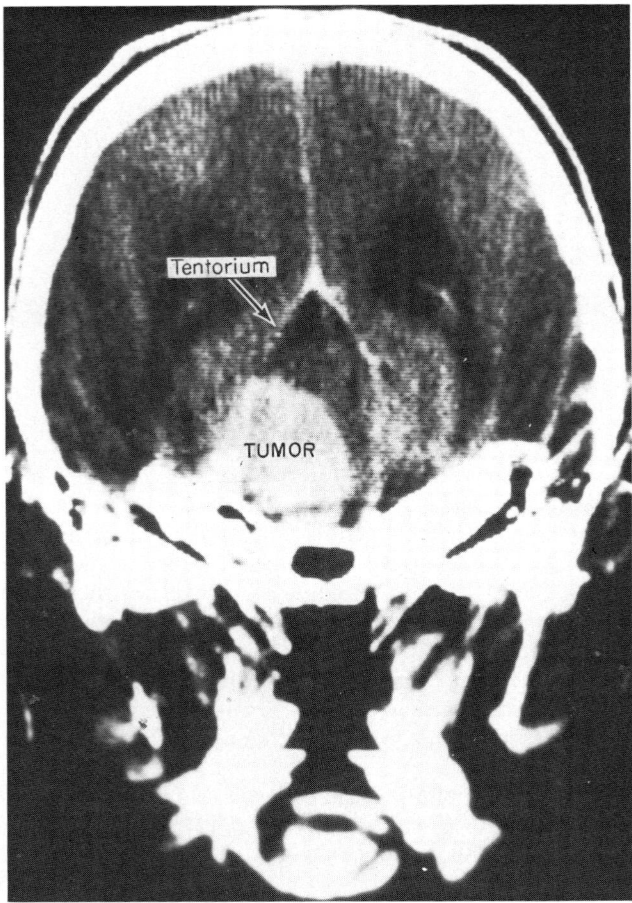

Fig. 56-1. Advantages of a coronal CT scan for clivus tumors. Precise relationships of the tumor to the tentorial edge are less clear on a horizontal CT scan than on a coronal CT scan, where it can be seen that most of tumor is beneath tentorial edge. In this instance the tumor was approached through the posterior fossa with grossly complete removal of the meningioma.

temporal bone in acoustic neuroma surgery are suitable for removing bone over the dural sinuses without injuring them and for skeletonizing the emissary veins so they can be coagulated before they are opened.

It is common for air embolism in clinically insignificant amounts to be detected by the Doppler monitor. Careful inspection of the surgical field does not always reveal a source, however. If the amount of air entering the bloodstream appears significant, the field should be covered and the wound further inspected area by area while the remaining field is covered with moist sponges. When cardiovascular changes occur, an atrial catheter, if available, can be used to aspirate the air. This is occasionally but not always helpful and the clinical value of an atrial catheter in the sitting position is not yet proven. The surgeon is not bothered by these distractions when the patient is in the horizontal position. Nevertheless, with an experienced anesthesia team the sitting position is still safe and can be advantageous with larger or the highly vascular lesions.

When a tentorial tumor is near the midline, the prone position is advantageous. When the tumor is laterally situated, the head is placed in a horizontal position, usually with the patient nearly supine.

A straight vertical scalp incision extending above and below the nuchal line permits a wide exposure (Figure 56-2).

The bony exposure primarily below the tentorium is extended up above the tentorium as necessary, bringing the supratentorial portion down through the tentorium if the supratentorial extension is not extensive (Figure 56-3).

For all of these approaches, the pin fixation provided by a Mayfield headrest is most convenient, since it permits the use of the Leyla Yarsargil self-retaining brain retractor, which is fixed to the operating table. I find the multiple connections that require tightening and loosening on other self-retaining brain retractors less convenient for microsurgery than the single-control tightening on the Leyla Yarsargil retractor, since the surgeon does not have to be diverted from the microscope to reposition the retractor.

For tumors that are laterally situated beneath the tentorium, I prefer the supine position with the head turned so that the midsagittal plane of the skull is nearly parallel to the floor. When working in the lateral recess of the posterior fossa in this position, brain retraction is nearly unnecessary, since gravity provides sufficient cerebellar retraction to permit a wide exposure of the angle once cerebrospinal fluid has been aspirated.

SURGICAL APPROACHES

Coronal CT scanning or reconstruction permits accurate judgment of the relative volumes of supratentorial and infratentorial tumors. If the major extent of the tumor is above the tentorium, the approach should be from above, beneath the temporal or occipital lobe, depending on how far posterior and medial the tumor is situated. If the tumor perforates the tentorium, removal of the portion below the tentorium can be carried out from above. An approach from above is also indicated if the occipital lobe is injured or atrophic. When the major or entire bulk of the tumor lies beneath the tentorium, an approach from below is advisable.

Staging the operation, performing a partial removal of the tumor, and returning subsequently to remove the remaining portion is a technique I have tried to avoid. It is clearly the surgeon's obligation to ensure that nothing, not even teaching residents, interferes with the completion of the operation in one stage when this is within the power of the principal surgeon. It is unusual that a tumor cannot be safely dealt with in one operation.

When the dural sinuses are infiltrated by tumor, the risk-to-benefit ratio of removing tumor from the sinuses needs to be carefully assessed. As such, tumor should be removed from the sinuses themselves as is consistent with safety. A severely compromised or occluded sinus can safely be sacrificed.[9] If the sinus rectus is patent, this should not be ligated. There usually is enough confluence in the region of the torcular to permit sufficient collateral venous drainage if a lateral sinus needs to be sacrificed. The more important consideration is preserving the large draining veins that drain the inferior surface of the temporal lobe. These should not be interfered with. If necessary, the lateral sinus can be ligated anterior to the vein of Labbé by expanding the bony exposure beneath the tentorium and the lateral sinus; the lateral sinus and the lateral portion of the tentorium can be retracted upward with the temporal lobe to avoid interfering with the important temporal venous drainage, as has been described by Malis (unpublished) and is discussed below in relation to clivus tumors.

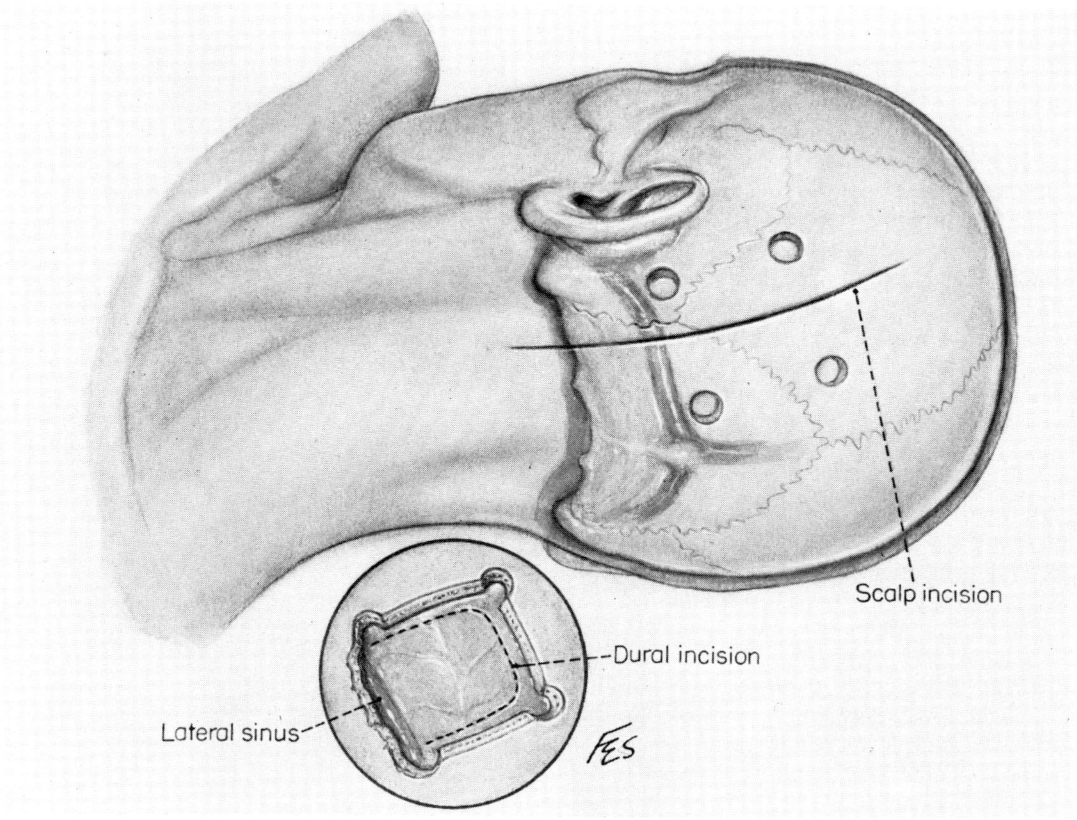

Fig. 56-2. Approach to a tumor of the tentorium mainly situated above the tentorium beneath the left occipital lobe with extension beneath the tentorium. The patient is in a supine position with the head turned to the right. A straight paramedium scalp incision is shown with the bone flap above the tentorium.

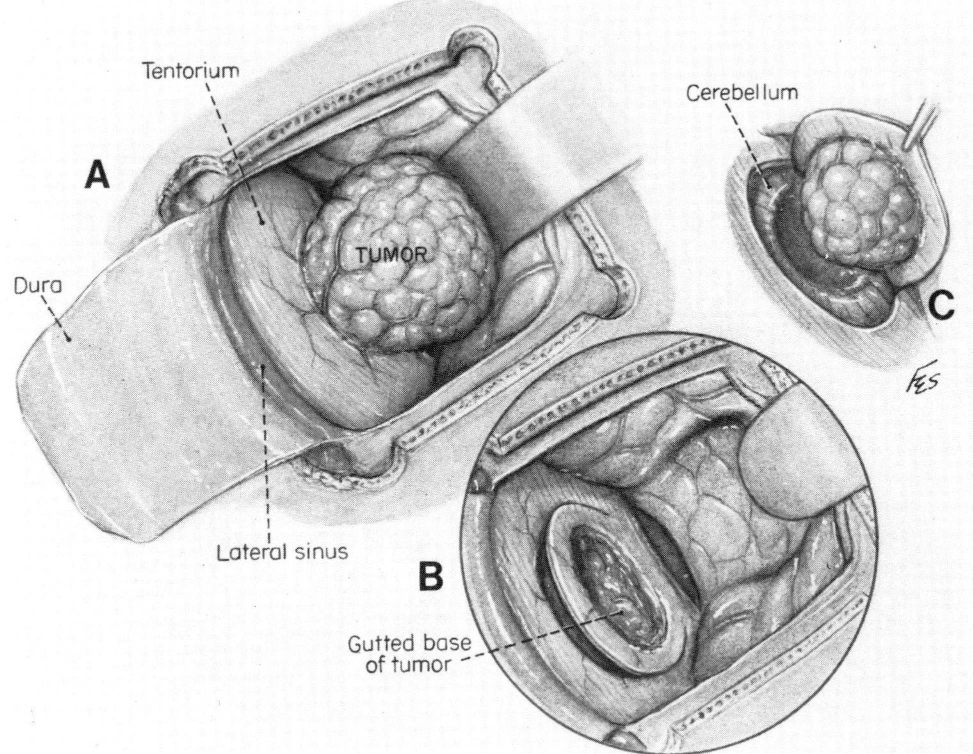

Fig. 56-3. Same orientation as Figure 56-2. (A) The dura is opened and reflected inferiorly. The left occipital lobe is elevated, avoiding bridging veins. Tumor is exposed and debulked. (B) The base of tumor is debulked. The tentorium is opened circumferentially around the base of the tumor. The small sinus at the edge of the tentorium is clipped and divided if necessary. (C) The tentorial flap is elevated, reflecting the inferior extension of the tumor off the cerebellum.

MICROSURGERY—RETRACTION—SPECIAL INSTRUMENTS

Microsurgery has had a tremendous impact on the safe removal of lesions of the tentorium and clivus. The technical advances related to microsurgery are discussed at length elsewhere in this volume. Before the widespread application of microsurgery, bone flaps and scalp incisions had to be large to permit adequate light in the depths of a deep wound. With microsurgical optics and lighting, adequate exposure can be provided with smaller incisions and bony openings.

Brain retraction techniques are nowhere more important than in dealing with lesions of the clivus and tentorium. A self-retaining retractor system is invaluable in microsurgery. The ideal system would permit free and easy shifting of the retractor from one portion of the field to another without delay in the operation and would maintain the position of the retractor without slipping. Microsurgery minimizes retraction and the exposure necessary to obtain well-lighted depth perception, allowing smaller bone flaps. The aspiration of cerebrospinal fluid from the cisterna and the occasional use of mannitol are appropriate aids. Retractor pressure on the brain should be minimal.

Instruments to gut the interior of the lesion more expeditiously can be helpful in decompressing the tumor and allow the surgeon to conserve energy for the more difficult removal of the capsule of the lesion from important structures. We have tested a variety of devices for this, including the Cavitron ultrasonic aspirator and the House-Urban rotary dissector. The Cavitron has been much improved and can be very helpful in debulking large lesions quickly and gently—justifying the considerable expense of this hardware to a department treating many tumors. The less costly House-Urban rotary dissector does permit the tumor to be gutted quite expeditiously and is not difficult for nurses to set up. It is particularly advantageous when dealing with a deep lesion in which there is not sufficient room to use the two-point coagulator and scissors to debulk the tumor in the standard way. Some have reported the laser helpful, but my own experiences with the laser have led me to feel it is much too slow in its present form to be practical, especially for the larger lesions where a dissecting aid is most needed. I therefore feel that, if available, the Cavitron is the best available adjunct for dissection.

CLIVUS TUMORS

Tumors arising purely from the clivus are unusual. Many cerebellopontine-angle meningiomas involve the lateral portions of the clivus, but these are much less difficult to deal with than those tumors that arise from the clivus itself. Tumors characterized as clivus meningiomas constituted 11 percent of the tumors in the Olivecrona series of posterior fossa meningiomas. Chordomas arise in this region as well. Clinically, in contrast to tentorial tumors, the lowest seven cranial nerves may be involved, and, if they are involved, usually are so at an early stage. The sixth nerve can be within the tumor itself. The basilar artery usually is displaced contralaterally, but occasionally it is posteriorly shifted. Disturbances of cranial nerves are common at the outset, including dysfunction of hearing and swallowing. Many of these lesions are inoperable, and the surgeon's judgment on whether a patient's symptoms can safely be alleviated and the long-term quality of life improved is perhaps the most critical phase of the operation for a clivus tumor.

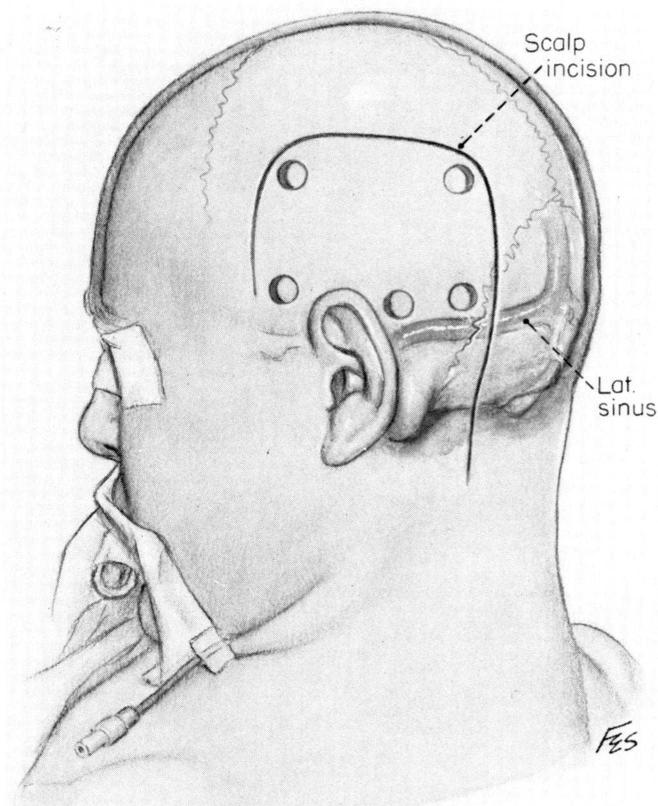

Fig. 56-4. Clivus meningioma. A combined supratentorial and infratentorial approach is usually not necessary but may be helpful in some instances. The patient is in the sitting position, the bone flap is above the lateral sinus with suboccipital squama to be rongeured away, exposing the lateral sinus. Preoperative angiography demonstrated the position of the vein of Labbé.

RADIOLOGIC FEATURES

The radiologic diagnosis usually should be based on CT scanning. The tumor borders in meningiomas should be round and lobulated. The lesions are fairly homogeneous. Ordinarily the meningiomas are enhancing lesions that may have calcium in them. With clivus chordomas, there is usually extensive destruction of the clivus itself. On CT scans, the tumor's appearance is less homogeneous. The differential diagnosis of clivus neoplasms includes nasopharyngeal carcinomas, cerebellopontine angle meningiomas, occasionally acoustic neuromas that extend medially, and tumors of the foramen magnum. The differentiation between a large aneurysm of the basilar artery and a clivus tumor should not be difficult with CT scanning, particularly if angiography is used when the clinical and radiologic diagnosis is obscure.

SURGICAL APPROACHES

Once surgery has been decided upon, clivus tumors should be categorized into four groups. Tumors involving the dorsum sellae should be approached beneath the temporofrontal junction. Tumors involving the upper portion of the clivus can best be exposed subtemporally if a major or complete resection appears feasible preoperatively. Tumors of the lower clivus are best reached from a lateral suboccipital approach through the cerebellopontine angle. For lesions of the mid-clivus, either the lateral suboccipital or the subtemporal approach is appropriate.

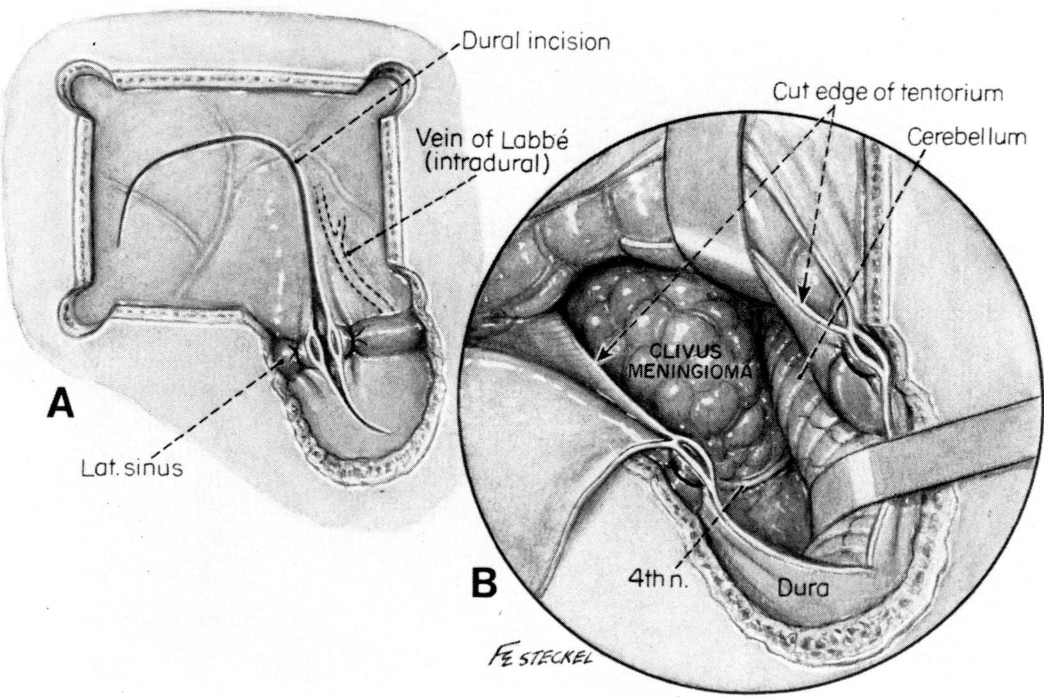

Fig. 56-5. (A) The lateral sinus is ligated anterior to the vein of Labbé. (B) The tentorium is incised through the tentorial edge. The lateral sinus, tentorium, and temporal and occipital lobes are elevated on a self-retaining retractor to expose the most medial portion of the cerebellopontine angle and clivus with minimal retraction of the cerebellum and no retraction of the brain stem. The fourth nerve can be seen coursing lateral to the tumor. This wide lateral approach can be a significant advantage in certain cases and permits gross complete removal of tumor in this instance.

An advantage of the posterior fossa suboccipital approach is that a wide bony decompression here is more effective than is a supratentorial bony decompression should the lesion prove to be inoperable. A combined supra- and infratentorial approach to the clivus has been discussed by Malis (unpublished). It provides a wide exposure of this region without interfering with important draining veins. Preoperative angiography is used to judge the venous drainage of the posterior temporal region. A combined temporal and suboccipital flap is turned down across the lateral sinus (Figure 56-4). The lateral sinus is ligated anterior to the vein of Labbé (Figure 56-5). At this point the venous drainage following ligation passes posteriorly through the lateral sinus to the torcular. The tentorium, lateral sinus, and temporo-occipital junction then are elevated on a self-retaining retractor after the tentorium has been divided medial to the ligated portion of the lateral sinus by extending the excision all the way through the tentorial hiatus; this is very useful in exposing tumors of this region. Special care is required to preserve the delicate fourth nerve passing across the field, usually lateral to the tumor.

For clivus chordomas, a complete resection of the tumor to effect a surgical cure is not possible. These tumors can be widely decompressed and irradiated. Judging which tumors are inoperable is perhaps the most critical part of the operation for lesions of the clivus. In elderly patients or those patients in generally poor health, extensive surgery is, of course, not advisable. If the symptoms relate mainly to hydrocephalus to a very significant degree, which is unusual, a shunt may be helpful. Not all of these lesions should be considered inoperable, as was formerly the case. The more favorable clivus chordomas can be decompressed through these approaches. The anterior approaches through the clivus are not practical for the extensive removal of intradural tumors of the clivus, although these anterior transclival approaches have been used to decompress extensive clivus chordomas.[10]

REFERENCES

1. Castellano F, Ruggiero G: Meningiomas of the posterior fossa. Acta Radiol (Suppl) 104, 1953
2. Markham JW, Fager CA, Horrax G, et al: Meningiomas of the posterior fossa: Their diagnosis, clinical features and surgical treatment. Arch Neurol Psychiatr 74:163, 1955
3. Campbell E, Whitfield RD: Posterior fossa meningiomas. J Neurosurg 5:131, 1948
4. Cushing H, Eisenhardt L: Meningiomas: Their Classification, Regional Behavior, Life History and Surgical End Results. Springfield, Ill, Charles C Thomas, 1938
5. d'Errico A: Meningiomas of the cerebellar fossa. J Neurosurg 7:225, 1950
6. Russell JR: Meningiomas of the posterior fossa. Surg Gynecol Obstet 96:183, 1953
7. McCarty CS: Surgical techniques for removal of meningiomas. Clin Neurosurg 7:103, 1951
8. Savorcardo M, Passerini A, Allegranza A: The hypodense meningioma: Report of two cases. Neuroradiology 16:558, 1978
9. Dandy WE: Removal of dural sinuses involved in tumors. Arch Surg 31:244, 1940
10. Cloward RB, Passarelli P: Removal of giant clival chordoma by an anterior cervical approach. Surg Neurol 11:129, 1979

CHAPTER 57
Surgical Management of Posterior Fossa Tumors

John Duckworth   Henry H. Schmidek

THE SURGICAL MANAGEMENT of masses located within the posterior fossa involves dealing with a diverse pathologic spectrum of lesions. The symptoms of these tumors are either the result of direct neuronal dysfunction or the consequences of obstructive hydrocephalus. Such interference with cerebrospinal fluid circulation is seen especially in the case of midline posterior fossa lesions but can be the initial feature of tumors situated anywhere within the posterior fossa.[1,2] This often results in the symptoms of raised intracranial pressure. Since the cranial sutures are not functionally fused until the second decade of life, the effect of raised intracranial pressure can be partially offset by expansion of the cranial volume and periods of symptomatic remission prior to diagnosis.[3] Expanding head size may be apparent before other symptoms of raised intracranial pressure are evident in infants.

The neurologic consequences of posterior fossa masses are dependent on their location and the age of the patient. Midline cerebellar masses produce truncal and gait ataxia with a broad-based unsteady gait and imperfect tandem walking, while hemispheric lesions give rise to limb ataxias manifested as dysmetria, abnormalities of rapid alternating movements, nystagmus, hypotonia, and hyporeflexia.[1] Intrinsic brain stem tumors will produce dysfunction of multiple and usually contiguous cranial nerves before the CSF pathways are obstructed.[4] Dysfunction of extraocular motility may be the result of the direct effect of the tumor on the brain stem and cerebellum.[4,5] Horizontal gaze paretic nystagmus is seen with lesions around the fourth ventricle, and upbeat nystagmus is seen with posterior fossa tumors and evidence of direct brain stem involvement. Vertigo is associated with laterally positioned tumors and may be disabling in severity. Compression or invasion of brain stem structures produces a variety of disturbances involving the cranial nerve nuclei and the motor and sensory pathways of the brain stem.

PATHOLOGY

The differential diagnosis is dictated by the patient's age, symptoms and signs, and the CT characteristics of the lesion (Table 57-1). A hemispheric tumor occurring in a child between 5 and 14 years of age is most likely a cerebellar astrocytoma, whereas medulloblastoma is a midline lesion that is more common in boys 3 to 7 years of age.[4,6] Children with ependymomas generally have hydrocephalus, intractable emesis, and

nystagmus and are usually younger than 5 years of age.[4,6–9] Dermoid tumors and arachnoid cysts are usually a problem of childhood and may produce mass effects as they enlarge in the quadrigeminal plate cistern, cerebellar vermis, or medial cerebellar hemispheres.[10–13] Dermoids typically produce direct cerebellar/brain stem dysfunction, while arachnoid cysts more often cause obstructive hydrocephalus.[13] Dandy-Walker malformations are rare lesions usually appearing before 1 year of age.[11,14] Fifty-five to 70 percent of cerebellar masses in adults are metastatic in origin, the figure being higher if the patient is over the age of 40 years. Cerebellar astrocytomas can occur sporadically in adults at any age, while cerebellar hemangioblastomas most frequently arise in patients between 30 and 50 years of age.[15] Medulloblastoma may appear in adults less than 30 years of age as a paramidline posterior fossa mass.[1]

PREOPERATIVE DIAGNOSTIC AND THERAPEUTIC MEASURES

Patients suspected of harboring a posterior fossa mass require an unenhanced CT scan to look for calcification, hemorrhage, hydrocephalus, and intracranial mass effect. Contrast enhancement raises the sensitivity of this study and a false-negative enhanced CT scan occurs in less than 1 percent of intrinsic, cerebellar, fourth ventricle, and brain stem lesions.[16]

The appearance on CT scans may be suggestive of the tumor's histologic type. Cerebellar astrocytomas are characterized by a large cystic component, the walls of which are composed of tumor tissue or which possess only an enhancing mural nodule of tumor.[17–20] In adults, such cystic lesions with mural nodules are likely to be cerebellar hemangioblastomas.[21] Medulloblastomas and ependymomas are usually centered in the fourth ventricle. Medulloblastomas have a heterogeneous CT density with variable contrast enhancement,[17,22,23] and calcify in dense ''clumps,'' while ependymomas calcify in small punctate aggregates.[17] Medulloblastomas calcify considerably less often than do the ependymomas; however, because of their more frequent occurrence, nearly 40 percent of calcific midline posterior masses in children are medulloblastomas.[17] Typically, both low and high grade brain stem gliomas are low density masses, with CT images enhanced only slightly with contrast; gliomas enlarge the brain stem and displace the fourth ventricle.[17]

A metastatic tumor is usually situated at the gray–white

OPERATIVE NEUROSURGICAL TECHNIQUES
ISBN 0-8089-1862-1

Table 57-1. Typical characteristics of posterior fossa masses

Primary Tumor	Age (years)	Signs/Symptoms	Location	CT Findings
Medulloblastoma	3–7	Obstructive hydrocephalus	Midline 4th ventricle	Homogeneous enhancement; calcifications absent or contiguous
Ependymoma	less than 5	Obstructive hydrocephalus	Midline 4th ventricle	4th ventricle floor; speckled calcification
Astrocytoma	5–14	Obstructive hydrocephalus	Cerebellar hemisphere	Cystic mass enhancing mural nodule
Brain stem glioma	3–9	Multiple bilateral contiguous central nervous dysfunction	Brain stem	Low density brain stem mass
Hemangioblastoma	30–50	Cerebellar dysfunction	Cerebellum	Cystic mass enhancing mural nodule
Dermoid	10–30	Cerebellar or brain stem dysfunction	Midline posterior fossa	Round midline low lesion
Arachnoid cyst	10–30	Obstructive hydrocephalus	Areas of subarachnoid space	Round midline low lesion
Metastatic cerebellar tumors	40–60	Cerebellar or brain stem dysfunction	Cerebellum/brain stem	Ring enhancing mass—gray–white junction; cerebellar cortex

interface of the cerebellar cortex and appears as a ringlike enhancing mass with prominent degrees of peritumoral edema.[24] The presence of more than one lesion is suggestive of metastases, although this appearance may be seen with hemangioblastomas. Low density, cystic, extra-axial lesions without an enhancing mural nodule suggest an epidermoid tumor or arachnoid cyst.[25,26] Cerebellar hemorrhages are high density lesions with edema that produce a shift of midline structures and may occur in pre-existing tumors, producing a disproportionate shift of the intracranial contents.[1] The findings on CT scans often provide a considerable amount of information about tumor size and location and frequently suggest its nature. Electroencephalography, radionuclide brain scanning, skull roentgenography, and ventriculography rarely provide additional diagnostically useful information. An angiogram may be required in an adult to assess the vascularity of a posterior fossa lesion or to locate potentially vascular lesions (e.g., hemangioblastoma).[21] Angiography is also useful in distinguishing Dandy-Walker malformations from arachnoid cysts.[11]

Lesions requiring further neuroradiologic investigation include masses within the brain stem and tumors extending into the subarachnoid space. When a lesion is peripherally situated or located within the brain stem or subarachnoid space, a CT scan may be misleading.[16] Metrizamide instilled into the subarachnoid space helps define lesions in and around the brain stem or cerebellum and is particularly sensitive at distinguishing intra-axial from extra-axial lesions and detecting subarachnoid spread of tumor.[27–29] Magnetic resonance imaging (MRI) is superior to computed tomography in its sensitivity at detecting a posterior fossa lesion, defining the displacement of normal structures, and demonstrating the extent of the pathologic process.[30–32] However, MRI cannot distinguish tumor from surrounding edema, although the use of intravenous gadolinium as a contrast-enhancing agent may be helpful in this regard.[32,33] Subarachnoid metrizamide-enhanced CT and MRI require a cooperative patient, and their use in children or disoriented adults may require sedation or general anesthesia.

The need for preoperative CSF shunting or external ventricular drainage in the case of an obstructive hydrocephalus secondary to a posterior fossa mass is a matter of judgment in a particular case and controversial when one attempts to generalize. Advocates of this as a standard approach cite a reduction in the perioperative and intraoperative morbidity as justification for placement of a CSF shunt[34,35]; however, most patients do not require either preoperative shunting or external ventricular drainage following the administration of corticosteroids.[36] The diversion of CSF is reserved for acutely ill patients with headache and vomiting unrelieved by corticosteroids and in immediate danger because of intracranial hypertension. Definitive treatment of the hydrocephalus involves removal of the tumor mass. Patients with partial tumor removal have a greater likelihood of requiring a permanent shunt than do those with total removal. The placement of a temporary external ventricular drain for postoperative management can be decided upon by the surgeon at the time of surgery.[37] McLaurin has reported no differences in the postoperative conditions of patients with preoperative shunts and those without shunts. Preoperative shunting lengthens hospitalization without improving outcome.[38]

SURGICAL MANAGEMENT

The surgical management of masses in the posterior fossa is dependent upon the patient's age, the suspected nature of the pathologic process, the mass of the tumor, and the patient's general condition. In all cases, patients are begun on dexamethasone in doses of 10 mg/kg every 6 hours 24 to 48 hours before surgery and prophylactic antibiotics just before the operation. Intubation must be accomplished with care, particularly in the presence of raised intracranial pressure.[39] The eyes are taped shut and ECG, Doppler, and temperature probes inserted, following which the head is immobilized in a Gardner three-point headrest.

The majority of cases are maintained under controlled mechanical ventilation rather than spontaneous respiration, which allows precise control of arterial PCO_2 levels, reduces venous bleeding, and may decrease the incidence of air embolism.[4,7,40,41,42] In the rare instances in which spontaneous ventilation is the preferable technique, it is accomplished with a shorter acting inhalation agent, and the rate of respiration is increased by altering the concentration of the carbon dioxide inhaled. This technique is sometimes useful during surgery in or on the brain stem.[39,42,43]

Operations in the posterior fossa can be performed with the patient in the seated position, the prone position, or the lateral recumbent position. The sitting position is used for surgical procedures in the posterior fossa because it affords the surgeon an eye-level visual approach to the posterior fossa contents, promotes venous drainage, and allows blood, CSF, and irrigating solutions to drain away from the operative field during the procedure.[4,7,40,44,45] These complications are minimized by positioning the head so neck flexion does not exceed 45 degrees. A child should be wrapped in a heated blanket and the temperature maintained with an external heat source. The lower extremities are wrapped to the thighs and elevated above the level of the pelvis to promote venous return. Surgery is conducted using both a cardiac Doppler monitor and measurement of the end tidal CO_2 levels to detect air embolization; arterial lines and a central venous catheter in the right atrium are also used. A three-point head pin fixation is used routinely to maintain the position of the head in adults. The patient is gradually elevated into the sitting position to prevent hypotension. Should this develop during the positioning of the patient, it can usually be resolved by lowering the patient's trunk a few degrees for a short time; if it persists, an inotropic medication such as dopamine may be necessary. After securing the headpiece to the table brackets, the neck is flexed 45 degrees (Figure 57-1). One should be able to slip one's hand comfortably between the patient's chin and neck to ensure against excessive neck flexion. The patient's arms should rest on pillows in his or her lap. The sitting position should be avoided in children under 4 years of age, generally in patients over 65 years of age, and in those patients with unstable cardiovascular function. In these patients the development of sudden hypotension from blood loss, redistribution of intravascular volume, small air emboli, or a combination of these can be catastrophic. The prone positions—fully prone, three-quarter prone, and lateral recumbent—are alternatives for surgery in the posterior fossa that reduce these dangers[41,42,46,47] (Figure 57-2). In the fully prone position the patient is placed on a bolster to allow free abdominal excursion and to avoid compression of the inferior vena cava. Pin fixation of the head is used in adult patients and in older children. In patients under 2 years of age, the head is positioned in a U-shaped headrest. One must be particularly careful to ensure that the eyes have no pressure placed on them by the headrest, both during positioning and when one has reached the final position. This is repeatedly checked during the operation. Special care must also be taken to secure the endotracheal tube, since in the prone position direct access to the airway is very difficult.

The patient is then placed in a minus Trendelenburg position of about 15 degrees to promote venous drainage.[47] The operative exposure chosen depends on the location and extent of the mass lesion. A midline posterior fossa craniectomy is suited for lesions situated on or close to the midline in the vermis or for operations on the cerebellar tonsils or in the

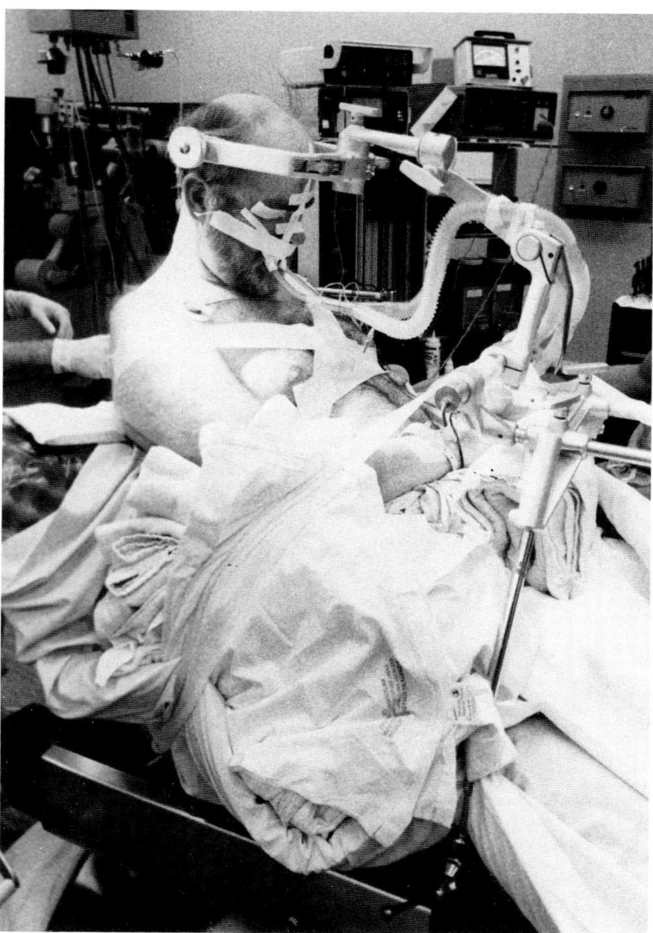

Fig. 57-1. Positioning of the patient for the sitting position. Proper neck flexion allows an eye-level view of the posterior fossa.

region of the foramen magnum. This approach, modified to extend to one side, is also often used in managing large space-occupying cerebellar lesions. A unilateral posterior fossa craniectomy is used in cases restricted to one cerebellar hemisphere. A more laterally situated craniectomy can be used for approaches to the cerebellopontine angle, and a combined supratentorial and infratentorial approach can be used for large tumors involving these compartments.

MIDLINE POSTERIOR FOSSA CRANIECTOMY

Lesions within the fourth ventricle, cerebellar vermis, and medial-cerebellar hemispheres are best approached through a bilateral midline exposure (Figure 57-3). A midline skin incision that extends from the inion to around the midcervical region is used, and hemostasis from these layers and subcutaneous tissue is accomplished by the application of Raney clips. The operation then proceeds in the midline by incising the avascular median raphe attached to the spinous processes. The occipital muscles are separated and cut with the cautery an inch from their insertion. The periosteum is cleared, exposing the middle half of the occipital bone. Because of the danger of air embolism, venous bleeding in muscle and bone should be controlled promptly; air emboli can occur in either the sitting or the prone

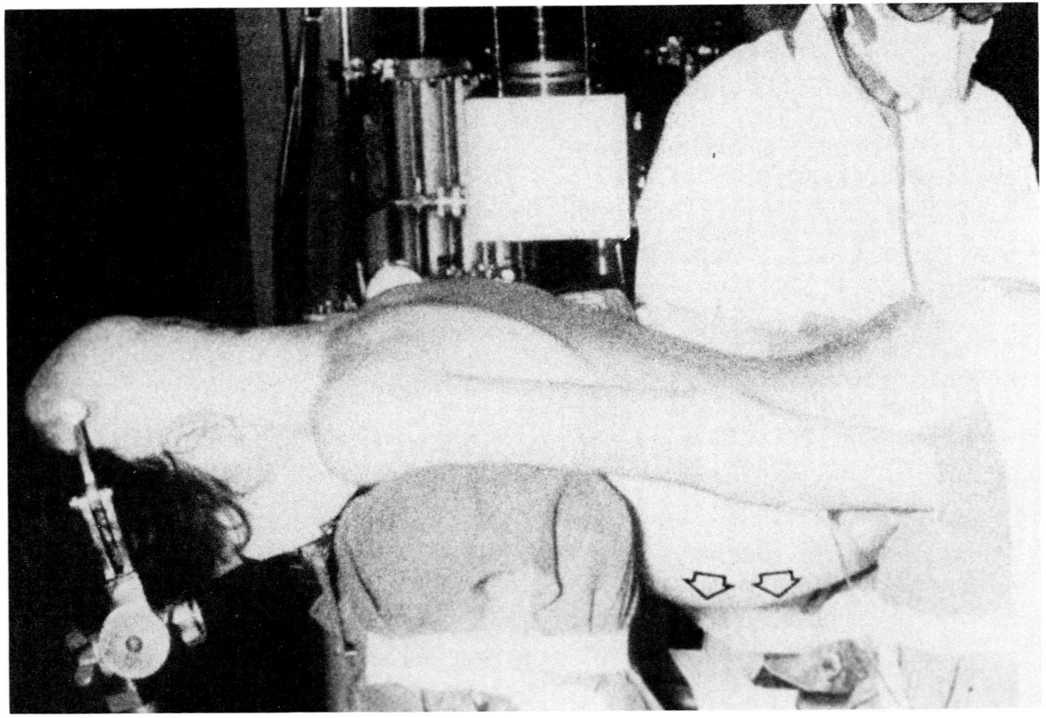

Fig. 57-2. The prone position for posterior fossa surgery. Note that the abdomen must lie free (open arrows) to avoid compression of the vena cava. (Reprinted from Humphreys RP, Creighton RE, Hendrick FB, et al: Advantages of the prone position for neurosurgical procedures on the upper cervical spine and posterior cranial fossa in children. Childs Brain 1:325, 1975. With permission from S. Karger AG, Publishers, Basel, Switzerland.)

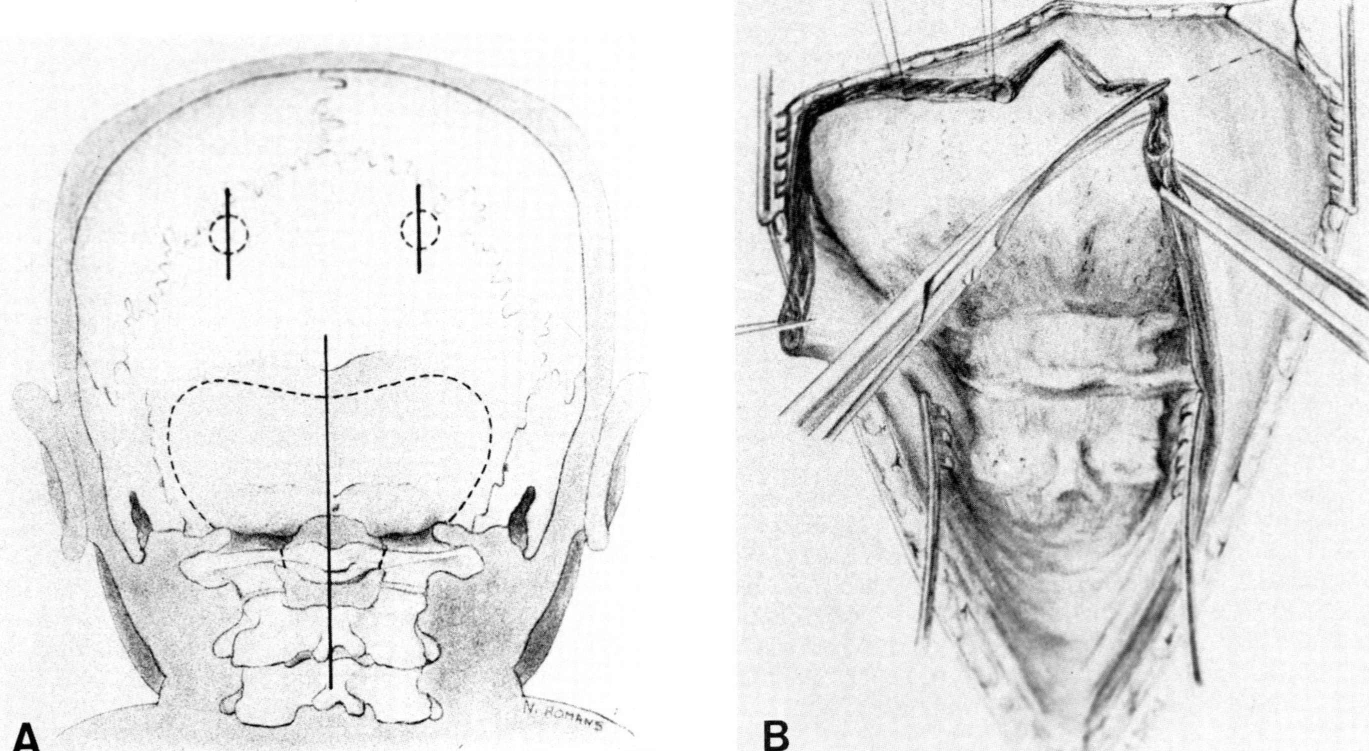

Fig. 57-3. These diagrammatic representations show the midline incision and suboccipital craniectomy. (A) The operative plan for the incisions (heavy lines) as well as the craniectomy and burr holes (dotted lines). (B) The actual operative exposure. (Reprinted from Matson DD: Neurosurgery of Infancy and Childhood, ed 2, 1969, pp 431, 432. Courtesy of Charles C Thomas, Publisher, Springfield, Illinois.)

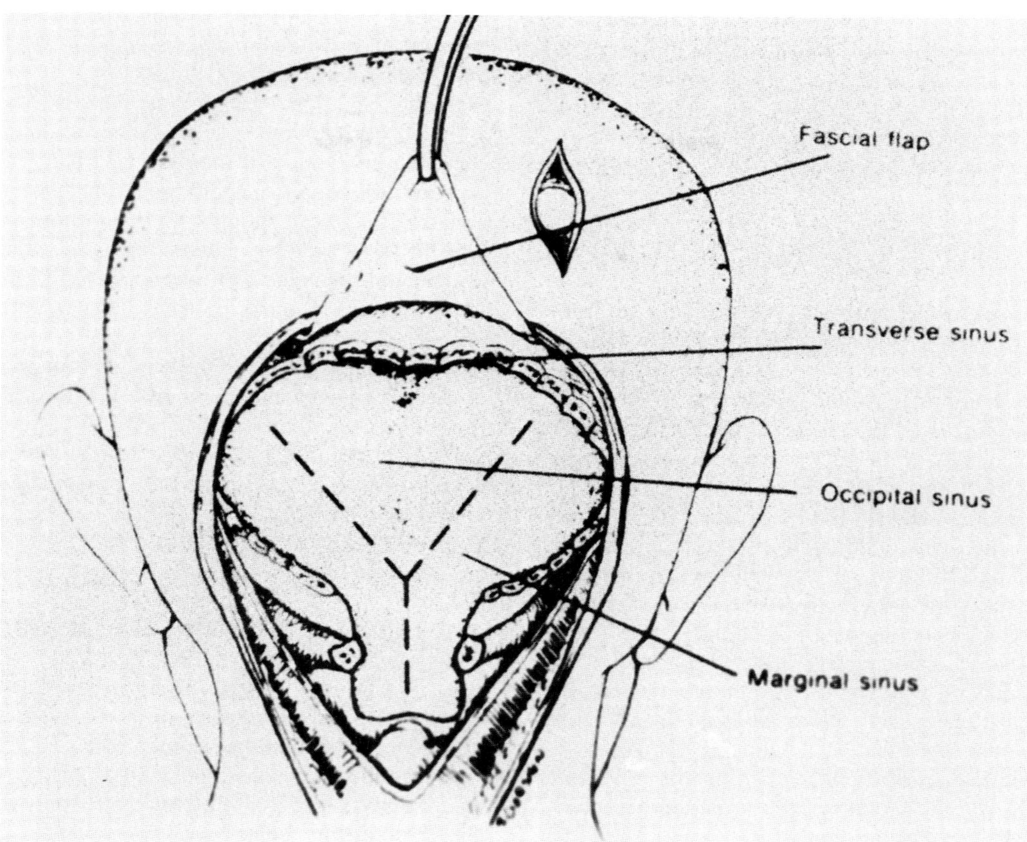

Fig. 57-4. Representation of the Y-shaped midline dural opening. The arch of C1 has been removed and a right occipital burr hole is present. (Reprinted from Epstein F: Pediatric posterior fossa tumors—Part II. Contemp Neurosurg 8(18):1. Copyright 1986 by Williams & Wilkins. With permission.)

position.[41,42] If these are detected, the operative field is flooded with saline and packed with wet gauze sponges. When the patient's condition is stable, a diligent search for the site of air entry should be accomplished, although often the source of the trouble is not pinpointed. Positive end-expiratory pressure (PEEP) will increase the venous bleeding and aid in the identification of the source of the air embolization but also reduces the chance for further air entry into the systemic circulation.

Exposure extends from the superior nuchal line and laterally to the mastoid process. The caudal exposure includes visualization of the arches of C1 and C2. The mastoid emissary veins are often encountered and are occluded by coagulation and the application of bone wax. The position of the vertebral artery and its relationship to the arch of C1 should be kept in mind.

In a patient with obstructive hydrocephalus and raised intracranial pressure, an occipital burr hole can be placed for ventricular drainage. The incision is placed 4 cm lateral to the midline and 6 cm above the inion on the right side (Figure 57-3). The lateral ventricle is cannulated by directing a ventricular catheter through the occipital burr hole in a trajectory toward the medial aspect of the orbit. Rapid ventricular drainage is avoided particularly if the intracranial pressure is significantly elevated, since it can cause the tearing of bridging cortical veins and the creation of a subdural hematoma. The intracranial pressure is gradually, over a period of 5 to 10 minutes, allowed to reach atmospheric levels. These drains can be left in position throughout the operation and retained until the patient is past the early postoperative period. They also can be used to

confirm that an obstructive hydrocephalus has been relieved; this is done by injecting fluid into them and watching for free passage of the fluid through the fourth ventricle.

The posterior fossa craniectomy involves placing burr holes in the occipital bone on either side of the midline below the inion. The craniectomy is enlarged to the foramen magnum with either high-speed drills or rongeurs. Dural attachments to the foramen magnum may be tenacious and require sharp dissection from the overlying bone. The occipital bone is particularly thick in the midline and a high-speed burr is used to thin this bone prior to its removal with rongeurs. In the case of a patient with clinical or radiographic evidence of tonsillar herniation, the arch of C1 and the yellow ligament between C1 and C2 are removed, allowing adequate decompression of the medulla and upper cervical spinal cord.

The dura is divided in a Y-shaped configuration (Figure 57-4). This opening will cross the occipital sinus and circular sinuses, which are cauterized and cut rather than obliterated with metallic hemoclips. Metallic clips will interfere with subsequent radiographic studies; plastic hemostatic clips are useful in this regard. The dura is then reflected laterally and the arachnoid is opened, permitting CSF drainage. This CSF pathway can be opened prior to opening the dura in cases where the posterior fossa appears tense and one wants to allow gradual reduction of the pressure coincident with carrying out the measures described to expose the contents of the posterior fossa. A midline craniectomy will expose the foramen of Magendie at the caudal end of the vermis. Lesions in or adjacent to the fourth ventricle (medulloblastoma, ependymoma) will often protrude from this foramina. Their exposure will require coagulating the vermis with bipolar forceps and splitting it to gain adequate exposure of the tumor and the floor of the fourth ventricle. It is imperative that the floor of the fourth ventricle be identified as the major regional landmark in attempting surgical removal of the tumor.

MEDULLOBLASTOMA

Medulloblastomas are reddish-gray, friable masses that frequently distend the vermis and protrude from the foramen of Magendie. These tumors are easily aspirated, and it is usually necessary to remove tumor between the cerebellar tonsils in order to identify the fourth ventricular outlet and the floor of the fourth ventricle. The region of the obex and subarachnoid space at the foramen magnum are gently packed with cottonoids to reduce the potential for seeding of the spinal subarachnoid space with tumor cells, which can occur during the course of tumor removal. Once the foramen of Magendie is identified, the vermis is split to identify the upper margin of the tumor. Tumor removal can be accomplished by gentle suction aspiration and coagulation with the bipolar cautery, laser vaporization, or, particularly expeditiously, with the Cavitron ultrasonic aspirator. Tumor removal is continued so that the lateral recesses of the fourth ventricle and aqueduct of Sylvius are visualized. It may not be possible to remove tumor adherent to the floor of the fourth ventricle without endangering the patient unnecessarily. In these cases the carbon dioxide laser can be used to vaporize residual neoplasm.[48] We attempt to accomplish surgical resection of this tumor type, although it may not be feasible because of invasion of eloquent areas of the nervous system. This approach is based on the improved 5-year survival statistics for patients having radical resections compared with patients having subtotal resections (40–60 percent and 30 percent, respectively).[48,49,50] Chang developed an operative staging system for medulloblastoma and showed that the size of the tumor has a direct influence on surgical resectability.[51] Patients with smaller tumors (T1) have a 75 percent 5-year survival, but patients with very large tumors (T4) do not survive to 5 years.[49] Other authors have been unable to confirm the prognostic value of this system, since some large tumors are resectable[52,53] and some small tumors have seeded the neuraxis before their diagnosis.[54,55] Generally, survival is probably better in children over 5 years of age,[48,52] in patients with less mitosis and necrosis in their tumors,[56] and in patients with the desmoplastic variant of medulloblastoma.[57] These impressions have not been confirmed by all investigators.[47,48]

Postoperative radiation is routinely administered following the surgery of medulloblastoma to eradicate microscopic deposits of tumor. In adults and older children approximately 3500 rad is given to the brain and spinal cord and a total of 5500 rad to the posterior fossa.[52–54,58,59] Because of concern about the possibility of intellectual and growth impairment,[60] the total craniospinal dose of radiation in young children is limited to 2500 rad following gross total tumor resection. In the cases of Tomita and McClone[54] there was a 100 percent 1-year survival rate with this protocol. Patients with subtotal tumor removal undergoing the same radiation schedule had a 44.4 percent 1-year survival.

Medulloblastoma tends to recur in the posterior fossa, although subarachnoid and systemic metastases are often the cause of further morbidity and mortality. Ventricular shunting has been implicated in the spread of these neoplastic cells beyond the neuraxis, and some authors therefore recommend the use of a millipore-type filter interposed in the shunt system until the radiation has sterilized the field.[47,48] This tactic is attended by a 25 percent incidence of shunt malfunction because of obstruction of the filter by tumor cells.[52] In addition, one author found no difference in the rate of systemic metastasis between patients with or without an interposed filter, a result challenged by another report in which 1 of 24 patients (4.2 percent) developed systemic metastases when a filter was interposed but 5 of 25 patients (20 percent) with nonfiltered shunts developed metastases.[48,61–63]

A contrast-enhanced cranial CT scan is performed postoperatively to document the extent of the surgical resection and the state of the ventricular system. This study is repeated at 3 months, 6 months, and then at yearly intervals. Myelography is performed prior to radiation therapy to identify silent "drop" metastases, which may require additional local irradiation.[54,64–66]

EPENDYMOMA OF THE FOURTH VENTRICLE

Ependymomas often arise in the region of the obex and frequently protrude into the upper cervical spinal canal, requiring a laminectomy of C1 and possibly C2 in addition to the posterior fossa craniectomy for their exposure. Ependymomas characteristically conform to the shape and surfaces of the space into which they grow.[6,7,67] Since most ependymomas of the fourth ventricle arise in the region of the hypoglossal and vagal trigone and are intimately adherent to underlying neural tissue, the complete removal of these tumors may not be possible, although the laser may be helpful in vaporizing residual tumor.

In contrast to medulloblastoma therapy, postoperative irradiation is limited to the structures of the posterior fossa and has been reported to improve survival even for tumors that appear histologically benign.[8,68,69,70] Histologic classification and tumor size are prognostic in a broad sense,[69,71] but biologic activity is difficult to predict, since there is no difference in 5-year survival between benign and malignant appearing ependymomas.[22,68–72] Subarachnoid metastases occur in approximately 5 to 10 percent of patients and are associated with the more malignant forms of this tumor.[68–71] The 5-year survival for patients with posterior fossa ependymomas is 20 to 30 percent,[69,70] falling to less than 15 percent for young children.[7,70,73]

POSTERIOR FOSSA CYSTS

A variety of midline cystic masses may be encountered in the posterior fossa, including extra-axial arachnoid cysts,[10,12,13,25,74] the cyst associated with the Dandy-Walker syndrome,[75] and dermoid cysts.[25] These lesions are symptomatic as a result of direct brain stem and cerebellar compression or obstructive hydrocephalus or both. It is important to differentiate these cysts from loculations of fluid associated with cystic tumors. Cyst fluid that is xanthochromic or has a protein content of greater than 20 mg/dl is unlikely to be associated with an arachnoid cyst or Dandy-Walker cyst. In this case the lesion is fully exposed, the cyst wall carefully examined, and multiple biopsy specimens obtained from the walls. Arachnoid cysts and Dandy-Walker cysts can usually be treated by cyst-peritoneal shunting.[76,77] The supratentorial hydrocephalus occasionally associated with these lesions persists in spite of satisfactory shunting and may require either a separate ventriculoperitoneal shunt or a ventricular catheter joined through a Y-connector to the cyst-peritoneal shunt.

Dermoid cysts located in the posterior fossa typically arise near the midline. These lesions are present from birth, although they may not be symptomatic until adult life, growing slowly into a cyst as sebaceous material and desquamated epithelium are discharged. Patients may have recurrent bouts of meningitis as a result of entrance of bacteria through a sinus tract or chemical inflammation from cholesterol leakage into the CSF. These cysts need to be completely excised along with the sinus tract that arises from the skin.[4,25]

UNILATERAL POSTERIOR FOSSA CRANIECTOMY

When the pathologic entity involves one cerebellar hemisphere, a unilateral exposure of that hemisphere is usually adequate. In this case the skin incision extends from approximately the top of the mastoid process to the external occipital protuberance and then caudally in the midline to an extent depending on the exposure desired (Figure 57-5). The exposure usually includes removal of the rim of the foramen magnum and the arch of C1. Several burr holes are placed off the midline and below the superior nuchal line and the intervening bone thinned with a high-speed drill and removed with rongeurs and bone punches. Exposure is from the midline superiorly to the edge of the transverse sinus and laterally to the mastoid process. The

mastoid air cells are closed with bone wax, and the dura is separated from the skull to prevent dural tears and the inadvertent opening of the transverse dural sinus. The craniectomy extends to the foramen magnum inferiorly. Before the dura is opened, a decision must be made whether the posterior fossa contents are under tension and thus require that the occipital horn be cannulated in order to relieve the intracranial pressure. Alternately, a large posterior fossa cyst whose location is known from the preoperative CT scan can be cannulated directly through an opening made in the posterior fossa dura.

CEREBELLAR ASTROCYTOMA

The cerebellar astrocytoma is the prototypical primary tumor of the cerebellar hemisphere. These tumors may be solid, cystic, or microcystic, and their location makes total excision the treatment of choice. If the posterior fossa is under significant tension, the cystic tumor should first be cannulated with removal of some of its xanthochromic fluid, following which the dura is opened and the mass exposed through a cerebellar corticectomy. If the tumor is solid, dissection is carried around its perimeter,[6,8] or it can first be debulked with the ultrasonic aspirator. In the case of a cystic tumor with a mural nodule, a total excision of the mural nodule should be carried out.[6] Removal of the wall of the cyst is not necessary.[3] The 5-year survival for cerebellar astrocytomas treated in this manner is about 85 percent.[3,4,7-9,78-81] Some pathologic characteristics of cerebellar astrocytomas are of prognostic significance: microcysts, leptomeningeal deposits, Rosenthal fibers, and oligodendroglial elements (Winston's type A) have a 94 percent 10-year survival rate, whereas patients with a tumor demonstrating perivascular rosette formation, a high degree of

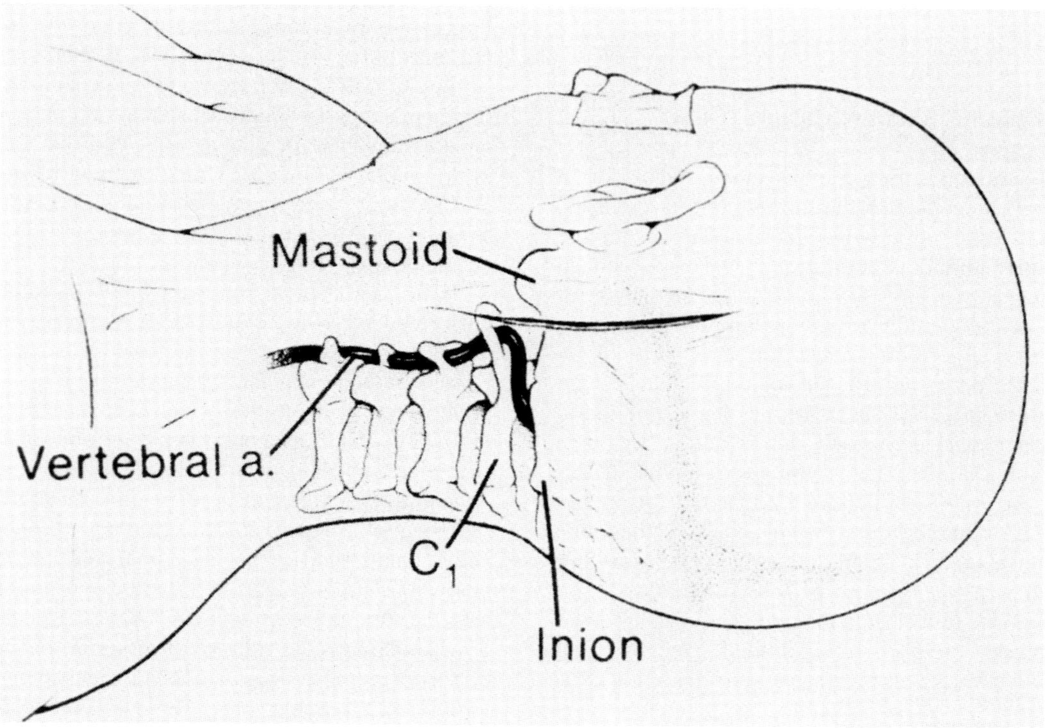

Fig. 57-5. The lateral incision for exposure of hemispheric lesions of the cerebellum. (Reprinted from Fiandaca MS, Tindall GT: Neurosurgical management of acoustic neuromas, part I. Contemp Neurosurg 7(20):1. Copyright 1985 by Williams & Wilkins. With permission.)

cellularity, necrosis, frequent mitosis, and calcifications have a 29 percent 10-year survival.[82] Solid cerebellar astrocytomas and cerebellar astrocytomas located in the midline have a significantly higher incidence of recurrence.[9,18] Every attempt should be made to affect total tumor removal with the first operation.

Following surgery, patients with type A tumors are subjected to CT or MRI studies at 6 months, 1 year, and then annually. Closer follow-up should be maintained for patients with solid or type B tumors, so that an asymptomatic recurrence can be detected and reoperation undertaken. Treatment of recurrent cerebellar astrocytoma is controversial because of the higher morbidity and mortality associated with treating recurrent disease.[78,80,83]

METASTATIC TUMORS OF THE CEREBELLUM

The course of patients with carcinomas of the breast, kidney, lung, or ovary is frequently complicated by solitary cerebellar metastases. These may be amenable to surgical resection, providing the patient with significant palliation. The cerebellar mass is removed if the primary site is slowly growing, so that survival by 3 to 6 months is expected if the cerebellar mass is removed.[84,85] The procedures for the surgical removal of metastatic masses from the cerebellum are the same as those for dealing with the cystic or solid cerebellar astrocytomas described above. In these cases postoperative fractionated whole brain radiation of 3000 rad is routinely administered to the brain in 2 weeks.[86,87] The 1-year survival after surgery and radiation in this situation is 32 to 45 percent for metastatic lung carcinomas, 45 to 63 percent for metastatic breast carcinomas, 30 to 52 percent for metastatic melanomas, and 31 to 30 percent overall for patients with metastatic lesions to the brain.[84,85,88] Only in the most unusual case is a patient with multiple metastatic lesions to the brain considered for surgical intervention.

CEREBELLAR HEMANGIOBLASTOMA

Cerebellar hemangioblastomas are vascular tumors often located in a cerebellar hemisphere. In three quarters of cases, the mass exists as a cystic tumor with a mural nodule. Complete removal of the tumor nodule is curative.[14,89,90] Ten percent of patients harbor more than one tumor mass in the posterior fossa, especially in association with von Hippel-Lindau disease.[90–92] Preoperative vertebral angiography is particularly important in patients potentially harboring cerebellar hemangioblastomas, both to judge the vascularity of the lesion and to define the location and size of each tumor nodule.[14,93] The arterial feeders known on the basis of the angiographic studies to be supplying the mass should be interrupted before an attempt is made to remove tumor tissue.[94] Even then one should try to remove them by going around the lesion rather than by piecemeal removal because of the potential of major hemorrhage. About one fourth of hemangioblastomas are solid tumors.[90] These masses are particularly difficult to remove and prone to invade the brain stem, making total excision impossible.[94,95]

In the case of a cystic lesion, a cortical incision is made into the cyst cavity following exposure of the cerebellum. Self-retaining retractors are used to hold the walls of the cyst apart, and a search is made for the mural nodule. This tumor will often appear as a mulberry-sized mass. The area surrounding the tumor is cauterized with bipolar forceps, the tumor drawn into the cyst cavity, and its base cauterized. These tumors do not have a true capsule to assist in the dissection.[9] If an obvious mural nodule is not encountered, one must carefully look for areas of discoloration or induration.[90] The appearance of these lesions can be quite variable, requiring careful correlation between the angiogram and the operative field to identify the nidus of tumor.[96]

In the case of a very large, solid hemangioblastoma that cannot be removed as a solitary mass, the surgeon should attempt to interrupt the tumor's arterial supply before trying to remove the lesion. Since the tumor's blood supply often arises from arterial branches passing through the tentorium, a combined supratentorial and infratentorial approach may be necessary (Figure 57-6) to interrupt the tumor's vascularity before the mass is removed, often in a piecemeal fashion. Tumor recurrence from undetected multiple or residual tumor is common and has a significantly higher mortality and morbidity, so that every reasonable attempt should be made at primary total tumor removal.[94] Patients with evidence of postoperative residual hemangioblastomas should receive radiation directed to the posterior fossa, and follow-up CT scanning should be performed every 6 months, so that if the mass enlarges or symptoms develop, its operative removal can again be attempted.

THE COMBINED SUPRATENTORIAL AND INFRATENTORIAL APPROACH TO POSTERIOR FOSSA TUMORS

Masses in the anterior and superior part of the cerebellum, high in the cerebellopontine angle, or involving the tentorial hiatus are difficult to expose (Figure 57-7), and the major arterial supply to these tumors may pass through the tentorium. Some tumors extend from the posterior fossa through the tentorial notch. In these cases, a combined laterally situated supratentorial and infratentorial approach may be needed to remove the lesions. Since this approach may require ligation of one lateral sinus, the preoperative contrast studies that provide information on the venous phase help to delineate the anatomy of the dural venous sinuses and to determine whether the ligation of the sinus ipsilateral to the side of the tumor is permissible.[97]

The combined supratentorial and infratentorial approach is performed following exposure of the occipital bone through a lateral skin incision. The incision is carried superiorly and curved into a standard craniotomy incision. An occipital craniotomy is then performed above the transverse sinus, following which the bone over the transverse sinus is thinned with a high-speed drill and then removed. If the main reason for exposing the tentorium is to be able to obliterate the tumor's blood supply, it may not be necessary to ligate the transverse sinus. In this case, the dural incisions are made above and below the sinus (Figure 57-7), and the superior dural flap is situated lateral to the vein of Labbé. This leaves a bridge of dura containing the transverse sinus. Superomedial retraction of the occipital lobe will expose the superior surface of the tentorium. Bridging veins from the cerebellar surface to the dura are cauterized and divided, exposing the inferior surface of the tentorium. It should then be possible to assess the characteristics of the tumor mass and to set about interrupting its

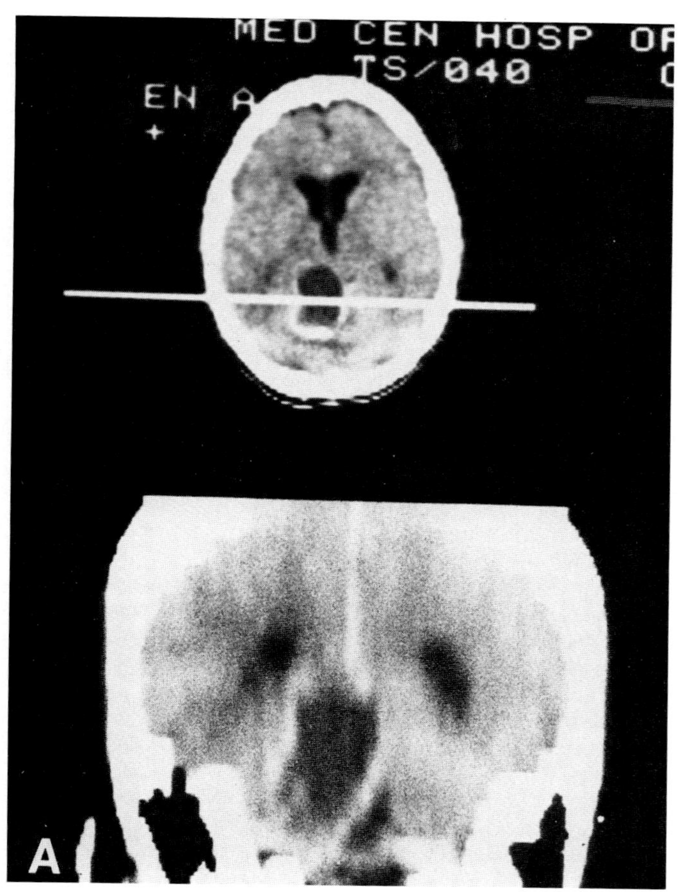

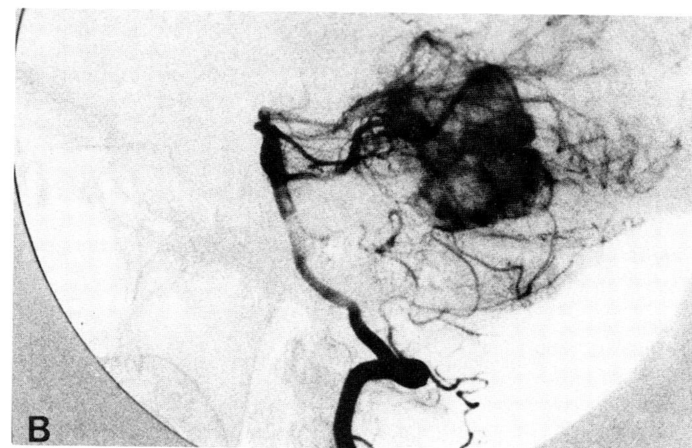

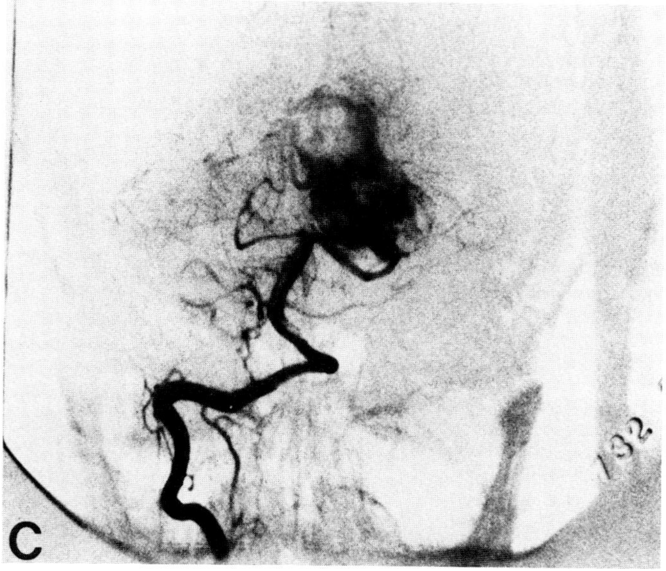

Fig. 57-6. This cystic cerebellar astrocytoma shows features that required a supra) and infratentorial craniotomy for removal. The CT scan (A) shows the bulk of the mass in the superior-medial portion of the posterior fossa, which was decompressed from below the tentorium. The angiogram (B,C) shows a generous vascular supply, which was best visualized and controlled through a supratentorial approach.

arterial feeders. The tumor mass below the tentorium is often debulked first. If additional exposure is needed, the tentorium is split, avoiding the deep veins, posterior cerebral artery, and cranial nerves III, IV, and VI at the incisura. Even greater exposure is provided by ligating and splitting the transverse sinus.[44,98]

Masses within the cerebellopontine angle are approached in either a sitting or prone position. We currently prefer to use the prone position with the head turned to the side by about 40 degrees, or, alternatively, the lateral recumbent position. With the exception of very large tumors, these lesions can generally be managed through a laterally situated craniectomy. In this case the skin incision is a long S-shaped incision 2 cm medial to the mastoid process. The incision may extend high enough to allow it to be used to place an occipital burr hole. Bleeding from the mastoid emissary veins may be troublesome and is controlled with bone wax and cautery. The occipital artery should be cauterized, ligated, and cut when it is encountered. The craniectomy extends from the lower edge of the transverse sinus to the foramen magnum, from the medial edge of the

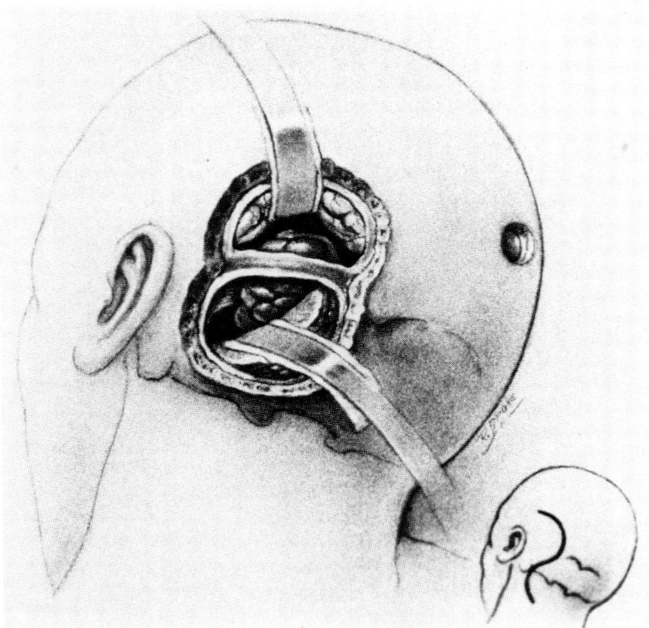

Fig. 57-7. Diagram of the dural opening for the combined supratentorial and infratentorial approach to lesions in the posterior fossa. (Reprinted from McCarty CS: The Surgical Treatment of Intracranial Meningiomas. 1961, p 48. Courtesy of Charles C Thomas, Publisher, Springfield, Illinois.)

sigmoid sinus about one half of the distance to the midline of the occiput. In the course of creating this exposure the mastoid air cells are usually opened and should be occluded with bone wax. A single burr hole is then placed and the remaining bone thinned with a high-speed air drill before its removal with rongeurs. After the dura is opened in a stellate fashion, a Jannetta retractor is adjusted to provide exposure of the tumor in the cerebellopontine angle coincident with the local removal of CSF.

We do not subscribe to the idea of leaving the dura open following surgery within the posterior fossa, but rather close it in a watertight manner. Small rents in the dura that cannot be closed are repaired with pericranial fascia taken from a site adjacent to the operative field. If larger pieces of fascia are needed, fascia lata or freeze-dried cadaver dura can be used, and the subarachnoid space is filled with saline before the dural repair is completed, following which the venous pressure is increased with a Valsalva's maneuver to confirm the watertightness of the closure. Failure to close the dura of the posterior fossa after surgery is associated with an increased incidence of aseptic meningitis,[99] especially in children, and can result in a protracted morbidity. The epidural space is drained with a Jackson-Pratt drain and the muscle and skin layers meticulously approximated. The postoperative management of patients after posterior fossa surgery is accomplished in an intensive care setting. Respiratory status must be carefully monitored and the endotracheal tube left in situ until the patient is awake, following commands, and able to exchange air and secretions adequately. External ventricular drainage is not used routinely unless there is an obstructive hydrocephalus unrelieved by the operation. We have on occasion found it useful to insert an epidural pressure switch outside the dura and below the bone at the craniectomy site to monitor the posterior fossa intracranial pressure, sometimes combining this with monitoring at the site

of the occipital burr hole to alert us of differential changes in pressure within the intracranial compartments.

ACKNOWLEDGMENT

The authors wish to thank Steven Wald, MD, for his comments and review of the manuscript.

REFERENCES

1. Gilman S, Bloedel JR, Lechteyberg R: Neoplasms, in Disorders of the Cerebellum. Philadelphia, FA Davis Co, 1981
2. Amici R, Avanzini G, Pacini L: Cerebellar Tumors. Monographs in Neural Science, vol 4. Basel, S. Karger, 1976
3. Cushing H: Experience with the cerebellar astrocytomas: A critical review of seventy-six cases. Surg Gynecol Obstet 52:129, 1931
4. Matson DD: Neurosurgery of Infancy and Childhood. Springfield, Ill, Charles C Thomas, 1969
5. Ojemann GA. Pathophysiologic basis of posterior fossa tumor signs and symptoms, in Buchheit WA, Truex RC Jr (eds): Surgery of the Posterior Fossa. New York, Raven Press, 1979
6. Koos WT, Miller MH: Intracranial Tumors of Infants and Children. St Louis, CV Mosby, 1971
7. Humphreys R: Posterior crania fossa brain tumors in children, in Youmans JR (ed): Neurological Surgery, vol 5. Philadelphia, WB Saunders, 1982, pp 2733–2758
8. Matson DD: Surgery of posterior fossa tumors in childhood. Clin Neurosurg 15:247, 1968
9. Russell DS, Rubinstein LJ: Pathology of Tumours of the Nervous System, ed 3. Baltimore, Williams & Wilkins, 1972
10. Osborn DR: Epidermoid and dermoid tumors: Radiology, in Wilkins RH, Rengachary SS (eds): Neurosurgery, vol 1. New York, McGraw-Hill, 1985, pp 662–667
11. Latorre E, Fortuna A, Occhipinti E: Angiographic differentiation between Dandy Walker cyst and the arachnoid cyst of the posterior fossa in the newborn infant and children. J Neurosurg 38:298, 1973
12. Little JR, Gomez MR, MacCarty CS: Infratentorial arachnoid cysts. J Neurosurg 39:380, 1973
13. Stein SC. Intracranial developmental cysts in children: Treatment by cystoperitoneal shunting. Neurosurgery 8:647, 1981
14. French BN: Midline fusion defects and defects of formation, In Youmans JR (ed): Neurological Surgery, vol 3. Philadelphia, WB Saunders Co, 1982, pp 1288–1298
15. Olivecrona H: The cerebellar angioreticulomas. J Neurosurg 9:317, 1952
16. Baker HL, Houser OW, Campbell JK: National Cancer Institute study: Evaluation of computed tomography in the diagnosis of intracranial neoplasms. I. Overall results. Radiology 136:91, 1980
17. Fitz CR: Neuroradiology of posterior fossa tumors. Clin Neurosurg 30:189, 1983
18. Naidich TP, Lin JP, Leeds NE, et al: Primary tumors and other masses of the cerebellum and fourth ventricle: Differential diagnosis by computed tomography. Neuroradiology 14:153, 1977
19. Zimmerman RA, Bilaniuk LT, Bruno L, et al: Computed tomography of cerebellar astrocytoma. AJR 130:929, 1978
20. Gol A: Cerebellar astrocytoma in children. Am J Dis Child 106:21, 1963
21. Seeger JE, Burke DP, Knake JE, et al: Computed tomographic and angiographic evaluation of hemangioblastoma. Radiology 143:97, 1982
22. Schwartz JD, Zimmerman RA, Bilaniuk LT: Computed tomography of intracranial ependymomas. Radiology 143:97, 1982
23. Zimmerman RA, Bilaniuk LT, Pahlajani H: Spectrum of medulloblastomas as demonstrated by computed tomography. Radiology 126:137, 1978

24. Gamache FW, Posner JB, Patterson RH: Metastatic brain tumors, in Youmans JR (ed): Neurological Surgery, vol 5. Philadelphia, WB Saunders, 1982, pp 2872–2898

25. Bracket CE, Rengachary SS: Arachnoid cysts, in Youmans JR (ed): Neurological Surgery, vol 3. Philadelphia, WB Saunders Co, 1982, pp 1436–1446

26. O'Brien MS, Tindall SC: Posterior fossa tumors in childhood: Unusual types, in "The Pediatric Section of the American Association of Neurological Surgeons" (eds): Pediatric Neurosurgery. New York, Grune & Stratton, 1982, pp 395–407

27. Glanz S, Geehr RB, Duncan CC, et al: Metrizamide-enhanced CT for evaluation of brainstem tumors. AJR 134:821, 1980

28. Chakeres DW, Kapila A: Brainstem and related structures: Normal CT anatomy using direct longitudinal scanning with metrizamide cisternography. Radiology 149:709, 1983

29. Mawad ME, Silver AJ, Hilal SR, et al: Computed tomography of the brainstem with intrathecal metrizamide. Part II. Lesions in and around the brainstem. AJR 140:565, 1983

30. Randell CP, Collins AG, Young IR, et al: Nuclear magnetic resonance imaging of posterior fossa tumors. AJR 141:489, 1983

31. McGinnis BD, Brady TJ, New PFJ, et al: Nuclear magnetic resonance (NMR) imaging of tumors in the posterior fossa. J Comput Assist Tomogr 7:575, 1983

32. Peterman SB, Steiner RE, Bydder GM, et al: Nuclear magnetic resonance imaging (NMR),(MRI) of brainstem tumours. Neuroradiology 27:202, 1985

33. Carr DH, Bydder GM, Brown J, et al: Intravenous chelated gadolinium as a contrast agent in NMR imaging of cerebral tumors. Lancet 1:484, 1984

34. Albright L, Reigel DL: Management of hydrocephalus secondary to posterior fossa tumors. J Neurosurg 46:52, 1977

35. Albright AL: The value of precraniotomy shunts in children with posterior fossa tumors. Clin Neurosurg 30:278, 1983

36. Epstein F, Murali R: Pediatric posterior fossa tumors: Hazards of the "preoperative" shunt. Neurosurgery 3:348, 1978

37. Papo I, Caruselli G, Luongo A: External ventricular drainage in the management of posterior fossa tumors in children and adolescents. Neurosurgery 10:13, 1982

38. McLaurin RL: Disadvantages of the preoperative shunt in posterior fossa tumors. Clin Neurosurg 30:286, 1983

39. Michenfelder JD, Gronert GA, Rehder K: Neuroanesthesia. Anesthesiology 30:65, 1969

40. Allen D, Kim HS, Cox JM: The anesthetic management of posterior fossa explorations in infants. Can Anesth Soc J 17:227, 1970

41. Meridy HW, Creighton RE, Humphreys RP: Complications during neurosurgery in the prone position in children. Can Anesth Soc J 21:445, 1974

42. Humphreys RP, Creighton RE, Hendrick FB, et al: Advantages of the prone position for neurosurgical procedures on the upper cervical spine and posterior cranial fossa in children. Childs Brain 1:325, 1975

43. Whitby JD: Electrocardiography during posterior fossa operations. Br J Anaesth 35:624, 1963

44. Kempe LG: Operative Neurosurgery, vol 1. New York, Springer-Verlag, 1968

45. Horowitz NH, Rizzoli HV: Postoperative Complications in Neurosurgical Practice. Baltimore, Williams & Wilkins, 1967

46. Bucy PC: Exposure of the posterior or cerebellar fossa. J Neurosurg 24:820, 1966

47. Hoffman HH, Hendrick EB, Humphreys RP: Management of medulloblastoma in childhood. Clin Neurosurg 30:226, 1983

48. Park TS, Hoffman HJ, Hendrick EB, et al: Medulloblastoma: Clinical presentation and management. Experience at the Hospital for Sick Children, Toronto, 1950–1980. J Neurosurg 58:543, 1983

49. Hiarisiadis L, Chang CH: Medulloblastoma in children: A correlation between staging and results of treatment. Int J Oncol Biol Phys 2:833, 1977

50. Raimondi A, Tomita T: Medulloblastoma in childhood. Comparative results of partial and total resection. Childs Brain 5:310, 1979

51. Chang CH, Housepian EM, Herbert C: An operative staging system and a megavoltage radiotherapeutic technic for cerebellar medulloblastoma. Radiology 93:1351, 1969

52. Berry MP, Jenkin DT, Keen CW, et al: Radiation treatment for medulloblastoma: A 21-year review. J Neurosurg 55:43, 1981

53. Silverman CL, Simpson JR. Cerebellar medulloblastoma: The importance of posterior fossa dose to survival and patterns of failure. Int J Oncol Biol Phys 8:1869, 1982

54. Tomita T, McLone DG: Medulloblastoma in childhood: Results of radical resection and low-dose neuraxis radiation therapy. J Neurosurg 64:238, 1986

55. Tomita T, McLone DG: Spontaneous seeing of medulloblastoma: Results of cerebrospinal fluid cytology and arachnoid biopsy from the cisterna magna. Neurosurgery 12:265, 1983

56. Kopelson G, Linggood RM, Kleinman GM: Medulloblastoma: The identification of prognostic subgroups and implications for multimodality management. Cancer 51:312, 1983

57. Chatty EM, Earle KM: Medulloblastoma: A report of 201 cases with emphasis on the relationship of histologic variants to survival. Cancer 28:977, 1971

58. Bloom HJ: Medulloblastoma in children: Increasing survival rates and further prospects. Int J Radiat Oncol Biol Phys 8:2023, 1982

59. Jereb B, Reid A, Ahuja RK: Patterns of failure in patients with medulloblastoma. Cancer 50:2941, 1982

60. Cumberlin RL, Luk KH, Wara WM, et al: Medulloblastoma: Treatment results and effects on normal tissues. Cancer 43:1014, 1979

61. Edwards MSB, Levin VA, Wilson CB: Chemotherapy of recurrent pediatric posterior fossa tumors. Clin Neurosurg 30:209, 1983

62. Hoffman HJ, Hendrick EB, Humphreys RP: Metastasis via ventriculoperitoneal shunt in patients with medulloblastoma. J Neurosurg 44:562, 1976

63. Kleinman GM, Hochberg FH, Richardson EP: Systemic metastases from medulloblastoma: Report of 2 cases and review of the literature. Cancer 48:2296, 1981

64. Deutsch M, Reigel DH: The value of myelography in the management of childhood medulloblastoma. Cancer 45:2194, 1980

65. Dorwart RH, Wara WM, Norman D, et al: Complete myelographic evaluation of spinal metastases from medulloblastoma. Radiology 139:403, 1981

66. Allen JC, Epstein F: Medulloblastoma and other primary malignant neuroectodermal tumors of the CNS: The effect of patient's age and extent of disease on prognosis. J Neurosurg 57:446, 1982

67. Courville CB, Broussalian SL: Plastic ependymomas of the lateral recess: Report of eight verified cases. J Neurosurg 18:792, 1961

68. Barone BM, Elvidge AR: Ependymomas: A clinical study. J Neurosurg 33:428, 1970

69. Dohrman GJ, Farwell JR, Flannery JT: Ependymomas and ependymoblastomas in children. J Neurosurg 45:273, 1976

70. Phillips TL, Shewe GE, Boldrey E: Therapeutic considerations in tumors affecting the central nervous system: Ependymomas. Radiology 83:98, 1964

71. Kricheff I, Becker M, Schneck SA, et al: Intracranial ependymomas: A study of survival in 65 cases treated by surgery and irradiation. AJR 91:167, 1964

72. Kricheff II, Becker M, Schneck SA, et al: Intracranial ependymoma: Factors influencing prognosis. J Neurosurg 21:7, 1964

73. Coulon RA, Till K: Intracranial ependymomas in children: A review of 43 cases. Childs Brain 3:154, 1977

74. Choux M, Raybaud C, Pinsard N, et al: Intracranial supratentorial cysts in children excluding tumor and parasitic cysts. Childs Brain 4:15, 1978

75. Hirsch JF, Pierre-Kann A, Renier D, et al: The Dandy-Walker malformation: A review of 40 cases. J Neurosurg 61:515, 1984

76. Anderson FM, Segall HD, Canton WL: Use of computerized tomography scanning in supratentorial arachnoid cysts: A report on 20 children and four adults. J Neurosurg 50:333, 1979

77. Andersen FM, Segall HD: Intracranial arachnoid cysts, in Pediatric Neurosurgery. New York, Grune & Stratton, 1968

78. Bruno L, Schut L, Bruce DA: Cerebellar astrocytoma, in Pediatric Neurosurgery. New York, Grune & Stratton, 1982, pp 367–374

79. German WJ: The gliomas: A follow-up study. Clin Neurosurg 7:1, 1961

80. Sheline GE: Radiation therapy of tumors of the central nervous system in childhood. Cancer 35:957, 1975

81. Carmel PW: Cerebellar tumors in childhood. Dev Med Child Neurol 14:809, 1972

82. Winston K, Gilles FH, Leviton A, et al: Cerebellar gliomas in children. J Natl Cancer Inst 58:833, 1977

83. Walker MD: Diagnosis and treatment of brain tumors. Pediat Clin North Am 23:131, 1976

84. Zulch KJ: Brain Tumors: Their Biology and Pathology. Berlin, Springer-Verlag, 1986, pp 490–498

85. Takakura K, Sano K, Shuntaro H, et al: Metastatic Tumors of the Central Nervous System. Tokyo, Igaku-Shoin, 1982

86. Gelber RD, Larson M, Borgelt BB, et al: Equivalence of radiation schedules for the palliative treatment of brain metastases in patients with favorable prognosis. Cancer 48:1749, 1981

87. Borgelt BB, Gelber RD, Kramer S: The palliation of brain metastases: Final results of the first two studies by the Radiation Therapy Oncology Group. Int J Radiat Oncol Biol Phys 6:1, 1980

88. Ransohoff J: Surgical management of metastatic tumors. Semin Oncol 2:21, 1975

89. Jeffreys R: Pathologic and haematological aspects of posterior fossa: Haemangioblastoma. J Neurol Neurosurg Psychiatry 38:112, 1975

90. Jeffreys R: Clinical and surgical aspects of posterior fossa: Haemangioblastoma. J Neurol Neurosurg Psychiatry 38:105, 1975

91. Melmon KL, Rosen SW: Lindau's disease: Review of the literature and a study of a large kindred. Am J Med 36:595, 1964

92. Soriya LW, Nijensohn DE, Miller RH: Multiple hemangioblastomas of the central nervous system. Minn Med 56:1059, 1973

93. Skucas J, Brinker RA: Cerebellar haemangioblastoma with a tentorial artery supply: Report of a case. Neuroradiology 3:113, 1971

94. Shige-Hisa O: Solid cerebellar hemangioblastoma. J Neurosurg 39:514, 1973

95. Sung PI, Chang CH, Harisiadis L: Cerebellar hemangioblastoma. Cancer 49:553, 1982

96. Silver ML, Hennigar G: Cerebellar hemangioma (hemangioblastoma): A clinicopathological review of 40 cases. J Neurosurg 9:484, 1952

97. Kapp JP, Schmidek HH: The Cerebral Venous System and Its Disorders. Orlando, Grune & Stratton, 1984, pp 581–623

98. Sato O: Transoccipital transtentorial approach for removal of cerebellar haemangioblastoma. Acta Neurochir 59:195, 1981

99. Carmel PW, Fraser RAR, Stein BM: Aseptic meningitis following posterior fossa surgery in children. J Neurosurg 41:44, 1974

CHAPTER 58

Transtemporal Approaches to the Posterior Cranial Fossa

Gale Gardner   Jon H. Robertson   W. Craig Clark

A VARIETY OF SURGICAL APPROACHES to the posterior cranial fossa are available through the temporal bone. Unlike craniotomies elsewhere, entry to the posterior fossa through the temporal bone imposes special problems for the surgeon if the internal carotid artery and sigmoid sinus, the seventh and eighth cranial nerves, and the specialized structures for hearing and balance are to be preserved. Nevertheless, the access routes through the temporal bone allow the neurosurgeon the opportunity to carry out a number of procedures more directly than with other traditional approaches. Clinical examples of this are the skull base approach for glomus jugulare tumor removal, the retrolabyrinthine approach for vestibular nerve section, and the translabyrinthine approach for acoustic tumor removal.

The intent of this chapter is not to provide a detailed description of the surgical techniques involved, but rather to provide the neurosurgeon with a concept of how the temporal bone can be used to provide a variety of avenues to approach the posterior fossa for specific purposes. The neurosurgeon, with otologic collaboration, can use these approaches singly and in combination in creative ways, to achieve the most ideal approach for a particular problem of the posterior fossa.

BASIC SURGICAL APPROACHES

The transtemporal approaches to the posterior fossa will be discussed in two groups, first the basic individual approaches, followed by combined approaches that have been used successfully by the authors.

SUBOCCIPITAL APPROACH

Cushing,[1] Dandy,[2] and others in the early decades of this century refined and developed the classic approach to the posterior fossa through the subocciput. Entry into the posterior fossa in this way avoids the neurovascular structures of the temporal bone. Relatively wide access to the posterior fossa is accomplished, but retraction of the cerebellum is required. It continues to be the basic approach for dealing with pathologic conditions in the posterior fossa. When applied to acoustic tumor surgery, maximal exposure is accomplished, while at the same time removal of tumors without intentional sacrifice of hearing and balance function is possible. The development of monitoring techniques using evoked response methodology has

greatly increased the practicality of this particular feature (Figure 58-1).

TRANSLABYRINTHINE APPROACH

Panse,[3] in 1904, reported his early efforts to approach the posterior fossa through the labyrinth. William House,[4] however, made the first successful use of this approach in the early 1960s. Earlier, House had attempted to remove acoustic tumors through a middle fossa approach, but turned to the translabyrinthine approach because of inadequate exposure and facial nerve problems. House described comparable surgical exposure and improved control of the facial nerve by drilling directly through the labyrinth and differentiating the superior vestibular nerve from the facial nerve at the lateral end of the internal auditory canal. He emphasized the value of the vertical crest of the internal auditory canal as a primary landmark.

The translabyrinthine approach provides a more direct anterolateral approach to the cerebellopontine angle (Figure 58-1). By removal of bone directly over the angle, less cerebellar retraction is required, and superior exposure of the facial nerve is possible (Figure 58-2). The value of this approach is primarily for the removal of posterior fossa tumors, but it can also be used for labyrinthectomy with associated sectioning of the vestibular nerves for severe vertigo. It can also be used for exposure of the entire intratemporal portion of the facial nerve.

The major disadvantage of the translabyrinthine approach is inadequate exposure of the inferior and posterior poles of large posterior fossa tumors.

MIDDLE FOSSA APPROACH

House[5] developed middle fossa access (Figure 58-1) to the internal auditory canal and adjacent structures in the late 1950s in an effort to remove foci of labyrinthine otosclerosis. Although House used this approach briefly for the removal of acoustic tumors, he soon directed his efforts to a translabyrinthine approach. A subtemporal craniectomy is performed. It is necessary to elevate the temporal lobe with a mechanical retractor in order to make the floor of the middle fossa available for precise bone removal (Figure 58-3). Exact placement of the craniectomy opening is important in this regard. Careful identification of specific landmarks, particularly the greater

OPERATIVE NEUROSURGICAL TECHNIQUES
ISBN 0-8089-1862-1

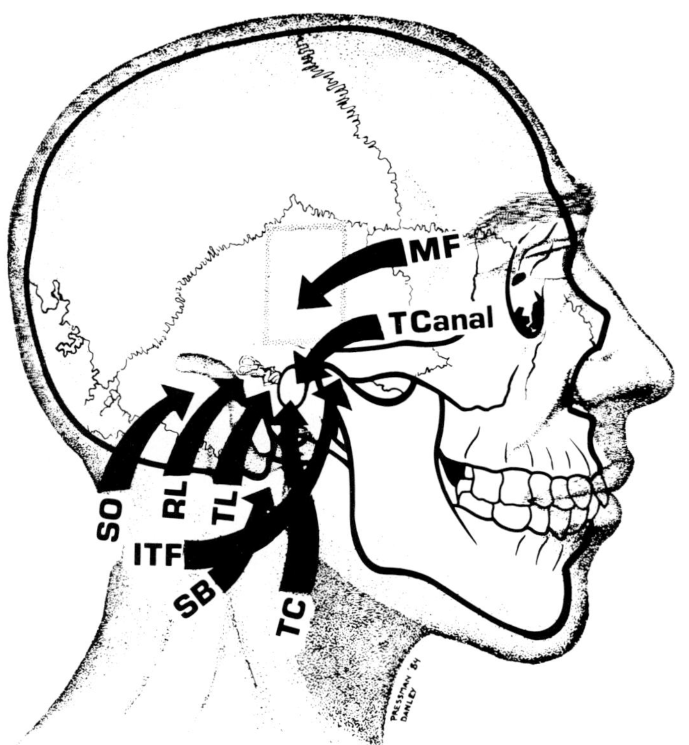

Fig. 58-1. Multiple approach routes through the temporal bone to the posterior fossa. SO = suboccipital; TL = translabyrinthine; TC = transcochlear; MF = middle fossa; RL = retrolabyrinthine; SB = skull base; ITF = infratemporal fossa; T Canal = transcanal.

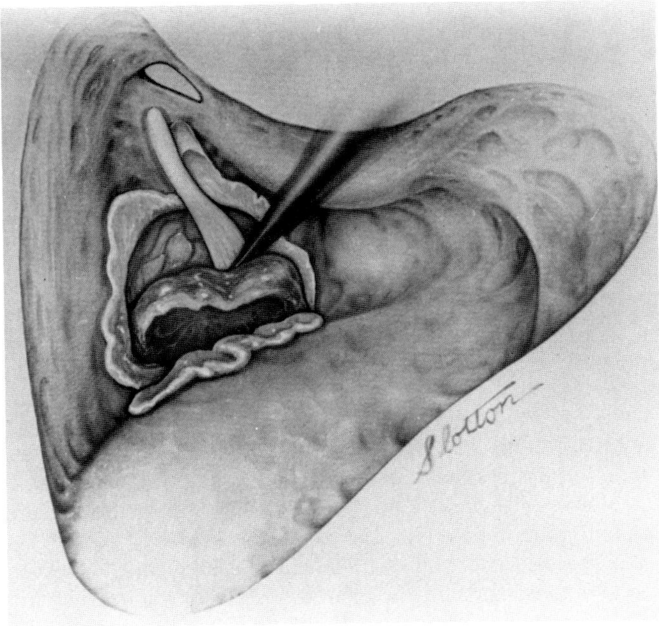

Fig. 58-2. Translabyrinthine approach. Note the surgical plane being developed between the tumor and the facial nerve. (Reprinted from Gardner G, Robertson JH, Clark WC: 105 patients operated upon for cerebellopontine angle tumors—experience using combined approach and CO_2 laser. Laryngoscope 93:1050, 1983. With permission.)

superficial petrosal nerve and arcuate imminence, allows bone removal from over the internal auditory canal and adjacent areas according to the requirement of the surgery being performed.

The primary value of this procedure is for the removal of tumors limited to the internal auditory canal, with only limited extension into the cerebellopontine angle. This approach can also be used for decompression of the labyrinthine and tympanic segments of the facial nerve, either for Bell's palsy or for removal of pathologic processes involving the facial nerve, such as facial nerve neuroma. The vestibular nerve fibers can be sectioned through the middle fossa, allowing preservation of hearing in conditions such as Meniere's disease. Tumors or other pathologic entities of the petrous apex can be approached through this route as well. Theoretically, this approach could be used for access to the horizontal portion of the internal carotid artery as well as the eustachian tube and temporomandibular joint.

The great advantage of the middle fossa approach is that it provides access to areas otherwise difficult to reach. Along with the suboccipital approach, it is unique in allowing removal of acoustic tumors with preservation of hearing. It is also unique in allowing access to the labyrinthine segment of the facial nerve without sacrifice of hearing. Disadvantages associated with this approach include the very narrow margin of error resulting from delicate bone drilling through such a restricted working area. Other problems include the necessity of working very close to the facial nerve, which is in the most superficial plane of the surgical field, the possibility of temporal lobe symptoms as a result of its retraction, and the very thin temporal lobe dura that is frequently present in patients over the age of 50 years.

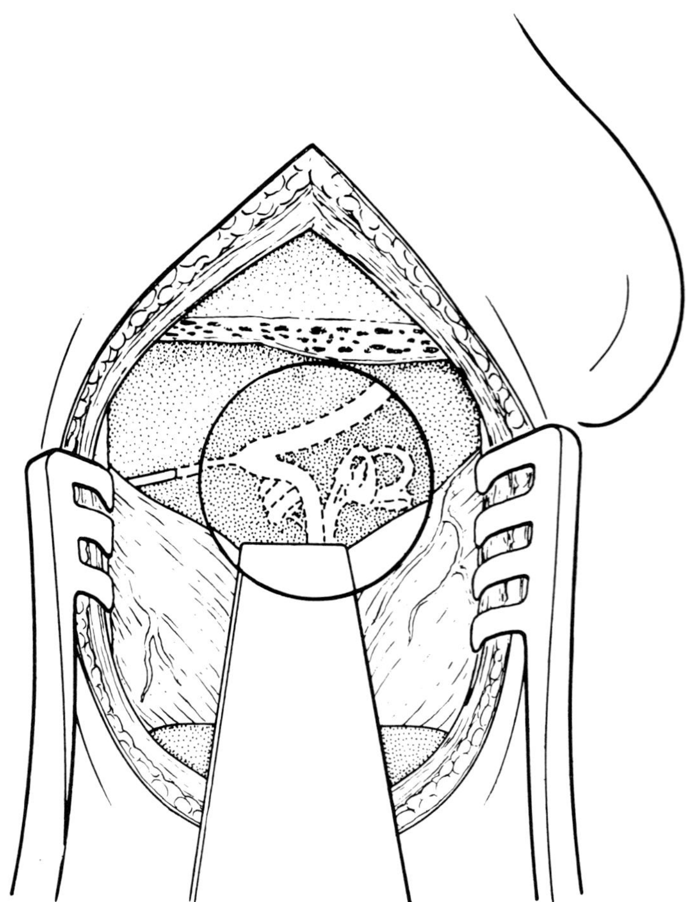

Fig. 58–3. Middle fossa approach. Note the facial nerve, cochlea, and semicircular canals seen through the bone. (Reprinted from Lee, Yanagasawa, Gardner: Surgical Atlas of Otology and Neuro-otology. Orlando, Fl, Grune & Stratton, 1983, p 318. With permission.)

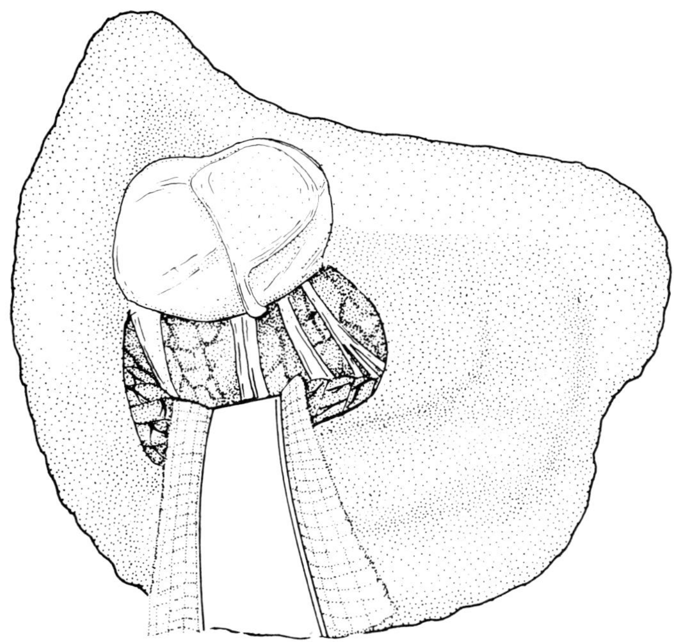

Fig. 58–4. Retrolabyrinthine approach. Note the dural flap containing the endolymphatic sac turned anteriorly. Cranial nerves V, VII, VIII, X, and XI are shown exposed. (Reprinted from Lee, Yanagasawa, Gardner: Surgical Atlas of Otology and Neuro-otology. Orlando, Fl, Grune & Stratton, 1983, p 318. With permission.)

RETROLABYRINTHINE APPROACH

The retrolabyrinthine approach to the posterior fossa is an alternative to the translabyrinthine and suboccipital approaches (Figure 58-1). It was first described by Hitselberger and Pulec[6] in 1972, and has been popularized by Norrell and Silverstein[7] in 1977. It is performed through the mastoid air cells, with elevation of a dural flap between the labyrinth and the sigmoid sinus (Figure 58-4). The concept of this procedure is to allow entry into the cerebellopontine angle anteriorly to the sigmoid sinus, with less necessity for cerebellar retraction. It was originally described as being useful for partial sectioning of the fibers of the sensory route of the fifth cranial nerve for trigeminal neuralgia. More recently it has been advocated for selective sectioning of the vestibular division of the eighth cranial nerve for vertigo. It has also been used on occasion for removal of small acoustic tumors in cases in which it was desirable to preserve hearing.

The major advantage that has been described is the direct access it provides to the cerebellopontine angle without sacrifice of hearing nor extensive cerebellar retraction. The major disadvantage of this approach is the limited exposure that may be available when the mastoid air space is contracted.

TRANSCANAL APPROACH

Silverstein[8] in 1977 described an approach to the internal auditory canal through the external auditory canal using a postauricular incision (Figure 58-1). It has been advocated as being of value for exploring the internal auditory canal, while sectioning the vestibular nerve for vertigo. Silverstein has felt that this approach enhances the ability of the otologic surgeon to detect a very small acoustic tumor that might otherwise not be identified. The major disadvantages of this approach are the risk to the facial nerve and the possibility of meningitis and cerebrospinal fluid leakage. In spite of the primary limitation of

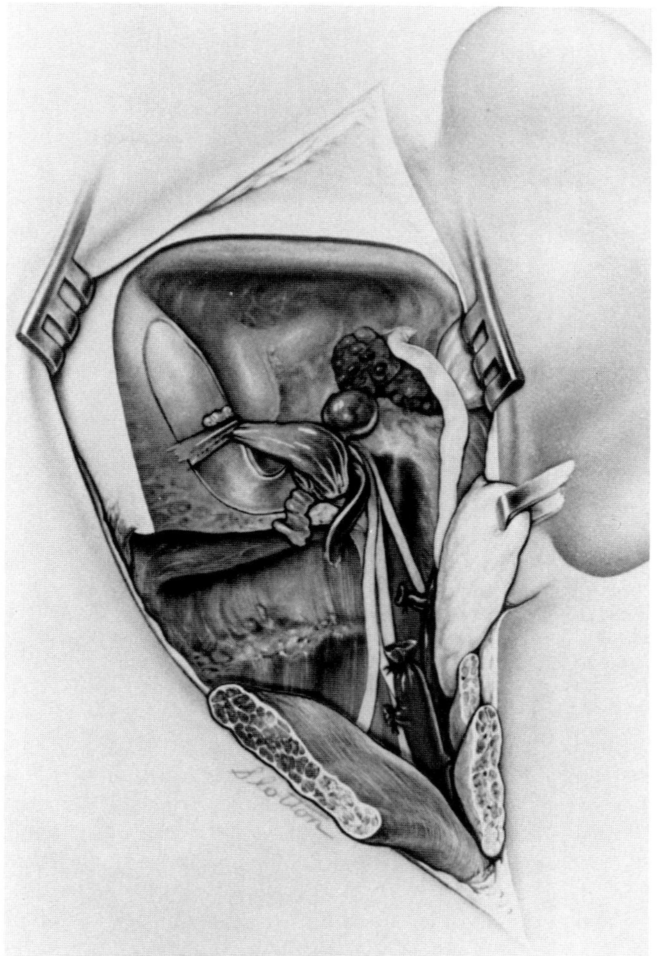

Fig. 58-5. Skull base approach. Note the jugular bulb and glomus jugulare tumor being dissected in continuity with the jugular vein and sigmoid sinus. The lower cranial nerves and internal carotid artery are visible. (Reprinted from Gardner G, Cocke EW, Robertson JT, et al: Combined approach surgery for removal of glomus jugulare tumors. Laryngoscope 87:677, 1977. With permission.)

limited operating space, Silverstein maintains that it provides a very direct and less complicated approach to the internal auditory canal.

SKULL BASE APPROACH

The details of the skull base approach are described elsewhere in this text. Gardner et al.[9] described the historic sequence of efforts culminating in this procedure in 1977. The purpose of this particular approach (Figure 58-1) is to allow direct and wide exposure of the jugular bulb area and the inferior portion of the cerebellopontine angle. The approach is accomplished by extensive soft tissue dissection in the upper neck and over the base of the skull, followed by removal of bone from over the jugular fossa and skull base areas. Its primary purpose is removal of glomus jugulare tumors, as well as other tumors involving the jugular fossa and skull base. In the case of a glomus jugulare tumor, we advocate removal of the tumor and jugular bulb in continuity with the adjacent internal jugular vein, the lateral wall of the sigmoid sinus, which is ligated, and any tumor extension within the posterior fossa (Figure 58-5). The external auditory canal is resected, the external meatus sutured, and the facial nerve transposed ante-

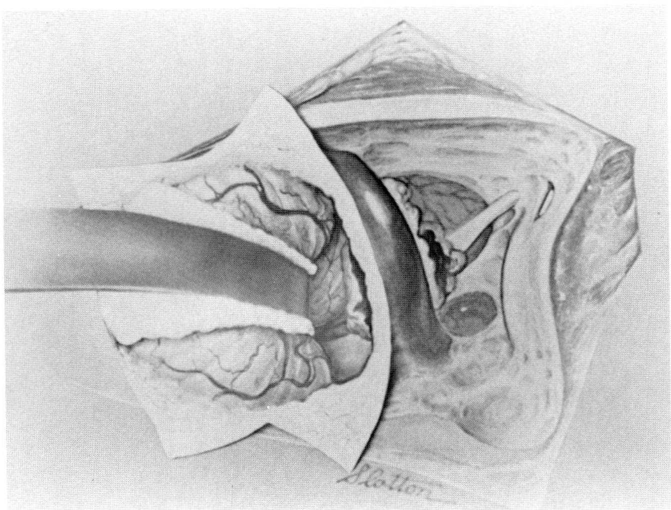

Fig. 58-6. Combined suboccipital-translabyrinthine approach. Note the cerebellum retracted to the left and the facial nerve in view anteriorly with the sigmoid sinus preserved and in an intermediate position. (Reprinted from Gardner G, Robertson JH, Clark WC: 105 patients operated upon for cerebellopontine angle tumors—experience using combined approach and CO_2 laser. Laryngoscope 93:1050, 1983. With permission.)

riorly out of the surgical field. The concept of the surgery is to allow direct vision of the tumor along with the adjacent neurovascular structures, so that en bloc removal of the tumor can be accomplished as opposed to piecemeal and subtotal removal.

The alternative approach through the subocciput fails to provide adequate exposure through the temporal bone, while traditional mastoid approaches have failed to provide exposure for extension of the tumor into the posterior fossa. By combining these two approaches, the skull base approach provides a comprehensive exposure of the entire tumor and provides the surgeon with an opportunity to accomplish total removal with visualization of adjacent structures.

The disadvantages associated with this procedure include the necessity of rerouting the facial nerve, with the likelihood that at least temporary facial paralysis will result postoperatively. Unless the tumor is quite small, hearing is sacrificed because of removal of the ear canal and middle ear structures. If major extension of the tumor occurs anteriorly, it is necessary to utilize infratemporal fossa exposure in order to achieve control over the internal carotid artery. Major problems associated with this procedure have been cerebrospinal fluid leakage and cranial nerve deficit resulting from damage to the vagus nerve.

COMBINED SURGICAL APPROACHES

SUBOCCIPITAL-TRANSLABYRINTHINE APPROACH

Because of relative disadvantages associated with the suboccipital and translabyrinthine approaches, there is a long history of efforts to combine the two. These efforts were basically unsuccessful until Maddox[10] in 1977 described a practical one-stage combined approach with preservation of the sigmoid sinus. We[11] have also contributed to the development of this procedure.

The purpose of the combined procedure is to gain maximal access to the cerebellopontine angle through the subocciput while retaining the advantages of internal auditory canal exposure and facial nerve identification through the labyrinth. This procedure is used for large or otherwise difficult posterior fossa tumors. This procedure is infrequently used because of the bias of the neurosurgeon in favor of the suboccipital approach and the bias of the otologic surgeon in favor of the translabyrinthine approach. The principle of this procedure, however, is that the boundary between the two components, the sigmoid sinus, is an artificial one. By being able to work alternatively both anterior and posterior to the sinus, the neurotologic surgeon achieves a wider operative field and better control of the anterior and posterior extents of the exposure (Figure 58-6).

TRANSCOCHLEAR APPROACH

Hitselberger and House[12] described the transcochlear approach (Figure 58-1) to the cerebellopontine angle and clivus in 1976. This involves an extension of the translabyrinthine approach anteriorly by drilling away the bone of the cochlea and exposing the dura over the petrous pyramid anteriorly to the internal auditory canal. In concept, it thereby allows increased exposure to the most anterior extent of the cerebellopontine angle. It is particularly useful in dealing with tumors such as meningiomas, primary cholesteatomas, and chordomas.

Disadvantages of this procedure include the necessity for removing the facial nerve from the fallopian canal and transposing it posteriorly (Figure 58-7), with the likelihood of at least temporary facial paralysis postoperatively. The procedure as described by Hitselberger and House is also disadvantaged by the very constricted operating area resulting from maintenance of the bony ear canal wall (Figure 58-8). This is overcome to some degree by a modification advocated by Gantz and Fisch[13] and described as a transotic approach in which the posterior bony ear canal is removed and the facial nerve not transposed. A major advantage of the transcochlear approach is control of the blood supply to a meningioma by being able to approach the dural base of the tumor before encountering the tumor itself.

INFRATEMPORAL FOSSA APPROACH

Fisch[14] in 1977 first described the infratemporal fossa approach to the skull base (Figure 58-1). We consider it to be a combination of approaches through the infratemporal fossa and skull base. Its particular advantage is exposure of the internal carotid artery.

Retraction or resection of the ramus of the mandible is accomplished in order to allow removal of bone over the petrous portion of the internal carotid artery. This exposure, combined with the skull base exposure, provides access for removal of glomus jugulare tumors involving the carotid artery. Even larger tumors and tumors of other types with greater anterior extension can be managed by extending this approach further anteriorly.

The major advantage of this approach is the extensive exposure that it provides in the region adjacent to the internal carotid artery. The major disadvantage is the necessity for transposition of the facial nerve and the necessity for resecting the ear canal with subsequent hearing loss.

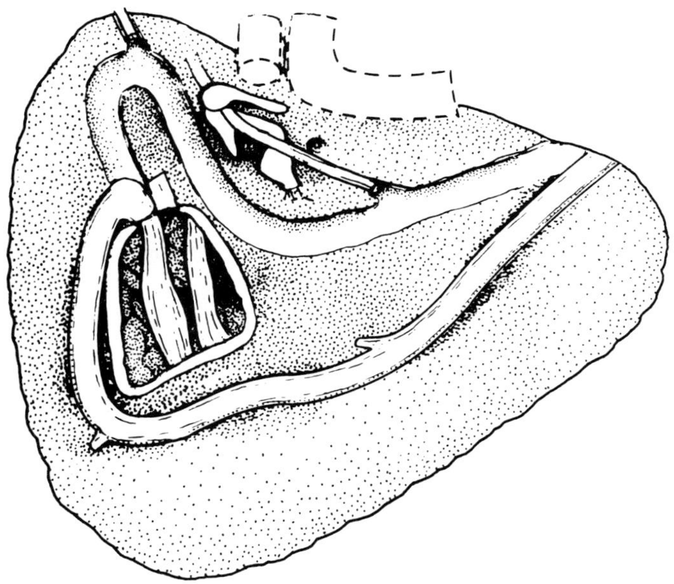

Fig. 58-7. Transcochlear approach. Note the facial nerve displaced posteriorly out of the fallopian canal with the seventh and eighth cranial nerves in view intracranially. The eustachian tube and junction of the horizontal and vertical segments of the internal carotid artery are seen anteriorly. The middle ear ossicles and chorda tympani are in an intermediate position. (Reprinted from Lee, Yanagasawa, Gardner: Surgical Atlas of Otology and Neuro-otology. Orlando, Fl, Grune & Stratton, 1983, p 318. With permission.)

MIDDLE FOSSA-INFRATEMPORAL FOSSA APPROACH

We have used a combination of the middle fossa and infratemporal fossa approaches for dealing with an en plaque meningioma of the middle fossa floor extending into the infratemporal fossa (Figure 58-9). Close et al.,[15] have reported

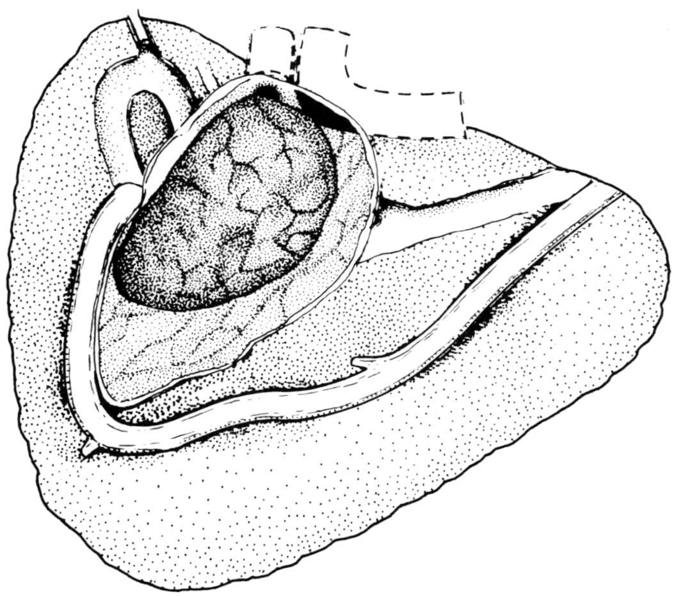

Fig. 58-8. Transcochlear approach with tumor exposed. Note that the bone of the middle ear, cochlea, and eustachian tube has been drilled away, allowing the tumor to be exposed. The anterior limit of dissection is the internal carotid artery. (Reprinted from Lee, Yanagasawa, Gardner: Surgical Atlas of Otology and Neuro-otology. Orlando, Fl, Grune & Stratton, 1983, p 318. With permission.)

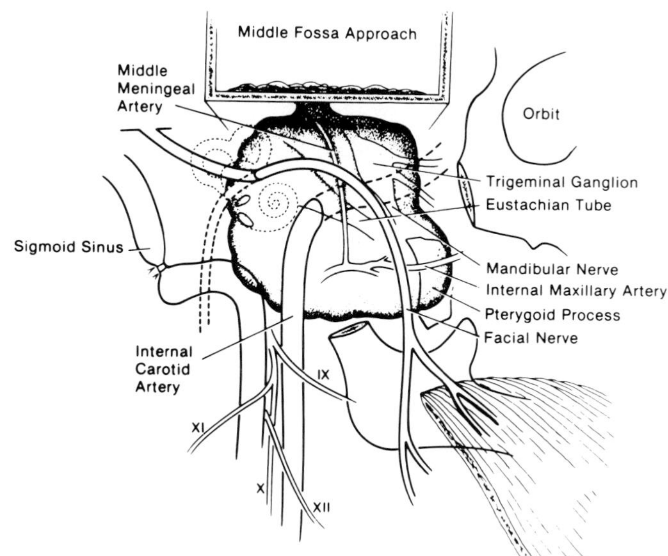

Fig. 58-9. Combined middle fossa-infratemporal fossa approach. Adjacent structures are shown. The facial nerve is displaced and the internal carotid artery is exposed. (Reprinted from Gardner G: Transtemporal approach to the cranial cavity. Am J Otol 6 (suppl):118, 1985. With permission.)

a similar procedure. This particular combination of approaches is a logical extension of either individual approach when the pathologic process involves both areas. The primary value of the approach is in the removal of tumors in this region, but it could conceivably be of value in providing wider access to the internal carotid artery.

CASE REPORTS

The following two case reports illustrate the use of combining the above approaches when faced with particular surgical problems.

Case 1. A 31-year-old white woman was referred to us in March, 1984, with complaints of tinnitus, hearing loss, and fullness in the left ear for 6 years. For 2 years she had noted swelling in the left zygomatic area. A myringotomy and placement of a ventilation tube had been performed in the involved ear in 1978 on two occasions. A CT examination had been within normal limits. Exploration of the left middle ear in July, 1982, had demonstrated a grayish mass within the middle ear space. Pathologic examination indicated this to be a meningioma. A CT examination showed no intracranial involvement, and a decision was made to observe the patient.

A 3–4-cm mass was noted to be present in the left temporal area in October, 1983. Again, CT examination did not demonstrate intracranial disease. One month later exploration was carried out through a frontotemporal craniotomy with identification and removal of a meningioma involving the temporalis muscle. No tumor was noted intracranially.

Re-exploration was carried out in February, 1984, after CT examination demonstrated a tumor involving the temporal fossa and sphenoid wing. The tumor was removed from the middle fossa floor, but it was difficult to establish a well-defined plane. Again pathologic examination showed this to be meningioma.

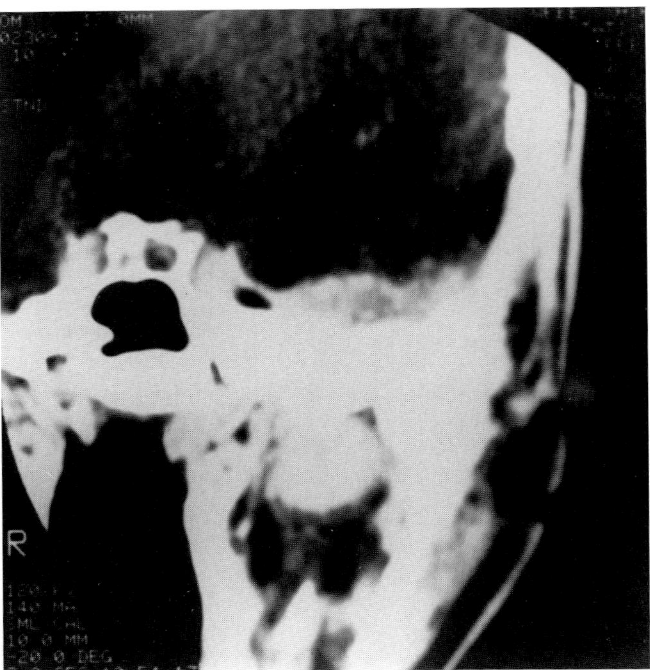

Fig. 58-10. En plaque meningioma. Note the inferior extension into the infratemporal fossa.

The patient had a mild and brief impairment of memory postoperatively.

When we first saw the patient in March of 1984, she showed no significant neurologic deficit. Cranial nerves were intact, and otoscopic examination showed a normal tympanic membrane. A very slight conductive hearing loss was present on the left, with normal neurosensory function. The CT examination showed abnormality of the floor of the left middle cranial fossa, with a nodular density present in the infratemporal fossa (Figure 58-10). Arteriography did not produce significant additional findings. We felt that this lesion represented an en plaque meningioma of the left temporal bone with inferior extension into the infratemporal fossa, as described by Nager.[16]

Surgery was performed in two stages. In May, 1984, through a left middle fossa exposure, the tumor was identified involving the middle fossa floor, with anterior and lateral extension and involvement of the middle ear space. A surgical drill was used to remove the entire floor of the middle fossa. Extension of the tumor into the middle ear was removed, with exposure of the facial nerve, the internal carotid artery, and the eustachian tube. Tumor was identified extending inferiorly into the infratemporal fossa, but exposure was not adequate for its removal, and a secondary procedure was planned.

Two weeks later, operating through a combined middle-infratemporal fossa approach, adequate exposure of the tumor was accomplished. The tumor was grayish-white in color, and measured 4–5 cm in greatest diameter. It involved the structures of the infratemporal fossa with extension anteriorly to the pterygoid plates and superiorly to the base of the skull. Total removal of the tumor was accomplished. The zygomatic arch was turned inferiorly during the procedure, then wired back into its normal position. The condyle of the mandible was removed to allow exposure.

Postoperatively the patient experienced no significant complications. She described improvement in the tinnitus with no change in hearing. There was no significant facial nerve dysfunction. The patient has remained asymptomatic without evidence of tumor recurrence.

Case 2. A 19-year-old white man was referred to us on September 4, 1984, with an 18-month history of hearing loss, pain, and ringing tinnitus involving the left ear, with dizziness of 1 year's duration. A CT examination had shown a 3.5-cm cerebellopontine angle tumor. Audiometry showed a very minimal sensorineural hearing loss with moderate impairment of speech discrimination. Auditory brain stem response audiometry had been within normal limits.

We felt that this tumor was probably an acoustic neuroma. Because the tumor extended markedly anteriorly, we elected to use a combined translabyrinthine-transcochlear approach in order to achieve maximal anterior exposure. We employed Fisch's transotic modification to avoid transposition of the facial nerve. The posterior bony ear canal wall was removed and the external meatus of the ear closed primarily. This combination of approaches was particularly helpful in allowing us to work anteriorly to the porus acusticus and to control the anterior extent of the tumor.

COMMENTS

Although these approaches to the posterior fossa through the temporal bone require special techniques because of the specialized structures involved, we feel that they provide the neurosurgeon with a flexibility of approach that is important in dealing with tumors of this area. We further believe that this type of surgery is still evolving and that additional innovations will be limited only by the imagination of those who perform this surgery.

Those who elect to perform this type of surgery will find it necessary to make a major commitment of time and effort in order to master the techniques involved. Because of the overlap of neurosurgery and otology in this area, collaboration of neurosurgeons and otologists is mandatory.

SUBOCCIPITAL APPROACH

The possibility of preserving hearing through the suboccipital approach has enhanced the value of this basic approach to the cerebellopontine angle. Questions regarding the validity of the concept of hearing preservation remain to be answered, however. Is the hearing that is preserved stable, or can it undergo regression in the future? Is the benefit of retained hearing worth the tinnitus and dizziness that may be retained and perhaps made worse? Is there a risk of leaving residual tumor within the retained cochlear nerve, and is this of long-term significance? Can intraoperative use of auditory evoked responses improve our ability to preserve hearing and perhaps allow us to achieve this with even larger tumors? Needless to say, these same questions apply also to the middle fossa approach.

TRANSLABYRINTHINE APPROACH

In the use of the translabyrinthine approach to the cerebellopontine angle, it is important to emphasize achieving a maximum of operating space before undertaking tumor removal. Unfortunately many neurosurgeons form their initial opinion of this approach based on the early efforts of a collaborating otologic surgeon. There frequently has been a tendency to abandon the translabyrinthine approach on the basis of such experiences, whereas continued experience will allow increased exposure. There are a number of minor but valuable maneuvers that allow maximizing surgical exposure through the labyrinth, but they must be mastered by the otologic surgeon over a considerable period of time, both in the dissection laboratory and in the operating room.

TRANSLABYRINTHINE-SUBOCCIPITAL APPROACH

An alternative to the above process is the use of the suboccipital approach as an additional exposure combined with the translabyrinthine approach. The greater exposure thereby afforded by the suboccipital approach can be utilized when necessary, while the particular advantages of translabyrinthine exposure are retained, including facial nerve identification and improved exposure of the internal auditory canal.

MIDDLE FOSSA APPROACH

Middle fossa surgery places major demands on the otologic surgeon. This is certainly not a procedure to attempt without having thoroughly mastered the techniques by working in a dissection laboratory. As with translabyrinthine surgery, there are seemingly small details that are of significant importance to the success of the surgery. An example of this is proper placement of the craniotomy to allow proper placement of the retractor, which in turn allows maximal exposure of the necessary landmarks. Unless this process is adhered to, significant complications can result. On the other hand, careful identification of landmarks allows the neurosurgeon to utilize this procedure in exposing areas that cannot be reached as effectively otherwise.

TRANSCANAL APPROACH

Neurosurgeons are not likely to become enthusiastic with working through such a small access area to the posterior fossa. Bleeding and other complications are likely to place more requirements on this approach than it can provide. It is therefore of limited value at this time.

SKULL BASE APPROACH

Our own experience with the surgical removal of glomus jugulare tumors has convinced us that the infratemporal fossa extension is rarely needed for satisfactory tumor removal. Retraction of the ramus of the mandible and removal of the bone over the vertical portion of the internal carotid artery provide satisfactory exposure of the tumor in this area in all but very rare circumstances. If adequate removal of bone from the skull base is carried out initially, and the tumor is fully exposed, the necessity of extended exposure anteriorly is diminished in most circumstances.

TRANSCOCHLEAR-TRANSOTIC APPROACH

Exposure of the anterior extent of the cerebellopontine angle by drilling away the cochlea is an important addition to this system of transtemporal approaches. Even as it is helpful to

extend the suboccipital approach anteriorly through the translabyrinthine approach, it is also helpful to extend the translabyrinthine approach further anteriorly by utilizing the transotic or transcochlear approach. This has great value when dealing with a cerebellopontine angle tumor in which the anterior pole is well beyond our line of vision. The modification suggested by Fisch has, in our experience, been particularly helpful, and we advocate its use. In case 2, the additional anterior exposure converted a very marginal exposure situation to one that was quite satisfactory.

INFRATEMPORAL FOSSA APPROACH

We consider the infratemporal fossa procedure to be primarily of value in dealing with extremely large glomus jugulare tumors and other tumors involving this portion of the skull base. For these purposes, we believe that development of this approach by Fisch was a major contribution to our ability to extend our operative efforts into those spaces adjacent to the anterior portion of the temporal bone.

MIDDLE FOSSA-INFRATEMPORAL APPROACH

Nager[16] has clarified how meningiomas of the temporal bone can extend through the middle fossa floor into the neck. Understanding this concept was critical to dealing with the tumor described in case 1.

CONCLUSIONS

The ability to approach the posterior cranial fossa in a variety of ways is advantageous to the neurosurgeon by allowing him or her more options in approaching and dealing with tumors in this area. The ability to drill away selected segments of the temporal bone without major sacrifice of function to achieve access for these procedures is a continuing and exciting challenge for both neurosurgeons and their otologic colleagues.

ACKNOWLEDGMENTS

The authors gratefully acknowledge the editorial assistance and word-processing skills of Ms. Florence M. Bruce and Mrs. Joan Wallis.

REFERENCES

1. Cushing H: Tumors of the Nervus Acousticus and the Syndrome of the Cerebellopontine Angle, ed 2. New York, Hafner, 1963
2. Dandy WE: An operation for the total removal of cerebellopontine (acoustic) tumors. Surg Gynecol Obstet 41:139, 1925
3. Panse R: Ein Gliom des Akustikus. Arch Ohrenheilk 61:251, 1904
4. House WF: Evolution of the transtemporal bone removal of acoustic tumors. Arch Otol 80:731, 1964
5. House WF: Middle cranial approach to the petrous pyramid: Report of 50 cases. Arch Otolaryngol 78:460, 1963
6. Hitselberger WE, Pulec JL: Trigeminal nerve (posterior root) retrolabyrinthine selection section—operative procedure for intractable pain. Arch Otolaryngol 96:412, 1972
7. Silverstein H, Norrell H: Retrolabyrinthine surgery: A direct approach to the cerebellopontine angle, in Silverstein H, Norrell H

(eds): Neurological Surgery of the Ear. Birmingham, Ala, Aesculapius, 1977, pp 318–322

8. Silverstein H: Transmeatal cochleovestibular neurectomy, in Silverstein H, Norrell H (eds): Neurological Surgery of the Ear. Birmingham, Ala, Aesculapius, 1977, pp 176–189

9. Gardner G, Cocke EW, Robertson JT, et al: Combined approach surgery for removal of glomus jugulare tumors. Laryngoscope 87:665, 1977

10. Maddox HE III: The lateral approach to acoustic tumors. Laryngoscope 87:1572, 1977

11. Gardner G, Robertson JH, Clark WC: 105 patients operated upon for cerebellopontine angle tumors—experience using combined approach and CO_2 laser. Laryngoscope 93:1049, 1983

12. House WF, Hitselberger WE: The transcochlear approach to the skull base. Arch Otolaryngol 102:334, 1976

13. Gantz BJ, Fisch U: Modified transotic approach to the cerebello-pontine angle. Arch Otolaryngol 109:252, 1983

14. Fisch U: Infratemporal fossa approach for extensive tumors of the temporal bone and base of the skull, in Silverstein H, Norrell H (eds): Neurological Surgery of the Ear. Birmingham, Ala, Aesculapius, 1977, pp 34–53

15. Close LG, Mickey BE, Semson DS, et al: Resection of upper aerodigestive tract tumors involving the middle cranial fossa. Laryngoscope 95:908, 1985

16. Nager GT, Heroy J, Hoeplinger M: Meningioma involving the temporal bone with extension to the neck. Am J Otolaryngol 4:297, 1983

CHAPTER 59

Tumors of the Cerebellopontine Angle: Clinical Features and Surgical Management

William A. Buchheit   Robert H. Rosenwasser

THE HISTORY of the surgery of the posterior fossa is essentially the history of acoustic neuroma surgery. Prior to the 20th century, occasional attempts at surgery within the cerebellopontine angle were carried out. These procedures were associated with extremely high mortality, and most people, including surgeons, considered the operations suicidal. After the turn of the century, improvements in anesthesia and surgical technique led to a marked reduction in the mortality and morbidity of neurosurgery in general and of surgery of the posterior fossa in particular. The mortality dropped from 85 percent in Henschen's cases reported in 1910[1] to 4 percent by Cushing[2] 22 years later. Progressive improvement in diagnostic and surgical techniques led to the modern era. Computed tomography and MRI scanning now make it possible to diagnose these tumors in their early stage of development, and microneurosurgical techniques allow surgeons to remove them with a consistently low mortality and morbidity. An operation that was once believed to be impossible is now performed daily. Nowhere has the progress of neurosurgery been so dramatically demonstrated as in surgery in the posterior fossa.

CLINICAL FEATURES

The clinical features of cerebellopontine angle lesions are uniquely specific. The proximity of multiple important structures permits the clinical diagnosis of a cerebellopontine angle mass with great certainty. On the other hand, the slow growth rates of these tumors make histologic differentiation practically impossible. Fortunately, diagnostic aids (discussed elsewhere) permit differentiation of tumor types with a high degree of reliability. A combination of clinical examination and specific neuroradiologic, audiologic, and neurophysiologic considerations allow a neurosurgeon to come to the operating room with an accurate preoperative diagnosis.

Acoustic neuromas are the most common cerebellopontine angle tumors and serve as a prototype for lesions in this area. A history of progressive unilateral hearing loss, usually over many months and sometimes even years, is the hallmark of these lesions, whose growth begins within the internal auditory canal. This growth is associated with tinnitus, in the usual case, and as the tumor enlarges and extends out of the internal auditory canal, the patient begins to complain of unsteadiness of gait and loss of balance. True rotational vertigo is rare.

The tolerance of the facial nerve to stretching and distortion from progressive growth of these lesions is a curiosity that has been observed over many years. The nerve usually maintains its functional capacity until the tumor reaches a very large size and even then, when difficulty with a nerve develops, it is usually mild. Total facial paralysis is rare and is seen only in the largest lesions. Presumably, a microvascular anomaly is the cause of the progressive neural dysfunction.

Involvement of the trigeminal nerve likewise occurs late and is seen primarily in tumors more than 3 cm in diameter. As the tumor grows upward into the superior aspect of the cerebellopontine angle, it encroaches upon the trigeminal nerve and produces diminution and, later, loss of the corneal reflex. Facial analgesia and anesthesia follow in slow progression. Anesthesia of the face, like seventh nerve palsy, is usually associated with only the largest tumors. Ticlike pain may occur, but this is infrequent.

Cerebellar signs and symptoms occur late and are usually preceded by signs and symptoms of trigeminal facial nerve dysfunction. Papilledema and hydrocephalus occur even later.

Unilateral hearing loss is the most consistent symptom in patients with acoustic tumors. Details of the audiologic manifestations are discussed in another chapter.

Next to acoustic neuromas, meningiomas are the most frequent tumors of the angle. These tumors have the same general size and symptoms of acoustic tumors with several exceptions. These lesions most frequently arise from the superior and anterior lip of the internal auditory canal and therefore are associated with early involvement of the seventh nerve, sparing the eighth nerve with associated hearing deficits. Involvement of the posterior root of the fifth nerve may lead to numbness of the face and ticlike symptoms. When they precede hearing loss, these symptoms tip the scales in favor of a diagnosis of meningioma or, less likely, a tumor of the trigeminal nerve.

Either a meningioma or an acoustic neuroma can grow downward toward the jugular foramen where they produce hoarseness, dysphagia, and dysphonia, as the ninth, tenth and eleventh nerves are compromised. Ataxia becomes prominent when the lesion distorts the cerebellum and the respective

OPERATIVE NEUROSURGICAL TECHNIQUES
ISBN 0-8089-1862-1

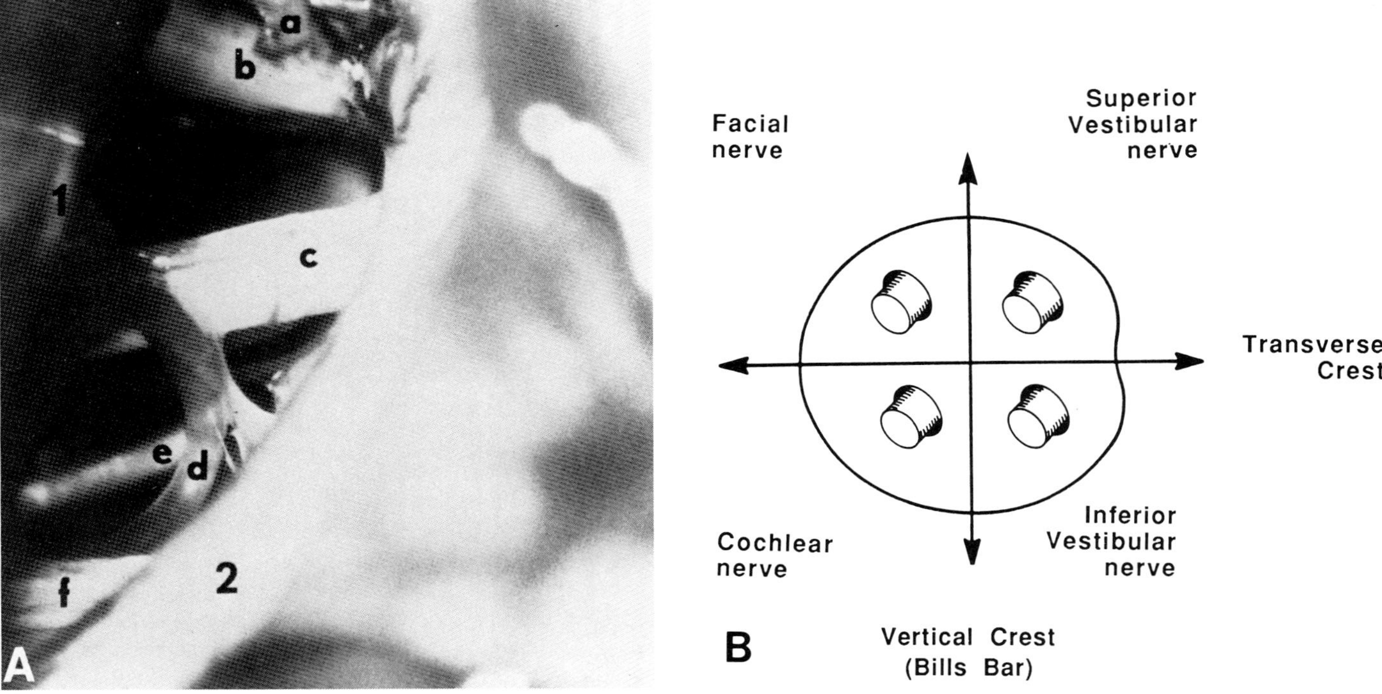

Fig. 59-1.   (A) The normal microsurgical anatomy of the right cerebellopontine angle. (1) Cerebellar retractor; (2) petrous bone; (a) petrosal vein; (b) trigeminal nerve; (c) seventh-eighth nerve complex; (d) anterior inferior cerebellar artery; (e) sixth nerve; (f) ninth-tenth-eleventh nerve complex. (B) Diagrammatic representation of the right internal auditory canal illustrating the positions of the neural elements.

cerebellar peduncle. Exceptionally large tumors may even lead to brain stem compression and pyramidal tract signs.

Those meningiomas that arise in the superior aspect of the cerebellopontine angle ultimately produce similar signs, but they are preceded by fifth nerve symptoms. When the tumor growth is in the direction of the tentorial incisura, early signs and symptoms of hydrocephalus and increased intracranial pressure may occur. Associated with these symptoms are upper pontine and midbrain signs including involvment of the third, fourth, and sixth cranial nerves.

Metastatic tumors of the angle occur less frequently than either meningiomas or acoustic neuromas but without prior knowledge of a primary tumor, the differentiation is practically impossible.

ANATOMY

The cerebellopontine angle is an inverted triangular cistern in which the fifth, seventh, and eighth cranial nerves, along with the anterior inferior cerebellar artery (AICA) and the superior petrosal vein, are located (Figure 59-1A). From a surgeon's viewpoint, the cistern is bounded laterally by the back wall of the petrous bone, medially by the pons, and cephalad by the tentorium, which forms the base of the triangle. This cistern communicates freely with the other cerebrospinal fluid spaces within the posterior fossa, including a small diverticulum that extends down into the porus acusticus.[3]

At the upper aspect of the cistern, the fifth nerve is a broad white band, extending from the lateral aspect of the pons into Meckel's cavity. At the upper posterior edge of this nerve is the petrosal vein, which drains from the superior aspect of the cerebellum to the superior petrosal sinus. This vein is usually 1

to 2 mm in diameter and at times may be made up of a cluster of veins.[4,5]

The seventh and eighth nerves course laterally from the pontomedullary junction to the internal auditory canal. They cross the cistern in what appears to be a single nerve, which is composed of four discrete nerves—the superior and inferior vestibular nerves, the cochlear nerve, and the facial nerve. When viewed from the suboccipital approach, the vestibular nerves form the posterior aspect or the portion closest to the surgeon. The facial nerve makes up the anterior superior portion within this bundle, and the cochlear division of the eighth nerve makes up the anterior inferior portion.[6] This is represented schematically in Figure 59-1B. When one looks into the posterior fossa from the extreme lateral aspect of a suboccipital approach, the sixth nerve is occasionally seen coursing from its origin at the pontomedullary junction to its entrance into the dura of the clivus (Dorello's canal). In situations in which the tumor has rotated and displaced the brain stem, this nerve may be confused with the seventh nerve, inasmuch as it exits on the same plane as the seventh nerve and enters the dura at the same level as the internal auditory canal.

The ninth, tenth, and eleventh nerves, although not specifically within the cerebellopontine angle cistern, are found immediately below its inferior margin. The most superior of these nerves, the ninth, is round and shiny and made up of a single filament. The tenth nerve consists of multiple filaments, which are flat, and the eleventh nerve is unique in having a spinal root traversing the foramen magnum.

The anterior inferior cerebellar artery has a variable location within the cistern. In acoustic tumors, this vessel is usually located in the arachnoid over the cleft between the cerebellum and the dome of the tumor.

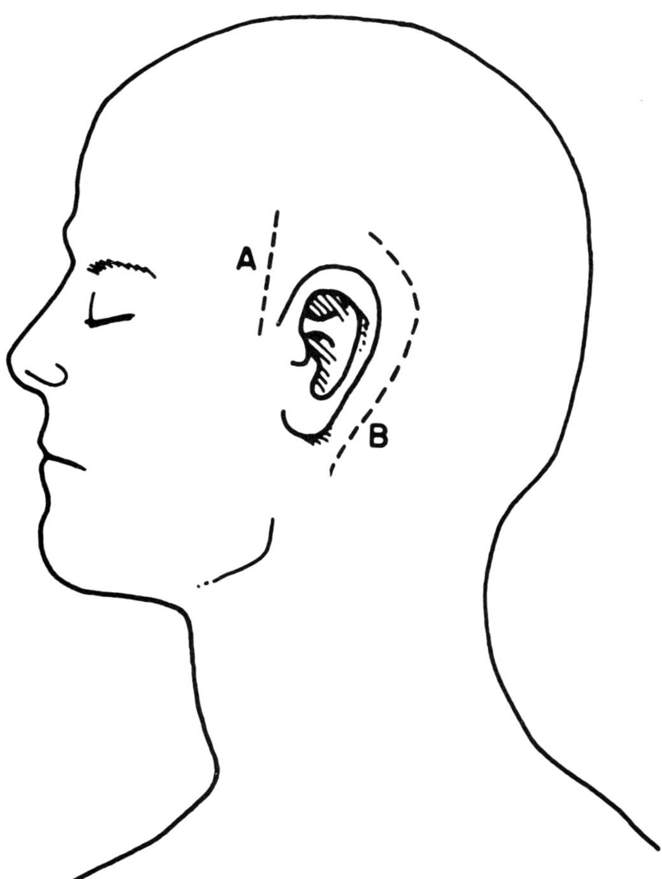

Fig. 59-2. Surgical incisions used for (A) the middle fossa approach and (B) the translabyrinthine approach to acoustic tumors.

OPERATIVE APPROACHES TO THE CEREBELLOPONTINE ANGLE

MIDDLE FOSSA APPROACH

The middle fossa approach, as described by House in 1961,[7] involves an extradural subtemporal approach with microsurgical unroofing of the internal auditory canal. This approach is limited to the excision of small intracanalicular tumors that have not escaped the confines of the internal auditory canal. It is usually performed in patients in whom audition remains at a functional level, providing a chance at preserving hearing.

The procedure is performed with the patient in the lateral position. A linear temporal incision is made from the zygomatic arch to the insertion of the temporalis fascia (Figure 59-2). A bone flap is fashioned as a square, two thirds anterior and one third posterior to the external auditory canal. Once the dura is elevated from the floor of the temporal fossa, the House-Urban retractor is secured in place. Several anatomic structures come into view as the dural dissection continues. First is the middle meningeal artery exiting the foramen spinosum. This landmark is used as the anterior limit of the point at which it has been grooved by the superior petrosal sinus. Care must be taken not to injure the geniculate ganglion or the greater superficial petrosal nerve, both of which lie unprotected by bone in about 5 percent of cases. The greater superficial petrosal nerve when followed posteriorly leads to the facial nerve. At this point in the operation, it is usually possible to identify the middle meningeal artery, the arcuate eminence, the greater superficial

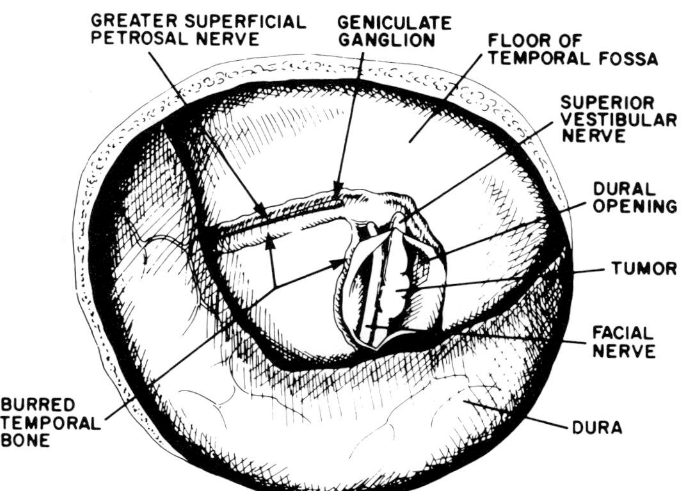

Fig. 59-3. The middle fossa approach. Schematic overall view of an intracanalicular acoustic neuroma.

petrosal nerve, and the facial hiatus. Bone removal over the auditory canal follows. It is easier to identify the internal auditory canal by following the facial nerve. The entire superior wall of the canal is exposed and removed (Figure 59-3). The lateral end of the internal auditory canal is dissected, and the vertical crest of bone separating the facial from the superior vestibular nerve (Bill's bar) is identified. The dura is opened along the posterior aspect of the internal auditory canal. The tumor is removed by first freeing it from the facial nerve and internal auditory canal, posterior to and beneath the facial nerve.

The search for the anterior inferior cerebellar artery is begun after a plane has been developed between the facial and cochlear nerves and the tumor. This artery is most likely to be spared from injury if it is identified early and dissected free from the tumor capsule.

A temporalis muscle graft is used to obliterate the defect in the internal auditory canal. The craniotomy and skin flap are then closed in the usual fashion.

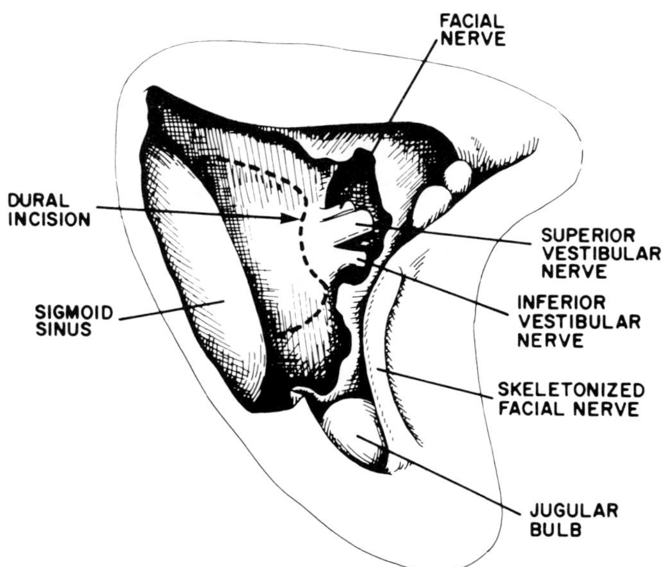

Fig. 59-4. The translabyrinthine approach. The landmarks and exposure seen during microscopic dissection.

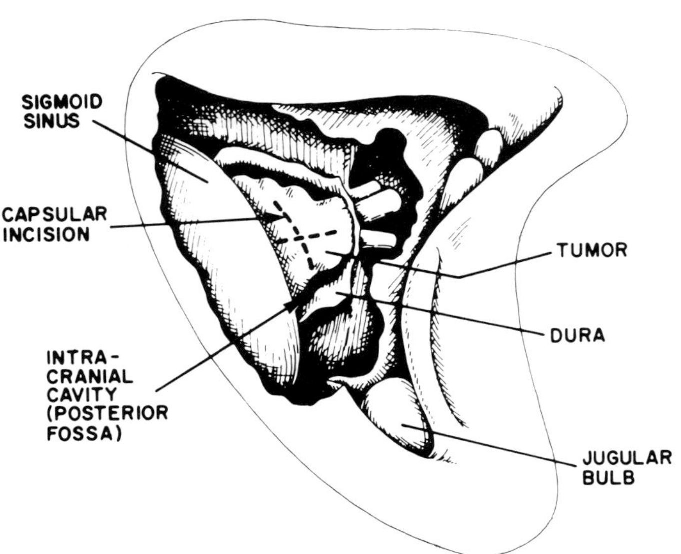

Fig. 59-5. The translahyrinthine approach. The dura has been entered and the tumor exposed. Tumor removal is begun by debulking the center of the tumor as illustrated.

TRANSLABYRINTHINE APPROACH

The microsurgical translabyrinthine approach was developed by House in 1964.[8] It exposes the dura of the posterior fossa in the retromeatal trigone (Trautmann's triangle) formed by the sigmoid sinus, jugular bulb, and superior petrosal sinus. This approach is usually reserved for patients with moderate-sized tumors (1.0 to 2.5 cm in diameter). Unfortunately, any preoperative auditory function is lost as a result of this approach.

The mastoid is exposed through an incision approximately 2 cm behind the ear (Figure 59-2). The mastoidectomy and labyrinthectomy are performed with a high-speed drill with a diamond burr under the operating microscope. The facial nerve is exposed and freed from the tumor in the vicinity of the porus acusticus.

Following bone removal (Figure 59-4), the dura in front of the sigmoid sinus is opened, and this opening is carried forward to the porus acusticus, exposing the tumor. Dissection around the tumor is carried superiorly and medially to free the cerebellum and then continued in the direction of the superior petrosal sinus and the anterior inferior cerebellar artery. Care must be taken to visualize the ninth, tenth, and eleventh nerves and to dissect them away from the lower pole of the tumor capsule. The tumor is then incised and removed in a piecemeal fashion (Figure 59-5). Further dissection is carried out between these neurovascular structures and the capsule as tumor removal continues.

After the tumor has been removed, the dural defect is covered with a temporalis muscle graft or fat. The soft tissues are closed in layers in the usual fashion.

POSTERIOR FOSSA TRANSMEATAL APPROACH

After induction of anesthesia, furosemide (40 mg) and mannitol (1–2 g/kg) are administered parenterally. With the patient in the lateral position, spinal drainage is used routinely to facilitate cerebellar relaxation.

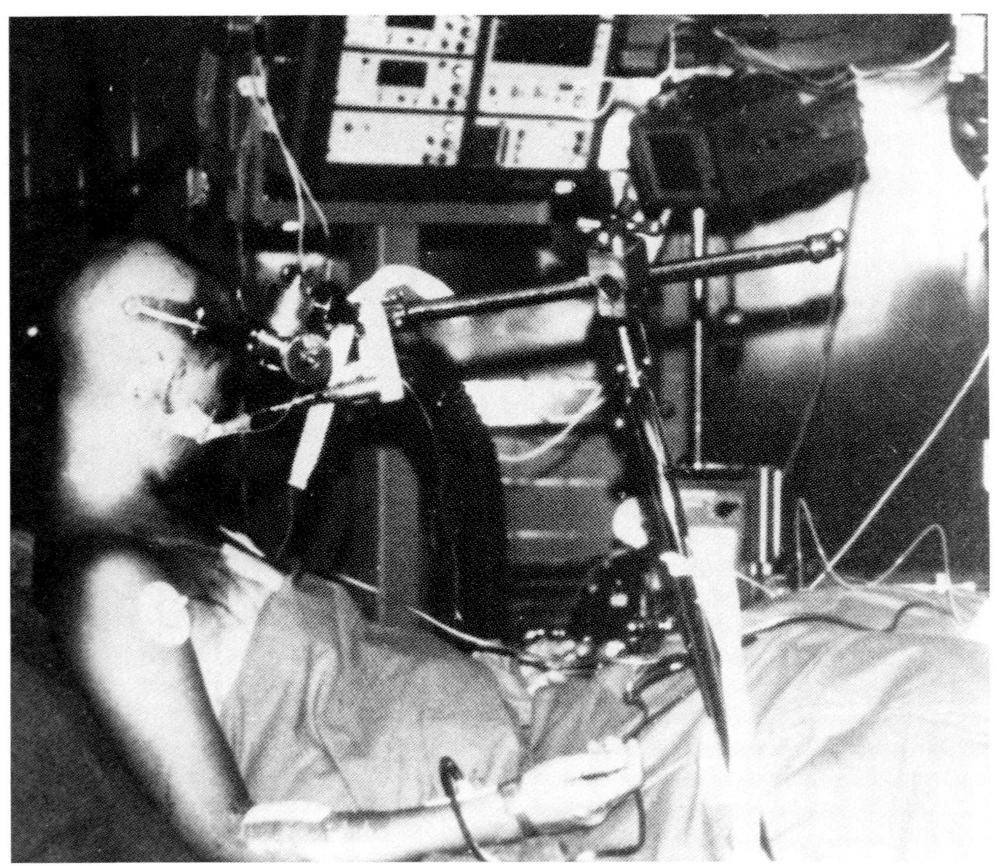

Fig. 59-6. The sitting position.

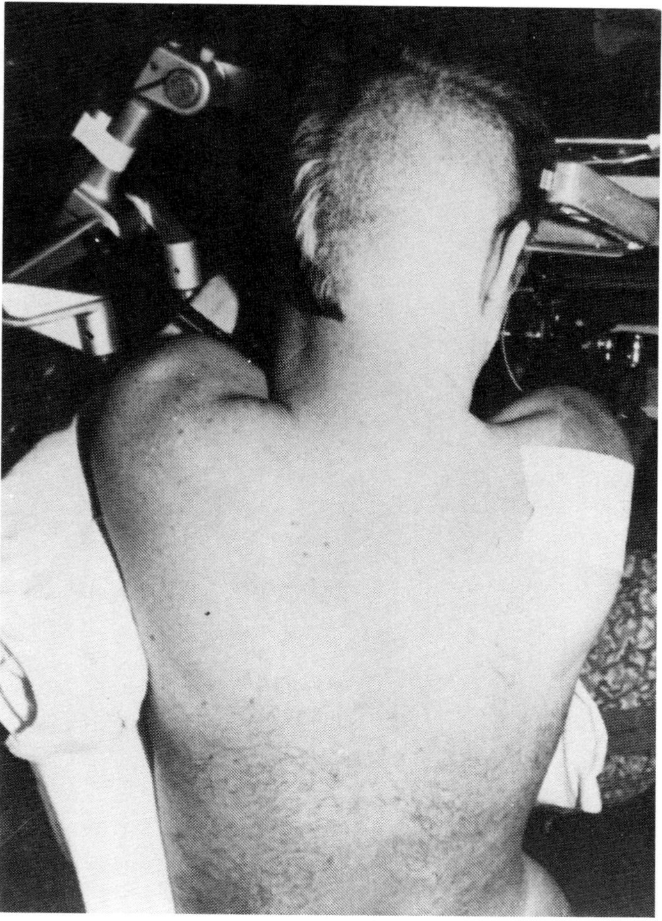

Fig. 59-7. The lateral position.

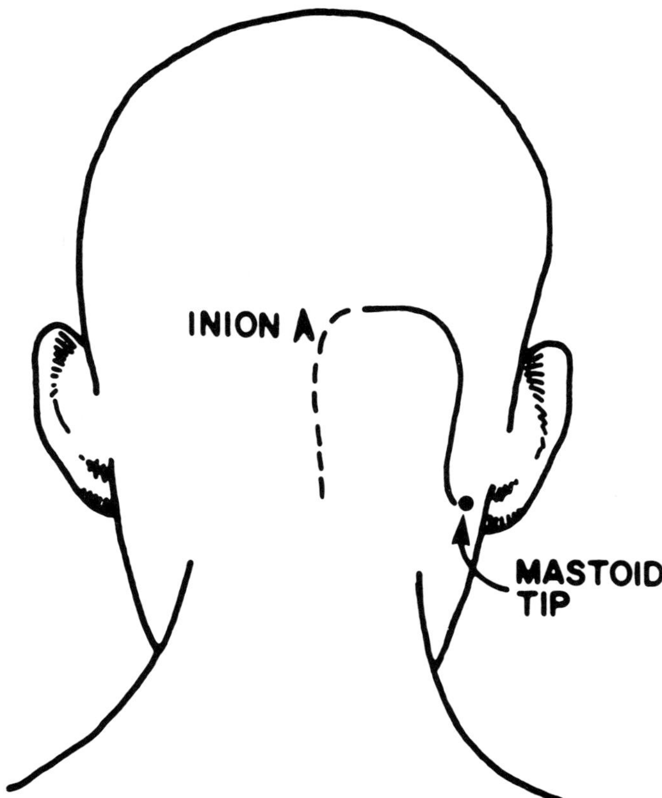

Fig. 59-8. Surgical incision. The standard incision used for cerebello-pontine angle tumors (solid line). Extension of the incision for large tumors (dotted line).

We have begun to operate on the majority of our patients using the lateral position, although occasionally the sitting position is still used (Figures 59-6 and 59-7).[9] The patient is placed on the operating table in the supine position with a roll under the shoulder ipsilateral to the tumor and the head is rotated contralateral to the tumor with the falx parallel to the floor. When the patient is in this position with the head slightly flexed, it is possible to operate at any angle without difficulty.

The positioning of the patient for the sitting position is begun by placing the head forward in the neutral position and then gently turning the head toward the side of the lesion. The cervical spine is flexed slightly and then stabilized with skull fixation.

With both the lateral and sitting positions, preoperative cervical spine films with flexion extension are obtained to identify those patients with spinal stenosis or spondylytic deformities. Once these are identified, the position is modified in such a way that it is safe for the patient.

Regardless of the position, the patient is prepared and draped in the usual fashion, and a modified "hockey-stick" incision is made (Figure 59-8). The horizontal limb of the skin incision is 2 cm above and parallel to the nuchal line, avoiding transection of the suboccipital muscles. The vertical or lateral limb of the incision is made over the mastoid process as far lateral as possible. The skin and muscle flap are turned down in the usual way. Care must be exercised in the region of C1 and the foramen magnum to avoid an aberrant vertebral artery, which may loop up unexpectedly into the cervical muscles.

The craniectomy should extend up to the edge of the sigmoid sinus, which corresponds roughly to the medial border of the petrous bone. If mastoid air cells are entered, they are ultimately sealed with bone wax. We are not at all reluctant to open these cells widely to gain exposure.

The dura is opened at the midpoint of the craniectomy and then further opened up to the edge of the transverse and sigmoid sinus. The final 1 to 2 mm of the dural incision is made with the aid of fiberoptic transillumination, the light being inserted into the subdural space making the edge of the sinus quite clear (Figure 59-9). The dura flaps are sewn back to expose the cerebellum, which is elevated to expose the cisterna magnum, which is then opened. With the cerebrospinal fluid drained, a self-retaining retractor is inserted and the cerebellar hemisphere elevated superiorly and medially. Most cerebellopontine angle tumors arise outside of the subarachnoid space, and their continued growth is associated with an involution or infolding of the arachnoid. This arachnoid plane provides a constant landmark to the surgeon and often forms a distinct double-layered cap, especially on the medial aspect between the tumor and the brain stem (Figure 59-10). This arachnoid membrane contains the important vessels and nerves of the cerebellopontine angle and serves as a cleavage plane for the dissection (Figure 59-11). This plane should be well established prior to beginning removal of the tumor.

The site of origin of the tumor determines the direction in which the lower cranial nerves will be displaced. In acoustic tumors, the seventh nerve is usually displaced anteriorly around the tumor on the side deep to the surgeon. On the other hand, with meningiomas that have originated from the superior lip of the internal auditory canal, the seventh nerve will be

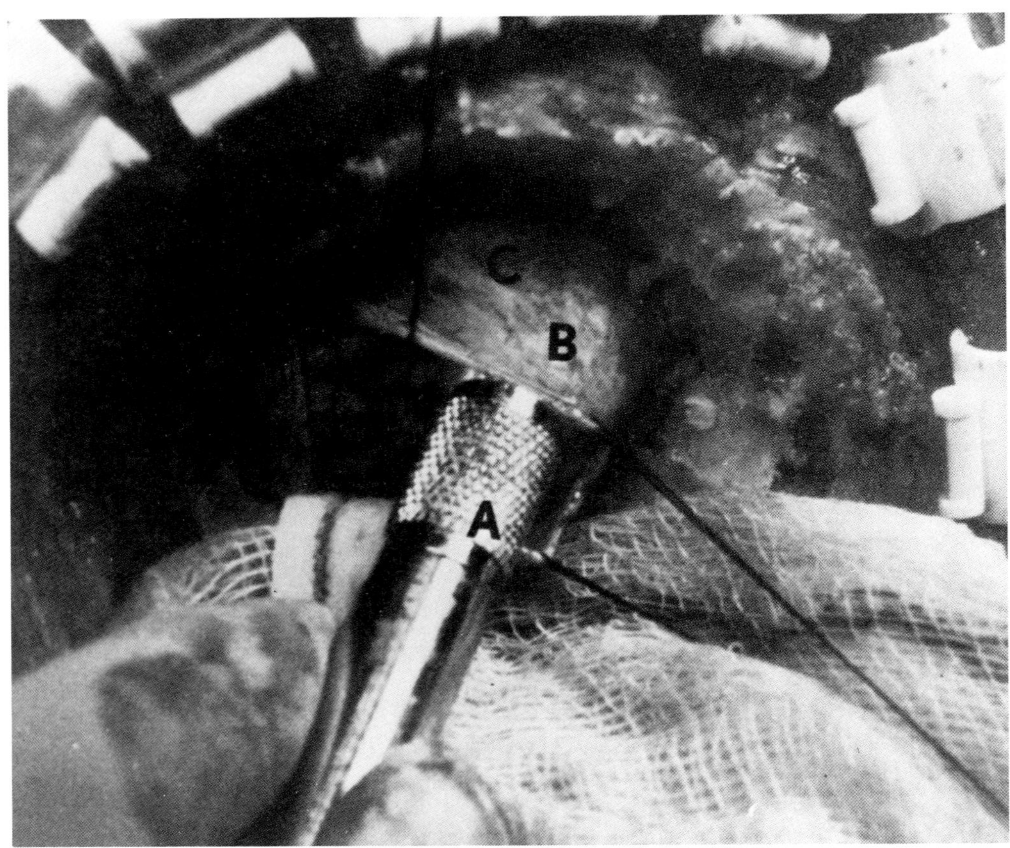

Fig. 59-9. Dural transillumination. (A) Fiberoptic light; (B) dura; (C) transverse sinus.

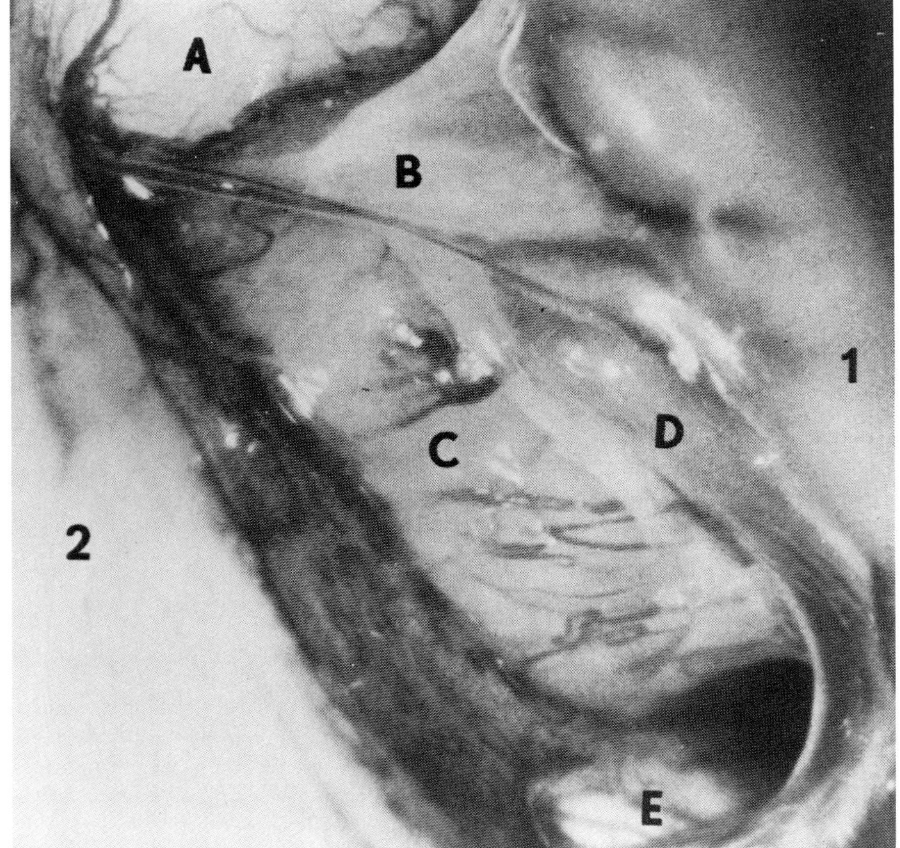

Fig. 59-10. Acoustic tumor. (1) Cerebellar retractor; (2) temporal bone; (A) tentorium; (B) CPA arachnoid; (C) acoustic tumor; (D) AICA; (E) ninth-tenth-eleventh nerve complex.

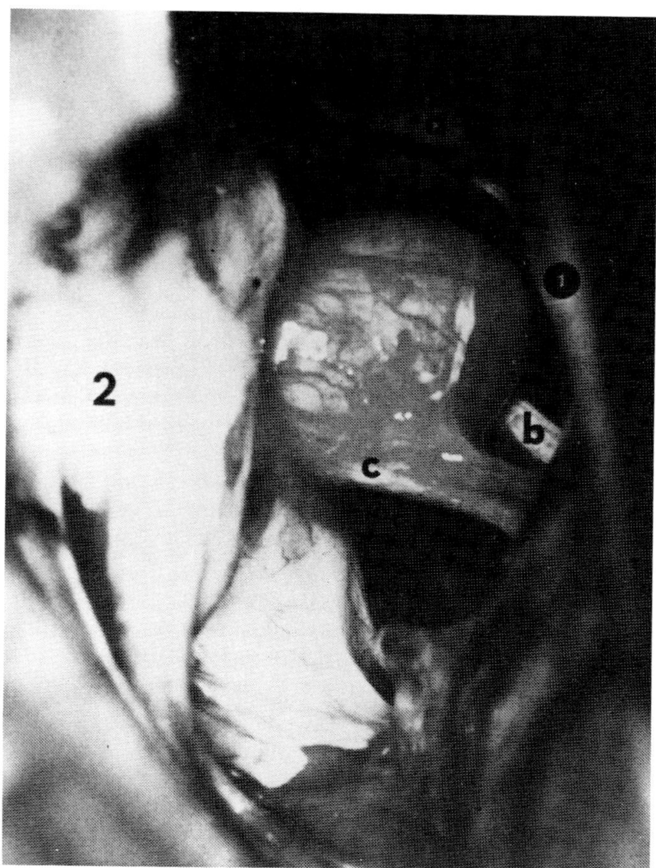

Fig. 59-11. Microscopic view of a small acoustic tumor. (1) Cerebellar retractor; (2) temporal bone; (a) fifth nerve; (b) seventh nerve; (c) eighth nerve and acoustic tumor.

displaced inferiorly and posteriorly toward the surgeon. Meningiomas of the clivus displace the nerves laterally over the tumor. In all circumstances, the location of the nerve can be confirmed with stimulation.

Once the landmarks have been identified, the tumor is reduced in size by internal decompression (Figure 59-12). Many of these tumors are soft, and it is possible to remove them with bipolar coagulation and aspiration. In others, it is necessary to use an ultrasonic aspirator or laser.[10] The decompression process allows the walls of the tumor to cave in and eventually converts a large tumor to a small one. As the walls of the tumor collapse, the arachnoid dissection allows mobilization of the cranial nerves, the anterior inferior cerebellar artery, and the brain stem. It is our preference to dissect first the medial aspect of the tumor along the cleavage plane between the tumor and the brain stem. If, however, one has difficulty locating the root exit zone of the seventh nerve at the brain stem, one can identify the nerve in the anteroinferior portion of the internal canal after drilling the superolateral wall of the porus. Dissection of the intracanalicular portion of the tumor then proceeds in a lateral to medial direction following the nerve toward the brain stem. In general, tumors are dissected with microscissors and an absolute minimum of traction. No attempt is made to remove the lesion in one piece. The final stage in the removal of an acoustic tumor is opening the internal auditory canal. The dura over the canal is removed with sharp dissection and coagulation. The canal is then unroofed, first with a cutting burr and then with a diamond burr. Once exposed, the dural lining of the porus is coagulated and the contents easily dissected.

Even with the large tumors, it is usually not necessary to remove the lateral third of the cerebellum to gain exposure, although we prefer this rather than hard retraction on the cerebellum. With small tumors, furosemide, mannitol, and

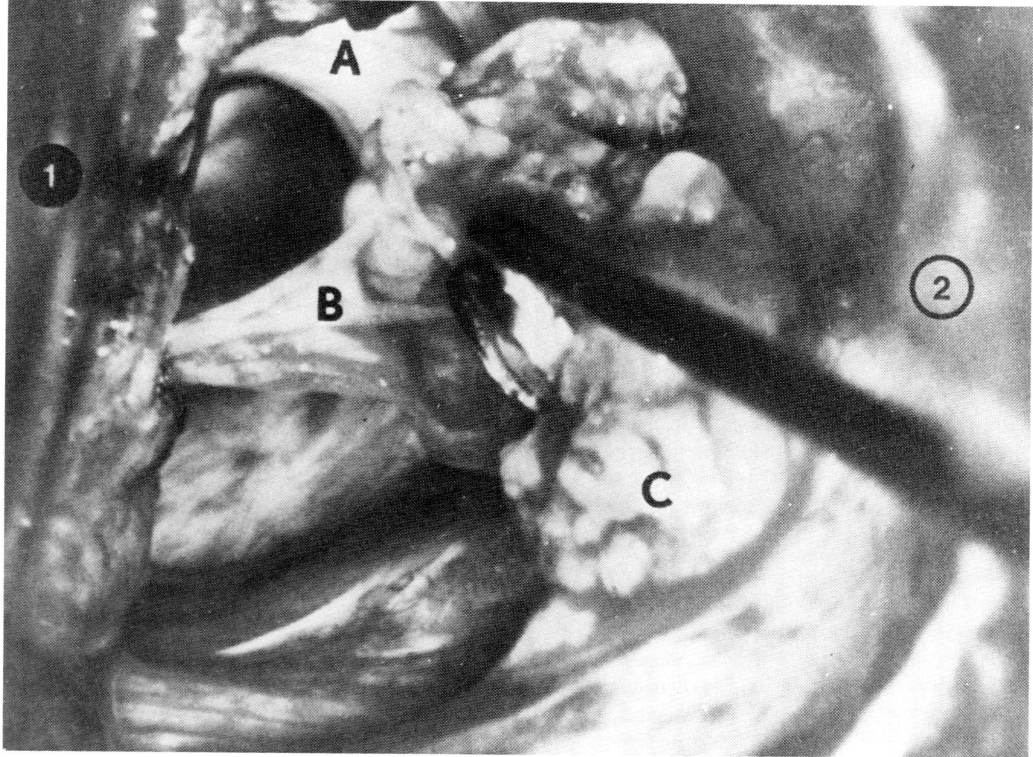

Fig. 59-12. Tumor excision. (1) Cerebellar retractor; (2) temporal bone; (A) fifth nerve; (B) seventh-eighth nerve complex; (C) acoustic tumor.

judicious elevation of the hemisphere are usually adequate to gain exposure. Once the tumor has been removed, meticulous hemostasis must be obtained and confirmed with jugular vein compression, a series of Valsalva's maneuvers, and stabilization of the blood pressure. Prior to closure, the integrity of the seventh nerve is demonstrated by electrical nerve stimulation and facial muscle recordings.[11] In the event that the nerve has been severed, intracranial anastomosis is attempted. Following this, the dura is closed over a Silastic subarachnoid pressure catheter for postoperative ICP monitoring and drainage, and then the scalp is closed.

OPERATIVE COMPLICATIONS

Complications related to surgery within the cerebellopontine angle can be divided into three distinct groups: those occurring during surgery, those occurring during the early postoperative period, and those occurring during the late postoperative period. The complications that occur during surgery can be further subdivided into anesthetic, surgical, and positional.

With the patient in the sitting position, the most common anesthetic complication is air embolization. Although this is usually not a serious problem, it has the potential of becoming a catastrophic one. Careful maintenance of hemostasis, beginning with the skin incision and continuing through wound closure, minimizes the risk. A Doppler precordial stethoscope and expiratory CO_2 monitor alert the anesthesiologist and the surgeon to the presence of air. When evidence of embolization occurs, the administration of nitrous oxide must be discontinued if it is being used and the anesthesiologist must simultaneously aspirate the air from the atrial catheter.[12] Occasionally, the site of the embolus is not apparent, and it may be necessary to pack the wound and stop the procedure until the condition is under control. In extreme cases, it is necessary to remove the patient from the sitting position or discontinue the operation.

The most serious complication of the sitting position is quadriplegia. Although the mechanisms of this complication are not clear, steps may be taken to minimize the risk. The most obvious precaution is careful positioning of the head and neck in skeletal fixation as described in the operative procedure. Preoperative cervical spine films are a necessity. It is possible that spinal cord ischemia leading to quadriplegia accounts for this complication, so the maintenance of blood pressure is measured by way of a transducer at the level of the neck so that accurate recordings of brain stem and spinal cord perfusion pressure are closely monitored.

Stretch injuries of the sciatic nerve and the brachial plexus are also a risk. The sciatic nerve may be injured if the patient's legs are straight on the operating table, with the hips flexed and knees extended. This position, over a period of several hours, may lead to neuropathy. This problem is easily avoided by flexing the knees to release the tension on the nerve. Similarly, the arms should not be allowed to hang, creating drag on the brachial plexus. This is easily avoided by securing the arms across the abdomen.

Hemorrhage during surgery in the angle is usually not a major problem. Occasionally, the petrosal vein is torn, and this can usually be managed with gentle packing with Gelfoam. Laceration of an artery is usually a tear in a small branch that likewise responds to packing. Either of these bleeding problems tends to be more troublesome than serious.

Cerebellar swelling occasionally occurs, usually from CO_2 retention or bleeding above the cerebellum. The former is easily managed by the anesthesiologist or, as with the latter, usually responds to irrigation and Gelfoam packs.

During the early postoperative period, monitoring of intracranial pressure aids in the detection of complications. A 35-mm Silastic catheter placed in the subdural space at the conclusion of the surgery and brought out through a stab wound accurately monitors posterior fossa pressure. This has proven to be a safe and reliable method in our hands, and so far we have experienced no serious complications as a result of it. If the posterior fossa pressure remains less than 15 mm Hg for 24 hours, the monitor is discontinued, and the catheter removed.[13]

Acute hydrocephalus may occur during the early postoperative period and a CT scan may be necessary to differentiate it from a postoperative hemorrhage.

Postoperative bacterial meningitis commonly occurs on the fifth postoperative day and is heralded by fever, leukocytosis, and nuchal rigidity. The diagnosis can only be made by spinal fluid analysis and a positive culture. Sterile meningitis can only be distinguished by culture and is a diagnosis of exclusion.

Cerebrospinal fluid leak may result from poor wound healing, increased intracranial pressure, wound infection, or mastoid air cells that have not been sealed. A clean, sharp incision, careful handling of the wound edges, and meticulous anatomic closure of the wound, including the dura, are logical steps that prevent postoperative complications. In spite of these measures, cerebrospinal fluid may still leak if intracranial pressure is elevated or if a wound infection develops. Unfortunately, a few simple stitches seldom control a CSF leak unless the increased intracranial pressure is controlled. In patients with hydrocephalus, a ventriculoperitoneal shunt may be necessary to stop the drainage. A more difficult problem occurs in patients with meningitis and hydrocephalus. In general, we prefer a ventriculostomy with instillation of intraventricular antibiotics until the cerebrospinal fluid is sterile; we then insert a shunt.

The surgeon must be alert for occult cerebrospinal fluid leak through the mastoid air cells that have been opened during the craniotomy or while the porus acusticus is being drilled. The fluid may drain from the mastoid cells into the middle ear and then through the eustachian tube down the pharynx or out the nose. We prefer a few days of external lumbar drainage, but if the leak persists beyond 3 or 4 days, the wound is usually re-explored.

Fifth nerve injury may occur. Within several days after surgery, the resultant corneal anesthesia may lead to corneal ulceration if proper eye care is not provided. Fifth nerve function should be evaluated as soon as the patient awakens from anesthesia, even when there is no suspicion of injury to the nerve. When the corneal reflex is diminished, the eye should be covered with a protective shield and artificial tears inserted every 4 hours. If the reflex is absent or if there is an associated facial palsy, it may be necessary to do a temporary tarsorrhaphy or insert an eyelid spring (Table 59-1).

Postoperative facial paralysis is of two types—one that occurs immediately after surgery and one that occurs 3 or 4

Table 59-1. Management of trigeminal lesions

Facial nerve intact: Observation
Facial nerve paralyzed: immediate tarsorrhaphy

Table 59-2. Management of facial paralysis

Facial nerve intact:
  Tarsorrhaphy
  Biofeedback
  Physical therapy
Facial nerve not intact:
  Tarsorrhaphy
  Cranial nerve anastomosis
  Static facial support (plastic surgery)

days after surgery. The immediate type is the result of either anatomic disruption of the nerve or, more frequently, contusion and axonotmesis. With the immediate type, a curious phenomenon of spurious facial function may occur for 24 to 48 hours. During this time, the eye closes and the face moves, but within several days the function disappears. The reasons for this are not clear. Regardless of the time frame, postoperative facial palsy impairs the blink reflex and must be dealt with as a potential serious problem. Seventh nerve function should be evaluated in the recovery room. If the face is paralyzed, the eye should be covered with a protective shield and artificial tears inserted every 4 hours. Our preference is for the oculoplastic surgeons to insert an eyelid spring rather than a tarsorrhaphy.

If there has been total disruption of the facial nerve during surgery, plans are made for a facial reanimation procedure (Table 59-2). Generally, we delay both of these procedures 3 to 4 months, sometimes longer, giving the patient time to recover from the brain operation. Details of the nerve anastomosis are presented elsewhere in this chapter.

BILATERAL ACOUSTIC TUMORS

Bilateral acoustic tumors are pathognomonic of central neurofibromatosis and often are associated with intracranial and intraspinal meningiomas. Deafness is a strong possibility in these patients, so prior to surgery they should be encouraged to learn lip reading; once this skill has been mastered, surgery can proceed.

We do not remove both tumors during the same operation, although initially a bilateral skin incision is made that is suitable for both operations. In general, the larger tumor is operated on first. Removal of the tumor is carried out with the technique outlined earlier in this chapter. The patient returns to the hospital for surgery on the second side only after there has been complete recovery from the first operation. This includes wound healing and facial nerve function. In the event of facial

nerve paralysis following the first operation, the second one is delayed until the nerve recovers or the face is reanimated by other means. In general, the smaller tumor is removed before the patient becomes deaf, since there is a possibility that some degree of existing hearing may be preserved.

FACIAL PARALYSIS

Several procedures have been developed to improve facial tone and motor function in patients with postoperative facial nerve paralysis. The choice of procedure is tailored to the individual case. The ideal treatment is intracranial end-to-end anastomosis of the facial nerve during the initial operation. Unfortunately, most often the nerve has been attenuated or destroyed, making this impossible. The alternatives then are hypoglossal-facial, spinal accessory-facial, or phrenic-facial nerve anastomosis. We prefer the hypoglossal-facial nerve anastomosis, particularly for patients who are not dependent upon speech for their livelihood.

TIMING OF SURGERY

The timing of surgery depends on the state of integrity of the facial nerve. If it is anatomically severed and cannot be repaired intracranially, it is our practice to wait 3 to 4 weeks,

Table 59-3. Acoustic neuromas: Preservation of nerve function

Size of Tumor	Number of Patients	Anatomically Preserved Postoperatively	
		Seventh Nerve	Eighth Nerve
>2 cm	134	101 (76%)	5 (3%)
1–2 cm	52	48 (92%)	15 (30%)
<1 cm	14	14 (100%)	10 (70%)

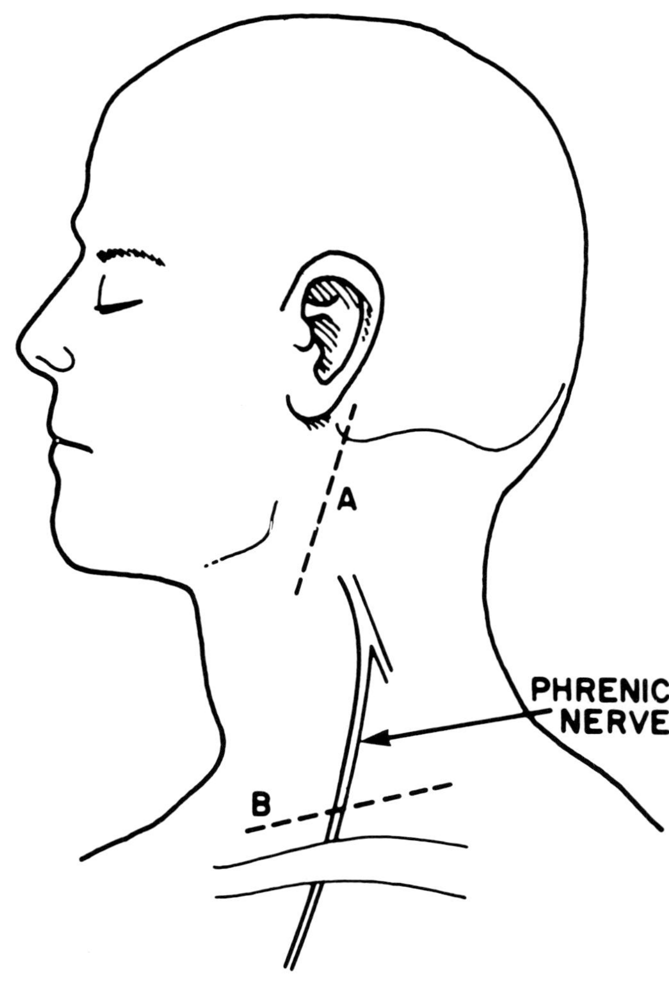

Fig. 59-13. Surgical incisions for (A) hypoglossal-facial nerve and spinal accessory-facial nerve anastomoses; (B) second incision used for the phrenic-facial nerve anastomosis.

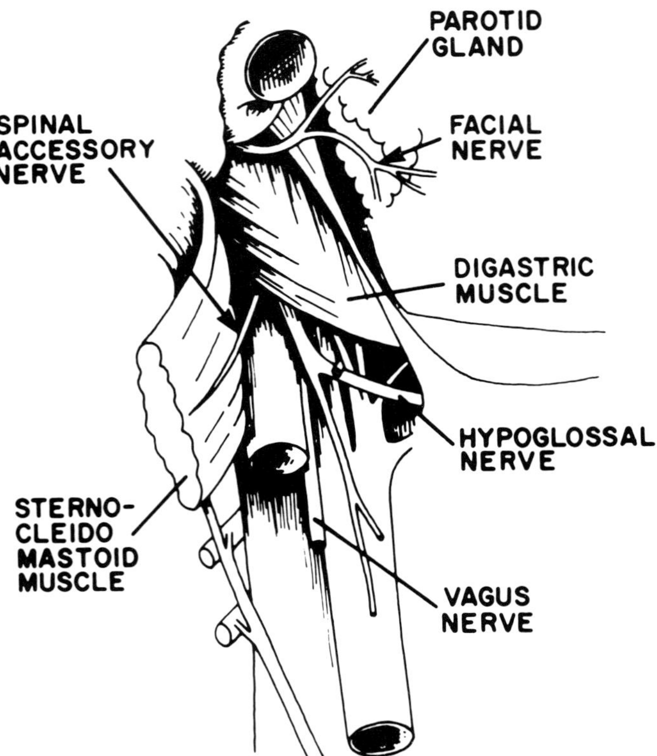

Fig. 59-14. Diagrammatic illustration of the anatomy and landmarks used for hypoglossal-facial nerve and spinal accessory-facial nerve anastomoses.

SURGICAL TECHNIQUE

Hypoglossal-Facial Nerve Anastomosis

Hypoglossal-facial nerve anastomosis is performed with the patient under general anesthesia, supine on the operating table, and the head turned to the contralateral side. The ear lobe is stitched up anteriorly, out of the operative field. A postauricular incision is made, from ½ inch above the tip of the mastoid down in front of the sternocleidomastoid muscle, for a length of approximately 10 cm (Figure 59-13). The skin and subcutaneous tissue are opened, and the fascia and platysmal muscles are then divided in a longitudinal fashion. The sternocleidomastoid muscle is identified and retracted laterally. Dissection continues superiorly and medially, and the cervical fascia is identified and opened. The posterior belly of the digastric muscle is identified and dissection is carried around it until the anteromedial tendinous portion is identified. The hypoglossal nerve is located underneath the posterior belly of the digastric muscle. It can be identified by following the descending ansa hypoglossi up until it meets with the hypoglossal nerve.

Attention is turned to the area of the mastoid tip. Using the periosteal elevator, the digastric muscle is partially separated from the periosteum of the mastoid process. The tip of the mastoid process is rongeured away, improving visualization of the area of the styloid process and the stylomastoid foramen. We prefer sharp dissection for the exposure of the facial nerve at its exit from the stylomastoid foramen (Figure 59-14). occasionally, one must go through the posterior portion of the parotid gland to identify this nerve. Once both the facial and hypoglossal nerves have been identified, the hypoglossal nerve is sectioned at the point at which it begins to branch.

The facial nerve is sectioned at the stylomastoid foramen. The distal end of the hypoglossal nerve is swung upward posteriorly, in contact with the proximal end of the facial nerve, adjacent to the posterior belly of the digastric muscle. Using microsurgical technique, the two ends are joined, using 10-0 Prolene (Ethicon, Inc., Somerville, NJ). Care must be taken to

then readmit the patient for hypoglossal-facial nerve anastomosis. If the nerve is anatomically and physiologically preserved during surgery but is without postoperative function, the anastomosis is generally not done for at least 2 years, since 90 percent of the patients on our service seem to have adequate, although delayed, functional facial nerve recovery.

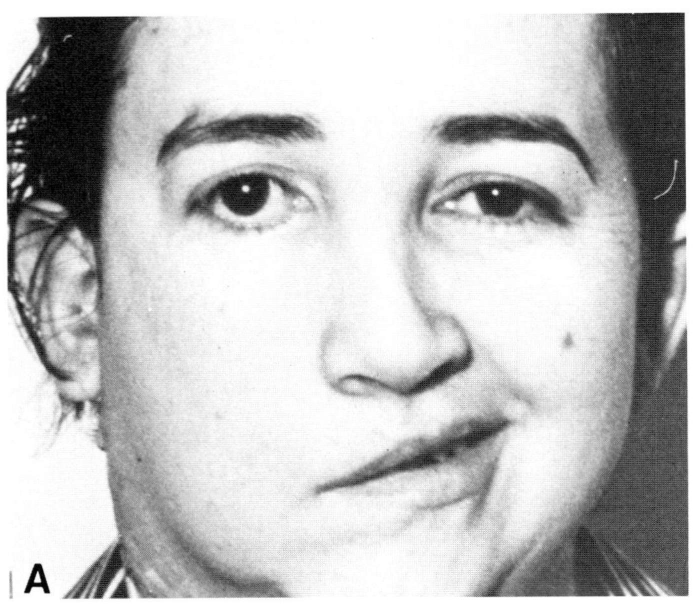

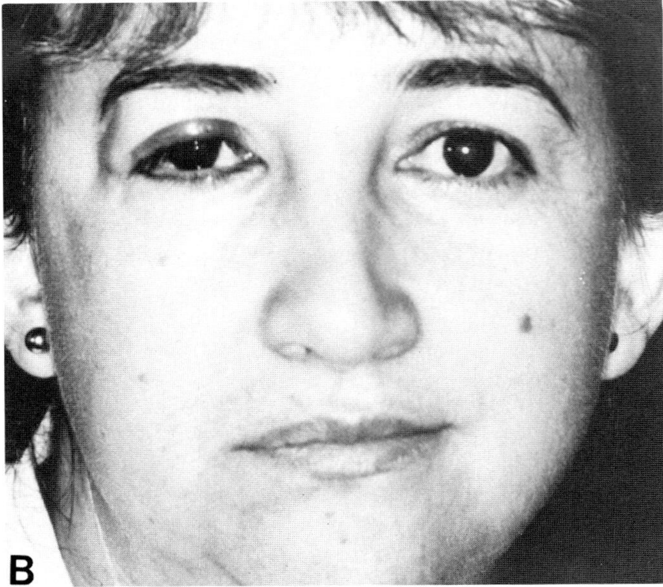

Fig. 59-15. (A) Preoperative photograph of a patient with facial paralysis after removal of a cerebellopontine angle tumor. (B) The same patient 6 months after a hypoglossal-facial nerve anastomosis.

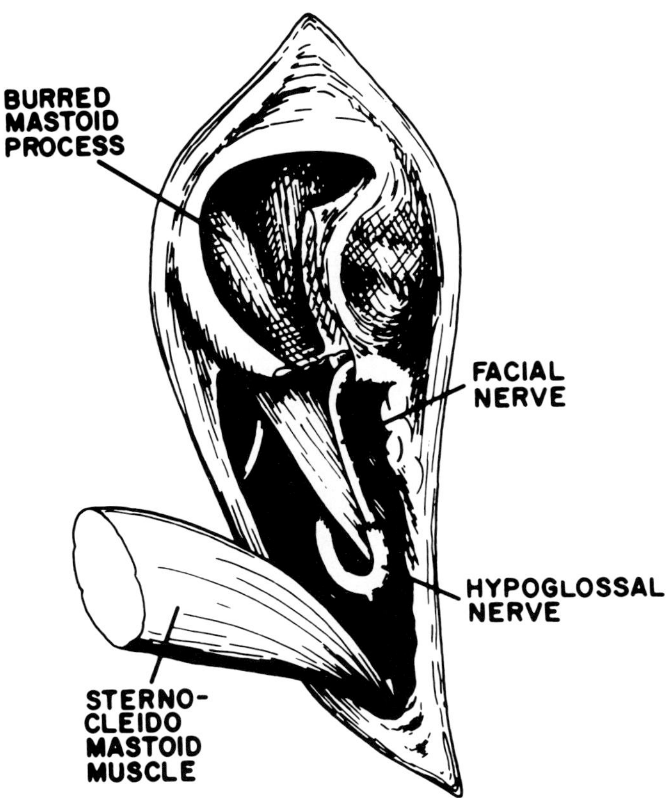

Fig. 59-16. Surgical alternative when an additional length of facial nerve is required.

periorly, and the anterior scalene muscle will then come into view. The phrenic nerve is in front of the anterior scalene muscle, underneath the fascia. Once it is identified, it is cut at the lowermost end of the anterior scalenus. The proximal end of the phrenic nerve is brought up underneath the sternocleidomastoid muscle and anastomosed to the facial nerve. It is recommended that the phrenic nerve be cut and brought up first, to help judge the length of facial nerve that will be needed to perform the anastomosis without tension. If there is trouble obtaining the needed length, it is always possible to perform a mastoidectomy and expose the facial nerve higher up at the stylomastoid foramen (Figure 59-16).

With these anastomotic procedures, satisfactory functional results are obtained in most cases. Recovery is not expected until at least 4 to 6 months after anastomosis. In some cases, it takes a year for the expected surgical results to occur.

ensure that the nerve is not angulated or under tension. After the anastomosis has been completed, the wound is closed in standard fashion. The results of facial reanimation have been quite satisfactory, based on the patient's opinion of cosmesis and eye closure (Figure 59-15A and B).

Spinal Accessory-Facial Anastomosis

The incision for spinal accessory-facial nerve anastomosis is identical to the one used for the hypoglossal-facial nerve anastomosis. The sternocleidomastoid muscle is identified and retracted laterally and inferiorly, exposing the posterior belly of the digastric muscle. The spinal accessory nerve can be identified entering the posterior aspect of the sternocleidomastoid muscle (Figure 59-14). To expose the distal end of the facial nerve, the technique described above is used. Once the facial nerve has been dissected at the stylomastoid foramen, the spinal accessory nerve is sectioned in its most distal portion, roughly where it enters the sternocleidomastoid muscle. The proximal spinal accessory nerve is swung around superiorly and posteriorly and anastomosed to the distal facial nerve.

Phrenic-Facial Nerve Anastomosis

Two incisions are used for phrenic-facial nerve anastomosis, one similar to the one described for the hypoglossal-facial nerve and the spinal accessory-facial nerve anastomoses in order to expose the distal facial nerve right at the stylomastoid foramen, and another placed approximately two fingerbreadths above the clavicle in the supraclavicular fossa (Figure 59-13). The sternocleidomastoid muscle is retracted medially and su-

REFERENCES

1. Henschen F: Ueber Geschwulste der hinteren Schadelgrube, insbesondere des Kleinhirnbruckenwinkels: Klinische und anatomische Studien. Jena, Gustav Fischer, 1910
2. Cushing H: The surgical mortality percentages pertaining to a series of two thousand verified intracranial tumors. Arch Neurol Psychiatry 27:1273, 1932
3. Portmann M, Sterkers JM, Charachon R, et al: The Internal Auditory Meatus: Anatomy, Pathology, and Surgery.
4. Hollinshead WH: Anatomy for Surgeons, ed 2, vol 1. The Head and Neck. New York, Harper & Row, 1968
5. Wilson M: The Anatomic Foundation of Neuroradiology of the Brain, ed 2. Boston, Little, Brown, 1972
6. Rhoton A Jr: Microsurgery of the internal acoustic meatus. Surg Neurol 2:311, 1974
7. House WF: Surgical exposure of the internal auditory canal and its contents through the middle cranial fossa. Laryngoscope 71:1363, 1961
8. House WF (ed): Monograph: Transtemporal bone microsurgical removal of acoustic neuromas. Arch Otolaryngol 80:597, 1964
9. Buchheit WA, Delgado TE: The surgical removal of acoustic neuromas, in Schmidek HH, Sweet WH (eds): Operative Neurosurgical Technigues: Indications, Methods, and Results. New York, Grune & Stratton, 1982, pp 637–648
10. Wald SL, Schmidek HH: The laser and ultrasonic aspirator in neurosurgery, in Schmidek HH, Sweet WH (eds): Operative Neurosurgical Techniques: Indications, Methods, and Results. New York, Grune & Stratton, 1982, vol 2, pp 1541–1550
11. Cushing H, Buchheit WA, Rosenholtz HR, Chrissian S: Intraoperative monitoring of facial muscle evoked responses obtained by intracranial stimulation of the facial nerve: A more accurate technique for facial nerve dissection. Neurosurgery 4:418, 1979
12. Smith WH, Harp JR: Anesthesia for neurosurgery in the sitting position, in Buchheit WA, Truex RC Jr (eds): Surgery of the Posterior Fossa. New York, Raven Press, 1979, pp 89–97
13. Rosenwasser RH, Kleiner L, Buchheit WA: ICP monitoring of the posterior fossa: Preliminary Report. J Neurosurg 1987 (in press)
14. Miller R: Meningiomas of the posterior fossa, in Buchheit WA, Truex RC Jr (eds): Surgery of the Posterior Fossa. New York, Raven Press, 1979, pp 99–110
15. Leksell L: A note on the treatment of acoustic tumors. Acta Chir Scand 137:763, 1971
16. Norlen G, Leksell L: Stereotactic treatment of acoustic tumors, in Szikle G (ed): Stereotactic Cerebral Irradiation. Amsterdam, Elsevier, 1979, pp 241–244

CHAPTER 60

Translabyrinthine Operation for the Removal of Acoustic Nerve Tumors

T. T. King   A. W. Morrison

LITTLE HAS HAPPENED since the last edition of this work to modify the view expressed then that the translabyrinthine operation for the removal of acoustic nerve tumors is not likely to establish a place in the neurosurgical repertoire, except in a few centers with a special interest in it. The reasons for this, discussed then, can be briefly reviewed. The origins of the operation's revival in the early 1960s,[1] more than 50 years after it was first attempted by Quix,[2] lay in a number of factors. First was the rather poor results obtained by the average, or even the most accomplished, neurosurgeon, who with a lesion deemed favorable on other grounds, could seldom reduce the mortality below 20 percent; morbidity was even more formidable.[3,4] Then, developments in audiology allowed diagnosis of a number of growths when symptoms were confined to the eighth nerve and the tumor small; and finally was the introduction of the operating microscope, and with it refined surgical instruments that established the surgery of the petrous bone on a new level. These factors combined to encourage ear-nose-and-throat (ENT) surgeons, led by House, to attack a lesion hitherto the province of neurosurgeons, and the early results, while open to criticism, which was both plentiful and bitter, suddenly raised expectations regarding what could be achieved in this difficult field. Preservation of the facial nerve in an appreciable proportion of cases was the most striking gain, but a steep reduction in morbidity and mortality was an even more important consequence.

Two of the factors mentioned above, early diagnosis and the operating microscope, were also available to neurosurgeons who were driven to improve their results. This they did, and the best results from the posterior fossa operation are at least equal to those achieved by the translabyrinthine procedure, which, since it involves an unfamiliar approach and more or less requires the coòperation of an ENT surgeon, has not appealed to neurosurgeons, who have, with a few exceptions,[5] rejected it.

ADVANTAGES AND DISADVANTAGES OF THE TRANSLABYRINTHINE OPERATION

The view of the present authors, based on experience with the present operation in over 300 cases (although not to the exclusion of the posterior fossa operation, which has been used in a further 50 or so cases, usually for special reasons), is that the translabyrinthine operation has certain advantages, and that these are sufficiently marked to make us favor it as a routine. There are, however, clear contraindications and certain obvious disadvantages to this procedure.

The principal advantage of the method is that it leads directly into the cerebellopontine angle, exposing the tumor without the need for retraction of the cerebellum at any stage (Figure 60-1A and B). In the posterior fossa approach, exposure of the cerebellar hemisphere is unavoidable, and some retraction is usually necessary, while the ninth, tenth, and eleventh nerves are also exposed from the beginning, and although both they and the cerebellar hemispheres are protected by cottonoids as far as possible, it may be difficult, over a prolonged period of time, to avoid some harm to them. The apex of the cerebellopontine angle, where the tumor reaches the trigeminal root and the tentorium near the hiatus, is more easily and directly approached through the labyrinth than through a posterior fossa craniectomy, from which it is remote. This directness of access is an advantage not only for the removal of small tumors confined to the meatus or the subarachnoid space of the angle, the removal of which becomes almost an extracerebral procedure analogous to the transsphenoidal operation for pituitary tumors, but is even more an advantage in the approach to large tumors, for it makes easier the turning of the tumor out of its nest in the cerebellum, middle cerebellar peduncle, and brain stem. Indeed, in spite of the commonly held view that such a restricted exposure, developed by an ENT surgeon, is only suitable for the removal of small growths, we have found that the larger the tumor (Figure 60-1A) the more the advantages are felt, while for small tumors it makes not a lot of difference which approach is used. Desgeorges and Sterkers[6] and Tator and Nedzeski[7] expressed a similar view, which is at variance with the opinion usually advanced by neurosurgeons.[8]

The approach gives extremely good exposure of the lateral end of the meatus, where the facial nerve can readily be found in the operation by reference to anatomic points in the petrous bone. This alone does not give the technique a big advantage over the posterior operation, in which finding the facial nerve either close to the brain stem or in the lateral part of the internal auditory meatus occasions little difficulty; but the ability to expose the whole length of the facial nerve and the petrous bone can be of considerable advantage if the tumor arises from the facial nerve itself and extends into the bone along the facial canal, as happens in about 2 percent of cases. In these uncommon cases, the true origin and extent of the tumor is probably not recognizable by the orthodox approach. Being able to

OPERATIVE NEUROSURGICAL TECHNIQUES
ISBN 0-8089-1862-1

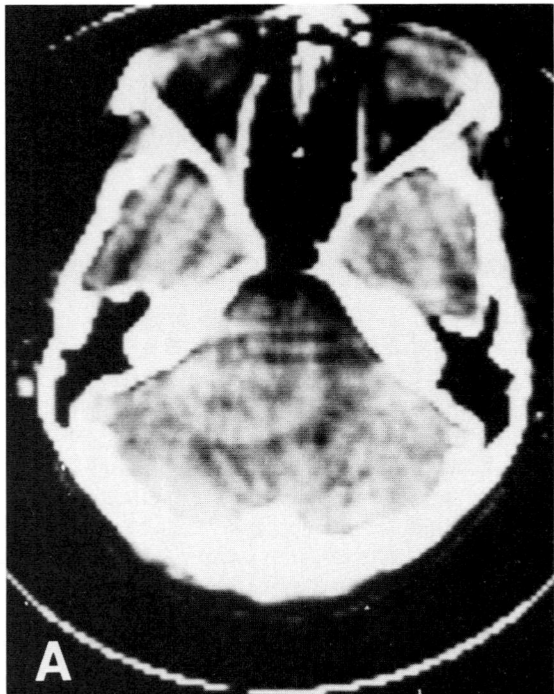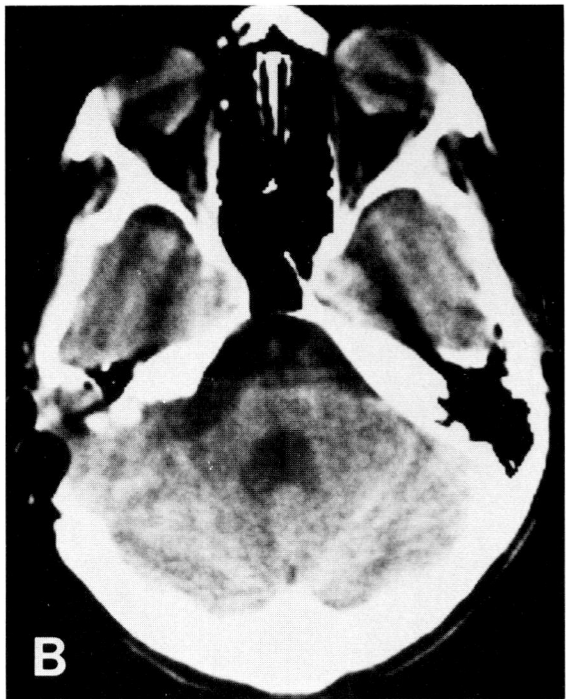

Fig. 60-1. (A) Enhanced scan of a large acoustic nerve tumor in a pregnant woman. (B) Enhanced scan 3 years postoperatively. The direction of surgical approach is indicated by the bone removal on the left of the picture.

expose the intrapetrous facial nerve and to mobilize it can also be of advantage if an end-to-end anastomosis or the insertion of a graft into it is attempted, since the exposure provides a longer distal segment with which to work.

A special circumstance favoring the translabyrinthine operation is re-operation for recurrent tumor previously attacked through the posterior fossa; in such instances it offers a fresh field through which to approach the cerebellopontine angle. Although acoustic nerve tumors remain the main target for the method, it can be used for other conditions, especially meningiomas at or medial to the porus acusticus.

There is some flexibility in the approach, since it can be extended into the middle fossa by division of the superior petrosal sinus and tentorium, a useful maneuver for dealing with meningiomas extending from the cerebellopontine angle into the middle fossa by penetrating the tentorium.[7,9] The apex of the petrous bone and the region of the clivus can also be approached by mobilizing the facial nerve out of its canal, turning it backwards, and then drilling away the cochlear and medial wall of the internal auditory meatus.[10] This can be used to approach epidermoid cysts in the petrous apex, provided the patient is already deaf, and may offer an improved exposure for the removal of meningiomas of the petrous apex and clivus, especially as it, too, can be extended through the tentorium.

Finally, setting the patient up on the table is very straightforward and the position is a comfortable one in which to operate. Both the sitting and the lateral positions have attached to them some risks; air embolism and hypotension in the former and damage to the inferior arm in the latter. Furthermore, in the lateral position, the patient's upper shoulder can hinder the surgeon's freedom of movement.

There are two contraindications. If hearing and speech discrimination are good and the tumor is small, the posterior fossa operation should be used because it is usually impossible to preserve hearing with the translabyrinthine procedure. The middle fossa approach of House is too restricted to be seriously considered in this sort of case. If there has been previous chronic infective ear disease, it is unwise to open the petrous bone widely, and the conventional operation is therefore to be preferred. Because the translabyrinthine dissection lengthens the operating time, this technique is not worth using if a subtotal removal has been decided upon because of the patient's age or infirmity.

Objections to the present technique are numerous and have been strongly presented in the past, but they are mainly relative and not so powerful as is usually thought. The unfamiliarity of the approach and the desirability of having an ENT colleague with whom one can work are probably the most important practical reasons for the lack of approval by neurosurgeons. The rather narrow access is, at first sight, a persuasive point against the method, although, as will be described below, the opening can be made wide enough to allow the removal of the largest tumors if the surgeon is familiar with the technique. The temporal bone dissection adds an hour or two to the duration of the operation, although if the ENT surgeon is inexperienced, it may extend the total operating time much more than this. The middle ear, potentially a source of infection, is opened, but in practice meningitis or wound infection has proved rare. The risks of a cerebrospinal fluid (CSF) leak postoperatively, fluid escaping from the cerebellopontine angle through the middle ear and eustachian tube to the nose, has been a major problem and is the biggest defect in the technique. This point will be dealt with later.

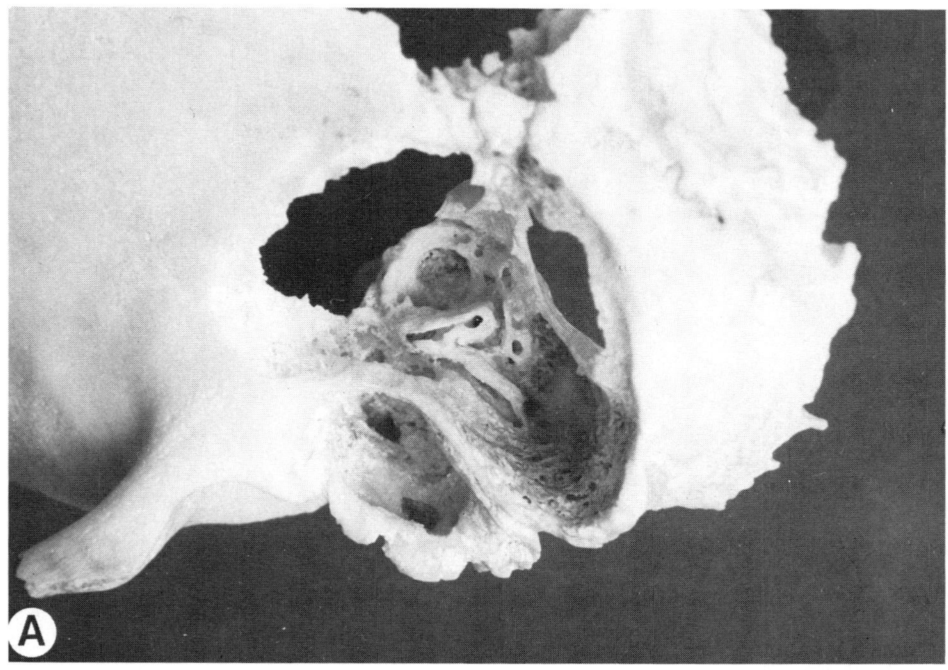

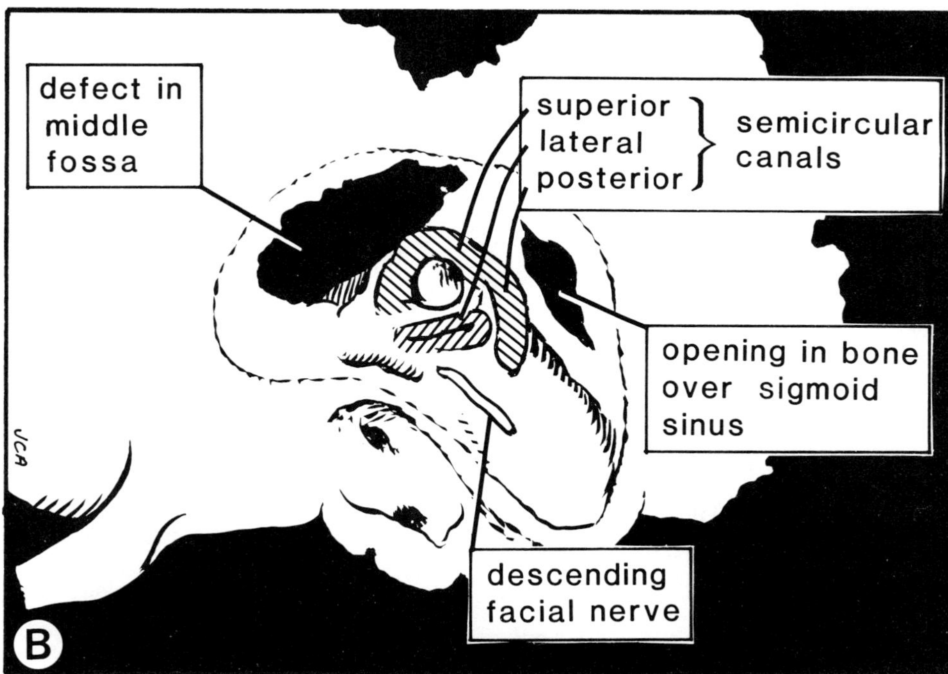

Fig. 60-2. (A) The semicircular canals dissected in a dry temporal bone and seen through the mastoid opening used for a translabyrinthine operation. (B) The portions of the superior, posterior, and lateral semicircular canals to be removed are cross-hatched. The facial canal has been opened to show its proximity to the anterior end of the lateral semicircular canal.

ANATOMY

It is impossible in the space available to cover the detailed anatomy of the petrous bone as it applies to this exposure. Excellent accounts are available elsewhere. All that can be attempted is a brief outline of the structures encountered in approaching the internal auditory meatus from the mastoid region.

Figures 60-2 and 60-3 show the semicircular canals dissected out in a dried temporal bone. The lateral semicircular canal is the first important landmark to be encountered after the mastoid cavity has been excavated and the epitympanic recess of the middle ear exposed, on the medial wall of which it forms a prominence. The facial nerve lies in bone below and anteriorly, and the two structures are in close proximity at the anterior end of the semicircular canal. As Figure 60-3 demonstrates, the semicircular canals and vestibule lie directly between the mastoid cavity and the internal auditory meatus and must be removed together with the endolymphatic duct and vestibule in order to expose the meatus.

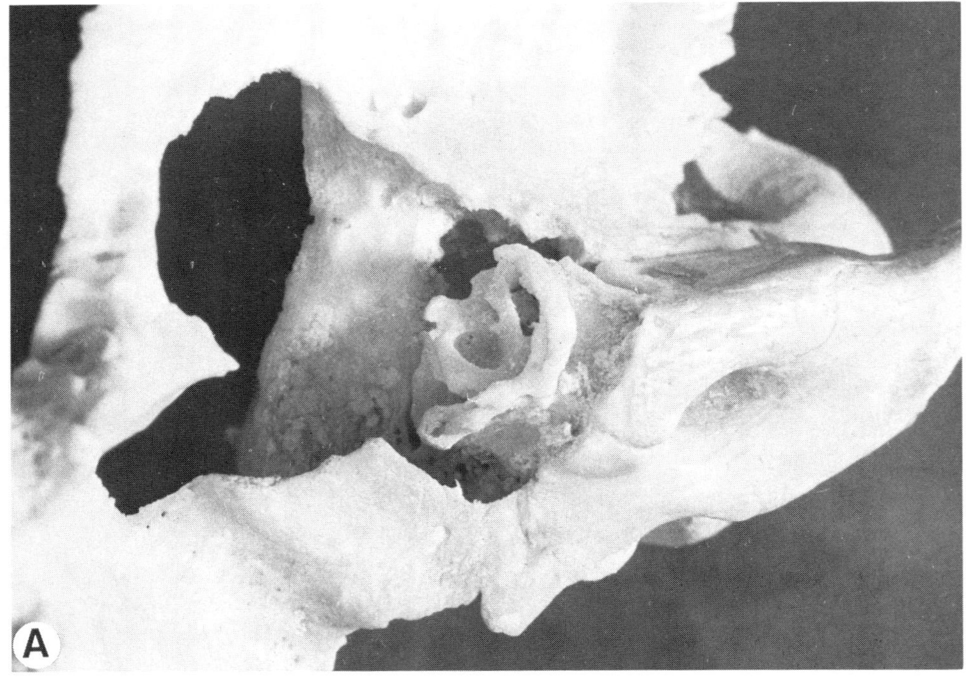

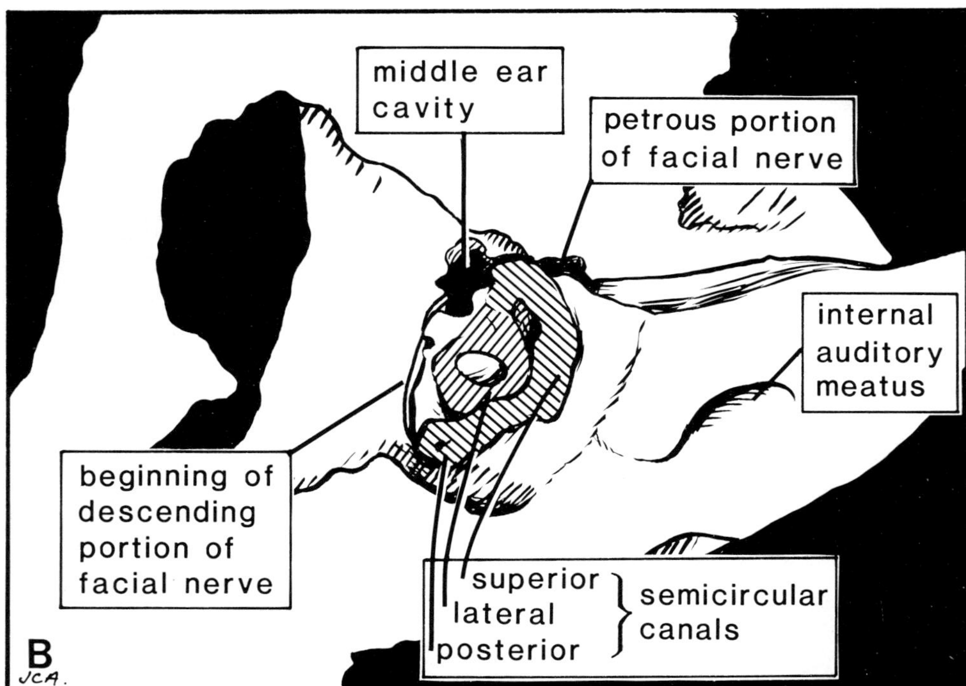

Fig. 60-3.   (A) The same dissection as shown in Figure 60-2, seen from above and behind. (B) Note how the whole of the semicircular canals needs to be removed in order to reach the internal meatus. The union of the posterior and superior canals to form the common crus leading to the vestibule is seen just lateral to the meatus.

The relationships of a tumor within the meatus and in the cerebellopontine angle vary within fairly restricted limits that depend on its size and probably depend also on the specific nerve from which it has arisen. A tumor occasionally will be entirely within the cerebellopontine angle, leaving the meatus empty, a finding that implies a proximal origin. The great majority of tumors, however, start on one of the vestibular nerves, usually the superior, in the subarachnoid space of the meatus, which they fill before extending into the cerebellopontine angle cistern. The direction in which the facial nerve is displaced varies, although in the majority of cases it lies along the anterior wall of the meatus and, at the porus, is displaced anteromedially on the capsule as well as running somewhat upward before finally turning downward and backward to the brain stem. Cushing,[11] in his Figure 178, illustrated this anatomic arrangement.

Less commonly, the nerve is pushed to the roof of the meatus and, from the porus, runs almost directly upward toward the top pole of the tumor, which may, in these circumstances, insinuate itself deep to it, toward the apex of the petrous bone, an arrangement that makes the nerve very vulnerable. Much rarer is displacement of the nerve inferiorly.

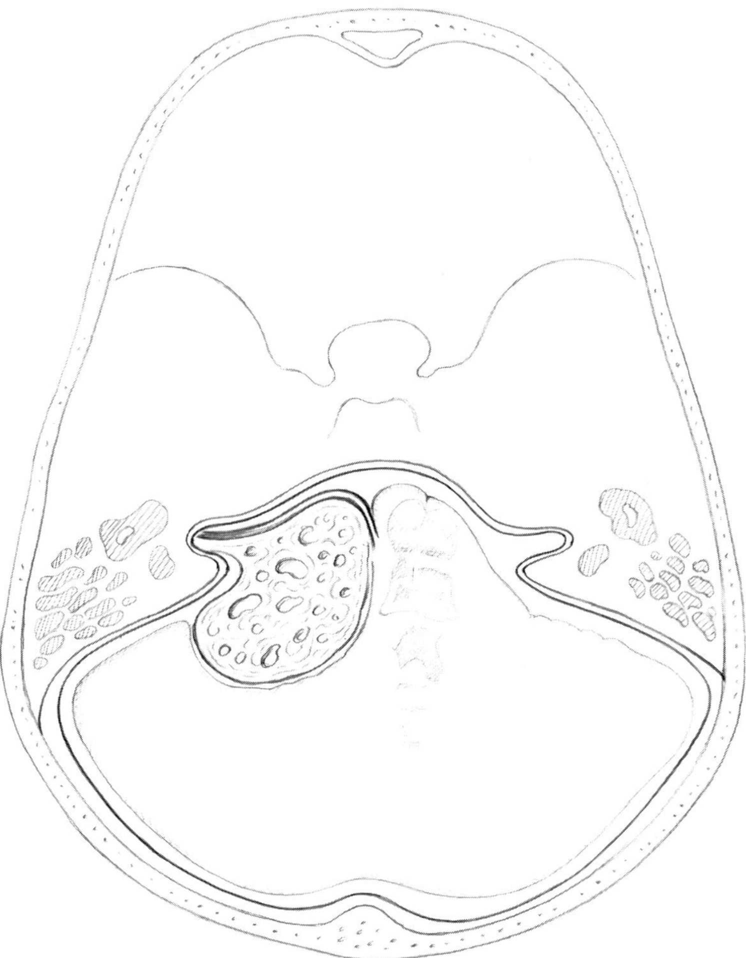

Fig. 60-4. Horizontal section of the posterior fossa through the internal auditory meatus to show the relationship of the tumor to the arachnoid (intermediate black line) plus the facial nerve stretched around its medial side.

These variations of position, combined with variations in the consistency and adherence of the tumor, are important obstacles to preserving the nerve. The invariability of the position of the nerve at the lateral end of the meatus where it enters the facial canal and is immediately exposed by the translabyrinthine operation makes this the best place to start the dissection.

While preservation of the nerve is aided by an understanding of its common relationship to the tumor, the total removal of the latter requires a grasp of how the tumor grows relative to the arachnoid (Figure 60-4). The tumor begins in the subarachnoid space in the meatus, which it fills; the arachnoid membrane thus becomes fused with the surface of the tumor. At the porus acusticus, the tumor balloons out into the cistern or, looked at in another way, the arachnoid funnels into the porus, sticking around its edges to the tumor and dura to produce a sort of hernial neck or constriction. On the medial side of the porus, the facial nerve is pressed against the arachnoid and maintains this relationship until it approaches the brain stem. When the tumor is dissected from the anterior wall of the meatus, the arachnoid has to be divided above and below the nerve in order to allow the growth to be freed and turned backward. The porus is a critical point in this dissection, because here it is easy to pass into the subdural space if care is not taken. The constricting ring of the arachnoid has to be divided laterally, and the dissection carried both upward and downward to the superior and inferior margins of the porus, the arachnoid being dissected off the surface of the tumor so that the plane between the two is developed. Except at points where the tumor lies in the subarachnoid space itself, e.g., at the lower and upper poles and just ventral to the brain stem, or where it lies against the facial or trigeminal nerve, or against the anterior surface of the cerebellum and the middle cerebellar peduncle and pons, it is in this plane, between arachnoid and tumor, that the dissection is carried out, and it is at the porus that it is most difficult yet important to start correctly. Much has been written about the relationship of the tumor to the arteries within the cerebellopontine angle, especially the anterior inferior cerebellar artery, the distal part of which is found just below the meatus; in cases of small growths, it is free in the subarachnoid space, and in larger ones it is stretched over the capsule. It is desirable, but not essential, to preserve the artery at this point; deeper in the exposure, when the brain stem is being approached, it is absolutely essential to avoid occluding arteries of any size. An ability to recognize a vessel and preserve it is more important than extensive knowledge of arterial anatomy, which is variable.

ANESTHESIA

General anesthesia with an endotracheal tube and controlled ventilation is used. The advantage of spontaneous respiration, which was once highly valued as a gauge that would

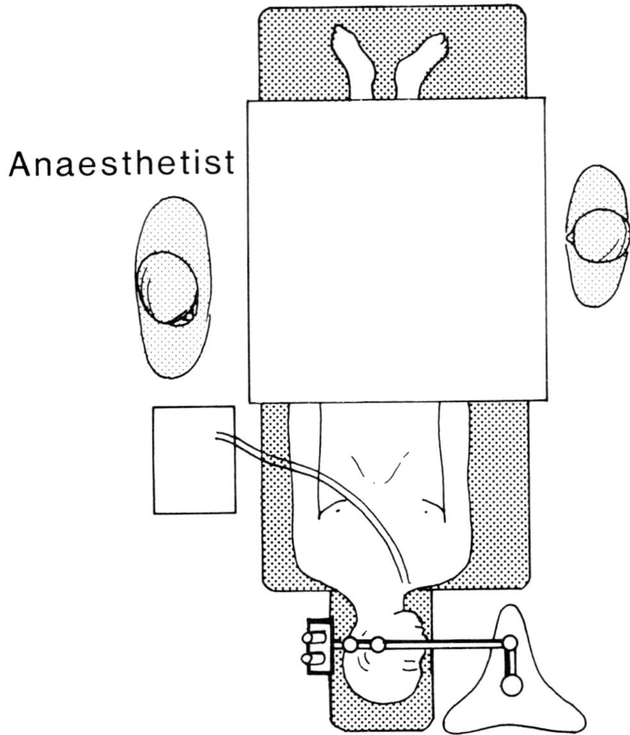

Fig. 60-5. Arrangement of the operating table, nurse, anesthetist, and microscope for a left translabyrinthine operation. Note that the position of the anesthetist and nurse is irrespective of the side of the operation, and that the cranial margin of the overhead table is level with the patient's costal margin. The instrument would be on the left side for an operation on the right.

warn the surgeon by its fluctuations that the brain stem was being disturbed, is now seen to be heavily offset by the more satisfactory respiratory exchange and operating conditions obtained by the anesthetist's taking over this function. The endotracheal tube needs to be securely fixed to the patient's face by strapping, so that it will not be displaced by readjustments of the head, which are often necessary during the petrous dissection.

An intravenous infusion is set up in the left arm, and an intra-arterial line is attached to a pressure monitor. This is best inserted into the dorsalis pedis artery, a safer site than the radial artery, although more difficult to cannulate. The continuous record of pulse and blood pressure thus obtained, together with an ECG, will provide a warning system at least as sensitive as that provided by monitoring spontaneous respirations. When the tumor is large, i.e., more than 2.5 cm in diameter, mannitol is given at the end of the bone dissection and therefore a urinary catheter should be inserted.

POSITIONING ON THE TABLE

The patient is placed supine, with the head on a flat headpiece. The rigid restraint offered by a skeletal clamp of the Gardner sort, while satisfactory for the intracranial part of the operation, makes the petrous portion awkward by preventing slight adjustments of position.

As a separate procedure at the beginning, a piece of fat about the size of one's thumb is taken from the right thigh, together with a 5-cm-square piece of fascia lata. These are put

into a small bowl of saline containing antibiotic and are covered and kept until the end of the operation, at which time they will be needed to fill the petrous cavity. The thigh wound is closed carefully in two layers, with care being taken to obliterate the dead space created by the removal of fat.

The head is now turned about 45 degrees to the opposite side. Excessive rotation should be avoided, because it might constrict the venous return to the neck and provide an unsuitable angle of approach for the translabyrinthine work. A stiff or short neck may make sufficient rotation difficult and may require elevating one shoulder with a pillow in order to get the head in the right position, but too much elevation is to be guarded against, since the shoulder will cause an embarrassing prominence that will obstruct the surgeon's hand on that side. The anesthetist is placed halfway down the table on the left side, and the surgical nurse on the right, irrespective of the side of the tumor. The overhead table is placed well toward the patient's feet, its upper edge being no further up than the costal margin. The surgeon should check this, since it is very irritating to find during the procedure that the table is too close to the head and is constantly hampering the operator. Tilting the top half of the table upward is useful in reducing venous pressure in the head.

The surgeon sits on an adjustable stool placed at the side of the head, thus working from behind the patient. The microscope, when introduced, is on the opposite side of the head, as illustrated, in order to give maximum maneuverability. Figure 60-5 shows the general geography of the operating room for an operation on the left side. For a right-sided tumor, the only alteration is in the position of the microscope, which is then a mirror-image of that shown. Because many movements of the microscope are required during the operation, a Contraves stand is a great boon, markedly reducing fatigue in the surgeon.

SURGICAL PROCEDURE

The scalp over the area of the incision is infiltrated with local anesthetic (1:200,000 adrenaline in 0.5 percent lignocaine), and the incision is scratched on the skin. Except in cases of intracanalicular tumors, we always mark out a frontal burr hole. In small growths (up to 2.5 cm in diameter), the dura is not opened, because the hole is intended to allow access to the ventricle only as an emergency measure in the event of a postoperative hemorrhage, when the frontal horn can then be tapped with a lumbar puncture needle and the intracranial pressure lowered while arrangements are made for returning to

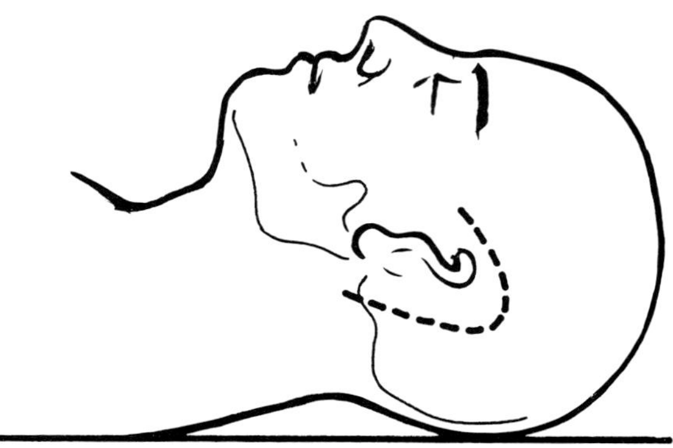

Fig. 60-6. Outline of a scalp incision. The head is rotated to the opposite side about 45 degrees.

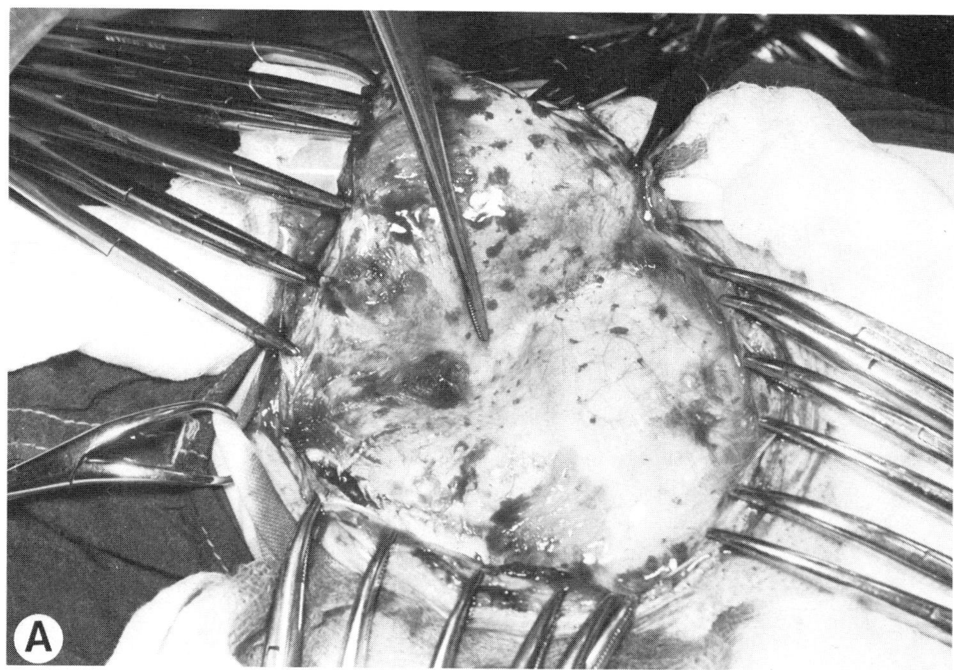

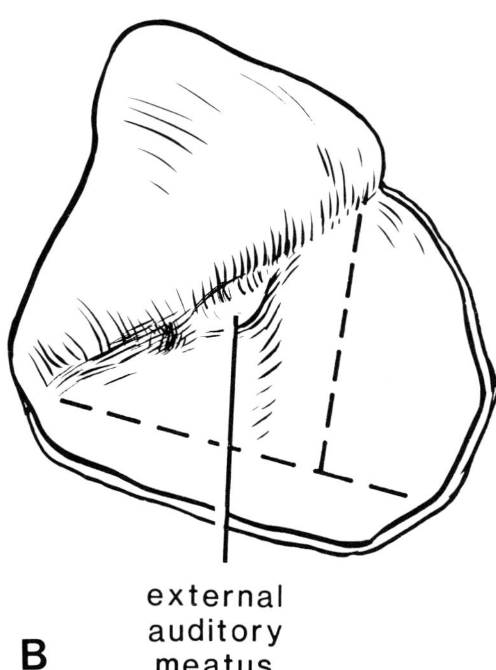

Fig. 60-7. (A) The scalp is reflected forward until the margin of the external auditory meatus is reached. (B) Dotted lines show the incision in the pericranium and temporalis muscle.

the operating room as rapidly as possible. In cases of large tumors, a catheter is inserted into the frontal horn and allowed to drain as the need for room is felt during the operation. House avoids ventricular drainage because of an unfortunate experience, when it led to intracranial hemorrhage, but, while recognizing this risk, we think it is small and acceptable because of the help CSF drainage can offer in an approach in which room is often at a premium.

The incision we use starts just below the tip of the mastoid

process, runs upward over its lateral surface about a finger's breadth behind the root of the pinna to a point 2 cm or so above and behind the tip of the pinna, then curves forward and downward over the temporalis muscle to finish two finger-breadths above the zygomatic arch (Figure 60-6). The anterior extension must allow for reflection of the flap far enough forward to expose the back of the external auditory meatus (Figure 60-7). This hockey-stick incision produces a flap somewhat larger than is necessary for the translabyrinthine opera-

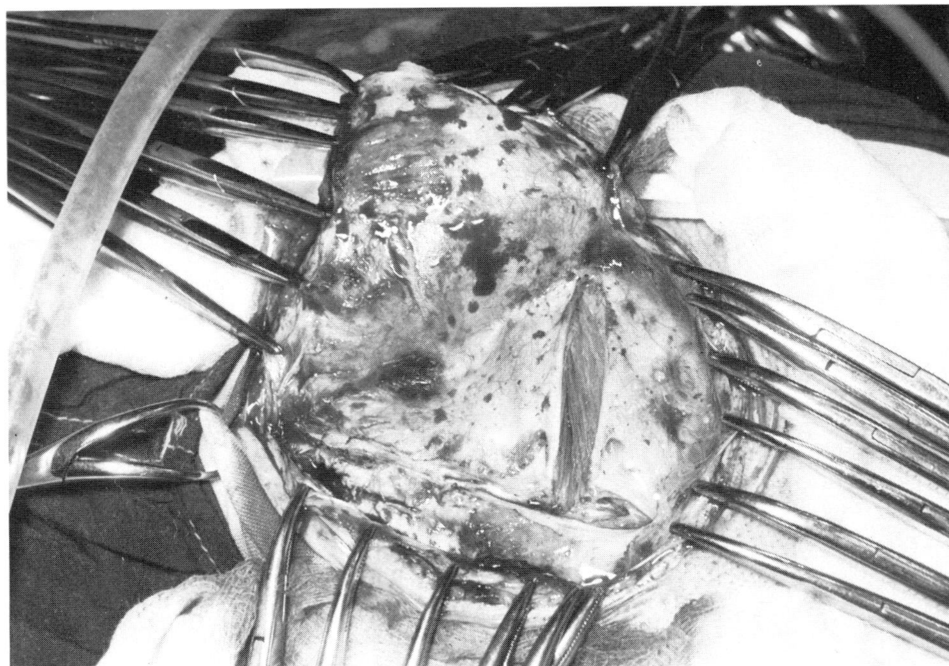

Fig. 60-8. The pericranial flaps are fashioned. The anterior triangular flap of fascia and temporalis muscle will be reflected forward to the external meatus and held, along with the scalp flap, by a self-retaining retractor.

tion, but it allows exposure of the temporal lobe and division of the superior petrosal sinus and even the tentorium. We no longer find these latter two steps necessary for acoustic nerve tumors, although they are still useful maneuvers in other circumstances, such as the removal of certain meningiomas. The rather generous exposure is also useful in keeping the galeal hemostats clear of the operative field.

The head is now draped, part of the pinna and the burr hole being in included in the field. The burr hole is made, if needed, is sutured up, and the scalp flap fashioned in the usual way. It is reflected forward until the root of the pinna is reached and the posterior and posterosuperior margins of the external auditory meatus are defined (Figure 60-7A and B). The scalp along the posterior margin of the exposure is reflected off the pericranium in a backward direction in order to allow access to the whole of the lateral surface of the mastoid. A vertical cut is made with the diathermy in the pericranium, reaching from the tip of the mastoid process to the upper end of the exposure, whence another cut is made, passing forward into the temporalis muscle above the ear (Figure 60-8A and B). The triangular flap thus produced anteriorly is turned forward, at first by diathermy and then using a sharp periosteal elevator, until the external auditory meatus is reached and its posterior and upper margins defined.

The posterior pericranial flap is also reflected backward for a short distance to expose the mastoid. The anterior flap is held forward, together with the scalp flap, both of which are covered with a piece of moist gauze, by a small, self-retaining retractor.

TRANSLABYRINTHINE DISSECTION

The translabyrinthine dissection is carried out by the otologist. Although House[12] insisted that there should be no division of labor and that both specialists should be able to do either part of the procedure, in ordinary practice where each surgeon has to deal with many other conditions, it does not seem practicable for a neurosurgeon to master completely the technique of a skilled temporal bone surgeon or that an otologist be required to operate on a large cerebellopontine mass.

The special equipment needed consists of a power drill designed for ENT work and powered by an electric motor mounted in the handle or by an air turbine, a variety of sizes of burrs (both cutting and diamond), and several sizes of suction tips provided with an extra channel through which continuous saline irrigation can be provided to cool the burr during the drilling (Figure 60-9). The suction tip is also valuable during the removal of the tumor, for the saline will wash away blood from the narrow crevice between the tumor and either the facial nerve or the brain, where the dissection is being developed. A fine instrument is used for this part of the operation, while the removal of bone dust during the petrous dissection demands a wider-bore tube. Fine otologic curettes, dissectors, and hooks are also needed.

The cortical opening is roughly the shape of a rather large keyhole (Figure 60-10A and B). The whole of the lateral cortex of the mastoid process is removed and the opening extended upward. Its anterior margin hugs the posterior border of the external meatus, and reaches as far forward above it as possible, before curving backward a centimeter or more above the level of the floor of the middle cranial fossa to meet the posterior border of the mastoid opening well posteriorly, the upward enlargement thus uncovering the dura over the lateral and undersurfaces of the temporal lobe, while posteriorly the sigmoid sinus will be divested of bone (Figures 60-11 and 60-12). In these two areas, extra room is thereby made available that is of critical importance, for by considerably increasing the superficial limits of the opening, the surgeon widens the arc through which both his or her line of vision is moved and the instruments inserted. Thus, by lifting up the temporal lobe dura, the operator can look from here well down to the inferior pole, and by retracting the sigmoid sinus backward and collapsing it, can

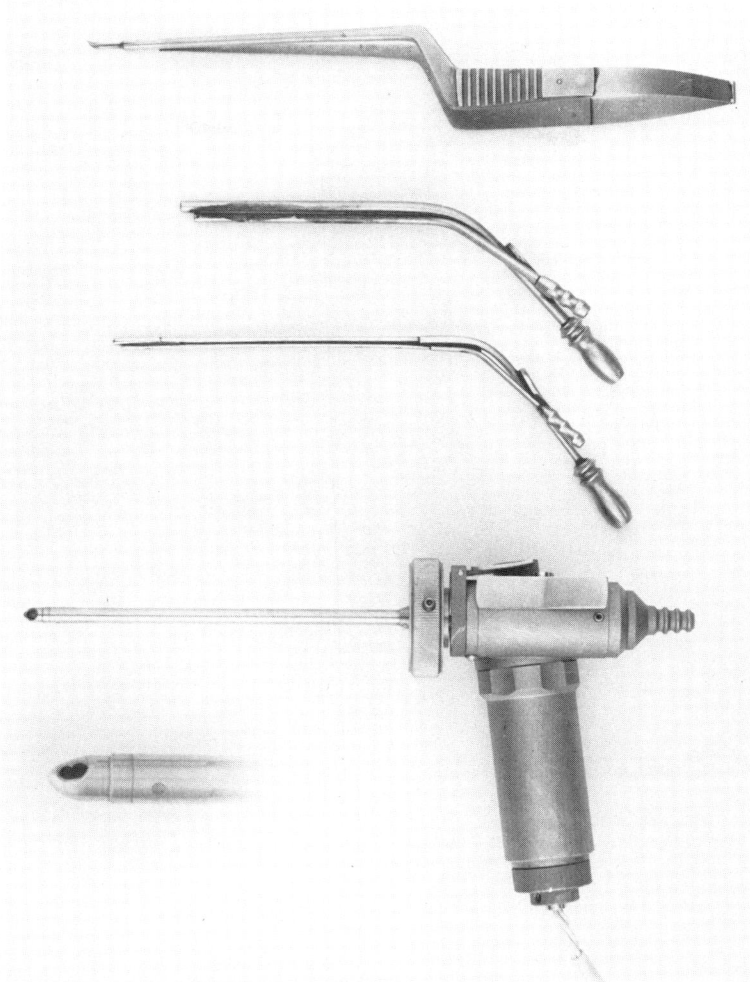

Fig. 60-9. Some instruments required for the translabyrinthine operation. From top: bayonet microscissors, large irrigating sucker tip for use in the bone dissection; fine irrigating sucker used in the removal of the tumor; House-Urban rotary dissector for gutting the tumor. Suction tubing is applied to the right-hand end of the dissector, the inner cannula of which is driven by an electric motor in the handle. The inset shows the tip of the dissector. The openings in the outer and inner cannulae are almost coincident, but the tooth on the cutting edge of the inner cannula is visible at the top of the opening.

look along the line of the posterior face of the petrous bone, medial to the meatus, up toward the trigeminal nerve and the tentorial hiatus. It is sometimes necessary to enlarge the superficial opening by further removal of bone in these two directions if, later in the operation, the surgeon is restricted by the bony edges.

With a large 6-mm cutting burr, the entire extent of the mastoidectomy opening is fashioned and the margins bevelled or saucerized to avoid overhanging edges. The mastoid process is hollowed out and, posteriorly, the air cells are removed until the cortical plate of bone overlying the sinus is exposed and thinned. It is not removed completely at this stage, lest bleeding obscure the deep dissection. Similarly, the inner table covering the dura of the middle fossa is exposed and the dissection is carried as far forward above the meatus as possible. The posterior and superior walls of the meatus are now followed with a cutting burr toward the middle ear cavity. The dissection is concentrated on the space between the upper meatus and the middle fossa until the mastoid antrum and aditus are reached.

The lateral semicircular canal is identified on the medial wall of the epitympanic recess, where it is the most important landmark to the labyrinth and facial nerve. Once it has been found, the position of the facial nerve below and parallel to its anterior part can be estimated, and the nerve skeletonized in its descending portion to form the anterior limit of the exposure here. The incus can be removed at this point, so that the tympanic cavity can be packed with fat later, but there are objections to this (see below). The mastoid cavity at this stage is limited by the posterior wall of the external meatus and the facial nerve anteriorly, the middle fossa plate above, and the sinus plate and sinodural angle posteriorly. Labyrinthectomy is now carried out, starting with removal of the lateral semicircular canal, the anterior end of which leads into the vestibule. Posteriorly, the dissection is carried along the superior petrosal sinus, which is left covered with a thin layer of bone for the moment, however, while the posterior and superior canals are followed medially until the crus commune is reached and the vestibule opened again. Behind and below, the dura of the posterior fossa is exposed, the vestibular aqueduct and endolymphatic sac are removed, and the jugular bulb identified. It is important to make as much room down here as possible,

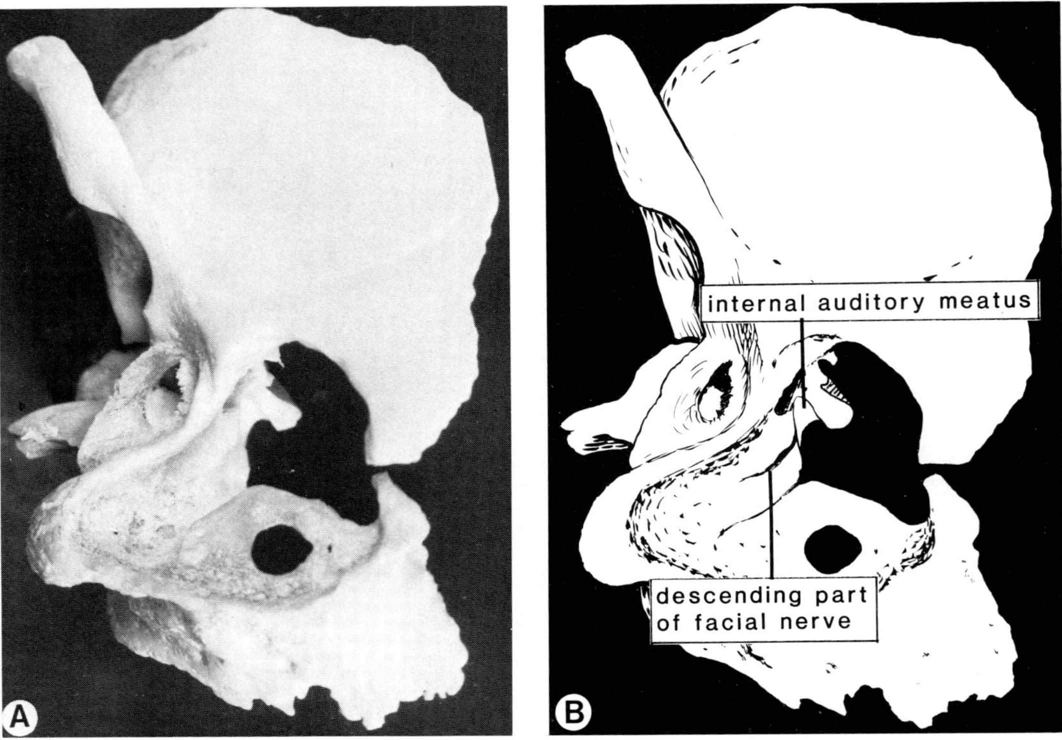

Fig. 60-10. (A) Dried temporal bone showing the extent of the dissection in the translabyrinthine operation. The bone covering the sigmoid sinus is not yet removed. (B) Note that the internal auditory meatus is seen almost axially and that the descending part of the facial nerve, which is left covered with bone, forms the anterior boundary of the exposure.

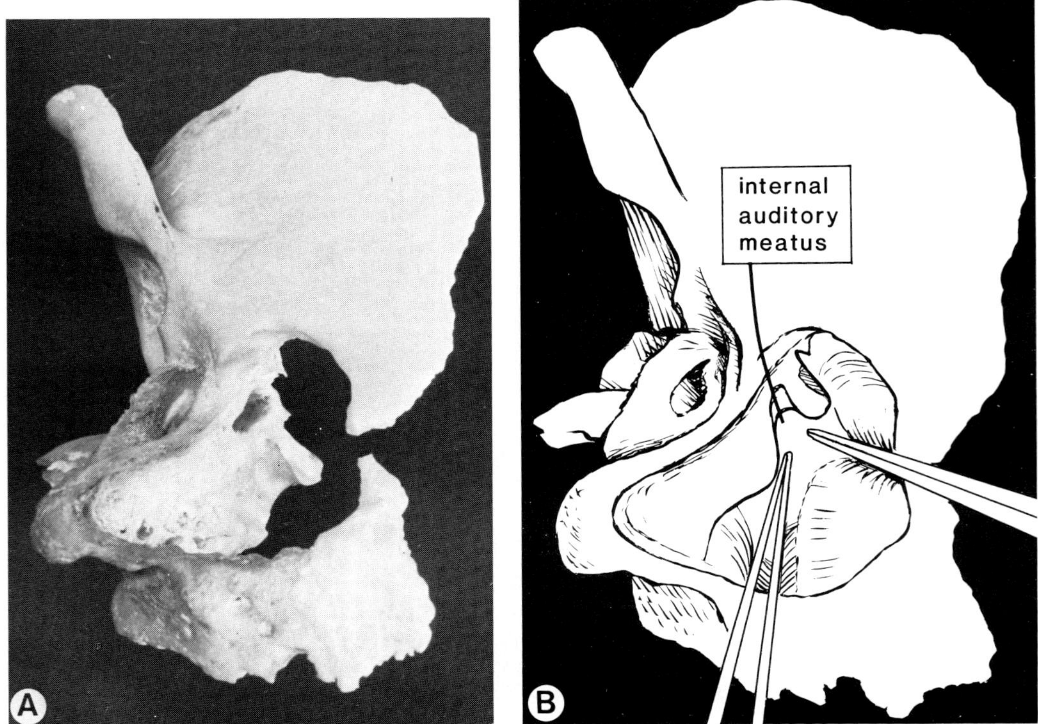

Fig. 60-11. (A) Same dissection as shown in Figure 60-10 but with the sinus plate removed. (B) By retracting the middle fossa dura and the sinus with the shafts of long instruments, the exposure is increased.

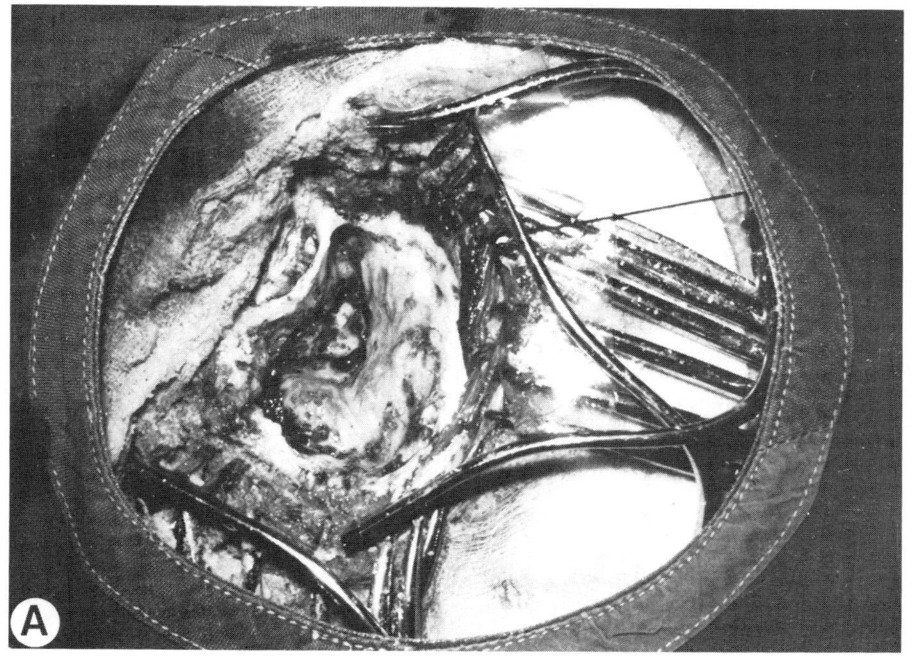

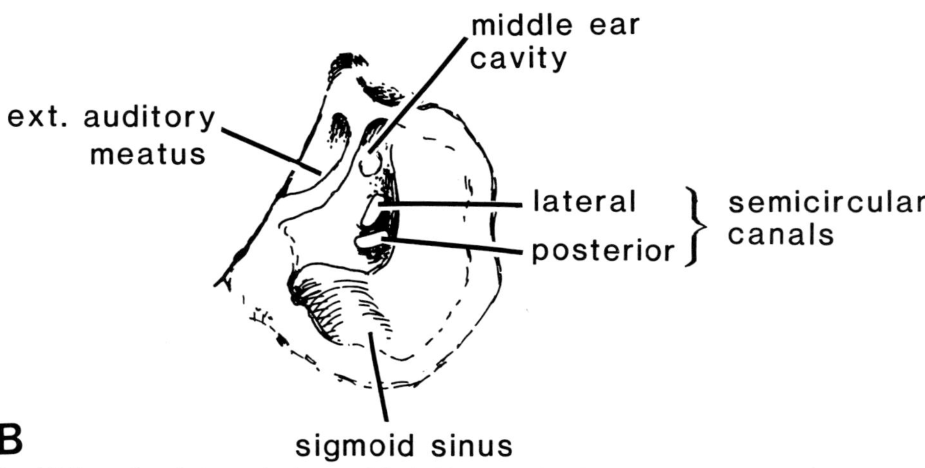

Fig. 60-12. (A) Operative photograph of a translabyrinthine operation. The superficial limits of the exposure are seen. The labyrinthectomy has not yet been carried out, but the lateral and posterior canals have been skeletonized. (B) Note that the sigmoid sinus is uncovered by removing the sinus plate and that the middle fossa dura is also extensively exposed.

since it is needed during the removal of the lower pole of the tumor.

The jugular bulb may come quite high,[12] even reaching the ampulla of the posterior canal.[12,13] It is wise to leave a layer of bone over it, since bleeding from it is a nuisance, although bleeding can be controlled with Surgicel or Gelfoam or, in difficult circumstances, a muscle pack. House, who fears the entry of Surgicel emboli into the venous system, advocates preliminary ligation of the internal jugular vein just below the skull base before packing the bulb with hemostatic material, but we have never found this measure necessary.

The internal auditory meatus is found immediately deep to the vestibule, and House recommends entering it by following the superior vestibular nerve. Once entered, it must be widely exposed by the removal of its posterior wall and as much of the superior and inferior walls as possible. A diamond burr is used because it is much less likely to damage the contents by catching on the edge of a ledge of bone and jumping; its

direction of rotation should be altered so that, should it jump, it will be directed away from the meatus. There is a limit to the amount of bone that can be removed above, between the roof of the meatus and the middle fossa, because progression medially and forward here leads eventually to the facial nerve, and the fear of damaging it should make the surgeon stop a little less than halfway across the roof of the internal auditory canal. The posterior wall is followed medially until the lateral lip of the porus is removed.

The otologic or bony part of the operation is now almost completed; only the removal of the thin layer of bone left over the sinuses and the posterior and middle fossa dura with curettes or fine rongeurs remains to be done.

The cavity resulting from this dissection is roughly pyramidal in shape, with its base at the cortical opening in the mastoid; three sides, the posterior fossa dura behind, the middle fossa above, and the petrous bone, middle ear cavity, and descending facial nerve anteriorly; and the internal meatus

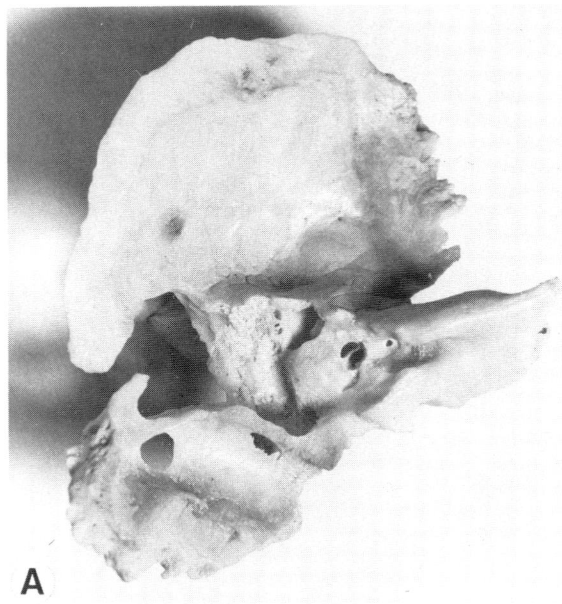

Fig. 60-13. (A) The same specimen as shown in Figures 60-9 and 60-10, from above and behind. (B) This shows how the bone removal extends from the meatus medially to the sigmoid sinus laterally (still covered with bone here) and from the jugular bulb below to the superior petrosal sinus and middle fossa dura above. The oval window seen through the opened vestibule gives the latter the appearance of a double opening.

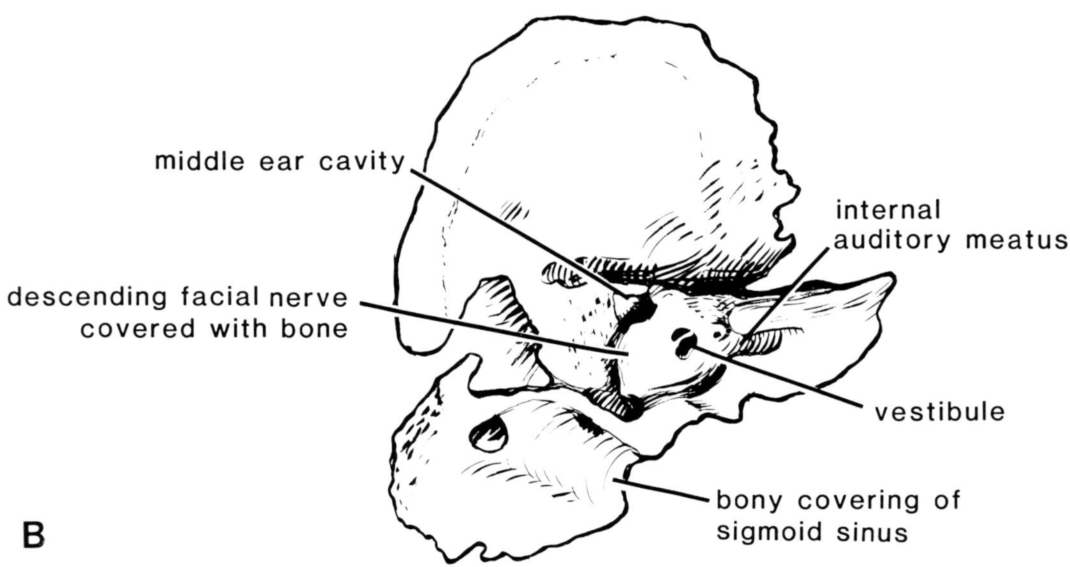

at its apex (Figures 60-10, 60-11, and 60-13). The size of the opening varies according to anatomic factors, the most important of which are the distance between the sigmoid sinus and the back of the external meatus (i.e., how far forward the sinus comes), how high the jugular bulb expands into the petrous bone, and how low the dura of the middle fossa reaches.

REMOVAL OF TUMOR

In tumors of all sizes, the next step is to open the dura of the meatus. Even in the smallest growth, this incision needs to be carried through the thickened dura at the porus and into the posterior fossa, although the extent to which the latter is exposed may vary somewhat according to the size of the mass lying in the cerebellopontine angle. In the meatus, the dura is often extremely thin, but it can be picked off the surface of the tumor with a sharp hook inserted in the appropriate plane. When the porus is reached, the dura becomes so thick, forming

a distinct constriction ring, that it needs to be divided with a sharp Jacobsen scissors. The incision then runs laterally across the posterior fossa dura and, as the sigmoid sinus is approached, splits into an upward and downward limb. For a full exposure of the posterior fossa, the upper limb should reach into the apex of the angle made by the superior petrosal sinus entering the sigmoid sinus, while inferiorly the other limb reaches to the edge of the bone exposure. Hitching stitches are placed on the dural flap superiorly and inferiorly (Figure 60-14), and also laterally (not illustrated), and the tumor will then be exposed in the meatus, and, if it is of a sufficient size, in the cerebellopontine angle, where it is covered with arachnoid that stretches from the porus to the edge of the cerebellum, just visible in the lateral part of the posterior fossa.

There are four steps to be carried out at this early stage:

1. Identify the facial nerve in the internal auditory meatus.
2. Free the tumor from its attachments to arachnoid and dura at the porus, thus making the whole mass more mobile.

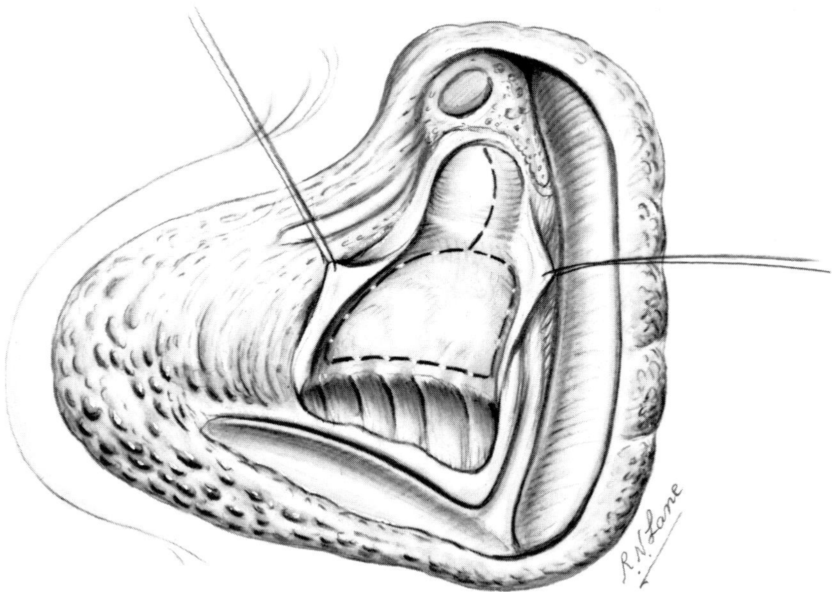

Fig. 60-14.   The operative exposure after the dura of the posterior fossa has been opened and retracted. The dotted line on the tumor in the meatus and angle indicates where the arachnoid is to be opened. Note the small exposure of the cerebellum.

3. Open the arachnoid and establish a plane between that membrane and the surface of the tumor at the meatus, and the porus, and in the cerebellopontine angle.
4. Start reducing in size the portion of the tumor that extends into the cerebellopontine angle.

The superior vestibular nerve is identified as it enters the bone at the lateral end of the meatus, is divided, and turned back, together with the lateral extent of the tumor. The facial nerve will then be picked up immediately anterior, and a vertical bar of bone separating the vestibular nerve from the facial nerve as it enters the petrous bone (Bill's bar) is easily palpable with a sharp hook and is a useful landmark. With the

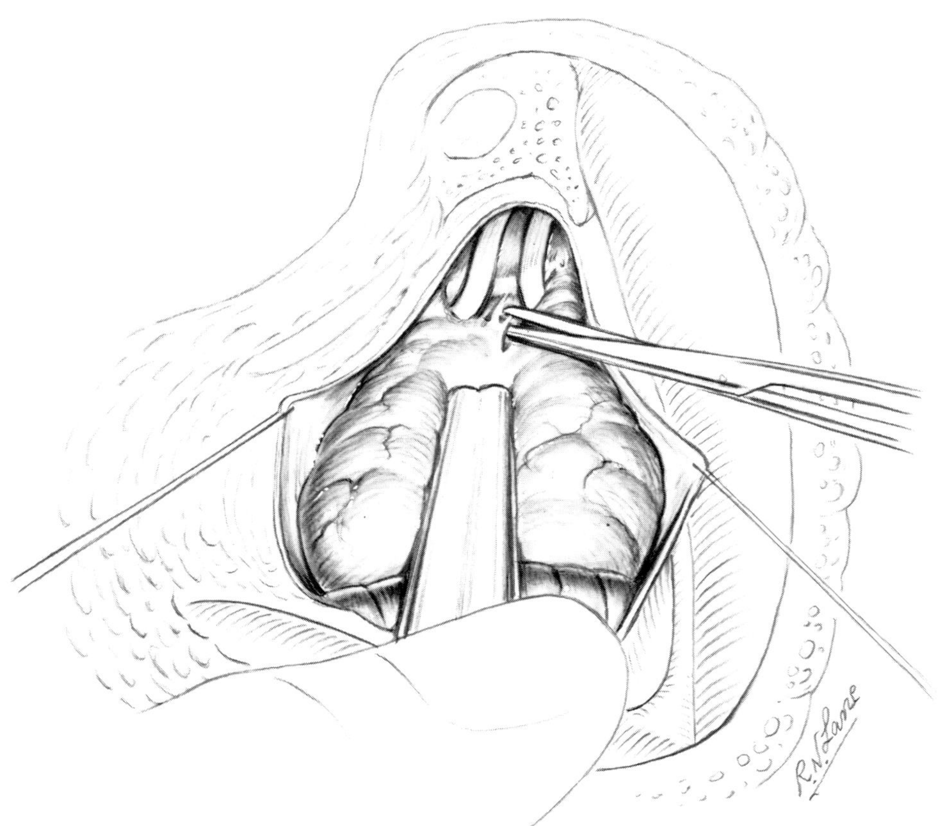

Fig. 60-15.   In this illustration the tumor, which has been retracted backward by the tip of a double-lumened irrigating sucker, has been separated from the facial and cochlear nerves in the internal auditory meatus.

tip of a fine irrigating sucker placed on a cottonoid square, the meatal tumor can be gently retracted backwards, and the arachnoidal strands binding it to the facial nerve above and below are divided with a fine microscissors (Figure 60-15). The advantages of doing this early are that the landmarks are all well defined at this stage and have not become obscured with blood, as tends to happen later, and the position of the facial nerve in the meatus is established. If the nerve lies along the anterior wall of the canal, it will usually be displaced directly medially at the porus and be relatively safe from damage when the upper and lower attachments to the porus are tackled later. On the other hand, if the nerve is found to lie along the upper margin of the meatus, it will, at the porus, be displaced upwards, be more superficial, and easily damaged. Indeed, a piece of tumor may pass medial to the nerve, and this anatomic arrangement makes the nerve vulnerable when the upper pole of the tumor is being mobilized, the nerve being encountered much earlier than expected. One disadvantage of mobilizing the tumor from the meatus early is that if the dissection is carried too far along the meatus, particularly if it passes beyond the level of the porus, it is very common for the plane between nerve and tumor to be lost because of the medial deviation of the nerve at this point. It is best, therefore, not to take the dissection more than about halfway to the porus, just far enough to identify the lie of the nerve. Its position should be marked with a small square of Silastic so that when, later, the dissection is resumed here, nerve can be more easily identified. It is, however, often difficult to define the nerve very clearly on returning to it because a certain amount of blood collects over it and it is usually necessary to resume the dissection by keeping very closely on the surface of the tumor rather than by formally defining the nerve, which would be at risk.

Freeing the tumor from the porus is accomplished by developing the plane between arachnoid and the neck of the tumor around the rim of the porus. Inferiorly, this can be done safely, since damage to the cochlear nerve is not of significance. Superiorly, the facial nerve may be at risk, especially under the circumstances just mentioned, and it may be necessary to avoid taking this dissection too far at this point. In favorable cases, though, even if it is impossible to free the tumor completely from the meatus at this stage, it should be possible to make the tumor considerably more mobile by dividing the arachnoid as far as one dares, having regard to the estimated position of the facial nerve.

The arachnoid incision in the cerebellopontine angle follows the outline marked in Figure 60-14, starting from the upper margin of the porus and passing upward under the tentorium, where the superior petrosal vein will usually be found encased in thickened membrane. Although no damage comes from dividing the vein, it is often possible in the case of smaller growths to separate it by means of sharp dissection from the upper portion of the tumor, thus running the arachnoid incision along its margin. Posteriorly, the incision turns downward, defining the plane between the cerebellar hemisphere and the posterior surface of the tumor, and inferiorly it turns forward to join the dissection already undertaken at the lower margin of the porus. The plane between the tumor and arachnoid can be developed below the meatus, toward the inferior pole of the tumor, and easily leads into the large cistern surrounding the medulla, the opening of which allows a flood of CSF to escape; this may provide further improvement in operative conditions even in cases where the lateral ventricle has been tapped already. Indeed, if any difficulties are being encountered be-

cause of lack of room in the posterior fossa, it is very valuable to carry out this maneuver of draining the medullary cistern as soon as the dura of the posterior fossa is opened.

The facial nerve has now been identified in the meatus, the tumor has been loosened from its attachment to the porus, and the correct plane between tumor and arachnoid has been identified around the margins of the part lying in the angle. It is now possible to start the removal of the tumor. This involves, in all large and in many medium tumors, gutting, or internally decompressing the tumor.

GENERAL DESCRIPTION—REMOVAL OF A LARGE TUMOR

If the tumor is small, confined to the meatus or just protruding into the angle, it may be possible to remove it in one piece. For larger growths, removal is achieved by reducing or shrinking the tumor, usually by removing a portion of its contents so that the adjacent capsule collapses, allowing the dissection to be extended, under direct vision around the far side of the tumor, where important structures, cranial nerves, the brain stem and its arteries, lie. Most of the time occupied in removing a large tumor is spent in gutting it as extensively as one dares at any particular stage and thereafter removing the mobilized segment.

It is a serious error to mobilize one portion of the tumor, pack the space between it and the brain with cottonoids, and then to leave them while the dissection is extended to another part, because, on returning, the surgeon will find that the cottonoids have become stuck with blood to brain and tumor, and it is very difficult to re-develop the plane. Mobilization of part of the tumor should be followed immediately by its piecemeal removal. The point of attack has to be changed progressively, and as the limits of mobilization are reached at one point, the surgeon moves to another. There are four main directions from which the deep part of the dissection can be made: (1) from the front or meatal side, along the facial nerve; (2) from above, under the tentorium, petrosal vein and, deeper in, the trigeminal nerve; (3) from behind, along the anterior surface of the cerebellum and the middle cerebellar peduncle; and (4) from below, in the cistern of the medulla and the ninth, tenth, and eleventh nerves.

The order of attack depends upon circumstances, with the surgeon taking the line of least resistance and with work shifted from one point, should difficulties be arising there, to another. When as much mobilization as is possible has been achieved in one part and the free piece of tumor removed, the point is best marked by leaving, not a cottonoid, but a small square of Silastic sheeting in the cleft between nervous tissue and the surface of the tumor, since this is much more easily located when the time comes to resume dissection. It is impossible to avoid leaving temporary cottonoids at certain points to control bleeding, but a conscious effort should be made to keep their number to a minimum. Reduction of its bulk not only allows the tumor gradually to be mobilized into the central and more superficial part of the wound, but is also helpful in preserving the facial nerve. The sharp deviation of this medially or upward at the porus and the difficulties that this may occasion in following the plane between the two have been mentioned. If the tumor is greatly reduced in bulk internally, the part of it that is pushing the nerve medially or upward will gradually collapse, bringing the nerve with it and making it more superficial while reducing the angle at which the nerve is deviated. Furthermore, a reduction in the stretching of the nerve around the surface of the tumor is also achieved, making the former less vulnerable to injury.

As the tumor is gradually reduced in size and the dissection proceeds further and further around its upper, lower anterior, and posterior poles, more and more attention is paid to developing the dissection along the facial nerve. We have found that the best chance of saving the nerve and avoiding temporary damage to it is to work from the porus to the brain stem, pushing reduced tumor backward and creeping along the surface of the nerve, which is not itself handled, with a scissors. If the plane is lost medial to the porus, which is a common occurrence, it may be possible to re-establish it by working above the porus toward the upper pole. If this portion of the tumor is gutted and carefully retracted downward with a sucker, the nerve can be recognized lying on the surface of the capsule deep to, and somewhat above, the porus. A plane can be developed between the two using a sharp hook, and this plane can then be extended laterally toward the porus until that sliver of tumor left on the nerve earlier has been freed from it. It is desirable to avoid coming upon the nerve from behind, where it enters the brain stem and, therefore, to avoid carrying the posterior dissection beyond the middle cerebellar peduncle, a point that is recognizable because here the tumor is in direct contact with white matter. Just beyond this point, as the tumor is lifted forward from behind, the brain stem is reached and the tumor seems to become adherent, because the cochlear nerve is attached to it. Troublesome bleeding can occur from veins[14] at this point. Unless the facial nerve has already been lost or the difficulties of preserving it are regarded as insuperable, dissection is stopped here and taken up again anteriorly along the nerve.

GUTTING

The usual technique is to define as large an area on the surface of the tumor facing the surgeon as possible, coagulating any vessels and cutting a window out of the tumor capsule in order to expose the substance of the tumor, which is then evacuated with a sucker, rongeurs, and a curette. The ease with which this can be done depends upon the tumor's consistency, which varies from something so soft that a sucker alone will remove it to a hardness that will defeat any technique except the use of a knife or scissors. The normal thing, however, is to find something a bit too hard to be sucked easily without preliminary fragmentation. Tumors vary in color from gray, which usually denotes toughness, to a characteristic yellow, which accompanies a very soft tumor; usually both colors and consistencies are present in one growth. With a tumor of average consistency, the contents can be broken up by opening and shutting the jaws of a pituitary rongeur repeatedly while sucking away the fragments thus freed with the other hand. It is wise not to shut the jaws of the rongeur completely with each bite, since this ensures that should the capsule be breached inadvertently, vessels on the surface will not be injured. The House-Urban rotary dissector is of great value at this stage. It consists of two concentric cannulae, one fitting exactly within the other, and each has an opening at the tip. The inner cannula is rotated by an electric motor in the handle, while suction is applied up the center of it. When the two openings are coincident, tumor is sucked into the lumen of the inner cannula and then amputated as the cannula rotates. Provided the tumor is relatively soft but not so soft that suction alone will remove it (in which case the machine would be superfluous), this instrument

works extremely well and greatly reduces time and effort on the surgeon's part. With an irrigating sucker in one hand to act as a sucker and as a retractor and also to provide a continuous flow of saline, and with the dissector in the other hand, equivalent to a pituitary rongeur and another sucker, the surgeon has in effect five instruments in the opening. The Cavitron (Cavitron Surgical Systems, Stamford, Connecticut) ultrasonic aspirator performs a similar function, but it is very bulky and extremely expensive. We have no experience in the use of the laser in this operation.

If the tumor is too hard for the above technique, the surgeon must resort to cutting a cone out of the tumor with a No. 15 scalpel blade, mobilizing the tumor beyond the edge of the hole, and cutting further wedges off with a knife. One might think that a hard tumor would be more difficult to reduce and to mobilize than a soft one, and this is partly true. A tough tumor consistency, however, has the advantage that the capsule can be grasped without breaking and can be drawn progressively toward the center of the cored-out area, whereas a soft tumor ruptures so easily that reliance has to be made on retracting it gently away from the brain with the tip of a sucker on a cottonoid. Even with this method, the surgeon may be hampered by a tendency for the surface to give way so that the sucker and cottonoid sink into it. Thus, slight differences of technique are required in these different circumstances. It should be added that an alternative method of applying gentle traction on a hard tumor is to stick a pair of sharp, fine forceps into it like a toothpick into a cocktail sausage. This technique can be used in tumors that are not quite tough enough to be grasped.

In all types of tumors, hemorrhage from the raw surface produced by gutting may be troublesome. Quite large bleeders may be encountered, and these require bipolar diathermy. Smaller hemorrhagic points will usually respond to the application of a temporary layer of Surgicel or to packing with cottonoids soaked in hydrogen peroxide. If constant oozing is a problem, it is helpful to have the anesthetist lower the blood pressure by using halothane or isoflurane. A drop in systolic blood pressure from 100 to 80 may make a surprising difference to operative conditions, and this level of hypotension can be safely maintained for many hours. Severe hypotension is unwise in this operation because of the long duration of the operation.

CHARACTERISTICS OF THE FOUR QUADRANTS OF THE DISSECTION

LOWER QUADRANT

The ease with which the medullary cistern can be entered here, even before any gutting of the tumor has been undertaken, has already been mentioned. A little gutting usually allows the lower pole to be lifted away from the ninth, tenth, and eleventh nerves, which are usually not seen very well, since they tend to lie out of sight just around the corner of the opening. The anterior inferior cerebellar artery is usually found lying on the capsule here and can be dissected off, its branches to the tumor being coagulated and divided. It is safe, however, to divide the main trunk at this point, if necessary, although it may merely postpone the difficulty, since the artery still has to be dissected off more deeply and anteriorly, where it is unsafe to occlude it. The medulla and the choroid plexus of the lateral recess will come into view relatively early in the operation, and when the

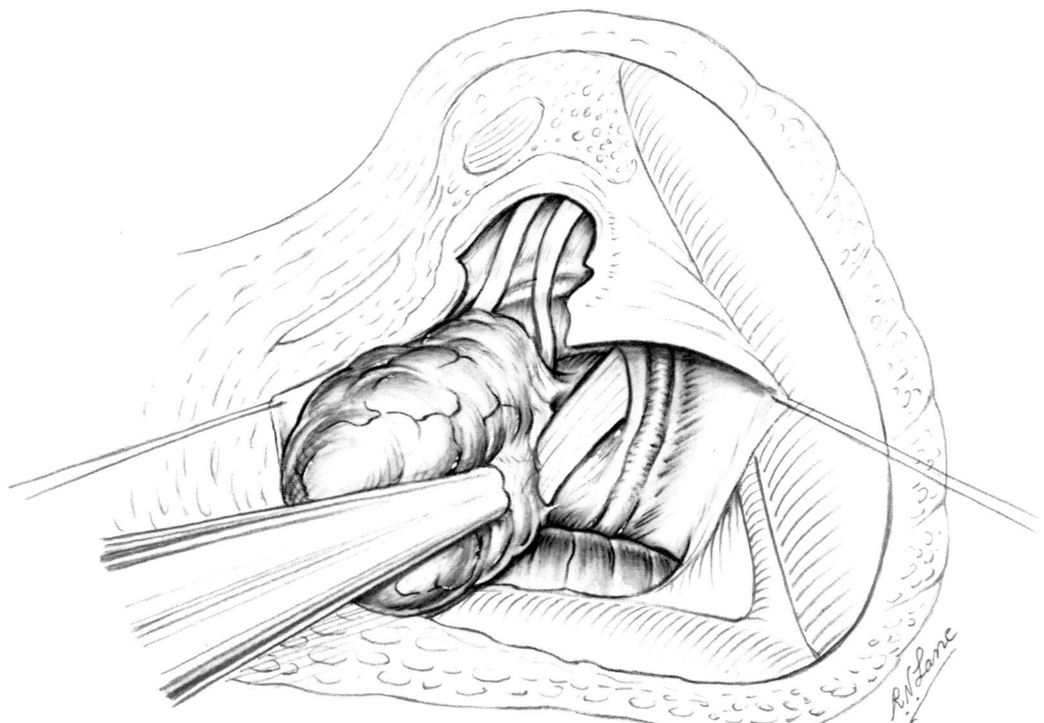

Fig. 60-16. Mobilization of the upper pole. The tumor has been freed from the upper porus and is retracted downward while being freed from the arachnoid by sharp dissection. In this case, the facial nerve has been displaced directly medially. The petrosal vein has been left intact, embedded in the arachnoid, and the fifth nerve is coming into view as the cistern around it has been entered.

latter is visible, this part of the dissection should be temporarily abandoned, since it is difficult to get much further up the brain stem until further reduction in the main bulk of the tumor has been effected. A piece of Silastic sheeting is left to mark the site of the medulla and choroid plexus.

UPPER QUADRANT

Whether the upper pole is attacked early depends upon whether the meatal dissection has established the position of the facial nerve. If it is known that the nerve lies directly medially, it is safe to work over the top of the growth, freeing it from the arachnoid under the tentorium and the petrosal vein. The trigeminal nerve is usually encountered quite deeply, gleaming white across the subarachnoid space to enter Meckel's cave (Figure 60-16). Further downward, it will be found in contact with the tumor, which usually can be lifted or retracted away from it easily; there is therefore little necessity for sharp dissection and none for actually handling the nerve, which ought to be avoided if recovery of sensory loss in the face is to be achieved. The pons will usually be reached when the nerve is followed down to its attachment to the brain stem, which will have been reached at both top and bottom ends of the dissection.

ANTERIOR QUADRANT

For tumors confined to the meatus or extending only a limited distance into the cerebellopontine angle, the main attack is made from the anterior aspect, for once the nerve has been traced to the brain stem or to the end of its attachment to tumor, which in small tumors may be well lateral to the brain stem, the main part of the operation has been completed and it is relatively easy to divide the remaining arachnoidal attachments and lift out the whole tumor. The method of separating tumor from nerve has already been described. As the plane is developed, the work often requires a high level of magnification, and a flow of irrigation from the sucker is extremely helpful in keeping the cleft clear of blood, which, even in small amounts, obscures vision. Great care is necessary to avoid leaving fragments of tumor on the nerve, for once this is started it will lead to an ever-increasing layer accumulating, until the surgeon suddenly realizes that the nerve has been completely lost and the dissection is being made inside the tumor. This is possible even with small tumors, but it is a real hazard with large ones, in which it is very likely to occur just medial to the porus, as mentioned previously.

POSTERIOR QUADRANT

The arachnoid between the cerebellum (very little of which is immediately visible through the exposure) and the tumor has been divided. The plane now developed, by retracting the tumor forward and dividing the bands of arachnoid that are stretched, is continued along the length of the posterolateral surface. As one gets deeper, the arachnoid disappears and the middle cerebellar peduncle is reached and, eventually, the brain stem and attachment of the cochlear nerve. When the brain stem has been reached at all points, there is usually a relatively small portion of tumor left, although great vigilance is necessary in mobilizing this final piece, for damage either to the anterior inferior cerebellar artery or the facial nerve can occur.

Most removals are completed working from above or from in front, turning the tumor downward or backward until the

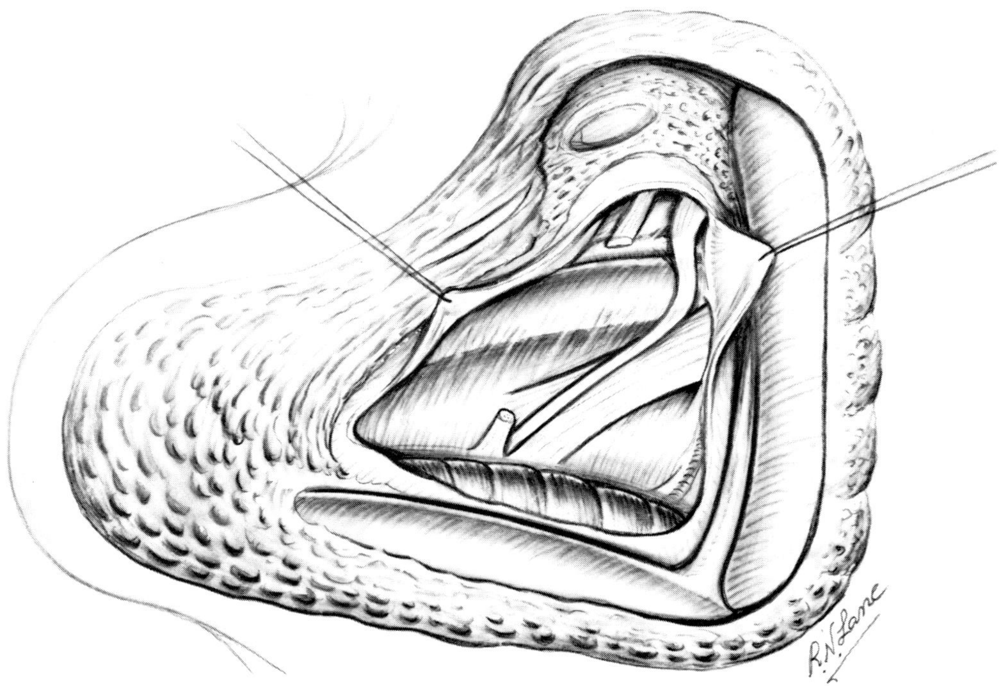

Fig. 60-17. The bed of the tumor. The facial nerve is illustrated as it most commonly is found, displaced medially and upward to overlie the fifth nerve before curving downward to reach the pontomedullary junction. In some cases, the nerve passes almost directly upward from the porus, thus lying more superficial than in this drawing, and consequently being more vulnerable.

central end of the facial nerve is completely free. The cochlear nerve, lateral to it, can then be divided. If the facial nerve has been destroyed at an earlier point, the removal of the tumor is thereby facilitated, although the clearing of the brain stem still demands care.

With the tumor removed, the field is inspected (Figure 60-17) and the function of the facial nerve, if still intact, is checked by stimulating it with a disposable nerve stimulator using a 2 A current. Objections that this may harm the nerve are not borne out in practice, and it is reassuring to know that the nerve will conduct from the brain stem to the periphery. The stimulator can first be applied to the nerve in the middle ear, through the bone, to ascertain that the nerve is capable of conduction with the level of stimulus being used, then in the meatus, and finally on the brain stem. Failure to get a contraction from the brain stem does not rule out recovery, but success guarantees it. Care must be taken not to confuse masseter contraction from stimulation of the trigeminal nerve with movement in the facial muscles.

HEMOSTASIS

Either before before or after testing of the facial nerve, the cottonoids left for temporary hemostasis on the brain stem are removed, and often a good deal of bleeding will occur. Venous bleeding offers little problem, since it is easily controlled by the application of small pieces of Gelfoam. If arterial bleeding is occurring from the brain stem, the bleeding usually comes from a side hole in an artery where a small tumor branch has been avulsed. It is unwise to coagulate such an artery, since infarction of the brain stem may be produced. Such bleeding can usually be stopped by the patient application of a muscle stamp held by a cottonoid pressed onto a piece of Silastic.

Repeated and prolonged packing of the wound with cottonoids and with cotton wool soaked in peroxide should be carried out while the anesthetist allows the blood pressure to rise to a normal level and completes a blood transfusion if this is deemed necessary. It is a good rule to delay the closure of the wound for at least half an hour, even in the most favorable cases, to ensure that the cavity is quite dry, since a postoperative hematoma in such an enclosed space is of extremely serious consequence.

CLOSURE

The dural opening into the posterior fossa cannot be sutured, and thus the petrous cavity connects the now-empty cerebellopontine angle cistern with the middle ear. A CSF leak through the latter, into the nose, is the most important single complication of the procedure, and we have not been able to devise an absolutely reliable method of preventing it. Hitherto, the incus has been removed early in the petrous dissection, and at the end the middle ear has been packed with muscle. However, it has become clear, during re-exploration of the cavity for postoperative CSF leaks, that in some cases CSF was entering the middle ear directly, and we have assumed that the stapes footplate was displaced so that the middle ear communicated with the vestibule, and thus with the cerebellopontine angle, directly through the oval window rather than through the mastoid antrum (Figure 60-15). Until recently, we have placed two layers of fascia over the surface of the petrous bone, centering them on the mastoid antrum tund holding them in place with fat grafts. However, postoperative leakage has continued to be a problem, and lately, having found that re-operation through the posterior fossa and the placing of a large graft across the dural defect and meatus from inside the cranial cavity seemed effective, we have tried to achieve the same effect primarily, by placing the graft on the inside of the dural defect rather than over the petrous bone, tacking it in place with three stitches above, below, and laterally, and glueing it with Tisseel (Immuno A.G. Vienna, Austria) over the meatus. A second graft has been placed over the petrous bone, as before, and the space between the two filled very loosely with fat. This technique has been promising so far, though it is more difficult and time-consuming than is the earlier method.

House[12] recommended packing the petrous cavity with strips of abdominal fat wedged tightly into place without any fascia lata. We have tried this once, but, probably because of the extensive exposure of the temporal dura we obtained, the packing stripped the dura from the middle fossa, producing a large extradural hemorrhage that, fortunately, was recognized before the operation was completed and was evacuated without ill effect.

The pericranial temporalis flap is re-sutured over the petrous cavity using Vicryl sutures, and the scalp is closed in two layers without a subgaleal drain. If a ventricular catheter has been used, it is spiggoted before the closure starts. Antibiotics are used postoperatively because of the length of the operation and the route through the middle ear. Dexamethasone is used in the usual dosage, even in cases of small tumor, for it may offer some protection against swelling of the facial nerve and delayed paralysis.

POSTOPERATIVE MANAGEMENT

If the facial nerve is anatomically intact at the end of the operation, the facial musculature should be tested as soon as the patient recovers from anesthesia. Where the nerve has been extensively dissected, total paralysis is immediately apparent in many cases. In some, however, a little movement is seen at this stage but disappears within a few hours. Definite contraction of some part of the ipsilateral facial musculature, however slight or transitory, is a sure indication of some eventual recovery and will encourage the surgeon and the patient during the long wait for this to occur. It is important to be careful in attributing movements of the ipsilateral face to preserved function, for some movement may be transmitted from the opposite side, and eye closure is often possible immediately postoperatively even if the face is totally paralyzed. One must look for definite local movement in some part of the face before accepting that conduction is still occurring in the nerve. The patient is returned to bed; the head end of the bed should be tilted upward 15 to 20 degrees, provided that the blood pressure is stable. The eye should be covered with a protective shield if the face is paralyzed, and methyl cellulose eye drops instilled three times a day thereafter. The usual neurosurgical observations are made every half-hour for the first 24 hours, and the drip is kept open until nausea has subsided and the patient can take oral fluids. Oral feeding can usually be started the next day and the patient allowed out of bed in 24 to 48 hours. The ventricular catheter is removed in 48 hours if the patient is well.

In cases in which the face is paralyzed, eye care is of great importance, especially if there is absence of the corneal reflex and facial analgesia. The patient should be provided with protective spectacles for use out-of-doors and should be warned to report back if the eye becomes red or painful, if it shows discharge, or if vision becomes blurred. At the follow-up, the patient should be reviewed for corneal ulceration and referred to an ophthalmologist at any suggestion of trouble. The sutures are removed from the cranial wound in 4 days and from the leg in 10.

POSTOPERATIVE COMPLICATIONS

The problems of facial paralysis have been dealt with, and if the nerve is thought to be intact anatomically, at least 6 months should be allowed to pass before a faciohypoglossal anastomosis is considered. Most nerves that are functionless immediately after surgery will take at least that long to recover, and a few may take longer.

HEMATOMA IN THE OPERATIVE CAVITY

If hemostasis is careful, hematoma is rare. It has occurred in our experience in 5 of 300 cases, and it seems most likely to afflict elderly patients. Prompt action is required. The intracranial pressure must be lowered by opening the ventricular catheter, if one is present, or by tapping the frontal horn through the burr hole; respirations and the airway must be protected by artificial ventilation with a mask or through an endotracheal tube; and the patient must be taken to the operating theater with the greatest speed, the wound reopened, and the clot evacuated.

House recommended reopening the wound in the ward or recovery room, and has a microscope and sterile kit beside the bed for this purpose. We have preferred to use the measures enumerated above, because a clot capable of producing deep unconsciousness, respiratory failure, and pulmonary edema can be relatively small and lie in the deepest part of the wound against the side of the pons. It is an anxious task to find one's way down to evacuate it, and one that requires the favorable circumstances provided in the operating room. As House's practice implies, there is no time to waste, since death can occur within half an hour of the first signs of trouble. Three of our five cases recovered, one died almost immediately, and the fourth, a man of 77, succumbed to pulmonary complications some time after the apparently successful evacuation. There is, of course, a considerable risk that damage to the cranial nerves or ataxia will result either from the clot or the attempts to evacuate it. Good vision with the microscope, a very fine sucker, copious irrigation, and a very patient evacuation will lessen the risk of damage to the brain or cranial nerves. Two extradural hematomas above the tentorium have been seen, the one already described, caused by too tight packing of the petrous cavity, the other in relation to the precautionary burr hole, in this instance placed in the parietal area without opening the dura. Neither was followed by any serious consequence.

CSF RHINORRHEA

As has been mentioned, CSF rhinorrhea[15] is the bane of the technique and occurs in up to 14 percent of cases. Although it is usually evident within a few days of operation, it may be delayed. The patient should be tested before discharge and on first follow-up by being placed in the head-down position. A warning should also be given about the importance of reporting any watery discharge from the ipsilateral nostril, especially if it occurs on leaning forward. The leak is usually so copious that there is no doubt of its nature, and testing the discharge for sugar is usually unnecessary. Prior to adopting the technique described above, we had a number of cases in which repeated replacements of the graft in the petrous cavity were unsuccessful. Then a new approach to the posterior fossa, with positioning of a new graft over the defect from within, was discovered to be effective. Leaks through the wound occur sometimes, but are easily dealt with by the use of a spinal drain, although this technique is not useful for leaks through the ear, which are merely concealed for the time being, recurring when the drain is removed.

OTHER SPECIAL COMPLICATIONS

In cases in which the temporal lobe is exposed, by division either of the petrosal sinus or of the entire tentorium, cortical damage may lead either to epilepsy or, on the dominant side, to dysphasia. These techniques, which we rarely use now, are described elsewhere.[7,9]

RESULTS

The most important series is that of House and his colleagues, the first 200 cases of which were presented in his Monograph II.[16] This report covers the period of development of the operation and the results are therefore not a fair indication of what can be achieved with this technique, although the results were used for this purpose by Di Tullio and his colleagues[17] in their tendentious paper. Luetje[18] presented the next 500 consecutive cases and, although his analysis includes 17 middle fossa and 13 transsigmoid operations, the figures may be taken to represent the best that have been presented, in terms of both quality and numbers.

Total removal was achieved in 93.4 percent of all cases: in 100 percent of small tumors confined to the meatus; in 97.6 percent of medium tumors extending 2.5 cm or less into the cerebellopontine angle but not distorting the brain stem; and in 85 percent of large growths. The operative mortality was 2.6 percent. In 96.6 percent of cases, the facial nerve was thought to be anatomically intact at the end of the operation, but not all the patients recovered function; 13.4 percent of the series were left with total paralysis (0 percent of patients with small growths, 10.4 percent of those with medium growths, and 21.4 percent of those with large growths). These are excellent figures, although criticism can be made of the incidence of partial removal, which, for the large tumors, looks appreciable. Partial removal is an unsatisfactory outcome, especially in medium or small tumors, in which, if a cure is not to be effected at such a favorable stage, the operation might just as well be deferred until the patient has serious symptoms. It appears, however, that of 21 patients who had a partial removal because of difficulties experienced during the operation, 14 had the removal completed at a second stage. This underlines an important point: if difficulties lead to the abandonment of the operation short of total removal, a second procedure should be undertaken unless there are strong reasons for not doing so, and it is sometimes surprisingly straightforward.

We[18] achieved total removal in 100 percent of 150 cases. We did not use the technique if elective partial removal had been decided upon preoperatively. In 3 cases, however, a second operation was required in order to complete the removal of very large and hemorrhagic tumors. The mortality was 2.5 percent, being nil in small tumors, 1.6 percent in medium tumors, and 2.7 percent in large tumors. We were not nearly so successful as the House group in preserving the facial nerve,

only achieving this in 54 percent of cases overall. With small tumors, the figure was 100 percent, and with medium tumors, 80 percent, rates that can be regarded as reasonably satisfactory, but only 20 percent of those with large tumors enjoyed preservation of the facial nerve. Since this report, we have improved our figures somewhat in a further 150 consecutive cases. Two deaths occurred, one from aspergillosis infection in a patient with a medium-sized tumor, and one, mentioned above, from a postoperative hematoma in a man of 77. In both cases, the facial nerve had been preserved. The overall mortality in the second group was thus 1.3 percent (1 percent for large tumors, 2 percent for medium tumors, and 0 percent for small). The facial nerve was preserved (in one case a graft was inserted that recovered) in 52 of 94 cases of large tumors (55 percent), and in all of 47 cases of medium and 9 cases of small tumors, bringing the overall rate to 72 percent. Preservation here means that some recovery took place. One would expect results to improve with experience, but it should be noted that the preservation of the facial nerve in large tumors was mainly achieved in the lower range of that category, and that it remains a rather difficult feat. It is impossible to be confident about it beforehand, since it is affected by factors that are unpredictable preoperatively, such as the position of the nerve and its degree of adherence to the tumor. Where the tumor is of very large size, a realistic preoperative assessment would be pessimistic.

The quality of recovery in the facial nerve needs some mention, for it is by no means always satisfactory. Attempts to grade degrees of recovery[19] quantitatively by assigning percentages to recovery are not very satisfactory, and a coarse, qualitative grading conveys more meaning. Total paralysis clearly represents failure; normal function is very satisfactory. Anything noticeably less than normal function is very apparent, especially to the educated eye and to the patient, and this must be deemed unsatisfactory with one exception. A very slight degree of weakness may persist, and, while precluding the description ''normal,'' may be reasonably satisfactory and may be described as good. Where there is pronounced weakness and an unsatisfactory cosmetic result, the retention of eye closure, because of its functional value, puts the result into a better category.

Prediction of the end result is usually possible soon after the operation. A complete paralysis immediately postoperatively means the face will take at least 6 months to recover and will do so very imperfectly with marked weakness and synkineses being very disfiguring features. If no weakness is evident when the patient wakes from the anesthetic or if weakness is slight or delayed, a fairly satisfactory outcome will ensue.

Some anxiety exists that preserving the facial nerve may lead to recurrence because small fragments of tumor have been left on the nerve in what is otherwise a total removal.[20] We have been able to keep in touch with about 70 percent of these patients and have seen only one recurrence. This was revealed on a scan done for headaches 7 years after the original operation. Since the tumor seemed asymptomatic, no action was taken until the patient developed trigeminal pain and numbness 1 year later, when the tumor was removed without relief of the facial pain. The patient subsequently proved to have a carcinoma of the skull base. The risk of recurrence after preservation of the facial nerve would therefore appear to be very low. The end results generally are very satisfactory, and over 90 percent of patients return to normal life. A great diminution in morbidity and mortality therefore has been the most striking advance in the treatment of acoustic nerve tumors since House's monograph in 1964.

REFERENCES

1. House WF (ed): Monograph. Transtemporal bone microsurgical removal of acoustic neuromas. Arch Otolaryngol 80:597, 1964
2. Quix F: Ein Fall von translabyrintharisch operiertem Tumor Acusticus. Verh Dtsch Otol Ges 21:245, 1912
3. King TT: Clinical presentation and treatment of tumors of the cervical nerves and spinal roots, in Dyck PJ, Thomas PK, Lambert EH, et al (eds): Peripheral Neuropathy, ed 2. Philadelphia, WB Saunders, 1984, pp 2204–2235
4. Block JM, Nathanson M: A review of acoustic neurinoma at the Mount Sinai Hospital. J Mount Sinai Hosp 30:217, 1963
5. Tator CH: Acoustic neuromas: Management of 204 cases. Can J Neurosci 12:353, 1985
6. Desgeorges M, Sterkers JM: La chirurgie des gros neurinomas de l'acoustique opérés uniquement par voie translabyrinthique: A propos de 50 cas. Neurochirurgie 30:255, 1984
7. Tator CH, Nedzelski JM: Facial nerve preservation in patients with large acoustic neuromas by a combined middle fossa transtentorial translabyrinthine approach. J Neurosurg 57:1, 1982
8. Long DM, Kennedy DW, Holliday MJ: Selecting a surgical approach for removal of acoustic schwannoma. Ear Nose Throat J 65:163, 1986
9. Morrison AW, King TT: Experiences with a translabyrinthine and transtentorial approach to the cerebello-pontine angle. J Neurosurg 38:382, 1973
10. House WF, De La Cruz A, Hitselberger WE: Surgery of the skull base: Transcochlear approach to the petrous apex and clivus. Otolaryngol Head Neck Surg 86:770, 1978
11. Cushing H: Tumors of the Nervus Acusticus and the Syndrome of the Cerebellopontine Angle. Philadelphia, WB Saunders, 1917
12. House WF: The translabyrinthine approach, in House WF, Luetje CM (eds): Acoustic Tumors, vol 2. Baltimore, University Park Press, 1979, pp 43–87
13. Wadin K, Wilbrand H: The topographic relations of the high jugular fossa to the inner ear. Acta Radiol (Diagn) 27:315, 1986
14. Rhoton AL: Microsurgical anatomy of the brainstem surface facing an acoustic neuroma. Surg Neurol 25:326, 1986
15. Tos M, Thomsen J: Cerebrospinal fluid leak after translabyrinthine surgery for acoustic nerve tumour. Laryngoscope 95:351, 1985
16. House WF: Monograph II: Acoustic neuroma. Arch Otolaryngol 88:576, 1968
17. Di Tullio MVJ, Malkasian D, Rand RW: A critical comparison of neurosurgical and otolaryngological approaches to acoustic neuromas. J Neurosurg 48:1, 1978
18. Luetje CM: Preface, in House WF, Luetje CM (eds): Acoustic Tumors, vol 11, Management. Baltimore, University Park Press, 1979, pp xiii–xiv
19. Brackmann DE, Barro DM: Assessing recovery of facial function following acoustic neuroma surgery. Otolargyngol Head Neck Surg 92:88, 1984
20. King TT, Morrison AW: Translabyrinthine and transtentorial removal of acoustic nerve tumors. Results in 150 cases. J Neurosurg 32:210, 1968

CHAPTER 61

Surgical Correction of Facial Palsy

David W. Leitner

THE SURGICAL CORRECTION of facial palsy, particularly after intracranial surgery for acoustic neuromas, is a difficult task. The harmonious interaction of the muscles contributing to normal facial expression is such that surgical restoration of these qualities can only be approximated by the techniques presently available. Treatment aims at achieving a static balance of these muscles, closure of the eyelids, and symmetry during voluntary and involuntary emotion.

Numerous procedures have been used to reanimate paralyzed facial muscles. These involve (1) the use of a peripheral nerve other than the injured ipsilateral seventh nerve to provide innervation for the denervated musculature; (2) transfer of a local or distant muscle, with or without nerve grafting, to provide the motor power for animation; or (3) static procedures to achieve balance. Aside from the selection of the appropriate procedures for a given case, perhaps the most vexing problem is the timing of any reanimation surgery. If a person has a facial paralysis of 1 or 2 years' duration, it is very probable that spontaneous animation will not return.[1] In such a case, surgical intervention would be the only means of reanimation. If the paralysis has existed for less than 1 year, however, there is the possibility that some element of function may return.[2]

In this situation, surgical intervention may be further delayed until it can be determined clinically and electromyographically whether or not facial nerve regeneration is occurring.[3]

The timing of surgery involves assessing the status of the injured facial nerve and the functional capabilities of its denervated musculature. To employ a reanimation technique that provides direct innervation to the facial muscles of the injured side requires muscle units that are capable of regaining their function after such reinnervation. The recuperative power of denervated muscle varies widely as to the period of time that can elapse beyond which muscle units no longer regain their contractile capability. While studies have demonstrated that the longer the period of denervation the less complete the recovery of muscle function, to date no specific limits have been determined.[4,5] Sunderland showed that good or complete functional recovery could occur for up to 12 months after denervation.[5] Measurements of the chronaxy of the facial muscles or electromyography can be of assistance in establishing whether or not there has been recovery or deterioration of the status of the muscles.[6,7]

METHODS OF SURGICAL TREATMENT

PERIPHERAL NERVE SURGERY

Cross-Facial Nerve Graft

Cross-facial nerve grafting, in which a nerve graft (usually the sural nerve) is routed from normal facial nerve funiculi to the affected funiculi on the contralateral side of the face, has been advocated by severals authors.[8–11] This procedure depends on the ability of the denervated muscle on the affected side to have the potential to regain its contractile capacity. The procedure is recommmended in situations in which the facial paralysis has been present for less than 12 to 18 months. The theoretical advantage of this type of procedure is that successful reinnervation of the existing facial muscles results in the same natural directions of contracture as seen on the nonparalyzed side. In addition, there is the potential that the use of the contralateral facial nerve will allow the patient to regain spontaneous, emotionally induced movements as well as conscious, premeditated facial animation.[12–14] Despite these potential benefits the procedure has not met with uniform success, particularly in older patients or in those patients with long-standing facial paralysis.[15,16] While there may be some loss of contractability of the contralateral musculature innervated by the donor seventh nerve funiculi, the effects of this type of neurectomy are minimal.

Nerve Transfers

If the hypoglossal nerve is intact and functional, it can be transferred to the ipsilateral facial nerve trunk or its branches to innervate the facial muscles.[17,18] The phrenic nerve and the descending cervicalis nerve also have been used for nerve transfer but to a much lesser extent than the hypoglossal nerves.[3,19] Hypoglossal facial nerve anastomosis provides a reliable means of establishing successful dynamic reconstruction. Conley and Baker reported that in 137 patients they had a 95 percent rate of return of facial muscle contraction.[20] The results depend upon the availability of potentially functioning facial muscles.

Among the drawbacks to the hypoglossal facial nerve transfer are moderate to severe tongue atrophy, which occurred in 78 percent of this series.[20] There is also the problem of mass movement of the facial muscles during chewing, deglutition, and talking.[20] As in the case of cross-facial nerve grafting, the question of whether or not emotional expression can be retained is debatable.

OPERATIVE NEUROSURGICAL TECHNIQUES
ISBN 0-8089-1862-1

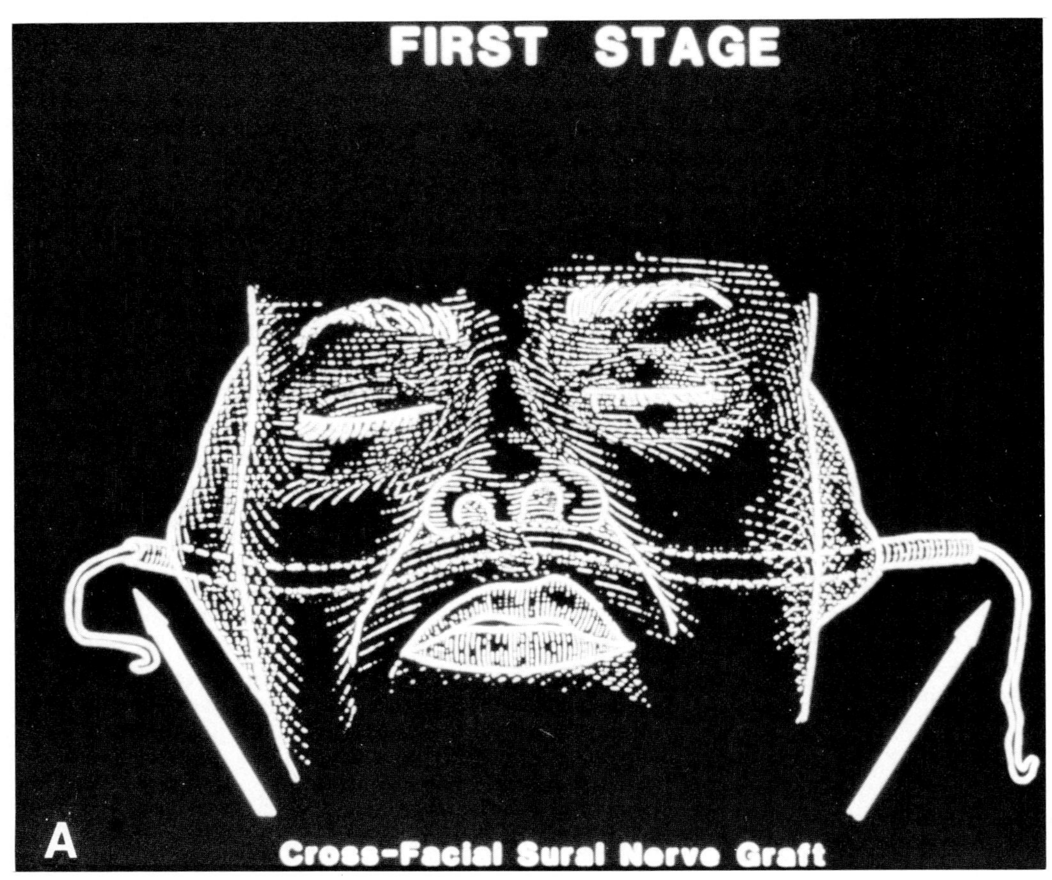

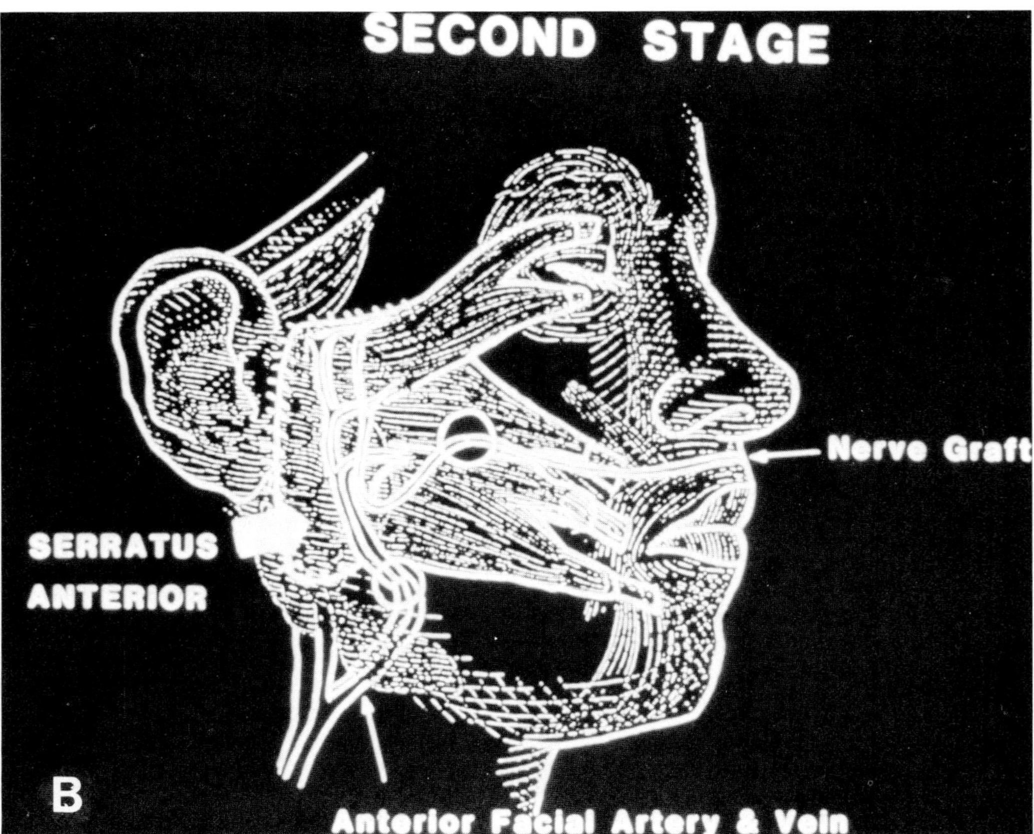

Fig. 61-1. (A) First stage cross-facial nerve graft. (B) Second stage microneurovascular muscle transplantation. (Courtesy of H. J. Buncke, M.D.)

DYNAMIC MUSCLE RECONSTRUCTION

Local Muscle Transfers

For facial paralysis in which there is little chance of re-establishing contraction of the in situ facial muscles (i.e., long-standing paralysis) and in which either the mandibular branch of the trigeminal nerve or the hypoglossi are intact, local muscle transfers can be used. The ipsilateral masseter muscle, which is innervated by the trigeminal nerve, can be used for a transfer to the region of the affected orbicularis oris. The muscle is detached from its insertion on the mandible while its origin at the zygoma is maintained. The neurovascular pedicle is maintained, the muscle split longitudinally, rotated anteriorly, and tunneled toward the orbicularis oris region beneath the skin, where it is attached to the orbicularis of the upper and lower lip to provide support and dynamic retraction of the oral commissure. Alternatively, because the size and arc of rotation of the masseter limit its applicability for reanimation to the oral commissure, the larger ipsilateral temporalis muscle can be used at the commissure of the mouth and to reanimate the upper and lower eyelid.[21] The temporalis muscle can be detached from its origin, elevated down to its insertion, and divided into four separate slips, which are then interdigitated with the fibers of the orbicularis oris and orbicularis oculi.

Another local muscle transfer that can be used for facial reanimation is that in which portions of the omohyoid, sternohyoid, and sternothyroid muscles are harvested with branches of the ansa cervicalis. These small muscle-nerve units are then transferred and imbedded into the substance of the musculature at the oral commissure.[22] Any subsequent muscular contraction at the commissure is the result of myoneurotization rather than the transfer of a contractile unit such as with the other muscle transfers.

Transfer of the larger muscles (i.e., masseter and temporalis) can provide good facial animation, but as with the peripheral nerve transfers, persistence and motivation is required of the patient to obtain facial movement by contraction of the appropriate muscles of mastication. The movement is a mass movement. In addition, there is some loss of mastication power when these transfers are used.

Distant Muscle Transfers

If local muscle transfers are not available or desirable, distant muscles or muscle groups can be transferred. Thompson suggested using a nonvascularized transfer of the extensor digitorum brevis muscle of the foot to the paralyzed side of the face.[23] The harvested muscle is placed on denervated facial musculature without any direct arterial or venous anastomosis. The nerve supply to the muscle, a branch of the anterior tibial nerve, is then sutured to a branch of the contralateral facial nerve. The muscle is then theoretically revascularized from the surrounding soft tissue. Freilinger used the same concept but preceded muscle transfer by a cross-facial nerve graft several months before the transfer so that the transplanted muscle would be innervated more rapidly.[24] The procedure produced very weak muscular activity.

With the development of microsurgical small vessel anastomosis the immediate revascularization of a transplanted muscle to the face became possible.[25,26] Harii first demonstrated this by transferring a portion of the gracilis muscle to the face after a cross-facial nerve graft.[27] This subsequently has also been done utilizing the pectoralis minor,[28] the latissimus dorsi,[29] or a portion of the serratus anterior muscle[30] as the muscle unit to be transferred to supply reanimation.

The use of a vascularized distant muscle transfer for unilateral facial paralysis is done in two stages. A cross-facial nerve graft is performed, and the distal end of the graft is positioned in the preauricular region on the paralyzed side (Figure 61-1). No attempt is made to connect the nerve to the existing facial musculature. Six to 10 months after the Tinel's sign has reached the distal stump of the nerve graft, the vascularized muscle transfer can be done (Figure 61-1B). A modification of a face lift/parotid incision is made on the paralyzed side of the face, and the recipient vessels and the distal stump of the cross-facial nerve graft are identified. The cheek is then undermined to provide space for the transferred muscle. The donor muscle and its neurovascular pedicle is simultaneously harvested. The muscle is then transferred to the face, and the microvascular repair of the vessels and nerves is completed. The muscle is anchored to the preauricular and mastoid regions, and the slips of the muscle are split and attached to the designated anatomic areas (i.e., oral commissure). Active contraction is usually seen in the transplanted muscle between 6 months and 1 year after the transfer.

The results of cross-facial nerve grafting and distant vascularized muscle transfer have varied. Reports of weak contraction, excessive contraction, bulkiness of the muscle, and mass movement have been made.[28,29,31,32] Despite these possible problems, the technique is becoming more widely accepted because no facial motor re-education is needed, as is the case with local transfers. With microvascular free tissue transfers there is no loss of intact facial reanimation on the treated side.

STATIC PROCEDURES

Various static techniques have been attempted to recreate facial symmetry. These procedures have been used to complement dynamic methods of reconstruction or as definitive treatment. Neurectomy or myomectomy on the contralateral side of the face have been advocated to produce balance with the paralyzed side of the face.[33,34] Facial and dermal slings have been used to elevate specific areas of the paralyzed face, but these frequently stretched over time.[35] Wedge resections of the lower eyelids, lateral canthoplasty, lid magnets, loading the lid with weights, and various froms of palpebral springs all have had varying levels of success in protecting exposed cornea.[3639]

CONCLUSION

It has been said that "in facial paralysis, joy, happiness, sorrow, shock, surprise, and all emotions have for their common expression the same blank stare."[40] The need to correct this "blank stare" has prompted generations of surgeons to pursue this goal by alternative methods. While a single procedure to recreate the natural harmony of emotion and the protective function produced by the facial musculature remains elusive, there are now at least options available to patients with unilateral facial paralysis. These surgical options can help to break the monotony of the "blank stare" and by doing so, provide an effect where once there was none.

REFERENCES

1. Seddon H: Three types of nerve injury. Brain 66:237, 1943
2. Sunderland S: Nerve and Nerve Injuries. Edinburgh, Churchill-Livingstone, 1972, Ch. 9

3. Freeman B: Facial palsy, in Converse J (ed): Reconstructive Plastic Surgery, ed 2, vol 3. Philadelphia, W.B. Saunders, 1977, Ch 36

4. Gutmann E, Young J: The reinnervation of muscle after various periods of atrophy. J Anat 78:15, 1944

5. Sunderland S: Capacity of reinnervated muscles to function efficiently after prolonged denervation. Arch Neurol Psychiatr 64:755, 1950

6. May M, Hardin W: Facial palsy: Interpretation of neurological findings. Laryngoscope 8:1352, 1978

7. Hughes G: Electroneurography: Objective prognostic assessment of facial paralysis. Am J Otol 4:73, 1982

8. Smith J: A new technique of facial animation, in Hueston J (ed): Transactions of the Fifth International Congress of Plastic and Reconstructive Surgery. Australia, Butterworth, 1971, p 83

9. Scarmella L: L'Anastomosi Tra I Due Nervi Facciali. Arch Otolagia 82:209, 1971

10. Andrel H: Reconstruction of the face through cross facial nerve transplantation in facial paralysis. Chir Plast 2:17, 1973

11. Fisch U: Facial nerve grafting. Otolaryngol Clin North Am 7:517, 1974

12. Andrel H: Cross face nerve grafting—up to 12 months of seventh nerve disruption, in Rubin L (ed): Reanimation of the Paralyzed Face. St. Louis, CV Mosby, 1977

13. Fisch U: Current surgical treatment of intratemporal facial palsy. Clin Plast Surg 6:377, 1979

14. Conley J: Myths and misconceptions in the rehabilitation of facial paralysis. Plast Reconstr Surg 71:538, 1983

15. Delbeke J, Thauloy C: Electrophysiologic evaluation of cross-facial nerve graft and treatment of facial palsy. Acta Neurochir 65:111, 1982

16. Tolhurst D, Bos K: Free revascularized muscle grafts in facial paralysis. Plast Reconstr Surg 69:760, 1982

17. Korte W: Ein Fall von Nervenpropfung des Nervus Fascialis auf den Nervus Hypoglossus. Dtsch Med Wochenschr 29:2 1903

18. Sargent P: Four cases of facial paralysis treated by hypoglossal facial anastomosis. Proc R Soc Med 12:69, 1911

19. Perret G: Results of phrenicofacial nerve anastomosis for facial paralysis. Arch Surg 94:505, 1967

20. Conley J, Baker D: Hypoglossal-facial nerve anastomosis for reinnervation of the paralyzed face. Plast Reconstr Surg 63:63, 1979

21. Rubin L: Reanimation of the Paralyzed Face. St. Louis, CV Mosby, 1977

22. Tucker H: Restoration of selective facial nerve function by the nerve-muscle pedicle technique. Clin Plast Surg 6:293, 1979

23. Thompson N: Autogenous free grafts of skeletal muscle. A preliminary experimental and clinical study. Plast Reconstr Surg 48:11, 1971

24. Freilinger G: A new technique to correct facial paralysis. Plast Reconstr Surg 56:44, 1975

25. Jacobson J, Suarez E: Microsurgery in anastomosis of small vessels. Surg Forum 9:243, 1960

26. Tamai S: Free muscle transplants in dogs with microsurgical neurovascular anastomosis. Plast Reconstr Surg 46:219, 1970

27. Mayou B, Watson J, Harrison D, et al: Free microvascular and microneural transfer of the extensor digitorum brevis muscle for the treatment of unilateral facial palsy. Br J Plast Surg 34:362, 1981

28. Harrison D: The pectoralis minor vascularized muscle graft for the treatment of unilateral facial palsy. Plast Reconstr Surg 75:206, 1985

29. Harii K: Treatment of long standing facial paralysis by combining vascularized muscle transplantation with crossface nerve grafting, in Buncke H, Furnas D (eds): Symposium on Clinical Frontiers in Reconstructive Microsurgery. St. Louis, CV Mosby, 1984, pp 159–171

30. Buncke H, Alpert B, Gordon L, et al: Free serratus anterior muscle transplantation for unilateral facial nerve paralysis. Presented at the American Association of Plastic Surgeons Meeting, Chicago, Illinois, 1984

31. Harii K, Ohmori K, Torm S: Free gracilis muscle transplantation with microvascular anastomosis for the treatment of facial paralysis. Plast Reconstr Surg 57:133, 1976

32. Harrison D, Mayou B: Extensor digitorum brevis and pectoralis major and minor muscles in the treatment of unilateral facial palsy, in Buncke H, Furnas D (eds): Symposium on Clinical Frontiers in Reconstructive Microsurgery. St. Louis, CV Mosby, 1984, pp 177–187

33. Niklison J: Contribution to the subject of facial paralysis. Plast Reconstr Surg 17:276, 1956

34. Rubin L, Lee G, Simpson S: Reanimation of the long-standing partial facial paralysis. Plast Reconstr Surg 77:41, 1986

35. Edgerton M, Wolfort F: The dermal flap canthal lift for lower eyelid support. Plast Reconstr Surg 43:42, 1969

36. Jelks G, Smith B, Bosniak S: The evaluation and management of the eye in facial palsy. Clin Plast Surg 6:397, 1979

37. Muhlbauer W, Sageth H, Viessman H: Restoration of lid function in facial palsy with permanent magnets. Chir Plast 1:295, 1973

38. Smellie G: Restoration of the blinking reflex in facial palsy by a simple lid load operation. Br J Plast Surg 19:279, 1966

39. Morel-Fatio D, Laladrie J: Palliative surgical treatment of facial paralysis. The palpebral spring. Plast Reconstr Surg 23:446, 1964

40. Bunnell S: Suture of the facial nerve within the temporal bone with a report of the first successful case. Surg Gynecol Obstet 45:7, 1927

CHAPTER 62

The Surgical Treatment of Primary Brain Stem Tumors

A. Konovalov   J. Atieh

BRAIN STEM TUMORS constitute about 5 to 15 percent of all intracranial tumors.[1-3] A frequency of up to 25 percent for these tumors has been noted in childhood and adolescence.[4,5] These numbers are higher if the thalamus is considered a part of the brain stem.[6-10]

Brain stem gliomas can be benign or malignant. Malignant brain stem gliomas are more common,[11-16] however, some authors have reported an equal frequency of malignant and benign tumors.[17-23]

Historically, all brain stem gliomas were considered to be infiltrative, characterized by a diffuse proliferation that causes enlargement or hypertrophy of the brain stem. Hoffman[13] reported a small series of caudal brain stem tumors that did not infiltrate the brain stem but expanded into the subarachnoid space and into the lumen of the fourth ventricle. These tumors can be well circumscribed and grow expansively within the brain stem.[24] Such nodular astrocytomas have been encountered in the cerebral aqueduct[25] and in the pineal region.[26] Study of these nodular tumors is very important because the successful removal of some types of brain stem tumors has recently been reported.[24,27-31]

Brain stem tumors are diagnosed mainly from clinical findings and computed tomographic (CT) and magnetic resonance imaging (MRI) examination. The CT scan with intravenous[32] or intrathecal[33,34] injection of contrast medium and especially the MRI scan[35] can demonstrate the presence and precise location of brain stem tumors.

The treatment of patients with primary brain stem gliomas is a controversial subject. Until recently, radiotherapy administered without biopsy or histologic study of the tumor was the principal form of treatment for patients with brain stem gliomas. Almost invariably the prognosis was bad and survival for longer than 1 year was so rare that Matson concluded: ''Should any patient with a clinical diagnosis of brain stem glioma still be alive as long as 18 months after diagnosis, with or without x-ray treatment, reinvestigation and probably surgical exploration is indicated, as some other lesion is probably present.''[36] In contrast, a number of reports cited the beneficial effect of radiation therapy[19,20,37,38] or chemotherapy[39] on some brain stem tumors.

Biopsy of brain stem tumors has been considered dangerous and unnecessary. This opinion continues to be shared by some authors.[40,41] In contrast, others consider it a safe approach that can be important in planning radio- or chemotherapy.[22,23,42]

When the tumor occludes CSF pathways different shunting procedures have been widely used.[21,43]

Isolated cases of long-term survival following aspiration of cystic components[44,45,46] or partial resection of extra-axial portions of brain stem gliomas,[47,48] in which radiotherapy is also given have been reported.

Recently, favorable results have been achieved with the radical removal of nodular intrinsic brain stem gliomas.[24,30,31,49,50] This success is the result of the use of the operating microscope, the laser,[31] and the ultrasonic aspirator.[30]

Attempts to remove malignant brain stem tumors have not changed the utterly unfavorable prognosis of this disease. This chapter of neurosurgery, which was described by Bailey[51] in 1939 as a ''pessimistic'' one, has just begun to develop and the possibility of surgical treatment of primary brain stem tumors is still open to question. The present report is meant to share our initial experience with the surgical removal of tumors of different parts of the brain stem.

MATERIALS AND METHODS

Quite recently treatment of brain stem gliomas at the Moscow Burdenko Institute of Neurosurgery has been limited to exploration, cyst aspiration, biopsy, or partial resection of extra-axial portions of the tumor with subsequent radiotherapy. Patients with obstructive hydrocephalus were treated with various CSF diversionary procedures. At the Burdenko Institute, however, there have been cases of caudal brain stem gliomas growing into the fourth ventricle that were successfully removed. These operations were performed by different surgeons and it is impossible to establish the exact extent of surgery; for this reason these cases are excluded from the present report.

Our experience is based on 38 cases in which radical removal of mostly nodular tumors in different parts of the brain stem were carried out. The patients consisted of 27 children (under 15 years of age) and 11 adults; 17 were males and 21 were females. All patients were operated upon during the last 4 years by the same surgeon (A.K.) using the same principles. In these cases the diagnosis was based on CT scans alone or in combination with MRI scans, and the extent of tumor removal in the majority of cases was subsequently assessed using these same methods.

OPERATIVE NEUROSURGICAL TECHNIQUES
ISBN 0-8089-1862-1

The tumors were located predominantly in the caudal brain stem (pons and medulla) in 16 patients, in the midbrain in 9 patients, and in the thalamus in 13 patients. However, these tumors often involved different parts of the brain stem; some pontine tumors spread into the midbrain and some midbrain tumors penetrated the thalamus and the pons or vice versa. In some cases, portions of the brain stem were involved (see Figure 62-29). For this reason and because the diencephalon is considered anatomically a part of the brain stem by some authors, we included thalamic tumors in our series. These lesions often grow into the midbrain and even into the pons.[6-10]

Thalamic tumors were also been included in the groups of brain stem gliomas reported by some authors.[38,41] In this chapter we did not include the results for patients with gliomas predominantly within the third ventricle, although these tumors can also be included among brain stem gliomas, since the techniques for the surgical removal of tumors in both locations have some specific features in common.

The histologic tumor types in the cases included:

1. Fibrillary astrocytoma (grade II): 24 patients.
2. Pilocytic astrocytoma (grade I): 4 patients.
3. Protoplasmic astrocytoma (grade II): 3 patients.
4. Subependymal giant cell astrocytoma (grade I): 1 patient.
5. Ganglioglioma (grade I-II): 2 patients.
6. Anaplastic (malignant) astrocytoma (grade III): 2 patients.
7. Astroblastoma (grade III-IV): 1 patient.
8. Primitive polar spongioblastoma (grade IV): 1 patient.

We also analyzed the pathologic characteristics of the lesions of 26 patients (only 3 of whom had been operated upon) with primary brain stem tumors who died at our Institute prior to the series under discussion. The purpose of this study was to determine the topographic variants of brain stem gliomas and to clarify their relationship to the neural structures. The histologic tumor types in this group of 26 patients were:

1. Fibrillary astrocytoma (grade II): 19 cases.
2. Pilocytic astrocytoma (grade I): 3 cases.
3. Protoplasmic astrocytoma (grade II): 3 cases.
4. Glioblastoma (grade IV): 1 case.

The topography of the tumor was investigated under the dissecting microscope and in 15 cases with serial microscopic sections of the entire brain stem including the tumor and stained with thionine, Spielmeyer's, Nissl's, or hematoxylin-eosin

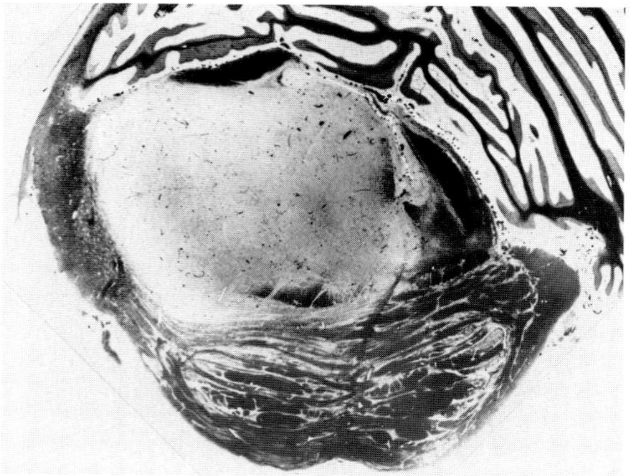

Fig. 62-1. Intratruncal caudal brain stem fibrillary astrocytoma. Spielmeyer's stain.

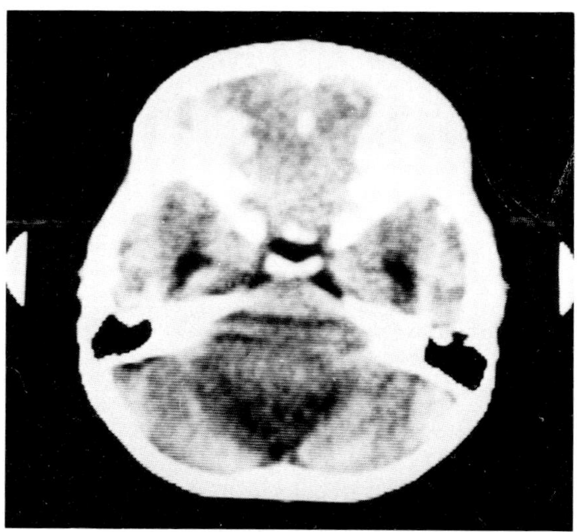

Fig. 62-2. A CT scan obtained after intravenous injection of contrast medium showing a hypodense zone caused by an intratruncal protoplasmic astrocytoma of the caudal brain stem (verified at surgery).

stains. These preparations allowed us to study the structure of the tumor and the relationship of the tumor and its margins to the adjacent brain tissue.

To determine the accuracy of CT and MRI scanning in the diagnosis of brain stem gliomas, in addition to the 38 patients undergoing surgery, we analyzed another 11 cases in which parapontine tumors were misdiagnosed as primary brain stem gliomas.

Auditory evoked potentials were assessed in 12 patients with caudal brain stem tumors and in 3 patients with thalamic and midbrain gliomas to assess brain stem function. In addition, somatosensory evoked potentials were also recorded in 3 patients with oral brain stem tumors. Intraoperative and post-operative monitoring of evoked potentials was used in some cases.

RESULTS AND DISCUSSION

Our data were analyzed with particular attention to the following:

1. The topography of the gliomas, which involved different parts of the brain stem.
2. The relationship of the tumor to the brain structures in cases of infiltrative or nodular growth.
3. Diagnosing brain stem gliomas and predicting the type of tumor growth (nodular or infiltrative) and its histology based on CT and MRI scans.
4. Defining the indications for direct surgical removal of primary brain stem gliomas and the surgical techniques to be used.
5. Evaluating the results of this surgery.

In view of the relatively few cases and the short follow-up, we consider the present report a preliminary one.

BRAIN STEM TUMORS—
ANATOMIC STUDIES

Based on our morphologic investigations and intraoperative observations, we developed the following categories of primary brain stem tumors:

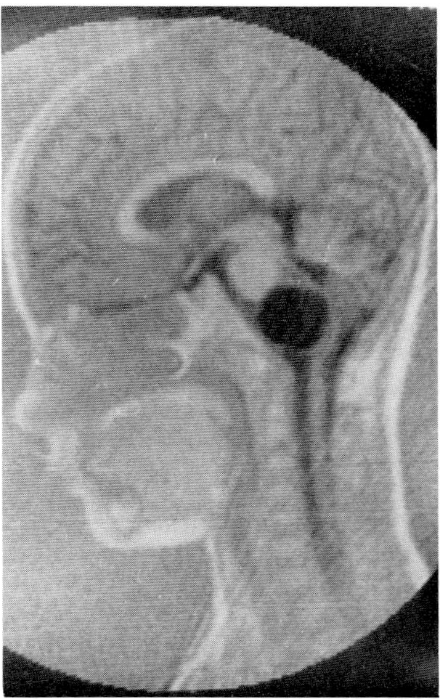

Fig. 62-3. A MRI scan demonstrating a cystic fibrillary astrocytoma localized within the medulla and lower pons. At surgery the tumor found to have an intratruncal location.

1. Tumors of the caudal portion of the brain stem (pons and medulla).
2. Midbrain tumors.
3. Thalamic tumors.

Caudal brain stem tumors can be further subdivided into:

1. Intratruncal tumors: tumors confined intrinsically to the brain stem tissue practically without exophytic components into the fourth ventricle or parapontine cisterns (Figures 62-1, 62-2, and 62-3).

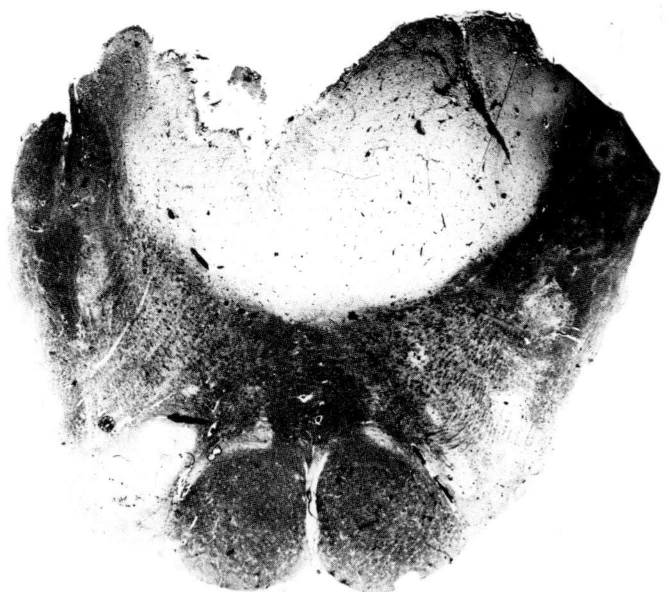

Fig. 62-4. A fibrillary astrocytoma arising from the tegmentum and filling the cavity of the fourth ventricle. The tumor has a well-defined border with the brain tissue. A thin (1–2 mm) zone of infiltration adjacent to the tumor nodule is visible. No brain stem structures within the tumor nodule were apparent under the microscope. Spielmeyer's stain.

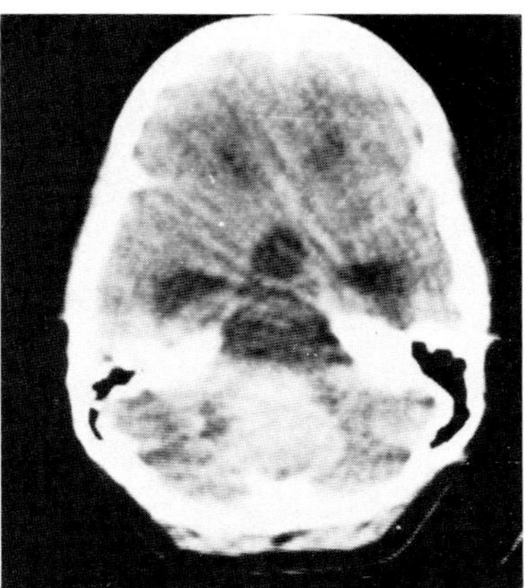

Fig. 62-5. A CT scan obtained after intravenous injection of contrast medium. Note the hyperdense zone caused by a fibrillary astrocytoma arising from the tegmentum of the caudal brain stem and filling the fourth ventricle. The tumor was verified at surgery.

2. Tumors arising from the tegmentum (the floor of the fourth ventricle) and forming nodules within the cavity of the fourth ventricle (Figures 62-4, 62-5, and 62-6). Often such tumors extend into the cisterna magna (c. cerebellomedullaris P.N.A.) through the foramen of Magendie, into the lateral pontine cistern through the foramen of Luschka, or into both.
3. Tumors involving half of the brain stem and filling the lateral pontine cistern (Figures 62-7 and 62-8). Such tumors are separated from the cavity of the fourth ventricle by a layer of brain stem tissue.

Midbrain tumors have three variants:

1. Tectal gliomas. The gliomas arise from the quadrigeminal plate and grow in the direction of the upper vermis and posterior third ventricle. The main part of the tumor occupies the quadrigeminal cistern (Figures 62-9 and 62-10). Large tumors of this variant may spread to the medial parts of the lateral ventricles and to the lateral portions of the ambient cistern.
2. Ventrally located tumors confined to one of the cerebral peduncles frequently spreading into the thalamus, into the pons, or into both. The most caudal portion of the tumor in such cases can be classified as caudal brain stem variants 1

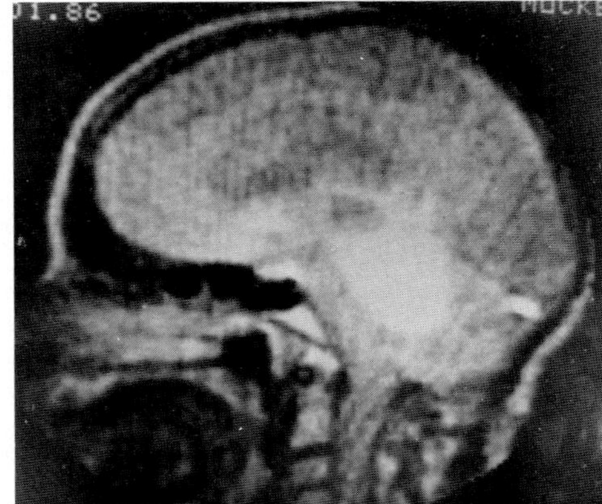

Fig. 62-6. A MRI scan showing a nodular protoplasmic astrocytoma of the caudal brain stem filling the fourth ventricle. At surgery the tumor was found to arise from the tegmentum of the pons and upper medulla.

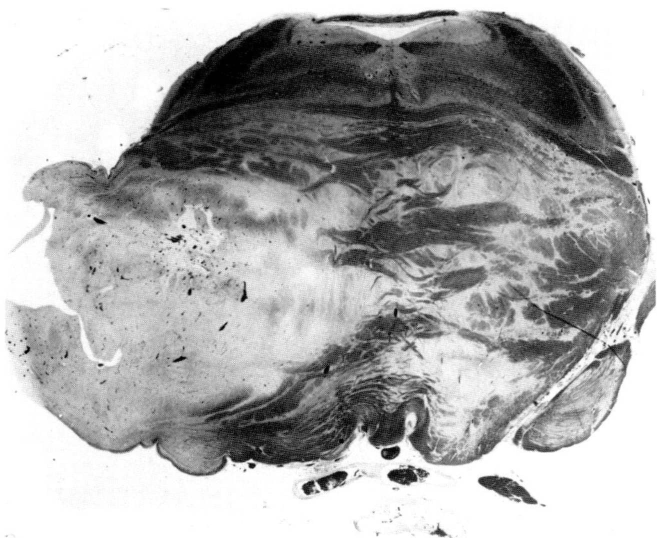

Fig. 62-7. A nodular pilocytic astrocytoma with a wide zone of infiltration. The tumor involves half of the caudal brain stem and forms a nodule in the lateral pontine cistern. Spielmeyer's stain.

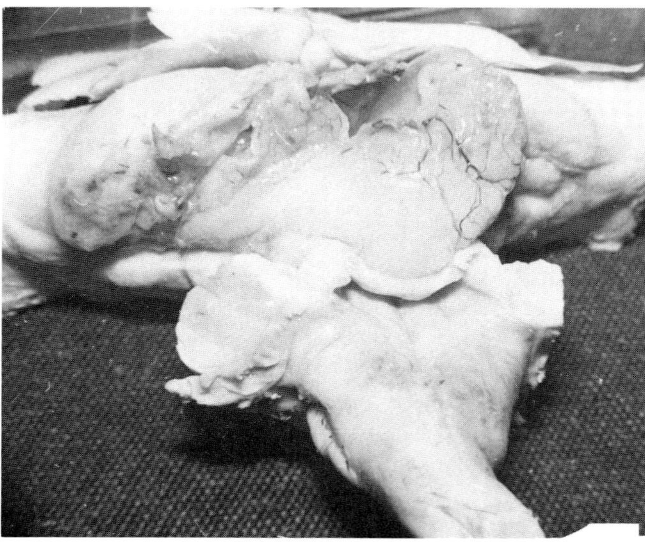

Fig. 62-9. A midbrain fibrillary astrocytoma filling the quadrigeminal cistern. The tumor arises from the tectum and displaces the anterior cerebral velum downward, which separates it from the cavity of the fourth ventricle.

or 3. These tumors may be large, with exophytic components filling the lateral parts of the ambient cistern and the lateral pontine cistern and may even spread into the medial portions of the middle cerebral fossa (Figures 62-11, 62-12, and 62-13).

3. Tumors of the cerebral aqueduct, which are relatively small and circumscribed (Figure 62-14) and do not penetrate the central gray substance. We only had autopsy examples of these tumors, but reports of their surgical removal exist in the literature.[45] It therefore is important to distinguish this variant of midbrain tumors.

Thalamic tumors can be divided into two variants:

1. Pulvinar gliomas (see Figures 62-20D and E) arise from the posterior portion of the thalamus and spread to the retrothalamic and quadrigeminal cisterns. Often such tumors grow into the midbrain. Tectal and pulvinar gliomas are often included among the group of pineal region or posterior third ventricle tumors.[52,53]

2. Gliomas of the middle and anterior thalamus, which usually spread into the basal ganglia (see Figures 62-20A, 62-32A and B), the cavity of the third ventricle (Figure 62-15), and the hypothalamus. Such tumors are often large and may spread into one cerebral peduncle and the pons (see Figures 62-28A, B, C, and D and 62-29).

We considered such detailed differentiation of brain stem gliomas essential, because tumors in different locations require different surgical approaches.

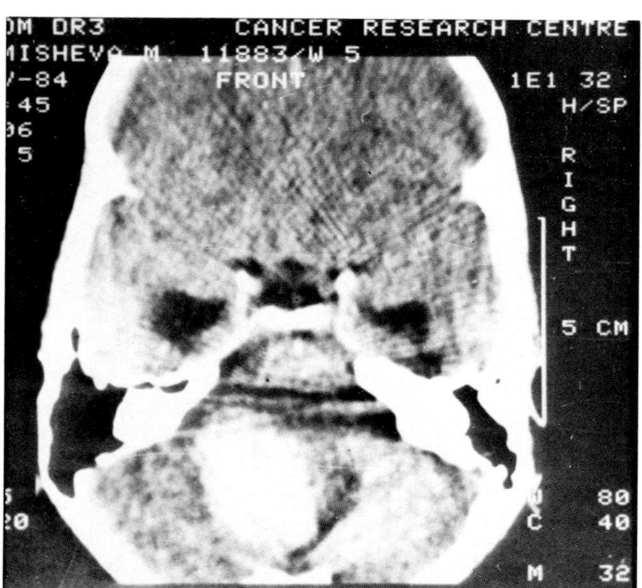

Fig. 62-8. A CT scan obtained after intravenous injection of contrast medium. There is a hyperdense zone caused by a pilocytic astrocytoma of the left half of the caudal brain stem. At surgery the tumor was found to fill the left pontine cistern.

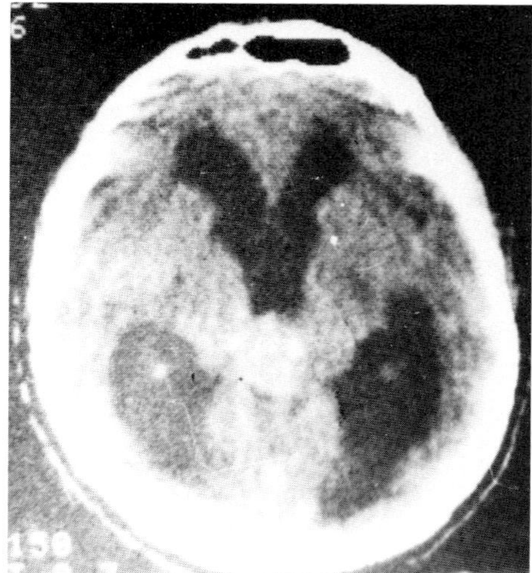

Fig. 62-10. A CT scan with enhancement. The hyperdense zone is a result of a dorsally localized midbrain (tectal) ganglioglioma.

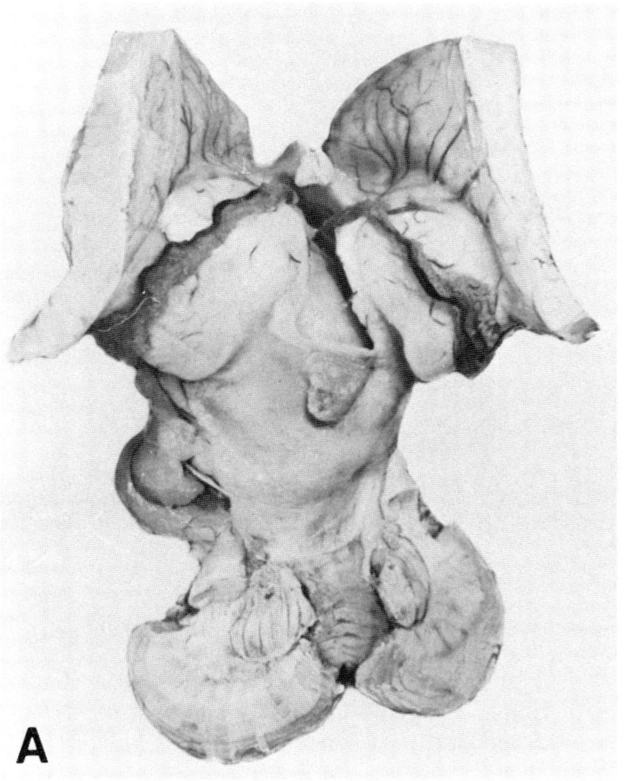

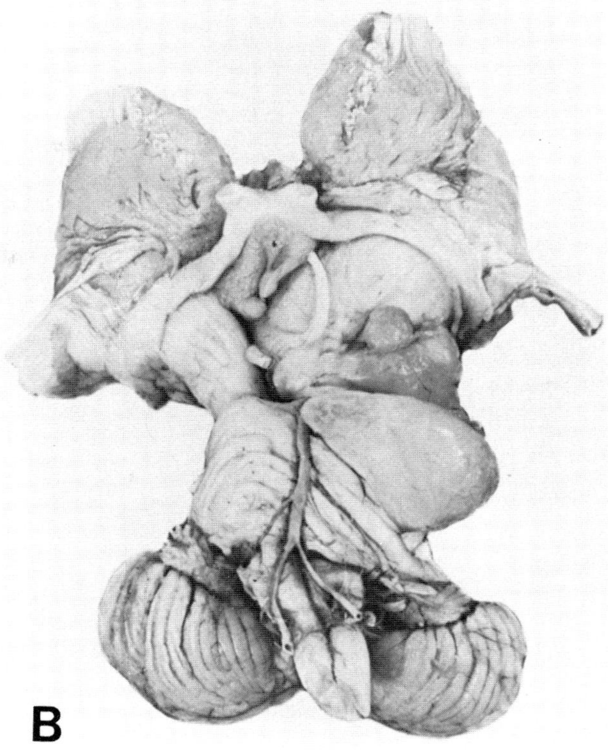

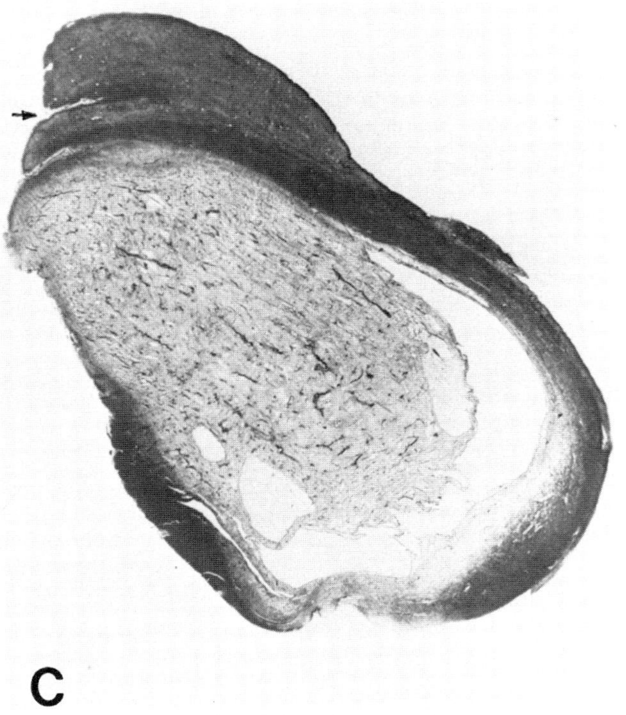

Fig. 62-11. A ventrally localized midbrain fibrillary astrocytoma. (A) The dorsal aspect of the brain stem; the enlarged left cerebral peduncle bulges into the cavity of the third ventricle. (B) The ventral aspect of the brain stem. The left oculomotor nerve is displaced medially and forward by the enlarged left cerebral peduncle. Exophytic components of the tumor fill the left half of the ambient cistern and deform the upper left half of the pons. (C) Microscopic section through the left cerebral peduncle at the level of the upper colliculi. The tumor occupies the interior parts of the left cerebral peduncle. It has a well-defined border with the brain tissue. Arrows: the cerebral aqueduct. Spielmeyer's stain.

TYPES OF GROWTH OF BRAIN STEM GLIOMAS

In making a decision about whether to remove a primary brain stem tumor, one of the important factors is to identify nodular forms that might be anatomically amenable to radical excision. Focal (nodular) brain stem gliomas are probably more frequent than is apparent from the literature.[13] No exact data about the frequency of nodular brain stem gliomas exists, but in 20 of 26 of our cases the tumor was a circumscribed nodule.

Our clinical, surgical, and morphologic data indicated that there are three growth types of brain stem gliomas:

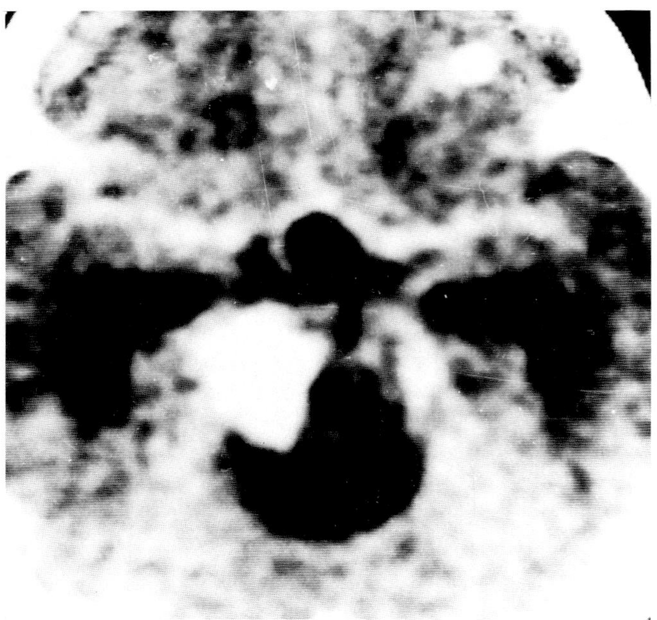

Fig. 62-12. A CT scan with enhancement. A cystic fibrillary astrocytoma of the left cerebral peduncle.

1. Nodular tumors with definite borders with the brain tissue.
2. Nodular tumors with a wide zone of infiltration into the adjacent brain tissue.
3. Infiltrative tumors.

The first growth type is characterized by a well circumscribed tumor with a tendency toward expansive growth. These tumors displace brain stem structures but do not seriously damage them. No brain elements are encountered within the tumor nodule (Figure 62-16). In some tumors of this type, a thin zone of infiltration (1–2 mm) adjacent to the tumor might exist (Figure 62-17).

The second growth type includes tumors with nodular growth and wide (about 5 mm) areas of infiltration (Figure 62-18). In such tumors a well-defined border exists between the nodule of the tumor (where tumor cell density is about 400,000/mm) and the zone of infiltration (with a relatively small amount of tumor cells) (Figure 62-18). This perifocal area may contain a zone of necrosis and dilated vessels with microcellular infiltration. Within this area are islands of tumor cells around the dilated vessels. In some instances we noted that the tumor invaded the brain tissue in a tongue-shaped manner (see Figure 62-7). In a few cases of this type we observed small colonies of tumor cells situated within the brain stem tissue distant from the main nodule and from each other. As in the first growth type, some portions of the tumor nodule of this growth type may have well-defined borders with the brain tissue.

In almost all cases of growth types I and II we observed an interesting phenomenon: the structure of the tumor might be different even at the same level of section, that is, near the portions of the tumor in which there were high amount of cells there were zones with low cellular density, small cysts, and necrosis (Figure 62-17).

As was previously mentioned, the tumor nodule of growth type I does not contain any neural elements; in contrast, in growth type II some elements of neural tracts (see Figure 62-1)

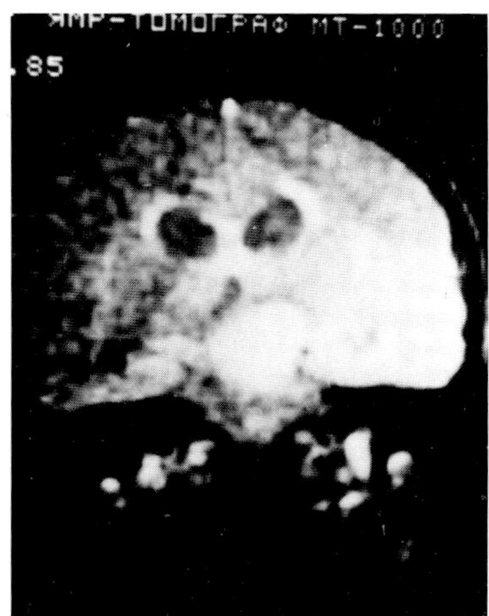

Fig. 62-13. A MRI scan, frontal section, showing a fibrillary astrocytoma of the left cerebral peduncle displacing the third ventricle medially.

or neurons can be found within the tumoral tissue (just near the zone of infiltration).

The third growth type is an infiltrative lesion. In these cases the tumor cells infiltrate between normal neural structures, separating them and producing a diffuse enlargement of the brain stem. It is difficult in such cases to define where the tumor ends and where neural structures begin, even with the operating microscope. This form of growth has been called "hypertrophy of the pons."[54] Fibrillary, pilocytic, and protoplasmic astrocytomas often grow in a type I or type II pattern although they can also be infiltrative.

Our classification is very schematic, and in some cases it may be quite difficult to differentiate tumors of the second and third growth types, although with the further development of the CT and MRI technology and with contrast enhancement it may soon be possible to differentiate between these types of lesions.

Focal circumscribed gliomas (growth type I and some growth type II) have a tendency to grow expansively, displacing nuclei and long tracts rather than destroying them. The direction of displacement of the neural structure depends upon the topographic variations of the tumor site. Thus, in cases of intratruncal gliomas of the caudal brain stem, dorsolateral displacement of the nuclei of the craniocerebral nerves occur, while the pyramidal tracts are displaced ventrolaterally. The caudal brain stem tumors of the second variant are characterized by ventrolateral displacement of the nuclei and tracts. Tumors affecting half of the caudal brain stem cause dorsomedial displacement of the nuclei and ventromedial displacement of the pyramidal tracts. These details require further study, but they must be kept in mind when a surgical approach is chosen.

Displacement of the midbrain and thalamic structures also occurs differently, depending upon the topographic variations of the tumor.

DIAGNOSTICS

Since the neurologic signs and symptoms of brain stem tumors are well known we will only evaluate those features that are important in the differentiation of focal and diffuse brain stem gliomas.

The relationship of the onset and duration of the illness to

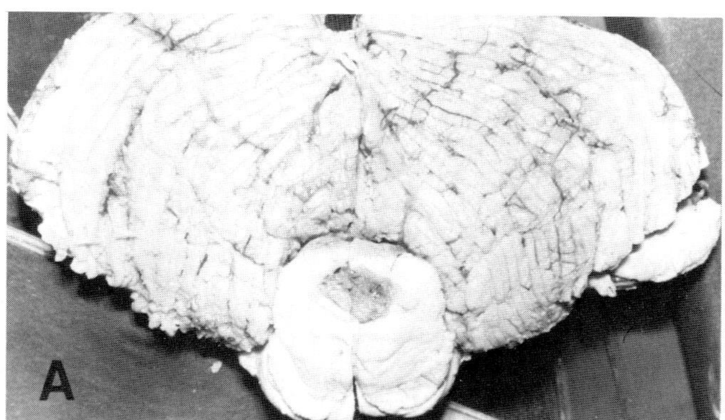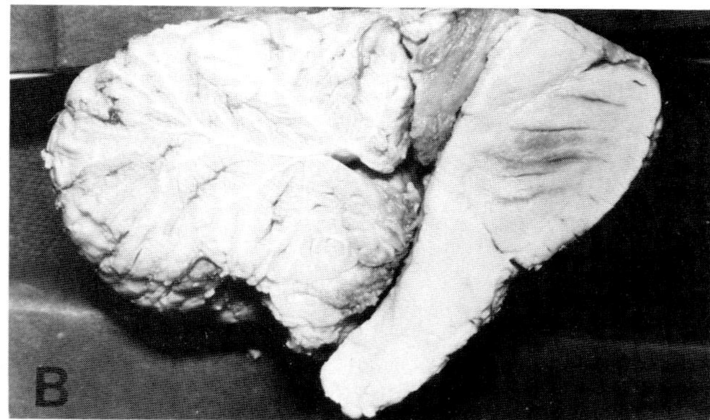

Fig. 62-14. A nodular fibrillary astrocytoma of the cerebral aqueduct. (A) Horizontal section. (B) Sagittal section.

the type of tumor growth is of some interest. Development of the tumor at an early age (under 4 years),[13] and its slow progression[24] are characteristics more typical of focal brain stem gliomas.

In our cases the development of the illness varied greatly. In the case of caudal brain stem tumors, patients had the tumors from 4 months to 13 years; for midbrain tumors it was 3 months to 26 years, and for thalamic tumors it was 5 months to 18 years.

Because in this study there were few (6 of 61) diffuse gliomas, we cannot compare them with focal gliomas. It should be mentioned, however, that we had cases of diffuse caudal brain stem tumor in which the tumor was present for 2 years before the diagnosis was established.

Focal brain stem tumors are more frequent in children than in adults (two thirds of our cases of nodular tumors occurred in children). The oldest patient was 59 years of age.

Although traditionally it is thought that intracranial hypertension is not common in patients with brain stem gliomas, the majority of our patients had evidence of raised intracranial pressure, and this was severe in over half of these cases (34 of 61). The incidence and degree of intracranial hypertension depends upon the location of the tumor. Midbrain, posterior thalamic, and caudal brain stem tumors extending into the fourth ventricle cause elevation of the intracranial pressure more often than tumors in other locations.

Clinical signs of unilateral damage of the craniocerebral

nerve nuclei and tracts in cases of focal caudal brain stem tumors were observed in 11 of 23 cases; however, this syndrome is not pathognomonic for focal gliomas because it is observed in some cases with diffuse tumors of the pons and medulla. This alternating syndrome is often observed in patients with tumors of one half of the caudal brain stem.

A quite rare and quite peculiar manifestation of thalamic and midbrain gliomas is persistent hyperkinesis of the contralateral extremities. In one such case hemilateral chorea was caused by a cystic fibrillary astrocytoma of the pons that spread into one cerebral peduncle and the thalamus. In two cases (one with a pulvinar anaplastic astrocytoma and the other with an anterior and midthalamic cystic ganglioglioma) athetosis was noted. Six patients had an atypical intension tremor of the extremities and in these patients the tumors were located in the anterior and middle thalamus (2 patients), the pulvinar (1 patient), the midbrain (2 patients), and the pons and cerebral peduncle (1 patient). One of these 6 patients had a ganglioglioma and the other 5 had fibrillary astrocytomas. All patients with hyperkinesis had brain stem tumors of the nodular type. Hyperkinesis caused by thalamic and midbrain tumors has also been noted by other investigators.[55–61]

There are a number of single observations in the literature of thalamic pain syndrome caused by thalamic tumors.[27,56–58,62–65] Among our cases only 1 patient exhibited intractable pain in the right hand and leg as a result of a large

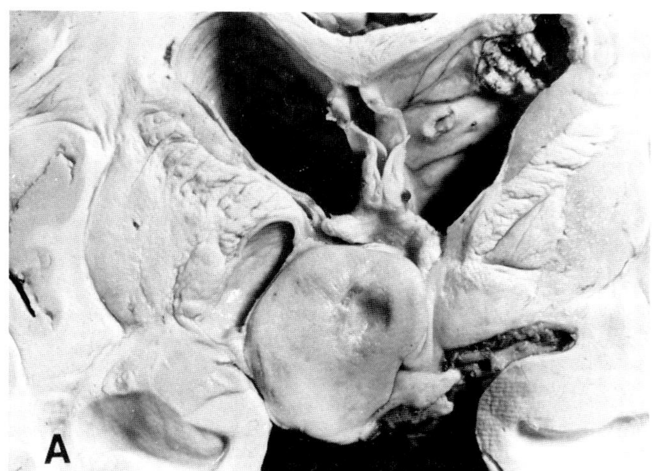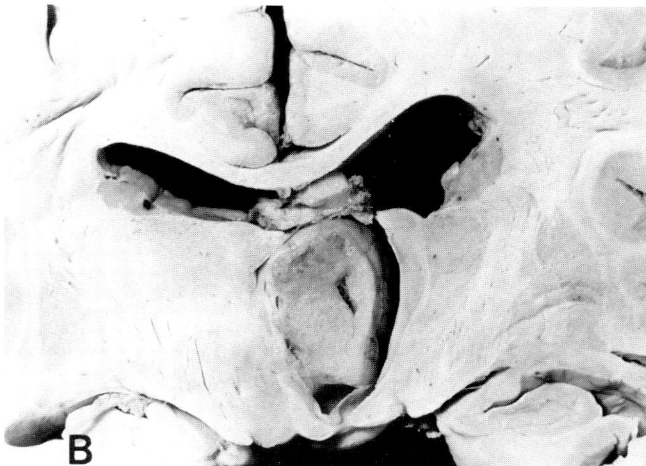

Fig. 62-15. A right thalamic fibrillary astrocytoma of the nodular type. (A) Frontal section anterior to the chiasm. The nodular tumor occupies the cavity of the fourth ventricle, displacing its floor and the chiasm downward. There is a cyst in the region of the interior capsule. (B) The tumor arises from the medial portions of the right thalamus.

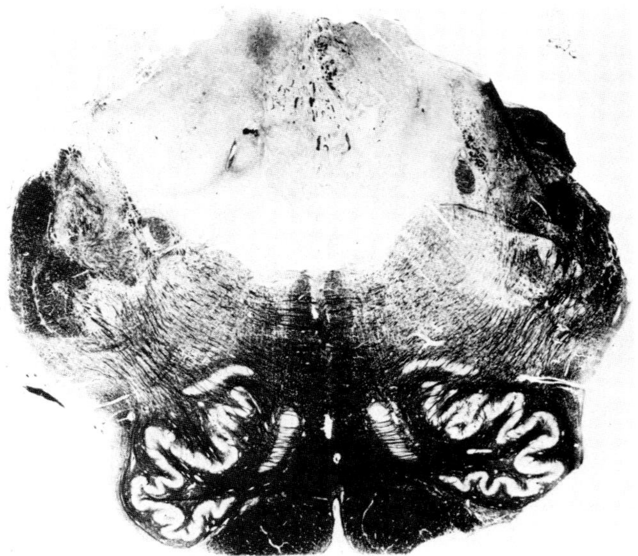

Fig. 62-16. A fibrillary astrocytoma arising from the tegmentum of the caudal brain stem. Note the well-defined border with the brain tissue. There are no brain structures within the tumor nodule and the tumor does not infiltrate the brain stem. The brain structures are displaced by the tumor. Spielmeyer's stain; original magnification × 25.

glioma of the anterior and middle portions of the left thalamus extending to the basal ganglia and hypothalamus.

EVOKED POTENTIALS

Evoked potentials are being used increasingly pre) and postoperatively in patients with brain stem tumors to monitor brain stem function. This study can also be recorded during surgery without undue prolongation of operating time and inconvenience to the surgeon. In addition, one report indicates that this method can be sensitive in detecting even subclinical lesions (a case of mesencephalic glioma[66]).

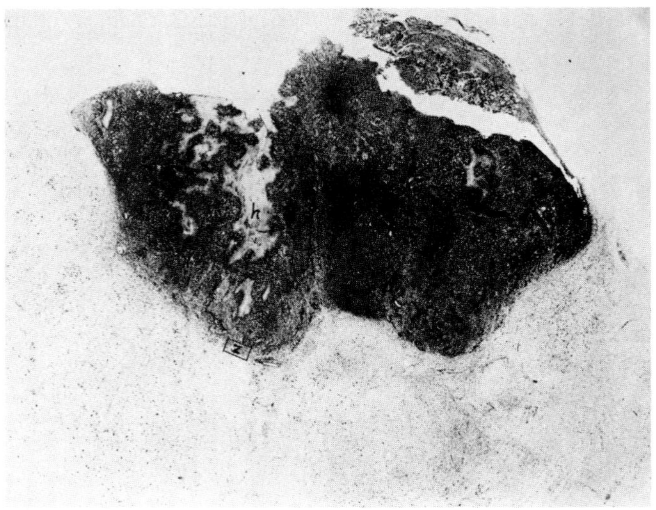

Fig. 62-17. A fibrillary astrocytoma with a well-defined border with the brain tissue. A small thin (1–2 mm) layer of infiltration can be seen just near the tumoral nodule (Z). A difference in structure (d,h) of the tumoral nodule at the same level of section is seen. Nissel's stain; original magnification: × 25.

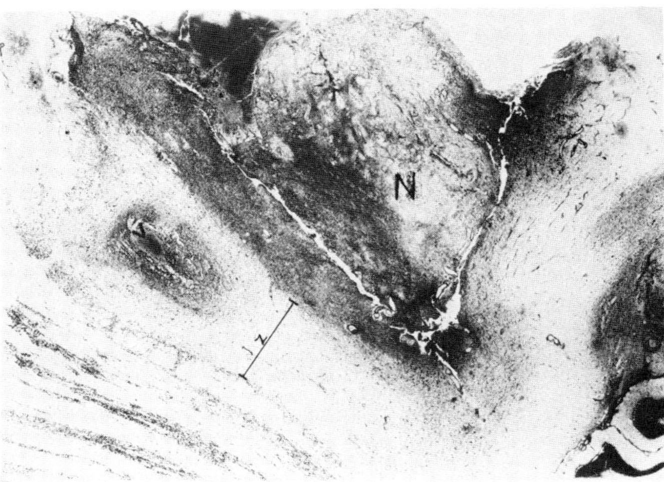

Fig. 62-18. A well-demarcated tumor nodule (N) associated with a wide (5 mm) zone of infiltration (Z). V = vessel. Nissl's stain; original magnification: × 25.

In 4 of 12 patients examined, brain stem auditory evoked potentials (BSAEPs) were normal. The tumor was located within the oral brain stem in 3 of these patients, and in one there was an intratruncal tumor of the medulla and lower pons.

Eight observations with pontine tumors were associated with BSAEP changes, characterized by prolongation of the interwave latency and a reduction of the IV and V components. When there was asymmetry of the BSAEP, the more pronounced changes were on the side of the lesion. Oh[67] reported possible lateralization of brain stem lesions by BSAEP.

Since the short latency evoked potentials were relatively resistant to anesthetic agents and independent of the arousal level of the patient and relatively unaffected by alterations in blood pressure and acid-base balance, they have been widely used for intraoperative monitoring during manipulation of the brain stem or to monitor the physiologic effects of tumor resection. We also consider this method to be important and informative in evaluating the function of the brain stem structures in the postoperative period.

CT AND MRI DIAGNOSIS

Computed tomography with intravenous and intrathecal administration of contrast is one of the best methods for diagnosing brain stem tumors, nevertheless, in 3 of 48 cases tumors were not disclosed by this method, an experience confirmed by Bilaniuk.[32] In some (especially caudal brain stem tumors), it was difficult or impossible to differentiate between primary brain stem and parapontine tumors (Figure 62-19).

A considerable number of our brain stem gliomas are isodense and do not enhance with contrast. In these cases the CT scan is an indirect guide to a mass lesion of the brain stem, revealing occlusive hydrocephalus or narrowing of the paratruncal cisterns. As a rule, however, a CT scan with intravenous injection of contrast medium showed hyperdense (up to 54 Hounsfield units), hypodense (up to 20 Hounsfield units), or heterogenous lesions. Additional information was gained in some cases by CT cisternography after intrathecal injection of contrast. This method was helpful in some cases in defining the exact location and extent of the tumor.

In 24 percent of cases it was possible to recognize cystic

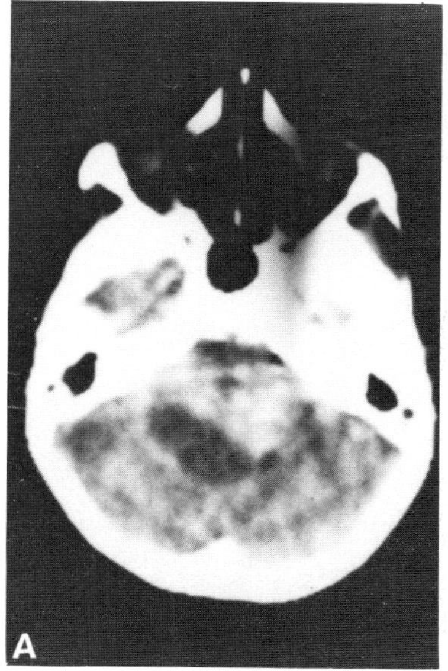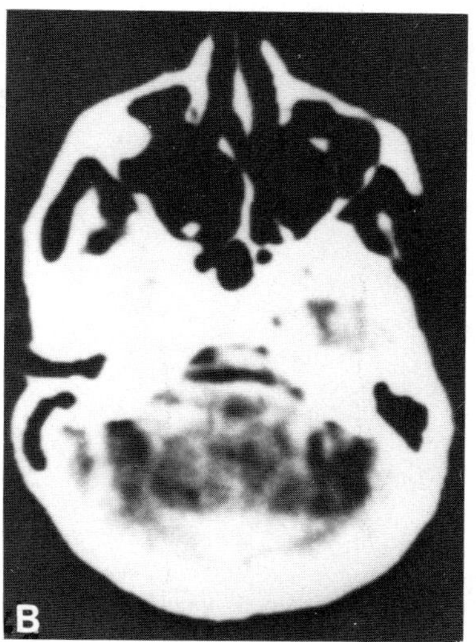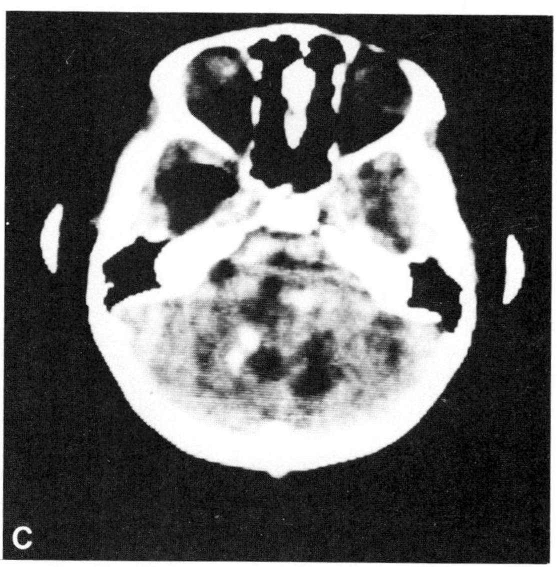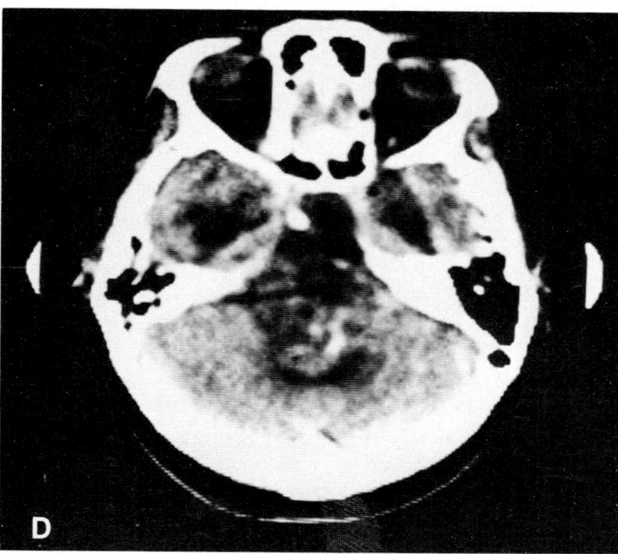

Fig. 62-19. Identical CT images of brain stem and paratruncal tumors after intravenous injection of contrast medium. (A) Fibrillary astrocytoma and (B) cystic acoustic neuroma. (C) Fibrillary astrocytoma and (D) epidermoid, invading the brain stem.

portions of the tumor. These cysts were of different sizes; the largest one was 76 mm by 45 mm. The tumor nodules also were of various sizes, in some cases 40 to 60 mm in diameter.

The CT scan appearance does not allow one to predict the histologic type of tumor or to differentiate between benign and malignant brain stem tumors, since approximately identical CT scans were seen in malignant and benign brain stem gliomas (Figure 62-20), and, conversely, tumors of identical histologic type often have a different CT scan appearance (Figure 62-21).

The importance of CT scans lies in the possibility of recognizing nodular and infiltrative brain stem gliomas. Of 44 cases in which the correct diagnosis of brain stem glioma was made from the CT scans, in 38 cases a recognizable border between the tumor and normal tissue could be seen on the CT scan, and this was subsequently confirmed by surgery or autopsy. It is problematic to differentiate between perifocal edema and the zone of tumor infiltration with the aid of CT

scans. In about half of the cases with nodular tumors at surgery or autopsy we observed an infiltrative zone of varying width around the tumor nodule. This zone appeared as an area of low density and was preoperatively thought to represent peritumoral edema.

Of 5 cases in which the CT scan showed an infiltrative tumor without any borders with the brain tissue, 3 were morphologically proven infiltrative and 2 were focal tumors. This discrepancy between the CT and morphologic findings is the result of the CT examination having been performed without intravenous contrast enhancement.

Some practice is needed to diagnose primary brain stem tumors and to detect their topographic variations on CT scans. That is why in our early CT studies decisions about tumor location were not always correct.

Our experience with MRI in evaluating brain stem gliomas is limited to 10 cases; nevertheless, some preliminary impres-

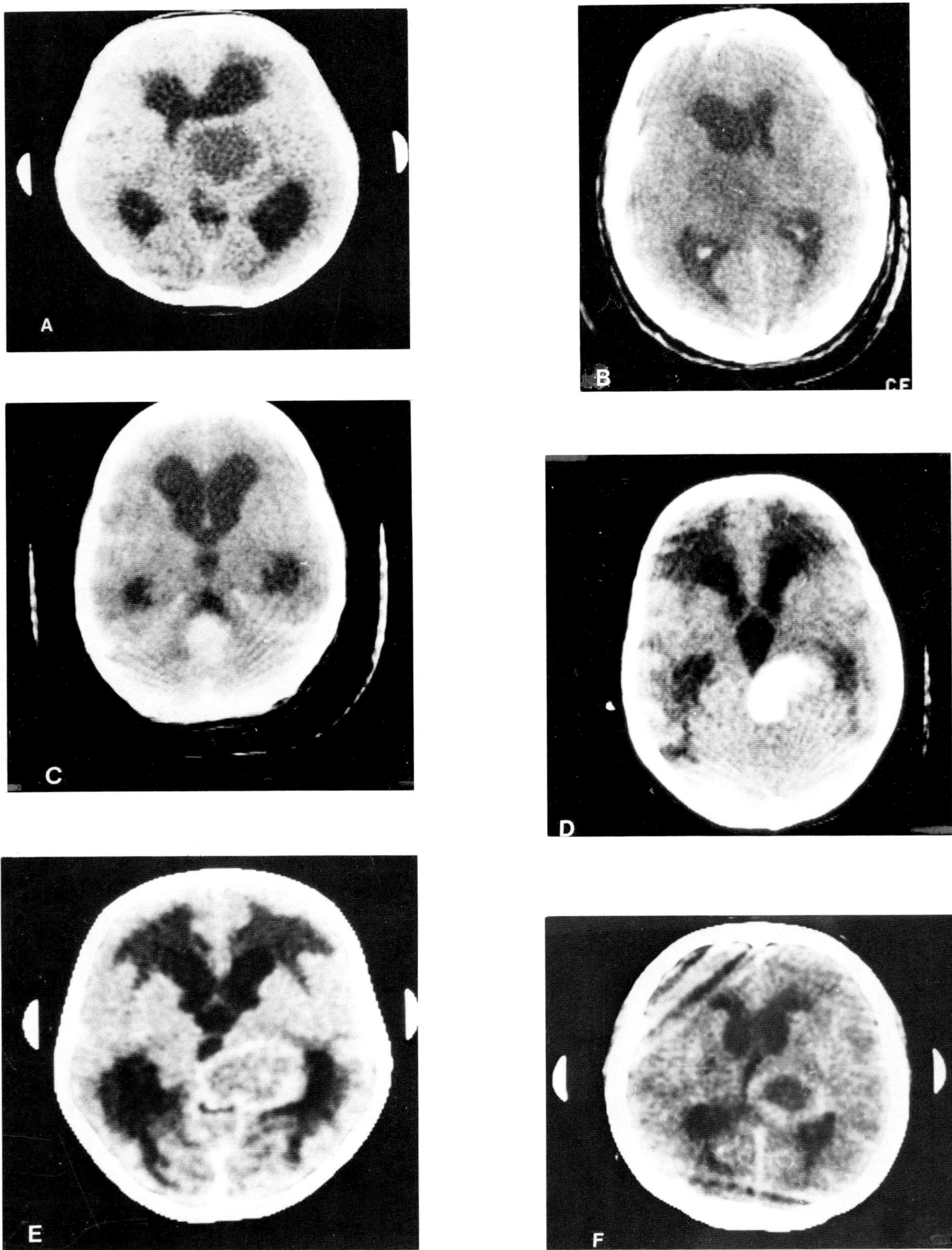

Fig. 62-20 (continued).

sions about its advantages are that MRI is better than CT in evaluating brain stem tumors, especially those involving the medulla and lower pons, a finding confirming that of Zimmerman.[35] Magnetic resonance imaging facilitates the recognition of tumors spreading along the brain stem axis and the differentiation of various topographic variations of tumor. In some cases MRI is helpful in detecting caudal brain stem gliomas that were misdiagnosed on the CT scans. In some cases MRI allowed better prediction of tumor size and growth (nodular or infiltrative) than the CT scan. In these cases the MRI scan resolved a ''CT-probable'' into a ''MRI-definite'' focal tumor (Figure 62-22).

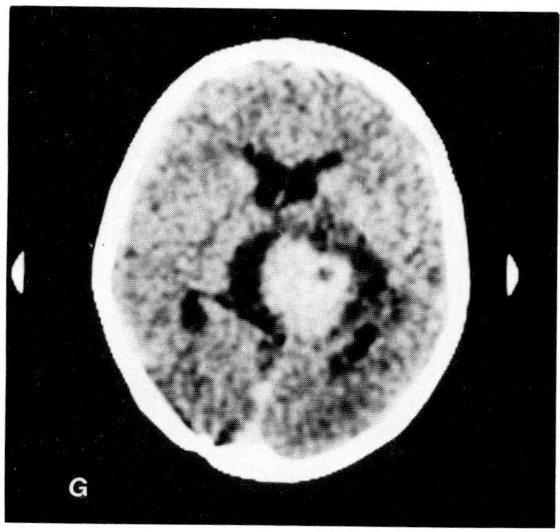

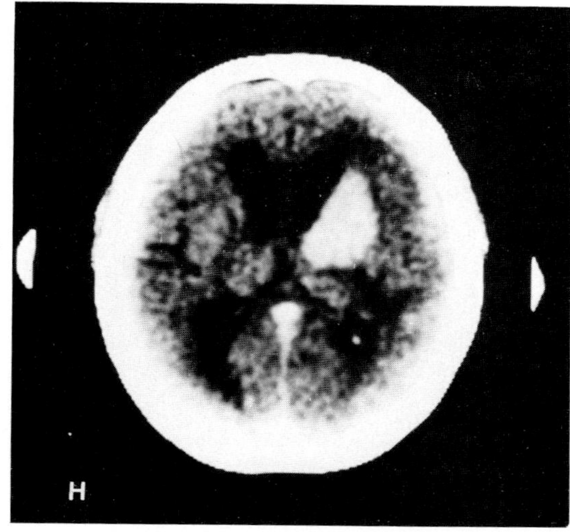

Fig. 62-20. Identical CT images (with intravenous enhancement) of benign and malignant brain stem tumors. (A,C,E,G) benign gliomas; (B) polar spongioblastoma; (D,F) anaplastic astrocytomas; (H) glioblastoma.

TREATMENT OF PATIENTS WITH BRAIN STEM TUMOR

This section is devoted to patients with predominantly focal brain stem tumors in whom a radical extirpation of the tumor was attempted. Shunt operations were not used, even if severe intracranial hypertension existed, hoping that radical removal of the tumor would restore the CSF circulation; however, 5 patients had been operated on elsewhere previously because of obstructive hydrocephalus, and in these cases ventriculocisternostomy or ventriculoatrial shunt procedures had been performed.

Three patients were operated upon 6 months to 2 years after decompressive operation, cyst evacuation, biopsy, or partial resection of their tumors. In 2 cases with cystic thalamic tumors a cyst aspiration through a stereotactic puncture or with the use of ventriculoscope had been performed several days before the direct operation.

Stereotactic biopsy was performed in 2 cases to determine preoperatively the histologic type of the tumor. In both cases, a correct histologic diagnosis was not made.

METHODS OF SURGICAL REMOVAL OF BRAIN STEM GLIOMAS

All patients are operated on under general anesthesia with muscle relaxants and artificial respiration. Different types of combined narcosis with neuroleptic analgesia and aterolgesia are used. The operations usually last between 4 and 8 hours.

Because different approaches are used, the patients are operated in various positions. For patients with a tumor in the caudal brain stem, the midbrain, and in some cases with posterior thalamic tumors, the sitting position is used (28 cases). In the majority of patients with thalamic tumors the supine position is used.

APPROACHES

Various surgical approaches are used according to the topographic and anatomic variations of the tumor within the different parts of the brain stem. Caudal brain stem tumors are exposed through a midline or retromastoid suboccipital approach to the posterior fossa (the last approach was used in caudal brain stem tumors of the third variant). In some cases in which such tumors invade the caudal medulla and the upper cervical cord, the posterior fossa craniectomy is supplemented by an upper cervical laminectomy.

In some cases in which caudal brain stem tumors spread to the midbrain, a combined approach to the posterior fossa and to the quadrigeminal cistern (suboccipital craniectomy and occipital craniotomy) is used (Figure 62-23).

The supratentorial occipital approach is used in cases of midbrain tumors with the side of the approach depending upon the predominant direction of tumor spread. In cases with midline tumors the craniotomy is done on the nondominant side. In all these cases a wide incision of the tentorium cerebelli is performed along the straight sinus.

Different supratentorial approaches are used in cases of thalamic tumors; occipital, supratentorial, transcallosal, and transcortical (through the anterior horn of the lateral ventricle). The surgical access in these cases depends upon the predominant location and direction of tumor growth.

The technique of tumor removal depends upon several factors; the first of these is whether the tumor had exophytic components or is located within the brain stem. The presence of cysts, which are encountered in some of our cases, usually facilitates the tumor removal; opening the cyst wall and evacuating its fluid contents provides a wide access to the solid parts of the tumor. It the tumor has no exophytic components to the paratruncal CSF spaces, we incise the brain stem. In some cases several incisions are made in the brain stem. The length of the incisions varies from 7 to 30 mm, and the locations of the brain stem incisions used in these cases are summarized in Figure 62-24.

The surgical microscope and microsurgical instruments were obligatory in the management of brain stem tumors. In the majority of our cases the solid portions of the tumor are removed with an ultrasonic aspirator. This instrument is useful, especially when the tumor is hard, but its large handpiece restricts the operative field. In some cases soft tumors are removed with a conventional aspirator and bipolar coagulation.

The degree of tumor removal depends upon the type of the

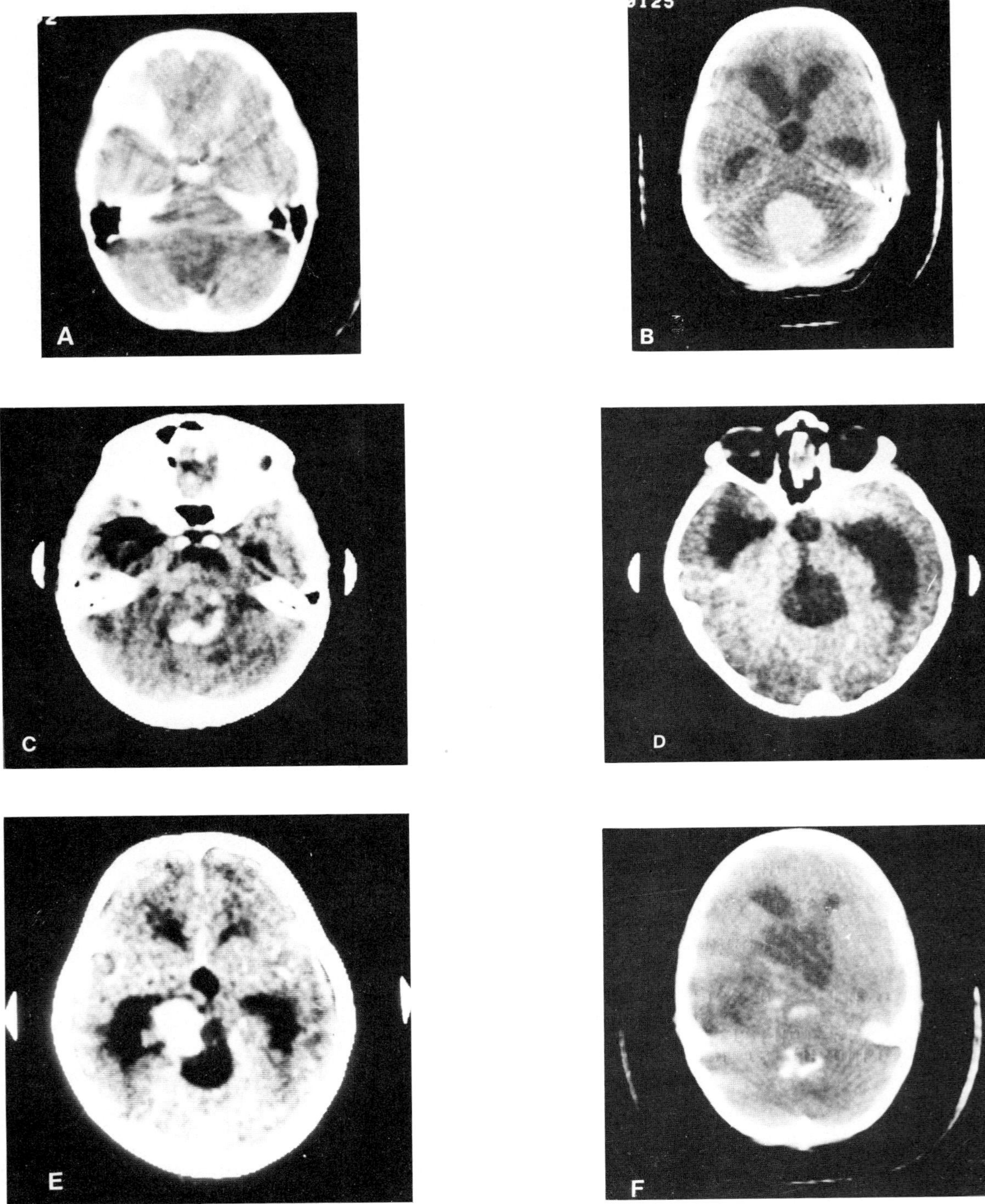

Fig. 62-21 (continued).

tumor growth—focal or infiltrative. Nodular (focal) tumors that have definite borders with the brain tissue (growth type I) are removed until only normal brain tissue is visible (19 cases). In focal tumors surrounded by a wide zone of infiltration (growth type II) the majority of the tumor is removed, but the infiltrative zone is left behind (16 cases). In these cases the postoperative CT and MRI scans reveals small fragments of unremoved tumor. In diffuse gliomas (growth type III) when a definite border between the tumor and brain tissue is absent under the microscope the major part of the tumor is left unresected (3 cases).

After the nodular tumors were removed, vessels and craniocerebral nerves located on the ventral and lateral aspects of the brain stem can be seen. Often at the beginning of the operation, because of gross deformation of the brain stem and the surrounding structures, it is difficult or impossible to determine the true topographic and anatomic relationships between the tumor and the brain stem, whereas by the end of the operation, after tumor removal, the brain stem and the surrounding structures return to their normal shape and position.

Most brain stem gliomas are relatively avascular, however, in some highly vascular cases the surgeon is obliged to coagu-

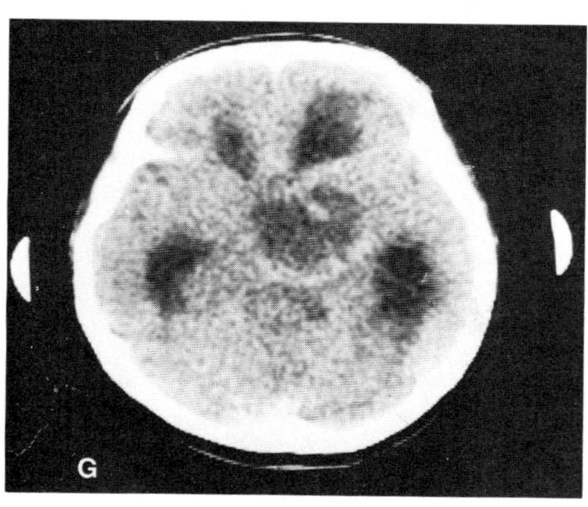

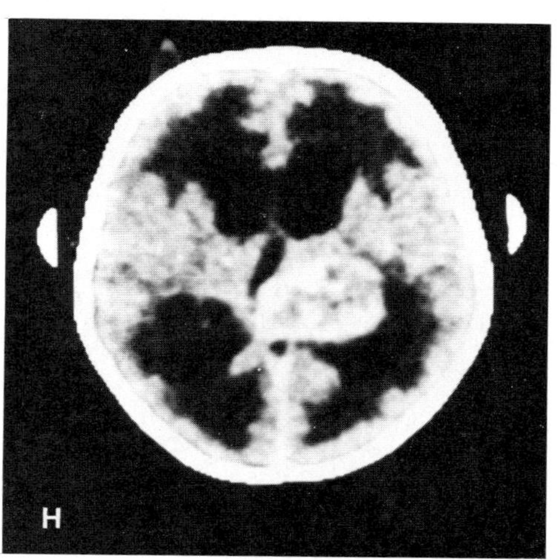

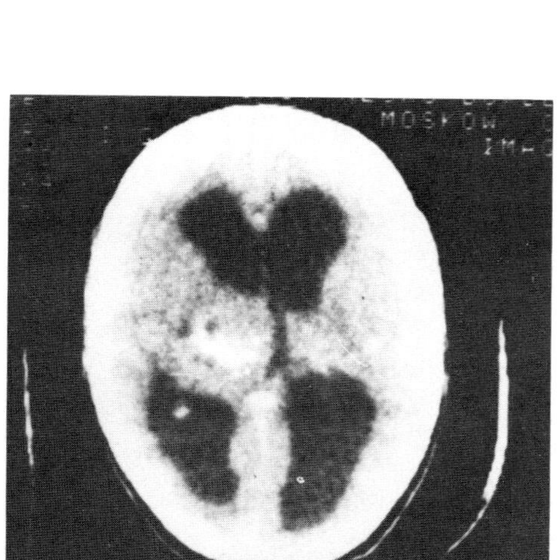

Fig. 62-21. CT scans of fibrillary astrocytomas in different parts of the brain stem. (A) hypodense caudal brain stem astrocytoma; (B) hyperdense caudal brain stem astrocytoma; (C) heterogeneous caudal brain stem astrocytoma (as a result of convoluted enhancement with the columnar density; (D) hyperdense midbrain astrocytoma; (E) hyperdense midline cyst; (F) heterogeneous midbrain astrocytoma (as a result of convoluted enhancement with the columnar density); (G) hypodense thalamic astrocytoma; (H) hyperdense thalamic lesion caused by necrosis; (I) heterogeneous thalamic astrocytoma (as a result of convoluted enhancement with the columnar density).

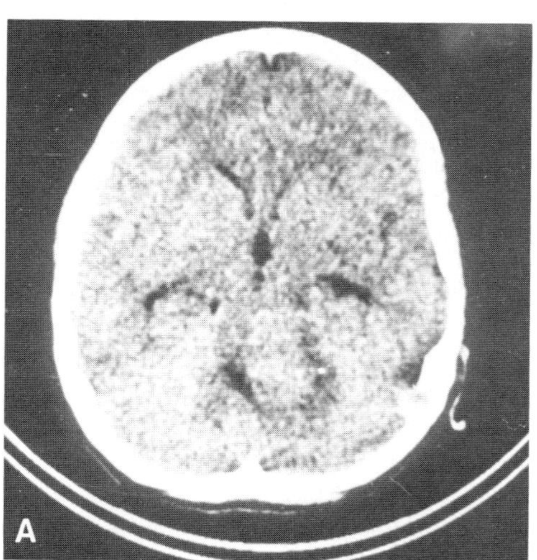

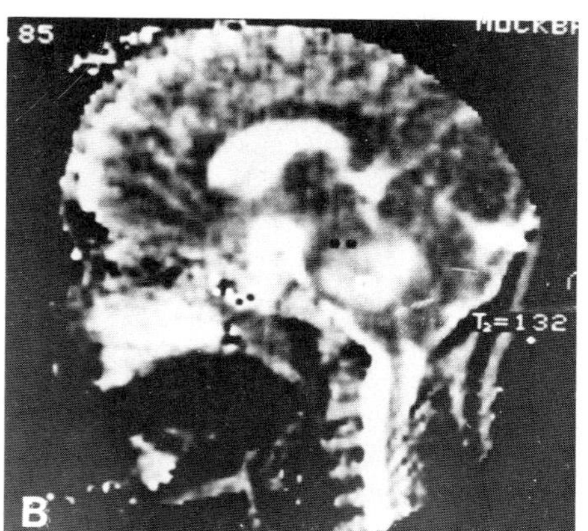

Fig. 62-22. A nodular pilocytic astrocytoma of the caudal brain stem (verified at surgery). (A) On the CT scan the lesion is a "probable" nodular tumor. (B) On the MRI scan the lesion is a "definite" nodular tumor.

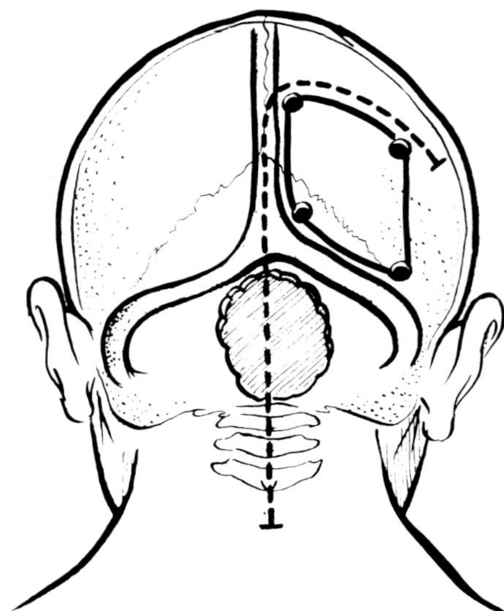

Fig. 62-23. The combined approach to the pineal region and to the posterior fossa.

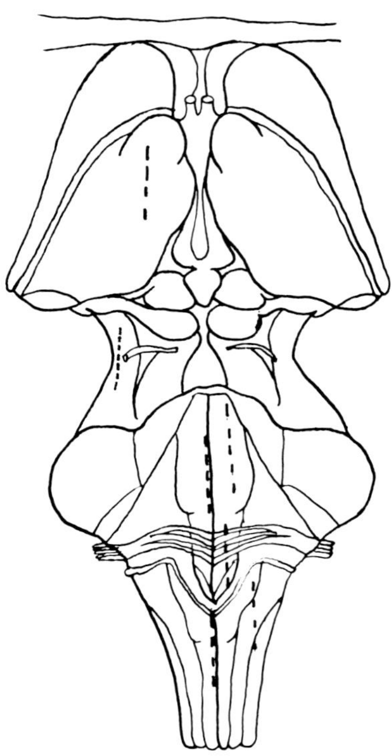

Fig. 62-24. The brain stem incisions (dotted lines) used for access to intratruncal tumors.

late and section quite sizable arterial and venous branches to remove the tumor. Because it is difficult to differentiate tumor vessels from normal brain stem vessels, we were afraid cutting such vessels might aggravate the local neurologic signs in the postoperative period. But in those patients in whom such techniques were necessary, there were no neurologic signs in the postoperative period that could be explained solely by insufficiency of the brain stem blood supply.

Special caution is necessary in removing tectal gliomas, because some branches of the superior cerebellar and posterior cerebral arteries may pass through the tumor. In removing these gliomas, as other pineal region tumors, such as pinealomas and germinomas, special care must be taken with the great cerebral, basal, and the internal cerebral veins because serious complications can result from their damage. In a patient with a tectal glioma, the great cerebral vein was found to be incorporated in the tumor and had to be coagulated and cut. Nevertheless, in the postoperative period there were no neurologic signs of venous circulatory disturbances. The patient died 1½ months after surgery from hemorrhage from the unremoved portions of the infiltrative tumor. The autopsy also did not reveal any signs of venous circulation disturbances in deep brain structures. Most probably, additional pathways of outflow had developed as a result of chronic (12 years duration) compression of the vein of Galen.

RESULTS

In the majority of cases with focal brain stem gliomas (19 cases) the tumor was totally or almost totally removed (up to the boundaries with normal brain tissue). In tumors with wide zones of infiltration (16 cases), total removal of the tumor was impossible; nevertheless the bulk of the tumor was removed.

Immediately after surgery (in 1–6 week period) 3 patients died; one with a caudal brain stem tumor and two with midbrain tumors. These cases were grade II fibrillary astrocytomas with a diffuse growth pattern.

The majority of cases exhibited a temporary aggravation of local neurologic signs in the postoperative period. In 5 cases the postoperative period involved disturbances of vital functions that required ICU care and artificial respiration for several weeks. Nevertheless, all these complications disappeared and in 2 to 3 months the condition of most of the patients was better than preoperatively. The signs of intracranial hypertension improved quite rapidly.

The neurologic signs and symptoms evident after surgery are summarized in Figures 62-25, 62-26, and 62-27 and will not be discussed in detail. Two aspects deserve mention: the neurologic consequences of brain stem incisions and the dynamics of hemihyperkinesis after tumor removal. Twenty-five incisions in the brain stem varying in length from 7 to 30 mm were used in 21 cases to expose the tumor. The brain stem incisions were made close to the tumor in an avascular zone where the brain tissue seemed to be thin and abnormal. It is quite difficult to identify those findings that might have been caused by a brain stem incision among the panoply of postoperative neurologic findings, nevertheless, in only 1 or 2 patients did such incisions appear to aggravate local neurologic signs. We agree with Entzian[24] that such incisions can be made without injury to the tracts and nuclei of the cranial nerves.

Eight patients undergoing resection of caudal brain stem gliomas abruptly developed cardiovascular disturbances: bradycardia, tachycardia, extrasystoles, or fluctuations in blood pressure. These disturbances were usually transitory and observed at the point in the operation at which the portions of the tumor adjacent to the surrounding tissue were removed. Incision of the brain stem surface did not produce any hemodynamic disturbances.

Hyperkinesis caused by brain stem tumors and especially its dynamics after surgery are of interest. In 9 patients there was preoperative hyperkinesis, the character of which has been discussed. In 8 of these patients, the hyperkinesis disappeared or improved after surgery: in 1 patient immediately after the

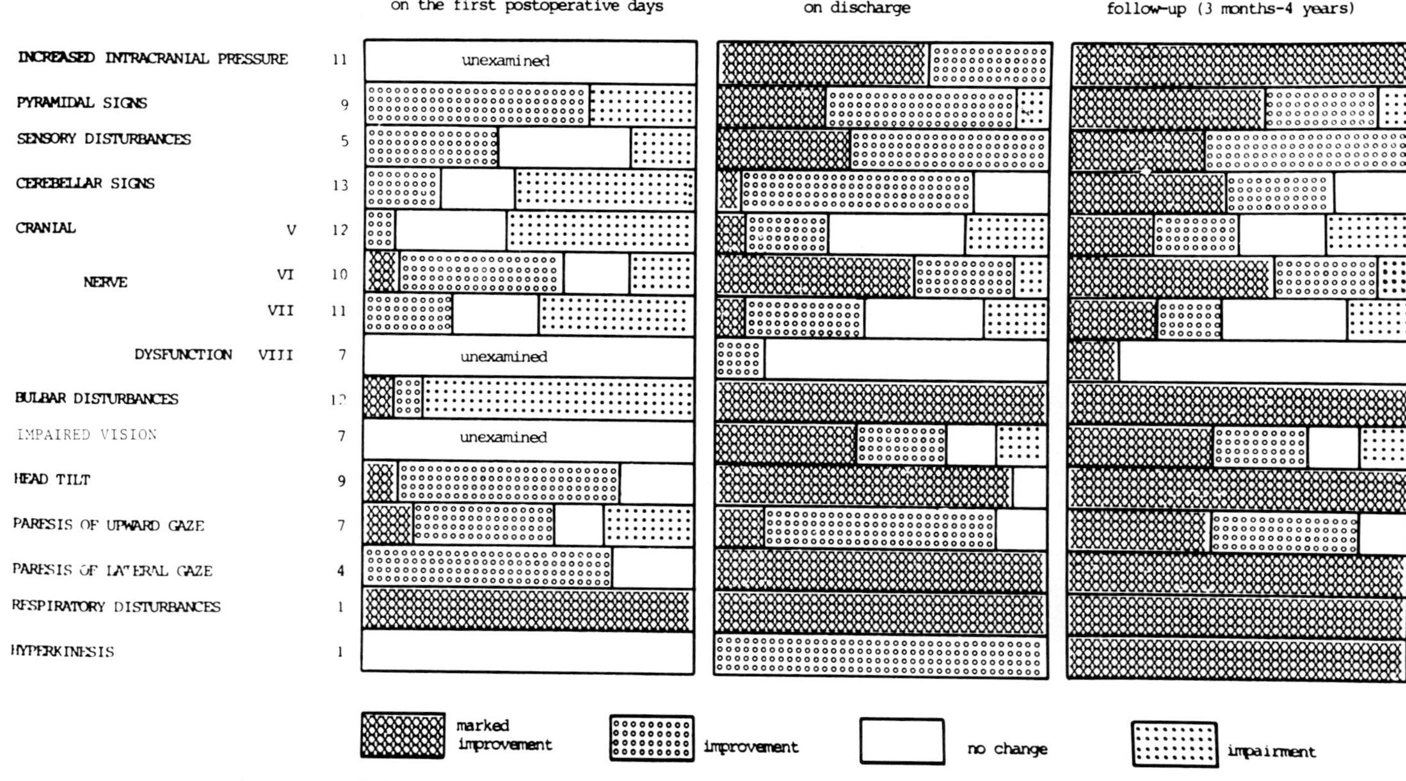

Fig. 62-25. Dynamics of preoperative clinical signs and symptoms in 15 patients with focal caudal brain stem gliomas treated by surgery.

DYNAMICS OF PREOPERATIVE CLINICAL SIGNS AND SYMPTOMS IN 7 OPERATED PATIENTS WITH FOCAL MIDBRAIN GLIOMAS

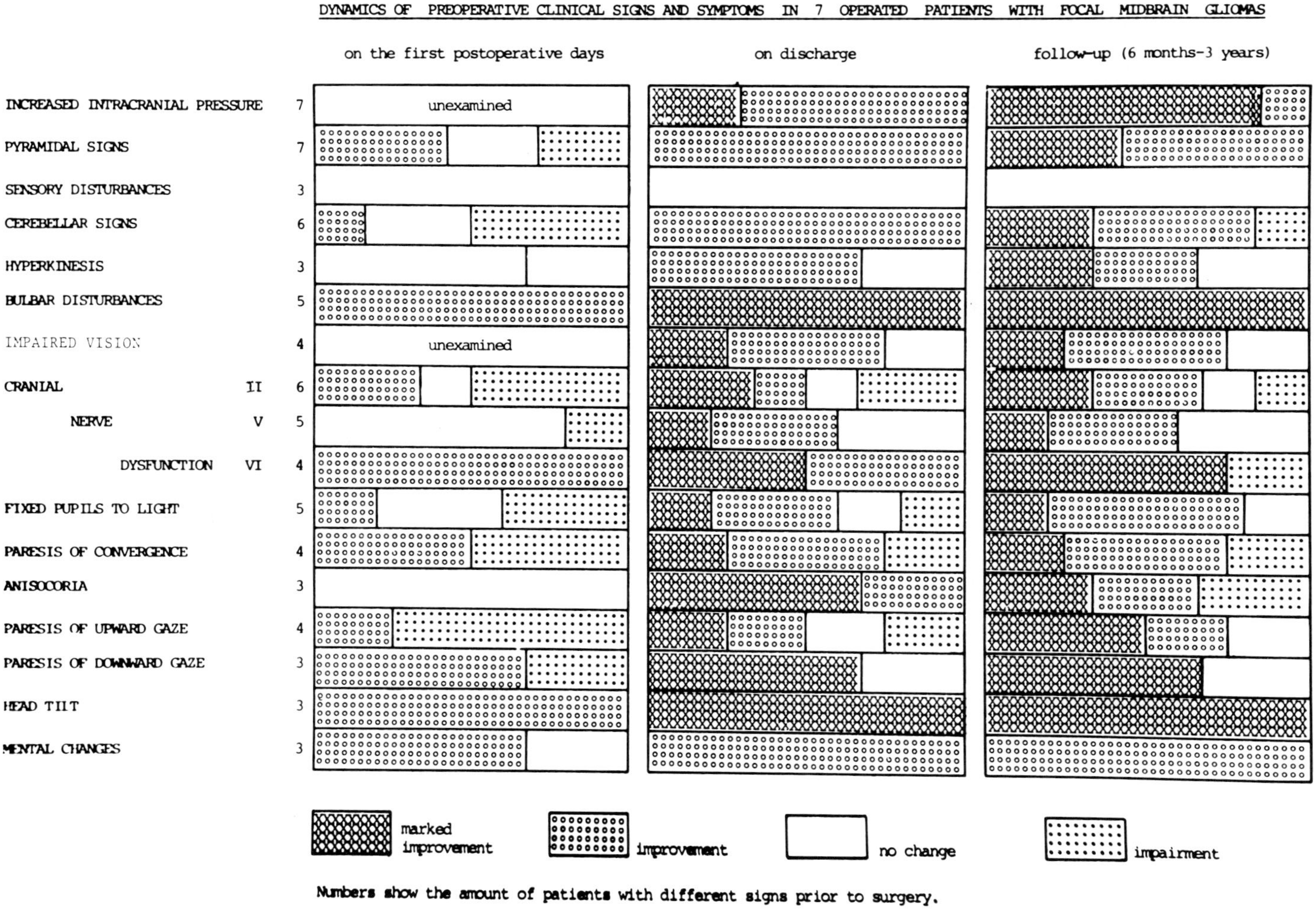

Fig. 62-26. Dynamics of preoperative signs and symptoms in 7 patients with focal midbrain gliomas treated by surgery.

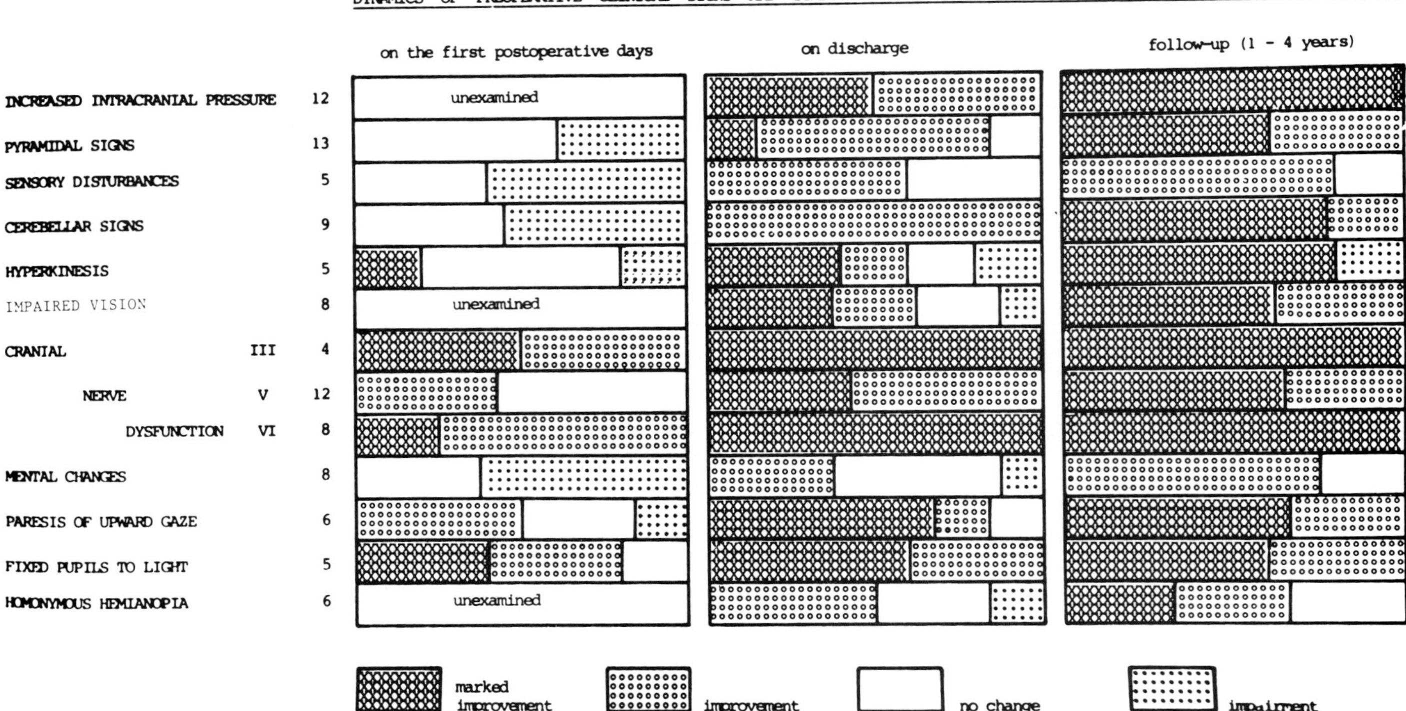

Fig. 62-27. Dynamics of preoperative clinical signs and sumptoms in 13 patients with focal thalamic gliomas treated by surgery.

operation, in 5 at discharge, in 2 within 7 months to 1½ years. In 1 patient there were no important changes in the severity of the hyperkinesis during a short postoperative follow-up period.

One patient with athetosis improved within a couple of days after removal of an anaplastic (grade III) pulvinar astrocytoma, but 1½ years later a coarse tremor appeared as a single sign of tumor recurrence. In contrast, another patient with a grade II fibrillary astrocytoma of the posterior thalamus, developed athetosis and hemiballism after surgery which were added to the preoperative coarse tremor. Within 1½ to 2 years all extrapyramidal disorders had nearly subsided. Based on these observations that hyperkinesis caused by brain stem gliomas often disappear following tumor removal, we suspect that the possible cause of the extrapyramidal disorders was the irritation of the brain stem structures responsible for muscle tone and organization of motor activity.

Radiotherapy is used in the postoperative period in patients with malignant tumors (2 patients) and with low grade astrocytomas with a wide zone of infiltration and were highly vascularized (2 patients). We are unable to draw any conclusions about the role of postoperative radiotherapy in the treatment of brain stem gliomas.

Of 35 patients who tolerated surgery, 28 were followed for 1 to 4 years (the other 7 patients were operated on within the past year). Twenty-two of 28 patients returned to work or school; 6 are still disabled. Signs of tumor recurrence were observed in 3 patients (2 with malignant tumors and 1 with a low grade astrocytoma) 6 months to 2 years postoperatively.

CASE REPORTS

The following case reports illustrate the fact that focal tumors of different portions of the brain stem not only could but should be removed.

Case 1. A 7-year-old girl was admitted to the Burdenko Institute of Neurosurgery with a 7-month history of headache and weakness in the left extremities. Severe intracranial hypertension, a left-sided hemiparesis with hyperactive tendon reflexes and extrapyramidal muscle tone, hemihypesthesia in the left half of the body, central paresis of the left facial nerve, bilateral paresis of the sixth nerve, and moderate mesencephalic signs were present.

The CT examination showed a cystic tumor in the right thalamus extending into the right cerebral peduncle and the right half of the upper pons with a definite border with the surrounding tissue (Figure 62-28A-E).

On February 16, 1984, a fibrillary astrocytoma was totally removed from the right half of the brain stem (the location of the tumor as determined at the operation is shown in Figure 62-29).

A small right fronto-parasagittal craniotomy was done extending through the midline. A transcallosal approach to the right lateral ventricle exposed the deformed base of its body. On splitting the superficial layers of the thalamus, just near the thalamostriate vein, a cystic cavity was entered beneath which a gray-yellow dense tumor was found. Its surface was clearly delineated and it was separated from the normal appearing brain tissue under the dissecting microscope. The tumor was removed from the thalamus, cerebral peduncle, and the upper pons with the ultrasonic aspirator until only normal brain tissue remained. Vessels passing through the tumor were coagulated and sectioned during tumor removal.

The patient tolerated the operation well. There was rapid resolution of the signs of intracranial hypertension. At discharge 3 weeks later the visual acuity was normal, the mesencephalic signs had disappeared, and the hemiparesis was less evident. A follow-up CT scan showed no residual tumor (Figure 62-28F-I). One year after the operation the patient was

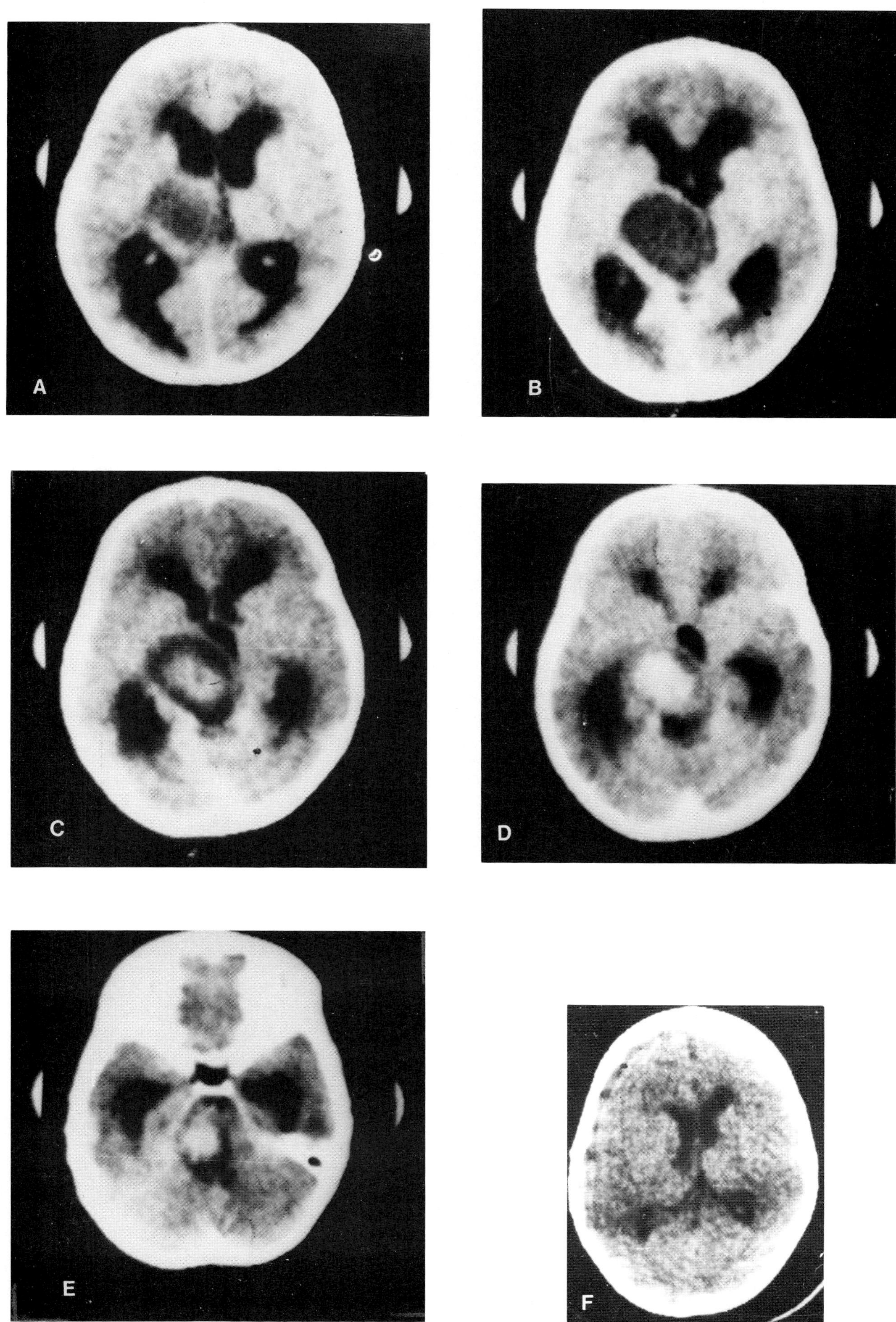

Fig. 62-28 (continued).

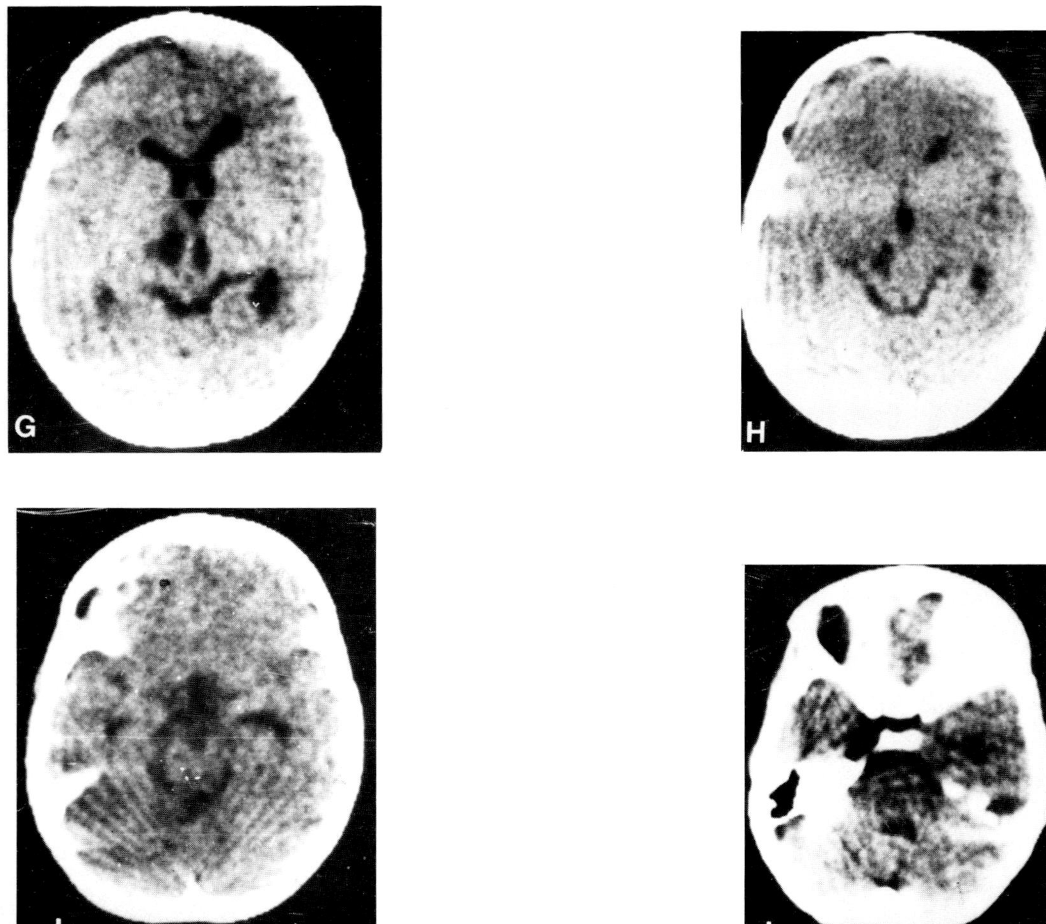

Fig. 62-28. (A–E) Preoperative CT scans show a large hypodense right thalamic lesion with hyperdense foci in the right cerebral peduncle and right half of the pons with definite margins. (F–J) Postoperative CT scans (3 weeks) after removal of a fibrillary astrocytoma of the right half of the brain stem. No residual tumor is seen.

symptom free except for left-sided hyperactive tendon reflexes and hemihypesthesia. She attends school and is doing well.

Case 2. A 15-year-old boy had a slowly progressing left hemiparesis of 7-years duration. Neurologic examination revealed an upward gaze palsy, bilateral paresis of the sixth cranial nerves, left spastic hemiparesis, hyperactive tendon reflexes of the left extremities with bilateral positive Babinski signs, left homonymous hemianopia, and bilateral papilledema. Craniography showed signs of high intracranial pressure. Neuropsychologic study disclosed moderate amnesic disturbances.

The CT examination revealed an extensive lesion of high density within the right thalamus extending to the right cerebral peduncle (Figure 62-30A, B, and C), small cystic and petrified lesions were seen within the tumor nodule, which had a definite border with the surrounding tissue. Lateral and anterior displacement of the inferior horn of the right lateral ventricle by the tumor were noted.

On April 6, 1982 a fibrillary astrocytoma was removed from the right thalamus and right cerebral peduncle (the location of the tumor is shown in Figure 62-31) through a craniotomy in the right parietotemporal area. On exposing the right lateral ventricle through a transcortical approach, the floor was noted to be

deformed and elevated. The prominence seemed to be caused by a tumor within the enlarged thalamus. A short incision of the superficial layers of the thalamus allowed visualization of a dense tumoral tissue 5 mm beneath the surface. The tumor nodule was gray in color, 5 cm in diameter, was clearly

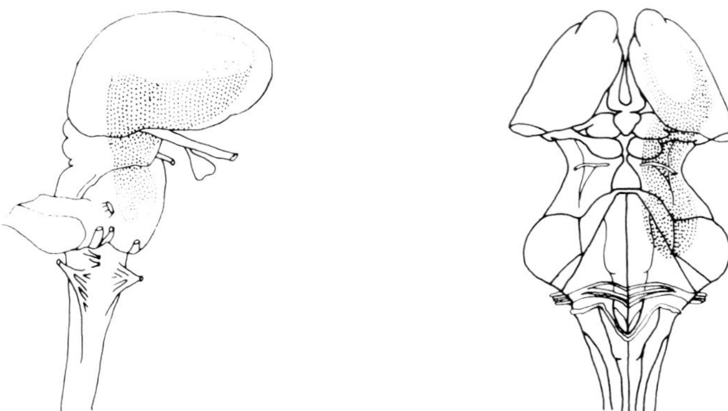

Fig. 62-29. The location of the tumor in case 1. Shaded area: the solid part of the tumor; open area: cystic part of the tumor.

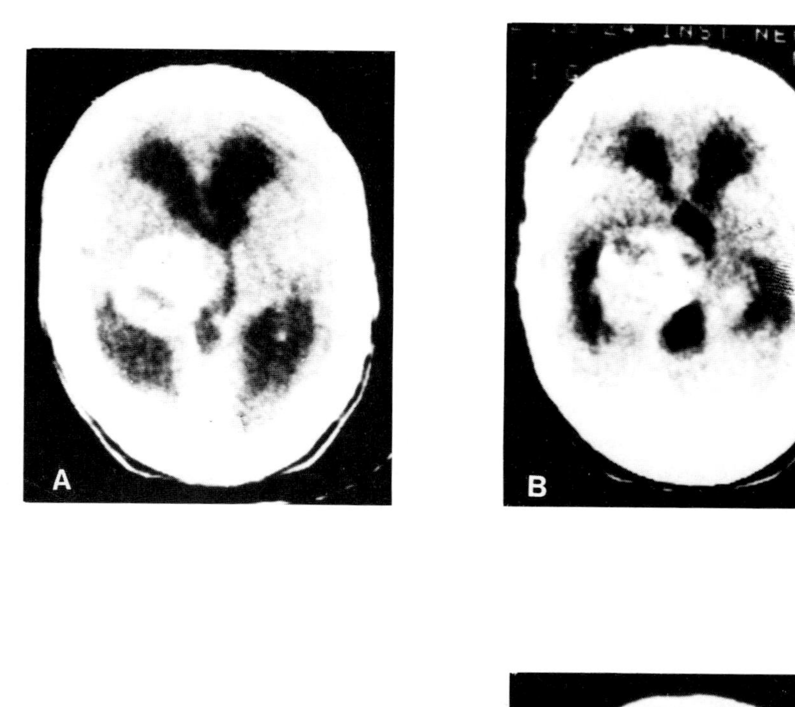
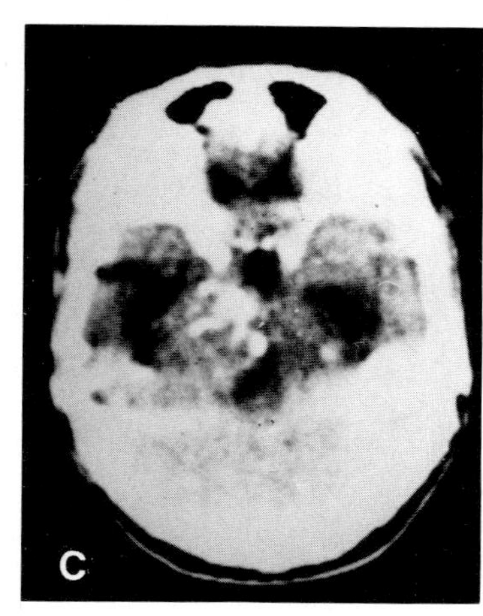
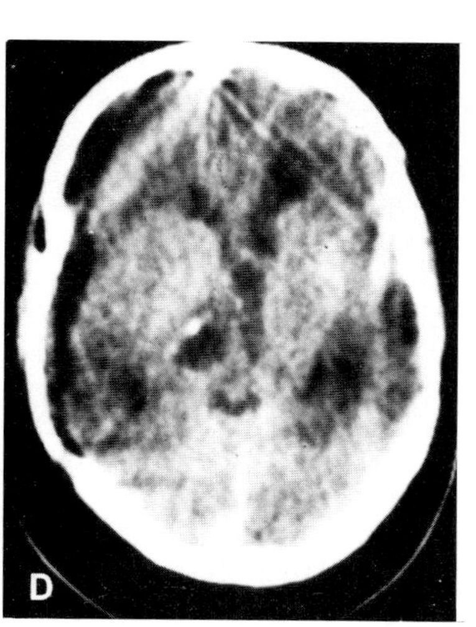
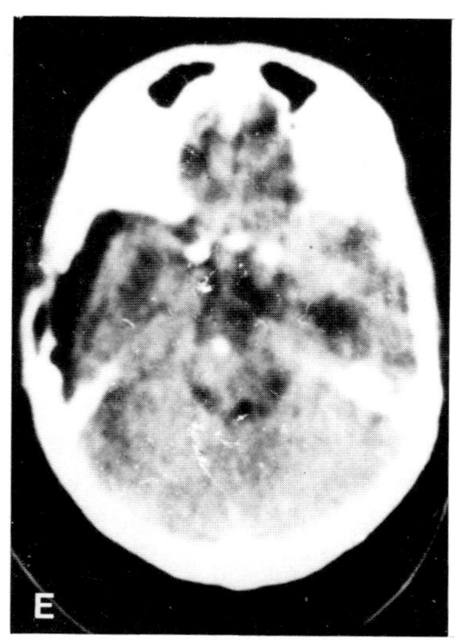
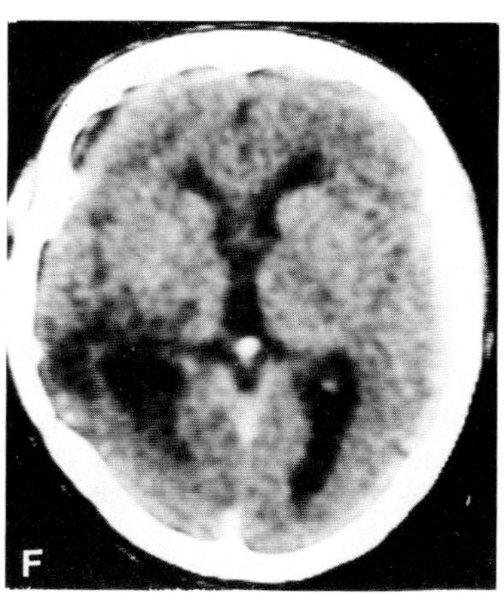
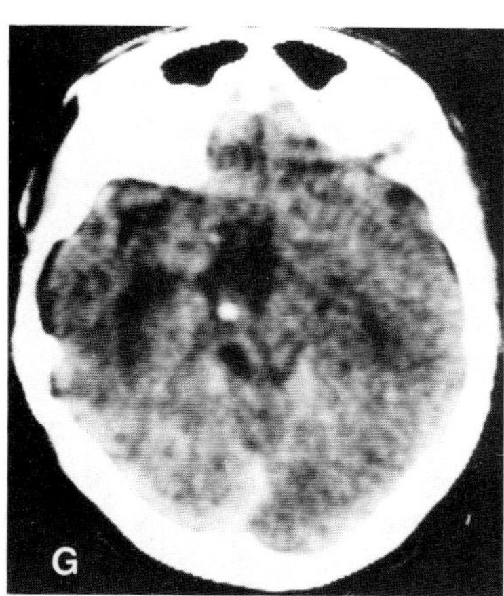

Fig. 62-30. Case 2. Enhanced CT scans obtained preoperatively (A,B,C), 3 weeks (D,E), and 4 years (F,G) after surgery. There was no tumor recurrence 4 years after the operation.

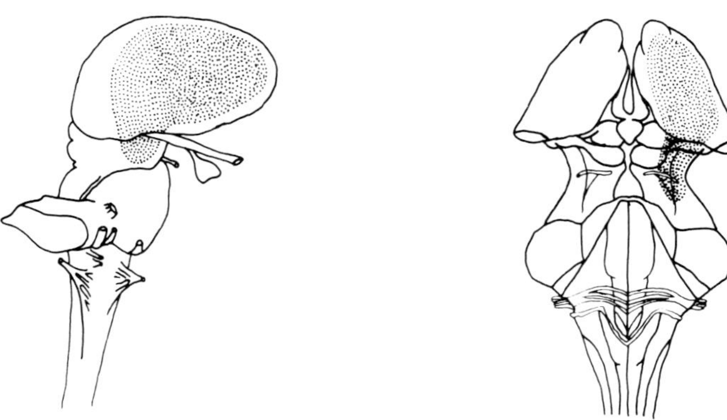

Fig. 62-31. The location of the brain stem tumor in case 2.

delineated, and could be separated from the normal tissue of the thalamus and the cerebral peduncle under the dissecting microscope. It contained small cysts and calcifications. After the tumor was removed, the base (floor) of the lateral ventricle regained its normal configuration.

The postoperative course was remarkably smooth. On discharge 3 weeks after the operation there was no papilledema, the patient could walk unaided, and the spasticity was less evident. A CT examination before discharge showed no residual tumor (Figure 62-30F and G).

Case 3. A 15-year-old boy was admitted with a history of headache for 2 years, weakness in the left extremities for 6 months, and diminished visual acuity for many weeks. Neurologic examination disclosed increased intracranial pressure, left-sided spastic hemiparesis with hyperactive tendon reflexes and positive Babinski sign, tremor in the left hand, left homonymous hemianopia, and diminished visual acuity (0.6 in each eye).

The CT examination following the intravenous injection of a contrast agent demonstrated a fairly defined and well-demarcated hyperdense tumor in the projection of the right thalamus, basal ganglia, and cerebral peduncle (Figure 62-32A, B, and C).

On June 22, 1983, a fibrillary astrocytoma was totally removed from the right thalamus and extending to the head of the caudate nucleus and the right cerebral peduncle (Figure 62-33). On exposing the right lateral ventricle through a transcortical approach to the anterior horn, no tumor within the ventricular cavity was seen. The floor and the lateral wall of the body of the lateral ventricle seemed to be deformed and were fungating into its cavity. A 2-cm incision in the deformed brain tissue 1 cm laterally to the foramen of Monro exposed a dense gray tumor 4 mm below the surface. The nodule of the tumor had well-defined borders with the surrounding brain tissue and was removed totally from the thalamus, the head of the caudate nucleus, and the right cerebral peduncle under the dissecting microscope. Two large veins passing through the tumor were coagulated and sectioned.

During the first 3 postoperative days the patient was alert, but on the fourth day he developed anisocoria and began to deteriorate; he became stuporous. Diminished hemispheric and regional brain blood flow (to 40 percent) developed with hyperemia in the zone of the right basal ganglia. The CT scan showed a hematoma in the bed of the removed tumor (Figure 62-32D, E, and F).

After reoperation in which the blood clot was removed, the patient's conscious state rapidly improved to normal and the anisocoria subsided. Examination of brain blood flow revealed normal parameters. The control CT scan showed no residual hematoma or tumor (Figure 62-32G, H, and I).

The patient was discharged 3 weeks later in good condition. Neurologic examination revealed regress of the intracranial hypertension, normal visual acuity (1.0 in each eye), and good visual fields. The hemiparesis and the tremor in the left hand became less evident.

Two years later the patient is symptom free except for mild pyramidal signs and mild tremor in the left hand. Now he attends school where he is doing well.

Case 4. A 13-year-old boy was admitted with a history of weakness in the right extremities for 10 months and bulbar disturbances for several weeks. Neurologic examination revealed hemiparesis as evidence of involvement of the base of the left brain stem, bilateral ptosis, difficulty in convergence, loss of upward gaze, and diminished pupillary reflexes to light. In addition, hyperkinesis in the right hand, severe bulbar symptoms, and signs of moderate intracranial hypertension were noted.

A CT scan (Figure 62-34A and B) and MRI scan (Figure 62-35A and B) showed a cystic tumor within the midbrain, with well-demarcated borders with the surrounding tissue.

On January 15, 1986 a fibrillary astrocytoma was radically removed from the left cerebral peduncle and upper pons (the location of the tumor is shown in Figure 62-36). On exposing the left portion of the ambient cistern through an occipital transtentorial approach to the quadrigeminal area, the left cerebral peduncle seemed to be enlarged and deformed. A tiny incision 1 cm long in an avascular area of the fungating cerebral peduncle disclosed a cystic cavity 2 to 3 mm beneath the brain tissue. The anterior wall of the cyst was formed by a yellowish-gray tumor, the posterior portions of which had a spongy texture and were severely vascularized. In contrast, the more anterior portions of the tumor were more dense. The tumor was radically removed with simple and ultrasonic aspirators from the left cerebral peduncle and the left half of the upper pons until the only normal brain tissue was apparent. Vessels passing through the tumor tissue were coagulated and sectioned.

After the tumor had been removed, the arachnoid was opened and the upper part of the basilar artery with its branches, the superior cerebellar and posterior cerebral arteries, and the left oculomotor nerve could be seen.

The postoperative course was remarkably smooth. In the first day the bulbar symptoms subsided, but the paresis of the right arm became worse. At discharge 3 weeks later, the patient was symptom free, except for a mild right-sided hemiparesis and a statokinetic tremor in the right hand.

The CT scan and MRI control scans before discharge showed a small area of residual tumor (Figure 62-34C and D; 62-35C and D), so a course of gamma radiation therapy (4550 rad) was given over 35 days. The patient tolerated the radiotherapy well.

Case 5. A girl, aged 9, was admitted complaining of weakness of the right extremities, disturbances of equilibrium, unsteady gait, dizziness, difficulties in swallowing, hoarseness, and vomiting. The disease had begun with paresis of the right foot 10 months prior to hospitalization.

Neurologic examination revealed severe brain stem cere-

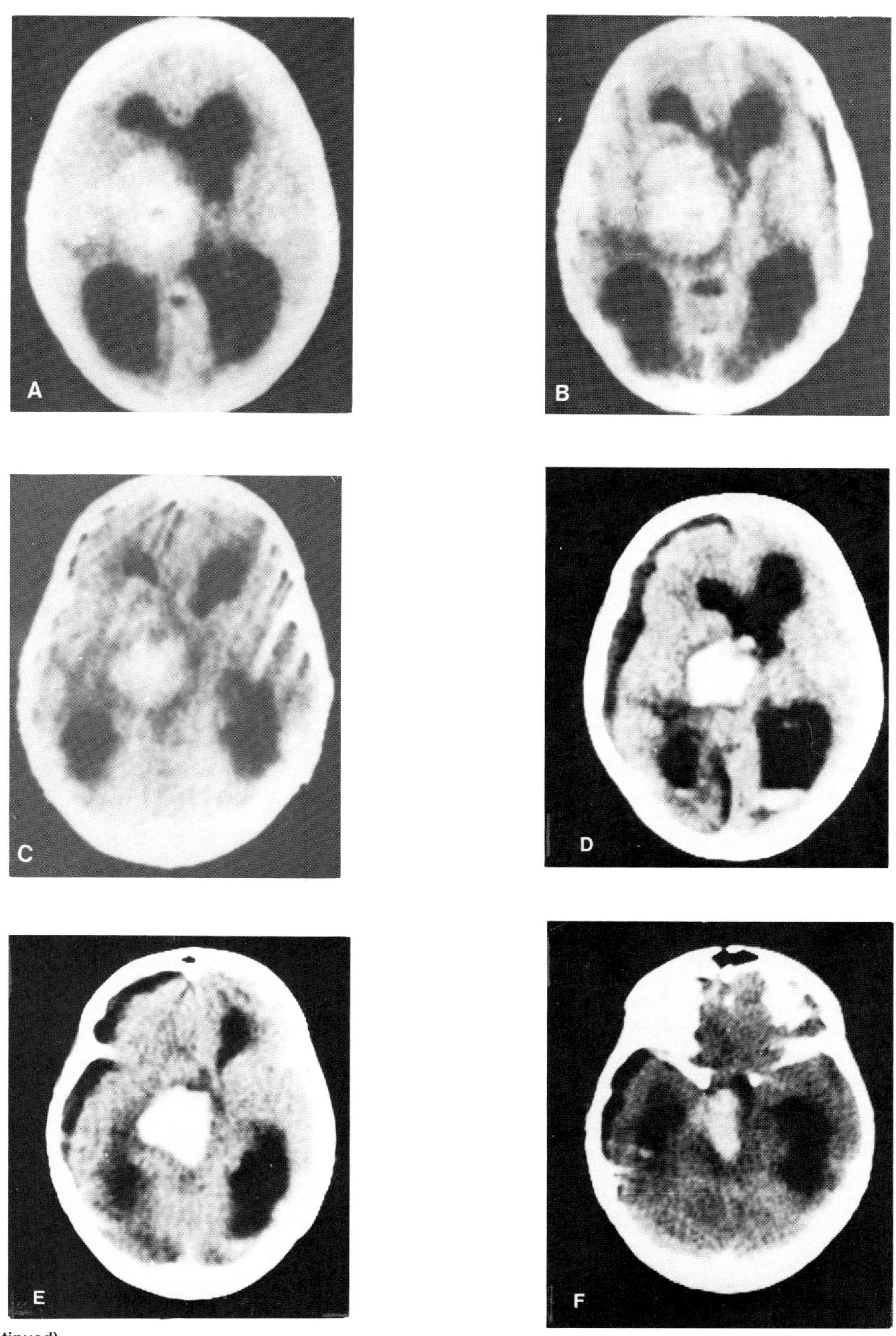

Fig. 62-32 (continued).

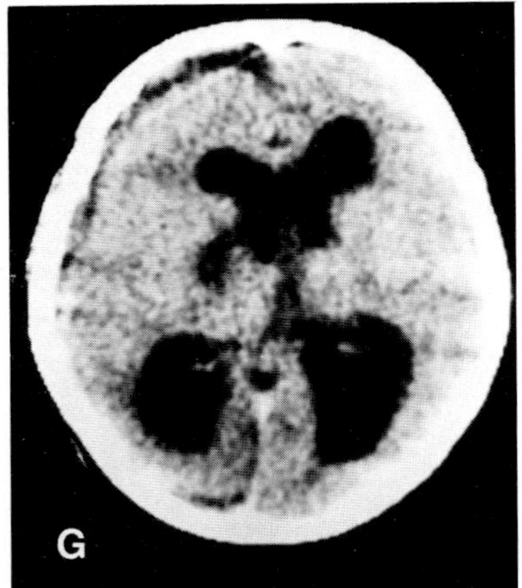 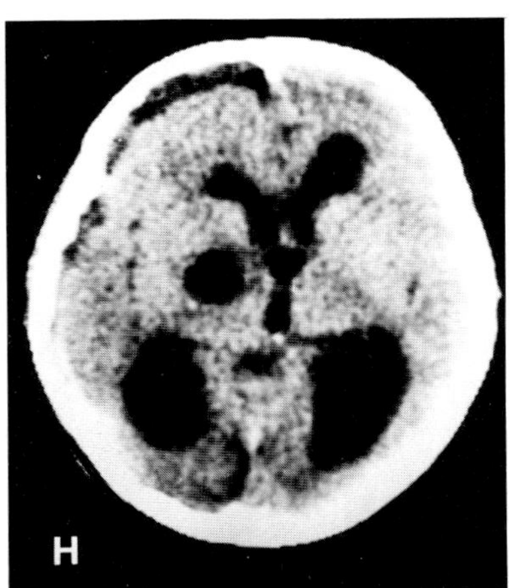 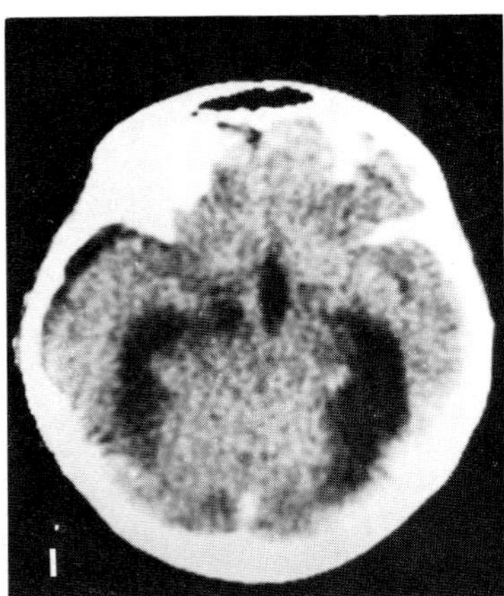

Fig. 62-32. (A,B,C) A well-circumscribed hyperdense fibrillary astrocytoma of the right thalamus extending to the head of the caudate nucleus and cerebral peduncle. (D,E,F) Hematoma in the bed of the removed tumor. (G,H,K) A CT scan after reoperation. No hematoma or residual tumor is apparent.

bellar, pyramidal, and bulbar signs. In addition there was hyperkinesis in the right hand (in the form of chorea). There was no papilledema. A recording of the brain stem auditory evoked potentials revealed prolongation of the interpeak latency, a low amplitude of all waves (especially the IV and V), and a prolongation of latency of all waves (Figure 62-37A). A CT scan indicated the presence of an infratentorial space-occupying lesion, probably within the pons and extending into the left cerebral peduncle and left thalamus (Figure 62-38A-E). The lesion, which was of low density, had a definite border with the surrounding tissue.

On June 4, 1985 a nodular benign grade I-II fibrillary astrocytoma was removed from the pons, the left cerebral peduncle, and the lower portion of the left thalamus (the location of the tumor site is presented in Figure 62-39).

A combined approach to the pineal region and to the posterior fossa was found to be suitable. Supratentorial craniotomy in the left occipital area was supplemented by a bilateral suboccipital craniectomy. A hockey-stick shaped skin incision was used (see Figure 62-23).

The occipital transtentorial approach allowed exposure and evacuation of a large cyst beneath which the enlarged left cerebral peduncle came into view. No further manipulations through this approach were attempted. After the fourth ventricle had been entered through the foramen of Magendie, the cranial portion of the ventricular floor seemed to be distended by an intrapontine mass. A tiny median incision 2 cm in length was made and a grayish spongy tumor was encountered at the depth of 2 to 3 mm beneath the brain tissue. The tumor nodule contained a number of sizable blood vessels, which where were coagulated and sectioned. The tumor was removed with the ultrasonic and conventional aspirators. This approach (through an incision of the oral portion of the fourth ventricular floor) allowed radical removal the tumor from the pons, the left cerebral peduncle, and the thalamus. The tumor was removed under the microscope until only normal brain tissue was apparent, after which the floor of the fourth ventricle returned to its normal shape and position. No hemodynamic disturbances during surgery were noted.

The patient tolerated the operation well and the postoperative course was remarkably smooth. On the first postoperative day the bulbar symptoms and the hyperkinesis subsided, but the hemiparesis became more evident. At discharge 5 weeks later, the patient was symptom-free except for a mild right-sided hemiparesis and mild ataxia. On discharge the CT scan showed no residual tumor (Figure 62-38F, G, and H). There was only CSF in the space of the removed tumor.

A follow-up study 10 months postoperatively showed that the patient was symptom-free. She attends school and studies dance. Her BSEP recording became nearly normal (Figure 62-37B).

Case 6. A 15-year-old girl was admitted complaining of headache, neck pain, and weakness in the right extremities. The disease had begun with headache 1 year before admission. Weakness of the right hand and leg developed gradually. Remission of these signs occurred during 6 months, but after a mild head injury they became worse. On admission the patient was alert and cooperative. The head was found to be tilted to the left and backward. There were signs of high intracranial pressure, profound right hemiparesis with increased reflexes on the right side, and bilateral Babinski responses and right hemi-hypesthesia of deep sensation. The corneal reflex was absent on the right. Bilateral lateral rectus paresis and right facial weakness were noted. She had bilateral horizontal and vertical

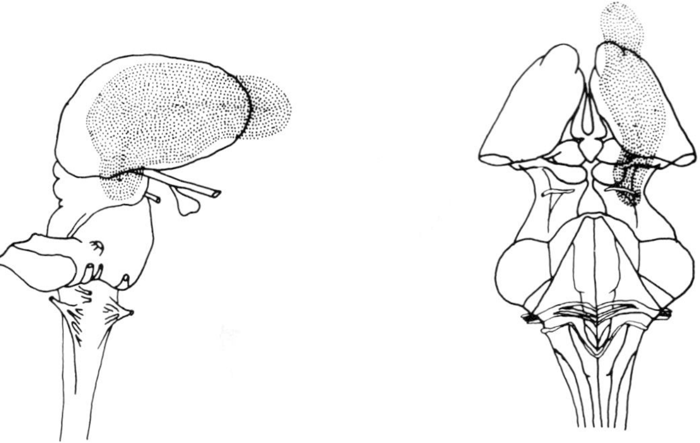

Fig. 62-33. Location of the tumor in case 3.

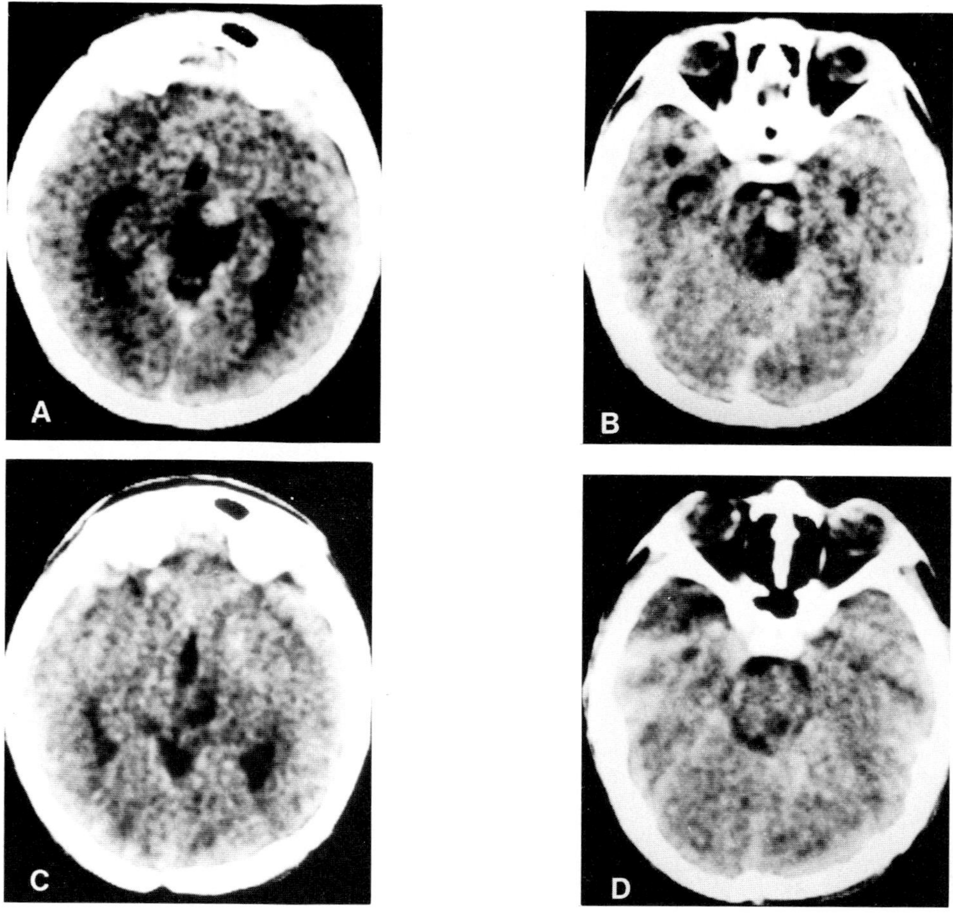

Fig. 62-34. (A,B) A cystic midbrain fibrillary astrocytoma extending to the upper pons. (C,D) Postoperative CT scans.

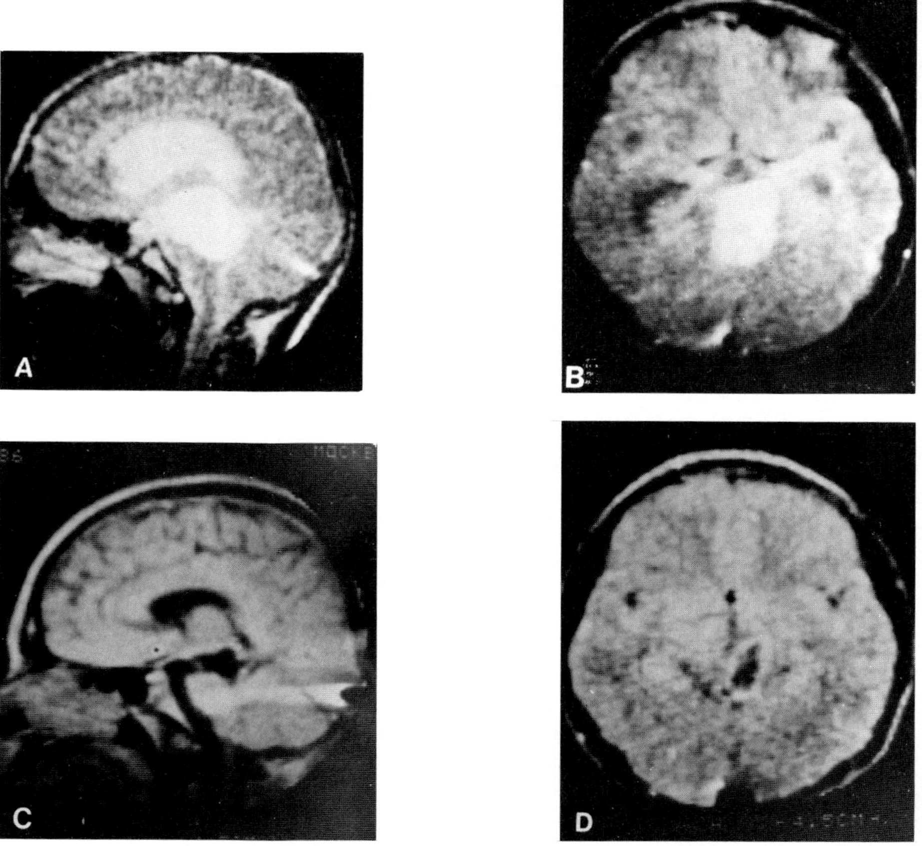

Fig. 62-35. MRI scans of a midbrain astrocytoma (case 4) (A,B) before and (C,D) after surgery.

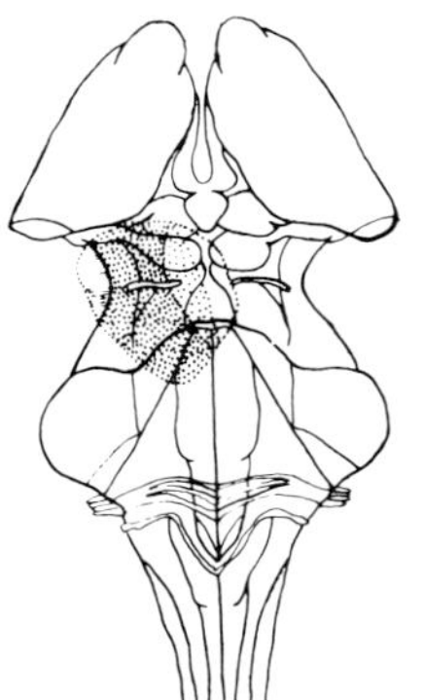

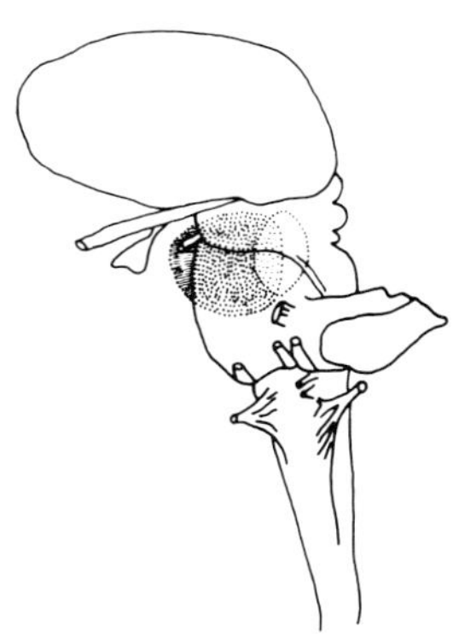

Fig. 62-36. Location of the tumor in case 4. Shaded area: intratruncal portion; cross-hatched area: exophytic portion; open area: cystic portion.

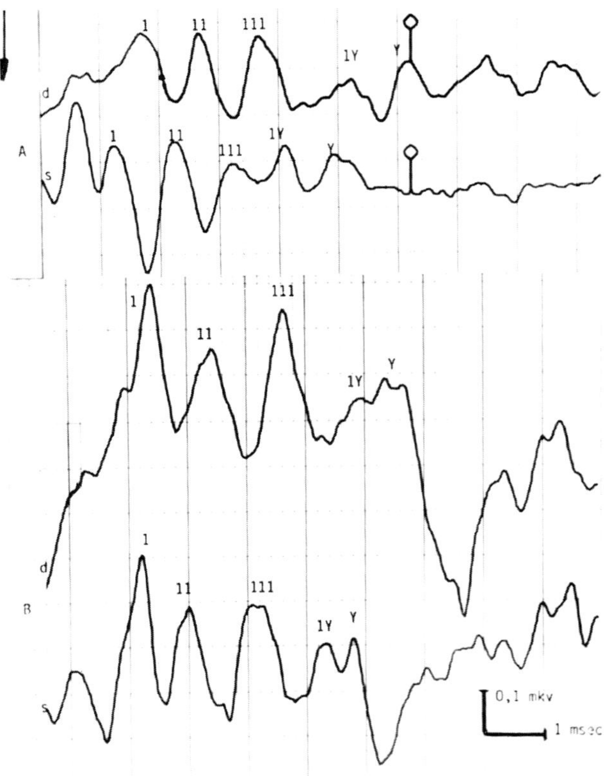

Fig. 62-37. (A) Prolongation of latency to wave V and prolongation of III-V and I-V interwave latency to 2.5 and 4.6 msec are apparent in the preoperative right BSAEP recording. Note the diminished amplitude of wave V in the preoperative left BSAEPs. (B) Ten months after surgery the interwave III-V and I-V latency of the right BSAEPs is normal (1.8 and 4.0 msec). The left BSAEPs are also normal.

nystagmus. The gag reflex was absent and the tongue deviated to the right.

A CT scan obtained after the intravenous injection of contrast medium revealed a well-demarcated lesion of heterogenous density within the lower fourth ventricle.

On March 14, 1985 a fibrillary astrocytoma was radically removed from the medulla and lower pons (the tumor location is presented in Figure 62-40). A suboccipital craniectomy supplemented by resection of the posterior part of the arch of the atlas revealed a deformed and enlarged medulla and lower pons (Figure 62-41A). The fourth ventricle was displaced upward. There were no extrinsic portions of the tumor, so a midline incision 3 cm length was performed on the most prominent part of the medulla.

At 2 mm under the brain tissue a cystic cavity was entered and its fluid contents evacuated. On inspecting the interior of the cyst, a delicate layer of tumorous tissue could be seen carpeting the wall. The tumor had a dense texture and was well-delineated from the normal brain tissue. Under the dissecting microscope the tumor was removed with the ultrasonic aspirator until only normal brain tissue was apparent. A temporary rise of the blood pressure was noted when the tumoral portion adjacent to the brain tissue was removed. After the tumor had been removed radically the caudal brain stem regained its normal configuration and it became possible to inspect the cavity of the fourth ventricle (Figure 62-41B).

The patient tolerated the operation well, but aggravation of the caudal brain stem symptoms occurred. At discharge 13 days later, the main preoperative and postoperative symptoms had improved. The CT examination on discharge did not reveal any residual tumor. One year after surgery the patient is symptom-free except for right hemihypesthesia and bilateral horizontal nystagmus. She attends school.

Case 7. A 5-year-old patient was admitted to the Burdenko Institute of Neurosurgery with a history of unsteady gait for 1 year, headache, dizziness, and vomiting for 6 months prior to admission. Neurologic examination disclosed signs of increased intracranial pressure. There were signs and symptoms of involvement of the right fifth (including the motor portion), sixth, seventh, and eighth cranial nerves. Moderate pyramidal, cerebellar, and bulbar signs were also evident.

A CT scan with intravenous contrast revealed a hyperdense, well-demarcated lesion in the right half of the posterior fossa (Figure 62-42A). A hypodense zone around the tumor nodule was considered to be a cystic portion of the tumor.

On December 8, 1983 a fibrillary astrocytoma of the right half of the pons and spreading to the right cerebellopontine cistern was radically removed (the scheme of the tumor site as seen during surgery is presented in Figure 62-43).

On exposing the right cerebellopontine angle through a retromastoid approach a large cyst was encountered and yellowish fluid was evacuated. In front of the cyst a dense tumor nodule was found filling the lateral pontine cistern and spreading to the tentorial incisure. The tumor arose from the right half of the pons, displaced the seventh and eighth and caudal nerve group downward. After the central and lateral portions of the tumor had been removed, its inferior apex was separated from the seventh, eighth, and caudal nerves and resected. The anterior aspect of the tumor was separated from the right cerebral peduncle and removed. The major portion of the tumor was located within the right half of the pons from which it was removed radically with the ultrasonic aspirator until only normal brain tissue was apparent. No hemodynamic disturbances were noted during surgery.

The postoperative course was remarkably smooth but signs

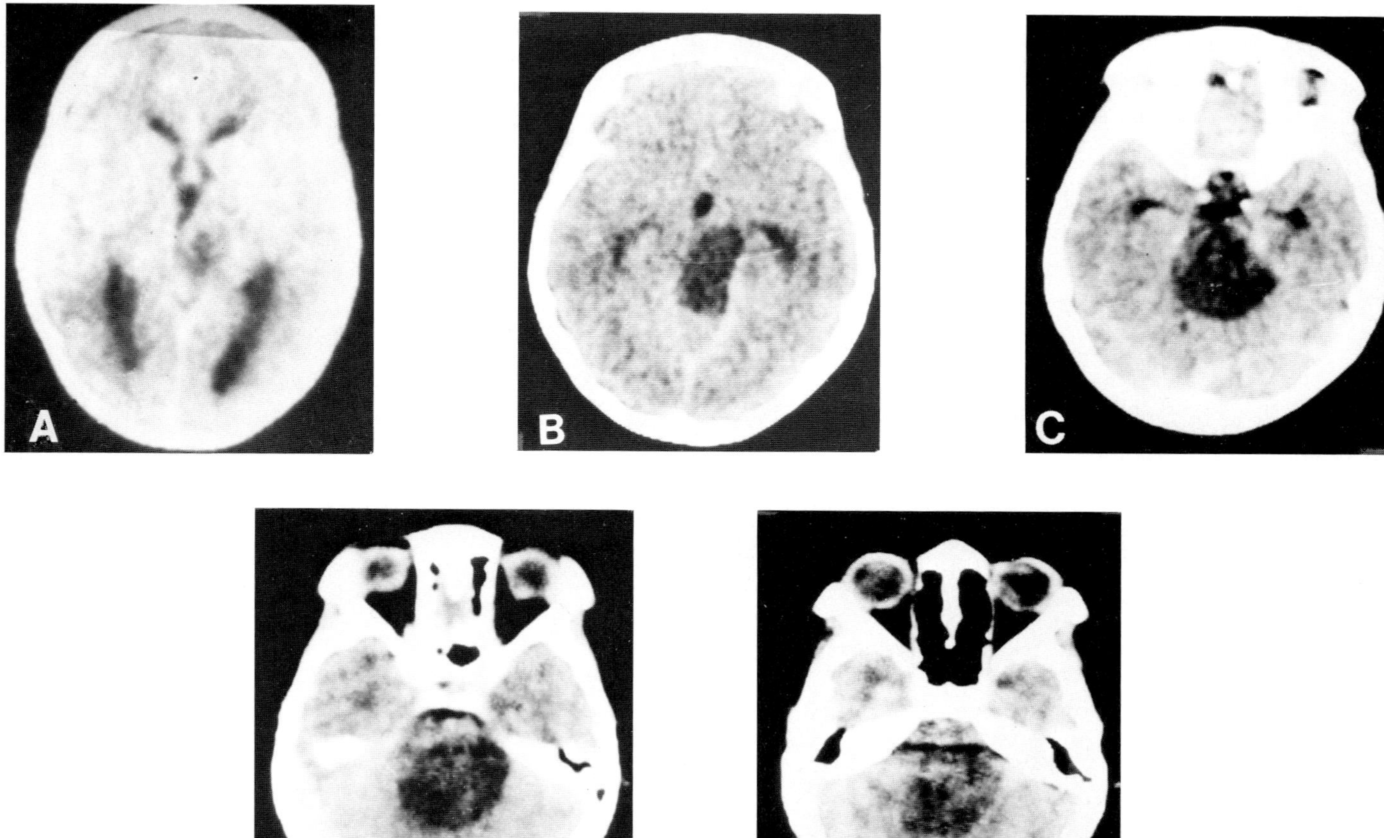

Fig. 62-38 (continued).

of damage to the right fifth and seventh nerves became more evident. The postoperative CT scan showed no residual tumor (Figure 62-42B). At discharge 20 days later, the intracranial hypertension had improved without any remarkable changes in the other symptoms. A follow-up study 2 years postoperatively showed that the patient was symptom-free except for deafness in the right ear (as before the operation). He attends school where he is doing quite well.

CONCLUSIONS

Our experience in surgical removal of primary tumors of different parts of the brain stem is relatively small (38 cases) and the follow-up period is so far limited (1 to 4 years). These conclusions are therefore only preliminary. Nevertheless, this experience has allowed us to conclude that focal brain stem tumors, which constituted the majority of our surgically treated cases (35 out of 38), not only can be, but should be removed, since the general condition and the neurologic status of most of our patients became better after surgery.

The operating microscope, microsurgical instrumentation, and ultrasonic aspirators make it possible to remove focal brain stem tumors radically with minimal damage to the surrounding brain tissue.

The majority of the patients with focal (nodular) benign brain stem gliomas tolerate the surgery comparatively well. In the postoperative period in some cases the local neurologic signs (and the vital functions in 5 patients) may be aggravated, but they gradually improve and by 3 to 6 months later the majority of the patients are better than before surgery. The tumor recurred in only 1 patient 2 years after surgery.

The result of surgery in the group with diffuse infiltrative brain stem tumors (even though they were histologically benign) is unfavorable. In these cases only partial removal of the tumor can be done, and these 3 patients died of hemorrhage from the unresected tumor.

Four patients had malignant gliomas. The postoperative course for these patients was stormy, and the tumor recurred in 2 patients after 7 months and 1½ years, respectively. All these patients are still alive but disabled.

In selecting patients for surgery we made attempts to exclude those patients with infiltrative gliomas and tumors with signs of malignancy, since there was no basis for hopeful outcome.

The favorable results obtained after surgical removal of focal gliomas of different parts of the brain stem should stimulate study of the different types of tumor growth and the possibility of differentiating between focal and infiltrative brain stem gliomas using CT and MRI scanning. In such cases important additional information can be gained from MRI. A wider experience is needed to define the diagnostic criteria for focal and infiltrative brain stem gliomas.

It is important to divide brain stem gliomas into three

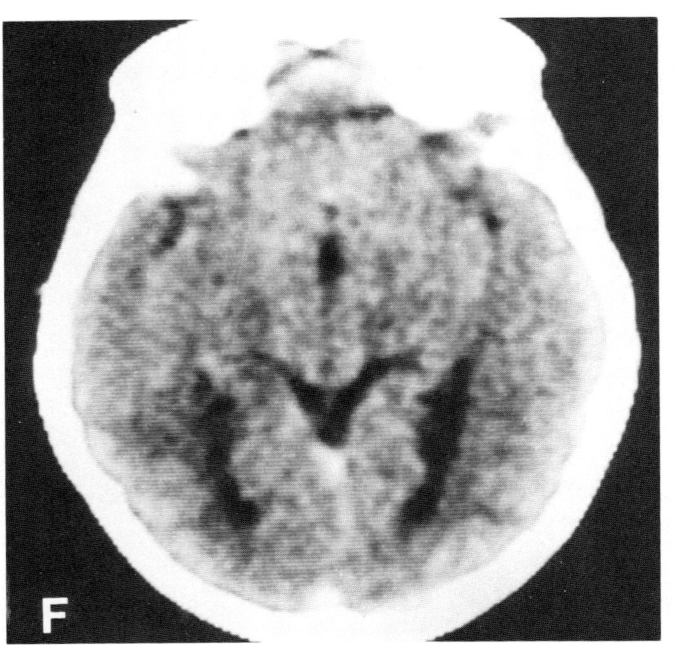

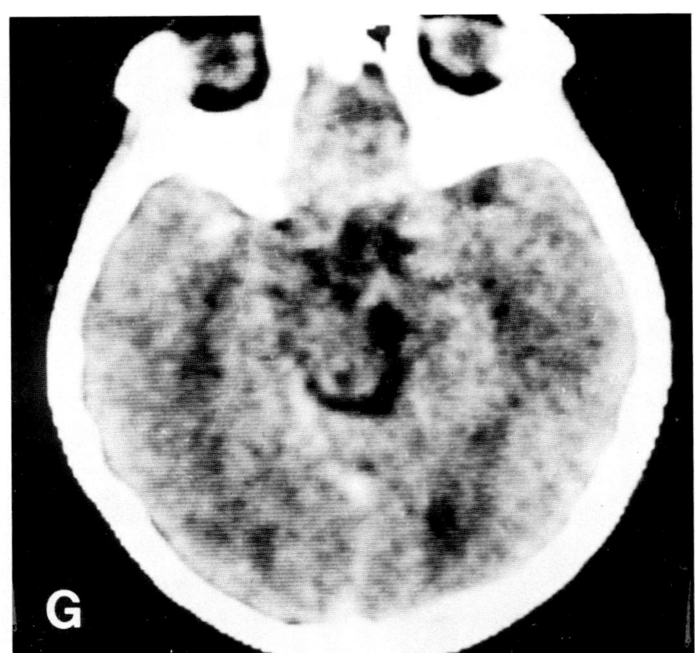

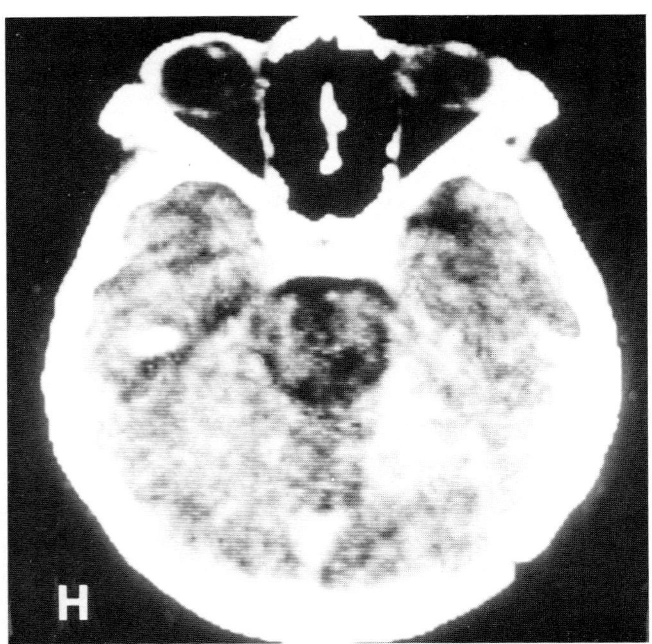

Fig. 62-38. Case 5. Enhanced CT scans. (A–E) preoperative; (F,G,H) postoperative.

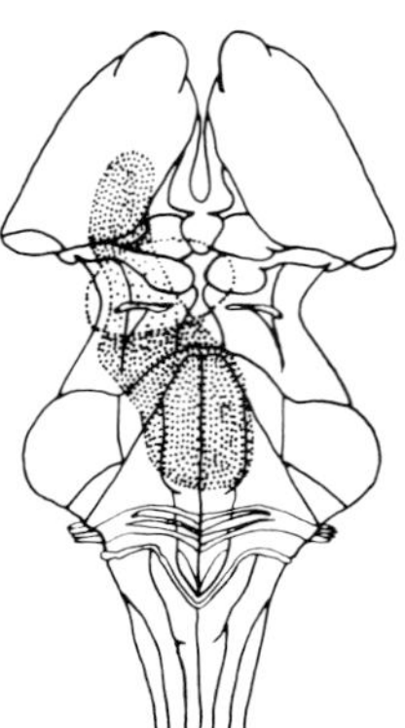

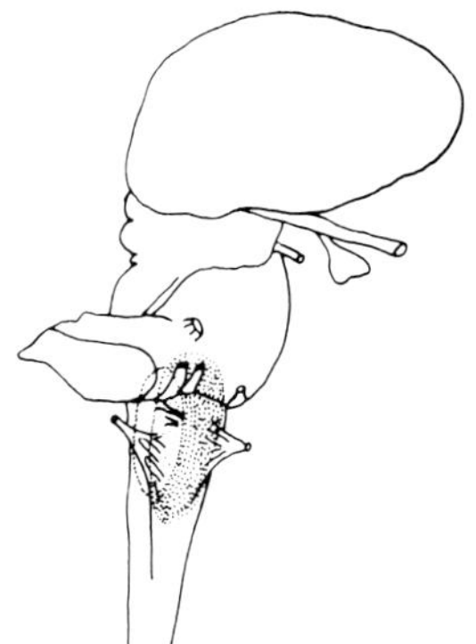

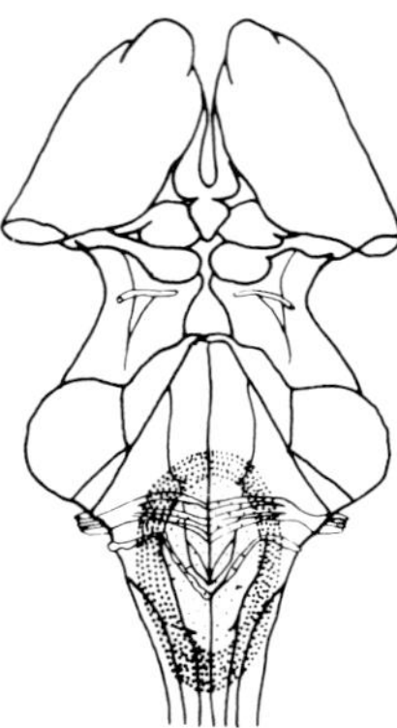

Fig. 62-39. Location of the tumor in case 5. Shaded area: intratruncal portion; open area: cystic portion.

Fig. 62-40. Location of the tumor in case 6. Shaded area: intratruncal portion; open area: cystic portion.

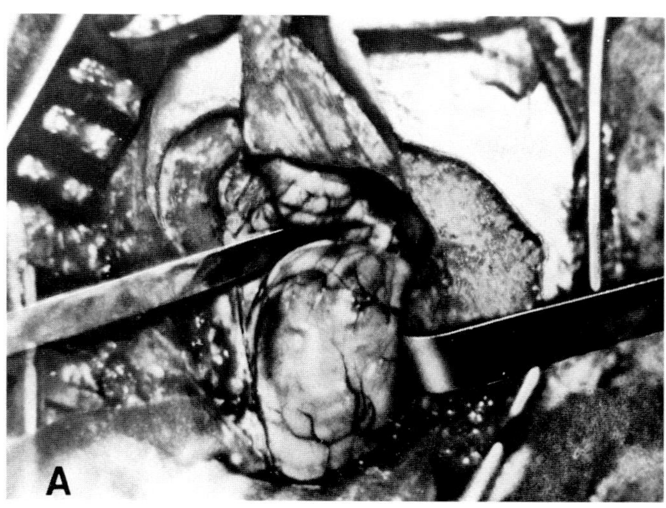
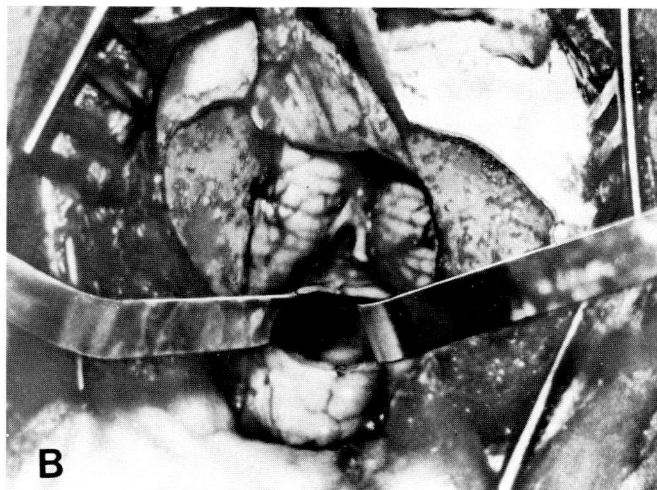

Fig. 62-41. Intraoperative photographs. (A) Intratruncal fibrillary astrocytoma of the medulla and caudal pons bulging into the fourth ventricle. The enlarged caudal brain stem is visible. (B) The spatulas are in the bed of the removed tumor.

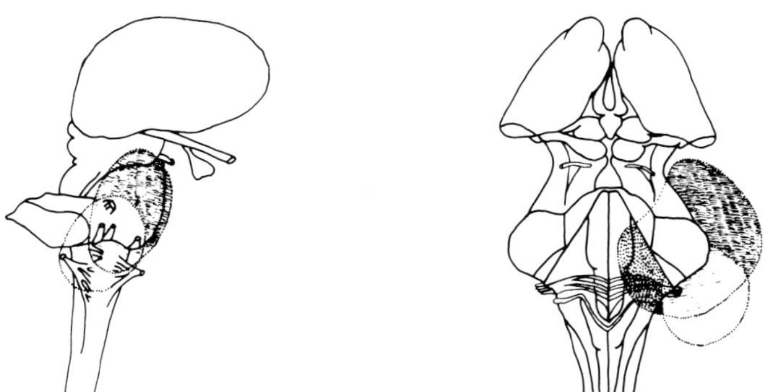

Fig. 62-42. Location of the tumor in case 7. Shaded area: intratruncal portion; cross-hatched area: extrinsic portion; open area: cyst.

groups (thalamic, midbrain, and caudal brain stem) and to identify different variations within each group. Such topographic and anatomic grouping is essential in choosing the suitable approach for direct surgical attack.

In spite of the fact that radiotherapy was widely used to treat patients with primary brain stem tumors, because the number of observations is still limited, no conclusive evidence about its effect on different gliomas and especially after tumor removal exists.

For many years the treatment of patients with brain stem gliomas was considered hopeless and hazardous. Only recently, as a result of rapid progress in diagnostic and surgical techniques, the development of neuroanesthesiology, postoperative intensive care, can this difficult neurosurgical problem be

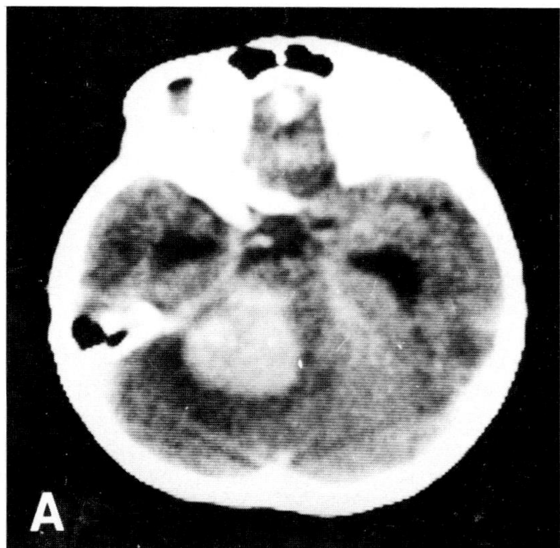
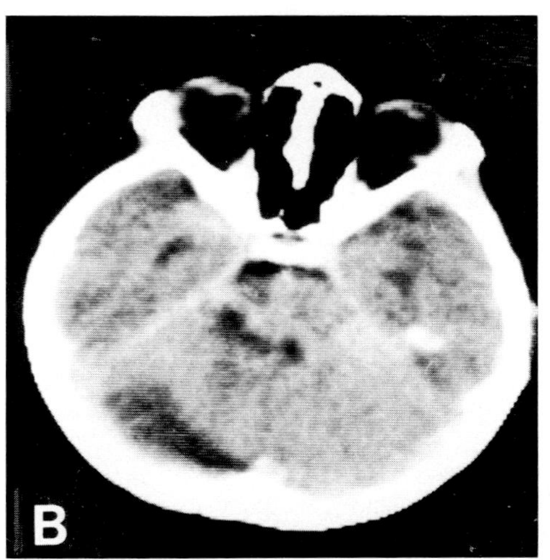

Fig. 62-43. Case 7. CT scans (A) before and (B) after surgery.

approached. The success noted in this chapter should stimulate further study and research in this area of neurosurgery.

ACKNOWLEDGMENTS

The authors wish to express their gratitude to Prof. S. M. Blinkov and Dr. M. V. Pucillo for their assistance in analyzing the morphologic data on the brain stem gliomas discussed in this chapter.

REFERENCES

1. Bouchard J, Pierce CB: Radiation therapy in the management of neoplasma of the central nervous system with special note in regard to children: Twenty years experience, 1938–1958. AJR 84:610, 1960

2. Whyte TR, Colby MY, Layton DD: Radiation therapy of brain stem tumors. Radiology 93:413, 1969

3. Greenberger JS, Cassady JR, Levene MB: Radiation therapy of thalamic, midbrain and brain stem gliomas. Radiology 122:463, 1977

4. Krenkel W: Prognostic and catamnestic studies of supratentorial and brainstem tumors in childhood, Bushe KA, Spoerri O, Shaw J (eds): Progress in Paediatric Neurosurgery. Stuttgart, Hippokrates Verlag, pp 22–28

5. Bruno L, Schut L: Survey of pediatric brain tumors, in Section of Pediatric Neurosurgery, American Association of Neurological Surgeons: Pediatric Neurosurgery: Surgery of the Developing Nervous System. New York, Grune & Stratton, 1982, pp 361–365

6. Rieley HA: An Atlas of the Basal Ganglia, Brain Stem and Spinal Cord. Baltimore, Williams, 1943, p 697

7. Sarkisov SA, Filimonova IN (eds): Atlas of the Brain Stem in Humans and Animals. Moscow, Brain Institute, 1947, (in Russian)

8. Blinkov SM, Smirnov NA: Brain displacements and deformations. New York, Plenum Press, 1971 pp 218

9. Schlesinger B: The Upper Brain Stem in the Human, Its Nuclear Configuration and Vascular Supply. Berlin, Springer-Verlag, 1976

10. Fix JD: Atlas of the Human Brain Stem and Spinal Cord. 1981

11. Russell DS, Rubinstein LJ: Pathology of Tumors of the Nervous System. London, Edward Arnold, 1971

12. Russell DS, Rubinstein LJ: Pathology of Tumors of the Nervous System, ed 4. Baltimore, Williams & Wilkins, 1977, pp 181–182

13. Hoffman HJ, Becker L, Craven MA: A clinically and pathologically distinct group of benign brain stem gliomas. Neurosurgery 7:243, 1980

14. Humphreys RP: Posterior cranial fossa brain tumors in children, in Youmans (ed) Neurological Surgery, vol 5. 1982, pp 2733–2758

15. Mantravadi RVP, Phatak R, Bellur S, et al: Brain stem gliomas. An autopsy study of 25 cases. Cancer 49:1294, 1982

16. Zemskaja AG, Lechinski BI: Brain Tumors of Astrocytic Type. Leningrad, Medicina, 1985, pp 28–29, (in Russian)

17. Lassman LP, Lond MB, Arjona VE, et al: Pontine gliomas of childhood. Lancet 1:913, 1967

18. Pantich HS, Berg BO: Brain stem tumors of childhood and adolescence. Am J Dis Child 119:465, 1970

19. Littman P, Jarrett P, Bilaniuk LT, et al: Pediatric brain stem gliomas. Cancer 45:2787, 1980

20. Kim TH, Chin HW, Pollan S, et al: Radiotherapy of primary brain stem tumors. Int J Radiat Oncol Biol Phys 6:51, 1980

21. Raimondi AJ, Tomita T: Hydrocephalus and infratentorial tumors. J Neurosurg 55:174, 1981

22. Albright AL, Price RA, Guthkeleah AN: Brain stem gliomas of children. A clinicopathological study. Cancer 52:2313, 1983

23. Bernstein M, Hoffman HJ, Halliday WC, et al: Thalamic tumors in children. Long-term follow-up and treatment guidelines. J Neurosurg 61:649, 1984

24. Entzian W Removal of intrapontomesencephalic spongioblastoma. Neurosurg Rev 6:67, 1983

25. Ho KL: Tumors of the cerebral aqueduct. Cancer 49:154, 1982

26. DeGirolami U, Armbrustmacher VW: Juvenile pilocytic astrocytoma of the pineal region. Report of a case. Cancer 50:1185, 1982

27. Arseni C: Tumors of the basal ganglia. Their surgical treatment. Arch Neurol Psychiatry 80:1824, 1958

28. Savchenko UN, Zinoviev AS: Favorable outcome after the resection of medulla astrocytoma. Zh Vopr Neirochirurg 6:56, 1971 (in Russian)

29. Mashiyama S, Mori T, Kamiyama K, et al: Total removal of glioma at the base of the fourth ventricle. Case report. Neurol Med Chir 22:855, 1982

30. Albright AL, Sclabassi RT: Use of the Cavitron ultronic surgical aspirator and evoked potentials for the treatment of thalamic and brain stem tumors of children. Neurosurgery 17:563, 1985

31. Epstein F, McCleary EL: Intrinsic brainstem tumors of childhood: Surgical indications. J Neurosurg 64:11, 1986

32. Bilaniuk LT, Zimmerman RA, Littman P, et al: Computed tomography of brain stem gliomas in children. Radiology 134:89, 1980

33. Glanz S, Geehr RB, Duncan CC, et al: Metrizamide-enhanced CT for evaluation of brainstem tumors. AJR 134:821, 1980

34. Mawad ME, Silver AJ, Hibl SK, et al: Computed tomography of the brain stem with intrathecal metrizamide. Part II: Lesions in and around the brain stem. AJR 140:565, 1983

35. Zimmerman RA, Bilaniuk LT, Packer R, et al: Resistive NMR of brain stem gliomas. Neuroradiology 27:21, 1985

36. Matson DD: Tumors of the posterior fossa, in Neurosurgery of Infancy and Childhood, ed 2. Springfield, Ill, Charles C Thomas, 1969, pp 410–479

37. Redmond JS: The roentgen therapy of pontine gliomas. AJR 86:644, 1961

38. Lee F: Radiation of infratentorial and supratentorial brainstem tumors. J Neurosurg 43:65, 1975

39. Fulton DS, Levin VA, Wava WM, et al: Chemotherapy of pediatric brainstem tumors. J Neurosurg 1981, 54:721, 1981

40. Cobb CA, Youmans JR: Glial and neuronal tumors of the brain in adults, in Youmans (ed): Neurological Surgery, vol 5. 1982, pp 2759–2835

41. Cassady JR, Eifel P, Balli JA: Progress and problems in the treatment of brain stem glioma, medulloblastoma and craniopharyngioma in childhood, in Amendola, Amendola (eds): Recent trends in Radiation Oncology and Related Fields. Amsterdam, Elsevier, 1983

42. Baghai P, Varies JK, Bechtel PC: Retromastoid approach for biopsy of brain stem tumors. Neurosurgery 10:574, 1982

43. Sandurskii IM: Treatment of brainstem tumors. Zh Vopr Neirochirurg 4:40, 1978 (in Russian)

44. Lassiter KRL, Alexander E, Davis CH, et al: Surgical treatment of brain stem gliomas: Case reports. J Neurosurg 34:719, 1971

45. Pool JL: Gliomas in the region of the brain stem. J Neurosurg 29:164, 1968

46. Schönmayr R, Agnoli AL: Brain stem tumors: Diagnosis and surgical treatment. Neurosurg Rev 6:57, 1983

47. Kunicki A: Some remarks on the mode of spread of primary benign brainstem tumors based on description of three cases. Zbl Neurochirurg 44:187, 1983

48. Kunicki A: Some remarks about the definite type of benign brain stem gliomas. Neurol Neurochir Pol 18:29, 1984

49. Konovalov AN, Atieh JH: Surgical treatment of caudal brain stem astrocytomas. Zh Vopr Neirochirurg 1986 (in press) (in Russian)

50. Konovalov AN, Larin AI, Mjavanadze GO: Three cases of successful removal of gliomas of the optic thalamus. Zh Vopr Neirochirurg 5:58, 1983

51. Bailey P, Buchanan DN, Bucy PC: Intracranial Tumors of Infancy and Childhood. Chicago, University of Chicago Press, 1939, pp 188–241

52. Greitz T: Tumors of the quadrigeminal plate and adjacent structures. Acta Radiol (Diagn) 12:513, 1972

53. DeGirolami U, Schmidek H: Clinicopathological study of 53 tumors of the pineal region. J Neurosurg 39:455, 1973

54. Kahn EA, Crosby EC, Dejonge BR: Tumors of the posterior fossa, in Correlative Neurosurgery, ed 2. Springfield, Ill, Charles C Thomas, 1969, p 206

55. Netsky MG, Strobos RRJ: Neoplasms within the midbrain. Arch Neurol Psychiatry 68:116, 1952

56. Kandel EI: In Problems of Modern Neurosurgery, vol 3. Moscow, 1959, pp 165–188 (in Russian)

57. Kandel EI: In Guide in Neurology, vol 5. 1961, pp 284–298

58. Tovi D, Schisano G, Liljeqvist B: Primary tumors of the region of the thalamus. J Neurosurg 18:730, 1961

59. Millichap JG, Miller RH, Backus RC: Intracranial tumors in childhood. JAMA 179:589, 1962

60. Hirose G, Lombroso CT, Eisenberg H: Thalamic tumors in childhood. Clinical, laboratory and therapeutic considerations. Arch Neurol 32:740, 1975

61. Arseni C, Horvath L, Dumitrescu L: Extrapyramidal syndromes in intracranial space-occupying processes in children. Eur Neurol 7:169, 1972

62. Clarke JM: The accurate localization of intracranial tumors, excluding tumors of the motor cortex, motor tract, pons and medulla. Brain 21:305, 1898

63. Smyth GE, Stern K: Tumors of the thalamus: A clinicopathological study. Brain 61:339, 1938

64. Hyndman OR, Van Epps C: Tumor of the thalamus. A ventriculographic entity. Arch Surg 39:792, 1939

65. Cheek WR, Taveras JM: Thalamic tumors. J Neurosurg 24:505, 1966

66. Erwin CW, Brendle A, Drake ME: Evoked potentials from the visual, auditory, and somastosensory systems, in Wilkins RH, Rengachary SS (eds): Neurosurgery, vol 1. New York, McGraw-Hill, 1985, pp 211–224

67. Oh SR, Kuba T, Soyer A, et al: Lateralization of brainstem lesions by brainstem auditory evoked potentials. Neurology 31:14, 1981

CHAPTER 63

Glomus Jugulare Tumors— Skull Base Surgery

Gale Gardner   James T. Robertson   Jon H. Robertson
Edwin W. Cocke, Jr.   W. Craig Clark

GLOMUS JUGULARE TUMORS, occurring at the base of the skull, frequently involving the lower cranial nerves, and occasionally extending into the posterior cranial fossa, can constitute a significant surgical problem for the neurosurgeon. The ideal method of treatment is surgical excision. This chapter will describe a surgical method that has been used successfully in 22 patients. We will also review the historical developments leading up to this procedure, the methods of diagnosis that we have employed, and present the results obtained in this study. Ancillary forms of management will also be discussed, and a case presentation made.

HISTORICAL REVIEW

The definitive work on glomus tumors was done by Guild[1] and Rosenwasser[2] in the early 1940s. Since that time, a continuing effort has been made by both neurosurgeons and otologists to accomplish total removal of glomus jugulare tumors. The unique problems associated with this tumor, which originates in the dome of the jugular bulb and involves the base of the skull, include inaccessibility to conventional surgical approaches, close proximity to important vascular and neurologic structures, and the vascular nature of the tumor itself. Whereas glomus tympanic tumors arising in the middle ear can usually be removed either through the ear canal or mastoid with a reasonable certainty of complete removal, such is not the case with a glomus jugulare tumor arising from the jugular bulb. All too often surgeons have found it necessary to compromise oncologic principles and remove the tumor piece by piece, accompanied by formidable bleeding and the risk of incomplete removal and damage to adjacent neurovascular structures.

As a result of this, over the years many authorities have recommended either limited surgery combined with radiation therapy or radiation therapy alone.[3-5] The typically slow growth of glomus tumors and their relative responsiveness to irradiation have supported this conclusion.

This approach has not been entirely satisfactory, however. The natural history of the tumor and its response to irradiation have been unpredictable and erratic.[6] While some tumors have grown slowly without treatment over a period of as long as 42 years,[7] others have in a short time frame destroyed the temporal bone and the base of the skull, extended into the neck, involved the cranial cavity, and occasionally metastasized elsewhere.[4]

Mortality has been reported to be between 9.4 and 22 percent.[4,7,8] As a result of this, a variety of surgical approaches have been developed over the past 35 years, having in common the goal of total removal of the tumor as a unit, usually with inclusion of the jugular bulb, based on wide exposure and relative hemostasis.

In 1949, Lundgren[9] suggested removal or coagulation of the jugular bulb in those instances in which a glomus tumor appeared to arise from the bulb. He was influenced in this by the earlier work of Seiffert,[10] who in 1934 had reported a case of an apparent glomus jugulare tumor[11] originating in the bulb and producing a jugular foramen syndrome. In this case he had explored the bulb and found an intraluminal tumor.

In 1951, Weille[12] discussed the surgical problems associated with removal of glomus tumors, and recommended making the assumption that they originate from the dome of the jugular bulb. He advised removal of bone from around the tumor to avoid trauma to and bleeding from the tumor. He did not recommend removal of the bulb, however, feeling that the risk of significant hemorrhage was too great.

Also in 1951, Seemes,[13] in Memphis, reported successfully removing a 2-cm glomus jugulare tumor from the jugular foramen through a suboccipital approach. The patient had complained of hearing loss and tinnitus, and a red discoloration of the involved tympanic membrane had been noted preoperatively, as well as involvement of cranial nerves IX–XII. Total removal of the tumor was accomplished from the posterior fossa. In a later personal communication (March 29, 1976), Semmes stated that no effort had been made to remove the tumor from the middle ear or mastoid. Rather, radiation therapy had been used preoperatively, and the patient was living and well 25 years later.

At approximately the same time, Bucy and Albernaz[14] reported on a patient who had had symptoms and findings of jugular foramen compression and hearing loss. Using a suboccipital approach, the lower cranial nerves appeared to be abnormal, but no tumor was visualized. Cardiorespiratory collapse occurred during closure and the patient expired. Autopsy showed a 1×2-cm tumor within the jugular foramen involving adjacent structures. Bucy felt that this tumor had arisen from the paragangli intravagali of the ganglion nodosum, but in a later personal communication (March 22, 1976) he acknowledged that it was entirely possible that the tumor may

OPERATIVE NEUROSURGICAL TECHNIQUES
ISBN 0-8089-1862-1

have been a glomus jugulare tumor since it originated within the jugular foramen. Bucy concluded that exposure of this tumor would have required resection of the base of the skull lateral to the jugular foramen and indicated that when faced with a similar problem, he would use such an approach.

In 1952, Capps[15] reported upon the cases of 5 patients having glomus jugulare tumors whom he had treated. In one case he described mobilizing the facial nerve, packing off the lateral sinus, ligating the upper end of the internal jugular vein, and attempting unsuccessfully to remove the jugular bulb. A stormy postoperative course resulted. Capps concluded that he would be reluctant to carry out such a procedure again, and instead had used radiation therapy on the remaining four cases in his series. He had not found the tumor to be as radioresistant as previously reported and described gratifying results in these cases.

In 1955, Williams[3] concluded, on the basis of his own experience as well as that of others, surgical treatment for these lesions was decreasingly popular, and that radiation therapy, either singly or combined with surgery, was preferable. In coming to this conclusion, Williams was influenced by the state of the art existing in diagnosis at the time. It was impossible, using the technology available, to differentiate precisely between a glomus tumor arising in the middle ear from one arising in the jugular bulb. Neither was it possible to know the size and location of these tumors with any degree of accuracy. While arteriography had recently become available,[16] subtraction technique[17] would not be available until 1916, Valvasorri[18] would not report on the use of polytomography until 1963, and Gejrot[19] would not report on retrograde jugularography until 1964. These advances in diagnostic technology would allow Kohut and Lindsay[20] in 1964 and McCabe[4] in 1969 to advocate careful assessment of the size and extent of glomus tumors as the basis for selecting the most appropriate form of treatment.

In 1958, Meacham and Capps[21] and Thoms[22] reported the removal of glomus jugulare tumors through the subocciput. Although Thoms believed that many of these lesions could be resected surgically in this way, he believed that if there was extensive involvement of bone, surgery was not feasible, and he preferred radiation therapy. Beginning in the early 1960s, a renewal of interest in complete surgical removal of glomus jugular tumors, including the jugular bulb, was noted. Gastpar[23] advocated removal of the jugular bulb when involved, including sacrifice of the facial nerve and labyrinth if necessary.

Michelson and Connolloy[24] in 1962 reported the case of a patient in whom they had used vascular occlusion and hypothermia to allow removal of a recurrent glomus jugulare tumor that involved the internal carotid artery. Bilaterial occlusion of the common carotid and vertebral arteries was employed for a period of 10 minutes. They felt that this technique would allow intracranial surgery to be accomplished in situations otherwise inoperable because of vascular involvement.

In 1963, Shapiro and Neues[25] reported the case of a patient who had previously undergone a radical mastoidectomy for glomus jugulare tumor, with later recurrence. They described using an extended incision, rerouting the facial nerve, exposing the hypotympanum and jugular bulb, and accomplishing complete tumor removal with minimal blood loss and no neurologic sequelae.

Gejrot, who had developed retrograde jugularography[19] and was therefore aware of the frequency of intraluminal jugular bulb involvement by these tumors, in 1965[26] described a procedure similar to Shapiro's. He performed a radical mastoidectomy; rerouted the facial nerve; exposed and opened the internal jugular vein, jugular bulb, and sigmoid sinus; and removed the tumor tissue in and around the bulb. He had performed four of these procedures. Several features of Gejrot's report were of particular significance. He believed that jugular bulb involvement was invariably present when a glomus tumor was present in the hypotympanum and concluded that removal of the bulb was a necessary part of any surgical procedure in these cases. He also described packing the sigmoid sinus superiorly, and then resecting the lateral wall of the sinus inferiorly to the level of the jugular bulb, thereby preserving the medial wall of the sinus and avoiding opening into the subarachnoid space. With control of the sigmoid sinus above and the internal jugular vein below, and the jugular bulb exposed, he described removing the tumor from both directions. His article included a photograph of a surgical specimen with intact tumor within the jugular vein.

In 1968, William House[27] described his experience with removal of glomus jugulare tumors with preservation of the bony ear canal and preservation of hearing. He described exposure of the jugular bulb through a combined neck and simple mastoidectomy approach. Leaving the facial nerve in place, he operated through the facial recess, which he extended inferiorly to expose the hypotympanum. He recognized the need for greater exposure at the base of the skull (personal communication, March 30, 1976). The experience of working with House stimulated one of us (GG) to begin a study to overcome this problem, which eventually led to the results reported in this chapter.

Portmann[28] also in 1968 described the removal in two stages of a large glomus jugulare tumor having intracranial extension, using a team approach with neurosurgical and otologic participation.

The 1970s and 1980s have seen continued and increasing interest in total removal of glomus jugulare tumors. In 1971, Kempe[29] described en bloc excision of tumors arising in the jugular foramen which involve both the temporal bone and the posterior fossa. His approach was similar to that described by Shapiro and Gejrot but in addition included a suboccipital craniectomy. Kempe did not, however, mention transposition of the facial nerve. He described the use of dural grafts when large tumors necessitated the resection of dura.

Also in 1971, Hilding and Greenberg[30] reported a single case of glomus jugulare tumor with intracranial extension in which they performed both a transtemporal and suboccipital approach. A radical mastoidectomy had been performed and the facial nerve rerouted. In addition, they had removed bone anteriorly from over the internal carotid artery through the glenoid fossa. The sigmoid sinus was ligated and the subocciput opened, followed by piecemeal removal of the tumor. Although the tenth cranial nerve was sacrificed because of tumor involvement, normal facial nerve function and normal hearing were preserved.

Spector, Maisel, and Ogura[6] in 1973 analyzed the results of their treatment for 46 patients having glomus tumors. They concluded that the treatment of choice was surgical and preferred Shapiro's technique of wide excision for those very large tumors involving the jugular foramen and skull base.

In 1974, Glasscock[31] described a combination of Shapiro's approach with that of House in which he preserved the posterior bony canal wall and utilized an extended facial recess approach. In most instances, it had not been necessary to transpose the facial nerve. In 1976, we first reported the surgical method we had developed for the management of this problem and that is described in this chapter.[32]

In 1977, Fisch[33] reported operating through the infratemporal fossa to remove glomus jugulare tumors and to expose the internal carotid artery on 12 patients. This exposure overcame the problem of internal carotid exposure within the temporal bone. In a later report,[34] Fisch elaborated upon this procedure, and described three basic approaches, depending upon the size and extent of the tumor. Fisch classified glomus tumors as being of four types:

Class A: Those tumors confined to the middle ear space.
Class B: Those tumors limited to the middle ear and mastoid without involvement of the infralabyrinthine space.
Class C: Those tumors involving the infralabyrinthine and apical spaces of the temporal bone: (1) tumors involving the jugular bulb and foramen but without significant involvement of the vertical segment of the carotid canal; (2) tumors invading the vertical segment of the carotid canal; and (3) tumors invading the horizontal segment of the carotid canal.
Class D: Those tumors extending intracranially and intradurally: (1) tumors extending intracranially less than 2 cm in diameter; (2) tumors greater than 2 cm in diameter; and (3) tumors that are inoperable.

Jackson et al.,[35] in 1982, elaborated upon their concepts and techniques, including a classification of tumors similar to that of Fisch.

Goldenberg,[36] in 1984, described the surgical anatomy of the skull base with an extensive literature review.

EPIDEMIOLOGY

Glomus tumors represent the most common neoplasm involving the middle ear, and with the exception of acoustic tumors, represent the most common neoplasm of the temporal bone.[37] They can occur at any decade of life, occur six times more frequently in women than in men, and produce symptoms that precede diagnosis from 1 month to 28 years.[38] Their most characteristic presentation is in women in middle life.[39] There have been only rare reports of multiple glomus tumors in the same patient.[40] McNeill and Milner[41] reported an incidence of bilateral glomus jugulare tumors. More commonly, glomus jugulare tumors occur in association with carotid body tumors or glomus vagali tumors, as well as with associated malignancies.[40] Although previous reports indicate a familial tendency in carotid body tumors,[42,43] this has not been as well demonstrated with glomus jugulare tumors. Goekoop[44] reported the incidence of glomus jugulare tumors in three sisters. Our series includes glomus jugulare tumors in a brother and sister.

ANATOMY AND PATHOLOGY

Glomus tumors are highly vascular. The blood supply is predominantly from the inferior tympanic branch of the ascending pharyngeal artery, with added supply from the posterior auricular artery via the stylomastoid branch, and from branches of the occipital, internal maxillary, vertebral, and internal carotid arteries.[45]

The histologic structure is indistinguishable from that of carotid body tumor. Large groups of polyhedral epithelioid chief cells are noted, with centrally located hyperchromatic nuclei and finely granular eosinophilic cytoplasm. Cells are arranged in clusters that are interspersed in a network of fibrous tissue, and are adjacent to thin-walled capillary vessels.[46]

Glomus jugulare tumors are locally invasive.[47] Metastasis is rare, occurring in under 10 percent of cases, with spread usually involving regional lymph nodes or the lung.[4,38,48-50] Tumor spread is along planes of least resistance, typically mastoid air cells, and along preformed pathways. Spector et al.,[51] have described pathways for central extension as being (1) along the eustachian tube into the nasopharynx and through foramina at the base of the skull; (2) along the carotid artery into the middle fossa space; (3) along the jugular vein or hypoglossal canal into the posterior fossa; (4) through the tegmen tympani to the middle fossa floor; and (5) through the round window of the labyrinth and extending through the internal auditory canal to the cerebellopontine angle. It is therefore not unusual for central nervous system invasion to occur in multiple sites.

Our own experience is that tumor extension into the posterior fossa occurs in two different ways, with resulting surgical significance. The less common form of extension is by direct herniation through the jugular foramen, utilizing the dural defect that is anatomically present. A more common extension, however, is by erosion of bone overlying the posterior fossa and extension into the fossa, pushing the overlying dura ahead of it. In this case, the intracranial tumor extension is extradural, while in the former instance it is intradural. In the case of extradural tumor extension, every effort should be made to take advantage of the protection afforded by the dura by preserving it. In the event of intradural extension, which we think is less common, greater risk is obviously involved.

Our experience has been that the primary tumor mass is centered in the jugular fossa, with the tumor filling the lumen of the jugular bulb, and appearing smooth and lobulated. We have noted a dissimilarity between the appearance of the tumor on x-ray studies preoperatively and after its removal. In contrast to the massive nature of the x-ray appearance and the appearance of the tumor during exposure at surgery, the specimen itself has appeared much smaller and less extensive. The smooth, lobulated primary tumor mass situated within the jugular bulb has a quite different appearance from the budding excrescences seen within the air cells of the mastoid air cell system. We have not noted any single, well-defined connection between the primary tumor mass and these extensions into the air cell system.

PHYSIOLOGY

The physiologic function of glomus bodies remains uncertain. While some investigators believe that they are similar to the carotid body and act as chemoreceptors sensitive to changes in oxygen and carbon dioxide tension,[52] others believe that they are functionally inert.[53] Anatomically, glomus bodies are considered part of the chemoreceptor system that includes the carotid body and the aortic body. Similar glomus tissue has been identified in the ciliary ganglion, the ganglion nodosum of the vagus nerve, and in or adjacent to the walls of large arteries, particularly the superior mesenteric artery and the femoral artery.[38] Lawson[54] has concluded that the glomus cell, which differentiates into an epithelioid-type cell, is a modified neuroblast of presumed neural crest origin. This neurogenic nature and its secretory capacity make it a true neurocrine[46] cell,

Table 63-1. Initial symptoms of glomus tumor patients

Symptoms*	Number of Cases	Mean Durations (Months)
Tinnitus	24	70
Hearing loss	20	110
Ear pain	17	40
Blockage	12	54
Dizziness	5	36

*In 13 patients two or three of these initial symptoms occurred simultaneously.

but the actual incidence of functional activity in glomus jugulare tumors is only approximately 1 percent.[55]

Considerable histochemical and ultrastructural evidence for catecholamine secretion in glomus jugulare tumors exists, even in those tumors that are endocrinologically silent.[56] Formaldehyde-induced fluorescence microscopy, chromatography, spectrofluorophotometry, and electron microscopy have been used to confirm the presence of catecholamines. Electron microscopy has demonstrated that the dense secretory granules found in the cytoplasm of glomus cells are the type of granules known to contain catecholamines.[56]

The biochemistry of catecholamines has been reviewed elsewhere.[57] Clinically, several studies have documented high levels of norepinephrine in functional glomus tumors.[56,58–60] Norepinephrine levels are elevated because glomus tumors lack the enzyme methyl transferase, and it is this enzyme that converts norepinephrine to epinephrine. Norepinephrine and epinephrine are metabolized to normetanephrine and metanephrine, respectively. Both of these products are converted to vanillylmandelic acid (VMA), which is excreted in the urine, along with lesser quantities of metanephrines. Screening a 24–hour urine collection for VMA and metanephrines allows the surgeon to avoid the surprise of a potentially lethal hypertensive crisis at the time of surgery.

CLINICAL MATERIAL

Thirty-six patients were treated by us for glomus jugulare tumors between June 20, 1972, and the present. The average age of these patients was 46 years when first seen by us. Twenty-one patients were female, and 15 were male. Seven patients were treated with surgery alone; 14 were treated with radiation therapy alone; and 15 were treated using a combination of radiation therapy and surgery.

DIAGNOSIS

A diagnosis of glomus jugulare tumor in this series of patients had been suspected on the basis of preceding symptoms (Table 63-1) and established by procedures listed in Table 63-2. Various combinations of cranial nerve dysfunction were noted preoperatively (Table 63-3). Arteriography and, particularly, computed tomography (CT) have become the definitive diagnostic methods we use.

Table 63-2. Positive findings

Finding	Number of Cases
Ear canal	36
Arteriography	32
Audiometry	24
Cranial nerves	21
Biopsy/venography	19
Plain x-ray studies	17
CT scans	16

COMPUTED TOMOGRAPHY

We most recently used the GE 9800 scanner to map out the extent of and to confirm the characteristics of glomus jugular tumors. Slices 1.5 cm apart are used. The contrast portion of the examination is carried out with a biphasic injection (bolus plus infusion) in order to maintain a high intravascular iodine content throughout the examination, and high resolution technique is used. Axial projections are obtained routinely; coronal projections are obtained if involvement of the internal carotid artery is suspected. Reformatted images are obtained to maximize three-dimensional visualization of the tumor.

ARTERIOGRAPHY

On the day after CT examination, transfemoral arteriography is performed with selective catheterization of the external and internal carotid and vertebral arteries and with selective injection of the external carotid as well as the feeding vessels, when this is possible. The arterial system is evaluated to confirm the characteristic tumor blush produced by a glomus tumor as well as to study the feeding vessels to establish possible candidacy for embolization. Intra-arterial digital subtraction is used as an adjunct to enhance the study.

DIFFERENTIAL DIAGNOSIS

Depending upon whether the presentation is otologic or neurologic, the clinician is faced with a variety of differential diagnoses.[61] If the presentation is otologic, certain other conditions must be excluded. The use of high-resolution computed tomography allows evaluation of the bony walls separating the jugular bulb and the carotid artery from the middle ear. If these

Table 63-3. Initial cranial nerve dysfunction

Cranial Nerves Involved	Number of Cases
VI, VII, VIII	1
VII, VIII	1
VII, VIII, IX, X, XI, XII	1
XII	1
VIII	10
VIII, IX, X, XI, XII	2
VII, VIII, X, XI, XII	2
X	1
VIII, X, XII	1
VII, VIII, X, XII	1
None	15
Total	36

bony walls are intact and in normal position, one can conclude that the lesion is limited to the middle ear and that vascular anomalies are not present.[62] Vascular anomalies that can mimic glomus tumors include congenital dehiscence of the bony jugular wall with protrusion of the jugular bulb into the hypotympanum,[63] aberrant carotid artery involving the middle ear,[53] persistent stapedial artery,[64] and aneurysm of the internal carotid artery presenting in the middle ear.[65]

If the presentation is neurologic, as in the case of a jugular foramen syndrome, one must exclude other causes such as neurilemmoma, primary cholesteatoma, cholesterol granuloma, chondrosarcoma, carcinoma, metastatic tumor, or meningioma.[66] The major differential is between glomus jugulare tumors and neurilemmomas.[67] Although both enhance with high resolution computed tomography, they have different angiographic appearances.[62]

Primary cholesteatomas and cholesterol granulomas have a similar appearance on CT, but can be differentiated on the basis of their varying degrees of density.[68]

Sarcomas and carcinomas of the temporal bone are often large, destructive masses, but they characteristically do not follow standard pathways of involvement.[69] Metastases, particularly renal and thyroid, may produce destructive vascular lesions similar to glomus jugulare tumors. Metastases, however, do not follow the typical routes of invasion and are clinically invasive, producing early multiple cranial nerve palsies.[70]

Meningiomas can occasionally occur in the inferior portion of the posterior fossa. Calcification of the tumor and hyperostosis of surrounding bone, which are visible on high resolution computed tomography, suggest this diagnosis, but not invariably. These lesions are quite vascular on arteriograms, and may obtain their blood supply from the ascending pharyngeal artery.[71]

The primary purposes for arteriography are (1) confirmation of diagnosis; (2) demonstration of arterial feeders; (3) exclusion of associated carotid body or glomus vagale tumors; and (4) assessment of candidacy for preoperative embolization.[62] Retrograde jugular venography was the procedure of choice for demonstrating blockage of the jugular bulb.[19] This procedure, however, was not suitable for demonstration of extraluminal tumor extension.[62] This information is now obtained either by means of a delayed venous-phase arteriogram or by intravenous injection using digital subtraction technique. Kinney and Modic[72] now rely on intravenous digital subtraction angiography when embolization is not being considered. Pluridirectional tomography demonstrates the bony extent of glomus jugulare tumors accurately but does not allow demonstration of intracranial extension. It is therefore rarely used as a primary diagnostic tool at this time, but rather is used to provide additional information in areas that are questionable on CT scans.[62]

High resolution computed tomography is therefore the diagnostic method of choice in the evaluation of glomus jugulare tumors. If the jugular plate is eroded, or if neurologic signs are present, the lesion may be outlined by axial and coronal cuts, with arteriography to confirm the diagnosis, demonstrate arterial feeders, demonstrate blockage of the jugular bulb, and indicate candidacy for possible embolization.[62] Because of the importance of the bony anatomy in the evaluation of glomus jugulare tumors, the role of magnetic resonance imaging is uncertain at this time, and high resolution computed tomography remains the diagnostic procedure of choice.

TREATMENT

SELECTION OF TREATMENT

We use a variety of treatment methods, singly and in combination, depending on the clinical circumstances. These methods include radiation therapy given preoperatively, postoperatively, or alone; embolization given preoperatively (or conceivably alone); and surgery, either alone or in combination with radiation therapy, embolization, or both. Surgery can involve the skull base approach with or without the use of additional approaches to extend the exposure, or the hypotympanotomy approach for a tumor that does not require resection of the jugular bulb.

RADIATION THERAPY

The role of radiation therapy in relation to surgery for the treatment of glomus jugulare tumors is controversial.[73] Opinion ranges between feelings that radiation therapy is of value[38,73,74] to feelings that it is contraindicated.[75] Cole[74] reported the long-term results with 20 patients having glomus jugulare tumors that showed no significant growth following treatment with 4000–5000 rad of radiation therapy. Cummings et al.[73] reported on a series of 45 patients who received a smaller amount of radiation therapy, with only three instances of recurrence or tumor progression.

The way in which radiotherapy affects tumor growth is not well understood. Fibrosis has been demonstrated, but an effect upon cellular or vascular components is doubtful.[38] Maruyami et al.,[76] studied patients angiographically before and after radiation therapy, and in spite of an excellent clinical response, they could demonstrate no changes radiographically.

We prefer not to use irradiation in very young patients but have found it useful otherwise. We discussed our use of it in an earlier article.[32] In patients having large tumors who are surgical candidates, we have used it in an attempt to reduce tumor vascularity to facilitate the surgical procedure. In elderly patients, or in those having a significant medical problem, we have used it alone and followed the patient on a long-term basis with repeated CT scans. If tumor growth recurs, we re-evaluate the patient's surgical candidacy in light of the tumor growth. We have also used radiation therapy postoperatively in several patients early in our experience when residual tumor was left on the internal carotid artery.

For preoperative therapy, we are currently administering 4500 rad in 5 weeks to tumor volume, using colbalt 60 radiation with superior/inferior wedge-paired fields. Isodose curves are chosen to give a margin of 1.0–1.5 cm on tumor volume. We usually schedule surgery 3 to 4 months after the completion of therapy. For x-ray therapy without surgery, we administer an additional 1000 rad, using the appropriate electron or photon energy, generally with a single opposed field.

We carried out comparative histologic studies on tumor tissue from 6 patients in our series who had received preoperative radiation therapy and 6 patients who had not. The endothelium of the blood vessels in the irradiated tumors showed radiation changes. Swelling of endothelial cells lining thrombi-containing vessels was the most consistent change distinguishing the irradiated tumors from the nonirradiated tumors. Swelling of endothelial cells was seen frequently in the specimens of those patients not having received radiation therapy. In one of the irradiated specimens, a portion of tumor was necrotic as a result of infarction, implying interference with blood supply to the tumor.

Two of the irradiated specimens showed changes in the tumor cells themselves. These changes consisted of focal disappearance of cells and the appearance of pyknotic nuclear and granular cytoplasm. These changes were not seen in the remaining specimens.

A comparison of the degree of fibrosis present in the irradiated specimens with those that were not irradiated failed to show any significant difference between the two groups. The nonirradiated specimens showed varying amounts of dense dehyalinized collagen traversing irregularly through the tumor in unpredictable patterns. The degree of fibrosis varied widely in both series. Our conclusion was that the changes noted in the endothelial cells were the primary manifestation of radiation effect, and that this correlated with the surgical impression that bleeding was substantially reduced in those patients who had received radiation. We felt that the short time interval (4–6 weeks) between the completion of irradiation and the time of surgery explained the absence of an increased amount of fibrosis in the irradiated specimens.

Prior to instituting radiation therapy, we have made it a practice to perform a biopsy of the tumor through the ear canal to be certain of the diagnosis. We have had no complications from this and have performed the procedure on an inpatient basis as a part of the initial diagnostic work-up.

EMBOLIZATION

Embolization of glomus jugulare tumors has two objectives: to decrease the vascularity of the tumor as a preoperative procedure, or to serve as a means of palliation where surgery is not indicated. Transfemoral catheterization of the specific vessel feeding the tumor is the preferred technique. Numerous materials, including muscle and clotted blood, have been used to embolize tumors, but the most commonly used material presently is Silastic spheres impregnated with barium. Gelfoam and isobutyl-2-cyanoacrylate (IBCA) also have been used but are more difficult to deposit within the tumor and may produce increased morbidity.

Pre-embolization angiography is essential in order to document all feeding vessels, which may include the ipsilateral internal carotid and the vertebral arteries as well as the branches of the external carotid artery.[77,78] Embolization of the internal carotid and the vertebral arterial supply to the tumor is rarely practical because the vessels supplying the tumor are quite small and because of the risk of intracranial embolization.

The catheter is positioned into the appropriate branch of the external carotid artery and the emboli are injected. The size of the embolus should be the smallest one that does not traverse the tumor and enter the venous circulation. One to three spheres are injected at a time, with films obtained frequently to determine the site of the material. Intermittent injections of contrast medium should be given to evaluate the effect of the emboli upon the vascularity of the tumor.

The primary risk of the procedure is embolization to intracerebral vessels and resulting cerebral ischemia. Reflux emboli into the internal carotid artery can occur even though the catheter is positioned into a branch of the external carotid. This primarily occurs because of spasm of the external carotid branch and the catheter being positioned too low in the selected vessel. Unusual anastomotic pathways between the external carotid and the internal carotid systems may be present[79] which

provide a source of entry of the embolus from the external carotid system into the intracerebral circulation. This is not likely to occur, however, if an embolus of the correct size is selected. Embolization of branches of the external carotid supplying normal structures rarely leads to ischemia because of the good collateral circulation in the head and neck.

Embolization of a glomus jugulare tumor can produce palliation, but the tumor will develop new sources of arterial flow. Isobutyl-2-cyanoacrylate may be the preferred embolic material if palliation is the goal because it will occlude smaller vessels deep within the tumor. There is an increased morbidity, however, because of the risk of embolization to the intracerebral circulation, other branches of the external carotid, and into the venous system. Also, IBCA is more difficult to use since the time of fixation is critical. The risk of venous embolization is increased if the material does not polymerize quickly enough. Conversely, if polymerization occurs too rapidly, the catheter may become glued to the vessel and very difficult to remove. Embolization using any material, but particularly IBCA, should be performed only by a radiologist experienced in the technique and in cooperation with a surgeon familiar with the complications that can occur and with their treatment.

We currently consider preoperative embolization for particularly large tumors in which there are major feeding vessels that appear to be favorable for subselective catheterization and no evidence of posterior fossa or internal carotid communication. We currently prefer Ivalon as the embolizing material. We would consider using embolization alone as palliation in a patient who is not a candidate for either surgery or radiation therapy but have not done so to this date.

PREOPERATIVE MEDICAL MANAGEMENT

Elderly patients with significant health problems or those suspected of having a catecholamine-secreting tumor are separately evaluated and managed medically by an internist who is familiar with the surgical procedure and routines. In addition to recognizing generalized medical problems, we are particularly anxious to identify anything that may exacerbate the expected airway problems after removal of large tumors and the likelihood of injury to the ninth and tenth cranial nerves. Chronic pulmonary disease, hiatal hernia, and other conditions that can compromise airway control and function are identified and managed to the extent possible. If this aspect of the patient's status is considered a likely problem postoperatively, it may influence us to perform a tracheostomy at the time of surgery.

We pay particular attention to cardiovascular and hypertensive disease and try to control them as much as possible. We determine whether hypertension is cardiovascular in nature or related to catecholamine secretion by obtaining 24-hour urinary studies for vanillylmandelic acid and metanephrine, free catecholamine, and 5-HIAA. Particular care must be taken to avoid certain medications and stress for 3 days before urine collection in order to avoid invalidation of the procedure.

If high levels of catecholamines are identified, we have treated the patient with an alpha blocker for 10 to 14 days preoperatively for its effect on norepinephrine and with a beta blocker for 24 hours preoperatively to avoid tachycardia during surgery. We have not encountered a serotonin-secreting tumor.

ANESTHESIA

Inclusion of an anesthetist who is knowledgeable and skilled in neuroanesthetic techniques has benefited our surgical procedure significantly. We have used one individual exclusively, so that he could become particularly familiar with the requirements of this surgery as well as to promote familiarity and ease of communication throughout the surgical team. With a variety of procedures being performed, both by the anesthetist and by the surgeons, coordination and communication are important in order to avoid the introduction of technical problems. As an example of this, our anesthetist has preferred that tracheostomy, if it is to be performed, be carried out at the end of the procedure rather than initially, so as to facilitate his control of the airway.

From an anesthetic point of view, we consider a number of other adjunctive procedures worthy of consideration. We use beta blockade, as mentioned previously, to avoid tachycardia during surgery. A blanket warmer, or an ''egg crate'' mattress, and TED stockings and Venodyne cuffs are placed preoperatively. An armoured endotracheal tube with 60-inch breathing circuits is used so as to avoid kinking and to allow maximal access to the head and neck area by the surgeons. Two large-bore 14-gauge IV needles are used. For monitoring we prefer an arterial line, a central venous pressure line via the basilic vein, temperature probe, Foley catheter, nerve stimulator, standard monitoring with ECG, cuff blood pressure, and precordial stethoscope. Moist eye pads are placed over the patient's eyes and moist towels over the exposed endotracheal tube and breathing tubes if the surgical laser is to be used.

For anesthetic induction and management, we have used nitrous oxide (narcotic technique). In the presence of an epinephrine- or serotonin-secreting tumor, anesthetic agents that are inconsistent with the secreted materials must be avoided. We have managed the effects of secreting tumors with nitroprusside and propranolol.

We prefer the patient to be as alert as possible at the end of the procedure so that his or her neurologic status can be assessed. Anesthetic management is directed toward accomplishing this. We have not found it necessary to use prolonged or profound muscle relaxation.

Anesthesia must therefore be carried out in anticipation of a prolonged surgical procedure, with the possibility of sudden and dramatic blood loss, the possibility of epinephrine- or serotonin-secreting effects, probable lower cranial nerve stimulation, possible posterior fossa exploration, and varying anesthetic requirements at various times during the procedure.

DENTAL

If a definite decision is made to resect the condyle of the mandible, dental evaluation before surgery facilitates postoperative temporomandibular joint rehabilitation and the maintenance of normal jaw motion and dental occlusion.

SURGICAL TECHNIQUE— SKULL BASE APPROACH

We reported our surgical technique previously.[32,80,81] Although this technique is unchanged in principle, certain changes in technique have been incorporated, which will be outlined here.

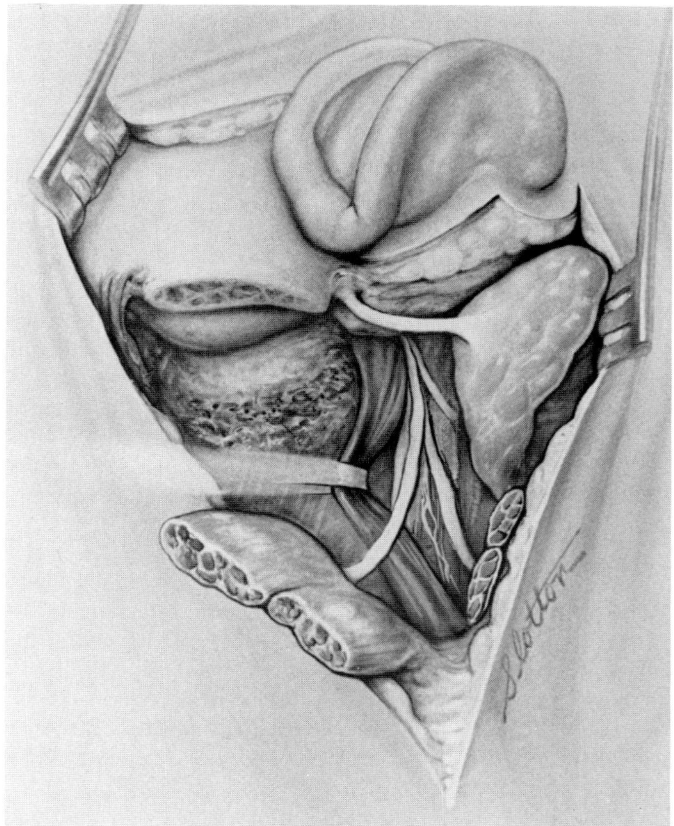

Fig. 63-1. Soft tissue exposure of the skull base, right side. Note the mastoid tip has been resected, the ear is turned upward, and the internal jugular vein is being retracted. The facial nerve is visible entering the parotid gland. (Reprinted from Gardner G, Cocke EW, Robertson JH, et al: Skull base surgery for glomus jugulare tumors. Am J Otol 6:127, 1985. With permission.)

Preoperative Adjunctive Procedures

If a very large tumor is present and difficulty with swallowing and aspiration is anticipated postoperatively, a KEO feeding tube is placed preoperatively or an esophagostomy is peformed. In older individuals in whom the facial nerve is mobilized, we ordinarily perform a tarsorrhaphy as the initial procedure after the patient enters the operating room.

Skull Base Exposure

A postauricular incision is extended into the neck. Skin flaps are elevated, and the ear canal transected at the bony-cartilaginous junction. Cartilage is resected from the membranous ear canal and the meatus closed permanently. The facial nerve is identified at the stylomastoid foramen and followed to its second bifurcation. A large musculoperiosteal flap consisting of the temporalis muscle, mastoid periosteum and subcutaneous tissue, and sternocleidomastoid muscle is outlined so that it is based inferiorly, and maintained for later use in closure. The tip of the mastoid is resected with a Gigli saw.

The neurovascular structures of the upper neck are identified. The soft tissue along the base of the skull between the posterior end of the digastric groove to the lateral lip of the jugular foramen is resected along with the styloid process and attached tendons. The posterior three fourths of the bony circumference of the jugular foramen is freed of soft tissue attachments (Figure 63-1). The tip of the lateral process of the first cervical vertebra is resected if necessary for exposure. If the tumor is large, the soft tissue is elevated from the glenoid fossa, and the condyle of the mandible retracted anteriorly or resected.

Temporal Bone Exposure

A simple mastoidectomy is performed with a high-speed drill and suction-irrigation. The mastoid and tympanic segments of the facial nerve are skeletonized. The posterior bony canal wall is removed. The facial nerve is bared of bone and elevated from the fallopian canal extending from the geniculate ganglion to the stylomastoid foramen. Continuity is established at the stylomastoid foramen with the earlier nerve dissection. A tangential groove is drilled through the bone of the anterior epitympanum to soft tissue depth as described by Fisch,[33] the facial nerve placed proximally within this groove and distally along the substance of the parotid gland, and sutured permanently in this position.

The sigmoid sinus is skeletonized and adjacent posterior fossa dura exposed anteriorly and posteriorly to the sigmoid. Using the skull base exposure achieved earlier, the bone of the base of the skull is removed between the posterior end of the digastric groove and the jugular foramen to the level of soft tissue, thereby skeletonizing the tumor mass or the jugular bulb. Care is take to avoid opening the horizontal or posterior semicircular canals or the cochlea, unless sensorineural function has been lost.

Anteriorly, the bony anterior wall of the tympanum and hypotympanum as well as the bone of the glenoid fossa is removed. The internal carotid artery is skeletonized from the level of the carotid foramen inferiorly to the genu of the artery adjacent to the cochlea and eustachian tube. The horizontal segment of the carotid can be skeletonized if necessary for exposure (Figure 63-2). The tumor mass in the middle ear is mobilized inferiorly in continuity with the primary mass in the hypotympanum. The tympanic membrane and bony meatal skin are included, or resected. The stapes is carefully protected.

Sigmoid-Jugular Control

A silk ligature is passed atraumatically through the dura adjacent to the sigmoid sinus and around the sinus, which is ligated, and the lateral wall is divided. The internal jugular vein is ligated and divided in the neck. Care is taken during ligation of the sigmoid and internal jugular vein that the ligatures are placed beyond any tumor extension that is present within the sinus or venous lumen.

Tumor Removal

The lateral wall of the sigmoid sinus is resected from the point of sinus ligation to the junction with the tumor or bulb. Working alternately from below and above, the tumor is mobilized. Very careful dissection is required in elevating the tumor from the medial wall of the jugular fossa and away from the lower cranial nerves. The Nd:YAG laser may be useful in removing large tumor masses. Bleeding from the inferior petrosal sinus is controlled by direct packing with Surgicel and bone wax (Figure 63-3).

Larger tumors often are attached to the internal carotid artery and can extend into the posterior fossa. Dura frequently may have been pushed medially by the tumor and can be preserved as the intracranial portion of the tumor is removed,

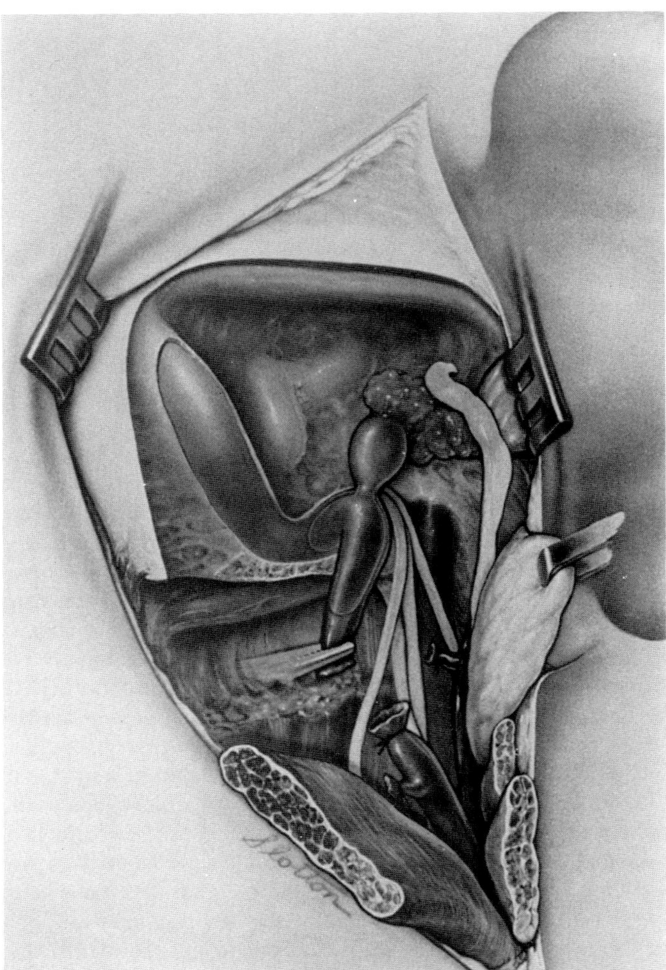

Fig. 63-2.   Tumor exposure. Note the sigmoid sinus and jugular bulb are exposed and the tumor is visible within the bulb. The internal carotid artery is visible to the right of (anterior to) the jugular bulb, the facial nerve has been mobilized anteriorly, and lower cranial nerves are in view. (Reprinted from Gardner G, Cocke EW, Robertson JH, et al: Skull base surgery for glomus jugulare tumors. Am J Otol :127, 1985. With permission.)

thereby minimizing the risk of postoperative CSF leakage. Less frequently there is no layer of dura between the tumor and the contents of the cerebellopontine angle.

Wound Closure

Remaining mucosa is removed from the middle ear and mastoid. Proplast is used to pack the opening of the eustachian tube. The facial nerve is maintained in its new anterior, soft tissue-based location. Abdominal wall fat is placed into the surgical defect. The previously prepared musculoperiosteal flap, inferiorly based, is placed over the fat, and the wound edges closed in layers. Hemovac drainage is used.

Postoperative Adjunctive Procedures

If a tracheostomy is felt to be needed, it is carried out at this point. If CSF leakage is anticipated, lumbar drainage is instituted. If aspiration is anticipated as a result of damage to cranial nerves 9 and 10, the vocal cord can be injected with Gelfoam or Teflon.

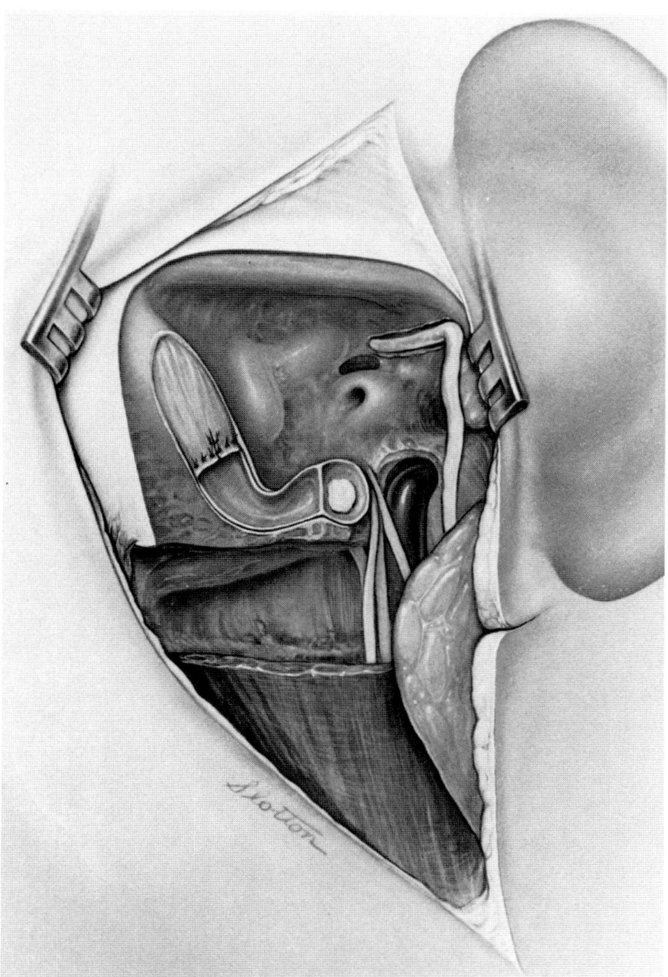

Fig. 63-3. Tumor removal. Note removal of the lateral wall of the sigmoid sinus and packing in the inferior petrosal sinus. The vertical segment of the internal carotid artery is exposed. The facial nerve has been placed anteriorly in a bony groove. (Reprinted from Gardner G, Cocke EW, Robertson JT, et al: Combined approach surgery for removal of glomus jugulare tumors. Laryngoscope 87:674, 1977. With permission.)

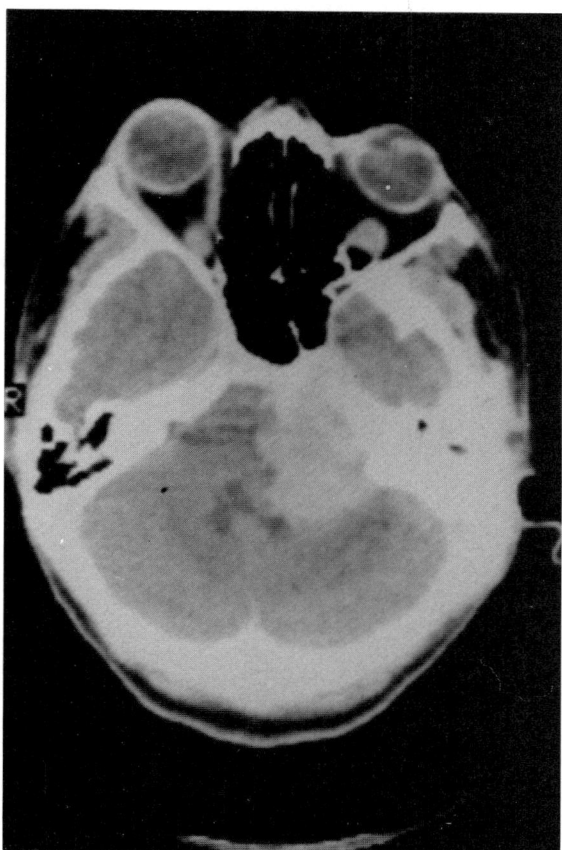

Fig. 63-4. A CT scan demonstrates posterior fossa extension. (Reprinted from Gardner G, Cocke EW, Robertson JT, et al: Combined approach surgery for removal of glomus jugulare tumors. Laryngoscope 87:676, 1977. With permission.)

ALTERNATIVE PROCEDURES

Small Tumors

Very small tumors extending no great distance from their origin in the jugular bulb can be managed more conservatively. If the tumor has arisen only on the dome of the bulb and the lumen of the bulb is free of tumor, tumor removal can be accomplished by a hypotympanotomy approach as described by Shambaugh[82] and Farrior.[83]

Alternatively, the previously described skull base approach can be used without sacrifice of the posterior canal wall and with retention of the middle ear structures as advocated by Glasscock.[84] Under these circumstances, the limited mobilization of the facial nerve described by Farrior,[85] in which only the mastoid segment of the nerve is temporarily elevated, can be used.

Very Large Tumors

Tumors extending well anteriorly with major involvement of the internal carotid artery are best managed by extending the skull base approach by using the infratemporal fossa exposure developed by Fisch.[33]

When there is significant tumor extension into the posterior fossa, particularly anterior to the level of the clivus, the skull base approach can be extended by utilizing the transcochlear approach developed by House and Hitselberger.[86]

POSTOPERATIVE CARE

Careful timing is necessary in deciding when to remove the Hemovac drainage tube and the tracheostomy and feeding tubes (if used) and when to attempt to feed the patient. If a tracheostomy has been performed, we prefer to use a plastic tube having an attached balloon initially, but switch to a metal tube as soon as possible to allow the patient to talk. Spinal drainage can be continued for several days, as necessary. Careful attention is given to the status of the cornea, in order to avoid exposure keratitis. Medical care is continued postoperatively.

CASE PRESENTATION

A 35-year-old woman was referred to us on April 20, 1984, with a 2-year history of dizziness, ringing tinnitus, and pain in the left ear and a 1-month history of hearing loss in the same ear. The patient's father had had a carotid body tumor.

Physical examination demonstrated a vascular-appearing mass in the inferior tympanum behind an intact tympanic membrane. There was a 68 dB sensorineural hearing loss with

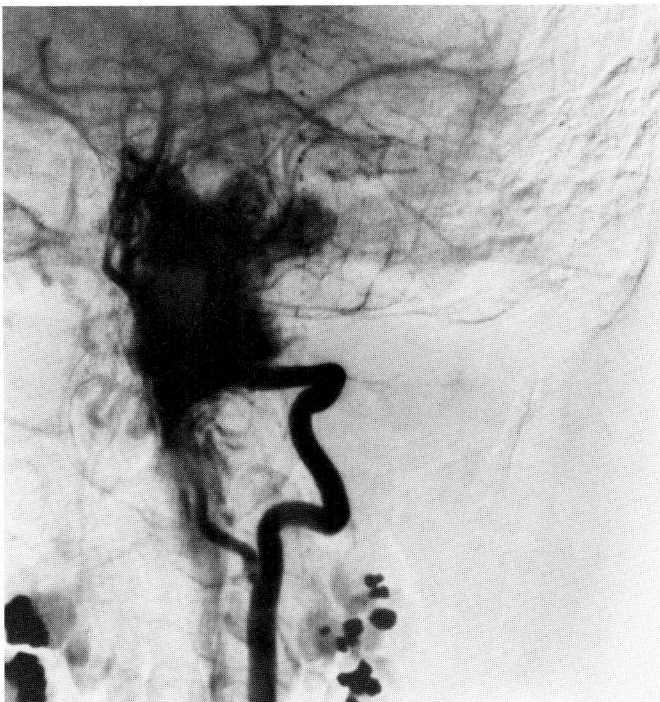

Fig. 63-5. An arteriogram shows tumor blush. (Reprinted from Cocke EW, Gardner G: The skull base—surgical treatment of glomus jugulare tumors, in Silver CE (ed): Atlas of Head and Neck Surgery. New York, Churchill Livingstone, 1986, p 153. With permission.)

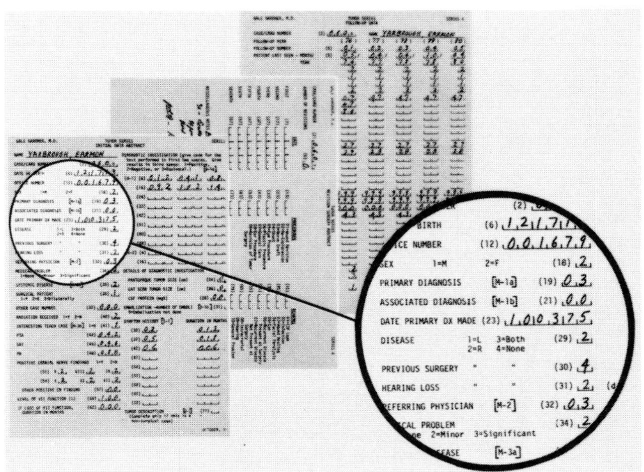

Fig. 63-6. Data worksheets are designed for systematic data collection. (Reprinted from Gardner G: Acoustic tumor management—combined approach surgery with CO=2 laser. Am J Otol 6:92, 1983. With permission.)

no significant speech discrimination present. Cranial nerves 10–12 demonstrated involvement. Temporal bone x-ray studies showed evidence of bone destruction of the left petrous pyramid.

Computed tomography (Figure 63-4) showed extensive destruction of the petrous portion of the left temporal bone with apparent tumor extension into the posterior fossa, the middle fossa, and the upper neck, with partial destruction of the first cervical vertebra and the clivus. Arteriography showed a marked tumor blush (Figure 63-5).

A biopsy specimen of the vascular-appearing middle ear lesion was obtained and proved to be a glomus tumor. A 50–mm rise in systolic blood pressure was noted when the tumor was manipulated. The patient was treated with 4500 rad of preoperative radiation therapy between April 27 and May 31, 1984. Catecholamine levels were found to be elevated on three occasions, and the patient was subsequently treated with appropriate alpha and beta blockers preoperatively.

Surgery was performed in August, 1984, using a combination of skull base, infratemporal fossa, and transcochlear approaches. The facial nerve was mobilized, but continuity not maintained, and the ends reapproximated at the completion of surgery. The sigmoid sinus was ligated, the condyle of the mandible resected, and the internal carotid artery skeletonized through the glenoid fossa. Because the tumor extended well anterior to the clivus, exposure was extended anteriorly using the transcochlear approach.

When exposure was satisfactory, and the tumor could be completely visualized, it was estimated to be 5 cm in diameter. The tumor had entered the posterior fossa directly through the jugular foramen, with no intervening dural layer. The Nd:YAG laser was used for the majority of tumor removal, together with conventional cup forceps. Four units of whole blood were replaced. The tumor was dissected away from the lower cranial nerves, which were felt to be preserved. No significant changes in blood pressure were noted during surgery.

The postoperative course was complicated primarily by CSF leakage and difficulty in swallowing. Wound revision was required, as well as tracheostomy, injection of the left vocal cord, and tarsorrhaphy. The spinal fluid leakage stopped after wound revision, and swallowing gradually became possible over a 2-month period. There was also a problem with left jaw function, but dental exercises controlled this promptly.

She was last seen in February, 1986. She had returned to work. Facial nerve function had not returned, but she was swallowing well, and no significant hoarseness was present.

RESULTS

Data accumulated during the treatment of the patients constituting this study were recorded on specially designed worksheets (Figure 63-6) based upon a systematic plan for collecting and recording of the data. Data processing with a Radio Shack TRS-80 Model II microcomputer and dBase-II software was used for data storage and retrieval. Analysis was accomplished using the SLM program.

Thirty-six patients were treated for glomus jugulare tumors between June 20, 1972, and 1986. The average age of these patients was 46 years. Twenty-one were women and 15 were men. Seven patients were treated with surgery alone; 14 were

Table 63-4. Follow-up status

Follow-up	Number of Cases
Seen within 12 months	23
Seen within 2 years	27
Seen within 3 years	28
Seen within 4 years	29
Seen within 5 years	32
Seen within 7 years	34
Deceased	2

Table 63-5. Surgical complications

Complications	Number of Cases
Death	0
CSF leak (persistent)	4
Meningitis	1
Dysphagia	11
Facial nerve lost	4

Table 63-7. Postoperative cranial nerve status in 21 patients

Cranial Nerve Dysfunction*	Number of Patients
Immediately postoperatively	
IX, X, XI, XII	3
X	2
IX, X	1
IX, XI	1
IX, X, XII	1
XI	1
XI, XII	1
None	11
Most recent follow-up	
IX, X, XI, XII	1
X	1
X, XII	1
XI	1
XII	1
None	16

*Excluding cranial nerves VII and VIII.

treated with radiation therapy alone: and 15 were managed using a combination of radiation therapy and surgery. The extent to which we have been able to achieve follow-up with these patients is indicated in Table 63-4.

Radiation therapy was given to 29 patients; preoperatively in 13, postoperatively in 2, and alone to 14 patients.

Surgical treatment was used in the treatment of 22 patients. The skull base approach was used in 17 patients, a more limited transmastoid approach in 2, a transcanal hypotympanotomy in two, and skull base approach combined with infratemporal fossa and transcochlear approaches in one. The surgery was unstaged in 13 patients and staged in 8. Average blood loss was between 3 and 4 units. Tumor removal was total or virtually total in 20 patients and subtotal in 1, the first patient in this series.

Thirty-four of the 36 patients are alive at this time. Two patients died of other causes unrelated to their glomus tumors.

Surgical complications are listed in Table 63-5 and other complications in Table 63–6. The postoperative cranial nerve status, as determined immediately postoperatively and at most recent follow-up, is shown in Table 63-7. Facial nerve function was graded as less than 80 percent postoperatively in 20 patients. Eleven patients continued to demonstrate facial nerve dysfunction to this degree, but 5 of them underwent surgery relatively recently. There have been two instances of tumor recurrence. One patient who initially underwent a hypotympanotomy approach developed a recurrence and subsequently had revision surgery through the skull base approach with apparently total removal. The second patient previously had skull base removal of her tumor, but it recurred in the posterior fossa and was removed subtotally through a suboccipital approach.

DISCUSSION

USE OF RADIATION THERAPY

We continue to use radiation therapy both for reduction of tumor vascularity preoperatively and for primary treatment of elderly and poor-risk patients. Having seen no firm evidence

Table 63-6. Postoperative complications

Complication	Number of Cases
Wound problem	5
Revision surgery	3
Recurrence of tumor	2
Radiation chondritis of auricle	1
Pulmonary embolism	1
Significant increase in size of tumor after irradiation	1

that radiation therapy actually reduces tumor size, we prefer surgical treatment. As our surgical experience has increased, we find that we use radiation therapy for preoperative reduction of tumor vascularity less frequently.

Nevertheless, we also recognize the major problems that can result from surgery, particularly in elderly patients. We have seen no major complications from the use of x-ray therapy and no significant tumor growth in any of the patients in whom it was primarily used and have been impressed with the quality of life in these patients. We therefore plan to continue its use in selected cases.

SURGICAL APPROACH AND EXTENSION

Based on our experience, we believe that a direct approach to these tumors through the skull base and mastoid provides excellent exposure for all but a small percentage of patients. Of the latter, depending upon the direction of tumor extension, additional exposure may be necessary. When anterior tumor extension produces major involvement of the internal carotid artery, the infratemporal fossa approach provides the additional exposure required. In the event of extension within the posterior fossa, particularly extreme anterior extension to the clivus, use of the transcochlear approach may be helpful, as demonstrated in the accompanying case report.

SURGICAL TECHNIQUES

We are no longer using a Fogarty catheter as a preliminary to imbricating the superior end of the sigmoid sinus but have instead adopted Fisch's[33] method of ligating the sigmoid. We have been pleased with this technique and have noted no resulting problem with CSF leakage.

Farrior's[85] report of removal of glomus tumors with preservation of the ear canal and middle ear structures, with mobilization of the facial nerve limited to the mastoid segment, is attractive. We plan to explore this, but only for smaller tumors. We continue to be pleased with the exposure provided for large tumors by removal of the posterior bony canal wall with primary closure of the external meatus.

Regardless of the operative strategy employed for facial nerve management, use of intraoperative electromyographic monitoring with direct silver electrode stimulation of the facial nerve should be a part of the routine operative effort toward facial nerve preservation.

BLEEDING

The vascularity of glomus jugulare tumors has always been one of the more persistent challenges of this surgery. A variety of techniques, including preoperative irradiation, embolization, and controlled hypotension, have been advocated as adjunctive measures to decrease blood loss. We have recently used both the cardon dioxide and Nd:YAG lasers as an aid to vaporization, coagulation, and hemostasis in these tumors, and have been pleased with the intitial results. The ultimate use of either of these lasers must, however, remain speculative until further experience has been acquired. Probably the greatest aid to decreased blood loss during the removal of these tumors is complete exposure of the tumor and careful, patient, meticulous operative dissection. We make every effort to use embolization for particularly large tumors having intracranial extension as a further attempt at hemostasis but wish to emphasize the potential for major complications if the embolizing material enters the internal carotid system.

CEREBROSPINAL FLUID FISTULAE

Postoperative cerebrospinal fluid leakage is best managed by prevention. Basically this consists of filling the operative space with adipose tissue and maintaining the integrity of the posterior fossa dura if at all possible. Closure of the external auditory canal, obliteration of the eustachian tube with Proplast, use of a large musculoperiosteal flap, and continuous lumbar spinal drainage are also helpful in avoiding CSF leakage. Any leakage that occurs must be managed aggressively, with wound revision performed early when required.

CRANIAL NERVE DYSFUNCTION

We feel that the major unsolved problem associated with this surgery is dysfunction of cranial nerves 9 and 10. Our approach in attempting to overcome this problem has been to achieve a wide exposure of the jugular bulb area by removal of bone and to carry out a very careful dissection of the tumor from the cranial nerves using magnification and microinstrumentation with continuous irrigation and suction. These measures have resulted in less difficulty with impairment of swallowing. We advocate performing a tracheostomy and esophagostomy or gastrostomy if severe cranial nerve dysfunction is anticipated or occurs. We also advocate early injection of a paralyzed vocal cord to reduce the likelihood of aspiration. We have recently tended to rely on the placement of small diameter Silastic feeding tubes for nutrition rather than esophagostomy or gastrostomy because swallowing impairments have been of shorter duration.

CONCLUSIONS

It is unfortunate that neurosurgeons and otolaryngologists have not read each other's literature more often in the past. While neurosurgeons have been dealing with glomus tumors at the base of the skull and within the cranial cavity with reasonable success for years, they have felt that involvement of the internal structures of the temporal bone has precluded surgery. Otologists meanwhile have achieved a similar degree of success with tumors involving the interior of the temporal bone, but have believed that for the most part intracranial extension and skull base involvement contraindicate surgery.

The missing key to total removal of the tumor from the neurosurgical point of view has been the inability to remove soft tissue at the base of the skull, to remove the temporal bone from the surface of the tumor, and to preserve the facial nerve. From the otologic point of view, the missing key has been the inability to control the sigmoid sinus, to deal with extension of the tumor into the posterior fossa, and to manage intracranial complications. By working together as a team, neurosurgeons and otologists can enhance their skills and thereby more effectively accomplish total removal of these large and challenging tumors.

ACKNOWLEDGMENT

To authors wish to thank Ms. Florence M. Bruce for her assistance in the preparation of the manuscript.

REFERENCES

1. Guild SR: A hitherto unrecognized structure, the glomus jugularis in man. Anat Rec 79 (Suppl 2):28, 1941
2. Rosenwasser H: Carotid body tumor of the middle ear and mastoid. Arch Otolaryngol 41:64, 1945
3. William H., Childs DS Jr, Parkhill EM, et al: Chemodectomas of the glomus jugulare (nonchromaffin paragangliomas) with especial reference to their response to roentgen therapy. Trans Am Otol Soc 43:264, 1955
4. McCabe BF, Fletcher M: Selection of therapy of glomus jugulare tumors. Arch Otolaryngol 89:156, 1969
5. Rosenwasser H: Glomus jugulare tumors. Long term tumors. Arch Otolaryngol 89:160, 1969
6. Spector GJ, Maisel RH, Ogura JH: Glomus tumors in the middle ear. I. An analysis of 46 patients. Laryngoscope 83:1652, 1973
7. Bickerstaff ER, Howell JS: The neurological importance of tumors of the glomus jugulare. Brain 76:576, 1953
8. Rosenwasser H: Long-term results of therapy of glomus jugulare tumors. Arch Otolaryngol 97:49, 1973
9. Lundgren N: Tympanic body tumors in the middle ear—Tumors of carotid body type. Acta Otolyaryngol 37:366, 1949
10. Seiffert A: Cited in Lundgren N: Tympanic body tumors in the middle ear—Tumors of carotid body type. Acta Otolaryngol 37:366, 1949
11. Berg NO: Tumors arising from the tympanic gland (glomus jugularis) and their differential diagnoses. Acta Pathol Microbiol Scand 27:194, 1950
12. Weille FL, Lane CS Jr: Surgical problems involved in the removal of glomus-jugulare tumors. Laryngoscope 61:448, 1951
13. Semmes RE: Discussion of paper by E Alexander Jr and S Adams. Tumor of the glomus jugulare. Follow-up study two years after roentgen therapy. J Neurosurg 10:672, 1953
14. Albernaz JG, Bucy PC: Nonchromaffin paraganglioma of the jugular foramen. J Neurosurg 10:663, 1953
15. Capps FCW: Glomus jugulare tumors of the middle ear. J Laryngol Otol 66:302, 1952
16. Riemenschneider PA, Hoople GD, Brewer D, et al: Roentgenographic diagnosis of tumors of the glomus jugularis. Am J Roentgenol Radium Ther Nucl Med 69:59, 1953
17. Ziedes de Plantes, cited in Kohut RI, Lindsay JR: GLomus jugulare tumors (new techniques for determining operability). Laryngoscope 75:750, 1965

18. Valvassori GE: Laminography of the ear—Normal roentgeno-graphic anatomy and pathologic conditions. AJR 89:1155, 1963

19. Gejrot T: Retrograde jugularography in the diagnosis of abnormalities of the superior bulb of the internal jugular vein. Acta Otolaryngol 57:170, 1964

20. Kohut RI, Lindsay JR: Glomus jugulare tumors (new techniques for determining operability). Laryngoscope 75:750, 1965

21. Meacham WF, Capps JM: Intracranial glomus-jugulare tumor with successful surgical removal. J Neurosurg 17:157, 1960

22. Thoms OJ, Shaw DT, Towbridge WV: Glomus jugulare tumor. Report of a case with surgical removal. J Neurosurg 17:500, 1960

23. Gastpar H: Die Tumoren des glomus Caroticum, glomus Jugulare-Tympanicum und glomus Vagale. Acta Otolaryngol (Suppl) 167, 1961

24. Michelson RP, Connolly JE: Removal of glomus jugulare tumor utilizing complete occlusion of the cerebral circulation. Laryngoscope 72:788, 1962

25. Shapiro MJ, Neues DK: Technique for removal of glomus jugulare tumors. Arch Otolaryngol 79:219, 1964

26. Gejrot T: Surgical treatment of glomus jugulare tumors. With special reference to the diagnostic value of retrograde jugularography. Acta Otolaryngol 60:150, 1965

27. House W: Panel discussion; BF McCabe, Moderator; H Rosenwasser, W House, RM Witten, C-A Hamberger. Management of glomus tumors. Arch Otolaryngol 89:170, 1969

28. Hamberger C-A, Wersall J (eds): Disorders of the Skull Base Region. New York, John Wiley & Sons, 1969, pp 297–298

29. Kempe L, VanderArk GD, Smith DR: The neurosurgical treatment of glomus jugulare tumors. J Neurosurg 35:59, 1971

30. Hilding DA, Greenberg A: Surgery for large glomus jugulare tumor. Arch Otolaryngol 93:227, 1971

31. Glasscock ME, Harris PF, Newsome G: Glomus tumors: Diagnosis and treatment. Laryngoscope 84:2006, 1974

32. Gardner G, Cocke EW, Robertson JT, et al: Combined approach surgery for removal of glomus jugulare tumors. Laryngoscope 87:655, 1977

33. Fisch U: Infratemporal fossa approach for extensive tumors of the temporal bone and base of the skull, in Silverstein H, Norrell H (eds): Neurological Surgery of the Ear. Birmingham, Ala, Aesculapius, 1977, pp 34–53

34. Fisch U, Fagan P, Valavanis A: The infratemporal fossa approach for the lateral skull base. Otolaryngol Clin North Am 17:513, 1984

35. Jackson CG, Glasscock ME, Nissen AF, et al: Glomus tumor surgery. The approach, results, and problems. Otolaryngol Clin North Am 15:897, 1982

36. Goldenberg RA: Surgeon's view of the skull base from the lateral approach. Laryngoscope 94 (Supp 36):1, 1984

37. House HP, House WF: Historical review and problems of acoustic neuromas. Arch Otolaryngol 80:601, 1964

38. Brown JS: Glomus jugulare tumors revisited. A ten year statistical follow-up of 231 cases. Laryngoscope 95:284, 1985

39. Glenner GG, Grimley PM: Tumors of the extra-adrenal paraganglion system, in Finninger HI (ed): Atlas of Tumor Pathology, Fascicle 9. Washington, DC, Armed Forces Institute of Pathology, 1974, pp 13–38, 61–66, 73–75

40. Spector GJ, Ciralsky R, Maisel RH: Multiple glomus tumors in the head and neck. Laryngoscope 85:1066, 1975

41. McNeill KA, Milner GA: Bilateral tumors of the glomus jugulare. J Laryngol Otol 69:430, 1955

42. Ghani GA, Sung YF, Per-Lee JH: Glomus jugulare tumors. Origin, pathology and anesthetic considerations. Anesth Analg 62:686, 1983

43. Kroll AJ, Alexander B, Cochios F, et al: Hereditary deficiencies of clotting factors VII and X associated with carotid body tumors. N Engl J Med 270:6, 1964

44. Rosen S: Glomus jugulare tumors of the middle ear with normal drum. Ann Otol Rhinol Laryngol 61:448, 1952 (Reference to Goekoop)

45. Robertson JT: Chemodectomas, in Wilkins RH, Rengachary SS (eds): Neurosurgery. New York, McGraw-Hill, 1985, pp 785–790

46. Rubenstein LJ: Tumors of the central nervous system, in Atlas of Tumor Pathology, Fascicle 6. Washington, DC, Armed Forces Institute of Pathology, 1972, pp 314–315

47. Stewart JP, Ogilivie RF, Sammon JDS: Tumors of the glomus jugulare and paraganglion juxtavagale of the ganglion nodosum. J Laryngol Otol 70:196, 1956

48. Davis JM, Davis KR, Hesselink JR, et al: Malignant glomus jugulare tumor. A case with two radiographic features. J Comput Assist Tomogr 4:415, 1980

49. El Fiky FM, Paparella MM: A metastatic glomus jugulare tumor. Am J Otol 5:197, 1984

50. Taylor DM, Alford BR, Greenberg SD: Metastases of glomus jugulare tumors. Arch Otolaryngol 82:5, 1965

51. Spector GJ, Druck NS, Gado MH: Neurologic manifestations of glomus tumors in the head and neck. Arch Neurol 33:270, 1976

52. Fuller AM, Brown HA, Harrison EG: Chemodectomas of the glomus jugulare tumor. Laryngoscope 76:218, 1966

53. Lapayowher MS, Liebman EP, Ronis ML, et al: Presentation of the internal carotid artery as a tumor of the middle ear. Radiology 98:293, 1971

54. Lawson W: The neuroendocrine nature of the glomus cells. An experimental, ultrastructural, and histochemical tissue culture study. Laryngoscope 90:120, 1980

55. Zak FG, Lawson W: The Paraganglionic Chemorecptor System. New York, Springer-Verlag, 1982, pp 276–285

56. Schwaber MK, Glasscock ME, Jackson CG, et al: Diagnosis and management of catecholamine secreting glomus tumors. Laryngoscope 94:1008, 1984

57. Axelrod J, Weinshilboum R: Catecholamines. N Engl J Med 287:237, 1972

58. Gardner G, Cocke EW, Robertson JH, et al: Skull base surgery for glomus jugulare tumors. Am J Otol (Suppl): 126–134, 1985

59. Levit SA, Sheps SG, Espinosa RE, et al: Catecholamine secreting paraganglioma of glomus jugulare region resembling pheochromocytoma. N Engl J Med 281:805, 1969

60. Farrior JB III, Hyams VJ, Beneke RH, et al: Carcinoid apudoma arising in a glomus jugulare tumor; review of endocrine activity in glomus jugulare tumors. Laryngoscope 90:110, 1980

61. Lo WW, Solti-Bohman LG, Lambert PR: High resolution CT in the evaluation of glomus tumors of the temporal bone. Radiology 150:737, 1984

62. Curtin HD: Radiologic approach to paragangliomas of the temporal bone. Radiology 150:837, 1984

63. Lloyd TV, Aman MV, Johnson JC: Aberrant jugular bulb presenting as a middle ear mass. Radiology 131:139, 1979

64. Guinto FC, Garrabrant EC, Radcliffe WB: Radiology of the persistent stapedial artery. Radiology 105:365, 1972

65. Stallings JO, McCabe BF: Congenital middle ear aneurysm of internal carotid. Arch Otolaryngol 90:39, 1969

66. Svien HJ, Baker HL, Rivers MH: Jugular foramen syndrome and allied syndromes. Neurology 13:797, 1963 67. Chakeres DW, LaMasters DL: Paragangliomas of the temporal bone. High resolution CT studies. Radiology 150:749, 1984

68. House JL, Brackmann DE: Cholesterol granuolomas of the cerebellopontine angle. Arch Otolaryngol 108:504, 1982

69. Bird CR, Hasso AN, Stewart CE, et al: Malignant primary neoplasms of the ear and temporal bone studied by high resolution computed tomography. Radiology 149:171, 1983

70. Dolan KD: Malignant lesions of the ear. Radiol Clin North Am 12:585, 1974

71. Newton TH: Abnormal external carotid artery, in Newton TH, Potts DG (eds): Radiology of the Skull and Brain. St. Louis, CV Mosby, 1974, pp 1280–1284

72. Kinney SE, Modic MT: The role of digital subtraction angiography in diagnosis of skull base lesions. Otolaryngol Head Neck Surg 92:151, 1984

73. Cummings BJ, Beale FA, Garrett PG, et al: The treatment of

glomus tumors in the temporal bone by megavoltage radiation. Cancer 53:2635, 1984

74. Cole JM: Glomus jugulare tumors of the temporal bone. Radiation of glomus tumors of the temporal bone. Laryngoscope 89:1623, 1979

75. Kempe LG: Glomus jugulare tumors, in Youmans JR (ed): Neurological Surgery, ed 2. Philadelphia, WB Saunders, 1982, pp 3285–3298

76. Maruyama Y, Gold LHA, Kieffer SA: Radioactive cobalt treatment of glomus jugulare tumors. Clinical and angiographic investigation. Acta Radiol Ther Phys Biol 10:239, 1971

77. Duncan W, Lack E, Deck MF: Radiological evaluation of paragangliomas of the head and neck. Radiology 132:99, 1979

78. Quisling G: Intrapetrous carotid artery branches: Pathological applications. Radiology 134:109, 1980

79. Lasjaunias P: Nasopharyngeal angiofibromas: Hazards of embolization. Radiology 136:119, 1980

80. Gardner G, Cocke EW, Robertson JT, et al: Glomus jugulare tumors—combined treatment: Part I. J Laryngol Otol 95:437, 1981

81. Gardner G, Cocke EW, Robertson JT, et al: Glomus jugulare tumors—combined treatment: Part II. J Laryngol Otol 95:567, 1981

82. Shambaugh GE Jr: Surgical approach for so-called glomus jugulare tumors of the middle ear. Laryngoscope 65:185, 1955

83. Farrior JB: Glomus tumors—postauricular hypotympanotomy and hypotympanotomy. Arch Otolaryngol 86:33, 1967

84. Glasscock ME, Harris P: Glomus tumors—diagnosis, classification, and management of large lesions. Arch Otolaryngol 108:401, 1982

85. Farrior JB: Infratemporal approach to skull base for glomus tumors: Anatomic considerations. Ann Otol Rhinol Laryngol 93:616, 1984

86. House WF, Hitselberger WE: The transcochlear approach to the skull base. Arch Otolaryngol 102:334, 1976

CHAPTER 64

Surgical Therapy of Diseases of the Extracranial Carotid Artery

Robert A. Ratcheson   Robert L. Grubb

THE VARIED AND COMPLEX DANGERS presented by atherosclerotic carotid artery bifurcation lesions are widely appreciated. Many of these lesions obstruct blood flow to the cerebral hemispheres, while others are hemodynamically insignificant but have the potential to produce ischemic cerebral damage as a result of distal embolization from diseased intima. Although both embolic and hemodynamic mechanisms play important roles in cerebral ischemia and infarction, embolization appears to be the dominant factor in the carotid system. These emboli may originate from focal accumulation of intimal lipid-laden smooth muscle cells surrounded by an intracellular matrix of lipid, collagen, elastic fibers, and proteoglycans, which become altered as a result of hemorrhage, calcification, cell necrosis, and thrombosis.[1] In the cervical carotid artery these lesions usually occur at or near the common carotid bifurcation. The etiology of the underlying disease, atherosclerosis, and the factors that render these lesions active remain poorly understood. At the present time, surgical therapy of these lesions offers the most direct and efficient mechanism to remove the source of cerebral emboli and restore cerebral blood flow when the lesion produces a critical stenosis. Treatment cannot be directed only toward removal of an anatomic abnormality, however, but must include consideration of the multiple problems introduced by the patient's physiological state and collateral cerebral circulation. In certain situations, a patient will be better served by treatment with anticoagulants or agents that suppress platelet aggregation. A number of conditions of nonatherosclerotic etiology affect the cervical carotid artery and may interfere with cerebral blood flow or serve as a nidus for thrombus formation and cerebral embolization. For many of these conditions, the role of surgical therapy is not well defined.

DIAGNOSIS AND PATIENT SELECTION

All angiographically identified carotid artery lesions do not represent a significant risk to an individual patient. The decision to perform carotid endarterectomy therefore must rely upon an accurate correlation of clinical symptomatology and angiographic findings, a thorough understanding of the influence of anatomic variations upon the cerebral circulation, and knowledge of the pathophysiology of extracranial and intracranial vascular occlusive disease. Medical and surgical factors that increase the risk of surgery must also enter into the decision whether to perform carotid endarterectomy or treat the patient medically.

INDICATIONS

The primary indication for carotid endarterectomy is the angiographic demonstration of a stenotic or ulcerated lesion in the extracranial carotid artery compatible with the patient's cerebrovascular symptomatology. Initial symptoms may include any and all of the spectrum of cerebral and ocular ischemia. Patients with amaurosis fugax, central retinal artery occlusion, carotid distribution transient ischemic attacks (TIAs), prolonged reversible ischemic neurologic deficits (PRINDs), and mild to moderate fixed neurologic deficits are at risk for further hemispheric ischemic damage. All patients having cerebrovascular symptoms should be evaluated as to their specific risk of stroke. Those patients at the greatest risk, including patients with frequent TIAs, stuttering stroke symptomatology, or acute onset of mild to moderate neurologic deficit, should be evaluated on an urgent basis. Patients having infrequent cerebral episodes are at unknown risk but should be evaluated without undue delay. The evaluation of each patient should include an assessment of surgical risk factors for carotid endarterectomy. At the present time, there is no noninvasive test that can reliably depict all the conditions of the cervical carotid artery that may be responsible for cerebral symptomatology. A number of diagnostic techniques under development may dramatically alter the approach to the patient threatened with cerebral infarction; however, in the authors' experience standard and intra-arterial digital subtraction cerebral angiography are the only reliable techniques to accurately demonstrate extracranial and intracranial vascular lesions. Medical evaluation searching for causes of cerebral symptoms other than extracranial and intracranial vascular disease should not delay definitive angiographic studies unless there is evidence to implicate such an etiology. In most instances the administration of intravenous heparin will prevent further ischemic episodes until angiography can be performed under optimal conditions. However, anticoagulation does not guarantee that a patient will not suffer additional symptoms and permanent sequelae. We prefer to perform angiography immediately after appropriate medical evaluation and computed tomographic scanning of the head. If stenosis with less than 1 mm of residual lumen or intraluminal thrombus is found, surgery is usually performed on an urgent basis. If ulceration or plaque formation is demon-

OPERATIVE NEUROSURGICAL TECHNIQUES
ISBN 0-8089-1862-1

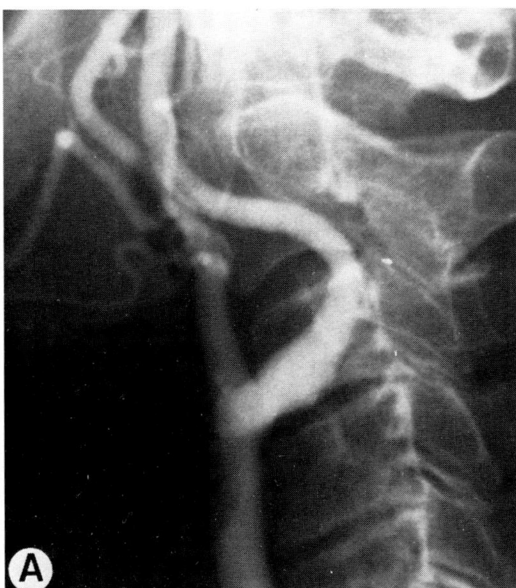 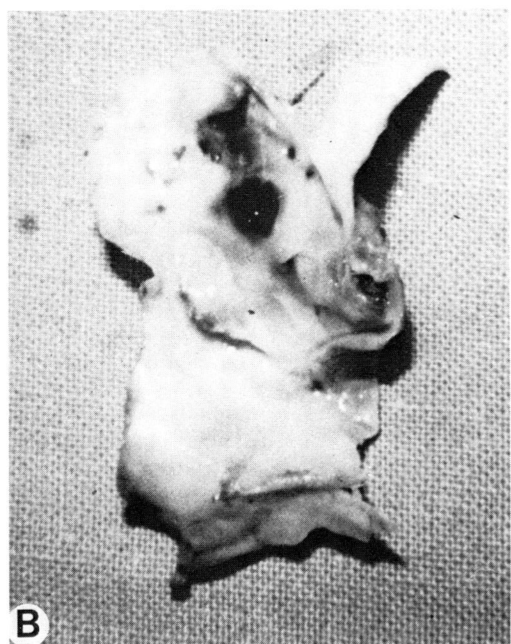

Fig. 64-1. (A) A left carotid angiogram of a patient with sudden onset of transient dysphasia and right arm weakness. Fairly smooth, shallow irregularities are visible near the carotid bifurcation. The patient was treated with warfarin but suffered a further episode of dysphasia and right arm clumsiness, which partially improved. (B) Surgically removed atheroma from the left carotid artery depicted in A. Intraluminal thrombus, not apparent on standard angiographic views, was found attached to an ulcer crater.

strated in the appropriate carotid artery, a patient without neurologic deficit will undergo surgery at the next elective opportunity. When the cervical carotid artery contains a nonstenotic lesion with only shallow ulceration, it is our preference to treat these patients with either warfarin anticoagulant therapy or anti-platelet aggregation agents. On occasion, despite adequate anticoagulation, such patients will have persistent symptoms and require carotid endarterectomy (Figure 64-1).

The indications for surgical therapy in a large group of patients, which include those with asymptomatic cervical bruits, asymptomatic angiographic lesions, and vertebrobasilar symptoms associated with carotid artery stenosis, are controversial. The natural history of patients with asymptomatic cervical bruits is not clearly defined,[2-6] and we do not recommend further investigation of these patients, preferring to closely follow their course and bruit. If a change in character of the bruit is noted, further study is advised. Recently, however, we have seen patients who not only harbor bruits but who have had intravenous digital subtraction angiograms, a test which has gained wide acceptance for outpatient screening. When high grade stenosis is suspected, consideration is given for definitive angiographic studies. Frequently, the neurosurgeon must also decide whether to treat an asymptomatic, angiographically demonstrated lesion found during investigation of a contralateral symptomatic lesion. With the exception of unusual circumstances, dictated by the pattern of collateral circulation or lesion accessibility, treatment should be directed toward the symptomatic side. Because the natural history of asymptomatic lesions is also not well defined,[7-11] we restrict surgery to those lesions having a residual lumen of 2 mm or less or lesions with evidence of multiple intraluminal irregularities that could produce eddy currents interrupting normal laminar blood flow and predisposing the vessel to further ulceration and thrombus formation. On occasion, patients with symptoms of vertebro-

basilar insufficiency will benefit from carotid endarterectomy if it is demonstrated that an insufficient posterior circulation blood flow may be augmented by removing a critical carotid stenosis. These patients must be carefully evaluated to determine the competence of the circle of Willis and collateral blood flow.

CEREBRAL ANGIOGRAPHY

Good quality angiography is an absolute necessity in the evaluation of patients for carotid endarterectomy. It is important that the origin of the cerebral vessels in the thorax and the cervical and intracranial distribution of the carotid arteries be well visualized. Neurologic consequences are not proportional to the size of a carotid lesion, and the angiographic appearance is often an unreliable predictor of the presence of active ulceration with shallow erosion of endothelium and the accumulation of thrombus and debris. The chances of a nonstenotic angiographic lesion containing active elements are higher if its presence can be correlated with appropriate clinical symptomatology. In our surgical experience, greater than 90 percent of the atherosclerotic plaques occurring in a carotid artery ipsilateral to a hemisphere affected by a TIA or monocular visual loss will be ulcerated and contain platelet aggregates and thrombus. When surgery is performed for asymptomatic cervical carotid lesions, irregularities identified angiographically are often found to be smooth and endothelialized.

PREOPERATIVE PREPARATION

Prior to surgery, the patient's cardiopulmonary status must be carefully evaluated. Detailed attention must be given to maintenance of adequate intravascular volume. During preoperative evaluation, patients may become hypovolemic as a consequence of fluid redistribution due to bed rest, the diuresis

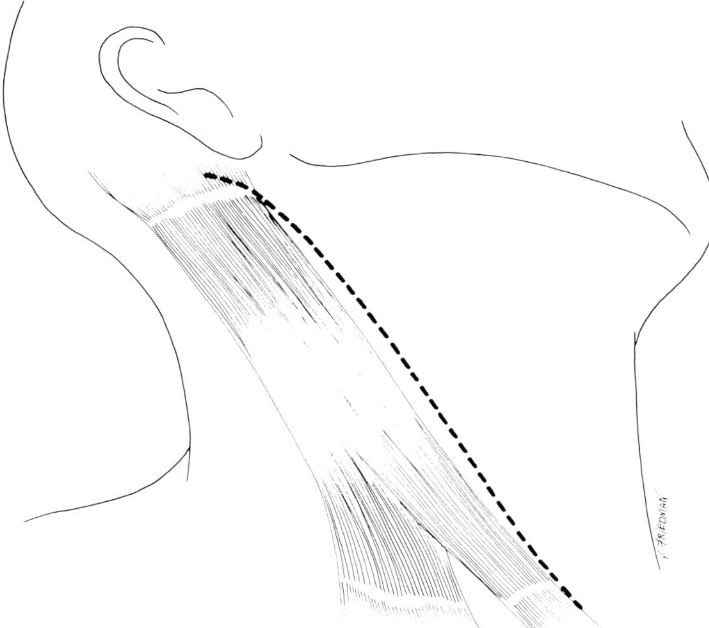

Fig. 64-2.   Position of the neck and location of the skin incision for carotid endarterectomy.

induced by hyperosmolar contrast agents administered for angiography and CT scanning, and the prohibition of fluid intake in preparation for these tests. In some instances, it is necessary to supplement patients with intravenous fluid or in select patients with severe cardiac disease we have found it advantageous to insert a Swan-Ganz catheter before the operation. Patients with severe chronic obstructive pulmonary disease, angina at rest, or recent myocardial infarction are treated with anticoagulant or platelet-suppressing agents rather than an operation, when possible.

SURGICAL MANAGEMENT

Satisfactory results following carotid endarterectomy have been reported with a variety of surgical techniques. The operation requires careful attention to technical details and certain specific principles are essential to achieve a consistently favorable outcome. It is important to adequately expose the distal internal carotid artery to enable direct visualization of the entire extent of an atheromatous plaque. The following technique has been used and continuously modified by the authors and neurosurgical residents who have assisted and, in turn, been assisted in the performance of this operation.

The operation is performed under ''balanced'' anesthesia by the intravenous administration of supplementary isoflurane and the inhalation of a mixture of 50 percent nitrous oxide and 50 percent oxygen. Atracurium or Vecuronium is administered for muscle relaxation. An arterial line is placed in the radial artery after an Allen test is performed. Nasotracheal intubation, which allows greater mobility of submandibular structures, is carried out when it is anticipated that high dissection will be required for distal exposure. Blood pressure is maintained at a normal or slightly elevated level throughout the procedure. Undesirable elevations of blood pressure are controlled by the administration of small amounts of isoflurane or nitroglycerin.

Phenylephrine is used to raise blood pressure when indicated. $PaCO_2$ is maintained in the normal range to avoid both the reduction of cerebral blood flow associated with hypocarbia and the theoretical possibility of luxury perfusion occurring around an ischemic area as a result of hypercapnia.

The patient is positioned with the head slightly extended and turned 45 degrees away from the side to be operated upon. The incision is made along the anterior border of the sternocleidomastoid muscle and can be extended to a point 1 cm posterior to the angle of the jaw, where it is gently curved toward the mastoid process (Figure 64-2). Careful attention is given to hemostasis during the dissection, since systemic anticoagulation will later be employed. The platysma is divided and sharp dissection is continued along the medial border of the sternocleidomastoid muscle until the carotid sheath is encountered. The sheath is entered with care taken to avoid manipulation of the bifurcation. The internal jugular vein is identified and dissection continued medial to the vein (Figure 64-3). The common facial vein and other large bridging veins may require double ligation and division. Dissection of the common carotid artery is performed with minimal disturbance of adjacent tissues to avoid injury to the recurrent laryngeal nerve. The artery is isolated with a right angle gallbladder clamp and secured with a Silastic tape passed through a rubber catheter. When use of an internal shunt is anticipated, an umbilical tape is placed about the artery proximal to the Silastic tape.

The carotid bifurcation is identified and 0.1 ml of 1 percent lidocaine is injected into the region of the carotid sinus nerve to prevent reflex bradycardia and hypotension as a result of sinus manipulation. The bifurcation is left undisturbed in its adventitial bed and the external carotid artery dissected free, isolated distally and secured with a Silastic tourniquet. The origin of the superior thyroid artery is exposed for a few millimeters, carefully avoiding the underlying superior laryngeal nerve (Figure 64-3). The superior thyroid artery is temporarily occluded by double wrapping with a 2-0 silk suture under

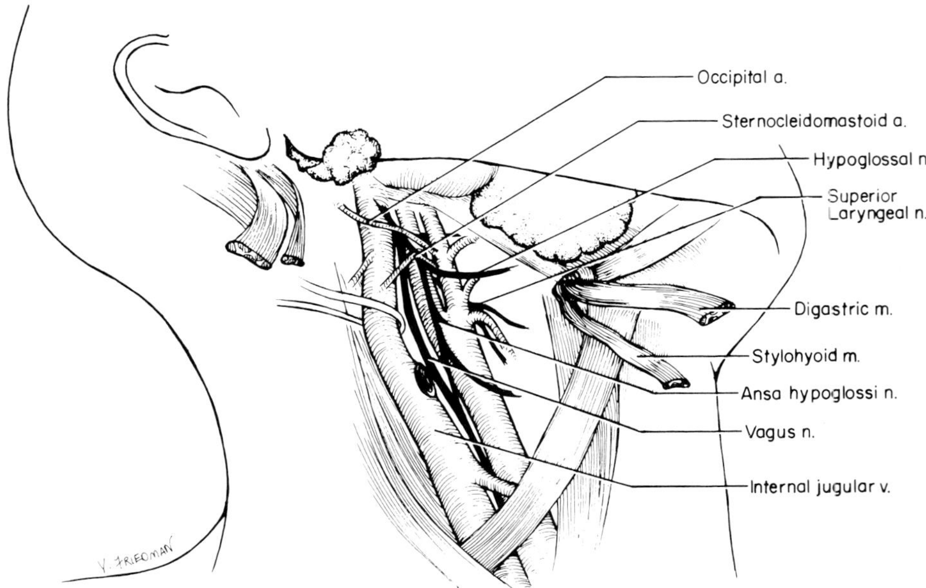

Fig. 64-3. Relationship of the carotid artery to adjacent vascular and neural structures.

tension. Other branches of the external carotid artery having a proximal origin can be handled in a similar fashion. In many instances, it is necessary to divide the ansa hypoglossi during distal exposure of the internal carotid artery in order to mobilize the hypoglossal nerve without traction. Division of the ansa hypoglossi is without clinical effect. In most cases, the internal carotid artery immediately distal to the carotid bulb is mobile and easily freed from surrounding tissue. However, just distal to the bifurcation the adventitia is often more adherent to the arterial wall, and it is helpful to initially enter the correct plane distal to the bulb. When the diseased segment of vessel extends beyond the bulb into the distal internal carotid artery, this segment may be more difficult to dissect free. As seen in Figure 64-3, the vagus nerve lies posterior and lateral to the carotid artery. In rare instances, however, its position may be anterior to the carotid where it is vulnerable to injury unless its presence is anticipated. It is often necessary to expose the lower pole of the parotid gland, which can be undermined and retracted superiorly to allow additional exposure. Care is taken to avoid entering the glandular stroma, since this can lead to postoperative sialorrhea. The marginalus mandibulae branch of the facial nerve, which supplies the lower lip, passes through the substance of the inferior pole of the parotid gland. Retraction of the inferior pole may produce paralysis of the homolateral lip, which is nearly always transient, usually clearing in 6 to 10 weeks. Additional exposure of the artery is facilitated by dividing the posterior belly of the digastric and rarely the stylohyoid muscle in addition to the sternocleidomastoid artery and vein, the so called "sling vessels," as they cross the hypoglossal nerve. These structures and branches of the occipital artery and vein may limit mobilization of the hypoglossal nerve superiorly and away from the vessel. It may be necessary to mobilize the occipital artery and occasionally to divide it in order to gain additional length. These maneuvers allow the internal carotid artery to be exposed to within 1 cm of the base of the skull. The digastric muscle is easily repaired if tagged at the time of division. Exposure of the internal carotid artery to the base of the skull can be achieved by use of an alternate

incision. This incision is begun at the midline, two fingerbreadths below the mandible, extended in a horizontal fashion over the anterior border of the sternocleidomastoid muscle, and then directed posteriorly and superiorly into the retromastoid area. Flaps are elevated beneath the platysma muscle superiorly and inferiorly. It is important to mobilize and preserve the mandibular branch of the facial nerve with the superior flap before beginning the deeper portion of the dissection to expose the carotid artery. With this incision, the parotid gland can be partially mobilized and dissection of the internal carotid artery to the base of the skull is facilitated. Even greater exposure of the distal internal carotid artery can be obtained by disarticulating the mandible,[12,13] but this is almost never required to adequately expose lesions of the carotid bifurcation and proximal internal carotid artery. The common, internal, and external carotid arteries are isolated away from the diseased segment of vessel to avoid embolization of friable plaque and thrombus (Figure 64-4A). At times, it is necessary to dissect free the posterior aspect of the bifurcation. When ulceration has penetrated the media and involves the posterior adventitia, the bifurcation must be mobilized in order to repair the artery. In some circumstances, adequate exposure can only be obtained by dividing the nerve to the carotid sinus with mobilization of the entire bifurcation. Dissection should be performed immediately adjacent to the carotid artery to avoid injury to the superior laryngeal nerve, which innervates the cricothyroid muscle and lies beneath the bifurcation and approximates the course of the superior thyroid artery (Figure 64-3). Injury to this nerve may result in mild hoarseness, loss of high-pitch phonation, and cough with subjective complaints of inability to clear the throat. When the internal carotid artery lies directly posterior to the external carotid artery, access to the internal carotid artery and the view of the surgical assistant can be improved by tilting the operating table to the contralateral side.

Following isolation of the artery and its major branches, the patient is given 5000 units of heparin intravenously. The external carotid artery is occluded with a large aneurysm clip

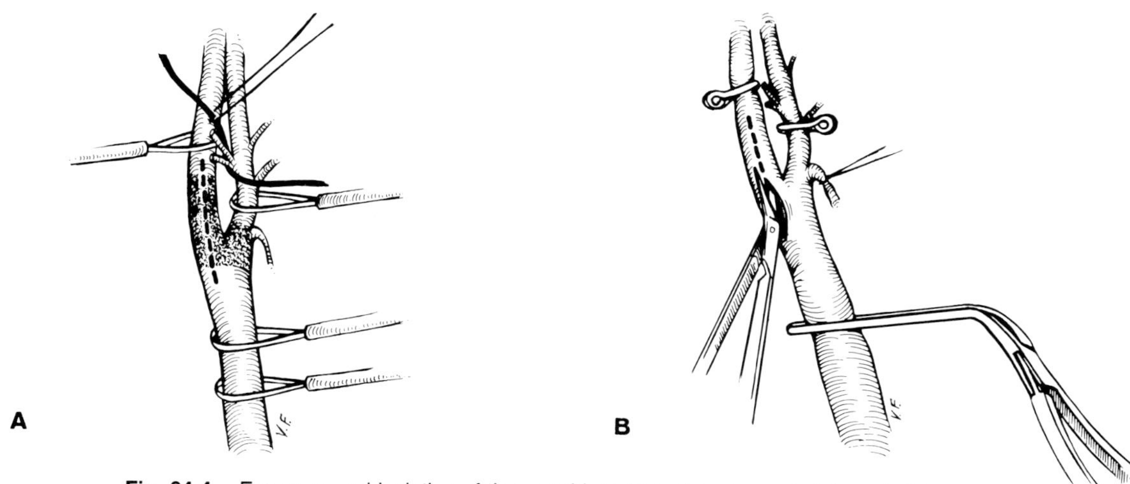

Fig. 64-4.　Exposure and isolation of the carotid artery and placement of the arteriotomy.

and the common carotid artery with an appropriately angled DeBakey vascular clamp.

An intraoperative shunt is not routinely used. In the past we have relied chiefly upon the angiographic evaluation of the circle of Willis and the intraoperative measurement of carotid artery stump pressure to aid in the selection of patients in whom to employ a shunt. We believe that in certain cases an intraoperative shunt provides an added margin of safety. Stump pressure is measured through a 23-gauge needle inserted into the common carotid artery just below the level of angiographically identified disease. When the mean pressure is below 40 mm Hg, a shunt is utilized during arterial occlusion if it does not interfere with dissection of the plaque. Currently, we also employ EEG and compressed spectral analysis monitoring but have developed no uniform preference since our experience has not documented any advantage to either technique for determining if a shunt should be used. The distal internal carotid artery is occluded with a large aneurysm clip and an incision made in the common carotid artery with a small scalpel blade beginning at the point in the common carotid artery where the stump pressure was measured. The arteriotomy is extended with an angled Pott's scissors (Figure 64-4B) into the internal carotid artery and carried through the involved area into the region of relatively normal intima (Figure 64-5A). If a shunt is to be used, one of appropriate size is chosen and inserted into the distal internal carotid artery. If back-bleeding about the shunt persists, the Silastic loop is gently tightened about the shunt. The shunt is back-bled, placed in the common carotid artery, and loosely secured by the Silastic loop placed around the common carotid artery. This will prevent vigorous bleeding and allow optimal positioning of the shunt, which can then be secured by tightening the umbilical tape (Figure 64-5B). On occasion, the ascending pharyngeal artery will originate from the posterior aspect of the distal common carotid artery, causing back-bleeding that may obscure the surgical field. This can be controlled by compression of the tissue lying between the internal and external carotid arteries without disturbing the bifurcation. With advanced atherosclerotic plaque formation, a well-defined plane demarcating atheromatous intimal changes from relatively uninvolved media can be visualized at the arteriotomy edge. With a small blunt dissector, the plane of dissection is usually carried distally into the internal carotid artery (Figure 64-5C). Often the plaque will end at the distal carotid bulb and feather off from normal intima, which is

adherent to the vessel wall. If the bifurcation is high, or atheroma extends beyond the bulb, as in Figure 64-6, it may be necessary when a shunt is used, to remove the shunt when the distal plaque is dissected from the arterial wall. During this period of time blood pressure should be elevated. Dissection of the intact plaque proceeds into the common and external carotid arteries. While in most cases separation of plaque from uninvolved media is facilitated by initial removal from the internal carotid artery, in some instances, often determined by the exact location of atheroma, it will be easier to start the dissection in the common carotid artery. Circumferential dissection about the plaque extending into the external carotid orifice defines a plane between diseased and normal arterial wall. The end of the external carotid plaque can often be blindly reached with a dissector. However, in most instances, it will be necessary to temporarily remove the occluding aneurysm clip from the external carotid artery in order to deliver the entire plaque. The plaque is separated from the common carotid media and sharply amputated (Figure 64-5D). It is important to maintain a single plane between the intima and media. This is best accomplished by starting the dissection on one side of the arteriotomy and by separating the plaque circumferentially. A right-angle blunt nerve hook can be very helpful in achieving this. The remaining cuff of intima, which may be thickened, will be pressed against the vessel wall by the force of the arterial flow. It is unnecessary to place tack-up sutures if the distal intima is adherent and not thickened. When the intima is not securely attached, simple longitudinal 7-0 silk sutures extending over the intimal cuff are placed with care being taken to avoid buckling the arterial wall (Figure 64-5E). When the atherosclerotic disease process produces shallow intimal ulceration with fibrin and thrombus accumulation, it may be considerably more difficult to determine the appropriate plane for dissection. In these cases, the use of magnification is very helpful. The distal extent of the plaque will not be prominent and it may be necessary to divide the intima using microscissors. After the plaque is removed, the artery is irrigated with heparinized saline and carefully inspected for any loose fronds of tissue. On occasion, ulcerations extend through the media to involve the adventitial layer. When the artery is of sufficient size, it may be possible to repair the vessel by plication without compromise of the lumen. If this is not feasible, a patch graft should be placed.

Closure is with a continuous 5-0 or 6-0 suture. Because of its handling characteristics, Proline (monofilament polypropyl-

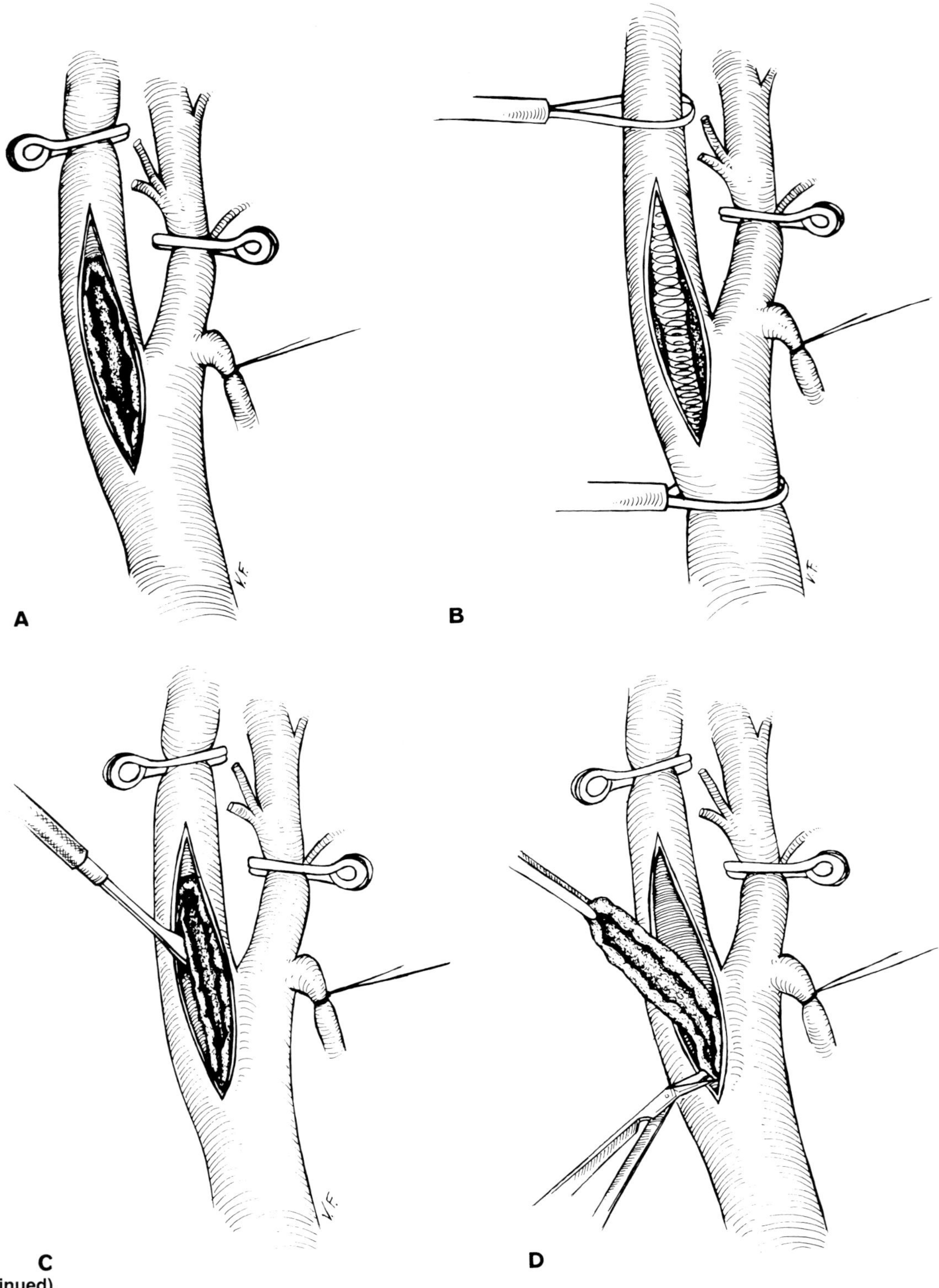

Fig. 64-5 (continued).

ene suture, Ethicon, Inc.) is preferred, but carries the disadvantage of requiring that a number of knots be placed to secure the ends. In the distal internal carotid artery the space between running stitches may be smaller than the bulk of the knot, interfering with a tight suture line. To ensure competency of the suture line the following technique is used. A suture is placed at the distal extreme of the arteriotomy and secured with two overhand knots. Another suture is placed immediately proximal to the first and also secured with two knots. Both ends of the

distal suture are then tied to the trailing end of the proximal suture. This same procedure is repeated at the proximal end of the arteriotomy. The arteriotomy is closed with the proximal suture beginning at the distal internal carotid artery. Individual stitches are placed close to each other, accurately approximating the layers of the arterial wall. The individual loops of suture have a tendency to roll over and it is essential that each loop be tightened perpendicular to the vessel wall to prevent leakage. Just before the closure is completed, the internal and common

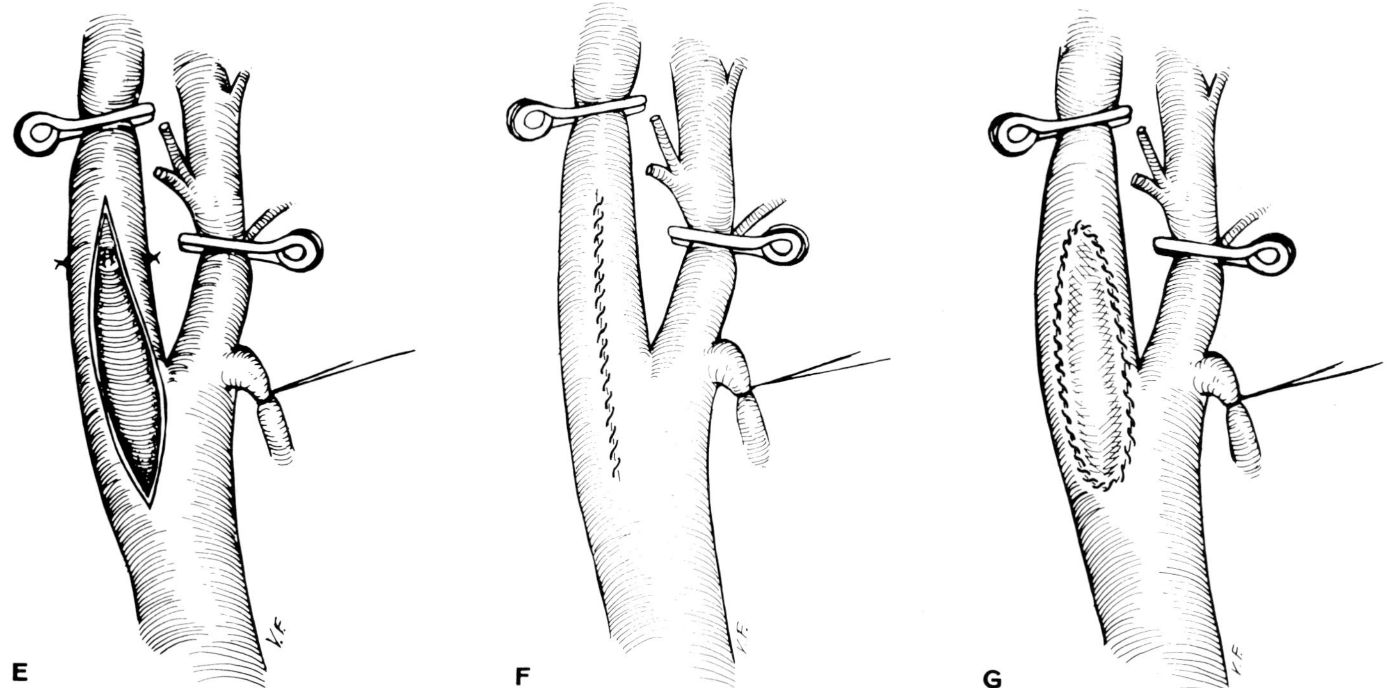

Fig. 64-5. Surgical procedures in carotid endarterectomy.

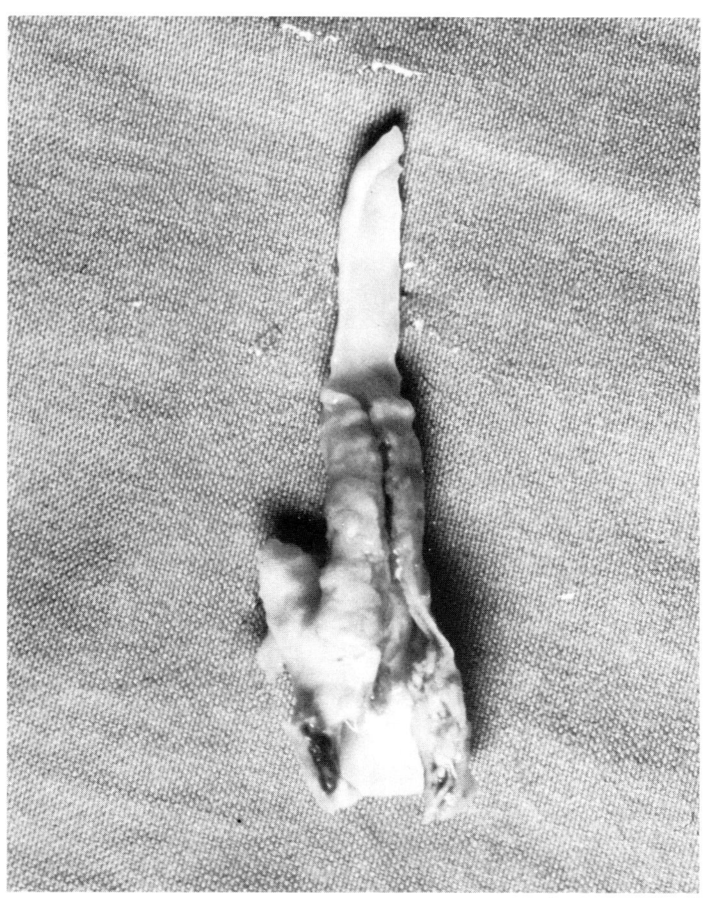

Fig. 64-6. Surgically removed atherosclerotic plaque that extended beyond carotid bulb.

carotid arteries are back-bled, the vessels again occluded, and closure completed by tying a final backhand stitch, utilizing the suture placed at the proximal end of the arteriotomy, to the running suture (Figure 64-5F). A shunt, when used, is removed before the final centimeter of the arteriotomy is closed. We do not routinely use a vein or synthetic patch for closure unless the internal carotid artery is particularly small and simple closure may compromise the lumen (Figure 64-5G). Placement of a graft is also effective in preventing kinks, which can occur as a result of the artery being removed from its bed. Occluding clamps are removed from the external carotid artery, followed by the common carotid artery, allowing any air and debris to be flushed up the external carotid system. The aneurysm clip is then removed from the distal internal carotid artery. Hemostasis is encouraged by holding warm abdominal lap pads over the suture line, followed by cold irrigation. In those instances in which brisk bleeding from the suture line is encountered, it may be necessary to seal the vessel with a 6-0 Proline suture passed through a Teflon pledget. This last maneuver has the potential to cause narrowing of the internal carotid artery and is best avoided by careful attention to the original closure. Hemostasis of the suture line will present little problem if sutures are placed close together and evenly spaced. A soft Silastic drain is inserted through an inferior stab wound, the platysma approximated, and skin closure completed. The heparin previously administered is not reversed.

Bilateral carotid endarterectomies should be staged at least 3 weeks apart. Before the second operation, the vocal cords and tongue should be checked for mobility, since bilateral vocal cord or hypoglossal nerve pareses are serious and disabling complications. Blood pressure lability, which can accompany bilateral endarterectomy, can be avoided by increasing the time between the two procedures and by sparing at least one of the nerves to the carotid sinus.

Restenosis of the carotid bifurcation following endarterectomy is caused by myointimal proliferation, which is thought to be secondary to technically inadequate vessel closure or the postoperative build-up of platelet aggregates at the suture line. Surgery for this condition is tedious and at times difficult because of perivascular scarring, which can interfere with distal control of the internal carotid artery. Control can be achieved by inserting a small balloon catheter beyond the stenotic area and inflating it to provide intraluminal occlusion. Often the obstructing lesion cannot be demarcated from uninvolved media; however, at times a plane can be initiated with sharp dissection and the tissue removed. A vein patch or one of microporous polytetrafluoroethylene is placed to enlarge the arterial lumen and encourage continued vessel patency.

POSTOPERATIVE CARE

Following the operation, particularly during the first 24 hours, the patient must be carefully monitored. Vital signs and neurologic status are checked frequently during the initial 6 hours and then every hour for the first 24 hours. Pain is rarely a problem and is easily controlled with codeine. More potent analgesics should be avoided since they may depress respiratory function. Arterial blood gases are routinely checked in the early postoperative period. Respiratory function must be carefully monitored, especially in those patients who have previously undergone a contralateral carotid endarterectomy. Bilateral procedures may result in the loss of carotid body function,

leaving the patient without compensatory respiratory and circulatory responses to hypoxia.[14] Pareses of the tenth and twelfth nerves can also contribute to postoperative respiratory problems. The operative area must be watched for the development of hematoma and airway obstruction. A hematoma that causes tracheal compromise and respiratory insufficiency requires immediate evacuation. The incidence of this complication can be decreased by connecting the wound drain to low pressure suction for 12 to 18 hours.

Arterial blood pressure changes and cardiac arrhythmias must be recognized and treated promptly because of the high incidence of coexistent coronary artery disease. Arterial blood pressure is maintained at normal or mildly elevated levels. Blood pressure is often labile following carotid endarterectomy as a result of carotid baroreceptor dysfunction,[15,16] and a significant number of patients will develop early postoperative hypotension, which will often respond to fluid replacement. More severe decreases must be corrected promptly to avoid carotid thrombosis. Intravenous fluids including colloid solutions and blood are used to expand systemic blood volume. If these measures fail, vasopressors are administered. Patients remain at bed rest for 18 to 24 hours before being allowed to sit up because of potential blood pressure instability. Even then, assuming the upright position can cause a significant fall in pressure. When the patient tolerates the sitting position, ambulation is begun. Some patients will develop hypertension in the postoperative period. Mild elevations are safely tolerated, but severe degrees must be vigorously treated, especially in patients who have suffered a recent cerebral infarction, to prevent the development of an intracerebral hemorrhage or cerebral edema.

Therapy of cerebrovascular atherosclerotic disease does not end with carotid endarterectomy. Long-term treatment with anti-platelet drugs, while not proven to be of benefit, is recommended. Risk factors, including cardiac disease, hypertension, diabetes mellitus, obesity, hyperlipidemia, and cigarette smoking must be reduced.

COMPLICATIONS

The complications of carotid endarterectomy are listed in Tables 64-1 and 64-2. The incidence of complications is low when attention is given to the details of patient selection, intraoperative management and postoperative care.[17,18]

The occurrence of a new neurologic deficit as a result of carotid endarterectomy is a serious complication. The majority of intraoperative deficits are thought to be the result of embolization from ulcerated atherosclerotic lesions during dissection and manipulation of the carotid artery. Intraoperative ischemia, either secondary to hypotension or inadequate collateral circulation during carotid occlusion, can also result in neurologic deficit. By avoiding decreases in blood pressure during anesthesia and using techniques to enhance cerebral perfusion, including induced hypertension and temporary intraluminal bypass, the incidence of cerebral ischemia is reduced. In the early postoperative period, neurologic deficit can be caused by cerebral emboli originating from platelet aggregates at the suture line and denuded media. Severe postoperative hypotension may predispose the vessel to this thrombus formation. If the patient develops a postoperative neurologic deficit, computed tomography and angiography should be performed immediately and the patient returned to the operat-

Table 64-1. Causes and rates of morbidity and mortality for carotid endarterectomy based on 575 procedures in 523 patients

Cause	Number	Percent
Perioperative mortality		
Myocardial infarction	4	0.7
Stroke	1	0.2
Other	3	0.5
Total	8	1.4
Neurologic worsening		
Transient	19	3.3
Permanent, ipsilateral		
Mild	4	0.7
Major	5	0.9
Permanent, secondary to hemorrhage into infarct		
Mild	3	0.5
Major	1	0.2
Neurologic deficit in other territory		
Transient	1	0.2
Mild	2	0.2
Major	1	0.2
Mortality and permanent major neurologic deficit		2.6
Permanent minor neurologic deficit		1.4

ing room to correct abnormalities such as occlusion of the carotid vessels, thrombus formation at the endarterectomy site, and dissection of a distal intimal flap that obstructs flow in the internal carotid artery. If angiography cannot be performed immediately and the CT scan does not reveal a cerebral hemorrhage, the patient should be returned directly to the operating room.

Figure 64-3 demonstrates the major cranial nerves and their branches, which are often encountered during exposure of the carotid artery. Others lie near the area of dissection. These include the hypoglossal, the vagus (with its superior and recurrent laryngeal branches), the marginal branch of the facial, and the cervical sympathetic trunk. Fortunately, postoperative pareses of these nerves are rarely permanent and their incidence can be greatly reduced by meticulous dissection techniques and avoidance of vigorous retraction.

Disruption and aneurysm formation occasionally occur after carotid endarterectomy. The incidence of these complications is higher when synthetic patch grafts are used to close the arteriotomy, especially if a deep wound infection occurs. Infection following carotid endarterectomy is rare.

Because of the high incidence of associated coronary artery disease, myocardial ischemia and cardiac arrhythmias are not infrequently encountered during and after carotid endarterectomy. Myocardial infarction is the leading single cause of operative mortality (Table 64-1).

Following surgery many patients experience headaches ipsilateral to the endarterectomy site.[19] These headaches are usually self-limited, rarely lasting more than a few days. An infrequent complication is postoperative seizures,[20] which are frequently focal in nature and associated with paroxysmal lateralizing epileptiform discharges on EEG recordings. These seizures are resistant to anticonvulsant therapy and have been attributed to restoration of flow in a previously ischemic zone representing a manifestation of reactive hyperemia.[21] Another likely explanation is cerebral embolization.[22] If seizures occur, cerebral angiography should be performed.

The complications we have encountered in a series of 575 procedures performed in 523 consecutive patients are listed in Tables 64-1 and 64-2. Of eight postoperative deaths, four were caused by myocardial infarction. New or increased permanent neurologic deficit following surgery was noted in 2.7 percent of patients. In 1.4 percent the deficits were mild.

Sundt and co-workers[23] have published an analysis of 1145

Table 64-2. Causes and rates of perioperative morbidity and mortality for carotid endarterectomy based on 575 procedures in 523 patients

Cause	Number	Percent
Myocardial infarction (nonfatal)	7	1.2
Pulmonary embolus	1	0.2
Transient seventh, tenth, eleventh, and twelfth cervical sympathetic nerves	29	5.0
Permanent vocal cord paralysis	5	0.9
Disruption of suture line	1	0.2
Re-exploration for neck hematoma	6	1.0
Wound infection	1	0.2
Asymptomatic intimal flap	2	0.2

carotid endarterectomies in which they related the rate of mortality and serious morbidity to preoperative risk factors. Neurologically stable patients without major medical or angiographically determined risks incurred no mortality or major stroke and a 1 percent group incidence of minor stroke. Neurologically unstable patients or those with associated major medical or angiographic risks suffered the highest rate of neurologic complications following operation, having a 3 percent group mortality and a 1.9 percent incidence of major and 1.3 percent incidence of minor stroke. In this large series, the rate of mortality and permanent major neurologic deficit was 2.5 percent.

OUTCOME OF CAROTID ENDARTERECTOMY

The long-term outcome of carotid endarterectomy is difficult to evaluate. The wide variation in severity of preoperative neurologic deficits and the natural history of improvement of strokes without treatment make it difficult to assess the role of endarterectomy in neurologic recovery. In selected patients with mild, stable strokes, carotid endarterectomy appears to lower the incidence of recurrent strokes and possibly has been responsible for improvement in neurologic function beyond that expected from the natural course of the disease.[24,25] The role of carotid endarterectomy in patients with TIAs is better defined. Carotid endarterectomy is effective in relieving symptoms of TIAs and lowering the incidence of stroke in selected patients.[26] The majority of late deaths in patients undergoing carotid endarterectomy are of cardiac origin. While at the present time no increase in survival rate of surgical patients compared with control patients can be demonstrated,[27] it is believed that the avoidance of stroke significantly improves the quality of life.

MISCELLANEOUS CONDITIONS AFFECTING THE EXTRACRANIAL CAROTID ARTERIES

TRAUMATIC INJURIES

Injuries to the carotid artery can result from penetrating or less frequently blunt trauma.[28,29] Penetrating neck wounds, usually the result of stab or missile injuries, most frequently involve the common carotid artery.[29] Findings of a local, at times pulsatile hematoma, may accompany the injury. Arteriovenous fistulas are not uncommon. A significant number of patients will demonstrate a related neurologic deficit.

Patients with hypotension as a result of blood loss from a suspected carotid artery injury require rapid resuscitation and immediate neck exploration to control hemorrhage. Tracheal intubation is essential, since airway compromise by external compression from hematoma or massive internal bleeding may occur. When bleeding is controlled and the airway not compromised, angiography should be performed to define the presence and extent of vascular injuries.[30,31] Information obtained from good quality angiograms may be crucial in planning the surgical approach to a correctable vascular injury. While some evidence indicates that early arterial repair in the presence of a neurologic deficit may lead to worsening of neurologic status,[32,33] many authorities advocate early exploration as essential to appropriate management.[34,35] Preoperative neurologic deficits

are often permanent.[29,34] While penetrating injuries are frequently tangential, perforation and complete transection of the carotid artery are also seen. The method of operative repair is dictated by the nature of the injury to the vessel. Necrotic portions must be resected and intimal flaps excised. With some tangential wounds, arteriorrhaphy or a vein patch graft may be sufficient for repair, especially when the common carotid artery is involved. End-to-end anastomosis of the artery using either a vein or synthetic graft is required to repair more extensive arterial injuries. A temporary shunt is seldom needed and may interfere with repair. Clots should be evacuated from the distal stump of the artery by back-bleeding or careful extraction with a Fogarty catheter. During repair heparin should be systemically administered. When the injured artery cannot be adequately exposed for repair, ligation may be necessary to control hemorrhage. The presence of coma before surgery is a grave prognostic sign.[34]

Blunt injuries of the carotid artery are uncommon, but when unrecognized are associated with a high incidence of severe neurologic complications.[28,29] Often there is no evidence of direct trauma to the neck and the frequent association with closed head injury may obscure recognition of the carotid injury.[36] Direct blunt trauma to the neck causing arterial damage frequently involves the carotid bifurcation, particularly in older patients with atheromatous disease. Extension and rotation of the neck as a result of head trauma may stretch the internal carotid artery over a transverse process of an upper cervical vertebra. Basilar skull fractures can disrupt the petrosal portion of the internal carotid artery, while intraoral trauma may be associated with injury to the internal carotid artery adjacent to the tonsillar fossa.

Suspicion of a blunt carotid artery injury may not arise until the patient develops focal neurologic symptoms, perhaps hours to weeks after the injury. Neck swelling or a Horner's syndrome often will be present and serve as an early clue. The diagnosis should be corroborated by angiography. Surgical management is indicated if an appropriate accessible lesion is found.

KINKING

The clinical importance of elongation with looping and kinking of the cervical carotid artery is obscure. Although a number of surgical techniques have been developed to deal with this phenomenon, most surgeons question the need for surgery in the majority of cases.[37] Kinking or buckling of the carotid artery is caused by atherosclerosis and is distinguished from coiling, which is thought to be a developmental abnormality.[38] Coiling in an exaggerated S-shaped curvature or circular configuration is caused by elongation and redundancy of the internal carotid artery and is often an incidental angiographic finding. Kinking, which consists of angulation of one or more segments of the artery, is usually associated with atherosclerotic disease at the carotid bifurcation. True kinking may, in rare instances, cause obstructive symptoms. In this situation, factors such as changes in neck position, blood pressure variation, and the presence of extracranial atherosclerotic occlusive disease may play a major role. In patients with recurrent cerebrovascular symptoms, resection of the kink should be considered only if it significantly reduces the arterial lumen and no other causative angiographic abnormality is found.[38,39,40] The head should be rotated during angiography to observe the effects upon the kink. Symptomatic kinking is surgically managed by resection of the involved segment of the internal carotid artery with end-to-end anastomosis. The difficulties encountered with unequal size of the ends may be overcome by use of a vein patch. At times, it is necessary to reimplant the distal internal carotid artery into the common carotid artery.[41]

ANEURYSMS

Nondissecting aneurysms of the extracranial carotid artery are rare but represent a serious entity having the potential of death or stroke from rupture, thrombosis, or embolism.[41,42] In the past, syphilis and pharyngeal infections were the predominate causes of these aneurysms, but today they are most often associated with trauma or atherosclerosis. They can occur following carotid endarterectomy, most frequently when a patch graft has been employed in closure.[43] Patients usually have a pulsatile cervical mass and bruit. These lesions should be resected. The involved arterial segment is excised and replaced with a synthetic or vein graft. A saccular aneurysm rarely can be transected through its stalk and the carotid artery directly repaired.

Dissecting extracranial carotid artery aneurysms constitute a group of lesions that usually occur above the carotid bifurcation.[44–47] Some cases are clearly related to a predisposing factor such as trauma, angiography, and fibromuscular dysplasia, but many have a spontaneous onset with an obscure etiology. The dissection can occur bilaterally, often forming pseudoaneurysms. Symptoms and signs are ascribed to three basic mechanisms: disruption of sympathetic fibers within the wall of the carotid artery, accumulation of thrombi on areas of intimal disruption leading to cerebral emboli, and reduction in cerebral blood flow as a result of stenosis or occlusion of the carotid artery.[44] Initial symptoms may include unilateral head and face pain associated with an ipsilateral Horner's syndrome,[47] TIAs, and stroke. The diagnosis is made by angiography.

A number of therapeutic approaches have been utilized in small groups of patients. Operative management includes segmental resection and grafting, thrombectomy and endarterectomy, dilatation, carotid ligation, and extracranial/intracranial bypass.[44,48] However, the distal extent of dissection in the majority of cases can make direct surgery hazardous and lead to undesirable clinical results. Patients surviving an extracranial carotid artery dissection often have a stable or improving course, although if aneurysmal changes are present, some evidence of the lesion may persist.[45] The recommended initial treatment is anticoagulation to prevent thromboembolic events. Serial angiography has shown that many of these lesions will resolve when treated in this manner.[49]

FIBROMUSCULAR DYSPLASIA

Fibromuscular dysplasia of the internal carotid arteries is often an incidental angiographic finding.[24] This condition is most commonly seen in women in their third and fourth decades. The lesions are frequently bilateral, nearly always located in the distal part of the cervical internal carotid artery extending to or beyond the base of the skull. The proximal 2.5 cm of the internal carotid is usually spared. There is a recognized association with fibromuscular hyperplasia of the renal arteries, hypertension, and multiple intracranial aneurysms. In

general, this condition is thought to have a benign course.[50] In older patients, associated atherosclerotic lesions near the carotid bifurcation are more likely to be the source of cerebrovascular symptoms. Surgical treatment should be directed toward the atherosclerotic plaque. In patients without associated lesions, symptoms of cerebrovascular insufficiency have been attributed to fibromuscular dysplasia. In these patients, surgical treatment will vary with the location of the lesion. In most cases, it is not possible to expose normal distal internal carotid artery with a cervical approach, and techniques of graded arterial dilation using instruments such as rigid biliary dilators,[51] coronary artery dilators,[52] small Fogarty catheters, and percutaneous transluminal angioplasty have been employed.[53,54,55] Satisfactory results have been reported in selected patients using these techniques.

SUMMARY AND CONCLUSIONS

In selected patients, carotid endarterectomy is a relatively safe and effective means of preventing cerebral infarction as a result of atherosclerotic occlusive and embolic disease of the extracranial carotid artery. Patients having a cerebral ischemic event and who have significant hemispheric neurologic function at risk should undergo computed tomography of the head and cerebral angiography following appropriate medical evaluation and determination of surgical candidacy. Among the factors influencing a decision to treat a patient surgically are the correlation of clinical and angiographic features, collateral cerebral circulation, and medical and surgical risk factors. Satisfactory surgical results require precise attention to technical details. Measures must be taken to avoid intraoperative embolization and ischemia and to ensure continued vessel patency by direct visualization of the distal extent of atheromatous involvement of the internal carotid artery. Rapid correction of postoperative abnormalities of cardiovascular and respiratory status will diminish the rate of serious complications during this period. The patient with atherosclerotic cerebrovascular disease must have continued treatment of identifiable risk factors following carotid endarterectomy.

REFERENCES

1. Ross R, Glomset, JA: The pathogenesis of arteriosclerosis, Part 1. N Engl J Med 295:369, 1976
2. Hammond JH, Eisinger RP: Carotid bruits in 1,000 normal subjects. Arch Intern Med 109:109, 1962
3. Heyman A, Wilkins WE, Heyden S, et al: Risk of stroke in asymptomatic persons with cervical arterial bruits: A population study in Evans County, Georgia. N Engl J Med 302:838, 1980
4. Mohr JP: Asymptomatic carotid artery disease. Stroke 13:431, 1982
5. Wolf PA, Kannel WB, Sorlie P, et al: Asymptomatic carotid bruit and risk of stroke. The Framingham study. JAMA 245:1442, 1981
6. Yatsu FM, Hart RG: Asymptomatic carotid bruit and stenosis. Stroke 14:301, 1983
7. Moore WS, Boren G, Malone JA, et al: Asymptomatic carotid stenosis: Immediate and long-term results after prophylactic endarterectomy. Am J Surg 138:228, 1979
8. Levin SM, Sondheimer FK, Levin JM: The contralateral diseased but asymptomatic carotid artery: To operate or not? An update. Am J Surg 140:203, 1980
9. Dixon S, Pais O, Raviola C, et al: Natural history of non-stenotic, asymptomatic ulcerative lesions of the carotid artery. A further analysis. Arch Surg 117:1493, 1982

10. Chambers BR, Norris JW: The case against surgery for asymptomatic carotid stenosis. Stroke 15:964, 1984

11. Durwood QJ, Ferguson GG, Barr HWK: The natural history of asymptomatic carotid bifurcation plaques. Stroke 13:459, 1982

12. Fisher DF, Clagett GP, Parker JI, et al: Mandibular subluxation for high carotid exposure. J Vasc Surg 1:727, 1984

13. Balagura, S, Carter JB, Gossett DL: Surgical approach to the high subcranial internal carotid artery. Neurosurgery 16:402, 1985

14. Wade JG, Larson CP Jr, Hickey RF, et al: Effect of carotid endarterectomy on carotid chemoreceptor and baroreceptor function in man. N Engl J Med 282:823, 1970

15. Bove EL, Fry WJ, Gross WS, et al: Hypotension and hypertension as consequences of baroreceptor dysfunction following carotid endarterectomy. Surgery 85:633, 1979

16. Tarlov E, Schmidek H, Scott RM, et al: Reflex hypotension following carotid endarterectomy: Mechanism and management. J Neurosurg 29:323, 1973

17. Thompson JE: Complications of carotid endarterectomy and their prevention. World J Surg 3:155, 1979

18. Dunsker SB: Complications of carotid endarterectomy. Clin Neurosurg 23:336, 1976

19. Messert B, Black JA: Cluster headache, hemicrania, and other head pains: Morbidity of carotid endarterectomy. Stroke 9:559, 1978

20. Wilkinson JT, Adams HP Jr, Wright, CB: Convulsions after carotid endarterectomy. JAMA 244:1827, 1980

21. Sundt TM, Houser OW, Sharbrough F, et al: Carotid endarterectomy: Results, complications, and monitoring techniques, in Thompson RA, Green JA (eds): Advances in Neurology, vol 16. New York, Raven Press, 1977, pp 97–119

22. Sundt TM: Extracranial occlusive cerebral vascular disease, in Wilson CB, Hoff JT (eds): Current Management of Neurologic Disease. New York, Churchill-Livingstone, 1980, pp 191–201

23. Sundt TM Jr, Sharbrough FW, Piepgras DG, et al: Correlation of cerebral blood flow and electroencephalographic changes during carotid endarterectomy. With results of surgery and hemodynamics of cerebral ischemia. Mayo Clin Proc 56:533, 1981

24. Thompson JE, Talkington CM: Carotid endarterectomy. Ann Surg 184:1, 1976

25. Weinbaum F, Riles TS, Lamparello PJ, et al: Results of carotid surgery for patients with permanent neurologic deficits. Circulation 70(Suppl 2):136, 1984

26. Whisnant JP, Sandok BA, Sundt TM Jr: Carotid endarterectomy for unilateral carotid system transient cerebral ischemia. Mayo Clin Proc 58:171, 1983

27. Toole JF, Janeway R, Choi K, et al: Transient ischemic attacks due to atherosclerosis: A prospective study of 160 patients. Arch Neurol 32:5, 1975

28. Krajewski LP, Hertzer NR: Blunt carotid artery trauma. Ann Surg 191:341, 1980

29. Rubio PA, Reul GJ Jr, Beall AC Jr, et al: Acute carotid artery injury: 25 years experience. J Trauma 14:967, 1974

30. Ledgerwood AM, Mullins RJ, Lucas CE: Primary repair vs. ligation for carotid artery injures. Arch Surg 115:488, 1980

31. O'Donnell VA, Atik M, Pick RA: Evaluation and management of penetrating wounds of the neck. The role of emergency angiograph. Am J Surg 138:309, 1979

32. Bradley EL III: Management of penetrating carotid injuries: An alternative approach. J Trauma 13:248, 1973

33. Samson DS: Cervical carotid injuries, in Clinical Neurosurgery, vol 29. Baltimore, Williams & Wilkins, 1981, pp 647–656

34. Unger SW, Tucker WS Jr, Mrdeza MA, et al: Carotid arterial trauma. Surgery 87:477, 1980

35. Karlin RM, Marks C: Extracranial carotid artery injury. Presented at the 11th Annual Meeting of the Society for Clinical Vascular Surgery, 1983, pp 225–227

36. Heilbrun MP, Ratcheson RA: Multiple extracranial vessel injuries following closed head and neck trauma: Case report. J Neurosurg 37:219, 1972

37. Perdue GD, Barreca JP, Smith RB, et al: The significance of elongation and angulation of the carotid artery: A negative view. Surgery 77:45, 1975

38. Desai B, Toole JF: Kinks, coils and carotids: A review. Stroke 6:649, 1975

39. Connolly JE: Discussion: Kinking of internal carotid artery. Am J Surg 134:88, 1977

40. Leipzig TJ, Dohrmann GJ: The tortuous or kinked carotid artery: Pathogenesis and clinical considerations. A historical review. Surg Neurol 25:478, 1986

41. Cooley DA, Wukasch DC: Techniques in Vascular Surgery. Philadelphia, WB Saunders, 1979, pp 20–44

42. Coleman PG, Kittle GF: Aneurysms of the common carotid artery. Surg Clin North Am 53:231, 1973

43. Smith RB III, Perdue GP, Collier RH, et al: Postoperative false aneurysms of the carotid artery. Am Surg 36:335, 1970

44. Friedman WA, Day AL, Quisling RG, et al: Cervical carotid dissecting aneurysms. Neurosurgery 7:207, 1980

45. Luken MG III, Ascherl GF Jr, Correll JW, et al: Spontaneous dissecting aneurysm of the extracranial internal carotid artery. Clin Neurosurg 26:353, 1978

46. Fisher CM, Ojemann RG, Roberson GH: Spontaneous dissection of cervico-cerebral arteries. Can J Neurol Sci 5:9, 1978

47. Hart RG, Easton JD: Dissections of Cervical and Cerebral Arteries. Neurol Clin 1:155, 1983

48. Ehrenfeld WK, Wylie EJ: Spontaneous dissection of the internal carotid artery. Arch Surg 111:1294, 1976

49. Mokri B, Sundt TM Jr, Houser OW, et al: Spontaneous dissection of the cervical internal carotid artery. Ann Neurol 19:126, 1986

50. Wells RP, Smith RR: Fibromuscular dysplasia of the internal carotid artery: A long term follow up. Neurosurgery 10:39, 1982

51. Morris GC, Lechter A, DeBakey ME: Surgical treatment of fibromuscular disease of the carotid arteries. Arch Surg 96:636, 1968

52. Ehrenfeld WK, Wylie EJ: Fibromuscular dysplasia of the internalcarotid artery. Arch Surg 109:676, 1974

53. Mullan S, Duda EE, Patromas NJ: Some examples of balloon technology in neurosurgery. J Neurosurg 52:321, 1980

54. Tsai FY, Matovich V, Hieshima G, et al: Percutaneous transluminal angioplasty of the carotid artery. AJNR 7:349, 1986

55. Jooma R, Bradshaw JR, Griffith HB: Intimal dissection following percutaneous transluminal carotid angioplasty for fibromuscular dysplasia. Neuroradiology 27:181, 1985

CHAPTER 65

Exposure of the Distal Internal Carotid Artery

Calvin B. Ernst

SINCE FIRST SUCCESSFULLY PERFORMED over three decades ago, the technique of carotid bifurcation endarterectomy has evolved; the procedure is now standardized and safe. That approximately 100,000 carotid endarterectomies were performed in the United States in 1983 is testimony to its widespread acceptance.[1] Less well standardized is exposure and reconstruction of the distal internal carotid artery, which is considered by some to be inaccessible. No doubt this is because of the infrequent need to correct lesions situated distally in the internal carotid artery; it was a requirement in less than 1 percent of patients treated by the Vascular Surgery Division at the Henry Ford Hospital. In addition, such arteries are inaccessible because they are situated deep in the body or are obscured by bone, e.g., the mandible in the case of the distal internal carotid artery. However, most seemingly inaccessible arteries can be exposed surgically; when this is not possible or prudent, reasonable therapeutic alternatives usually are available.

LESIONS REQUIRING EXPOSURE OF THE DISTAL CAROTID

Almost all carotid bifurcation lesions requiring surgical correction are atherosclerotic in origin. Conversely, lesions requiring exposure and reconstruction of the distal carotid are rarely atherosclerotic and most commonly include traumatic lesions, aneurysms (either true, false, or mycotic), and fibromuscular dysplastic stenoses and kinks (Table 65-1). On occasion an atherosclerotic plaque originating at the carotid bifurcation may extend up to the base of the skull, beyond the limits of standard bifurcation endarterectomy and for which distal exposure will be required. The management of arterial complications of radiation therapy or the need for resection of benign or malignant neoplasms may require exposure of the distal carotid for reconstruction or ligation. Although rare, since a false aneurysm after a standard endarterectomy usually involves the accessible bifurcation, distal exposure may be required for repair, particularly if the pseudoaneurysm is large. The tendency of a thin-walled infected or mycotic aneurysm to rupture or for luminal contents to dislodge during dissection also mandates exposure of the distal carotid to successfully manage such lesions.

ALTERNATIVES TO DISTAL EXPOSURE

For certain distal fibromuscular dysplastic lesions complicated by elongation and flow-reducing kinks or stenoses, an alternative to direct repair is proximal internal carotid resection, transluminal dilation of the stenosis, and anastomosis to foreshorten and straighten the vessel (Figures 65-1 and 65-2).

Certain extenuating circumstances may preclude carotid reconstruction, and the only available prudent alternative is distal ligation. Indications for ligation include radiation-induced arteriomalacia or necrosis, unreconstructible penetrating wounds, inaccessible aneurysms that act as a source of microemboli, a friable infected aneurysm, and unreconstructible carotid dissections. Under such circumstances, safety of ligation without subsequent development of a stroke must be assured. Recent data suggest that a systolic stump pressure of 70 torr implies adequate intracranial collateral circulation and is an index for safe ligation. Systolic stump pressures less than 70 torr are associated with a 50 percent risk of stroke.[2] Alternative revascularization procedures such as extracranial-to-intracranial bypass must be used under such circumstances.[3]

TECHNIQUE OF EXPOSURE OF THE DISTAL CAROTID

ANESTHESIA

Before anesthesia is induced, a cannula is inserted in the radial artery of the nondominant arm to obtain blood samples for blood gas measurements and for continuous monitoring of systemic blood pressure. Nasotracheal intubation is required in anticipation of the need for mandibular manipulation to facilitate exposure of the distal carotid. Furthermore, the depth of anesthesia must be closely modulated to ensure interpretable electroencephalographic (EEG) monitoring if this monitoring method is used during carotid occlusion. After adequate anesthesia is established, mandibular subluxation is performed.

MANDIBULAR SUBLUXATION

Ipsilateral mandibular subluxation is performed in conjunction with an oral surgeon. In dentate patients circummandibular-transnasal wiring is preferred to hold the mandible in the subluxed position.[4] In edentulous patients, $3/32$-inch threaded Steinmann pins are inserted obliquely into the mandible and

OPERATIVE NEUROSURGICAL TECHNIQUES
ISBN 0-8089-1862-1

Table 65-1. Lesions requiring exposure
of the distal carotid artery

Distal extension of atherosclerotic bifurcation disease
Trauma
Fibromuscular dysplasia
Congenital loops or kinks
Aneurysm: true, false, mycotic
Postirradiation arteriomalacia
Neoplastic involvement

maxilla, secured by wires, and then encased in methylmethacrylate to provide external fixation to hold the mandible subluxed. The Steinmann pins are placed into the contralateral maxillary alveolar process with a drill. The first pin should be placed 1 to 2 cm above the crest of the alveolar ridge and angled toward the angle of the mandible of the opposite side. The placement is stopped when the tip of the pin is felt protruding through the palatal mucosa. A second pin is inserted into the ipsilateral mandible 1 to 2 cm inferior to the alveolar crest and angled toward the angle of the mandible of the opposite side. The pins are cut so 1 to 2 cm protrude, and a loop of 25-gauge wire is used to secure the two pins after the temporomandibular joint is subluxed on the side of the carotid to be exposed. Gentle anterior pressure subluxes the mandible anteriorly from the temporomandibular fossa while are the pins are secured by tightening the wire with a wire twister. Gentle steady pressure is required so the discal and capsular ligaments are not overly stretched or injured. Once maximum subluxation has been produced, the wire is twisted down tightly. Gauze coated with petroleum jelly is placed around the pins and the adjacent oral mucosa. With the wired pins holding the mandible in an anterior position, methylmethacrylate is placed over the gauze to encase the pins and wire and provide further stabilization. When the carotid reconstruction is completed, the methylmethacrylate and pins are removed and the mandible is restored to its anatomic position.

Either of these mandibular subluxation methods converts the triangular operative field at the distal carotid artery into a rectangular one. The rectangular space provides an additional 2 cm of critical operating room and exposure of the distal carotid (Figures 65-3 and 65-4).

Others have suggested longitudinal osteotomy of the vertical ramus of the mandible, rotating the temporomandibular joint segment outward to provide retromandibular exposure (Figure 65-5).[5,6] This requires exposing the angle of the mandible and incising and elevating the periosteum on its superficial and deep surfaces up to the mandibular notch between the coronoid and condyloid processes. It is important to place the osteotomy posterior to the entrance of the inferior alveolar nerve and artery where they enter the foramen on the medial aspect of the mandible so that the posterior mandibular segment can he rotated outward (Figure 65-5). After the carotid reconstructive procedure is completed, the mandibular segments are reduced and wired together. Although it is helpful to know it, this technique is rarely required; I prefer the less complex subluxation techniques.

After the subluxation maneuvers have been performed, the patient is positioned with the head turned to the opposite side and the neck slightly extended. The operating table is placed in a 15-degree reversed Trendelenburg position to minimize ve-

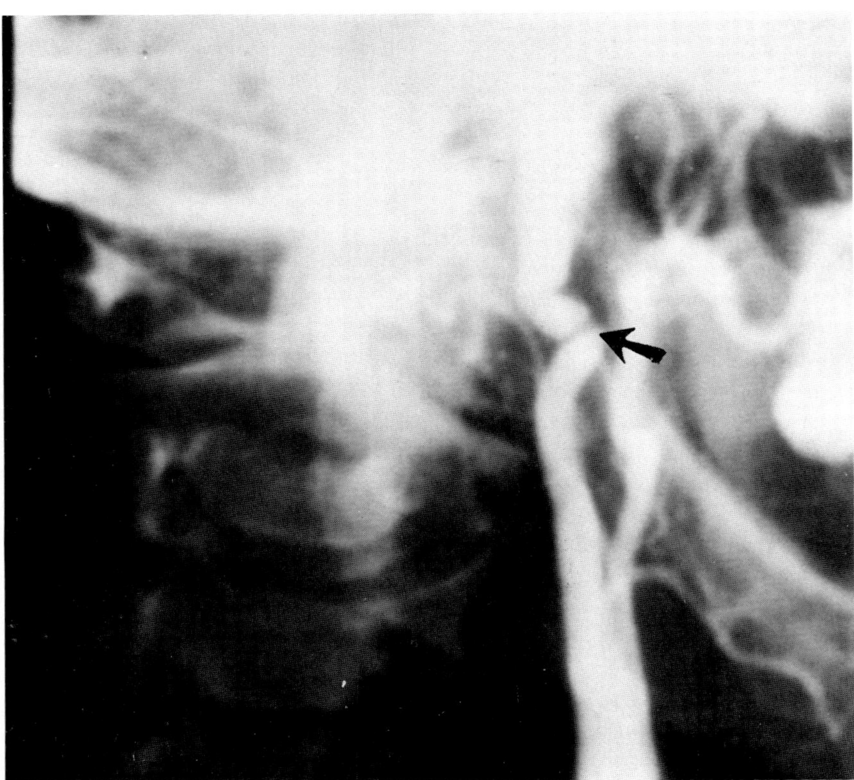

Fig. 65-1. An arteriogram demonstrating preocclusive fibrodysplastic stenosis of the distal internal carotid artery (arrow). Note the typical location of the lesion, several centimeters distal to the carotid bifurcation, close to the base of the skull. (Reprinted from Ernst CB: Exposure of inaccessible arteries. Part I: Carotid and arm exposure. Surgical Rounds 8:21, 1985. With permission.)

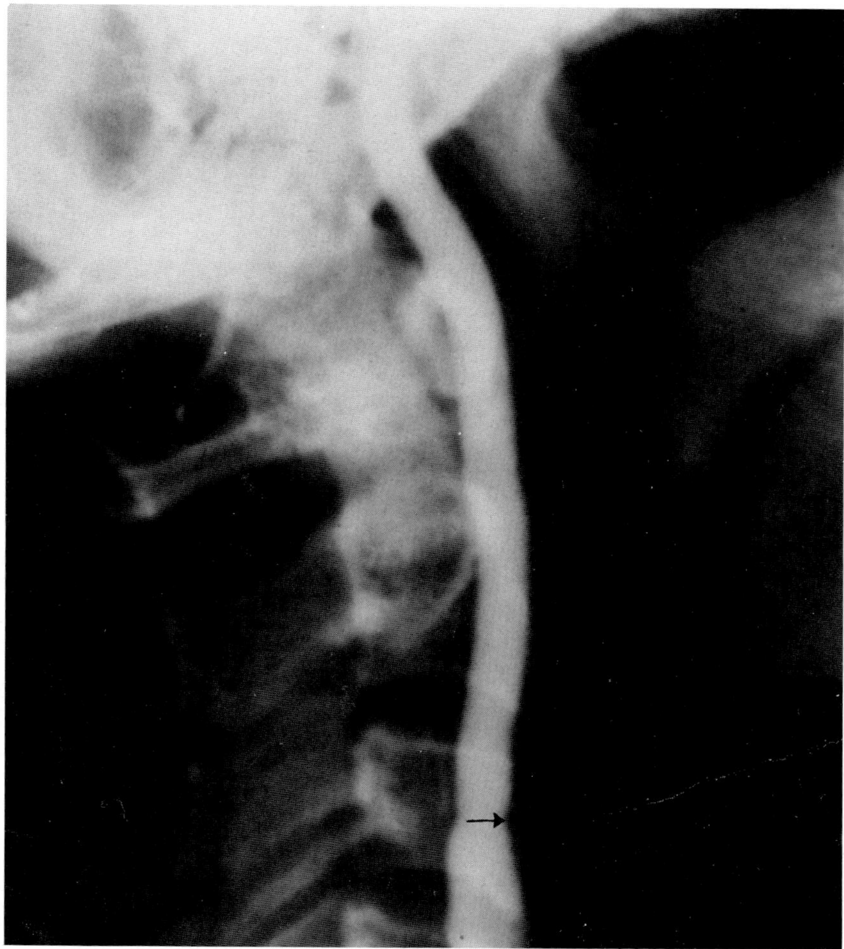

Fig. 65-2.   A postoperative arteriogram of the patient in Figure 65-1 documenting satisfactory dilation of the fibrodysplastic stenosis. A proximal end-to-end anastomosis (arrow) was performed after open transluminal dilation and resection of a 1-cm segment of redundant carotid artery. (Reprinted from Ernst CB: Exposure of inaccessible arteries. Part I: Carotid and arm exposure. Surgical Rounds 8:21, 1985. With permission.)

nous engorgement. The face, neck, and upper chest are prepared and draped. It is important to include the ear in the operative field in the event the incision must be extended cephalad either anterior or posterior to the ear. Also, if autogenous vein reconstruction is anticipated, either as a patch or as a replacement conduit, the groin must be prepared and draped for saphenous vein harvesting.

CAROTID DISSECTION AND EXPOSURE

Exposure of the distal internal carotid artery is best obtained through a longitudinal incision anterior to the sternocleidomastoid muscle (Figure 65-5). Preauricular or retroauricular extension of the incision may be required. The tip of the parotid gland can be mobilized anteriorly or, alternatively, it can be divided if the tip is relatively small. After the sternocleidomastoid muscle is mobilized and retracted posteriorly, the carotid sheath is incised and the carotid bifurcation is dissected, starting with the common carotid artery, which is encircled with a length of PE-90 polyethylene tubing to allow atraumatic traction. The external carotid artery is mobilized next; the superior thyroid artery is ligated when necessary. The interval between the internal and external carotid vessels is incised and the proximal external carotid artery is encircled with PE-90

tubing, which is threaded through an 8-cm segment of 18F Robinson catheter. This will later serve for external carotid snare occlusion. If hypotension or bradycardia occur during carotid sinus manipulation, 1 to 2 ml of 1-percent Xylocaine is injected into the adventitia of the carotid bifurcation to block the baroreceptor mechanism. The carotid sinus nerve is preserved. Traction on the polyethylene catheters allows gentle, atraumatic, no-touch dissection of the remainder of the carotid bifurcation while the internal carotid artery is mobilized.

After the vagus, hypoglossal, and glossopharyngeal (carotid sinus) nerves are identified, dissection proceeds toward the base of the skull. The decendens hypoglossi branch of the hypoglossal nerve can serve as a marker to the hypoglossal nerve; the decendens is usually divided 0.5 cm from the main trunk. Subluxation of the temporomandibular joint stretches the hypoglossal nerve and digastric muscle; consequently, the hypoglossal nerve can be situated slightly cephalad to its normal location than when subluxation is not employed. Division of the posterior belly of the digastric muscle and the styloglossus, stylopharyngeus, and stylohyoid muscles exposes the underlying internal carotid artery. If necessary, the styloid process can be excised after the mastoid insertion of the sternocleidomastoid muscle is divided. Styloid process excision is rarely required but it can provide additional exposure if the

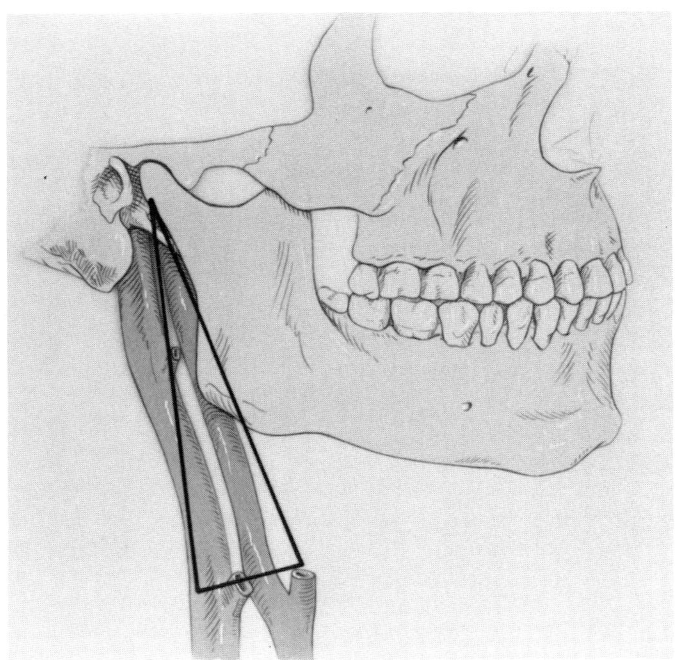 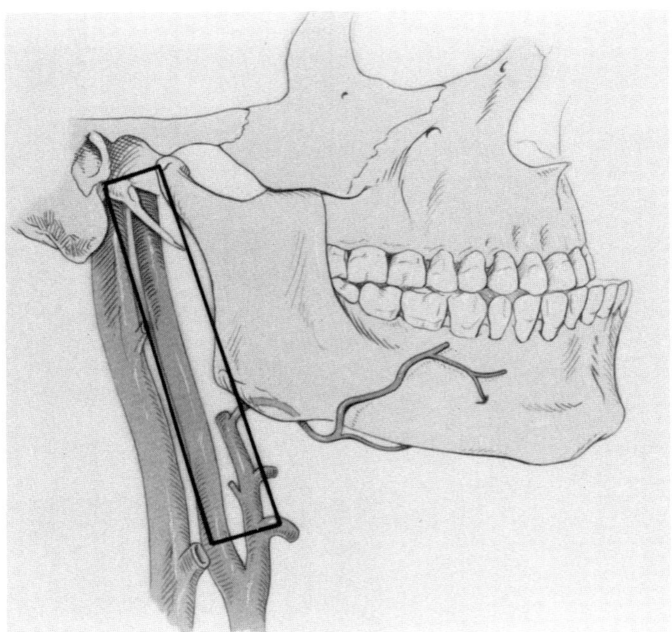

Fig. 65-3. The mandible in its anatomic position. The triangular outline illustrates the field of exposure of the distal internal carotid artery limited by vertical ramus of mandible. (Reprinted from Fisher DF Jr, Clagett GP, Parker JI, et al: Mandibular subluxation for high carotid exposure. J Vasc Surg 1:727–733, 1984. With permission.)

Fig. 65-4. The mandible in a subluxed position showing conversion of the triangular operative field into a rectangular one, thereby gaining an additional 2 cm of exposure of the distal carotid. (Reprinted from Fisher DF Jr, Clagett GP, Parker JI, et al: Mandibular subluxation for high carotid exposure. J Vasc Surg 1:727–733, 1984. With permission.)

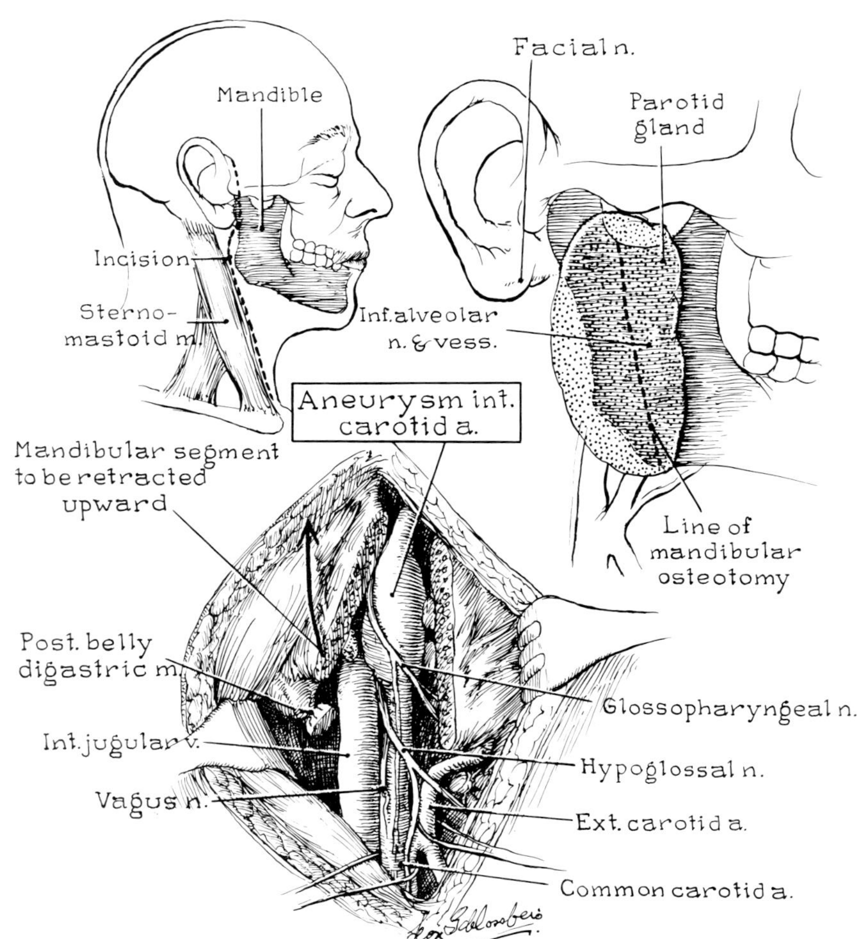

Fig. 65-5. Exposure of the distal internal carotid artery. The skin incision is anterior to the sternocleidomastoid muscle with cephalad extension anterior to the ear (upper left). Line of mandibular osteotomy (upper right). The mandibular osteotomy is completed and the posterior segment of the mandible is rotated outward and up, facilitating distal carotid exposure (bottom). (Reprinted from Ernst CB: Exposure of inaccessible arteries. Part I: Carotid and arm exposure. Surgical Rounds 8:21, 1985. With permission.)

process is a large structure. Care must be taken to protect the vagus, glossopharyngeal, and facial nerves during this dissection. Similarly, the spinal accessory nerve is vulnerable when the sternocleidomastoid muscle is mobilized and the styloid process exposed.

During dissection of the distal internal carotid, many delicate veins must be carefully ligated. Avulsion or tearing of such vessels causes troublesome bleeding. Such bleeding obscures the nerves, which subsequently can be damaged in pursuit of hemostasis. In addition, the occipital artery overlies the internal carotid artery as it courses posteriorly and must be ligated and divided. Similarly, small branches from the external carotid artery to the sternocleidomastoid muscle must be ligated. The use of electrocautery is discouraged when the region of the hypoglossal nerve is being dissected. Mobilization and inferior traction and displacement of the hypoglossal nerve along with division of the above-noted muscles, particularly the digastric and the stylopharyngeus, provide ready access to the suprahypoglossal segment of the distal internal carotid artery.

After carotid reconstruction, the wound is closed without drainage. Deep structures are not reapproximated. Interrupted sutures are placed in the platysma layer and staples are used on the skin. After the skin is closed, the mandibular retaining devices are removed and the mandible is gently replaced in its normal position.

COMMENT

The dissection described here permits exposure of all but the distal 1 cm of the internal carotid artery before it enters the skull. Nonetheless, carotid reconstruction by graft interposition requires an adequate distal segment for application of the distal vascular clamp and sufficient remaining length for anastomosis. Additional space is available for distal suturing if the vessel is unencumbered by a distal vascular clamp. This is facilitated by a No. 3 Fogarty intraluminal occlusion balloon catheter threaded into the distal artery and gently inflated. If EEG monitoring or stump pressure measurements suggest that an inlying shunt is necessary, a Pruitt-Inahara balloon shunt has proved helpful. Balloon shunting or balloon occlusion is particularly useful if exposure of the distal carotid is required for trauma where expeditious hemostasis is of prime concern.

Complications of extended distal carotid exposure mainly are nerve injuries, which can be avoided by clear knowledge of anatomy and meticulous dissection.[7] The most commonly injured are nerves XII, X, VII, and IX. Surprisingly, temporomandibular joint problems are rare.[4] Some patients have complained of transient discomfort over the temporomandibular joint and a few noted gingival soreness that rapidly subsided.

A potential complication of unilateral mandibular subluxation is contralateral compression of the carotid sheath between the angle of the mandible and the transverse vertebral process.[8] This can result in compression of the vagus nerve or compromise of flow in the contralateral carotid. Under such circumstances, collateral flow during carotid occlusion may be impaired. It therefore is suggested that EEG monitoring be used under such circumstances to detect impaired carotid flow and the necessity of intraluminal shunting.

Occasionally, even with various bone resection or dislocation manuevers, the distal internal carotid defies exposure and alternatives to direct repair or even ligation are required. However, the majority of distal internal carotid lesions can be treated definitively by meticulous, extended dissection and vigorous mandibular retraction. A few lesions require mandibular subluxation or resection techniques, and fewer still require carotid ligation.

REFERENCES

1. Rutkow IM, Ernst CB: An analysis of vascular surgical manpower requirements and vascular surgical rates in the United States. J Vascular Surg 3:74, 1986
2. Ehrenfeld WK, Stoney RJ, Wylie EJ: Relation of carotid stump pressure to safety of carotid artery ligation. Surgery 93:299, 1983
3. Samson DS, Gewertz BL, Beyer CW, et al: Saphenous vein interposition grafts in the microsurgical treatment of cerebral ischemia. Arch Surg 116:1578, 1981
4. Fisher DF Jr, Clagett GP, Parker JI, et al: Mandibular subluxation for high carotid exposure. J Vascular Surg 1:727, 1984
5. Ernst CB: Exposure of inaccessible arteries. Part I: Carotid and arm exposure. Surgical Rounds 8:21, 1985
6. Welsh P, Pradier R, Repetto R: Fibromuscular dysplasia of the distal cervical internal carotid artery. J Cardiovasc Surg 22:321, 1981
7. Hertzer NR, Feldman BJ, Beven EG, et al: A prospective study of the incidence of injury to the cranial nerves during carotid endarterectomy. Surg Gynecol Obstet 151:781, 1980
8. Stanley JC: Discussion of Fisher DF Jr, Clagett GP, Parker JI, et al: Mandibular subluxation for high carotid exposure. J Vasc Surg 1:733, 1984

CHAPTER 66
Surgical Management of Extracranial Lesions of the Vertebral Artery

Edward F. Downing

THE PROBLEM OF VERTEBROBASILAR INSUFFICIENCY long has been overshadowed by the problem of carotid insufficiency. The unqualified acceptance[1] of this attitude is no longer acceptable, however. The dogmatic attitudes of the neurologic world have contributed to this state of affairs, which, in our experience, is not justified.

Sorenus in 98 AD described what is known today as vertebrobasilar insufficiency in his syndrome of dizziness, tinnitus, and ataxia. It was not until 1955, however, that Millikan and Siekert[2] further elucidated the modern-day syndrome of vertebrobasilar insufficiency in their classical paper. The first successful vertebral artery endarterectomy was done in 1959 by DeBakey et al.[3] and by Cate and Scott.[4] Since then, references to this procedure in the literature have been scanty.[5–7] Natali et al.[8] reported 13 cases, and Cormier and Laurian[9] reported the treatment of 119 vertebral elongations. In 1968, Morris et al.[10] reported on 365 vertebral reconstructions out of 2900 extracranial reconstructive operations. In our material vertebral operations form approximately 10 percent of the total carotid operations.

There are certain distinguishing characteristics of the symptoms produced by extracranial vertebral artery disease compared with those produced by occlusive disease of the intracranial vertebral and basilar arteries. The symptoms produced by extracranial disease are almost uniformly reproducible by mechanical maneuvers of the cervical spine and are almost exclusively mechanical in nature. In the management of extracranial vertebral disease, there are two key indications for surgical treatment:

1. The isolated posterior circulation, meaning no contribution to the vertebrobasilar system is made from the posterior communicating arteries on either side. It has been well demonstrated by Drake (personal communication) that both vertebral arteries can be ligated in the cervical region if there is adequate collateral circulation from the posterior communicating arteries from the carotid circulation.
2. Symptoms that can be reproduced by mechanical maneuvers. Our experience is limited to patients who fulfill these two criteria and has resulted in the routine alleviation of the patient's symptoms.

Muller et al., Greitz,[11] 1966, and the American Joint Study[12] all have shown that stenosis and occlusion of the vertebral artery is approximately two thirds as common as occlusion of the internal carotid artery. This also has been confirmed by the work of Hutchinson and Yates. Stenosis at the origin of the vertebral artery has a much greater significance in the development of symptoms than lateral osteophytes, which I have never seen produce vertebrobasilar symptoms. The tortuosities in stenosis of the vertebral artery are still not sufficiently appreciated, even though Rieben has shown by flow studies in the vertebral artery that a mechanical effect on the speed of flow is produced by movements of the head and cervical spine.[1] This obstruction or even interruption of blood flow can be more severe when there is stenosis and tortuosity of the vertebral artery, thus this finding is of importance in the illness. It is the author's opinion that operable causes of vertebrobasilar insufficiency at the proximal segment of the vertebral artery bear much more attention.

CLINICAL CONSIDERATIONS

In our experience of over 50 cases of vertebrobasilar insufficiency, dizziness has been present in 80 percent of the patients; ataxia in 45 percent; bilateral visual disturbance in 40 percent; and motor sensory changes in 25 percent. Headaches, drop attacks, and mental changes rarely have been present.

Before invasive investigation of patients with symptoms of vertebrobasilar insufficiency is performed, a cardiac etiology of the symptoms is ruled out. All patients in our series have been investigated with arch aortography and four-vessel, selective retrograde cervical and intracranial arteriography. It is mandatory that views of the origin of both vertebral arteries be obtained, preferably with 104 Cine radiography, as it is that views of the intracranial vertebral and basilar circulation along with bilateral internal carotid series be obtained in order to determine the patency of the posterior communicating arteries. We have elected not to operate on any patient in whom the posterior communicating arteries were patent unless the symptoms, in our opinion, were embolic in origin, which has been rare. The pathology in this series consists of the following types of lesions.

1. Severe atherosclerotic stenosis of the origin of the vertebral artery.
2. Extraluminal compression of the vertebral origin, producing severe stenosis from fibromuscular bands.
3. Bilateral, second-portion vertebral stenosis from extraluminal compression of the arteries caused by hypertrophied scalene muscles (some have questioned whether

OPERATIVE NEUROSURGICAL TECHNIQUES
ISBN 0-8089-1862-1

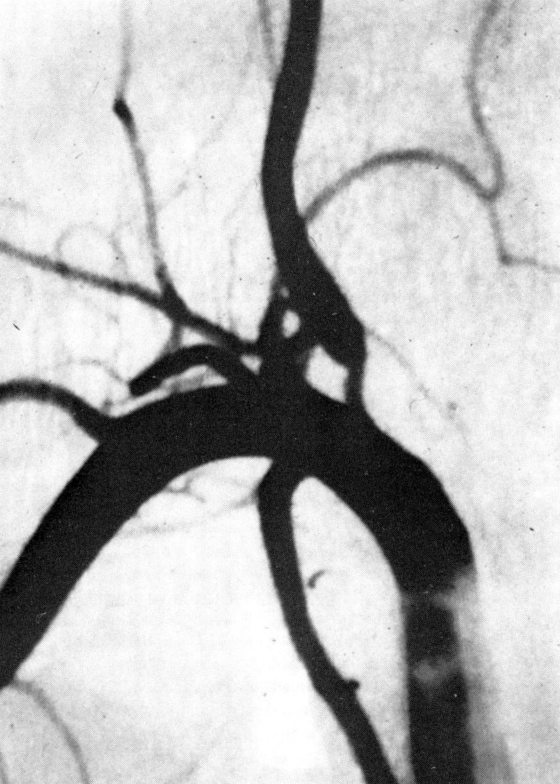

Fig. 66-1. A severe occlusive lesion at the origin of the vertebral artery. Note the hourglass shape.

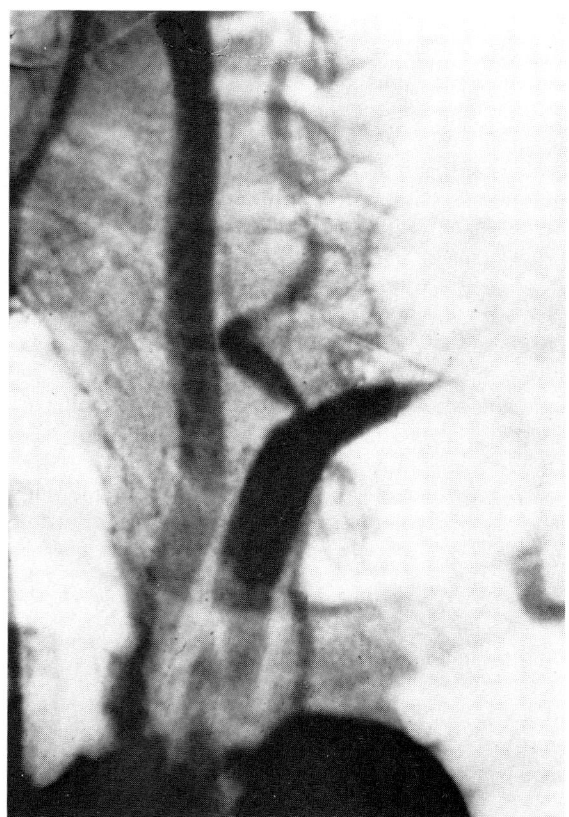

Fig. 66-2. Stenosis at the origin of the vertebral artery from extraluminal fibromuscular bands.

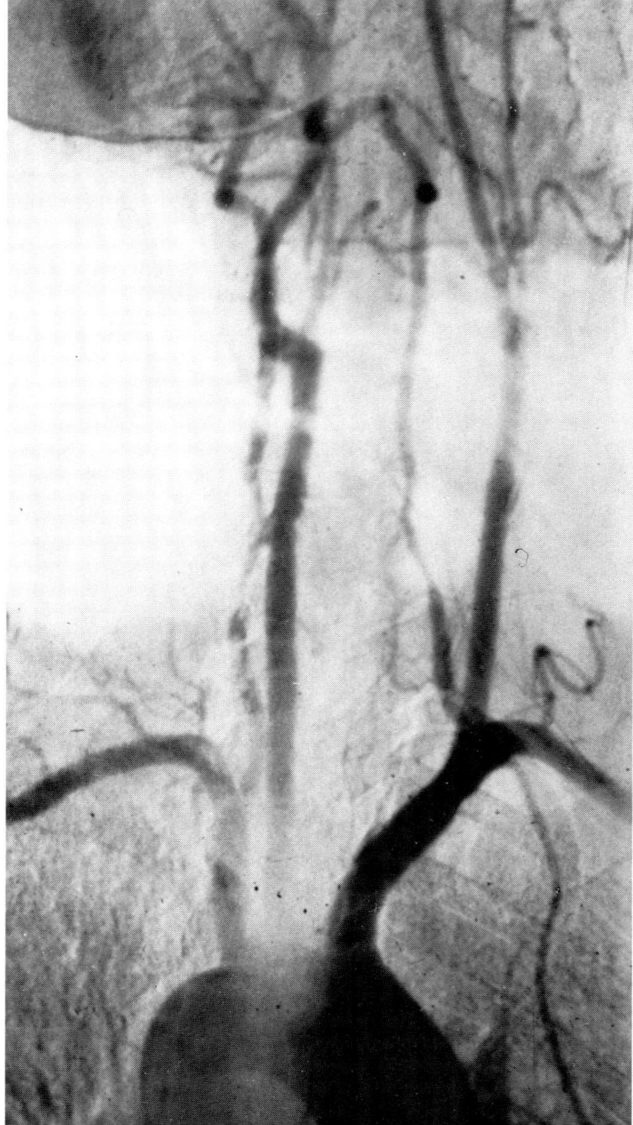

Fig. 66-3. Bilateral stenosis of the second portion of the vertebral artery.

this may be an early form of fibromuscular hyperplasia of the vertebral artery).

4. Combined, severe, ulcerative occlusive disease of the proximal subclavian and vertebral origin.
5. Subclavian steal syndrome.

We have tended not to operate on unilateral stenotic lesions of the vertebral origin when the contralateral vertebral artery has been widely patent unless the stenotic lesion was subtotal in character. If the unilateral vertebral lesion has been subtotal in character and the contralateral vertebral artery has been widely patent, we have recommended endarterectomy on the basis of preventing impending occlusion of the vertebral artery, which in our experience has been the most common cause of the Wallenberg syndrome.

Figure 66-1 illustrates the most common cause of symptomatic extracranial vertebral stenosis, that being an hourglass-shaped, severe, occlusive lesion at the origin of the vertebral artery. This represented over 80 percent of the patients in our

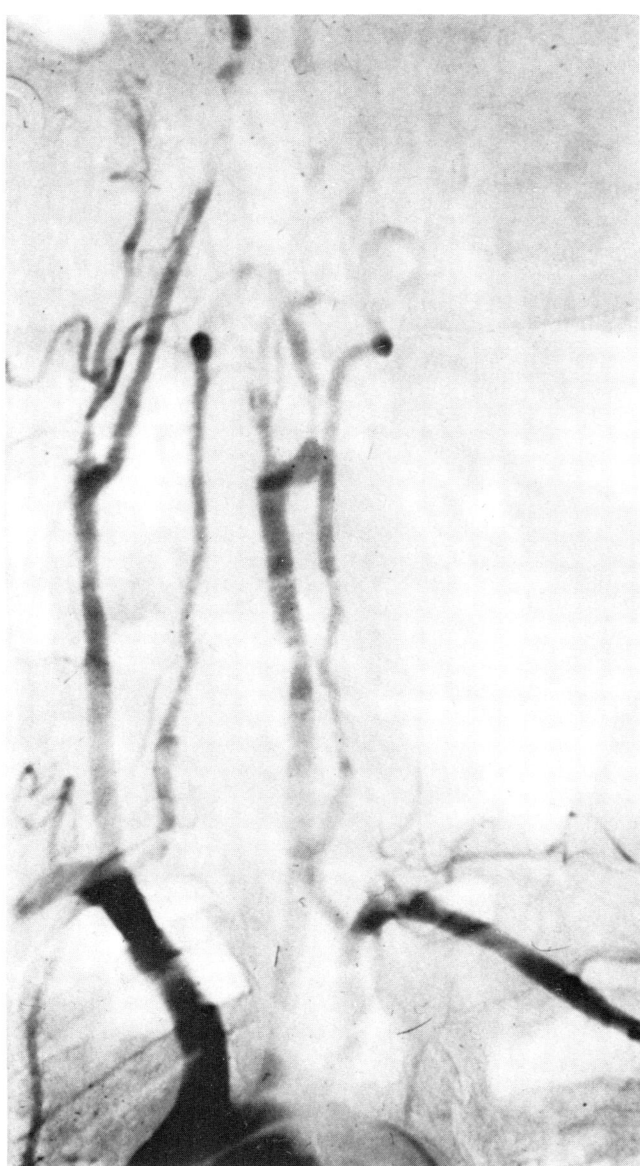

Fig. 66-4. A postoperative angiogram of the patient in Figure 66-3 after extraluminal decompression of the vertebral arteries.

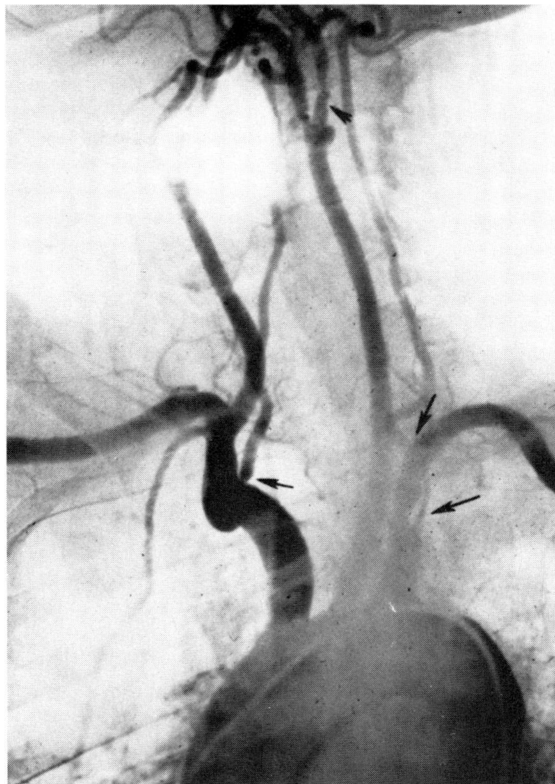

Fig. 66-5. Stenosis of the origin of the vertebral artery combined with severe ulcerative stenotic disease of the proximal subclavian artery.

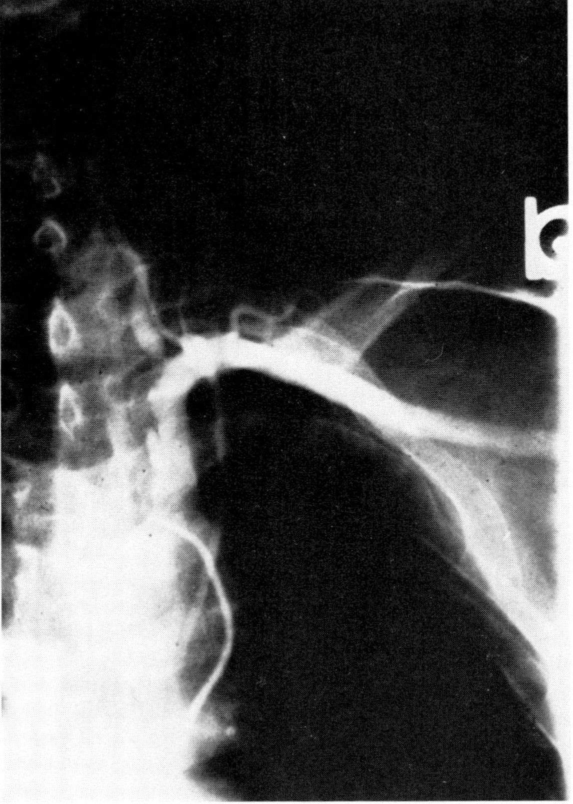

Fig. 66-6. Stenosis of the origin of the vertebral artery combined with severe ulcerative stenotic disease of the proximal subclavian artery.

series. We have treated this lesion with transsubclavian vertebral artery endarterectomy.

Figure 66-2 represents stenosis of the origin of the vertebral artery from extraluminal fibromuscular bands. You will note that this differs from the atherosclerotic narrowing of the origin of the vertebral artery in that the narrowing of the artery is from one side only, always the medial side, as opposed to the hourglass-type constriction, which is secondary to intraluminal atherosclerotic plaquing. Careful evaluation of this angiographic configuration has led us to this conclusion. The surgical treatment for this lesion is simply a scalenotomy, with care being taken to be sure that all of the fibromuscular bands of the posterior aspect of the posterior scalene muscle has been lysed. After this has been done, care must be taken to palpate with vascular forceps to be sure that there is not an intraluminal atherosclerotic plaque, which in our experience has not been present. This thesis has been verified with postoperative angiography and with intraluminal inspection of the vertebral arteries.

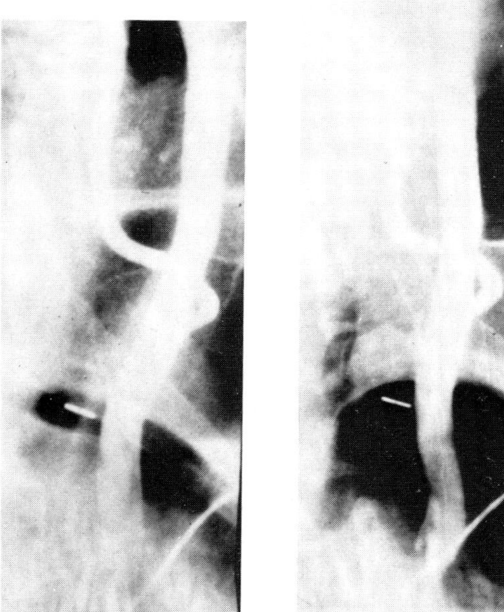

Fig. 66-7.   Postoperative angiograms of the patient in Figures 66-5 and
66-6 after end-to-side anastomosis of the vertebral artery to the common carotid.

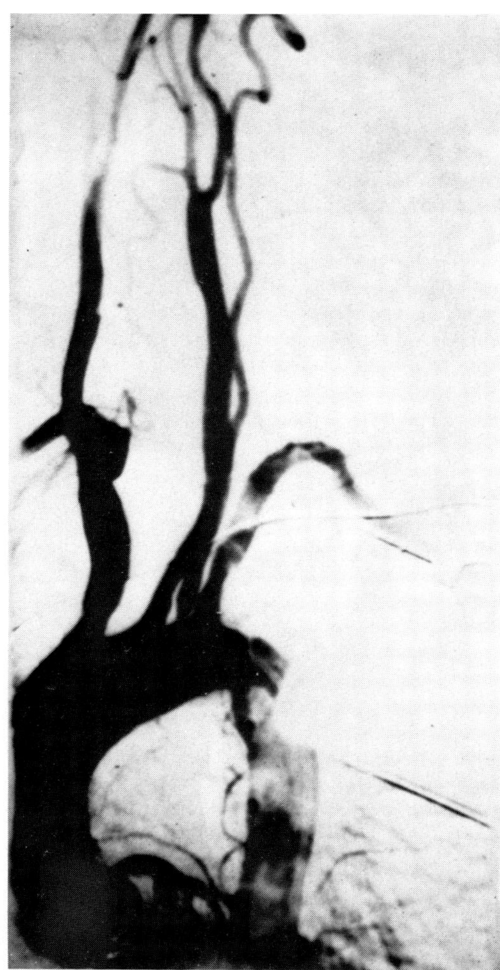

Fig. 66-8.   Severe stenosis of a left vertebral artery that arises from the
aortic arch.

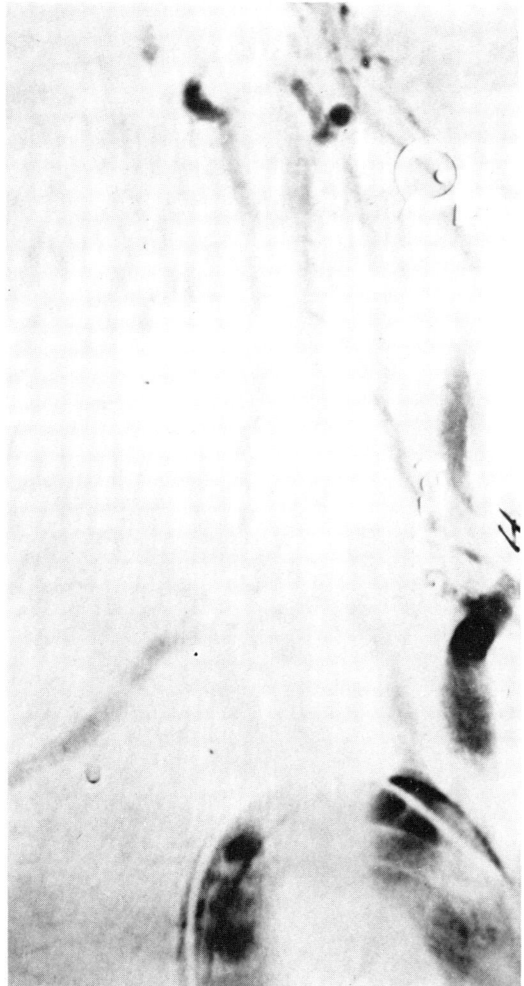

Fig. 66-9.   A subtraction arch study of a subclavian steal.

Figure 66-3 represents bilateral stenosis of the second portion
of the vertebral artery, just proximal to the entrance into the
transverse foramen. We have seen 3 such cases and all have been
present in extremely short, stocky, and muscular individuals. The
symptoms have been uniformly reproducible by simply extending
the neck. It is interesting to note that all 3 of these patients were
timber cutters. This type of lesion has been treated with bilateral
extraluminal decompression of the vertebral artery from its origin
to its entrance into the transverse foramen.

Figure 66-4 is the postoperative angiogram of the condition
in Figure 66-3 after extraluminal decompression of both vertebral arteries. Some people have suggested this could be treated
simply by intraluminal dilatation; however, we have had no
experience with that procedure.

Figures 66-5 and 66-6 represent stenosis of the vertebral
origin combined with severe ulcerative stenotic disease of the
proximal subclavian. Because an endarterectomy at the origin of
the vertebral artery in this situation would only form a funnel to
channel emboli to the basilar circulation from the proximal
subclavian, we have treated this lesion with amputation to the
vertebral artery at its origin and end-to-side anastomosis to the
ipsilateral common carotid artery. The postoperative angiogram of
the end-to-side vertebral-to-common carotid anastomosis of the
patient shown in Figures 66-5 and 66-6 is shown in Figure 66-7.

Figure 66-8 represents a patient who had severe stenosis of

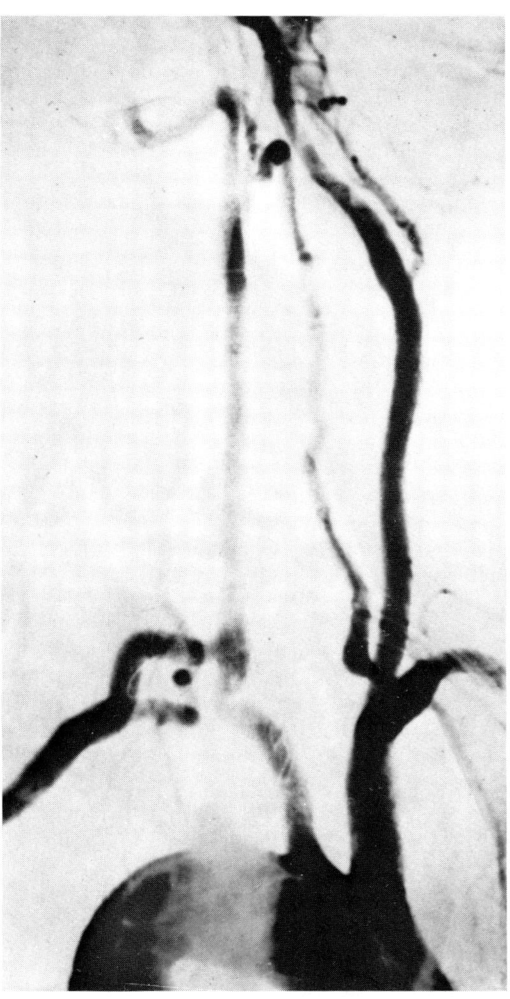

Fig. 66-10. A postoperative angiogram of the patient in Figure 66-9 after treatment by an extrathoracic common carotid-to-subclavian artery bypass graft.

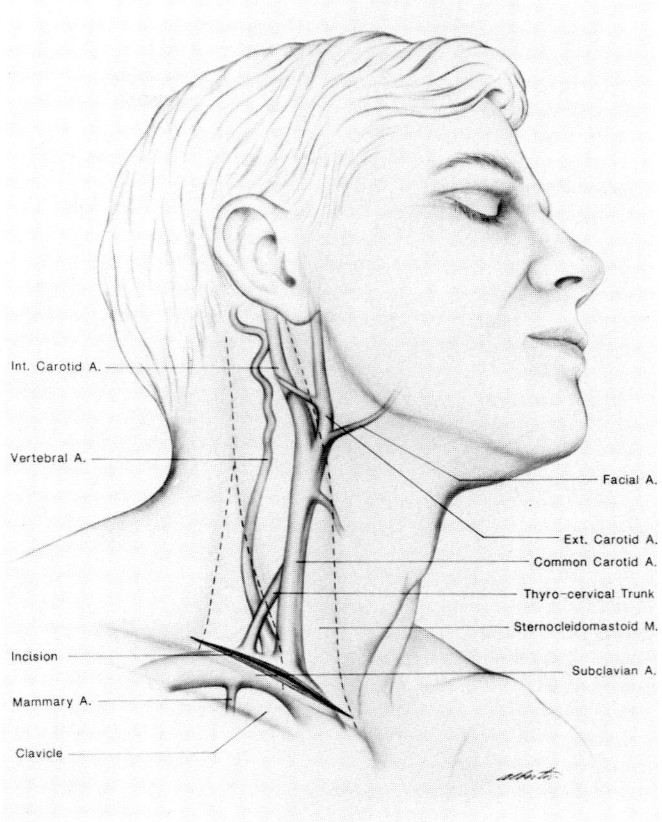

Fig. 66-11. The line of incision for vertebral endarterectomy.

the origin of the left vertebral artery that arose from the aortic arch. The right vertebral artery was totally occluded and there were no posterior communicating arteries present. This patient also was treated with vertebral amputation and end-to-side anastomosis of the left vertebral artery into the left common carotid artery with alleviation of symptoms.

Figure 66-9 is a subtraction arch study of a subclavian steal. Figure 66-10 shows the postoperative angiogram of this patient after he was treated by an extrathoracic common carotid-to-subclavian bypass graft.

OPERATIVE CONSIDERATIONS

VERTEBRAL ENDARTERECTOMY

In my opinion, one of the main reasons that vertebral endarterectomy has not become as popular as carotid endarterectomy has been the uniformly poor results produced in the 1960s. The reasons for these results are two-fold. (1) The early surgical attempts at vertebral artery reconstruction were focused directly on the vertebral artery at its origin. The vertebral artery is a very thin artery once the atherosclerotic plaque is removed and does not lend itself well to direct surgery

at all. (2) The suture material used in the early operations was large in size.

The surgical approach[13,14] that I have chosen to use in this series avoids both of these problems. The approach has been an indirect approach through the subclavian artery across from the vertebral orifice, and 7-0 suture material is used. Figure 66-11 shows the skin incision, which consists of a 10-cm incision parallel to and just above the clavicle from the sternal notch laterally. The entire sternocleidomastoid muscle must be taken down just adjacent to its insertion on the clavicle. This is done by doubly clamping the sternocleidomastoid once it has been completely dissected free by blunt dissection with four large, curved Kelly clamps. The muscle then is sectioned with the cutting current and the ends are coagulated with the coagulating current. The medial and lateral halves of the muscle are individually mattress sutured with 0 silk suture, both distally and proximally. These sutures then are left long, and the muscles are allowed to retract. Figure 66-12 shows the exposure after the sternocleidomastoids have been transected with the internal jugular vein coming into view, which on some occasions may have to be ligated because of its position in the wound. It usually can be retracted out of the way, along with the phrenic nerve, which runs anterior to the anterior scalene muscle. The scalene fat pad has been removed at this point to allow visualization of the scalene muscle, the phrenic nerve, and the brachial plexus. The phrenic nerve generally is retracted either medially or laterally with a 0.25-inch Penrose drain, with care being taken to retract as little as possible. The scalene muscles then are completely transected. Figure 66-13

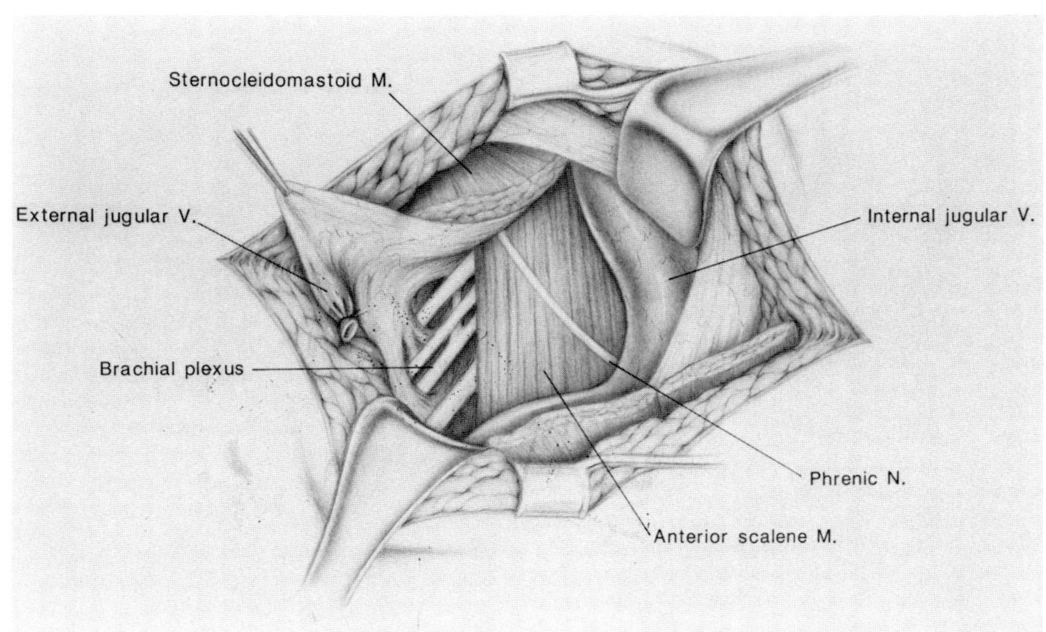

Fig. 66-12. The exposure for vertebral endarterectomy after the sternocleidomastoid muscle has been transected and the internal jugular vein is visible.

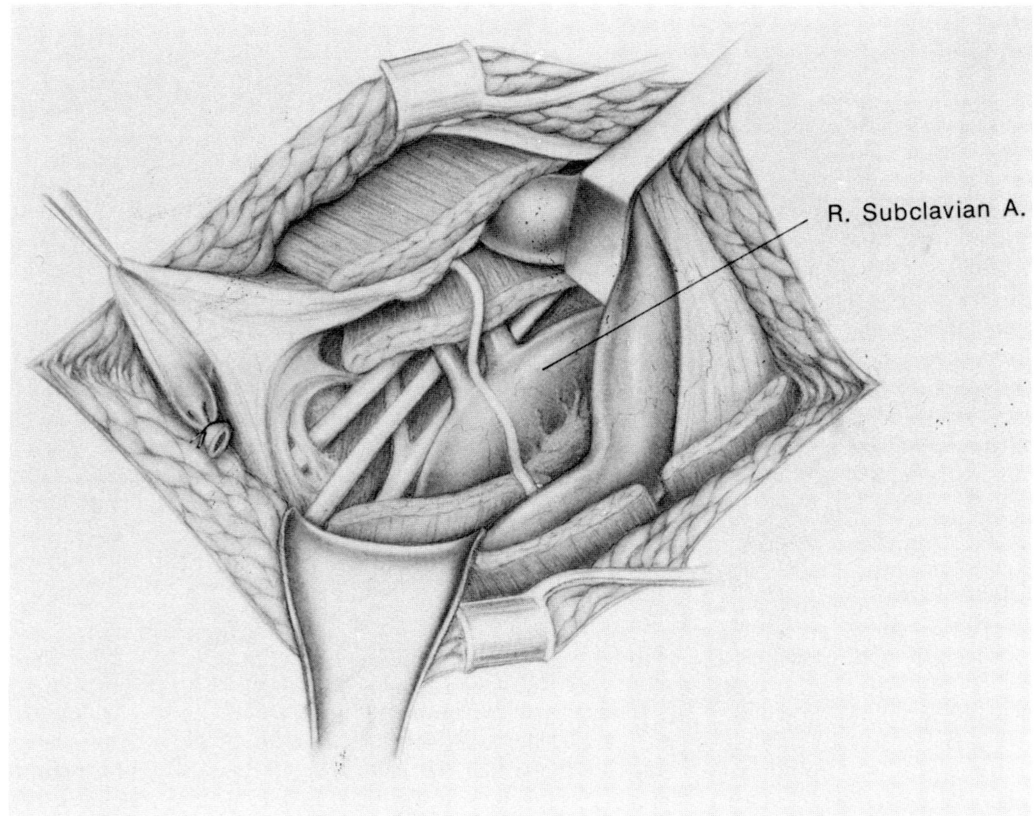

Fig. 66-13. The exposure after transection of the scalene muscle. The dome of the subclavian artery is visible.

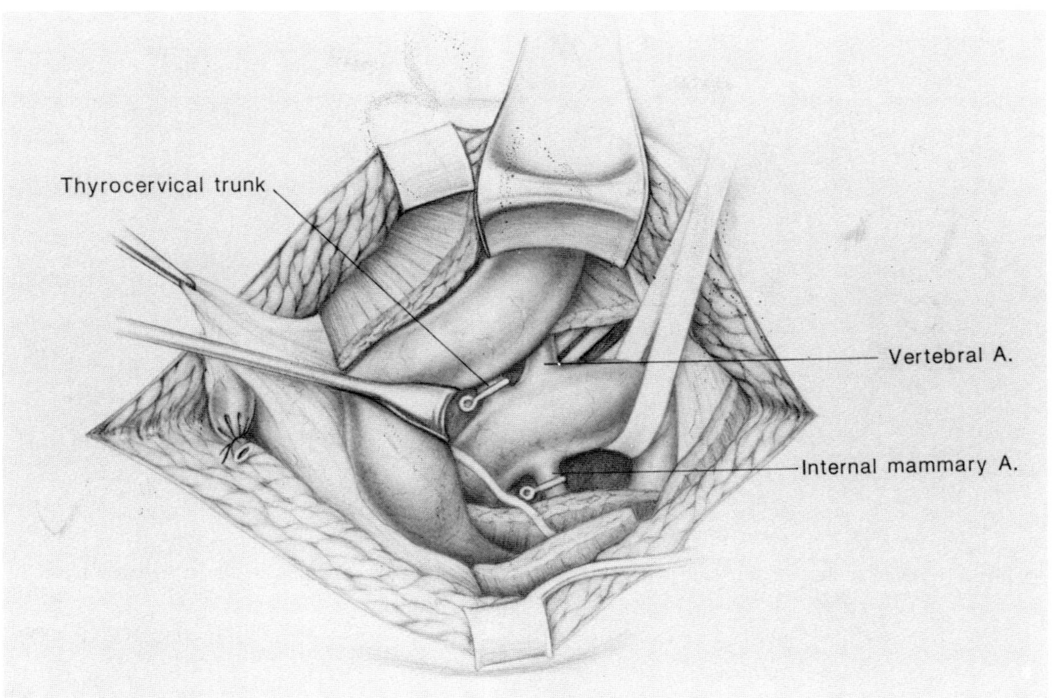

Fig. 66-14. The dissection continues along the dome of the subclavian artery, the thyrocervical trunk artery, the internal mammary artery, and the vertebral artery.

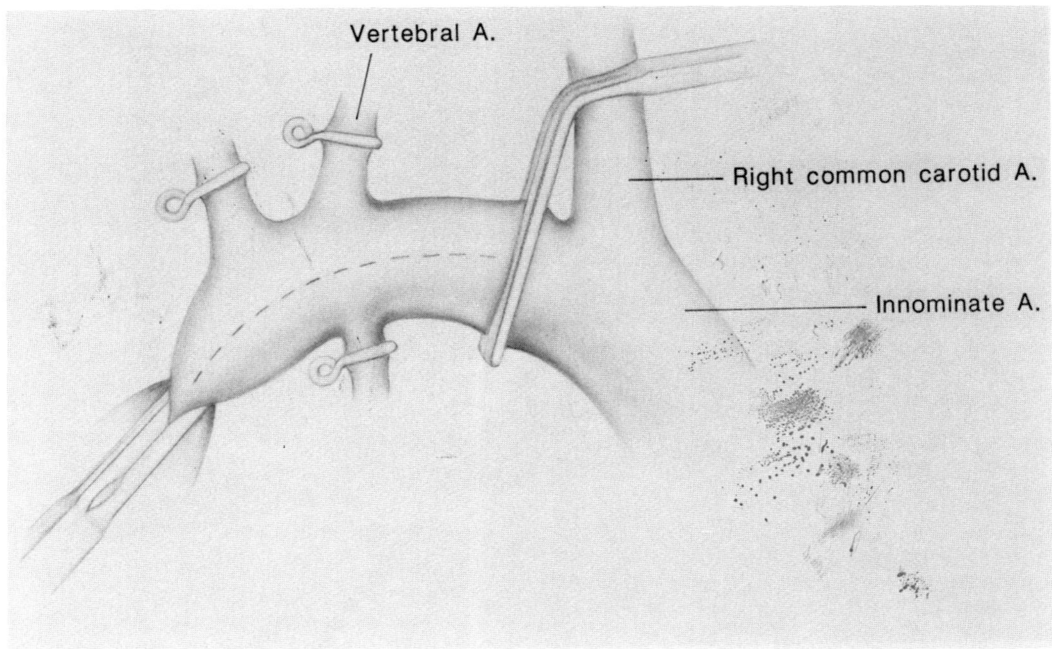

Fig. 66-15. The line of incision in the subclavian artery opposite the origin of the vertebral artery.

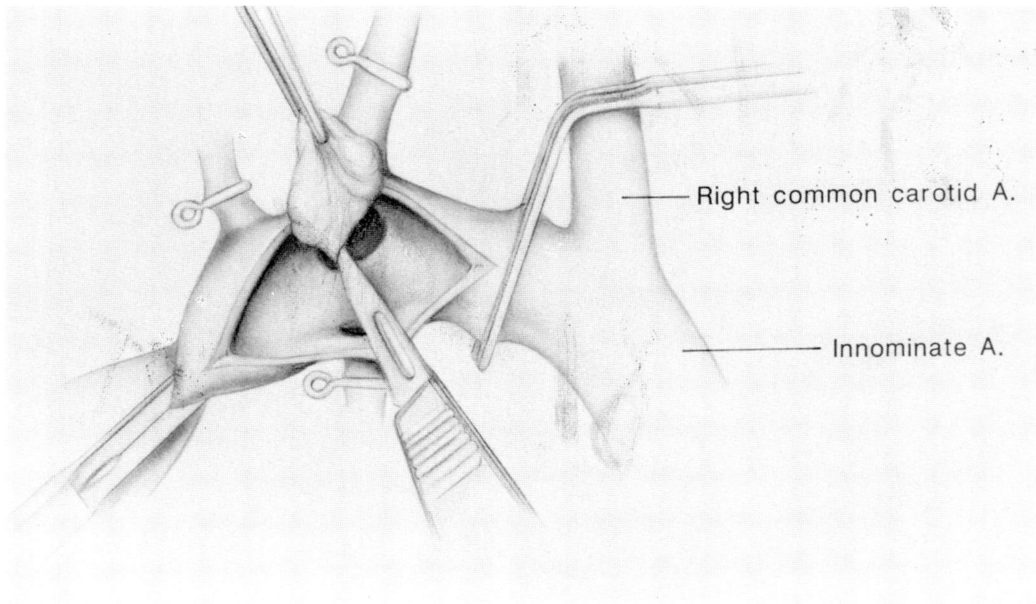

Fig. 66-16.   Tenting sutures are placed in the subclavian artery and a No. 11 blade is used to excise the plaque in the origin of the vertebral artery.

shows the scalene muscles after transection with the dome of the subclavian artery coming into view. The dome of the subclavian artery then is exposed along with the thyrocervical trunk (Figure 66-14), the internal mammary artery, and the origin of the vertebral artery. It is necessary to reflect the subclavian approximately 2.5 cm proximal to the origin of the vertebral artery and approximately 2.5 cm distal to the thyrocervical trunk or internal mammary, whichever is the most distal. Once this exposure is obtained, the patient is fully heparinized. The vertebral artery then is dissected free for approximately 3 cm, which will always be distal to the plaque. The plaque is always situated at the origin and is always very short in nature, as opposed to the rather long plaque of the internal carotid origin. The internal mammary artery, the thyrocervical trunk, and the distal vertebral artery then are temporarily occluded with Scoville aneurysm clips, following which the proximal subclavian and distal subclavian arteries are temporarily occluded with large, angled, vascular occlusion

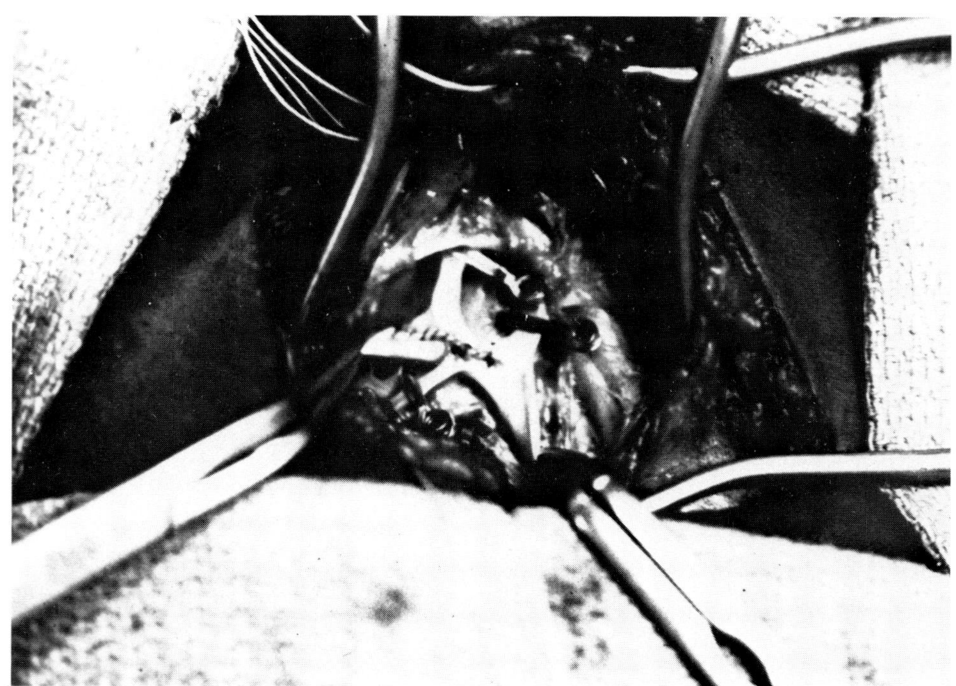

Fig. 66-17.   The operative field after the plaque has been removed and the subclavian artery closed with 7-0 Prolene sutures.

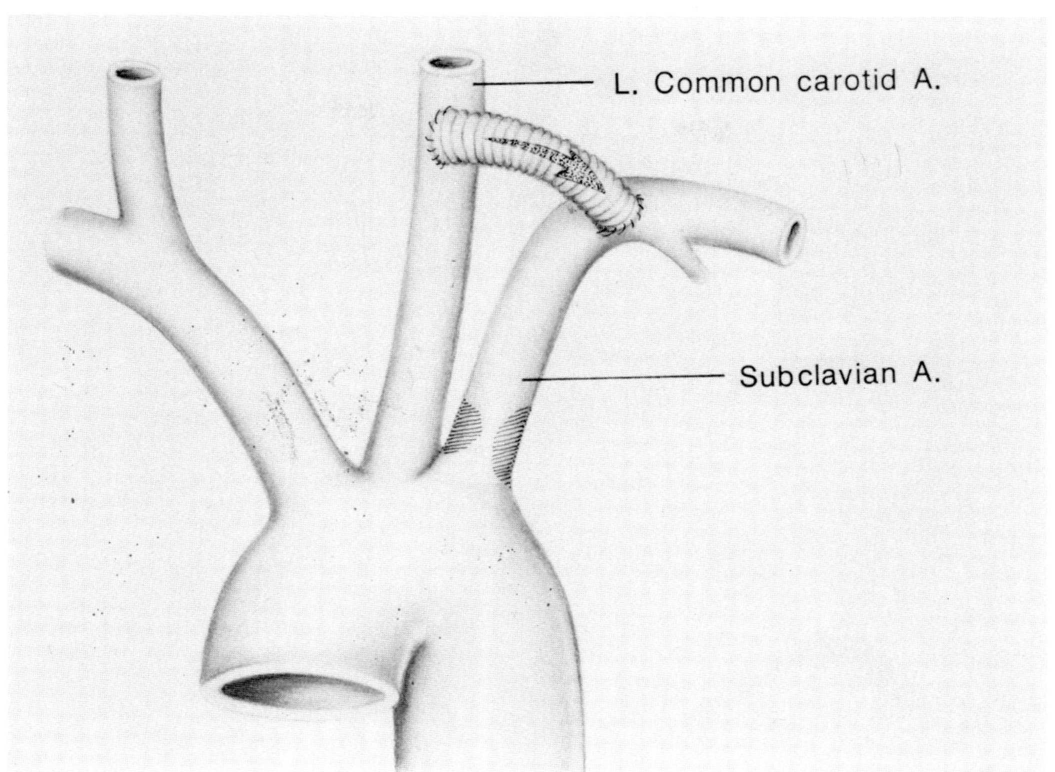

Fig. 66-18. A diagram of the technique of extrathoracic common carotid-subclavian artery bypass for the treatment of subclavian steal.

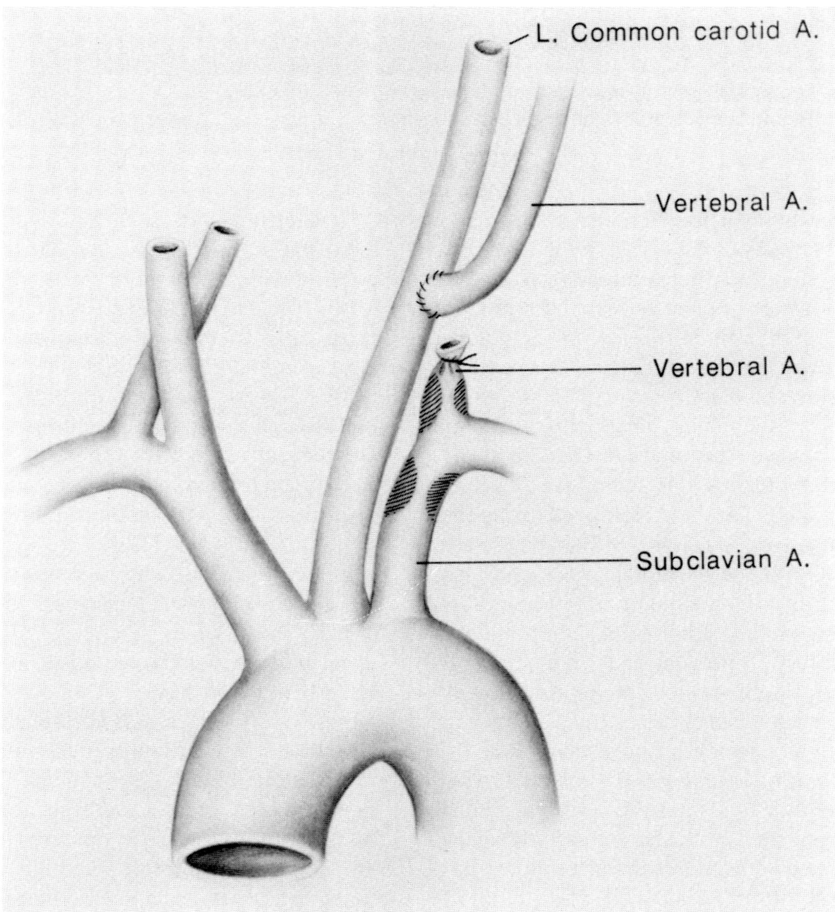

Fig. 66-19. The operative technique for combined subclavian-carotid stenosis.

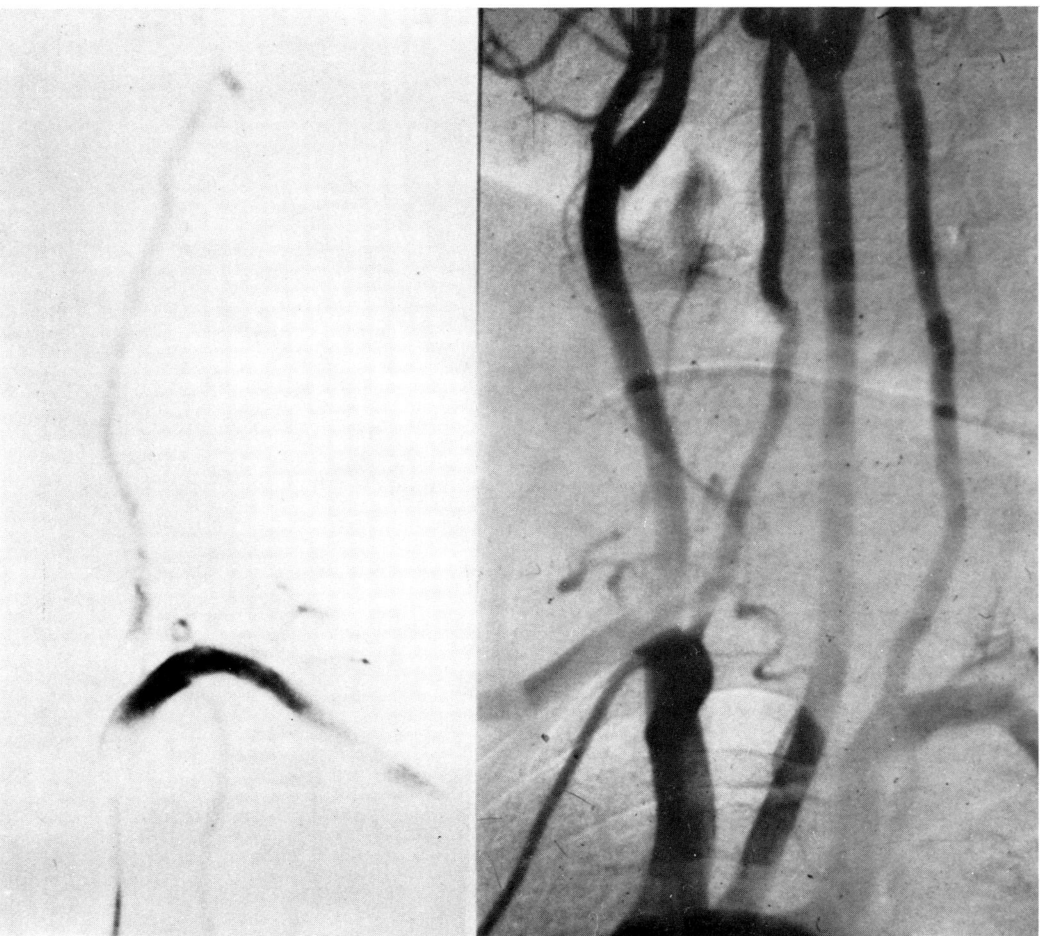

Fig. 66-20. (Left) Subtotal occlusion of the origin of the left vertebral artery is visible in this preoperative angiogram. (Right) A postoperative angiogram demonstrates a widely patent vertebral orifice.

clamps (Figure 66-15), following which a 2-cm incision is made in the subclavian artery just opposite the origin of the vertebral artery. After this has been done, tenting sutures are placed in each leaf of the subclavian artery (Figure 66-16) and a No. 11 blade is used to make a circumferential incision in the plaque around the origin of the vertebral artery. Then, with careful teasing with a small dissector, the plaque is removed in toto by the intussusception, pull-down technique. The fact that lesions of the vertebral origin are always short and are situated at the origin of the vertebral artery makes this technique feasible. After the funnel-shaped plaque has been removed from the origin of the vertebral artery, care is taken to be sure there are no loose intimal tags distally in the vertebral artery and also distally in the subclavian artery. Occasionally it will be necessary to use tacking sutures in the rather thick atheromatous plaque in the subclavian artery to prevent distal dissection. If tacking sutures are needed, double-armed, No. 6 arterial silk sutures are used. After the plaque has been removed along with all intimal tags and the intimal edges have been taken care of, the arteriotomy is closed with a running 7-0 Prolene suture. Figure 66-17 shows the operative field after the vertebral plaque has been removed and the subclavian closed with a 7-0 Prolene suture before removal of the clamps. After the arteriotomy has been closed, the vertebral artery is opened first to allow back-bleeding into the operative site. This also is done after the plaque is removed before the arteriotomy is closed.

After the vertebral has flooded the operative site and hemostasis of the suture line has been ascertained, the temporary Scoville aneurysm clip is placed back on the vertebral artery. The clamps then are removed from the subclavian artery proximally, then distally, followed by removal of the aneurysm clips from the internal mammary, the thyrocervical trunk, and, lastly, the vertebral artery. A 0.25-inch Penrose drain is brought out through a stab wound and the sternocleidomastoid muscles are reconstructed with the 0 silk sutures that previously had been placed in a mattress fashion at the beginning of the operation. After these sutures have been tied, approximately six additional 0 silk sutures are used to reconstruct the sternocleidomastoid. The platysma and the subcuticular layers then are closed with 4-0 Tycron and the skin is closed with Steri-strips. The drain is removed 12 hours postoperatively. The usual clamp time of the vertebral artery has been approximately 15 to 20 minutes; however, on one occasion, a clamp time of 35 minutes was necessary in the absence of the contralateral vertebral artery without producing any ischemia.

Postoperatively, the patients are treated with aspirin and Persantine on a long-term basis and the operative anticoagulation is not reversed. This operative procedure has not produced any new ischemic attacks and has relieved preoperative symptoms that were mechanically reproducible in every occasion. It has been my experience that temporary diaphragmatic paralysis has been present almost uniformly but has never persisted for

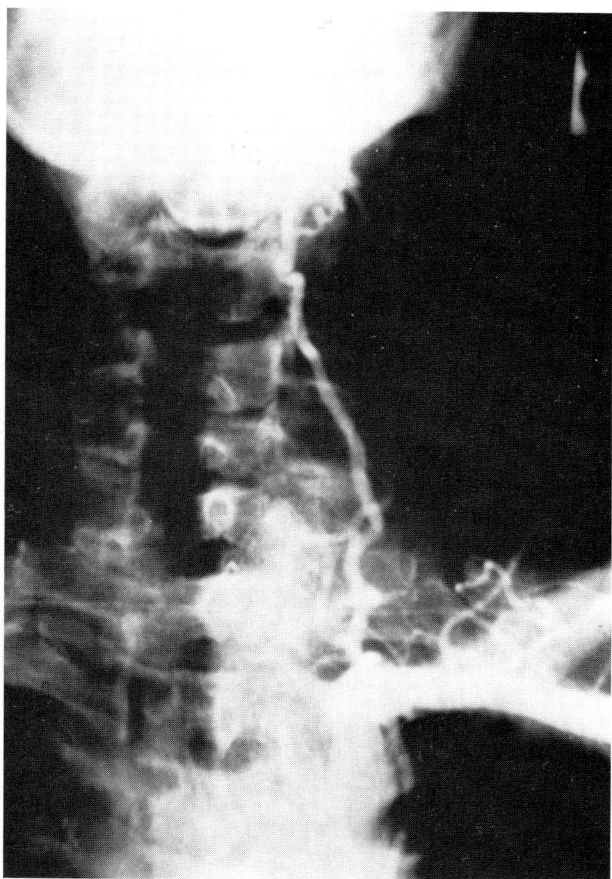

Fig. 66-21. Bilateral occlusion of the internal carotid arteries and the vertebral arteries was noted in this patient who was undergoing studies because of asymptomatic bruits noticed before coronary bypass surgery. Note that the left vertebral artery has been reconstituted via muscular branches of the left thyrocervical trunk.

more than 6 weeks and has never produced any symptoms. The only complication that we have encountered has been a thoracic duct fistula, which required reoperation and ligation. When operating on the left side, the thoracic duct must be adequately ligated to prevent this complication.

SUBCLAVIAN STEAL

The recommended surgical procedure of choice for the treatment of subclavian steal syndrome[15,16] is the extrathoracic common carotid-subclavian bypass. Figure 66-18 illustrates the operative technique for this procedure. Story (personal communication) and Fein[17] have advocated treatment of the subclavian steal by end-to-side, vertebral-to-common carotid anastomosis. Long-term follow-up results are not available at this time for this variation of treatment, and until they are available, the extrathoracic bypass is the procedure of choice. There are certain technical points that must be vividly adhered to, however, in order to avoid complications with this procedure. When the bypass graft is manastomosed to the common carotid artery, either an exclusion clamp should be used or a temporary internal bypass should be placed in the common carotid artery in order to avoid occluding this artery more than a minute or two while the anastomosis is being made. This is an extremely important technical consideration because the dele-

terious results of early repairs of subclavian steal syndrome were almost uniformly related to ischemia in the carotid distribution from prolonged clamping of the carotid artery.

COMBINED SUBCLAVIAN-CAROTID STENOSIS

The surgical approach[18] to combined subclavian-carotid stenosis is exactly the same as for a vertebral endarterectomy down to the exposure of the vertebral origin. After the vertebral origin has been exposed, the common carotid artery, which is immediately adjacent, is exposed. The vertebral artery is amputated at its origin with a 2-0 silk ligature (Figure 66-19). Distally, the vertebral artery is temporarily occluded with a Scoville aneurysm clip, and a small vascular exclusion clamp is used to partially occlude the common carotid artery, following which a vertical arteriotomy is made and an end-to-side anastomosis is completed in a running fashion with 7-0 Prolene sutures after two corner anchoring sutures have been placed. After the end-to-side anastomosis has been completed, the temporary clip on the distal vertebral artery is removed to allow flooding of the operative site to test the anastomosis. After this has been done and the anastomosis has been ascertained to be adequate, the partial exclusion clamp is removed from the common carotid artery. By using the partial exclusion clamp, flow in the common carotid is not been interrupted at all. The closure from this point on is exactly the same as in the previously described vertebral endarterectomy procedure.

Figure 66-20 illustrates preoperative and postoperative angiograms of a tightly stenotic lesion of the vertebral origin. The left side of the figure demonstrates a subtotal occlusion of the origin of the left vertebral artery, and the right side of the figure represents a postoperative angiogram showing the widely patent vertebral orifice.

Many patients have asymptomatic vertebral stenotic disease, which is incidentally found on angiograms performed for other reasons. Figure 66-21 represents a patient who was studied because of asymptomatic bruits before a coronary artery bypass and was demonstrated to have bilateral occlusion of the internal carotid arteries and bilateral vertebral artery occlusion with reconstitution of the left vertebral artery via the muscular branches of the left thyrocervical trunk. This patient illustrates why extracranial vertebral artery reconstruction surgery should not be recommended for any patient who is asymptomatic or whose symptoms cannot be reproduced by mechanical maneuvers. If these operative indications are adhered to, the postoperative results strongly suggest that a more active, aggressive attitude should be adopted toward reconstructive surgery of the vertebral artery.

REFERENCES

1. Rieben FW: Zur Orthologie und Pathologie der Arteria Vertebralis. Sitzungsberichte der Heidelberger Akad. Wiss., math-nat. Kl. Berlin, Springer-Verlag, 1973, pp 95–132
2. Millikan CH, Siekert G: Studies in cerebrovascular disease: I. The syndrome of intermittent insufficiency of the basilar arterial system. Proc Staff Meet Mayo Clin 30:61, 1955
3. DeBakey ME, Crawford ES, Cooley DA, et al: Surgical considerations of occlusive disease of innominate, carotid, subclavian, and vertebral arteries. Ann Surg 149:690, 1959
4. Cate W, Scott RH Jr: Cerebral ischemia of central origin: Relief by

subclavian-vertebral artery thromboendarterectomy. Surgery 45:19, 1959
5. Berguer R, Audaya LV, Bauer RB: Vertebral artery bypass. Arch Surg 3:976, 1976
6. Castaigne P, Lhermitte F, Gautier JC, et al: Arterial occlusions in the vertebrobasilar system: a study of 44 patients with postmortem data. Brain 96:133, 1973
7. Fisher CM, Gore I, Okalie N, et al: Atherosclerosis of the carotid and vertebral arteries-extracranial and intracranial. J Neuropathol Exp Neurol 24:455, 1965
8. Natali J, Maraval M, Kiefer E: Surgical treatment of stenosis and occlusion of the internal carotid and vertebral arteries. J Cardiovasc Surg 13:4, 1972
9. Cormier JM, Laurian C: Surgical management of vertebral-basilar insufficiency. J Cardiovasc Surg 17:205, 1976
10. Morris GC Jr, Crawford ES, DeBakey ME: The vertebral artery in cerebral anoxia, in de la Camp B, Linder HF, Trede M, et al (eds): Joint Meeting, Munich, 1968, Berlin, Springer-Verlag, 1969, pp 42–49
11. Hutchinson EC, Acheson J: Strokes, Natural History, Pathology, and Surgical Treatment. London, WB Saunders, 1975
12. Marshall J: The Management of Cerebrovascular Disease, ed 3. Oxford, Blackwell, 1976
13. Ruel GL, Cooley DA, Olson SK, et al: Long term results of direct vertebral artery operations. Surgery 96:854, 1984
14. Tevenet A, Rutolo C: Surgical repair of vertebral artery stenoses. J Cardiovasc Surg 25:101, 1984
15. Editorial: A new vascular syndrome—"The Subclavian Steal." N Engl J Med 265:912, 1961
16. North RR, Fields WS, DeBakey ME, et al: Brachial-basilar insufficiency syndrome. Neurology 12:810, 1962
17. Fein JM: Vertebral artery transposition for vertebrobasilar insufficiency. Presented at the 50th Meeting of the American Association of Neurological Surgeons, Boston, April, 1981
18. Diaz FG, Ausman JI, De-Los-Reyes RA, et al: Surgical reconstruction of the proximal vertebral artery. J Neurosurg 61:874, 1984
19. Kajima N, Tamaki N, Fugita K, et al: Vertebral artery occlusion at the narrowed scalenovertebral angle, mechanical vertebral compression in the distal first portion. Neurosurgery 16:672, 1985

CHAPTER 67

Direct Brain Revascularization

Robert M. Crowell   Jafar J. Jafar

INDICATIONS FOR SURGERY

SUPERFICIAL TEMPORAL artery-middle cerebral artery (STA-MCA) anastomosis was developed to bypass areas of occlusive disease that are not amenable to direct surgery. It was first performed by Donaghy and Yasargil in 1967 using microsurgical techniques.[1,2] Refinements in techniques have included the use of interrupted sutures for greater precision,[3] use of the angular branch of the MCA for maximum flow,[4] and linear incision over the STA to avoid scalp flap necrosis. More recently Little and colleagues have recommended interposition of a saphenous vein segment ("short vein graft") between the STA and an MCA branch to provide high flow revascularization.[5]

Since STA-MCA bypass often improves collateral circulation distal to an inaccessible occlusive lesion,[6,7] it is reasonable to expect the procedure might protect against future ischemic infarction. It has also been suggested that bypass might enhance fragmentation of emboli penetrating the MCA territory. Bypass also carries risk of stroke or death, however, and the procedure might enhance passage of emboli via the external carotid artery or increase the chance of proximal occlusion by diminishing the pressure gradient across a stenosis.

Speculative debate regarding rationales for and against STA-MCA bypass has been reduced sharply by the emergence of controlled data.[8] The Extracranial-Intracranial Bypass Study assessed in controlled, randomized fashion the impact of STA-MCA bypass on stroke and death in patients with stenosis or occlusion of the MCA or internal carotid artery and recent related TIA or stroke. A total of 1495 patients from 71 centers was randomly allocated to best medical therapy (including antiaggregant therapy) or medical therapy plus STA-MCA bypass. Follow-up averaged 55.8 months without loss of a single case. Technical proficiency was high in that 96 percent of bypasses were angiographically patent, and the risk of major stroke or death was about 3 percent.

The major conclusion of the study was that STA-MCA bypass did not reduce the risk of ischemic stroke in the groups studied. Nor did any subgroup enjoy a benefit from surgery; in fact, MCA stenosis and siphon stenosis had statistically superior results with medical treatment. It is therefore difficult to recommend bypass for patients such as those included in the EC-IC Bypass Study.[9]

However, there still may be a responsive subgroup that could be defined physiologically.[10] There is some evidence that altered metabolism (oxygen extraction fraction) may indicate a favorable candidate for bypass.[7,11] A careful investigation will be needed to establish a role for bypass in these cases. Moreover, the EC-IC Bypass Study provides no direct data

regarding several categories of patients with occlusive cerebrovascular disease. Further investigation will be needed to define the place of bypass surgery in these special groups. Since basal arterial occlusive disease (including moyamoya cases) causes substantial neurologic complications, STA-MCA bypass has been recommended for these patients (Figure 67-1).[12–14] There may be a role for bypass in patients with ICA or MCA stenosis with TIA or stroke despite maximum medical therapy. The role of bypass remains uncertain for amaurosis fugax with ICA occlusion,[15] chronic cerebral ischemia,[16,17] and dementia caused by multiple cerebrovascular occlusions.[18] Bypass may also have a role when medical therapy fails to halt TIAs.

The use of emergency STA-MCA bypass grafting has been assessed and the reports from the literature indicate mixed results.[19–21] In most reported cases, the conditions have been far from ideal with a long delay between the onset of symptoms and surgery or the presence of occlusive material in the lenticulostriate branches. A recent report showed some encouraging results,[22] but this approach remains unproved.

Bypass grafts seem helpful in preventing ischemia when planned internal carotid artery (ICA) occlusion is done for a giant ICA aneurysm in the presence of poor collateral supply (Figure 67-2).[2,23–26] Since many patients tolerate carotid occlusion without bypass, the precise role of bypass in this setting has not yet been fully defined. Cerebral blood flow studies can help select aneurysm cases for bypass (Figure 67-3; Table 67-1) In exceptional cases of basal tumor with high operative risk of MCA compromise, an initial STA-MCA bypass can protect against ischemia.

SUPERFICIAL TEMPORAL ARTERY-MIDDLE CEREBRAL ARTERY BYPASS

PREOPERATIVE EVALUATION

The preoperative medical evaluation for STA-MCA bypass is similar to that for carotid endarterectomy. The keystone for planning a bypass operation is three-vessel angiography to delineate cerebrovascular occlusions, collateral circulation, and potential bypass vessels. Delayed films in some cases may show reconstitution of the carotid siphon with reflux to the upper cervical ICA, a sign that suggests the carotid occlusion may be opened surgically. Multiple filling defects in MCA branches suggest embolic occlusions that probably cannot be helped by STA-MCA anastomosis. Poor collateral circulation to a symptomatic hemisphere suggests a hemodynamic mechanism. Careful study of the angiogram usually permits identification of the

OPERATIVE NEUROSURGICAL TECHNIQUES
ISBN 0-8089-1862-1

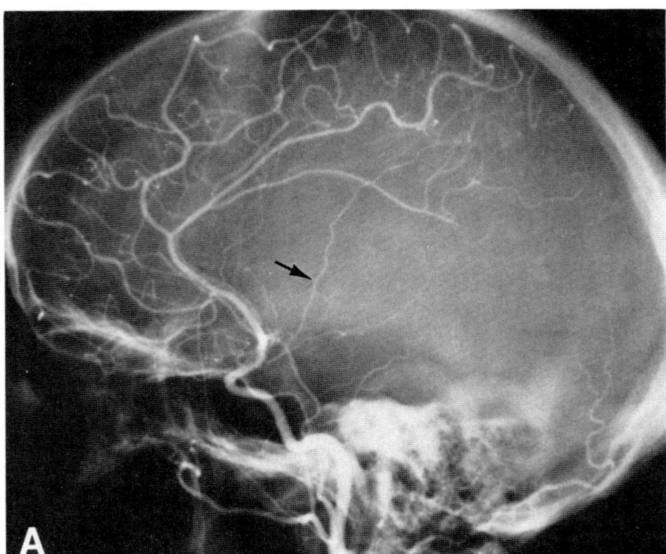 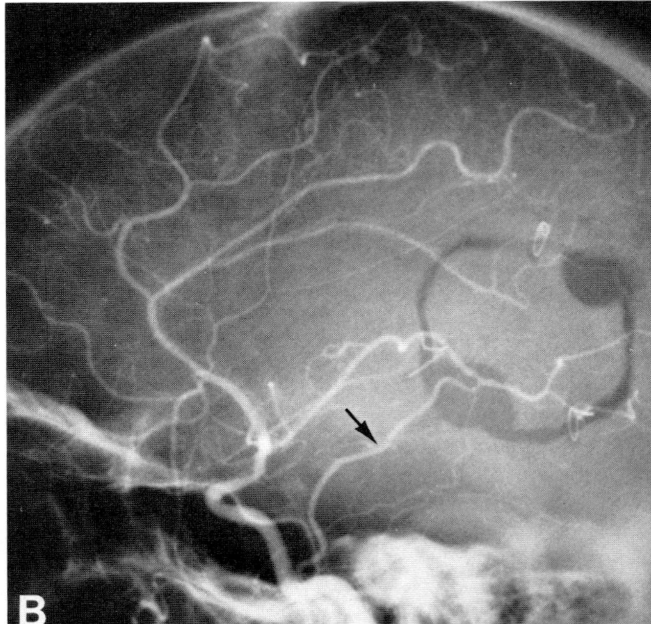

Fig. 67-1. Moyamoya disease with occlusion of the middle cerebral artery. (A) Before bypass; (B) after STA-MCA bypass. Note the increase in diameter of the STA (arrows).

best vessels for anastomosis. Failure to opacify MCA branches by collateral routes need not imply lack of a suitable recipient branch for the operation. The larger STA branch, usually the frontal, is selected, and when this is less than 1 mm in diameter, the occipital artery may be chosen instead.[27] In the setting of a tiny STA and a proximally branching occipital artery, a short vein graft can be interposed between the STA or the occipital artery and the MCA recipient branch.[5] Studies of regional cerebral blood flow and metabolism may help establish the indications for revascularization (Figure 67-3).[28]

If the patient is on heparin, this is stopped at least 8 hours before the operation. Many patients are on aspirin, dipyridamole, or both. Generally, we prefer to stop these drugs several days before the operation. However, some surgeons prefer to maintain antiplatelet therapy through the operative period. This does increase the risk of intraoperative oozing, which may require platelet transfusion for hemostasis. Antihypertensive medication is maintained since cerebral hemorrhage can result from postoperative hypertension.[29] Diphenylhydantoin is begun the day before surgery to ensure prophylactic blood levels of this anticonvulsant medication in the immediate postoperative period.

ANESTHESIA

Premedication is kept to a minimum. The patient's legs are wrapped with Ace bandages. General endotracheal anesthesia is used; usually enflurane is chosen or a balanced technique with nitrous oxide, Innovar, and a muscle relaxant. Controlled ventilation is preferred to maintain the arterial PCO_2 in the range of 35–40 torr. Precordial electrodes provide continuous ECG monitoring. Arterial blood pressure is monitored continuously with a radial artery catheter. Infusions of colloid, phenylephrine, or nitroprusside are used to maintain blood pressure in the normal range of the individual patient during induction and surgery. Oxacillin is administered prior to inci-

sion and for 24 hours postoperatively in divided doses of 2 g every 6 hours.

OPERATIVE TECHNIQUE

Positioning

Before the induction of anesthesia, the operative area is shaved and the STA course marked with a marking pen because the pulse may be harder to delineate after induction. Sometimes a Doppler probe is needed to trace the vessel. The patient lies supine with the head turned to the opposite side. The table is flexed slightly to bring the head above heart level. A small roll serves to elevate the shoulder on the operative side. The head is flexed and held in a Mayfield-Kees three-point skeletal fixation headrest. The operating table may need to be tilted with the "side" adjustment to bring the temporal squama parallel to the floor.

Instruments

Several microsurgical instruments are essential for this operation. The Wild operating microscope is preferred with a 300-mm objective. The stereoscopic binocular observer tube is attached to the microscope via the small beam splitter. The assistant is positioned on the left (for a right-handed surgeon) to allow free access by the scrub nurse to the surgeon's dominant hand. A No. 5 Dumont jeweler's forceps adapted for bipolar coagulation is needed for precise hemostasis near bypass vessels. A similar forceps and Heifetz curved scissors serve well to prepare the small arteries for anastomosis. Kleinert-Kees miniature clips are ideal for temporary occlusion of cortical arteries with minimal trauma. A 10-mm straight Heifetz clip is satisfactory for temporary occlusion of the STA origin. Miniature Gelpi retractors are helpful in maintaining satisfactory exposure. A curved Heifetz microscissors is used to fashion the cortical arteriotomy. Fine Silastic tubing (0.25 inch outside diameter) serves as an MCA stent during surgery. The anastomosis is

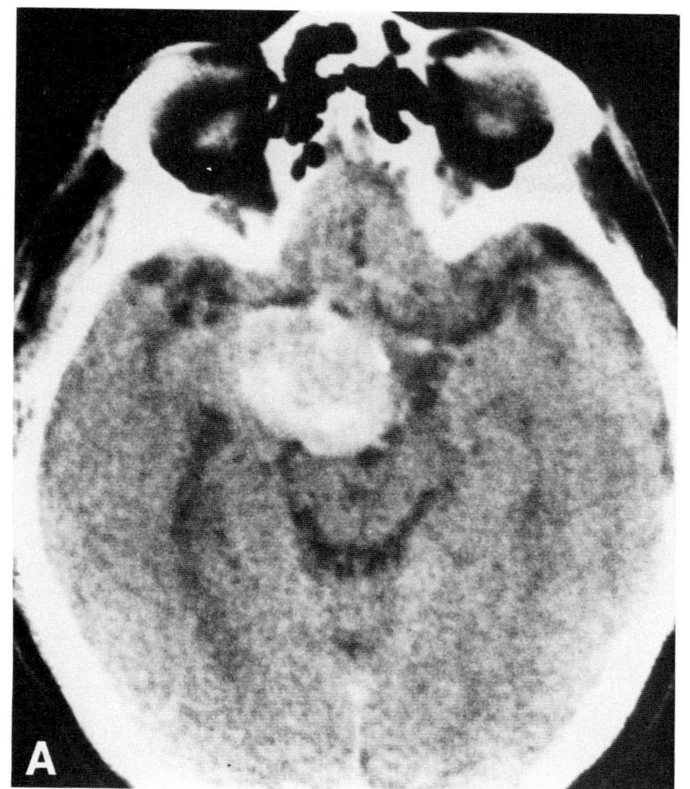
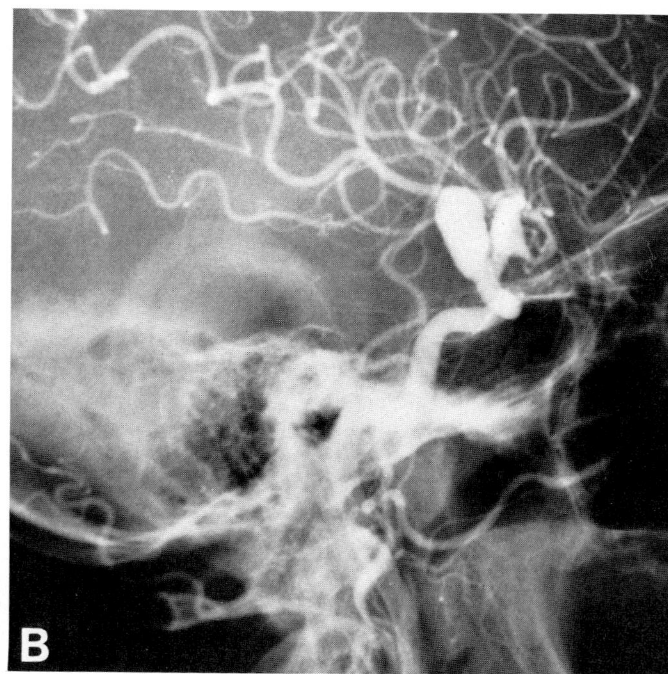
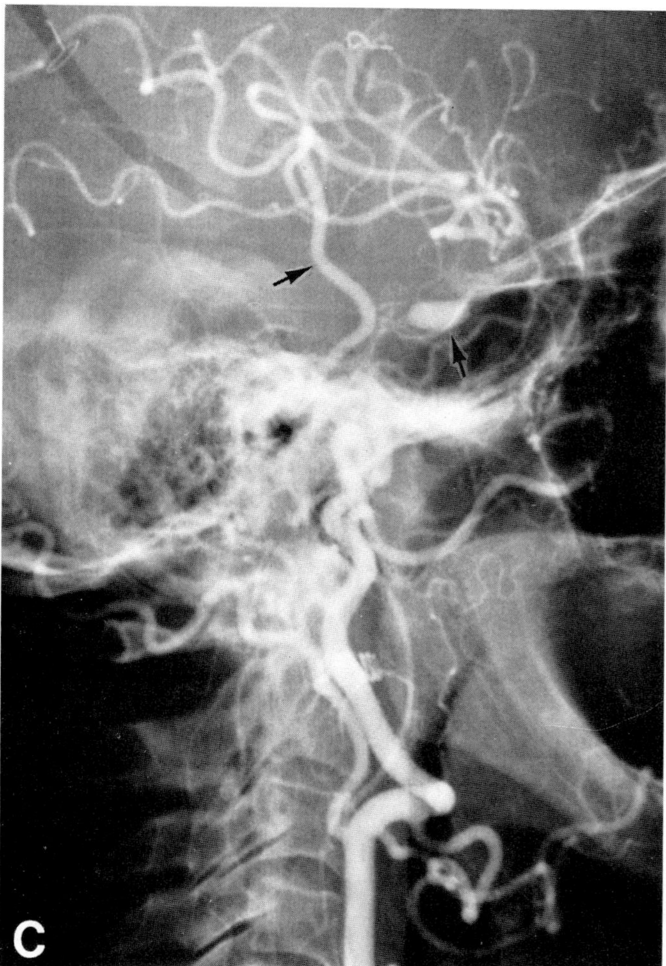

Fig. 67-2. Giant internal carotid artery aneurysm. (A) A CT scan revealing the true size of the aneurysm. (B) A right lateral internal carotid angiogram showing the lumen of the aneurysm. (C) After STA-MCA bypass with balloon occlusion of the right internal carotid artery (arrows).

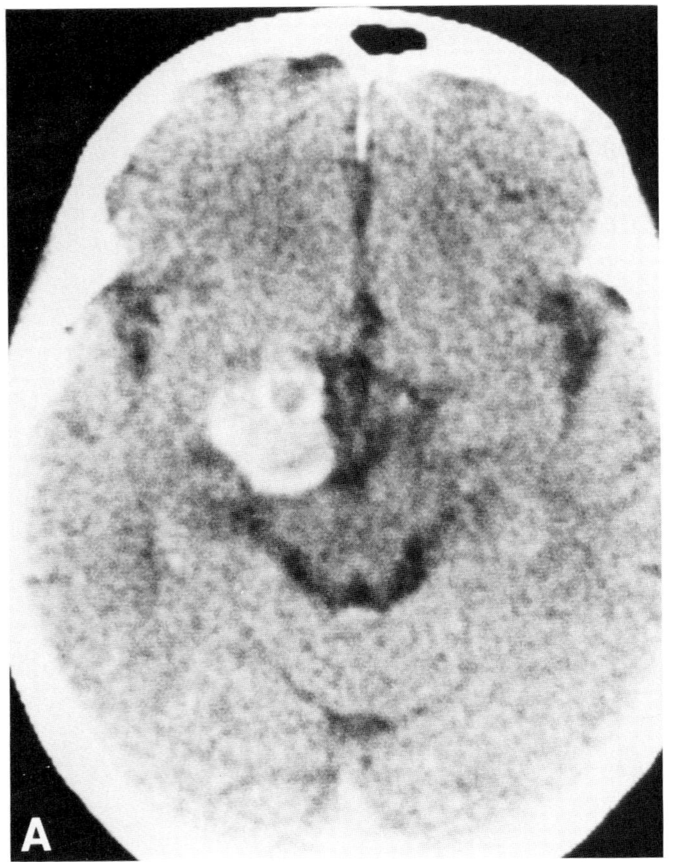

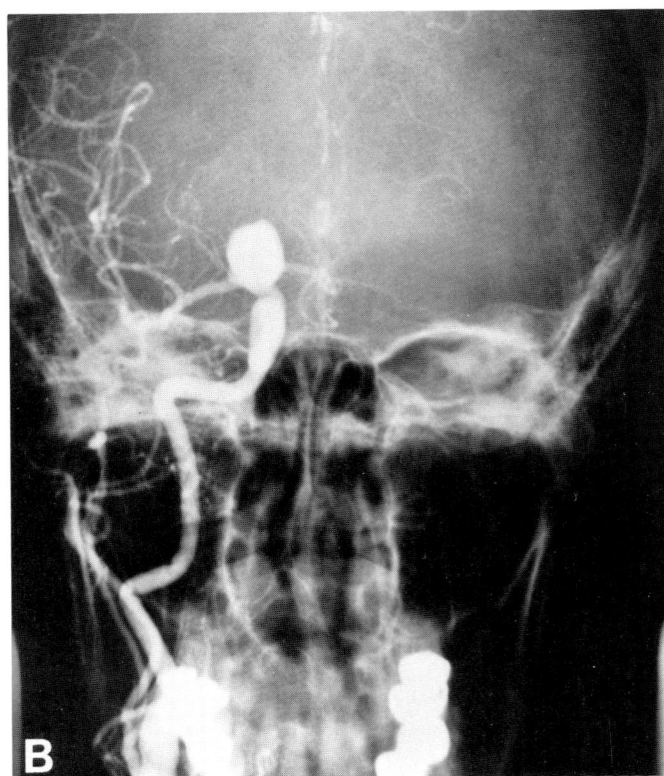

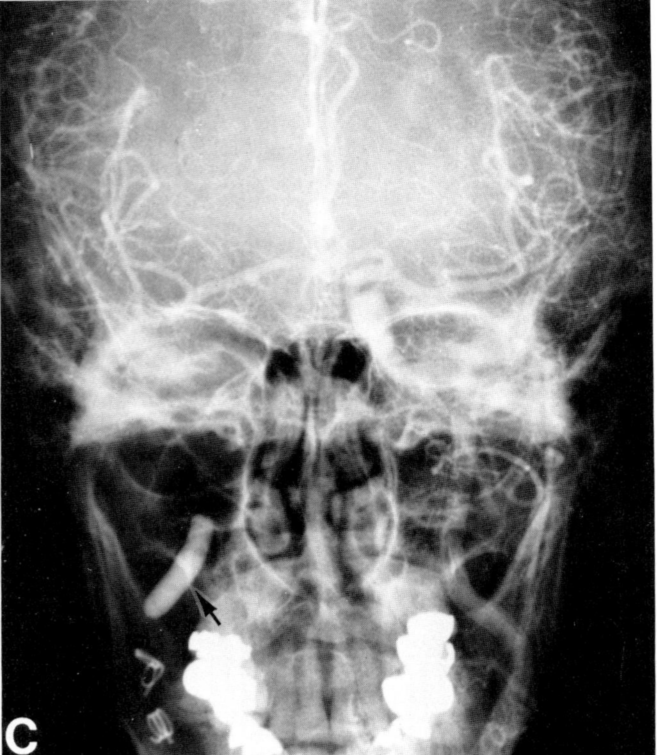

Fig. 67-3. Giant right internal carotid aneurysm. (A) A CT scan revealing the size of the aneurysm. (B) An angiogram showing the lumen of the aneurysm. (C) After detachable balloon occlusion of the right internal carotid artery (arrow) with cross filling of the right MCA via the anterior communicating artery on left carotid angiogram. The patient had adequate CBF on test balloon occlusion.

Table 67-1. The use of cerebral blood flow studies to determine whether the collateral blood supply is adequate before balloon detachment in the treatment of giant intracranial aneurysms

Patient	Aneurysm Site	Preocclusion CBF (>40 ml/100 g/min)	Test occlusion CBF (>40 ml/100 g/min)	Other Treatment
R.H.	Ophthalmic	+	− (37)	EC-IC bypass
W.K.	ACoA	+	reversible hemiplegia	−
M.S.	Ophthalmic	+	+	−
J.H.	Cavernous	+	− (37) (neurologically intact)	Mannitol*
M.S.	Supraclinoid	+	+	−
B.L.	Ophthalmic	+	+	−
E.S.	Cavernous	+	+	−

A CBF of >40 ml/100 g/min during test occlusion indicates adequate collateral blood supply.
*The patient was placed on intravenous mannitol and the CBF improved to >40 ml/100 g/min; the mannitol was then tapered off uneventfully 3 days later. A repeat CBF study showed a CBF of >40 ml/100 g/min.

performed with a curved 8-inch Rhoton needle holder and 9-0 monofilament nylon suture on a BV-6 needle (Ethicon).

Exposure

Before preparation of the scalp, the STA course is scratched into the skin over the previous pen marking. The position of the MCA recipient branch is determined from the angiogram and is likewise marked. When a pterional or other approach to an intracranial aneurysm or tumor is needed in conjunction with a bypass, a modified flap as shown in Figure 67-4 may provide exposure for all contemplated surgical procedures. Although one might anticipate ischemia at the tips of the flaps, we have not experienced this problem.

When a craniotomy is made, we prefer to turn the scalp and bone flaps under loupes and headlight illumination. No local anesthetic is injected, and skin clips are used with care. Care is taken to avoid injury to the STA, which is meticulously dissected with a mosquito hemostat. The larger branch, usually the frontal, is preserved for anastomosis, and the smaller is ligated and divided (Figure 67-5). The temporalis muscle is exposed by reflecting scalp flaps. The temporalis incision is planned to permit compression-free routing of the graft to the MCA branch for anastomosis. The craniotomy is made over a point 6 cm above the external auditory meatus to optimize chances for a large MCA branch being exposed (Figure 67-6). Once the dura is opened, the microscope is swung into the field.

When no other intracranial surgery is contemplated, we prefer linear incisions in contrast to a scalp flap (Figure 67-4). Linear incisions permit rapid STA preparation and avoid the scalp necrosis that can occur with a flap. One or two linear incisions may be needed, depending on the STA branch selected and occasionally on the MCA branch chosen. Most frequently the frontal branch of the STA and the angular branch of the MCA are the largest and thus the best arteries available for anastomosis (Figure 67-4A). The angular branch can be used with safety even on the dominant hemisphere. Occasionally, the posterior branch of the STA (Figure 67-4B) or a frontal branch of the MCA will be selected for bypass (Figure 67-4C).

When a cutdown technique is used, the initial incision is made over the STA with the microscope at 16×. The surgeon's arms are supported on either side with portable Mayo stands. The seated surgeon and assistant link arms to provide comfortable access for all four hands into the operative site. Subcutaneous injection of local anesthetic is omitted. The initial incision with a No. 15 blade is made over the distal STA down to

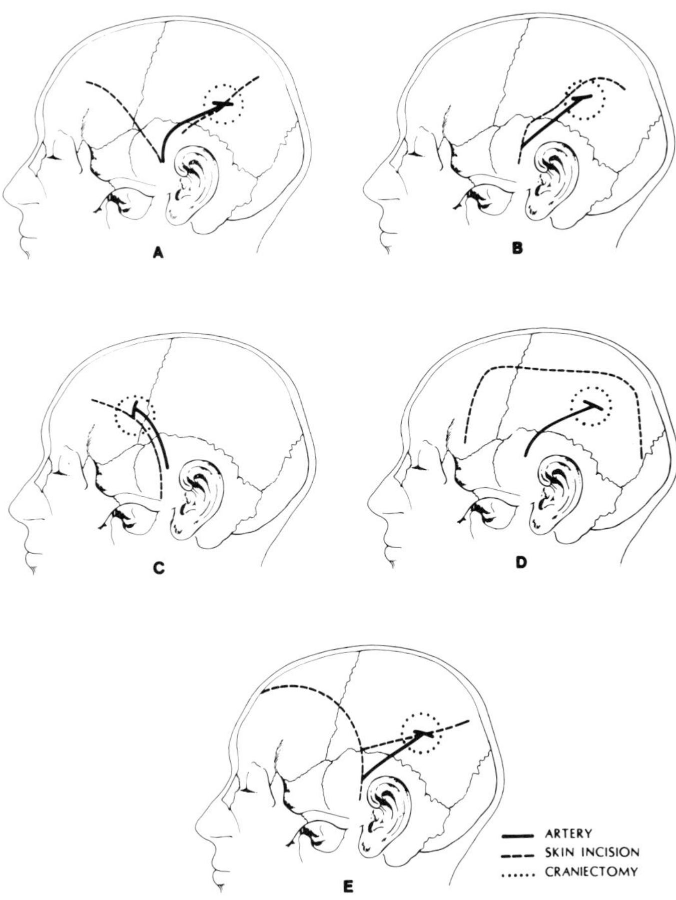

Fig. 67-4. STA-MCA bypass. A variety of approaches can be used for specific circumstances. (A) Most commonly, two linear incisions permit anastomosis of the largest branches, namely the frontal branch of the STA and the angular branch of the MCA. (B) Sometimes a parietal branch of the STA is larger and is therefore used. (C) Occasionally the frontal STA is joined to a frontal branch of the MCA. (D) A scalp flap gives the widest perusal and selection of the STA branches; also, a double bypass can be performed with this exposure. (E) When a craniotomy for an aneurysm is to be used, a T-shaped incision can be used for the bypass.

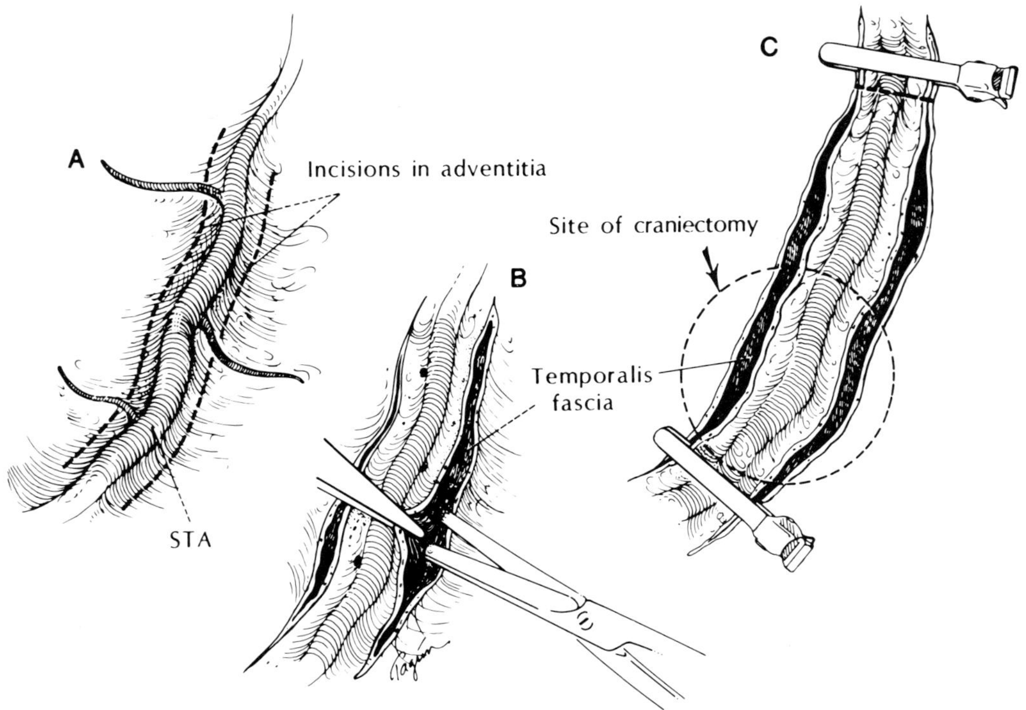

Fig. 67-5. STA-MCA bypass technique: Preparation of the STA. (A) Exposure; (B) undermining; (C) mobilization.

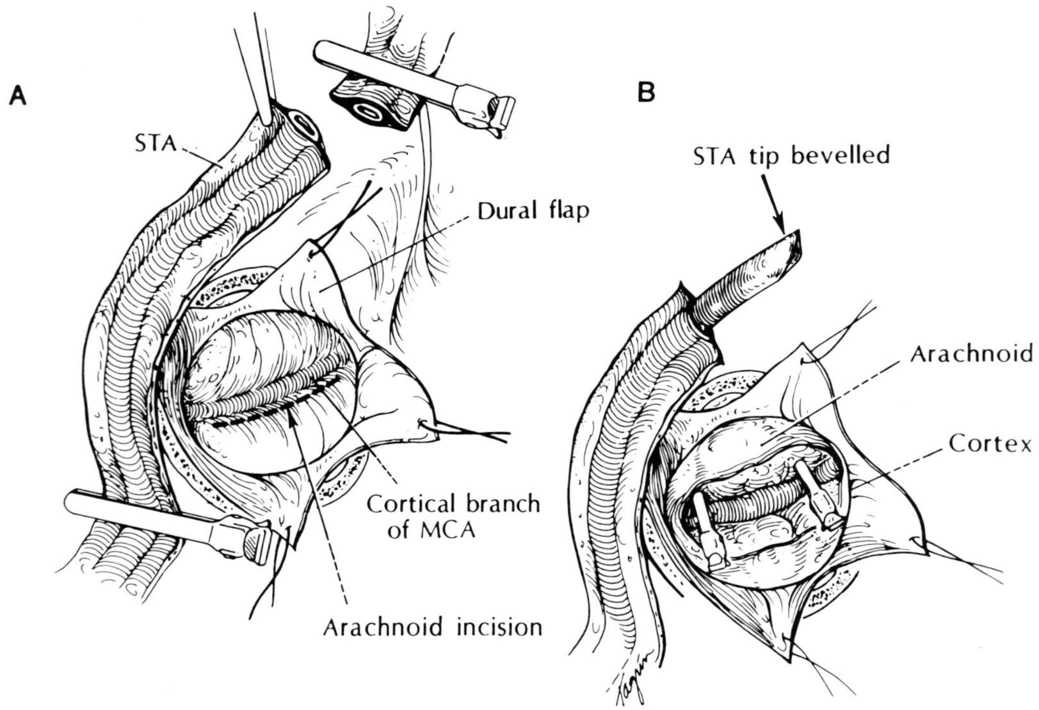

Fig. 67-6. STA-MCA bypass technique: Preparation of vessels. (A) A craniotomy and opening of the dura expose the cortical branch of the MCA. The STA is cut to the proper length. (B) The arachnoid is opened and clips are applied. The tip of the STA is freed of adventitia and tailored.

the subcutaneous fat to avoid injury to the STA trunk. Then the surgeon and assistant elevate the scalp tissue with Adson forceps, and the plane just superficial to STA is developed with Metzenbaum scissors. When the proper plane is chosen, the STA is readily exposed over a length of 8 to 10 cm.

STA Preparation

For the flap technique, the STA is identified just deep to galea. Often an appropriate branch can be traced retrograde from the scalp incision. The STA is isolated by sharp dissection down to fat and hair follicles, where a plane is established superficial to the vessel. Some adventitia is left in place. Small bleeders are coagulated with bipolar cautery away from the STA. Branches larger than 0.5 mm are divided between 6-0 silk ligatures. To facilitate this dissection, the surgeon uses a knife and forceps and the assistant uses a sucker and bipolar cautery. When a cutdown technique is used (Figure 67-4A-C), small scalp flaps are elevated on either side of the STA. The adventitia is incised with a No. 15 knife blade approximately 2 mm to each side of the STA down to the temporalis fascia. A few spreading movements with the Metzenbaum scissors develop a plane between the STA and the temporalis fascia, thus completing isolation of the vessel. After exposure of the MCA recipient branch (described below), the STA is cut to an adequate length. This is usually 8 cm and includes a bit of extra length to facilitate suturing of the back wall. The artery is occluded with a Heifetz clip and divided. Heparinized saline is flushed into the STA via a No. 20 Medicut catheter. This irrigation flushes out blood and helps identify bleeders for coagulation. When a large proximal side branch is available, an irrigation catheter can be tied into the branch to permit intermittent STA irrigation during anastomosis and bypass pressure measurement after completion of the graft. Irrigation of the STA with saline serves to clear bits of clot and to identify gaps that require additional stitches.

The tip of the STA is then freed of adventitia over a 1-cm length. The tip is beveled in a fish-mouth fashion to maximize the anastomotic opening (Figure 67-6B). If the intima should separate from the muscularis, a second effort at beveling usually is associated with adherence of the two layers of the artery. After the STA tip is prepared, flow is measured by letting the artery bleed into a beaker for a specific length of time. The artery is again flushed with heparinized saline.

In some patients, the STA segment must be led from one incision to another. A tunnel is prepared by blunt dissection between the galea and temporalis fascia. The STA tip is pulled through the tunnel with a terminal silk tie. Twists and kinks in the STA segments are carefully avoided.

MCA Preparation

The angular branch of the MCA generally is used, lying about 6 cm rostral to the external auditory canal. When the frontal STA is used, the angular branch is exposed through a separate incision (Figure 67-4A). The temporalis muscle is opened with cutting cautery, which also can be used to elevate the periosteum.

A small craniotomy flap, about 7 cm in diameter, is fashioned over the recipient artery with the power drill and craniotome. We have found this method faster and safer than either craniectomy or trephine. Bone edges are waxed and the dura opened in a cruciate fashion. Additional bone can be removed (especially inferiorly) if no suitable recipient branch is identified. When a suitable vessel is exposed, three drill holes are made in the bone edge for eventual bone flap replacement, and dural to pericranial sutures are placed.

The arachnoid next to the MCA is cut with microscissors under 25× magnification. Tiny side branches can be coagulated with the bipolar cautery on low power and cut as needed to prepare a 1-cm length of artery. One or two larger side branches can be preserved by using temporary clips. A strip of rubber dam is placed under the MCA to protect the cortex.

Final preparation of the MCA is achieved at 25× magnification with the prepared STA tip in full view. Kleinert-Kees clips are placed on the MCA branch at least 10 mm apart. A slender oval arteriotomy, the same length as the STA tip width, is made in the MCA with one or two snips of the microscissors (Figure 67-7A). The vessel is irrigated with heparinized saline. A stent of fine Silastic tubing is inserted into the vessel.

Anastomosis

The STA tip is positioned against the MCA opening with the tip aimed backward toward the MCA origin to promote flow throughout the territory of the MCA. A needle holder and jeweler's forceps are used to place interrupted 9-0 nylon sutures in each corner (Figure 67-7B). Forceps are used primarily as a counter pressor during suturing, and the vessel wall is handled as little and as gently as possible. Squeezing the intima is particularly avoided. An additional six to eight interrupted sutures are placed in the front wall (Figure 67-8A), and these are tied down after all have been placed to give maximum accuracy. Bites are a bit larger on the STA side to promote slight eversion and intima-to-intima apposition. Sutures must accurately include the intima of the STA, which may be thickened and separated from the muscularis. Inside-to-outside passage of the needle through the STA is recommended when an intimal flap threatens. Sutures are placed slightly closer together near the corner, where leaks are more common. Keeping the area dry facilitates suture handling. Keeping the needle in view on the rubber dam minimizes time lost in searching. Some surgeons advocate a running suture technique routinely, but in our hands interrupted stitches have provided superior precision and maximum ostial width.

The STA is reflected aside to reveal the back wall of the anastomosis. The front wall suture line is inspected from inside to confirm accurate suture placement. Six to eight interrupted sutures then are used to complete the back wall (Figure 67-8B). Before the last two sutures are tied, the stent tube is gently removed and the three vascular limbs opened briefly to check flow and expel air. The final sutures are tied down.

The distal MCA clip is removed first and then the proximal. Utilizing 25× magnification, the suture line is inspected for leaks. A major area of leak requires a stitch; suture line ooze will stop without additional sutures. The rubber dam is folded over the suture line, and pressure applied with a cottonoid for 1 to 2 minutes. In some cases, a collar of Gelfoam can secure suture line hemostasis. Finally, the STA clip is removed to begin augmented cerebral blood flow. Graft pressures can be measured when a suitable side branch of STA has been cannulated. Graft flow can also be estimated with an electromagnetic flow probe, but great care must be exercised to avoid injury to the STA by the flow probe. Graft patency can be assessed with real-time Doppler ultrasonography.

Closure

The dura is loosely approximated with 4-0 sutures. A Gelfoam pledget is used to cover the exposed dura and surround the distal STA segment. After the graft is routed

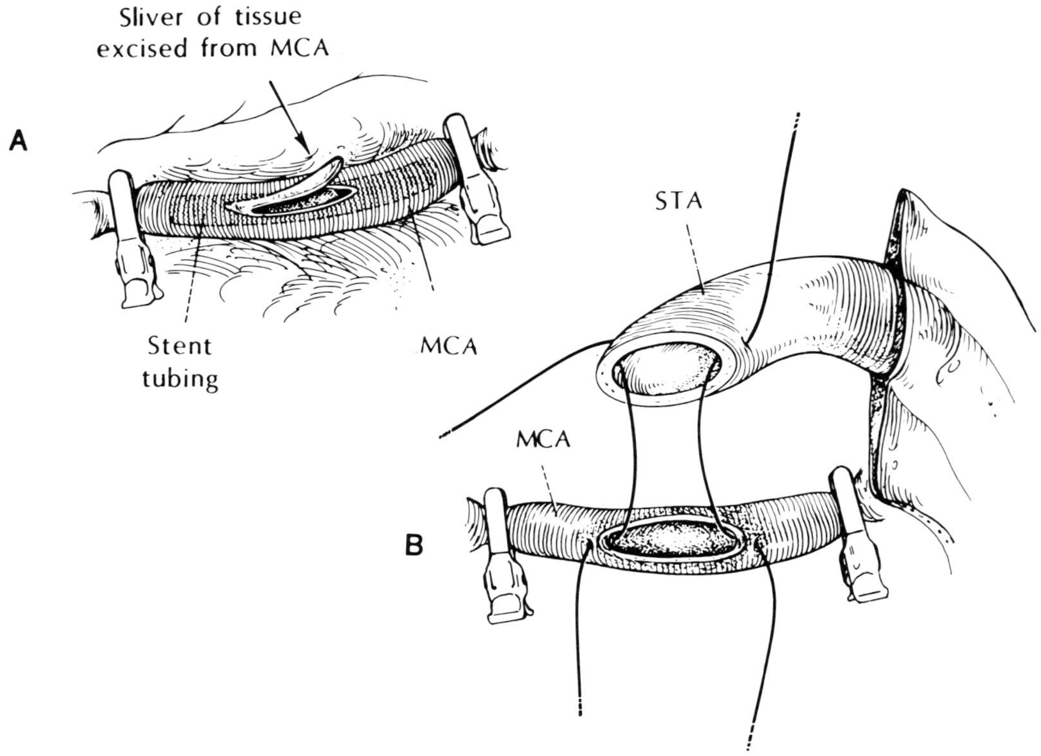

Fig. 67-7. STA-MCA bypass technique: Arteriotomy. (A) A sliver of the MCA is excised with scissors and a stent is inserted. (B) Interrupted corner sutures appose the STA to the MCA.

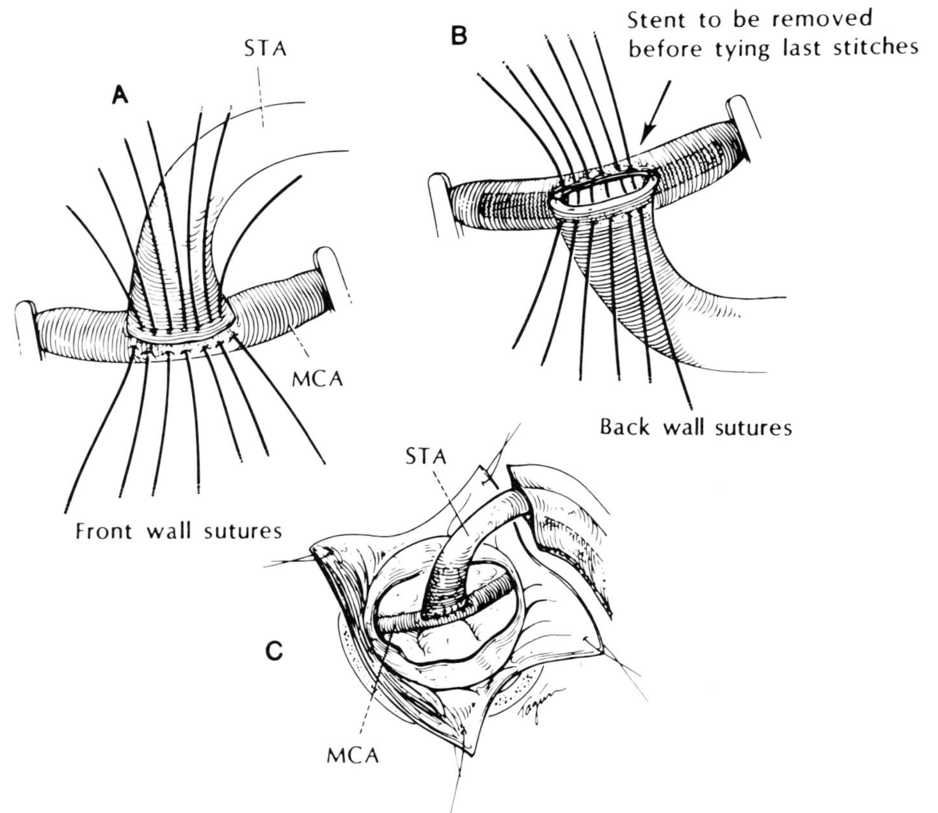

Fig. 67-8. STA-MCA bypass technique: Anastomosis. (A) Interrupted sutures are placed in the front wall; the sutures are tied after all have been placed. (B) The back wall sutures are placed. The front wall suture line is inspected and the stent is removed before the last sutures are tied. (C) The completed anastomosis.

smoothly and without kinking, the bone flap is trimmed with rongeurs to avoid contact with the STA and then wired in place. The temporalis muscle and fascia are approximated as separate layers with interrupted 3-0 coated Vicryl. Great care is taken to avoid compression of the graft. The wound is irrigated with Bacitracin solution and closed with 3-0 interrupted coated Vicryl to the galea and continuous nylon to the skin. When scalp edge viability is in question, closure with interrupted 5-0 nylon without tension offers the best chance of avoiding necrosis. A small dressing is applied together with a warning sign against pressure and a mark to indicate the point to check for pulse in the superficial temporal artery.

POSTOPERATIVE MANAGEMENT AND COMPLICATIONS

Blood pressure is carefully monitored with the aid of a radial artery catheter and is maintained in the normal range for the individual patient with infusions of colloids, pressors, or nitroprusside. Patients are gradually mobilized after 48 hours and blood pressure controlled with oral agents as needed. Diphenylhydantoin (300 mg/day) is used. Aspirin (300 mg) and dipyridamole (25 mg) are given twice daily for 6 months. Careful management of risk factors continues indefinitely.

If the patient is not doing well in the immediate postoperative period, a CT scan is performed; if this does not clarify the problem, angiography is done.

Major complications of this procedure include intraoperative graft thrombosis with either acute or late stroke, subdural hematoma, and intracerebral hemorrhage.[2,29–31] Less serious complications include transient neurologic worsening, wound infection, seizures, scalp edge necrosis, and myocardial ischemia.

Blue-black discoloration of the graft suggests intraoperative thrombosis. To confirm this, a suture or two must be removed. If clot is encountered and removed, a search is made for a technical error, such as an intimal flap or narrowing. Although efforts at correction are usually futile, we have on one occasion been able to reestablish flow and achieve angiographic patency.

Angiography is performed after 1 week to assess patency of the anastomosis in those patients who do not develop complications. Patency in our published series was documented angiographically in 45 of 49 grafts studies (see Figure 67-1B). Technical errors led to thrombosis in two cases. In one, the first in the series, insufficient attention was paid to the course of the graft through the muscle and bone. Compression of the graft by these structures led to asymptomatic thrombosis. In the other patient, the STA segment was cut too short and there was tension on the suture line. Although an initial angiogram showed only minor irregularity at the anastomotic site, occlusion occurred 3 months later and was associated with a mild stroke. In two other cases, intraoperative thrombosis occurred without neurologic sequelae.

Delayed strokes can occur despite a functioning bypass graft.[30] This happened in three of our cases. In two, occlusion of a previously markedly stenotic intracranial internal carotid artery occurred after surgery. Mild strokes resulted in both these patients despite improved filling of the MCA via the graft, compared with the immediate postoperative studies. In the other patients, a mild stroke occurred in the face of a functioning graft and poor collateral circulation. We have observed internal carotid occlusion once without symptoms. In these cases, STA-MCA bypass may have promoted ICA occlusion, protected against infarction, or both. Complete occlusion of distal carotid stenosis following establishment of STA-MCA bypass graft has also been reported by others.[32,33]

A patient occasionally will continue to have TIAs following a bypass procedure. This may indicate that the mechanism of ischemia is other than that postulated preoperatively. For example, following ICA occlusion, the mechanism of TIAs may be external carotid artery stenosis or distal stump embolization rather than a hemodynamic problem, and a bypass therefore could be ineffectual. Alternatively, the bypass may be occluded, providing no additional collateral circulation to the brain. Another possibility is the inducement of occlusion in a previously stenotic internal carotid artery as discussed above. In order to evaluate the precise mechanism and symptomatology in this situation, cerebral angiography is required. In one of our patients, episodes of numbness in the left face presumably related to severe distal ICA stenosis persisted following superficial temporal artery-middle cerebral bypass. Cerebral angiography confirmed continued patency of the stenotic vessel and good filling of the bypass graft into the middle cerebral circulation. The patient was treated with aspirin and Persantine but the episodes persisted. Approximately 1 year later, the patient suffered a moderate right cerebral hemisphere stroke, which cleared to a mild deficit. Cerebral angiography at that time disclosed occlusion of the internal carotid artery with newly enhanced filling of the middle cerebral territory via the graft. An appropriate cerebral infarction was demonstrated on a CT scan. This case has persuaded us that should TIAs persist after bypass graft and antiplatelet therapy, strong consideration of Coumadin therapy should be entertained.

RESULTS

Our experience with 50 grafts in 45 patients has been reported.[34] Patency has been high (92 percent), serious complications infrequent (4 percent), and there have been no deaths directly attributable to surgery. Similar results have been reported by others.[1–4,31,35–37]

OTHER MIDDLE CEREBRAL REVASCULARIZATION

SHORT VEIN GRAFT

Little et al.[5] reported good results after interposition of a saphenous vein segment between the STA and a cortical branch of the MCA. The vein segment of 5 to 10 cm is irrigated with heparin and aligned so that subsequent flow occurs in the direction of the valves. The ends of the vein graft are freed of adventitia to facilitate suturing. An end-to-side anastomosis of the vein to the cortical artery is carried out using continuous 9-0 nylon for the back wall and interrupted 10-0 nylon for the front wall. A temporary clip across the vein graft near the anastomosis then permits removal of temporary clips from the cortical recipient artery. Full heparinization is carried out to prevent thrombosis at the cortical anastomosis. An end-to-side anastomosis of the vein to the STA trunk above the zygoma is accomplished in similar fashion. After all clamps are opened, heparin is reversed with protamine sulfate. In 19 cases, angiography demonstrated a 90 percent patency rate, and no patient experienced recurrent TIAs. Cerebral blood flow studies suggest a substantial increment in collateral circulation.

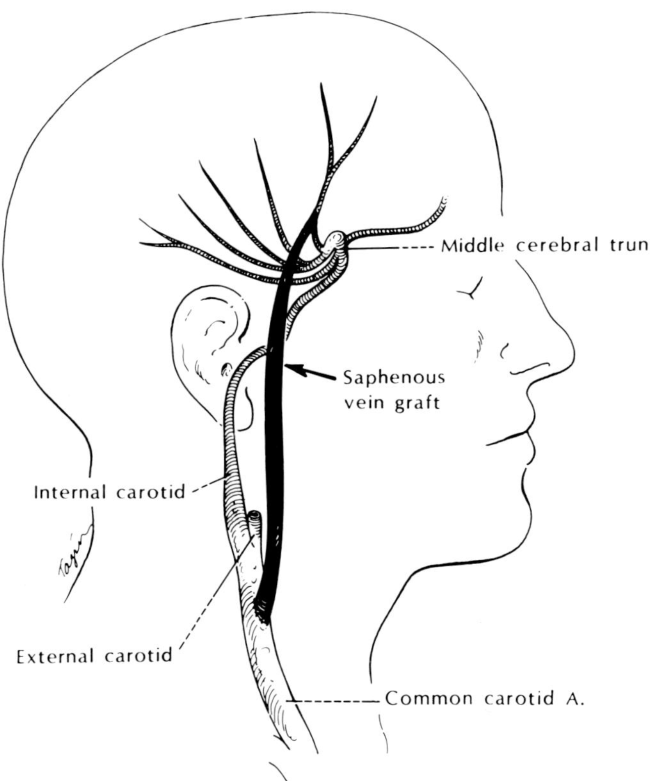

Fig. 67-9. Long graft. A free graft of saphenous vein is interposed between the external carotid artery and a branch of the MCA. Long grafts give high-flow revascularization of the anterior circulation, but indications remain uncertain.

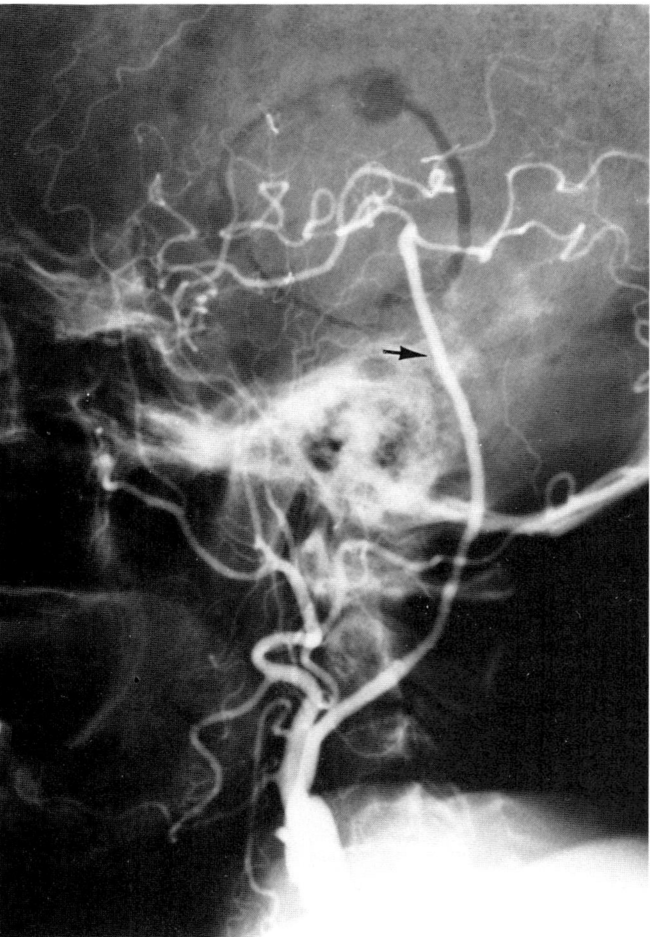

Fig. 67-10. Left lateral carotid angiogram showing an external carotid-MCA saphenous vein bypass graft (arrow).

LONG VEIN GRAFTS

To provide immediate high flow revascularization, free grafts have been interposed between an artery in the neck and a recipient intracranially.[38] The subclavian, common carotid, and external carotid arteries have served as donor arteries; the supraclinoid, internal carotid, and cortical MCA have been used as recipient arteries.[33,39–43] Recent reports indicate good patency rates with low complication rates, but indications have not been established.

When immediate high flow is needed or suitable cranial donor arteries are lacking, we have performed saphenous vein interposition between the external carotid and cortical MCA. Two teams of surgeons work simultaneously, one to prepare the carotid bifurcation and perform the craniotomy, the other to harvest the saphenous vein (about 12 cm ending at the constriction near the knee)(see below for details). The end-to-end proximal anastomosis is done under the operating microscope with 7-0 nylon interrupted sutures. Full heparinization is used during cross-clamping, and after the proximal anastomosis is completed a Heifetz clip is applied to the vein near the anastomosis and the carotid clamps are removed. The vein is routed through a channel drilled in the occipital bone (or over the zygoma) to the craniotomy site, with care taken to avoid compression or redundancy (Figure 67-9). A pen mark made on the saphenous vein in its original site helps to avoid a twist in the final site. A side branch near the proximal anastomosis is useful for irrigation through the graft. The distal vein ostium, which should be about 3 or 4 mm in diameter, is bevelled back toward the MCA origin. End-to-side anastomosis is carried out

with 9-0 monofilament nylon. A running suture technique may be useful, especially for the back wall. Intermittent irrigation through a side branch helps clear clots and identify leakage sites. Protamine sulfate serves to reverse heparinization. Care must be taken to avoid postoperative hypertension, which can lead to hemorrhage. Dramatic angiographic filling can be achieved with long grafting (Figure 67-10).

OTHER PROCEDURES

When the STA is inadequate, the occipital artery can sometimes be used.[27] Whether this vessel is adequate can be determined from the angiogram; in some cases the artery is small or bifurcates early into small distal branches. Palpation and a Doppler probe can be used to help mark the artery's course. Direct cutdown on the occipital artery provides the best exposure. Careful sharp dissection is needed to free the vessel from surrounding dense adhesions. Exposure and preparation of the MCA branch and anastomosis are completed as in STA-MCA bypass.

Ordinarily, the middle meningeal artery is too small to be useful for revascularization. Occasionally, the artery may be large enough for grafting when it is enlarged as a result of the presence of a meningioma.[44] When no suitable recipient vessel can be identified, the STA can be laid directly on the cortex.[45] This approach has recently been adapted for moyamoya disease.[46] The pedicle of the uninterrupted STA is inserted through a strip craniectomy to be sewn to the cut edges of the dura mater. Striking STA-MCA anastomoses have been shown angiographically. The procedure has several advantages: it can be done quickly in small children, the cranial defect is small, and the STA remains intact with small risk of thrombosis.

Several authors have recommended placement of vascularized omental grafts directly on the brain to add vascular supply.[47–49]

VERTEBROBASILAR REVASCULARIZATION

OCCIPITAL ARTERY-POSTERIOR INFERIOR CEREBELLAR ARTERY (OCCIPITAL-PICA) BYPASS

The technical feasibility and relative safety of occipital to PICA bypass have been established.[50,51] Impressive angiographic filling of the vertebrobasilar circulation has been demonstrated following this operation. However, the clinical indications for this procedure are not yet defined.

General anesthesia is required with strict attention to maintenance of normal blood pressure throughout the procedure. The lateral position seems to provide adequate exposure and avoids the danger of cerebral ischemia inherent in the sitting position. A modified hockey-stick incision, rising high in the midline above the inion, provides adequate length for the occipital artery and access to the caudal PICA loop (Figure 67-11). To avoid scalp edge necrosis, no clamps are placed on the flap edge. The occipital artery, which is invested in dense fascia, must be freed up by meticulous sharp microdissection. A suboccipital craniectomy, with removal of the posterior rim of the foramen magnum and a hemilaminectomy of C1, allows exposure of the cerebellar tonsils. The caudal loop of the PICA, which is localized angiographically, is dissected free of arachnoid and supported by a sling of rubber dam stitched to extracranial soft tissues.

The anastomosis is completed much like an STA-MCA bypass graft. The tip of the occipital artery is cleared of adventitia and bevelled. A clip is placed on the caudal loop of the PICA, an oval window is excised, and a small stent is inserted. Anastomosis is done with interrupted 10-0 monofilament nylon sutures. The occipital artery is bevelled back toward the origin of the PICA in order to promote vertebrobasilar perfusion. Compression of the graft during closure of the wound must be carefully avoided.

In a report of 22 patients, it was noted that the primary problem with the operative procedure was marginal neurologic status prior to operation leading to respiratory complications from preoperative impairment of the cranial nerves.[51] Only two patients had a permanent increase in neurologic deficits (unilateral hearing loss and homonymous hemianopia). The same general complications noted with STA-MCA grafts were also encountered with this procedure.

INTERPOSITION VEIN GRAFT TO POSTERIOR CEREBRAL ARTERY

For basilar artery occlusive disease, direct revascularization may offer effective protection against stroke when TIAs continue in spite of anticoagulation. The larger caliber of the posterior cerebral artery in many patients makes this an attractive vessel for anastomosis. Use of a saphenous vein graft

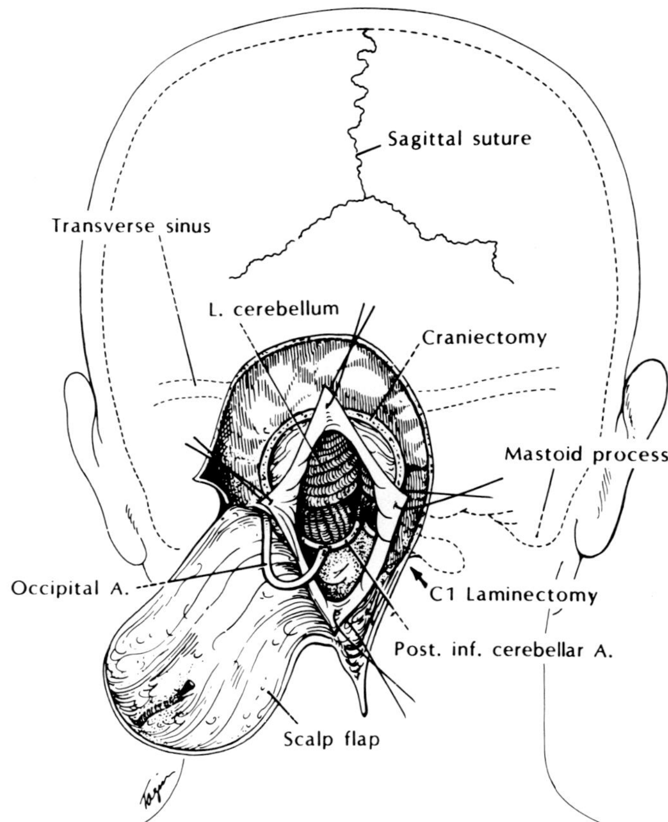

Fig. 67-11. Occipital-PICA graft. A suboccipital craniectomy and a C1 laminectomy provide exposure of the caudal loop of the PICA. Anastomosis of the occipital artery to the PICA provides new collateral to the posterior circulation.

between the external carotid and the proximal posterior cerebral artery has been reported.[43] This procedure provides a high blood flow to the distal basilar artery. Experience has shown that patency is high and morbidity small. The procedure can be considered in cases of vertebrobasilar TIAs associated with bilateral intracranial vertebral occlusive disease,[52] especially when terminal vertebral obstruction obviates occipital artery-PICA bypass.

Under general anesthesia, the patient is positioned supine with a roll under the shoulder and with the head turned fully and held in the three-point head holder. The sitting position is avoided and great care is taken throughout surgery to maintain normal to slightly elevated blood pressure in an effort to avoid vertebrobasilar ischemia and infarction. The temporal and cervical regions are prepared and draped in a single field. The medial thigh and calf (the left is more convenient) are shaved, prepared, and draped. Two teams of surgeons simultaneously expose the carotid bifurcation and harvest the saphenous vein.

The saphenous vein is harvested beginning 1 cm anterior to the medial malleolus. It is convenient to dissect adventitia from the vein and to cut the skin with a Metzenbaum scissors. The vessel is followed distal to its narrowing at the knee, a narrowing which helps minimize the discrepancy in diameter with the posterior cerebral artery. Side branches are divided between 4-0 silk ligatures and several prominent branches near the ankle are saved long for later irrigation. The superficial aspect of the vessel is marked in situ with a marking pen to help avoid twists in final positioning. Patency is maintained until the vessel is cross-cut, removed, and immediately irrigated in an antegrade

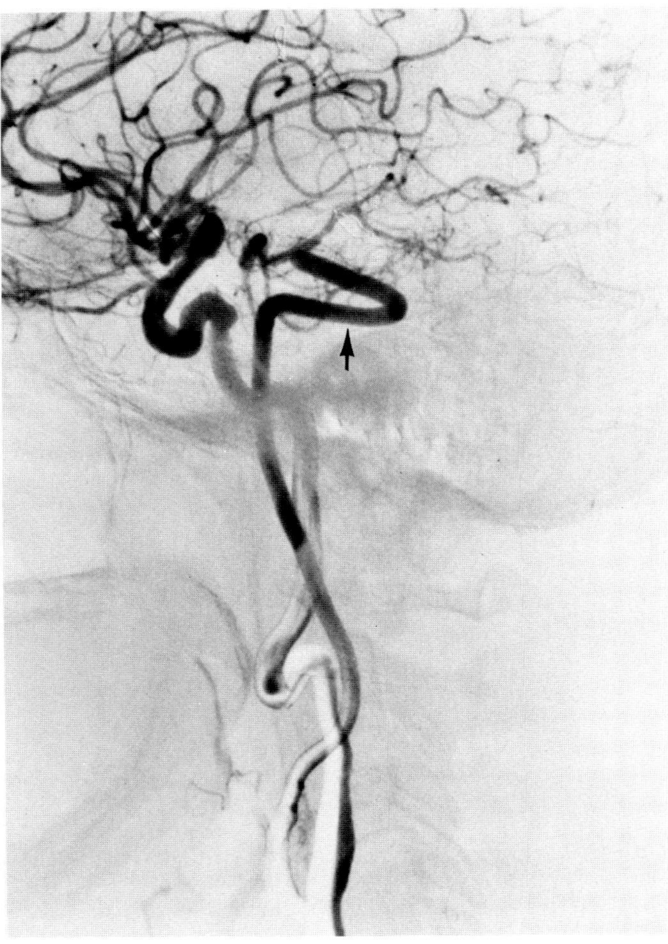

Fig. 67-12. Left external carotid artery to posterior cerebral artery saphenous vein graft. Episodes of upper limb paralysis and bilateral ophthalmoplegia caused by bilateral vertebral occlusion were eliminated by revascularization.

end is cross-cut at 90 degrees, avoiding valves. A side branch is catheterized with a 20-gauge Medicut catheter for intermittent irrigation with heparinized saline.

For the proximal anastomosis, we give the patient 7000 units of heparin intravenously before cross-clamping the external carotid artery. At a convenient point, usually just before the first major bifurcation, the vessel is cross-cut at 90 degrees. If there is substantial atheroma, a limited endarterectomy is warranted. Under the operating microscope, an end-to-end anastomosis is performed between the ECA and the saphenous vein graft. We prefer interrupted 6-0 Prolene, about 6 stitches on each side, without the need for a stent. On one occasion, we used a diagonal cut of the vessels to minimize diameter discrepancy, but this usually is not a problem.

Length is checked and the distal graft cross-cut at 90 degrees. During the distal anastomosis, intermittent irrigation through the side branch serves to clear small clots, identify leaks and clear the field. Under the microscope, the PCA lateral to the brain stem is dissected free over at least 1 cm. It is usually possible to preserve all side branches. The vessel is cross-clamped with Sugita temporary clips. With the graft in the field as a guide, an arteriotomy is made in the PCA using a No. 11 blade. The anastomosis is fashioned with interrupted 9-0 nylon, about 6 stitches for each side with a small Silastic stent. Completion of the back wall is aided by deviation of the graft with a cottonoid toward the temporal lobe. Before tying the last stitch, flow in the PCA is checked and brief flow through the graft is permitted to blow out debris and air. The final stitch is tied, and all clips are removed, thus establishing graft flow. At this point after surgery, blood pressure is carefully held in the range normal for the individual patient. Protamine sulfate is given (70 mg intravenously) to reverse the effect of heparin. Wounds are closed in routine fashion, with care to avoid compression of the graft.

Experience with four such grafts has been encouraging. All patients had bilateral intracranial vertebral disease. Two patients with disabling frequent TIAs have had no further such TIAs (Figure 67-12). One patient with two prior infarctions and multiple TIAs as a result of bilateral vertebral occlusion has had occasional minor TIAs but no infarction in 3 years of follow-up. A patient with bilateral vertebral occlusions and multiple cerebral and cerebellar infarcts suffered a progressive stepwise decline despite anticoagulants. We performed bypass reluctantly and found organized thrombus in the PCA, removal of which led to a fairly good proximal backflow without distal backflow. We ligated the PCA distal to the completed anastomosis to avoid propagation of clot. The patient improved promptly after surgery only to revert to his former status when the graft occluded 3 days after surgery, probably as a result of the pre-existing intra-luminal thrombus. The other three grafts have remained patent 1 to 3 years postoperatively.

fashion with heparinized saline. Vigorous high-pressure irrigation, which could expand the graft and exaggerate diameter discrepancy, is avoided. The graft is placed in heparinized saline until anastomosis.

While the saphenous vein is being harvested, the carotid bifurcation is exposed. Since the head is turned more than usual, the surgeon should be prepared to dissect deeper beneath the sternomastoid muscle. A complete freeing of the external carotid artery is needed about 3 cm above its origin. The common carotid, external, and internal carotid arteries are controlled with tapes. Through a linear (''tic'') incision, a small temporal craniotomy is fashioned, such as used in exposure of a basilar bifurcation aneurysm. In order to slacken the brain for retraction, Mannitol is administered (100 g intravenously), and spinal fluid withdrawn via the previously placed spinal subarachnoid catheter. The temporal lobe is gently elevated with a self-retaining retractor to expose the posterior cerebral artery lateral to the brain stem. Using a Kelly clamp, a tunnel is made from the cranial to the cervical incision, routing superficial to the zygoma with care to avoid the branches of the facial nerve.

With care taken to avoid twisting, the saphenous vein graft is pulled from the cervical wound through the subcutaneous tunnel to the cranial wound with a 0 silk tied to the narrowed rostral end. This end is brought close to the PCA to judge appropriate graft length. Some redundancy makes the distal anastomosis easier and does not cause problems. The cervical

REFERENCES

1. Donaghy RMP, Yasargil MG: Micro-Vascular Surgery. Stuttgart, Georg Thieme Verlag, 1967.
2. Yasargil MG: Microsurgery Applied to Neurosurgery. Stuttgart, Georg Thieme Verlag, 1968.
3. Reichman OH, Davis DO, Roberts TS, et al: Anastomosis between STA and cortical branch of MCA for the treatment of occlusive cerebrovascular disease, in Marei FT (ed): Reconstructive Surgery of Brain Arteries. Budapest, Akademiai Kiado, 1974.
4. Chater N, Popp J: Microsurgical vascular bypass for occlusive

cerebrovascular disease: Review of 100 cases. Surg Neurol 6:115, 1976.

5. Little JR, Furlan AJ, Bryerton B: Short vein grafts for cerebral revascularization. J Neurosurg 59:384, 1983.

6. Schmiedek P, Gratzel O, Spetzler R, et al: Selection of patients for extra-intracranial arterial bypass surgery based on rCBF measurements. J Neurosurg 44:303, 1976.

7. Powers WJ, Martin WR, Herscovitch P, et al: Extracranial ±intracranial bypass surgery. Hemodynamic and metabolic effects. Neurology 34:1168, 1984.

8. The EC/IC Bypass Study Group: Failure of extracranial-intracranial arterial bypass to reduce the risk of ischemic stroke. Results of an international randomized trial. N Engl J Med 313:1191, 1985.

9. Editorial: Extracranial to intracranial bypass and the prevention of stroke. Lancet 2:1401, 1985.

10. Gibbs JM, Wise RJS, Leenders KL, et al: Evaluation of cerebral perfusion in patients with carotid artery occlusion. Lancet 1:310, 1984.

11. Grubb RL, Ratcheson RA, Raichle ME, et al: Regional cerebral blood flow and oxygen utilization in superficial temporal-middle cerebral artery anastomosis patients. J Neurosurg 50:733, 1979.

12. Amine AR, Moody RA, Meeks W: Bilateral temporal-middle cerebral artery anastomosis for moyamoya syndrome. Surg Neurol 8:3, 1977.

13. Karasawa J, Kikichi H, Furtuse S, et al: Treatment of moyamoya disease with STA-MCA anastomosis. J Neurosurg 49:679, 1978.

14. Quest DO, Correll JW: Basal arterial occlusive disease. Neurosurgery 17:937, 1985.

15. Kearns TP, Siekert RG, Sundt TM Jr: The ocular aspects of bypass surgery of the carotid artery. Mayo Clin Proc 54:3, 1979.

16. Holbach K-H, Wassmann HW, Hoheluchter KL, et al: Reversibility of the chronic post-stroke state. Storke 7:296, 1976.

17. Holback K-H, Wassmann HW, Hoheluchter KL, et al: Differentation between reversible and irreversible post-stroke changes in brain tissue: Its relevance for cerebrovascular surgery. Surg Neurol 7:325, 1977.

18. Ferguson GG, Peerless SJ: Extracranial-intracranial arterial bypass in the treatment of dementia and multiple extracranial arterial occlusion. Presented at the Twenty-sixth Annual Meeting of the Congress of Neurological Surgeons, New Orleans, October 28, 1976.

19. Crowell RM: Emergency STA-MCA bypass for acute focal cerebral ischemia, in Schmiedek P, et al (eds): Microneurosurgical Anastomoses for Cerebral Ischemia. Berlin, Springer-Verlag, 1977.

20. Crowell RM, Olsson Y: Effect of extracranial-intracranial vascular bypass graft on experimental acute stroke in dogs. J Neurosurg 38:26, 1973.

21. Crowell RM, Jafar JJ: Emergency cerebral revascularization. Clin Neurosurg 33:281, 1986.

22. Diaz FG, Ausman JI, Mehta B, et al: Acute cerebral revascularization. J Neurosurg 63:200, 1985.

23. Ammerman BJ, Smith DR: Giant fusiform middle cerebral aneurysm: Successful treatment utilizing microvascular bypass. Surg Neurol 7:255, 1977.

24. Gelber BR, Sundt TM Jr: Treatment of intracavernous and giant carotid aneurysms by combined internal carotid ligation and extra) to intracranial bypass. J Neurosurg 52:1, 1980.

24. Crowell RM, Olsson Y: Direct brain revascularization, in Schmidek H, Sweet H (eds): Current Techniques of Operative Neurosurgery. New York, Grune & Stratton, 1978.

25. Spetzler RF, Shuster H, Roski RA: Elective extracranial-intracranial arterial bypass in the treatment of inoperable giant internal carotid artery aneurysms. J Neurosurg 53:22, 1980.

26. Sundt TM Jr, Piepgras DG: Surgical approach to giant intracranial aneurysms: Operative experience with 80 cases. J Neurosurg 51:731, 1979.

27. Spetzler RF, Chater N: Occipital artery-middle cerebral artery anastomosis for cerebral artery occlusive disease. Surg Neurol 2:235, 1974.

28. Tan WS, Jafar JJ, Abejo R, et al: Regional cerebral blood flow assessment prior to balloon detachment in the treatment of intracranial giant aneurysms. Acta Neuroradiol (in press)

29. Heros RC, Nelson PB: Intracerebral hemorrhage after microsurgical cerebral revascularization. Neurosurgery 6:371, 1980.

30. Reichman OH: Complications of cerebral revascularization. Clin Neurosurg 23:318, 1976.

31. Yasargil MG, Krayenbhul HA, Jacobson JH: Microneurosurgical arterial reconstruction. Surgery 67:221, 1970.

32. Furlan AJ, Little JR, Dohn DF: Arterial occlusion following anastomosis of the superficial temporal artery to middle cerebral artery. Stroke 11:91, 1980.

33. Iwabuchi T, Kudo T, Hatanaka M, et al: Vein graft bypass in treatment of giant aneurysm. Surg Neurol 12:463, 1979.

34. Crowell RM, Olsson Y: Direct brain revascularization, in Schmidek H, Sweet H (eds): Current Techniques of Operative Neurosurgery. New York, Grune & Stratton, 1978.

35. Samson DS, Boone S: Extracranial-intracranial (EC-IC) arterial bypass: Past performance and current concepts. Neurosurgery 3:79, 1978.

36. Sundt TM Jr, Siekert RG, Piepgras DG, et al: Bypass surgery for vascular disease of the carotid system. Mayo Clin Proc 51:677, 1976.

37. Tew JM Jr: Reconstructive vascular surgery for prevention of stroke. Clin Neurosurg 22:264, 1975.

38. Woringer E, Kunlin J: Anastomose entre la carotide primitive et la carotide intra-cranienne on la Sylvienne par greffon selon la technique de la suture suspendue. Neurochirurgie 9:181, 1963.

39. Lougheed WM, Marshall BM, Hunter M, et al: Common carotid to intracranial internal carotid bypass venous graft. J Neurosurg 34:114, 1971.

40. Samson DS, Boone S: Extracranial-intracranial (EC-IC) arterial bypass: Past performance and current concepts. Neurosurgery 3:79, 1978.

41. Spetzler RF, Rhodes RS, Roski RA, et al: Subclavian to middle cerebral artery saphenous vein bypass graft. J Neurosurg 53:465, 1980.

42. Story JL, Brown WE Jr, Eidelberg E, et al: Cerebral revascularization: Common carotid to distal middle cerebral artery bypass. Neurosurgery 2:131, 1978.

43. Sundt TM Jr, Piepgras DG, Houser OW, et al: Interposition saphenous vein grafts for advanced occlusive disease and large aneurysms in the posterior circulation. J Neurosurg 56:205, 1982.

44. Miller CF II, Spetzler RF, Kopaniky DJ: Middle meningeal to middle cerebral arterial bypass for cerebral revascularization. Case report. J Neurosurg 50:802, 1979.

45. Ausman JI, Moore J, Chou SN: Spontaneous cerebral revascularization in a patient with STA-MCA anastomosis. J Neurosurg 44:84, 1976.

46. Matsushima Y, Fukai N, Tanaka K, et al: A new surgical treatment of moyamoya disease in children: A preliminary report. Surg Neurol 15:313, 1980.

47. Goldsmith HS, Duckett S, Chen WF: Prevention of cerebral infarction in the monkey by omental transposition to the brain. Stroke 9:224, 1978.

48. Henschen C: Operative revascularisation des zirkulatorisch geschadigten Gehirns durch aufulage gestielter Muskellapen Encephalo-myo-synangiose. Langenbecks Arch Klin Chir 264:392, 1950.

49. Yonekawa Y, Yasargil MG: Brain vascularization by transplanted omentum: A possible treatment of cerebral ischemia. Neurosurgery 1:256, 1977.

50. Khodadad G: Occipital artery-posterior inferior cerebellar artery anastomosis. Surg Neurol 5:225, 1976.

51. Sundt TM Jr, Piepgras DG: Occipital to posterior inferior cerebellar artery bypass surgery. J Neurosurg 48:916, 1978.

52. Caplan LR: Vertebrobasilar occlusive disease, in Barnett HJM, Stein BM, Mohr JP, Yatsu FM (eds): Stroke. New York, Churchill Livingstone, 1986, pp 549–620

CHAPTER 68

Surgical Management of Moyamoya Disease

Tsuneyoshi Eguchi   Kazuo Ugajin

THE JAPANESE WORD *MOYAMOYA* denotes a nebulous or hazy state. For example, the word denotes the smoke of a cigarette hanging in the air in a quiet room. In this chapter, moyamoya is used for the angiographic appearance of a specific type of abnormality of blood vessels.

Kudoh first described the occlusions of the vessels of the circle of Willis known as moyamoya disease 30 years ago. Since that time the cause of the disease has not been elucidated. Pathologically it results from stenosis or occlusion of cerebral vessels due to fibrous thickening of the intima, mainly of the terminal portions of the internal carotid arteries (Figure 68-1 and Color Plate 68-1).[1] The disease can be congenital or acquired in nature. It has been known as Willis' circle occlusion, cerebral juxtabasal telangiectasia, and cerebral arterial rete, but because of its unique angiographic appearance, it is now commonly called moyamoya disease.

The diagnosis of moyamoya disease depends on a characteristic finding on cerebral angiograms: the "moyamoya" pattern—an image similar to a puff of cigarette smoke—in addition to the stenosis or occlusion of the cerebral vessels as described above. It has recently been noted that the narrowing or closure of the arteries also frequently extends to the vertebrobasilar system.[2] Table 68-1 indicates the diagnostic criteria for this disease proposed by the Japanese Ministry of Health and Welfare.

EPIDEMIOLOGY AND ETIOLOGY

Initially it was thought that this disease was confined to the Japanese people; however, it now been reported to occur in non-Japanese patients in several other countries.[3–6] The disease characteristically affects females more frequently. Nishimoto reported 518 cases in Japan before 1973, and 389 cases from 1976 through 1978, and found the ratio of afflicted males to females to be 1:1.52 in these 907 cases. There are two peaks in age distribution, one below age 10 and another in the third decade; these peaks correspond with the juvenile and adult forms of the disease. Ischemic symptoms herald the illness in its juvenile form; intracranial bleeding the adult form. The mortality rate is 2.7 percent in children and 11.1 percent in adults, with an average of 7.6 percent; most deaths are caused by intracranial bleeding.

There are four types of moyamoya disease: hemorrhagic, epileptic, ischemic with infarction, and transient ischemic at-tack (TIA). In juveniles, the infarction and TIA types of the disease each account for about 40 percent of cases of juvenile moyamoya disease or about 80 percent of the total number of cases. In contrast, the hemorrhagic type accounts for 65 percent of the total number of cases of adult moyamoya disease, suggesting that the mechanism of illness differs in the different age groups (Table 68-2).[7,8]

Congenital malformation, acquired occlusion, or a combination of the two have been proposed as causes of the disease, but no clear-cut etiology has yet been determined. The mode of onset differs between the juvenile and the adult forms of the disorder, and the abnormal basal vascular net is more readily developed in children than in adults. Kudoh[9] and Nishimoto[7] presented a follow-up study in which some of the epileptic or infarction variants of the disease present in childhood recurred later as the hemorrhagic type; thus, the findings change as patient age increases. It is believed that in the first decade the stenosis or occlusion develop at the terminal portion of internal carotid artery. As the collateral circulation develops these arteries weaken, resulting in rupture of the collateral vessels in the third decade.

Moyamoya disease can also be congenital as shown by the following: It is prevalent among people of Japanese origin; 12 percent of cases show a strong familial tendency[10]; monozygotic twins occasionally have moyamoya disease[11,12]; this disease is sometimes found in combination with other congenital malformations, e.g., cerebral aneurysm,[13] arteriovenous malformation,[14] fibromuscular dysplasia,[15] Down's syndrome,[16,17] von Recklinghausen's disease,[18] syndactylia,[19] or primitive trigeminal artery[20]; and a considerable number of patients demonstrate immune deficiency.[10] Kitahara reported a relatively high incidence of positive histocompatibility antigens: HLA-AW24, BW46, BW54, and natural T cell toxic autoantibody, or NTA. Natural T cell toxic autoantibody is closely related to autoimmunity.[10]

The acquired nature of moyamoya disease is supported by the following evidence. When arteriosclerosis or trauma leads to the closure of the main cerebral arteries, an abnormal vascular net may develop (Figure 68-2) as a collateral circulation.[21,22]

Kodama et al. sensitized dogs with foreign protein and could demonstrate exfoliation of the intima, thickening of the intimal wall, rupture and telescoping of the elastica interna, thinning of the muscle layer, and necrosis of the media. These findings are similar to those of moyamoya disease and not found

OPERATIVE NEUROSURGICAL TECHNIQUES
ISBN 0-8089-1862-1

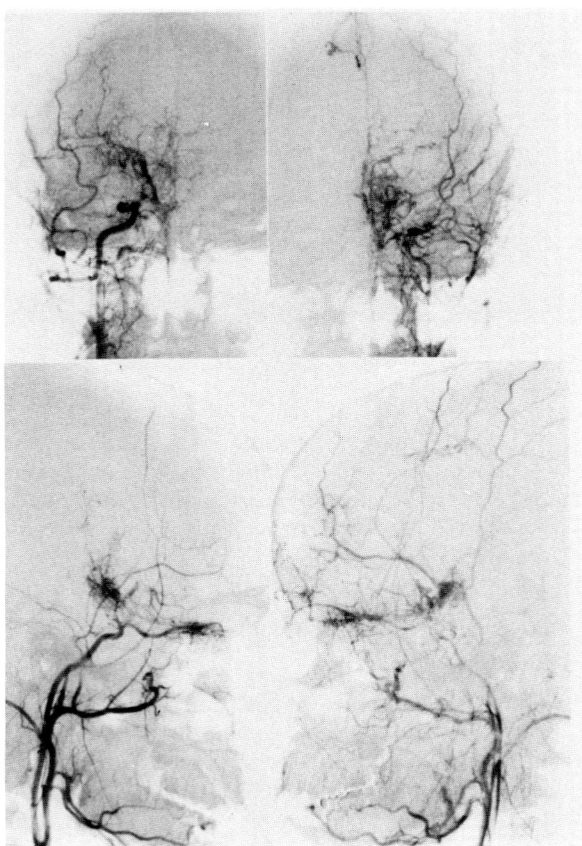

Fig. 68-1. Typical moyamoya disease, seen here in a 9-year-old girl. Upper row: AP views of the right and left hemispheres. Lower row: right and left lateral views. Each internal carotid artery is closed at its terminal portion (siphon). An abnormal vascular net (moyamoya) is seen in the basal area.

in arteries of the distal arterial tree. They observed an increase in the terminal fibers of the sympathetic nerves from the superior cervical ganglion (SCG) in these basal vessels, suggesting that chronic sympathetic stimulation resulted in these pathologic findings.[24]

PATHOLOGY OF MOYAMOYA DISEASE

FINDINGS ON CEREBRAL ANGIOGRAMS

The occlusion in the bilateral internal carotid arteries and the abnormal vascular network of basal arteries serving as a collateral circulation differ in the juvenile and adult forms of the disease. Suzuki classified these findings into 6 phases, and stressed that these phases are aspects of one disease and are of an acquired nature (Figure 68-3).[25]

Mishkin and Schreiber enumerated the varying capacities of the following vessels to form collateral circulation in the following decreasing order: the circle of Willis, parenchymal anastomosis, leptomeningeal collaterals, and transdural cortical anastomosis.[26] These pathways constitute the collateral circulation in moyamoya disease.

The abnormal basal vascular network seen on angiograms consists of dilated parenchymal anastomoses in a basal moyamoya and transdural cortical anastomoses in an ethmoidal[27] or

vault[28] moyamoya. The main vessel supplying an ethmoidal moyamoya is the ophthalmic artery. A vault moyamoya involves a meningeal artery, with contributions from the superficial temporal and occipital arteries with their reverse flow.

An ethmoidal or vault moyamoya is an important collateral circulation, since it develops and increases with increasing age. Insufficient collateral circulation through these vessels can result in mental retardation; the long-term prognosis may be guarded when the disease develops as a result of insufficient collateral circulation in childhood.[29] Takahashi et al. believe that the "adult" form of moyamoya disease should be classified as a transitional form of the juvenile disease when an ethmoidal or vault moyamoya is well developed.[29]

FINDINGS ON COMPUTED TOMOGRAPHIC SCANS

In the ischemic form of moyamoya disease, CT scans may not demonstrate any abnormality within hours of onset other than cerebral atrophy or dilatation of cerebral ventricles if the ischemic process is chronic. In the later stage of infarction, CT scans show an area of low density, mostly in the cortical or subcortical areas. Rarely, a low density area will be seen in the basal ganglia.

When the symptoms of moyamoya disease begin with intracranial bleeding, a characteristic high density abnormality is present on the CT scan, particularly in the paraventricular or intraventricular regions.

FINDINGS IN CEREBRAL CIRCULATION

Many reports indicate that in adults there is rarely an abnormality in regional cerebral blood flow (rCBF) unless cerebral infarction occurs, whereas low flow is often seen in children.[30,31]

Three-dimensional rCBF measurement with xenon-enhanced CT showed low rCBF in the cortical area, particularly in the frontal and temporal regions; the thalamus and basal ganglia had abnormally high rCBF, indicating that the abnormal vascular net increases the rCBF.[32] Gotoh et al., on the other hand, showed that rCBF was normal in the basal ganglia in which moyamoya vessels were present, and concluded that the moyamoya vessels act only as a pathway of collateral circulation.[33]

The response of rCBF to hypercapnia is disturbed in moyamoya disease, but the response to hypocapnia produced by hyperventilation is normal. Carbon dioxide loading does not increase the rCBF as it does in a normal subject; hyperventilation lowers the rCBF as it does in a normal subject. Autoregulation is disturbed in most cases.[34] This strange response to carbon dioxide can be explained as follows: Because a reaction against cerebral ischemia is induced by stenosis or occlusion of the main vessels, other vessels, including the abnormal basal vascular net, become maximally dilated.[35] Additional carbon dioxide loading is unable to increase the dilatation of the affected cerebral arteries further, but the cerebral vessels still retain the ability to constrict in response to hypocapnia, thus decreasing rCBF.

A 33-year-old male developed left hemiplegia 4 months prior to admission. His CT scan (Figure 68-4) showed a low density area in the frontal, temporal, and parietal regions on the right side. Moyamoya disease was diagnosed angiographically.

Table 68-1. Diagnostic guide to moyamoya disease

I. A. The onset of disease spans all age groups but it is more frequent in the young and in females.
    B. The symptoms and course are varied. It can be found accidentally. The course can be transient. The symptoms can be minor or serious or those of fixed neurologic manifestations.
    C. It takes the form of an ischemic disease in juveniles, intracranial bleeding in adults.
    D. In the juvenile form, hemiplegia, monoplegia, sensory abnormality, involuntary movements, headache, or convulsions appear repeatedly as an ictus; these sometimes appear alternatively on the left or right side. Some patients manifest mental retardation or fixed neurologic abnormalities. However, bleeding episodes in juveniles are rare.
    In the adult form some patients may have what appears to be the juvenile form but most show the sudden onset of bleeding episodes in the cerebral ventricles, subarachnoid and intracerebral parenchyma. Many patients improve, but fixed neurologic abnormalities remain. Some become seriously ill and die.

II. Cerebral angiography is mandatory for diagnosis and will show the following:
    A. The end of the intracranial internal carotid artery or the adjacent anterior and middle cerebral arteries are stenosed or obstructed.
    B. An abnormal vascular net is observed near the stenosed artery in the arterial phase.
    C. These findings are present bilaterally.

III. The cause of the disease is unknown.

IV. Pathologic findings suggesting the diagnosis:
    A. Intimal thickening around the end of the internal carotid artery and resultant stenosis or obstruction are present bilaterally.
    B. The fibrous thickening of the intima, telescoping lamina elastica interna, and thinning of the media with various degrees of stenosis and obstructions are often present in the anterior, middle, and posterior communicating arteries, i.e., the circle of Willis.
    C. Many small vessels (perforating and anastomosing branches) are present around the circle of Willis.
    D. A netlike collection of small vessels is often seen in the pia mater.

Adapted from Nishimoto A: Moyamoya disease. Neurol Med Chir (Tokyo) 19:221, 1979.

The terminal portion of the internal carotid artery was obstructed on the right and stenotic on the left. The patient's rCBF studies showed low flow in the frontal, temporal, and parietal areas on the right (Color Plate 68-2). Carbon dioxide loading tests showed a disturbance of carbon dioxide response in the thalamus and basal ganglia (Color Plate 68-2A and D). The distribution of red corpuscles labeled with [99] showed an increase in regional cerebral blood volume (rCBV) in the area of low density on the right in the same slice as that in which the CT scan indicated "compensatory" dilatation of vessels; obstruction of the terminal internal carotid artery was also shown in the same hemisphere. The right cerebral hemisphere showed an increase in red corpuscles (increase in rCBV, Color Plate 68-2B). It was determined that the cerebral vessels were dilated to a significant degree in the right hemisphere, including the thalamus and basal ganglia.

Fluorescein angiography was employed by Takeuchi et al. to study the epicerebral microcirculation of moyamoya disease. These investigators demonstrated a variegated pattern resulting from multiple collateral pathways arising in response to obstruction of the main stem artery.[36] Eguchi et al. observed early venous filling on angiograms (Figure 68-5) and an increase in pial vessels and the presence of red cortical veins (Color Plate 68-3A and B). They concluded that an arteriovenous shunt, the phenomenon of luxury perfusion in ischemic regions, or a reduction of oxygen consumption might exist in the area of the brain affected by a moyamoya.[37]

Table 68-2. Clinical types of moyamoya disease

Clinical Sign	Children	Adults	Total
Hemorrhage	7 (5)*	152 (65)	159 (41)
Seizure	22 (14)	13 (6)	35 (9)
Completed stroke	61 (39)	43 (18)	104 (27)
TIAs	61 (39)	15 (6)	76 (20)
Other	4	11	15
Total	155	234	389

*Numbers in parentheses are percentages of total.
Adapted from Nishimoto A, Ueta K, Onbe H: Cooperative study on moyamoya disease in Japan. Proceedings of the 10th Japanese Conference on Surgery of Cerebral Stroke. Tokyo, Nyuron-sha, 1981, pp 53–58.

ELECTROENCEPHALOGRAPHIC (EEG) FINDINGS

In children, hyperventilation in moyamoya disease induces significant slow wave activity.[38] Kodama observed that the slow waves appearing after hyperventilation differed from those of build-up during hyperventilation in that they were fewer in frequency and more irregular in pattern. In addition, between the build-up waves and the post-hyperventilation slow waves there was a period without slow waves. He named this second period of slow waves "re-build-up" and thought the re-build-up period was useful in screening for moyamoya disease.[39]

Suzuki et al. thought that this re-build-up period derived from the ischemic hypoxia of moyamoya disease overlapping inhibited respiration following hyperventilation (hypoxic hy-

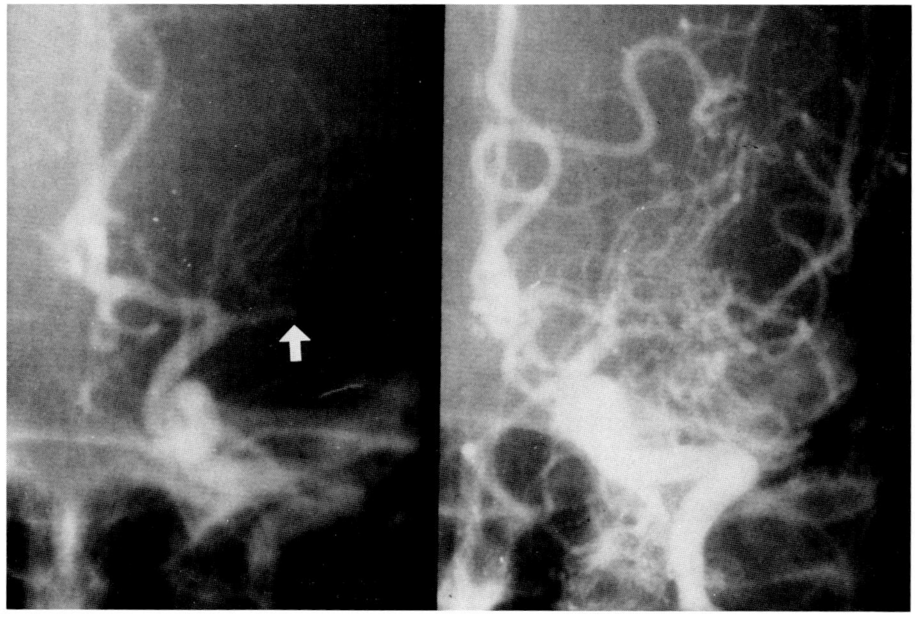

Fig. 68-2. Development of moyamoya vessels in a 2-year-old boy who developed right hemiparesis as a result of an angiographically verified left middle carotid artery occlusion (arrow) without moyamoya vessels. Many newly developed moyamoya vessels were observed in follow-up angiograms taken 6 years later.

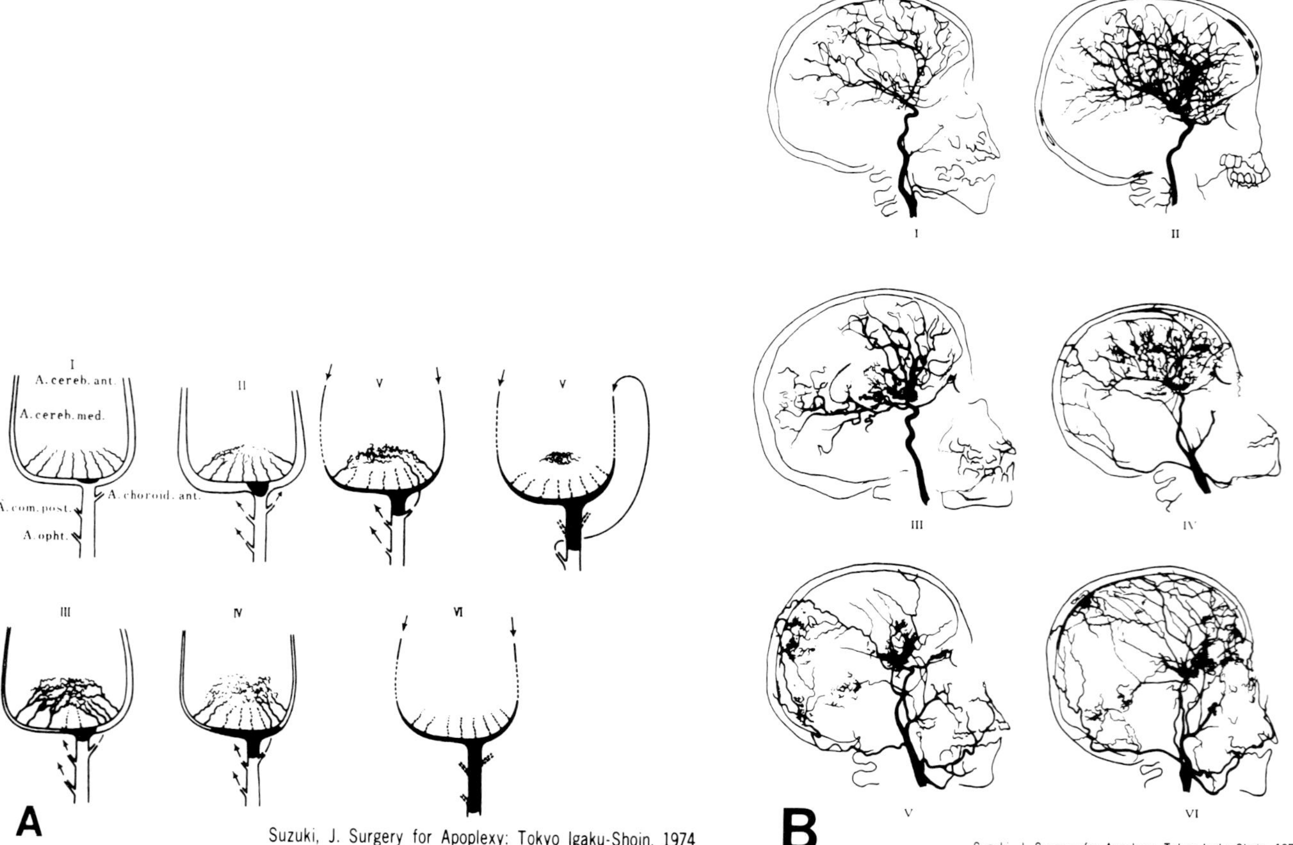

Fig. 68-3. Proposed mechanism of cerebrovascular moyamoya disease. I. Process begins as narrowing of the carotid fork. The vascular pattern is otherwise normal. II. As narrowing progresses, significant poststenotic dilatation is observed intracranially. III. As the narrowing advances further, nebulous (moyamoya) vessels begin to appear, mainly in the area of perforating branches, the diameter of which clearly increases. IV. As obstruction advances, every perforating branch closes, resulting in temporary relapse of symptoms. The thick component of moyamoya vessels gradually begins thinning. The disease process is also oriented to the cerebral base. V. First the middle cerebral artery disappears, then the anterior cerebral artery. VI. As obstruction advances further, it involves the posterior communicating and ophthalmic arteries. The blood supply to the brain via the internal carotid artery ceases and the blood inflow continues only through external and vertebral arteries.

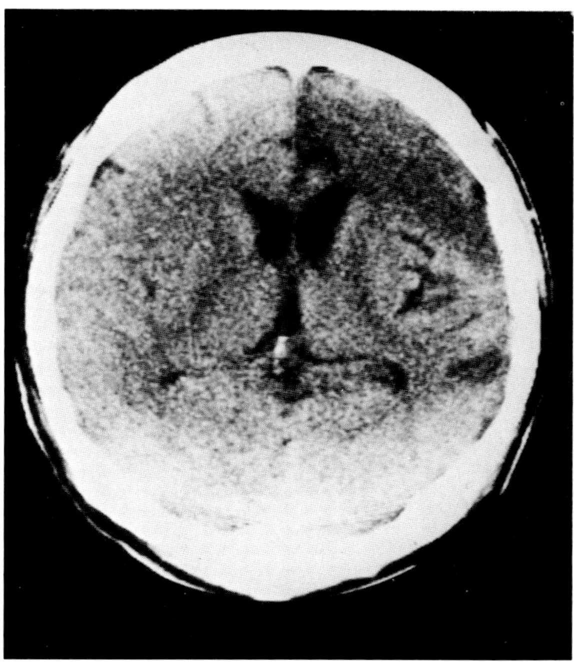

Fig. 68-4. A CT scan of moyamoya disease. The right and left internal carotid arteries are stenotic. An area of low density is apparent on right frontal and temporal areas.

poxia).[40] Takahashi et al. observed through angiography a decrease in the number of basal moyamoya vessels and in the diameter of cortical arteries during the re-build-up period.[41]

THERAPY

Since the etiology of moyamoya disease is not clear, treatment is symptomatic.

Yoshii stated that the improvement seen in the EEG in response to 5-percent carbon dioxide inhalation might suggest a better clinical prognosis.[42] Although various medications have been tried, their effect is not rapid. They consist of cerebral vessel dilators, stimulants of cerebral metabolism, anticonvulsants, steroids, and vitamin C. Also included are antiplatelet agents[43] and calcium antagonists.[44]

Surgical treatment involves (1) durapexis—placing a piece of dura with viable vessels onto the cortical surface[45]; (2) cervical perivascular sympathectomy or superior cervical ganglionectomy[46]; (3) encephalomyosynangiosis (EMS) (Figure 68-6)[47]; (4) superficial temporal-middle cerebral artery anastomosis (Figure 68-7)[48]; (5) omentum transplantation[49,50]; and (6) encephaloduroarteriosynangiosis (EDAS).[51]

The use of cervical perivascular sympathectomy or of superior cervical ganglionectomy is based on the hypothesis that moyamoya disease is related to sympathetic dysfunction. Encephalomyosynangiosis (EMS) and EDAS do not require anastomotic technique. Superficial temporal-middle cerebral artery (STA-MCA) anastomosis is effective only if the diameter of the recipient artery is large enough to supply the required blood flow in the early postoperative period. Omentum transplantation requires laparotomy but is able to supply blood flow for a large area, including the territory of the anterior and posterior cerebral arteries. The EMS procedure involves the possibility of compressing the cerebral cortex, thus inducing postoperative convulsions.

These operations are indicated for transient ischemic attack, reversible ischemic neurologic deficit, minor completed strokes, and convulsions resulting from ischemia. Recently, surgical revascularization has also been performed in select cases of the hemorrhagic type of moyamoya disease.

In the case of extracranial-intracranial (EC/IC) bypass, a large collateral circulation is created, thus reducing the load of the collateral flow through dilated and weakened moyamoya vessels. The moyamoya vessels may therefore occlude and reduce the danger of rupture and resultant bleeding. The decrease in moyamoya vessels has been observed through conventional cerebral angiography[37,52] (Figure 68-8) and radioisotope (RI) angiography.[53,54]

Using angiography, Karasawa et al. followed 8 patients who had undergone bypass surgery for more than 3½ years. Three months after the anastomosis, all the branches of the middle cerebral artery were visualized as a result of the surgical

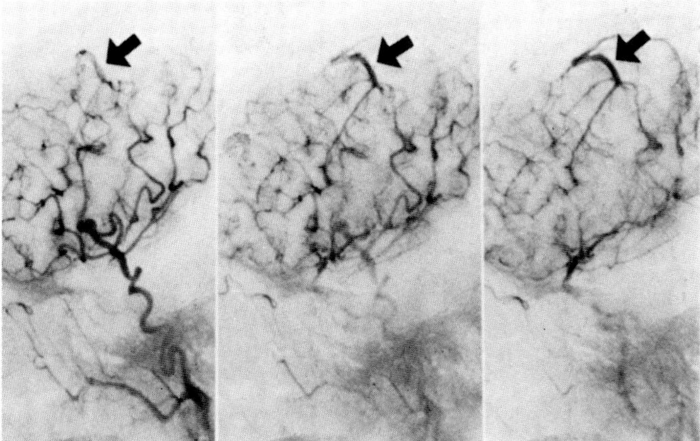

Fig. 68-5. Angiographical indication of early venous filling. In moyamoya disease, it is thought that the blood circulation in the brain is slow; because of this slow circulation, the veins of the brain appear in a very late stage in angiograms. We observed, however, in some of our cases, an early venous filling of the internal cerebral vein, the basal vein of Rosenthal, and the ascending cortical vein (arrow). In the brains of those affected by moyamoya disease, there must be some areas in which the blood circulation is rather fast.

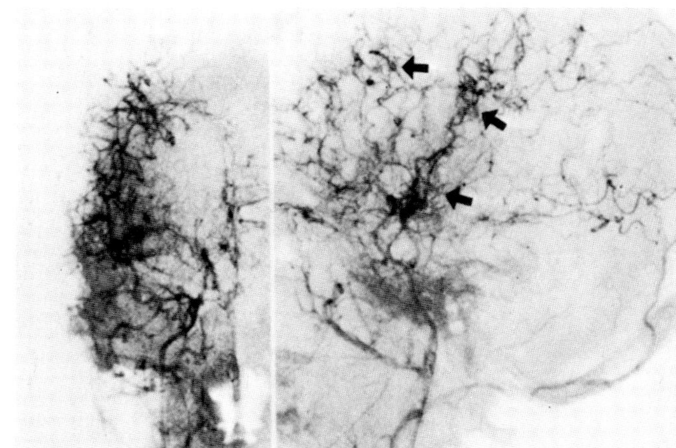

Fig. 68-6. A 9-year-old girl in whom moyamoya disease began as TIAs. Cerebral angiogram obtained 10 months after EMS. External carotid injection. Left: PA view. Right: lateral view. The cerebral arteries are visualized via spontaneous revascularization (arrows) from the temporal muscle.

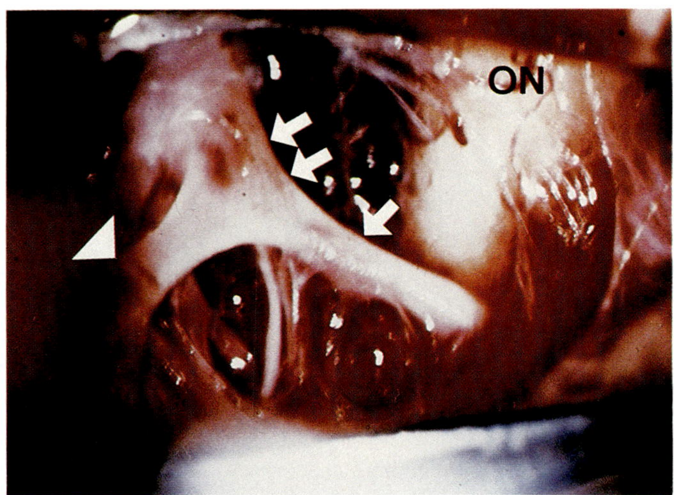

Color Plate 68-1. A 36-year-old man. Intraoperative photograph of the carotid fork. At age 10, this patient's ictus began as TIAs with left hemiplegia. Intracerebral bleeding heralded illness this time. Intracerebral hematoma was removed. The left internal carotid artery (double arrows), left middle carotid artery, M1 (arrowhead), and left anterior carotid artery, A1 (single arrow), are stenosed; dilated perforators are also seen. ON = optic nerve.

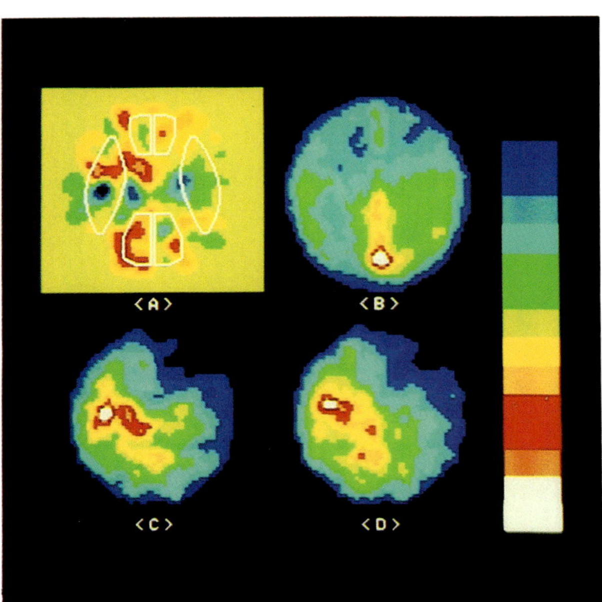

Color Plate 68-2. (A, C, and D) rCBF images. (C) rCBF while subject is at rest, eyes closed. Low flow is observed in the right frontal, temporal, and parietal areas. (D) rCBF with carbon dioxide loading after Diamox injection. No significant increase in rCBF is observed. Note the decrease in the thalamus and basal ganglia. (A) Subtraction image, D minus C. (B) Cerebral blood volume (^{99m}Tc-labeled RBCs). Although the blood flow decreases in the right cerebral hemisphere where the internal carotid artery is obstructed (per cerebral angiography), the blood volume increases, indicating that the cerebral arteries are dilated in order to compensate for ischemia.

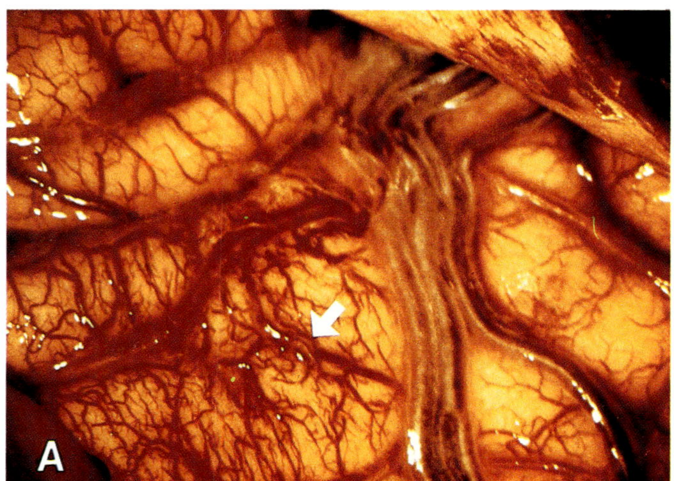

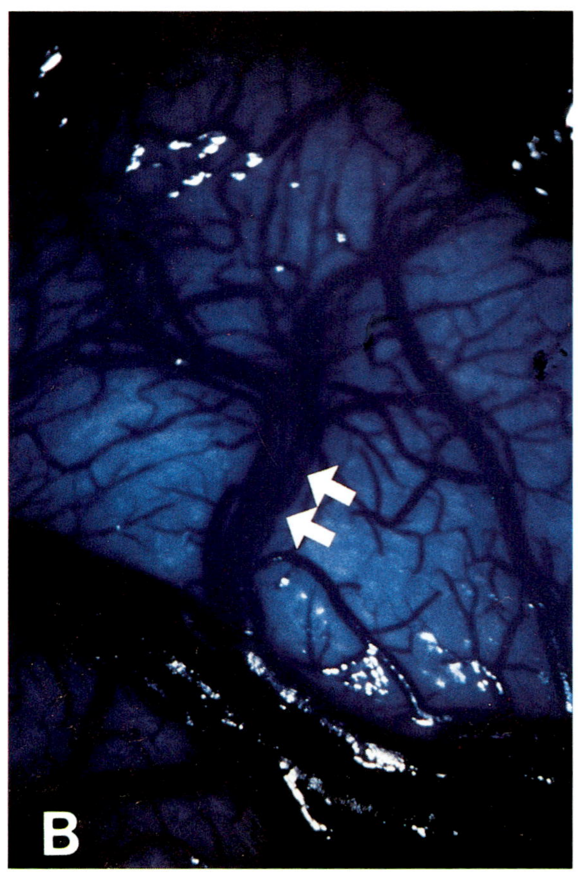

Color Plate 68-3. Increase in number of pial vessels and red cortical veins. On the cortical surface, an increase in the number of pial vessels is observed (A, arrow), as is an increase in the number of red cortical veins (B, arrow), in which the arterial and venous blood showed a laminar flow. An arteriovenous shunt, a phenomenon of luxury perfusion, or reduction of oxygen consumption might exist in the brains of those affected by moyamoya disease.

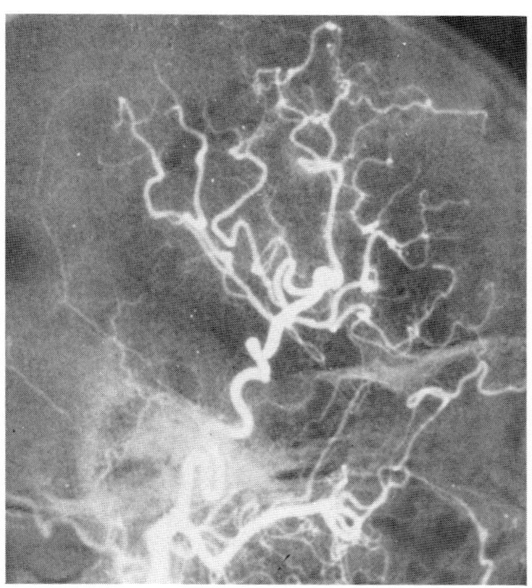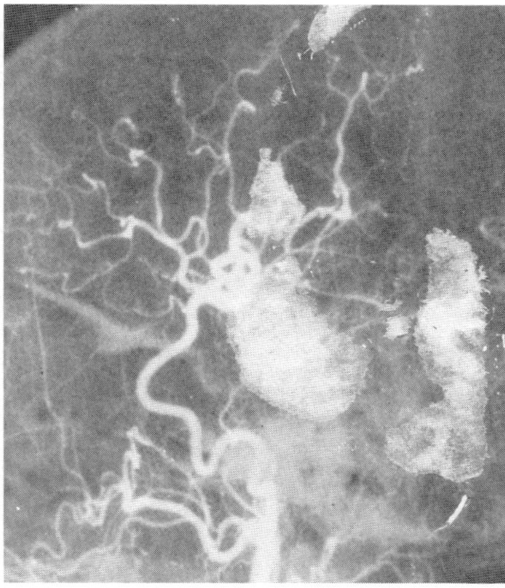

Fig. 68-7. A 39-year-old woman in whom moyamoya disease began as intraventricular hemorrhage. Cerebral angiogram after STA-MCA anastomosis. Lateral views. Left: right-sided injection. Right: left-sided injection.

anastomosis and spontaneous anastomosis of the middle meningeal artery. Later, the anastomosis closed, and a fine vascular net developed in situ through which flow to the middle cerebral artery was visualized.[52] They determined that the pathologic process was also progressing in the cortical branches of the middle cerebral artery.[55]

Takemoto, Koike, and others evaluated the effectiveness of STA-MCA anastomosis using vascular imaging with ^{99m}Tc-labeled red blood cells (RBC) (RI angiography). They observed early and significant RI activity in the abnormal basal vascular network, but this activity appeared very late in the area of the anterior and middle cerebral arteries; postoperatively, the ac-

tivity decreased in the basal area, increased in the area of the middle cerebral artery (MCA), and showed no increase in the anterior cerebral artery (ACA) territory. They calculated the local mode of transit time (MOTT) and found an improvement in the cortical circulation.[53,54] These findings coincide with the finding that angiographic visualization of cortical vessels, mainly of the MCA, improves, and that the abnormal basal vascular network decreases.

When preoperative and postoperative CBF, the cerebral metabolic rate of oxygen consumption ($CMRO_2$), and the cerebral metabolic rate of glucose consumption (CMRGl) were measured, Mitsugi et al.,[56] obtained the following results. The CBF increased until the second postoperative day, decreased in

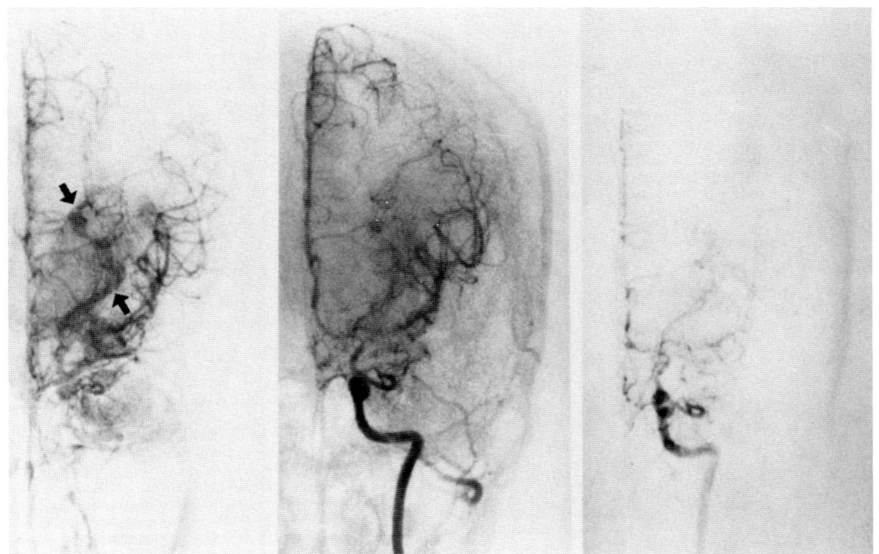

Fig. 68-8. A 15-year-old girl affected by moyamoya disease in whom symptoms began with subarachnoid hemorrhage. Left: moyamoya vessels as visualized preoperatively (arrows). Center: the moyamoya vessels are seen to have diminished 1 week after STA-MCA anastomosis. Right: 3 months after the operation the moyamoya vessels have disappeared.

the following month, and then increased again, reaching aplateau (higher than the preoperative values) by the third month. The CMRO$_2$ and CMRGl showed higher values after the sixth postoperative month.[56]

Takahashi et al. observed EEG changes and found a worsening during the first week after the operation. Improvement was then observed after the third month until the EEG status was better than that observed preoperatively.[57] These findings led to the practice of a unilateral operation followed by surgery on the remaining side 3 months later in cases in which bilateral operations were required.

The STA-MCA anastomosis procedure or EMS will improve posterior basal moyamoyas. Miyamoto called this diminution of a moyamoya the indirect redistribution effect.[2] Waga observed the disappearance of a cerebral aneurysm of the posterior choroidal artery accompanying moyamoya disease when bilateral STA-MCA anastomosis and EMS were performed and concluded that the surgical revascularization of the anterior circulation reduced the load on a basal moyamoya of the posterior circulation.[58]

The PaCO$_2$ should be maintained at about 45 mm Hg in order to avoid hypocapnia during general anesthesia. Arterial hypotension should also be avoided. These measures are of greatest importance in juvenile cases.[59,60]

SURGICAL RESULTS

Kasai followed 31 juvenile and 17 adult patients treated by cervical perivascular sympathectomy or superior cervical ganglionectomy from 6 months to 12 years. Improvement was observed in 61.3 percent and 47.1 percent of the juvenile and adult patients, respectively. He stated that these extracranial procedures should be the first surgical methods tried before other methods are employed.[61]

Karasawa et al. reported on 69 cases—53 juvenile and 16 adult—followed for 4½ years. Significant improvement, i.e., disappearance of TIAs and recovery of neurologic deficit except for homonymous hemianopia or mental disturbance, was seen in 50.7 percent of the patients. Good results, i.e., fewer episodes of TIAs, disappearance of minor neurologic deficits with occasional TIA attacks, or improvement of major neurologic deficits, were achieved in 31.9 percent of the patients. Of the remaining patients, 10.1 percent showed minimal improvement of major deficits; 4.3 percent had an unaltered status; 1.4 percent worsened; and 1.4 percent died. An evaluation of daily life activities (ADL evaluation) showed excellent results (complete return to previous activity) in 50.7 percent of patients; good results (return with some minor limitations) in 34.8 percent; fair results (able to maintain self-care, but social life difficult) in 11.6 percent; and poor results (unable to maintain self-care) in 1.4 percent. Most of the 8 ''fair'' cases showed mental disturbance.[62] It is believed that surgical intervention should be carried out before mental disturbance becomes manifest. The STA-MCA anastomosis procedure or EMS did not improve visual acuity or field defect. Although omentum transplantation was attempted in an effort to improve circulation in a large area, including the territory of the posterior cerebral artery, and in an effort to improve visual acuity or field defect, its effectiveness is uncertain at this time.

The EDAS procedure in juvenile cases is simple. It does not disturb the anastomosis already present and does not compress the cerebral cortex, thus minimizing postoperative convulsion. Matsushima reported on 10 cases treated by this method with follow-ups of 21 to 51 months. The TIAs disappeared in all cases; motor ability improved in 4 cases. Mental disturbance did not diminish in any cases.[63]

These reports indicate that moyamoya disease is a progressive ailment; surgical procedures should be considered before mental disturbance becomes apparent.

REFERENCES

1. Kudoh T (ed): A Disease with Abnormal Intracranial Vascular Networks—Spontaneous Occlusion of the Circle of Willis. Tokyo, Igaku Shoin, 1967
2. Miyamoto S, Kikuchi H, Karasawa J, et al: Study on the vertebrobasilar system in "Moyamoya" disease. Brain Nerve (Tokyo) 36:491, 1984
3. Gadoth N, Hirsch M: Primary and acquired forms of Moyamoya syndrome. A review and three case reports. Israel J Med Sci 16:370, 1980
4. Meriwether RP, Barnett HG, Echols DH: Moyamoya disease as a cause of subarachnoid hemorrhage in a negro patient. J Neurosurg 44:620, 1976
5. Peh WCG, Kwok RK: Moyamoya disease in Singapore. Ann Acad Med Singapore 14:71, 1985
6. Taveras JM: Multiple progressive intracranial arterial occlusions: A syndrome of children and young adults. AJR 106:235, 1969
7. Nishimoto A, Ueta K, Onbe H: Cooperative study on Moyamoya disease in Japan. Proceedings of the 10th Japanese Conference on Surgery of Cerebral Stroke. Tokyo, Nyuron-sha, 1981, pp 53–58
8. Nishimoto A: Moyamoya disease. Neurol Med Chir (Tokyo) 19:221, 1979
9. Kudo T, Fukuda S: Spontaneous occlusion of the circle of Willis. Sinkei Shinpo (Tokyo) 20:170, 1976
10. Kitahara T, Semba A, Yamaura A, et al: Genetical and immunological analysis on Moyamoya disease. Proceedings of the 10th Japanese Conference on Surgery of Cerebral Stroke. Tokyo, Nyuron-sha, 1981, pp 27–30
11. Kashihara M, Oki H, Sasaki K, et al: Adult identical twins with Moyamoya disease. Neurol Surg (Tokyo) 12:1425, 1984
12. Sonobe M, Takahashi S, Urakawa Y, et al: "Moyamoya" disease found in identical twins. Neurol Surg (Tokyo) 8:1183, 1980
13. Furuse S, Matsumoto S, Tanaka Y, et al: Moyamoya disease associated with a false aneurysm—Case report and review of the literature. Neurol Surg (Tokyo) 10:1005, 1982
14. Kayama T, Suzuki S, Sakurai Y, et al: A case of Moyamoya disease accompanied by an arteriovenous malformation. Neurosurg 18:465, 1986
15. Terasawa K, Yamaguchi Y, Ishihara O, et al: Moya-moya disease associated with fibromuscular dysplasia of renal artery. No To Hattatsu (Tokyo) 15:350, 1983
16. Ichiba N, Murakawa S, Ohtahara S: A case of Down's syndrome with "Moyamoya" disease: A consideration on the fibromuscular dysplasia. No To Hattatsu (Tokyo) 16:487, 1984
17. Nishimura M, Takakura H, Ieshima A, et al: A case of Down's syndrome with Moya Moya disease. No To Hattatsu (Tokyo) 17:71, 1985
18. Chono Y, Ueno K, Nunomura M, et al: Von Recklinghausen's disease associated with occlusion of bilateral middle cerebral artery, Moyamoya phenomenon, and an anterior communicating artery aneurysm. Report of an autopsy case. Neurol Med Chir (Tokyo) 25:209, 1985

19. Kato Y, Kurokawa T, Hasuo K, et al: Moyamoya disease with a developmental anomaly of the mesenchyme. Eur J Pediatr 144:93, 1985

20. Kwak R, Kadoya S: Moyamoya disease associated with persistent primitive trigeminal artery. Report of two cases. J Neurosurg 59:166, 1983

21. Fukawa O, Aihara H, Wakasa H: Middle cerebral artery occlusion with Moyamoya phenomenon. Second report: Report of an autopsy case. Neurol Surg (Tokyo) 10:1303, 1982

22. Yamada K, Hayakawa T, Ushio Y, et al: Cerebral arterial dolichoectasia associated with Moyamoya vessels. Surg Neurol 23:19, 1985

23. Takebayashi S, Matsuo K, Kaneko M: Ultrastructural studies of cerebral arteries and collateral vessels in Moyamoya disease. Stroke 15:728, 1984

24. Kodama N, Fujiwara S, Kasai N, et al: The experimental study on causal genesis of Moyamoya disease—Correlation with immunological reaction and sympathetic nerve influence for vascular changes. Proceedings of the 10th Japanese Conference on Surgery of Cerebral Stroke. Tokyo, Nyuron-sha, 1981, pp 17–26

25. Suzuki J: Cerebral Moyamoya disease, in Suzuki J (ed): Surgery of Stroke. Tokyo, Igaku Shoin, 1974, pp 291–302

26. Mishkin MM, Schreiber MN: Collateral circulation, in Newton TH, Potts DG (eds): Radiology of the Skull and Brain. Angiography. St. Louis, CV Mosby, 1974, pp 2344–2374

27. Suzuki J, Kodama N: Cerebrovascular "moyamoya" disease. Second report: Collateral routes to forebrain via ethmoid sinus and superior nasal meatus. Angiography 22:223, 1971

28. Kodama N, Fujiwara S, Horie Y, et al: Transdural anastomosis in Moyamoya disease—Vault moyamoya. Neurol Surg (Tokyo) 8(8):729, 1980

29. Takahashi A, Fujiwara S, Suzuki J: Long-term follow-up angiography of Moyamoya disease—Cases followed up from childhood to adolescence. Neurol Surg (Tokyo) 14:23, 1986

30. Nagao T, Nukui H, Miyagi O, et al: Cerebral hemodynamics in cases with "Moyamoya" disease. Neurol Med Chir (Tokyo) 22:707, 1982

31. Ogawa A, Kogure T, Fujiwara S, et al: Regional cerebral blood flow on Moyamoya disease—Study with ^{133}Xe intravenous injection method. Proceedings of the 10th Japanese Conference on Surgery of Cerebral Stroke. Tokyo, Nyuron-sha, 1981, pp 189–194

32. Suzuki R, Tsuruoka S, Hiratsuka H, et al: Cerebral circulation in pediatric patients with Moyamoya disease. Tomographic cerebral blood flow map obtained by Xenon-enhanced computerized tomography. Neurol Med Chir (Tokyo) 25:969, 1985

33. Gotoh F, Ebihara S, Sakai F, et al: Cerebral circulation and metabolism of occlusion of circle of Willis (part 3). Study of moyamoya disease. Ministry of Health and Welfare, Japan, 1980, pp 65–71

34. Ohta H, Ito Z, Suzuki A, et al: Regional cerebral blood flow in Moyamoya disease evaluated by ^{133}Xe intracarotid injection method. Proceedings of the 10th Japanese Conference on Surgery of Cerebral Stroke. Tokyo, Nyuron-sha, 1981, pp 167–173

35. Uemura K, Yamaguchi K, Kojima S, et al: Regional cerebral blood flow on cerebrovascular "Moyamoya" disease—Study by ^{133}Xe clearance method and cerebral angiography. Brain Nerve (Tokyo) 27(4):385, 1975

36. Takeuchi S, Ishii R, Tsuchida T, et al: Cerebral hemodynamics in patients with Moyamoya disease. A study of the epicerebral microcirculation by fluorescein angiography. Surg Neurol 21:333, 1984

37. Eguchi T, Oka H, Suzuki I, et al: Angiographical early venous filling, red cortical vein, intraarterial pressure and CBF values in Moyamoya disease. Proceedings of the 10th Japanese Conference on Surgery of Cerebral Stroke. Tokyo, Nyuron-sha, 1981, pp 273–280

38. Yoshii N, Kudo T: Electroencephalographical study on occlusion of the Willis arterial ring. Clin Neurol (Tokyo) 8:301, 1968

39. Kodama N, Aoki Y, Hiraga H, et al: Electroencephalographic findings in children with Moyamoya disease. Acta Neurol 36:16, 1979

40. Suzuki J, Ohyama H, Niizuma H, et al: Simultaneous recording of EEG, tcPO₂, tcPCO₂ and respiration curve in pre- and posthyperventilation periods of juvenile moyamoya disease—Mechanism of build up and re-build up. Study of Moyamoya disease. Ministry of Health and Welfare, Japan, 1983, pp 124–135

41. Takahashi A, Fujiwara S, Suzuki J: Cerebral angiography following hyperventilation in Moyamoya disease—In reference to the "rebuild up" phenomenon on EEG. Neurol Surg (Tokyo) 13:255, 1985

42. Yoshii N, Samejima H, Mizokami T, et al: Long term followup study of "Moyamoya Disease" (occlusion of circle of Willis) with drug therapy. Proceedings of the 10th Japanese Conference on Surgery of Cerebral Stroke. Tokyo, Nyuron-sha, 1981, pp 12–15

43. Albala MM, Levine PH: Platelet factor 4 and beta thromboglobulin in Moya-Moya disease. Am J Pediatr Hematol Oncol 6:96, 1984

44. McLean MJ, Gebarski SS, Goldstein GW, et al: Response of Moyamoya disease to Verapamil (Letter). Lancet 1:163, 1985

45. Tsubokawa T, Kikuchi M, Asano S, et al: Surgical treatment for intracranial thrombosis, case report of "Durapexia." Neurol Med Chir (Tokyo) 6:428, 1964

46. Suzuki J, Takaku A, Kodama N, et al: An attempt to treat cerebrovascular moyamoya disease. Childs Brain 1:193, 1975

47. Karasawa J, Kikuchi H, Furuse S, et al: A surgical treatment of "moyamoya" disease. "Encephalo-myo synangiosis." Neurol Med Chir (Tokyo) 17(part 1):29, 1977

48. Karasawa J, Kikuchi H, Furuse S, et al: Treatment of moyamoya disease with STA-MCA anastomosis. J Neurosurg 49:679, 1978

49. Kikuchi H, Karasawa J, Takahashi N: EC/IC bypass surgery for occlusive cerebrovascular lesion. Neurol Med Chir (Tokyo) 20:115, 1980

50. Yonekawa Y, Handa H: Surgical treatment of occlusive cerebrovascular disease. Brain Nerve (Tokyo) 32:239, 1980

51. Matsushima Y, Fukai N, Tanaka K, et al: A new surgical treatment of Moyamoya disease in children: A preliminary report. Surg Neurol 15:313, 1981

52. Karasawa J, Kikuchi H, Kobayashi K, et al: Evaluation of angiographical changes after ST-MC anastomosis in "Moyamoya" disease. Proceedings of the 10th Japanese Conference on Surgery of Cerebral Stroke. Tokyo, Nyuron-sha, 1981, pp 313–317

53. Koike T, Kikuchi H, Karasawa J, et al: Evaluation of radioisotope studies after surgical treatment in "Moyamoya" disease. Proceedings of the 10th Japanese Conference on Surgery of Cerebral Stroke. Tokyo, Nyuron-sha, 1981, pp 318–322

54. Takemoto M, Motoki M, Yoshioka J, et al: Follow up study of Moyamoya disease with Tc-RBCs vascular imaging. Proceedings of the 10th Japanese Conference on Surgery of Cerebral Stroke. Tokyo, Nyuron-sha, 1981, pp 301–305

55. Kobayashi K, Takeuchi S, Tsuchida T, et al: Encephalomyosynangiosis (EMS) in Moyamoya disease. Neurol Med Chir (Tokyo) 21:1229, 1981

56. Mitsugi T, Kikuchi H, Karasawa J, et al: Evaluation of CBF studies, changes of CBF and cerebral metabolism after surgical treatment in "Moyamoya" disease. Proceedings of the 10th Japanese Conference on Surgery of Cerebral Stroke. Tokyo, Nyuron-sha, 1981, pp 323–327

57. Takahashi N, Kikuchi H, Karasawa J, et al: Evaluation of EEG changes after surgical treatment in the children with "Moyamoya" disease. Proceedings of the 10th Japanese Conference on Surgery of Cerebral Stroke. Tokyo, Nyuron-sha, 1981, pp 334–339

58. Waga S, Tochio H: Intracranial aneurysm associated with Moyamoya disease in children. Surg Neurol 23:237, 1985

59. Bingham RM, Wilkinson DJ: Anesthetic management in Moya-Moya disease. Anesthesia 40:1198, 1985

60. Kuro M, Karasawa J, Kuriyama Y, et al: Anesthetic management of "Moyamoya" disease in children. Proceedings of the 10th Japa-

nese Conference on Surgery of Cerebral Stroke. Tokyo, Nyuron-sha, 1981, pp 207–211

61. Kasai N, Fujiwara S, Kodama N, et al: Surgical treatment in Moyamoya disease. Proceedings of the 10th Japanese Conference on Surgery of Cerebral Stroke. Tokyo, Nyuron-sha, 1981, pp 221–224

62. Karasawa J, Kikuchi H: Surgery of cerebrovascular disease.

"Moyamoya" disease. Japanisch-deutsche medizinische Berichte 29:367, 1984

63. Matsushima Y, Tomita H, Takei H, et al: Changes in symptoms after encephaloduroarteriosynangiosis (EDAS) in pediatric Moyamoya disease, in Spetzler RF, Carter LP, Selman WR, et al (eds): Cerebral Revascularization for Stroke. Stuttgart, Georg Thieme Verlag, 1985, pp 578–583

CHAPTER 69

Posterior Fossa Revascularization

James I. Ausman
Dante F. Vacca
Carl E. Shrontz
Randy Gehring

Fernando G. Diaz
R.A. de los Reyes
Jeffrey E. Pearce

THE SYNDROME of vertebrobasilar insufficiency (VBI) was brought to the attention of clinicians in 1946 with the publication of a report on a series of patients selected at autopsy with basilar artery occlusion by Kubik and Adams.[1] Subsequently, a number of reports appeared that attempted to further define the symptomatology, incidence, pathology, natural history, and treatment of VBI.[2,3] The incidence of VBI has been reported to be approximately half that of symptomatic anterior circulation ischemia.[4] As in the anterior circulation, atherosclerosis is by far the most common disease process affecting the posterior circulation.[3] Atherogenic stenotic and occlusive lesions have been described from the vertebral origins to the posterior cerebral arteries,[5] however, precise clinical localization has been rarely possible prior to angiography.[6] The natural history of these various pathologic lesions remains unknown and speculative, except, perhaps, for basilar occlusion, for which the mortality ranges from 44 to 70 percent within 14 weeks after angiographic diagnosis.[2,7,8] The best available information at present for transient ischemic attacks (TIAs) referable to the posterior circulation (in an un-angiogrammed population) is an infarction risk of 35 percent over 4 years.[4]

Pathophysiologic mechanisms in VBI include, singly or in combination, hypoperfusion, arterial emboli, penetrating branch disease, thrombosis, vessel wall disease, and hypercoagulation.[2,3] Treatment strategies must take these into consideration, as well as taking into consideration the anatomy of the disease. A number of studies have reported the efficacy of coumadin in reducing the incidence of infarction in a population of patients with clinical VBI.[9,10] In these trials, however, the diagnosis was not confirmed by angiography and the patients were not randomized into treatment and control groups. Similarly, no study has shown antiplatelet agents to be beneficial in decreasing the incidence of stroke in a randomized population of patients with angiographically demonstrated vertebrobasilar disease.[2,3]

The continued refinements in neuroradiology have made complete visualization of the vertebrobasilar circulation possible with minimal morbidity and mortality.[2] Progress in microvascular techniques, neuroanesthesia, and instrumentation has enabled surgeons to bypass stenotic and occlusive lesions at all levels of the vertebrobasilar system. In this chapter, we will describe the surgical technique and review our experience with the following posterior fossa revascularization procedures: (1) vertebral to carotid transposition (VCT); (2) distal vertebral endarterectomy (DVEA); (3) occipital artery to posterior inferior cerebellar artery (OA-PICA) bypass; (4) occipital artery to anterior inferior cerebellar artery (OA-AICA) bypass; and (5) superficial temporal artery to superior cerebellar artery (STA-SCA) bypass

SURGICAL INDICATIONS

In general, patients who are considered candidates for posterior fossa revascularization are individuals who have had ongoing symptoms of VBI. Patients undergoing posterior fossa revascularization at Henry Ford Hospital have nearly all been treated with antiplatelet agents and most have also been treated with coumadin or heparin and have remained refractory to these medical interventions. The diagnosis of VBI is suspected when patients have at least two of the following symptoms, or with signs of posterior circulation ischemia: vertigo or dizziness, dysarthria, diplopia, dysphagia, bilateral visual field complaints or deficits, ataxia, mono) to quadriparesis, mono) to quadrihypesthesia, alternating paresis or hypesthesia, and perioral numbness. Most patients we evaluate have four or more of these symptoms and signs. Chronic dizziness and so-called ''drop attacks'' occurring in the absence of other symptoms are rarely, if ever, a feature of VBI.[2,3] Many of our patients have a mild to moderate fixed neurologic deficit indicative of previous infarction in addition to recurrent TIAs. A substantial number of patients have crescendo TIAs or stroke in evolution and are considered clinically unstable.

Once the diagnosis is suspected by history and physical examination, blood work, including a complete blood count and coagulation profile, an electrocardiogram, and a CT scan of the head with and without intravenous contrast are obtained. An echocardiogram, electroencephalogram, otologic evaluation, and Holter monitoring are obtained if suggested clinically. If these fail to disclose a nonvascular cause of the patient's symptoms, we proceed with complete, selective, 4-vessel cerebral angiography, utilizing subtraction and magnification techniques. Regional cerebral blood flow (rCBF) measurements applied to the posterior fossa have been difficult to interpret secondary to artifactual contamination from the cervico-occip-

OPERATIVE NEUROSURGICAL TECHNIQUES
ISBN 0-8089-1862-1

ital musculature and naso-oropharynx.[11] As rCBF techniques improve, they may provide valuable additional information in the evaluation of patients with VBI. Newer diagnostic modalities such as positron emission tomography and magnetic resonance imaging may allow physiologic determination of reversible ischemia and aid in the selection of patients for revascularization.

The decision to intervene surgically is based on the synthesis of all obtained data, and primarily on the patient's clinical course, the angiographic demonstration of an appropriate hemodynamically significant lesion, and the absence of significant contribution of blood flow from the anterior circulation across the posterior communicating arteries. The surgical procedure required for revascularization is directed by the anatomy of disease. Absolute contraindications to revascularization include acute established infarction and severe, fixed neurologic deficits secondary to remote infarction. Relative contraindications include multiple and advanced systemic disease, including cardiopulmonary disease, diabetes mellitus, cancer, and hepatic and renal insufficiency.

PREOPERATIVE PREPARATION

At bedtime the evening before surgery, the patient receives intravenous fluids and 1 g cefazolin intravenously, and 4 mg dexamethasone orally. If the patient is scheduled for an STA-SCA bypass, that patient is loaded with diphenylhydantoin orally. On call to the operating room, the patient receives 1 g cefazolin and 4 mg dexamethasone intravenously, and 60 mg codeine, 100 mg seconal, and 0.2 mg glycopyrrolate intramuscularly. Patients take their pre-admission medications as usual, with a small sip of water.

The patient is then taken to the preoperative holding area, where an arterial line is placed for continuous blood pressure monitoring. If the patient has a history of significant cardiopulmonary disease or is elderly and suspected of having limited cardiopulmonary reserve, a Swan-Ganz pulmonary artery catheter is inserted. The patient's head and neck are then shaved. The patient is transported to the operating room and transferred to the operating table. ECG leads are placed and cardiac activity, blood pressure, and central cardiac pressures are continuously displayed. General anesthesia is induced and maintained with barbiturates, narcotics, and isoflurane. A reinforced endotracheal tube is utilized for DVEA, OA-PICA and OA-AICA bypasses. Blood pressure is carefully monitored and maintained at preoperative values with intravenous fluids and pressors as required to avoid a drop in cerebral perfusion pressure. An esophageal stethoscope/temperature monitor is placed along with a Foley urinary catheter to closed drainage. A lumbar spinal drain is placed if the patient is to have a STA-SCA bypass.

All patients are positioned in a horizontal fashion, thereby minimizing the potential for hypotension, air embolism, and surgeon fatigue that are associated with the sitting position. As the patient is positioned, pressure points are carefully padded. A Doppler ultrasound probe is then used to trace the course of the STA or OA as required. Concurrently, the operating microscope is being prepared, utilizing the 12.5× eyepieces and 250-mm objective. The patient is then prepared and draped in a sterile manner. The initial incision and subsequent dissection is achieved with the Shaw electric scalpel and bipolar cautery, which allows nearly bloodless surgery.

VERTEBRAL TO CAROTID TRANSPOSITION (VCT)

The most common site of disease in the vertebral artery is at its origin.[5] Angiographic findings in patients considered candidates for VCT indicate severe proximal vertebral stenosis with contralateral vertebral occlusion, hypoplasia, or severe stenosis. Symptomatic subclavian steal syndrome is also a surgical indication. A number of surgical procedures have been devised to reconstruct these lesions, including endarterectomy and interposition vein grafting.[11] However, these operations were often technically difficult and fraught with intraoperative and postoperative complications, including vertebral artery occlusion, lymphoceles, chyle cysts and fistulas, phrenic nerve paresis, pneumothorax, and vocal cord paralysis. In 1972, Edwards and Wright described the VCT procedure,[13] which we believe to be the safest and most effective approach to lesions of the proximal vertebral artery. When necessary, this technique also allows simultaneous carotid endarterectomy.[14]

OPERATIVE TECHNIQUE

The patient is positioned supine, with the neck slightly extended. A transverse cervical incision is made from the midline to the lateral border of the sternocleidomastoid (SCM) at the inferior-most natural skin crease 1.5 to 3.0 cm above the clavicle. The platysma is incised transversely, and subsequent dissection undercutting superiorly exposes the medial border of the SCM. The SCM is dissected laterally and the strap muscles medially, exposing the jugular vein. The jugular vein is then retracted laterally and the common carotid artery is exposed on entering the carotid sheath. The carotid artery is retracted laterally, exposing the posterior cervical fascia. Palpation of the carotid tubercle identifies the C6 transverse process, and facilitates dissection of the vertebral artery just below the inverted V formed by the insertions of the anterior scalene and longus colli muscles onto the tubercle. In most cases, a large vein lies superficial to the vertebral artery, and this must be dissected free and retracted. The vertebral artery is then exposed proximally to its origin. Utmost care is required at this point to identify and ligate or coagulate, with bipolar coagulation, lymphatic vessels draining into the subclavian vein. When the procedure is performed on the right side, care must be taken to avoid injury to the recurrent laryngeal nerve, which is most often located below the origin of the inferior thyroid vein.

Following complete dissection of the vertebral artery, the patient is given 5000 units of heparin intravenously. After a ligature and permanent clip are placed at the origin and a temporary clip at the level of the foramen transversarium of the vertebral artery, it is transected proximally. Back bleeding from the vertebral artery is then checked. The artery is then irrigated with heparinized saline. On exceptional occasions, it may be necessary to resect the anterior surface of the C6 foramen transversarium with rongeurs and to dissect the vertebral artery further distally in order to gain length needed to complete the anastomosis. With this maneuver, one must be careful to avoid injury to possible radicular branches. Also, in this instance, the periarterial venous plexus must be carefully bipolared and divided before vertebral mobilization. If atherosclerotic plaque involves the proximal vertebral artery, it is gently excised with eversion of the artery over the plaque until totally removed. A fishmouth arteriotomy is made at the proximal vertebral artery. The patient is then given 250 mg thiopental and 100 mg lidocaine

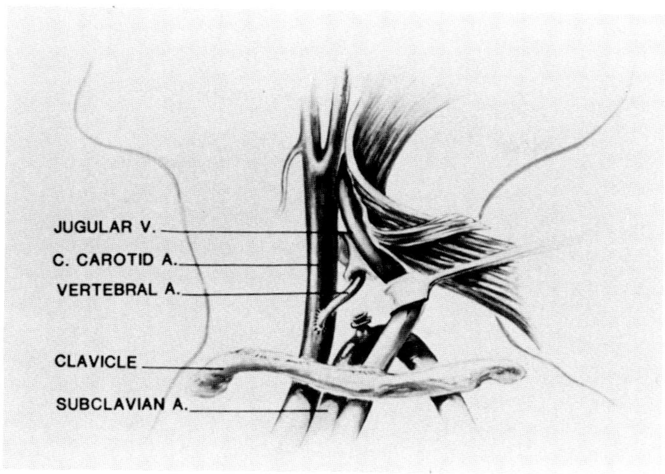

Fig. 69-1. Vertebral to carotid transposition (VCT).

intravenously. A segment of ipsiltaeral common carotid artery is isolated between two vascular clamps, and with a 4- or 5-mm arterial punch, a circular arterectomy is made in the medial wall. Heparinized saline irrigation is used to evacuate the isolated blood. An end-to-side anastomosis is then performed under magnification, with suturing of the posterior wall first and then of the anterior wall with running 6-0 or 7-0 monofilament nylon. Before the anastomosis is completed, generally within 20 to 30 minutes, air bubbles are removed by sequentially releasing all three clamps. When the anastomosis is finally completed,

Table 69-1. Vertebral to carotid transposition

	Number of Patients
Total	107
Angiographic patency	
Patent	84
Occluded	2
Not determined	20
Postoperative course	
Well	101
Died	
Third month postop	1
Second month postop	1
Major perioperative infarction	1
Persistent VBI	3
Postoperative complications	
Transient Horner's syndrome	50
Transient unilateral vocal cord paralysis	5
Phrenic nerve paresis	2
Wound infection	1
Wound hematoma	1
Chyle cyst	1
Transient upper brachial plexus palsy	1

flow is initially directed to the external carotid, then all clamps are removed. After hemostasis is achieved, closure is accomplished in layers over a Jackson-Pratt drain brought out through a separate stab incision and connected to closed bulb suction. The drain is removed in 12 to 24 hours (Figures 69-1 and 69-2).

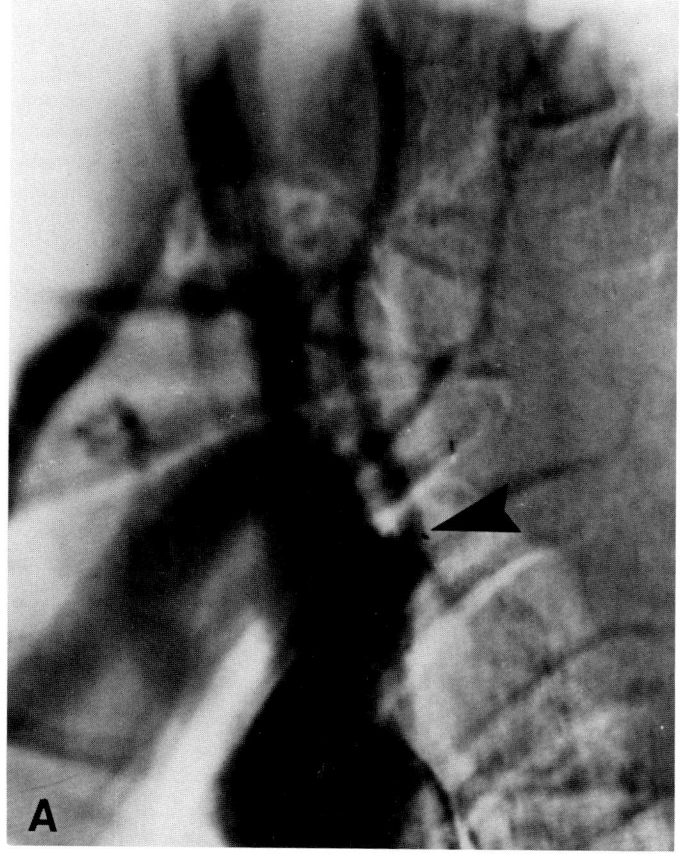

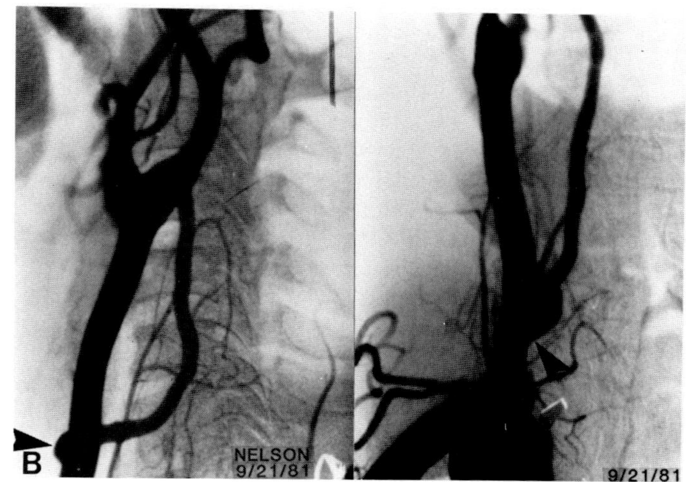

Fig. 69-2. (A) Preoperative angiogram. Arrow indicates area of vertebral artery origin stenosis. (B) Postoperative VCT angiogram.

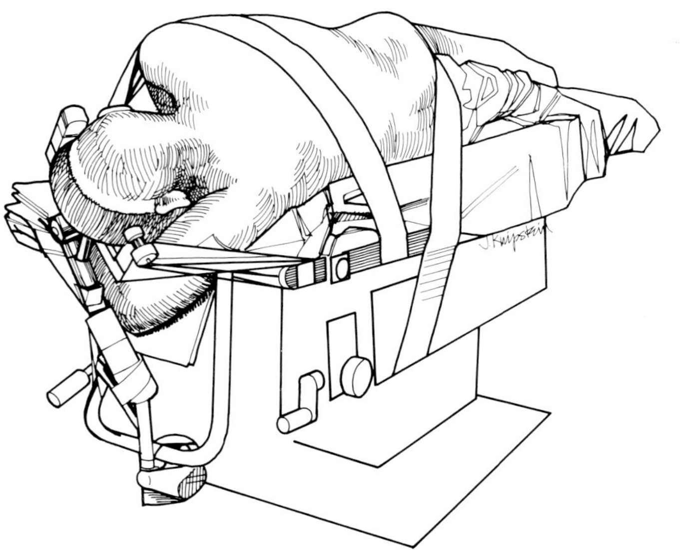

Fig. 69-3. The three-quarters prone position. (Reprinted from Ausman JI, Diaz FG, de los Reyes RA, et al: Microsurgery for atherosclerosis in the distal vertebral and basilar arteries, in Rand RW: Microneurosurgery, ed 3. St. Louis, C.V. Mosby Co., 1985. With permission.)

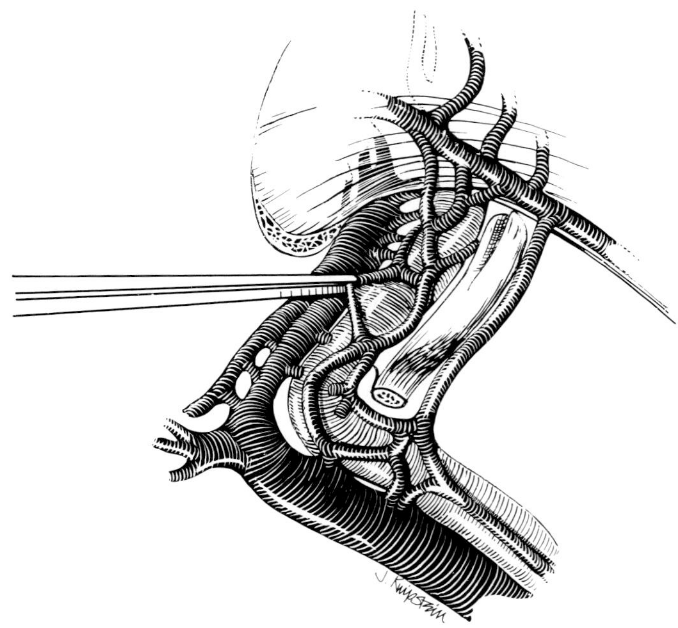

Fig. 69-4. Dissection of the distal vertebral artery perivenous plexus. (Reprinted from Ausman JI, Diaz FG, de los Reyes RA, et al: Microsurgery for atherosclerosis in the distal vertebral and basilar arteries, in Rand RW: Microneurosurgery, ed 3. St. Louis, C.V. Mosby Co., 1985. With permission.)

For more distal disease of the second portion of the vertebral artery, a VCT may still be possible, although it is technically more difficult and requires meticulous dissection of the artery as it courses through several foramina transversaria. Otherwise, a saphenous interposition vein graft is utilized from the common or external carotid arteries.[15] Another possibility is an anastomosis using a branch of the external carotid artery.[16,17]

RESULTS

Since July 1980, we have performed 107 VCT procedures; these are summarized in Table 69-1. Simultaneous carotid endarterectomy was performed in 34 patients who had significant stenosis of their ipsilateral internal carotid arteries. Postoperative mortality occurred in one patient who had a combined VCT/CEA and was quadriparetic upon awakening from anesthesia. The patient deteriorated and expired a few days later. Emergency angiography had revealed wide patency of the internal carotid artery and VCT. Postmortem examination revealed bilateral parieto-occipital infarctions. A second death occurred unexpectedly 2 months postoperatively and was caused by cerebral infarction in a patient who had previously been doing well. The VCT had been demonstrated to be patent postoperatively. No postmortem examination was obtained. Significant morbidity included a right hemispheric infarct with dense left hemiparesis in one patient after a right VCT. Three patients had persistent VBI. One patient, after demonstration of an occluded VCT and persistent symptoms, is presently scheduled for an OA-PICA bypass. The only other patient of ours to have an occlusion of his VCT with persistent symptoms underwent subsequent OA-AICA bypass and is now doing well. Another patient had persistent symptoms despite demonstrated patency of his VCT and underwent an STA-SCA bypass with good results.

Of the 107 patients, 103 (two requiring subsequent EC-IC procedures) became entirely asymptomatic or have had a significant reduction in the frequency, severity, and number of symptoms previously experienced. Postoperative complications were transient and resolved with appropriate treatment except for a few examples of persistent Horner's syndrome.

DISTAL VERTEBRAL ENDARTERECTOMY

Distal vertebral endarterectomy is designed for stenosing atherosclerotic disease of the distal second, third, and fourth segments of the vertebral artery. Angiographic indications include severe distal vertebral stenosis with contralateral vertebral occlusion, hypoplasia, or severe stenosis.

OPERATIVE TECHNIQUE

For this procedure, the patient is placed in a three-quarters prone position, operated side down, with the patient's head flexed and maintained in three-point fixation (Figure 69-3). The course of the OA is marked in case an OA-PICA bypass may be required. We believe this position offers several advantages in addition to those afforded by its being horizontal, as previously discussed. These include ideal positioning should OA-PICA bypass be required; optimal exposure and alignment of the vertebral artery along the surgeon's line of site toward the brain stem; a relatively wide area in which the assistant can work, thus facilitating active participation; and decreased thoracic and abdominal pressure, thereby decreasing venous bleeding.

A midline incision is extended inferiorly from the inion to the C5 spinous process. Dissection continues down to the spinous processes and occipital bone, and is carried laterally along the laminae to the articular facets. The vertebral artery is palpated and dissected atop C1, and followed proximally to the foramina transversarium of C1. The C2 nerve root is identified and divided just lateral to where it passes over the vertebral

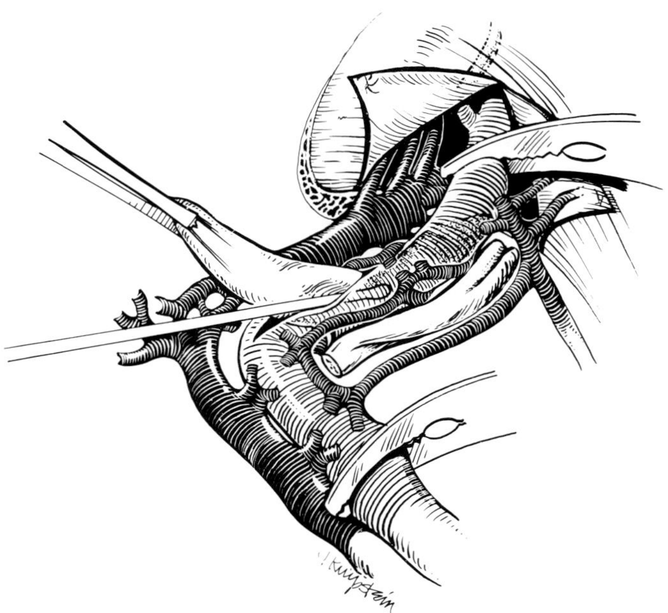

Fig. 69-5. Distal vertebral endarterectomy (DVEA). (Reprinted from Ausman JI, Diaz FG, de los Reyes RA, et al: Microsurgery for atherosclerosis in the distal vertebral and basilar arteries, in Rand RW: Microneurosurgery, ed 3. St. Louis, C.V. Mosby Co., 1985. With permission.)

artery in order to avoid injury to a possible radicular artery running with the nerve, deep to it, to the spinal cord. Using a small Kerrison rongeur, the vertebral artery at the C1 foramen is unroofed. The artery is dissected proximally to the superior aspect of the C2 transverse process. Meticulous dissection with bipolar cautery and microscissors under magnification of the periarterial venous plexus prevents copious venous bleeding (Figure 69-4).

A suboccipital craniectomy is then performed at the foramen magnum where the vertebral artery enters the dura. The venous plexus is dissected from C1 to this point, thereby completing exposure of the third portion of the artery. The dura just above the artery is opened, exposing the fourth portion of the artery and posterior fossa contents. A tethering dural band is resected as the artery enters the intradural space. The dentate ligament adjacent to the eleventh cranial nerve is sectioned. The patient is then given 5000 units heparin, 250 mg thiopental, 100 mg lidocaine, and 25 g mannitol intravenously, for brain protection, 5 minutes before clamps are placed.

Vascular clamps are placed proximal and distal to the plaque. If the lesion extends beyond the PICA origin, a temporary clip is used to occlude PICA at its origin. With a No. 11 blade, a longitudinal arteriotomy is made and extended as necessary with microscissors. Backflow is momentarily checked and blood is washed away with heparinized saline. The plaque is then circumferentially dissected using Penfield and microdissectors. Positioning allows the surgeon to view distal plaque dissection intraluminally, thereby facilitating complete excision of the plaque and removal of luminal tags with microbiopsy forceps. The vessel is then closed with a running 7-0 Prolene suture. The clamps are sequentially relaxed before final closure to eliminate air bubbles, and the area is irrigated with heparinized saline. With completion of the suture line, the clamps are removed to re-establish flow. The wound is closed tightly in multiple layers (Figures 69-5 and 69-6).

RESULTS

Allen et al., in 1981, first reported an intracranial DVEA.[18] Theoretically, this procedure would be preferable to an extracranial-intracranial (EC-IC) bypass for revascularization, since the largest possible channel of flow would be established. The procedure is, however, technically demanding, and plaque at the distal vertebral artery is often difficult to dissect. To date,

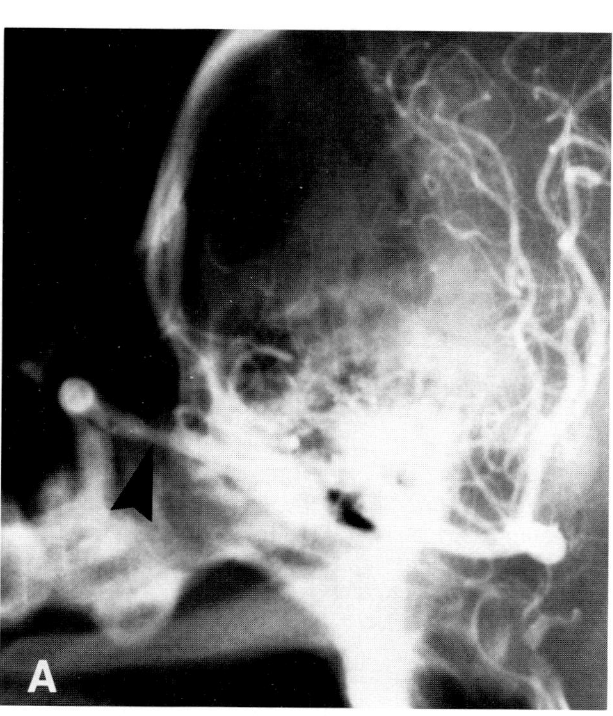

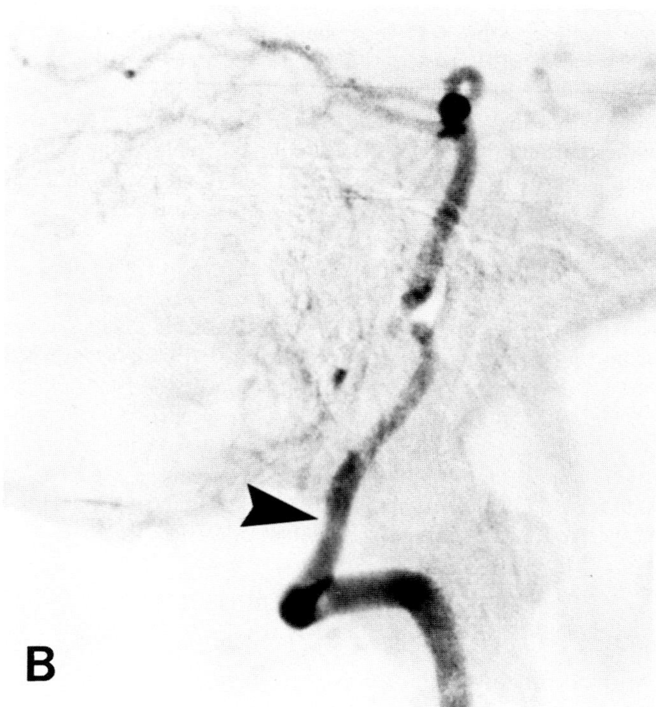

Fig. 69-6. (A) Preoperative angiogram. Arrow indicates area of distal vertebral artery stenosis. (B) Postoperative DVEA angiogram.

Table 69-2. Distal vertebral endarterectomy

	Number of Patients		
	DVEA	Distal Vertebral Artery Ligation	Distal Vertebral Artery Closed Without Endarterectomy
Total number of patients	3	1	1
Angiographic patency			
Patent	2		1
Occluded	1		
Postoperative course			
Well	3		
Major perioperative infarction		1	
Well after OA-PICA bypass			1
Postoperative complications			
Wallenberg syndrome		1	
Incisional CSF leak, bacterial meningitis			1

we have attempted DVEA in 5 patients (Table 69-2). In one patient, the plaque was discovered to be eroding into the arterial wall and the vessel had to be ligated. In another, the plaque was found to extend over too long a segment to be resected, a condition which was not appreciated on the preoperative angiogram. The arteriotomy was closed.

The procedure was completed in 3 patients, and postoperative angiography revealed wide patency in two and occlusion in one. Symptomatology decreased in these 3 patients postoperatively. There were no deaths. Postoperative complications included a Wallenburg syndrome in the patient requiring vertebral ligation, who was incapacitated by the event, and an incisional CSF leak with meningitis in one patient, which resolved spontaneously with continuous lumbar CSF drainage and antibiotics. The patient whose arteriotomy was closed without attempted resection of the plaque subsequently underwent an OA-PICA bypass and had symptom resolution. The patient whose endarterectomy occluded is an interesting case. This patient had a prophylactic right superficial temporal artery to middle cerebral artery (STA-MCA) bypass for right internal carotid occlusion, before the planned DVEA, because the patient's right hemisphere was supplied only via a large right posterior communicating artery. We felt that the patient's VBI was secondary to a "steal" phenomenon of the right anterior circulation. The fact that the patient was improved symptomatically despite occlusion at the endarterectomy site, and that a friable atherosclerotic plaque was found at surgery, represents indirect evidence for embolization, rather than hypoperfusion, as the pathophysiological mechanism of VBI in this paient.

OCCIPITAL ARTERY TO POSTERIOR INFERIOR CEREBELLAR ARTERY BYPASS

In 1976, Ausman et al. reported the first EC-IC bypass to the posterior circulation.[19] Angiographic findings in patients considered candidates for this procedure include bilateral distal vertebral (but proximal to PICA) disease, whether severe, lengthy stenosis, or occlusion. However, since the vertebral artery is more commonly diseased distal to the PICA, to the vertebrobasilar junction, this procedure is not often indicated and a more distal EC-IC bypass is required.

OPERATIVE TECHNIQUE

Initially, we positioned patients in the seated position, but we now utilize either the three-quarters prone or the lateral positions. The head is flexed and maintained in three-point fixation. The ultrasonic Doppler is used to trace the course of the OA from the mastoid over the back of the head. The incision is then made directly over the OA, which forms a lazy S shape extending inferiorly from the vertical portion of the artery and then swings laterally at the point of perforation of the artery through the posterior cervical fascia towards the mastoid; the incision is then directed inferiorly to the C3 level. With microdissection, the OA is exposed along its entire length from the mastoid to the occipital convexity. Once the necessary length of artery has been exposed, approximately 10 cm, the incision is carried down to the periosteum on either side of the artery, providing a 2) to 3-mm connective tissue cuff. Side branches are all ligated or cauterized and transected. The continuity of the OA is maintained proximally and distally. The OA is then wrapped with papavarine-soaked cottonoids and retracted. The suboccipital muscles are then incised and retracted, thereby exposing the area of the foramen magnum and the arch of C1. A unilateral suboccipital craniectomy is performed from the foramen magnum to the transverse sinus, and from the midline to the medial edge of the mastoid. It is usually not necessary to take the arch of C1. The dura is opened and the cisterna magna is drained of CSF, thereby allowing the cerebellum to fall away by its own weight.

The perimedullary portion of PICA is then identified and a segment of either the rostral or caudal branches devoid of perforating vessels is dissected and isolated. The OA is then transected distally after a temporary clip is placed proximally. The lumen is then irrigated with heparinized saline. The length required to perform the anastomosis to PICA is determined, and the distal 1.5 cm of the OA is freed of adventitia. A bevelled, fishmouthed stoma is then prepared at the distal OA. The patient is then given 250 mg thiopental, 100 mg lidocaine, and 25 g mannitol intravenously 5 minutes before clamping. The segment of PICA chosen is isolated with a small rubber dam beneath and between temporary clips. A longitudinal arteriotomy equal in length to the OA stoma is made with microscalpel and microscissors, and a small polyethylene stent may be placed inside the isolated PICA segment.

With 10-0 nylon suture on a half-circle needle, the anastomosis is begun in either an interrupted or continuous fashion, both of which are satisfactory. The anastomosis with interrupted sutures is begun by fixing first the heel of the OA stoma to one of the apices of the PICA arteriotomy. The distal tip of the stoma is then sutured to the opposite apex, and two more anchoring sutures are placed in the midposition on each anastomotic surface. Once the anastomotic surface has been divided into four quadrants, each is then closed with interrupted sutures. The stent is removed before the last 2 or 3 sutures are tied.

The anastomosis with continuous suture is started by securing the two apices as previously described, and then continuing these two individual sutures in a through-and-

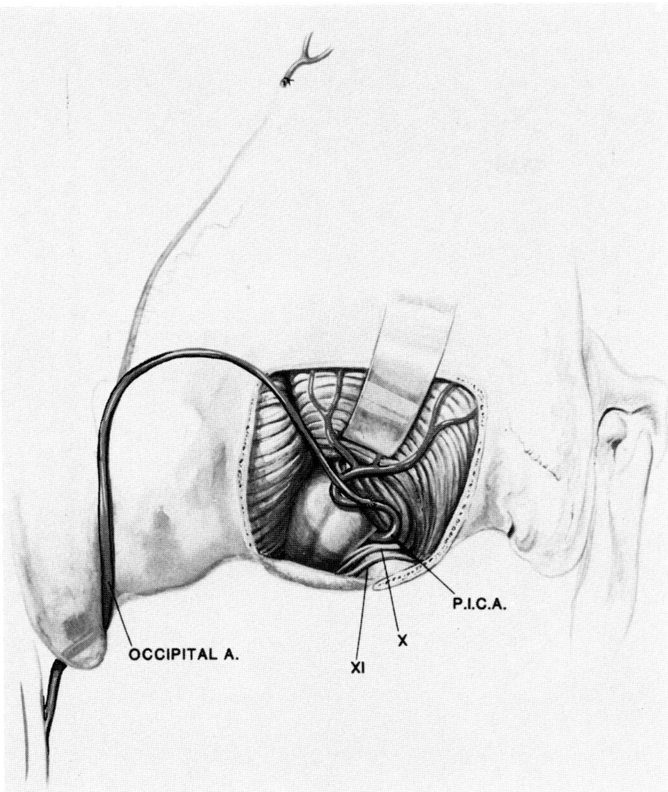

Fig. 69-7. Occipital artery to posterior inferior cerebellar artery (OA-PICA) bypass. (Reprinted from Ausman JI, Diaz FG, de los Reyes RA, et al: Microsurgery for atherosclerosis in the distal vertebral and basilar arteries, in Rand RW: Microneurosurgery, ed 3. St. Louis, C.V. Mosby Co., 1985. With permission.)

through fashion on either side of the anastomotic surface. Meticulous technique is required if one is to avoid loose portions of the suture line. The two ends of different sutures must not be tied together, as this provides for a rigid purse-string. We prefer the continuous suture technique to limit clamp time.

With completion of the anastomosis, the temporary clips are removed serially, from the PICA first and then from the OA. The small amount of bleeding usually encountered at the anastomotic site is controlled by packing the surface with absorbable gelatin sponge or cotton. Occasionally, one or two additional sutures are required to stop the bleeding, but whenever possible we avoid this, as strictures may result at the anastomosis. Once hemostasis is assured, the dura is closed except for a small dural opening where the OA passes. The wound is then closed tightly in layers (Figures 69-7 and 69-8).

RESULTS

As of November 1974, we have performed 16 OA-PICA bypasses, which are summarized in Table 69-3. There was one postoperative death, early in our experience, in a patient who expired the following morning secondary to congestive heart failure and pulmonary edema. Fluid status and hemodynamic variables have subsequently been carefully monitored in our postoperative patients. Another patient, who had a stroke in evolution, had persistent severe neurologic deficits postoperatively and died 6 weeks later of massive pulmonary embolism. Severe incapacitating infarction occurred in one patient, who, on initial presentation was clinically unstable, and who developed left hemiparesis perioperatively. The preoperative angiogram had revealed a right internal carotid occlusion. The patient was taken to the operating room 2 days later for a right STA-MCA bypass. The patient became hemiplegic after this second procedure. Two patients had persistent symptoms and postoperative angiography revealed nonpatent anastomoses. Both subsequently underwent STA-SCA bypass and are presently doing well. One patient was lost to follow-up. Of 16 patients, 12 became asymptomatic or markedly improved. One of these patients died 4 years postoperatively from myocardial infarction. Postoperative complications were, for the most part, transient. Incisional CSF leaks and cases of bacterial meningitis resolved with continuous lumbar CSF drainage and antibiotics.

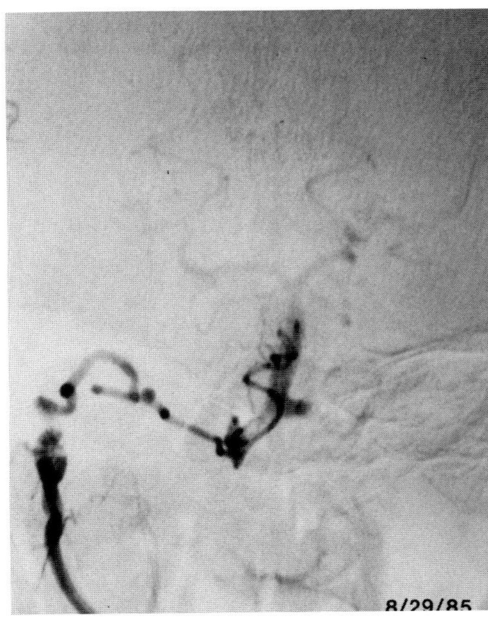

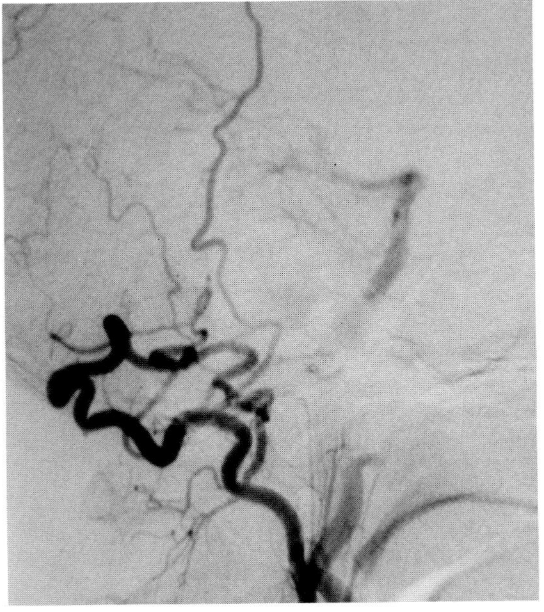

Fig. 69-8. Postoperative OA-PICA bypass visualization via selective external carotid angiogram.

Table 69-3. Occipital artery to posterior inferior cerebellar artery bypass

	Number of Patients	
	Clinically Stable	Clinically Unstable
Total number of patients	13	3
Angiographic patency		
Patent	8	2
Occluded	2	1
Not determined	3	
Postoperative course		
Well	9	1
Persistent VBI 2 degrees to occluded bypass: well after STA-SCA bypass	2	
Major perioperative infarction		1
Died 1 day postop	1	
Died 6 weeks postop		1
Lost to follow-up	1	
Postoperative complications		
Incisional CSF leak	2	
Bacterial meningitis	1	1
Aseptic meningitis	3	
Transient ataxia	2	
Persistent ataxia	1	
Congestive heart failure	1	
Pulmonary embolism		1
Aspiration/sepsis		1

OCCIPITAL ARTERY TO ANTERIOR INFERIOR CEREBELLAR ARTERY BYPASS

This procedure is utilized in patients whose cerebral angiograms have disclosed severe basilar artery stenosis or occlusion proximal to the AICAs, or have disclosed bilateral, severe,

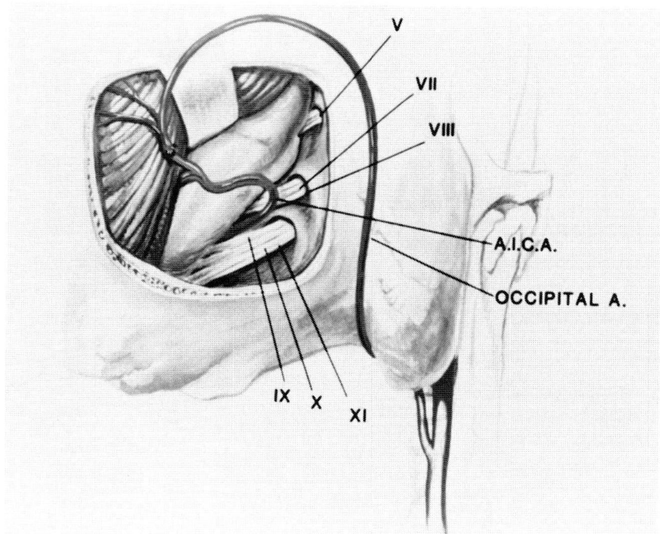

Fig. 69-9. Occipital artery to anterior inferior cerebellar artery (OA-AICA) bypass. (Reprinted from Ausman JI, Diaz FG, de los Reyes RA, et al: Microsurgery for atherosclerosis in the distal vertebral and basilar arteries, in Rand RW: Microneurosurgery, ed 3. St. Louis, C.V. Mosby Co., 1985. With permission.)

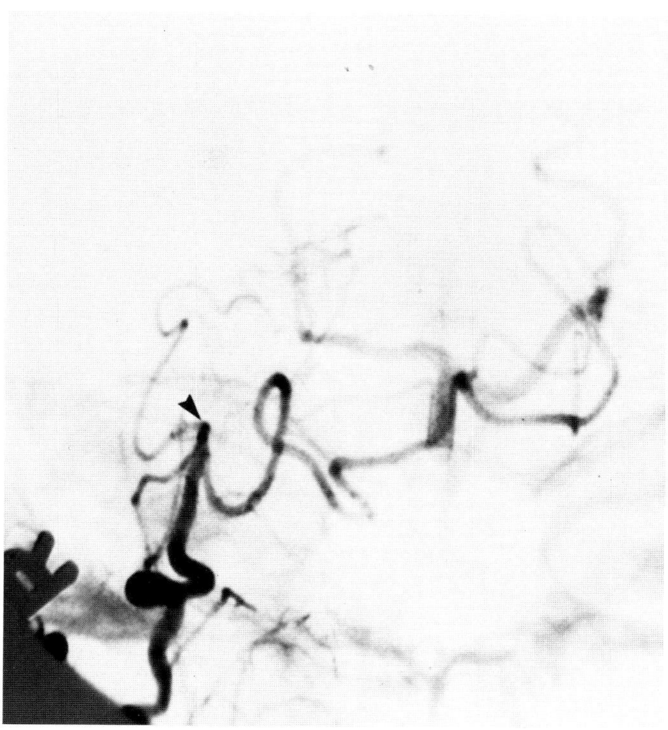

Fig. 69-10. Postoperative OA-AICA bypass visualization via selective external carotid angiogram.

distal (to PICA) vertebral artery stenosis, occlusion, or hypoplasia.

OPERATIVE TECHNIQUE

For this procedure, the patient is placed in the lateral decubitus position and the head is flexed and secured in three-point fixation. The dissection of the OA and exposure of the posterior fossa contents are essentially the same as that for the OA-PICA bypass. After draining CSF from the cisterna magna, the cerebellum is gently retracted medially with self-retaining retractors, in order to expose the seventh and eighth cranial nerves. The prepontine portion of AICA is identified as it extends to the anterior cerebellar surface from just in front of the foramen of Luschka. At this location, AICA has divided into rostral and caudal branches. In order to avoid confusion with a rostral branch of PICA, the arterial segment chosen for anastomosis must be followed to its level of origin. The largest segment devoid of brain-stem perforators is chosen for the anastomotic site. Performing the anastomosis too proximally requires excessive cerebellar retraction and may compromise PICA-AICA pial collaterals, resulting in ischemia and possible infarction. Once the site of the OA-AICA anastomosis is chosen, it is completed as previously described for the OA-PICA bypass. The wound is then closed tightly in layers (Figures 69-9 and 69-10).

RESULTS

We have performed 19 OA-AICA bypasses since February 1980; these are summarized in Table 69-4. Postoperative mortality occurred in one patient, who had a stroke in evolution and was quadriparetic before surgery. Patency of this anastomosis was not determined, and the patient died 2 days later. Our other

Table 69-4. Occipital artery to anterior inferior cerebellar artery bypass

	Number of Patients	
	Clinically Stable	Clinically Unstable
Total number of patients	13	6
Angiographic patency		
Patent	12	4
Not determined	1	2
Postoperative course		
Well	12	3
Died		
Second month postop		1
Third month postop		1
Mild infarction		
Nine months postop	1	
Twelve months postop	1	
Recurrent VBI 2 years postop: major infarction after DVEA		1
Debilitated	1	
Postoperative complications		
Incisional CSF leak	2	2
Bacterial meningitis	1	1
Transient unilateral cord paralysis	2	
Obstructive hydrocephalus/ temporary ventriculostomy	2	
Bacterial ventriculitis	1	
Tension pneumothorax/ARDS	1	
Dysphagia		1
Aspiration/sepsis		1
Vocal cord paresis/ tracheostomy		1

death occurred 4 months postoperatively in a patient who had been unstable at presentation. The patient's moderate neurologic deficits, present preoperatively, persisted, and he also developed several postoperative complications, including incisional CSF leak requiring re-exploration, bacterial meningitis, vocal cord paralysis requiring tracheostomy, dysphagia, aspiration, and sepsis, which was the terminal event. Patency of the anastomosis was not determined.

One patient made a remarkable recovery from several life-threatening postoperative complications, including acute obstructive hydrocephalus requiring ventriculostomy, tension pneumothorax, ARDS, bacterial ventriculitis, and sepsis. At the time of his discharge, the patient was generally weak and debilitated but had no new neurologic findings or persistent symptoms. Postoperative angiograms have not yet been obtained.

Recurrent symptoms developed in our first patient 2 years postoperatively, and attempted DVEA at that time resulted in vertebral ligation and a disabling Wallenburg syndrome. Mild neurologic deficits occurred secondary to infarction in 2 patients postoperatively. One patient developed mild ataxia secondary to a presumed vermian infarct one year postoperatively, and the other developed a mild Wallenburg syndrome 9 months postoperatively, secondary to occlusion of a previously stenotic distal vertebral artery. Bypasses were patent in both patients and they are presently doing well.

Fifteen patients became asymptomatic or were significantly improved postoperatively. Excluding the complicated postoperative courses of the 2 patients described above, the remaining postoperative complications were, in general, transient. The incisional CSF leaks and cases of bacterial meningitis resolved with continuous lumbar CSF drainage and antibiotics. One patient required a shunting procedure for a posterior fossa arachnoid cyst postoperatively. The shunt was later removed and the patient is doing well.

SUPERFICIAL TEMPORAL ARTERY TO SUPERIOR CEREBELLAR ARTERY BYPASS

A STA-SCA bypass is required for revascularization when severe basilar artery stenosis or occlusion occurs distal to the AICAs. Others have bypassed, using the STA or interposition vein grafts from the external carotid artery, to the posterior cerebral artery,[20,21] however, we prefer the SCA, since collateral circulation is more extensive from this artery. Also, should vascular occlusion occur, we believe the possible cerebellar deficit would be less disabling than an occipital lobe deficit. Anatomic studies have shown the perimesencephalic SCA to average 1.3 mm in outer diameter and to be devoid of perforators, which makes this vessel well suited for anastomosis.[22]

OPERATIVE TECHNIQUE

After placement of a lumbar CSF drain, which is required for this procedure to allow temporal lobe retraction, the patient is placed in a semilateral position so that the right side of the head is up and parallel to the floor and the right body elevated. The course of the larger STA branch is traced using the Doppler ultrasound. A minimum length of 15 cm is required for the procedure. The incision is made directly over the STA, beginning just above the zygoma, and is extended superiorly. The STA is dissected as previously described for the OA, with as much length as possible being obtained. The proximal and distal ends of the dissected artery remain in continuity, and the artery is wrapped in papavarine-soaked cottonoids and retracted. The temporalis muscle is incised and retracted, thereby exposing the temporal bone. Centered on the ear, a temporal craniotomy is performed such that the inferior extent is flush with the floor of the middle cranial fossa and extends a minimum of 3 cm on each side of the external auditory meatus.

To allow temporal lobe retraction, the patient is given 25 g mannitol before the initial incision, and 150–200 ml of CSF is drained before the dura is opened. After opening the dura, the temporal lobe is elevated with a self-retaining retractor. Throughout the procedure, the minimal amount of temporal lobe retraction necessary is used, because of the possibility of compromising pial collaterals, in addition to causing postoperative swelling and seizures. Care must be taken to preserve temporal veins in order to prevent postoperative swelling.

The arachnoid at the tentorial incisura is opened, thereby exposing the perimesencephalic SCA. Taking care to avoid injury to the fourth cranial nerve, exposure is enhanced by incising the tentorium from 2 cm posterior to its insertion on the posterior clinoid, with the incision directed toward the petrous apex. The two flaps of the tentorium are then reflected laterally and sutured back to the dura.

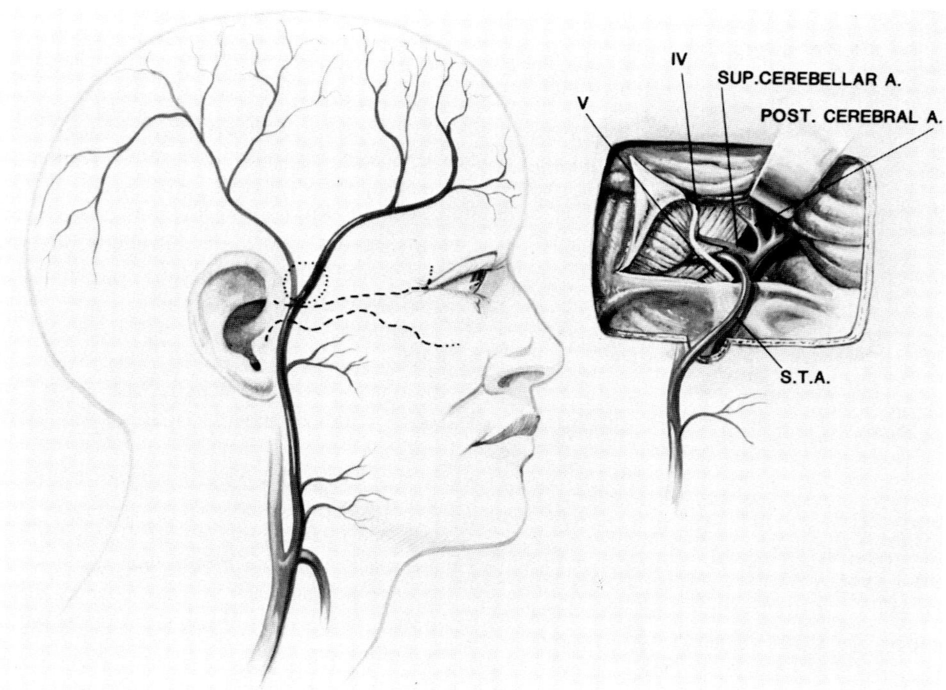

Fig. 69-11. Superficial temporal artery to superior cerebellar artery (STA-SCA) bypass. (Reprinted from Ausman JI, Diaz FG, de los Reyes RA, et al: Microsurgery for atherosclerosis in the distal vertebral and basilar arteries, in Rand RW: Microneurosurgery, ed 3. St. Louis, C.V. Mosby Co., 1985. With permission.)

The rostral and caudal branches of the SCA are explored, and the largest of these, without perforators, is carefully dissected and isolated. The distal end of the STA is now transected and an atraumatic, temporary clip is placed at its base. The distal, bevelled, fishmouthed stoma is prepared as previously described. The patient is given 250 mg thiopental and 100 mg lidocaine intravenously 5 minutes before clamping. The chosen segment of SCA is isolated between 2 vascular clips lying over a rubber dam. The STA is then brought down to the recipient vessel, and an end-to-side anastomosis is completed as previously described. The STA should be long enough that it lies in the temporal fossa without tension.

Once the anastomosis is completed, the clips are removed from the SCA and then from the STA. Once hemostasis is assured, the dura is closed except for the small dural defect where the STA passes. The bone flap is replaced and the wound is then closed tightly in layers (Figures 69-11 and 69-12).

RESULTS

Since April 1977, we have performed 38 STA-SCA bypasses; the results are summarized in Table 69-5. Postoperatively, there were 4 deaths. Two of these patients had stroke in evolution. Basilar artery thrombosis was demonstrated angiographically in both patients, who died within 3 weeks after surgery. One patient had subarachnoid hemorrhage secondary to a leaking anastomosis and died on the third postoperative day. The other patient died 2 weeks postoperatively secondary

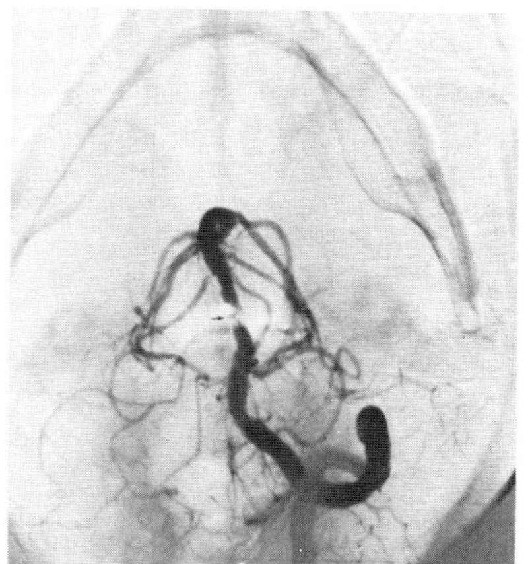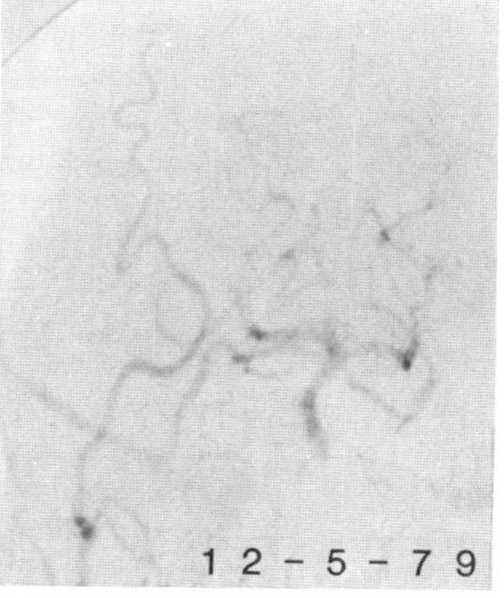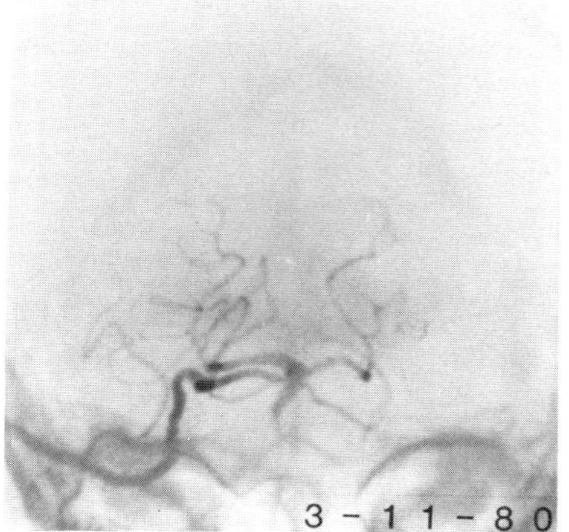

Fig. 69-12. Postoperative STA-SCA bypass visualization via selective external carotid angiogram.

Table 69-5. Superficial temporal artery to superior cerebellar artery bypass

	Number of Patients	
	Clinically Stable	Clinically Unstable
Total number of patients	24	14
Angiographic patency		
Patent	24	13
Occluded		1
Postoperative course		
Well	19	6
Died		
Third week postop	1	2
Second week postop	1	
Five months postop		1
Major perioperative infarction		3
Recurrent VBI		2
Four years postop	1	
Persistent vertigo	2	
Postoperative complications		
Transient fourth nerve palsy	8	1
Seizures	6	1
Mild neurologic deficit	3	1
Incisional CSF leak	2	1
Moderate neurologic deficit	1	
Bacterial meningitis	1	1
Wound infection	1	1
Removal of infected bone flap	1	1
Evacuation of subdural collection	1	1
Pulmonary embolism	1	
Transient radio nerve palsy	1	
Scalp necrosis	1	
Cerebellar hematoma	1	
Partial third nerve palsy		1
GU sepsis		1
Transient dysphagia		1
Vocal cord paresis/temporary tracheostomy		1

to basilar artery thrombosis. This patient had done very well initially and was discharged after angiography had demonstrated luxuriant filling of the distal basilar artery and its branches. A fifth patient remained asymptomatic for 4 months postoperatively before expiring from a cerebral infarction. The exact cause of death was not determined in this patient.

Incapacitating infarction occurred in 3 patients perioperatively, all of whom had stroke in evolution. Five patients had continuing symptoms. Meniere's disease and degenerative cerebellar disease were subsequently diagnosed as being responsible for persistent vertigo in 2 patients; both had patent anastomoses. A third patient developed worsening basilar stenosis despite a patent anastomosis. The remaining 2 patients with recurrent symptoms, one of whom remained asymptomatic for 4 years postoperatively, had patent anastomoses but demonstrated poor retrograde flow to the basilar artery.

Twenty-four patients became asymptomatic or were significantly improved postoperatively. Postoperative complications included mild to moderate neurologic deficit in 5 patients: mild ataxia, homonymous hemianopsia, mild right hemiparesis with bilateral homonymous hemianopsia, and slight worsening of preoperative hemiparesis in 2 patients. Other postoperative complications were transient for the most part. One incisional CSF leak required intracranial repair. Both subdural collections were surgically drained and infected bone flaps were removed in 2 patients. Transient temporal lobe swelling is common secondary to operative retraction, and often resulted in postoperative seizures prior to prophylactic, preoperative Dilantin loading. A small intracerebellar hematoma resolved spontaneously in one patient, leaving no residual deficit. Scalp necrosis in one patient required a plastic surgery procedure. Vocal cord paralysis required temporary tracheostomy in one patient.

POSTOPERATIVE MANAGEMENT

With completion of the procedure, the patient is taken to the recovery room where neurologic status and hemodynamic variables are carefully monitored. Blood pressure is strictly maintained at preoperative values with intravenous fluids and pressors, if necessary. Anesthesia time is generally 8 to 10 hours, and these patients are therefore relatively slow to wake up postoperatively. Once satisfactory progress is documented in the recovery room, the patient is taken to the surgical intensive care unit. Intravascular volume is expanded to high normal as guided by central pressures. Except for post-VCT patients, we generally leave these patients intubated overnight and extubate the following morning. Cefazolin is continued for 24 hours postoperatively, and the dexamethasone is maintained at 4 mg every 6 hours until the patient is transferred to the general neurosurgical ward, where it is rapidly tapered. The patient continues to take 325 mg of aspirin each day. These patients are kept at bed rest in the intensive care unit with the head of the bed elevated to a maximum of 30 degrees.

Patients are generally transferred to the ward on the third or fourth postoperative day, where they are slowly and cautiously allowed to ambulate and resume normal activities. Any neurologic deterioration is evaluated by physical examination, assessment of hemodynamic status, review of pertinent laboratory values, CT scans of the head, electroencephalograms, if indicated, and, when necessary, emergency angiography. Further intervention is directed by the results of these studies. Careful, repeated inspection of the wound is necessary to detect early CSF leaks that will require continuous lumbar CSF drainage, or reoperation if a leak does not seal spontaneously. Seizures, often subclinical, have been common after STA-SCA bypasses, and these patients are now maintained on Dilantin for 6 to 12 months postoperatively. Essentially all patients undergo selective external carotid angiography to visualize the bypass, or selective vertebral angiography in the case of DVEA, before discharge from the hospital. We now obtain outpatient venous digital subtraction angiography to evaluate our postoperative VCTs. Sutures are removed in 6 weeks.

CONCLUSION

In this chapter, we have presented our rationale for the evaluation and selection of patients who may benefit from posterior fossa revascularization. These individuals have had multiple repeated TIAs indicative of posterior circulation ischemia, and most have been refractory to our best medical therapy, namely systemic anticoagulation. In the presence of a hemodynamically significant lesion(s) as demonstrated by angiography, we believe these individuals are at high risk for future infarction. The revascularization procedures required are directed by the anatomy of atherosclerotic disease, and these procedures have been described. The procedures are technically much more demanding than are anterior circulation EC-IC anastomoses, and require considerable skill to complete.

Mortality and significant neurologic morbidity in our series has occurred primarily in that subset of patients who were clinically unstable at presentation. Operating on such individuals often represents a desperate attempt to salvage viable, ischemic tissue from inevitable infarction, as these patients continue to deteriorate despite maximal medical therapy. Most postoperative morbidity has been transient and has become less common with increasing experience. Our longest follow-up has been 8 to 10 years, but most patients have been followed postoperatively considerably less than this. We have demonstrated enlargement and increased flow through these anastomoses on repeated, follow-up angiography in a number of patients, which suggests a process of maturation.[23]

There obviously is a great need to further define the natural history of the specific anatomic disease and pathophysiologic processes responsible for symptoms that we lump under the heading of VBI. Only with this understanding will we be able, in the future, to make rational decisions regarding therapeutic options. For the present, we believe posterior fossa revascularization offers a favorable alternative for patients with brainstem ischemia refractory to medical interventions.

REFERENCES

1. Kubik CS, Adams RO: Occlusion of the basilar artery: A clinical and pathological study. Brain 69:73, 1946
2. Ausman JI, Shrontz CE, Pearce JE, et al: Vertebrobasilar insufficiency: A review. Arch Neurol 42:803, 1985
3. Caplan LR: Vertebrobasilar occlusive disease, in Barnett HJM, Mohr JP, Stein BM, et al (eds): Stroke: Pathophysiology, Diagnosis and Management, vol 1. New York, Churchill Livingstone, 1986, pp 549–619
4. Cartlidge NEF, Whisnant JP, Elveback LR: Carotid and vertebral basilar transient cerebral ischemic attacks. Mayo Clin Proc 52:117, 1977
5. Fisher CM, Gore I, Okabe N, et al: Atherosclerosis of the carotid and vertebral arteries: Extracranial and intracranial. J Neuropathol Exp Neurol 24:455, 1965
6. Duffey PE, Jacobs GB: Clinical and pathological findings in vertebral artery thrombosis. Neurology 8:862, 1958
7. Thompson JR, Simmons CR, Hasso AN, et al: Occlusion of the intradural vertebrobasilar artery. Neuroradiology 14:219, 1978
8. Archer CR, Hornstein S: Basilar artery occlusion: Clinical and radiological correlation. Stroke 8:383, 1977
9. Millikan CH, Siekert RG, Shick RM: Studies in cerebrovascular disease. III. The use of anticoagulant drugs in the treatment of insufficiency or thrombosis within the basilar arterial system. Proc Staff Meet Mayo Clin 30:116, 1955
10. Whisnant JP, Cartlidge NEF, Elveback LR: Carotid and vertebralbasilar transient ischemic attacks: Effects of anticoagulants, hypertension, and cardiac disorders on survival and stroke occurrence— A population study. Ann Neurol 3:107, 1978
11. Juge 0, Meyer JS, Sakai F, et al: Critical appraisal of cerebral blood flow measured from brainstem and cerebellar regions after ^{133}Xe inhalation in humans. Stroke 10:428, 1979
12. Berguer R, Bauer RB: Vertebral artery reconstruction. Ann Surg 193:441, 1981
13. Edwards WH, Wright RS: A new surgical technique for relief of subclavian stenosis. Hosp Pract 7:78, 1972
14. Diaz FG, Ausman JI, de los Reyes RA, et al: Surgical reconstruction of the proximal vertebral artery. J Neurosurg 61:874, 1984
15. Clark K, Perry MO: Carotid vertebral anastomosis: An alternate technique for repair of the subclavian steal syndrome. Ann Surg 163:414, 1966
16. Pritz MB, Chandler WF, Kindt GW: Vertebral artery disease: Radiological evaluation, medical management, and microsurgical treatment. Neurosurgery 9:524, 1981
17. Corkill G, French BN, Michas C, et al: External carotid-vertebral artery anastomosis for vertebrobasilar insufficiency. Surg Neurol 7:109, 1977
18. Allen GS, Cohen RJ, Preziosi TJ: Microsurgical endarterectomy of the intracranial vertebral artery for vertebrobasilar transient ischemic attacks. Neurosurgery 8:56, 1981
19. Ausman JI, Lee MC, Klassen AC, et al: Stroke: What's New? Cerebral revascularization. Minn Med 59:223, 1976
20. Spetzler RF: Extracranial-intracranial arterial anastomosis for cerebrovascular disease. Surg Neurol 11:157, 1975
21. Sundt TM, Piepgras DG: Extracranial to intracranial bypass grafting: Posterior circulation, in Wilkins RH, Rengachary SS (eds): Neurosurgery, vol 2. New York, McGraw-Hill, 1985, pp 1281–1292
22. Shrontz CE, Dujovny M, Ausman JI, et al: Vertebrobasilar reconstruction: Microanatomical considerations. Surg Forum 36:506, 1986
23. Park TS, Dacey RG, Jane JA, et al: Donor artery changes following anastomosis. Va Med 107:108, 1980

CHAPTER 70

Treatment of Intracerebral Vascular Lesions with Balloon Catheters

Gerard M. Debrun

INTERVENTIONAL NEURORADIOLOGY has become a specialty of its own within the last 10 years. Some neuroradiologists are devoting their entire professional activity to this field; this is becoming increasingly necessary in order to master all the techniques now available. This chapter will describe the materials, techniques, and indications for interventional procedures in the treatment of fistulae, brain or spinal cord arteriovenous malformations (AVMs), aneurysms, and malignant gliomas.

MATERIALS AND TECHNIQUES

DETACHABLE BALLOONS

There are two detachable balloons currently available commercially: Silastic balloons (Bard Parker, Lincoln Park, NJ) and latex balloons (Ingenor Laboratories, Paris, France).

Silastic Balloon

The Silastic balloon[1-4] has a valve mechanism, and is available in diameters of either 4 mm or 8 mm (inflated) and 1 mm and 2 mm (uninflated), respectively. Although a balloon with a maximum inflated diameter of 8 mm is sufficient for the treatment of a large variety of problems, it is sometimes too small for permanently occluding a vessel that is 8 mm or more in diameter, for occluding a fistula with a large tear and a large cavernous sinus, or for totally occluding a giant aneurysm. This balloon is not tied over the microcatheter, which makes it easier to detach but also easier to lose in the wrong position than is a balloon tied to the catheter. The balloons are inflated with iso-osmolar, water-soluble iodinated contrast medium and remain inflated for weeks or months.

Latex Balloon

There are two types of latex balloons. The first has been in use for over 10 years and has been described in many previous publications.[5-10] This balloon is a fingerlike latex sleeve with a narrow channel and a small distal teatlike chamber in which a metallic marker can be lodged. Between the narrow channel and the small distal teat there is a wider chamber that constitutes the balloon when inflated. A tiny, flexible catheter enters the balloon through the narrow portion of the sleeve, and a latex thread firmly ligates the balloon over the catheter at the level of

the narrow channel (Figure 70-1). As a result, it is almost impossible to lose this balloon, but it is more difficult to detach than is the Silastic balloon. Because of the risk of dislodging the balloon from its position when detaching it from the catheter, it is usually safer to use a coaxial catheter, which is slid up to the balloon and holds it in place while the inner catheter is removed. The coefficient of elasticity of latex is twice that of Silastic, and there are therefore many different sizes and shapes of latex balloons. These balloons range in size from inflated diameters of 4 mm to 30 mm and therefore can be used in all neurologic circumstances in which their usage is appropriate, including the treatment of giant aneurysms and large cavernous sinuses.

These balloons are sold in sets of 12 with 4 coaxial delivery catheter systems, 1 or 2 introducing catheters of 8F and 9F, and the various stopcocks and adapters needed for one procedure. The latex threads are included; the balloon has to be tied onto the catheter on the day of the procedure or immediately before it is used. The balloon can be sterilized either before or after it is attached to the catheter. The type of sterilization used on these devices is important, because the elasticity of the latex can be modified. Cold gas sterilization below 40°C is acceptable before the balloon is attached. This type of sterilization has to be done immediately before the balloon is used. Sterilization by immersing the balloon in Cidex solution for 15 minutes is another way to deal with this difficult problem. Placement of the balloons and threads in a box containing formaldehyde tablets is a third way to sterilize them, although this is not generally considered to be acceptable.

Latex balloons can be inflated with either iso-osmolar iodinated contrast agent or with a polymerizing substance. When inflated with contrast, they slowly deflate over a period of weeks or months; when inflated with a polymerizing substance, they retain their size and shape, depending on the capacity of the balloon and the dead space of the catheter. With a single-lumen catheter, the balloon is initially filled with contrast and is then deflated. When the polymerizing substance is injected, a quantity of contrast remaining in the dead space of the tubing is re-introduced into the balloon, partially filling it. To inflate the balloon entirely with polymerizing substance, a double-lumen catheter is used. The choice between the two ways of filling the balloon depends on whether a permanent or transient occlusion is to be accomplished with the balloon of that particular size.

OPERATIVE NEUROSURGICAL TECHNIQUES
ISBN 0-8089-1862-1

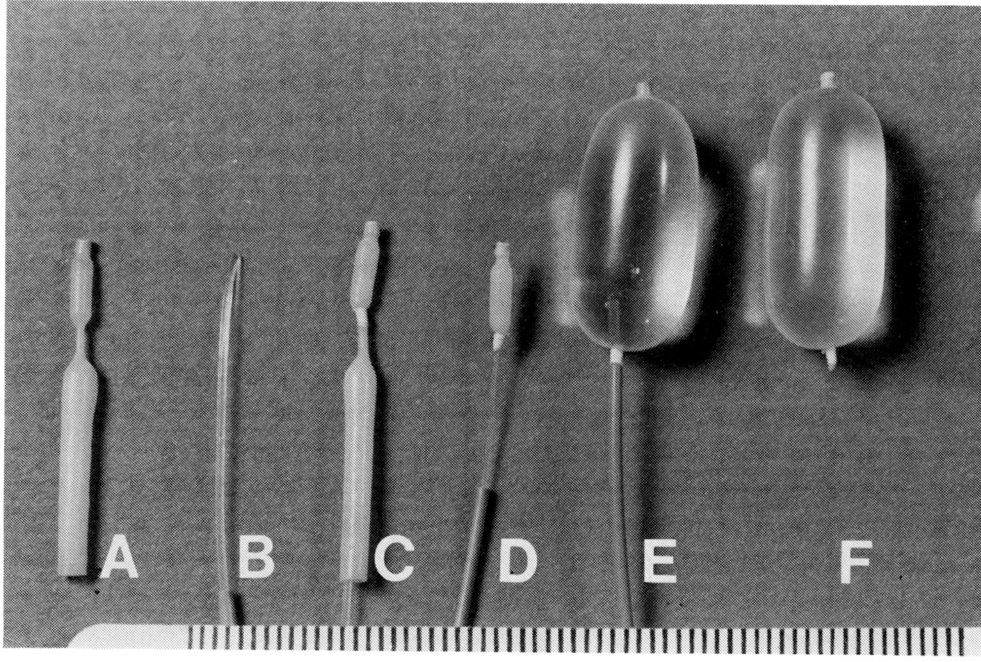

Fig. 70-1. Latex detachable balloon material. Scale: 1 mm between each graduation. (A) One latex sleeve. Metallic marker inside the tip. (B) Small Teflon tubing (0.4 × 0.6 mm). (C) The Teflon tubing is pushed into the sleeve and reaches its tip. The sleeve is tied over the tubing with a latex thread. The proximal end of the sleeve below the arrow will be cut. (D) The balloon is ready to be inflated. The coaxial tubing is visible. (E) The coaxial tubing is slid over the Teflon tubing and reaches the inflated balloon at the level of the ligature. (F) The Teflon tubing is pulled down until the balloon is detached. The latex thread ligature closes the aperture of the balloon, which is self-sealing when inflated with water-soluble iodine contrast.

CALIBRATED-LEAK BALLOONS

When it became possible to reach the most distal cerebral vessels with latex balloons, some were made with a distal hole to allow selective chemotherapeutic infusion.[10] Later, a Silastic calibrated-leak balloon was used to inject liquid polymerizing substances in brain.[11] The Silastic balloon was considered dangerous and was replaced by latex balloons.[12] Latex balloons have better adaptability to the size of the vessel in which they are inflated, thereby decreasing the risk of vessel dissection. Currently, Ingenor Laboratory makes three different sizes of latex calibrated-leak balloons, which are glued to the tip of very flexible Siltane tubing. This catheter is coiled into a plastic injection chamber and propelled with saline through a 7F introducer catheter previously positioned in the internal carotid or vertebral artery (Figure 70-2). There is a small metallic cylinder inside the tip of the catheter that can be seen fluoroscopically without inflating the balloon with contrast medium. Different types of small catheters allow vessels of less than 1 mm internal diameter to be selectively catheterized. This goal can also be accomplished by using open-end guide wires that slide over the microsteerable guide wires with torque control.

EMBOLIC AGENTS

A variety of materials have been used to embolize blood vessels. These agents are either solid particles or liquid substances that solidify.

Solid Particles

The first particles used in the embolization of branches of the external carotid artery were pieces of Gelfoam. Gelfoam particles can be used in various sizes, ranging from powder to large cubes. If the powder particles are too small, there is a risk of their crossing the capillary barrier. Another consideration is that even with larger particles, the vessels embolized with Gelfoam recanalize. Embolization of a lesion with Gelfoam should be considered a presurgical maneuver, after which surgical resection is carried out within a few days. Gelfoam has to a large extent been replaced by particles of plastic sponge of polyvinylalcohol foam (PVA). These particles are prepared in a range of sizes, from 150μ to 250μ, from 250μ to 500μ, and from 500μ to 1 mm. Some people have tried to obtain smaller particles with a blender, but this technique introduces particles 1μ in size, which can pass through the capillary barrier. It therefore is necessary to calibrate the particles obtained by blender technique by passing them through a filter of the desirable size. There is a substantial incidence of vessel recanalization following embolization with PVA. Several other solid materials have also been tried for embolization, including Silastic spheres, pieces of lyophilized dura mater, or autologous clots. More recently, selective embolization of the nidus of brain AVMs has been done with pieces of surgical nylon thread[13] or with PVA and collagen.[14]

Liquid Substances that Solidify

The ideal polymerizing substance must be of low viscosity, must solidify quickly in a controllable way, and must be

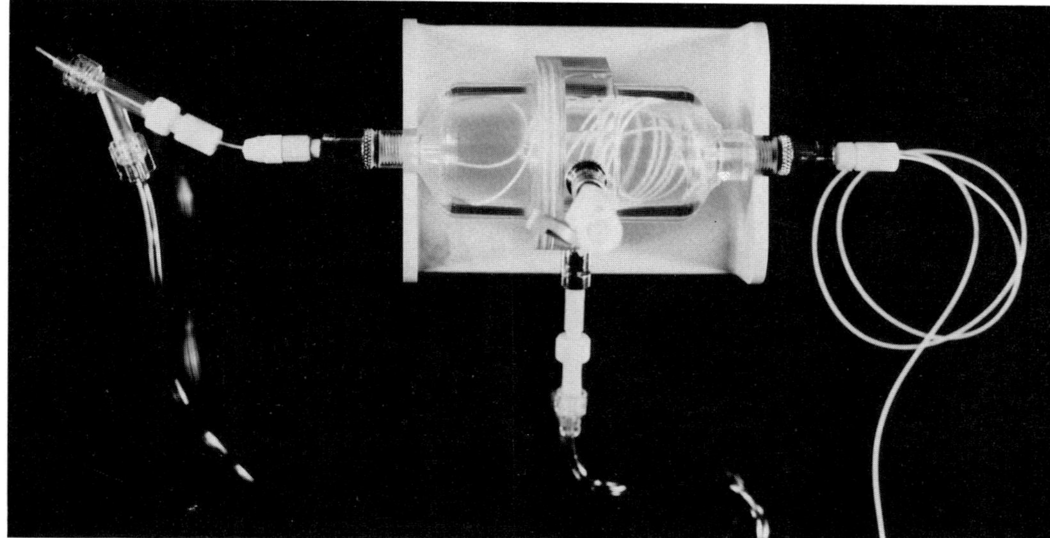

Fig. 70-2. Calibrated leak balloon catheter. The catheter is coiled into the chamber filled with saline. A Tuohyborst adapter holds the catheter at each extremity and prevents leakage of saline. A transparent side arm distal to the left Tuohyborst adapter allows injection of iodine contrast and also allows angiography. This side arm is connected to the introducing catheter in the groin. The lateral entry into the chamber allows injection of saline, which will propel the catheter outside the chamber.

nontoxic and noncarcinogenic. Silicone oil polymerizes when a catalyst is added and it is radiopaque. A cast of silicone is seen on the roentgenograms. The speed at which this substance polymerizes allows embolization of tumors but is too slow for use with a high-flow system such as an AVM.

Isobutyl 2-cyanoacrylate (bucrylate) is an acrylic substance that can be mixed with Pantopaque and tantalum powder; it solidifies within several seconds, although solidification can be retarded by the addition of glacial acetic acid to the solution.[15] When injected into normal tissues in experimental models, infarction and tissue necrosis have been induced; however, it is well tolerated if it remains confined to the abnormal vascular network of the nidus of an AVM or to the lumen of its vessels. The inflammatory reaction with macrophages seen in some pathologic specimens is probably caused by the bucrylate having reached functional brain tissue. Recent reports indicate that the nidus of an AVM previously embolized with bucrylate can recanalize.[16] In spite of these disadvantages, bucrylate remains the liquid agent of choice for the embolization of brain AVMs and of some other types of AVMs. Recent unpublished data also mention a carcinogenic effect associated with bucrylate injected into the peritoneal cavity of rats, although no report of cancer in humans related to the use of bucrylate has ever been published. Nevertheless, the follow-up of the first patients treated with bucrylate is still too short to yield conclusive results.

Pure ethanol is used in certain situations in which flow is very slow, such as certain cavernomas of the face, where the ethanol can be injected directly into the lesion. There are ongoing experiments that seem to demonstrate that pure ethanol can be combined with other embolic agents, such as collagen. However, the tremendous edema and inflammatory reaction induced by the injection of pure alcohol has to be kept in mind whenever it is used for an intracranial lesion, because of the risk of suddenly raising the intracranial pressure.

CATHETERS AND GUIDE WIRES

A wide variety of catheters and guide wires have been developed. It is possible to work with microcatheters of 0.1 mm inside and 0.3 mm outside diameter. Any type of balloon can be attached to the tip. Small Silastic catheters have been abandoned in the vasculature of patients without inducing any symptoms. This happened initially as a complication in a few cases of brain AVM in which the tip of the catheter became embedded in the bucrylate and could not be removed. None of these patients developed neurologic complications related to the presence of the tube, which sometimes went from the aorta to the brain and was finally epithelialized by the wall of the vessel. There have also been a few cases of carotid cavernous fistulae or cavernous aneurysms treated with a Fogarty catheter, with the balloon completely occluding the internal carotid artery. However, control angiograms showed in these very unusual cases that the balloon had moved either into the cavernous sinus (in the case of the fistula) or into the aneurysm with complete recanalization of the internal carotid artery. These patients live with 5F Fogarty catheters in their internal carotid arteries without obvious symptoms. These observations have initiated the concept that the microcatheter could be left in place in cases of multiple tortuosities of the vessel when great difficulty in detaching the balloon is encountered.

Open-end guide wires can be used as catheters for embolization. With the combined use of microsteerable guide wires, it is possible to reach branches of the fifth to tenth subdivisions of the main artery and to achieve superselective delivery of embolic agents.

The angioplasty balloon catheters used for peripheral vessels have been used by several investigators for angioplasty of subclavian stenosis, vertebral origin stenosis, fibromuscular dysplasia of the carotid arteries, weblike stenosis of the carotid artery, and, more recently, atheromatous stenosis of the internal carotid artery. However, the indications for balloon

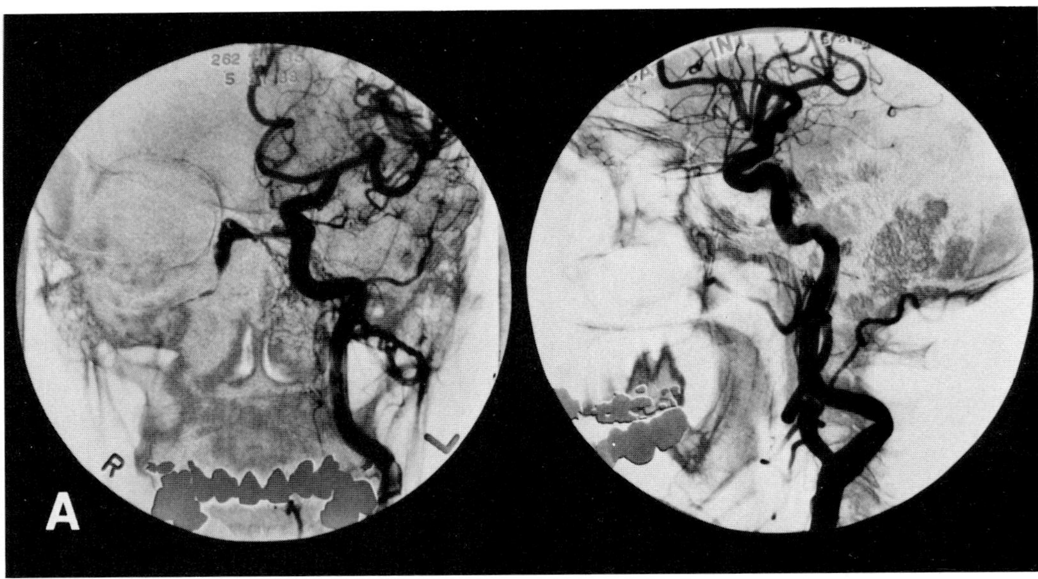

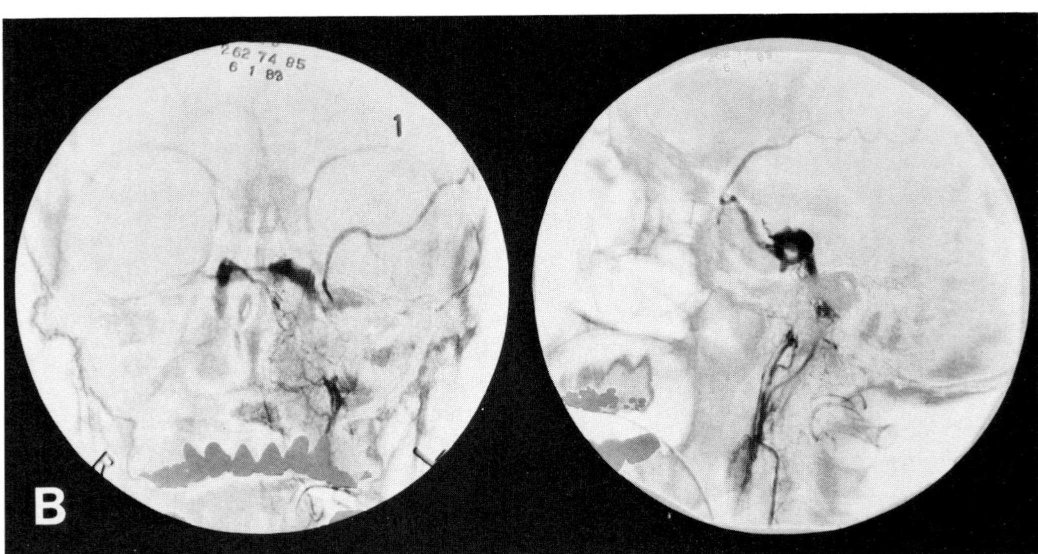

Fig. 70-3. Traumatic carotid cavernous fistula. (A) Lateral view: anterior, posterior, and inferior venous drainage of the cavernous sinus. (B) AP view: the cavernous sinus drains to the contralateral side as well.

angioplasty versus surgery and the follow-up results for these patients are still poorly known and will not be considered in this chapter.

FISTULAE

Fistulae are divided into two groups of lesions that require type-specific treatment. True fistulae, with a single communication between an artery and a vein, are the triumph of the detachable balloon technique, whereas (often multiple) fistulae with an abnormal network or rete between the artery and the vein must be treated with solid particles or liquid agents.

CAROTID CAVERNOUS FISTULAE

Traumatic Carotid Cavernous Fistulae

Clinical Presentation. Patients with traumatic carotid cavernous fistulae (CCF) become symptomatic immediately or shortly after a severe craniofacial injury. The development and the importance of the arterialization of the superior ophthalmic vein and the predominance of the venous drainage of the fistula anteriorly are responsible for the proptosis and chemosis. Because of the aberrant venous drainage of the fistula, the proptosis and chemosis may be absent (if the venous drainage is totally posterior, with a tear on the C5 or C6 portion of the carotid artery) or contralateral (if the venous drainage of the ipsilateral cavernous sinus is totally relegated to the other cavernous sinus through a huge coronal vein). Partial or complete sixth or third nerve palsy is frequent. Vision is usually normal and remains so for a long period. The rare cases in which the ocular venous pressure is above 45 mm Hg should, however, be considered an emergency, since the patient may lose vision abruptly. Retro-orbital pain or facial anesthesia are consequent on the involvement of the fifth nerve. A loud bruit can be heard over the eye.

Diagnostic Work-up. The diagnostic work-up includes an ipsilateral carotid angiogram showing the geometry of the carotid bifurcation (anticipation of potential difficulties during

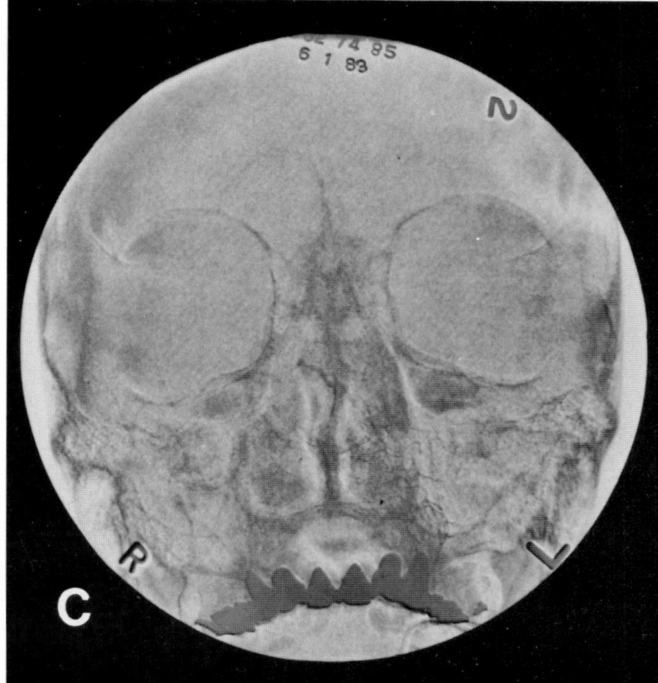
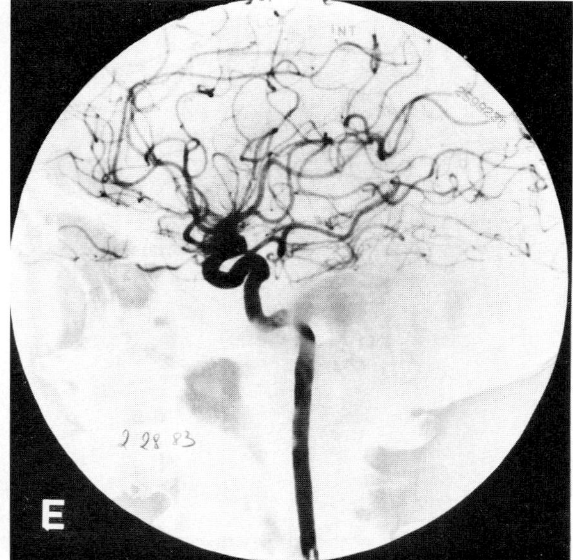
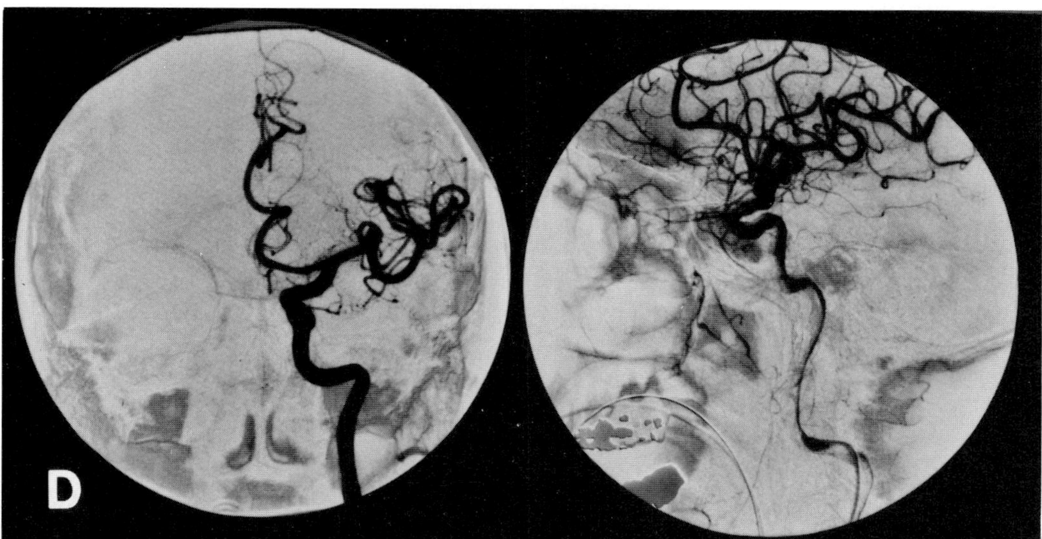

Fig. 70-3. (C) Vertebral angiogram with compression of the carotid artery. The location of the fistula is precisely determined. (D) Angiogram after detachment of one balloon in the cavernous sinus. The fistula is totally occluded. The carotid siphon shows some narrowing in its C5 portion at the level of the tear. (E) Control angiogram 3 months later. Normal internal carotid artery.

treatment), the normality of the external carotid artery (which almost never is involved in the arterialization of the cavernous sinus in this type of traumatic CCF), and the type of venous drainage of the fistula. The neuroradiologist must systematically look for anterior venous drainage through the superior and inferior ophthalmic veins and then the facial vein; for inferior venous drainage through the pterygoid venous plexus; for posterior venous drainage through the superior and inferior petrosal sinuses and the internal jugular vein (the detachable balloon technique can be performed through the jugular vein and the inferior petrosal sinus when the fistula is low and posterior with a predominant posterior venous drainage); for upper venous drainage through the sylvian vein; and for con-

tralateral venous drainage on anteroposterior views, where the subtracted films often show filling of both superior ophthalmic veins.

It is also mandatory to note the importance of the steal effect of the fistula.[17] In rare cases, the steal is complete and there is no filling of the internal carotid artery beyond the level of the fistula. If these patients have no neurologic symptoms, it is proof that the circle of Willis is widely open. However, a bed-rest compression test of the ipsilateral carotid artery, which should be done in every case of traumatic CCF, could well induce a contralateral hemiplegia after 20 to 30 seconds of compression; this hemiplegia regresses as soon as the compression is stopped. This phenomenon needs to be interpreted

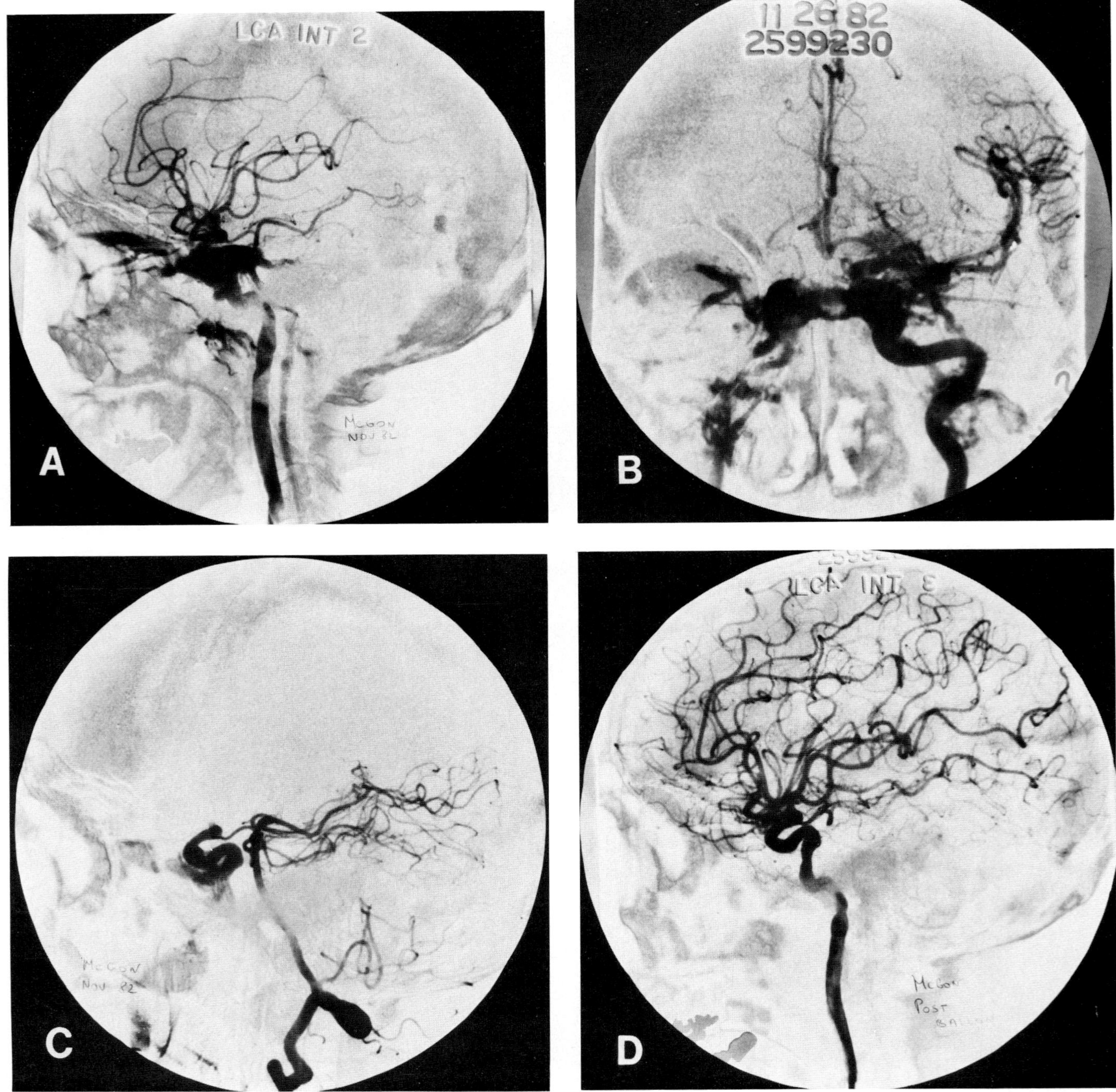

Fig. 70-4. Spontaneous carotid cavernous fistula of the dural type. (1) Left internal carotid angiogram showing reflux of contrast into the left external carotid meningeal branches from the carotid siphon filling the right cavernous sinus. There is partial thrombosis of the left cavernous sinus. (B) Selective angiogram of the left ascending pharyngeal artery showing filling of both cavernous sinuses. (C) Embolization of the left ascending pharyngeal artery with bucrylate. (D) Left internal carotid angiogram showing reflux of contrast into the external carotid. There is no filling of the fistula.

correctly. It means that during the compression, the fistula is stealing enormous amounts of blood from the circle of Willis; this is what jeopardizes the vascularization of the ipsilateral hemisphere. The confirmation of this interpretation is proven by the fact that the patient will tolerate prolonged compression of the ipsilateral carotid after closure of the fistula tear with a balloon inflated in the cavernous sinus.

This complete steal phenomenon also has an important therapeutic implication, because it has been said that this is proof that the internal carotid artery is totally interrupted and that the treatment should be complete occlusion of the carotid artery with a balloon.[10] In fact, these cases should be treated exactly the same as cases in which there is partial steal and the carotid artery is visible beyond the fistula. The quality of the repair of the carotid artery can be as good as in any other case. It simply means that the tear is probably wide and that a large balloon will be necessary to occlude the fistula. It is almost certain that a Silastic balloon, which cannot be inflated to a diameter of more than 8 mm, is too small for this type of fistula and will fail to occlude it totally. This is the main reason for preferring latex balloons to Silastic ones in the treatment of traumatic CCFs. This will not be true when larger Silastic balloons become available.

After all diagnostic and therapeutic information on the ipsilateral carotid artery has been obtained, the diagnostic work-up must be directed to the contralateral internal carotid artery. An anteroposterior projection angiogram is sufficient. If the anterior communicating artery induces opacification of the A1 and M1 segments of the other side, a compression test is not necessary. If there is no cross flow, it is necessary to repeat the AP injection with compression of the carotid artery on the side of the fistula.

The last step of the diagnostic work-up is an angiogram of the vertebral artery with compression of the carotid artery on the side of the fistula. This lateral view will almost invariably demonstrate the location and the size of the tear on the carotid siphon. Another way to document the size and location of the fistula is to use a double-lumen catheter and to occlude the internal carotid artery for a few seconds below the fistula. The injection of contrast through the second lumen of the catheter distal to the inflated balloon will provide this information.

Treatment of Traumatic CCFs. There are three main routes for the treatment of traumatic CCFs (Figure 70-3): (1) the arterial route; (2) the venous route; and (3) the direct surgical approach of the cavernous sinus.

The Arterial Route. The majority of traumatic CCFs can be treated intra-arterially.[8,18,19] In most cases, an 8F or 9F sheath will be positioned into the femoral artery and an 8F or 9F thin-wall catheter will be advanced into the internal carotid artery. When the aortic arch and the carotid arteries are too tortuous, it is necessary to reach the carotid artery by direct puncture of the neck. The wide lumen of the 8F or 9F catheter allows easy introduction of any size balloon, up to 3 mm in uninflated diameter. Each balloon has a metallic marker inside that shows immediately when the balloon reaches the tip of the 9F catheter. The balloon catheter is gently pushed up and the balloon slightly inflated. The balloon follows the curves of the carotid artery through the petrous bone and appears in the cavernous area. It is sucked by the flow of the fistula into the cavernous sinus. It then is inflated until complete closure of the fistula is achieved.

A perfect result is apparent on a digital subtraction arteriogram if: (1) the balloon is in the cavernous sinus, that is, outside the carotid siphon on at least one projection[20]; (2) the fistula is totally occluded without the slightest filling of the cavernous sinus on the arterial phase (filling on the late venous phase is physiologic); and (3) the internal carotid blood flow is preserved with no or minimal narrowing of the lumen. The balloon, which is inflated with iso-osmolar iodinated contrast medium, can be detached at that time, or it can be deflated and refilled with a polymerizing substance. There is no strict rule in using one or the other means of filling the balloon, but the advantages and disadvantages of each method must be understood. There is the risk that a balloon inflated with iodinated contrast may shrink and deflate rather quickly, which could result in recurrence of the fistula (if the balloon deflates within 48 hours after treatment) or which could result in the development of a false venous aneurysm (if the deflation occurs more slowly). These disadvantages are offset by an advantage; if an oculomotor nerve palsy occurs as a result of compression of the nerve by the inflated balloon, rapid recovery should be expected. A balloon inflated with silicone will maintain its size permanently. The frequency of recurrence of the fistula and of false venous aneurysm is diminished. Conversely, the disad-

vantage is that if oculomotor nerve palsy develops, recovery may take more time.

The Venous Route. In the rare case in which the venous drainage is mainly or exclusively posterior and inferior through the inferior petrosal vein and the jugular vein, the fistula can be approached in a retrograde manner.[8,21] The technical difficulties, however, are often high and it is probably better to reserve the venous route for possible failure and to treat the fistula through the arterial route. When the superior ophthalmic vien (SOV) is large and arterialized and when the arterial route has failed, direct puncture or surgical exposure of the SOV is an excellent alternative.[22]

The Direct Surgical Approach to the Cavernous Sinus. In cases in which the carotid artery was ligated, clamped, or divided several years earlier for the treatment of a traumatic CCF, but the artery failed to close, surgical ligation of the internal carotid artery intracranially is not always enough to obliterate the fistula. In such cases or in the rare case in which the internal carotid artery is reconstituted through an embryologic vessel such as a trigeminal or a hypoglossal artery, it is possible to surgically expose the cavernous sinus area,[23–27] to repair the tear of the artery, or to use electrothrombosis or thrombogenic wires, or to puncture the Parkinson triangle, and to introduce into the cavernous sinus a detachable balloon that will be inflated under fluoroscopic control in the operating room until the fistula is closed.[8] Digital subtraction angiography in the operating room is very useful in demonstrating the quality of treatment.

Results of Treatment After closure of the fistula, the proptosis and chemosis improve quickly, and the eye looks normal 1 month after treatment. The bruit over the eye disappears. Such a result is obtained in 99 percent of patients. The preservation of carotid blood flow can be obtained in 90 percent of cases. It is not clear if the 10 percent of patients in whom the internal carotid artery is permanently occluded should have been treated by the surgical approach to the cavernous sinus or the SOV with detachment of the balloon into the cavernous sinus. The reasons for failure to preserve the carotid artery rarely include an inability to enter the cavernous sinus; rather, they usually involve the existence of a large tear, so large that the balloon bulges through the tear and stenoses or totally occludes the carotid artery.

Complications are rare, and most are transient. Oculomotor nerve palsies can occur in up to 20 percent of cases, usually as a result of damage to the sixth nerve. They always improve in a few months, and rarely result in a permanent partial deficit. It is, however, difficult to determine the true percentage of the oculomotor nerve palsies induced by treatment; certain reports mention a 100 percent incidence of oculomotor nerve palsies before treatment. Other permanent neurologic deficits are exceptional, but infarction resulting from ischemic or embolic complications, usually in very old persons, has been reported. The rate of recurrence or incomplete closure of the fistula after treatment is low, although it is higher in those cases in which Silastic balloons are used than in those cases in which latex balloons are used, since the available Silastic balloons are often too small, even if several balloons are used. A second treatment is curative in all these cases.

There are very few articles mentioning follow-up of these patients.[8,28] Most of these patients are lost to follow-up and do not undergo a control angiogram 1 year after treatment. It is,

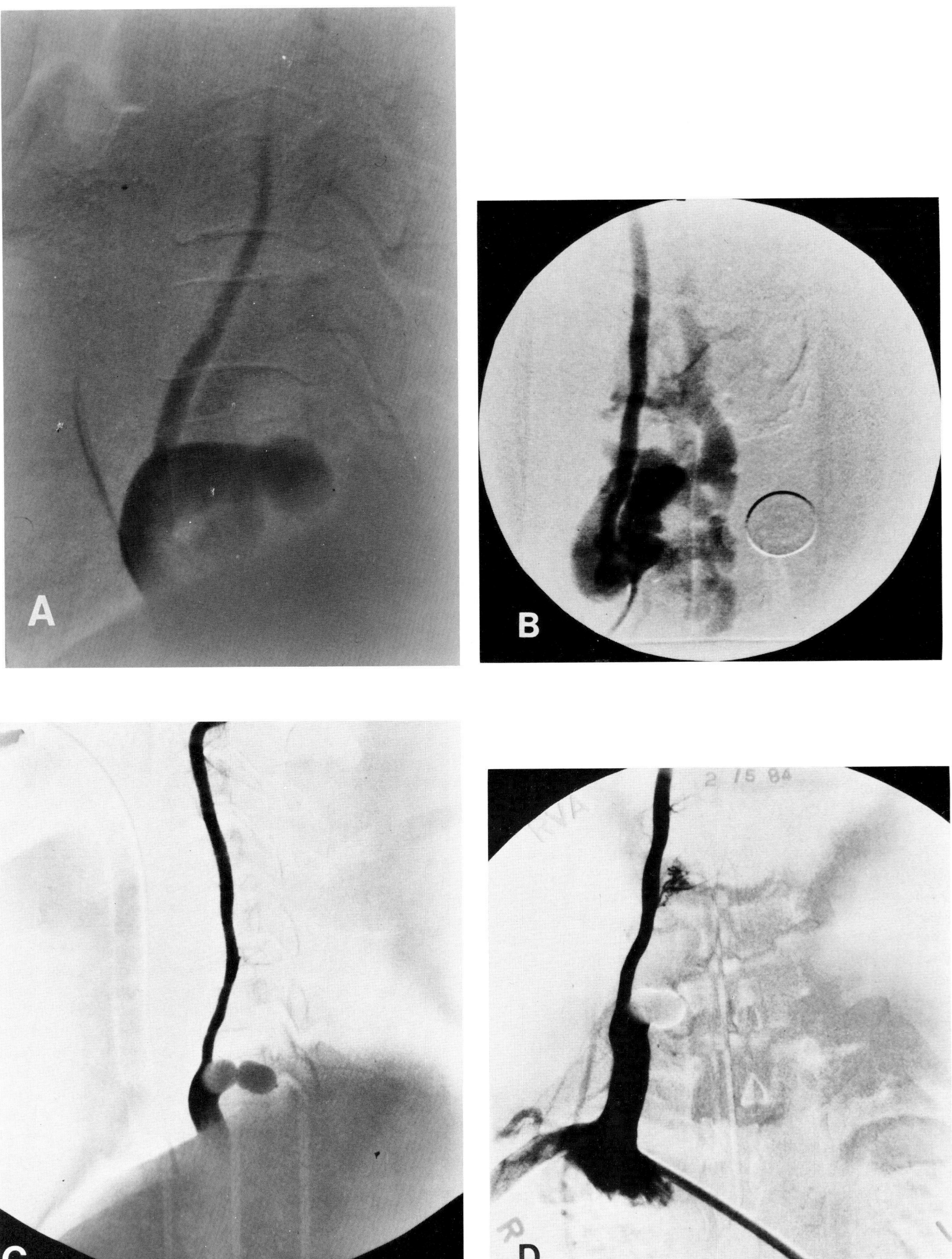

Fig. 70-5. Vertebral fistula. (A) Lateral angiogram of right vertebral artery. Note the large fistula. (B) AP view of the same patient. (C) Occlusion of the fistula with 2 balloons detached in the vein. Preservation of vertebral flow. (D) AP view of the same patient after treatment.

however, very important to know the quality of repair of the carotid artery. In one report,[8] a false venous pouch was noted in up to 50 percent of the patients treated. It usually is a small bulging of the artery into the cavernous sinus at the level of the tear of the artery. Most patients are asymptomatic; only those with a large pouch were symptomatic (oculomotor nerve palsy, retro-orbital pain) and had to be treated with permanent occlusion of the carotid artery. They all were eventually cured.

When it is decided to permanently occlude the internal carotid, it is important to be sure that the fistula is completely closed. The best way to be sure is probably to detach two balloons, one above and one below the fistula. In a few cases, the artery was totally occluded below the fistula, but the tear was incompletely closed and the fistula continued to be filled in a retrograde manner from the circle of Willis. These patients must be operated upon and must have intracranial carotid ligation below the ophthalmic artery.

Spontaneous Carotid Cavernous Fistulae

Most spontaneous CCFs are dural AVMs (Figure 70-4). A few of them are secondary to rupture of a pre-existing cavernous aneurysm and should be treated accordingly. The dural type of CCF can be divided into three subtypes: (1) fistulae with abnormal feeders from the carotid siphon and from the branches of the external carotid artery—the most frequent type; (2) fistulae with feeders from the carotid siphon to the cavernous sinus but a normal external carotid artery—very rare[29]; or (3) fistulae with feeders coming only from the external carotid branches—also very rare.

Type 1 is often seen in elderly women and is often bilateral. Spontaneous cure can ensue, and it is reasonable to wait several months before treating them and then only if they are symptomatic. In addition to tinnitus, the patients have mild chemosis and proptosis and sixth nerve palsy. The diagnostic work-up should always include both internal carotid angiograms and selective angiography of both the ascending pharyngeal artery and the internal maxillary artery. This last trunk reaches the cavernous area through the middle meningeal or accessory meningeal artery or through the artery of the foramen rotundum.

Treatment is difficult.[30] The size of the feeders connecting the carotid siphon to the cavernous sinus is rarely large enough to accept the passage of any type of balloon. In a few cases, however, it has been possible to enter the cavernous sinus with a small balloon.

Most often the treatment must be limited to the embolization of the external feeders. With the new technology of microcatheters and guide wires, it is now possible to catheterize the feeders very distally and to avoid the dangerous collaterals to the cranial nerves or to the intracranial circulation. Solid particles or liquid agents can be used; liquid agents give better clinical results but are more dangerous. Obliteration of the CCF is not always obtained in one sitting with embolization, so additional attempts may be necessary. A surgical approach to the cavernous sinus or the SOV or stereotactic irradiation of the cavernous sinus are the two best alternatives for preserving carotid blood flow.

VERTEBRAL FISTULAE

Vertebral fistulae can be congenital or traumatic, including the iatrogenic cases[9] (Figure 70-5). The traumatic cases are often secondary to gunshots, and the tear in the artery rarely allows preservation of vertebral blood flow. They can be treated with detachable balloons, with care taken to ensure that the fistula is well occluded and does not fill through the contralateral vertebral artery (this should always be checked before the first balloon is detached). If the tear is on the straight portion of the vertebral artery, below C2, it is possible to block the artery with Gianturco coils, which do as well as detachable balloons. If the fistula is above C2, it is more risky to advance the coil at the right place; detachable balloons are much safer.

In iatrogenic cases the fistula is always below C3 and can usually be treated with a detachable balloon with good preservation of vertebral flow. The congenital cases include the cases in which there is no obvious explanation for the presence of the fistula and there is no way to prove that the fistula is truly congenital. In addition to the abnormal communication between the vertebral artery, which is usually at the level of C1, and the vertebral venous plexus, it is always necessary to look for other feeders. The occipital artery, the deep cervical artery, and the ascending cervical artery may reach the fistula, either at the level of the vertebral fistula, or separately into the venous plexus. In the first situation, it is possible to treat the fistula through the occipital artery. In the second situation, the vertebral fistula must be occluded first with a detachable balloon, and then each accessory feeder must be occluded. These fistulae can usually be obliterated with detachable balloons and vertebral blood flow preserved. Large balloons, up to 30 mm, may be necessary. Even when the balloon is inflated with iodinated contrast, progressive deflation of the balloon does not seem to induce any false venous aneurysm when observed at the level of the cavernous sinus.

EXTERNAL CAROTID FISTULAE

External carotid fistulae[31] can be either traumatic or congenital. It is very easy and elegant to occlude the fistula with a detachable balloon. So far the treatment has been successful and without complications.

FISTULAE WITHIN BRAIN AVMS

One of the most recent and important findings is that of direct communication between an artery and a vein inside an AVM in addition to the usual network of abnormal vessels interposed between an artery and a vein in the remainder of the AVM. These fistulae have to be blocked either with a detachable balloon or with a liquid agent that solidifies very quickly. The technique of embolization of brain AVMs will be discussed later in this chapter.

DURAL FISTULAE

Dural fistulae are true AVMs, and it is important to consider them as such for therapeutic purposes. In addition to the spontaneous CCF, the most frequent dural fistula involves the sigmoid sinus. It is increasingly accepted that this is an acquired disease.[32–34] It is exceptional in children. It is often heralded by episodes of headache, fever, papilledema with normal-sized ventricles as demonstrated by computed tomographic (CT) scanning, and acute neurologic deficit secondary to hemorrhagic infarction associated with cerebral venous thrombosis.[35,36] This symptomatology means that the course of the disease is not always benign, and that the angiograms often shows partial obstruction of the sigmoid sinus on the side of the AVM. The patients also frequently complain of tinnitus.

The angiographic work-up includes bilateral vertebral angiograms, bilateral internal carotid angiograms, and bilateral selective angiography of the occipital artery, ascending pharyngeal artery, posterior auricular artery, middle meningeal artery, and accessory meningeal arteries. There is always a collateral network of abnormal vessels invading the wall of the sigmoid sinus. The patients who develop an important network of cortical venous drainage with increased cerebral venous pressure are at risk of cerebral venous infarctions and should be treated as well as those who have progressive decreased vision.

The inflammatory and progressive thrombotic process may induce spontaneous cure of the lesion. At that time, the delayed phase of the carotid or vertebral angiogram shows complete occlusion of the ipsilateral sigmoid sinus. Obliteration can be surgical,[37] or through embolization with particles or with liquid agents delivered very close to the nidus, which is possible with the new microtechniques. Several attempts at embolization may be required in order to cure the lesion. However, when the tentorial and meningeal vessels from the carotid siphon and the vertebral artery are largely participating in the network of abnormal vessels around the sigmoid sinus, embolization of the external carotid feeders is usually insufficient to occlude the malformation, and surgical excision is a better alternative. Other dural AVMs include those around the vein of Galen, the superior longitudinal sinus, and the cavernous sinus.

ANEURYSM OF THE VEIN OF GALEN

Aneurysm of the vein of Galen is in fact a congenital malformation of the deep venous sinuses associated with a giant aneurysmal dilatation of the vein of Galen.[38] The shunt is either of the fistulous type or of the AVM type. The fistulous type includes those cases in which the dominant symptom is cardiac failure at birth, which kills the newborn unless aggressive therapy is undertaken. One or several arteries, including the choroidal vessels or the pericallosal arteries, drain directly into the vein of Galen. The AVM type includes those cases in which the patient survives after birth and develops progressive hydrocephalus. There is a network of abnormal vessels between the dilated vein of Galen and the feeding arteries.

The fistulous type should be treated as a fistula. The fistula can be occluded with a detachable balloon or with liquid agents. The treatment must be done through the femoral artery.[39] A more recent alternative consists of puncturing the straight sinus at the torcular and advancing a catheter to the vein of Galen.[40] Gianturco coils of different sizes and lengths are packed into the vein. Complete obliteration of the vein of Galen is not desirable; it is safer to stage the procedure and to occlude it completely in two or three sittings separated by one or several weeks. The clinical improvement is spectacular with a tremendous decrease of heart failure.

The AVM type of fistula can be treated with solid particles or with liquid agents. The associated hydrocephalus is surgically treated.

TREATMENT OF BRAIN AVMS WITH EMBOLIZATION

The management of brain AVMs is difficult because each case has it own peculiarities. The alternatives are: (1) conservative treatment; (2) surgical resection; (3) embolization; (4) embolization followed by surgical resection; (5) radiation therapy; and (6) radiation therapy following incomplete embolization or incomplete surgical resection. The indications for each of the alternatives depend on what is known of the natural history of the disease,[41-43] on the clinical status of the patient, and on unpredictable factors such as personal experience, the conservative or aggressive nature of the referring physician, and, finally, the decision of the patient.

Patients who have bled, who have uncontrollable seizures, and who have progressive neurologic deficits are candidates for some kind of treatment in which the risks of morbidity and mortality are considered to be less dangerous than is the natural history. Embolization in the treatment of an AVM is still debated, and the indications for and the long-term results of embolization are still unknown. Embolization can be considered either as a complete treatment, if complete obliteration of the AVM can be obtained, or as an incomplete treatment, if the AVM is only partially obliterated. In this situation, complete obliteration of the malformation can be obtained in a certain number of cases if surgical resection or radiation therapy is technically possible. Also, embolization can be done either with solid particles or with liquid agents.

Embolization with solid particles has been done with different materials, including detachable balloons,[10] Silastic spheres,[44,45] or particles of PVA[46] or Gelfoam. Detachable balloons should probably be reserved for occlusion of a true fistula inside an AVM and not used for the proximal occlusion of the feeders, which might momentarily reduce the steal effect of the AVM; recanalization and growth of underdeveloped feeders will recreate the same pathologic situation.

Embolization with Silastic spheres is still preferred by some.[41] The lesion cannot be completely obliterated, but a substantial decrease in the steal effect can be obtained; however, this effect is transient. It is extremely important that the geometry of the vessels and their size be studied before consideration is given to the use of particles.[44,47] The ratio of the diameter of the feeders of the AVM to the diameter of the normal carotid vessels has to be at least 4 to 1, otherwise the particles may stray into normal cortical vessels. It is also mandatory that the geometry and the size of the main trunks at the bifurcation of a common trunk be considered in a case of a pericallosal AVM. The direction of the internal carotid artery usually is prolonged into the middle cerebral artery, and the A1 segment of the anterior cerebral artery makes a sharp angle from the carotid bifurcation. It is therefore almost certain that several particles will enter the M1, even if the A1 has the same caliber as M1. In this particular case, it is possible to temporarily occlude the origin of M1 with an inflated balloon, while the particles are injected into the internal carotid artery. The same concept can be used for a thalamic AVM when one wants to protect the distal middle cerebral artery. An inflated balloon can occlude the MCA distal to the origin of the lenticulostriate arteries, and the particles can be injected into the internal carotid artery if there is no large posterior communicating artery or large anterior cerebral artery.

Even with the best geometry and preferential flow of the feeders of the AVM compared with the vessels of the normal brain, it is almost impossible to avoid the straying of some particles because the hemodynamic changes induced by the first particles increase the likelihood of such an event. It is also difficult to prevent particles from passing through the AVM and reaching the lungs. It is recommended that the clinician choose the size of radiopaque particles that seems appropriate to the size of the vessels of the nidus of the AVM and that one or two particles be injected and followed with control fluoroscopy to determine that they have lodged in the AVM. If they are not visible in the brain, they are probably already in the lungs. Two particles of larger diameter can then be injected and checked, and so on until the size of the particles is such that they stay in the nidus. The inner diameter of the catheter, however, limits the maximum diameter of the particles that can be used. For Silastic spheres, this maximum diameter is 4 mm. If particles of less than 3 mm and more than 2 mm are too small to lodge in the nidus, this is proof that the size of the communications is enormous, that there are probably true fistulae inside the AVM, and that other techniques are better suited to treating such a case.

Two situations are amenable to particle embolization (but do not contraindicate the use of liquid agents). One is a situation involving AVMs causing progressive neurologic deficit, where the steal effect of the malformation is considered to be responsible for the symptomatology. The other situation involves large AVMs in which resection in one operation would be risky because of possible breakthrough phenomenon. In this situation, presurgical embolization decreases the steal and improves the circulation of the surrounding brain, making surgical resection in one operation possible. A rare indication is a case in which there are thalamic or brain stem AVMs with multiple feeders in which it is dangerous to embolize the AVMS with liquid agents.

The complications induced by embolization with solid particles are rarely severe. In 50 percent of cases, the endpoint of the embolization is heralded by some neurologic deficit,[44] indicating that one or several particles are occluding normal cortical vessels. These neurologic deficits are usually transient.

Benati and his team[13] have recently used pieces of 3-0 nylon surgical thread injected through Silastic tubing. Each feeder of the AVM is selectively catheterized and the tip of the tubing is positioned close to the nidus. This technique has proven to be very effective in reducing the size and the steal effect of the AVM, which becomes amenable to surgical resection. The technique seems to be very safe with no mortality and very low morbidity.

EMBOLIZATION WITH LIQUID AGENTS

Silicone was used to treat a few cases of brain AVMs several years ago, but it is not a good liquid agent because the time required for polymerization is not short enough to avoid a large amount of it reaching the venous system. Ethanol, pure or in solutions of differing concentrations, has been considered as a potential sclerosing agent. A major inconvenience is that this agent induces a tremendous inflammatory reaction and enormous edema, with a resultant risk of decompensating the patient. More experimental data must be collected before this liquid agent can be offered as a reasonable treatment.

Embolization with bucrylate has been extensively used during the last decade.[48–56] Its viscosity is very low, and it can be rendered radiopaque by mixing it with tantalum powder and iophendylate. This has two advantages. The first advantage is

that one is able to precisely monitor the injection of bucrylate using digital subtraction television. The second adavntage is an increase in the time of polymerization by a few seconds, allowing more time to control the injection of bucrylate and to withdraw the calibrated leak balloon before it is glued within the cast of solidified bucrylate. By adding a small amount of glacial acetic acid to the bucrylate,[15] it is possible to increase the time of solidification even more, which is useful in slow-flow situations. Few people use bucrylate in its pure and nonradiopaque form[50,51]; most prefer to see where the bucrylate goes during the injection and to stop the injection either when the liquid agent has reached the vein draining the AVM, when the bucrylate ceases to move forward and starts to embed the balloon, or when it reaches normal collaterals.

EMBOLIZATION WITH BUCRYLATE USING A CALIBRATED LEAK BALLOON

There are several precautions that increase the safety of embolization with bucrylate (Figure 70-6). The first precaution involves bringing the calibrated leak balloon as close as possible to the nidus of the AVM. This prevents the injection of bucrylate into normal cortical branches coming out of the feeder. We emphasize that the balloon should be brought close to but not into the nidus, because the abnormal vessels of the nidus are very fragile and could burst when the balloon is inflated. The second precaution involves the choice of appropriate diameter of the latex calibrated-leak balloon. This diameter is compared with that of the feeder to be catheterized, being sure that the inflated balloon will never over-distend the feeder. The third precaution involves carrying out selective angiography when the balloon is in good position. This allows one to see which area of the AVM is injected and to measure the speed with which the contrast flows through the AVM. The time measured from the injection of the contrast to the beginning of filling of the drainage vein indicates the solidification time that should be chosen for the bucrylate. The fourth precaution involves carrying out an amytal test by injecting 30 mg of amytal through the calibrated-leak balloon and testing for any neurologic deficits in the following minutes. If present, such a deficit should be considered a contraindication to embolization of this given feeder.

By sticking to these rules, complications will be few. The dissection of a feeder, which has happened in the past when balloons were too big for the size of the feeder, is now a rare complication. Glueing the balloon into the cast of bucrylate is still a potential risk, but certainly happens now only rarely to experienced teams. There is no reported clinical complication related to the permanent implantation of a calibrated leak balloon catheter that could not be removed after the injection of bucrylate. Careful measurement of the speed of opacification of the feeding artery and the draining vein has permitted individualization of drainage sectors within an AVM. Some feeders are directly connected to a draining vein, with almost instantaneous filling of the vein.[59] In this situation, an extremely fast polymerization time should be chosen or the fistula should be closed with a detachable balloon. Other feeders may irrigate a much slower sector of the AVM, and a delayed time of polymerization can be used. A knowledge of these phenomena has certainly decreased the rate of complications, the amount of bucrylate reaching the draining vein of the AVM, and at the same time improved the obliteration of the malformation.

By staging the embolization in several sittings separated by

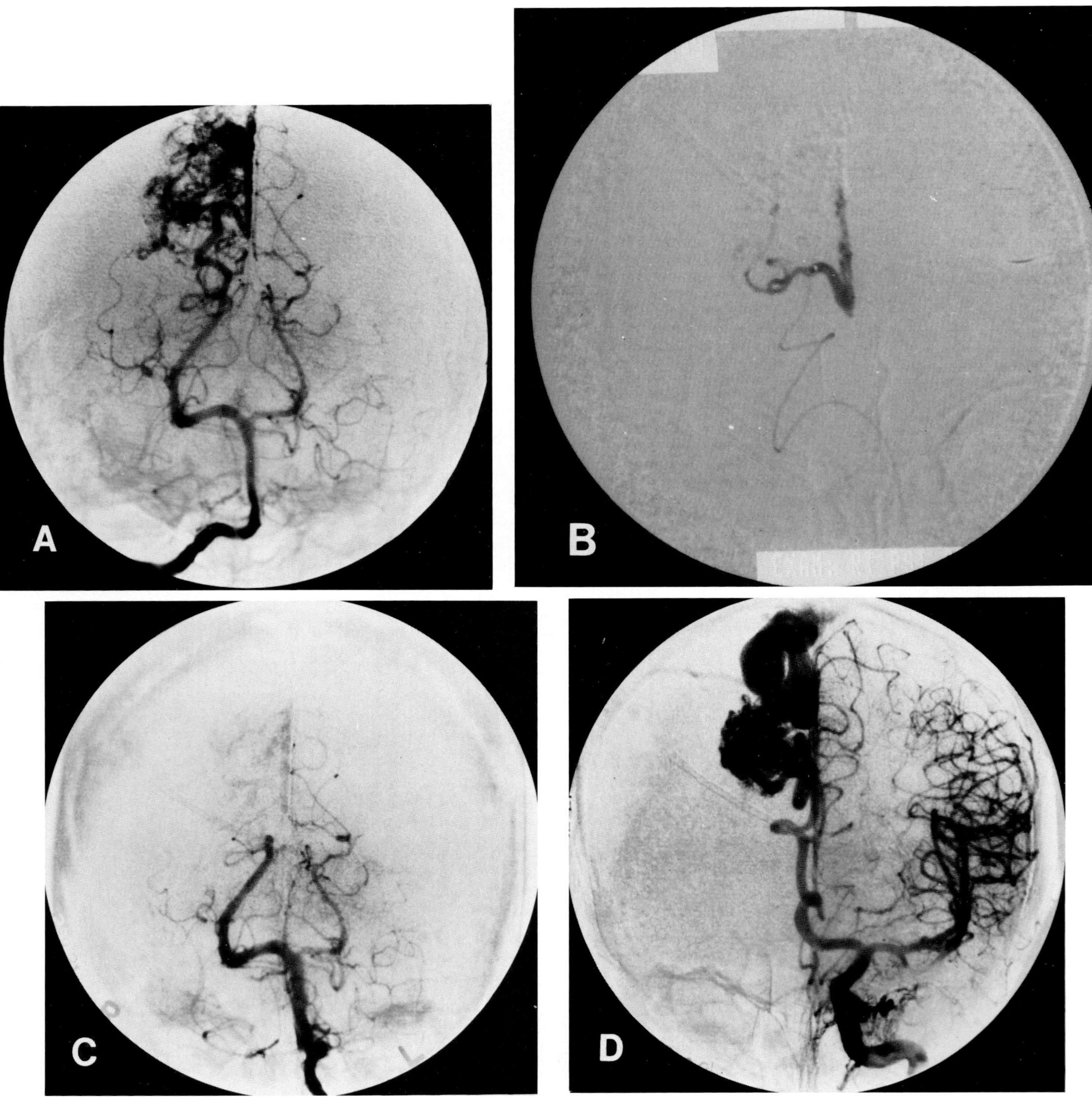

a few weeks rather than embolizing as many feeders as possible at one stage, a certain number of severe complications, such as swelling of the AVM and hemorrhagic infarction of the nidus and of the surrounding brain tissue, can be avoided. This complication becomes a possibility when the venous output of the AVM has been obliterated, while some arterial feeders are still filling the AVM. The neurologic complications usually resolve. However, permanent neurologic deficits have been noted in 10 to 20 percent of patients in some series, although most of the deficits were mild. The mortality rate is between 1 and 4 percent. It should be noted that most of the AVMs included in these statistics were very large AVMs that could not be resected without a much higher risk of mortality and morbidity, on the order of 10 percent and 40 percent, respectively.

An indication for embolization with a calibrated-leak balloon is the presence of deep arterial feeders coming out of the pericallosal or posterior cerebral arteries. Choroidal and lenticulostriate feeders have also been embolized by different teams, but more information is needed about the results and the risks of these embolizations.

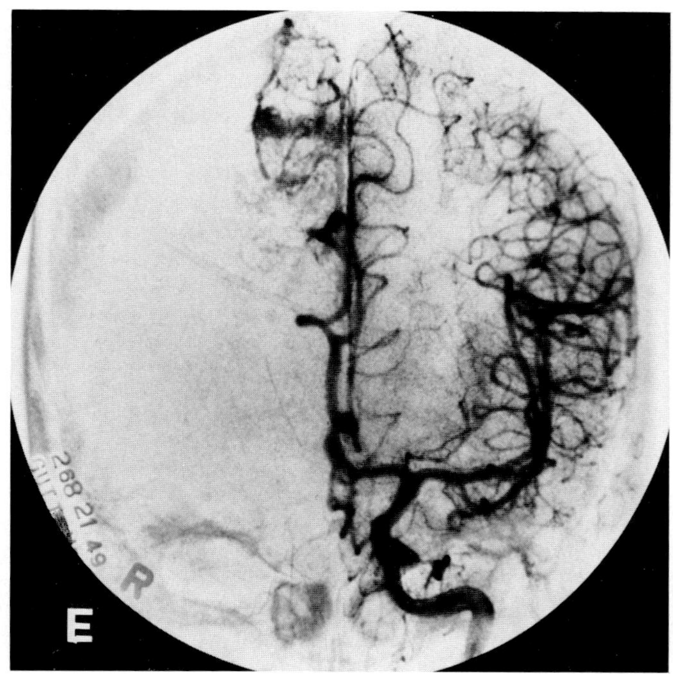

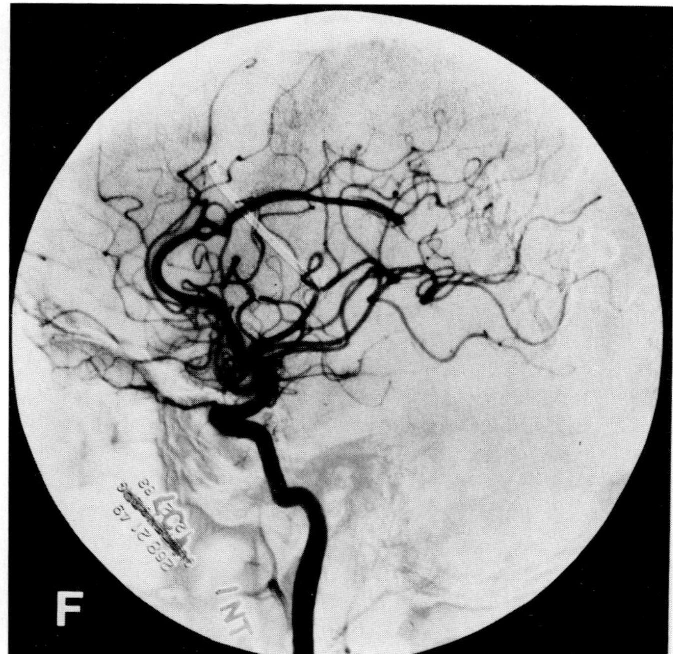

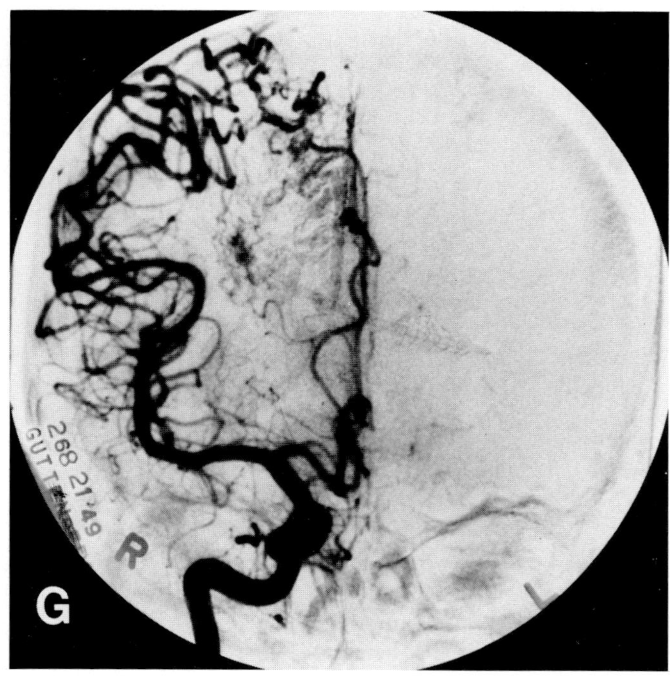

Fig. 70-6. (E) Left carotid angiogram after embolization of the pericallosal with bucrylate. (F) Lateral view of the left carotid artery. No filling of this parasagittal portion of the AVM. (G) Right carotid angiogram. Watershed area fed by cortical branches of the right MCA. The patient underwent total resection of his AVM, and had a good recovery with minor residual right-leg weakness.

INTRAOPERATIVE EMBOLIZATION

Injection of bucrylate can be done at surgery after exposure of one feeder. The best indication for this technique is the presence of the cortical feeders, which are easily exposed without any dissection of the brain tissue. This type of embolization has been extensively used by certain teams,[48,50,51,53] either exclusively[51] or in conjunction with intra-arterial calibrated-leak technique.[49,50,53] It seems that teams that have experience with both techniques use intraoperative embolization less today than in the past. One of the main reasons is that it appears to be safer to stage the embolization, and it is difficult to have more than one intraoperative sitting accepted by the patient. Also, improvements in the calibrated-leak balloon technique and the increased skill of the interventional neuroradiologist are other explanations for the decreased use of intraoperative embolization.

RESULTS

Five percent of brain AVMs embolized with bucrylate are completely obliterated. This low figure is the result of the fact that small AVMs with only a few feeders, which can be occluded by embolization, are usually resected or irradiated. Ninety-five percent are only partially obliterated, but 40 percent of them are totally resected after the last embolization. It is too soon to know if some of the partially obliterated AVMs treated with radiation therapy will be cured at 2 years. Very few have been treated with this combination of therapies, and none of them are cured at this time.

ANEURYSMS

The treatment of symptomatic berry aneurysms is usually synonymous with surgical clipping of the neck of the aneurysm (Figure 70-7). However, certain Soviet physicians[57] have a tremendous experience with occlusion of aneurysms with detachable balloons. More recently, there is some evidence that giant unclippable aneurysms are not the only ones that can be treated with balloon occlusion.[58–61] Our available data deal with giant unclippable aneurysms of the cavernous area or of the distal internal carotid. Very few cases involving the vertebrobasilar system have been treated with balloon occlusion.

Giant aneurysms rarely bleed, but usually compress the surrounding neurologic structures. Because the mass effect of the aneurysm is the cause of the symptoms, it seems illogical to inflate a balloon inside the sac in order to try to preserve the parent artery. Furthermore, the neck of these aneurysms is usually very wide, 5 mm or more, and a spherical balloon inflated inside the sac will bulge through the neck and will narrow or occlude the lumen of the parent artery. Also, unsuspected difficulties have been experienced in a certain number of cases treated by saccular occlusion. This has increased the rate of embolic complications. It is also well known that an aneurysm will be obliterated by intrasaccular balloon occlusion if 100 percent of the neck of the aneurysm is occluded. If the slightest leak persists at the level of the neck, with a small crescent of contrast visible between the inflated balloon and the wall of the aneurysm, no clot will form and there will be no spontaneous occlusion of the sac; conversely, there will be progressive enlargement of the neck and it will finally become necessary to permanently block the parent artery with a balloon occluding the neck as well. For all these reasons, the accepted treatment for these giant unclippable aneurysms is permanent occlusion of the parent artery with detachable balloons. The best result is obtained when the balloon that occludes the artery also occludes the neck of the aneurysm. The width of the neck, however, is often such that the balloon does not stay in the artery; rather, it protrudes into the neck and finally migrates into the aneurysm. When this happens, there are two alternatives. The first is to detach the first balloon into the aneurysm and to detach a second one in the parent artery at the level of the neck. This second balloon cannot migrate into the aneurysm, which is already filled with the first balloon. The second alternative is to detach two balloons in the artery, one beyond the neck and one below the neck. For the treatment of carotid ophthalmic aneurysms, it is necessary to occlude the origin of the ophthalmic artery with the balloon. The occlusion of the carotid artery below the ophthalmic artery could induce complete thrombosis of the aneurysm but also could induce partial thrombosis, as the ophthalmic artery fills in a retrograde manner from the distal internal carotid after permanent occlusion of the proximal internal carotid.

Permanent occlusion of the internal carotid artery should be effected only after a battery of tests has shown that the patient will tolerate it. Rather than the simple compression test of the carotid artery in the neck at bed rest, which could be difficult to interpret correctly, the first test is contralateral carotid angiography and vertebral angiography with ipsilateral compression of the carotid artery in the neck. These angiograms will demonstrate the size of the anterior and posterior communicating arteries and the quality of filling of the ipsilateral middle cerebral territory. Cerebral blood flow measurements should be correlated with the angiograms whenever the equipment is available.

There are two categories of patients. There are those patients with very poor collateral circulation who become symptomatic after 20 to 30 seconds of occlusion of the carotid artery. Their aneurysms cannot be treated without an external carotid-middle cerebral artery bypass followed by permanent occlusion of the carotid artery with a detachable balloon. Even in this situation, the occlusion test should be done and the balloon detached after 15 minutes of occlusion of the carotid artery if the patient is still neurologically intact. There are also those patients, the majority, who have apparently good collateral circulation for whom one can predict good tolerance of the occlusion of the carotid artery. These patients should also have the 15-minute occlusion test before detachment of the balloon. This treatment is usually done with the patient awake and fully heparinized and with permanent blood-pressure monitoring through an intra-arterial line. Particularly in older patients, it is mandatory to maintain the blood pressure slightly above the baseline figures. There is medical debate regarding whether or not to maintain the patient on anticoagulant therapy for 1 month after permanent occlusion of the carotid artery. It is commonly accepted practice to keep the patient on aspirin for a few days before and 1 month after treatment.

In spite of all these precautions, clot emboli or ischemic complications have not disappeared. Most statistics include the first cases treated with this technique, for which the rate of complications was relatively high, but not higher than the rate for those treated by surgical means. The reports of the most recent series mention no mortality and approximately 5 percent morbidity. Basilar unclippable aneurysms are much more difficult to treat. There are a few cases of occlusion of a basilar tip aneurysm with a detachable balloon[60,61]; in these cases the results have either been good or very poor. Some basilar trunk aneurysms have been treated with permanent occlusion of both vertebral arteries with good clinical results. It is too early to know the efficiency of the detachable balloon technique for treating berry aneurysms of the anterior communicating artery or middle cerebral artery that cannot be treated surgically.

SPINAL CORD AVMS AND FISTULAE

There are four different types of AVMs of the spinal cord: (1) anterior AVMs; (2) posterior AVMs; (3) small fistulae within the dura; and (4) large intradural fistulae.

ANTERIOR AVMS

Since the anterior spinal arteries supply four fifths of the spinal cord with blood, any AVM on one of these arteries jeopardizes the cord by the steal effect or by intramedullary hemorrhage. The AVM is often extra) and intramedullary. When surgical resection is not attempted, careful embolization of the anterior spinal artery feeding the AVM can be done with solid particles. The embolization should be interrupted as soon as the nidus of the AVM is occluded in order to protect the many tiny perforating medullary arteries coming off the anterior spinal artery.[62–68] The embolization is also safer when the spinal cord angiogram shows normal anterior spinal arteries above and below the AVM. Monitoring with evoked potentials helps in testing the tolerance of the feeders of the AVM to occlusion.[69] It is not totally reliable.[70]

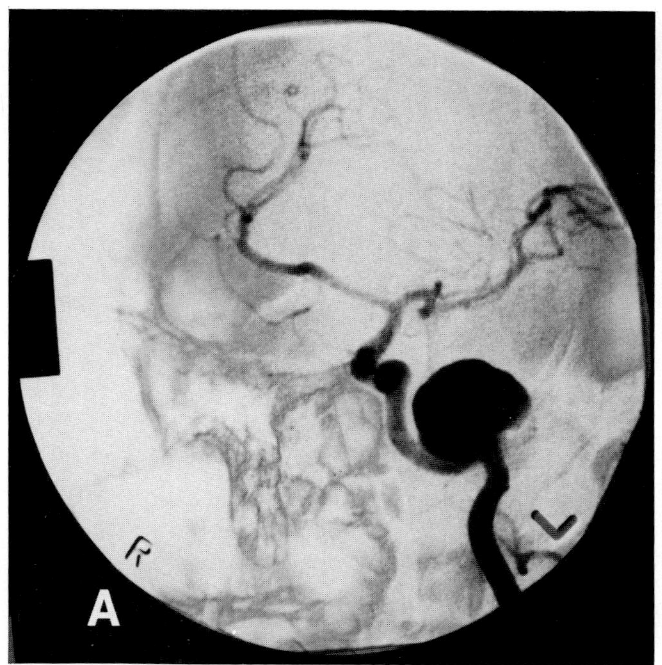

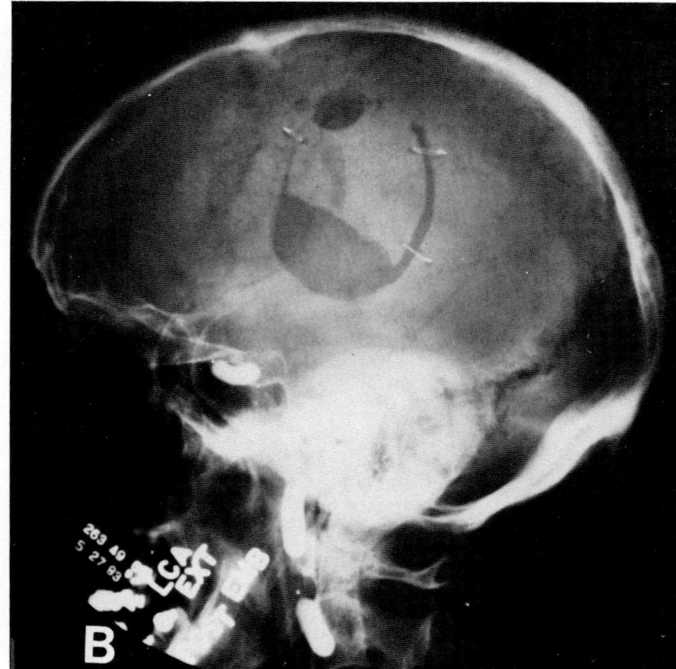

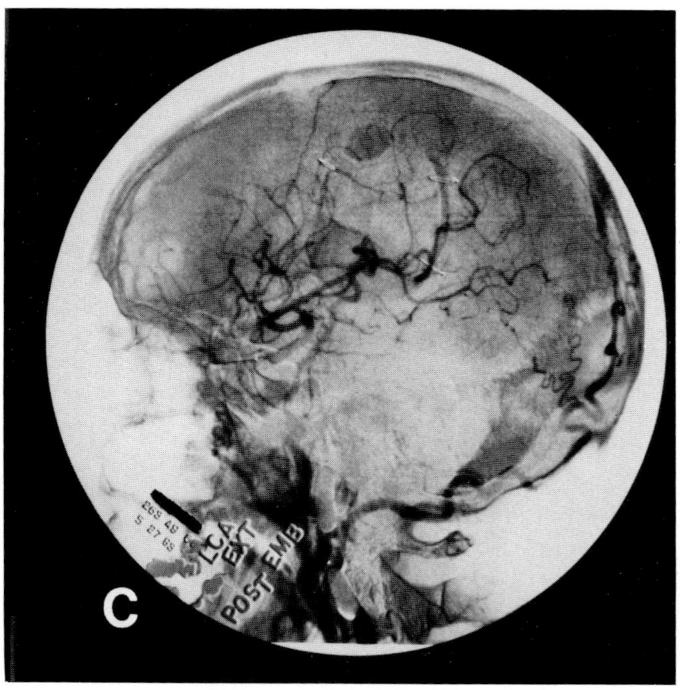

Fig. 70-7. Giant unclippable intrapetrous aneurysm. (A) Left carotid angiogram—left giant intrapetrous aneurysm with wide neck. (B) Trapping of the aneurysm with 3 detachable balloons. The upper one occludes the horizontal C4 portion of the carotid siphon above the aneurysm. The two other balloons occlude the carotid artery in the neck below the aneurysm. (C) The patient underwent EC-IC bypass before permanent occlusion of the internal carotid artery. The left external carotid angiogram obtained after balloon occlusion of the internal carotid shows the nice filling of the left MCA.

POSTERIOR AVMS

Posterior AVMs are fed by posterolateral spinal arteries that normally supply one fifth of the cord posteriorly. This means that the prognosis for these AVMs is usually better than for the anterior AVMs, even when they invade the cord. Also, surgical resection or embolization can be done with less risk than is true for resection or embolization of anterior AVMs. In fact, this division between anterior and posterior AVMs is not always sharply demarcated, and anterior spinal cord AVMs that also receive their blood supply from posterior lateral spinal arteries are frequent. In juveniles, the malformation can be more complex and may involve the vertebrae and the soft tissues.

SMALL FISTULAE WITHIN THE DURA

Small fistulae within the dura have been individualized recently,[71–73] and were confused with posterior AVMs in the past. The patients are predominantly men in their fifties or sixties. Progressive paraplegia or cauda equina syndrome associated with lumbar pain is the usual presentation. When a myelogram is done, abnormal tortuous vessels are demonstrated running over the cord, posteriorly more often than anteriorly. Selective injection of all the intercostal and lumbar arteries and of the sacral arteries shows that one of these arteries is enlarged and drains into a dilated vein that starts precisely where the artery perforates the dura. The vein reaches the conus and drains into the venous plexus, running over the

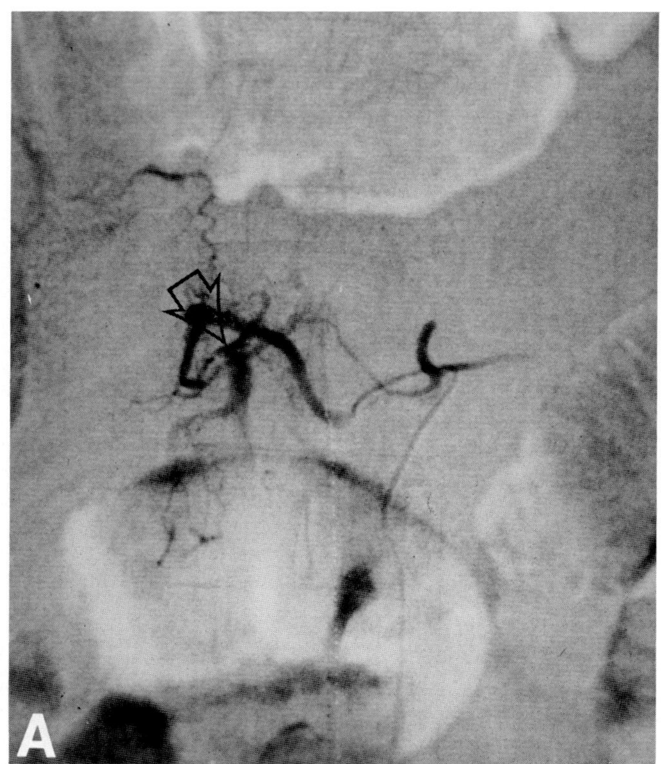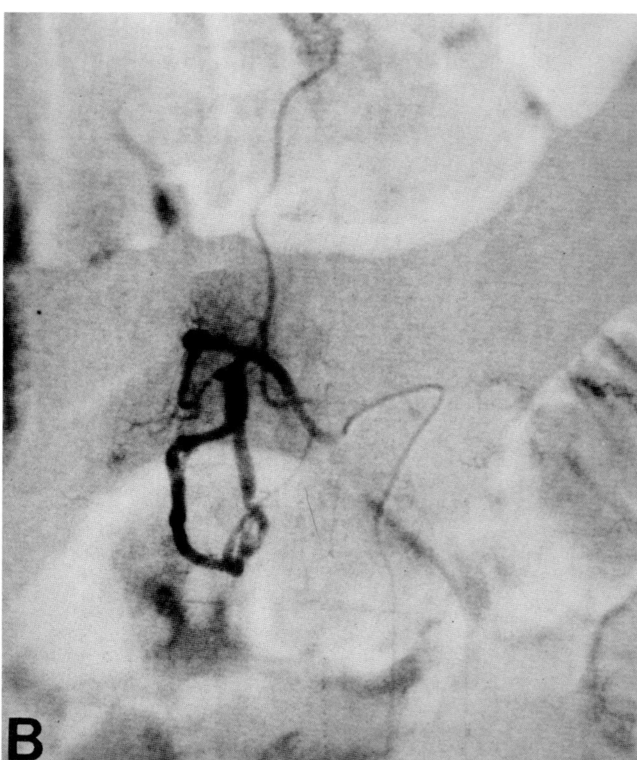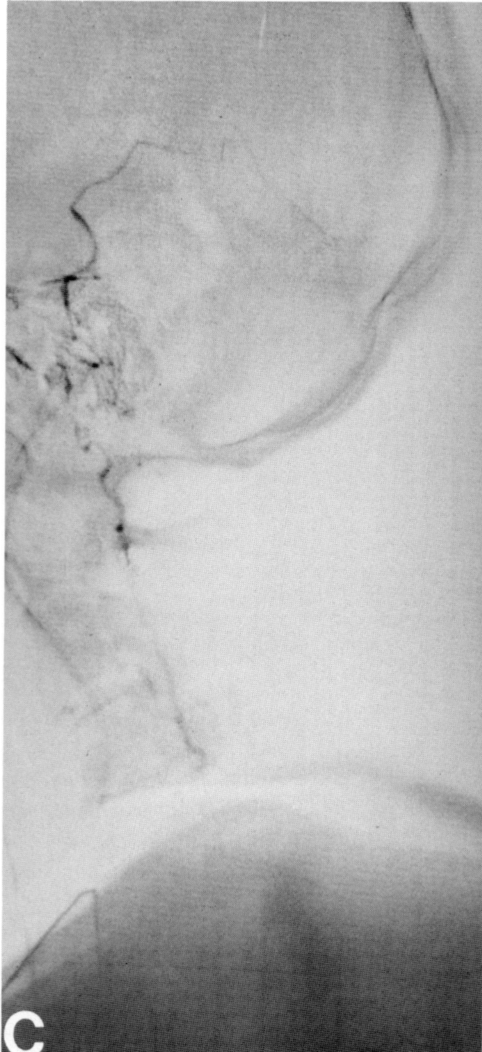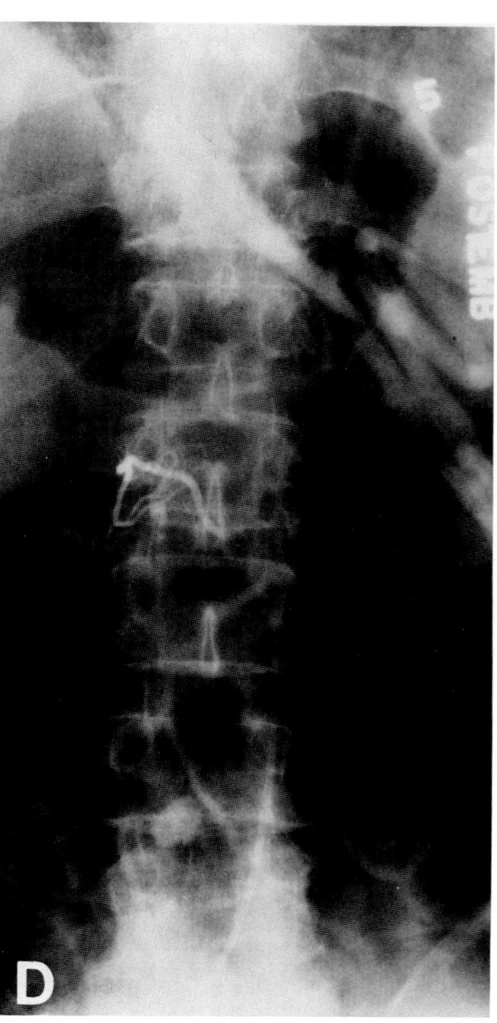

Fig. 70-8. Spinal dural fistula with medullary venous drainage in a 60-year-old man with progressive paraplegia. Selective angiography of the first right lumbar artery. The fistula (A, arrow) drains into a large extramedullary vein that finally reaches the perimedullary venous plexus (B), and can be followed up to the posterior fossa (C). (D) Embolization of right L1 with bucrylate. The injection of bucrylate was interrupted as soon as the fistula was occluded. There was good clinical improvement.

posterior surface of the cord. The tortuous vessels seen on the myelogram are the loops of this venous plexus. The arterialized venous plexus can be followed upward, often up to the posterior fossa where it drains into the straight sinus or the pontomesencephalic veins. Before there was an understanding that there was a direct communication between an artery and a vein within the dura, the draining posterior venous plexus running up over the cord was considered to be the AVM and was treated as such by surgical resection or by extensive embolization. The result was usually catastrophic. Today, these patients can be cured either by surgical resection or by embolization limited to the fistula within the dura[72,73] (Figure 70-8). The treatment has the best chance of improving the status of the patient if it is done before the patient has reached the stage of complete paraplegia.

LARGE INTRADURAL SPINAL CORD FISTULAE

Large intradural spinal cord fistulae are exceptional and only a few reports of cases have been published.[74–76] One anterior spinal artery is enormously dilated and drains directly into a large vein. The treatment has to be either surgical or blockage of the fistula with a detachable balloon.

SELECTIVE INFUSION OF CHEMOTHERAPEUTIC AGENTS

Nitrosourea has been extensively used as a chemotherapeutic adjunct in the treatment of brain gliomas. It has been administered either intravenously or into the cervical internal carotid artery. The boundary between systemic toxicity and target activity is very light. When injected into the cervical internal carotid artery, side effects on the eye, including pain, redness, decreased vision, or even unilateral blindness, have been reported. The use of a calibrated leak balloon positioned above the ophthalmic artery during the infusion of nitrosourea avoids these complications.[77] However, nitrosourea is not the ideal drug for the treatment of glioblastomas. Its systemic side effects and its toxicity to the normal brain make its use very difficult. It is our hope that new chemotherapeutic agents, less toxic and more effective on the tumor, will be found and selectively delivered into the tumoral vessels with the calibrated leak balloon technique.

REFERENCES

1. Ahn HS, White RI, Kumar AJ: Carotid cavernous fistulae—Intravascular treatment with a self-sealing detachable balloon: Radiology 149:583, 1983
2. Norman D, Newton TH, Edwards MS: Carotid cavernous fistulae: Closure with detachable silicone balloons. Radiology 149:149, 1983
3. Tsai FY, Hieshima GB, Mehringer CM: Delayed effects in the treatment of carotid cavernous fistulae. AJNR 4:357, 1983
4. White RI, Barth KH, Kaufman SL: Therapeutic occlusion with detachable balloons. Cardiovasc Intervent Radiol 3:229, 1980
5. Berenstein A, Kricheff II, Ransohoff J: Carotid cavernous fistulae—Intraarterial treatment. AJNR 1:449, 1980
6. Debrun G, Lacour P, Caron JP, et al: Experimental approach to the treatment of carotid cavernous fistulae with an inflatable and isolated balloon. Neuroradiology 9:9, 1975
7. Debrun G, Lacour P, Caron JP, et al: Inflatable and released balloon technique. Experimentation in dog—Application in man. Neuroradiology 9:267, 1975
8. Debrun GM, Lacour P, Vinuela F, et al: Treatment of 54 traumatic carotid-cavernous fistulae. J Neurosurg 55:678, 1981
9. Debrun G, Legre J, Kasbarian M, et al: Endovascular occlusion of vertebral fistulae by detachable balloons with conservation of the vertebral blood flow. Radiology 130:141, 1979
10. Serbinenko FA: Balloon catheterization and occlusion of major cerebral vessels. J Neurosurg 41:125, 1974
11. Kerber C: Balloon catheter with a calibrated leak. A new system for superselective angiography and occlusive catheter therapy. Radiology 120:547, 1976
12. Debrun GM, Vinuela FV, Fox AJ, et al: Two different calibrated-leak balloons: Experimental work and application in humans. AJNR 3:407, 1982
13. Benati A, Beltramello A, Mashio A: Combined embolization of intracranial AVMs with a multipurpose mobile-wing microcatheter system. Indications and results in 58 cases. Paper presented at the 25th Annual Meeting of the ASNR, New York, May 11, 1987
14. Strother CM, Kikuchi K, Morless A: The use of polyvinyl alcohol particles and gluteraldehyde cross-linked collagen (Angiostat) in the treatment of intracranial arteriovenous malformations. Paper presented at the 25th Annual Meeting of the ASNR, New York, May 11, 1987
15. Spiegel SM, Vinuela FV, Goldwasser JM, et al: Adjusting the polymerization time of isobutyl-2 cyanoacylate. AJNR 7:109, 1986
16. Klara PM, George ED, McDonnell DE, et al: Morphological studies of human arteriovenous malformations: Effects of isobutyl 2-cyanoacylate embolization. J Neurosurg 63:421, 1985
17. Sbeith IA, O'Laoire SA: Traumatic carotid-cavernous fistula due to transection of the intracavernous artery. J Neurosurg 60:1080, 1984
18. Negoro M, Kageyama N, Ishiguchi T: Cerebrovascular occlusion by catheterization and embolization: Clinical experience. AJNR 4:362, 1983
19. Scialfa G, Valsecchi F, Scotti G: Treatment of vascular lesions with balloon catheters. AJNR 4:395, 1983
20. Graeb DA, Robertson WD, Lapointe JS, et al: Avoiding intraarterial balloon detachment in the treatment of posttraumatic carotid-cavernous fistulae with detachable balloons. AJNR 6:602, 1985
21. Manelfe C, Berenstein A: Treatment of carotid cavernous fistulas by venous approach. J Neuroradiol 7:13, 1980
22. Uflacker R, Lima S, Ribas GC: Carotid cavernous fistulas: Embolization through the superior ophthalmic vein approach. Radiology 159:175, 1986
23. Hosobuchi Y: Electrothrombosis of carotid cavernous fistula. J Neurosurg 41:76, 1975
24. Dolenc V: Direct microsurgical repair of intracavernous fistula. J Neurosurg 38:99, 1973
25. Mullan S: Experiences with surgical thrombosis of intracranial berry aneurysms and carotid cavernous fistulae. J Neurosurg 41:657, 1974
26. Parkinson D: Carotid cavernous fistula: Direct repair with preservation of the carotid artery. Technical note. J Neurosurg 38:99, 1973
27. Isamat, Ferrer E, Twose J: Direct intracavernous obliteration of high flow carotid cavernous fistulas. J Neurosurg 65:770, 1986
28. Debrun G: Treatment of traumatic carotid-cavernous fistula using detachable balloon catheters. AJNR 4:355, 1983
29. Bradac GB, Bender A, Curio G, et al: Report of two cases of spontaneous direct carotid-cavernous fistula. Neuroradiology 27:436, 1985
30. Vinuela F, Fox AJ, Debrun GM: Spontaneous carotid-cavernous fistulae: Clinical, radiological, and therapeutic considerations. Experience with 20 cases. J Neurosurg 60:976, 1984
31. Ahn HS, Kerber CW: Embolisation therapeutique d'une fistule carotide externe—Sinus caverneux chez le nourrisson: J Neuroradiol 10:261, 1983
32. Chaudhary MY, Sachdev VP, Cho SH, et al: Dural arteriovenous

malformation of the major venous sinuses: An acquired lesion. AJNR 3:13, 1982

33. Kazuo K, Taneda M: Angiographic disappearance of multiple dural arteriovenous malformations. J Neurosurg 60:1275, 1984

34. Seeger JF, Gabrielsen TO, Giannotta SL, et al: Carotid-cavernous sinus fistulae and venous thrombosis. AJNR 1:141, 1980

35. Fardoun R, Adam Y, Mercier P, et al: Tentorial arteriovenous malformation presenting as intracerebral hematoma. J Neurosurg 55:976, 1981

36. Sakaki S, Fujita H, Kohno K, et al: Dural arteriovenous malformation in the posterior fossa associated with intracerebellar hematoma. J Neurosurg 60:1067, 1984

37. Sundt TM, Piepgras DG: The surgical approach to arteriovenous malformations of the lateral and sigmoid dural sinuses. J Neurosurg 59:32, 1983

38. Raybaud CA, Hald JK, Strother CM: Aneurysms of the vein of Galen. Embryological, anatomical and angiographic considerations. ASNR 23rd Annual Meeting, New Orleans, 1985

39. Berenstein A, Epstein F, Choi IS: The role of embolization in the management of the vein of Galen malformations. Presented at the ASNR 23rd annual meeting, New Orleans, 1985

40. Parker MJ: Embolization of aneurysms of the vein of Galen with coils and through venous approach. Treatment of two cases, included in lecture "Neurosurgical correlation: Carotid cavernous fistulae, AVMs and giant aneurysms." Presented at the 3rd Interventional Radiology Seminar, Disneyworld (Epcot Center), Orlando, Florida, 1985

41. Luessenhop AJ, Rosa L: Cerebral arteriovenous malformations: Indications for and results of surgery, and the role of intravascular techniques. J Neurosurg 60:14, 1984

42. Graf CJ, Perret GE, Torner JC: Bleeding from cerebral arteriovenous malformations as part of their natural history. J Neurosurg 58:331, 1983

43. Jane JA, Kassell NF, Torner JC, et al: The natural history of aneurysms and arteriovenous malformations. J Neurosurg 62:321, 1985

44. Wolpert SM, Stein BM: Factors governing the course of emboli in the therapeutic embolization of cerebral arteriovenous malformations. Radiology 131:125, 1979

45. Wolpert SM, Barnett FJ, Prager RJ: Benefits of embolization without surgery for cerebral arteriovenous malformations. AJNR 2:535, 1981

46. Scialfa G, Scotti G: Superselective injection of polyvinyl alcohol microemboli for the treatment of cerebral arteriovenous malformations. AJNR 6:957, 1985

47. Patronas NJ, Marx WJ, Duda EE, et al: Microvascular embolization of arteriovenous malformations. Predicting success by cerebral angiography. AJNR 1:459, 1980

48. Cromwell LD, Harris AB: Treatment of cerebral AVMs. Combined neurosurgical and neuroradiological approach. AJNR 4:366, 1983

49. Debrun GM, Vinuela FV, Fox AJ, et al: Embolizations of cerebral arteriovenous malformations with bucrylate. Experience in 46 cases. J Neurosurg 56:615, 1982

50. Pevsner PH, Doppman JL: Therapeutic embolization with a microballoon catheter system. AJNR 1:171, 1980

51. Samson D, Ditmore QM, Beyer CW: Intravascular use of IBCA for intracranial AVMs. Neurosurgery 8:43, 1981

52. Bank WO, Kerber CW, Cromwell LD: Treatment of intracerebral AVMs with IBCA. Initial clinical experience. Radiology 139:609, 1981

53. Fox AJ, Girvin JP, Vinuela FV: Rolandic arteriovenous malformations: Improvement in limb function by IBC embolization. AJNR 6:575, 1985

54. Vinuela FV, Debrun GM, Fox AJ: Dominant hemisphere AVMs. Therapeutic embolization with IBCA. AJNR 4:959, 1983

55. Vinuela FV, Fox AJ, Debrun GM, et al: Progressive thrombosis of brain arteriovenous malformations after embolization with isobutyl 2-cyanoacylate. AJNR 4:1233, 1983

56. Vinuela FV, Debrun GM, Fox AJ, et al: Dominant-hemisphere arteriovenous malformations: Therapeutic embolization with isobutyl-2-cyanoacylate. AJNR 4:959, 1983

57. Romodanov AP, Shcheglov VI: Intravascular occlusion of saccular aneurysms of the cerebral arteries by means of a detachable balloon catheter, in Advances and Technical Standards in Neurosurgery, vol 9. Berlin, Springer-Verlag, pp 25–49

58. Berenstein A, Ransohoff J, Kupersmith M: Transvascular treatment of giant aneurysms of the cavernous carotid and vertebral arteries. Surg Neurol 21:3, 1984

59. Vinuela FV, Fox AJ, Debrun GM, et al: Preembolization superselective angiography: Role in the treatment of brain arteriovenous malformations with isobutyl-2 cyanoacylate. AJNR 5:765, 1984

60. Halbach VV, Higashida RT, Hieshima GB: Treatment of intracranial aneurysm with mass effects by transvascular balloon embolization. Paper presented at the 25th annual meeting of the ASNR, New York, May 11, 1987

61. Hieshima GB: Transcatheter treatment of intracranial aneurysms. Lecturer at the 25th annual meeting of the ASNR, New York, May 11, 1987

62. Djindjian R: Embolization of angiomas of the spinal cord. Surg Neurol 4:411,420, 1975

63. Doppman JL, DiChiro G, Ommaya AK: Percutaneous embolization of spinal cord AVMs. J Neurosurg 34:48, 1971

64. Horton JA, Latchaw RE, Gold LHA, et al: Embolization of intramedullary arteriovenous malformations of the spinal cord. AJNR 7:113, 1986

65. Margolis MT, Freeny PC, Kendrick MM: Cyanoacylate occlusion of a spinal cord arteriovenous malformation. J Neurosurg 51:107, 1979

66. Riche MC, Melki JP, Merland JJ: Embolization of spinal cord vascular malformations via the anterior spinal artery. AJNR 4:378, 1983

67. Theron J, Cosgrove R, Melanson D, et al: Spinal arteriovenous malformations: Advances in therapeutic embolization. Radiology 158:163, 1986

68. Ausman JI, Gold LH, Tadavarthy SM, et al: Intraparenchymal embolization for obliteration of an intramedullary AVM of the spinal cord. J Neurosurg 47:119, 1977

69. Berenstein A, Young W, Ransohoff J: Somatosensory evoked potentials during spinal angiography and therapeutic transvascular embolization. J Neurosurg 60:777, 1984

70. Ginsburg HH, Shetter AG, Rauzens PA: Postoperative paraplegia with preserved intraoperative somatosensory evoked potentials. J Neurosurg 63:296, 1985

71. Kendall BE, Logue V: Spinal epidural angiomatous malformations draining into intathecal veins. Neuroradiology 13:181, 1977

72. Merland JJ, Riche MC, Chiras J: Intraspinal extramedullary arteriovenous fistula draining into the medullary veins. J Neuroradiol 7:271, 1980

73. Symon L, Kuyama H, Kendall B: Dural AVMs of the spine. Clinical features and surgical results in 55 cases. J Neurosurg 60:238, 1984

74. Djindjian R: L'Angiographie de la Moelle Epiniere (Angiography of the Spinal Cord). Paris, Masson, 1970

75. Heros RC, Debrun GM, Ojemann RG, et al: Direct spinal arteriovenous fistula: A new type of spinal AVM. J Neurosurg 64:134, 1986

76. Riche MC, Scialfa G, Gueguen B, et al: Giant extramedullary arteriovenous fistula supplied by the anterior spinal artery: Treatment by detachable balloons. AJNR 4:391, 1983

77. Debrun GM, Davis KR, Hochberg FH: Superselective injection of BCNU through a latex calibrated-leak balloon. AJNR 4:399, 1983

Index

Abscess. *See specific sites and diagnoses*
Accident, emergency care, 19
Acoustic neuroma, 705–708
  anatomy, 687–689
  anesthesia for, 689–690
  cerebellopontine angle, 673–674
  cerebrospinal fluid rhinorrhea with, 702–703
  closure, 701–702
  differential diagnosis, 572
  four quadrants dissection, 699–701
  gutting procedure, 699
  hematoma with, 702
  hemostasis, 701
  patient positioning, 690
  postoperative complications, 702–703
  postoperative management, 702
  postradiosurgery complications, 521
  removal, 696–699
  results, 703
  stereotactic radiosurgery, 520–521
  surgical management, 690–692
  translabyrinthine dissection, 692–696
  translabyrinthine operation, 685–704
Acoustic tumor (bilateral), 681
Acquired immune deficiency syndrome, 419, 422
Acromegaly, 299
  stereotactic radiosurgery, 518
ACTH assay, in pituitary adenoma, 300
Adult respiratory distress syndrome, with acute head injury, 27–28
Affective disorders
  surgery for, 1057–1060
  surgical anatomy, 1058
  surgical controversies, 1059–1060
  surgical indications, 1060
Air embolism, in tentorium tumor, 648
Alloplastic grafting materials, for skull defects, 11, 14–16
Alpha fetoprotein, in intracranial germ cell tumor, 398
Amnesia, after transcallosal interfornicial approach to third ventricle, 389–390
Amphotericin B, in fungus infection, 90
Amyotrophic lateral sclerosis, 1352, 1354, 1355
Analgesia, implanted electrode brain stimulation for, 1089–1095
Anaphylaxis, from chymopapain chemonucleolysis, 1437, 1438, 1440
Anesthesia. *See also specific diagnoses and procedures*
  anatomophysiologic factors in children, 103–116
  for head injury, 113–114
  for neuroradiographic procedures, 112–113
Anesthetic agents
  for children, 104
  epidural infusion for intractable pain, 1145

Aneurysm, 1003–1007. *See also specific sites*
  age factor, 1003, 1005
  arteriography in, 1004, 1006
  asymptomatic, 1006
  bleeding potential, 1004
  clinical parameters, 1004, 1006
  computed tomography in, 1004, 1006
  diagnosis, 1003–1004
  electroencephalography in, 1004, 1006
  hypertension and, 1003, 1006
  incidence, 1003, 1006
  intraoperative ultrasonography visualization, 217
  laser occlusion, 226
  multiple, 1003, 1006
  nonsurgical management, 1006
  risk of rupture, 1005
  ruptured, 1004, 1005
  sex factor, 1003
  site, 1003
  subarachnoid hemorrhage with, 1004, 1005
  surgical criteria, 1005
  surgical morbidity, 1005
  surgical treatment, 1005, 1006
  unruptured, 1005–1006
Aneurysm (giant)
  internal carotid artery at anterior communicating region, 1026
  at middle cerebral artery, 1026
  of vertebrobasilar circulation, 1026
Aneurysm (intracerebral)
  balloon catheter management, 831–832
  traumatic, 991–995
Aneurysm (unclippable), 1023–1034
  aneurysmorrhaphy in, 1032–1033
  angiography, 1029–1030
  balloon occlusion, 1024, 1033
  computed tomography, 1029–1030
  configuration factor, 1029–1030
  deep hypotension in, 1030, 1032
  evaluation at surgery, 1030–1033
  indirect procedures, 1033
  ingenious clip techniques, 1033
  intra-aneurysmal thrombosis, 1033
  preoperative evaluation, 1023–1030
  Sendai cocktail, 1032
  site factor, 1023
  size factor, 1025–1029
  temporary proximal occlusion or trapping, 1030–1032
  wrapping of, 1032
Aneurysmorrhaphy, 1032–1033
Angiography
  in arterial aneurysm, 1011, 1013
  in anterior communicating artery aneurysm, 940, 949, 951, 953
  in anterior skull base tumor, 612
  in arteriovenous malformation, 523–525, 900, 902, 1011, 1017

  in anteroinferior dural venous fistula, 849–854
  in bacterial intracranial aneurysm, 997, 998–999
  in carotid artery lesion, 753, 754, 757
  in carotid cavernous fistula, 846
  in carotid ophthalmic aneurysm, 918, 925, 927
  in cerebellar hemangioma, 660
  in cervical spondylosis, 1332
  in Chiari malformation with hydromelia, 1316
  in clivus and basioccipital region tumor, 638
  in craniopharyngioma, 356
  in dural fistula, 828
  in dural sinus malformation, 861
  in gunshot wounds of head, 38–39
  in internal carotid artery aneurysm, 837, 930
  in intracerebral hemorrhage, 885
  in intramedullary spinal cord tumor, 1490, 1492
  in medial sphenoid wing meningioma, 538
  in meningioma, 550–551, 564–566, 572
  in middle cerebral artery aneurysm, 957, 970
  in moyamoya disease, 798–801, 803
  in olfactory groove meningioma, 540
  in optic nerve decompression, 270
  in spine tumor, 1526–1527
  in STA-MCA bypass, 783, 791
  in suprasellar germinoma, 398
  in suprasellar meningioma, 531
  in tentorium tumor, 647
  in traumatic aneurysm, 991, 992
  in traumatic carotid cavernous fistula, 822, 825
  in unclippable aneurysm, 1029–1030
  for vertebrobasilar insufficiency, 808, 810, 812
Angiography (digital), with stereotactic intra-axial tumor resection, 481, 483
Ankle clonus, stimulation management, 1056–1057
Ankylosing spondylitis, 1300–1303
  atlantoaxial subluxation, 1303
  cauda equina syndrome, 1303
  intraspinal ossification, 1303
  pachymeningitis, 1303
  spinal fracture/dislocation, 1302–1303
  stress fracture, 1303
Annulus of Zinn, 235, 236
Anterior communicating artery aneurysm, 939–955, 1032
  anesthesia, 940
  aneurysm neck dissection, 945–946
  aneurysm obliterating, 946–948
  aneurysm rupture management, 946
  angiography, 940, 949, 951, 953

Anterior communicating
    artery aneurysm (continued)
  bipolar neck cauterization, 948
  brain tension reduction, 941
  carotid balloon occlusion, 951
  case reports, 949–952
  cerebral blood flow studies, 939, 949, 950,
      951, 954
  clipping alternatives, 946–948
  closure, 948
  complications, 954
  computed tomography in, 939, 949, 952
  controlled hypotension in, 941
  deterioration with, 939, 940
  dome aspiration, 948
  exposure, 942–943
  incision, 941–942
  indirect surgical attack, 948–949, 954
  ligature placement, 948
  magnetic resonance imaging in, 939
  medical management, 939–940
  microsurgical dissection, 944–945
  patient positioning, 941
  periarterial hematoma removal, 950–951
  postoperative management, 949
  preoperative management, 939
  reinforcement with muslin, 948
  results, 952–953
  surgical technique, 941–949
  temporary clipping and cerebral
      protection, 945, 954
  vasospasm with, 941, 954
Anterior lumbar discectomy/interbody
    fusion, 1421–1436
  abdominal ileus with, 1431
  anticoagulation therapy after, 1427
  case reports, 1431–1434
  complications, 1428–1431
  computed tomography, 1423
  contraindications, 1423
  donor site disturbance, 1429–1430
  electromyography, 1423
  impotence with, 1430–1431
  indications for, 1421–1422
  infection with, 1431
  intraoperative hemorrhage, 1431
  metrizamide myelography for, 1423
  postoperative hematoma, 1431
  postoperative management, 1426–1428
  pseudoarthrosis with, 1428–1429
  radiography, 1422, 1427–1428
  results, 1434–1435
  technetium 99 bone scan, 1423
  technique, 1423–1426
  thermography, 1423
  thromboembolism with, 1428, 1430
  urinary tract disturbance with, 1430
  venography for, 1423
Anterior skull base tumor
  angiography, 612
  computed tomography, 611
  craniofacial resection, 609–618
  radiography, 611
Antibiotic prophylaxis
  in cerebrospinal fluid leakage, 61, 62
  with missile injury, 52
Anticholinergic agents, in torticollis, 1262
Anticoagulation therapy
  after anterior lumbar discectomy, 1427

  in carotid artery lesion, 753, 756, 760
Anticonvulsants
  in cerebral glioma, 435–436
  in missile injury, 52
  in torticollis, 1262
  in tuberculoma, 82
Antidepressants, in torticollis, 1262
Antituberculosis agents
  in tuberculoma, 81–82
  in tuberculous meningitis, 84
Arachnoid cyst
  extra-axial, 658–659
  reconstruction technique, 331
Argon laser, 223–224, 226
Arnold-Chiari malformation, posterior fossa
    decompression, 111
Arterial aneurysm (cerebral)
  angiography, 1011, 1013
  case reports, 1013–1017
  preoperative stereotactic calculations,
      1011–1012
  stereotactic clipping, 1009–1022
    indications/contraindications, 1012–1013
    instrumentation, 1010–1011
    results, 1013–1017
    technique, 1012
Arteriography
  in aneurysm, 1004, 1006
  in arteriovenous malformation, 905, 908
  in glomus jugulare tumor, 742, 744
  in pineal tumor, 403
  after proton beam therapy, 911–912
  in scalp/skull tumor, 604
  in spinal cord arteriovenous malformation,
      1501, 1502, 1506
  in vertebrobasilar insufficiency, 771–775
Arteriosclerotic vascular disease, lumbar
    sympathectomy for pain and
    ulceration, 1278
Arteriovenous malformation
  angiography, 523–525
  case reports, 525–526
  cerebellar, 908
  cerebellopontine angle-brain stem, 908
  in children, 109
  computed tomography, 523, 526
  dural, 908
  embolization in, 905, 906, 908, 909
  intraoperative ultrasonography
      visualization, 217
  intraventricular, 908
  magnetic resonance imaging, 523, 905
  postoperative evaluation, 908–909
  preoperative evaluation, 905–906
  radiation therapy, 906
  radiosurgery results, 526–528
  recurrent hemorrhage after radiosurgery,
      528
  stereotactic radiosurgery, 521–528
  stereotactic resection, 489
  surgical management, 906–908
  with tumor, 909
Arteriovenous malformation (cerebral), 899,
    905–910
  angiography, 1011, 1017, 1018
  arteriography, 905, 908
  block resection, 901
  with bucrylate and calibrated leak balloon,
      829–830

  case reports, 1019–1021
  computed tomography, 905
  direct coagulation and obliteration, 900
  embolization management, 828–831, 903,
      911
  fistula with, 827
  headache with, 914
  hemorrhage with, 905, 913–914
  intraoperative embolization, 830–831
  liquid agent embolization, 829
  marginal resection, 900–901
  natural history, 899
  neurologic deficit with, 914
  operative staging, 902
  postoperative management, 902
  preoperative evaluation, 900
  preoperative stereotactic calculations,
      1011–1012, 1018
  proton beam therapy, 911–915
  regional cerebral blood flow in, 1018
  results, 831, 903, 911–912
  steal effect, 829
  stereotactic clipping, 1009–1022
    indications/contraindications, 1012–
      1013
    instrumentation, 1010–1011
    results, 1017–1021
    technique, 1012
  surgical access difficulty, 902–903
  surgical complications, 901
  surgical risk, 899–900
  surgical technique, 900–901
Arteriovenous malformation (spinal cord),
    832–835, 1497–1506
  anatomy, 1498–1500
  anterior vs. posterior, 832–833
  arteriography, 1501, 1502, 1506
  balloon catheter management, 832–833
  clinical presentation, 1500
  computed tomography, 1501
  diagnosis, 1500–1501
  embolization, 1502
  glomus, 1504–1505
  juvenile (diffuse), 1505
  long dorsal, 1503–1504
  myelography, 1500–1501
  natural history, 1500
  radiography, 1500–1501
  results, 1505–1506
  with small dural fistula, 833, 835
  somatosensory evoked potentials, 1501
  surgical excision, 1502–1503
  types, 1499–1500
Aspirator, ultrasonic surgical, 226–227
Astrocytoma
  cystic pilocytic of cerebral hemispheres,
      431–432
  grades 3 and 4, 431
  intramedullary spinal cord, 175–185, 1490,
      1495
  intraoperative ultrasonography
      visualization, 216
  malignant, 182, 184, 185
  optic nerve, 239
  stereotactic resection, 487–488
  supratentorial grade, 1–2, 431
Atherosclerosis, carotid artery bifurcation
    lesions, 753, 757
Axonotmesis, 1584

Back pain (low), anterior lumbar discectomy and interbody fusion for, 1421–1436
Backlund biopsy instrument, 467–468
Bacterial endocarditis, aneurysm with, 997–1001
Bacterial intracranial aneurysm, 997–1001
    angiography, 997, 998–999
    clinical manifestations, 997–998
    computed tomography, 998
    culture in, 997–998
    diagnosis, 998–999
    incidence, 997
    medical treatment, 999
    multiple, 999–1000
    sites, 998
    surgical treatment, 999–1000
Ballism, stereotactic surgery for, 1053
Ballistics
    of gunshot wounds, 37
    missile injury relation, 49–50
Balloon catheter
    calibrated-leak balloon, 820
    catheter and guide wires available, 821–822
    detachable balloon, 819
    embolic agents with, 820–821
    instrumentation, 819–822
    in intracerebral vascular lesion management, 819–836
    latex balloon, 819, 820
    silastic balloon, 819, 820, 824
Balloon embolization, 873
Balloon occlusion, of unclippable aneurysm, 1024, 1033
Basilar-anterior inferior cerebellar artery aneurysm, 984–986
Basilar artery aneurysm, 973–989
    anesthesia, 973–974
    monitoring techniques, 973–974
    patient positioning, 974
    subtemporal approach, 975
    surgical technique, 975–979
    unclippable, 1026–1029, 1031
Basilar artery occlusive disease, interposition vein graft to posterior cerebral artery, 793
Basilar bifurcation aneurysm, 979–982
    giant/bulbous, 983
Basioccipital region. *See* Clivus and basioccipital region
Biliary tract, splanchnicectomy for pain, 1276
Biologic markers, in pineal tumor, 403
Biopsy. *See also* Stereotactic biopsy; *specific diagnoses*
    Backlund instrument, 467–468
    with Brown-Roberts-Wells stereotactic frame, 475–480
    computed tomography in, 463–474
    free-hand computed tomography techniques, 463
    magnetic resonance imaging in, 463–474
Bischof's myelotomy, 1177–1184
    circular griseotomy, 1181, 1183
    complications, 1182–1183
    exploration, 1178–1179
    indications for, 1178
    lateral longitudinal, 1179–1180
    lesion production, 1179–1181

    in lower limb spasticity, 1177–1184
    posterior longitudinal, 1180
    postoperative care, 1182
    preoperative management, 1178
    results, 1182–1183
    technical factors, 1177
Bladder function, with spinal dysraphism, 166
Blast injury, 51
Body temperature regulation, in children, 106, 108
Bone chips, with missile injury, 50
Bone grafts, for skull defects, 11
Boston Brace, 193
Brachial plexus avulsion, dorsal root entry zone thermocoagulation for pain, 1170–1171, 1173–1174
Brachial plexus injury
    closed, 1578–1581
    computed tomography, 1578
    infraclavicular, 1578
    myelography, 1578
    open wounds, 1577–1578
    pain management, 1581
    radiation neuropathy, 1580
    radiography, 1578
    supraclavicular, 1578
    surgical technique, 1580
Brachycurietherapy, 491, 499–502
    indications for, 507–512
    results, 507
Bracing, in scoliosis, 191–194
Brain abscess, 72–74
    computed tomography in, 73
    intraoperative ultrasonography visualization, 217
Brain biopsy, 419–422
    complications, 421–422
    indications for, 419
    intraoperative ultrasonography in, 219
    legal/moral/ethical considerations, 419
    operative techniques, 419–421
    preferred sites, 420
    results, 420
Brain lesion
    computed tomography, 215–217
    intracranial ultrasonography, 215
    normal vs. pathologic ultrasonography visualization, 215–216
    preoperative localization, 215
Brain metastasis, intraoperative ultrasonography visualization, 217
Brain revascularization (direct), 783–795
Brain stem auditory evoked potentials, in brain stem tumor, 716
Brain stem glioma, 709–737
    anatomic categories, 710–714
    computed tomography in, 716–718
    diagnosis, 714–716
    growth types, 713–714
    histology, 710
    magnetic resonance imaging in, 716–718
    postoperative neurological signs, 722
    postoperative radiotherapy, 724, 735
    removal, 719–722
    results, 722–724
    sites, 710
    surgical approach, 719–722
    symptomatology, 714–716

Brain stem tumor, 709–737
    case reports, 724–733
    caudal, 711
    computed tomography in, 716–718
    evoked potentials in, 716
    hyperkinesis with, 722, 724
    magnetic resonance imaging in, 716–718
    midbrain, 711–712
    thalamic, 712
    treatment, 719
Brain stimulation
    for cancer pain, 1047
    for denervation pain, 1049
    electrode implantation for, 1039, 1041–1043
    with implanted electrodes for analgesia, 1089–1095
    periventricular/periaqueductal area, 1041–1042
    sites for, 1041–1043
    somatosensory system, 1042–1043
Brain tumor, stereotactic biopsy with radionuclide implantation, 491–514
Brown-Roberts-Wells stereotactic frame, 475–480, 1037
    biopsy with, 476–477
    cases, 477–478
    complications, 478
    computed tomography with, 477
    instrumentation, 477
    postoperative care, 478
    potential applications, 478
    results, 477–478
    target localization, 475–476
    target selection, 475–476
Brown-Roberts-Wells stereotactic system, 466–467
Bucrylate, as embolic agent, 821
Burr holes, exploratory, 22
Bypass grafts. *See specific procedures*

Campotomy, for movement disorder, 1051
Cancer pain. *See also* Pain (intractable)
    ablative procedures for, 1043
    of cervical and craniofacial region, 1079–1088
    commissural myelotomy for, 1185–1190
    intraventricular morphine for, 1077–1088
    management of, 1043
    narcotics for, 1043
    neurosurgical management, 1043–1047
    percutaneous cordotomy for, 1191–1205
    percutaneous electrode implantation for, 1047
    percutaneous rhizotomy in, 1125–1127
    spinal sensory rhizotomy for, 1209, 1211
Canthotomy, lateral, 254
Carbon dioxide laser, 223, 224, 225
    in meningioma surgery, 559
    wet-field, 226
Carotid artery
    in dural venous sinus lesions, 872–873
    trapping procedure, 872–873
Carotid artery (extracranial), 753–764
    aneurysms, 763
    angiography, 753, 754, 757
    anticoagulation, 753, 756, 760
    asymptomatic lesions, 754

Carotid artery (extracranial) *(continued)*
  atherosclerosis, 753, 757
  computed tomography, 753
  embolization, 753
  fibromuscular dysplasia, 763
  kinking, 762–763
  lesion diagnosis, 753–755
  lesion symptomatology, 753–755
  traumatic injury, 762
Carotid artery aneurysm, subarachnoid
      hemorrhage with, 917, 918, 927
Carotid cavernous fistula
  angiography in, 846
  anterior approach, 846
  balloon catheter management, 822–827
  balloon embolization, 873
  with basilar skull fracture, 21–22
  classification, 845
  embolization, 873
  lateral approach, 846–847
  percutaneous jugular approach, 847
  posterior approach, 847
  preoperative planning, 846
  results, 847
  superficial temporal artery catheterization,
      846
  thrombosis technique, 845–847
  thrombosis via positive current, 873
Carotid cavernous fistula (spontaneous), 827
  dural subtypes, 827
  embolization management, 827
Carotid cavernous fistula (traumatic), 822–
      827
  angiography, 822, 825
  arterial approach, 825
  clinical presentation, 822
  diagnosis, 822–825
  direct surgical approach, 825
  results, 825, 827
  steal effect, 823–824
  venous approach, 825
Carotid endarterectomy, 765–769
  anesthesia, 755
  bilateral, 760
  closure, 757–760
  complications, 760–761
  indications for, 753–754
  intraoperative shunt, 757
  patient positioning, 755
  postoperative care, 760
  preoperative preparation, 754–755
  restenosis management, 760
  results, 762
  risk factors, 753
  technique, 755–760
Carotid fistula (external), balloon catheter
      management, 827
Carotid ligation, for internal carotid artery
      aneurysm, 1025
Carotid occlusion, for internal carotid artery
      aneurysm, 1023
Carotid ophthalmic aneurysm, 917–928
  anatomy, 917
  anesthesia, 918
  angiography, 918, 925, 927
  brain tension reduction, 918
  case report, 927
  cerebral blood flow studies, 918, 927
  cervical carotid occlusion for, 925

  clinoid process removal, 921–922
  computed tomography, 917–918
  contralateral aneurysm clipping, 924–925
  controlled hypotension in, 918–919
  dissection, 922
  extubation, 919
  incision, 919
  magnetic resonance imaging, 917
  medical management, 917–918
  microsurgical dissection, 921
  obliteration, 923–924
  patient positioning, 919
  postoperative management, 925, 927
  pterional (frontotemporal) craniotomy
      exposure, 920
  results, 927
  STA-MCA bypass in, 927
  superior hypophyseal, 925
  surgical technique, 919–925
  symptomatology, 917
  vasospasm management, 919
  wound closure, 925
Carpal tunnel syndrome, 1583–1584
  medial palmar cutaneous nerve and, 1586
  surgical management, 1585–1588
Catecholamines, in glomus jugulare tumor,
      744
Caudal brain stem tumor, 711
  symptomatology, 714–716
Cauda equina syndrome, 1303
Causalgia, 1271, 1272
  lower extremity, 1277–1278
  sympathectomy for, 1049
Cavitron ultrasonic surgical aspirator, 178,
      184, 650
  in craniofacial resection, 613
Central nervous system cyst, toxin-leaking,
      373–374
Central nervous system infection, 79–91
Central retinal artery occlusion, with
      radiofrequency rhizotomy, 1141–1142
Cerebellar artery (anterior inferior)
      aneurysm, 984–986
Cerebellar artery (superior) aneurysm, 983–
      984
Cerebellar astrocytoma
  computed tomography, 660
  magnetic resonance imaging, 660
  surgical management, 659–660
Cerebellar hemangioblastoma
  angiography, 660
  computed tomography, 660
  radiation therapy, 660
  surgical management, 660
Cerebellar metastasis, surgical management,
      660
Cerebellopontine angle
  anatomy, 674
  middle fossa approach, 675
  posterior cranial fossa transmeatal
      approach, 676–680
  surgical approaches, 675–680
  translabyrinthine approach, 676
Cerebellopontine angle tumor, 673–683
  clinical features, 673–674
  surgical approaches, 675–680
  surgical complications, 680–681
Cerebral angiography, anesthesia for, 112
Cerebral artery (posterior) aneurysm, 984

Cerebral blood flow (regional)
  in arteriovenous malformation, 1018
  in moyamoya disease, 798–799, 803
  in vertebrobasilar insufficiency, 807–808
Cerebral contusion, with acute head injury,
      24
Cerebral palsy, stereotactic surgery for, 1054
Cerebritis, with fungus infection, 89
Cerebrospinal fluid
  with intraventricular hemorrhage, 119
  in suprasellar germinoma, 398
  morphine injections, 1078–1088
Cerebrospinal fluid drainage
  catheter management, 62–63
  complications, 62
  infection prevention, 62
  technique, 62
Cerebrospinal fluid fistula, 57–69
  with basilar skull fracture, 21
  diagnosis, 58–60
  external drainage, 62
  extralabyrinthine, 61
  with glomus jugulare tumor, 750
  high-pressure vs. low-pressure, 61
  intralabyrinthine, 61
  with missile injury, 53
Cerebrospinal fluid leakage, 57–69
  anatomic considerations, 60–61
  anterior fossa craniotomy, 63–64
  antibiotic prophylaxis, 61, 62
  cerebrospinal fluid shunt in, 66
  contrast studies, 60
  craniotomy for, 63
  dural repair for, 110
  epidemiology, 58
  etiology, 58
  extracranial surgical approach, 65–66
  facial fracture reduction with craniotomy,
      65
  glucose concentration, 59
  in gunshot wound of head, 45
  headache with, 59
  immunofixation technique in, 60
  intensive care for, 61
  lumbar drainage in, 66
  management with sella turcica
      reconstruction, 324–325
  meningitis with, 58, 61, 63
  methylmethacrylate repair, 66
  middle fossa craniotomy, 64–65
  patient position, 61
  in pituitary adenoma, 306
  pneumocephalus with, 58
  posterior fossa craniotomy, 65
  postoperative, 58
  radiography in, 59
  radioisotope scan in, 59–60
  reservoir sign, 59
  in sella turcica surgery, 304–305, 306
  site delineation, 58, 59, 60–61
  spinal, 66–67
  surgical indications, 63
  surgical management, 63
  target sign, 59
  tissue adhesives in, 66
  traumatic vs. spontaneous (nontraumatic),
      57–58, 60–61
Cerebrospinal fluid rhinorrhea
  with acoustic nerve tumor, 702–703

posthypophysectomy, 348
  as postoperative complication, 331, 333
Cerebrospinal fluid shunt, in cerebrospinal
  fluid leakage, 66
Cervical deformity, after laminectomy in
  children, 1509
Cervical disc excision (anterior)
  in cervical myelopathy, 1339–1341
  in cervical radiculopathy, 1337–1339
  in cervical spondylosis, 1327–1342
  complications, 1335–1337
  fusion with, 1335, 1337
  procedure, 1333–1335
  surgical anatomy, 1332–1333
  surgical indications, 1327–1329
Cervical disc herniation, 1347–1358
Cervical disc herniation (lateral), 1347–1351
  clinical manifestations, 1347
  complications, 1351
  diagnosis, 1348
  incidence, 1347
  nonsurgical treatment, 1348
  patient selection for surgery, 1348
  radiography, 1348
  results, 1351
  surgical treatment, 1348–1351
Cervical fracture-dislocation, skeletal
  traction in, 1449–1451
Cervical laminectomy, postoperative spinal
  deformity in children, 1509
Cervical meningocele, 158
Cervical radiculopathy
  anterior cervical disc excision in, 1327
  anterolateral disc excision results, 1337–
    1339
Cervical rhizotomy, percutaneous
  electrothermo-coagulation technique,
  1211–1216
Cervical rhizotomy (anterior), in torticollis,
  1263
Cervical spinal cord injury
  anesthesia, 1451, 1452
  anterior fusion, 1453–1461
  anterolateral approach to upper spine,
    1461–1462
  posterior fusion, 1464–1466
  pulmonary considerations, 1452
  transoral odontoid resection and fusion,
    1462–1464
  in children, 175
Cervical spine fusion
  anterolateral approach to upper spine,
    1461–1462
  transoral odontoid resection with fusion,
    1462–1464
Cervical spine fusion (anterior)
  in middle/lower spine injury, 1454–1461
  in upper spine injury, 1453–1454
Cervical spine fusion (posterior), 1471–1480
  in atlantoaxial fracture-dislocation, 1464
  lateral facet, 1467–1468
Cervical spondylosis
  angiography, 1332
  anterior cervical disc excision in, 1327–
    1342
  computed tomography, 1332
  diagnosis, 1329–1332
  dysphagia with, 1328–1329
  myelography, 1332

radiography, 1329–1332
  surgical anatomy, 1332–1333
  surgical complications, 1335–1337
  surgical management, 1333–1335
  vertebral artery compression with, 1329
Cervical spondylotic myelopathy, 1351–1357
  anterior cervical disc excision in, 1327–
    1328
  anterolateral disc excision results, 1339–
    1341
  clinical manifestations, 1352
  complications, 1354–1355
  diagnosis, 1352
  incidence, 1351–1352
  nonsurgical treatment, 1352
  pathogenesis, 1351–1352
  radiography, 1352
  surgical approaches, 1352–1353
  surgical indications, 1352
  surgical results, 1355–1357
  surgical technique, 1353–1354
Cervicothoracic junction epidural tumor
  (metastatic), 1555–1557
Chemonucleolysis, 1419, 1437–1441
  anaphylaxis with chymopapain, 1437,
    1438, 1440
  anesthesia, 1439
  with chymopapain, 1437–1441
  complications, 1440
  failures, 1440
  indications for, 1438
  in intervertebral disc disease, 1443–1448
  needle placement, 1439–1440
  patient positioning, 1438–1439
  postoperative course, 1440
  radiography, 1438, 1439
  technique, 1438–1440
Chemotherapy
  with balloon catheter management of
    intracerebral vascular lesion, 835
  in cerebral glioma, 448
  in intracranial metastasis, 455, 456, 460,
    461
  in pineal region tumor, 399
  for pineal tumor, 404–405
Chiari malformation with hydromelia
  angiography, 1316
  diagnosis, 1309–1316
  cerebrospinal fluid shunting in, 1326
  clinical factors, 1308–1309
  computed tomography, 1313
  magnetic resonance imaging, 1311
  microsurgical technique, 1316–1317
  myelography, 1313–1316
  percutaneous cyst needling, 1326
  radiography in, 1309–1316
  surgical management, 1316–1317
  surgical results, 1317
  terminal ventriculostomy for, 1326
  treatment alternatives, 1326
Chiari II malformation, 123
Children. *See also* Neonate, *specific
    childhood conditions*
  anesthesia management, 103–116
  computed tomography in, 1509
  head injury in, 113–114
  holo spinal cord widening, 1495
  intracranial pressure in, 103, 106
  magnetic resonance imaging in, 1509

myelography in, 1509
  neuroradiographic procedures for, 112–
    113
  postoperative care, 107
  preoperative assessment, 106
  spinal cord injury, 114–115
  spinal deformity after neurosurgery, 1509–
    1513
Chordoma
  of clivus, 651
  of clivus and basioccipital region, 635–
    636, 637, 645
Choreoathetosis, stereotactic surgery for,
  1055
Chymopapain, 1437–1441
  anaphylaxis, 1437, 1438
  chemistry, 1437
  pharmacology, 1437
  toxicity, 1437, 1440
Chymopapain chemonucleolysis, 1419
  adverse reactions, 1443–1444
  in intervertebral disc disease, 1443–1448
  mortality, 1443
Cingulate gyrus
  anatomy, 1069–1070
  physiologic factors, 1069–1070
Cingulotomy, for cancer pain, 1047
Cingulotomy (stereotactic)
  for chronic pain, 1069–1075
  equipment, 1071
  patient selection, 1070–1071
  postoperative management, 1073
  for psychiatric disorder, 1069–1075
  results, 1072–1075
  technique, 1071–1072
Circle of Willis, moyamoya disease of, 797–
  806
Cisternography
  metrizamide, 60
  radioisotope, 60
Clivus
  anatomy, 635
  embryology, 635
Clivus and basioccipital region tumor, 635–
  646
  angiography in, 638
  chordoma, 635–636, 637, 645
  clinical presentation, 637
  computed tomography in, 639
  extradural anterior approaches, 642–643
  extradural posterolateral approaches, 644
  intradural approaches, 640–642
  magnetic resonance imaging in, 639–640
  meningioma, 637, 645
  radiography, 637–640
  surgical approach, 640–644
  surgical approach selection, 645
  transbasal approach, 644
  transoral median labiomandibular
    approaches, 643–644
  transsphenoidal approach, 643
Clivus tumor, 650
  chordoma, 651
  classification, 650–651
  computed tomography, 650
  radiography, 650
  surgical approaches, 650–651
Clonogenic assay, in intracranial metastasis,
  456

Cluster headache (chronic migrainous neuralgia)
  glycerol injection for, 1136
  radiofrequency heating for, 1136
Coagulation disorders, with acute head injury, 30
Cobalt 60 Gamma Unit, 515–529
Commissural myelotomy, 1185–1190
  for cancer pain, 1044
  postoperative care, 1187
  results, 1187, 1189
  technique, 1185–1187
Common peroneal nerve compression, 1596
Computed tomography
  in acute head injury, 19
  in aneurysm, 1004, 1006
  in anterior communicating artery aneurysm, 939, 949, 952
  for anterior lumbar discectomy, 1423
  in anterior skull base tumor, 611
  in arteriovenous malformation, 523, 526, 905
  in bacterial intracranial aneurysm, 998
  in brachial plexus injury, 1578
  in brain abscess, 73
  in brain lesion localization, 215, 216, 217
  in brain stem tumor, 716–718
  in carotid artery lesion, 753
  in carotid ophthalmic aneurysm, 917–918
  in cerebellar astrocytoma, 660
  in cerebellar hemangioblastoma, 660
  in cerebral glioma, 432–433, 436, 444, 445
  in cerebrospinal fluid leakage, 59
  in cervical spondylosis, 1332
  in cervical spondylotic myelopathy, 1352
  in children, 113, 1509
  in clivus and basioccipital region tumor, 639, 650
  in craniofacial abnormality, 135
  in craniopharyngioma, 355–356, 357
  in cysticercosis, 86, 94, 98
  data transposition to stereotactic films, 463–464
  in dural fistula, 827
  in dural sinus malformation, 861
  in exophthalmos, 229
  free-hand techniques, 463
  in fungus infection, 89
  in glomus jugulare tumor, 742, 743
  in gunshot wounds of head, 38
  in internal carotid artery aneurysm, 837, 930
  in intracerebral hematoma, 890–891
  in intracerebral hemorrhage, 881, 884–886
  in intracranial metastasis, 457–458, 459
  in intramedullary spinal cord tumor, 1490
  in intraorbital tumor, 238
  for intraventricular morphine injection, 1079
  in lateral ventricle tumor, 583
  in lesion localization and biopsy, 463–474
  of lumbar intervertebral disc, 1393, 1394
  in medial sphenoid wing meningioma, 537–538
  in medulloblastoma, 658
  in meningioma, 549–550, 564, 571–572
  in metastatic spine tumor, 1516, 1520
  in middle cerebral artery aneurysm, 957, 958, 968
  in missile injury, 49, 54

in moyamoya disease, 798
in olfactory groove meningioma, 540
in optic glioma, 279
in optic nerve decompression, 270
in orbit pathology, 249, 250, 251
in Paget's disease, 1304
in pineal tumor, 403
in posterior fossa tumor, 653–654
in Rathke's cleft cyst, 373, 374
in rheumatoid arthritis, 1296
in scalp/skull tumor, 604
of sella turcica, 300–301, 356
in spinal cord arteriovenous malformation, 1501
in spinal cord astrocytoma, 176, 177, 184
in spinal dysraphism, 168
in spine trauma, 1449
in spine tumor, 1525, 1526, 1527, 1528, 1530
with stereotactic biopsy, 495–498, 502
stereotactic frame modification for, 464–466
with stereotactic intra-axial tumor resection, 481–490
in stereotactic surgery, 463, 1061–1062
in subdural hematoma, 33–35
in suprasellar cyst, 375
in suprasellar germinoma, 398
in suprasellar meningioma, 531
in synostosis, 126–127, 130, 132, 133
in tentorium tumor, 647, 648
in thoracolumbar fracture, 1481, 1483, 1484–1485
in traumatic aneurysm, 991, 993
in trigonal meningioma, 597
in tuberculoma, 80–81
in tuberculosis meningitis, 84
in unclippable aneurysm, 1029–1030
in vertebrobasilar insufficiency, 807
Computer analysis, for stereotactic resection, 483–484, 485, 486
Contusion, with missile injury, 51
Cordis Brain State Analyzer, 177
Cordotomy
  for cancer pain, 1043–1044
  percutaneous, 1191–1205
Cordotomy (open)
  anesthesia, 1158
  anterolateral, spinal cord anatomy and, 1156
  bilateral, 1155–1156, 1163
  bladder dysfunction after, 1163
  corticospinal tract anatomy and, 1156–1157
  dentate insertion variations and, 1157
  dysesthesias after, 1165
  electrophysiologic monitoring, 1158
  failures, 1164
  indications for, 1155–1156
  instrumentation, 1157–1158
  for intractable pain, 1155–1168
  mortality, 1164
  patient positioning, 1159
  postoperative complications, 1163
  postoperative hypotension, 1163, 1165
  postoperative sleep apnea, 1163
  postoperative weakness, 1163, 1165
  preoperative preparation, 1157–1158
  respiratory complications, 1164
  results, 1163–1164

sexual dysfunction after, 1165
spinal cord width variations and, 1157
spinothalamic tract anatomy and, 1156
unilateral, 1155, 1159–1163
Coronal synostosis
  complications, 131
  diagnosis, 130
  lateral canthal advancement, 131
  results, 131
  surgical technique, 131
Corpus callostomy
  commissurotomy results, 1247–1249
  commissurotomy technique, 1244–1247
  complications, 1248
  for epilepsy, 1243–1250
  neuropsychological effects, 1248–1249
Cortical resection
  anesthesia for, 1225
  complications, 1232–1233
  for epilepsy, 1223–1234
  incision, 1226
  partial temporal lobectomy, 1223–1234
  patient positioning, 1226
  postoperative care, 1232
  results, 1233–1234
Corticosteroids
  in cerebral glioma, 435
  in intracranial metastasis, 453, 461
  in missile injury, 51
  in orbit pathology, 251
  in spinal cord compression, 1541
  in subdural hematoma, 33
  in tuberculoma, 82
Costotransversectomy, in thoracic disc herniation, 1367–1371
Cotrel-Dubousset fixation, in scoliosis, 201–202
Cranial nerve(s), nociceptive afferents, 1165–1166
Cranial nerve disorders, 1097–1109, *See also specific diagnoses*
Cranial nerve injury
  with basilar skull fracture, 21
  after stereotactic radiosurgery, 521
Cranial nociceptive tract (descending), medullary tractotomy of, 1165–1166
Cranial suture, histology, 125
Craniofacial abnormality, 134–137
  classification, 135
  complications, 137
  computed tomography in, 135
  diagnosis, 135
  genetic factor, 135
  hypertelorism with, 137
  LeFort III midface advancement, 137
  radiography in, 135
  results, 137
  treatment, 135
Craniofacial repair, anesthesia for, 111–112
Craniofacial resection
  for anterior skull base tumor, 609–618
  Cavitron ultrasonic tumor aspirator in, 613
  complications, 616–617
  for epidermoid cancer, 609
  for nasal tumor, 611
  for paranasal sinus tumor, 609
  patient selection, 612
  postoperative management, 615–616
  preoperative evaluation, 612
  results, 617

for salivary gland tumor, 609
skull base reconstruction in, 615
technique, 612–615
Craniopharyngioma, 349–379
angiography, 356–357
calcification removal, 363
in children, 109
clinical presentation, 355
computed tomography, 355–356, 357
desmopressin acetate in, 365
endocrine management, 364–365
extracerebral removal, 359–360
growth characteristics, 349–355
growth direction, 349–352
growth rate, 349
histology, 352–354
lateroposterior transpetrosal-transtentorial
approach, 362
magnetic resonance imaging, 355–356
metabolic management, 364–365
microscopic features, 352–355
pituitary stalk sacrifice in, 363
pterional approach, 362
radiation therapy, 368–372
radical surgery, 357–368
radiography, 355–357
reconstruction technique, 331
removal of bone anterior to sella, 360
reservoir drainage system for, 364
results, 365–367, 369
retrochiasmal removal, 360–362
sequelae, 365
shunting procedures, 364
site, 349–352
size/cystic content relation to operation
type, 362–363
small tumor management, 367–368
stereotactic radiosurgery, 515–516
suboccipital approach, 364
subtemporal approach, 362
transcallosal approach, 364
transcorticoventricular approach, 364
transfrontal approach, 358–359
transsphenoidal approach, 317–318, 363–
364
visual deficit, 355
Cranioplasty
brain protection factor, 12
complications, 14
cosmetic considerations, 12
indications for, 12, 14
infection with, 14
methyl methacrylate for, 11, 14–16
technique, 14–16
Craniosynostosis, 125–134. *See also specific
deformities*
anatomy, 125–126
anesthesia for, 111
associated abnormalities, 125
pathophysiology, 125–126
preoperative evaluation, 125–126
Craniotomy
basic trauma, 22–23
for cerebrospinal fluid leakage, 63
exploratory burr holes, 22
for neonate, 117–119
Craniovertebral junction abnormality, 1281–
1293
anatomy, 1281–1282
anterior transoral-transpharyngeal

approach, 1288–1292
diagnosis, 1284
embryology, 1281–1282
immobilization management, 1285
posterior decompression for, 1287
posterior fusion for, 1285–1287
radiography, 1284
surgical procedures for, 1281
surgical results, 1292
surgical technique, 1285–1292
symptoms, 1282–1284
Curietherapy, 491, 499–503
indications for, 507–512
Currarino triad, 160
Cushing's disease, 299–300
stereotactic radiosurgery, 516–518
Cyanoacrylate tissue adhesive, in
cerebrospinal fluid leakage, 66
Cysticercosis, 85–88, 93–102
cerebrospinal fluid blockage with, 98, 99
in chiasmatic region, 98
clinical features, 86, 93–94
computed tomography in, 86, 94, 98
cysts (*Cysticercus cellulosae*), 93
diagnosis, 86, 94–95
diagnosis, 94–95
drug therapy, 87
epidemiology, 93
incidence, 85
increased intracranial pressure with, 98
management, 87
medical management, 95
pathology, 85–86, 93
prognosis, 95
racemose lesions, 96
seizures with, 95, 96
serology, 94–95
spinal, 98
surgical approaches, 98–99
surgical indications, 95–96
surgical management, 87–88, 95–99
Taenia solium transmission, 93
of ventricular pathways, 96
Cysticercus cellulosae, 93

Dandy-Foerster operation, 1054
Dandy-Walker malformation, 121, 123, 658–
659
Decompression, in cerebral glioma, 436,
442–443
Decompression laminectomy, in metastatic
spine tumor, 1519–1523
Denervation pain, 1042
stimulation therapy for, 1049
Dermal sinus pore, 166
Dermoid cyst, posterior fossa, 658–659
Descending cranial nociceptive tract. *See
Medullary tractotomy*
Desmopressin acetate, in
craniopharyngioma, 365
Dexamethasone suppression test, 300
Diabetes insipidus, 300, 398
with pituitary adenoma, 307
posthypophysectomy, 348
Diabetic retinopathy, stereotactic thermal
hypophysectomy for, 345–348
Diastematomyelia, 164–165
surgery for, 169–170

Dinorphin, 1078
Diplomyelia, 165
Disc distention test, 1343–1345
Discography, 1343–1345
for anterior lumbar discectomy, 1422–1423
Discometry, 1343
Disseminated intravascular coagulation, with
acute head injury, 27
Distal vertebral endarterectomy
results, 811–812
technique, 810–811
for vertebrobasilar insufficiency, 810–812
Dopaminergic agents, in torticollis, 1262
Dorsal column stimulation, for denervation
pain, 1049
Dorsal root entry zone, anatomy, 1169
Dorsal root entry zone thermocoagulation,
1169–1175
at conus, 1173
electrophysiologic control, 1173
indications for, 1170–1172
patient selection, 1170–1172
physiologic basis, 1169–1170
results, 1173–1174
technique, 1172–1174
Dorsal spinal cord stimulation, electrode
implantation for, 1039
Dura tear repair, 110
Dural arteriovenous malformation (lateral/
sigmoid sinuses), 855–862
craniotomy, 856
embolization, 855
patient positioning, 855
preoperative embolization, 855
scalp flap, 855
sinus ligation, 856–857
soft-tissue dissection, 855
surgical technique, 855–859
Dural fistula
angiography, 828
anteroinferior dural, 849–854
balloon catheter management, 827–828
computed tomography, 827
Dural sinus laceration, 875–879
anatomy, 876–877
diagnosis, 875
exposure, 875
patient positioning, 875
surgical preparation, 875
surgical technique, 877–879
Dural sinus malformation
angiography, 861
arterial supply, 861
bridging veins, 861
closure, 859
computed tomography, 861
diagnosis, 861
magnetic resonance imaging, 861
pathogenesis, 860
pathophysiology, 860
results, 859
symptomatology, 859–860
technical considerations, 861
venous drainage, 861
Dural sinus repair, with penetrating missile
injury, 53
Dural venous fistula (anteroinferior)
case reports, 850–854
obliteration, 849–854
transvenous approach, 849–854

Dural venous sinuses
  abnormal vascular channel elimination, 872–873
  abnormal vascular communication management, 872–873
  compressive obstruction control, 863, 868
  dural tunnel construction, 865
  embolization for abnormal vascular communication, 873
  hemorrhage control, 863
  intima-lined stent placement, 868, 871
  normal flow reinstitution, 868–876
  replacement graft, 868
  surgical management, 863–874
  trapping for abnormal vascular communication, 872–873
Dwyer instrumentation, in scoliosis, 203–204
Dysphagia, with cervical spondylosis, 1328–1329
Dystonia (adult-onset), 1261, 1269
  medical treatment, 1261
  peripheral denervation in, 1268
  surgical management, 1268
Dystonia musculorum deformans, stereotactic surgery for, 1053

Electric current thrombosis, 873
Electrical stimulation
  in scoliosis, 191–194
  with temporal lobectomy, 1229–1230
Electrocorticography, in temporal lobectomy, 1227
Electrode brain stimulation
  for analgesia, 1089–1095
  electrode internalization, 1094–1095
  implantation procedure, 1090–1094
  patient selection, 1089
  postimplantation care, 1094
  postoperative constant point screening, 1094
  results, 1095
Electroencephalography
  in aneurysm, 1004, 1006
  in epilepsy, 1224
  in infantile hemiplegia, 1235–1236
  in meningioma, 551
  in moyamoya disease, 799, 801, 804
  with stereotactic surgery, 1038
Electrolyte balance, with acute head injury, 29–30, 114
Electromyelography
  in compressive nerve lesions, 1584, 1585
  in thoracic outlet syndrome, 1592
Electromyography
  for anterior lumbar discectomy, 1432
  in cervical disc herniation, 1348
  in cervical spondylotic myelopathy, 1352
  in peripheral nerve injury, 1567, 1571
  in torticollis, 1263–1264
Electroneuroprosthesis, 1062–1064
Electronic stimulators (implantable), 1039
  implantation technique, 1039–1040
Electrophysiologic monitoring, for open cordotomy, 1158
Electrothermocoagulation (percutaneous), of spinal nerve trunk/ganglion/rootlets, 1207–1221
Embolic agents
  for intracerebral vascular lesion

management, 820–821
  liquid substances that solidify, 820–821
  solid particles, 820
Embolization
  in arteriovenous aneurysm, 905, 906, 908, 909
  in arteriovenous malformation, 828–831, 903, 911
  in atherosclerotic carotid artery lesion, 753
  in carotid cavernous fistula, 873
  in dural arteriovenous malformation, 855
  of glomus jugulare tumor, 744
  for meningioma, 551–553
  for spinal cord arteriovenous malformation, 1502
  in spine tumor, 1526
Encephalocele
  frontal nasal, 121
  intraorbital, 239
  occipital, 120–121
Encephaloduroarteriosynangiosis, in moyamoya disease, 802, 804
Encephalomyosynangiosis, in moyamoya disease, 802, 804
Endocrine factor
  in craniopharyngioma, 364–365
  in pituitary adenoma, 299–300, 305
  in sella turcica lesion, 299–300
  in third ventricle tumor, 398
Endorphins, 1078
Endoscopy (neurologic), 423–430
  operative procedures, 426
  optical system, 425–428
  preoperative procedures, 425
  prospectus, 424–425
  stereotactic protocol, 428–430
Endotracheal intubation, in children, 104
Enkephalins, 1078
Ependymoma, intramedullary spinal cord, 1490
Epidermoid cancer, craniofacial resection for, 609
Epidural cervical stimulation, in torticollis, 1262
Epidural hematoma, with acute head injury, 23
Epidural implantation systems
  availability, 1147–1148
  complications, 1149–1152
  for intractable pain, 1147–1148
Epidural tumor (metastatic)
  anterior decompression and vertebral body replacement, 1548–1559
  bone compression factor, 1543–1544
  bone grafting in, 1547–1548
  cell type factor, 1541
  of cervicothoracic junction, 1555–1557
  complications, 1560
  corticosteroids response factor, 1541
  functional prognosis, 1541
  incidence, 1539
  location, 1539, 1541–1542
  of lumbar spine, 1559
  morbidity, 1560–1561
  mortality, 1560
  neurologic deterioration with, 1541
  pathophysiology, 1540
  posterior decompression and instrumentation, 1545–1548
  postoperative care, 1548, 1553

pretreatment neurologic status, 1541
  radiation therapy, 1542, 1543, 1560
  radioresistance, 1543
  with spinal cord compression, 1539–1562
  spinal instability factor, 1543–1544
  surgical indications, 1543–1544
  surgical management, 1543–1559
  surgical techniques, 1544–1559
  survival, 1540–1541
  symptomatology, 1539
  therapy alternatives, 1542
  therapy selection, 1542
  of thoracic spine, 1553–1555
  thoracic wall excision, 1553
  of thoracolumbar spine, 1557–1559
  vertebral body replacement technique, 1552–1553
Epilepsy
  in children, 110
  clinical investigation, 1224
  corpus callosum section for, 1243–1250
  cortical resection for, 1223–1234
  electroencephalography in, 1224
  neuropsychologic examination in, 1224
  operative procedure for corpus callostomy, 1244–1247
  patient positioning, 1226
  postoperative care, 1232
  preoperative preparation, 1225
  radiography in, 1224
  stereotactic surgery for, 1060–1061
  surgical complications, 1232–1233
  surgical criteria, 1223–1224
  surgical indications, 1243–1244
  surgical results, 1233–1234, 1247–1249
Epsilon-aminocaproic acid, 931
Esthesioneuroblastoma, 611
Ethambutal, 81
Ethanol, as embolic agent, 821
Ethmoidectomy (external), in optic nerve decompression, 270
Exophthalmos
  in adults, 229
  bilateral, 229–233
  in children, 229
  computed tomography in, 229
  differential diagnosis, 229–233
  unilateral, 229–233
Extralemniscal myelotomy, for cancer pain, 1044
Extraocular muscles, 236
Extrapyramidal system, in movement disorders, 1050–1051
Extrathoracic common carotid-subclavian bypass, 781

Facial fracture, with cerebrospinal fluid leakage, 65
Facial neuralgia (atypical), glycerol injection for, 1136
Facial neuralgia (post-traumatic), glycerol injection for, 1136
Facial pain, percutaneous rhizotomy/microvascular decompression complications, 1139–1143
Facial pain (atypical), trigeminal rhizotomy for, 1120–1121
Facial pain (intractable), percutaneous rhizotomy for, 1111–1123

Facial palsy
cross-facial nerve graft, 705
dynamic muscle reconstruction, 707
local/distant muscle transfer in, 707
nerve transfer in, 705
neurectomy/myomectomy for, 707
peripheral nerve surgery, 705
static procedures for, 707
surgical correction, 705–708
Facial paralysis, surgical management, 681–683
Fawn's tail, 166
Fiberoptic endoscopy, 423–430
Fibrillation potentials, in peripheral nerve injury, 1567
Fibrin clot adhesives, in cerebrospinal fluid leakage, 66
Firearms, ballistic data, 37
Fistula. *See specific sites*
Flucytosine, in fungus infection, 90
Fluid balance
with acute head injury, 29–30, 114
in children, 105–106
Fluorescein scan, in cerebrospinal fluid leakage, 59
Fourth ventricle ependymoma
radiation therapy, 658
surgical management, 658
Frontal lobectomy
in cerebral glioma, 436–439
exposure, 437–438
patient positioning, 437
postoperative deficits, 439
Frontal nasal encephalocele, 121
Frontotemporal approach, to clivus, 640
Functional neurosurgery, 1035–1068. *See also specific disorders*
chronic stimulation techniques, 1039–1040
indications for, 1040–1057
stereotactic techniques, 1035–1039
Fungus infection, 79, 88–90
cerebritis with, 89
computed tomography, 89
diagnosis, 89
drug therapy, 90
granuloma with, 89
management, 90
pathology, 89
surgical management, 90

Gadolinium-diethylenetriamine pentaacetic acid, 280, 550
Gelfoam, as embolic agent, 820
Germ cell tumor
alpha fetoprotein in, 398
human chorionic gonadotropin in, 398
Germinoma. *See also specific sites*
chemotherapy, 399
suprasellar, 397
Genetic factor
in craniofacial abnormality, 135
in moyamoya disease, 797
in myelomeningocele, 151
in synostosis, 126
Gigantism, 299
Glasco Coma Scale, in subdural hematoma, 33
Glioblastoma multiforme, 431

Glioma. *See also specific diagnoses*
intraoperative ultrasonography visualization, 217
preoperative assessment, 432
Glioma (intracranial), 431–450
anticonvulsants in, 435–436
biopsy in, 436
chemotherapy, 448
computed tomography, 432–433, 436, 444, 445
corticosteroids in, 435
decompression in, 436, 442–443
frontal lobectomy in, 436–439
immunotherapy, 448
intraoperative management, 436
Karnofsky rating in, 444–445
magnetic resonance imaging, 433
neuropsychologic testing, 434–435
occipital lobectomy in, 441–442
postoperative care, 443–444
preoperative management, 435–436
radiation therapy, 448
radiography, 432–433
reoperation for, 444–446
surgical alternatives, 436
survival rates, 436
temporal lobectomy in, 439–441
visual fields in, 433–434
Glomus jugulare tumor, 739–752
anatomy, 741
anesthesia in, 745
arteriography, 742, 744
biochemistry, 742
bleeding with, 750
case, 747
cerebrospinal fluid fistula with, 750
classification, 741
clinical material, 742
complications, 749
computed tomography, 742, 743
cranial nerve dysfunction, 742, 750
dental evaluation, 745
diagnosis, 742–743
differential diagnosis, 742
embolization, 744
epidemiology, 741
pathology, 741
postoperative management, 746, 747
preoperative medical management, 744
preoperative procedures, 745
radiation therapy, 739, 743–744, 749
results, 748–749
sigmoid-jugular control, 746
skull base approach, 745–746
skull base exposure, 745–746
small tumor management, 747
surgical approach, 749
surgical approach review, 739–741
surgical technique, 749–750
symptoms, 742
temporal bone exposure, 746
treatment selection, 743
tumor removal, 746
very large tumor management, 747
wound closure, 746
Glossopharyngeal neuralgia, 1108–1109
percutaneous rhizotomy for, 1121–1122, 1125–1127
Glucose (CSF), in cerebrospinal fluid leakage, 59

Glycerol chemoneurolysis, in trigeminal neuralgia, 1098
Glycerol injection (retrogasserian)
for atypical facial neuralgia, 1136
biological effects, 1134–1136
for cluster headache, 1136
complications, 1131
hemorrhagic diasthesis with, 1133
mechanism of action, 1134–1136
for multiple sclerosis, 1134
results, 1129–1133
for post-traumatic facial neuralgia, 1136
technique, 1133–1134
in trigeminal neuralgia, 1129–1137
Grafts. *See specific reconstruction techniques*
Granuloma, with fungus infection, 89
Griseotomy, radiofrequency, 1181
Growth hormone, in pituitary adenoma, 299
Gunshot wounds
ballistic data, 37
of brachial plexus, 1578
Gunshot wounds (head), 37–48
angiography, 38–39
bacterial contamination, 38, 43
bone fragment removal, 39
case reports, 41–44
cerebrospinal fluid leakage with, 45
computed tomography, 38
debridement, 39, 40, 43
diuretics preoperatively, 39
exit wound, 39
hemostasis, 39, 40
laceration and crushing, 37–38
neurologic deficit, 38
postoperative care, 47–48
preoperative evaluation, 38
prognosis-wound type relation, 45
radiography, 38–39
retained bone management, 45, 47
shock waves, 38
with spent bullet, 44–45
surgical pathology, 37–38
surgical technique, 39–41
temporary cavitation, 38
watertight closure, 39–40

Håkanson procedure, 1129
results, 1129–1133
Harrington rod instrumentation, 198
Harrington-rod thoracolumbar spine fusion, 1475–1478
Head injury
anesthesia for, 113–114
in children, 113–114
gunshot wound management, 37–48
nonoperative management, 114
optic nerve lesion with, 269
Head injury (acute). *See also specific lesions*
blood pressure management, 25
coagulopathy with, 30
complications, 25–30
computed tomography in, 19
emergency room care, 19
fluid and electrolyte management, 29–30
gastrointestinal complications, 30
infection with, 26–27
intracranial pressure monitoring with, 25–26, 27

Head injury (acute) (continued)
    postoperative management, 24–25
    preoperative care, 19
    respiratory complications, 27–29
    seizures with, 30
    specific injury management, 20–24
    surgical management, 19–31
    traumatic mass lesion, 22–24
    triage for, 19, 20
    ventilatory assistance with, 27–29
Headache
    with arteriovenous malformation, 914
    with cerebrospinal fluid leakage, 59
Hearing, electroneuroprosthesis, 1063
Hearing loss
    in Meniere's disease, 1251
    after stereotactic radiosurgery, 521
Hemangioblastoma, intramedullary spinal
        cord, 1492, 1495–1496
Hemangioma (cavernous) stereotactic
        resection, 489
Hematoma. See also specific lesions
    with acoustic nerve tumor, 702
    with missile injury, 51
Hematoma (intracerebral)
    case reports, 893–897
    computed tomography, 890–891
    preoperative calculations, 890–891
    results, 892
    stereotactic evacuation, 889–898
    stereotactic instrumentation, 889–890
    surgical technique, 891
    with traumatic aneurysm, 991
Hemiballism, stereotactic surgery for, 1053
Hemifacial spasm, 1105–1108
    Jannetta microvascular decompression,
        1106–1108
    results, 1108
    surgical complications, 1108
Hemiplegia (infantile)
    electroencephalography, 1235–1236
    etiology, 1235
    hemispherectomy for, 1235–1241
    homonymous hemianopsia with, 1235,
        1236
    mental retardation with, 1236
    neurologic aspects, 1236
    radiography in, 1236
    seizures with, 1235
Hemispherectomy (cerebral), 1235–1241
    behavior modification, 1239
    clinical aspects, 1235
    hemianopsia and, 1235, 1236
    hemosiderosis with, 1236
    intellectual status results, 1239
    intracranial pressure complications, 1238
    late complications, 1236, 1240
    patient selection, 1235–1236
    postoperative care, 1238
    preoperative preparation, 1237
    results, 1239–1240
    socioeconomic status postoperative, 1239–
        1240
    technique, 1237–1238
Hemorrhage. See specific sites
    with arteriovenous malformation, 913–914
Hemosiderosis, with cerebral
        hemispherectomy, 1236
Hemostatis
    with laser, 226

in meningioma surgery, 558, 560
Herpes simplex encephalitis, 419
Herpes zoster
    dorsal root entry zone thermocoagulation
        for pain, 1171–1172, 1174
    medical management, 1172
    postherpetic neuralgia, 1049
Hibbs spine fusion, 1473
Holo spinal cord widening, 1495
Homonymous hemianopsia, 1235, 1236
Horsley-Clark stereotactic apparatus, 491,
        492, 494, 1035, 1037
House-Urban rotary dissector, 650
Human chorionic gonadotropin, in
        intracranial germ cell tumor, 398
Huntington's chorea, stereotactic surgery
        for, 1052–1053
Hydrocephalus, 141–150. See also Shunting
        procedure
    in children, 110
    clinical findings, 141–142
    endoscopy in, 423
    in intracranial metastasis, 459
    with missile injury, 53
    with myelomeningocele, 119
    in neonate, 119
    pathophysiology, 141
    with spinal cord astrocytoma, 182
    after stereotactic radiosurgery, 521
    surgical shunting indications, 141
    surgical treatment, 142–150
    with tuberculous meningitis, 83–85
    ventricular drainage, 573
Hydromyelia, with Chiari malformation,
        1307–1326
Hyperhidrosis, 1271, 1272
Hyperkinesis, with brain stem tumor, 722,
        724
Hypertelorism, 137
Hypertension, aneurysm and, 1003, 1006
Hypertensive hematoma, stereotactic
        evacuation, 889–898
Hypoglossal-facial nerve anastomosis, 682–
        683
Hypoglossal nerve, transfer in facial palsy,
        705
Hyponatremia, with acute head injury, 30
Hypophysectomy. See also Stereotactic
        thermal hypophysectomy
    reconstruction technique, 331
    replacement therapy, 347–348
    transsphenoidal approach, 315–316
Hypotension (controlled)
    in anterior communicating artery
        aneurysm, 941
    in carotid ophthalmic aneurysm, 918–919
    in children, 107
    in unclippable aneurysm, 1030, 1032
Hypothermia (induced)
    in children, 108
    in neonate, 117
    in saccular aneurysm, 839, 841

Immunofixation technique, in cerebrospinal
        fluid leakage, 60
Immunotherapy
    in cerebral glioma, 448
    in intracranial metastasis, 460

Impedance monitoring, in percutaneous
        cordotomy, 1195, 1198
Implantable electronic stimulators, 1039
Implantable systems, for intractable pain,
        1145–1153
Indigo carmine scan, in cerebrospinal fluid
        leakage, 59–60
Infection. See also specific diagnoses
    with acute head injury, 26–27
    with skull fracture, 14
Infratemporal fossa approach
    to clivus, 644
    to posterior cranial fossa, 668, 671
Infratentorial approach, to posterior fossa
        tumor, 660–662
Intercostal nerve denervation, percutaneous
        electrothermocoagulation technique,
        1215–1216
Interfornicial approach, to third ventricle,
        382, 389
Internal carotid artery
    complications of distal exposure, 769
    distal exposure, 765–769
    distal exposure alternatives, 765
    dissection, 767
    lesions requiring distal exposure, 765
    reconstruction, 769
Internal carotid artery aneurysm,
        angiography in, 930
    at anterior choroidal artery, 929, 930, 932
    at carotid bifurcation, 929, 930, 931, 932,
        1025
    carotid ligation, 1025
    carotid occlusion for, 1023
    clipping procedure, 934–935
    computed tomography, 930
    diagnosis, 930–931
    paraclinoid, 1032
    at posterior communicating artery
        junction, 929, 930, 931–932, 1025
    preoperative management, 931
    results, 935–936
    subarachnoid hemorrhage with, 929, 930,
        931, 936
    supraclinoid, 930
    surgical anatomy, 931
    surgical management, 929–955
    surgical procedure, 932–935
    symptoms, 929–930
Internal carotid artery aneurysm
        (intracavernous), 837–844
    angiography, 837
    computed tomography, 837
    developmental vs. traumatic, 837
    diagnosis, 837
    direct surgical repair, 839–842
    epistaxis with, 837, 838
    hemorrhage control, 838–839
    hypothermia in, 839, 841
    radiography, 837
    treatment, 837–842
Intervertebral disc (cervical)
    disc distention test, 1343–1345
    discography, 1343–1345
    discometry, 1343
Intervertebral disc (lumbar)
    anesthesia selection, 1380
    computed tomography, 1393, 1394
    degeneration, 1393
    epidural fat management, 1388–1389

excision, 1390
exploratory surgery, 1379
free disc fragments, 1391
herniation pathology, 1393
interlaminar surgery, 1390
interspace dissection, 1387
lesion site confirmation, 1380
microsurgical discectomy, 1399
myelography, 1375–1376, 1393, 1394
nerve root anomalies, 1392
nerve root damage, 1388–1389, 1394
neurological changes evaluation, 1375, 1393
procedure selection, 1380
prognostic factors, 1377
root tension management, 1390
sciatica and, 1393
subperiosteal dissection, 1385–1387
surface landmarks, 1384
surgery—historical development, 1379–1380
surgery—predictive score card, 1376–1378, 1393
surgical contraindications, 1377, 1379
surgical criteria, 1375
surgical field inspection, 1390
surgical incision, 1384–1385
surgical positioning, 1382–1384, 1394
wound closure, 1392
Intervertebral disc (thoracic)
costotransversectomy, 1367–1371
excision technique, 1367–1374
transthoracic (transpleural) approach, 1371–1374
Intervertebral disc disease
anterior lumbar discectomy and interbody fusion for, 1421–1436
chymopapain chemonucleolysis in, 1443–1448
diagnosis, 1422–1423
Intervertebral disc herniation, intraoperative ultrasonography visualization, 221
Intra-axial tumor
approach alternatives, 484–485
stereotactic definition of approach, 485
stereotactic resection, 481–490
volume interpolation, 483–484
Intracerebral hematoma, with acute head injury, 24
Intracerebral hemorrhage, 881–888
angiography, 885
classification, 881
clinical presentation, 881–882
computed tomography, 881, 884–886
diagnosis, 884–885
etiology, 881
general management, 885
postoperative care, 887
primary, 881
prognosis, 884–885
subependymal/intraventricular in infants, 884
surgical management, 885–887
surgical technique, 887
symptomatic, 882–884
Intracranial infection, 71–77
Intracranial extradural abscess, 71
Intracranial lesion, stereotactic biopsy, 495–498
Intracranial pressure

with acute head injury, 25–26, 27
anesthesia management and, 103, 106
in children, 103, 106
with head injury, 114
with hemispherectomy, 1238
with intraventricular hemorrhage, 119
with missile injury, 51, 52
in subdural hematoma, 34
with synostosis, 125–126
Intracranial subdural abscess, 71–72
Intracranial tumor
approach, 239
stereotactic radiosurgery, 515–529
Intracranial tumor (deep-seated), stereotactic resection, 481–490
Intramedullary spinal cord astrocytoma
anterior subarachnoid spinal fluid loculation, 182
in children, 175–185
clinical presentation, 175
computed tomography in, 176, 177, 184
congenital, 184
focal, 177
holocord, 176, 184, 185
hydrocephalus with, 182
magnetic resonance imaging in, 177, 184
malignant, 182
neurodiagnostic evaluation, 176, 184
postoperative morbidity relation to segmental location, 184
radiation therapy for, 180, 185
results, 184
rostral or caudal tumor fragment, 181–182
surgical complications, 181–184
surgical procedure for, 177–180
transcutaneous ultrasonography in, 177, 184
Intramedullary tumor, with syringomyelia, 1307, 1326
Intraneural artery, in peripheral nerve repair, 1564
Intraorbital tumor, 235–244
anatomy, 235–238
anesthesia, 239
case selection, 238–239
closure, 243
complications, 244
computed tomography in, 238
diagnosis, 238
instrumentation, 239
lateral orbital approach, 243
magnetic resonance imaging in, 238
medial orbit approach, 241
operative procedure, 240–244
polytomography in, 238
postoperative care, 244
preoperative management, 239
tarsorrhaphy in, 244
Intraspinal infection, 71–77
Intraspinal tumor, postoperative kyphosis/scoliosis in children, 1509–1513
Intraventricular hemorrhage, in premature infant, 119
Iontophoresis, in torticollis, 1262
Isoflurane, in children, 108
Isobutyl-2-cyanoacrylate, 744
Isoniazid, 81–82

Jannetta microvascular decompression anesthesia for, 1099

complications, 1104–1105
for glossopharyngeal neuralgia, 1108–1109
for hemifacial spasm, 1106–1108
instrumentation, 1101–1102
positioning for, 1099
postoperative considerations, 1103–1104
preoperative evaluation, 1099
results, 1104–1105
surgical procedure, 1099–1103
for trigeminal neuralgia, 1097–1098
Jugular foramen syndrome, 743

Karnofsky rating, 444–445
Kidney disease, with myelomeningocele, 151
Krönlein procedure, 270
Kyphosis, 187–211. See also Scoliosis
classification, 187
after intraspinal tumor surgery in children, 1509–1513
natural history, 190–191
after radiation therapy in children, 1509

Labbé's vein, 857, 861
Labyrinthectomy, in Meniere's disease, 1255
Labyrinthine disorders. See also specific diagnoses
nonsurgical treatment, 1254
Labyrinthitis (chronic)
nonsurgical treatment, 1254
pathophysiology, 1254
Lacrimal gland tumor, 264–265
Lambdoid synostosis, 132–133
complications, 133
diagnosis, 132
lambdoid synostectomy, 132–133
results, 133
surgical technique, 132–133
Laminectomy, in spinal cord injury, 1466–1467
Laminectomy (decompressive), in Paget's disease, 1305
Laryngoscopy, in children, 104
Laser technology, 223
aneurysm occlusion, 226
argon, 223–224, 226
biologic effects, 223–225
carbon dioxide, 223, 224, 225
clinical applications, 225–226
with computer-assisted stereotactic resection, 485–486
evaluation, 223
hemostasis, 226
in meningioma surgery, 559
Nd:YGA, 223, 226
neoplasm excision, 223–228
pain surgery, 226
perspectus, 226
physics, 223
stereotactic laser microsurgery, 226, 1062
systems, 225
techniques, 225
tissue bonding, 226
wet-field carbon dioxide, 226
Later particle agglutination test, in tuberculous meningitis, 84
Lateral femoral cutaneous nerve entrapment, 1593
Lateral osteotomy approach, to spine tumor, 1535–1536

Lateral sinus, dural arteriovenous
   malformation, 855–862
Lateral ventricle meningioma (trigonal)
   computed tomography in, 597
   surgical approaches, 597–599
Lateral ventricle tumor, 583–596
   approaches, 583
   case report, 592–595
   computed tomography in, 583
   postoperative care, 592
   preoperative studies, 583
   surgical complications, 591–592
Lateral ventricle tumor (frontal horn), 589–
      591
   anatomy, 589–590
   surgical approach, 590–591
   transcallosal approach, 590–591
Lateral ventricle tumor (midbody), 588–589
   anatomy, 588
   surgical approach, 588–589
   transcallosal approach, 588–589
Lateral ventricle tumor (temporal horn), 591
   anatomy, 591
   surgical approach, 591
Lateral ventricle tumor (trigonal), 583–588
   anatomy, 584
   approaches, 584–588
   lateral temporal parietal lobe incision, 584
   middle temporal gyrus incision, 584
   occipital lobectomy, 585
   superior parietal occipital incision, 585
   transcallosal approach, 585–586
   transtemporal horn occipital temporal
      gyrus incision, 586–587
Lateroposterior transpetrosal-transtentorial
      approach, to craniopharyngioma, 362
LeFort III midface advancement, 137
Leksell stereotactic system, 464–465, 492,
      1037
Limbic system surgery, 1069–1070
Lipoma, transpinal, 163, 170–172
Lipomyelomeningocele, 163
Lobectomy. *See specific approaches*
Localization technique
   computed tomography in, 463–474
   magnetic resonance imaging in, 463–474
Low back pain, stimulation management,
      1049
Lower extremity causalgia, lumbar
      sympathectomy for, 1277–1278
Lumbar disc excision (microsurgical)
   advantages/disadvantages, 1397
   patient selection, 1395
   postoperative care, 1396–1397
   results, 1397
   preoperative preparation, 1395
   procedure rationale, 1395
   technique, 1395–1397
Lumbar disc herniation
   chymopapain chemonucleolysis, 1437–
      1441
   microsurgical disc excision, 1395–1397
Lumbar drainage, in cerebrospinal fluid
      leakage, 66
Lumbar epidural tumor (metastatic), 1559
Lumbar interbody fusion (posterior)
   biochemical considerations, 1401–1405
   closure, 1410
   complications, 1414–1415

decortication with, 1404, 1408
   epidural hemostasis with, 1406
   exposure, 1405–1406
   grafting, 1402–1403, 1404–1405, 1408–1410,
      1418
   indications for, 1401
   for lumbar spondylosis, 1401–1420
   patient positioning, 1405
   posterior motion segment preservation,
      1403
   postoperative care, 1410, 1412
   pseudoarthrodesis with, 1414
   results, 1415–1417
   surgical pitfalls, 1412–1414
   technique, 1405–1410
   total discectomy with, 1403–1404, 1406–
      1408
   unigraft concept, 1404–1405
Lumbar meningocele, 158–159
Lumbar rhizotomy
   fifth lumbar denervation, 1217–1220
   percutaneous electrothermocoagulation
      technique, 1216–1220
Lumbar shunt, spinal complications after,
      1510
Lumbar spinal deformity, surgical treatment,
      1511–1512
Lumbar spine fusion, 1473
   extraperitoneal, 1474–1475
Lumbar spine injury, anterior lateral
      approach, 1468
Lumbar spondylosis
   anatomic alignment changes with, 1401
   instability categories, 1401
   posterior lumbar interbody fusion in,
      1401–1420
   postoperative care, 1410, 1412
   radiography, 1403
   surgical results, 1415–1417
Lumbar sympathectomy, 1277–1279
   anatomy, 1277
   complications, 1279
   indications for, 1277–1278
   results, 1279
   surgical technique, 1277–1279
Lumbosacral spine fusion, 1474

Magnetic resonance imaging
   anesthesia for, 113
   in anterior communicating artery
      aneurysm, 939
   in arteriovenous malformation, 523, 905
   in brain stem tumor, 716–718
   in carotid ophthalmic aneurysm, 917
   in cerebellar astrocytoma, 660
   in cerebral glioma, 433
   in cerebrospinal fluid leakage, 59
   in cervical spondylotic myelopathy, 1352
   in Chiari malformation with hydromyelia,
      1311
   in children, 1509
   in clivus and basiocciptial region tumor,
      639–640
   in craniopharyngioma, 355–356
   in dural sinus malformation, 861
   in intraoribital tumor, 238
   in lesion localization and biopsy, 463–474
   in meningioma, 550, 566–567, 572

in metastatic spine tumor, 1517
   in optic glioma, 279–280
   in pineal tumor, 403
   in posterior fossa tumor, 654
   in rheumatoid arthritis, 1296, 1301
   in sella turcica lesion, 301
   in spinal cord astrocytoma, 177, 184
   in spinal dysraphism, 168
   in spine trauma, 1449
   in spine tumor, 1525, 1526
   with stereotactic biopsy, 495–498, 502
   stereotactic frame modification for, 464–
      466
   with stereotactic intra-axial tumor
      resection, 481–490
   in stereotactic surgery, 463
   in tentorium tumor, 647
Mandibular subluxation, with distal internal
      carotid artery exposure, 765–767, 769
Marcus-Gunn pupil, 269, 270
Mauer's triad, 837
Mebendazole, in cysticercosis, 87
Medial nerve, intraneural artery, 1564
Medial palmar cutaneous nerve, in carpal
      tunnel syndrome, 1586
Medial sphenoid wing meningioma, 537–539
   angiography, 538
   computed tomography, 537–538
   presentation, 537–538
   radiography, 537–538
   results, 539
   surgical technique, 538–539
Median nerve entrapment, 1585–1588
   anterior interosseous syndrome, 1588
   conservative management, 1585
   diagnosis, 1585
   pronator syndrome, 1588
   proximal forearm, 1586–1587
   surgical management, 1586
Mediolongitudinal myelotomy. *See*
      Commissural myelotomy
Medullary tractotomy
   anatomic basis, 1165–1166
   anesthesia, 1166–1167
   for cancer pain, 1045
   complications, 1167–1168
   indications for, 1166
   instrumentation, 1166
   for intractable pain, 1165–1168
   patient positioning, 1167
   results, 1167–1168
   technique, 1167
Medulloblastoma
   computed tomography, 658
   postoperative radiation therapy, 658
   recurrence, 658
   surgical management, 658
Meniere's disease, 1251–1259
   labyrinthectomy in, 1255
   nonsurgical treatment, 1254
   pathophysiology, 1251
   streptomycin sulfate ablation of vestibular
      nerve, 1259
   surgical treatment, 1255–1258
   vestibular nerve transection in, 1251–1259
Meningeal carcinomatosis, 460
Meningioma
   angiography, 550–551, 564–566, 572
   bone flap elevation, 557–558

carbon dioxide laser surgery, 559
cerebellopontine angle, 673–674
of clivus and basioccipital region, 637, 645
computed tomography, 549–550, 564, 571–572
differential diagnosis, 572
dural opening, 558
encephalography in, 551
excision, 559
exposure, 558–559
hemostasis, 558, 560
histology, 547–548
intraoperative ultrasonography visualization, 217
magnetic resonance imaging, 550, 566–567, 572
myelography, 572–573
NdYAG laser surgery, 559
optic nerve, 235, 236, 239, 241
patient positioning, 556
postoperative care, 561
preoperative embolization, 551–553
preoperative evaluation, 547–553
preoperative preparation, 553
prognosis, 547–548
radiation therapy, 551
radiography, 548–551, 564–567, 571–573
recurrence, 547
scalp incision, 556–557
sites, 547
of skull base, 627, 629
stereotactic radiosurgery, 519
surgical principles, 556–561, 567–570, 575–581
surgical treatment, 551
ultrasonic aspiration, 559
ventriculography, 573
wound closure, 560
Meningioma (cerebellopontine angle), 572
computed tomography, 572
magnetic resonance imaging, 572
surgical technique, 578–579
Meningioma (convexity), 555–562
classification, 555
coronal, 555
occipital, 556
pararolandic, 555
parietal, 555
postcoronal, 555
precoronal, 555
symptomatology, 555–556
temporal, 555–556
Meningioma (falx), 563–570
angiography, 564–566
excision, 569
exposure, 569
radiography, 564–567
surgical principles, 567–570
Meningioma (foramen magnum), surgical technique, 578–579
Meningioma (parasagittal), 563–570
angiography, 564–566
bone flap, 567, 569
computed tomography, 544
dural opening, 569
excision, 569
exposure, 569
magnetic resonance imaging, 566–567
patient positioning, 567

radiography, 564–567
sagittal sinography, 566
scalp incision, 567
site, 563
surgical principles, 567–570
symptomatology, 563–564
Meningioma (posterior fossa), 571–582
anesthesia, 574
angiography, 572
classification, 571
computed tomography, 571–572
magnetic resonance imaging, 572
myelography, 572–573
obstructive hydrocephalus control, 573
patient positioning, 574–575
radiography, 571–573
site-symptoms relationship, 571
surgical approach, 575–581
surgical technique, 575–581
ventriculography, 573
Meningioma (posterior petrous ridge), surgical technique, 575–578
Meningioma (tentorium cerebelli), surgical technique, 575–578
Meningitis. *See also* Tuberculous meningitis
with cerebrospinal fluid leakage, 58, 61, 63
Meningitis (chemical), with Rathke's cleft cyst, 373–374
Meningocele
anterior sacral, 159–161
anterolateral spinal, 158–161
cervical, 158
intrasacral, 159–161
lumbar, 158–159
posterior spinal, 157–158
thoracic, 158–159
Meningocele manqué, 164
surgery for, 169
Mental retardation, with infantile hemiplegia, 1236
Mesencephalotomy, for cancer pain, 1045–1046
Metastasis (intracranial), 451–462
biopsy in, 454, 457, 459
chemotherapy, 455, 456, 460, 461
clonogenic assay, 456
combined surgical and radiation therapy, 454
computed tomography in, 457–458, 459
corticosteroids in, 453, 461
differential diagnosis, 459
distribution, 451
immunotherapy, 460
incidence, 451
latency of, 451–452
leptomeningeal, 451, 460
lesion characteristics, 451
mortality and morbidity, 456
origin, 451
postoperative complications, 456
primary tumor factor, 459
radiation therapy, 453–454, 460, 461
results, 455, 456
shunt for hydrocephalus, 459
solitary and accessible, 458–459
solitary vs. multiple, 451
stereotactic biopsy in, 457
surgical indications, 458–459
surgical management, 454–458

terminal illness, 461
treatment modalities evaluation, 452–453
Metastatic tumor (intra-axial), stereotactic resection, 488–489
Methylmethacrylate
in cerebrospinal fluid leakage repair, 66
for skull implant, 11, 14–16
spine fusion, 1522–1523
Metopic synostosis, 133–134
complications, 134
diagnosis, 133
"floating forehead," 134
metopic syntectomy, 134
results, 134
surgical treatment, 133–134
Metrizamine, computed tomography enhancement, 176, 184, 1332
Metrizamine cisternography, 60
Metrizamide instillation, in posterior fossa tumor, 654
Metrizamide myelography, 1518
for anterior lumbar discectomy, 1423
Microslad, for stereotactic resection, 486
Microvascular decompression
for facial pain, complications, 1139–1143
for glossopharyngeal neuralgia, 1108–1109
for hemifacial spasm, 1107
Microvascular replantation
in scalp avulsion, 6–9
for trigeminal neuralgia, 1097–1098
Midbrain, stereotactic surgery, 472
Midbrain tumor, 711–712
symptomology, 714–716
Middle cerebral artery aneurysm, 957–971, 1026, 1032
angiography, 957, 970
at bifurcation, 959
computed tomography, 957, 958, 968
giant aneurysm, 963–967
patient positioning, 959–960
postoperative care, 968, 970
preoperative medication, 957–958
proximal, 959
results, 970
sites, 959
somatosensory evoked response monitoring, 967–968
subarachnoid hemorrhage with, 957, 958, 970
surgery timing, 958–959
surgical approach, 959
surgical procedure, 960–963
temporary vascular occlusion in, 967–968
at trifurcation, 962–963
Middle cranial fossa approach
to cerebellopontine angle, 675
to posterior cranial fossa, 665–666, 671
Middle fossa-infratemporal fossa approach, to posterior cranial fossa, 669, 671
Milwaukee Brace, 193
Missile injury (penetrating), 49–55
antibiotic prophylaxis with, 52
anticonvulsants in, 52
ballistics factor, 49–50
blast injury with, 51
bone chips, 50
bone fragment management, 52
bone fragment replacement, 53–54
bullet track factor, 50

Missile injury (penetrating) *(continued)*
  cerebrospinal fluid fistula with, 53
  computed tomography in, 49, 54
  contusions, 51
  corticosteroids in, 51
  debridement, 52
  dural sinus repair, 53
  explosive bullets management, 53
  hematoma with, 51
  hydrocephalus with, 53
  intracranial pressure with, 51, 52
  issues, 49
  migrating metallic fragments, 52–53
  nutrition with, 51–52
  pathophysiology, 50
  skull fracture with, 51
  strategic considerations, 54
  surgical principles, 51
  tangential injury, 51
  velocity factor, 50
Morphine test, 1089–1090
Morphine therapy, opioid system and, 1077–1078
Morphine therapy (intraventricular)
  for cancer pain, 1077–1088
  case reports, 1079–1085
  cerebrospinal fluid injection, 1078–1088
  computed tomography, 1079
  instrumentation, 1079, 1086
  patient selection, 1079
  results, 1079, 1086
  surgical technique, 1079
Movement disorders
  extrapyramidal system in, 1050–1051
  neurosurgical management, 1050–1057
  stereotactic surgery for, 1051
Moyamoya disease, 797–806
  angiography, 798–801, 803
  computed tomography, 798
  electroencephalography, 799, 801, 804
  encephaloduroarteriosynangiosis in, 802, 804
  encephalomyosynangiosis in, 802, 804
  epidemiology, 797–798
  etiology, 797–798
  genetic factor, 797
  medical management, 801
  omentum transplantation in, 801
  regional cerebral blood flow in, 798–799, 803
  results, 804
  pathology, 798–801
  STA-MCA anastomosis in, 802, 804
  surgical management, 801–804
  sympathectomy in, 801, 804
  transient ischemic attacks with, 797, 801, 804
  types, 797
Multiple sclerosis
  retrogasserian glycerol injection for, 1134
  stimulation management, 1055–1056
  trigeminal neuralgia with, 1105
  trigeminal rhizotomy in, 1120
Muscle reconstruction, in facial palsy, 707
Mycobacterium tuberculosis, 79–85
Myelocystocele, 166
  terminal, 158
Myelography
  anesthesia for, 112

  in brachial plexus injury, 1578
  in cervical disc herniation, 1348
  in cervical spondylosis, 1332
  in cervical spondylotic myelopathy, 1352
  in Chiari malformation with hydromyelia, 1313–1316
  in children, 1509
  in intramedullary spinal cord tumor, 1492
  of lumbar intervertebral disc, 1375–1376, 1393, 1394
  in meningioma, 572–573
  in metastatic spine tumor, 1517–1518
  in Paget's disease, 1304, 1305
  in rheumatoid arthritis, 1296
  in spinal cord arteriovenous malformation, 1500–1501
  in spine tumor, 1526
  in third ventricle tumor, 398
Myelomeningocele, 151–162
  anesthesia for, 111
  closure-site reconstruction, 156–157
  concurrent care considerations, 151
  demographic factor, 151
  genetic factor, 151
  with hydrocephalus, 119
  kidney disease with, 151
  postnatal care, 152–154
  postoperative care, 156
  spinal deformity with hydromyelia and malfunction shunt, 1510–1511
  surgical closure technique, 154–157
  survivals, 151–152
  treatment criteria, 152
Myelotomy (longitudinal-Bischof's), 1177–1184
  for cancer pain, 1044
  commissural, 1185–1190
Myofascial syndrome, trigger point blocks for, 1049

Nasal cavity tumor
  craniofacial resection for, 611
  patient selection, 612
  preoperative evaluation, 612
Nasal structures, reconstruction techniques, 331–337
Nasopharyngeal cancer, percutaneous rhizotomy for pain, 1125–1127
Needlescope, 424
Nelson's syndrome, stereotactic radiosurgery, 518
Neodymium:ytterium argon garnet laser, 223, 226
  in mengioma surgery, 559
Neonate
  Chiari II malformation, 123
  Dandy-Walker malformation, 121, 123
  frontal nasal encephalocele, 121
  head trauma, 119–120
  hydrocephalus in, 119
    with myelomeningocele, 119
  intraoperative considerations, 117–119
  intraventricular hemorrhage in, 117
  neurosurgical management in, 117–123
  occipital encephalocele, 120–121
  positioning precautions, 117
  temperature regulation in, 117
  vein of Galen malformation, 120

  venipuncture in, 117
Neoplasm
  laser excision, 223–228
  ultrasonic surgical fragmentation, 227
Nerve conduction velocity, in peripheral nerve injury, 1567
Nerve graft, in facial palsy, 705
Nerve root microvascular lysis, in torticollis, 1262
Nerve transfer, in facial palsy, 705
Neural decompression, in thoracolumbar fracture, 1481, 1482, 1483
Neuralgia, spinal sensory rhizotomy for, 1211
Neurapraxia, 1584
Neurocysticercosis, 79, 93–102
Neurofibroma, 1603–1605
  optic nerve, 239, 243
  surgical indications, 1604
Neurofibromatosis. *See* Von Recklinghausen's disease
Neurologic deficit, with arteriovenous malformation, 914
Neurolysis, in peripheral nerve injury, 1572
Neuroma, with peripheral entrapment neuropathy, 1585
Neuromuscular blockade, in children, 104–105
Neuromuscular disease, scoliosis and, 191
Neuropsychologic testing, in cerebral glioma, 434–435
Neurotmesis, 1584
Neurotransmitters, 1070
Niclosamide, 87
Nitroprusside (sodium), in children, 107–108
Nucleus pulposus, chemonucleolysis with chymopapain, 1437–1441
Nutrition, in penetrating missile injury, 51–52

Occipital artery–anterior inferior cerebellar artery bypass
  in vertebrobasilar insufficiency, 814–815
  results, 814–815
  technique, 814
Occipital artery–middle cerebral artery bypass, 792–793
Occipital artery–posterior inferior cerebellar artery bypass, 793
  results, 813
  technique, 812–813
  in vertebrobasilar insufficiency, 810, 812–814
Occipital encephalocele
  anesthesia for, 110–113
  in neonate, 120–121
Occipital lobectomy
  in cerebral glioma, 441–442
  exposure, 441–442
  patient positioning, 441–442
Occipital transtentorial approach, to pineal region, 411–418
Occlusive cerebrovascular disease
  direct brain revascularization, 783–795
  interposition vein graft to posterior cerebral artery, 793
  long vein grafts, 792

occipital artery–middle cerebral artery bypass, 792–793
occipital artery–posterior inferior cerebellar artery bypass, 793
short vein graft, 791
STA-MCA bypass for, 783–791
vertebrobasilar revascularization, 793–794
Odontoidectomy, transoral, 1289
Olfactory groove meningioma
  angiography, 540
  computed tomography, 540
  presentation, 539–540
  radiography, 540
  results, 545
  surgical technique, 541–545
Oligodendroglioma, 432
  stereotactic resection, 488
Omentum transplantation, in moyamoya disease, 802

Ommaya reservoir, 219
Ophthalmic artery, 236–237
Opthalmic artery aneurysm. *See* Carotid ophthalmic aneurysm
Opthalmic vein, 237
Ophthalmologic testing, in cerebral glioma, 433–434
Opiates
  epidural infusion for intractable pain, 1145–1147
  epidural system availability, 1147–1148
  epidural therapy complications, 1149–1152
  epidural therapy results, 1148–1149
  indications for epidural implantation systems, 1147
  preparation for epidural administration, 1147
Opioid system, morphine therapy and, 1077–1078
Optic glioma, 235, 239, 241, 279–298
  calcification, 279
  case reports, 280–282, 290–293
  chiasma/optic nerve/brain involvement, 279, 287–295
  computed tomography in, 279
  cystic component, 289
  diagnosis, 279–286, 287–288
  diagnostic controversies, 280–286
  with edema/without neoplastic invasion, 288–289
  exophytic tumor growth, 289–290
  hemorrhagic component, 289
  hypothalamic invasion, 293–294
  magnetic resonance imaging, 279–280
  of one optic nerve, 285–286
  partial vs. complete resection, 288–290
  radiation therapy, 295
  spontaneous regression, 284–285
  surgery for, 286–295
  visual evoked potentials in, 280
Optic nerve, 235
  sphenoethmoid approach, 269–277
  visual deficit after head trauma, 269
Optic nerve decompression
  angiography, 270
  case reports, 272–276
  computed tomography, 270
  external ethmoidectomy approach, 270

indications for, 271–272
  Krönlein procedure, 270
  sphenoethmoid approach, 270–271
  surgical requirements, 269
  transantralethmoidal approach, 270
  transantrosphenoidal approach, 270
  transfrontal craniotomy approach, 269–270
  transsphenoidal approach, 270, 275
Optic nerve lesions, with radiofrequency rhizotomy, 1140–1141
Optic nerve tumor, 235
  approach, 238, 239, 241–243
  radiation therapy, 239
Orbit
  anatomy, 235
  arterial supply, 236–237
  nerve supply, 237–238
  venous drainage, 236–237
Orbit pathology
  anterior approach, 248, 251–252, 261–264
  computed tomography, 249, 250, 251
  contrast media in diagnosis, 249–250
  contrast orbitography, 250–251
  corticosteroids in, 251
  instrumentation, 252
  lacrimal gland tumor, 264–265
  lateral approach, 247–248, 249, 252–253
  lateral canthotomy, 254
  lateral orbitotomy, 254–261
  microsurgical approaches, 245–267
  noninvasive vs. invasive diagnostic procedures, 249
  postoperative complications, 266
  radiography, 250
  superior approach, 251
  surgical anatomy, 245–249
  surgical approaches, 251–265
  surgical complications, 265–266
  surgical indications, 252
  venography, 250
Orbital surgery, 235–244
Orbitography (contrast), in orbit pathology, 250–251
Orbitotomy, lateral, 254–261
Osteoma, intraorbital, 239
Osteomyelitis
  of skull, 71
  of spine, 76–77
Owl percutaneous cordotomy electrode, 1194–1195

Pachymeningitis, 1303
Packing substances
  for pituitary fossa, 321
  for sphenoidal sinus, 322
Paget's disease, 1303–1305
  computed tomography in, 1304
  decompressive laminectomy in, 1305
  medical management, 1304–1305
  myelography in, 1304, 1305
  spinal cord compression, 1303–1304
Pain
  anatomy of, 1040–1041
  deep-brain stimulation for, 1041–1043
  denervation, 1042
  functional neurosurgery for, 1040–1050
  laser surgery for, 226
  lower body segments/thoracic region,

commissural myelotomy for, 1185–1190
  nociceptive vs. deafferentation, 1191, 1199
  pathways of, 1041
  perception of, 1041
Pain (chronic). *See also specific syndromes*
  indications for surgery, 1047
  management, 1047–1050
  medication addiction and, 1048
  multiple management factors, 1048
  patient classification, 1047–1048
  patient selection for stereotactic cingulotomy, 1071
  postcingulotomy management, 1074
  psychopathology with, 1048–1049
  sympathectomy for, 1049
  stereotactic cingulotomy for, 1069–1075
  trigger point blocks for, 1049
Pain (intractable)
  dorsal root entry zone thermocoagulation for, 1169–1175
  epidural anesthetic infusion for, 1145
  epidural morphine therapy complications, 1149–1152
  epidural morphine therapy results, 1148–1149
  epidural opiate infusion for, 1145–1147
  implantable systems for management of, 1145–1153
  implanted electrode brain stimulation for, 1089–1095
  medullary tractotomy for, 1165–1168
  morphine test for, 1089–1090
  open cordotomy for, 1155–1168
  paramedian, midline, bilateral: bilateral cordotomy for, 1156
  types of, 1040–1050
  unilateral somatic cancer: unilater cordotomy for, 1155
  unilateral visceral: bilateral cordotomy for, 1155–1156
Painful disc syndrome, 1327
Pallidotomy
  in dystonia, 1268
  in torticollis, 1262–1263
Pan synostosis, 134
Pancreas cancer, splanchnicectomy for pain, 1275
Pancreatitis, splanchnicectomy for, 1275
Pan-hypopituitarism, 300
Papaya latex, 1437
Papilledema, 235
Para-aminosalicylic acid, 81
Paranasal sinus tumor
  craniofacial approach, 609
  patient selection, 612
  preoperative evaluation, 612
Paranasal structures, reconstruction techniques, 331–337
Paraplegia, scoliosis and, 191
Paraplegia (traumatic), dorsal root entry zone thermocoagulation for pain, 1172, 1174
Parasite infection, 93–102. *See also specific diagnoses*
Parkinson's disease
  campotomy for, 1052
  stereotactic procedures for, 1051, 1052
  thalamotomy for, 1052

Pattern visual evoked potentials, 280
Percutaneous cordotomy, 1191–1205
  analgesia maintenance, 1200
  anesthesia for, 1194, 1195, 1199
  bilateral, 1192, 1199, 1202
  complications, 1202–1203
  cord structure identification, 1198
  dermatome level factor, 1192
  impedance monitoring, 1195, 1198
  instrumentation, 1194–1195
  lateral high cervical, 1191
  lateral spinothalamic tract identification,
      1196–1198, 1200
  lesion making, 1198
  lesion tailoring, 1199
  local pathology factor, 1192–1193
  for midline pain, 1192
  nociceptive vs. deafferentation pain factor,
      1191, 1199
  in nonmalignant disease, 1201
  vs. open procedure, 1193
  pain location factor, 1192
  pain persistence after, 1200–1201
  pain recurrence, 1201–1202
  pain relief results, 1199, 1202
  patient positioning, 1194
  patient selection, 1191
  physiologic localization, 1195–1198
  postcordotomy dysesthesia, 1200–1201
  postoperative care, 1199
  preoperative preparation, 1194
  radiographic localization in, 1195, 1198
  respiratory function factor, 1192
  results, 1199–1203
  surgical technique, 1193–1199
  technique selection, 1193
Percutaneous electrode implantation, 1040
  for cancer pain, 1047
Percutaneous electrothermocoagulation, of
      spinal nerve trunk/ganglion/rootlets,
      1207–1221
Percutaneous rhizotomy
  for cancer pain, 1125–1127
  commentary, 1125–1127
  for facial pain, complications, 1139–1143
  in trigeminal neuralgia, 1125–1127
Percutaneous trigeminal neurolysis, 1097–
      1098
Periaqueductal gray matter, stimulation site
      in pain control, 1089, 1091, 1094
Periorbita, 235–236
Peripheral denervation
  in dystonia, 1268
  results, 1266–1267
  surgical technique, 1264–1266
  in torticollis, 1263–1268
Peripheral entrapment neuropathy, 1583–
      1597
  classification, 1584
  common peroneal nerve compression,
      1596
  compression and, 1583
  compressive lesions, 1584–1596
  electromyelography, 1584, 1585
  ischemia and, 1583
  lateral femoral cutaneous nerve, 1593
  median nerve, 1585–1588
  neurolysis, 1585
  neuroma with, 1585

  posterior tibial nerve, 1593
  radial nerve entrapment, 1589–1590
  suprascapular nerve, 1590–1591
  surgical management, 1585
  thoracic outlet syndrome, 1591–1593
  ulnar nerve compression, 1588–1589
Peripheral nerve(s)
  anatomy, 1563–1564
  blood supply, 1564
  degeneration/regeneration, 1565–1566
  injury mechanism, 1564–1565
Peripheral nerve injury
  anesthesia, 1570
  complete transection, 1572
  compression lesion, 1572
  diagnosis, 1566–1568
  electromyography in, 1567, 1571
  epineurial suture, 1573
  fascicular/group fascicular repair, 1573–
      1574, 1575
  fibrillation potentials, 1567
  with fracture/dislocation, 1570
  grafting in, 1574, 1575
  injection, 1572
  magnification requirements, 1571
  microsurgical instrumentation, 1571
  nerve conduction velocity, 1567
  neurolysis in, 1572
  patient positioning, 1570
  postoperative management, 1575
  radiation injury and, 1572
  resection length criteria, 1572–1573
  results variables, 1575–1577
  sensory testing, 1566
  sudomotor function, 1568
  surgical indications, 1568–1570
  surgical technique, 1572
  suture material, 1571
  sympathectomy for sequela, 1272
  Tinel's sign, 1566–1567
  tourniquet management, 1570–1571
Peripheral nerve lesions, classification, 1584
Peripheral nerve surgery, in facial palsy, 705
Peripheral nerve tumor, 1599–1610
  biopsy, 1606–1607
  classification, 1599
  clinical diagnosis, 1599
  extrinsic compressive, 1608
  extrinsic invasive, 1608
  intraoperative diagnosis, 1599
  malignant, 1605–1607
  neurofibroma, 1603–1605
  postoperative care, 1608–1609
  schwannoma, 1599–1603
  Von Recklinghausen's disease, 1605
Phantom limb pain, stimulation
      management, 1049
Photoradiation therapy, 226
Phrenic–facial nerve anastomosis, 683
Physiotherapy, in torticollis, 1267
Pig tape worm, 79
Pineal region, occipital transtentorial
      approach, 411–418
Pineal region tumor, 397–399
  associated syndromes, 397
  benign vs. malignant, 397
  chemotherapy, 399
  neuro-ophthalmologic examination, 398
  radiation therapy, 399

  sterotactic radiosurgery, 518–519
  suprasellar germinoma, 397
  surgical management, 398–399
  symptomatology, 397
  third ventricle lesion, 398
  tumor markers in, 398
Pineal tumor
  arteriography in, 403
  biologic markers in, 403
  chemotherapy, 404–405
  classification, 404–405
  clinical features, 402
  computed tomography, 403
  diagnosis, 402–404
  incidence, 401
  magnetic resonance imaging in, 403
  occipital transtentorial approach, 411–418
  posterior fossa approach, 405–407
  radiation therapy, 404–405
  radiography in, 403
  site distribution, 401
  supracerebellar approach, 401–409
  surgical alternatives, 401–402
  surgical complications, 407–408
  surgical criteria, 403–404
  surgical indications, 401
  surgical results, 408
  surgical technique, 405–407
  therapeutic alternatives, 404
  ventriculography in, 403
Pituitary adenoma, 299–307
  ACTH assay in, 300
  cerebrospinal fluid leak, 306
  dexamethasone suppression test, 300
  diabetes insipidus with, 307
  endocrine function in, 299–300
  endocrine results, 305
  empty sella complication, 330
  ghost sella complication, 330–331
  growth hormone level, 299
  intrasella, 325–326
  pan-hypopituitarism with, 300
  postoperative considerations, 305
  radiofrequency electrode application,
      302
  sella turcica reconstruction, 325–326
  serum prolactin, 299
  sinusitis with, 306
  suprasellar extension with, 326–329
  surgical complications, 306–307
  surgical identification, 305
  surgical results, 305–306
  transsphenoidal approach, 299–307, 309–
      319
  visual results, 306
Pituitary fossa
  anchored intradural packing, 323–324
  cerebrospinal fluid leakage management,
      324–325
  combined extradural-intradural packing,
      324
  extradural packing, 324
  packing substances, 321
  reconstruction complications, 333–334
  reconstruction techniques, 321–337
  simple intradural packing, 323
  transsphenoidal approach, 321–337
Pituitary gland, transethmoidal
      sphenoidotomy approach, 339–343

Pituitary microadenoma
  sella turcica reconstruction, 325
  transsphenoidal approach, 314
Pituitary stalk, sacrifice in
    craniopharyngioma, 363
Pituitary tumor (hypersecreting), stereotactic
    radiosurgery, 516–518
Pneumocephalus, with cerebrospinal fluid
    leakage, 58
Pneumography, of sella turcica, 356
Polymethyl methacrylate, 1530
Polytomography, in intraorbital tumor, 238
Polyvinyl alcohol foam, for embolization,
    552, 820
Pons, stereotactic surgery, 472
Positioning. *See also specific diagnoses and
    procedures*
  of children, 105, 106
Positive-end-expiratory pressure, in acute
    head injury, 27–28
Positron emission tomography, 433
Posterior cerebral aneurysm, 973–989. *See
    also* Basilar artery aneurysm
  anesthesia, 973–974
  anterior-projecting, 983
  monitoring techniques, 973–974
  patient positioning, 974
  posterior-projecting, 982–983
Posterior cranial fossa
  case reports, 669–670
  infratemporal fossa approach, 668, 671
  middle fossa approach, 665–666, 671
  middle fossa–infratemporal fossa
      approach, 669, 671
  retrolabyrinthine approach, 667
  skull base approach, 667–668, 671
  suboccipital approach, 665, 670
  suboccipital–translabyrinthine approach,
      668, 671
  transcanal approach, 667, 671
  transcochlear approach, 668, 671
  translabyrinthine approach, 665, 670–671
  transmeatal approach to cerebellopontine
      angle, 676–680
  transtemporal approaches, 665–672
Posterior fossa approach, to pineal tumor,
    405–407
Posterior fossa craniectomy
  midline, 655–658
  unilateral, 659
Posterior fossa cyst, surgical management,
    658–659
Posterior fossa revascularization, 807–818
  indications for, 807–808
Posterior fossa tumor, 653–664
  cerebrospinal fluid diversion, 654
  in children, 109
  combined supratentorial and infratentorial
      approach, 660–662
  computed tomography, 653–654
  diagnosis, 653–654
  magnetic resonance imaging, 654
  metrizamide instillation, 654
  midline posterior fossa craniectomy, 655–
      658
  neurologic consequences, 653
  pathology, 656
  patient positioning, 655
  surgical management, 654–659

symptomatology, 653
Posterior tibial nerve entrapment, 1593
Postherpetic neuralgia
  stimulation management, 1049
  surgical management, 1049
Praziquantel, 87
Prefrontal lobotomy, 1057, 1069
Prematurity, intraventricular hemorrhage
    with, 119
Premedication, for children, 106
Prolactin (serum), in pituitary adenoma, 299
Prolactinoma, 299
Proptosis, 235, 238
Proton beam therapy
  arteriography after, 911–912
  for arteriovenous malformation, 911–915
  complications, 912, 914
  hemorrhage with, 913–914
  incubation period with, 913
  ionizing event with, 913
  lesion tissue changes from, 912
  response variation, 914
  risk, 914
  tissue histology, 912–913
Pseudoarthrosis, with spine fusion, 1478,
    1480
Psychiatric disorder
  patient selection for stereotactic
      cingulotomy, 1070–1071
  postcingulotomy management, 1073–1074
  prefrontal lobotomy, 1069
  stereotactic cingulotomy for, 1069–1075
Psychosurgery, 1057–1060
Psychotrophic drugs, 1070
Pterional approach
  in craniopharyngioma, 362
  to sella turcica, 303–304
Pyrazinamide, 81

Quadriplegia, electroneuroprosthesis for,
    1062–1063

Radial nerve entrapment, 1589–1590
Radiation therapy. *See also specific
    modalities*
  in arteriovenous malformation, 906
  brachial plexus neuropathy and, 1580
  in brain stem glioma, 724, 735
  in cerebellar hemangioblastoma, 660
  in cerebral glioma, 448
  contact radiation devices, 504–507
  in craniopharyngioma, 368–372
  for fourth ventricle ependymoma, 658
  for glomus jugulare tumor, 739, 743–744,
      749
  in intracranial metastasis, 453–454, 460,
      461
  in intramedullary spinal cord tumor, 1496
  in medulloblastoma, 658
  in meningioma, 551
  in metastatic epidural tumor, 1542, 1543
  in metastatic spine tumor, 1515, 1522,
      1560
  for optic glioma, 295
  in optic nerve tumor, 239
  in pineal region tumor, 399
  for pineal tumor, 404–405

postradiation kyphosis/scoliosis in
    children, 1509
peripheral nerve injury and, 1572
for spinal cord astrocytoma, 180, 186
in spine tumor, 1526, 1527, 1530, 1531
Radiofrequency electrode, in pituitary
    adenoma resection, 302
Radiofrequency griseotomy, in lower limb
    spasticity, 1181
Radiofrequency heating
  for cluster headache, 1136
  for trigeminal neuralgia, 1134
Radiofrequency rhizotomy
  central retinal artery occlusion with, 1141–
      1142
  optic nerve lesions with, 1140–1141
Radiofrequency thermocoagulation, in
    trigeminal neuralgia, 1098
Radiography. *See also specific procedures*
  in anterior lumbar discectomy, 1422, 1427–
      1428
  in anterior skull base tumor, 611
  in brachial plexus injury, 1578
  in cerebral glioma, 432–433
  in cerebrospinal fluid leakage, 59
  in cervical disc herniation, 1348
  in cervical spondylosis, 1329–1332
  in cervical spondylotic myelopathy, 1352
  in Chiari malformation with hydromyelia,
      1309–1316
  in chymopapain chemonucleolysis, 1438,
      1439
  in clivus and basioccipital region tumor,
      637–640
  in clivus tumor, 650
  in craniofacial abnormality, 135
  in craniopharyngioma, 355–357
  in craniovertebral junction abnormality,
      1284
  in epilepsy, 1224
  in gunshot wounds of head, 38–39
  in infantile hemiplegia, 1236
  in internal carotid artery aneurysm, 837
  in intramedullary spinal cord tumor, 1488–
      1490
  in lumbar spondylosis, 1403
  in medial sphenoid wing meningioma, 537–
      538
  in meningioma, 548–551, 564–567, 571–573
  in metastatic spine tumor, 1516–1518,
      1520, 1522
  in olfactory groove meningioma, 540
  in orbit pathology, 250
  in percutaneous cordotomy, 1195, 1198
  in pineal tumor, 403
  in rheumatoid arthritis, 1296
  in scalp/skull tumor, 604
  in scoliosis, 191
  in sella turcica lesion, 299, 300–301
  in spinal cord arteriovenous malformation,
      1500–1501
  in spinal dysraphism, 167–168
  in spinal sensory rhizotomy, 1211, 1215,
      1216, 1220
  of spine in children, 1509
  in spine tumor, 1526–1527, 1528
  with stereotactic surgery, 1037–1038
  in suprasellar germinoma, 398
  in suprasellar meningioma, 531

Radiography (continued)
  in synostosis, 125, 126, 130, 132, 133
  in tentorium tumor, 647
  for third ventricle lesion, 382, 391–392
  in thoracolumbar fracture, 1483
  in tuberculoma, 80–81
  in vertebrobasilar insufficiency, 771–775
Radioisotope scan
  in cerebrospinal fluid leakage, 59–60
  in spine tumor, 1526, 1528
Radionuclide implantation
  indications for, 507–512
  nuclides for, 500
  permanent (curietherapy) technique, 491,
    499–503
  results, 507
  stereotactic biopsy with, 491–514
  temporary (brachycurietherapy) technique,
    491, 499–502, 503–504
Radiosurgery, stereotactic, 515–529
Rathke's cleft (epithelial) cyst, 349, 372–374
  chemical meningitis with, 373–374
  computed tomography, 373, 374
Renal pain, splanchnicectomy for, 1275
Retrolabyrinthine approach, to posterior
    cranial fossa, 667
Revascularization. See specific sites and
    procedures
Reye-Johnson syndrome, anesthesia
    management, 115
Rheumatoid arthritis, 1295–1306
  anterior atlantoaxial subluxation, 1295–
    1301
  C1-C2 fusion for subluxation, 1296–1300
  computed tomography in, 1296
  diagnostic studies, 1296
  lumbar spine involvement, 1300
  magnetic resonance imaging in, 1296, 1301
  myelography in, 1296
  radiography in, 1296
  subaxial subluxation, 1299–1300
  subluxation presentation, 1295–1296
  subluxation stabilization in, 1296
  thoracic spine involvement, 1300
  vertical atlantoaxial subluxation, 1300–
    1301
Rhizotomy. See specific procedures
Rhinopharyngeal tumor, of skull base, 630,
    633
Rhodes-Glenn stereotactic system, 467
Riechert-Mundinger stereotactic system,
    464–465, 495
Rifampicin, 81–82
Rigidity, stereotactic surgery for, 1051

Sacral meningocele
  anterior, 159–161
  intrasacral, 159–161
Sacral rhizotomy, percutaneous
    electrothermocoagulation technique,
    1217–1220
Sagittal sinography, 566
Sagittal sinus, dural laceration, 875–879
Sagittal synostosis, 126–130
  complications, 130
  diagnosis, 126–128
  midline sagittal crainectomy, 128–129
  pi procedure, 129

results, 130
  surgical management, 128–130
  surgical technique, 129–130
  vault remodeling, 129–130
Salivary gland tumor, craniofacial resection
    for, 609
Saphenous vein graft, to posterior cerebral
    artery, 793–794
Scalp
  anatomy, 1
  circulation, 1, 3
  congenital aplasia, 5
  innervation, 1
  vasculature, 1
Scalp avulsion
  anatomy, 7
  microvascular replantation, 6–9
  vascular/coagulation status after
    replantation, 9
Scalp burn
  electrical, 6
  thermal, 6
Scalp defect. See also specific defects
  assessment, 1
  back cutting, 4
  flaps available, 3
  free skin grafts, 2–3
  local attached flaps, 3
  management principles, 1–2
  reconstructions available, 2
  repair technique, 4
  rotation flaps, 3
  tissue expansion in reconstruction, 4–5
Scalp laceration, 5, 20
Scalp tumor, 601–607
  arteriography, 604
  case report, 602–603
  computed tomography, 604
  postoperative management, 606
  preoperative management, 603–604
  radiography, 604
  surgical management, 604–606
Schwannoma, 1599–1603
  anesthesia, 1600
  instrumentation, 1601
  patient positioning, 1600–1601
  surgical management, 1601–1603
Sciatic nerve, intraneural artery, 1564
Sciatica, 1393
  chymopapain chemonucleolysis, 1437–
    1441
Scoliosis, 187–211
  anterior surgical approach, 195–196, 202–
    204
  bone graft in, 197–198
  bracing in, 191–194
  classification, 187
  complications of therapy, 205–206
  congenital, 187
  Cotrel-Dubousset fixation, 201–202
  diagnostic evaluation, 191–192
  Dwyer instrumentation, 203–204
  electrical stimulation in, 191–194
  etiology, 187
  fusion procedures, 194–195, 197–198
  Harrington rod instrumentation, 198
  with hydromyelia with shunt malfunction
    in myelomeningocele, 1510–1511
  idiopathic, 187, 190–191, 195

incidence, 190
  after intraspinal tumor surgery in children,
    1509–1513
  mechanical complications, 206
  natural history, 190–191
  neurologic complications, 206
  neuromuscular development and, 191
  nonoperative treatment, 191–194
  paraplegia and, 191
  posterior surgical approach, 196–198
  postoperative management, 204–205
  after radiation therapy in children, 1509
  radiography, 191
  segmental instrumentation, 200
  spinal cord monitoring, 207
  spinal fracture and, 191
  surgical approaches, 195–196
  surgical indications, 194–195
  surgical treatment, 194–204
  transpedicle fixateurs, 202
  tumor and, 191
  Wisconsin system, 201
Seizures. See also Epilepsy
  with acute head injury, 30
  with cysticercosis, 95, 96
  with infantile hemiplegia, 1235, 1237, 1238,
    1239, 1240
Sella turcica
  computed tomography, 356
  empty sella complication, 330
  floor closure, 321–322
  ghost sella complication, 330–331
  pneumography, 356
  reconstruction techniques, 321–337
  transsphenoidal approach, 309–319
Sella turcica lesion, 299–307
  cerebrospinal fluid leak with, 304–305, 306
  classification, 299
  computed tomography in, 300–301, 356
  endocrine factor, 299–300
  intraoperative bleeding, 304
  magnetic resonance imaging in, 301
  postoperative considerations, 305
  preoperative evaluation, 299
  radiography, 299, 300–301
  subfrontal approach, 303
  subtemporal approach, 304
  surgical complications, 304
  surgical results, 305–306
  transcranial approach, 302–303
  transethmoid approach, 302
  transsphenoidal approach, 301–304
  visual examination, 299, 301
Sendai cocktail, 1032
Sex factor, in aneurysm, 1003
Sheldon-Jacques tumorscope, 430
Sheldon tumorscope, 427
Shunting procedure
  for craniopharyngioma, 364
  for hydrocephalus, 142–152
  intraoperative ultrasonography with, 219
  postoperative care, 148
  preoperative preparation, 143
  shunts available, 143
  technique, 143
  with transcallosal approach, 386
Sigmoid sinus, dural arteriovenous
    malformation, 855–862
Silicone oil, as embolic agent, 821

Sinusitus, with pituitary adenoma, 306
Sleep apnea, after open cordotomy, 1163
Somatomedin C, 299
Somatosensory evoked potentials
    in middle cerebral artery aneurysm, 967–968
    in spinal cord arteriovenous malformation, 1501
    in spinal cord astrocytoma, 177
    in thoracolumbar fracture, 1482
Skeletal traction, in cervical fracture-dislocation, 1449–1451
Skin abnormality, with spinal dysraphism, 166
Skull osteomyelitis, 71
Skull base approach
    to glomus jugulare tumor, 745–746
    to posterior cranial fossa, 667–668, 671
Skull base tumor. *See also* specific lesions
    clivus removal, 625, 626
    closure, 625–626
    combined approaches, 626
    exposure, 622–623
    meningeal repair, 623–624
    meningioma, 627, 629
    mucosal plane preservation, 621–622
    preoperative management, 619, 621
    removal, 624–625
    of rhinopharyngeal origin, 630, 633
    skull base repair, 625
    surgical indications, 627–633
    transbasal approach, 619–633
    true bone tumor, 630
Skull defect, 11–17. See also Cranioplasty
    in children, 11–12
    complications, 14
    cosmetic considerations, 11
    grafting materials, 11
    infection with, 14
    preoperative evaluation, 11–14
    repair principles, 11–14
    from trephine, 14
    ventricular migration with, 12
Skull fracture
    basilar, 21–22
    depressed, 20–21
    with missile injury, 51
    parasellar saccular aneurysm with, 837
Skull traction, in cervical fracture dislocation, 1449
Skull tumor, 601–607
    case reports, 601–602
    computed tomography, 604
    postoperative management, 606
    preoperative management, 603–604
    radiography, 604
    surgical management, 604–606
Spasticity
    stereotactic surgery for, 1054–1055
    stimulation management, 1055–1056
Spasticity (lower limb)
    Bischof's myelotomy for, 1177–1184
    radiofrequency griseotomy, 1181
Sphenoethmoid approach
    disadvantages, 275
    to optic nerve, 269–277
    in optic nerve decompression, 270–271
Sphenoidal sinus, packing and closure, 322

Sphenoidotomy, approach to pituitary, 339–343
Spiegel-Wycis apparatus, 1037
Spina bifida, 163–173
Spina bifida occulta
    dermal sinus with, 165, 166
    with spinal dysraphism, 166
Spine
    anterior atlantoaxial subluxation, 1295–1301
    degenerative changes, 1343–1344
    atlantoaxial subluxation, 1295–1299
    growth and development, 189–190
    osteomyelitis, 76–77
    in Paget's disease, 1303–1305
    radiography in children, 1509
    subaxial subluxation, 1299–1300
    vertical atlantoaxial subluxation, 1300–1301
Spine anomaly, cerebrospinal fluid leakage with, 66–67
Spine fracture, scoliosis and, 191
Spine fracture (thoracolumbar), 1359–1365
    decompression and stabilization, 1361–1365
    transthoracic approach, 1361–1365
Spine fusion
    Cotrel-Dubousset fixation, 201–202
    extraperitoneal, 1474–1475
    Harrington rod instrumentation, 198
    Harrington-rod thoracolumbar, 1475–1478
    Hibbs technique, 1473
    intertransverse, 1474
    in intervertebral disc disease, 1421–1436
    after laminectomy, 198
    lateral extrapleural, 1474–1475
    lumbar spine, 1473
    methyl-methacrylate, 1522–1523
    posterior cervical spine, 1471–1480
    posterolateral, 1474
    postoperative care, 1478
    pseudoarthrosis with, 1478, 1480
    in scoliosis, 194–195, 197–198
    segmental instrumentation, 200
    thoracic spine, 1473
    transpedicle fixateurs, 202
    Wisconsin system, 201
Spine trauma, 1449–1469
    anesthesia in, 1451, 1452
    anterior cervical approach, 1453–1461
    anterolateral cervical approach, 1461–1462
    anterolateral lumbar approach, 1468
    cardiovascular considerations, 1451–1452
    computed tomography in, 1449
    laminectomy in, 1466–1467
    magnetic resonance imaging, 1449
    posterior approach, 1464–1466
    posterior lateral approach, 1467–1468
    pulmonary consideratons, 1452
    surgical management, 1452–1468
    thoracoabdominal approach, 1468
    transoral odontoid approach, 1462–1464
    ventilatory assistance in, 1452
Spine tumor, 1525–1537
    angiography, 1526–1527
    biopsy, 1527–1528
    clinical presentation, 1525–1526
    computed tomography, 1525, 1526, 1527, 1528, 1530

    corticosteroid therapy, 1525, 1526, 1527, 1528
    incidence, 1525
    laminectomy in, 1528–1529
    lateral osteotomy approach, 1535–1536
    magnetic resonance imaging in, 1525, 1526
    myelography, 1526
    neurological deficits with, 1526
    neurological salvage, 1527, 1528
    pain relief, 1528
    postoperative care, 1534, 1536
    preoperative assessment, 1528
    presurgical embolization in, 1527
    radiation vs. surgical treatment, 1515, 1522
    radiation therapy, 1526, 1527, 1530, 1531
    radiography, 1526–1527, 1528
    radionuclide scan in, 1526, 1528
    stabilization in, 1527, 1529, 1533
    surgical approach, 1528–1536
    surgical goals, 1525, 1527
    surgical indications, 1527
    surgical results, 1536
    thoracolumbar region approach, 1534–1535
    tissue diagnosis, 1527–1528
    transabdominal approach, 1535
    transthoracic approach, 1530, 1532, 1535
    vertebral body resection, 1529–1534
Spine tumor (metastatic), 1515–1524
    anterior spinal canal decompression, 1523–1524
    clinical presentation, 1515–1516
    complications, 1524
    computed tomography, 1516, 1520
    decompression laminectomy in, 1519–1523
    magnetic resonance imaging, 1517
    methyl-methacrylate fusion in, 1522–1523
    myelography, 1517–1518
    postoperative care, 1524
    preoperative evaluation, 1518–1519
    preoperative preparation, 1518–1519
    radiography, 1516–1518, 1520, 1522
    results, 1524
Spinal accessory–facial nerve anastomosis, 683
Spinal cord biopsy, intraoperative ultrasonography in, 222
Spinal cord compression
    corticosteroids in, 1541
    from epidural metastasis, 1539–1562
Spinal cord decompression, in epidural metastatic tumor, 1545–1548
Spinal cord injury, anesthesia for, 114–115
Spinal cord lesion
    intraoperative ultrasonography, 219–222
    normal vs. pathologic ultrasonography visualization, 219–222
Spinal cord stimulation
    for cancer pain, 1047
    electrode implantation for, 1039–1040
Spinal cord tethering, 163, 166
Spinal cord tumor, 1487–1507
    astrocytoma, 175–185
    in children, 175–185
    scoliosis and, 191
Spinal cord tumor (extramedullary), intraoperative ultrasonography visualization, 220–221
Spinal cord tumor (intramedullary), 1487–1497

Spinal cord tumor *(continued)*
angiography, 1490, 1492
clinical presentation, 1487
computed tomography, 1490
diagnosis, 1488–1490
intraoperative ultrasonography
visualization, 221–222
myelography, 1492
postoperative care, 1497
radiation therapy, 1496
radiography, 1488–1490
results, 1497
surgical management, 1490–1497
surgical pathology, 1490
Spinal deformity, 187–211. *See also specific
diagnoses*
classification, 187
with hydromyelia with shunt malfunction
in myelomeningocele, 1510–1511
fusion operation for, 1511
after lumbar shunt, 1510
after neurosurgery in children, 1509–1513
prevention after neurosurgery in children,
1509–1510
stabilization procedures, 1511–1512
Spinal dysraphism (occult), 163–173
bladder function with, 166
clinical presentation, 166–167
computed tomography, 168
diagnosis, 167–168
follow-up, 172
magnetic resonance imaging, 168
pathology, 163–166
radiography in, 167–168
results, 172
skin abnormalities with, 166
with spina bifida occulta, 166
spine abnormalities with, 166
surgical indications, 167–168
surgical technique, 168–172
Spinal extradural abscess, 74–75
Spinal intramedullary abscess, 75–76
Spinal meningocele
anterolateral, 158–161
posterior, 157–158
Spinal nerves, rootlets, ganglion, trunk
anatomy, 1207–1208
Spinal sensory rhizotomy
anatomy, 1207–1209
anesthesia, 1211, 1215
cervical procedure, 1211
diagnostic paravertebral block, 1209
indications for, 1209
intercostal nerve denervation, 1215–1216
patient preparation, 1211
patient selection, 1209
physiology, 1207–1209
posterior rhizotomy extent, 1209–1211
radicular arteries in, 1208–1209
radiography, 1211, 1215, 1216, 1220
thoracic procedure, 1211–1215
Spinal subdural abscess, 75
Splanchnicectomy,
anatomy, 1274–1275
for biliary tract pain, 1275
for cancer pain, 1044–1045
complications, 1277
indications for, 1275
for pancreas cancer pain, 1275
for renal pain, 1276

results, 1277
surgical technique, 1276–1277
Spondylotic myelopathy, 1351–1357
Stereotactic atlas, 1036–1037
Stereotactic biopsy, 463–474
in cerebral glioma, 436
computed tomography with, 495–498, 502
consecutive procedures after, 498–499
of intracranial lesion, 495–498
in intracranial metastasis, 457
with magnetic resonance imaging, 495–
498, 502
with radionuclide implantation, 491–514
results, 498
Stereotactic Bragg peak proton beam
therapy, in arteriovenous
malformation, 911–915
Stereotactic head holder, 481–482
Stereotactic instrumentation, 491–495, 1035,
1037
Brown-Roberts-Wells apparatus, 1037
Leksell's apparatus, 492, 1037
Horsley-Clarke apparatus, 491, 492, 494,
1035, 1037
Riechert-Mundinger apparatus, 495
Spiegel-Wycis apparatus, 1037
Talairach apparatus, 491–492
Todd-Wells apparatus, 1037
types, 1037
Stereotactic laser microsurgery, 226
Stereotactic radiosurgery, 515–529
Stereotactic resection, 481–490
accessory instruments, 486
clinical experience, 487–488
computer analysis, 483–484, 485, 486
data acquisition, 481
instrumentation, 485–486
for large deep-seated tumor, 489–490
for metastacic tumor, 488–489
microslad for, 486
patient rotation for, 485
stereotactic frame for, 485–486
surgical approach definition, 485
surgical planning, 484–485
surgical procedure, 486–487
for vascular malformation, 489
Stereotactic retractors, 486
Stereotactic surgery. *See also* Cingulotomy
(stereotactic); *specific diagnoses*
arterial aneurysm clipping, 1009–1022
arteriovenous malformation clipping,
1009–1022
with Brown-Robert-Wells frame, 475–480
clipping indications/contraindications,
1012–1013
clipping instrumentation, 1010–1011
clipping operation results, 1013–1021
clipping technique, 1009–1010, 1012
computed tomography in, 463, 1061–1062
computed tomography data transposition
to film, 463–464
development of, 1057–1058
electrode insertion, 1038
electroencephalography with, 1038
electroneuroprosthesis, 1062–1064
as functional neurosurgery modality,
1035–1039
hematoma evacuation results, 892
indications for, 467–468
instrumentation, 889–890

in intracerebral hematoma, 889–898
with laser, 1062
lesion production, 1038–1039
lesion site, 470–471
magnetic resonance imaging in, 463
of midbrain and pons, 472
for motor disorders, 1051
preoperative calculations, 1011–1012
Presbyterian-University Hospital
(Pittsburgh) technique, 468–472
radiography with, 1037–1038
results, 470–472
stereotactic atlas, 1036–1037
technique, 891
ventrolateral nucleus lesion, 1051
Stereotactic system
Brown-Roberts-Wells, 466–467, 1037
CT-compatible, 467
device alternatives, 464
frame modification for CT and MRI, 464–
466
Rhodes-Glenn, 467
Leksell, 464–465, 492, 1037
Todd-Wells, 464, 466, 1037
Stereotactic thermal hypophysectomy, 345–
348
anesthesia, 345
complications, 348
indications for, 345
patient preparation, 345
postoperative management, 347–348
procedure, 345–347
replacement therapy, 347–348
Stimulation techniques (chronic), 1039–1040.
See also specific diagnoses
Storz pediatric-type Hopkins endoscope, 426
Streptomycin
in tuberculoma, 81
in tuberculous meningitis, 84
in vestibular nerve ablation, 1258–1259
Stroke, 881–888. *See also* Intracerebral
hemorrhage
direct brain revascularization, 783
posterior fossa revascularization, 807
Subarachnoid hemorrhage
with aneurysm, 929, 930, 931, 936, 1004,
1005
with anterior communicating artery
aneurysm, 939, 954
with carotid ophthalmic artery aneurysm,
917, 918, 927
with middle cerebral artery aneurysm,
957, 958, 970
Subclavian-carotid stenosis, 781
Subcutaneous electrode implantation, 1039,
1040
Subdural hematoma, 33–35
acute, chronic, subacute, 33
with acute head injury, 24
anesthesia management, 34
computed tomography in, 33–35
corticosteroids in, 33
diagnosis, 33
intracranial pressure monitoring, 34
postoperative complications, 35
preoperative management, 33
surgery for acute condition, 33–35
surgery for chronic condition, 35
Subfornicial approach, to third ventricle,
381–382

Subfrontal approach, to sella turcica, 303
Suboccipital approach
    to clivus, 642
    to craniopharyngioma, 364
    to posterior cranial fossa, 665, 670
    to vertebral junction aneurysm, 986
Suboccipital craniectomy, with upper
        cervical laminectomy for Chiari
        malformation, 1317
Suboccipital-translabyrinthine approach, to
        posterior cranial fossa, 668, 671
Subtemporal approach
    to AICA aneurysm, 984
    to basilar artery aneurysm, 975
    to clivus, 640–642
    to craniopharyngioma, 362
    to sella turcica, 304
    to superior cerebellar artery aneurysm,
        984
Sudomotor function, in peripheral nerve
        injury, 1568
Superficial temporal artery–middle cerebral
        artery bypass, 783–791
    anastomosis, 789
    anesthesia, 784
    angiography, 783, 791
    in carotid ophthalmic aneurysm, 927
    closure, 789, 791
    complications, 791
    exposure, 787
    instrumentations, 784, 787
    long vein grafts, 792
    MCA preparation, 789
    in moyamoya disease, 801–804
    patient positioning, 784
    postoperative management, 791
    preoperative evaluation, 783–784
    results, 791
    short vein graft in, 791
    STA preparation, 789
    technique, 784–791
Superficial temporal artery–superior
        cerebellar artery bypass
    results, 816
    technique, 815–816
    in vertebrobasilar insufficiency, 808, 813
Supracerebellar approach, to pineal region
        neoplasms, 401–409
Suprascapular nerve entrapment, 1590–1591
Suprasellar cyst, 349, 375
    computed tomography, 375
Suprasellar germinoma, 397
    angiography, 398
    cerebrospinal fluid cytology, 398
    chemotherapy, 399
    computed tomography, 398
    radiography, 398
    symptoms, 397
Suprasellar meningioma
    angiography, 531
    approach, 532
    computed tomography, 531
    presentation, 531
    radiography, 531
    results, 536–537
    surgical technique, 532–535
Supratentorial approach, to posterior fossa
        tumor, 660–662
Sympathetic nervous system, 1271–1280
Sympathectomy, 1271–1280

    for causalgia, 1049
    lumbar, 1277–1279
    in moyamoya disease, 801, 804
    preganglionic, 1271–1272
    splanchnicectomy, 1274–1277
    upper thoracic ganglionectomy, 1271–1274
Synostosis, 125. See also specific
        deformities
    computed tomography, 126–127, 130, 132,
        133
    etiology, 126
    genetic factor, 126
    intracranial pressure with, 125–126
    radiography, 125, 126, 130, 132, 133
    surgical indications, 126
    syndromes with, 126
Syringobulbia, 1307
Syringomyelia, 1307–1326. See also Chiari
        malformation with hydromelia
    hydrodynamic theory for, 1307
    intramedullary tumor with, 1307, 1326
Syringomyelic cord syndrome, 1307–1326
    cyst formation with, 1308
    pathology, 1308

Taenia solium, 79, 93
Talairach stereotactic apparatus, 491–492
Tarsorrhaphy, in intraorbital tumor, 244
Technetium 99 bone scan, for anterior
        lumbar discectomy, 1423
Temperature regulation, in neonate, 117
Temporal lobectomy
    in cerebral glioma, 439–441
    cortical resection in, 1231–1232
Temporal lobectomy (partial)
    anatomic considerations, 1230–1231
    closure, 1232
    complications, 1232–1233
    electrical stimulation study in, 1229–1230
    electrocorticography in, 1227
    for epilepsy, 1223–1234
    postexcision recording, 1232
    postoperative care, 1232
    results, 1233–1234
Temporary vascular occlusion in middle
        cerebral artery aneurysm, 967–968
Tentorium tumor, 647–651
    air embolism in, 648
    anesthesia, 647
    angiography, 647
    computed tomography, 647, 648
    diagnosis, 647
    instrumentation, 650
    magnetic resonance imaging, 647
    microsurgery, 650
    radiography, 647
    retraction technique, 650
    surgical approaches, 648
    surgical positioning, 647–648
Teratoma, intramedullary spinal cord tumor,
        1496
Terminal ventriculostomy, for Chiari
        malformation with hydromelia, 1326
Thalamic glioma, 710
Thalamic pain syndrome, 715–716
Thalamic tumor, 712
    symptomatology, 714–716
Thalamotomy
    for cancer pain, 1046–1047

    in dystonia, 1268
    for Parkinson's disease, 1052
    in torticollis, 1262–1263
Thalamus, stimulation site in pain control,
        1089, 1092, 1094
Thermocoagulation, of dorsal root entry
        zone, 1169–1175
Thermography, for anterior lumbar
        discectomy, 1423
Thoracic epidural tumor (metastatic), 1557–
        1559
    anterior decompression and vertebral
        body replacement, 1548–1559
    high thoracic spine approach, 1553
Thoracic lateral extrapleural spine fusion,
        1474–1475
Thoracic meningocele, 158–159
Thoracic outlet syndrome, 1591–1593
    electromyelography, 1592
    etiology, 1591–1592
    surgical management, 1591–1593
    symptoms, 1592
Thoracic rhizotomy, percutaneous
        electrothermocoagulation technique,
        1211–1215
Thoracic spinal cord tumor, in children,
        175–176
Thoracic spinal deformity, surgical
        treatment, 1511–1512
Thoracic spine fusion, 1473
    lateral facet, 1467–1468
Thoracolumbar fracture, 1481–1486
    approach, 1483
    burst fracture, 1481, 1482, 1485
    classification, 1481
    complications, 1484
    computed tomography, 1481, 1483, 1484–
        1485
    grafting in, 1483, 1484
    immobilization management, 1483
    neural decompression in, 1481, 1482, 1483
    postoperative management, 1484
    preoperative management, 1481–1483
    radiography, 1483
    somatosensory evoked responses in,
        1482
    spine stabilization in, 1483–1484
    surgical management, 1483–1484
    unstable vs. stable, 1481
Thoracolumbar Harrington-rod spine fusion,
        1475–1478
Thoracolumbar spine fusion, 1464–1466
Thoracolumbar spine injury
    posterior spine fusion in, 1464–1466
    thoracoabdominal approach, 1468
Third ventricle
    lesions encountered, 381
    surgical approaches, 381–382, 389
    transcallosal approach, 381–387
    transcallosal interfornicial approach, 389–
        395
    preoperative evaluation of lesion, 382
Third ventricle colloid cyst, intraoperative
        ultrasonography visualization, 218
Third ventricle lesion, stereotactic resection,
        489
Third ventricle tumor (posterior)
    endocrine function in, 398
    myelography in, 398
    surgical management, 398–399

Thrombosis technique, for carotid cavernous fistula, 845–847
Tic convulsif, 1108
Tinel's sign, 1566–1567
Tissue adhesives, in cerebrospinal fluid leakage, 66
Tissue aspiration, ultrasonic, 226–227
Tissue bonding, with laser, 226
Tissue expander, in scalp reconstruction, 4–5
Todd-Wells stereotactic system, 464, 466, 1037
Torticollis
    anterior cervical rhizotomy in, 1263
    iontophoresis, 1262
    muscle resection in, 1263
    physiotherapy in, 1267
    selective peripheral denervation in, 1263–1268
    surgical management, 1262
Torticollis (spasmodic), 1261–1268
    conservative treatment, 1261–1262
    Dandy-Foerster operation for, 1054
    electromyography in, 1263–1264
    epidural crevical stimulation in, 1262
    frontal capsular adversive pathway interruption, 1262
    medical treatment, 1262
    nerve root microvascular lysis, 1262
    pallidotomy in, 1262–1263
    stereotactic surgery for, 1053–1054
    thalamotomy in, 1262–1263
Transantralethmoidal approach, in optic nerve decompression, 270
Transantrosphenoidal approach, in optic nerve decompression, 270
Transbasal approach
    to clivus, 644
    closure, 625–626
    goals, 619
    hazards, 619
    indications for, 627–633
    limits, 626
    meningeal repair, 623–624
    mucosal plane preservation, 621–622
    skull base exposure, 622–623
    to skull base tumor, 619–633
Transcallosal approach
    cingulate gyrus exposure, 383
    closure with, 386
    corpus callosum exposure, 383
    to craniopharyngioma, 364
    foramen of Monro in, 382–386
    to frontal horn lateral ventricle tumor, 590–591
    intraventricular exposure, 384
    to midbody lateral ventricle tumor, 588–589
    patient positioning, 382
    shunt with, 386
    surgical procedure, 382
    to third ventricle tumor, 381–387
    to trigonal lateral ventricle tumor, 585–586
Transcallosal interfornicial approach
    advantages, 391
    anatomy, 390–391
    bone flap with, 392–393
    choroid plexus in, 395
    cingulate gyri in, 393
    complications, 389–390

corpus callosum in, 393
    dural incision, 393
    lateral ventricle entry, 394
    patient positioning, 392
    physiology, 390–391
    preoperative planning, 391–392
    results, 389
    risk factors, 390–391
    septum pellucidum in, 395
    surgical technique, 392–395
    to third ventricle, 389–395
    transcalvarial entry, 392–393
Transcanal approach, to posterior cranial fossa, 667, 671
Transcervical approach, to clivus, 642
Transcochlear approach, to posterior cranial fossa, 668, 671
Transcorticoventricular approach, to craniopharyngioma, 364
Transcranial approach, to sella turcica, 302–303
Transethmoid approach, to sella turcica, 302
Transethmoidal sphenoidotomy
    advantages, 339
    approach to pituitary, 339–343
    complications, 339
    contraindications, 339
    disadvantages, 339
    indications, 339
    preoperative evaluation, 339–340
    procedure, 342–343
    technique, 340–342
Transforaminal approach, to third ventricle, 389
Transfrontal approach
    to craniopharyngioma, 358–359
    to third ventricle, 381
Transfrontal craniotomy approach, for optic nerve decompression, 269–270
Transient ischemic attacks
    direct brain revascularization, 783, 791, 794
    with moyamoya disease, 797, 801, 804
    posterior fossa revascularization in, 807
Translabyrinthine operation
    for acoustic nerve tumor, 685–704
    acoustic nerve tumor removal, 696–698
    advantages/disadvantages, 685–686
    anatomy, 687–689
    anesthesia for, 689–690
    at cerebellopontine angle, 676
    cerebrospinal fluid rhinorrhea with, 702–703
    dissection, 692–696
    four quadrants dissection, 699–701
    gutting procedure, 699
    hematoma with, 702
    hemostasis, 701
    closure, 701–702
    patient positioning, 690
    at posterior cranial fossa, 665, 670–671
    postoperative complications, 702–703
    postoperative management, 702
    procedure, 690–692
    results, 703
Transoral approach, to clivus, 642–643
Transoral median labiomandibular approach, to clivus, 643–644
Transoral odontoid resection and fusion, in cervical spinal cord injury, 1462–1464

Transoral-transpharyngeal approach, to craniovertebral junction abnormality, 1288–1292
Transpedicle fixateurs, in scoliosis, 202
Transsphenoidal approach, 299–307
    to clivus, 643
    complications, 319
    to craniopharyngioma, 363–364
    hemitransfixion incision, 309
    indications for, 309
    operative procedure, 309–318
    in optic nerve decompression, 270, 275
    patient positioning, 309
    risk factors, 334–335
    to sella turcica, 301–304, 309–319, 321–337
    sublabial incision, 309
Transtemporal approaches
    case reports, 669–670
    infratemporal fossa, 668, 671
    middle fossa, 665–666, 671
    middle fossa-infratemporal fossa, 669, 671
    to posterior cranial fossa, 665–672
    retrolabyrinthine, 667
    skull base, 667–668, 671
    suboccipital, 665, 670
    suboccipital-translabyrinthine, 668, 671
    transcanal, 667, 671
    transcochlear, 668, 671
    translabyrinthine, 665, 670–671
Transtemporal horn occipital temporal gyrus incision, to trigonal lateral ventricle tumor, 586–587
Transthoracic approach
    to spine tumor, 1530, 1532, 1535
    to thoracic spine, 1361–1365
Transthoracic (transpleural) approach, to thoracic intervertebral disc, 1371–1374
Transvenous approach, to anteroinferior dural venous fistula, 849–854
Transverse sinus, dural laceration, 875–879
Traumatic aneurysm, 991–995
    angiography, 991, 992
    computed tomography, 991, 993
    intracerebral hematoma with, 991
    surgical management, 991–994
    symptomatology, 991
Traumatic mass lesions, 22–24
Tremor, stereotactic surgery for, 1051–1052
Trephine defects, 14
Triage, for acute head injury, 19, 20
Trigeminal nerve injury, after stereotactic radiosurgery, 521
Trigeminal neuralgia, 1097–1105
    herpes simplex with, 1119
    Jannetta microvascular decompression procedure, 1097–1098
    medical management, 1097, 1111, 1117
    microvascular decompression for, 1111
    motor paresis with, 1119
    with multiple sclerosis, 1105
    ocular complications, 1117, 1119
    patient evaluation, 1111
    percutaneous rhizotomy for, 1111–1120, 1125–1127
    percutaneous rhizotomy/microvascular decompression complications, 1139–1143
    percutaneous trigeminal neurolysis, 1097–1098
    radiofrequency heating for, 1134

recurrence, 1119
retrogasserian glycerol injection, 1129–1137
sensory complications, 1117, 1119
surgical management, 1097–1105
surgical procedures comparison, 1119–1120
surgical results, 1116–1117
Trigeminal rhizotomy
for atypical facial pain, 1120–1121
electrode locatization for, 1115–1116
hemorrhage with, 1139–1140
lesion production, 1116
for multiple sclerosis, 1120
percutaneous technique, 1112–1116
for trigeminal neuralgia, 1111–1120
Tuberculoma
age factor, 80
anticonvulsants in, 82
antituberculosis agents, 81–82
clinical features, 80
computed tomography, 80–81
corticosteroids in, 82
incidence, 79
location, 79
pathology, 80
radiography, 80–81
results, 83
sex factor, 80
surgical management, 82–83
treatment, 81
Tuberculosis, 79–85
Tuberculous meningitis, 83–85
antituberculosis agents, 84
computed tomography, 84
diagnosis, 84
hydrocephalus with, 83–85
later particle agglutination test in, 84
results, 85
surgical management, 84–85
ventriculoatrial/ventriculoperitoneal shunts in, 84
Tumor. See specific diagnoses and sites
Tumor markers, in pineal region tumor, 398
Tumorscope, 424, 427

Ulnar nerve compression, 1588–1589
Ultrasonic surgical aspirator, 226–227
applications, 227
biologic effects, 227
in meningioma surgery, 559
neoplasm fragmentation, 227
system, 227
Ultrasonography (intraoperative), 213–222
biopsy guide for, 215
in biopsy procedures, 219, 222
in brain lesion localization, 215
equipment, 214
equipment sterilization, 214
history, 213–214
intracranial, 215
intraspinal, 219–222
7.5-MHz crystal for, 213–214
normal brain tissue visualization, 215–216
normal spinal cord tissue visualization, 219–220
pathologic brain tissue visualization, 215–216

pathologic spinal cord tissue visualization, 220–222
techniques, 214–215
Ultrasonography (transcutaneous), in spinal cord astrocytoma, 177, 184
Upper extremity, sympathetic denervation, 1271
Upper thoracic ganglionectomy, 1271–1274
anatomy, 1271–1272
for causalgia, 1271, 1272
complications, 1273–1274
for hyperhidrosis, 1271, 1272
indications for, 1272
results, 1273
surgical approach, 1272
surgical technique, 1272–1273

Vascular disorders, in children, 109
Vascular lesions (intracerebral)
balloon catheter management, 819–836
chemotherapy infusion, 835
embolic agents for, 820–821
Vascular malformations, stereotactic resection, 489
Vasoglossopharyngeal neuralgia, percutaneous rhizotomy in, 1121–1122, 1125–1127
Vein of Galen aneurysm
balloon catheter management, 828
in children, 109
Vein of Galen lesion, occipital transtentorial approach, 411–418
Vein of Galen malformation, 120
Venipuncture, in neonate, 117
Venography
for anterior lumbar discectomy, 1423
in orbit pathology, 250
Venous fistula, anteroinferior dural, 849–854
Venous hypertension, with anteroinferior dural fistula, 849
Ventilation management
in children, 104
with head injury, 27–29, 114
in spine trauma, 1452
Ventricular drainage, for obstructive hydrocephalus, 573
Ventricular migration, with skull defect, 12
Ventriculography
anesthesia for, 113
in meningioma, 573
in pineal tumor, 403
Ventriculoperitoneal shunt, in tuberculous meningitis, 84–85
Ventrolateral nucleus, stimulation lesion production, 1051
Vertebral artery (extracranial), 771–782
Vertebral artery compression, with cervical spondylosis, 1329
Vertebral artery endarterectomy, 771–782
technique, 775–781
Vertebral body replacement, in epidural metastatic tumor, 1552–1553
Vertebral to carotid transposition
results, 810
technique, 808–810
for vertebrobasilar insufficiency, 808–810
Vertebral column
embryology, 189
fracture-dislocation, 1449–1469

Vertebral fistula, balloon catheter management, 827
Vertebral junction aneurysm, 986
Vertebrobasilar insufficiency, 771–782
arteriography, 771–775, 808, 810, 812
cerebral blood flow (regional) measurement in, 807–808
clinical evaluation, 771–775
computed tomography, 807
distal vertebral endarterectomy for, 810–812
OA-AICA bypass in, 814–815
OA-PICA bypass for, 810, 812–814
pathology, 771–772, 774
posterior fossa revascularization in, 807–818
postoperative management, 817
preoperative preparation, 808
radiography, 771–775
results, 818
STA-SCA bypass for, 808, 813, 815–817
surgical indications, 772
symptoms, 771, 772
vertebral to carotid transposition for, 808–810
Vertebrobasilar revascularization, 793–794
Vertebrobasilar system aneurysm, 973–989
Vertigo
in chronic labyrinthitis, 1254
medical ablation of vestibular nerve in, 1258–1259
in Meniere's disease, 1251
nonsurgical treatment, 1254
surgical treatment, 1255–1258
in vestibular neuritis, 1251, 1254
Vestibular nerve ablation, with streptomycin sulfate, 1258–1259
Vestibular nerve transection
cerebellopontine angle (posterior fossa approach), 1258
complications, 1258
internal auditory canal (middle fossa) approach, 1256–1258
in Meniere's disease, 1251–1259
procedure, 1256–1258
results, 1258
Vestibular neuritis
nonsurgical treatment, 1254
pathophysiology, 1251, 1254
Vietnam Head Injury Study, 49
Vision, electroneuroprosthesis, 1063
Visual deficit
in craniopharyngioma, 355
after head trauma, 269
Visual evoked potentials, 280
with head trauma, 269, 270
Visual examination, in sella turcica lesion, 299, 301
Visual fields, in cerebral glioma, 433–434
Volume interpolation, for intra-axial tumor, 483–484
Von Hippel-Lindau disease, 660
Von Recklinghausen's disease, 158, 1605

Wada intra-arterial sodium amytal test, 433
Wallenberg syndrome, 772
Weapons, ballistic design-injury relation, 50
Wisconsin system, of spine fusion, 201
Wounds. See Gunshot wounds; specific sites

Operative Neurosurgical Techniques

Indications, Methods and Results

Second Edition

Operative Neurosurgical Techniques

Indications, Methods and Results

Second Edition

Volume II

Edited by

Henry H. Schmidek, M.D., F.A.C.S.
Division of Neurosurgery
Department of Surgery
New England Deaconess Hospital
Harvard Medical School
Boston, Massachusetts

and

William H. Sweet, M.D., D.Sc.
Department of Neurosurgery
Massachusetts General Hospital
Harvard Medical School
Boston, Massachusetts

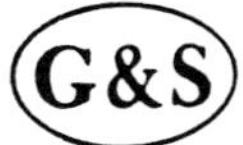

GRUNE & STRATTON, INC.

Harcourt Brace Jovanovich, Publishers
Orlando   New York   San Diego   London
San Francisco   Tokyo   Sydney   Toronto

Grune & Stratton, Inc.
Orlando, Florida   32887

Distributed in the United Kingdom by
Grune & Stratton, Ltd.
24/28 Oval Road, London NW 1

Library of Congress Catalog Number 87-082817
International Standard Book Number 0-8089-1862-1
Printed in the United States of America
87 88 89 90   10 9 8 7 6 5 4 3 2 1

Contents

1. **Surgery of the Scalp**
   Peter C. Linton and David W. Leitner   1

2. **Repair of Defects of the Skull**
   Michael S. Olin   11

3. **Surgical Management of Acute Head Injuries**
   George F. Gade and Donald P. Becker   19

4. **Surgical Management of Acute and Chronic Subdural Hematoma**
   J. Douglas Miller   33

5. **Surgical Management of Gunshot Wounds of the Head**
   Maurice I. Saba   37

6. **Penetrating Missile Injuries of the Head**
   Eugene D. George and T. Forcht Dagi   49

7. **The Management of Cerebrospinal Fluid Leaks**
   T. Forcht Dagi and Eugene D. George   57

8. **Surgical Management of Intracranial and Intraspinal Infections**
   R. Lewis Wright   71

9. **A Surgical Management of Tuberculosis, Cysticerocis, and Fungal Infections of the Central Nervous System**
   R. Bhatia and P. N. Tandon   79

10. **Neurosurgical Aspects of Neurocysticercosis**
    Francisco Escobedo   93

11. **Anesthetic Considerations and Techniques in Pediatric Neurosurgical Patients**
    Mounir N. Abou-Madi and Davy Trop   103

12. **Management of Neurosurgical Problems in the Neonate**
    R. Michael Scott   117

13. **Surgical Management of Craniosynostosis and Craniofacial Abnormalities**
    Steven L. Wald and Henry H. Schmidek   125

14. **Surgical Management of Hydrocephalus**
    Mel. H. Epstein   141

15. **Surgical Management of Meningoceles and Myelomeningoceles**
    A. Loren Amacher   151

16. **Occult Spinal Dysraphism: Recognition and Surgical Management**
    Paul H. Chapman   163

17. **Spinal Cord Tumors in Children**
    Fred J. Epstein and Jeffrey H. Wisoff   175

18. **Current Surgical Management of Scoliosis and Kyphosis**
    Morey S. Moreland   187

19. **Intraoperative Ultrasonography in Neurosurgery**
    Robert A. Kane, Daniel H. O'Leary, and Ernest S. Mathews   213

20. **The Laser and Ultrasonic Aspirator in Neurosurgery**
    Steven L. Wald and Henry H. Schmidek   223

21. **The Differential Diagnosis and Investigation of Unilateral and Bilateral Exophthalmos**
    Don C. Bienfang   229

22. **Intraorbital Tumors**
    Edgar M. Housepian   235

23. **Anterior and Lateral Microsurgical Approaches to Orbital Pathology**
    Melvin G. Alper and Phil A. Aitken   245

24. **Sphenoethmoid Approach to the Optic Nerve**
    Robert A. Sofferman   269

25. **Gliomas of the Anterior Visual Pathways**
William H. Sweet, Shirley H. Wray, and Paul F. New   279

26. **Surgical Management of Seller and Parasellar Lesions**
Peter Black and Nicholas T. Zervas   299

27. **Transsphenoidal Approach to Lesions in and about the Sella Turcica**
Edward R. Laws, Jr.   309

28. **Techniques of Reconstruction of the Sella and Related Structures**
Renata Spanziante, Enrico de Divitiis, and Paolo Cappabianca   321

29. **Transethmoidal Approach to the Pituitary**
Charles W. Cummings and Jonas Johnson   339

30. **Stereotactic Thermal Hypophysectomy**
Nicholas T. Zervas   345

31. **Craniopharyngiomas (With a note of Rathke's Cleft or Epithelial Cysts and on Suprasellar Cysts)**
William H. Sweet   349

32. **Transcallosal Approach to Tumors of the Third Ventricle**
Bennett M. Stein   381

33. **Transcallosal Interiornicial Exposure of Lesions of the Third Ventricle**
Michael L. J. Apuzzo   389

34. **Considerations in the Management of Masses in the Pineal Region**
Henry H. Schmidek   397

35. **Supracerebellar Approach for Pineal Region Neoplasms**
Bennett M. Stein   401

36. **The Occipital Transtentorial Approach to the Pineal Region**
Kemp Clark   411

37. **Brain Biopsy: Indications, Methods, and Complications**
Anthony Salerni, Steven Wald, and Henry H. Schmidek   419

38. **Neurologic Endoscopy**
C. Hunter Shelden, Skip Jacques, and Harold R. Lutes   423

39. **Surgical Management of Intracranial Gliomas**
Carrie L. Walters and Henry H. Schmidek   431

40. **Surgical Management of Intracranial Metastasis**
Perry Black   451

41. **Localization and Biopsy of Intracranial Lesions with Computed Tomography and Magnetic Resonance Imaging**
Robert J. Coffey and L. Dade Lunsford   463

41C. **Commentary: Stereotactic Techniques Using the Brown-Roberts-Wells Stereotactic Frame**
Peter Black   475

42. **Computed Tomographic and Magnetic Resonance Imaging Based Stereotactic Resection of Deep-Seated Intracranial Tumors**
Patrick J. Kelly   481

43. **Stereotactic Biopsy and Implantation of Radionuclides Guided by Computed Tomographic and Magnetic Resonance Imaging for Therapy of Brain Tumors**
F. Mundinger   491

44. **Stereotactic Radiosurgery with the Cobalt 60 Gamma Unit in the Surgical Treatment of Intracranial Tumors and Arteriovenous Malformations**
Ladislau Steiner   515

45. **Surgical Management of Olfactory Groove, Suprasellar, and Medical Sphenoid Wing Meningiomas**
Robert G. Ojemann and Karl W. Swann   531

46. **Preoperative Evaluation and Management of Meningiomas**
Robert E. Maxwell and Shelly N. Chou   547

47. **Convexity Meningiomas and General Principles of Meningioma Surgery**
Robert E. Maxwell and Shelly N. Chou   555

48. **Parasagittal and Falx Maningiomas**
Robert E. Maxwell and Shelly N. Chou   563

49. **Posterior Fossa Meningiomas**
Robert E. Maxwell and Shelley N. Chou   571

50. **Surgical Management of Lateral Intraventricular Tumors**
Dennis D. Spencer, William Collins, and Kimberlee J. Sass   583

51. **Surgical Approaches to Intraventricular Meningiomas of the Trigone**
Cecil L. Jun and Stephen L. Nutik   597

52. **Surgical Management of Extensive Tumors Involving the Skull and the Scalp**
Howard A. Richter   601

53. **Craniofacial Resection**
Narayan Sundaresan   609

54. **The Transbasal Approach to Tumors Invading the Base of the Skull**
Patrick J. Dermone   619

55. **Surgical Treatment of Tumors of the Clivus and Basloccipital Region**
R. B. Snow and R. R. Patterson, Jr   635

56. **Surgical Management of Tumors of the Tentorium and Clivus**
Edward Tarlov   647

57. **Surgical Management of Posterior Fossa Tumors**
John Duckworth and Henry H. Schmidek   653

58. **Transtemporal Approaches to the Poster Cranial Fossa**
Gale Gardner, Jon H. Robertson, and W. Craig Clark   665

59. **Tumors of the Cerebellopontine Angle: Clinical Features and Surgical Management**
William A. Buchheit and Robert H. Rosenwasser   673

60. **The Translabyrinthine Operation for the Removal of Acoustic Nerve Tumors**
T. T. King and A. W. Morrison   685

61. **Surgical Correction of Facial Palsy**
David W. Leitner   705

62. **The Surgical Treatment of Primary Brain Stem Tumors**
A. Konovalov and J. Atieh   709

63. **Glomus Jugulare Tumors—Skull Base Surgery**
Gale Gardner, James T. Robertson, Jon H. Robertson, Edwin W. Cocke, Jr., and W. Craig Clark   739

64. **Surgical Therapy of Diseases of the Extracranial Carotid Artery**
Robert A. Ratcheson and Robert L. Grubb   753

65. **Exposure of the Distal Internal Carotid Artery**
Calvin B. Ernst   765

66. **Surgical Management of Extracranial Lesions of the Vetebral Artery**
Edward F. Downing   771

67. **Direct Brain Revascularization**
Robert M. Crowell and Jafar J. Jafar   783

68. **Moyamoya Disease**
Tsuneyoshi Eguchi and Kazuo Ugajin   797

69. **Posterior Fossa Revascularization**
James I. Ausman, Fernando G. Diaz, Dante F. Vacca, R. A. de los Reyes, Carl E. Shrontz, Jeffrey E. Pearce, and Randy Gehrig   807

70. **Treatment of Intracerebral Vascular Lesions with Balloon Catheters**
Gerard M. Debrun   819

VOLUME II

71. **Surgical Management of Internal Carotid Artery Aneurysms within the Cavernous Sinus**
Dwight Parkinson   837

72. **Techniques of Thrombosis of Carotid Cavernous Fistulae**
John F. Mullan   845

73. **Commentary on the Transvenous Treatment of Anterioinferior Duval Venous Fistulae**
Henry H. Schmidek and Joseph R. Madsen   849

74. **The Surgical Approach to Arteriovenous Malformations of the Lateral and Sigmoid Dural Sinuses**
Thoralf M. Sundt, Jr., David G. Piepgras, and Glenn S. Forbes   855

75. **Surgical Management of Lesions of the Dural Venous Sinuses**
R. M. Peardon Donaghy   863

76. **Surgical Management of Dural Sinus Lacerations**
John P. Kapp   875

77. **Surgical Management of Intracerebral Hemorrhage**
David G. Pieparas and Michael J. Redmond   881

78. **Stereotactic Evacuation of Intracerebral Hematomas**
Edward I. Kandel and Vjacheslav V. Peresedov   889

79. **Cranial Arteriovenous Malformations**
Alfred J. Luessenhop   899

80. **Surgical Management of Cranial Arteriovenous Malformations**
Francis W. Gannoche, Jr. and Russell H. Patterson, Jr   905

81. **Proton Beam Therapy for Aeteriovenous Malformations of the Brain**
Raymond N. Kjellberg   911

viii   CONTENTS

82. Surgical Treatment of Carotid Ophthalmic Aneurysms
Jafar J. Jafar, Robert M. Crowell, and Roberto Heros   917

83. Surgical Management of Aneurysms of the Internal Carotid: Posterior Communicating, Anterior Choroidal, and Bifurcation Aneurysms
Henry H. Schmidek   929

84. Surgical Treatment of Anterior Communicating Artery Aneurysms
Robert M. Crowell and Jafar J. Jafar   939

85. Surgical Management Aneurysms of the Middle Cerebral Artery
Lindsay Symon   957

86. Surgical Techniques of Posterior Cerebral Aneurysms
Sidney J. Peerless and Charles G. Drake   973

87. Surgical Management of Traumatic Aneurysms
Dwight Parkinson   991

88. Surgical Management of Bacterial Intracranial Aneurysms
Robert G. Ojemann   997

89. Treatment of Multiple and Asymptomatic Aneurysms
Ronald Brisman   1003

90. Stereotactic Clipping of Arterial Aneurysms and Arteriovenous Malformations of the Brain
Edward I. Kandel and Vyacheslav V. Peresedov   1009

91. Management of Unclippable Aneurysms
Roberto C. Heros   1023

92. Functional Neurosurgery
Philip L. Goldenberg   1035

93. Treatment of Intractable Psychiatric Illness and Chronic Pain by Stereotactic Cingulotomy
H. Thomas Ballantine and Ida E. Giriunas   1069

94. Intraventricular Morphine in the Treatment of Pain Secondary to Cancer
Alberto Lenzi, Giuseppe Galli, and Giovanni Marini   1077

95. Analgesia Induced by Brain Stimulation with Chronically Implanted Electrodes
Yoshio Hosobuchi   1089

96. Surgical Management of Disorders of the Lower Cranial Nerves
Ronald I. Apfelbaum   1097

97. Percutaneous Rhizotomy in the Treatment of Intractable Facial Pain (Trigeminal, Glossopharyngeal, and Vagal Nerves)
John Tew, Jr. and Harry van Loveren   1111

97C. Commentary: Percutaneous Rhizotomy
William H. Sweet   1125

98. Tetrogasserian Glycerol Injection as Treatment for Trigeminal
William H. Sweet   1129

99. Complications of Percutaneous Rhizotomy and Microvascular Decompression Operations for Facial Pain
William H. Sweet and Charles E. Poletti   1139

100. Intraspinal and Intraventricular Implantable Systems and Agents for Long-Term Relief of Cancer Pain
Charles E. Poletti, William H. Sweet, Henry H. Schmidek, and Robert N. Pilon   1145

101. Open Cordotomy Medullary Tractomy
Charles E. Poletti   1155

102. Dorsal Root Entry Zone Thermocoagulation
D. G. T. Thomas   1169

103. Longitundinal (Bishof's) Myelotomy
Leslie P. Ivan   1177

104. Commisural Myelotomy
John E. Adams, Robert Lippert, and Yoshio Hosobuchi   1185

105. Percutaneous Cordotomy: The Lateral High Cervical Technique
Ronald R. Tasker   1191

106. Percutaneous Electrothermocoagulation of Spinal Nerve Trunk, Ganglion, and Rootlets
Sumio Uematsu   1207

107. Surgery of Epilepsy—Current Technique of Cortical Resection
Robert R. Hansebout   1223

108. Cerebral Hemispherectomy: Indications, Methods, and Results
Theodore Rasmussen   1235

109. Section of the Corpus Callosum for Epilepsy
David W. Roberts   1243

110. Selective Vestibular Nerve Transection in the Treatment of Meniere's Disease
Richard R. Gacek   1251

111. Surgical Management of Spasmodic Torticollis and Adult-Onset Dystonia with Emphasis on Selective Denervation
Claude M. Bertrand   1261

112. **Surgery of the Sympathetic Nervous System**
Russell W. Hardy, Jr. and Janet W. Bay   1271

113. **Craniovertebral Abnormalities and their Treatment**
John C. VanGilder and Arnold H. Menezes   1281

114. **Surgical Treatment of Rheumatoid Arthritis, Ankylosing Spondylitis, and Paget's Disease with Neurologic Deficit**
Ghaus M. Malik and James L. Sanders, Jr.   1295

115. **Microsurgery of Syringomyelia and Syringomyelic Cord Syndrome**
Albert L. Rhoton, Jr.   1307

116. **Anterior Cervical Disc Excision in the Treatment of Cervical Spondylosis**
Henry H. Schmidek and Donald A. Smith   1327

117. **Cervical Discography, Discometry, Cervical Disc Distention Test**
William H. Sweet and Henry H. Schmidek   1343

118. **Posterior Operations for Cervical Disc Herniation and Spondylotic Myelopathy**
James C. Collias and Melville P. Roberts   1347

119. **The Transthoracic Approach to the Thoracolumbar Spine for Decompression and Spinal Stabilization**
Henry H. Schmidek   1359

120. **Transthoracic Disc Excision**
Frederic A. Simeone and Ralph Rashbaum   1367

121. **Lumbar Disc Excision**
Bernard Finneson   1375

121C. **Commentary: Lumbar Disc Excision**
Edward Tarlov   1393

122. **Microsurgical Lumbar Disc Excision**
Robert E. Harbaugh   1395

122C. **Commentary: Microsurgical Lumbar Discectomy**
Richard L. Saunders   1399

123. **Posterior Lumbar Interbody Fusion**
Paul M. Lin   1401

124. **Anterior Lumbar Discectomy and Interbody Fusion: Indications and Technique**
J. Leonard Goldner, Kenneth E. Wood, and James R. Urbaniak   1421

125. **Chemonucleolysis**
Walter William Whisler   1437

125C. **Commentary: Chymopapain**
Charles A. Fager   1443

126. **Surgical Management of Trauma to the Spine**
David Yashon   1449

127. **Techniques of Fusion in the Cervical, Thoracic, and Lumbar Spine**
Robert C. Cantu   1471

128. **Surgical Management of Thoracolumbar Fractures: Indications, Methods, Results**
Carrie L. Walters and Henry H. Schmidek   1481

129. **Surgical Management of Spinal Cord Tumors and Arteriovenous Malformations**
Kalmon D. Post and Bennett M. Stein   1487

130. **Spinal Deformities Following Neurosurgical Procedures in Children**
Edwin G. Fischer and John E. Hall   1509

131. **Metastatic Tumors of the Spine**
Eugene A. Quindlen   1515

132. **Surgical Approaches to Primary and Metastatic Tumors of the Spine**
Narayan Sundaresan, George V. DiGiacinto, and James E. O. Hughes   1525

133. **The Management of Malignant Epidural Tumors Compressing the Spinal Cord**
Tzony Siegal and Tali Siegel   1539

134. **Surgery of the Peripheral Nerves and Brachial Plexus**
Robert D. Leffert   1563

135. **Surgical Management of Peripheral Entrapment Neuropathy**
Henry A. Young   1583

136. **Peripheral Nerve Tumors**
Alan R. Hudson, Fred Gentili, and David Kline   1599

The complete index appears following chapters 70 and 136.

Contributors

Mounir N. Abou-Madi, M.B., Ch.B., F.R.C.P.(C), Department of Anesthesiology, Montreal Neurological Hospital and Institute, and McGill University, Montreal, Quebec, Canada

John E. Adams, M.D., Department of Neurological Surgery, University of California, San Francisco, San Francisco, California

Phil A. Aitken, M.D., Division of Ophthalmology, University of Vermont College of Medicine, Burlington, Vermont

Melvin G. Alper, M.D., Departments of Ophthalmology and Neurological Surgery, The George Washington University School of Medicine and the Washington Hospital Center, Washington, D.C.

A. Loren Amacher, M.D., Department of Neurosurgery, University of Connecticut, Farmington, Connecticut

Ronald I. Apfelbaum, M.D., Division of Neurosurgery, University of Utah Health Sciences Center, Salt Lake City, Utah

Michael L. J. Apuzzo, M.D., Department of Neurological Surgery, University of Southern California School of Medicine, Los Angeles, California

J. Atieh, M.D., Burdenko Institute of Neurosurgery, Moscow, Union of Soviet Socialist Republics

James I. Ausman, M.D., Ph.D., Department of Neurological Surgery, Henry Ford Hospital, Detroit, Michigan

H. Thomas Ballantine, M.D., Department of Neurological Surgery, Massachusetts General Hospital, Boston, Massachusetts

Janet W. Bay, M.D., Department of Neurological Surgery, Cleveland Clinic Foundation, Cleveland, Ohio

Donald P. Becker, M.D., Division of Neurosurgery, School of Medicine, University of California at Los Angeles, Los Angeles, California

Claude M. Bertrand, M.D., Division of Neurosurgery, Hospital Notre Dame and University of Montreal, Montreal, Quebec, Canada

R. Bhatia, M.S. (Surg), M.Ch. (Neuro), Department of Neurosurgery, All India Institute of Medical Sciences, New Delhi, India

Don C. Bienfang, M.D., Department of Ophthalmology, Brigham and Women's Hospital, Boston, Massachusetts

Perry Black, M.D., Department of Neurosurgery, Hahnemann University, Philadelphia, Pennsylvania

Peter McL. Black, M.D., Neurosurgical Service, Brigham and Women's Hospital, Boston, Massachusetts

Ronald Brisman, M.D., Department of Neurological Surgery, College of Physicians and Surgeons of Columbia University, Neurological Institute of New York, New York, New York

William A. Buchheit, M.D., Department of Neurosurgery, Temple University Health Science Center, Philadelphia, Pennsylvania

Robert C. Cantu, M.D., Neurosurgical Service, Department of Surgery, Emerson Hospital, Concord, Massachusetts

Paolo Cappabianca, M.D., Department of Functional Neurosurgery, Institute of Neurosurgery, University of Naples, Naples, Italy

Paul H. Chapman, M.D., Department of Neurological Surgery, Massachusetts General Hospital and the Harvard Medical School, Boston, Massachusetts

Shelly N. Chou, M.D., Ph.D., Department of Neurosurgery, University of Minnesota Hospitals, Minneapolis, Minnesota

Kemp Clark, M.D., Division of Neurological Surgery, Southwestern Medical School, The University of Texas Health Science Center at Dallas, Dallas, Texas

W. Craig Clark, M.D., Ph.D., Department of Neurosurgery, University of Tennessee-Memphis, Memphis, Tennessee

Edwin W. Cocke Jr., M.D., Department of Otolaryngology and Maxillofacial Surgery, University of Tennessee-Memphis, Memphis, Tennessee

Robert Coffey, M.D., Department of Neurological Surgery, University of Pittsburgh School of Medicine, Pittsburgh, Pennsylvania

James C. Collias, M.D., Department of Neurosurgery, Hartford Hospital, Hartford, Connecticut, and Division of Neurosurgery, University of Connecticut School of Medicine, Farmington, Connecticut

William F. Collins, M.D., Section of Neurological Surgery, Yale University School of Medicine, New Haven, Connecticut

Robert M. Crowell, M.D., Department of Neurological Surgery, University of Illinois College of Medicine, Chicago, Illinois

Charles W. Cummings, M.D., Department of Otolaryngology, University of Washington, Seattle, Washington

T. Forcht Dagi, M.D., Lt. Col. M.C., Neurosurgical Service, Walter Reed Army Medical Center, Washington, DC

Enrico De Divitiis, M.D., Department of Functional Neurosurgery, Institute of Neurosurgery, University of Naples, Naples, Italy

R. A. de los Reyes, M.D., Department of Neurological Surgery, Henry Ford Hospital, Detroit, Michigan

Gerard M. Debrun, M.D., Neuroradiology Section, The Johns Hopkins Hospital and the Johns Hopkins University School of Medicine, Baltimore, Maryland

P. J. Derome, M.D., Service de Neuro-Chirurgie, Centre Medico-Chirurgical Foch, Suresnes, France

Fernando G. Diaz, M.D., Ph.D., Department of Neurological Surgery, Henry Ford Hospital, Detroit, Michigan

George V. DiGiacinto, M.D., Division of Neurosurgery, St. Luke's-Roosevelt Hospital Center, and Department of Neurological Surgery, College of Physicians and Surgeons of Columbia University, New York, New York

R. M. Peardon Donaghy, M.D., Division of Neurosurgery, University of Vermont College of Medicine, Burlington, Vermont

Edward F. Downing, M.D., Neurological Institute of Savannah, Savannah, Georgia

Charles G. Drake, M.D., Division of Neurosurgery, University of Western Ontario University Hospital, London, Ontario, Canada

John W. Duckworth, M.D., Division of Neurosurgery, University of Vermont College of Medicine, Burlington, Vermont

Tsuneyoshi Eguchi, M.D., Division of Neurological Surgery, Kameda General Hospital, Kamogawa, Japan

Fred J. Epstein, M.D., Division of Pediatric Neurosurgery, Department of Neurosurgery, New York University Medical Center, New York, New York

Mel H. Epstein, M.D., Department of Clinical Neurosciences, Brown University, and the Department of Neurosurgery, Rhode Island Hospital, Providence, Rhode Island

Calvin B. Ernst, M.D., Division of Vascular Surgery, Henry Ford Hospital, University of Michigan Medical School, Detroit, Michigan

Francisco Escobedo, M.D., Instituto Nacional de Neurologia y Neurocirugia, Mexico City, Mexico

Charles A. Fager, M.D., Department of Neurosurgery, Lahey Clinic Medical Center, Burlington, Massachusetts

Bernard E. Finneson, M.D., Low Back Pain Clinic, Crozer-Chester Medical Center, Chester, Pennsylvania, and Department of Neurosurgery, Hahnemann University, Philadelphia, Pennsylvania

Edwin G. Fischer, M.D., Department of Neurosurgery, Children's Hospital and Department of Surgery, Harvard Medical School, Boston, Massachusetts

Glenn S. Forbes, M.D., Department of Radiology, Mayo Clinic, Rochester, Minnesota

Richard R. Gacek, M.D., Department of Otolaryngology and Communication Sciences, State University of New York Health Science Center at Syracuse, Syracuse, New York

George F. Gade, M.D., Division of Neurosurgery, School of Medicine, University of California at Los Angeles, Los Angeles, California

Giuseppe Galli, M.D., Department of Neurosurgery, University of Brescia and the Regional General Hospital, Brescia, Italy

Francis W. Gamache Jr., M.D., Division of Neurological Surgery, Cornell University Medical College, New York, New York

Gale Gardner, M.D., Department of Otolaryngology and Maxillofacial Surgery, University of Tennessee-Memphis, Memphis, Tennessee

Randy Gehring, M.D., Department of Neurological Surgery, Henry Ford Hospital, Detroit, Michigan

Fred Gentili, M.D., Division of Neurosurgery, University of Toronto, Toronto, Ontario, Canada

Eugene D. George, M.D., Col. M.C., Neurosurgical Service, Walter Reed Army Medical Center, Washington, D.C.

Philip L. Gildenberg, M.D., Ph. D., Division of Neurosurgery, University of Texas Mecical School, Houston, Texas

Ida E. Giriunas, R.N., Department of Neurological Surgery, Massachusetts General Hospital, Boston, Massachusetts

J. Leonard Goldner, M.D., Department of Orthopaedic Surgery, Duke University School of Medicine, Durham, North Carolina

Robert L. Grubb, M.D., Department of Neurology and Neurological Surgery, Washington University School of Medicine, St. Louis, Missouri

John E. Hall, M.D., Department of Orthopedics, Children's Hospital, and Department of Orthopedics, Harvard Medical School, Boston, Massachusetts

Robert R. Hansebout, M.D., F.R.C.S.(C), Department of Surgery, McMaster University, St. Joseph's Hospital, Hamilton, Ontario, Canada

Robert F. Harbaugh, M.D., Section of Neurosurgery, Dartmouth-Hitchcock Medical Center, Hanover, New Hampshire

Russell W. Hardy Jr., M.D., Department of Neurological Surgery, Cleveland Clinic Foundation, Cleveland, Ohio

Roberto C. Heros, M.D., Department of Neurological Surgery, Massachusetts General Hospital, Boston, Massachusetts

Yoshio Hosobuchi, M.D., Department of Neurological Surgery, University of California, San Francisco, San Francisco, California

Edgar M. Housepian, M.D., Department of Neurological Surgery, Neurological Institute of New York, College of Physicians and Surgeons of Columbia University, New York, New York

Alan R. Hudson, M.D., Division of Neurosurgery, University of Toronto, Toronto, Ontario, Canada

James E. O. Hughes, M.D., Division of Neurosurgery, St. Luke's-Roosevelt Hospital Center, and Department of Neurological Surgery, College of Physicians and Surgeons of Columbia University, New York, New York

Leslie P. Ivan, M.D., F.R.C.S.(C), Division of Neurosurgery, School of Medicine, Faculty of Health Sciences, University of Ottawa, Ottawa, Ontario, Canada

Skip Jacques, M.D., Advanced Neurosurgical Laboratory, Huntington Medical Research Institutes, California Institute of Technology, Pasadena, California

Jafar J. Jafar, M.D., Department of Neurological Surgery, University of Illinois College of Medicine, Chicago, Illinois

Jonas Johnson, M.D., Department of Otolaryngology, University of Pittsburgh, Pittsburgh, Pennsylvania

Cecil L. Jun, M.D., Department of Neurosurgery, Kaiser-Permanente Medical Center, Redwood City, California

Edward I. Kandel, M.D., D.Sc., Neurosurgery Clinic, Institute of Neurology, Moscow, Union of Soviet Socialist Republics

Robert A. Kane, M.D., Department of Radiology, New England Deaconess Hospital, Boston, Massachusetts

John P. Kapp, M.D., Department of Neurosurgery, State University of New York, Buffalo, New York

Patrick J. Kelly, M.D., Department of Neurological Surgery, Mayo Clinic, Rochester, Minnesota

T. T. King, F.R.C.S., Department of Neurosurgery, The London Hospital, Whitechapel, London, England

Raymond N. Kjellbeg, M.D., Department of Neurological Surgery, Massachusetts General Hospital, Boston, Massachusetts

David Kline, M.D., Division of Neurosurgery, Louisiana State University, Baton Rouge, Louisiana

A. Konovalov, M.D., Burdenko Institute of Neurosurgery, Moscow, Union of Soviet Socialist Republics

George Krol, M.D., Department of Radiology, Memorial Sloan-Kettering Cancer Center and Cornell University Medical Center, New York, New York

Edward R. Laws Jr., M.D., Department of Neurologic Surgery, Mayo Clinic, Rochester, Minnesota

Robert D. Leffert, M.D., Department of Orthopedic Surgery and Department of Rehabilitation Medicine, Massachusetts General Hospital, and Harvard Medical School, Boston, Massachusetts

David W. Leitner, M.D., Assistant Professor of Surgery, Division of Plastic Surgery, University of Vermont College of Medicine, Burlington, Vermont

Alberto Lenzi, M.D., Department of Neurosurgery, University of Brescia and the Regional General Hospital, Brescia, Italy

Paul M. Lin, M.D., Jenkintown, Pennsylvania

Peter C. Linton, M.D., Associate Professor of Surgery, Division of Plastic Surgery, University of Vermont College of Medicine, Burlington, Vermont

Robert Lippert, M.D., Department of Neurological Surgery, University of California, San Francisco, San Francisco, California

Alfred J. Luessenhop, M.D., Division of Neurosurgery, Georgetown University Hospital, Washington, D.C.

L. Dade Lunsford, M.D., Departments of Neurological Surgery and Radiology, University of Pittsburgh School of Medicine, Pittsburgh, Pennsylvania

Harold R. Lutes, O.D., Advanced Neurosurgical Laboratory, Huntington Medical Research Institutes, California Institute of Technology, Pasadena, California

Joseph R. Madsen, M.D., Department of Neurological Surgery, Massachusetts General Hospital, Boston, Massachusetts

Ghaus M. Malik, M.D., Department of Neurological Surgery, Henry Ford Hospital, Detroit, Michigan

Giovanni Marini, M.D., Department of Neurosurgery, University of Brescia and the Regional General Hospital, Brescia, Italy

Ernest S. Mathews, M.D., Department of Neurosurgery, New England Deaconess Hospital, Boston, Massachusetts

Robert E. Maxwell, M.D., Ph.D., Department of Neurosurgery, University of Minnesota Hospitals, Minneapolis, Minnesota

Arnold H. Menezes, M.D., Division of Neurosurgery, University of Iowa, Iowa City, Iowa

J. Douglas Miller, M.D., Ph.D., F.R.C.S., F.A.C.S., F.R.C.P.E., Department of Surgical Neurology, University of Edinburgh, Edinburgh, Scotland

Morey S. Moreland, M.D., Department of Orthopaedics and Rehabilitation, University of Vermont College of Medicine, Burlington, Vermont

A. W. Morrison, M.D., Department of Otolaryngology, The London Hospital, Whitechapel, London, England

John F. Mullan, M.D., Neurological Surgery, The University of Chicago Medical Center, Chicago, Illinois

F. Mundinger, M.D., Abteilung Stereotaxie and Neuronuklearmedizin, Neurochirurgische Universitätsklinik, Freiburg, Federal Republic of Germany

Paul F. New, M.D., Neuroradiology Section, Massachusetts General Hospital, Boston, Massachusetts

Stephen L. Nutik, M.D., Ph.D., Department of Neurosurgery, Kaiser-Permanente Medical Center, Redwood City, California

Daniel H. O'Leary, M.D., Department of Radiology, New England Deaconess Hospital, Boston, Massachusetts

Robert G. Ojemann, M.D., Department of Neurological Surgery, Massachusetts General Hospital and Department of Surgery, Harvard Medical School, Boston, Massachusetts

Michael S. Olin, M.D., Department of Neurosurgery, St. Joseph Hospital, Providence, Rhode Island

Dwight Parkinson, M.D., Department of Surgery, The University of Manitoba, Winnipeg, Manitoba, Canada

Russel H. Patterson Jr., M.D., Division of Neurosurgery, The New York Hospital-Cornell Mecical Center, New York, New York

Jeffrey E. Pearce, M.D., Department of Neurological Surgery, Henry Ford Hospital, Detroit, Michigan

Sidney J. Peerless, M.D., Division of Neurosurgery, University of Western Ontario University Hospital, London, Ontario, Canada

Vyacheslav V. Peresedov, M.D., Neurosurgery Clinic, Institute of Neurology, Moscow, Union of Soviet Socialist Republics

David G. Piepgras, M.D., Department of Neurosurgery, Mayo Clinic, Rochester, Minnesota

Robert N. Pilon, M.D., Department of Anesthesia, Athens General Hospital, Athens, Georgia

Charles E. Poletti, M.D., Department of Neurological Surgery, Massachusetts General Hospital, Boston, Massachusetts

Kalmon D. Post, M.D., Department of Neurological Surgery, College of Physicians and Surgeons of Columbia University, New York, New York

Eugene A. Quindlen, M.D., Department of Neurological Surgery, University of South Alabama College of Medicine, Mobile, Alabama

Ralph Rashbaum, M.D., Division of Neurosurgery, University of Pennsylvania School Medicine, and Pennsylvania Hospital, Philadelphia, Pennsylvania

Theodore Rasmussen, M.D., Montreal Neurological Institute and Hospital, Montreal, Quebec, Canada

Robert A. Ratcheson, M.D., Division of Neurological Surgery, Case-Western Reserve University, University Hospitals of Cleveland, Cleveland, Ohio

Michael J. Redmond, M.D., Department of Neurological Surgery, Mayo Clinic, Rochester, Minnesota

Albert L. Rhoton Jr., M.D., Department of Neurological Surgery, University of Florida College of Medicine, Gainesville, Florida

Howard A. Richter, M.D., Division of Neurosurgery, Lankenau Hospital and the Thomas Jefferson Medical College, Philadelphia, Pennsylvania

David W. Roberts, M.D., Section of Neurosurgery, Dartmouth-Hitchcock Medical Center, Hanover, New Hampshire

Melville P. Roberts, M.D., Division of Neurosurgery, University of Connecticut School of Medicine, Farmington, Connecticut, and Hartford Hospital, Hartford, Connecticut

James T. Robertson, M.D., Department of Neurosurgery, University of Tennessee-Memphis, Memphis, Tennessee

Jon H. Robertson, M.D., Department of Neurosurgery, University of Tennessee-Memphis, Memphis, Tennessee

Robert H. Rosenwasser, M.D., Department of Neurosurgery and Physiology, Temple University Health Science Center, Philadelphia, Pennsylvania

Maurice I. Saba, M.D., Division of Neurosurgery, American University Hospital of Beirut, Beirut, Lebanon

Ved Sachdev, M.D., Department of Surgery, Mount Sinai Medical Center and Mount Sinai Medical School, New York, New York

Anthony Salerni, M.D., Division of Neurosurgery, University of Vermont College of Medicine, Burlington, Vermont

James L. Sanders Jr., M.D., Department of Neurological Surgery, Henry Ford Hospital, Detroit, Michigan

Kimberlee J. Sass, Ph.D., Section of Neurological Surgery, Yale University School of Medicine, New Haven, Connecticut

Richard L. Saunders, M.D., Section of Neurosurgery, Dartmouth-Hitchcock Medical Center, Hanover, New Hampshire

Henry H. Schmidek, M.D., Department of Surgery, New England Deaconess Hospital, and Harvard Medical School, Boston, Massachusetts

R. Michael Scott, M.D., F.A.C.S., Department of Neurosurgery, New England Medical Center Hospitals and Tufts University, Boston, Massachusetts

C. Hunter Shelden, M.D., Advanced Neurosurgical Laboratory, Huntington Medical Research Institutes, California Institute of Technology, Pasadena, California

Carl E. Shrontz, M.D., Department of Neurological Surgery, Henry Ford Hospital, Detroit, Michigan

Tali Siegal, M.D., Spinal Surgery Unit, Beilinson Medical Center, Petah Tivka, and the Department of Oncology and Neurology, Hadassah University Hospital, Jerusalem, Israel

Tzony Siegal, M.D., D.M.D., Spinal Surgery Unit, Beilinson Medical Center, Petah Tivka, and the Departments of Oncology and Neurology, Hadassah University Hospital, Jerusalem, Israel

Frederick A. Simeone, M.D., Division of Neurosurgery, University of Pennsylvania School of Medicine, and Pennsylvania Hospital, Philadelphia, Pennsylvania

Donald A. Smith, M.D., Division of Neurosurgery, University of Vermont College of Medicine, Burlington, Vermont

Robert B. Snow, M.D., Ph.D., Division of Neurosurgery, The New York Hospital-Cornell Medical Center, New York, New York

Robert A. Sofferman, M.D., Division of Otolaryngology, University of Vermont College of Medicine, Burlington, Vermont

Renato Spaziante, M.D., Department of Functional Neurosurgery, Institute of Neurosurgery, University of Naples, Naples, Italy

Dennis D. Spencer, M.D., Section of Neurological Surgery, Yale University School of Medicine, New Haven, Connecticut

Bennet M. Stein, M.D., Department of Neurosurgery, Neurological Institute of New York, Columbia-Presbyterian Medical Center, New York, New York

Ladislau Steiner, M.D., Stockholm, Sweden

Narayan Sundaresan, M.D., Division of Neurooncology, St. Luke's-Roosevelt Hospital Center and Department of Neurological Surgery, College of Physicians and Surgeons of Columbia University, New York, New York

Thoralf M. Sundt Jr., M.D., Department of Neurosurgery, Mayo Clinic, Rochester, Minnesota

Karl Swann, M.D., Department of Neurological Surgery, Massachusetts General Hospital, Boston, Massachusetts

William H. Sweet, M.D., D.Sc., D.H.C., Department of Neurological Surgery, Massachusetts General Hospital and the Department of Surgery, Harvard Medical School, Boston, Massachusetts

Lindsay Symon, T.D., F.R.C.S., F.R.C.S.E., Gough-Cooper Department of Neurological Surgery, Institute of Neurology, University of London, National Hospital, London, England

P. N. Tandon, M.S., F.R.C.S.(E), Department of Neurosurgery, All India Institute of Medical Sciences, New Delhi, India

Edward Tarlov, M.D., Department of Neurosurgery, Lahey Clinic Medical Center, Burlington, Massachusetts

Ronald R. Tasker, M.D., Division of Neurosurgery, Toronto General Hospital, and Department of Surgery, University of Toronto, Toronto, Ontario, Canada

John M. Tew Jr., M.D., Department of Neurosurgery, University of Cincinnati College of Medicine, Cincinnati, Ohio

D. G. T. Thomas, M.A., F.R.C.P.(Glas.), F.R.C.S.(Ed.), Department of Neurological Surgery, Institute of Neurology, The National Hospital, London, England

Davy Trop, M.D., F.R.C.P.(C), F.A.C.A., Department of Anesthesiology, Montreal Neurological Hospital and Institute and McGill University, Montreal, Quebec, Canada

Sumio Uematsu, M.D., Department of Neurosurgery, The Johns Hopkins University School of Medicine, Baltimore, Maryland

Kazuo Ugajin, M.D., Division of Neurological Surgery, Kameda General Hospital, Kamogawa, Japan

James R. Urbaniak, M.D., Department of Neurosurgery, Duke University School of Medicine, Durham, North Carolina

Dante F. Vacca, M.D., Department of Neurological Surgery, Henry Ford Hospital, Detroit, Michigan

Harry R. van Loveren, M.D., Department of Neurosurgery, University of Cincinnati College of Medicine, Cincinnati, Ohio

John C. VanGilder, M.D., Division of Neurosurgery, University of Iowa, Iowa City, Iowa

Steven L. Wald, M.D., Division of Neurosurgery, University of Vermont College of Medicine, Burlington, Vermont

Carrie L. Walters, M.D., Division of Neurosurgery, University of Vermont College of Medicine, Burlington, Vermont

Walter William Whisler, M.D., Ph.D., Department of Neurosurgery, Rush Medical College and Presbyterian-St. Luke's Hospital, Chicago, Illinois

Jeffrey H. Wisoff, M.D., Division of Pediatric Neurosurgery, Department of Neurosurgery, New York University Medical Center, New York, New York

Kenneth E. Wood, M.D., Department of Orthopaedic Surgery, Duke University School of Medicine, Durham, North Carolina

Shirley H. Wray, Neuroophthalmology Service, Massachusetts General Hospital, Boston, Massachusetts

R. Lewis Wright, M.D., Department of Neurosurgery, Stuart Circle Hospital and St. Mary's Hospital, Richmond, Virginia

David Yashon, M.D., Department of Neurosurgery, Ohio State University and St. Anthony's Hospital, Columbus, Ohio

Henry A. Young, M.D., Augusta, Georgia

Nicholas T. Zervas, M.D., Department of Neurological Surgery, Massachusetts General Hospital and the Department of Surgery, Harvard Medical School, Boston, Massachusetts

Surgical Management of Internal Carotid Artery Aneurysms within the Cavernous Sinus

Dwight Parkinson

SYMPTOMATIC SACCULAR ANEURYSMS of the internal carotid artery within the cavernous sinus can be either of developmental or traumatic origin. The developmental variety probably slightly outnumber the traumatic variety in occurrence, but together they total less than 5 percent of all intracranial aneurysms.[1–5] It is estimated that an equal number of asymptomatic aneurysms are found incidentally during angiography that is performed for other purposes, and still others may be overlooked at autopsy because they lie extradurally and are collapsed. The developmental variety occurs more frequently in females than in males, with a female-to-male ratio of 14:3, and this variety is also predominant in groups over the age of 50 years.[2] These aneurysms may be related to the normal branches of the parasellar carotid. Posteriorly, and above the sixth nerve, they should arise from the meningohypophyseal departure[6]; if below and posteriorly, they should arise from a persistent trigeminal remnant[7,8]; and if laterally placed, they might arise from the artery of the inferior cavernous sinus departure[6]; however, we have never been able to prove these relationships.

DIAGNOSIS

Traumatic parasellar saccular aneurysms usually are associated with a basal skull fracture,[2,9] and may even be the residue of a spontaneous closure of a carotid fistula.[10,11] When present, Maurer's[12] triad of "unilateral blindness, orbital fracture, and delayed massive epistaxis following head injury" is diagnostic. Many such cases have been reported (Vandellen JR: personal communication, September, 1980),[13,14] but usually one of the triad is missing.[15–19] Vandellen added an interesting observation, that there may be a fluid level in the sphenoid sinus or an opaque sphenoid sinus, and also pointed out that relatively minor trauma may produce a fracture in the sphenoid area, with damage to the carotid. Even more significantly, he noted a case with delayed intracerebral hematoma that caused a deterioration preceded by epistaxis.

The diagnosis of either type of aneurysm—traumatic or developmental—depends upon a suspicion that such a lesion may be present. Without epistaxis, there is no reliable bedside differentiation between an aneurysm and any other mass in this region.[20–37]

The signs and symptoms are anatomically logical.[16,21,22,31,38–42] Involvement of the first division of the fifth cranial nerve and of the third, fourth, and sixth cranial nerves is the earliest and most common sign.[43] Pain in the second division of the fifth nerve is less common, and involvement of the optic nerve and the third division of the fifth nerve is far less common.[44] Still less common again are exophthalmos, orbital venous engorgement, and intracranial mass effect.[45,46]

Jefferson's[18,47] classic description of the signs and symptoms remains relatively unchallenged. The occasional finding of a small pupil in association with a third-nerve palsy has been explained as being a result of the net of sympathetic nerves around the carotid being stretched or otherwise disturbed by the aneurysm.[18,47–51] We believe this net around the carotid represents a sympathetic supply to, rather than from, the arterial wall.[52,53] Our work indicates that the largest residue of this sympathetic nerve, after supplying the carotid and other structures, then joins the sixth nerve, runs with it a few millimeters, and leaves to join the first division of the fifth nerve.[52–55] The small pupil probably results from interruption of this nerve of sympathetic continuation.[53,56] To date, there are no reports of altered patterns of sweating caused by involvement of the various divisions of the fifth cranial nerve.

The skull roentgenograms are abnormal in a very high percentage of symptomatic aneurysms. Erosion of the anterior clinoid, erosion of the lateral sphenoid sinus wall, and curvilinear calcification are the most frequent abnormalities.[32,57,58]

Although computed tomographic (CT) scans are used more frequently for all intracranial diagnosis than is angiography,[10,27,35,59–63] and although with their higher resolution they are able to pick up and better delineate parasellar lesions,[62] angiography remains the definitive procedure. This study should demonstrate each carotid individually and be supplemented with cross-compression to better evaluate the presence or absence of an adequate anterior communicating artery. These studies also exclude the rare case of bilateral intracavernous aneurysms.[36,45,63]

TREATMENT

The first recorded surgical approach to an intracavernous aneurysm was that of Birley and Trotter,[64] who in 1928 ligated both the internal and external carotid arteries. Demoris and Lana-Peixoto[63] reported treating bilateral aneurysms by ligating

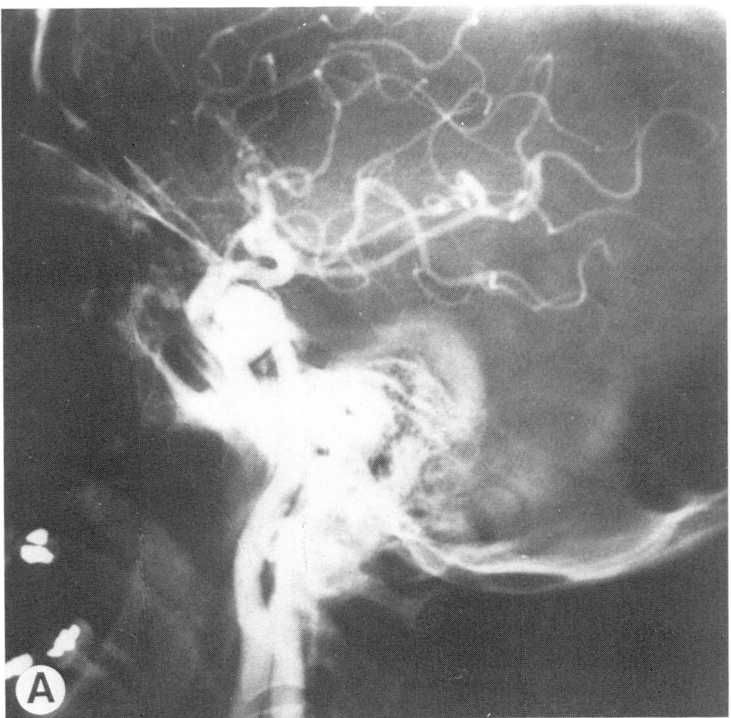

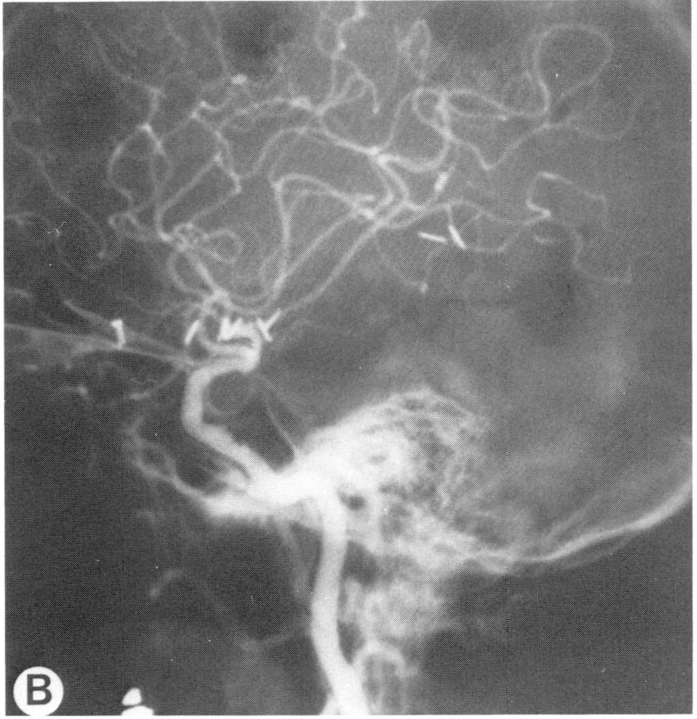

Fig. 71-1. (A) Preoperative and (B) postoperative angiograms demonstrating repair of a saccular aneurysm that had burst posteriorly and superiorly to become a fistula. (Reprinted from Parkinson D: Aneurysms of the cavernous sinus, in Pia HW, Langmaid C, Zierski J (eds): Cerebral Aneurysms: Advances in Diagnosis and Therapy. Berlin, Springer-Verlag, 1979, pp 80–81. With permission.)

one internal carotid artery and partially occluding the opposite one 3 years later, with no ill effects.

Although most of the traumatic aneurysms and virtually all of the developmental sacs never bleed, the neurosurgeon's skill will be challenged to the utmost when confronted with an exsanguinating epistaxis. Initially, the hemorrhage must be brought under control.[12,41,65] During digital compression of the cervical carotid arteries, one must watch carefully for signs of cerebral ischemia and of ipsilateral retinal ischemia. If the hemorrhage persists with adequate digital compression, any retinal or hemispheric ischemia might be due to a steal,[66] and the carotid artery distal to the bleeding aneurysm must be

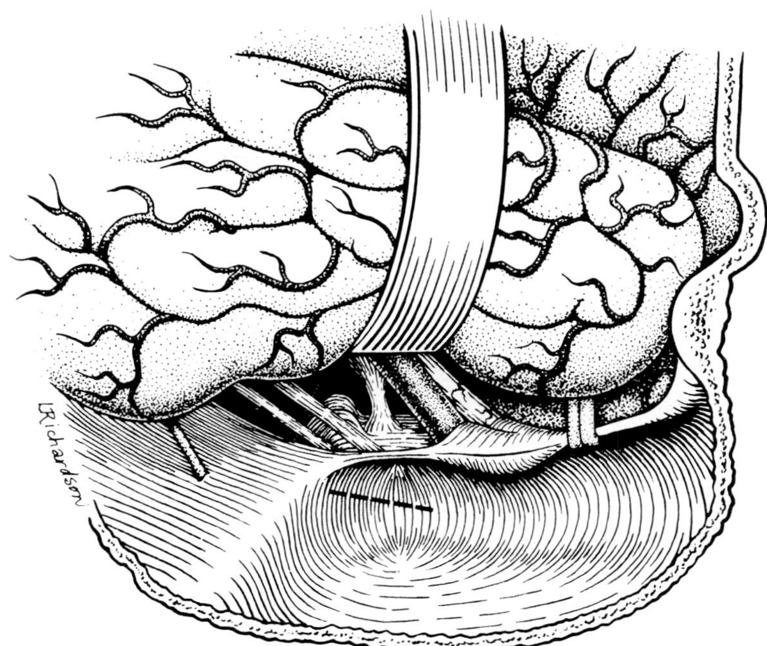

Fig. 71–2. A drawing of the right middle fossa. The dashed line shows the site and slope of the incision of the triangular space. Note that it does not parallel the slope of the third and fourth nerves as the brain is elevated, but, rather, the slope those nerves would follow if the brain were not elevated.

brought under control. If the hemorrhage persists without evidence of retinal or hemispheric ischemia, the steal is neurologically innocuous, and probably results from the intracranial anastomosis of the meningohypophyseal arteries.[67] If the hemorrhage is brought under control and leaves no neurologic or visual deficit during digital compression (whether continuous or intermittent), one is relatively safe in ligating the internal carotid as a finite procedure. If, however, the hemorrhage stops during digital compression, and there is hemispheric or visual impairment, the surgeon faces a dilemma. In either case, we would favor exposing the common and internal and external carotid arteries under local anesthesia, and determining whether the hemorrhage can be controlled and function preserved by clamping the common carotid artery or, preferably, the internal carotid artery by itself, leaving the external carotid collateral to supply circulation to the retina. Faced with a positive Matas test, but with the hemorrhage under control, a preliminary extracranial-intracranial bypass should be considered.

Although it has not yet been reported, it should be possible to get a guided balloon into the hemorrhaging opening[9] in order to control the aneurysmal hemorrhage and preserve the blood flow through the carotid artery.

Proximal ligation remains the treatment of choice for both traumatic and developmental saccular aneurysms within the cavernous sinus.[17,33,63,65,66,68–70] The clipping of the supraclinoid in addition to proximal ligation has been advocated, with the hope of further decreasing the turgor of the aneurysm, and thus diminishing or reversing the disturbance of the cranial nerve. Two authors have plicated the aneurysm after trapping the carotid artery, in an effort to accomplish decompression of the cranial nerves.[3,68]

Until about 7 years ago, our treatment was ligation and trapping, but as we developed more confidence in our use of profound hypothermia with complete circulatory arrest while working on the direct repair of carotid cavernous fistulae,[6,71–74] it occurred to us that we should attempt the direct repair of one of these aneurysms. We have now repaired the aneurysm and successfully established a normal continuity of the carotid in 3 patients, one of whom subsequently died. Each patient had an intraoperative angiogram that confirmed satisfactory reconstruction of the carotid lumen with normal patency of that vessel (Figure 71-1A and B).

DIRECT SURGICAL REPAIR

As with all surgical procedures, exposure is the first and most important consideration. Profound hypothermia provides a very excellent reduction in brain volume, but in addition, we place the patient in a lateral position to allow for spinal drainage as the exposure is developed. Mannitol is of questionable value in conjunction with cardiopulmonary bypass, although we have used this aid before starting the bypass. Once the dura is opened, it is of utmost importance to avoid bruising the temporal lobe.

Once the dural wall is exposed, the third nerve is identified as it appears over the free margin of the tentorium (Figure 71-2). This nerve should be clearly in view during the placement of the incision in the lateral wall of the cavernous sinus and during the retraction and development of the next layer.[6] This exposure should not be attempted without first verifying the landmarks many times on cadavers (Figures 71-3 and 71-4). It is better to incise the dura of the lateral wall of the cavernous sinus low rather than high, since injury to a few fibers of the first division of the fifth nerve is of less importance than the risk of cutting the third or fourth nerves. As indicated in Figures 71-5 and 71–6, the triangular space is widened by any mass within it, which also obliterates the venous channels.[72,75-78] The sixth nerve is always pushed laterally and downward, parallel to the

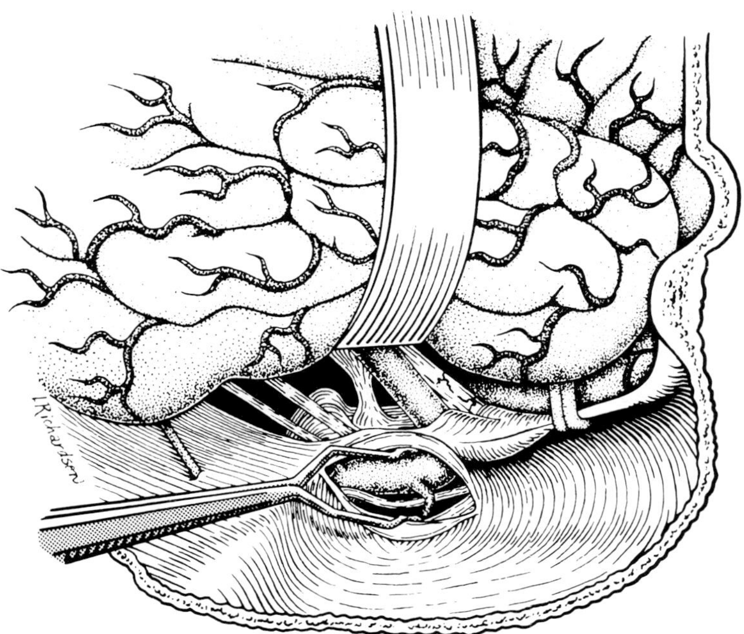

Fig. 71-3.   A drawing showing the exposure of normal structures through the incision. The third and fourth nerves are elevated within the upper dural margin, and the first division of the fifth nerve is visible in the down-turned lower margin. The sixth nerve is visible within the space parallel to the first division of the fifth nerve.

first division of the fifth nerve. Therefore, if no evidence of the first division of the fifth nerve is seen after incising the dura, the surgeon is probably well above both it and the sixth nerve, since it is almost impossible to be inferior to the first division of the fifth nerve. If some fibers of the fifth nerve are noticed when the dural incision is made, they should be brushed inferiorly before the incision is enlarged.[73]

The attenuation of the dura that is caused by the bulge of the intracavernous aneurysm often allows the first division of the fifth nerve to be seen through the dura. If not, it can often be felt by rubbing the blunt handle of the scalpel up and down in a vertical fashion[73]; the small ridge created by this nerve is palpable to the transverse of the knife handle. By centering at the point at which the third nerve appears over the horizon, the incision can be safely extended forward for 1 cm parallel to the course of the third and fourth nerves. It must be remembered that with elevation of the temporal lobe, the third and fourth nerves assume a more vertical course, and it is the normal course that the incision must parallel, which is almost the slope of the free margin of the tentorium (Figure 71-2). If any fibers of the fifth nerve appear in the incision, they should be brushed inferiorly with the handle of the knife. Once the incision is 1 cm long, it can be extended forward by separating the fibers with a blunt hook; this minimizes the risk of cutting the third and

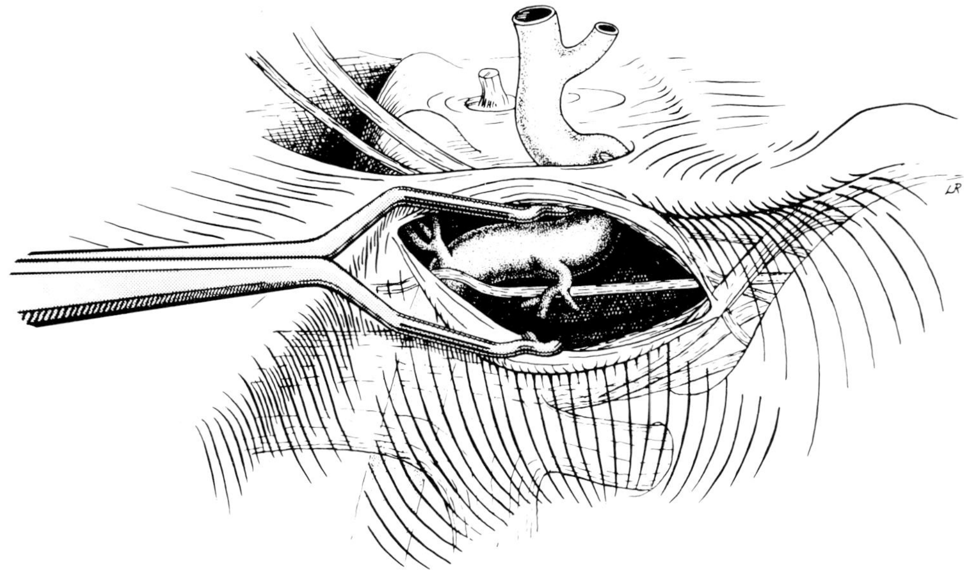

Fig. 71-4.   A drawing giving an enlarged view of the exposure. The continuation of the first division of the fifth nerve and the third and fourth nerves, along with the second and third divisions of the fifth nerve below, are ghosted-in.

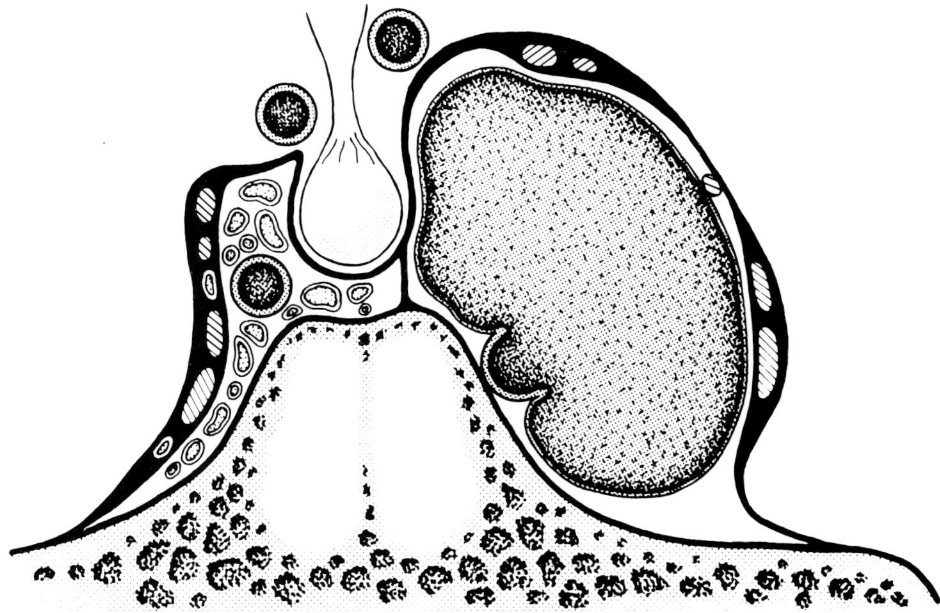

Fig. 71-5.   A diagram of a coronal section, indicating how the triangular space is widened by an aneurysm or by any mass on the right, and also how the venous channels are obliterated. The cross-hatched areas from above downward represent the third, fourth, and sixth nerves, and the first and second divisions of the fifth nerve. On the left, the venous channels in the dural wall and within the parasellar space have a stippled center and plain walls.

fourth nerves above or the sixth nerve and first division of the fifth nerve as they converge to approach the superior orbital fissure. Posteriorly, there is no risk of cutting the cranial nerves, since they course farther apart in this area, but there is a risk of penetrating into the posterior fossa. It is always safe to expose posteriorly over a blunt hook, until the circumference of the aneurysm is sufficiently developed. Next, the dura should be separated up and down 2–3 mm, in order to expose the surface of the aneurysm, thus further ensuring against damage to the cranial nerves.

The aneurysm is opened after hypothermia and circulatory arrest have been induced. This is a safe procedure; however, the continued oozing of heparinized blood at the operative site when the circulation is restarted is a real problem that can be overcome only by waiting out the reversal of heparinization as the patient is warmed and the pump discontinued.

Technically, the aneurysmal site is best reinforced with a flap taken from the medial wall (Figure 71-7) using 6-0 sutures in the arterial wall. This also avoids incising a cranial nerve, as the nerves will be pushed up or down and laterally. The defect in

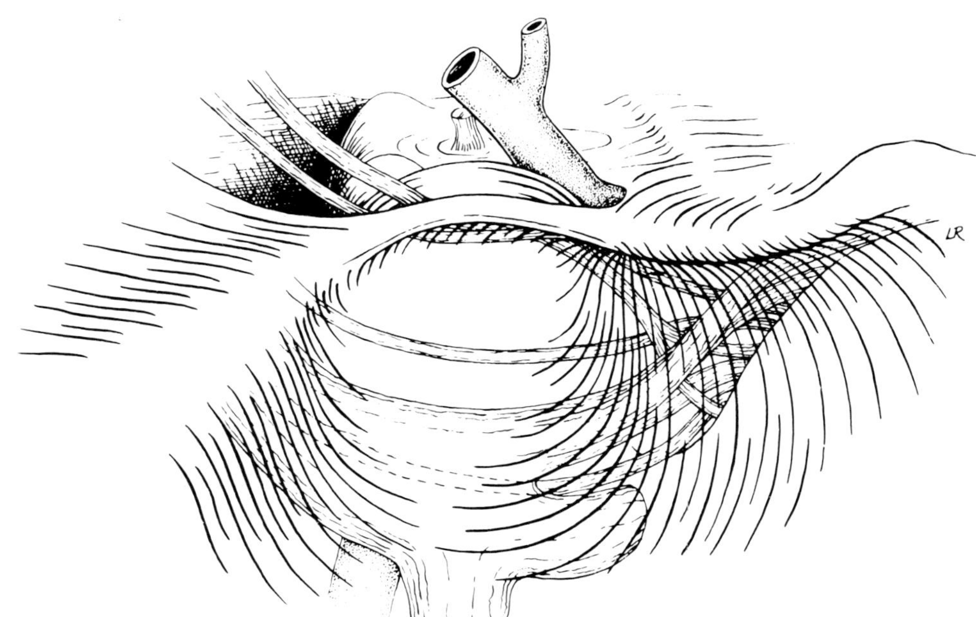

Fig. 71-6.   A drawing demonstrating the lateral aspect and showing the widening of the triangular space with the third and fourth nerves again at the top, and the sixth nerve and first division of the fifth nerve bowed laterally and slightly downward.

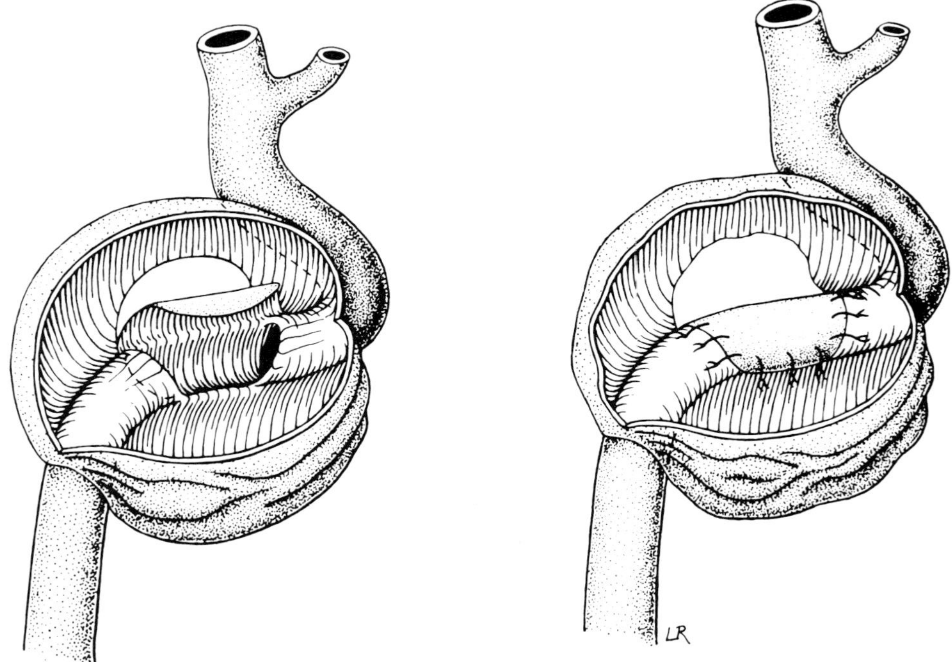

Fig. 71-7. A diagram of the repair procedure. A flap cut from the medial wall is rolled down and sutured. The remainder of the aneurysm wall is left in situ. The repair site is then packed lightly with Gelfoam and muscle, and the dural incision is closed.

the medial wall is patched with Gelfoam. We do not attempt to further remove the aneurysmal sac, as this would risk avulsing one of the cranial nerves. The area of repair on the carotid wall then is lightly packed with Gelfoam or muscle, and the dural incision is closed with 4-0 Mersaline suture. The illumination and magnification of the operating microscope is of immense value throughout the procedure. We do not heparinize our patients postoperatively.

This procedure could be accomplished by trapping the carotid artery without circulatory arrest, but we have been concerned about leaving an occluding clip or ligature on the carotid artery for any length of time for fear of causing an intimal lesion, which then might lead to thrombus formation. This may well be an unrealistic fear. If this operation were attempted by means of trapping alone, without circulatory arrest, one would have to contend with the minimal but obscurant retrograde bleeding from the meningohypophyseal and the ophthalmic arteries. This should be easily controlled with a small pledget in the proximal and distal mouths of the aneurysmal opening.

We have never seen an aneurysm in this location with a neck to which a clip could be applied. All those aneurysms we have treated had enlarged the connection with the lumen in the manner diagrammed in Figure 71-7. Some aneurysms possibly could be clipped—we just have not seen one. If the aneurysm could be clipped, this approach would not require any form of vascular occlusion, only the assurance that the cranial nerves had been brushed aside before the clip was applied.

REFERENCES

1. Alajouanine T, Thurel R, Nehlil J, et al: L'aneurysme due siphon-carotidien et son retentissement osseaux (reunion du trou optique et de la fente sphenoidale). Rev Neurol 92:249, 1955

2. Brihaye J, Mage J, Verhiest G: Aneurysme traumatique de la carotide interne dans sa portion supraclinoidienne. Acta Neurol Psychiatr Belg 54:411, 1954

3. Nakahara A, Asakura T, Kawabatake H, et al: A giant aneurysm of the internal carotid artery treated by intracranial direct surgery with a special reference to the anatomical relationship between the cavernous sinus and the internal artery. Neurol Surg 3:783, 1975

4. Parkinson D, West M: Traumatic intracranial aneurysms. J Neurosurg 52:11, 1980

5. Verbruggen A: Subarachnoid hemorrhage. Miss Valley Med J 77:95, 1955

6. Parkinson D: A surgical approach to the cavernous portion of the carotid artery. Anatomical studies and case report. J Neurosurg 23:474, 1965

7. Drake CG: Subdural hematoma from arterial rupture. J Neurosurg 18:597, 1961

8. Parkinson D, Shields C: Persistent trigeminal artery: Its relationship to the normal branches of the cavernous carotid. J Neurosurg 40:245, 1974

9. Serbinenko FA: Balloon catheterization and occlusion of major cerebral vessel. J Neurosurg 41:125, 1974

10. Lombardi G, Passerini A, Migliavacca F: Intracavernous aneurysms of the internal carotid artery. AJR 89:361, 1963

11. Taptas J N: Etiologie et pathogenie des exophtalmies d'origine vasculaire dites exophtalmies pusatiles. Arch Ophtal 10:22, 1950

12. Maurer JJ, Mills M, German WJ: Triad of unilateral blindness, orbital fractures and massive epistaxis after head injury. J Neurosurg 18:837, 1961

13. Ming-Ying Liu, Chung Jen Shih, Yeou Chih Wang, et al: Traumatic intracavernous carotid aneurysm with massive epistaxis. Neurosurgery 17:569, 1985

14. Shallat RF: Traumatic intracavernous aneurysm. Neurosurgery 8:569, 1981

15. Beadles CF: Aneurysms of the larger cerebral arteries. Brain 30:285, 1907

16. Bonnet P, Bonnet I: Le syndrome du trou dechire anterieur, symptomatique de l'aneurysme de la carotide intracranienne. Rev Otoneuroophtalmol 27:22, 1955

17. Davis RAD, Wetzel N, Davis L: An analysis of the results of treatment of intracranial vascular lesions by carotid artery ligation. Ann Surg 143:641, 1965

18. Jefferson G: Concerning injuries, aneurysms, and tumors involving the cavernous sinus. Trans Ophthalmol Soc UK 73:117, 1953

19. Weinberger LM, Adler FH, Grant FC: Primary pituitary adenoma and the syndrome of the cavernous sinus. A clinical and anatomic study. Arch Ophthalmol 24:1197, 1940

20. Barr HWK, Blackwood W, Meadows SP: Intracavernous carotid aneurysms—a clinical pathological report. Brain 94:607, 1971

21. Bartholow R: Aneurysms of the arteries at the base of the brain: Their symptomology, diagnosis, and treatment. Am J Med Sci 64:375, 1872

22. Cogan DG, Mount HTJ: Intracranial aneurysms causing ophthalmoplegia. Arch Ophthalmol 70:757, 1963

23. Foix M: Syndrome de la paroi externe du sinus caverneux. Ophthalmoplegie unilaterale a marche rapidement progressive. Bull Mem Soc Med Hop Paris 36:1355, 1920

24. Glasauer FE, Tandan PN: Trigeminal neurinoma in adolescents. J Neurol Neurosurg Psychiatry 32:562, 1969

25. Godtfredsen E, Lederman M: Studies on the cavernous sinus syndrome. 2. Diagnostic and prognostic roles of ophthalmo-neurological signs and symptoms in malignant nasopharyngeal tumors. Acta Neurol Scand 41:51, 1965

26. Krayenbuhl H: Primary tumors of the fifth cranial nerve: Their distinction from tumors of the gasserian ganglion. Brain 49:337, 1936

27. Legre J, Dufour M, Debaene A, et al: Signes angiographiques des tumeurs de la region due sinus caverneux. Neurochirurgie 19:29, 1973

28. Love JG, Woltman HW: Trigeminal neuralgia and tumors of the gasserian ganglion. Proc Staff Meet Mayo Clin 17:490, 1942

29. Malis LI: Tumors of the parasellar region. Adv Neurol 15:281, 1975

30. McGrath P: The cavernous sinus: Anatomical survey. Aust NZ J Surg 47:601, 1977

31. Sakalas R, Harbison JW, Vines FS, et al: Chronic sixth nerve palsy, initial sign of a petrous apex cavernous sinus tumor. Arch Ophthalmol 93:186, 1975

32. Trobe J D, Glaser JS, Post JD: Meningiomas and aneurysms of the cavernous sinus. Neuroophthalmologic features. Arch Ophthalmol 96:457, 1978

33. Trotter W: Symptoms of malignant tumors of the nasopharynx. Lancet 1:1277, 1911

34. Waga S, Kikuchi H, Handa J, et al: Cavernous sinus venography. AJR 109:130, 1970

35. White JC, Ballantine HT: Intrasellar aneurysms simulating hypophyseal tumors. J Neurosurg 18:34, 1961

36. Wilson CB, Myers FK: Bilateral saccular aneurysms of the internal carotid artery in the cavernous sinus. J Neurol Neurosurg Psychiatry 26:174, 1963

37. Zuzulia YA, Romodanov SA, Patsko YV: Diagnosis and surgical treatment of benign craniobasal tumors involving the cavernous sinus. Acta Neurochir (Suppl) 28:287, 1979

38. Bronner A, Brini A, Risse JF, et al: Painful ophthalmoplegia and syndrome of the cavernous sinus (optalmoplegie douloreuse et syndrome du sinus caverneaux d'orgine inflammatoire). N J Fr Ophtalmol 2:49, 1979

39. Hamby WB: Carotid Cavernous Fistulae. Springfield, Ill, Charles C Thomas, 1966

40. Holmes T: Aneurysms of the internal carotid artery in the cavernous sinus. Trans Pathol Soc London 12:61, 1860–1861

41. Seftel DM, Kolson H, Gordon BS: Ruptured intracranial carotid artery aneurysm with fatal epistaxis. Arch Otolaryngol 70:52, 1959

42. Unsoldt R, Saffron AB, Saffron E, et al: Metastatic infiltration of nerves on the cavernous sinus. Arch Neurol 37:59, 1980

43. Meadows SP: Intracavernous aneurysms of the carotid artery. Arch Ophthalmol 62:566, 1959

44. Jefferson G: Compression of the chiasma, optic nerves, and optic tracts by intracranial aneurysms. Brain 60:444, 1937

45. Nukui H, Imai S, Fukumachi A, et al: Giant aneurysms of the internal carotid within the cavernous sinus associated with an aneurysm of the basilar artery. Neurol Surg 3:479, 1977

46. Jefferson G: Extrasellar extensions of pituitary adenomas. Proc R Soc Med 38:433, 1940

47. Jefferson G: On the saccular aneurysms of the internal carotid artery in the cavernous sinus. Br J Surg 26:267, 1938

48. Jefferson G: Trigeminal neurinomas with some remarks on the malignant invasion of the gasserian ganglion. Clin Neurosurg 1:11, 1955

49. Rucker CW: The causes of paralysis of the third, fourth, and sixth cranial nerves. Am J Ophthalmol 61:1293, 1966

50. Raeder JG: Paratrigeminai paralysis of oculo-pupillary sympathetic. Brain 47:149, 1924

51. Talosa E: Periarteritic lesion of the carotid syphon with the clinical features of a carotid intraclinoid aneurysm. J Neurol Neurosurg Psychiatry 17:300, 1954

52. Johnston JA, Parkinson D: Intracranial sympathetic pathways associated with the sixth cranial nerve. J Neurosurg 39:236, 1974

53. Parkinson D: Bernard, Mitchell, Horner syndrome and others? Surg Neurol 11:211, 1979

54. Parkinson D, Johnson JA, Chaudhuri A: Sympathetic connections to the fifth and sixth cranial nerves. Anat Rec 191:221, 1978

55. Sunderland S, Hughes ESR: The pupilloconstrictor pathway and the nerves to the ocular muscles in man. Brain 39:301, 1946

56. McKinney J, Acree T, Soltz SE: Syndrome of ruptured aneurysm of intracranial portion of internal carotid artery. Bull Neurol Inst NY 5:247, 1936

57. Post M, Glaser JS, Trobe J D: Radiographic diagnosis of cavernous meningiomas and aneurysms with a review of the neuro-vascular anatomy of the cavernous sinus. CRC Crit Rev Diagn Imaging 12:1, 1979

58. Jefferson G: Discussion of the value of radiology in neurosurgery. Proc R Soc Med 29:1169, 1936

59. Chase NE, Taveras J M: Carotid angiography in the diagnosis of extradural parasellar tumors. Acta Radiol (Diagn) 1:214, 1963

60. Laun A: Survey of traumatic aneurysms, in Pia HW, Langmaid C, Zierski J (eds): Cerebral Aneurysms: Advances in Diagnosis and Therapy. Berlin, Springer-Verlag, 1979, pp 364–375

61. Lloyd GAS: The localization of lesions in the orbital apex and cavernous sinus by frontal venography. Br J Radiol 45:405, 1972

62. Chiu M, Tucker W, Hudson A, et al: High resolution CT of Meckel's cave. Neuroradiology 27:403, 1985

63. Demoris JV, Lana-Peixoto MA: Treatment by bilateral carotid ligation. Surg Neurol 9:379, 1978

64. Birley JL, Trotter W: Traumatic aneurysm of the intracranial portion of the internal carotid artery. Brain 51:184, 1928

65. Voris HC, Basile JXR: Recurrent epistaxis from aneurysm of the internal carotid artery. J Neurosurg 18:841, 1961

66. Adson AW: Surgical treatment of vascular diseases altering function of eyes. Am J Ophthalmol 25:824, 1942

67. Parkinson D: Collateral circulation of cavernous carotid artery: Anatomy. Can J Surg 7:251, 1964

68. Vandelen J R: Intercavernous traumatic aneurysms. Surg Neurol 13:203, 1980

69. Tindall GT, Goree JA, Lee JF, et al: Effect of common carotid ligature on size of internal carotid aneurysms and distal intracarotid and retinal artery pressures. J Neurosurg 25:503, 1966

70. Tytus JS, Ward AL: The effect of cervical carotid ligation on giant intracranial aneurysms. J Neurosurg 33:184, 1970

71. Parkinson D: Transcavernous repair of carotid cavernous fistula. J Neurosurg 26:420, 1967

72. Parkinson D: Carotid cavernous fistula, in Vinken PJ, Bruyn GW (eds): Handbook of Clinical Neurology, vol 12. Amsterdam, North-Holland, 1972

73. Parkinson D: Carotid cavernous fistula: Direct repair with preservation of carotid artery. J Neurosurg 38:99, 1973

74. Parkinson D: Carotid cavernous fistula, direct approach with repair

of fistula and preservation of the artery, in Morley TP (ed): Current Controversies in Neurosurgery. Philadelphia, WB Saunders, 1976, pp 237–249

75. Bedford MA: Cavernous sinus. Br J Ophthalmol 52:41, 1966

76. Solassol A, Zidane C, Slimane-Taleb S, et al: The veins of the cavernous sinus in the four month old human fetus. C A Assoc Anat 149:1009, 1970

77. Thomas JE, Yoss RE: The parasellar syndrome. Problems in determining etiology. Mayo Clin Proc 45:617, 1970

78. Winslow J B: Exposition Anatomique de la Structure du Corps Humain, vol 2. London, Prevost, 1734, p 31

79. Parkinson D: Aneurysms of the cavernous sinus, in Pia HW, Langmaid C, Zierski J (eds): Cerebral Aneurysms—Advances in Diagnosis and Therapy. Berlin, Springer-Verlag, 1979, pp 79–82

CHAPTER 72

Techniques of Thrombosis of Carotid Cavernous Fistulae

John F. Mullan

THE SPONTANEOUS MORTALITY associated with carotid cavernous fistulae is low and results mainly from occasional nasal hemorrhage (3 percent). The incidence of neurologic deficit, in the form of hemiplegia or aphasia, is also low. Progressive ocular complications (70 percent), up to and including blindness, do occur.[1] Treatment therefore should be designed to prevent these ocular problems but should not invoke any measure traditionally prone to mortality, hemiplegia, or aphasia. Traditional treatment, which involves some form of occlusion of the carotid artery, therefore is conceptually undesirable and inadequate. Either the fistulous connection or the total venous sac must be shut off by a procedure that is virtually free from any risk of mortality, hemiplegia, or aphasia.

Detailed study of patients with fistulae has shown that each is different and that safe occlusion must be individually planned and may involve a variety of approaches and a variety of occlusive techniques.

The thrombogenic materials are:

1. Copper-clad steel needles
2. Phosphor bronze wire (0.005 mm in diameter)
3. Occlusive balloons
4. Conventional thrombogenic material (Gelfoam, oxidized cellulose, cotton).

It should be noted that an electric current is not advised in any instance.

Approaches to the carotid cavernous sinus are:

1. Anterior
2. Lateral
3. Posterior
4. Percutaneous transjugular

The types of fistulae that have been encountered are:

1. Radiologically visible fistulous connections. This is ideal and can be dealt with by stereotactic or direct insertion of copper-clad steel needles into the fistula, using the lateral approach.
2. Fistulae that drain exclusively anteriorly into the ophthalmic vein. This group directs its entire force into the orbit and produces severe orbital problems. It is the simplest to deal with. By the anterior approach, the point of junction between the ophthalmic vein and the sinus is entered, and the sinus is packed with conventional thrombogenic material. In some of these in which there is very little cavernous sinus component and the artery opens almost directly into the ophthalmic vein, copper-needle insertion might be adequate.
3. Fistulae that drain exclusively posteriorly. The posterior approach is a difficult one. Parkinson's triangle is devoid of nerves but the carotid artery lies in its depth, which is a problem for needle and wire insertion. We have used: (a) Direct insertion of wire or needles below and behind the third nerve, avoiding the artery by means of intraoperative angiography. (b) Direct insertion of thrombogenic material into the superior petrosal sinus and thence into the posterior cavernous sinus. The superior petrosal sinus is not always adequately developed. (c) Percutaneous retrograde insertion of an occlusive balloon via the jugular vein. The inferior petrosal sinus is not always adequately developed.
4. Large fistulae of long standing. These are relatively simple to manage. Their specific problem is that the carotid cannot be visualized initially by intraoperative angiography. They are approached by the lateral route. Wire is first inserted intradurally into the safe anterior inferior corner. Alternatively, the anterior inferior corner is packed by the anterior extradural approach. When this corner is occluded, the artery begins to show up on the arteriogram and further wire insertion can be carried out close to the artery, as indicated. These large fistulae may require 80 or more feet of wire.
5. Smaller recent fistulae draining in all directions. These usually require a combination of several approaches. They may be difficult.
6. Bilateral fistulae. These are approached as unilateral fistulae, one at a time.
7. Fistulae with an intolerance to carotid compression. It is believed that fistulae with this problem are not as dangerous as intact carotids with the same problem. Since carotid cavernous fistulae carry little spontaneous mortality or hemispheric morbidity, however, it seems unjustifiable to ever take any risk of hemispheric insufficiency. Therefore, in bilateral instances in which the contralateral side was treated by carotid occlusion, and in unilateral cases intolerant to compression, all risk of carotid spasm must be avoided. Copper needles, which might cause carotid spasm if inserted flush with the artery, should either be avoided or inserted at a few millimeters distance from the artery, even if a small pouch persists.

OPERATIVE NEUROSURGICAL TECHNIQUES
ISBN 0-8089-1862-1

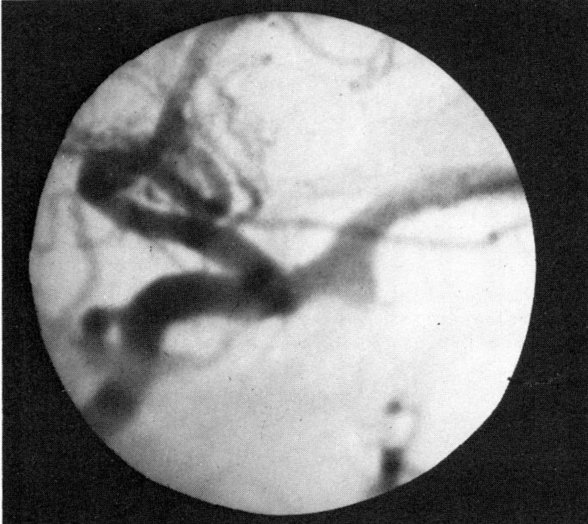

Fig. 72-1. This fistula drains almost entirely anteriorly.

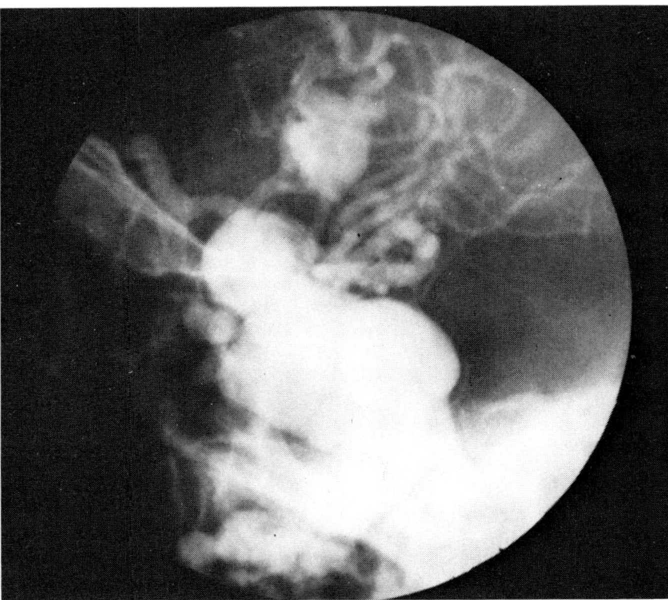

Fig. 72-3. A fistula of 6 years' duration with a greatly distended sinus and distended middle cerebral veins. The carotid is obscured by the sinus.

PROBLEMS

Two have been encountered:

1. Occlusion of the posterior exit from the sinus, before the anterior exit is sealed, exacerbates orbital symptoms and demands immediate attention.
2. Occlusion of both anterior and posterior exits without obliteration of the middle results in a central aneurysm, with resulting temporary nerve paralysis. This too requires further treatment once the condition is recognized.

Therefore, in planning the attack upon the fistula, the sequence and extent of each thrombogenic measure should be carefully determined. In general, it is desirable to complete unilateral occlusion in one stage, but staged occlusion is possible, either deliberately or if the initial procedure fails to achieve a complete result.

TECHNICAL DETAILS

SUPERFICIAL TEMPORAL ARTERY CATHETERIZATION

Angiography is necessary for the lateral, posterior, and transjugular approaches but not for the anterior approach. The essential components are use of intraluminal and perivascular papaverine; clear delineation of the lumen so that the catheter is not misplaced in the wall; secure anchoring of the catheter to the artery wall and surrounding deep tissues so that the catheter cannot possibly become displaced; and continuous heparinized irrigation.

Use of a carotid needle or catheter for angiography is not recommended during a prolonged operative procedure. The superior thyroid artery is a better alternative.

ANTERIOR APPROACH

Through a simple low temporal craniotomy, the region of the foramen rotundum is located anteriorly in the extradural space. This guides the operator into the inferior orbital fissure. The bone between the superior and inferior orbital fissures is drilled out. The arterialized vein is seen running down from the roof of the orbit to the inferior fissure. Its presence at the point of entry into the sinus is confirmed by aspiration with a tuberculin syringe and fine needle. This point is entered with a fine scalpel, and the sinus is gently packed with Gelfoam, oxidized cellulose, or cotton. These materials have different degrees of rigidity and are used in combination to secure gentle packing of the anterior sinus. The bulk depends upon the size of the cavernous distention. Care should be taken that the packing does not slide anteriorly into the vein instead of into the sinus (Figures 72-1 and 72-2).

LATERAL APPROACH

Through the low temporal craniotomy, the dura is opened and the temporal lobe is elevated after lumbar drainage and administration of mannitol. Radiologic markers are placed on

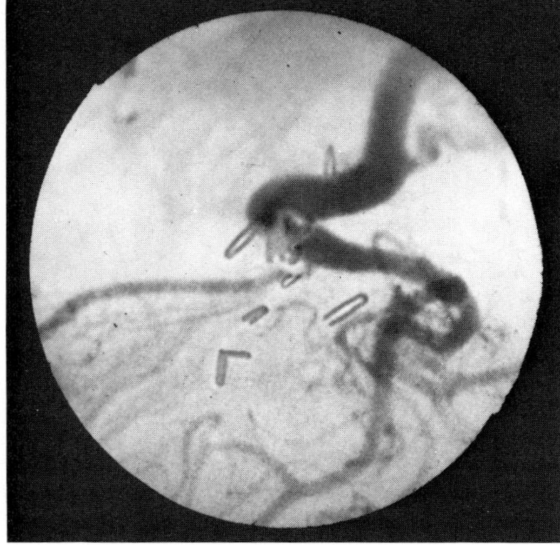

Fig. 72-2. This fistula occluded by packing the connection between ophthalmic vein and cavernous sinus.

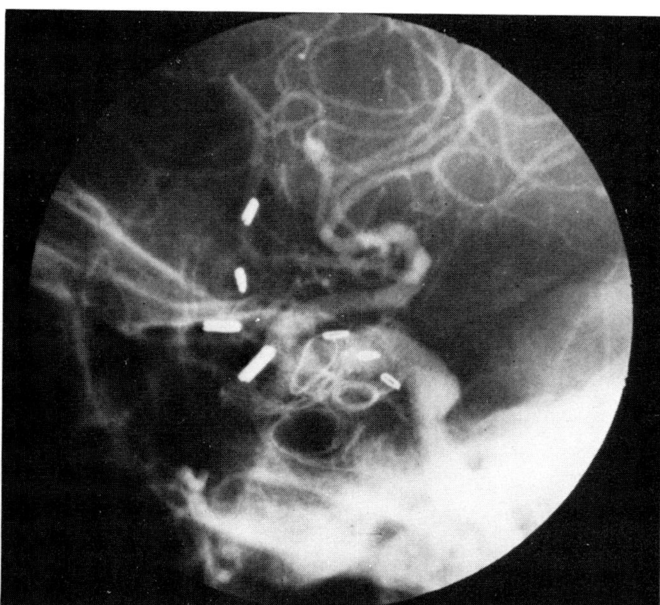

Fig. 72-4. A cavernous sinus occluded by wire inserted first into the anterior inferior corner. The three posterior clips are dural markers.

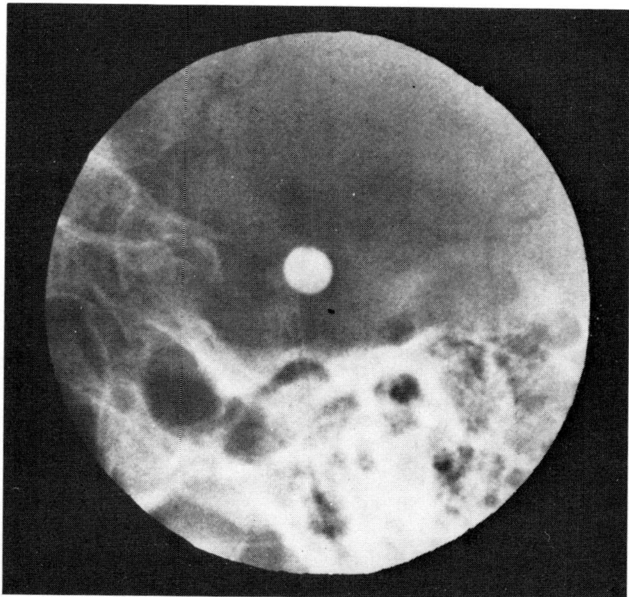

Fig. 72-5. Percutaneous transjugular, transinferior petrosal sinus insertion of a balloon catheter. This is applicable to some fistulae from the region of the meningohypophyseal artery.

the dura along the presumed path of the artery. Metal clips can be sewn to the dura. After angiography, phosphor-bronze is inserted, by the method previously described,[2] through a point in the dura that is radiologically free from artery. If the artery is not defined on the initial angiogram, wire is inserted anteroinferiorly (or the anteroinferior corner is packed by the anterior extradural approach, as already described). Wire insertion is completed when resistance prevents further entrance. Thrombosis may be completed at this point or may require further minutes, hours, days, or, in one instance, even 3 months. Usually it is complete within an hour (Figures 72-3 and 72-4).

POSTERIOR APPROACH

The posterior approach also requires intraoperative angiography. It too is intradural. Wire or needles are inserted behind the radiographically outlined artery and below the visually identified third nerve. If conventional packing material is used, greater temporal retraction is necessary. The superior petrosal sinus is entered several millimeters behind its exit from the cavernous sinus, and the material is packed forward in a gentle manner. This has resulted in a temporary sixth-nerve palsy on one occasion.

PERCUTANEOUS JUGULAR APPROACH

A No. 5 Fogarty catheter has been used successfully. A No. 3 proved to be flexible. The catheter enters the lateral sinus preferentially. Appropriate manipulation usually guides it into

the inferior petrosal sinus, but this attempt has not always been successful (Figure 72-5).

COMBINED APPROACH

In most instances more than one approach is necessary for each individual fistula.

RESULTS

In a previous study, 7 cases were reported and the techniques of stereotactic insertion of copper needles and craniotomy insertion of thrombogenic wire were described.[2] One temporary sixth-nerve palsy was encountered. We have since treated 17 additional patients. There was one temporary sixth-nerve palsy. In another recent patient the fistula was temporarily converted into an aneurysm. A partial ophthalmoplegia became complete and has again been resolved. There was no mortality and no sign of insufficiency of hemispheric blood flow in any patient.

REFERENCES

1. Hamby WG: Carotid Cavernous Fistula. Springfield, Ill, Charles C Thomas, 1966
2. Mullan S: Experiences with surgical thrombosis of intracranial berry aneurysms and carotid cavernous fistulas. J Neurosurg 41:657, 1974

CHAPTER 73

Commentary on the Transvenous Treatment of Anteroinferior Dural Venous Fistulae

Henry H. Schmidek   Joseph R. Madsen

WHILE SOME DURAL FISTULAE are amenable to resection of the nidus of their shunt, those in the vicinity of the cavernous sinus, categorized as anteroinferior lesions by Kempe,[1] pose a unique challenge. These fistulous short-circuits receive their primary arterial supply from meningeal feeders arising from the external carotid artery (ECA) or from one or both internal carotid arteries (ICAs). These lesions become symptomatic because of local venous hypertension involving structures within the orbit, notably the retina and extraocular muscles (Figure 73-1). The correction of the venous hypertension by obliteration of these fistulae forms the pathophysiologic principle of the transvenous approach which was pioneered by Mullan and described in the preceding chapter.

Our limited experience with the surgical approach for these lesions has been with progressively symptomatic dural fistulae, which produce ophthalmic venous hypertension and massive distension of the ophthalmic veins. This is the presentation in cases of dural arteriovenous fistula involving the anteroinferior group of venous sinuses. In contradistinction to the classical carotid-cavernous fistulae, which involve a major communication from the internal carotid artery to the cavernous sinus arising secondary to trauma or the intracavernous rupture of an ICA aneurysm, the arterial supply of these dural fistulae arises from relatively small dural arteries.[2,3] Hence, these lesions have flow rates which, angiographically gauged, are lower than the more common traumatic carotid-cavernous fistulae, as well as the majority of far more prevalent intracranial arteriovenous malformations. Angiographic studies demonstrate that the fistula occurs between meningeal branches of the internal carotid artery, external carotid artery, and the cavernous sinus. The most frequent tributary from the internal carotid artery is the meningohypophyseal trunk and its branches (Figure 73-2). A fistula involving this vessel is situated proximally and posteriorly in the cavernous sinus. For shunts within the cavernous sinus, additional arterial supply can derive from the middle meningeal artery, the distal internal maxillary artery, and ascending pharyngeal branches of the external carotid artery. The venous drainage from the cavernous sinus includes the superior ophthalmic vein, with anteriorly directed flow resulting from high intracavernous pressure, thrombosis of the posterior drainage pathways, or both (Figure 73-3). Occlusion of the posterior route may be important in the conversion of asymp-

tomatic fistulae into symptomatic lesions, and result in redirecting the relatively high-pressure venous outflow anteriorly into the orbital veins.[4]

The clinical presentation of these dural fistulae typically involves middle-aged female patients with proptosis, paresis of the extraocular muscles, episcleral vascular congestion, elevated intraocular pressure, and only occasionally with a retro-orbital bruit. There is a potential for visual loss as a result of retinopathy secondary to retinal vascular congestion, glaucoma, or retinal hemorrhage.

Spontaneous closures of these fistulae have been reported, as well as the anecdotal use of estrogens to hasten this process. In the face of a worsening clinical situation refractory to

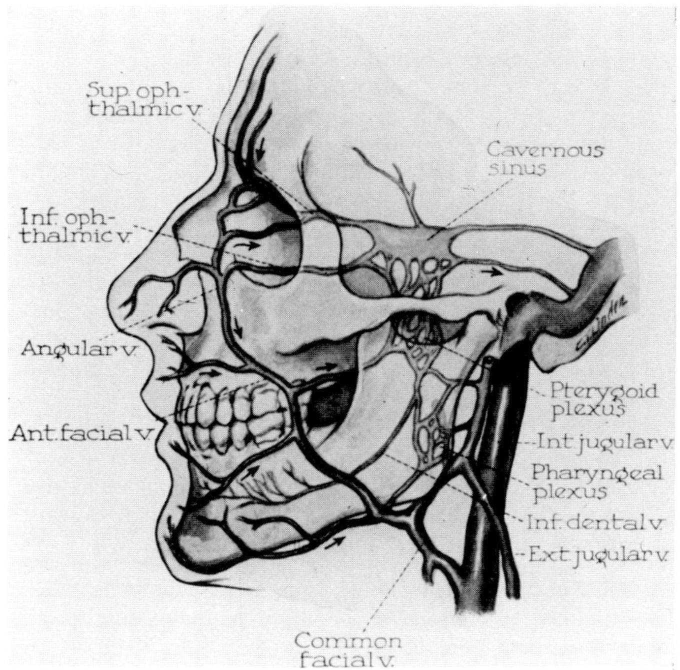

Fig. 73-1. Diagrammatic representation of anterior craniofacial venous drainage. This diagram does not show the confluence of the superior and inferior ophthalmic veins prior to entry into the cavernous sinus. (Reprinted from Thorek P: Anatomy in Surgery. With permission.)

OPERATIVE NEUROSURGICAL TECHNIQUES
ISBN 0-8089-1862-1

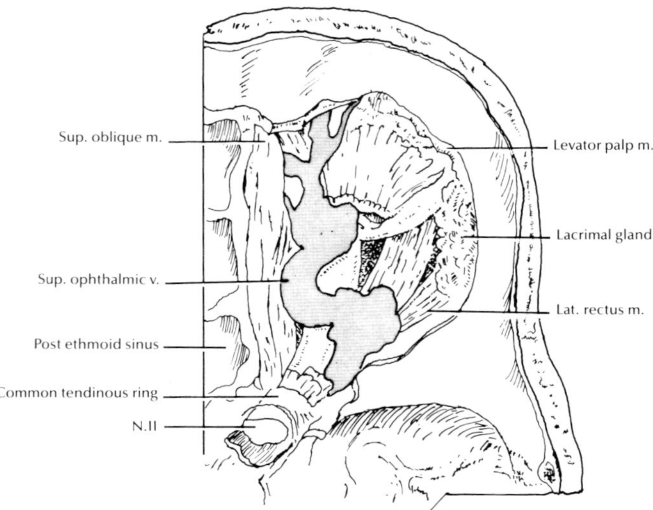

Fig. 73-2. Meningeal branches of the internal carotid artery which can contribute to arteriovenous fistulae. (Reprinted from Kempe L: Venous aneurysms and dural venous malformations, in Kapp JP, Schmidek HH (eds): The Cerebral Venous System and its Disorders. Orlando, Grune & Stratton, 1984.)

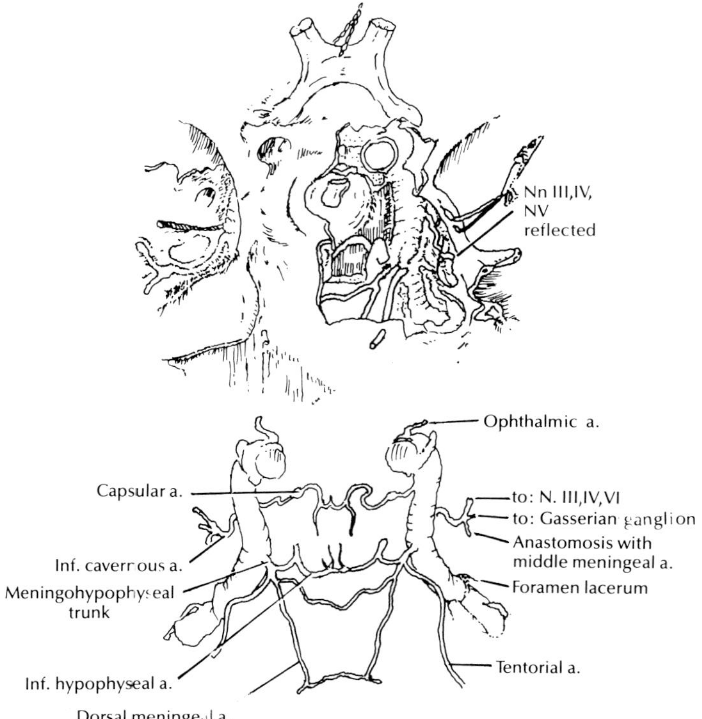

Fig. 73-3. Enlarged superior ophthalmic vein representing orbital and cavernous sinus venous hypertension. (Reprinted from Kempe L: Venous aneurysms and dural venous malformations, in Kapp JP, Schmidek HH (eds): The Cerebral Venous System and its Disorders. Orlando, Grune & Stratton, 1984).

medical treatment for glaucoma, however, the hope for fortuitous thrombosis of the fistula is less satisfactory than a direct attack on the lesion. Attempts at fistula closure using the conventional techniques of interventional radiology (Chapter 70), are in our experience only partially successful in closing the fistulous openings because of the multiplicity of the involved arterial branches. The direct obliteration of the intracavernous fistula without sacrificing the patency of the internal carotid artery, protecting the eye from the effects of the venous hypertension, represents the surgical goal. To interrupt the fistula within the cavernous sinus using Mullan's technique involves the retrograde packing of the ipsilateral cavernous sinus through its dilated superior ophthalmic vein, thrombosing the sinus and secondarily obliterating its arterial feeders.

With respect to alternative therapeutic options of carotid ligation or selective embolization, Mullan indicates five situations favoring direct venous obliteration[5]:

1. ICA-supplied fistula, with flow volume too small to permit balloon occlusion of the fistula while sparing carotid flow.
2. Combined ICA and ECA-supplied fistula, where embolization of ECA vessels alone would not close the entire fistula.
3. Recurrent fistula following prior carotid ligation or trapping procedures.
4. Bilateral independent fistulae, where the carotid sparing venous occlusion is indicated on at least one side.
5. Any case where the risk of ischemic complications from carotid ligation is high, including advanced age or known or suspected contralateral atheromatous disease.

The technical maneuvers required to accomplish these goals involve a pterional craniotomy and exposure of the foramen rotundum in the middle cranial fossa. Anterior and medial to this foramen one locates the inferior margin of the superior orbital fissure and defines the junction of the inferior orbital fissure and the site where the superior ophthalmic vein emerges from the orbit into the anterior-most part of the cavernous sinus. This vein is identified and its nature is confirmed by its aspiration with a 26-gauge needle. The superior ophthalmic vein is then opened between sutures on one aspect, and the cavernous sinus is packed using cotton, oxidized

cellulose, or Gelfoam. The structure most prone to damage during the packing is the sixth cranial nerve, and care is taken to pack gently enough not to damage this structure. When packing is completed as gauged by the resistance encountered, the superior ophthalmic vein is obliterated with hemoclips and divided. Our experience in three cases of anteroinferior dural venous fistulae with massively enlarged orbital veins and ocular symptomatology has impressed us with the value of this technique.

Our interest in this approach began with the experience of seeing a patient following conventional management of this type of problem. This 52-year-old woman experienced the spontaneous onset of unilateral exophthalmos, lateral rectus palsy, and raised intraocular pressure. No bruit was present on repeat examinations. Investigations included carotid and vertebral angiography. These studies demonstrated a dural arteriovenous fistula involving the right cavernous sinus. The fistulous communication received its arterial supply from branches of both external carotid arteries (meningeal branches of the internal maxillary arteries), and from both vertebral arteries (anterior meningeal maxillary arteries), and from both vertebral arteries (anterior meningeal branches). The fistula drained into the basal vein, straight sinus, and superior sagittal sinus and anteriorly into the superior ophthalmic vein. On five separate occasions selective embolizations were performed using the techniques of superselective angiography without significant reduction in the fistulous openings or in the patient's complaints (Figure 73-4). Subsequently, on separate occasions, the external carotid arteries were embolized and ligated with intraoperative angiographic monitoring of the fistula's appearance. Following the second operation there was a reduction of the intraocular

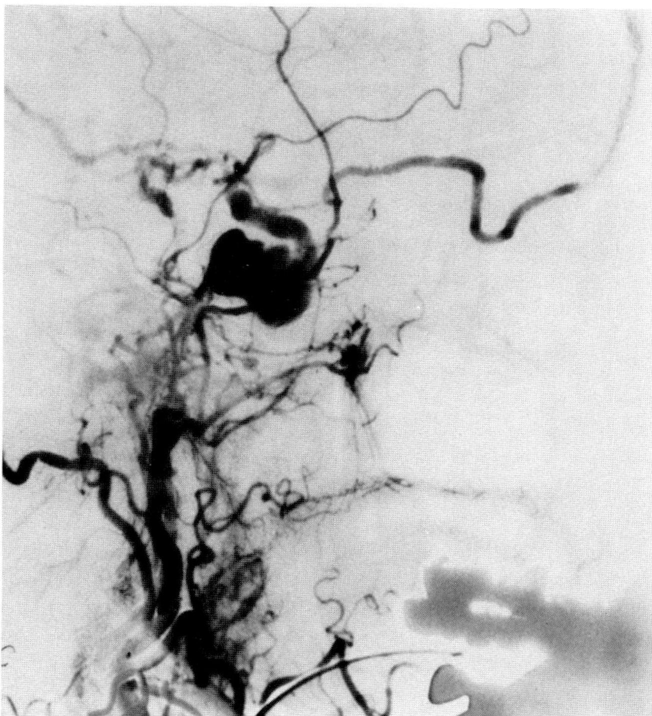

Fig. 73-4.   Selective external carotid artery injection following multiple previous unsuccessful embolization attempts to obliterate a fistula.

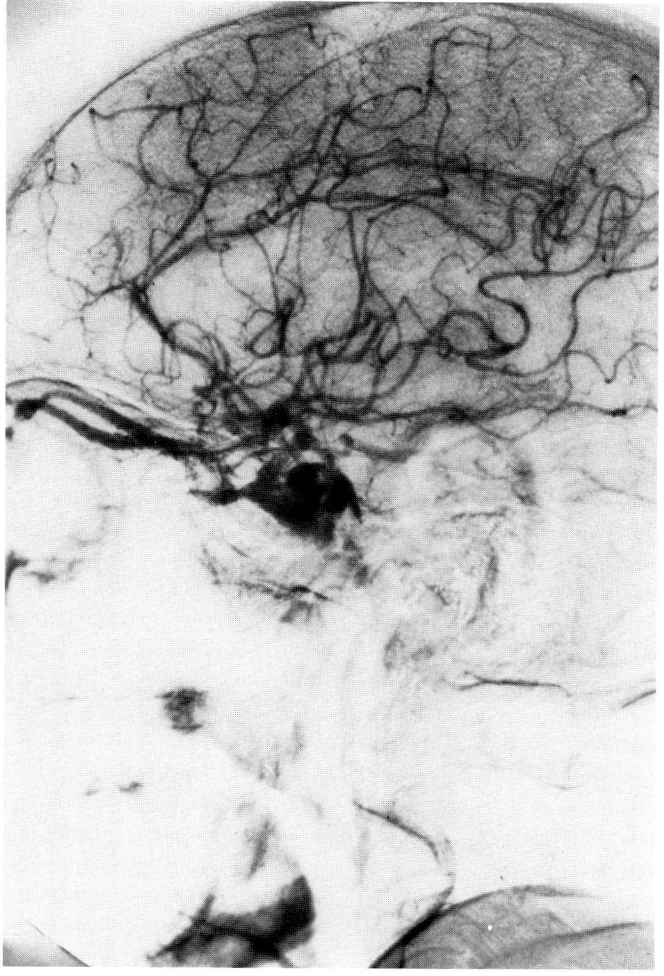

Fig. 73-5.   Preoperative lateral view of carotid angiogram showing the fistula of the cavernous sinus region draining into the superior ophthalmic veins.

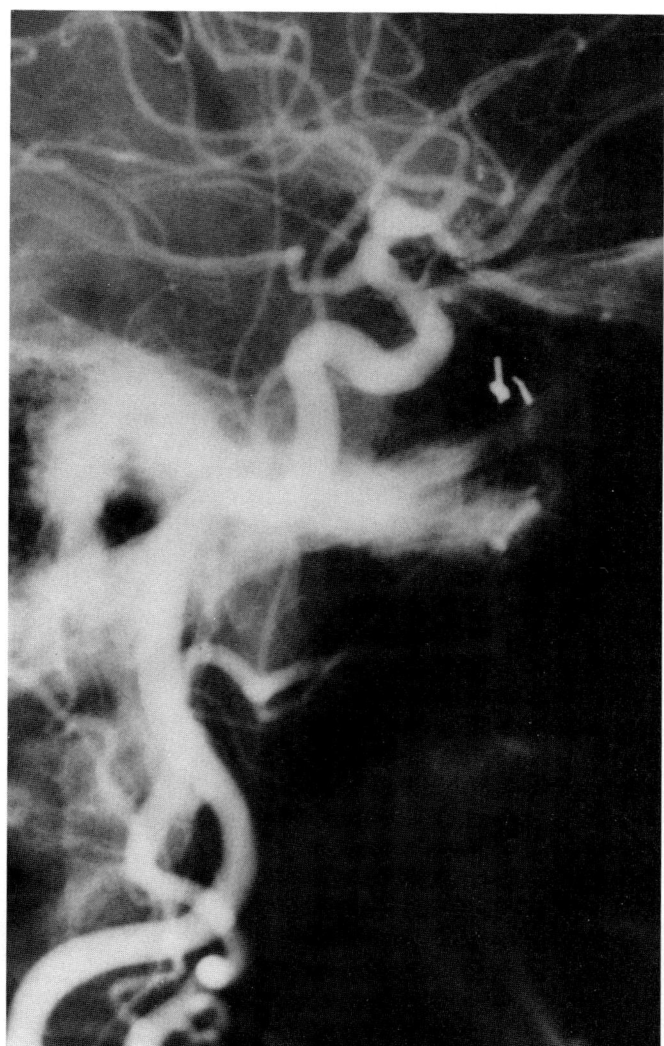

Fig. 73-6.   Postoperative lateral view of carotid angiogram (of same patient shown in Figure 73-6), showing obliteration of fistula with preservation of the patency of the ICA.

pressure to normal levels but no change in lateral rectus function during serial examinations over a 4-year period.

This case is characteristic of the cases of dural fistulae of the anteroinferior group in the following respects: the spontaneous onset, the absence of a bruit, the insidious progression with increasing levels of intraocular pressure, and the blood supply from meningeal branches of the carotid and vertebral circulations. This case also illustrates that although significant technologic advances have been made over the last decade in invasive neuroradiology allowing for the superselective catheterization of small intracranial vessels, the multiple embolizations carried out in this case by a highly experienced angiographer at a major teaching hospital failed to obliterate the fistula. The surgical interruption of the majority of the fistula's blood supply by sequential ligation of both external carotid arteries after their intraoperative embolization normalized the intraocular pressure but did not correct a longstanding lateral rectus palsy.

The next case was that of a 71-year-old woman who struck her head against a kitchen cabinet 6 weeks before she became symptomatic. She was in otherwise excellent health, but then

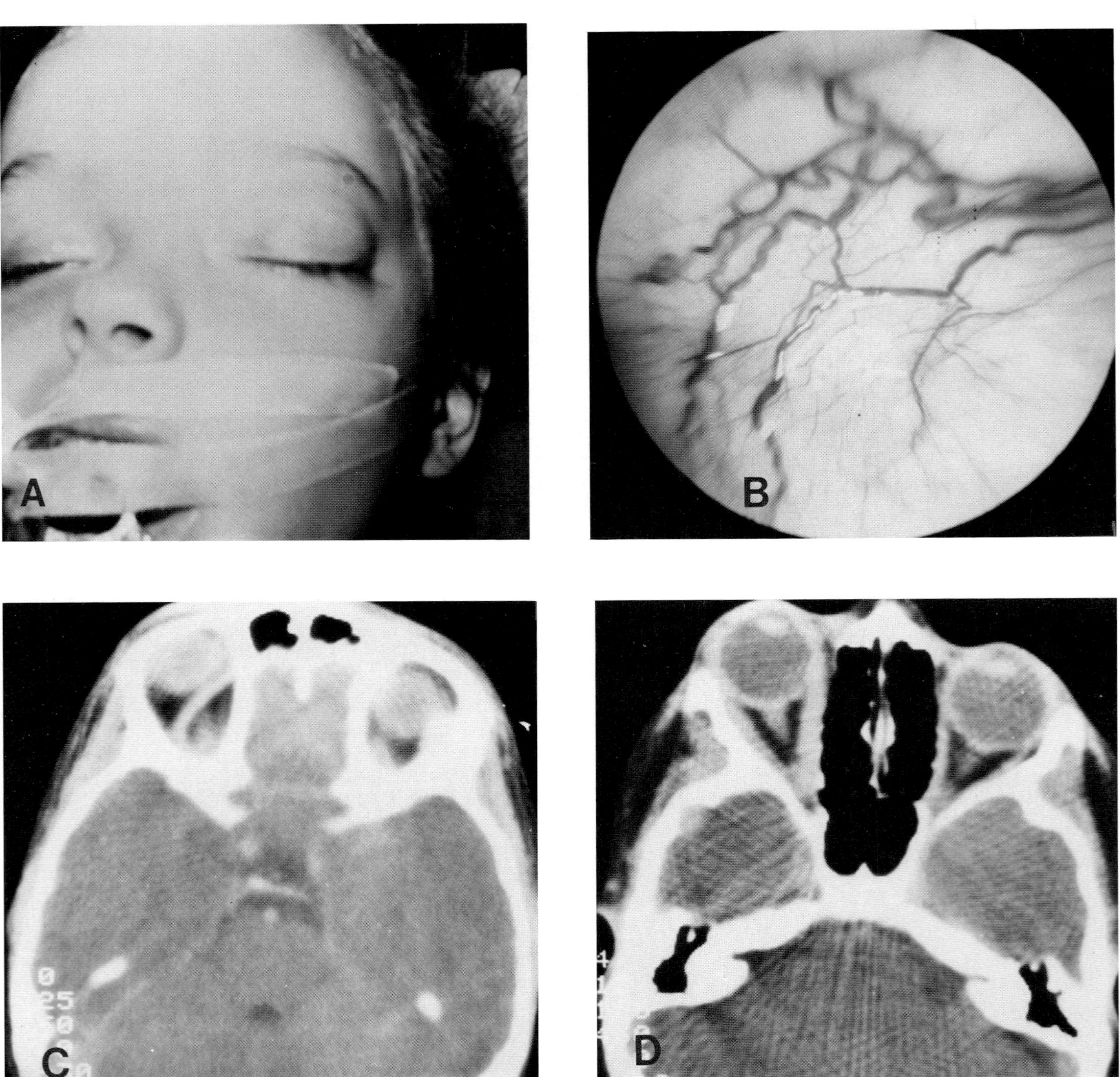

Fig. 73-7.   Clinical and radiographic presentation of anteroinferior venous fistulae with orbital venous hypertension. (A) Proptosis. (B) Dilated episcleral vessels. (C,D) CT scans, highlighting dilated superior ophthalmic vein (in C), and proptosis with swollen extraocular muscles (D). (E,F) Arteriographic views of fistula draining into cavernous sinus, superior ophthalmic vein, and angular vein.

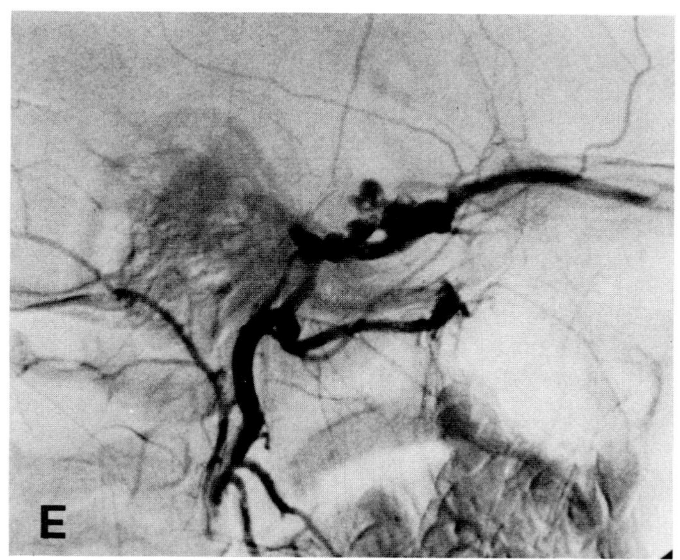

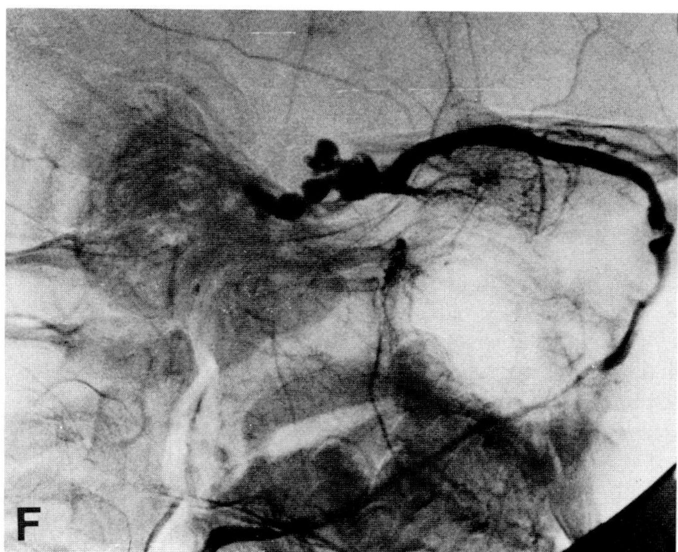

Fig. 73-7

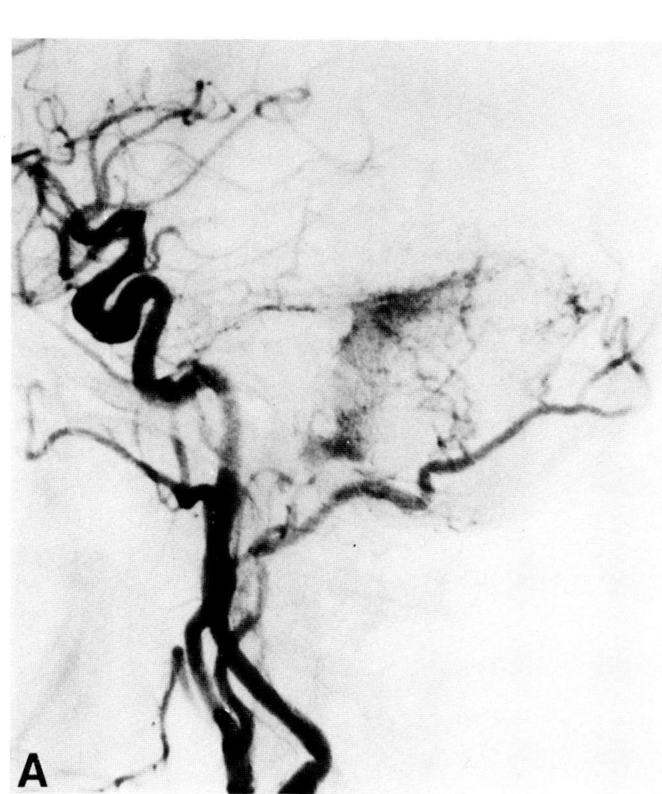

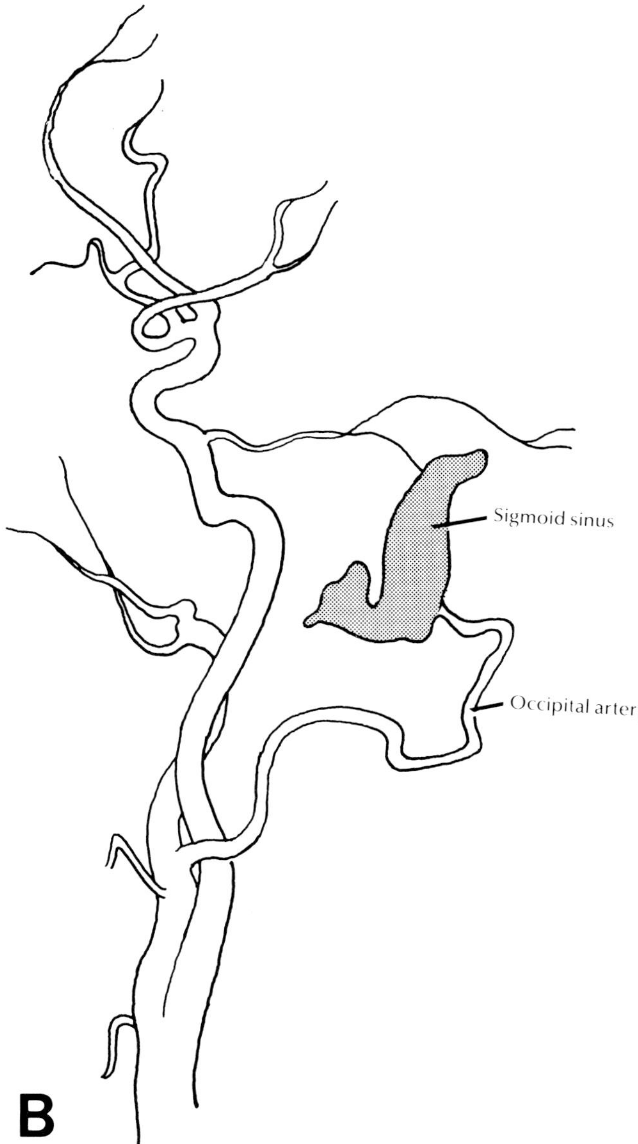

Fig. 73-8. Dural fistula involving the transverse sinus. (A) Angiographic findings. (B) Schematic representation of fistula.

developed diplopia and unilateral exophthalmos. A unilateral retro-orbital bruit was present. Angiography showed an antero-inferior dural arteriovenous fistula being fed by meningeal branches of the internal carotid artery in the cavernous sinus and draining into the superior ophthalmic veins (Figure 73-5). The fistula and its venous drainage were obliterated through a pterional craniotomy. By the fifth postoperative day the patient was entirely asymptomatic, neither bruit nor proptosis was present, and there was a full range of extraocular movements. Postoperative angiography demonstrated a patent internal carotid artery and elimination of the fistula (Figure 73-6).

Another case occurred subsequently in a child. Four months after sustaining a left temporal skull fracture crossing the middle meningeal groove, a 7-year-old, otherwise healthy girl began to have unilateral, left-sided redness and puffiness of her eye and eyelid (Figure 73-7A,B). The severity of these symptoms varied, but visual acuity and intraocular pressure were normal until 11 months after the trauma. The patient then began to experience diplopia, increasing left periorbital swelling, and a significantly elevated unilateral intraocular pressure. A left-sided proptosis, episcleral injection, and a retro-ocular bruit were now present. Visual acuity and fields remained normal. A contrast-enhanced CT scan showed an enlarged superior ophthalmic vein and marked swelling of the extraocular muscles unilaterally (Figure 73-7C, D). A large maxillary artery entering a fistula centered at the site of the middle meningeal groove fracture was demonstrated angiographically. The fistula drained into the cavernous sinus, and anteriorly into the dilated superior ophthalmic vein (Figure 73-7E,F). The studies of the opposite ICA and vertebral systems did not show any contribution from these vessels into the fistula. At surgery a massively dilated middle meningeal artery was identified and ligated, following which the still distended superior ophthalmic vein was identified, opened, packed, and obliterated in the manner previously described. The patient's

clinical improvement was apparent within days of surgery with elimination of the bruit and reversion of all ocular findings to normal by the time of the first postoperative visit 4 weeks later.

In contrast to these cases, a second broad category of dural arteriovenous fistulae are the posterosuperior group of lesions; those involving the superior and inferior sagittal sinuses, transverse-sigmoid sinuses, or occipital sinus (Figure 73-8). In such cases the symptomatology tends to be less mild and may include headache, retromastoid tinnitus, bruit, intracranial hypertension, subarachnoid hemorrhage, and hypopituitarism. The flow through these lesions is rapid and may arise from pial or dural arterial feeders or both. Because they do not disappear spontaneously and because attempts to obliterate them by embolization of feeding arterioles have been disappointing, the concept of radical excision, in which the involved segment of the transverse or sigmoid sinus is isolated from all arterial input and removed, has arisen. This is now considered an appropriate procedure in the management of this condition in symptomatic patients, and is described by Sundt in Chapter 74.

REFERENCES

1. Kempe L: Venous aneurysms and dural venous malformations, in Kapp JP, Schmidek HH (eds): The Cerebral Venous System and Its Disorders. Orlando, Grune & Stratton, 1984

2. Aminoff MJ: Vascular anomalies in the intracranial dura mater. Brain 96:601, 1973

3. Newton TH, Hoyt WF: Dural arteriovenous shunts in the region of the cavernous sinus. Neuroradiology 1:71, 1970.

4. Grove AS Jr: The dural shunt syndrome: Pathophysiology and clinical course. Ophthalmology 90:31, 1983

5. Mullan S: Carotid-cavernous fistulas and intracavernous aneurysms, in Wilkins RH, Rengachary SS (eds): Neurosurgery, vol 2. New York, McGraw-Hill, 1986

The Surgical Approach to Arteriovenous Malformations of the Lateral and Sigmoid Dural Sinuses

Thoralf M. Sundt Jr.   David G. Piepgras
Glenn S. Forbes

ARTERIOVENOUS MALFORMATIONS of the lateral and dural sinuses are uniquely interesting since they have been proved to be acquired lesions developing from a previously thrombosed sinus.[1] It is not our purpose here to discuss the pathogenesis, symptomatology, or natural history of these lesions; these aspects of the illness have been discussed and reported previously.[2–12]

In this chapter, we will focus on the surgical approaches and techniques for their obliteration, which were originally reported in the *Journal of Neurosurgery* in 1983.[12] Our experience is based on 41 cases collected over a period of 13 years. Clinical and radiographic characteristics of the case material are summarized in Tables 74-1 and 74-2.

PREOPERATIVE EMBOLIZATION

It is our current practice to diminish blood flow through these very vascular lesions by preoperative embolization 1 to 2 days before the anticipated date of surgery. This has resulted in a dramatic reduction in the amount of bleeding during the operative procedure. There is obviously an inherent risk with this technique, but in the hands of skillful angiographers and with careful monitoring it has proved in our experience to be amazingly safe.

It is beyond the scope of this chapter to discuss in detail the techniques for embolization of these malformations. Careful analysis of the preoperative angiograms is necessary. This includes assessment of the size and number of feeding vessels, the routes of access for therapeutic catheterization, the degree of flow through the shunt, which determines the type of occlusive agent to be used, and potential patent communications between the external carotid and vertebral basilar systems. Good communication between surgeon and angiographer is mandatory in assessing the risks versus the benefits for different embolization methods for the overall management of the patient.

Pre- and postembolization angiograms of a patient undergoing embolization before surgery are illustrated in Figures 74-1 and 74-2. Although the malformation appears to be well oblit-

erated from embolization alone, we are reluctant to accept this as a treatment per se, because our experience is that large malformations recur after embolization alone. When the malformation recurs, the circulation has been driven into the internal structures of the brain and dura, making excision extraordinarily difficult.

SURGICAL TECHNIQUES

POSITIONING THE PATIENT

The patient can be positioned semi-prone, as was the patient in the illustrative case (Figure 74-3). Or the patient can be placed supine with the head turned sharply (see Figure 74–5A). In either case, it is necessary that the surgeon have ready access to the region between the inion and the mastoid. A malleable lumbar spinal needle is placed for later drainage of cerebrospinal fluid (CSF).

SCALP FLAP

The incision used is shaped much like a question mark (Figures 74-3 and 74-5A). There is more than average bleeding from the scalp margins that must be controlled and secured well to prevent troublesome or unnoticed blood loss during the remainder of the case. The scalp flap is reflected to its base, exposing the mastoid process, and the occipital margin is retracted to the inion. In so doing, a greatly enlarged occipital artery and posterior auricular artery are doubly ligated and divided, along with many of their branches. In some instances, the major blood supply to the malformation has thereby been interrupted.

SOFT-TISSUE DISSECTION

After the scalp flap is reflected, the deep cervical fascia and nuchal musculature are incised with a cutting current just below their insertion onto the occipital bone. Invariably, a number of large feeding and draining vessels are encountered here, and these require coagulation or even clipping. The pericranium is

OPERATIVE NEUROSURGICAL TECHNIQUES
ISBN 0-8089-1862-1

Table 74-1. Frequency of the most common clinical symptoms and signs of AVMs of the lateral and sigmoid dural sinuses in 41 patients

Symptom or Sign	Number of Cases
Pulsatile tinnitus	37
Bruit	36
Headache	21
Impaired vision	11
Papilledema	7

now incised and stripped away from the bone along the path for the craniotomy (see Figure 74-5B).

CRANIOTOMY

The craniotomy is effected using the cutting bit of the air drill (Figures 74-4 and 74-5B). This is a very important step, and considerable care and thought are required to avoid potentially catastrophic bleeding. The craniotome should not be used here, since a laceration of the highly vascular dura or sinus (both of which are quite adherent to the bone) could produce a fatal hemorrhage—analogous to the rupture of an intracranial aneurysm before the bone plate is elevated. The air drill must be held at an angle of approximately 30 degrees to the bone; if it is held vertically it tends to drill through the bone. As the craniotomy is deepened, the drill bit is switched for a smaller one that allows better visualization in the depth of the cut and lessens the risk of a dural tear. The dura can be visualized through a thin layer of bone when the craniotomy has been carried to a sufficient depth. The surgeon is now in position to elevate the bone plate.

Before the bone is removed, preparations should be made for the possibility of a major loss of blood in a very short time. This is variable and seemingly is related to the amount of venous drainage that has developed from the arteriovenous malformation (AVM) through the diploë of the bone. We have found it helpful to lower the blood pressure and to start a rapid transfusion of blood at the time the bone plate is elevated. In spite of the above measures, the rapid loss of blood can be shocking to the patient and staggering to the surgeon. We have calculated blood loss to approach 300 ml/minute on several occasions. Although the loss is great, it can usually be slowed and controlled by digitally compressing a large piece of Surgicel, reinforced with a surgical sponge packing, over the entire expanse of the exposed dura. The margins are then gradually enlarged as the pack is withdrawn, and bleeding points are individually arrested with bipolar coagulation until the pack is removed (Figures 74-5C and D). As indicated, preoperative embolization greatly reduces this bleeding.

Table 74-2. Frequency of sinus thrombosis associated with AVMs of the lateral and sigmoid dural sinuses

Type of Occlusion	Number of Cases
Occlusion of ipsilateral sinus	16
Thrombus, ipsilateral sinus	4
Thrombus, contralateral sinus	2
Bilateral sinus occlusions	2

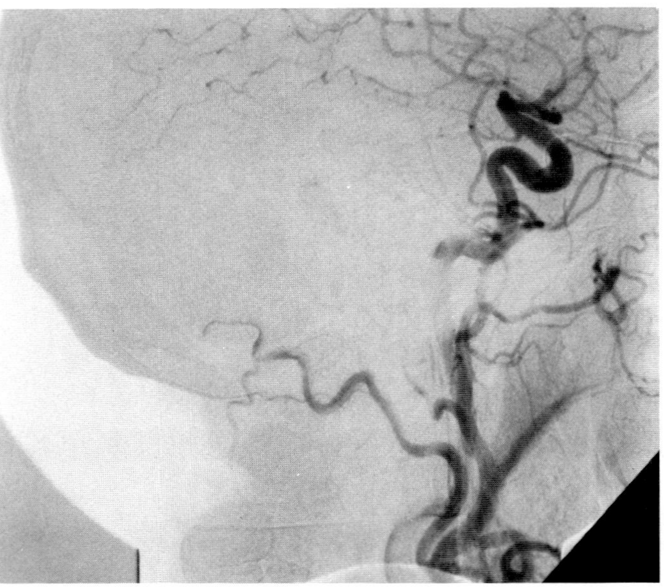

Fig. 74-1. A preoperative lateral angiogram demonstrating a dural arteriovenous malformation involving the right lateral sinus. The primary blood supply to the malformation is derived from branches of the occipital artery.

SINUS LIGATION

After good hemostasis is achieved, the margins of the dura are firmly affixed to the margins of the craniotomy with tacking sutures placed about 2 cm apart. These numerous sutures are

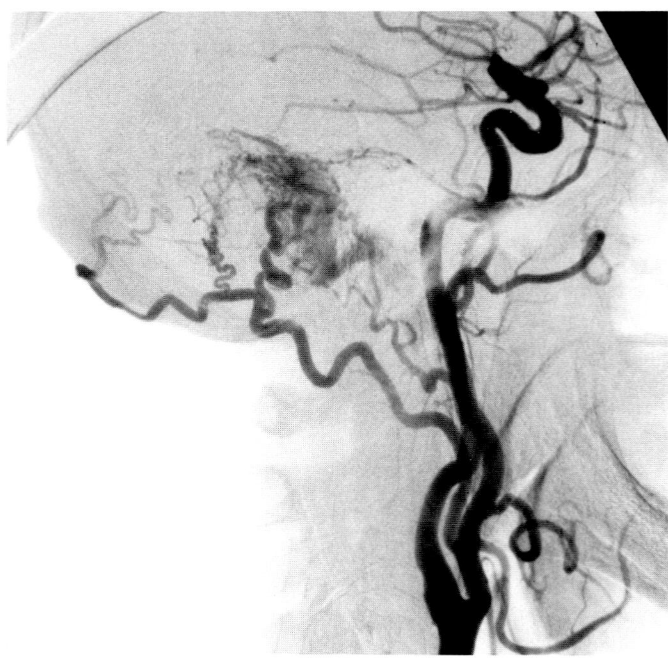

Fig. 74-2. Postoperative angiogram demonstrating: (1) occlusion of the arteriovenous malformation at the capillary shunting level, with preservation of the normal occipital artery; (2) closure of the shunting component of the posterior branch of the middle meningeal artery from occlusion at the capillary level (this would not happen if the occipital artery were ligated proximal to the shunt; in that case, the collateral supply from the meningeal circulation would continue); and (3) maintenance of the normal remaining external carotid artery and internal carotid artery branches.

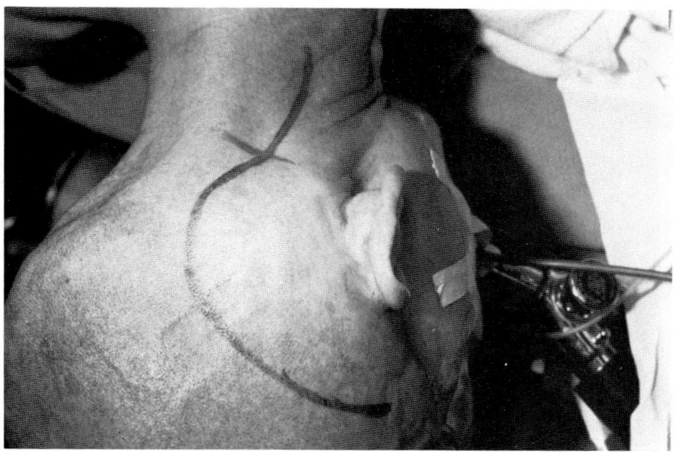

Fig. 74-3.   A curvilinear scalp incision extending inferior to the lateral sinus. It is shaped so that this structure can be exposed, with retraction, from the petrous bone to the torcular.

required to obliterate the epidural space, which is more vascular than normal because of its participation in the drainage pattern of the AVM.

The lateral sinus lies in the middle area of the craniotomy (Figure 74-5E). Two dural incisions are made parallel to the long axis of the sinus, one superior to and the other inferior to the sinus. These are enlarged by secondary incisions vertical to them, so that two Ts are created above and below the sinus (Figure 74-5E). Then 30 to 40 ml of CSF is withdrawn through the malleable needle previously placed in the lumbar spinal space. Bridging veins off the occipital pole and superior cerebellum are coagulated with the bipolar coagulator and are divided.

Two curved hemostats are next placed with an intervening distance of at least 1.5 cm across the sinus, followed by two more if necessary, lateral and medial, respectively, to the first pair (Figure 74-5F). The sinus is now cut with curved scissors (Figure 74-5F). The medial sinus is closed with a running suture, and these hemostats are removed.

RESECTION OF THE AVM

The lateral hemostats are used to elevate the sinus and its AVM from the wound (Figure 74-5G). With minimal retraction of the occipital lobe and superior cerebellum, the tentorium is exposed and incised bit by bit with curved scissors. The traction applied to the hemostats securing the cut edge of the lateral sinus places tension on the tentorium. Large feeding dural vessels are best controlled with small hemostatic clips. In this manner, the sinus is isolated from the dura overlying the cerebellum and occipital lobe, and from the tentorium (Figure 74-5G).

This brings us to the epicenter of the AVM, which invariably is located at the junction point between the lateral and sigmoid sinuses. The chief source of bleeding now seems to be the petrous bone itself from large feeding arteries contained in it. Some of these bleeding points can be arrested with the cutting current of the Bovie unit, but others are best handled with Surgicel or Avitene packed firmly into the vascular channels. In spite of the major bleeding that continues to develop as the bone is removed, it is necessary to resect the margins of petrous bone adjacent to the anterior surface of the proximal one third of the sigmoid sinus to be certain that the arterial supply to the AVM has been interrupted. This is best accomplished using a diamond burr on the air drill (Figure 74-5H).

Earlier in our experience, we attempted to resect the sigmoid sinus, but later we found this to be unnecessary if we opened it and securely occluded it by packing it tightly with Surgicel (Figure 74-5I). This has the distinct advantage of leaving a cuff of dura, which allows sufficient purchase for a tight homologous dural or fascia lata graft closure, a matter of some importance in avoiding the possibility of CSF leaking through resected mastoid air cells (Figure 74-5I).

VEIN OF LABBÉ

Bridging veins that are red can be divided with relative impunity, since they are draining the AVM rather than the brain. Those that are black must be respected, and this is

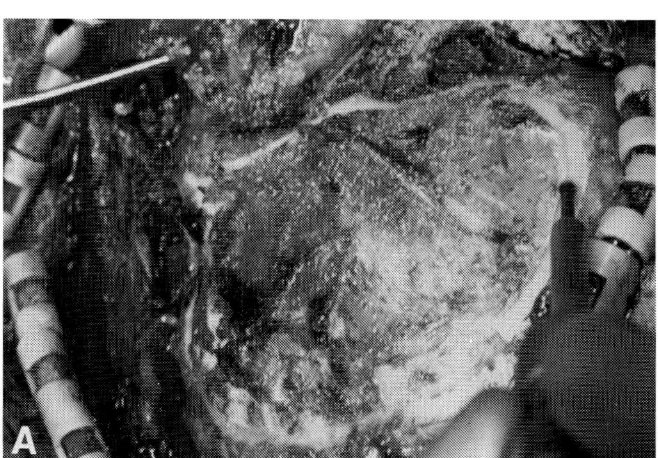

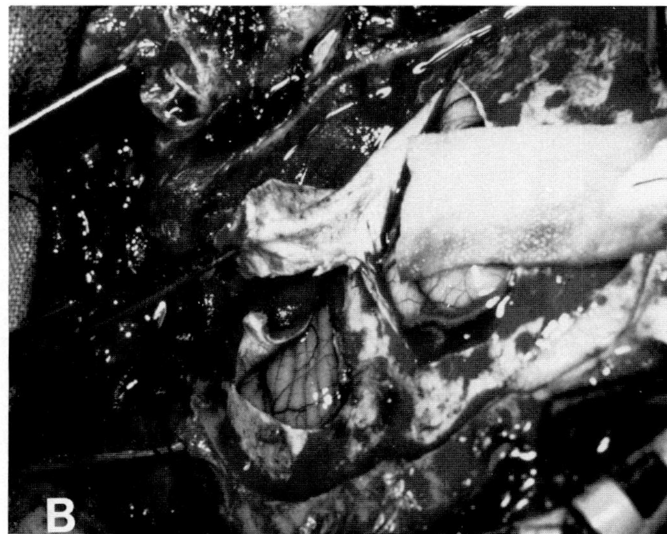

Fig. 74-4.   (A) Craniotomy is performed using a high-speed air drill. It extends above and below the lateral sinus and from the petrous bone almost to the midline. The proximal portion of the sigmoid sinus is visible through this craniotomy. (B) The dura is opened above and below the lateral sinus to facilitate resection of this structure.

Skin incision
Bone excision
MAYO ©1982
A
Mastoid portion temporal bone
Post. auricularis a. ligated
Occipitalis a. ligated
MAYO ©1982
B
Elevation of bone flap
Cavernous sinus
Transverse sinus
Int. jugular v.
Thrombus
MAYO ©1982
C
D
Occipital lobe
Cotton strip
Incisions in dura
Thrombus
Transverse sinus
Cerebellar hemisphere
Dura retracted
MAYO ©1982
E
Schematic view from above...
Petrous portion of temporal bone
Foramen magnum
Tentorium
Thrombus
MAYO ©1982
Transverse sinus (cut)
F

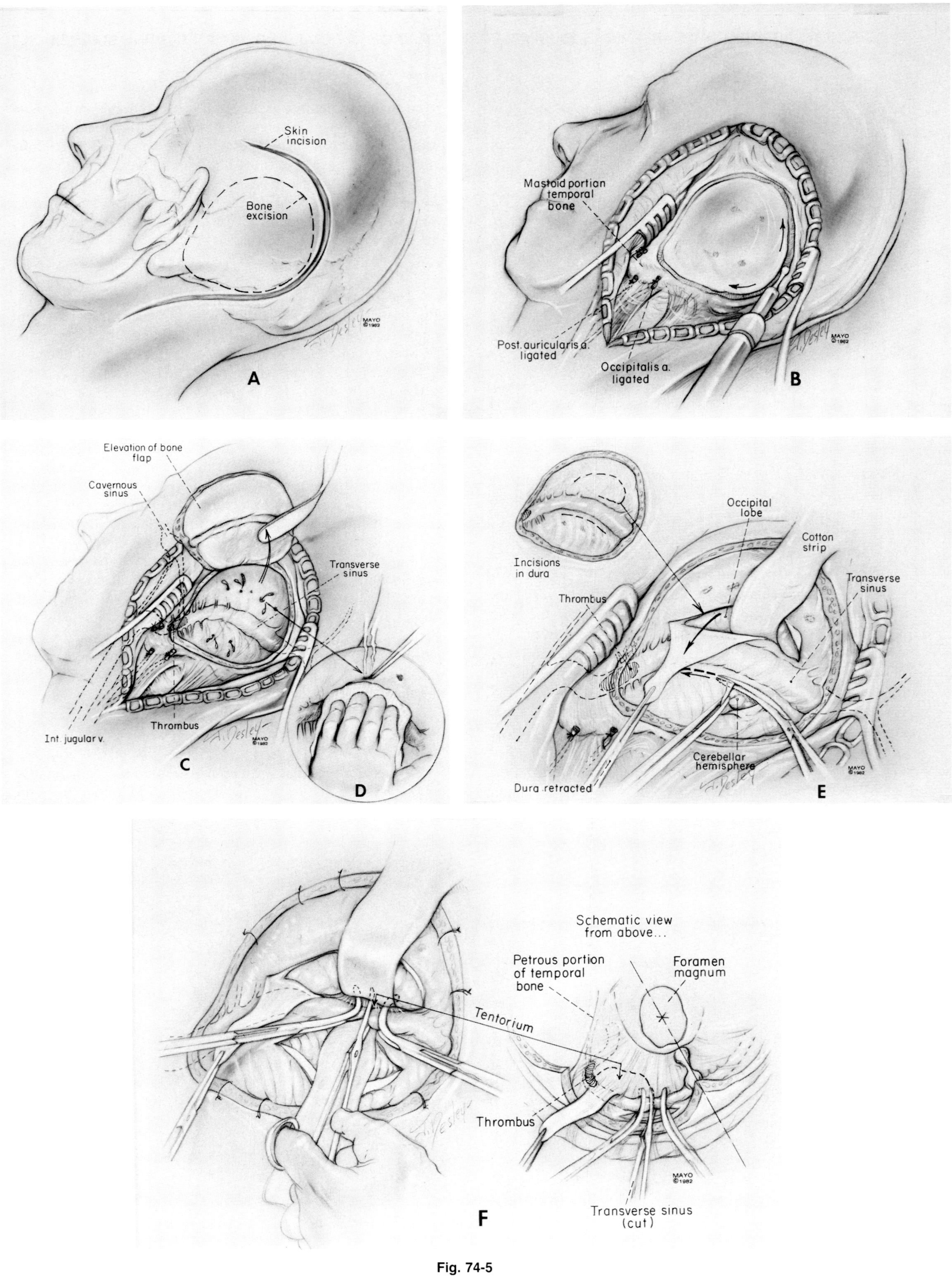

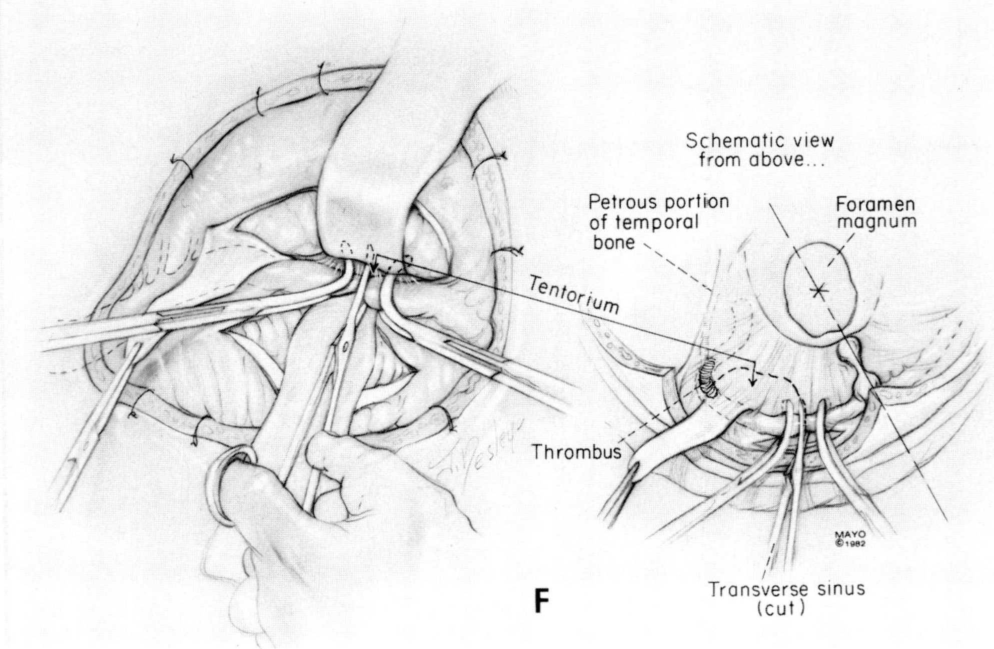

Fig. 74-5

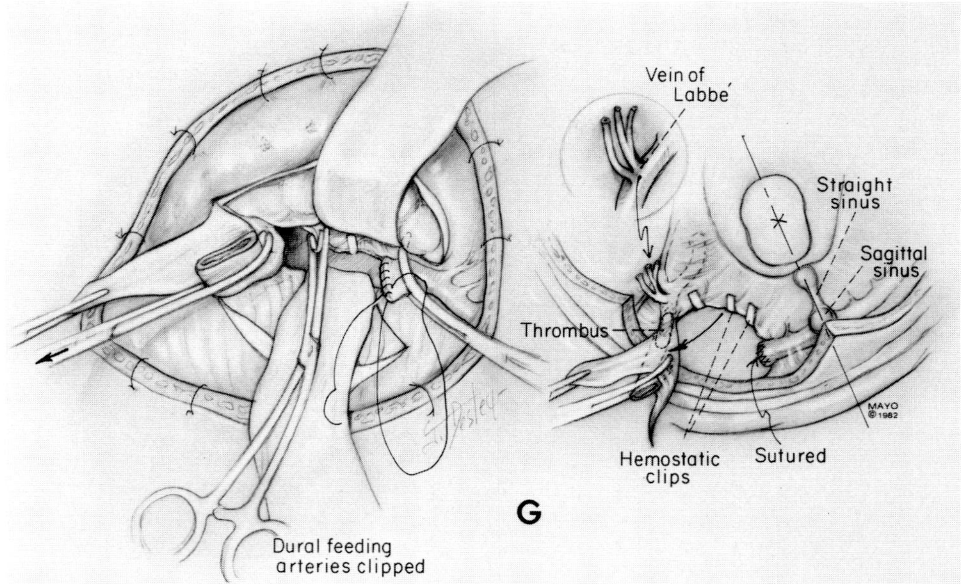

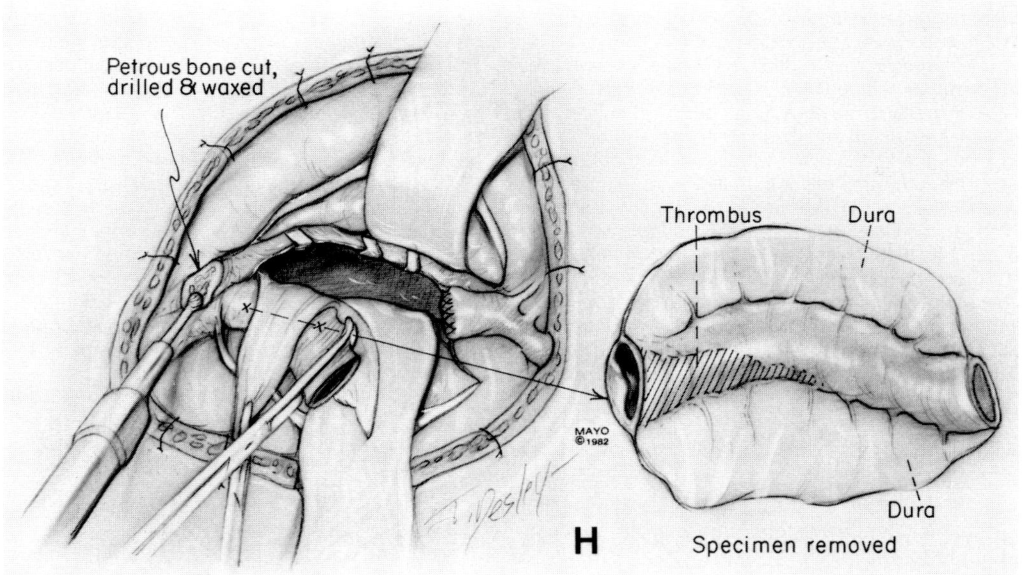

Fig. 74-5

particularly true of the vein of Labbé, which fortunately rarely interferes (see Discussion).

CLOSURE

The dura is replaced with a homologous dural graft or a piece of fascia lata. The bone plate is wired to the skull with 4 or 5 wires. The scalp is closed with a single layer of vertical mattress sutures.

OPERATIVE RESULTS

There were 36 excellent, 1 good, and 2 poor results in the group, along with 2 deaths. Two poor results were in patients who did not recover the use of their vision, both having been legally blind from chronic papilledema prior to surgery. Two patients died. One of these deaths was the result of a cardiac arrest related to blood loss; this occurred in the only infant in the series. The infant had a torcular malformation that was different from the other malformations in both its pathogenesis and magnitude. It was the only congenital malformation in the series. The other death occurred in a patient with a high flow arteriovenous malformation that was producing a progressing deficit and that had been operated on and embolized previously. The usual external carotid system supply was replaced with multiple dural vessels arising from the internal carotid and vertebral arteries. When the bone plate was elevated, a torrent of blood followed and the patient exsanguinated. Compression of the convexity dura was of no avail, as the entire dura overlying the posterior aspect of the petrous bone was simply a pulsating arterial sinus.

DISCUSSION

SYMPTOMATOLOGY

Although this has been reviewed previously, and it was not the purpose of this chapter to discuss the clinical presentation of these cases, a few brief comments are necessary for com-

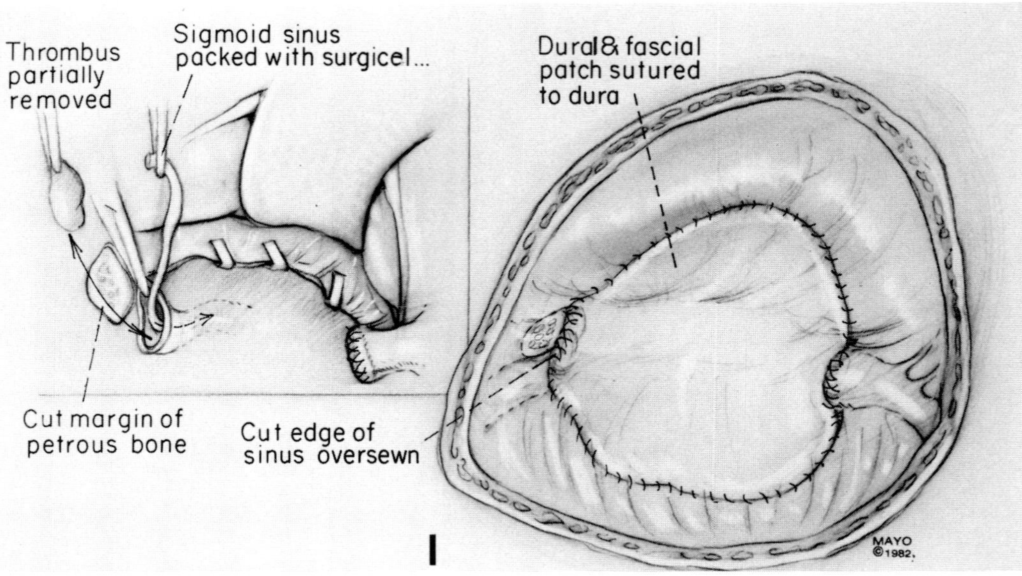

Fig. 74-5. (A) Schematic representation of the skin incision and area of bone to be excised. (B) The bone plate is elevated using an air drill that is held at a 30-degree angle to prevent perforation of the dura. The area of osteotomy is gradually increased peripherally around the margin of the bone plate until the dura is just barely visible through a thin layer of cortical bone. The bone plate is then elevated using a periosteal elevator. (C and D) After removal of the bone plate, dural bleeding can be profuse. This is controlled with bipolar coagulation of bleeding points and a large piece of Gelfoam that is placed over the entire expanse of exposed dura and held in place with uniform digital compression. The margins of the dura are then gradually exposed, as the packing is retracted and bleeding points individually coagulated. (E) Preparations are made for excision of the lateral sinus by opening the dura above and below the lateral sinus with incisions that parallel the long axis of the sinus. (F) After the dura has been opened, it is tacked up to the margins of the craniotomy securely with multiple, closely placed, dural tacking sutures. The sinus is then incised between 2 hemostats occluding the sinus proximally and distally. (G) The medial portion of the sinus is closed with a running dural suture. The lateral portion of the sinus containing the arteriovenous malformation is elevated from the wound using a hemostat and is excised from the tentorium. Major bleeding points on the tentorium are best controlled with hemostatic clips. In patients with a large vein of Labbé, it is occasionally possible to save this vein by carrying the incision directly into the sinus itself and then closing the sinus with a running suture so that the vein of Labbé can drain into the superior petrosal sinus. (H) The AVM is excised as far lateral as the petrosal bone, and a considerable portion of the petrosal bone is removed with a high-speed air drill. Bleeding from this area can be profuse, but is controlled with cauterization of the bone using the cutting current of the Bovie coagulator and bone wax. Examination of the excised specimen will often reveal a thrombus in situ. (I) Following excision of the lateral sinus at its junction point with the sigmoid sinus, the sigmoid sinus is packed with Surgicel and then closed with a running suture to the dural or fascial patch.

pleteness. A bruit that is annoying to some patients and incapacitating to others is usually present. This condition is not, however, invariable, and some report no noise. Headaches are the next most common complaint. These are relatively nonspecific in character. They may be caused by intracranial hypertension. Other symptoms of increased intracranial pressure (ICP) include visual obscurations, dimness in vision, and blindness. Papilledema may be present on examination. Two primary causes for symptoms of increased ICP and the findings of papilledema should be considered. One cause is simply the impairment of venous runoff because of associated major sinus occlusion, and the other cause is an increase in ICP as a result of high flow into the draining sinuses, with an elevation in the intrasinus pressure. Retrograde flow was a common finding in patients with AVMs of the lateral sinus. A retrospective analysis of the case material has revealed that, invariably, patients with papilledema either had associated sinus occlusions or an AVM of a magnitude sufficient to produce retrograde flow with or without an occluded sinus.

Focal neurologic symptoms have included classic transient ischemic attacks and seizures. Both have been attributed to increased venous pressure in the area of the AVM. Spontaneous subarachnoid hemorrhage (SAH) is uncommon in our experience.

PATHOGENESIS AND PATHOPHYSIOLOGY

Houser et al. presented convincing evidence that these are acquired lesions evolving from organization and vascularization of a previously thrombosed sinus.[1] According to this hypothesis, the sinus thrombosis is the primary event, be it spontaneous or traumatic. Subsequently, the clot in the sinus undergoes organization and, in the process, develops a dural blood supply with the potential for communicating with the patent portion of the sinus. The gradual hypertrophy of these vessels ultimately results in a dural AVM. Sequential angiograms have documented the progression of a thrombosed sinus to a dural AVM, and the concurrence of an occluded sinus and dural AVM in our experience is common.

If this theory is correct, and we believe that it is, then surgery will ultimately be required in most cases, since the AVM will continue to enlarge and progressively increase the intracranial venous pressure, producing the symptomatology discussed briefly above. Nevertheless, those affected are often elderly patients with other ailments, and a delay in surgery with a period of observation to follow the progression of the illness is acceptable. Insofar as SAHs are uncommon, they do not create emergency situations. If the signs of increased ICP become present, surgical intervention is mandatory.

DIAGNOSTIC STUDIES

Computed tomographic (CT) scans are usually normal, although some prominence of vessels in the region of the lateral sinus is sometimes seen on an enhanced scan. Magnetic resonance imaging (MRI) may prove to be more useful than CT, since abnormal flow phenomena in venous channels can sometimes be seen; however, this has not been established in clinical series. Angiography performed specifically for the purpose of evaluating a possible AVM clearly establishes the diagnosis. This angiography may include delayed venous-phase filming, subselective catheterization of potential feeders, vertebral as well as carotid injections, and contralateral vessel study to assess potential collateral supply.

ARTERIAL SUPPLY

In primary (unoperated or untreated) AVMs, the arterial blood supply is derived from 5 general sources: (1) the occipital artery and its major branches; (2) in large or recurrent cases, perforating branches arising from the ascending pharyngeal or posterior auricular artery are often present. These result in a vascularized petrous bone; (3) meningeal arteries in the dura overlying the cerebellum; (4) branches of the middle meningeal artery in the dura of the temporal and occipital lobes; and (5) branches of the meningohypophyseal artery in the tentorium. The occipital artery is usually the dominant feeder.

In recurrent cases, the occipital and more superficial dural arteries have been ligated and the blood supply has been driven deeper, much as it is in parenchymal AVMs that have had partial and inadequate resection. There seems to be a particular propensity for the dura overlying the posterior aspect of the petrous bone to become the primary zone of supply. This creates a very dangerous situation, since control of this bleeding is extraordinarily difficult. It may represent an indication for profound hypothermia.

VENOUS DRAINAGE AND BRIDGING VEINS

These AVMs often drain primarily through the opposite lateral sinus if the sigmoid sinus is occluded (although sometimes both sigmoid sinuses are occluded). In other instances, the exact source of drainage is not clear from the angiogram, and in these cases one should expect the drainage to be via the diploë of the overlying bone.

The secondary runoff can be composed of various routes involving the superior petrosal sinus, the epidural space and hence flow to the diploë, and bridging veins. Thus, with removal of the bone plate and ligation of the medial portion of the lateral sinus, the venous drainage has in many instances been largely compromised. Although this increases bleeding from the AVM, it is unavoidable. In any case, by this point in the procedure, in unoperated (but not recurrent) cases of AVMs, the major blood supply has been interrupted.

Prior to the operation, it behooves the surgeon to examine in great detail the venous drainage of the temporal and occipital lobes. It is virtually impossible to preserve major perforating veins from the lateral occipital pole or posterior temporal lobe. Fortunately, however, the occlusion of the sigmoid sinus followed by the development of the AVM has interfered with the normal venous drainage, and major functional bridging veins are uncommon, as the venous drainage has sought and found other avenues of escape. The reverse is, in fact, often the case

with reversal of flow and presence of red veins. These, as indicated previously, can be severed with impunity.

The vein of Labbé is a vessel of special importance. In aneurysm surgery, it is a maxim that this vein should be preserved if at all possible.

In dural AVM cases, it is usually not prominent, perhaps because it never was large, explaining in part the low flow through the nondominant sinus (thought to be a major factor in cases of spontaneous occlusion of a lateral sinus). If the vein of Labbé is prominent, it should be preserved if possible and allowed to drain into the superior petrosal sinus. Obviously, in this situation a radical resection of the sinus must be substituted with a less ambitious undertaking in which the dural supply and petrous bone are still resected, but in which a total resection of the sinus is replaced by a subtotal resection (see the legend to Figure 74-5G). In these cases, the margin of the sinus serving the superior petrosal sinus is preserved, allowing a reversal of flow and thus drainage from the vein of Labbé through the petrosal sinus.

TECHNICAL NOTES

The notorious vascularity of these malformations leads one to consider the possibility of placing the patient in a sitting position. In our judgment, this is ill-advised. The sitting position for this operation is hazardous, since the wide-open venous channels in the diploë make a major air embolism almost a certainty.

The second temptation is to attempt a piecemeal resection of the bone (in effect making a craniectomy), using rongeurs, rather than elevating the bone as a single plate. Not only does this result in a less satisfactory cosmetic result but, more importantly, the bleeding is greater since the exposure and isolation of the arterial inflow and venous runoff are more difficult to control.

Embolization through the external carotid artery may be a definitive form of treatment in those cases with exclusively external carotid artery feeders. Embolization, however, may provide only transient improvement and ultimately compound the problem for the reasons cited above. It should be undertaken cautiously and the patients followed rather closely thereafter. In those cases in which the age of the patient or other medical conditions mitigate against excision of the lesion, embolization is a reasonable approach. Fine particulate emboli or perhaps even tissue adhesives are useful in these cases, because it is necessary to occlude the finest distal branches of the lesion rather than simply to obstruct the major feeding arteries. Embolization may be a consideration in selected, extremely vascular lesions as a preoperative treatment in an attempt to reduce some of the blood supply immediately before the operation.

Every attempt should be made to excise the malformation as completely as possible with the initial procedure. The 5 cases with recurrence were technically a great deal more difficult than the primary lesions, and the 2 deaths were in patients in this group. It is our experience that recurrent lesions are more difficult pirmarily because the primary blood supply to the malformation is no longer from the external carotid artery but rather from deep branches originating from the internal carotid artery.

We have not found the operating microscope particularly helpful in this procedure because of the extraordinary vascularity of the lesions and the size of the operative field. Magnification loupes have, however, been most helpful.

REFERENCES

1. Houser OW, Campbell JK, Campbell RJ, et al: Arteriovenous malformation affecting the transverse dural venous sinus—An acquired lesion. Mayo Clin Proc 54:651, 1979
2. Aminoff MJ: Vascular anomalies in the intracranial dura mater. Brain 96:601, 1973
3. Handa J, Yoneda S, Handa H: Venous sinus occlusion with a dural arteriovenous malformation of the posterior fossa. Surg Neurol 4:433, 1975
4. Hugosson R, Bergstrom K: Surgical treatment of dural arteriovenous malformation in the region of the sigmoid sinus. J Neurol Neurosurg Psychiatry 37:97, 1974
5. Kosnik EJ, Hunt WE, Miller CA: Dural arteriovenous malformations. J Neurosurg 40:322, 1974
6. Kuhner A, Krastel A, Stoll W: Arteriovenous malformations of the transverse dural sinus. J Neurosurg 45:12, 1976
7. Lamas E, Lobato RD, Esparza J, et al: Dural posterior fossa AVM producing raised sagittal sinus pressure. Case report. J Neurosurg 46:804, 1977
8. Magidson MA, Weinberg PE: Spontaneous closure of a dural arteriovenous malformation. Surg Neurol 6:107, 1976
9. Newton TH, Cronqvist S: Involvement of dural arteries in intracranial arteriovenous malformations. Radiology 93:1071, 1969
10. Nicola GC, Nizzoli V: Dural arteriovenous malformations of the posterior fossa. J Neurol Neurosurg Psychiatry 31:514, 1968
11. Obrador S, Soto M, Silvela J: Clinical syndromes of arteriovenous malformations of the transverse-sigmoid sinus. J Neurol Neurosurg Psychiatry 38:436, 1975
12. Sundt TM Jr, Piepgras DG: The surgical approach to arteriovenous malformations of the lateral and sigmoid dural sinuses. J Neurosurg 59:32, 1983

CHAPTER 75

Surgical Management of Lesions of the Dural Venous Sinuses

R. M. Peardon Donaghy

TRAUMA OF THE DURAL SINUSES of a severity sufficient to warrant surgical consideration is more common in military situations than in civilian life, but the occurrence nonetheless is common enough to merit familiarity with the forms of therapy.[1] On occasion, therapy could prove lifesaving.

Although there are five single and six sets of paired venous sinuses within the cranium,[2,3] only one of the former—the superior longitudinal or superior sagittal sinus—and two of the latter—the cavernous and the lateral or transverse sinuses—have a frequency of trauma and a specificity of therapy sufficient to suggest individual consideration.

The aims of surgical interference include:

1. The control of hemorrhage.
2. The elimination of compressive obstruction.
3. The reinstitution of normal blood flow.
4. The elimination of abnormal vascular communications.

In general, a venous channel can be sacrificed during surgery and not repaired or reconstituted if there is adequate venous drainage of the area by an alternate route. The superior longitudinal sinus ordinarily can be ligated with impunity along the anterior one third of its course, for example, but ligation in the posterior two thirds, especially posterior to the rolandic fissure, is likely to lead to increasing intracranial pressure, often with alarming rapidity (Figure 75-1).[3–5] If the patient's condition permits, presurgical evaluation of venous drainage and its pattern in the area can be accomplished by angiography. If the patient's condition does not permit such presurgical examination, such information can be gained by intraoperative sinography. In performing sinography, care must be taken to confine the contrast medium to the interior of the sinus, since the medium may be an intense irritant to the cerebral cortex.

A corollary to the above general principle is that the loss of a large venous drainage channel that serves an area that does not have other drainage facilities may portend a grave emergency. A lateral or transverse sinus should not be occluded unless there is adequate drainage from the opposite side. Likewise, should a cervical wound cause injury to an internal jugular vein, the vein should not be permanently ligated until patency of the opposite internal jugular vein has been confirmed or provision made for whatever bypass procedure will allow for adequate drainage.[6,7]

CONTROL OF HEMORRHAGE

Puncture wounds or small openings into a major sinus usually do not pose a severe problem since the wound is small, bleeding is at venous pressure, and, if the bleeding occurs on the external surface of the sinus, it is often tamponaded against the skull. Moreover, since bleeding usually occurs at a fracture line, the site is apparent.

Simple puncture or short linear tears can be sutured directly (Figures 75-2 and 75-3). Larger or irregular tears may require patching. The adjacent dura is an excellent source of patch material (Figures 75-4, 75-5, and 75-6).

ELIMINATION OF COMPRESSIVE OBSTRUCTION

A rare situation but one of great danger to the patient can occur when a small amount of bleeding occurs between the fracture line and the external surface of the sinus. If the clot exerts enough pressure upon the sinus to obstruct it and the dura does not strip away from the skull sufficiently to relieve it, intracranial pressure may develop very rapidly if the sinus has no adequate collateral drainage. There may not be enough time for angiography, and the lesion may not be demonstrable in other studies. The essential thing is to keep this danger in mind. Immediate decompression at the fracture site may be lifesaving. Once decompressed, flow in the sinus should be confirmed before the wound is closed, lest thrombus within the sinus remain unrecognized. Flow in the sinus can be confirmed by aspirating at the site, or by angiography or sinography.

On occasion one may find the sinus totally disrupted or even a portion of the sinus avulsed. A clot may be dislodged in exploring the wound, allowing for brisk hemorrhage from the open sinus ends. A maneuver that has been of great value is to quickly control the hemorrhage by inserting a finger beneath the sinus and exerting pressure outward against the intact skull while an assistant performs the same maneuver at the opposite end of the wound (Figures 75-7, 75-8, and 75-9). Care should be exercised not to tear bridging veins. The maneuver should not be done blindly except in the most urgent of circumstances. Adequate washing and suction usually provide acceptable visibility.

Once the hemorrhage is controlled, we have found it expedient to introduce a siliconized vascular T-tube, with each

OPERATIVE NEUROSURGICAL TECHNIQUES
ISBN 0-8089-1862-1

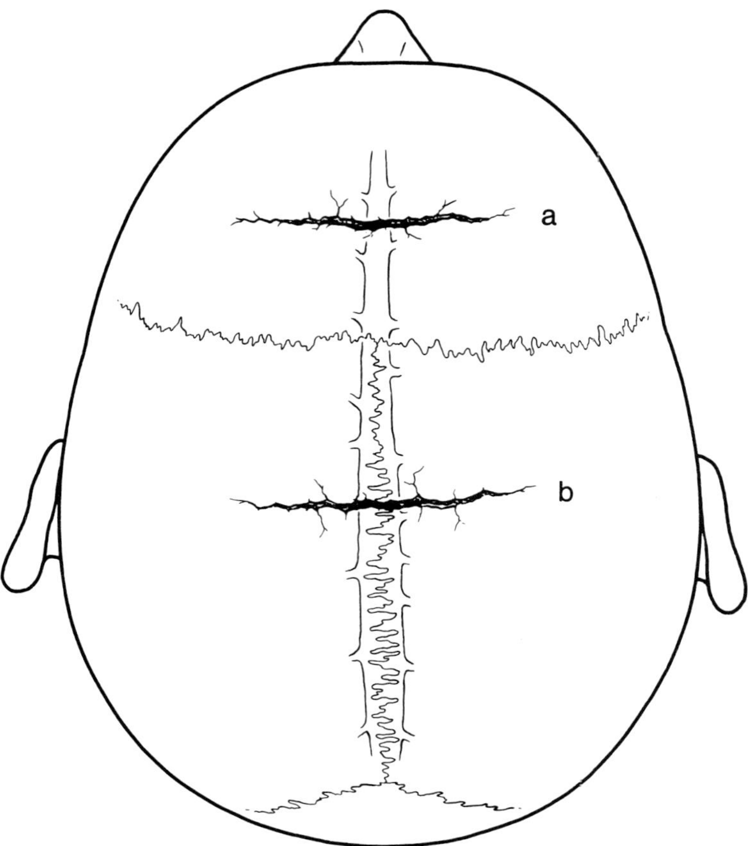

Fig. 75-1. The sinus beneath fracture A probably can be ligated safely if it is damaged beyond easy repair. The sinus beneath fracture B probably cannot be ligated without serious consequences. The surgeon should be prepared to handle a disrupted sinus before embarking upon exploration.

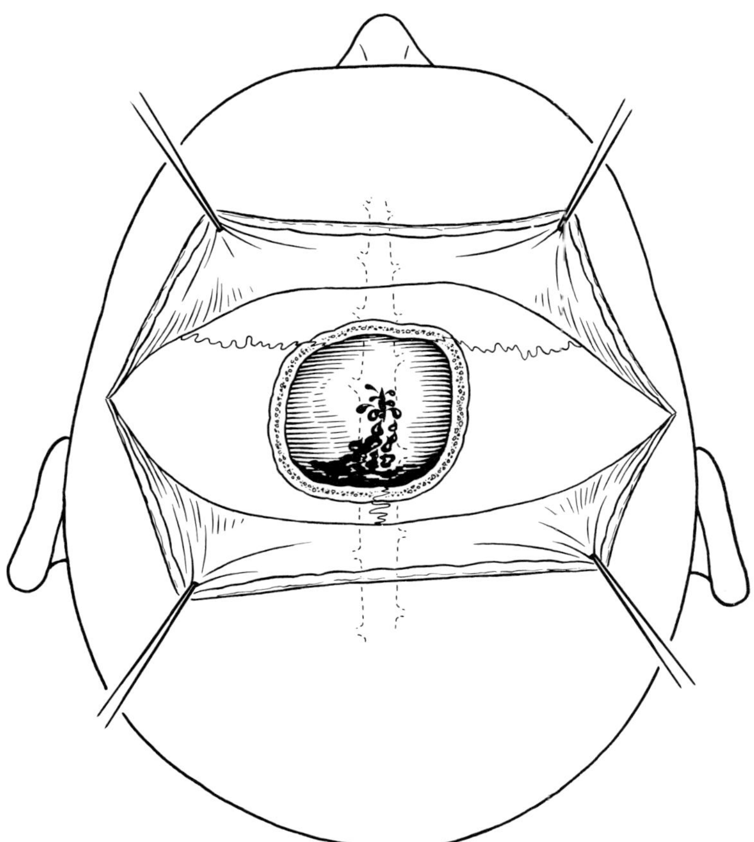

Fig. 75-2. Bleeding from a small rent in a sinus.

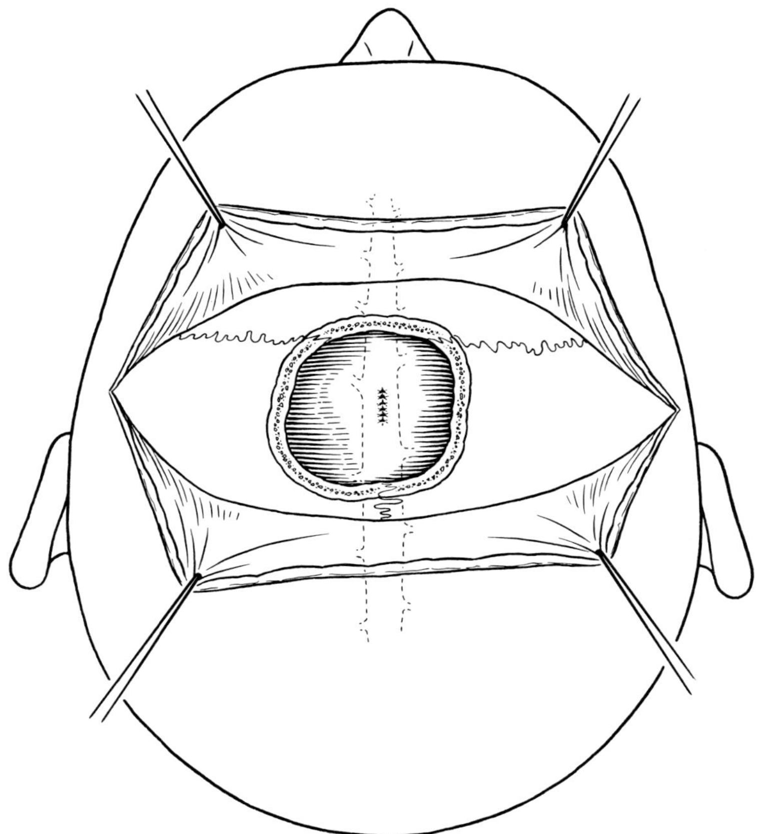

Fig. 75-3. Repair of a linear rent by direct suture.

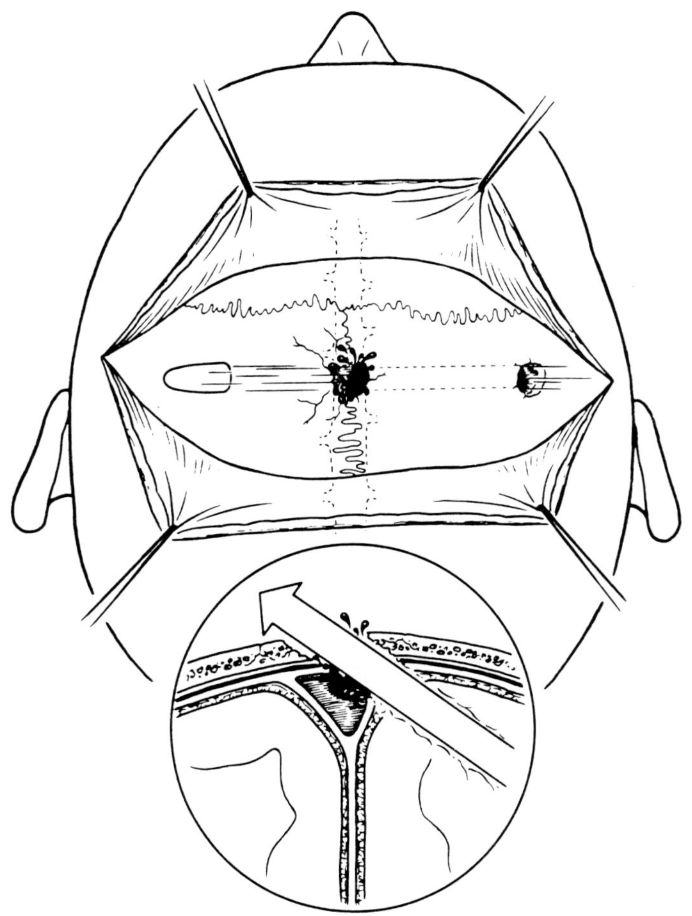

Fig. 75-4. Loss of a portion of a sinus wall from a gunshot wound.

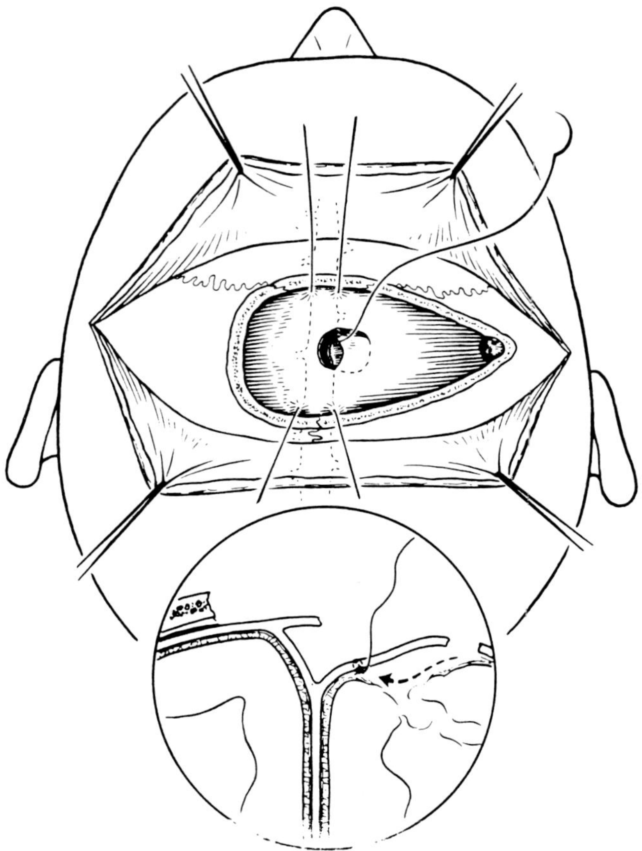

Fig. 75-5. Patch of a sinus wall using adjacent dura.

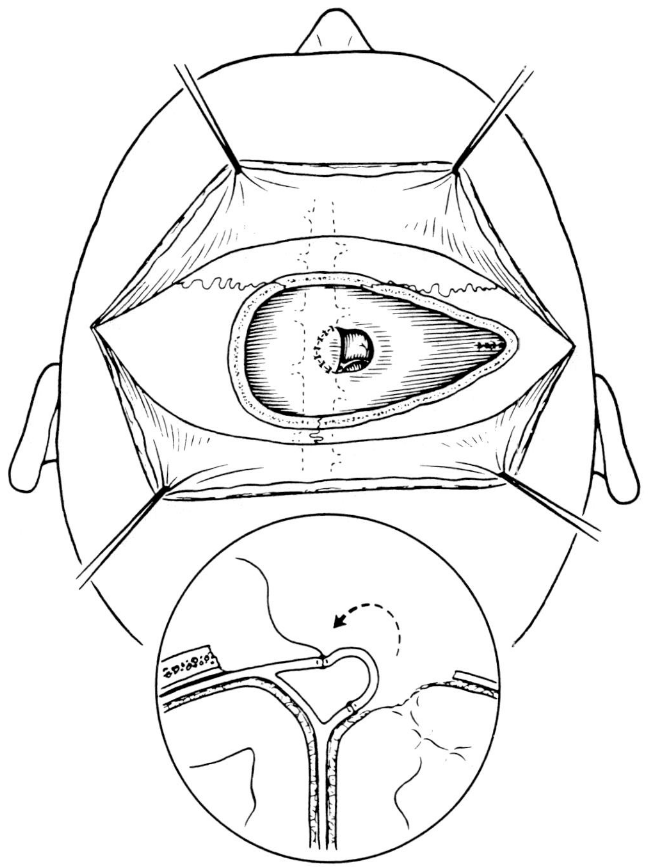

Fig. 75-6. Completed patch of the sinus in Figure 75-5.

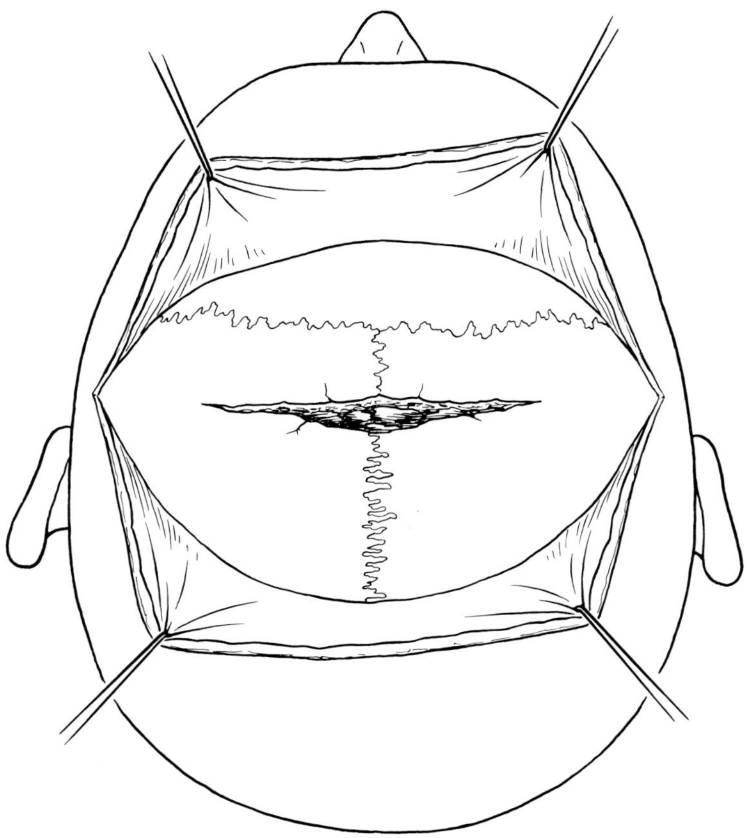

Fig. 75-7. A wide fracture line, warning the surgeon that the underlying sinus may be extensively torn.

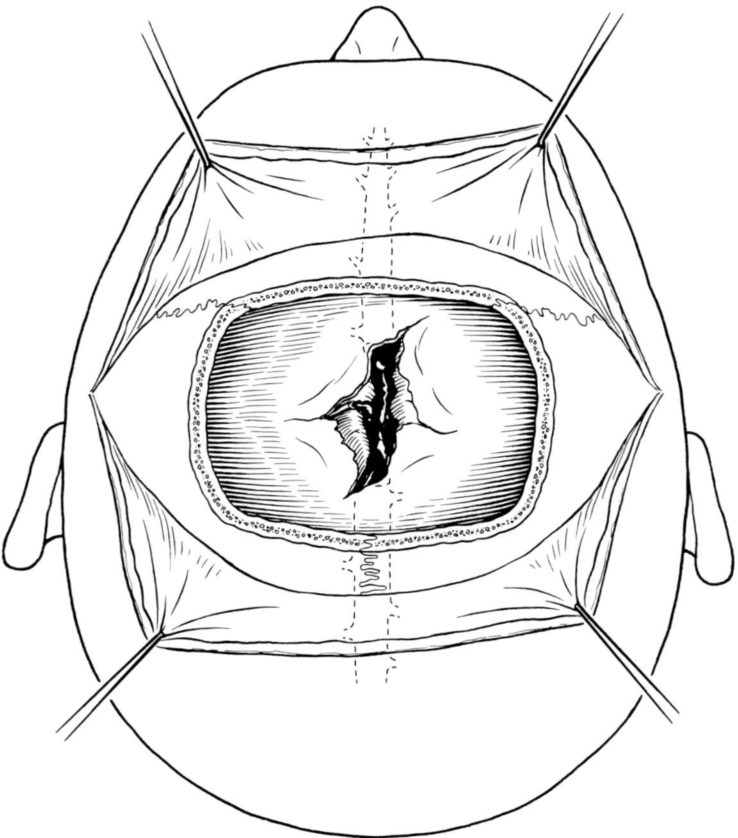

Fig. 75-8. Exposed sinus revealing a clot at the torn sinus ends and at the mouth of a torn bridging vein.

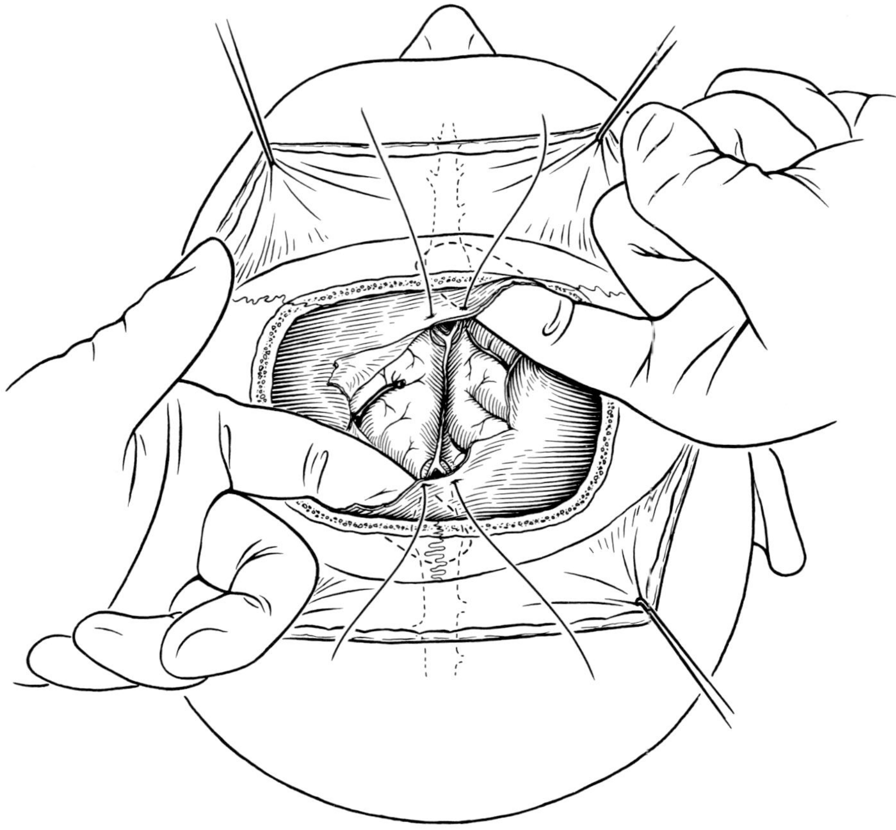

Fig. 75-9.   Maneuver for control of hemorrhage following expulsion of a clot.

end secured in the sinus by a single encircling suture (Figures 75-10, 75-11).

Flow is now re-established in the sinus. Flow can be monitored in either direction, and the T-tube can be used to introduce heparin or for sinography. Most important, the acuteness of the emergency has been met and one can now plan the reconstruction or replacement if this is necessary.[8,9]

REINSTITUTION OF NORMAL FLOW

Several techniques are available for reinstituting normal flow.

DURAL TUNNEL

If the missing segment is short (1.00-1.25 cm), a dural tunnel can be fashioned to bridge the defect (Figure 75-12). The advantages of the dural tunnel are (1) the dura is an autogenous tissue, and (2) it is locally available. The disadvantages are (1) the procedure is time-consuming and flow in the sinus is interrupted during the suturing of the graft; (2) the graft does not have an intimal lining; and (3) dura from some surface must be sacrificed.

VENOUS REPLACEMENT GRAFT

A graft of the required length can be obtained from a vein of an extremity. The advantages of this graft are (1) long defects can be bridged; (2) the tissues are autogenous; and (3) it is a

vascular structure and has an intimal lining. The disadvantages are (1) it is time-consuming and flow is interrupted while the graft is being placed; (2) it is not locally available and an additional and separate incision must be made in the arm or leg; (3) the vein contains valves that must be removed or at least the segment must be oriented so that it allows flow in the proper direction; and (4) the vein does not have stiff walls as does the sinus and hence may collapse if negative pressure develops within the sinus.[10] The adventitia, however, can be sutured to surrounding dura or periosteum to lessen the likelihood of this problem (Figure 75-13).

REPLACEMENT BY AN INTIMA-LINED STENT

A section of siliconized vascular T-tube is cut of sufficient diameter to just fit inside the orifice of the open sinus and that is slightly longer than the defect.[9] Holes are cut at intervals through the walls of the stent. A piece of vein from an extremity, slightly longer than the stent, is passed through the stent and the ends are folded back over the end of the stent and held by a ligature at each end.

The disadvantages of the method are (1) the stent wall itself is a foreign body and one is reluctant to introduce a foreign body into a wound. The foreign material is not in contact with the bloodstream, however. (2) The valves must be removed from the vein segment that lines the stent or at least the stent must be so oriented to allow flow in the proper direction past the valves. The advantages of the method are (1) the lining of the stent is vascular and autogenous; (2) placing the stent into

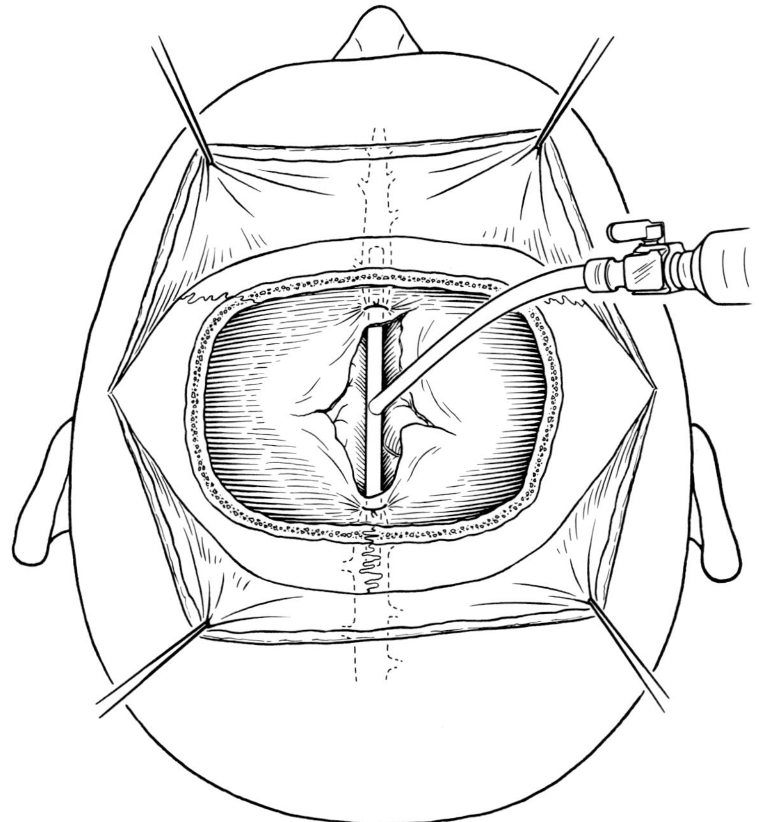

Fig. 75-10. A siliconized vascular T-tube in a sinus.

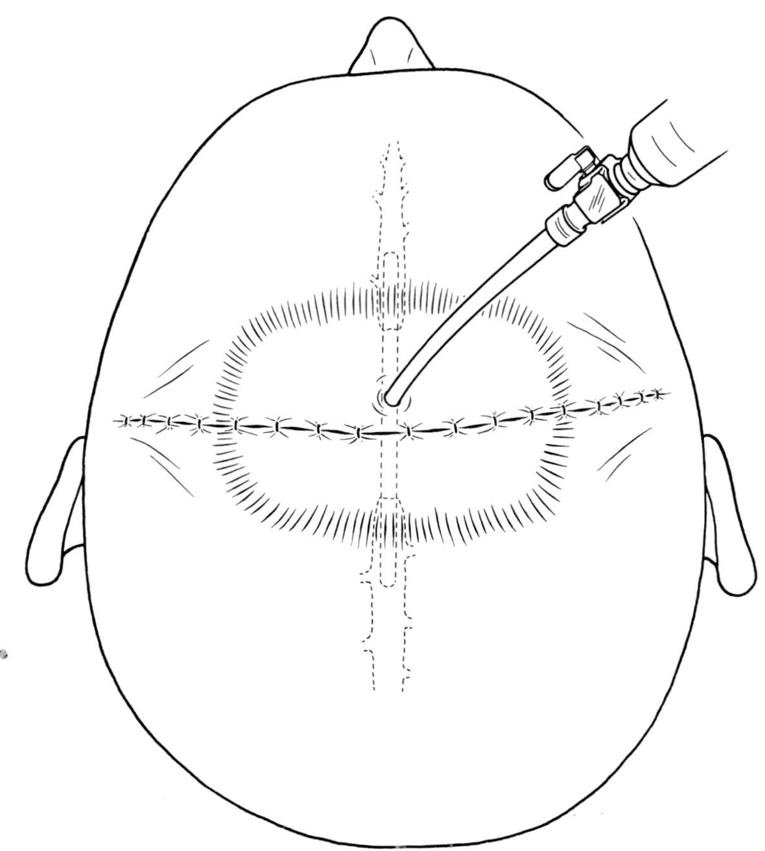

Fig. 75-11. The wound is closed following introduction of the T-tube.

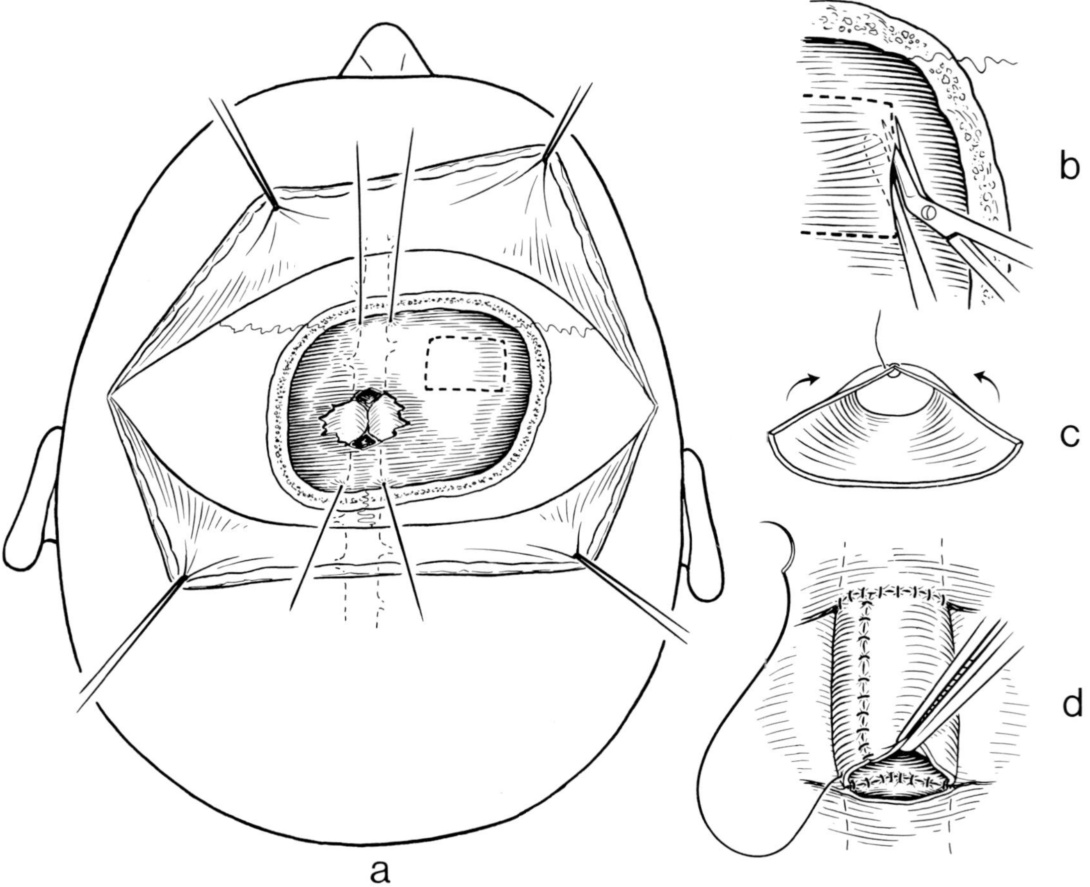

Fig. 75-12. Formation of a dural tunnel. (a) Sinus disruption. The dural flap is outlined on the right. (b) Raising the dural flap. (c) Forming the dural tunnel. (d) Completing the dural tunnel.

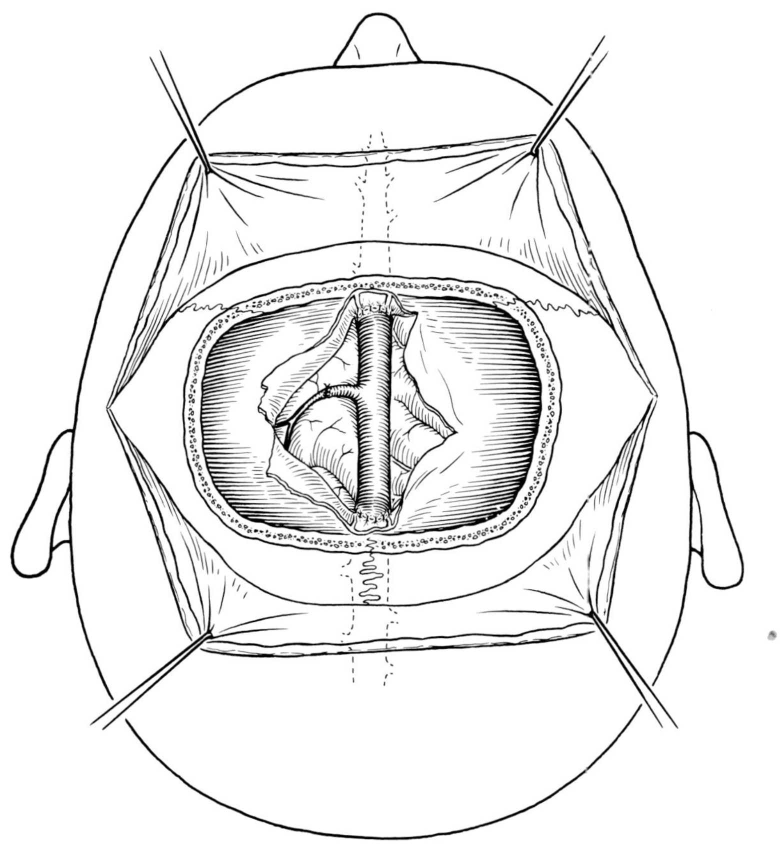

Fig. 75-13. A vein graft in place, bridging a long sinus defect.

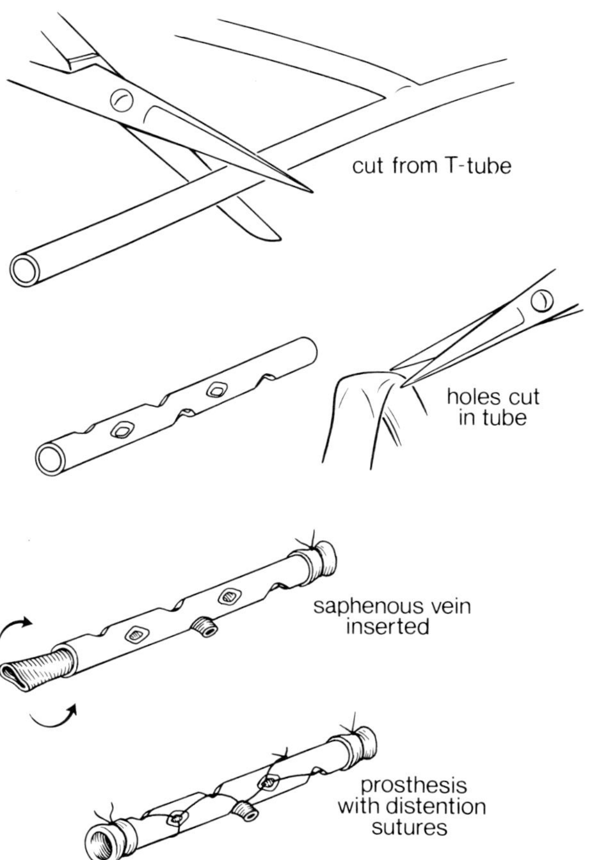

Fig. 75-14. Formation of an intima-lined stent.

the sinus to replace the T-tube already in place can be done in a very few minutes, and, hence, flow is interrupted for a very short time; and (3) the segment will not collapse since the lining of the vein is held by traction sutures over the wall of the stent and through the holes in the stent wall to the adventitia of the graft segment (Figures 75-14, 75-15, and 75-16).

Based upon observations of Sawyer and Pate,[11–13] Mullan,[14] and Schwartz (personal communication), a technique was developed to help prevent thrombosis in the relatively slow-flowing sagittal sinus after grafting or the introduction of a prosthesis.

After completion of the graft or positioning of the prosthesis, three platinum wires (.003 inch) are sutured into the sinus at either end of the graft or prosthesis so that a portion of the wire is in contact with the bloodstream within the sinus. The ends of the wire are left long. A third wire is similarly placed in the center of the graft or prosthesis. Fine polyethylene tubing is placed over the wire to provide insulation from the tissue, and the three wires are twisted together at their free ends and attached to the negative pole of a 9-V battery.

A similarly insulated wire is attached to the positive pole of the battery and soldered at its other end to a chest electrode (a U.S. 25-cent piece) that is attached to the chest wall by adhesives with an ECG conducting gel between the 25-cent piece and the skin. The position of the chest electrode is changed daily to prevent skin irritation beneath it.

By this means a negative current is provided at the intima of the sinus for 5 to 7 days. After that time the wires are removed from the sinus under direct vision by reopening the skin incision.

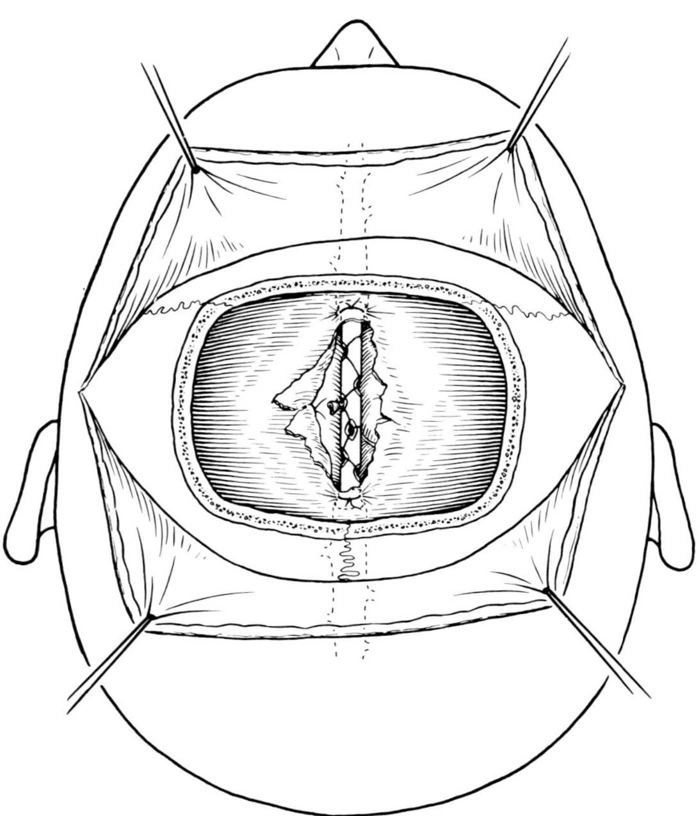

Fig. 75-15. Stent in place following removal of a temporary T-tube.

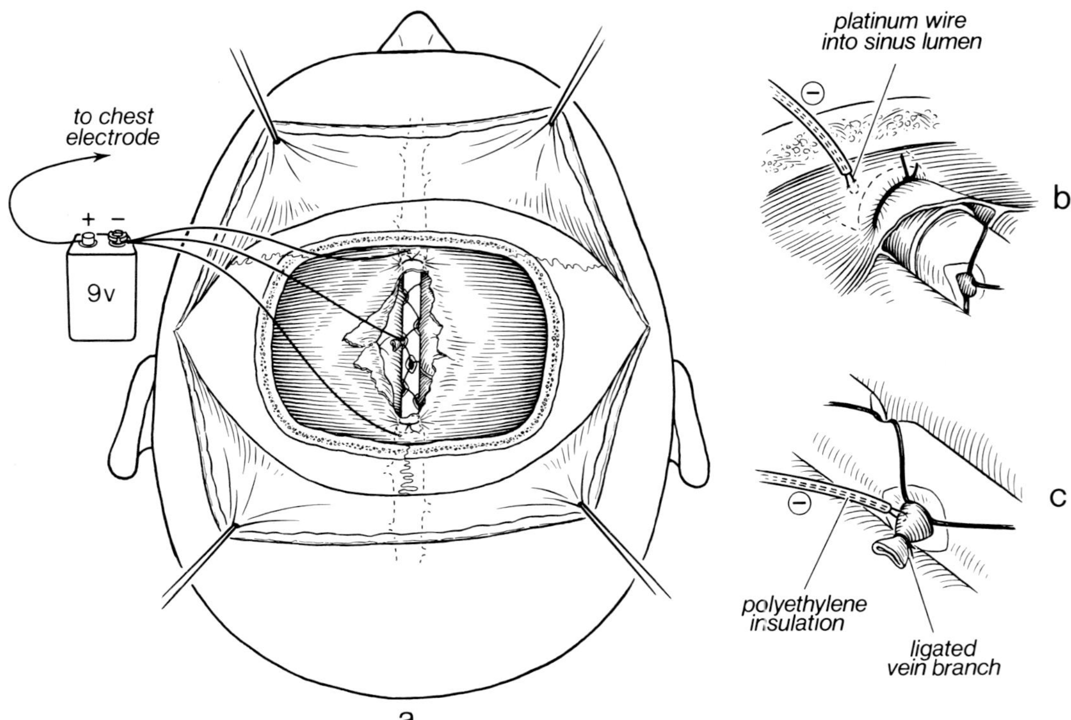

Fig. 75-16. Apparatus to provide 5 to 7 days of continuous negative current to the sinus intima.

ELIMINATION OF ABNORMAL VASCULAR COMMUNICATIONS

The most common example of an abnormal vascular communication is the artery-vein communication seen in trauma to the wall of the internal carotid artery during its course through the cavernous sinus. This is not an infrequent complication of injuries to the frontal area. This complication may not occur at the time of the initial trauma but becomes apparent when a pulsating exophthalmos develops on the injured site, resulting in an audible bruit over the area and swelling and chemosis of the conjunctiva. The mechanism is simply that the carotid artery has begun to leak, but since it is encased at its point of rupture within the various venous channels of the cavernous sinus, it bleeds within the dural confines of the sinus. Hence, patients do not bleed to death since they are bleeding into their own bloodstream, albeit from an arterial to a venous structure. The fact that the venous structure of the sinus now contains blood at close to arterial pressures accounts for most of the symptomatology. The distention of the venous components of the sinus and back pressure upon the orbital veins give rise to the proptosis of the eye with swelling and chemosis of the conjunctiva. The jet of arterial blood in the carotid artery into the venous structure of the cavernous sinus accounts for the bruit.

THERAPEUTIC CHOICES

Nonsurgical Choices

There is no satisfactory nonsurgical answer to the problem of an abnormal vascular communication. This opinion is based upon a history of the disorder. Although in a small number of such cases the communication sealed spontaneously, in the greater proportion there was gradually increasing proptosis and conjunctival edema, paralysis of the extraocular muscles, and diminished vision. Useful function of the ipsilateral eye is frequently lost (20 percent).

Surgical Choices

Ligating the cervical carotid artery reduces the arterial pressure in the carotid artery at the site of the arterial tear, hence favoring thrombosis and sealing of the communication. The advantages of this procedure are (1) it is simply and easily performed; (2) it does not require craniotomy; and (3) it can be performed under local anesthesia. The disadvantages are (1) it has a high failure rate. Because of retrograde flow in the distal internal carotid artery, the syndrome may persist. It may be somewhat less severe or may slowly worsen. (2) It is often accompanied by significant complications such as embolism or ischemia, resulting in neurologic deficit such as hemiplegia.

Trapping has perhaps been the most widely used method of surgical therapy, at least until very recent years. It consists of ligating either the internal carotid artery or the common carotid artery in the neck and the intracranial internal carotid artery, thus trapping the leaking area between the occlusions and reducing flow and pressure at the site of communication, thereby promoting thrombosis at this site.

The relative popularity of this method is not because it is without risk but rather because there has been a fair measure of success with it and because it is the least complicated of a number of procedures that have complication rates. This procedure, along with the newer procedures, also has a significant failure rate, however. In the case of trapping, failure may be caused by collateral flow via the ophthalmic arteries, hypophyseal vessels, small communicators from the opposite side, or persistent trigeminal arteries.

To perform trapping, the internal or common carotid artery is exposed in the neck. An umbilical tape is placed about it so that a tourniquet or an arterial clamp, such as a Selverstone or Crutchfield, can be applied.

If the patient is being operated upon under general anesthesia, the vessel is allowed to remain fully open until the patient has recovered from the anesthesia. Then the vessel is occluded, either slowly or rapidly depending upon the preference and experience of the surgeon. The patient is continuously monitored and if untoward symptoms develop, the device can be immediately released. (Not all neurologic deficits recover on release, but many do.) When the vessel is completely closed, the patient is monitored for 24 to 48 hours. If no untoward symptoms develop, the external portion of the clamp can be disconnected and the vessel permanently ligated. Some prefer to ligate doubly and to section the vessel; others leave it in continuity. The common carotid artery is preferred as the ligation site by many neurosurgeons. The approach is easier and is alleged to have a lower complication rate than the internal carotid approach, although it also is alleged to have a higher failure rate.

The intracranial clipping of the internal carotid artery then can be performed as a second operation if the communication persists. Such clipping should be proximal to the posterior communicating artery to allow the circulation of that vessel to remain in continuity with the distal internal carotid, the anterior choroidal artery, and the anterior and middle cerebral arteries of that side.

Some surgeons prefer to do both the cervical operation and the craniotomy at the same time because they feel there is a lower incidence of embolization that way. This depends largely on the surgeon's experience. It is difficult to argue with a high success rate in the hands of an individual and improper to advocate persistence in the face of misfortune.

The following procedures have been performed but no series was of great size, and extensive experience is not available. The interested reader is encouraged to consult the reference literature or to seek the advice of the innovator.

With the advent of the cervical carotid to intracranial internal carotid shunt, a method was presented for trapping the carotid and cavernous fistula[15] while at the same time preserving blood flow to the distal internal carotid. Such procedures have so far been unsuccessful for technical reasons, but simulated surgery in the laboratory has an established success rate.[16–18] Theoretically, the success rate should be higher than in surgery for atherosclerotic disease since the distal internal carotid is not involved because of disease and since most artery-vein communications occur in young people who have good vessels in general except for the lesion that was induced by trauma.

Embolization. In 1940, Mixter (personal communication) considered closing a carotid cavernous fistula by introducing a piece of muscle marked by a small silver clip, and attached to a long suture, into the cervical carotid artery and allowing it to enter the carotid siphon, with the thought that it would be sucked into the orifice of the communication and thus block it. Should it have passed beyond the site, it could have been recovered by traction upon the suture. There had been no laboratory preparation for this procedure and Mixter never did use it, but he did a good deal of thinking about it. In more recent years, however, embolization has been tried with muscle, Gelfoam, etc.[19–21]

Balloon Embolization. Serbinenko devised and successfully used a catheter with a detachable balloon that he introduces into the cervical carotid. Then, under roentgenographic control, he guides the balloon to the carotid rent and releases it from the catheter, allowing it to plug the communication.[22,23]

Use of a Balloon in the Venous Channel. Mullan reported using a balloon that he introduces into the venous channels leading to the sinus,[24] and Wright and Donaghy (unreported case), after unsuccessfully attempting to catheterize a series of cadavers via the superior petrosal sinus, did introduce such a balloon into the cavernous sinus via the ophthalmic veins. Although the balloon deflated, thrombosis occurred in the venous channels secondary to foreign body effect. Proptosis and extraocular movement improved, although the patient did not recover his sight.

Thrombosis via Positive Current. Mullan, using the experience of Sawyer,[11,13] devised a method of introducing positive electric current into the venous structures leading from the sinus, thus promoting thrombosis.[24]

Parkinson reported an elegant procedure based upon his anatomic research on the structure of the cavernous sinus.[25–27] In his procedure, the sinus is opened under cardiac arrest and the internal carotid artery rent is identified and repaired under direct vision. This procedure goes to the very heart of the problem. There is no question that the surgery is one of great magnitude, but the fact that it was conceived and then applied with some success testifies to the magnitude of the problem it was designed to correct.

REFERENCES

1. Kapp JP, Gielchinsky I: Management of combat wounds of the dural sinus. Surgery 71:913, 1972
2. Piersal GA (ed): Human Anatomy, ed 8. Philadelphia, JB Lippincott, 1923, pp 867-874
3. Browder J, Browder A, Kaplan H: The venous sinuses of the cerebral dura mater. Arch Neurol 26:175, 1972
4. Kaplan HA, Browder J: Atresia of the rostral superior sagittal venous channels. Neurosurgery 38:602, 1973
5. Browder J, Kaplan HA: Venous drainage following ablation or occlusive isolation of the rostral superior sagittal sinus. Surg Neurol 1:245, 1973
6. Troup H, Tarkkanen J: Continuous recording of the sigmoid sinus pressure after radical neck dissection. J Laryngol Otol 82:1013, 1968
7. Fitz-Hugh GS, Robins RB, Craddock WD: Increased intracranial pressure complicating unilateral neck dissection. Laryngoscope 76:893, 1966
8. Kapp JP, Gielchinsky I, Petty C, et al: Internal shunt for use in reconstruction of dural sinuses: technical note. J Neurosurg 35:351, 1971
9. Donaghy RMP, Wallman LJ, Flanagan ME, et al: Sagittal sinus repair. J Neurosurg 38:244, 1973
10. Bonnal J, Brotchi J: Surgery of the superior sagittal sinus in parasagittal meningiomas. J Neurosurg 48:935, 1978
11. Sawyer PN, Pate JW: Bio-electric phenomena as an etiologic factor in intravascular thrombosis. Am J Physiol 175:103, 1953
12. Sawyer PN, Pate JW, Weldon CS: Relations of abnormal and injury electric potential differences to intravascular thrombosis. Am J Physiol 175:108, 1953
13. Sawyer PN, Pate JW: Electrical potential differences across the normal aorta and aortic grafts of dogs. Am J Physiol 175:113, 1953
14. Mullan S: Experience with surgical thrombosis of intracranial berry aneurysm and carotid cavernous fistula. J Neurosurg 41:657, 1974
15. Woringer E, Kunlin J: Anastomose entre la carotide primitive et la

carotide intra-cranienne ou la sylvienne par greffon selon la technique de la suture suspendue. Neurochirurgie 9:181, 1963

16. Maroon J, Donaghy RMP: Experimental cerebral revascularization with autogenous grafts. J Neurosurg 38:172, 1973

17. Shields CB: Autogenous artery and vein grafts in common carotid suproclinoid carotid anastomoses. J Microsurg 1:114, 1979

18. Lougheed WM, Marshall BM, Hunter M, et al.: Common carotid to intracranial internal carotid bypass venous graft: Technical note. J Neurosurg 34:114, 1971

19. Mixter, WJ: Personal communication, 1940

20. Treatment of carotid-cavernous fistula consisting of one stage operation by muscle embolization of the fistula's carotid segment, in Donaghy RMP, Yasargil MG (eds): Microvascular Surgery. Stuttgart, Georg Thieme Verlag, 1967, pp 151-167

21. Brooks B: The treatment of traumatic arteriovenous fistula. South Med J 23:100, 1930

22. Ohta T, Nishimura S, Kikuchi H, et al: Closure of carotid-cavernous fistula with polyurethane foam embolus: Technical note. J Neurosurg 38:107, 1973

23. Serbinenko FA: Balloon catheterization and occlusion of major cerebral vessels. J Neurosurg 41:125, 1974

24. Picard L, Lepoire J, Montaut J, et al: Endoarterial occlusion of carotid-cavernous sinus fistulas using a balloon-tipped catheter. Neuroradiology 8:5, 1974

25. Mullan S, Brown FD, Patronas NJ: Treatment of carotid-cavernous fistulas by cavernous sinus occlusion. J Neurosurg 50:131, 1979

26. Wright S, Donaghy RMP: Unreported case.

27. Parkinson D: A surgical approach to the cavernous sinus portion of the carotid artery. Anatomical studies and case report. J Neurosurg 23:474, 1965

28. Parkinson D: Transcavernous repair of carotid-cavernous fistula. Case report. J Neurosurg 26:420, 1967

29. Parkinson D: Carotid cavernous fistula. Direct repair with preservation of the carotid artery. Technical note. J Neurosurg 38:99, 1973

CHAPTER 76

Surgical Management of Dural Sinus Lacerations

John P. Kapp

LACERATIONS OF THE DURAL VENOUS SINUSES are associated most commonly with missile wounds, and confront the neurosurgeon with the special problems of massive hemorrhage and cerebral edema secondary to venous obstruction. Patients with dural sinus injuries are usually unstable, and referral over long distances to specialized centers is rarely practical.

DIAGNOSIS AND PREPARATION

Surgery will be greatly facilitated if a dural sinus injury is suspected preoperatively and suitable preparation is made for this contingency. There is no specific syndrome associated with damage to the anterior half of the superior sagittal sinus. Paresis and spasticity of the legs are characteristic of injuries to the midportion of the sagittal sinus. More posterior lesions involving the superior sagittal sinus or torcular are frequently associated with cortical blindness or coma. Transverse sinus lesions are not associated with any distinct clinical features. The outflow of the torcular is essentially unilateral in 24 percent of cases. In 16 percent, the right transverse sinus is predominant, and in 8 percent the left transverse sinus is predominant. Occlusion of a dominant transverse sinus would produce a clinical picture similar to occlusion of the posterior portion of the superior sagittal sinus or torcular. A wound or depressed fracture over the sinus, a skull fracture crossing a sinus, especially one radiating from an entry wound, or the trajectory of either a missile or bone fragment crossing a sinus should alert the surgeon to the possibility of a dural sinus injury.[1]

Preparation for dural venous sinus repair begins with positioning the patient on the operating table. Elevation of the head so that the sinus lesion is uppermost helps in reducing blood loss. The patient may be hypovolemic, however, and circulatory collapse can occur when the patient is placed in the reversed Trendelenburg position. I have had one death immediately after placing a patient with a transverse sinus wound in the head-up position. This experience prompts the recommendation that the head-up position should never be used in patients who are hypotensive and should be used with great trepidation for other patients with normal blood pressure but in whom an unknown quantity of blood has been lost from a venous sinus wound. The possibility of air embolism must be kept in mind if one chooses to elevate the head, and every effort must be made to prevent the entry of air into the venous system. Most venous sinus wounds requiring repair can best be handled with the patient in the prone position on the operating table.

Before turning the patient prone, a segment of greater saphenous vein should be taken from the proximal thigh. A segment of sufficient length (about 20 cm) should be taken so that multiple strips of opened vein will be available. Branches are ligated with fine silk as the vein is separated from the subcutaneous tissue. A Horsley cannula is inserted into the distal end of the graft and secured with a circumferential ligature. The graft is immediately flushed with heparinized saline after removal. The Horsley cannula can be left in place to ensure proper orientation of the graft. Hydrostatic dilatation of the graft is accomplished by pinching the proximal end of the graft with gloved fingers and gently distending the graft with heparinized saline. Major points of leakage from the graft may be closed with 5–0 atraumatic suture. Since the graft will be oriented in the direction of flow, removal of the valves is not necessary.

A segment of intravenous tubing with the distal adapter removed is inserted into the proximal stump of the saphenous vein, threaded into the inferior vena cava, and secured with a suture. This large line greatly facilitates rapid transfusion should it become necessary. The groin wound then is closed. If the condition of the patient does not permit a delay of this magnitude and the prone position is required for the cranial surgery, a portion of greater saphenous vein below the knee can be removed by a second surgical team after the craniectomy has begun.

Exposure of both sides of the sinus both proximal and distal to the operative area is essential. In trauma cases this can best be accomplished by placing multiple cranial perforations side by side around the margin of the proposed craniectomy with a power perforator and connecting them with a rongeur. Power craniotomes, or even Gigli saws, which can pass subdurally through a dural laceration and cut the dura, should be avoided. The injured area of the sinus, if not actively bleeding when the bone is removed, should be left undisturbed until the exposure is completed.

Once the area has been adequately exposed, the extent of injury to the sinus can be assessed and a suitable procedure planned according to the nature of the lesion. The immediate problem is the control of hemorrhage and the establishment of a dry operative field. At this point the unique anatomy of the

OPERATIVE NEUROSURGICAL TECHNIQUES
ISBN 0-8089-1862-1

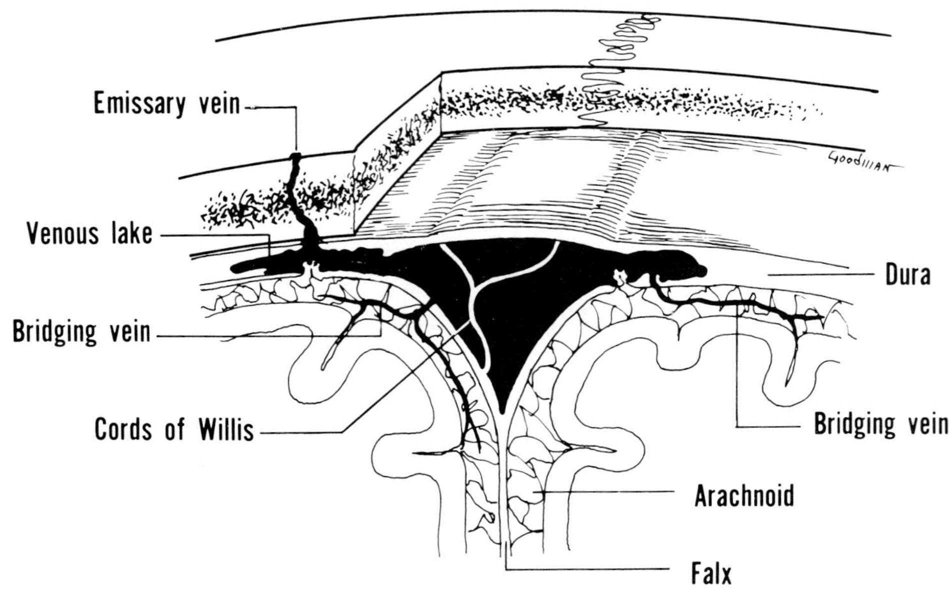

Fig. 76-1.   A cross-section of the superior sagittal sinus showing the relationship of the dural layers, the entering veins, the venous lakes, and the cords of Willis.

dural venous sinuses dictates the techniques for control of hemorrhage and repair.

ANATOMY

The sagittal and transverse sinuses are formed by the triangular space where the outer and inner leaves of the dura split to form the falx and tentorium, respectively. The wall of the sinus is half the thickness of the adjoining dura. Firm attachment of the triangular sinus at each corner maintains the patency of the lumen of the sinus, even in the face of a negative venous pressure within the sinus. The corners of the sinus adjoining the convexity dura are often not regular, but extend laterally between the leaves of the dura to form venous lakes. Bridging veins from the cerebral cortex and pacchionian gran-

ulations may enter these venous lakes rather than enter the sinus directly. Finally, the lumen of the sinus may be transversed by fibrous bands, or "cords of Willis" (Figure 76-1).

Each of these peculiarities in the anatomy of the sagittal and transverse sinus has its technical implication. The wall of a sinus is thin and nonelastic and cannot be sutured under tension. The sinus is difficult to occlude with external clamps or tourniquets, because mobilization of the sinus by division of the dura adjacent to the sinus may interrupt bridging veins or open venous lakes. The cords of Willis may present an obstruction to the passage of suction catheters of shunts within the sinus.

To avoid confusion, the heart will be used as a reference point to define direction of flow. Thus, in the normal sagittal sinus, blood flows in a distal to proximal direction. The trian-

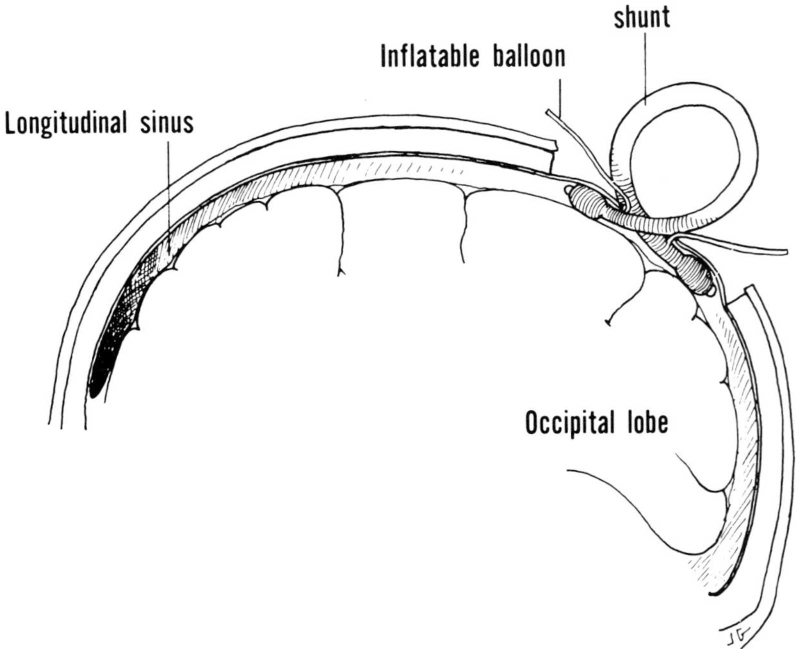

Fig. 76-2.   A shunt in place within the superior sagittal sinus.

gulated sinuses adjacent to the skull will be considered to have an outer wall and right and left walls in the case of the sagittal sinus, or outer and superior and inferior walls in the case of the transverse sinus.

TECHNIQUE

The major departure from established techniques of vascular surgery necessitated by the peculiar anatomy of the dural sinus is a method for occluding the sinus from within, by the use of balloon catheters and shunts, rather than by using methods for control of hemorrhage that require mobilization of a segment of the sinus. A large (No. 7) Fogarty catheter is most suitable for sinus occlusion, since it will fill the lumen of the sinus and remain soft enough to conform to the triangular contours while inflated.

In areas where preservation of blood flow is critical (i.e., the posterior portion of the sagittal sinus and a dominant transverse sinus), a special shunt that uses the principle of internal occlusion can be made (Figure 76-2). This shunt can be constructed from a pediatric anode endotracheal tube, which is made of latex molded around a wire coil to prevent buckling. The adapter ends of the tube are cut off, and two short pediatric tracheostomy tube cuffs are placed on the tube as close to each end as possible. The entire assembly is siliconized by applying a thin layer of Dow-Corning high-vacuum silicone stop-cock grease to both the lumen and the exterior surface. The shunt is washed and gas-sterilized before use.

One should be prepared for brisk bleeding when the bone overlying the sinus is removed. If the sinus is obstructed by clot, brain tissue, or bone fragments, there will be brisk bleeding from the dura distal to the obstruction. This can be reduced by covering the area with fibrin foam (Gelfoam) soaked in thrombin solution. The injured area, if not actively bleeding, should be left undisturbed until the situation can be assessed.

Bleeding from the injured area can be controlled by applying digital pressure over the sinus proximal and distal to the laceration, especially if the laceration is small. A Fogarty catheter can be introduced through the laceration and directed distally in the sinus. Inflation of the balloon within the sinus will control distal bleeding. Digital pressure over the proximal sinus is usually sufficient to control bleeding and prevent air embolism (Figure 76-3). The lumen of the sinus may be difficult to identify because of extensive damage. If this is the case, a small sinotomy may be made distal to the lesion and the Fogarty catheter inserted into the lumen of the sinus and inflated. Damaged veins in the area of injury will require coagulation. Intact veins emptying into he disrupted sinus, if in a critical area, should be left intact. The bleeding that occurs from these veins during sinus repair can be tolerated, and there is a distinct possibility that they would thrombose if occluded by temporary vascular clips.

Ligation of the damaged sinus may be elected when the injury is in a noncritical area and primary suture repair would result in stenosis of such magnitude that postoperative thrombosis would be expected. Ligation also should be considered when the distal venous flow is insignificant because of damage to the bridging cortical veins. The areas that have been considered noncritical are the portion of the superior sagittal sinus anterior to the entrance of the rolandic veins, the nondominant transverse or sigmoid sinus, the inferior sagittal

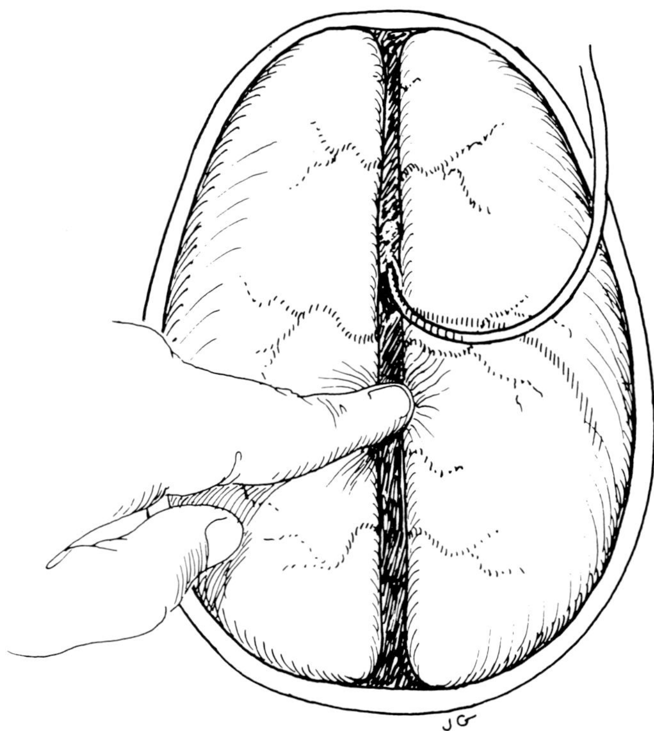

Fig. 76-3. Use of a Fogarty catheter and digital pressure to control bleeding from small dural sinus lacerations.

and straight sinus, and the minor sinuses on the floor of the skull.

The surgeon should never convert a minor problem into a major one. Conventional methods for dural sinus repair are entirely adequate and effective in many cases, especially in the small lacerations that usually are associated with noncompound skull fractures. These methods include primary suture repair of the sinus, or coverage of small sinus defects with fascia or dura.

The exact amount a sagittal or transverse sinus can be stenosed without compromising blood flow is unknown. I have assumed that stenosis of 50 percent was acceptable, and that primary suture repair would succeed provided the sinus was stenosed no more than 50 percent. Most often, dural lacerations involve a lateral corner of a sinus and the outer sinus wall can be sutured to a lateral sinus wall without tension (Figure 76-4). Lacerations of an outer sinus wall may not be directly suturable without tension, especially if even minimal debridement of the edges of the laceration is necessary. Because the wall consists of only a single leaf of the dura, sutures tend to pull out with even minimal tension, thus leaving a frayed edge that may require further debridement. In these cases, one usually can incorporate a small roll of pericranium, temporalis fascia, or dura into the suture line to complete closure without tension.

In areas of the superior sagittal sinus posterior to the rolandic vein, the torcular, and the dominant transverse sinus, where one or more walls have been extensively damaged so that primary repair after adequate debridement either is impossible or would produce critical stenosis, autogenous vein grafts appear to be the most physiologic and suitable replacement. Other tissues, notably pericranium and dura, have been used with success (Hester RW: Personal communication, 1980).[2] Arterial grafts have been tried in experimental animals, and have been found to be less suitable than veins because of progressive fibrosis and contraction of the graft.[3] There is more

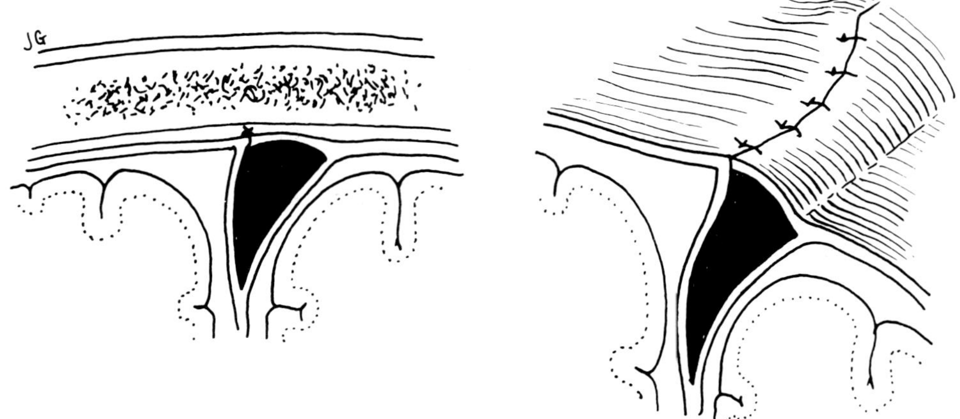

Fig. 76-4. Repair of injury to a lateral corner of the sinus by primary suture of the lateral leaf to the outer leaf of the sinus with 50 percent stenosis of the lumen.

experience with autogenous vein as a material for replacement of dural sinuses as well as for grafting in other parts of the venous system.[4] Securing the vein segment usually does not add greatly to the magnitude of the procedure, since the vein can be obtained when the large venous cutdown is done.

After adequate exposure of the injured area of sinus is obtained, foreign material, bone fragments, and clots are removed from the lumen of the sinus. The cords of Willis within the sinus may obstruct insertion of a sucker tip or shunt. They may be broken by applying gentle pressure with a large metal sucker tip. The lumen of the sinus is irrigated with heparinized saline, the anatomy of the lesion is defined, and, if the shunt is not already in place, it is inserted at this time. Contused and destroyed intima and frayed edges are debrided. The previously prepared vein graft is opened and oriented so that valves, if present in the graft, will not impede flow. A 5-0 Tevdek or other nonabsorbable vascular suture is placed to approximate the end of the graft to the end of the defect. One side and the ends of the graft are sutured into the defect with a continuous suture (Figure 76-5). The remainder of the graft is tailored to fit the defect, and the second suture line is partially completed with a continuous suture to a point where the opening will allow easy removal of the shunt. Interrupted sutures are placed to close the remaining defect that has admitted the shunt but not tied (Figure 76-6). The shunt is removed, a large-bore sucker is passed in each direction within the sinus to remove clots, and the preplaced sutures are tied down to complete the suture line (Figure 76-7).

At completion of the procedure, every effort should be made to attach the repaired segment of sinus to the dura on three sides to prevent its collapse if intrasinus pressure becomes negative. This may be accomplished on one or more sides simply by dural closure. The remaining sides should be attached to the dura under proper tension, using interrupted atraumatic vascular sutures placed through the sinus walls, and dural grafts of pericranium or temporalis fascia of proper size. Subgaleal collections of fluid may apply external pressure to the grafted segment, causing it to collapse and possibly thrombose. Therefore, hemostasis should be as complete as possible. The use of a soft suction drain (such as a Jackson-Pratt drain) in the subgaleal space may be advisable.

I have not used the operating microscope for dural sinus repair. Use of the microscope adds time to the procedure and limits the accessibility of the assistant. Hemostasis is rarely complete during repairs, since veins entering the sinus at the injured segment usually continue to bleed, making time and assistance critical factors in successful repair. Finally, the sagittal and transverse sinuses are not microscopic structures. Sutures need not be placed at extremely close intervals as is done in a superficial temporal-middle cerebral artery anastomosis, since one is working in a low-pressure system. Accurate approximation of endothelial surface to endothelial surface is

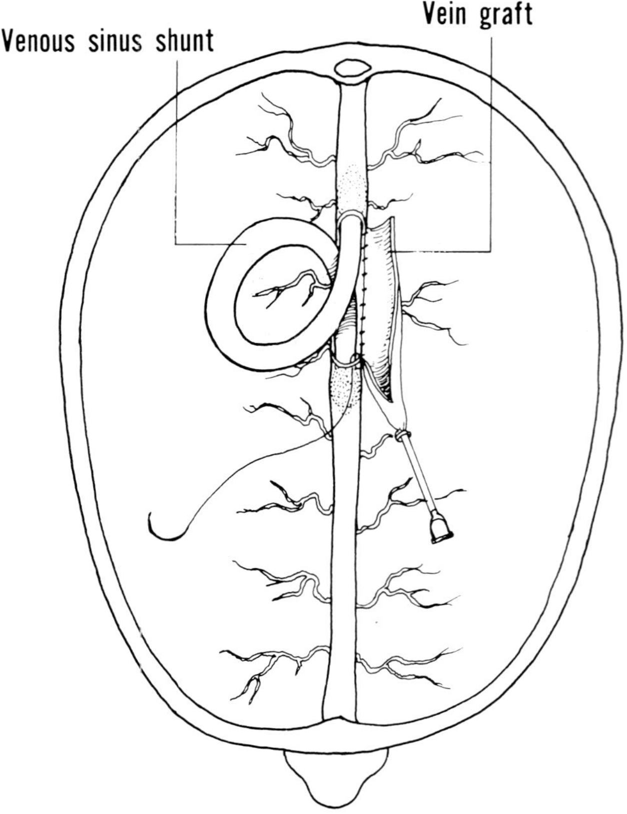

Fig. 76-5. Repair of an extensive sinus defect with an autogenous vein graft. A Horslely cannula in the distal end of the vein maintains correct orientation of the graft and serves as a handle. A continuous suture has been placed to secure one edge of the graft to an edge of the defect.

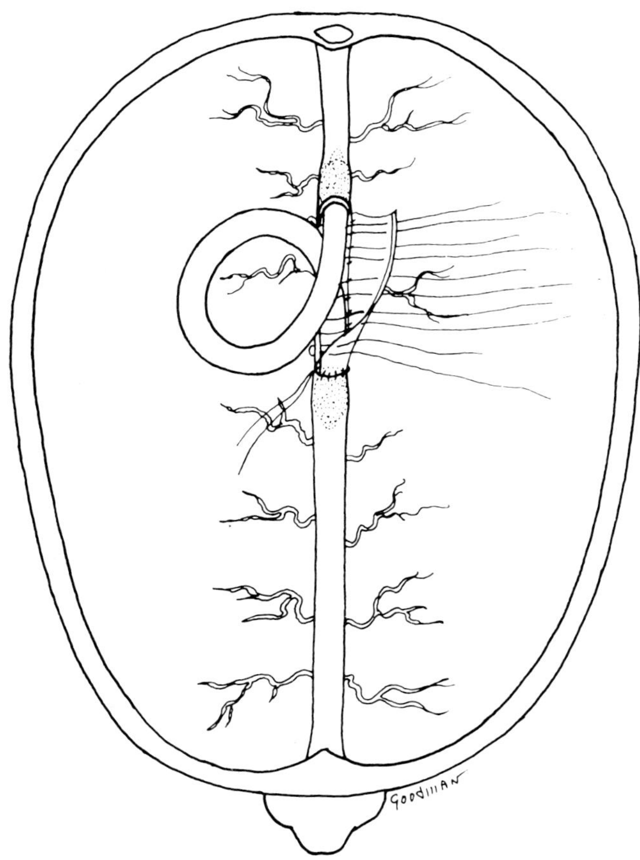

Fig. 76-6. Interrupted sutures have been preplaced to approximate the other edge of the graft to the edge of the defect after the shunt is removed.

important, but this can be done without the aid of the surgical microscope.

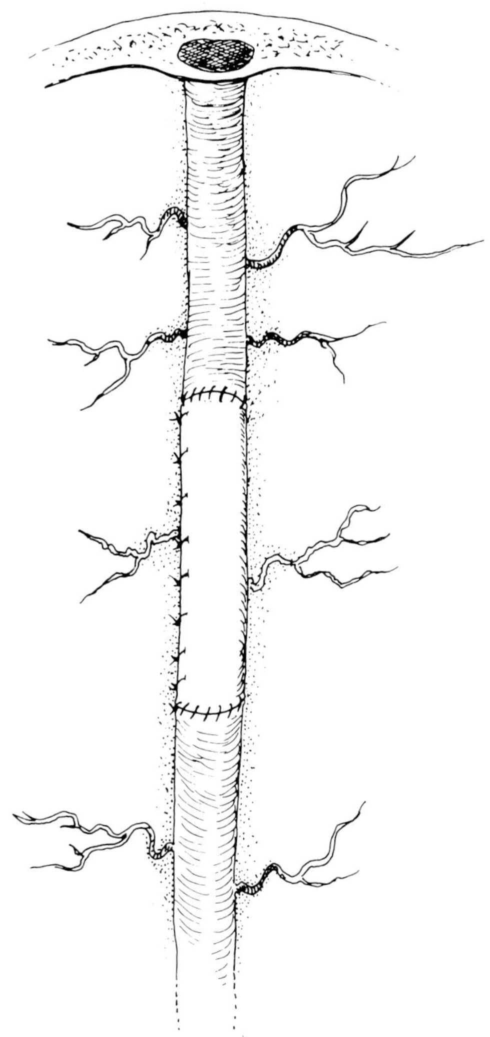

Fig. 76-7. The autogenous vein graft sutured in place.

SUMMARY

The following seven points are recommended for successful management of dural sinus lacerations:

1. Correct preoperative diagnosis.
2. Preparation for sinus repair or reconstruction, including patient positioning, a large intravenous line, and removal of a vein segment for possible use as a graft.
3. Adequate exposure of both sides of the sinus proximal and distal to the laceration.
4. Proximal and distal control of hemorrhage, occluding the sinus from within by inflating a balloon when necessary, and using a shunt in critical areas to prevent venous stasis and cerebral edema.
5. Debridement of frayed and severely contused sinus wall.
6. Accurate approximation of endothelial surfaces, using fine vascular suture material.
7. Reconstruction of areas involving extensive tissue loss in critical sinuses with autogenous vein grafts.

By following this management plan, dural sinus injuries can be managed in a relatively bloodless field, brain swelling secondary to venous stasis during repair can be eliminated, and high postoperative patency rates can be anticipated.

REFERENCES

1. Kapp JP, Schmidek HH: The Cerebral Venous System and Its Disorders. Orlando, Fl, Grune & Stratton, 1984
2. Kempe LG: Operative Neurosurgery, vol 1. New York, Springer-Verlag, 1968, pp 142–144
3. Sindou M, Mazoyer J, Fischer G, et al: Experimental bypass for sagittal sinus repair. J Neurosurg 44:325, 1976
4. Hiratzka LF, Wright CB: Experimental and clinical results of grafts in the venous system. A current review. J Surg Res 25:542, 1978

CHAPTER 77

Surgical Management of Intracerebral Hemorrhage

David G. Piepgras   Michael J. Redmond

STROKE IS THE THIRD MOST COMMON CAUSE OF DEATH in the United States after coronary heart disease and cancer, accounting for 11 percent of all deaths.[1,2] The annual incidence of spontaneous intracerebral hemorrhage is approximately 15 per 100,000.[3] The relative gravity of the problem of intracerebral hemorrhage is evident from its high morbidity and mortality: a 1-month survival rate of only 17 percent compared with 35 percent for subarachnoid hemorrhage and 73 percent for stroke resulting from cerebral thrombosis.[4]

CLASSIFICATION

Intracerebral hemorrhages can be classified as "symptomatic"—those caused by the rupture of an aneurysm or arteriovenous malformation (AVM), related to a known hematologic disorder or cerebral mass lesion—and "primary" intracerebral hemorrhages—those hemorrhages for which such underlying causes cannot be determined. Excluded from both of these categories are the relatively common traumatic and preterm neonatal intracerebral hemorrhages.

PRIMARY INTRACEREBRAL HEMORRHAGE

The large majority of spontaneous intracerebral hemorrhages fall into the "primary" category, with hypertension most often implicated as the contributing factor. Ransohoff[5] stated that hypertension is the cause in over 90 percent of single, sizable intracerebral hemorrhages; however, McCormick and Rosenfield,[6] in a prospective autopsy study, concluded that hypertension could be incriminated in only 25 percent of their patients with massive spontaneous intracerebral hemorrhages. Furlan et al.,[3] reviewing cases in an essentially white population over the past 20 years, found an 81 percent frequency of hypertension in their patients with primary intracerebral hemorrhage.

Although the exact pathologic lesion of hypertensive intracerebral hemorrhage remains a subject of discussion among neuropathologists, there is evidence to incriminate a degenerative process specific to small cerebral arteries, now described as lipohyalinosis[7] or fibrinoid necrosis.[8] The distribution of these changes match those sites at which the greatest incidence of intracerebral hemorrhage and lacunar infarcts occur. Consistent with this, sites of predilection for hypertensive intracerebral hemorrhage have been identified, with ap-

proximately half occurring in the striate body, 15 percent in the thalamus, 10 to 15 percent in the pons, 10 percent in the cerebellum, and 10 to 20 percent in the cerebral white matter.[5,9,10] The hemorrhage can be massive and fatal or small with good recovery. It is characteristic of an intracerebral hemorrhage to dissect along tissue planes and tracts, separating and compressing the nervous tissue rather than destroying it. Extension into the ventricular system has been stated to be common, and according to Fisher,[10] occurs in 90 percent of the cases. This estimate was made in the era before computed tomography (CT), however, and was undoubtedly based on findings of bloody cerebrospinal fluid or at autopsy. Interestingly, a series of CT studies in patients with gangliothalamic and lobar hematomas showed intraventricular or cisternal blood in only 9 percent and 20 percent of cases, respectively.[11]

CLINICAL PRESENTATION

The onset of symptoms in a patient with a primary intracerebral hemorrhage typically occurs abruptly while the patient is awake and active; prodromal symptoms are not typical.[10] Neurologic deficit develops progressively as the hemorrhage increases, usually becoming maximal in hours to days. Headache occurs in one half to two thirds of the patients and is commonly lateralized to the side of the hemorrhage. A declining level of consciousness occurs as the hemorrhage extends directly into the brain stem or because of increased intracranial pressure and secondary involvement of the brain stem.

For a more detailed review of the syndromes related to intracerebral hemorrhages at the various sites of predilection, see the excellent monographs of Fisher.[10,12] Emphasis should be placed, however, on the clinical profile of cerebellar hemorrhage inasmuch as correct diagnosis may be difficult early in its course and delayed treatment may prove fatal.[13] An acute complex of symptoms, including headache, nausea and vomiting, and inability to walk or stand, with signs of gait or appendicular ataxia, ocular disturbances, and peripheral facial palsy, should suggest the diagnosis, which can be readily confirmed by CT scan. These hemorrhages characteristically originate in or near one of the dentate nuclei where branches of the cerebellar arteries anastomose.[14] Extension of the hemorrhage into the vermis or opposite hemisphere can occur, and rupture into the fourth ventricle is not uncommon (Figure 77-1).

The causes of primary brain hemorrhage other than hyper-

OPERATIVE NEUROSURGICAL TECHNIQUES
ISBN 0-8089-1862-1

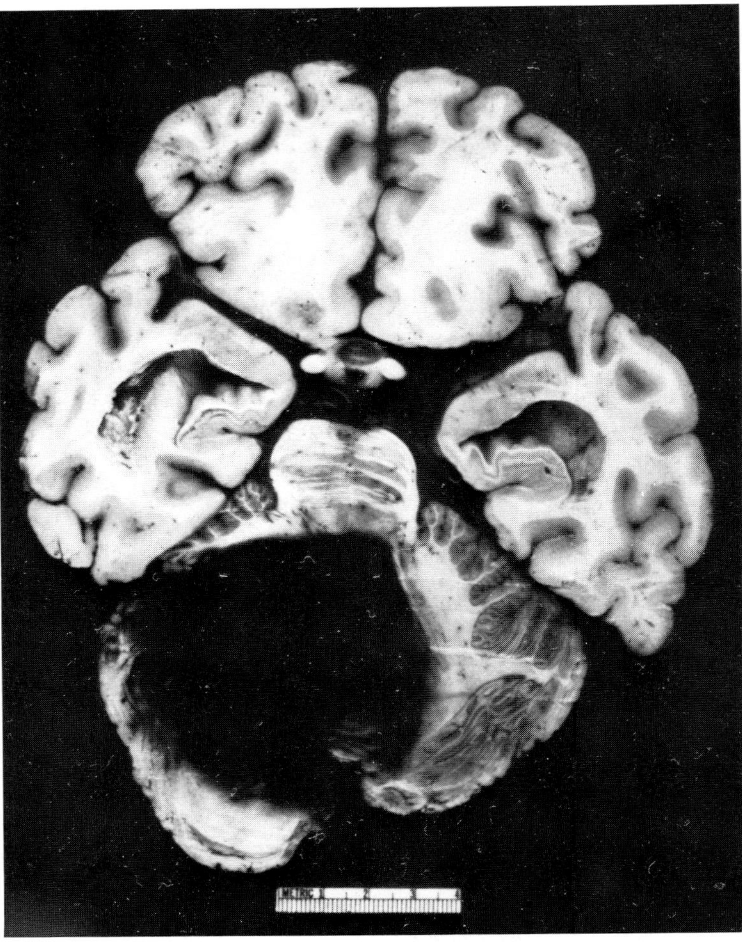

Fig. 77-1. A transverse section of brain showing massive hemorrhage of the cerebellar hemisphere with midline extension and rupture into the fourth ventricle.

tension and anticoagulants rarely are defined. Cerebral amyloid angiopathy has been recognized as a rare but important cause in aged patients.[8,15,16,16A] The occurrence of single or multiple intracerebral hemorrhages in elderly, perhaps demented, nonhypertensive patients suggests amyloid angiopathy. In contrast to hypertensive hemorrhages, hematomas secondary to amyloid angiopathy tend to be near the cortical surface in the parietal and occipital lobes.[16] Amyloid angiopathy has also been implicated as the cause of cerebral hemorrhage after shunting procedures for what was clinically considered a normal pressure hydrocephalus.[17]

SYMPTOMATIC INTRACEREBRAL HEMORRHAGE

Symptomatic intracerebral hemorrhages most commonly are caused by aneurysms, arteriovenous malformations, or blood dyscrasias, but the bleeding also can be caused by a brain tumor or sepsis, or can be secondary to liver disease or other systemic illnesses. Intracerebral hemorrhages occurring in the anterior sylvian fissure and adjacent regions of the frontal and temporal lobes commonly are caused by middle cerebral or, less likely, internal carotid artery aneurysms (Figure 77-2). Hematomas in the interhemispheric fissure and the medial aspect of the frontal lobe suggest an aneurysm of the anterior

communicating artery as the source of bleeding. Intraventricular extension of the hemorrhage can occur from any aneurysmal site, but probably is more common in aneurysms of the anterior communicating and internal carotid arteries.[18] Lobar intracerebral hemorrhages may be primary (hypertensive), but their occurrence should always raise the question of the underlying vascular abnormality, particularly an AVM (Figure 77-3). Most underlying vascular lesions will be apparent on a contrasted CT scan or angiogram, but even if they are not visible on these studies, an occult vascular malformation may be the source and may be diagnosed only in a later angiogram[19] or at surgery or autopsy.

Spontaneous intracerebral hemorrhage may be the first symptom of a previously unsuspected cerebral neoplasm, but more commonly this develops acutely on a background of known malignancy or a course indicative of a progressive focal cerebral lesion. Although neoplasms account for only 2 to 3 percent of intracranial hemorrhage in series reported by Locksley[20] and Russell,[21] Scott[22] found primary or metastatic tumors as the cause in 10 percent of 80 patients operated on for spontaneous intracerebral hemorrhage. A wide spectrum of neoplasms producing intracerebral hemorrhage have been reported, the more common primary tumors being gliomas, angiomas, and meningiomas, and metastases including melanomas, bronchogenic carcinomas, and chorioepitheliomas.[5,22]

Massive intracerebral hemorrhage can occur in acute leu-

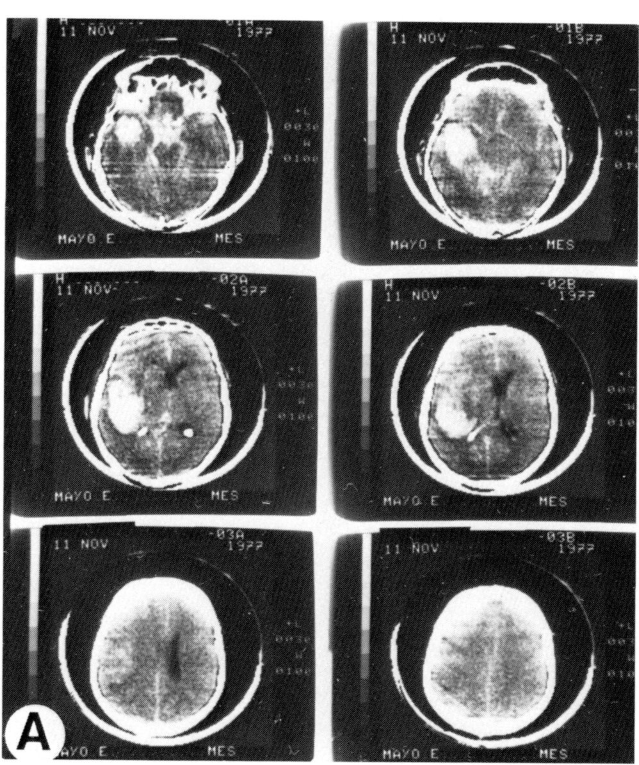

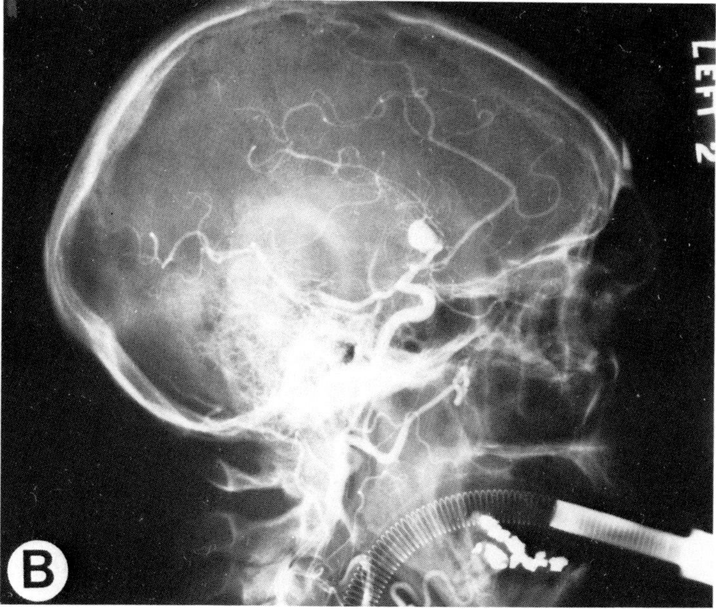

Fig. 77-2.   (A) A CT scan showing a left temporal intracerebral hemorrhage. (B) A lateral angiogram of the left carotid of the same patient, showing a large aneurysm of the left middle cerebral artery with elevation of the sylvian vessels caused by the temporal hematoma mass.

kemias, particularly in association with extreme leukemic leukocytosis or "blast crisis." Hemorrhage probably results from a combination of cerebral vascular insults including perivascular infiltration by blast cells, an elevated blood viscosity, and microcirculation thrombosis and vasodilatation. In an attempt to prevent this complication, Dearth et al.[23] advised emergency cranial radiation as well as other therapeutic measures for any patient with acute leukemia who has a leukocyte count exceeding 100,000/mm³.

Intracranial hemorrhage is the leading cause of death in hemophiliac patients and poses a special challenge to the neurosurgeon. Approximately half of these hemorrhages are subdural or epidural. Intracerebral hemorrhage and its operative treatment have carried a high mortality in these patients and led Silverstein to state in 1960 that "the only worthwhile indication for surgical intervention in the treatment of intracranial hemorrhage in hemophiliacs is bleeding limited to the sub- or epidural spaces."[24] Since that time dramatic improvement in replacement therapy and methods for neutralization of factor VIII inhibitors have allowed hematologists to render even the severe hemophiliac hemostatically competent so that the hemorrhage can be managed in accordance with basic neurosurgical principles. More recent series, therefore, show a marked improvement in the results of management of

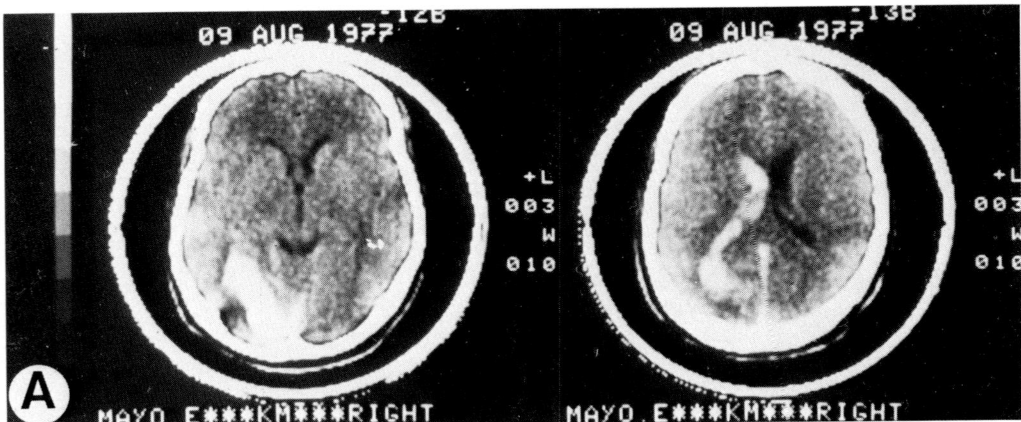

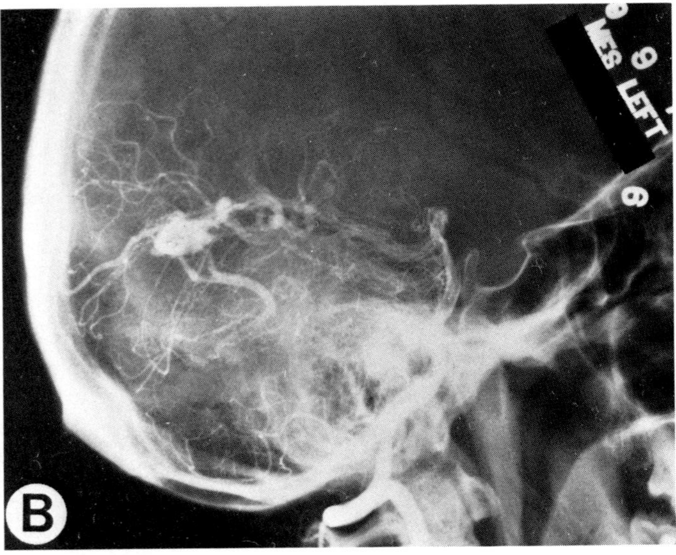

Fig. 77-3. (A) A CT scan demonstrating a hemorrhage of the left occipital lobe with intraventricular extension. (B) A lateral angiogram of the left vertebrobasilar system in the same patient. There is a moderate-sized occipital AVM filling from the left posterior cerebral artery and draining into the transverse sinus.

intracranial hemorrhage including intracerebral hematoma.[25,26] See specific authoritative references for guidelines on replacement therapy and operative management of hemophiliac patients.[26–28]

An entirely separate category of intracerebral hemorrhage is the subependymal and intraventricular hemorrhages (SEH-IVH), which occur in preterm and, less frequently, full-term infants. With improved clinical recognition of the syndrome and, particularly, absolute diagnosis with CT scanning, SEH or IVH or both are now known to occur in 40 percent to 50 percent of newborn infants of less than 35 weeks gestation who require intensive care for more than 24 hours.[29] The majority of infants with SEH-IVH survive; Ahmann et al.[30] found a mortality rate of 28 percent in premature infants conforming to the above criteria, with hemorrhage the primary cause of death in 75 percent.

The onset of the hemorrhage typically occurs in the first several days of life, with a mean age of 38 hours.[31] Cases occurring in older infants have been recognized, although the etiology of the hemorrhage in these cases probably is different.[32] The hemorrhages are thought to arise from the periventricular germinal matrix area secondary to congestion, thrombosis, and disruption of the weakly supported capillaries and veins in this region.[29] In addition to prematurity, factors associated with high risk for SEH-IVH include hyaline membrane hypoxia, mechanical ventilation, and rupture of alveoli. It

has been postulated that increased central venous pressure and decreased cerebral venous return caused by mechanical ventilation or rupture of alveoli leads to disruption of the germinal matrix microvasculature, which is already damaged by hypoxia and ischemia.[29] Clinical symptoms may be an abrupt deterioration with progression to death, or a stuttering course of deterioration followed by stabilization and improvement. A bulging fontanelle, seizures, decreased muscle tone, and abnormal eye signs may also be present. Of the infants surviving IVH, progressive hydrocephalus develops in about 20 percent, particularly in those infants who had more severe hemorrhages. This may resolve spontaneously or with medical management including serial lumbar punctures. In the study of Ahmann et al.,[30] shunting was eventually required in only 2 of 12 patients.

DIAGNOSIS AND PROGNOSIS

Prior to CT the diagnosis of intracerebral hemorrhage was made on the basis of clinical features aided by x-ray or echoencephalographic evidence of midline structure shift, a cautious lumbar puncture, and cerebral angiography. In spite of these measures, a "diagnostic impasse" sometimes existed "in as many as 30 percent of the patients presenting with acute cerebrovascular episodes"[33] for whom the critical difference between hemorrhage and infarction could not be readily distinguished, and expeditious treatment was therefore compromised. Now, CT scanning allows rapid diagnosis of intracerebral hemorrhage, and, in addition to being the most definitive diagnostic test, also gives information regarding the exact site, extent, and possibly the cause of the hemorrhage, considerations that substantially affect the prognosis and management. Computed tompgraphic scanning after contrast infusion may be very helpful in demonstrating the source of the intracerebral hemorrhage, particularly in cases of vascular malformation, tumors, and occasionally aneurysms. Although most cases of gangliothalamic hemorrhage are primary, Weisberg has advised contrasted CT for patients less than 40 years of age: those without a history of hypertension; those in whom maximal neurologic deficit developed after 4 hours or longer; those with prodromal symptoms; those with a history of neoplasm, endocarditis, or blood dyscrasia; and, last, those whose noncontrasted CT scans had an atypical appearance.[11] Contrast examination is likewise indicated in all cases of lobar hemorrhage, cerebellar hemorrhage in young or nonhypertensive patients,[11,19] and the rare cases of multiple spontaneous intracerebral hematomas.[34]

Computed tomography is very useful in following cases of intracerebral hemorrhage, particularly those managed nonsurgically or in an expectant fashion (Figure 77-4). Liquefaction and resorption of intracerebral hematomas may occur over several weeks,[33] while blood usually is cleared from the ventricles within 2 weeks.[18] Also, delayed development of communicating hydrocephalus is best diagnosed by CT.

Although some have advocated angiography in all cases of intracerebral hemorrhage to be treated surgically,[13] we would not consider this necessary in cases where there is a typical clinical and CT picture for primary intracerebral or cerebellar hemorrhage or in patients whose condition is deteriorating so rapidly that a delay in surgery seems contraindicated. Angioigraphy is strongly indicated where hypertension is not clearly the cause and in all cases of lobar hemorrhage. Even if negative in the acute phase, follow up angiography and CT scans after several months may be to diagnose underlying tumor or vascular malformation.[34A]

In an analysis of the CT scans of 300 patients with nontraumatic intracranial hemorrhage, Weisberg found 283 with intracerebral hemorrhage, 12 with subarachnoid bleeding, and only 5 with exclusively intraventricular hemorrhage.[11] The overall mortality in this series was 26 percent, similar to that of another series of intracerebral hemorrhage diagnosed with CT,[35] and markedly better than the 83 percent 1-month mortality for cases of cerebral hemorrhage reported by Whisnant[4] before the advent of CT diagnosis. This difference in mortality can be accounted for in part by the present-day CT diagnosis of milder cases of intracerebral hemorrhage previously misdiagnosed as ischemic stroke or subarachnoid hemorrhage. Thalamic-ganglionic hemorrhage was present in 232 of Weisberg's cases,[11] 81 percent of these being hypertensive patients. The mortality for patients with thalamic-ganglionic hemorrhage without ventricular extension was 25 percent, but rose to 70 percent for those with ventricular extension. The mortality in patients with lobar hematomas was 20 percent with or without extension of the hemorrhage into the ventricular system. Ropper et al. found a 12 percent mortality in 26 cases of lobar hemorrhage,[19] whereas Kase et al.[35A] recorded a 32 percent mortality in their series.

Extensive intraventricular hemorrhage caused by extension from a thalamic-ganglionic hypertensive hemorrhage or aneurysm rupture usually carries a grave prognosis. Little et al.[18] found an overall mortality of 83 percent in adult patients with intraventricular hemorrhage and a 100 percent mortality in those with "massive" extension into the ventricles. The latter group typically had sudden profound coma and neurologic deficits of pontomedullary dysfunction and died within 48 hours. A second group of patients in the series of Little et al. developed sudden focal cerebral or cerebellar disturbance and secondary brain stem dysfunction; in these the mortality was 88 percent. A smaller group of patients with intraventricular hemorrhage had relatively mild symptoms and signs and followed a benign course with no mortality directly related to the hemorrhage.

In another recent series of patients with intraventricular hemorrhage diagnosed by CT, de Weerd[36] found an overall mortality of 53 percent, which rose to 63 percent if the hemorrhage extended into all ventricles and dropped to 38 percent if there was limited ventricular extension. Of the latter subgroup in de Weerd's series, i.e., limited ventricular extension of the hemorrhage, 38 percent also survived with no disability.[36]

As in other series,[18,37,38,38A] de Weerd found a close correlation between the clinical condition of the patient on admission and prognosis.[36] This fact has already been alluded to earlier in this chapter in reference to cerebellar hemorrhage. In the review of Ott et al.,[39] two thirds of the patients suffering from cerebellar hemorrhage were responsive on admission, but one half were comatose within 24 hours and 75 percent within 1 week of onset. With surgical intervention the mortality for cerebellar hemorrhage was only 17 percent if the patients were operated on while they were still in a responsive condition, but this rose to 75 percent for unresponsive patients. The prognosis for cerebellar hemorrhage in children has been found to be better than for adults despite the severity of the initial condition.[40,41]

MANAGEMENT

GENERAL MEASURES

With the widespread availability of CT, the diagnosis of intracerebral hemorrhage can now be readily established and early specific treatment initiated. The airway should be secured with intubation, if necessary, to avoid hypoxia and hypercarbia. Close observation of vital signs, neurologic status, and ventilation, pulmonary toilet, and fluid balance usually dictate the need for intensive care nursing of the acutely ill patient. If a coagulopathy is present, particularly one brought on by anticoagulant therapy, it should be expeditiously corrected with appropriate blood component transfusions and reversal medications. Hypertension should be treated aggressively[42] with intravenous infusions of nitroprusside for rapid reduction and optimal control of blood pressure in cases of extreme elevation, or intramuscular hydralazine hydrochloride when the need for a reduction in blood pressure is less acute. Anticonvulsant medication has been advocated in all cases of supratentorial intracerebral hematoma by some authors.[34A] If there is evidence of increased intracranial pressure (ICP), treatment with urea, mannitol, or furosemide may be indicated and placement of an intracranial pressure (ICP) monitor should be considered to guide this therapy. Such monitoring and treatment may permit adequate control of intracranial hypertension in certain cases so that surgery can be avoided. If the elevation of intracranial pressure becomes refractory to medical treatment, surgery may be indicated.[43,44]

SURGICAL THERAPY

The indications for and timing of surgical intervention for intracranial hemorrhage have been contentious. In 1961, McKissock et al.[45] published the results of a controlled clinical trial that compared the benefits of surgical therapy with those of aggressive conservative management. The overall mortality was 65 percent for the surgically treated group and 51 percent for the nonsurgically treated patients. The authors concluded: "We have been unable to demonstrate any benefit from surgery in regard to either mortality or morbidity."[45]

A uniform surgical management for primary intracerebral hemorrhage, including angiography and surgery within 24 hours on all patients with a demonstrable intracerebral hematoma mass, major focal neurologic deficit, and a depressed level of consciousness or signs of brain stem involvement, was reported by Luessenhop et al. in 1967.[37] Their overall mortality was 37 percent, and it was 32 percent for the surgically treated patients, considerably better than that reported by McKissock. In 7 of the 12 surgically treated patients who died and in several survivors, reaccumulation of a hematoma occurred and was considered the most important surgical complication. The operative mortality was 89 percent in capsular hemorrhage cases compared with 4 percent in those with lobar hematomas. Patients not moribund on admission had an operative mortality of only 8 percent.

Kaneo et al.[38] recently reported remarkable success with early evacuation of laterally situated hypertensive basal ganglia hemorrhages, stressing the importance of surgery within 7 hours of ictus and microsurgical technique. Other authors have not concurred in this[38A,45A] or advocated a less urgent, or even delayed, elective evacuation of the intracerebral hematoma, citing higher mortality rates in patients on whom surgery was performed earlier.[46–49,49A] This approach can be supported to some degree with the observations of Papo[43] and Janny et al.,[44] who monitored intracranial pressure in a series of patients with intracerebral hemorrhage and found that the intracranial pressure in these patients was generally only moderately elevated (less than 33 mm Hg) shortly after the ictus and gradually became normal over several weeks. After the surgical evacuation of the hematomas, there was a rapid but only temporary reduction in pressure, followed by an increase to its preoperative level.[44] Except in the most mildly and most severely affected patients, no definite correlation was found between ICP and clinical condition or outcome.[43,44A] Such findings indicate that the damaging effects of intracerebral hemorrhage are caused more by the disruption of the brain by the hemorrhage than the secondary intracranial hypertension, and that the beneficial effect of evacuating a hematoma may be due more to the reduction in local tissue pressures and improved microcirculation than the reduction in the increased intracranial pressure. More recent experimental studies suggest that intracerebral hemorrhage rapidly induces secondary brain tissue edema, hemorrhage, and necrosis, which can be minimized or halted by hematoma evacuation within six hours.[50] Clinical experiences in certain patients such as exemplified in Figure 77-4 attest to the edemogenic properties of intracerebral blood.

In the final decision-making process regarding operative versus conservative management of a patient with intracerebral hemorrhage, the surgeon must consider multiple factors includ-

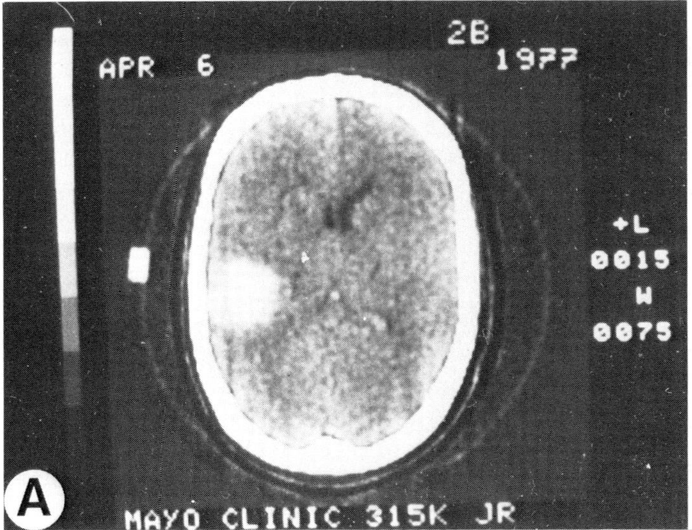

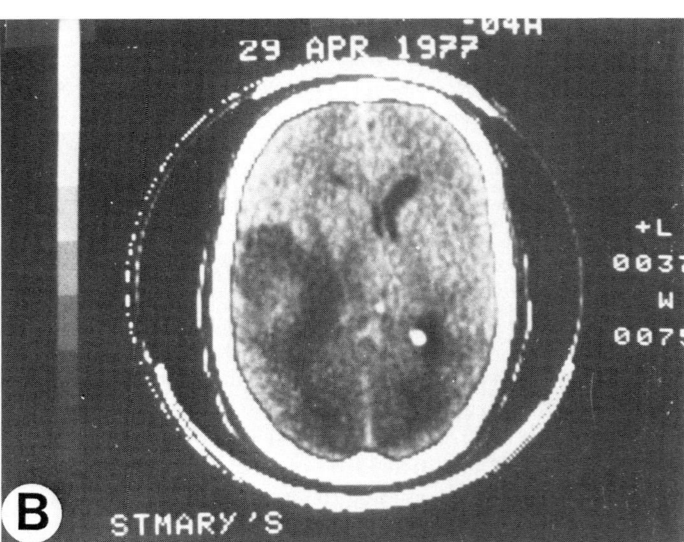

Fig. 77-4. (A) A CT scan demonstrating a moderate-sized, acute, primary, left posterotemporal intracerebral hemorrhage in a young man. His only neurologic deficit was moderate aphasia, and conservative therapy was elected. (B) A CT scan of the same patient 3 weeks later. The hematoma has liquefied, but there is now extensive surrounding edema with midline shift. The patient showed increased aphasia and papilledema, which resolved after craniotomy and evacuation of the liquefied clot.

ing the clinical condition of the patient, particularly the severity and progression of neurologic deficits, and the site and extent of the hemorrhage as indicated on CT scans and the question of quality of survival rather than simply survival.[38A,45A,50A] Patients of advanced age and poor nutritional status or those who have co-existent major life-threatening medical problems are not usually candidates for surgical intervention. The patient with an extensive basal ganglia hemorrhage who is deeply comatose with severely depressed or absent brain stem reflexes and faltering vital signs should also not be subjected to operation. Conversely, those patients who have a small hemorrhage causing stable neurologic deficit and little alteration in their level of consciousness can be expected to do well without surgery.

Ten to 50 percent[5,37] of the patients with intracerebral hemorrhage will be between these two extremes, however, and should be considered for surgery. If their level of consciousness is deteriorating or the lateralized deficit increasing, emergency surgery may be indicated. If there is a pronounced focal neurologic deficit or stable depression of level of consciousness and a significant mass exists caused by an intracerebral hematoma, especially one that is lobar or subcortical in location, evacuation of the clot should be carried out at the earliest convenient time.[34A,35A] When predominantly intraventricular hemorrhage is present and there is significant obtundation or evidence of increased intracranial pressure, ventricular drainage may be helpful but an open evacuation of a solid clot also may need to be considered.[34A,51]

Special mention should be made regarding the management of cerebellar hemorrhage, since its course is unpredictable and it can produce rapid deterioration and death. With this in mind, Ott et al.[39] advised immediate surgery for all patients with intracerebellar hemorrhage who are seen in the first 48 hours after ictus and for most patients within a week of onset. In an analysis of patients with cerebellar hemorrhage confirmed by CT scan, Little et al.[52] concluded that immediate evacuation of the hematoma was indicated if there was evidence of brain stem compression, hydrocephalus, or if the hematoma was larger than 3 cm. Ojemann[53] advised immediate evacuation of all large hematomas even when the neurologic status is stable and there is hydrocephalus and neurologic compromise. Although rare, evacuation of brain stem hematomas may be indicated in selected cases.[54,55]

OPERATIVE TECHNIQUE

Evacuation of an intracerebral hemorrhage should be carried out through a full craniotomy that is adequate enough to expose the limits of the hematoma and that also makes it possible to identify and deal with unsuspected pathologic processes that might be present, such as a tumor, vascular malformation, or aneurysm. The cavity of the hematoma should be entered through a cortical incision that provides the most direct access yet the least injury to vital cortical areas, tracts, or blood vessels. The hematoma is evacuated with gentle suction and irrigation and forceps. Leaving some clot attached to the walls may be preferable to an overly aggressive removal with resultant injury to the adjacent brain or small vessels. Attention should be given during the removal to identifying a likely source for the hemorrhage such as an occult vascular malformation or a tumor, and suspicious-looking tissue fragments should be saved for thorough histologic examination. Magnification and illumination with the operating microscope are particularly helpful during evacuation and exploration of cavities of deep hematomas approached through a limited cortical incision. In rare instances a single artery may be identified as the source of hemorrhage and bleeding controlled with a clip or coagulation. Bleeding from the cavity walls can be controlled by temporarily applying cottonoid patties and hemostatic gelatin sponge, gauze, or fibrillar collagen.

Irrigating the cavity of the hematoma with a gentle saline lavage will reveal persistent bleeding sites. Meticulous hemostasis must be achieved and Ojemann[56] has advised temporarily elevating the blood pressure to hypertensive levels to help visualize any possible recurrent bleeding site.

Small series of stereotaxic and endoscopic evacuation of intracerebral hematomas have been reported with impressive results in selected cases.[57,58,59] The development of imaginative equipment and techniques has allowed removal of extensive, acute clots which was not possible utilizing simple cannulation and aspiration. Recurrent hemorrhage remains a significant complication even with this technology and more experience is necessary before it can be advocated for general use over more standard approaches.

POSTOPERATIVE CARE

Postoperative care should follow routine neurosurgical principles. Blood pressure control should be continued to avoid severe hypertension. Extensive cerebral edema may be associated with acute intracerebral hemorrhage;[50] steroids may be of benefit in its treatment and these should not be discontinued prematurely.[34A]

Neurologic deterioration in the early postoperative period suggests hematoma reaccumulation, whereas delayed deterioration, particularly in cases of intraventricular hemorrhage, may be the result of hydrocephalus. Fortunately, computed tomography has greatly facilitated the diagnosis of these conditions as well as more routine follow-up of intracerebral hemorrhages.

REFERENCES

1. Wolf PA, Dawber TR, Thomas HE, et al: Epidemiology of stroke. Adv Neurol 16:5, 1977
2. Kurtzke JF: Epidemiology of cerebrovascular diseases, in Siekert RG (ed): Cerebrovascular Survey Report for Joint Council Subcommittee on Cerebrovascular Disease, National Institute of Neurological and Communicative Disorders and Stroke and National Heart and Lung Institute. Rochester, Minn, Whiting, 1976, pp 213–242
3. Furlan AJ, Whisnant JP, Elveback LR: The decreasing incidence of primary intracerebral hemorrhage: A population study. Ann Neurol 5:367, 1979
4. Whisnant JP, Fitzgibbons JP, Kurland LT, et al: Natural history of stroke in Rochester, Minnesota, 1945 through 1954. Stroke 2:11, 1971
5. Ransohoff J, Derby B, Kricheff I: Spontaneous intracerebral hemorrhage. Clin Neurosurg 18:247, 1971
6. McCormick WF, Rosenfield DB: Massive brain hemorrhage: A review of 144 cases and an examination of their causes. Stroke 4:946, 1973
7. Fisher CM: Cerebral miliary aneurysms in hypertension. Am J Pathol 66:313, 1972
8. Okazaki H, Reagan JT, Campbell RJ: Clinicopathologic studies of primary cerebral amyloid angiopathy. Mayo Clin Proc 54:22, 1979
9. Freytag E: Fatal hypertensive intracerebral hematomas: A survey of the pathological anatomy of 393 cases. J Neurol Neurosurg Psychiatry 31:616, 1968
10. Fisher CM: Clinical syndromes in cerebral thrombosis, hypertensive hemorrhage, and ruptured saccular aneurysm. Clin Neurosurg 22:117, 1974
11. Weisberg L: Computerized tomography in intracranial hemorrhage. Arch Neurol 36:422, 1979
12. Fisher CM: Clinical syndromes in cerebral hemorrhage, in Fields WS (ed): Pathogenesis and Treatment of Cerebrovascular Disease. Springfield, Ill, Charles C Thomas, 1961, pp 318–342
13. Rossi GF, Maira G: Comments on chapters 28 and 29. Adv Neurol 25:305, 1979
14. Freeman RE, Onofrio BM, Okazaki H, et al: Spontaneous intracerebellar hemorrhage. Diagnosis and surgical treatment. Neurology 23:84, 1973
15. Jellinger K: Cerebrovascular amyloidosis with cerebral hemorrhage. J Neurol 214:195, 1977

16. Rengachary SS, Racela LS, Watanabe I, et al: Neurosurgical and immunological implications of primary cerebral amyloid (congophilic) angiopathy. Neurosurgery 7:1, 1980

16A. Kase C: Intracerebral hemorrhage: Common nonhypertensive causes. Current Concepts of Cerebrovascular Disease, Stroke 20:19, 1985.

17. Torack RM: Congophilic angiopathy complicated by surgery and massive hemorrhage: A light and electron microscopic study. Am J Pathol 81:349, 1975

18. Little JR, Blomquist GA, Ethier R: Intraventricular hemorrhage in adults. Surg Neurol 8:143, 1977

19. Ropper AH, Davis KR: Lobar cerebral hemorrhages: Acute clinical syndromes in 26 cases. Ann Neurol 8:141, 1980

20. Locksley HB, Sahs AL, Sandler R: Report on the cooperative study of intracranial aneurysms and subarachnoid hemorrhage. Section 3 Subarachnoid hemorrhage unrelated to intracranial aneurysm and A-V malformations: A study of associated diseases and prognosis. J Neurosurg 24:1034, 1966

21. Russel DS: The pathology of spontaneous intracerebral hemorrhage. Proc R Soc Med 47:689, 1954

22. Scott M: Spontaneous intracerebral hematoma caused by cerebral neoplasms. Report of 8 verified cases. J Neurosurg 42:338, 1975

23. Dearth JC, Fountain KS, Smithson WA, et al: Extreme leukemic leucocytosis (blast crisis) in childhood. Mayo Clin Proc 53:207, 1978

24. Silverstein A: Intracranial bleeding in hemophilia. Arch Neurol 3:141, 1960

25. Van Trotsenburg L: Neurological complications of haemophilia, in Brinkhaus KM, Hemker HC (eds): Handbook of Hemophilia, part 1. New York, American Elsevier, 1975, p 389

26. Gilchrist GS, Piepgras DG: Neurologic complications in hemophilia, in Hilgartner MW (ed): Hemophilia in Children. Littleton, Mass, Publishing Sciences Group, 1976, p 79

27. Hilgartner MW: Current therapy, in Hilgartner MW (ed): Hemophilia in Children. Littleton, Mass, Publishing Sciences Group, 1976, p 151

28. Olsen ER: Intracranial surgery in hemophiliacs. Arch Neurol 21:401, 1969

29. Dykes FD, Kazzara A, Ahmann P, et al: Intraventricular hemorrhage: A prospective evaluation of etiopathogenesis. Pediatrics 66:42, 1980

30. Ahmann PA, Lazzara A, Dykes FD, et al: Intraventricular hemorrhage in the high risk pre term infant: Incidence and outcome. Ann Neurol 7:118, 1980

31. Tsiantos A, Victorin L, Reilier JP, et al: Intracranial hemorrhage in the prematurely born infant. J Pediatr 85:854, 1974

32. Mitchell W, O'Tuama L: Cerebral intraventricular hemorrhages in infants: A widening age spectrum. Pediatrics 65:35, 1980

33. Feindel W: Management of intracerebral hemorrhage. Adv Neurol 25:293, 1979

34. Weisberg L: Multiple spontaneous intracerebral hemorrhages. Clinical and computerized tomographic correlations. Neurology 311:897, 1981

34A. Ojemann R, Heros R: Spontaneous Brain Hemorrhage. Stroke 14:468, 1983.

35. Kinkel WR, Jacobs L: Computerized tomography in cerebrovascular disease. Neurology 26:924, 1976

35A. Kase C, Williams J, Wyatt D, et al: Lobar intracerebral hematomas: Clinical and CT analysis of 22 cases. Neurology 32:1146, 1982.

36. de Weerd AW: The prognosis of intraventricular hemorrhage. J Neurol 222:45, 1979

37. Luessenhop AJ, Shevlin WA, Ferrero AA, et al: Surgical management of primary intracerebral hemorrhage. J Neurosurg 27:419, 1967

38. Kaneo M, Tokomi K, Yokoyama T: Early surgical treatment for hypertensive intracerebral hemorrhage. J Neurosurg 46:579, 1977

38A. Waga S, Yamamota Y: Hypertensive putaminal hemorrhage: Treatment and results. Is surgical treatment superior to conservative one? Stroke 14:480, 1983.

39. Ott KH, Kase CS, Ojemann RG, et al: Cerebellar hemorrhage: Diagnosis and treatment. A review of 56 cases. Arch Neurol 31:160, 1974

40. Erenberg G, Rubin R, Shulman K: Cerebellar haematoma caused by angiomas in children. J Neurol Neurosurg Psychiatry 35:304, 1972

41. Kazmiroff PB, Weichsel ME, Grinnel V, et al: Acute cerebellar hemorrhage in childhood: Etiology diagnosis and treatment. Neurosurgery 6:524, 1980

42. Meyer J, Bauer R: Medical treatment of spontaneous intracranial hemorrhage by use of hypotensive drugs. Neurology 12:36, 1962

42A. Duff T, Aveni S, Levin A, et al: Nonsurgical mnanagement of spontaneous intracerebral hematoma. Neurosurgery 9:387, 1981.

43. Papo I, Janny P, Caruselli G, et al: Intracranial pressure time course in primary intracerebral hemorrhage. Neurosurgery 6:504, 1979

44. Janny P, Colnet G, Georget A, et al: Intracranial pressure with intracerebral hemorrhages. Surg Neurol 10:371, 1978

44A. Ropper AH, King R: Intracranial pressure monitoring in comatose patients with cerebral hemorrhage. Arch Neurol 44:725, 1984

45. McKissock W, Richardson A, Taylor J: Primary intracerebral hemorrhage: A controlled trial of surgical and conservative treatment in 180 unselected cases. Lancet 2:221, 1961

45A. Kanno T, Sano H, Shinomiya T: Role of surgery in hypertensive intracerebral hematoma. J Neurosurg 61:1091, 1984

46. Paillas JE, Alliez B: Surgical treatment of spontaneous intracerebral hemorrhage: Immediate and long-term results in 250 cases. J Neurosurg 39:145, 1973

47. Tedeschi G, Bernini FP, Cerillo A: Indications for surgical treatment of intracerebral hemorrhage. J Neurosurg 43:590, 1975

48. Cautico W, Adib S, Gaston P: Spontaneous intracerebral hematomas. J Neurosurg 22:569, 1965

49. Benes V, Koukolik F, Obrovska D: Two types of spontaneous intracerebral hemorrhage due to hypertension. J Neurosurg 37:509, 1972

50. Suzuki J, Ebina T: Sequential changes in tissue surrounding ICH, in Pia HW, Langmaid C, Zierski J (eds): Spontaneous Intracerebral Haematomas, Advances in Diagnosis and Therapy. New York, Springer-Verlag, 1980, pp 121–128

50A. Volpin L, Cerevellini P, Colombo F, et al: Spontaneous intracerebral hematomas: A new proposal about the usefulness and limits of surgical treatment. Neurosurgery 15:663, 1984.

51. Pia HW: The surgical treatment of intracerebral and intraventricular haematomas. Acta Neurochir 27:149, 1972

52. Little JR, Tubman DE, Ethier R: Cerebellar hemorrhage in adults: Diagnosis by computerized tomography. J Neurosurg 48:575, 1978

53. Ojemann RG: Comments in Kazimiroff PB, Weichsel E, Grinnel V, Young RF: Acute cerebellar hemorrhage in childhood: Etiology, diagnosis and treatment. Neurosurgery 6:524, 1980

54. Cioffi FA, Tomasello F, D'Avanzo R: Pontine hematomas. Surg Neurol 16:13, 1981

55. Murphy M: Successful evacuation of acute pontine hematoma. J Neurosurg 37:224, 1972

56. Ojemann RG, Mohr JP: Hypertensive brain hemorrhage. Clin Neurosurg 23:220, 1975

CHAPTER 78

Stereotactic Evacuation of Intracerebral Hematomas

Edward I. Kandel   Vjacheslav V. Peresedov

THE SURGICAL TREATMENT of spontaneous, nontraumatic, intracerebral hemorrhage caused by hypertension and cerebral arterioscerosis has been developing over the past three decades,[1-5] yet many important problems remain to be resolved. Different and sometimes opposite points of view exist about the indications and contraindications for surgery, the timing of the operations, and surgical techniques in the management of these problems. The postoperative mortality varies from 15 to 80 percent, the latter rate being seen in patients operated on in deep coma and with medial thalamic hemorrhages; however, there are grounds for suggesting that early evacuation of the hematoma should increase the patients' chances for surviving and for making a functional recovery as well.

Traditionally, intracerebral hemotomas are removed following craniotomy and corticectomy performed under direct vision. Although not technically difficult, the operative procedure carries a high risk in the most severe cases, and many neurosurgeons believe that the operation is contraindicated if the patient is comatose.

Past attempts to remove hematoma radically using a less traumatic technique than craniotomy have included attempts to aspirate the hematoma through a burr hole. Unfortunately, within a few hours after the onset of the stroke the hematoma consists of both liquid blood (about 20 percent of its volume) and dense clots (about 80 percent). Attempts to remove a hematoma even through a cannula of large diameter were unsuccessful because evacuation of dense clots was practically impossible. The attempted stereotactic aspiration of intracerebral hematoma through a cannula was also found to be ineffective and was not accepted in practice.[6] This situation stimulated the search for a less traumatic, safer method of removing intracerebral hematomas. The development of CT investigation in neurosurgery opened up new possibilities for using the sterectactic technique in the treatment of spontaneous intracerebral hemorrhages.

A new principle of stereotactic evacuation of these hematomas was proposed by Backlund and von Holst,[7] who described its successful clinical use in only one case. The authors used an instrument consisting of a cannula 4 mm in diameter containing a mandrel-like Archimedes' screw which the surgeon rotated manually. The propeller-like action of the screw fragments the dense blood clots. A conventional surgical aspirator is connected with the outer end of the cannula and small pieces of clot are then aspirated into the bottle. This device has some substantial shortcomings. The digital rotation of the screw by the surgeon is not convenient and it is practically impossible to carry

on this maneuver for a long time. Higgins and Nashold[8] have modified this device by adding a thin tube along the cannula. This tube allows one to maintain the vacuum when the cannula lumen is occluded by clot and to inject a saline through the tube into the hematoma cavity. We used this device on three patients, on two of them twice.

Broseta[9] reported the application of a similar device in 16 patients with hypertensive hematomas. Eleven of them were in a comatose state, and penetration of blood into the ventricles occurred in nine cases. The postoperative mortality was extremely high (81 percent). Two patients died from recurrent hemorrhage.

For the stereotactic evacuation of intracranial hematomas we have constructed a new patented piece of improved equipment which is a further development of the Backlund and von Holst apparatus. We began to use our method in the clinic in 1979 and published our first results between 1982 and 1984.[10,11,12]

The central element of our device is a stainless steel cannula 17 cm long with an outer diameter of 3.6 mm and an opening on the distal end (Figure 78-1). The cannula is introduced into the hematoma cavity stereotactically. There are two changeable pivots for the cannula. The first pivot is a metallic pin with a blunt tip. The second pivot is a thin stainless steel Archimedes' screw for destruction of densely coagulated clots. The tip of the screw is 1.5 mm shorter than the open end of the cannula according to our experimental data (see below). It is important that the screw occupies only 7 percent of the space inside the cannula. This is several times less than in Backlund's device. This thin screw markedly increases the effectiveness of the aspiration.

The opening for the plastic tube connected with the aspirator is located not on the side of the outer cannula end, as in Backlund's device, but on the axis of the cannula. The "straight flow" removal of clots prevents the development of blocking inside the cannula.

The screw is connected with a minature electric engine on the outer end of the device with changeable screw speeds from 50 to 200 rpm. The transparent plastic tube on the outer end of the cannula connects it with the glass bottle graduated in milliliters. The second tube connects the bottle with a conventional surgical aspirator which removes the fragmented clots. The degree of the aspirator vacuum may be changed up to 2 atmospheres.

Before its clinical use this device was tested in a series of animal and technical experiments. The aim of the first experi-

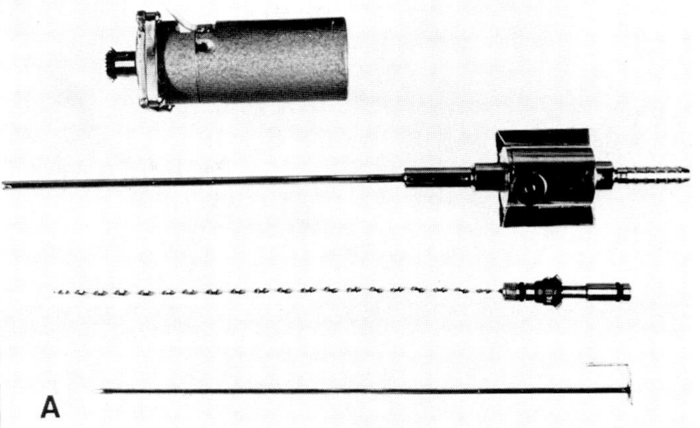

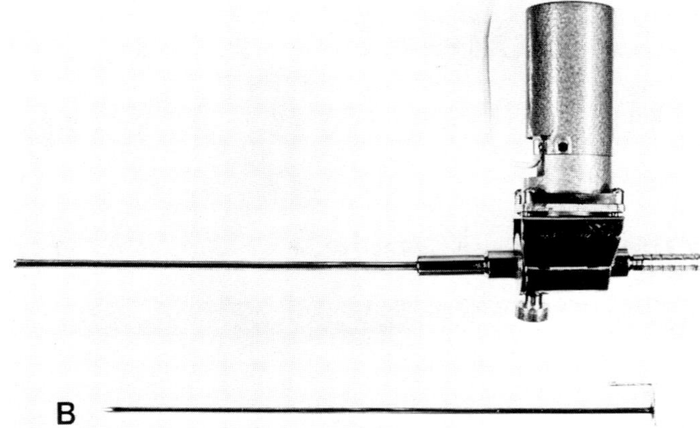

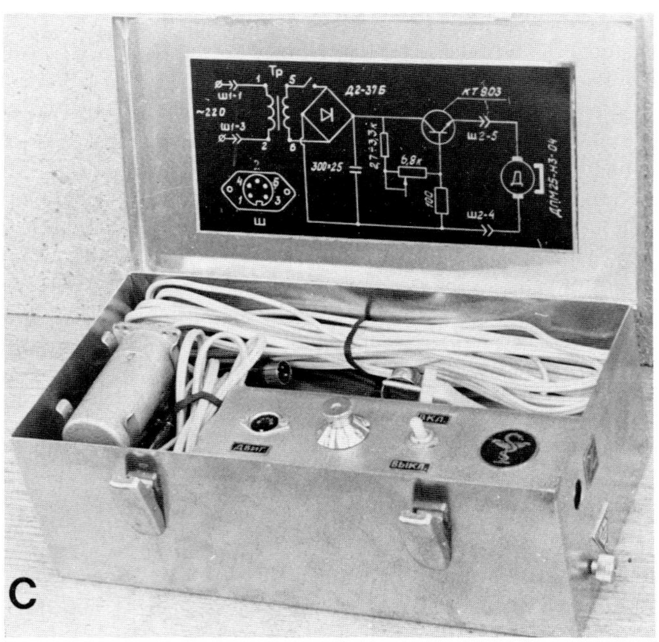

Fig. 78-1. The device for stereotactic evacuation of intracerebral hematomas shown disassembled (A), assembled (B), and collected in a case (C).

ments on rabbit brains was to determine the optimal speed of rotation of the screw and optimal vacuum of the aspirator. Small trephinations were made under general anesthesia, the dura incised, and the cannula tip introduced into the rabbit brain for 5 to 6 mm. With the aspirator vacuum at less than 0.5 atmosphere there is no aspiration of the brain tissue. Damage of tissue is absent at screw speeds from 60 to 200 rpm, but the optimal speed is about 100 rpm.

The device was also tested on stored human blood and clotted without preservatives to investigate the optimal parameters for the suction of blood clots. The optimal speed of rotation for dense clots is up to 120 rpm, for less dense clots about 80 rpm. The vacuum needs to be at approximately 0.2 to 0.3 atmosphere.

A second series of experiments was conducted to determine the relationship between the tips of the cannula and the screw. It was shown that the optimal variant is when the screw tip is 1.5 to 2 mm shorter than the cannula tip. In that case damage to the brain tissue during aspiration is prevented and aspiration is more effective.

PREOPERATIVE CALCULATIONS

Before surgery, we analyzed CT scans to assess the size and location of the intercerbral hematoma, its x-ray density, the degree of associated brain edema, the mass effect of the hematoma, and the penetration of the blood into the ventricles. To exclude the presence of an arterial aneurysm or AVM, cerebral angiography was also performed.

The volume of the hematoma is estimated based on the CT scan. The planimetric method allows one to calculate the hematoma area on each scan, multiplying the area by the thickness of the scan (8 mm in our scanner) and summing up all scans on which the hematoma is seen. Another way to estimate the volume of the hematoma is as the volume of an ellipsoid by the formula: $V = 4/5\ a \times b \times c$, where a, b, and c are the hemiaxes of the ellipsoid. The difference in the results obtained by these two estimations of the hematoma volume is small. The results are multiplied by 3.5 to obtain the actual volume of the hematoma.

One next transfers the information regarding the contours of the hematoma from the CT scans to the plain x-ray films in both projections taken in the operating room accorrding to the routine stereotactic technique. It is important that these films be taken in the perpendicular position of the base plane of scanning to both films. For this the base plane of the CT scan is checked by metallic marks attached to the patient's head. Using TV control with electronic amplifiers the base plane is positioned perpendicular to both stereotactic plain films.

A target point (or points) is then selected within the hematoma on the scans for introduction of the cannula to the desired points. We used to choose a point 1 to 2 cm posterior to the center of the hematoma, assuming that during the stereotactic aspiration in the supine position the clots would sink toward the cannula because of gravity. In the presence of a very large hematoma we sometimes aspirate 2 to 3 parts of the hematoma, and in such cases we choose several target points on the plain films.

Selection of the burr hole location depends on the site and volume of the hematoma. Generally, we place the burr hole near the coronal suture. In the case of deep-lying hematomas the cannula trajectory is decided after review of Schaltenbrand and Bailey's stereotactic atlas.

OPERATIVE TECHNIQUE

As a rule, the operation is performed under general endotracheal anesthesia, although we sometimes use neuroleptanalgesia. In most comotose patients it is possible to carry out the operation under local anesthesia.

Preoperatively the sagittal line and the point of its crossing with the coronal suture are marked on the patient's head. The burr hole site is measured from both marks. The patient's head is then placed on the special headrest and fixed in the stereotactic frame (Figure 78-2). After making a skin incision 4 cm long the burr hole is made using a coronal trephine 25 mm in diameter to expose the dura. The dura is incised and the stereotactic apparatus including the device for aspiration is installed in the burr hole. A second burr hole is made on the opposite side, also near the coronal suture, and a silicone

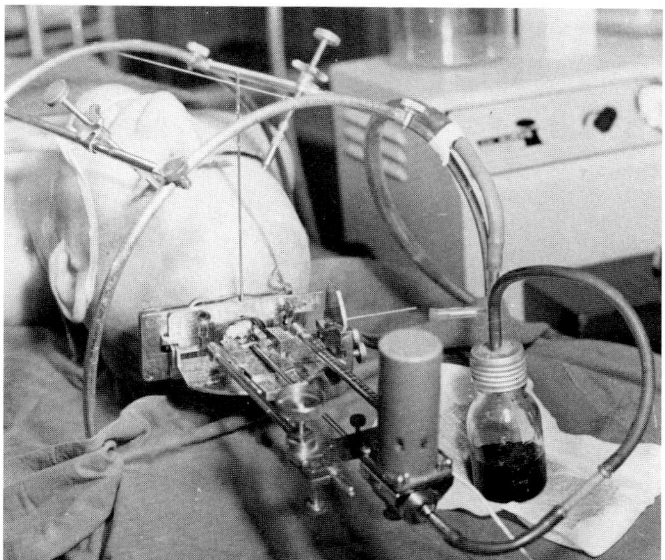

Fig. 78-2. General view of the operation.

catheter is introduced into the ventricle for continuous monitoring of intraventricular pressure intraoperatively and postoperatively. Plain films in both projections are taken by routine stereotactic technique.

Stereotactic calculations are carried out on both films, and angles of correction in degrees are transferred to the axes of the stereotactic apparatus. The aspiration cannula with the first stylet inside is introduced into the preselected target point in the hematoma (Figure 78-3). After reaching the point the stylet is removed from the cannula and replaced by a thin catheter. If aspiration by an ordinary syringe yields dark liquid blood, the catheter is removed and the Archimedes' screw is introduced into the cannula. The next step is decreasing the usually high intracranial pressure by withdrawing CSF from the ventricle on the other side while monitoring intraventricular pressure and decreasing it to 15 to 20 torr (Figure 78-4). In many cases the pressure in the contralateral ventricle diminished sharply to near zero or even to negative figures. In this event the ventricle pressure was increased to 15 to 18 torr by the introduction of saline.

The electric motor and aspirator are switched on with preselected speed and vacuum level. Experiments have shown the optimal speed of the motor is about 100 rpm and aspirator vacuum level is about 0.2 atmosphere. Dark bits of clot pass through the transparent tube to the graduated bottle at a speed of about 2 to 4 meters per minute. The effectiveness of hematoma evacuation can be controlled by judging the quantity of liquid blood and clot in the vessel.

According to the speed of the removal of clot it is possible to vary the rpms of the motor and the vacuum level of the aspirator. When the quantity of clots in the bottle is a few milliliters less than the hematoma volume estimated before the operation the motor and aspirator are switched off. After hematoma removal is completed, one must wait 10 to 15 minutes to be sure that there is no fresh bleeding. There was no such complication in our cases.

Unlike Backlund's technique, we usually try to achieve practically total evacuation of the hematoma, leaving only a few milliliters of blood in the cavity. If it is not possible to remove the hematoma completely initially or if recurrent bleeding is diagnosed postoperatively the operation may be repeated.

There is no need to pump air into the cavity of the partially removed hematoma or into the lateral ventricle to control the degree of evacuation.[8] Air spontaneously enters the cavity of the hematoma as its content is evacuated and is clearly visible on CT scans and on standard skull roentgenograms.

The screw is removed from the cannula and replaced by a balloon catheter, which is inflated with saline and left in the hematoma cavity for prevention of recurrent bleeding. The degree of inflation is governed by the pressure in the contralateral ventricle. The quantity of saline introduced into the balloon varies from 6 to 24 ml. The cannula is then withdrawn from the brain and the stereotactic apparatus removed. The balloon catheter is fixed to the skin and the wound is sutured. The catheter is left in place with the outer end closed for 3 to 4 days for control of the intracavitary pressure. During this period the pressure is gradually diminished by removal of a few milliliters of the saline from the balloon. After 3 to 4 days of observation the balloon is withdrawn. Control CT scans are performed immediately after the operation and on the following and subsequent days.

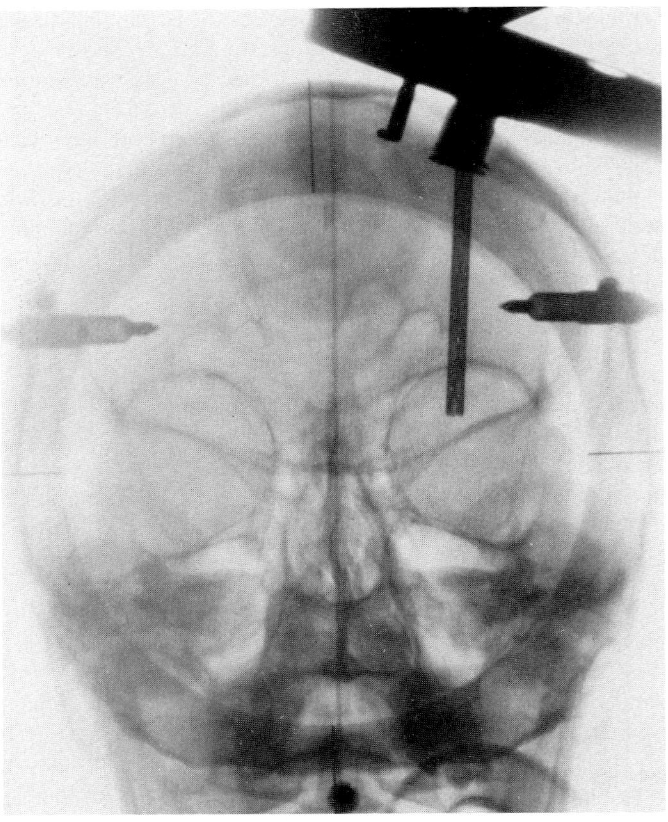

Fig. 78-3. Cannula of the device introduced stereotactically into an intracerebral hematoma.

CLINICAL RESULTS

During the last 4 years we have used this technique 60 times in 56 patients (29 men and 27 women) aged 27 to 64 years. Spontaneous intracerebral hemorrhages due to arterial hypertension and cerebral arteriosclerosis were observed in 54 cases, aneurysmal intracerebral hematoma in one case, and one case of hematoma associated with an AVM. In four cases stereotactic aspiration was performed twice. Stereotactic aspiration was performed 41 times in first 3 days after the hemorrhage, 15 times in 4 to 9 days, and in 4 cases 3 weeks after hemorrhage.

Nearly all the patients were admitted in a grave condition; 20 were in stupor and 36 were comatose. All the patients rapidly developed severe neurologic deficits; complete or near complete hemiplegia, hemianesthesia, aphasia, hemianopsia, and so forth. In some patients cardiovascular and respiratory disorders occurred. The majority of patients had high blood pressure.

Preoperative CT scans disclosed hematomas of the basal ganglia-thalamus-internal capsule in 23 cases; of the globus pallidus and putamen in 29 cases; and of the medial thalamus in 4 cases. Massive penetration of blood into the ventricular system was noted in 62 percent of cases. Brain edema was present in different degrees. The hematoma volume varied from 24 to 120 ml (less than 30 ml in 9 cases, 30 to 50 ml in 14 cases, more than 50 ml in 33 cases).

In all but five cases the hematomas were found to have been removed totally by postoperative CT control carried out immediately after surgery. It is important to note that in the majority of cases it was also possible to remove practically all of the clot from the ventricles. The patients' condition in the postoperative period was usually critical, as before the operation, and as usual after prevention of spontaneous hemorrhages. All patients required long periods of intensive care. Within a few days after surgery repeat hemorrhages developed in 7 patients,[4] in whom total removal had been confirmed initially by CT investigation. Four of these patients were reoperated upon by the same method and two of these patients survived.

There were 12 fatalities (21 percent) which occurred anywhere between 3 and 14 days after surgery. All but one of these patients was comatose before operation. The causes of mortality were recurrent hemorrhages in 5 cases, pulmonary thromboembolism in 4 cases, and renal insufficiency or myocardial infarction in 3 cases. Nine patients out of the 12 who died were operated on early, in the first 3 days after the stroke. It is interesting that fatal outcomes from recurrent hemorrhages took place after early operations (up to 3 days after onset), but from pulmonary embolism after delayed operations (from 3 to 7 days).

A follow-up of 44 patients from 2 months to 4 years after operation has shown that in 38 cases the neurologic deficit disappeared or improved to varying degrees. Eleven patients made an essentially complete recovery and are working full or part time or do work at home. Twenty-seven patients have a residual hemiparesis but can walk with a cane and are relatively independent. Six patients are bedridden. There was not a single case of recurrent hemorrhage during follow-up.

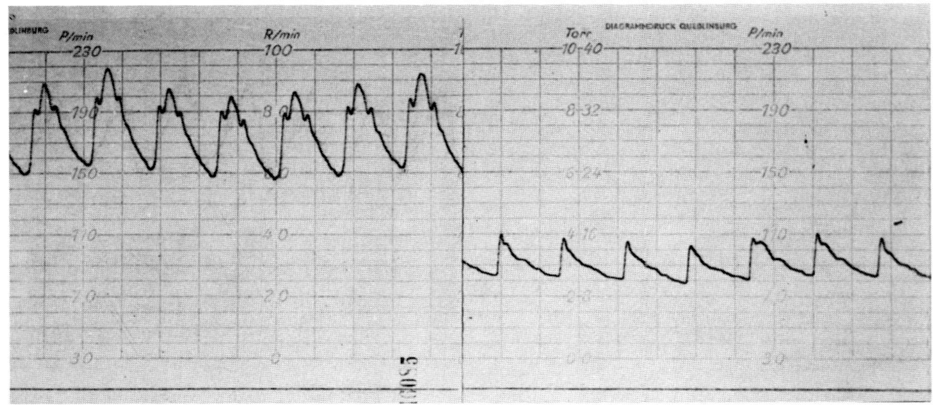

Fig. 78-4. Pressure monitoring in the contralateral ventricle during the stereotactic aspiration of hematoma. Note the sharp decrease in pressure after the aspiration from 34 to 14 mm Hg.

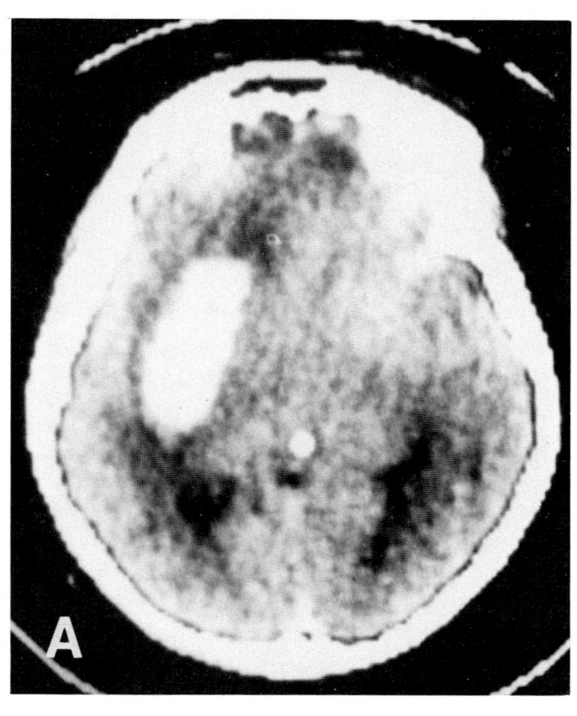

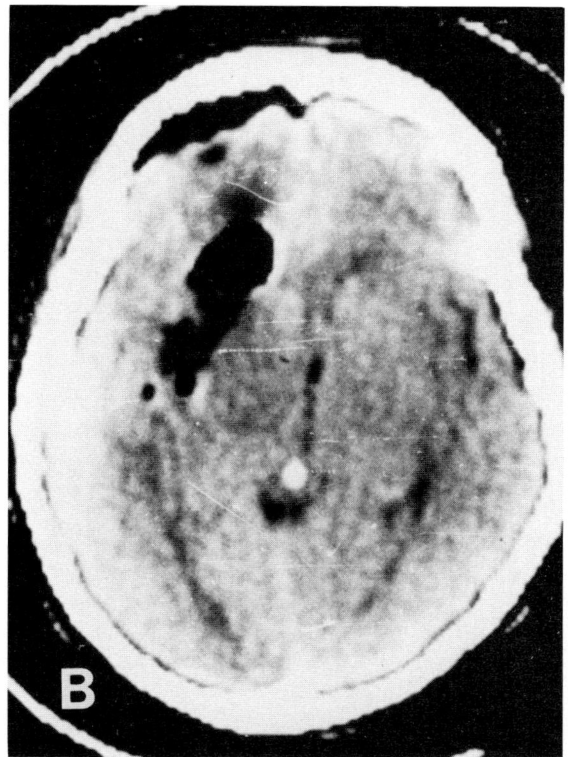

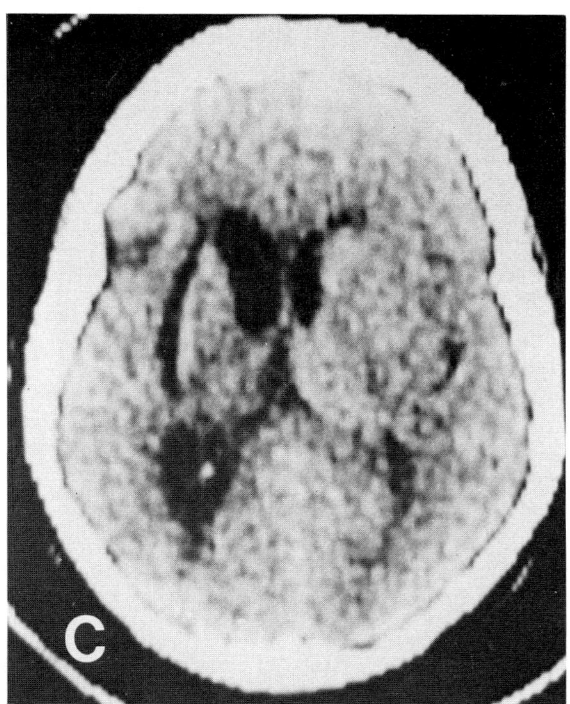

Fig. 78-5. A CT scan of the intracerebral hematoma in a lateral location (volume 65 ml). (A) Before the operation. (B) Immediately after surgery. The cavity fills with air. (C) One year after surgery. A small cystic strip remains in the site of the hematoma.

CASE REPORTS

Two cases with the total stereotactic evacuation of hypertensive hematomas with good functional recovery are described.

Case 1. A 51-year-old woman with long-standing arterial hypertension was admitted to our clinic 20 hours after the development of deep stupor with right-sided hemiplegia and aphasia. The CSF was very bloody. CT scans disclosed a hematoma estimated to have a volume of 65 ml located in the left hemisphere lateral to the internal capsule (Figure 78-5A). Complete stereotactic aspiration of the hematoma was carried out (Figure 78-5B). Five days after surgery, active movements appeared in the right extremities and the patient began to speak a few words. Relatively rapid neurologic recovery took place in the next 2 months. One year after the operation only slight hemiparesis and mild sensory aphasia remained. The patient could walk with a cane. CT scans performed 1 year after surgery show a small cystic strip in the site of the hematoma.

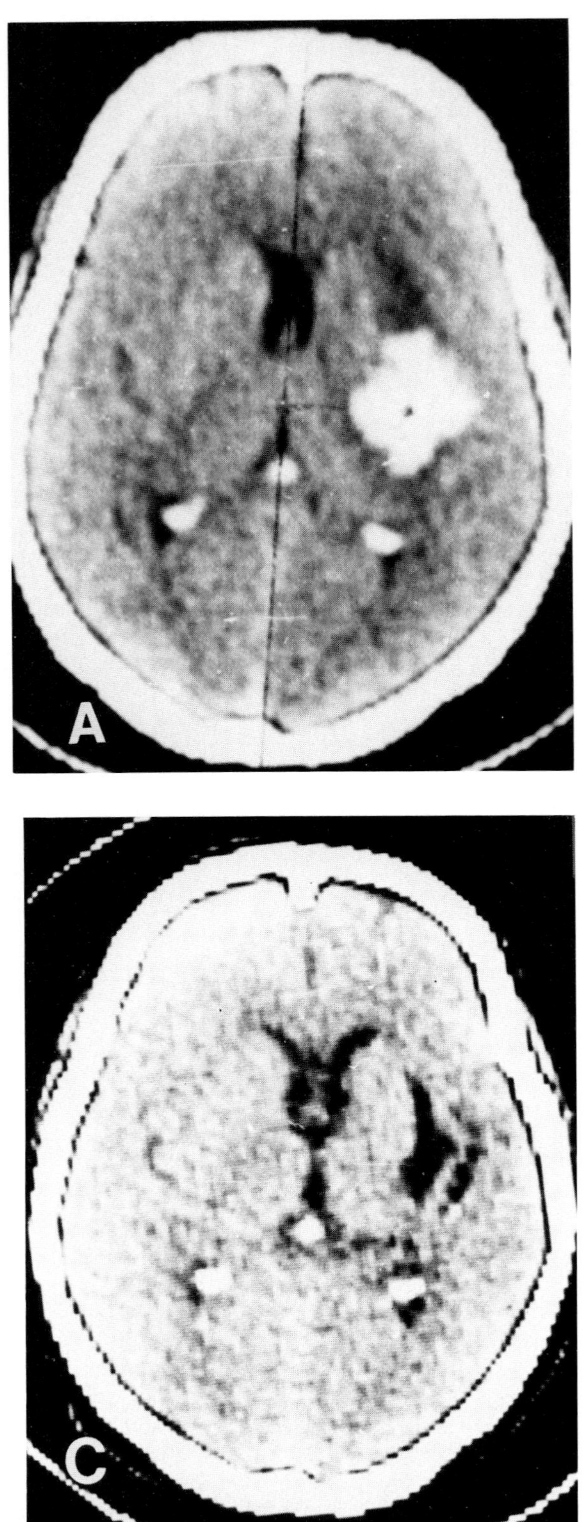

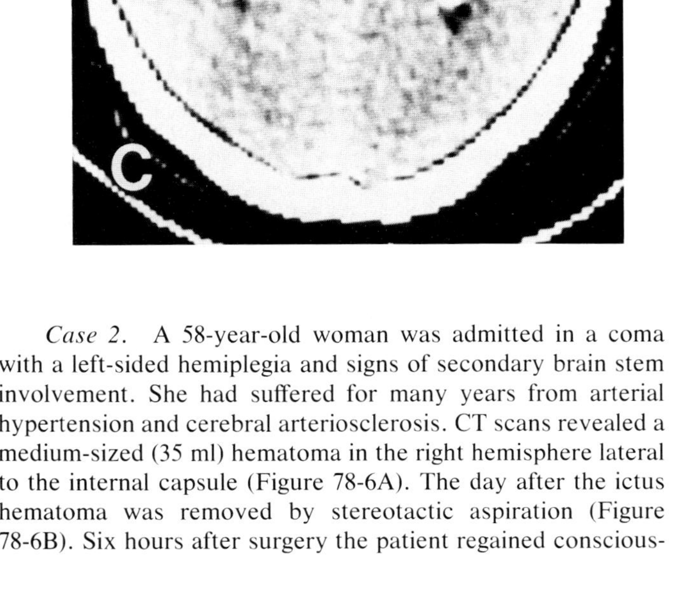

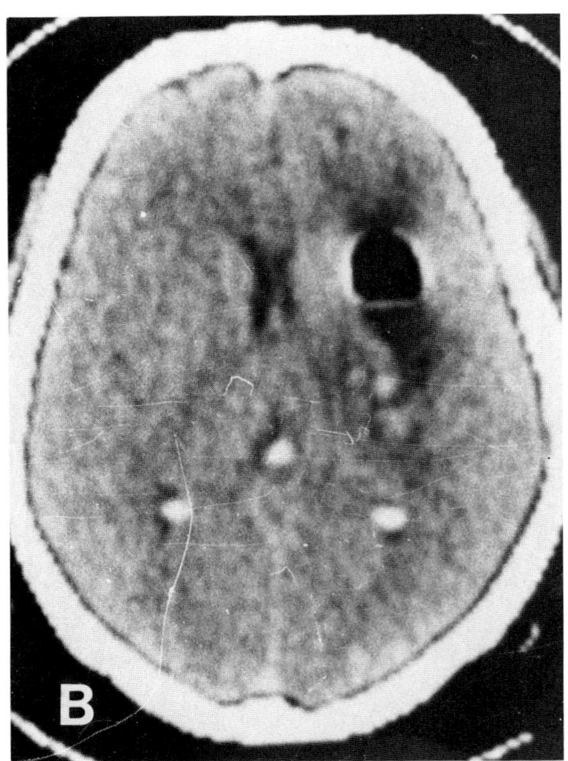

Fig. 78-6. A CT scan of the intracerebral hematoma in a lateral location (volume 35 ml). (A) Before, (B) immediately after stereotactic evacuation, (C) two years after surgery. A small cyst remains in the site of the hematoma.

Case 2. A 58-year-old woman was admitted in a coma with a left-sided hemiplegia and signs of secondary brain stem involvement. She had suffered for many years from arterial hypertension and cerebral arteriosclerosis. CT scans revealed a medium-sized (35 ml) hematoma in the right hemisphere lateral to the internal capsule (Figure 78-6A). The day after the ictus hematoma was removed by stereotactic aspiration (Figure 78-6B). Six hours after surgery the patient regained conscious-

ness and voluntary movements in the left arm and leg reappeared. Two years after surgery the strength and movements in the left extremities are normal and the (Figure 78-6C) patient is fully independent.

Although medial (thalamic) hemorrhages are associated with an extremely high mortality (up to 80 to 90 percent) and poor prognosis the following case illustrates the exception after stereotactic removal of this type of hematoma.

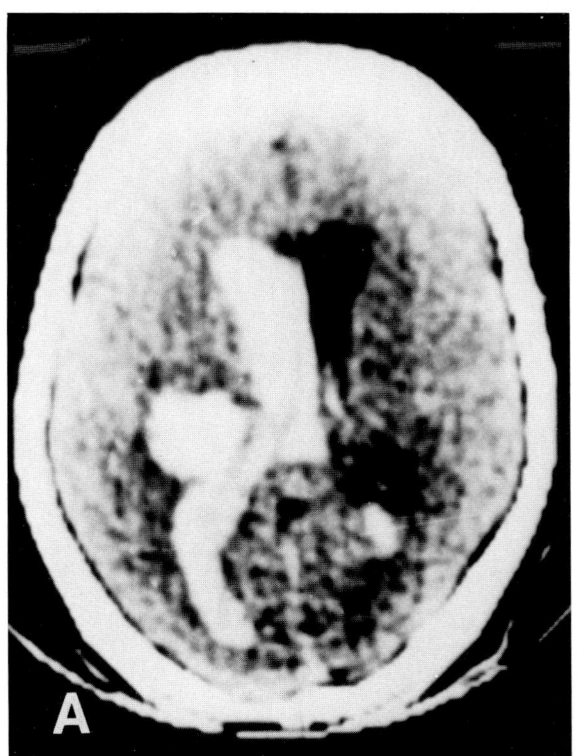
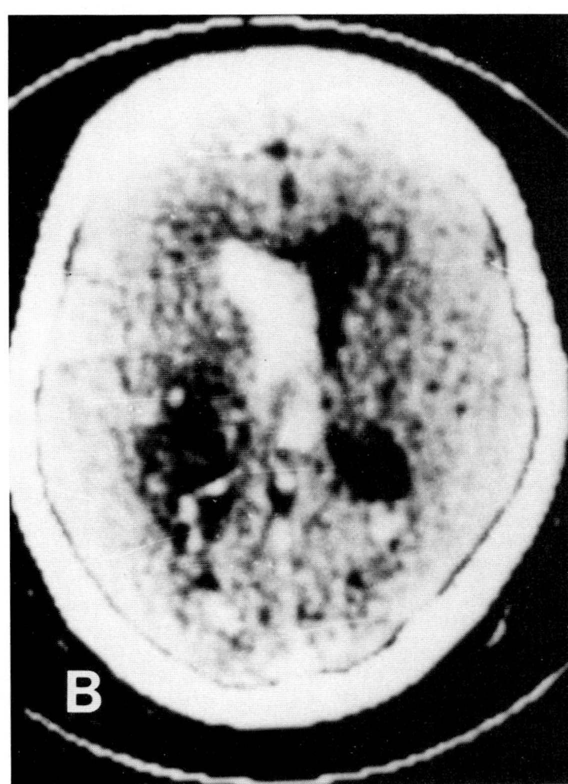

Fig. 78-7. A CT scan of the intracerebral hematoma in a medial location (volume 25 ml) with massive penetration of blood into left lateral and third ventricles. (A) Before, (B) after total evacuation of the hematoma and partial removal of blood from the ventricles.

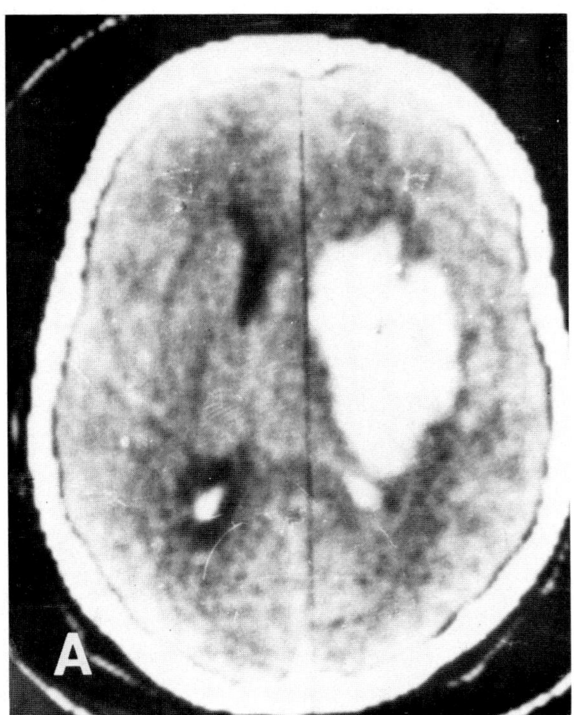
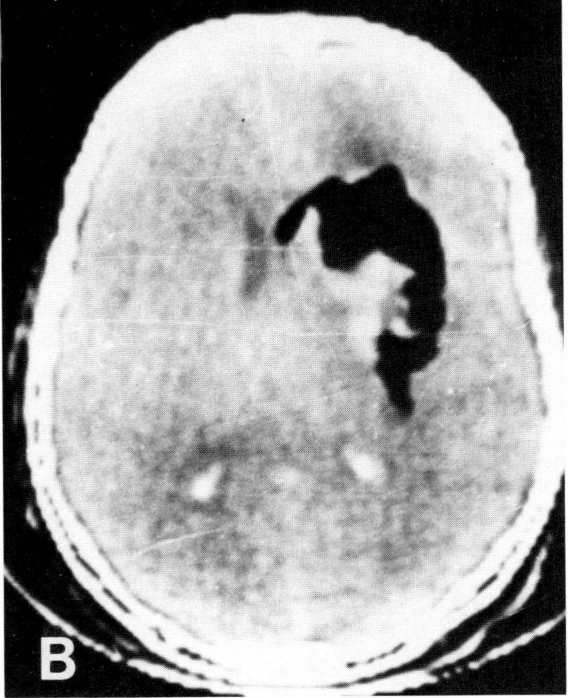

Fig. 78-8. A CT scan of a very large intracerebral hematoma in mixed locations (volume 87 ml). (A) Recurrent hematoma 3 days after operation, (B) after nearly total evacuation of the recurrent hematoma.

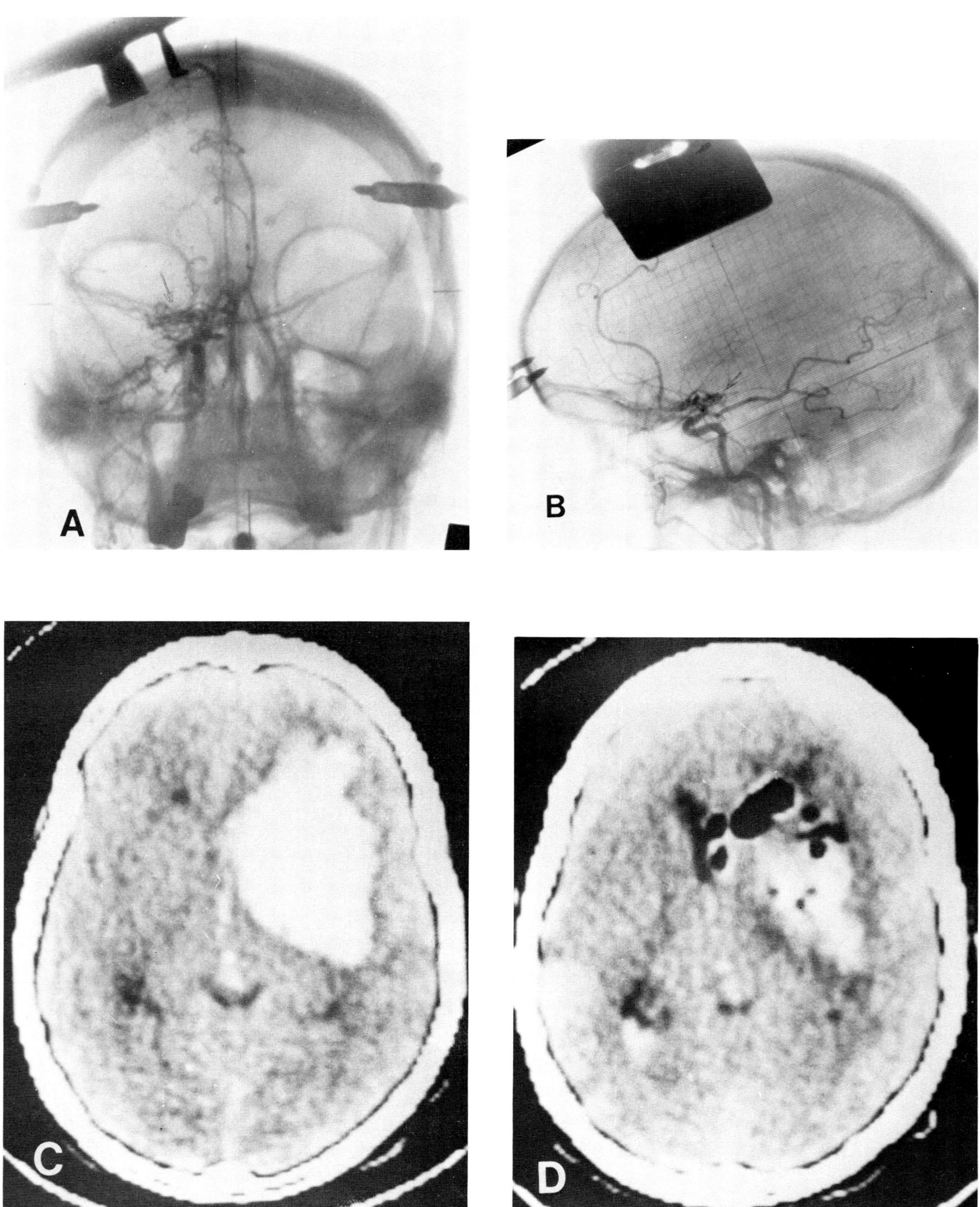

Fig. 78-9. A small arteriovenous malformation with intracerebral hematoma (volume 70 ml). (A) AP angiogram. Note the small AVM (arrow), the shift of the anterior cerebral artery to the left, and marked spasm of the middle cerebral artery. (B) The AVM on the lateral angiogram (arrow). (C) A CT scan before, (D) after subtotal stereotactic aspiration of the intracerebral hematoma.

Case 3. A 53-year-old woman with long standing arterial hypertension suddenly developed a right-sided hemiplegia with aphasia. She was admitted to our clinic in a stuporous state. CT investigations disclosed a relatively small hematoma (24 ml) in the left thalamus with involvement of the internal capsule (Figure 78-7A). Massive hemorrhage filled the lateral and third ventricles. Stereotactic total evacuation of the hematoma and partial removal of the blood from the lateral ventricle were carried out on the third day after the stroke (Figure 78-7B). Two weeks after surgery movements in the right extremities and spontaneous speech began to reappear. Two-and-a-half years after surgery only mild right-sided hemiparesis and slight motor aphasia have remained. She walks with a cane.

The following case shows successful stereotactic aspiration of recurrent hemorrhage shortly after the first operation in a patient in critical condition.

Case 4. A 42-year-old woman with long-standing renal arterial hypertension was admitted to our clinic in coma, without pupillary light reaction, and bilateral pathologic reflexes. A hematoma measuring about 90 ml in volume was demonstrated in the region of internal capsule and adjacent structures (Figure 78-8A). Subsequently, the hematoma was completely removed stereotactically 18 hours after the onset of the stroke. The patient improved rapidly, regained consciousness, and responded to simple commands. Three days later, after a temporary rise of blood pressure to 210/130 mm Hg her condition suddenly worsened and she became deeply stuporous. Repeated CT investigations disclosed a recurrent hematoma of the same volume in the same location. A second stereotactic aspiration of the hematoma was performed immediately with complete removal of the clot (Figure 78-8B). The next day the patient was again conscious, but remained on a respirator for about 3 weeks. Her condition continued to improve gradually, and 1½ years after surgery the patient has a major hemiparesis but can walk with assistance.

Higgins and Nashold[8] expressed the opinion that intracerebral hematomas due to the rupture of arterial aneurysms and AVMs should not be removed stereotactically. Based on our experience in two such cases, we believe that there may be a place for this to be performed in selected cases. This operation is indicated when the one-stage open removal of the hematoma and occlusion of the aneurysm is too dangerous because of the critical condition of the patient for other reasons. Obviously the stereotactic aspiration of the hematoma has to be performed with extreme care so as not to precipitate repeat bleeding. In these cases the hematoma should probably only be partially removed.

Two illustrative cases which demonstrate the possibilities of stereotactic evacuation of hematomas developing after rupture of arterial aneurysms or AVMs are presented.

Case 5. A 27-year-old man was admitted in critical condition after a sudden subarachnoid-parenchymatous hemorrhage. The patient was in a deep stupor with left-sided hemiplegia and advanced brain stem syndrome "swimming movements" anddivergence of the eye, bilateral pathologic reflexes, cardiovascular and respizatory disorders requiring the patient be on a respirator. Angiography disclosed a small aneurysm of the middle cerebral artery and CT scans revealed a large hematoma (volume 55 ml) deep in the right hemisphere. After a few hours, stereotactic evacuation of 35 ml of dark blood and clot was performed. The part of the hematoma near

the aneurysm was not removed. The patient's condition improved gradually. One month later he began to walk. Follow-up angiography failed to show the aneurysm probably due to its spontaneous thrombosis. One year after surgery the patient has a mild hemiparesis and is able to walk without a cane.

Case 6. A 43-year-old woman without known arterial hypertension suddenly developed a left hemiplegia and stupor. Bloody CSF was found on the next day after the stroke and a small AVM was disclosed angiographically near the main trunk of the right middle cerebral artery (Figure 78-9A, B). Severe spasm associated vasespasm was noted in the affected artery. The right anterior cerebral artery was shifted markedly to the opposite side. A CT scan showed a 70-ml hematoma in the frontal and temporal lobes with extravasation of blood into the third ventricle (Figure 78-9C). Two days after the onset of symptoms stereotactic removal of 50 ml of the main part of the hematoma was carried out. One third of the hematoma was left adjacent to the AVM (Figure 78-9D). During the operation angiography was carried out. The next day the patient was alert and had active movement on her left side. She began to walk 2 weeks after surgery. By 1 month the movements in the left arm and leg had returned completely. The patient rejected a second operation for the removal of the AVM. There have been no recurrent hemorrhages in the 2 years of follow-up.

Recurrent bleeding after the aspiration of hematoma by any existing method is the most dangerous surgical complication, the prevention of which remains an important unsolved problem. Recurrence of hemorrhage occurred in 13 percent of our cases of stereotactic aspiration performed in the early period after the stroke. CT studies done within a few hours of surgery showed that the hematoma cavity does not collapse immediately after aspiration of the clot.

To reduce this very serious and relatively frequent complication we inflated a Silastic balloon which is introduced into the cavity of hematoma after its evacuation. Using this technique there have been no recurrent hematomas in our, as yet, limited experience.

We disagree the that the total evacuation of spontaneous hematomas is not recommended.[7] Our experience has shown that it is both possible and advisable to remove practically the entire hematoma, leaving only a few milliliters of blood in its cavity. There is no evidence that complete removal of the hematoma increases the risk of recurrent bleeding; although one certainly must be very careful with the aspiration of hematomas secondary to aneurysmal rupture. In such cases the clot near the aneurysm must not be disturbed.

CONCLUSION

Our experience with stereotactic evacuation of spontaneous and aneurysmal intracerebral hemorrhages has shown that this method is effective and offers substantial advantages over conventional surgical treatment. It affords the possibility of total or practically total evacuation of all kinds of intracerebral hematomas of different volume and location, including those with aneurysmal hemmorrhage. It also offers the possibility of removing blood clots from the cerebral ventricles. The method enables aspiration of clots of any density through a cannula of small diameter. Since the operation is less traumatic and safer, the method can be used in patients who are in a grave condition.

REFERENCES

1. Luessenhop AS, Shevlin WA, Ferrero AA, et al: Surgical management of primary intracerebral hemorrhage. J Neurosurg 27:419, 1967

2. McKissock V, Richardson A, Taylor J: Primary intracerebral hemorrhage: A controlled trial of surgical and conservative treatment in 180 cases. Lancet 2:221, 1961

3. Paillas JE, Alliez B: Surgical treatment of spontaneous intracerebral hemorrhage. Immediate and long-term results in 250 cases. J Neurosurg 39:145, 1973

4. Romodanov AP, Pedachenko GA: [Hemorrhagical Stroke.] Kiev, Zdorowje, 1971

5. Vigouroux RP, Gondin-Olivera S, Guillemain P: The choice of the management in spontaneous brain hematomas (258 cases from Marseille's neurosurgeons since CT scan use), in 7th European Congress of Neurosurgery, Brussels, Belgium, Abstracts, 1983, p 132

6. Benes V, Vladyka V, Zvérina F: Stereotaxic evacuation of typical brain hemorrhage. Acta Neurochir 13:419, 1965

7. Backlund EO, von Holst H: Controlled subtotal evacuation of intracerebral hematomas by sterotactic technique. Surg Neurol 9:99, 1978

8. Higgins AC, Nashold BS: Stereotactic evacuation of large intracerebral hematoma. Appl Neurophysiol 43:96, 1980

9. Broseta J, Gonzalez-Darder J, Barcia-Szlorio JL: Stereotactic evacuation of intracerebral hematomas. Appl Neurophysiol 49:443, 1982

10. Kandel EI, Peresedov VV: [A new method of stereotactic removal of intracranial hemorrhages,] in Proceedings of the Third All-Union Congress of Neurosurgery, Tallin, 1982, pp 49–50

11. Kandel EI, Feresedov VV: Stereotaxic evacuation of spontaneous intracerebra hematomas. J Neurosurg 62:206, 1985

12. Peresedov VV, Kandel EI: [Device for the stereotactic evacuation of intracerebral hematomas.] Vopr Neurokhir 6:53, 1983

CHAPTER 79

Cranial Arteriovenous Malformations

Alfred J. Luessenhop

THE RECENT important advances in the management of cerebral arteriovenous malformations (AVMs) include the application of microsurgical techniques for deep, critically located lesions; continuing innovations and perfections of intravascular techniques for occluding AVMs; a better understanding of the anatomy and hemodynamics of the lesions; and, finally, a better appreciation of their natural history, so the course for an untreated patient is now reasonably predictable. Despite these advances, however, not all cerebral AVMs fall within our therapeutic domain. Some are diffuse throughout a cerebral hemisphere without a focal concentration of artery-to-vein shunting. Others extend through the basal ganglia, internal capsule, and thalamus, within the territories of most or all of the penetrating arteries from the circle of Willis. Finally, even for somewhat smaller AVMs, when diagnosed in later life, the surgical risks, though small, may still exceed the risks of the remaining natural course.[1]

It is estimated that approximately 70 to 80 percent of all cerebral AVMs are treatable with the objective of total elimination at the time of initial diagnosis.[2] It is the responsibility of the neurosurgeon to judge accurately the surgical risks and possible benefit in each case. Many of the mortalities and severe morbidities associated with this surgery stem from the neurosurgeon's overestimation of his or her technical expertise and a lack of appreciation of the natural course of the disease. In this chapter important points in the natural history, which must be known by all neurosurgeons, will be outlined initially, followed by comments about surgical risks that arise when a broad range of these lesions are operated upon.

NATURAL HISTORY

Because cerebral AVMs are congenital, the natural history commences at birth rather than at the time of diagnosis.[1,2] The lesion is not static. There is now considerable evidence of a continuous process of change, mostly during the first two decades of life. This is a gradual transformation from a diffuse vascular aberration to a more discrete one with greater shunting and more extensive incorporation of enlarged draining veins.[1] In later life more subtle changes ensue, with smaller lesions becoming slightly larger and, from time to time, larger lesions becoming smaller when demonstrated angiographically. Rarely there is spontaneous thrombosis.

Toward the end of the second decade of life AVMs become progressively more symptomatic, with the appearance of seizures, neurologic deficits, and spontaneous bleeding. By the end of the fourth decade approximately 80 percent of all AVMs will have become symptomatic and diagnosed. Throughout an individual's lifetime the average rate for spontaneous bleeding is 2 to 3 percent per year, which is the same as that for saccular aneurysms.[3] In contrast to aneurysms, however, there is no increased risk of early rehemorrhage, but there is evidence that the bleeding rate does increase to approximately 6 percent throughout the first year after a hemorrhage. By our best estimates, each clinically evident hemorrhage carries a 10 percent mortality and a 30 percent morbidity, which is more favorable than the rates for aneurysms.[2,4]

Gradual neurologic deterioration may be associated with large hemispheric lesions or somewhat smaller lesions extensively involving the deeper hemispheric structures. When this commences after the second decade of life, progression is usually slow; there may be long intervals of stability. Even in the absence of intervening hemorrhage, this progression may lead to neurologic disability over many years, but only rarely is there progression to a severe hemiparesis or disabling aphasia.[1]

When headache becomes the dominant clinical symptom, it usually persists throughout the patient's lifetime, and when severe it may by itself force a decision for surgery.[1] Only rarely do seizures become a management problem. It must be pointed out that surgery for seizures alone, as for many other lesions, is not uniformly effective.

SURGICAL RISK

Surgical risk depends upon the overall size of the AVM, its location, and the degree of shunting. Of these considerations, the most significant is the size of the lesion. For lesions with a maximum angiographic spread of less than 2 cm, the surgical risk is generally very small except for lesion located in absolutely critical areas. With increasing size the surgical risk steadily increases, and when the maximum spread approaches 6 cm the operative mortality may reach 10 percent by present techniques and in the hands of very experienced neurosurgeons.[2,5] It therefore is reasonable to consider nearly all lesions under 2 cm in size as candidates for surgery even when the lesion is found incidentally. Arteriovenous malformations between 2 and 4 cm in size are usually operable, but greater consideration must be given to location. The large lesions require careful consideration of the natural risk of the untreated lesion compared with the risk of surgery. In particular, the age of the patient must be considered, since this determines the remaining years of exposure to the risk.[2,4]

It may be possible to excise critically located lesions of intermediate or large size without producing a new neurologic

OPERATIVE NEUROSURGICAL TECHNIQUES
ISBN 0-8089-1862-1

deficit, and occasionally it may be possible to reverse a pre-existing deficit.[6,7] Mostly this is achieved with AVMs with rather discrete nidi. However, the neurosurgeon cannot always depend upon this, for even the most careful dissection requires sacrifice of functional cerebral tissue in the marginal vascular interspaces. This must be taken into account when considering whether an AVM can be treated surgically. The decision might be whether the creation of a modest persisting deficit is better than the continuing risk of future hemorrhage.[2,8,9]

When there is extensive diversion of blood flow to the AVM and considerable enlargement of the feeding arteries, circulatory breakthrough can ensue when these arteries are interrupted.[10,11] This may be predictable from the angiograms when these feeding arteries have a long course and there is a paucity of filling of intervening normal arteries. Overall, severe circulatory breakthrough occurs in only 2 to 3 percent of cases, and this incidence can be minimized further by the use of hypotension both during and after surgery.[10,11]

PRESURGICAL EVALUATION

The surgeon must be completely familiar with the angiographic anatomy of the AVM, and the major feeding and draining vessels must be carefully mapped. The films should be as close to normal size as possible so the angiographic picture accurately depicts the anatomy the surgeon will encounter. Feeding arteries should be inspected for aneurysms because these may require clipping during excision of the AVM.[12]

If possible, the surgery should be performed under elective conditions, particularly in the case of larger AVMs. If there is a recent adjacent intracerebral hematoma, the surgery should be delayed until this is almost absorbed and the surrounding edema has subsided.[13] Occasionally, removal of a fresh hematoma is necessary. For larger AVMs it may be best to remove the hematoma and leave the AVM for removal at a second stage. If small, the AVM should be removed simultaneously. Angiograms should be obtained after the clot has been absorbed because hematoma can distort the natural anatomy and extent of an AVM.

SURGICAL TECHNIQUE

As for most intracranial procedures, the patient should receive steroids preoperatively, and mannitol should be given as the craniotomy commences. Brain shrinkage facilitates identification of abnormal vessels as they branch into the malformation. Moderate hypotension should be used at key points during the exposure and dissection.

The patient should be positioned on the operating table to place the malformation above the highest point of venous drainage. The craniotomy should permit wide exposure of the surface of the AVM and the associated feeding and draining vessels. At least 20 percent of the larger convexity AVMs have dural arterial contributions. These arteries are interrupted on the dural surface before the dura is opened.

Some degree of magnification is mandatory for AVM surgery.[5,7,9,14] For large hemispheric convexity AVMs magnifying loupes are usually adequate. This allows more rapid viewing of separate areas around the margins of the AVM and is adequate for the size of the vessels usually encountered. The higher magnification of an operating microscope becomes nec-

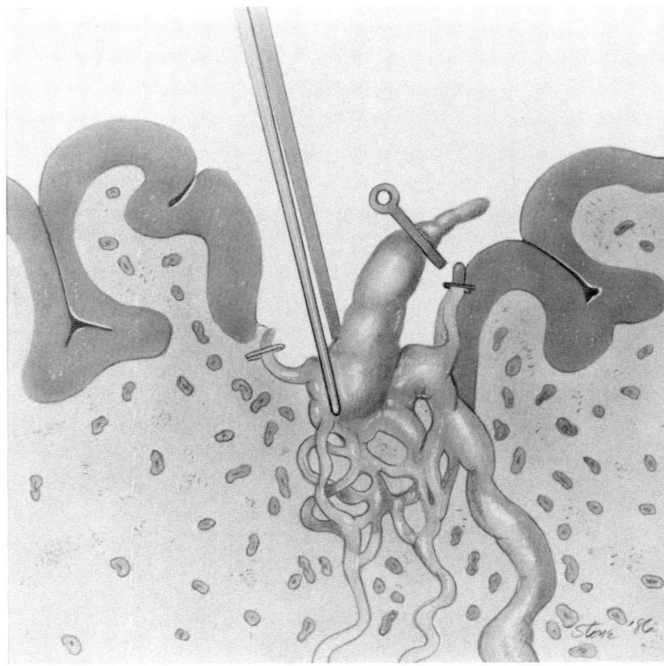

Fig. 79-1. Bipolar coagulation of an AVM in situ. The superficial draining vein is followed to the nidus, then the entire lesion is coagulated with minimal disturbance of the surrounding brain. This is feasible in some lesions up to 2 cm in diameter.

essary for the deeper, critically situated AVMs. Furthermore, the operating microscope has the advantage of coaxial illumination of sites deep beneath the cortical surface.

Basically, there are three techniques for the obliteration or excision of cerebral AVMs. The first and easiest is direct coagulation of the entire lesion. The second is marginal resection and is the standard technique for the larger AVMs. The third is block resection, which can be employed in situations where adjacent brain can be sacrificed without risk of increased neurologic deficit. All of these techniques may be necessary to some degree in any given lesion.

DIRECT COAGULATION AND OBLITERATION

Direct coagulation and obliteration is least likely to damage or destroy surrounding viable brain tissue. The adjacent feeding arteries on the brain surface are interrupted with clips, and the entire vascular mass is gradually coagulated (Figure 79-1). Draining veins on the cortical surface subsequently are interrupted and used as a stem to guide the coagulation.[14] I have become increasingly impressed that lesions up to 2 or 3 cm in diameter on the cortical surface or even deep within a sulcus can be handled in this fashion. Deeper AVMs do require retraction of the adjacent brain to produce an adequate exposure, but destruction of cerebral tissue remains minimal.

MARGINAL RESECTION

In larger AVMs the center or nidus of the lesion consists of bulbous intercommunicating channels that create a space-taking effect on the surrounding brain tissue. Much of the surface of an AVM can be a thin-walled vascular sac, but always at some sites the margin will consist of intertwined vascular

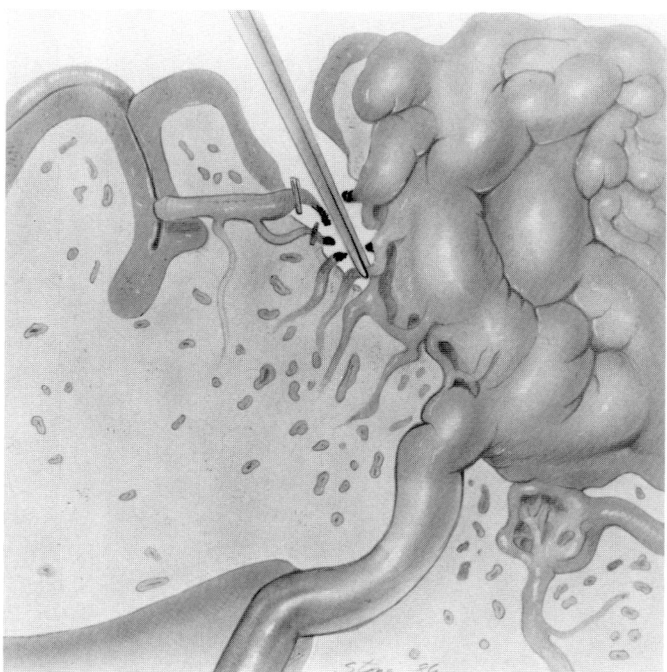

Fig. 79-2. Marginal resection along the dilated venous sacs. The plexus of smaller vessels along the margin is coagulated and clipped.

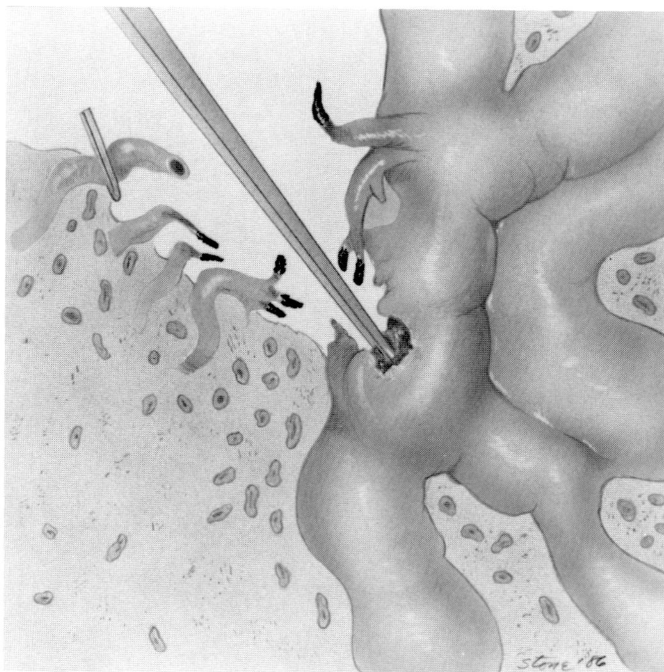

Fig. 79-3. Bipolar coagulation of the wall of the venous sacs may lead to rupture and bleeding that is difficult to control.

channels of smaller diameter. Initially, the feeding arteries are interrupted at sites as close to the AVM as feasible.[2,6,7,15] A plane of cleavage then is established along the margins; this cleavage is gradually deepened by suction and interruption of the feeding arteries and draining veins, either by simple coagulation or by clipping and coagulation (Figure 79-2). Major draining veins on the surface are left intact until the bulk of the lesion can be removed en bloc. Both the adjacent brain tissue and the AVM itself are periodically retracted to open the surrounding groove and to minimize the amount of cerebral tissue damaged by suction. The groove should be equal around the entire AVM, at least initially, and the surgeon should not shift from one site in the groove to another without first achieving complete hemostasis.

The most difficult part of this dissection is interruption of the deeper feeding arteries at the apex (or deepest extent) of the AVM.[9,15] Retraction exposure is least effective here, and there is a tendency for these deep arteries to retract into the white matter even when there is only minimal edema. Throughout the dissection the degree of persisting arterial feeding can be estimated by the rate of filling of the venous sacs after they are gently compressed. The venous drainage generally remains red until nearly all arterial feeders are interrupted.

In addition to the problems of interruption of the deep arterial contribution, three additional problems may be encountered in marginal resection. The first of these stems from a failure to differentiate between the walls of dilated venous sacs and marginal participating vessels of smaller diameter. Coagulation of the lateral wall of the sac will occasionally lead to its rupture (Figure 79-3). At times it is extremely difficult to stem the ensuing bleeding, and the use of large clips across the margins may be the only solution. The dissection process sometimes must be hastily accelerated to interrupt the remaining participating arteries.

The second problem is retraction of incompletely coagu-

lated or clipped arteries into the surrounding edematous white matter. Bleeding from these vessels becomes difficult to discern, and suction removal of additional brain tissue may become necessary (Figure 79-4). With further retraction regional cerebral edema may accelerate and obliterate the plane of cleavage altogether. If this becomes severe, it may be wise to terminate the procedure after hemostasis has been established. Severe edema may require the removal of excessive amounts of cerebral tissue, which defeats the purpose of the technique.

The third problem is circulatory breakthrough.[10,11] The likelihood of this complication can be estimated from the preoperative arteriograms, and presurgical embolization may be helpful in preventing it. Characteristically, this problem begins shortly after the dissection commences; the adjacent cortex begins to swell, the surface arteries dilate, and, when severe, areas of focal hemorrhage appear on the cortex. Management involves instituting profound hypotension and securing hemostasis along the margins of the AVM. The bone flap should be removed to afford as much decompression as possible, and hypotension should be continued for 4 to 7 days. The formation of postoperative hematomas adjacent to the AVM is likely.

BLOCK RESECTION

In a block resection the plane of cleavage is distant from the walls of the dilated venous sacs and the number of bridging vessels to be interrupted is fewer, and therefore the possibility of rupturing the wall of important venous sacs is considerably reduced (Figure 79-5). This technique is applicable only to those AVMs in which the immediately surrounding brain is expendable without fear of significant functional interference, e.g., those lesions near the tips of the frontal or temporal lobes.

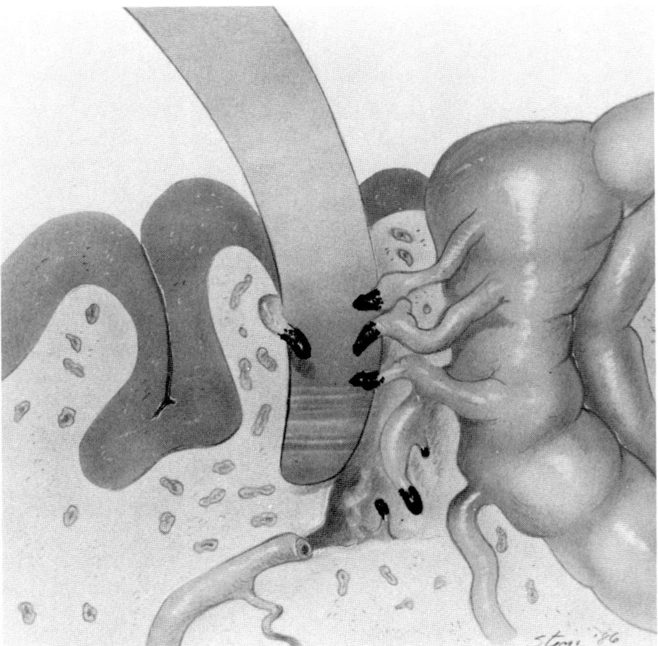

Fig. 79-4.   During marginal resection, edema of the adjacent brain may lead to retraction of an incompletely coagulated feeding artery into the white matter. Hemostatic control requires further sacrifice of adjacent white matter.

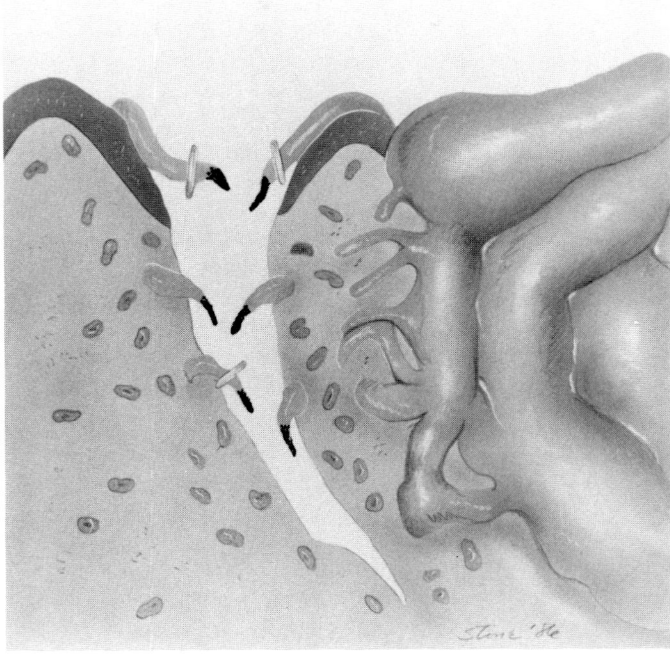

Fig. 79-5.   Resection distant from the nidus requires interruption of fewer participating arteries and veins and minimizes the risk of rupture of the nidus and retraction of participating vessels.

POSTOPERATIVE MANAGEMENT

Irrespective of the tediousness of the surgery or the exasperation caused by the bleeding, the surgeon must never leave active bleeding at the time of closure, since this will always lead to the formation of a large hematoma throughout the bed of resection. This is the most important postoperative complication and can occur even when there is excellent hemostasis at the time of closure. The walls of the feeding arteries are thinner than normal and they tend to dilate in the immediate postoperative period, allowing for renewed bleeding from apparently adequately coagulated stumps. Although this is a factor, most cases of rebleeding and hematoma formation in the immediate postoperative period are associated with the presence of residual portions of the AVM. It is wise to obtain a CT scan within the first day after surgery to identify and assess the extent of a hematoma. There should be no hesitation to reopening the craniotomy should the hematoma appear to be significant. Cerebral angiography should be repeated before reoperation to demonstrate any residual portions of the AVM that might require further dissection.

A moderate degree of hypotension should be maintained in the immediate postoperative period. This will reduce the likelihood of delayed circulatory breakthrough and allow the occluded feeding arteries to re-establish normal autoregulation. The time necessary for this to occur is not known, but 4 to 7 days is a reasonable estimate.

Routine postoperative cerebral angiography should be performed within 1 to 2 weeks after resection. These studies usually will show segmental enlargement of many of the occluded feeding arteries. At times, the determination whether or not total removal of the AVM has been effected is difficult, particularly when these occluded arteries are relatively small and immediately adjacent to the original AVM. If there is

uncertainty, angiography should be repeated after 1 or 2 months, allowing time for these arteries to revert to normal caliber. If residual AVM is clearly present, reoperation should be carried out a week or two after the initial surgery. Previously placed clips can be used as landmarks to direct the surgeon to the site of the residual lesion. It is important that the patient be aware of this possibility and agree to reoperation during the initial discussions regarding the events that may transpire in an attempt to cure the problem. It is likely that residual portions of an AVM have the same potential for future rebleeding as the original AVM.

OPERATIVE STAGING

Planned operative staging is usually indicated for large AVMs with major arterial supplies from distant sites such as the middle, posterior, and anterior cerebral circulations. In other patients with large AVMs, it may be advisable to stage the surgery when marginal resection will require many hours of retraction of the normal surrounding brain. Such a situation can lead to edema, particularly when a certain degree of breakthrough is superimposed. It is always best to anticipate this.

AVMs WITH DIFFICULT SURGICAL ACCESS

In contrast to AVMs on the hemispheric convexities, AVMs of the medial and undersurfaces of the hemispheres, those in the posterior fossa,[16] and those immediately adjacent to or within the ventricular system require special consideration. Visualization of the presenting portion of the AVM is at an oblique angle, and the establishment of a groove around the lesion is more difficult.[15] It also may be necessary to sacrifice major draining veins before the feeding arteries can be seen. In some, particularly in the medial temporal lobe or temporal fissure, preservation of the continuity of adjacent arteries is necessary to prevent infarction of brain tissue in their distal territories.[17]

Most of the larger AVMs on the medial surfaces, however, have both surface and deep venous drainage, and sacrifice of the superficial drainage before exposure is usually compensated for. Also, despite the obliquity of the exposure, marginal resection, at least in part, is frequently possible. Furthermore, many of the AVMs on the medial surfaces are relatively small and the technique of total coagulation in situ is applicable. As the coils of thin-walled veins gradually collapse, the deep and surface feeding arteries become visible for clipping.

For most of the AVMs extending through the corpus callosum, it is nearly always possible to interrupt the pericallosal feeders proximally without risk of creating a neurologic deficit. This leaves only the choroidal arterial contributions to be dealt with after the corpus callosum is divided.[15,18,19]

Arteriovenous malformations within or adjacent to the ventricular system and in the choroid plexus can be approached transcallosally and gradually coagulated in situ. Other small lesions in the medial trigonal area can be approached through a cortical incision in the temporal lobe, which affords an interventricular exposure.

INTRAVASCULAR TECHNIQUES AS ADJUNCTS TO SURGICAL EXCISION

Intravascular techniques have an important role in the management of cerebral AVMs, both as the sole method of management and as an adjunct to planned surgical excision.[2,20,21] For very large AVMs with progressive neurologic deterioration either by circulatory diversion (steal) or progressive enlargement of venous sacs that compress adjacent brain, embolization alone is very useful. In suitable cases this will reduce the size of the venous sacs and create a higher perfusion pressure for the adjacent brain. As an adjunct to surgery embolization has three roles:[2,21]

1. For AVMs in which there is a high likelihood of circulatory breakthrough when the major feeding arteries are acutely interrupted, presurgical embolization will gradually reduce the degree of shunting and restore a normal perfusion pressure to the surrounding brain. Some degree of normal autoregulation will be established by the time of surgery 4 to 6 days later.
2. General reduction in the size of large AVMs to facilitate marginal resection and reduce the number of associated vascular channels that require interruption.
3. Occlusion of major feeding arteries for which there would be poor access before the nidus of the AVM is encountered. Mostly these are AVMs of the medial occipital lobe, predominantly in the territory of the posterior cerebral artery.

When presurgical embolization is planned, direct surgery should take place within a few days. A longer interval allows time for a collateral arterial supply to develop, which may introduce greater surgical difficulties.

SURGICAL RESULTS

By present techniques it can be anticipated that surgical excision of small or medium-sized AVMs (under 3 cm in angiographic diameter) on the cerebral convexities can be done with extremely low morbidity and mortality. Arteriovenous malformations of the same size but located on the medial surfaces may produce slightly greater mortality and morbidity, but in general are nearly always operable. Arteriovenous malformations in these categories constitute at least one half of all those encountered. For the larger AVMs in multiple arterial territories, a significant degree of surgical mortality and morbidity can be anticipated. Careful judgment is necessary for this group of AVMs, for if operative mortality approaches 10 percent it is unlikely that the neurosurgeon is doing better than natural history.[5]

REFERENCES

1. Luessenhop AJ: Natural history of cerebral arteriovenous malformations, in Wilson CB, Stein BM (eds): Current Neurosurgical Practice: Intracranial Arteriovenous Malformations. Baltimore, Williams & Wilkins, 1984, pp 12–23
2. Luessenhop AJ, Rosa L: Indications for and results of surgery, and the role of intravascular techniques. J Neurosurg 60:14, 1984
3. Graf CJ, Perret GE, Torner JC: Bleeding from cerebral arteriovenous malformations as part of their natural history. J Neurosurg 58:331, 1983
4. Michelsen WJ: Natural history and pathophysiology of arteriovenous malformations. Clin Neurosurg 26:307, 1979
5. Parkinson D, Bacher G: Arteriovenous malformations. Summary of 100 consecutive supratentorial cases. J Neurosurg 53:285, 1980
6. Stein MS: Arteriovenous malformations of the cerebral convexities, in Wilson CB, Stein BM (eds): Current Neurosurgical Practice: Intracranial Arteriovenous Malformations. Baltimore, Williams & Wilkins, 1984, pp 156–183
7. Stein MS: General techniques for the surgical removal of arteriovenous malformations, in Wilson CB, Stein BM (eds): Current Neurosurgical Practice: Intracranial Arteriovenous Malformations. Baltimore, Williams & Wilkins, 1984, pp 143–155
8. Amacher AL, Allcock JM, Drake CG: Cerebral angiomas: The sequelae of surgical treatment. J Neurosurg 37:571, 1972
9. Drake CG: Cerebral arteriovenous malformations: Considerations for and experience with surgical treatment in 166 cases. Clin Neurosurg 26:145, 1979
10. Luessenhop AJ, Ferraz FM, Rosa L: Estimate of the incidence and importance of circulatory breakthrough in the surgery of cerebral arteriovenous malformations. Neurol Res 4:177, 1982
11. Spetzler RF, Wilson CB, Weinstein P, et al: Normal perfusion pressure breakthrough theory. Clin Neurosurg 25:651, 1978
12. Wilkins RH: Multiple aneurysms and associated arteriovenous malformations, operative considerations, in Hopkins LN (ed): Clinical Management of Intracranial Aneurysms. New York, Raven Press, 1982, pp 193–200
13. Pia HW: The acute treatment of cerebral arteriovenous angiomas associated with hematomas, in Pia HW, Gleave JRW, Grote E, et al (eds): Cerebral Angiomas. Advances in Diagnosis and Therapy. New York, Springer-Verlag, 1975, pp 155–177
14. Malis LI: Arteriovenous malformations of the brain, in Youmans JR (ed): Neurological Surgery, vol 3. Philadelphia, WB Saunders, 1982, pp 1786–1806
15. Wilson CB, Martin NA: Deep supratentorial arteriovenous malformation, in Wilson CB, Stein BM (eds): Current Neurosurgical Practice: Intracranial Arteriovenous Malformations. Baltimore, Williams & Wilkins, 1984, pp 184–208
16. Martin NA, Stein BM, Wilson CB: Arteriovenous malformations of the posterior fossa, in Wilson CB, Stein BM (eds): Current

Neurosurgical Practice: Intracranial Arteriovenous Malformations. Baltimore, Williams & Wilkins, 1984, pp 209–221

17. Heros RC: Arteriovenous malformations of the medial temporal lobe. Surgical approach and neuroradiological characterization. J Neurosurg 56:44, 1982

18. Yasargil MG, Jain KK, Antic J, et al: Arteriovenous malformation of the anterior and middle portion of the corpus callosum: Microsurgical treatment. Surg Neurol 5:67, 1976

19. Yasargil MG, Jain KK, Antic J, et al: Arteriovenous malformation of the splenium of the corpus callosum: Microsurgical treatment. Surg Neurol 5:5, 1976

20. Cromwell LD, Harris AB: Treatment of cerebral arteriovenous malformations. A combined neurosurgical and neuroradiological approach. J Neurosurg 52:705, 1980

21. Luessenhop AJ, Presper JH: Surgical embolization of cerebral arteriovenous malformations through internal carotid and vertebral arteries. Long-term results. J Neurosurg 42:443, 1975 J Luessenhop

Surgical Management of Cranial Arteriovenous Malformations

Francis W. Gamache, Jr.   Russel H. Patterson, Jr.

INTRACRANIAL VASCULAR MALFORMATIONS have been classified by McCormick[1,2] as telangiectases, varices, cavernous malformations, venous malformations, and arteriovenous malformations (AVMs). Some of the clinical and pathologic distinctions are summarized in Table 80-1.

Approximately 20 percent of strokes are associated with hemorrhage. Of these, the ratio of parenchymal brain hemorrhage to subarachnoid hemorrhage is approximately 3:1. Rupture of an AVM accounts for only 10 percent of the cases of subarachnoid hemorrhage.

Hemorrhage is the first sign of an AVM in approximately 50 percent of the cases. Small AVMs tend to bleed and rebleed more than large ones, and the hematoma associated with a small AVM is likely to be larger than one associated with a large AVM. Seizures are a sign of an AVM in approximately one third of the cases, and perhaps 10 percent of patients with an AVM have a hemorrhage associated with a seizure.[2,4–6]

Although AVMs are not a cause of classical migraine headache, they can produce a headache accompanied by an unusual premonitory aura that lasts into the phase of the headache or even comes on after the onset of the headache. Arteriovenous malformations also have been blamed for progressive neurologic deficit, but this is relatively uncommon (i.e., 20 percent of cases or less). A progressive deficit seems more common in those cases that involve the brain stem or those that are large enough to produce a progressive hemodynamic steal.[5]

Approximately 80 percent of AVMs are detectable on an unenhanced computed tomogram, and almost all of them will be revealed on an enhanced scan.[8,9] Magnetic resonance imaging (MRI) scans usually provide an excellent image of AVMs and reveal the shape and extent of the malformation and its relationship to normal anatomic structures in the brain (Figure 80-1).[10] Arteriovenous malformations can be situated anywhere in the brain, and their frequency in a given region approximates the ratio of the mass of the region with respect to the whole brain.

A subgroup of intracranial AVMs is composed of dural AVMs. The relationships between anatomic location together with venous drainage and the propensity for hemorrhage has been described by several authors.[11–14] The carotid cavernous lesions are more benign than dural lesions draining into the transverse or sigmoid sinuses. Surgical intervention is tempered accordingly.[13,14]

PREOPERATIVE EVALUATION

Complete multivessel arteriography is the single most important aid in both diagnosing and planning surgery for the patient with an AVM. Since adequate treatment of the patient requires that the anomaly in its entirety be obliterated, a complete arteriogram is necessary to document each and every feeder vessel. The angiogram also may reveal associated abnormalities such as tumor or aneurysm. Since 15 percent of AVMs are supplied by branches of the external carotid artery, preoperative studies should include information regarding the arteries that normally supply the extracranial compartment in addition to those supplying the intracranial compartment. Complete arteriography also includes such techniques as magnification, subtraction, rapid-sequence exposure, and multiview radiography in order to obtain maximum arteriographic information.[15] Digital subtraction angiography can be especially helpful since it permits the most rapid filming sequences possible and requires less contrast agent than conventional angiography.

In addition to providing information about the morphology of an AVM, the neuroradiologist has assumed an important role in their treatment as well.[16] Many AVMs may be embolized preoperatively and significantly devascularized with Gelfoam, polyurethane sponge, silicone pellets, or cyanoacrylate glues.[17–23] Recently, some concerns have been raised about the potential carcinogenicity of the cyanoacrylate glues; thus their future availability for use is in doubt.[24] For AVMs with one or two major feeders, the feeders occasionally may be occluded just before surgery with the aid of an intravascular detachable balloon, as described by Debrun (see Chapter 70).[25] Inherent in all of these techniques is the risk that the development of collaterals, given sufficient time, will erode the gains made by embolization. Because of this, surgery should follow an embolization procedure within a few weeks. The hope is that the preoperative embolization will help the surgeon by devascularizing the mass, making removal easier and therefore safer for the patient. Embolization alone occasionally obliterates an AVM, but most often a few feeders remain. Partial embolization does not reduce the chances of recurrent hemorrhage, so surgery is almost always required. Embolization of vascular malformations carries significant risks, with a 4 percent mortality and 13 percent morbidity even in experienced hands.[26,27] Sometimes the venous side of the anomaly is occluded prematurely when the arterial side is still patent, which

OPERATIVE NEUROSURGICAL TECHNIQUES
ISBN 0-8089-1862-1

Table 80-1. Classification of vascular malformations according to McCormick[1]

Telangiectasis: A small conglomeration of thin-walled capillaries separated by normal parenchyma. It is common in the pons or at the junctions of gray and white matter and is only occasionally associated with hemorrhage.

Varix: A dilated anomalous or normal vein that is usually a singular structure with normal surrounding parenchyma. It occasionally is responsible for massive hemorrhage.

Cavernous malformation: A mass of sinusoidal vascular spaces; commonly a small mass in the cerebrum, with associated calcium and with no parenchyma between vessels. It is an infrequent lesion in the brain that occasionally ruptures. Angiography may reveal only mass effect and no pathologic circulation.

Venous malformation: A mass of abnormal vessels, generally small, with no direct arterial feeders but with a central draining vein. The abnormal vessels are separated by relatively normal parenchyma. This is one of the most common of the vascular malformations in the nervous system; only rarely is it a source of hemorrhage. However, cerebellar venous malformations appear to bleed and rebleed more frequently than venous malformations located elsewhere.[3]

Arteriovenous malformation: A mass of abnormal vessels with enlarged arterial feeders and large draining veins. The anomalous vessels may have the histologic characteristics of arteries or veins. The mass tends to be wedge-shaped with a broad base on the cortical surface and the apex pointing to the ventricle. The parenchyma surrounding the abnormal vessels is commonly gliotic. This lesion is the most likely of the five forms of vascular malformation to hemorrhage; it can be found in any anatomic location within the nervous system.

---

may precipitate a hemorrhage. A feeding artery may also supply normal brain; if it is occluded by an embolus, a cerebral infarction may result. Particulate emboli may reflux out of a feeding artery and into a normal brain artery with the same consequence. Occasionally, the fine catheter used for this superselective work will be glued inadvertently in the artery. Fortunately, the now permanently implanted catheter is sometimes well tolerated in the brain. Neurosurgeons may find that operating on a malformation which is hardened by cyanoacrylate increases the difficulty of the surgery. Since the mass is no longer pliant, retraction of the mass transmits pressure to normal brain possibly leading to increased cerebral edema in the postoperative period.

SURGICAL TECHNIQUES EMPLOYED IN THE MANAGEMENT OF AVMS

The ideal treatment of all AVMs is complete obliteration. Lesser measures, such as partial embolization and interruption of major feeding arteries, reduce the AVM only temporarily and offer very little protection from hemorrhage. Consequently, excision remains the primary form of therapy, although specialized radiation techniques appear to be useful in the management of some small AVMs. The principles of surgery, while common knowledge, are nevertheless worth reiterating.

The craniotomy always should be large enough to expose and allow access to all the major arterial feeders and draining veins. The dura should be reflected in a careful manner so as to avoid injury to any underlying adherent vessels from the AVM. In the case of cerebral AVMs, frequently all that is seen on the surface of the brain is a red draining vein. In such a case, the arachnoid around the vein should be dissected free and the vein traced into the brain parenchyma until the malformation is encountered. Usually this can be accomplished with the removal of little or no normal cortex.

The operating microscope is a considerable help in AVM surgery, and with experience few surgeons would wish to undertake these formidable operations relying on only the naked eye or loupes. Initial dissection begins in the gliotic plane between the normal brain and the AVM. As the dissection is carried around the anomaly, large arteries will be encountered which appear to enter the AVM. Prior to dividing such an artery, it is prudent to trace the vessel to ensure the vessel in question truly ends in the AVM rather than ending perhaps more distally to supply the AVM on the one side and eloquent brain on the other. Consequently, large arteries may have to be sacrificed late in the dissection after their destinations have been clearly identified. On the other hand, coagulation of the small "feeders" with their associated cork-screw tangles can be performed early in the procedure with safety. Needless to say, at least one large draining vein should be saved until the end, and careful study of the venous anatomy preoperatively is important in planning surgical strategy.[28]

Remaining close to the AVM in the gliotic plane is easy to advise, but sometimes difficult to follow in practice. The surgeon may be easily misled between coils of vessels into the core of the AVM, which he or she realizes only when pathologic tissue is found on both sides of the plane of dissection.

Choroidal feeders pose another challenge. Most malformations extend to the cerebral ventricle to receive an enlarged choroidal artery and give off a draining choroidal vein. Since these vessels are deep and under the mass of the malformation, they are often difficult to visualize until late in the dissection and may be difficult to control since they are difficult to coagulate and tear quite easily. Thus, the ventricle should be packed with cottonoids to prevent blood from filling the ventricles in the event of profuse bleeding. Persistence eventually leads to control of the choroidal vessels, which represents a giant step toward completion of the operation.

After the malformation has been removed, the bed of the anomaly should be carefully inspected for possible residual pathologic vessels. Such vessels may appear as loops of large vessels or small capillaries which give the gliotic brain a Swiss cheese appearance. In any case, these vessels must be removed. Raising venous pressure by bilateral simultaneous jugular compression or raising arterial pressure through the use of a vasopressor such a phenylephrine have been helpful in identifying residual AVM. Since the most feared complication of this surgery is postoperative hemorrhage, as from residual AVM, some authors have stressed the use of intraoperative serial arteriography.[29] In our experience, a disastrous hemor-

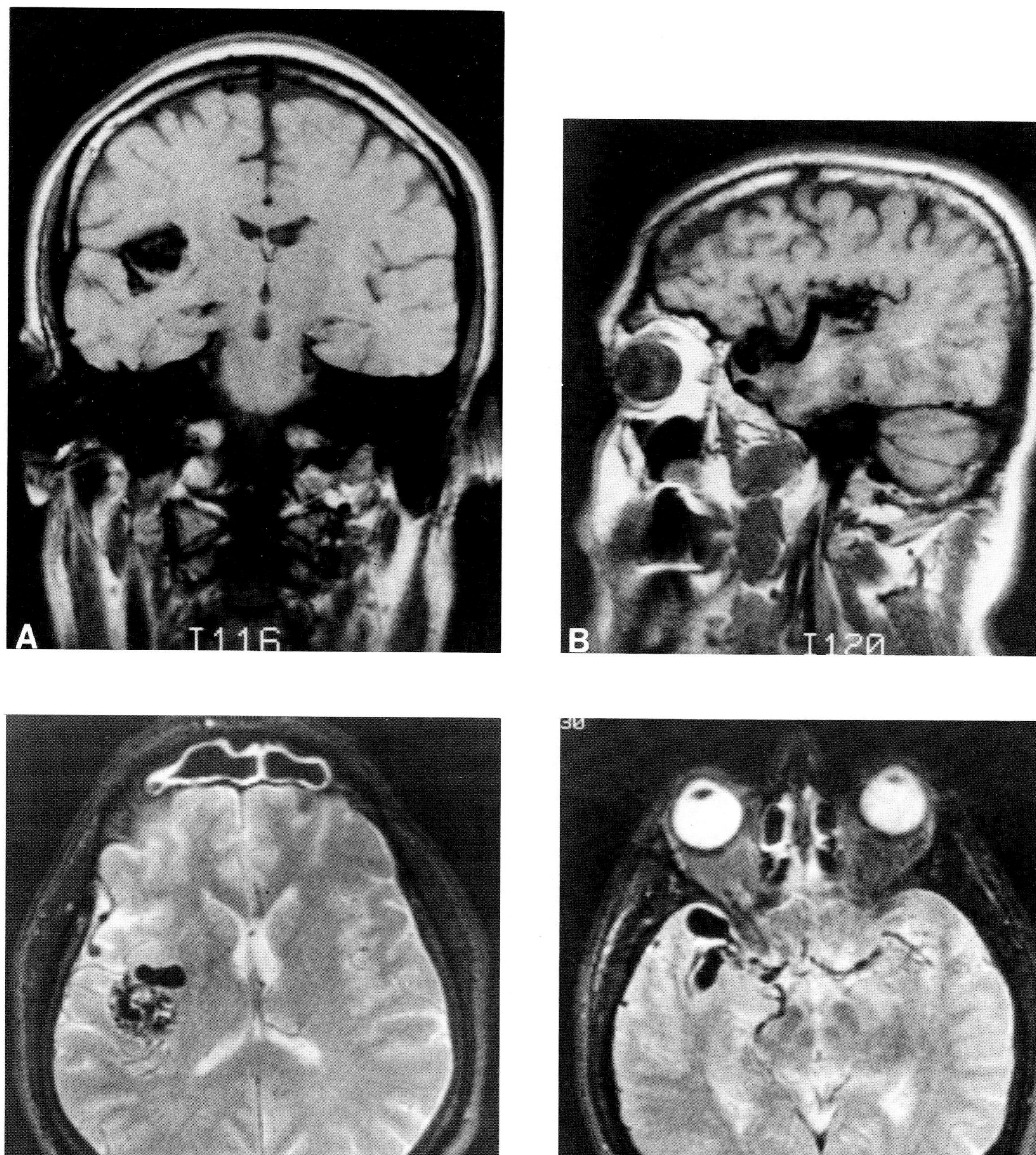

Fig. 80-1. T1 and T2 weighted MRI scans of a brain in a middle-aged man complaining of headaches. A right sylvian fissure AVM was clearly delineated by MRI. (A) The relationship of the lesion to the sylvian fissue, ventricular system, and nearby basal ganglia is evident. (B) A huge draining vein is evident on the sagittal view. (C) Brain tissue with essentially normal signal intensity surrounds the lesion. (D) A prominently enlarged carotid artery and large draining veins are obvious on the axial view.

rhage complicating recovery has not occurred when manipulation of arterial and venous pressures had failed to produce hemorrhage at the conclusion of resection. While it is prudent to line the AVM cavity with oxidized cellulose, topical hemostatic agents by themselves are not an adequate safeguard from rebleeding from residual AVM.

Some have proposed beginning the attack on an AVM by cannulating and embolizing major feeding arteries under direct vision.[22,27,30] After cannulating the artery, an angiogram is taken to confirm that the artery supplies the AVM exclusively and not brain. Then the embolic material, usually cyanoacrylate glue and Pantopaque in a 50:50 mixture, is injected. This strategy reduces the vascularity of the AVM at the price of either turning part of it into a hard mass, which may be difficult to remove, or gluing or encasing a possibly important nutrient artery from normal brain to the AVM.

In order to remove an AVM from an eloquent area of brain, some surgeons recommend operating under local anesthesia and identifying speech and motor areas by electrically stimulating the cerebral cortex.[27,31] Feeding arteries can be temporarily clamped and a speech and or motor deficit tested prior to permanent division.[27] This is a reasonable approach to the problem, but comparable results can be obtained by careful microdissection of the malformation with preservation of all major arteries until the surgeon is certain they supply only the malformation.

Some surgeons have recommended staged microsurgical excisions combined with barbiturate coma,[32] clamping of the ipsilateral cervical internal carotid artery,[33] or temporary vascular clips placed close to the AVM in combination with mannitol and fluorochemicals.[34] Results obtained using such adjuncts do not appear to differ significantly from those obtained using more classical techniques. In addition, a drawback of staged surgical procedures is possible hemorrhage from a fresh surgical bed which contains residual AVM intentionally left for treatment at a future date.

After the operation is over, systemic arterial blood pressure must be carefully monitored to help avoid a sudden elevation in blood pressure that might trigger a postoperative hemorrhage. Whether or not a syndrome of malignant brain edema exists after excision of a large anomaly remains a matter of dispute.[35]

ARTERIOVENOUS MALFORMATIONS IN SPECIFIC LOCATIONS

DURAL

Intracranial AVMs nestled primarily in the dura usually involve the cavernous sinus or the transverse-sigmoid sinus. The lesions involving the cavernous sinus appear more clinically benign, demonstrate a higher propensity for spontaneous thrombosis, and frequently are treatable by embolization alone.[13]

Dural AVMs draining into the transverse-sigmoid sinus carry a worse prognosis without treatment. Careful evaluation of the pattern of venous drainage may reveal significant retrograde drainage into cortical veins because of various degrees of sinus thrombosis or high shunt volume.[23] Preoperative embolization followed by careful interruption of the dura near the venous sinuses is a workable strategy. Patent major sinuses and veins should be preserved to prevent venous infarction.

After the intracranial portion of the AVM is removed, the dura which has been excised should be replaced with a graft. Consideration may need to be given to the need for special scalp flaps, as for example when the scalp is involved as well.[36–39] Particular problems and techniques associated with treatment of lesions involving the transverse-sigmoid sinus and the cavernous sinus have been reviewed recently.[12,13]

INTRAVENTRICULAR

Intraventricular lesions generally are supplied primarily by choroidal vessels. After standard craniotomy the ventricle is exposed either by incising the corpus callosum or through the depths of a sulcus. After the foramen of Monro has been adequately packed off with cottonoids, the standard principles of excision then may be employed to remove the intraventricular lesion. Yasargil et al. have described the microsurgical excision of AVMs involving both the corpus callosum and the ventricle.[40] Stein has described the surgical approach to AVMs involving the nearby limbic system.[41]

CEREBELLAR LESIONS

Cerebellar AVMs generally are amenable to excision via a wide suboccipital craniectomy and application of the principles outlined for cerebral AVMs. Some posterior fossa AVMs involve the lateral or sigmoid sinuses. If division of one of the major sinuses is anticipated, the best test for the safety of the maneuver is to obstruct the sinus temporarily and observe the brain. When sectioning or retracting the tentorium, care should be exercised to avoid tearing the draining veins.

CEREBELLOPONTINE ANGLE-BRAIN STEM AVMS

Cerebellopontine angle lesions generally peel off of the cerebellum, brain stem, and cranial nerves as long as care is exercised to remain within the plane separating the AVM from normal brain. Some of these lesions, like AVMs of the spinal cord, sit in the subarachnoid cisterns or on the pial surface of the brain. Other AVMs, however, infiltrate the brain stem, in which case they are not removable, except perhaps by using circulatory arrest under deep hypothermia. It is here that radiation therapy either with heavy particles or with the gamma knife finds a role in management. Even then there is risk to functional nerve tissue. Cerebellopontine angle AVMs sometimes have to be approached by a combination subtentorial-supratentorial exposure. This approach provides satisfactory access to posterior cerebral and superior cerebellar arterial feeders, and as well allows adequate handling of vessels that may be straddling the tentorium. Even in experienced hands, the morbidity and mortality from surgical treatment of posterior fossa AVMs is generally higher than for supratentorial lesions.[40,42] Detailed descriptions of surgical technique can be found in the literature.[5,40,43–47]

POSTOPERATIVE EVALUATION

Just as the morphology of the AVM cannot be documented without complete arteriography, neither can surgical cure be documented without arteriography. Residual lesions may be treated with follow-up surgery, additional embolization, and perhaps in some cases with the aid of radiation therapy.[48] Postoperative MRI is also useful in evaluating residual AVM as well as postoperative hydrocephalus.[10]

SPECIAL CONSIDERATIONS

Currently, embolization, either flow-directed or by means of craniotomy or high energy treatment, as for example from proton beam, cobalt 60, or conventional x-rays, may supplement surgical excision of AVMs. Complete obliteration of an AVM with embolization alone occurs infrequently (10 percent of cases) and usually involves small lesions with one or two feeders. Such lesions are often amenable to surgical excision. On the other hand, through preoperative embolization the vascularity of the AVM is reduced and the need for blood transfusion is frequently reduced as well.[26,49] Similarly, surgery may be useful in reducing the size of a very large "unresectable" lesion into one that is of a size amenable to radiation therapy. For a residual mass 50 mm or less in size (preferably 25 mm or less), embolization or high energy treatment may finish off the AVM.[48,50,51] Unfortunately, high energy therapy totally obliterates the AVM in a variable percentage of patients (i.e., 20 to 80 percent) and thrombosis of the AVM usually takes 12 to 24 months to occur.[49–51] During the 12- to 24-month period following radiotherapy, rebleeding may occur. Such therapy is not the solution for lesions greater than 50 mm in size. Nevertheless, for lesions in surgically inaccessible locations (i.e., basal ganglia, thalamus, intra-axial brain stem) embolization or radiotherapy may be necessary.

Arteriovenous malformations occasionally are associated with a tumor or with aneurysms. In the case of the associated tumor, the AVM can be treated first and the tumor removed either at the same or a second operation. In the case of associated aneurysms, the aneurysms are best treated during the primary attack or just preceding the primary attack on the arteriovenous malformation. Such lesions are often but not always located in the circulation proximal to the AVM. When they are located proximal to the AVM, they may be dealt with at the same operation. When an aneurysm is located in another area of the cerebral circulation, however, it should be treated first, unless there is clear-cut information (such as a computed tomogram) documenting hemorrhage from the AVM. A recent review by Gamache et al. summarizes the experience in this regard.[52,53]

REFERENCES

1. McCormick WF: The pathology of vascular ("arteriovenous"') malformations. J Neurosurg 24:807, 1966
2. McCormick WF, Hardman GM, Boulter TR: Vascular malformation "angiomas" of the brain with special reference to those occurring in the posterior fossa. J Neurosurg 28:241, 1968
3. Rothfus WE, Albright AL, Caset KF, et al: Cerebellar venous angioma: "Benign" entity? AJNR 5:61, 1984
4. Paterson JH, McKissock W: A clinical survey of intracranial angiomas with special reference to their mode of progression and surgical treatment. A report of 110 cases. Brain 79:233, 1956
5. Gamache FW Jr, Patterson RH Jr: Infratentorial arteriovenous malformations, in Fein J, Flamm E (eds): Cerebrovascular Surgery. New York, Springer-Verlag, 1985, pp 1117–1137
6. Perret G, Nishioka H: Report on the cooperative study of intracranial aneurysms and subarachnoid hemorrhage VI. Arteriovenous malformations. J Neurosurg 25:467, 1966
7. Wilkins RH: Natural history of intracranial vascular malformations: A review. Neurosurgery 16:421, 1985
8. Pressman BD, Kirkwood JR, Davis DO: Computerized transverse tomography of vascular lesions of the brain. Part I. AJR 124:208, 1975
9. Terbrugge K, Scotti G, Eitheir R, et al: Computed tomography in intracranial arteriovenous malformation. Radiology 122:703, 1977
10. Kucharczyk W, Lemme-Pleghes L, Uske A, et al: Intracranial vascular malformations: MR and CT imaging. Radiology 156:383, 1985
11. Malik GM, Pearce JE, Ausman JI, et al: Dural arteriovenous malformations and intracranial hemorrhage. Neurosurgery 15:332, 1984
12. Obrador S, Soto M, Silvela J: Clinical syndromes of arteriovenous malformations of the transverse-sigmoid sinus. J Neurol Neurosurg Psychiatry 38:436, 1975
13. Vinuela F, Fox AJ, Debrun GM, et al: Spontaneous carotid cavernous fistulas: Clinical, radiologic, and therapeutic considerations. Experience with 20 cases. J Neurosurg 60:976, 1984
14. Sundt TM Jr, Piepgras DG: The surgical approach to arteriovenous malformations of the lateral and sigmoid dural sinuses. J Neurosurg 59:32, 1983
15. Debrun G, Chartres A: Infra and supratentorial arteriovenous malformation. A general review. Neuroradiology 3:184, 1972
16. Cromwell LD, Harris AB: Treatment of cerebral arteriovenous malformation. A combined neurosurgical and neuroradiological approach. J Neurosurg 52:705, 1980
17. Dubois PG, Kerber CW, Heinz ER: Interventional techniques in neuroradiology. Radiol Clin North Am 17:515, 1979
18. Djindjian R, Cophignon J, Theron J, et al: Embolization by superselective arteriography from the femoral route. Review of 60 cases 1. Technique, Indications, Complications. Neuroradiology 6:20, 1973
19. Kerber CW: Catheter therapy: Fluoroscopic monitoring of deliberate embolic occlusion. Radiology 125:538, 1977
20. Kricheff I, Madayag M, Braumstein P: Transfemoral catheter embolization of cerebral and posterior fossa arteriovenous malformations. Radiology 103:107, 1972
21. Wolpert SM, Stein BM: Catheter embolization of intracranial arteriovenous malformations as an aid to surgical excision. Neuroradiology 10:73, 1975
22. Fox AF, Girvin JP, Vinuela F, et al: Rolandic arteriovenous malformations: Improvement in limb function by IBC embolization. AJNR 6:575, 1985
23. Lasjaunias P, Terbrugge K, Chin M: Dural AVM. Neurosurgery 16:435, 1985
24. Vintners HV, Lundie JM, Kaufman JC: Long term pathological follow-up of cerebral arteriovenous malformations treated by embolization with bucrylate. N Engl J Med 314:477, 1986
25. Debrun G, Lacour P, Caron JP: Balloon arterial catheter techniques in the treatment of intracranial disease, in Krayenbuhl H (ed): Advances and Technical Standards in Neurosurgery, vol 4. Vienna, Springer-Verlag, pp 131–145
26. Fox A: Presented at the 25th annual meeting of the American Society of Neuroradiology, New York City, May 10–15, 1987
27. Girvin JP, Fox AJ, Vinuela F, et al: Intraoperative embolization (IBC) of cerebral arteriovenous malformations in the awake patient. Clin Neurosurg 31:188, 1984
28. Jomin M, Lesoin F, Lozes G: Prognosis for arteriovenous malformations of the brain in adults based on 150 cases. Surg Neurol 23:362, 1985
29. Parkinson D, Bachers G: Arteriovenous malformations. Summary of 100 consecutive supratentorial cases. J Neurosurg 53:285, 1980
30. Vlahovitch B, Fuentes JM: Embolization of cerebral angiomas by cerebral catheterization of cortical arteries. Neuroradiology 11:243, 1976
31. Garretson NH: Surgery of arteriovenous malformations. Presented

at the Sixth Joint Meeting on Stroke and Cerebral Circulation, Los Angeles. Feb. 12–14, 1981

32. Sang H: Microsurgical excision of paraventricular arteriovenous malformations. Neurosurgery 16:293, 1985

33. Bonnal J, Born JD, Hans P: One stage excision of high flow arteriovenous malformations. J Neurosurg 62:128, 1985

34. Suzuki J, Onuma T, Kayama T: Surgical treatment of intracranial arteriovenous malformation. Neurol Res 4:191, 1982

35. Day AL, Friedman WA, Sypert GW, et al: Successful treatment of the normal perfusion pressure breakthrough syndrome. Neurosurgery 11:625, 1982

36. Fernandez-Urdanibia J, Silvela J, Soto M: Occipital dural arteriovenous malformations. Neuroradiology 7:57, 1972

37. Houser OW, Baker HC, Rhoton AL, et al: Intracranial dural arteriovenous malformations. Radiology 105:55, 1972

38. Kosnik EJ, Hunt WF, Miller CA: Dural arteriovenous malformations. J Neurosurg 40:322, 1974

39. Manaka S, Izawa M, Nawata H: Dural arteriovenous malformations treated by artificial embolization with liquid silicone. Surg Neurol 7:63, 1977

40. Yasargil MG, Jain KK, Antic J, et al: Arteriovenous malformations of the splenium of the corpus callosum: Microsurgical treatment. Surg Neurol 5:5, 1976

41. Stein B: Arteriovenous malformations of the medial cerebral hemisphere and the limbic system. J Neurosurg 60:23, 1984

42. Drake CG, Friedman AH, Peerless SJ: Posterior fossa arteriovenous malformations. J Neurosurg 64:1, 1986

43. Drake CG: Surgical removal of arteriovenous malformations from brain stem and cerebellopontine angle. J Neurosurg 43:661, 1975

44. Patterson RH Jr, Fraser RA: Vascular neoplasms of the brainstem: A place for profound hypothermia and circulatory arrest. Adv Neurosurg 3:425, 1975

45. Samson D, Batjer H: Arteriovenous malformations of the cerebellar vermis. Neurosurgery 16:341, 1985

46. Aoki N: Combined occipital transtentorial and infratentorial supracerebellar approach in the Concorde position for the treatment of an arteriovenous malformation in the upper vermis: Case report. Neurosurgery 17:815, 1985

47. Salcman M, Nudelman RW, Bellis EH: Arteriovenous malformations of the superior cerebellar artery: Excision via an occipital transtentorial approach. Neurosurgery 17:749, 1985

48. Steiner L, Leksell L, Greitz T, et al: Stereotactic radiosurgery in intracranial arteriovenous malformations. Acta Neurochir (Suppl) 21:195, 1974

49. Drake CG: Arteriovenous malformations of the brain. The options for management. N Engl J Med 309:308, 1983

50. Kjellberg RN, Hanamura T, Davis KR, et al: Bragg-peak proton beam therapy for arteriovenous malformations of the brain. N Engl J Med 309:269, 1983

51. Yamada F, Fukuda S, Matsumoto K, et al: Effect of radiotherapy on dural arteriovenous malformation: Long term follow-up study and clinical evaluation. Neurol Med Chir 24:591, 1984

52. Gamache FW Jr, Drake CG, Peerless SJ, et al: Arteriovenous malformations associated with intracranial aneurysms. Presented at the 50th anniversary meeting of the American Association of Neurological Surgeons, Boston, April 8, 1981

CHAPTER 81

Proton Beam Therapy for Arteriovenous Malformations of the Brain

Raymond N. Kjellberg

ARTERIOVENOUS MALFORMATIONS are congenital anomalies that enlarge slowly during life.[1-3] The lesions manifest themselves clinically when they produce intracranial bleeding, seizures, progressive neurologic deficits, headache, and other clinical phenomena.[4]

Patients whose lesions are considered inaccessible to conventional therapies are those in whom the malformation is large, centrally located, or lying in the speech areas of the dominant cerebral hemisphere or in the brain stem. It is mainly this group of patients who have come within our purview. Patients also have sought to avoid the risk of craniotomy and excision by electing proton beam therapy.

Bragg peak proton beam therapy has been used during the past 20 years for the treatment of arteriovenous malformations (AVMs) of the brain. Most of these patients were considered unsuitable for surgical excision or embolization. One or two years are required for the effects of proton beam therapy to develop. Following this "incubation period," hemorrhage, particularly lethal hemorrhage, is substantially reduced. Seizures, progressive neurologic deficits, and headaches are normally arrested or improved. Lethal complications of the therapy have not been encountered, and functional complications were substantially reduced after we had an opportunity to evaluate our prior experience and alter the method.

We have performed 717 procedures for AVMs in 709 patients using stereotactic Bragg peak proton beam therapy (Table 81-1). This report is based on that experience. We have followed 92 percent of these patients for more than 2 years.

The stereotactic method is used to direct the Bragg peak of the proton beam to the AVM. Doses used in proton therapy cannot be easily compared with conventional fractioned x-ray dose schedules because of the difference in the interval of exposure, the volume exposed to ionization, and the extent to which tissue necrosis is to be achieved or avoided in therapy.[5,6]

THERAPY

Preparation for treatment involves medical, neurologic, and neuro-ophthalmologic CT scanning and bilateral carotid and vertebral angiography.

Stereotactic Bragg peak proton beam therapy for arteriovenous malformations is performed under local anesthesia in a single session lasting about 1½ hours. The patient's head is secured by skeletal fixation with drill rods in the outer table of the calvaria (Figure 81-1). Orthogonal x-ray films in the anteroposterior and lateral views precisely localize the aiming point in three planes of space within the volume of the malformation. The volume to be irradiated is established from angiograms. We seek to identify the "small vessel" component of the AVM as the target volume and avoid targeting dilated arteries within this target volume. Beam diameters from 7 to 50 mm are selected and modified to conform to the size and shape of the target volume. We have determined isoeffective doses for various beam diameters, which vary from 5000 rad for 7-mm beams to 1050 rad for 50-mm beams. Brain exposed before injury (stroke, open excision) has slightly lower tolerances in relatively more sensitive subjects.

The first of our patients with an arteriovenous malformation was treated on February 26, 1965. Our current report is based on 20 years of follow-up observation on 709 cases. The mean age of the patients at treatment was 31.1 years (S.D. + 11.5 years).[13]

Hemorrhage was the first symptom in 44 percent of patients, seizures in 32 percent, headaches in 11 percent, and progressive neurologic deficit (PND) in 11 percent. Other symptoms may develop later.

RESULTS

CLINICAL FOLLOW-UP

Of 709 patients treated, 389 patients underwent therapy 2 or more years ago, and we have follow-up data on 92 percent of them (Table 81-1).

ARTERIOGRAPHIC FINDINGS

Following proton beam therapy, the changes in the subsequent arteriograms ranged from total obliteration of the AVM to no evident change. In 20 percent of patients the malformation was totally obliterated. In 56 percent of patients the AVM was reduced by 50 percent or more, and in 13 percent it was unchanged. The arteriographic change usually involved the small vessel component of the AVM. Enlarged feeding arteries

OPERATIVE NEUROSURGICAL TECHNIQUES
ISBN 0-8089-1862-1

Table 81-1. Patients with arteriovenous malformations treated by proton beam therapy

Patients treated (as of 9/30/85)	709
Number of procedures	717
Number of patients followed up	443
Number of patients followed for 2 years or more after treatment	389

and draining veins were not included in the volume of tissue treated by Bragg peak proton beam. However, because the small vessel component was reduced, dilated arteries and veins returned to more normal calibers (Figures 81-2 through 81-5).

LESION TISSUE CHANGES ATTRIBUTABLE TO THERAPY

We had access to three pathologic specimens from patients treated by proton beam therapy. The lumens of nearly all of the vessels in the specimens, which grossly resembled balls of twine, were either totally occluded or greatly reduced. The walls were extremely thick, and the normal layers could no longer be distinguished in many of the larger arteries and veins. Elastic tissue, endothelial cells, smooth muscle cells, and adventitial fibroblasts were replaced by homogeneous collagenous material. Some vessels were patent, even in areas where most others were occluded. Where the vascular malformation abutted the pia-arachnoid, there was marked thickening of the meninges. Strands of collagen and fibroblastic connective tissue also extended into the cerebral cortex.

COMPLICATIONS

Four major complications occurred in our first 12 patients. Four moderate complications occurred in patients 13 to 73. In patients 74 to 709, two mild complications occurred (Table 81-2). As a result of these observations, the dose was revised so that patients now are treated with ionization doses below those that earlier produced complications.

No patient treated with Bragg peak proton beam irradiation died of procedure-related causes; there have been no infections, no procedure-related hemorrhages, no thromboembolic events, and no persistent anesthetic complications.

DISCUSSION

Histologically, endothelial cells of the AVM that are injured by the proton beam are provoked to deposit subendothelial collagen and hyaline, and as a result the lumens of the "small vessels" of the AVM become smaller and the flow rate and "steal" are reduced. Furthermore, the subendothelial collagen and hyaline thicken the walls of the small vessels of the AVM. We are convinced that the threshold of this effect occurs at a smaller dose in the AVM embryonic small vessels than in normal capillaries. We infer from our experience that normal capillaries are unaffected by the ionization doses used. Our evidence for this inference is that many of the patients with basal ganglia-thalamic AVMs have not suffered from any consequences of ionization of the corticospinal pathways (and other neurologically active zones), which would have inevitably occurred were there no differential in the threshold at which the ionization endotheliitis occurs.

Regarding our current thinking about the nature of ionizing

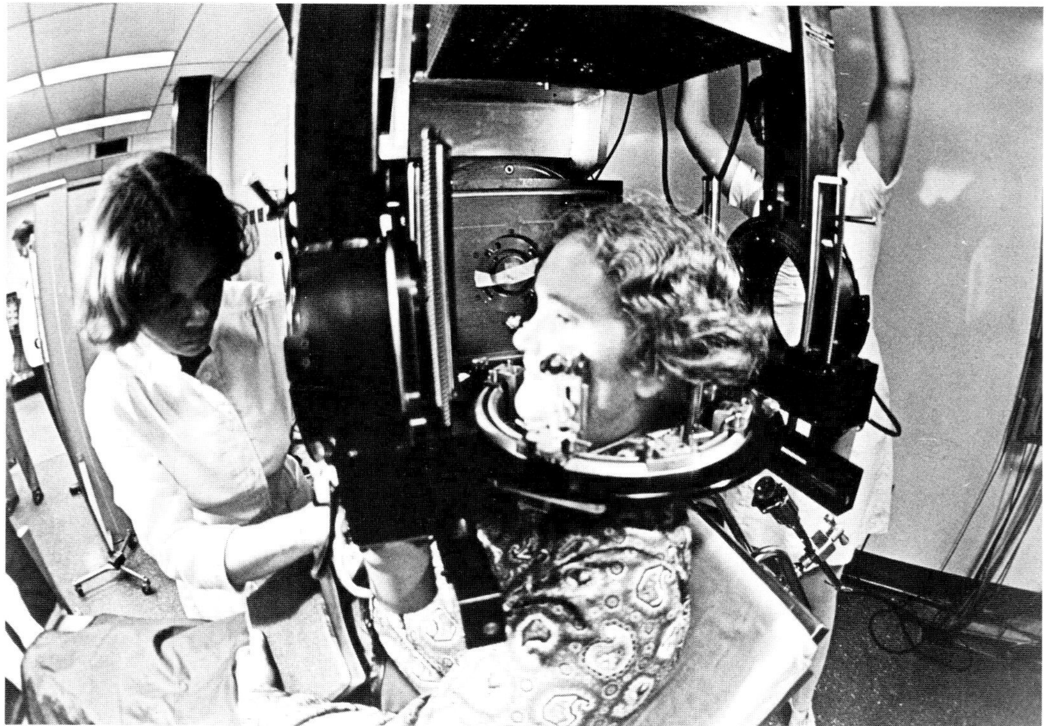

Fig. 81-1. Patient in the stereotactic instrument of the proton beam therapy machine. The instrument is applied under local anesthesia with the patient awake. The AVM target is localized with the aid of orthogonal Polaroid x-ray films. The proton beam comes from the background of the photograph and is measured by a calibrated nitrogen ion chamber. The variable water absorber controls the depth of penetration of the Bragg peak of the proton beam so that the Bragg peak falls within the target volume of the AVM.

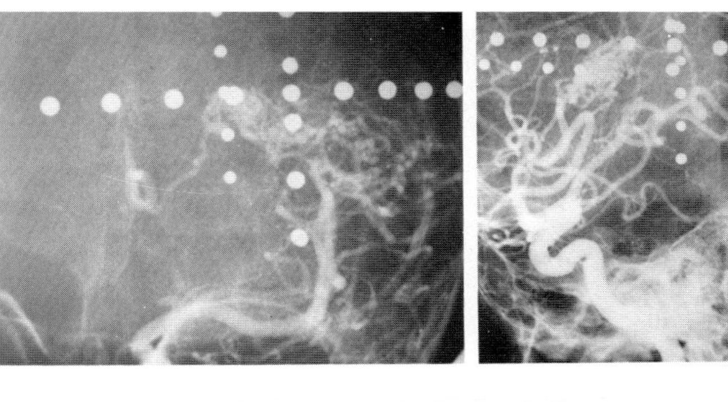

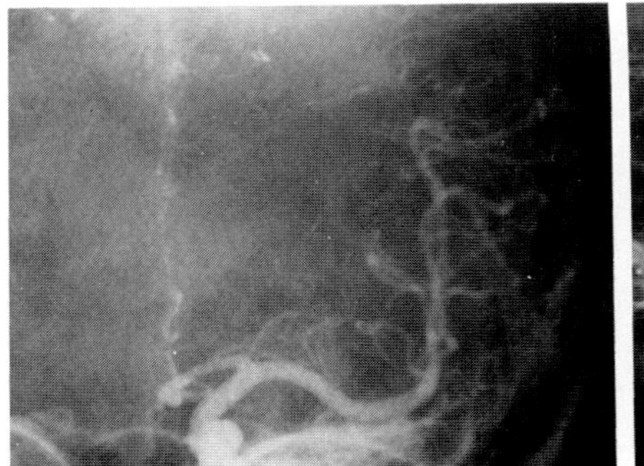

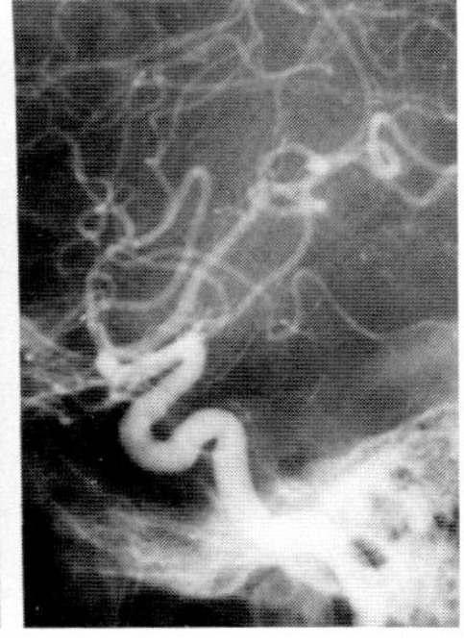

Fig. 81-2. A 21-year-old man had a left thalamic AVM that hemorrhaged and was without residual deficits. Two years after proton beam therapy he had had no further hemorrhage and his angiogram showed complete obliteration of the AVM.

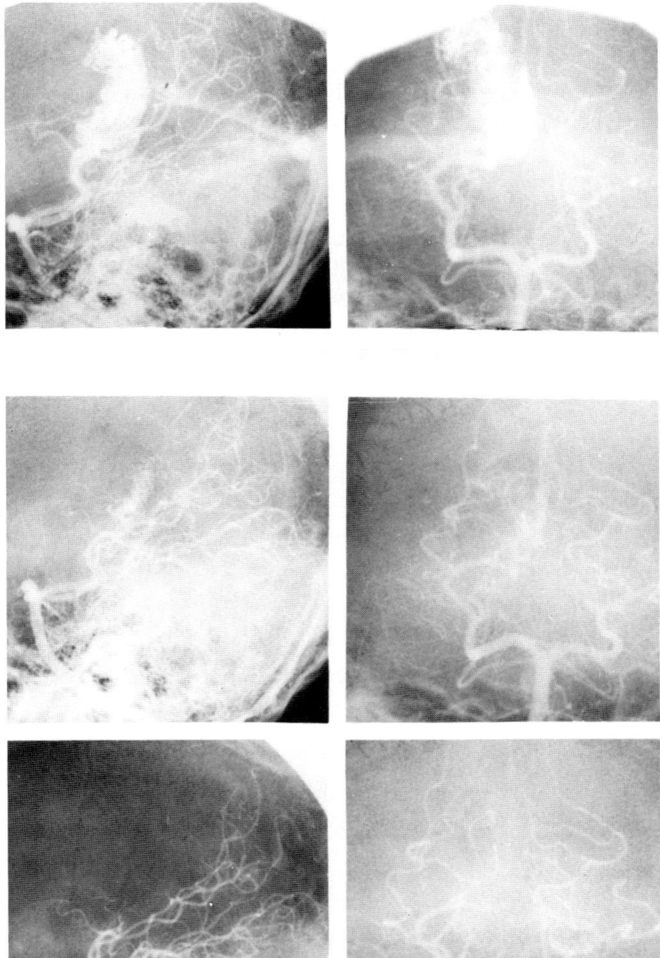

Fig. 81-3. A 22-year-old male teacher had a right retrosplenial AVM that hemorrhaged and suffered a slight residual memory deficit. His AVM was reduced about 96 percent angiographically 2.1 years after proton beam treatment and was completely gone 7.2 years after treatment. He continued working.

events that take place which lead to the effects we have ascribed to them, the entry of a proton into the nucleus of the endothelial cell of the AVM small vessel produces an ionization.[7] The ionizing event produces a break or a "sticky place" in the DNA. The replicative or metabolic function of this point on the DNA chain is inactivated. This replicative or metabolic function may not be called upon for some time. Furthermore, a single break or "sticky place" does not totally disable the cell. Many such breaks must accumulate (integrate) for the cell to become sick; this is called endotheliitis. The sick endothelial cell induces the formation of collagen and hyaline in the subendothelial space, leading to narrowing or occlusion of the lumen of the AVM small vessel and thickening of its walls.

Proton beam therapy has no evident immediate effect and infrequently is any clinical response evident during the first 12 months after the procedure. This interval can be referred to as the "incubation period." During this interval, hemorrhages, including lethal hemorrhages, can occur, and seizures and progressive neurologic deficits can advance. Such clinical findings seem to parallel the course of symptoms with untreated AVMs. Between 12 and 24 months after treatment, clinical improvement becomes evident. The improvement in some cases continues after the 24-month posttreatment interval.

Death from hemorrhage is the most serious outcome of a patient harboring an AVM. Death from brain hemorrhage occurred in 8 patients less than 2 years after proton beam treatment at intervals of 0.5, 1, 9, 11, 12, 13, 15, and 18 months after therapy. Death following elective craniotomy occurred in three patients 2.9, 3.3, and 4.1 years after proton beam therapy. We consider this mortality during the first year as a result of bleeding to be compatible with the mortality of untreated AVMs. One patient with a massive AVM that nearly filled one

hemisphere arrived at our hospital with extremely elevated intracranial pressure and in end-stage cerebral decompensation. Proton beam therapy, a shunt, and various open procedures did not interrupt his downhill course. One young patient who had both cerebral and oronasal AVMs died of hemorrhage of his nasal-facial AVM. One patient bled and died 4.6 years after treatment. We regard this as a failure of therapy. Although the majority of this patient's AVM had undergone collagenous and hyaline sclerosis, the bleeding appeared to originate from vessels at the margin of the sclerotic mass. We appreciate that small vessels may exist in an AVM that are beyond the resolution of current state-of-the-art angiography. If we did not see these vessels on the angiogram, we did not account for them in determining the volume to be treated. For patients followed beyond the 24-month interval after therapy, this patient's death represents a 0.27 percent total mortality as a result of AVM hemorrhage during the total 18-year interval for those followed 2 years or more. This result suggests that proton beam therapy confers protection from death caused by hemorrhage.

Of the patients dying of cerebral hemorrhage less than 2

years after treatment, three were initial hemorrhage patients, two patients initially had seizures, and three patients initially had headaches. No patient whose initial symptom was a progressive neurologic deficit died among those we followed.

The rate of further bleeding in patients with hemorrhage has been reported to be between 3.7 and 6.25 percent/year;[4,8,9] in our patients the rate was 7.25 percent/year before treatment. In the 1966 Cooperative Study of Intracranial Aneurysms and Subarachnoid Hemorrhage,[4] the mortality from further bleeding was 0.9 percent/year, but no patient who initially had seizures died of bleeding. In the recent restudy of these patients, overall bleeding and death as a result of bleeding were carefully analyzed.[10] Their experience and ours can be regarded as compatible. In other studies, the annual rates in "conservatively treated" unselected patients were 1.3 percent,[11] 1.6 percent,[9] and 1.4 percent.[8]

The pretreatment rebleeding rate of 7.25 percent/year for our patients was compared with the bleeding rate 2 years after therapy. The P values were determined by both the binomial and Poisson methods. We had 1022 patient years of follow-up in this group. The binomial method showed a statistically significant difference, with a P value of 0.002, and the Poisson method showed a statistically significant difference at a P value of 0.0003.

The second most important liability incurred by patients with arteriovenous malformations is neurologic deficit and disability. This can occur as a result of hemorrhage or nonhemorrhagic progressive deficit caused by the AVM. Hemorrhage occurred as a first symptom in 44 percent of our patients; of these, 55 percent were left with a fixed neurologic deficit. If we excluded the patients who died in the first 18 months, two fixed neurologic deficits as a result of hemorrhage occurred after proton beam treatment in the remaining patients.

In patients who first have seizures as an initial symptom, management of the seizures is often effectively achieved with anticonvulsant medication, and such patients are not necessarily candidates for therapy. However, if the seizures are uncontrolled, if bleeding occurs, or if the presence of an untreated lesion provokes anxiety or depression, we recommend proton beam therapy.

Headaches alone infrequently lead to studies that reveal an arteriovenous malformation. If headache is found to be associated with an AVM, treatment is considered only if the headache is severe and disabling. The development of hemorrhage, seizures, or progressive neurologic deficit, as was the case in two thirds of our patients with headache as a first symptom, strengthens the indication for therapy. Progressive neurologic deficit appears to develop slowly but intractably worsen. We favor early treatment of patients with this condition, even though therapy may fail in some of them.

Another problem inherent in this method is the variability in response to ionization by different individuals. We must operate at or below the one percentile range for necrosis for reasons previously expressed. Additionally, we recognize that these low doses lead us to provide ineffective therapy for those patients who are comparatively ionization resistant. Lowering the dose increases the possibility of failure. Patients are therefore advised that further treatment may be recommended 2 or more years after the first treatment. On balance, the results obtained in the first 709 patients encourage us to continue with this mode of therapy, emphasizing therapy for patients who are untreatable by other means.

Proton beam therapy appears to be associated with a low

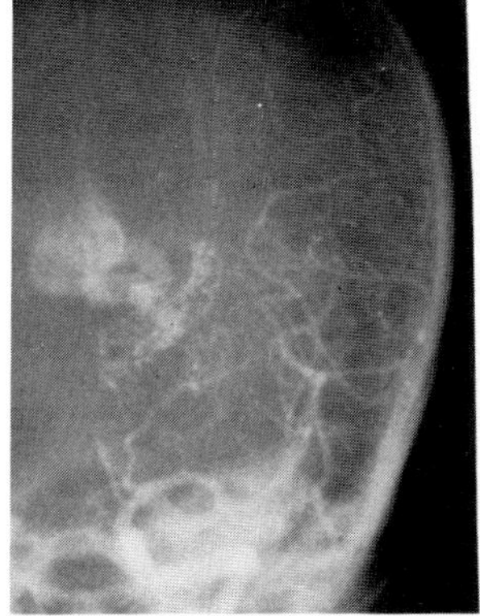
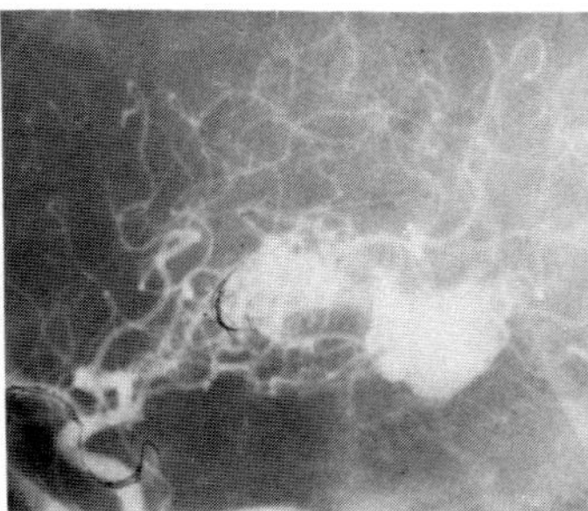
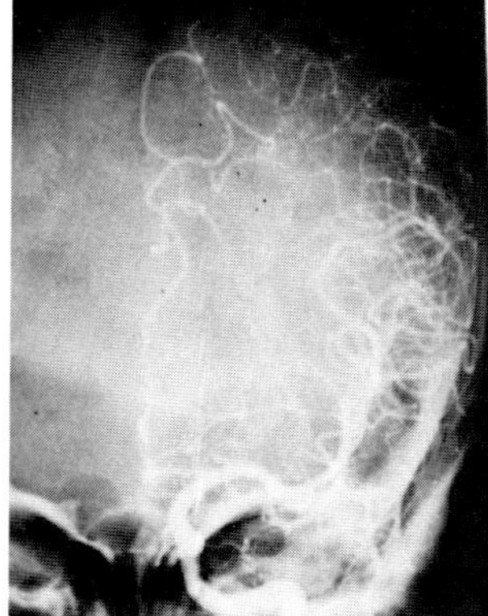
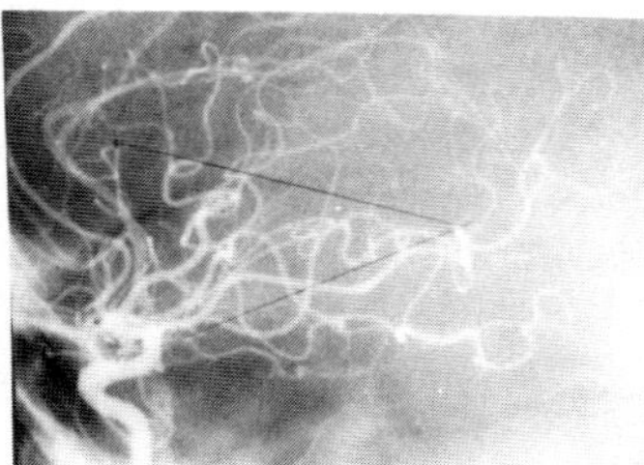

Fig. 81-4.   A 39-year-old woman had a left posterior thalamic AVM that bled and was left with a mild right hemiparesis and memory deficit. She bled a second time 3 years later. Her AVM was completely gone angiographically 1 year after proton beam therapy. At 6.3 years after treatment, digital subtraction angiograms reconfirmed the absence of the AVM. Her mild deficits continued.

risk. We have not observed procedure-related mortality, hemorrhages, sepsis, or thromboembolic events. Since revision of our first dosimetry technique, we have not seen any new procedure-induced persistent deficits in the past 20 years. Considering that injured brain might have a lower threshold for injury than normal brain,[12] we revised the dosimetry schedule to below the one percentile isoeffective-dose line for patients who had prior neurologic deficits. Only two complication have occurred since 1978. Thus, after accounting for early incubation period deaths (1.1 percent), subsequent stroke deficits, complications (currently 0.5 percent), and other untoward events, the remaining patients, over 90 percent of those treated, retain full vigor and function, which has been preserved into the 20 years of follow-up to date.

Table 81-2. Complications of proton beam treatment for AVMs

Patient Number	Severe Complications	Moderate Complications
1–12	4	0
13–73	0	4
74–709	0	2

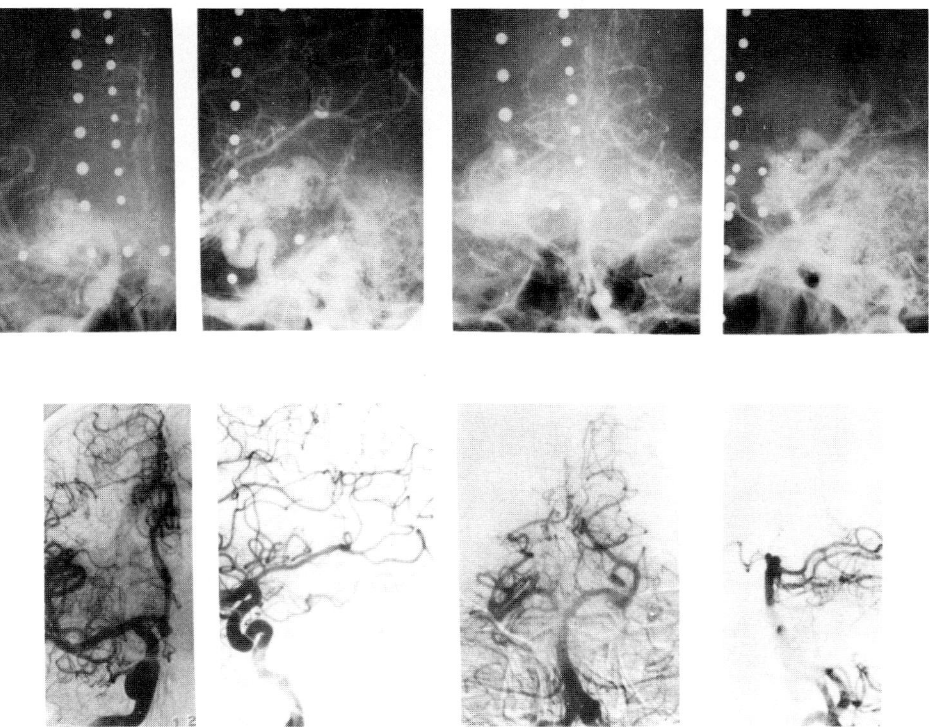

Fig. 81-5.   This 53-year-old surgeon had temporal lobe seizures for over 20 years. At 2.1 years after proton beam therapy, the AVM was completely gone and his seizures and behavior improved.

REFERENCES

1. Olivecrona H, Ladenheim J: Congenital Arteriovenous Aneurysms of the Carotid and Vertebral Arterial Systems. Berlin, Springer Verlag, 1957
2. Padget DH: The cranial venous system in man in reference to development. Adult configuration and relation to the arteries. Am J Anat 98:307, 1956
3. Russell DS, Rubenstein LJ: Pathology of Tumors of the Nervous System, ed 4. Baltimore, Williams & Wilkins, 1977, pp 116–145
4. Perret G, Nishioka H: Arteriovenous malformations. An analysis of 545 cases of craniocerebral arteriovenous malformations and fistulae reported to the cooperative study. J Neurosurg 25:467, 1966
5. Kjellberg RN: Isoeffective dose parameters for brain necrosis in relation to proton radiosurgical dosimetry, in Szikla G (ed): Stereotactic Cerebral Irradiations. Amsterdam, Elsevier, 1979, pp 157–166
6. Kjellberg RN: Radiobiology, dosimetry, and stereotactic technique for Bragg peak proton radiosurgical procedures. Proceedings of the First International Seminar on the Use of Proton Beams in Radiation Therapy, Moscow, 1977, vol 2. Moscow, Moskva AtomnzAat, 1979, pp 69–83
7. Hall EJ: Radiobiology for the Radiologist, ed 2. Hagerstown, Md, Harper and Row, 1958
8. Forster DMC, Steiner L, Hakanson S: Arteriovenous malformations of the brain. A long term clinical study. J Neurosurg 37:562, 1972
9. Paterson JH, McKissock W: Intracranial angiomas. A clinical study of intracranial angiomas with special reference to their mode of progression and surgical treatment: A report of 110 cases. Brain 79:233, 1956
10. Graf J, Perrett GE, Torner JC: Bleeding from cerebral arteriovenous malformation as part of their natural history. J Neurosurg 58:331, 1983
11. Troupp H, Marttila I, Halonen V: Arteriovenous malformations of the brain. Prognosis without operation. Acta Neurochir 22:125, 1970
12. Gilbert HA, Kagan AR (eds): Radiation Damage to the Nervous System: A Delayed Therapeutic Hazard. New York, Raven Press, 1980, pp 1, 36, 50, 183

CHAPTER 82

Surgical Treatment of Carotid Ophthalmic Aneurysms

Jafar J. Jafar   Robert M. Crowell   Roberto Heros

CAROTID OPHTHALMIC ANEURYSMS arise from the internal carotid artery just distal to the ophthalmic artery origin. They account for 5.4 percent of all intracranial aneurysms. A female preponderance has been observed.[1–3] The age of onset is the same as for other intracranial aneurysms. There is an unusual preponderance of multiple intracranial aneurysms in association with carotid ophthalmic aneurysms.

ANATOMY

The ophthalmic artery is the first branch of the internal carotid artery as it exits from the cavernous sinus in 90 percent of the cases. In 10 percent, the ophthalmic artery arises from the intracavernous portion of the internal carotid artery.[4] At this point, the internal carotid artery is inferolateral to the optic nerve just medial to the anterior clinoid process. The ophthalmic artery usually arises from the superior portion of the internal carotid artery and heads towards the optic canal beneath the optic nerve.

Carotid ophthalmic aneurysms may point: (1) medially beneath the optic nerve; (2) laterally beneath the anterior clinoid process; (3) superomedially above the optic nerve; or (4) within the cavernous sinus.

PRESENTATION

The most common initial symptom of an ophthalmic artery aneurysm is subarachnoid hemorrhage. Progressive decrease in visual acuity is the second most common symptom. Rarely do ophthalmic artery aneurysms produce seizures or pituitary or hypothalamic dysfunction. When the diagnosis of subarachnoid hemorrhage is suspected, the first step is to obtain a computed tomographic (CT) scan without and with contrast.[5] This test may establish the diagnosis by showing blood in the basal cisterns, the interhemispheric fissure, or within the brain tissue. In some cases, the aneurysm may be visualized with the infusion study. A magnetic resonance imaging study (MRI) may be helpful in showing giant aneurysms and in elucidating the anatomy (Figure 82-1). Lumbar puncture may be used to

Portions of this chapter have appeared in Ojemann RG, Crowell RM: Surgical Management of Cerebrovascular Disease. Baltimore, Williams & Wilkins, 1983.

diagnose subarachnoid hemorrhage if there is no evidence of a mass lesion and no blood is demonstrated on the CT scan.

All patients with subarachnoid hemorrhage should undergo screening tests for clotting function, including prothrombin time (PT), partial thromboplastin time (PTT), and platelet count. An electrocardiogram may show abnormalities related to subarachnoid hemorrhage. Complete blood counts, serum electrolytes, and osmolarity should be determined as baseline values.

Management is guided by the clinical status, cerebral blood flow, and CT findings. Symptomatic intracranial hematomas may require emergency surgical evacuation. Patients with symptomatic hydrocephalus may need emergency external ventricular drainage.

MEDICAL THERAPY

A standard medical regimen is instituted for stable patients without mass lesions.

1. Bed rest.
2. Fluid administration aimed at maintaining normovolemia; serum electrolytes are checked serially, as is serum osmolarity and intake and output.
3. Pulmonary support, which includes intubation and ventilation if needed.
4. Elastic stockings or pneumatic compression boots.
5. Epsilon-aminocaproic acid (Amicar, 36 g/day intravenously).
6. Anticonvulsants (diphenylhydantoin, 300 mg/day).
7. Stool softeners.
8. Blood pressure is controlled; trimethaphan camsylate or sodium nitroprusside may be used to lower elevated systolic blood pressure to about 150 torr (if drowsiness or neurologic deficits are absent).
9. Haloperidol (Haldol, 2 mg I.M. every 3–4 hours) may be given for agitation.
10. Dexamethasone (4 mg IV every 6 hours) if cerebral swelling is present.
11. Cimetidine (300 mg by mouth or IV every 6 hours) to decrease gastric acidity.

Metabolic studies and CT scan are re-checked on an emergency basis should the patient deteriorate. Electrolyte

OPERATIVE NEUROSURGICAL TECHNIQUES
ISBN 0-8089-1862-1

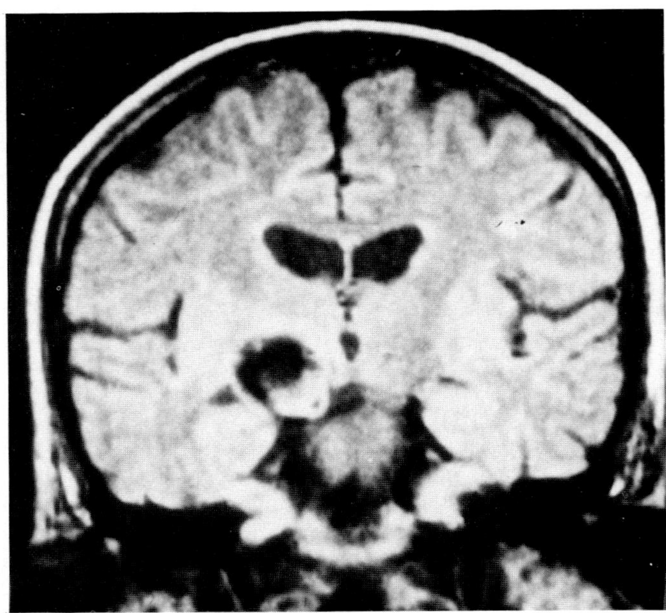

Fig. 82-1. A MRI scan revealing a giant right carotid-ophthalmic artery aneurysm.

imbalance may require correction. The CT scan may reveal hydrocephalus, focal cerebral ischemia, or edema. Progressive hydrocephalus requires an external ventricular drainage with subsequent ventriculoperitoneal shunting for relief of symptoms. Angiography is performed if a clear explanation for deterioration is not found.

All patients suffering from subarachnoid hemorrhage undergo xenon 133 cerebral blood flow studies (CBF). This test helps in the timing of surgery and in selection of patients for hyperperfusion therapy. Whenever significant spasm is demonstrated on angiograms, a cerebral blood flow study is repeated every 3 days until it becomes normal, when surgery is judged appropriate despite angiographic spasm.

In case the lesion points medially, a contralateral approach may be best. For this approach, a pre-fixed chiasm could obscure the lesion. The position of the chiasm can be assessed by reference to a negative image on CT scan when there is extensive basal hemorrhage, or by metrizamide cisternography.

ANGIOGRAPHY

If the patient is in good condition (Hunt grade I or II),[6] we proceed with immediate angiography. If a carotid-ophthalmic aneurysm is found with no evidence of spasm and normal CBF, we operate as soon as possible. When the patient is in poor condition (grade III or IV), if there is spasm on the angiogram, or if CBF is decreased, we wait 10 days to repeat the studies and reconsider surgery. When there have been two hemorrhages, we tend to operate early even if there is a minor deficit or minor spasm.

Transfemoral selective 4-vessel cerebral angiography is preferred. Studies should begin with the vessel that is suspected of harboring the bleeding lesion. If an ophthalmic artery aneurysm is disclosed, special views must be obtained for complete characterization of the sac, its neck, and the relationship to the internal carotid and ophthalmic arteries. Standard AP and lateral projections may require supplementary views, including base, oblique, or off-lateral projections. Subtraction views are often helpful in visualization of the ophthalmic artery. In case the aneurysm proves unapproachable and is best treated by an indirect procedure, views of the carotid bifurcation, external carotid, superficial temporal artery, and collateral circulation to the carotid territory will be required.

ANESTHESIA

The patient is premedicated with Decadron, 4 mg, triazolam, 2 mg IM, and glycopyrrolate, 0.2 mg IM at 6 AMthe day of surgery. In the induction room, an intravenous route is established. A catheter is inserted into the radial artery for continuous monitoring of arterial pressure. Such monitoring is particularly important during induction, when wide swings of arterial pressure can occur. The placement of a central venous pressure catheter is deferred until the patient is under anesthesia. In patients who do not have a suitable vein, the internal jugular or subclavian vein is catheterized. Pressors and antihypertensive agents are available for infusions; phenylephrine (Neosynephrine, 10 mg in 250 ml of 5-perent dextrose in water) and sodium nitroprusside (50 mg in 250 ml of dextrose in water shielded with foil) serve well for these needs.

INDUCTION

Once all preparations are complete, a slow induction is carried out with preparation of over 10 minutes or more before induction. Sodium thiopental (3 mg/kg) is given intravenously after an initial preoxygenation. Once the patient is deeply drowsy, a mask is applied and the patient breathes a mixture of nitrous oxide and oyxgen. Then isoflurane is given through the mask, and ventilation is controlled. Before intubation, a muscle relaxant (pancuronium, 0.1 mg/kg) is given intravenously. A twitch monitor is applied to the ulnar nerve in order to monitor the completeness of neuromuscular blockade. An additional increment of sodium thiopental is given intravenously just before intratracheal intubation. Lidocaine (1 mg/kg) is given intravenously 1 minute before intubation. Ideally, the blood pressure is in the range of 100 torr systolic at this point.

When the patient is stable and well anesthetized, laryngoscopy is executed with gentle endotracheal intubation. In case of a sustained rise of blood pressure, further increments of sodium thiopental are given intravenously, and the concentration of isoflurane may be increased temporarily. Controlled ventilation is maintained with an arterial PCO_2 in the range of 34, as demonstrated by frequently sampled arterial blood gases. The arterial blood gases likewise provide a frequent check on the adequacy of oxygenation.

REDUCTION OF BRAIN TENSION

All patients are given 100 g of mannitol intravenously while the bone flap is being turned. This usually gives excellent relaxation of the brain. Dexamethasone (4 mg IV) is continued every 4 hours. For giant lesions, a spinal subarachnoid catheter can be used to withdraw cerebral spinal fluid (CSF).

CONTROLLED HYPOTENSION

Careful communication between the neuroanesthesiologist and the surgeon is crucial to control of hypotension.[7] For pharmacologic control of blood pressure during surgery, the dialogue is of particular importance. Induced hypotension is used to slacken the aneurysm during dissection in order to decrease the likelihood of intraoperative rupture. In most patients, the blood pressure is maintained at about 100 torr during the initial exposure. Once the aneurysm is in view, the pressure is dropped further, to about 90 torr systolic. During critical dissection of the neck of the aneurysm, deep hypotension rarely may be required (systolic blood pressure of 60 torr or a mean arterial blood pressure of about 40 torr).

Most patients tolerate this brief type of hypotension without postoperative sequelae. In the normal brain, autoregulation maintains local CBF down to mean arterial blood pressures of about 40 to 45 torr. In patients with subarachnoid hemorrhage, however, autoregulation may be lost in some zones. Moreover, in some elderly patients and in those with ischemic heart disease, prolonged and deep hypotension may not be well tolerated by the brain, heart, or kidneys.

Several techniques of controlled hypotension are available. Moderate hypotension can be achieved simply by increasing the concentration of inspired isoflurane in many cases. In most cases, an additional agent, such as sodium nitroprusside, will be required to further diminish the blood pressure. Trimethaphan camsylate also may be used for this purpose.

We recently have obviated the need for deep hypotension in most cases by utilizing temporary clips under mannitol protection as described by Suzuki.[8] For giant carotid-ophthalmic aneurysms, proximal control requires exposure of the internal carotid artery in the neck.

VASOSPASM

Care should be taken not to lower the blood pressure in patients with vasospasm, either suspected or proven by angiography. Once the aneurysm is obliterated, cerebral perfusion is maximized by volume expansion with colloid and packed cells if necessary. In cases in which vasospasm is noted or suspected, the patient is placed on a mannitol regimen, 100 g intravenously every 8 hours.[9] Blood pressure is elevated to about 160 torr systolic by use of a pressor if necessary.

EXTUBATION

Toward the conclusion of the procedure, the anesthetic is managed in such a fashion that the muscle relaxant will have worn off, and the patient can be extubated and awakened in the operating theater. This approach, which is guided by twitch monitoring, permits early assessment of neurologic function postoperatively.

OPERATIVE TECHNIQUE

POSITIONING AND PREPARATION

The approach in most instances is ipsilateral to the carotid-ophthalmic artery aneurysm. Occasionally, for a lesion that points medially or inferiorly from the internal carotid artery, a contralateral craniotomy will provide the best visualization of the sac and its neck. In the case of bilateral ophthalmic aneurysms, careful selection of the most appropriate site for craniotomy may permit direct attack on both lesions from one side.

After the induction of anesthesia, the patient is positioned supine with the head slightly elevated. For most cases, the head is turned about 45 degrees, the zygoma uppermost and the vertex depressed slightly below the horizontal plane. In patients with limited mobility of the neck, a small roll is placed under the shoulder. The Mayfield-Kees three-point clamp is then applied after the scalp sites are prepared with an antibiotic solution. Additional increments of sodium thiopental (50 mg IV) are given just before this painful stimulation. Protective plastic shields are placed across the eyes. The proposed incision site is shaved and sterile towels are draped to wall off the area. Either elastic bandages or pneumatic compression boots are used on the lower extremities to help prevent thrombophlebitis. The scrub nurse stands on the surgeon's right side (for a right-handed surgeon) with the instrument table over the patient's chest and abdomen.

INCISION

In most cases, an incision just behind the hairline is preferred, proceeding from the widow's peak in a curvilinear fashion to a point just above the zygoma in front of the tragus. The superficial temporal artery is palpated and marked. The incision should lie posterior to the root of the superficial temporal artery in order to preserve the structure with the flap. Occasionally in bald individuals or in cases in which additional exposure is desired for another aneurysm, an alternative incision may be planned, utilizing a wrinkle high in the forehead or a coronal incision extending across the midline.

Both the surgeon and the assistant use magnifying loupes and headlights during the initial stages of the procedure. Local anesthesia (lidocaine, 1 percent with 1/400,000 epinephrine) is injected along the incision except near the superficial temporal artery. The incision is begun anteriorly and cuts to but not through the periosteum. Care is taken to avoid injury to the superficial temporal artery, particularly near its root. The posterior branch of this artery is dissected free and divided between 3-0 silk ligatures, thus permitting the trunk and frontal branch of the vessel, which might be needed for later cerebral revascularization, to be reflected forward with the soft tissue flap.

Hemostasis is obtained by applying hemostatic clips to both margins of the skin incision. Next, the temporalis fascia is incised with a knife and the temporalis muscle is opened with the cutting cautery. A branch of the deep temporal artery is regularly encountered within the muscle, and this must be cauterized accurately in order to avoid troublesome bleeding later. The periosteum is swept off the skull with a periosteal elevator just to the edge of the orbit, and the muscle is reflected from the skull, including the superior temporal line, with the cutting cautery, until the zygomatic process of the frontal bone is approached. The soft tissue flap is folded over a sponge to prevent ischemic compression, protected with a Bacitracin-soaked sponge, and held in place with silk sutures placed into the muscle and attached by rubber bands to the drapes.

A final maneuver that permits maximal visualization beneath the muscle is the application of Cushing retractors to the muscle along the zygomatic process of the frontal bone, with tension applied to these retractors by rubber bands and Allis clamps attached to the drapes. This approach provides excellent exposure once the bone flap is removed.

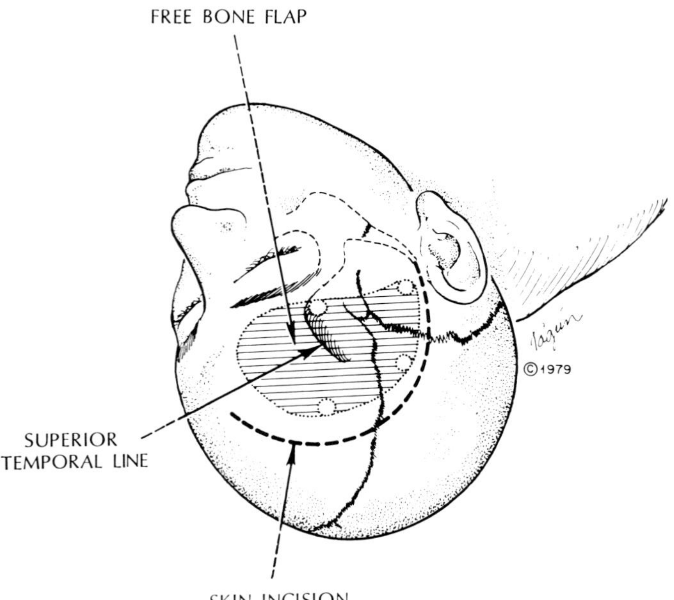

Fig. 82-2. Exposure of the lesion via a pterional craniotomy. An incision behind the hairline permits a small frontotemporal craniotomy. The frontal lobe then is gently elevated.

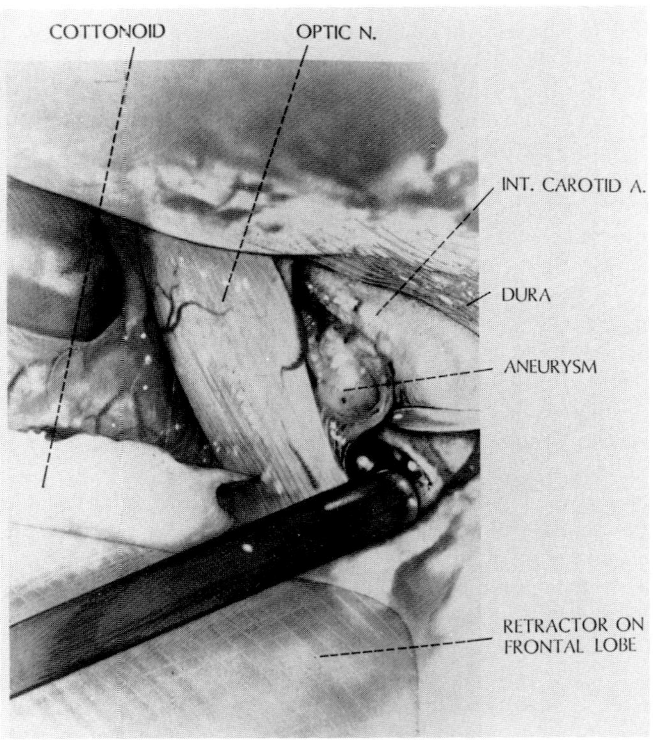

Fig. 82-3. Approach to carotid-ophthalmic aneurysm. A right pterional craniotomy offers exposure of this aneurysm of the right side. Dissection has established distal control of the internal carotid artery. The optic nerve and the anterior clinoid process hide the proximal neck of the lesion.

INITIAL EXPOSURE

A pterional (frontotemporal) craniotomy permits satisfactory exposure of carotid-ophthalmic artery aneurysms (Figure 82-2).[10,11] A free pterional bone flap is turned with the power drill and craniotome. The initial burr hole is placed just behind the zygomatic process of the frontal bone and below the end of the superior temporal line. Additional burr holes are placed in the low temporal and posterior frontal regions. The unsightly depression of an inferomedial frontal burr hole can be eliminated by the use of a curved bony cut with the craniotome. The dura is separated from the inner table of the skull with a No. 3 Penfield. The craniotome cut is begun along the floor of the anterior fossa, proceeding medially about 3 to 4 cm, and then curving in an easy arch posterior to the high temporal burr hole. It is good to angle this soft curve slightly, beveling outward to provide a nice seating for the bone flap when it is replaced. Another saw cut with the craniotome is made between the superior and inferior temporal burr holes. Finally, the keyhole and the inferior temporal burr hole are connected using ronguers. A portion of the lateral sphenoid ridge is preserved with the bone flap, which is finally broken off by means of prying it with a periosteal elevator. The bone flap is carefully peeled off the dura, and the middle meningeal artery is then identified, coagulated, and cut. Bony edges are waxed for hemostasis. Additional bone is ronguered from the lateral sphenoid ridge. Care is taken at this point to avoid injury to structures in the superior orbital fissure. Frequently, a small arterial branch to the dura in this region must be coagulated. These maneuvers effectively level the sphenoid ridge between the frontal and temporal bones, thus creating an unobstructed access to the anterior clinoid area.

In some cases, the inner table of bone that forms the floor of the anterior fossa over the orbit will be characterized by mountainous irregularities, impeding the view. In such cases, a high-speed drill can be used to smooth the area. If a small opening into the orbit occurs, it is closed with wax and Gelfoam. If additional access is needed along the floor of the anterior fossa behind the orbit, the inner table of bone at the edge of the craniotomy just anterior to the keyhole also can be removed with a rongeur without compromising the cosmetic appearance of the outer table.

In some cases, a very prominent and lateral frontal sinus may be encountered with the saw cut or bony removal. If this occurs, the mucosa should be removed, the sinus packed with Bacitracin-soaked Gelfoam, and the opening covered with a small flap of pericranium dissected from the back of the scalp and stitched to the adjacent dura. Next, a fine drill point is used to create burr holes for wires to hold the flap in place at the time of closure. Dura-to-pericranial sutures of 4-0 Neurolon are placed around the periphery of the bony opening in order to achieve epidural hemostasis. Tiny strips of Surgicel are inserted into the epidural space as needed. Bacitracin-soaked sponges are placed over the skin edge and over all exposed tissue except the dura.

During this stage, the surgeon can regularly determine whether the brain is slack. If this is not the case, measures must be taken to obtain adequate slackness. The PCO_2 may need adjustment, additional dehydration may be required, or CSF may need to be drained. Occasionally, ventricular puncture will be needed to obtain a slack brain.

A linear dural incision is made approximately 6 to 8 mm above the inferior margin of the bony opening, with inferior turning at the frontal and temporal corners. The inferior dural flap is tacked up over the bone edge, avoiding a buckle at the center of the flap, which could interfere with intradural visualization.

At this point, the Greenberg retractor posts are attached to the three-point headrest and the Greenberg retractor is mounted. Under loupe magnification, a medium-width, hand-

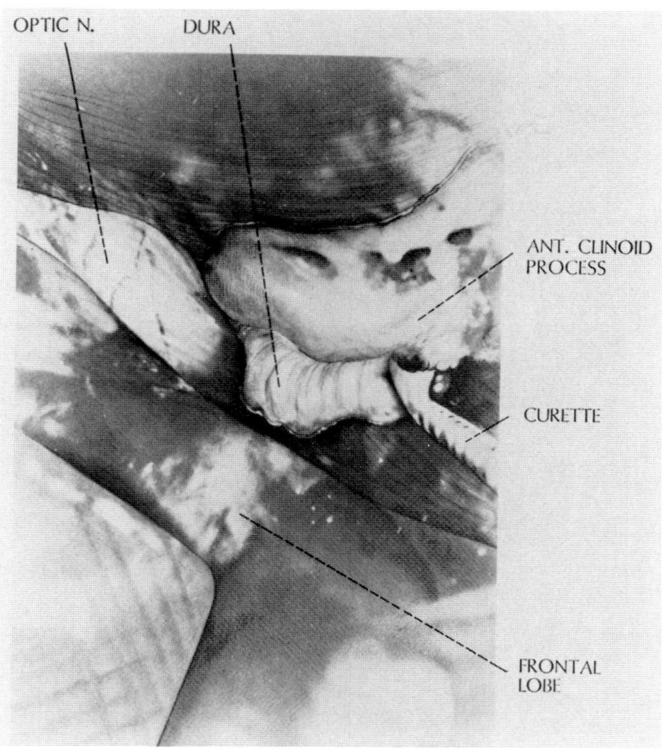

Fig. 82-4. Exposing the anterior clinoid process. After incision of the dura, a microcurette is used to dissect the dural flap off the clinoid process.

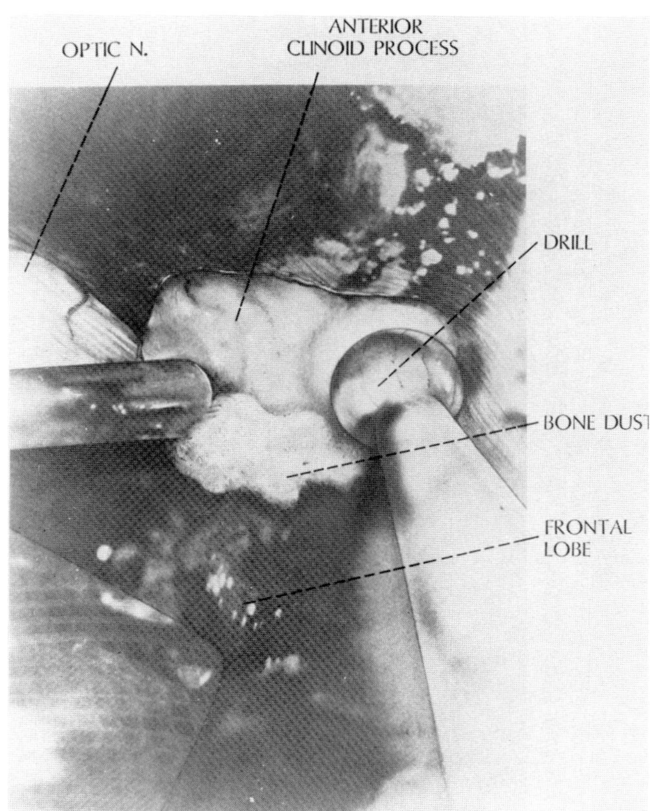

Fig. 82-5. Removal of the anterior clinoid process. A high-speed drill weakens the clinoid process medially and laterally (as shown). The resulting fragment of bone is dissected free of soft tissue and removed.

held brain retractor is used to gently elevate the frontal lobe. A sucker on a cottonoid can be used to gradually remove any CSF that may appear inferior to the frontal lobe. The retractor is slowly advanced just in front of the edge of the sphenoid wing.

The olfactory tract, an important landmark, will come into view, and following this a few millimeters posteriorly will lead the surgeon to the optic nerve. Since the frontal lobe may be adherent to the aneurysm, no efforts should be made to expose the internal carotid artery at this stage. Time should be spent allowing further CSF to drain. It is most important that the brain be so slack that only mild retraction is needed for adequate exposure.

Next, a protective layer of Telfa, pre-cut to the proper shape, is placed like a rug over the exposed frontal lobe down to the olfactory tract. At this point, the Greenberg self-retaining retractor system holding a posted retractor blade bent to about 60 degrees is placed to elevate the frontal lobe. The retractor should take a low profile so as to give easy access to the infrafrontal cleft.

Next, a narrow hand-held retractor is used to carefully elevate the temporal lobe. Temporal-tip bridging veins are coagulated and divided. Once the temporal tip is free, a covering of Telfa is placed and the lobe held posteriorly with a slender retractor blade fixed on the Greenberg apparatus. The two retractor blades should be separated by only several millimeters at right angles to each other.

Up to this point, the combination of loupe magnification and headlight illumination has been used for maximal mobility with adequate visualization. From this point, however, the operating microscope is used to maximize illumination and visualization of critical structures.

MICROSURGICAL DISSECTION

We use the Wild microscope with a 300-mm objective lens, 12.5× eye pieces, and variable-angle binocular tubes for microsurgical dissection. The visual image is channeled by a 50:50 small beam splitter to an observer tube on one side and a unified adapter for video and intermittent film photography on the other side. A clear video image projected on a monitor in a corner of the operating theater provides involvement in the microsurgical action for all members of the microsurgical team, including the scrub nurse and anesthesiologist.

Under microsurgical vision, the frontal lobe is gently elevated in order to expose the internal carotid artery and the anterior clinoid process (Figure 82-3). In some cases, the aneurysm may need gentle dissection from the frontal lobe. Controlled hypotension is appropriate in these circumstances. In many cases, the surgical sequence involves removal of the anterior clinoid process to facilitate dissection and clipping of the aneurysm.

REMOVAL OF THE CLINOID PROCESS

In order to remove the anterior clinoid process, the overlying dura must be removed (Figure 82-4).[11,12] A coated Penfield No. 4 dissector and monopolar electrocautery at low current are used to coagulate a semicircular path over the clinoid process medially to laterally. Great care must be exercised to avoid injury to the optic nerve, which may lie under the dura uncovered by bone in this area. Lateral coagulation must be terminated at the edge of the cavernous sinus. The resulting flap of dura is incised with a No. 15 knife blade. The resulting flap of

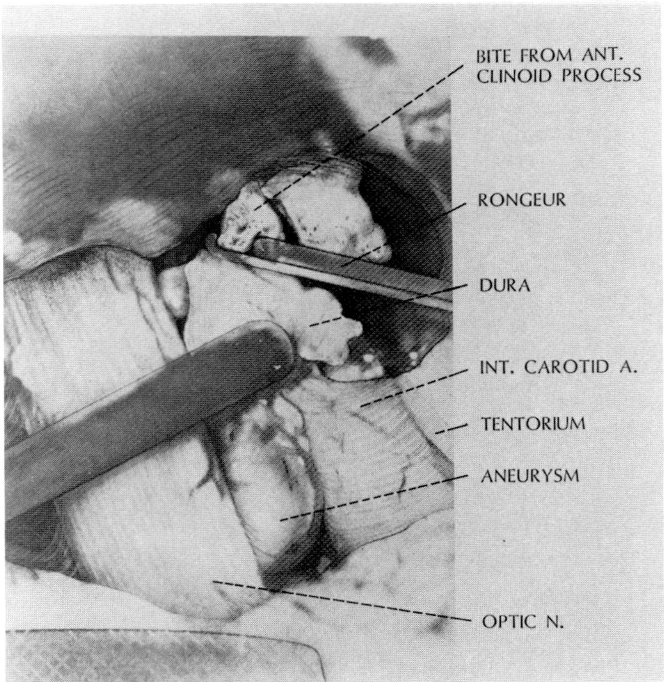

Fig. 82-6.   Ronguering of additional bone. A microantrostomy punch is used to gain additional access to the proximal internal carotid artery.

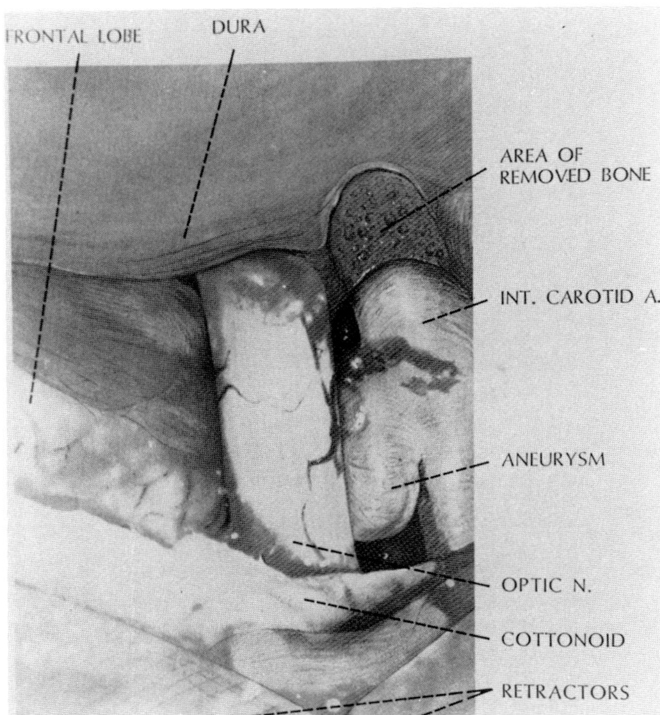

Fig. 82-7.   Exposing the proximal neck of the aneurysm. With the anterior clinoid process removed, the proximal internal carotid artery and the neck of the aneurysm can be freed. The ophthalmic artery (not seen) lies just proximal and medial to the neck of the aneurysm in this case.

dura may be conveniently elevated with a fine angled microcurette. This flap of dura lies over the internal carotid artery, thus protecting it during subsequent drilling.

The anterior clinoid process next is removed with a high-speed drill with an angled handpiece and a diamond burr (Figure 8-25). The surgeon can conveniently control this instrument with the right hand, resting the wrist firmly while a fine stream of irrigation is directed onto the drill point from a microirrigator held by the assistant (12 ml syringe with a 22-gauge plastic catheter).

The clinoid process can be isolated by drilling its medial and lateral bony supports. Usually one drill spot accurately placed on either side of the process will achieve this goal. Once underlying soft tissue is encountered, drilling is redirected slightly superiorly or inferiorly until each buttress—lateral and medial—is weakened. Then a 5-0 straight bone curette is used to gradually fracture and mobilize the resulting anterior clinoid fragment. This is accomplished with utmost care and control in order to avoid abrupt movement of the fragment and possible injury to nearby structures. The 5-0 curette and microcurettes are used to dissect the fragment free from underlying soft tissue. If the bony exposure seems inadequate, additional drilling can be used to widen the field of view. A fine microantrostomy punch can be used for additional bony removal, if space permits (Figure 82-6).

It should be noted that paranasal sinus mucosa may in some cases extend into bone in this area. If mucosa is encountered, the overlying bone opening must be gently waxed. If bleeding from soft tissue occurs, tiny amounts of Surgicel and Gelfoam can be used for hemostasis.

DISSECTION OF THE ANEURYSM

Once the anterior clinoid process is removed, the protective function of the small dural flap no longer applies and it is removed. The surgeon next obtains proximal and distal control

of the internal carotid artery (Figure 82-7). In many cases, the distal control is straightforward. The posterior communicating artery and anterior choroidal artery provide a distal boundary for dissection. Proximal control usually is a greater challenge. At this point in the procedure, because of the threat of rupture of the aneurysm, the blood pressure is lowered to about 90 torr systolic. This level of hypotension is well tolerated for up to 1 hour by most patients. The internal carotid artery is freed proximal to the aneurysm. Often a microdissector serves nicely for this dissection. Dense arachnoid bands can be electrocoagulated with the bipolar cautery and cut sharply. Dura may be opened laterally with cauterization and sharp dissection, with the cavernous sinus as the end point. Every effort should be made to visualize and spare the ophthalmic artery, which usually arises from the internal carotid artery just proximal to the neck of the aneurysm. If the ophthalmic artery is not seen, the proximal neck of the aneurysm must be completely dissected and visualized before application of the clip in the area.

In many cases in which the lesion projects superiorly, gentle deflection of the lesion posteriorly with the sucker will permit passage of a fine dissector proximal to the neck and medially as far as the optic nerve or beneath it. Gentle lateral deflection of the aneurysm may permit dissection of the medial aspect of the aneurysm from the optic nerve. Lesions that point medially beneath the optic nerve will require gentle deflection of the nerve medially and superiorly in order to isolate the aneurysm neck.

Only occasionally, when preoperative studies suggest difficulty in obtaining proximal control (e.g., giant aneurysm), do we expose the internal carotid artery for extracranial control.

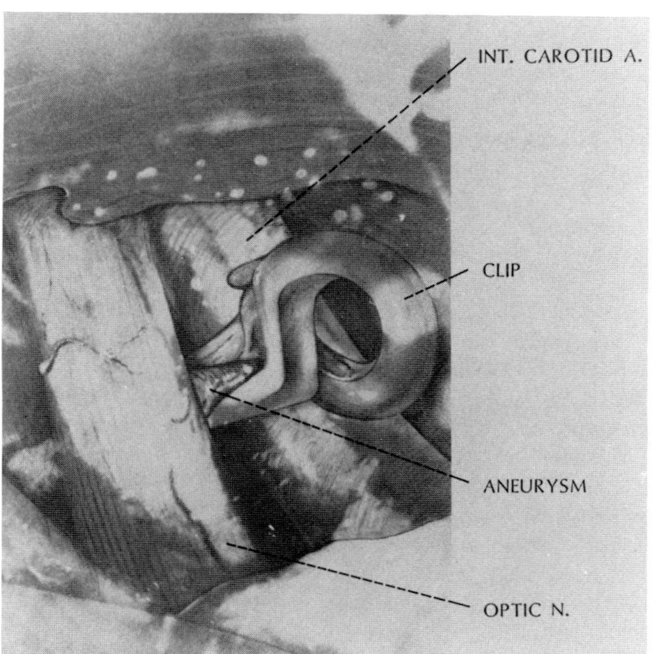

Fig. 82-8. Clipping of the aneurysm. A narrow-bladed clip is placed across the neck of the aneurysm and flush with the internal carotid artery. The origin of the ophthalmic artery is just lateral to the tips of the clip.

OBLITERATION OF THE ANEURYSM

Once the neck of the aneurysm is completely freed and the ophthalmic artery separated from it, obliteration of the aneurysm can be carried out (Figure 82-8). This can be accomplished in many cases without substantial manipulation of the sac or neck, and thus moderate hypotension (systolic pressure around 80-90 torr) provides adequate reduction of tension in the lesion. Occasionally, a particularly thin-walled lesion or one requiring substantial manipulation for clipping presents a greater danger of rupture; in these circumstances, 100 g of mannitol is given intravenously 15 minutes before the application of temporary clips proximal and distal to the aneurysm. At the same time, the systolic blood pressure is elevated to the 160–170 torr level in order to enhance collateral circulation. This usually will give about 45 minutes of time in which to dissect the aneurysm and apply a permanent clip.

Various types of clips can be used to obliterate the aneurysm. The blade length is chosen to provide just enough length to fully cross the neck. Often the available space between the internal carotid artery, the bony skull, and the optic nerve dictates use of the narrowest blade available. Frequently this feature favors a Yasargil or, more commonly, a Sugita clip, because of their narrow blades; the Sugita clip is preferred because it has a wider aperture when fully opened. The shape of the clip generally is either straight or slightly curved, with the concave aspect of the curve applied smoothly to the conforming aspect of the internal carotid artery. The angle of application generally is lateral to medial. Occasionally, a right-angled fenestrated Sugita clip may be required to obliterate the aneurysm. A Sano variable angle clip applier is very useful in tailoring the clip application.

In most cases, the sac is deflected distally with a fine sucker in order to visualize the neck and ophthalmic artery during application of the clip. The tips of the clip are held just wide enough to encompass the neck, and are advanced slowly with a slightly axial rotational movement to minimize friction against the lesion. Once the clip is seen to project just beyond the neck, the blades are slowly closed, with constant observation of resulting effects on the aneurysm and adjacent structures. The applicator is maintained on the clip hub, and if adverse effects are evident (incomplete neck obliteration, encroachment of the optic nerve or ophthalmic artery), the clip is satisfactorily repositioned or removed. If the clip position seems adequate, the hub of the clip is released and the applicator removed. Occasionally this may prove difficult with the Yasargil clip, because these clips can be hard to release. It is worth testing release outside the wound before clip application.

If difficulty is encountered after clip application, the clip applicator can be opened widely by placing the third and fourth fingers within the handle of the applicator and gently forcing the two handles away from each other. No such problem is encountered with the use of the Sano clip applier. Once the clip is in place and released, the adequacy of clipping should be carefully checked. By deflecting the aneurysm dome slightly, the complete obliteration of the neck with the tips of the clip extending beyond can be confirmed. Furthermore, the internal carotid artery and ophthalmic artery must be free of deformation or kinking, and the optic nerve should not be excessively deformed. Minor contact between the clip and the nerve is common. When significant displacement of the nerve is caused by the clip, further dissection of the nerve and even the chiasm may permit a gentle sloping displacement with limited infringement on the nerve. Reapplication of the clip in some cases may be necessary in order to avoid unsatisfactory deformation of the optic nerve.

For some aneurysms with broad necks, electrocoagulation can narrow the neck and set the stage for clipping (Figure 82-9). For this maneuver, the bipolar cautery is set at low current, and the blades of the cautery forceps are positioned fully across the neck of the lesion. Low current is applied and the forceps tips are gently squeezed and released repeatedly. Continuous irrigation is applied during this maneuver. The process is continued until the neck gradually shrinks, becoming whiter and thicker. If the bipolar cautery tips are only partially across the neck, perforation of the aneurysm is possible.

Cauterization may thicken a reddened aneurysmal neck. In situations in which application of the forceps tips requires hazardous manipulation of the aneurysm, a brief burst of hypotension may slacken the lesion and diminish the hazard.

For other aneurysms with broad necks, a ligature may safely obliterate the lesion or set the stage for clipping. A fine ligature passer can facilitate positioning of a 3-0 silk ligature. Alternatively, the ligature can be placed with forceps anterior to the lesion, and then the suture retrieved medially to the lesion with gentle deflection of the aneurysm. This latter method may minimize manipulation of the aneurysm during ligature placement. A surgeon's knot is placed and gradually tightened with two hemostats, the tips of which are applied to the suture within 1 to 2 mm of the knot in order to avoid unwanted torque on the neck. Sometimes the knot can be tied down firmly, obliterating the neck. More commonly, the ligature narrows the neck of the aneurysm and sets the stage for clipping.

Unusual situations occasionally are encountered. A Sundt clip-graft might be helpful, possibly with a window for the ophthalmic artery. In other instances, a right-angled fenestrated Sugita clip may be required, allowing the carotid artery to pass through the aperture and obliterating the neck of the aneurysm

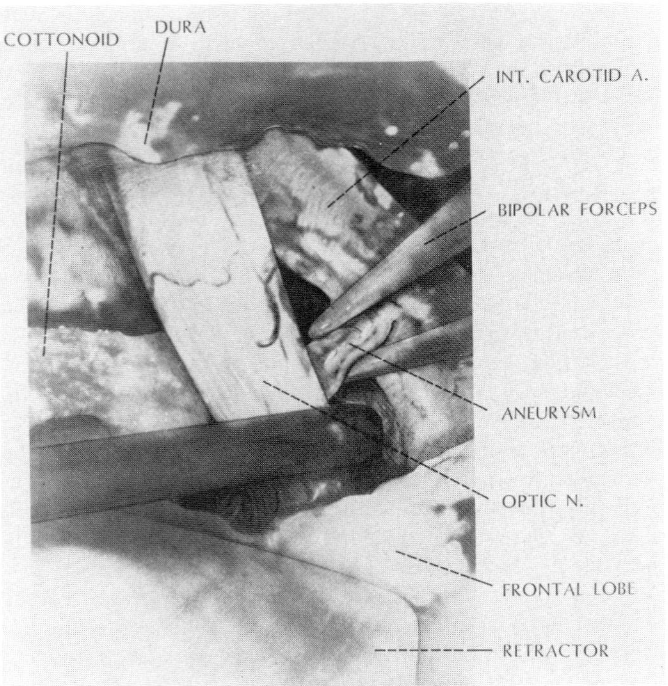

Fig. 82-9. Preparation of the neck of the aneurysm. Bipolar cautery is applied to the neck of the aneurysm to strengthen and shrink it. Forceps tips cross the neck completely and avoid the nearby ophthalmic artery. Low current is utilized to avoid spasm to native arteries.

(Figure 82-1). Sometimes, when obliteration cannot be achieved safely, the lesion can be reinforced with muslin.

Another maneuver that is occasionally of help in large aneurysms is puncturing the aneurysm with a 20-gauge butterfly needle connected to the suction system. This will allow collapse of the aneurysm and facilitate its clipping.

When multiple aneurysms are present, consideration must be given to the accessibility of the remaining lesion(s) once the initial clip is placed. It is best to clip the bleeding lesion first, but accessibility must be considered. Often, the lesion positioned deepest in the field is dealt with first, thus retaining visualization of the more superficial lesion(s). Features of the clip employed, including size, angle, and route of application, will influence the accessibility of secondary aneurysms. In general, the smallest possible clip is used, in order to conserve precious space in a narrow field.

In the special case of bilateral ophthalmic aneurysms, the contralateral lesion is dealt with first, in order to permit satisfactory access to both lesions. It is difficult and hazardous to drill the anterior clinoid process with a carotid aneurysm clip nearby, but on occasion we have done this successfully.

CLIPPING OF CONTRALATERAL OPHTHALMIC ANEURYSMS

Occasionally, an ophthalmic aneurysm can be treated through a contralateral frontotemporal craniotomy (Figure 82-10).[3] This approach may suggest itself in the case of bilateral ophthalmic aneurysms, or when the aneurysm projects inferiorly or medially. In the exposure of the contralateral lesion, the retraction will be deep. Removal of CSF by a subarachnoid

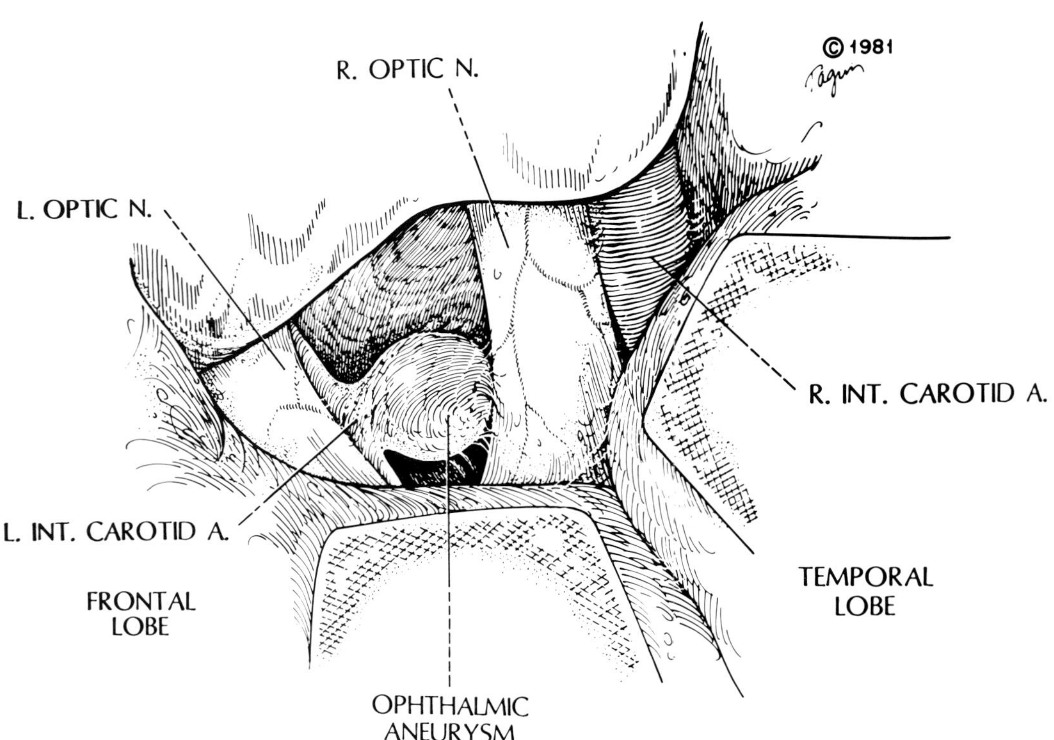

Fig. 82-10. Exposing a contralateral carotid-ophthalmic aneurysm. Through a right pterional craniotomy, a left carotid-ophthalmic aneurysm, which points medially, has been exposed. In this case, an aneurysm of the right internal carotid-posterior communicating artery was clipped after the left carotid-ophthalmic lesion was obliterated.

catheter can be useful in this circumstance. Extra care must be taken to avoid tearing of one or both olfactory tracts at the cribriform plate. As the frontal lobes are elevated, the arachnoid attachments to the optic nerves and chiasm are severed sharply. The contralateral proximal internal carotid artery comes into view inferior to the optic nerve. In this area, the contralateral ophthalmic artery aneurysm may be visualized projecting inferiorly and medially from its origin. The neck is freed and the ophthalmic artery is preserved. A straight clip just long enough to do the job obliterates the neck.

Occasionally, the bony tuberculum sella will have to be removed in order to expose the proximal aneurysmal neck. Coagulation and reflection of the dura for this task will permit drilling of the obstructing bony prominence. Usually, only a small amount of bone has to be removed. Care must be taken to avoid entry into the sphenoid sinus; careful obliteration of the opening is carried out with bone wax if such should occur.

SUPERIOR HYPOPHYSEAL ANEURYSMS

We have encountered 5 patients with aneurysms arising at the origin of the superior hypophyseal artery who had subarachnoid hemorrhage. Angiographically, these aneuryms superficially mimicked posterior communicating artery aneurysms (Figure 82-11). On close scrutiny of the angiogram, however, the origin was discovered to be near the anterior clinoid process. At surgery, they were all found to arise from the carotid artery proximal to the posterior communicating artery and directed posteromedially beneath the optic nerve. The operative technique involved is similar to that for carotid-ophthalmic artery aneurysms. The angled-aperture Sugita clips were ideal in all five of our cases. In all these cases, obtaining proximal control also necessitated drilling of the anterior clinoid.

CLOSURE

After satisfactory clipping of the aneurysm, the blood pressure is gradually returned to the normal level for that patient, generally in the range of 125 torr systolic. The area of the aneurysm is carefully observed under the operating microscope for signs of bleeding. In the rare instance of inadequate hemostasis in the area of the aneurysm, adjustment of the clip may be necessary in order to achieve the required hemostasis. When the field is dry, the retractors are removed and strips of Surgicel are placed over the areas of retraction. The dura is closed and tented to the bone flap. The bone flap is wired in place with 28-gauge stainless steel wires. Appropriate closure of the soft tissue then is done.

INDIRECT OPERATION

Some lesions cannot be effectively obliterated by direct attack. These can be predicted from the angiogram if the lesion projects below the level of the ophthalmic artery into the cavernous sinus. In some cases, this circumstance can be ascertained only at the time of surgery. For such aneurysms, the safest approach may be cervical carotid occlusion. Formerly, common carotid occlusion with a gradual occluding clamp was the procedure of choice. Recent reports indicate that the safest approach may be internal carotid occlusion with or without cerebral revascularization. Studies of cerebral blood flow may be helpful in determining the need for an STA-MCA bypass.[13] At the present

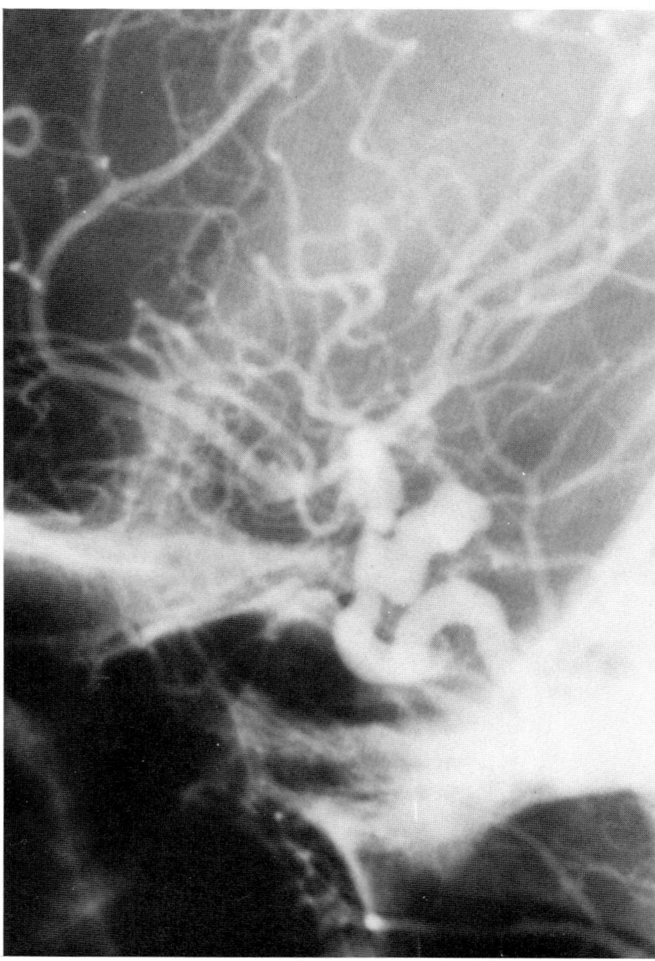

Fig. 82-11. A superior hypophyseal artery aneurysm. Note its origin under the anterior clinoid process and its posteromedial direction.

time, we achieve internal carotid artery occlusion with the transfemoral detachable balloon technique. We perform the balloon occlusion under cerebral blood flow control in the angiography suite. After balloon occlusion of the cervical internal carotid artery, the patient is heparinized for 3 days.

POSTOPERATIVE MANAGEMENT

The patient is treated prophylactically against vasospasm at the conclusion of the procedure. The central venous pressure is brought to 10 cm of water with colloid if there is no cardiac contraindication. The blood pressure is maintained in the range of 120 to 140 torr with volume and pressors as required. Medications include Decadron (4 mg q6h IV), which is tapered after 3 days, an antacid, and Dilantin (300 mg/day). The use of elastic stockings or pneumatic compression boots is continued.

In the event of neurologic deterioration, an immediate CT scan is performed in order to look for an intracranial hematoma, hydrocephalus, or cerebral edema. Appropriate treatment is instituted if one of these conditions is found. An angiogram is performed if the CT fails to disclose an adequate explanation for the deterioration. If a vascular occlusion by the clip is disclosed, adjustment of the clip might be indicated. More commonly, cerebral vasospasm may be demonstrated. If significant vasospasm is seen, additional treatment is indicated. The cen-

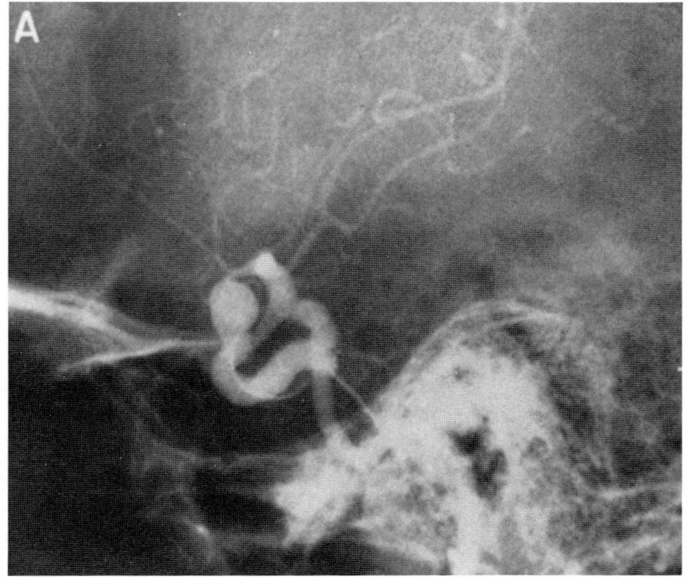

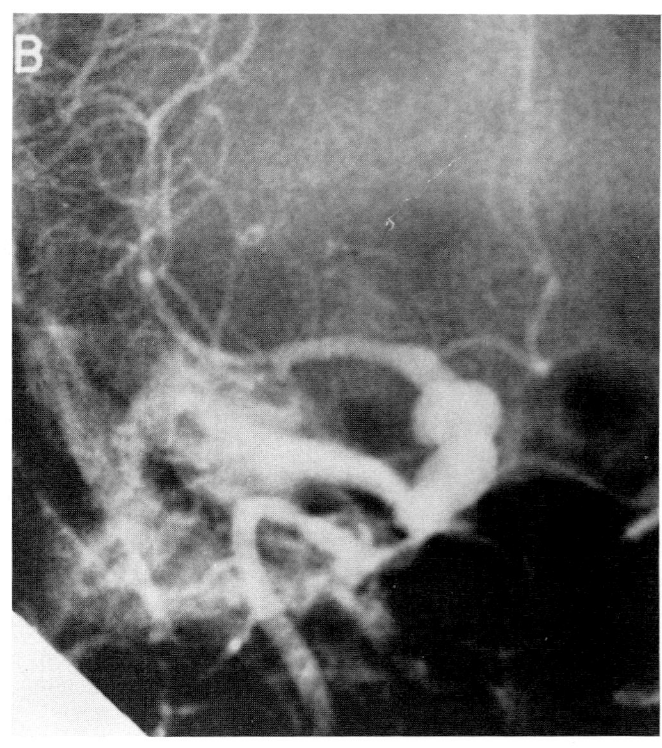

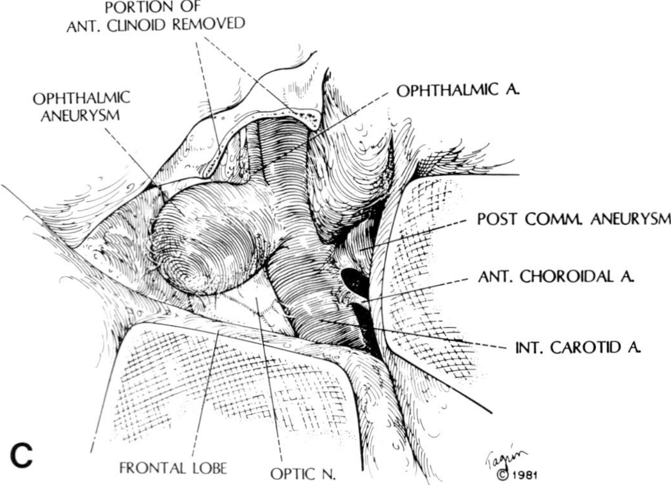

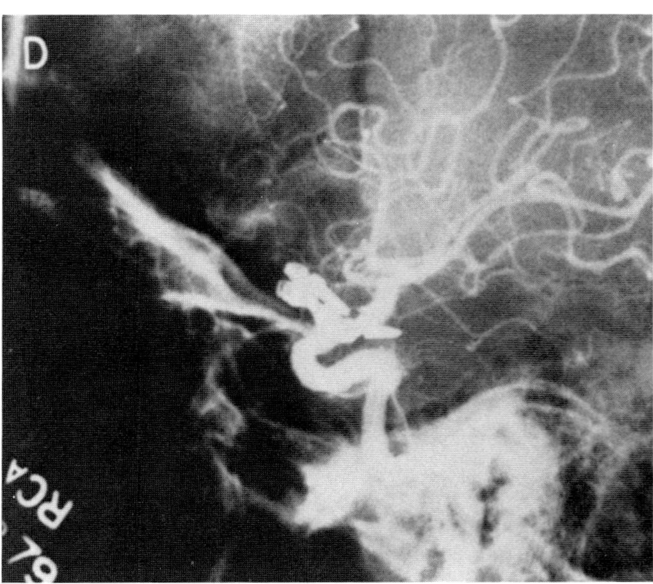

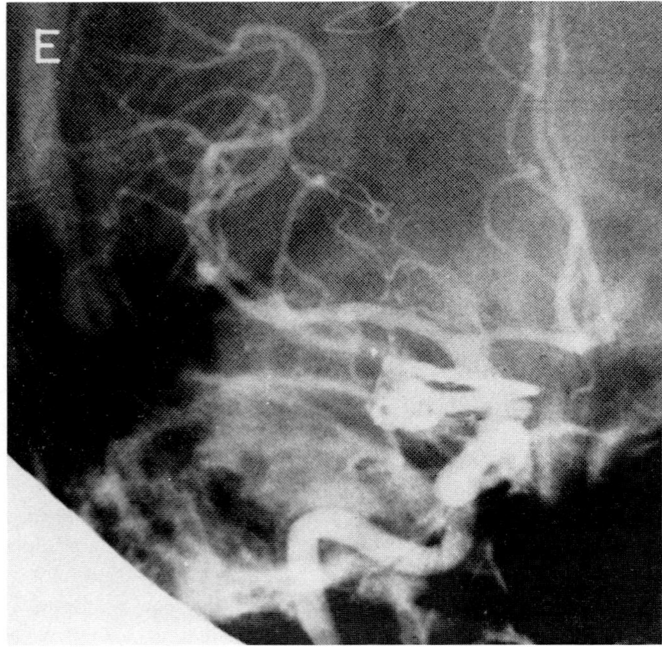

Fig. 82-12. Illustrative case: Clipping of right carotid-ophthalmic and posterior communicating aneurysms. (A and B) Preoperative right lateral carotid angiogram demonstrates both lesions and the ophthalmic artery. (C) Sketch depicting removal of the anterior clinoid process in order to expose the proximal carotid-ophthalmic aneurysm. The relation of lesion to the optic nerve and the ophthalmic artery is demonstrated. After dissection of the neck, a clip was placed across the neck, thus sparing the ophthalmic artery. (D and E) Postoperative right lateral carotid angiogram shows obliteration of the aneurysms and preservation of the native arteries.

tral venous pressure should be elevated to the range of 10 to 12 cm with colloid, and systolic blood pressure should be increased to the range of 160 to 180 torr systolic (dopamine or Neosynephrine can be used for this purpose). The mannitol regimen is instituted.[9]

Postoperative angiography is recommended in most cases in order to ascertain the adequacy of aneurysm obliteration and maintenance of normal vasculature.

ILLUSTRATIVE CASE

A 54-year-old right-handed woman experienced a severe, sudden headache with brief loss of consciousness. Initial evaluation showed a normal neurologic evaluation. Her blood pressure was 180/100, and a lumbar puncture showed grossly bloody spinal fluid. On transfer, the neurologic examination was normal save for restlessness. A medical program was instituted, including Amicar and blood pressure control. The patient became slightly confused; CT scan showed mild ventricular enlargement.

Lumbar puncture on day 12 showed an opening pressure of 390 mm of CSF with clear xanthochromic fluid. The mannitol regimen was instituted. Angiography on day 14 showed spasm of the right internal carotid artery with a right ophthalmic artery aneurysm and a right internal carotid-posterior communicating artery aneurysm (Figure 82-12A). There was moderate hydrocephalus. A CBF study performed was normal.

On day 17, a right frontotemporal craniotomy was performed for clipping of the aneurysms (Figure 82-12B). Postoperatively, the patient was intermittently confused, with gradual return to normal mentation. Angiography 10 days after surgery showed obliteration of both aneurysms (Figure 82-12C).

RESULTS

DIRECT APPROACH

The approach to ophthalmic aneurysms described above has produced good results (Table 82-1). In 15 patients, 87 percent experienced excellent results (no deficit) or good results (minimal deficit). In a single case there was ipsilateral blindness after clipping of a giant aneurysm, and another patient developed a wound infection that required removal of an infected bone flap. These cases were listed as poor results, although in fact neither patient had any postoperative restriction of activities. In all 15 cases, obliteration of the ophthalmic artery aneurysm was possible by direct intracranial surgery. These results are comparable to those reported by others.[3,15–17]

INDIRECT APPROACH

We have obliterated 4 surgically unclippable ophthalmic artery aneurysms with transfemoral intravascular detachable balloon occlusion of the internal carotid artery. This was done under cerebral blood flow (CBF) control. During temporary occlusion, if the CBF remained above 40 ml/100 gm/min, then the balloon was detached and the artery permanently occluded. After occlusion, the patients were heparinized for 3 days in an attempt to prevent distal emboli. All these patients had excellent results.

DISCUSSION

Carotid-ophthalmic aneurysms deserve separate consideration by virtue of their distinct anatomy, presentation, and surgical management.[3,12,14–17] These lesions typically arise from the internal carotid artery just distal to the origin of the ophthalmic artery. Aneurysms of the ophthalmic artery itself are very rare. Complete angiography, with oblique and off-lateral views and subtraction technique, can be helpful in defining the anatomy, but often surgical exploration will be needed in order to determine the position of the neck of the aneurysm and its suitability for clipping.

Direct attack with microsurgery offers the best results. For lesions of less than giant size, results are comparable with those achieved with aneurysms in other sites. Removal of the anterior clinoid process for most lesions facilitates proximal control and sets the stage for clipping.

For giant-sized lesions and for grade 3 and 4 patients with subarachnoid hemorrhage secondary to a ruptured carotid-ophthalmic artery aneurysm, the mortality and morbidity are still high.[18] It is sometimes necessary, particularly for giant aneurysms, to consider special approaches such as cervical internal carotid occlusion. By virtue of their proximal location, carotid-ophthalmic aneurysms are accessible to transvascular obliteration with detachable balloon catheter methods. We have found CBF studies performed during temporary occlusion of the internal carotid artery to be quite reliable and helpful in determining whether an STA-MCA bypass is needed or not.[13]

Cerebrovascular spasm may lead to cerebral infarction, either before or after the surgery.[19] Preoperative and postoperative vasospasm can be minimized by delaying surgery for about 10 days after subarachnoid hemorrhage and by the prophylactic use of the mannitol regimen.[9] If proved vasospasm should become symptomatic, elevation of cardiac output and cerebral perfusion seems to restrict cerebral damage.

The biggest problem is the subarachnoid hemorrhage patient who never reaches the operating room.[20] Probably two thirds of all subarachnoid hemorrhage victims suffer devastating or fatal hemorrhages that could not be reversed. Perhaps newer techniques, such as digital subtraction angiography or magnetic resonance imaging can identify some of these lesions before hemorrhage. Prophylactic surgery might be justified in some asymptomatic patients in order to avert unheralded catastrophic bleeding.[21]

REFERENCES

1. Locksley HB: Report on the cooperative study of intracranial aneurysms and subarachnoid hemorrhage. Section V, part 1. Natural history of subarachnoid hemorrhage, intracranial aneurysms and arteriovenous malformations: Based on 6368 cases in the cooperative study. J Neurosurg 25:219, 1966
2. Sengupta RP: Management of large and giant aneurysms. Neurosurg Rev 5:173, 1982
3. Yasargil MG, Gasser JG, Hodosh RM, et al: Carotid aneurysm: Direct microsurgical approach. Surg Neurol 8:155, 1977

Table 82-1. Results of 15 cases of carotid-ophthalmic aneurysm treated by direct intracranial surgery

Aneurysm Grade	Results (%)				
	Excellent	Good	Poor	Death	Total
1–2	10 (67)	3 (20)	2 (13)	0	15

4. Rhoton AL, Homi AS, Renn WH: Microsurgical anatomy of the sellar region and cavernous sinus, in Claser JS (ed): Neuro-ophthalmology Symposium of the University of Miami, 1977, pp 75–105

5. Davis KR, New PFJ, Ojemann RG, et al: Computed tomographic evaluation of hemorrhage secondary to intracranial aneurysm. AJR 127:143, 1976

6. Hunt WE, Hess RM: Surgical risk as related to time of intervention in the repair of intracranial aneurysms. J Neurosurg 28:14, 1968

7. Aitken RR, Drake CG: A technique of anesthesia with induced hypotension for surgical correction of intracranial aneurysms. Clin Neurosurg 21:107, 1974

8. Suzuki J, Yoshimoto T, Takamasa K: Surgical treatment of middle cerebral artery aneurysms. J Neurosurg 61:17, 1984

9. Jafar JJ, Johns LM, Mullan SF: The effect of mannitol on cerebral blood flow. J Neurosurg 64:754, 1986

10. Krayenbuhl HA, Yasargil MC, Flamm ES, et al: Microsurgical treatment of intracranial sacular aneurysms. J Neurosurg 37:678, 1972

11. Yasargil MC, Fox JL: The microsurgical approach to intracranial aneurysm. Surg Neurol 3:7, 1975

12. Drake CG, Vanderlinden RG, Amacher AL: Carotid-ophthalmic aneurysm. J Neurosurg 29:24, 1968

13. Jafar JJ, Tan W, Abejo R, et al: Balloon occlusion of giant intracranial aneurysms under cerebral blood flow control. (in preparation)

14. Sundt TM Jr, Murphy F: Clip grafts for aneurysms and small vessel surgery. Part 3: Clinical experience in intracranial carotid artery aneurysms. J Neurosurg 31:59, 1968

15. Ferguson GG, Drake CG: Carotid-ophthalmic aneurysm. Visual abnormalities in 32 patients and the results of treatment. Surg Neurol 16:1, 1981

16. Ferguson GG, Drake CG: Carotid-ophthalmic aneurysm. The surgical management of those cases presenting with compression of the opt c nerves and chiasm alone. Clin Neurosurg 27:263, 1980

17. Guidetti B, LaTorre E: Carotid-ophthalmic aneurysms. A series of 16 cases treated by direct approach. Acta Neurochir 22:289, 1970

18. Ferguson GG: Carotid-ophthalmic artery aneurysms, in Wilkins RH, Rengachary SS (eds): Neurosurgery. New York, McGraw-Hill, 1985, pp 1385–1393

19. Fisher CM, Roberson GJ, Ojemann RG: Cerebral vasospasm with ruptured saccular aneurysm—The clinical manifestations. Neurosurgery 1:245, 1977

20. Drake CG: Perspective on cerebral aneurysms. Stroke 11:124, 1980

21. Jane JA, Winn HR, Richardson AE: The natural history of intracranial aneurysms: Re-bleeding rate during the acute and long time period and implications for surgery management. Clin Neurosurg 24:176, 1977

Surgical Management of Aneurysms of the Internal Carotid: Posterior Communicating, Anterior Choroidal, and Bifurcation Aneurysms

Henry H. Schmidek

FOLLOWING THE INTRODUCTION of cerebral angiography, which allowed the diagnosis of an intracranial aneurysm to be established and provided detailed information concerning its specific anatomic features, the era of planned surgical management of these lesions was inaugurated. It was soon discovered that aneurysms arising from the supraclinoid internal carotid artery are common and amenable to surgical treatment. In 1933, Norman Dott[1] became the first to operate on a cerebral aneurysm demonstrated by cerebral angiography. The patient was a 23-year-old woman who experienced a severe headache and progressive left oculomotor nerve palsy. The aneurysm, a 7-mm lesion attached by a narrow neck to the inferior aspect of the junction of the left internal carotid artery with its posterior communicating branch, was treated by cervical carotid ligation on March 24, 1933. The patient made an excellent recovery generally and of her oculomotor nerve function. In 1936, Walter Dandy[2] began to treat aneurysms of the internal carotid artery in or near the cavernous sinus by a trapping procedure that involved ligation of the involved vessel proximal and distal to the aneurysm. He then introduced directly occluding the neck of a saccular aneurysm intracranially while preserving the parent artery. This was first carried out in a 43-year-old chronic alcoholic with a paralysis of the oculomotor nerve. Based on clinical findings alone, and without angiographic studies, the patient was operated on and a pea-sized aneurysm found projecting from the outer wall of the internal carotid artery adjacent to the posterior communicating artery. The aneurysm arose by a narrow neck, projected beneath the tentorial dura, and was attached to the oculomotor nerve. A silver clip was placed across the neck of the sac flush with the wall of the internal carotid artery, obliterating the sac completely. The aneurysm was then thrombosed with electrocautery. Within 3 days, the patient's ptosis and extraocular movements began to improve; and in 7 months there was complete return of all oculomotor nerve functions.[2] In the 50 years since these pioneering efforts, a major activity of the neurosurgical community has been directed to characterizing the natural history of cerebral aneurysms and to their perioperative and intraoperative management to reduce the morbidity associated with these

phases of a patient's care. This chapter will discuss our current medical and surgical treatment of cerebral aneurysms as practiced on my neurosurgical service and will address those factors specifically related to internal carotid aneurysms (ICAs) arising at the level of the posterior communicating artery, anterior choroidal artery, and carotid bifurcation of which the surgeon should be aware.

Aneurysms of the supraclinoid carotid artery present in patients of any age. They have been described within the first days of life,[3] and have been successfully operated on within the first month of age. Although uncommon in the pediatric population, cerebral aneurysms often exist in association with bacterial endocarditis, chronic lung infections, polycystic kidney disease, aortic coarctation, Marfan's or Ehler-Danlos syndrome, and familial aneurysms, so one must maintain a particular suspicion of the possibility of these lesions being present in these settings. Although ten times less common than arteriovenous malformations, cerebral aneurysms in children are more prone to rupture and account for approximately one third of the cases of spontaneous subarachnoid hemorrhage in children between the ages of 4 and 15 years. The vast majority of patients have subarachnoid hemorrhage, and the clinical features are as those in adults. Probably less than 5 percent of the aneurysms in children produce a mass effect.[4] Both adults and children may become symptomatic with aneurysmal expansion that produces headache, retro-orbital or facial pain, or compression of the optic pathways. It is among the aneurysms of the internal carotid artery–posterior communicating artery junction and with aneurysms at the carotid bifurcation that the highest incidence of warning signs exists before aneurysmal rupture. In a retrospective review, such warnings are described in 69.2 percent of the internal carotid artery–posterior communicating artery cases and 60 percent of the carotid bifurcation aneurysms.[5] In these cases the complaints are related to head or facial pain or mass effect on cranial nerves.

Most of the aneurysms of the internal carotid artery distal to the ophthalmic artery are discovered after they rupture. In 40 percent of the patients, an oculomotor palsy develops, sometimes immediately and sometimes within a few days of the

OPERATIVE NEUROSURGICAL TECHNIQUES
ISBN 0-8089-1862-1

ictus. Before subarachnoid hemorrhage, ipsilateral retro-orbital and frontal head pain occurs in about one fourth of the patients. The pain may exist for months or years before the aneurysm ruptures or produces an oculomotor palsy. In many cases oculomotor palsy appears within 2 weeks of the onset of pain, and in these patients, oculomotor palsy is often the only sign of disease. It has been found that the overall incidence of oculomotor palsy is 38 percent in patients with carotid–posterior communicating artery aneurysms. Hook and Norlen[7] and Odom[8] cited 36 percent and 42 percent, respectively. When the oculomotor nerve is affected by an aneurysm, paresis is usually complete with involvement of the levator, extraocular muscles, and the pupillary sphincter. A nontraumatic oculomotor palsy with pupillary involvement is, until proven otherwise, an aneurysm or tumor.[9] The oculomotor nerve is usually compressed where it enters the dura at the posterior end of the cavernous sinus. Visual defects may rarely occur in conjunction with these aneurysms and result from compression of the optic tract, thereby producing a contralateral homonymous hemianopia and pallor of the optic discs. Mental derangements may arise when the aneurysm compresses the mamillary bodies or the blood supply to the diencephalon, or pituitary insufficiency when the aneurysm grows into the sella turcica.

Aneurysms that arise at the carotid bifurcation frequently present as a subarachnoid hemorrhage in conjunction with an orbitofrontal or temporal lobe intracerebral hematoma. They may grow without rupturing and mimic a suprasellar tumor. This can produce a bitemporal field defect; or, if the aneurysm expands posteriorly and medially, it can compress an optic tract; if it expands posteriorly and inferiorly, it can compress the oculomotor nerve.

The aneurysm discovered as an incidental finding revealed during the angiographic investigation of cerebral ischemia and head trauma is an increasingly common phenomenon and its optimal management remains unresolved.[8] Taking into consideration the patient's general condition, the familial history, particularly of aneurysms or subarachnoid hemorrhage, psychologic make-up, the specific characteristics as to aneurysm site and location, and the anticipated technical ease of obliterating the lesion, the patient is presented with the option of deferring surgical intervention until a change in the size of the lesion is manifested clinically or by annual angiography, or of having the operation performed electively. Given a favorable array of variables, my preference is for early surgical isolation of the aneurysm from the circulation (see the chapter by Mount and Brisman).

DIAGNOSTIC EVALUATION

After appropriate general medical and laboratory studies, all patients suspected of harboring an intracranial aneurysm are studied by computed tomographic (CT) scanning and four-vessel cerebral angiography. In the patient without a prior subarachnoid hemorrhage, these studies are completed within days of admission, whereas in a patient with a subarachnoid hemorrhage, the studies are performed within hours of hospitalization.

The CT scan performed with and without infusion of Renografin (Squibb & Sons, Inc., Boston, Mass) gives evidence about intracerebral, subdural, or intraventricular hemorrhage (their location and dimensions), the extent and location of bleeding into the basal cisterns, the localization of the ruptured aneurysm in the presence of multiple aneurysms, and information concerning ventricular size and hemorrhage and the extent of cerebral edema or infarction. On occasion the aneurysm can be seen adjacent to the anterior clinoid process—particularly if it is over 1.0 cm in diameter. Although Scotti et al.[10] concluded that the diagnosis of subarachnoid hemorrhage was possible in all cases when a CT scan was performed within 5 to 7 days after subarachnoid hemorrhage, this was not found to be the case in 12 percent of the series of Mizukami et al.[11] of 111 cases of subarachnoid hemorrhage, suggesting that it is not always possible to diagnose the subarachnoid hemorrhage with CT scanning alone. Hayward[5] reported the relationship between CT findings and the localization of ruptured aneurysms and concluded that the aneurysm could be determined in 68 percent of those arising from the internal carotid artery.

The CT scan may be of predictive value in anticipating the development of cerebral vasospasm after aneurysmal hemorrhage. In the study by Mizukami and his colleagues,[11] the presence or absence of cerebral vasospasm was judged in 75 cases in which surgical treatment was not performed before the 15th day after the hemorrhage. Cerebral angiography was repeated between days 5 and 14, this being the time frame when the presence of cerebral vasospasm was most likely to be present. When a significant collection of blood was present in the subarachnoid space, cerebral vasospasm was confirmed angiographically in 84 percent of the cases in the first 4 days after subarachnoid hemorrhage, in 75 percent of the cases in 5 to 7 days, and in 86 percent in the second week. In 8 cases where this finding was not present on CT scan after subarachnoid hemorrhage within 4 days of the ictus, no vasospasm was seen. No relationship was found between the presence of cisternal blood and cerebral vasospasm when a CT scan was performed after day 5 of the disease.

If CT scanning allows the diagnosis of subarachnoid hemorrhage to be made, and particularly if there is a mass effect and shift of brain between intracranial compartments, a lumbar puncture is not performed. If the diagnosis is in doubt, and occasionally to relieve an unremitting headache, a lumbar puncture will be performed in a patient who is awake and alert.

Cerebral angiography is usually performed under sedation and local anesthesia by the femoral route using standard catheter techniques. All four cerebral vessels are visualized, and oblique, basal, and cross-compression views are performed as indicated. The detailed anatomy of all aneurysms is further delineated with magnification and subtraction studies. This allows assessment of the degree of atherosclerosis, the size, site, and configuration of the aneurysm, and the presence of other lesions, and provides a baseline for evaluating the vessels for vasospasm.

In cases with a supraclinoid carotid aneurysm, the angiograms are studied specifically to assess whether the ipsilateral posterior communicating artery is an essential blood supply to the posterior cerebral artery territory and to the neck of the aneurysm, as well as the exact relationship of the posterior communicating artery. Anterior choroidal artery aneurysms usually arise from the inferior wall of the supraclinoid carotid artery and project downward. In these cases one needs an accurate assessment of the aneurysm's specific configuration, since they are often a diffuse dilatation of the wall of the carotid artery extending toward the carotid bifurcation, with the anterior choroidal artery incorporated in this dilatation. As a result, the aneurysm may not be amenable to direct clipping. One should therefore be prepared to reinforce rather than clip the aneurysm. Aneurysms arising at the carotid bifurcation can be extremely difficult to delineate angiographically, although these are usually small lesions with a discrete neck that can be clipped. To find and characterize these lesions, it is particularly important to have oblique and subtraction studies to find the aneurysm among the vessels present at the termination of the carotid artery.

In patients in whom no lesion is discovered to account for the subarachnoid hemorrhage, repeat four-vessel cerebral angiography is performed 2 to 3 weeks after the first studies. Should this study also fail to clarify the situation, the remote possibility exists that the subarachnoid hemorrhage was caused by a spinal tumor or malformation.

PREOPERATIVE MANAGEMENT

The preoperative management following aneurysmal subarachnoid hemorrhage is designed to provide symptomatic relief and reduce the tendency to re-hemorrhage. The program involves bedrest, mild analgesics, anticonvulsants, steroids (dexamethasone 8–10 mg IV every 6 hours), antacids, and epsilon-aminocaproic acid (EACA) at a dose of 36 g/day (i.e., 1.5 g/hour intravenously). Although there is suggestive evidence of a causal relationship between complications of thrombosis, cerebral vasospasm, hydrocephalus and myopathy, and EACA therapy, we have not been impressed with the incidence of these problems on this service and continue to use this agent. The systolic blood pressure is maintained at normotensive levels. A variety of agents are used for this purpose including furosemide, hydralazine, chlorpromazine, trimethaphan camphorsulfonate, and sodium nitroprusside, with progression from agents such as furosemide to sodium nitroprusside as required by the situation. These agents are used in an intensive care unit setting, allowing continuous nursing supervision and continuous arterial pressure monitoring.

The timing of surgical intervention depends on the patient's overall and neurologic condition and the appearance on CT scan, particularly of widespread hemorrhage in the basal cisterns. The patient in good condition, without massive cisternal blood and without angiographic evidence of vasospasm, is operated on within 1 to 2 weeks of admission, under optimal circumstances with the most experienced anesthetic, surgical, and nursing team available.

Patients are transferred to our neurosurgical service days or weeks after their subarachnoid hemorrhage; if the patient is obtunded and significant vasospasm is present angiographically, surgical intervention is deferred until repeat angiography no longer demonstrates the presence of such vasospasm, and the patient is maintained on the medical regimen described above.

If the patient is in good condition, without angiographic evidence of vasospasm on the contrast study performed before surgery, an operation is performed soon after admission when optimal circumstances are available to the patient.

In patients with profound neurologic deficits without an intracerebral hematoma and secondary to vasospasm, an epidural pressure switch is inserted and an attempt is made to maintain the intracranial pressure under 20 torr using mannitol, furosemide, hyperventilation, and ventricular drainage. Treatment is continued until the intracranial pressure remains under 20 torr without these agents. The patients are intubated and hyperventilated to a $pCO = 2$ of 25–30 torr and are fully supported to maintain their metabolic, cardiovascular, and respiratory function. Surgical intervention is reserved for those patients who can be weaned off this program and who have the potential for a useful existence.

In patients whose problem is complicated by an intracerebral hemorrhage, those patients who are undergoing neurologic deterioration but who are potentially salvageable and useful individuals are subjected to immediate surgery. At the time of surgery the hemorrhage is removed and the aneurysm dealt with definitively if this is technically feasible.

SURGICAL ANATOMY

The internal carotid artery has four segments: cervical, intrapetrosal, intracavernous, and supraclinoid. The supraclinoid segment begins as the artery emerges from the cavernous sinus and passes medial to the anterior clinoid process. This portion of the artery extends upward and the ophthalmic, posterior communicating, and anterior choroidal arteries arise from this segment. The most frequent site of internal carotid artery aneurysms is at the posterior communicating artery junction, with aneurysms arising at the internal carotid artery–anterior choroidal junction and the bifurcation of the internal carotid artery being uncommon. Aneurysms arising distally on these arteries are rare, although investment of the aneurysm and the vessel by arachnoid may create the impression that the aneurysm appears to arise from the artery directly.

The posterior communicating artery arises from the posteromedial surface of the internal carotid artery and runs backward for 5 to 10 mm to anastomose with the posterior cerebral artery. The posterior cerebral artery varies greatly in size from being rudimentary to occasionally being so large that the posterior cerebral artery appears to be arising from the internal carotid rather than from the basilar artery. It is frequently larger on the left side. This vessel may constitute the main source of blood to the posterior cerebral artery. If this artery fills predominantly from the basilar artery, its occlusion is associated with little risk; whereas if the posterior communicating artery fills primarily from the posterior communicating artery, its occlusion may result in a major cerebral infarction.

POSTERIOR COMMUNICATING ARTERY

The posterior communicating artery gives rise to 4 to 12 branches. These branches supply the genu and anterior one third of the posterior limb of the internal capsule, the anterior one third of the thalamus, and the walls of the third ventricle. This vessel also gives off branches to the optic tract, the optic chiasm, the cerebral peduncle, and the tuber cinereum, and terminates as the anterior thalamo-perforating artery.

Aneurysms that arise at the junction of the carotid and posterior communicating arteries can be globular, elongated, multilobular, or irregular in shape. They also can vary greatly in size, although aneurysms greater than 2.5 cm in diameter are rarely seen at this location.

The most common type of aneurysm arising at the posterior communicating artery–internal carotid artery junction projects posterolaterally (86 percent) and involves the oculomotor nerve in about one third of the cases. The aneurysm frequently overlies the origin of the posterior communicating artery. In the presence of multiple aneurysms, there is a 65 percent chance of one of the aneurysms being situated at this site. Since these aneurysms are most likely to bleed freely into the basal cisterns, they are also the most likely to produce a communicating hydrocephalus, a complication encountered in approximately one third of patients after subarachnoid hemorrhage resulting from an aneurysm in this location.

In a smaller group of patients, the aneurysm is directed posterolaterally and extends above the tentorial edge. These are a more difficult group to approach since retraction of the temporal lobe may result in their premature rupture. Although it is uncommon for posterior communicating arteries to be associated with an intracerebral hemorrhage, it is in this subgroup of cases that temporal lobe hemorrhages occur.

Medially situated aneurysms arising at the internal carotid artery–posterior communicating artery junction occur in 3.6 percent of the cases and tend to extend beneath the optic nerve and produce visual symptoms, subarachnoid hemorrhage, or both. These lesions are approached by mobilizing the frontal and temporal lobes, gaining exposure of the internal carotid artery proximal and distal to the aneurysm.[6]

ANTERIOR CHOROIDAL ARTERY

The anterior choroidal artery is, next to the middle cerebral artery, the most important vascular supply to the internal capsule. The artery originates a few millimeters above the posterior communicating artery from the posterior surface of the internal carotid artery. This vessel may arise as two separate arteries or as a single trunk that divides a short way from its origin. It is often larger on the left side, and takes a course along the optic tract, around the cerebral peduncle to the lateral geniculate body, where its main branches enter the choroid plexus of the inferior horn of the lateral ventricle and anastomoses with branches of the posterior choroidal artery. In its course it supplies branches to the optic tract, the cerebral peduncle, and the base of the brain. These branches terminate in the lateral geniculate body, the tail of the caudate nucleus, and the posterior two thirds of the posterior limb of the internal capsule as far as the dorsal limit of the globus pallidus. The infralenticular and retrolenticular portions of the internal capsule are also vascularized by branches of the anterior choroidal artery.

Although occlusion of this artery does not invariably lead to a profound deficit, its injury may result in a contralateral hemiplegia, hemianesthesia, hemianopia, stupor, and death. Many aneurysms arising from the supraclinoid internal carotid artery involve this vessel in their wall, especially if the aneurysm is larger than 5 mm in size. This vessel is at risk with any surgical procedure in the vicinity of the supraclinoid internal carotid artery. There is also a tendency for aneurysms to co-exist at this location, which may not be appreciated preoperatively. Clinically, these aneurysms may be indistinguishable from the internal carotid artery–posterior communicating artery aneurysm, even to involvement of the oculomotor nerve. In addition, since the anterior choroidal artery can be attached to the fundus of a posterior communicating aneurysm, this artery must be identified before the aneurysm is clipped.

The anterior choroidal aneurysm usually projects from the inferior aspect of the internal carotid artery 3 to 6 mm proximal to the carotid bifurcation and projects laterally, whereas the anterior choroidal artery itself curves medially. The aneurysm will often obscure the origin of the anterior choroidal artery. There is usually an angle of separation, however, between the parent vessel and the aneurysm, which should allow a clip to be applied to the aneurysmal neck without injuring the anterior choroidal artery.

Internal carotid artery bifurcation aneurysms represent about 5 percent of intracranial aneurysms, and often produce a frontal intracerebral hemorrhage. The aneurysms may be difficult to delineate angiographically since they are often small and hidden by other vessels. Morphologically, the aneurysms represent either a direct continuation of the internal carotid artery trunk or possess a broad-based origin that incorporates the junction of the internal carotid artery and anterior cerebral arteries or the internal carotid artery–middle cerebral artery junction and include parts of the main trunk of the anterior or middle cerebral artery. The majority of these lesions project superiorly or superiorly and ventrally beneath the orbitofrontal lobe in the area of the anterior perforated substance. Only occasionally does the aneurysm arise from the dorsal aspect of the carotid bifurcation. Most of these aneurysms are of the same dimensions as encountered elsewhere along the carotid artery. Giant aneurysms are exceptional at this site. The dome of the aneurysm is usually covered by frontal lobe or may be located in the sylvian fissure. Among aneurysms of the supraclinoid internal carotid artery, these aneurysms are the most likely to present with an associated intracerebral hemorrhage. Exposure of these lesions requires delineation of the vessels at the bifurcation, the lenticulostriate vessels, and the anterior choroidal artery, which is best accomplished by dissection along the anterior and inferior margins of the major vessels while leaving the fundus, which is usually buried in the frontal lobe, alone.

OPERATIVE PROCEDURE

Craniotomy is performed under general endotracheal anesthesia, usually with a "balanced technique," controlled ventilation, and continuous monitoring of electrocardiogram, blood gases, arterial pressure, and urinary output. The patient is brought to the operating room under atropine-droperidol sedation, and with a functioning intravenous line, is anesthetized and gently intubated without raising the blood pressure and before insertion of the central venous pressure and arterial lines and Foley catheter. Neither spinal fluid drainage nor hypothermia is used. It is important that the radial artery catheter be calibrated to reflect the blood pressure at the level of the head since the operating table is flexed. The patient is in a supine position, the head is shaved and turned 15 to 20 degrees away from the side of the aneurysm, and then the position is maintained in the three-point headrest. The arms and legs are protected with an egg-crate mattress and blankets, and both ends of the operating table are flexed to facilitate the venous return.

The operation is begun with the patient receiving mannitol (1.5 g/kg), furosemide (20–40 mg IV), Decadron (25 mg IV), and Kefzol (1.0 g IV).

An aneurysm tray is available on a separate Mayo stand and consists of the entire spectrum of Yasargil, Scoville, Sugita, Drake, Mayfield, Heifetz, and Sundt clips and applicators so that the surgeon can choose the optimal configuration from this collection. The tray also includes muslin and plastics to allow alternatives to clipping the aneurysm should this tactic be preferable.

The preferred operating microscope is the Zeiss OPMI 6

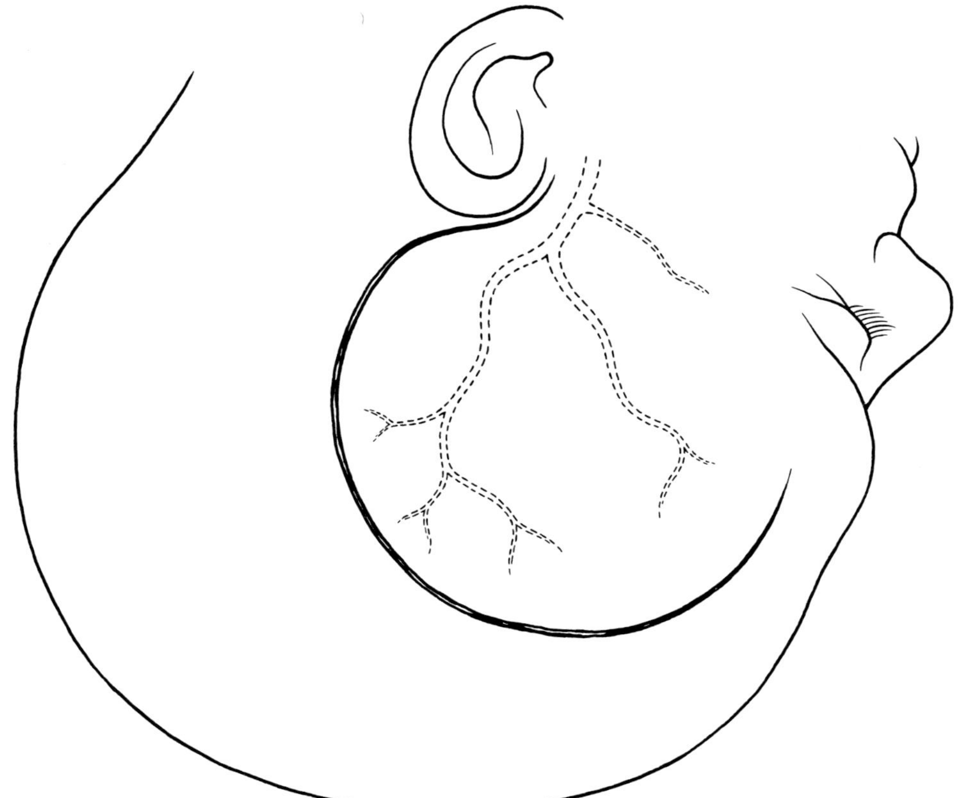

Fig. 83-1. Frequently used skin incision for the pterional approach to the internal carotid artery, posterior communicating artery, and carotid bifurcation.

set up on the Contraves stand, which allows the microscope to be suspended almost weightlessly and adjustments to be made effortlessly.

After the skin is cleansed with Betadine and alcohol, a small scalp flap is made that extends from the zygomatic process of the temporal bone and curves anteriorly to intersect the hairline at approximately the midpoint of the superior orbital ridge, taking into account the position of the frontal branch of the facial nerve (Figure 83-1). Separate skin and muscle flaps can be reflected; however, an osteoplastic bone flap is cosmetically preferable in the frontotemporal area. A frontotemporal craniotomy is fashioned flush with the anterior cranial fossa, and the dura is gradually separated to allow removal of the lateral one third of the greater wing of the sphenoid with an air drill (Figure 83-2). Before inserting the dural tenting sutures, the baseplate of the Yasargil self-retaining retractor is positioned on the superior and medial aspect of the bony opening, and microfibrillar collagen is inserted beneath the bone edges to control epidural bleeding along with the tenting sutures.

If an intracerebral hematoma is covering the frontal and temporal areas, the dura is not opened until the brain is pulsating freely. If the brain is still tense after the administration of mannitol, furosemide, and hyperventilation, the hematoma is gently cannulated and a few cubic centimeters of blood removed. This maneuver will often make it possible to open the dura without the brain herniating through the opening. Occasionally it is necessary to cannulate the lateral ventricle before opening the dura if the brain remains tense when there is no intracerebral hemorrhage.

The dura is opened to allow exposure to the lateral aspect of the frontal lobe and anterior temporal lobes. The exposed brain is covered with wet Gelfoam.

The initial intradural exposure of supraclinoid ICA aneurysms is along the sphenoid ridge to the anterior clinoid process. By retracting the frontal lobe or the temporal tip or both with a ½- to 1-inch Silastic-coated retractor, dissection is carried down to the optic nerve using operating telescopes allowing 3.5–4.5× magnification in conjunction with fiberoptic headlight illumination. With gentle retraction, the optic nerve is exposed and the arachnoid is opened over the carotid artery and the optic nerve with a sharp knife, allowing aspiration of cerebrospinal fluid to provide additional exposure. The retractor then is fixed in position; if necessary, a second Silastic-coated retractor can be introduced to gain additional exposure.

It is only at this phase of the operation that the operating microscope needs to be introduced. The microscope is used until the aneurysm is clipped. It is then removed and the operation proceeds with loupes. Further dissection is carried out at 6–16× magnification. Unless contraindicated by the patient's general condition, the patient's blood pressure can be lowered slowly to a mean of 60–80 mm Hg by deepening the level of anesthesia, infusing intravenous sodium nitroprusside, or both. This technique increases the flaccidity of the aneurysm and decreases its tendency to rupture with manipulation. We do not, however, use this technique in about one half of our cases, and often find that the aneurysm can be clipped without lowering the blood pressure.

The internal carotid artery is identified with respect to its bifurcation and inferiorly along the internal carotid artery to the aneurysm. Dissection is continued until the upper and lower borders of the aneurysmal neck and the proximal internal

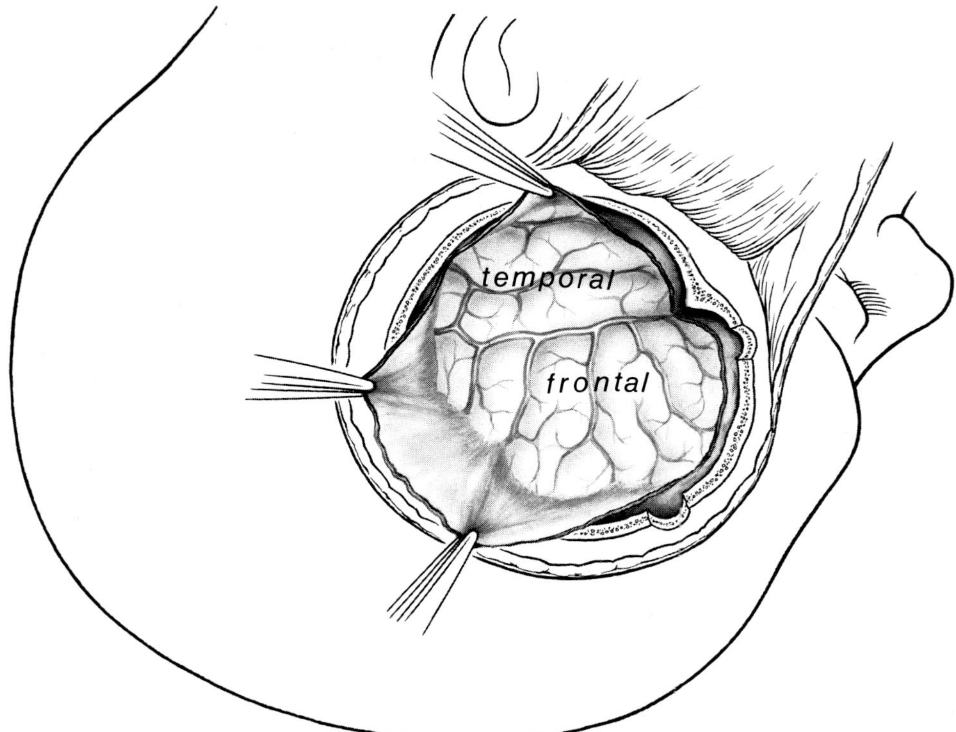

Fig. 83-2.   Craniotomy after opening dura and exposing brain surface of the frontal and temporal lobes.

carotid artery can be seen (Figures 83-3 and 83-4). This provides proximal and distal control of the vessel in the event of bleeding. The application of temporary clips to the carotid artery is not routinely used. The arachnoid around the vessel and the aneurysmal neck is gently cut, and a passage that is free of vessels is developed on either side of the neck. Often the vessels adjacent to the aneurysm blend with the arachnoid covering the aneurysm so that it is crucial to dissect beyond this arachnoidal layer while preserving the vessels in it. Before clipping the neck, one must know the location of the anterior choroidal and posterior communicating arteries. The clip is applied and if necessary reapplied several times to ensure preservation of these vessels. The aneurysm is occluded immediately adjacent to the parent vessel to prevent recurrence of the aneurysm proximal to the clip. The majority of aneurysms can be obliterated with a suitable Yasargil or Sugita clip. Before applying a clip to the aneurysmal neck, one must test the clip and applicator to ensure that the clip can be released from its holder with minimal force.

If the aneurysm is seen to extend below the tentorium, additional exposure is achieved by coagulating and dividing the veins at the temporal tip and gradually retracting the tip of the temporal lobe posteriorly to expose the proximal internal carotid artery and the aneurysm.

If the aneurysmal sac projects above the tentorium and is buried in the temporal lobe, retraction is limited to the frontal lobe, exposing the aneurysmal neck without disturbing the lesion further.

Aneurysms arising from the carotid bifurcation are frequently encased in dense adhesions between the aneurysm, the anterior and middle cerebral arteries, and vessels entering the anterior perforated substance. One or more vessels may be incorporated in the aneurysm, and clip occlusion may compromise major arterial trunks. Dissection is carried along the internal carotid artery up toward the bifurcation, staying along the anterior and inferior margin of the anterior and middle cerebral arteries while trying to identify the lenticulostriate vessels and anterior choroidal artery.

After clipping or reinforcement of a carotid aneurysm, the basal cisterns are irrigated of all free blood; if vasospasm is seen, a 2.5 percent papaverine solution can be applied topically on cotton pledgets to the affected vessels. If an intracerebral hemorrhage is present, enough of the clot is removed before exposing the aneurysm to carry out the dissection; it is not until after the aneurysm has been clipped that the majority of the clot is removed. In the patient with an oculomotor nerve palsy, the aneurysm can be aspirated after clipping to further reduce the pressure against this nerve. No attempt is made to dissect the aneurysm from the nerve. Third-nerve palsy can be expected to resolve with improvement in ptosis within a few months, followed by an increasing range of extraocular movements and the return of pupillary reactivity.

If the aneurysm cannot be obliterated with a single clip, several alternatives are available to the surgeon, including attempting to place several clips across the aneurysm; dissecting out both the neck and fundus and wrapping the entire lesion in surgical or muslin gauze, which is then impregnated with cyanoacrylate; or relying on graduated cervical carotid occlusion.

If the aneurysm detaches from the parent artery during dissection, leaving a hole in the artery, this can be dealt with either by using a Sundt clip on the carotid artery or alternatively by using a Silastic T-tube, introduced through the hole in the artery to provide continued flow while the defect is repaired using microsurgical techniques.

Intraoperative angiography can be performed at this stage to confirm the adequacy of the clip placement while it is still possible to conveniently reapply a malpositioned clip, thus

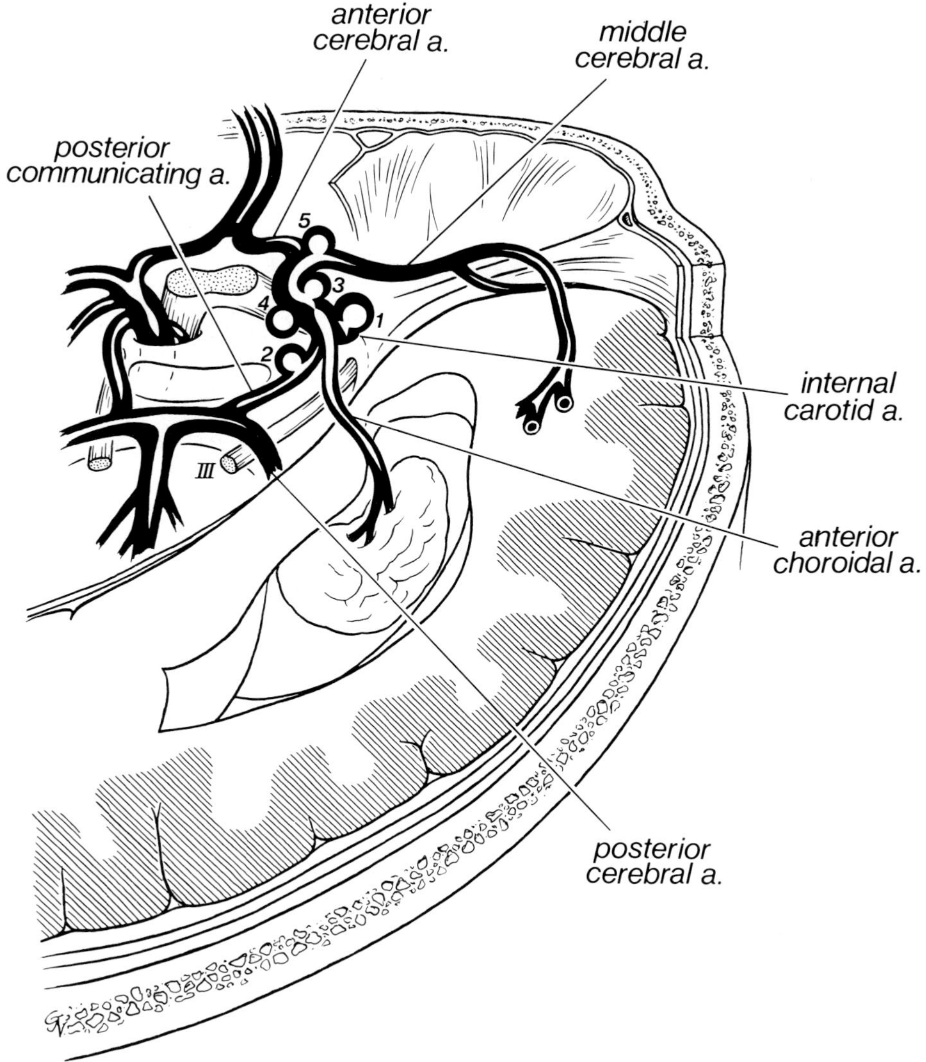

Fig. 83–3.   Schematic diagram indicating the sites of the internal carotid artery aneurysms and the regional anatomy of the structures surrounding these lesions.

sparing the patient the experience of another angiogram under local anesthesia before discharge. This is not necessary if the aneurysm is either aspirated or opened after clipping.

Once the aneurysm is clipped, the blood pressure is brought to normotensive levels and the adequacy of hemostasis is confirmed. Epsilon-aminocaproic acid (Amicar) is discontinued. The cisterns are filled with saline, the retractors are removed, and the dura is closed. If there is any difficulty in approximating the dural edges, a dural graft is inserted. A pressure switch is then placed in the epidural space to allow constant monitoring of the intracranial pressure, along with a medium-sized Jackson-Pratt drain (Heyerschulte, Inc., Worcester, Mass), which is emptied hourly. Postoperative antibiotics are continued until the drain and the switch are removed. The bone flap is reapproximated to assure a good cosmetic result, and the galea and skin are closed as separate layers. The incision and exit sites of the drain and switch are covered with an antibiotic ointment and a dressing is applied.

Postoperatively, the patient is maintained on much the same regimen as preoperatively, and dexamethasone, phenytoin, and codeine are continued. The intracranial pressure is kept under 20 torr. A baseline CT scan is performed to

estimate the extent of cerebral edema and to establish whether there are hemorrhages or hydrocephalus. The blood pressure is maintained at normotensive levels except when cerebral vasospasm arises, and is documented angiographically. This complication is treated by vascular expansion. Anticonvulsants are routinely continued after surgery, and in most cases the patient is examined by postoperative angiography before discharge, unless the aneurysm has been aspirated or opened intraoperatively.

RESULTS

There are many reports of aneurysms managed surgically in which the morbidity and mortality in a given series was less than 10 percent, creating the impression that, as a result of current microsurgical techniques and surgical virtuosity, the problems attending the management of these lesions have to a large extent been mastered. These reports reflect the results in a highly selected population of cases referred to centers of acknowledged excellence in the surgical care of aneurysms. The overall morbidity and mortality rate of patients admitted to

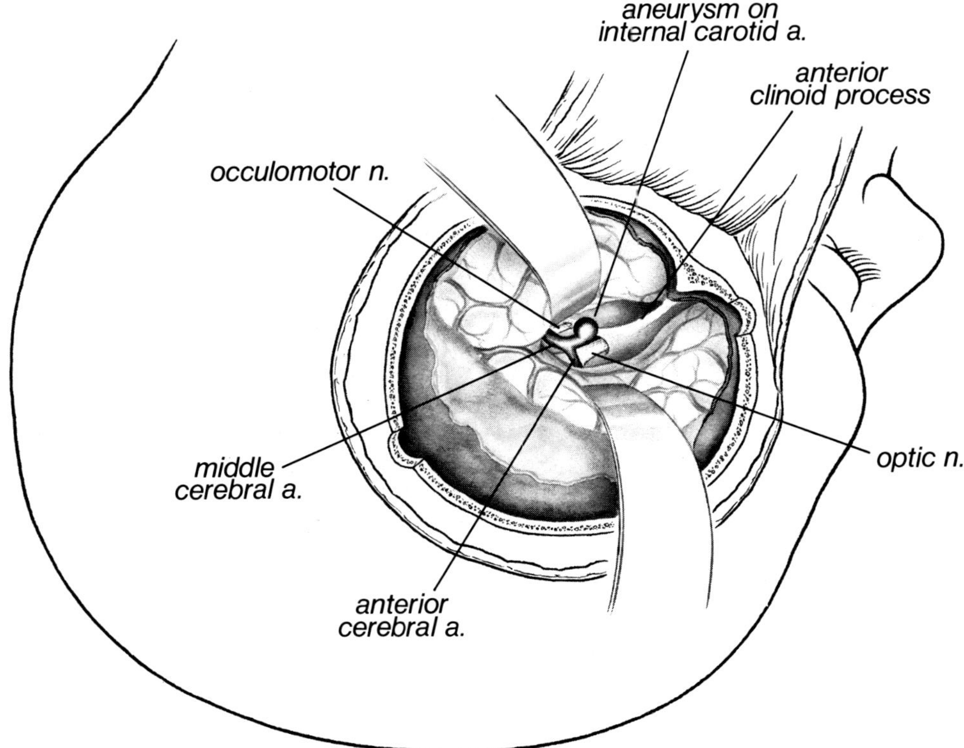

Fig. 83-4.   Final exposure of the left internal carotid artery, anterior and middle cerebral arteries, optic nerve, and an aneurysm of the internal carotid artery.

our neurosurgical unit with subarachnoid hemorrhage resulting from a proven intracranial aneurysm and followed from the first day of hemorrhage to 90 days is considerably higher, in spite of the exemplary medical and surgical care. The results attending the management of aneurysmal subarachnoid hemorrhage have been corroborated in the the Cooperative Aneurysm Study by Adams, Kassell et al.,[12] which analyzed the experience of neurosurgeons at 11 participating institutions who managed 249 patients admitted within 3 days of subarachnoid hemorrhage and on whom surgery was not performed sooner than 12 days after the most recent subarachnoid hemorrhage. Management consisted of bedrest, anticonvulsants, sedation, analgesics,

epsilon-aminocaproic acid at 36 g/day, and steroids, as well as mannitol as indicated. A total of 158 patients were treated operatively. Among the cases in good neurologic condition, 13 were subjected to carotid ligation and 116 to intracranial operations; among the cases considered as poor risks, 4 had carotid ligation, 20 intracranial surgery, and in the entire series 5 patients had both carotid ligation and intracranial surgery. Assessment of the overall results of the 235 cases on whom data were available shows 46 percent had a favorable outcome, 17.9 percent an unfavorable outcome, and 36.2 percent died. These results included a 55.7 percent favorable outcome and a 28.7 percent mortality among patients in good condition, although the procedure-related mortality attending intracranial surgery was 8.8 percent.

In the Cooperative Aneurysm Study, 50 patients had an aneurysm of the internal carotid artery (32 were on the middle cerebral artery, 54 were on the anterior cerebral complex, 20 were vertebrobasilar, and 63 demonstrated multiple aneurysms). The results for this group of cases are show in Table 83-1.

These results suggest, in comparison with the entire population of cases in the study, that aneurysms of the internal carotid artery are a prognostically favorable subgroup, although these cases are still associated with a 38 percent mortality within 90 days of the subarachnoid hemorrhage and a 13 percent mortality for those cases managed by intracranial surgery. Carotid ligation is not associated with any deaths in this report but has the disadvantage of a late re-bleeding rate of about a 7 percent even when the carotid ligation was successful, and a significant morbidity that mediates against its routine use except for aneurysms within the cavernous sinus and those

Table 83-1.   Mortality from internal carotid artery aneurysms in patients admitted 0 to 3 days after subarachnoid hemorrhage

	Total Number of Patients	Died	Percent
14-Day mortality (preoperative)	50	9	18
14-to-90-day mortality			
Not treated surgically	15	8	53
Intracranial surgery	16	2	13
Carotid ligation	8	0	0
Both	2	0	0
Total mortality (0–90 days)	50	19	38

aneurysms whose configuration may preclude direct intracranial occlusion.

REFERENCES

1. Dott NM: Intracranial aneurysms: Cerebral arterio-radiography; surgical treatment. Med J (Edinburg) 40:219, 1933
2. Dandy WE: Intracranial aneurysm of the internal carotid artery cured by operation. Ann Surg 107:654, 1938
3. Okawara SH: Warning signs prior to rupture of an intracranial aneurysm. J Neurosurg 38:575, 1973
4. Gelber BR, Sundt TM Jr: Treatment of intracavernous and giant carotid aneurysms by combined internal carotid ligation and extra to intracranial bypass. N Neurosurg 52:1, 1980
5. Hayward RD, O'Reilly GV: Intracerebral haemorrhage: Accuracy of CT scanning in predicting underlying aetiology. Lancet 1:1, 1976
6. Fisher CM, Kistler JP, Davis JM: Relation of cerebral vasospasm to subarachnoid hemorrhage visualized by computerized tomographic scanning. Neurosurgery 6:1, 1980
7. Hook D, Norlen G: Aneurysms of the internal carotid artery. Acta Neurol Scand 40:200, 1964 8. Odom GL: Ophthalmic involvement in neurological vascular lesions, in Smith JL (ed): Neuro-ophthalmology. Springfield, Ill, Charles C. Thomas, 1964
9. Overgaard J, Riishede J: Multiple cerebral saccular aneurysms. Acta Neurol Scand 41:363, 1965
10. Scotti G, Ethier R, Melancon D, et al: Computed tomography in the evaluation of intracranial aneurysms and subarachnoid hemorrhage. Radiology 123:85, 1977
11. Mizukami M, Takemae T, Tazawa T, et al: Value of computerized tomography in the prediction of cerebral vasospasm after aneurysm rupture. Neurosurgery 7:583, 1980
12. Adams HP, Kassel NF, Torner JC, et al: Early mangement of aneurysmal subarachnoid hemorrhage. J Neurosurg 54:141, 1981
J Schmidek (Ch 83) leg Legends

CHAPTER 84

Surgical Treatment of Anterior Communicating Artery Aneurysms

Robert M. Crowell   Jafar J. Jafar

ANTERIOR COMMUNICATING ARTERY ANEURYSMS account for 28 percent of intracranial aneurysms.[1] They often result in subarachnoid hemorrhage (SAH). Often the subarachnoid hemorrhage is a minor "warning leak" causing severe headache and a stiff neck. Sometimes SAH produces neurologic deficits ranging from minor to profound. By virtue of its location, the anterior communicating aneurysm is liable to hemorrhage upward into the third ventricle and hypothalamic region. Damage in these areas can be associated with memory disturbance (particularly for recent events), abulia, inappropriate secretion of antidiuretic hormone,[2] symptomatic hydrocephalus, or autonomic instability with unstable pulse and blood pressure. Alternatively, the aneurysm may rupture laterally, spilling blood into the cisterns surrounding the internal carotid and middle cerebral arteries or directly into the parenchyma, including the internal capsule.

Delayed complications are common with these lesions. Bleeding into the basal cisterns and third ventricle frequently causes hydrocephalus, which may become symptomatic and require shunting. Delayed deterioration may be related to vasospasm: spasm of the anterior cerebral arteries may cause lower-limb paresis or abulia; spasm of the internal carotid and middle cerebral arteries may lead to hemiparesis.

In rare instances, anterior communicating aneurysms reach giant size and compress visual pathways, the hypothalamus, or the internal capsule. In such instances, the patient presents has visual symptoms, mental disturbance, or hemiparesis.

PREOPERATIVE MANAGEMENT

INITIAL EVALUATION

When the diagnosis of SAH is suspected, the first step is a computed tomographic (CT) scan of the brain, with and without contrast. This test may confirm the diagnosis by demonstrating blood in the basal cisterns, interhemispheric fissure, ventricles, or adjacent brain tissue. In some cases, the aneurysm may be visualized with the infusion study. A magnetic resonance imaging study (MRI) may be of help to show giant aneurysms and to elucidate the anatomy (Figure 84-1). Lumbar puncture can be

Portions of this chapter appeared in Ojemann RG, Crowell RM: Surgical Management of Cerebrovascular Disease. Baltimore, Williams & Wilkins, 1983.

used when the diagnosis has not been established by CT scan, but only if there is no evidence of increased intracranial pressure.

All patients with subarachnoid hemorrhage should undergo screening tests of clotting function, including prothrombin time (PT), partial thromboplastin time (PTT), and platelet count. An electrocardiogram (ECG) may show abnormalities related to SAH. A complete blood count and serum electrolytes and serum osmolarity should be determined as baseline values. Psychometric testing, when possible, provides a quantitative parameter so that mental status can be characterized and followed.

All patients suffering from SAH undergo xenon 133 cerebral blood flow studies (CBF). This test helps in the timing of surgery and in selection of patients for hyperperfusion therapy. Whenever significant spasm is demonstrated on angiography, a cerebral blood flow study is repeated every 3 days until it becomes normal, when surgery is judged appropriate despite spasm.

Early management is guided by the clinical status of the patient, the CT findings, and the cerebral blood flow studies. For cases of symptomatic intracranial hematoma, emergency surgical evacuation is advisable. For those patients with symptomatic hydrocephalus, emergency external ventricular drainage may reverse the clinical symptomatology.

MEDICAL MANAGEMENT

MEDICAL REGIMEN

For stable patients without mass lesions or hydrocephalus, a standard medical regimen is instituted. This includes the following:

1. Bedrest.
2. Administration of fluids in an attempt to maintain normal circulating volume and central venous pressure.
3. Elastic stockings or pneumatic compression boots.
4. Epsilon-aminocaproic acid (Amicar, 36 g/day IV).
5. Anticonvulsants (diphenylhydantoin, 300 mg/day).
6. Stool softeners (Colace, 100 mg b.i.d.).
7. For agitation, haloperidol (Haldol, 2 mg IM every 2 to 4 hours).
8. For hypertension, trimethaphan camsylate or sodium

OPERATIVE NEUROSURGICAL TECHNIQUES
ISBN 0-8089-1862-1

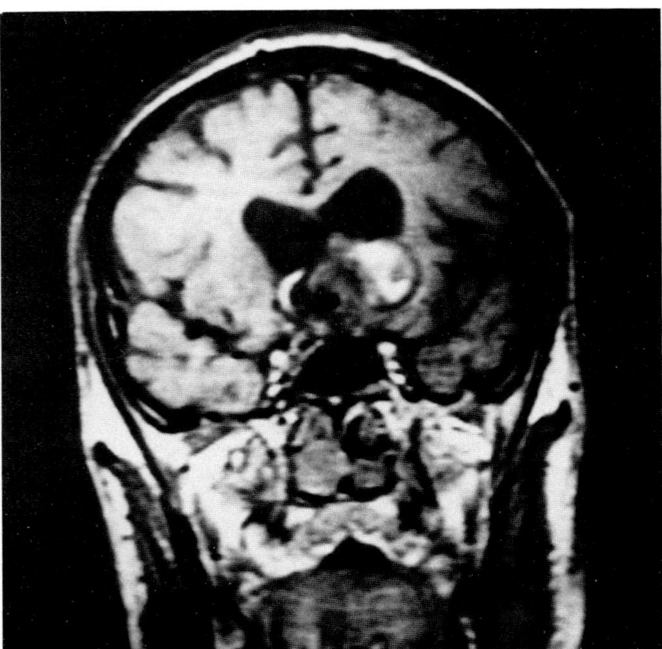

Fig. 84-1. A giant anterior communicating artery aneurysm as seen on a MRI scan.

nitroprusside to bring the systolic blood pressure below 150 torr without causing drowsiness or neurologic deficits.

9. Dexamethasone (4 mg IV q6h) to reduce cerebral swelling in symptomatic patients.
10. Cimetidine (300 mg PO or IV q6h).
11. Codeine for headache (30–60 mg PO or IM q3-4h).

DETERIORATION

Should a patient deteriorate, metabolic studies and CT scans are conducted on an emergency basis. Electrolyte imbalance may require correction. The CT scan may reveal hydrocephalus or focal cerebral ischemia or edema. Progressive hydrocephalus requires external ventricular drainage and subsequent shunting for relief of symptoms. If a clear explanation for the deterioration is not found, angiography is performed. If angiography discloses a significant degree of vasospasm (grade 3–4), a program of therapy is begun, and cuff arterial pressure, radial artery pressure, and central venous pressure are monitored. The intravascular volume is increased with colloid or packed cells to achieve a central venous pressure of 10 to 12 cm of water. The patient is started on mannitol (100 g q8h as a continuous IV drip).[3] Cautious elevation of blood pressure is produced with volume and pressors.[4]

TIMING OF SURGERY

The timing of angiography and surgery is determined by the clinical condition as judged by the Hunt classification,[5] as well as by the cerebral blood flow studies. For patients in good condition (grades 1–2) who have normal cerebral blood flow studies, angiography is carried out immediately, with surgery performed as soon as possible if no spasm is demonstrated. For patients in poor condition (grades 3–4), angiography is deferred about 2 weeks after subarachnoid hemorrhage.

ANGIOGRAPHY

Angiography must demonstrate the sac and neck, their relationship to the parent arteries, and the direction in which the lesion points. Satisfactory visualization will often require both oblique and base views. To ensure visualization of the anterior communicating artery and both precommunal (A1) anterior cerebral arteries, cross-compression of one carotid artery is occasionally needed during injection of the contralateral internal carotid artery. The posterior circulation should be visualized in order to exclude multiple lesions. Subtraction techniques are often useful in the delineation of complex vascular anatomy in this area.

ANESTHESIA

The patient is premedicated with 4 mg dexamethasone, triazolam, 2 mg intramuscularly, and glycopyrrolate, 0.2 mg intramuscularly at 6 AM the day of surgery. In the induction room, an intravenous route is established. This is preferably a large-bore plastic cannula, but in many patients receiving Amicar therapy, suitable veins are hard to identify. Rather than agitate such patients with repeated venipuncture efforts, it is better to place a small-gauge needle intravenously and then establish two large-bore intravenous routes after the patient is anesthetized.

In rare cases, no intravenous line can be established, and mask induction of anesthesia may be the best initial maneuver. A catheter is introduced into the radial artery for continuous monitoring of arterial pressure. Such monitoring is particularly important during induction, when wide swings of arterial pressure can occur. A central venous pressure line is always inserted. Pressor and hypotensive agents are available for infusion; phenylephrine (Neosynephrine, 10 mg in 250 ml of 5-percent dextrose in water) and sodium nitroprusside (50 mg in 250 ml of 5-percent dextrose in water shielded with tin foil) serve well for these needs.

INDUCTION

Once all preparations have been made, a slow induction is carried out, with preparation over 10 minutes or more before intubation. Sodium thiopental (3 mg/kg) is given intravenously after an initial preoxygenation. Once the patient is deeply drowsy, a mask is applied and the patient breathes a mixture of nitrous oxide and oxygen. Isoflurane is then given through the mask and ventilation is controlled. Before intubation, a muscle relaxant (pancuronium, 0.1 mg/kg) is given intravenously. A twitch monitor is applied to the ulnar nerve in order to monitor the completeness of neuromuscular blockade.

An additional increment of sodium thiopental is given intravenously just before intratracheal intubation. The blood pressure is in the range of 100 torr systolic at this point. Laryngoscopy is carried out and the vocal cords are sprayed with a local anesthetic solution. Further oxygenation with isoflurane administered through a mask is carried out. The blood pressure response to laryngoscopy is noted; if a substantial hypertensive response occurs, an additional increment of sodium thiopental, additional isoflurane, or both is administered.

Once stable and well anesthetized, laryngoscopy is carried out with gentle endotracheal intubation of the patient. In the case of a sustained rise in blood pressure, further increments of sodium thiopental are given intravenously and the concentration of isoflurane may be increased temporarily. The cuff of the endotracheal tube is inflated and checked to ensure that it adequately prevents leaks. The tube is then taped in place. Controlled ventilation is preferred, with arterial PCO_2 maintained in the range of 30 torr, as demonstrated by frequently sampled arterial blood gases. The arterial blood gases likewise provide a frequent check on the adequacy of oxygenation.

REDUCTION OF BRAIN TENSION

All patients receive 100 g mannitol intravenously while the bone flap is being turned; in many cases, this is preceded by Lasix, 20 mg intravenously. This usually relaxes the brain nicely. Dexamethasone, 4 mg intravenously, is continued every 4 hours.

In many cases of anterior communicating aneurysm, a lumbar subarachnoid spinal catheter is quite helpful. After the induction of anesthesia, such a catheter (22-gauge polyethylene tubing) can be introduced via a Touhy needle. Only a small amount of fluid is allowed to escape at the time of introduction. The catheter is led in such a fashion that additional fluid can be removed by the anesthesiologist upon request.

CONTROLLED HYPOTENSION

Careful communication between the neuroanesthesiologist and the surgeon is crucial.[6] Of particular importance is the pharmacologic control of blood pressure during surgery. Controlled hypotension is used to slacken the aneursym during dissection in order to decrease the likelihood of intraoperative rupture. In most patients, the systolic blood pressure is maintained at about 100 torr during the initial exposure. Once the aneurysm is in view, the pressure is further dropped to about 90 systolic. During critical dissection of the neck of the aneurysm, deep hypotension may rarely be used to prevent rupture (systolic blood pressure of 60 torr or a mean arterial blood pressure of about 40 torr). Most patients tolerate this brief hypotension without postoperative sequelae. In patients with subarachnoid hemorrhage, however, autoregulation may be lost in some zones, and in some elderly patients, prolonged hypotension may not be well tolerated by the brain, heart, and kidneys. In such cases, levels of controlled hypotension can be moderated.

In many cases, moderate hypotension can be achieved simply by increasing the concentration of inspired isoflurane. Sodium nitroprusside often will be required in order to further diminish the blood pressure. Formerly, we often used hypotension, but now use it only occasionally. We recently have obviated the need for deep hypotension in most cases by utilizing temporary clips under mannitol protection as described by Suzuki (see below).[7]

VASOSPASM

In patients with vasospasm suspected or proven by angiography or cerebral blood flow, care is taken not to lower the blood pressure. Once the aneurysm is obliterated, cerebral perfusion is maximized by volume expansion with colloid and packed cells if necessary. In cases in which vasospasm is noted or suspected, the patient is placed on a mannitol regimen, 100 g intravenously every 8 hours.[3] Blood pressure is elevated to about 160 torr systolic, using a pressor if necessary.

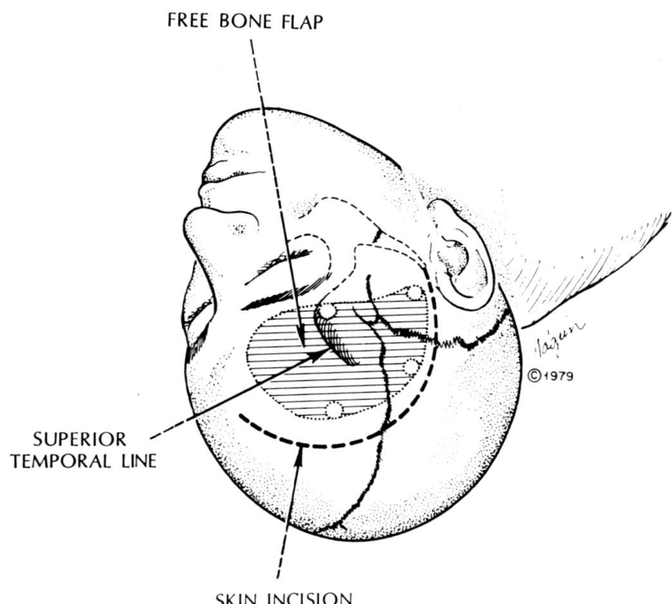

Fig. 84-2. Incision and pterional craniotomy. The skin incision is just behind the hairline and the anterior branch of the superficial temporal artery. Key burr hole lies just behind the zygomatic process of the frontal bone and inferior to the superior temporal line. Often 3 burr holes are sufficient.

OPERATIVE TECHNIQUE

POSITIONING AND PREPARATION

In most cases, the approach is from the right side. The head is turned to the left about 60 degrees, with the zygoma uppermost and the vertex depressed slightly below the horizontal plane. In some cases, a small roll is placed under the right shoulder of patients with limited mobility of the neck. Indications for a left subfrontal approach include an additional left-sided aneurysm, a large anterior communicating artery aneurysm pointing sharply toward the right, or a large dominant left A1 feeder with no right A1 visualized on the angiogram.

The scalp sites are prepared with an antibiotic solution, and then the Mayfield-Kees three-point headrest is applied. Additional increments of sodium thiopental (50 mg IV) are given just before this painful stimulation.

Protective plastic shields are placed across the eyes. The proposed incision site is shaved, and sterile towels are placed to wall off the area. Elastic bandages or pneumatic compression boots are used on the lower extremities to help prevent thrombophlebitis. The operating table then is positioned in the operating room; the anesthetist and anesthesia equipment are situated at the patient's left side, below shoulder level to provide satisfactory room for the operating microscope. The scrub nurse stands on the patient's right side, with the instrument table over the patient's chest and abdomen.

INCISION

After the operative site has been prepared, the incision is marked with a marking pen (Figure 84-2). In most cases, an incision just behind the hairline is preferred, proceeding from the widow's peak curvilinearly to a point just above the zygoma in front of the tragus. The superficial temporal artery is palpated

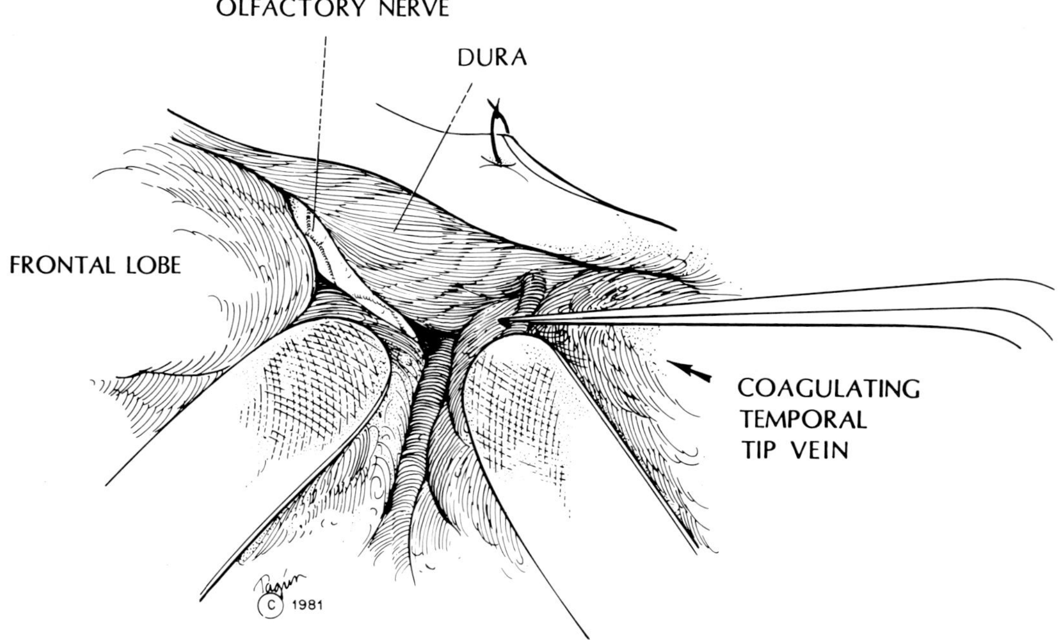

Fig. 84-3. Elevation of the frontal lobes. This is done gradually, with suction removal of CSF. The olfactory tract leads back to the optic nerve. Temporal bridging veins are coagulated and cut near the cortex.

and marked. The incision should lie posterior to the root of the superficial temporal artery in order to preserve this structure with the flap. Occasionally in bald persons or in cases in which additional exposure is desired for another aneurysm, an alternative incision may be planned, using a wrinkle high in the forehead or a coronal incision extending across the midline.

Both the surgeon and the assistant use magnification loupes and headlights during the initial phases of the procedure. Local anesthesia (1-percent lidocaine with 1:400,000 epinephrine) is injected along the incision, except near the superficial temporal artery. The incision is begun anteriorly and cuts down to but not through the periosteum. Care is taken to avoid injury to the superficial temporal artery, particularly near its root. The posterior branch of this artery is dissected free and divided between 3-0 silk ligatures, thus permitting the trunk and frontal branch of the vessel, which might be needed for later cerebral revascularization, to be reflected forward with the soft tissue flap.

Hemostasis is obtained by applying hemostatic clips to both margins of the skin incision. Next, temporalis fascia is excised with a knife and the temporalis muscle is opened with the cutting cautery. A branch of the deep temporal artery is regularly encountered within the muscle, and this must be cauterized accurately in order to avoid pesky bleeding later. The periosteum is swept off the skull with a periosteal elevator just to the edge of the orbit, and the muscle, including the superior temporal line, is reflected from the skull with the cutting cautery until the zygomatic process of the frontal bone is approached. The soft tissue flap is folded over a sponge to prevent ischemic compression and is protected with a sponge soaked in Bacitracin; it is held in place with silk sutures sewn into the muscle and attached by rubber bands to the drapes.

A final maneuver, which permits maximum visualization beneath the muscle, is the application of a Cushing retractor to the muscles along the zygomatic process of the frontal bone. Tension should be applied to these retractors by attaching rubber bands and Allis clamps to the drapes. This approach provides excellent exposure once the bone flap is removed.

INITIAL EXPOSURE

A free peritoneal bone flap is turned with the power drill and craniotome[7] (Figure 84-2). The critical burr hole is placed just behind the zygomatic process of the frontal bone and below the anterior end of the superior temporal line. Additional burr holes are placed in the frontal and the temporal regions, the latter just at the superior temporal line. The unsightly depression of an inferomedial frontal burr hole can be eliminated by making a curved bony cut with the craniotome.

Dura is separated from the inner table of the skull with a No. 3 Penfield dissector. The craniotome cut is made, starting along the floor of the anterior fossa proceeding medially about 3 to 4 cm and then curving in an easy arch posterior to the high temporal bone. It is advisable to angle this soft curve slightly, beveling outward in order to provide nice seating for the bone flap when it is replaced. The lateral sphenoid ridge is preserved with the bone flap, which is finally broken off by prying with a periosteal elevator. The bone flap is gently peeled off the dura and the meningeal artery is identified, coagulated, and cut.

Bony edges are waxed for hemostasis. Additional bone is rongeured from the lateral sphenoid ridge. Care is taken at this point to avoid injury to structures in the superior orbital fissure. A small arterial branch to the dura in this region frequently must be coagulated. These maneuvers level the sphenoid ridge effectively between the frontal and temporal bones, thus creating unobstructed visual access to the anterior clinoid area. In some cases, a high-speed drill can be used to smooth the area. If there is a small opening into the orbit, it should be plugged with Gelfoam or bone wax.

If additional access is needed along the floor of the anterior fossa behind the orbital ridge, the inner table of bone at the edge of the craniotomy just anterior to the keyhole can also be

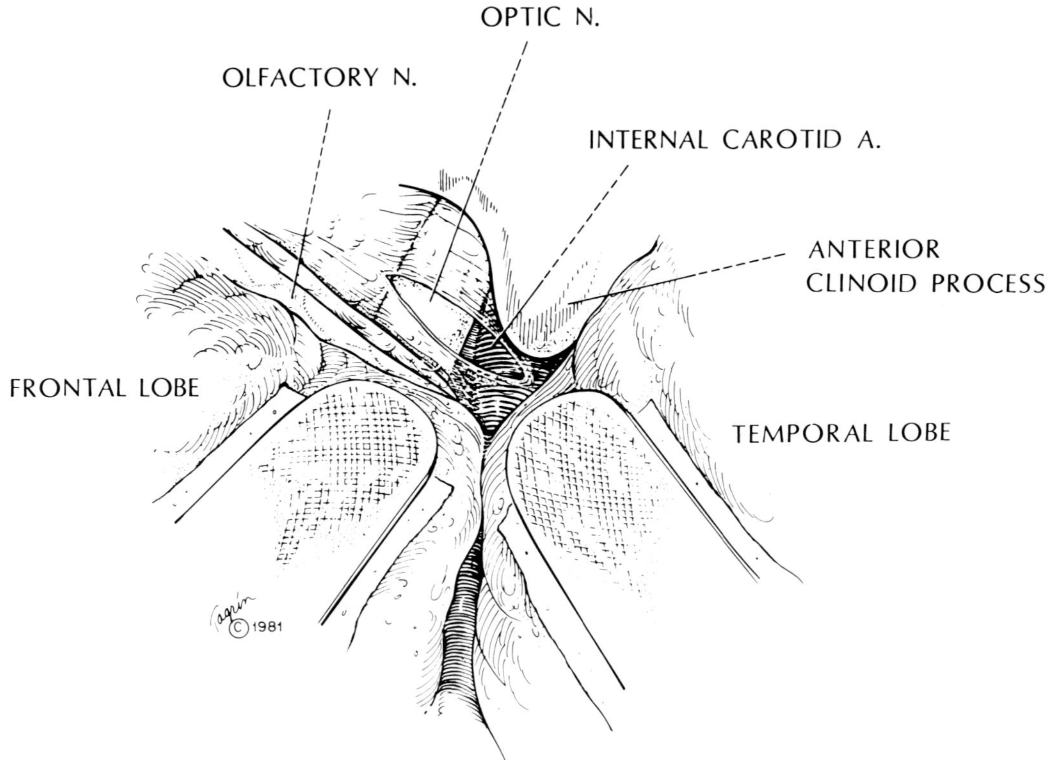

Fig. 84-4.　Incision of the arachnoid. Under the microscope, a sharp hook is used to open the arachnoid over the internal carotid artery and the optic nerve. This permits further elevation of the frontal lobe.

removed with the rongeur without compromising the cosmetic appearance of the outer table. In some patients, a very prominent and lateral frontal sinus may be encountered with the saw cut or bone removal. If this occurs, the mucosa should be removed and the sinus should be packed with Gelfoam soaked in Bacitracin, and the opening in the bone should be covered with a flap of pericranium tissue dissected from the back of the scalp and then sewn to the adjacent dura. Next, the wire-pass drill is used to create holes for wires to hold the flap in place at the time of closure. Sutures of 4-0 silk, attaching the dura to the pericranial tissue, are placed around the periphery of the opening of the bone in order to achieve epidural hemostasis. Tiny strips of Surgicel are inserted in the epidural space as needed. Bacitracin-soaked sponges are placed over the edges of the skin and over all exposed tissue except the dura.

During this phase, the surgeon can readily determine whether the brain is slack. If it is not, then measures must be taken to obtain adequate slackness; the PCO₂ may need adjustment, additional dehydration may be required, and at this stage the anesthesiologist is instructed to withdraw 75 ml of CSF slowly. If the subarachnoid catheter is not working, it occasionally will be necessary to puncture the ventricle in order to obtain a slack brain.

A linear dural incision is made approximately 6 to 8 mm above the inferior margin of the bony opening with inferior turning at the frontal and temporal corners. The inferior dural flap is turned up flush with the bone edge and is held with tacking sutures under tension. Care should be taken to avoid a buckle in the center of this flap, which could interfere with intradural visualization.

The surface of the brain under loupe magnification is inspected for evidence of subdural hematoma, subarachnoid hemorrhage, or cerebral infarction. A medium-width, hand-held brain retractor is used to gently elevate the frontal lobe (Figure 84-3). A sucker on a cottonoid can be used to gradually remove CSF that may be inferior to the frontal lobe. The retractor is advanced slowly just in front of the edge of the sphenoid wing.

The olfactory tract, an important landmark, will come into view, and following this a few millimeters posteriorly will lead to the region of the optic nerve (Figure 84-3). The arachnoid usually is thin and the optic nerve and carotid artery can be visualized, but at times the arachnoid may be relatively thick and obscure these structures. The arachnoid is opened using the fine, right-angled hook and a microdissector or microscissors. Time should then be spent allowing further CSF to drain. It is most important that the brain be so slack that only mild retraction is needed for adequate exposure.

Next, a protective layer of Telfa pre-cut to the proper shape is rolled like a rug over the exposed frontal lobe down to the olfactory tract. At this point, the Greenberg self-retaining retractor system holding a posted retractor blade is placed to elevate the frontal lobe. The retractor should take a low profile in order to give easy access to the infrafrontal cleft. Next, a narrow, hand-held retractor is used to carefully elevate the temporal lobe. Temporal tip bridging veins are divided (Figure 84-3). Once the temporal tip is free, a covering of Telfa is placed and the lobe is held posteriorly with a slender retractor blade fixed on the Greenberg apparatus. The two retractor blades should be separated by only several millimeters at right angles to each other.

Up to this point, the combination of loupes and headlight illumination has been used to allow maximum mobility with adequate visualization. From this point, however, the surgical operating microscope is used to maximize illumination and visualization of critical structures.

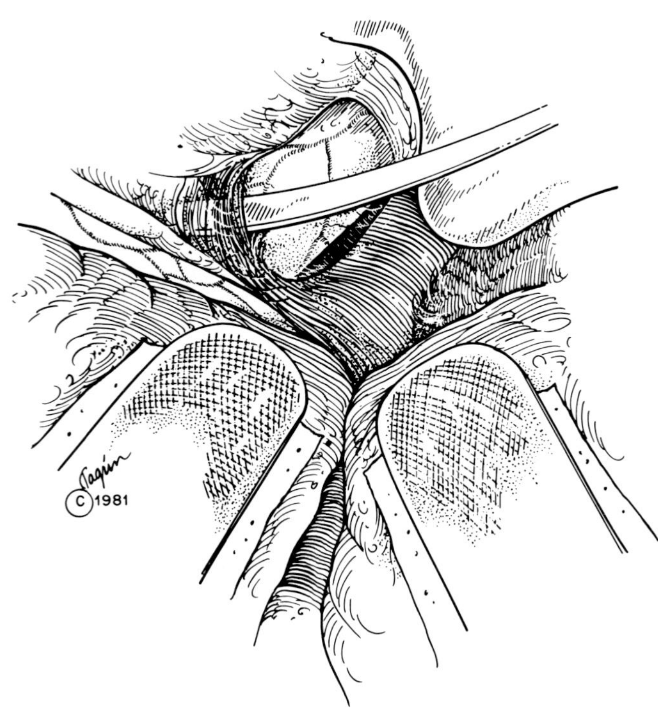

Fig. 84-5. Dissection of the right A1 artery. The anterior border of the vessel is freed of the arachnoid with a Rhoton No. 6 dissector and microscissors.

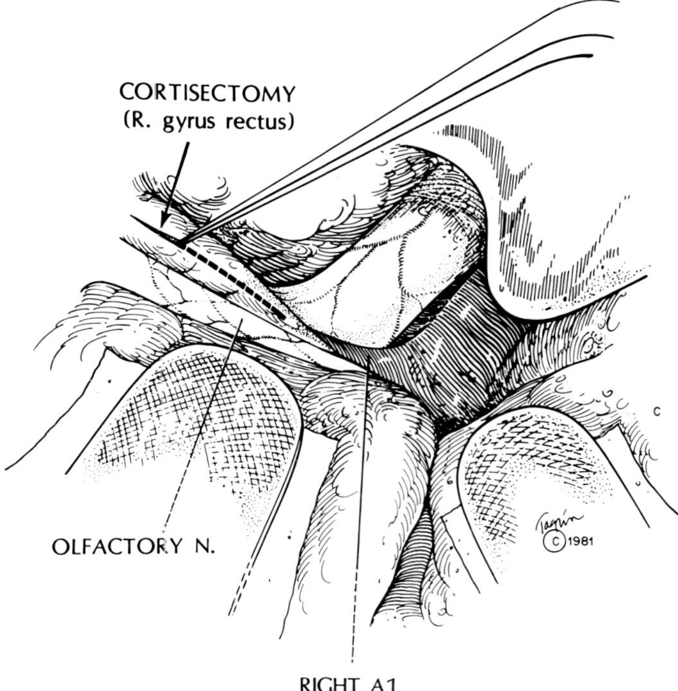

Fig. 84-6. Gyrus rectus corticectomy. Bipolar cauterization and incision of the pia over 1–1.5 cm. Care must be taken to place the corticectomy over the aneurysm site (usually near the medial edge of the optic nerve).

MICROSURGICAL DISSECTION

We use the Wild microscope with a 300-mm objective lens, 12.5× eyepieces, and a variable-angle binocular tube for microsurgical dissection. The visual image is channelled by a 50:50 small beam splitter to an observer tube on one side and a unified adapter for video and intermittent still photography on the other side. A clear image projected on a monitor in the corner of the operating theater provides access to the microsurgical action for all members of the microsurgical team, including the scrub nurse and anesthesiologist.

Dissection begins on the internal carotid artery (Figure 84-4). The surgeon opens the cistern of the internal carotid artery further using a 16-gauge sucker in the left hand and a fine arachnoid hook in the right, permitting free egress of CSF. With a fine dissector, the internal carotid is followed distally. In some cases, the right A1 anterior cerebral artery takeoff can be visualized and the anterior edge of this vessel followed medially toward the aneurysm (Figure 84-5). This procedure leads right to the aneurysm and avoids an excessively large gyrus rectus incision.

In other cases, however, the internal carotid artery segment is long and the anterior cerebral origin is high and posteriorly placed. In such instances, excessive frontal retraction would be needed to see the origin of A1, and it is wisest to proceed directly to gyrus rectus corticectomy. A controlled sucker device is helpful in providing adequate low-level suction without the danger of suction injury to important structures. Retraction at this point involves not only elevation of the frontal lobe and olfactory tract, but also a gentle lifting of the lobe away from the interhemispheric fissure. Only when the brain is slack can this type of critical retraction be obtained and held. The direction of view at this point proceeds from temporally quite

medially, facilitated by marked leftward turning of the head. If the head is not turned far enough up to the left, the surgeon will bend to the right in an awkward fashion.

A corticectomy is made in the gyrus rectus[8] just medial to the olfactory tract, beginning at the optic nerve and extending anteriorly for about 1.5 cm (Figure 84-6). The incision is deepened until the pia arachnoid over the A1 segment first and then the interhemispheric fissure is reached. This protection overlying the aneurysm is left intact. The arachnoid overlying the right A1 anterior cerebral artery is opened (Figure 84-7).

Once the right A1 anterior cerebral artery is visualized, it is wise to bring the blood pressure into the range of 90 to 100 torr systolic in most patients. Branches of this vessel, which may include Heubner's artery, should be preserved. The A1 segment is followed distally to the anterior communicating artery and then to the right A2 anterior cerebral artery.[8] If possible, the aneurysm is avoided at this stage.

Dissection proceeds with a combination of blunt dissection and a fine microdissector and microscissors for cutting the arachnoid after electrocoagulation. Next, the left A2 anterior cerebral artery is identified in the interhemispheric fissure (Figure 84-8). The angiograms are checked to determine whether the left A2 anterior cerebral artery is anterior or posterior to its right-sided counterpart, then the vessel is sought in the appropriate direction. Once the left A2 is identified, it can be followed retrograde to the left A1 anterior cerebral artery.

Careful scrutiny of the angiogram and knowledge of anatomic variance guide the dissection. Important normal variants include: (1) a hypoplastic A1 segment; (2) (multiple) reduplicated anterior communicating arteries; and (3) a persistent artery to the corpus callosum from the anterior communicating

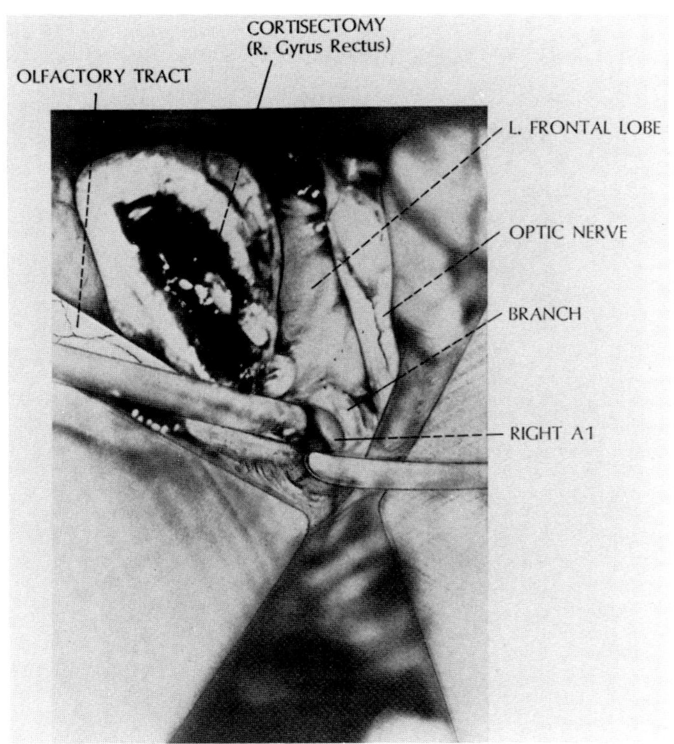

Fig. 84-7. Dissection of the right A1 artery through the corticectomy. The microscope has been directed more medially. Suction and bipolar cauterization remove the cortex down to the interhemispheric pia-arachnoid. With a fine dissector, the pia-arachnoid is removed from the right A1 artery and the neck of the aneurysm.

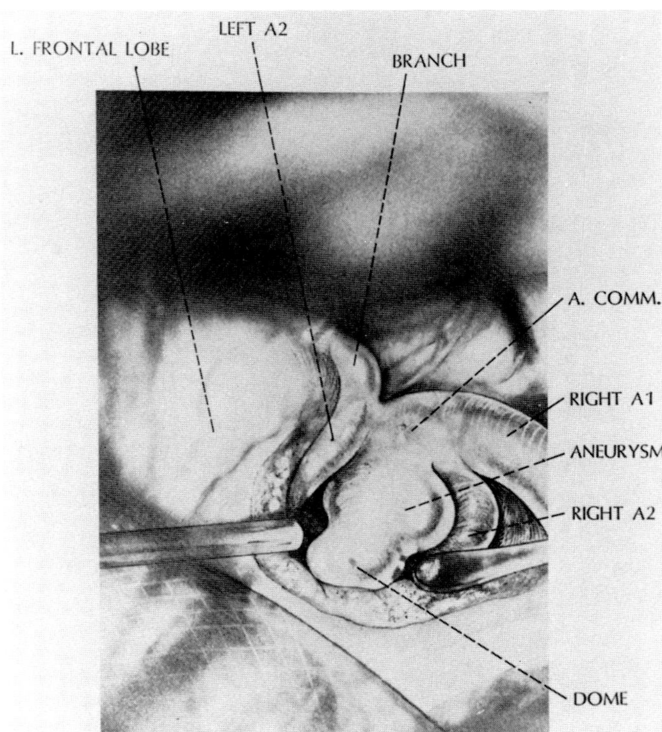

Fig. 84-8. Dissection of an aneurysm. Proceeding clockwise, the surgeon frees up the right A1 and A2 arteries, then the left A2 and A1 arteries. Finally, the aneurysm is encircled, and the dome and neck are completely dissected.

artery. The aneurysm almost always arises from the junction of the larger A1 and anterior communicating artery.

As the surgeon seeks to identify the left anterior cerebral artery segments, significant retraction of the aneurysm is often needed. This is best accomplished by leaving pia-arachnoid overlying the lesion, with retraction applied by the suckers through an intervening cottonoid. The surgeon should seek to identify and free all major arterial trunks before working on the aneurysm. Dissection then proceeds with a microdissector or the combination of cautery and division of adhesive bands.

The avenue of attack depends on the direction in which the aneurysm projects. For the lesion that projects straight up from the anterior communicating artery, the left A1 anterior cerebral artery may be most accessible ventrally. In this situation, the anterior portion of the aneurysm and frontal lobe are gently reflected superiorly and back, permitting sharp dissection of the aneurysm neck away from the superior surface of the chiasm and both optic nerves. In this way, the ventral aspect of the anterior communicating artery and the left A1 anterior cerebral artery may be identified.

When the lesion projects forward, as is most common, access to the left A1 is easiest from behind the lesion. When the aneurysm points posteriorly next to the perforant branches, dissection of the ventral neck may be directed ventral to A2 in order to avoid a tear in the neck. In any event, encirclement of the lesion is required. At this stage, it is wise to leave in place any small, potentially important arterial branches that are adherent to the dome of the lesion.

TEMPORARY CLIPPING AND CEREBRAL PROTECTION

A particularly thin-walled lesion or one requiring substantial manipulation for clipping presents a greater than usual danger of rupture. For these situations (perhaps a quarter of cases), we use temporary clipping. For cerebral protection, 100 g of mannitol is given intravenously 15 minutes before the application of temporary clips proximal and distal to the aneurysm. At the same time, systolic blood pressure is elevated to the 160–170-torr level in order to enhance collateral circulation.[7] This will give about 45 minutes of time to dissect the aneurysm and apply a permanent clip. (Temporary clips can be released every 5 minutes for even greater protection, as suggested by Drake.)

DISSECTION OF THE NECK OF THE ANEURYSM

A sucker, with or without a cottonoid, is used to reflect the lesion to one side, and a fine dissector or microscissors frees the neck from adherent structures. When visualization permits, sharp dissection is preferable. Usually the microscope provides identification of a cleavage plane right to the edge of the neck. It is wise to dissect a bit up on the dome initially, in case of a tear in the neck itself, which can be disastrous. It is necessary to reflect the lesion to ensure preservation of the perforating branches of the anterior communicating artery (Figure 84-9). These vessels are often adherent to the ventral posterior wall of the aneurysm and must be carefully separated from it.

In many cases, direct reflection of the aneurysm anteriorly while peering over the right A2 artery will give the needed view.

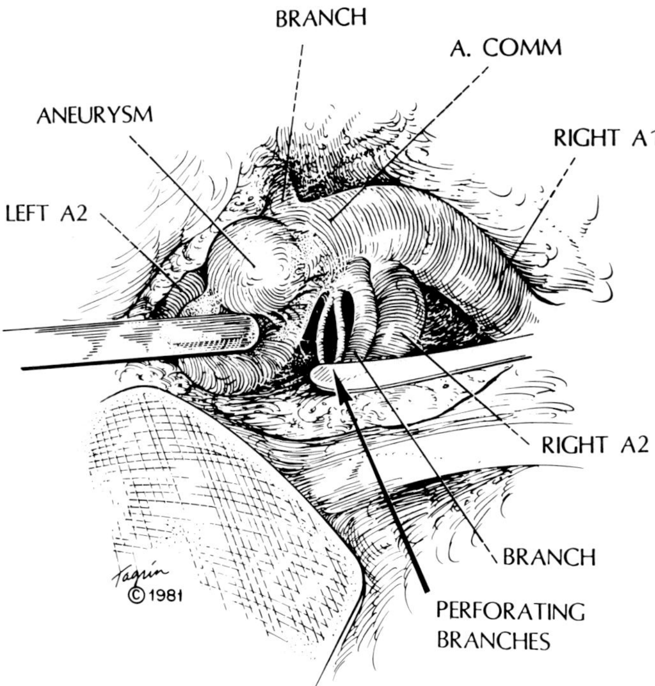

Fig. 84-9. Dissection of perforating branches. These crucial vessels emerge from the anterior communicating artery and proceed posteriorly to the hypothalamus. They must be gently freed from the aneurysm and excluded from clipping.

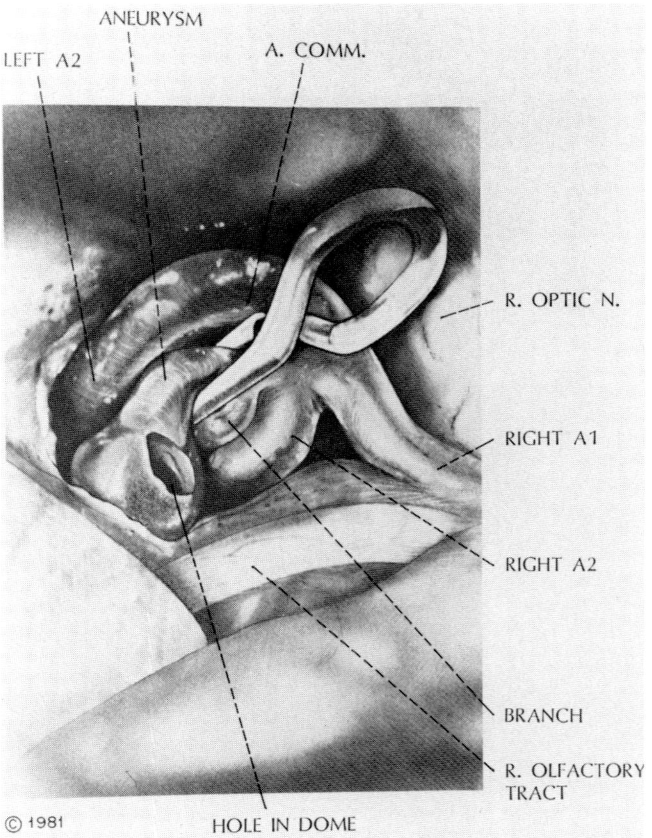

Fig. 84-10. Clipping the aneurysm. The entire lesion is obliterated, with preservation of the trunk and perforating arteries. The aneurysm is opened to prove the adequacy of clipping.

In some instances, however, for the posteriorly or posteroinferiorly directed lesion, a reflection of the aneurysm and the right A2 arteries superiorly will give a nice view of the ventral aspect of these structures and of their plane of separation from the perforators. In a similar fashion, forward rotation of a downward-pointing lesion may help free adherent branches.

Whatever the technique, the primary aim is clear cleavage between the ventroposterior aspect of the aneurysm and the numerous vertical perforating arteries emanating from the posterior aspect of the anterior communicating artery. It is particularly important that this be achieved before clipping of the aneurysm, because visualization of these perforators during application of the clip is frequently difficult or impossible. Occasionally, preservation of these perforators is inconsistent with complete obliteration of the aneurysm. On two such occasions, we have purposely occluded a single perforator, then maintained perfusion with mannitol and hyperperfusion, and were pleased to note no deficit.

Finally, adherent arterial branches overlying the dome of the aneurysm can be dissected free. Such branches may yield to blunt dissection with a right-angled hook or with a ball dissector. In some cases, in which the actual visualization of the arachnoid bands is possible, sharp dissection with scissors may be preferred. With temporary clips, the aneurysm may be aspirated in order to ease dissection. If aneurysmal rupture occurs at this point, the problem can be controlled, since the aneurysm neck has essentially been completely dissected.

ANEURYSMAL RUPTURE

In case of aneurysmal rupture at any point during dissection, deliberate action is necessary. Initially, the bleeding should be controlled with suction. In some cases, this can be accomplished

with a fine sucker (No. 16) or a large sucker (No. 7 or No. 1). Very careful direction of the sucker tip to the precise point of bleeding should be attempted to clear the field of blood entirely. Then precise coagulation with the bipolar cautery or application of a bit of Surgicel or muscle compression for a few minutes may seal a minor leak. When hemostasis can be obtained in this fashion, it is best to direct dissection to another corner and return to the area of hemorrhage at a later time.

In other cases bleeding is brisker. When the neck is prepared, direct application of a clip may be appropriate. If this stops the bleeding, inspection determines the adequacy of clipping. If clip position is good, accept it as final. If the position is not ideal, the clip is regarded as preliminary, permitting complete dissection of the lesion and subsequent repositioning. When the neck is not ready to be clipped, temporary clips are applied to both A1 and A2 arteries that have already been dissected. Hypertension and mannitol are used for cerebral protection. This maneuver may permit continued dissection, with final application of the clip to the neck of the lesion. In all events, the surgeon must proceed in an orderly fashion with temporary hemostasis, precise visualization of the source of hemorrhage and its relation to critical structures, and then accurate clipping.

OBLITERATION OF THE ANEURYSM

In the majority of cases, a *metal aneurysm clip* is the best solution (Figure 84-10). Once the lesion has been completely dissected and the relationship of its neck is defined (to sur-

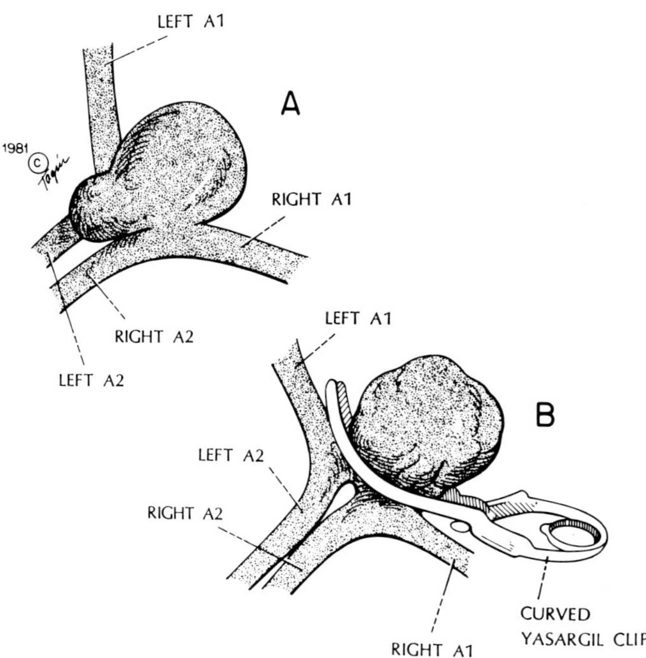

Fig. 84-11. Problem: Posterior bulge. A sucker gathers up the bulge for inclusion in a curved Yasargil clip.

rounding critical structures including the perforating arteries), the surgeon can judge what technique will best obliterate the lesion. We have usually used a Sugita or Yasargil clip. The long, straight Sugita clip is particularly effective for upward-pointing lesions. Because of the angle of the application, the variable-angle Sano clip applier frequently is most useful. The Sugita clip is also useful for lesions with a wide neck, because of its narrow blade and wide-opening jaws. The Yasargil clip is used for lesions with necks smaller than 5 mm.

Often a projecting lobe can be gathered up with the sucker tip into the jaws of a Sugita or Yasargil clip (Figure 84-11). When release is difficult with the Yasargil or Sugita clips, it can be facilitated by distracting the handle blades of the clip applier with the third and fourth fingers placed inferiorly.

Occasionally, a *fenestrated Sugita clip* may be needed,[9] with the aperture enclosing either the right or left A1 anterior cerebral artery segments (Figure 84-12). Sometimes a slight curve or even a very abrupt curve will be handy to approximate an aneurysm neck. At times, the force of two clips may be needed to ensure complete closure of a thick aneurysmal wall. A Sundt booster clip or an obliquely applied Sugita clip serves this purpose nicely.

In the case of giant anterior communicating aneurysms, the Sugita clip or the Drake clip (up to 30 mm) may provide the only accurate and adequate clipping. Precise application of the clip is required. The clip is advanced gently with tiny axial rotational wiggles to reduce drag. Generally it is possible to visualize one of two blades as it advances. The clip is advanced until the tips are just behind the opposite side of the neck, as previously calculated, and as actually visualized in most cases. If significant resistance is encountered, one should stop and remove the clip. Adequate dissection with freeing of arachnoid attachments will eliminate significant resistance, which could lead to perforation of the lesion with the clip.

In case of an aneurysm with a paper-thin neck, *temporary clipping* may be needed just at the time of clip application. If only 2 or 3 minutes are needed, special cerebral protection

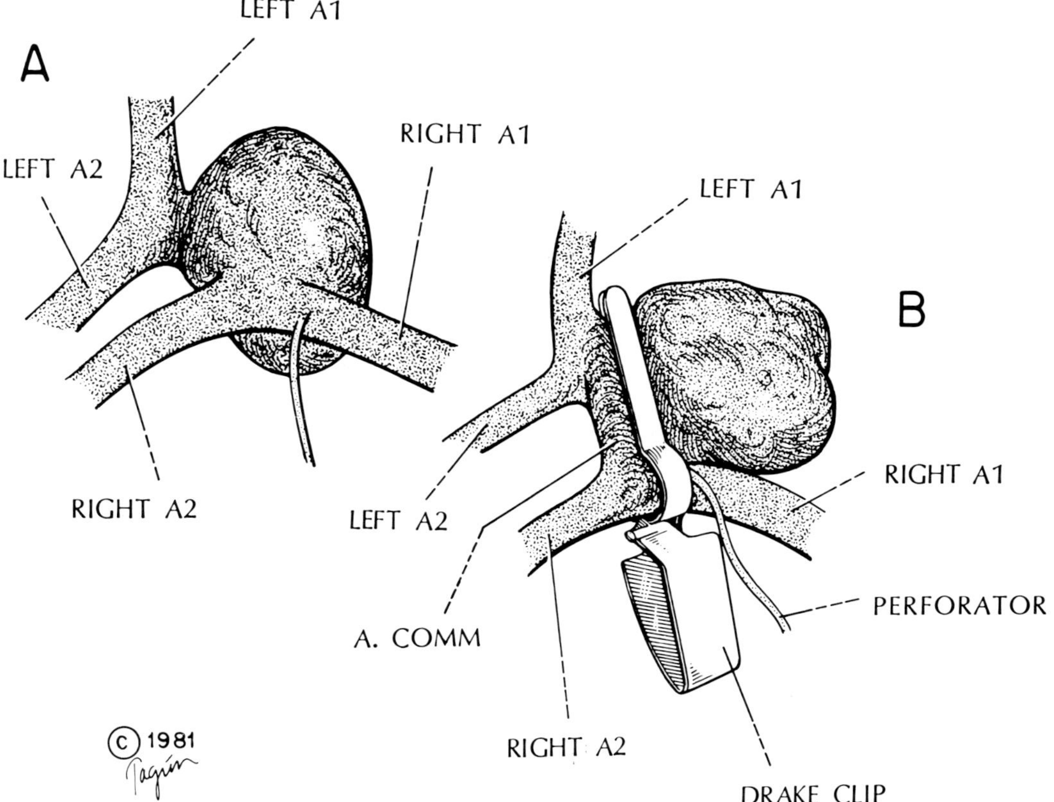

Fig. 84-12. Problem: Common wall for aneurysms and right A1 artery. A fenestrated clip opens the right A1 and perforant arteries.

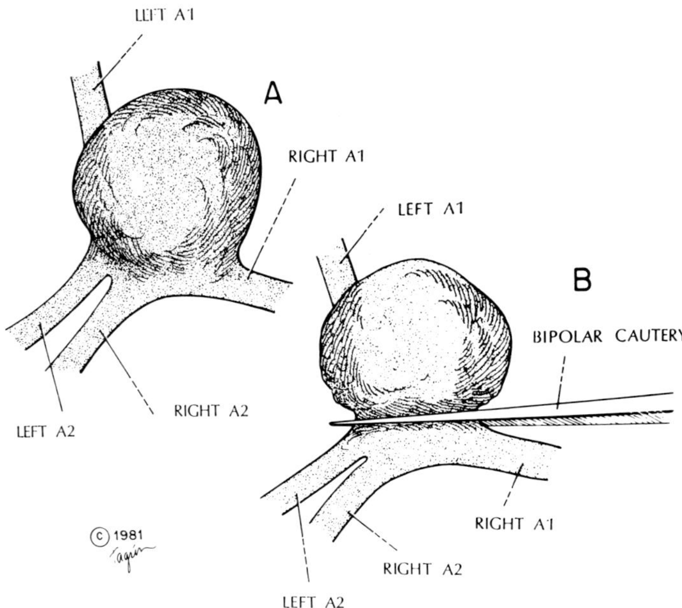

Fig. 84-13. Problem: Broad base. Bipolar cauterization of the neck excludes all native arteries.

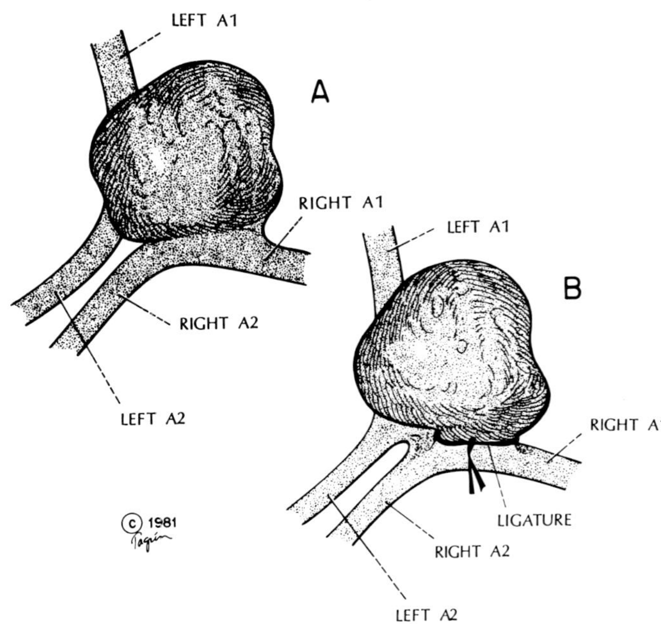

Fig. 84-14. Problem: Broad base. A ligature narrows the base to permit clipping.

seems unnecessary. After clip application, one must check the adequacy of clipping and the condition of the native circulation. The clip tips must be visualized beyond the opposite edge of the lesion, and the entire aneurysm should be obliterated. Both anterior cerebral arteries and the anterior communicating artery with its perforating vessels must be maintained intact. If these criteria are not satisfied, the clip may need repositioning, even multiple repositioning to obtain a satisfactory application.

Satisfactory clipping of the lesion can be proven by *aspiration of the dome* of the aneurysm with a 25-gauge spinal needle (Figure 84-10). If bleeding from the aneurysm persists after the needle perforation, further obliteration will be needed. Finally, the surgeon should be satisfied that, as retractors are removed, the clip will not produce dangerous torque on the aneurysmal neck or produce compression of the optic nerve or brain.

In some cases, *bipolar cauterization of the neck* of the aneurysm may be helpful (Figure 84-13). This technique, initiated by Yasargil, can narrow the neck for easier clipping. In addition, it may thicken the neck, eliminating dangerous thin spots in the area. Laboratory practice is helpful in learning the technique, and several technical pointers may be useful. Broad forceps tips are preferred. The bipolar cautery should be set low, with prior testing of its electrocautery effect. The blades of the forceps should pass completely across the neck of the lesion since there is a danger that the points may cause electrocautery damage to the neck. As current is applied, very gentle pressure and release are applied several times. Ideally, a slow coagulation with whitening and thickening of the neck is produced without charring or sudden effects. The area of the coagulation should be continuously irrigated while it is being performed. In some cases, the coagulation may completely obliterate the neck, but more commonly a simple thickening without total obliteration of the neck will be achieved.

Sometimes a *ligature* helps, particularly in lesions with a wide neck or in cases in which it is difficult to decide on a clear area for a clip (Figure 84-14). Generally 3-0 silk is best. A variety of ligature passers are available. Often where space is

limited, the ligature can be placed deep to the lesion with fine forceps. The surgeon then reflects the lesion to the opposite side, searching for the ligature beyond the lesion's neck and retrieving it gently with a forceps. After the ligature is placed about the neck of the lesion, a surgeon's knot is fashioned and gently pulled taut. In some cases, the neck can be obliterated totally by these maneuvers. In most cases, the ligature narrows the neck for subsequent clipping.

Rarely, a lesion here defies clipping and ligation. In such instances, *reinforcement with muslin* may be the safest technique. However, this material must be kept off the optic nerves in order to avoid neuropathy.[10] In case of optic arachnoiditis, steroid therapy and scar removal may improve vision.

After the aneurysm is obliterated, Surgicel is applied to the edges of the corticectomy. At this point, the neuroanesthetist gradually raises the blood pressure to the normal level for that patient. The surgeon carefully checks to make certain that hemostasis at the aneurysm site is adequate.

CLOSURE

Irrigation is carried out with saline. When the brain is slack, substantial saline can be added to fill the subdural space. The dura is closed. Surgicel is placed in the epidural space for hemostasis. The bone flap is wired in place with 28-gauge stainless wire sutures, and the dura is apposed to the bone flap with a central tenting suture. The muscle, galea, and skin are closed with appropriate sutures.

INDIRECT OPERATION

Some giant aneurysms cannot be effectively obliterated by direct attack. This circumstance can be predicted from the angiogram in some cases, but it usually can be ascertained only at the time of surgery. For such aneurysms, the Odom procedure is the safest approach.[11] This entails placing a clip on the dominant A1 artery, with occlusion of the cervical carotid artery on the opposite side. Formerly, common carotid occlusion with a gradual occluding clamp was the procedure of choice. Recent reports indicate that the safest approach may be occlusion of the internal carotid artery with a detachable balloon, with or without cerebral revascularization.

Studies of cerebral blood flow can be helpful in determining the adequacy of collateral circulation. At the present time, we achieve internal carotid artery occlusion with a percutaneous transfemoral detachable balloon technique. We perform the balloon occlusion under cerebral blood flow control in the angiography suite. After balloon occlusion of the cerebral internal carotid artery, the patient is heparinized for 3 days.

POSTOPERATIVE MANAGEMENT

The patient is treated prophylactically against vasospasm at the completion of the procedure. The central venous pressure is brought to 10 cm H_2O with colloid if there is no cardiac contraindication. The blood pressure is maintained in the range of 110 to 140 torr systolic with volume and pressors as required. Medications include dexamethasone, 4 mg q6h IV, which is tapered off after 3 days, an antacid, and Dilantin, 300 mg/day. The use of elastic stockings or pneumatic compression boots is continued until the patient is ambulatory.

In the event of neurologic deterioration, a CT scan is performed immediately in search of an intracranial hematoma, hydrocephalus, or cerebral edema. Appropriate treatment is instituted if one of these conditions is found. An angiogram is performed if the CT fails to disclose an adequate explanation for the deterioration. If a vascular occlusion by the clip is disclosed, adjustment of the clip might be indicated. More commonly, cerebral vasospasm may be demonstrated. If significant vasospasm is seen, additional treatment is indicated. The central venous pressure should be elevated to the range of 10 to 12 cm with colloid, and systolic blood pressure should be increased to the range of 160–180 torr systolic. (Dopamine or Neosynephrine can be used for this purpose.) The mannitol regimen is instituted.

Postoperative angiography is not recommended in cases in which the aneurysm has been aspirated and maintenance of normal vasculature has been ascertained during surgery. If there is a question regarding completeness of clipping or vascular occlusion, then angiography is warranted.

ILLUSTRATIVE CASES

USE OF CBF STUDIES, MANNITOL/HYPERTENSION, AND DELAYED SURGERY

Case 1. This 64-year-old, right-handed woman experienced a sudden extraocular severe bifrontal headache. Five minutes later, she had a brief syncopal episode. On admission to a local hospital, a lumbar puncture showed blood in the subarachnoid space. Past medical history was remarkable for hypertension and 2 myocardial infarctions. Physical examination on transfer demonstrated a blood pressure of 150/90 and a normal neurologic examination. Her neck was remarkably stiff.

A CT scan showed a small amount of blood in the basal cisterns and interhemispheric fissure, suggesting an anterior communicating artery aneurysm. The patient was placed on a regimen of Amicar and blood pressure control. The cerebral blood flow study revealed decreased blood flow throughout the

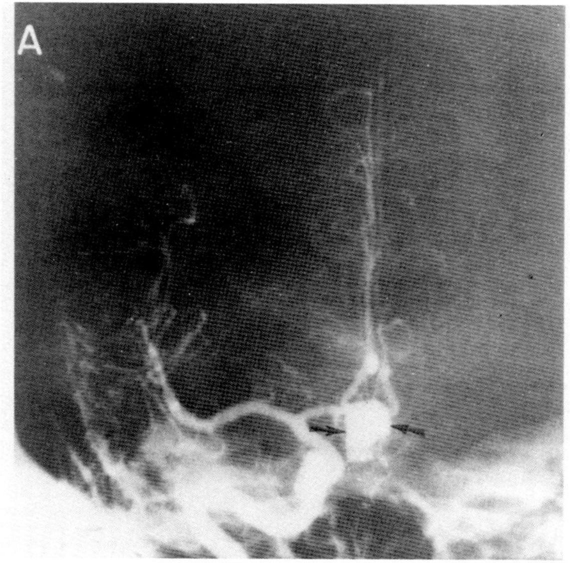

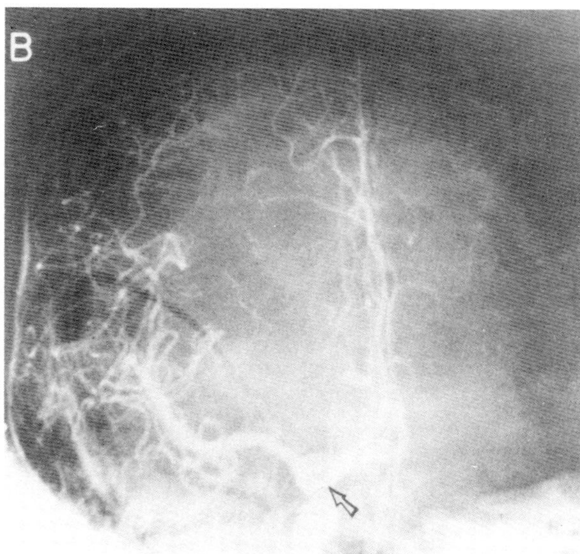

Fig. 84-15. Case 1: Typical clipping of an aneurysm. (A) A preoperative angiogram shows the aneurysm pointing downward (closed arrows). (B) A postoperative angiogram shows a Yasargil clip (open arrow) obliterating the aneurysm.

brain. A cerebral angiogram study showed an anterior communicating artery aneurysm with moderate spasm of the anterior cerebral and left middle cerebral arteries. Because of the spasm and low cerebral blood flow, surgery was delayed.

On the fifth day after subarachnoid hemorrhage, the patient developed dysphasia and drift of her right upper extremity. Hyperperfusion therapy and mannitol were initiated. The patient gradually improved, but was left with a mild dysphasia. On day 14, the patient had another cerebral blood flow study which was normal, and a repeat angiogram revealed marked improvement in vasospasm (Figure 84-15A).

Subsequently, a frontotemporal craniotomy was carried out. Through a gyrus rectus approach, the aneurysm was dissected free and clipped with a curved Yasargil clip. A reduplicated anterior communicating artery was noted. After surgery, the patient was initially bright and awake, but gradually became drowsy and dysphasic. Dopamine was infused with

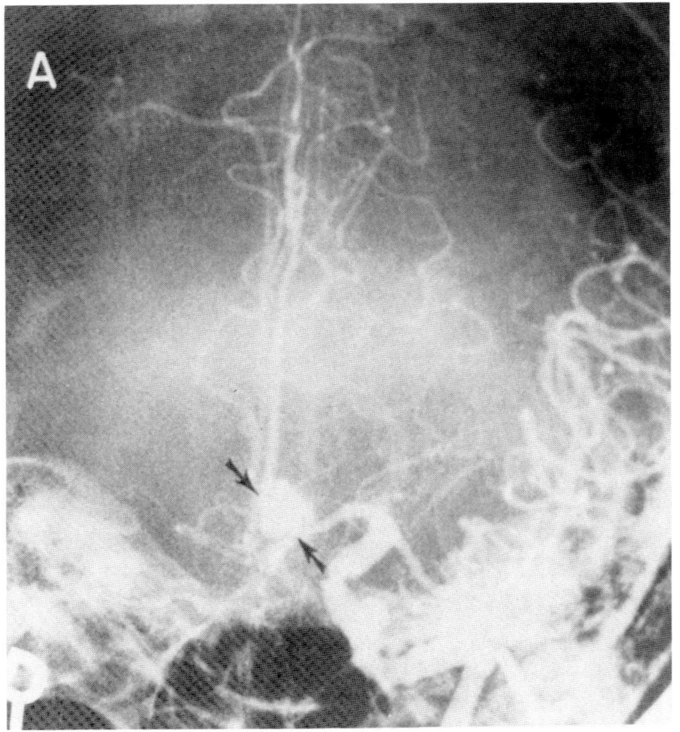

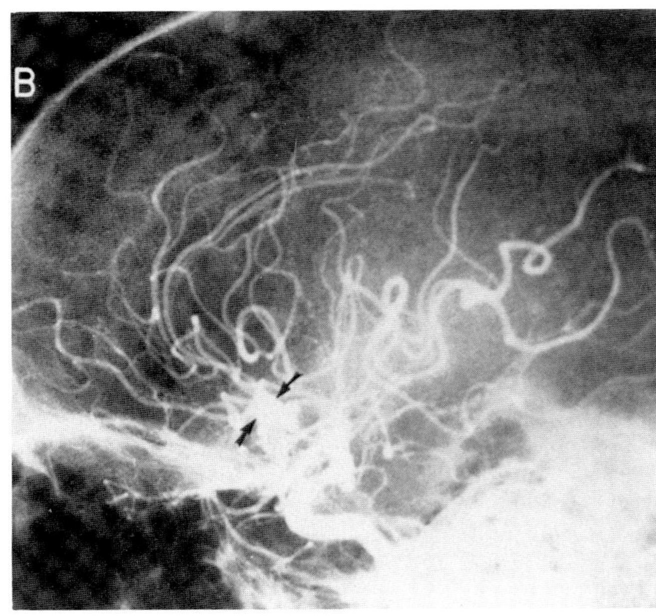

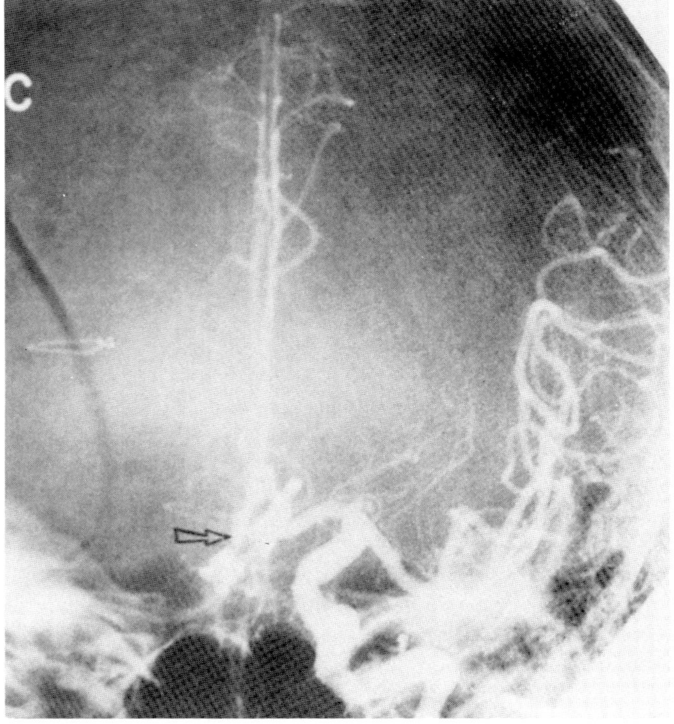

Fig. 84-16. Case 2: Some unusual features. (A and B) A preoperative left carotid angiogram shows an aneurysm pointing anteriorly (closed arrow). At surgery clot was found around arteries shown angiographically to be in spasm. (C and D) A postoperative left carotid angiogram shows a Drake clip (open arrow) encircling the present A2 artery.

elevation of the blood pressure to the range of 150 to 170 torr systolic. Mannitol was given. The patient improved markedly with regard to mental status. She made a gradual complete recovery of speech and motor function. Postoperative angiography 10 days later disclosed complete obliteration of the aneurysm and no residual vasospasm (Figure 84-15B).

Comment: This case illustrates how vasospasm can cause worsening neurologic deficits. Cerebral blood flow studies and hyperperfusion therapy before and after surgery reversed deficits. We prefer to delay surgery until neurologic status is normal with improving angiographic vasospasm.

SPINAL DRAINAGE IMPROVES CLINICAL STATUS; REMOVAL OF PERIARTERIAL HEMATOMA

Case 2. This 59-year-old, right-handed woman passed out and awoke a few minutes later. Within 1 hour, she experienced the onset of bioccipital headache and neck pain. At a local hospital, the neurologic examination showed a left Babinski sign and mild drowsiness. A lumbar puncture revealed grossly bloody cerebrospinal fluid, xanthochromia, and an opening pressure of 18 mm of CSF.

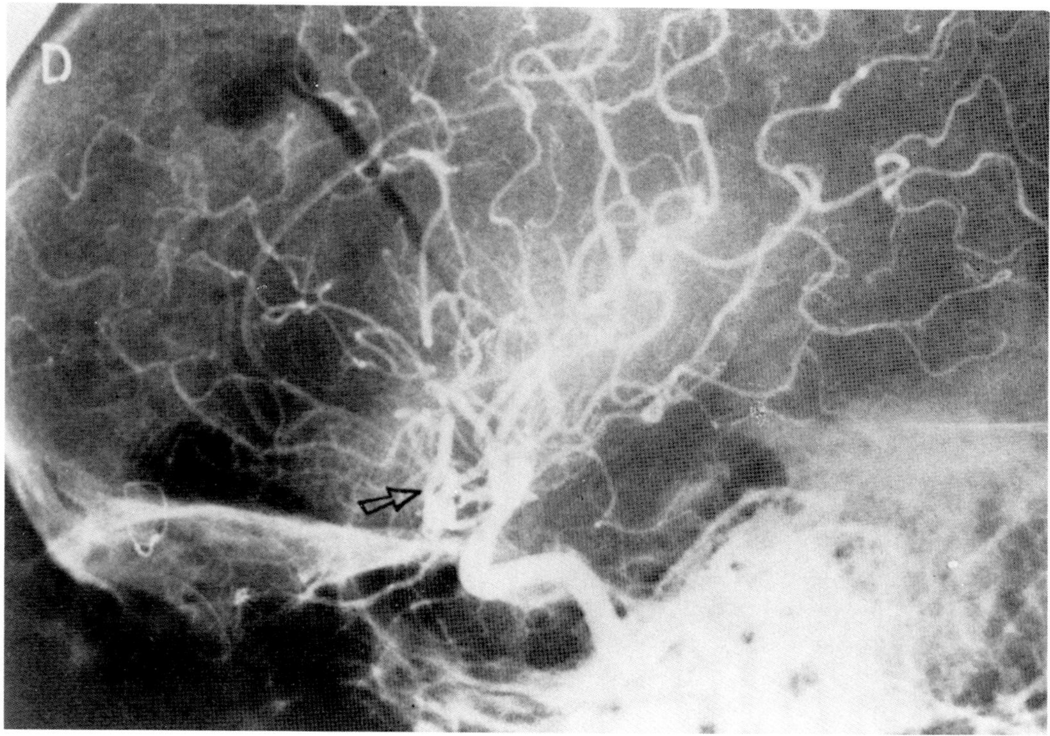

Fig. 84-16 (cont.)

Neurologic examination at the time of transfer, 24 hours after the onset of illness, showed no deficits, and the blood pressure was 159/88 torr. A CT scan showed blood in the basal cisterns. The patient was placed on a medical program including epsilon-amninocaproic acid, blood pressure control, and sedation. There was mild intermittent confusion, progressing to marked obtundation on day 7. Angiography performed at that time showed a multilobular anterior communicating artery aneurysm with severe internal carotid artery spasm bilaterally and slow distal flow. The ventricles were enlarged. Continuous spinal drainage was instituted with prompt improvement of the mental status to the point of spontaneous discussion of her own illness.

On the 17th day, the angiogram was repeated, and diminished vasospasm was noted (Figure 84-16A and B). The cerebral blood flow study at this time was normal.

On the 18th day, a right frontotemporal craniotomy was performed. An extensive subarachnoid clot was removed from around the right and left internal carotid arteries, and the distal left cerebral artery A1 segment. A Drake clip was used to obliterate the aneurysm, with the aperture encircling the right A2 segment and perforating vessels. There was mild postoperative obtundation, with return to preoperative status by 3 days.

Over the 3 weeks following the operation, there was waxing and waning abulia and memory abnormality; her gait was normal. A lumbar puncture showed an opening pressure of 88 mm, and a CT scan showed moderate ventricle enlargement, somewhat greater than was true preoperatively. The patient gradually improved spontaneously. Angiography 1 month after surgery showed obliteration of the aneurysm, with mild right A1 vascular narrowing (Figure 84-16C and D). Four months after surgery, the patient had returned to an entirely normal mental status.

Comment: Early CT scans showed a large amount of subarachnoid clot and predicted later serious spasm. The case of this patient illustrates how hydrocephalus and vasospasm may together lead to deterioration. Prompt angiography confirmed both diagnoses and spinal drainage improved the clinical status, setting the stage for surgery. At operation, a clot was found adherent to the two arteries that were in spasm on the angiogram. Experience in 25 operated cases confirms that a subarachnoid clot must be present locally to cause arterial spasm.

CAROTID OCCLUSION WITH DETACHABLE BALLOON AND CBF STUDIES FOR GIANT ANTERIOR COMMUNICATING ANEURYSM

Case 3. This 60-year-old, right-handed man suffered from subarachnoid hemorrhage 10 years prior to his present admission. At that time, an angiogram revealed a giant anterior communicating artery aneurysm (Figure 84-17A). A right internal carotid artery Selverstone clamp was placed in the neck occluding the right internal carotid artery. Two years prior to admission, the patient experienced massive SAH with a right subdural hematoma leading to coma for 3 weeks, with eventual partial recovery. Twenty-one days prior to his present admission, the patient passed out. A lumbar puncture revealed grossly bloody cerebrospinal fluid. A repeat angiogram revealed enlargement of the anterior communicating artery aneurysm, which was fed mainly by the left carotid system (Figure 84-17B and C). He had a large posterior communicating artery perfusing the right side of the brain. Upon transfer to our hospital, he was mentally slow with moderate dysphasia. He also had bilateral Babinski signs.

Because the patient had demonstrable posterior communicating arteries on the angiogram, we elected to treat him by occluding the left internal carotid artery. He was taken to the

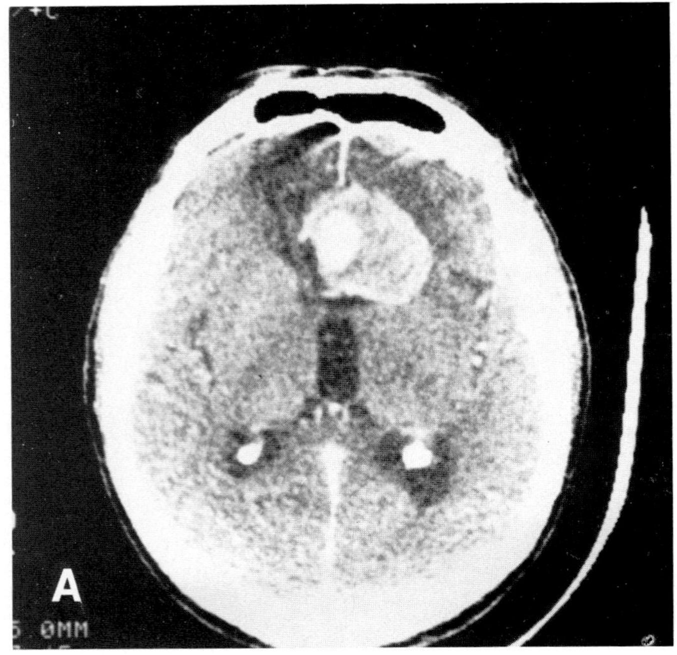

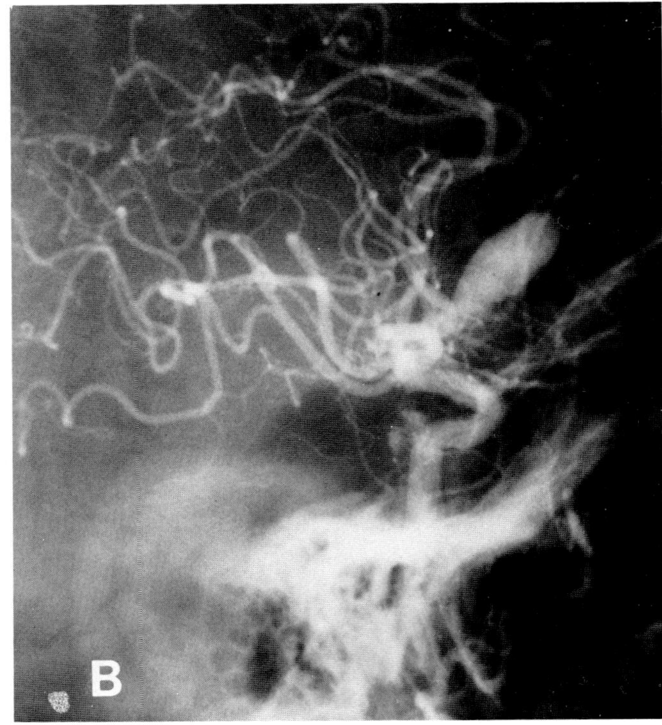

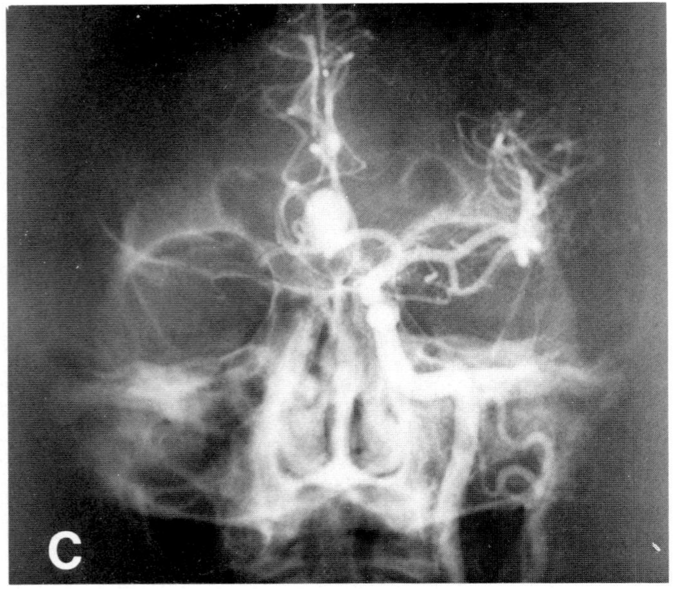

Fig. 84-17. Case 3: Giant unclippable anterior communicating artery aneurysm fed mainly by the left internal carotid artery. (A) CT scan. (B and C) Pre-occlusion angiogram.

angiography suite, where, under cerebral blood flow control, his left internal carotid artery was occluded with a detachable balloon.

After occlusion, the patient's cerebral blood flow remained adequate (50 ml/min/100 gm). A repeat angiogram revealed marked diminution of the aneurysm lumen, and this was confirmed on CT scans. A repeat CT scan 1 year later failed to reveal any residual lumen. The patient has improved to a mild dysphasia.

Comment: This case illustrates the difficulty in treating large, unclippable lesions. It also serves to elucidate the usefulness of the indirect method for treating these giant lesions with a detachable balloon under cerebral blood flow control.

RESULTS

The approach described above has produced satisfactory results in our hands. We have reported 53 consecutive anterior communicating artery aneurysms treated according to this program and surgical technique.[12] Surgical results in this series are presented in Table 84-1. Overall, 38 of 41 patients in grades I-II preoperatively (92 percent) had outcomes that were either excellent (normal) or good (minor disability, working status unchanged). There were two cases in this category that were judged as poor results (5 percent). One patient, despite a normal neurologic examination and extensive drug therapy over a 2-year period, had persisting disabling anxiety that made his

Table 84-1. Results of surgery on aneurysms of the anterior communicating artery

Condition	Result				
	Excellent	Good	Poor	Died	Total
Grades I-II	28 (68%)	10 (24%)	2 (5%)	1 (2%)	41
Grades III-IV		5 (45%)	5 (45%)	1 (9%)	11
Total	28 (54%)	15 (29%)	7 (14%)	2 (4%)	52

Table 84-2. Complications of surgery on aneurysms of the anterior communicating artery

Complication	Number of Patients
Morbidity	
Anxiety	1
Blindness OD	1
Temporary leg paresis	1
Pulmonary embolus	1
Bilateral femoral head necrosis	1
Total	5 (9.6%)
Mortality	
Myocardial infarction	1
Grade IV, never awoke	1
Total	2 (3.8%)

return to work impossible. In one other case, there was immediate blindness in the right eye following the surgery, possibly related to intraoperative injury to the optic nerve vasculature; there was no improvement in vision over a 1-year follow-up.

Among the 41 patients in the "good" category, we encountered a single death, in a 47-year-old engineer who underwent uneventful clipping of anterior communicating artery and internal carotid artery aneurysms only to suffer a fatal postoperative myocardial infarction.

Results in poor-risk patients were satisfactory in a smaller percentage. Among 11 patients judged grade III-IV preoperatively, 5 (45 percent) enjoyed a good result, with no excellent results. Five additional cases (45 percent) enjoyed good results because of preoperative neurologic deficits that persisted after surgery. There was a single death in a patient who was deeply comatose with an intracerebral hematoma from a ruptured anterior communicating artery aneurysm.

Postoperative angiography was performed in 48 cases. Total obliteration of the aneurysm was demonstrated in every case. "Slipped clips" were not observed. In two instances, the right A1 anterior cerebral artery was narrowed, and in another instance occluded, by the clip; none of these patients were symptomatic. Otherwise, native arterial supply was intact. We have stopped performing routine postoperative angiography on patients who have had an uneventful clipping and intraoperative aspiration of the aneurysm.

COMPLICATIONS

As shown in Table 84-2, microsurgical obliteration of anterior communicating artery aneurysms was associated with complications in 5 cases (9.6 percent) and associated with death in 2 (3.8 percent).

Neurologic complications included temporary left-leg weakness due to a delayed right A2 cerebral embolus, presumably from the clip site. Multiple clip applications were required, and minimizing the number of applications probably reduces the likelihood of this problem. In another patient, unilateral blindness probably resulted from direct clip pressure or compromise of vascularity. Clip repositioning was considered too risky. In another case, disabling anxiety (without other signs) occurred after surgery, possibly related to frontobasal irritation.

Nonneurologic complications included a pulmonary embolus requiring vena cava interruption. In another patient,

bilateral femoral head necrosis was noted, apparently related to high-dose steroid therapy. Bilateral total hip replacement was curative.

Death occurred in 2 patients. One patient, operated on acutely for hematoma while in deep coma, never awoke. Another patient, who came through surgery without deficit, suffered a fatal myocardial infarction 5 days after surgery.

Although we have not accumulated enough experience with early surgery for a definitive statement, our impression is that good grade patients with small lesions pointing anteriorly without vasospasm can be operated early with good results. We still prefer to delay surgery in the face of poor clinical condition, vasospasm, diminished CBF, or a particularly difficult lesion.

DISCUSSION

Early surgery has gained support. There is a solid rationale. Prompt obliteration of the aneurysm eliminates potential rebleeding. Epsilon-aminocaproic acid, reported to reduce rebleeding, does so, but at a cost of increased complications from ischemia and hydrocephalus, with no net gain. When the aneurysm is secured early on, vigorous hypertensive therapy can be pursued if vasospasm develops later. This rationale is backed by encouraging data: all major controlled studies report that the results of early surgery are as good as or better than those attained by delayed operation.[13–16]

There are, however, problems. Ljunggren's data indicate that anterior communicating aneurysms are associated with worse results than are carotid or middle cerebral aneurysms after early surgery.[17] This is in accordance with the common experience that it is more difficult to operate on anterior communicating lesions, and perforator occlusion can lead to dyskinetic abulia. Nonetheless, some good results from early surgery in this group have been reported,[13,16] and we have some successful personal experiences as well.

Which anterior communicating aneurysms do well with early surgery? Precise data are unavailable. Our current recommendation is for early surgery only in cases with grade I-II clinical condition, small anteriorly directed aneurysms, absence of vasospasm, and proof of normal CBF and intracranial pressure, though we put special emphasis on normal CBF as a guide to the timing of surgery.

Prophylactic surgery is the principal hope for future reduction of devastation from intracranial aneurysms. In about half of the 26,000 annual cases of SAH in the United States, the patients die before medical attention.[18] Thus, only detection and obliteration prior to rupture can help these patients. Many aneurysms can be detected noninvasively by CT or MRI scanning, especially those unruptured lesions of over 1 cm, which are most likely to rupture. Ultrasonography may eventually detect unruptured aneurysms.

In patients over 40 years of age, with a relatively increased likelihood of aneurysms, screening may eventually be feasible, especially as costs of medical imaging diminish. Once an aneurysm is detected, prophylactic surgery may be considered. The risk is low in patients with a solid medical condition and non-giant aneurysms, including anterior communicating lesions.[19]

Surgery is clearly warranted in patients with lesions 1 cm or larger. Extension of these concepts may reduce the present health havoc wrought by SAH from intracranial aneurysms. It is now clear that all patients should have normal intravascular volume status as a prophylaxis against vasospasm.

Diagnosis of impending or actual vasospasm still depends on angiography, but CBF studies may be a helpful harbinger. We are currently testing CBF diagnosis of vasospasm against angiography.

Treatment of established symptomatic vasospasm includes expansion of intravascular volume with vigorous hypertension in cases where the aneurysm has been repaired. Note that early surgery can thus be helpful in dealing with vasospasm. Initial treatment suggests that mannitol infusion can improve CBF and clinical status in patients with symptomatic vasospasm.[3,7]

Temporary clipping appears to be superior to intraoperative hypotension to "defuse the bomb." Substantial experience in several centers indicates a lack of local thromboses, greatly enhanced ability to dissect and obliterate even paper-thin lesions, and good clinical outcomes. For brief temporary clipping (a step we usually employ), no special steps toward cerebral protection appear necessary. On the other hand, for extensive dissection of a large lesion requiring 30 minutes or more, cerebral protection is compulsory. Several measures have been recommended. Mannitol given prior to temporary clipping has been advocated by Suzuki. Hypertension can bolster collateral supply. Drake suggests opening the temporary clips every five minutes (or more often). Using all these maneuvers, we have occluded various arteries, including the anterior communicating complex, for up to 45 minutes without new deficits. We now favor this approach for dissecting the thin-walled, more threatening lesions, which constitute perhaps a quarter of all aneurysms of the anterior communicating artery.

Indirect operation is still a good choice in selected cases, especially cases of giant lesions, and particularly in poor surgical candidates. Many giant aneurysms can be thrombosed by Hunterian ligature of the parent artery.[20] When both anterior cerebral arteries fill only from one side, ligature of that internal carotid artery very likely will lead to aneurysmal thrombosis.[11] When the aneurysm fills from both carotid arteries, bilateral ligature may be needed, as in the Odom procedure, which interrupts the larger A1 artery and the contralateral internal carotid artery. Recent experience suggests that balloon catheter technique can occlude the internal carotid artery without surgery, and CBF measurement can identify candidates with suitable collateral circulation. Unsuitable candidates may be used to artificially boost marginal collateral circulation until natural enhancement can develop.

Cerebrovascular vasospasm remains a major problem, causing symptoms in about 35 percent of hospitalized cases of SAH.[21] Calcium channel blockade as prophylaxis seems rational, and initial results with nimodipine are promising,[22–24] but definitive results are awaited. We are in the process of evaluating a new calcium channel blocker (Sandoz PY 108-068) to combat vasospasm, and preliminary results are encouraging. A multi-center trial of a related long-acting calcium channel blocker is underway.

REFERENCES

1. Sahs AL, Perret GE, Locksley HB, et al: Intracranial Aneurysms and Subarachnoid Hemorrhage. Philadelphia, JB Lippincott, 1969
2. Sakaku A, Shindo K, Tanaka S, et al: Fluid and electrolyte disturbances in patients with intracranial aneurysms. Surg Neurol 11:349, 1979
3. Jafar JJ, Johns LM, Mullan SF: The effect of mannitol on cerebral blood flow. J Neurosurg 64:754, 1986
4. Kassell NF, Peerless SJ, Durward QJ, et al: Treatment of ischemic deficits from vasospasm with intravascular volume expansion and induced arterial hypertension. Neurosurgery 11:337, 1982
5. Hunt WE, Hess RM: Surgical risk as related to time of intervention in the repair of intracranial aneurysms. J Neurosurg 28:14, 1968
6. Aitken RR, Drake CG: A technique of anesthesia with induced hypotension for surgical correction of intracranial aneurysms. Clin Neurosurg 21:107, 1974
7. Suzuki J, Yoshimoto T, Takamasa K: Surgical treatment of middle cerebral artery aneurysms. J Neurosurg 61:17, 1984
8. Vander Ark GD, Kempe LG, Smith DR: Anterior communicating aneurysms: The gyrus rectus approach. Clin Neurosurg 21:120, 1974
9. Sugita K, Kobayashi S, Kyoshima K, et al: Fenestrated clips for unusual aneurysms of the carotid artery. J Neurosurg 57:240, 1982
10. Carney PG, Oatey PE: Muslin wrapping of aneurysms and delayed visual failure. A report of three cases. J Clin Neuro-Ophthalmol 91, 1983
11. Odom GL, Tindall GT: Carotid ligation in the treatment of certain intracranial aneurysms. Clin Neurosurg 15:101, 1968
12. Crowell RM, Ojemann RG: Surgical treatment of anterior communicating artery aneurysms, in Schmidek HH, Sweet WH (eds): Operative Neurosurgical Techniques. New York, Grune & Stratton, 1982, pp 829–854
13. Kassell NF: Cooperative study on timing of aneurysm surgery. Presented at the Annual Meeting of the American Association of Neurological Surgeons, Atlanta, Ga, April 1985
14. Ljunggren B, Saveland H, Brandt L, et al: Early operation and overall outcome in aneurysmal subarachnoid hemorrhage. J Neurosurg 62:547, 1985
15. Auer LM: Acute operation and preventive nimodipine improve outcome in patients with ruptured cerebral aneurysms. Neurosurgery 15:57, 1985
16. Weir B, Aronyk K: Management and postoperative mortality related to time of clipping for supratentorial aneurysms: A personal series. Acta Neurochir 63:135, 1982
17. Ljunggren B, Brandt L: Timing of aneurysm surgery. Clin Neurosurg 33:159, 1985
18. Drake CG: Perspective on cerebral aneurysms. Stroke 11:124, 1980
19. Wirth FP: Surgical treatment of incidental intracranial aneurysms. Clin Neurosurg 33:125, 1986
20. Drake CG: Ligation of vertebral (unilateral or bilateral) or basilar artery in the treatment of large intracranial aneurysms. J Neurosurg 43:255, 1975

21. Post KD, Flamm ES, Goodgold A, et al: Ruptured intracranial aneurysms. Case morbidity and mortality. J Neurosurg 46:290, 1977

22. Allen GS, Ahn HS, Preziosi TJ, et al: Cerebral arterial spasm—A controlled trial of nimodipine in patients with subarachnoid hemorrhage. N Engl J Med 308:619, 1983

23. Auer LM, Ito Z, Suzuki A, et al: Prevention of symptomatic vasospasm by topically applied nimodipine. Acta Neurochir 63:297, 1982

24. Ljunggren B, Brandt L, Saveland H, et al: Outcome in 60 consecutive patients treated with early aneurysm operation and intravenous nimodipine. J Neurosurg 61:864, 1984

CHAPTER 85

Surgical Management of Aneurysms of the Middle Cerebral Artery

Lindsay Symon

ANEURYSMS OF THE MIDDLE CEREBRAL ARTERY have for long had a somewhat sinister reputation. There was indeed a suggestion in the first detailed analysis of large numbers of cases presented by McKissock and his colleagues[1] that female patients with middle cerebral artery aneurysms had a notably poor operative prognosis, scarcely different from that for conservative management. This has not proved to be the case, since with the advent of modern microsurgical methods, most surgeons agree that direct intracranial surgical intervention for aneurysms of the middle cerebral artery is both justified and indicated. One might suppose that because of the evocative nature of the area of the cortex that is supplied by the middle cerebral artery more of these aneurysms would fall into grades 3 or 4 of the classification of Hunt and Hess[2] than might be the case for supratentorial aneurysms as a whole. A comparison of 101 middle cerebral artery aneurysms with the remainder of 450 supratentorial aneurysms in my own series reveals that this is not the case. About one third of the middle cerebral artery aneurysms were in grade 3, which is about the same percentage as that for the total series. About one fifth of them were in grade 4; again, a statistic similar to that for the series as a whole (Table 85-1). No detectable difference in the behavior of middle cerebral artery aneurysms between male and female patients was apparent in my series nor in those presented in recent publications. It is interesting to note that the proportion of the total series—just over 20 percent—is similar to that in Suzuki's series of 1000 supratentorial aneurysms, 174 (17.4 percent) of which were in the distribution of the middle cerebral artery.[3] It is clear that this is a less common aneurysm than the others of the anterior circle and therefore a large surgical experience has been slower to accumulate. The techniques to be described in this chapter concerning the management of these lesions have been standard in the Department of Neurological Surgery of the National Hospital, London, for many years.

ESSENTIAL INVESTIGATIONS

Subarachnoid hemorrhage may well be a surgical emergency in the neurosurgical unit. It is, however, essential that the general condition of the patient be investigated before any form of surgical intervention for the aneurysm is attempted. Such investigation need not be time consuming but should include a coagulation profile, a full blood count, determination of serum electrolyte and blood urea levels, chest x-ray films, and an evaluation of the cardiovascular status of the patient, with particular attention being given to ascertaining whether the hypertension that may well accompany subarachnoid hemorrhage existed before the hemorrhage. These are factors that will weigh heavily in the decision to attempt surgical obliteration of the lesion.

It is my practice to proceed to computed tomographic (CT) scanning within a few hours of the patient's hospitalization. The extent of the subarachnoid hemorrhage can be judged by quantifying the amount of blood present in the basal cisterns. This finding may be of predictive value in relation to the subsequent development of cerebral vasospasm.[4,5] The presence or absence of a low-density lesion is suggestive of cerebral infarction (which, of course, will appear a few days later) or of an appreciable intracerebral hematoma.

With a typical history and clinical findings suggestive of subarachnoid hemorrhage (stiff neck, mild hemiparesis, and the presence of blood as determined from the CT scan), the necessity for lumbar puncture may be questioned. It is my practice, however, to perform a lumbar puncture to confirm the subarachnoid hemorrhage unless this test has been previously performed at the referring hospital with convincing results.

Cerebral angiography is a mandatory investigation before surgery. With the advent of high-quality CT scanning, some controversy exists about the necessary extent of such angiography. At the National Hospital, angiography is performed by retrograde femoral catheterization under general anesthesia and by highly skilled radiologists. It is worthwhile to visualize the entire carotid circulation to delineate both the distribution and the extent of the vasospasm and the presence of other lesions, including aneurysms. In young patients in good general condition, vertebrobasilar angiography is also performed, whereas in elderly patients (60–70 years of age) with a convincing middle cerebral hemorrhage and a middle cerebral artery aneurysm at the appropriate site as demonstrated by carotid angiography, vertebral angiography is omitted.

PREOPERATIVE MEDICATION

Personal preference rather than scientific analysis is an important determinant in the choice of medications used before surgery. Many surgeons place all patients with subarachnoid hemorrhage on antifibrinolytic agents. This has not been the practice at the National Hospital; I prefer early surgery to a

Table 85-1. Preoperative grade in 92 patients with middle cerebral artery aneurysms with recent subarachnoid hemorrhage

Grade	Number of Cases
1	20
2	27
3	31
4	16
5	1

delay in preventing rehemorrhage of the aneurysm (Table 85-2). Patients with subarachnoid hemorrhage are placed on a moderate dose of steroid (e.g., 4 mg of dexamethasone every 6 hours) as soon as they are admitted. This dosage is continued until 48 hours after surgery. Patients also are routinely placed on oxacillin (1 g every 6 hours) beginning 24 hours before surgery and continuing for 5 days thereafter. Anticonvulsants (usually diphenylhydantoinate; 100 mg three times a day) are started on admission. Sodium valproate (Epilim), 500 mg three times a day, is substituted if the patient is allergic to Dilantin. Blood levels of these anticonvulsants are estimated during hospitalization, and this medication is maintained for 12 months after surgery, and then is gradually discontinued over a period of 6 to 8 weeks.

THE TIMING OF SURGERY

Intracranial pressure, cerebral blood flow, and, most recently, conduction time within the central nervous system itself[6] all have been used in determining the appropriate time for surgery after a subarachnoid hemorrhage.

Although the latter technique is being developed in the neurological surgery unit of the National Hospital, the decision of when to operate is still made on clinical grounds. Patients in grades 1 to 3 (Hunt classification) undergo angiography as soon as it is convenient. If the aneurysm neck appears difficult to clip, arteriograms of the highest quality will be necessary and should include multiple oblique views. A skilled angiographer therefore must be available. It is unlikely that the best-quality films will be obtained in the middle of the night.

The patient is allowed to recover from the angiographic session for 24 hours, and, provided he or she has been stable and there are no other major contraindications to surgery, the patient then is ready for the operation. Severe hypertension and the presence of an unstable or fluctuating neurologic condition should prompt caution.

Table 85-2. The timing of surgery after hospitalization in 62 patients with middle cerebral artery aneurysms and recent subarachnoid hemorrhage

Days After Admission	Number of Patients
0-5	21
6-10	35
11-15	18
16-21	8
21-60 +	13

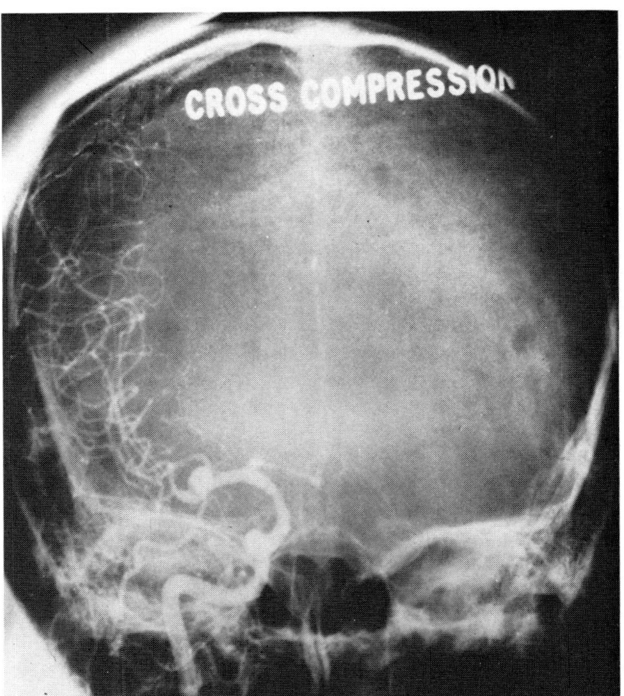

Fig. 85-1. A typical aneurysm of the middle cerebral artery in the crotch of the first bifurcation.

Patients in grades 4 and 5 are not subjected to surgery until their condition has improved, save in the circumstance of a massive hematoma. In these instances the hematoma will have been apparent on the CT scans, and some concern may be expressed over the propriety of angiography in view of the serious condition of the patient. If the situation of the hematoma suggests the possibility of an underlying rupture of the middle cerebral artery aneurysm, angiography before evacuation of the hematoma is mandatory. Rupture of the aneurysm in the course of evacuation of the hematoma may prove impossible to control with safety if some prior knowledge of the regional vascular anatomy is not available. At the same time, the obliteration of the aneurysm in a patient in such poor condition is hazardous and should not be attempted unless it is forced upon the surgeon by disastrous rupture in the course of limited evacuation of the intracerebral hemorrhage. Evacuation of the hemorrhage should be made through a linear incision above and in front of the ear. This incision may be extended to a classical aneurysm flap around the outer end of the sphenoid wing if necessary at the time, or by preference at a later date. The temporal mass is removed through a linear corticectomy. Should the hematoma lie deep within the internal capsular area, then a tentative evacuation is probably unjustified, and the patient should be treated by medical supportive measures alone. In most circumstances it is better to improve the general condition of the patient with steroids, to avoid the use of dehydrating agents such as mannitol, and to avoid induced hypotension. Surges of excessively high blood pressure are controlled by beta-blocking agents such as propranolol (10–20 mg t.d.s, IM). A seriously ill patient with a large intracerebral hematoma may improve quite remarkably over a few days, and the outlook for radical surgery under these circumstances is not nearly so grave. If evacuation of the hemorrhage is unavoidable in order to save the life of the patient, the prognosis is extremely grave and must be communicated to the relatives in these terms.

The referral pattern to the National Hospital is such that

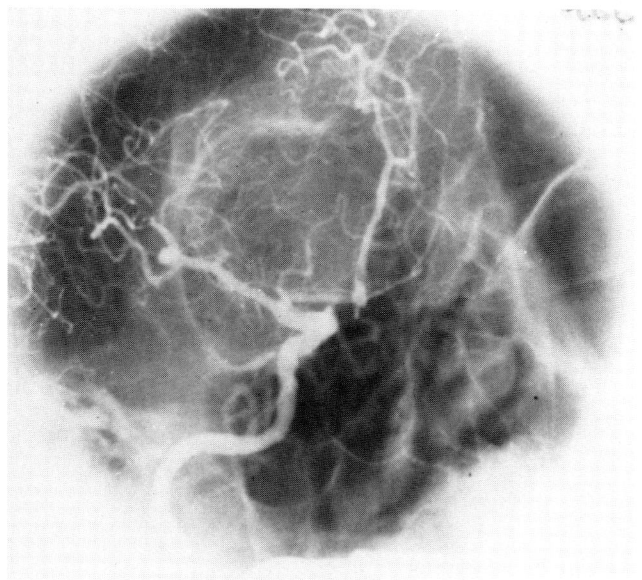

Fig. 85-2. Oblique views may help to elucidate the anatomy as in this oblique view of a typical bifurcation aneurysm of the middle cerebral artery.

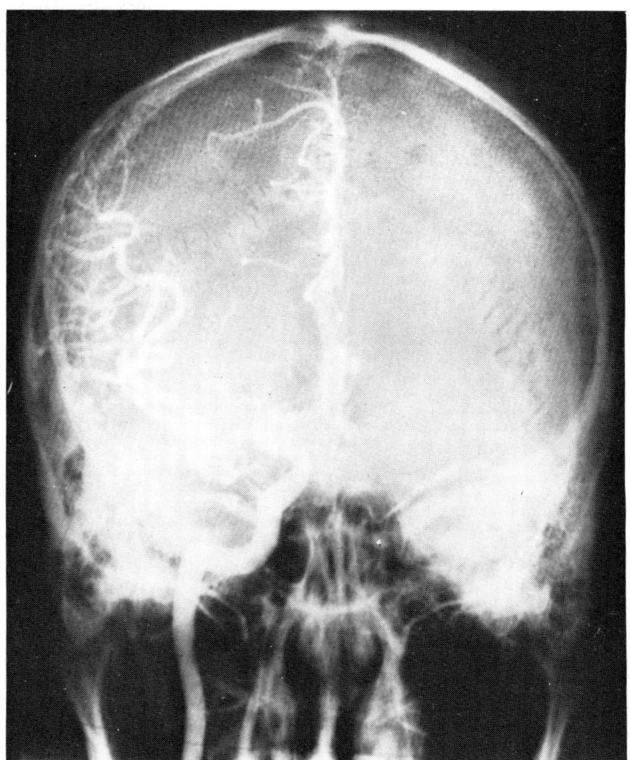

Fig. 85-3. A middle cerebral artery aneurysm that is slightly more proximal, arising at the origin of the proximal temporal branch.

patients are seldom admitted on the day of the hemorrhage, i.e, on day 1. Patients are commonly admitted on day 2, investigated on day 3, allowed to rest on day 4, and operated upon the fifth day after hemorrhage. In some circumstances, it is possible to operate within 48 hours of the hemorrhage if the condition of the patient is excellent and recovery from angiography is prompt.

THE SURGICAL PROCEDURE

PLANNING THE APPROACH

Two approaches to middle cerebral artery aneurysms can be used. The approach depends on the angiographic characteristics of the aneurysm. Commonly, a middle cerebral artery aneurysm will arise in the crotch of the bifurcation or trifurcation of the middle cerebral artery (Figures 85-1 and 85-2). These lesions are quite distal in the sylvian fissure and distal to the segment of the middle cerebral artery from which the perforating branches arise, and they are often partially embraced by the insular branches of the distal middle cerebral artery. For these aneurysms an approach through a resection of the superior temporal gyrus is preferred.

When the aneurysm arises from the more proximal part of the middle cerebral artery, often in association with a premature origin of the anterior temporal branch (Figures 85-3 and 85-4), a more restricted approach through the sylvian fissure, as classically advocated by Yasargil[7] and Lougheed,[8] is more appropriate and effective. These two approaches will be described in detail.

POSITIONING THE PATIENT

The position of the patient for both approaches is the same. The patient is positioned on his or her back with the head turned well to the side opposite the aneurysm. A frontotemporal flap is

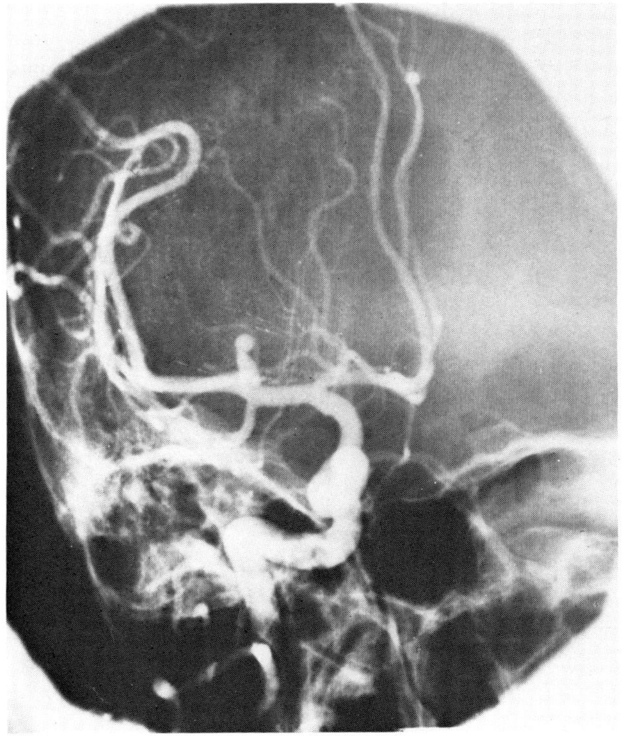

Fig. 85-4. An unusual aneurysm of the middle cerebral artery arising opposite the first, very proximal bifurcation, close to the segment bearing the perforators.

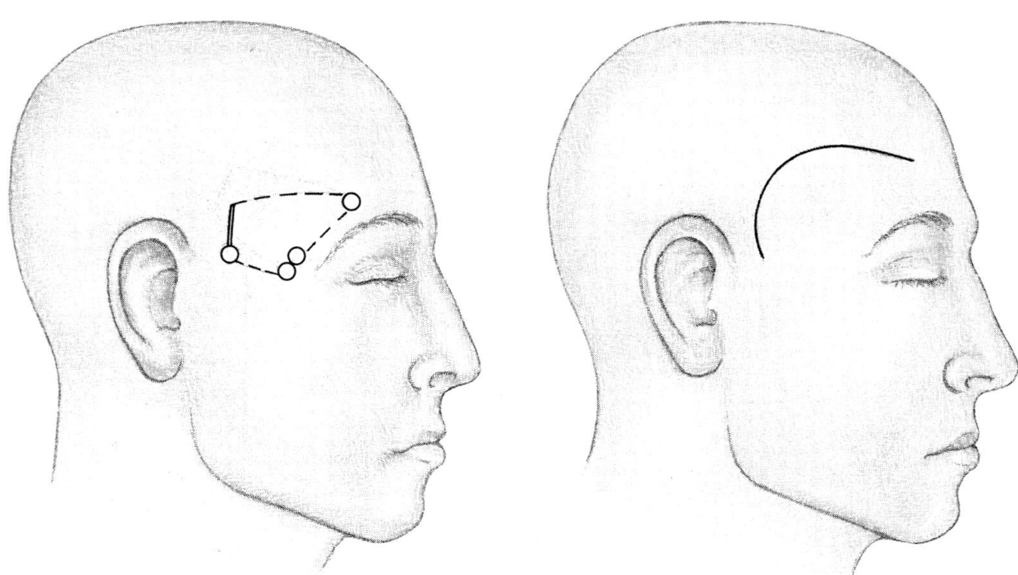

Fig. 85-5. The position of the scalp flap and bone flap for exposure of middle cerebral artery aneurysms.

marked out around the outer end of the sphenoid wing (Figure 85-5). The scalp flap is turned back in a single layer, and an effort is made to preserve the frontalis branch of the facial nerve in the base of the flap. Although this nerve is frequently stretched in the flap resection, the exposure should not be cramped in an attempt to avoid it. Since the healing of this flap is remarkably good, a more cosmetic flap can be attempted. If the anterior burr hole is appropriately filled in, a small lateral "worry" line will be the only sign visible below the hairline. The frontalis branch of the facial nerve will recover in about 6 months even if it is severed.

The base of the scalp flap can be held down by tension sutures to allow the muscle incision to be made close to the frontal process of the zygomatic bone. The muscle incision is carried down through the temporal fossa to expose the lateral aspect of the temporal fossa and the groove between the frontal and temporal fossae. The muscle incision is carried anteriorly to just above the superior temporal line, then sloped back to the rear of the scalp flap. The bone flap can be cut through three burr holes. One of these, which I have referred to as a "spectacle" burr hole and which McCartney has described as a "key-hole" burr hole (personal communication), opens both the frontal and temporal fossae, and allows the outer end of the sphenoid wing to be bitten off with sharp rongeurs. A small extension of the anterior part of the key-hole toward the floor of the frontal fossa allows the anterior saw cut to be kept low. An anterior burr hole and a burr hole fairly low posteriorly, which again may be extended with De Vilbis rongeurs to allow an adequately sized bone flap to be turned, will allow the bone flap to be broken down on the anterior part of the temporalis muscle within the temporal fossa, and avoids the necessity for subtemporal decompression. The outer end of the sphenoid wing should be rongeured away. If the spectacle burr hole was appropriately placed, little bone removal is necessary in most cases and no great bony defect will be visible postoperatively, which means that the extensive depression in the anterior temporal fossa that is sometimes seen will not occur. The bone flap should be held back with retention sutures, duroperiosteal sutures should be inserted to preserve hemostasis, and the appropriate self-retaining retractor inserted. The post bearing a

double arm for the Yasargil retractor can be placed at the posterosuperior aspect of the flap. The dura is opened through a triradiate incision that is started subfrontally and slopes down into the anterior temporal fossa. A silk suture is passed under the middle meningeal artery and is anchored to the intermuscular septum in the temporal muscle. The muscle incision commonly ends at about the level of the meningeal artery. A re-entrant incision posteriorly along the line of the sylvian fissure allows the dura to be held up in three flaps, which are sufficiently wide to ensure adequate extradural hemostasis and to prevent bleeding into the intracranial space. Continuous drainage of cerebrospinal fluid is not used. If the intracranial tension appears to be unduly high, an attempt can be made to tap the frontal horn of the lateral ventricle. This is usually fairly straightforward; the line of the frontal horn of the lateral ventricle is continuous with the line of the curve of the anterior temporal fossa, and if the patient's head is in the appropriate position, the floor of the frontal fossa will certainly be sloping a little away from the surgeon. Such measures to control intracranial pressure can be taken before the dural flap is opened, but if the patient is in reasonable clinical condition, these measures usually are unnecessary, and adequate control of intracranial tension is commonly obtained by a fairly rapid dissection down the subfrontal region under direct vision, gentle retraction of the brain from in front of the sphenoid wing, and opening of the arachnoid of the basal cisterns over or anterior to the optic nerve. It should be remembered that dissection of the sylvian fissure at this stage carries a risk of premature rupture of the aneurysm, particularly an aneurysm that faces anteriorly, and dissection to control intracranial pressure aimed at the carotid artery should stay as far away from the aneurysm as possible. At this stage subfrontal self-retaining retraction can be placed for a moment or two, and the terminal carotid artery can be defined under the operating microscope. This will usually allow a clip to be placed on the terminal carotid artery should severe rupture of the aneurysm occur before adequate control of the proximal middle cerebral artery is possible. The route of progression from this point depends on the detailed anatomy of the aneurysm.

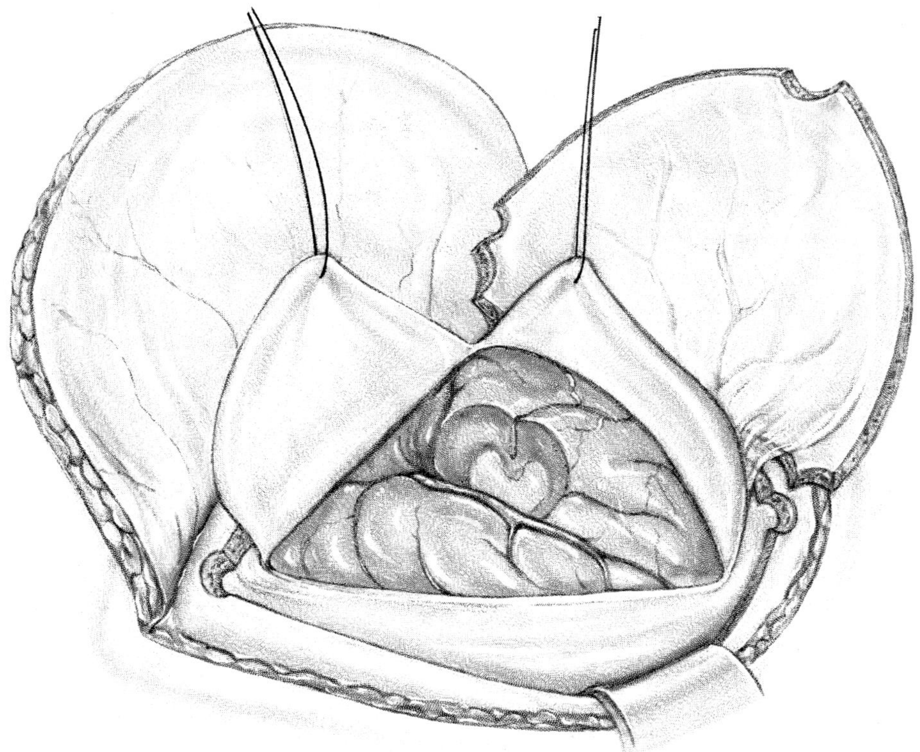

Fig. 85-6. The approach to a trifurcation aneurysm. The position of the reflected scalp and bone flap is shown, although this would normally be covered by cottonoid strips. The dural flaps are shown elevated to maintain hemostasis. The proximal ½ inch or so of the superior temporal gyrus is being resected.

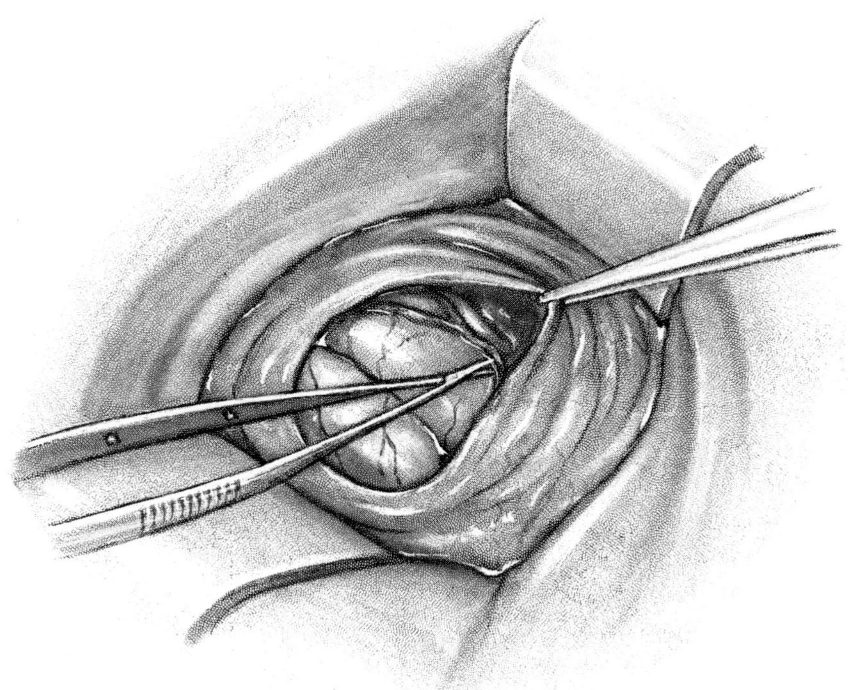

Fig. 85-7. Self-retaining retraction has been placed on the upper and lower banks of the dissection and the view is under high magnification. The arachnoid over the insula has been opened and definition of the distal middle cerebral branches is under way.

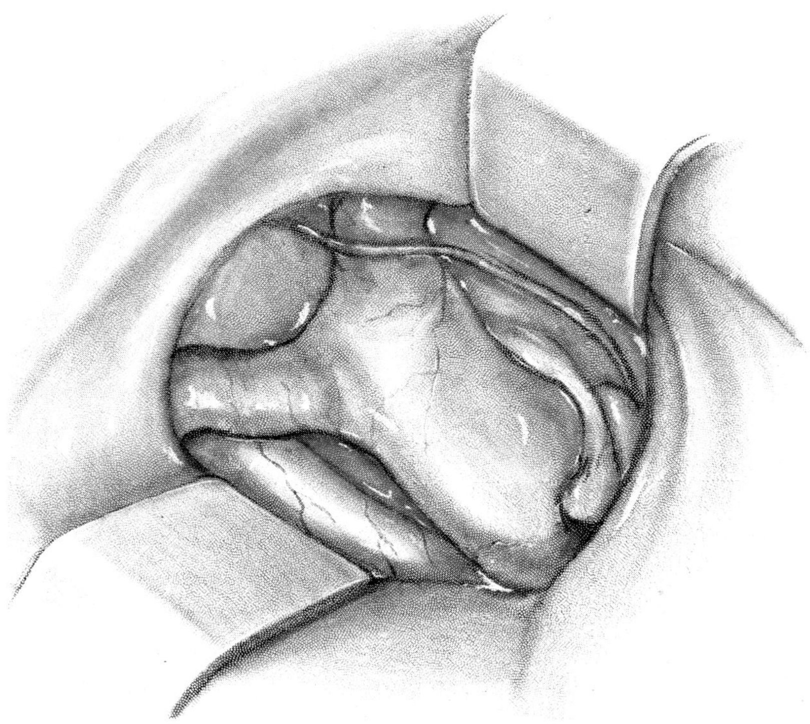

Fig. 85-8. The trifurcation of the middle cerebral artery has been exposed and the distal middle cerebral branches are shown, one on the lower bank of the insula and one running posteriorly. The slightly unusual middle cerebral aneurysm points posteriorly and with a crossing vein is just evident. (Figures 85-8, 85-9, and 85-10 were made from a video tape of the actual dissection of the aneurysm shown in Figure 85-10.)

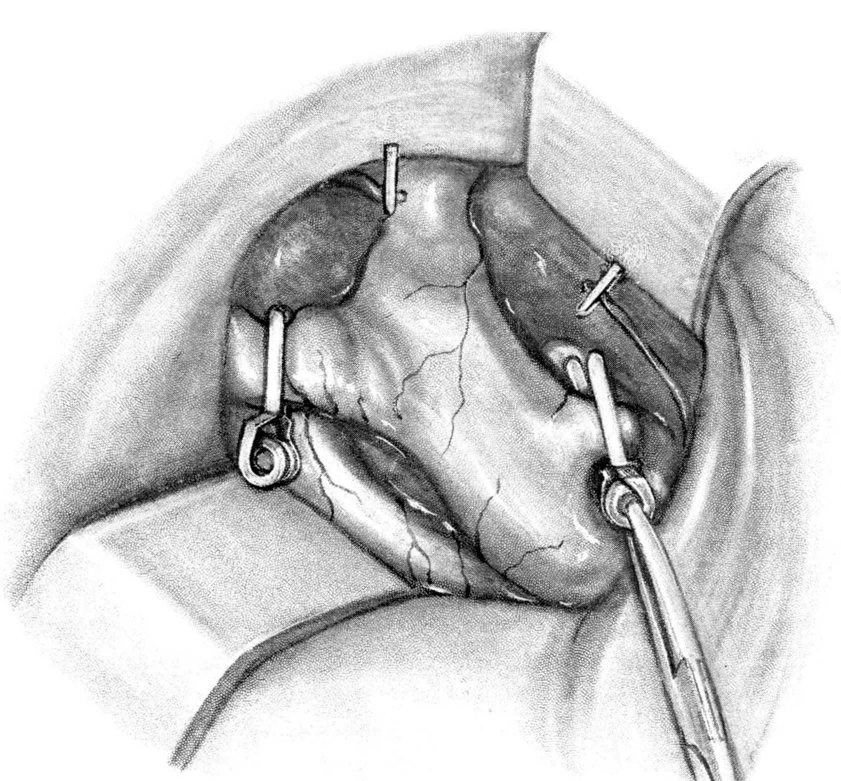

Fig. 85-9. A further stage in the dissection. A temporary clip has been placed on the proximal middle cerebral artery just proximal to the bifurcation. The definitive aneurysm clip has been placed on the neck of the aneurysm.

MIDDLE CEREBRAL ARTERY ANEURYSMS AT THE TRIFURCATION

For aneurysms of the trifurcation of the middle cerebral artery, the inner end of the sylvian fissure is opened and the terminal carotid artery is identified. The anterior ½ inch of the superior temporal gyrus is resected (Figure 85-6), the resection staying below, that is, inferior to the pia of the sylvian fissure. As the dissection deepens, hemorrhage within the sylvian fissure usually becomes apparent in the case of a recently ruptured aneurysm. The major branches of the middle cerebral artery are identified on the surface of the insula and deep to the pia with careful microscopic dissection before the sylvian fissure or the arachnoidal spaces of the insula are opened (Figure 85-7). At any point, of course, a hematoma in the temporal lobe may be entered. The admitted disadvantage of this approach is that the fundus of the aneurysm is reached before its neck. Should the aneurysm rupture, temporary occlusion of the carotid artery may sufficiently reduce the hemorrhage to enable the surgeon to dissect and occlude the aneurysm. This has never been necessary in any of my cases, but would be contemplated if severe hemorrhage were to occur at this stage in the procedure. More commonly, the clot is entered and the branches of the middle cerebral artery embracing the aneurysm can be dissected without difficulty. It is usually wise to pass down through the temporal lobe below the aneurysm and to re-enter the fissure just proximal to the trifurcation and identify the proximal middle cerebral artery at this point, which is distal to the segment bearing the perforators. The most common potential hazard in dissecting middle cerebral artery aneurysms is damage to the segment of the middle cerebral artery that bears the perforators, and it is dissection of a difficult aneurysm embraced by the branches of the trifurcating middle cerebral artery through the fissure that is most likely to result in stretch and rupture of these vessels. With the approach through the superior temporal gyrus, the segment of the middle cerebral artery bearing the perforators is left undisturbed. With control of the proximal middle cerebral artery thus assured should it be necessary, more resolute dissection of the branches of the middle cerebral artery and the aneurysm embraced by these branches can continue (Figure 85-8). Quite frequently, adhesion between the emergent branches and the fundus of the aneurysm is fairly dense over the portion of the fundus where the most recent hemorrhage has occurred and rather less dense over the older part of the aneurysm close to its neck, where the wall is often rather sturdier and the main branches can be dissected from the fundus with greater ease and less risk. Rather than undergo repetitive leak and rupture of the fundus, however, a proximal clamp can be placed on the middle cerebral artery without hesitation for periods of up to 10 minutes. Such proximal occlusion has been used at the National Hospital for some years in cases of recent subarachnoid hemorrhage without evident sequelae (Figures 85-9 and 85-10) and a more detailed description of the technique follows. The increasing use of electrophysiologic monitoring may well place this rule of thumb on a more eclectic basis.

Commonly, the neck of the aneurysm can be occluded with a straight or curved clip. My preference is the Scoville-type clip, which can be readily manipulated and is easy to apply and remove. At the National Hospital, Scoville clips have been curved by the instrument makers to the appropriate degrees of curvature necessary to meet most circumstances. Unfortu-nately, these are not commercially available. The Suzuki-type clip is equally good, however. I have not found the Yasargil clips, although admittedly excellent instruments, as attractive as the Scoville clips because they are more difficult to remove and replace as a result of the design of the clip-applicator forceps. Likewise the older type of Mayfield clip applicator is now so clumsy that it obscures a good deal of the microscopic field. The attraction of the Scoville clip is that it can be placed and replaced with an artery forceps, which is a much smaller instrument.

The neck of the aneurysm can be coagulated if it seems likely to result in a more ready application of a clip. Not infrequently there is an aneurysmic bulge on the opposite side of the trifurcation of the middle cerebral artery, making it impossible to completely occlude the aneurysm. Under these circumstances, the major portion on one side can be clipped and the bulge on the other side can be wrapped with gauze or muslin or reinforced with acrylic or some other suitable plastic.

The Scoville clip can be anchored in place with a drop of acrylic placed on the curved spring shank. This not only prevents the clip from coming off, but also, by expanding within the curve of the shank, tightens the force of the clip. No clip disruption has been apparent over a 10-year period using this maneuver, despite the dire warnings of electrolytic danger.[9] It is, of course, necessary to make absolutely certain that the position is ideal before the clip is fixed, since once it is fixed, it is impossible to remove it.

THE MANAGEMENT OF GIANT ANEURYSMS OF THE MIDDLE CEREBRAL ARTERY

The experience with giant aneurysms of the middle cerebral artery at the National Hospital is based on 15 aneurysms measuring an inch in diameter or more, 9 of which qualify as giant in being space-occupying lesions partially occupied by thrombus. Most of these patients had recently had multiple

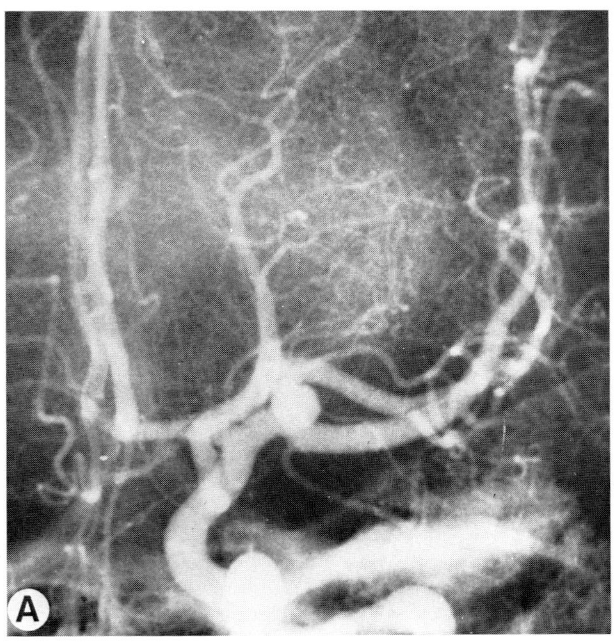

Fig. 85-10

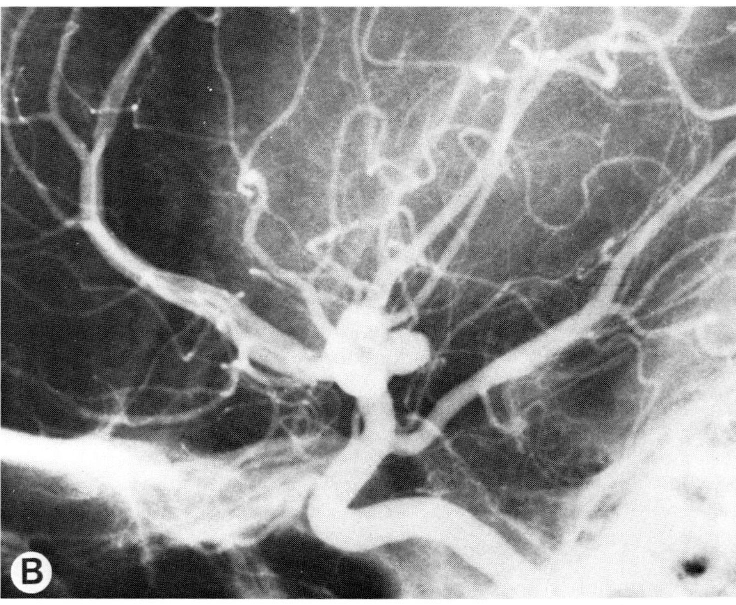

Fig. 85-10. (A and B) Anteroposterior and lateral angiograms of a middle cerebral aneurysm, the dissection of which was depicted in the preceding figures. This is a slightly unusual lesion, arising from a proximal bifurcation and pointing backward. Anterior dissection would have proved extremely difficult. Above all, this is the indication for approach through the superior temporal gyrus.

subarachnoid hemorrhages and were operated upon to prevent further bleeding. Two patients were operated upon because of recurrent episodes of hemiparesis, and subarachnoid hemorrhage had occurred only in the remote past. One aneurysm was associated with a recent subarachnoid hemorrhage and was simply a large aneurysm unoccupied by clot. The remainder were diagnosed as a result of CT scans for a variety of hemispheral symptoms, mild hemiparesis, parkinsonian features, or epilepsy.

In the operative management of giant aneurysms, temporary occlusion of the middle cerebral circulation is almost inevitable while the neck is being defined. The aneurysm that is

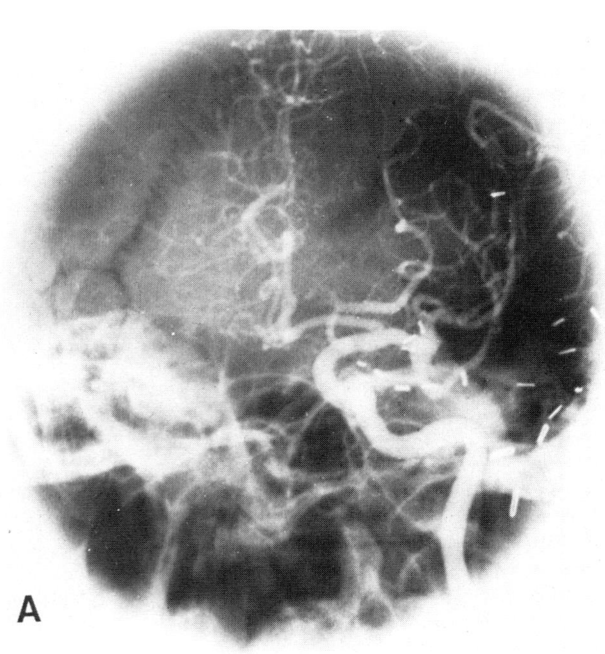

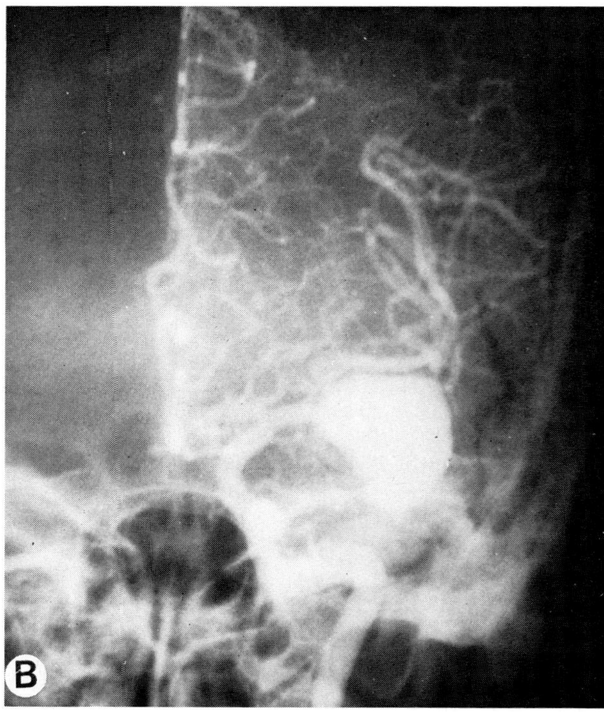

Fig. 85-11. (A) A giant middle cerebral aneurysm that caused subarachnoid hemorrhage. (Reprinted from Subarachnoid hemorrhage from intracranial aneurysm and angioma, in Ross Russell RW (ed): Cerebral Arterial Disease. New York, Churchill Livingstone, 1976. With permission.) (B) The giant aneurysm after ligation.

visualized can be very much smaller than the actual aneurysm as defined either by vascular displacement or from the CT scan, and, therefore, at some stage the aneurysm may have to be opened and the clot evacuated in order to make the wall amenable to the fashioning of a neck and the application of a ligature or clip. This is particularly true if the aneurysm is a space-occupying lesion, since occlusion of its neck alone will not relieve the mass effect. Figure 85-11 demonstrates an aneurysm that had bled recurrently over the previous 2 months, and Figure 85-12 shows an aneurysm that had bled in the remote past and was acting as a space-occupying lesion. Many surgeons now feel it wise to fashion a superficial temporal artery-middle cerebral artery anastomosis before tackling the aneurysm itself. The alternative method of management, which has

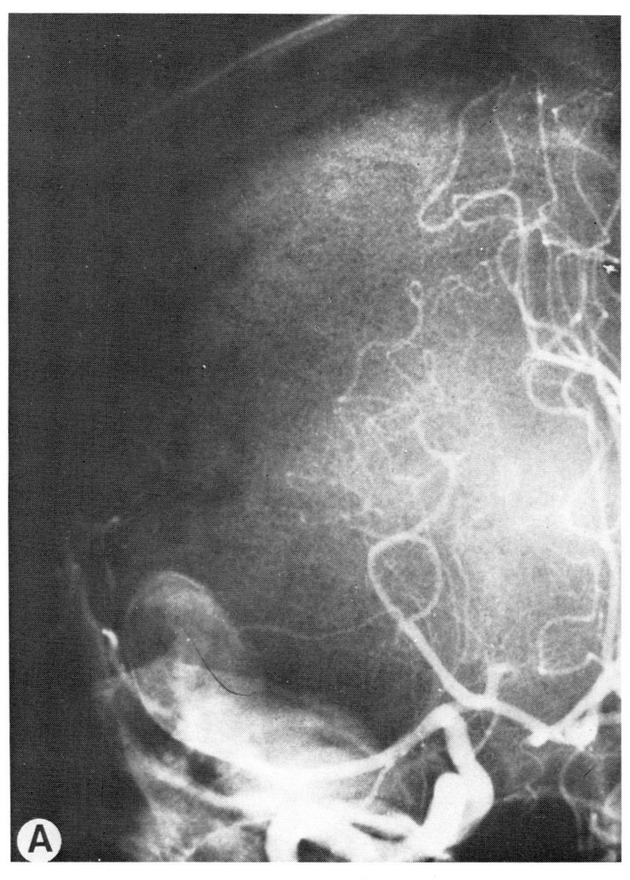

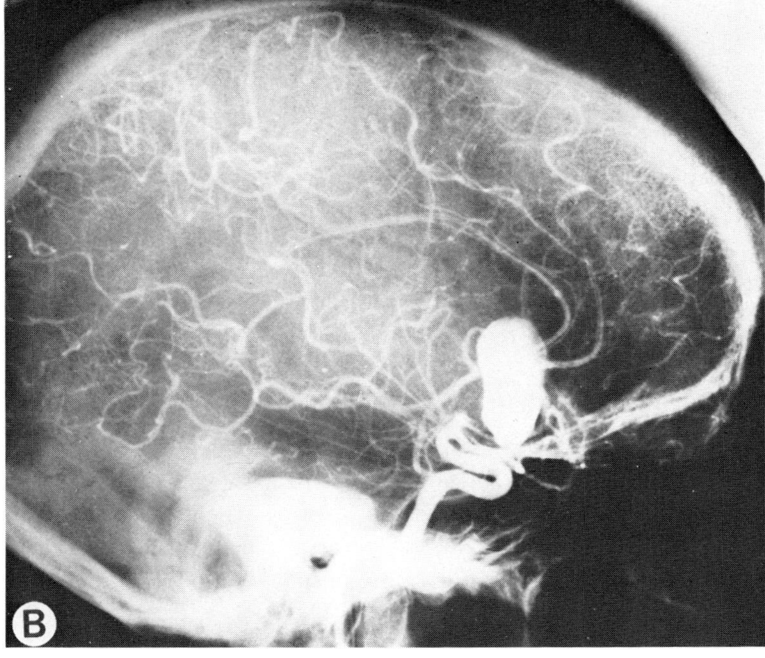

Fig. 85-12

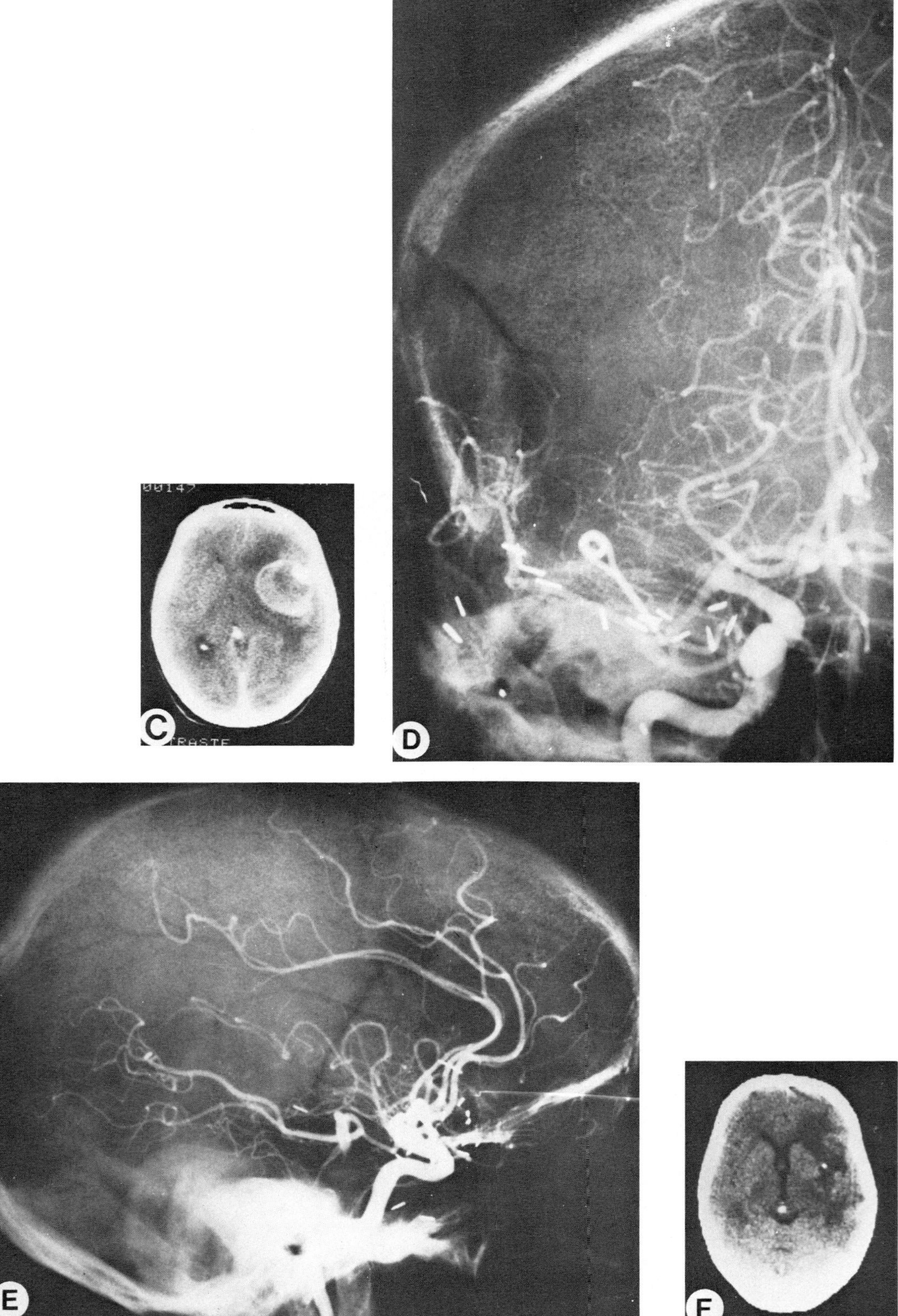

Fig. 85-12. (A and B) Anteroposterior and lateral angiograms and (C) a CT scan of a giant middle cerebral aneurysm that had bled in the remote past and was causing hemiparesis and raised intracranial pressure. A surrounding low density in the distribution of the middle cerebral artery is evident, and slow collateral filling of the distal middle cerebral distribution was evident on later phases of the angicgram. (D and E) Anteroposterior and lateral angiograms and (F) a CT scan made 2 months postoperatively. Imprcved filling of the distal middle cerebral field is evident. The fact that the lesion had a narrow neck is evidenced by its occlusion with a single Scoville clip, and the extent of postoperative low density is shown on the CT scan. The patient's hemiparesis had by this time disappeared and there were no signs. Fortunately, the lesion was in the nondominant hemisphere.

been used in all of my cases, is to depend upon the collateral circulation to sustain the field of the middle cerebral artery during transient periods of occlusion. In larger aneurysms, slow filling of the distal middle cerebral circulation can be seen from leptomeningeal collaterals in the preoperative angiograms, and it has therefore appeared likely that the partial obstruction of the distal middle cerebral circulation caused by the aneurysm had evoked appreciable collateral circulation. The patient whose lesion is shown in Figure 85-12 is a middle-aged woman. She withstood 45 minutes of proximal and distal occlusion of the middle cerebral artery while the aneurysm neck was dissected, the aneurysm opened, the clot evacuated, and a clip placed on the much-reduced neck. The relationship of the perforating vessels, as shown on the diagram, was determined from preoperative angiograms, and this portion of the sac was dissected with great care, although quite frequently the wall of such an aneurysm within the brain comes away very cleanly. The same cannot be said for the walls of giant aneurysms toward the base of the brain, because they often become extremely adherent to structures in the subarachnoid space, other parts of the circle of Willis, the optic nerves, and so forth. Within the brain, however, they often can be dissected quite rapidly. Another giant aneurysm (Figure 85-13) required sacrifice of the anterior temporal branch with proximal and distal occlusion of the middle cerebral artery, including the perforating segment, for 6 minutes and 30 seconds, while the neck dissection was completed. This aneurysm was occluded by a single Scoville clip once the sacrifice of the anterior temporal branch was accepted. No hemiparesis developed, and, this being a dominant hemisphere lesion, the preoperative dysphasic defect present as a result of the last hemorrhage was no worse and gradually improved to normal in the postoperative period.

In the case of a third giant aneurysm (Figure 85-11), the proximal middle cerebral artery was occluded for 20 minutes while the sac was dissected from the distal branches and the neck was ligated. Again, some retrograde collateral filling was evident on the preoperative angiograms and no neurologic deficits resulted from the procedure.

A NOTE ON TEMPORARY VASCULAR OCCLUSION AND SOMATOSENSORY EVOKED RESPONSE MONITORING

I have practiced temporary vascular occlusion for the past 15 years. A review of 185 consecutive cases[10] operated on by me in the 5-year period between January, 1980 and January, 1985, compared 66 cases in which temporary occlusion of main vessels had been employed with 119 patients without occlusion. The longest occlusion time for patients with an excellent outcome was 23 minutes for the A1 segments, 40 minutes for the middle cerebral artery, 27 minutes and 44 seconds for the internal carotid artery, and 13 minutes and 30 seconds for the basilar artery. There was no significant difference in the outcome in terms of mortality or postoperative grade when the two groups of patients were compared.

In an endeavour to increase the safety of temporary arterial occlusion, we have rountinely used somatosensory evoked response recording[11] over the past 6 years. Over a 150 cases have now been recorded in this way, and the technique is of particular utility in relation to middle cerebral artery aneurysms.

Temporary clipping varied in duration from 1 minute to 15 minutes and 50 seconds, and in 7 cases produced no significant changes in conduction time following temporary vascular occlusion. No postoperative morbidity was seen in any of these cases. There was some significant change on the affected side in 6 of 12 cases, 2 of whom showed significant prolongation in central conduction time within a few minutes following middle cerebral occlusion. Both of them, however, showed rapid recovery of conduction to the immediately preceeding level within 5 minutes following release of the clip and showed no postoperative neurologic deficit.

In 4 cases, the cortical peak (N_{20}) disappeared within 4 minutes of occlusion of the middle cerebral artery (Figure 85-14). In these cases recovery of the N_{20} peak occurred in 3 minutes and 25 seconds, 14 minutes, 45 minutes, and 1 hour and 30 minutes following recirculation, respectively. Postoperative morbidity was associated in 3 of these 4 cases although it was fully recoverable in 2. As a result of assessment of cases with temporary vascular occlusion of the internal carotid artery or middle cerebral artery, it would appear that the rapidity of disappearance of the evoked response as originally indicated by Branston et al.[12] is the most reliable predictor of outcome. Up to now no postoperative morbidity has been seen in any case of middle cerebral artery occlusion in which there has been no conduction time abnormality. Six of our 13 patients showed significant abnormality in conduction time within 4 minutes following temporary occlusion and the time course of decline of the N_{20} was similar to that following acute middle cerebral artery occlusion in baboons indicating that the cortical blood flow had been rapidly reduced to less than the critical level (the electrical threshold) in these cases. Three of these 4 cases showed postoperative morbidity, which was completely recoverable in 2. In 1 case the N_{20} peak disappeared within 2 minutes after occlusion of the artery and recovered 3 minutes after the release of occlusion lasting 8 minutes. This

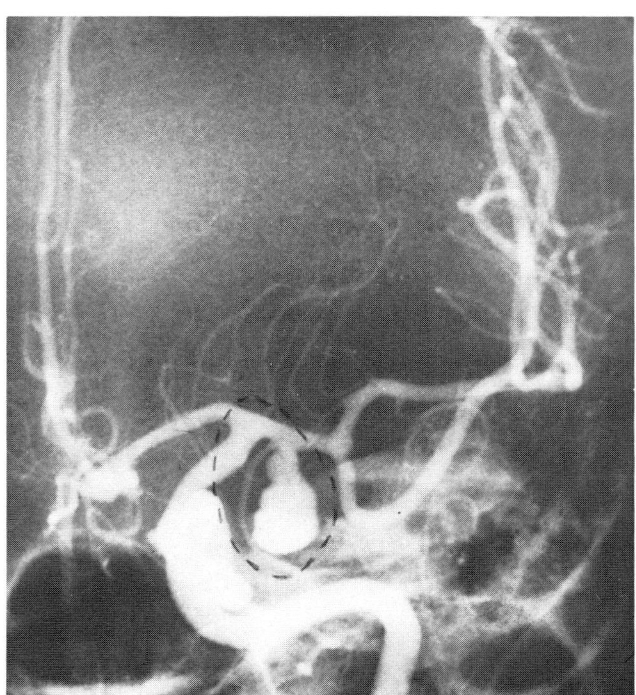

Fig. 85-13. A giant aneurysm that bled recurrently in the months preceding surgery. Only the center of the lesion was visualized. The approximate size of the actual aneurysm is indicated by the dotted line.

patient developed a mild dysphasia incompletely resolving over 2 weeks. The longest period of middle cerebral occlusion without neurologic deficit in this series was 15 minutes and 50 seconds, but a previous case in which electrophysiologic recording was not performed, already referred to in this chapter, sustained occlusion for 45 minutes without postoperative deficit.

In middle cerebral artery aneurysms particularly, therefore, assessment of the somatosensory evoked response is a worthwhile technique, and the surgeon may safely assume that provided the evoked response persists for a period of 3 to 4 minutes after the occlusion is applied, even though it subsequently disappears, it is likely that the degree of ischemia is not sufficient to produce permanent infarction and that periods of occlusion between 10 to 15 minutes may be safely practiced, If the evoked response remains constant throughout the procedure despite middle cerebral occlusion, then an infinite time is probably available. If, however, the conduction disappears rapidly within 2 to 3 minutes following temporary vascular occlusion, it is likely that dense ischemia has been produced in the distal territory and occlusion of under 10 minutes is probably all that is safe. Evidence of this is given in the case of a giant aneurysm in which occlusion for 6 minutes and 30 seconds was occupied by gross postoperative neurology which fortunately proved transient and resolved completely within 48 hours (Figure 85-15).

POSTOPERATIVE CARE

The postoperative care of patients with aneurysms of the middle cerebral artery differs little from the general postoperative management of other aneurysm patients. These aneurysms differ from others above all because hemipareses are common in the postoperative period as a result of the phenomenon of reduced perfusion (which we term ''vasospasm'') that afflicts the highly evocative cortex. In recent years, the induction of hypertension with metaraminol and a high fluid load (an added 500 to 1000 ml of 10-percent Dextran 40 in 24 hours) have been used to overcome transient postoperative deficits once the clip is safely in place.[13,14] Intraoperative monitoring of central conduction time has proved of increasing value while temporary clips are in place on the middle cerebral artery. Full steroid therapy is maintained for 48 hours postoperatively and then tapered off over the next few days. The regimen of added Dextran is maintained for 5 postoperative days, and the patient is allowed to get up on the fifth postoperative day. Continuous closed subgaleal suction drainage is maintained for 2 days postoperatively, but no other attempt is made to drain cerebrospinal fluid.

A CT scan is routinely obtained on all aneurysm patients on the night of the operation whether or not they are well. This will indicate whether brain swelling has occurred, and, should transient neurologic signs develop, is of value in deciding whether artificial hypertension will be used. Where transient hemiparesis develops in the postoperative period and is unattended by a shift on the CT scans, induced hypertension is certainly safe. If brain swelling already exists, however, induced hypertension should be used with caution, since transudation of fluid into an already swollen brain can occur and

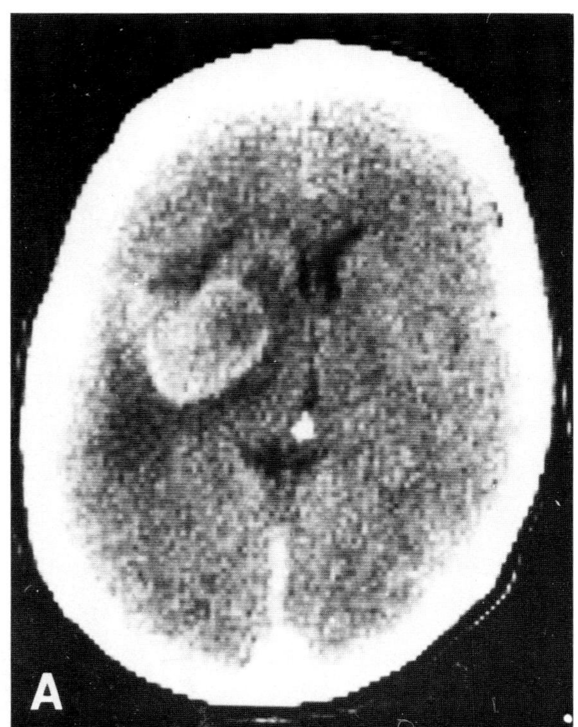

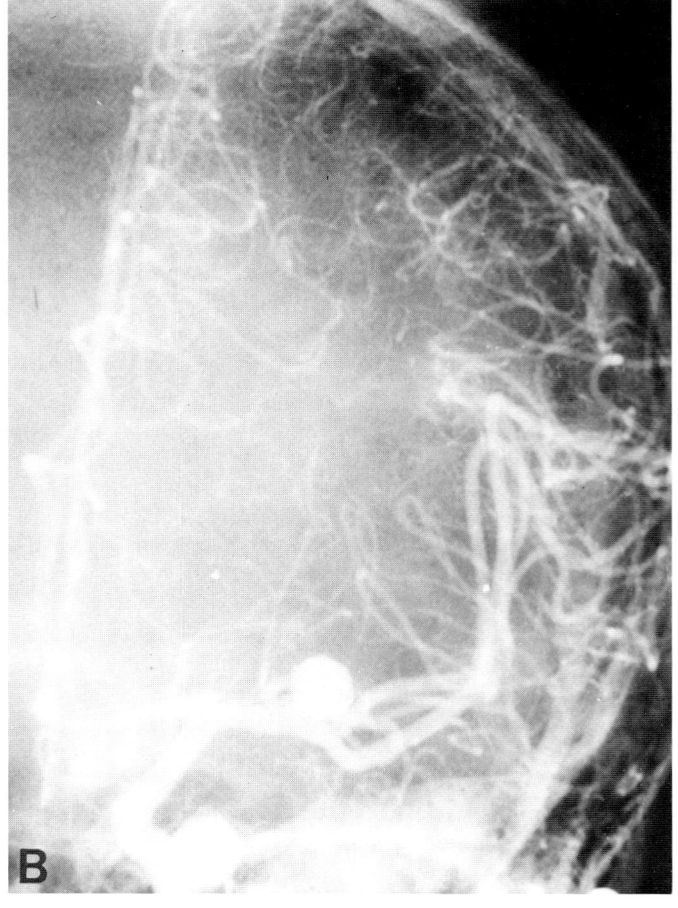

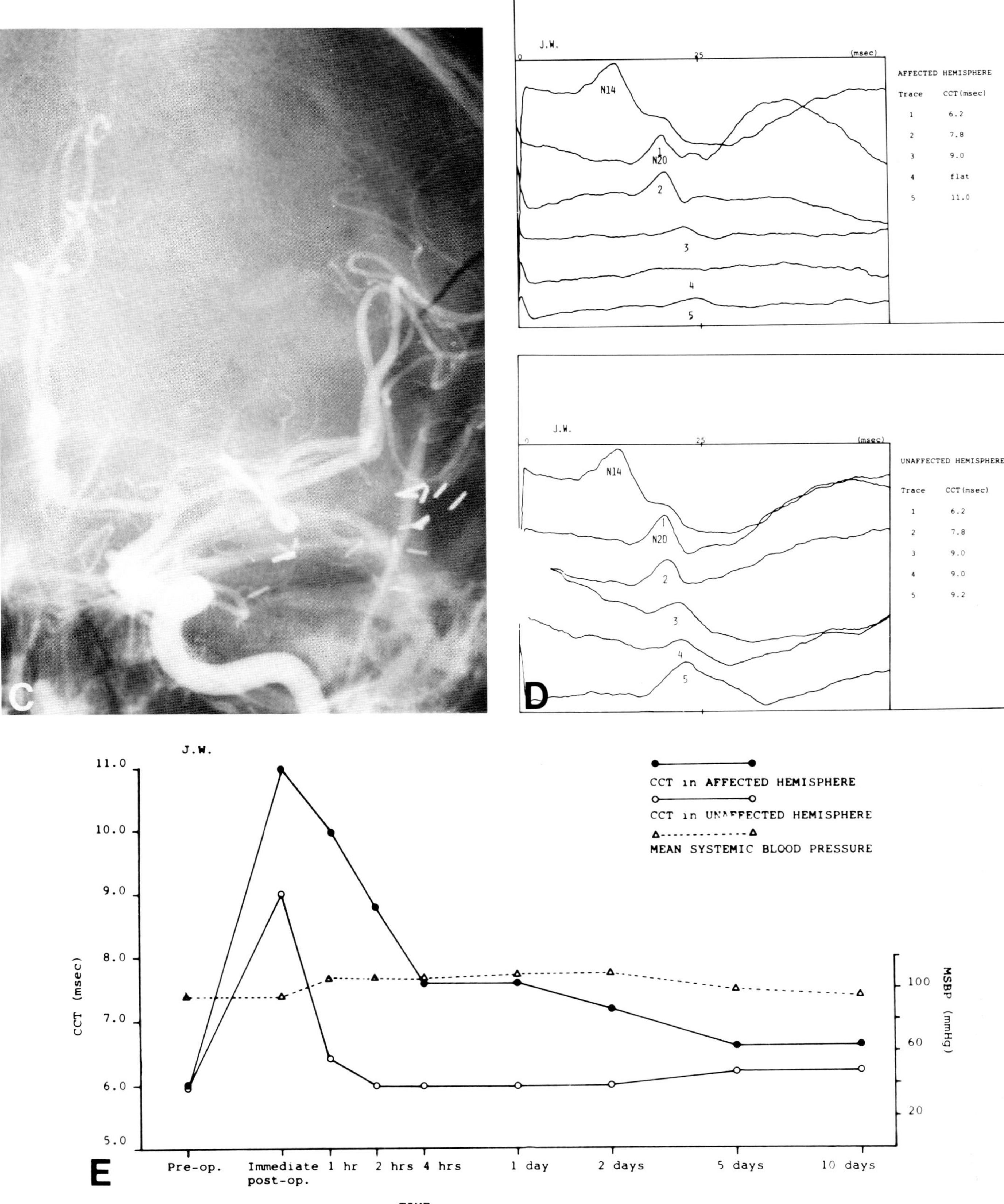

Fig. 85-14. (A) An enhanced CT scan of a giant middle cerebral aneurysm. (B) Preoperative AP arteriogram. The opacified segment of the aneurysm is as usual small. The bulk can to some extent be inferred by the displacement of perforating vessels. (C) Postoperative AP angiogram. The aneurysm has been occluded by a single clip. (D) Perioperative evoked response recordings show in the upper panel recording from the affected hemisphere. Trace 4 the N_{20} peak is no longer recognizable. The contralateral hemisphere in the lower panel shows appreciable delay in conduction due in this case to considerable influence of the anesthetic, halothane in a concentration of between 0.5 and 1.5 percent. (E) The profile of central conduction in the two hemispheres over the few days succeeding operation. The unaffected hemisphere showed a rapid return to normal conduction with the dissipation of anesthesia, but the affected hemisphere remained prolonged, although it had returned to normal by the 5 day assessment. The patient woke aphasic and extending the right side but showed a progressive recovery over the next few hours. By 24 hours postoperatively his neurologic status was normal, and psychometric testing postoperatively showed him to have retained his extremely high premorbid IQ. He returned to normal function as a school teacher.

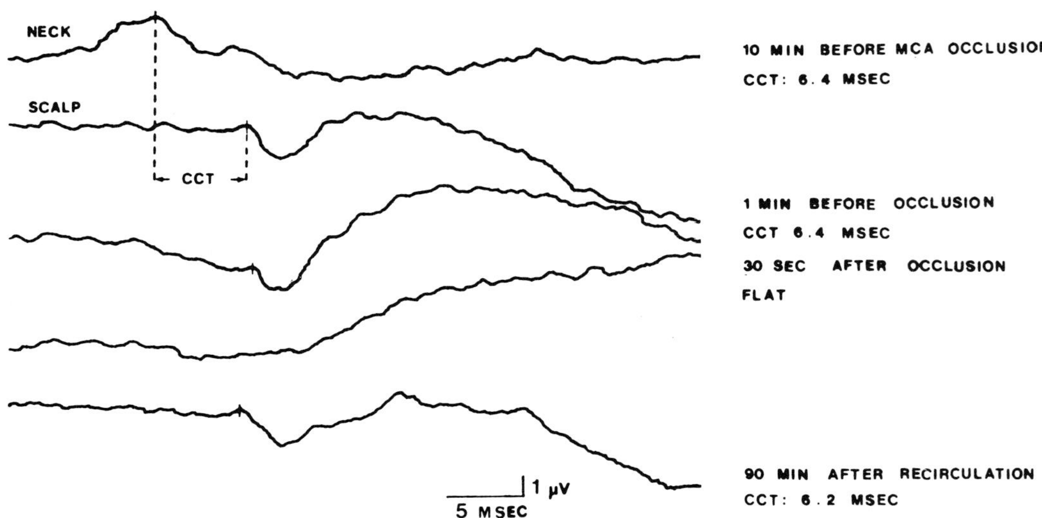

Fig. 85-15.   Recording of evoked potentials in the neck and skull during the occlusion of a middle cerebral artery aneurysm. The N_{20}, much suppressed by anesthesia, is still detectible for occlusion but has disappeared together with the later cortical waves 30 seconds after occlusion. At 90 minutes after recirculation the CCT had returned to normal values. The patient showed a moderate contralateral hemiparesis which fully recovered over the next 10 days.

cause the patient's state to worsen. Under these circumstances, dehydrating agents rather than induced hypertension may be the only method open to the surgeon. Monitoring of intracranial pressure[15] may be of value in controlling a difficult situation here. For many years it was the routine practice in this clinic to perform postoperative angiography. With the advent of the operating microscope, this has no longer been thought necessary, and angiography is performed only rarely now after operations for middle cerebral aneurysms. Where a pouch of aneurysm has had to be left, however, postoperative angiography is of value, since it will prove to be a useful baseline should further hemorrhage occur.

angiography before the evacuation of the clot, and, because the aneurysm was in the clot, also was subjected to clipping of the aneurysm. If this case is excluded, the total mortality of 4.2 percent would be 3.2 percent and the morbidity, including one unacceptable result, would be 4.6 percent.

There is little justification for urgent clipping of aneurysms in grade-5 patients. It certainly will not improve the patient's prospects, and probably brings aneurysm surgery into poor repute. If the patient can be persuaded to improve by judicious evacuation of the clot or by steroid management alone, then delayed surgery presents a more attractive prospect.

RESULTS

This chapter is based on my personal series of operations for aneurysms of the middle cerebral artery. Of a total of 450 anterior circle aneurysms with recent subarachnoid hemorrhage, there were 95 aneurysms of the middle cerebral artery. The grades and times of surgery are shown in Table 85-2. Three of the giant aneurysms were operated upon long after from any hemorrhage and are not included in this table.

An endeavor was made to operate on aneurysms early, thus 56 were operated upon in the first 10 days, 74 in the first 15 days, and 82 in the first 21 days. Only 21 were operated upon in the first 5 days, however, because of delay in referral.

There was 1 death in the patients operated on in grades 1 through 3, which gives an operative mortality of 1.3 percent. The total operative mortality, including three additional deaths, two in grade 4 and one in grade 5, is 4.2 percent. Unacceptable morbidity occurred in one grade-4 patient, who was confused and suffering from appreciable hemiparesis preoperatively and was densely hemiplegic postoperatively. Thus, the total morbidity (dead or unacceptably disabled) for the series was 5.3 percent. In one case, the patient had a grade 5 aneurysm with a large clot extending in all limbs. The patient was subjected to

REFERENCES

1. McKissock W, Richardson A, Walsh LS: Middle cerebral artery aneurysms. Further results in the controlled trial of conservative and surgical treatment of ruptured intracranial aneurysms. Lancet 2:417, 1962
2. Hunt WE, Hess RM: Surgical risk as related to time of intervention on the repair of intracranial aneurysms. J Neurosurg 38:14, 1968
3. Suzuki J, Kodama N, Fujiwara S, et al: Surgical treatment of middle cerebral artery aneurysms: From the experience of 174 cases, in Suzuki J (ed): Cerebral Aneurysms. Tokyo, Neuron Publishing Co., 1979, pp 278–283
4. Fisher CM, Kistler MD, Davis JM: Relation of cerebral vasospasm to subarachnoid hemorrhage visualized by computerized tomographic scanning. Neurosurgery 6:1, 1980
5. Bell BA, Kendall BE, Symon L: Computerized tomography in aneurysmal subarachnoid hemorrhage. J Neurol Neurosurg Psychiatry 43:522, 1980
6. Symon L, Hargadine J, Zawirski M, et al: Central conduction time as an index of ischemia in subarachnoid hemorrhage. J Neurol Sci 44:95, 1979
7. Yasargil MG, Fox JL: Microsurgical approach to intracranial aneurysms. Surg Neurol 3:7, 1975
8. Lougheed WM, Marshall BM: Measurement of the anterior circu-

lation by intracranial procedures, in Youmans (ed): Neurological Surgery. Philadelphia, WB Saunders, 1973, pp 731–767

9. McFadden JT: Tissue reactions to standard neurosurgical metallic implants. J Neurosurg 36:598, 1972

10. Jabre A, Symon L: Temporary vascular occlusion during aneurysm surgery. Surg Neurol 27:47, 1987

11. Momma F, Wang AD, Symon L: Effects of temporary arterial occlusion on somatosensory evoked responses in aneurysm surgery. Surg Neurol 27:343, 1987

12. Branston NM, Symon L, Crockard HA, et al: Relationship between the cortical evoked potential and local cortical blood flow following acute middle cerebral artery occlusion in the baboon. Exp Neurol 45:195, 1974

13. Kosnick EJ, Hunt WE: Postoperative hypertension in the management of patients with intracranial aneurysms. J Neurosurg 38:14, 1976

14. Symon L: Disordered cerebrovascular physiology in aneurysmal subarachnoid hemorrhage. Acta Neurochir 41:7, 1978

15. Kassell N F, Peerless SJ, Durward OJ, et al: Neurological deterioration from cerebral vasospasm: Treatment with induced arterial hypertension, in Wilkins RH (ed): Cerebral Arterial Spasm. (Proceedings of the 2nd International Workshop, 1979.) Baltimore, Williams & Wilkins, 1979, pp 665–672

CHAPTER 86

Surgical Techniques of Posterior Cerebral Aneurysms

Sydney J. Peerless   Charles G. Drake

IT IS ONLY RECENTLY that neurosurgeons have been able to attack aneurysms of the vertebral-basilar circulation with the same safety and assurance with which they attack aneurysms arising from the carotid circulation. The reasons for this late development are many. Aneurysms arising from the posterior circulation are relatively uncommon, amounting to less than 15 percent of all aneurysms of the brain, giving few surgeons the opportunity to gain the necessary experience and confidence in exploring the confined space in front of the cerebellum. The late refinement of routine vertebral angiography resulted in only a few of these lesions being diagnosed, and then only when the aneurysms had grown to giant size and presented as tumors. Before 1950, a few large masses of unknown nature were explored, found to be thrombosed aneurysms, and shelled out and secured with proximal vessel ligation by Dandy, Tonnis, Falconer, Poppen, and Logue.[1–5] Schwartz is credited with the first deliberate, direct attack on an aneurysm in the cerebello-pontine angle.[6] His dramatic description of controlling the bleeding and trapping the sac that was buried in the pons is memorable—the more so when one considers that the procedure was carried out without magnification, and with the crude clips and instruments available at that time. The patient did well.

At the time of Drake's original report of his own experience with 4 patients with aneurysms of the basilar bifurcation, there was considerable skepticism as to the value or safety of direct surgical attack on aneurysms of the posterior circulation. Of the 47 cases reported to that time, 14 had been treated indirectly with vertebral artery ligation, and almost half of the remainder were peripheral aneurysms arising distally on branches of the vertebral or basilar artery. The 10 aneurysms arising at the basilar bifurcation proved to be technically unapproachable; fewer than half were clipped, and the remainder were packed.[7] Jamieson emphasized his discouragement in his index report of the direct surgical treatment of 19 aneurysms of the vertebro-basilar system. Ten of his patients had died and only 4 of the survivors were employable.[8]

Although a note of optimism was evident in Drake's 1965 paper describing the treatment of aneurysms of the basilar trunk, the safe treatment of aneurysms of the basilar artery remained elusive.[9] The first 7 patients with aneurysms of the terminal basilar artery had not done well; 4 died, 1 was severely disabled, and only 2 returned to normal life. It was at this time that Drake realized the importance of identifying and sparing the tiny perforating vessels arising from the terminal basilar

artery and proximal posterior cerebral arteries. It was evident that these small arteries, which were vital to the irrigation of the hypothalamus, midbrain, and pons, were often adhering to the posterior wall of the sac and were surrounded by old blood and adhesions and were frequently difficult, if not impossible, to visualize in the confined space of the exposure.

At this time, there was a dramatic improvement in the technology of neurosurgery. The operating microscope, new fine instruments and clips, and the refinements of modern neuroanesthesia, including profound hypotension, all were combined to bring about a remarkable improvement in results. In 1968, Drake reported 12 additional cases with no direct operative deaths and 10 good results.[10]

In the past 2 decades, our experience has grown to more than 1400 cases, and contemporary results are comparable with the results of treatment of aneurysms of the anterior circulation. Poor results today are almost entirely limited to patients harboring giant aneurysms or those who are in a poor clinical state before the operation (Figure 86-1).

ANESTHESIA END MONITORING TECHNIQUES

It would be improper not to mention some of our anesthetic and monitoring techniques, in that so much of the success of the actual technical procedure of approaching an aneurysm begins with the preparation of the patient and with careful, moment-to-moment assessment of patient condition during the procedure. Patients are brought to the operating room lightly sedated and with an accurate assessment of that patient's fluid balance. An arterial line is installed, usually with a flexible needle in the dorsalis pedis or radial artery, where the arterial pressure can be continuously monitored. The patient is induced gently with pentothal, paralyzed, and then intubated with an armored tube. The anesthetic technique is basically an assisted controlled ventilation in most instances, using halothane, nitrous oxide, or a narcotic technique, depending on the preference of the anesthetist; the recent tendency is toward isoflurane. The anesthetic is kept generally light, with meticulous monitoring of blood gases in order to maintain the PCO_2 in the range of 40 to 45 torr, and the PO_2 in excess of 100 torr.

The success of the procedure largely depends upon adequate intracranial relaxation. For this reason, we routinely give 1 g/kg of 20-percent mannitol, increasing this to 2 g/kg if we

OPERATIVE NEUROSURGICAL TECHNIQUES
ISBN 0-8089-1862-1

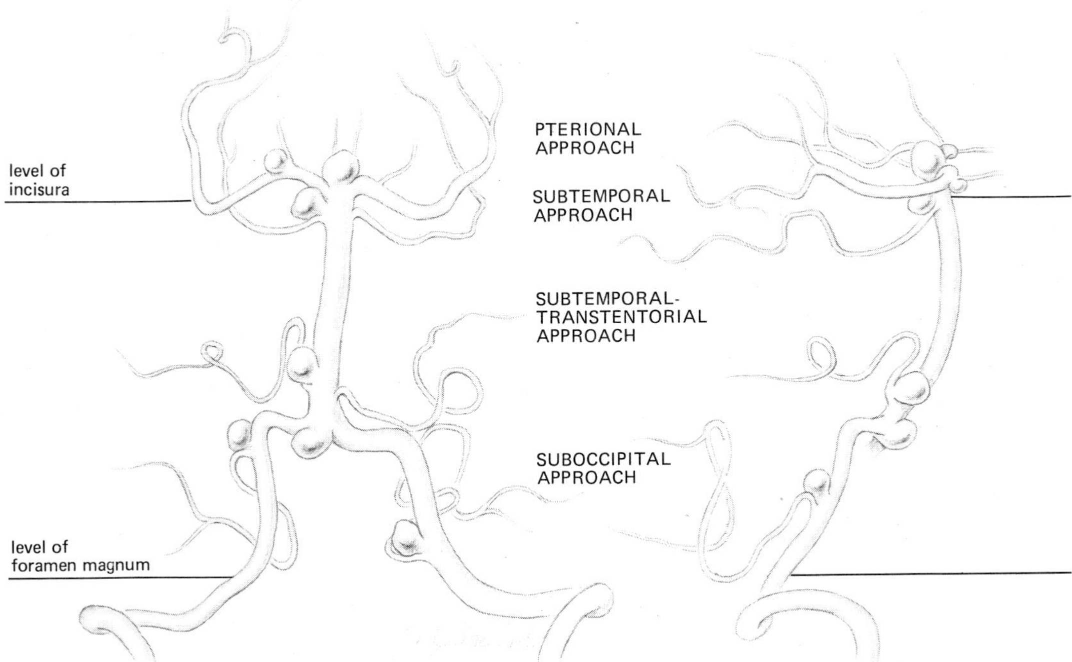

Fig. 86-1.   Common sites of posterior circulation aneurysms. The level of the tentorial incisura and foramen magna is depicted at the usual site of the aneurysms relative to these fixed points. The surgical approaches to aneurysms of various regions is noted.

contemplate temporary occlusion of a major intracranial vessel. Furosemide (1 mg/kg) is given intravenously shortly after induction and the administration of mannitol. While the patient is being positioned, the anesthetist uses a Touhy needle to insert a lumbar subarachnoid catheter (PE 100) into the lumbar subarachnoid space, and attaches this tubing to a closed collection bag. The lumbar subarachnoid drain is kept clamped until the dura is opened, at which time cerebrospinal fluid (CSF) drainage is commenced to add to the intracranial relaxation.

We frequently use intentional hypotension during the dissection and clipping of the aneurysm. The anesthetist prepares for this by connecting the transducer from the arterial line, at a level equal to the height of the brain, to an electronic monitor that gives systolic, diastolic, and mean pressures. Hypotension is induced by deepening the isoflurane anesthesia. Systemic arterial pressures of 50 to 60 torr are routinely used during the initial dissection around the aneurysm, and when manipulation of the aneurysm itself or application of the clip begins, the pressure is lowered to 40 to 45 torr. It has been our experience that these low pressures are routinely well tolerated for 30 to 40 minutes and have rarely been responsible for significant problems when prolonged for 60 to 90 minutes.

In recent years, we have frequently come to rely on temporary occlusion of the parent (basilar or vertebral) artery as a means to soften the aneurysmal sac while dissecting and preparing the neck for clipping. The new small, temporary clips designed by Suzuki and Sugita are admirable for this purpose, not only for their reliably soft closing pressures, but also for their relative ease of application and removal. The temporary clip must have a gentle closing pressure (less than 40 g) to prevent injury to the parent vessel, and it should not occlude any perforating vessels. Of course, before application of a temporary proximal clip, the patient should be normotensive and should receive an additional bolus of 1 g/kg 20-percent

mannitol. Under these circumstances, temporary occlusion of the basilar artery for up to 10 minutes is well tolerated. Occasionally, we have occluded the basilar artery for more than 1 hour, with 6 or 7 occlusions of 10 minutes each interspersed with periods of reperfusion.

With the patient positioned, the anesthetist begins meticulous monitoring of fluid balance, ECG, systemic arterial blood pressure, and blood gases. Occasionally we will employ brain retractor pressure monitoring, EEG, evoked potential, and intraoperative cerebral blood flow (CBF) monitoring in unique situations of giant aneurysms, or when we anticipate prolonged interruption of focal cerebral blood flow.[11]

POSITIONING

Almost all aneurysms of the basilar artery above the anterior inferior cerebellar arteries can be approached through the lateral decubitus, or "park bench," position. In that we normally aim to approach the aneurysm under the nondominant temporal lobe, the patient is placed on his or her left side, with a sandbag under the left axilla to elevate the shoulder from the table and provide free respiratory excursion of the chest. The back and chest of the patient are supported by rests attached to the table, and the head is fixed in a three-point pin headrest. The alignment of the head is critical for the subtemporal approach. The anteroposterior (AP) axis should be precisely parallel to the floor, and the sagittal plane of the head tipped 15 degrees toward the floor. The head does not move relative to the body following fixation in this position, but the whole table may be tipped head up or head down or rotated from one side to the other as necessary to gain further visual access to the upper basilar artery (Figure 86-2).

In our initial experience with aneurysms of the upper

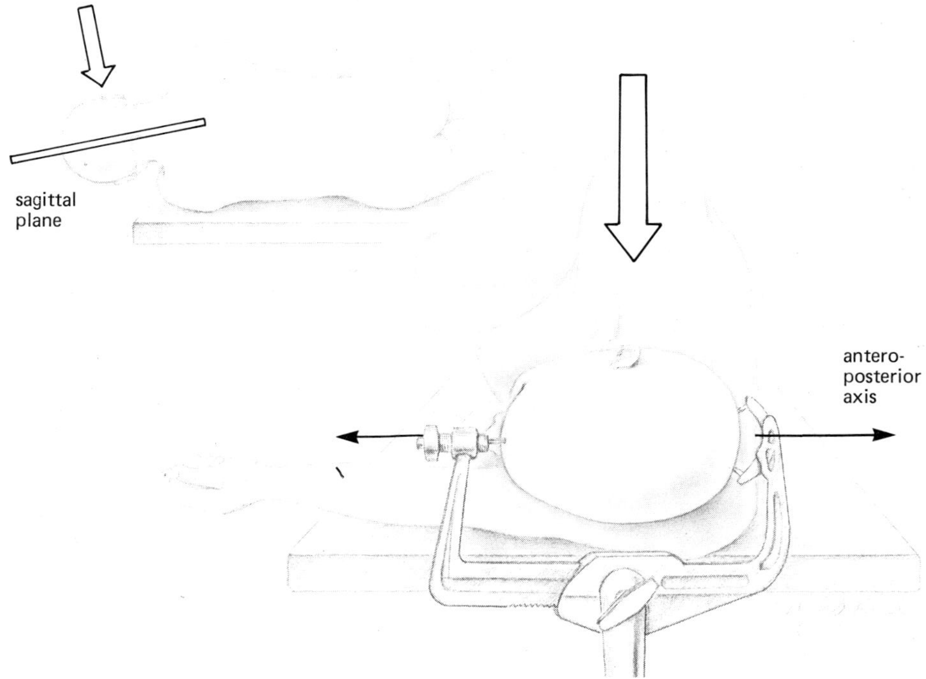

Fig. 86-2 Patient position for the subtemporal approach. Note that the anterior posterior access of the head is fixed parallel to the floor, and that the sagittal plane is tipped 15 degrees to the perpendicular. The open arrow shows the starting position of the operating microscope.

basilar artery, we routinely turned sizeable temporal bone flaps. In our more recent 1000 cases, this has proved unnecessary. As will be seen by the orientation drawings, the aim of the exposure is to get as close to the base of the skull as possible at the junction of the anterior and middle thirds of the temporal lobe, where the temporal lobe has already begun to turn upward following the convex floor of the middle cranial fossa. Little is gained by fashioning a large bone flap up over the lateral surface of the temporal lobe or posteriorly, except in circumstances in which it is necessary to divide the tentorium in order to gain access to the middle portions of the basilar artery (Figures 86-3, 86-4, and 86-5).

We now routinely make a linear incision extending vertically upward, curving slightly backward at its upper extent, and originating at the zygomatic process of the temporal bone approximately one finger's width anterior to the ear. After the

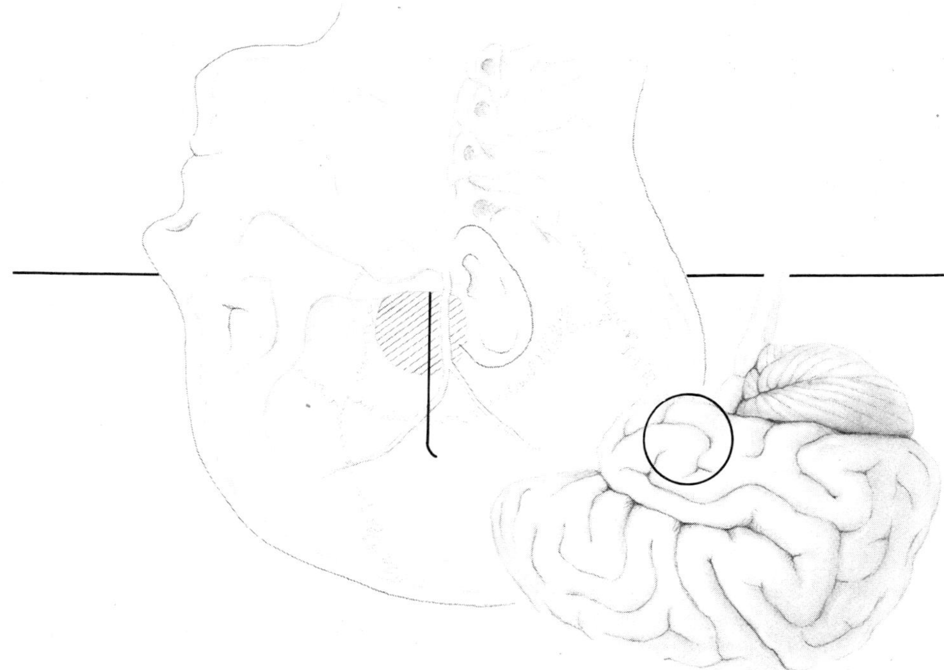

Fig. 86-3. Subtemporal approach. Relationship of scalp incision and craniectomy to skull and brain landmarks.

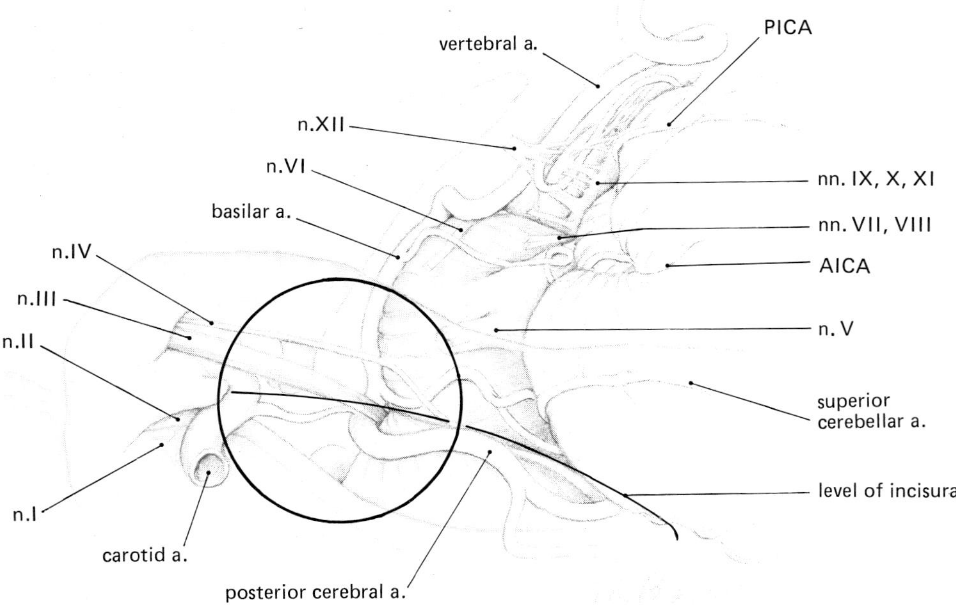

Fig. 86-4.   An overview of the anatomy of the vertebral basilar circulation as seen from the subtemporal approach. The circle depicts the size of the craniectomy.

skin, subcutaneous tissue, and galea are divided, the temporalis fascia and muscle are divided 5 mm on either side of the vertical incision at the level of the zygomatic process. With the soft tissue held apart by a tic retractor, a single burr hole in the squamous portion of the temporal bone is enlarged with rongeurs, forming a somewhat pear-shaped opening that is widest at the base, with bone nibbled away down to the floor of the middle cranial fossa. The main stem and posterior branch of the superficial temporal artery are preserved in the posterior aspect of the scalp flap, but often the anterior branch of this vessel must be divided (Figure 86-6).

The dura is opened in a triangle with the base. The main stem and posterior branch of the superficial temporal artery are preserved in the posterior aspect of the scalp flap, but often the anterior branch of this vessel must be divided (Figure 86-6).

The dura is opened in a triangle with the base inferior, and is sutured up to the overlying soft tissue so as not to obscure the view at the base. At this point, the lumbar subarachnoid drain is opened and CSF removal is begun. A slack brain is essential. The combination of the osmotic and loop diuretic and the removal of CSF is usually sufficient to produce excellent intracranial relaxation. If the brain remains full, however, and gentle retraction of the temporal lobe does not easily expose the middle intracranial fossa, it is imperative to wait, elevate the head, remove more CSF, check to ensure that the ventilation parameters are adequate, and wait again until adequate reduction of the intracranial contents has been achieved. If, with time, the brain continues to remain full, it may be advisable to abandon the procedure and return another day. Cerebral edema is the most likely cause for a persistently swollen and tight brain. Most maneuvers on the operating table will not adequately relieve this, and further retraction and manipulation run a high likelihood of aggravating the edema in the postoperative period.

With the brain relaxed, the surface of the temporal lobe should be covered with a compressed sheet of Gelfoam. With a hand-held retractor, the undersurface of the temporal lobe is inspected for the position of bridging veins. The vein of Labbé is usually seen just beyond the posterior limits of the craniectomy. It should, when visualized, be covered with several strips of Gelfoam and must be protected at all costs against rupture. Similarly, bridging veins at the tip of the temporal lobe seen just beyond the anterior limits of the bony removal should also be protected. Small bridging veins, from the undersurface of the temporal lobe to the tent, can be coagulated and divided with impunity; the larger veins on the surface, however, should never be sacrificed, because of the danger of producing venous swelling or infarction.

With further retraction, the uncus of the temporal lobe is gently elevated and the free edge of the tentorium comes into view. A Greenberg or Yasargil self-retaining retractor should now be fixed without excessive retractor pressure. With this retractor in place, and with a 2- to 3-mm gap visible between the uncus and the free surface of the tent, it is likely that the retractor will not need to be moved again. The position of the tip of the retractor is important. It should just touch the uncus and its overlying arachnoid and be centered at about the midpoint of the concave curve of the free edge of the tent. Positioning the retractor anterior or posterior to this will lead the surgeon forward into the interpeduncular fossa and posterior clinoid, or will lead backward onto the cerebral peduncle, instead of directly medially onto the terminal basilar artery (Figure 86-7).

It is almost always necessary at this point to pass a 4-0 silk suture through the free edge of the tentorium and to tie it back into the floor of the middle cranial fossa. This maneuver provides 3 to 5 mm more exposure by rolling back the free edge of the tentorium. Only rarely will it be necessary to divide the tent in the exposure of aneurysms of the distal end of the basilar artery.

At this point, the operating microscope should be brought into position and, under 10–16× magnification, the operator focuses on the layer of arachnoid covering the uncus and cerebral peduncle, passing onto and under the free edge of the

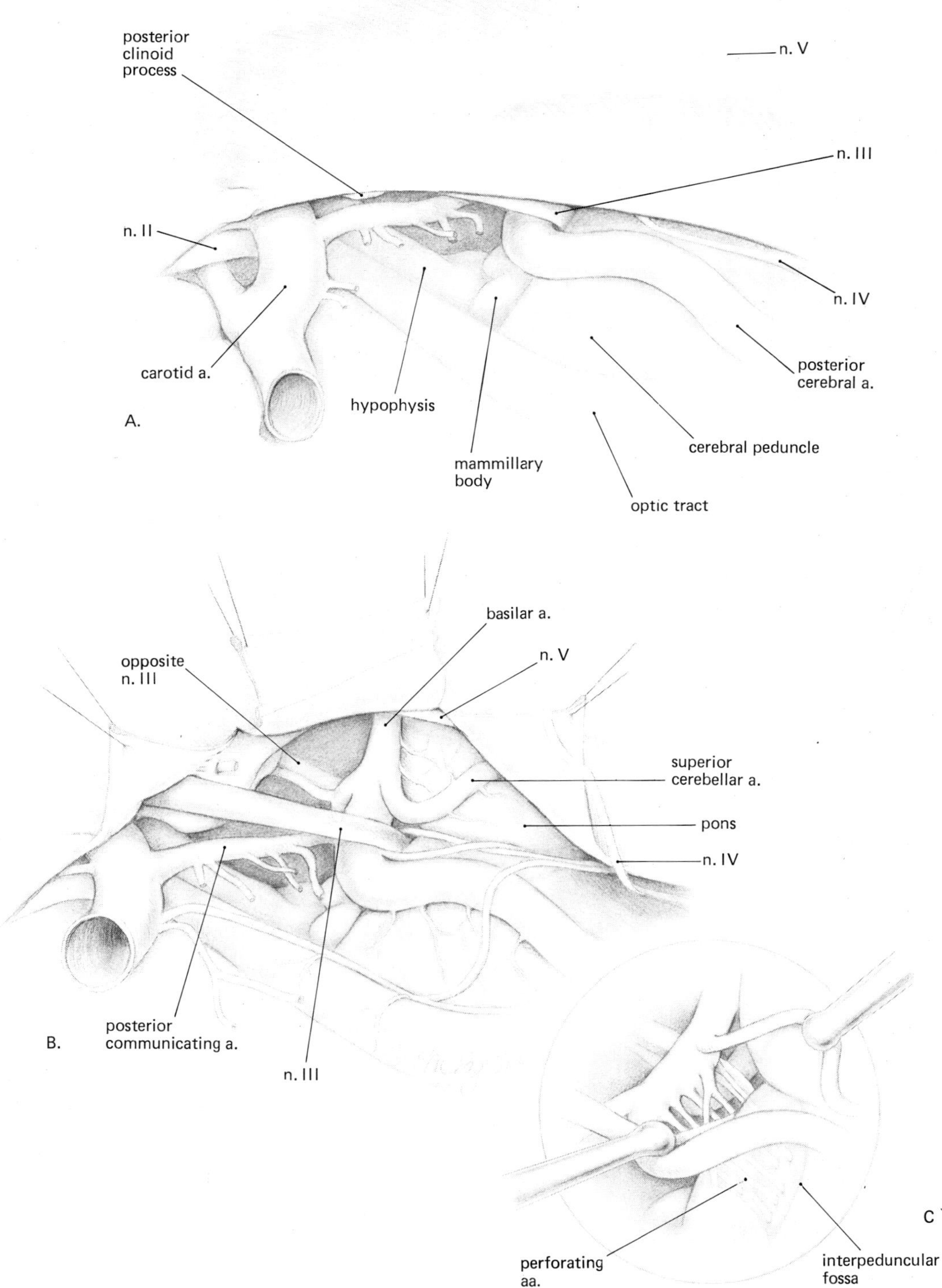

Fig. 86-5.　Microscopic anatomy of the interpeduncular fossa and its contents. (A) Uncus and hippocampal gyrus of temporal removed and intact. (B) Tentorium divided and retracted. (C) Terminal basilar artery drawn out of interpeduncular fossa to show perforating artery.

tentorium. It is usually possible to identify the oculomotor nerve at this point, coming up from the depths under the uncus and piercing the arachnoid in the anterior aspect of the exposure to enter its cavernous compartment. The trochlear nerve will also be seen posteriorly in the exposure, lying beneath the arachnoid and turning inferiorly underneath the tentorium. Popular textbooks of anatomy often depict the trochlear nerve passing between layers of the tentorium at this site, but it does

not. It remains within its arachnoid layer, attached to the undersurface of the tentorium for about 2 cm, and swings in an arc laterally forward and then medially toward the cavernous sinus.

The initial arachnoid incision should then be made by picking up the arachnoid covering the side of the peduncle superior to the trochlear nerve and inferior to the uncus. This incision is extended forward below the course of the third

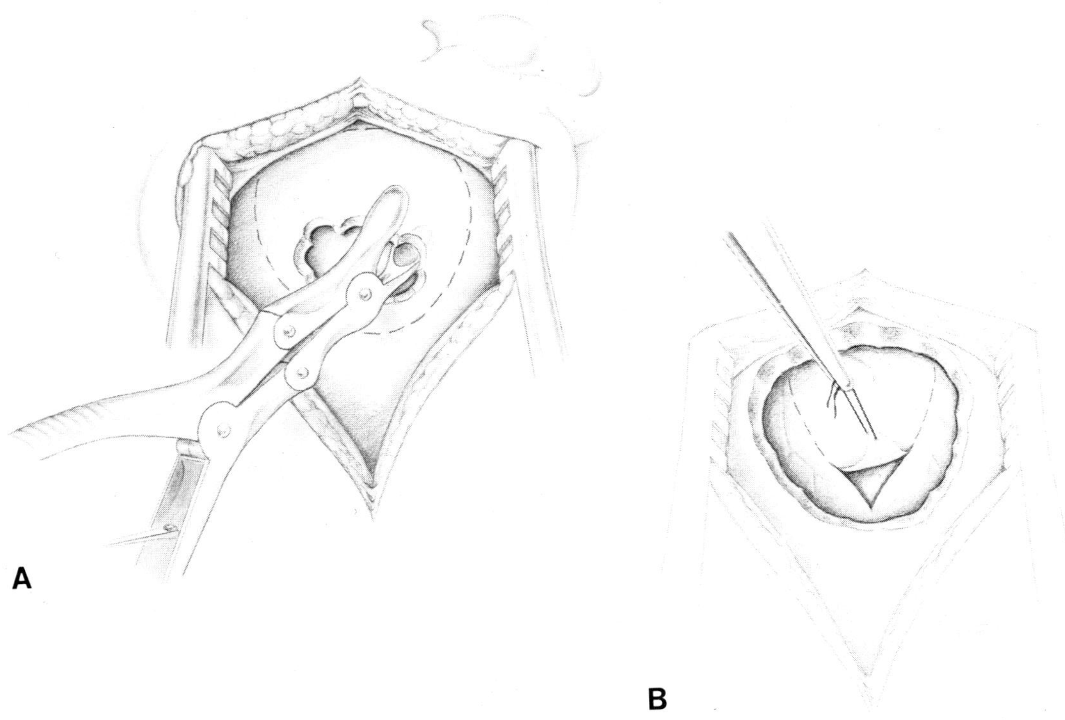

Fig. 86-6.　Subtemporal approach. Operative procedure. (A) Exposure of dura. (B) Dural incision.

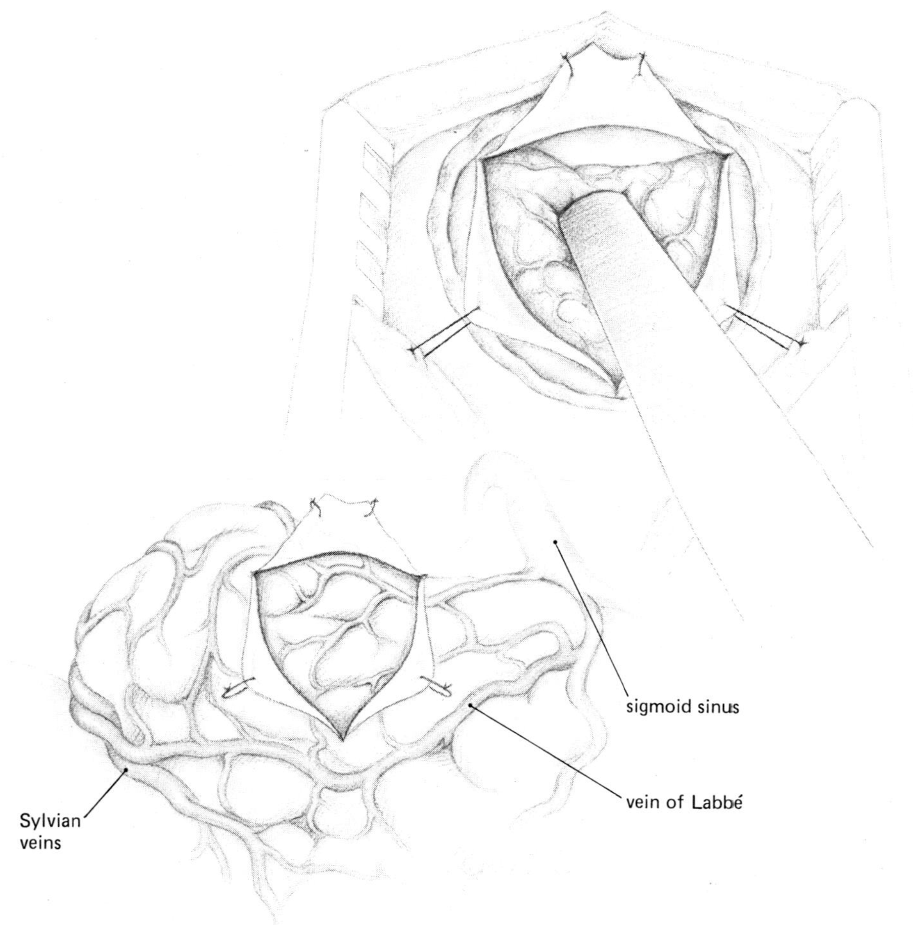

Fig. 86-7.　Subtemporal approach. Retraction of temporal lobe and temporal lobe veins.

nerve. This arachnoid is a rather thick and complex structure, dividing anteriorly to form a band running medially across the interpeduncular fossa known as the membrane of Lilliequist. This band of arachnoid should also be sharply divided across the front of the pons to permit the removal of clot in the interpeduncular fossa and to permit visualization of the opposite oculomotor nerve and posterior cerebral artery (Figures 86-8 and 86-9).

At this stage, the inexperienced surgeon will often be surprised if he or she is unable to see the posterior cerebral artery. This vessel, of course, follows a compound curved course, bending upward laterally, forward, and then turning backward, and is usually obscured by the third nerve, the uncus, and the mesial portion of the temporal lobe as it winds its way back around the midbrain. Branches of the superior cerebellar artery are readily apparent at this stage as they wind around the peduncle, and these branches can be followed medially to the basilar artery. The surgeon must now have a clear mental picture of the anatomy gained from knowledge of the normal anatomy and by study of the angiograms, so that he or she can readily identify the structures in the depths of the exposure. It is usually best to begin removal of the blood clot in the region along the lateral aspects of the basilar artery between the superior cerebellar and the origin of P1. Once the wall of the basilar artery is in view, dissection can be carried out in that plane anteriorly and posteriorly, removing clot with suction and forceps and working from the base of the presumed neck of the aneurysm and distally toward the fundus (Figure 86-10).

BASILAR BIFURCATION ANEURYSMS

Basilar bifurcation aneurysms may be small (up to 1.5 cm in diameter), bulbous (1.5–2.5 cm in diameter), or giant (greater than 2.5 cm in diameter). These aneurysms may point forward, directly upward, or backward. For each size and orientation, there are special problems in dissection and clipping. The position of the basilar bifurcation relative to the posterior clinoid is also an important variable to be considered in one's approach to these aneurysms. Most often, the bifurcation lies precisely at the level of the posterior clinoid, but in some cases it may be several millimeters or up to 1 cm below the clinoid, and in others, the basilar artery is elongated, with the bifurcation lying some distance above the clinoid. With aneurysms arising from the basilar bifurcation located at the level of the posterior clinoid, the approach from this point will be quite straightforward. A high bifurcation will require further retraction of the uncus and, indeed, may be preferentially approached from the frontotemporal exposure after splitting of the sylvian fissure. The low-lying basilar bifurcation is particularly hazardous, in that the interpeduncular space narrows to the apex of a cone, making manipulation and visualization difficult around the bulging belly of the pons and, with the thin dome of the fundus, obscuring the surgeon's path to the neck.

With an aneurysm of average size and in the middle position, it is preferable at this stage to begin the dissection on the anterior surface of the aneurysm. By following the surface of the basilar artery anteriorly sund superiorly, the origin of the P1 artery on the right side will be identified, as well as the anterior aspect of the neck of the sac. The neck of the sac and the termination of the basilar artery are gently retracted backward into the interpeduncular fossa and, with further removal of clot, the opposite (left) P1 artery will be exposed and

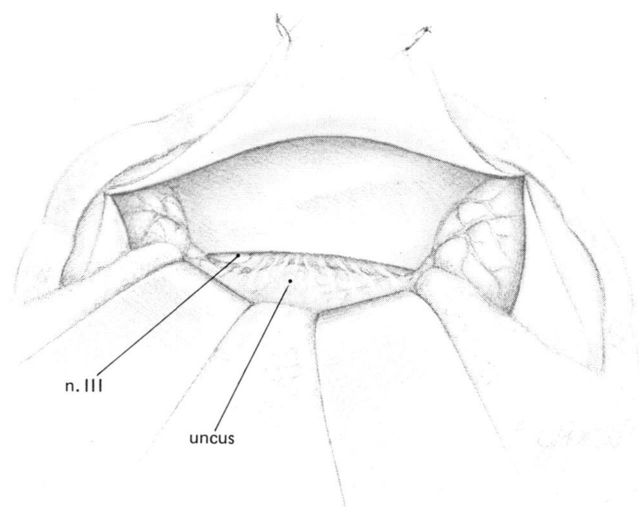

Fig. 86-8. Subtemporal approach. Retraction of temporal lobe to expose edge of tentorium and first layer of arachnoid.

visualized through a layer of arachnoid, with the left oculomotor nerve passing forward. One must use this maneuver cautiously with aneurysms pointing forward, for they are often fused to the clivus at the site of rupture; rough handling can tear away this point of junction and cause troublesome bleeding.

It is important to emphasize at this point that the termination of the basilar artery is usually widened and ectatic at the base of aneurysms arising from the bifurcation. One must have an appreciation of this variation in anatomy and identify the origin of the P1 artery precisely, lest one mistake the terminal basilar artery for a portion of the sac and position the clip dangerously low, resulting in occlusion of the terminal basilar artery. Furthermore, the distal basilar artery and the origin of both posterior cerebral arteries forms a V-shaped structure as viewed from the front, making the neck of these aneurysms quite narrow. This often comes as a surprise when the aneurysm is exposed in the operating room, in that the conventional angiographic projections of this area commonly superimpose the P1 artery and the neck of the aneurysm, giving the appearance of a spuriously wide base. Bearing this in mind, care must be taken to prevent placement of a clip with blades that are too long, as this would risk narrowing or occluding the opposite P1 artery. Moreover, the base of the aneurysm is narrower from front to back than from side to side, making application of the clip from the side somewhat safer, in that properly positioned clip blades are least likely to crimp the origins of the P1 artery.

After exposure of the front side of the aneurysm, dissection should be directed to the right lateral and posterior aspect of the aneurysm. Here the goal is to define the posterior aspect of the sac and, more importantly, to identify and separate the perforators that arise from the proximal, posterior portion of the P1 artery and that normally stream backward over the sac of the aneurysm to enter the posterior perforated substance and peduncle. These perforators are small vessels, often branching once or twice before penetrating the pia covering the brain. It is essential that each of these vital vessels be preserved, and any amount of time taken to separate these vessels from the sac can be justified. Often these perforators will have to be separated with a sharp hook, or, after they have been stretched, by sharply dividing with a knife the fibrous bands fusing them to the sac. One must remember that the perforators are paired,

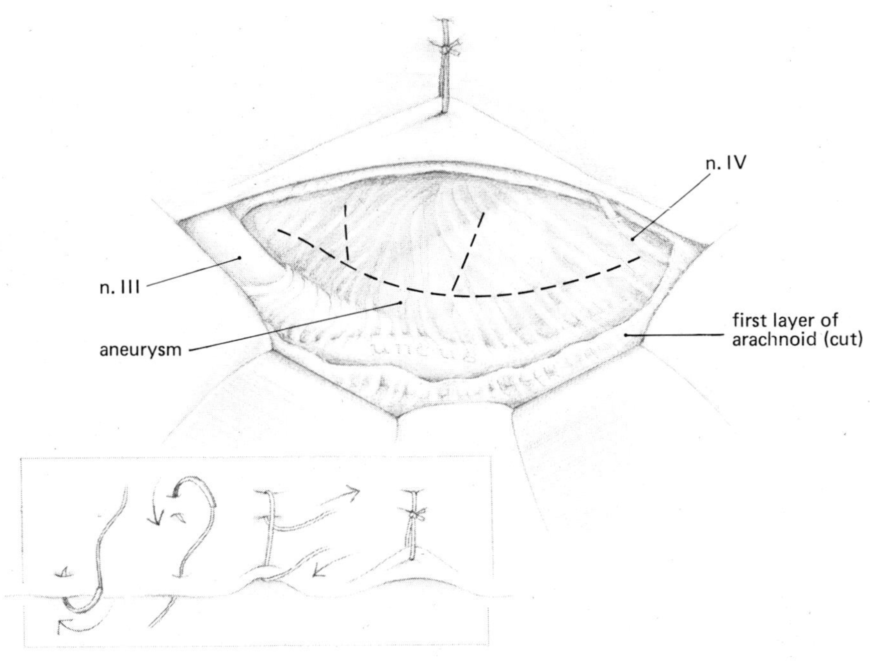

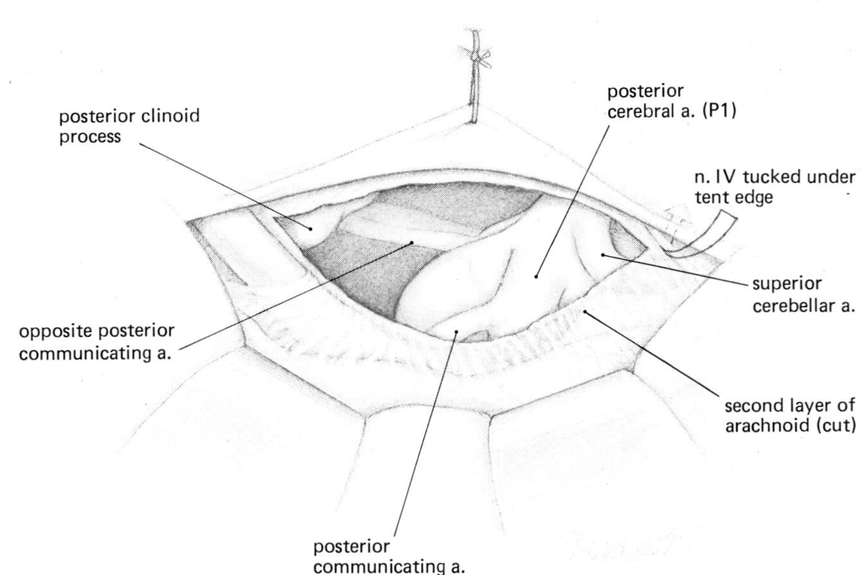

Fig. 86-9. (A) Subtemporal approach. First layer of arachnoid has been removed, showing the intact second layer. Tentorial edge has been sutured into the middle fossa. Inset depicts technique of suturing tentorium. (B) Second layer of arachnoid and membrane of Lillequist has been divided in order to expose the terminal basilar artery and bifurcation aneurysm. Note that the fourth cranial nerve has been tucked back under the edge of the tentorium.

with 2 to 6 vessels arising from each P1 artery, making it necessary to displace the terminal basilar artery and the sac away from the interpeduncular fossa and to dissect across the midline to visualize the perforators on the far side, as well as those more readily seen on the near side. Displacement of the whole of the terminal basilar complex away from the interpeduncular fossa during periods of hypotension can be achieved by using a relatively wide blade dissector.

It is important to emphasize that before any clip is placed, the origin of both of the P1 arteries must be identified on both the right and left sides. This is accomplished by looking across the front of the basilar artery and across the back, and then all the perforators arising from both of the P1 arteries passing backward and upward must be seen and separated from the sac. Occasionally, with a low or highly placed basilar bifurcation, one may momentarily confuse the opposite superior cerebellar artery with the posterior cerebral artery. To inadvertently place the clip blades proximal to the origin of the opposite P1 artery is, of course, disastrous and can be avoided by identifying the opposite oculomotor nerve and recalling that this structure

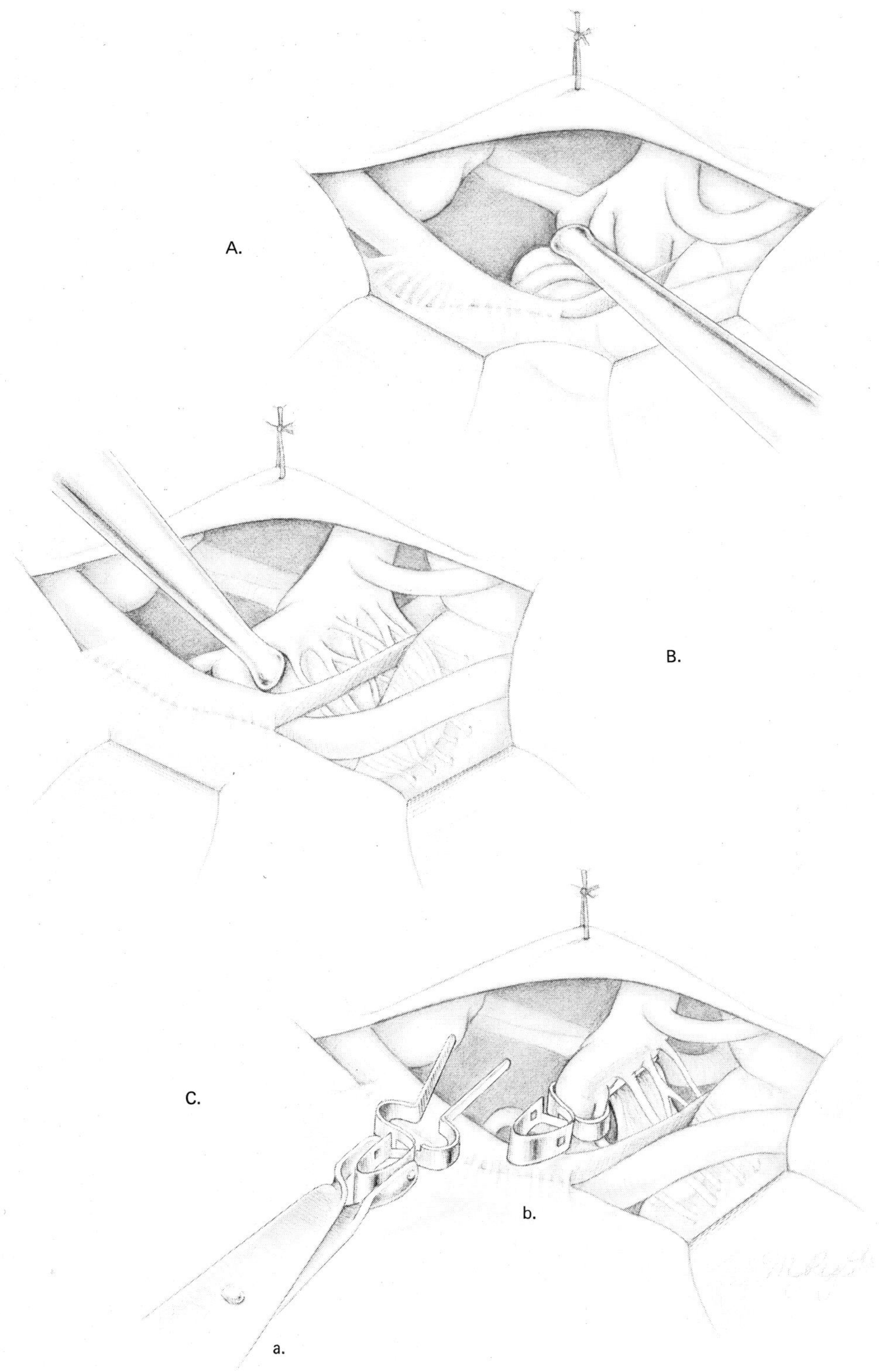

Fig. 86-10. Subtemporal approach. Exposure and clipping of a basilar bifurcation aneurysm. (A) Dissector compressing anterior belly of aneurysm in order to expose opposite P1, posterior communicating artery, and oculomotor nerve. (B) Microdissector displacing the right P1 anteriorly in order to display perforators on side wall of aneurysm. (C) a = Drake aperture clip; b = an aperture clip in place, occluding neck of aneurysm and encircling right P1 and one perforator in the aperture.

always runs between the superior cerebellar and posterior cerebral arteries. The absolute confirmation of this anatomy on both the near and far sides is fundamental to the success of the procedure.

In most instances, the dissection can be confined to the neck of the basilar bifurcation aneurysm and the adjacent proximal posterior cerebral arteries and their perforating branches. It is rarely necessary and, indeed, hazardous to extend the dissection up onto the body or fundus, for the wall is almost always thinner in this region and is the site of the original rupture; it will bleed again if not handled with care.

With the neck defined, the decision is now made regarding the type of clip to be used and its placement. For aneurysms that point forward or backward from the bifurcation, a simple straight clip may suffice after the sac is displaced away from the P1 arteries and, in the case of posterior projecting aneurysms, working the blades under the perforators. The more common aneurysm, however, projects directly upward in the line of the basilar artery and the origins of the P1 artery and cannot be secured with a simple straight or angled clip. For this reason, we have developed the aperture clip designed to enclose the P1 artery and, if necessary, adjacent perforators within the aperture, permitting the clip blades to compress only the neck of the aneurysm. Successful use of this clip depends on precise choice of the correct blade length, as blades that are too long will narrow or occlude the origin of the P1 segments of the posterior cerebral artery, and blades that are too short will permit continued filling of the aneurysm. We have frequently found it necessary to cut and file the ends of the clips in order to ensure the precise blade length necessary for the job. A common error is to use a clip blade that is too long.

After placing the clip, one should not breathe a sigh of relief and step back. This is perhaps the most critical part of the procedure, a time when the surgeon must quickly inspect both the anterior and posterior surfaces of the neck to ensure that the P1 segments are not kinked, and to see that all perforators are entirely free. If there is any suspicion that a perforator is trapped or kinked by the clip, or that the origins of the P1 artery are narrowed, the clip should be removed immediately, further dissection accomplished, and the clip reapplied. Commonly, the clip will have to be positioned and repositioned several times before a precise and accurate placement is achieved. Then the dome of the aneurysm should be punctured with a needle and its contents aspirated, and with the added room afforded by the collapsed sac, the whole anatomy can be reviewed and perfect positioning of the clip guaranteed.

One must recall that the height of the basilar bifurcation varies considerably. Most often, the bifurcation is at or just above the level of the dorsum sellae. Occasionally it is higher, reaching the apex of the interpeduncular cistern and tucked in behind the mamillary bodies. Rarely, the bifurcation may be higher still, with the aneurysm indenting the floor of the third ventricle and posterior hypothalamus. The higher the placement of the bifurcation, the more temporal lobe retraction will be required, and retraction of the peduncle or mamillary body may even be necessary to expose the bifurcation and perforators. Retraction of these structures with a small spatula is normally well tolerated.

As noted above, an aneurysm that is very high is often best approached through the so-called pterional exposure, utilizing splitting and separation of the sylvian fissure.[12] With a moderately high bifurcation, it will occasionally be necessary to dissect above the oculomotor nerve in the space between the oculomotor nerve and the hippocampal gyrus. In this situation, it is sometimes necessary to enclose the oculomotor nerve along with the P1 segment in the aperture of the clip, a maneuver that is well tolerated by this hardy nerve.

If the bifurcation is unusually low (at the base of the dorsum sellae or even lower), the exposure is considerably more difficult and hazardous. The interpeduncular fossa is cone-shaped, with the apex pointing downward into the groove of the pons, forcing the surgeon to gain visual access around the belly of the pons in the depths of the wound. This line of sight can be enhanced by retracting the temporal lobe somewhat more posteriorly, in order to view the anterior aspect of the pons and the pontomesencephalic junction. Although division

of the tent may be used, it frequently does not improve the exposure at this site because both the trigeminal and the trochlear nerves cross the sight line and obscure the view.

Angled aperture clips are often essential for dealing with these low-placed aneurysms. It should also be remembered that the sylvian approach to basilar bifurcation aneurysms is quite unsuitable for these low-lying lesions in that it is impossible to see over the obstruction of the dorsum sellae. It should also be remembered that angiograms taken in the Townes projection usually show the P1 segments as entirely separate from the neck of the aneurysm and coming out almost straight laterally from the side of the basilar artery. The course of the posterior cerebral artery is complex, however, coursing forward and upward before it turns outward to cross above the oculomotor nerve and before swinging around the peduncle under the cover of the hippocampal gyrus. With this angiographic view in mind, the surgeon is often surprised, particularly when faced with a large or bulbous aneurysm, to see from the lateral exposure what appear to be the P1 segments and their perforators arising directly out of the sac. This is rarely if ever true, but underlines the necessity of carefully dissecting between the P1 artery and the sac on both the near and far sides, in order to clearly define the lowermost portion of the neck to be clipped. This anomalous appearance of vessels arising from the side wall of the aneurysm is particularly prominent when the terminal basilar artery is ectatic.

POSTERIOR-PROJECTING ANEURYSMS

Although the angiographic appearance of posterior-projecting aneurysms would suggest that they would be the most difficult and dangerous to expose, as a group they have proven to be quite suitable for direct surgical treatment. With these aneurysms, it is usually necessary to work both above and below the third nerve to gain access to the neck. Often the perforators are fairly readily dissected from the neck, but are densely adherent more distally on the dome, where they can and should be left untouched. With posterior-projecting aneurysms, one can readily visualize the opposite P1 artery across the front of the aneurysm and, with the position of the neck in view, it is then possible to work a fine sucker between the basilar artery and the crus with the left hand and gently draw the basilar artery forward, displacing the terminal basilar artery and the sac out of the interpeduncular fossa. Dissecting with a fine spatula in the right hand, it is then possible to see the perforators that have been stretched, and to separate them from the neck on both the near and far sides. The fundus of this aneurysm is usually never seen, as it is buried high up in the interpeduncular fossa; and in that it is covered with brain stem, it is probably more secure and less likely to rupture. Because of the backward displacement of this aneurysm away from the curve of the posterior cerebral artery, one is frequently able to secure the neck with a simple straight clip, which, when placed across the neck and partially closed, allows excellent visualization across the back of the neck before final placement. A particular hazard with this aneurysm is the portion of the fundus bulging downward below the level of the neck posteriorly. This configuration makes blind application of the clip blades on the posterior aspect of the aneurysm hazardous, as the inferior blade of the clip could pierce the sac. By beginning the dissection low on the back surface of the basilar artery at the origins of the superior cerebellar arteries and working distally, however, one will usually encounter this rolled-over portion of the fundus, allowing it to be separated from the parent vessel and tipped upward before the clip blades are applied.

ANTERIOR-PROJECTING ANEURYSMS

Anterior-projecting are the least common of the basilar bifurcation aneurysms, which is unfortunate in that they are the most straightforward with which to deal. The anterior-projecting aneurysm projects upward and forward from the line of the basilar artery, with the fundus usually placed above the dorsum sellae, free of the interpeduncular fossa and mamillary bodies. In the same way, the aneurysm is usually free of the posterior cerebral arteries and perforators, and only passing attention need be given to these structures in the definition of the terminal basilar anatomy. These aneurysms are, however, frequently fused to the dura of the dorsum and clivus, and care must be taken in the displacement of the aneurysm backward for fear of tearing away this attachment, which is usually at the site of rupture and, therefore, thin and friable. It is also important not to confuse this aneurysm with the bi-lobed, bulbous sac that typically has an upward- or backward-projecting sac as well as the more obvious forward-projecting portion. In contrast, these bi-lobed lesions are among the most complex and difficult aneurysms to deal with because of their bulk, as well as the unusually wide and deformed terminal basilar artery.

GIANT OR BULBOUS BASILAR BIFURCATION ANEURYSMS

Most giant or bulbous aneurysms of the basilar bifurcation project vertically and are always associated with a widened terminal basilar artery, giving the appearance that the posterior cerebral arteries are arising out of the neck and proximal fundus. As a group, these aneurysms are hazardous, in that they are difficult to expose and technically demanding to clip. The exceptional bulk of the aneurysm filling the interpeduncular cistern and deforming the parent and branch vessels makes definition of the anatomy difficult and at times impossible. It is usually necessary to firmly indent the waist of the sac anteriorly and posteriorly to visualize the neck, and often it must be held indented while the clip is being positioned. Again, it is important to clearly identify the opposite P1 artery and its perforators before the clip is finally placed. It is frequently necessary to manipulate the clip into place with the left hand while holding perforators off with a small dissector in the right hand.

Another major concern with this aneurysm is that, frequently, the neck of the aneurysm and the terminal ectatic basilar artery are firm and yellow with atherosclerosis. Instead of being soft and pliable, the neck and terminal basilar artery are solid and often calcified, and as the clip blades are closed, the clip tends to slide down and occlude the terminal basilar artery or the atherosclerotic plaque fractures, and fragments are driven into the P1 segments. If the clip does slip downward because of the firmness of the wall and the mass of the sac above, it may be necessary to place a clip high up across the body of the sac to occlude the fundus and permit its aspiration, and to then seat a smaller clip more precisely across the neck. It is always safer, however, to clip these aneurysms somewhat more distally than at the actual neck, since considerable narrowing several millimeters proximal to the clip is the rule as the

blades approximate the firm wall, and this may impede flow through the P1 segments or the proximal perforators.

If the dilatation and ectasia of the terminal basilar artery are extensive, the entire vessel and its major branches will be involved in the aneurysmal dilation, making it impossible to secure the neck with a clip without occluding or seriously stenosing the orifice of one or both posterior cerebral arteries. In this situation, consideration must be given to proximal basilar artery occlusion as the only definitive form of treatment, particularly if generous posterior communicating arteries are known to be present.

SUPERIOR CEREBELLAR ARTERY ANEURYSMS

Superior cerebellar artery aneurysms arise at the distal carina of the origin of the superior cerebellar artery. The aneurysm almost always projects laterally forward or backward, with the fundus embedded in the peduncle. As the sac enlarges, it usually occupies the whole of the length of the basilar artery between the distal carina of the superior cerebellar artery and the proximal origin of the posterior cerebral artery. The fundus frequently has an intimate association with the oculomotor nerve, and often stretches this nerve above or below the sac, as well as indenting the peduncle on that side.

Unless they are unusually large, these aneurysms can be dealt with in a relatively straightforward manner. The subtemporal exposure gives excellent visualization of the neck, and as there are no perforators arising off the segment of the basilar artery between the superior cerebellar and posterior cerebral arteries or off the superior surface of the superior cerebellar artery, the clip can be placed across the neck with concern only for preserving the integrity of the basilar artery and encompassing the whole of the neck between the blades. As noted, these aneurysms normally project laterally and, as a consequence, one is faced with approaching the left-pointing aneurysm under the dominant temporal lobe. In our experience, this represents an additional and real hazard to the patient. When this aneurysm reaches large or giant proportions, the superior and anterior surface of the sac will be in direct contact with the perforators arising off the P1 artery. These should be identified and spared, as in the case of basilar bifurcation aneurysms. The larger aneurysms pointing toward the left side may be approached from the right, working across the midline and over the top of the basilar artery, for the basilar artery is usually deflected toward the right side as the sac enlarges (Figure 86-11).

Superior cerebellar aneurysms are best dissected first on their anterior surface, again defining the plane of the basilar artery and the origins of the superior cerebellar and posterior cerebral arteries. It is then necessary to work on the distal and proximal surface of the sac to provide room for the clip blades. It is preferable to work a curved clip blade from the superior and anterior surface downward, following the curve of the interior surface of the posterior cerebral artery and the lateral wall of the basilar artery as the clip blades are closed. In this way, one is able to locate the tips of the clip precisely, in order to ensure that they are not impinging on the origin of the superior cerebellar artery. The fundus of the aneurysm can then be punctured and aspirated, and quick inspection of the posterior surface can be carried out to ensure that perforators from the P1 artery have not been picked up by the posterior blade.

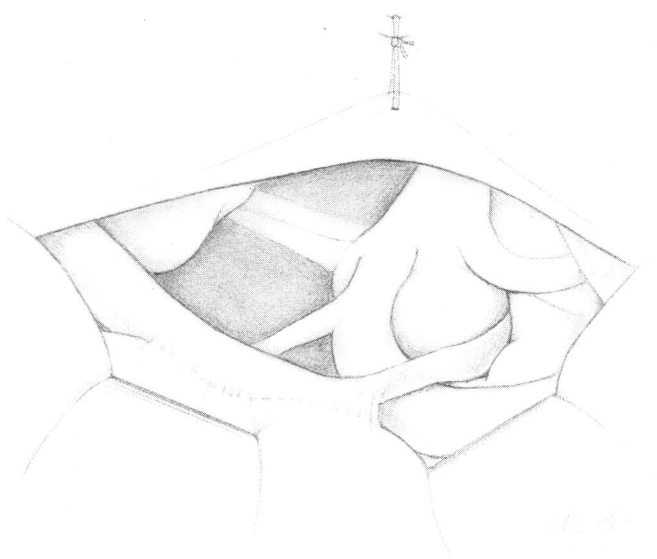

Fig. 86-11.   Subtemporal approach to show superior cerebellar artery aneurysm in situ. Note that the third cranial nerve is displaced over the dome of the aneurysm.

One must be cautious, particularly with larger aneurysms, that the clip does not slide medially and kink the basilar artery. Of course, care should always be taken to avoid injuring the third nerve by these manipulations and, indeed, it may be necessary to encircle the nerve in a curved aperture clip so that it is not deformed or compressed by the clip itself.

POSTERIOR CEREBRAL ARTERY ANEURYSMS

Aneurysms arise typically at four sites along the course of the posterior cerebral artery: first, at the origin of the large perforating branches of the P1 artery; second, at the junction of the posterior communicating artery and the P1 artery; third, at the origin of the anterior and posterior occipital temporal arteries along the side of the brain stem; and, finally, at the terminal branching of the vessel into its parietal and calcarine arteries. The most common sites are at the origin of the posterior communicating artery and at the first major branching at the side of the brain stem.

The more proximal aneurysms are usually dealt with in exactly the same manner as are aneurysms of the terminal basilar artery. They generally are easy aneurysms to dissect in that they are relatively lateral and generally are situated a few millimeters away from the major perforators going to the peduncle. These perforators must be identified in the case of large or giant aneurysms, and separating these aneurysms from the neck may provide a technical challenge. The most distal aneurysms are frequently hidden under the hippocampal gyrus and require retraction relatively posteriorly and, occasionally, require resection of a small portion of the gyrus. This is almost always necessary with those aneurysms lying in the mouth of the choroidal fissure. As with any aneurysm, the purpose is to secure the neck while maintaining normal flow through the parent and branching vessels in the region. Tiny posterior cerebral artery perforators are a lesser problem, except for the

segment that winds around the midbrain and normally gives rise to several circumferential vessels that must be seen and preserved. More distally (i.e., beyond the emergence of the major temporal branch of the posterior cerebral artery), it is usually acceptable and quite safe to trap a large aneurysm.

In our experience, the posterior cerebral artery has perhaps the richest potential for collateralization of any of the major cerebral arteries. In 27 cases in which we have deliberately or inadvertently occluded the posterior cerebral artery, we have noted only one case of a persistent field defect as a result of occipital infarction. One must be exceptionally cautious, however, not to occlude the vessel proximal to the posterior choroidal arteries, for ischemia and infarction in the territory of these vessels can be devastating. Deliberate occlusion of the P1 or proximal P2 segments is therefore most satisfactorily accomplished using the microtourniquet technique in an awake patient.

BASILAR-ANTERIOR INFERIOR CEREBELLAR ARTERY (AICA) ANEURYSMS

Like most aneurysms, the AICA aneurysm usually arises at the distal carina of the origin of the anterior inferior cerebellar artery and basilar artery. It is not rare, however, for these aneurysms to arise on the proximal side of this junction. This variation in the usual aneurysm anatomy should be ascertained from angiograms, for the position of the AICA may radically alter one's approach to this aneurysm. Most often, the AICA aneurysm projects laterally, but it may project forward and be firmly adherent to the clivus, or it may even point backward and be buried in the pons or pontomedullary junction. The dome of the aneurysm usually has a close relationship to the abducens nerve.

The approach to these aneurysms depends largely upon their size and configuration, for they can be reached from either above via the subtemporal transtentorial route or from below by a suboccipital craniotomy. Generally, the whole of the basilar artery down to the vertebral junctions may be exposed through the tentorium. It is the size and shape of aneurysms at the trunk of the basilar artery that determines one's approach. For example, an AICA aneurysm originating from the midpoint of the basilar artery with the dome projecting upward and the AICA arising from its proximal surface may be more safely approached by the suboccipital route. Similarly, trunk aneurysms arising from the proximal crotch of the AICA and pointing laterally and downward and buried into the medulla are often more safely visualized and clipped subtemporally through the tentorium. These aneurysms lie in a narrow and confined space some distance from either the approach from above or below. It is usually in the surgeon's (and patient's) best interest to see the aneurysm neck and the critical branch of origin first rather than be faced with the walled fundus obscuring the neck. For this reason, we prefer to plan the approach that will most readily bring the neck into view. Usually these aneurysms lie at about the junction of the middle and lower thirds of the clivus and close to the midline, but they may vary by as much as 2 cm above or below this point, and may be placed laterally as far as the cerebellopontine angle (Figure 86-12).

When exposing this aneurysm with a subtemporal, transtentorial approach, it is necessary to turn a moderately sized temporal bone flap that is centered to permit a direct line

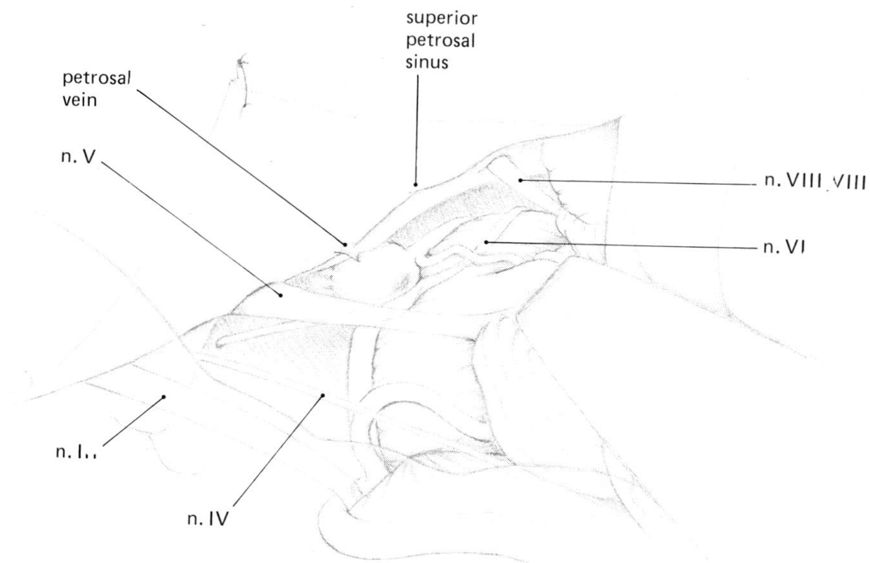

Fig. 86-12. Subtemporal transtentorial approach showing an AICA aneurysm in situ. The retractor is on the anterior edge of the cerebellum.

of sight down the posterior slope of the petrous bone. The vein of Labbé will be in the middle or anterior third of this exposure and must be protected and spared. With elevation of the temporal lobe, the free edge of the tentorium is exposed in its posterior part, and it can be divided by placing a hook about 1 to 1.5 cm behind the attachment of the trochlear nerve. Using the hook to firmly lift the tentorium, and touching it with the monopolar coagulator, the tent is divided in steps, almost to the junction of the petrosal and lateral sinuses. The anterior leaf of tentorium is then picked up with a 4-0 silk suture and stitched forward into the middle fossa. Immediately upon reflection of the tent, the arachnoidal roof in the posterior fossa will come into view. Piercing this arachnoid will be the pertrosal vein, which should be coagulated and divided immediately. Deep to the arachnoid, the trochlear and trigeminal nerves will be seen. The arachnoid should be carefully opened just lateral to the trigeminal nerve and a narrow retractor blade slipped into this opening, gently elevating the anterior superior margin of the cerebellar hemisphere. With further deepening of the retractor, the pons will be gently elevated, exposing the facial and cochlear nerves just lateral to the retractor blade and crossing the cerebellopontine angle. At this point, the abducens nerve will be seen just at the tip of the retractor as a thin, slack structure coursing upward to gain the cavernous sinus. Gentle removal of clot and CSF will expose the basilar artery and the aneurysm. It is usually necessary to separate the sixth nerve from the aneurysm, but, as noted, this nerve has a lot of slack as it passes from the brain to the cavernous sinus, allowing it to be displaced either forward toward the clivus or back toward the pons to clear the neck of the aneurysm. As with the third nerve, if it is handled gently, the abducens nerve usually regains its normal function within about 3 months.

Again, it is wise to begin the dissection proximal or distal to the aneurysm on the basilar artery, removing clot and debris until the adventitia of this vessel is clearly in view. Staying within this plane, the dissection is continued toward the neck of the aneurysm, removing the clot packed into this narrow space in front of the pons. It should be recalled that the AICA usually

leaves the basilar artery and then courses inferiorly in a path parallel to the main trunk of the basilar artery before turning laterally to wind around the pons. With a sizeable aneurysm, the origin of the AICA usually will not be seen initially from the transtentorial approach, but obviously must be clearly identified before any attempt is made to place the clip. More often than not, its original course will be quite free of the aneurysm, but it may occasionally be firmly adherent to the inferior side and have to be dissected free from the neck and body of the sac. This maneuver can be facilitated by gently grasping the neck of the aneurysm in bipolar forceps, tipping the sac forward toward the clivus to expose the AICA, and allowing it to be sharply removed from the side wall of the aneurysm. Inasmuch as these aneurysms are frequently pointing forward and are adherent to the clivus, the identification of the basilar artery, the AICA, and clumps of perforating vessels arising from the posterior surface of the basilar artery is quite straightforward. If, however, the sac is displaced laterally or backward into the pons, then this maneuver of grasping the neck and rolling the sac out of its bed will be essential. Certainly, application of a clip in this narrow, confined space is always awkward, since the clip mechanism and applier obscure the surgeon's view at the critical moment of closure. For this reason, it is important to remove the applicator quickly and to inspect the position of the blades in order to ensure precision in their placement; only absolute accuracy should be accepted. Minor narrowing of the origin of the AICA, entrapment of mid-basilar perforators, or partial stenosis of the basilar artery will almost always herald disaster.

Only occasionally have we encountered aneurysms arising from the trunk of the basilar artery between the AICA and the SCA, presumably at the sites of the short or long circumferential pontine vessels or even the trigeminal artery. These aneurysms usually are approached by the transtentorial route, but are difficult to expose in that they usually are partially hidden by the full belly of the pons, and more superficially the approach is guarded by the fleshy mass of the trigeminal nerve. This aneurysm usually requires gentle lateral retraction of the fifth nerve and simultaneous medial retraction of the belly of the pons for exposure. Pontine retraction should always be intermittent and all the small arterials irrigating the pons must be spared.

As a general rule, exposure of the high basilar trunk aneurysm is more safely accomplished through the subtemporal-transtentorial route, in that manipulation and retraction on the fourth, fifth, and sixth cranial nerves usually is well tolerated and has an excellent potential for full recovery. In contrast, the suboccipital exposure requires dissection between the ninth, tenth, and eleventh cranial nerves, and damage to these nerves is almost always associated with significant morbidity, and not infrequently mortality, secondary to aspiration and pneumonia.

Many years ago, we attempted to expose these aneurysms through the transoral-transclival approach. This exposure is always distressingly confined, usually puts the fundus of the aneurysm between the operator and the parent vessel, and runs the very real risk of postoperative meningitis. A subtemporal or suboccipital approach is much more satisfactory, making the transoral exposure unnecessary.

VERTEBRAL JUNCTION ANEURYSMS

Vertebral junction aneurysms are uncommon even in our series. They are commonly associated with anomalous development of the vertebral artery. For example, one vertebral artery terminating at the posterior inferior cerebellar artery, duplication of the proximal basilar artery, fenestration of the proximal basilar artery, or congenital absence of one vertebral artery.

Normally, the two vertebral arteries join just at or below the junction of the middle and inferior thirds of the clivus. With anomalous development, however, this point of junction may be considerably higher or lower and can be displaced well off the midline. In our experience, an equal number of these aneurysms have been approached from the subtemporal and suboccipital exposure. The decision in any one patient is therefore dependent on the size and configuration of the aneurysm more than on the absolute position of the origin of the neck. The difficulty of treating this aneurysm lies not with identification of perforating vessels, which are usually either not present or so small as to be of little consequence at this site, but rather with the extreme importance of being able to deal with the neck of the aneurysm in the very confined space of an exposure from either above or from below and to ensure at the same time the patency of the basilar and vertebral arteries when the clip is finally placed. One must be cautious not to choose a clip that is too long, and to identify the position of the tips of the clip with certainty once the clip is seated and in place. This aneurysm is always awkward and difficult to expose. Once again, great care must be taken to avoid injuring the lower cranial nerves when manipulating instruments around the front of the brain stem, and care taken to recall the importance of starting the dissection well proximal along the vertebral artery. Once the plane of the adventitial surface of the vertebral artery has been reached, it is important to stay precisely in this plane, removing a clot and debris piecemeal as one proceeds distally along the parent vessel toward the neck of the vertebral aneurysm.

These aneurysms arise from the vertebral artery usually at the distal crotch or the origin of the posterior inferior cerebellar artery and, less frequently, on the proximal side of the origin of this vessel. Rarely, these aneurysms arise quite separate from the PICA either proximal or distal to unnamed perforators coursing to the lateral side of the medulla and, occasionally, from the origin of the anterior spinal artery. It will be recalled that the length, caliber, and configuration of the vertebral artery, as well as the site of origin of the PICA, is extraordinarily variable. We have seen PICA aneurysms situated in the foramen magnum and even as low as the first denticulate ligament and as high as the middle of the clivus. We have also encountered aneurysms arising from the left vertebral artery lying in the right cerebellopontine angle. The aneurysms typically are lying quite free in the subarachnoid space, although they are intimately associated with a lower cranial nerve, but they may, particularly when they reach large or giant proportions, be buried within the medulla or inferior pons.

Aneurysms of the PICA typically have an intimate association with the hypoglossal nerve, often splitting this nerve or having the nerve firmly fused to the side wall or neck of the sac. Also, these aneurysms typically originate not only from the vertebral artery but also from the proximal portion of the PICA, giving this vessel the appearance of arising out of the lateral wall of the sac, which indeed it partially does, having at least a portion of its origin involved in the aneurysmal dilatation. This configuration is important to recognize, for it is essential that the placement of the clip protect the origin of the posterior cerebellar artery.

Vertebral artery aneurysms usually are approached through a unilateral suboccipital exposure, with the patient in the lateral or park bench position and with the face turned slightly toward the floor (Figure 86-13). This position usually gives a good exposure of the aneurysm without any concern of air embolism, and it is favored by the anesthetist in that it gives good access to the endotracheal tube and is a position that ensures easy ventilation and a stable cardiovascular system. A midline or lateral paramedian incision is used, with care taken to preserve the occipital nerve and to remove bone as far laterally as the mastoid air cell. The rim of the foramen magnum will be removed in most instances, but in high-lying vertebral artery aneurysms this may not be necessary. Extreme lateral or medial approaches are unnecessary, as these aneurysms usually lie in close proximity to the lateral medulla, and the PICA usually projects posteriorly and upward (Figure 86-14). After the cisterna magna is opened and CSF is removed, the retractor is placed to gently elevate the cerebellar tonsil medially and slightly upward off the medulla to expose the ninth, tenth, and eleventh nerves. With this initial retraction, the caudal loop of the PICA and the beginning intracranial course of the vertebral artery will come into view. It is at this level that the dissection should begin with magnified vision. The vertebral artery is followed distally under the emerging cranial nerve, and by staying in the plane of the vessel, one will come upon the origin of the PICA, which usually arises off the superior and slightly lateral side of the vessel and is usually placed proximal to the neck of the aneurysm. It will be remembered that the vertebral artery runs somewhat medially under the medulla, and it may therefore be necessary to gently retract the medulla to gain the necessary exposure. We have found it useful to have the patient under light general anesthesia at this stage, and breathing spontaneously, so that a measure of the gentleness of medullary retraction can be gauged by the persistence of spontaneous respirations.

With the vertebral artery, the origin of the PICA, and the neck of the aneurysm exposed, it is important to carry the dissection beyond the aneurysm, in order to identify the distal vertebral artery or the origin of the basilar artery in order to

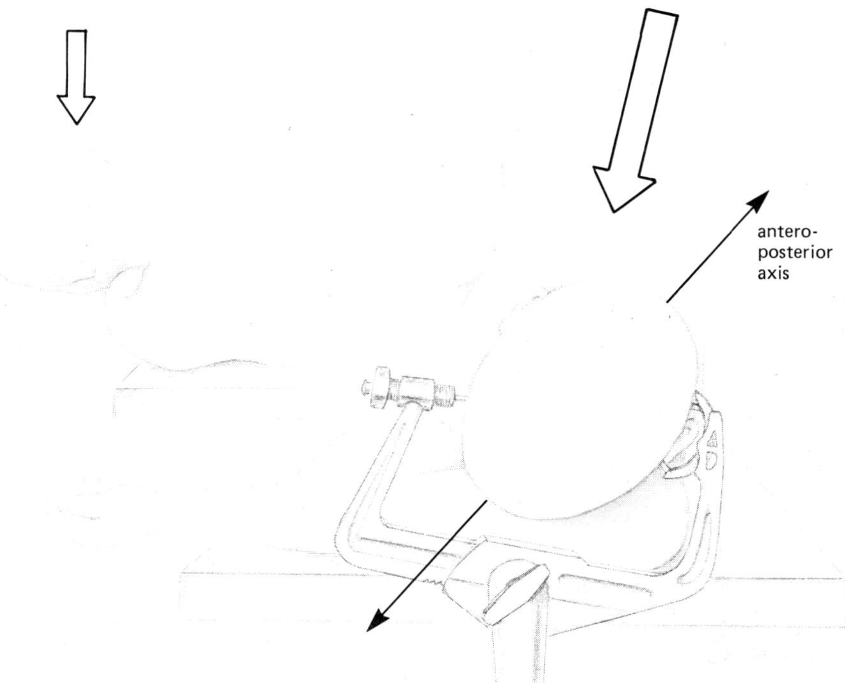

Fig. 86-13.   Suboccipital approach. Note the lateral decubitus, or "park bench" position, with the face turned toward the floor. The open arrow depicts the direction of the microscope.

gain an appreciation of the position of the structure and the total width of the aneurysm neck. The hypoglossal nerve usually is on the far side of the neck, but may be on the near side or even split by the dome of the aneurysm, and very frequently needs to be manipulated up off the neck to allow adequate clip placement (Figure 86-15). We have often found it useful to narrow the neck of this type of aneurysm with bipolar cautery, taking care to avoid contact with the fibers of the vagus and spinal accessory nerve. It is also frequently useful to use aperture clips to enclose the PICA or even both PICAs and the vertebral artery, recognizing that the PICA often takes at least part of its origin from the side wall of the neck. Once again, it is important to stress that the dissection to approach this aneurysm must take place between the pharyngeal filaments of

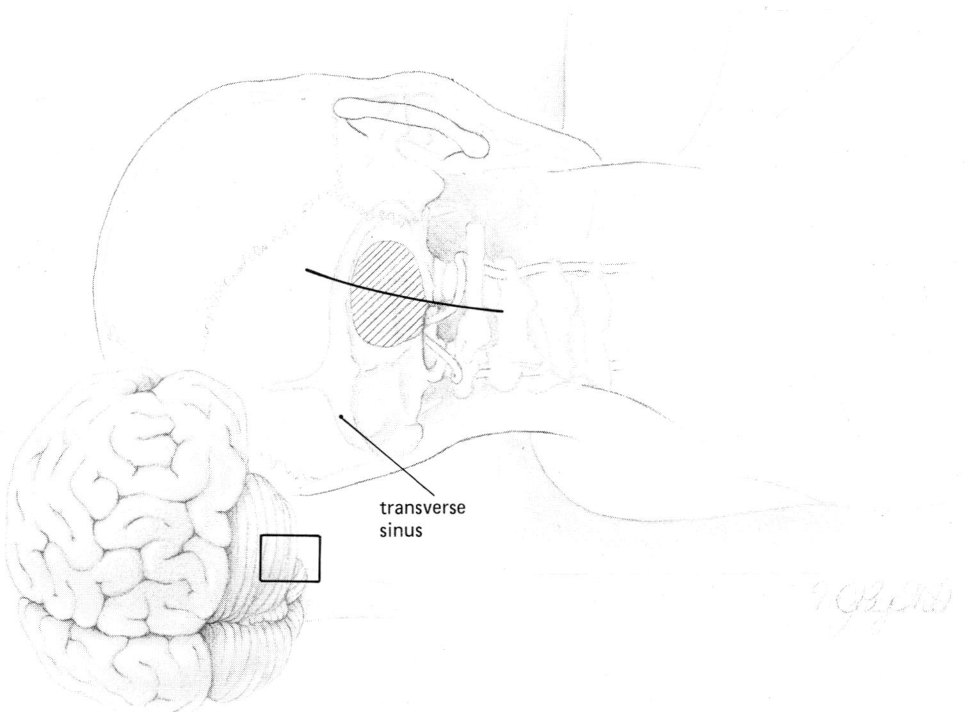

Fig. 86-14.   Suboccipital approach. Relationship of incision and craniectomy to skull and brain landmarks.

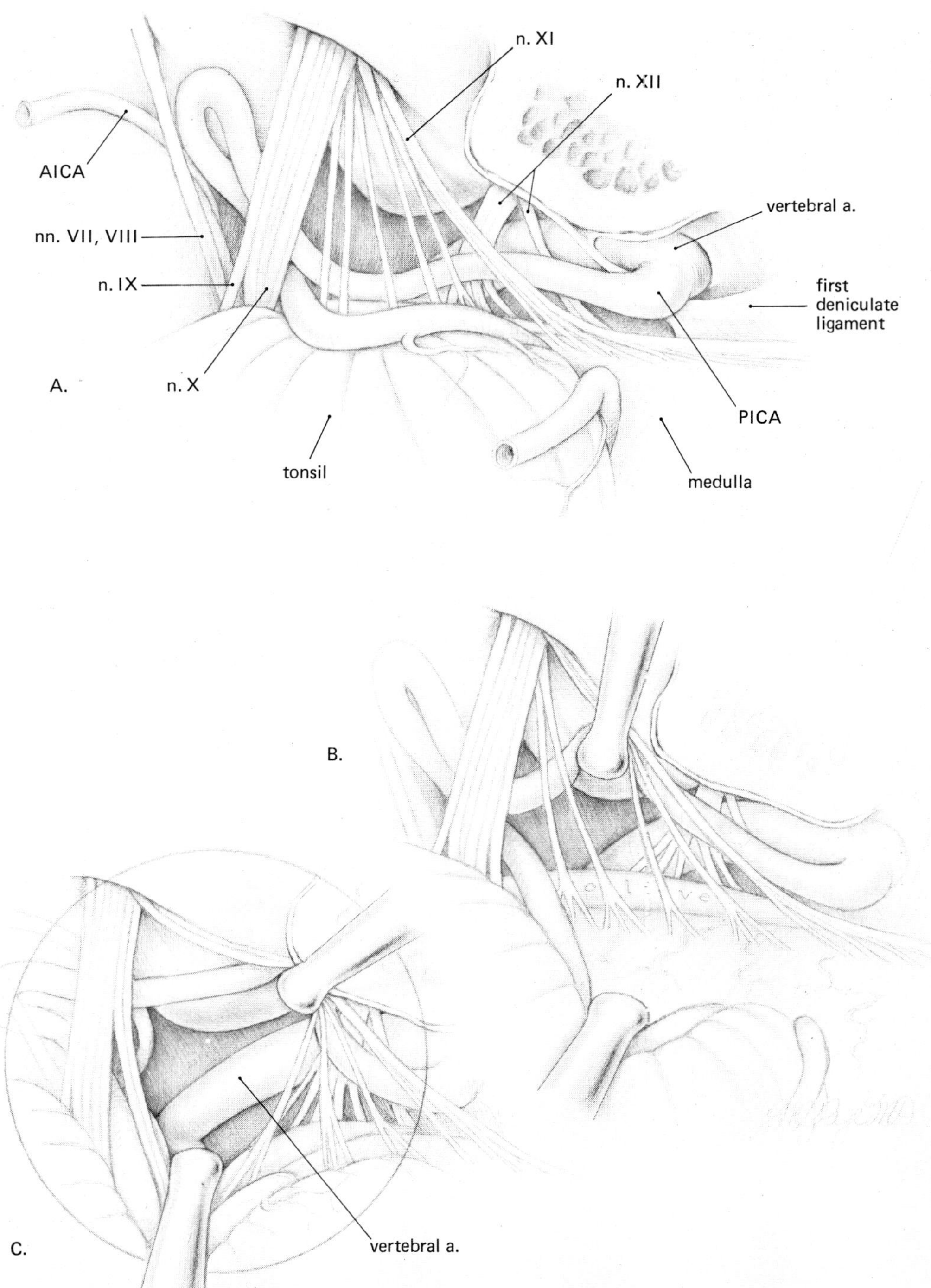

Fig. 86-15.   Suboccipital approach, to expose the right vertebral artery. (A) Microscopic anatomy. (B) Disssectors displacing an unusually long rostral loop of the PICA in order to expose the inferior olive. (C) Filaments of lower cranial nerves, displaced, show distal vertebral artery.

the eleventh and the lower fibers of the tenth cranial nerves, and that these fibers must be protected at all costs before their injury brings about distressing and dangerous postoperative complications.

CONCLUSIONS AND RESULTS

The evolution of these surgical techniques for aneurysms of the vertebral basilar system has resulted in increasingly satisfactory results as our surgical expertise has grown and has been supported by refinements in neuroradiology and neuro-anesthesia. It is now possible to attack aneurysms on the vertebral basilar system and to anticipate results as good as results obtained on aneurysms of the anterior circulation. In 625 cases of smaller aneurysms in the posterior circulation, we have experienced a surgical mortality of 3.2 percent, which included our earliest endeavors with these aneurysms, as well as patients in poor condition. The risks and complications of surgical attack on large aneurysms increases proportionately with the size of the lesion, but even so, in 1400 of our surgical cases we have achieved excellent or good results in 85 percent, an overall surgical mortality of 5.3 percent, and an overall management morbidity of 10 percent. Overall, the basilar bifurcation is the most hazardous site for both large and small aneurysms of the posterior circulation, and it needs to be stressed again that it is the inadvertent rupture or occlusion of perforators of the P1 artery, or occlusion of the terminal basilar artery by the clip or atheroma, that accounts for most of the mortality and morbidity. It is essential to be completely familiar with the anatomy and to accept only precise and accurate placement of the clip in every case. With technical experience and uniform excellence in neuroanesthesia, most, if not all, saccular aneurysms of the vertebral basilar system will be amenable to direct surgical treatment.

REFERENCES

1. Dandy WE: Intracranial Arterial Aneurysms. Ithaca, NY, Comstock, 1944
2. Tonnis W: Zur Behandlung Intrakraniellar Aneurysmen. Arch Klin Chir 189:474, 1937
3. Falconer MA: Surgical treatment of spontaneous intracranial hemorrhage. Br Med J 1:790, 1958
4. Poppen JL: Vascular surgery of the posterior fossa. Proc Congr Neurol Surg 6:198, 1969
5. Logue V: Posterior fossa aneurysms, in Shillito J, Mosberg WH (eds): Clinical Neurosurgery, vol 11. Baltimore, Williams & Wilkins, 1964, pp 183–207
6. Schwartz HG: Arterial aneurysms of the posterior fossa. J Neurosurg 5:312, 1948
7. Drake CG: Bleeding aneurysms of the basilar artery. Direct surgical management in four cases. J Neurosurg 23:230, 1961
8. Jamieson KG: Aneurysms of the vertebrobasilar system. Surgical intervention in 19 cases. J Neurosurg 21:781, 1964
9. Drake CG: Surgical treatment of ruptured aneurysms of the basilar artery. Experience with 14 cases. J Neurosurg 23:457, 1965
10. Drake CG: Further experience with surgical treatment of aneurysms of the basilar artery. J Neurosurg 29:372, 1968
11. Peerless SJ: Pre and post-operative management of intracranial aneurysms, in Clinical Neurosurgery, vol 26. Baltimore, Williams & Wilkins, 1978
12. Yasargil MG, Antic J, Laciga R, et al: Microsurgical pterional approach to aneurysms of the basilar bifurcation. Surg Neurol 6:83, 1976

CHAPTER 87
Surgical Management of Traumatic Aneurysms

Dwight Parkinson

TRAUMATIC INTRACRANIAL ANEURYSMS are exceedingly rare.[1–76] Excluding intracavernous carotid aneurysms, Laun et al.[35] collected 73 cases from the world literature, including 3 from their own total of 450 aneurysms. We have collected 13 cases among our last 6000 head injuries. In this series there were 281 extracerebral hematomas and 112 traumatic intracerebral hematomas. Considering this incidence of the intra- and extracerebral hemorrhage, it is evident that the rarity of traumatic aneurysms is not because the intracranial arteries are well protected from trauma. These aneurysms may result from blunt or penetrating head trauma,[13,14,16,20,25,40] (including iatrogenic penetrations[1,7,12,25,29,31,34,42,43,47,48,50,51,69,70]) and over 90 percent occur in association with a skull fracture.[23,26,58,59,63] Occasionally the aneurysm is partially trapped in the fracture line.[8,23,30,33] Aneurysms of the pericallosal artery probably arise after these arteries are injured by the edge of the falx.[44] For the traumatic saccular aneurysms in the parasellar regions, see chapter 71. Vandellen (personal communication, September, 1980) reported a case in which there was a delayed intracerebral hematoma associated with a traumatic, parasellar, carotid aneurysm and also delayed massive epistaxis.

Infratentorial traumatic aneurysms constitute no more than 5 percent of the total reported.[6,15,47,49] Saccular and arteriovenous aneurysms of the middle meningeal artery are surprisingly few considering the intimate relationship between this artery and bone.[21,27,29,30,33,35,36,42,46,47,53,67,71]

Some authors have categorized saccular traumatic aneurysms into either "true" or "false,"[8,11,23,31] and "mixed" or "dissecting" types.[57,68] Their criteria for a so-called "true" traumatic aneurysm is disruption of the arterial wall with only the adventitia left intact.[12,17,41,50] This differs from the true saccular aneurysm, which contains both intima and adventitia in its wall. Their "false" aneurysms result from full-thickness lacerations that are occluded by hematoma, which subsequently organizes and excavates to leave a saccular defect with none of the normal arterial structures in the wall.[12,19,21,48,49,54,72] "Mixed" aneurysms result from the posttraumatic rupture of a "true" aneurysm, which produces a secondary "false" aneurysm,[12] and a "dissecting" aneurysm results from the formation of a false lumen between the intima and the elastica.[57,68,73,74]

SIGNS AND SYMPTOMS

The cases of delayed apoplexy following head injury that were reported by Bollinger[75] may well have been the result of traumatic aneurysms, although his explanation for these cases was focal brain softening and delayed hemorrhage from the unsupported and injured blood vessels. Aside from persistent headache (not always present) and the delayed deterioration following head injury,[38] there are few clinical features that point to the diagnosis, which can only be established by angiograms of the common carotid artery.[12,17,23,34,47,48,51,64,76] These aneurysms usually enlarge progressively, but occasionally they may decrease in size or even spontaneously disappear.[6,12,17,23,34,48]

The angiographic features differentiating the traumatic from the common saccular aneurysm are:

1. Delayed filling and emptying of the aneurysmal sac (Figure 87-1).
2. A peripheral location of the aneurysm at a site other than a branching point (Figure 87-2).
3. Irregular contour (Figure 87-2).
4. The absence of a neck (Figure 87-2).[8,12,33,62,63,73]

The increasing reliance on CT scanning and the decreasing use of angiography in evaluating the patient with a head injury will result in an unfortunate number of these aneurysms being missed. Early diagnosis is most important. Patients diagnosed after rupture have a mortality almost three times as high as those diagnosed before rupture.[23] The surgical mortality recorded in the literature averages 24 percent, while the untreated cases have a mortality approaching 50 percent.[47] Because of the superficial nature of these lesions, the operative mortality should be negligible and result from the extent of the associated brain damage sustained with the original trauma. Unfortunately, they are rarely recognized until their presence is heralded by delayed deterioration, by which time the salvage rate is halved. Earlier recognition can only be accomplished by a higher degree of suspicion and the increased use of angiography.

TREATMENT

The treatment is surgical. Although superficial, most of these lesions are frequently invisible beneath the surface, and may be difficult to find, particularly if associated with a large intracerebral hematoma. If the aneurysm is not immediately

OPERATIVE NEUROSURGICAL TECHNIQUES
ISBN 0-8089-1862-1

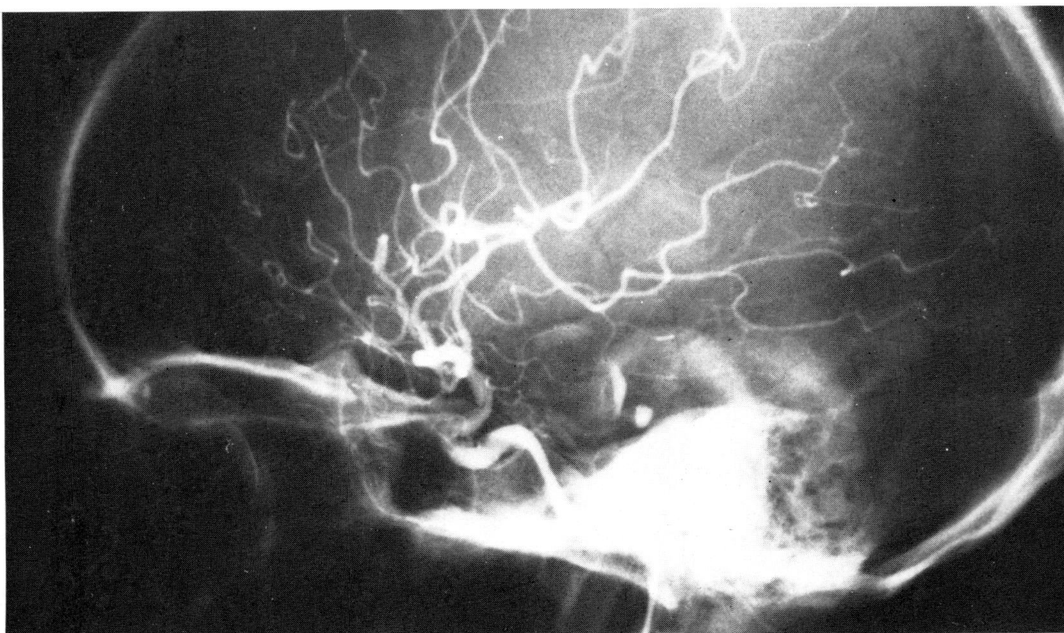

Fig. 87-1. A right carotid angiogram. The lower arrow points to a meniscus in a false aneurysm on the posterior branch of the middle meningeal artery. A second smaller globular false aneurysm can be seen behind and beneath the arrow tip. The upper arrow indicates a wide stellate temporal-parietal fracture. (Reprinted from Parkinson D: Traumatic intracranial aneurysms. J Neurosurg 52:11–20, 1980. With permission.)

apparent, it is located very easily by placing one or two metallic clips in the suspected area for reference, and then performing an intraoperative angiogram, whereupon the relationship of the sac to these clips becomes immediately evident.[77] This saves time and the unnecessary destruction of tissue. The arteriovenous malformations usually are easier to find lying within the dura associated with a fracture line. Intraoperative angiography provides the surgeon with the immediate assurance that the lesion has been obliterated (Figure 87-3).

In the future, some of the saccular lesions possibly will be amenable to excision with direct repair of the cerebral artery by graft or end-to-end anastomosis,[78] but at this time, obliteration has only been accomplished by clipping or coagulating the parent vessel as it enters the aneurysm (see Figures 87-1 and 87-2).

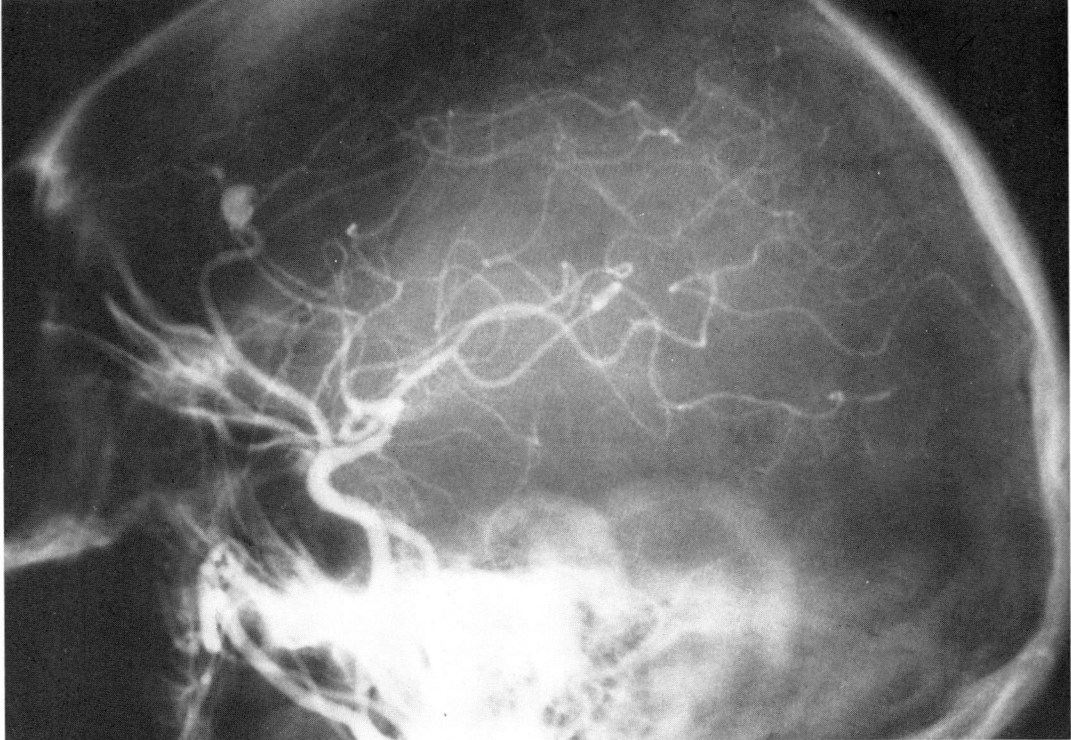

Fig. 87-2. A traumatic aneurysm on the callosal artery. The artery presumably was damaged by impingement against the edge of the falx.

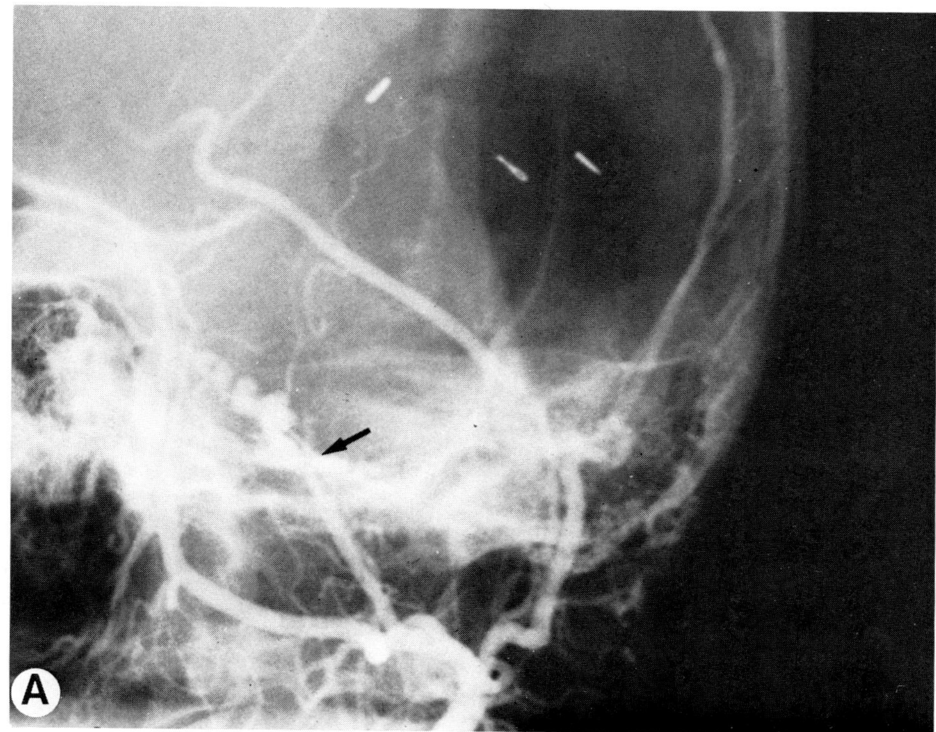

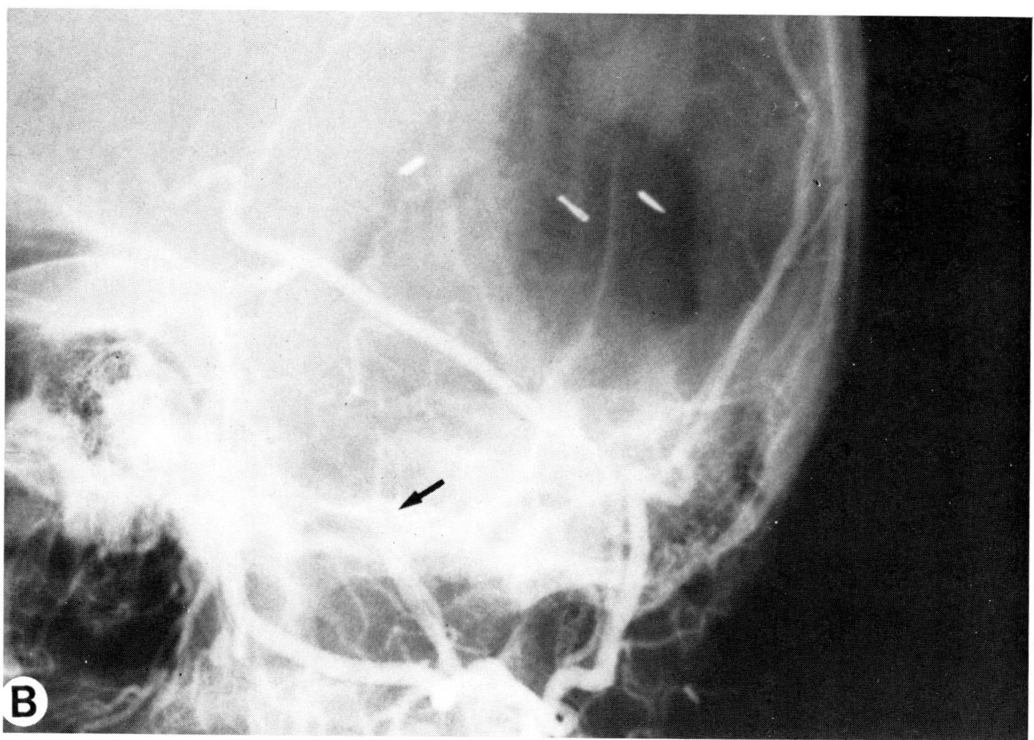

Fig. 87-3. (A) An intraoperative angiogram (oblique view). The black arrow points to an arteriovenous fistula coming from the middle meningeal artery. (B) An intraoperative angiogram of the same case in A showing the site of obliteration of the arteriovenous fistula, which was accomplished by embolization and cautery. (Reprinted from Parkinson D: Traumatic intracranial aneurysms. J Neurosurg 52:11–20, 1980. With permission.)

The recognition of these potentially fatal lesions rose significantly during the era of angiography, with a corresponding decrease in the mortality rate. Now the number of angiograms done annually for head injuries is rapidly approaching zero being replaced by the CT scan.[55] It is unlikely that this trend is going to be reversed unless there were to be a large series of deaths caused by delayed hemorrhage from proven traumatic aneurysms (proven at autopsy). Because of the rarity of the situation, this is unlikely to occur and one or two deaths would be considered ''acceptable'' in any large series. One has to ask, ''acceptable to whom—the hospital administration, the medical staff or the patient who dies or his lawyer?'' It is probably advisable that any head injury that deteriorates and is found to have a clot that did not exist on admission or one that has recurred after removal should also have an angiogram.

REFERENCES

1. Acosta C, William PE Jr, Clark K: Traumatic aneurysms of the cerebral vessels. J Neurosurg 36:531, 1972

2. Alexander E Jr, Adams JE, Davis CH Jr: Complications in the use of temporary intracranial arterial clip. J Neurosurg 20:810, 1963

3. Ameli NO: Aneurysms of the middle meningeal artery. J Neurol Neurosurg Psychiatry 28:175, 1965

4. Araki C, Handa H, Handa J, et al: Traumatic aneurysm of the intracranial extradural portion of the internal carotid artery. Report of a case. J Neurosurg 23:64, 1965

5. Asari S, Nakamura S, Yamada O, et al: Traumatic aneurysm of peripheral cerebral arteries. Report of two cases. J Neurosurg 46:795, 1977

6. Bank WO, Nelson PB, Drayer BP, et al: Traumatic aneurysm of the basilar artery. AJR 130:975, 1978

7. Barrett JH, Lawrence VL: Aneurysms of the internal carotid artery as a complication of mastoidectomy. Arch Otolaryngol 72:366, 1960

8. Benoit BG, Wortzman G: Traumatic cerebral aneurysms. Clinical features and natural history. J Neurol Neurosurg Psychiatry 36:127, 1973

9. Bergstrom K, Hemmingsson A: False cortical aneurysm in subdural haematoma following head injury without fracture. Acta Radiol (Diagn) 14:657, 1973

10. Birley JL, Trotter W: Traumatic aneurysm of the intracranial portion of the internal carotid artery. Brain 51:184, 1928

11. Brihaye J, Mage J, Verhiest G: Aneurysme traumatique de la carotide interne dans sa portion supraclinoidienne. Acta Neurol Psychiatr Belg 54:411, 1954

12. Burton C, Velasco F, Dorman J: Traumatic aneurysm of a peripheral cerebral artery. Review and case report. J Neurosurg 28:468, 1968

13. Carothers A: Orbitofacial wounds and cerebral artery injuries caused by umbrella tips. JAMA 239:1151, 1978

14. Chadduck WM: Traumatic cerebral aneurysm due to speargun injury. Case report. J Neurosurg 31:77, 1969

15. Cockrill HH Jr, Jimenez JP, Goree JA: Traumatic false aneurysm of the superior cerebellar artery simulating posterior fossa tumor. Case report. J Neurosurg 46:377, 1977

16. Courville CB: Traumatic aneurysm of an intracranial artery. Description of a lesion incident to a shotgun wound of the skull and brain. Bull Los Angeles Neurol Soc 25:48, 1960

17. Cressman MR, Hayes GJ: Traumatic aneurysm of the anterior choroidal artery. Case report. J Neurosurg 24:102, 1966

18. Drake CG: Subdural haematoma from arterial rupture. J Neurosurg 18:597, 1961

19. Eichler A, Story JL, Bennett DE, et al: Traumatic aneurysm of a cerebral artery. Case report. J Neurosurg 31:72, 1969

20. Ferry DJ Jr, Kempe LG: False aneurysm secondary to penetration of the brain through orbitofacial wounds. Report of two cases. J Neurosurg 36:503, 1972

21. Fincher EF: Arteriovenous fistula between the middle meningeal artery and the greater petrosal sinus. Case report. Ann Surg 133:886, 1951

22. Finkemeyer H: Ein sackchenformiges Aneurysma der A. cerebri media als postoperative Komplikation. Zentralbl Neurochir 15:302, 1955

23. Fleischer AS, Patton JM, Tindall GT: Cerebral aneurysms of traumatic origin. Surg Neurol 4:233, 1975

24. Go KG, Penning L, Oen TS: Acute subdural haematoma in connection with angiographically demonstrated traumatic rupture of a cortical cerebral artery (presenting as false aneurysm). Report of two cases. Neuroradiology 2:107, 1971

25. Goald HJ, Ronderos A: Traumatic perforation of the intracranial portion of the internal carotid artery with eleven-day survival. Case report. J Neurosurg 18:401, 1961

26. Handa J, Shimizu Y, Matsuda M, et al: Traumatic aneurysm of the middle cerebral artery. Am J Roentgenol Radium Ther Nucl Med 109:127, 1970

27. Handa J, Shimizu Y, Sato K, et al: Traumatic aneurysm and arteriovenous fistula of the middle meningeal artery. Clin Radiol 21:39, 1970

28. Handel SF, Perpetuo FOL, Handel CH: Subdural hematomas due to ruptured cerebral aneurysms: Angiographic diagnosis and potential pitfall for CT. AJR 130:507, 1978

29. Higazi I, El-Banhawy A, El-Nady F: Importance of angiography in identifying false aneurysm of the middle meningeal artery as a cause of extradural hematoma. Case report. J Neurosurg 30:172, 1969

30. Jackson DC, du Boulay GH: Traumatic arterio-venous aneurysm of the middle meningeal artery. Br J Radiol 37:788, 1964

31. Jackson FE, Gleave JRW, Janon E: The traumatic cranial and intracranial aneurysms, in Vinken PJ, Bruyn GW (eds): Handbook of Clinical Neurology, vol 24. Amsterdam, North-Holland, 1976, pp 381–398

32. Krauland W: Zur Entstehung traumatischer Aneurysmen der Schlagadern am Hirngrund. Schweiz Z Pathol Bakt 12:113, 1949

33. Kuhn RA, Kugler H: False aneurysms of the middle meningeal artery. J Neurosurg 21:92, 1964

34. Lassman LP, Ramani PS, Sengupta RP: Aneurysms of peripheral cerebral arteries due to surgical trauma. Vasc Surg 8:1, 1974

35. Laun A: Survey of traumatic aneurysms, in Pia HW, Langmaid C, Zierski J (eds): Cerebral Aneurysms: Advances in Diagnosis and Therapy. Berlin, Springer-Verlag, 1979, pp 364–375

36. Locksley HB: Report on the cooperative study of intracranial aneurysms and subarachnoid hemorrhage. Section V, Part 1. Natural history of subarachnoid hemorrhage, intracranial aneurysms and arteriovenous malformations. Based on 6,368 cases in the cooperative study. J Neurosurg 25:219, 1966

37. Lukin R, Chambers A: Traumatic aneurysm of peripheral cerebral artery. Neuroradiology 8:1, 1974

38. Mann KS, Yue CP, Ngan H: Traumatic intracranial aneurysms and fistula associated with epidural hematoma. J Neurol Neurosurg Psychiatry 49:1085, 1986

39. Martinez SN, Bertrand C, Thierry A: Les faux an [acutee] vrismes posttraumatiques. Can J Surg 9:397, 1966

40. Maurer JJ, Milis M, German WJ: Triad of unilateral blindness, orbital fractures and massive epistaxis after head injury. J Neurosurg 18:837, 1961

41. Melvill RL, De Villiers JC: Peripheral cerebral arterial aneurysms caused by stabbing. S Afr Med J 51:471, 1977

42. Menezes AH, Graf CJ: True traumatic aneurysm of anterior cerebral artery. Case report. J Neurosurg 40:544, 1974

43. Nakamura K, Tsugane R, Ito H, et al: Traumatic arteriovenous fistula of the middle meningeal vessels. J Neurosurg 25:424, 1966

44. Nakstad P, Nornes H, Hauge HN: Traumatic aneurysms of pericallosal arteries. Neuroradiology 28:335, 1986

45. Overton MC III, Calvin TH Jr: Iatrogenic cerebral cortical aneurysm. Case report. J Neurosurg 24:672, 1966

46. Paillas JE, Bonnal J, Lavieille J: Angiographic images of false aneurysmal sac caused by rupture of median meningeal artery in the course of traumatic extradural hematomata. Report of 3 cases. J Neurosurg 21:667, 1964

47. Parkinson D, West M: Traumatic intracranial aneurysms. J Neurosurgery 52:11, 1980

48. Perret G, Nishioka H: Report on the cooperative study of intracranial aneurysms and subarachnoid hemorrhage. Section VI. Arteriovenous malformations. An analysis of 545 cases of craniocerebral arteriovenous malformations and fistulae reported to the cooperative study. J Neurosurg 25:467, 1966

49. Petty JM: Epistaxis from aneurysm of the internal carotid artery due to a gunshot wound. Case report. J Neurosurg 30:741, 1969

50. Raimondi AJ, Yashon D, Reyes C, et al: Intracranial false aneurysms. Neurochirugia 11:219, 1968

51. Rumbaugh CL, Bergeron RT, Talalla A, et al: Traumatic aneurysms of the cortical cerebral arteries. Radiographic aspects. Radiology 96:49, 1970

52. Sachdev VP, Drapkin AJ, Hollin SA, et al: Subarachnoid hemorrhage following intranasal procedures. Surg Neurol 8:122, 1977

53. Sadar ES, Jane JA, Lewis LW, et al: Traumatic aneurysms of the intracranial circulation. Surg Gynecol Obstet 137:59, 1973

54. Salmon JH, Blatt ES: Aneurysm of the internal carotid artery due to closed trauma. J Thorac Cardiovasc Surg 56:28, 1968

55. Salazar FJ, Vaquero J, Sola GR, et al: Traumatic false aneurysms of the middle meningeal artery. Neurosurgery 18:200, 1986

56. Schechter MM: Angiography in head trauma. Clin Neurosurg 12:193, 1966

57. Sezimir CB, Occleshaw JV, Buxton PH: False cerebral aneurysm. Case report. J Neurosurg 29:636, 1968

58. Seftel DM, Kolson H, Gordon BS: Ruptured intracranial carotid artery aneurysm with fatal epistaxis. Arch Otolaryngol 70:54, 1959

59. Shaw CM, Foltz EL: Traumatic dissecting aneurysm of middle cerebral artery and carotid-cavernous fistula with massive intracerebral hemorrhage. Case report. J Neurosurg 28:475, 1968

60. Smith DR, Kempe LG: Cerebral false aneurysm formation in closed head trauma. Case report. J Neurosurg 32:357, 1970

61. Smith S: On the difficulties attending the diagnosis of aneurism being a contribution to surgical diagnosis and medical jurisprudence. Am J Med Sci 66:401, 1873

62. Stehbens WE: Pathology of the Cerebral Blood Vessels. St. Louis, CV Mosby, 1972, pp 452–455

63. Taylor PE: Delayed postoperative hemorrhage from intracranial aneurysm after craniotomy for tumor. Neurology 11:225, 1961

64. Teal JS, Bergeron RT, Rumbaugh CL, et al: Aneurysms of the petrous or cavernous portions of the internal carotid artery associated with nonpenetrating head trauma. J Neurosurg 38:568, 1973

65. Thompson JR, Harwood-Nash DC, Fitz CR: Cerebral aneurysms in children. Am J Roentgenol Radium Ther Nucl Med 118:163, 1973

66. Umebayashi Y, Kuwayama M, Handa J, et al: Traumatic aneurysm of a peripheral cerebral artery: Case report. Clin Radiol 21:36, 1970

67. Weaver DF, Gates EM, Nielsen AE: Traumatic intracranial vascular lesions producing late massive nasal hemorrhage. Trans Am Acad Ophthalmol Otolaryngol 65:759, 1961

68. White JC, Sayre GP, Whisnant JP: Experiemenial destruction of the media for the production of intracranial arterial aneurysms. J Neurosurg 18:741, 1961

69. Wilson CB, Cronic F: Traumatic arteriovenous fistulas involving middle meningeal vessels. JAMA 188:953, 1964

70. Amagasa M, Onuma T, Suzuki J: Pseudoaneurysm of the cortical artery associated with chronic subdural hematoma: A consideration on traumatic middle cerebral artery aneurysm. No Shinkei Geka 15(1):81–86, 1987

71. Amagasa M, Onuma T, Suzuki J, et al: Traumatic anterior cerebral artery aneurysms: Experiences in 4 cases and review of the literature. No Shinkei Geka 14(13): 1585–1592, 1986

72. Hayashi A, Oda M, Sekino T, et al: Traumatic aneurysm occurring after surgical procedure of large cerebral aneurysm. No Shinkei Geka 14(7):881–885, 1986

73. Salazar-Flores J, Vaquero J, Garcia-Sola R, et al: Traumatic false aneurysms of the middle meningeal artery. Neurosurgery 18(2): 200–203, 1986

74. Rahimizadeh A, Abtahi H, Daylami MS, et al: Traumatic cerebral aneurysms caused by shell fragments: Report of four cases and review of the literature. Acta Neurochir (Wien) 84(3–4): 93–98, 1987

75. Pertuiset B: Predictability of outcome in neurological surgery. Acta Neurochir (Wein) 82(3–4): 73–91, 1986

76. Inagawa T, Takeda T, Taguchi H, et al: Traumatic middle meningeal arteriovenous fistula caused by three-point skull fixation: Case report. J. Neurosurg 60(4):853–855, 1984

77. Yamaura A, Makino H, Hachisu H, et al: Secondary aneurysm due to arterial injury during surgical procedures. Surg Neurol 10:327, 1978

78. Pakarinen S: Arteriovenous fistula between the middle meningeal artery and the sphenoparietal sinus. A case report. J Neurosurgery 23:438, 1965

79. Voris HC, Basile JXR: Recurrent epistaxis from aneurysm of the internal carotid artery. Case report with cure by operation. J Neurosurg 18:841, 1961

80. Smith KR, Bardenheier JA III: Aneurysm of the pericallosal artery caused by closed cranial trauma. Case report. J Neurosurg 29:551, 1968

81. Wolman L: Cerebral dissecting aneurysms. Brain 82:276, 1959

82. Bollinger O: Uber traumatische Spat Apoplexie; ein Bietrag zum Lehre von der Hirnerschutterung. Festschr Rud Virchow 2:457, 1891

83. Leslie EV, Smith BH, Zoll JG: Value of angiography in head trauma. Radiology 78:930, 1962

84. Parkinson D, Legal J, Holloway AF, et al: A new combined neurosurgical headholder and cassette changer for intraoperative serial angiography. Technical note. J Neurosurg 48:1038, 1978

85. Dolenc V: Treatment of fusiform aneurysms of the peripheral cerebral arteries. Report of two cases. J Neurosurg 49:272, 1978

CHAPTER 88
Surgical Management of Bacterial Intracranial Aneurysms

Robert G. Ojemann

SINCE THE DESCRIPTION of an aortic aneurysm associated with bacterial endocarditis by William Osler in 1885,[1] the term "mycotic" aneurysm has been used to designate any aneurysm that developed following an infection in the wall of an artery. Until a few years ago almost every publication concerning intracranial "mycotic" aneurysms reported a bacterial cause for the aneurysm, usually in association with endocarditis. Reports of aneurysms related to meningitis and cavernous sinus thrombophlebitis as well as true mycotic (fungal) aneurysms now have appeared.[2] The designation "bacterial intracranial aneurysm," should be used for those aneurysms that result from bacterial infection.[3] It is suggested that all types of aneurysms caused by infection be grouped under the heading of infectious intracranial aneurysms.[2]

Several publications have reviewed the subject of bacterial intracranial aneurysms.[2–6] In one, 85 cases found at angiography, surgery, or autopsy between 1954 and 1978 were summarized.[3] In another, infectious intracranial aneurysms documented by angiography and reported in the 20 years from 1959 through 1978 were analyzed.[2] This included 53 patients with bacterial intracranial aneurysms associated with definite or probable endocarditis,[2–32] 5 cases caused by meningitis,[33–36] 7 cases related to cavernous sinus thrombophlebitis,[30,35,37,38] and 5 fungal aneurysms.[39–43] Subsequently, further reports of patients with bacterial aneurysms documented by angiography brought the total number of cases through 1980 to 81.[5,44–52]

CLINICAL MANIFESTATIONS

The majority of bacterial intracranial aneurysms occur in patients with subacute bacterial endocarditis, some of whom have associated congenital heart disease or rheumatic heart disease. In a few patients with bacterial intracranial aneurysms, a diagnosis of endocarditis is not established. These patients usually have had a history of infection such as pharyngitis or infected laceration, or they are drug addicts.

The aneurysms are caused by infected emboli reaching the cerebral circulation and are most often located on a distal branch of an intracranial artery, usually a branch of the middle cerebral artery. This tends to differentiate this type of aneurysm from the more common developmental aneurysm that usually is

found on the circle of Willis or the proximal middle cerebral artery.

Neurologic problems are frequent in patients with bacterial endocarditis and may be the initial symptoms.[15,53,54] Jones et al.[15] found neurologic symptoms in 29 percent (110 of 385) and Pruitt et al.[53] in 39 percent (84 of 218) of patients with bacterial endocarditis. The majority of patients have evidence of cerebral embolism with infarction, but hemorrhage (subarachnoid or intracerebral) and infarction followed by hemorrhage may occur. A few patients have had brain abscess or meningitis. Occasionally, headache has been noted without evidence of hemorrhage.[17]

Intracranial bacterial aneurysms occur in 4 to 10 percent of patients with bacterial endocarditis.[3] The incidence may be even higher since some aneurysms are asymptomatic. Multiple aneurysms occur in up to 20 percent of the patients with an aneurysm, but the true figure is unknown since very few patients have had full angiographic studies. The lesions may occur at any age.

When a patient with endocarditis develops a bacterial aneurysm it usually produces signs and symptoms of subarachnoid or intracerebral hemorrhage. Patients without a previous diagnosis of bacterial endocarditis may have the onset of hemorrhage from a bacterial aneurysm as the first manifestation of the disease. Another clinical group are those patients who first have symptoms and signs of cerebral ischemia but are found to have an aneurysm when the neurologic deficit caused by the infarct is investigated by angiography, or who initially have clinical evidence of cerebral infarction and then days to weeks later develop a subarachnoid or intracerebral hemorrhage from an aneurysm.[53] Recurrent hemorrhage occurs, but the incidence is unknown.

In the reports of the 81 patients we reviewed with bacterial aneurysms caused by endocarditis and documented by angiography, 65 had enough clinical information to determine the probable initial neurologic event that led to the angiogram. This was definite or probable hemorrhage in 42, infarction in 16, infarction followed by hemorrhage in 5, and headache without hemorrhage in 2 (Table 88-1). In the 16 patients with ruptured aneurysms reported by Pruitt et al.,[53] 8 had a history suggesting embolization and infarction before the hemorrhage. At angiography an occluded vessel often was found in association with the aneurysm.

The most frequent organism cultured in patients with bacterial aneurysms caused by endocarditis has been the strep-

Portions of this chapter are reprinted with permission from Ojemann RG, Crowell RM: Surgical Management of Cerebrovascular Disease. Baltimore, Williams & Wilkins, 1983.

OPERATIVE NEUROSURGICAL TECHNIQUES
ISBN 0-8089-1862-1

Table 88-1. Clinical presentation of 81 patients with bacterial intracranial aneurysms associated with definite or probable endocarditis and documented by angiography, 1959–1980

Finding	Number of Patients
Hemorrhage	42
Infarction	16
Infarction followed by hemorrhage	5
Headache without hemorrhage	2
Not enough information	16
Total	81

tococcus (Table 88-2). *Staphylococcus,* however, has become a more common organism in the reports during the past few years. In some cases no organisms can be isolated from the blood culture because of effective prophylactic treatment or the use of broad spectrum antibiotics in patients with a febrile illness. In spite of the improvement in the recovery rate from infectious endocarditis because of the effective use of antibiotics, the incidence of neurologic complications of the disease has not been significantly reduced.[17,37] It is important to note that aneurysms can develop and hemorrhage can occur in a patient who is receiving adequate antibiotic treatment.

DIAGNOSTIC STUDIES

When there is evidence to suggest subarachnoid hemorrhage in a patient with bacterial endocarditis, a computed tomographic (CT) scan followed by cerebral angiography should be done. It has been suggested that the presence of cerebral embolization during the course of bacterial endocarditis is a strong indication for cerebral angiography.[23]

The CT scan should be done with and without contrast enhancement. It may localize the aneurysm either directly or by demonstrating adjacent hematoma. The extent of intracerebral or intraventricular hemorrhage is determined. Associated changes in adjacent cerebral tissue caused by edema, infarction, or abscess and the degree of hydrocephalus will be seen.

Angiography is the definitive study in outlining the location and relationship of the aneurysm to the parent vessel (Figures

Table 88-2. Bacteria cultured from specimens in 81 patients with bacterial intracranial aneurysms associated with definite or probable endocarditis and documented by angiography, 1959–1980

Bacteria	Number of Patients
Streptococcus	36
Staphylococcus	15
Pseudomonas	2
Enterococcus	1
Corynebacterium	1
Cardiobacterium	1
Multiple	4
No growth	10
No information	11

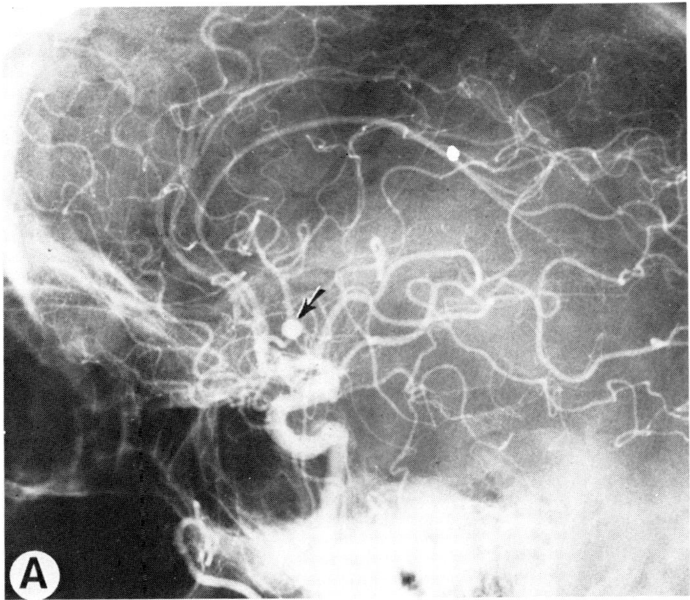

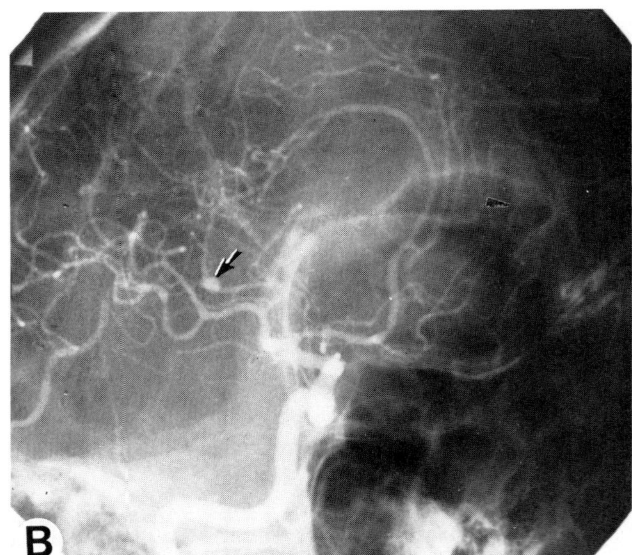

Fig. 88-1.   Lateral (A) and oblique (B) angiograms showing a bacterial intracranial aneurysm (arrows) on a distal branch of the middle cerebral artery. Between 75 and 80 percent of these aneurysms occur on a distal branch of the middle cerebral artery.

88-1A and B). If the diagnosis of associated subarachnoid hemorrhage is in doubt or if meningitis is suspected, a lumbar puncture is indicated after the CT scan has been done.

The predominant involvement of the middle cerebral artery and a distal intracranial branch when any artery is involved is striking (Table 88-3). In the 71 patients in which the site of the angiographically proven bacterial aneurysms was definitely established on the initial angiogram, 64 had at least one aneurysm on a distal branch of an intracranial artery and in 55 a middle cerebral artery branch was involved. Very few patients have had complete angiographic studies, so the true incidence of multiple aneurysms is unknown.

In 27 patients who had not had surgery, follow-up angiography was performed within a few days to 8 months after the first study, but usually within 2 to 8 weeks. A few patients had more than one follow-up study. In 8 patients a new aneurysm

Table 88-3. Findings on the initial angiogram in 81 patients with bacterial intracranial aneurysms associated with definite or probable endocarditis, 1959–1980

Location of Aneurysm	Number of Patients
Single	
Distal middle cerebral artery	44
Distal anterior cerebral artery	3
Distal posterior cerebral artery	4
Proximal intracranial artery	7
Middle cerebral artery—unspecified	3
Total	61
Multiple	
Distal middle cerebral artery only	4
Distal middle cerebral artery and other vessels	7
Combinations not including middle cerebral artery	2
Unspecified	2
Total	15
No aneurysm seen	5
Occluded artery in addition to aneurysm	13

was found; 3 of these had a normal initial angiogram. At the time of the last angiographic study, the aneurysm was no longer visualized in 8, was smaller in 5, unchanged in 4, larger in 6, and in 4 a new aneurysm was found but no further study was reported. Seven other patients had postoperative angiography. The original aneurysm was gone in all cases, but 1 patient had a new aneurysm on the distal middle cerebral artery that had ruptured.

TREATMENT

A program of treatment for patients with bacterial intracranial aneurysms can be outlined based on a review of the literature.[2,3,5,11,28,53,55] Medical treatment should include the administration of appropriate intravenous antibiotics and the correction of the responsible cardiac lesion if indicated. It has been recommended that the cardiac operation be done before repair of the intracranial aneurysm, unless the patient is threatened by mass effect from a hematoma, to remove the source for further emboli and correct any hemodynamic problem.[55]

The place of surgical treatment has been discussed in recent reports. Bingham[11] reviewed 45 cases of bacterial intracranial aneurysms of all types where it was thought that adequate antibiotic treatment had been given and where angiography had been done. He concluded that there did not appear to be a clear-cut advantage to surgery plus antibiotics over antibiotics alone. Twenty patients received antibiotic treatment only, but 3 died from hemorrhage while under treatment. In the 25 patients who had combined antibiotic and surgical treatment, 6 died, but most of these were poor risk patients. In fact, he noted that the mortality associated with a definitive surgical procedure for a bacterial intracranial aneurysm on a distal arterial branch appears to be quite low if one eliminates the poor risk surgical candidates. The deaths in this series were the result of cardiac or other medical problems and fatal hemorrhage from a second previously undiagnosed aneurysm. He

recommended an operation only if the aneurysm enlarged or did not change in size after 6 weeks of antibiotic therapy. Bohmfalk et al.[3] reviewed reports of 17 patients who had surgical removal of bacterial aneurysms of distal arterial branches. There was no mortality. He also noted 6 patients in the literature who did not develop hemorrhage until after completion of their antibiotic treatment for endocarditis. Cantu et al.[4] reported an autopsy series of 5 patients in whom death was caused by rupture of a bacterial aneurysm; all had been receiving intensive antibiotic therapy at the time of the hemorrhage.[4] Pruitt et al.[53] reported 9 patients who were adequately treated with antibiotics before aneurysmal ruptures. Frazee et al.[5] concluded that patients with a diagnosis of bacterial endocarditis who develop sudden severe headache, focal neurologic signs, or symptoms or seizures should undergo serial angiography every 7 to 10 days throughout their hospitalization. If an aneurysm is identified, it should be excised whenever possible. Morawetz and Karp noted that new aneurysms may appear and existing ones enlarge during the first 4 to 6 weeks of antibiotic therapy and these changes do not mandate surgery but surgical intervention is indicated after intracerebral or subarachnoid hemorrhage or when an aneurysm enlarges after the completion of a full course of antibiotic therapy.[55]

The results of a review of the literature of 81 patients who had angiography because of a neurologic symptom and were found to have a bacterial aneurysm are outlined in Table 88-4. In 30 patients treated with antibiotics where the outcome was known, 13 died. Elective surgery was done in 29 patients; 2 died, but in both instances they recovered from the surgery only to die of rupture of a second unrecognized aneurysm. As would be expected in situations where emergency surgery was required, usually because of an intracranial hematoma that had caused a serious neurologic deficit, the results were worse.

In planning the surgical treatment, it is important to remember that these aneurysms have an inflamed, friable wall that may easily fragment. In the peripheral lesions, the aneurysm can be excised with the small vessel from which it arises, usually with little or no neurologic deficit. The less common proximal or less accessible lesions may present a more serious technical problem. Treatment with antibiotics may allow the arteritis to resolve and some reparative fibrosis to take place in the wall of the aneurysm and the parent artery. The lesions then can be handled more safely at surgery.[28] If surgery is needed for a proximal lesion, a bypass graft may be required as the initial procedure.

A single aneurysm on a distal branch of the middle cerebral artery associated with subarachnoid or intracerebral hemorrhage should be excised if the medical condition of the patient is stable. For bacterial aneurysms on the proximal arterial trunks, unruptured aneurysms or those involving arteries whose excision is very likely to cause a serious neurologic deficit, a program of antibiotics and serial angiography is indicated. How often the angiogram should be done has not been established and has ranged from one to several weeks.[5,55–57] If the aneurysm is larger at follow-up angiography, surgery is indicated. If it is the same size or smaller, the antibiotic treatment should be continued. Angiography is repeated at an appropriate interval and again when antibiotic treatment is completed. If the aneurysm does not disappear after treatment or at any time becomes larger, surgery usually is considered.

The literature does not give a definitive answer to the question of what to do with the patient when multiple bacterial aneurysms are found. A review of 15 reported cases of multiple

Table 88-4. Treatment and results in 81 patients with bacterial intracranial aneurysms associated with definite or probable endocarditis and documented by angiography, 1959–1980

Treatment	Results			
	Recovered*	Died	No Information	Total
Antibiotics	17	13	1	31
Elective surgery†	27	2	—	29
Emergency surgery†	8	6	—	14
No treatment	1	1	1	3
No information	—	—	4	4

*Some patients who recovered from their neurologic illness subsequently died of a cardiac cause and some were left with a neurologic disability.
†Patients who had surgery also received antibiotics.

bacterial aneurysms caused by a variety of factors including meningitis revealed that 11 were treated nonsurgically and none died as a direct result of this treatment.[5] Analysis of reports of 10 patients with multiple bacterial aneurysms seen on angiography and related to established or probable endocarditis revealed that 7 were treated by antibiotics alone with only 1 death.[2] This was a patient who also was a heroin addict and who had a brain abscess and infarction. There is no explanation for the findings of a low mortality rate with antibiotic therapy alone compared with the higher mortality rate for patients treated nonsurgically with a single aneurysm. We have already noted, however, that 2 patients who had recovered from elective surgery for removal of a single aneurysm subsequently died because of hemorrhage from a second unrecognized aneurysm. Frazee et al.[5] proposed that if multiple aneurysms are unilateral, they should be excised at one operation wherever possible, and if they are bilateral, the largest aneurysm or the one presumed to have bled should be excised and the patient then followed by angiography. Another plan is to treat the patient with antibiotics and repeat the angiogram at 2-week intervals and when therapy is completed. If the lesions become larger or do not disappear after treatment, surgery may be indicated.

At the time of surgery the neurosurgeon may encounter not only an intracerebral hematoma or an area of infarction but also a brain abscess. In the series of cases reviewed 5 patients had associated brain abscess.

CONCLUSIONS

Even though there has been progress in the diagnosis and treatment of bacterial endocarditis, neurologic symptoms are frequent and bacterial aneurysms are a cause of morbidity and mortality. CT scans and angiography are indicated in patients suspected of having a bacterial intracranial aneurysm. The finding of an aneurysm on a distal intracranial arterial branch, especially of the middle cerebral artery, is strongly suggestive of an infectious etiology. A single bacterial aneurysm on a distal branch of the middle cerebral artery that has ruptured should be excised if the medical condition of the patient is stable. A bacterial aneurysm that is enlarging or does not disappear after antibiotic treatment also should be excised whenever possible. A definitive plan for treating unruptured bacterial aneurysms, those involving proximal arterial trunks, and multiple bacterial aneurysms has not been established.

REFERENCES

1. Osler W: Gulstonian lectures on malignant endocarditis. Lancet 1:415, 459, 505, 1885
2. Ojemann RG: Infectious intracranial aneurysms, in Fein J, Flamm E (eds): Cerebrovascular Surgery, vol 3. New York, Springer-Verlag, 1985, pp 1047–1060
3. Bohmfalk GL, Story JL, Wissinger JP, et al.: Bacterial intracranial aneurysm. J Neurosurg 48:369, 1978
4. Cantu RC, LeMay M, Wilkinson HA: The importance of repeated angiography in the treatment of mycotic-embolic intracranial aneurysms. J Neurosurg 25:189, 1966
5. Frazee JG, Cahan LD, Winter J: Bacterial intracranial aneurysms. J Neurosurg 53:633, 1980
6. Hourihane JB: Ruptured mycotic intracranial aneurysm. A report of three cases. Vasc Surg 4:21, 1970
7. Agnoli A, Bettag W: Endokarditis und subarachnoidalblutung. Z Neurol 199:295, 1971
8. Alajouanine T, Castaigne P, Lhermitte F, et al: Cerebral arteritis of bacterial endocarditis: Its late complications. JAMA 170:1858, 1959
9. Amine ARC: Neurosurgical complications of heroin addiction: Brain abscess and mycotic aneurysm. Surg Neurol 7:385, 1977
10. Bell WE, Butler C II: Cerebral mycotic aneurysms in children. Two case reports. Neurology 18:81, 1968
11. Bingham WF: Treatment of mycotic intracranial aneurysms. J Neurosurg 46:428, 1977
12. Gilroy J, Andaya L, Thomas VJ: Intracranial mycotic aneurysms and subacute bacterial endocarditis in heroin addiction. Neurology 23:1193, 1973
13. Harrison MJG, Hampton JR: Neurological presentation of bacterial endocarditis. Br Med J 2:148, 1967
14. Ishikawa M, Waga S, Moritake K, et al: Cerebral bacterial aneurysms: Report of three cases. Surg Neurol 2:257, 1974
15. Jones HR Jr, Siekert RG, Geraci JE: Neurologic manifestations of bacterial endocarditis. Ann Intern Med 71:21, 1969
16. Katz RI, Goldberg HI, Selzer ME: Mycotic aneurysm. Case report with novel sequential angiographic findings. Arch Intern Med 134:939, 1974
17. Kaufman SL, White RI, Harrington DP, et al: Protean manifestations of mycotic aneurysm. AJR 131:1019, 1978
18. King AB: Successful surgical treatment of an intracranial mycotic aneurysm complicated by a subdural hematoma. J Neurosurg 17:788, 1960
19. Laguna J, Derby BM, Chase R: Cardiobacterium hominis endocarditis with cerebral mycotic aneurysm. Arch Neurol 32:638, 1975
20. Matson DD: Intracranial arterial aneurysms in childhood. J Neurosurg 23:578, 1965
21. McNeel D, Evans RA, Ory EM: Angiography of cerebral mycotic aneurysms. Acta Radiol (Diagn) 9:407, 1969
22. Morin MA, Talalla A: Angiography for mycotic aneurysm (letter). N Engl J Med 281:1249, 1969
23. Moskowitz MA, Rosenbaum AE, Tyler HR: Angiographically monitored resolution of cerebral mycotic aneurysms. Neurology 24:1103, 1974
24. Ng KK, Wong WK, Skene-Smith H: Ruptured mycotic intracranial aneurysm. Australas Radiol 19:255, 1975
25. Noonan JA, Wilson CB, Spencer FC, et al: Cerebral and cardiac complications from bacterial endocarditis. A successfully managed case with unusual complications. Am J Dis Child 116:666, 1968

26. North-Coombes D, Schonland MM: Cerebral mycotic aneurysm. A case report. S Afr Med J 48:1808, 1974

27. Pool JL, and Potts DG: Aneurysm and Arteriovenous Anomalies of the Brain. New York, Harper and Row, 1965, pp 60–62

28. Roach MR, Drake CG: Ruptured cerebral aneurysms caused by micro-organisms. N Engl J Med 273:240, 1965

29. Schold C, Earnest MP: Cerebral hemorrhage from a mycotic aneurysm developing during appropriate antibiotic therapy. Stroke 9:267, 1978

30. Tanemura H, Sakai N, Yamamori T, et al: Intracranial mycotic aneurysm-report of a case. Neurol Surg 5:871, 1977

31. Yarnell PR, Stears J: Intracerebral hemorrhage and occult sepsis. Neurology 24:870, 1974

32. Ziment I, Johnson BL Jr: Angiography in the management of intracranial mycotic aneurysms. Arch Intern Med 122:349, 1968

33. Harrison MJG, Hampton JR: Neurological presentation of bacterial endocarditis. Br Med J 2:148, 1967

34. Ojemann RG, New PFJ, Fleming TC: Intracranial aneurysms associated with bacterial meningitis. Neurology 16:1222, 1966

35. Suwanwela C, Suwanwela N, Charuchinda S, et al: Intracranial mycotic aneurysms of extra-vascular origin. J Neurosurg 36:552, 1972

36. Sypert GW, Young HF: Ruptured mycotic pericallosal aneurysm with meningitis due to Neisseria meningitides infection. Case report. J Neurosurg 37:467, 1972

37. Lansky LL, Maxwell JA: Mycotic aneurysm of the internal carotid artery in an unusual intracranial location. Dev Med Child Neurol 17:79, 1975

38. Shibuya S, Igarashi S, Amo T, et al: Mycotic aneurysms of the internal carotid artery. Case report. J Neurosurg 44:105, 1976

39. Ahuja GK, Jain N, Vijayaraghaven M, et al: Cerebral mycotic aneurysm of fungal origin. J Neurosurg 49:107, 1978

40. Davidson P, Robertson DM: A true mycotic (Aspergillus) aneurysm leading to fatal subarachnoid hemorrhage in a patient with hereditary hemorrhagic telangiectasia. Case report. J Neurosurg 35:71, 1971

41. Horten BC, Abbott GF, Porro RS: Fungal aneurysms of intracranial vessels. Arch Neurol 33:577, 1976

42. Mahaley MS, Spock A: An unusual case of intracranial aneurysm, in Smith JL (ed): Neuroophthalmology, vol 4. St. Louis, CV Mosby, 1968, pp 148–166

43. Visudhiphan P, Bunyaratavej S, Khantanaphar S: Cerebral aspergillosis. Report of 3 cases. J Neurosurg 38:472, 1973

44. Almazan V, Pulpin A, Galnan D, et al: Mycotic aneurysm secondary to bacterial endocarditis. Arch Inst Cardiol Mex 48:1224, 1978

45. Grinberg M, Lage SH, DeAlmcida GG: Infective endocarditis, cerebral mycotic aneurysm and meningeal hemorrhage. Arq Bras Cardiol 32:257, 1979

46. Jara FM, Lewis JF, Magilligan DG: Operative experience with infective endocarditis and intracerebral mycotic aneurysm. J Thorac Cardiovasc Surg 80:28, 1980

47. Maly Z: Paraventricular hemorrhage from a mycotic aneurysm. Cesk Neurol Neurochir 41:394, 1978

48. Nishimura T, Aoko N, Aruga T, et al: Case of mycotic aneurysm after open heart surgery. No Shinkei Geka 7:371, 1979

49. Sato T, Sakuta Y, Suzuki J, et al: Successful surgical treatment of intracranial mycotic aneurysm with brain abscess. Acta Neurochir 47:53, 1979

50. Shillito J Jr: Strokes in children. Clin Neurosurg 23:185, 1976

51. Simmons KC, Sage MR, Reilly PL: CT of intracerebral hemorrhage due to mycotic aneurysm-case report. Neuroradiology 19:215, 1980

52. Valadares JB, DeSouza MT, Hankinson J, et al: Multiple intracranial mycotic aneurysms—Case report. Arq Neuropsiquiatr 37:311, 1979

53. Pruitt AA, Rubin RH, Karchmer AW, et al: Neurologic complications of bacterial endocarditis. Medicine 57:329, 1978

54. Lerner PI: Neurologic complications of infective endocarditis. Med Clin North Am 69:385, 1985

55. Morawetz RB, Karp RB: Evolution and resolution of intracranial bacterial (mycotic) aneurysms. Neurosurgery 15:43, 1984

56. Leipzig TJ, Brown FD: Treatment of mycotic aneurysms. Surg Neurol 23:403, 1985

57. Pootrakul A, Canter LP: Bacterial intracranial aneurysms: Importance of sequential angiography. Surg Neurol 17:429, 1982

CHAPTER 89
Treatment of Multiple and Asymptomatic Aneurysms

Ronald Brisman

THERE IS GENERAL AGREEMENT in the neurosurgical community that symptomatic aneurysms should be treated, usually by a direct surgical approach. In patients with multiple aneurysms, the important issues are the methods for determining which aneurysm has ruptured and which of the asymptomatic aneurysms should be treated surgically.

INCIDENCE

The incidence of patients who have more than one aneurysm ranges from 5 percent (an operative series from 1953)[1] to 33.5 percent.[2] In older angiographic series (1950–1960) in which arteriography was incomplete, incidences of 7 to 9 percent were noted.[3–5] In later angiographic series (1965–1980) with more complete but not always four-vessel angiographic studies a higher incidence (16 to 19 percent) of multiplicity was noted,[6,7] as was the case in our own series of 197 patients with multiple aneurysms treated between 1958 and 1980 (Neurological Institute of New York [NINY], 1980), which represents 19 percent of our total number of aneurysm cases.

Autopsy studies have tended to indicate a higher incidence of multiple aneurysms. In one such study, McCormick found that 26 percent of aneurysm patients had more than one aneurysm.[8] He included aneurysms that were 2 mm or more in size, but indicated that there was an artifact at autopsy caused by both lack of perfusion and fixation, which made the aneurysm appear at least 30 to 60 percent smaller than in vivo.

A recent study, which reports the highest incidence of multiplicity (33.5 percent) is an angiographic review in which aneurysms 1 mm in greatest dimension or larger were included.[2]

SEX

Although there is a slight tendency for single bleeding aneurysms to occur more frequently in women (56 percent) than in men,[7] there is a much greater preponderance of women (80 percent, NINY 1980) in series of patients with multiple aneurysms.[2,9,10] The female-to-male ratio increases as the number of aneurysms increases[2,9]; in one series, multiple aneurysms were five times more common in women, but in patients with three or more aneurysms, the female-to-male ratio rose to 11:1.[2] This sex predilection on the part of multiple aneurysms reflects the fact that most aneurysms in patients with multiple aneurysms are on the internal carotid artery and women are much more likely than men to have internal carotid artery aneurysms.[7] Anterior communicating artery aneurysms, which occur less frequently in patients with multiple aneurysms, are seen more often in men.

LOCATION

The internal carotid artery is the most common site for aneurysms in clinical series of patients with multiple aneurysms (Table 89-1). The middle cerebral artery is the second most frequent location, and the anterior communicating artery is the least likely supratentorial location. Bilateral symmetrical aneurysms occur in approximately 49 percent of those patients with multiple aneurysms (NINY 1980).

MULTIPLICITY OF ANEURYSMS

Most patients (74 percent) with multiple aneurysms will have two aneurysms. Approximately 17 percent will have three aneurysms. Between 7 and 9 percent will have four or more aneurysms.[11]

AGE AND HYPERTENSION

In one study, no interaction between the age of the patient and the number of aneurysms could be demonstrated.[10] There may be exceptions in certain subgroups. Aneurysms are less frequently seen in young patients (20 years of age and younger) than in older patients, males predominate, and multiple aneurysms are encountered less commonly.[12] In another report, hypertensive males and females (younger than 55 years of age) were more likely to have multiple aneurysms than normotensive patients. Using a logistic-regression analysis, one group of investigators was able to show that the most important factor in multiplicity was the presence of hypertension (greater than 145/95 mm Hg).[10] A different group, using slightly lower blood pressure values to define hypertension (140/90 mm Hg), was unable to detect an association between hypertension and multiplicity of aneurysms.[13]

DIAGNOSIS

Two diagnostic considerations are of major importance in patients with multiple aneurysms: (1) an awareness that a patient with an intracranial aneurysm may have more than one

OPERATIVE NEUROSURGICAL TECHNIQUES
ISBN 0-8089-1862-1

Table 89-1. Location of Aneurysms in Patients with Multiple Aneurysms

Location	NINY 1980*		Cooperative Study 1966, Cases of Double Aneurysms	
	Number of Aneurysms	Percentage of Total	Number of Aneurysms	Percentage of Total
Internal carotid†	309	65	428	48
Middle cerebral	89	19	265	30
Anterior communicating/cerebral	45	9	165	18
Posterior circulation	32	7	40	4
Total	475	100	898	100

* All cases of multiple aneurysms.
† Includes 30 intracavernous aneurysms.

aneurysm and that thorough four-vessel angiography is necessary to find these aneurysms; and (2) a need to determine which aneurysm is symptomatic and which is asymptomatic.

WHICH ANEURYSM HAS RUPTURED?

The most common symptom in patients with intracranial aneurysms is subarachnoid hemorrhage (SAH); this was the case in 74 percent of patients with multiple aneurysms (NINY 1980). Computerized tomography and arteriography are the most useful diagnostic tests for determining which aneurysm has ruptured. When these are used in conjunction with EEG and clinical findings, the ruptured aneurysm can be determined in more than 95 percent of cases.[2]

COMPUTERIZED TOMOGRAPHY

Computerized tomographic (CT) scanning should be done within 24 hours after subarachnoid hemorrhage is suspected because it will frequently (68 percent[14] to 90 percent[15]) confirm the presence of intracranial blood and will often (50 percent[16]) localize the source of bleeding. Unenhanced CT scans show the greatest density of subarachnoid blood in the cistern that is closest to the bleeding aneurysm.[17] Extravasated blood has a density of 70–90 Hounsfield units (35–45 EMI units), and is usually no longer recognizable on CT scans between 6 and 10 days after the hemorrhage.[15]

The CT scan is of greatest additional help in localizing the ruptured aneurysm when there is a small hematoma that does not cause vascular displacement on arteriograms. This occurs most often with anterior communicating artery aneurysms that form hematomas on the anterior interhemispheric fissure and medial inferior frontal lobe. Hayward and O'Reilly showed how the presence of a hematoma in the cavum of the septum pellucidum or corpus callosum could be taken "as an absolute indication of an anterior cerebral complex aneurysm," which they were able to diagnose correctly in 27 out of 27 cases. Middle cerebral artery aneurysms usually could (in 20 of 24 cases) be identified if the associated hematoma followed the curve (comma shape) of the sylvian fissure.[18]

Contrast-enhanced CT scans are helpful in visualizing approximately 30 percent of intracranial aneurysms.[14] Except for indicating the larger aneurysm in cases with multiple aneurysms, enhancement does little to show which aneurysm has bled.

ARTERIOGRAPHY

Arteriograms are often helpful in identifying the ruptured aneurysm. Wood found that a mass associated with hematoma or an edematous cerebral infarct was the most reliable arteriographic indication that an aneurysm had ruptured.[19] He found that greater size was the most frequent finding among aneurysms that had bled in patients with multiple aneurysms; it occurred in 87 percent of cases.[19] He regarded spasm as less reliable evidence that an aneurysm had bled, and felt that only moderately or severely localized spasm in association with a mass was a useful indicator; it was present in 57 percent of patients. Another sign of rupture was the observation, during successive examinations over a period of time, of an increase in the size of the aneurysm and the development of loculations.

Nehls found that irregularity of contour was more important than size in identifying the site of rupture; the presence of a nipple-sign was highly reliable.[2] The more irregular aneurysm bled in 93 percent (28 of 30 cases), and the larger aneurysm bled in only 83 percent (30 of 36 cases).

ELECTROENCEPHALOGRAPHY

Electroencephalograms (EEGs) were helpful in identifying which aneurysm has ruptured in 62 percent[2] of patients with multiple aneurysms. The EEG can be particularly helpful in cases with bilateral middle cerebral artery aneurysms, where it is more likely to provide localizing information and may sometimes do so even when CT scans and arteriograms do not provide definitive information.[2,20]

CLINICAL PARAMETERS

Clinical findings such as focal deficit, localized pain, or cranial nerve palsy occasionally can provide additional localizing assistance, although in one series they were helpful in only 7 percent of patients.[2]

PROBABILITY OF BLEEDING

The anterior communicating artery is the site with the highest rate of rupture.[2] In an autopsy series, aneurysms of the anterior communicating artery, when present, were the ones to rupture 75 percent of the time regardless of the type of combinations with other aneurysms.[19] Middle cerebral artery aneurysms ruptured infrequently (27 percent).[2] This may be explained by the tendency for smaller aneurysms to occur on the middle cerebral artery and smaller aneurysms (less than 6 mm in diameter) are less likely to rupture.[2,19,21]

SURGICAL TREATMENT

THE RUPTURED ANEURYSM

There is general agreement that the treatment of patients with multiple intracranial aneurysms should first be directed at the aneurysm that has ruptured, since this aneurysm poses the greatest immediate risk to the patient. Once the patient's clinical condition has improved and severe vasospasm has subsided, direct intracranial surgery usually is indicated. Microvascular techniques are used to expose the aneurysm and to clip the neck, or, when this is not possible, to wrap the aneurysm with muslin (sometimes with the addition of plastic spray). Extracranial carotid ligation is done less often and only for carotid aneurysms that cannot be treated intracranially. One is especially reluctant to ligate the extracranial carotid artery if there is also a contralateral intracranial aneurysm.

THE UNRUPTURED ANEURYSM

The surgical management of asymptomatic aneurysms is more controversial than that of symptomatic aneurysms. Less enthusiasm for surgical treatment has been expressed in the British literature[22–24] than in the North American[3,6,25–29] or the French[30,31] literature, where an increasing number of authors are recommending surgical treatment. This is because of the improved surgical results with microsurgery and the greater awareness of the persistent risk from an originally asymptomatic aneurysm. One of the few opponents of surgical treatment for asymptomatic aneurysms[32] has revised his opinion in the light of further evidence[33] and now recommends that they be operated upon. A British surgeon with a very large personal experience with intracranial aneurysms recently has also changed his policy and now operates on asymptomatic aneurysms in cases of angiographically proven multiple aneurysms.[34]

Although the question posed is usually whether or not to operate on asymptomatic aneurysms, a more appropriate consideration focuses on which asymptomatic aneurysms should be treated surgically. Most neurosurgeons would agree that a 9-mm aneurysm at the junction of the internal carotid and posterior communicating arteries in a 30-year-old patient should be operated upon and that a 2-mm basilar tip aneurysm in a 75-year-old patient with severe heart disease should not. In between these extremes there are areas of disagreement. Individual decisions in situations that are not so obvious can be resolved by balancing the risk factors associated with the natural history of a particular aneurysm with the possibility of complications during definitive surgical management.

There are various estimates of the likelihood of rupture of an asymptomatic aneurysm. According to some, usually with small series and short follow-ups, this rarely occurs.[7,22,23,35] One study indicates an extremely high annual risk (5 percent) of fatal subarachnoid hemorrhage from an originally asymptomatic aneurysm; this is based on an unrealistically low estimate (0.5 percent) of the prevalence of asymptomatic aneurysms, which was determined angiographically.[36] When the more valid figures derived from autopsy of a 5 percent prevalence of intracranial aneurysms and 21,000 yearly cases of aneurysmal bleeding are used, a more realistic estimate (0.4 to 0.5 percent) of the annual risk of bleeding from an asymptomatic aneurysm for 40) to 65-year-old patients is derived.[37]

Higher risk figures are obtained from clinical series of patients with multiple aneurysms, which indicate that 10 to 17 percent[6,27,32] of patients with angiographically demonstrated asymptomatic aneurysms will have SAHs and 40 percent[27] of these will be fatal. Based on an average follow-up of 5 years, the yearly risk of hemorrhage is between 1 percent[38] and 2 percent.[11]

Perhaps the greater apparent risk of SAH from an asymptomatic aneurysm in a patient with multiple aneurysms is that some of the aneurysms that were thought to be asymptomatic were really aneurysms that had ruptured originally and were therefore more likely to hemorrhage again than a truly asymptomatic aneurysm. Another explanation is that the patients with multiple aneurysms may have asymptomatic aneurysms that are larger than those in the autopsy series.

The size of an aneurysm is important in determining the chances of it hemorrhaging again. Although one group of investigators found that asymptomatic aneurysms 10 mm or larger were most likely to rupture,[39,40] others demonstrated that aneurysms 6 mm or greater in diameter also have a substantially greater chance of hemorrhaging again.[21,41] Smaller aneurysms may bleed, but they are much less likely to do so.

A patient's age at the time of diagnosis influences the yearly risk for hemorrhaging as well as the cumulative risk. A 50-year-old patient with an asymptomatic aneurysm has an estimated risk of rupture for each of the next 5 years (0.57) that is more than ten times that of a 25-year-old (0.051).[37] The younger patient has a greater cumulative life-time risk of rupture, which for a 20-year-old patient (16.6 percent) is more than three times that of a 60-year-old (4.7 percent).[37]

The risks of subsequent bleeding from an originally asymptomatic aneurysm have to be balanced against the possible morbidity of definitive surgical treatment. As a result of advances in microsurgical technique, intracranial treatment of an asymptomatic aneurysm can be performed effectively with very low morbidity or mortality when the surgical team is skilled in aneurysm surgery. A number of series confirm that such surgery can be done with a morbidity of approximately 5 percent and a mortality of less than 1 percent.[6,26,27,29,42,43]

Certain factors increase the chances for operative morbidity. In addition to major medical illness, these include symptoms of cerebral ischemia, large aneurysm size, and less accessible location.[42] In one study, operative morbidity with aneurysms less than 5 mm in diameter was 2.3 percent; with those 6 to 15 mm in diameter it was 6.8 percent; and with those 16 to 24 mm in diameter it was 14 percent.[42] The operative morbidity in relation to the location of the aneurysm on the artery was 4.8 percent for internal carotid-posterior communicating artery aneurysms; 8.1 percent for middle cerebral artery aneurysms; 11.8 percent for ophthalmic artery aneurysms; 15.5 percent for anterior communicating artery aneurysms; and 16.8 percent for carotid bifurcation aneurysms.[42]

The decision of whether to treat an asymptomatic aneurysm surgically should be individualized based on the patient's age and general medical condition, the aneurysm's size and location, and the patient's choice when realistic risks of surgery versus nonsurgery are carefully explained. Surgery should usually be recommended to most patients who are younger than 55 years of age and who have surgically accessible asymptomatic intracranial aneurysms that are larger than 5 mm in greatest diameter.

If the asymptomatic and symptomatic aneurysms are on the same side, they both can be treated during the initial craniotomy. Multiple aneurysms of the same internal carotid artery sometimes can be clipped separately; however, it may be helpful to apply a clip with its jaws parallel to the long axis of the internal carotid artery.[44] If multiple aneurysms are on opposite sides, then a separate craniotomy should be done, usually several weeks after the symptomatic aneurysm has been treated.

NONSURGICAL MANAGEMENT OF ASYMPTOMATIC ANEURYSMS

If a decision is made not to operate on an unruptured aneurysm and the patient has systemic hypertension, it is particularly important to treat the patient with antihypertensive medication. This may lessen the chance of subsequent enlargement or rupture of the aneurysm. If the patient's blood pressure is normal, the patient should undergo regular blood pressure determinations so that hypertension can be detected early and treated. The correction of hypertension in any patient with an aneurysm, whether ruptured or not, can possibly prevent the development of multiple aneurysms. Medical hypotensive therapy has been advocated for normotensive as well as hypertensive aneurysm patients[45] and has been used on those patients with multiple aneurysms in whom some of the asymptomatic aneurysms were not treated surgically.[46]

It is desirable to perform repeat arteriography on patients with a small, asymptomatic aneurysm that is not treated surgically because enlargement of the aneurysm may make subsequent rupture more likely and may lead the neurosurgeon to recommend surgery before the hemorrhage occurs. Follow-up arteriography should be done approximately 6 to 12 months after the initial diagnosis and again a few years later if no interval change is noted.

SUMMARY

INCIDENCE OF MULTIPLE ANEURYSMS

Twenty-six percent of patients with intracranial aneurysms have multiple aneurysms if aneurysms that are 2 mm or greater in diameter are counted. The incidence is 33 percent if aneurysmal enlargements of 1 to 2 mm are included.

CLINICAL FEATURES

Eighty percent of patients with multiple aneurysms are women. In clinical series, the internal carotid artery is the most frequent location and the anterior communicating-anterior cerebral artery is the least likely site. Most patients with multiple aneurysms (70 to 75 percent) will have only two aneurysms. Bilaterally symmetrical aneurysms occur in approximately 49 percent of patients with multiple aneurysms.

ANGIOGRAPHY

Four-vessel angiography, usually via the femoral route, is the most definitive way to study patients who may have intracranial aneurysms. In patients with subarachnoid hemorrhage and multiple aneurysms, the more irregular or larger aneurysm is more likely to have ruptured.

COMPUTERIZED TOMOGRAPHY

A CT scan obtained within the first few days of subarachnoid hemorrhage will often identify the source of the bleeding.

ELECTROENCEPHALOGRAPHY

If the aneurysm that has ruptured cannot be determined from arteriograms, CT scans, and clinical findings, an EEG recording may be helpful, especially in patients with bilateral middle cerebral artery aneurysms.

TREATMENT

It is most important to identify and treat by intracranial surgery the aneurysm that has ruptured, because if it is left untreated, it poses the greatest risk to the patient of another hemorrhage—which often is fatal. Asymptomatic aneurysms that can be reached through the initial exposure should be treated at the same time.

SURGERY FOR ASYMPTOMATIC ANEURYSMS

A decision about which asymptomatic aneurysms require further surgery is based on a balance of risk factors. A larger aneurysm is more likely to rupture, and a younger patient has a greater cumulative risk for such a rupture if the aneurysm is not treated surgically. Although generally low, surgical morbidity is increased if the aneurysm is very large or relatively inaccessible. Surgery for asymptomatic aneurysms should be recommended to most patients younger than 55 years of age who have surgically accessible asymptomatic aneurysms that are larger than 5 mm in greatest diameter.

NONSURGICAL MANAGEMENT

Hypertension should be treated medically. Patients with small, asymptomatic aneurysms that have not been surgically treated should be followed with repeat arteriography.

REFERENCES

1. Norlén G, Olivecrona H: The treatment of aneurysms of the circle of Willis. J Neurosurg 10:404, 1953
2. Nehls DG, Flom RA, Carter LP, et al: Multiple intracranial aneurysms: Determining the site of rupture. J Neurosurg 63:342, 1985
3. Hamby WB: Multiple intracranial aneurysms. J Neurosurg 16:558, 1959
4. Poppen JL, Fager CA: Multiple intracranial aneurysms. J Neurosurg 16:581, 1959
5. Björkesten G, Troupp H: Multiple intracranial arterial aneurysms. Acta Chir Scand 118:387, 1960
6. Moyes PD: Surgical treatment of multiple aneurysms and of incidentally discovered unruptured aneurysms. J Neurosurg 35:291, 1971
7. Sahs AL, Perret GE, Locksley HB, et al: Intracranial Aneurysms and Subarachnoid Hemorrhage. A Cooperative Study. Philadelphia, JB Lippincott, 1969, p 50 8. McCormick WF: Intracranial arterial aneurysm: A pathologist's view. Stroke 8:15, 1973
9. Andrews RJ, Spiegel PK: Intracranial aneurysms. Age, sex, blood pressure, and multiplicity in an unselected series of patients. J Neurosurg 51:27, 1979
10. Østergaard JR, Høg E: Incidence of multiple intracranial aneurysms. Influence of arterial hypertension and gender. J Neurosurg 63:49, 1985

11. Brisman R: Management of multiple and asymptomatic aneurysms, in Fein JM, Flamm ES (eds): Cerebrovascular Surgery, vol 3. New York, Springer-Verlag, 1985, pp 983–995

12. Hourihan MD, Gates PC, McAllister VL: Subarachnoid hemorrhage in childhood and adolescence. J Neurosurg 60:1163, 1984

13. McCormick WF, Schmalstieg EJ: The relationship of arterial hypertension to intracranial aneurysms. Arch Neurol 34:285, 1977

14. Modesti LM, Binet EF: Value of computed tomography in the diagnosis and management of subarachnoid hemorrhage. Neurosurgery 3:151, 1978

15. Scotti G, Ethier R, Melancon D, et al: Computed tomography in the evaluation of intracranial aneurysms and subarachnoid hemorrhage. Radiology 123:85, 1977

16. Almaani WS, Richardson AE: Multiple intracranial aneurysms: Identifying the ruptured lesion. Surg Neurol 9:303, 1978

17. Lim ST, Sage DJ: Detection of subarachnoid blood clot and other thin, flat structures by computed tomography. Radiology 123:79, 1977

18. Hayward RD, O'Reilly GVA: Intracerebral hemorrhage. Accuracy of computerized transverse axial scanning in predicting the underlying etiology. Lancet 1:1, 1976

19. Wood EH: Angiographic identification of the ruptured lesion in patients with multiple cerebral aneurysms. J Neurosurg 21:182, 1964

20. Beatty RA, Richardson AE: The value of electroencephalography in the management of multiple intracranial aneurysms. J Neurosurg 80:150, 1969

21. McCormick WF, Acosta-Rua GJ: The size of intracranial saccular aneurysms. An autopsy study. J Neurosurg 88:422, 1970

22. Kendall BE, Lee BCP, Claveria E: Computerized tomography and angiography in subarachnoid haemorrhage. Br J Radiol 49:488, 1976

23. McKissock W, Richardson A, Walsh L, et al: Multiple intracranial aneurysms. Lancet 1:628, 1964

24. Paterson A, Bond MR: Treatment of multiple intracranial arterial aneurysms. Lancet 1:1802, 1978

25. Drake CG, Girvin, JP: The surgical treatment of subarachnoid hemorrhage with multiple aneurysms, in Morley TP (ed): Current Controversies in Neurosurgery. Philadelphia, WB Saunders, 1976, pp 274–278

26. Mount LA, Brisman R: Treatment of multiple intracranial aneurysms. J Neurosurg 85:728, 1971

27. Mount LA, Brisman R: Treatment of multiple aneurysms—symptomatic and asymptomatic. Clinical Neurosurgery, vol 21. Baltimore, Williams & Wilkins, 1974, pp 166–170

28. Pool JL, Potts DG: Aneurysms and Arteriovenous Anomalies of the Brain. Diagnosis and Treatment. New York, Harper and Row, 1965, p 287

29. Samson DS, Hodosh RM, Clark WK: Surgical management of unruptured asymptomatic aneurysms. J Neurosurg 46:781, 1977

30. Pouyanne H, Banayan A, Guerin J, et al: Les anévrysmes sacculaires multiples du système carotidien supra clinoidien. Étude anatomoclinique et thérapeutique. Neurochirurgie 19(suppl 1), 1978

31. Pouyanne H, Riemens V, Guerin J, et al: Les anévrysmes sacculaires multiples du système carotidien. Indications et résultats de l'abord direct. Neurochirurgie 16:25, 1970

32. Heiskanen O, Marttila I: Risk of rupture of a second aneurysm in patients with multiple aneurysms. J Neurosurg 82:295, 1970

33. Heiskanen O: Risk of bleeding from unruptured aneurysms in cases with multiple intracranial aneurysms. J Neurosurg 55:524, 1981

34. Shephard RH: Ruptured cerebral aneurysms: Early and late prognosis with surgical treatment. A personal series, 1958–1980. J Neurosurg 59:6, 1988

35. Zacks DJ, Russell DB, Miller JDR: Fortuitously discovered intracranial aneurysms. Arch Neurol 87:89, 1980 36. DuBoulay GH: Some observations on the natural history of intracranial aneurysms. Br J Radiol 38:721, 1965

37. Dell S: Asymptomatic cerebral aneurysm: Assessment of its risk of rupture. Neurosurgery 10:162, 1982

38. Winn HR, Almaani WS, Berga SL, et al: The long-term outcome in patients with multiple aneurysms. Incidence of late hemorrhage and implications for treatment of incidental aneurysms. J Neurosurg 59:642, 1988

39. Wiebers DO, Whisnant JP, O'Fallon WM: The natural history of unruptured intracranial aneurysms. N Engl J Med 804:696, 1981

40. Wiebers DO, Whisnant JP: Natural history of intracranial aneurysms. Correspondence. N Engl J Med 305:99, 1981

41. Ferguson GG, Peerless SJ, Drake CG: Natural history of intracranial aneurysms. Correspondence. N Engl J Med 305:99, 1981

42. Wirth FP, Laws ER Jr, Piepgras D, et al: Surgical treatment of incidental intracranial aneurysms. Neurosurgery 12:507, 1988

43. Salazar JL: Surgical treatment of asymptomatic and incidental intracranial aneurysms. J Neurosurg 58:20, 1980 44. Jefferson A: The significance for diagnosis and for surgical technique of multiple aneurysms of the same internal carotid artery. Acta Neurochir 41:23, 1978

45. Slosberg PS: Nonoperative management of ruptured intracranial aneurysms. Clin Neurosurg 21:90, 1974

46. Post KD, Flamm ES, Goodgold A, et al: Ruptured intracranial aneurysms. Case morbidity and mortality. J Neurosurg 46:290, 1977

Stereotactic Clipping of Arterial Aneurysms and Arteriovenous Malformations of the Brain

Edward I. Kandel　　　　　　Vyacheslav V. Peresedov

GREAT ADVANCES in the surgery of cerebral arterial aneurysms and arteriovenous malformations (AVMs) have been achieved during the past two decades as a result of the development of microsurgical techniques and modern anesthesiologic methods. In spite of that remarkable progress, however, many problems remain unsolved. In the case of arterial aneurysms, a direct attack very often is technically difficult because of the possibility of serious complications and mortality from rupture or arterial spasm. The risk to the patient increases greatly in acute stages of subarachnoid hemorrhage (SAH), in the presence of arterial spasm, or in cases of cerebral infarction, which may be aggravated by the surgery.

Total extirpation of AVMs is a most adequate method of their management. Only a radical operation can relieve a patient from the continuous threat to life from subarachnoid-parenchymatous hemorrhages and epileptic seizures. In the past 15 years microsurgical technique has significantly increased the possibilities for radical removal of AVMs and had improved the results of surgical treatment. At the same time there are many unsolved problems in the surgery of AVMs.

We have summarized the large series of AVMs reported in the literature. These data indicate that only one half of the hemispheric malformations were totally extirpated. In the other half of the cases radical extirpation was impossible because of the giant size of the AVMs or its location in the deep or functionally import regions of the brain.

One half of patients harboring AVMs are doomed to gradual deterioration as a consequence of epileptic fits and increasing neurologic deficit. The patients live under the constant threat of intracranial hemorrhage, which may end fatally. When a direct attack is too dangerous or impossible, the problem of palliative surgical treatment arises.

Palliative operations for AVMs which cannot be totally removed have been performed for several decades. The main operation is a ligation or clipping of the arteries supplying the AVM. In the 1950s some neurosurgeons expressed the opinion that the operation is not effective. Indeed, in many cases after the exclusion of arteries, an increase in the diameter of other small vessels feeding the malformation was noted. In the last decade the experience with artificial embolization of AVMs has shown that exclusion of afferent vessels allows one to diminish substantially the volume of blood supply, and consequently, the

AVM volume. This has resulted in decreasing the seizure rate and risk of intracranial bleeding. Many neurosurgeons now recommend performance of open clipping of afferent arteries in inoperable AVMs of the basal ganglia, brain stem, and posterior fossa.

Our contribution in dealing with this problem consists of using stereotactic techniques to obliterate vessels feeding AVMs and cerebral aneurysms. The first attempts at applying the stereotactic method for the visual clipping of the feeding vessels of deep-seated and poorly accessible AVMs were made about 25 years ago.[1,2] Following the performance of a standard flap craniotomy, a stereotactic device was applied to the skull and a thin probe was introduced toward the AVM. After the probe touched its nidus, a routine approach to the lesion was performed using the probe as a guide. The clipping of vessels and the removal of the AVM was made ad oculus. Four cases with deep AVMs successfully removed in this way were reported.[2] The stereotactic method was used exclusively to locate the aneurysm, while all subsequent manipulations including clipping of the arteries were carried out under the direct visual control using ordinary clip holders.

Almost two decades ago the technique of magnetic thrombosis of the arterial aneurysms was developed. Alksne and Rand[3] using a stereotactic method introduced a magnetic cannula 6 mm in diameter at the dome of the arterial aneurysm. After the wall was punctured with a fine needle, an iron suspension was injected into the aneurysm with the objective of producing intra-aneurysmal thrombosis. The results of stereotactic occlusion of anterior communicating artery aneurysms by means of an iron-acrylic mixture introduced into the carotid was reported.[4] Complete thrombosis of aneurysms was shown in 17 of 22 patients.

Mullan[5] produced stereotactic intra-aneurysmal thrombosis by inserting several fine needles into the aneurysmal sac, after which direct electric current was applied. The results were generally considered to be satisfactory. However, the series included four postoperative deaths directly attributed to the procedure while in 8 cases the aneurysm showed incomplete obliteration.

Four patients with anterior communicating-anterior cerebral arterial aneurysms were operated by Samotokin and Hilki,[6] who introduced electrodes stereotatically into aneurysms and

OPERATIVE NEUROSURGICAL TECHNIQUES
ISBN 0-8089-1862-1

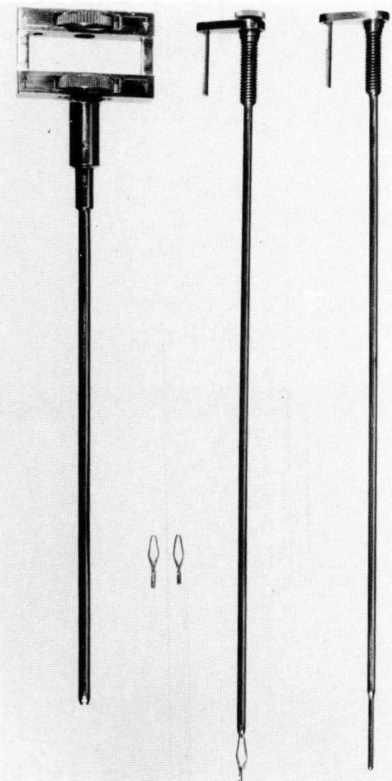

Fig. 90-1. The clipping device shown unassembled. (Right) The tube with a special structure at the outer end for controlling clip movements. (Center) Second (working) pivot with attached closed clip fixed in the grip on the pivot tip and two clips of different size separately. (Left) First (guide) pivot with thin terminal segment.

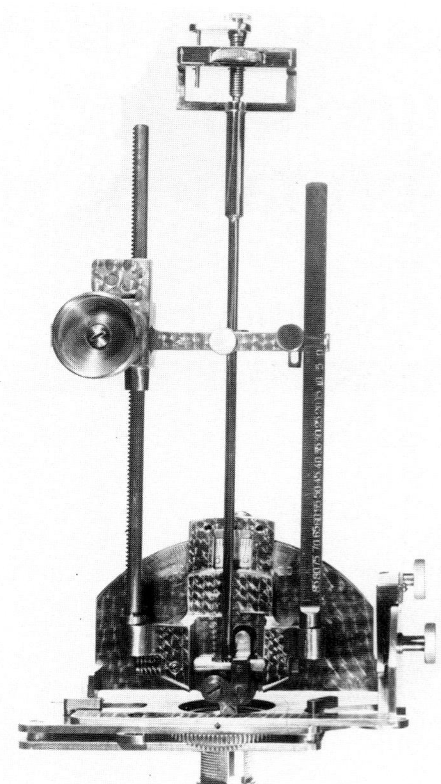

Fig. 90-2. The device for stereotactic clipping combined with the stereotactic apparatus.

followed this by anodal electrolysis for 1 to 3 hours. In all cases aneurysm volume was reduced by 30 to 40 percent, but complete thrombosis was not achieved. One case of successful stereotactic thrombosis of an anterior communicating arterial aneurysm and another case of stereotactic electrocoagulation of a single vessel feeding a small AVM of an 8-year-old child have also been reported.[7,8]

In spite of these reports the stereotactic management of arterial aneurysms and AVMs is a seldom used technique and was not put into common neurosurgical practice. The situation prompted us to propose a new approach to the problem and to develop "pure" stereotactic clipping of any vessel or aneurysmal neck without performance of a craniotomy but rather through an ordinary burr hole. It was our hope that this method would allow the surgery of arterial aneurysms and AVMs to be performed more safely.

STEREOTACTIC CLIPPING

We began to develop the method of stereotactic clipping of arterial aneurysms and AVMs in 1971; we used the technique in clinical practice for the first time in 1973. The technique has many a priori advantages. The stereotactic method allows one to reach the target in deep parts of the brain with minimal trauma to the cerebral tissue and without retraction-related complications such as brain edema. This technique also eliminates the necessity of manipulating the vessels of the circle of Willis, thereby probably reducing the risk of vasospasm. There is no need to release the aneurysm from adhesions, which frequently leads to aneurysmal rupture.

The development of the new technique has prompted the creation of a device that permits access of the clip to the vessel or the aneurysmal neck with the help of stereotactic technique. The method was used clinically only after extensive testing of the technical equipment and many animal experiments. The equipment consists of a stereotactic apparatus[13] and a special device that allows placement of a clip at the aneurysmal neck or vessel stereotactically through a burr hole, opening of the clip very close to the vessel, then closing it around the neck. One must be able in case of complications or incorrect placement to remove the clip and put in on another part of the vessel, controlling the degree of compression during the procedure. Moreover, all clip movements inside the brain must be controlled by the extracerebral part of the device (patented in the USSR, United States, West Germany, England, Canada, France, and Japan). This consists of several parts (Figure 90-1). The main part is a stainless steel thin-walled tube 17 cm long with an outer diameter of 3.2 mm. Inside the tip of the tube there is a conical narrowing, which opens the clip. At the outer end of the tube there are a rectangular shackle graduated in millimeters and two nuts. These control the opening and closing of the clip and disconnecting it from the device after it has been applied to the vessel or aneurysm. The tube of the device is adapted to our stereotactic apparatus (Figure 90-2).

There are also two interchangeable metal units, which I call pivots, that are inserted consecutively into the tube. Their diameters fit exactly into the tube's inner diameter. The first, a (guide) stylet, has a short, thin terminal segment that protrudes from the end of the tube for several millimeters. The length of the segment is equal to the distance from the end of the tube to

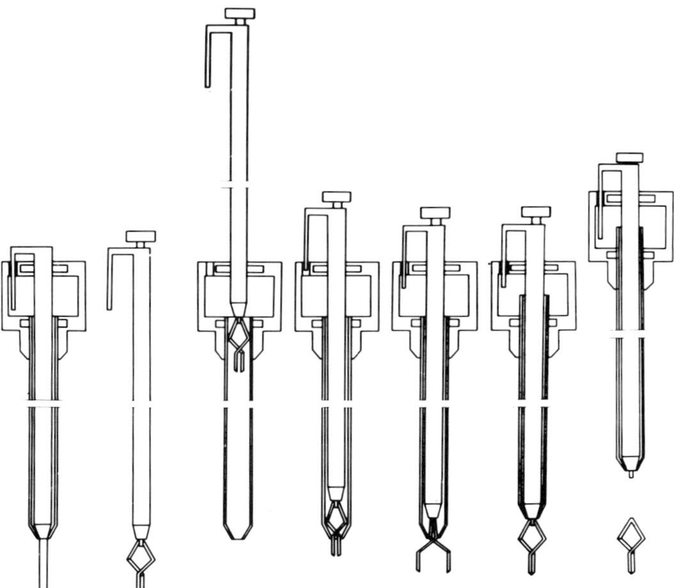

Fig. 90-3. Schematic representation of the principle of the action of the clipping device (see text).

the ends of the clip blades when they are opened to their fullest extent. This stylet or "guide pivot" is installed in the tube, which is introduced stereotactically toward the target point. Once the target has been reached, the guide stylet is removed, and a second unit with a special clip fixed on its tip is inserted into the tube. The outer end of the second unit has a scale graduated in millimeters that corresponds to the distance between the clip blades as they open inside the brain. The principle of action of the device, consecutive introduction of both units (pivots) and phases of clip opening and squeezing are shown schematically in Figure 90-3.

Special removable stainless-steel clips have been constructed for use with this device. The length of the clips ranges from 10 to 17 mm, and their weight from 80 to 140 mg. They are of crossing-spring type with parallel blades and can be used to clip vessels from 1 to 7 mm in diameter. It is important to note that the blades of a clip loaded into the 3-mm tube may be opened to a distance of about 8 mm without loss of spring property. The clips are made of biologically inert, highly elastic and anticorrosive steel consisting of 18 percent chromium, 9 percent nickel, and 9.5 percent titanium.

Our clips are flat springs with a squeezing force (40–45 g/mm^2) that is constant because it depends on the clip spring features and does not depend on the surgeon's hand force. The parallel blades of the clip and the clip length prevent its slipping.

Reliable clipping demands that the clip blades totally close the vessel lumen. Our experience has shown that to accomplish this the clip blades have to exceed the margins of the vessel for about 1 mm.

The clips are constructed so that after closing only the blade tips are in contact; there is a tiny space between both blades. Based on the angiographic studies the surgeon chooses a suitable clip before the operation depending on the diameter of the artery or size of the aneurysmal neck to be clipped. The clip is attached to the tip of the second or "working" pivot before it is inserted into the tube. The loop of the clip is fixed in the grip of the working pivot. As the clip passes through the conical narrowing at the end of the tube, the shoulders of the loop are squeezed and the blades are open as they emerge from the tube. When the clip loop moves past the narrow portion of the tube, the blades of the clip are closed by the spring action of the loop. To release the clip, one has to press the button on the control structure. After that the grip is opened and the clip is released. The consecutive stages of stereotactic clipping are presented schematically in Figure 90-4.

The construction of the device enables removal of the clip after its application to the vessel. Rotation of the button on the control structure once again fixes the clip in the grip, and by returning the clip loop into the tube, the clip blades are opened, and can again be put into the tube.

PREOPERATIVE CALCULATIONS

After the diagnosis of aneurysm or AVM is established, preoperative calculations are made based on angiograms in both projections. The aim of the calculations is (1) to select the point of clipping (target point) of the feeding artery (or arteries) or the aneurysmal neck; (2) to determine the position of the burr hole; and (3) to determine the plane of approach for the open clip.

The target point must be chosen in accordance with several factors. In aneurysms, the target point is the middle of the neck, which has to be relatively long and narrow. The diameter of the neck at the target point is carefully measured so the degree of clip opening can be determined. Sometimes it is difficult to determine the target point because the neck is poorly visible in one or both projections. In such cases oblique angiograms are helpful.

In the case of AVMs the selection of the target point is more difficult. We have experience with clipping anterior and middle cerebral arteries and their branches. The target in AVMs can be at any point along the feeding artery (arteries). As a rule, however, a point is selected beyond the last normal distal branch of the artery close to the nidus of the lesion. This target

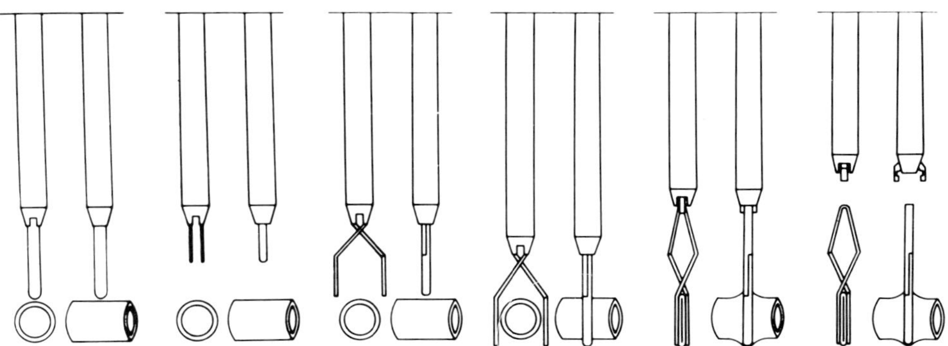

Fig. 90-4. Consecutive stages of the clipping of a vessel by the device (see text).

is probably safer and more effective because the proximal branches supplying the normal brain tissue remain patent. In many instances, clipping a feeder close the the AVM may be dangerous because of the possibility of damaging angiomatous tissue or large draining veins, and we therefore prefer to clip the arteries 4 to 6 cm and in rare cases even 8 cm from the nidus. Our experience has shown that clipping the hypertrophic feeding vessel quite proximal to the AVM yields good results without producing a new neurologic deficit, probably because these arteries supply only the AVM and not normal brain tissue.

Before each operation, the trajectory of the device through different subcortical structures is analyzed with the aid of the Schaltenbrand and Bailey stereotactic atlas. The aim of the analysis is to avoid damage to functionally important cerebral structures. It is necessary to know in which brain structures the clip blades will be opened near the aneurysmal neck or vessel.

The determination of an adequate clip opening is an important element of preoperative calculations. Dense adhesions, tend to develop around the aneurysmal sac and neck after SAH and firmly join the aneurysm and surrounding brain tissue and vessels. Disturbing these adhesions may cause the aneurysm to rupture. In our series of cases there were no such complications but for safety it is necessary to choose the correct size of the clip. The clip's open blades must not touch the aneurysmal sac and there should be some space between the blades and the sac (about 0.5 to 0.7 mm). Moreover, excessively opening the blades may disturb nearby vessels. For instance, if the aneurysmal neck has an outer diameter of 3 mm, the opening of the clip should be 4.5 mm. We measure the inner diameter of the neck or vessel on angiograms using a magnifying glass graduated with 0.1 mm marks. After correction of the x-ray divergence we get the real inner diameter. Assuming that the neck wall has a thickness of about 0.5 mm, we add 1 mm to the figure of the inner diameter.

After the target point is chosen, two decisions have to be made: determination of the burr hole location and the plane of clip opening. To achieve this we transfer the target point and vessel axis to the drafting board and make the geometric calculations. The task of the calculation is to determine the mutual location of such geometric elements as the axis of the artery or aneurysmal neck which should be clipped, the plane of clip opening, and the axis of the clipping device.

The location of the plane of clipping (or the plane of opening of the clip blades) is very important because the plane and axis of the vessel have to be nearly perpendicular. This position creates the optimal condition for clipping and practically excludes slipping of the clip.

In choosing the site of the burr hole, which determines the location of the line of approach, one has to pay attention the (1) portion of the brain through which the tube will pass does not involve functionally important areas; (2) the best angle of approach is 90 degrees, but it must not be less than 45 degrees. If it is less than that critical value, the clip may slip. In that case it is necessary to change the location of the burr hole; (3) the angle of inclination depends upon the construction of the stereotactic apparatus (in the case of our apparatus the angle must not be more than 20 degrees).

OPERATIVE TECHNIQUE

The operation is carried out with the patient under general anesthesia or neuroleptanalgesia with routine premedication. The patient's head is placed in the supine position of the stereotatic head-holder and fixed rigidly with two sharp pins.

A sagittal line, the point of its crossing with the coronal suture, the preselected center of the burr hole and the plane of clip opening are drawn on the patient's skull. A catheter is inserted percutaneously into the ipsilateral extracranial carotid artery for intraoperative angiography.

A skin incision 4 to 5 cm long is preferably near the coronal suture. A 25-mm opening is made with a trephine and the dura incised. Our stereotactic apparatus with the clipping device attached is then fixed in the burr hole. The guide stylet or pivot is inserted into the device. Anteroposterior and lateral plain films are taken, and the preselected target point is transferred from the peroperative angiograms to the films. Ordinary stereotactic calculations are made for the correct orientation of the clipping device. The calculations have to be made carefully because the effectiveness of the clipping depends on the accuracy with which the target point can be reached. Two angles of correction in both projections are calculated and then are transferred to the protractors of the stereotactic apparatus.

Under the control of an image intensifier with a television monitor, the tube is introduced into the brain in the correct direction to the depth at which the tip of the guide pivot touches the target point. The guide pivot is replaced by the working pivot, which carries a clip of the appropriate size.

A control angiogram is performed. The target point on the preoperative angiograms is then transferred to the newly obtained angiograms. If the tip of the tube is at the correct point, the clipping device is oriented in the required plane for clip opening, as calculated before the operation. By turning a ring on the shackle on the outer end of the device, the clip is pushed out of the tube and is opened in the immediate vicinity of the aneurysmal neck or its artery of origin. The distance between the clip blades in millimeters is checked on the scale. After the blades are opened to the required extent under TV control, another angiogram is performed. If this shows the clip to be in the correct position it is carefully and slowly introduced a little deeper and applied to the vessel or aneurysmal neck. Coincident with these maneuvers the blood pressure is lowered to 50 to 60 mg Hg by intravenous administration of Arfonad. Further turning of the ring pushes the clip past the tapered end of the tube and it closes. The next angiogram should verify effective clipping of the aneurysm.

Immediately after this procedure the patient is awakened so that function of the contralateral extremities and speech can be assessed. If these functions are satisfactory, neuroleptanalgesia is repeated and the blood pressure is increased gradually. The clip is released from the pivot by pushing a button on the outer end of the device. Under television control, the tube is withdrawn from the brain.

The stereotactic apparatus is released and removed. The bone plug is replaced and the wound is closed. This operation requires an average of 1.5 to 2 hours. If it is necessary to clip two or more vessels, the entire procedure can be repeated as required.

INDICATIONS AND CONTRAINDICATIONS
TO STEREOTACTIC CLIPPING

The possibilities of stereotactic clipping have not yet been fully investigated because the indications and timing of stereotactic clipping of arterial aneurysms and AVMs have not been completely established. The indications for this alternative treatment depend in each particular case on the evaluation of numerous factors: the location and size of the aneurysm, the size of the neck, the patient's condition, the presence of arterial vasospasm, and the time interval since the onset of the subarachnoid hemorrhage.

In general, this technique is advisable in carefully selected cases of arterial aneurysms and in cases of giant or deep-seated AVMs when direct attack may be dangerous or technically impossible. As a rule, the stereotactic clipping of the AVMs is palliative, but in cases of small AVMs fed by a single artery this technique may be a method of radical treatment.

Below we shall present the main factors in connection with indications for stereotactic clipping.

In arteral aneurysms:

1. Supraclinoid aneurysms, aneurysms of internal carotid bifurcation and the anterior cerebral artery.
2. Clipping of dominant anterior cerebral artery (A1) in anterior communicating aneurysms and also the trunk of the anterior cerebral artery in aneurysms of this artery. The possibility of the stereotactic clipping of arterial aneurysms of other locations has not been established.

Our experience has shown the stereotactic clipping did not cause arterial spasm and also did not increase it, if it was present before the operation. This confirms the possibility of clipping arterial aneurysms stereotactically even in the presence of marked arterial spasm and the critical condition of the patient. This conclusion has to be judged as preliminary because further experiences must be gained.

The absence of a neck, and also giant aneurysms, are contraindications to the method.

In AVMs:

1. AVMs of any size supplied by anterior and middle carebral arteries and its branches. The clipping of the posterior cerebral artery supplying AVMs and aneurysms of vertebrobasilar system is apparently impossible.
2. AVMs supplied by one or several hypertrophied branches of the abovementioned arteries. In so-called ''scattered'' type of blood supply by many small feeding arteries the use of the method is not indicated.

CLINICAL RESULTS

To date we have performed 59 stereotactic clipping operations on 56 patients: 24 operations for arterial aneurysms and 34 operations for AVMs.

ARTERIAL ANEURYSMS

Twenty-three patients with arterial aneurysms (10 men and 14 women) aged from 22 to 53 years were operated upon by this technique. Before the operation 9 patients had one, and 15 had two or more subarachnoid hemorrhages. Supraclinoid aneurysms were disclosed in 16 cases (9 on the right and 7 on the left side); aneurysms of the anterior communicating artery in 6; aneurysm of the internal carotid bifurcation in 1; and aneurysm of the anterior cerebral artery at the origin of frontopolar artery in 1. The volume of the aneurysms varied from 250 to 900 mm^3.

The patients were operated on at different times after SAH ranging from 3 days to 11 months. The condition of the patients before the operation varied from good without any complaints (15 patients) to deep stupor (5). Twelve of 24 patients had no neurologic symptoms. In the remaining 12 patients there were marked meningeal signs, third nerve palsy, local pain in the

fronto-orbital region, hemiparesis or hemiplegia, disturbances of sensation, or pupil edema.

In the majority of cases (14 of 24) vasospasm involving neighboring arteries was seen on the angiograms. In 7 cases, including 5 patients in grave condition, a severe diffuse arterial spasm narrowing the vessels more than 50 percent of their normal diameter occurred. In other cases, the spasm was mild and involved mainly the supraclinoid internal carotid artery.

Sixteen supraclinoid aneurysms, which are the most common of all intracranial aneurysms, were of different size. Their neck and sac were directed mainly posteriorly, ventrally, and laterally. The diameter of the neck varied from 2.2 to 3.5 mm. The narrow neck of the majority of supraclinoid aneurysms makes them particularly suitable for stereotactic clipping. All supraclinoid aneurysms were successfully clipped.

Below are two illustrative cases.

Case 1. A 49-year-old woman was admitted to our clinic following two severe subarachnoid hemorrhages 17 months and 1 month previously. Her general condition was satisfactory, but she had paralysis of the left third nerve, mild right hemiparesis, and a mild sensorimotor aphasia. Angiograms demonstrated a bilobed supraclinoid saccular aneurysm, 14 × 7 mm in size on the lateral projection, arising from the left internal carotid (Figure 90-5A, B). The neck of the aneurysm was narrow. There was a mild spasm of the left carotid artery. Stereotactic clipping of the aneurysmal neck was carried out under general anesthesia. The stereotactic apparatus with the clipping device was installed in a burr hole, and a catheter was percutaneously introduced into the left common carotid. The target point (aneurysmal neck) was transferred from angiograms to the plain films and stereotactic calculations were made. The second pivot with a compressed clip in the tip reached the target 76 mm from the cortex. The clip was placed on the aneurysmal neck, and its correct positioning was confirmed angiographically.

The patient was awakened for several minutes to allow testing of the strength of movement in the contralateral limbs and no changes were noted. The angiograms showed that the aneurysm neck had been clipped and that there was no filling of the aneurysm. The operation lasted 1 hour and 40 minutes. There were no postoperative complications and no neurologic changes. The patient was ambulated 3 days after surgery and her aphasia and third nerve paralysis disappeared completely soon after the operation.

Angiograms performed 2 weeks after surgery demonstrated that the aneurysm was no longer present (Figure 90-5C). Eight years later the patient's condition is neurologically intact and she is working full-time.

Case 2. A 38-year-old woman suddenly experienced severe headaches and vomiting with a disturbance of consciousness followed 2 weeks later by sharp left orbitofrontal headaches and a total left third nerve palsy. An aneurysm on the internal carotid at its junction with the posterior communicating artery was demonstrated angiographically. The size of the aneurysm in the lateral projection was 11 × 7 mm. Stereotactic clipping of the neck of the aneurysm, which was located at a depth of 77 mm from the cortex, was performed (Figure 90-6A).

The patient's postoperative course was uneventful. The patient was up and walking 4 days after operation. A repeat angiogram disclosed that the aneurysm had been successfully clipped (Figure 90-6B). Mild spasm of the middle cerebral

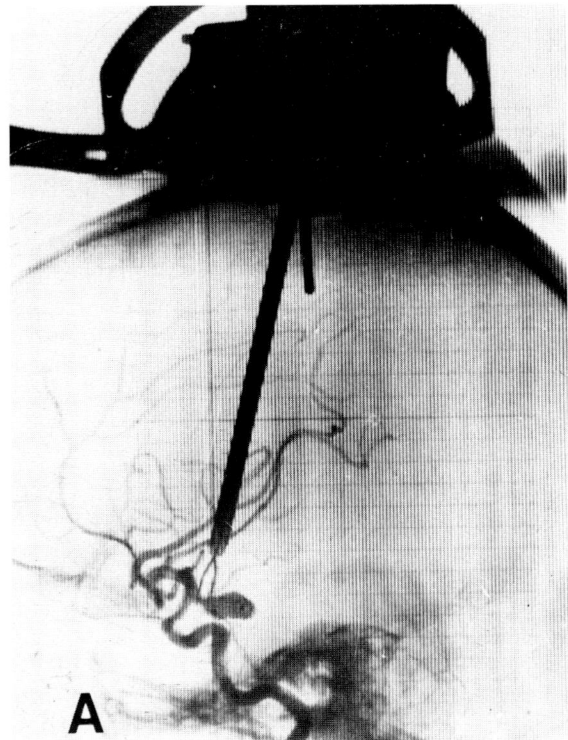

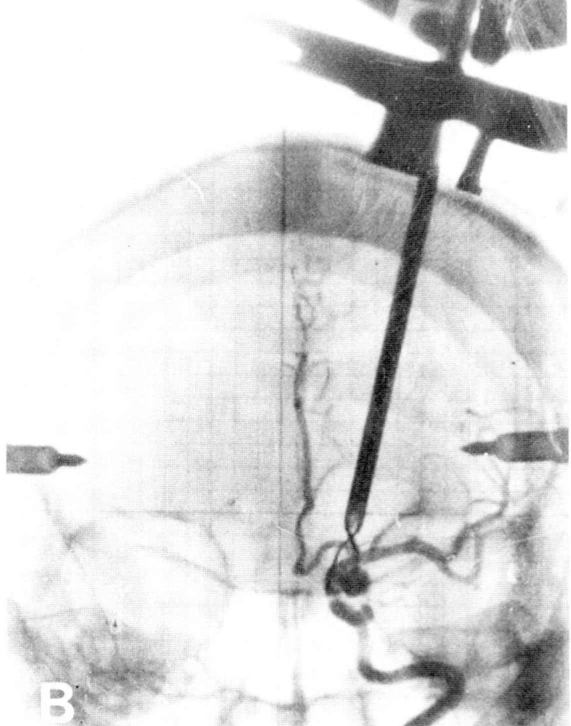

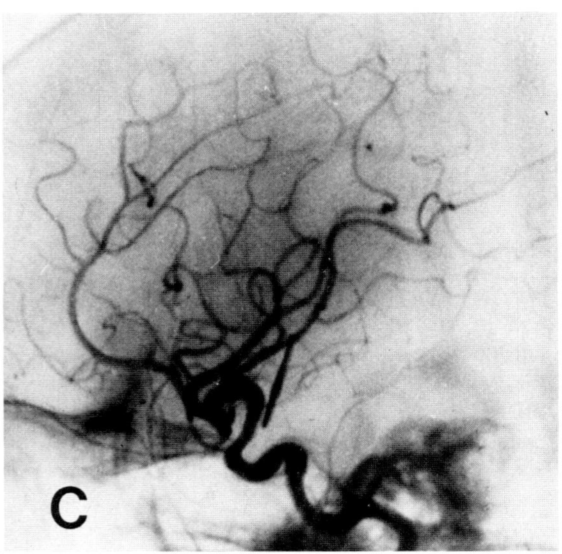

Fig. 90-5. Angiograms showing the supraclinoid internal carotid aneurysm during stereotactic clipping (A, B) and 2 weeks after operation (C).

artery disappeared. In the 4 years since surgery the third nerve function has recovered completely. No further rebleeding has occurred. The patient works on a part-time basis.

Aneurysms of the internal carotid bifurcation are an important surgical problem. The approach and direct attack on these aneurysms are associated with many technical difficulties. The following example illustrates the possibility of successful stereotactic clipping of such an aneurysm.

Case 3. A 48-year-old man suddenly developed severe headaches without impairment of consciousness. About 1 month later the headaches and pain in the right eye recurred followed 5 days later by left-sided hemiplegia. On admission to our clinic the patient was in bad general condition with a

hemiplegia, decreased muscular tone, and pathologic reflexes. Angiography disclosed a saccular aneurysm at the internal carotid artery bifurcation and marked spasm of the internal carotid and its main branches (Figure 90-7A). The neck of the aneurysm was 2.5 mm in diameter. Stereotactic clipping of the aneurysm was performed (Figure 90-7B) at a target depth 77 mm from the cortical surface.

There were no complications after the operation. Movements on left extremities gradually returned. The patient began to walk 3 weeks after the operation. A follow-up examination 2 years later showed light hemiparesis and good general condition.

In spite of remarkable improvements in the results of a direct attack on aneurysms of the anterior communicating

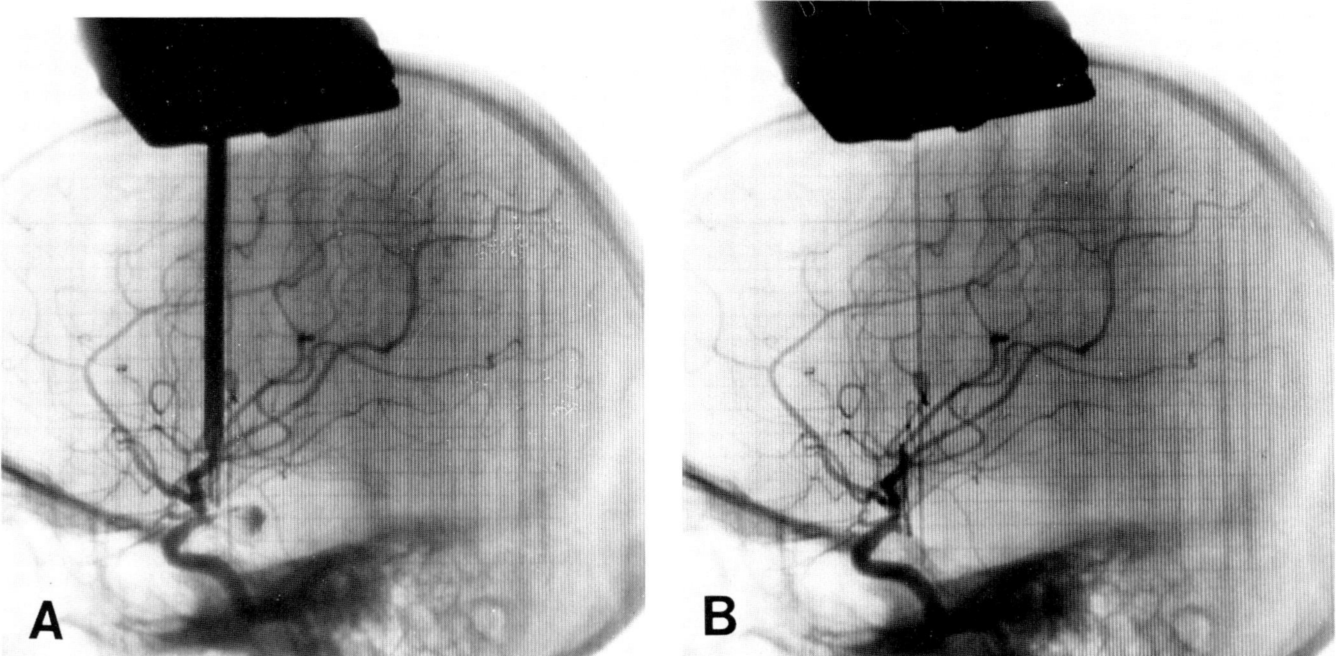

Fig. 90-6. Stereotactic operation on a supraclinoid aneurysm. Before (A) and after (B) stereotactic clipping.

artery by the microsurgical approach, the technical difficulties and rate of complications remain serious problems. However, because of special anatomic conditions of the region, the stereotactic clipping of the neck of such aneurysms is currently impossible, although in the future it may be done in exceptionally rare cases.

Several neurosurgeons have proposed the open clipping of the dominant anterior cerebral artery in the treatment of anterior communicating aneurysms. This operation may be done by the stereotactic method. In those cases in which the anterior communicating aneurysm is filled from a single (dominant) anterior cerebral artery, the clipping of the A1 segment of this artery may lead to a sharp decrease of pressure in the aneurysm and its thrombosis.

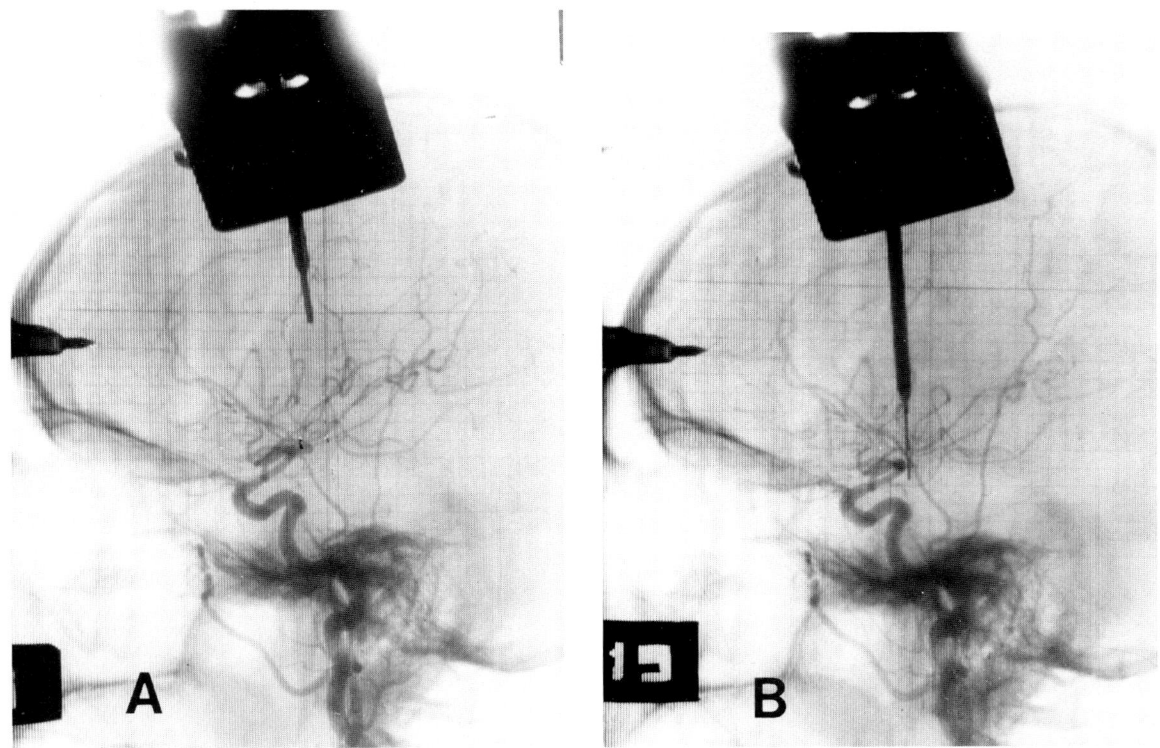

Fig. 90-7. Aneurysm of the internal carotid bifurcation before (A) and after (B) stereotactic clipping.

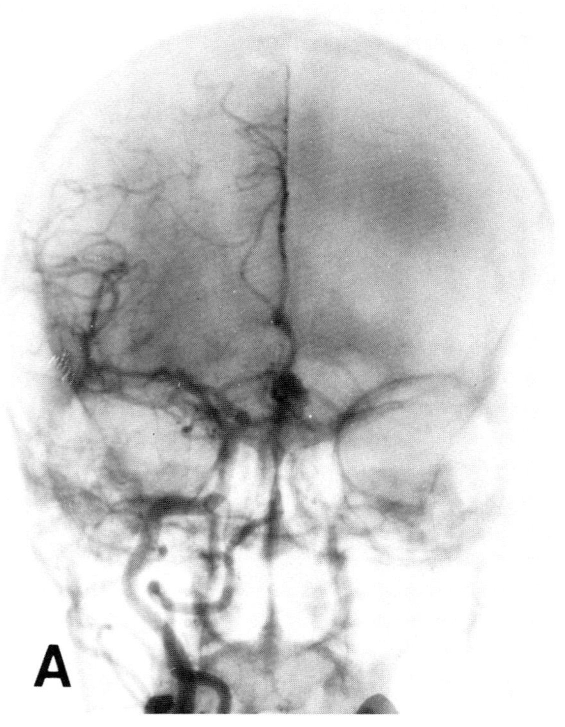

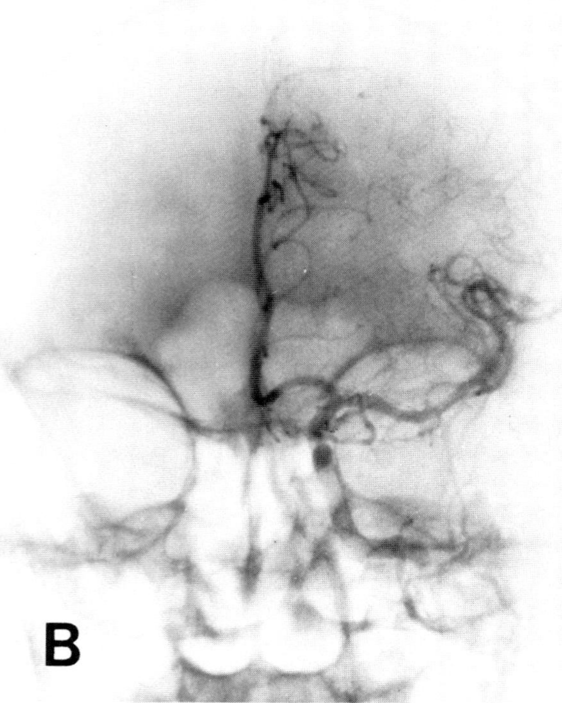

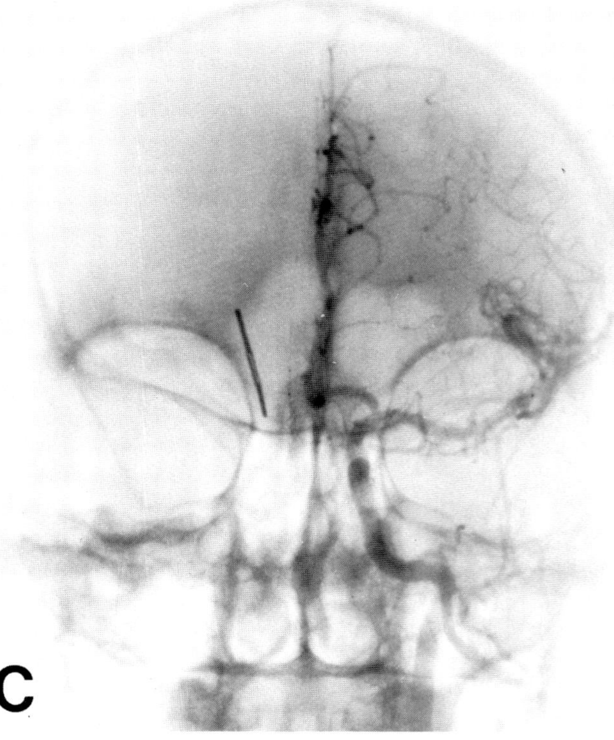

Fig. 90-8. (A) Right-sided carotid angiogram showing an anterior communicating artery aneurysm before operation; (B) left-sided carotid angiogram; the aneurysm is not filling; (C) left-sided carotid angirograms after operation showing filling of both anterior cerebral arteries without filling of the aneurysm.

The reports in the literature show that open clipping of the dominant anterior cerebral artery is an effective method of management of anterior communicating aneurysms, especially when the clipping of their neck is technically impossible; however, the postoperative mortality is reported to be 12 to 15 percent.

We have performed stereotactic clipping of the dominant anterior cerebral artery in 6 cases of anterior communicating aneurysms. One patient required a second operation. Below we present an illustrative case.

Case 4. A 50-year-old woman began to suffer from sudden headaches and repeated vomiting, and on one occasion she

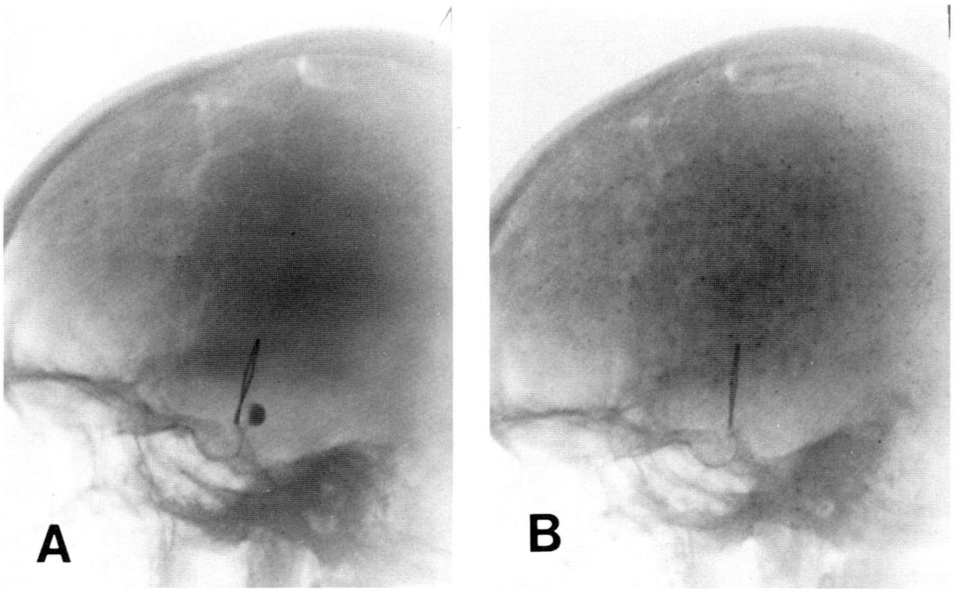

Fig. 90-9. X-ray films obtained 2 hours after stereotactic clipping of the supraclinoid aneurysm (A) and 4 hours after clipping (B).

lost consciousness for 3 hours. Initially, she showed signs of meningeal irritation and also slight pyramidal signs on the right side and hemorrhagic spinal fluid. After admission to our clinic 3 weeks later, she complained of a headache, but her general condition was good.

Right-sided angiography disclosed a large saccular aneurysm of the anterior communicating artery (Figure 90-8A). Left carotid angiography showed no filling of the aneurysm (Figure 90-8B). The aneurysmal neck was not clearly visible. Since stereotactic clipping of the neck seemed technically impossible, clipping of the dominant right anterior cerebral artery was performed. A subsequent left carotid angiogram showed that the right anterior cerebral artery was clipped and the aneurysm no longer filled (Figure 90-8C). A follow-up examination 6 years later found the patient to be in excellent health, asymptomatic, and working full-time.

Our limited experience has shown that stereotactic clipping of the dominant A1 is technically feasible. Repeat angiography in our 5 cases (in one case it was not done for technical reasons) has shown that in 4 cases the aneurysms were no longer filled, and in one case, it filled from the other side although it had not do so before surgery.

Stereotactic clipping was performed in one case of a peripherally situated aneurysm of the frontopolar artery. The clipping of the A2 segment of the anterior cerebral artery successfully excluded this aneurysm from the circulation.

Three of 24 patients (13 percent) died after stereotactic clipping of their arterial aneurysms. Two patients with supraclinoid aneurysms were operated on in grave condition and expired on the 4th and 5th days after surgery from pulmonary thromboembolism. The third patient died on the third postoperative day after successful clipping of the supraclinoid aneurysm from an unexpected rupture of a second lesion, an AVM in the same hemisphere; this AVM was not visible on the preoperative angiograms.

Angiographic studies were performed in all cases during the operation, about 1 month after surgery, and (in 16 cases) from 1 to 6 years later. It is interesting to note that the contrast medium remains in the aneurysmal sac immediately after clipping and is sometimes visible on the plain films (Figure 90-9). Postoperative angiography has shown that all clipped aneurysms were excluded from circulation. Long-term follow-up in 19 patients (two cases were lost to follow-up) from 6 months to 10 years confirmed the absence of repeated subarachnoid hemorrhages in all cases.

Stereotactic clipping of arterial aneurysms does not increase the arterial spasm if it existed preoperatively, and does not cause it if it was absent before surgery. There was no rupture of the aneurysms during or after surgery and brain edema did not develop. It should be emphasized that stereotactic clipping is a low stress operation which the patients endure easily so that the majority of patients were ambulatory 2 to 3 days after surgery.

ARTERIOVENOUS MALFORMATIONS

We have performed 34 stereotactic operations in 32 patients with AVMs: 91 men and 13 women aged from 13 to 52 years. The period of time from the onset of the illness to the operation varied greatly, from several months to 30 years. Intracranial hemorrhage was the main clinical sign in 18 patients, seizures in 9, and severe headache in 5.

Fifteen patients were admitted in good general condition, 14 were in fair condition, and 3 patients were in bad condition. Hemiparesis of varying severity, meningeal signs, motor aphasia, and memory disturbances were present in some of the cases. Neurologic deficit was, as a rule, the consequence of previous subarachnoid-parenchymatous hemorrhages.

The first angiogram was performed on the side of the supposed AVM. If the lesion was disclosed, an angiogram of the other side was made to check the participation of contralateral arteries in AVMs blood supply.

The volume of the AVMs varied widely, from 8.4 to 198 cm^3. The AVMs were of small and middle size (up to 20 cm^3) in 7 cases, large (up to 100 cm^3) in 17, and gigantic (more than 100

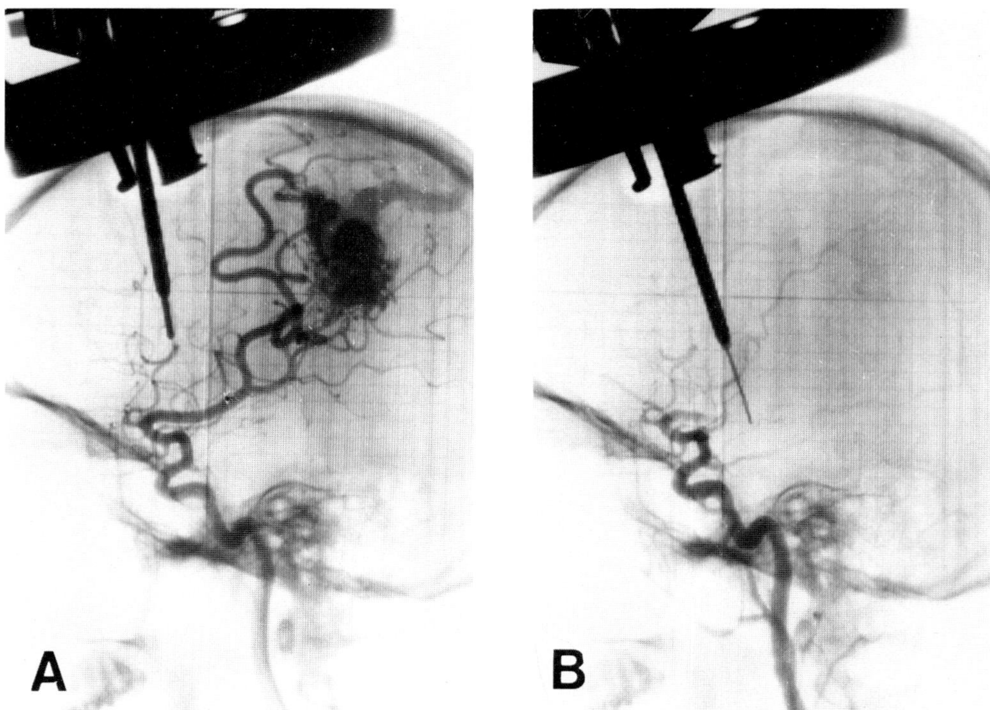

Fig. 90-10. Angiograms showing a large AVM supplied by a hypertrophic branch of the middle cerebral artery during the operation (A). After clipping of the main trunk of the artery (B) the aneurysm did not fill.

cm^3) in 8. Fourteen AVMs were located in the right hemisphere, 10 in the left, 5 in region V and V3, and 3 in the medial frontobasal regions.

In all 32 of our cases the feasibility of total surgical extirpation of the AVMs was determined. For this purpose not only the volume and source of blood supply of the AVM were taken into account, but also its relationship to the functionally important brain structures. The Schaltenbrand and Bailey stereotactic atlas was used for the evaluation of these factors. This method made it possible to determine the brain structures involved by the AVM, which is of paramount importance for deciding the possibility of its radical removal.

Large and giant AVMs in 25 of 32 cases involved to different degrees the central area, one or two brain lobes, the mesencephalon, the thalamic nuclei, and the subthalamic region. The majority of them had a multichannel blood supply from several arterial systems. In half of the cases the supply was from arteries of both hemispheres. Proceeding from such analysis, one may conclude that 25 of these AVMs were inoperable in the sense of complete extirpation. In four cases total removal was apparently possible but connected with great risk, and only in three AVMs was it possible to perform complete excision. Therefore, stereotactic clipping is, first and foremost, a method of treatment of radically inoperable AVMs. However, in certain selected cases this method can ensure total extirpation of an AVM, and in such cases, it may be regarded as a radical method of treatment.

Since the location of the burr hole determines the path of the cannula, it is necessary to choose a trajectory at a safe distance from the AVM and its draining veins. The target point and the center point of the burr hole were connected by lines on both films. With the aid of the stereotactic atlas one must be convinced that the cannula will not damage functionally important structures.

The preoperative geometric calculations showed that the angle of approach (the angle between the axis of the tube and the axis of the clipped vessel) in all our operations on AVMs was from 58 to 88 degrees, much more than the "critical level" when the danger of clip slippage exists. The diameter of the clipped arteries was from 2 to 6 mm.

All operations on AVMs were performed under general intratracheal anesthesia or neuroleptanalgesia. The arterial pressure was lowered before clipping to 50–60 torr. The depth of the clipped arteries from the brain surface varied from 30 to 83 mm. The operating time was from 2 to 3 hours.

There were no serious permanent complications and no fatality in these 34 operations. Only once did the clip slip from the artery, but 1 week later the operation was repeated and the clip was set correctly. No increase of neurologic deficit was noted postoperatively in any case. All patients tolerated the operation well and began to walk 3 to 4 days after surgery.

It is known that total and regional cerebral blood flow (CBF) in the presence of the AVMs is substantially increased. As our previous study has shown the high total CBF in hemispheric AVMs correlated well with the lesion's size and is from 16 to 300 percent more than normal. As our data have shown, the total cerebral CBF increased by 33 to 222 percent and regional CBF by 50 to 290 percent. In the case of large and giant AVMs, the CBF was also substantially increased in the other hemisphere. The same study disclosed that after surgery the CBF in half of the patients decreased practically to normal, and in the other half it was sharply diminished. One may conclude that CBF studies demonstrate one of the objective criteria of the effectiveness of AVM stereotactic clipping.

Repeat angiography was performed in all cases an average of 3 weeks after surgery (excluding three cases), and in 18 patients in a follow-up period from 1 to 7 years. These data have shown that in 5 patients the AVMs were excluded completely,

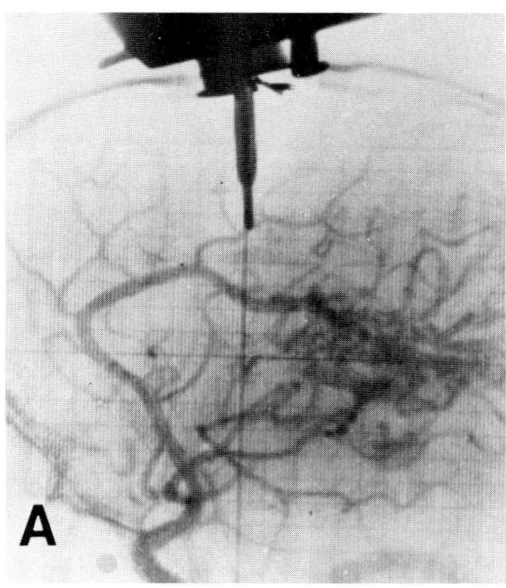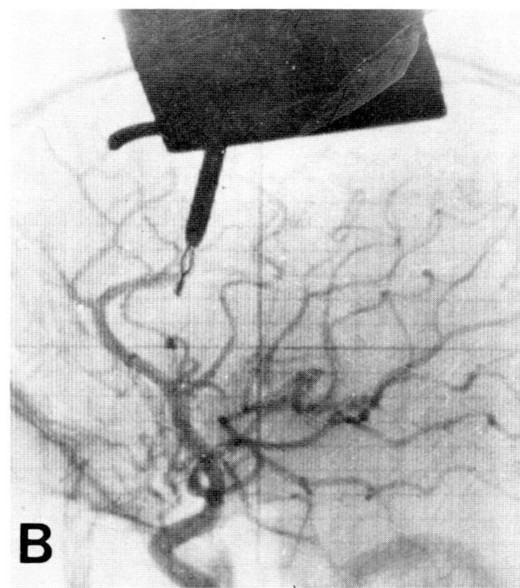

Fig. 90-11. Angiograms of an AVM supplied mainly by the pericallosal artery during the operation (A). After stereotactic clipping of the artery the aneurysm did not fill (B).

in 20 patients the volume of the AVMs was diminished in varying degrees, and in 7 cases the volume did not change because the AVM was filling from other channels.

A favorable clinical effect was observed in all patients during the period of follow-up (6 months to 12 years). There was no repeat or primary intracranial hemorrhage. The generalized or focal seizures disappeared in 7 patients and became much less frequent in two. Motor and sensory disturbances which were the consequence of intracerebral hemorrhages disappeared gradually. Hemiparesis to various degrees persisted in 5 cases. The severe and pulsating headache disappeared immediately after surgery in all 5 patients. Speech disturbances were restored completely in 1 patient and became minimal in 2 others.

Below we present several illustrative examples of long-term results after stereotactic clipping of AVMs of different size and location.

AVMs fed by the middle cerebral artery are very common. The radical removal of the AVM from the central part of the hemisphere is undoubtedly associated with a high risk of serious functional disturbances. The following case illustrates successful stereotactic clipping of the main trunk of the middle cerebral artery substantially proximal to an AVM.

Case 5. A 21-year-old woman suddenly developed sharp headaches and increased weakness in her right extremities. She then lost consciousness for 20 hours. Upon admission her right arm was paralyzed, and there was severe paresis of the right leg, severe motor aphasia, marked papilledema, and bloody CSF.

Angiography demonstrated a large AVM (4 × 3 × 2.5 cm) located in the parietofrontal region and supplied by hypertrophic branches of the left middle cerebral artery (Figure 90-10A). Stereotactic clipping of the main trunk of the artery was performed (Figure 90-10B). The diameter of the trunk at the target point was 3.5 mm; the distance from the surface was 58 mm. A control angiogram disclosed parctically complete elimination of the AVM from the circulation. The postoperative

course was free of complications. A severe neurologic deficit disappeared in 1 month. More than 4 years after the operation the patient was in good condition without any complaints. There was no recurrent bleeding.

AVMs supplied mainly by the pericallosal artery are frequent in neurosurgical practice. The artery may be either the single feeder of the AVM or supply it in combination with other arteries. These AVMs are frequently located deep in the corpus callosum and are often marginally accessible to radical extirpation. The following case illustrates the possibility of clipping the pericallosal artery, which supplied an inoperable AVM of the corpus callosum and basal ganglia.

Case 6. A 13-year-old boy suffered several intraventricular hemorrhages during the 4 years before admission. He was admitted 3 weeks after the last hemorrhage. Angiography disclosed a large AVM involving the corpus callosum, the deep medial cerebral structures and the posterior part of V3. The aneurysm was supplied mainly by the right pericallosal artery and, to a lesser extent, by branches of the right middle and both posterior cerebral arteries (Figure 90-11A). The deep bilateral location of the aneurysm made it inoperable.

Successful stereotactic clipping of the main feeder of the aneurysm, the pericallosal artery, was performed. Subsequent angiography showed that the AVM no longer filled through the artery (Figure 90-11B). In comparison with the preoperative investigation, the CBF markedly decreased. There were no postoperative complications. During 8 years of follow-up there were no epileptic seizures or intracranial hemorrhages. The patient is in good condition. He is now working at a factory.

In certain cases of AVMs of the anterior cerebral artery, the technical difficulties are connected with the fact that the trajectory of the cannula will be too close to the nidus of the AVM or great draining veins creating a potential danger of major damage. In such a case we use the approach to the anterior cerebral artery through the contralateral (''healthy'') hemisphere eliminating the possibility of disturbing the AVM vessels. Below we describe such a case.

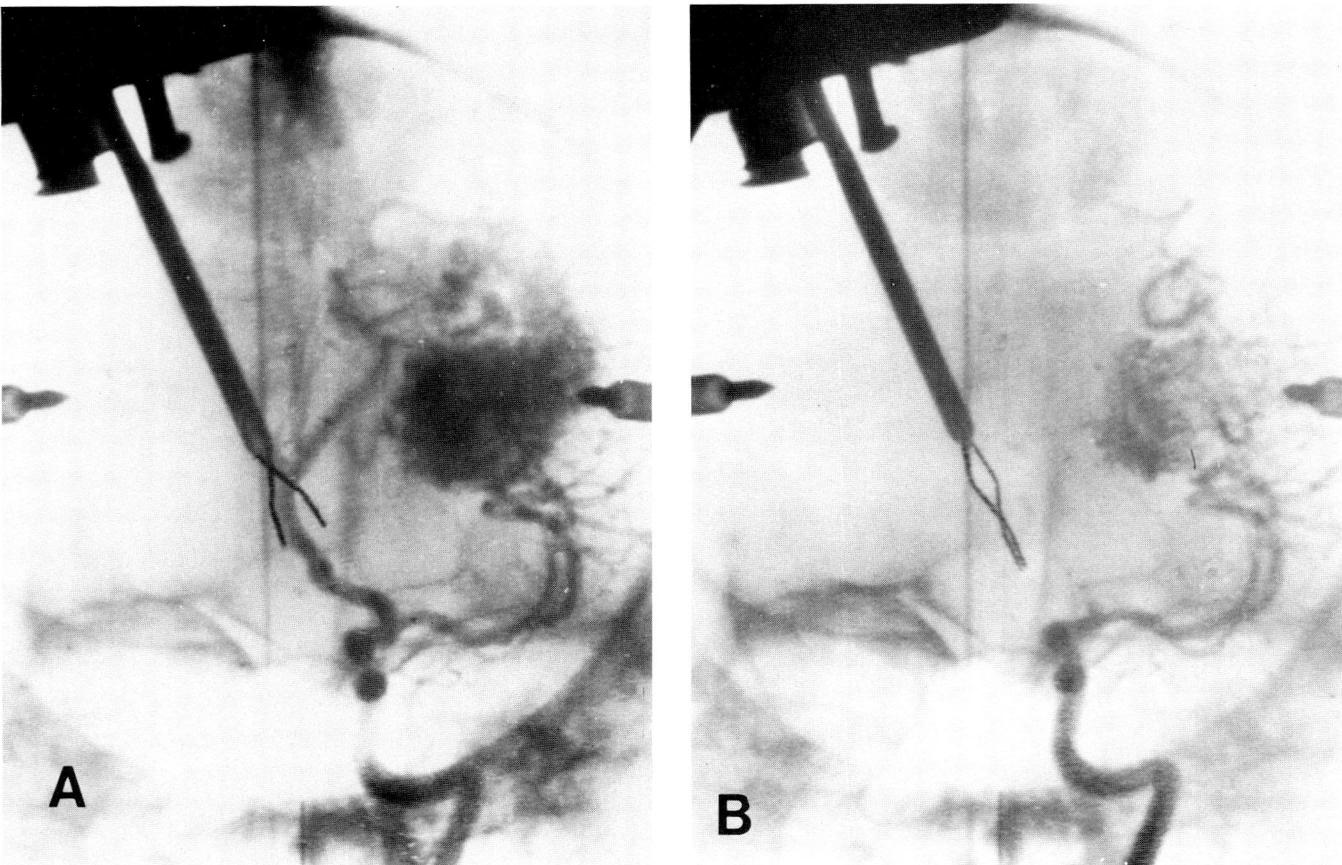

Fig. 90-12.   Angiograms showing the large AVM fed by a hypertrophied anterior cerebral artery before stereotactic clipping from the contralateral side (A) and after clipping (B).

Case 7.   A 33-year-old woman was admitted a few months after sudden severe headaches with loss of consciousness and coma for about 24 hours. After coming out of the coma, paralysis of the right arm and severe paresis of the right leg were noted.

Four-vessel angiography disclosed a large AVM (about 6 cm on the lateral view) fed by a hypertrophied anterior cerebral artery (Figure 90-12A). The malformation was located in the left frontal lobe and was encircled by many large draining veins. The burr hole was put on the contralateral side near the coronal suture. The pericallosal artery was clipped stereotactically. Control angiography showed filling of only a small part of the AVM supplied by small branches of the middle cerebral artery (Figure 90-12B). Two years after the operation the patient's condition is quite good. There is mild right-sided hemiparesis without recurrent hemorrhages.

Besides the anterior and middle cerebral arteries, stereotactic clipping of the deep-seated arterial branches supplying AVMs located in the lateral ventricles and paraventricular regions is also technically possible. Below is an example of successful clipping of the anterior choroidal artery feeding a small AVM in the lateral ventricle.

Case 8.   A 29-year-old man suffered a severe subarachnoid-parenchymatous hemorrhage into the left hemisphere. A severe right-sided hemiparesis and the meningeal syndrome were prominent at admission.

Angiography disclosed a small AVM in the anterior part of the right lateral ventricle (Figure 90-13A). The AVM was supplied by the anterior choroidal artery, which was clipped stereotactically. Intraoperative angiography revealed non-filling of the AVM (Figure 90-13B). Only slight hemiparesis remains 2 years after the operation.

The next case is important for the evaluation of the clipping method. In this case, the method was used to manage an AVM that undoubtedly could have been completely removed by classic open surgery. It is known that AVMs supplied by one feeder are relatively rare. Their total extirpation usually can be achieved without great technical difficulties. Nevertheless, to study the possibilities of stereotactic clipping, we employed it in few cases in which the AVM was radically operable. It should be emphasized that stereotactic clipping totally eliminated the AVM from the circulation. An illustrative case is described below.

Case 9.   A 26-year-old man was admitted to our clinic several hours after a single subarachnoid-parenchymatous hemorrhage. Pronounced hemiparesis gradually disappeared. Angiography showed a small AVM (23 cm^3) in the right parietotemporal region. There was only one small feeding branch from the middle cerebral artery (Figure 90-14A). There were no complications in the postoperative period. Control angiography 3 weeks after the operation showed the complete exclusion of

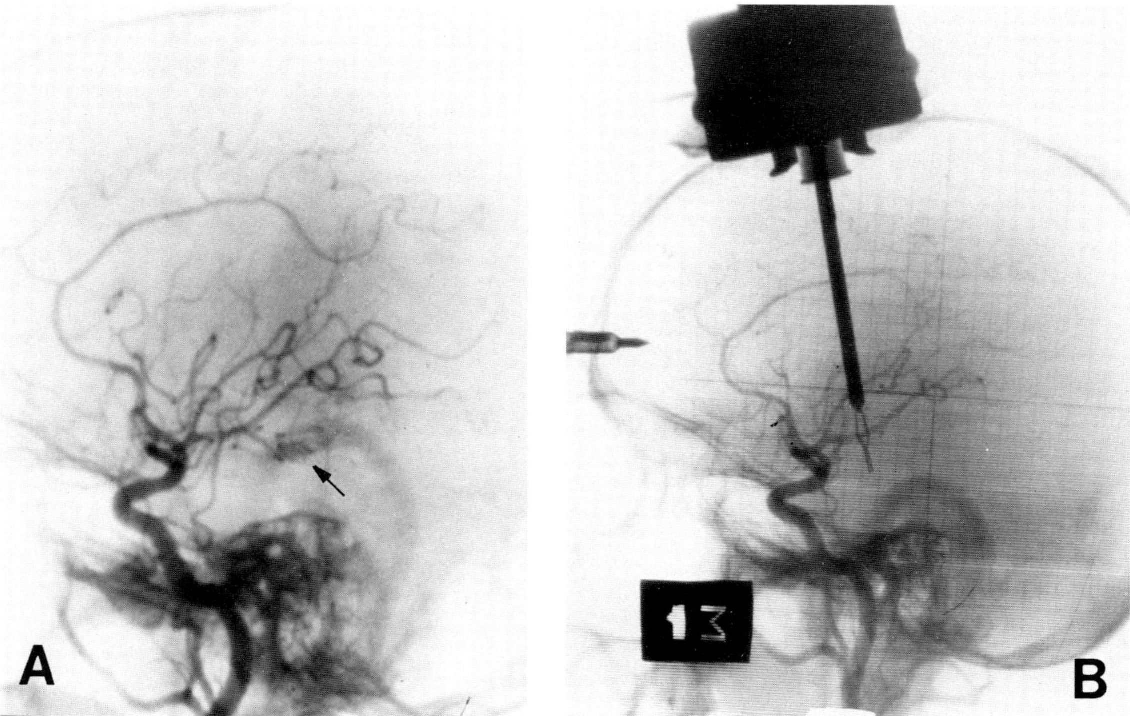

Fig. 90-13. Angiograms showing a small AVM in the anterior part of the right lateral ventricle supplied by the anterior choroidal artery (A). Intraoperative angiography revealed non-filling of the AVM (B).

the malformation (Figure 90-14B). It is important to note that the second ''normal'' branch of the middle cerebral artery, which was located very close to the first branch supplying the AVM, remained intact. Postoperative CBF studies demonstrated a return to normal values. About 8 years after surgery the patient is in good condition without a neurologic deficit. He is working full-time. Intracranial hemorrhage has not recurred.

CONCLUSIONS

The technique of stereotactic treatment of cerebral arterial aneurysms and AVMs is undoubtedly not universally applicable. As with all new surgical methods careful studies are needed regarding the indications and modifications of the technique. At the present stage of its development this technique has the

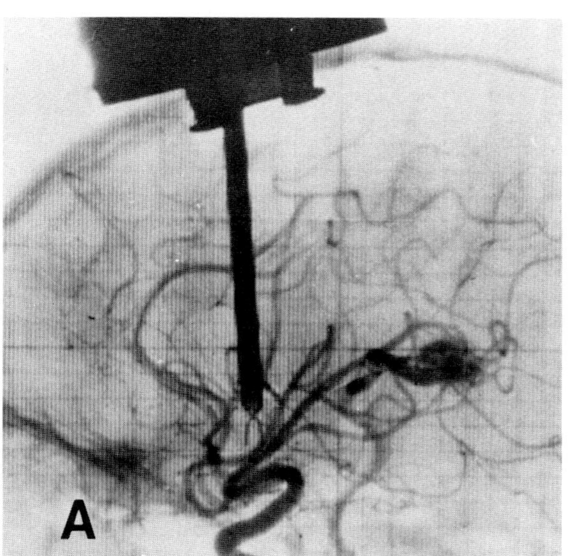

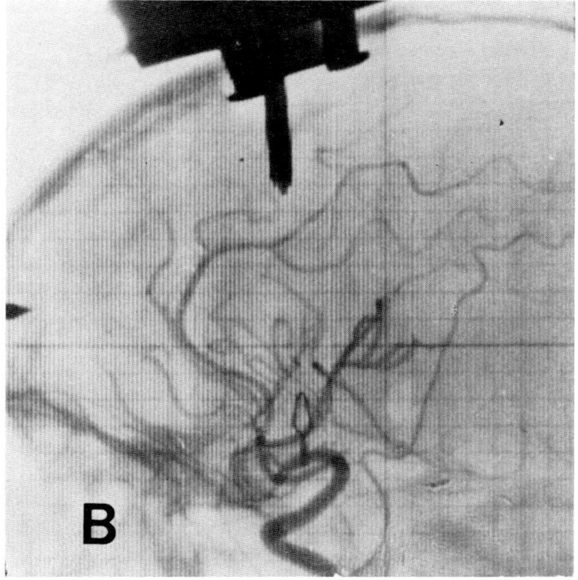

Fig. 90-14. A small AV aneurysm supplied by only one branch of the middle cerebral artery just before (A), and after (B) stereotactic clipping operation. The aneurysm was totally excluded from the circulation.

traumatic and safer than direct attack by the open approach. It results in less complications and can be used in the presence of arterial spasm after subarachnoid hemorrhage.

REFERENCES

1. Guiot G, Rougerie J, Sachs M, et al: Repérage stéréotaxique de malformations vascularies profondes intracérébrales. Semin Hop Paris 36:1134, 1960
2. Riechert T, Mundinger P: Combined stereotaxic operation for treatment of deep-seated angiomas and aneurysm. J Neurosurg 21:358, 1964
3. Alksne JE, Rand RW: Current status of metallic thrombosis of intracranial aneurysms. Prog Neurol Surg 3:212, 1969
4. Alksne JE: Stereotaxic occlusion of 22 consecutive anterior communicating artery aneurysms. J Neurosurg 52:790, 1980
5. Mullan S: Experiences with surgical thrombosis of intracranial berry aneurysms and carotid cavernous fistulas. J Neurosurg 41: 657, 1974
6. Samotokin BA, Hilko VA: [Aneurysms and Arteriovenous Fistulas of the Brain.] Leningrad, Meditsina, 1973
7. Cahan LD, Rand RW: Stereotaxic coagulation of a paraventricular arteriovenous malformation. Case report. J Neurosurg 39:770, 1973
8. Rand RW, Mosso JA: Treatment of cerebral aneurysms by stereotaxic ferromagnetic silicone thrombosis. Bull Los Angeles Neurol Soc 38:21, 1972
9. Kandel EI, Peresedov VV: [Stereotactic clipping of an arterial aneurysm of the brain.] Vopr Neirokhir 39:13, 1974,
10. Kandel EI, Peresedov VV: Stereotaxic clipping of arterial aneurysms and arteriovenous malformations. J Neurosurg 46:12, 1977
11. Kandel EI, Peresedov VV: Stereotaxic clipping of arterial and arteriovenous aneurysms of the brain. Acta Neurochir Suppl 30:405, 1980
12. Kandel EI, Peresedov VV: Stereotactic clipping of arterial aneurysms and arteriovenous malformations of the brain, Schmidek HH, Sweet WH (eds): Operative Neurosurgical Techniques: Indications, Methods, and Results, vol 2. New York, Grune & Stratton, 1982, pp 771–781

CHAPTER 91
Management of Unclippable Aneurysms

Roberto C. Heros

THE IDEAL FORM of management for any intracranial aneurysm is direct surgical clipping of its neck. Not infrequently, however, the aneurysm cannot be clipped because of its size, location, or configuration. In general, whether an aneurysm can be clipped or not is determined either before intracranial exploration from studying the arteriograms and CT scans, or at intracranial exploration after the surgeon has had a chance to directly view the anatomy. We will consider these situations separately.

PREOPERATIVE DETERMINATION OF INABILITY TO CLIP AN ANEURYSM

The decision that a particular aneurysm cannot be clipped can be made preoperatively on the basis of its location, size, or configuration as determined from the radiographic studies.

LOCATION

Inability to clip an aneurysm because of its location is usually the result of the aneurysm being located extradurally on the internal carotid artery; i.e., on the petrous or cavernous segment of the internal carotid artery. With aneurysms of the petrous segment of the internal carotid artery, such a determination is usually straightforward. This is also the case with aneurysms of the cavernous segment of the internal carotid artery. However, with some aneurysms of the clinoid region, it is not clear whether the aneurysm is intradural or extradural. Multiple angiographic views sometimes are required to identify the precise origin of the neck. In general, the anterior clinoid is a reliable landmark if it is well defined radiographically; it is probably more reliable than the origin of the ophthalmic artery. If the neck is above the base of the anterior clinoid process on lateral views, the aneurysm is generally intradural and can be reached intracranially by drilling off the anterior clinoid process. The converse is the case when the neck is below the base of the anterior clinoid. The ophthalmic artery usually originates from the carotid artery in the general area of the base of the anterior clinoid process. Therefore, if the neck of the aneurysm is distal to the ophthalmic artery, it usually can be clipped; however, the origin of the ophthalmic artery is somewhat more variable than the anterior clinoid and this is why it is not a reliable landmark.[1]

Techniques have been developed to approach aneurysms of the clinoid region and aneurysms that are even lower and completely intracavernous by a combined epidural and subdural direct approach.[2,3] Direct techniques have also been used to deal with aneurysms of the petrous segment of the internal carotid artery.[4,5] In general, these direct approaches to the cavernous sinus and to the petrous segment of the internal carotid artery should be used only in centers with a special interest in these techniques, since ordinarily these aneurysms can be dealt with effectively by indirect methods. In the case of aneurysms in the region of the anterior clinoid, an intracranial exploration is in order if there is any doubt.

Carotid Occlusion for Aneurysms of the Internal Carotid Artery

The surgeon is faced with a number of choices once he or she decides to occlude the carotid artery to treat an aneurysm. Table 91-1 gives a general outline of the choices available.

The most important decision is whether to occlude the common or the internal carotid artery. The surgeon then must decide whether to occlude the artery acutely with a simple ligature or to place a clamp on the artery for delayed abrupt occlusion or gradual occlusion. If the choice is to occlude the internal carotid artery, there is the option of doing it with a detachable balloon instead of directly. Again, if the internal carotid has been chosen for occlusion, a decision must be made whether or not to perform a preliminary extracranial-to-intracranial (EC-IC) bypass graft. In both cases, internal or common carotid ligation, there is the option of trapping the aneurysm by occluding the artery intracranially, usually below the posterior communicating artery in cases of proximal aneurysms. This subject is obviously too complex to be discussed here in great detail and it has been reviewed by me in several other publications.[6–9]

From a review of the literature as well as from personal experience, several opinions have been formed. Ligation of the common carotid is safer than ligation of the internal carotid. Even though it would appear that ligation of the internal carotid is more effective in the treatment of internal carotid aneurysms, a thorough review of the literature indicates that both procedures (internal and common carotid ligation) have about the same incidence of rehemorrhage and about the same incidence of subsequent aneurysmal thrombosis, i.e., they are about equally effective. When initially tolerated, abrupt ligation is as safe as gradual occlusion; however, about 20 percent of the patients do not tolerate abrupt ligation. For these patients, the choices are to attempt gradual occlusion, which will be toler-

OPERATIVE NEUROSURGICAL TECHNIQUES
ISBN 0-8089-1862-1

Table 91-1. Choices available for treating unclippable aneurysms of the internal carotid artery

Occlusion of common carotid 　Ligature; abrupt occlusion 　Clamp 　　Acute occlusion 　　Gradual occlusion	with or without trapping
Occlusion of internal carotid 　Ligature; abrupt occlusion 　Clamp 　　Acute occlusion 　　Gradual occlusion 　Detachable balloon	with or without EC-IC with or without trapping

ated by some in spite of the fact they cannot tolerate abrupt occlusion, or to recommend an EC-IC procedure followed by occlusion of the internal carotid. There is a group of patients (between 10 and 15 percent) who can tolerate neither abrupt nor gradual occlusion. For this group of patients, the only alternative is a preliminary EC-IC procedure followed by occlusion of the internal carotid.

Balloon occlusion of the internal carotid artery initially was thought to be a very safe form of treatment of these aneurysms, since by placing the balloon close to the origin of the aneurysm problems with thrombosis and subsequent embolism of the internal carotid could be avoided. However, we have encountered problems with emboli from thrombi and from the balloon itself in cases treated in this manner.[10]

Based on these premises, we developed the decision tree roughly outlined in Figure 91-1. We first perform complete cerebral angiography with cross-compression studies and with a period of test occlusion to determine whether the patient appears to have sufficient collateral circulation to tolerate carotid occlusion. If the patient has inadequate collateral circulation or does not tolerate the test occlusion during angiography, we recommend an EC-IC bypass procedure followed by occlusion of the internal carotid artery. We prefer to occlude the carotid artery by the balloon technique with the patient awake, since in this manner it can be determined if the bypass graft is open, and, if this is the case, one can proceed with another period of test occlusion. If this is tolerated, the balloon can be detached.

If the patient has adequate collateral circulation, we expose the carotid artery in the neck and measure the stump pressure and then subject the patient to a period of temporary occlusion while he or she is being tested clinically (if the patient is awake, which we prefer) or while the EEG is being recorded (if the patient is asleep). If the patient has a very low stump pressure (less than 30 torr) and test occlusion is not tolerated (e.g., the awake patient develops clinical symptoms or the EEG changes markedly in the sleeping patient), we plan an EC-IC bypass followed by occlusion of the internal carotid artery by balloon. If the stump pressure is very low but the patient tolerates the test occlusion or if the patient has adequate stump pressure but does not tolerate test occlusion, we plan to occlude the common carotid artery gradually with a clamp over the next several days. If there is adequate stump pressure and test occlusion is well tolerated, we proceed with abrupt ligation of the common carotid, usually by ligating the artery with three silk ligatures placed just below the bifurcation.

Patients who have symptoms of rapidly progressive visual loss or brain compression should probably be treated by a trapping procedure with decompression of the aneurysmal mass after occlusion of the internal carotid below and above the aneurysm with or without an EC-IC procedure, depending on the collateral circulation.

This is a very simplified scheme and each patient needs to

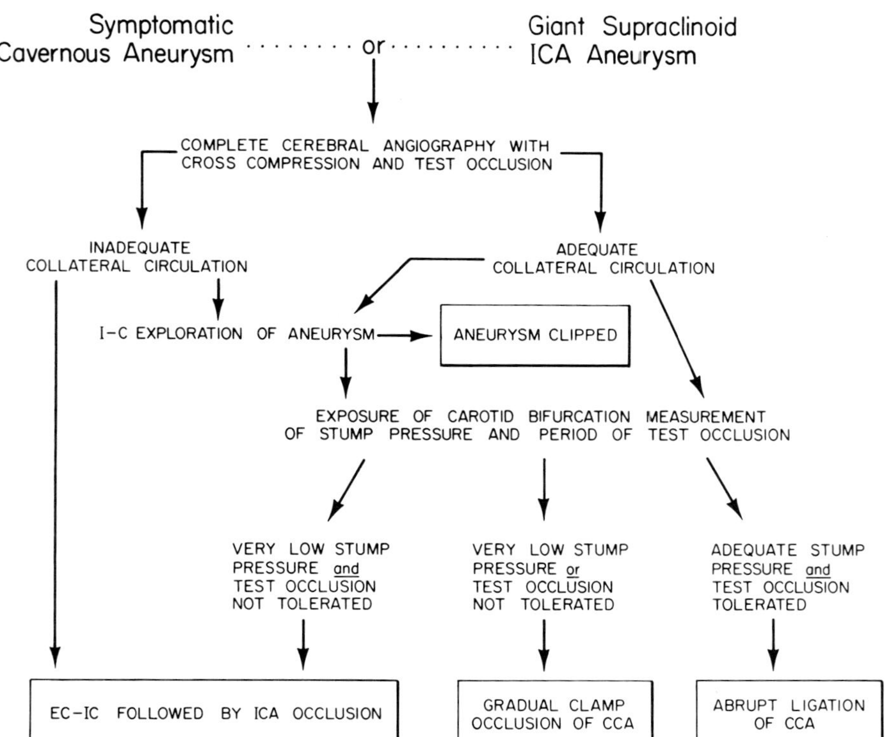

Fig. 91-1. Decision tree for determining if an aneurysm can be clipped.

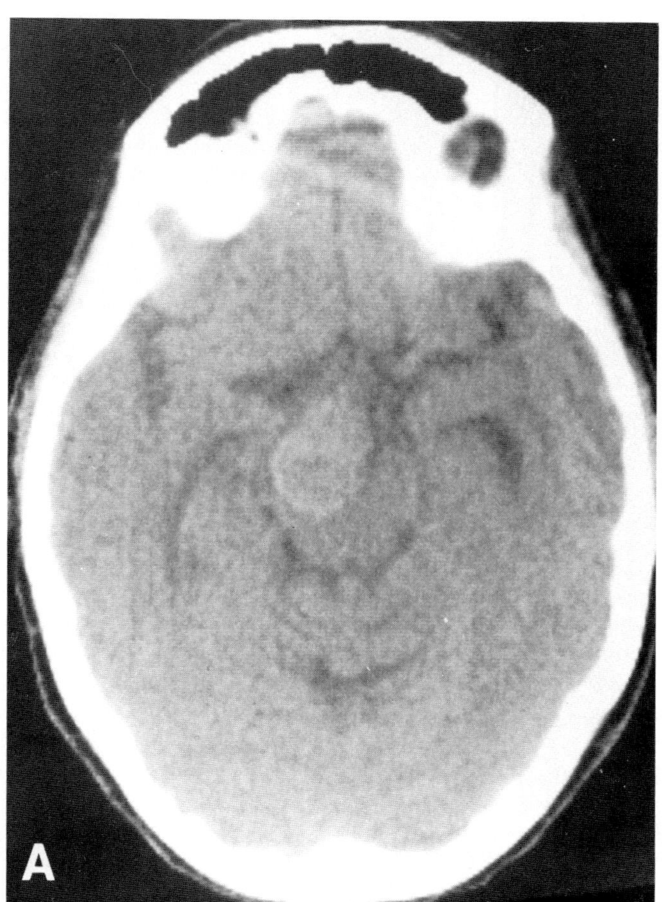
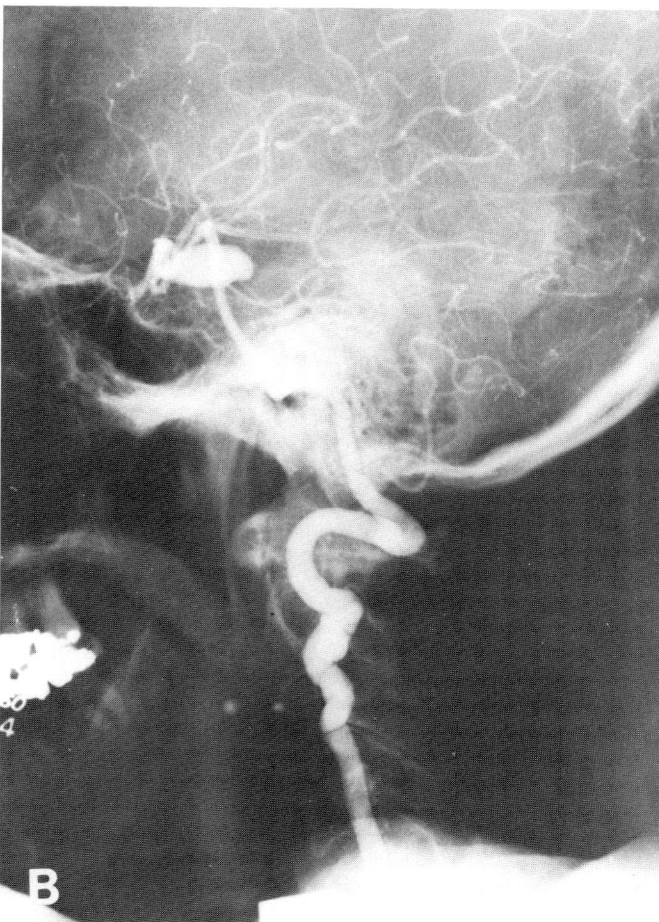

Fig. 91-2. A patient with a large right posterior communicating aneurysm treated 5 years earlier by ligation of the right common carotid. On examination the patient had signs of brainstem compression. The aneurysm was explored, clipped, and excised successfully. (A) A CT scan showing the partially thrombosed aneurysm. (B) A left vertebral arteriogram showing filling of the aneurysm through the posterior communicating artery.

be considered individually, but in general we have found this to be a helpful scheme in decision making. It should be apparent that we use EC-IC procedures only in a very few patients who do not seem to tolerate the immediate effects of carotid occlusion. We do not use this procedure on a prophylactic basis since we are skeptical about the value of this procedure in preventing future ischemic problems. Our skepticism has been reinforced by the generally negative results of the recently reported international cooperative study on bypass procedures.[11] This area is still relatively controversial, and many other surgeons favor a prophylactic bypass procedure whenever the carotid artery is to be ligated intentionally.

SIZE

The second major reason for deciding without intracranial exploration that an aneurysm cannot be clipped is because the aneurysm appears to be too large to accept the clip. Here, again, intracranial exploration is in order if there is any doubt, since not rarely an aneurysm that appears too large to accept a clip on the radiographic studies will be found to have a clippable neck at surgery (Figure 91-2). The available alternatives will be discussed separately for each major site of aneurysm development.

For aneurysms of the internal carotid artery, carotid ligation is a very effective form of therapy. Carotid ligation tends to

be most effective for the more proximally located aneurysms (those on the petrous and cavernous segments). This is almost certainly because there is less potential for collateral circulation at this level. Carotid ligation is still effective for aneurysms above the ophthalmic artery, but because of a potential for collateral circulation through the ophthalmic artery, the likelihood of thrombosis of the aneurysm is slightly less in the paraclinoid region than for aneurysms located more proximally. There is less chance of successfully treating aneurysms in the area of the origin of the posterior communicating artery and the anterior choroidal artery with carotid ligation because of the potential for continued filling through the posterior communicating artery (see Figure 91-1). There is an even smaller chance of successfully treating aneurysms at the bifurcation of the internal carotid artery by carotid ligation because there is the added potential for collateral flow in a retrograde fashion through the anterior cerebral artery. However, even in this location, carotid ligation can be quite effective in promoting aneurysmal thrombosis (Figure 91-3).

Giant aneurysms of the anterior communicating region usually produce either visual symptoms from compression of the chiasm and optic nerves or subarachnoid hemorrhage. They occasionally can grow to a very large size without producing optic compression if they project forward and upward. This latter type of aneurysm can mimic a large basal tumor such as an olfactory groove meningioma and produce dementia and

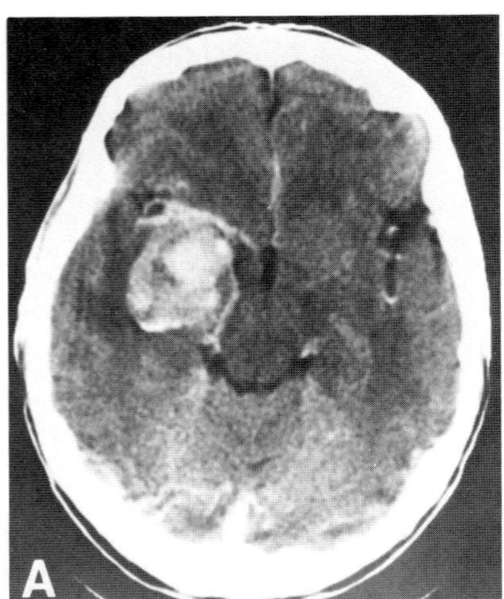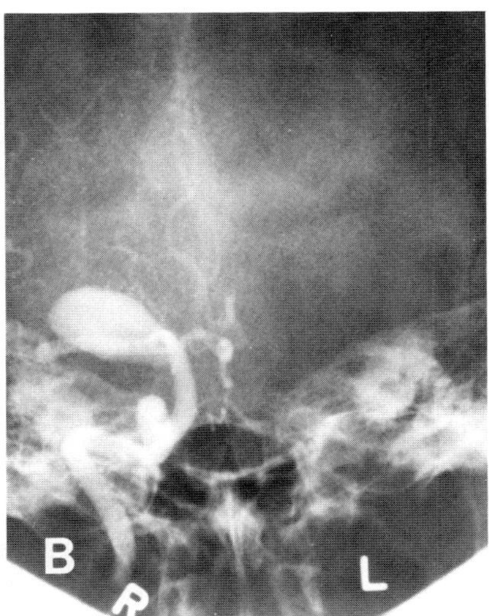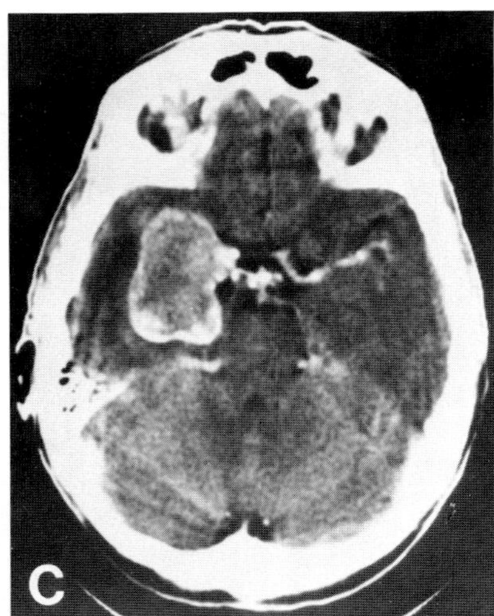

Fig. 91-3.   A patient with a giant, partially thrombosed aneurysm of the right carotid bifurcation that was treated successfully by ligation of the common carotid. (A) A pre-operative CT scan (enhanced). (B) An AP carotid arteriogram showing partial filling of the aneurysm. (C) A postoperative CT scan (plain) showing thrombosis (high-density—no further enhancement) of the previously patent portion of the aneurysm.

signs of increased intracranial pressure.[6,12,13] Carotid ligation is, in general, not effective for anterior communicating aneurysms and it cannot be recommended as adequate treatment for these lesions. The first indirect procedure that was recommended for anterior communicating aneurysms is the so-called "Logue" procedure, which essentially consists of proximal ligation of the dominant anterior cerebral artery, i.e., the artery that fills the aneurysm primarily.[14] This operation is effective, but even when applied to smaller aneurysms, it has an ischemic complication rate of between 10 and 20 percent. Care must be taken to place the clip in such a manner that it does not injure the perforating vessels from the anterior cerebral artery or the recurrent artery of Heubner, which runs in close approximation to the anterior cerebral artery. Tindall and Odom offered a modification of this procedure that consists of ligation of the dominant cerebral artery at its origin and ligation of the contralateral common carotid.[15,16] This procedure may be of help in those cases in which the aneurysm fills about equally from both sides. We have had no significant experience with either of these procedures as primary treatment for giant anterior communicating aneurysms, mainly because we have seen only a few of these patients and they all have been treated either by clipping or by aneurysmorrhaphy under temporary occlusion of both anterior cerebral arteries.

Giant aneurysms of the middle cerebral artery also cannot be treated effectively with carotid ligation. Most frequently, these aneurysms produce either subarachnoid hemorrhage or a mass effect (lateralizing hemispheric signs, temporal lobe epilepsy, or headaches or papilledema). Less commonly they produce abrupt ischemic events as a result of emboli from an intra-aneurysmal clot or compression of adjacent vessels or extension of the clot into the main lumen of the middle cerebral artery. The approach to these aneurysms most often should include aneurysmorrhaphy to relieve the mass effect. If they are going to be treated only indirectly, however, the only treatment available is occlusion of the proximal middle cerebral artery. The occlusion should be as close to the aneurysm as possible to preserve perforating vessels. In our opinion, planned occlusion of the middle cerebral artery should always be preceded by a bypass graft, since the chances of a patient tolerating occlusion of the main stem of the middle cerebral artery without a

significant neurologic deficit is probably less than 10 percent. In fact, we prefer to use a "high flow" bypass graft, being somewhat skeptical about the ability of a simple superficial temporal artery bypass to provide enough blood to sustain the middle cerebral circulation. A saphenous vein graft, usually from the external carotid or the subclavian artery, is our preferred approach (Figure 91-4). There must be free communication between the division of the middle cerebral artery to which the bypass graft is anastomosed and the other division. If one of the divisions is occluded, either iatrogenically or by the aneurysm, then the bypass graft must be anastomosed to both major divisions of the middle cerebral artery; that is, to a branch above the sylvian fissure and to a branch below the sylvian fissure for practical purposes.[17,18]

The treatment of giant aneurysms of the vertebrobasilar circulation is a highly specialized area of neurosurgical treatment that should be reserved for a few centers. For aneurysms of the top of the basilar artery, the indirect procedure of choice is ligation of the basilar artery just below the superior cerebellar arteries. It rarely is possible to ligate the basilar artery between the superior cerebellar and the posterior cerebral arteries, since with giant aneurysms this area is usually already involved in the neck of the aneurysm. Drake introduced the "tourniquet technique" for ligation of the basilar and middle cerebral arteries.[19] In this technique the tourniquet is placed around the artery at surgery and the patient is allowed to wake up completely; occlusion then is attempted later that day or the next day percutaneously with the patient awake. This is usually done in the angiography suite so that the occlusion can be monitored radiographically.

A prerequisite for attempting distal basilar occlusion is an adequate collateral circulation, which usually means at least one normal-sized posterior communicating artery as demonstrated by the Allcock maneuver (injection of a vertebral artery while each internal carotid artery is temporarily occluded).[19] The question of whether to perform a prophylactic EC-IC bypass procedure whenever the basilar artery is to be ligated remains open. This has only been necessary on a few occasions in the very large series from London, Ontario.[19,20] Others have preferred to use a bypass graft, usually a saphenous vein graft to the proximal posterior cerebral artery, whenever basilar

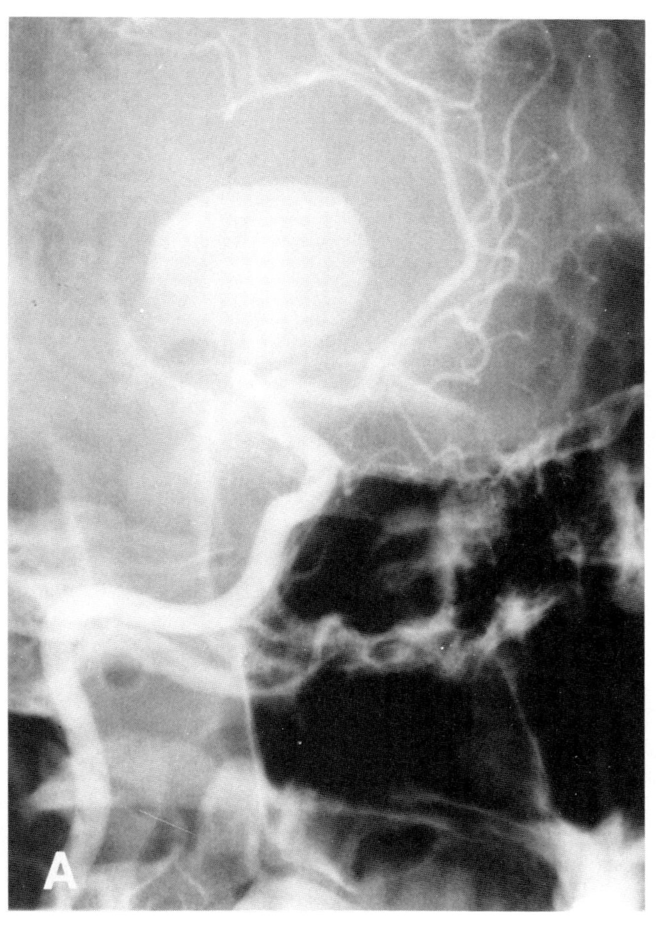

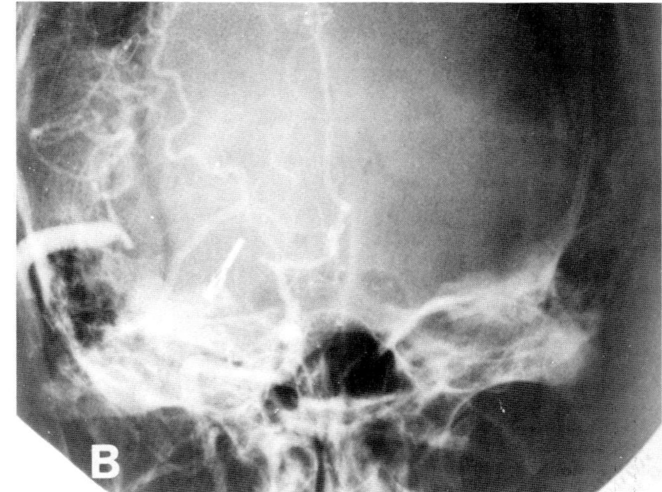

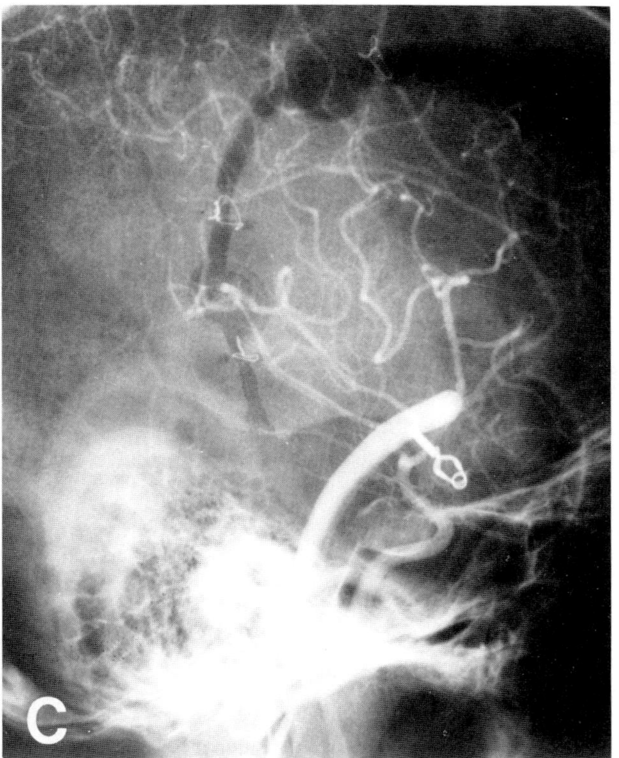

Fig. 91-4. A patient with temporal lobe epilepsy and a giant right middle cerebral aneurysm that could not be clipped at exploration. The aneurysm was treated successfully by a saphenous vein EC-IC bypass and occlusion of the middle cerebral artery. (A) A preoperative oblique right carotid arteriogram. (B) A postoperative AP right carotid arteriogram showing the patent vein graft and the surgically occluded right middle cerebral artery. There is no filling of the aneurysm. (C) A postoperative lateral right carotid arteriogram. The entire middle cerebral territory and the right anterior cerebral territory are filled by the vein graft.

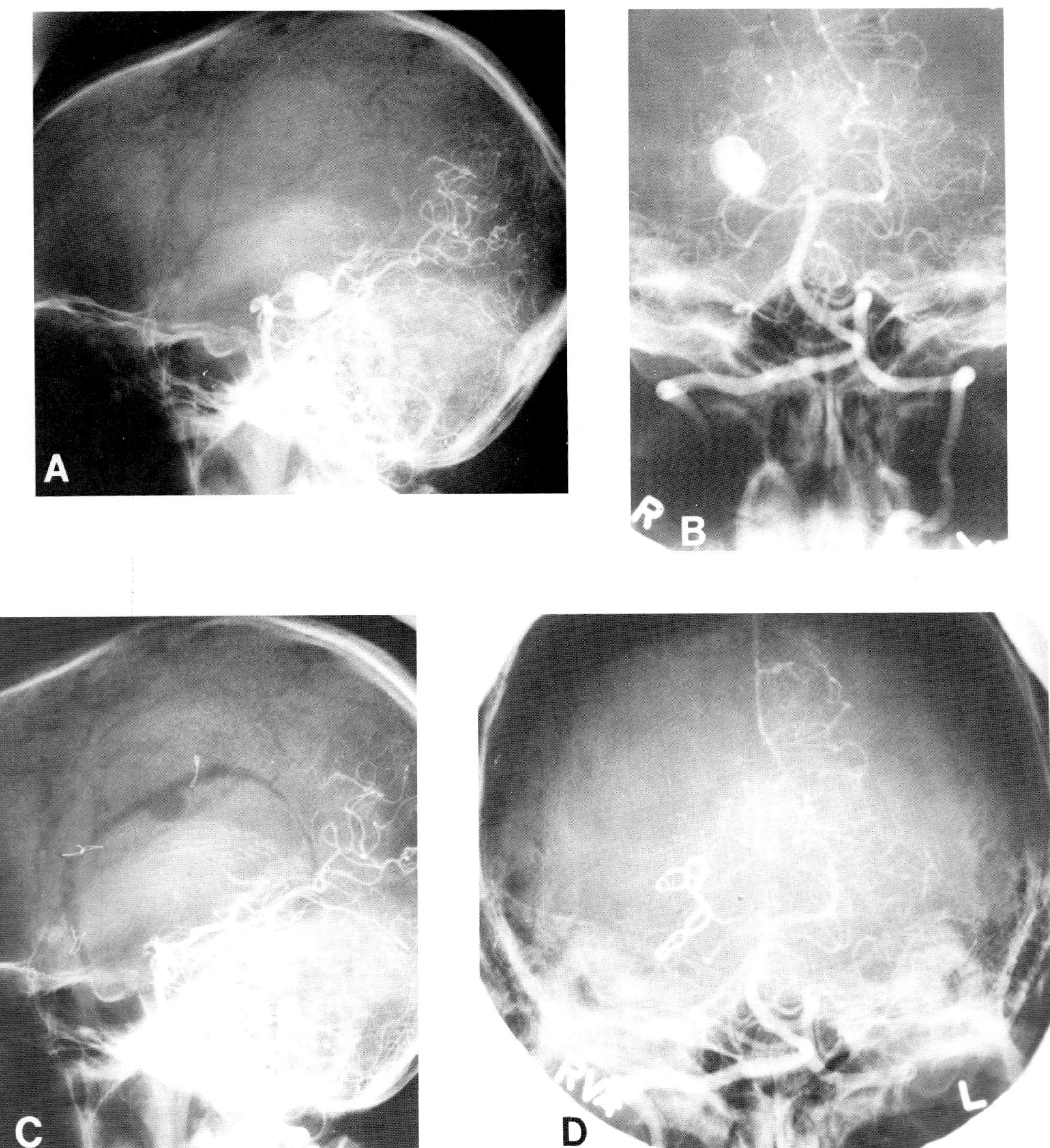

Fig. 91-5. A patient with brainstem compression from a giant, partially thrombosed fusiform aneurysm of the posterior cerebral artery. At surgery the aneurysm was fusiform, involving a segment of the posterior cerebral artery about 2 cm in length. The arterial lumen was reconstructed with two Sugita-Drake clips applied from opposite directions. After clipping, flow through the posterior cerebral artery was excellent. The patient did well postoperatively, but an arteriogram done routinely 1 week later showed thrombosis of the artery and the aneurysm. The collateral circulation must have been adequate to prevent a neurologic deficit. (A, B) Preoperative lateral and AP vertebral arteriograms showing only the patent portion of the aneurysm. (C, D) Postoperative lateral and AP vertebral angiograms showing no filling of the aneurysm but thrombosis of the posterior cerebral artery (AP view), which was clinically asymptomatic. Note some "kinking" or angulation of the clips, which at surgery had been placed in a straight line.

occlusion is planned.[21] One word of caution: the planned arterial occlusion should be performed very soon after the bypass graft is established, particularly if it is a high-flow type of graft such as a saphenous vein graft. If the parent artery is left open and there is additional flow from the bypass graft, the aneurysm is likely to rupture. This happened to one of our patients with a giant aneurysm of the top of the basilar artery in whom we established a saphenous vein bypass graft to the proximal posterior cerebral artery and placed a tourniquet around the distal basilar artery for later occlusion. The night after surgery, before the intended occlusion of the basilar artery by tourniquet, the patient suffered a fatal rupture of her previously

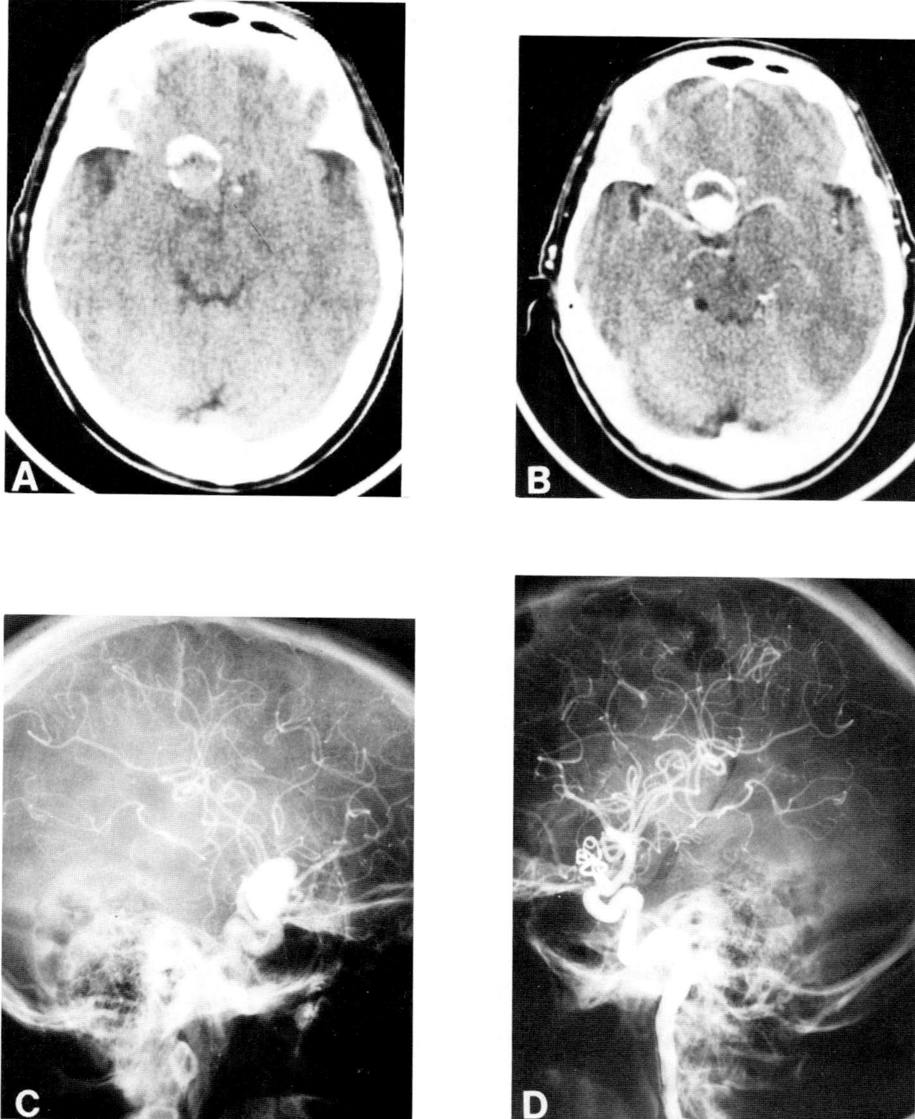

Fig. 91-6. A patient with a giant right paraclinoid aneurysm producing visual loss. After thorough drilling of the anterior clinoid and unroofing of the optic nerve the aneurysm could be clipped satisfactorily, but postoperatively the patient's vision was worse in that eye. (A) A plain CT scan showing heavy calcification of the aneurysm. (B) An enhanced CT scan showing that the aneurysm is partially thrombosed. (C) A lateral right carotid arteriogram showing the patent portion of the aneurysm. (D) A postoperative right carotid arteriogram showing satisfactory clipping of the aneurysm with two Sugita clips.

intact aneurysm.[22] In an early report of his experience with 42 giant basilar bifurcation aneurysms, Drake treated 14 patients by basilar artery occlusion. The results were good in 7.[19]

Aneurysms of the basilar trunk and the vertebrobasilar junction can be treated by unilateral or bilateral vertebral ligation. Unilateral vertebral ligation is usually well tolerated provided there is a patent contralateral vertebral artery of at least moderate size. Bilateral vertebral occlusion is extremely dangerous unless there is extraordinarily good collateral flow to the basilar artery from the carotid circulation.[19,20] Vertebral artery occlusion usually should be done intracranially or just as the artery enters the skull in the sulcus arteriosum of C1. If the vertebral ligation is carried out proximally, the usually abundant collateral circulation from muscular branches in the neck will keep the distal vertebral artery and possibly the aneurysm patent.

CONFIGURATION

The third major reason for deciding a priori to treat an aneurysm by an indirect method is the configuration of the aneurysm as seen on angiograms or CT scans. This decision is frequently made when the aneurysm is fusiform in appearance. In most instances, these aneurysms cannot be clipped; if treated at all, they must be treated by an indirect method. Indirect methods, however, are rarely successful for these aneurysms because the aneurysm involves a large segment of the parent vessel and in order to eliminate the aneurysm from the circulation successfully, the entire segment of the vessel involved by the aneurysm must be trapped or excised. This is rarely tolerated in the supraclinoid carotid, middle cerebral, or basilar arteries. Very important perforators come from these vessels, and the loss of a large segment of these arteries is not tolerated.

In the posterior cerebral and vertebral arteries, however, it is occasionally possible to trap a fusiform aneurysm without untoward effects. It should be noted that presently some fusiform aneurysms can be treated successfully by reconstruction of the vessel wall with specially designed clips. The right-angle fenestrated Sugita clip is especially helpful in these cases.[23] However, this can be done only exceptionally in those rare fusiform aneurysms with a soft arterial wall. Most of the fusiform aneurysms are related to atherosclerosis, and the arterial wall is hard and gritty and not amenable to clipping. Even after what appears to be successful surgical "reconstruction" of a long arterial segment, thrombosis can occur postoperatively from "kinking" of the usually complicated clip assembly (Figure 91-5).

In addition to fusiform aneurysms, partially thrombosed aneurysms, particularly when they contain calcium in the wall, are frequently thought to be unclippable a priori. Here again, intracranial exploration is necessary if there is any hope at all of clipping the aneurysm, because even when the base of the aneurysm appears heavily calcified, the aneurysm sometimes has a clippable neck at surgery (Figure 91-6).

Computed tomographic scans may indicate the presence of a giant aneurysm and arteriograms reveal what appears to be a "serpentine" aneurysm, which essentially means that there is a long, narrow lumen along the aneurysm leading to an important distal branch.[24] True serpentine aneurysms represent a special form of fusiform aneurysm and they cannot be clipped. The angiographic appearance can be misleading, however. In one of our cases, intracranial exploration was carried out to decompress what appeared to be a serpentine aneurysm. At surgery, the aneurysm was found to have a neck that could be ligated, and, contrary to the appearance on the preoperative arteriograms, there was no vessel coming from its dome. The aneurysm was ligated and completely resected without untoward effect (Figure 91-7).

DETERMINATION OF AN INABILITY TO CLIP AN ANEURYSM AT SURGERY

Not infrequently, the surgeon determines directly at intracranial surgery that the aneurysm cannot be clipped. Once again, this can be a result of the size of the aneurysm, its location (i.e., it was thought that the aneurysm was intradural and even after the anterior clinoid process is removed, the neck is actually extradural, in the cavernous sinus, and cannot be reached), or its configuration (i.e., heavy calcification in the base, partial thrombosis, branches coming off distally in the neck, or a relationship to visual structures). In these instances, the surgeon has several options: deep hypotension; temporary proximal occlusion or trapping; wrapping; aneurysmorrhaphy; the use of multiple or specialized clips; thrombosis or balloon occlusion; or indirect procedures.

DEEP HYPOTENSION

Not infrequently an aneurysm that appears impossible to clip upon first inspection may become soft and pliable enough to accept a clip under deep hypotension (i.e., a mean systemic pressure of 35 to 45 torr for several minutes or mean pressures of 45 and 55 torr if a more prolonged period of hypotension is necessary). To achieve these levels of hypotension it is necessary for the patient to be in good cardiovascular condition. It is best to avoid such levels of hypotension in elderly patients or in patients with evidence of preoperative vasospasm. Also, we prefer to avoid deep hypotension in any patient who is not in good preoperative neurologic condition under the assumption that patients in higher neurologic grades may have a dysautoregulated brain that will not tolerate hypotension.

When deep hypotension is to be used, the first requirement is an experienced anesthesiologist. This technique is not to be used by the general anesthetist without specialized neurosurgical experience. If volatile anesthetics are used, moderate hypotension can be achieved simply by increasing the anesthetic concentration; however, deep levels of hypotension cannot usually be achieved in this manner. When such levels are required, rapidly reversible agents must be used.[25] Our favorite agent has been sodium nitroprusside. The primary drawback of nitroprusside is cyanide toxicity, but this is not a problem when the agent is used for a short period of time. Fast, reliable, and extremely controllable levels of hypotension can be achieved with nitroprusside.

Nitroglycerin is just as effective in some patients, but we have found that approximately 50 percent of patients do not respond as well to nitroglycerin. Ganglionic blockers are also effective but we prefer not to use them because they can cause postoperative drowsiness and pupillary irregularity, which can interfere with the neurologic examination.[25]

One precaution to be kept in mind when deep hypotension is used is to be careful with subsequent hypertension in these patients. In our early experience, we had the tragic occurrence of a massive intracerebral hemorrhage when we artificially raised the blood pressure to higher than normal levels to check for hemostasis before closing the craniotomy in a patient who had been subjected to a rather prolonged period of intraoperative hypotension. We attributed this catastrophe to the fact that after a period of relatively deep hypotension, the brain became dysautoregulated and therefore subsequent hypertension caused hemorrhage.

TEMPORARY PROXIMAL OCCLUSION OR TRAPPING

For many years, neurosurgeons have used temporary proximal ligation or trapping of the artery in emergency situations such as a major rupture of the aneurysm during dissection. Such a maneuver has saved many lives but it has also resulted in much neurologic morbidity. This is because in many instances the surgeon was not prepared for temporary occlusion and the patient may have been hypotensive or dehydrated. Also, there is no time for "protective" measures to be undertaken under such circumstances. In addition, it is clear that temporary arterial occlusion is particularly dangerous at a time when the aneurysm is bleeding massively. In these instances, the aneurysm usually continues to bleed from retrograde collateral flow and, because the surgeon's suction is the path of least resistance, a good deal of the collateral circulation is suctioned away instead of perfusing the brain. It is far better to perform temporary proximal occlusion or trapping under controlled circumstances. This has been recommended by Suzuki for many years,[27,26] but it has only recently been adopted widely in aneurysm surgery. We have found this technique extremely useful and although we initially used it only for giant aneurysms or other large or complicated aneurysms that appeared very difficult to clip otherwise, we presently use it almost routinely for all large and complicated aneurysms, including most aneurysms at the top of the basilar artery.

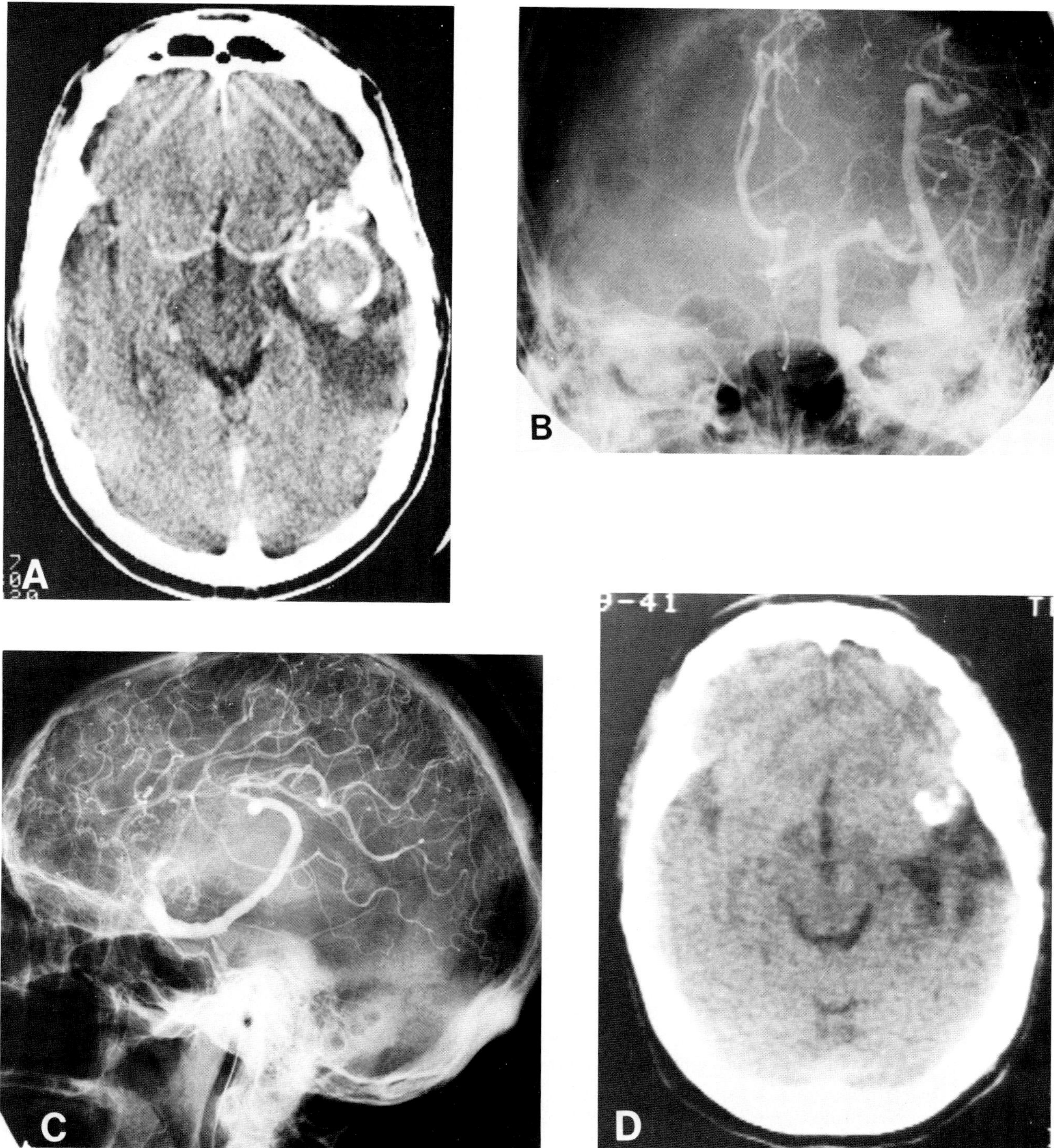

Fig. 91-7. A patient with a history of remote subarachnoid hemorrhage and progressive aphasia. The aneurysm, which initially was thought to be a "serpentine" aneurysm, was successfully ligated and excised at surgery. There was no vessel coming off the dome of the aneurysm. (A) A preoperative CT scan showing the giant, calcified, mostly thrombosed left middle cerebral aneurysm with a small residual lumen ("target sign"). (B) A left AP carotid arteriogram showing an elongated residual aneurysmal lumen suggestive of a "serpentine" aneurysm. (C) A left lateral carotid arteriogram suggesting that there is a vessel coming off the distal end of the elongated residual lumen. At surgery this vessel was adherent to the aneurysm, but it was not within it and could be separated and spared. The aneurysm could be excised without untoward effect. (D) A postoperative CT scan showing a low density area in the bed of the excised aneurysm and a residual area of calcification anteriorly that was found at surgery to be separate from the aneurysm and probably related to a previous hemorrhage.

Several points must be kept in mind when planning to use temporary arterial occlusion. It is important not to use concomitant hypotension in this situation. We usually keep the patient normotensive but others prefer to temporarily raise the pressure artificially. This can be useful if prolonged periods of arterial occlusion are contemplated. It is very important to use only low pressure clips for temporary occlusion, since it has been clearly shown that the normal and high pressure clips used for permanent aneurysmal occlusion can cause significant arterial damage, even when used for a short period of time, in normal blood vessels.[28] Several of the lines of aneurysm clips currently available include special low-force temporary clips, which are adequate for this purpose (the temporary Yasargil and Sugita clips, which we have found to very useful, are marked by a golden head or shank on the clip).

The operative approach frequently must be slightly altered when using temporary arterial occlusion. For example, if the aneurysm is a paraclinoid aneurysm where there is no possibility of intracranial proximal occlusion, the carotid bifurcation can be exposed in the neck in order to gain proximal control.[9] Others have suggested that digital carotid compression by the anesthesiologist is sufficient; however, this requires an anesthesiologist with considerable experience in this specific maneuver, and the technique is not reliable enough to be recommended for general use. It may be difficult to achieve proximal control in cases of basilar top aneurysms in which the basilar bifurcation is relatively low. It then may be necessary not only to retract the edge of the tentorium, as is done routinely for subtemporal exposure, but also to cut the tentorium for some distance. In these instances, it is important to divide the tentorium behind the insertion of the fourth nerve. Extreme care must be taken not to injure this very fragile structure.

In cases of middle cerebral aneurysms approached by opening the sylvian fissure peripherally or through the superior temporal gyrus, the aneurysm is frequently encountered before proximal control has been achieved. However, one can usually work around the base of the aneurysm without disturbing the dome and achieve proximal control by exposing a small segment of the distal M1 before proceeding with complete aneurysmal dissection.[29]

With anterior communicating aneurysms, we routinely approach the aneurysm from the side of the dominant A1 (the parent vessel from which the aneurysm fills predominantly). With this technique, we always have proximal control of at least the major afferent vessel before aneurysmal dissection. It is also very frequently possible to achieve control of the contralateral A1 by working in front of and under the aneurysm if the aneurysm projects superiorly or by working behind the aneurysm if the aneurysm projects anteriorly and inferiorly. Suzuki routinely uses a bifrontal approach in order to achieve easy control of both A1s and both A2s before aneurysmal dissection.[30]

Another important consideration when temporary arterial occlusion is to be used is the duration of occlusion. Suzuki routinely uses periods of 20 to 30 minutes, and he feels that periods as long as 40 minutes are quite safe provided that special measures are taken to ''protect'' the brain during the time of temporary occlusion.[27,31] These long periods are required if the entire dissection of the aneurysm is planned under temporary occlusion. However, if as much of the dissection is done as appears safe to do and temporary occlusion is reserved for the final critical phase of dissection and clip application, it is rarely necessary to exceed periods of 5 to 8 minutes of temporary occlusion. We recommend the latter technique and, in addition, we recommend that if longer periods are necessary, it may be preferable to use repeated short periods of occlusion rather than one prolonged period.

Another important consideration is the use of ''protective'' agents during temporary occlusion. Suzuki had popularized the use of the ''Sendai cocktail.''[31] This consists of a large bolus of mannitol together with perfluorochemicals and free radical scavengers such as vitamin E. Barbiturates have also been used frequently for this purpose. They can be used as a bolus infusion (i.e., 200–300 mg of pentobarbital) immediately before temporary occlusion. There is experimental evidence that bar-

biturates in this setting are helpful.[32] There is always a concern about producing hypotension with this maneuver, which is exactly the opposite of the desired effect. However, with experience the anesthesiologist can avoid this difficulty by having the patient well hydrated and by using vasopressors if necessary. When using short-acting barbiturates, the problem of drowsiness after surgery is usually not serious, although it is a concern in obese patients who sequester much of the drug in their fatty tissues. In general, we recommend using either a bolus of mannitol or a bolus of barbiturates just before the temporary occlusion; however, this may not be necessary if only a short period of occlusion, such as 4 or 5 minutes, is anticipated. The use of either or both agents is preferable if longer periods are contemplated.

WRAPPING

The technique of aneurysmal wrapping has been discussed in detail in the previous edition of this text.[33] In general this technique is possible and effective only in middle cerebral artery aneurysms that can be completely dissected circumferentially. We have never been able to completely dissect an unclippable aneurysm of the anterior communicating complex, the paraclinoid region, or the basilar artery. With microsurgery, it has become increasingly clear that most of the aneurysms that were previously wrapped can actually be clipped and that what appear to be vessels coming off the dome of the aneurysm are actually vessels coming off the neck and simply adhering to the dome. These can be dissected away from it with care under higher magnification.[29]

We therefore have had essentially no experience with aneurysmal wrapping during the last several years except for partial wrapping and reinforcement of small segments of aneurysms that are left out of the clip in order to avoid kinking of the parent vessel or compromise of one of the major divisions. In these cases, we use muslin gauze and alpha-aron glue. It is clear, however, that none of the available glues are either totally safe or perfectly effective.[34]

ANEURYSMORRHAPHY

An aneurysm that appears to be too large to be clipped occasionally can be clipped after simple decompression of the fundus by continuous suction through a small needle introduced directly into the aneurysm, as suggested by Flamm.[35] In other instances, aneurysmorrhaphy will allow the blind pouch to be clipped or sutured after the bulk of the aneurysm has been removed. This is particularly true in cases in which there is a hard atherosclerotic plaque at the neck of the aneurysm or in which there is partial thrombosis that will make it impossible or dangerous to attempt to clip the aneurysm because of the risk of embolization into the parent artery. Obviously, complete trapping of the aneurysm is necessary before aneurysmorrhaphy. The period of trapping is usually longer than the short periods required for clipping. The use of some form of protection therefore is necessary. There has been some experience with cardiopulmonary bypass under these circumstances but except for the results in one center,[36] the morbidity with this technique has been significant.[19]

When aneurysmorrhaphy is to be carried out, we prepare the patient with volume expansion and increase the blood pressure with pressor agents. We then give the patient a bolus of mannitol (50 g) and a large bolus of barbiturates (300–500 mg). In addition, a constant infusion of barbiturates is maintained during the period of trapping. Others have suggested performing a bypass graft in anticipation of a prolonged period of trapping for aneurysmorrhaphy even though it is anticipated that the parent vessel will be spared.[21]

The technique of aneurysmorrhaphy is very difficult and cannot be described in detail here. Extreme caution must be used in removing the atheroma in the area of the neck, particularly if there is heavy calcification. The most important thing is not to be too aggressive in this respect because there may be no neck left to close. This happened to us on one occasion in which it was necessary to sacrifice the parent artery with resultant hemiplegia and aphasia.[37] We have found that the Cavitron ultrasonic aspirator (CUSA) is particularly useful in rapidly removing the intra-aneurysmal clot, which is usually very thick and organized and cannot be removed by simple suction.

Some form of monitoring of brain function during the prolonged period of arterial occlusion necessary for aneurysmorrhaphy is useful. We have frequently used EEG but the number of standard leads that can be placed around the larger craniotomy that is necessary for these cases is limited. Others have monitored cortical excitability[38] and cortical blood flow by thermodilution[39] and have found these techniques useful.

MULTIPLE CLIPS, TANDEM CLIPS, BOOSTER CLIPS, ULTRALONG CLIPS

Many aneurysms that initially appear unclippable can be clipped by using ingenious techniques such as tandem application of multiple clips, taking advantage of such features as the flexibility offered by the Drake fenestrations, which have been thoughtfully incorporated in the Sugita clips.[19,23] Some of these techniques, long advocated by Drake, have been beautifully illustrated in a recently published surgical atlas.[40]

The possibilities available with newly developed clips are simply too varied to be described or illustrated in detail, and the surgeon must improvise constantly because each aneurysm is slightly different. It is therefore extremely important to have an array of clips available. It also may be useful to have a sterile strong wire cutter and a diamond drill that can be used to shorten clips to the precise size necessary.[40]

Sundt has introduced special "booster" clips that can be applied over the initial clip to exert extra force at its tips in order to deal with the not infrequent situation of a clip that keeps opening up with each systole because it is not strong enough to occlude the aneurysmal neck.[41] The "ultra-long" clips developed by Sugita are also very useful for this purpose.[42]

INTRA-ANEURYSMAL THROMBOSIS OR BALLOON OCCLUSION

We have had no experience with the very specialized techniques of surgical thrombosis of intracranial aneurysms by direct or stereotactic injection of hair or wire with or without the addition of electrical induction.[43,44] These techniques are complicated and carry significant morbidity and therefore should be reserved to very specialized centers where the techniques are being refined.

Likewise, we have had no experience with occlusion of the aneurysmal lumen itself by a detachable balloon placed inside the aneurysm by either direct transmural injection or by intra-luminal catheterization.[45–47] Again, the morbidity of these procedures has been too high for them to be generally adopted at this time.[47]

INDIRECT PROCEDURES

When it appears impossible to do anything directly with the aneurysm, the surgeon must resort to an indirect method of treatment by arterial occlusion as described in detail in the previous section. When to do this is a matter of exquisite surgical judgment. No rules can be given to indicate when it is too dangerous to attempt one of the direct methods of dealing with the aneurysm and therefore the surgeon may be better off to abandon the direct attempt in favor of an indirect method. Not infrequently the surgeon becomes "committed" to direct occlusion of the aneurysm or at least to complete trapping of the aneurysm when a major rupture ensues during the attempted direct approach. Still, as has been emphasized by Drake,[19] no indirect method is as satisfactory as direct occlusion of the aneurysm when such is possible.

REFERENCES

1. Nutik S: Carotid paraclinoid aneurysms with intradural origin and intracavernous location. J Neurosurg 48:526, 1978
2. Dolenc VV: A combined epi- and subdural direct approach to carotid ophthalmic artery aneurysms. J Neurosurg 62:667, 1985
3. Dolenc VV: Direct microsurgical repair of intracavernous vascular lesions. J Neurosurg 58:842, 1983
4. Glasscock ME, Smith PG, Whitaker SR, et al: Management of aneurysms of the petrous portion of the internal carotid artery by resection and primary anastomosis. Laryngoscope 93:1445, 1983
5. Sarwar M: Abducens nerve paralysis due to giant aneurysms in the medial carotid canal. J Neurosurg 46:121, 1977
6. Heros R: Giant intracranial aneurysm, in Long DM (ed): Current Therapy in Neurological Surgery. Philadelphia, B.C. Decker, 1985, pp 80–84
7. Heros RC: Surgical management of large paraclinoid aneurysms. Contemp Neurosurg 12:1, 1983
8. Heros RC: Thromboembolic complications after combined internal carotid ligation and extra-to-intracranial bypass. Surg Neurol 21: 75, 1984
9. Heros RC, Nelson PB, Ojemann RG, et al: Large and giant paraclinoid aneurysms: Surgical techniques, complications and results. Neurosurgery 12:153, 1983
10. Swann KW, Heros RC, Debrun GM, et al: Inadvertent middle cerebral artery embolism by a detachable balloon: Management by embolectomy. Case report. J Neurosurg 64:309, 1986
11. The EC-IC Bypass Study Group. Failure of extracranial-intracranial arterial bypass to reduce the risk of ischemic stroke. N Engl J Med 313:1191, 1985
12. Sarwar M. Batnitzky S, Schecter MM. Tumorous aneurysms. Neuroradiology 12:79, 1976
13. Alksne JR, Smith RW: Stereotactic occlusion of 22 consecutive anterior communicating artery aneurysms. J Neurosurg 52:790, 1980
14. Logue V: Surgery in spontaneous subarchnoid hemorrhage. Operative treatment of aneurysm of the anterior cerebral and anterior communicating artery. Br Med J 1:473, 1956
15. Tindall BT, Odom GL: Treatment of intracranial aneurysm by proximal carotid ligation. Prog Neurol Surg 3:66, 1969
16. Tindall GT, Kapp J, Odom LG, et al: A combined technique for treating certain aneurysms of the anterior communicating artery. J Neurosurg 33:41, 1970
17. Gelber BR, Sundt TM: The treatment of intracavernous and giant

carotid aneurysms by combined internal carotid ligation and extra-to intracranial bypass. J Neurosurg 52:1, 1980

18. Spetzler RF, Schuster H, Roski R: Elective extracranial-intracranial artery bypass in the treatment of inoperable giant aneurysms of the internal carotid artery. J Neurosurg 53:22, 1980

19. Drake C: Giant intracranial aneurysms: Experience with surgical treatment in 174 patients. Clin Neurosurg 26:12, 1979

20. Drake C: Ligation of the vertebral (unilateral or bilateral) or basilar artery in the treatment of large intracranial aneurysms. J Neurosurg 43:255, 1975

21. Sundt TM Jr, Piepgras DG: Surgical approach to giant intracranial aneurysms. Operative experience with 80 cases. J Neurosurg 51:731, 1979

22. Swearingen B, Heros RC: Fatal rupture of a thrombosed giant basilar artery aneurysm. Surg Neurol 23:299, 1985

23. Sugita K, Kobayashi S, Kyoshima K, et al: Fenestrated clips for usual aneurysms of the carotid artery. J Neurosurg 57:240, 1982

24. Segal HD, McLaurin RL: Giant serpentine aneurysm. Report of two cases. J Neurosurg 46:115, 1977

25. Albin MS: Neuroanesthesia and aneurysmal surgery, in Hopkins LM, Long DM (eds): Clinical Management of Intracranial Aneurysms. New York, Raven Press, 1982, pp 263–272

26. Onuma T, Suzuki JL: Surgical treatment of giant intracranial aneurysms. J Neurosurg 51:33, 1979

27. Yoshimoto T, Suzuki J: Intracranial definitive aneurysm surgery under normothermia and normotension—utilizing temporary occlusion of major cerebral arteries and preoperative mannitol administration.

28. Dujovny M, Wakenhut N, Kossovsky N, et al: Minimum vascular occlusive force. J Neurosurg 51:662, 1979

29. Heros RC, Ojemann RG, Crowell RM: Superior temporal gyrus approach to middle cerebral artery aneurysms: Technique and results. Neurosurgery 10:308, 1982

30. Suzuki J, Kodama N, Ebina T, et al: Surgical treatment of anterior communicating artery aneurysms: From the experiences of 346 cases, in Suzuki J (ed): Cerebral Aneurysms. Tokyo, Neuron Publishing Co., 1979, pp 238–243

31. Suzuki J, Tanaka S, Yoshimoto T: Suppression of brain swelling with mannitol and perfluorochemicals—an experimental study. Acta Neurochir 58:149, 1981

32. Selman WR, Spetzler RF, Roessman R, et al: Barbiturate-induced coma therapy for focal cerebral ischemia: Effect after temporary and permanent MCA occlusion. J Neurosurg 55:220, 1981

33. Selverstone B: Coating of intracranial aneurysms with nontoxic adherent plastics, in Schmidek HH, Sweet WH (eds): Operative Neurosurgical Techniques: Indications, Methods and Results, vol 2. New York, Grune & Stratton, 1982, pp 949–955

34. Chou SN, Ortiz-Suarez HJ, Brown WE: Techniques and material for coating aneurysms, in Wilkins RH (ed): Clinical Neurosurgery, vol 21. Baltimore, Williams & Wilkins, 1974, pp 182–193

35. Flamm ES: Suction decompression of aneurysms. Technical note. J Neurosurg 54:275, 1981

36. Silverberg GD, Reitz BA, Team AK: Hypothermia and cardiac arrest in the treatment of giant aneurysms of the cerebral circulation and hemangioblastoma of the medulla. J Neurosurg 55:337, 1982

37. Heros RC, Kolluri S: Giant intracranial aneurysm presenting with massive cerebral edema. Neurosurgery 15:572, 1984

38. Eisenberg HM, Turner JW, Terodale G, et al: Monitoring of cortical excitability during induced hypotension in aneurysm operations. J Neurosurg 50:595, 1979

39. Carter LP, Erspamer R, White WL, et al: Cortical blood flow during craniotomy for aneurysm. Surg Neurol 17:203, 1982

40. Sugita K: Microsurgical Atlas. Tokyo, Springer-Verlag, 1985

41. Sundt TM Jr, Piepgras DG, Marsh WR: Booster clips for giant and thickening aneurysms. J Neurosurg 60:761, 1984

42. Sugita K, Kobayashi S, Inoue T, et al: Characteristics and use of ultralong aneurysm clips. J Neurosurg 60:145, 1984

43. Hosobuchi Y: Direct surgical treatment of giant intracranial aneurysms. J Neurosurg 51:743, 1979

44. Mullan S: Experiences with surgical thrombosis of intracranial berry aneurysms and carotid cavernous fistulas. J Neurosurg 41:657, 1974

45. Debrun G, Lacour P, Caron JP, et al: Detachable balloon and calibrated lead balloon techniques in the treatment of cerebral vascular lesions. J Neurosurg 49:635, 1978

46. Serbinenko FA: Balloon catherization and occlusion of major cerebral vessels. J Neurosurg 41:125, 1974

47. Debrun G, Fox A, Drake, et al: Giant unclippable aneurysms: Treatment with detachable balloons. AJNR 2:167, 1981

CHAPTER 92

Functional Neurosurgery

Philip L. Gildenberg

FUNCTIONAL NEUROSURGERY is that aspect of neurosurgery that acts to change neurophysiologic function by surgical means. To discuss the indications for such procedures it is necessary to consider alternate nonsurgical treatments as well.

The usual modalities by which function of the nervous system can be changed are ablation and stimulation of specific sites. Ablation, or the production of a lesion, is accomplished by the application of heat, cold, electrical energy, or radiation. Radiation also can be used either by local insertion of a radioisotope or by focusing large amounts of radiation on a small field within the nervous system. Temporary or permanent functional changes of the nervous system also may follow application of a chemical or pharmacologic agent, which can be administered on a short-term basis by injection or on a long-term basis by the use of a chemode, i.e., an implanted reservoir from which minute quantities of an agent may leech over a protracted period of time. The present discussion will concentrate primarily on ablation and stimulation procedures in clinical use.

Classically, functional neurosurgery has concerned conditions in which the function of the nervous system has become defective, so that restoration of normal function or obliteration or modification of symptoms that represent an abnormal expression of nervous system function is desirable. Thus, the problems with which functional neurosurgery have been most involved have been intractable pain, movement disorders, disorders of muscle tone, affective disorders, and epilepsy.

Through the present time, the best we have been able to accomplish with functional neurosurgery has been the alleviation of symptoms. However, techniques presently under investigation may make it possible to treat the disease itself by replacing deficient neurotransmitters through the stereotactic insertion of tissues that produce those transmitters. Similar techniques may make it possible some day to repair interrupted pathways by the injection of embryonal tissue.

STEREOTACTIC SURGERY

Stereotactic surgery involves techniques whereby an apparatus is employed to direct an electrode to an intracerebral target to alter the function of structures deep within the brain with minimal damage to overlying structures. Before the advent of stereotactic surgery, it was necessary to ablate a structure under direct vision.

In 1908, Horsley and Clarke[1] devised a technique that allowed an electrode to be introduced into specific subcortical structures in experimental animals. Their technique required the preparation of an atlas, which pictured brain slices in a measured relationship to landmarks on the skull of the animal, to ensure that the electrode would consistently reach a point in space that had a specific relationship to the landmarks.

To accomplish this, three planes at right angles to each other are employed to form a system of Cartesian coordinates. The horizontal or basal plane is the plane that intersects both external auditory canals and the inferior orbital ridge. The experimental apparatus is fashioned to secure the head of the animal by means of ear plugs placed in the auditory canals and tabs that rest on the inferior orbital ridges, thus aligning the head with the horizontal plane. The second plane, at right angles to the basal plane, lies in the midsagittal plane of the brain. The third plane lies at right angles to the first two, and also passes through the external auditory canals. Thus, a given point in space can be defined as lying X millimeters to the right or left of the midsagittal plane, Y millimeters in front of the interaural plane, and Z millimeters above the basal plane, and only one point in space can satisfy this description. It is thereby possible to identify the coordinates of a given anatomic structure from an atlas of brains sliced parallel to one of the reference planes and a measured distance from that plane; the relationship to the other planes is indicated by millimeter scales along the borders of the brain slices.

With the Horsley-Clarke apparatus it became possible to introduce an electrode into a subcortical structure with a reasonable degree of certainty, without destroying the overlying tissue. Modifications of this device are standard tools essential for neurophysiologic investigations.

Attempts to apply this system to humans were difficult. Since there is great variability between the landmarks on the skull and anatomic structures, accuracy of the system did not approach that required for clinical use.

In 1947, Spiegel et al.[2] related the coordinate system to internal landmarks within the human brain, allowing stereotactic techniques to be applied to humans. Originally, they took as their landmarks the foramen of Monro and the pineal gland, as seen on pneumoencephalograms.

The system currently in use is based on improved radiologic techniques. In this system the basal plane passes through a line drawn between the anterior and posterior commissures at right angles to the midsagittal plane. The third reference plane is at right angles to these two planes, and either passes through the posterior commissure or through the midpoint of the intercommissural line (Figure 92-1). Some authors use a line between the posterior commissure and the foramen of Monro.

OPERATIVE NEUROSURGICAL TECHNIQUES
ISBN 0-8089-1862-1

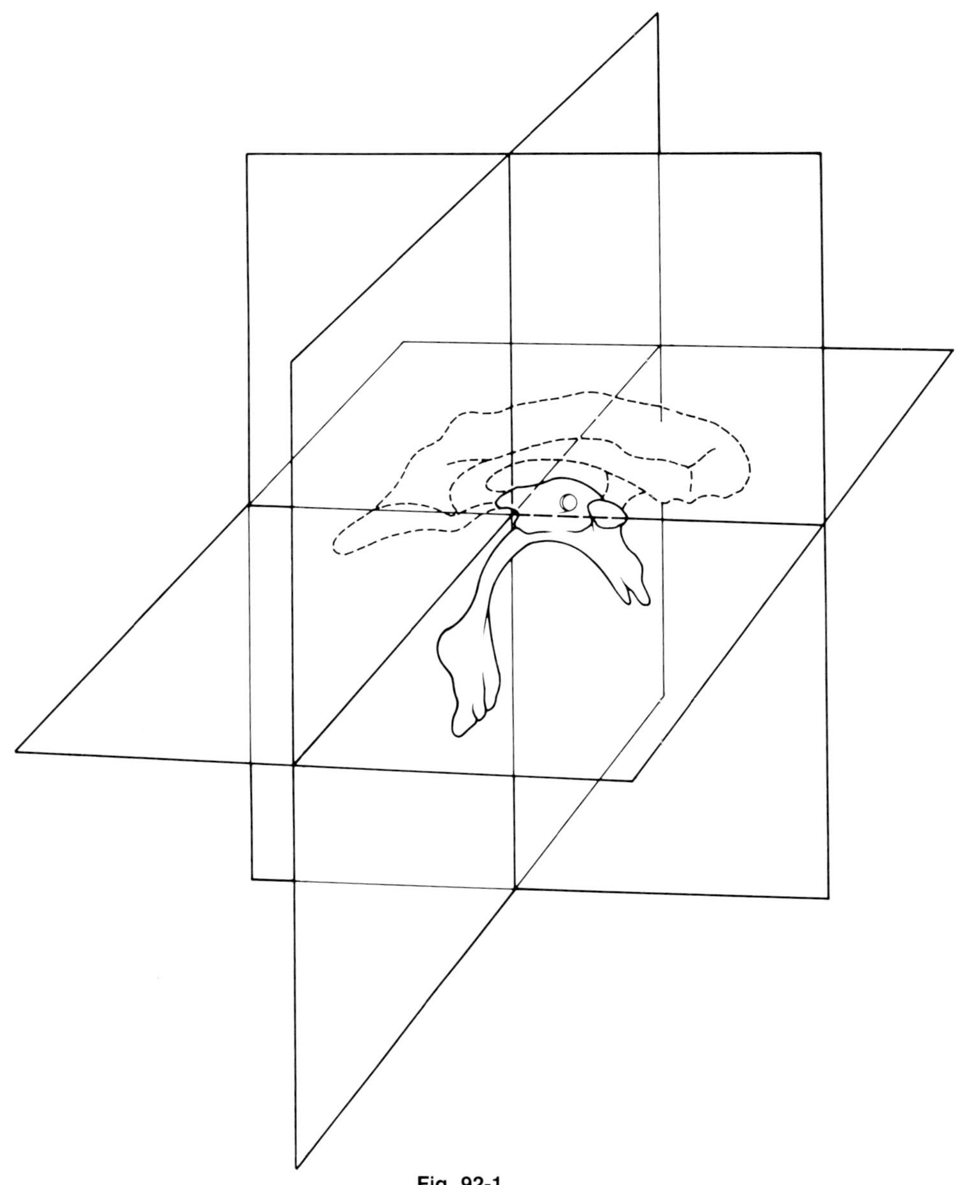

Fig. 92-1.

Landmarks are visualized by a pneumoencephalogram performed just before surgery, or by instilling air or, more frequently, contrast material through a ventriculostomy inserted during surgery.

Several techniques are presently under development which may make it possible to determine the coordinates of functional stereotactic landmarks based on landmarks visualized by CT scanning or magnetic resonance imaging.[3]

STEREOTACTIC ATLAS

Several atlases of the human brain have been published. The first, that of Spiegel and Wycis, published in 1952,[4] is still quite useful. One of the more widely used, however, is that of Schaltenbrand and Bailey,[5] which consists of beautifully enlarged photographs of brain slices with overlays outlining anatomic structures. The excellent atlas by Talairach et al.[6] is used by many Europeans, and recently some atlases have been specifically directed to the diencephalon[7–9] or the brain stem and cerebellum.[10]

A key factor in the use of stereotactic atlases is the considerable variability between brains. The coordinates obtained from a stereotactic atlas provide only approximations of where a given anatomic structure is most likely to be found. For this reason, most atlases include variability tables so that corrections in coordinates can be made for a patient whose brain does not have the same general characteristics as the representative sections appearing in the atlas.

Most recently, stereotactic atlases are digitized and stored in a three-dimensional configuration in a computer. Programs have been devised that allow not only identification of specific structures and anatomic variability, but also artificial distortion of the atlas to conform to the configuration of structures such as the thalamus, theoretically increasing the accuracy even more.[11,12]

Consequently, one must differentiate between anatomic accuracy and stereotactic or mechanical accuracy. A well-constructed stereotactic apparatus can bring the tip of an electrode to within 1 mm of a specific coordinate. Whether the desired anatomic structure lies at that coordinate is a reflection

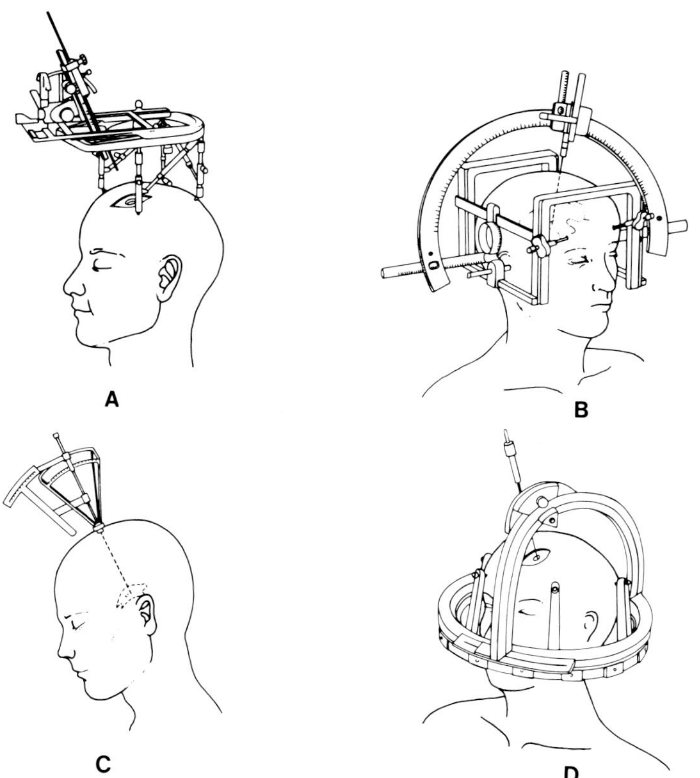

Fig. 92-2. The three basic types of stereotactic apparatus.

of anatomic variability, and this factor must be considered in every stereotactic procedure. Consequently, physiologic verification of the location of the electrode tip by recording or stimulation techniques is necessary whenever possible.

TYPES OF STEREOTACTIC APPARATUS

There are four basic types of stereotactic apparatus (Figure 92-2). The most common is the arc type (C), in which the target point lies at the center of an arc along which the electrode holder moves. The electrode approaches the brain in a direction perpendicular to the tangent of the arc, so that it is always directed toward a target point at the center of that arc. If the electrode is advanced from the arc by a distance equal to the radius of the arc, the electrode is accurately guided to the target point. If the arc is positioned so that the desired anatomic target point coincides with the mechanical target point at the center of the arc, the electrode can be advanced to the desired structure.

The three most widely used commercially available stereotactic apparatuses use the arc principle.[13] The Leksell apparatus[14] has a coordinate system radiologically indicated on a rectangular frame attached to the patient's head; the coordinate system of the frame can be related to the reference planes on the x-ray films. The arc is attached to the rectangular frame so the center of the arc lies at the desired coordinate where the anatomic target is most likely located. The Riechert apparatus[15] has a basal ring to which the patient's head is secured, and the arc is positioned in relation to the basal ring so that the target point lies at the appropriate coordinates. The Todd-Wells apparatus[16] works in a reciprocal fashion. The system of arcs is in constant relation to the frame of the apparatus and the patient's head is moved in order to bring the anatomic structure to the mechanical target point.

The rectilinear type of stereotactic apparatus is based on the same principle as the Horsley-Clarke[1] and Spiegel-Wycis[2] devices (A). It provides individually for the longitudinal and vertical movements of the electrode by simple linear mechanical adjustments. Most of the rectilinear apparatuses that presently are available also provide for sagittal and transverse angle adjustments so that the electrode can be aimed and advanced to the target point along a predetermined trajectory. The center of the arc of the angular adjustment, however, does not coincide with the target point.

The aiming type of stereotactic apparatus consists of a ball joint screwed into a burr hole (B). The angles of insertion of an electrode can be adjusted and the depth of insertion of the electrode controlled so the probe can be pointed to the target and advanced into it. Since it is difficult to secure an apparatus to the edge of a burr hole, however, distortion occurs as the device is manipulated, and since angular adjustments generally are less accurate than linear adjustments, a device that depends totally on angular adjustments tends to be less accurate.

A new system is based on a complex principle of interlocking arcs, the Brown-Roberts-Wells stereotactic apparatus.[17,18] The settings for the four arcs are calculated after entering into a computer the coordinates of the target and the fiduciaries of an aiming device which can be seen on each slice of a CT scan. Although it was designed primarily for use with a CT scanner, it can also be used for functional neurosurgery, either by means of a floor stand, which makes it possible to aim the system in relationship to Cartesian coordinates related to the ventricular system, or with several techniques (which are still investigational) that relate the functional stereotactic target to anatomic structures that can be seen on CT or MRI scans.

RADIOLOGIC CONSIDERATIONS

Several radiologic considerations are crucial to stereotactic surgery. Since x-rays emanate from their source in a radial fashion rather than in parallel rays, parallax and magnification may distort the stereotactic measurements. To minimize the effects of parallax (the distortion that occurs when an object is looked at obliquely), the reference planes of the stereotactic apparatus or the brain must be aligned with the central beam of the x-ray source. This is accomplished by attaching radiopaque markers to the apparatus or to the patient's head so that superimposition of those markers on the x-ray picture verifies proper alignment.

Since the x-ray beams are radial rather than parallel, x-ray images are magnified, depending on the distance between the x-ray source and the head compared to the distance between the head and the cassette. Magnification can be minimized by holding the x-ray tube at a long distance from the subject so that the rays are more nearly parallel when they reach the subject. Systems using a shorter tube-to-cassette distance require that the magnification be measured, and the actual distances can be calculated. A radiopaque centimeter scale is positioned in the midsagittal plane or plane of reference and appears on the x-ray film so that magnification can be measured. It must be remembered, however, that cerebral structures closer to the x-ray tube will have a larger magnification than those closer to the cassette, and these differences also must be corrected.

Techniques presently being developed will allow stereotactic penetration of anatomic structures based on their direct visualization or their relationship to landmarks visualized on CT or MRI scanning. These techniques generally employ an apparatus designed particularly for CT stereotactic biopsy and follow somewhat different radiologic principles. However, such systems are not sufficiently developed to have been adopted for general use at the time of this writing and will not be discussed here.

PROCEDURE

Most functional stereotactic procedures are performed under local anesthesia so accuracy in the placement of the electrode in the proper anatomic structure can be tested and the effects of stimulation or lesion production assessed during the procedure.[19]

After the head is shaved, the apparatus is secured to the patient's head, using local anesthesia at the contact points.

The third ventricle is visualized by a pneumoencephalogram, with air instilled just before surgery, or through a burr hole with a ventricular catheter placed to instill air or contrast material. Conray or Pantopaque (metrizamide) have been used successfully but must be used with caution. If air is used, it may be necessary to instill the air under controlled pressure to visualize the posterior commissure.

Anteroposterior (AP) and lateral x-ray films are taken. The midline of the third ventricle is determined in relation to the coordinate system of the apparatus so that appropriate lateral corrections can be made.

The anterior and posterior commissures are identified on the lateral x-ray films, and a line is drawn between the two. The intended target point, determined from an atlas, is measured from those reference lines and marked on the AP and lateral x-ray studies.

The apparatus is adjusted by a series of progressive approximations. Some arc-type apparatuses have an indicator that is visualized on the AP or lateral films to designate the mechanical target point. With other apparatuses it is necessary to secure a probe in the electrode holder and advance that probe until it just touches the scalp or burr hole; a line is drawn on the AP and lateral x-ray films through and beyond the image of the probe to indicate the trajectory. The apparatus is readjusted to bring the electrode trajectory to the intended coordinates. Another pair of AP and lateral x-ray films is taken to determine whether the adjustment is accurate. Finer and finer adjustments are employed until the electrode carrier is accurately pointed to the target.

Depending on the procedure, the ventriculostomy burr hole may be used to insert the electrode, or a second may be made. The dura is coagulated and incised, and the electrode is advanced to the intended target point. Anteroposterior and lateral films are taken with the electrode in position to verify the accuracy of electrode placement.

When the electrode is at the proper coordinates, it is usually desirable and necessary to employ physiologic verification to ensure that the proper anatomic structure has been impaled. If the intended target has identifiable electrical activity, such as the amygdala, depth EEG recording can provide verification. Indeed, it may be advantageous to perform such recordings as the electrode is advanced to the target point so that the appropriate change in spontaneous electrical activity can signal entrance into the desired structure. An area of abnormal electrical activity or cessation of electrical activity may characterize the target structure and may be used as a physiologic marker.

Single units have been successfully recorded during stereotactic surgery. This is of considerable research interest, but because the population of cells sampled is quite small, single-unit recording may not be of general clinical help during surgery, except for the recording of bursts of spontaneous activity synchronous with tremor during thalamotomy.[20] There is a great deal of extraneous electrical noise when attempts are made to record with a microelectrode or semi-microelectrode. Changes in the level of this noise can be employed to determine when the electrode is moving through the interface from one structure to another and to demonstrate that the thalamus has been entered.[20,21]

If the electrode is to be inserted into a specific somatosensory relay nucleus, such as the ventral posterolateral nucleus or the intralaminar nucleus of the thalamus, potentials evoked by stimulation of peripheral nerves are helpful indicators that these structures have been entered.

Without employing elaborate recording equipment, or in an operating room where the electrical environment is not favorable for intraoperative recording, considerable information can be obtained from stimulation. Tasker et al.[22] have produced maps based on the subjective response of patients to stimulation as an electrode is advanced within the thalamus. Contralateral motor responses can be helpful in indicating the proximity of an electrode to the internal capsule and the distribution of motor fibers therein.[23] Extraocular movements may indicate an electrode approach that is too close to oculomotor fibers.

Attempts have been made to define borders of anatomic structures by measuring electrical impedance. This can be helpful in identifying when the ventricle has been entered, but the difference of impedance between the subnuclei is not adequately specific to be helpful.

Perhaps the most gratifying physiologic test for proper electrode placement is the influence that mechanical introduction of the electrode into the proper target may have on abnormal movements. For example, patients with Parkinsonian tremor may have an abrupt cessation of tremor as the electrode reaches its target, and these patients generally have a good result when the lesion is made at that point.

If the lesion is to be made by freezing, it is possible to have a temporary cessation of activity when the area is cooled only slightly.[24] The size of the cryoprobe is large, however, and may produce suppression of activity by its insertion alone. Since brain tissue is an excellent insulator, the steep thermal gradient confines the reversibly cooled tissue to a very narrow radius.

Once the electrode is inserted to the proper target, a lesion may be produced by local ablation, or a chronic stimulating electrode may be inserted.

Several methods are used to produce lesions within the central nervous system. The most common employs a radiofrequency current, a rapidly alternating current of 50,000 to 2,000,000 Hz. As this current passes through the tissue adjacent to the electrode, where the current concentration is greatest, it sets ions oscillating at frequencies where the friction produces heat within the tissues. If the heat produced exceeds 45°–50°C, a permanent lesion results. A thermistor is built into the electrode tip to monitor the temperature so the strength of the radiofrequency current can be adjusted to produce a controlled lesion. The maintenance of 80° C for 60 to 90 seconds will produce a consistent and predictable lesion. The size of the lesion may be varied by using electrodes of different sizes, with larger electrodes distributing the current and heat more widely.[25]

An alternate means of producing a lesion is with a cryoprobe. Typically, the metallic probe contains several thermistors at the tip that feed back to a system of valves to allow the circulation of liquid nitrogen through the probe to cool the tissue to a predetermined level.[24] Tissue frozen at $-70°C$ for 3 minutes produces a consistent lesion.[26] The cryoprobe is less versatile than the radiofrequency electrode, precluding stimulation or recording through the probe. In addition, probes are not available to produce extremely small lesions.

Direct current now is rarely used for the production of lesions because of its inherent danger. A sudden interruption or change in current flow can cause damaging stimulation to the patient's brain and heart. Nevertheless, the use of direct current is of historical importance, since it was used both by Horsley and Clarke[1] and then by Spiegel and Wycis.[2] It is still used in research laboratories and occasionally for producing small discrete lesions in stereotactic surgery, since it is possible to produce a much smaller controlled lesion. Perhaps the best and most thorough discussion of the use of direct current to produce lesions in the brain appeared in Horsley and Clarke's original article on stereotaxis in 1908.[1]

CHRONIC STIMULATION TECHNIQUES

To accomplish chronic stimulation, or stimulation that can be applied over weeks or months, it is necessary to control the stimulation externally with a source of sufficient power. The requirements for stimulation often are complex, so that flexibility in stimulation parameters is required. Until recently, it was only possible to stimulate the nervous system chronically through percutaneous wires directly attached to an externally powered and controlled electronic stimulator. The risk of infection and the undesirability of having wires pierce the skin make such systems impractical.

A change that revolutionized functional neurosurgery was the development of implantable electronic stimulators powered and controlled from external sources. The key was radiofrequency coupling of an external power supply and control unit with an internalized radio receiver attached by subcutaneous leads to an electrode. The internal device is activated by electronic power transmitted in the radiofrequency control signal through the skin.

The implanted radio receiver converts the radiofrequency signal to individual impulses, the characteristics of which are dependent on the transmitted signal. The hand-held radio transmitter is connected to a disc-shaped antenna that can be taped to the skin overlying the subcutaneously implanted radio receiver. The carrier frequency is selected to minimize interference or inadvertent stimulation from incidental radio signals.[27] Such stimulation has been applied to stereotactically implanted electrodes within the brain, or electrodes inserted over the anterior lobe of the cerebellum,[28] or other neural structures, such as peripheral nerve or spinal cord.

Stimulation applied to nervous tissue does not mimic the physiologic activity of the stimulated structure. The stimulation parameters have been empirically determined, and may be in the range of usual discharge frequencies of a structure, may be frequencies that block rather than stimulate the structure, or may exert their effect by releasing regional transmitter substances.

Each type of neural tissue stimulated requires a different electrode design and a somewhat different technique for implantation.

IMPLANTATION TECHNIQUE

The radio receiver is housed in a subcutaneous pocket, usually situated below the clavicle or on the side of the abdomen so that the patient can hold the antenna against it while using the other hand to adjust the stimulation parameters. It is convenient to implant the stimulator just below the clavicle in women so that the antenna can be held by the brassiere strap.[29]

A subcutaneous pocket is created through a 5–7-cm skin incision, and is packed with wet sponges during the remainder of the dissection. A subcutaneous tunnel is made so that the leads from the radio receiver can be passed to the electrode site. A vascular mandrel or special instrument may be used to create the tunnel from an incision over the stimulation site to the receiver pocket. A Penrose drain is passed through the tunnel, and the electrodes or connecters are placed in the end of the Penrose drain and secured with umbilical tape. As the drain is pulled through the tunnel, the lead wires are drawn through the tunnel, and the Penrose drain is removed.

For deep-brain stimulation, the electrode consists of a multi-contact wire electrode that is stereotactically inserted into the brain.[30] The electrode is secured to a burr hole cover specifically designed for this purpose. Most deep-brain stimulating electrodes come with four contacts, and the best two contacts are selected for optimal stimulation. The procedure can be done in two stages, with expendable lead wires emerging through the scalp for a period of direct electrode stimulation on a trial basis. When permanent internalization is desired, the electrode lead wires are tunneled under the scalp to a site where they connect with the lead wires that are tunneled from the radio receiver, ordinarily housed at the infraclavicular site. The connectors lie beneath the scalp positioned so they are not uncomfortable.

Dorsal cord-stimulating electrodes were originally designed to be implanted through a one or two-level laminectomy.[29] Originally the electrode was sutured in the subarachnoid space within the dura just behind the dorsal columns, following which a watertight dural closure was attempted. There was a high incidence of cerebrospinal fluid leak and decreasing stimulation intensity, however, as presumably the electrodes became surrounded by fibrous tissue, so the electrodes were later implanted in the subdural space, without opening the arachnoid. Despite this improvement, late electrode failure sometimes occurred within 2 years, with the development of fibrous tissue around the electrode. The technique evolved by which a pocket was formed within the dura in which the electrode was sutured (endodural placement), which appeared to offer a slight advantage over the subdural or subarachnoid placement. It now appears that it is acceptable to suture the electrode epidurally, minimizing complications while still achieving adequate stimulation.

Recent developments have facilitated implantation of dorsal cord-stimulating electrodes. Percutaneous electrodes are available that can be passed into the epidural space under fluoroscopic guidance and local anesthesia.[31] The percutaneous electrode consists of a flexible insulated wire, usually the appropriate size to fit through an 18-gauge Tuohy needle. The distal 3 to 5 mm of the wire are uninsulated and form the electrode contact. Some electrodes have four separate contacts over the distal 2 cm. The pair of contacts providing the most satisfactory sensation can either be selected during a trial period of stimulation or, with some types of transmitters, may be selected electronically. The end of the wire left protruding has a bare contact to which a connector can be attached, or it may have a small extension wire that is several inches long. In the latter case the entire electrode wire is placed subcutaneously, and the extension wires are brought out through a stab wound. To convert the electrodes to a permanently implanted system, if that is desired, the extension wires are cut off, and the electrode wires themselves (which have remained in a protected subcutaneous position) are connected to the lead wires from the radio receiver.

The percutaneous electrode wires are implanted under fluoroscopic guidance. For lower extremity pain, a midthoracic placement is best. For thoracic or upper extremity pain, an upper thoracic or cervical placement may be attempted. The patient is placed in the prone position on the x-ray table. A small stab wound is made in the skin in the midline at the site of the electrode insertion. Either a monopolar system may be used with a stimulator that incorporates the indifferent electrode, or two percutaneous electrodes wires can be inserted approximately 1 level apart to form a bipolar system. The Tuohy needle is inserted into the epidural space in the midline. The electrode wires are inserted through the needle and are threaded up several segments. A stiffening wire within the electrode can be used to help guide the electrode to the proper position. When the electrode is in the correct position, the needle is removed, leaving the electrode in place.

A stimulator is attached to the lead wires so the effects of stimulation may be tested while the patient is still on the table. The electrodes are advanced, withdrawn, or repositioned until the sensation is projected to the proper area, which may take some experimentation. When the sensation is appropriate, the ends of the wire are buried in a subcutaneous pocket for later attachment under general anesthesia to a subcutaneous radio receiver.

One problem with percutaneous electrodes has been migration of the electrodes as the patient moves. If the electrode migrates to a nerve root sleeve, the sensation may be projected along the distribution of that nerve at a voltage that is too low to obtain optimal pain relief from cord stimulation. This problem has been obviated by the use of sigma-shaped percutaneous electrodes. These electrodes are straight when inserted, but when a stiffening wire is removed, they assume a curved sigma shape, which holds them in midline position in the epidural space.

INDICATIONS FOR FUNCTIONAL NEUROSURGERY

PAIN

Types of Pain

Any neurosurgeon who deals with patients with intractable pain must recognize that different types of pain require entirely different approaches. Unfortunately this all-too-obvious rule is all too frequently neglected to the disadvantage of the patient and physician. One may consider that there are three types of pain of clinical importance—acute pain, cancer pain, and chronic pain.

Acute pain is an appropriate physiologic response to tissue damage or potential tissue damage. Because acute pain is temporally self-limited, the appropriate approach is to treat the pain with analgesics and rest. The major effort is directed to treating the underlying cause of the pain. If this is done, the pain ordinarily will go away, the analgesics can be stopped, and the patient can return to his previous activities.

Cancer pain may be considered to be continually recurrent acute pain. Treatment involves the aggressive use of analgesics or narcotics. Neurosurgical management usually involves ablation or interruption of pain pathways and, occasionally, chronic stimulation.

Patients with cancer usually are anxious or depressed. Treatment also must be directed to the emotional welfare and stability of the patient in a comprehensive fashion. Tranquilizers benefit the anxiety, antidepressants may be helpful, and hypnotics may serve to secure the patient adequate rest.

Chronic pain may be defined as pain that lasts more than 3 to 6 months and that has no useful biologic purpose. The original cause may have left some residual damage or may have healed. Analgesics, particularly narcotics, may complicate the picture with a superimposed addiction, may contribute to depression, and are not appropriate for chronic pain. Patients with chronic pain frequently are depressed and regressed, and the psychologic aspects of the patient's problems often are more significant than the actual physical impairment. The pain may be perpetuated by psychiatric considerations, so that neurosurgical procedures are most often doomed to failure.

There is little use for ablative neurosurgical procedures in the management of chronic pain, and stimulation procedures are useful only in a small, well-selected group of patients.

The key to neurosurgical management of chronic pain does not lie in the technical aspects of surgical operations. The key is in patient selection. Any neurosurgeon who takes the responsibility for managing patients with pain also must take the responsibility for evaluating and attending to the multitude of psychiatric problems that surround a patient in a state of pain. It behooves the neurosurgeon dealing with chronic pain to have alternate nonsurgical methods of management available, either personally or through close colleagues.

Anatomy of Pain

Pain is a complex sensation, in contradistinction to other sensory modalities. The pathways concerning the perception of pain are multiple,[32] and it is the interaction of these pathways that allows the sensation of pain to come to consciousness. Because of the complexity of the system, pain can be modified by numerous factors, such as mental concentration, emotional tone, and whether one anticipates feeling pain or not.

Most of the information we have about ascending pain pathways relates to acute pain. The perception of chronic pain is far more complex, and may not always involve pain pathways.

A noxious stimulus is defined as one that has the potential to produce tissue damage and physiologically results in the perception of acute pain in the conscious subject. The pathologic condition that produces acute pain often is related to tissue damage, such as a laceration or fracture, inflammation, or tearing of tissue, and may produce acute pain when it reaches the threshold of the small peripheral nerve fibers. Large nerves, as a rule, have a lower threshold to natural and electrical stimulation so that stimulation strong enough to stimulate small fibers is also suprathreshold for the larger nerve fibers that relate to somatic sensations other than pain.

The sensory nerves enter the spinal cord via the segmental roots. Melzack and Wall[33] have described a gate or neurophysiologic arrangement at the dorsal root entry zone, that determines whether the pain pathways will fire. Because of this gating mechanism, there is competition between the large and small nerve fibers to determine whether the pain pathways fire. If the stimulus is mild or nonpainful so that the large fibers predominate, the gate will remain closed. If the intensity of the stimulus increases to the point where the small fibers predominate, the gate opens and pain is perceived.

Because pain perception depends in part on the balance between the large and small fibers, one can treat pain either by decreasing the firing of a small fiber (as with local anesthetic) or by increasing the firing of a large fiber (when you rub it, it feels better). Hence, it is possible to increase the firing of large cells by applying a nonpainful stimulus peripherally or by stimulating the dorsal columns of the spinal cord, in which case the impulse proceeds downward in a retrograde fashion (in addition to upward) to help close the gate at each spinal segment. There is further evidence that similar gating mechanisms occur higher in the nervous system, as in subthalamic levels of the brain stem.[34,35]

For the purposes of explaining ablative procedures useful in the treatment of pain, particularly cancer pain, one might consider that there are at least three ascending pain pathways that may fire when the gate is opened to conduct the sensation of pain to the brain, where it is perceived.

The neospinothalamic tract, or lateral spinothalamic tract, is the best known. The cells of origin lie in the posterior horn just anterior to the substantia gelatinosa, cross the midline in the anterior white commissure within a few segments, and ascend in the contralateral anterolateral quadrant of the spinal cord through the medial lemniscus to the ventral posterolateral nucleus of the thalamus. Because pain sensation running in this tract is separate from other somatosensory modalities that ascend primarily in the dorsal columns, and because the other tracts in the anterolateral quadrant of the spinal cord can be sacrificed with minimal neurologic impairment, this pathway is a convenient target for the neurosurgical treatment of cancer pain. Interruption of this pathway results in analgesia in the area of the body represented, that is, a loss of ability to perceive pain on the contralateral body below the level of the lesion. All of the sensory modalities from the body are intermingled in the ventral posterolateral (and ventral posteromedial) nucleus of the thalamus, where they synapse in a somatotopic array with neurons, which then project to the primary somatosensory area of the postcentral gyrus of the cortex. It appears that pain is brought to consciousness at thalamic levels or below, since interruption of this final neuron or the cortex may not alleviate the pain, although it may distort it or make it less localized.

The paleospinothalamic tract involves the same peripheral and spinal neurons as the neospinothalamic tract. The spinal neurons, however, give off collaterals to the reticular formation at the pons and midbrain levels to form the multisynaptic paleospinothalamic pathway, which ascends to those areas concerned with emotion, the hypothalamus, the intralaminar nuclei of the thalamus, the centrum medianum and parafascicularis nuclei, and the limbic lobe, which includes the cingulate gyrus, the hippocampus, and the amygdala.[36] Projection is bilateral, so that a lesion on one side may affect pain on either side of the body, but the manner in which the pain is affected is somewhat different than after a neospinothalamic tract lesion. The pain from a metastatic lesion may be gone after a lesion is made in either intralaminar nucleus, but if the patient

is tested with a pin, acute pain sensation remains intact, and there is no detectable analgesia by usual methods of testing.

The archispinothalamic system is far less defined. There appears to be a multisynaptic pathway ascending in the spinal cord through the reticular formation to perhaps the same areas of the diencephalon and cerebrum as the paleospinothalamic tract, including the limbic system. There is no good anatomic demonstration of the location of this pathway within the spinal cord, but recent evidence suggests that, at least in some patients, this multisynaptic pathway may ascend as a relatively compact bundle somewhere near the central canal.[37] Interruption of this pathway at spinal levels may provide the same type of relief as a lesion of the paleospinothalamic pathway, that is, relief of pain without corresponding analgesia.

Curiously, a lesion in the limbic lobe, such as an interruption of the cingulate gyrus, may be of help in managing certain types of pain. The patient may appear to be comfortable and may no longer require narcotics; when asked, however, he may relate that the pain still exists, "but it doesn't bother me anymore." Thus, a lesion in the limbic system may relieve the suffering associated with the pain without relieving the pain itself.

In addition to the ascending pain pathways, there is a descending pain system, which appears to be related to the inhibition of pain. It was discovered in rats that stimulation of the area around the aqueduct at midbrain levels produced analgesia, so that the rats did not respond to noxious stimuli, so-called stimulation-produced analgesics (SPA).[38,39] It was verified in patients that stimulation just lateral to the posterior wall of the third ventricle and the periaqueductal gray matter may lead to relief from chronic pain or cancer pain, but not produce analgesia,[30,40,41] as discussed in the chapter by Hosobuchi in this text.

Deep-Brain Stimulation

A number of sites have been found that produce analgesia when stimulated. The most effective are in the ventrolateral periaqueductal gray matter[42] and the gray matter just lateral to the third ventricle in the region of the posterior commissure.[41,43] In humans, the duration of pain relief may exceed the period of stimulation by hours.[41,44]

Studies suggest that opiate analgesia and stimulation-produced analgesia have so many similar characteristics that the two may operate by a common mechanism.[45,46] The most effective sites for stimulation-produced analgesia are basically those where opiate receptors have been found, particularly in the periaqueductal gray matter. There is considerable cross-tolerance between stimulation-produced analgesia and opiate analgesia, in that patients tolerant to morphine may lose the pain-relieving effects of deep-brain stimulation.[38] Also, naloxone, which is a specific narcotic antagonist, partially blocks stimulation-produced analgesia.[44,47]

It has been demonstrated that stimulation in the periventricular and periaqueductal area causes the release of endorphins into the ventricular fluid.[41] These are the same endorphins that produce analgesia when injected into certain brain sites in experimental animals, the action of which can be blocked by narcotic antagonists such as naloxone.[48] Interestingly, stimulation-produced analgesia and stimulation-produced pain relief in patients also can be blocked by naloxone, which suggests that such analgesia may depend on the release of endorphins.[38]

The procedure of chronic deep-brain stimulation of the

Table 92-1.

Procedure	Clinical indication	Target	Landmark	Coordinates (mm) AP	Lateral	Depth
Deep-brain stimulation	Pain	Periventricular gray	Post. comm.	A1	6	−2 to −3
Deep-brain stimulation	Denervation pain, face	VPM	Mid AC-PC	P8	8	+3 to +5
Deep-brain stimulation	Denervation pain, body	VPL	Mid AC-PC	P9	10 to 12	+2 to +5
Deep-brain stimulation	Denervation pain, body	Post. limb int. capsl.	Post. comm.	0	25	+1 to +2
Mesencephalotomy	Pain	Medial lemniscus	Post. comm.	P5	5 to 10	−5
Basal thalamotomy	Pain	Extralemniscular fibers	Post. comm.	A1	12	0 to +11
				A4	11	+2 to +13
Medial thalamotomy	Pain	Intralaminar-CM nu.	Post. comm.	A9	9	+2 to +13
Dorsomedian thalamotomy	Pain	Dorsomedial nu.	Post. comm.	A4	4	+2 to +10
VL thalamotomy	Affective disorders Tremor Dystonia	VL (V.o.p) nu.	Mid AC-PC	P2	11.5	+3
VL thalamotomy	Rigidity	VL (V.o.a) nu.	Mid AC-PC	A2	9.5	+3
V.i.m thalamotomy	Tremor	V.i.m. nu	Post. comm.	A5	15	0
Campotomy	Tremor Rigidity Dystonia Cerebral palsy Seizures	Forel's field	Mid AC-PC	0	6	−2
Pallidotomy	Hemiballism Cerebral palsy Salaam convulsions	Globus pallidus	Ant. comm.	P2	10	0
Cingulotomy	Pain Obsessive-compulsion	Cingulum	Ant. horn	P30	Lat. edge	+5
				P30	8 medial to lateral edge	+5
	Anxiety			P18	Lateral edge	+5
	Depression			P18	8 medial to lateral edge	+5
Anterior capsulotomy	Obsessive-compulsion	Ant. limb of int. capsule	Ant. clinoid	A15	6	+10
				A15	6	+15
				A15	14	+10
Amygdalotomy	Temporal lobe seizures Salaam convulsions	Amygdala	Tip of temporal horn	A5	5 medial to lateral edge	3 above inferior border

periventricular gray matter involves the stereotactic insertion of four-contact stimulating electrodes, as elaborated in the chapter by Hosobuchi and earlier in this chapter. The usual target point (Table 92-1) lies about 1 mm posterior to the posterior commissure, 2 to 3 mm below the posterior commissure, and 2 to 3 mm lateral to the wall of the third ventricle (usually 6 mm lateral to the midline), although there is not complete agreement about those specific coordinates.[31,41] The electrode is secured to the burr hole with a special burr hole cover. The four contacts of the electrodes are connected to a special adaptor with four leads that are pulled through a needle hole in the scalp just above the ear. The incision at the burr hole is sutured. The following days or weeks can be used to test different stimulus parameters in order to determine whether the patient has pain relief from stimulation, and the optimal stimulus parameters and electrode

combination to obtain such relief. When this has been accomplished, the system is internalized, usually under general anesthesia. The scalp incision is re-opened, the protruding wires are cut off, and the special adaptor is removed. A radio receiver is placed in a pocket below a clavicle and the lead wire is tunneled to emerge at the scalp incision. The two leads from the receiver are connected to the two leads of the electrode that have been selected to provide optimal stimulation, and the connection is sealed with Silastic and the incisions closed.

In addition to stimulation of the periventricular system producing pain relief, chronic deep-brain stimulation of the somatosensory system may afford relief of denervation pain. Electrodes are inserted into either the ventral posterior nucleus of the thalamus or the posterior limb of the internal capsule. It is hypothesized that the pain is the result of deprivation of diencephalic or cortical sensory areas from the inhibitory influences of the normally occurring sensory input. Substituting electrical stimulation for that absent sensory input may provide the patient with pain relief.

The coordinates for the somatosensory targets vary, depending upon the area of the body involved, because of the somatotopic distribution of fibers. For facial pain, the target is in the ventral posteromedial nucleus of the thalamus, and the initial coordinates are 8 mm posterior to the midpoint of the intercommissural (AC-PC) line, 8 mm lateral and 3 to 5 mm above the intercommissural line.[30,43] For pain in the extremities, the target is in the ventral posterolateral nucleus, and the coordinates are 9 mm posterior to the midpoint of the intercommissural line, 10 to 12 mm lateral and 2 to 5 mm above the (AC-PC) line. Alternatively, the electrode can be placed in the posterior limb of the internal capsule, in the coronal plane of the posterior commissure, 25 mm lateral and 1 to 2 mm above the AC-PC line.[30]

The electrodes should be inserted under local anesthesia so that stimulation can be applied and the coordinates adjusted as physiologically indicated.

Management of Cancer Pain

Patients with cancer who complain of pain deserve a comprehensive program. Not only must the pain be dealt with specifically, but the emotional changes that accompany both the pain and a terminal illness must be recognized and managed.

In addition to attention to the patient's emotional welfare, the initial phase in the management of patients with cancer pain is pharmacologic. Analgesics should be given, the type and amount depending upon the amount of pain and tolerance. The patient's prognosis should be taken into account when prescribing narcotics. If the patient is expected to live for a long time, pain medications must be alternated or the dosage increased cautiously so that tolerance does not interfere prematurely with pain relief. The only narcotics that are absorbed well by mouth are codeine and methadone. If other narcotics are used orally, their dosage must be appropriate to that route of administration. For patients with severe pain who are in the advanced state of malignancy, methadone or one of the newer long-lasting oral morphine preparations can be extremely useful analgesics.

Morphine may provide prolonged relief of cancer pain when administered directly to the central nervous system. Techniques have been devised to provide repeated small doses of morphine in the spinal epidural space and sometimes also into the ventricle, but such techniques are beyond the scope of this chapter and will be discussed in Chapter 100.

All narcotics are depressant drugs. This may compound significantly the emotional depression that results from the disability and the realization that an illness is terminal. Depression must be recognized and treated. Psychiatric counseling can sometimes be of help, particularly when it involves groups of cancer patients and their families. Antidepressant medication, such as the tricyclic antidepressants, may be extremely helpful, but must be given in sufficient dosage and for at least several weeks before their effect can be assessed. If the antidepressants are given at bedtime, their immediate sedative effect can also help ensure that the patient will get adequate rest.

Anxiety frequently accompanies depression in cancer patients. Again, psychiatric care or tranquilizers may be of benefit, but one must caution that the latter may increase depression, particularly when they are used in combination with narcotics. If tranquilizers are added to the patient's program, it is often possible to decrease the dose of narcotics, which may prolong their effectiveness. It is important to recognize that patients who are anxious or depressed may request narcotics for the soporific effects rather than the analgesic, and tranquilizers may be more effective and more appropriate for that use.

Patients who are fatigued tolerate pain less well, so that pain and anxiety may be considerably increased unless adequate sleep is obtained. Rather than relying solely on narcotics to ensure adequate sleep, hypnotics, especially nonbarbiturate sedatives, may be a beneficial addition to the overall program.

The principle of functional neurosurgical management of cancer pain is that interruption of the ascending pain pathways by ablative procedures may afford pain relief. The choice of procedure is determined by the distribution of the cancer pain more than its specific characteristics. The following general rules apply to the selection of procedures:

1. The most caudal or peripheral procedure that affects the entire area of pain is preferable.
2. If a patient has a minor pain in an area other than the major pain, one can anticipate an increase in the minor pain when the major pain is alleviated.
3. The less change in sensory function the better; a cordotomy usually is superior to multiple rhizotomies, since it leaves the patient with normal somatosensory sensation except for pain.
4. You should not talk a patient into having a pain procedure.
5. Be sure the patient is told of potential side-effects in detail and in advance—pain is forgotten once it is relieved, and side-effects that may have seemed minor before surgery become extremely distressing.
6. Anticipate disappointment; patients often blame all of their disability on the pain, but if the pain is alleviated and they still feel seriously ill and weak, they must acknowledge they are ill; such patients remember how they felt before the pain began, often months before, and may unrealistically expect to be returned to that vigorous state.

Various ablative procedures will be considered in ascending anatomic order.

Sensory rhizotomy involves the section of dorsal roots. Because almost every area of the body is innervated by multiple segments, it is necessary to section several roots in order to obtain relief. Consequently, almost the only indication for sensory rhizotomy in patients with cancer pain is a case in which a specific nerve or plexus of nerves is infiltrated by tumor. Before performing the surgery, it may be possible to evaluate the patient's response to a rhizotomy by blocking those nerve roots to be cut. Since sensory rhizotomy results in a loss of all modalities of sensation, the area is left insensitive, which many patients find even less tolerable than their original pain. An extremity should never be denervated completely, since the loss of proprioception feedback may cause the extremity to flail about involuntarily.

Cordotomy involves interrupting the lateral spinothalamic tract within the spinal cord. It can be done by exposing the spinal cord by laminectomy at a level above the innervation of the affected area and incising the anterolateral quadrant of the spinal cord under direct vision, or by introducing an electrode into the spinal cord at cervical levels, using a percutaneous technique as described in Chapter 105.

Cordotomy is perhaps the most widely used neurosurgical procedure for the treatment of cancer pain. It is particularly useful if the pain is unilateral, and is generally better for somatic than visceral pain. If the pain involves a lower extremity, cordotomy can be performed at either a thoracic or cervical level, but if the pain involves the upper extremity, a high cervical cordotomy must be done. Because a lesion above the C_4 level also affects fibers concerned with respiration, high cervical cordotomy can be performed only unilaterally with safety. Cordotomy is performed far less frequently since the development of techniques for chronic epidural administration of morphine.

Cordotomy often fails to secure relief of midline pain when the spine or perineum is involved, and is particularly poor for midline pelvic pain. Risk includes weakness of the extremities ipsilateral to the lesion. If bilateral cordotomy is performed, there is a risk that bladder function will be affected, particularly if the bladder innervation is already compromised from a pelvic tumor. Some patients complain of dysesthesia in the area that become analgesic, but this does not occur often with cancer patients. Both bladder dysfunction and postcordotomy dysesthesia are less common after percutaneous cordotomy than after surgical cordotomy.[49]

Commissural myelotomy (see Chapter 104) involves bisecting the spinal cord to interrupt the fibers going to the lateral spinothalamic tract as they decussate in the anterior white commissure. Classically, it is necessary to interrupt the commissural fibers throughout those dermatomes involved with the sensation of pain. Commissural myelotomy has been found to be especially valuable for bilateral or midline pain, particularly secondary to pelvic cancer, and has achieved renewed popularity recently as microneurosurgical techniques have become available.[50,51]

It has been observed many times that patients have pain relief in excess of what would be anticipated from the area of analgesia that develops after commissural myelotomy.[50–55] Indeed, it is possible to have excellent pain relief with no detectable analgesia. This observation led to the consideration that the archespinothalamic pathway may ascend in a discrete bundle near the center of the spinal cord, that it may inadvertently be interrupted by the commissural myelotomy, and that the pain relief without analgesia may be a result of the interruption of this pathway, which has not yet been described anatomically.[56] This led to the development of procedures specifically designed to interrupt this theoretical pathway. When performed stereotactically at the cervicomedullary junction, the procedure has been called extralemniscal myelotomy, and when performed under direct surgical exposure at thoracic levels it has been given the name of limited myelotomy.

In extralemniscal myelotomy, the electrode is inserted under stereotactic control in the midline between the posterior arch of C1 and the foramen magnum, with the patient's neck flexed.[57–59] As the electrode is advanced through the midline of the spinal cord, low-current stimulation is applied to map somatotopic distribution of the fibers in the posterior columns. As the electrode is moved progressively toward the center of the cord, the sensation is projected progressively down the legs, and when it stops, it indicates that the tip of the electrode lies anterior to the posterior columns. It is at that point that a lesion is made.[59,60]

Excellent relief of pain throughout the entire body has been reported with this procedure, especially in cancer patients, with minimal complications, even though no objective analgesia may be detected postoperatively. The procedure requires the use of a stereotactic apparatus that allows penetration of the spinal cord with the head flexed, such as the Hitchcock or Leksell apparatus.

Because of the difficulty in performing this procedure with the more commonly available stereotactic apparatuses, and because it seemed reasonable to attempt interruption of this same pathway at lower levels in the spinal cord when the pain was confined to the pelvis, the procedure of limited myelotomy was developed.[61,62] This procedure has been found to be particularly helpful in patients with visceral pain of pelvic distribution, especially patients with rectal carcinoma. To date there have been no complications. There have been no posterior column symptoms, even immediately after surgery, as one often sees with extensive commissural myelotomy, and no leg weakness.

One interesting side-effect is that some of the patients with successful pain relief have great difficulty discontinuing narcotics following the procedure. They may have severe withdrawal symptoms, including sleeplessness, agitation, diarrhea, and generalized body pains, which is the opposite effect of the one seen after intralaminar thalamotomy or cingulotomy, which is characterized by easy discontinuation of narcotics. Overall, 75 percent of the patients have successful relief of cancer pain after limited myelotomy once they have gotten through the initial week of narcotic withdrawal, and none has demonstrated an area of analgesia.

Limited myelotomy is performed under general anesthesia with the patient in the prone position. A T9 or T10 laminectomy is done in order to expose the spinal cord at approximately the twelfth thoracic dermatome. It is desirable to make the lesion above the entry of the lumbosacral segments, but to avoid the midthoracic levels where the blood supply is poorest. The midline is identified under the operating microscope and a 5-mm vertical incision is made in the pia at the midline. A small blunt microdissector is introduced until the infolded pia of the anterior median fissure is palpated, usually at a depth of 6 mm. With the blunt dissector, a mechanical lesion is made in the center of the spinal cord for a length of 5 to 7 mm, slightly less than one segment. Alternatively, the dissector may be removed and a percutaneous cervical cordotomy electrode inserted into the center of the spinal cord and a lesion made, using the same parameters as for a percutaneous cordotomy. The intent is to interrupt a pathway that theoretically ascends near the central canal of the spinal cord, so it is not necessary to interrupt a significant number of commissural fibers.

Splanchnicectomy (Chapter 112) can be used for abdominal visceral pain. Pain sensation from the abdominal viscera is, to a large extent, transmitted via splanchnic nerves to the sympathetic chains and from there through the spinal cord to join the pain-conducting systems. If the cancer is confined to the abdominal viscera and does not extend below the descending colon, excellent pain relief may result from sympathetic denervation of the abdomen. Because the various abdominal sympathetic plexuses consist of a multitude of fine fibers that are extremely difficult to dissect, it is more convenient and more reliable to interrupt the sympathetic innervation just above the diaphragm.

Splanchnicectomy is perhaps the most effective procedure for pain resulting from carcinoma of the pancreas. Indeed, since pain is usually the presenting symptom and since pancreatic resection for pain relief is not usually possible, splanchnicectomy may be done at the same time as the laparotomy when tissue diagnosis is made. Under the same anesthetic, the patient is turned to the prone position and a splanchnicectomy is performed.

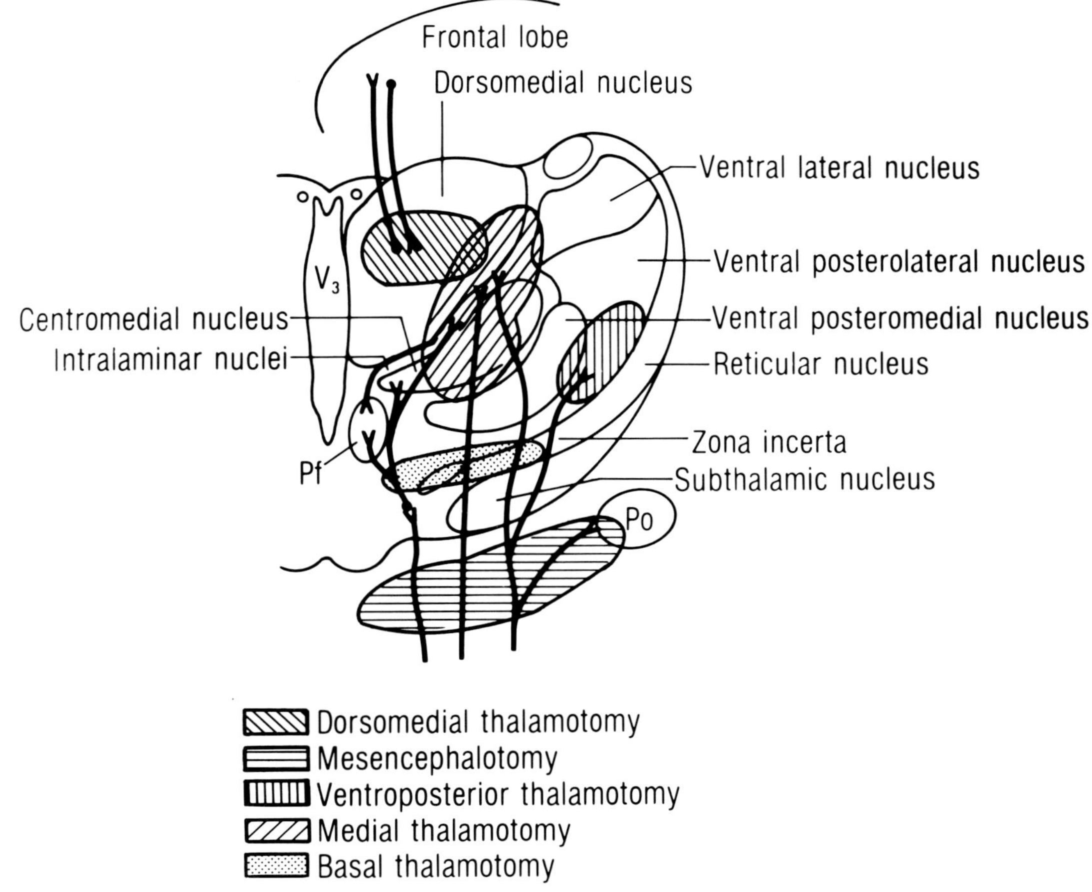

Fig. 92-3.

Medullary tractotomy involves interrupting the spinothalamic tract above spinal levels. Pain involving the head, face, or neck is obviously too high to be managed by cordotomy. The innervation of the head, however, is arranged so that pathways concerned with the perception of pain are separated from pathways involved with other modalities. Pain information that enters through the trigeminal nerve descends in the descending tract of the trigeminal nucleus as far as the upper cervical levels, where it synapses in a manner similar to that of the substantia gelatinosa in the spinal cord. This descending trigeminal tract can be interrupted in the medulla where it lies just below the posterolateral surface. This is best done with suboccipital craniotomy and direct visualization of the medulla, although certain types of stereotactic apparatus allow electrodes to be introduced through the foramen magnum to perform medullary tractotomy.

If the procedure is done with open surgery, the landmarks are somewhat indefinite, so that it may be necessary to operate under local anesthesia and to use local electrical stimulation. The lesion is made at the level of the obex. The anterior edge of the lesion is in the line of emergence of the spinal accessory nerve rootlets. The posterior border of the cut is at the lateral edge of the nucleus cuneatus, but the small groove showing the division between the nuclei may be poorly delineated. To achieve total analgesia of the mouth area, the lesion should begin ventrally, in the spinothalamic tract, and extend dorsally well into the fasciculus cuneatus.

If medullary tractotomy is performed stereotactically, the procedure is done under local anesthetic with the patient in the prone or sitting position, depending upon which stereotactic apparatus is used.[59] The electrode is angled craniad 30 degrees and is introduced 6 mm from the midline and 4 mm deep within the cord. It is necessary to use a fine electrode, 0.5–0.6 mm, since the pia may be quite firm in this area and pressure on the medulla may be uncomfortable and distort the anatomy. Once the pia has been entered, verification of the position of the electrode is obtained by electrical stimulation at 50 Hz. If the electrode lies within the tract, sensation should be projected to the face at a low stimulating current. The dorsal border of the descending trigeminal tract may be defined by the homolateral responses from the fasciculus cuneatus, and the ventral border by the contralateral responses from the spinothalamic tract. In addition to cancer pain, this procedure has been helpful to patients with postherpetic neuralgia and anesthesia dolorosa.

Because of the potential side-effects of medullary tractotomy, and because the pain may involve more than the area innervated by the trigeminal nerve, it may be preferable to use stereotactic mesencephalotomy for head and neck pain (Figure 92-3). Since patients with cancer pain often have widespread pain throughout the body, mesencephalotomy is often preferred over medullary tractotomy if either is indicated.[63]

It is preferable to make the burr hole more dorsal for mesencephalotomy than for stereotactic thalamotomy. A burr hole 2 cm behind the interaural plane will allow insertion of the electrode approximately parallel to the fibers of the medial lemniscus within the brain stem to afford maximal opportunity for interrupting those fibers without affecting surrounding structures.[64] The coordinates are 5 mm posterior to the posterior commissure, 5 mm below that structure, and 5 to 10 mm from the midline (Table 92-1).[65]

Great care must be taken to avoid pyramidal tract fibers or oculomotor fibers. If the electrode is too low or a bit medial, stimulation at 50 Hz may produce abrupt medial deviation of the eye and pupillary constriction. If the electrode is too far lateral or anterior, stimulation at 5 Hz may cause involuntary movement of the contralateral extremities.

This suggests the two most common untoward side-effects from mesencephalotomy-diplopia and contralateral weakness. Since it is necessary to interrupt lemniscal fibers, which are the extension of the lateral spinothalamic tract, it is necessary to obtain analgesia in the area of pain in order to effect pain relief. It may be necessary to reposition the electrode by stimulating at 50 Hz and noting the patient's perception of projected sensation to the appropriate part of the body to ensure effective analgesia. It is generally inadvisable to perform mesencephalotomy bilaterally, for it can leave the patient at risk from loss of the protective influence of pain sensation throughout the body.[66]

There are several types of thalamotomy for pain relief. The convergence of the various pathways that relate to the different aspects of pathologic pain makes it possible to tailor the lesion within the thalamus to the needs of a given patient (Figure 92-3). In the past, the lesions were directed to the posterior nuclei of the thalamus. A theoretical risk of producing a lesion in the ventral posterior nuclei is that it could produce a thalamic syndrome, which generally contraindicates the use of that procedure. It is more efficient, however, to interrupt the lemniscal fibers as they ascend into that nucleus through the mesencephalon, which is described as mesencephalotomy. The nonspecific fibers, concerned with the paleospinothalamic and archispinothalamic systems, ascend to the medial portion of the thalamus, where they may be interrupted without sacrificing the lemniscal pathways. Such lesions may afford pain relief without significantly altering somatic sensation.

Basal thalamotomy involves the production of a small discrete lesion to interrupt the extralemniscal fibers as they ascend toward the intralaminar nuclei, the centrum medianum, and the parafascicular nucleus. Medial thalamotomy involves the production of a somewhat larger lesion to interrupt these same fibers at their termination in the intralaminar nuclei and centrum medianum. Although it was originally hoped that basal thalamotomy would produce longer-lasting and more complete pain relief more efficiently than intralaminar thalamotomy, the results following these two procedures are comparable. Indeed, perhaps the best chance for pain relief is produced with an intralaminar lesion extended to the same level as the basal thalamotomy, which does not appear to carry with it any greater risk.

The final type of thalamotomy for pain relief is the dorsomedian thalamotomy, which involves the production of a lesion in the dorsomedian nucleus to interrupt the origin of those fibers that project to the frontal lobe. This is the same thalamic lesion that has been employed for the treatment of affective disorders. Successful alleviation of pain also has been reported with bilateral lesions in the centrum medianum, the effect of which would be similar to that seen after medial thalamotomy.[65] In addition, lesions of the intralaminar nuclei have been successfully combined with lesions of the parafascicular complex for successful pain relief without analgesia.[67,68]

Stimulation at 50 Hz should be employed before production of a lesion. In basal thalamotomy, look for extraocular movements that might indicate that the electrode is too deep and encroaching on the oculomotor fibers, which lie just below the level of the basal thalamotomy lesions. Specific projection of pain sensation to the opposite side of the body may indicate that the electrode is slightly lateral and encroaching on the lemniscal fibers; although this would not compromise the result, it may cause an unnecessary sensory loss.

The medial-basal thalamotomy is done unilaterally, generally on the side opposite the greatest pain, and a dorsomedian thalamotomy may be done at the same sitting. If necessary, the second side can be done in 3 to 6 weeks. Results for cancer pain have been good; early pain relief was generally reported in 80 to 90 percent of the cases. Although medial-basal thalamotomy has also been employed for pain of benign origin, it has only a 30 to 35 percent long-term success rate for chronic pain,[69,70] so it is best avoided except for cancer pain.

Dorsomedian thalamotomy may be used alone for cancer pain.[71] The effects are similar to frontal leukotomy or cingulotomy, which have also been recognized as helpful for cancer pain. Since there is little additional risk, and conceivably potentially better results by combining the intralaminar with the dorsomedian nucleus lesion, there appears to be little advantage to performing dorsomedian thalamotomy alone for cancer pain.

Consequently, the recommended lesion for thalamotomy for treatment of cancer pain is a medial thalamotomy with a lesion in the intralaminar nuclei so that the lesion extends downward to combine with a basal thalamotomy lesion. If the patient has a great deal of emotional turmoil associated with the cancer, the lesion may be further extended medially into the dorsomedian nucleus to produce a combined dorsomedian thalamotomy as well.

The coordinates for the combined medial-basal thalamotomy (Table 92-1) require placing the burr hole somewhat more medial than usual, at approximately 2 cm from the midline, so the electrode can be introduced at an angle of 5 degrees to the sagittal plane. The electrode should be introduced perpendicular to the intercommissural line. After the stereotactic apparatus is positioned so the electrode is directed at the proper trajectory, the electrode should be brought into contact with the skull. It may be necessary to make a second burr hole at that point or to extend the ventriculostomy burr hole, which should be done rather than compromising the angle of insertion of the electrode.

Three separate insertions should be used, with several lesions at different depths at each insertion site. A small electrode is used so the lesion is narrow. The first coordinate lies 1 mm anterior to the posterior commissure, 12 mm lateral, and at the level of the intercommissural line. After one lesion has been made at that level, the electrode is withdrawn 3 to 4 mm to make a second lesion, and perhaps even a third (depending upon the length of the active portion of the electrode) so that the lesions extend from the level of the intercommissural line to a point 11 mm above. The electrode then is withdrawn and reinserted 4 mm anterior to the posterior commissure, 11 mm lateral, and 2 mm above the intercommissural line, and a series of lesions is made to extend from the +2 level to the +13. The third insertion is made 9 mm anterior to the posterior commissure and 9 mm lateral, with the lesion extending from 2 mm above the intercommissural line to 13 mm above the intercommissural line.[59,70]

A lesion of the dorsomedial nucleus can be made with a somewhat larger electrode at 4 mm anterior to the posterior commissure and 4 mm lateral, so the lesion extends from 2 to 10 mm above the intercommissural line. The proximity to the insertion site for the medial-basal thalamotomy facilitates combining these two procedures.

Relief of suffering often can be obtained by interrupting the limbic system rather than interrupting or ablating the pain pathway itself. There are several areas where lesions can be conveniently made to afford pain relief for cancer patients. Such a procedure should be considered in patients with widespread metastatic disease, pain, and emotional turmoil who become drug dependent. Although these procedures may cause a slightly dulled affect in the initial postoperative period, the medication requirement is generally so much less than preoperatively that the net effect is one of reduced mental impairment.

If it is desired to make a lesion in the limbic system, cingulotomy may be the procedure of choice.[72,73] The technique of cingulotomy is presented in the section on surgery for affective disorders.

Although chronic stimulation techniques are more often used for chronic pain, they can be considered helpful for cancer pain as well, particularly if there is concurrent neuropathic or denervation pain.

Spinal cord stimulation can be helpful for some patients with cancer pain, if it is not too severe. A percutaneous trial of stimulation may be helpful for patients with moderate pain from such problems as lumbosacral plexus involvement. The risks are minimal, and if satisfactory pain relief is not obtained, the percutaneous electrodes can be removed and other measures considered.

Deep-brain stimulation can be of value, particularly for patients with widespread pain of metastatic disease and patients with pain involving the head and neck. The contraindications would include those patients who have open and potentially infected lesions of the head, which may expose the patient to undue risk of infection from the implanted device. The details of the use of deep-brain stimulation are covered in Chapter 95.

Management of Chronic Pain

Chronic pain has been defined, for purposes of management, as pain that has persisted for at least 3 to 6 months, has defied attempts at treatment by ordinary means or treatment of underlying etiology, and serves no useful biologic purpose.

Although chronic pain is not primarily treated surgically, it is necessary to present an overview of its management to demonstrate the contrast in approach, instruct the surgeon about alternate means of treatment to allow better judgment for the selection of patients for surgery (or a conservative program), and to put in context those few chronic pain conditions for which a surgical procedure may be indicated.

An informal inquiry of six neurosurgeons who are leaders in the field of pain management revealed that only 1 to 15 percent of the patients referred to them for pain management were subjected to some sort of procedure. In contrast, several neurosurgeons with private general neurosurgery practices responded to this same question by indicating that 85 to 90 percent of their patients referred for the management of pain were subjected to a procedure. Even assuming that the patient population was different because more intractable pain patients were referred to neurosurgeons in a pain clinic, one must assume that many patients who had surgery at the hands of a neurosurgical generalist would not have had surgery had they been referred to neurosurgeons who were more sophisticated in the management of chronic pain. Part of this difference may be because of the availability of a chronic pain management program in their repertoire.

Several features are common to the majority of the chronic pain patients who have presented at our pain clinic.[74–76] Most stated that the current pain was similar to their initial pain, which was usually associated with an acute medical problem or injury, but worse following many medical or surgical attempts at relief. They offered medical histories of treatment failures freely and in great detail, often with considerable relish. All had tried numerous medications, and most were addicted to narcotics, but they continued to take medication that they admitted did not offer either significant or long-lasting relief, but just ''to take the edge off'' the pain. Significantly, all said their pain complaints were urgent or emergency problems. Not only did they describe willingness to undergo any treatment aimed at pain relief, but frequently tried to manipulate the physician into inappropriate or excessive procedures. Finally, and importantly, many claimed they had no other problem and that everything would be fine if only the doctor would take their pain away. The patient's daily life was organized around, and defined by, the pain; the pain explained all difficulties of living.

Although the chronic pain patient moved in an exaggerated, guarded fashion, on physical examination, the described disability was generally in excess of that warranted by objective physical findings.

Pervading the presentation was a sense of urgency and expectation that the physician would institute a definitive treatment in which the patient would have little responsibility, but which would make the pain suddenly and, almost magically, disappear. Such a presentation may be appropriate for acute pain but not chronic pain.

In addition to the usual chronic pain patient described above, there are several categories of pain patients the surgeon must be aware of in order to direct the program appropriate to a nonsurgical approach. Pain may be a symptom of depression. A small group of patients may have a delusional symptom of psychosis. Such patients generally are identifiable by their bizarre behavior, which can be seen only if the physician looks closely. Pain may be a symptom of anxiety, particularly anxiety about an illness, such as cardiac disease or cancer. Pain may be a symptom of hysterical neurosis, in which the pain is an attempt to resolve personal conflict that the patient cannot deal with in a healthy way; often the description of pain may relate to the underlying personal conflict, and the benefits gained by the disability may allow the patient to avoid that conflict. Patients with chronic pain frequently have unresolved grief, in which case the pain may allow identification with the lost loved one, either by the type of pain, the manner in which the pain presented, or the timing of the onset or exacerbation of the pain.

Another group of chronic pain patients is made up of those whose personality indicates a need to suffer. These patients have a life-long history of multiple surgeries of many kinds, frequent personal disasters (which always seem to occur just when everything is going well), and multiple unsuccessful doctor-patient relationships. Although this group constitutes only a moderate portion of chronic pain patients, they present repeatedly to multiple physicians, frustrating many and standing out because virtually any treatment program is doomed to failure.

Most chronic pain patients are both depressed and regressed by the time they are referred to a neurosurgeon. Depression is usual for patients who are disabled from any cause for as long as 6 months. Although it is a normal reaction to an abnormal situation, it must be managed successfully for the patient to progress from the stage of disability to that of rehabilitation.

Regression is an exaggeration of the dependency that begins during the acute phase of the patient's illness. As the patient withdraws more and more from normal activities and responsibilities, it becomes more and more difficult, both psychologically and physically, to resume these activities later. Frequently, the dependency state is reinforced by the patient's caretaker, usually the spouse, who may receive considerable psychologic gain from keeping the patient in a regressed and dependent attitude.

Most patients are addicted to inappropriate medications at the time they present for management of their chronic pain. All analgesics are designed for acute pain, virtually all produce both tolerance and addiction, most have depression as a significant side-effect, and none works for chronic pain.

Many patients are suffering from recurrent withdrawal by the time they present to the neurosurgeon. They are firmly addicted to a pain medication, usually containing a narcotic. They go through a regular cycle every few hours. They take their pain medication, but several hours later begin to go into withdrawal. As a consequence of the withdrawal, they become anxious, agitated, and, as part of the withdrawal, their pain perception becomes intensified, so their pain becomes worse. After watching the clock anxiously, they take their pain medication again at the prescribed time (or before), and find that the medication "takes the edge off the pain." They are treating the withdrawal rather than the pain, and at the same time are perpetuating the narcotic dependency. Several hours later the pattern is repeated, and the pain perception becomes intensified so that another dose of medication is taken.

The management of any patient with chronic pain should take all of these factors into account. Indeed, before making a final decision to subject a patient with chronic pain to a neurosurgical procedure, such as implantation of a stimulator, the patient should have the opportunity to participate in a chronic pain program. Many patients who may initially appear to be candidates for stimulators may find so much relief from nonsurgical means that an invasive procedure is not appropriate. Other patients may appear to be emotionally stable, but on closer inspection over time may prove to have such significant psychopathology that any procedure should be considered only with reluctance. Still other patients may be laying so much of the blame for their personal problems on their pain symptom that it becomes obvious they would neither be less disabled nor satisfied, regardless of the effectiveness of the pain-relieving procedure.

Little in the way of pain management can be accomplished unless and until both the patient and the treating physician exchange the goal of pain relief for that of rehabilitation. The attitude of the patient must be redirected from one aimed at having someone else take the pain away to one aimed at coping with the physical problem and abandoning disability as a way of life, following which, in most cases, the pain becomes significantly ameliorated.

A comprehensive chronic pain program should include the following:[76]

1. Neuropsychologic evaluation, concentrating mainly on the patient's disability and how he copes with various stresses, including pain. Neuropsychologic tests are usually worthless for identifying what proportion of the patient's pain is primarily organic and what proportion may be primarily psychologic. Realistic goals must be set, both in regard to the patient and the place of the patient within the family.

2. Withdrawal of medication can usually best be accomplished abruptly, except for barbiturates and diazepam. It should be explained to the patient beforehand that he will feel lousy for several days, during which time the pain will be intensified, but that following that the pain may be significantly relieved. A period of withdrawal is also accompanied by sleeplessness, since chronic administration of pain medication may disrupt the normal diurnal sleep cycle, and many pain patients have been on sedatives. No sleep medications should be given during this stage, since they interfere with resumption of a normal sleep cycle.

3. Treatment of depression should include both pharmacologic and psychiatric means. Discontinuation of pain medications and tranquilizers is an important part of the treatment of depression, as is the addition of tricyclic antidepressants, which may have a direct effect on chronic pain as well.

4. Treatment of regression can best be managed by forcefully encouraging the patient toward self-care, generally using behavior modification techniques. Rather than always instructing the patient to do less and less, the patient should be encouraged to do more and more. It is important to involve the spouse or caretaker in the treatment of regression, since often the spouse's psychologic needs may be met by keeping the patient dependent.

5. Resocialization involves encouraging the patient to regain social contacts and recreational activities.

6. Remobilization should be done gradually and progressively. A program of progressive exercises that start at a very simple level, such as the Royal Canadian Air Force Exercise Program, will allow the patient to begin to exercise at a tolerated activity level.

7. Physical therapy is usually directed to the physical conditioning program. Such local modalities as heat and massage may help muscle spasm, and gentle stretching exercises can improve mobilization.

8. Transcutaneous stimulation can be of help, particularly in the initial phase when the patient is beginning to remobilize. It is not a pain program in itself, however, and is much more effective when incorporated into an overall program.

9. Specific techniques can be taught to lessen pain perception and to allow the patient to relax without the use of drugs, such as biofeedback and relaxation training.[77]

A final word of caution should be said about the manipulative patient. Many chronic pain patients have more experience than their physician in directing their program, and those patients who have a psychologic need to suffer or for the treatment to fail will often manipulate the physician into fulfilling these prophecies. The key to managing a manipulative patient is to make it understood from the start that manipulation will not be tolerated and that the physician, not the patient, is in charge of the program. When the patient recognizes that manipulation will not accomplish its usual end, it will usually cease.

There are several procedures that are extremely helpful in the management of a few selected patients with chronic pain. The most common procedure in that category is one of trigger point blocks,[78] which may be a valuable adjunct to the treatment of myofascial syndrome. Although that syndrome has been defined variously, we can consider it to be a localized area of muscle pain and spasm secondary to a tearing injury. It commonly occurs at the origin of the back muscles at the sacral crest, the medial portion of the iliac crest and posterior iliac spine, the lower posterior cervical area, the suboccipital muscles, or the site of a laminectomy, fusion, or bone graft donor. Although the process is usually localized, the painful muscle spasm may spread to adjacent muscles and cause the pain to radiate up and down the back. In addition, the pain may be referred along the involved dermatome, but can be differentiated from radicular pain because both the radiating and local pain may be alleviated by a local trigger point block.

The trigger points of a myofascial syndrome can be identified at physical examination by a report of pain on deep muscle palpation, particularly in the locations described above, or by the palpation of localized muscle spasm or nodularity. When such a trigger point, or multiple points, are identified, the skin should be marked with a pen so the pattern can be visualized and the trigger points treated.

Treatment of trigger points may be begun by the patient with a conservative program that involves application of local heat (a bathtub or shower being preferable to a heating pad), local massage, and gentle stretching exercises. Many patients find that they can break up the pattern of muscle spasm by steady, deep, local, digital pressure several times a day.

If the patient is unable to manage the myofascial pain, physical therapy several times a week can be incorporated into the program. In addition to the modalities above, the use of a local vibrator may help break up the pattern of muscle spasm.

A series of trigger point blocks may be done for both diagnostic and therapeutic purposes. In order to identify the trigger points, 1 ml of 1 percent lidocaine is injected into each point and may be combined with triamcindone, 40 mg. A 22-gauge ½-inch needle is used, and, as the needle enters the trigger point, the physician can feel the sudden penetration of a fascial plane or the palpation of bony attachment, as the patient reports the sudden exacerbation of the pain. Alleviation of the pain on injection of a local anesthetic is diagnostic, particularly if consistent on repeated blocks.

If diagnostic blocks are successful, a series of weekly or biweekly blocks with local anesthetic is undertaken. If the pain recurs promptly after each block in the series, a longer-acting local anesthetic such as bupivacaine may be substituted. If the patient still has recurrence after six or eight local anesthetic blocks but has excellent temporary relief from each series of blocks, phenol blocks may afford a long-term benefit. Five hundred milligrams of phenol crystals are dissolved in 5 ml of saline for a 10 percent concentration, and 1 ml of that solution is injected at each trigger point, with a maximum of 5 ml in any given weekly session.

Causalgia is treated primarily with sympathectomy (Chapter 112). If pain persists following sympathectomy, however, extralemniscal or limited myelotomy may be of benefit. Cingulotomy may also be beneficial, but experience has shown that relief of chronic pain, from whatever cause, is usually limited to 2 to 4 months.

Denervation-type pain may be treated by dorsal column stimulation or deep-brain stimulation, either in the periventricular or somatosensory areas. Since dorsal column stimulation can be evaluated percutaneously and carries less risk, that procedure should be tried first. If dorsal column stimulation is unsuccessful, or if the pain involves the face, deep-brain stimulation may be attempted (see Chapter 95). For denervation pain, electrodes should be inserted both in the periventricular area and the appropriate somatosensory area, as described above, and the appropriate leads selected by a trial of stimulation.

Postherpetic neuralgia remains an enigma. Approximately 50 percent of the patients respond to transcutaneous stimulation, however, if encouraged to persist in trying various electrode placements. If the pain is justifiably severe and relief is not obtained from transcutaneous stimulation, percutaneous dorsal column stimulation may be tried, but, again, without anticipating more than a 50 percent chance of success. It has been reported that postherpetic intractable pain cases respond well to extralemniscal myelotomy[59] or lesions of the dorsal root entry zone.[79] If the face is involved, it may be necessary to perform intralaminar or basal thalamotomy.

The most common chronic pain problem is that of low back pain. Many patients can avoid this chronic problem with appropriate management of their acute injury. It is disheartening how many patients appear at the Chronic Pain Clinic having had a laminectomy for what was described as a classic myofascial syndrome. Unless a patient presents with classic signs and symptoms of herniated lumbar or cervical disc, a myofascial syndrome should be evaluated with appropriate trigger point blocks.

The patient with chronic low back pain should undergo a chronic pain program as described above before any decision is made about a procedure. Trigger point blocks may be usefully combined with a long-term physical therapy program. After the depression, regression, and drug dependency are brought under control, the patient can be evaluated more objectively for response to transcutaneous stimulation, and later to dorsal column stimulation, if necessary. With a strict selection protocol, few patients will have dorsal column stimulators implanted, but the long-term success rate is high in those who are candidates.

I have been discouraged by the long-term effects of ablative procedures for chronic low back and leg pain. Although the short-term results are excellent with a number of procedures (such as rhizotomy, microsurgical decompression, radiofrequency rhizotomy, and interruption of pain pathways), pain relief rarely lasts longer than 2 to 4 months.

Phantom limb pain presents a particularly challenging problem. Many, if not most, patients with phantom limb pain have a great deal of emotional involvement in their physical disability, and should undergo a chronic pain clinic evaluation as the initial step in management. If the pain is actually local tenderness secondary to neuroma formation, resection of the nerve proximal to the neuroma may be helpful, whereas searching through dense scar tissue to find a neuroma is rarely rewarding. Transcutaneous stimulation can be extremely helpful for many patients with phantom limb pain, as can dorsal column stimulation or peripheral nerve stimulation.

It is of the utmost importance that the surgeon reserve the option of telling the patient that there is nothing to offer if there is nothing that stands a reasonable chance of success. Chronic pain patients are notorious for manipulating physicians into

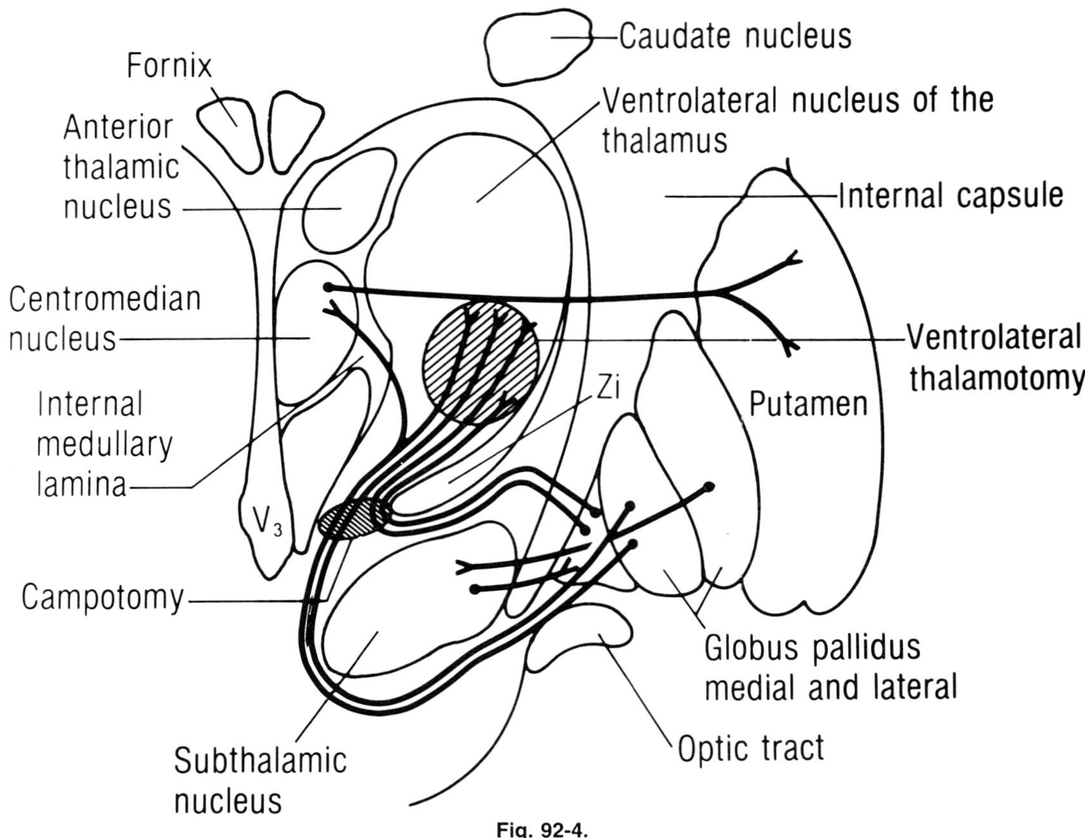

Fig. 92-4.

procedures against their better judgment, which, more often than not, results in an increase of the problem. When confronted directly, however, most patients accept this news gracefully. They should be admonished that there is no acceptable treatment for their problem and discouraged from traveling from physician to physician looking for a magical cure.

MOVEMENT DISORDERS

Anatomy of Motor Control

Most of the movement disorders of functional neurosurgical interest concern the extrapyramidal system, which consists of two interlocking circuits that are important from the stereotactic standpoint.

One concerns the basal ganglia and the thalamus. Fibers from the putamen enter the globus pallidus; both internal and external pallidum feed into the ventral-anterior nucleus of the thalamus by way of several pathways. The lenticular fasciculus runs above the subthalamic nucleus, and the ansa lenticularis runs below the subthalamic nucleus to join together in Forel's field H. These two pathways ascend together as the thalamic fasciculus (H1) to the ventral-anterior nucleus of the thalamus.

Note that virtually the entire outflow of both the internal and external pallidum funnels together into a compact bundle as it traverses Forel's field H, where the maximum number of fibers can be interrupted with the smallest lesion (Figure 92-4). From the thalamus, there are connections to the supplementary motor cortex. Connections within the cortex lead to fibers that project to the caudate nucleus, which in turn projects back to the putamen to complete the putamen-globus pallidus-thalamus (ventral anterior)-cortex-caudate-putamen circuit.

There is a second interlocking circuit that links the cerebellum to the basal ganglia. The major outflow from the cerebellum is via the dentate nucleus, which projects to the red nucleus. Some fibers synapse in the red nucleus and others pass directly through joining fibers that originate in the red nucleus to end in the ventrolateral nucleus of the thalamus. The area of the thalamus involved abuts with the area that receives fibers from the globus pallidus. The ventrolateral nucleus projects to the primary and secondary motor cortex. Cortical efferent fibers descend through the internal capsule to end in the pontine nuclei. Neurons that originate in those nuclei project to the cortex of the cerebellum in a somatotopic distribution. Cerebellar cortical fibers then synapse in the dentate nucleus to

Table 92-2.

Ventral-anterior nucleus (VA)	Nucleus lateropolaris (L. po)
Ventrolateral nucleus (VL) (ventral half)	Nucleus ventro-oralis anterior (V.o.a) Nucleus ventro-oralis posterior (V.o.p) Nucleus ventrointermedius (V.im)
Ventral-posterolateral nucleus (VPL)	Nucleus ventrocaudalis externa (V.c.e)
Ventral-posteromedial nucleus (VPM)	Nucleus ventrocaudalis interna (V.c.i)

complete the second cerebellum-dentate-ruber-thalamus (ventrolateral)-cortex-pontine nuclei-cerebellum motor-control circuit.

It is in the area of the thalamus where these two circuits juxtapose that stereotactic lesions are made for the treatment of involuntary movement and tremor.

Much of the stereotactic literature relates to the Hassler nomenclature of thalamic nuclei, and may be confusing to those not familiar with that system. Different criteria are used for the delineation of Hassler's nuclei and subnuclei than for the Walker terminology above, so that it is not possible to correlate them entirely, but several generalizations can be made that clarify the relationship sufficiently for the purposes of stereotactic surgery (Table 92-2).[80]

The ventral-anterior nucleus is called the nucleus lateropolaris (L.po). According to Hassler, some fibers run directly from the external lamina of the globus pallidus to the L.po, and additional fibers are carried by way of the thalamic fasciculus (H1). Cortical projections are primarily to the supplementary motor area.

The ventrolateral nucleus is divided into several subnuclei in the Hassler classification. The ventral half of the ventral-lateral nucleus is divided into the nucleus ventro-oralis anterior (V.o.a) and the nucleus ventro-oralis posterior (V.o.p), and the intermediate nucleus between these nuclei and the ventral-posteromedial and ventral-posterolateral nuclei is called the nucleus ventrointermedius (V.im).

There is evidence that the V.im receives input from the vestibular nuclei and projects to area 3a of the sensory motor cortex. It has been reported that a 5–7-Hz rhythm can be recorded from the base of the V.im. Although it has been suggested that this is the pacemaker of the tremor of Parkinson's disease, some patients may get excellent relief of tremor with only minor involvement of the V.im by the lesion, suggesting that the bursting activity may be from a bundle traveling through the V.im to the V.o.p.[81,82] Some authors, however, feel that V.im is the specific target for tremor.[83,84]

The nucleus ventro-oralis anterior (V.o.a) receives axons going from the internal lamina of the globus pallidus through the thalamic fasciculus (H1) to the secondary motor cortex, so that, in some definitions, the V.o.a might actually be included in the dorsal part of the ventral-anterior nucleus. It appears to be involved in slow, specialized movements or turning of the trunk. The usual effect of stimulation of the V.o.a (as well as the V.o.p) is an increase in amplitude of the tremor of Parkinson's disease, especially at low stimulus rates (5 Hz). Tremor may be blocked by stimulation of the V.o.p, however, and if the current is sufficiently high, such a blockage may occur because of the spread of the current to the V.o.p., even though the tip of the electrode is in the V.o.a. The rate of rapidly alternating movements of the arm may be slowed by 50-Hz stimulation of the V.o.a, and stimulation of the V.o.a may cause ocular movements, with conjugate turning of the eyes to the opposite side, opening of the eyes, and possibly mydriasis.

The nucleus ventro-oralis posterior (V.o.p) is the main relay of the nucleus for input from the dentato-rubro-thalamic system to the primary motor cortex, area 4. This system controls rapid, sudden movements. Since the V.o.p may be the site of the rhythmic discharges that control the 5–7-Hz tremor of Parkinson's disease, it may be possible to record bursting activity at that frequency. Stimulation at 50 Hz may block the tremor, perhaps by interfering with the generation of these burst discharges.

The ventral-posterolateral nucleus (VPL) is referred to as the nucleus ventrocaudalis externa (V.c.e), and the ventral-posteromedial nucleus (VPM) is the nucleus ventrocaudalis interna (V.c.i). The anatomic definitions of these nuclei are the same in both the Walker and Hassler nomenclature, but, according to Hassler, the nucleus ventrocaudalis is also divided into an anterior and posterior part, with duplicate somatotopic representation, with proprioception relayed to the V.c.p and a tactile homunculus in the V.c.a.[81]

Despite the appearance of an ultrascientific rationale, one must simplistically recognize that most stereotactic procedures for motor disorders involve interruption of the interlocking pathway described above, usually somewhere between the globus pallidus and the thalamus or within the thalamus, and targets have been determined empirically. Historically, the first targets for Parkinson's disease were in the globus pallidus. With more experience, the target moved to the neighborhood of the ventrolateral nucleus of the thalamus. Since fibers between these two areas must funnel through the ansa lenticularis and Forel's field, they likewise became targets. There have been many opinions about which specific coordinates are best for which symptoms, but the areas are so close and anatomic confirmation by autopsy so limited that only a few definitive statements can be made.

Autopsy confirmation indicates that improvement of rigidity of Parkinson's disease can be correlated with a lesion involving the V.o.a or H1, confirming that interruption of the pallidothalamic connections are optimal for the improvement of rigidity.[59,85] Relief of tremor, however, correlates more closely with coagulation of the V.o.p, which involves the dentato-thalamic fibers. Both of these symptoms respond to a lesion in Forel's field, tremor responding more consistently than rigidity.[86,87] Bradykinesia does not appear to be affected as much, regardless of the placement of the lesion. Gait disturbances of various types may be treated by ablation of the V.o.a.[85]

Management of Movement Disorders

Coordinates may be determined by a consideration of specific symptoms. In order to produce a lesion in the ventrolateral nucleus (V.o.a) for treatment of rigidity, the electrode might be directed to the following coordinates: 2 mm anterior to the midpoint of the intercommissural (AC-PC) line, 9.5 mm lateral, and 3 mm above the AC-PC line. If there is tremor present, it may be increased by stimulation at 5 Hz. Stimulation at 50 Hz may slow the speed of arm movements at low voltage, and at higher voltage may decrease tremor. Conjugate movement of the eyes may occur.

In order to produce a lesion in the ventrolateral nucleus (V.o.p) or V.im for treatment of tremor, insert the electrode to the coordinates 2 mm posterior to the mid AC-PC line, 11.5 lateral and 3 mm above the AC-PC line. It may be possible to record rhythmic discharges at the same frequency as the tremor, particularly with a microelectrode or semimicroelectrode. Stimulation at 50 Hz may block the tremor. There is evidence that the most effective site within the V.o.p. is that which lies just anterior to the somatosensory representation in the V.c.a of the body part affected.[82]

A lesion in Forel's field H (campus Foreli) is called campotomy, and may be used for either tremor or rigidity.[86,87] The coordinates are at the mid AC-PC line, 6 mm lateral, with the tip of the electrode 2 mm below the AC-PC line (Figure 92-4). There is no characteristic electrical activity from that area. Stimulation at 5 Hz should assure that the pyramidal tract is not being encroached upon. Stimulation at 50 Hz may cause an increase in the tremor. If the electrode is too close to oculomotor fibers, medial deviation of the ipsilateral eye and mydriasis may be seen, in which case the electrode should be raised 1 or 2 mm and tested with stimulation once again.

Parkinson's Disease

Parkinson's disease is the most common motor disorder for which stereotactic surgery is used. Indeed, the popularization of stereotactic surgery occurred during the time that large numbers of patients were available, many with postencephalitic Parkinson's disease after influenza epidemics, and medical management was only marginally successful. As a large portion of the resident population was treated, and as L-dopa therapy provided relief for many other patients, the reservoir of patients for stereotactic surgery dropped.[13]

Parkinson's syndrome consists of a multitude of signs and symptoms. Although the most dramatic and obvious is the characteristic tremor, it is usually not the most disabling, since it occurs at rest and very often lessens or stops on intention. Bradykinesia, however, is usually the disabling feature of the disease. It is often associated with rigidity, and the resultant paucity of movements may make the patient "a prisoner in his own body." The postural changes that occur with Parkinson's syndrome are so characteristic that the diagnosis may be made even before the appearance of other signs. The patient stands with shoulders and head thrust forward. The kyphosis is fixed, so that the head remains suspended above the pillow when the patient is lying supine. Adding to the postural abnormality is the absence of associated movements, such that the arms no longer swing on walking, indicating that automatic arm and leg coordination is absent. Vegetative symptoms complete the characteristic picture: a masklike face, oily skin, and excessive accumulation of saliva in the mouth.

It must be recognized that although L-dopa works quite well for bradykinesia, it may have little effect on tremor, or may even make the tremor worse. In contrast, stereotactic surgery works exceedingly well against tremor and moderately well against rigidity, but may have little effect on bradykinesia. Consequently, many patients with both bradykinesia and tremor are candidates for stereotactic surgery plus L-dopa management. Also, as patients are treated with L-dopa for 3 to 5 years, many become intolerant to the medication, or the symptoms begin to break through once again, and these patients may still benefit from stereotactic surgery. Further, the response to L-dopa may be much better following a stereotactic lesion than before, and L-dopa-induced tremor and involuntary movements occur less frequently in limbs contralateral to prior stereotactic procedures.[88]

Consequently, the recommendation at present is for the following in sequence:

1. If bradykinesia is the major problem, a course of medical management should be pursued.
2. If the patient does not respond to medication or becomes intolerant to the medication, stereotactic surgery should be considered.
3. If the patient still has significant bradykinesia following stereotactic surgery, L-dopa should be tried once again in gradually escalating doses in hopes that its benefit may become enhanced.
4. If tremor is the major problem, a brief course of medical management should be tried.
5. If the patient does not respond promptly to modest doses of medication, stereotactic surgery is indicated.
6. If tremor is still a problem following stereotactic surgery, a medical program should be tried once again.
7. If the patient has symmetrical bilateral tremor, the dominant side should be operated on first to give the patient maximum rehabilitation from a unilateral procedure.
8. If it is necessary to perform stereotactic surgery on the second side, either because of bilateral tremor or because tremor on the asymptomatic side emerges afterward, a minimum of 6 to 12 weeks should elapse before the second side is done.
9. If lesions are made on both sides, every attempt should be made to make asymmetrical lesions to minimize the risk of side-effects affecting mentation or verbalization. In no case should bilateral campotomy be performed, because of a risk of mutism.

The contraindications for stereotactic surgery in patients with Parkinson's disease are related to the age and general health of the patient. The possibility of a successful result begins to decrease with patients over the age of 60, and certainly with patients over the age of 65. Older patients who have become debilitated from a long-term disability may succumb to pneumonia or other complications during the initial week following surgery, when the patient may be quite sedated from the lesion.

One can anticipate satisfactory relief of tremor in 80 to 85 percent of selected patients. The chance of neurologic complications or worsening of symptoms is approximately 4 percent, and is more likely to occur in older patients.

Essential tremor, or familial tremor, may be quite disabling, since it is a tremor of intention. The more the patient tries to stop the tremor, the worse the tremor becomes. It may not be apparent or disabling until adulthood or middle years, and may affect many members of a single family. It may respond to a medical program, particularly relaxants, but usually does not.

On the other hand, stereotactic campotomy or thalamotomy may result in immediate and dramatic relief of the tremor. The target is the same as for the tremor of Parkinson's disease (vide supra) (Figure 92-4).

Tremor may be the result of other etiologies, such as a stroke or head trauma. Because one is dealing with a nervous system that is not intact, and the damage to other parts of the motor system cannot be known, the results of stereotactic surgery are less predictable. Nevertheless, if the tremor is disabling enough and the patient is willing to risk the uncertain result, stereotactic surgery may be indicated. One must also warn the patient that the possibility of side-effects is also somewhat unpredictable and that previously resolved weakness or paralysis may return.

Stereotactic surgery can be used for selected patients with Huntington's chorea, and indeed this was the first use of stereotactic surgery for motor disorders.[89] Huntington's chorea is a familial disease marked by progressive mental deterioration and choreiform movements associated with degeneration of the caudate nuclei. It is important to select patients for stereotactic surgery critically, to be sure that it is the motor impairment and not the mental deterioration that is the cause of the patient's disability. Because the condition is progressive, the long-term prognosis remains poor, but it may be possible to allow the patient 6 months or a year of independence or self-care, provided his mental status is adequate. One must caution, however, that performing unilateral lesions or making a lesion in the dominant hemisphere may increase problems with mentation in patients who are functioning at a borderline level, so the procedure is not entirely without risk.

The target is either Forel's field or the ventrolateral nucleus, as it is for other nonspecific movement disorders. Symmetrical lesions should not be made bilaterally, especially in this group of patients who have impaired neurologic reserve to compensate for the lesions. Results in most patients can be gratifying, with marked decrease in choreiform movements immediately upon production of the lesion.

Hemiballism is of stereotactic interest from two standpoints. First, it has been reported as a rare complication of subthalamic stereotactic lesions, and second, hemiballism occurring after stroke may be successfully treated with stereotactic surgery.

Ballism consists of involuntary hurling, irregular, frequently violent movements of the shoulder and proximal arm, which may occur after a lesion of the subthalamic nucleus. Ordinarily, hemiballism is the result of a localized problem and consequently unilateral. There is some evidence that a partial destruction of the subthalamic nucleus may lead to ballism, but it does not occur if the nucleus is completely destroyed.

The postsurgical incidence has been reported to range from 0.3 to 9.0 percent,[90] with one series reporting 4 cases out of 4866 stereotactic surgeries.[91] This author has never seen a case following the production of a stereotactic lesion, but has participated in the treatment of several cases that occurred spontaneously, presumably following a localized stroke.

Indications for surgery in patients with spontaneous hemiballism follow the general rules for stereotactic intervention. The symptoms must be severe enough to justify the procedure, and since ballistic movements of any magnitude are invariably disabling, this criterion is often met. The patient must not be disabled from other neurologic problems, although the stroke that caused ballism may also cause other neurologic problems. Hemiballism is frequently of a transient nature so that surgery should not be contemplated unless the problem has been stable for at least 2 to 3 months.

The treatment of ballism consists of destroying the same part of the ventrolateral nucleus or Forel's field that is the general target for other movement disorders. Earlier reports also indicated successful relief of hemiballism following lesions of the medial part of the globus pallidus, and a satisfactory result can be anticipated from either target.[92]

Dystonia musculorum deformans (torsion spasm) is a progressive condition characterized by torsion of the trunk muscles with asymmetrical spasm, spasticity, and contractures of the extremities, leading to profound immobility.

The results of ventrolateral thalamotomy for dystonia musculorum deformans are somewhat unpredictable, but approximately 50 percent can be improved by stereotactic surgery. Some patients may have dramatic alleviation of virtually all symptoms, and improvement may last for many years. Others may have minimal or no improvement, even though the presenting picture may have appeared to be the same. Many patients will have a moderate or modest improvement, but become disabled once again as the progressive nature of the disease overtakes the improvement.[26]

Early treatment for dystonia musculorum deformans was pallido-ansotomy, or a lesion in the globus pallidus and associated ansa lenticularis.[93] Currently, a lesion in Forel's field or the posterior half of the ventrolateral nucleus is recommended (Figure 92-4). A peculiarity of this condition is that the improvement may not be apparent for several weeks after the lesion is made, and may be progressive for several months thereafter. Consequently, one should initially make a generous lesion extending from Forel's field[92] into the ventrolateral nucleus,[94] and, if necessary, repeat or enlarge the lesion at 3-month intervals as long as it appears that progress is being made. Since the condition may involve primarily the trunk, it may be necessary to make bilateral lesions before any response is seen. It is recommended that the first lesion be placed on the side opposite the greater muscle spasm, particularly if extremities are affected, or, if the spasm is equal bilaterally, on the dominant side. Usually a contralateral lesion is necessary some time later, and working on the nondominant side allows the surgeon to be more generous in the size of the second lesion.

It is important that the patient recognize the unpredictability of results in this condition, and certainly a pessimistic projection should be presented. It must be recognized that there is no other available treatment, however, so many patients are desperate by the time they reach the stereotactic surgeon.

Spasmodic torticollis may be confused with the early stages of dystonia but certainly constitutes a separate disease. It may be distinguished in that it occurs more often in adults and is confined only to the neck and possibly the trapezius muscles. It may involve tilting or rotation of the head to one or the other side, or symmetrical extension (retrocollis). It may be intermittent and clonic in nature, or it may be steady and tonic.

Many patients with spasmodic torticollis have significant emotional problems, and there is considerable disagreement about what constitutes satisfactory management. The literature is loaded with single reports of a multitude of medications, but rarely do second validating reports appear. More or less mutilating procedures may be advocated.

Although there have been several reports of beneficial results from stereotactic surgery, this author has not been encouraged. Subsequent modifications may provide the key to successful alleviation of torticollis by stereotactic surgery, but it is premature to suggest that we have the answer at the present time.[95]

Consequently, a comprehensive stepwise program has been developed for patients with spasmodic torticollis.[96] They are admitted to the Chronic Pain Unit for an evaluation period of approximately 2 weeks. The initial step is a thorough psychiatric evaluation and psychometric testing. Half of the patients who have been referred fail this initial part of the evaluation and prove to be sufficiently unstable so that major surgical procedures or the use of implanted stimulators would be contraindicated.

It is important to establish goals early in the program. Some torticollis patients have considerable neck pain and are distressed from the continual pulling sensation. Others have minimal discomfort but are self-conscious about the abnormal head position. The individual program should be directed toward alleviating the specific problem the patient finds distressing.

Patients are given training in relaxation techniques.[77] An occasional patient who has torticollis secondary to an emotional reaction to a specific psychiatric problem may benefit sufficiently from psychiatric therapy so that nothing further need be done.

Biofeedback is helpful in a very small number of patients. If the pulling sensation or muscle pain is the major problem, electromyographic biofeedback of the involved cervical muscles may be helpful. If abnormal head position is the major complaint, visual biofeedback may be employed—the patient stands in front of a mirror on which a cross has been taped and attempts to align the nose and brows with it.

All patients in the program undergo a trial of transcutaneous stimulation (TENS). Various electrode positions are tried, with both electrodes over the more involved sternocleidomastoid muscle, with one over that muscle and the other in a neutral position, with one on each side of the neck, etc. Although only a few patients respond extremely well to transcutaneous stimulation, it is such a benign procedure that a trial is warranted for every torticollis patient being considered for an invasive procedure.

Those patients who remain candidates after psychiatric evaluation, who are not sufficiently improved by a conservative program, and who can tolerate stimulation and the apparatus of TENS may be considered for dorsal cord stimulation.

The major advantage of dorsal cord stimulation is that it is possible to evaluate the patient with a percutaneously inserted subarachnoid electrode in a reasonably convenient and safe manner, and, indeed, two thirds of the patients thus evaluated have responded satisfactorily. Another advantage of dorsal cord stimulation for the management of spasmodic torticollis is that no complications have been reported with its use.

For the percutaneous trial, the subarachnoid space is entered with a Tuohy needle introduced at the C2 level, just as in percutaneous cervical cordotomy. The electrode is threaded down to the C5 level and the needle removed, leaving the electrode in place. The patient may be up and about while a trial of stimulation is carried out over 5 to 8 days. Since only a monopolar system is employed, a transcutaneous stimulating electrode can be used as the indifferent electrode and taped to a neutral position at the base of the neck.

Stimulation frequencies up to 1500 Hz should be tried. It has been found empirically that most patients respond better to frequencies greater than 1100 Hz. It may be that the therapeutic effect is the result of depolarization of the proprioceptive nerve roots as they enter the cervical spinal cord, with resultant abolition of abnormal tonic neck reflexes.

If the patient responds to stimulation through the percutaneous electrode, the system can be converted to a permanent implanted device. Because it is difficult to obtain satisfactory placement of a percutaneous epidural electrode in patients whose neck is turning, surgically implanted electrodes have been employed. Epidural placement after a C1 laminectomy has been found to be effective. It may be necessary to order a modified transmitter to provide the stimulus frequency that has been found to be most effective. Other investigators recommend proceeding directly to a surgically implanted stimulator with no percutaneous trial.[97]

For the one third who do not respond to dorsal cord stimulation or who are opposed to trial stimulation for any reason, the classical Dandy-Foerster operation is recommended.[98] This involves section of the anterior roots of C1, C2, and C3 bilaterally, both spinal accessory nerves, and possibly section of the anterior of root C4 on the more involved side.[99]

A suboccipital craniectomy is performed, along with a laminectomy from C1 through C4. The dura is opened, and, under the operating microscope, the procedure is begun at the lowest root to be sectioned. The dentate ligament is cut from its attachment to the dura at each level, the anterior roots are identified, accompanying radicular arteries are dissected free

and preserved, and the anterior roots are cut. It is important to identify the C1 nerve roots accurately, since failure to section all of the fibers precludes a good result. There is usually not a posterior root to C1, and the anterior root may extend in a downward direction where it may be obscured by the vertebral artery.

The usual procedure is to section the spinal accessory nerves intradurally at the same sitting, but one must recognize that that denervates the trapezius as well as the sternocleidomastoid muscle. If the patient would be disabled by shoulder weakness, it may be more desirable to section the innervation of the sternocleidomastoid muscles selectively through separate incisions in the neck.

If an intradural section of the spinal accessory nerves is done, it should be done as far laterally as possible as the nerve enters the jugular foramen. The lower-most fibers of the vagus nerve can be seen joining the spinal accessory nerve laterally, and they should be included in the section, since they are actually spinal accessory fibers. Even at that, 50 percent of the patients demonstrate some remaining innervation of sternocleidomastoid muscles if an electromyogram is done several days after surgery. This remaining innervation should be looked for routinely, and if it exists, the spinal accessory nerve should be sectioned in the neck.

The procedure to section the spinal accessory nerve peripherally is done with the patient in the supine position. A diagonal incision is made at the anterior border of the sternocleidomastoid muscle just below its attachment to the skull. Alternately, a more cosmetically satisfactory result can be obtained by allowing the skin incision to fall into a natural crease, but this compromises the exposure somewhat. Dissection is carried out on the undersurface of the sternocleidomastoid muscle. The spinal accessory nerve can usually be found entering that muscle at the point where the lateral mass of the C2 vertebra can be palpated. The branch to the trapezius muscle usually comes off just before it enters the body of the sternocleidomastoid muscle. If not, dissection can be carried into the muscle in an attempt to separate the sternocleidomastoid fibers selectively, if that is desired. Each branch can be identified with the use of an intraoperative nerve stimulator.

The potential side-effects of the Dandy-Foerster operation involve primarily damage to the brain stem (which may follow damage to small radicular arteries) such as dysphagia, vestibular symptoms, unsteadiness, or even failure to regain consciousness after surgery. The mortality rate is reported between 1 and 4 percent. The usual potential complications of posterior fossa surgery in the sitting position must be considered, of course, such as venous air embolism or hypotension.

Eighty percent of the patients have satisfactory improvement following this procedure. There is surprisingly little loss of mobility of the neck, but loss of trapezius power may cause weakness of the shoulders.

Cerebral palsy does not lend itself readily to neurosurgical management. Although there are some aspects of the motor disorders of cerebral palsy, spasticity in particular, that may be somewhat alleviated by functional neurosurgery, the major motor disabilities involved with choreoathetosis are only minimally affected, if at all.

On the other hand, the spasticity that accompanies cerebral palsy may respond to one of several functional neurosurgical manipulations, either ablation or stimulation. A number of reports in the late 1960s encouraged the feeling that dentatotomy might be useful for the treatment of spasticity of cerebral palsy.[100–102] The effect decreased with long-term follow-up, however, so that it is not often used today. Nevertheless, a 30 percent improvement in spasticity was generally reported, with perhaps facilitation of nursing care in 50 percent of the patients.[101] The operation was relatively direct, with the coordinates being related to a fourth ventriculogram (although the coordinates of the dentate nucleus per se caused some disagreement). The operation was safe with surprisingly little risk of cerebellar or motor impairment.

Stereotactic thalamotomy or pallidotomy has been tried with patients with choreoathetosis, with mixed results.[103]

There is a stimulation procedure worthy of note. Chronic cerebellar stimulation (CCS) has been employed for spasticity of cerebral origin in cerebral palsy patients, but has not obtained widespread acceptance. It was observed[104] that stimulation of the anterior lobe of the cerebellum may inhibit decerebrate rigidity in experimental animals, presumably because of a descending inhibitory influence on the myotatic reflex arc. Because a similar mechanism of increase in segmental activity is involved in spasticity of cerebral palsy origin,[105,106] a technique was developed to stimulate the anterior lobe of the cerebellum in cerebral palsy patients.

The technique of implantation involves performing a small craniectomy or two craniectomies on either side of the midline just below the transverse sinus. The dura is opened parallel to the sinus and flat cerebellar electrodes are inserted; the electrodes are mounted on a Silastic pad that is the approximate length required to position the electrodes anteriorly. There are two different models, one with a single channel and the other with two separate channels requiring the implantation of two separate receivers, that seem to work equally well. The dura is closed.

The same type of radio receiver is implanted in a infraclavicular pocket for chronic cerebellar stimulation as for other implanted stimulating devices. A subcutaneous tunnel is passed to the incision overlying the suboccipital area.

Various types of stimulation have been employed, and it appears that intermittent stimulation may provide the best effect. The radio transmitter especially devised for cerebellar stimulation has the option of such duty cycles built into it so that it can be programmed to stimulate and rest at several-minute intervals. It is necessary to try various parameters for each patient to find the optimal program.

There has been considerable concern about whether the stimulation of the cerebellum causes damage, particularly to the Purkinje cells. One early report[107] indicated significant damage underlying the electrodes, but later reports[108] were not in agreement. It appears that there may have been artifacts associated with the size of the electrode and current densities in the original study, and later studies indicate there is a significant safety factor in the use of chronic cerebellar stimulation.[108] Aside from that concern, there have been no significant complications reported. One technical problem is the occasional leakage of cerebrospinal fluid along the leads, but this can be prevented by applying a purse-string suture along the tract at the time of the initial surgery.

Although chronic cerebellar stimulation was originally intended to alleviate the spasticity of cerebral palsy, there have been reports of subjective improvement in choreoathetosis as well.[105] Such improvement has not, however, been completely documented. Basically, it may be said that patients look the same but may be able to perform better. Patients who walk only with assistance may be able to walk with crutches, speech or

swallowing may be significantly improved, and care may be easier. Attempts at documenting the magnitude and the mechanism of improvement have yielded inconclusive results.[106]

Nevertheless, some patients with cerebral palsy appear to have benefited from chronic cerebellar stimulation, even those whose major disability was choreoathetosis. Its use might be recommended for those patients with good mentation who could improve their motor activities with some improvement in spasticity or choreoathetosis.

It can be generalized that stereotactic lesions have a similar effect to chronic cerebellar stimulation in cerebral palsy, that is, patients look the same but may perform better. Indeed, in taking motion pictures of a number of cerebral palsy patients before and after stereotactic surgery, it was difficult to see any difference. Their performance record, however, as documented on the film, demonstrated a significant increase in motor facility.

The target point was originally defined as being in the globus pallidus, but the present recommendation is to make the primary lesion in Forel's field. If a second lesion is going to be made a lesion on the second side 3 months later, it can be made in the medial portion of the globus pallidus, at the origin of the ansa lenticularis. The target point may be 2 mm posterior to the anterior commissure, 10 mm lateral, and at the level of the intercommissural line. If stimulation produces visual sensations, the electrode should be withdrawn 1 mm. If low-frequency stimulation produces motor effects, the electrode is too close to the internal capsule and should be moved 2 mm lateral.

It is important to remember that patients with cerebral palsy have not had the opportunity to acquire a repertoire of patterned motor behavior. Even if the spasticity or abnormal movements are obviated, it is still necessary to work intensively with this group of patients to train the released muscles to do those things that would have developed automatically, an approach to "habilitation" rather than rehabilitation.

Spasticity may respond quite well to functional neurosurgery, depending on the origin of the problem. In general, one should consider whether the spasticity is of cerebral or spinal origin. Cerebral causes for spasticity include cerebral palsy, stroke, and degenerative disease. Spinal causes of spasticity include spinal cord injury, spinal cord tumor, cervical canal stenosis, and some spinal degenerative diseases. Multiple sclerosis may be a combination of cerebral and spinal spasticity, but there is generally a sufficient spinal component so that remarks concerning spinal etiology of spasticity may be taken to include multiple sclerosis.

Because the spasticity that accompanies hemiplegia after a stroke generally does not have an underlying pattern of normal motor control, functional neurosurgical procedures are not ordinarily recommended. On the other hand, spasticity of spinal origin may often be dealt with successfully, particularly the spasticity that may accompany a spinal degenerative disease such as multiple sclerosis.

Patients with multiple sclerosis may respond quite dramatically to dorsal cord stimulation. The mechanism for such response is not known, but one may theorize that it is the stimulation of a descending inhibitory pathway. Stimulation at relatively modest frequencies, 28 to 120 Hz, may allow significant improvement in function, not only of the extremities, but of the bowel and bladder as well. In fact, even though stimulation is applied to the cervical area, some patients experience improvement in speech.

Because evaluation with a percutaneous or subarachnoid

electrode is quite simple, any patient with multiple sclerosis who is impaired by spasticity but still has underlying motor control and good mentation may be considered a candidate for dorsal cord stimulation.

An epidural electrode can be inserted for cervical stimulation by performing a puncture in the midline at or near the T1 level and threading the electrode upward. Because symptoms may vary from day to day, a trial of stimulation should last for at least several days. It is not uncommon for stimulation for several hours to be followed by improvement in spasticity for several days, and such an observation should not necessarily be interpreted as coincidental spontaneous remission. Stimulation is well tolerated, and it does not appear that the use of stimulators is associated with exacerbation or acceleration of the multiple sclerosis. If stimulation provides a beneficial effect, the radio receiver can be implanted and the entire system internalized.

Spasticity after partial spinal cord injury may be managed with an approach similar to that used for multiple sclerosis, but spasticity below the level of a complete spinal cord functional transection is different both in mechanism and management.

The indication for treatment of spasticity after complete spinal cord injury concerns not the injury itself but the occurrence of complications. Patients with spastic contractures of extremities for whom rehabilitation has become difficult or impossible may benefit from improved ability to position and move more advantageously. Patients whose position in bed is limited because of spastic contractures may develop decubiti, which can be managed only by resolving the spasticity to position the patient to lie off the ulcers.

One must consider the distribution of the spasticity that must be alleviated. Patients with spinal cord injury may have spasticity particularly of muscle groups on one side of a joint, leading to contracture of that joint (in contrast to patients with cerebral palsy who may have a multitude of patterns of spasticity of individual muscle groups that may prohibit full use of extremities).

Determination is made as to which muscle or groups require decreased hypertonicity, and ideally this pattern is verified by electromyography. If a single hypertonic muscle can be identified as the cause of the specific problem, treatment with 40 percent alcohol injection to the motor points is fairly simple and may be quite effective. If the problem involves a group of muscles with partial denervation, the nerve supplying that muscle group may be blocked with lidocaine as a temporary test, and, if effective, the lesion may be made permanent by injection of 6 to 10 percent phenol in saline. If the spasticity involves several muscle groups, particularly if they are unilateral, surgical or chemical rhizotomy may be considered.[109] If sensory loss already exists, a dorsal rhizotomy may be effective, without producing the atrophy of a lower motor neuron lesion. Alternatively, a rhizotomy involving some but not all of the anterior root may provide sufficient relief.

Sensory rhizotomy as an open surgical technique for the treatment of spasticity involves a multiple-level laminectomy to expose the spinal cord at the appropriate levels, with due attention to the discrepancy between the vertebral level and the level of the spinal nerve roots. In order to verify that the appropriate nerve roots are identified, electromyographic electrodes should be placed in the appropriate muscles, as well as adjacent muscle groups, prior to surgical draping, so the response to electrical stimulation of the exposed anterior roots can guide the surgeon to section only the appropriate spinal roots. It is necessary to separate the dentate ligament from its attachment to the dura to rotate the cord slightly to gain access to the anterior root. Care should be taken to avoid radicular arteries if preservation of spinal cord activity or segmental reflex patterns is desired.

Radiofrequency rhizotomy, as described elsewhere, may also be used to treat spasticity. It may be extremely difficult, however, to position the patient with contractures for the optimal x-ray control that this procedure requires.

One of the factors in deciding the manner in which spasticity of the lower extremities might be attacked is the function of the patient's bladder. If the patient has a contracted bladder in continual spasm, there may be an advantage to treating the spasticity of the bladder as well by one of the injection techniques. If the patient has a reflex bladder that is operating in optimal fashion with periodic evacuation, one would wish to avoid compromise of bladder function and would want to consider a longitudinal or Bischoff's myelotomy[110,111] (see Chapter 103). If the spasticity of the lower extremities is extensor and provides the patient with some weight-bearing capabilities that are best left preserved, yet problems exist with spasticity of the bladder, one might consider a presacral neurectomy or rhizotomy of the S2, S3, and S4 roots by radiofrequency current or injection.

If less selective treatment of spasticity is desired, however (either to include sacral segments or if it is not critical whether or not sacral segments are included), the simple technique of hot saline injection might be considered. This procedure can be done only on patients with complete functional transection of the spinal cord who have no sensation below the level of the injury. Saline at 80° C is instilled into the subarachnoid space in order to destroy the nerve roots and possibly an isolated spinal cord segment. Because both temperature and volume are controlled, the saline cools as it mixes with cerebrospinal fluid so that the functioning cord at higher levels is protected.

The procedure can be done in the patient's room. A basin of saline with a thermometer is placed on a hot plate. Lumbar puncture is performed at L3 or L4. When a free flow of spinal fluid is obtained, a volume of saline is instilled. For a midthoracic lesion, 10 ml of saline can be rapidly injected. If spasticity persists, an additional 10 to 20 ml can be injected after several minutes. The spasticity may return totally or in part over the next few days, in which case the procedure is repeated. Interestingly, when two injections are performed within several days, there is much less likelihood of return of spasticity after the second injection. If spasticity persists, the volume can be adjusted accordingly.

If a more selective injection is desired, for unilateral effect only, for instance, intrathecal phenol can be used. The patient is placed in the lateral position on the myelogram table. A lumbar puncture is performed and 1 ml of Pantopaque is instilled. The table is tilted so that the Pantopaque is centered at the center of the roots the surgeon wants to affect. Phenol crystals are dissolved in Pantopaque, 100 mg/ml. If 2 nerve roots are to be treated, 3 ml can be used, and if 4 nerve roots, 6 ml can be used. The phenol-Pantopaque is instilled and the table readjusted as necessary to position the Pantopaque over the involved roots. The patient is allowed to remain in that position for 10 to 15 minutes, and the Pantopaque is removed.

A unique use of functional neurosurgery may be employed to break the pattern of ankle clonus in a patient who is otherwise ambulatory. A peripheral nerve stimulator, as used for pain treatment, can be implanted on the common peroneal nerve. Stimulation produces sufficient reciprocal inhibition between the antagonistic muscles so voluntary movement can be maintained as the pattern of clonus is broken up. The stimulus intensity and rate are adjusted to produce nonpainful sensation and sustained, slightly tonic dorsal flexion and eversion of the foot.[112,113] The frequency, duration, and amplitude of the stimulus train must be established for each patient. In general, the amplitude must be large enough to produce an H wave, the train duration must be greater than 400 msec, and the frequency must be from 30 to 50 Hz.

DEVELOPMENT OF STEREOTACTIC SURGERY

The history of the development of stereotactic surgery originally involved surgery for affective disorders. Indeed, it was dissatisfaction with classical prefrontal lobotomy[114,115] that motivated Spiegel and Wycis[2,92] to develop the techniques for human stereotactic surgery, and the first reported stereotactic patients were treated for affective disorders. One must also put into context that the indications for psychiatric surgery of any type were much broader at that time, before the development of tranquilizers.

HISTORICAL PERSPECTIVE

The original techniques of open or semiblind prefrontal lobotomy were relatively nonselective in that they interrupted the fibers to the frontal area concerned with intellectual function, along with those fibers involved with regulation of emotions.[116–118] The original stereotactic target for affective disease was the dorsomedian nucleus of the thalamus, from which those frontal projecting fibers of emotional importance originate, but not those of intellectual function.[71,92,119] Even as techniques became more refined and selective during the 1950s and 1960s, precise interruption of only the desired tracts remained uncertain.

Although it has been more than 35 years since it has been demonstrated that psychosurgery can be performed with significantly less risk to intellect than the original nonselective procedures,[117,120] there are those who have lobbied against the use of psychosurgery, without acknowledging the progress and refinements that have occurred in that field since the introduction of stereotactic and selective techniques.

Approximately 15 years ago, a movement was instigated to ban psychosurgery,[121] and a discussion of the present status of psychosurgery must examine that controversy. Four unsubstantiated allegations were made:

1. Psychosurgery was not an effective means of treatment for psychiatric conditions.
2. Psychosurgery resulted in intolerable mental deficits.
3. Psychosurgery was being used (or misused) as a social or political tool.
4. Psychosurgery was selectively used against minorities.

To investigate these allegations, the National Commission for the Protection of Human Subjects of Biomedical and Behavioral Research was formed. Not only were all four allegations proven false, but the evidence gathered to investigate these allegations demonstrated that psychosurgery was reasonably safe and effective.[122]

Despite the favorable findings of the Commission, the furor provoked by this political controversy has significantly wounded the field of psychosurgery. Although there may be a gradual increase in procedures over the past few years, it is estimated that the present rate of psychosurgery is only 10 to 15 percent what it was two decades ago, even though no other significant advances in psychiatric care have provided alternate forms of treatment for the group of patients that was formerly treated with psychosurgery. This low level of activity, plus perhaps the reluctance of some investigators to perform research in the area, has significantly slowed progress in the field. Nevertheless, surgery is still indicated for many patients with affective disorders, and may be their only chance of improvement.

As part of the effort to evaluate psychosurgery, the Commission reviewed the extent to which psychosurgery was being practiced in the United States, and extensively reviewed the literature. Perhaps most significantly, a contract was let for a group of experts not involved with individual patients to perform a retrospective and prospective neuropsychologic examination of patients undergoing cingulotomy for a variety of psychiatric problems. This examination, representing a reasonably well-controlled and most objective review of the potential side-effects and neurologic function following cingulotomy for affective disorders (as well as pain), detected no lasting deficits in behavioral capacities from surgery,[123,124] but considerable subjective benefit.

In summary, the Commission recommended that "psychosurgery be used only to meet the health needs of individual patients and then only under strict limitations and controls, with added safeguards when the patient is a prisoner, a minor, or in a mental institution."[122] The Commission also noted that the safety and efficacy of specific neurosurgical procedures for the treatment of particular disorders, however, have not been demonstrated to the degree that would permit such procedures to be considered "accepted" practice. It was recognized that degrees of expertise and ancillary psychiatric facilities varied from one neurosurgeon to another, and it was felt that the decision for psychosurgery should be in the hands of a competent team. For this reason, as well as to assure that psychosurgery would not be misused, the Commission recommended that a board, similar to the institutional review boards that evaluate experimental protocols, be available at institutions where psychosurgery is contemplated, to evaluate protocols and procedures (but not make decisions about the case of individual patients) and that the composition and procedures for review of psychosurgical programs be recommended by the Department of Health, Education and Welfare (now the Department of Health and Human Services).[122] Even though a decade has passed since these recommendations were made, they were not enacted, partly because of the decrease in activity in the field.[125]

The Commission suggested that it was still appropriate to call psychosurgery experimental, not because it did not have demonstrated safety and effectiveness, but because there were still sufficient unknowns regarding the field. Accordingly, anyone who assumed the responsibility of using this treatment should likewise assume the responsibility of maintaining available records of well-controlled observations for the further advancement of the field, a recommendation that would be appropriate for most surgical procedures.

As a general rule, it should be stressed that surgery should be considered for the treatment of affective disorders only after an extensive period of psychiatric and pharmacologic management has verified that no other treatment is satisfactory. Since the indications for psychosurgery hinge on psychiatric rather than neurosurgical diagnosis, it should be considered only upon recommendation of one or preferably several psychiatrists who have personally evaluated the patient. A thorough search for underlying pathology, particularly epilepsy, should precede any psychosurgical procedure. Surgery might be considered before an extensive course of electroconvulsive therapy (ECT), since there is evidence that stereotactic procedures result in less permanent neurologic deficits than ECT.[122,123] The only exception to the recommendation for a prolonged period of psychiatric management involves those patients who are so suicidal that they would likely not survive a prolonged evaluation.

Much of the evaluation of the effectiveness of surgery for affective disorders involves the subjective impression of the examiner. Except for neuropsychologic testing to evaluate untoward side-effects, there exist few objective criteria to evaluate the efficacy of any given procedure. Nevertheless, there is some consistency in the subjective reports of both patients and physicians that allow conclusions to be drawn about the effectiveness of particular procedures for specific psychiatric problems.

There is some disagreement about the relationship between psychosurgery and surgery for chronic pain. Many patients who present with a chief complaint of intractable pain may benefit from psychosurgery, particularly cingulotomy, but the duration of benefit is often limited. Such patients ordinarily have such obvious and severe emotional problems associated with their pain that, in this group of patients, cingulotomy very often might be recommended for their affective problems alone. With this in mind, the rule otherwise stands that there is little role for ablative procedures in the management of chronic intractable pain, although it may be useful to treat cancer pain.

ANATOMY OF SURGERY FOR AFFECTIVE DISORDERS

The portion of the brain concerned with regulation and expression of emotions is generally referred to as the limbic system. As might be anticipated from the system that controls such a basic aspect of behavior as emotion, it consists, to a large extent, of the philogenetically old type of cortical tissue that encircles the inner part of the cerebral hemispheres-hence, the name "limbic" or border. This cortex has interconnections with other structures, such as the hypothalamus, the anterior thalamic nuclei, the cingulate gyrus, the fornix, the mammillary bodies, and the hippocampus, all of which constituted the original Papez limbic circuit.[126] This system has been expanded to include the cortex of the orbitofrontal area, the insula, and the anterior temporal lobes, along with their connections to the amygdala and the dorsomedian nucleus of the thalamus.[127]

The limbic system, as currently defined, consists of two circuits—the medial limbic circuit and the basolateral circuit[128]—and sometimes a third circuit referred to as the defense reaction circuit.[129]

The medial limbic circuit, or Papez circuit, is the medial frontal cortex-cingulate-hippocampal-fornix-mammillary-anterior thalamic-frontal cortex circuit and has rich connections with the reticular activating system.[130] It passes from the septal nuclei via the cingulum bundle in the cingulate gyrus to the hippocampus of the temporal lobe. Fibers pass from the hippocampal gyrus by way of the fornix to the mammillary body, and then via the mammillo-thalamic tract to the anterior nucleus of the thalamus. Fibers project from that nucleus via the anterior thalamic radiation to the orbito-frontal cortex, which projects back to the cingulum to close the circuit. Affective and autonomic responses have been obtained from stimulation of this circuit.[112,130] In addition to the involvement of this circuit with emotions, parts of the circuit are concerned with memory, such as the hippocampus, the fornix, and the mammillary bodies.[131]

The basolateral or lateral limbic circuit lies outside the brain stem and involves the orbital cortex with its cortical connections to the anterior temporal cortex, which radiates in turn to the amygdala, which serves in this case as the outflow from the temporal neocortex. Projections run from the amygdala to the dorsomedial nucleus of the thalamus, and from there to the orbital cortex to complete the orbito-frontal cortex-temporal-amygdala-dorsomedial thalamic-frontal circuit.

Thus, as in the motor-control system, we have two circuits that involve adjacent (but in this case not overlapping) areas of the thalamus, whose efferent conducting systems are comparable, forming a massive linked system.[131]

The defense reaction circuit connects those areas of the brain concerned with generation of emotion to the areas concerned with the visceral responses to emotion, such as fight or flight.[129] It involves connections from the hypothalamus via the stria terminalis to the amygdala, and from the amygdala back to the hypothalamus.

Since the amygdala serves as one of the major outflow tracts from the temporal cortex, it may propagate seizure activity from the temporal lobe to other areas where such abnormal activity might be expressed. If a temporal lobe seizure involves behavioral abnormalities, as is common, a lesion in the amygdala may interrupt the expression of that abnormal behavior.[132–136]

Since the limbic system is more of a functional than an anatomic unit and is defined experimentally, to a large extent, by response to stimulation, it is not surprising that simulation in humans may produce identifiable reactions that allow localization of electrode placement. Although most stereotactic surgery is performed on conscious and cooperating patients, the patient population for surgery for affective disorders sometimes makes it necessary to perform such surgery under general anesthesia. Nevertheless, awake patients are able to report the effects of stimulation,[137] which are very often emotional in nature, that is, a feeling of well-being or a feeling of anxiety and tension. Although there may be no response to stimulation in approximately half the cases, when a response does occur, it provides good verification of electrode placement.

If there is a response on stimulation of the fibers between the thalamus and the orbital cortex within the anterior limb of the internal capsule, it is likely to be a positive response, or a feeling of well-being.[137] Likewise, as one might expect, a similar response may be obtained from stimulation of the genu of the corpus callosum. Of those patients who respond to stimulation of the cingulum, half may report a "negative" feeling, or one of dysphoria, or some other strange or ill-defined sensation, but it is uncommon for a positive response to occur.[138] Stimulation of the amygdala may produce a range of aggressive responses, such as a desire to attack the examiner, or swearing or destructive behavior.[139] One must comment, however, that the characteristic depth electroencephalogram that may be recorded from the amygdala often provides accurate localization without stimulation.

Interestingly, patients undergoing stimulation under local

anesthesia rarely have autonomic or visceral responses, except perhaps secondary to a physical response. Under general anesthesia, however, stimulation of the cingulate gyrus or mesial-frontal projections usually causes apnea with less constant changes in pulse, blood pressure, and forearm blood flow.[130,140,141]

SURGICAL MANAGEMENT OF AFFECTIVE DISORDERS

Disagreement about the technique of psychosurgery may stem from several sources, including the following:

1. Psychosurgery as originally practiced involved blind sectioning of fibers projecting to large areas of the frontal lobes. The areas affected were diffuse and inconsistent, both because of the poor control over anatomic landmarks and the variable effect of interrupting blood supply. Although there was significant benefit to many patients, it was often at the expense of significant deterioration of mentation. At that time, however, before the advent of tranquilizers, there was often no alternate pharmacologic therapy available.[142]
2. Psychiatric diagnosis has been and remains imprecise. Even though many conditions for which there are psychosurgical indications are well defined, difference in nomenclature between countries or during different decades makes it difficult to compare ideas and results.[125]
3. Most neurosurgeons who report their experience with psychosurgery tend to report the effect of a single procedure on patients in several diagnostic categories. There is no extensive well-controlled study to compare the effects of various procedures on matched patients. Consequently, it is impossible to designate with certainty which procedure may be more effective for a particular condition, although it can generally be stated that interrupting the limbic system at any accessible point in its circuit may provide similar results. Authors who use different procedures may draw opposite conclusions.[143,144]
4. Many studies are poorly controlled and rely on such general assessments as "generally improved" or "quality of life improved." The duration of follow-up varies significantly, as does the completeness of follow-up. Often the operating surgeon may be the only one to assess the results, a problem common to many therapeutic studies. Although there are several good attempts at prospective studies with managed controls, it is difficult to obtain sufficient patients in the control groups to make meaningful comparison possible. Despite those shortcomings, however, results are generally in agreement in those studies that are well controlled.[145]
5. Early studies, before the availability of tranquilizers, concentrated on schizophrenic patients who remained management problems even though they were hospitalized. Presently, many such patients are being managed successfully by medical means, and the emphasis of psychosurgery is on specific behavioral disorders, rather than schizophrenia. In general discussions about psychiatric treatment of emotional illness, all too often there is insufficient distinction made between those early imprecise procedures and indications and the present-day procedures, which involve limited interruption of specific pathways.

Conditions that are generally agreed to be indications for psychosurgery are those characterized by a stereotyped and excessive emotional response, that is, depression,[46,146-149] chronic anxiety or tension state,[149] obsessive-compulsive states,[150] and perhaps the depressive component of manic-depressive disorder.[46]

There is considerable disagreement as to whether surgery is the appropriate treatment for aggression. The type of aggressiveness and violence for which one might consider the surgery used for epilepsy is "personal violent behavior, unwarranted and usually unprovoked acts that directly attempt to, or actually do, injure or destroy another person or thing. This does not include violence consistently organized for a political motive."[151] Most such patients have epilepsy,[152] and even those who are not classified as such have a high incidence of abnormal EEG or postoperative seizures. The implication is, of course, that the type of aggression that responds to stereotactic surgery is that associated with temporal lobe seizures, and the procedure of choice is amygdalotomy. This is in contrast to the early literature in which prefrontal lobotomy was employed in unmanageably aggressive schizophrenic patients, in which case it might have rendered the patients less aggressive or violent, but it did not have a beneficial effect on the schizophrenia itself.[116]

Some authors[153,154] attempt to interrupt the autonomic component of such aggressive behavior by producing lesions in the posterior hypothalamus. Although they report beneficial results in 80 percent or more of their patients, this procedure is not generally accepted, so that we might recommend, for the purpose of this presentation, to consider explosive aggression as a component of temporal lobe epilepsy for which amygdalotomy or temporal lobectomy would be the procedure of choice,[155] as has been found in one controlled study comparing both procedures.[156]

There has been even greater controversy concerning the use of surgery for the treatment of "hedonia," sexual delinquency, pedophilia, homosexuality, or sexual violence, with "good results" from anterior hypothalamotomy for all except homosexuality.[157-159] The indications for such surgery are both controversial and ill defined. Patients included in these series have generally been confined because of legal difficulties emanating from their behavior, but it is not always clear whether it was the sexual component of their behavior or their generally unacceptable behavior that was the problem, and whether truly voluntary consent can be given by patients so incarcerated.[160] Since the diagnoses are not defined in a standard fashion, a neurosurgeon from Sweden pointed out, when hearing of these results, "What's considered hypersexuality in Germany may be normal behavior in Sweden."

One may find it acceptable to use the same target point for obsessive-compulsive state, anxiety, and depression; that is, cingulotomy is the procedure most likely to give beneficial results in all three conditions with minimal chance of undesirable side-effects,[142] even though there are favorable reports on the use of anterior capsulotomy for these same conditions.[161-163]

There have been numerous cingulotomy techniques described in the literature, some with open surgery, some with relatively freehand insertion of electrodes, and some stereotactic. Since stereotactic surgery provides the best opportunity for the accurate placement of a controlled lesion with the greatest safety, that is the procedure of choice and the technique that will be presented primarily (see Table 92-1).[130]

A ventriculostomy is performed as sufficient air is introduced to demonstrate the anterior horn and roof of both lateral ventricles. On the lateral x-ray film, a vertical line, approximately at right angles to the intercommissural line, is drawn 3 cm behind the tip of the frontal horn. The first lesion is made on a vertical line 3 cm posterior to the tip of the frontal horn and 5 mm above the roof the ventricle at the lateral-most border of the ventricle. A second lesion is made 8 mm medial to this. Another pair of lesions are made 12 mm anterior to the first pair, for a total of four lesions on each side.[129,140] A relatively large electrode should be used, since it is desirable to interrupt as much of the cingulate bundle as possible. Lesions are made bilaterally at one sitting, since unilateral lesions are frequently not effective and bilateral lesions are well tolerated.

Alternately, target points for cingulotomy can be made 3 to 4 cm behind the tip of the lateral ventricle, 5 mm lateral to the midline, and both 1 and 2 cm above the roof of the ventricle.[148] Single lesions can be made at these points, if they are relatively large, that is, 1 cm in diameter. Other authors[120,164] report similar procedures, but all are designed to interrupt the cingulate bundle at various sites.

For the first 7 to 10 days postoperatively, the patient may exhibit anergia, lack of drive, and lack of initiation of conversation.[149,165] Although this initial appearance may be distressing, it is only temporary, and bears no relationship to the final clinical result. During the remainder of the first 3 weeks, the patient may show some increased irritability and verbal aggressiveness, but this gradually settles down so that many patients have achieved their final clinical results in 4 to 6 weeks.

If an adequate clinical result is not obtained after waiting a minimum of 6 to 12 weeks, lesions may also be made in the fibers extending between the thalamus and the orbital cortex as they pass through the anterior limb of the internal capsule, a so-called anterior capsulotomy or medial prefrontal leukotomy. The coordinates for these lesions are on a vertical line 1.5 cm anterior to the base of the anterior clinoid process. Three lesions are made in the form of a triangle with its apex superior. At 6 mm from the midline, one lesion is made 1 cm above the floor of the anterior fossa and a second lesion 1.5 cm above the floor of the anterior fossa. A single lateral lesion is made 14 mm from the midline and 1 cm above the floor of the anterior fossa.[130]

For those surgeons who would still prefer an open rather than a stereotactic operation, the following technique is described,[165] although others may be equally satisfactory.[166] Bilateral trephine openings are made 2.5 cm from the midline and 13 cm above the glabella. The dura is opened, and a brain needle is passed vertically until it touches the orbital plate. A core of brain tissue is dissected along the brain needle for a width of 1.5 cm. The ventricle may either be traversed or a subependymal dissection can be performed if the ependyma separates easily. Dissection continues along the tract of the brain needle through the inferior part of the cingulate gyrus, and is carried medially until the gray matter on the mesial surface of the frontal lobe is encountered and inferiorly until the subfrontal cortex is seen. The inferior portion of the dissection is entirely medial to the brain cannula, since the fibers to be interrupted are just below the mesial cortex, and the lateral fibers should be preserved.

There is some opinion[144] that obsessive-compulsive patients do better if the primary procedure is an anterior capsulotomy, but statistical comparisons suggest that cingulate lesions are preferable.[167]

It has been suggested that schizophrenic patients who are unmanageable because of a great deal of anxiety and tension may benefit from a lesion in the genu of the corpus callosum, interrupting the pathways between the two frontal lobes, a procedure called a mesoloviotomy.[168] Although results are encouraging, the procedure has not been widely adopted.

EPILEPSY

The surgical management of epilepsy is discussed in Chapter 107. It might be appropriate, however, to review briefly the role of stereotactic surgery in the management of epilepsy (see also Gildenberg in Frost).[169]

Regardless of the surgical approach contemplated, depth electrode recording for the localization of the epileptogenic focus may be helpful, particularly when the surface electroencephalogram is inconclusive. It may be possible to obtain evidence for laterality of a temporal lobe focus, even though surface recording may show bilateral discharges,[40,170] or to identify the focus critically, so the location, shape, and extent of a resection can be tailored to an individual patient.

It is not uncommon for a seizure not to present itself during a random electroencephalographic recording session, in which case it may be necessary to perform prolonged monitoring. Since seizure activity may be particularly apparent at night or during the induction of sleep, a sleep recording may demonstrate a focus that is not otherwise apparent. There are a group of patients who fail to demonstrate sufficient interictal abnormal activity to localize the epileptogenic focus without recording an actual seizure. Other patients may not demonstrate a focus, even with prolonged sleep recording, and others still may show so much bilateral epileptogenic activity that the localization of the focus becomes obscured. In all these cases, the origin of the epileptic activity may become apparent with recording from implanted electrodes over several days or several weeks.

Epidural or subdural electrodes usually consist of several electrodes mounted on a Silastic strip, which are inserted through a small craniectomy or burr hole underneath the temporal lobe, particularly under the mesial part or at the temporal tip. The electrode wires are brought out through the scalp so direct connections can be made for recordings.

A subcortical electrode may provide more precise information about the origin of epileptic activity, particularly if prolonged recordings are made to capture the profile of a seizure. Propagation of abnormal activity from one electrode site to another can provide definite localization, particularly when the seizure activity begins in one temporal lobe and projects contralaterally or involves subcortical structures, such as the globus pallidus or thalamus.[93]

There are several types of depth electrodes for recording. The most practical are those with multiple contacts, which consist of several wires bound together to form a number of separate contacts.[171] Coordinates are selected to distribute the electrode array throughout a representative portion of the temporal lobes, and four or five electrodes may be implanted on each side. Some stereotactic apparatuses, such as the Talairach apparatus, allow implantation of the electrodes from laterally, for direct access to the temporal areas.[170] If multiple electrodes are used, particularly in the temporal areas or in the area of the sylvian fissure, it is helpful to refer to an angiogram to position the electrodes to minimize the risk to vascular structures.

The electrode wires are brought out through a stab wound or scalp incision so that direct contact can be made for EEG recording. The impedance is not very dissimilar to that of scalp electrodes and remains stable for many months, so no special electronic arrangements need be made for depth recording.

Either single- or multi-contact electrodes can be used. They should be directed stereotactically to areas of suspicion, particularly the mesial temporal lobes, common sites for seizure activity where surface recordings are less accurate. Recordings can be performed directly from the amygdala or the hippocampus. Coordinates are generally determined by the configuration of the electrodes and related to a ventriculogram demonstrating the temporal horn. Ordinarily, multiple electrodes are inserted in a single session, either separately or through a single burr hole over the convexity. At least several days should be allowed before recordings are begun, since the trauma of insertion may change the electrical activity. Usually, sufficient information can be obtained from recording sessions performed over 1 to 2 weeks, but electrodes have been left for many weeks with reasonable safety.

There are some situations in which stereotactic lesions can prevent the propagation of seizure activity and consequently prevent the development of clinical seizures. Patients who cannot be satisfactorily managed with medication and whose focus is not sufficiently localized to be considered for temporal lobectomy may respond to a stereotactic subcortical lesion.

Some authors recommend stereotactic ablation as the procedure of choice over temporal lobectomy, suggesting that there is less risk of undesirable side-effects, such as amnesia, paresis, aphasia, hemianopsia, or the development of Kluver-Bucy syndrome.[92,171]

Temporal lobe seizure activity may depend on the amygdala for its propagation, and may be precipitated by stimulation of that structure,[172–174] so that stereotactic amygdalotomy may be used for temporal lobe epilepsy, especially lesions of the medial portion of that nucleus.[136,175] The amygdala can be identified readily by its characteristic electrical activity on insertion of the electrode, and relatively large lesions can be made with minor side-effects. The coordinates from which to begin the search are 5 mm anterior to the tip of the temporal horn, 5 mm medial to the lateral edge of the temporal horn, and 3 mm above a line drawn as an extension of the inferior border of the temporal horn.[176] Further confirmation of the relationship of the electrode to the amygdala may be obtained from a CT scan (vide infra).

Some authors recommend lesions in the hippocampus, which can be made most conveniently by introducing an electrode into the longitudinal axis of this gyrus,[6,177] provided the individual stereotactic apparatus allows that approach.

Because epileptogenic foci are frequently multiple, beneficial effects of such lesions may be only transient, with recurrences most frequent at about 6 months to 1 year. Success can be regained, however, by repeating the stereotactic surgery, enlarging the lesion, or interrupting a different structure within the circuit of propagation. Amygdala lesions may be combined with hippocampal lesions[170] or with unilateral interruption of the fornix[132,178] or anterior commissure.[179] A section of the fornix alone may provide specific interruption of the hippocampofugal fibers to control temporal lobe epilepsy.[180] There is interesting evidence that bilateral lesions in Forel's field H may interrupt the propagation of epileptogenic impulses originating in the cortex and basal ganglia,[181] but these effects may be only transitory and may be associated with speech disturbances if they are bilateral. Such lesions may be considered, however, in patients with seizures of diffuse origin who are intractable to other treatments.

Salaam convulsions, also called akinetic seizures, static seizures, drop seizures, nodding spasm, or propulsive petit mal, can usually be treated satisfactorily with a lesion in the globus pallidus, sometimes combined with a lesion in the amygdala.[92,182]

In resistent cases, the ventral-anterior nucleus of the thalamus may be added to the amygdala, fornix, and anterior commissure in order to obtain relief of grand mal seizures, if combined with temporal lobe or centrencephalic foci.[132]

APPLICATIONS

CT-Guided Stereotactic Surgery

A new era in stereotactic surgery has just begun with the marriage of stereotaxis and computed tomographic (CT) scanning. It has become possible to insert a probe or biopsy forceps into almost any lesion that can be seen on CT scan. Although these techniques may require the use of special apparatus,[1,183–189] it is possible to calculate stereotactic coordinates directly from the CT scan for use with any stereotactic apparatus (vide infra).

Swedish neurosurgeons have been leaders in this field, to the point where 45 percent of the neurosurgery being conducted at one neurosurgical center is stereotactic in nature.[177]

Stereotactic coordinates can be calculated directly from CT scan performed on a GE 8800 scanner with ScoutView capabilities as follows.[190]

The ScoutView produces an image similar to an AP or a lateral skull x-ray film and can be manipulated on the console of the scanner. On the lateral ScoutView it is possible to reproduce lines that indicate the planes at which each of the slices was scanned. By relating these indicator lines to the lateral x-ray film taken at the time of the stereotactic procedure, the Z axis or vertical axis can be defined. The X and Y axes can be read directly from the individual CT slices.

Although relating the ScoutView to the lateral x-ray film introduces some inaccuracy, it has been calculated that the mechanical accuracy of this system is within 3 mm, and abscesses less than 1 cm have been aspirated with great reliability. Since the system does not relate to the usual stereotactic landmarks identified in various atlases, however, it has not been used for functional stereotactic surgery, but can be used to verify cingulotomy or amygdalotomy lesion placement.

A CT scan of the head is made in the usual fashion, care being taken to avoid moving the head between the CT scanning and the ScoutView.[191] The target within the lesion to be biopsied or cannulated is identified on the appropriate slice, and any number of targets in various slices may be calculated. The slice that is closest to the majority of targets is taken as the "zero slice." The zero slice is displayed on the CT console and the distance from the most anterior bone shadow to the most posterior bone shadow is measured and then bisected, and the cursor placed at that midpoint in the midline, which becomes the zero point for the measurement of the X and Y coordinates. If a target lies in the zero plane, the AP and lateral distances are measured from the zero point to the target point, and noted. If one wishes to determine the X and Y coordinates on other slices, the cursor is placed at the zero point and the display is changed to the slice demonstrating the second target point without moving the cursor. The zero point is where the cursor is displayed on the new slice, and the AP and lateral measurements can be made from that point, and all of the measurements and slice numbers noted.

The patient then is arranged for stereotactic surgery in the usual fashion, depending on which stereotactic apparatus is used. AP and lateral x-ray films are taken and compared to the ScoutView. On the ScoutView, a reference plane is selected near the base of the skull, which intersects identifiable landmarks, such as the inion, the roof of the orbit, etc. A line representing this plane is then drawn on the lateral x-ray film so that the identical reference plane is established.

Since the slice number of each target is known, and since the distance between slices is also known from the scanning program, lines representing the slices containing the targets are drawn on the lateral x-ray film parallel to and the appropriate distance above the reference plane. The zero plane is also drawn in similar fashion; the distance between the most anterior and most posterior bony shadow is bisected on the zero plane, so that the zero point is established on the lateral x-ray film. A line is drawn perpendicular to those planes through the zero point, giving the zero point on the lateral x-ray film on each of the slices of interest. For each target, the line representing the appropriate slice is selected, and the previously derived anterior or posterior measurement is marked on that line the appropriate distance from the zero point, which denotes the target on the lateral x-ray film. The cannula is then directed to that target, the distance from the midline already having been derived from the CT scan.

If the target is an anatomic lesion, such as a tumor or abscess, additional accuracy can be obtained by measuring impedance or electrical activity. The same device can be used to measure impedance as is used to confirm penetration of the spinal cord or ventricle, and may be particularly helpful in entering fluid-filled cavities. There may be so much fluctuation in impedance, however, as the electrode advances through the tissue that a clear demarcation of the tumor edge may not be evident, particularly if the tumor is infiltrative. In that case, the monitoring of electrical activity may be more accurate. As the edge of the tumor or mass is approached, the frequency of the spontaneous electrical activity may decrease, with the amplitude remaining the same or sometimes increasing. As the lesion is entered, electrical silence or a marked attention of amplitude may occur.

Biopsy of intracranial lesions, particularly tumors, can be both safe and diagnostic.[192–195] The popularity[196] of biopsy has increased rapidly over the past few years because of the ability to identify on CT scan deep lesions, which invite biopsy, the recognition that biopsy of deep tumors can be safe and accurate,[194,195] and the ability to diagnose diffuse neurologic conditions by chemical or enzymatic techniques[192] has led to renewed interest in that technique. The equipment should be integrated, so that the variety of electrodes, biopsy forceps, or biopsy screws can all be inserted through the same cannula, after the cannula is advanced to the target. For most purposes the cannula need not and should not be more than 2.0 to 2.5 mm in diameter. If only a small amount of tissue is available, a smear preparation may provide the diagnosis of tumor.[194] With the increasing incidence of AIDS patients, many of whom have a variety of intracranial lesions[197] that defy diagnosis by noninvasive techniques, stereotactic biopsy is becoming increasingly important in the management of that condition.

Not only can the stereotactic tissue diagnosis be helpful in anticipating the needs of an open surgical procedure, but repeated biopsies may be taken to assess the efficacy of radiation therapy or chemotherapy.

CT localization and biopsy of intracranial lesions are discussed in other chapters, as is stereotactic hypophysectomy.

Stereotactic aspiration of brain abscesses has been found to be particularly effective. With the possibility of demonstrating multiple abscesses on CT scan, each abscess in turn can be aspirated, irrigated, and, if desired, infused with antibiotic. Aspiration of an intracerebral hematoma is facilitated when an irrigating cannula is used, through which a clot can be propelled by a rotating helical mandrel[198,199]

A colloid cyst of the third ventricle can be aspirated. Once the wall is disrupted and the normal ventricular fluid pathway is opened, the cyst usually will not recur.

Radioisotopes can be introduced through the same cannula as biopsy is taken. Sophisticated computerized techniques for selection of the appropriate radioisotope and plotting the distribution of radiation have been developed, but these techniques are so specialized that they should be attempted only in a few centers.[194,200]

There are situations in which it is desirable to combine stereotactic and open surgery, such as the retrieval of a foreign body. The patient may undergo stereotactic surgery in order to introduce a probe to the site of the foreign body along a trajectory that would be appropriate for direct surgical removal. The probe remains in place while the surgeon follows along the probe to find the target. Optionally, a section of loose-fitting Silastic tubing can be fitted around the probe before insertion, advanced to the target point, and left in place as the probe is withdrawn. The tubing can then serve as a marker for the surgeon as the foreign body or other small deep-seated target is dissected.

This technique also can be used to approach deep vascular lesions along the optimal trajectory, or to identify feeding vessels. It is necessary to transform angiographic information to CT scan or to the AP and lateral x-ray films taken at the time of stereotactic surgery in order to establish the coordinate of the appropriate vessels, and a probe or Silastic marker can then be left in place in order to direct surgery to the vascular lesion.

More recent techniques have married stereotactic surgery with the use of a laser.[193] With the head secured in a stereotactic apparatus, the optimal approach to a deep-seated lesion can be made stereotactically.[201,202] A core of brain tissue is removed to provide access to the lesion, at which point a laser is used under direct vision to vaporize it. Associated techniques allow the three-dimensional computer reconstruction of the tumor mass, as visualized on CT, angiography, or MRI, so the laser might be directed by computer to provide a relatively complete removal of even irregularly shaped, deep-seated masses. Although these techniques are early in development and are not yet generally employed, they undoubtedly will become more widespread in the future, demonstrating how stereotactic surgery will impact more and more significantly on the general field of neurosurgery.[203]

Electroneuroprostheses

An additional application of functional neurosurgery that is not readily classified with any of the above but that nevertheless represents a useful technique is that of diaphragm pacing. An electronic stimulator, similar to those used for dorsal cord stimulation or peripheral nerve stimulation, is implanted to stimulate the phrenic nerve to drive respiration artificially. It can be helpful in the management of high cervical quadriplegic patients, patients with failure of central regulation of ventilation, and an occasional patient with chronic obstructive pulmonary disease. It is important that the phrenic nerves and diaphragm be functional, as well as the lungs. Patients with injuries at middle levels of the cervical spinal cord may have lower motor neuron lesions of the phrenic nerve, and consequently would not benefit from phrenic nerve stimulation. A patient whose injury is confined to levels C3 or above, however, may be maintained for long periods on diaphragm pacing, obviating the need for endotracheal intubation and positive pressure respiration.

In order to assess viability of the phrenic nerve, an electrode can be inserted percutaneously along the anterior border of the scalene muscle, where the phrenic nerve will be located just medial to the brachial plexus. A brisk, contraction of the diaphragm of several centimeters on stimulation assures sufficient function of the nerve to attempt chronic stimulation.

The implanted portion of the system is similar to that used for peripheral nerve or dorsal cord stimulation. The transmitter, however, generates a coded signal that is modulated by a continuous series of pulse trains. Each train corresponds to an inspiration period and is adjustable in duration from 1.2 to 1.45 seconds in adults and from 0.5 to 0.8 seconds in infants. The respiratory rate is adjustable from 12 to 24 breaths per minute for adults and 12 to 40 breaths per minute in infants. Because smooth contraction of the diaphragm is necessary, the pulse train is tailored to provide a gradually increasing contraction. The amplitude of the first pulse in the train is relatively small, with a gradual increase until the final pulse, similar to a ramp type of stimulation. Otherwise the transmitter is essentially the same as those used for other purposes.

Unilateral stimulation generally is sufficient to provide adequate tidal volume in adults. Because of the relatively smaller volume of an infant's lung, however, and because of the mobility of the mediastinum, it is necessary to use bilateral stimulation in infants, which necessitates the installation of a second receiver and electrode. The transmitter for bilateral stimulation allows either simultaneous or alternating stimulation.[171,204,205]

Attempts at reproducing bladder function electrophysiologically had, until recently, been directed to the bladder or peripheral innervation. Although contraction of various bladder muscles could be obtained, coordinating contraction of various parts of the bladder with other pelvic activities that constitute normal bladder emptying was not seen. It has been well recognized that paraplegic patients may develop reflex bladder emptying, however, wherein coordinated micturition can occur through the segmental reflex patterns that exist in the isolated lower end of the spinal cord. This led Nashold[206] to investigate a manner by which reflex micturition could be initiated with electrical stimulation. It was found that in many paraplegic patients stimulation of a localized site between the S1 and S2 segments of the conus medullaris can cause a well-organized reflex bladder emptying. Such electromicturition can be applied on a chronic basis by inserting the same type of radio receiver used for other types of central nervous system stimulation, connected to a Silastic cuff bearing two electrodes that are implanted into the proper sites in the conus. Not only is excellent bladder pressure obtained by stimulation, but the pattern of contraction simulates normal micturition and results in almost complete bladder emptying. Although only a limited group of paraplegic patients are candidates for such bladder

prostheses, it should be considered the best possible form of bladder management for those patients.

As an additional indication for the use of functional neurosurgery, one can look to the future in which electronic circuits may substitute for entire systems that are no longer functioning. An example of that, which is not yet developed to practical application, is artificial vision for the blind by electrical stimulation of the visual cortex.[207] It has been recognized that direct stimulation of the visual cortex leads to the perception of lights at specific points in the visual field related to the area of the cortex that is stimulated, so-called phosphenes.

This led Brindley and Lewin to a pioneering experiment, in which they inserted an 81 subdural electrode array in a blind patient.[208] They could indeed produce phosphenes at specific visual field sites, although they were not sufficient to form useful images. This encouraged Dobelle[207] to pursue physiologic investigations in hopes of perfecting the technique. Since production of phosphenes can be detected only by the individual, it was necessary to use human subjects. Patients who had occipital lobes exposed for any reason, such as tumor or resection, were operated upon under local anesthesia so the area could be stimulated to map the production of phosphenes. Electrodes and stimuli were developed to stimulate over long periods with maximum safety to the underlying cortex. The consistency of the anatomic distribution of phosphene-producing points was investigated. This culminated in the implantation of electrode arrays in several blind patients.

Up to the present, stimulation is done by direct linkage to electrodes through the scalp. The television camera and computer are large and not portable, so the technique has not yet become practical. As many of the physiologic problems are solved, however, the further development of subminiature television cameras and implantable computers may provide a practical visual prosthesis. The ultimate goal is for a miniature television camera to look at the environment, convert the image by computer into a pattern, and have that pattern of phosphenes produced by selective stimulation of several of the electrodes in the area over the visual cortex, producing, in effect, artificial vision.

Perhaps even more futuristic is the auditory prosthesis described by the same group.[209] Multi-contact electrodes were threaded into the scala tympani of the cochlea of deaf volunteers. These were connected to leads that penetrated the skin over the mastoid area and led to a connector that was accessible externally. A computer-controlled stimulator was attached to the connector so that various amplitudes, frequencies, and combinations of electrodes could be stimulated to produce various sounds. The subjects could control many of the parameters of stimulation in search of stimulus characteristics that might be useful to convey information. Pitch could be controlled either by location of the activated electrode or by the frequency of stimulation. As anticipated, loudness could be controlled by the amplitude of stimulation. Various wave forms and electrode configurations change the sensation. Although simple melodies could be discriminated, speech could not be successfully simulated. Subjective sensations remained stable over a long period, and there was no problem with scar tissue or infection of the cochlea. Although these findings were preliminary, the results were encouraging from the standpoint of developing an auditory prosthesis. As additional work continues in the area it may become possible to substitute an electronic component for other end-organs that may have become damaged from injury or disease.

The history of electroneuroprostheses began as long ago as 1953, when Wendell Krieg suggested chronic stimulation of the nervous system for vision in blind patients, cochlear or auditory stimulation for deaf patients, and stimulation of motor pathways for the treatment of paralysis.[210] These "implausible" and futuristic ideas are indeed coming to pass, and the next decade will provide a significant turning point for the field of neurosurgery to replace function when a cure is not possible.

However, we are on the threshold of a new field of stereotactic surgery which may, indeed, represent our first ability to cure neurologic disease rather than merely treat symptoms. In those conditions characterized by a decrease in neurotransmitters in specific nuclei, such as Parkinson's disease, it may soon be possible to replace the deficient neurotransmitters by stereotactic transplantation of tissue producing the deficient transmitter. The first tentative steps have already been taken in a limited number of patients in whom a homograft of adrenal tissue producing dopamine was stereotactically implanted into the ventricle adjacent to the basal ganglion. Although it was demonstrated that dopamine was produced, the transependymal absorption may have caused some modest improvement in neurologic function.[211]

Of greater futuristic implication, it has been demonstrated that injured neurons within the central nervous system do indeed have the ability to regenerate, and that transplanted fetal neurons may promote restitution of lost neurologic function.[212] The implication for the management of head and spinal cord injury are immense, but there is a long journey before clinical applicability will be developed. Nevertheless, the future of functional neurosurgery over the next few decades promises to be one of exciting and significant new developments.

REFERENCES

1. Horsley V, Clarke RH: The structure and function of the cerebellum examined by a new method. Brain 31:45, 1908
2. Spiegel EA, Wycis HT, Marks M, et al: Stereotaxic apparatus for operations on the human brain. Science 106:349, 1947
3. Kall BA, Kelly PJ, Goerss S, et al: The computer as a stereotactic surgical instrument. Appl Neurophysiol 48:89, 1985
4. Spiegel EA, Wycis HT: Stereoencephalotomy, Part 1. New York, Grune & Stratton, 1952
5. Staltenbrand G, Bailey P: Introduction to Stereotaxis with an Atlas of the Human Brain. Stuttgart, Georg Thieme, 1959
6. Talairach J, David M, Tournoux P, et al: Atlas d'anatomie Stéréotaxique. Paris, Masson, 1957
7. Andrew J, Watkins ES: A Stereotaxic Atlas of the Human Thalamus. Baltimore, Williams & Wilkins, 1969
8. Emmers R, Tasker RR: The Human Somesthetic Thalamus. New York, Raven Press, 1975
9. Van Buren JM, Borke RC: Variations and Connections of the Human Thalamus. 2. Variations of the Human Diencephalon. New York, Springer-Verlag, 1972
10. Afshar F, Watkins ES, Yap JC: Stereotaxic Atlas of the Human Brainstem and Cerebellar Nuclei. New York, Raven Press, 1978
11. Kelly PJ, Kall BA, Goerss S: Methodology and clinical experience with computed tomography and a computer resident stereotactic atlas. Neurosurgery (in press)
12. Hardy TL, Koch J, Lassiter A: Computer graphics with computerized tomography for functional neurosurgery. Appl Neurophysiol 46:193, 1983
13. Gildenberg PL: Survey of stereotactic and functional neurosurgery in the United States and Canada. Appl Neurophysiol 38:31, 1975
14. Leksel L: Stereotaxis and Radiosurgery. An Operative System. Springfield, Ill, Charles C Thomas, 1971
15. Riechert T: Stereotactic Brain Operations. Bern, Hans Huber, 1980
16. Todd EM: Todd-Wells Manual of Stereotaxic Procedures. Randolph, Mass, Codman and Shurtleff, 1967
17. Brown RA: A computerized tomography-computer graphics approach to stereotaxic localization. J Neurosurg 50:715, 1979
18. Roberts TS, Brown R: Technical and clinical aspects of CT-directed stereotaxis. Appl Neurophysiol 43:170, 1980
19. Gildenberg PL: Stereotactic surgery, in Frost EAM (ed): Clinical Anesthesia in Neurosurgery. New York, Butterworth, 1984, pp 293–315
20. Narabayashi H, Ohye C: Importance of microstereoencephalotomy for tremor alleviation. Appl Neurophysiol 43:222, 1980
21. Fukamachi A, Ohye C, Saito Y, et al: Estimation of the neural noise within the human thalamus. Acta Neurochir [Suppl] 24:121, 1977
22. Tasker RR, Hawrylshyn P, Rowe IH, et al: Computerized graphic display of results of subcortical stimulation during stereotactic surgery. Acta Neurochir [Suppl] 24:85, 1977
23. Hardy TL, Bertrand G, Thompson CJ: The position and organization of motor fibers in the internal capsule found during stereotactic surgery. Appl Neurophysiol 42:160, 1979
24. Cooper IS, Lee ASJ: Cryostatic congelation. J Nerv Ment Dis 133:259, 1961
25. Gildenberg PL (ed): Radiofrequency lesion making procedures. Appl Neurophysiol 39:69, 1976/77
26. Cooper IS: Involuntary Movement Disorders. New York, Hoeber, 1969
27. Gildenberg PL (ed): Safety and clinical efficacy of implanted neuroaugmentive devices. Appl Neurophysiol 40:69, 1977/78
28. Gildenberg PL: The use of pacemakers (electrical stimulation) in functional neurological disorders, in Rasmussen T, Marino R (eds.): Functional Neurosurgery. New York, Raven Press, 1979, pp 59–74
29. Sweet WH, Wepsic JG: Stimulation of the posterior columns of the spinal cord for pain control: Indications, technique and results. Clin Neurosurg 21:278, 1974
30. Adams JE: Technique and technical problems associated with implantation of neuroaugmentive devices. Appl Neurophysiol 40:111, 1977/78
31. North RB, Fischell TA, Long DM: Chronic dorsal column stimulation via percutaneously inserted epidural electrodes. Appl Neurophysiol 40:184, 1977/78
32. Willis WD: The Pain System. The neural basis of nociceptive transmssion in the mammalian nervous system, in Gildenberg PL (ed): Pain and Headache, vol 8. Basel, S. Karger, 1985
33. Melzack R, Wall PD: Pain mechanisms: A new theory. Science 150:971, 1965
34. Basbaum AI, Fields HL: Endogenous pain control mechanisms: Review and hypothesis. Ann Neurol 4:451, 1978
35. Gildenberg PL, Murthy KSK: Influence of dorsal column stimulation upon human thalamic somatosensory-evoked potentials. Appl Neurophysiol 43:8, 1980
36. Mehler WR: Some neurological species differences—a posteriori. Ann NY Acad Sci 167:424, 1969
37. Gildenberg PL, Hirshberg RM: Limited myelotomy for the treatment of intractable pain. Neurochir (Suppl):66, 1981
38. Mayer DJ, Hayes RL: Stimulation-produced analgesia: Development of tolerance and cross-tolerance to morphine. Science 188:941, 1975
39. Reynolds DV: Surgery in the rat during electrical analgesia induced by focal brain stimulation. Science 164:445, 1969
40. Nashold BS Jr, Wilson WP, Boone E: Depth recordings and stimulation of the human brain: A twenty year experience, in Rasmussen T, Marino R (eds): Functional Neurosurgery. New York, Raven Press, 1979, pp 181–195

41. Richardson DE, Akil H: Pain reduction by electrical brain stimulation in man. II. Chronic self administration in the periventricular gray matter. J Neurosurg 47:184, 1977

42. Mayer DJ, Liebeskind JC: Pain reduction by focal electrical stimulation of the brain: An anatomical and behavioral analysis. Brain Res 68:73, 1974

43. Hosobuchi Y, Adams JE, Rutkins B: Chronic thalamic stimulation for the control of facial anesthesia dolorosa. Arch Neurol 29:158, 1973

44. Hosobuchi Y, Adams JE, Linchitz R: Pain relief by electrical stimulation of the central gray matter in humans and its reversal by naloxone. Science 197:183, 1977

45. Mayer DJ, Price DD: Central nervous system mechanisms of analgesia. Pain 2:379, 1976

46. Sweet WH, Obrado S, Martin-Rodriguez JG (eds): Neurosurgical Treatment in Psychiatry, Pain and Epilepsy. Baltimore, University Park Press, 1977

47. Akil H, Mayer DJ, Liebeskind JC: Antagonism of stimulation-produced analgesia by naloxone, a narcotic antagonist. Science 191:961, 1976

48. Snyder SH: Opiate receptors and internal opiates. Sci Am 236:44, 1977

49. Gildenberg PL: Percutaneous cervical cordotomy. Clin Neurosurg 21:246, 1974

50. Cook AW, Kawakami Y: Commissural myelotomy. J Neurosurg 47:1, 1977

51. King RG: Anterior commissurotomy for intractable pain. J Neurosurg 47:7, 1977

52. Armour D: Surgery of the spinal cord and its membranes. Lancet 1:691, 1927

53. Broager B: Commissural, sagittal myelotomy for pains in the lower half of the body of 22 patients. Acta Neurol Scand 48:258, 1972

54. Sourek K: Commissural myelotomy. J Neurosurg 31:524, 1969

55. Wertheimer P, Lecuire J: La myelotomie commissurale posteriure. A propos de 107 observations. Acta Chir Belg 52:568, 1953

56. Hitchcock ER: Stereotactic myelotomy. J R Soc Med 67:771, 1974

57. Hitchcock ER: Stereotactic cervical myelotomy. J Neurol Neurosurg Psychiatry 33:224, 1970

58. Hitchcock ER: Stereotaxis of the spinal cord. Conf Neurol 34:299, 1972

59. Schvarcz JR: Spinal cord stereotactic techniques re trigeminal nucleotomy and extralemniscal myelotomy. Appl Neurophysiol 41:99, 1978

60. Schvarcz JR: Functional exploration of the spinomedullary junction. Acta Neurochir [Suppl] 24:179, 1977

61. Gildenberg PL, Hirshberg R: Limited myelotomy for the treatment of cancer pain. Appl Neurophysiol (in press)

62. Gildenberg PL, Hirshberg R: Treatment of cancer pain with limited myelotomy. Med J St Jos Hosp (Houston) 16:199, 1981

63. Spiegel EA, Wycis HT: Mesencephalotomy in the treatment of "intractable" facial pain. Arch Neurol 69:1, 1953

64. Nashold BS Jr: Extensive cephalic and oral pain relieved by midbrain tractotomy. Conf Neurol 34:382, 1972

65. Voris HC, Whisler WW: Results of stereotaxic surgery for intractable pain. Conf Neurol 37:86, 1975

66. Spiegel EA, Wycis HT: Stereoencephalotomy, Part II. New York, Grune & Stratton, 1962

67. Mark VH, Ervin FR, Hackett TP: Clinical aspects of stereotactic thalamotomy in the human. Part I. Arch Neurol 3:17, 1960

68. Mark VH, Ervin FR, Yakovlev PI: Stereotactic thalamotomy. Arch Neurol 8:528, 1963

69. Spiegel EA, Wycis HT, Szekely EG, et al: Combined dorsomedial, intralaminar and basal thalamotomy for relief of so-called intractable pain. J Int Coll Surg 42:160, 1964

70. Spiegel EA, Wycis HT, Szekely EG, et al: Medial and basal thalamotomy in so-called intractable pain, in Knighton RS, Dumke PR (eds): Pain. Boston, Little, Brown, 1966, pp 503–517

71. White JC, Sweet WH: Pain and the Neurosurgeon. Springfield Ill, Charles C Thomas, 1969

72. Foltz EL, White LE Jr: Rostral cingulotomy and pain "relief," in Knighton RS, Dumke PR (eds): Pain. Boston, Little, Brown, 1966, pp 469–491

73. Hurt RW, Ballantine HT Jr: Stereotactic anterior cingulate lesions for persistent pain: A report of 68 cases. Clin Neurosurg 21:334, 1974

74. DeVaul RA, Faillace LA: Persistent pain and illness insistence. A medical profile of proneness to surgery. Am J Surg 135:828, 1978

75. Gildenberg PL, DeVaul RA: Management of chronic pain refractory to specific therapy, in Youmans JR (ed): Neurological Surgery, ed 2. Philadelphia, WB Saunders, 1981, pp 3749–3768

76. Gildenberg PL, DeVaul RA: The Chronic Pain Patient. Evaluation and Management. Basel, S. Karger, 1985

77. Jacobson E: Modern Treatment of Tense Patients. Springfield Ill, Charles C Thomas, 1970

78. Travell J: Myofascial trigger points: Clinical view, in Bonica JJ, Albe-Fessard D (eds): Advances in Pain Research and Therapy, vol 1. New York, Raven Press, 1976, pp 919–926

79. Nashold BS, Ostdahl RH: Dorsal root entry zone lesions for pain relief. J Neurosurg 51:59, 1979

80. Hassler R, Mundinger F, Riechert T: Stereotaxis in Parkinson Syndrome. Berlin, Springer-Verlag, 1979

81. Hassler R, Mundinger F, Riechert T: Pathophysiology of tremor at rest derived from the correlation of anatomical and clinical data. Conf Neurol 32:79, 1970

82. Kelly PJ: Microelectrode recording for the somatotopic placement of stereotactic thalamic lesions in the treatment of parkinsonian and cerebellar intention tremor. Appl Neurophysiol 43:262, 1980

83. Oyhe C, Hirai T, Miyazaki M, Shibazaki T, Nakajima H: V.im thalamotomy for the treatment of various kinds of tremor. Appl Neurophysiol 45:275, 1982

84. Tasker RR, Siqueira J, Hawrylyshyn P, Organ LW: What happened to V.im thalamotomy for Parkinson's disease? Appl Neurophysiol 46:68, 1983

85. Mundinger F, Riechert T: Die stereotaktischen Hirnoperationen zur Behandlung extrapyramidaler Beregungsstörungen (Parkinsonismus und Hyperkinesen) und ihre Resultate Postoperative und Langzeitergebnisse der stereotaktischen Hirnoperationen bei extrapyramidal-motorischen Bewegongsstörungen. Teil B. Fortschr Neurol Psychiatr 31:69, 1963

86. Spiegel EA, Wycis HT, Szekely EG, et al: Campotomy in various extrapyramidal disorders. J Neurosurg 20:871, 1963

87. Spiegel EA, Wycis HT, Szekely EG, et al: Stimulation of Forel's field during stereotaxic operations in the human brain. EEG Clin Neurophysiol 16:537, 1964

88. Kelly PJ, Gillingham FJ: The long-term results of stereotaxic surgery and L-dopa therapy in patients with Parkinson's disease. A 10–year follow-up study. J Neurosurg 53:332, 1980

89. Spiegel EA, Wycis HT: Pallido-thalamotomy in chorea. Arch Neurol Psychiatry 64:495, 1950

90. Hoff A, Woringer E, Hamou I: Postoperative hemiballismus. Neurochirurgia 11:1, 1968

91. Mundinger F, Reichert T: Die stereotaktischen Hirnoperationen zur Behandlung extrapyramidaler Bewegungsstörungen und ihre Resultate. Fortschr Neurol Psychiatr 31:1, 1963

92. Spiegel EA: Guided Brain Operations. Basel, S. Karger, 1982

93. Spiegei EA, Wycis HT: Stereoencephalotomy, Part II. New York, Grune & Stratton, 1962

94. Cooper, IS: Involuntary Movement Disorders. New York, Hoeber, 1969

95. Gildenberg PL, Tasker RR: Spasmodic torticollis. Contemp Neurosurg 4:1, 1982

96. Gildenberg PL: A comprehensive program for spasmodic torticollis. Appl Neurophysiol 44:233, 1981

97. Waltz JM, Andreesen WH: Multiple lead spinal cord stimulation: Technique. Appl Neurophysiol 44:30, 1981

98. Hamby WB, Schiffer S: Spasmodic torticollis: Results after cervical rhizotomy in 50 cases. J Neurosurg 31:323, 1969

99. Hernesniemi J, Laitinen L: Late results of surgical treatment of spasmodic torticollis. Neurochirurgie 23:123, 1977

100. Heimburger RF, Whitlock CC: Stereotaxic destruction of the human dentate nucleus. Conf Neurol 26:346, 1965

101. Siegfried J: Neurosurgical treatment of spasticity, in Rasmussen T, Marino R (eds): Functional Neurosurgery. New York, Raven Press, 1979, pp 123–128

102. Zervas N: Long term view of dentatectomy in dystonia musculorum deformans and cerebral palsy. Acta Neurochir [Suppl] 24:49, 1977

103. Spiegel EA, Wycis HT, Baird HW: Effect of thalamic and pallidal lesions upon involuntary movements in choreoathetosis. Trans Am Neurol Assoc 75:234, 1950

104. Sprague JM, Chambers WW: Control of posture by reticular formation and cerebellum in the intact anesthetized and unanesthetized and in the decerebrated cat. Am J Physiol 176:52, 1954

105. Davis R, Gray E, Kudzman J: Beneficial augmentation following dorsal column stimulation in some neurological diseases. Appl Neurophysiol 44:37, 1981

106. Penn RD, Gottlieb GL, Agarwal GC: Cerebellar stimulation in man. Quantitative changes in spasticity. J Neurosurg 48:779, 1978

107. Gilman S, Dauth GW, Tennyson V, et al: Chronic cerebellar stimulation in the monkey. Preliminary observations. Arch Neurol 32:474, 1975

108. Davis R, Gray E: Technical factors important to dorsal column stimulation. Appl Neurophysiol (in press)

109. Dimitrijevic MR, Sherwood AM: Spasticity: Medical and surgical treatment. Neurology 30:19, 1980

110. Bischof W: Die longitudinale myelotomie. Zentralbl Neurochir 11:79, 1951

111. Bischof W: Zür dorsalen longitudinalen myelotomie. Zentralbl Neurochir 28:123, 1967

112. Nauta, WJH: The problem of the frontal lobe: A reinterpretation. J Psychiatr Res 8:167, 1971

113. Vodovnik L, Kralj A, Stanic U, et al: Recent applications of functional electrical stimulation to stroke patients in Ljubljana. Clin Orthop 131:64, 1978

114. Freeman W: Frontal lobotomy in early schizophrenia. Long follow-up in 415 cases, in Hitchcock E, Laitinen L, Vaernet K (eds): Psychosurgery. Springfield, Ill, Charles C Thomas, 1972, pp 311–321

115. Freeman W: Frontal lobotomy in early schizophrenia: Long follow-up in 415 cases. Br J Psychiatry 114:1223, 1971

116. Flor-Henry P: Progress and problems in psychosurgery. Curr Psychiatr Ther 17:283, 1977

117. Freeman W, Watts JW: Psychosurgery. Springfield, Ill, Charles C Thomas, 1942

118. Mitchell-Heggs N, Kelly D, Richardson AE: Stereotactic limbic leucotomy: Clinical, psychological and physiological assessment at 16 months, in Sweet WH, Obrador S, Martin-Rodriquez JG (eds): Neurosurgical Treatment in Psychiatry, Pain and Epilepsy. Baltimore, University Park Press, 1977, pp 367–379

119. Hackett TP, White JC, Sweet WH: Leukotomy for the relief of pain: The selection of cases and psychological hazards, in Knighton RS, Dumke PR (eds): Pain. Boston, Little, Brown, 1966, pp 461–467

120. Livingston KF: The frontal lobes revisited. The case for a second look. Arch Neurol 20:90–95, 1969

121. Breggin PR: The return of lobotomy and psychosurgery. Congressional Record 118(26): Feb 24, 1972

122. National Commission for the Protection of Human Subjects of Biomedical and Behavioral Research. Report and Recommendations. Psychosurgery, Washington DC, DHEW Publications No. (05) 77–0001, 1977

123. Teuber HL, Corkin S, Twitchell TE: A study of cingulotomy in man. DHEW Publications No. (OS) 77–0002, 1977

124. Teuber JL, Corkin S, Twitchell TF: Study of cingulotomy in man: A summary, in Sweet WH, Obrador S, Martin-Rogriguez JG (eds): Neurosurgical Treatment in Psychiatry, Pain and Epilepsy. Baltimore, University Park Press, 1977, pp 355–362

125. Ballantine HT Jr, Giriunas IE: Advances in psychiatric surgery, in Rasmussen T, Marino R: Functional Neurosurgery. New York, Raven Press, 1979, pp 155–164

126. Papez JW: A proposed mechanism of emotion. Arch Neurol Psychiatry 38:725, 1937

127. Yakovlev PI: Motility behavior in the brain: Stereodynamic organization in neural coordinates of behavior. J Nerv Ment Dis 107:313, 1948

128. Livingston K: Neurosurgical aspects of primary affective disorders, in Youmans JR (ed): Neurological Surgery, vol 3, Philadelphia, WB Saunders, 1973, pp 1881–1900

129. Kelly D: Psychosurgery and the limbic system. Postgrad Med J 49:825, 1973

130. Richardson A: Stereotactic limbic leukotomy: Surgical technique. Postgrad Med J 49:860, 1973

131. Turner E: Custom psychosurgery. Postgrad Med J 49:834, 1973

132. Bouchard G, Kim YK, Umbach W: Stereotaxic methods in different forms of epilepsy. Conf Neurol 37:232, 1975

133. Heimburger RF, Whitlock CC, Kalsbeck JE: Stereotaxic amygdalotomy for epilepsy with aggressive behavior. JAMA 198:741, 1966

134. Mark V, Sweet WH, Ervin FR: The effect of amygdalotomy on violent behavior in patients with temporal lobe epilepsy, in Hitchcock E, Laitinen L, Vaernet K (eds): Psychosurgery. Springfield, Ill, Charles C Thomas, 1972, pp 139–155

135. Mempel E: The effect of partial amygdalectomy on emotional disturbances and epileptic seizures. Polish Med J 10:969, 1971

136. Narabayashi H, Nagao T, Saito Y, et al: Stereotaxic amygdalotomy for behavior disorders. Arch Neurol 9:1, 1963

137. Laitinen LV: Emotional responses to subcortical electrical stimulation in psychiatric patients. Clin Neurol Neurosurg 81:148, 1979

138. Richardson DE: Stereotaxic cingulomotomy and prefrontal lobotomy in mental disease. South Med J 65:1221, 1972

139. Hitchcock ER, Cairns V: Amygdalotomy. Postgrad Med J 49:894, 1973

140. Kelly D, Richardson A, Mitchell-Heggs N: Stereotactic limbic leucotomy: Neurophysiological aspects and operative technique. Br J Psychiatry 123:133, 1973

141. Richardson AE, Kelly D, Mitchell-Heggs N: Lesion site determination in stereotactic limbic leukotomy, in Sweet WH, Obrador S, Martin-Rodriguez JG (eds): Neurosurgical Treatment in Psychiatry, Pain and Epilepsy. Baltimore, University Park Press, 1977, pp 363–365

142. Sweet WH: Treatment of medically intractable mental disease by limited frontal leukotomy—justifiable? N Engl Med 289:1117, 1973

143. Ballantine HT Jr, Levy BS, Dagi TF, et al: Cingulotomy for psychiatric illness: Report of 13 years' experience, in Sweet WH, Obrador S, Martin-Rodriguez JG (eds): Neurosurgical Treatment in Psychiatry, Pain and Epilepsy. Baltimore, University Park Press, 1977, pp 333–353

144. Kullberg G: Differences in effect of capsulotomy and cingulotomy, in Sweet WH, Obrador S, Martin-Rodriguez JG (eds): Neurosurgical Treatment in Psychiatry, Pain and Epilepsy. Baltimore, University Park Press, 1977, pp 301–308

145. Teuber HL, Ball J, Klett CJ, et al: Veterans Administration study of prefrontal lobotomy. J Clin Exp Psychopath Quart Rev Psychiatr Neurol 20:205, 1959

146. Bailey HE, Dowling JL, Davies E: Cingulotractotomy and related procedures for severe depressive illness (Studies in depression: IV), in Sweet WH, Obrador S, Martin-Rodriguez JG (eds): Neurosurgical Treatment in Psychiatry, Pain and Epilepsy. Baltimore, University Park Press, 1977, pp 229–251

147. Ballantine HT Jr, Cassidy WL, Brodeur J, et al: Frontal cingulotomy for mood disturbance, in Hitchcock E, Laitinen L, Vaernet K (eds): Psychosurgery. Springfield, Ill, Charles C Thomas, 1972, pp 221–229

148. Ballantine HT Jr, Cassidy WL, Flanagan NB, et al: Stereotaxic anterior cingulotomy for neuropsychiatric illness and intractable pain. J Neurosurg 26:488, 1967

149. Lopez-Ibor JJ, Lopez-Ibor A: Selection criteria for patients who should undergo psychiatric surgery, in Sweet WH, Obrador S, Martin-Rodriguez JG (eds): Neurosurgical Treatment in Psychiatry, Pain and Epilepsy. Baltimore, University Park Press, 1977, pp 151–162

150. Orthner H, M ü ller D, Roeder F: Stereotaxic psychosurgery. Techniques and results since 1955, in Hitchcock E, Laitinen L, Vaernet K (eds): Psychosurgery. Springfield, Ill, Charles C Thomas, 1972, pp 377–390

151. Mark VH, Nevelle R: Brain surgery in aggressive epileptics. Social and ethical implications. JAMA 226:765, 1973

152. Vaernet K, Madsen A: Lesions in the amygdala and the substantia innominata in aggressive psychotic patients, in Hitchcock E, Laitinen L, Vaernet K (eds): Psychosurgery. Springfield, Ill, Charles C Thomas, 1972, pp 187–194

153. Rubio E, Arjon V, Rodriguez-Burgos F: Stereotactic cryohypothalamotomy in aggressive behavior, in Sweet WH, Obrador S, Martin-Rodriguez JG (eds): Neurosurgical Treatment in Psychiatry, Pain and Epilepsy. Baltimore, University Park Press, 1977, pp 439–444

154. Schvarcz JR, Droillet R, Rios E, et al: Stereotaxic hypothalamotomy for behavior disorders. J Neurol Neurosurg Psychiatry 35:356, 1972

155. Vaernet K, Madsen AL: Stereotaxic amygdalotomy and basofrontal tractotomy in psychotics with aggressive behavior. J Neurol Neurosurg Psychiatry 33:858, 1970

156. Barcia-Salorio JL, Broseta J, Roland P, et al: Stereotactic amygdalotomy versus posteromedial hypothalamotomy in the treatment of behavioral disorders in epilepsy. Appl Neurophysiol (in press)

157. Dieckmann G, Hassler R: Unilateral hypothalamotomy in sexual delinquents. Conf Neurol 37:177, 1975

158. M ü ller D, Roeder F, Orthner H: Further results of stereotaxis in the human hypothalamus in sexual deviations: First use of this operation in addiction to drugs. Neurochirurgia 16:113, 1973

159. Roeder F, Orthner H, Müller D: The stereotaxic treatment of pedophilic homosexuality and other sexual deviations, in Hitchcock E, Laitinen L, Vaernet K (eds): Psychosurgery. Springfield, Ill, Charles C Thomas, 1972, pp 87–111

160. Rieber I, Sigusch V: Psychosurgery on sex offenders and sexual "deviants" in West Germany. Arch Sex Behav 8:523, 1979

161. Crow HJ, Cooper R, Phillips DG: Controlled multifocal frontal leukotomy for psychiatric illness. J Neurol Neurosurg Psychiatry 24:353, 1961

162. Smith JS, Kiloh LG, Boots JA: Prospective evaluation of prefrontal leukotomy: Results at 30 months follow-up, in Sweet WH, Obrador S, Martin-Rodriguez JG (eds): Neurosurgical Treatment in Psychiatry, Pain and Epilepsy. Baltimore, University Park Press, 1977, pp 217–224

163. Ström-Olsen R, Carlisle S: Bi-frontal stereotactic tractotomy. A follow-up study of its effects on 210 patients. Br J Psychiatry 118:141, 1971

164. Martin WL, McElhaney ML, Meyer GA: Stereotactic cingulotomy: Results of psychological testing and clinical evaluation preoperatively and postoperatively, in Sweet WH, Obrador S, Martin-Rodriguez JG (eds): Neurosurgical Treatment in Psychiatry, Pain and Epilepsy. Baltimore, University Park Press, 1977, pp 381–386

165. Bailey HR, Dowling JL, Davies E: Studies in depression, III: The control of affective illness by cingulotractotomy. A review of 150 cases. Med J Aust 2:366, 1973

166. Scoville WB: Selective cortical undercutting as a means of modifying and studying frontal lobe function in man. J Neurosurg 6:65, 1949

167. Bingley T, Leksel L, Meyerson BA, et al: Long-term results of stereotactic anterior capsulotomy in chronic obsessive-compulsive neurosis, in Sweet WH, Obrador S, Martin-Rodriguez JG (eds): Neurosurgical Treatment in Psychiatry, Pain and Epilepsy. Baltimore, University Park Press, 1977, pp 287–299

168. Laitinen LV: Stereotactic lesions in the knee of the corpus callosum in the treatment of emotional disorders. Lancet 1:472, 1972

169. Gildenberg PL: Surgery for seizures, in Frost EAM (ed): Clinical Anesthesia in Neurosurgery. New York, Butterworth, 1984, pp 265–278

170. Talairach J, Bancaud J: Stereotactic approach to epilepsy. Prog Neurol Surg 5:297, 1973

171. Glenn WWL, Hogan JF, Phelps ML: Ventilatory support for the quadriplegic patient with respiratory paralysis by diaphragm pacing. Surg Clin North Am 60:1055, 1980

172. Bancaud J, Talairach J, Morel P, et al: La corne d'Ammon et le noyau amygdalien: effets cliniques et eletriques de leur stimulation chez l'homme. Rev Neurol 115:329, 1966

173. Chapman W: Studies of the periamygdaloid area in relation to human behavior. Res Publ Assoc Nerv Ment Dis 36:258, 1958

174. Weingarten S, Charlow DG, Holmgren E: The relation of hallucination to the depth structures of the temporal lobe. Arch Neurol [Suppl] 24:199, 1977

175. Narabayashi H, Mizutani T: Epileptic seizures and stereotaxic amygdalotomy. Conf Neurol 32:289, 1970

176. Heimburger RF: Stereotaxic coordinates for amygdalotomy. Conf Neurol 37:202, 1975

177. Nádvornik P, Sramka M, Gajdosová D, et al: Longitudinal hippocampectomy. Conf Neurol 37:404, 1975

178. Mundinger F, Becker P, Groebner E, et al: Late results of stereotactic surgery of epilepsy predominantly temporal lobe type. Acta Neurochir Suppl 23:177, 1976

179. Schaltenbrand G, Spuler H, Nadjmi M, et al: Die stereotaktische behandlung der epilepsien. Conf Neurol 27:111, 1966

180. Hassler R, Riechert T: über einen Fall von doppelseitiger Fornicotomie bei sogenannter temporaler Epilepsie. Acta Neurochir 5:330, 1957

181. Jinnai D, Nishimoto A: Stereotaxic destruction of Forel H for treatment of epilepsy. Neurochirurgia 6:164, 1963

182. Spiegel EA, Wycis HT, Baird HW: Pallidotomy and pallidoamygdalotomy in certain types of convulsive disorders. AMA Arch Neurol Psychiatry 80:714, 1958

183. Bergströ m M, Boë thius J, Eriksson L, et al: Head fixation device for reproducible position alignment in transmission CT and positron emission tomography. Technical note. J Comput Assist Tomogr 5:136, 1981

184. Brown R: A computerized tomography-computer graphics approach to stereotaxic localization. J Neurosurg 50:715, 1979

185. Greitz T, Bergström M: Stereotactic procedures in computer tomography, in Newton TH, Potts DG (eds): Radiology of the Skull and Brain. Technical Aspects of Computer Tomography. St. Louis, CV Mosby, 1981, pp 4286–4296

186. Jacques S, Shelden CH, McCann GD, et al: Computerized three-dimensional stereotaxic removal of small central nervous system lesions in patients. J Neurosurg 53:816, 1980

187. Koslow M, Abele MG, Griffith RC, et al: Stereotactic surgical system controlled by computed tomography. Neurosurgery 8:72, 1981

188. Rosenbaum A, Lunsford LD, Perry J: Computerized tomography guided stereotaxis. A new approach. Appl Neurophysiol 43:172, 1980

189. Rushworth RG: Stereotactic guided biopsy in the computerized tomographic scanner. Surg Neurol 14:451, 1980

190. Gildenberg PL, Kaufman HH, Murthy KSK: Calculation of stereotactic coordinates from the computed tomographic scan. Neurosurgery 10:580, 1982

191. Kaufman HH, Gildenberg PL: New head-positioning system for use with computer tomographic scanning. Neurosurgery 7:147, 1980

192. Kaufman HH, Catalano LW: Diagnostic brain biopsy, a series. Neurosurgery 4:129, 1979

193. Kelly PJ, Alker GJ Jr: A method for stereotactic laser microsurgery in the treatment of deep seated CNS neoplasms. Appl Neurophysiol 43:210, 1980

194. Mundinger F, Ostertag C, Birg W, et al: Stereotactic treatment of brain lesions: biopsy, interstitial radiotherapy (Ir-192 and I-125) and drainage procedures. Appl Neurophysiol (in press)

195. Ostertag CB, Mennel HD, Kiessling M: Stereotactic biopsy of brain tumors. Surg Neurol 14:275, 1980

196. Gildenberg PL, Franklin PO: Survey of CT-guided stereotactic surgery. Appl Neurophysiol 48:477, 1985

197. Levy RM, Bredesen DE, Rosenblum ML: Neurological manifestations of the acquired immuno-deficiency syndrome (AIDS): Experience at UCSF and review of the literature. J Neurosurg 62:475, 1985

198. Backlund E, von Holst H: Controlled subtotal evacuation of intracerebral hematomas by stereotactic technique. Surg Neurol 9:99, 1978

199. Higgins AC, Nashold BS Jr: Modification of instrument for stereotactic evacuation of intracerebral hematoma: Technical note. Neurosurgery 7:604, 1980

200. Szikla G (ed): Stereotactic Cerebral Irradiation. Amsterdam, Elsevier/North Holland, 1979

201. Gildenberg PL: Computerized tomography and stereotactic surgery, in Spiegel EA (ed): Guided Brain Operations. Basel, S. Karger, 1982

202. Kelly PJ, Kall BA, Goerss S, Earnest F: Present and future developments of stereotactic surgery. Appl Neurophysiol 48:1, 1985

203. Kelly PJ: Computer-assisted stereotaxis: New approaches for the management of intracranial intra-axial tumors. Neurology 36:535, 1986

204. Glenn WWL: Diaphragm pacing: Present status. Pace 1:357, 1978

205. Glenn WWL, Hogan JF, Loke JSO, et al: Ventilatory support by pacing of the conditioned diaphragm in quadriplegia. N Engl J Med 310:1150, 1984

206. Nashold BS Jr, Friedman H, Grimes J, et al: Electromicturition in the paraplegic: An electroneuroprosthesis to control voiding, in Fields WS (ed): Neural Organization and Its Relevance to Prosthetics. New York, Intercontinental Medical Book Corp, 1973, pp 349–368

207. Dobelle WH, Quest DO, Antones JL, et al: Artificial vision for the blind by electrical stimulation of the visual cortex. Neurosurgery 5:521, 1979

208. Brindley GS, Lewin WS: The sensation produced by electrical stimulation of the visual cortex. J Physiol (Lond) 196:479, 1968

209. Eddington DK, Dobelle WH, Brackmann DE, et al: Auditory prostheses research with multiple channel intracochlear stimulation in man. Ann Otol Rhinol Laryngol [Suppl] 53:5, 1978

210. Krieg WJS: Electroneuroprosthesis. History and forecast. IMJ 136:1, 1969

211. Backlund, EO, Granberg PO, Hamberger B, et al: Transplantation of adrenal medullary tissue to striatum in parkinsonism. First clinical trials. J Neurosurg 62:169, 1985

212. Proceedings of the Colloquium of the Use of Embryonic Cell Transplantation for Correction of CNS Disorders. Appl Neurophysiol 47:6, 1984

Treatment of Intractable Psychiatric Illness and Chronic Pain by Stereotactic Cingulotomy

H. Thomas Ballantine, Jr.   Ida E. Giriunas

INTRACRANIAL SURGERY for the treatment of psychiatric illness and chronic pain has been under scrutiny and criticism since 1936, when the Portugese neurologist, Egas Moniz, reported the results of frontal lobotomies performed by him and his neurosurgical colleague, Almeida Lima, on 20 institutionalized, severely ill psychiatric patients. Because of this controversy, we have included in this chapter pertinent details about the history of psychiatric surgery, the rationale for its performance, and the preoperative safeguards we employ to make certain that surgical intervention is appropriate and that informed consent is obtained.

In his paper, Moniz stated that 14 of 20 patients (70 percent) had shown worthwhile improvement, which led others to embrace this innovative method of treating psychiatric patients. One of the most enthusiastic (destined later to become overly enthusiastic)[1] of those who embraced this treatment modality was the neuropsychiatrist, Walter Freeman, of Washington, D.C. Three months after Moniz published his original paper, Freeman, with the neurosurgical assistance of James Watts, performed the first prefrontal lobotomy in the United States.

In 1942, Freeman and Watts published a monograph titled "Psychosurgery" that encompassed their initial experiences with 80 prefrontal lobotomies. Subsequently, they observed that some psychiatric patients who also complained of unbearable pain were free of that complaint postoperatively. They became increasingly impressed by this finding, and in the second edition of their book, published in 1950, the title was changed to "Psychosurgery: In the Treatment of Mental Disorders and Intractable Pain."[2]

Early on, however, complications and undesirable side effects of this radical procedure were being reported. Tooth and Newton[3] reviewed 10,365 operations performed between 1943 and 1954. They confirmed that the rate of improvement was about 70 percent, but they also reported a 6 percent mortality rate and a 1 percent epilepsy rate, and reported that 1.5 percent of the patients had loss of social control, often characterized by inappropriate behavior and obscene speech.

These complications of the standard prefrontal lobotomy led to a search for an operation that could confer the same benefit with much less risk. Restricted frontal leukotomies, such as bilateral inferior leukotomy, bimedial leukotomy, and orbital gyrus undercutting, had their proponents. Then, in 1948, at the suggestion of John Fulton of Yale, Cairns in England and LeBeau in France moved away from the frontal lobes and began to perform open anterior cingulectomies.

The introduction of stereotactic surgery revolutionized psychiatric surgery, and today open operations are rare. In 1961, Foltz and White[4] reported the outcomes of stereotactic cingulotomies carried out for intractable pain. Encouraged by their results, we began in 1962 to employ a modification of their technique for the treatment of psychiatric illness as well as pain.

THE CINGULATE GYRUS: ANATOMIC AND PHYSIOLOGIC CONSIDERATIONS

The cingulate gyri, along with the parahippocampal gyri, are located on the medial surfaces of the cerebral hemispheres and form a "limbus," or border. This region and the structures it surrounds are often termed the "limbic lobe" of the brain. In 1937, J.W. Papez published an important paper under the title: "A Proposed Mechanism of Emotion."[5] He postulated that the gyri cinguli, the hypothalamus, and the hippocampus, and their interconnections constituted the "anatomic basis of the emotions." Over the next 4 decades, the Papez theory was greatly enlarged to include a myriad of anatomic entities that, taken together, form the limbic system. Figure 93-1 illustrates diagrammatically this complex arrangement.

It has been theorized that the central pathways of the emotions and the responses to them might be as follows: sensory stimuli, both external and internal, are assembled at the brain stem and travel to the hypothalamus (Figure 93-1). From there, they may pass to the anterior thalamic nuclei (AT), and thence to the cingulum via the anterior thalamic radiations (ATR). From the cingulum, stimuli can be transmitted back to the hippocampus, the mammillary bodies, the anterior thalamic nuclei via the mammilothalmic tract (MTT), and from there back to the cingulum and hippocampus.

The output from this reverberating circuit is transmitted to the frontal lobes by way of several connections, the most important of which is the cingulum. In this way, the limbic system may, in the words of Papez, "add emotional coloring to the psychic process."

In similar fashion, "psychic processes with emotional

OPERATIVE NEUROSURGICAL TECHNIQUES
ISBN 0-8089-1862-1

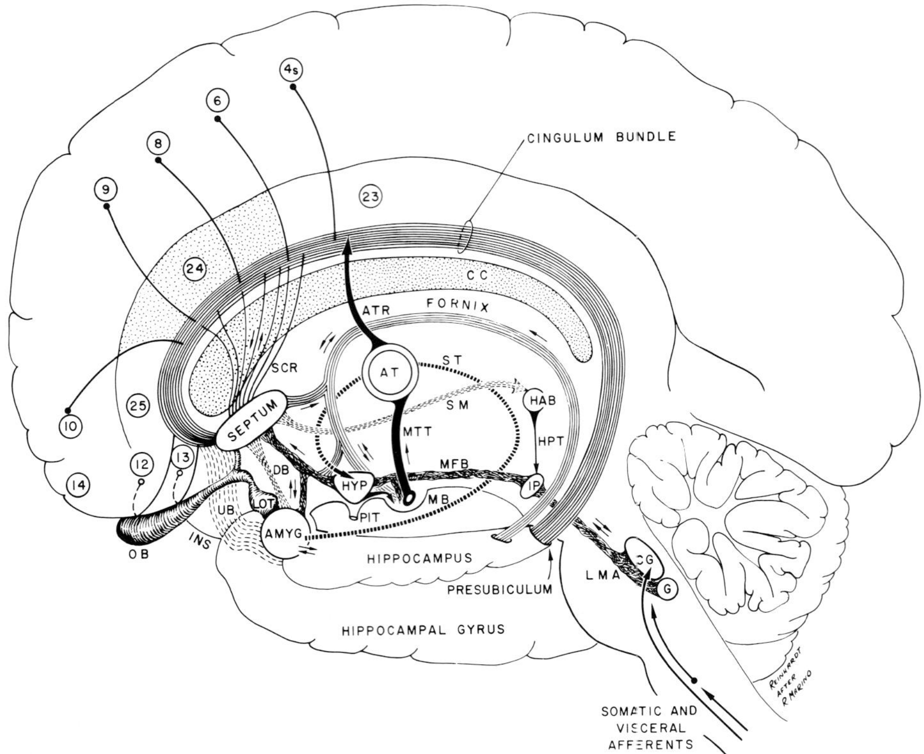

Fig. 93-1. Schematic model of the limbic system. HYP = hypothalamus; AT = anterior thalamus; ATR = anterior thalamic radiations; MTT = mammillothalamic tract. (Reprinted from Ballantine HT Jr, Cassidy WL, Flanagan NB, et al: Stereotaxic anterior cingulotomy for neuropsychiatric illness and intractable pain. J Neurosurg 26:488–495, 1967. With permission.)

coloring'' can be transmitted back to the limbic system, and these efferent stimuli will affect the thought processes, feelings, and behavior that are unique for each individual. Although this theoretical construct may require significant modification, it is unlikely that the important role of the cingulum in the complex interplay of cognition and affect will be diminished in the future.

Neuroscientists have delineated an interrelationship between cortex, limbic system, and brainstem reticular activating system. Neurotransmitters, (e.g., norepinephrine and serotonin), neuromodulators (e.g., GABA, somatostatin), and aberrant electrical neurophysiology (e.g., kindling) all mediate this complex plastic system that appears to be responsible for the activities associated with thinking, mood, and behavior. Medications[6] aimed at either enhancing neurotransmitter synthesis, inhibiting the inactivation of it, or effecting receptor sensitivity are being successfully used in the treatment of, and in furthering our knowledge and understanding of, central nervous system function.

Psychotropic drugs have proven helpful in the treatment of depression snd other psychistric illnesses, and have been shown to activate receptor sensitivity and neurotransmitter concentration. For instance, the tricyclics prevent neurotransmitter re-uptake of serotonin and norepinephrine at the synapse, thereby increasing neurotransmitter concentration at the receptor site and down-regulating beta receptor sensitivity.

These findings have encouraged many physicians to believe that alterations in neurotransmitters at the neuronal synapses play a leading, if not exclusive, role in the cause of psychiatric disorders. Our knowledge of the central biochemical correlates of these illnesses is, however, rudimentary, and there are still patients (about 20 percent of the severely mentally ill) who gain little or no benefit from currently available therapeutic modalities.

An observation by ourselves and others, that maximum improvement following limbic system surgery may not be obtained for several months, has led to our hypothesis that the lesions not only affect the neuronal pathways, but also influence neurotransmitter concentrations.

CRITERIA FOR THE SELECTION OF PSYCHIATRIC PATIENTS

It is the usual practice at our institution to accept for evaluation any person who is chronically disabled by a psychiatric illness that has not responded satisfactorily to all currently available therapies (psychotherapy, behavior modification techniques, medications, electroconvulsive therapy (ECT), etc.). The duration of the illness can be of less importance than its severity. In a highly suicidal patient who has not responded to treatment, evaluation for early cingulotomy should be considered. A diagnosis of an affective disorder indicates a better prognosis than does a diagnosis of personality disorder or schizophrenia. However, carefully selected cases of those suffering from these latter two conditions, those in whom depression, anxiety, or obsessions are very prominent accompanying symptoms, those who are not severely deteriorated, are likely to benefit by having the psychiatric conditions modified by cingulotomy.

All patients being considered for cingulotomy must be under psychiatric treatment and referred by a written statement from the treating psychiatrist, who agrees to be responsible for postoperative psychiatric care. Similarly, the patient must agree to return to the referring psychiatrist with the understanding that cingulotomy is an adjunct to, but not a substitute for, careful psychiatric management.

In addition to the above, both the patient and the psychiatrist must fulfill the following specific criteria before being accepted for evaluation by a screening group at the Massachusetts General Hospital (MGH):

1. The referring psychiatrist must complete a form devised by the MGH psychiatrists that will provide the referring psychiatrist with detailed information concerning the patient's past history, present illness, family history, and all prior treatments.
2. To clarify points in the patient's past history, copies of the patient's records are collected and distributed to those involved in the evaluation process.
3. The patient is required to have someone near and dear to him or her who agrees to give emotional support before, during, and after the hospitalization for surgery.
4. The patient, along with the aforementioned "support" person, must be fully informed of the risks and benefits of the cingulotomy, must understand them, and must give consent for the operation.

The MGH evaluation consists of an electroencephalogram (EEG), computed tomographic (CT) scan, a cortical function test, and independently conducted examinations of the patient and perusal of the patient's records by the operating surgeon, a neurologist, and a psychiatrist in an outpatient setting unless the illness is so severe as to make outpatient evaluation impossible. Neither the psychiatrist nor the neurologist is involved in the care of the patient pre) or postoperatively, so that their opinions will be completely impartial.

All three evaluators must agree that the patient meets the criteria, that the cingulotomy is indicated, and that the requirements of informed consent are fulfilled.

Contraindications are few. Patients with pronounced hysterical or sociopathic personalities do not do well, even if presenting symptoms are appropriate. Elderly patients are at an increased risk of postoperative confusion and operative complications, but cingulotomy is likely to have fewer side effects than are long courses of ECT or high dosages of psychotropic drugs.

CRITERIA FOR SELECTION OF CHRONIC PAIN SYNDROME PATIENTS

Criteria for selection of chronic pain syndrome patients are very similar to those for the psychiatric patients, in that any patient who is chronically disabled by severe pain and who has had limited or negligible response to pain-relieving procedures, such as surgery for the removal of the presumed cause of the pain, nerve blocks, pain clinic trials, psychotropic drug trials, etc., is accepted for evaluation. Cingulate surgery is, however, definitely contraindicated for those individuals with pronounced hysterical or sociopathic traits.

Most patients can be managed by the operating neurosurgeon or the local referring physicians so that, unless there is a severe depressive component to the illness, pre- or postoperative psychiatric care is not required. Therefore, referrals from local physicians for pain management are accepted.

The patient completes a detailed pain questionnaire that includes a pain drawing, a visual analogue scale of pain severity, a life history, a McGill-Melzack pain questionnaire, a list of 52 questions probing the patient's personality and the influence it has on the illness, a check-off list of 132 adjectives used to describe feelings about himself or herself, and a check-off list (known as SCL-90-R) of 90 problems by which a pain patient might be troubled.

Patients not previously treated with psychotropic drugs are given a trial of medications such as doxepin 150–300 mg at night, with clonazepam 1.5–3.0 mg in divided doses during the day.

The MGH evaluation of chronic pain patients follows the pattern delineated for the psychiatric patients. It is, however, permissible for the screening neurologist and psychiatrist to be involved in the care of these individuals before and after cingulotomy.

A close relative or friend who will provide emotional support is also required for these patients and, again, both must be fully informed of the risks and benefits and must give consent.

Limbic system surgery should be undertaken, when indicated, in both the psychiatric and pain patients before their support systems (family unit and social environment), employment opportunities, and personality functions have been significantly and perhaps irreversibly damaged by chronic and/or severe dysfunction.

EQUIPMENT FOR STEREOTACTIC ANTERIOR CINGULOTOMY

The equipment used for stereotactic anterior cingulotomy includes: a radiofrequency lesion (RFL) generator with thermistor controls; a gas-sterilized Ballantine thermistor cingulotomy set; and x-ray equipment. The cingulotomy set contains:

1. Two 17G Ballantine ventricular needles with stylets. (The needles are insulated except for the distal centimeter.)
2. One thermistor probe.
3. One connecting cable for thermistor to RFL generator.

The x-ray equipment includes:

1. Fluoroscopy unit with C-arm and image intensifier.
2. Four x-ray cassettes.
3. Plastic headband embedded with lead beads situated at 1-cm intervals.
4. Centimeter ruler with adjustable gauge.
5. Radiolucent headpiece for operating table.
6. Plastic head holder.

SURGICAL TECHNIQUE

Under local or general endotracheal anesthesia, the patient is placed supine on an operating table that is equipped with a radiolucent headpiece and an x-ray cassette holder. The head is placed in a plastic holder that allows access to the frontal region, and is elevated to a 30-degree angle by flexing the table. A 4 × 10 cm area of the scalp, just behind the frontal hairline, is shaved. The center of this area is at the midline and 9.5 cm posterior to the nasion. After the midline is accurately identified, cross-hatches are scratched on the scalp 9.5 cm posterior to the nasion and 1.5 cm to either side of the midline. Stab wounds are made through the scalp at these points, through

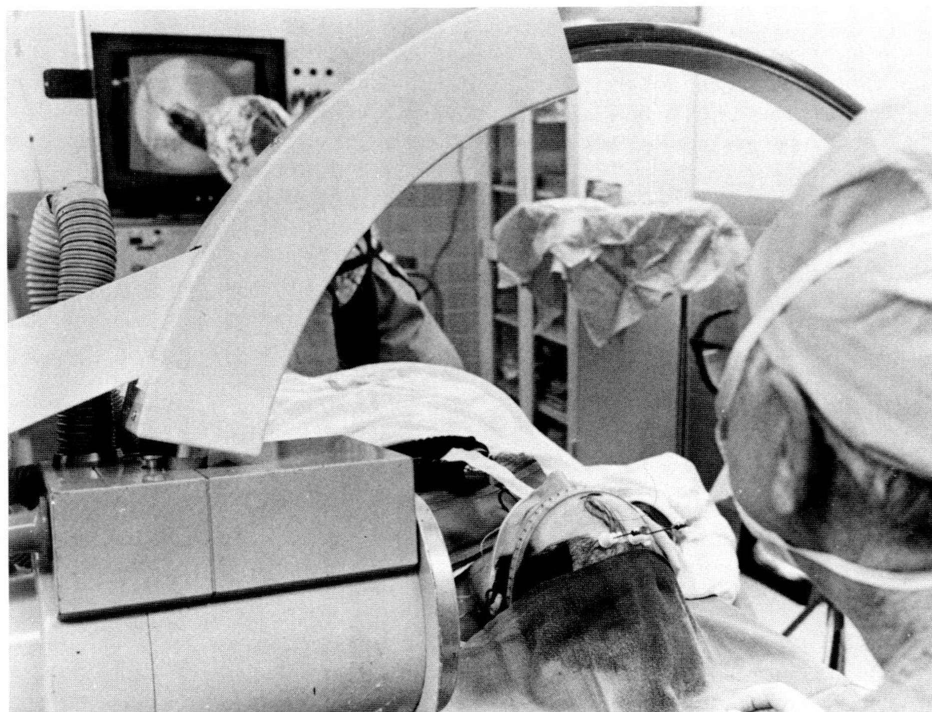

Fig. 93-2. Stereotactic cingulotomy. Arrangement of the patient, the surgeon, the plastic headband, the C-arm fluoroscope and screen. The needle electrodes are in position. The radiofrequency generator is at the surgeon's right.

which the skull is also marked with twist drill holes. The scalp is incised transversely through the points on the scalp. Bilateral burr holes are made at the twist drill holes, and the dura and the cortex beneath the burr holes are lightly cauterized. A ventricular needle is introduced to a depth of about 2 cm in an attempt to be certain that no subcortical bleeding will be encountered during the introduction of the electrodes. The wound is then closed.

A plastic headband with embedded lead beads situated at 1-cm intervals is placed around the head over the orbital ridge, above the ears and around the occiput (Figure 93-2) to enable calculation of the amount of magnification of the fluoroscopic image.

Specially designed 17-gauge ventricular needles, electrically insulated except for the distal centimeter, are introduced into the lateral ventricles by angling the needles toward the external auditory meatus on the lateral view and 7 mm from the midline on the frontal view. To adequately visualize the anterior horns and the roofs of the lateral ventricles, 6 ml of air is required in each one. This can usually be accomplished by introducing 12 ml of air through one ventricular puncture. Using intermittent fluoroscopic localization, and marking the targets on the fluoroscopic screen, the needles (now being used as thermistor-equipped electrodes) are first positioned bilaterally 1 cm above the roof of the lateral ventricles, 2.5 cm posterior to the anterior tips, and 0.7 cm on either side of the midline. After the first lesions are made, the electrodes are lowered 1 cm, without changing the lateral and anteroposterior position. Lesions are made by the application of a radiofrequency current that heats the electrode tip to 85°C for 100 seconds at each position. The lesion volume is about 1 cm in diameter and 2 cm in vertical height, the inferior border being at a point about 1

mm above the lateral ventricular shadow. (Figures 93-3 and 93-4 are roentgenograms showing the electrodes in place, and Figures 93-5 and 93-6 are from a CT scan showing the necrotic areas.) The air is withdrawn after the lesions are completed, and the wound is covered with a simple dressing. The length of the entire procedure is approximately 1.5 to 2.0 hours.

Repeat cingulotomies do not generally require an incision, and can usually be done under local anesthesia following preoperative medication of 5 mg of droperidol intramuscularly and 10 mg of diazepam orally. This provides heavy sedation, but the patient is arousable. The areas of the burr holes are shaved and sterilized. The scalp is punctured with a 15-gauge needle, through which the electrodes can be inserted. If the interval since the first operation is more than a year, the inner table of the skull may have regenerated and a twist drill puncture is necessary. A limited ventriculogram is required, after which the electrodes are positioned as before, but 1 cm anterior to the previous lesions.

SAFETY

In our series of 714 cingulotomies performed on 474 patients, there have been no deaths and no infections. Two hemiplegias have occured secondary to acute subdural hematomas caused by laceration of cortical arteries during introduction of the ventricular needles. One patient made a complete recovery after evacuation of the clot; the other remains hemiplegic. One male patient, aged 40, developed a chronic subdural hematoma at the site of his left burr hole, which required evacuation 4 weeks after his cingulotomy. He made a complete recovery, suffered a relapse in his depression,

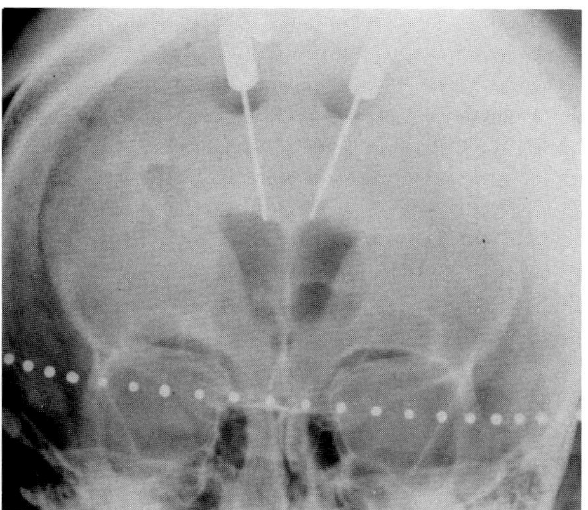

Fig. 93-3. Anteroposterior view of the electrodes during cingulotomy. The lead beads embedded in the headband are 10 mm apart.

underwent a second procedure without incident, did well, but had another relapse 4½ years later and underwent a third cingulotomy. Six weeks after this last cingulotomy, he developed another chronic subdural hematoma, again at the site of his left burr hole. It required evacuation and recovery was again complete without neurologic deficit.

Convulsions have occurred in 5 of our patients, but have been easily controlled with phenytoin. There have been no permanent neurologic, behavioral, or intellectual deficits as a result of the cingulate lesions themsleves.

IMMEDIATE POSTOPERATIVE MANAGEMENT

Postoperatively, these patients are usually nauseated and develop headache, cervical pain, and fever of 100–102°F, which is caused by the introduced air and the red blood cells in the cerebral spinal fluid from the ventricular puncture, and also by the resolution of the lesion's necrotic tissue. Also, it is not

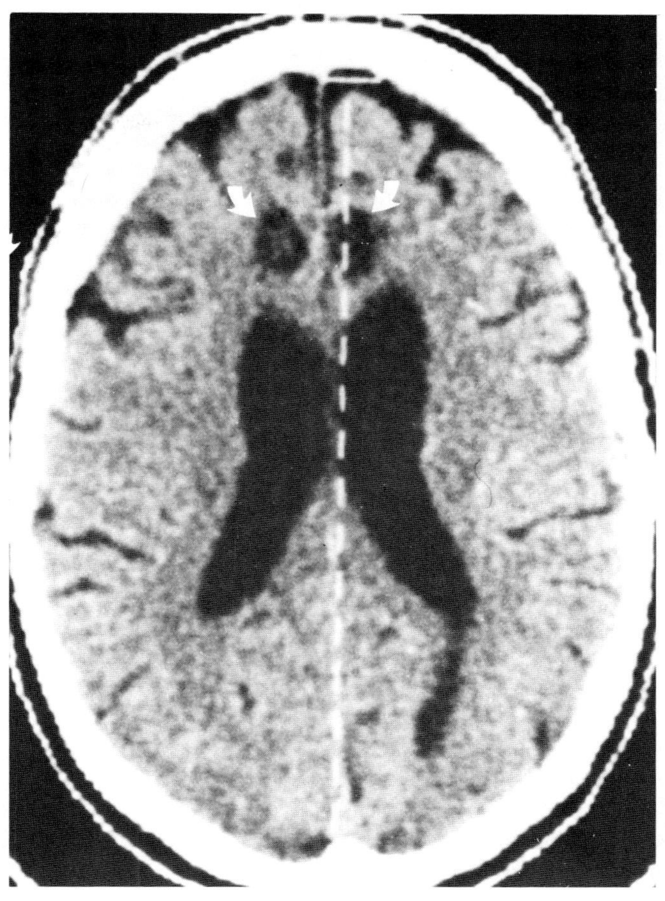

Fig. 93-5. A CT scan (axial view) showing bilateral cingulate lesions (arrows).

uncommon for these patients to have bladder dysfunction (either incontinence or retention). All of these side effects are treated with appropriate medication, and usually clear within 4 days. Psychiatric patients are maintained on their preoperative psychotropic medications, but usually at lower doses postoperatively than preoperatively. Chronic pain patients are given non-narcotic analgesics along with appropriate psychotropic therapy. They do not suffer narcotic withdrawal symptoms.

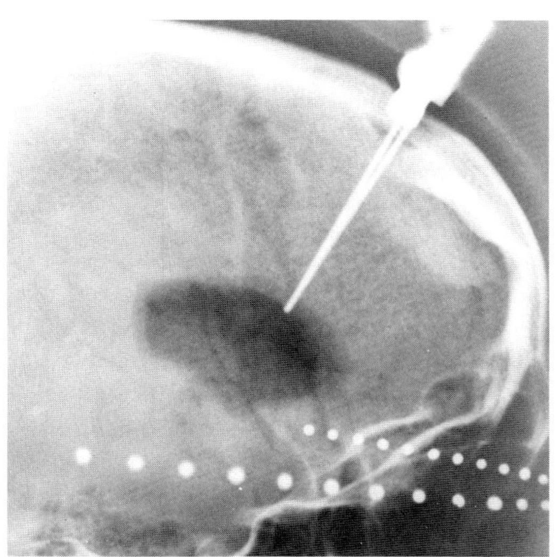

Fig. 93-4. Lateral view of the electrodes during cingulotomy.

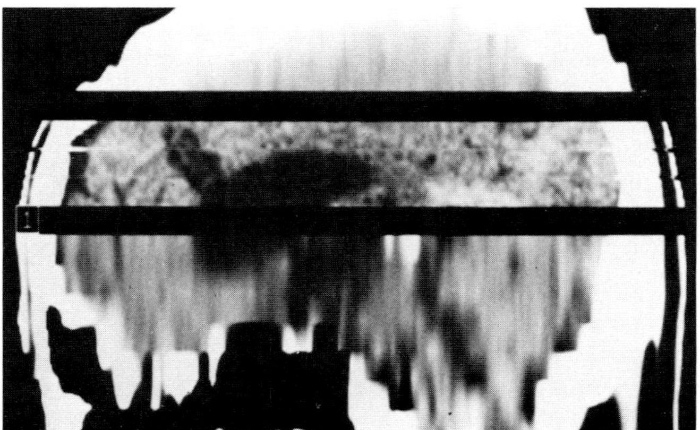

Fig. 93-6. A CT scan (sagittal reconstruction) showing cingulotomy lesions.

LONG-TERM POSTOPERATIVE MANAGEMENT

PSYCHIATRIC MANAGEMENT

Most of our patients require careful, long-term psychiatric management. We ask their psychiatrists to see them weekly at first, adjusting their medications and treating them as they would any of their very sick psychiatric patients, since we consider cingulotomy not an instant cure, but rather an adjunct to good psychiatric care. Medications (often at lowered doses), psychotherapy, and ECT, which gave only temporary or partial relief preoperatively, are often very effective postoperatively.

The psychiatric status is usually cyclic, with gradual improvement occurring over a period of 1 month to 5 years. For the first 4 months, the low periods of these cycles are often lower than they were preoperatively. We believe this is caused by a discouragement factor, a feeling that "the operation failed and now there is nothing left," or "I felt normal for a while; I cannot go through the anguish of my illness again!" The suicidal risk at this stage is high, and hospitalization is often required to protect and treat the patient.

The high periods of the cycles can occasionally result in hypomania. Lithium and often a neuroleptic are required to prevent the attack from becoming increasingly serious. If the symptom is unrecognized and denied by the patient, however, it could become so severe that hospitalization would also be required during the acute stage.

Family members or close friends are essential in the management of these patients, especially during the low and high periods of their cycles, for it is they who may be required to alert the psychiatrist to the abnormal behavior.

Of the psychiatric patients we have categorized in the "well" status, 45 percent underwent more than one cingulotomy. We are, however, reluctant to perform a double set of lesions at the first operation, because not every patient requires it, and we feel that the absence of emotional and cognitive deficits in our series is due largely to the staging of the lesions. It is therefore our practice to repeat the cingulotomy after 3 months if there has been no response to the first cingulotomy.

CHRONIC PAIN PATIENTS

Chronic pain patients generally run a smooth postoperative course. Within 5 to 7 days postoperatively, they are often able to tolerate their pain without narcotic analgesics and are discharged from the hospital on a psychotropic medication regimen with non-narcotic analgesics when needed. They are usually managed by the operating neurosurgeon if the depressive component of their illness is not too severe. Slow, steady improvement is concurrent with their physical and social rehabilitation, and maximum improvement seems to occur within 3 to 6 months. The assistance of family and friends in the rehabilitation process is invaluable. It is of interest that only 9 percent of the 23 chronic pain patients who were categorized as "well" required more than one operation.

EFFICACY

A study of 198 psychiatric patients operated upon during a 20-year period and followed from 2 to 22 years (mean, 8.6 years) was recently completed. One hundred twenty of the psychiatric patients carried a diagnosis of affective disorder (unipolar or bipolar depression, or schizoaffective disorder), 14 suffered from disabling anxiety, 32 from obsessive-compulsive disorders, 11 suffered from schizophrenia, and 21 fell into a "miscellaneous" category. All of the patients were disabled preoperatively; 43 percent (86 patients) had suicidal ideation, and 26 percent (52 patients) had made suicide attempts.

In assessing the postoperative status of this group, we limited worthwhile improvement to include only those patients who were well or functioning normally on medication and/or psychotherapy, or who were no longer critically ill and suicidal, but still had recurring, disabling psychiatric symptoms. Using these criteria, we placed 62 percent of our patients in the satisfactorily improved group. Another 17 percent, who remained severely disabled but required less medication, spent less time in hospitals, required less psychiatric supervision, and were easier to manage than was true preoperatively, were felt to have shown only slight postoperative improvement. The best results have been attained in patients diagnosed as having affective or anxiety disorders.

We have also reviewed the postoperative status of 123 patients who underwent cingulotomy for pain. Thirty-five of them had terminal cancer, and for the first 3 postoperative months, 20 (57 percent) obtained satisfactory pain relief. Ten patients lived more than 3 months, and pain relief was sustained in only two.

The 98 patients with noncancerous chronic pain have been followed for 1 to 21 years (mean, 7 years). There were no deaths or complications in this group, and only three were lost to follow-up. Severe, constant pain refractory to all the usual therapies constituted the primary indications for cingulotomy. All of those with chronic back pain had undergone one or more laminectomies. In the entire series, 19 percent were addicted to narcotics and 58 percent were diagnosed as suffering from one or more of the following psychiatric disorders: affective, anxiety, and personality.

The patients have been grouped as shown in Table 93-1.

In judging whether or not the operation had conferred a worthwhile benefit, we used the following criteria: (1) the patient no longer complained of pain and required no medication; or (2) the patient was symptom-free on minor psychotropic drugs; or (3) the patient was comfortable on a regimen of minor psychotropic drugs and non-narcotic analgesics. Except for the "failed back" patients, the numbers in the other categories are too small to be of other than anecdotal value in reference to perceived benefit. Five of 6 patients with chronic abdominal pain were usefully improved, as were 3 of 5 patients with phantom limb pain. The operation appeared to have been of little or no help to patients suffering from tabetic, thalamic, or postherpetic pain.

On the other hand, 45 (74 percent) of 61 patients with chronic low back pain appeared to have obtained benefit from cingulotomy, and in 38 (62 percent) the result was satisfactory. It is again of interest that the operation was of more benefit to females than to males (77 percent versus 47 percent). Four males in this group committed suicide postoperatively; three of the four carried an additional diagnosis of clinical depression.

If a satisfactory postoperative status is attained after cingulotomy for chronic pain of nonmalignant origin, this status is usually permanent. This finding stands in marked contrast to the fading of pain relief in patients who have been operated upon for intractable cancer pain.

Table 93-1. Patients with noncancerous chronic pain treated by cingulotomy

Locus or Cause of Pain	Number of Patients
Low back	62 (1 not followed)
Abdomen and flank	7 (1 not followed)
Unknown cause	6
Miscellaneous	
Herpetic	6
Headache	3
Thalamic	3
Facial neuralgia	1
Phantom limb	5
Tabetic and "spinal"	2
Upper extremity (trauma)	3 (1 not followed)
Total	23

DISCUSSION

Although we have limited this chapter to cingulotomy, there are other approaches to the limbic system; chief among these are subcaudate tractotomy, limbic leukotomy, and anterior capsulotomy. The operative techniques and the reported results have been delineated elsewhere;[7] but it should be noted that anterior capsulotomy and limbic leukotomy are said to yield better postoperative outcomes than does cingulotomy in cases of obsessive-compulsive neurosis. It is because of this diversity of approaches that we prefer the term "limbic system surgery" to either "psychiatric surgery" or "psychosurgery." Indeed, psychosurgery is thought by most of the general public and many physicians to refer exclusively to the outmoded and rejected prefrontal lobotomy. This semantic confusion has retarded progress and limited the acceptance and application of surgical therapy for mental illness.

In 1986, 50 years after its initial acceptance and 27 years after Moniz was awarded the Nobel prize for its introduction, limbic system surgery remains controversial. It is imperative, therefore, that every possible precaution be taken to ensure that psychiatrically ill patients be chosen for operation only after all other generally accepted therapies have failed, that thorough preoperative evaluation be performed, and that informed consent has been obtained.

SUMMARY AND CONCLUSIONS

We have presented the operative technique employed in performing 714 bilateral anterior stereotactic cingulotomies on 474 patients. There have been no deaths or infections. There is no evidence of impairment of cognition or "emotional tone" as a result of cingulate interruption. Two patients became hemiplegic and one developed chronic subdural hematomas postoperatively. Five patients each reported 1 postoperative seizure. Subsets of 198 psychiatric and 123 chronic pain patients have been intensively evaluated over a mean follow-up period of 8.6 and 7 years, respectively. The clinical status of 79 percent of the psychiatric patients improved postoperatively, and 62 percent had achieved a satisfactory status at the time of evaluation. In the series of chronic pain patients, 73 percent showed improvement, and in 62 percent the operation was felt to have been definitely worthwhile.

We conclude from this experience that stereotactic cingulotomy is relatively safe and effective. It should be available to the severely mentally ill who are failures of nonoperative therapies, particularly those who suffer from affective disorders. Similarly, it should be considered as a last resort for certain patients with intractable pain. Our experiences with the treatment of the "failed back syndrome" lead us to conclude that cingulotomy offers a better and safer chance for amelioration of pain than do other destructive operations such as nerve root ablation or cordotomy.

REFERENCES

1. Shutts D: Lobotomy: Resort to the Knife. New York, Van Nostrand Rheinhold, 1982, pp 117–179
2. Freeman WL, Watts JW: Psychosurgery: In the Treatment of Mental Disorders and Intractable Pain, ed 2. Springfield, Ill, Charles C Thomas, 1951, pp 353–374
3. Tooth GC, Newton MP: Leucotomy in England and Wales 1942–1954. Reports on Public Health and Medical Subjects, no. 104. London, Her Majesty's Stationery Office, 1961
4. Foltz EL, White LE Jr: Pain "relief" by frontal cingulotomy. J Neurosurg 19:89, 1962
5. Papez JW: A proposed mechanism of emotion. Arch Neurol Psychiatry 38:725, 1937
6. Bernstein JG: Neurotransmitters and receptors in pharmacopsychiatry, in Bernstein JG (ed): Clinical Psychopharmacology, ed 2. Massachusetts, John Wright-PSG, Inc., 1984, pp 59–74
7. Ballantine HT Jr: Neurosurgery for behavioral disorders, in Wilkins RH, Rengachary SS (eds): Neurosurgery. New York, Elsevier/North-Holland, 1985, pp 2527–2537

CHAPTER 94

Intraventricular Morphine in the Treatment of Pain Secondary to Cancer

Alberto Lenzi   Giuseppe Galli   Giovanni Marini

OVER THE PAST 15 YEARS, biochemical studies, however fragmentary, have shown us that within the "human ecosystem" interdependent relationships exist between the somatic and vegetative nervous system, between neuromodulators and hormones, and also between psychic activity and the immune system.[1-3]

This ecosystem appears to have been fashioned over the course of evolution into a definite structure, the ultimate goal of which is preservation of the human species against polymorphous external aggressions. Anthropologic studies have further heightened the awareness that environmental stress can heavily influence the onset of many otherwise classically idiopathic diseases like cancer. Cancer, in fact, could very well be the end result of an imbalance between aggressive external forces and internal defense mechanisms, in which a great many factors interact in unknown proportions, producing an interference of congenital and acquired elements (either causal or voluntary), sometimes due to proneness, sometimes conditioned.

Within this complex meshwork of factors, pain is a warning signal of acute changes occurring in the physiologic homeostasis; and pain is also an epiphenomenon signalling the progressive and chronic deterioration of multiple organic systems whose balanced functions ensure physical and psychological well-being.[46]

In the treatment of pain secondary to cancer, our prime objective is to achieve analgesia for as long as possible, using methods that provide long-lasting pain relief and, in addition, require limited surgery and create minimal injury to the nervous system's structure.[7,8]

The techniques that allow the slow infusion of microdoses of morphine into the cerebrospinal fluid (CSF) not only fulfill these requirements, they also make it easier for family members to handle a patient's pain over long periods of time.

MORPHINE THERAPY AND THE OPIOID SYSTEM

The analgesic effects of morphine are for the most part due to its central actions. Morphine does not significantly influence the response threshold of the nerve endings, nor the conduction of stimuli by peripheral nerves. Nevertheless, it remains rather difficult to define which centers of the nervous system are responsible for analgesia and behavioral responses.

Many of a brain's structures involved with pain perception and modulation are affected by morphine, yet the drug's effects on the spinal cord, the limbic system, and the periventricular and periaqueductal grey matter seem to constitute the very neurophysiologic basis of its analgesic efficacy.

The biochemical activity of opioids in providing pain relief in cancer management has been elucidated as a result of two important discoveries: the identification of specific receptors for exogenous opiates within the central nervous system; and the detection of endogenous peptide-type substances with effects similar to those of morphine. This began when Pert and Snyder of the United States, and Terenius of Sweden, identified the precise location of binding sites with a high affinity for opioids in the fragments of cell membrane obtained from rat brain and from the intestines of guinea pigs.[9,10]

Subsequently, many others were able to measure the density and the actual distribution of these receptors in the brain and spinal cord.[11] Classically, it has been held that there are two distinct pathways involved in the perception of pain. An acute, localized pain (which is hardly diminished by opioids) is conveyed through a monosynaptic route that is phylogenetically recent, and this pain travels up the ventral spinothalamic tract and enters the ventral lateral nucleus of the thalamus, from which the neurons project out into the primary somatosensory area. Conversely, deeper pain (which is efficaciously alleviated by opioids) is conveyed through phylogenetically older, multisynaptic routes.

These multisynaptic routes are made up of groups of cells with multiple and widespread interconnections; they are interconnected by unmyelinated fibers having low conduction speed. This paleospinothalamic pathway travels up the spinal cord to reach the brain, and makes two important "integration stops" along the way: one at the periaqueductal gray matter level, and the second in the median area of the thalamus. The map of opioid receptor distribution corresponds to the distribution of the paleospinothalamic pathways of pain. Although a high density of receptors is also present in the amygdala, in the corpus striatum, and in the hypothalamus, regions of the brain that act together in processing the emotional components of pain. Maximum receptor density is found in the substantia gelatina of the spinal cord, and also in proximity of the substantia gelatina of the spinal trigeminal nucleus.

In 1976, Martin et al. hypothesized the existence of three receptor subtypes, μ, κ, and σ, with initials matching those of the agonist types, i.e., morphine, ketocyclazocine, and N-allilnormetazocine.[12,13]

OPERATIVE NEUROSURGICAL TECHNIQUES
ISBN 0-8089-1862-1

Other authors report a fourth receptor, δ, specifically antagonized by D-ala-met-enkephalin. The pharmacologic picture induced by common exogenous opiates (i.e., morphine, pentazocine, and buprenorphine) appears to be the algebraic sum of the different agonist/antagonist effects carried out vis-a-vis specific receptors.[13,14]

In 1975, Hughes and Kosterlitz[15] were able to isolate and identify the first two analgesic peptides, met-enkephalin and leu-enkephalin, in pig brain. Soon thereafter, β-endorphin was identified, a peptide with 31 amino acids that has a structure similar to that of the met-enkephalin within it. In 1979, for the first time, Chavkin and Goldstein[16] described dinorphin, a peptide with 13 amino acids that includes the leu-enkephalin structure.

Today, three major families of endogenous opiates are recognized.[17] Pro-opio-melano-cortin derivatives are the first major family of endogenous opiates. Their prime elements are β-endorphin, ACTH, and g-MSH. β-Endorphin is maximally concentrated in the adeno-hypophysis, and is present in lesser amounts in the hypothalamus, in the amygdala, in the periaqueductal gray matter, and in sympathetic ganglia. β-Endorphin is a very powerful agonist for μ receptors and a relatively good one for δ receptors. Polypeptides derived from pro-opio-melano-cortin play a complex yet complementary role in the body's reaction to stress. In such situations, all the polypeptides derived from this precursor are released simultaneously. Correlations between neurons containing β-endorphin, the hypothalamus, and periaqueductal gray matter all confirm the role of β-endorphin as filter/modulator of spinal pains. Projections towards the median area of the hypothalamus confirm the role of β-endorphin in regulating the hypophysis function in such a way as to maintain the body's homeostasis punctually and continuously.

Proenkephalin A derivatives are the second major family of endogenous opiates. Their prime elements are met-enkephalin and, to a certain extent, leu-enkephalin. Maximum concentration is observed in the limbic system, in the median area of the thalamus, in the amygdala, and in the substantia gelatina of the spinal cord. Enkephalin has a preferential sensitivity for δ receptors, and in part for μ receptors. Enkephalin directly acts on the cell containing these specific receptors via an inhibitory mechanism. Enkephalin released from the cell containing it triggers an increase in sodium conduction through the cell membrane, thereby partially depolarizing it. When an impulse then reaches the nerve ending, the net depolarization it engenders results inferior. Hence, release of the excited mediator is proportionally less. The next receiving cell undergoes proportionally less stimulation. Thus, moment by moment, these inhibiting actions control the ascending pain pathways from the spinal cord to the brain. Substance P is considered to be the mediator of nociceptive stimuli. Enkephalins therefore act as modulators by way of presynaptic inhibitory mechanisms that manage the release of substance P in the spinal cord (Jessel and Iversen, 1977).

Proenkephalin B derivatives are the third major family of endogenous opiates. Their prime element is dinorphin,[18,19] which is most concentrated around the neurohypophysis and the spinal cord. These polypeptides tend to bind with κ receptors, and, at the spinal cord level, they develop an intense analgesic effect. In addition to being present in the intestinal tract and medullary tract of the adrenal gland, they are also contained in different types of neurons of the central nervous system.[14,20,21] While classical types of neurotransmitters (e.g., norepinephrine) hold an enzymatic synthesis at the nerve endings, are released following tonic stimuli, and undergo an enzymatic degradation or uptake, neuropeptides are produced at ribosome level in the form of long protein precursors; they are released intermittently and tend to have a long-lasting effect without uptake. Thus, the classical neurotransmission system carried out by excitation or by postsynaptic inhibition of the cell acts as an emergency signal indicating rapid changes within the organism; the neuropeptide system, in contrast, has the role of maintaining a continuous basic environment of optimal well-being and the progressive adaptation to varying input conditions in order that the cell may rapidly return to optimal well-being. Classic peptides and neurotransmitters can coexist within the same neurons, even when confined to different compartments.[22] This coexistence, in fact, has led us to believe that peptides as regulators of nervous functions are of vital importance.

At the posterior horn of the spinal cord are located the primary sensory neurons containing substance P, somatostatin, gastrin, and cholecystokinin; spinal interneurons containing enkephalin, substance P, and neurotensin; and descending systems containing substance P, enkephalin, and serotonin. It is clear that all these play an important integrator/modulator role in afferent sensory impulses, which generally occur in this region with the fundamental presence of neuropeptides. Neuropeptides also execute a vital modulating role in hypophysis and endocrine activity via hypothalamic release or inhibitive factors of incretion.

As was mentioned earlier, the human body reacts to situations of stress by releasing, from the same precursor, three functionally distinct peptides: β-endorphin, ACTH, and g-MSH. Recent studies conducted by Panerai highlighted the fact that a state of analgesia maintained normally and continuously is the result of a balance and modulated interaction, at the receptor level, of endogenous agonist/antagonist opiates, among which are cholecystokinin and TRH.[21]

MORPHINE INJECTIONS INTO THE CEREBROSPINAL FLUID

Since the early 1980s, microdose morphine injection into the cerebrospinal fluid (CSF) has progressively acquired a fairly well-defined place in cancer pain therapy. This trend displaces a preference for ablative techniques, which neurosurgeons had previouly used to control pain of this kind, whereas general practitioners and internists often treated pain with ad libitum administration of oral or intramuscular morphine, resulting in tolerance and progressive impairment of mental faculties. Administered parenterally or orally, opiates undergo rapid metabolic inactivation by the liver.[23–25] Only a small portion of the drug reaches the specific central nervous system (CNS) receptors and, therefore, attains an analgesic effect of limited quality and duration. Conversely, morphine injected into the CSF bypasses the blood-brain barrier, and reaches specific receptor sites immediately, thus making small doses of drug particulary effective.

For many years, fear of respiratory depression[26–29] hindered the general acceptance of this technique. Following proof, however, that intrathecal morphine provides intense analgesia in rats, several authors tested the effects in humans of morphine administered directly into the CSF at the extradural or subarachnoid level.[30,31] In 1981, Leavens[32] reported the use of intraventricular injections of morphine in four cancer patients. Our current series includes 50 patients receiving intraventricular morphine therapeutically, 119 patients receiving morphine in the spinal CSF, and 119 patients receiving morphine administered via catheter into the spinal extradural space.

The present chapter reports our experience with 50 patients suffering from neoplastic pain syndromes of the cervical and craniofacial regions. In these cases, microdoses of morphine were injected into the ventricular fluid through a catheter connected to a subcutaneous reservoir. We believe this type of drug administration offers a good way of assessing the advantages and disadvantages of the technique, even in comparison to the spinal, subarachnoid, and extradural routes.

PATIENT SELECTION

We chose patients with a presumptive life expectancy of about 6 months in whom neurosurgical procedures (e.g., thermorhizotomy, chemical rhizotomy) had either become ineffective, as a result of progression of the neoplastic illness or were not indicated. All patients in this series underwent a full trial of standard analgesic regimen, both medical and surgical, and radiotherapy.

SURGICAL TECHNIQUE

A computed tomographic (CT) scan of the brain is performed in order to examine the morphology and dimensions of the cerebral ventricles and to exclude CNS involvement by the patient's disease. Subsequently, the patient is operated on in the supine position, with the neck moderately flexed. Local anesthesia is used. A right frontal arch-shaped incision is made, and a burr hole is placed 2 cm from the midline and 6 cm above the superciliary arch. The dura is opened and the right frontal horn cannulated with a ventricular needle, and fluid is withdrawn. The ventricular needle is then replaced with a Silastic ventricular catheter (6–8 cm), connected to a 1.5-ml reservoir (Cordis Italia, Milano, Italy) (Figure 94-1) that is placed beneath the galea. To ensure that the system is functioning perfectly, patent CSF is aspirated from the reservoir prior to skin closure.

When opiates are to be administered, the skin is disinfected repeatedly, and the reservoir tapped transcutaneously with a 25-gauge needle connected to a 2.5-ml syringe. Half a milligram to 1 mg of morphine hydrochloride diluted in 1 ml of a 5-percent glucose solution is injected while washing the inner part of the system with CSF to guarantee dispersion of the drug throughout the ventricle.

CASE SUMMARIES

Table 94-1 summarizes the type and site of the tumor in our series of 50 cases as well as the distribution, duration, and rhythm of the neoplastic pain attacks. The table also summarizes previous therapies. In 39 of 50 patients, the tumor was limited to the head and neck, tongue, larynx, parotid gland, pharynx, palatine-tonsil, and oral cavity. In 4 of another 12 cases, the tumor involved the pulmonary apex (cases 4, 7, 16, and 29) or the breast (case 7), with extension into the brachial plexus. Case 34 was that of a patient suffering from bronchiogenic cancer that metastasized to the bodies of the fourth and fifth vertebrae. In 2 patients suffering from kidney tumor (cases 12 and 13), metastases reached cranial bones, causing pain in this region. Patient 18 had thyroid cancer with multiple bony metastases, and patient 33 had melanoma with multiple bony and subcutaneous metastases.

Almost all of these patients had received minor analgesic drugs (acetylsalicylic acid, ketoprofen, noramidopyrine), the efficacy of which decreased over time. Methylprednisolone was also administered occasionally. Nine patients received analgesic therapy with morphine syrup, with poor results or unacceptable side effects. Ten patients received pentazocine as needed, often many times a day. This therapy influenced the quality of the subsequent intraventricular morphine usage because of the appearance of a more or less high toxicodependence.

Of 50 patients, 44 were male and 6 were female. The mean age was 53 years. The pain classification, continuous or intermittent, was influenced, in our opinion, by the patient's personality. The pain syndrome had an average duration of 2.13 months. The use of intraventricular morphine must not begin too early, because management of these patients for long periods is difficult because of the risk of sepsis, respiratory depression, and increasing drug tolerance. Conversely, therapy must not be deferred unduly when either the general clinical condition of the patient is largely compromised or the overuse of major analgesic drugs (morphine, pentazocine) has already caused a dependence that is difficult to manage.

In the first 9 patients of this series, an Ommaya reservoir was used. This was replaced by the reservoir (Figure 94-1) prepared by Cordis Italia, which includes a 1.5-ml Silastic reservoir with a metal base and a ventricular catheter connected to it at a right angle; the catheter length varies from 6 to 8 cm.

Following introduction of this system, the patients are kept hospitalized for a 5 to 7 days, while the drug is administered and the patient monitored with respect to response and possible side effects experienced. For home treatment, a relative or a visiting nurse can be taught how to administer the drug. All patients are monitored weekly at the hospital if possible, otherwise by phone from their homes.

RESULTS

Pain relief is classified as excellent (80–100 percent pain decrease), good (40–80 percent), fair (20–40 percent), and bad (less than 20 percent). Table 94-2 summarizes the initial and final doses of morphine, the time from morphine administration to onset of analgesia, analgesia quality, and side effects. The table also includes some short notes indicating the impressions and emotional evaluations of relatives, useful in underlining the efficacy of treatment, which was sometimes very good.

We administered a single dose of morphine hydrochloride, 1 mg in 1 ml of a 5-percent glucose solution, to the first patients. Analgesia, sometimes excellent (100 percent relief of pain), appeared in 5 to 30 minutes and lasted 24 to 48 hours. We later decided to decrease the initial test dose to 0.5 mg/day. This dosage represents the initial minimal dose necessary to obtain analgesia that is effective for 24 hours with very few or no side effects. Recently, as the table shows, we started to use 0.25 mg/24 hours as the initial dose.

The best results, from the point of view of both analgesia and subjective well-being, are obtained in patients never previously treated with opioids or other major analgesic drugs. Pentazocine in particular leads rapidly to a dependence, and, in cases 10, 17, and 29, greatly influenced the outcome. The most encouraging result was observed in patient 18 (survival 104 days), whose pentazocine dependence was eliminated, although with difficulty. On the other hand, intraventricular morphine was completely ineffective for patient 7. In this subject, an

Table 94–1. Origin and characteristics of pain and previous therapies

Case	Age, Sex	Etiology of Pain, Site of Tumor	Distribution, Duration of Pain	Previous Cancer-specific Treatment	Previous Analgesic Treatment
1	45, M	Tonsils, local invasion	Soft palate, pharynx, neck; 2 mo, continuous	Local resection	Minor analgesic drugs
2	50, M	Rhinopharynx, local invasion	Orofacies, neck; 3 mo, continuous	Biopsy, radiotherapy	ACTH, methylprednisolone
3	42, M	Tongue, local invasion	Oropharynx, soft palate; 3 mo, intermittent	Biopsy, radiotherapy	ACTH, methylprednisolone
4	57, M	Pulmonary apex, diffusion to brachial plexus	R arm, R cervical region, R chest wall; 1 mo, continuous	Biopsy, radiotherapy	Minor analgesic drugs
5	63, M	Tonsils, local invasion	Tongue, oropharynx, soft palate; 2 mo, continuous	Biopsy, chemotherapy	Morphine syrup
6	56, M	Pharynx, local invasion	orofacies, neck; 5 mo, intermittent	Biopsy, radiotherapy, chemotherapy	Methylprednisolone, pentazocine
7	56, F	L breast, diffusion to brachial plexus	Upper L chest, axillary cavity, L arm, L neck; 2 mo, continuous	Mastectomy, radiotherapy	Minor analgesic drugs, alcoholic hypophysectomy
8	62, M	Tongue	Oropharynx, neck; 1 mo, continuous	Biopsy, radiotherapy	Minor analgesic drugs
9	61, M	Larynx, local invasion	Oropharynx, ear, R mastoid region; 3 mo, intermittent	Local resection, tracheostomy	Minor analgesic drugs
10	45, M	Tongue, local invasion	Oropharynx; 2 mo, continuous	Biopsy, radiotherapy	Minor analgesic drugs, pentazocine occasionally
11	64, M	Soft palate, local invasion	Orofacies, pharynx, neck; 1 mo, continuous	Biopsy, radiotherapy	ACTH, methylprednisolone
12	60, M	Kidney, multiple metastases (cranium, lungs)	Generalized; 16 mo, continuous	Nephrectomy	Morphine syrup, minor analgesic drugs
13	73, M	Kidney, multiple metastases (liver, pancreas, jaw bone)	Generalized, more severe in facial/neck region; 1 mo, intermittent	Nephrectomy	Morphine syrup
14	69, M	Tongue, local invasion	Oropharynx, R ear, neck; 2 mo, continuous	Biopsy, radiotherapy	Minor analgesic drugs, pentazocine occasionally
15	73, M	L maxillary sinus, local invasion	Orofacies, neck, L hemicranium; 4 mo, intermittent	Local resections repeatedly	Minor analgesic drugs
16	64, M	Pulmonary apex, multiple cranial metastases	Generalized; 1 mo, intermittent	Biopsy, chemotherapy	Minor analgesic drugs
17	46, M	Tongue, local invasion	Orofacies, R hemicranium, R neck; 3 mo, continuous	Local resection, radiotherapy	Pentazocine
18	36, M	Thyroid gland, multiple cranium/jaw metastases	Generalized (neck, cranium); 5 mo, continuous	Local resection, radiotherapy	Morphine syrup, pentazocine

19	59, M	Tongue, local invasion (jaw)	Orofacies, cranium, R neck; 9 mo, continuous	Local resections repeatedly, radiotherapy, chemotherapy	Morphine syrup
20	42, M	Jaw, local invasion	Orofacies, cranium, neck; 4 mo, continuous	Biopsy, radiotherapy	Morphine syrup
21	62, M	Pharynx, local invasion	Oropharynx, occipital; 2 mo, intermittent	Biopsy, radiotherapy	Minor analgesic drugs
22	77, F	Skin of the neck, local invasion	Face, L neck; 2 mo, intermittent	Biopsy, radiotherapy	Minor analgesic drugs
23	59, M	Pharynx, local invasion	Oropharynx, R neck; 5 mo, continuous	Biopsy, radiotherapy	Minor analgesic drugs
24	62, F	Tongue, local invasion (jaw)	Orofacies, neck; 5 mo, continuous	Local resection, radiotherapy	Minor analgesic drugs
25	50, F	Pharynx, local invasion	Oropharynx, neck, R hemicranium; 2 mo, intermittent	Biopsy, radiotherapy	Minor analgesic drugs, morphine syrup
26	57, M	Larynx, local invasion	Neck, face, occipital area; 7 mo, continuous	Local resection, radiotherapy	Minor analgesic drugs
27	52, M	Tongue, local invasion	Orofacies, cranium; 2 mo, intermittent	Biopsy, radiotherapy	Minor analgesic drugs
28	60, M	Oral cavity	Orofacies, L neck; 3 mo, continuous	Biopsy, radiotherapy, partial resection of the jaw	Minor analgesic drugs
29	50, M	R pulmonary apex, diffusion to brachial plexus	R neck, R arm, R chest wall; 7 mo, continuous	Biopsy, radiotherapy	Minor analgesic drugs, pentazocine daily
30	62, M	Larynx, pulmonary metastases	Orofacies, neck, occipital & thoracic areas; 9 mo, continuous	Local resection, radiotherapy, chemotherapy	Morphine syrup, minor analgesic drugs
31	54, F	C-2 body, oropharynx invasion	Craniofacies, L neck; 8 mo, continuous	Biopsy, radiotherapy	Minor analgesic drugs, pentazocine
32	64, M	Pharynx, local invasion	Cranium, oropharynx, L neck; 9 mo, continuous	Local resection, radiotherapy	Minor analgesic drugs
33	51, F	skin, multiple bone/subcutaneous metastases	Generalized; 5 mo, continuous	Local resection, radiotherapy, chemotherapy	Minor analgesic drugs, epidural morphine
34	56, M	Bronchia, metastases to C-4, C-5 bodies	Occipital, cervical, thoracic areas; 6 mo, continuous	Biopsy, radiotherapy, laser therapy	Pentazocine daily, morphine syrup
35	59, M	L maxillary sinus, local invasion	L orofacial, cervical, occipital areas; 11 mo, continuous	Biopsy, radiotherapy	Minor analgesic drugs, L thermorhizotomy
36	70, M	Pharynx, local invasion	Oropharynx, R neck; 9 mo, continuous	Local resection, radiotherapy, chemotherapy	Minor analgesic drugs, pentazocine
37	67, M	R parotid, local invasion	R orofacies, neck; 9 mo, continuous	Biopsy, radiotherapy	Minor analgesic drugs
38	65, M	Larynx, local invasion	Oropharynx, R neck; 11 mo, intermittent	Biopsy, radiotherapy	Minor analgesic drugs

Table 94-1 (continued)

Case	Age, Sex	Etiology of Pain, Site of Tumor	Distribution, Duration of Pain	Previous Cancer-specific Treatment	Previous Analgesic Treatment
39	69, M	Pharynx, local invasion	Cranium, oropharynx, neck 3 mo, continuous	Surgical resection, radiotherapy, chemotherapy	Minor analgesic drugs, bruprenorphine
40	66, M	Pharynx, local invasion	Orofacies, neck 4 mo, continuous	Surgical resection, radiotherapy	Minor analgesic drugs, pentazocine
41	34, M	Thyroid, C2 body metastasis	Oropharynx, neck, 1 mo, intermittent	Biopsy, radiotherapy	Minor analgesic drugs, buprenorphine
42	56, M	Pharynx, local invasion	Oropharynx, neck 4 mo, continuous	Biopsy, radiotherapy	Minor analgesic drugs, pentazocine
43	46, M	Rectum cancer, R lung bone metastases	R thorax, L shoulder, neck, occiput, 12 mo, continuous	Surgical resection, radiotherapy	Minor analgesic drugs, buprenorphine
44	56, M	Prostate gland, multiple bone metastases	Generalized, cranium, orofacies 7 mo, intermittent	Biopsy, chemotherapy	Minor analgesic drugs, pentazocine
45	59, M	Tongue, local invasion	Neck, orofacies, occiput, 3 mo, intermittent	Biopsy, radiotherapy, chemotherapy	Minor analgesic drugs
46	53, M	Pharynx, local invasion	Orofacies, cranium, L neck 3 mo, continuous	Radiotherapy, biopsy, chemotherapy	Minor analgesic drugs
47	64, M	Tongue, local invasion	Occiput, R neck, orofacies, 10 mo, continuous	Surgical resection, radiotherapy	Minor analgesic drugs
48	58, M	Larynx, local invasion, diffusion to R brachial plexus	Neck, R arm polyrhizopathy, 3 mo, continuous	Surgical resection, radiotherapy, chemotherapy	Minor analgesic drugs, buprenorphine
49	57, M	Tongue, local invasion	Orofacies, neck, 3 mo, continuous	Surgical resection, radiotherapy	Minor analgesic drugs
50	61, M	Tongue, local invasion	Orofacies, R neck, 2 mo, continuous	Surgical resection, radiotherapy	Minor analgesic drugs, buprenorphine

Table 94-2. Results of intraventricular morphine in neoplastic patients

Case	Intraventricular Morphine (mg/hr)		Duration of Treatment (d)	Analgesia		Final Evaluation	Side Effects	Notes during Treatment
	Initial dose	Final dose		Onset (min)	Quality			
1	1/24	1/24	32	10–15	Excellent	Excellent	None	No pharmacological association
2	1/48	1/48	29	10–15	Good	Excellent	None	Minor analgesic drugs occasionally
3	1/48	1 + 1/24	274	5–10	Excellent	Excellent	Somnolence initially	Oral feeding; body weight increase social life almost normalized; death without anguish
4	1/24	1.5/24	39	10–15	Excellent	Excellent	Constipation initially	Lucid mind, euphoria, no knowledge of imminent death
5	1/24	1/24	26	10–20	Good	Good	Emesis	Minor analgesic drugs occasionally
6	1/24	1/24	47	10–15	Excellent	Excellent	Emesis, itching	Only antiemetic drug
7	1/24	1 + 1/24	45	30	Poor	Poor	None	Treatment completely ineffective; previous alcohol neuroadenolysis
8	0.5/24	1.5/24	93	5–10	Excellent	Excellent	Emesis occasionally	Lucid mind, quiet, participation in social life; death without anguish
9	1/48	1.5/24	99	10–15	Excellent	Excellent	Emesis, itching initially	Quiet, euphoria, partial participation in social life
10	1/48	1/24	49	10–15	Excellent	Good	None	Pentazocine occasionally
11	0.5/24	1/24	67	5–10	Excellent	Excellent	Respiratory depression during the 3rd dosing, reversed by naloxone	3rd dosing wrongly overdosed
12	1/24	1/24	24	10–15	Good	Good	Disorientation, confusion	General condition very bad
13	0.5/24	1/24	47	5–10	Excellent	Excellent	None	Lucid mind, quiet, reasonable self-sufficiency
14	0.5/24	1/24	21	10–15	Excellent	Excellent	None	Quiet, oral feeding resumed
15	0.5/24	1/24	292	5–10	Excellent	Excellent	Urinary retention initially, dizziness	Treatment interrupted after 5 doses weekly treatment for 2 mo; then1 mg/24 hr
16	1/24	1/24	5	10–15	Good	Poor	None	General condition very bad
17	1/24	0.5 + 0.5/24	29	20–25	Good	Good	Emesis	Pentazocine
18	0.5/24	1/24	104	5–10	Excellent	Excellent	None	Pentazocine abstinence initially; then quiet, euphoria until death without anguish
19	0.5/24	1/24	4	15–20	Good	Good	Emesis, somnolence	Stupor, general condition very bad
20	0.5/24	1/24	195	5–10	Excellent	Excellent	Emesis for 2 d	Lucid mind, quiet, social life almost normalized; death without anguish

Table 94-2 (continued)

Case	Intraventricular Morphine (mg/hr)		Duration of Treatment (d)	Analgesia		Final Evaluation	Side Effects	Notes during Treatment
	Initial dose	Final dose		Onset (min)	Quality			
21	0.5/24	0.5/24	238	5–10	Excellent	Excellent	None	After the 1st dose, analgesia for 2 mo; then treatment on request
22	0.5/24	1/24	249	5–10	Excellent	Excellent	Emesis initially	Lucid mind, quiet; death without anguish
23	1/24	1/24	16	15–20	Good	Good	Disorientation, stupor	General condition very bad
24	0.5/24	1/24	31	10–15	Excellent	Excellent	None	Lucid mind, quiet; death without anguish
25	1/24	1/24	25	15–20	Good	Good	None	Death without anguish
26	0.5/24	0.5/24	34	15–30	Good	Good	Disorientation, confusion	Late treatment; condition very bad
27	0.5/24	1 + 1/24	217	5–10	Excellent	Excellent	None	Lucid mind, quiet, euphoria occasionally, death without anguish
28	1/24	1/24	85	5–10	Excellent	Excellent	None	Quiet, pain-free until last 3 d
29	0.5/24	0.5/24	23	15–20	Excellent	Good	Somnolence, confusion	Pentazocine; death from transtentorial hernia due to occipital metastases
30	0.5/24	1 + 1/24	89	5–10	Excellent	Excellent	Itching initially	Lucid mind, quiet; death without anguish
31	0.5/24	0.5/24	19	15–20	Excellent	Good	emesis initially, somnolence, disorientation	Late treatment; condition very bad

32	0.5/24	1/24	47	10–15	Good	Good	Emesis initially	Trigeminal hyperalgic anesthesia after thermorhizotomy; tricyclic drugs
33	0.5/24	1 + 1/24	24	10–15	Excellent	Good	Constipation	Lucid mind, pain-free, but anguish
34	0.5/24	0.5/24	19	5–10	Excellent	Excellent	None	Lucid mind, quiet; sudden death while sleeping
35	0.5/24	0.5/24	137	5–10	Excellent	Excellent	None	Social life almost normalized. Pain-free until the death
36	0.5/24	0.5/24	56	5–10	Excellent	Excellent	Constipation	Oral feeding, quiet, lucid mind. Death without anguish
37	0.5/24	0.5/24	67	5–10	Excellent	Excellent	None	Social life almost normalized. Lucid mind.
38	0.5/24	0.5/24	35	5–10	Excellent	Excellent	None	Quiet, lucid mind. Pain free.
39	0.5/24	1/24	97	5–10	Excellent	Excellent	None	Quiet, pain-free until death
40	0.25/24	0.5/24	13	10–15	Good	Good	Somnolence	General condition very bad
41	0.5/24	0.5/24	79	5–10	Excellent	Excellent	None	Lucid mind, death without anguish
42	0.25/24	0.5/24	25	10	Good	Good	Sedation, somnolence	Pain-free until death
43	0.25/24	1/24	76	5–10	Excellent	Excellent	Nausea, vomiting	Quiet, pain-free
44	0.25/24	—	—	5	Excellent	—	Constipation	Follow-up note possible
45	0.25/24	0.5/24	27	10	Excellent	Excellent	Sedation	Quiet, death without anguish
46	0.25/24	—	—	10	Good	—		Follow-up not possible
47	0.25/24	0.25/24	3	10	Good	Poor	Somnolence, mental, depression, anorexia	Treatment interrupted
48	0.25/24	0.5/24	43	5–10	Excellent	Excellent	None	Lucid mind, self-sufficiency until death
49	0.25/24	0.5/24	39	5–10	Excellent	Excellent	Sedation	Pain-free, death without anguish
50	0.25/24	0.25/24	27	10–15	Good	Good	None	Lucid mind, liveliness

alcohol hypophysectomy had been performed previously to relieve pain.

In 7 cases (12, 16, 19, 23, 26, 31, and 40), treatment was performed at an advanced stage, when the patients' general condition was poor, analgesia ineffective, and mentation impaired, thereby making evaluation of the therapy impossible.

Two subjects (15 and 21), after the first dosages, had long periods of excellent analgesia. When their pain recurred, it was easily controlled by the infrequent administration of intraventricular morphine.

The most frequent side effects encountered are vomiting and itching at the beginning of the treatment; constipation appears occasionally. Loss of orientation and mental confusion are characteristically encountered among patients who underwent late operation. We believe that their mental activities were impaired by this treatment. In one patient (case 43), treatment was interrupted after 3 days because of side effects (drowsiness, anorexia, moodiness) becoming intolerable.

One patient (case 11) experienced respiratory depression due to overdosage, but this was controlled promptly with naloxone.[6,10,14] In three patients (cases 46, 48, and 49), follow-up was impossible.

The best results were observed in those patients whose presumptive survival time and general condition were good, and who had never been treated with opioids or major analgesic drugs. Many subjects could renew their social lives and sometimes return to manual and intellectual jobs; moreover, those in whom therapy was most efficacious died without anguish.

DISCUSSION

Our experience shows that neoplastic pain of the cervical and craniofacial regions can be efficaciously controlled with microdoses of morphine injected in the ventricular fluid. In our opinion, this therapy represents a considerable improvement in the treatment of neoplastic pain of this type. Analgesia obtained by administering microdoses of morphine intraventricularly appears quickly (within 5 to 30 minutes) and is long-lasting (24 to 48 hours) when a dose of 0.5 mg is administered. The decrease of analgesic effect over the weeks or months of treatment is managed by either adjusting the inter-dose intervals, or by increasing the daily dosage, but never exceeding a total of 2 mg/24 hours. We have not observed morphine dependence among our patients on this program. The therapeutic results are usually clearly positive or negative, and when ineffective, e.g., patient 7, the administration of doses of 2.5–5.0 mg/24 hours did not change the ineffectiveness of this form of treatment.

With treatment, the quality of life of many of our patients improved greatly, and often the patient described an absence of pain, not merely a dulling of the pain as generally happens with morphine administered by other routes. In many patients, mentation was normal for a long period, and sometimes until death. Other patients were often euphoric, a condition we believe to be due both to the excellent quality of analgesia, removing anxiety and depression, and perhaps to the release of central inhibitory mechanisms.

We consider intraventricular morphine to be a therapeutic procedure specific for neoplastic pain of the cervical and craniofacial regions. Because of the technical ease of administration, the lack of major side effects, and the high quality of pain relief, this form of treatment can be extended to patients with pain from multiple bony metastases at the cervical and craniofacial regions, because morphine administered in the spinal fluid is often without efficacy, perhaps because of its excessive dilution.

Over the past few months, we have become all the more convinced that, vis-à-vis consistently valid analgesic effects, there have been some handicaps impeding the full acceptance and success of intrathecal and intraventricular morphine therapy in microdoses as a method of pain reduction.

Recently, to further improve our results, we have chosen to match therapy with life expectancy, and, moreover, to strive for an improvement in the patient's quality of life. We can identify three subpopulations among our patients: those with a short, medium, or long life expectancy. The short-term group includes patients with a probable survival of 2 to 3 weeks. In these patients, a spinal extradural catheter is used to provide daily doses of morphine (1–3 mg) at fixed intervals. In the second group, with a probable life expectancy of 1 to 2 months, and with pain localized at the soma, a subarachnoid catheter is placed at L3-L4 or L4-L5 through a Tuohy needle (14 gauge); after tunneling, the catheter is then connected to a metal-base reservoir that is inserted subcutaneously on the anterior chest wall.

In the case of craniofacial and cervical pain involving cranial nerves V through IX and the first cervical roots unilaterally or bilaterally, an intraventricular catheter is inserted through a right frontal burr hole into the lateral ventricle. Among these patients, a relative or nurse is carefully taught to inject the subcutaneous reservoir transcutaneously. This procedure requires meticulous asepsis and skill to avoid damage to the implanted system.

Patients in the third group have a life expectancy of more than 2 months. For this group, we suggest use of a multidose manually operated pump to deliver the morphine, rather than daily repeat injections of a reservoir. The latter technique is difficult to manage over long periods, because of the risk of sepsis, risk of damage to the system, and often the need for a nurse to administer drugs.

The pump used for this purpose has a simple manual control, allows multidoses (120 therapeutic doses at a normal regime of 1 mg morphine per single administration), is easily reloaded, and last, is relatively inexpensive ($1000).

Since December 1985, in collaboration with Cordis-Europa, the Department of Neurosurgery at the University of Brescia has been using this system, which comprises a spinal catheter (76 cm) connected to a 6.5 × 1.5 cm pump weighing 44 g.

The pump includes (Figures 94-2 and 94-3) a loading system composed of a Silastic dome placed between two buttons with which to periodically supply more drugs. Below it is a unidirectional valve to avoid drug reflux from the reservoir. The reservoir is a silicone-reinforced polyester membrane fixed to the sealing ring in polysulfonate. At the time of insertion, this position below the check valve is loaded with twelve 1-centigram vials of morphine hydrochloride. In full regime, the reservoir can hold up to 12 ml of narcotic, which equals 120 mg of morphine, equal to 120 therapeutic doses. The administration technique relies on 2 buttons, which are to be pushed in sequence; the first is lateral, the second medial. The first button tranfers the desired amount of drug (e.g., 0.1 ml = 1 mg) from the reservoir to the catheter; the second, via progressive bolus, effects the actual administration of the drug into the CSF.

An incorrect maneuver, like the inversion of sequence, repeated depression of the same button, or the simultaneous depression of both buttons, will not permit proper administra-

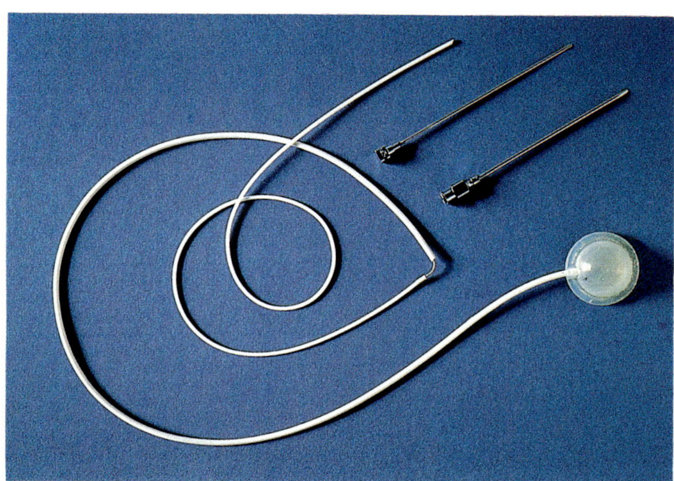

Fig. 94-1. The ventricular needle replaced with a ventricular catheter (6–8cm) and connected to a 1.5 ml reservoir (Cordis Italia, Milano Italy) is placed beneath the galea.

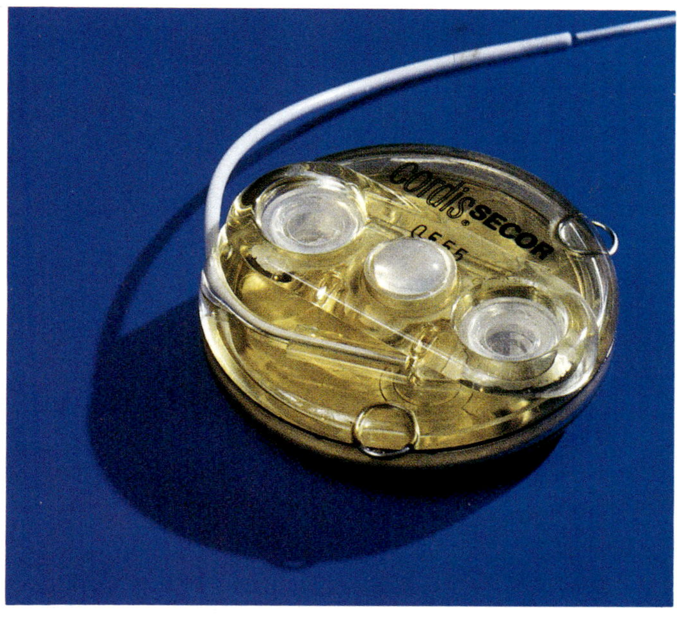

Fig. 94-2. A spiral catheter (76 cm) is connected to a 6.5 x 1.5 cm pump weighing 44 g. The pump includes a loading system composed of a Siasto dome placed between two buttons.

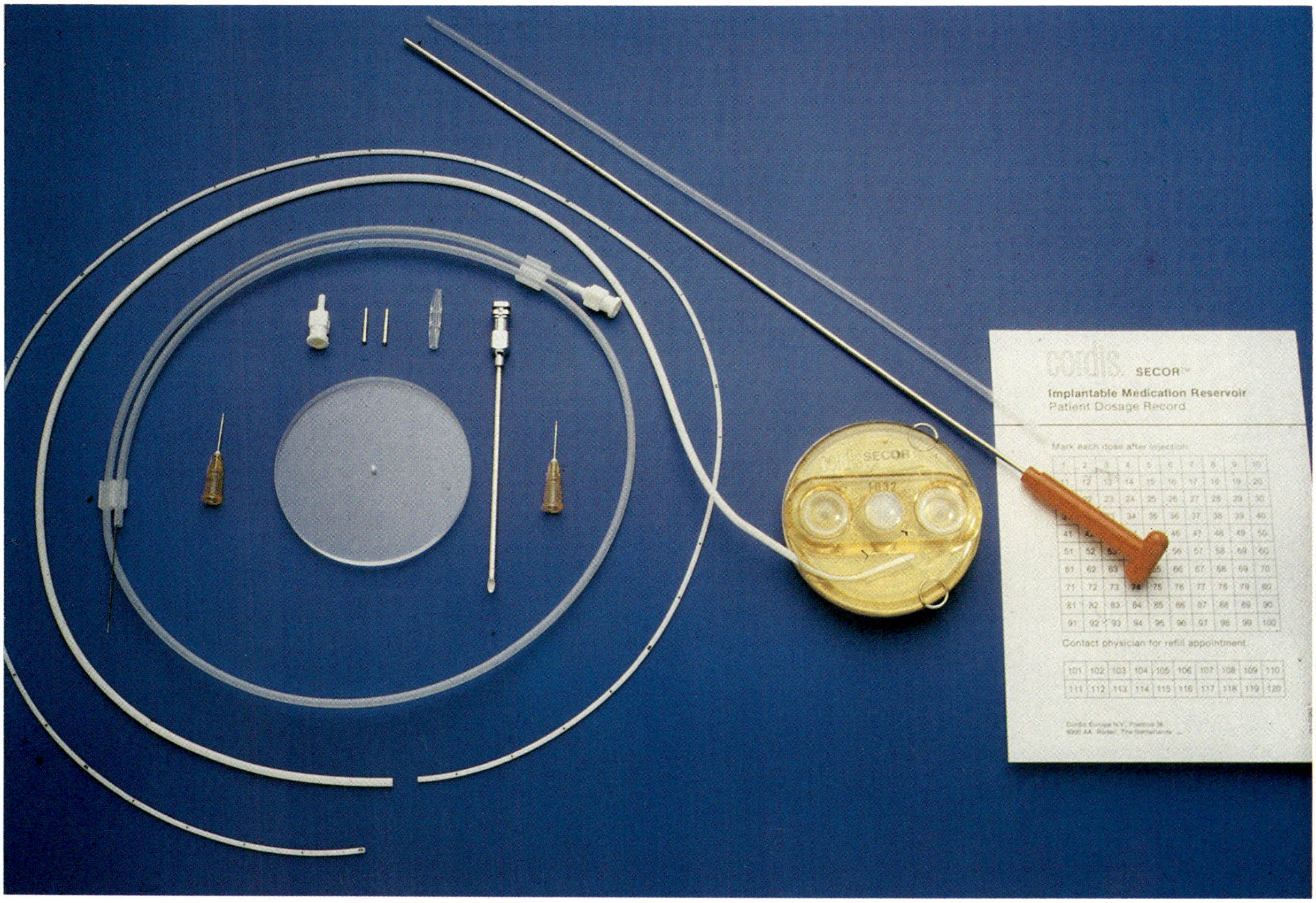

Fig. 94-3. Below the pump is a unidirectional valve that helps avoid drug reflux from the reservoir. The reservoir is a silicone-reinforced polyester membrane fixed to the sealing ring in polysulfonate.

tion because of the system's unidirectional flow arrangement. The spinal catheter (76 cm) is made of radiopaque Silastic. This material is inserted in the subarachnoid space at L3-L4 or L4-L5 through a Tuohy needle (14 gauge). The catheter is connected to the pump and is inserted subcutaneously on the anterior chest wall.

In the case of ventricular morphine therapy using a Secor pump, we suggest placement of the pump just below the clavicle.

CLINICAL MATERIAL

To date, we have used this system in 8 cases, and are impressed by the safety, simple use, and reliability of this pump. We have not encountered drug overdosage, incorrect administration, breakdown of parts or system failure, or skin breakdown or CSF infection.

The first patient in whom we used this system had a rectal cancer with local recurrence and involvement of the sacrum. The system was implanted December 12, 1985, and has been operating continously for the last 9 months. The pump was reloaded 4 times. The initial dose was 1 mg morphine per day. From the third month onward, dosage was increased to 2 mg morphine/day. Analgesia, which initially was reported as being 100 percent, now remains at more than 80 percent. The patient is attentive, can walk around the house, takes walks in the garden, and cares for himself to a limited extent.

The second patient, a 75-year-old man with prostatic cancer and multiple bony metastases to the lumbar dorsal spine and the pelvis, and with metastases to both lungs and multiple costal fractures, had a system implanted February 27, 1986. Seven months later, the patient, although bedridden, was pain-free. The pump has been reloaded 3 times since its insertion.

The third patient, a 56-year-old man, has a plastocytoma involving C5, L5, the right shoulder, right tibia, pelvis, and sternum. A system that was implanted August 11, 1986 provided total pain relief during the first several weeks following its usage, but now is judged as providing relief of 80 percent of his pain.

The fourth patient, a 44-year-old man with carcinoma of the pancreas and liver metastases, had a system implanted June 28, 1986. The pump was reloaded on September 13, 1986. The patient even came personally to the hospital for supplies. He is pain-free on 2 mg morphine/day, even though severely cachectic (weight 43 kg) and intensely icteric.

CONCLUSIONS

The manually controlled pump we have been using allows relatively easy administration of drugs into the CSF, optimal analgesic effect (since one can vary both dosage and frequency of administration), reduced side effects (a result achieved by using microdoses of morphine), and a reduced risk of infection compared with systems requiring transcutaneous injection. The need to sequentially depress the 2 buttons (lateral and medial) for drug administration makes the presence of a professional nurse unnecessary, yet is somewhat complicated for the patient to handle alone, so that another person is present when the drug is given, thus avoiding the risk of intentional overdosage.

REFERENCES

1. Cannon WB: The James Lange theory of emotion. Am J Psychol 39:106, 1927
2. De Wied D: Hormonal influence on motivation learning and memory processes. Hosp Pract 11:123, 1976
3. Lazarus RS, Averill JR, Opton EM: Toward a cognitive theory of emotion, in Arnold M (ed): Feeling and Emotions. New York, Academic Press, 1970
4. Pancheri P, Biondi M: Psicologia e Psicosomatica dei Tumori. Rome, La Goliardica, 1979
5. Reich W: La Biopatia del Cancro. Milan, Sugar Co., 1976
6. Scarpa A: Etnomedicina. Milan, Lucisano, 1980
7. Selye H: Stress. Torino, Einaudi, 1957
8. Gianasi GC, Caruso GC: Dolore e psiche, psiche e cancro. Algos 2:46, 1985
9. Pert CB, Snyder SH: Opiate receptor: Its demonstration in nervous tissue. Science 179:1011, 1973
10. Terenius L: Endogenous peptides and analgesia. Ann Rev Pharmacol Toxicol 18:189, 1978
11. Lord JAH, Waterfield AA, Hughes J, et al: Endogenous opioid peptides: Multiple agonist and receptors. Nature 267:495, 1977
12. Martin WR, Eades CG, Thompson JA, et al: The effect of morphine and nalorphine-like drugs in the non dependent and morphine-dependent chronic spinal dog. J Pharmacol Exp Ther 197:517, 1976
13. Wood PL: Multiple opiate receptors: Support for unique mu, delta and kappa sites. Neuropharmacology 21:487, 1982
14. Brunello M, Volterra A, Di Giulio AM, et al: Modulation of opioid system in C57 mice after repeated treatment with morphine and naloxone: Biochemical and behavioral correlates. Life Sci 34:1669, 1984
15. Hughes J, Smith TW, Kosterlitz HW, et al: Identification of two related pentapeptides from the brain with potent opiate agonist activity. Nature 258:577, 1975
16. Chavkin C, Goldstein A: Demonstration of a specific dynorphin receptor in guinea-pig ileum myenteric plexus. Nature 291:591, 1981
17. Volterra A, Brunello N, Racagni G: Recettori degli oppiacei e peptidi oppioidi endogeni. Algos 2:23, 1985
18. Chavkin C, James IF, Goldstein A: Dynorphin is a specific endogenous ligand for the k-opioid receptor. Science 215:413, 1982
19. Wards SJ, Portoghese PS, Takemori AE: Improved assays for the assessment of k- and delta-properties of opiate ligands. Eur J Pharmacol 80:351, 1982
20. Imura H, Nakai Y, Nakao K, et al: Biosynthesis and distribution of opioid peptides. J Endocrinol Invest 6:139, 1983
21. Panerai AE: Sistemi peptidergici nella modulazione del dolore. Algos 3:50, 1986
22. Hokfelt T, Johansson O, Lijungdahl A, et al: Peptidergic neurones. Nature 284:515, 1980
23. Boerner U, Abbott S, Roe RL: The metabolism of morphine and heroin in man. Drug Metabol Rev 4:39, 1975
24. Wikler A: Sites and mechanism of action of morphine and related drugs in the central nervous system. Pharmacol Rev 2:435, 1950
25. Van Ree JM: Multiple brain sites involved in morphine antinociception. J Pharm Pharmacol 29:765, 1977
26. Davies GK, Tolhurst-Cleaver CL, James TL: CNS depression from intrathecal morphine (letter). Anesthesiology 52:280, 1980
27. Glynn CJ, Mther LE, Cousin MJ: Spinal narcotics and respiratory depression. Lancet 2:356, 1979
28. Boas RA: Hazards of epidural morphine. Anesthetist 2:3, 1977
29. Davies GK, Tolhurst-Cleaver CL, James TL: Respiratory depression after intrathecal narcotics. Anaesthesia 35:180, 1980
30. Lazorthes Y, Gouarderes C, Verdie GC, et al: Analgesie par injection intrathecale de morphine. Neurochirurgie 26:159, 1980
31. Pilon RN, Baker AR: Chronic pain control by means of an epidural catheter. Cancer 37:903, 1976
32. Leavens ME, Hill CS Jr, Cech DA, et al: Intrathecal and intraventricular morphine for pain in cancer patients: Initial study. J Neurosurg 56:241, 1982

CHAPTER 95
Analgesia Induced by Brain Stimulation with Chronically Implanted Electrodes

Yoshio Hosobuchi

OVER THE PAST DECADE electrical stimulation has been applied in two subcortical sites to produce analgesia in humans. First, the somatosensory areas—the medial lemniscus, the sensory nuclei of the thalamus (the posterior ventralis medialis and lateralis; PVM and PVL, respectively), and the posterior limb of the internal capsule—were stimulated for the control of deafferentation pain.[1] The periaqueductal and periventricular gray matter (PAG and PVG, respectively) then were selected as the stimulation site for pain originating from peripheral noxious stimuli.[2]

The focus of this discussion is on PAG stimulation and thalamic stimulation. The following sections describe the selection of patients for the electrical stimulation procedure, the electrode implantation technique, and the final coupling of the brain electrode to a radiofrequency receiver unit after an appropriate trial of various permutations of the electrode contacts is made to achieve successful pain control.

PATIENT SELECTION

Patients who are experiencing severe and chronic intractable pain that cannot be controlled by medication, including opiates in large doses, may be considered candidates for the electrical stimulation procedure. Patients with deafferentation pain respond best to stimulation of the thalamic region, whereas those with pain of peripheral origin are candidates for stimulation of the PAG. Patients suffering from pain secondary to cancer, however, generally are poor candidates for PAG stimulation, since the efficacy of this stimulation depends greatly upon the nutritional status of the patient.

Over the past 5 years, I have used a morphine test: (1) to differentiate patients with pain of peripheral origin from those with deafferentation pain; and (2) to determine the presence or absence of tolerance to opiates in patients being considered for electrical stimulation of deep brain structures.[3] Making these distinctions accurately is critical for the success of subcortical stimulation for pain control, because: (1) deafferentation pain that is not responsive to opiates responds better to thalamic stimulation than to PAG stimulation, and (2) patients who have developed tolerance to the analgesic effect of opiates manifest cross-tolerance to the analgesic effect of PAG stimulation.[3] Unless this tolerance is reversed before further therapy is attempted, PAG stimulation will not provide satisfactory pain control.

MORPHINE TEST

The analgesic efficacy of opiates in the individual patient is tested in the following way: Opiate analgesics are withheld for 12 hours before the test. During the testing period, the patient lies recumbent in a hospital bed. Base-line respiration, pulse rates, and blood pressure measurements are made before testing begins and are carefully monitored from the beginning of the test until at least 2 hours afterward.

A base-line assessment of the pain level is made by the patient using a subjective visual analogue scale of 0 (no pain) to 10 (maximum pain). Morphine sulfate (up to 30 mg intravenously) is administered in divided doses over a period of 35 to 45 minutes. Administration is done in a double-blind manner; the placebo is normal saline. At intervals of 5 to 10 minutes after the first injection of morphine, the degree of pain relief is assessed by the patient using the visual analogue scale. If the patient is suffering from chronic low-back pain, his or her ability to endure straight-leg raising can be used concurrently as an objective measurement of pain relief (Figure 95-1).

After reporting relief of pain from the morphine, or after having received 30 mg of morphine, the patient is given naloxone, an opiate antagonist. If the effect of the morphine is reversed when naloxone is administered, the probability of successfully providing analgesia by PAG stimulation is high, since the analgesia induced by PAG stimulation also is reversible with naloxone. Generally, the patient suffering from deafferentation pain caused by a neuronal lesion proximal to dorsal root ganglia either experiences no relief from 30 mg of morphine or the relief mainly is due to the euphoric effect of the morphine and is not dose-dependent; it therefore requires a considerably high intravenous dose of naloxone to reverse the pain relief induced. In contrast, if the source of the patient's pain lies distal to the dorsal root ganglia (examples would include some types of deafferentation pain, such as peripheral neuropathy), then the degree of pain relief reported by the patient will reflect a more or less dose-dependent correlation with the amount of morphine administered. In this case, the analgesic effect of morphine is always reversed by a small dose of naloxone (less than 1 mg) (Figure 95-2). If the patient undergoing the morphine test has developed tolerance to the analgesic effect of morphine, the relief from pain is partial, though it is generally dose-dependent (Figure 95-2). Tolerance at such a stage often can be reversed by the administration of oral loading doses of the

OPERATIVE NEUROSURGICAL TECHNIQUES
ISBN 0-8089-1862-1

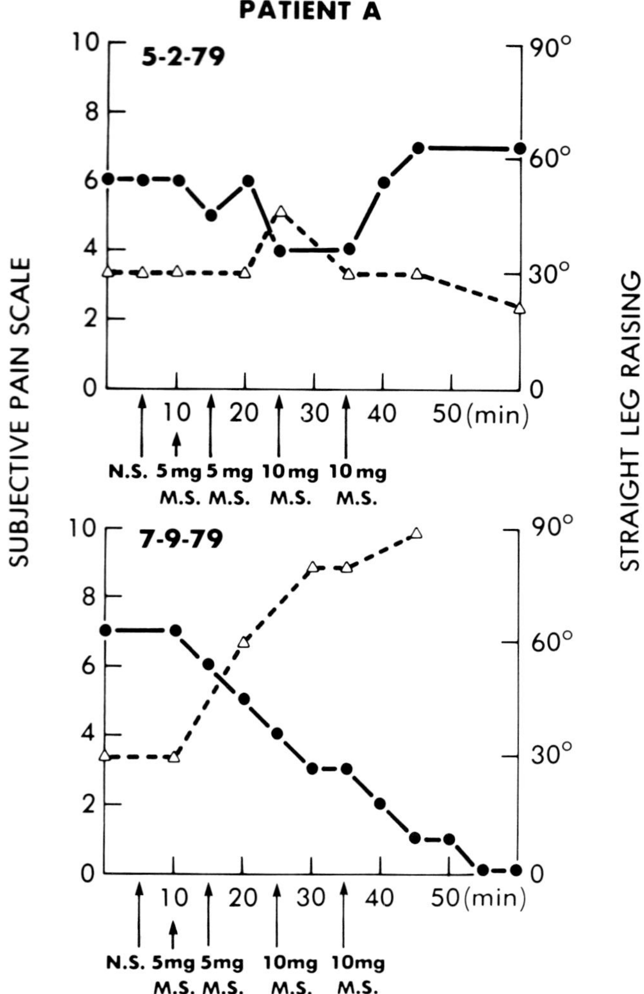

Fig. 95-1. A graph of the reactions of a patient with chronic pain to 30 mg of morphine sulfate administered in intravenous boluses over 35 minutes. The first test (upper) represents the presumed opiate-tolerant state; the later test (lower) shows the effect of tolerance reversal after several weeks of dietary loading with L-tryptophan. The abscissas represent time in minutes (N.S. = placebo bolus of normal saline; M.S. = bolus of morphine sulfate); on the ordinates are represented the patient's subjective evaluation of pain on a scale of 0 to 10 (left) (O--O) and the patient's tolerance of straight-leg raising in degrees from the horizontal (right) (A--A). (Reprinted from Hosobuchi Y, Lamb S, Baskin D: Tryptophan loading may reverse tolerance to opiate analgesics in humans: A preliminary report. Pain 9:161–169, 1980. With permission.)

serotonin precursor, L-tryptophan (4 g daily) over a period of a few weeks (see Figure 95-1).

Defining the tolerance of a patient to the analgesic action of opiates on the basis of responses to an intravenous 30-mg dosage of morphine is arbitrary; if a higher dose is given to these opiate-tolerant individuals, they may continue to have relief from pain. Nevertheless, if the patient shows only partial pain relief with 30 mg of morphine given intravenously within the duration of 30 to 45 minutes (that is to say, if the analgesic response is not reduced beyond the level of 3 on the visual analogue scale), withholding surgery for electrode implantation is advised until this tolerance is reversed by loading doses of L-tryptophan. After taking L-tryptophan (4 g daily) for a period of 2 to 6 weeks, patients usually report increasing analgesic efficacy of the opiate, and their demand for opiate analgesics decreases.

An obvious pitfall of the morphine test is that the pain may arise from mixed lesions (e.g., a chronic low-back problem concurrent with arachnoiditis and radiculopathy). In such circumstances, a second morphine test made after the period of L-tryptophan loading can differentiate between the components of the pain (e.g., patients may experience total relief from the back pain, but none or only partial relief from a burning pain in the legs or feet).

IMPLANTATION OF THE ELECTRODES

The electrode that currently is available commercially is made of pure platinum. It consists of four wires that are entwined, terminating with the individual wires separated from one another to form four 1-mm-long loops (0.8 mm in diameter). These constitute four separate contact points. They are 2 mm apart, as measured from the midpoint of each contact. The electrode contact points are labeled 0, 1, 2, and 3 by the manufacturer; 0 is the most inferior contact point. The loop of the most inferior contact (0) facilitates the insertion of the electrode into the central gray matter by encircling the tip of the special tool that is used to insert the electrode into the brain.

The implantation of the electrode is accomplished by means of a stereotactic neurosurgical procedure. Local scalp anesthesia is used. A standard stereotactic apparatus (such as the Leksell, Riechert-Mundinger, or Todd-Wells apparatuses) serves satisfactorily for this operation, although I prefer to use the Leksell apparatus.

The patient is placed in the semi-sitting position on a specially designed operating table. The head is shaved, washed with Betadine soap and water, and painted with Betadine solution. The head rests on a small suboccipital cup support. First, the stereotactic head frame is positioned and supported using calibrated ear plugs, and the midline of the apparatus (Z axis) is carefully approximated to the midsagittal plane of the head. Three entry zones on the scalp are selected for the placement of three skull pins that will be screwed into the outer table of the skull. These scalp areas are generously infiltrated with local anesthetic. The hole for the anterior skull pin is placed just behind the hairline of the forehead (for naturally bald patients. this site is approximated as closely as possible). The other two sites are positioned approximately 4 cm behind each external auditory meatus. A guiding tube that pierces the scalp is inserted at each of these three sites, and is firmly fixed to the pericranium. Then, a skull pin is inserted into each of the three guiding tubes and is screwed into the outer table of the skull using a special drill.

The surgeon must, at this point, make sure that the frame is firmly fixed to the patient's skull. The head and frame then are partially draped, leaving the patient's face exposed. The location for two separate scalp incisions are marked so as to bisect the coronal suture on each side, 2.5 cm from the midline, and the scalp is infiltrated with local anesthetic. Bilateral, paramedian, pericoronal burr holes are made 1 cm anterior to the coronal sutures and 2.5 cm from the midline. It is critical that the burr holes be made in precisely this location. (In the case of brachycephalic or dolichocephalic patients, the burr holes are moved in either an anterior or posterior direction so that the line connecting the burr holes to the posterior commissure will form an angle of 60 to 70 degrees to the intercommissural line.) Since the target points in either the PAG or the sensory thalamic nuclei are located within 5 mm of the X and Y

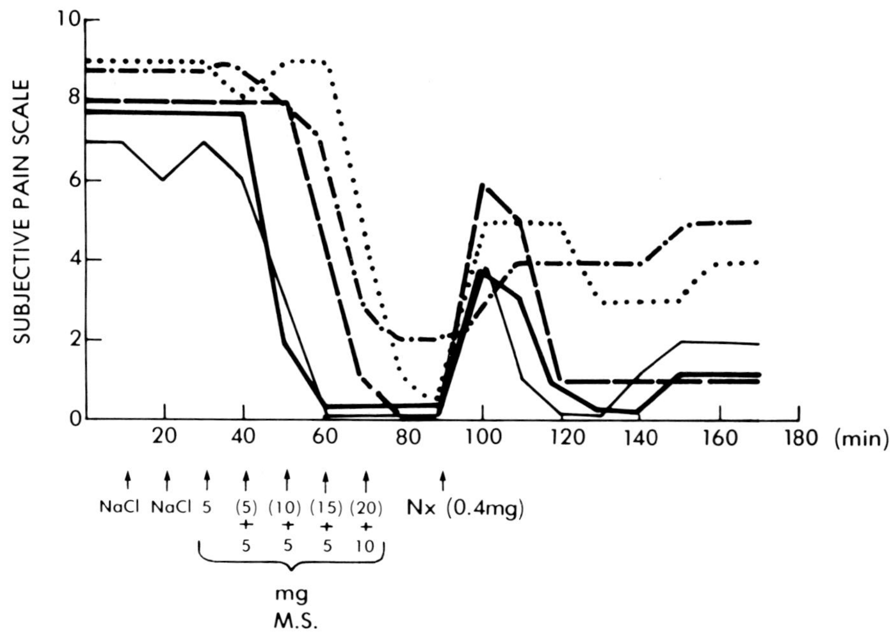

Fig. 95-2. A graph of the analgesic response of 5 patients with chronic pain from arachnoiditis to 30 mg of morphine sulfate administered in intravenous boluses over 70 minutes, followed at 90 minutes by an intravenous bolus of the opiate antagonist naloxone. The abscissa represents time in minutes (NaCl = placebo bolus of normal saline; M.S. = bolus of morphine sulfate; Nx = naloxone); on the ordinate are represented the patients' subjective evaluation of pain on a scale of 0 to 10.

axis (the anteroposterior (AP) axis and ventrodorsal axis), this trajectory offers the maximum probability of the electrode contact points being placed in the region that will produce therapeutically effective stimulation.

After the burr holes are appropriately placed, the dura of the right burr hole is opened in cruciate fashion and is coagulated. The cortical surface is inspected carefully so that a major sulcus is not encountered in the trajectory. The surface of a gyrus is cauterized, a small cortical incision is made using a No. 15 blade, and the right lateral ventricle is cannulated with a Scott cannula. The tip of the cannula is aimed toward the contralateral angle of the mandible so that the catheter can be advanced to the third ventricle through the foramen of Monro. At this time 2 ml of air is introduced into the ventricle, and x-ray films (AP and lateral views) are obtained to verify the location of the catheter. If necessary, the catheter positioning and x-ray exposure factors are corrected. Ventriculograms then are obtained in the AP and lateral projections using 3 ml of Conray contrast medium mixed with 7 ml of ventricular cerebrospinal fluid (CSF). These ventriculograms should delineate the foramen of Monro, the third ventricle, and the anterior and posterior commissures.

In my opinion the use of the computed tomography (CT) scan in combination with the stereotactic apparatus for the electrode implantation procedure is unjustifiable, not only because of the expense of the CT scanning process, but more importantly because CT scanning cannot provide the surgeon with information sufficient for accurately determining the site of implantation of the electrode.

TARGET

Periaqueductal gray or periventricuiar gray. For X and Y coordinates, the iter of the aqueduct is selected (Figure 95-3). The laterality of the Z coordinate is therefore not influenced by

the width of the third ventricle, as the target is caudal to this structure. The shape of the aqueduct is oblong in the ventral and dorsal axis at the iter, and the laterality of the target is determined by the ventral-dorsal diameter of the aqueduct at the iter, which is almost always less than 2 mm. Consequently, in most cases, the target laterality (Z coordinate) is 3 mm from the midline for the insertion tool. Since the electrode is always inserted in a position lateral to the insertion tool, the tip of the electrode usually lies 2.5 to 3.5 mm lateral from the midline of the iter of the aqueduct. The target point is marked on the ventriculogram; this point is projected perpendicularly to the reference scale of the frame, and the X, Y, and Z coordinates are calculated.

Implantation may be performed either unilaterally or bilaterally, although in my experience better analgesia is produced (by a 9 to 1 ratio) when the electrode is implanted in the left, rather than the right, PAG. Since there is no way to determine whether a patient will respond better with the electrode implanted in the left side or the right, and since bilateral implantation does not appear to produce greater morbidity, I routinely implant electrodes bilaterally to increase the chance of finding the optimal pair of contact points for stimulation that will produce the most effective analgesia.

After correct unilateral or bilateral X, Y, and Z coordinates, either unilaterally or bilaterally, for the prospective site(s) of implantation have been obtained, side bars are attached to the frame at the appropriate Y coordinate. The dura of the left burr hole is opened and the cortical surface is prepared as described earlier. The insertion tool is placed through the trajectory stage of the frame and is adjusted to ensure that the tip of the tool will hit the target point accurately. The arc is attached to the frame by clamping it to the side bar at the predetermined X and Z coordinates.

The scalp posterior to the burr holes then is infiltrated with a local anesthetic, and is penetrated with a 14-gauge needle with

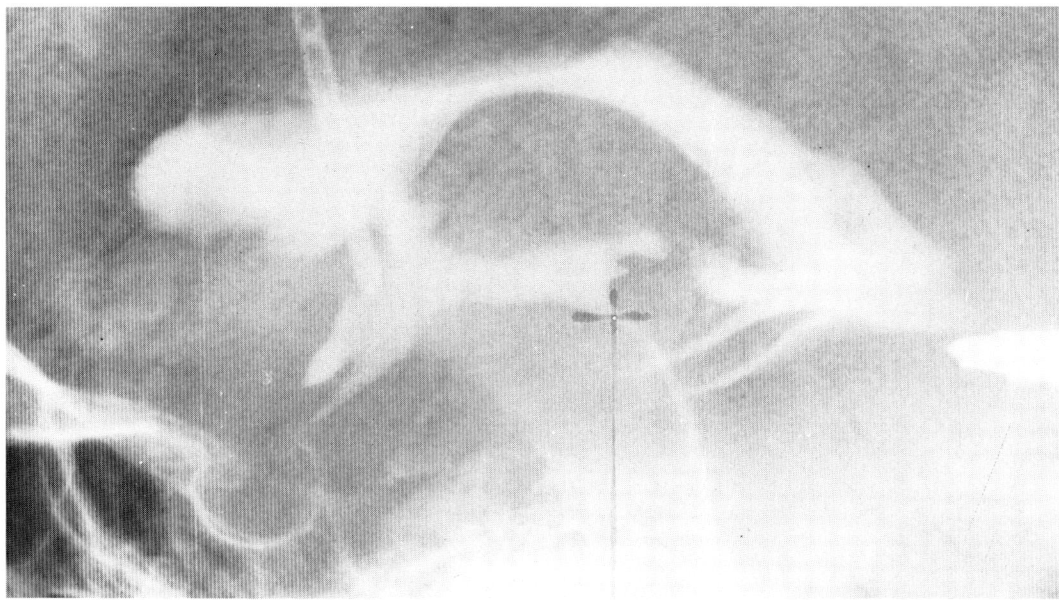

Fig. 95-3. A Conray ventriculogram, lateral view. The cross indicates the target point for the PAG electrode.

its stylet in place. The needle is inserted approximately 5 cm posterior to the burr holes and is passed subgaleally to each burr hole. The stylet then is removed from the needle. The percutaneous extension of the electrode is passed through the needle shaft from the site of the burr hole to the hub of the needle; as the extension appears from the needle hub, the needle is carefully withdrawn from the scalp. The connector of the electrode to the percutaneous extension is taped (with Steri-strips) to the self-retaining retractor on the burr-hole incision.

The electrode now is inserted. The tip of the insertion tool is placed within the terminal loop of the electrode. The electrode always should be lateral to the insertion tool to avoid unnecessary damage to the posterior medial thalamus and hypothalamus by a leukotomy-type injury created by the angle between the insertion tool and the electrode. The surgeon holds the electrode close to the insertion tool using blunt forceps, and the assistant advances the insertion tool into the brain. It is very important to avoid excessive tension of the electrode against the insertion tool because this will uncoil the second contact point, which might alter the distance between the first contact or loop to the second contact or possibly break the loop.

When the insertion tool reaches the target point, the electrode is disengaged from the tool by very gentle clockwise and counterclockwise rotation of the tool around approximately 45 degrees. Excessive and vigorous rotation of the tool should be avoided because it will dislodge the electrode from the target. The insertion tool is withdrawn from the brain. The electrode is temporarily fixed to the edge of the burr hole by a small ball of bone wax, and the burr hole is covered with a wet cotton ball.

Test stimulation is delivered between the most distant pair of contact points, using the most inferior contact point as the cathode. The settings for test stimulation are pulse duration—0.5 msec; frequency—50 Hz; and amplitude starting at 1 V and gradually increasing. At about 6 to 8 V, the patient invariably reports oscillopsia or an inability to initiate ocular movement. I have found that the suppression of conjugate upward gaze during stimulation is the most reliable physiologic determinant

to assure correct placement of the electrode. Although pain relief is effected at a much lower amplitude, I do not use a demonstration of the analgesic efficacy of PAG stimulation in the operating room as a determinant of accurate electrode placement, since, under the stress of surgery under local anesthesia, the patient may perceive the pain to be alleviated when in fact it is not.

The same procedure is repeated to implant the electrode on the right side.

After both electrodes are implanted and after electrical stimulation induces a satisfactory ocular response, the cortex is covered with Gelfoam and the electrodes are fixed to the edge of the burr holes with cranioplastic material. A subgaleal pocket is developed and the extra length of electrode connector and percutaneous extension cable are inserted into it; the wounds then are closed in two layers. The final confirmation of electrode localization usually is made at this stage; however, if the surgeon is not certain that the electrode is situated optimally (for example, if the expected ocular response is not obtained), then confirmatory x-ray films (AP and lateral views) must be made before the electrode is fixed to the burr holes by cranioplasty (Figures 95-4A and B). Correction of the electrode position can be made by removing the electrodes, re-examining the coordinates, and reinserting the electrodes. Multiple trials of electrode insertion are unquestionably inadvisable since with each trial the risk of ocular palsy or possible intracerebral or intraventricular hemorrhage is increased.

Sensory thalamic nuclei (PVM, PUL). The basic coordinates for the sensory nuclei of the thalamus are obtained from the Schaltenbrand-Bailey stereotactic atlas. The widest coronal dimension of the nuclei is approximately 10 mm posterior to the midpoint of the line joining the anterior and posterior commissures (AC-PC line). The face area of the nucleus presents medially, starting 9 to 11 mm laterally at 2 mm below the level of the AC-PC line; the arm and leg area are located further laterally, 2 to 3 mm apart. The dimensions and location of the sensory thalamic nuclei vary considerably among individuals according to the length of the AC-PC line and the width of the third ventricle.

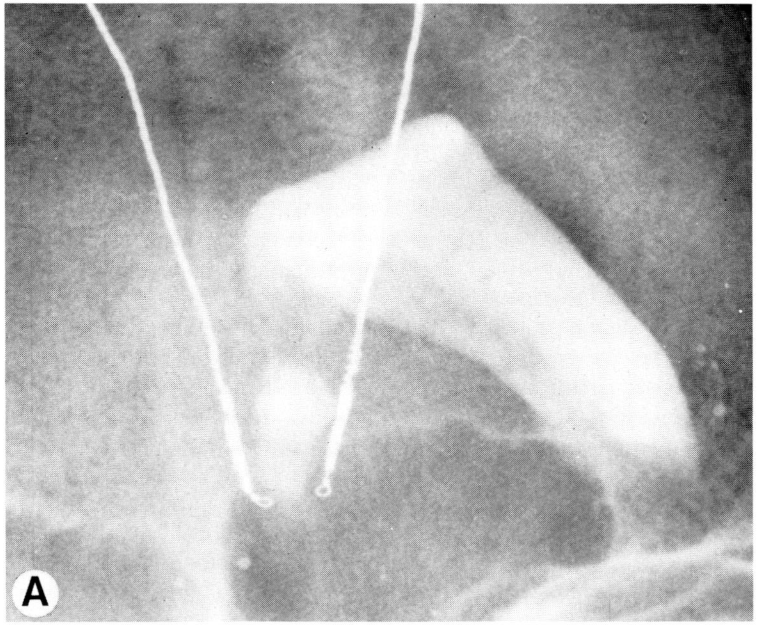

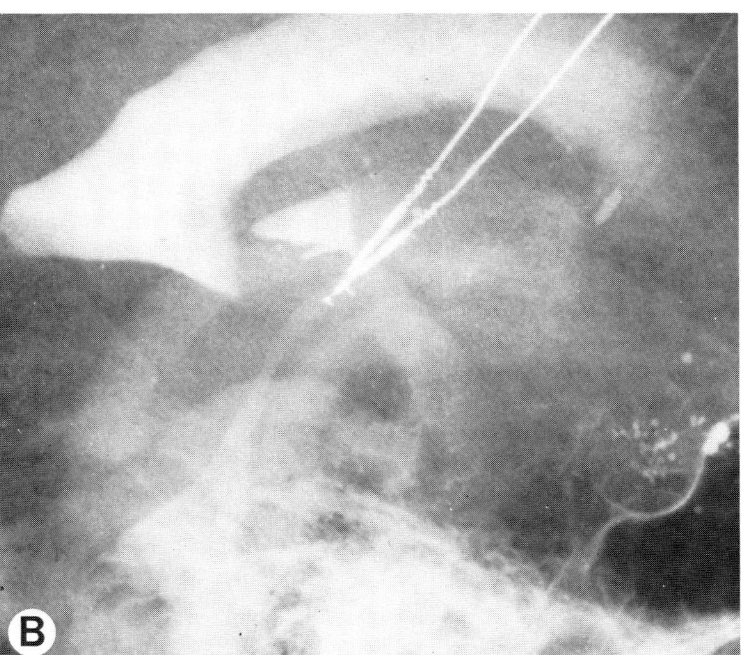

Fig. 95-4.   Bilaterally implanted PAG electrodes. Postoperative Conray ventriculograms in the (A) AP and (B) lateral views show the appropriate relationship of the electrodes to the iter of the aqueduct.

Exploratory stimulation of the target area with a monopolar electrode, 0.8 mm in diameter with a 2 to 3 mm exposed tip, is advised. The exploratory stimulation begins 5 mm proximal to the target point, extending perhaps 5 to 7 mm beyond the target point along the same trajectory.

The patient reports the area in which he experiences paresthesia in order to guide the surgeon in placing the stimulation electrode at the point where optimal induced paresthesia is obtained. In cases of deafferentation pain the most crisp response of induced paresthesia in the desired area of the body usually is obtained at the boundary of the gray and white matter or where the medial lemniscus enters the sensory nuclei; therefore, impedance monitoring also may be useful.

If induced paresthesia is not experienced in the desired area of the body, the surgeon must withdraw the monopolar electrode and replace it either medially or laterally, and often 2 to 3 mm posteriorly—especially in cases of pain in the lower extremity. It therefore is not unusual for the final coordinates of the target point to deviate 2 to 3 mm in any direction (X, Y, or Z) from the target initially calculated on the basis of the ventriculogram and the stereotactic atlas.

The insertion of the electrode follows essentially the same procedure as that described for the PAG target, except that the surgeon has to move the trajectory of the insertion tool 1 mm medially to ensure that the most inferior contact point of the permanent electrode rests in the correct target area. Placement of the electrode is reaffirmed by stimulation of the most distant pair of contacts, using the most inferior contact as the cathode. The stimulation settings of 0.5-msec pulse duration, 50- to 100–Hz frequency, and 1 to 3 V should induce pleasant paresthesia in the region of the body involved with deafferentation pain. The electrodes are fixed to the burr holes by cranioplasty, and confirmatory x-ray films (AP and lateral) are obtained. The wound is closed as described above.

POSTIMPLANTATION PATIENT CARE

After electrode implantation surgery, patients often complain of headache, nausea, and occasionally, in the case of PAG implantation, diplopia; in addition, they feel their original pain. To control the pain at this stage, the administration of a short-acting opiate analgesic, such as meperidine (Demerol) administered intramuscularly, is perferred in order to avoid masking an altered level of consciousness that would signify possible intracerebral or intraventricular hemorrhage. Dexamethasone (Decadron) rarely is used unless the patient complains of significant diplopia. Compazine is given intramuscularly to control nausea and vomiting if they occur.

On very rare occasions a patient may have a seizure 4 to 8 hours after surgery. This is thought to be a consequence of the circulation of potentially epileptogenic contrast medium (Conray) from the ventricular system out into the subarachnoid space over the convexities. Despite the relative infrequency of this complication (in about 2 percent to 3 percent of patients), it is wise to start the administration of Dilantin 24 hours before the implantation surgery. To ensure rapid washout of the Conray from the CSF, patients should be well hydrated. If the patient cannot maintain adequate oral fluid intake, intravenous fluid therapy is continued.

POSTOPERATIVE SCREENING OF THE CONTACT POINTS

Because of the usual postoperative headache and nausea, it may not be possible to start trial stimulation through the percutaneous extension for 2 to 3 days after surgery. When the patient recovers from the acute discomfort of the operation and is able to walk, screening of the various pairs of contact points begins in order to identify the most effective pair of contact points through which stimulation best relieves the original pain.

The most inferior contact point (contact point 0) should be in the optimal anatomic position. Over 80 percent of the patients find 0 to be the most effective cathode, although the anode may vary. Occasionally 1, 2, or 3, rather than 0, is the more effective cathode. The patients are provided with a polarized cable to connect the percutaneous extension to a battery-operated stimulator for self-stimulation. They then are instructed in the use of the self-stimulation device.

Patients receiving PAG stimulation are given a timer so that the duration of their self stimulation is strictly limited to 15 to 20 minutes for each session. The biphasic stimulation settings for PAG stimulation are 25–Hz frequency, 0.5–msec pulse duration, and one half of the voltage that induces apparent oscillopsia in the individual patient. (For example, if the patient reports oscillopsia starting at 8 V, then 4 V should produce pain relief without causing any other neurologic or psychologic alterations.) Stimulation should be limited to no more than 15 to 20 minutes for each session, and should be used no more frequently than every 4 to 6 hours.

In the case of patients using stimulation of the sensory nuclei of the thalamus, the stimulation settings are 0.5-msec pulse duration, 50- to 100-Hz frequency; the voltage is that at which the induced paresthesia is not unpleasantly strong. The stimulation is biphasic and must be administered in ramp fashion; the optimal duration of the ramp envelope is 20 to 30 seconds. Patients must be carefully apprised of the significance of ramp stimulation, since the stimulator occasionally may malfunction and, failing to produce ramp mode, may not produce a therapeutic effect. In such a circumstance the patient should realize that the stimulator must be readjusted.

Patients are provided with a self-assessment sheet on which to rate the efficacy of the stimulation from each particular pair of contact points. The pain is assessed on a subjective scale of 0 to 10, 0 denoting "no pain" and 10 denoting pain that the patient can barely tolerate. They are instructed to note the severity of the pain before and after brain stimulation. If stimulation does not provide adequate pain relief, or if they still have postoperative headache, they are allowed to use analgesics; but they must record the time and dosage, the reason for the need of the analgesic, and the extent of the relief obtained from the medication.

In over 90 percent of patients the efficacy of brain stimulation in controlling chronic pain becomes apparent within 7 to 10 days of their initial identification of a specific pair of contact points. In some cases, however, arriving at the optimal efficacy may require more time. When the decision is delayed, it usually is because of uncertainty about whether or not the most effective pair of contact points has been selected, or because the patient's pain is related to the type or extent of his daily activities. In such situations patients are encouraged to return home while they continue the screening process. In all cases an additional 2 to 3 weeks of trial stimulation provides an answer. While the electrodes are externalized through the percutaneous extension, it is essential that the wound through which the percutaneous extension exits is kept clean by daily swabbing with hydrogen peroxide, and that local applications of antibiotic ointment are used to prevent scalp infection. If the patient is discharged from the hospital for further screening at home, a family member is fully instructed in how to care for the wound(s).

INTERNALIZATION OF THE ELECTRODE

When the most effective pair of contact points for analgesic brain stimulation has been identified, the patient is ready for internalization of the electrode, which will be connected to a radiofrequency receiver for transcutaneous self-stimulation.

Since this surgical procedure is primarily performed subcutaneously, it is done under general anesthesia. The percutaneous extension wires from the electrodes are cut flush with the skin before skin preparation is undertaken. The head is turned to the side opposite the site where the receiver will be placed, and is supported by a horseshoe-type of headrest. Since the percutaneous extension communicates from the skin surface to the subgaleal plane, there is a potential risk of subgaleal infection. It is therefore our custom to administer tobramycin (1.5 g/kg) and vancomycin (15 mg/kg) intravenously before making a skin incision. Antibiotic therapy every 8 hours is continued for the first 48 hours postoperatively.

After draping the patient, a 5-cm transverse subclavicular incision is made, and a subcutaneous pocket is created for the radiofrequency receiver. A 3-cm incision is made over the mastoid process, and a subcutaneous tunnel is developed from this wound to the subclavicular wound using a specially designed metal bar to which a sharp, arrowheadlike tip can be attached. Care is taken to avoid perforating the apex of the lung or tearing the anterior branch of the external jugular vein. The "arrowhead" tip then is replaced with a specially designed attachment into which the ends of the extension cable from the receiver can be secured. The extension cable connector is enclosed within this device and is delivered subcutaneously into the mastoid wound. The burr hole incision is reopened and the procedure is repeated to bring the extension connector up to the burr hole wound.

The residual cables exiting from the connector nearest to the brain electrode, which previously exited percutaneously, are cut flush with the tips of the pins of this connector and are discarded. The silicone covering on the two pins to be connected is carefully stripped. The surgeon then places a protective plastic connector boot on the lead, connects the appropriate pins and tightens the connector screws, and pulls this protective boot over the entire connection. By convention, the negative pole of the conductor is identified with a white sleeve by the manufacturer. The protective boot assembly is filled with type-A silicone medical adhesive, which is provided by the manufacturer to create a water-tight seal. The three wounds are well irrigated with saline and closed in two layers. The extra lead wire is pulled through to the subclavicular end and is placed in the subcutaneous pocket with the radiofrequency receiver.

EXPECTED RESULTS AND FOLLOW-UP

Postoperatively, the patient starts self-stimulation within 2 or 3 days and is discharged from the hospital within 5 to 7 days. If the patients have been selected properly, the stereotactic placement of the electrodes is correct, and appropriate contact pairs of the electrodes have been identified after thorough testing, then the majority of patients should obtain good relief of pain from transcutaneous stimulation and should require no further use of opiate analgesics.[5] For patients who have PAG electrodes, it is of paramount importance that they receive L-tryptophan (4 g orally each day) to avoid their developing a tolerance to PAG stimulation. If a tolerance develops, the patient is instructed to refrain from stimulation for at least 2 weeks. By the end of this period, the analgesic efficacy of PAG stimulation usually has returned. Further details about the management of tolerance to stimulation is beyond the scope of this chapter; readers are referred to the previous publications cited below.[4-6]

REFERENCES

1. Hosobuchi Y, Adams JE, Rutkin B: Chronic thalamic stimulation for the control of facial anesthesia dolorosa. Arch Neurol 29:158, 1973
2. Hosobuchi Y, Adams J E, Linchitz R: Pain relief by electrical stimulation of the central gray matter in humans. Science 197:183, 1977
3. Hosobuchi Y, Lamb S, Baskin D: Tryptophan loading may reverse tolerance to opiate analgesics in humans: A preliminary report. Pain 9:161, 1980
4. Hosobuchi Y, Wemmer J: Disulfiram inhibition of development of tolerance to analgesia induced by central gray stimulation in humans. Eur J Pharmacol 43:385, 1977
5. Hosobuchi Y: Dietary supplementation with L-tryptophan reverses tolerance to analgesia induced by periaqueductal gray stimulation in humans, in Way EL (ed): Endogenous and Exogenous Opiate Agonists and Antagonists. New York, Pergamon Press, 1980, pp 375–378
6. Hosobuchi Y: Subcortical electrical stimulation for control of intractable pain in humans. Report of 122 cases (1970–1984). J Neurosurg 64:543, 1986

CHAPTER 96

Surgical Management of Disorders of the Lower Cranial Nerves

Ronald I. Apfelbaum

A NUMBER OF CLINICAL SYNDROMES have been correlated with cross compression of specific cranial nerves at their exit or entrance to the brain stem. The paradigm of these syndromes is trigeminal neuralgia or tic douloureux. Dandy first observed the frequent occurrence of arterial channels, veins, or neoplasms compressing the trigeminal nerve in the posterior fossa and wrote in 1932 that these, he believed, were the cause of tic douloureux.[1] Similarly, in the motor equivalent of this problem—hemifacial spasm—Gardner and Sava[2] described vascular compressive lesions in over half of the patients they operated upon via the posterior fossa.

It was not until Jannetta[3,4] applied the operating microscope to the systematic study of these problems, however, that the truly remarkable incidence of compression of the entry or exit zone of the brain stem root of these nerves was appreciated. In several large series, compressive lesions have been demonstrated in over 94 percent of the patients.[5–7] Furthermore, Jannetta has devised an operative technique to displace these vessels from the nerve without sacrificing neural integrity and has been successful in relieving the clinical syndrome in the vast majority of patients treated. In this chapter we will attempt to discuss the individual syndromes and the specific operative techniques that can be used in treating them.

TRIGEMINAL NEURALGIA

Trigeminal neuralgia is a condition characterized by a very stereotyped clinical syndrome. Patients suffering from this problem exhibit brief, extremely intense paroxysms of pain confined entirely to one or more divisions of the trigeminal nerve. These attacks may be triggered by light cutaneous stimuli, usually, but not exclusively, within the trigeminal territory. The pain typically is described as an electric shocklike sensation or an intense stabbing feeling. The most common areas of involvement are in the second and third divisions, usually anteriorly, in the region about the mouth. The dental area is especially prone to be the site of the symptoms, and for this reason many patients undergo unnecessary dental surgery without achieving satisfactory relief. The pain typically is most pronounced during the day and most patients will be pain-free or have markedly decreased episodes during the night. Patients will guard their face, refuse to allow it be touched, will avoid shaving, washing, applying makeup, eating, chewing, and brushing their teeth, since all of these maneuvers may provoke

the attacks. A characteristic clinical sign is often made by the patient who, in describing the pain, will rapidly fling open his hand to indicate the rapid paroxysmal nature of the jolts of pain.

Approximately 50 percent of those afflicted will respond to diphenylhydantoin (Dilantin)[8] in a dose of 300 mg/day, and up to 80 percent of the patients will obtain pain relief with Tegretol.[8,9] This medication has numerous side effects and must be administered carefully. We recommend starting Tegretol at 100 mg b.i.d. and increasing it by 100 mg every other day until pain control is achieved or toxicity develops. An average dose might be 800 mg/day in four divided doses, but some patients can tolerate, and will require, two to three times as much. Our patients are instructed to take this medication on a full stomach and to have a monthly blood count made so that hematologic toxicity can be detected. In this manner, good control of the pain can be achieved in the vast majority of patients. Surgery is reserved for those who become refractory to medical treatment or who develop side effects that necessitate discounting the medication.

We have chosen to restrict this surgery to patients who have demonstrated a typical clinical picture as outlined above. Trigeminal neuralgia is an amazingly consistent disease and a similar history will be obtained from almost every patient truly suffering from this problem. A history of sustained pain that is not paroxysmal must be questioned carefully. At times, patients will describe frequent repetitive jabs of pain as one prolonged attack. This does not preclude the diagnosis of trigeminal neuralgia. A slowly developing pain that builds in intensity, lasts for variable periods of time (often hours to days), and then subsides, however, is not characteristic of this problem. The most common mistake in diagnosis in our experience has been misdiagnosing trigeminal neuralgia for chronic cluster syndrome (Horton's cephalalgia). This and other atypical facial and trigeminal neuralgias respond much less satisfactorily to this type of surgery, and its indications in these conditions is not yet clear.

In addition to meeting the specific clinical picture, patients selected for this surgery also, we feel, should have had an adequate trial of medical therapy and the syndrome proven impossible to control. At this juncture, it is our practice to explain fully the Jannetta microvascular decompressive operation as well as the procedure for selective percutaneous lesioning of the trigeminal nerve, either with radiofrequency, thermal coagulation, or glycerol chemoneurolysis. The patient is asked to choose between these procedures after a clear explanation of

OPERATIVE NEUROSURGICAL TECHNIQUES
ISBN 0-8089-1862-1

Table 96-1. The relative benefits and risks of percutaneous trigeminal neurolysis and microvascular decompression of the trigeminal nerve for the treatment of trigeminal neuralgia

Procedure	Benefits	Risks/Drawbacks
Percutaneous trigeminal neurolysis (radiofrequency thermocoagulation or glycerol chemoneurolysis)	Safe, well tolerated despite age or infirmity Brief hospitalization Repeated easily if needed	Treats symptoms, not cause Destructive; permanently alters facial sensation Risk of corneal anesthesia Dysesthetic sequelae—at times severe (denervation hyperpathia) Increased recurrences with passage of time
Microvascular decompression	Spares the nerve; patient returned to normal No numbness No dysesthesia No corneal anesthesia Treats apparent cause; may be curative	Craniectomy required; general anesthesia required Increased risk of serious, even lethal complications Should be limited to healthy patients younger than 65 years

the relative benefits and risks of each as detailed in Table 96-1 has been made. In essence then, they are asked to decide between permanent partial alteration of facial sensation and the potential for the development of dysesthetic sequelae, corneal anesthesia, or both versus the Jannetta procedure, which offers the likelihood of pain relief without neural destruction and thus avoids dysesthetic sequelae and corneal anesthesia. They are cautioned, however, that the percutaneous lesioning is a safer procedure that avoids the risks of anesthesia and surgery. It is made clear to them that these risks include potentially fatal complications. In addition, they are made aware of the risks of injury to the underlying brain or adjacent neural structures.

In Table 96-2 we have delineated the experience with these factors in our personal series. This agrees with the published literature for the most part,[10–16] although we seem to have had a higher incidence of undesirable facial numbness and dysesthetic sequelae with radiofrequency lesioning than do some of the larger series in the literature. Our series, however, may be more representative of what one can expect if one does not perform a very large number of these procedures (i.e., more than 25 per year).

We feel that the Jannetta microvascular decompressive operation is the procedure of choice for the treatment of typical trigeminal neuralgia in an otherwise healthy patient who for the most part is less than 65 years of age. *The decision, however, must be made by the patient after he or she is fully informed about both of these procedures, since the patient, not the*

Table 96-2. Relative risks of percutaneous trigeminal neurolysis and microvascular decompression of the trigeminal nerve for the treatment of trigeminal neuralgia (complications noted in our personal series)

Procedure	Complication	Percentage of Patients Affected
Percutaneous trigeminal neurolysis:		
Radiofrequency thermocoagulation	Death	1
	Altered facial sensation	100
	Corneal hypesthesia (> mild)	18
	Corneal ulceration	2
	Dysesthesia	20
	Anesthesia dolorosa	4.5
	Cranial nerve palsies	1
	Brain abscess	1
Glycerol chemoneurolysis	Altered facial sensation	25
	Corneal hypesthesia (> mild)	8
	Dysesthesia	5
Microvascular decompression	Death	1.0
	Cerebellar hematoma	1.6
	Stroke	0.6
	Cranial nerve palsies:	
	Fourth	4.3 (all transient)
	Seventh	1.6 (most transient)
	Eighth	3.0

surgeon, is the one who ultimately accepts the risks and the possible sequelae.

PREOPERATIVE EVALUATION

Patients who elect to undergo this procedure are evaluated in the routine fashion used for any patient about to undergo general anesthesia, that is, routine hospital laboratory testing, a chest x-ray film, and an electrocardiogram are obtained and reviewed. If the patient is older than 55 years or so, or if there is any question about underlying medical problems, a complete medical evaluation also is obtained before proceeding with surgery. We obtain a computed tomographic (CT) scan with contrast augmentation before surgery to detect possibly unrecognized neoplasms or arteriovenous malformations. It has not been our practice, however, to obtain cerebral angiograms. While certainly the cerebral vessels can be delineated in this manner, the exact localization of the nerves is not determined and a difference of a few millimeters in positioning totally alters the intracranial situation. We thus feel that the information obtained by a routine angiogram is not helpful enough to warrant the small but never absent risk of angiography.

ANESTHESTIC CONSIDERATIONS

A number of varied anesthetic techniques are applicable to this type of surgery and we make no attempt to influence the anesthesiologist in the choice of agents; rather, we prefer to rely upon the anesthesiologist's experience and expertise in the selection of the agent and technique that he or she prefers to use for each individual patient. We do feel that it is necessary, however, to have the patient paralyzed and on controlled ventilation. This is done for two reasons: (1) it minimizes motion in the field, which is greatly magnified by the operating microscope, and (2) it prevents the patient from developing a gasp reflex should a small amount of air embolization occur. This reflex occurs with only a tiny entrainment of air and can rapidly result in a massive air embolism.[17]

To detect air embolization, a Doppler precordial detector and ultrasonic monitor are used. This detector must be carefully placed on the right side of the heart and its position confirmed by the intravenous injection of a small bolus of air at the beginning of the procedure. We prefer to operate with our patients in the sitting position. In this position the incidence of air embolization is higher than in the park bench or lateral decubitus position, but in any position in which the heart is higher than the head, air embolization can occur. The Doppler precordial detector is extremely sensitive[18] and will detect even the most minute amounts of air. This allows the anesthesiologist to raise the venous pressure and prevent the further entrainment of air thereby avoiding the serious sequelae of massive air embolization. End tidal CO_2 monitoring is also used to enhance our ability to detect air emboli.

The effectiveness of these methods of detection is such that we have abandoned the use of central venous pressure (CVP) catheters for this type of surgery.[19] The CVP catheter was originally inserted to allow the aspiration of air trapped in the right atrium. The initial entrainment of small amounts of air, however, does not sequester in the atrium but rather passes through the heart into the pulmonary circulation. If it is detected at its earliest stages, raising the venous pressure to prevent further entrainment is sufficient. As such, the CVP catheter provides no useful margin of safety and rather is associated with its own set of complications, which we have chosen to avoid.

Fraser (personal communication) has suggested the use of positive end-expiratory pressure (PEEP). In this manner the venous pressure can be raised almost to the level of the head thus creating the physiologic equivalent of having the patient supine while in the sitting position. This should prevent any air entrainment and add a further margin of safety. The level of the venous pressure can be adjusted to avoid seriously raising intracranial venous pressure with its associated increased intracranial pressure.

We routinely use osmotic agents (e.g., mannitol; approximately 1g/k) to minimize cerebral retraction. This is given as a rapid infusion about 15 minutes before the start of the skin incision. When using this medication it is necessary, of course, to place a Foley catheter to accommodate the diuresis that occurs intraoperatively.

As in all neurosurgical anesthesia, it is desirable for the patient to have as smooth an induction as possible, and, even more important that the termination of anesthesia be effected in such a manner that the patient is allowed to awaken gradually and not buck on the endotracheal tube.

POSITIONING

As indicated above, we prefer to place the patient in the sitting position for this procedure. This position offers a great many advantages to the patient and the surgeon. It can be easily achieved in patients of any physiognomy and produces a relaxed operative field with the structures in their normal anatomic relationships. It has advantages for the anesthesiologist in that it avoids chest compression, allows good ventilation, and allows good access to the patient. Cerebrospinal fluid flows out of the wound, and if any bleeding occurs, it can be washed clear with irrigation and the point of the bleeding delineated and controlled with bipolar cautery. This eliminates the need, for the most part, for using suction during this operation. Suction, we feel, is one of the most dangerous instruments that can be used in the posterior fossa because of the great potential risk of inadvertent suctioning and injury of cranial nerves, other neural structures, or small blood vessels. The positioning steps are detailed in Buchheit and Delgado's chapter on the suboccipital approach to removal of acoustic neuromas. We achieve this position using a pin-fixation head holder for rigid fixation of the head. The patient is placed with his head rotated 15 to 30 degrees to the ipsilateral side and the head flexed gently (Figure 96-1). There should be ample room for placing one or two fingers beneath the patient's chin and at no point should the patient's neck be under tension. The elevation of the back of the table is such that the patient is actually in a semi-sitting or slouch position most of the time, although higher elevation of the back rest may be necessary in older patients with a stiff and less flexible neck. If the surgeon has experience and is more comfortable with other positions such as the lateral or park bench position, they certainly can be employed successfully for this procedure. Thus, the actual choice should be determined by the preference of the operating surgeon.

OPERATIVE PROCEDURE

After the patient is satisfactorily anesthetized and positioned as described above, the operative table is also angled 15 to 20 degrees so that the surgeon approaches the patient at an

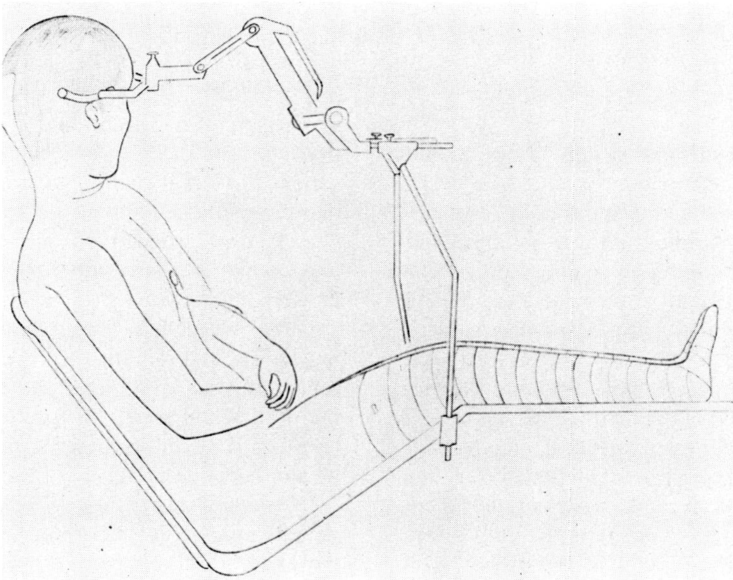

Fig. 96-1. Positioning of the patient for the semi-sitting position. Note the rotation of the head to the same side as the surgery (in this case to the patient's left), the support of the head in the pin-fixation holder, the use of elastic wraps on the legs and elevation of the legs to minimize pooling and hypotension, and the use of the Doppler precordial detector for early detection of air embolism.

angle of approximately 45 degrees from the midline. The hair is shaved only from the posterior quadrant of the head on the affected side and routine preparation and draping is performed. The incision is a vertical paramedian incision (Figure 96-2) located 3 to 5 mm medial to the mastoid notch. This depression can best be identified by locating the mastoid process and then palpating along its medial side. For exposure of the trigeminal nerve, we use a linear incision approximately 7 to 8 cm in length centered two thirds above and one third below the mastoid

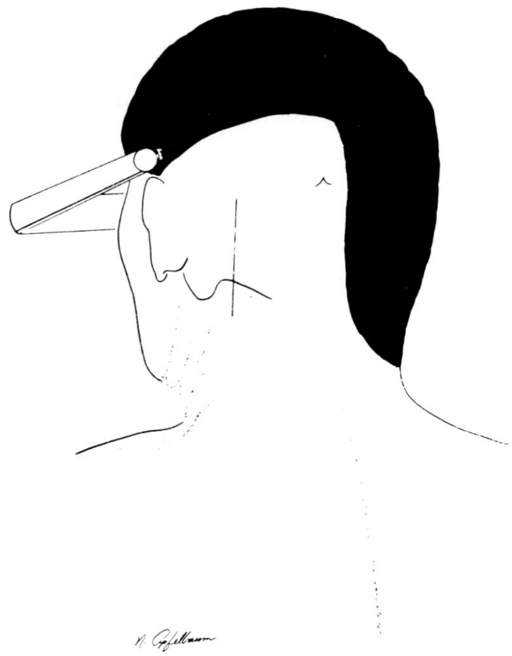

notch. *As with all microsurgery, when a limited exposure is used, the exposure must be targeted precisely.*

The scalp is routinely infiltrated with a 1:200,000 epinephrine solution if there is no anesthetic contraindications to its use. This decreases bleeding significantly. After incision of the skin, hemostasis is achieved with Dandy clamps secured to the drapes with elastic bands. Electrocautery then is used to divide the occipital muscle mass down to the occipital bone. Care is taken not to extend this incision too far inferiorly for fear of injuring the vertebral artery. The posterior auricular branch of the external carotid artery often is encountered and divided by this exposure. The muscle mass then is stripped from the posterior surface of the occipital bone. Care must be taken not to strip too far laterally in order to avoid having the incision centered too far laterally, since the degree of stripping of the muscle mass determines the localization of the exposure once the self-retaining retractor is placed. Any bridging emissary veins are coagulated and their openings in the bone sealed with bone wax.

A modified Weitlander retractor that serves as a base for a self-retaining brain retractor (Codman & Shurtleff, Inc., Randolph, Mass.) which then is placed (Figure 96-3). This must be secured by placing a gauze sponge through the loops of the handle and clipping it to the drape above the patient's head in order to provide good three-point fixation and thus achieve adequate stability for the retractor arm. A burr hole then is made and enlarged into a circular craniectomy defect (Figure 96-4). It should extend superiorly to the transverse sinus and laterally to expose the sigmoid sinus. This often carries it over mastoid air cells, which are thoroughly waxed at the completion of the craniectomy. Care is taken to displace the dura as the rongeuring proceeds in order to avoid entering the dura or the venous sinuses. Bridging veins also may be encountered and will have to be coagulated. If an opening is made into a venous emissary channel, it usually can be sealed readily with a small piece of Surgical covered with a cottonoid. A circular

Fig. 96-2. Localization of the paramedian retromastoid incision. Note that it is placed slightly medial to the mastoid notch and centered about two thirds above and one third below the notch.

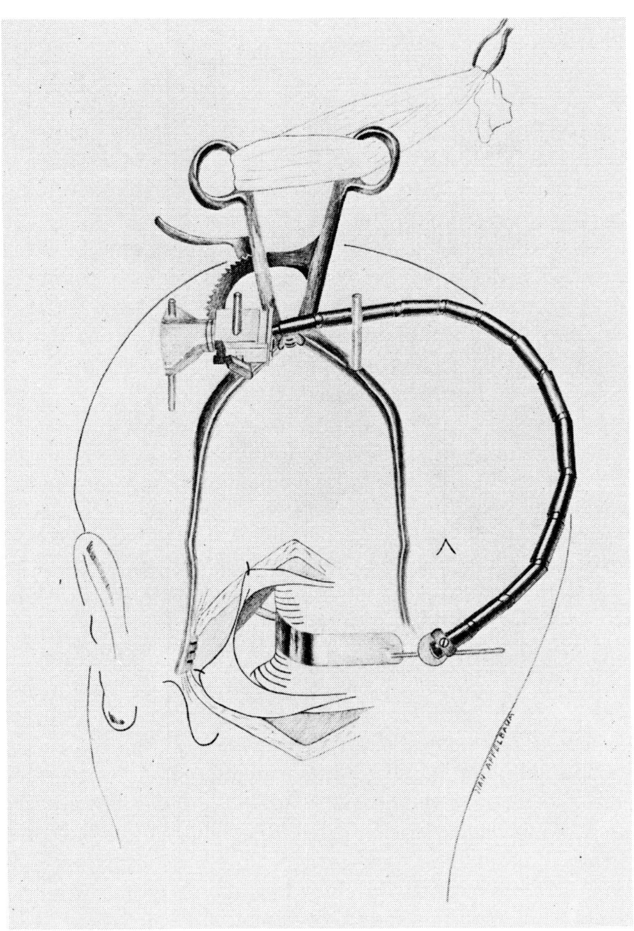

Fig. 96-3. This sketch demonstrates the use of the special cerebellar retractor. Note the fixation of the handle of the retractor with a gauze sponge looped through the rings and clamped to the drapes to provide stable three-point fixation. Note also the positioning of the flexible arm into a gentle arc that avoids sharp kinks. The dura has been opened and the cerebellum retracted to expose the petrosal vein bridging from the superior lateral margin of the cerebellum to the petrosal sinus at the junction of the tentorium and the petrous bone. This structure must be coagulated and divided.

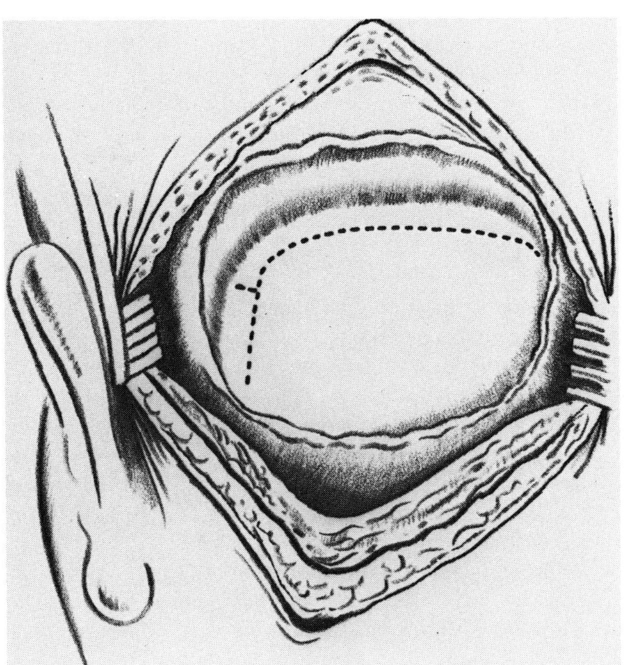

Fig. 96-4. Localization of the craniectomy defect and dural opening. Note the lateral placement adjacent to both the sigmoid sinus (superiorly) and the transverse sinus (laterally).

craniectomy defect measuring approximately 2.5 to 3 cm in diameter is thus created.

It cannot be emphasized too strongly that it is necessary to place this craniectomy superior and lateral enough, as determined by the venous sinuses, in order to achieve a proper exposure. The dura then is opened in an inverted L-shaped manner paralleling these channels and only a few millimeters from them (Figure 96-4). The dura can be "teed" at the superior corner to increase the exposure. It then is secured with tenting sutures superiorly and laterally to retract the sinuses slightly and complete the exposure.

Occasionally, adhesions or bridging vessels are encountered along the superior posterior margin of the cerebellum along the transverse sinus. These must be divided sharply to free the cerebellum. The Flex-bar retractor arm (Codman & Shurtleff) then is placed on the retractor base. This should be positioned in such a way that a gentle arch is negotiated and sharp kinks and bends are avoided (see Figure 96-3). Its tension is adjusted so that it remains in any position in which it is placed but can be readily moved without undo force. A specially shaped retractor blade is used (Codman & Shurtleff). This has

an elongated finger at its superior margin. The purpose of this finger is to allow deeper retraction in the vicinity of the trigeminal nerve but avoid retracting too deeply over the seventh and eighth nerves and thus avoid injury to these structures. A narrow retractor blade could achieve the same depth of exposure superiorly but might dig into the cerebellum. The initial exposure is at the superior lateral margin of the cerebellum. This is retracted in a medial to inferomedial direction and the operating microscope is brought into use.

We use a 275-mm objective on the operating microscope. This allows sufficient working distance between the objective end of the microscope and the patient for the insertion of microsurgical instruments while bringing the surgeon slightly closer to the operating field than is possible with a 300-mm objective. The latter, however, can be satisfactorily employed provided the surgeon is not endowed with overly short arms. Our standard procedure is to set up the operating microscope with the stereoscopic binocular observer tube for the surgical assistant on the surgeon's left. An optical switch photo adaptor (Designs for Vision, Inc., New York, NY) that accommodates a 35-mm still camera and a color television camera is placed on the right side port of the beam splitter.[20] These take up little space and provide no impediment to free access between the surgeon and the surgical scrub nurse who is placed on the surgeon's right. This position is used routinely for all cases regardless of whether the exposure is on the right or left side of the patient. It allows for a standardized operative set-up and excellent access between the surgeon and the nurse. We prefer this position to the use of an overhead table with the nurse placed high because it requires less reaching by either the surgeon or the nurse and allows a freer flow of instruments and better assistance by the nurse. Parenthetically, this same position and same incision is quite satisfactory and is our preferred choice for any exposure into the cerebellopontine angle.

Before placing the microscope, an arm rest is brought into

position. This is a Mayo stand, modified, as suggested by Malis, by removing the top and replacing it with a 6 × 18-inch piece of metal. This is padded, covered with a plastic sheet, and then covered with sterile drapes. Its height can be independently adjusted from the operating table to provide adequate support for the surgeon's arms.

With the microscope in place, the cerebellum is gently retracted medially and the petrosal vein identified (see Figure 96-3). This usually is encountered approximately two thirds of the way from the dura to the trigeminal nerve, but great variability exists and it may be absent or positioned very close to the nerve. It often consists of two channels that form a Y-type bifurcation just before entering the dura. The petrosal vein is coagulated and then divided sharply. This is best accomplished by dividing it partially to be sure that it is totally coagulated before completing the division, since once it is divided, it tends to retract out of sight, and if it is not fully coagulated, the control of bleeding could present a serious technical problem. The retractor then can be advanced, staying close to the tentorium, which should be relatively horizontal in the operative field. Variations in this view can be corrected with the use of the Trendelenburg control of the operating table. Staying high one advances above the seventh and eighth nerves without disturbing them or opening the arachnoid above them. This exposes the arachnoid overlying the trigeminal nerve. If any bleeding is encountered while retracting the cerebellum, it immediately should be suspected that a dorsal bridging vein from the cerebellum to the tentorium may have been torn. Removing the retractor and depressing the cerebellum slightly will allow inspection of this area and control of this problem before proceeding. This is an infrequent occurrence, but the surgeon must be aware of its possibility.

The arachnoid overlying the fifth nerve then must be opened sharply and widely to expose this area. This may be difficult because of the depth at which the work is being done and because of the narrow exposure. At times the arachnoid is quite thin and translucent and can be easily punctured and teased free; at other times, it is thick and opaque and must be sharply dissected. A great deal of care must be taken to avoid tugging on underlying structures. The trigeminal nerve usually will be easily identified at this point once the arachnoid is opened, and the neurovascular relationships at the brain stem then can be identified.

It must be emphasized that the site of the pathologic condition is *at* the brain stem. Vessels impinging distally on the nerve usually are not the cause of the problem. Table 96-4 details our findings. The usual situation involves the superior cerebellar artery looping down in front of the nerve and then emerging from the nerve dorsally at the point where the nerve exits from the stem (Figure 96-5A and B). I feel that it is quite important to open the arachnoid widely in order to allow a full inspection of the entire circumference of the nerve at the stem. Indeed, the first vessel seen may not be the only vascular channel involved in the neurovascular compression, for in a significant number of cases (25) multiple vessels have been encountered. It is also necessary to open the arachnoid anterior to the nerve to allow proper placement of the prosthesis.

The fourth nerve is a thin, delicate structure in the arachnoid above the fifth nerve, usually just below the tentorium. Great care must be taken to avoid injuring this nerve. This is one of the reasons that sharp rather than blunt dissection of the arachnoid is recommended. In addition, there may be small vascular channels traversing the subarachnoid space to the brain stem that might be injured by dissection of this arachnoid unless it is carried out quite carefully.

The Jannetta microsurgical instruments (V. Mueller & Co., Chicago, Ill) are our preference for this procedure, but other neurosurgical instruments that are of sufficient length and properly fashioned to allow adequate vision are certainly useful. Various microsurgical scissors including the Kurze left and right pistol grip scissors (V. Mueller) as well as straight and angled bayonetted microscissors also are employed. Once the arachnoid is opened fully and the area inspected completely, the exact nature of the compression can be determined. We have often found a microdental mirror (V. Mueller) to be useful in inspecting the region anterior to the nerve to be sure that channels were not being missed. This exposure is carried out directly over the seventh and eighth nerves, and their presence must be kept in mind at all times in order to avoid traumatizing them during the dissection or when inserting or removing instruments. The arterial loops then are carefully dissected free of the nerve (Figure 96-6).

When the superior cerebellar artery is the problem, the intent is to elevate it to a horizontal rather than a vertical loop and displace it up and away from the nerve. Small branches going to the brain stem may have been carried down with this vessel as it is gradually elongated, and normally these will not present any problem in the elevation of the vessel as long as their position is kept in mind and they are not injured. Venous channels above or below the nerve are dissected away from the nerve and are coagulated and divided. To facilitate this, small up-and-down angled bipolar forceps have been developed (Codman & Shurtleff) and have proven their usefulness by coagulating these structures safely while avoiding the spread of current to the adjacent neural structures. In the case of vessels compressing the nerve inferiorly, they must be displaced further inferiorly away from the nerve. In all cases, it is important to avoid kinking the arterial channels as they are repositioned.

To secure these vessels free of the nerve, a small prosthesis is inserted between the artery and nerve. We have used for this purpose Ivalon synthetic polyvinyl formyl alcohol foam sponge material (Unipoint Industries, High Point, NC) that has been safely used as a biologic implant for the last 30 years. This material comes packed in formalin and must be washed carefully to remove any trace of this preservative. It then can be cut into small blocks and autoclaved. Before its use, it must be soaked for about 10 minutes in a saline solution to rehydrate it and allow it to become soft and pliable. A small block of the material is then carved to fit between the artery and nerve. We usually fashion this as a saddle-shaped structure to fit completely over the nerve and extend both anterior and posterior to it to lock it in place (Figure 96-7A and B). A groove cut on its superior surface then cradles the artery. In this manner, i.e., interlocked between the artery and nerve, it effectively alters the arterial force vectors and creates a satisfactory decompression. It must be wide enough to extend from the petrous bone to the brain stem but not wide enough to cause any compression. In the case of a vessel inferior to the nerve, a similar type of sponge with a longer posterior element is fashioned, and this posterior element is inserted inferior to the nerve between the artery and vein. In this manner an adequate decompression can be achieved.

Another suitable prosthetic material is shredded Teflon felt. This material, or a felt patty, is often used in cardiac surgery. It can be shredded by grasping and tearing it with two hemostats to create a soft prosthesis resembling a cotton ball. It

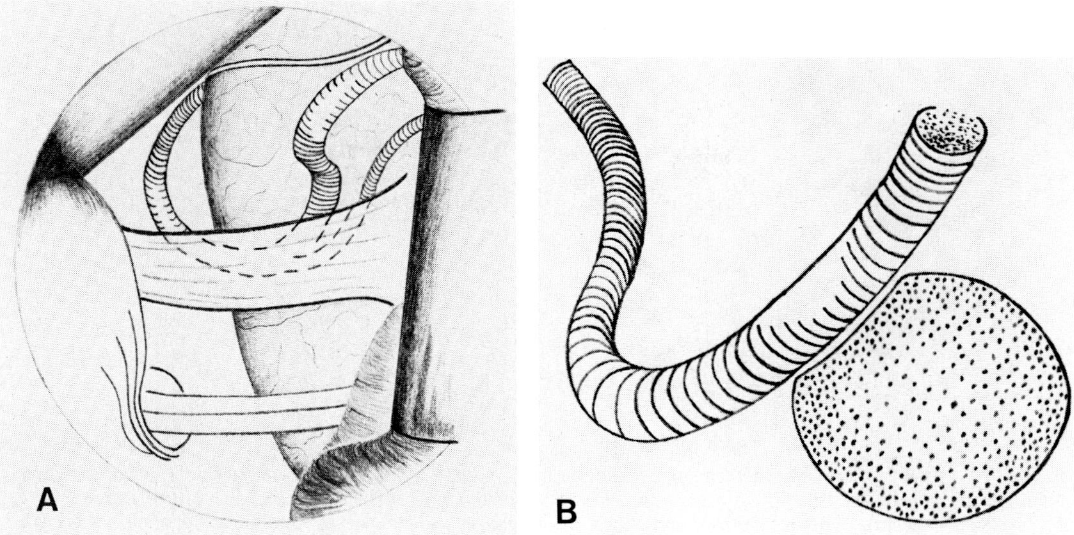

Fig. 96-5. (A) Typical findings in trigeminal neuralgia of the left side. An elongated superior cerebellar artery is looping down and cross-compressing the root entry zone of the trigeminal nerve from an anterior and superior direction. Note the thin fourth nerve just above the superior cerebellar artery and the relative positions of the seventh and eighth nerves below them. The arachnoid has been opened widely to visualize these structures. (B) Schematic lateral view showing the superior cerebellar artery coursing from the anterior (left) to the posterior (right) and impinging on the anterior and superior surfaces of the nerve at the brain stem.

does not have to carved but rather is gently interposed between the nerve and artery with enough being used to ensure a good decompression. It is somewhat easier to place but may produce a slightly higher aseptic meningeal reaction (headache and sterile CSF pleocytosis), which is self-limiting and essentially benign but may prolong postoperative recovery by a few days. We use this in trigeminal nerve surgery when tight subarachnoid space make this technically easier. In the case of seventh and eighth nerve decompressions, it may be the preferable material because of the more difficult anatomy in this area and the greater sensitivity of the eighth nerve to any compressive forces.

On two occasions, we created a sling using a partial thickness of the tentorium that was looped down around the vessel and reattached to the tentorium with a small suture. This was effective but technically much more difficult than inserting the sponge prosthesis. If venous channels alone are encountered, no prosthesis is required. The vessels, however, are both coagulated and divided. Coagulation alone shrinks them, which creates even more tension on the nerve and allows for potential recanalization. If a tumor is encountered, it of course is removed. In many cases the tumor itself is displacing a vessel against the nerve, but tumors, as the sole etiologic agent, have been encountered as well.

If visible spasm is produced in these vessels by the surgical manipulation, a small piece of Gelfoam soaked in papaverine solution is placed on them for a few minutes to lyse the spasm. The operative field then is irrigated and the retractor removed. The cerebellum should be inspected at this point to be sure that no surface bleeding has been produced. We routinely place a piece of Gelfoam over the surface of the cerebellum and then effect a water-tight dural closure using continuous and interrupted 4-0 Nurolon sutures (Ethicon, Inc., Somerville, NJ). The water-tight closure minimizes the chance of a subsequent cerebrospinal fluid leak; it also promotes a smooth postoperative course. Wound closure then is effected in layers using various grades of Nurolon or Vicryl (Ethicon) sutures. A small light surgical dressing is applied.

POSTOPERATIVE CONSIDERATIONS

Patients are nursed in the semi-sitting position for the first 24 hours and are observed carefully for any alterations in neural function. One must be especially alert to signs of pressure in the posterior fossa, since postoperative intracerebellar hematomas have occurred in our experience and have been responsible for patient mortality.

We routinely place our patients on dexamethasone (Decadron) before surgery and continue it for the first 24 hours. If no problems have occurred, it is discontinued at that time.

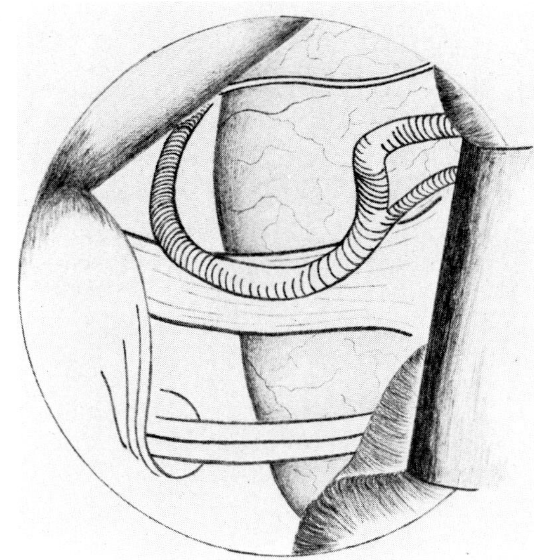

Fig. 96-6. A sketch demonstrating the view after the superior cerebellar artery has been dissected from the axilla of the trigeminal nerve.

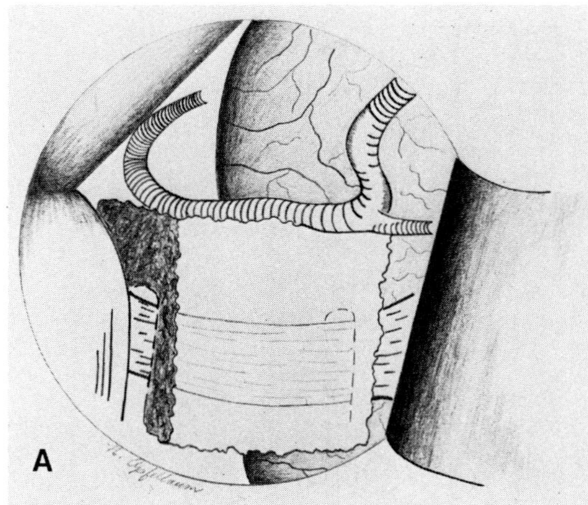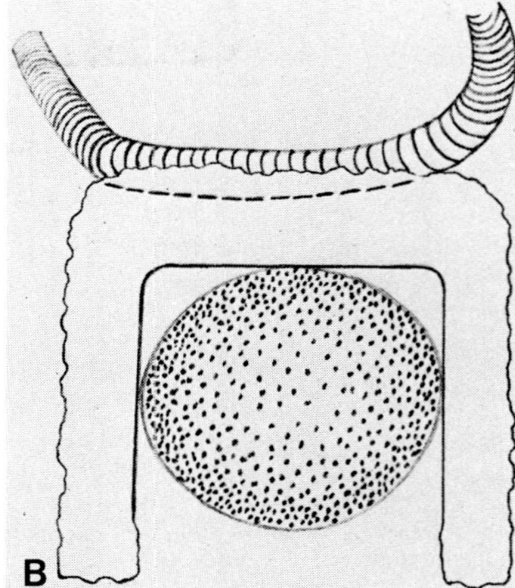

Fig. 96-7. (A) An Ivalon sponge prosthesis is inserted as a saddle around the trigeminal nerve, which elevates the superior cerebellar artery to a more horizontal course and prevents its reapposition to the nerve. (B) A schematic lateral view of the relationship between the artery, sponge, and nerve. Anterior is left, posterior is right.

Patients are allowed out of bed and begin oral intake on the first postoperative day. The Foley catheter is removed at that time, and intravenous feeding is discontinued as soon as the patient is able to achieve an adequate oral intake. The surgical dressing is removed on the second postoperative day.

Most patients have a significant postoperative headache, similar to that experienced after a pneumoencephalogram. We routinely prescribe mild narcotic analgesics (such as 60 mg codeine sulfate) and do not feel that this medication precludes adequate observation of the patient in the postoperative period. Antiemetics are used if necessary. The headache usually will subside within the first day or two, but on occasion it may persist for several weeks. Most patients convalesce rapidly from this procedure and are ready for discharge by the fifth postoperative day, following suture removal. The majority of patients will prefer another week or two at home for further convalescence. During that time their activities are not restricted; instead they are encouraged to gradually increase their activities to the limits of their tolerance. A mild oral analgesic may be prescribed during this period if required.

OPERATIVE RESULTS AND COMPLICATIONS

The results of this procedure, in our personal experience, correspond closely with those of Jannetta and are detailed fully as indicated in the references.[7,21] In summary (Table 96-3), the procedure has been effective in relieving the pain of trigeminal neuralgia in approximately 94 percent of the patients. The operative findings are detailed in Table 96-4. The majority of the patients awaken from the anesthesia without the pain but a number will continue to have postoperative pain for a few days or even a few weeks. The pain, however, will be clearly less than that present immediately before surgery and will gradually taper off. In an occasional patient Dilantin or Tegretol may be restarted if necessary and then tapered within a few days to a few weeks.

In follow-up of 300 consecutive patients operated upon over a 10-year period (Table 96-5), with an average follow-up of 63 months, the pain has been totally controlled in 63.2 percent of these patients. Another 5.6 percent of patients have had, at some time or another, the recurrence of one or more jabs of pain. These usually have been single jabs or isolated occurrences and have not progressed on to more severe recurrences. None of these patients have required the reinstitution of medication. Thus, 68.8 percent of our patients can be considered as having an excellent result.

In another 18.9 percent of patients the pain has recurred to the extent that medication has been necessary but they have been able to be completely controlled with the reinstitution of medication. All of these patients were refractory to medication before surgery, and many are now being controlled on minute doses of Tegretol (such as 100 mg once or twice a day). Most of

Table 96-3. Results of percutaneous trigeminal neurolysis and microvascular decompression of the trigeminal nerve in the treatment of trigeminal neuralgia (author's personal series of 10 years)

Procedure	Total Number of Patients	Relieved (%)	Dysesthesia (%)	Corneal Ulceration/ Hypesthesia (%)
Percutaneous trigeminal neurolysis:				
Radiofrequency	30	90	20	2/18
Glycerol	73	94.5*	5	0/10
Microvascular decompression	300	94	0*	0/0 +

* Some patients required several procedures.
\+ In patients in whom the nerve was not intentionally sectioned.

Table 96-4. Operative findings in 300 consecutive patients undergoing microvascular decompression for trigeminal neuralgia

Operative Finding	Number of Patients
Arterial channels—alone or with veins	235
Venous channels only (1 with AVM)	45
Tumor (5 with arteries; 5 tumors only)	10
Negative exploration	10

Table 96-5. Long-term results in treatment of trigeminal neuralgia in 300 patients with microvascular decompression (10-year experience, average duration of follow-up: 63 months)

Result	Percentage of Patients	
No pain	63.2	Excellent (68.8%)
Rare pain, no medication	8.6	
Pain; medically controlled	18.9	Improved
Pain; refractory	12.9	Failure

these patients (78 percent) feel that the procedure was quite beneficial to them although they obviously are a worrisome group because of the concern that they will become more severely afflicted in the future. In our experience, however, this usually has not been the case and, indeed, almost 50 percent of these patients have been able to discontinue the medication and remain pain-free or have so little pain that they do not feel they need medication. These patients represent a satisfactory but less than perfect result. They certainly have been helped by the procedure.

In an additional 12.9 percent of patients severe recurrences have occurred that have been refractory to medical control. These instances indeed are failures of the procedure and have necessitated an additional, usually destructive procedure to achieve relief. They rarely start as mild (controllable) pain, but rather are usually refractory form the onset.

The significant complications in our series are detailed in Table 96-2. As can be seen, deaths have occurred on three occasions, emphasizing again the need for careful patient selection and information. The remainder of the other complications have for the most part been self-limited. An incidence of fourth-nerve palsy of 4.3 percent represents the most frequent cranial nerve complication. In each of these cases the diplopia has subsided, usually within a few weeks, but on occasion it has lasted for several months (average 2.7 months). Facial nerve palsy has occurred in 5 patients and hearing loss in 10. The facial nerve palsy has been self-limited and resulted in good to satisfactory recovery in each case, although recovery has taken up to 6 months. Hearing loss was mild in 4 patients and severe in 6. Patients who develop a hearing loss usually do not recover their hearing, although one of our patients did. This type of hearing loss must be distinguished from modest decreases in hearing that many patients experience immediately after surgery from fluid behind the eardrum (presumably tracking in through the mastoid area). This is a benign, self-limited process that will clear spontaneously within a few weeks.

Occasionally, patients will experience nonpainful twinge-like feelings in the face that are often described as a ''zippy'' feeling. It is not painful but often produces great anxiety in the patient who fears it is a harbinger of a return of pain. These feelings are frequent in our experience. They usually subside with the passage of time and do not appear to indicate a potential for return of pain. The patient therefore should be so reassured.

CONCLUSION

The Jannetta microvascular procedure, as detailed above, has proved to be an effective means of treating trigeminal neuralgia for the vast majority of patients selected for this procedure. It offers the hope of being curative for most patients by treating the apparent cause of the problem rather than just the symptoms. If offers the major advantage of sparing neural function, thereby avoiding facial sensory loss with its subsequent sequelae as well as anesthesia dolorosa or other dysesthetic sensations and corneal anesthesia, but it carries with it a small but real risk of serious sequelae including death. It therefore should not be undertaken lightly by either the patient or the surgeon. While not a terribly difficult operative technique, it requires significant microsurgical experience and skill since it is an operation in a wound of great depth through a limited exposure. *It is basically an unforgiving operation in which there is little room for error in either judgment or technique.*

TRIGEMINAL NEURALGIA AND MULTIPLE SCLEROSIS

Trigeminal neuralgia (and glossopharyngeal neuralgia) can be a symptom of multiple sclerosis or of other demyelinating diseases. Trigeminal neuralgia will occur in 1 to 3 percent of the patients afflicted with multiple sclerosis, and 1 to 3 percent of the patients in a large series of trigeminal neuralgia will be found to suffer from multiple sclerosis. The clinical pictures are identical, and it is only the presence of neurologic dysfunction in other areas of the nervous system that alerts the surgeon to the demyelinating process. The site of pathologic process appears to be identical in these patients; namely, at the root entry zone of the nerve. In multiple sclerosis, however, the cause is intrinsic rather than extrinsic; namely, a demyelinating plaque rather than a vascular channel that compresses the nerve. The Jannetta microvascular decompression operation therefore offers no benefit to these patients, and a neural destructive procedure must be employed.

Should a patient be explored and a negative exploration be encountered at the root entry zone, it is recommended that a partial section of the nerve be performed. In the case of the trigeminal nerve, the posterior inferior one third to two thirds of the nerve may be sectioned. This usually will provide good pain relief with only modest sensory loss. If the diagnosis is known in advance, radiofrequency lesioning is recommended.

HEMIFACIAL SPASM

The motor analogue of trigeminal neuralgia is hemifacial spasm. Patients with this condition suffer with repetitive, painless paroxysmal twitching of the muscles of the face. Classically, this starts in the muscles about the eyes and progresses

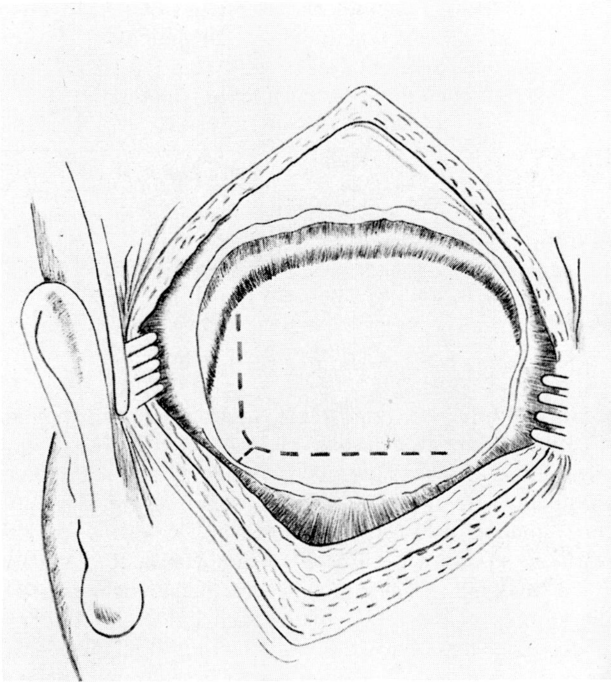

Fig. 96-8. The craniectomy defect and dural opening for exposure of the lower cranial nerves, such as for treatment of hemifacial spasm. Note that the bony opening is carried down lower to reach the point where the occipital bone slopes directly away from the surgeon. The dura is then opened in an L-shaped manner close to the lateral and inferior margins of the craniectomy.

slowly and insidiously to involve the lower and midfacial musculature and, when severe, occasionally will spread to involve both the corrugator of the forehead as well as the platysma muscle on the anterior neck. At times, severe sustained contractures lasting for several seconds will occur. The patient cannot voluntarily relax, so the contractures result in a grotesque disfigurement with forced closure of the eye and a tight grimace of the mouth.

This condition is often misdiagnosed as an emotional problem and, indeed, like many neurologic problems, it will become worse during periods of emotional stress. While initially these symptoms primarily have a cosmetic impact, they can have profound influence on an individual's life by altering self-image, affecting relationships with others, and seriously altering career potential. In addition, the repetitive frequent eye closures may alter an individual's ability to read, drive a car safely, etc. With progression of the condition, mild facial motor weakness may be noted between spasms and hearing may be moderately impaired.

Unlike trigeminal neuralgia, no medical treatment has been effective in relieving this problem. While partial division of the facial nerve has been advocated by some,[22,23] it is not a very effective procedure for hemifacial spasm, and as the condition progresses, it would involve continuous additional destruction until facial paresis and finally a facial palsy occurred.

The differential diagnosis of this condition includes several major entities. Emotional and nervous tics differ from hemifacial spasm in their multifocal presentation that involves multiple muscles, which are innervated by various nervous territories rather than being confined solely to the territory of a unilateral facial nerve. Blepharospasm is a bilateral forced contracture of the musculature about the eye. It differs from hemifacial spasm in being bilateral and involving only the musculature about the eye rather than presenting as a steady progression down the face. It appears to have a totally different etiology and is not thought to respond to this type of surgery.

More closely mimicking hemifacial spasm are the synkinetic movements that may occur following aberrant regeneration of the facial nerve after a Bell's palsy. A history of an antecedent Bell's palsy with these movements developing upon regeneration of the nerve will be most helpful in excluding it. Synkinetic movements develop with regeneration of the nerve and not as a late finding some time after adequate recovery from a Bell's palsy. Facial myokymia also must be considered in the differential. These undulating wormlike movements associated with intrinsic brain stem pathology have a distinct electromyographic pattern and can be separated by this type of evaluation. The association of other cranial nerve defects may help in the differential as well.

INDICATIONS

Patients who are in reasonably good health and less than approximately 65 years of age are potential candidates for this type of surgery. They must be adequately informed of the potential risks, which are of the same type and magnitude as detailed above for trigeminal neuralgia. The specific cranial nerves that are at jeopardy in this type of surgery are primarily the seventh and eighth nerves and the literature[24] indicates a 5 to 8 percent incidence of either facial palsy or hearing loss or both developing after this procedure. Patients who develop facial palsy may well recover at least to a satisfactory functional degree, but patients who lose their hearing are unlikely to recover it. As with any type of surgery, the patient must be fully informed of these risks in order to be able to make an adequate decision whether to proceed.

Preoperative and anesthetic considerations as well as patient positioning are identical to that described above for trigeminal neuralgia.

OPERATIVE PROCEDURE

The surgical incision is placed in the same location as that described for trigeminal neuralgia and is approximately the same length, but is centered slightly lower so that it is approximately half above and half below the mastoid notch. The exposure of the occipital bone and the craniectomy then are performed exactly as detailed above. The craniectomy (Figure 96-8) is carried up close to, but does not definitely have to expose, the transverse sinus. It is important, however, that it be lateral enough to expose the sigmoid sinus and be carried down far enough to reach the floor of the posterior fossa. At this point the bone is usually fairly thin and curves to extend almost straight away from the surgeon. It is important to not leave a lip on this area that will prevent the free egress of cerebrospinal fluid.

The dura is opened in an L-shaped or reversed-L-shaped manner paralleling the sigmoid sinus and the floor of the posterior fossa fairly close to these structures and, again, "teed" as necessary and secured with tenting sutures to widen the exposure.

The same type of self-retaining retractor system is used; however, a flat rectangular-shaped blade is used. This is placed beneath the cerebellum, and the cerebellum is elevated at its inferior lateral margin. The operating microscope, configured exactly as described above, is brought into use at this juncture. Under magnified vision, the cerebellum is gently elevated and a cottonoid strip is placed along its medial inferior edge. This acts as a wick that facilitates the drainage of cerebrospinal fluid and prevents it from welling up in the operative field. With elevation of the cerebellum, the retractor can be advanced anteriorly under direct vision until the spinal part of the eleventh cranial nerve comes into view. The arachnoid at this area is opened sharply, which allows further elevation of the cerebellum and exposure of the remaining nerves of the jugular foramen (Figure 96-9). Occasionally, minute bridging veins will have to be coagulated and divided to effect this exposure. Once the ninth cranial nerve, which is usually slightly separated from the tenth and eleventh nerves, is identified, the exposure is carried medially by sequentially dividing the arachnoid (using sharp dissection) between the ninth nerve and the cerebellum.

It should be noted that no attempt is made at this point to even identify the seventh and eighth nerves at the porus acusticus (although they often may be in view) at this point. They are not followed from the porus acusticus medially to the brain stem. To do so will increase the risk of injury to the eighth nerve. Rather, the dissection is carried out just above the ninth nerve, and by sharply dividing the arachnoid, the cerebellum is gently elevated. Proceeding laterally to medially in this manner, the choroid plexus emanating from the lateral recess of the fourth ventricle will soon come into view. Elevating this will expose the root entry zone of the seventh and eighth nerves at the brain stem.

Two techniques are helpful in this visualization: to increase the exposure superiorly toward the seventh and eighth nerves, the operating table is rotated forward using the Trendelenburg control. This minimizes the retraction that is necessary. It also helps to replace the retractor blade with a special retractor blade (Codman & Shurtleff) that has an elongated process in its center. This "finger" can be advanced up under the choroid plexus to elevate it and improve the visualization. This is a difficult area in which to work and one in which it is hard to be comfortable. The origins of the seventh and eighth nerves from the brain stem were depicted diagrammatically in Chapter 59. With the alterations in this position that occur with the patient's head flexed and the table tilted forward, the facial nerve will be visible in front of the eighth nerve with its origin slightly inferior. The facial nerve usually has a slightly grayish color compared with the pure white of the eighth nerve. The individual components of the eighth nerve normally are not appreciated as separate nerves but rather run together as a compact bundle.

It is in this region where the seventh nerve leaves the brain stem that the site of cross compression will be found. Several different vessels have been encountered in our experience (Table 96-6). The anterior inferior cerebellar artery may loop up against the nerve and then extend either laterally or inferiorly. The posterior inferior cerebellar artery likewise can loop up to compress this area before taking a more inferior course. On occasion, an ectatic vertebral artery will cause the same problem. On one occasion an indentation of the nerve was noted but no definite vascular channel was found. On closer inspection, however, an exostotic protuberance from the floor of the posterior fossa was noted, and when the retractor was gently released, it could be seen that this protuberance mated with the indentation on the nerve. In this instance, the protuberance was removed with a high-speed diamond drill to effect relief.

When a vessel is encountered, it must be carefully dis-

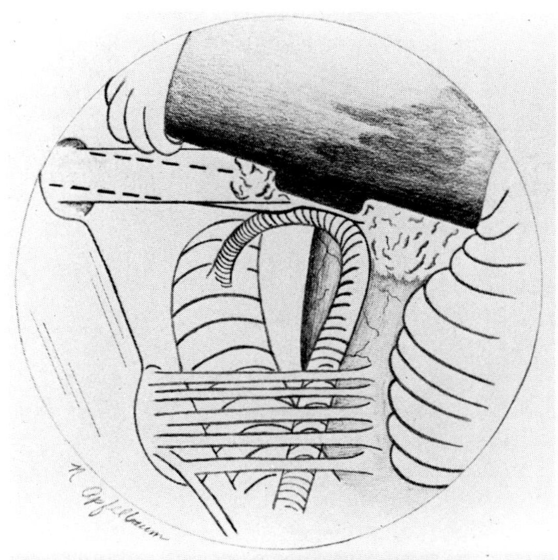

Fig. 96-9. A sketch demonstrating the view on exposure of the lower cranial nerves by elevation of the cerebellum. Inferiorly the spinal portion of the eleventh nerve ascends to enter the jugular foramen joined by the fibers of the ninth, tenth, and the cranial portion of the eleventh nerves. Anterior to these the vertebral artery, which gives off an elongated, tortuous posterior inferior cerebellar artery, is visible. This vessel loops cephalad before changing direction. At the apex of its loop it is indenting and cross-compressing the root entry zone of the seventh nerve, which lies slightly inferior but primarily anterior to the eighth nerve. The retractor is elevating both the cerebellum and the choroid plexus, which is emanating from the lateral recess of the fourth ventricle. This marks the root entry zone of the seventh and eighth nerves and at times obscures them.

sected free of the nerve, and a place must be found for it that will relieve the pressure on the nerve at the same time not kink or compromise the vessel. Many times small tethering branches to the brain stem limit the degree of displacement that can be achieved. One must always be aware of the possible presence of small branches along the medial side of the vessel going to the stem, especially at the apex of loops. After carefully dissecting the vessel free of the nerve and using the utmost in precautions not to manipulate either the seventh or eighth nerves, an Ivalon sponge prosthesis is fashioned to fit between the two. This often takes on a complicated shape because of the limited access in this area and the necessity of accommodating a number of different structures. We try to interdigitate it between the

Table 96-6. Operative findings in 53 consecutive patients undergoing microvascular decompression for treatment of hemifacial spasm

Cause of Compression of Seventh Nerve	Number of Patients
Loop of AICA	26
Loop of PICA	18
Vertebral artery—	1
Associated with AICA origin	3
Associated with PICA origin	3
Venous channel	1
Bony exostosis	1
Total	53

Table 96-7. Complications in 53 consecutive patients undergoing microvascular decompression for the treatment of hemifacial spasm

Complication	Number of Patients
Brain stem stroke—quadriplegia	1
Supratentorial stroke (good recovery; some residuae)	1
Transient supratentorial dysfunction	2
Facial weakness:	
Trace (resolving)	3
Moderate (resolved fully with 3 months)	1
Severe (resolved fully within 3 months)	2
Hearing loss (moderate)	1
Focal seizures (immediately postop in 1; at 6 months in other)	2

vessels and often fashion protuberances on the prosthesis to fit within the loops of the vessel to help anchor it in place. Alternatively, shredded Teflon felt can be used. This is softer and easier to manipulate in place. It may be less likely to compress the adjacent nerves and also less likely to compromise the vessel and its branches.

Various other prostheses have been used by surgeons employing the Jannetta procedure. Our personal experience has been primarily with Ivalon, and, more recently, with shredded Teflon felt, both of which have proved quite satisfactory. Absorbable materials, such as Gelfoam, should be avoided because the vessel may return to its compressive position against the nerve when they are absorbed. Similarly, material such as muscle, which is easier to insert, has on occasion led to recurrences as the muscle atrophied under the continued arterial pulsations and again allowed the artery and nerve to come into contact.

Once a satisfactory decompression of the nerve is achieved, spasm is lysed with topical papaverine, the area irrigated, and the retractor removed while the effects that releasing retraction has on the vascular anatomy are carefully observed. The closure and postoperative care are identical to that used in treating patients with trigeminal neuralgia.

OPERATIVE RESULTS AND COMPLICATIONS

In 53 consecutive cases, a cause of compression was identified in each situation. No negative explorations were encountered. The specific causes of compression are detailed in Table 96-6.

Hemifacial spasm was relieved in all of these patients. In 40 patients relief occurred immediately or within the first few days after surgery. At 2 weeks, a smaller subgroup of 9 patients had significant improvement in their hemifacial spasm, while the remaining 4 patients had about 50 percent reduction. At the 6 month point, 48 were completely resolved and the remaining 5 had only rare residual twitches. We have had recurrences in 16 patients. Eleven of these were mild, with 8 resolving spontaneously, 2 were moderate with 1 resolving and the other worsening to significant, and 3 were significant but 1 resolved. We have reoperated upon the 1 patient who suffered a recurrence at 5

months and whose spasms progressively increased to their preoperative level. A technically unsatisfactory prosthesis was replaced and this effected full resolution of his facial spasms. In long-term follow-up, 47 patients are excellent and 4 are good (rare residual twitches), while one each are rated fair (50 percent improvement) and poor.

Complications with this procedure are detailed in Table 96-7. Hearing has been compromised in 1 patient to a moderate degree. No patients have had an immediate postoperative facial palsy, but 2 have had delayed palsies that developed about 1 week after surgery. In each case these have recovered to normal in 2 to 6 months, respectively. One moderate facial paresis developed 1 week postoperatively and resolved in 3 months. Transient trace facial weakness has been detected in 3 other patients on careful examination. A severe brain stem stroke left one patient quadriplegic. Another patient had a supratentorial stroke but made a good recovery after a stormy course including neurogenic pulmonary edema and a gastrointestinal hemorrhage.

CONCLUSION

The Jannetta microvascular decompression as applied to the treatment of hemifacial spasm offers even more convincing results than those obtained in the treatment of trigeminal neuralgia. This is true because of the total lack of alternative forms of therapy and because of the very visible and graphic effects of the surgical procedure. The procedure, however, will always carry with it a small but significant risk of serious sequelae and, like the same procedure for trigeminal neuralgia, should not be undertaken lightly. It is a more difficult procedure than the decompression of the trigeminal nerve. Its potential benefits thus must be weighed carefully in this nonlethal, painless condition. Again, the basically unforgiving nature of this procedure cannot be emphasized too strongly.

TIC CONVULSIF

Cushing[25] described a few patients suffering from the combined clinical picture of trigeminal neuralgia and hemifacial spasm, a condition that he termed tic convulsif. These patients appear to have both entities, and it is appropriate to explore the root entry zone of both the seventh and fifth cranial nerves and to anticipate vascular channels on both nerves. It is conceivable that only one nerve will be effected because of anomalous innervation, but the safest course would be to explore both nerves.

GLOSSOPHARYNGEAL NEURALGIA

Glossopharyngeal neuralgia is a condition that is exactly analogous to trigeminal neuralgia but occurs in the territory of the ninth cranial nerve. Patients so afflicted experience lancinating spasms of pain in the posterior tongue and throat that usually are triggered by talking and swallowing. It is a much rarer condition than trigeminal neuralgia but otherwise appears to be identical in its behavior. Like trigeminal neuralgia, it usually can be controlled medically, and surgical intervention is infrequently required.

The Jannetta microvascular decompressive technique is equally applicable to this condition as it is to trigeminal neuralgia. The preoperative considerations and alternatives are the same. The operative exposure is the same as the one detailed for the seventh cranial nerve with the modification that the root entry zone of the ninth cranial nerve is inspected and decompressed. This is accomplished by following the superior surface of the ninth nerve back to the brain stem and then visualizing this area, working between the seventh and eighth nerves above and the ninth nerve below or between the fascicles of the ninth and tenth nerves.

Because of the rarity of this condition, experience is limited, but the results appear to parallel closely that of trigeminal neuralgia.

REFERENCES

1. Dandy WE: The treatment of trigeminal neuralgia by the cerebellar route. Ann Surg 96:787, 1932
2. Gardner WJ, Sava GA: Hemifacial spasm—a reversible pathophysiologic state. J Neurosurg 19:240, 1962
3. Jannetta PJ: Arterial compression of the trigeminal nerve at the pons in patients with trigeminal neuralgia. J Neurosurg 26:159, 1967
4. Jannetta PJ: Observations on the etiology of trigeminal neuralgia, hemifacial spasm, acoustic nerve dysfunction and glossopharyngeal neuralgia. definitive microsurgical treatment and results in 117 patients. Neurochirurgia 20:145, 1977
5. Jannetta PJ: Microsurgical approach to the trigeminal nerve for tic douloureux. Prog Neurol Surg 7:180, 1976
6. Apfelbaum RI, Kirk M, Terra AM: Microvascular decompression of the trigeminal nerve for the treatment of trigeminal neuralgia. J Neurosurg Nurs 10:77, 1978
7. Apfelbaum RI: The Jannetta microvascular decompressive operation for treatment of trigeminal neuralgia (in preparation)
8. White JC, Sweet WH: Pain and the Neurosurgeon; Medical Treatment of Trigeminal Neuralgia. Springfield, Ill, Charles C Thomas, 1969, p 169
9. Rasmussen P, Riishede J: Facial pain treated with carbamazepine (Tegretol). Acta Neurol Scand 46:385, 1970
10. Tew JM, Keller JT: The treatment of trigeminal neuralgia by percutaneous radiofrequency technique. Clin Neurosurg 24:557, 1976
11. Siegfried J: 500 percutaneous thermocoagulations of the gasserian ganglion for trigeminal pain. Surg Neurol 8:126, 1977
12. Jannetta PJ: Treatment of trigeminal neuralgia by suboccipital and transtentorial cranial operations. Clin Neurosurg 24:538, 1976
13. Lunsford LD, Apfelbaum RI: Choice of surgical therapeutic modalities for treatment of trigeminal neuralgia: Microvascular decompression, percutaneous retrogasserian thermal or glycerol rhizotomy. Clin Neurosurg 32:319, 1985
14. Lunsford LD: Treatment of tic douloureux by percutaneous retrogasserian glycerol injection. JAMA 248:449, 1982
15. Häkanson S: Trigeminal neuralgia treated by the injection of glycerol into the trigeminal cistern. Neurosurgery 9:638, 1981
16. Nugent GR: Technique and results of 800 percutaneous radiofrequency thermocoagulations for trigeminal neuralgia. Appl Neurophysiol 45:504, 1982
17. Adornato DC, Gildenberg PL, Ferrario CM, et al: Pathophysiology of intravenous air embolism in dogs. Anesthesiology 49:120, 1978
18. Frost EA: Anesthesia for neurosurgical procedures in the sitting position. Weekly Anesthesiology Update, Lesson 4, vol 1, 1977
19. Apfelbaum RI, Duncalf D, Phillips PL: Is central venous catheterization necessary for neurosurgical procedures in the sitting position? Presented at the annual meeting of the American Association of Neurological Surgeons, New York, 1980
20. Apfelbaum RI, Neurosurgical applications of video techniques. Clin Neurosurg 28:246, 1981
21. Apfelbaum RI: Surgery for tic douloureux. Clin Neurosurg 31:351, 1984
22. German WJ: Surgical treatment of spasmodic facial tic. Surgery 11:912, 1942
23. Scoville WB: Partial extracranial section of seventh nerve for hemi-facial spasm. J Neurosurg 31:106, 1969
24. Jannetta PJ, Abbasy M, Maroon J, et al: Etiology and definitive microsurgical treatment of hemifacial spasm. J Neurosurg 47:321, 1977
25. Cushing H: The major trigeminal neuralgias and their surgical treatment based on experiences with 332 gasserian operations. Am J Med Sci 160:157, 1920

Percutaneous Rhizotomy in the Treatment of Intractable Facial Pain (Trigeminal, Glossopharyngeal, and Vagal Nerves)

John M. Tew, Jr.   Harry van Loveren

TRIGEMINAL NEURALGIA

THE SURGICAL TREATMENT of trigeminal neuralgia continues to stimulate controversy despite the fact that this condition has been recognized and treated surgically for centuries. A totally satisfactory method of treatment has never been devised. Section of a peripheral branch of the trigeminal nerve was probably the earliest form of surgical therapy. Later, intracranial section of peripheral branches,[1,2] ganglion resection,[3] and retrogasserian rhizotomy were developed.[4–6] Some questioned the need for destructive procedures[7–10] and developed techniques for decompressing or compressing the posterior rootlets.

Peripheral procedures still are effective for the temporary control of chronic trigeminal pain, particularly as an early measure that provides the patient an opportunity to test the effect of sensory deprivation.[11,12]

Based upon the original observations of Dandy,[13] Jannetta[14] popularized the theory that trigeminal neuralgia was caused by compression of the trigeminal root entry zone to the brain stem by vascular structures. The efficacy of microvascular decompression has been established, although the recurrence rate associated with this operation demonstrates that it is not a "curative" procedure.[15]

The tactic of electrocoagulation of the trigeminal nerve originally was proposed by Kirschner in 1932.[16] Despite a report of favorable results,[17] this procedure gained no practitioners in this country until Sweet refined the technique[18,19] with the following modifications: (1) use of a short-acting anesthetic agent, which permits the patient to awaken rapidly for sensory testing during the operation; (2) use of a reliable radiofrequency current for production of the lesion; (3) use of electrical stimulation for precise localization; and (4) use of temperature monitoring for precise control of lesion configuration. This procedure has been extremely safe and has gained considerable acceptance as a method for partially destroying the sensory root.

PATIENT SELECTION

All patients with trigeminal neuralgia are subjected to a trial of medical therapy beginning with carbamazepine. Lioresal and phenytoin are drugs of second choice. The 75 percent of patients who fail to achieve long-term relief with medical therapy either because of the recurrence of pain or the development of toxic side effects are candidates for percutaneous rhizotomy. As a guideline we refer to Garvan and Siegfried,[20] who advocated that patients whose pain is only partially controlled after 1 year of drug therapy and patients who still require medication after consuming over 3000 tablets of a single drug be considered for surgery.

Posterior fossa exploration and possible microvascular decompression is offered to patients who are less than 60 years of age and without medical contraindication to general anesthesia. This procedure is recommended to patients who have primary involvement of the ophthalmic division to avoid the complications of corneal analgesia. Computed tomography or magnetic resonance imaging will exclude the rare patient with a tumor as a cause of trigeminal pain.[21] Angiography is not routinely used, since we have found it a poor predictor of neurovascular compression.

If surgical treatment is elected, the patient and family are required to read and listen to a full explanation of current procedures available for the control of trigeminal neuralgia. Frequently, the patient is advised to discuss results with others who have undergone major trigeminal surgery. This tactic reinforces the patient's understanding and appreciation of possible undesirable sensory loss. Differential sensory block enables the patient to experience the effect of sensory deprivation and may aid in the decision concerning operation for atypical facial pain.

A well-educated patient is better able to accept side effects, thus greatly reducing the incidence of postoperative disappointment. It has been our policy to let the informed patient make his or her own decision regarding the mode of treatment. If the patient elects a destructive procedure, such as electrocoagulation, he or she is encouraged to indicate the degree of sensory deficit he or she would like to acquire. While partial sensory loss is associated with a higher incidence of recurrence, patients usually are not reluctant to undergo repeat percutaneous rhizotomy.

OPERATIVE NEUROSURGICAL TECHNIQUES
ISBN 0-8089-1862-1

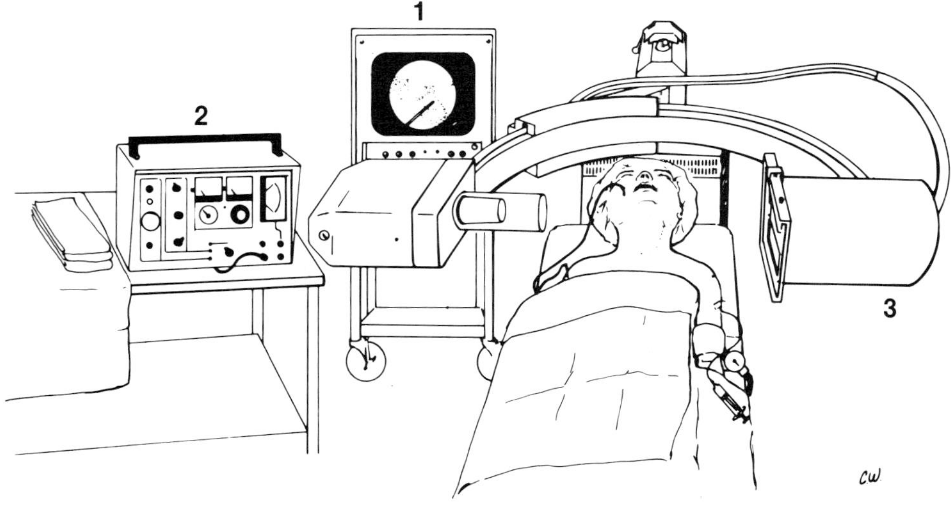

Fig. 97-1. The operative arrangement used for stereotactic rhizotomy of the trigeminal nerve. 1 = image intensifier; 2 = radiofrequency generator; 3 = C-arm cine radiographic unit.

TECHNIQUE—PERCUTANEOUS TRIGEMINAL RHIZOTOMY

The rationale for electrocoagulation of the trigeminal rootlets is based on the premise that differential thermal destruction of the small unmyelinated and finely myelinated fibers that conduct pain can be achieved.[22,23] The procedure is conducted in the radiographic suite (Figure 97-1).

The patient is anesthetized with an intravenous injection of 30–50 mg methohexital (Brevital, Eli Lilly & Co., Indianapolis, Indiana). A standard 100-mm length 20-gauge cannula and stylet are placed in the retrogasserian portion of the trigeminal nerve. Placement is by free-hand manipulation, but a guiding device as designed by Kirschner can be used. Three anatomic landmarks are chosen on the face (Figure 97-2): (1) a point 3 cm anterior to

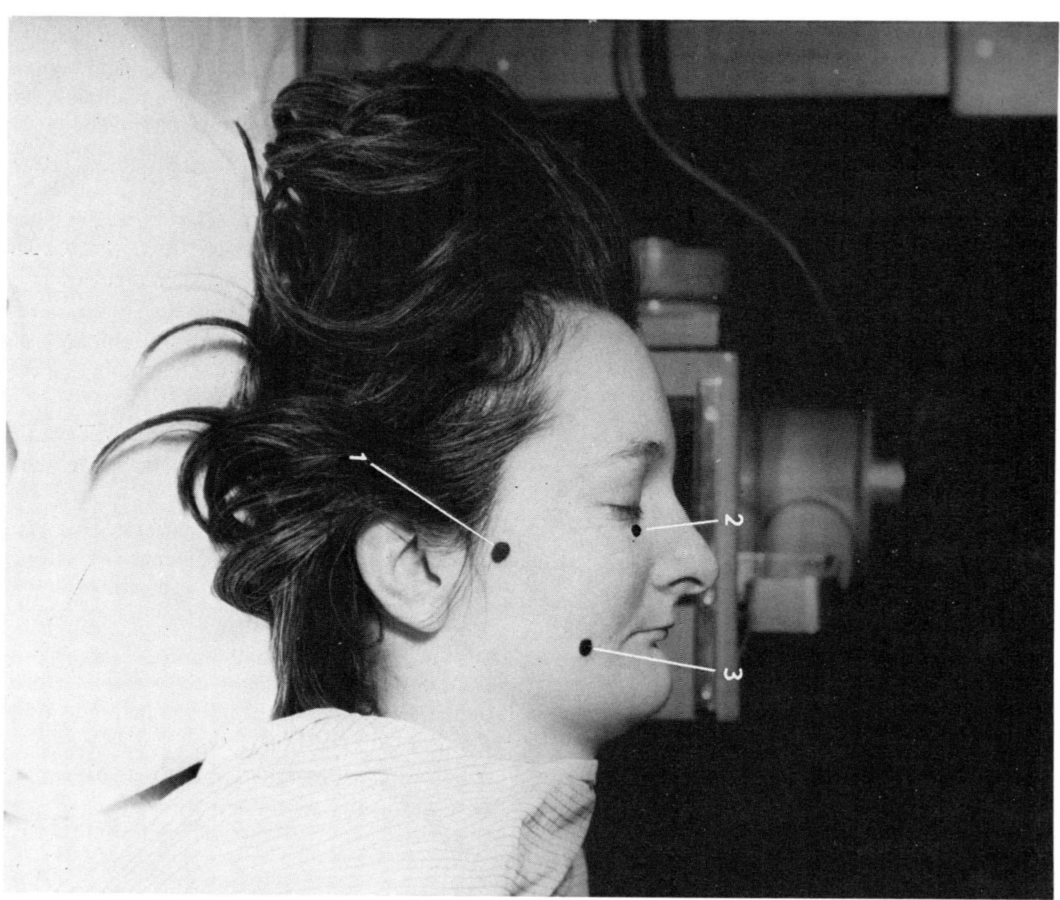

Fig. 97-2. Anatomic landmarks for electrode placement.

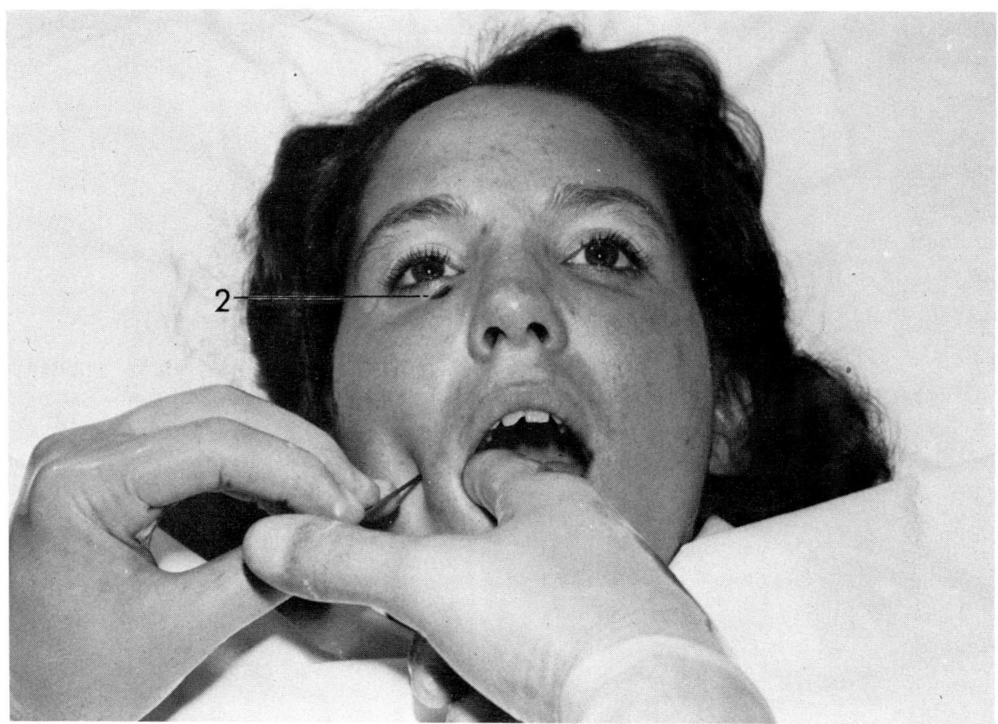

Fig. 97-3. Needle placement according to the technique of Härtel.

the external auditory meatus; (2) a point beneath the medial aspect of the pupil; and (3) a point 2.5 cm lateral to the oral commissure. The first two points indicate the site of the foramen ovale and the third is the point at which the needle penetrates the skin of the jaw. The anterior approach to the foramen ovale, as advocated by Härtel,[24] is used (Figure 97-3). Radiographic control has been reported to be of value, and we have used the image intensifier in a lateral plane as an effective method of localizing the needle.[25] Using the landmarks described, however, we have been able to penetrate the foramen ovale on the first attempt in most cases and after a simple adjustment in all instances.

The index finger of a gloved hand is placed just inferior to the lateral pterygoid wing, and the electrode is directed into the

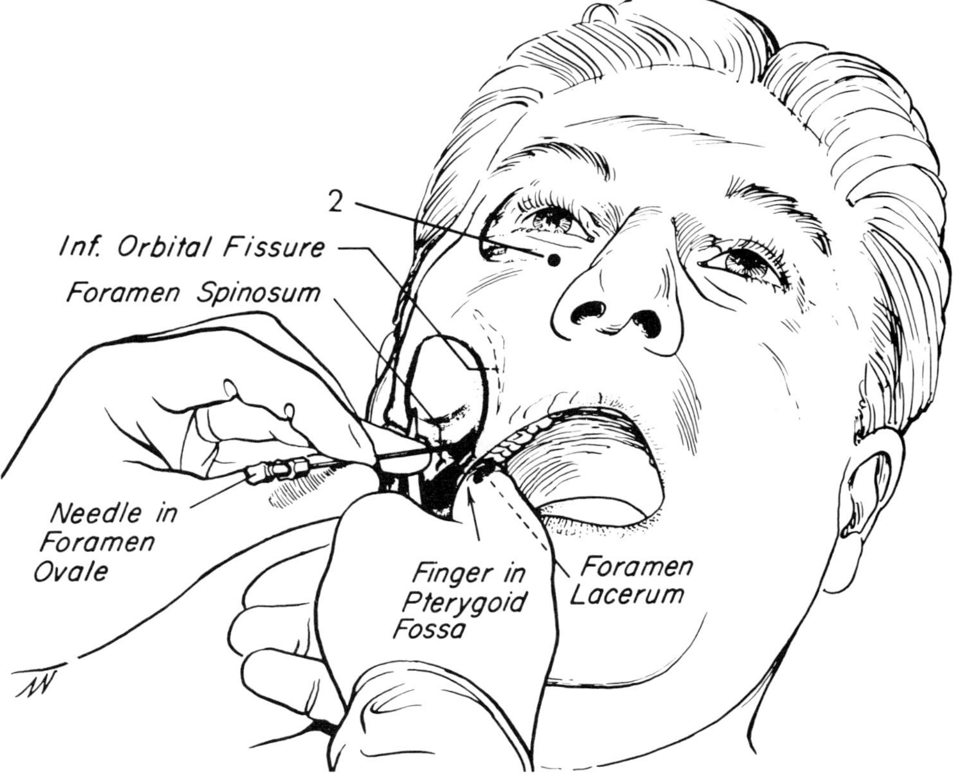

Fig. 97-4. Free-hand placement of the electrode. The guiding finger touches the pterygoid wing.

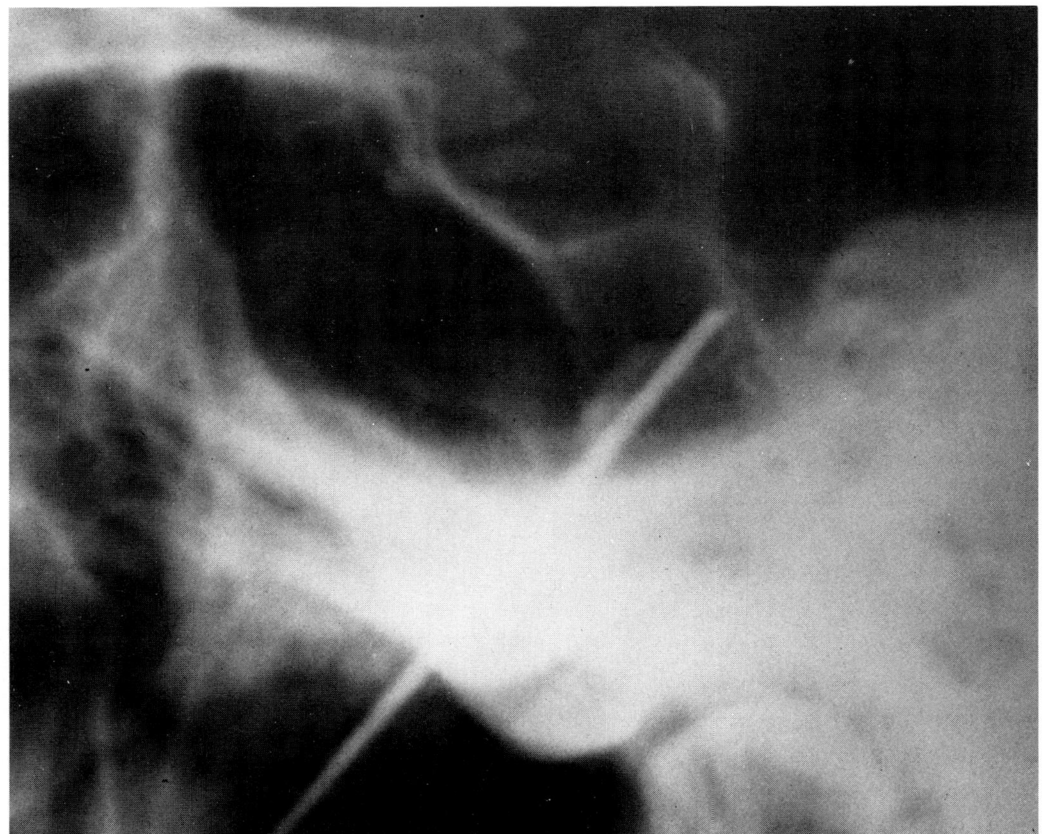

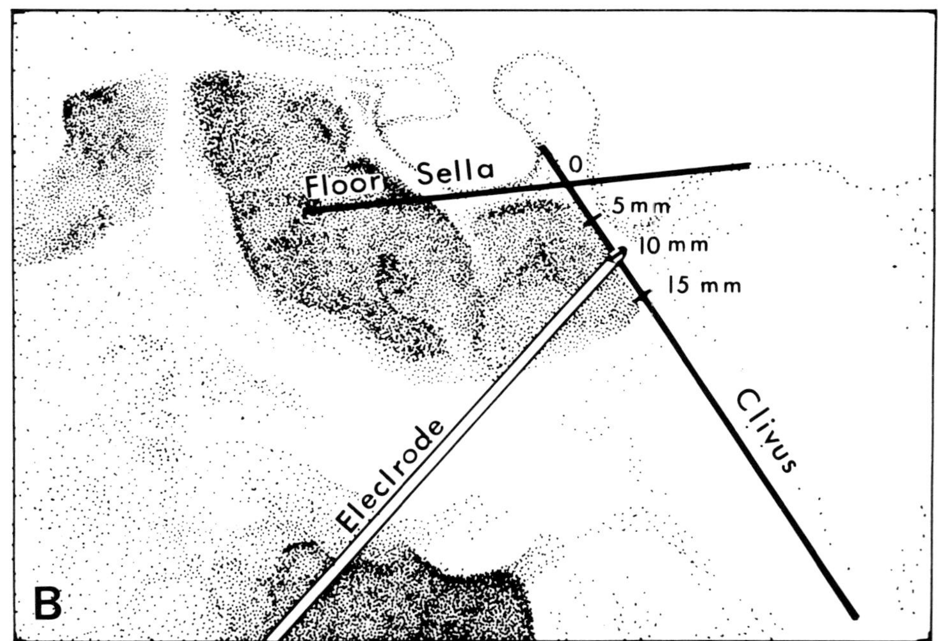

Fig. 97-5.   (A) A submento-vertex roentgenogram confirming electrode placement in the foramen ovale. (B) The ideal trajectory of the electrode (5–10 mm below the intersection of a line drawn from the floor of the sella turcica to the clival line).

medial portion of the foramen ovale (Figure 97-4). If the needle enters the posterolateral aspect of the foramen, it may not lie within the dural investment of the trigeminal ganglion and, if advanced, probably will not reach the maxillary or ophthalmic divisions of the rootlet of the nerve. As the electrode is advanced, an oral airway is placed between the patient's jaws to prevent the patient from involuntarily biting the finger guiding the electrode. Intravenous methohexital is injected as the foramen is neared. Entrance of the needle into the foramen is signaled by a wince and a brief contraction of the masseter muscle, indicating contact with the mandibular sensory and motor fibers. Before the electrode is advanced any further, a

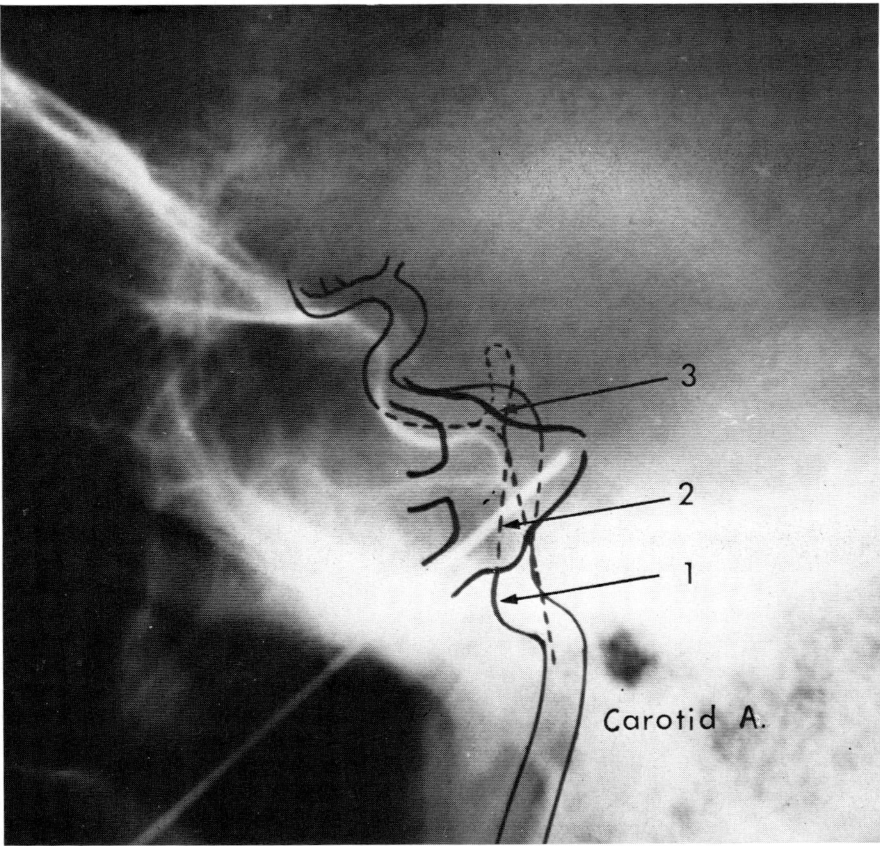

Fig. 97-6. A composite illustration demonstrating the relationship of the carotid artery to the trigeminal ganglion and posterior rootlets. Note the location of three points of possible carotid penetration.

second series of roentgenograms is obtained to confirm proper placement of the electrode (Figures 97-5A and B). The stylet is withdrawn to determine whether the carotid artery has been penetrated. In our experience, this has occurred on only two occasions.

If the carotid artery is penetrated, the needle should be withdrawn promptly and manual pressure applied over the posterior pharyngeal space. The procedure should be discontinued and the patient allowed to recuperate for 24 to 48 hours. Ischemic complications, such as hemiparesis, have resulted from puncture of the internal carotid artery.[26] If deviated laterally, the electrode can penetrate the cartilaginous covering of the foramen lacerum and puncture the carotid artery. If the electrode is directed posterolaterally, it can pierce the carotid artery at its entrance into the petrous bone. Finally, Rish[26] noted that after the electrode passes through the foramen ovale, it can penetrate the carotid artery. This can occur if the electrode is directed anteriorly and medially into the area of the cavernous sinus (Figure 97-6). Our anatomic studies illustrate that the carotid artery frequently is devoid of bony covering immediately ventral to Meckel's cave.

Electrode Localization

The cannula is calibrated in order to permit extrusion of the electrode in 1-mm increments. When the electrode is fully inserted into the cannula, the curved tip extends 5 mm beyond the end of the cannula and projects 3 mm perpendicular to the axis of the electrode. The cannula is insulated so that only the extruded portion of the electrode (0–5 mm) is conductive. The electrode can be rotated through a 360-degree axis for stimulation and lesion production.

Final placement of the electrode tip is determined by the response to electrical stimulation. A current of precisely 0.2 to 0.3 V at 50 to 75 cycles/second will reproduce the paroxysmal bouts of pain reminiscent of trigeminal neuralgia. Stimulation at higher voltage (1.0 to 2.0 V) may be required in patients who have had previous intracranial rhizotomy or repeated alcohol injections. The response evoked serves as a reliable indicator of the probe temperature required to produce a lesion.

After the cannula reaches the trigeminal cistern, stimulation should elicit a paroxysm of pain in the mandibular distribution. Lateral roentgenograms obtained at that time will indicate whether the tip of the electrode lies at a point 4 to 5 mm external to the profile of the clivus. If the needle is advanced 5 mm, its tip should lie at the level of the clivus, where stimulation will elicit paresthesias in the second-division rootlets. The electrode tip should not be advanced more than 8 mm deep to the profile of the clivus, since it can injure the abducens nerve in this region. Manipulation (rotation about its axis) of the curved electrode permits stimulation of different portions of the nerve (Figures 97-7 A, B, and C). Rotation of the electrode tip cephalad provides better access to the fibers of the ophthalmic division, while caudal rotation contacts the mandibular fibers. This maneuverability permits precise anatomic localization in the sensory root. If the electrode contacts the motor root, stimulation results in masseter contraction; lateral rotation of the electrode prevents the production of a lesion that could result in motor paresis. Although a straight electrode was used

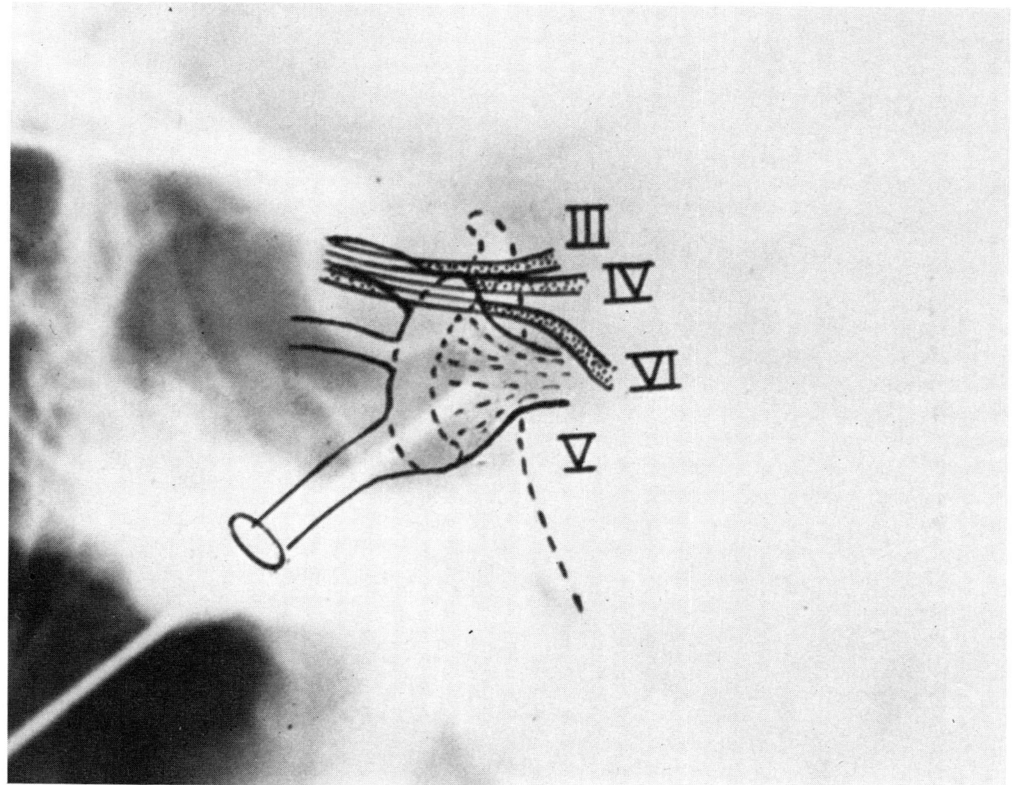

Fig. 97-7. (A) Composite illustration demonstrating the relationship of the trigeminal rootlets to the profile of the clivus. With the electrode tip at −5 mm, the third division is stimulated; at 0, the second division, and at +5 mm deep to the clivus, the first division fibers are stimulated. (B) An illustration of the trigeminal rootlets and the newly developed curved electrode with thermocouple, which is capable of producing lesions in any of the three divisions from a single position. (C) New curved electrode system, which is capable of lesion production and temperature measurement throughout the trigeminal root from a single position.

in our first 700 cases, the advantages of the curved-tip electrode described above have obviated the straight electrode technique.

Lesion Production

The geometry of the lesions varies with the medium; reproducible lesions are 5 × 5 × 4 mm and are eccentric with orientation toward the curve of the electrode. The electrode tip measures 0.5 mm in diameter. A thermocouple sensor is located at the tip of the electrode and provides calibration accuracy of ±2°C over the range of 30°–100°C.

Additional intravenous anesthetic is administered, and a preliminary lesion is produced at 60°C for 60 seconds. A facial blush usually appears at this point and helps to localize the region of the nerve root undergoing thermal destruction.[27] When the patient has fully awakened, careful sensory testing of the face is conducted. Repeat lesions are produced until the desired effect is achieved. Generally, sequential lesions of 90-second duration are made by increasing the temperature 5°C with each lesion. When analgesia is approached, great care is exercised to avoid overshooting the desired result, which includes preserving the sense of touch. After a partial lesion has been produced, it is frequently possible to complete the lesion without additional anesthetic agent. The pain associated with production of the lesion is reduced because a lower temperature is required to make an effective lesion and the curvature of the electrode avoids contact with the dura, which is the principal source of pain reception in this region. This tactic is particularly

valuable when partial sensation of a cornea or other trigeminal divisions are to be preserved.

Once the desired degree of sensory loss has been achieved, the patient is observed for an additional 15 minutes to determine if a fixed lesion has been produced. If the examination indicates a stable level of analgesia, the distribution and degree of deficit are determined by careful sensory testing. Touch perception is recorded in grams of pressure, using calibrated Von-Frey hairs. Masseter, pterygoid, facial, and ocular muscle functions are recorded. The patient then is returned to his or her room and observed for 24 hours. During this period the patient is informed of the necessity for eye care, of avoiding jaw strain, and of the consequences of facial analgesia.

RESULTS

At the time of this report 1100 patients have been treated surgically by percutaneous stereotactic rhizotomy. The straight electrode was used in the initial 700 operations. The curved electrode was used in subsequent cases with some modification of tactic and technique. The average follow-up period for all patients has been 8 years with a range of 1 to 18 years (Table 97-1). The mean age of onset was 57 years with a range of 10 to 95 years. The mean age at time of surgery was 65 years with a range of 25 to 97 years. Sixty-two percent of the patients were women and 60 percent had pain located on the right side. The most common area of involvement in this series was the combination of the second and third divisions. Twenty-nine

Table 97-1. Characteristics of 950 patients selected for electrocoagulation*

		Percent of Patients
Average age (years)	65	
Sex	62% female	
Side of coagulation		
Right		60
Bilateral		5
Division of trigeminal nerve involved		
V-1		1
V-2		16
V-3		15
V-1, V-2		15
V-2, V-3		40
V-1, V-2, V-3		13

* Patients with multiple sclerosis excluded.

percent of patients had a significant degree of pain in the first division but in only 12 percent of patients was pain isolated to the first division.

The disease had been present for an average of 8 years and was characterized by increasingly severe episodes of paroxysmal pain and progressively shorter periods of remission. Thirty-five percent of patients had undergone a previous operation, including nerve avulsion, alcohol injection, subtotal rhizotomy, ganglionectomy, microvascular decompression, or percutaneous rhizotomy. Although approximately one third of patients had an unnecessary dental extraction or manipulation after the onset of trigeminal neuralgia, 4 percent developed the disorder immediately after dental extraction. Four percent of patients had multiple sclerosis as the presumed cause of their trigeminal neuralgia. The incidence of bilateral involvement was 18 percent in patients with multiple sclerosis and 5 percent in patients without multiple sclerosis. All patients had been subjected to a rigorous trial of medical therapy with either carbamazepine (Tegretol), lioresal (Baclofen), or diphenylhydantoin (Dilantin).

Table 97-2. Long-term results of percutaneous stereotactic rhizotomy in 950 patients*

Result	Percent
Excellent (no tic pain, dysesthesias, or troublesome paresthesias	65
Good (no tic pain, minor dysesthesia/paresthesia)	27
Fair (no tic pain, moderate dysesthesia/paresthesia)	5
Poor (no tic pain, major dysesthesia/paresthesia)	1
Failure (immediate)	2
Recurrence	
Minor (no medications required)	5
Moderate (restart medications)	4
Severe (requiring surgery)	5
Total	14

* Average follow-up, 8 years. Includes patients undergoing multiple percutaneous stereotactic rhizotomies; subjective rating determined by patient.

Table 97-3. Complications in 950 cases of percutaneous rhizotomy*

Complication	Percentage
Masseter weakness†	18
Pterygoid weakness	9
Dysesthesia/paresthesia (minor)	20
Dysesthesia/paresthesia (major)	3
Diplopia	
Oculomotor	0.2
Trochlear	0.5
Abducens	0.8
Keratitis	3.0
Meningitis	0.3

* Includes patients undergoing multiple percutaneous rhizotomies.
† Nearly all nerve palsies (motor root and extraocular) represented axonotmesis and resolved within 6 months.

Initial effective relief was obtained in 92 percent of the patients treated with carbamazepine and in approximately 50 percent of the patients treated with diphenylhydantoin. Lioresal has not been used as a first-line drug. Seventy-five percent of patients eventually required a surgical procedure because of recurrence of pain or increasing side effects of medical therapy.

A response to follow-up was obtained for 950 patients (Table 97-2). At the time of evaluation, 92 percent reported excellent or good results. Five percent reported fair results because of undesirable side effects, and 1 percent reported poor results because of severe denervation dysesthesias. In 2 percent of patients, the procedure failed; usually these were patients with significant preoperative denervation.

SIDE EFFECTS

Sensory

Troublesome numbness and paresthesias as a result of the inherent sensory deficit proved to be the most consistent adverse side effect with both the straight and curved electrode technique. In our early experience with the curved electrode, the incidence of this side effect was reduced to zero. With a longer experience and utilization of the curved electrode in more complicated and recurrent cases, this problem is re-emerging. The overall incidence of major paresthesias (numbness that is troublesome or disturbing) is 3 percent (Table 97-3). Commonly, an intermittent crawling, burning, or itching sensation was described. Most patients readily adjusted to the sensory deficit, and the paresthesias usually diminished with time. The more active and mentally alert the patient, the fewer the disturbances of sensation reported. Older patients were more prone to this complication. Constant, severe dysesthesias in an anesthetic or analgesic zone (anesthesia dolorosa) rarely occurred with the straight electrode and have not occurred at all with the curved electrode technique.

Ocular

Ocular complications, including neurogenic keratitis or corneal abrasion, developed in 3 percent of patients. Thirty percent of this group had corneal analgesia rather than anesthesia, indicating that touch perception in the absence of pain perception does not necessarily protect against corneal ulceration. The corneal lesion was reversed in all patients by early

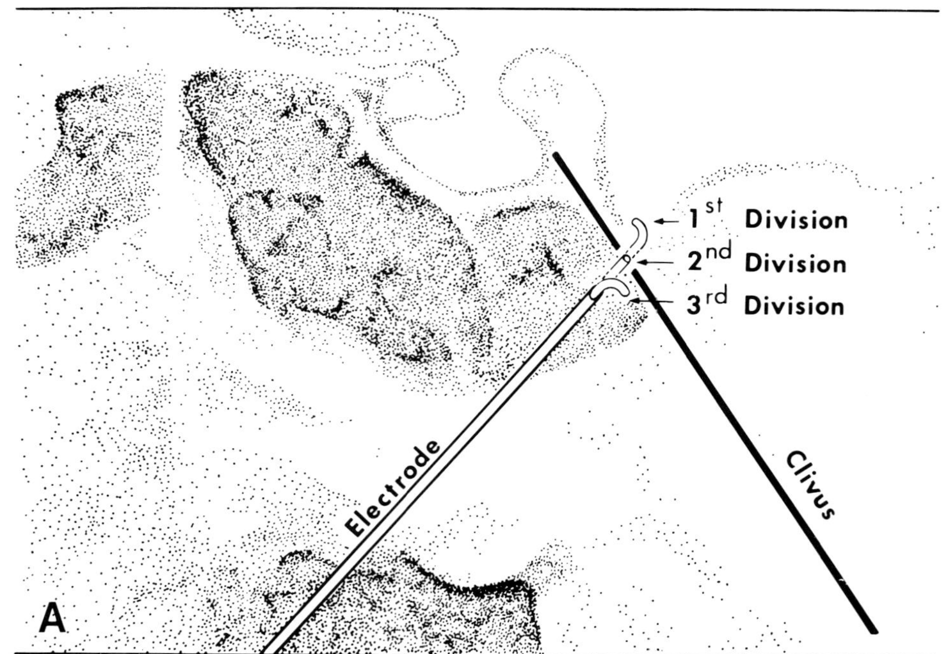

1st Division
2nd Division
3rd Division
Electrode
Clivus
A

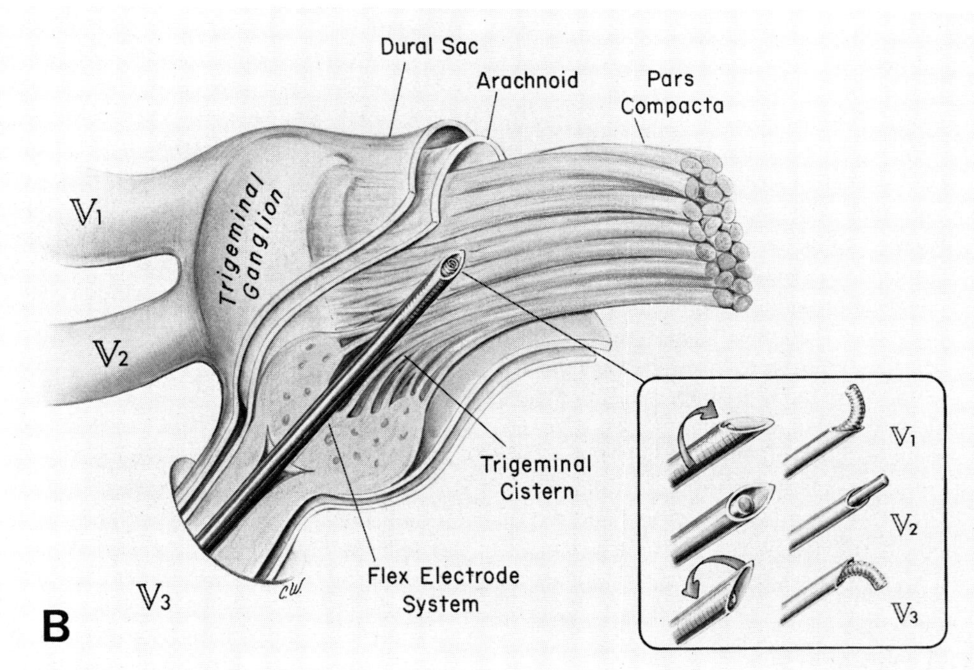

Dural Sac
Arachnoid
Pars Compacta
Trigeminal Ganglion
V1
V2
V3
Trigeminal Cistern
Flex Electrode System
V1
V2
V3
B

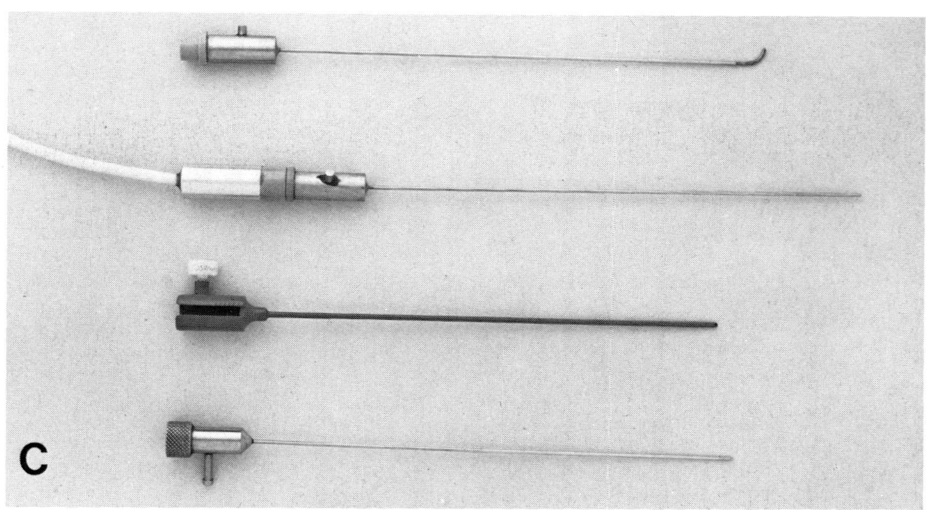

C

ophthalmologic treatment. Application of a soft contact lens, meticulous eye care, and occasional tarsorrhaphy prevented permanent visual loss.

Transient diplopia occurred in 2 percent of patients. The abducens nerve in the lateral dural wall of the cavernous sinus was the most commonly injured nerve, followed in order of frequency by the trochlear nerve and the oculomotor nerve (Figure 97-8). The most persistent diplopia was 4 months in duration. This complication was generally encountered when a lesion was created in the ophthalmic division.

Motor Paresis

Paresis of muscles innervated by the motor root of the trigeminal nerve occurred in 19 percent of patients. The motor root lies medial to the ganglion and can be avoided by rotating the curved electrode laterally if stimulation produces masseter contraction. Thus, the incidence of immediate postoperative muscle paresis was reduced from 24 percent to 13 percent by use of the more mobile curved electrode. In most instances the deficit was partial and transient.

Herpes Simplex

Lesions of herpes simplex were noted in 3 percent of patients. Since most were not examined more than 48 hours postoperatively, this figure is undoubtedly low.

Recurrence of Trigeminal Neuralgia

As the technique has become more refined, our strategy for its application has altered. The ease with which the procedure can be repeated allows production of a "light" sensory lesion as initial treatment: hypalgesia or analgesia in the primary division affected; hypalgesia in divisions secondarily affected or divisions harboring trigger zones. As this group of patients is followed, their recurrence rate is expected to rise (currently 14 percent), but the rate of troublesome dysesthesias (3 percent) remains low.

DISCUSSION

The role of percutaneous stereotactic rhizotomy in the treatment of trigeminal neuralgia has been investigated and discussed by numerous authors. Our long-term results with 950 patients responding to follow-up and treated by stereotactic rhizotomy using a straight electrode and subsequently the curved electrode are presented. In spite of the extensive experience of many neurosurgeons, there continues to be a high rate of undesirable side effects in patients treated by this procedure (Table 97-4) . Mild to moderate paresthesias and burning sensations were recorded in 93 percent of patients in one series.[28] Burchiel recently reported 15 percent mild paresthesias and 4 percent severe paresthesias.[29] Apfelbaum[30] reported 11 percent severe paresthesias which were sometimes as troublesome as the disease itself and for which there is no effective treatment. Sweet and Wepsic[31] reported loss of trigeminal motor function in 43 percent of patients, and in 40 percent of those, the motor loss was severe. Nugent reported motor weakness in 43 percent of his patients.[32]

In our experience the most troublesome side effects have been sensory paresthesias and trigeminal motor weakness. This

Table 97-4. Comparison of side effects

Reference	Number of Cases	Pares-thesias %	Anesthesia Dolorosa (%)	Motor Root Weakness (%)
Apfelbaum[30]	48	*	12	2
Burchiel[29]	78	15	4	*
Menzel[28]	315	93	2	50
Nugent	65	*	5	43
Sweet[31]	274	2	1	43
Tew	950	22	1	18

* Not reported.

report details our results in a group of 950 patients followed for 1 to 18 years (average: 8 years). The rate of recurrence, reoperation, and subsequent complications is expected to increase with extended follow-up. The application of new tactics and new technology, such as the curved electrode, has kept morbidity statistics at a level acceptable for continued use of the procedure. Glycerol rhizotomy has theoretical appeal as a mechanism for relief of pain without sensory loss; however, recent data suggest that this technique may likewise be destructive and sensory denervation a requisite to avoid recurrence.[33] Microvascular decompression will relieve trigeminal neuralgia but it has a recurrence rate equivalent to that of percutaneous rhizotomy.[15] Since trigeminal neuralgia is a benign condition, this operation must be avoided in patients with significant risk factors for craniotomy. The success of the procedure does not necessarily validate its theoretical framework. Microvascular decompression may well represent a form of subtle, chronic injury of the trigeminal sensory root. Peripheral neurectomy of any of the three peripheral branches of the trigeminal nerve must be a part of the armamentarium of all surgeons who would treat this condition.

COMPARISONS OF PERCUTANEOUS RHIZOTOMY WITH OTHER MAJOR SURGICAL PROCEDURES

Percutaneous rhizotomy can be compared with other major surgical procedures on the basis of complications and incidence of recurrent pain. No attempt was made to compare our results with all the series reported; only those that appeared to be representative were selected. Follow-up for percutaneous rhizotomy has not been as long as that for intracranial rhizotomy; therefore, recurrence data may not be comparable. Data for mortality and morbidity should be significant, however (Table 97-5).

Analysis indicates that the percutaneous approach is associated with the lowest mortality and morbidity. Recurrence rates compare favorably with those following intracranial rhizotomy, if analogous portions of the root are destroyed in both operations. Facial palsy has been eliminated, but ocular palsy occurs more frequently than in any other major procedure. The incidence of troublesome numbness ranks favorably with that reported for other forms of rhizotomy. This major side effect, however, has been eliminated in decompression proce-

---

Fig. 97-8 (A–C). A lateral roentgenogram demonstrating the course of the oculomotor, abducens, and trochlear nerves and their relationship to the trajectory of the electrode. The tip of the electrode should not extend more than 8 mm deep to the profile of the clivus.

Table 97-5. Analysis of comparative techniques and results in 2480 cases
of percutaneous rhizotomy

Technique	Number of cases	Recurrence Rate (%)	Surgical follow-up (years)	Relief of Pain* (%)	Complications (Percent of Patients)							
					Mortality	Ataxia	Corneal Ulcer	Facial Palsy	Ocular Palsy	Motor Palsy	Paresthesia	Anesthesia Dolorosa
Percutaneous rhizotomy												
Tew	950	14	8	98	0	0	2	0	2	18	22	1
Sweet and Wepsic[18]	274	22	4	91	0	0	NR (1 patient blind)	0	0	43	2	1
Menzel et al.[28]	315	80	12	97	0	0	0	0	NR	50	93	2
Decompression												
Svien and Love[9]	100	84	4	24	1.0	0	0	NR	0	0	0	0
Transtemporal rhizotomy												
Peet and Schneider[46]	553	14	8	95	1.6	NR	15	6	NR	NR	55	4
Posterior fossa rhizotomy												
Dandy[47]	88	NR	2	100	2.0	NR	0	1	2	0	0	0
Vascular decompression												
Jannetta[14]	200	4.5	4	98	0.5	2	0	0	1	0	0	0

NR = Not reported.
* = immediately postoperative.

dures. Temporal decompression is associated with a prohibitive recurrence rate, but vascular decompression, as described by Jannetta,[14] appears to provide an attractive alternative to percutaneous rhizotomy, particularly in young patients. As more experience is gained with this method, the incidence of successful pain relief and the freedom from recurrence can be better defined.

PERCUTANEOUS COAGULATION IN OTHER PAINFUL CONDITIONS

MULTIPLE SCLEROSIS

A review of several series indicates that approximately 1 percent of patients suffering from multiple sclerosis will develop trigeminal neuralgia.[34] Another perspective is that 4 percent of patients with trigeminal neuralgia have evidence of multiple sclerosis. A cause-and-effect relationship is generally accepted based on the identification of sclerotic myelin plaques on the trigeminal sensory root and descending trigeminal nucleus in several patients with this combination of disorders.[35] We have encountered 40 such patients, who constitute 4 percent of the entire group. Although trigeminal neuralgia was the initial symptom of multiple sclerosis in 5 percent of the tic-multiple sclerosis group, signs and symptoms of multiple sclerosis preceding the onset of trigeminal neuralgia had been overlooked. There is no difference in technique or results utilizing the percutaneous method in patients with multiple sclerosis. There is always concern that pain may be caused by a central plaque not amenable to rhizotomy, but experience has not borne out these fears. Special consideration, however, should be given to tactic. The tic-multiple sclerosis patient group has a greater tendency toward bilateral trigeminal neuralgia. Every effort should be made to preserve the motor root, thus preserving options for future contralateral treatment.

ATYPICAL FACIAL PAIN

Atypical facial pain is a "wastebasket" diagnostic category that includes psychological disorders with facial somatization, atypical trigeminal neuralgia, dental neuralgia, neuralgia of other regional nerves (e.g., sphenopalatine, Sluder's neuralgia), postherpetic neuralgia, vascular syndromes (cluster headache, lower facial migraine), TMJ dysfunction, and an endless list of real and imaginary diagnoses.[36–39] Denervation of the region of the face that harbors the pain will benefit less than 20 percent of patients in this category and another 20 percent will be wors-

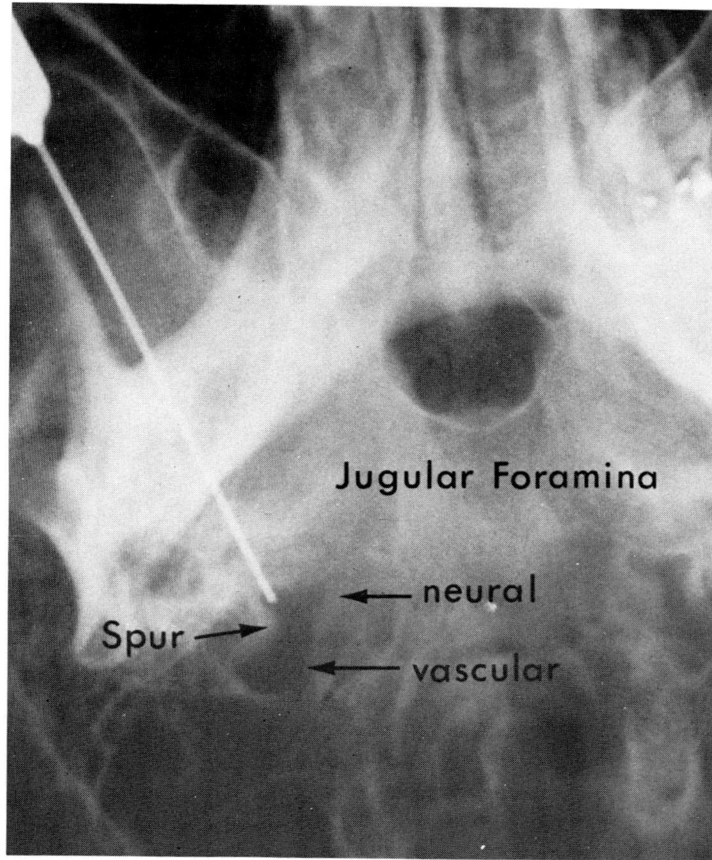

Fig. 97-9.   Needle penetrating the neural portion of the jugular foramen. Note the bony spur that divides the neural from the vascular portion.

ened by the addition of paresthesias and dysesthesias to their original complaint. We have performed percutaneous stereotactic rhizotomy on 62 such patients. The majority of patients are eliminated as surgical candidates by a failure to obtain relief from a test block of the trigeminal ganglion with 0.3 ml 0.75 percent Marcaine anesthetic. Pain caused by regional invasive tumors or carcinoma can be controlled by this technique.

VAGOGLOSSOPHARYNGEAL NEURALGIA

The incidence of glossopharyngeal neuralgia to trigeminal neuralgia is approximately 1:100 in this series. Initial therapy must be with agents documented to affect trigeminal neuralgia (e.g., carbamazepine, lioresal). Primary surgical therapy consists of an intradural section of the glossopharyngeal nerve and the upper one third of the vagal rootlets.[40] Percutaneous radiofrequency neurolysis of the glossopharyngeal nerve in the external nervus portion of the jugular canal was first reported by Tew (1977).[41] Safe penetration of the jugular foramen and physiologic identification of the glossopharyngeal nerve was discovered inadvertently during early experience with percutaneous rhizotomy for trigeminal neuralgia. Subsequent anatomic studies elucidated appropriate facial and bony landmarks that facilitate safe, reproducible penetration of the jugular foramen. Stimulation parameters for physiologic localization are required during clinical application of the procedure.[42] A free-hand technique guided by lateral fluoroscopy is used similar to that described for trigeminal neuralgia. A basal view of the skull demonstrates that the pars nervosa of the jugular foramen is in

a direct line with and posterior to the foramen ovale (Figure 97-9). The electrode entry point is 2.5 cm lateral to the oral commissure. The general target is the intersection of two planes: a sagittal plane through the pupil and a coronal plane through a point 3 cm anterior to the tragus of the ear (Figure 97-2). The specific target on the intersection line requires a caudal inclination of the electrode 14 degrees below the trajectory to the foramen ovale (Figure 97-10). On true lateral fluoroscopic images the jugular foramen is situated immediately posterior to the temporomandibular joint and anterior to the occipital condyle. The trajectory in the sagittal plane carries the electrode medial to the orifice of the carotid canal. Carotid artery penetration should be avoided but is not associated with significant complications unless penetration is unrecognized and attempts at lesion generation inside the artery are made. Physiologic localization is accomplished by stimulation with 100 to 300 mV current using a 1-msec square wave plus at 10 to 75 Hz. This will result in pain in the ear and throat. Higher current level stimulation produces cough and contraction of the sternocleidomastoid.

The procedure is performed in the radiography suite and small doses of methohexital (Brevital) are administered intravenously during painful parts of the procedure. Utilizing the Tew tic curved electrode (Radionics, Inc., Burlington, Massachusetts) with thermocouple tip, thermal lesions of the rootlets are started at 60°C for 90 seconds and repeated at 5° increments until the tonsillar pharynx is analgesic and previous triggers fail to reproduce glossopharyngeal pain.

Because of sensory denervation of the ipsilateral gag reflex

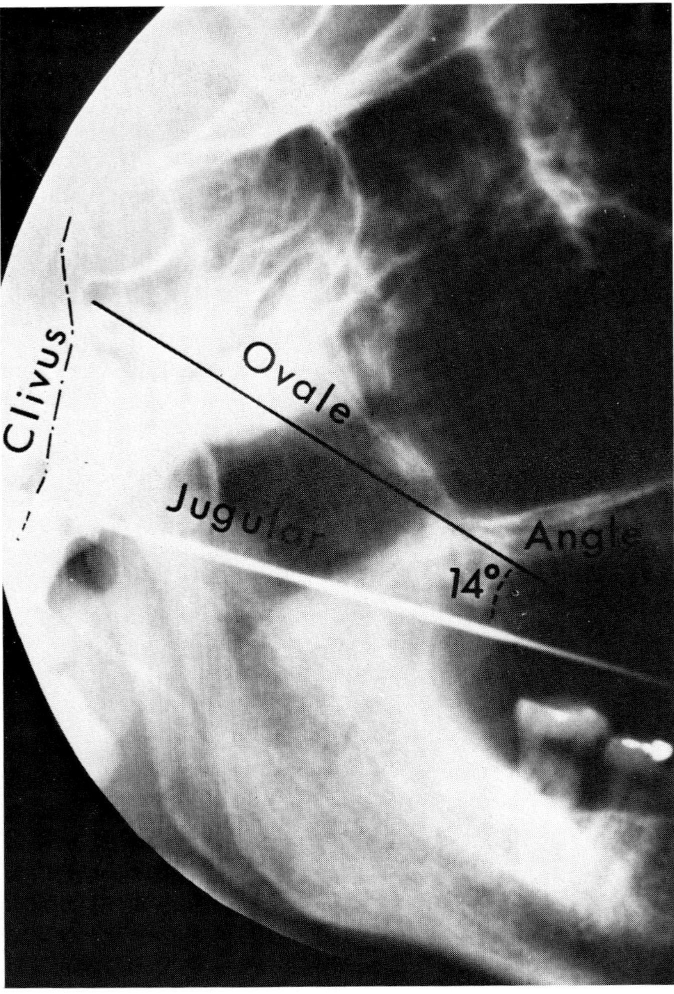

Fig. 97-10. A composite illustration demonstrating the trajectory of approaches to the foramen ovale and jugular foramen. The sagittal plane is identical for both procedures.

and possible paralysis of the ipsilateral vocal cord, this procedure has been largely restricted to patients with secondary neuralgia resulting from neoplasm. Modification of physiologic monitoring during lesion generation has allowed application of this technique to patients with idiopathic glossopharyngeal neuralgia.[43] Hypotension or bradycardia during a reversible heating test before lesion production or during lesion production indicates spread to vagal fibers and requires repositioning of the electrode tip. Selective preservation of vocal cord innervation can thereby be accomplished. A lateral percutaneous approach has also been described.[44]

Complications consist mainly of denervation of the gag reflex and vocal cord paralysis in patients with idiopathic neuralgia. There is a single report of syncope and cardiac arrest during lesion generation, presumably the result of activation of a vagal reflex.[45]

CONCLUSION

Percutaneous rhizotomy of the trigeminal nerve is a safe, elegant procedure in experienced hands. The benign nature of disorders treated by this technique demands a procedure of similar low morbidity and negligible mortality. The recurrence rate for procedures applied to trigeminal neuralgia are similar whether considering percutaneous stereotactic rhizotomy, open rhizotomy, microvascular decompression, or chemical neurolysis. Recurrence is not a significant problem with percutaneous stereotactic rhizotomy because the procedure is easily repeated and the success rates is similar to that of the initial procedure. Acceptance of a higher recurrence rate will allow creation of less severe lesions with a reduction of denervation paresthesias and dysesthesias. The application of percutaneous rhizotomy in other types of facial pain has also been described. Radiofrequency rhizotomy is a destructive procedure and therefore not the theoretically ideal treatment for any condition. Its widespread application underscores the deficient state of current strategies for treating facial pain.

REFERENCES

1. Hartley F: Intracranial neurectomy of the second and third divisions of the fifth nerve. NY J Med 55:317, 1892
2. Krause F: Resection des Trigeminus innerhalb der Schädelhöhle. Arch Klin Chir 41:821, 1892
3. Krause F: Entfernung des Ganglion Gasseri und des Central daron gelegnen trigemenusstammes. Dtsch Med Wochenschr 19:341, 1893
4. Horsley V: Remarks on the various surgical procedures devised for the relief or cure of trigeminal neuralgia. Br Med J 2:1139, 1891
5. Spiller WG, Frazier CH: The division of the sensory root of the trigeminus for the relief of tic douloureux. Univ Pa Med Bull 14:341, 1901
6. Spiller WG, Frazier CH: An experimental study of the regeneration of the posterior spinal root. Univ Pa Med Bull 16:126, 1903
7. Shelden CH, Pudenz RH, Freshwater D, et al: Compression rather than decompression for trigeminal neuralgia. J Neurosurg 12:123, 1955
8. Taarnhoj P: Decompression of the trigeminal root. J Neurosurg 11:299, 1954
9. Svien HS, Love JG: Results of decompression operation for trigeminal neuralgia four years plus after operation. J Neurosurg 16:653, 1959
10. Gardner WS: Concerning the mechanisms of trigeminal neuralgia and hemifacial spasm. J Neurosurg 19:947, 1962
11. Harris W: Alcohol injection of the gasserian ganglion for trigeminal neuralgia. Lancet 1:218, 1912
12. Harris W: An analysis of 1433 cases of paroxysmal trigeminal neuralgia (trigeminal-tic) and the end results of gasserian alcohol injection. Brain 63:653, 1940
13. Dandy WE: Concerning the cause of trigeminal neuralgia. Am J Surg 24:447, 1934
14. Jannetta P: Microsurgical approach to the trigeminal nerve for tic douloureux, in Progress in Neurological Surgery, vol 7. Basel, S. Karger, 1976, pp 180–200
15. van Loveren H, Tew JM, Keller JT, Nurre MA: A 10-year experience in the treatment of trigeminal neuralgia: A comparison of percutaneous stereotaxic rhizotomy and posterior fossa exploration. J Neurosurg 57:757, 1982
16. Kirschner M: Elektrocoagulation des ganglion gasseri. Zentralbl Chir 47:2841, 1932
17. Kirschner M: Zur behandlung der Trigeminusneuralgie. Med Wochenschr 89:235, 1942
18. Sweet WH, Wepsic SG: Controlled thermocoagulation of trigeminal ganglion and results for differential destruction of pain fibers. J Neurosurg 39:143, 1974
19. White JC, Sweet WH: Pain and the Neurosurgeon. Springfield, Ill, Charles C Thomas, 1969
20. Garvan NJ, Siegfried J: Trigeminal neuralgia—earlier referral for surgery. Postgrad Med J 59:435, 1983

21. Bullett E, Tew JM, Boyd J: Intracranial tumors in patients with facial pain. J Neurosurg 64:865, 1986

22. Letcher FS, Goldring S: The effect of radiofrequency current and heat on peripheral nerve action potential in the cat. J Neurosurg 29:42, 1968

23. Brodkey JS, Miyazaki Y, Ervin FR, et al: Reversible heat lesions with radiofrequency current. J Neurosurg 21:49, 1964

24. Härtel F: über die intracranielle Injektionsbehandlung der Trigeminusneuralgie. Med Klin 10:582, 1914

25. Tator CH, Rowed DW: Fluoroscopy of foramen ovale as an aid to thermocoagulation of the gasserian ganglion. J Neurosurg 44:254, 1976

26. Rish BL: Cerebrovascular accident after percutaneous thermocoagulation of the trigeminal ganglion. J Neurosurg 44:376, 1976

27. Gonzalez G, Onofrio BM, Ken FW: Vasodilator system of the face. J Neurosurg 42:696, 1975

28. Menzel J, Piotrowsin W, Penzholz H: Long-term results of gasserian ganglion electrocoagulation. J Neurosurg 42:140, 1975

29. Burchiel KJ, Steege TD, Howe JF, et al: Comparison of percutaneous radiofrequency gangliolysis and microvascular decompression for the surgical management of tic douloureux. Neurosurgery 9:111, 1981

30. Apfelbaum RI: A comparison of percutaneous radiofrequency trigeminal neurolysis and microvascular decompression of the trigeminal nerve for the treatment of tic douloureux. Neurosurgery 1:16, 1977

31. Sweet WH, Wepsic JG: Controlled thermocoagulation of trigeminal ganglion and rootlets for differential destruction of pain fibers. Part 1. Trigeminal neuralgia. J Neurosurg 40:143, 1974

32. Nugent GR, Berry B: Trigeminal neuralgia treated by differential percutaneous radiofrequency coagulation of the gasserian ganglion. J Neurosurg 40:517, 1974

33. Sweet WH: The treatment of trigeminal neuralgia (tic douloureaux). Current concepts. N Engl J Med 315:174, 1986

34. Rushton JG, Olafson RA: Trigeminal neuralgia associated with multiple sclerosis. Report of 35 cases. Arch Neurol 13:383, 1965

35. Lazar ML, Kirkpatrick JB: Trigeminal neuralgia and multiple sclerosis: Demonstration of the plaque in an operative case. Neurosurgery 5:711, 1979

36. Engel GL: Primary atypical facial neuralgia: An hysterical conversion symptom. Psychosom Med 13:375, 1951

37. Engel GL: "Psychogenic" pain and the pain-prone patient. Am J Med 26:899, 1959

38. Fay T: Atypical facial neuralgia, a syndrome of vascular pain. Ann Otol Rhinol Laryngol 41:1030, 1932

39. Keller JT, van Loveren H: Pathophysiology of the pain of trigeminal neuralgia and atypical facial pain: A neuroanatomical perspective. Clin Neurosurg 32:275, 1985

40. Tew JM, van Loveren H, Thomas G: Glossopharyngeal and geniculate neuralgia, in Youmans J (ed): Youmans Textbook of Neurosurgery (in press)

41. Tew JM Jr: Percutaneous rhizotomy in the treatment of intractable facial pain (trigeminal, glossopharyngeal, and vagal nerves), in Schmidek HH, Sweet WH (eds): Current Techniques in Operative Neurosurgery. New York, Grune & Stratton, 1977, pp 409–426

42. Lazorthes Y, Verdie J: Radiofrequency coagulation of the petrous ganglion in glossopharyngeal neuralgia. Neurosurgery 4:512, 1979 43. Isamat F, Ferran E, Acebes JJ: Selective percutaneous thermocoagulation rhizotomy in essential glossopharyngeal neuralgia. J Neurosurg 55:575, 1981

44. Saker G, Ori C, Baratto V, et al: Selective percutaneous thermolesions of the ninth cranial nerve by lateral cervical approach: Report of eight cases. Surg Neurol 20:276, 1983

45. Ori C, Salar G, Giron G: Percutaneous glossopharyngeal thermocoagulation complicated by syncope and seizures. Neurosurgery 4:427, 1983

46. Peet MM, Schneider RD: Trigeminal neuralgia. J Neurosurg 9:367, 1952

47. Dandy WE: Operation for cure of tic douloureaux, partial section of the sensory root at the pons. Arch Surg 18:687, 1929

Commentary: Percutaneous Rhizotomy

William H. Sweet

Tew and Lazorthes et al. independently in 1977 described their percutaneous radiofrequency techniques and results in the management of both idiopathic or "essential" vagoglossopharyngeal neuralgia and of cancer pain in this area.[1,2] Significant discrepancies in the directions for aiming the electrode characterize a number of the published accounts and make clear the major reliance we all place on the initial radiographic localization before stimulation.

It has been much more difficult for me to place an electrode tip properly for this objective than to get into Meckel's cave for the management of trigeminal pain. The tip must lie in or just below the pars nervosa of the jugular foramen, preferably in its anterolateral part where the upper vagal and glossopharyngeal fibers typically lie. Possibly this account may help the novice.

My principal difficulty has been in identifying with certainty the pars nervosa, and my neurorodiologic colleague, Dr. Paul New, and I have needed to use fluoroscopy with a standing image as well as films for this purpose. The bony spur intruding into the jugular foramen, which separates the larger lateral opening for the jugular bulb from the smaller medial opening for the ninth, tenth, and eleventh nerves, is the key to orientation. On the way into this destination one would prefer to miss the trigeminal third division and especially the internal carotid artery below its entrance into the petrous portion of the temporal bone. Figures 97-12A and B, views of a skull, show the black electrode shaft in proper position passing medial to both the mandibular branch and the artery. To position the electrode properly, it is best inserted only about 5 mm lateral to the labial commissure and 5 mm below the labial intercommissural line. Note that the hypoglossal foramen is further posterior in the same trajectory. In Figure 97-12B the skull is rotated a little more to the opposite side in order to make the critical bony spur more evident. I recommend deliberately aiming more medial than the pars nervosa at first, toward the innocuous broad expanse of the undersurface of the body of the sphenoid bone. Figure 97-13A illustrates the preliminary position of the electrode tip medial to the pars nervosa on bone. Figures 97-13B, C, and D are different projections in progressively increasing flexion, taken without changing the position of the electrode at the site where the successful lesions were made. They illustrate the fact that once the jugular foramen is spotted a variety of projections will show it. Viewed laterally, the electrode shaft was in line with the upper border of the tragus. Viewed in the sagittal plane, it was pointing in a line 9 mm lateral to the medial border of the lacrimal caruncle—representative of the measurements for the proper position. In order to go by the lateral pterygoid plate, the electrode may also have to pass below the middle of the foramen ovale. To my surprise, this usually has evoked no sensation referable to the third trigeminal division. In this patient, who had vagoglossopharyngeal neuralgia, stimulation at electrode placement in the lateral portion of the pars nervosa yielded a buzzing in the side of the throat and in front of the upper part of the pinna at 0.17 V of a square-wave signal at 50/sec. At 41°C there was burning in the ear canal.

Because of the reports of Lazorthes[2] of 3 cases of temporary vocal cord paralysis and dysphagia and of Tew[1] of 2 cases of vocal cord paralysis, I have sought to make these lesions in smaller increments and with the patient less obtunded than for trigeminal lesions. Hoarseness and swallowing then can be checked during making of the lesion as well as after it has been produced. The patient in Figure 97-13 is an example of this. During the two hours of intermittent radiofrequency heating, the temperature of the 20-gauge electrode with a 5-mm bare tip was finally kept at 105°C for 3 minutes, during which time no Brevital was required. After this degree of heating, the highest I have ever used, the patient had hypalgesia of the ipsilateral soft palate and oral pharynx but not of the tonsillar fossa. Not until the next day did some slight hoarseness and dysphagia develop. Some hoarseness, if she did much talking, and modest dysphagia persisted for 6 months. The pain remained relieved at 100 months, although she has recovered normalgesia on pinprick testing.

As with trigeminal radiofrequency heating, continuous electrocardiography and intra-arterial monitoring of blood fluid pressure are advisable.[4] Although dangerous blood pressure rises are less likely than with retrogasserian radiofrequency heating, the reverse changes of bradycardia and hypotension even to the point of cardiac arrest are much more frequent and demand prompt cessation of the heating. Thus, hypotension or bradycardia to a level less than half of the preoperative value occurred during 6 of the 11 procedures described in Ori et al.[5] Syncope in 2 of their patients followed a serious drop in pulse rate and blood pressure and one of the 2 required cardiac massage because of asystole and a convulsive seizure. It is apparent that one must promptly give intravenous atropine and replace the electrode to combat these vagal effects. Happily there were no permanent sequelae. Possibly their decision to use only fentanyl and no brief intravenous anesthetic agent plus a lateral approach transfixing the pars nervosa from lateral to

OPERATIVE NEUROSURGICAL TECHNIQUES
ISBN 0-8089-1862-1

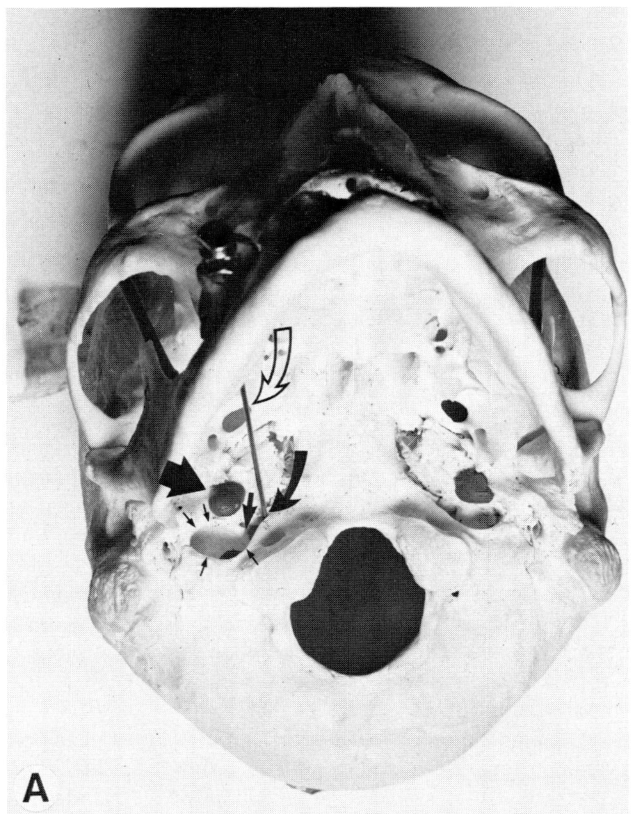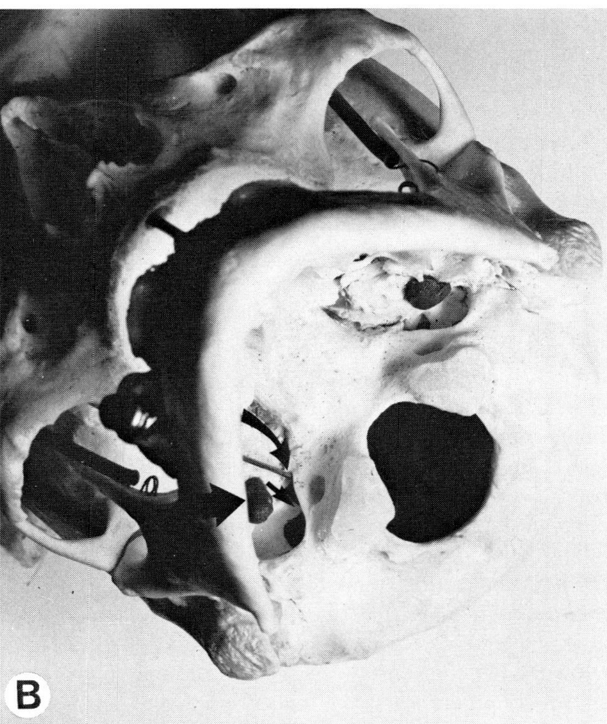

Fig. 97-12. Basal views of the skull with an electrode tip in the pars nervosa of the jugular foramen. (A) Slight rotation of the skull away from the side of the electrode in the head-extended position. Open curved arrow: electrode shaft overlying the medial corner of the foramen ovale. Closed curved arrow: electrode tip in medial corner of the pars nervosa. Large black arrowhead: internal carotid artery. Small black arrowhead: bony spur separating the pars nervosa for the jugular bulb from the smaller pars nervosa for the ninth, tenth, and eleventh nerves and associated ganglia.. Small arrows: margins of the pars nervosa. (B) More marked rotation of the skull with no extension of the head. Arrows are as in A. The bony spur is more obvious.

medial led to so many of these problems. Observing careful precautions, Isamat et al. maintained normal phonation and swallowing while relieving 4 patients with the idiopathic disorder.

The lateral cervical approach may be required if tumor at the base of the skull lies anterior to the jugular foramen.

Typically the glossopharyngeal fibers lie anterior and lateral to the upper vagal rootlets in the pars nervosa of the foramen, the orientation to guide replacement of the electrode if vagal motor responses occur. Despite my occasional use of much higher temperatures than the 75°C used by Isamat et al.[4] or the 65°C for 2 minutes used by Salar et al.,[6] we have had no significant postoperative problems with phonation or swallowing in 5 patients. There are now at least 7 reports of a satisfactory initial reduction of pain in 27 patients with tumors, and more complete relief in 18 with the "essential" disorder. Those with facial pain as well from their tumors have also required a retrogasserian radiofrequency lesion.[1–4,6–8] My patient with oropharyngofacial cancer pain was not helped. Those with the idiopathic disease do not require major analgesia throughout the throat and ear canal to be relieved. This is fortunate because neither the RF lesions nor indeed open rhizotomies of cranial nerve IX and the upper rootlets of X are likely to yield extensive analgesia. Of the 6 idiopathic patients

of Giorgi and Broggi, only one was a complete failure requiring open operation and the only one of their 11 patients who had persistent dysphagia was one of 5 who also had a tumor.[8] Repetition of the procedure in the event of initial failure or recurrence has been readily done.

It is impossible to enter the intracranial cavity via the approach to the jugular foramen. Hence, there have been no intracranial hemorrhages from the procedure as have followed retrogasserian rhizotomy and none is likely to occur. Moreover, oropharyngeal dysesthesias do not follow such lesions—open or percutaneous.

A dural sleeve may encase the rootlet bundle down into the jugular foramen, as attested by my obtaining CSF at this site in 3 patients. Moreover, the lower ganglion of IX, the petrous ganglion of Anderch, lies in the jugular foramen and the lower or nodose ganglion of the vagus lies below the jugular foramen so that one is making a lesion at or central to the cells of origin of the afferent fibers in both nerves. This probably accounts for the encouraging recurrence rate to date in the idiopathic group. Thus, Giorgi and Broggi reported 3 patients free of pain at 3, 4, and 5 years and 2 with recurrences at 2 and 3 years. Of my four such cases relief persists at 1 and 8 years in two with recurrences now controlled by medication in the other two.

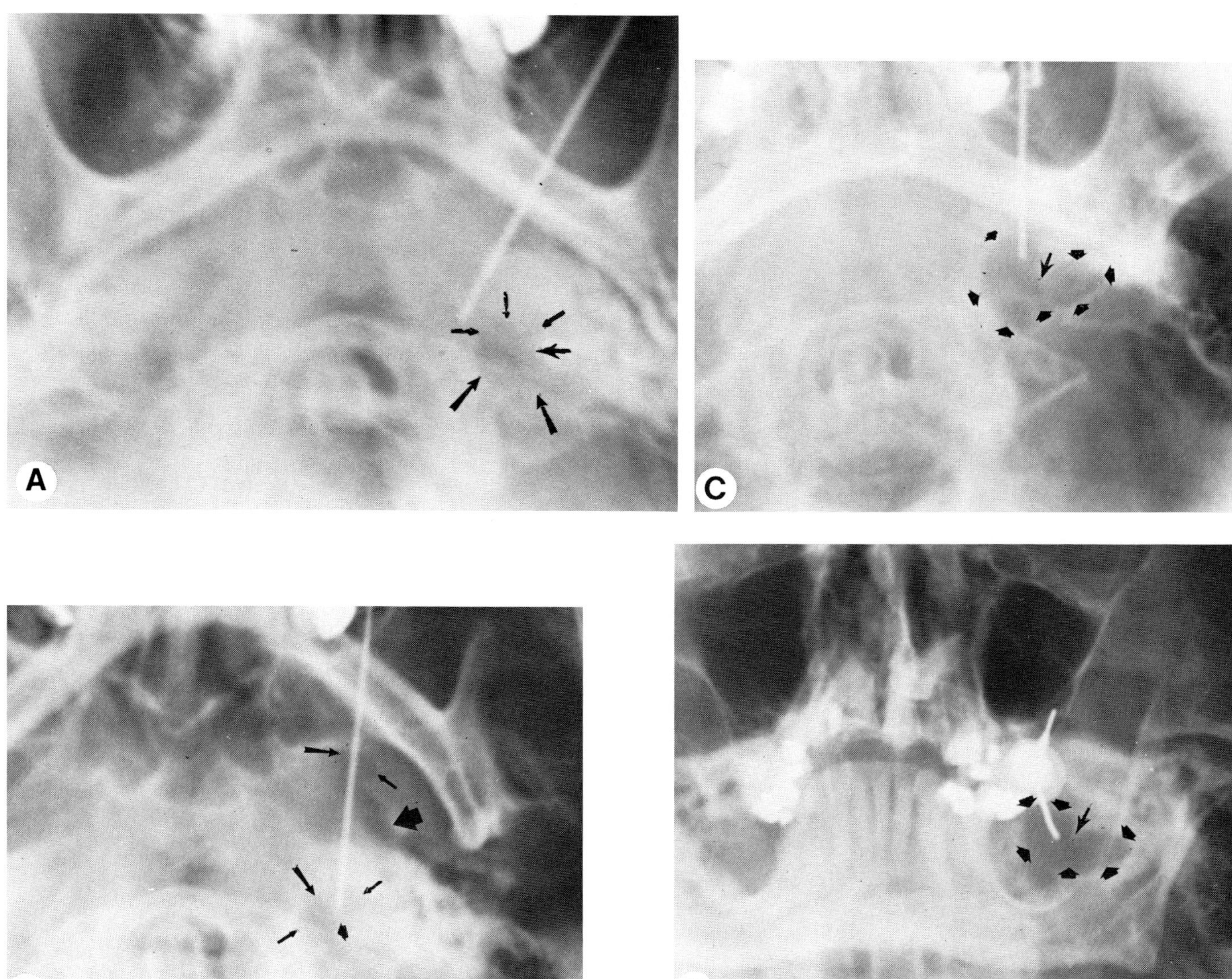

Fig. 97-13. (A) An electrode tip against the base of the body of the sphenoid bone medial to the pars nervosa of the foramen. (B,C,D) The electrode tip in position for lesion in the lateral part of the pars nervosa. Three projections in progressively less extension. (B) Shaft overlies approximately the middle of the foramen ovale. Arrows in A and B outline the pars nervosa; the two anterior arrows in B indicate the medial and lateral margins of the foramen ovale. Large arrowhead: opening for internal carotid artery. Arrowheads in C and D outline visible margins of both the pars nervosa and the pars venosa, with the small arrow pointing to the bony spur that divides the two portions.

REFERENCES

1. Tew JM: Percutaneous rhizotomy in the treatment of intractable facial pain (trigeminal, glossopharyngeal, and vagal nerves), in Schmidek HH, Sweet WH (eds): Current Techniques in Operative Neurosurgery. New York, Grune & Stratton, 1977

2. Lazorthes Y, Verdie JC: Traitement par thermocoagulation percutané des nevralgies trigeminales et glosso-pharyngiennes. Bull Group Rec Sci Stomotol Odontol 20:297, 1977

3. Lazorthes Y, Verdie JC: Radiofrequency coagulation of the petrous ganglion in glossopharyngeal neuralgia. Neurosurgery 4:512, 1979

4. Isamat F, Ferran E, Acebes JJ: Selective percutaneous thermocoagulation rhizotomy in essential glossopharyngeal neuralgia. J Neurosurg 55:575, 1981

5. Ori C, Salar G, Giron GP: Cardiovascular and cerebral complications during glossopharyngeal nerve thermocoagulation. Anaesthesia 40:433, 1985

6. Salar G, Ori C, Baratto V, et al: Selective percutaneous thermolesions of the ninth cranial nerve by lateral cervical approach: Report of eight cases. Surg Neurol 20:276, 1983

7. Arias MJ: Percutaneous radiofrequency thermocoagulation with low temperature in the treatment of essential glossopharyngeal neuralgia. Surg Neurol 25:94, 1986

8. Giorgi C, Broggi G: Surgical treatment of glossopharyngeal neuralgia and pain from cancer of the nsaopharynx. A 20-year experience. J Neurosurg 61:952, 1984

CHAPTER 98

Retrogasserian Glycerol Injection as Treatment for Trigeminal Neuralgia

William H. Sweet

IN 1975, HÅKANSON PIONEERED the use of glycerol within Meckel's cave for the treatment of trigeminal neuralgia, stating that his technique produced no significant sensory loss and no corneal anesthesia, painful dysesthesia, or involvement of other cranial nerves.[1]

TECHNIQUE OF HÅKANSON

The patient is seated in a rotatable chair with radiography available both by fluoroscopy and film. Premedication is with 1 ml oxicon with 1 ml scopolamine plus 5 mg droperidol (Dripdol). Half this dose is used for elder or debilitated patients. Local anesthesia alone was given to 74 of the first 75 patients. A 22-gauge lumbar puncture needle, outside diameter 0.7 mm, penetrates the skin well lateral to the labial commissure. Cerebrospinal fluid must be obtained. If fluoroscopy and film show the needle tip to be approximately in the correct position, but no CSF appears, Håkanson leaves that needle in position and places another needle in what he thinks is a more correct spot. Figure 98-1 illustrates a position that is too far lateral for the original needle. Usually, the shaft must go through the medial half of the foramen ovale. This film also illustrates the next step of Håkanson's procedure, in which he injects less than 1 ml of concentrated metrizamide (300 mg/ml). Fluoroscopy shows the contrast medium filling the cistern and running back through the porus trigemini into the cerebellopontine angle. The relationship of the cerebrospinal fluid (CSF) space with the rootlets to the subdural space in the cisterna trigeminalis and to the subarachnoid space beneath the temporal lobe is demonstrated by Håkanson's diagram in Figure 98-2. Films taken after the injection of the metrizamide may demonstrate that the needle is in the subarachnoid space below the temporal lobe, or, as shown in Figure 98-3A, in the subdural space of the cistern. Placement in the subdural space is more evident as the metrizamide passes through the porus trigemini and lines the subarachnoid space behind the clivus (Figure 98-3B). Håkanson found that previous open trigeminal operations in the middle cranial fossa often damaged the trigeminal cistern so that the metrizamide would leak out of it. Figure 98-4 shows the contrast medium lying medial to the needle tip in the cistern and below one cluster of metal clips marking the site of the previous open operation. When, as occurred rarely, Håkanson was unable to secure CSF, he made a selective thermal lesion. Having verified the proper position of the needle tip, he then emptied the metrizamide into the posterior fossa by removing the syringe and extending the patient's head for several minutes. If the patient had no third-division trigger zone, however, Håkanson sought to leave a little of the heavy metrizamide (specific gravity 1.329), which will in turn form a layer below the CSF (specific gravity 1.007). He adjusts the amount of glycerol to the volume of the cistern, estimating from the metrizamide picture that the total amount of glycerol to be injected into the cistern varies from 0.2 to 0.4 ml. Figures 98-5A, B, and C illustrate the marked variation in size and configuration of the normal cistern. (In one of Håkanson's cases, the metrizamide film revealed a small benign tumor here.) In cases with first- or second-division neuralgia, Håkanson injects up to 0.25 ml; his 22-gauge needle shaft contains about 0.05 ml. He does not examine facial sensibility during the procedure or at once after the procedure. Once an injection is complete, the patient is kept sitting in bed with the head flexed for another hour in order to keep the glycerol mainly in the cistern. Håkanson has mixed tantalum dust with the glycerol before injection in most cases, so that later films show the exact size of the cistern in order to facilitate a future injection therein.

Whisler and Apfelbaum also recommend routine fluoroscopy,[2,3] to which Gomori and Rappaport[4] have added the tactic of speeding up penetration of the foramen ovale by placing a small radiopaque marker 3 cm lateral to the labial commissure at the site of needle penetration of the skin. The head is positioned for a submentovertex view with slight contralateral obliquity, and under fluoroscopy the marker is projected to overlie the foramen ovale. This, they say, enables the operator to direct the needle straight down toward the foramen, aided by intermittent fluoroscopic feedback.

RESULTS

Increasing experience with the agent has led to discrepancy in appraisals of the value of the method. Håkanson, and Lunsford, an early proponent, continue to favor it. Håkanson has described "about 350 cases with no anesthesia dolorosa or painful dysesthesia."[5] Seventy-eight percent of his first 100 patients followed for a mean of 3.8 years were pain free after 1 or more injections.[6] Of Lunsford's 225 patients, 65 percent remained pain free at follow-ups as long as 3 years, a few having required a repeat procedure.[3] Only 6 percent developed annoy-

OPERATIVE NEUROSURGICAL TECHNIQUES
ISBN 0-8089-1862-1

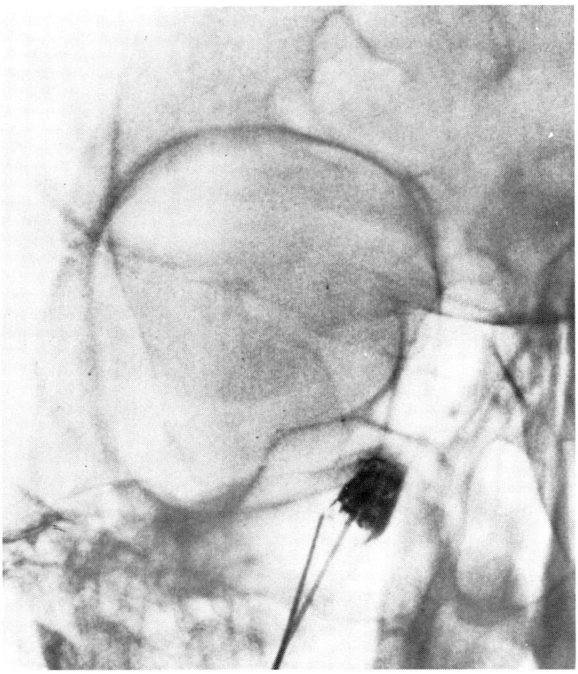

Fig. 98-1. Sagittal view of the right side of the skull with two needles through the foramen ovale, illustrating Håkanson's method of leaving in position one 22-gauge needle that has failed to yield CSF from the trigeminal cistern. The first needle was too far lateral. Metrizamide was injected into the more medial needle within the cistern. (Reprinted from Håkanson S: Treatment of trigeminal neuralgia by injection of glycerol into the trigeminal cistern. Neurosurgery 9:638-649, 1981. With permission.)

ing facial sensations and only 1 percent (2 patients) had major dysesthesias. Apfelbaum's figures for his 73 cases are similar, with 3 cases of corneal anesthesia and 90-percent relief after the initial 1 or 2 procedures. Recurrence took place in 23 percent after an average follow-up of 15 months—or a 66-percent figure for those remaining pain free.[3] There was one fatal outcome in their 298 cases; a 77-year-old patient who suffered a myocardial infarction in the recovery room. Others encouraged by the results include Dieckmann,[7] who had only 1 of 51 patients with lasting dysesthesias and 78 percent who were pain free at 1 to 4 years.[6] Arias describes 100 patients, with excellent results on virtually all scores (Table 98-1,) and as sequelae only 2 aseptic meningeal reactions.[8] Burchiel and Carson each prefer glycerol to radiofrequency (RF) lesions.[9,10] Waltz et al., in 58 cases, have had few sequelae: they report 7 aseptic meningitides, 13 with "decreased corneal reflex" and 1 cranial nerve palsy—"all transient".[11] They describe no dysesthesias. Their rate of failure to stop the pain was 17 percent after 1 or 2 injections. After a 1–32-month follow-up, their recurrence rate was also 17 percent.

Qualified endorsements come from two services, as described here.

Saini's large experience of 412 cases has yielded 55 (13 percent) with dysesthesias; 14 (3.4 percent) with anesthesia dolorosa; and none with keratitis—on the whole not really encouraging.[12,13] Beck et al., in 58 patients, had 21 percent treatment failures and 1 patient with lasting total trigeminal anesthesia and loss of corneal reflex; the most encouraging feature was absence of dysesthesias (Table 98-1).[14]

We report here the results described in published papers, and those of which we learned in a poll we took by correspondence, to which 110 neurosurgeons replied. At least 7 other

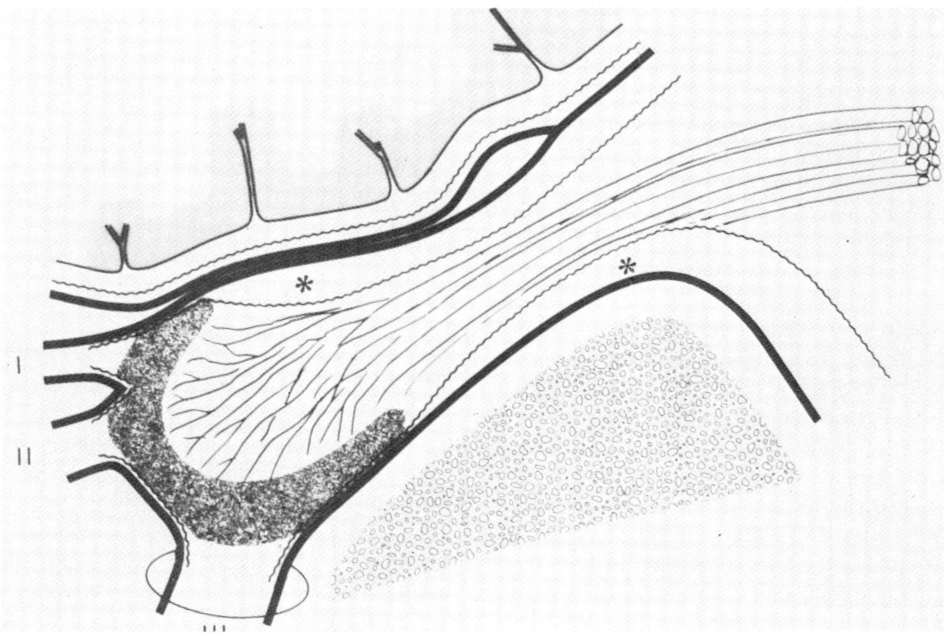

Fig. 98-2. Diagram of Håkanson illustrating the possibility of the subdural space of the trigeminal cistern being expanded by injection into it of contrast material. Asterisks in this space and below wavering lines indicate arachnoid membrane and within solid lines indicate dura. Subarachnoid and subdural spaces below temporal lobe are also indicated. (Reprinted from Håkanson S: Treatment of trigeminal neuralgia by injection of glycerol into the trigeminal cistern. Neurosurgery 9:638–649, 1981. With permission.)

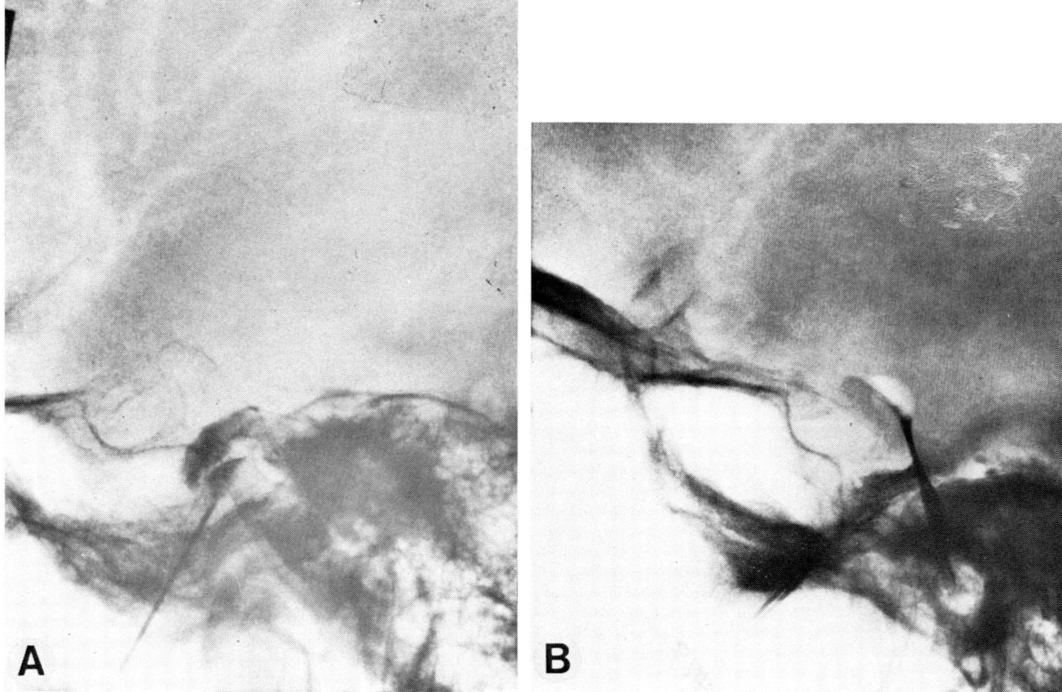

Fig. 98-3. Lateral views of the middle third of the base of the skull. (A) The metrizamide lies in two zones—one above and one below the rootlet zone. That this was in fact a subdural placement is more conclusively shown in (B), in which following extension of the head the metrizamide is seen closely applied to the full length of the clivus.

services have become dissatisfied for some combination of the following reasons:

1. Too many early failures and later recurrences.[15–22] Recurrence rates at 3 years were 40 percent for Fraioli, 57 percent for Price, and 20 percent at 1 to 3 years for Takusagawa. In our series, 15 percent with initial failures were supplemented by 28 percent with significant recurrences; 10 percent required medication and 18 percent reoperation at from 4 months to 4 years, with an average recurrence time of 1.8 years. Our rates of failure to achieve relief after one or more attempts at RF lesions come to less than 0.5 percent, this percentage mainly due to the 3 patients in whom we could not traverse completely the canal of the foramen ovale with our electrode. Our recurrence rate from this RF procedure after follow-ups of from 2½ to 7 years was 22 percent; it increased to 28 percent after follow-ups of from 4½ to 9 years.

2. Dysesthesias and major sensory loss. Håkanson's contention that these are not seen has not been confirmed. Corneal anesthesia occurred in 7 percent and dysesthesias in 21 percent of Price's cases.[19] Corneal sensation to cotton, initially normal, was reduced as a late finding in 10 (12 percent) of our patients to a level of 0–²/₁₀. In one patient, the sensation dropped from ⁵/₁₀ in the early postoperative period, to 0 at 1 month, where it remained. One of Fraioli's patients also had the delayed development at 1 month of a complete ipsilateral trigeminal anesthesia with keratitis.[15]

The worst experience regarding "painful dysesthesia" was that of Takusagawa—it occurred in 35 percent of 136 patients with a successful injection; in 2 it reached the level of anesthesia dolorosa; 3 had neuroparalytic keratitis.[22]

Igarashi et al. injected 0.15–0.6 ml glycerol in 27 patients,

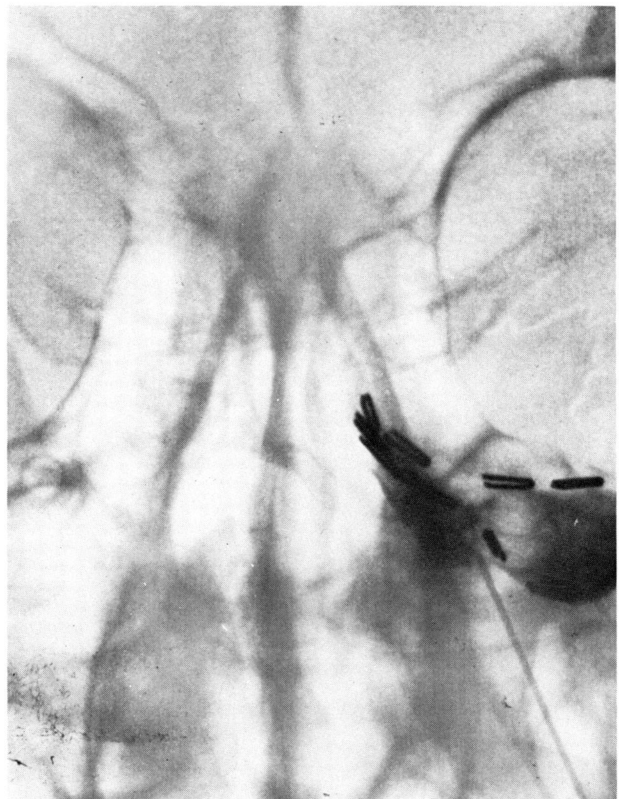

Fig. 98-4. Sagittal view of the skull near the midline. The numerous metal clips mark the site of a previous open operation to "decompress" trigeminal rootlets. The metrizamide has flowed medially away from the tip of the needle (and inferior to the medial group of clips). (Courtesy of S. Håkanson.)

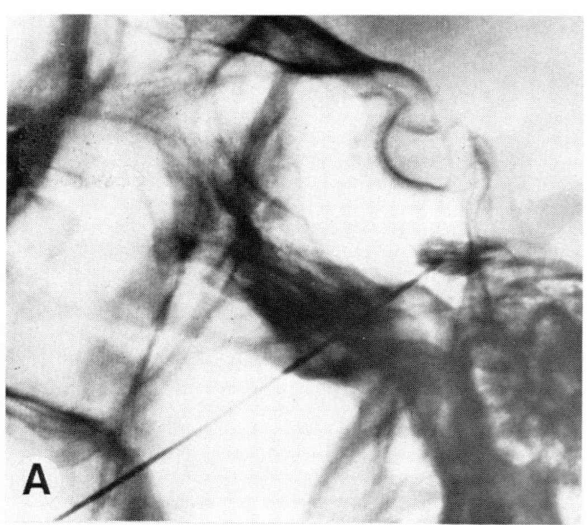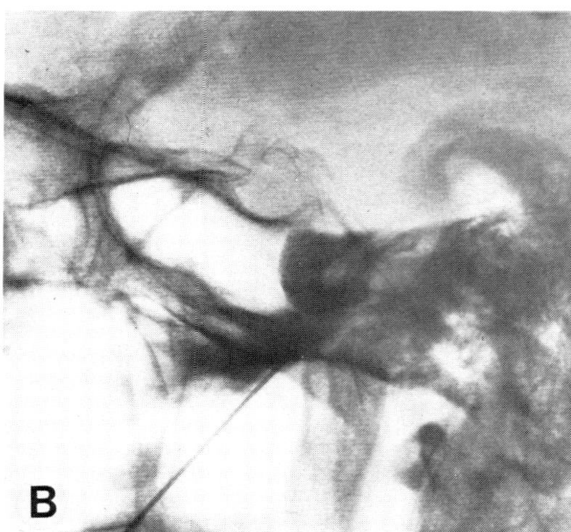

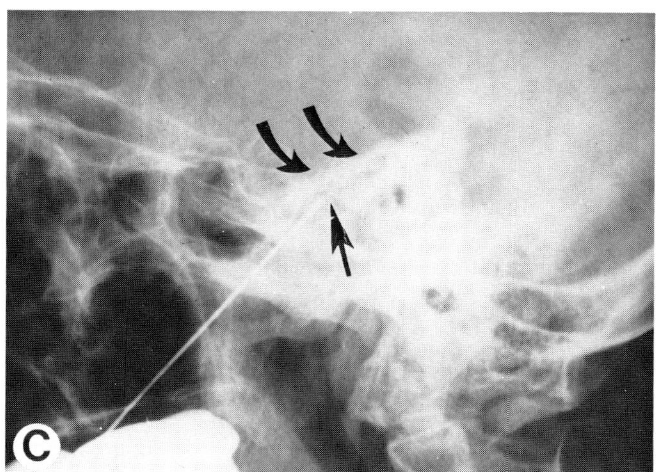

Fig. 98-5. Lateral views of the middle one third of the base of the skull showing (A) a small cistern, (B) a large cistern, and (C) an elongated cistern with irregular borders (the straight arrow points to the tip of the needle electrode; the curved arrows point to the top of the metrizamide shadow in the trigeminal cistern), Our case Ellen B. All normal variations. (A reprinted from Håkanson S: Treatment of trigeminal neuralgia by injection of glycerol into the trigeminal cistern. Neurosurgery 9:638-649, 1981. With permission.) (B courtesy of S. Håkanson.)

Table 98-1. Discrepant results of glycerol treatment for trigeminal neuralgia

	Number of Patients	Percentage Virtually Pain Free	Initial Failure (%)	Recurrent Pain Controlled with Drugs (%)	Recurrence (%)	Dysesthesia (%)	Late corneal anesthesia (%)	Followup
Håkanson (1983)	150	77	4	19	31	0	0	1–6 years; average 2½ years
Lunsford (1985)	62	66	13	19	21	3.2	0	3–18 months
Arias (1986)	100	95 (1–3 operations)	10		10	0	0	6–36 months; average nearly 2 years
Takusagawa-Fukushima (1985)	122	58	10	16	42	35	"keratitis" 3 patients	1–3 years
Beck et al. (1986)	58	72	21	7	11	0	2	2–40 months; average 18 months
Sweet-Poletti (1986)	80	52	14	10	33	20	16	1–7 years; average 2.8 years

producing initial dysesthesias in 81 percent; these persisted with hypalgesia at 8 weeks in 30 percent.[23] Of Laitinen's patients, 2 had the bitter experience of hypesthesia and dysesthesia in all 3 divisions plus no relief of the original pain; one of them had 2 injections.[17] We and Maxwell find that the patients may find the horizontal position and intermittent general anesthesia for an RF lesion preferable to the 1-hour, head-flexed, sitting position for glycerol.[18]

When no sensory loss occurs after the 0.4 ml maximum permissible injectate suggested by Håkanson, the tendency to inject more glycerol should probably be resisted. We have seen one patient in whom the first neurosurgeon injected 1.5 ml in 0.1-ml increments over 10 minutes, producing minutes later total ipsilateral trigeminal hypalgesia, but followed by intense constant pain with, at first, control of the provokable tic pains. The neurosurgeons, Lunsford and Jannetta, found at exploration 8 months later markedly atrophic trigeminal rootlets in the posterior fossa "compatible with prior injury." Severe hypalgesia dolorosa in V2 and analgesia dolorosa in V3 persisted 2 years later.

Extra-trigeminal morbidity has been minor or controllable. One case of extraocular palsy has been reported from each of 3 services. Blood pressure fluctuations during the procedure have included a patient of Fischer whose level went to 240/100 at once after glycerol was placed in the cistern. Subsidence to a normal level took 20 minutes.[24] Marked blood pressure rises with glycerol have also been noted by Young[25]; in one of his patients, the first drop of glycerol provoked such severe periorbital pain that he discontinued the procedure. Contrariwise, one of Patrick's patients had a marked fall in blood pressure related to a burst of pain in the sitting position.[26]

OUR CURRENT TACTICS

In our poll of 110 neurosurgeons of the world, we learned of 11 intracranial hemorrhages related to the needle-electrode puncture for RF lesion or glycerol injection, and 10 intracerebral hematomas distant from the needle electrode.[21]

The possibility of a hemorrhagic diathesis was suggested by the fact that many of these older patients have been on a wide variety of medications for years, and we have lately found that over 10 percent of them have an increased bleeding time greater than 9.5 minutes. Hence, we now check this, as well as prothrombin and partial thromboplastin times and platelet counts, before one of these needle-electrode procedures or an intracranial operation.

We agree with Lunsford that preoperative atropine to counteract vasovagal reactions and an anxiolytic and antiemetic agent such as droperidol (intravenously) are advisable. The patient lies supine during needle placement. Nausea has been enough of a problem in the sitting, head-flexed position so that we may supplement the initial 1.25–2.5 mg droperidol with 5–10 mg Compazine before raising the patient to the sitting position. Recent findings of dramatic increases of blood pressure during electrode placement, and, much less often, during glycerol administration, as already mentioned, have led us to use constant monitoring of blood pressure during the procedure, supplemented by intravenous sodium nitroprusside as needed to prevent such rises.[27]

In an effort to decrease the numbers of early failures, dysesthesias, and corneal anesthesias, we have modified the technique in three ways.

1. We test for physiologic responses to electrical stimulation in order to place the needle electrode to the best advantage, as we do for making an RF lesion. We seek to assure that the CSF is coming from the tip in the trigeminal cistern by adjusting it until the threshold for sensory response to pulses of 1 msec at 50 cycles/sec is 0.04–0.2 V, and that to gentle RF heating it is from 40° to 48°C—the lower the better. The electrode is adjusted so that the reference of sensation is confined to the lowest division harboring a trigger zone, i.e., the third division if both the second and third divisions contain trigger zones.

2. We use the physiologic responses of the patient to the injection as evidence that the glycerol is actually going into the trigeminal cisternal CSF rather than into the cisternal subdural space or the CSF under the temporal lobe. We inject only if a drop of CSF emerges from the needle with the patient sitting immediately prior to the placement of the glycerol syringe. The sensory responses are either of nonpainful paresthesias in a few patients, or, much more frequently, painful dysesthesias, usually evoked by the first drops of glycerol. In the sitting position in which the injection is made, it is not easy to maintain immobile the needle electrode so that no portion of the bevel lies in the subdural space, permitting some of the glycerol to lie subdurally. In fact, in one of our early patients, the flabby facial tissues allowed the needle to slip below the foramen ovale when she sat up with her head flexed. Now we have one person hold the needle electrode in its desired position for the several minutes required until the injection is finished.

In our experience, the glycerol has penetrated more readily into the first than the third division. Even keeping the patient's head fully flexed and leaning markedly toward the side of the lesion has not consistently solved this problem of securing third-division involvement. In the one patient in whom facial sensations did not occur during injection, the preinjection thresholds for electrical stimulation were also high; there was no immediate sensory loss and no relief of pain. We conclude that we failed here to make a cisternal CSF injection. (The other 11 failures did show varying degrees of early trigeminal sensory loss.) That we are usually securing an effective placement of the glycerol is indicated by the fact that in the 70 percent of our 70 cases with early relief, the relief was complete within less than 1 day, and in 27 percent more it occurred in less than 5 days. In 2 patients only was relief accomplished after a longer interval than this (at 3 and 6 weeks). Lunsford, in 62 patients, had a median latency to relief of 5 days, with a 21-day maximum.[28] Severe enough pain has been provoked during or shortly after the glycerol injection so that we keep the needle of a syringe loaded with brevital lying in the sidearm of the intravenous line, ready for instant use. When we are seeking to avoid first-division loss, we use first-division reference of sensation as an indication to withdraw slightly the electrode, so that subsequent increments cause sensation only in lower divisions.

Arias, in a comparative study of 100 cases (50 injected by each method), has also demonstrated that sensory examination during the procedure is preferable to metrizamide cisternography.[8] His tempo of injection is even slower than ours, with a wait of 1 to 5 minutes for sensory testing after each 0.05-ml increment of glycerol. He adds the useful feature of testing for correct position of the needle tip by insisting on trigeminal paresthesias or pain after the first 0.05 ml into the cistern, presumably correcting the position until this occurs. He seeks to place the needle tip at the profile of the middle third of the clivus as seen in the lateral radiograph. He finds that the preferable position of the head is a 40-degree flexion for first-division pain, 25-degree flexion for the second division, and almost erect for the third division. He keeps the patient in the appropriate position usually for an additional hour after the final drop of glycerol, decreasing this, however, if the sensory loss is greater than 30 percent. His report of excellent results urges serious consideration of the details of his technique. There has been only 1 aseptic meningeal reaction in our 83 procedures, and none in his 56 without metrizamide cisternography.

3. The promptness with which major sensory loss may develop has led us to do a sensory examination for sensitivity to pinprick after each drop of glycerol injected from 0.15 to the maximum 0.4 ml (the 10-cm shaft of a 20-gauge needle holds almost exactly 0.1 ml). We hoped that pouring the glycerol out of the trigeminal cistern by placing the patient horizontal within 20 minutes of the development of first-division analgesia would eliminate corneal anesthesia as a sequel, since many of the patients have major fading of their analgesia within the first weeks. Thus, the corneal sensation to cotton was lost in 10 (12 percent) of our patients later on the day of the procedure, and was graded 1–2/10 in another 7 patients (9 percent). By the next day or within a few months, 8 of these 17 patients had recovered some corneal sensation. Although 5 others lost some corneal sensation from levels of 5–10/10 in the early postoperative period, sensation dropped to 0 in only one of these. However, of the 4 patients who were allowed to maintain first-division analgesia by keeping glycerol in the cistern for about 20 minutes, there was recovery from the associated corneal anesthesia in only one; all four 4 had only 0.2–0.25 ml injected. Of the 23 procedures at which the glycerol was left in the cistern less than 15 minutes after the development of analgesia in the trigger areas or in the first division, no patient experienced corneal anesthesia, and any early decrease in corneal sensation did not persist. Hence, we not only recommend careful monitoring of the sensation throughout the drop-wise injection, but are tentatively concluding that limiting first-division analgesia to 10 minutes or less is likely to result in a greatly reduced incidence of corneal sensory loss. We think that a decision as to the dose of glycerol is more soundly based on the evolving sensory loss than on an estimate of the size of the trigeminal cistern.

COMPARISON BETWEEN RADIOFREQUENCY HEATING AND GLYCEROL

The most cogent data we have are in our 40 patients for whom, after radiofrequency heat or glycerol lesions were made at the first session, the other modality was used either for the recurrence or after failure of the first method. The sensations after the heating were worse in 6 patients; those after glycerol were worse in 14. No difference was noted by 6. The glycerol failed to give initial relief in 9 of these 40, the heating in 2. Of our 80 patients treated with 83 glycerol sessions, initial relief of pain occurred within 2 weeks after 70 procedures, i.e., 12 (14

percent) were complete failures. We have less than 2 percent complete failures after single RF lesions.

No dysesthesias or paresthesias at all followed 45 percent of our 70 initial successes with glycerol; and in another 20 percent, dysesthesias and paresthesias were brief and mild. Modest dysesthesias lasting from weeks to 1½ years occurred in 15 percent, and in the remaining 20 percent the dysesthesias have persisted, at times worsening, for follow-ups lasting as long as 7 years. All of these 20 percent have required medication for treatment; 2 are in the anesthesia dolorosa category of major severity. These persistent dysesthesias requiring medication have not been eliminated in subsequent cases by using small doses of glycerol for shorter periods. Thus, four of the patients in this category were limited, respectively, to 0.15 ml for 6½ minutes, 0.2 ml for 23 minutes, and 2 patients were each limited to 0.25 ml, for 4 and 5 minutes. In each instance, exposure to glycerol was stopped after analgesia had been present throughout the skin of the first 2 trigeminal divisions and, in three of the four, in the third division as well, for the specified number of minutes after the final drop of glycerol. Consequently, we are not as optimistic about controlling the problem of dysesthesias as we are about reducing the incidence of corneal sensory deficit by detailed sensory testing and reduction of the exposure time to glycerol.

Although the loss of corneal sensation, once produced, is not as likely to recover after an RF lesion as after glycerol administration, the locus and initial extent of sensory loss are more controllable with the RF heating.

We have discussed with Lunsford the major discrepancy in incidences of significant dysesthesia, and he has suggested that we may be injecting into the ganglia. We regard this as unlikely, since we have in 58 percent of our procedures injected with the needlepoint at or behind the profile of the clivus in the lateral view, and always only after CSF is obtained from the sitting patient's needle immediately before injection. Moreover, there has been minimal resistance to the injection.

MULTIPLE SCLEROSIS

Of Lunsford and Bennett's 12 patients, there was a poor result in only one,[29] whereas 3 of 4 of the multiple sclerotics of Beck et al. were failures.[14] We had failures in only 2 of our 10 procedures on these patients, with 5 recurrences at times ranging from 6 months to 2 years (average: 1.3 years); 3 patients enjoyed continuing relief at 2, 2, and 4 years.

BIOLOGICAL EFFECTS AND PROBABLE MECHANISM OF ACTION OF GLYCEROL

In our second edition (Chapter 71), we summarized the evidence that, despite a number of features suggesting a tissue protectant, especially a cryoprotectant, effect, pure glycerol is toxic to many tissues. Baxter and Schacherl found it to be as destructive to cord and nerve roots when injected intrathecally as is absolute alcohol.[30] More recently, Lunsford, Bennett, and Martinez demonstrated that a single drop (0.05 ml) of pure glycerol injected mainly into the second division of 4 cats, just behind the gasserian ganglion, provoked deterioration of evoked responses at epidural cervical 2 recording electrodes, as well as severe myelin destruction and axonal degeneration.[31]

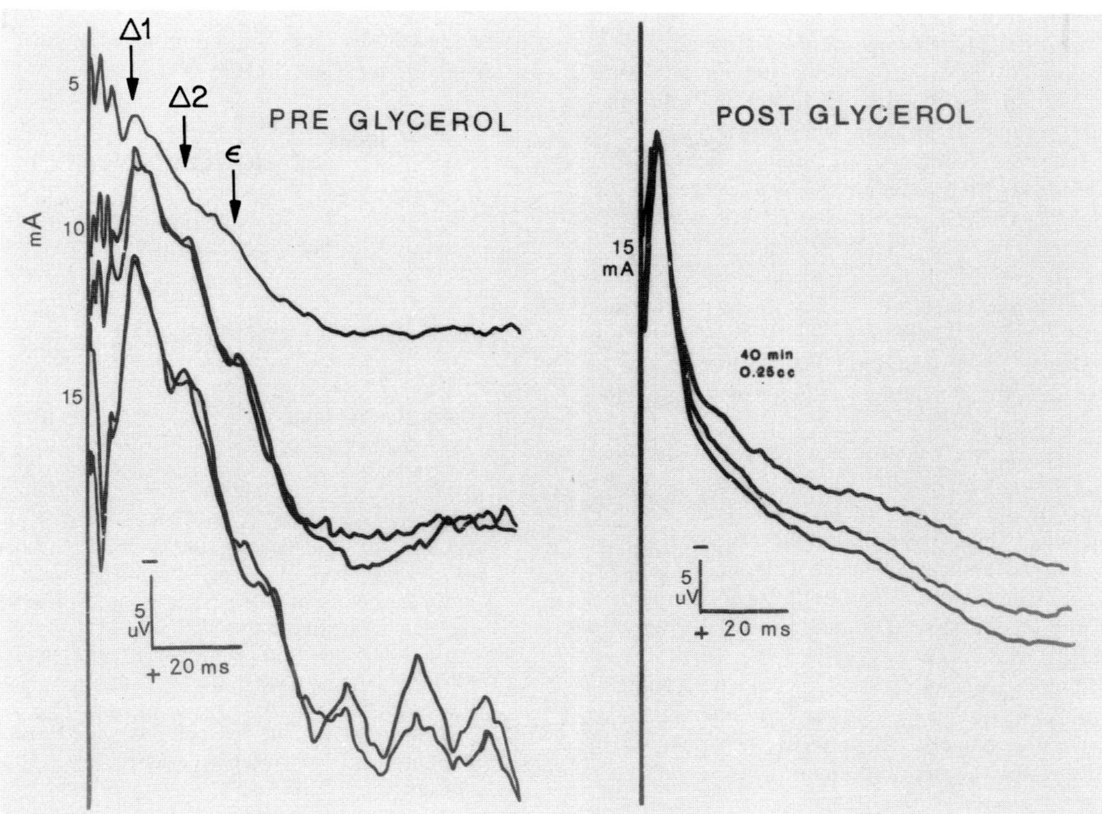

Fig. 98-6.   Glycerol trigeminal root potential (TRP). TRP in second trigeminal division before and after injection of glycerol. Electrical potentials evoked in right trigeminal rootlets of a patient with predominantly second-division, but also some first-division, location of trigger zones. The stimulating electrodes were 2 tiny platinum needles inserted into the skin of the cheek about 1 cm apart, to which were applied pulsed signals at the milliamperages indicated on the ordinates. The recording needle-electrode was a 20-gauge needle insulated except for its terminal 5 mm, lying in the second trigeminal division rootlets as indicated by the reference of tingling in nostril and upper lip upon stimulation at 0.05 V with a square wave stimulus at 50 cycles/sec, and a burning at the same sites upon heating with an RF current to 45.5°C. The point of the needle electrode lay in CSF 8 mm behind the profile of the clivus, as seen in the lateral view of the skull—probably in the posterior part of Meckel's cave. At this site, a total of 0.25 ml of pure glycerol was injected in 0.05-ml increments, producing second-division analgesia to pinprick shortly after the last injection, spreading by 16 minutes to all of the second-division skin and nasal mucosa. The oral mucosa and all of the first- and third-division areas were unaffected. The glycerol was left in Meckel's cave with the patient sitting for 42 minutes after the injection was complete, during which time the post-injection tracings were obtained. At the height of the analgesia as well as thereafter the patient was always able to localize the touch of a wisp of tissue paper through all three trigeminal divisions of the skin, nasal mucosa, and tongue, and had normal corneal sensation. By the following day the analgesia had faded to hypalgesia. There was no clear-cut sensory deficit at 3 months or at 38 months and no recurrence of pain. Each of the eight tracings represents the average response to 256 stimuli delivered in about 40 seconds. The left panel depicts the preinjection finding. At the top is the electrical response to one group of sweeps at 5 milliamperes (mA). Only an A-beta deflection is present. The stimuli evoked "a quivering sensation," but no pain. At 10 mA, two groups of 256 stimuli in each evoked "some pain" correlated with the first appearance of three more A deflections, labeled delta-1, delta-2, and epsilon, with no later deflection. At 15 mA, two groups of 256 stimuli evoked "severe pain" that was made a little more tolerable by administration of 0.1 mg fentanyl and 5 mg droperidol (intravenously) 70 minutes earlier. The pain was correlated with higher amplitude delta-1, delta-2, and epsilon deflections, plus a new tripartite group of C-wave deflections with conduction velocities of 1–2 m/sec. The right panel shows three groups of 256 stimuli, all at 15 mA; none of these caused any pain, and there are no deflections beyond A-beta, which, however, remains substantial. We have similar tracings following RF heat lesions.

(They obtained no electrophysiologic measures of C-fiber activity and identified no selective C-fiber changes in their histologic preparations.) However, in the histologic appraisal of Rengachary et al. of the effects of both topical application and intraneural injection of glycerol to the rat sciatic nerve, myelin disintegration and axonolysis occurred with "myelinated and unmyelinated fibers being affected at random."[32]

In his original paper, Håkanson suggests that "defective nerve fibers supposed to be involved in the trigger mechanism, are particularly sensitive to glycerol and are affected selectively."[1] Burchiel and Russell present supportive evidence for this view from animal studies.[33] In rats with experimentally induced saphenous neuromas, loss of the spontaneous action potential produced from the neuroma was the earliest electrophysiologic change noted upon topical application of glycerol. This was followed next by loss of conduction in C fibers and, later (upon experimentation with higher concentrations of glycerol), by a similar loss in A-fibers. Igarashi et al.

have recorded contralateral C5-C6 somatosensory potentials in humans before and after glycerol injection for trigeminal neuralgia.[34] In those patients with second-division pain who were relieved by the injection, the Negative 10 deflection dropped to 38 percent of its original amplitude, whereas those patients afflicted in the second division who secured no relief had a minimal decrease in Negative 10 amplitude to 86 percent of the original. These observations suggest that a reduction in normal parameters of conduction is correlated with an improved chance for relief. Essentially the reverse findings are, however, described by Bennett and Lunsford.[29] They found that normal N20 latencies after glycerol "were associated with pain relief in most cases," whereas recurrent pain was "more likely to develop in those trigeminal neuralgia patients whose evoked potential remained abnormal."

In our Chapter 71, we described the effect of cisternal glycerol, in a patient with trigeminal neuralgia, upon the trigeminal root potential evoked by painless and painful stimulation of the trigeminal skin. Glycerol (0.3 ml) produced in one patient second-division clinical analgesia without anesthesia, and eliminated the A-delta epsilon and bipartite C-fiber deflections of the compound action potential recorded from the relevant trigeminal rootlets in Meckel's cave. Figure 98-6 depicts similar tracings from another patient, in whom elimination of a tripartite C-wave and A-delta epsilon deflections was correlated again with analgesia to pinprick, preservation of touch, and cessation of the neuralgic pain. This second case emphasizes that a temporary inhibition of conduction in pain fibers may be followed by a protracted relief of the neuralgic pain.

CONCLUSION

At present, we offer the glycerol option only to those with trigger areas in the first division, major apprehension regarding dysesthesias, multiple sclerosis, or a desire to repeat glycerol when recurrence develops after an otherwise happy result from the first procedure. We take care to point out, however, that even with short periods of glycerol in the cistern, some patients may be very annoyed by the new sensations.

POST-TRAUMATIC FACIAL NEURALGIA; ATYPICAL FACIAL NEURALGIA; CHRONIC MIGRAINOUS NEURALGIA (CLUSTER HEADACHE)

The glycerol method was found ineffective for post-traumatic neuralgia in all 6 of Dieckmann's patients.[7] In atypical facial neuralgia in the 6 cases of Price, in the 2 of ours, and in 7 of the 8 of Waltz et al., the relief was unsatisfactory.[19,11] We agree with Lunsford and Apfelbaum that glycerol injection has no role in this disorder. In Ekbom's 6 cases of chronic migrainous neuralgia, 3 injections were given to one patient, and 2 injections to each of 5 others.[35] A major first-division trigeminal loss in three was followed by relief for 11 months or less. A marked decrease in facial sensation occurred on re-injection, with relief for 9, 18, and 47 months. A slight sensory loss only in the other 3 patients was followed by partial and short-lasting relief. Waltz et al. thought that 4 of their 5 patients with "cluster headache" had partial relief so that they could be

controlled medically. Our own results with RF lesions are much better than these.[36] It is our impression that the glycerol method is unsuitable for these 3 types of problems.

ACKNOWLEDGEMENT

Dr. Sweet wishes to thank the Neuro-Research Foundation for its support during the preparation of the manuscript.

REFERENCES

1. Håkanson S: Treatment of trigeminal neuralgia by injection of glycerol into the trigeminal cistern. Neurosurgery 9:638, 1981
2. Whisler WW, Hill BJ: A simplified technique for injection of the gasserian ganglia, in Voris HC, Whisler WW (eds): Treatment of Pain. Springfield, Ill, Charles C Thomas, 1975, pp 61–74
3. Lunsford LD, Apfelbaum RI: Choice of surgical therapeutic modalities for treatment of trigeminal neuralgia: Microvascular decompression, percutaneous retrogasserian thermal or glycerol rhizotomy. Clin Neurosurg 32:319, 1985
4. Gomori JM, Rappaport ZH: Transovale trigeminal cistern puncture: Modified fluoroscopically guided technique. Am J Neuroradiol 6:93, 1985
5. Håkanson S: Personal communication, February 8, 1984
6. Håkanson S: Retrogasserian glycerol injection as a treatment of tic douloureux, in Bonica JJ, et al (eds): Advances in Pain Research and Therapy, vol 5. New York, Raven Press, 1983, pp 927–933
7. Dieckmann G, Veras G, Sogabe K: Retrogasserian glycerol injection or percutaneous stimulation in the treatment of typical and atypical trigeminal pain. Abstracts of the 8th International Congress of Neurological Surgery, Toronto, July 7–13, 1985, p 142
8. Arias MJ: Percutaneous retrogasserian glycerol rhizotomy for trigeminal neuralgia. A prospective study of 100 cases. J Neurosurg 65:32, 1986
9. Burchiel K: Personal communication, December 10, 1985
10. Carson B: Personal communication, 1985
11. Waltz TA, Dalessio DJ, Ott KH, et al: Trigeminal cistern glycerol injections for facial pain. Headache 25:354, 1985
12. Saini SS: Injection treatment of trigeminal neuralgia with special reference to the use of anhydrous glycerol. Neurology India 29:31, 1981
13. Saini SS: Personal communication from R. Bhatia, December 11, 1985
14. Beck DW, Olson, JJ, Urig EJ: Percutaneous retrogasserian glycerol rhizotomy for treatment of trigeminal neuralgia. J Neurosurg 65:28, 1986
15. Fraioli B, Ferrante, L, Santoro A, et al: Recent progress in the treatment of trigeminal neuralgia: Glycerol into the trigeminal cistern and percutaneous gasserian compression by means of Fogarty's catheter. Acta Neurochirurgica 33:507, 1984
16. Fraioli B, Cantore G: Personal communication, December 12, 1985
17. Laitinen LV: Personal communication, December 17, 1985
18. Maxwell R: Personal communication, December 12, 1985
19. Price D: Material presented at the 8th International Congress of Neurological Surgery, Toronto, July 7–13, 1985
20. Siegfried J: Personal communication, 1985
21. Sweet WH, Poletti CE: Complications of standard treatments for trigeminal neuralgia. Presented at the meeting of the American Association of Neurological Surgeons, Denver, Colorado, April 13–17, 1986
22. Takusagawa Y, Wakiya K, Fukushima T: Treatment of trigeminal neuralgia by percutaneous gasserian ganglion glycerol injection. Abstracts of the 8th International Congress of Neurological Surgery, Toronto, July 7–13, 1985, p 143

23. Igarashi S, Suzuki F, Iwasaki I, et al: Glycerol injection method for trigeminal neuralgia. No Shinkei Geka 13:267, 1985

24. Fischer EG: Personal communication, December 3, 1985

25. Young RF: Personal communication, December 10, 1985

26. Patrick BS: Personal communcation, December 16, 1985

27. Sweet WH, Poletti CE, Roberts JT: Dangerous rises in blood pressure upon heating of trigeminal rootlets; Increased bleeding times in patients with trigeminal neuralgia. Neurosurgery 17:843, 1985

28. Lunsford LD: Trigeminal neuralgia: Treatment by glycerol rhizotomy, in Wilkins RH, Rengachary SS (eds): Neurosurgery, vol 3. New York, McGraw-Hill, 1985, pp 2351–2356

29. Bennett MH, Lunsford LD: Percutaneous retrogasserian glycerol rhizotomy for tic douloureux. Part 2. Results and implications of trigeminal evoked potential studies. Neurosurgery 14:431, 1984

30. Baxter DW, Schacherl U: Experimental studies on the morphological changes produced by intrathecal phenol. Can Med Assoc J 86:1200, 1962

31. Lunsford LD, Bennett MH, Martinez AJ: Experimental trigeminal glycerol injection. Electrophysiologic and morphologic effects. Arch Neurol 42:146, 1985

32. Rengachary SS, Watanabe IS, Singer P, et al: Effect of glycerol on peripheral nerve: An experimental study. Neurosurgery 13:681, 1983

33. Burchiel KJ, Russell LC: Glycerol neurolysis: Neurophysiological effects of topical glycerol application on rat saphenous nerve. JNeurosurg 63:784, 1985

34. Igarashi S, Suzuki F, Koyama T: Trigeminal sensory evoked potential in retrogasserian glycerol injection for trigeminal neuralgia. No Shinkei Geka 12:1349, 1984

35. Ekbom K: Treatment of cluster headache by retrogasserian glycerol. Presentation to International Cluster Headache Group, Hammersmith Hospital, London, September 1984

36. Sweet WH: Periodic (chronic) migrainous neuralgia; (chronic) cluster headache. Abstracts of the Combined Meeting of the Society of British Neurological Surgeons, Society of Neurosurgeons of South Africa, and Sociedad Luso-Espanola de Neurocirugia, Granada, April 29–May 1, 1985, pp 137–141

Complications of Percutaneous Rhizotomy and Microvascular Decompression Operations for Facial Pain

William H. Sweet   Charles E. Poletti

CONVERSATIONS WITH COLLEAGUES suggested that the sequelae of the most commonly used operations for trigeminal neuralgia may occur more frequently than is indicated by the published experiences of those of us who, with happy outcomes, have gone on to do large series of cases. Neurosurgeons describing the risks of the operations to candidates for the procedures in question have, of course, cited the nature and percentages of only the published complications. The problem as to the general validity of such data came to the fore when a neurosurgeon asked one of us to testify in his behalf when one of his patients died from an intracranial arterial subarachnoid hemorrhage occurring during a percutaneous radiofrequency (RF) rhizotomy and another's patient had a permanent major disability from a basal ganglionic hemorrhage related to a microvascular decompression.

We made personal inquiries of other neurosurgeons which revealed that several of their patients had had intracranial hemorrhages related to RF rhizotomies. These led to our confirmation of reports that mere placement of the needle-electrode into the nerve, ganglion and root,[14] as well as subsequent heating in the unconscious anesthetized patient often caused either severe bradycardia and asystole or conversely and much more often a major rise in arterial blood pressure plus tachycardia. We have also found that many trigeminal neuralgia patients have abnormal bleeding tendencies probably related to their heavy medication.

The careful examination of the records by WHS and discussions with the two aforementioned neurosurgeons revealed no intimation of negligence, but the case of the second neurosurgeon was settled by the insurance company during the trial for hundreds of thousands of dollars after the plaintiff's case had been presented and before any of us defense witnesses had testified. One basis for this insurance company's decision appeared to be that the defendant neurosurgeon, well-versed in microsurgical techniques, nevertheless had this unfortunate result in his second operation for microvascular decompression. The plaintiff's attorneys took the position, untenable in our view, that the neurosurgeon had a duty to make it clear to his patient that the operation in his less experienced hands would be more hazardous than the figures published by experienced surgeons. These events convinced us that it would be fruitful for doctors, patients, and even defense attorneys to have more information on the global experience with our operations. As a pilot study, we wrote to 200 neurosurgical friends (50 abroad) indicating the basis for the study and requesting data from them on complications on their services or of which they knew following percutaneous RF or glycerol lesions or microvascular decompression. To this burdensome request 140 neurosurgeons, to whom we are most grateful, replied.

The responses with respect to glycerol lesions have been included in Chapter 98.

COMPLICATIONS OF PERCUTANEOUS RF TRIGEMINAL RHIZOTOMIES

These are the data from 91 services, nearly all not previously reported: 29 services gave their entire numbers of rhizotomies, totaling over 7000. Of lesser complications there were 18 patients with neuroparalytic keratitis, 8 with aseptic meningeal reactions (negative cultures), and 5 with carotid-cavernous fistulas. In 3 of these 5 cases the Nugent type of blunt electrode protruding beyond the sharp pointed needle was used to make the heat lesion. There were 18 temporary oculomotor palsies and at least 1 that was permanent; this last lesion was later shown to be caused by placement of the electrode in the inferior orbital fissure, there having been no pre-lesion roentgenogram. A seizure occurred during the procedure in 2 patients and in 1 a transient postoperative psychosis developed. In 8 patients brief asystolic periods developed during needle-electrode placement or lesion production despite the patient's unconsciousness under intravenous anesthetic. These have been properly prevented from recurring by the use of intravenous atropine.

Hemorrhages might well have been related to increased bleeding times not only because of the high doses of varied drugs for the facial pain—trigeminal neuralgia in the great majority—but also because these older patients were often on anticoagulant drugs related to cardiac or cerebrovascular disease. Of 130 of our recent patients the bleeding time was abnormal at greater than 9 1/2 minutes in 16.2 percent (''surgicutt'' method).

RADIOFREQUENCY RHIZOTOMY FOR FACIAL PAIN

(Nearly all trigeminal neuralgia—Major complications not previously reported from 91 services)

Optic Nerve Lesions

1 in recovery room developed pupillary dilatation, subhyaloid hemorrhage, permanent blindness ipsilateral to lesion.

1 transient ipsilateral amblyopia as lesions being made.

4 permanent complete blindness at once after RF lesions. In 1 case total internal and external ophthalmoplegia, nerves III, IV and VI as well. In another case (with severe multiple sclerosis for 7 years) third division paresis accompanied the blindness. In 1 of the 2 cases who developed only blindness without extraocular motor paresis only 2 lesions were made totalling 1½ minutes at 75°C.

In at least 3 of the above 4 cases after electrode placement there was second division pain upon electrical stimulation—taken as adequate evidence of correct position of the electrode. Apparently no confirmatory roentgenograms were taken in 2 of the 4 cases because of technical failure of the radiographic equipment. Morley (personal communication, April 25, 1986) finds it unnecessary to ''resort to x-ray control for placement of the needle.'' However, we recommend: Make no lesion unless the desired responses at low threshold to electrical stimulation are accompanied by roentgenograms which in both lateral and sagittal views show the electrode shaft through the foramen ovale and the electrode tip in the expected position. We have at least 5 patients in whom the electrode shaft entered the middle fossa via an opening anterior to the foramen ovale, yet the much too anterior point gave rise on stimulation to first or second division paresthesias. In another case WHS obtained 16 ml

Trigeminal Neuralgia—Microvascular Decompression (Reports From 49 Services)

Number of Cases	Complications—Cases not previously published
	Virtually no complications 9 services
20	3 early recurrences; pain stopped when displaced Ivalon sponge replaced; 0 complications
~150	''no major complications or deaths''
~15	0 significant complication
9	0 complications
24	0 complications
—*	0 complications
''a few''	0 complications
3	0 complications
—	10 days postoperatively sudden ispilateral sensory loss with later recovery
	Moderate Complications 19 services
—	1 temporary bilateral deafness; 1 marked intraoperative cerebellar swelling → permanent VIII with mild ataxia
26	1 CSF leak → reop closure; 1 ipsilateral ataxia temporary
—	1 *contralateral* complete deafness permanent
72	2 cerebellar hematomas, removed, patients well; temporary—1 IV; 1 VI; 1 VII; 1 ataxia
—	some mild permanent gait disturbance; 2 temporary diplopias
~70	1 lasting total ipsilateral deafness; 1 shoulder dislocation (no previous shoulder problems)
—	1 supratentorial subdural hematoma, recovery; 2 VII, 1 VIII, all partial
24	2 permanent complete ipsilateral deafness; 1 temporary VII
—	1 permanent VII paresis
''several hundred''	2 partial deafness; 1 cerebellar edema → reoperated temporary diplopia and ataxia; 1 CSF rhinorrhea
—	temporary VI paresis
20	1 complete anesthesia all 3 V divisions, uneventful operation
20/yr	2 diplopia; some ''ataxias or other cerebellar findings''; some ''permanent gait disturbances''
5	1 painful dysesthesia—moderate
—	1 decadron-sensitive aseptic meningitis; symptoms recurred when decadron stopped—duration ~ 2 months
—	1 subdural hematoma at operative site—removed—recovery 1 aseptic meningeal reaction—cleared 10 days 1 laceration sigmoid sinus—2 liter blood loss—normal recovery
~50	1 lasting corneal anesthesia, 1 CSF leak requiring reoperation; 2 transient VIII; 1 laceration transverse sinus—operation aborted
—	several lower cranial nerve paralyses
—	lower cranial nerve palsies

Trigeminal Neuralgia (*continued*)

Number of Cases	Complications—Cases not previously published
	Major Complications 24 services
—	1 lasting disabling brain stem stroke; 1 CSF leak—protracted infection—recovery; 3 lasting palsies—2 VII, 1 VII and VIII
~14	1 pontine venous thrombosis—many petrosal veins coagulated at operation; decerebrate postures all 4 limbs—almost complete recovery
~10	1 temporary IV; 1 delayed cerebellar hematoma and hypertension 3 + weeks postoperatively—death
—	1 cerebellar subdural hematoma → death
—	1 "venous thrombosis and hemorrhagic infarction of cerebellum" second postoperative day
—	1 case V root in a nest of veins—all coagulated and cut → coma → death
~70	1 "moderate" brain stem stroke, minor residual; 1 disabling brain stem stroke
—	1 basilar artery rupture during operation; death
—	"occasional case" of posterior fossa hemorrhage, cerebellar hemorrhage, cerebellar infarction, VII or VIII lesion
—	thrombosis contralateral middle cerebral artery intraoperatively; death second day
2	1 intraoperative contralateral basal ganglionic hemorrhage—permanent total disability. (Transverse sinus entered during operation.)
—	2 serious strokes
"several"	1 meningitis → vasculitis → hemorrhage → death; 1 lasting complete ipsilateral deafness
111	1 cerebellar infarct → death; 1 severe lasting dementia; 2 hematomas → 1 acute epidural; 1 chronic subdural both recovered; 11 significant lasting cranial nerve injuries; 11 other lesser complications with recovery
—	1 cerebellar infarct → reoperated → polymicrobial meningitis → death in healthy 59-year-old woman
—	awoke after event-free operation with complete loss of cranial IV, V, VI, VII, VIII, severe ipsilateral ataxia, contralateral increased weakness and clumsiness; 2 years later same + anesthesia dolorosa
"very infrequently"	1 death pontine infarction
~30	excellent surgeons—2 deaths, males 1 age 31, 1 age 50, uneventful operations; post mortems: necrosis of cerebellum and brain stem—due to occlusion petrosal veins
15	multiple intraoperative intracerebral hemorrhages—confirmed at autopsy 6 days postoperatively, female age 55
"very few"	1 totally disabling "reactive meningitis"; at reoperation "chronic hypertrophic meningitis" involving many cranial nerves; impossible to remove sponge at trigeminal nerve
30	excellent surgeon—2 postoperative deaths in 2 healthy patients circa 50 years of age after smooth, uneventful operations
—	1 protracted wound infection, final recovery; 2 VII and 1 VII and VIII, all lasting; 1 disabling cerebellar and brain stem stroke
50	1 early postoperative death—cerebellar hematoma; 1 chronic bilateral frontal subdural hematoma with recovery
~125	2 deaths in 48 hours postoperatively: 1 superior cerebellar and post-cerebral infarcts—female late 50s 1 quadriplegia followed by coma—female "embittered family refused autopsy." Both operations uneventful
	1 left hemiplegia after left microvascular decompression—nearly normal by 6 weeks—female
	1 left hemiparesis left hemisensory deficit and left homonymous hemianopia; only the hemiparesis recovered—male aged 64 yrs

*A dash indicates no total number of cases stated.

clear colorless CSF at the electrode site. Stimulation evoked a throbbing in the cheek bone at 0.30 V, 50 cycles/sec 1 sigma pulse duration, and heating to 48°C elicited "warmth" in the cheek bone. The films revealed the needle point to be in the pars nervosa of the jugular foramen!

Central Retinal Artery Occlusion

1 diabetic

Dangerous, Disabling or Fatal Sequelae

1 myocardial infarct 4 days postoperatively—died—91-year-old patient

1 myocardial infarct developed during procedure when excessive dose of vasodilator drug, given to prevent rise of systolic pressure during lesion, was followed by hypotension of 24 mm Hg for 1½ min—complete recovery

7 intracerebral (usually temporal lobe) abscesses: 1 permanent mental impairment; 3 died

21 bacterial meningitides: 1 death in a patient whose symptoms began 1 week postopertively—late start of therapy; no other sequelae

19 hemorrhages (focal intracranial): 1 infratemporal subdural hematoma—needle puncture inferior temporal vein; removed recovery; 3 ipsilateral intratemporal lobe: 2 died, 1 disabled (reported earlier); 15 intracerebral probably unrelated to site of electrode—8 died; 4 major residual sequelae (1 caused by thrombocytopenia); 3 transitory hemiplegias

Recommend: Preoperative studies re coagulopathy including bleeding times, monitoring of blood pressure during procedure, with intravenous nitroprusside or other vasodilator to preclude excessive rise in blood pressure.

1 arterial puncture by needle-electrode followed by hemiparesis lasting 4 days.

5 arterial subarachnoid hemorrhages from needle-electrode; 2 full recovery; 3 died—1 with needle through infraorbital foramen into anterior cerebral artery; one 80-year-old woman brisk bleeding at needle placement—stopped—lesion made—6 hours later massive subarachnoid hemorrhage posterior and middle fossas bilaterally.

Recommend: Stop procedure at once if arterial bleeding produced—even if from extracranial internal carotid resume only days later when puncture site healed. We have used a 20-gauge needle-electrode—cross-sectional area 0.63 mm^2 in preference to a 19-gauge needle with a cross-sectional area of 0.95 mm^2. We have never had a sequel to arterial puncture with the 20-gauge electrode.

It is worth noting that there are at least six services in each of which well over 1000 percutaneous retrogasserian trigeminal procedures have been performed without any lasting major extratrigeminal complication (Broggi, Nugent, Siegfried, Sweet, Taren, Tew). It is easy to take a casual attitude toward the procedure because of its simplicity. The achievement of consistent success without sequelae demands scrupulous attention to detail.

TRIGEMINAL NEURALGIA— MICROVASCULAR DECOMPRESSION (REPORTS FROM 49 SERVICES)

Summary: 9 services reported essentially no complications; the 2 largest series with these results were 24 and circa 150 cases. No deaths and only moderate lasting sequelae were the experiences of 17 services. In the 9 of these reporting their numbers of operated cases, the figures varied from 5 to "several hundred." From 24 services came accounts of permanently disabling sequelae or deaths in 29 cases. The 2 largest series were of 111 and circa 125 cases. The next largest series was of 50 cases. The 2 most discouraging series involved 3 technically competent distinguished neurosurgeons, who had 4 deaths in 60 patients, all in "healthy" individuals, 3 in their 50s and 1 aged 31, all following "smooth, uneventful operations."

CONCLUSION

Although we think that one can almost eliminate by appropriate precautions the major complications and deaths from percutaneous operations, we recommend mentioning these risks to patients. How to reduce the risk of microvascular decompression is not so obvious. Perhaps the most clear-cut warning is that coagulation of essential veins draining the brain stem probably led to a major infarct in 4 cases. Should significant blood loss occur if the transverse sinus is opened, one should consider aborting the procedure. Even if the neurosurgeon has enough experience to emphasize only his own results, he would be well advised to describe to patients the possibility of a fuller range of complications than were seen in the best series.

ACKNOWLEDGMENT

The authors wish to express their gratitude to the Neuro Research Foundation for its support during the preparation of the manuscript.

ADDENDUM

Since the foregoing manuscript was submitted, the Executive Boards of the American Association of Neurological Surgeons and the Congress of Neurological Surgeons have decided to set up a central office to which neurosurgeons are invited to submit reports of their complications of all neurosurgical procedures. The understanding is that the medical data only will be transcribed and the original letter destroyed to preclude its origin being traced by anyone. The complications of each procedure will be published at appropriate intervals so that the fuller information on them will be available to the whole profession. The news letters of both the AANS and the Congress will describe the appropriate course of action remaking such reports when the machinery for handling the data has been set up.

Awareness of the major hemorrhages due to vascular puncture during percutaneous rhizotomy has led me to develop a technique less likely to provoke them. The most obvious change is to use a smaller needle-electrode, e.g., a 22-gauge shaft—area .43 sq mm, versus a 20-gauge electrode—area .64 sq mm or the Nugent-Berry electrode 18-gauge—area 1.25 sq mm. Until recently there was no temperature measuring device available that could be incorporated into the stilet for a 22-gauge shaft. Dr. Eric Cosman of the Radionics Instrument Company has now remedied this with a thermocouple which, via a thermocouple adapter unit he supplies, operates in conjunction with his main stimulating-lesioning device. Although only 6 of the 18 reported hemorrhages from percutaneous rhizotomy causing death or disabling sequelae were caused by vascular puncture, these were all probably due to placement of the needle-eelctrode into the brain. This can happen in two ways: (1) via some other opening than the foramen ovale and (2) via the proper target foramen, i.e., ovale.

The wrong foramina which are the most difficult to avoid are inconstantly present small openings for emissary veins only a few millimeters distant from the foramen ovale. I have now entered the more frequently occurring of these two foramina nine times. The first eight times this was without incident and was followed by replacement of the electrode and making of an appropriate lesion at the same session. The radiographic appearances in the first five cases were published in 1976 and were described as due to penetration of an unnamed foramen. However, the ninth time I produced a left intratemporal hemorrhage. Luckily, complete recovery from the evoked aphasia occurred in two weeks. The episode stimulated me to a more careful search, and I found at least three famous anatomical texts—Gray, Testut and Paturet—which describe a small "foramen or canal of Vesalius"—anterior and/or medial to ovale. Paturet alone of the three describes a second small opening posterior to the lateral third of ovale which he calls the innominate foramen or canaliculus of Arnold. I have seen the canal of Vesalius on the left side only in two of six skulls I have examined and found it large enough to admit an 18-gauge needle in one and a 19-gauge needle in the other. In the lateral radiographs of these skulls the electrode lies opposite the shadow of the sella turcica as was the case in seven of the nine in vivo cases. In the other two the shaft projected in front of the sella turcica and might have been in the inferior orbital fissure. In all nine cases the needle probably penetrated the temporal lobe. Professor de Rougemont describes having pierced the innominate foramen, probably with similar invasion of the temporal lobe.

Entry into the foramen lacerum has been reported, and is likely to puncture the internal carotid artery, a mishap that can also occur if the inferior bony wall of the intrapetrous internal carotid canal is absent. Direct entry into the desired middle to medial part of the foramen ovale can be achieved by the use of fluoroscopy, although I find this much more tedious than the free hand method with orientation by external landmarks I have used for 22 years. I have gone over to fluoroscopy with a 22-gauge electrode in a further effort to reduce the chance of a serious hemorrhage from electrode puncture. Details are given in a chapter in the new edition of Youmans.

It is also easily possible to enter temporal lobe or midbrain via the foramen ovale if the trajectory is too high or too far posterior. This can be avoided by using the fluoroscopic unit in the lateral view as one advances the electrode by small increments.

Since the percutaneous method inevitably involves a risk of intratrigeminal morbidity, one does well to maximize the avoidance of significant extratrigeminal morbidity, the main advantage of this tactic.

REFERENCES

1. Abou-Madi M, Trop D, Morin L, et al: Anesthetic considerations in percutaneous radiofrequency coagulation of the gasserian ganglion. Canad Anesth Soc J 31:255, 1984
2. Kehler CH, Brodsky JB, Samuels SI, et al: Blood pressure response during percutaneous rhizotomy for trigeminal neuralgia. Neurosurgery 10:200, 1982
3. Knitza R, Olbermann M, Fischer F, et al: Kreislaufverhalten, Blutgase, Säure- Basen- und Stoftwechselveränderungen unter Neuroleptanalgesie mit und ohne Betarezeptorenblocker bei der Elektrokoagulation des Ganglion Gasseri. Anaesthesist 27:213, 1978
4. Sweet WH, Poletti CE, Roberts JT: Dangerous rises in blood pressure upon heating of trigeminal rootlets; increased bleeding times in patients with trigeminal neuralgia. Neurosurgery 17:843,1985

Intraspinal and Intraventricular Implantable Systems and Agents for Long-Term Relief of Cancer Pain

Charles E. Poletti
Henry H. Schmidek

William H. Sweet
Robert N. Pilon

THE USE OF IMPLANTABLE SYSTEMS for the long-term focal delivery of neuropharmacologic agents to the central nervous system will probably represent a major therapeutic advance. Systems are now in use to administer opiates directly to the spinal cord for the treatment of intractable pain and are being or may also be used for the delivery of hormones, neurotransmitters, antibiotics, anticoagulants, oncolytic agents, and other compounds targeted to the epidural space, cerebrospinal fluid, neuraxis, or bloodstream.[1-3] In the management of pain states this approach has the advantage of avoiding both the systemic effects associated with high-dose narcotics and of the problems associated with the surgical destruction of portions of the nervous system. The nondestructive stimulation of the dorsal columns of the cord is usually ineffective in relieving pain associated with malignant disease.[4]

LONG-TERM INFUSION OF EPIDURAL LOCAL ANESTHETICS FOR INTRACTABLE PAIN

Attempts to control pain by means of a permanently placed subcutaneously implanted epidural system, allowing repeated intermittent injections of a local anesthetic, were first reported by Pilon and Baker in 1976.[5] The patient, a 52-year-old woman, five years after a sigmoid colectomy for adenocarcinoma, was debilitated by unilateral pain in the low back and buttock secondary to sacral metastases. The pain was largely unrelieved both by radiotherapy and unilateral thoracic cordotomy. Six months postoperatively the patient developed intractable pain on the other side, but refused a cordotomy on the second side, becoming instead dependent on large, frequent dosages of dihydromorphinone (Dilaudid) for pain relief. In order to control her pain, an epidural catheter was placed percutaneously and threaded beneath the skin to a subcutaneous reservoir. One week following the operation, the reservoir was injected with local anesthetic. Over the next 4½ months 50 injections were delivered in this way into the reservoir, and immediate pain relief was obtained shortly thereafter. About 20 injections were performed by the patient's husband at home. By adjusting the amount and concentration of the drug, it was consistently possible to achieve pain relief while motor function was intact. No complications were associated with this mode of therapy in the 4½-month period of its use. Control of bladder and bowel function was maintained and 34 cultures of fluid aspirated before injection of the agent from the reservoir were negative for bacterial growth. Throughout this period the patient was able once again to function as a housewife.

Based on this initial experience, two of the authors (HHS and RNP) then used this technique in 3 other patients with intractable pain caused by pelvic cancer invading the lumbosacral plexus and spine. In each of these cases the epidural catheter was positioned at open operation through a semi-hemilaminectomy with intraoperative radiographic confirmation of the catheter's position. The Silastic catheter was then connected subcutaneously to a specially designed system incorporating an on-off valve and an enlarged plastic reservoir with a 20-ml volume. Bupivacaine hydrochloride (Marcaine) 0.35 percent, without epinephrine, was injected through the system into the epidural space. In each case it was possible to achieve consistent pain relief for 6 to 12 hours following a single injection of this agent. The system was used for 3 weeks, 1 month, and 3 months, respectively, in these 3 patients. In none of these cases was any problem encountered from either malfunction of the system, infections, or adverse reaction to the local anesthetic agent. The patients were freed from the use of oral or injectable narcotics, and the systems remained in continuous use until the deaths of the patients. Postmortem examination in two cases revealed neither evidence of epidural infection nor of epidural scar tissue formation either around the catheter or in the adjacent dura.

LONG-TERM EPIDURAL INFUSION OF OPIATES FOR PAIN

Recently our interest has shifted from the use of local anesthetic agents in the epidural space[6] to the use of narcotics to control cancer pain. Although local anesthetics can successfully provide chronic pain relief, they block nonselectively the conduction of the nerve action potentials by reducing the amount and rate of development of the early transient increase in the permeability of the neural membranes to sodium ions normally produced by slight depolarization of the membrane. In view of this, specific relief of pain without interference with other myelinated nerve fiber function is difficult to achieve consistently, although motor and autonomic blockade in our patients was minimal.[9] With the identification of the opiate receptors in the more posterior cells of the dorsal horns of the spinal cord[10–19] and the demonstration of pain relief using focally administered opiates, without inducing sensory, motor, or autonomic dysfunction,[15,17,18,20–23] these agents have now supplanted the use of local anesthetic agents for epidural administration in our patients.

Opiate receptors are richly distributed in laminae I and II of the dorsal horn of the spinal cord, in the peri-4th-ventricular, and in the periaqueductal gray matter.[14] Narcotics show both nonspecific and stereo-specific binding to tissues, i.e., the l-rotatory form binds whereas the d-rotatory form does not. Specific binding at opiate receptor sites is more tenacious, but is reversed by naloxone, which competes for the specific receptor sites.[16] The duration of action of the usual 0.4 to 0.8 mg dose of IV naloxone is limited to 1 to 4 hours and so opiates with strong binding characteristics and long durations of action may re-establish their effects some hours after a reversal dose of naloxone.[24] Radioimmunoassay studies after epidural introduction of morphine, methadone, and β-endorphin in humans reveal absorption into both the CSF and the blood stream, but the peak concentrations in CSF are 50 to 500 times greater than those in the blood plasma, and 12 hours later are 10 to 20 times those in the plasma.[25,26] The intraspinal narcotics, whether introduced intrathecally or epidurally, pass from the cerebrospinal fluid into the lipid phase of the spinal cord. The narcotics need penetrate the dorsal surface of the cord only to a depth of about 1 mm to reach Rexed's laminae I & II in the dorsal horn from the spinal subarachnoid space. Autoradiographs in dogs have shown that lidocaine injected in the dorsal epidural space penetrates preferentially into the dorsal periphery of the cord.[9] Because all these agents spread cephalad in the CSF, they can penetrate the floor of the fourth ventricle to reach the opiate receptors in such structures as the locus coeruleus concerned with central reflex control of respiratory and cardiovascular functions. The degree of lipid solubility of a given agent is a major determinant of the rate of transfer from cerebrospinal fluid to the substance of the spinal cord. Hence the speed of onset of neural effects, the duration of sojourn of the agent in the CSF, the distance of its travel cephalad in the CSF, the speed of its washout from the lipid neuraxis and subsequent elimination in the blood are all related to its lipid solubility. The strength of receptor binding will also determine the duration of action once the agent has diffused into the substance of the spinal cord. Thus, the clinical effects of the various narcotics can be predicted, to a large degree, by knowledge of their lipid-solubility and their specific opiate-receptor binding proclivity.[27]

In short-term studies in volunteers of thoracic and lumbar epidural injections of narcotics highly soluble in lipids, such agents as methadone and hydromorphone (Dilaudid) have been found to produce segmental pain relief with relatively little depression of respiration. Sympathetic activity is unaffected, while a segmental loss to cold and pin sensation can be detected. Lumbar epidural injections of 10 mg of morphine have produced the following effects:[28]

1. Initial segmental pain relief mainly confined to the lower limb.
2. Urinary retention.
3. Cephalad spread of pain relief—after 3 to 4 hours—to involve the upper limb.
4. Gradual depression of CO_2 response curve.
5. Persistence of pain relief and respiratory depression for 16 to 22 hours.

Our results show that the effects of rostral spread of the drug are greatly reduced by using lower doses in smaller volumes.

Likewise epidural meperidine (Demerol) 100 mg in 10 ml has relieved severe pain completely for 4 to 20 hours. Lower doses, 30 mg in 6 ml, gave similar durations of complete relief to cancer patients. None of them had any detectable change to objective sensory, motor, or sympathetic tests.[21] Larger doses of morphine, well above those required for pain relief, have produced objective analgesia to pin prick. Ten patients given 20 mg of morphine intrathecally in a hyperbaric solution and placed in a 40-degree head-up position did develop an analgesic level ranging from T1 to T6.[29]

Numerous clinical studies of short-term intraspinal narcotics for postoperative, obstetrical, and cancer pain have been published in the past 2 to 3 years.[3,28,30–35] Different methodologies have made it difficult to compare results, but in general the clinical results have confirmed the animal data.[37] Pain relief is dramatically profound, predominantly segmental, and prolonged when the drug exhibits strong receptor binding and low lipid solubility (e.g., morphine). Drugs with high lipid solubility and weak receptor binding, such as fentanyl, have a rapid and intense segmental effect, but as they quickly wash out the therapeutic effects are short-lived. Some severe acute pain may be more difficult to control than chronic pain. Thus, relief from cancer pain may be achieved with quite small doses of intraspinal narcotics.

The side effects of epidural opiates are common and dose-dependent and include:[38]

1. Nausea and vomiting occurring 4 to 6 hours after epidural morphine and reversed by naloxone.
2. Pruritus in 80 percent of patients after 10 mg of epidural morphine and after fentanyl. This is widespread, poorly relieved in antihistaminics, although completely relieved by naloxone.
3. Urinary retention.
4. Respiratory depression as the agent flows cephalad with CSF into the medullary subarachnoid space and ventricular systems.[39–44] The depression of respiratory sensitivity from epidural morphine follows the rostral spread of pain relief, reaching its peak at the sixth to tenth hour. A number of clinical cases have been published of delayed, profound, and prolonged respiratory depression after administration of morphine directly in the subarachnoid space. Though less frequent, this may also occur with epidural morphine, especially when applied in the cervical region. Late respiratory depression is the most serious of the complications and may be life-threatening many hours after the patient has returned to his or her room; appropriate monitoring is therefore required. Intravenous naloxone promptly reverses the respiratory depression, but repeated doses may be needed. 0.4 mg is a common initial dose.
5. The syndrome of opiate withdrawal occurred in patients whose large systemic doses of morphine were stopped

when tiny doses of intraspinal morphine controlled the pain.[45]

We prefer the epidural to the intrathecal route for the administration of narcotics, since there is less chance of respiratory depression, and a possible infection is less dangerous in the epidural space than in the spinal fluid.

PREPARATION OF AGENTS FOR EPIDURAL ADMINISTRATION

Although we and others have given fentanyl, meperidine, and Dilaudid epidurally, morhine sulphate is the agent with which there is the most experience. The drug should be used without preservatives. Pure morphine sulfate powder is dissolved in water, filtered, and autoclaved for 5 minutes at 121°C. We use 2 mg/ml during initial evaluation of the agents via a percutaneously placed catheter. Higher concentrations are used in the chronic systems and have the advantage that the system need be refilled less frequently.

CURRENT INDICATIONS FOR IMPLANTATION OF CHRONIC EPIDURAL ANALGESIC SYSTEMS

Epidural morphine may be effective in the management of chronic pain, even in relatively low doses. The initial trials were confined to patients with cancer, and only those patients were selected in whom systemic narcotics in doses high enough to provide pain relief also left the patient obtunded and/or with other significant known side-effects of these agents. It is easier to minimize the risk of respiratory depression from a bulbar effect if the patient's cancer pain is confined to the legs, pelvis, and lower abdomen. The patients choose this approach to the control of their pain as an alternative to destructive surgical procedures such as cordotomy or myelotomy. Because of a higher incidence of respiratory depression among aged and debilitated patients, some physicians prefer to exclude these patients from this treatment; however other therapies are also more hazardous for them. Because of the relatively high risk of infection associated with these implanted foreign bodies, patients with immunosuppression may also be excluded. Some patients do not obtain relief with epidural narcotics, and hence are not candidates for a permanent surgical implant. Hence all of our patients selected for study undergo a trial of epidural morphine, often through a temporary catheter placed in the epidural space under local anesthesia. Adjacent colostomies or urethrostomies are not contraindications.

IMPLANTABLE SYSTEMS CURRENTLY AVAILABLE

Success of short-term clinical trials for pain control led us to the design of systems that offer the patient the benefit of long-term self-administration of epidural morphine while at home—systems 1, 2, and 3.[3] A fourth system, used more recently,[3,35,37] has been developed by the Infusaid Corporation (Sharon, Mass.). A fifth system, developed by NASA and just beginning clinical trials, embodies computerized telecommunication control of the pump.

DESCRIPTION OF FOUR CURRENTLY AVAILABLE IMPLANTABLE SYSTEMS

1. A partially externalized Broviac or Hickman catheter system[34,46–53] has been used extensively in children and adults for long-term right atrial intravenous administration of chemotherapeutic agents and for hyperalimentation. Even in severely immunosuppressed patients the infection rate has been reported to be only about 8 percent. Exit tracts from the indwelling Broviac catheters tend to seal in 6 months, permitting clean rather than sterile occlusive dressing, and allow normal activity. A midlumbar injection of a large volume of fluid (10 ml rather than 2 ml) into the Broviac catheter usually carries metrizamide cephalad in the normal epidural space to the upper thoracic region. The partially indwelling system thereby offers the potential of producing pain relief at higher spinal levels with the injection of additional fluid, which acts as a vehicle to carry the morphine higher in the epidural space (Figure 100-1).

2. The system in the 4 patients reported here, who were maintained on chronic epidural bupivacaine, consists of a reservoir with a capacity of 20 ml, a one-way valve system, and an on-off switch.[5] This allows two doses of bupivacaine hydrochloride (Marcaine) to be given with a single percutaneous injection into the reservoir, since 16 to 20 ml of bupivacaine hydrochloride remains in the system and can subsequently be emptied by compression. A more simple tactic has been used by Lazorthes et al.,[54] who have repeatedly injected morphine directly through the skin into a subcutaneously implanted reservoir in 9 patients.

3. A completely indwelling system[3] that also allows morphine self-administration with a potentially lower risk of infection, no wound care, and reservoir refilling only every 2 to 12 months uses a Holter Silastic ventricular catheter placed through a semi-hemilaminectomy into the epidural space, and attached to a PBC-500 cc Silastic-coated blood pack (Figure 100-2). This pack functions as a reservoir for 300 mg to 3 g of morphine in 300 ml of saline. The reservoir outlet tubing is connected to a Hakim high pressure pump valve assembly, and an on-off valve. These components are joined by subcutaneous Silastic tubing to the distal end of the epidural catheter and are secured in position. Postoperatively, the patient learns to self-administer the epidural morphine, pressing shut the intervalvular component of the tubing; each compression injects 0.1 ml into the epidural space. On a regimen of 2 mg of epidural morphine twice daily, one of our cases, previously reported,[3] was able to perform her chores for the 7 months until her death from the progression of her malignant disease.

4. A more complicated alternative totally implantable system[1,37] consists of an implantable automatic pump reservoir that continuously infuses morphine into the epidural space at a relatively constant rate (Figure 100-3). The Infusaid implantable infusion pump was originally developed by the University of Minnesota's Biochemical Engineering Department for the administration of heparin.[55] The system has also been used for the administration of insulin and chemotherapeutic agents. The pump is a flat, cylindrical structure, 3 cm thick, 9 cm in diameter, made of titanium, stainless steel, and silicone rubber, and weighs 180 g with a capacity of 47 ml. The infusion rate is adjustable between 0.5 and 6 ml per day. A disadvantage of the system is that the flow rate may be significantly increased by elevated body temperature or decreased atmospheric pressure. In addition, the patient might become drowsy and unaware of respiratory depression; yet the pump would automatically con-

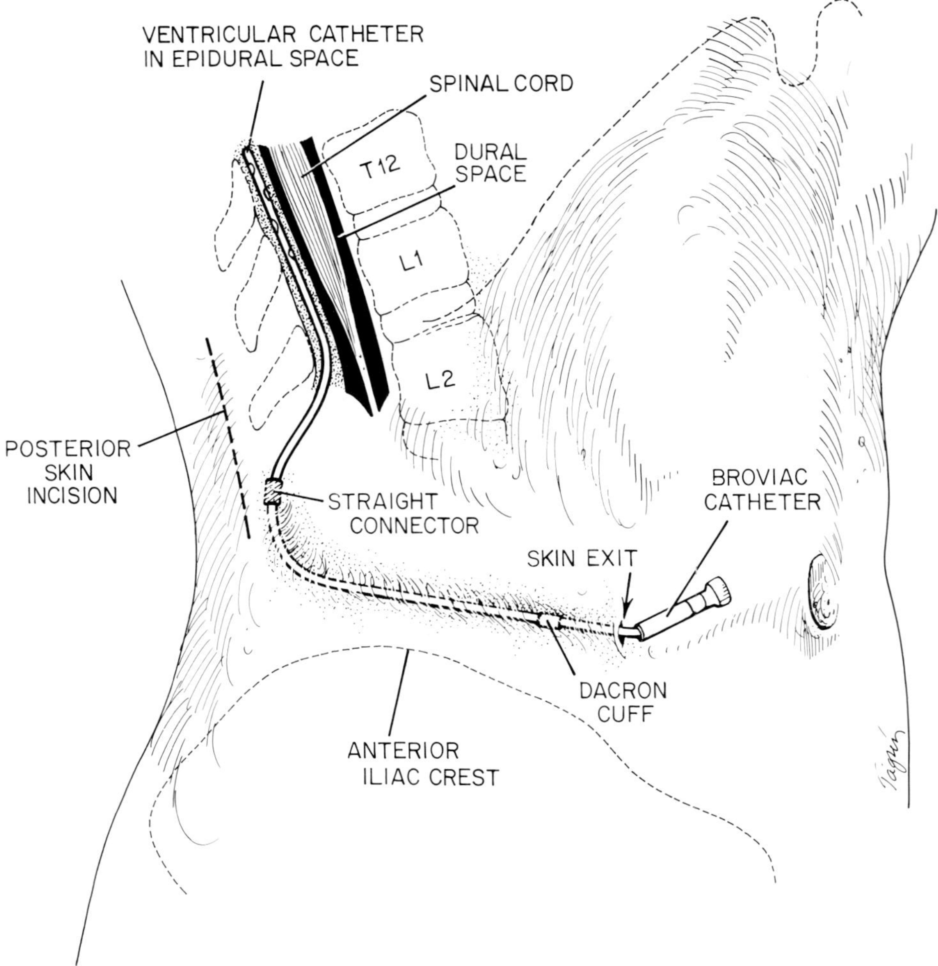

Fig. 100-1.   The partially indwelling Broviac catheter system for long-term administration of morphine into the epidural space. After healing, the skin exit wound requires clean rather than sterile dressing.

tinue the now dangerous infusion of more morphine. This system has been demonstrated to be effective for pain control in animals,[37] and its usage for pain control in humans has recently been reported by Onofrio[35] and is reported by Saunders and Coombs in this volume. The current cost of the device is $2700. It is implanted in a subcutaneous pocket in the abdominal wall and the Silastic outlet catheter is placed in the spinal epidural space. The pump has continued to work properly for years in experimental animals. In the treatment of chronic pain states, the drug must be replenished every 1 to 2 months. This is done by injecting the agent percutaneously through a self-sealing septum. This action simultaneously recharges the pump's intrinsic energy source, allowing continued infusion at a constant and precise flow rate. The system requires no catheter flushing or dressing changes. Subsequent to implantation the patient may be able to return to a normal existence. At the present this pump has not received approval from the Federal Drug Administration for use to administer intraspinal opioids.

INITIAL RESULTS OF LONG-TERM SPINAL MORPHINE THERAPY

The first 2 patients to receive long-term epidural morphine therapy for intractable pain obtained very satisfactory relief from their cancer with 2 mg b.i.d. delivered to the lumbar epidural space.[3] On this regimen both patients stopped their high doses of systemic narcotics, became fully alert, showed no withdrawal symptoms, and returned home with markedly increased functional activity. The patient with the completely indwelling system for self-administration (see Figure 100-2) became fully ambulatory, doing her own shopping until a month before her death 7 months later. During this period the large reservoir was refilled in the office once. The second patient, with a long-term externalized catheter (see Figure 100-1) was less ambulatory, and, living at a distance, was cared for by his family and a visiting nurse during the 6 months until his death, without requiring return to the hospital for reservoir refills. The amount of morphine required, 2 mg b.i.d., remained constant.

In the third patient to receive long-term spinal morphine, Onofrio and colleagues[35] used continuous constant infusion of morphine into the lumbar subarachnoid space, which provided satisfactory relief of pain with only 0.62 to 1.8 mg of morphine a day. Again, this patient obtained good pain relief, even in the postoperative period, stopped systemic narcotics, showed no sedation of his mental status, and returned home able to walk again. The segmental relief of pain afforded even by intrathecal lumbar morphine is well exemplified in this patient. He experienced apparently ''normal'' severe pain at the dentist while maintaining very satisfactory relief from his sacral chordoma.

Intrathecal bolus injections of morphine in short-term human trials by Wang provided single dose relief for 15 hours,

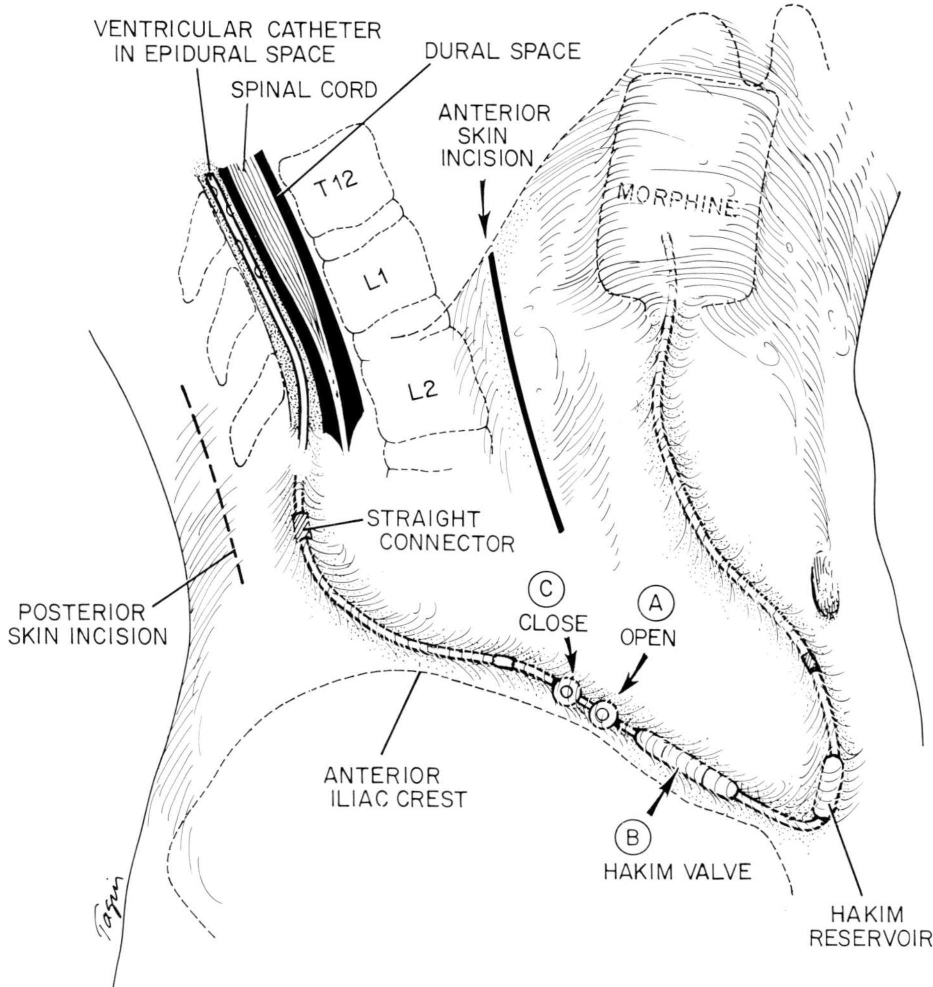

Fig. 100-2. Completely indwelling catheter system consisting of a morphine reservoir, one-way valves in tandem permitting pumping by intermittent compression of intervalvular tubing, and an on-off valve for long-term administration of morphine into the epidural space. For operation the on-off valve is opened (A), the Hakim valve is pumped 20 times (B), delivering 2 ml of morphine, and the on-off valve is then closed (C).

with the elapsed time from the instillation of the drug until its maximum effect ranging from 15 to 45 minutes; repeated injections afforded highly reproducible results.[22,36]

Because the surgery required for implantation of chronic delivery systems is relatively minor compared with most neurosurgical procedures, we expect larger series to continue to show low operative mortality and morbidity.

POTENTIAL COMPLICATIONS

The most serious of the complications to date is respiratory depression. To minimize this possibility we recommend initial measurement of respiratory reserve whenever indicated and frequent monitoring of respiratory rate and pupil size to provide warning of depression. If intrathecal or high epidural administration is occurring, an apnea alarm and serial blood gases give added safety for the first few days of administration. In the higher risk situations, a continuing intravenous line, plus naloxone and a ventilation mask and bag near at hand, are advisable. Lazorthes et al.,[54] however, found that "bolus" administration of 1 ml of a hyperbaric (10 percent glucose) solution containing 3 to 7 mg morphine even into the lumbar

intrathecal space is not hazardous if the patient is kept "semi-sitting" for 12 hours after the injection.

Common to the implantation of any foreign-body system is the increased risk of infections. This risk appears to be especially high for either partially externalized systems (see Figure 100-1) or for systems requiring frequent percutaneous injections to refill the drug reservoir and reactivate the pump (see Figure 100-3). Potentially, a system with a reservoir capacity of 5000 mg (500 ml—10 mg/ml) (see Figure 100-2), delivering morphine into the intrathecal space, might provide pain relief for years without refilling. As sepsis may present the principal limitation to long-term usage, we believe such systems should be designed to be capable of very infrequent filling. This must be balanced against the risk of a massive dose if the reservoir were ruptured or punctured. We must weigh these factors, as we are now trying out these systems in patients with severe "benign" pain of nonlethal cause—e.g., phantom limb, postherpetic neuralgia, postcordotomy dysesthesias, lumbar arachnoiditis, severe chronic pancreatitis, etc.

The second major limitation to the long-term usage of spinal opiates is the potential problem of tachyphylaxis and tolerance. This occurred so rapidly in 3 of our patients with benign pain that it was clearly inadvisable to implant a totally

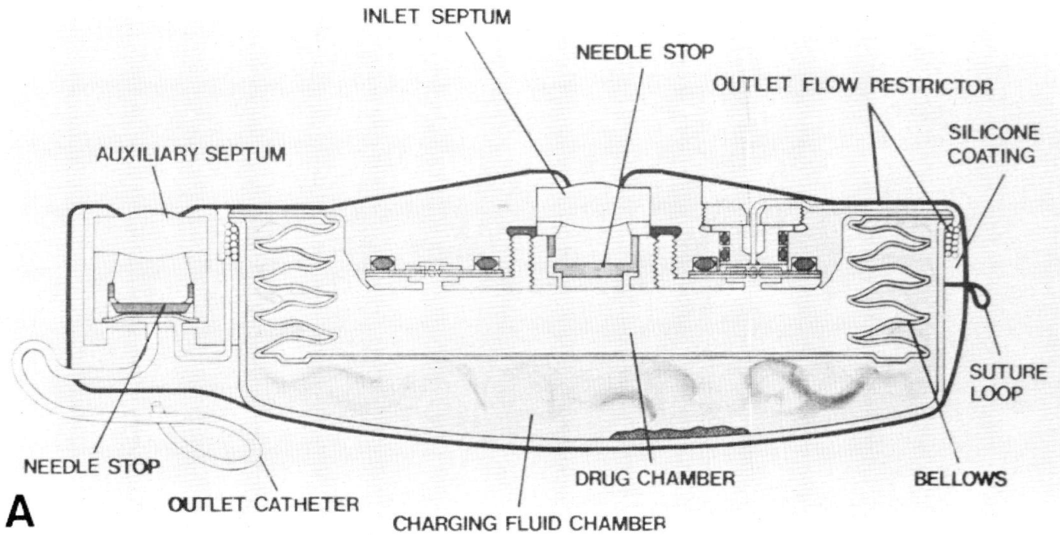

MODEL NO.	DIAMETER (mm)	THICKNESS (mm)	RESERVOIR VOLUME (ml)	EMPTY WEIGHT (gm)
100	87	28	47	187
200	87	23	32	172
400	~	28	47	208
500	87	20	22	165

B

Fig. 100-3.   The Infusaid pump system. (A) Model 400. (B) Model comparisons (typical valves).

subcutaneous system. Of the 6 patients treated by Coombs et al.,[56] the daily morphine requirement to provide sustained pain relief increased in 3 of them from the initial 1 to 4 mg per day over a 28-week period to 20 to 30 mg/day. In the other 3 the increase was to 4 to 8 mg/day. Results in the initial patients reported are encouraging.[3,35,57] Of the first three patients reported from this country, only one[3] appeared to develop some tolerance: over a 6–month period the dose was increased by 0.5 mg daily every 2 months (2.0 mg b.i.d. to 3.5 mg b.i.d.). Lazorthes and colleagues,[57] after implanting reservoirs in 9 cancer patients with pain in the lower limbs and lower torso, did not encounter excessive tolerance in follow-ups from 1 to 8 months.

There may be three ways to reduce the tendency to develop tachyphylaxis in the spinal opiate receptors: First, as Yaksh and colleagues[58] pointed out, the continuous application of constant minimal doses of the opiate may reduce the tendency to tachyphylaxis by eliminating the higher peak concentrations and increased degrees of receptor activation incident to bolus injections. Secondly, there is preliminary evidence in 3 patients[20] that a single injection of epidural lidocaine may restore the opiate receptor and its associated membrane-modifying mechanism to its original sensitivity, permitting return to the originally low therapeutic morphine doses. A third possibility is offered by recent data suggesting multiple specific opiate receptors that probably have independent mechanisms and hence low cross-tolerance. Accordingly, one would hope that once one set of receptors develops tolerance to high doses of morphine, a second pain suppressor agent could be used in low doses to activate another type of receptor that has not yet developed tolerance. While this new set is being activated, the receptor set that had developed tolerance would have time to recover spontaneously its original low dose sensitivity. β-endorphin may meet these requirements, but is at present prohibitively expensive.[59] A much cheaper likely candidate has been proposed by Yaksh, namely D-ala^2-d-leu^5-enkephalin (DADL). Whereas morphine binds more to the μ type of opiate receptors, the enkephalins bind preferentially to such receptors of the δ type. Yaksh and colleagues have shown no cross-tolerance to the enkephalin analogue DADL once such tolerance to intrathecal morphine has developed in rats. Moreover the DADL analogue degrades much more slowly than either the natural leu- or met-enkephalin; hence it raises the threshold to noxa for longer periods. Umansky et al.[60] have shown that after 2 weeks of high daily intrathecal injections in cats, it causes no significant histologic changes in the spinal cords or nerve roots.

Another potential impediment to extended long-term usage of these implanted delivery systems—probably less of a threat, however, than sepsis or tolerance—is malfunction of the system itself. Mechanically the complicated Infusaid pump has a life expectancy of 5 years. Perhaps simpler systems using shunt components (see Figure 100-2) might last even longer. Implantable pump systems with electronic battery-powered elements, such as the one currently being developed by NASA, will require surgery for battery replacement analogous to cardiac pacemakers. There again each change will increase the probability of infection. In addition to mechanical system failure, we anticipated a second possible source of system malfunction namely, scarring around the epidural catheter resulting in plugging it, or dural thickening preventing passage of morphine into the CSF and spinal cord. Neither of these occurred, however, in our patients with prolonged indwelling epidural catheters delivering xylocaine or morphine.[3-5] At autopsy, as mentioned earlier, there was no evidence of dural thickening or epidural scarring adjacent to the Silastic catheter.

These considerations of our potential ability to minimize sepsis, tolerance, and system malfunction seem encouraging. We are having an improved delivery system made, consisting of a 500-ml reservoir with two drug compartments for alternating activation of different opiate receptor sets, combined with a simple, reliable one-way valve system powered by external pressure applied by the patient himself for a long period without refilling. For people suffering from severe pain, especially those who are fully ambulatory with a variety of activities, we believe there is a great psychological value in systems that permit patient control with active self-administration. In fact, knowing that relief is readily available in some cases has decreased the usage.

The most encouraging aspect, however, of the future potential of focally applying opiates to the spinal cord rests in the remarkable specificity and efficacy of activating spinal opiate receptors. The effect is so circumscribed that pain relief is obtained without detectable interference with any other spinal cord system. There is no alteration of autonomic function such as changes in blood pressure regulation or bladder dynamics, and none in somatic motor function, In addition, not only is there no detectable alteration of proprioception, light touch, or thermal discrimination, but, most surprising, there is no apparent increase in the threshold for noxious pin pricks. These data again suggest, as do those from midline myelotomies, that the spinal cord may have two discrete neural systems, one for mediating severe chronic pain and perhaps also visceral pain, and another for mediating cutaneous acute pain perception. It is interesting that activation of the opiate receptor near threshold levels inhibits the former system but not the latter. Lastly, it is encouraging that segmental spinal opiate receptor activation rarely elicits subjective dysesthesias (except for itching) and does not depress mental alertness.

Accordingly, we envisage this application of surgically implantable systems for the chronic focal administration of pharmacologic agents to have a promising future especially for patients with intractable pain in the lower torso or lower limbs. Faced with the alternatives of systemic narcotic doses impairing their mental status or destructive major neurosurgical operations, we are finding that many patients already prefer to try this promising, relatively low-risk new therapeutic option.

Ninety-six head and neck cancer patients treated with intraventricular morphine were initially reported by 5 different investigators: Marini (35 cases),[61] Martin-Rodriquez (20 cases),[62] Lobato (17 cases),[63] Leavens (16 cases),[64,65] and Roquefeuil (8 cases).[66]

All of these investigators agree that intraventricular morphine is markedly effective in alleviating pain associated with cancer of the head and neck, but also the torso and limbs. Of the 96 patients, 70 were judged to have very good or excellent (80 to 100 percent) pain relief; 18 obtained significant to good relief (40 to 80 percent); and only 4 patients—all from Leavens series of 16 patients—were deemed to have no significant relief. (Four of the 96 patients were too ill in the postoperative period for reliable assessment.) This degree of pain relief was maintained until the patient's death, on the average of 3 months later. It seems clear that intraventricular morphine is markedly effective even in this very sick and terminal group of cancer patients.

The dose required was usually low, 2 mg/day, and tolerance in almost all the patients was either absent or insignificant. For instance, in Marini's series 34 patients all maintained the same degree of pain relief with no more than 2 mg/day, even in a patient who lived 9 months. A few patients maintained relief with as little as 0.10 mg/day. That tolerance to remarkable high doses can occur in some individuals is attested to by a patient of Leavens who survived 19 months postoperatively; before he died, to maintain pain relief, this patient tolerated 36 mg/day of intraventricular morphine.

The side effects of intraventricular morphine overall have been judged not to be serious, to have a short duration, and a low incidence. Respiratory depression, surprisingly, was detected in only 2 of the 96 patients. In one of these patients, 1 mg of intraventricular morphine produced 4 hours of respiratory depression; interestingly, naloxone then eliminated the respiratory suppression but did not reverse the analgesic effect. This patient subsequently maintained excellent pain relief without respiratory suppression from only 0.25 mg/day. In the second patient, very debilitated, an intraventricular injection of 9.5 mg morphine decreased respirations to 4/min. This is the patient who subsequently obtained excellent pain relief, without respiratory depression, with only 0.1 mg of morphine a day. For these reasons, most neurosurgeons administering intraventricular morphine recommended starting with a low dose, i.e., 0.24 mg and observing their patients in an ICU until a stable regimen of intraventricular morphine is being tolerated without respiratory suprression.

Only 1 infection was reported in the 96 patients. This patient became febrile and developed meningeal signs. The CSF culture was negative and the signs of infection cleared on antibiotics after removal of the reservoir and catheter. In all but 4 cases the morphine was injected via a needle passing through the skin into a 1-ml reservoir lying in a burr hole and attached to the ventricular catheter. The mean total number of injections per patient were approximately 135 (1–2 times/day for 3 months). In 4 instances, in order to facilitate self-injection by the patient, a larger reservoir was placed over the sternum and connected to the frontal ventricular catheter shunt tubing. Since morphine is stable at body temperature it is not necessary to flush the system with each injection.

Minor side effects, occasionally distressing, however, to the patient and his or her family, occur quite commonly, i.e., in 25 to 50 percent of patients. Typically, these subside within the first week of intraventricular morphine. Vomiting, nausea, urinary retention, hallucinations, confusion, dysphoria, dizziness, and pruritis occur frequently. In contrast, euphoria, also a common side effect, was found in all 5 series to help the patient, by counteracting the depression associated with dying from cancer.

In conclusion, intraventricular morphine warrants consideration especially in patients with cancer of the orofacial region, neck and shoulders. For these patients placing a ventricular catheter with an attached reservoir seems preferable to hypophysectomy, medullary tractotomy, or cordotomy especially in patients with bilateral disease. Intraventricular morphine also alleviates pain in patients with cancer in the torso and legs in whom spinal morphine has lost its effectiveness even at high doses.

The future for intraventricular analgesics seems quite promising. Improved delivery systems will further minimize the infections and new agents may be found to elicit pain relief without side effects. Somatostatin, 25 μg/hr intraventricularly, kept a 64-year-old man with bilateral cancer of the tongue, pain free. As with spinal somatostatin, this analgesic effect of intraventricular somatostatin was not reversed with naloxone.[67] Such compounds also offer promise in patients whose opiate receptors—spinal or central—have become tolerant to morphine.

ACKNOWLEDGMENT

The authors are grateful to the NeuroResearch Foundation for its support in the preparation of the manuscript.

REFERENCES

1. Blackshear PJ, Rohde TD, Prosl F, et al: The implantable infusion pump: A new concept in drug delivery. Med Prog Technol 6:149, 1979
2. Cohen AM, Kaufman S, Wood W, et al: Regional hepatic chemotherapy using an implantable drug infusion pump. Am J Surg (in press)
3. Poletti CE, Cohen AM, Todd DP, et al: Cancer pain relieved by long-term epidural morphine: Two case reports with permanent indwelling systems for self administration. J Neurosurg 55:581, 1981
4. Winkelmuller W, Dietz H, Stolke D: The clinical value of dorsal column stimulation. Adv Neurosurg 3:225, 1975
5. Pilon RN, Baker AR: Chronic pain by means of an epidural catheter. Cancer 37:903, 1976
6. Bromage PR: Epidural Analgesia. Philadelphia, WB Saunders, 1978
7. Strichartz GR: The inhibition of sodium currents in myelinated nerve by quaternary derivatives of lidocaine. J Gen Physiol 62:37, 1973
8. Taylor RE: Effect of procaine on electrical properties of squid axon membrane. Am J Physiol 196:1071, 1959
9. Bromage PR, Joyal AC, Binney JC: Local anesthetic drugs: Penetration from the spinal extradural space into the neuraxis. Science 140:392, 1963
10. Atweh SF, Kuhar MJ: Autoradiographic localization of opiate receptors in rat brain. I. Spinal cord and lower medulla. Brain Res 124:53, 1977
11. Cavillo O, Henry JL, Neuman RS: Effects of morphine and naloxone on dorsal horn neurones in the cat. Can J Physiol Pharmacol 52:1207, 1974
12. Kitahata LM, Kosaka Y, Taub A, et al: Lamina-specific suppression of dorsal-horn unit activity by morphine sulfate. Anesthesiology 41:39, 1974
13. Lamotte C, Pert CB, Snyder SH: Opiate receptor binding in primate spinal cord: Distribution and changes after dorsal root section. Brain Res 112:407, 1976
14. Pert CB, Kuhar MJ, Snyder SH: Opiate receptor: Autoradiographic localization in rat brain. Proc Natl Acad Sci USA 73:3729, 1976
15. Yaksh TL, Rudy TA: Analgesia mediated by a direct spinal action of narcotics. Science 192:1357, 1976
16. Yaksh TL, Rudy TA: A dose ratio comparison of the interaction between morphine and cyclazocine with naloxone in rhesus monkeys on the shock titration test. Eur J Pharmacol 46:83, 1977
17. Yaksh TL, Huang SP, Rudy TA: The direct and specific opiate-like effect of met-enkephalin and analogues on spinal cord. Neuroscience 2:593, 1977
18. Yaksh TL: Analgetic actions of intrathecal opiates in cat and primate. Brain Res 153:205, 1978
19. Yaksh TL, Else RP: Release of methionine-enkephalin immunoreactivity from the rat spinal cord in vivo. Eur J Pharmacol 63:359, 1980
20. Chayen MS, Rudick V, Borvine A: Pain control with epidural injection of morphine. Anesthesiology 53:338, 1980
21. Cousins MJ, Mather LE, Glynn CJ, et al: Selective spinal analgesia. Lancet 1:1141, 1979
22. Wang JK, Naus LA, Thomas JE: Pain relief by intrathecally applied morphine in man. Anesthesiology 50:149, 1979
23. Yaksh TL, Rudy TA: Chronic catheterization of the spinal subarachnoid space. Physiol Behav 17:1031, 1976
24. Goodman LS, Gilman A: The Pharmacological Basis of Therapeutics. New York, MacMillan, 1975, p 274
25. Andersen HB, Chraemmer-Jorgenson B, Engquist A: Morphine kinetics following peridural or spinal appiication. Pain (suppl 1), S250, 1981
26. Max M, Inturris CE, Gradinski P, et al: Epidural opiates: Plasma and cerebrospinal fluid (CSF) pharmacokinetics of morphine, methadone and Beta-endorphin. Pain (suppl 1), S122, 1981
27. Snyder, SH: Opiate receptors and internal opiates. Sci Am 236:44, 1977
28. Bromage PR: State of art: Extradural and intrathecal narcotics. American Society of Anesthesiologists' Refresher Course Outline 136:1, 1981
29. Samii K, Feret J, Harari A, et al: Selective spinal analgesia. Lancet 1:1142, 1979
30. Baraka A, et al: Intrathecal versus epidural morphine for obstetric analgesia. Anesthesiology 54:136, 1981
31. Behar M, Magora F, Olshwang D, et al: Epidural morphine in treatment of pain. Lancet 1:527, 1979
32. Bromage PR, Camporesi E, Chestbut D: Epidural narcotics for postoperative analgesia. Anesth Analg 59:473, 1980
33. Ebert J, Varner PD: The effective use of epidural morphine sulfate for postoperative orthopedic pain. Anesthesiology 53:257, 1980
34. Graham JL, King R, McCaughey W: Postoperative pain relief using epidural morphine. Anaesthesia 35:158, 1980
35. Onofrio BM, Yaksh TL, Arnold PG: Continuous low-dose intrathecal morphine administration in the treatment of chronic pain of malignant origin. Mayo Clin Proc 56:516, 1981
36. Wang J K: Analgesic effect of intrathecally administered morphine. Anesthesist 2:3-B, 1977
37. Cohen AM, Wood WC, Bamberg BS, et al: Continuous canine epidural morphine analgesia with an implanted drug infusion pump. J Surg Res 32:32, 1982
38. Boas RA: Hazards of epidural morphine. Anaesth Intensive Care 8:377, 1980
39. Baskoff JD, Watson RL, Muldoon SM: Respiratory arrest after intrathecal morphine. A case report. Anesthesiol Rev 7:12, 1980
40. Christensen V: Respiratory depression after extradural morphine. Br J Anaesth 52:841, 1980
41. Davies GK, Tolhurst-Cleaver CL, James TL: Respiratory depression after intrathecal narcotics. Anaesthesia 35:1080, 1980
42. Glynn CJ, et al: Spinal narcotics and respiratory depression. Lancet 2:356, 1979
43. Liolios A, Andersen FH: Selective spinal analgesia. Lancet 2:357, 1979
44. Scott DB, McClure J: Selective epidural analgesia. Lancet 1:1410, 1979
45. Tung AS, Tenicela R, Winter PM: Opiate withdrawal syndrome following intrathecal administration of morphine. Anesthesiology 53:340, 1980
46. Bottino J, McCredie KB, Groschel DHM, et al: Long-term intravenous therapy with peripherally inserted silicone elastomer central venous catheters in patients with malignant diseases. Cancer 43:1937, 1979
47. Broviac JW, Cole JJ, Scribner BH: A silicone rubber arterial catheter for prolonged parenteral alimentation. Surg Gynecol Obstet 136:602, 1973
48. Heimbach DM, Ivey TD: Technique for placement of a permanent

home hyperalimentation catheter. Surg Gynecol Obstet 143:634, 1976

49. Hickman RO, Buckner CD, Clift RA, et al: A modified right atrial catheter for access to the venous system in marrow transport recipients. Surg Gynecol Obstet 148:871, 1979

50. Hurtubise MR, Bottino JC, Lawson M, et al: Restoring patency of occluded central venous catheters. Arch Surg 115:212, 1980

51. Ponsky JL, Gauderer MWL: Expanded applications of Broviac catheter. Arch Surg 115:324, 1980

52. Thomas JH, MacArthur RI, Pierce GE, et al: Hickman-Broviac catheters. Indications and results. Am J Surg 140:791, 1980

53. Thomas M: The use of the Hickman catheter in the management of patients with leukaemia and other malignancies. Br J Surg 66:673, 1979

54. Lazorthes Y, Gouarderes C, Verdie JC, et al: Analgesie par injection intrathecale de morphine. Neurochirurgie 26:159, 1980

55. Chapleau CE, Robertson JJ: Spontaneous cervical carotid artery dissection: Outpatient treatment with continuous heparin infusion using a totally implantabie infusion device. Neurosurgery 8:83, 1981

56. Coombs DW, Saunders RL, Gaylor MS, et al: Continuous chronic pain relief by intraspinal narcotics inf used via an implanted reservoir. (in preparation)

57. Lazorthes Y, Siegfried J, Gouarderes C, et al: PVG stimulation versus intrathecal morphine in cancer pain. Pain (suppl 1), S29, 1981

58. Yaksh TL: Personal communication, 1982

59. Oyama T, Matsuki A, Taneichi T, et al: β-endorphin in obstetric analgesia. Am J Obstet Gynecol 137:613, 1980

60. Umansky F, Richardson EP, Sweet WH: Histologic studies of spinal cords and roots after intrathecal injections of D-Ala^2-D-leu^5-enkephalin in cats. Presented to the American Pain Society, Miami, October 29–31, 1982

61. Marini G, Lenzi A, Galli G: Intraventricular morphine for treatment orofacial and neck neoplastic pain. Presented to the combined meeting of Egyptian and Italian Neurosurgical Societies, Friday, March 16, 1984, Cairo

62. Martin-Rodriguez P: Personal Communication to Dr. W.H. Sweet, April 9, 1984

63. Lobato RD, Madrid JL, Fatela LV, et al: Intraventricular morphine for control of pain in terminal cancer patients. J Neurosurg 59:627, 1983

64. Leavens ME, Hill CS Jr, Cech DA, et al: Intrathecal and intraventricular morphine for pain in cancer patients: Initial study. J Neurosurg 56:241, 1982

65. Leavens M: Intraventricular morphine for the pain of cancer. Presented at the Houston Pain Symposium, Houston, Texas, April 6, 1984

66. Roquefeuil B, Benezech J, Batier CL, et al: Intéret de l'analgésie morphine par voie ventriculaire dans les algies rebelles néoplastiques. A propos de 8 cas dont 4 avec auto-administration. Neurochirurgie 29:135, 1983

67. Chrubasik J, Meynadier J, Ackerman E, et al: Somatostatin, A potent analgesic. Lancet 2:1208, 1984

CHAPTER 101

Open Cordotomy Medullary Tractotomy

Charles E. Poletti

INDICATIONS FOR OPEN CORDOTOMY

GENERAL: CANCER PAIN BELOW T5

We have become progressively inclined to perform cordotomy operations only on patients suffering from medically intractable cancer pain whose longevity appears limited to less than 3 years. This is because of the relatively high incidence of failures 1 to 2 years after cordotomy operations and the increasing late frequency of post-cordotomy painful dysesthesias. The significant instance of unavoidable complications—including motor weakness and bladder and sexual dysfunction—are further arguments against using the operation, especially bilaterally, in patients with benign disease. Accordingly, we have been reluctant to perform cordotomies on patients with peripheral nerve or spinal cord injuries, herpetic neuralgia, or chronic calcific pancreatitis, no matter how severely afflicted. With selected cancer patients, however, the operation often relieves the patient from suffering and excessive narcotics. For these individuals the operation should be done as a priority option. If delayed too long, the operation may not arrest or reverse extensive suffering and debilitation. For patients with markedly limited life spans a percutaneous cordotomy is often selected.

The use of cordotomy operations is further limited by progressive decreases in the level of analgesia during the first 6 months following the operation. Often within 3 weeks postoperatively the level has fallen three to six segments and at 6 months the level may have lowered a total of six to eight segments. Thus, most surgeons agree that even with high cervical cordotomies many patients may have no significant hypalgesia above T2-T3. Following a T2-T3 thoracic cordotomy, the level of significant permanent hypalgesia or analgesia usually is about T10. Consequently, one can usually count on a year of analgesia six to eight levels below the operation. A further consideration is that often during these postoperative 6 months in which the level of analgesia is falling, the cancer is progressing to higher levels. This is an important consideration before performing the cordotomy.

More important than determining the site of the referred pain is localizing the cancerous lesion producing the pain. For instance, a recent patient with prostatic cancer and severe, deep lateral flank pain on the right side appeared to be a good candidate for unilateral open thoracic cordotomy until a body computed tomographic (CT) scan revealed a single metastasis eroding the right half of the T12 vertebra. On further direct questioning, the patient finally admitted to pain in the corresponding left lateral flank. In this case unilateral cordotomy was no longer an option. We believe each cordotomy operation should be individually designed based primarily on the location of the cancerous lesion producing the pain.

UNILATERAL SOMATIC CANCER: UNILATERAL CORDOTOMY

Unilateral cordotomies are most effective for cancer not invading the viscera and for cancer located away from the midline and at or below the lower cervical region. Thus, excellent potential candidates are patients with cancer confined to the legs, the hips, the lateral retroperitoneal pelvic and abdominal space, the chest wall (e.g., breast cancer and Pancoast's tumor), and perhaps the lower brachial plexus. For disease below T8 we select a T2 unilateral thoracic cordotomy, which carries a lower risk than cervical cordotomy.

For the arms, as for the neck, nasopharyngeal, and facial cancer, a medullary tractotomy is worth considering instead of cordotomy, although the operative mortality and incidence of postoperative dysesthesias is slightly higher. An open C2-C3 cordotomy combined with a C2, C3 and C4 dorsal rhizotomy may relieve severe pain in the brachial plexus, upper extremity, shoulder, and neck.[1] We favor open C2-C3 cordotomy, occasionally combined with rhizotomy, over a C1-C2 percutaneous cordotomy because of the marked anatomic variations at C1-C2 and the belief that consistently more complete, uncomplicated lesions with higher permanent levels of analgesia can be obtained using our open technique at C2-C3.

UNILATERAL VISCERAL PAIN: BILATERAL CORDOTOMY

In general, whenever a significant component of the pain is caused by disease invading the viscera, bilateral deep cordotomies are required for satisfactory relief of suffering. Often the visceral pain from extensive cancer of the pancreas, intestine, colon, rectum, cervix, or uterus, and especially stomach and esophagus may be mediated by splanchnic nerves entering the spinal cord as high as T1. Many of these visceral nociceptive afferents do not cross to the other side of the spinal cord. Accordingly, in these patients the best chance of satisfactory results rests with the highest bilateral cervical cordotomies advisable, i.e., C1-C2 percutaneous or C2-C3 open

OPERATIVE NEUROSURGICAL TECHNIQUES
ISBN 0-8089-1862-1

cordotomy combined with an open contralateral C5-C6 cordotomy.

PARAMEDIAN, MIDLINE, AND BILATERAL CANCER: BILATERAL CORDOTOMY

Whenever the cancer is close to the midline, unilateral cordotomy has a high probability of not securing prolonged relief. These patients very often become aware of severe contralateral pain shortly after surgery. Accordingly, it should be emphasized that even for paramedian cancers it is wise to perform a bilateral cordotomy.

When bilateral cordotomies are indicated, an open cordotomy is performed at two levels, rather than a unilateral percutaneous cordotomy followed by an open operation.

ALTERNATIVES TO BILATERAL CORDOTOMY

Whenever open bilateral cordotomies are indicated, one should seriously consider various alternative operations that are available: A midline myelotomy operation may have a higher incidence of pain relief for bilateral pain in the arms, shoulders, and neck as well as pain from bilateral visceral or extensive midline disease. In addition, midline myelotomies, compared with bilateral cordotomies, have a significantly lower incidence of later postcordotomy dysesthesias and bladder dysfunction, sleep apnea, and motor weakness.

Recently Hitchcock[2,3] and Schvarcz[4-6] independently have pioneered central medullary myelotomies for high bilateral disease using stereotactic techniques. These appear promising but require special expertise.

Recently my colleagues and I developed a technically very simple nondestructive operation for intractable cancer pain in which a spinal epidural catheter is implanted for long-term administration of morphine.[7] Using three administration systems, we demonstrated for the first time that direct spinal narcotics can be employed on a chronic basis for effective pain relief.

SPINAL CORD ANATOMIC VARIATIONS AND ANTEROLATERAL CORDOTOMY

The goal of anterolateral cordotomy is to create a lesion in fibers ascending in the spinothalamic tract (STT) that carry nociceptive input from one side of the body caudal to the level of the lesion. Marked anatomic variations of the spinal cord, however, frequently impede optimal lesioning of the STT. Four major areas of anatomic variation that concern the surgeon are: (1) the course of the STT; (2) the course of the corticospinal tract (CST); (3) the position of the dentate insertion; and (4) the width of the spinal cord. Thus, in cordotomy as in aneurysm surgery, the individual patient's anatomy must be identified or analyzed. It often may be necessary to perform a variation of the standard operation in order to maximize the probability of satisfactory results for each individual.

STT ANATOMY AND VARIANTS

In some individuals the STT does not appear to decussate at all. In these patients a standard anterolateral cordotomy produces ipsilateral analgesia. Fortunately these cases are rare.

Most individuals, however, probably have a number of uncrossed nociceptive fibers. Perhaps these permit the recovery of pain following cordotomy. In particular, the nociceptive fibers mediating visceral pain in many cases do not decussate fully, but instead ascend on both sides of the spinal cord. This should encourage the surgeon toward bilateral cordotomies when visceral pain is felt to be significant.

Normally the vast majority of the nociceptive fibers do decussate, following two predictable patterns. First, the "sacral" fibers are positioned most posterolaterally and superficially. The more rostral fibers from the lumbar, thoracic, and cervical regions ascend to assume their course more anteromedially and deeper (Figure 101-1). The sacral fibers may lie immediately anterior to the base of the normally positioned dentate (Figure 101-1). The cordotomy lesion therefore should first reach as far dorsally as the equator of the spinal cord, usually at the base of the dentate insertion. Beginning the lesion 1 to 2 mm anterior to this point in some individuals results in sparing the sacral fibers.

A second relatively predictable pattern reflects the observation that pain from the superficial part of the body is relayed by fibers close to the surface of the spinal cord. Progressively deeper are the fibers mediating our sense of temperature, deep pain, and, finally, visceral pain (Figure 101-1). Accordingly, the lesion must extend deep to the anterolateral surface of the cord, especially in patients with visceral disease. In most patients, a depth of 5 mm is required, even in the cervical region.

Perhaps most important, the lesion should include the medial and anterior portion of the anterior quadrant. It is often in this portion of the spinal cord that fibers from the anterior commissure may ascend five to six segments or more before extending far enough laterally to assume their "classical" position in the "lateral" STT. In contrast, fibers from the dorsal horn appear to cross to the anterior commissure almost immediately, i.e., at the same level or at most within one to two segments. Yet these same fibers may then ascend for five to eight segments before "crossing" fully to form the "lateral" STT. Thus, the "anterior" STT in humans consists of ascending fibers gradually coursing laterally to form the "lateral" STT. Accordingly, a lesion in the lateral anterior quadrant, albeit deep, may produce analgesia extending rostrally only eight or more segments below the lesion. In contrast, a lesion of the anterior quadrant extending to the midline may in some individuals produce analgesia to within one segment of the lesion. Thus, especially in cervical cordotomies where a primary goal is a high permanent level of analgesia, we recommend extending the lesion at least 1 to 2 mm anterior to the most medial exiting fibers of the ventral root, i.e., within 1 to 2.5 mm of the anterior spinal artery (see Figure 101-7). A lesion only as far anteriorly as the ventral root may yield a satisfactory level of analgesia in only 80 percent of patients. The technique to be described, in fact, usually permits a lesion of the entire anterior quadrant extending immediately to the midline anterior pial septum and anterior spinal artery. This lesion, we believe, produces the highest level of analgesia feasible—usually within two and occasionally within one segment.

CORTICOSPINAL TRACT ANATOMY AND VARIATIONS

Rarely the CST does not decussate at all. Instead it descends uncrossed in the anterolateral quadrant of the cord. In these rare individuals an anterolateral cordotomy would be

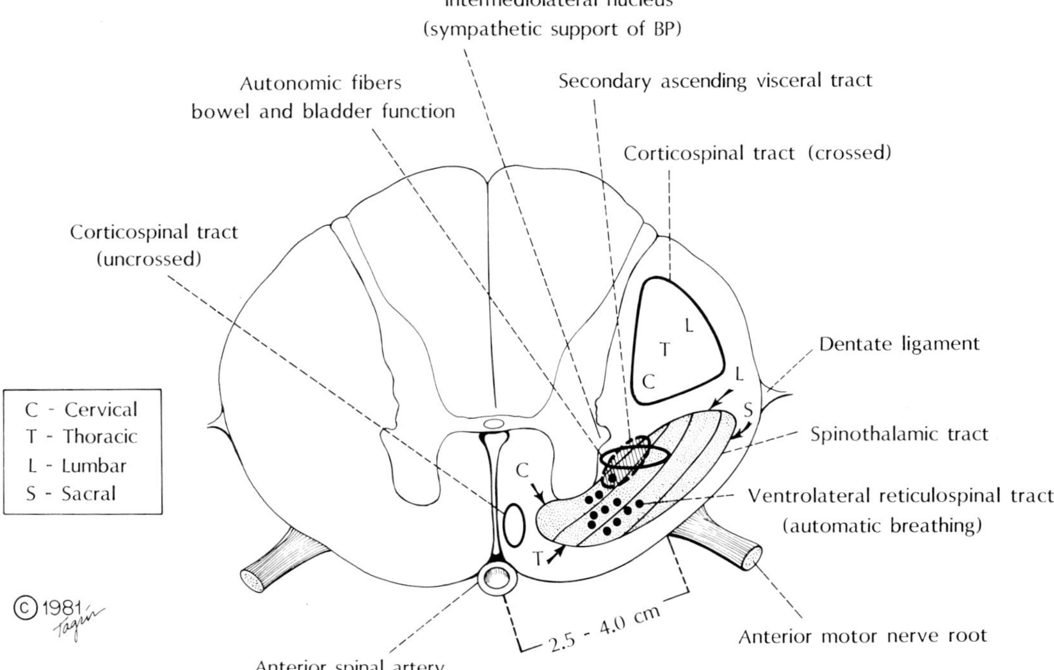

Fig. 101-1. The spinal cord at T3 with the axon tracts relevant to making lesions of the STT. Just dorsal to the equator of the cord is the descending CST. The lesion should start about 1 mm anterior to the anterior limit of the CST. The entire STT is shown, including the "anterior" and "lateral" components. It should be emphasized that intermingled within the STT fibers are other ascending and descending tracts. These of necessity must be lesioned to obtain a complete lesion of the STT. These tracts intermingled at least in part with the STT include the ventrolateral reticulospinal tract, which is responsible for nonvoluntary breathing, the descending autonomic fibers for bladder and bowel sphincter control, the ascending visceral tract, and sympathetic fibers just anterolateral to their origin in the intermedolateral nucleus. In the anteromedial aspect of the cord is the uncrossed CST adjacent to the midline septum and the anterior spinal artery. Note also that the distance from the medialmost exiting motor rootlet to the anterior spinal artery and midline varies from 2.0 to 3.5 mm.

expected to produce contralateral plegia as these aberrant tracts are believed to finally cross near the segment of their termination on the lower motor neuron. In addition, the data of Yakovlev and Rakic[8] indicates that these abnormal patterns of the CST are probably more common than we like to believe. It seems reasonable to assume there may be associated abnormalities or displacements of the normally adjacent STT.

Frequently, however, even in normal individuals the decussating pyramidal fibers may not be fully crossed and back into the posterior aspect of the cord until the caudal half of C2. Accordingly, we are inclined to do our cervical cordotomies at C3. A C4-C5 level of analgesia, as discussed above, may still be feasible by extending the lesion to the midline. Clearly when the decussation is abnormally low, careful stimulation and monitoring—even at C3—is necessary to avoid a lesion of the CST.

DENTATE INSERTION VARIATIONS

The dentate ligament is formed by the joining of a component of the ventral and dorsal spinal cord pia. Usually these join to form the dentate at the equator of the cord just anterior to the anterior extent of the CST and just posterior to the posterior extent of the sacral fibers of the SST. In a number of cases, however, as Sweet[9] has noted, the dentate origin may form anterior or posterior to this equatorial line. When it is anterior to its most common position, a lesion beginning at the dentate and extending anteriorly may not lesion nociceptive fibers from the sacrum. In cases of a posterior dentate a lesion beginning just anterior to the dentate clearly has a high probability of

producing an ipsilateral motor deficit. Accordingly, the lesion should begin at the equator of the cord, irrespective of the position of the dentate. Because the equator of the rotated cord is difficult to judge we again stress physiologic stimulation and monitoring, preferably with the patient awake.

SPINAL CORD WIDTH VARIATIONS

The width of the spinal cord appears to vary as well, both in the thoracic and cervical regions. This is especially true in patients with advanced cancer. In one of our patients, for instance, extensive pelvic cancer invaded the lumbosacral plexus bilaterally, producing significant sensory deficits and virtual paraplegia. In this patient the spinal cord at T2 under the microscope measured a total width of 5.2 mm. Obviously it would have been injudicious to try to cut the anterior quadrant to a depth of 4 to 5 mm, especially since at the time we were still using a cordotomy knife, not a blunt instrument capable of palpating the anterior midline septum adjacent to the anterior spinal artery. Accordingly, we recommend measuring the width of the spinal cord in each case and using that specific dimension to determine the approximate depth of the lesion.

PREOPERATIVE PROCEDURE

PREPARATIONS AND SPECIAL INSTRUMENTS

All patients are advised of the complications of cordotomy operations. When awakening the patient during the operation appears appropriate, the details and alternatives are discussed

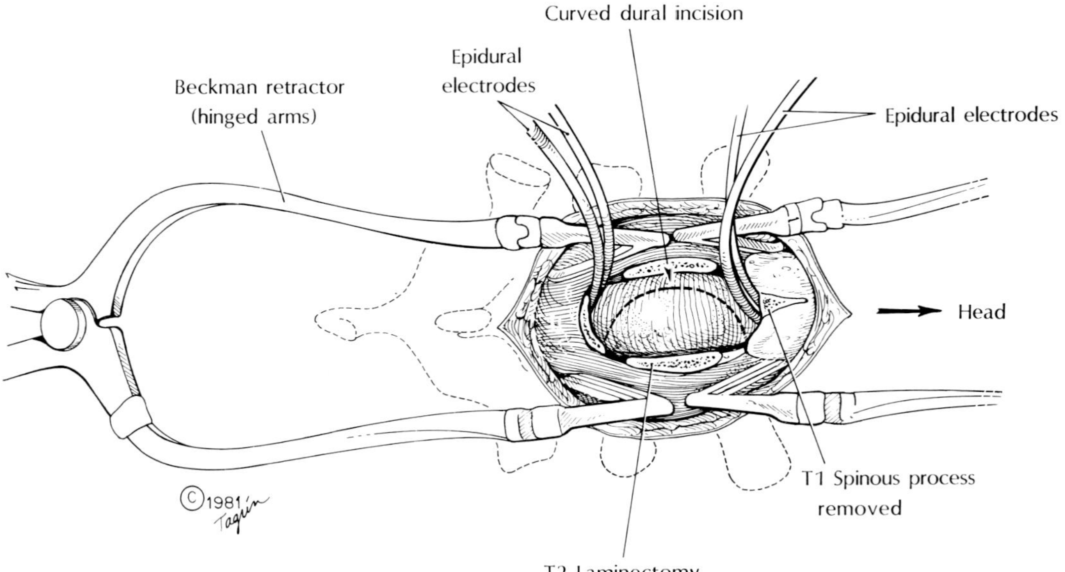

Fig. 101-2. The spinous processes of T1, T2, and T3 are exposed. The T1 and T2 processes are removed. A complete bilateral laminectomy at T2 is shown extending far laterally on the side of the lesion. The rostral and caudal yellow ligaments are excised. The bipolar epidural electrodes are then inserted in the midline rostrally and caudally for recording sensory evoked potentials from bilateral peroneal stimulation. The projected dural incision is shown by the dotted line.

with the patient, both by the surgeon and the anesthesiologist. If there is any suspicion of impaired pulmonary function contralateral to the planned lesion, then a comprehensive series of pulmonary function tests are done. When there is impaired motion of the contralateral hemidiaphragm, a unilateral cervical cordotomy may trigger fatal postoperative respiratory complications by interrupting the exclusively ipsilateral descending projections of the ventrolateral reticulospinal tract (Figure 101-1). The patient is wrapped with Ace bandages from the toes to the thigh to minimize the resulting operation-induced orthostatic hypotension. This is especially important when bilateral lesions are planned.

ELECTROPHYSIOLOGIC MONITORING EQUIPMENT (EMG)

Because of the marked potential variability in the location within the spinal cord of both the lateral spinothalamic tract and the corticospinal tracts, we conclude that intraoperative electrophysiologic stimulation of the spinal cord combined with dorsal column-evoked responses and EMG recording are useful. In order both to stimulate in the anterior quadrant to identify the STT in the awakened patient and later to stimulate while making the lesion to warn of nearby CST fibers, we use a 45-degree Jacobsen ball that is insulated except over the distal half of the ball and at the end of the handle. A standard stimulator is attached to the uninsulated end of the handle, preferably a simulator that is capable of constant current stimulation at 2–100 Hz. For measuring dorsal column potentials evoked by peroneal or median nerve stimulation, we use a Nicolet signal averager with bipolar epidural recording electrodes. This technique is described elsewhere.[10] Especially in cases in which wake-up anesthesia is not used, we monitor CST function by stimulating as the lesion is being made while looking for motor responses and elicited EMG recordings distally. A

small dental mirror on a malleable shaft is used to visualize the anterior spinal artery while making the lesion.

OPERATIVE PROCEDURES

ANESTHESIA

With the improved techniques of wake-up anesthesia supplemented by local infiltration of the wound, we have discontinued the use of only local anesthetics for cordotomy operations. Wake-up anesthesia offers the opportunity of identifying the SST by stimulation, of monitoring bilateral motor function as the lesion is being made, and, finally, of testing the extent of the induced sensory deficit before it is too late to enlarge the lesion. A third technique for having an awake patient following the initial cordotomy incision has recently been described.[11] With this new technique, segmental analgesia is produced (C4–T8) by blocking the dorsal roots using a single injection of epidural bupivacaine. Since normal spinal cord function is preserved and the T2 laminectomy easily tolerated, the patient remains fully awake and cooperative for testing sensory and motor function distal to T8 after the cordotomy lesions are produced.

The operative technique described here is designed especially to maximize the probability of obtaining an optimal lesion without subjecting the patient to being awake during surgery. The goal in this technique is making as large a lesion as feasible in the anterior quadrant without lesioning the CST. Dorsally the lesion extends to within 1 to 2 mm of the CST, medially to the midline anterior septum and all the way anteriorly and anterolaterally. If there is a dominant variant of the CST in the anteromedial aspect of the spinal cord, it is identified by the stimulus at the top of the Jacobsen ball. As a result, our last 7 patients have been operated on under continuous general anesthesia and all have had an initial contralateral distal hemianalgesia rising to within 2 segments of the complete anterior quadrant cordotomy without any detectable motor weakness.

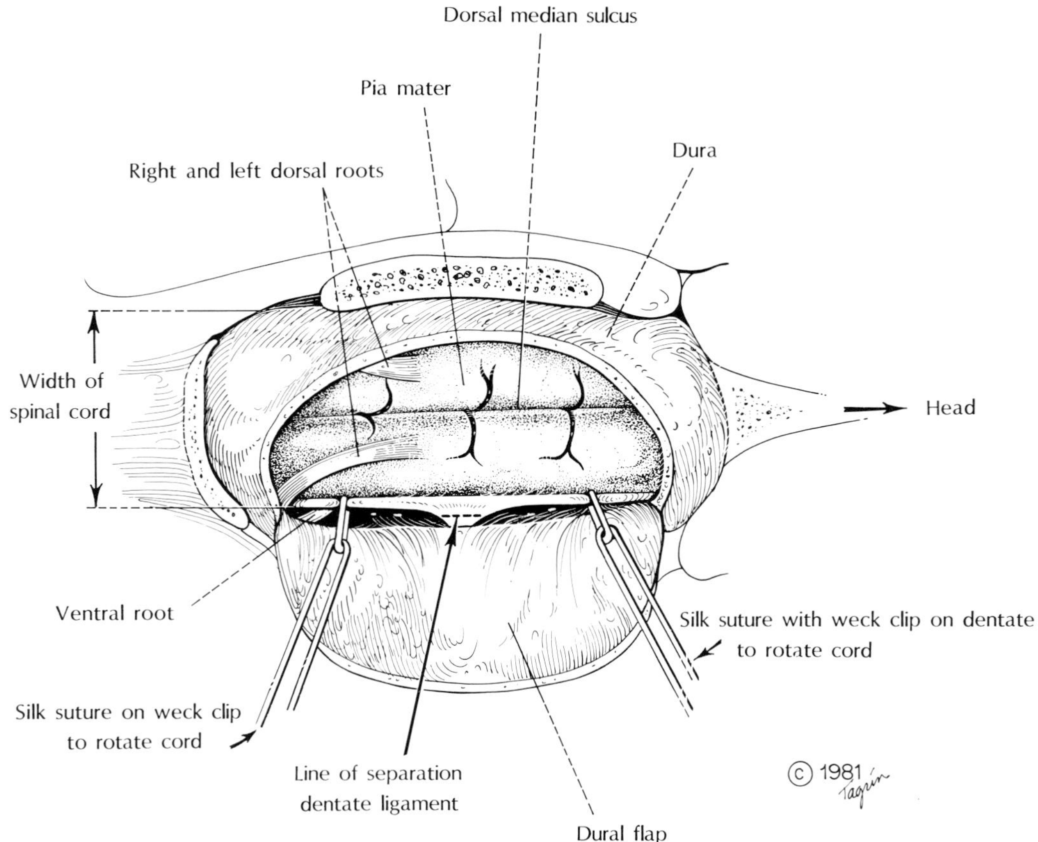

Fig. 101-3. The dura is opened. The microscope is brought into the field. The arachnoid is dissected bilaterally. The dura contralaterally is retracted to permit direct measurement of the width of the spinal cord. Weck clips with silk sutures are applied to the dentate as shown. The arachnoid around the dorsal roots is dissected, freeing the roots to their exit point.

POSITION

For unilateral cordotomy with wake-up anesthesia, the patient can be placed in the swimmer's position with the thorax rotated 45 degrees up from horizontal. With the spinal cord rotated 45 degrees, the operating microscope can be focused almost vertically and the cord viewed from a transverse direction. When bilateral lesions are anticipated, or in cases in which wake-up anesthesia is not employed, the patient should be placed prone. Especially for cervical cordotomies the head is placed in a neutral position to decrease tethering of the cord, which may occur with too much flexion. For cervical operations, the head is held in a three-pin headrest whereas during upper thoracic operations the head is allowed to rest on a doughnut headrest. The fully bandaged legs should be elevated on blankets and the table set in moderate reverse Trendelenburg position. With the patient in this position, a decrease in blood pressure following bilateral lesions will indicate, as noted by Sindou,[12] that the depth and dorsal extent of the lesion are satisfactory.

UNILATERAL CORDOTOMY PROCEDURE

A relatively long skin incision is made in order to provide wide lateral retraction of the skin and paraspinal muscles. This affords a view from a lateral angle of the anterior quadrant of the rotated cord.

For unilateral upper thoracic lesions the T2 and T3 laminae are exposed, while bilateral upper thoracic lesions call for exposure of the laminae of T2, T3, and T4. A complete laminectomy is done extending fully laterally on the side of the planned lesion. Next, the yellow ligament above and below the laminectomy is removed, exposing the inferior edge of the rostral lamina and the superior edge of the caudal lamina. The bipolar electrodes for recording evoked potentials from bilateral peroneal nerve stimulation are inserted in the midline epidural space rostrally and caudally (Figure 101-2).

The dura is then opened in a semicircular fashion extending far enough laterally to allow direct visualization of the contralateral side of the spinal cord (Figure 101-3). This permits exact measurement of the width of the spinal cord. The microscope is brought into the field. The arachnoid is opened for optimal visualization. The width of the cord is measured precisely under the microscope and a piece of bone wax is used to mark half of the cord width from the tip of the Jacobsen ball. This measurement will be used during lesioning to gauge the depth of cordotomy and to allow the tip of the Jacobsen ball to reach the midline. Once the cord width has been measured, the arachnoid opening is extended laterally over the dentate ligament.

Traction of the dorsal or ventral roots during rotation of the cord may result in painful dysesthesias postoperatively. The dorsal rootlets should therefore be freed from the cord to their point of exit or to the limit of the exposure. If necessary, the dorsal root should be cut to facilitate rotation, rather than risk a traction injury with postoperative hyperesthesia. As previously mentioned, in cervical cordotomies White and Sweet suggest performing bilateral rhizotomies of the three accessible

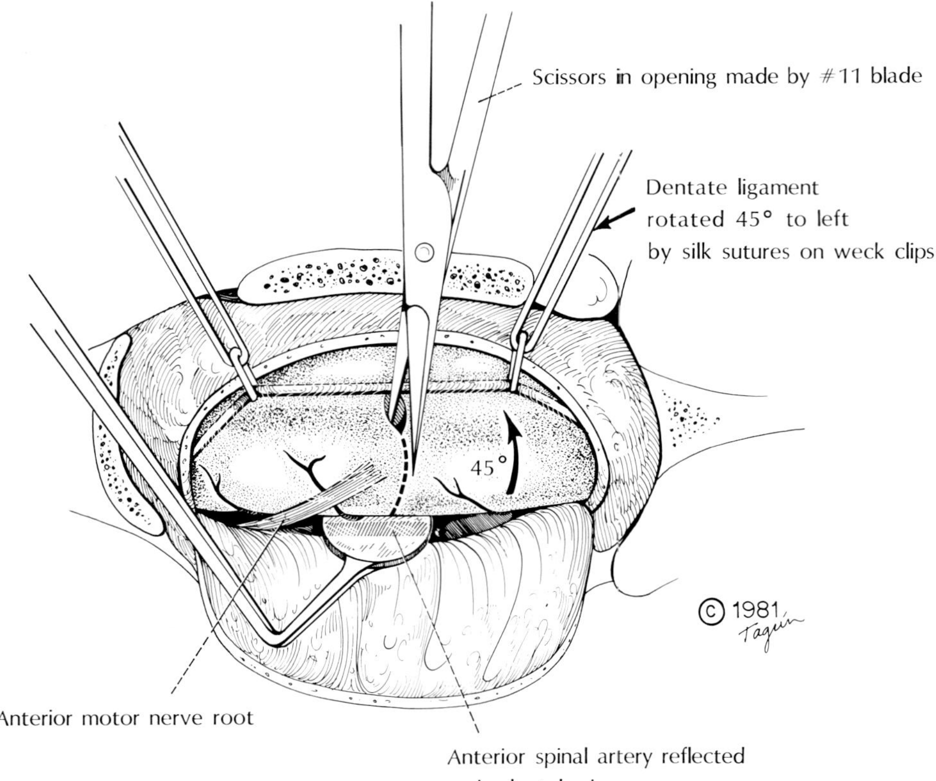

Fig. 101-4. The dentate ligament lateral attachment has been cut. Traction is applied on the silk sutures attached by Weck clips to the dentate until the cord is rotated 45 degrees. A small dental mirror is placed ventrolaterally to permit visualization of the anterior midline septum and the course of the anterior spinal artery. The microscissors are placed into the hole made in the pia just anterior to the equator of the cord. These are used to cut the pia arachnoid around the anterior quadrant to within 1 to 2 mm of the anterior midline septum. This is usually about 2 mm anterior to the medialmost exiting ventral rootlet.

dorsal roots in order to raise the level of analgesia and to decrease the postoperative incisional pain. Other workers have found that rhizotomies do not improve the results of the cordotomy.[13]

With the roots freed or cut, the cord is then rotated 45 degrees. To rotate the cord a 4-0 silk suture is placed in two Weck clips, which are in turn placed on the dentate ligament (Figure 101-4; see also Figure 101-3). The silk sutures are then used to put traction on the Weck clips and the dentate for rotating the cord. If the patient is under local anesthesia and experiences pain as the cord is rotated, the dorsal root should be cut. Alternatively, cerebrospinal fluid should be aspirated and a small cottonoid soaked in 10 percent cocaine applied selectively to the posterior root(s). If the root is sufficiently mobilized beforehand, however, pain during rotation is rarely elicited. With careful microsurgical dissection, the intact dentate insertion usually is strong enough to rotate the cord. If not, traction may be applied directly on the anterior root to rotate the cord. One should not be afraid to rotate the cord too far. If the anterior spinal artery along the anterior midline cannot be satisfactorily viewed, the dentate above and below the level of interest can be cut, permitting the cord to be rotated as much as 90 degrees. Electrophysiologic monitoring electrodes offer additional safety features, but we have not found their use to be mandatory if the techniques above are followed as described. Once the cord is rotated 45 degrees, a small dental mirror on a malleable handle may be used to visualize the exact course of the anterior spinal artery in the anterior midline septum, and the

medial limit of the exit of the ventral rootlets (Figures 101-4, 101-5). At the most avascular part of the exposed anterior quadrant the tip of a No. 11 blade is inserted into the equator of the spinal cord. As noted, this is usually located immediately under the dentate insertion. The exact site of the dentate attachment can be established by observation and blunt palpation on the dentate insertion in a dorsal-to-ventral manner. Microsurgical scissors are placed in the small hole made in the pia by the No. 11 blade (Figure 101-4). Only the pia arachnoid is then cut with the microscissors around the anterior quadrant of the cord. Cutting the pia with sharp scissors decreases the chance of avulsing the dentate attachment. Small pial vessels may be cauterized with bipolar microforceps. We incise the pia to a point 2 mm anterior to the medialmost exit of the ventral root, which should be at least 1 mm from the anterior spinal artery. An advantage of making the pial cut initially before lesioning the tracts is that the natural shape of the cord is subsequently preserved while the instrument is being inserted. Cutting the pia with a knife tends to distort the anatomy of the cord, making an accurate lesion difficult and placing indirect traction on adjacent vascular and neural structures.

With the incision in the pia, the cord is ready for cordotomy. Clearly, in making the spinal cord lesion the two principal cautions are to avoid transecting the cortical spinal tract, and to avoid damage to the anterior spinal artery and its main branches. The cortical spinal tract is particularly vulnerable to damage during cordotomy procedures and as mentioned previously, anatomic variations limit the surgeon's ability to

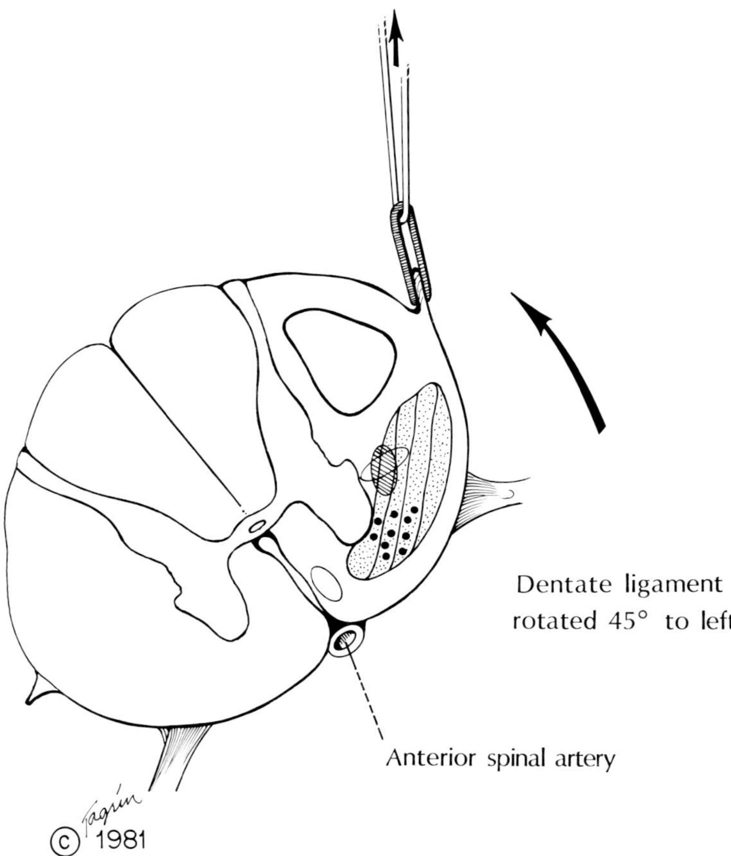

Fig. 101-5. The orientation of the relevant tracts within the cord once it has been rotated 45 degrees.

execute an adequate lesion without the possibility of damaging the motor system.

In making the lesion, our operative technique is unique in that it employs the use of a blunt Jacobsen ball to simultaneously stimulate while making the lesion. The stimulator is attached to the end of the handle of the Jacobsen ball instrument. A ground electrode is inserted in the paraspinal muscles. Stimulation parameters are set for 1-msec pulses delivered at 1.5 V. This stimulus will elicit responses in the cortical spinal tract with motion in the ipsilateral arm or leg in the asleep, unparalyzed patient when the ball tip approaches within 1 mm of the CST. This blunt-tipped instrument permits a safe traverse of the anterolateral cord all the way to the medial septum while the proximity of the instrument to the cortical spinal tract dorsally is concurrently monitored by looking for stimulation-evoked motor responses. Although the Jacobsen ball is a blunt instrument, it does not distort the very soft tissue of the cord. It has been our experience, particularly with midline myelotomies, that the Jacobsen ball is fully satisfactory for transecting spinal cord tracts.

The Jacobsen ball is inserted at the equator of the cord at the dorsalmost limit of the pial opening and is directed into the transverse axis of the cord until the bone wax indicates that the ball is halfway across the width of the cord. Since the spinal cord has been rotated 45 degrees, the tip of the Jacobsen ball is also angled 45 degrees. Thus, during this initial motion the shaft of the instrument is held vertically (Figure 101-6A and B). Usually the transverse diameter of the cord in the upper thoracic region is approximately 10 mm and thus initially an incision to a depth of approximately 5 mm is indicated. In the

cervical region the cord may be as wide as 16 mm, in which case an incision to 8 mm is permissible. As mentioned previously, however, the size of the cord may vary. We have seen a cord width as small as 5.2 mm in the thoracic region, presumably because of atrophy of the dorsal columns and descending cortical spinal tracts. In that particular case it was necessary to insert the ball to only 2.5 mm in order to place the lesion at the center of the cord. As the ball passes near the gray of the anterior horn, an ipsilateral trapezius contraction may be obtained during cervical cordotomy and contraction of intercostal muscles during thoracic cordotomy. The presence of distal ipsilateral motor responses indicates that the stimulating Jacobsen ball is too close to the descending cortical spinal tract and must be directed more anteriorly. This is most frequently necessary when working in the cervical region, where the motor fibers may not be exclusively dorsal to the equator of the cord. Once the ball is in the center of the cord (Figure 101-6B), it is drawn directly anteriorly along the palpable medial septum to the anteromedial corner of the anterior quadrant. The ball is then drawn laterally along the pia for about 1 to 2 mm until it exits from the cord at the most anteromedial extent of the pial incision (Figure 101-7). The ball should be drawn flush against the pia of the midline septum and the anterior quadrant. The pia is firm and can be readily palpated safely from inside the cord with the Jacobsen ball. There may be marked anatomic variation in the anteromedial portion of the anterior quadrant with a large uncrossed corticospinal tract. Should this be the case, one would expect contralateral motor responses in this region from the Jacobsen ball. We have not yet encountered such a case. Should this occur, it seems prudent to skirt this tract when

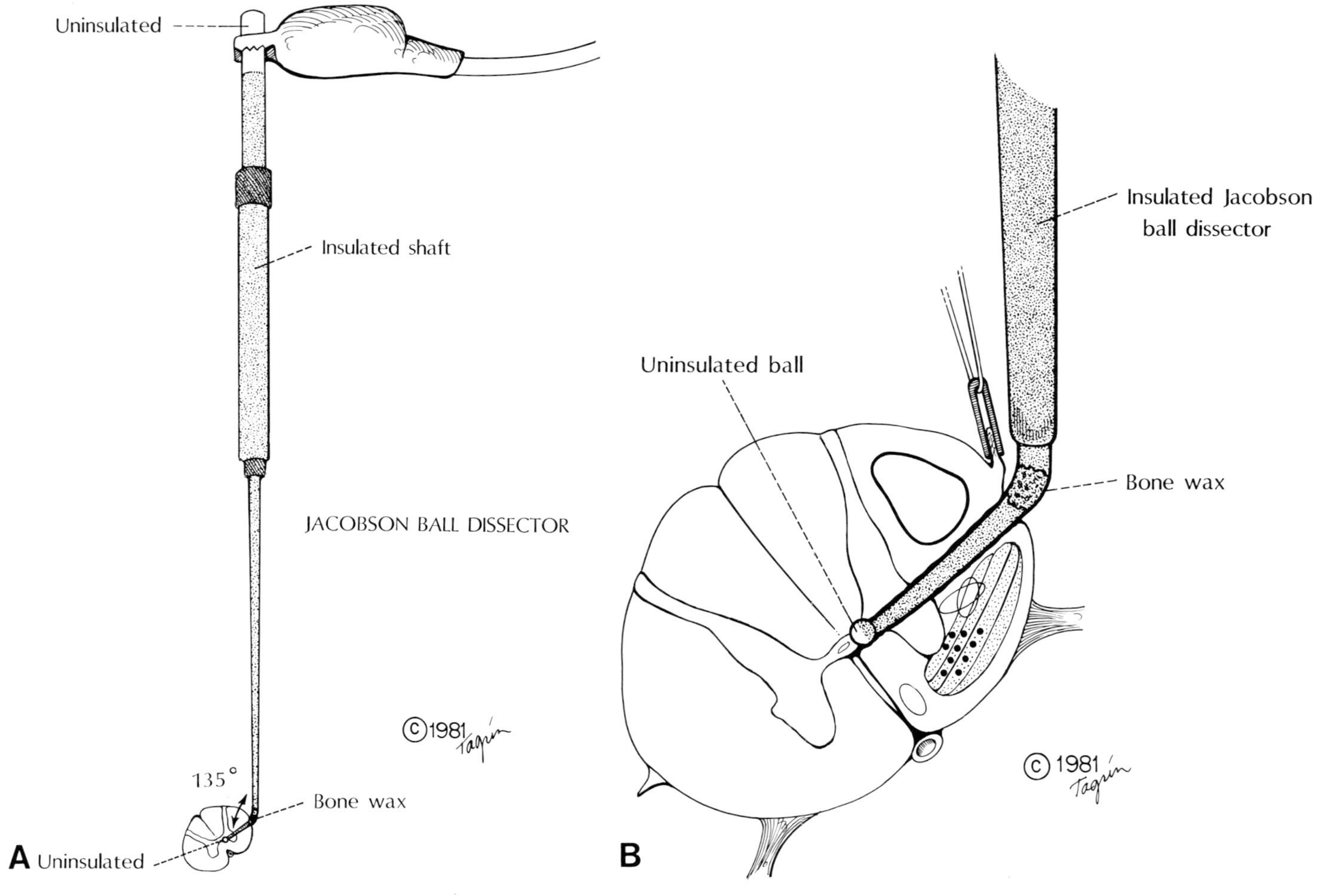

Fig. 101-6. (A) The 45-degree Jacobsen ball tip has been inserted just anterior to the equator of the cord and, while stimulating, is slowly advanced in the transverse axis of the cord until the tip reaches the midline (i.e., until the distal part of the bone wax marker on the tip is flush against the lateral aspect of the cord). The tip should pass far enough dorsally to include the intermedolateral nucleus and all the tracts depicted in Figure 101-1 except for the crossed CST. (B) An enlarged view of the Jacobsen ball instrument after the initial insertion. Note that the distal half of the Jacobsen ball is uninsulated. Should this pass closer than 1 mm to the CST during its insertion into the cord, ipsilateral motor responses will be elicited. In this case the ball should be redirected more anteriorly. From this position the ball is then slowly directed 90 degrees anteriorly, palpating the midline septum.

making the first lesion. The ball tip of the Jacobsen instrument usually can be seen as it comes out of the pia, but, it necessary, there is usually ample room to insert the mirror in order to see exactly where the ball exits. If it exits as planned, there is a very high probability that a satisfactory lesion was performed.

It is important, as shown in Figure 101-7, to make the lesion as close as possible to the midline septum. This is especially important in the cervical region, where recently crossed fibers may lie close to the septum for many levels before assuming a more lateral and dorsal position. Hardy[14] believes that an incision extending to the midline can raise the level of resulting analgesia virtually to the level of the lesion.

Selective cervical cordotomies, i.e., partial lesions of the anterolateral quadrant, are not recommended for two reasons: first, cancer may spread to wider areas, and second, the topological distribution of the spinal thalamic tract does not appear to be sufficiently specific for reliable results.

It should be stressed that in the cervical region the anterior spinal artery is usually 4.5 to 5.0 mm from the center of the exit zone of the anterior nerve root. A lesion 2 mm from the midline will still be 2.5 to 3.0 mm away from the center of the exiting ventral root. Except for the danger of entry into the anterior spinal artery, there does not appear to be any disadvantage to making an incision in the medial anterior quadrant as well. We have not seen a case of contralateral motor weakness caused by transection of the uncrossed descending motor tracts.

In summary, when making the initial lesion, an attempt should be made to transect virtually the entire anterior quadrant of the cord from the equator anteriorly, extending to the midline.

Following the initial cordotomy lesion, the patient may be awakened in order to test the extent of the resulting analgesia as well as the integrity of motor function. Before awakening, Xylocaine should be injected profusely into the paraspinal muscles. When the patient awakens, pain may originate from traction on a dorsal root. This can be blocked with Xylocaine or cocaine.

With the patient awake, it is advisable to test for deep visceral pain as well as for pin-prick perception. This is especially important for patients who have a significant portion of their disease lying in deep structures of the pelvis. Both legs should also be tested for motor strength since the pyramidal tracts may not be crossed, in which case the contralateral limbs may be supplied by the spinal tract in the anterior medial quadrant with the lesion.

If the level of analgesia does not reach far enough cephalad, the lesion should be extended medially and anteriorly to include fibers adjacent to the anterior midline septum. A lesion resulting in a level of analgesia that is not sufficiently caudal, e.g., sparing the perineum and sacral distribution, should be extended closer to the equator and thus closer to the crossed cortical spinal tract. Further extensions of the initial cordotomy lesion can be made with the patient awake as transection of the spinothalamic tract is not perceived as a painful stimulus. This permits functional monitoring of the motor system as well, while extending the lesion.

Upon achieving a satisfactory distribution of analgesia, the patient is reanesthetized for closure. The Weck clips on the dentate are cut free, the cord allowed to return to normal position, and the wound closed.

BILATERAL CORDOTOMY PROCEDURE

Bilateral high cervical cordotomies are not performed because of the high risk of sleep apnea and other complications. If bilateral analgesia is necessary, a percutaneous or open cordotomy can be done unilaterally at C2 or C3 with a contralateral cordotomy at C5-C6 performed by the posterior or anterior approach through the C5-C6 disc space. Usually when contralateral analgesia at a high level is not mandatory, a percutaneous cordotomy will be done at C2 on one side followed by a contralateral open thoracic cordotomy at T2 or T3.

When a lower bilateral level of analgesia is satisfactory, a bilateral operation should be performed in one stage in the upper thoracic region—with one lesion at T2 and the other contralateral at T4. For this operation the laminae at T2 and T4 are each removed as well as the spinous process of T3. The rest of the procedure is as described above. If a previous unilateral cordotomy has been done at T3 and it becomes evident later that a contralateral lesion is indicated, it can be made at the lower margin of T1 as early as 5 to 7 days postoperatively.

POSTOPERATIVE PRECAUTIONS

POSTOPERATIVE SLEEP APNEA

Following C2-C3 cordotomies the patient should be placed postoperatively in the intensive care recovery room, especially because of the danger of sleep apnea. When sent back to the floor, the patient should be monitored continuously with an apnea alarm, and tidal volume should periodically be checked. The nursing staff must be alert to the potential need for prompt respiratory assistance. The potential for sleep apnea may persist for a week postoperatively, after which time these precautions can be relaxed. If sleep apnea occurs after unilateral cervical cordotomies, the patient virtually always recovers after an adequate period of assisted support.

POSTOPERATIVE WEAKNESS

At the first sign of motor weakness postoperatively, we administer high-dose steroids and maintain the blood pressure if necessary to prevent any hypotension.

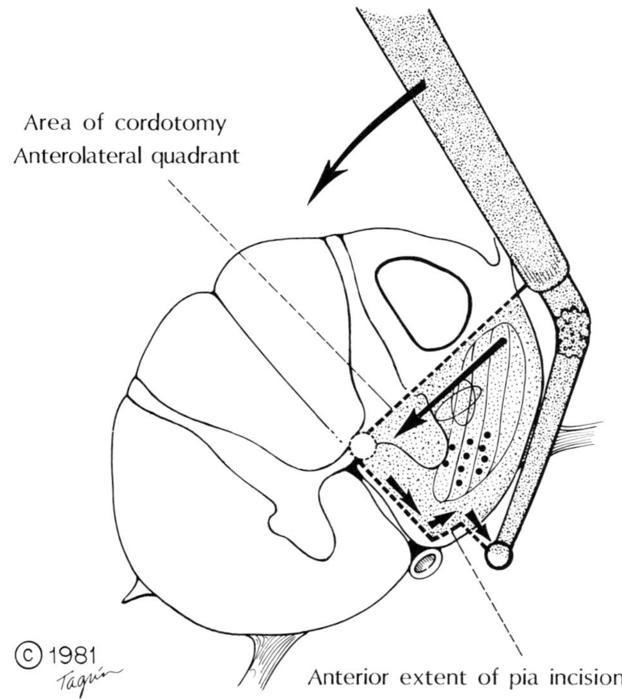

Fig. 101-7. The tip of the Jacobsen ball has been brought 90 degrees anteriorly, palpating along the midline septum until the pia on the anterior aspect of the cord is felt. The ball is then drawn laterally along the pia until it exits from the cord at the medialmost extent of the pial incision previously made with the microscissors.

POSTOPERATIVE HYPOTENSION

When bilateral lesions are done, the blood pressure must be monitored as the patient begins to mobilize—raising the head off the bed, dangling the feet, and walking. Toe-to-groin Ace wraps may be used with fluid loading and antihypotensive drugs as needed. The decrease in blood pressure—even with bilateral lesions—as well as orthostatic hypotension, gradually clears and is only a problem if unrecognized. A single episode of severe hypotension may render the blood supply significantly compromised, particularly to the upper thoracic cord. This ischemia may extend the lesion to the adjacent corticospinal tract.

POSTOPERATIVE URINARY RETENTION

If a Foley catheter has been placed before a bilateral procedure, a cystometrogram should be done several days postoperatively before the catheter is removed.

OPERATIVE RESULTS

The incidence of pain relief 3 months postoperatively varies from 54 to 90 percent with the average being 75 percent.[1,15–19] After 18 months the rate of relief falls to approximately 50 percent and stabilizes for another several years. It is generally agreed that the incidence of pain relief is greater in those patients with postoperative paresis and sphincter disturbance, suggesting a direct relation between the degree of pain relief and the extent of the lesion.

A T3 cordotomy, according to Taren et al.,[20] should be expected to produce a postoperative sensory level up to T4-T5, including postoperative loss of superficial pain, temperature, deep pain, visceral pain, and itch. The permanent level, however, usually settles at T7-T10. After cervical cordotomies, Grant and Wood[21] report an average permanent level of analgesia or hypalgesia only up to T5.

In some of our cases satisfactory and persisting relief of pain is achieved without superficial cutaneous analgesia. This dissociation between pain relief and cutaneous analgesia is seen commonly in midline myelotomies and characterizes certain thalamic lesions. Although the neurophysiologic explanation is not clear for the spinal cord, we propose that there may be two fiber systems involved, namely, in addition to the spinothalamic tract carrying acute pain perception, there also may be a midline multineuronal ascending system in the central gray matter of the spinal cord. This latter system may modulate a patient's ability to suppress chronic pain.

OPERATIVE FAILURES AND RECURRENCE OF PAIN

OPERATIVE FAILURES

The most common causes of failure to achieve satisfactory analgesia following cordotomy are:

1. Failure to cut close enough to the equator of the cord so there is sparing of the sacral representation in the spinal cord.
2. Failure to cut deep in the anterior quadrant. This may produce a satisfactory level of cutaneous analgesia without adequate relief of deep and visceral pain. Accordingly, in order to make sure the deep fibers carrying deep somatic visceral pain are severed, one should test these intraoperatively with wake-up anesthesia. A satisfactory test for visceral pain is a Foley balloon inflated within the bladder.
3. Insufficient extension of the lesion anteriorly and medially. This results in a level of analgesia many segments below the level of the cordotomy.
4. Failure to cut the anterior quadrant decisively. This produces an incomplete lesion with limited and patchy analgesia.
5. Performing a unilateral cordotomy when a bilateral procedure was indicated.
6. Subsequent spread of the cancer above the level of analgesia. If this is anticipated, a higher cordotomy should be done initially.
7. Anatomic variability of the spinal cord, resulting in an unsatisfactory lesion.

RECURRENCE OF PAIN WITH FADING OF ANALGESIA

If the level of analgesia falls and islands of recovered nociception occur within a few days postoperatively, the spinothalamic fibers in the periphery of the lesion have probably been bruised but not severed. The first postoperative drop in analgesic level may be caused by recovery from the direct injury of the surgery and the drop during the first week may be the result of recovery from edema and swelling. This may explain the two-to-five segment drop in the analgesic level during the first 2 postoperative weeks. In an excellent review on long-term follow-up of cordotomy patients, Grant and Wood[21] found both islands and large areas of returned sensation commencing even within a few months. It is conceivable that this

recovery of pain perception is caused by collateral regeneration of new synaptic terminal[5] in short-chain internuncial neurons taking over the previous function of the long spinothalamic tract. Four years after cordotomy, White and Alexander[22] found 54 percent of cordotomy patients to have recovered pain perception; subsequent higher anterolateral cordotomies generally proved unsuccessful in reinstituting analgesia. In addition to the hypothesis of collateral sprouting, long-term fading of postcordotomy analgesia may be explained by altered synaptic and membrane excitability in pre-existing potentially alternate nociceptive pathways. Indeed, in addition to first-order neurons ascending to medullary nuclei from the posterior columns, other neurons send efferent projections from the segmental gray matter. These may be partially responsible for conducting impulses concerned in the abnormal reference of pain. Partial support for this alternate pathway lies in the fact that stimulation of the dorsal column during midline myelotomy is often reported as painful by the awake patient.

Another hypothesis explaining the return of pain perception is that intrasegmental polysynaptic complexes form from collaterals of the crossing spinothalamic tract fibers. These may separate near the midline from the crossing spinothalamic tract fibers ascending in the spinal periaqueductal central gray matter to the reticular formation. Support for this hypothesis lies in the fact that relief of pain is experienced after midline commissural myelotomy or central myelotomy often not associated with cutaneous analgesia.

Accordingly, we believe that post cordotomy recovery of pain perception is less likely caused by spinal cord or thalamic axonal sprouting than by altered trans-synaptic excitability in pre-existing potentially alternate nociceptive pathways.

OPERATIVE COMPLICATIONS

MORTALITY

The mortality in various series reported in the literature varies from 3 to 21 percent.[1,15,16,17] The mortality is higher for unilateral cordotomies in the cervical region involving malignant disease and still higher for bilateral cervical cordotomies. The postoperative mortality clearly is higher in cancer patients than in patients with benign disease.

RESPIRATORY COMPLICATIONS

Some authors indicate that respiratory complications are the most serious concern in high cervical cordotomies. In the past, sleep apnea has been a frequent cause of death. Voluntary control of respiration is mediated by the cortical spinal tract, but subconscious ipsilateral respiratory movements are controlled by pathways descending deep in the centrolateral part of the spinal cord. This descending unilateral respiratory pathway is called the ventrolateral reticulospinal tract. Its fibers are, at least in part, intermingled with the fibers of the lateral spinothalamic tract (see Figure 101-1). Unilateral destruction of this pathway results in little functional respiratory loss unless contralateral respiratory function is poor. Accordingly, even for unilateral C2-C3 cordotomies, the function of the contralateral diaphragm should be evaluated preoperatively. Bilateral lesions clearly produce a high incidence of sleep apnea and death.

POSTCORDOTOMY HYPOTENSION

Intraoperatively there may be a sudden drop in blood pressure immediately after a cordotomy lesion has been made. Sindou[12] makes the point that such a drop in pressure assures the surgeon that the lesions have been made deep enough and far enough dorsally to assure lesioning of the fibers carrying visceral pain. In unilateral thoracic cordotomies, this drop is moderate and evanescent. The blood pressure usually returns to its normal level by the end of wound closure. Following bilateral lesions it may be marked and protracted, lasting well into the postoperative period.

Blood pressure is maintained by spinal sympathetic pathways that descend partially intermingled with the ascending STT (see Figure 101-1). Stimulation of these fibers elevates the blood pressure and the pressure within the bladder.[23] Unlike respiratory complications, blood pressure is seldom a cause of death or serious morbidity unless the patient is in a sitting position.

As noted, hypotension in the postoperative period may produce ischemia, especially in the thoracic region, thereby enlarging the surgical lesion and causing a new motor deficit.

MOTOR WEAKNESS

Assuming the cortical spinal tract has a relatively normal anatomy, the two principal causes of ipsilateral motor weakness following cordotomy are a lesion extending too far posteriorly that damages the crossed cortical spinal tract, and an extension too far anteromedially that damages the anterior spinal artery with resulting ischemia. A third possible mechanism is borderline ischemia accentuated by intra- or postoperative hypotension. The fact that the upper thoracic cord is especially susceptible to such ischemic damage may explain why there is a higher incidence of paresis after thoracic cordotomy compared with the cervical procedure.

The literature indicates that the incidence of paresis or paralysis following unilateral cordotomy varies from 0 to 11 percent,[16,17,24] whereas the incidence following bilateral cordotomies can run as high as 24 percent.[17] The incidence of permanent motor deficits is clearly much higher in bilateral lesions. We believe that the implementation of stimulation techniques as described decreases the incidence of paresis.

BLADDER DYSFUNCTION

Urinary bladder dysfunction after cordotomy is frequent. Following unilateral cordotomy this complication is relatively infrequent (0 to 8 percent).[1,16,24] This disturbance usually lasts only a few days and responds well to medical management. Following bilateral cordotomies, either cervical or thoracic, the incidence of urinary dysfunction is much higher and its duration is often permanent.

When a cordotomy is done for sacral pain, sphincter disturbances are particularly likely to occur. Nathan and Smith,[25,26] having studied the physiology of micturition and defecation, concluded that both the descending and ascending fibers responding to distention and the desire to relax sphincters are assembled in a narrow band almost crossing the equator of the cord opposite the central canal. Figure 101-1 clearly shows the high risk of bowel and bladder disturbance if a bilateral cordotomy is performed for sacral pain with the incision made close to the equator.

SEXUAL DYSFUNCTION

Sweet claims that the fibers involved in sexual sensation and function lie so close to those for pain (see Figure 101–1) that sexual function is almost always impaired after unilateral cordotomy and permanently impaired after bilateral cordotomy. Taren et al.[20] report that after section of the anterolateral tracts erection and ejaculation may still occur, but sexual sensation at the moment of orgasm is lost. Sexual potency does not seem to be disturbed with unilateral cordotomy but is almost always lost following the bilateral procedure.

DYSESTHESIAS

The abnormal sensations that may arise immediately after cordotomy, or as long as months after the operation, are sometimes divided into two groups: (1) referred sensations; and (2) dysesthesias.

Postoperatively, soreness of the skin and pain with girdle distribution may develop at or above the level of the lesion. This usually persists only for a few weeks and may be related to undue traction of the dorsal roots when the cord was rotated.

Referred sensations may be elicited by stimulation within the analgesic area in approximately 25 percent of patients. These sensations may be felt by the patient as noxious; they are poorly localized and often referred contralaterally. After bilateral cordotomy the sensations may be referred to an area above the level of analgesia as well as to areas of escape within the analgesic zone.

More serious are the severe constant painful dysesthesias referred to levels below the cordotomy. Their onset is usually delayed, occurring with increasing frequency as the postoperative period lengthens. Post cordotomy dysesthesias become a serious problem in approximately 6 percent of patients after 2 to 3 years. As noted, cordotomy at a higher level is not effective.

MEDULLARY TRACTOTOMY OF THE DESCENDING CRANIAL NOCICEPTIVE TRACT

ANATOMIC BASIS

The primary nociceptive afferents from the fifth, seventh, ninth, and tenth cranial nerves all descend in the medulla adjacent to each other forming the descending cranial nociceptive tract (DCNT).

Nature, in a degree of consideration for pain patients unparalleled in its design of the central nervous system, permits the neurosurgeon to interrupt virtually all orofacial primary nociceptive afferents by means of a single small ipsilateral lesion in the lateral dorsal medulla. Orofacial nociceptive cranial afferents, whether they enter via the fifth,, seventh, ninth, and/or tenth cranial nerves all descend in a compact tract, travelling caudally in the dorsolateral aspect of the medulla. At the level of the obex this tract is bounded dorsally by the nucleus cuneatus and ventrally by the contralateral ascending spinal thalamic tract (STT). The most superficial fibers of the tract, however, do not lie on the surface of the brain stem but are covered by the external arcuate fibers. (These fibers, important for coordination, arise from cells in the accessory cuneate nucleus and project to the cerebellum). The DCNT is 2 to 2.5 mm deep, with its ventral margin formed by the spinal trigeminal nucleus caudalis. In addition, the fibers within the tract have a very distinct topographic localization: descending in the most ventral portion of the descending trigeminal tract are fibers from the first trigeminal division. Immediately ventral to these fibers are the exiting motor fibers of the eleventh cranial nerve. In turn, just ventral to these exiting motor fibers of eleventh nerve are the ascending fibers of the contralateral STT. Dorsal to the descending nociceptive fibers of the first trigeminal division are the fibers from the second trigeminal division, with the fibers from the third trigeminal division next. In turn, just dorsal to these nociceptive fibers of the trigeminal third division are the primary nociceptive fibers from the seventh nerve's nervus intermedius and, most dorsally, the descending nociceptive fibers of the ninth and tenth nerves. Finally, just dorsal to the descending tenth nociceptive fibers are the ascending ipsilateral proprioceptive fibers to reach the nucleus cuneatus.

Accordingly, a surgical lesion made from the dorsal limit of the ascending contralateral STT, i.e., at the line demarcated by the exiting motor rootlets of the eleventh cranial nerve, dorsally to the ventral limit of nucleus cuneatus, will transect first the nociceptive fibers from V-1, followed by those from V-2, V-3, VII, IX, and X. If the lesion extends too far ventrally it will transect fibers from the contralateral STT; if too far dorsally, fibers entering nucleus cuneatus.[1] In order to sever all the fibers from each nerve the lesion must extend to a depth of 3 to 3.5 mm. In making such a lesion the overlying external arcuate fibers will, of necessity, be transected as well. Interrupting these fibers accounts for the postoperative truncal and gait ataxia.

Rowbotham, in 1938, was the first to take advantage of this configuration of the descending trigeminal nociceptive tract by performing, successfully, a trigeminal medullary tractotomy in a patient suffering from severe migrainous neuralgia involving the distribution of the first trigeminal division. It was not until 1942, however, when based on clinical observations and interpretations of Cajal's neuroanatomic drawings, that Sweet recognized that the spinal descending nociceptive tract included not only nociceptive fibers descending from the trigeminal nerve but also nociceptive fibers descending from the seventh nervus intermedius and the ninth and tenth nerves. Based on these observations, Sweet, in 1945, demonstrated that a single, slightly larger lesion in the dorsolateral medulla could interrupt virtually all primary nociceptive fibers from ipsilateral orofacial regions.

This medullary tractotomy of the DCNT, made dorsal to the exiting roots of the eleventh nerve, should be distinguished from a medullary tractotomy of the contralateral ascending STT, made just ventral to the exiting roots of the eleventh nerve. This operation, first performed by J. C. White, can be used to obtain contralateral analgesia to a dermatomal level as high as C2. This medullary tractotomy appears to be particularly appropriate for patients suffering from cancer invading the contralateral brachial plexus.

INDICATIONS FOR DCNT TRACTOTOMY

Even with the advent of intraventricular morphine we believe there continues to be an occasional patient in whom a unilateral lesion of the DCNT is the best available treatment. In our experience these patients are most likely to be suffering from a slow-growing indolent cancer affecting only one side of the face and oropharynx; or a very occasional patient suffering from extremely severe periodic migrainous neuralgia unrespon-

sive to conservative regimens and having failed a retrogasserian trigeminal rhizotomy. In these patients suffering from severe periodic migrainous neuralgia occasionally an avulsion of the greater and lesser superficial petrosal nerve has also already been made, especially in patients with marked autonomic changes: tearing, unilateral hyperhidrosis, hemicranial flush, and nasal mucosal engorgement. Another possible operation for patients suffering from periodic migrainous neuralgia has been to section the primary nociceptive afferents in the seventh nervus intermedius as well as the nociceptive fibers entering the ninth nerve and the rostral rootlets of the tenth. However, as shown by Bischoff's very meticulous microdissections, all pain fibers entering the VII-VIII root entry zone are, in fact, not confined to the discrete nervus intermedius. For, not only may afferent nociceptive fibers course among the efferent motor fibers of the seventh nerve, but they may also travel within the afferents of the body of the eighth nerve. Accordingly, in patients with severe, acute disseminated periodic migrainous neuralgia, a lesion of the DCNT may be indicated. Patients with periodic migrainous neuralgia, whose symptoms are confined to V-1 and V-2, as is typically the case, and who are unresponsive to cafergot and all other medical regimens, are almost certainly candidates first for a percutaneous retrogasserian trigeminal rhizotomy. Therefore, it is only patients who have a recrudescence of pain following this initial surgical procedure or spread of pain to nontrigeminal distributions that may be candidates for lesions of the DCNT.

An advantage of a DCNT tractotomy over a rhizotomy of V-1 and V-2 is that the tractotomy produces analgesia without anesthesia and invariably when made at the rostrocaudal level of the obex preserves corneal sensation. Since the midline portion of the dura and the posterior fossa is innervated by afferent pain fibers entering the VII-VIII complex, IX, and X, it is also an advantage of the tractotomy to denervate these structures in patients with periodic migrainous neuralgia referred to the deep occipital region.

DCNT TRACTOTOMY: OPERATIVE PROCEDURE

Instrumentation

The only special instrument used, in addition to the standard microneurosurgical array, is the Jacobsen ball dissector described above for use in open cordotomies. If the patient is awake, the tip of the ball can be stimulated to determine physiologically when the lesion has extended ventrally past V-1 fibers into the fibers of the contralateral spinal thalamic tract, thus helping to determine the ventral limit of the V-1 descending pain fibers. Similarly, the tip of the Jacobsen ball may be used to record evoked responses obtained by stimulating the dorsal column afferents from the median nerve. The sudden appearance of large evoked responses obtained by median nerve stimulation should indicate the approximation of the tip of the Jacobsen ball to the ascending dorsal fibers in nucleus cuneatus, as the lesion is extended rostrally from V-3 through VII, IX, and X fibers reaching nucleus cuneatus.

Anesthesia

One can use either sustained general or wake-up anesthesia. Satisfactory wake-up anesthesia, however, may be difficult after a prolonged exposure of the posterior fossa, especially when this is combined with a C1 and C2 laminectomy in those patients in whom a dorsal rhizotomy of C1 and C2 is also desired. Accordingly, Sweet, on several occasions, has done the suboccipital and upper cervical exposure in one operation and then returned for a second stage operation in which the wound was merely reopened and the dura opened and the patient promptly awakened after the initial lesion in the DCNT was made. Using this technique the patient may be fully satisfactorily awakened and extubated for detailed sensory testing. The patient is then put back to sleep briefly using intravenous Brevital to make any required enlargement of the lesion. In our last two cases, however, both with extremely severe periodic migrainous neuralgia, this author has preferred to use sustained general anesthesia and the techniques described below for obtaining a fully satisfactory DCNT tractotomy.

Patient Position and Operative Technique

The patient is placed half-way between a lateral and prone position with the head turned 45 degrees to the floor. The side of the anticipated tractotomy is placed uppermost, i.e., for a right-sided lesion the patient is placed with the left shoulder on the table and nose turned down to the left toward the floor. The head of the bed is elevated 20 to 30 degrees and the head flexed forward bringing the chin to within two finger-breadths from the sternum. The head is held in this position with a three-point skeletal fixation headrest.

A vertical midline incision is made from the low occipital region down to the upper cervical region. This is extended caudally in those patients in whom a concomitant dorsal rhizotomy of C1, 2 and 3 is planned. A craniectomy in the mid and low suboccipital region is made in the midline and slightly more to the side of the lesion. If just a tractotomy is planned a laminectomy of C1 is not necessary. The dura is opened by an incision begun over the cerebellum and cerebellar tonsil on the side of the anticipated lesion. The incision is then carried down to the midline at the cervicomedullary junction and caudally at least to the level of C1—further if a rhizotomy is planned.

The microscope is then brought into the field and angled rostrally towards the inferior limit of the fourth ventricle. Retractors are placed on either side and are used to retract the cerebellar tonsils dorsolaterally until the obex is seen directly. To do this the vermis does not have to be split. The cerebellar tonsil is then retracted further on the side of the anticipated lesion. (This will be, as noted, the cerebellar tonsil on the upper side in that the patient has been positioned so that the side of the lesion is upward).

A lesion of the DCNT may be made as far as 10 mm rostral to the obex, as advocated by Kunc, or at 2 mm below the obex as advocated by us. The more rostral tractotomy tends to make a slightly denser lesion for people with severe cancer pain, however, it also produces more discoordination and ataxia. (The more rostral lesion interrupts more nociceptive fibers from cranial nerves VII, IX, and X but also lesions more external arcuate fibers). Using microsurgical techniques we have been satisfied with the density of our lesions made 2 mm caudal to the obex. The lesion is made in a plane transverse to the brain stem on the lateral dorsal side of the medulla extending ventrally and dorsally. The line of demarcation between the most ventral descending fibers of V-1 and the most dorsal fibers of the contralateral STT is clearly defined on the surface of the medulla by the point of exit of the roots of the eleventh cranial nerves. Accordingly, the cerebellar tip should be retracted in order to visualize at least one emerging rootlet of the eleventh

nerve rostral and another root caudal to the anticipated transverse level of the lesion. These may be stimulated, even in the asleep patient, to be sure they represent motor fibers of the eleventh. A line is drawn between these two exiting rootlets and that line marks the ventral extent of the lesion. Dorsally the distinct prominences of nucleus gracilus, adjacent to the obex, and further laterally, of nucleus cuneatus can be seen. The lateral extent of the surface presentation of the eminence of nucleus cuneatus should mark the dorsal-medial extent of the projected incision. Any small surface blood vessels may be teased to either side of the projected incision or bipolaring very gently. The incision is begun by using the No. 11 blade to make a very small opening in the pia-arachnoid at the lateral extent of the eminence of the nucleus cuneatus. The microsurgical scissors are then used to incise the pia-arachnoid, going laterally and anteriorly until the incision reaches the line drawn between the two exiting eleventh nerve rootlets. At this point, if the patient has been awakened, the nerves to be cut may be stimulated by mechanical pressure, as characterizes the sensitivity of these primary nociceptive afferents. Both Kunc and Sweet have used needles or sharp nerve hooks to stimulate either the fibers of the DCNT or the proprioceptive fibers ascending to nucleus cuneatus. The patient may refer the sensations to a very focal area permitting discrimination between V-1, V-2, and V-3 descending fibers. When the fibers of nucleus cuneatus are stimulated mechanically, sensations are referred to the ipsilateral arm, neck and back of the head. (Proprioceptive fibers from the lower portions of the body ascend to nucleus gracilus.) If the patient is awake the lesion is extended ventrally until there is some nociceptive sensory loss in the contralateral distal lower extremity. The lesion is extended dorsomedially until there is some reference of sensation to the ipsilateral dorsal columns. The lesion should only be made to a depth of 3 mm. This is done in the current technique by putting a small piece of bone wax 3 mm up the shaft of the Jacobsen ball, and then inserting the instrument only to that depth dorsally. As in the anterior quadrant of the spinal cord, there is very little resistance even to the relatively blunt tip of the Jacobsen ball. Similarly, there is scarcely any bleeding obtained by this complete DCNT tractotomy. We recommend that the lesion extend ventrally at least partially into the contralateral STT and dorsally into the ascending proprioceptive fibers. This enhances the probability of a complete lasting lesion of the DCNT as the initial lesion tends to fade in the postoperative period.

Currently, as mentioned we are relying on these microsurgical techniques to make the tractotomy lesion with the patient under sustained general anesthesia. Additional guidance should be obtained in the future using advanced electrophysiologic techniques.

A medullary tractotomy of the contralateral ascending STT uses the same position and exposure. However, the incision begins just ventral to the exiting rootlets of the eleventh nerve and extends more ventrally.[1,27]

COMPLICATIONS, SIDE EFFECTS, RESULTS, AND THOUGHTS FOR THE FUTURE

Clearly, this DCNT tractotomy is a major operative procedure and carries a mortality and morbidity greater than that of percutaneous trigeminal rhizotomy or percutaneous glossopharyngeal rhizotomy. The worst side effect is the inevitable degree of difficulty in walking produced by this lesion. Patients almost invariably in the immediate postoperative period suffer from incoordination and lateral pulsion. As noted, this is less the case for lesions done caudal to the level of the obex. Usually by 1 month after the operation the degree of discoordination has cleared sufficiently for people in most walks of life to have normal function. Dysesthesias as seen following spinal lesions of the STT have not been a consistent problem following these lesions of the DCNT.

The degree of pain relief tends to be commensurate with the extent of the analgesia produced by the lesion. Thus, lesions producing lasting analgesia throughout the distribution of the cranial nerves has a high probability of relieving pain of either cancer or migrainous origin. Including a dorsal rhizotomy of C1, C2 and C3 increases the results in those patients whose migrainous neuralgia is not confined to orofacial regions. It is of interest that the pain of periodic migrainous neuralgia is eliminated by the DCNT tractotomy while the autonomic symptoms, which are characteristic of periodic migrainous neuralgia, may often persist. Several of our patients with extremely severe periodic migrainous neuralgia who were suicidal in spite of intensive medical and psychiatric therapy and failed radiofrequency trigeminal lesions have been markedly relieved by a DCNT tractotomy. As noted, orofacial cutaneous and mucosal and corneal touch sensation is functionally preserved.

REFERENCES

1. White JC, Sweet WH: Pain and the Neurosurgeon. Springfield, Ill, Charles C Thomas, 1969, pp 69, 629
2. Hitchcock ER: Stereotactic myelotomy. Proc R Soc Med 67:771, 1964
3. Hitchcock ER: Stereotactic cervical myelotomy. J Neurol Neurosurg Psychiatry 33:224, 1970
4. Schvarcz JR: Stereotactic extralemniscal myeiotomy. J Neurol Neurosurg Psychiatry 39:53, 1976
5. Schvarcz J R: Functional exploration of the spinomedullary junction. Acta Neurochir (suppl) 24:179, 1977
6. Schvarcz J R: Spinal cord stereotactic techniques re: trigeminal nucleotomy and extralemniscal myelotomy. Appl Neurophysiol 41:,99, 1978
7. Poletti CE, Cohen AM, Todd DP, et al: Clinical pain relieved by long-term epidural morphine: two case reports with permanent indwelling systems for self-administration. J Neurosurg 55:581, 1981
8. Yakovlev PI, Rakic P: Patterns of decussation of bulbar pyramidal tracts on two sides of the spinal cord. Trans Am Neurol Assoc 91:366, 1966
9. Sweet WH: Recent observations pertinent to improving anterolateral cordotomy. Clin Neurosurg 23:80, 1976
10. Macon JB, Poletti CE: Conducted somatosensory evoked potentials during spinal surgery. Part 1. Technical aspects. J Neurosurg (In press)
11. Cowie RA, Hitchcock EA: The late results of anterolateral cordotomy for pain relief. Acta Neurochir 64:39, 1982
12. Sindou M: Personal communication, June, 1981
13. Grunert VP, Sunder-Plassmann MS: Ergebnisse der zerikalen chordotomie mit und ohne rhizotomie bei konservitiv therapieresistenten schmerzen im Schulter-Arm-Bereich. Zentralbl Neurochir 46:267, 1985
14. Hardy D, LeClereq TA, Mercky F: Microsurgical selective cordotomy by the anterior approach, in Handa H (ed): Microsurgery. International Symposium on Microsurgery, Baltimore, University Park Press, 1973
15. Brihaye J, Retif J: Comparison of the results obtained by anterolateral cordotomy at the dorsal level and at the cervical level. Neurochirurgie 7:258, 1961
16. Diemath HE, Heppner F, Walker AE: Anterolateral chordotomy for relief of pain. Postgrad Med J 29:485, 1961
17. Nathan PW: Results of antero-lateral cordotomy for pain in cancer. J Neurol Neurosurg Psychiatry 26:353, 1963
18. Dautenhahn D, Reynolds A, Darby R, et al: Thoracic epidural analgesia for open cordotomy. Anesth Analg 63:1036, 1984
19. Jack T, Lloyd J: Long-term efficacy of surgical cordotomy in intractable nonmalignant pain. Ann R Coll Surg Engl 97–102, 1983
20. Taren DA, Kahn EA, Humphrey T: The surgery of pain, in Kahn EA, Crosby EC, Schneider RC, et al (eds): Correlative Neurosurgery. Springfield, Ill, Charles C Thomas, 1969
21. Grant FC, Wood FA: Experiences with cordotomy. Clin Neurosurg 5:38, 1957
22. White JC: Anterolateral cordotomy—its effectiveness in relieving pain of non-malignant disease. Neurochirurgia 6:83, 1963
23. Kerr FW, Alexander S: Descending autonomic pathways in the spinal cord. Arch Neurol 10:249, 1964
24. McKissock W: Second International Congress of Neurological Surgeons. International Congress Series No. 36 E27. Amsterdam, Excerpta Medica, 1961
25. Nathan PW, Smith MC: Spinal pathways subserving defecation and sensation from the lower bowel. J Neurol Neurosurg Psychiatry 16:245, 1953
26. Nathan PW, Smith MC: The centrifugal pathway for micturition within the spinal cord. J Neurol Neurosurg Psychiatry 21:177, 1958
27. Poletti CE, Ojemann RG: Stereo Atlas of Operative Microneurosurgery. Reel 19, View 3, pp 264–265, 1985

CHAPTER 102

Dorsal Root Entry Zone Thermocoagulation

D.G.T. Thomas

PAIN ASSOCIATED WITH DEAFFERENTATION following brachial plexus avulsion, pain consequent to herpes zoster infection of the spinal dorsal root ganglia, or pain resulting from traumatic paraplegia are all conditions difficult to control by drug treatment, by sympathectomy, by rhizotomy, by cordotomy, or by neurostimulation. Radiofrequency coagulation of the dorsal root entry zone (DREZ) has shown positive results in the treatment of these conditions. The exact mode of action of this procedure remains to be clarified, but it may be the result of destruction of pain-generating centers within the spinal cord, of a rebalancing of inhibitory and excitatory inputs within the damaged cord, or of interruption of ascending or descending local reflex pathways in the cord.

PHYSIOLOGIC BASIS

The concept of using neurosurgical lesions in the treatment of chronic pain is well established. Dorsal rhizotomy,[1-3] anterolateral cordotomy,[4] and commissural myelotomy[5] are examples. The physiologic basis upon which these methods depend is the division of a nociceptive pathway between the periphery of the nervous system and the brain, specifically in the dorsal roots or the crossed spinothalamic pain pathways. Melzack and Wall[6] in 1965 proposed the ''gate theory'' of pain control. In this theory, inhibitory influences of the lemniscal fibers modulated pain, and this modulation was proposed to take place at the entrance of the nociceptive fiber to the dorsal horn.

The DREZ consists anatomically of the central part of the dorsal spinal roots, Lissauer's tract, and the superficial layers of the dorsal horn, where the afferent fibers synapse with the cells of the spinothalamic tract. On entering the spinal cord, the nociceptive small myelinated A-delta and the unmyelinated C fibers are positioned in the lateral part of the posterior rootlet.[7] They penetrate the medial part of Lissauer's tract, which lies adjacent to the posterior lateral part of the dorsal horn. They proceed to reach the posterior horn itself directly, or through an ascending or descending connecting pathway over 2 spinal segments. The dorsal horn may be divided on the basis of cytoarchitecture into laminae, the Rexed laminations, and the nociceptive afferents that relay onto the marginal cells of lamina I or neurones of the nucleus proprius of lamina IV and V. From here, the ascending spinothalamic pathway ascends. The A-beta fibers, which lie medially in the root on entry to the cord, form long axons ascending in the dorsal columns, as well as

short collaterals that enter the substantia gelatinosa, that is, lamina II and III. Within the lateral part of the tract of Lissauer, there are local intersegmental reflex pathways connecting different levels of the substantia gelatinosa. The basis of the gate control of nociceptive input lies in these anatomic connections, because, in physiologic terms, the effect of stimulation of the nociceptive afferents is to produce substance P at the dendrites of the spinothalamic cells, and this can be inhibited by stimulation of the large lemniscal fibers and their collaterals with production of metencephalin in the substantia gelatinosa. The local segmental reflexes mediated via Lissauer's tract may inhibit or excite transmission of nociception, while the descending fibers of the reticulospinal tract may have further inhibitory effects. When the large lemniscal primary afferents in the peripheral nerve or in the posterior roots are lost, the loss of their inhibitory effect can result in excessive firing of dorsal horn neurones, causing deafferentation hyperactivity. Destruction of these firing neurones may reduce the nociceptive inpulses generated in the spinothalamic pathways, while destruction of the medial part of Lissauer's tract could diminish the regional excitability of nociceptive afferents.

Surgical lesions of the DREZ have been developed by Sindou[8,9] and Nashold,[10-11] with the aim of treating pain. Sindou's procedure of radicellotomie posterieure, or selective posterior rhizotomy (SPR), involves cutting the lateral small fiber component of each posterior rootlet as it enters the DREZ, by making an incision to a depth of 2 mm from the lateral aspect of the posterolateral sulcus. The incision is in to the medial part of Lissauer's tract, and is angled at 45 degrees. At its depth, the incision is at the apex of the dorsal horn, recognizable by a gray-brown color. The physiologic basis of this procedure is the selective destruction of the small nociceptive fibers that are grouped laterally in the rootlet, together with the destruction of the medial, excitatory, part of Lissauer's tract, with a consequent reduction in the hyperactivity of the spinothalamic pathways. In addition, the procedure aims to preserve the medial lemniscal fibers of the posterior rootlets as well as the lateral, inhibitory, intersegmental pathways in the lateral part of Lissauer's tract. This method is particularly suitable for preserving tactile and proprioceptive functions where posterior rhizotomy for pain is desired in cases in which the nerve roots are intact, as in a carcinomatous infiltration of the brachial plexus or in painful spasticity, and may be useful in treating, or avoiding, the onset of deafferentation pain.

Nashold's method is based on the coagulation of the

OPERATIVE NEUROSURGICAL TECHNIQUES
ISBN 0-8089-1862-1

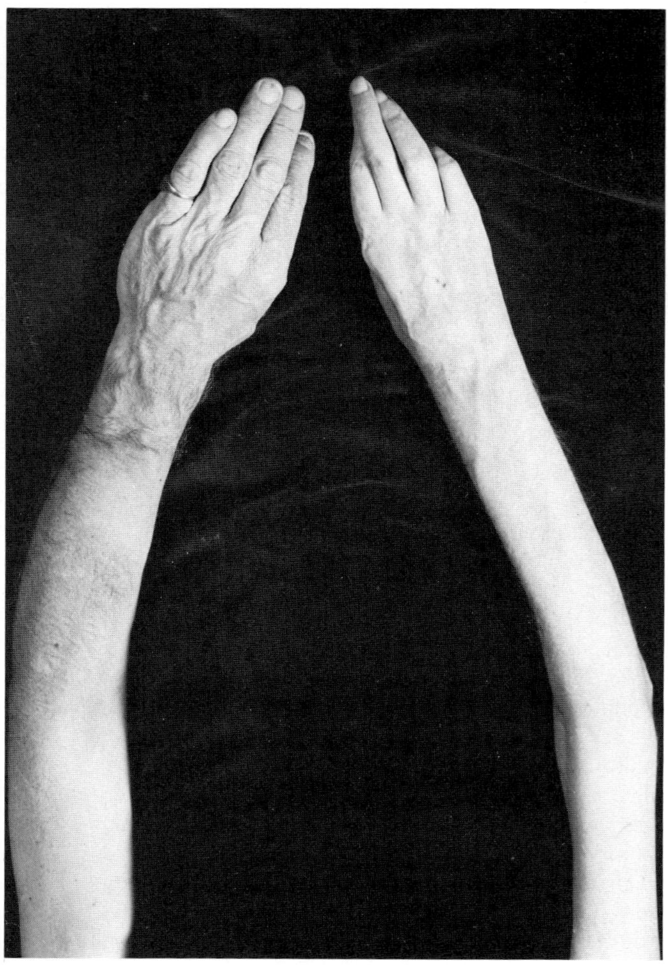

Fig. 102-1. Flail, wasted, deafferentated arm contrasted with normal, uninjured limb in brachial plexus avulsion.

posterior part of the dorsal horn, including substantia gelatinosa, and probably also the medial part of the tract of Lissauer, in order to control deafferentation pain (caused presumably by inappropriate impulses arising in these regions), by destruction of these regions. The practical aspects of this procedure will be discussed in detail below. In principle, however, the lesion in this case is made by heat passing from a 2-mm radiofrequency coagulation electrode, which is passed into the spinal cord from the posterolateral sulcus at an angle of 25 degrees, usually at the site of a totally avulsed posterior root. The physical principle underlying the creation of a thermal lesion in the DREZ by this method is that a radiofrequency voltage is applied between the ''active'' coagulation electrode and a ''dispersive'' electrode of much larger size. The body tissue completes the electrical circuit, and radiofrequency current flows. An electric field is generated and heating occurs close to the active electrode, where ions of the electrolytes in the target tissue are oscillating at radiofrequency and dissipating their energy in frictional heat. The shape of the isotherms created around the electrode is ellipsoidal, and tissue within the 45°C isotherm will be irreversibly denatured.[12] Data from animal and experimental studies, as well as human material in anterolateral cordotomy, indicate that a 2.0-mm electrode with a tip diameter of 0.25 mm will create a lesion about 2.0 mm wide and 2 to 3 mm deep, when heated to 70–75°C for 15 to 30 seconds.[12] Laser surgery has been used as an alternate method of destruction of DREZ[13] by cutting a narrow channel to a depth of 2 mm through use of microsurgical control.

INDICATIONS AND PATIENT SELECTION

The principal areas in which thermocoagulation of the DREZ, described by Nashold, may be indicated are neurogenic pain due to brachial plexus traction injuries, postherpetic neuralgia, and painful paraplegia. These indications will be discussed in detail. Microsurgical selective posterior rhizotomy in the DREZ, described by Sindou, may also be useful in the treatment of deafferentation pain, and in some cases of cancer pain in which the distribution is well localized, in postamputation pain, in peripheral nerve injury, and in painful hyperspastic hemiplegia or paraplegia[3,9,14,15]. Such uses of rhizotomy will not, however, be further discussed in this chapter on radiofrequency thermocoagulation.

PAIN IN AVULSION OF THE BRACHIAL PLEXUS

Severe traction forces on the limbs and limb girdles, as seen particularly in motorcyclists who have been involved in traffic accidents, can avulse the anterior and posterior spinal roots of the brachial or lumbosacral plexus from the spinal cord, causing chronic intractable pain in probably 20 percent of cases. Gunshot wounds can cause similar lesions. The pain experienced by patients with avulsion of the brachial plexus is highly characteristic. It is constant, burning or crushing.[16] In addition, there is often a severe shooting paroxysmal pain of agonizing intensity, which may come at unpredictable intervals. About 90 percent of patients with avulsions develop pain, which generally develops soon after injury—within days or weeks—although the exact timing may be masked by associated head injury and amnesia. Sometimes the pain may not begin until 3 months after injury. In the first year, the pain becomes tolerable in 25 percent of those affected, and by 3 years it has reached tolerable levels in about 70 percent. In the remaining cases, the pain remains a prominent feature, adding to the patient's physical disability. Physical rehabilitation, and the use of splints to control the flail limb, help recovery, as does distraction by the provision of work or hobbies. Transcutaneous electrical stimulation, in the root of the neck above the lesion and in the inner arm in a T2 root distribution, may be very beneficial. Drug treatment with the anticonvulsant drugs carbamazepine or valproate sodium may be useful, as may be the use of antidepressants that offer an analgesic effect, as does amitriptyline.[16]

Patients who have had a trial of conservative methods, including transcutaneous stimulation and drug treatment, and who continue to experience desperately severe pain, are candidates for DREZ thermocoagulation. The patient should be psychologically stable and be able to appreciate the possibility of failure of the operation to achieve pain relief, as well as the possibility of neurologic complications. It may be useful to interview the relatives as well as the patient to help to determine the impact of pain on the patient's life, as well as to inform all concerned of the seriousness of the surgery. Full notes of the description of the nature and severity of the pain before the operation are essential, so that, if necessary, the patient may be reminded of the once-desperate condition in the event of an unsatisfactory result.

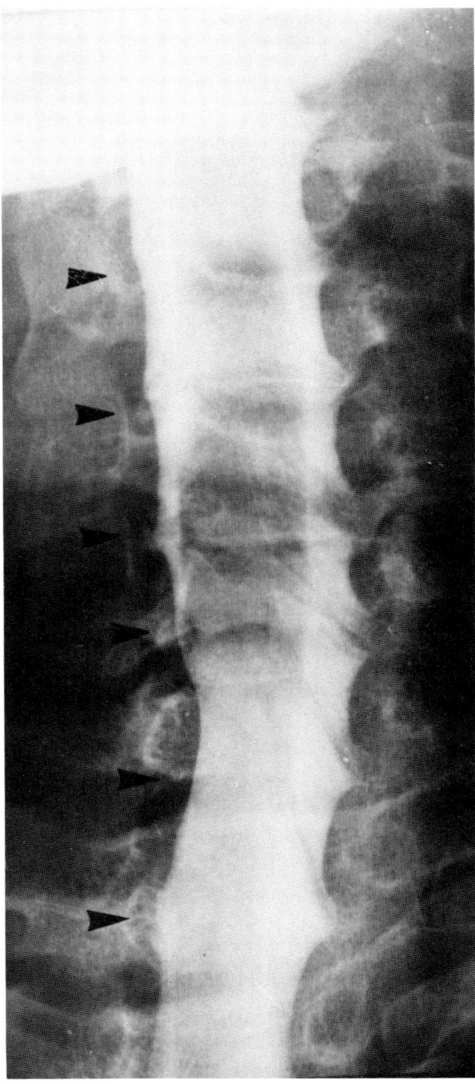

Fig. 102-2. Cervical myelogram in brachial plexus avulsion. Varying degrees of root damage with cord displacement at lower level.

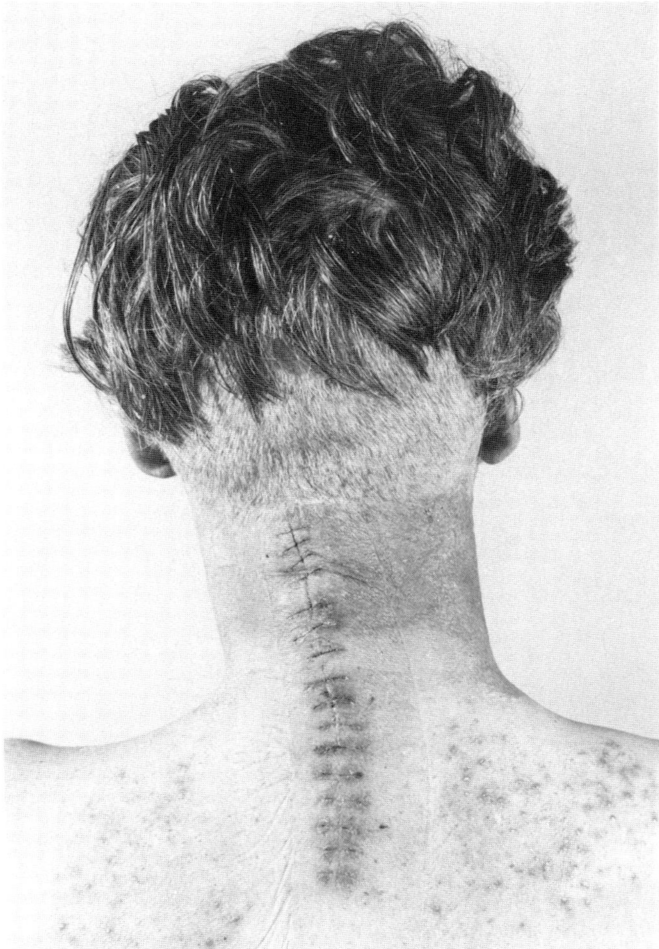

Fig. 102-3. Incision for cervical laminectomy in radiofrequency coagulation of DREZ for brachial plexus avulsion.

Preoperative Clinical Assessment and Investigation

In the early phase of management of brachial plexus avulsion, a distinction between partial and complete lesion is important, as ruptures of the C5-C7 roots are amenable to treatment by nerve grafting in an attempt to restore function at the shoulder and elbow. A patient with a complete lesion clinically, who suffers from severe pain, without Tinel's sign in the neck, with the presence of sensory action potentials associated with the presence of anaesthesia in the relevant digits, and with meningoceles on myelography,[17] as well as Horner's syndrome and paralysis of the proximal muscles (rhomboids, latissimus dorsi, and seratus anterior), is strongly suggestive of avulsion of the roots (Figures 102-1 and 102-2). However, positive Tinel's sign in the neck and absence of sensory conduction and sparing of proximal muscles, together with a normal myelogram, suggest probable rupture distal to the dorsal root ganglia. Early surgical exploration may be necessary to confirm the exact nature of the lesion, whether partial or complete and whether pre) or postganglionic. If the patient has not had myelography in the early postinjury phase, this is indicated as part of the preoperative assessment in order to anticipate the presence of large meningoceles that may affect the surgical approach (Figures 102-3 and 102-4), as well as to assess the extent of the root loss preoperatively.[17]

PAIN IN POSTHERPETIC NEURALGIA

Herpes zoster infection of a dorsal root ganglion of a spinal nerve root is associated with acute pain and a vesicular cutaneous rash in a dermatomal distribution. Generally, the pain settles as the rash resolves, but in about 10 percent of cases the pain persists.[18] The incidence of such postherpetic neuralgia increases with age, so that over 50 percent of patients aged 80 or over may experience lasting postherpetic neuralgia. The pain has two components, one superficial and one deep. The former is described as burning or aching and is made worse by light touch in the areas around the anesthetic, healed, scarred skin. The deep pain is paroxysmal and gripping, not associated with triggering factors. In addition, there may be severe itching in the affected area, which itself can feel subjectively swollen or tightly constricted. The original inflammatory process spreads both distally and centrally, and the effects pathologically include decrease in the number of large myelinated fibers in the

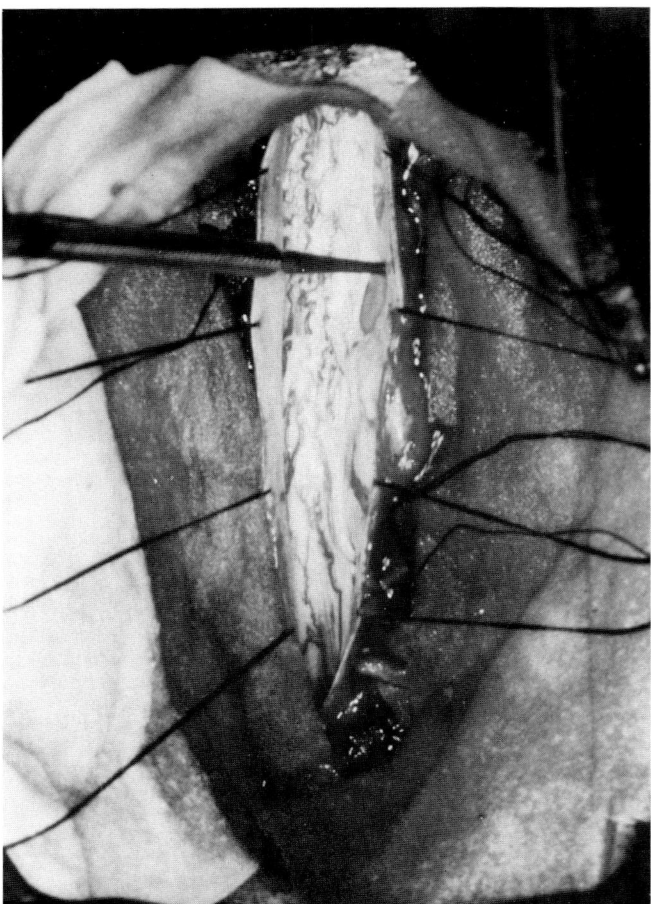

Fig. 102-4. Intradural exposure of cervical spinal cord in brachial plexus avulsion. Dissector indicates site of a pseudomeningocele. There is moderate hemiatrophy of the cord, with relatively poor blood supply and arachnoid adhesions.

peripheral nerve, and inflammation in the spinal meninges as well as within the dorsal horn of the spinal cord.

Medical Treatment and Patient Selection

Treatment of the initial attack of herpes zoster with topical idoxuridine[19] or systemic steroids[20] appears to reduce the incidence of postherpetic neuralgia. The established condition may prove very resistant to treatment. Physical measures such as cooling or transcutaneous stimulation may be beneficial.[21] Drug treatment with amitriptyline,[22–24] with carbamazepine,[25] or with chloroprothixene[26,27] may be successful. These measures, however, fail in a significant fraction of patients, who are then left with severely distressing postherpetic neuralgia. Generally, lesional surgery by means of peripheral neurectomy, ganglionectomy, dorsal rhizotomy, or percutaneous cordotomy have had only limited success in the treatment of this condition. DREZ thermocoagulation has been found to be an effective surgical treatment in many patients in spite of patient age and infirmity.[28,29] It is probably reasonable to wait at least 12 months following the acute attack before proceeding to surgery. Although the operation appears to carry less risk of neurological complications in the postherpetic cases than in the avulsion cases, it is important to fully document the severity of the patient's pain, as well as the patient's understanding of the possible risks of the surgery, as mentioned above.

CHRONIC PAIN IN TRAUMATIC PARAPLEGIA

Patients with spinal cord injury may experience chronic pain at or around the site of the original injury, and this may be due to spinal instability or other mechanical factors in the bones and joints. A second type of central pain may be experienced in the deafferentated areas, often starting early after injury and consisting of burning or tingling feelings in the anaesthetic limbs or trunk.[30] Another type of pain, triggered by touch and experienced in the anaesthetic areas, may be tingling or lancinating in nature. Pain due to mechanical factors can be treated by various procedures, including facet injection and spinal fusion. However, DREZ thermocoagulation at and for 2 to 3 segments above the spinal level may be beneficial, particularly for treatment of the triggered pain.[31] As in the cases of avulsion or postherpetic pain, the procedure is a serious one and should be done only for severe, intractable symptoms.

SURGICAL TECHNIQUE

Patients are operated on, by the author, under general anesthesia in a prone position.[32,33] In the most usual case, that of brachial plexus avulsion, it is possible to determine the spinal levels accurately by palpation of the prominent C7 vertebra when the patient is positioned with the neck flexed, and by subsequent palpation of the C2 or C1 vertebrae during the course of laminectomy. In the dorsal region, x-ray control preoperatively is useful, obtaining the cord level by adding 2 + from D1 to D6, and 3 + from D6 to D10. The identification of levels at the conus, or by physiologic methods, will be considered below. In the case of brachial plexus avulsion injury, full laminectomy from C4 to T1, inclusive, is performed (Figures 102-2 and 102-4). Alternatively, for nonavulsion cases, hemilaminectomy with preservation of the spinous processes may be satisfactory. The procedure may also be performed while the patient is in the sitting position.[11]

Certain technical details of the laminectomy are important. Hemostasis is achieved during the course of the exposure and laminectomy, and then the wound is sealed with lintine to exclude skin and muscle prior to dural opening. A dispersive earth electrode is implanted in the superficial muscle, and this can take the form of a 10-cm solid metal disposable lumbar puncture needle. The dura is opened to expose the C5-T1 spinal segments, or, alternatively, the appropriate thoracic or lumbar sacral outflow, and is then retracted with stay sutures. The arachnoid, if it has not already been opened, is dissected to expose the spinal cord. The operating microscope is introduced and used to provide both illumination and magnification (in the range of from 10× to 25× x). The next step, in the case of root avulsion, is to identify the posterolateral sulcus, which is the DREZ. Usually, there is a moderate to severe arachnoiditis, with adhesions between the spinal cord and its coverings. When this is dissected, universally in the avulsion cases, an atrophy of the cord on the side of injury is seen, often with displacement or rotation to the contralateral side caused by pseudomeningoceles (Figure 102-4). Usually, but not always, the pseudomeningoceles may have been anticipated on the basis of the preceding myelogram. In some cases, they may be very extensive cysts spreading to the supraclavicular region. Visual inspection of the cord may reveal the posterolateral sulcus at the appropriate site. Palpation with a metal dissector gently over the posterolateral surface of the cord will often distinguish the sulcus if it cannot be visualized. It is useful to observe the normal, contralateral, cord, where the intact posterior rootlets indicate the DREZ. It is also useful to inspect the rootlets at C4 and T2, above and below the damaged levels, in order to help in identification of the posterolateral sulcus. In the case of postherpetic neuralgia, the affected rootlets are often wasted and atrophic and slightly affected by arachnoiditis, features which may be identified under the microscope. In cases of traumatic paraplegia, preoperative myelography together with inspection at the time of surgery shows the level of trauma, and there is usually a degree of arachnoiditis at and above this level.

Once the appropriate spinal level has been identified, and the sulcus between the posterior and lateral columns confidently defined, it is possible to proceed to the radiofrequency thermocoagulation lesions of the specific target areas. Various techniques have been described for making the radiofrequency thermocoagulation (70 mA for 15 seconds[11] or 40 mA for 15 seconds,[34] with 0.5-mm-diameter electrodes). Currently, however, the optimum radiofrequency method involves the use of the 2-mm, 0.25-mm-diameter thermocouple active electrode (Radionics Inc., Burlington, Massachusetts), starting at 0 current and gradually increasing this to give a temperature of 70–75°C, which is held constant for 15 seconds and then switched off with removal of the electrode.[35] When the system is first set up prior to lesions in the cord, it is appropriate to test the impedance in the system—impedance should be in the region of 450 to 700 ohm—and to make sure that all the electrical connections are properly cleaned. The lesions are made with return of the current setting to 0 between each one, and withdrawal and cleaning of the electrode. In the cases of brachial plexus avulsion from C5 to T1, approximately 20 to 24 lesions placed 2 mm apart, made with the electrode held by hand under the microscope, are usually required. Typically, the current required to obtain a temperature of 70–75°C is 45 mA in the cervical region, whereas in the dorsal region it may be 25 mA. It is the temperature in the thermocouple-monitoring electrode that is the most accurate means of obtaining consistency in the lesions. In the dorsal region, for postherpetic neuralgia over the affected root level and one segment above and below, or in cases of paraplegia for the level of the lesion and 2 segments above, fewer lesions may be necessary. For some lesions in the dorsal region and in the conus, however, up to 50 lesions may be necessary. If bleeding occurs after puncture of the cord, this will generally stop on application of a pattie or absorbable surgical gauze. Occasionally, bipolar diathermy may be necessary to stop bleeding. It is usually possible, however, to avoid bleeding of this kind by ensuring that the electrode is not passed through significant vessels seen on the cord surface under the operating microscope.

SPECIAL ASPECTS OF DREZ
AT THE CONUS

Exposure by laminectomy of T10, T11, T12, and L1 may be necessary in order to fully expose the level of the conus. Electrical evoked potentials measured after stimulation of the nerve roots as they pass through the spinal foramina can be used to record in the conus the appropriate site for DREZ lesion for a particular root.[29] Anatomically, the last dentate ligament is approximately at the L5 segmental level, while the S1 root area is approximately 1 cm above the point where the filum terminale joins the conus.

Following the radiofrequency coagulations of the DREZ,

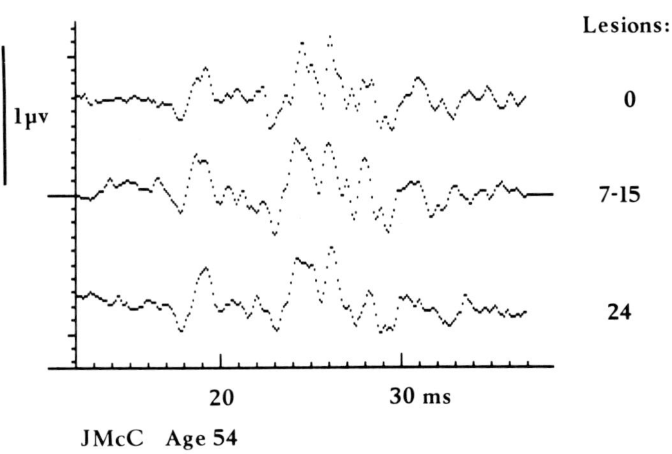

Fig. 102-5. Conducted spinal cord potentials recorded preoperatively before, during, and after 24 DREZ thermocoagulation lesions.

the dura is tightly closed and the laminectomy wound closed in a routine fashion, if necessary with subcutaneous drainage.

It is the author's practice to start drug treatment with dexamethasone prior to surgery, with a loading dose of 12 mg, and continuing at a dose of 4 mg every 6 hours in adults. This may be tapered off a few days later in the postoperative period, and is intended to limit the effects of edema due to surgery and lesion-making.

ELECTROPHYSIOLOGIC CONTROL
OF DREZ LESIONS

Perioperative conducted spinal cord potentials have been measured by tibial nerve stimulation at the knee and monopolar recording at C3 and T3 extra) and intradurally (Figure 102-5). Pre- and postoperative cortical somatosensory evoked potentials have also been recorded with posterior tibial nerve stimulation at the ankle, and with bipolar scalp recording (Figure 102-6). Subclinical damage was detected in some patients with avulsion of the brachial who were tested preoperatively. However, no immediate perioperative changes were found, which may indicate that long tract impairment and neurologic complications may be due not to surgical lesions, but rather to ischemic or inflammatory processes set in motion by surgery. The postoperative outcome with regard to neurologic complications, or to pain relief, was not predicted by preoperative somatosensory evoked potentials. There is a correlation, however, between somatosensory potential deterioration postoperatively and development of neurologic deficits in the lower limbs.[36] At present, the author is not using routine perioperative electrophysiologic control.

RESULTS

Complete abolition of pain is possible in brachial plexus avulsion cases in approximately one third of patients, with very significant pain improvement in an additional one third. Some patients are able to recognize that there has been pain relief in the first few hours after surgery. More commonly, because of pain from the laminectomy wound and because of postoperative analgesia and sedation, it may take days for patients to reach a stable state and to report on the degree of relief of their pain. Generally, if there is pain relief in the early postoperative

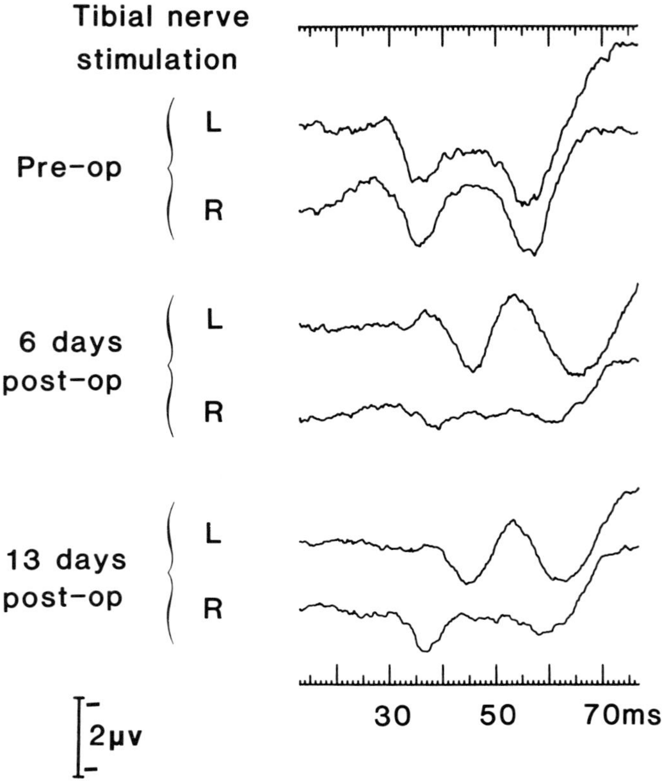

Fig. 102-6. Pre- and postoperative cortical somatosensory evoked potentials in a case of DREZ thermocoagulation in the right cervical region.

period, and provided that this remains stable over the first 3 to 6 months, then the relief will persist long-term. In several published series, pain improvement has been reported in the range of 60 to 80 percent of cases of brachial plexus avulsion.[11,13,32,33,37] However, temporary neurologic deficits have been reported in up to 50 percent of patients operated upon,[11,32,33,37] although with the improvement in electrode technology and lesion-making this figure has been reduced.

About 5 to 10 percent[33,38] of patients will have some permanent neurologic complication from the procedure. This may take the form of weakness and ataxia in the ipsilateral lower limb associated with sensory loss in the upper part of the trunk on the side of the lesion. Impotence has been reported as a rare complication.[16] There is often local pain persisting in the region of the laminectomy. A successful outcome in terms of improvement, or complete relief, of postherpetic pain is also found in about 60 percent of cases, with probably a smaller likelihood of neurologic complications.[28] Improvement in post-paraplegic pain is probably achieved in 50 to 60 percent of cases.[31] Even in those treated for postparaplegic pain, there can be neurologic complications in the spinal cord below the level of a complete lesion, with upset to automatic bladder function temporarily or even permanently. For a significant majority of patients with desperately severe pain of these three types, however, DREZ lesion offers a beneficial form of treatment in spite of these complications.

REFERENCES

1. Abbe R: A contribution to the surgery of the spine. Med Rec 35:149, 1889
2. Bennett WH: A case in which acute spasmodic pain in the left lower extremity was completely relieved by subdural division of the posterior roots of certain spinal nerves. Med Chir Trans 72:339, 1889
3. Sindou M, Fischer G, Mansuy L: Posterior spinal rhizotomy and selective posterior rhizotomy, in Krayenbuhl H, Maspers PE, Sweet WH (eds): Progress in Neurological Surgery, vol 7. Berlin, S. Karger, 1976, pp 201–250
4. Spiller WG, Martin E: The treatment of persistent pain of organic origin in the lower part of the body by division of the anterolateral column of the spinal cord. JAMA 58:1489, 1912
5. Leriche R: La chirurgie de la douleur. Paris, Masson, 1940
6. Melzack R, Wall PD: Pain mechanisms. A new theory. Science 150:971, 1965
7. Sindou M, Quoex C, Balleydier C: Fiber organization at the posterior spinal cord-rootlet junction in man. J Comp Neurol 153:15, 1974
8. Sindou M: Etude de la jonction radiculo-médullaire postérieure. La radicellotomie postérieure sélective dans la chirugie de la douleur. MD Thesis 173. Lyon, 1972
9. Sindou M, Fischer G, Goutelle A, et al: La radicellotomie postérieure sélective. Premiers resultats dans la chirugie de la douleur. Neurochirugie 20:391, 1974
10. Nashold BS, Urban B, Zorub DS: Phantom pain relief by focal destruction of the substantia gelatinosa of Rolando. Adv Pain Res Ther 1:959, 1976
11. Nashold BS, Ostdahl RH: Dorsal root entry zone lesion for pain relief. J Neurosurg 51:59, 1979
12. Cosman ER, Nashold BS, Ovelman-Levitt J: Theoretical aspects of radiofrequency lesions in the dorsal root entry zone. Neurosurgery 6:945, 1984
13. Levy WJ, Nutkiewicz A, Ditmore QM, et al: Laser-induced dorsal root entry zone lesions for pain control. J Neurosurg 59:884, 1983
14. Sindou M, Lapras C: Neurosurgical treatment of pain in the Pancoast-Tobias syndrome: Selective posterior rhizotomy and open anterolateral C2-cordotomy. Adv Pain Res Ther 4:199,1982
15. Sindou M, Millet MF, Mortamis J, et al: Results of selective posterior rhizotomy in the treatment of painful and spastic paraplegia seconcary to multiple sclerosis. Appl Neurophysiol 45:335, 1981
16. Wynn PCB: Pain in avulsion of the brachial plexus. Neurosurgery 15:960, 1984
17. Murphey F, Hartung W, Kirlin JW: Myelographic demonstration of avulsing injury of the brachial plexus. AJR 58:102, 1947
18. de Morgan JM, Kierland RR: The outcome of patients with herpes zoster. AMA Arch Dermatol 75:193, 1957
19. Juel-Jenson BE: Herpes simplex and zoster. Br Med J 1:406, 1973
20. Elliott FA: Treatment of herpes zoster with high dose prednisone. Lancet 2:610, 1964
21. Nathan PW, Wall PD: Treatment of post herpetic neuralgia by prolonged electrical stimulation. Br Med J 3:645, 1974
22. Taub A: Relief of post herpetic neuralgia with psychotropic drugs. J Neurosurg 39:235, 1973
23. Watson CP, Evans RJ, Reed K, et al: Amitriptyline versus placebo in post-herpetic neuralgia. Neurology 32:671, 1982
24. Woodforde JM, Dwyer B, McEwen BW, et al: Treatment of postherpetic neuralgia. Med J Aust 2:869, 1965
25. Gerson GR, Jones RB, Luscombe DK: Studies on the concomitant use of carbamazepine and domipramine for relief of post herpetic pain. Postgrad Med J 53 (suppl 4):104, 1977
26. Farber GA, Burks JW: Chlorprothixene therapy for herpes zoster neuralgia. South Med J 67:808, 1974
27. Nathan PW: Chlorprothixene (Taractan) in post-herpetic neuralgia and other severe chronic pains. Pain 5:367, 1978

28. Friedman AH, Nashold BS: Dorsal root entry zone lesions for the treatment of postherpetic neuralgia. Neurosurgery 15:969, 1984

29. Friedman AH, Nashold BS: Dorsal root entry zone lesions for the treatment of postherpetic neuralgia. Neurosurgery 15:969, 1984

30. Melzack R, Loeser JD: Phantom body pain in paraplegics: Evidence for a central "pattern generating mechanism" for pain. Pain 4:195, 1978

31. Nashold BS, Bullitt E: Dorsal root entry zone lesions to control central pain in paraplegics. J Neurosurg 55:414, 1981

32. Thomas DGT, Sheehy JPR: Dorsal root entry zone lesions (Nashold's procedure) for pain relief following brachial plexus avulsion. J Neurol Neurosurg Psychiatry 46:924, 1983

33. Thomas DGT, Jones SJ: Dorsal root entry zone lesions (Nashold's procedure) in brachial plexus avulsion. Neurosurgery 15:966, 1984

34. Nashold BS: Technical note: Modification of DREZ lesion technique. J Neurosurg 55:1012, 1981

35. Nashold BS: Current status of the DREZ operation. Neurosurgery 15:942, 1984

36. Jones SJ, Thomas DGT: Assessment of long sensory tract conduction in patients undergoing dorsal root entry zone coagulation for pain relief, in Schwann J, Jones SJ (eds): Spinal Cord Monitoring. Berlin, Springer-Verlag, 1985, pp 266–273

37. Samii M, Moringlane JR: Thermocoagulation of the dorsal root entry zone for the treatment of intractable pain. Neurosurgery 15:953, 1984

CHAPTER 103

Longitudinal (Bischof's) Myelotomy

Leslie P. Ivan

THE MAIN FEATURES OF SPASTICITY arise from the exaggerated stretch reflex and the exaggerated flexor withdrawal. Any surgical procedure that can disrupt the reflex arcs participating in these two basic spinal reflexes would relieve muscle spasm and flexor withdrawal reflexes. The methods listed in Table 103-1 all relieve spasticity, but each has some disadvantage. Posterior rhizotomy has no lasting effect and produces complete sensory denervation in the segments involved, thus predisposing these areas to the development of pressure sores. Intrathecal alcohol injection gives temporary relief only and may aggravate the bladder problem. Intrathecal phenol injection is somewhat unpredictable in its effects, and even a satisfactory injection has the same disadvantage as alcohol. Cordectomy is a major procedure and its finality makes both the patient and the surgeon uneasy. Cauda equina transection, besides having the same finality as cordectomy, has the disadvantages of both anterior and posterior rhizotomy. Anterior rhizotomy is followed by severe muscle wasting and exposure of bony prominences, which increases the risk of pressure sores either in the ischial region from sitting or in the lower extremities of patients who wear braces.

Bischof's myelotomy, on the other hand, produces permanent flaccidity without loss of muscle bulk and, except for segmental analgesia, should not affect other sensory modalities. With accurate technique, all long tracts, including the pyramidal tract, should remain intact following myelotomy. An important feature of longitudinal myelotomy is that after the operation there is no late recurrence of spasticity because the short propriospinal pathways and the long collaterals were disrupted (Figure 103-1). This disruption eliminates the influx of afferent impulses from higher and lower segments, which is the suggested cause of failure in some of the other methods.

Bischof[1] first described his procedure in 1951 and called it longitudinal lateral myelotomy. No response to his paper can be found in the medical literature until 1955 when Weber[2] reported

The work appearing in this chapter was supported by grants from the Medical Research Council of Canada, from the Ontario Crippled Children's Society, and from the Multiple Sclerosis Society of Canada.

Art work and photography were done by the Department of Medical Communication, Faculty of Medicine, University of Ottawa, and by the Department of Medical Illustration, Children's Hospital of Eastern Ontario.

The adjustable electrodes, the spinal cord gauges, and the special knives were developed by Mr. G. Zellerman, Accurate Surgical Instruments Co., Toronto, Ontario.

Special thanks are due to Maureen Melrose for assembling the references and editing the manuscript and to Lise Riffel for the numerous retypings.

OPERATIVE NEUROSURGICAL TECHNIQUES
ISBN 0-8089-1862-1

the use of this technique in 2 patients, with good results. Nadvornik,[3] in 1961, reported 1 such case and commented favorably on the procedure. In 1962, Tonnis and Bischof[4] gave an account of 20 cases with a follow-up time of 2 to 8 years. Our papers with Paine and Hunt,[5,6] in 1966 and 1967, appear to be the first North American accounts of this operation. The procedure gained popularity in Canada, and the Canadian experience was summarized by Moyes in 1969.[7] Since then, several reports from various countries have been published,[8–12] with all authors commenting favorably on the method.

TECHNICAL CONSIDERATIONS AND MODIFICATIONS

The original Bischof's myelotomy involves separating the spinal cord longitudinally into an anterior and posterior half between the L1 and L5 segments, to which unilateral separation between S1 and S3 can be added to decrease bladder spasticity. Bischof suggested severing the cord into an anterior and posterior half incompletely in order to leave the pyramidal tracts intact on both sides (Figure 103-2). Later Pourpre, in 1960,[14] and Bischof, in 1967,[15] suggested an approach through the posterior median fissure (Figure 103-3).

A further search for the ideal procedure resulted in the use of an L-shaped knife by the author, and this procedure was called *circular griseotomy* (Figure 103-4), which worked well in animal experiments (Figure 103-5). During laboratory trials it became obvious that both mechanical and radiofrequency destruction can be used (Figure 103-6). It was recognized that for the relief of spasticity the effective part of the surgery is *disruption of pathways inside the gray matter. That is why the term griseotomy (cutting the gray) was proposed.*[8,16]

In experiments on 43 dogs (Table 103-2), my colleagues and I made the following observations: lateral longitudinal myelotomy, circular griseotomy, T-griseotomy, and radiofrequency lesions would all relieve spasticity; however, myelotomy on intact animals caused more paraplegia than any of the other procedures. Radiofrequency heat could reduce or eliminate spasticity, provided the lesions were made close to each other (4 mm apart), at least two lesions per segment. This would indicate that to achieve segmental relief of spasticity of the lower limbs in human beings, at least 14 to 18 radio frequency lesions should be made on each side in the equatorial line of the cord. The target area is within the gray matter in lamina 6 and 7 of Rexed (Figure 103-7).

Table 103-1. Procedures for the relief of spasm

Procedure	Described By
Posterior rhizotomy	Foerster (1910)
Intrathecal alcohol	Dogliotti (1930)
Intrathecal phenol	Suvansa (1931)
Cordectomy	MacCarty (1948)
Transection of cauda equina	Meriowsky (1950)
Anterior rhizotomy	Munro (1945)
Myelotomy	Bischof (1951)

INDICATIONS FOR MYELOTOMY

Myelotomy can best be used for patients suffering from spasticity of the lower limbs that is of such a degree that the spasms interfere with sitting in a wheelchair or lying comfortably in bed and when there are some cord functions that are advantageous to preserve. *Without further refinement of the present technique, myelotomy should not be performed on patients who are able to walk.* In some patients the use of braces or the ability to walk may be restored following successful myelotomy, and it is possible to retain voluntary emptying of the bladder if this was preserved in the original injury or disease.

If the patient has severe pain in the lower limbs, which is not infrequent in spastic conditions, relief of this pain might be an additional indication for this type of procedure.

PREOPERATIVE MANAGEMENT

Routine laboratory studies, x-ray films of the lumbosacral spine, urodynamic studies, exact charting of muscle strength, muscle tone, reflexes and sensory functions, and also measurement of the degree of contractures are required.

Most patients already have indwelling catheters. If not, a catheter should be inserted before surgery. During surgery, electrocystometrography can be performed to ascertain whether bladder tone was reduced sufficiently.

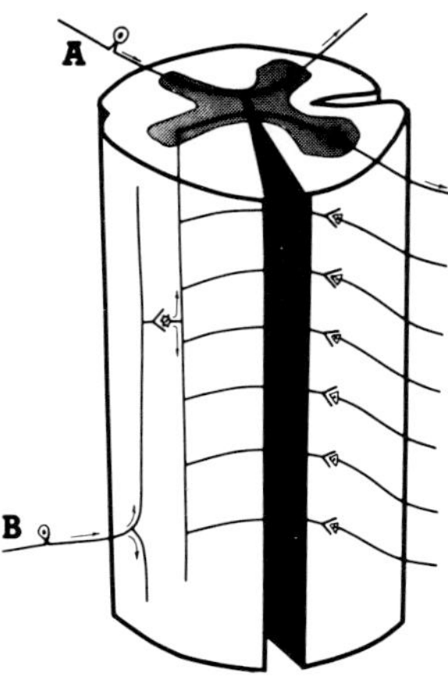

Fig. 103-1. Schematic representation of the original concept of Bischof's myelotomy. (A) Monosynaptic reflex arc. (B) Reflex collaterals with ascending and descending branches to motor neurons.

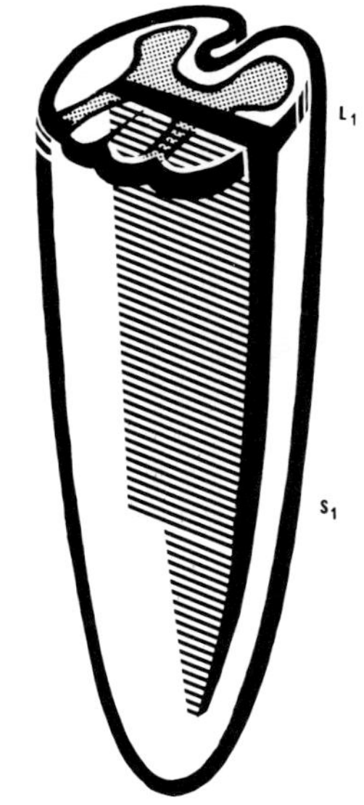

Fig. 103-2. Bischof's myelotomy. The original procedure.

OPERATIVE EXPLORATION

The surgery is always performed under general endotracheal anesthesia. The patient is positioned prone on the operating table, with semiflexion in hip and knee joints, and draped in such a way that an observer can report movements when nerve root stimulation is done during surgery.

The spinous processes are counted from C7 and the count double-checked by counting them from the L5 vertebra. The T10 vertebra is marked, and after the patient's back is cleansed with surgical soap and Betadine scrub, the operative field is draped between the T7 and L3 spinous processes. An incision is marked between the T9 and L2 spinous processes, and the subcutaneous tissue and paraspinal muscles are infiltrated with physiologic saline. The incision is made in the midline, and, through subperiosteal dissection, the T9, T10, T11, T12, and L1 vertebrae are exposed (Figure 103-8). A laminectomy is done on the T10, T11, T12, and L1 vertebrae. After the dura is opened, the conus medullaris should be at the caudal part of the

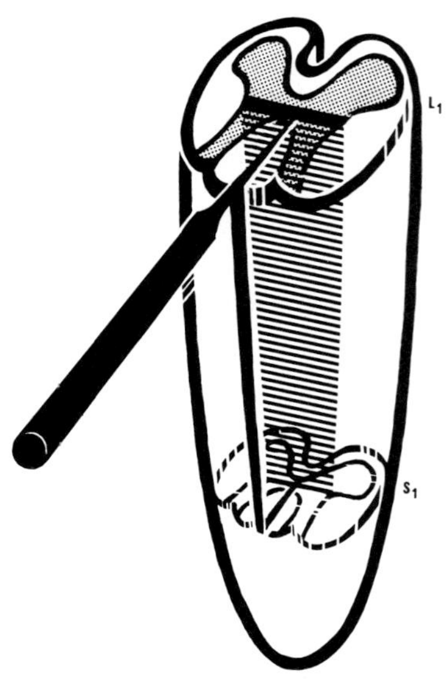

Fig. 103-3. Technique for T-griseotomy.

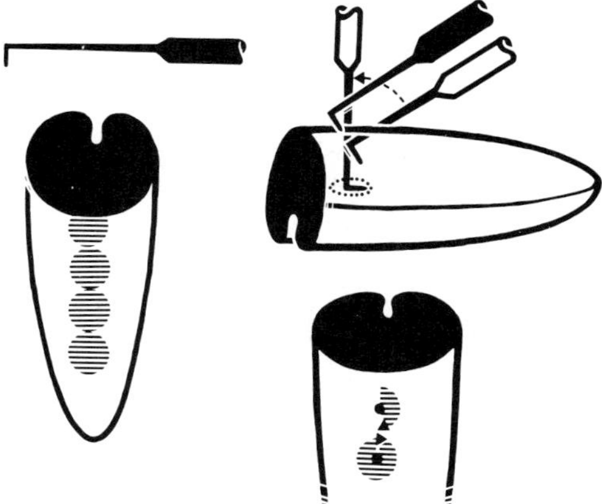

Fig. 103-4. Technique of circular griseotomy. An L-shaped instrument is inserted through the posterior midline sulcus and rotated 360 degrees in the equatorial plane of the cord.

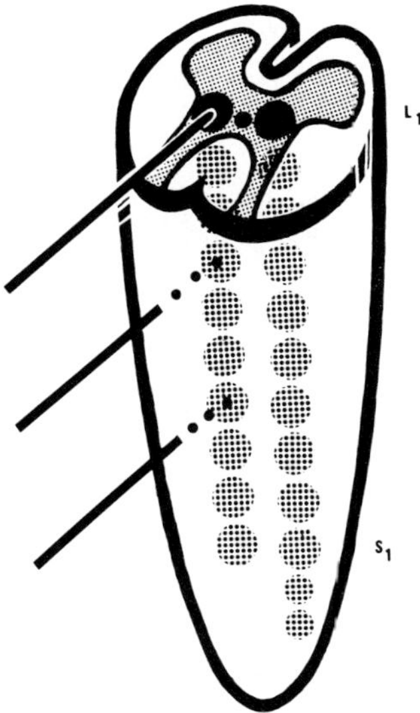

Fig. 103-6. Radiofrequency griseotomy. Radiofrequency heat microlesions within the gray matter made with a 0.5-mm bare-tip electrode through the posterior approach.

operative field and at least 80 mm of spinal cord should be visible. Holding sutures are placed in the dura, while the operative field is kept bloodless with the usual placement of cotton pledgets (Figure 103-9).

Using a nerve stimulator with a 2–7-V, 1-msec current, the T12 and S1 nerve roots should be identified. This is done by rotating the cord slightly and placing the stimulating electrode on the motor root of T12 while an observer identifies contraction of the lower abdominal muscles. Contraction can sometimes be felt by the operating surgeon through the draping. The S1 nerve root is usually the thickest of the cauda equina fibers, and when the motor root of S1 is stimulated, the foot should move into plantar flexion. After these two landmarks are identified (the distance between them varies between 55 to 70 mm), the surgeon should prepare the cord and instruments for the lesion-making procedure. The width and AP diameter of the cord are measured with a spinal cord gauge (Figure 103-10). The total length of the cord subject to lesion-making is also measured (Figure 103-9)

LESION PRODUCTION

Four methods of lesion-making will be described. The first three depend upon mechanical instruments that are used laterally on the cord or through a posterior approach. The fourth depends upon radiofrequency heat and is done posteriorly.

LATERAL LONGITUDINAL MYELOTOMY

Lateral longitudinal myelotomy is the original method of Bischof (Figure 103-11). In preparation for the myelotomy the cord is rotated sideways after the last three denticulate ligaments are cut. Some surgeons use a No. 11 blade or a keratome;[17] others, such as myself, use a slightly less sharp and smaller instrument (Figure 103-12). If it is difficult to rotate the cord, it can be transfixed with three 20-gauge needles to make it easier to rotate and find the cutting plane. An incision then is made slowly just anterior to the attachment of the denticulate ligament in the equatorial line of the cord, in such a way that about 2.5 mm of the cord is saved on the opposite side. This can be determined accurately by measuring the width of the cord (which may vary anywhere between 6 to 10 mm) and marking the knife with a hemoclip or a small piece of bone wax. The cutting (in a length of 55 to 70 mm) is done in small segments, because the space between the anterior and posterior roots

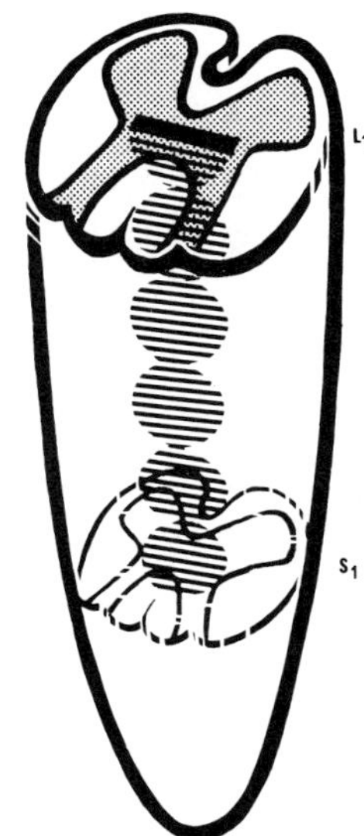

Fig. 103-5. The end result of circular griseotomy: a series of circular cuts within the gray matter.

Table 103-2. Segmental relief of spasticity

Group	Number of Dogs	Postoperative Paraplegia	Percentage
1. Lateral longitudinal myelotomy	4	4	100
2. Circular griseotomy	14	4	28
3. Radiofrequency griseotomy	25	10	40
Total	43	18	

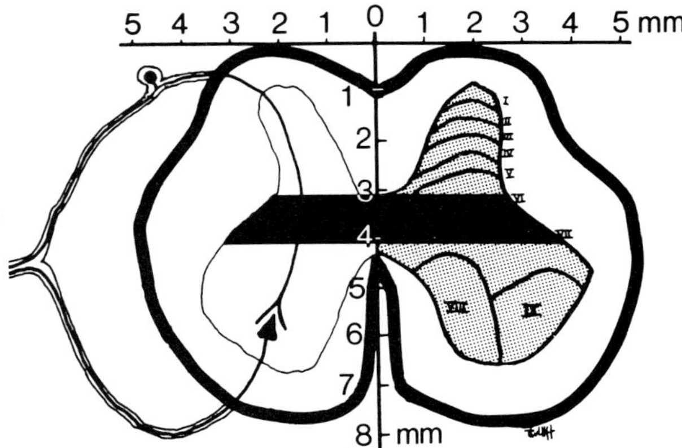

Fig. 103-7. The target area (blackened between 3 and 4 mm) within the gray matter for the relief of spasticity. The roman numerals indicate the laminar structure of the gray matter according to Rexed. The arabic numerals are reference points in millimeters.

prevents a continuous incision. Usually some blood begins to ooze in the line of the incision; the bleeding, however, stops when the wound is irrigated and small cotton pledgets are placed. When the oozing stops, the dura is closed with interrupted 0000 black silk sutures, and the muscle layer with 0 silk or 0 chromic catgut. The fascia, subcutaneous tissue, and the skin are closed with sutures, according to the surgeon's routine. There is no need for a drain.

POSTERIOR LONGITUDINAL MYELOTOMY

Posterior longitudinal myelotomy was first described by Pourpre, in 1960,[14] who called it *Myelotomy en Croix;* the author termed it *T-griseotomy* (Figure 103-3). After the exposure described previously and after nerve stimulation and measurements, the posterior median sulcus of the cord is identified under magnification and, avoiding injury to the dorsal vein, the posterior median fissure is entered to a depth half that of the AP diameter of the cord with an L-shaped knife. Separation is made in the usual myelotomy plane, 3 mm on each side, sideways from the midline. The final myelotomy is

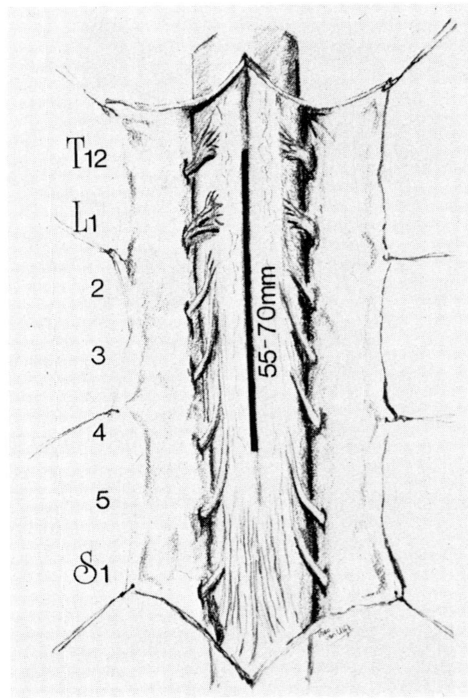

Fig. 103-9. Artist's concept of the exposed cord indicating the length of the cord between L1 and S1 segments.

reached by proceeding with the separation in small sections to avoid injuring the usually tortuous dorsal vein. At the end of this procedure a T-shaped cleavage is left in the cord for a length of 55 to 70 mm. Slight oozing is easily controlled by irrigation with physiologic saline and by placement of small cotton pledgets. The wound is closed as previously described.

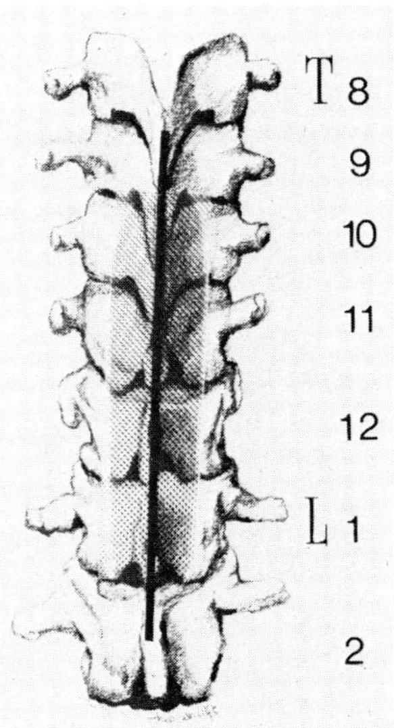

Fig. 103-8. Schematic drawing showing the extent of the incision and laminectomy.

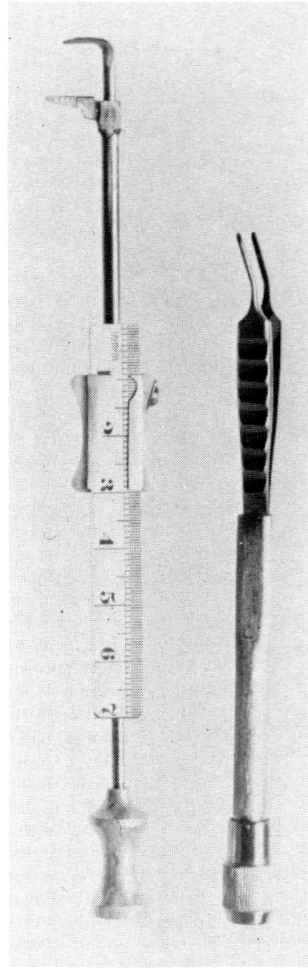

Fig. 103-10. Spinal cord gauges for measuring the width and AP diameter of the cord.

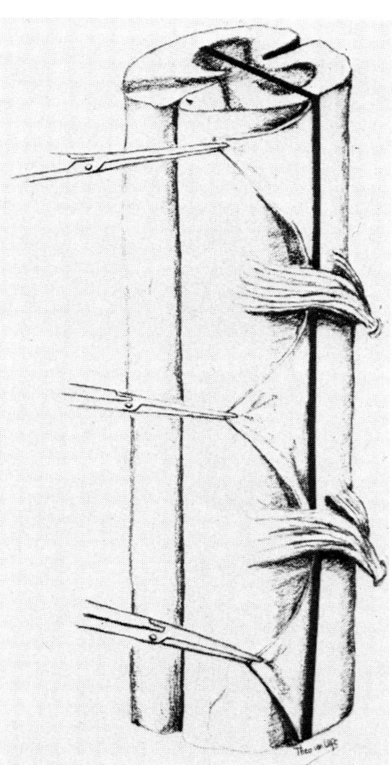

Fig. 103-11. A drawing showing the rotation of the cord and the plane of incision at the attachment of the dentate ligaments.

CIRCULAR GRISEOTOMY

Circular griseotomy (Figures 103-4 and 103-5) was used with a stereotactic attachment in animal experiments. A free-hand method was used by the author in 5 patients with good results, except for 1 patient who had unilateral recurrence of

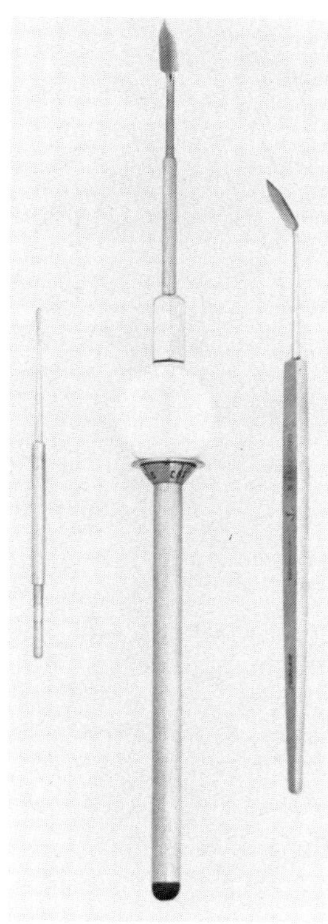

Fig. 103-12. Instruments used for the incision of the cord in lateral longitudinal myelotomy.

spasticity. A somewhat similar method was described by Yamada et al.,[18] who reported excellent results in 14 patients, 5 of whom were able to walk following the procedure (Figure 103-13).

RADIOFREQUENCY GRISEOTOMY

After several years of experimentation and the development of suitable electrodes, radiofrequency griseotomy was performed on 5 adults. The technique depends upon the same exploration as the previous procedures. Special electrodes with adjustable tips are used (Figure 103-14). Fourteen to 18 pairs of lesions are necessary to obtain satisfactory results (Figure 103-15). The tip of the needle should be inserted 2 mm from the midline on each side, and a pair of lesions should be made at each 4-mm distance along the posterior aspect of the cord. Depending upon the measurement of the cord, the half millimeter bare tip of the electrode should reach a depth of 3 to 4 mm (Figure 103-16). Using the Radionics lesion-maker with a test-lesion setting of 100 mA, 50-mA 10-sec-effective radiofrequency lesions are made at each insertion. Care should be taken to use a clean electrode for each lesion.

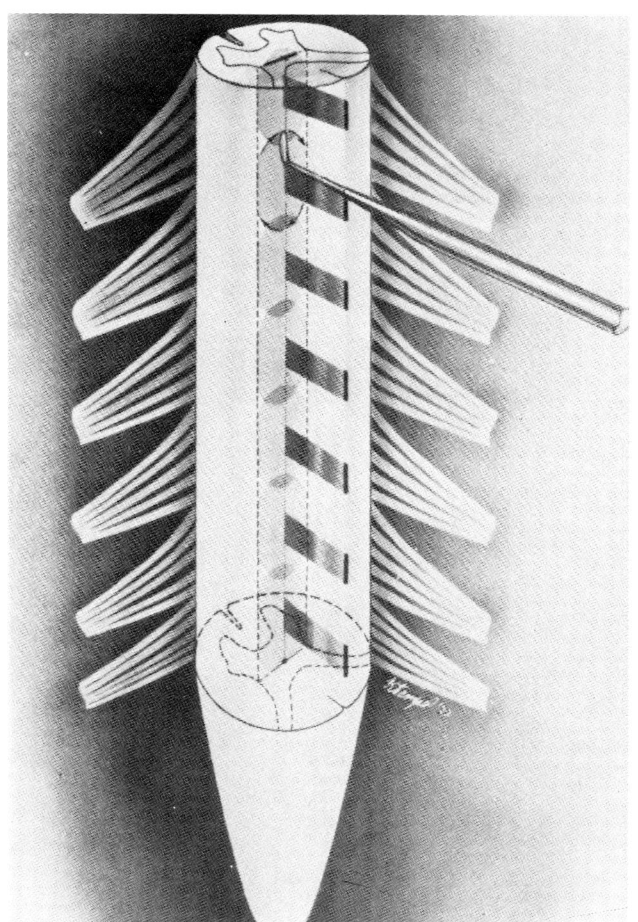

Fig. 103-13. Drawing illustrating the procedure described by Yamada and colleagues. (Reprinted from Yamada S, Perot PL, Ducker TB, et al: Myelotomy for control of mass spasms in paraplegia. J Neurosurg 45:683–690, 1976. With permission of the author and editor.)

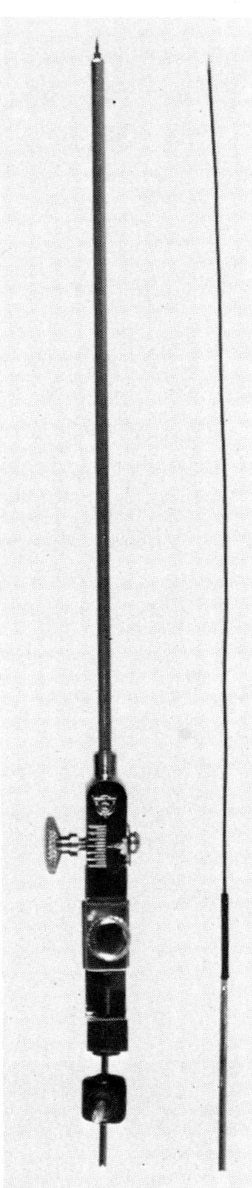

Fig. 103-14. Adjustable needle electrode with 0.5-mm bare tip. Depending on the AP diameter of the cord, the penetrating portion of the electrode can be adjusted with 0.5-mm accuracy.

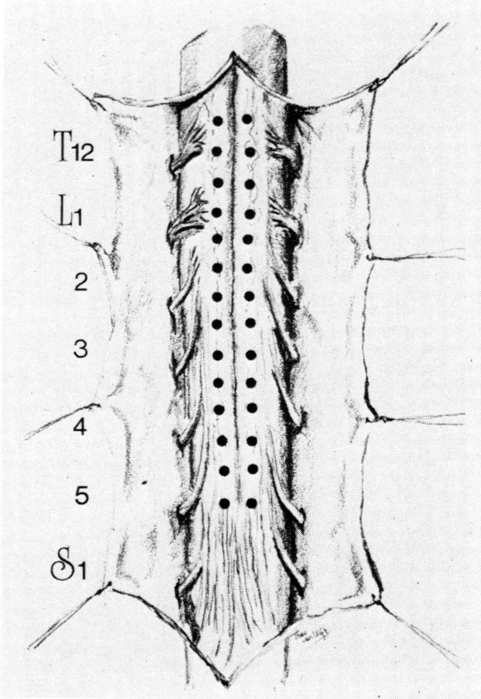

Fig. 103-15. Points of penetration on the dorsal aspect of the cord for radiofrequency griseotomy. The distance between the lesions is 4 mm, both in the craniocaudal and lateral directions.

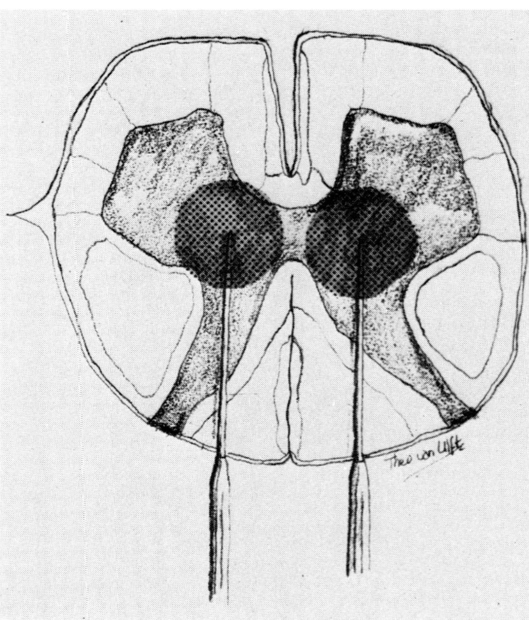

Fig. 103-16. Schematic drawing of the cord with two electrodes in position showing the approximate area of radiofrequency heat destruction in the intermediate gray matter.

POSTOPERATIVE CARE

After surgery, the patient should be turned hourly. Physiotherapy can be started on the day after surgery, Patients are able to take solid food 24 hours after surgery, although in some cases paralytic ileus may be a complicating factor. In case of pre-existing pressure sores in the sacral areas, prophylactic antibiotic treatment is justifiable to prevent wound infection. A week after surgery, wheelchair routine may start and, if the patient's condition permits, the learning of self-transfer from bed to wheelchair can be started. In case there are remaining useful functions, ambulation with long braces can be attempted 3 or 4 weeks after surgery.

RESULTS AND COMPLICATIONS

Most reports agree that myelotomy is one of the best available procedures for the permanent relief of spasticity. The question is, which type of myelotomy should be performed to ensure that spasticity recurs less frequently and a greater number of patients can ambulate after surgery? Unfortunately, on the basis of the available literature, including the author's material, this question cannot be answered with certainty.

The great majority of case reports comment on the original Bischof's method.[7,8,10,11,19,20] It appears that with unilateral longitudinal myelotomy, spasticity recurs on the opposite side to the cord incision in about 20 percent of the cases.[21]

Posterior commissural myelotomy (myelotomy en croix or T-griseotomy), on the other hand, seems to have definite advantages compared with the original Bischof's method.[14,19-21] There have been only about 26 cases reported in all of the medical literature. The author's single experience showed that this was a time-consuming procedure, but the patient had good relief of spasticity; movements in the ankle joint were preserved on both sides. The papers by Laitinen and Singounas[9] from Finland, reporting on the results in 9 patients, and Benedetti

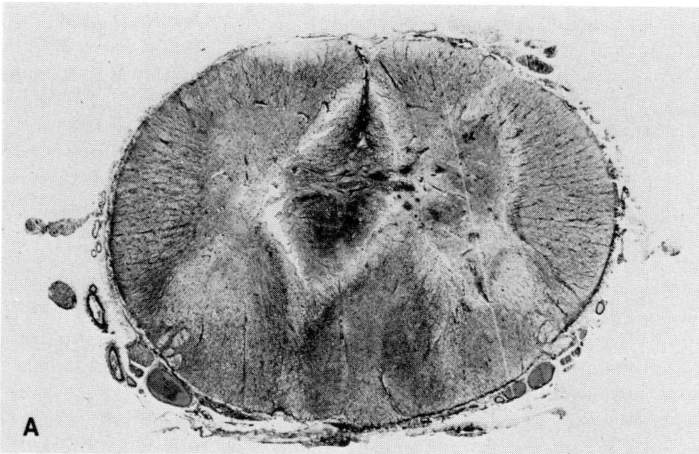

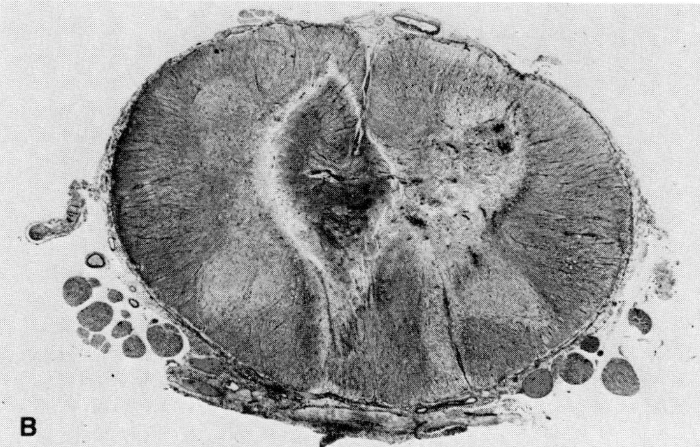

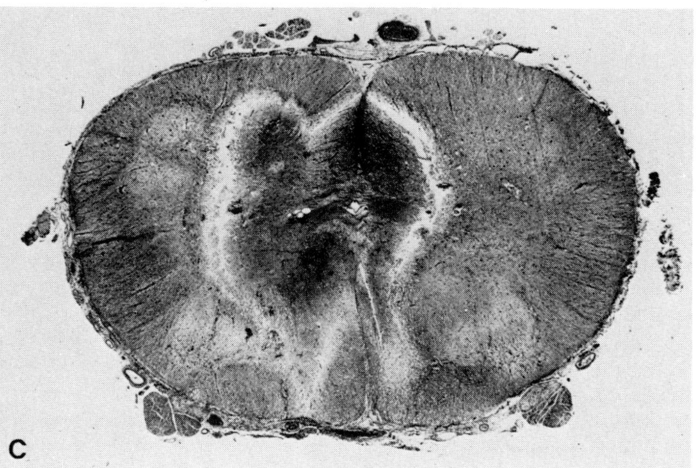

Fig. 103-17. Histologic appearance of human spinal cord 2 days after radiofrequency griseotomy. Death was the result of pulmonary embolism. Note the lesions, which are considerably larger than expected from egg-white experiments.

and Carbonin[22] from Italy, reporting on the results in 12 patients, give a very favorable impression of this method. The use of the microscope should further enhance the precision and value of this form of myelotomy.

Circular griseotomy appeared to be a feasible procedure in animal experiments and in patients.[18] Refinement of the instrumentation and adapting it for the characteristics of the human spinal cord may make this a very valuable technique in the hands of someone who has access to a large number of patients.

A variation of this procedure was suggested by Padovani,[23] who reported good results in 8 patients. Dorsal longitudinal myelotomy using Yamada's modification was performed by Fogel et al. in seven patients[25] and they conclude that "dorsal longitudinal myelotomy is not successful in the treatment of spasticity in the spinal-injured patient."

Radiofrequency griseotomy worked very well in animal experiments and was performed five times on patients by the author. The last 3 patients treated by this method had excellent results. One of the patients who died because of pulmonary embolism (the only fatality among 26 patients) provided us with a spinal cord specimen (Figure 103-17). Histologic examination showed that the lesions surprisingly were bigger than predicted from egg-white experiments. The radiofrequency lesions of the cord were entirely bloodless, but the selectivity of the method cannot be judged from the small number of cases.

My colleagues and I have frequently found that a contracture that appeared fixed clinically may disappear entirely under general anesthesia. A slight degree of contracture after myelotomy may resolve spontaneously. In a few cases we combined myelotomy with tenotomy of the hamstring muscles.

In my material, which consists of 26 cases, only 1 patient could walk with braces after surgery.

Spasticity recurs in about 20 percent of the cases. In half of these the recurrence is insignificant and not disturbing. In about 10 percent of the cases, re-operation or intrathecal alcohol injection should abolish the remaining spasticity.

For those neurosurgeons who have an occasional case, probably the original unilateral longitudinal myelotomy is the most suitable method. For those who see many cases, a variety of modifications are available, as discussed earlier.

From the purely experimental circular griseotomy through the proved radiofrequency griseotomy to the quite well-accepted posterior commissural myelotomy, there are a variety of lesion-making methods. With the development of ultrasound and laser, a wide field of experimentation remains open. The target to be destroyed within the gray matter, corresponding roughly to lamina 6 and 7 of Rexed, is well established;[16,24] it is the intermediate gray matter around the equatorial plane of the cord.

REFERENCES

1. Bischof W: Die longitudinale myelotomie. Zentralbl Neurochir 11:79, 1951
2. Weber W: Die Behandlung der spinalen Paraspastik unter besonderer Berucksichtigung der longitudinalen Myelotomie (Bischof). Med Monatsschr 9:510, 1955
3. Nadvornik P: Effect of longitudinal myelotomy on spasticity of lower limbs and urinary bladder. Sb Ved Pr Lek Sak Karlovy Univ 2:77, 1959, abstracted, Excerpta Med VIII 14:3876, 852, 1961
4. Tonnis W, Bischof W: Ergebnisse der lumbalen Myelotomie nach Bischof. Zentralbl Neurochir 23:120, 1962
5. Ivan LP, Paine KWE, Hunt TE: Experience with Bischof's myelotomy. Can J Surg 10:191, 1967
6. Paine KW, Ivan LP, Hunt TE: The Bischof myelotomy for treatment of spasticity in paraplegics. Proc Annu Clin Spinal Cord Inj Conf 15:72, 1966
7. Moyes PD: Longitudinal myelotomy for spasticity. J Neurosurg 31:615, 1969
8. Ivan LP, Wiley JJ: Myelotomy in the management of spasticity. Clin Orthop 108:52, 1975
9. Laitinen L, Singounas E: Longitudinal myelotomy in the treatment of spasticity of the legs. J Neurosurg 35:536, 1971

10. Schirmer M, Barz D, Wenker H: Longitudinal myelotomy—indication and resuits. Acta Neurochir 31:308, 1975
11. VanderArk MC, Kempe G L: Longitudinal myelotomy in spastic paraplegia. Milit Med 134:608, 1969
12. Virozub ID, Chipko SS: Our experience with 60 patients undergoing frontal myelotomy for severe spasticity. Vopr Neurochir 27:21, 1976 (Russian), cited from Dietrich J, Sonntag M: Behandlungergebnisse nach longitudinaler Myelotomie bei Paraspastik der Beine. Psychiatr Neurol Med Psychol 31:353, 1979
13. Guido LJ: Myelotomy in the treatment of spasticity. J Fla Med Assoc 65:98, 1978
14. Pourpre MH: Traitement neuro-chirurgical des contractures chez les paraplégiques post traumatiques. Neurochirurgie 6:229, 1960
15. Bischof W: Zur dorsalen longitudinalen Myelotomie. Zentralbl Neurochir 2:21, 1975
16. Ivan LP: The segmental relief of spasticity. Read before the 7th Canadian Congress of Neurological Sciences, Banff, 1972
17. Asenjo A: Neurosurgical Techniques. Springfield, Ill, Charles C Thomas, 1963
18. Yamada S, Perot PL, Ducker TB, et al: Myelotomy for control of mass spasms in paraplegia. J Neurosurg 45:683, 1976
19. Galanda M, Nadvornik P, Frohlich F: Contribution to surgical treatment of spasticity in spinal cord injuries (critical remarks to longitudinal myelotomy). Bratisl Lek List 61:589, 1974
20. Dietrich J, Sonntag M: Results of treatment of leg paraspasm cases following longitudinal frontal myelotomy. Psychiatr Neurol Med Psychol 31:353, 1979
21. Gonsette R, André-Baliseaux G: Contribution au traitement neurochirurgical de la spasticité des membres inférieurs dans la sclérose en plaque. Acta Neurol Psychiatr Belg 63:460, 1963
22. Benedetti A, Carbonin C: Resultats de la myelotomie lombaire dans la paraplégies spastiques avec contractions musculaires—Observations preliminaires chez douze malades. Neurochirurgie 23:347, 1977
23. Padovani R, Tognetti F, Pozzati E, et al: Treatment of spasticity by means of dorsal longitudinal myelotomy and lozenge-shaped griseotomy. Spine. 7:103, 1982
24. Fever H, Horner TG, De Myer WE, et al: Anatomical and histological lesiors in Bischof's myelotomy in dogs. Surg Forum 23:438, 1972
25. Fogel JP, Waters RL, Mahomar F: Dorsal Myelotomy for Relief of Spasticity in Spinal Injury Patients. Clin Orthop 192:137–144, 1985

CHAPTER 104
Commissural Myelotomy

John E. Adams   Robert Lippert   Yoshio Hosobuchi

COMMISSURAL OR MEDIOLONGITUDINAL MYELOT-OMY was first performed for the relief of pain by Armour in 1927.[1] The rationale for this operation is obviously based upon the traditional concept that finely myelinated and unmyelinated fibers of the lateral division of the dorsal root, which subserve nociception, cross in the anterior commissure of the spinal cord at the level of or up to three segments cephalad to their point of entry into the spinal cord. Thus, by sectioning the anterior commissure over several segments, the neurosurgeon theoretically should be able to bilaterally denervate relevant segments of the body from nociceptive input. This potential ability to relieve bilateral segmental pain during a single operation without compromising the function of the descending or ascending long tracts presents obvious advantages over bilateral anterolateral spinal tractotomy at either the high thoracic or high cervical level. The naturally occurring model for spinal commissurotomy, of course, is the cystic lesion of syringomyelia, where the pathologic process interrupts the same decussating fibers as the surgeon does with a knife, producing a result that is clinically identical insofar as the segmental loss of nociception is concerned.

The operation has enjoyed moderate popularity in European centers,[2–5] but until recently rarely has been performed in the United States.[6] It is perhaps noteworthy, however, that the introduction of the operating microscope has encouraged a revival of this operative procedure for the relief of intractable pain. This is no mere coincidence, since in spite of earlier successes achieved without benefit of the operating microscope, it is clear that both the success achieved without and prevention of postoperative complications are greatly enhanced by the microsurgical technique.

We have employed commissural myelotomy primarily to relieve intractable bilateral pain in the lower abdomen, pelvis, perineum, and lower extremities. Most patients have suffered from malignant disease, but we have employed the procedure in patients whose pain was of nonmalignant origin, such as in patients suffering from chronic adhesive arachnoiditis, trauma to the spinal column, etc. The majority of patients have had pain involving the lower segments of their body, but in a minority the pain has originated in the middle or upper thoracic region.

TECHNIQUE

The position of the incision in a caudad cephalad plane is dictated by the highest segment involved in the painful process. The myelotomy must extend at least three cord segments above this level. Thus, if the pain extends as high as the L1 derma-tome, it will be necessary to carry the myelotomy as high as the tenth thoracic segment in the cord.

General anesthesia usually is employed, although the operation can be done under local anesthesia. The patient is placed in the prone position, since there is nothing to be gained by employing either the lateral or sitting position. A skin marker is placed over the designated spinous process, which is then verified by an intraoperative x-ray film. After the laminectomy has been completed, if there is any doubt regarding the level, another intraoperative film can be taken.

After the appropriate laminectomy has been performed and the dura has been opened, the operating microscope is positioned and, at a magnification of four- to sixfold, the midline sulcus of the dorsal surface of the spinal cord is identified. This is accomplished by identifying the midline dorsal vein and the fine arachnoidal septum. With microdissection, the midline dorsal vein is coagulated with bipolar forceps throughout the length of proposed incision (Figure 104-1). It also may be necessary to coagulate one or two very small arterial radicals that may cross the midline. King[7] has stressed the advisability of preserving not only the midline dorsal vein but even the smallest arterial branch. We have not, however, encountered any deleterious effects after coagulation of these small vessels. The length of the proposed incision is thus prepared, varying from 2.5 to 4 cm, depending upon the extent of the body area involved in the painful syndrome.

Two methods have been used to carry out the section of the anterior commissure. Either an iridectomy knife or a No. 12 Bard-Parker blade held in a hemostat is used to penetrate the upper end of the median sulcus to a depth of 6 to 7 mm. The knife is then passed in a caudad direction, maintaining its position strictly in the midline, as viewed in the microscopic field, until the full length of the planned incision has been achieved (Figure 104-2).

An alternative method that is sometimes employed is to develop the median incision through the pia-arachnoid with sharp section and then, with a blunt microdissector, to penetrate the midline cord through the anterior commissure, with gentle bilateral retraction of the incision to give visualization throughout.

At the present time we employ the former technique in most cases because we feel that the open technique involves more manipulation of the cord and consequently more risk of damage to the posterior columns and the lateral funiculus.

King[7] prefers the open technique to ensure complete section of the anterior commissure, as well as to avoid coagulation of any blood vessels.

OPERATIVE NEUROSURGICAL TECHNIQUES
ISBN 0-8089-1862-1

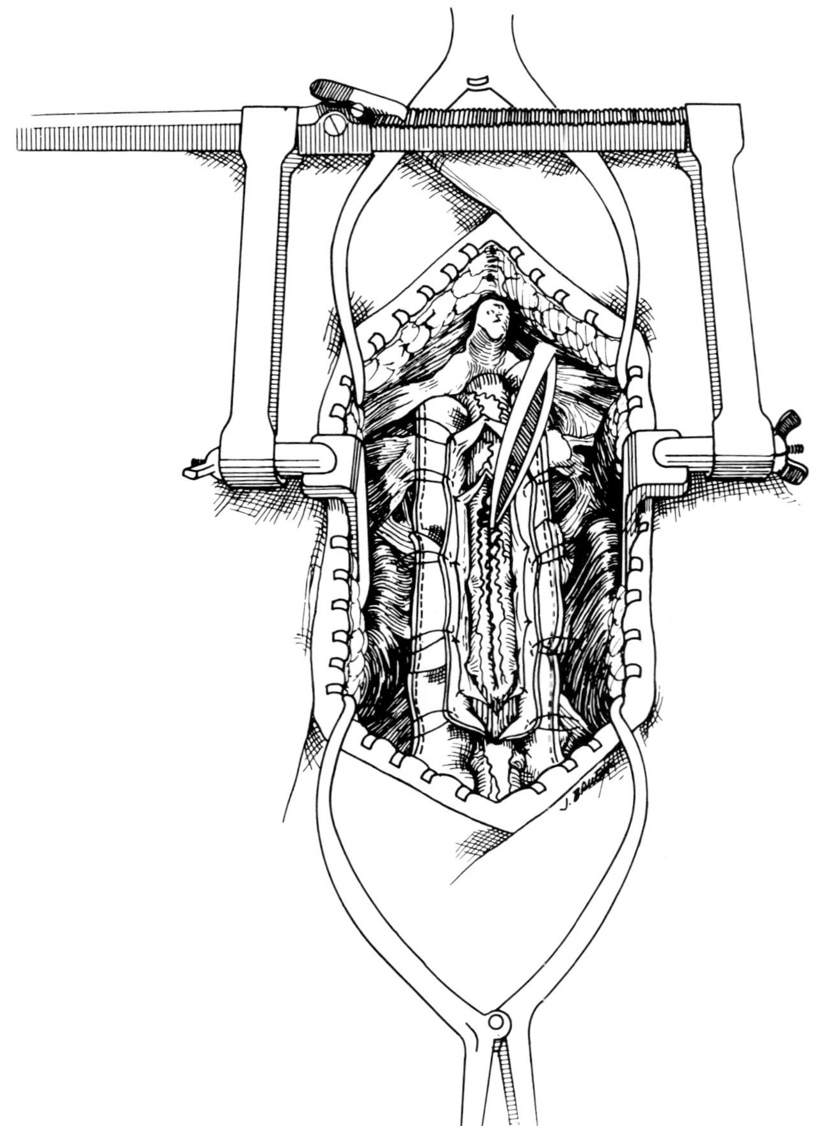

Fig. 104-1. Drawing of bipolar coagulation of the midline dorsal vein.

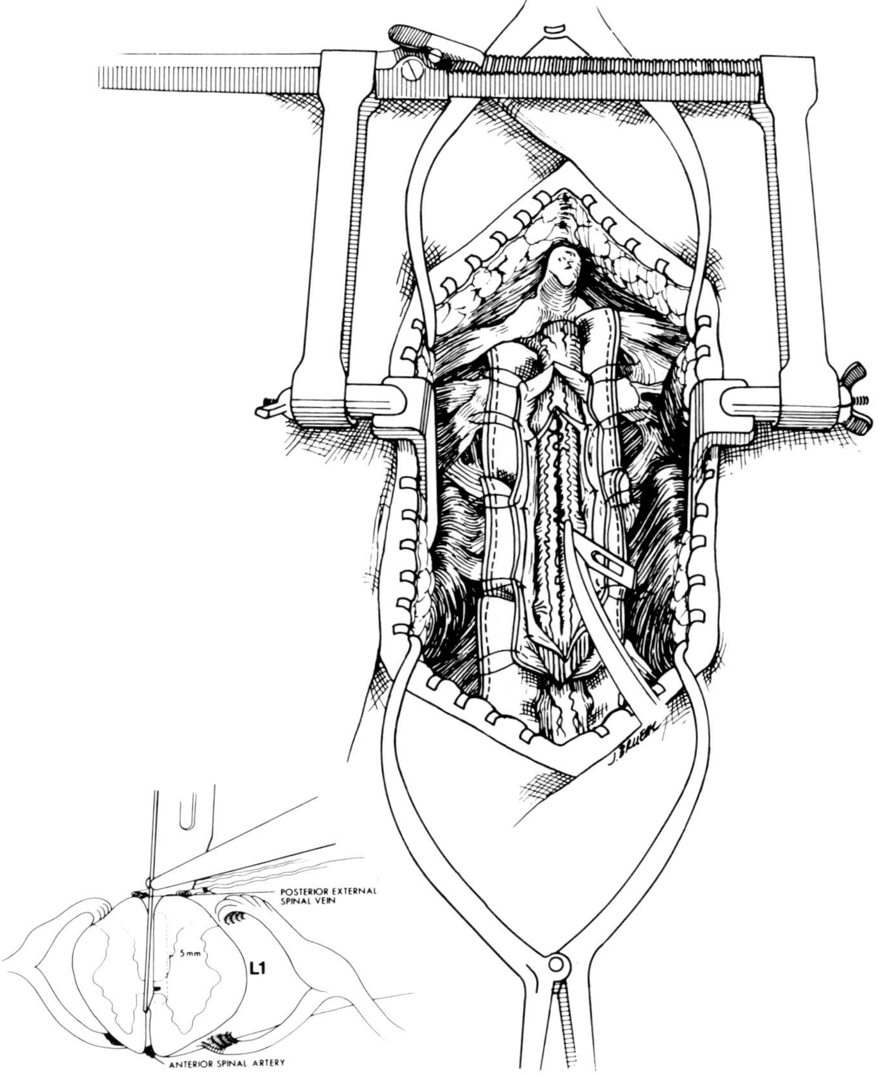

Fig. 104-2. Illustration of technique of blind resection through the midline of the spinal cord.. Diagrammatic representation of the section of the coronal plane (inset).

Table 104-1. Results of commissural myelotomy according to etiology in 24 patients

Diagnosis	No. of patients	Relief Complete	Partial	None	Bladder	Leg weakness	Persistent dysesthesia	Comments
Carcinoma of:								
Rectum and colon	7	5	1	1	1	1	3	Pain due to pelvic extension
Cervix and uterus	4	3	1	—	—	1	—	Pain due to pelvic extension
Bladder	1	1	—	—	—	—	1	Pain due to pelvic extension
Breast	1	—	1	—	—	—	—	Metastatic to lumbar spine and pelvic mass
Prostate	3	2	1	—	—	—	—	Metastic disease to the lumbar spine
Lung	2	—	1	1	1	—	—	Metastatic to the thoracic spine and sternum
Osteogenic sarcoma	1	1	—	—	—	—	—	Metastatic to the lumbar sacral spine
Transverse myelitis	1	—	1	—	—	—	—	Girdle chest pains
Medulloblastoma	1	1	—	—	—	—	—	Metastatic to cauda equina
Paraplegia traumatic	1	1	—	—	—	—	—	Burning leg pain
Multiple sclerosis	1	1	—	—	—	—	—	Constant sacral pain plus painful flexor spasms
Sacral Chordoma	1	—	1	—	1	—	—	—
Total	24	15	7	2	3	2	4	

POSTOPERATIVE CARE

Postoperative mobilization and ambulation are dictated, to some extent, by the primary disease but can occur as early as the first or second postoperative day. Catheterization may be necessary, but often is not.

RESULTS

Our results with 24 patients who have undergone this procedure are summarized in Table 104-1 and 104-2. Table 104-1 gives the results in terms of the etiology of the painful syndrome. For simplicity, the clinical result has been designated as either complete, partial, or no relief of pain. In Table 104-2 the same data are tabulated in terms of the anatomic site of pain. Since many patients had pain involving more than one area of the body, the number of pain locations represented is greater than the actual number of patients operated upon.

There were no deaths in this series and complications were not serious. Bladder function that was normal preoperatively was altered in 3 patients, 2 of whom became unable to void and were discharged with a catheter in place. One patient developed partial incontinence. Weakness of the legs, present in 2 pa-

Table 104-2. Results of commissural myelotomy according to anatomic site of pain

Location of pain	No. of patients	Relief Complete	Partial	None	Bladder	Motor loss	Persistent dysesthesia
Chest	2	1	—	1	1	—	—
Lumbosacral spine	3	2	1	—	—	—	—
Rectum and perineum	11	7	3	1	1	1	3
Buttock	2	1	1	—	1	—	—
Legs and hips	10	7	3	—	—	1	4
Suprapubic	1	1	—	—	—	—	1
Testicular	1	—	1	—	—	—	—
Total	30	19	9	2	3	2	8

tients, appeared to be a lower motor neuron disturbance and was interpreted as being a result of damage to anterior horn cells in appropriate segments. Paresthesias or dysesthesias were temporarily encountered in most patients, but disappeared within a few days in all but 4. This complication was interpreted as being the result of trauma to posterior columns of the cord. In the 4 patients in whom these symptoms persisted, there also was a concomitant loss of position sense in the lower extremities; this did not, however, interfere significantly with ambulation.

From these results, it can be seen that commissural myelotomy should be considered in the treatment of intractable pain when that pain is primarily bilateral or involves midline structures of the body. With the advent of the operating microscope and newer microsurgical techniques, it appears to be a relatively safe procedure. In this regard the operation was abandoned after its introduction into this country primarily because of the fear of injury to the anterior spinal artery.[8] This has not occurred in any of our cases.

In the series reported in the United States, commissural myelotomy has been performed primarily in lower segments of the cord for midline pain involving the pelvis or for bilateral lower extremity pain. In Europe and in England, however, the operation has been employed more frequently for midline or bilateral truncal pain as well as for pain involving the lower cervical areas and the upper extremities.[4]

The sensory loss following commissural myelotomy is extremely variable. In our cases no reproducible pattern was evident. The loss of awareness to pain and temperature might erratically involve the appropriate segments, but in some instances there was only minimal loss of acute pain and temperature sensation, even though there was complete relief from chronic pain. This has been the experience of all surgeons who have performed this operation.

DISCUSSION

As yet, there is no adequate explanation for the relief of pain obtained by this procedure. To consider that section of the decussating fibers in the anterior commissure is the sole explanation appears to be too simplistic, especially in view of the vagaries of the resultant sensory loss. Sourek[4] has hypothesized that the relief of pain is due to the involvement of two sensory systems that subserve nociception. These are the slow conducting anterolateral system and the more rapidly conducting mediodorsal system. Hitchcock[9] has produced profound and extensive analgesia following a stereotactically placed small midline lesion in the anterior commissure at either the medullary cervical junction or at the C1-2 level. He suggests that not only the pain relief but also the extensive analgesia produced by lesions at this site may be the result of interruption of decussations of both direct and crossed pain pathways ascending close to the gray matter of the spinal cord, or are possibly the result of interruption of fibers in the spinal cervical tract (Morin), which decussate in the high cervical area.

CONCLUSIONS

On the basis of our experience and a review of the literature, it would appear that spinal commissurotomy has now become a relatively safe and effective procedure. It should be seriously considered as a method to manage intractable pain related to midline structures of the body, or bilateral pain. It may well become the procedure of choice for rectal and perineal pain. At the present time, however, we still would recommend the use of other procedures for the relief of unilateral pain.

REFERENCES

1. Armour D: Surgery of the spinal cord. Lancet 2:691, 1927
2. Guillian J, Mazars G, Movillae V: La myelatomie commissurale. Presse Med 49:666, 1945
3. Neansery B, Lecuire J, Acassat L: Technique de la myelatomie commissurale posterieure. J Chir 60:206, 1944
4. Sourek K: Commissural myelotomy. J Neurosurg 31:524, 1969
5. Wertheimer P: Posterior commissural myelotomy for relief of pain. Acta Chir Belg 54:28, 1946
6. Lippert RS, Hosobuchi Y, Nielsen SL: Spinal commissurotomy. Surg Neurol 2:373, 1974
7. King RB: Anterior Commissurotomy for intractable pain. J Neurosurg 47:7, 1977
8. Putnam JJ: Myelotomy of the commissure. Arch Neurol Psychiatry 32:189, 1934
9. Hitchcock E: Stereotactic cervical myelotomy. J Neurol Neurosurg Psychiatry 33:224, 1970

CHAPTER 105

Percutaneous Cordotomy: The Lateral High Cervical Technique

Ronald R. Tasker

CORDOTOMY, first performed by Spiller and Martin[1] following the preparatory observations of Spiller[2] and Schuller,[3] remains the most satisfactory neurosurgical operation for the relief of chronic pain. This is particularly so as elaboration of the technique has progressively lessened morbidity and enhanced accuracy. Foerster[4] and Stookey[5] introduced the open high cervical approach, Mullan[6] the percutaneous high cervical approach, and Mullan et al.[7] and Rosomoff et al.[8] the direct current and radiofrequency lesion-making methods, respectively. Onofrio[9] added myelography, Gildenberg et al.[10] monitoring of electrical impedance, and Taren et al.[11,12] the correlation of both these modalities with physiologic studies, an area first pursued by Sweet et al.[13] Physiologic identification of target site has been further elaborated by Hitchcock et al.[14] and Tasker et al.[15,16]

Percutaneous cordotomy by the lateral high cervical approach performed according to a rigorous protocol is a low-risk, highly predictable procedure, the treatment of choice for most patients suffering from unilateral or bilateral nociceptive pain below the fourth cervical dermatome.

INDICATIONS AND PATIENT SELECTION

TYPE AND SEVERITY OF PAIN

Recourse to surgery to treat chronic pain presupposes the following:

1. That a major psychogenic element, usually a magnification syndrome, is not present.
2. That the cause of the pain is known and primary therapy exhausted.
3. That simpler treatment has failed.
4. That disability from the pain, rather than from other problems resulting from the primary disease, and the patient's life expectancy warrant the risk of surgery with its expectations of success.

Disability from pain can be assessed by physical examination with reference to impact on work, recreation, sleep, and drug intake, as well as by having the patient grade suffering on a 0-to)10 scale.

DEAFFERENTATION PAIN

Not all patients meeting these criteria are candidates for percutaneous cordotomy. Neurosurgeons long ago noticed that cordotomy was more effective in the treatment of patients with cancer than it was in others, so that one may still see references to "benign" and "malignant" pain as if there were something inherently different between the two. It is not the benign or malignant nature of the pain that matters, but whether nociceptive pathways are being stimulated continually or whether the pain is the result of destruction of the nervous system, whether by cancer or "benign" disease. Cordotomy can be equally effective in treating the pain of a pathological fracture or of osteoarthritis and equally a failure in the pain of brachial plexus avulsion or destruction of the brachial plexus by metastatic carcinoma.

There is ever-increasing awareness of a concept originally popularized by Livingston,[17] but forgotten in intervening years, that damage to somatosensory structures in the peripheral or central nervous system may set in motion a series of central changes that, once established, persist despite isolation of the original pathologic condition from the brain, a concept that was first pressed on us as we reviewed our experience with percutaneous cordotomy.[18] It is now customary to refer to such pain problems, including painful neuropathy, postherpetic neuralgia, the pain of spinal cord lesions, and thalamic pain, as deafferentation pain syndromes, as distinct from nociceptive pain.[15,16,19–21] Although the pathophysiology of such deafferentation pain is unknown, a reasonable hypothesis is that it is caused by deafferentation neuronal hypersensitivity, possibly in the reticulothalamic system and lateral thalamic or cortical neurons with which they are connected.[22]

Such pain is typically dysesthetic or causalgic in quality, may be accompanied by hyperpathia or allodynia, and is often delayed in onset. Its distribution is usually related to total or partial, particularly spinothalamic, somatosensory loss caused by the nervous lesion. In some patients, no clinically detectable sensory loss may be present in association with lesions that could reasonably have been expected to produce it; presumably sensory loss is subclinical in such cases. Such pain tends to be reduced by barbiturates but not by opiates, and though often relieved by proximal local anesthetic blockade of the nervous system, it is usually unaffected by destructive lesions at the same site. It is important to remember that the pain caused by cancer, for which cordotomy is most often performed, is usually the result of compression of lumbosacral, less often of brachial, plexus, and must be regarded as one end of a spectrum. Early on, while only compression occurs, only nociceptive pain exists and cordotomy can be expected to succeed. As time passes, plexus destruction manifested by

OPERATIVE NEUROSURGICAL TECHNIQUES
ISBN 0-8089-1862-1

reflex changes, wasting, and weakness, and sensory loss with deafferentation is added. At this stage, cordotomy will dissect out and relieve the nociceptive pain, leaving the deafferentation element behind. In the late stages of cancerous destruction, however, little nociceptive pain may remain, deafferentation pain alone persisting. Now cordotomy will be a complete failure.

CONDITION OF PATIENT

Few patients are too ill to withstand percutaneous cordotomy. Children and those unlikely to be cooperative may be successfully operated upon under general anesthesia despite reservations expressed when our experience was less.[23]

LOCATION OF PAIN

Pain in Higher Dermatomes

Since cordotomy by any means usually achieves a level of analgesia several dermatomes below the level of the surgery, pain in the C5 dermatome remains the most rostral that can be reliably relieved by high cervical percutaneous cordotomy.

Respiratory Function

The Solitary Lung. The relationship of cordotomy to respiratory dysfunction has been well studied.[24–32] Respiratory function in the cervical cord is dependent upon the cortico spinal tract for voluntary breathing and the reticulospinal tract for unconscious automatic breathing. Respiratory embarrassment from corticospinal damage is virtually unheard of after percutaneous cordotomy, and good criteria are available in the operating room for avoiding damage to the corticospinal tract. But if the reticulospinal pathway is damaged and that structure cannot be recognized by any physiologic means at the time of surgery, postoperatively the patient will be able to breathe upon cue but will hypoventilate when distracted or asleep, leading to carbon dioxide accumulation and eventual respiratory arrest. Since reticulospinal respiratory drive is transmitted only ipsilaterally, respiratory function is at risk when cordotomy is contemplated on the side of a solitary functioning lung, say after pneumonectomy, phrenic paralysis, or major pulmonary parenchymatous dysfunction, or combinations of these. Such a patient, deprived of automatic respiration on his one sound side, cannot support himself on the defective lung alone. The patients at risk are those with pain in the upper chest and arm in whom the highest possible level of analgesia must be sought. The reticulospinal tract serving the diaphragm, as indicated by Hitchcock and Leece,[28] lies between the cervical dermatomes of the spinothalamic tract and the ventral horn, where it is certain to be severed by a cordotomy achieving a high enough level of analgesia to produce pain relief in the shoulder, lower neck, and upper arm. Low anterior cervical open or percutaneous cordotomy[33–35] is of no use in such patients, since the level of analgesia is not high enough to be useful.

Bilateral Cordotomy. Given two adequately functioning lungs, no harm ensues if the reticulospinal tract is severed by cordotomy on one side only; the other will carry on adequately. Even in the case of moderately severe bilateral parenchymatous pulmonary disease, such is the case. Unfortunately, there appears to be no quantitative assessment that will identify the

problem patient preoperatively. One must be wary of severing the reticulospinal tract even unilaterally (that is, achieving high levels of analgesia) in patients with severely impaired respiratory function. When bilateral cordotomy is required even in patients with healthy lungs, *bilateral* reticulospinal damage (i.e., bilaterally high levels of analgesia) must be avoided. If pain affects such high dermatomes bilaterally, a rare situation, effective bilateral cordotomy cannot be safely accomplished, but as long as one reticulospinal tract serving an adequately functioning lung is spared, bilateral cordotomy can be performed with impunity. This can usually be accomplished by tailoring the level of analgesia on one or both sides to avoid the cervical dermatomes, as will be described below. Or else one can consider the low anterior open microscopic or percutaneous cervical cordotomy for the second side.[33,35]

Midline Pain

Midline or bilateral lumbar, abdominal, pelvic, and especially burning perineal pain in the absence of limb pain is best treated warily by cordotomy for two reasons.[36] First, the operation must often be bilateral, with all that that entails, despite the satisfactory experience recorded by Ischia et al.[37] with unilateral cordotomy in patients with bilateral pain. But most important, despite adequate bilateral analgesia, such pain, particularly perineal pain, may persist postoperatively. Failure of bilateral cordotomy, with persistence of pain, will be a certainty if the pain is dysesthetic or causalgic and related to clinically demonstrable sensory loss in the lower sacrococcygeal dermatomes. It is then clearly an example of deafferentation pain. But even in the absence of clinically demonstrable sensory loss, and even when the pain may not be dysesthetic or causalgic, the pain may still have a basis in deafferentation. It is our experience that pelvic manipulations, whether in the form of surgery or of radiation, commonly lead to persistent perineal discomfort even in the absence of recurrent or persistent disease, a condition colorfully labelled "phantom anus pain syndrome" by Boas.[38] Since such pelvic manipulations could easily damage the delicate innervations subserved by the minute lower sacral or coccygeal nerves without obvious clinically detectable sensory loss, we agree with Boas that such perineal pain is best considered a potential example of deafferentation pain not likely to be relieved by cordotomy.

In view of the risks and uncertainties of bilateral cordotomy in such patients, should surgery be required, the author prefers a trial of chronic epidural infusion of morphine. There is also evidence[39–41] that percutaneous high cervical commissurotomy, a procedure whose mechanism is unknown, may also be useful in such patients.

LOCAL PATHOLOGY

Although a theoretical restriction to percutaneous cordotomy,[23] local upper cervical spinal or cord pathology has never prevented the procedure in 380 consecutive procedures performed by the author. In several patients, the occipital-C1 interspace, rather than the C1-C2 space, was chosen to bypass anomalous bony impediments to cord access. In one patient with ankylosing spondylitis and a fixed 45-degree deformity of the cervical spine, a special wooden support for the neck was constructed.[23] In only one patient out of 380 procedures did repeated attempted cordotomy fail to achieve analgesia, suggesting anomalies of neuroanatomy such as rotation of the cord

Table 105-1. Cordotomy techniques

Open	Cervical	High Posterior
		Low Anterolateral
		Low Anterior
	Thoracic	High Posterior
Percutaneous	High Cervical	Lateral
		Dorsal
	Low Cervical	Anterior

described by Morley[42] and seen several times by the author at open laminectomy. No instances of unexpected paralysis or ipsilateral analgesia were seen.[43–46] On occasion, as illustrated by us,[23] the physiologically determined position of the spinothalamic tract lay far anterior or far posterior to the expected position, even when rotation of the neck and parallax were eliminated.

CHOICE OF CORDOTOMY TECHNIQUE

A variety of open and percutaneous approaches to cordotomy have been proposed, the open techniques being recently modified by the introduction of the operating microscope as listed in Table 105-1.

OPEN VERSUS PERCUTANEOUS CORDOTOMY

Whereas open cordotomy has the theoretical advantages of not requiring specialized instruments or skills and of being possible when local pathologic conditions might prevent the percutaneous approach, its greater morbidity and mortality and lesser accuracy (as compared to percutaneous cordotomy) in the absence of physiologic control virtually eliminates the open procedure from the neurosurgeon's armamentarium today,[23,47] except when repeated failure to locate the spinothalamic tract by percutaneous techniques suggests an unresolvable anomaly. And even then there are reports of unexpected results attributed to anomalous anatomy, even with the spinal cord visualized at open cordotomy.[43–46]

A comparison of the results of 113 open cordotomies done by various surgeons on 100 patients at the Toronto General Hospital with the author's first 141 percutaneous procedures done on 112 consecutive patients prior to April 1, 1973, assessed at the time of hospital discharge,[23] gives some idea of the difference in results, as shown in Table 105-2. For various reported series of open cordotomy,[23] mortality varied from 4 to 13.5 percent, paresis from 2 to 11 percent, increased bladder dysfunction from 3 to 23 percent, and pain relief from 52 to 67 percent. Kühner,[48] in a recent review, demonstrated obvious superiority of the percutaneous technique, which fails to justify his " . . . préférence au geste ouverte et micro-chirurgicale pour une douleur du membre inférieur afin d'éviter l'hémiplégie," as well as his preference for open cordotomy for bilateral or midline pain below D5.

The author has performed one open low anterior microsurgical cordotomy since learning the percutaneous method.

CHOICE OF PERCUTANEOUS TECHNIQUE

The author has no experience with the high dorsal cervical technique for percutaneous cordotomy[26,49] and, except for some early cases, has exclusively used the lateral high cervical

Table 105-2. Open versus percutaneous cordotomy, Toronto General Hospital

Percent	Open		Percutaneous	
	Uni-lateral	Bilat-eral	Uni-lateral	Bilat-eral
Relief of pain for which cordotomy performed	84	53	96	86
Mortality	6	16	0	3
Significant paresis	15	39	0	0
Worsening bladder function	2	25	6	21

approach. The high level of analgesia achieved, and the ease of repeated tiny incremental repositionings of the electrode without the need to first traverse the firm disc or a segment of the spinal cord, make the procedure simpler, more direct, and more easily controlled.

The low anterior cervical approach does have one advantage,[33–35] despite the awkwardness of having to traverse the cervical disc. When only a low level of analgesia is required, and there is concern for automatic respiration as discussed above, it offers an alternative to open operation or the demands of using the lateral high cervical approach with the absolute requirement of avoiding high levels of analgesia.

Table 105-3 lists the indications for 380 consecutive percutaneous cordotomies up to the end of December, 1985. Data until June, 1976 appear on the left, data from June, 1976 to December, 1985 on the right. The earlier group of data was quoted in the previous edition of this book.[50]

TECHNIQUE

Success in percutaneous cordotomy depends upon appropriate anesthesia, radiographic identification of the position of the electrode, monitoring of the depth of penetration of the cord by the measurement of electrical impedance, physiologic identification of the lateral spinothalamic tract, and avoidance of

Table 105-3. Indications for 380 consecutive percutaneous cordotomies to end of December, 1985

	To End June, 1976 (%)	To End December, 1985 (%)
Carcinoma		
Cervix	20.0	27.3
Rectum	18.8	11.4
Lung	8.1	3.4
Breast	5.5	1.1
Colon	4.7	18.2
Other	25.2	18.2
Sarcoma	4.8	8.0
Spinal Cord Trauma	6.4	5.7
"Failed Back"	1.3	2.3
Other Noncancerous	5.2	3.4
Records Lost	0.0	1.1

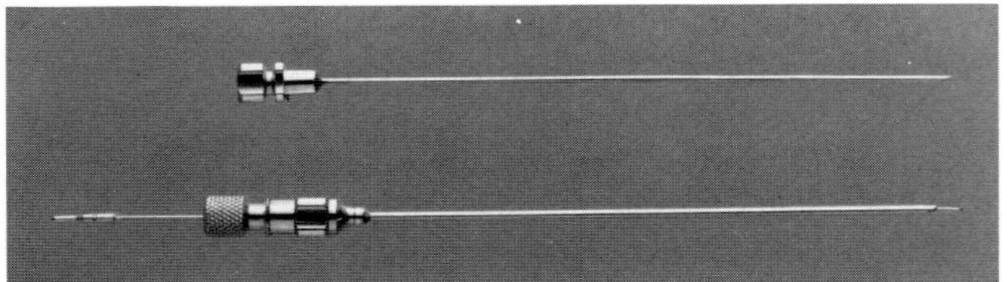

Fig. 105-1. The Owl cordotomy electrode (Diros Technology, Inc., Toronto, Canada). A 0.4-mm, electrolytically sharpened stainless steel wire projects 2 mm beyond shrunk-fit Teflon tubing, which in turn projects 2 mm beyond the tip of a thin-walled, 18-gauge lumbar puncture needle when the assembly is locked.

important adjacent structures, together with controlled, reproducible lesion-making using the radiofrequency current. The procedure is greatly facilitated by the use of suitable back-up equipment such as the Owl cordotomy system (Diros Technology, Toronto, Canada). It is essential to abide by a rigorous stepwise protocol in the conduct of the operation.

PREOPERATIVE PREPARATION

The patient is brought to the operating room without presedation but having received his or her regular dose of analgesic medication so that he or she will be able to cooperate accurately during physiologic testing.

ANESTHESIA

Although percutaneous cordotomy is ideally performed under neurolept analgesia, which we have used for functional neurosurgery since the early 1960s,[51] in the very young, confused, or apprehensive patient this procedure can be safely and effectively performed under general anesthesia as well, as will be described below.

Neurolept analgesia enables the patient to lie comfortably still during the 45 minutes to 2 hours that the procedure requires, and permits brief periods of more intense levels of analgesia repeatedly on demand without losing the capability of repeated re-arousal of the patient for physiologic testing.

Analgesia is achieved by the intravenous administration of the short-acting narcotic fentanyl citrate, which is pushed to the limit of respiratory suppression—a rate of 12 breaths/minute. Sedation is added as necessary by the separate intravenous administration of droperidol (2.5–5.0 mg) and diazepam (1 mg), drugs that must be used sparingly because of cumulative sedative effects. Alternatively, intravenous injections of small amounts of thiopental sodium (75–150 mg) may be used to achieve brief narcosis, especially during introduction of the needle in lesion-making.

POSITIONING

Percutaneous cordotomy is facilitated by carefully positioning the patient in the supine position. The dorsal margin of the upper cervical spinal canal should lie horizontally in order to trap contrast medium in the operative area. The patient's head and neck should be placed in a strictly anteroposterior position and the cordotomy electrode introduced as precisely horizontally as possible in order to minimize problems with tip localization caused by parallax and to simplify interpretation of physiologic data. Biplanar radiologic control is achieved with the use of a portable C arm image intensifier at the head of the operating table, arranged to provide a true lateral projection of the upper cervical spine. A portable x-ray unit placed beside the head of the table will provide a true AP view of the region of the odontoid, which will allow one to follow the progress of the needle. Again, rectilinear positioning minimizes errors resulting from parallax. It is essential that the image on the image intensifier be arranged with its attitude identical to that of the actual patient's neck.

THE CORDOTOMY ELECTRODE AND BACKUP SYSTEM

The Owl percutaneous cordotomy electrode manufactured by Diros Technology consists of an 0.4-mm stainless steel wire insulated with shrinkfit Teflon tubing so that its electrolytically sharpened tip projects 2 mm beyond the tubing. The electrode is introduced through a thin-walled, 18-gauge lumbar puncture needle into which it locks so that 2 mm of insulation in turn projects beyond the end of the needle, as shown in Figure 105-1. The 2-mm length of bare tip is critical for measurement of impedance, and determines the depth to which the cord is penetrated. Further, too deep penetration of the cord is impeded by the resistance of the Teflon tubing, producing a palpable resistance to the fingers of the surgeon. Back-up electronics are provided by the Owl universal RF system shown in Figure 105-2, which compactly provides controls and read-

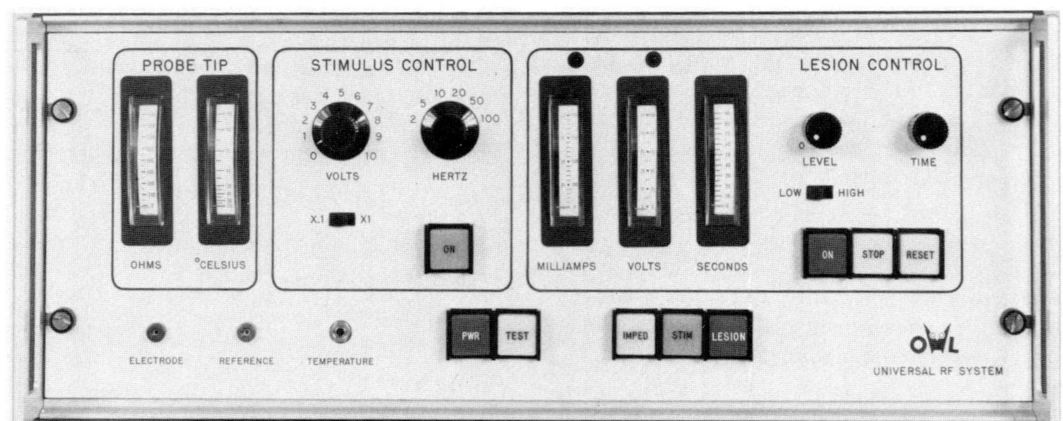

Fig. 105-2. The Owl Universal RF System (Diros Technology, Inc., Toronto, Canada) for measuring electrical impedance, providing electrical stimulation at 2–100 Hz, 0–10 volts, making radiofrequency lesions, and for monitoring electrode-tip temperature. The low output level must always be used for cordotomy.

outs for measuring electrical impedance producing stimulation at 2–100 Hz at voltages up to 10 V and regulating the duration and strength of the radiofrequency current used in lesion-making. Optionally, the temperature of the electrode tip can be monitored using a special electrode shown in Figure 105-3. The electrode is used in the monopolar mode by employing a 23-gauge, 1.5-inch intramuscular needle inserted in the ipsilateral deltoid muscle as an indifferent electrode.

RADIOLOGIC LOCALIZATION

Once adequate anesthesia and positioning have been achieved and the indifferent electrode inserted, the side of the neck contralateral to the patient's pain is suitably prepared and draped. Using the three-dimensional mechanical stage of the Owl cordotomy system, the lumbar puncture needle through which the electrode is to be introduced is positioned strictly horizontally so as to impinge on the patient's skin at the center of the C1-C2 space as seen in the lateral projection on the screen of the image intensifier. After the soft tissues have been injected with local anesthetic, they are penetrated with the needle, always horizontally, until a sense of resistance is felt by the surgeon and a twinge of pain by the patient, as, first, the ligamentum flavum, and then the dura, are sequentially penetrated. To attempt to infiltrate these structures with local anesthetic is unwise because of the risk of accidentally producing a high spinal anesthesia. Should this accident occur, only respiratory support need be given until the block wears off in approximately 45 minutes possibly with anticonvulsant coverage. It is helpful to warn the patient in advance of each maneuver anticipated to cause pain, and to have the anesthetist increase the depth of analgesia temporarily.

Keeping the needle horizontal and the tip centered in the C1-C2 space, since this is the expected location of the dentate ligament and dorsal margin of the lateral spinothalamic tract, the needle is advanced cautiously until, on withdrawal of the stylet, a flow of cerebrospinal fluid occurs. Once this happens, the needle must not be advanced further, and several cubic centimeters of insoluble positive contrast medium, such as that used for myelography, are now shaken in a 10-cc syringe, along with a similar quantity of cerebrospinal fluid, and injected into the subarachnoid space to outline the dentate ligament as shown in Figure 105-4. The dentate ligament should appear as a line of contrast medium in approximately the mid-anteroposterior plane of the spinal canal. The dentate ligament may, however, be displaced considerably, either anteriorly or posteriorly, and additional confusing lines of contrast medium may also be seen. The dorsal limit of the subarachnoid space is nearly always seen dorsally, and contrast medium also may be trapped on the ventral and dorsal root lines or upon the ventral margin of the cord itself. The contralateral dentate ligament may be outlined, either by itself or in addition to the ipsilateral one, adding to the confusion. If the dentate ligament is not visualized, it should be first established that the lumbar puncture needle is not positioned too far dorsally, and an additional injection should be made. It sometimes may be necessary to forcibly inject a small volume of emulsion mixed with air to achieve suitable visualization. In a quarter of the patients, the dentate ligament cannot be outlined despite every attempt, and localization of the needle must be based on other criteria, as listed below.

The procedure may also be performed in a similar fashion in the occipital-C1 space, where ipsilateral facial paresthesias

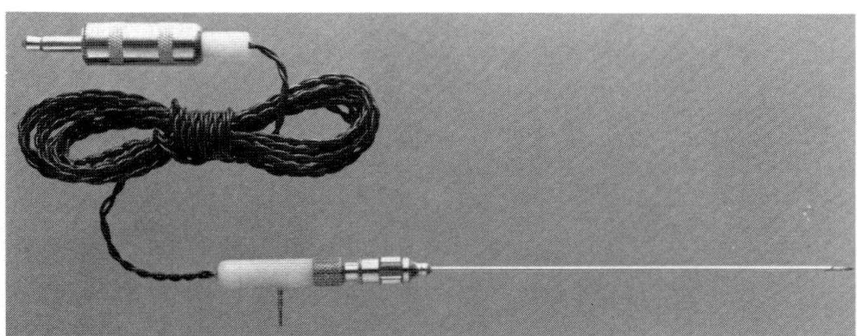

Fig. 105-3. Optional cordotomy electrode (Diros Technology, Inc., Toronto, Canada), capable of temperature monitoring during lesion-making.

may be elicited, in addition to responses described below, from stimulation of the ascending tract or spinal nucleus of the trigeminal nerve.

Once the dentate ligament has been adequately identified, the cordotomy electrode is locked into the lumbar puncture needle, thereby avoiding the loss of cerebrospinal fluid and contrast medium. The whole needle assembly with a projecting 2-mm bare tip is now advanced toward the anterior margin of the dentate ligament under radiological and impedance control until: (1) a sense of gritty resistance is felt by the surgeon's fingers; (2) the patient feels a sharp pain in the ipsilateral neck; (3) the impedance rises (see below); and (4) the tip of the electrode comes to lie at or just beyond the middle of the odontoid in the AP x-ray film. With increasing experience, the AP x-ray film is required less often.

IMPEDANCE MONITORING

As the needle electrode assembly is advanced, the electrical impedance about its tip is followed on the panel of the Owl universal RF system. As the tip impales the cord, the impedance rises sharply from approximately 400 to 500 ohms characteristic of spinal fluid to over 1000 ohms, as shown in Figure 105-5. The electrode should not be advanced any further once these criteria for cord penetration have been met, since further penetration carries the tip too deep and adds an unnecessary third dimension to calculation of electrode position. Furthermore, deeper penetration forces the Teflon tubing and lumbar puncture needle into the cord, increasing the risk of complications and disrupting further impedance readings in this area. Should the cord be accidentally impaled through and through, however, the operation should be continued in the usual way though impedance may be unreliable. Postoperatively, the patient should be monitored with particular care. Should the needle electrode assembly fail to impale the cord, but, rather, slip dorsal or ventral to it, the proper criteria for penetration, including impedance rise, will not be met. When the electrode impinges on the opposite side of the spinal canal, the AP x-ray flim will disclose the faulty position, the patient will report contralateral cervical pain, impedance will rise, and the electrode tip may be damaged.

PHYSIOLOGIC LOCALIZATION

Once the needle has appropriately penetrated the cord at the anterior margin of the dentate ligament, its position in the lateral spinothalamic tract must be confirmed physiologically using threshold electrical stimulation in trains of negative square waves of 3 msec at 2 and 100 Hz. Table 105-4 lists the

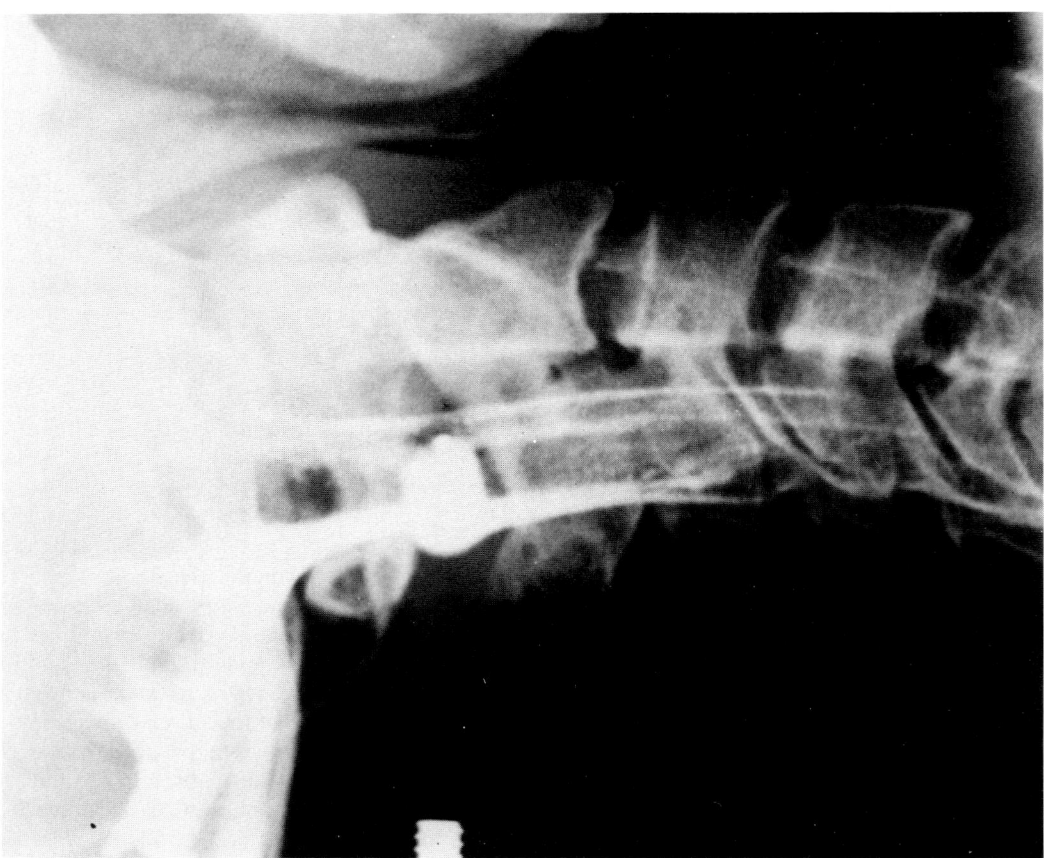

Fig. 105-4.   Lateral x-ray film taken with C-arm image intensifier, showing, outlined with contrast medium from anterior to posterior, the anterior cord margin, the dentate ligament, the dorsal root line, and the dorsal margin of subarachnoid space with a cordotomy electrode positioned in spinothalamic tract in the C1-C2 interspace.

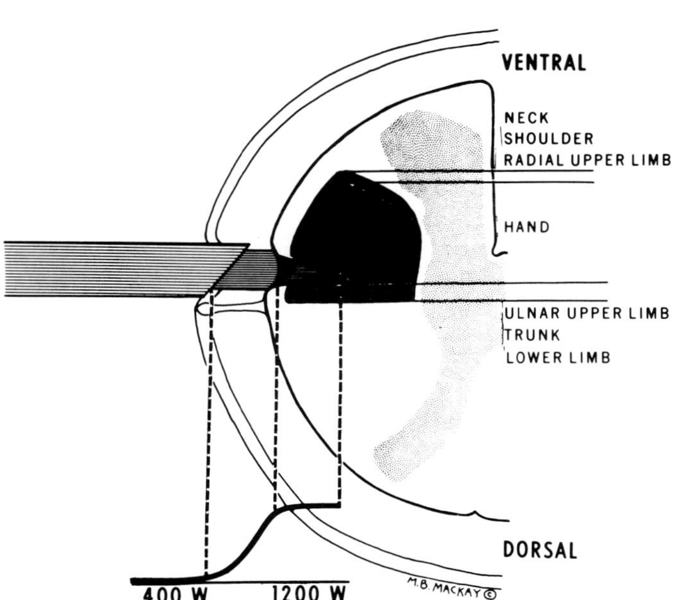

Fig. 105-5.   Diagrammatic representation of percutaneous cordotomy at C1-C2 by the lateral approach, illustrating the manner of penetration by the electrode-LP needle assembly, the accompanying impedance changes, the location of spinothalamic tract (shaded) with reference to other structures, and the anteroposterior order of somatotopic representation within the tract.

criteria for identification of structures found in the spinal cord at C1-C2. Only responses in the anterior horn, corticospinal tract, and lateral spinothalamic tract are usually seen. It is difficult to explain why motor effects are obtained when the spinothalamic tract is stimulated at 2 Hz. Possibly these motor effects represent activation of local cord reflexes. Similarly, ipsilateral sensory effects obtained at 100 Hz, presumably when the electrode is located in the corticospinal tract, are startling and may represent subclinical motor effects, activation of afferent pathways within the lateral columns, or possibly activation of muscle afferent pathways. If the stimulation strength is slightly increased, actual tetanization may occur.

Identification of the Lateral Spinothalamic Tract

Table 105-5 presents in more detail the effects elicited by stimulation at 2 Hz in our most recent 136 percutaneous cordotomies at sites where effective lesions were made. Threshold averaged 2.6 V. The responses consisted of contractions in the ipsilateral muscles innervated by cervical roots in 96.4 percent of the sites. Contralateral sensory effects were recorded during 2-Hz stimulation at 23.1 percent of the sites. Of the motor responses occurring during 2-Hz stimulation of the lateral spinothalamic tract, 86.6 percent affected the muscles of the neck. In 33.6 percent, the upper extremity was affected, usually along with neck muscles.

Table 105-6 presents the types of responses elicited by threshold stimulation at 100 Hz at effective lesion sites in our most recent 136 patients. Threshold averaged 0.40 V using the

Table 105-4. Physiologic identification of cord structures at C1-C2

Structure Stimulated	Effect of Electric Stimulation	
	2 Hz	100 Hz
Anterior horn	2-Hz twitches in ipsilateral C1-C2 myotomes	Tetanization of ipsilateral C1-C2 myotomes
Corticospinal tract	2-Hz twitches of any ipsilateral musculature below head	Tetanization of any ipsilateral musculature below head sometimes preceded by paresthetic effects in same area
Lateral spinothalamic tract	Usually 2-Hz twitches of ipsilateral muscles innervated by cervical roots sometimes with contralateral sensory effects	No motor effect. Contralateral temperature-coded, rarely paresthetic or painful effect below neck
Descending tract, caudal nucleus of V (rarely encountered)	Ipsilateral trigeminal sensory effects	Ipsilateral trigeminal paresthesiae
Dorsal columns (virtually never encountered)	Ipsilateral sensory effects below neck	Ipsilateral paresthesiae below neck

Owl system. Responses consisted of a feeling of heat or warmth in 35.1 percent of cases, coolness or cold in 16.2 percent, burning in 28.2 percent, pain in 6.8 percent, and isolated paresthesias in 1.7 percent. Thus, in our most recent 136 cordotomies, induction of contralateral hot, warm, cool, or cold effects was elicited at 51.3 percent of sites, compared with 94 percent in our previous 244 cordotomies, at the expense of an increase in burning and painful effects from 5 to 35 percent and of indescribable effects from 0 to 12 percent. Paresthetic effects constituted 1 percent in the earlier series and 1.7 percent in the later series.

The explanation for this difference may reflect an increasing awareness of the significance of the patients' reporting burning, as contrasted with warmth, heat, or cold, leading to

Table 105-5. Threshold motor responses at 2 Hz in spinothalamic tract; most recent 136 cordotomies

Response (All Ipsilateral)	Percent	
Trapezius	39.8	
Trapezius and other neck, shoulder girdle muscles	1.2	
Trapezius and forearm	10.8	
Trapezius and other upper limb	3.6	59.0
Trapezius and other neck, shoulder girdle, upper limb	2.4	
Trapezius, lower limb	1.2	
Posterior nuchal muscles	10.8	
Posterior nuchal and other girdle, neck	2.4	20.4
Posterior nuchal and upper limb	7.2	
Sternomastoid	1.2	
Lateral nuchal muscles	6.0	
Upper limb only	9.6	
No motor response	3.6	

more precise documentation. For we have been impressed by the fact that macrostimulation of the brain stem reticulothalamic system in patients with deafferentation syndromes commonly elicits a sensation of pain and burning,[19,22] while in patients not suffering from deafferentation pain, this area is insensitive to stimulation. Stimulation of the spinothalamic tract in the brain stem yielded a sensation of heat, cold, or burning in the former, more often heat or cold in the latter, groups of patients.

It was estimated that 65 (26.6 percent) of our first 244 cordotomies were performed on patients with contralateral deafferentation pain, 40 of whom had accompanying nociceptive pain. In the current 136, 30.6 percent were considered to have a contralateral deafferentation pain syndrome preoperatively, and a further 7.1 percent developed it postoperatively, for a total of 37.7 percent, which is a difference inadequate to explain the different stimulation phenomenon between the two series. These observations cast doubt on the significance of our earlier observations[19] of differences between contralateral sensory effects at 100-Hz stimulation in cord in the spinothalamic tract in patients with deafferentation and in those with nociceptive pain. We had reported that in the deafferentated sample of patients, hot, warm, cool, and cold effects were found in 28 percent, burning in 24 percent, and paresthesias in 38 percent.

Ipsilateral sensory effects elicited during 100-Hz stimulation are acceptable only if they accompany typical temperature-coded contralateral effects, and care should be exercised to

Table 105-6. Threshold sensory responses at 100 Hz in spinothalamic tract; most recent 136 cordotomies

Response (All Contralateral)	Percent
Hot	27.4
Warm	7.7
Burning	28.2
Cold, cool	16.2
Paresthetic	1.7
Pain	6.8
Not described	12.0

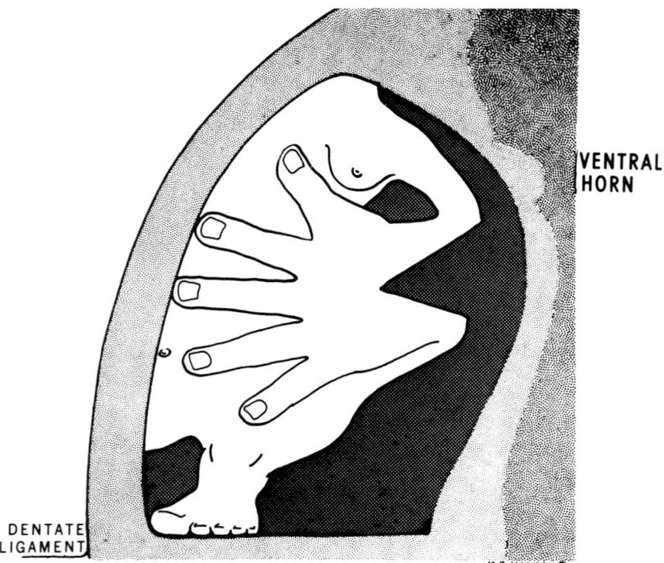

Fig. 105-6. Diagrammatic representation of the spinothalamic homunculus at C1-C2 in the spinal cord.

ensure that they do not represent subclinical motor effects, arising in corticospinal tract, by watching for tetanization as supra-threshold stimulation is delivered. Contralateral sensory effects involved the upper extremity exclusively in 54.5 percent of the most recent 136 cases, the lower extremity in 31.3 percent, both in 14.1 percent. Although the location of these sensory effects did not closely match that of analgesia induced by a lesion at the same site, the analgesia tended not to extend into the upper cervical dermatomes when the sensory effects were restricted to the lower limb. Extensive analgesia usually resulted when lesions were made in sites where stimulation-induced effects were perceived in the hand. (See the section on tailoring the lesion, below.)

Dorsoventral somatotopy within the lateral spinothalamic tract could be demonstrated readily by sequentially stimulating from the dentate ligament to the ventral horn when the dermatomal level of the induced sensory effects progressed from sacral to cervical[52] (Figure 105-6). Similar progression of the level of analgesia is seen if lesions are made progressively more ventrally or if lesions are progressively enlarged. Contralateral sensory effects referred only to the neck or trunk, particularly centrally, are uncertain indicators of satisfactory positioning. Although lesions have occasionally been made at sites where such responses were obtained and other localizing criteria had been met, unsatisfactory or suspended levels of analgesia often resulted.

In summary, provided that radiologic and impedance criteria have been met, it can be assumed with confidence that the electrode lies in the spinothalamic tract at a site where a lesion will be effective and safe when threshold stimulation at 2 Hz and 2.6 V induces 2-Hz contractions in the ipsilateral cervical myotomes and at 100 Hz at 0.4 V contralateral temperature-coded sensory effects. An ipsilateral motor effect induced at 2 Hz involving other than cervical myotomes, or any tetanization induced at 100 Hz, contraindicates lesion-making. Although unusual thresholds can be compatible with satisfactory positioning, caution must be exercised when extreme deviations are noted, especially if other criteria have not been met.

Identification of Structures Other than the Spinothalamic Tract

Table 105-4 lists the physiologic criteria for positioning in the anterior horn, where lesions are not dangerous, and in the corticospinal tract, where lesions may produce paresis. It is of interest that patients who develop postoperative paresis, virtually always in the ipsilateral leg, are nearly always those in whom the contralateral sensory effect obtained during 100-Hz stimulation at the lesion site was referred to the lower extremities. This reflects the proximity of spinothalamic leg fibers on one side to corticospinal leg fibers on the other. This paresis is virtually always reversible, provided that 100-Hz stimulation did not induce tetanization of the ipsilateral leg.

If criteria for suitable localization are not achieved, it must be decided whether the electrode lies dorsal or ventral to the lateral spinothalamic tract, whereupon very small, appropriate potitional adjustments must be made sequentially, repeating all the steps in the protocol until satisfactory positioning is achieved.

MAKING THE LESION

Lesion-making using the technique described is painful because of involvement of the pia. Once a lesion has been made, however, further enlargement at the same site is not painful. In preparation for lesion-making, the patient either should be briefly anesthetized with thiopental sodium, or else given maximal doses of fentanyl citrate. Lesion size is determined by the duration and level of current flow and the temperature achieved at the lesion site. The author has not used temperature monitoring, but suitable electrodes are available for the purpose, as shown in Figure 105-3. A minimal lesion is produced with the Owl equipment when 25 mA flows for at least 20 to 40 seconds of the 60 seconds during which current is delivered. It is best to start lesion-making at minimal levels, assessing the results at the end of each 60 seconds of current flow, gradually increasing current for a further 60 seconds until the desired level of analgesia is achieved or current fall-off occurs.

Analgesia is usually first observed with the Owl system after 30 mA flows for at least 20 to 30 seconds. Fall-off often occurs with currents in the 40–60 mA range, following which the lesion at that site can no longer be enlarged. If analgesia is still inadequate when fall-off occurs, the electrode may be advanced minimally deeper into the cord and the lesion repeated, but usually a new electrode placement is necessary, as is rigorous follow-through of the whole above-described protocol. Once a lesion has been made, such repetition of the whole process is more difficult, since impedance measurements and stimulation effects may be disrupted. In our first 244 cordotomies, single lesions were made in 6.2 percent, 2 in 22 percent, and 3 or more in 16.7 percent of procedures. Pursuing too high a current flow initially should be avoided for fear of producing sudden vaporization at the lesion site with current fall-off in less than 20 to 30 seconds, in which case a lesion is inadequate and cannot be enlarged. If lesion-making is performed with the patient conscious, ipsilateral leg power is simultaneously tested by having the patient perform straight leg raising. No one who is able to hold the leg off the bed at the conclusion of the procedure has developed persistent significant paresis.

POSTOPERATIVE CARE

Special postoperative care is usually not required. The patient is kept flat in bed for 24 hours to guard against post-lumbar puncture headache. Analgesics are necessary for postoperative headache and neck pain. Modification of preoperative analgesic needs must match changes in the patient's postoperative level of pain and must anticipate problems with narcotic withdrawal. The patient should be helped when first getting out of bed postoperatively in case of paresis, a problem that usually responds to appropriate physiotherapy in a few days. Following bilateral cordotomy, and in patients who had respiratory problems preoperatively, it is important to monitor vital signs and blood gases for about 3 days in order to detect evidence of hypercapnia or hypoxia, warning of incipient respiratory failure. Should such failure be detected, the patient should be transferred to an intensive care area with facilities for ventilatory support. Such respiratory decompensation usually reverses within 1 to 2 weeks under ventilatory assistance.

CORDOTOMY UNDER GENERAL ANESTHESIA

Seven of our 380 cordotomies have been performed under general anesthesia, either because of the patient's youth or the patient's lack of cooperation. Three of these were on the second side. One was done in a patient in whom four procedures failed to induce any analgesia. One resulted in a low level of analgesia and partial pain relief. Five produced adequate levels of analgesia and good pain relief. The only complication in these seven procedures was one instance of worsening of pre-existing urinary incontinence after bilateral surgery. One of these patients, who suffered from metastatic melanoma of brain and spine and who was paraplegic at the time of bilateral cordotomy, died a few days after the second procedure.

If the cordotomy is to be performed under general anesthesia, the anesthetist must avoid persistent muscular paralysis. The procedure can then be performed following the whole protocol outlined above, with the exception that the contralateral sensory effects must be observed during 100-Hz stimulation.

BILATERAL CORDOTOMY

Of the first 244 cordotomies, 17.9 percent, and of the most recent 136 cordotomies, 15.4 percent, were performed on the second side, three under general anesthesia. Results and complications are described below. Avoidance of respiratory damage has been described. The author is unaware of any method of avoiding the impairment of bladder function.

TAILORING THE LESION

In bilateral cordotomy, the need to avoid bilateral high levels of analgesia has been reviewed, and in this respect only physiologic criteria are useful. First and most important, the lesion must be cautiously and incrementally enlarged, with serial checks of the levels of analgesia. But some prediction of analgesic level can be made from the somatotopic site of the contralaterally induced sensory effects during 100-Hz stimulation. In our most recent 136 cordotomies, if stimulation at 100 Hz invoked a sensation in the contralateral upper limb, the analgesia resulting from a lesion at that site rose into at least the middle cervical dermatomes in 55.6 percent of cases. If, however, the sensory effects were referred to the lower limbs only, 38.7 percent achieved at least mid-cervical levels of analgesia. If sensory effects were felt in both upper and lower limbs, the chances were even of achieving high or lower levels of analgesia.

Looking retrospectively, it is evident that 100-Hz stimulation at lesion sites yielding high levels of analgesia had produced sensory effects in the contralateral upper limb in 61.2 percent, the lower limb in 24.5 percent, both in 14.3 percent of cases. For sites yielding low analgesic levels, these data were 48.0 percent, 38.0 percent, and 14.0 percent, respectively.

Second-sided cordotomy should not be attempted under general anesthesia if it is essential to avoid high levels of analgesia.

RESULTS

PAIN RELIEF

It is unfortunate that most reported experience with cordotomy fails to differentiate patients with nociceptive and deafferentation pain, those undergoing unilateral and bilateral surgery, and what is meant by relief or recurrence of pain, or by success or failure. Cordotomy is technically successful if it achieves persistent adequate levels of analgesia in the region of the patient's pain. Recurrence of pain can be expected in the short term, with fading or falling of the level of analgesia in the early postoperative period. Pain persistence or recurrence after technically successful cordotomy results from development of new pain as the disease progresses above the level of the analgesia, from new pain ipsilateral to the lesion, and from the persistence or appearance of deafferentation pain below the level of adequate analgesia. In our experience, spontaneous deafferentation pain in all or in part persists in 67 percent of patients below adequate levels of analgesia at the time of the patient's latest follow-up, though hyperathia and allodynia may disappear. New or increasing pain ipsilateral to the lesion may be the result of unmasking after the relief of more severe contralateral pain, of severing of inhibitory pathways, or, as Nathan suggests, through a physiologic phenomenon based on the spinal cord, possibly employing the dorsal columns, which he calls reference.[53,54] Nathan believes that such reference of pain is caused by the opening of new pathways; it led to the old teaching never to perform open cordotomy unilaterally because of the near-inevitability of ipsilateral pain postoperatively. Finally, post-cordotomy dysesthesia may develop below the level of analgesia or even of hypalgesia.

Long-term recurrence of pain after originally technically successful cordotomy is of great interest. Most cordotomies are performed in patients with cancer who survive on average only a few months. In the majority of patients surviving cordotomy for a long time, however, the level of analgesia may fade after years, when the operation may be repeated, recapturing analgesia and pain relief.[50] This effect has been noted by Lipton[55] and Nathan.[54]

Finally, when percutaneous cordotomy is performed bilaterally, it consists of two separate procedures performed in the same patient, often with too short an interval to permit full assessment of the results on each side separately. For this reason, the results of bilateral cordotomy obey the P-squared rule, and are not directly comparable to the results of unilateral procedure.

Recent Literature

Meglio and Cioni[56] reported 79 percent complete relief of pain after percutaneous cordotomy with a 3-week follow-up. Lahuerta et al.[57] reported complete relief in 64 percent, and partial in 23 percent in a selected group of 100 out of 181 patients. Kühner[48] reported 59 percent long-term excellent results in 138 procedures. Siegfried et al.[58] reported 75 percent significant pain relief, but with recurrence likely within 6 to 12 months. Lipton[55] reported 75 percent complete, 8 percent almost-complete pain relief. Lorenz,[59] in reviewing 3000 reported percutaneous cordotomies, found that 75 to 96 percent resulted in fairly good or excellent results. Ischia et al.[60] reported 47 percent complete, 12.5 percent partial pain relief after 36 bilateral cordotomies out of a series of 540.

Personal Experience

Complementing earlier reports,[15,16,18,23,47,50,61] we have reviewed all our 380 percutaneous cordotomies performed according to a consistent protocol up to the end of December, 1985, excluding the first 29 attempted by various methods.

Technical Success Locating the Spinothalamic Tract. The procedure was abandoned in 17 cases (4.5 percent) short of lesion-making. Four of these procedures were not repeated because they themselves were already repeat procedures and physiologic studies did not augur well for an improved result. Nine of the 14 were successfully repeated. Thus, 4 (1.0 percent) were abandoned without locating the spinothalamic tract and without a lesion ever being made. In other words, in 99 percent of patients in whom 380 cordotomies were attempted, the spinothalamic tract was located.

Achieving Adequate Analgesia. Out of these 376 operations during which the spinothalamic tract was located and lesioned, 10 (2.6 percent) had to be repeated within a few days to a few weeks because of fading or falling levels of analgesia, three following surgery by other than the author. In one of these latter 3 cases, the author was unable to induce any analgesia despite three more attempts on the same and the opposite sides, suggesting anomalous anatomy. Thus, a further 0.8 percent of the total group of procedures, all in one patient, failed to achieve analgesia at the outset.

Maintaining an Adequate Level of Analgesia in Follow-up. Of our earlier 244 cases, 37.6 percent were followed up to the time of hospital discharge only, 62.4 percent beyond that time. Of the subsequent 136, 81 percent were followed to death, longer than 1 month postoperatively, or else had demonstrated failure by the time of last follow-up. Sixty-four percent were followed beyond one month. In 19 percent, follow-up was less than 1 month and the patient known to have survived longer than a month.

Although only 2 percent of the 380 procedures resulted in no analgesia being attained eventually in the short term in that particular patient, this did not imply persisting adequate analgesia. Mention has been made of the 2.6 percent of procedures repeated within days to a few weeks because of failing and falling levels of analgesia. Of our earlier 244 cases, 92.5 percent had adequate levels of analgesia into their post-discharge follow-ups, while 94.5 percent of the subsequent 136 procedures led to adequate analgesia at the patient's latest follow-up available. In one of these procedures (0.7 percent), too low a level of analgesia resulted in no relief and the procedure was not repeated. Five (3.7 percent) more resulted in fading levels and failure to relieve pain. Two of these (1.5 percent) were successfully repeated, one (0.7 percent) with partial success.

Physiologic Success: The Problem of Failure to Relieve Pain Despite Adequate Analgesia. Achieving adequate levels of persisting analgesia does not guarantee relief of pain. Progressive disease may produce new pain outside the range of that for which the cordotomy was done. Ipsilateral pain and deafferentation pain, the lateral not amenable to cordotomy, has been discussed. It is, however, rare for pain that is truly nociceptive to persist below a level of adequate analgesia.

Of our first 244 cordotomies, 88 percent resulted in complete relief, 94.4 percent in significant relief, of the nociceptive pain for which the cordotomy was done at the time of discharge from hospital. Seventy-one percent resulted in complete relief, 82.3 percent in significant relief, of that pain at post-discharge follow-up. For the 65 of these 244 patients with deafferentation pain, these figures were 70.6 percent complete, 78.4 percent significant, relief at the time of discharge from hospital, but 33.3 percent complete, 50.0 percent partial, relief at the time of post-discharge follow-up.

Again, these data apply only to the pain contralateral to the lesion towards which the cordotomy was directed. By the time of post-discharge follow-up, 6.2 percent of these patients had developed new pain, presumably from progression of their disease above their adequate levels of analgesia. New or worsening pain ipsilateral to the lesion was experienced by 40.7 percent of these patients. Pain was demonstrated below a solid level of analgesia, pain that had features of deafferentation pain, in 13.7 percent of these patients. What was deemed to be post-cordotomy dysesthesia appeared in 8.6 percent, in half of them to a significant degree. Post-cordotomy dysesthesia had been recognized in only 1.5 percent of patients at the time they were discharged from hospital.

The data have been analyzed somewhat differently in our latest 136 patients. For unilateral procedures, including the first side of bilateral operations, at the time of latest available follow-up, 74.5 percent resulted in complete, 87.8 percent significant, relief of the pain for which the cordotomy had been done. Table 105-7 lists the data concerning postoperative pain in all 136 of these patients at the time of latest follow-up. Mention has already been made of technical failure. Table 105-7 deals with what we have called physiologic failure. First, only 32.7 percent of these patients were totally free of any pain at all, of whom 22.4 percent had short follow-ups. Total long-term relief of all pain after cordotomy is exceptional. A total of 12.2 percent enjoyed incomplete relief of the pain for which the cordotomy was done, nearly always because of inadequate depth or levels of analgesia. Two percent developed pain postoperatively above the level of their original pain, and 40.8 percent developed new or worsening pain ipsilateral to the cordotomy.

The interesting group is the 39.8 percent with persisting pain below a level of adequate analgesia. In 6.1 percent, the original pain persisted and may have been of the deafferentation type from the outset. In 33.7 percent, the pain differed from that present preoperatively, appeared to be dysesthetic in character, and in all but one patient matched neurologic deficit, usually including sensory loss, which had usually been present preoperatively. These figures considerably exceed the 13.7 percent incidence of postoperative deafferentation pain noted in the earlier 244 cases. Perhaps the currently more vigorous oncological therapy brings cordotomy to bear on patients in more advanced stages of their disease than has previously been the case.

These data reflect on the concept of post-cordotomy dysesthesia. Post-cordotomy dysesthesia can be classified as follows:

1. Dysesthesia in the distribution of the C-2 root on the side of the cordotomy.
2. Dysesthesia in all or part of the area rendered hypoalgesic or analgesic by the cordotomy.
3. Dysesthesia in the same area as the preoperative nociceptive pain of which it forms a "ghost."
4. Dysesthesia in an area of preoperative sensory loss.
5. Dysesthesia in an area corresponding to the distribution of a root or nerve with clinically detectable preoperative motor but not sensory damage.
6. Dysesthesia in an area corresponding to roots or nerves developing neurologic defects postoperatively from advancing disease.
7. Dysesthesia as a persisting deafferentation pain not relieved by cordotomy.

Type 1 pain is usually short-lived. Type 2 pain is true post-cordotomy dysesthesia—pain caused by the deafferentation induced by the cordotomy. Only 1 percent of our most recent 136 patients showed this type of pain, although in the earlier 244 we calculated that 1.5 percent had true post-cordotomy dysesthesia at discharge, 8.6 percent, at follow-up significant half.

We would suggest that consideration be given to the following hypothesis: that types 3, 4, 5, 6, and 7 pain may not be examples of post-cordotomy dysesthesia, but rather of deafferentation pain not capable of relief by cordotomy. We suggest that a large percentage of apparent cases of post-cordotomy dysesthesia are in fact not caused by the cordotomy, but rather by the deafferentation induced by the cancer. Of course, post-cordotomy dysesthesia induced by the cordotomy alone could accompany such pain or such neurologic defects, and would be difficult to distinguish from this type of deafferentation.

Comparison with Published Data. Ischia et al.[37] reported 81.1 percent relief of pain for which the cordotomy was performed in a selected 36 patients. However, 63.3 percent developed ipsilateral pain, while 13.9 percent continued to have pain or developed recurrent pain below a level of adequate analgesia, in some of whom deafferentation pain was considered. In another report, Ischia et al.[62] found 47.8 percent of 46 patients undergoing unilateral cordotomy had developed postoperative ipsilateral pain, 4.3 percent new pain, presumably above the level, 8.7 percent pain below the level of adequate analgesia thought to be deafferentation in type. In a review of 103 selected patients undergoing cordotomy for cervicothoracic pain caused by cancer, Ischia et al.[63] found adequate analgesia in 92.4 percent, ipsilateral pain in 56.3 percent, pain above the level of analgesia in 3.9 percent, and pain below a level of analgesia in 6.8 percent, this last pain thought to be deafferentation in type. Ipsilateral pain was commonest if the original pain was thoracic rather than located in the neck or shoulder.

Cordotomy in Nonmalignant Disease. Thirty-nine of the 380 cordotomies were performed in 25 patients for pain that was

Table 105-7. Pain following 136 most recent cordotomies to December 31, 1985

Type of Pain	Percent	Comment
No pain anywhere	32.7	22.4% short survival or follow-up
Partial relief of pain for which cordotomy performed	12.2	1% also with pain above level 2% also with ipsilateral pain
New pain above level of analgesia	2.0	1% also had dysesthetic pain below level
Ipsilateral new or worse pain	40.8	7.1% also had contralateral dysesthetic pain 2.0% dysesthetic
Persistent pain below adequate level of analgesia	6.1	1% etiology of pain uncertain 2% pain from cord injury 3.1% pain dysesthetic in quality but no neurologic defect
Dysesthetic pain below adequate level of analgesia different to preop pain	33.7	17.3% preoperative sensory loss in pain area 8.2% neurologic deficit without sensory loss in pain area 7.1% postoperative, not preoperative neurologic deficit in pain area 1.0% no preoperative or postoperative neurologic deficit in pain area

not caused by cancer, as listed in Table 105-8. Six procedures were repeated on the same side, 7 patients underwent bilateral procedures. For patients with pain caused by cord lesions, success was related to 3 factors: level of the original cord lesion that caused the pain; its completeness; and whether the patient suffered from steady pain alone below the level of sensory loss, or from steady pain plus exacerbations of sharp pain as well, of which the exacerbations of pain were the more severe. Table 105-9 illustrates that patients with incomplete low lesions who suffer from exacerbations of usually severe, sharp pain, typically shooting into the legs, are good candidates for cordotomy when such patients are compared with those who have high complete lesions and steady pain. Possibly the sharp, intermittent pain in the patients with incomplete lesions is really a nociceptive, rather than a deafferentation, phenomenon, caused by, say, scarring.

Recurrence of Pain After Cordotomy. Relief of pain after cordotomy is not forever. Probably as Lipton[55] and Nathan[54] suggest, if the patient lives long enough, the pain will always recur. Out of 23 of the author's patients, with pain caused by

Table 105-8. Percutaneous cordotomy
in 25 patients not suffering from cancer

Cause of pain	Percent	Percentage with significant pain relief
Spinal cord trauma	64	56.3
"Failed back"—with arachnoiditis and paraparesis	12	
Thoracic disc—paraplegia	4	
Pathological fracture NYD, paraparesis	4	42.9
Thorotrast myelogram, paraparesis	4	
Spina bifida	4	
Cerebral palsy, skeletal pain	4	
? Brachial plexus avulsion	4	100

Table 105-9. Factors influencing success
in cordotomy for pain from cord lesions

	Percent	
	Significant Relief*	Failure
Level:		
Cord	64.7	35.3
Conus-Cauda	83.0	17.0
Severity:		
Complete	55.6	44.4
Partial	80.0	20.0
Pain Type:		
Steady	54.5	45.5
Steady and exacerbations	83.3	16.7

* Usually of exacerbations which are more severe.

lesions of the spinal cord, who underwent percutaneous cordotomy, and out of 8 more undergoing open cordotomy, pain was observed to recur in 8 after 21, 13, 7, 6, 5, 4, 1.1, and 1 years, respectively, and in one more patient with cerebral palsy and musculoskeletal pain, after 4 years. This phenomenon was in each case associated with fading of the cordotomy-induced analgesia, an analgesia that was restored by repeating the cordotomy in 5 patients after 21, 7, 6, 5, and 4 years for those with spinal cord injury, and after 4 years in the patient with cerebral palsy. Although the level of analgesia was restored, pain relief was recaptured at least in the short term in the patient with cerebral palsy, in the paraplegics after 5 and 21 years, but not achieved in the other 3 patients, two with traumatic paraplegia, one 1 with arachnoiditis after multiple spinal injury. Lipton[55] has written to me that "I have even seen a cordotomy which had lasted for just over 10 years suddenly disappear in a matter of a week and the patient seemed absolutely normal as far as temperature, touch and pain were concerned on the previously cordotomized side." He adds that he has often repeated the cordotomy successfully in such cases, and has even done so on a third occasion, although only half of these procedures yielded a good result. There is no known scientific explanation for such observations, for, to this author's knowledge, regeneration in the spinothalamic tract has never been demonstrated.

Pain Relief after Bilateral Cordotomy. Of our earlier 244 procedures, 17.9 percent were performed on the second side, 91.5 percent of which resulted in significant bilateral relief (of the pain for which the procedures had been done) at the time of discharge from hospital. At the time of post-discharge follow-up, 71.4 percent had enjoyed such relief. Comparable figures for unilateral cordotomy were 96.3 and 82.7 percent, respectively, the discrepancies explained by the P-squared rule.

Twenty, or 14.7 percent, of the later 136 procedures were performed on the second side, three under general anesthesia, at intervals of up to 7 days in 20 percent, 1 week to 1 month in 30 percent, 1 to 6 months in 40 percent, and over 6 months in 10 percent. Cause of the pain in these bilaterally operated patients was similar to that in the unilateral group. Complete bilateral relief of the pain for which the cordotomies were done was achieved at the time of latest follow-up in 75 percent, significant relief in 90 percent. Follow-up results after the second-sided

operation showed relief lasting: less than 1 month in 35 percent; 1 to 2 months in 45 percent; 3 to 6 months in 3 percent; and 1 year in 5 percent.

COMPLICATIONS

Published Data

The complications of percutaneous cordotomy, prevention of which have been discussed, consist chiefly of respiratory failure, paresis and ataxia, bladder dysfunction, post-cordotomy dysesthesia, bowel dysfunction, hypotension, Horner's syndrome, and local pain.

Patients undergoing cordotomy are often terminally ill so that in most series, a number of patients die within a few days to weeks postoperatively from their disease, though they appear statistically as postoperative deaths. Death caused by cordotomy is usually always the result of respiratory decompensation. Similarly, many cordotomy patients are bedridden and remain so because of disease-induced paralysis, often associated with disease-induced incontinence, so that the effect of cordotomy on limb and visceral function may be unassessable. Many authors regard Horner's syndrome inevitable[57,60] or even a necessary requirement of good cordotomy, but this is not the author's experience.

Ischia et al.[62] recorded an apparently 10.1 percent incidence of paresis, 7.2 percent of bladder dysfunction, in 69 patients undergoing unilateral cordotomy. Ischia et al.[63] recorded a 4.2 percent incidence of respiratory failure in 103 selected patients undergoing unilateral cordotomy for pain caused by cancer in the cervicothoracic region, essentially patients with pulmonary cancer and Pancoast syndrome, a high-risk group, as explained above. Of these patients, 31.1 percent had transient, 1 percent permanent, paresis; 8.7 percent had bladder dysfunction. Lahuerta et al.[57] report 6 deaths in 100 selected patients in the first week from respiratory failure—5 in patients with carcinoma of the lung with unilateral cordotomy, the other after bilateral cordotomy. This matches the discussion we have outlined above. Sixty-nine percent had paresis, persistent in 4 percent, and 19 percent experienced bladder dysfunction, persistent in 3 percent. Twenty-six percent had suffered from headache or ipsilateral neck pain, 6 percent from dysesthesia, and 6 percent from contralateral limb weakness, a strange observation. Kühner[48] reported a 4 percent mortality, 2 percent incidence of paresis, 2.6 percent incidence of respiratory failure, 3 percent incidence of sphincter disturbance, and 20 percent incidence of dysesthesia after unilateral percutaneous cordotomy. There was a 10 percent mortality, 12 percent incidence of sphincter disturbance, 20 percent incidence of respiratory dysfunction, and a 40 percent incidence of hypotension after bilateral procedures. Lipton[55] found all his patients weak for a few days postoperatively. Forty percent showed minor weakness on testing, of whom half had trouble walking, and 8 percent of all patients remained disabled for a month. Two percent apparently suffered permanent disabling weakness.

Ischia et al.[60] reported 36 bilateral cordotomies, of whom four died in the first week after the second-sided procedure, all apparently from their disease, none from respiratory dysfunction. Of these patients, 36.1 percent had transient, 1.8 percent more permanent, paresis; 6 percent experienced worsening of bladder function after unilateral, 58 percent after bilateral, procedures. These figures, however, appear higher than usual since they are quoted on the basis of patients at risk for these complications, excluding those who had bladder incontinence or were bedridden by paresis at the time of the surgery. Of the patients included in this series, 36.1 percent had hypotension, and all suffered from Horner's syndrome. Koulousakis and Nittner[64] report 27 percent mortality within 2 weeks of bilateral cordotomy in 22 patients, in all but one due to respiratory failure. Sixty-seven percent of these patients who died also had paresis, and 83 percent had high levels of analgesia up to C2-C3 unilaterally or bilaterally, again underlining issues discussed above. Over 6 coagulations (an enormous number!) on one side was likely to lead to complications.

Personal Series

Table 105-10 lists the major and Table 105-11 the lesser complications recorded in our 380 percutaneous cordotomies up to December 31, 1985. There was an overall 0.3 percent mortality after unilateral procedures, 1.6 percent after bilateral procedures, attributable to surgery, all from respiratory difficulties, all in the earlier 244 cases. Two patients of the latest 136 died within 1 month of surgery, one 9 days after a bilateral operation, the other 11 days after a unilateral procedure. Both were terminally ill at the time of surgery, the first dying with

Table 105-10. Major complications of percutaneous cordotomy (%)

Complication	Unilateral		Bilateral	
	First 244	Last 136	First 244	Last 136
Death	0.5	0	2.4	0
Temporary respiratory failure	0.5	0	4.9	0
Significant persistent paresis	0.5	2	0	5
Persistent worsening of bladder function*	3.7	2	7.5	10
Other†	0.5	0	0	5‡

* Many already incontinent preoperatively.
† Acute hydrocephalus.
‡ Pulmonary emboli.

metastatic melanoma of brain and spine, the second being bedridden and paraplegic.

Eight-tenths percent of unilateral and 1.6 percent of bilateral procedures resulted in permanent limb paresis, while 2.9 percent of unilateral and 18.8 percent of bilateral procedures overall resulted in worsening of bladder function. However, one patient on a catheter was able after a bilateral cordotomy and a transurethral resection of prostate to resume voluntary voiding.

Lesser complications consisted of minor or transient usually lower limb paresis in 16.8 percent of unilateral and 28 percent of bilateral procedures; and minor or transient bladder dysfunction in 6.6 percent of unilateral and 9.4 percent of bilateral cordotomies. Horner's syndrome was common, but usually transient. Respiratory difficulties did not occur in our most recent 136 cases.

CONCLUSION

Cordotomy by the lateral high cervical percutaneous route, if performed according to a rigid protocol, is the most effective procedure available to the neurosurgeon for the relief of chronic

Table 105-11. Lesser complications of percutaneous cordotomy (%)

Complication	Unilateral			Bilateral		
	1st 244			1st 244		
	At Discharge	At Follow-up	Last 136	At Discharge	At Followup	Last 136
Respiratory	1.6	0.5	0	2.4	0	0
Transient, minor paresis	21.2	8.8	15.0	22.0	2.5	40.0
Transient, minor bladder dysfunction	7.3	7.7	5.0	24.0	2.5	10.0*
Bowel dysfunction	1.0	3.2	1.0	9.5	0	5.0*
Hypotension	1.6	0.5	2.0	9.5	5.0	0
Horner's syndrome†	28.6	13.2	20.0	12.2	5.0	40.0
Ipsilateral neck or head pain	3.1	1.6	7.0	0	0	5.0
Meningismus	1.0	0	0	0	0	0
Restless leg syndrome	0.5	0.5	1.0	0	0	0
Hoarseness ? cause	0	0	1.0	0	0	5.0

* Transient.
† Nearly always transient.

pain at the expense of very low morbidity. But to avoid disappointment demands a clear understanding of its limitations.

REFERENCES

1. Spiller WG, Martin E: The treatment of persistent pain of organic origin in the lower part of the body by division of the anterolateral column of the spinal cord. JAMA 58:1489, 1912
2. Spiller WG: The occasional clinical resemblance between caries of the vertebrae and lumbothoracic syringomyelia and the location within the spinal cord of the fibres for the sensations of pain and temperature. Univ Penn Med Bull 18:147, 1905
3. Schuller A: über operative Durchtrennung der Ruckenmarkstrange (Chordotomie). Wien Med Wochenschr 60:2292, 1910
4. Foerster 0: über die Vorderseiten—Strangdurchschneidung. Arch Psychiat Nerv Krankh 81:707, 1927
5. Stookey B: Chordotomy of the second cervical segment for relief from pain due to recurrent carcinoma of the breast. Arch Neurol Psychiatry 26:443, 1931
6. Mullan S, Harper PV, Hekmatpanah J, et al: Percutaneous interruption of spinal-pain tracts by means of a strontium-90 needle. J Neurosurg 20:931, 1963
7. Mullan S, Hekmatpanah J, Dobben G, et al: Percutaneous, intramedullary cordotomy utilizing the unipolar anodal electrolytic system. J Neurosurg 22:548, 1965
8. Rosomoff HL, Carroll F, Brown J, et al: Percutaneous radiofrequency cervical cordotomy. Technique. J Neurosurg 23:639, 1965
9. Onofrio BM: Cervical spinal cord and dentate delineation in percutaneous radiofrequency cordotomy at the level of the first to second cervical vertebrae. Surg Gynecol Obstet 133:30, 1971
10. Gildenberg PL, Zanes C, Flitter MA, et al: Impedance monitoring device for detection of penetration of the spinal cord in anterior percutaneous cervical cordotomy. Technical note. J Neurosurg 30:87, 1969
11. Taren JA, Davis R, Crosby EC: Target physiologic corroboration in stereotaxic cervical cordotomy. J Neurosurg 30:569, 1969
12. Taren JA: Physiologic corroboration in stereotaxic high cervical cordotomy. Confin Neurol 33:285, 1971
13. Sweet WH, White JC, Silverstone B, et al: Sensory responses from anterior roots and from surface and interior of spinal cord in man. Trans Am Neurol Assoc 75:165, 1950
14. Hitchcock ER, Tsukamoto Y: Distal and proximal sensory responses during stereotactic spinal tractotomy in man. Ann Clin Res 5:68, 1973
15. Tasker RR, Organ LW: Percutaneous cordotomy. Physiological identification of target site. Confin Neurol 35:110, 1973
16. Tasker RR, Organ LW, Smith KC: Physiological guidelines for the localization of lesions by percutaneous cordotomy. Acta Neurochirurgica Suppl 21:111, 1974
17. Livingston WK: Pain Mechanisms: A Physiologic Interpretation of Causalgia and its Related States. New York, Plenum Press, 1976
18. Tasker RR: Percutaneous cordotomy. Compr Ther 1:51, 1975
19. Tasker RR: Deafferentation, in Wall PD, Melzack R (eds): Textbook of Pain. Edinburgh, Livingstone, 1985, pp 119–132
20. Tasker RR, Organ LW, Hawrylyshyn P: Deafferentation and causalgia, in Bonica JJ (ed): Pain. Raven Press, New York, 1980, pp 305–329
21. Tasker RR, Tsuda T, Hawrylyshyn P: Clinical neurophysiological investigation of deafferentation pain, in Bonica JJ, et al (eds): Advances in Pain Research and Therapy. New York, Raven Press, 1983, pp 713–737
22. Tasker RR: Pain due to central nervous system pathology (central pain), in Bonica JJ (ed): Management of Pain in Clinical Practice, ed 2. (in press)
23. Tasker RR: Open cordotomy. Prog Neurol Surg 8:1, 1977
24. Belmusto L, Brown E, Owens G: Clinical observations on respiratory and vasomotor disturbances as related to cervical cordotomies. J Neurosurg 201:225, 1963
25. Belmusto L, Woldring S, Owens G: Localization and patterns of potentials of the respiratory pathways in the cervical spinal cord in the dog. J Neurosurg 22:277, 1965
26. Crue BL, Todd EM, Carregal EJA: Posterior approach for high cervical percutaneous radiofrequency cordotomy. Confin Neurol 30:41, 1968
27. Fox JL: Localization of the respiratory pathway in the upper cervical spinal cord following percutaneous cordotomy. Neurology 19:1115, 1969
28. Hitchcock E, Leece B: Somatotopic representation of the respiratory pathways in the cervical cord of man. J Neurosurg 27:320, 1967
29. Mullan S, Hosobuchi Y: Respiratory hazards of high cervical percutaneous cordotomy. J Neurosurg 28:291, 1968
30. Nathan PW: The descending respiratory pathway in man. J Neurol Neurosurg Psychiatry 26:487, 1963
31. Rosomoff HL, Krieger AJ, Kuperman AS: Effects of percutaneous cervical cordotomy on pulmonary function. J Neurosurg 31:620, 1969
32. Tenicela R, Rosomoff HL, Feist J, et al: Pulmonary function following percutaneous cervical cordotomy. Anesthesiology 29:7, 1968
33. Cloward RB: Cervical chordotomy by the anterior approach. Technique and advantages. J Neurosurg 21:19, 1964
34. Collis JS Jr: Anterolateral cordotomy by an anterior approach. Report of a case. J Neurosurg 20:445, 1963
35. Lin PM, Gildenberg PL, Polakoff PP: An anterior approach to percutaneous lower cervical cordotomy. J Neurosurg 25:553, 1966
36. Tasker RR: Surgical approaches to the primary afferent and spinal cord, in Fields HH, et al (eds): Advances in Pain Research and Therapy, vol 9. New York, Raven Press, 1985, pp 799–824
37. Ischia S, Luzzani A, Ischia A, et al: Subarachnoid neurolytic block (L5 S1) and unilateral percutaneous cervical cordotomy in the treatment of pain secondary to pelvic malignant disease. Pain 20:139, 1984
38. Boas RA: Phantom anus pain syndrome, in Bonica J, et al (eds): Advances in Pain Research and Therapy, vol 5. New York, Raven Press, 1983, pp 947–950
39. Hitchcock ER: Stereotactic cervical myelotomy. J Neurol Neurosurg Psychiatry 33:224, 1970
40. Schvarcz JR: Stereotactic high cervical extralemniscal myelotomy for pelvic cancer pain. Acta Neurochir Suppl 33:431, 1984
41. Schvarcz JR: Spinal cord stereotactic techniques re trigeminal nucleotomy and extralemniscal myelotomy. Appl Neurophysiol 41:99, 1978
42. Morley TP: Congenital rotation of the spinal cord. J Neurosurg 10:690, 1953
43. Sherman IC, Arieff AJ: Dissociation between pain and temperature in spinal cord lesions. J Nerv Ment Dis 108:285, 1948
44. Stookey B: Human chordotomy to abolish pain sense without destroying temperature sense. J Nerv Ment Dis 69:552, 1929
45. Voris HC: Ipsilateral sensory loss following cordotomy. Report of a case. Arch Neurol Psychiatry 65:95, 1957
46. Voris HC: Variations in the spinothalamic tract in man. J Neurosurg 14:55, 1957
47. Tasker RR: The merits of percutaneous cordotomy over the open operation, in Morley TP (ed): Current Controversies in Neurosurgery. Philadelphia, WB Saunders, 1976, pp 496–501
48. Kühner A: La cordotome percutanée. Sa place actuelle dans la chirurgie de la douleur. Anesth Anals 38:357, 1981
49. Hitchcock ER: An apparatus for stereotactic spinal surgery. A preliminary report. J Neurosurg 31:386, 1969
50. Tasker RR: Percutaneous cordotomy—The lateral high cervical technique, in Schmidek HH, Sweet WH (eds): Operative Neurosurgical Techniques, Indications, Methods, and Results. New York, Grune & Stratton, 1982, pp 1137–1153

51. Tasker RR, Marshall BM: Analgesia for surgical procedures performed on conscious patients. Can Anaesth Soc J 12:29, 1965.

52. Tasker RR: Somatotopographic representation in the human thalamus, midbrain, and spinal cord. The anatomical basis for the surgical relief of pain, in Morley TP (ed): Current Controversies in Neurosurgery. Philadelphia, WB Saunders, 1976, pp 485–495

53. Nathan PW: Reference of sensation at the spinal level. J Neurol Neurosurg Psychiatry 19:88, 1956

54. Nathan PW: Results of antero-lateral cordotomy for pain in cancer. J Neurol Neurosurg Psychiatry 26:353, 1963

55. Lipton S: Percutaneous cervical cordotomy. Acta Anaesthesiologica Belgica 32:81, 1981, with additional personal communications

56. Meglio M, Cioni B: The role of percutaneous cordotomy in the treatment of chronic cancer pain. Acta Neurochir 59:111, 1981

57. Lahuerta T, Lipton S, Wells JCD: Percutaneous cervical cordotomy: Results and complications in a recent series of 100 patients. Ann R Coll Surg Engl 67:41, 1985

58. Siegfried J, Kühner A, Sturm V: Neurosurgical treatment of cancer pain. Recent results. Cancer Res 89:148, 1984

59. Lorenz R: Methods of percutaneous spinothalamic tract section, in Krayenbuhl H (ed): Advances and Technical Standards in Neurosurgery, vol 3. Vienna, Springer-Verlag, 1976, pp 123–145

60. Ischia S, Luzzani A, Ischia A, et al: Bilateral percutaneous cervical cordotomy: Immediate and long-term results in 36 patients with neoplastic disease. J Neurol Neurosurg Psychiatry 47:141, 1984

61. Tasker RR, Evans RJ: Experience with percutaneous cordotomy. Can J Surg 16:1, 1973

62. Ischia S, Luzzani A, Ischia A, et al: Role of percutaneous cervical cordotomy in the treatment of neoplastic vertebral pain. Pain 19:123, 1984

63. Ischia S, Ischia A, Luzzani A, et al: Results up to death in the treatment of persistent cervico-thoracic (Pancoast) and thoracic malignant pain by unilateral percutaneous cervical cordotomy. Pain 21:339, 1985

64. Koulousakis A, Nittner K: Bilateral C1-C2 cordotomies. Can complications be avoided? Appl Neurophysiol 45:500, 1982

Percutaneous Electrothermocoagulation of Spinal Nerve Trunk, Ganglion, and Rootlets

Sumio Uematsu

SELECTIVE SURGICAL INTERRUPTION of posterior roots was first carried out by both Abbe[1] and Bennett[2] in 1889. This technique was later extended to sections of anterior roots for the treatment of motor disorders. The open surgical technique limits its applicability to some debilitated patients, however. Therefore, efforts have been made to develop a less traumatic rhizotomy technique. Scoville[3] described a simplified approach for extradural spinal sensory rhizotomy. Dogliotti[4] proposed injecting ethanol alcohol via lumbar puncture into the subarachnoid space, while Maher[5] advocated the use of phenol solution. These hypobaric solutions must be injected with extreme caution, however, since their penetration is likely to be unpredictable and C-fibers as well as the larger myelinated fibers may be destroyed.[6]

Electrothermocoagulation of the gasserian ganglion for trigeminal neuralgia was introduced by Kirschner.[7] It was later abandoned because of the high complication rate resulting from the uncontrolled effect of the diathermy current. In October, 1965, Sweets introduced an advanced technique for electrothermocoagulation of the trigeminal ganglion. Accumulated clinical experience has shown that it is possible to alleviate pain and still preserve proprioception and motor function in the trigeminal nerve.[8] Based on physiologic studies, it has been assumed that the less myelinated pain fibers were more easily destroyed by heat than were the larger fibers. A preliminary histologic study, however, revealed indiscriminate destruction of both small and large fibers rather than selective destruction of smaller, less myelinated ones. In my opinion, it is therefore logical to believe that the proportional destruction of nerve fibers increases the pain threshold but also preserves enough fibers for satisfactory proprioception and motor function (Figure 106-1).

Our first percutaneous radiofrequency spinal rhizotomy was carried out in 1971 on an 18-year-old girl with spastic paraplegia caused by a spinal cord injury. Bilateral L1, L2, and L3 roots were denervated to reduce spasticity of the hip joints. The first successful result with this technique encouraged us to expand its use to other spinal levels to treat pain and motor disorders. Possibly it also could be used to treat spasmodic torticollis[10] and cerebral palsy[11] by differential denervation of sacral rootlets.[12] The application of this technique to the release of spastic bladder was advocated in the previous chapter by this author. Young et al.[20] reported their successful results, the details of which are described in the appropriate section of this chapter.

The technique is relatively simple and definitely less invasive than surgical open rhizotomy. Its success, however, depends heavily upon the availability of a fluoroscopic x-ray monitor for precise stereotactic introduction of the probe into the intervertebral foramen. The procedure should be carried out under local anesthesia. Careful observation of the response to electrical stimulation and the assessment of sensory and motor functions during the entire period of the procedure are essential to avoid undesirable complications.

ANATOMY AND PHYSIOLOGY

ROOTLETS, GANGLION, AND TRUNK

Each spinal nerve arises from the cord through two roots: a posterior sensory and an anterior motor root. These roots traverse the subarachnoid sac, penetrate the dura, and reach the intervertebral foramen, where the posterior roots swell into the spinal ganglion, which contains the cells of origin of sensory fibers, Distal to the ganglion, the posterior and anterior roots unite and emerge from the intervertebral foramen of a mixed spinal nerve or common nerve trunk, which contains both sensory and motor fibers (Figure 106-2).

Each nerve root has the following five parts, based upon its meningeal covering and relationship to the intervertebral foramina.

1. Subarachnoid
2. Subdural
3. Extradural
4. Intraforaminal
5. Extraforaminal

Dural and arachnoid sleeves surround both the anterior and posterior nerve roots. The nerves may sometimes be separated or fused, but the arachnoid membranes are definitely separated by the dura and each root is surrounded by its own extension of the subarachnoid space. The subarachnoid space stops at the proximal end of the ganglion on the posterior roots and in the corresponding portion on the anterior roots. At this termina-

OPERATIVE NEUROSURGICAL TECHNIQUES
ISBN 0-8089-1862-1

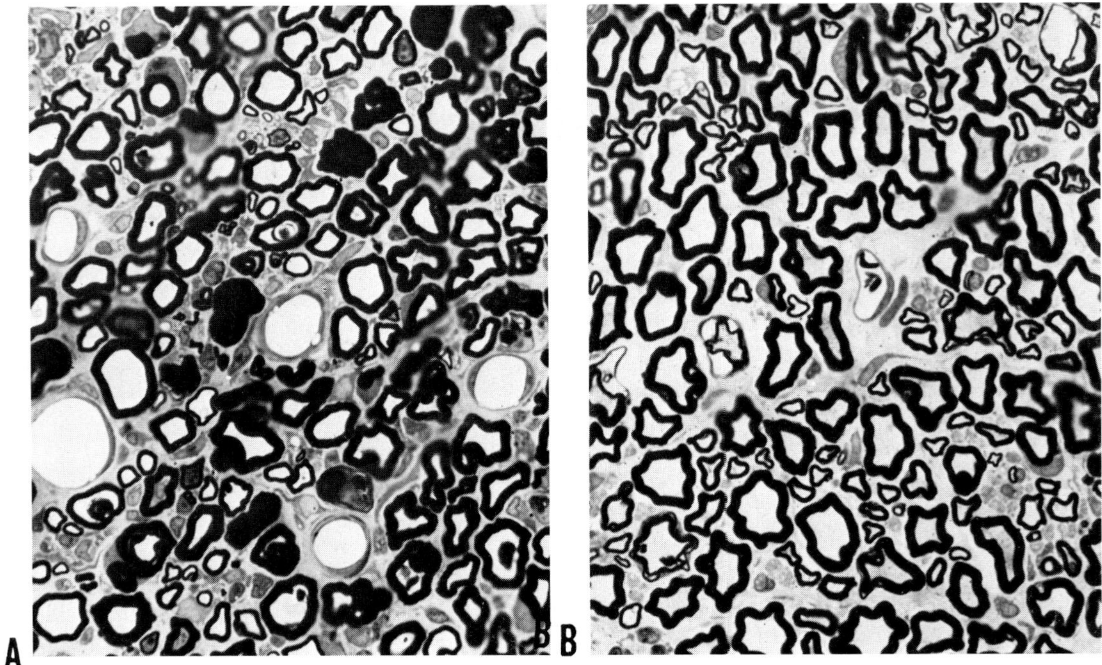

Fig. 106-1. Radiofrequency thermocoagulation of the sciatic nerve of a cat. (A) Section taken at the site of the heat lesion. Note the indiscriminate effect of the heat on both the small and large myelinated fibers. The wall of the capillaries is well preserved. (B) Control, proximal portion of same nerve, away from the heat lesion. Phosphotungstic acid hematoxylin stain; original magnification: ×750.

tion, there are three meningeal layers, which blend with connective tissue of the peripheral nerves. The subarachnoid space is not believed to be continuous with either the perineural space or the lymphatic channels, but the subdural space is thought to be continuous with connective tissue of the peripheral nerves.

The posterior roots are, as a rule, thicker than the ventral ones and vary with the size of their respective ganglia. The only exception is the first cervical nerve, the dorsal root of which is greatly reduced and often missing. The largest spinal nerves are the lower cervical and the first thoracic, which form the great nerve for the upper limbs and upper sacral nerve for the lower limbs. The smallest in size are the coccygeal nerve roots. Cervical nerve roots diminish in size from below and upward.[13]

RADICULAR ARTERY

Most of the 62 embryologic radicular arteries regress during the course of development, and in the adult only six to eight functioning arteries supply the anterior while between 10

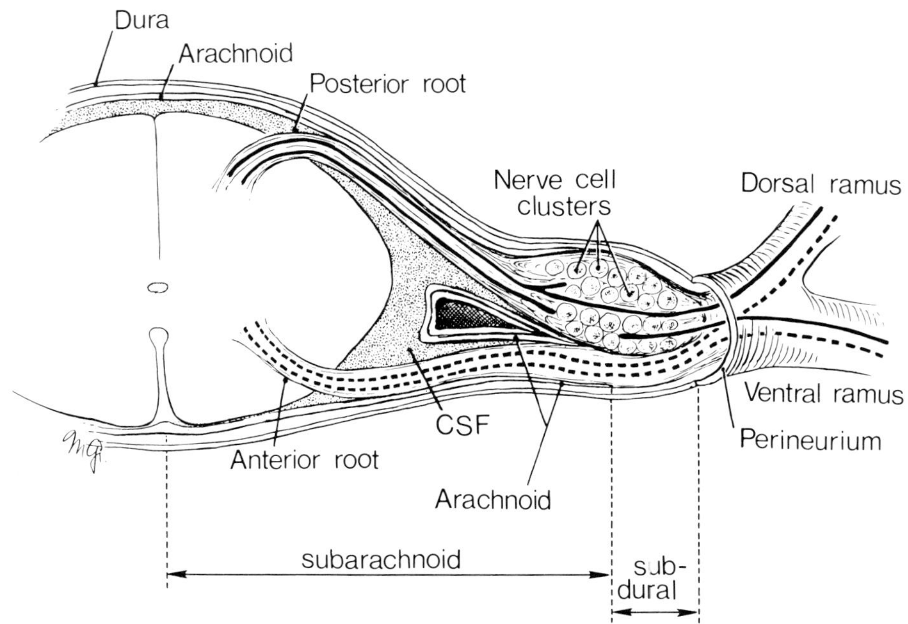

Fig. 106-2. Rootlets, ganglion, and trunk. The subarachnoid space stops at the proximal end of the ganglion.

and 23 functioning arteries supply the posterior spinal artery. The radicular arteries that actually supply the spinal cord are called *radiculomedullary arteries*. They perfuse the cord via two terminal branches; the anterior and posterior radicular arteries (Figure 106-3).

The anterior radicular arteries run in the intervertebral foramina on the anterior surface of the dural investment of the spinal roots and remain extradural until they reach the lateral border of the dural sheath proper. At this point they give off short to medium dural arteries. The anterior radicular arteries then pierce the dura anterior to, and slightly below, the nerve. The arteries then run upward at an angle that depends on the spinal level, always remaining anterior to the plane of the dentate ligament. The posterior radicular arteries in general run along the superior border of the nerve sheath, piercing the dura through the same opening as a nerve passing between the sensory nerve filaments, to reach the posterior spinal arteries, always remaining posterior to the plane of the dentate ligament.

The blood supply of the spinal cord may be jeopardized in certain transitional regions where its arterial supply is derived from two different sources. Because the upper third of the spinal cord is supplied primarily by the anterior spinal artery, an occlusion of the C2 or C3 radicular artery, or an occlusion of the vertebral artery, can be revascularized effectively by the retrograde flow from the basilar artery. The inferior two thirds, including the cervical enlargement, are supplied by a large artery, usually arising from the deep cervical artery, supplemented by a second artery, which is a branch of the first intercostal artery. In the presence of an obstruction of the subclavian artery, or an occlusion of the radicular artery at the interspace of C7 and C8, the only possible blood circulation comes from the contralateral subclavian system. The upper segment of the thoracic spinal cord, on the other hand, depends upon the radicular branches of the intercostal arteries. If one or more of the parent intercostal vessels is compressed, segments of the spinal cord, T1-4, cannot be adequately maintained by the small branches of the anterior spinal artery. For this reason, thoracic segment T1-4, particularly T4, is considered a vulnerable area in the distribution of the anterior spinal artery. The posterior surface of the cord most susceptible to vascular insult is also in segment T1-4. Cord segment T11 and L1, in which the blood supply depends upon the Adamkiewicz artery, is an equally vulnerable region. Any vascular injury may result in necrosis of an entire segment of the cord.

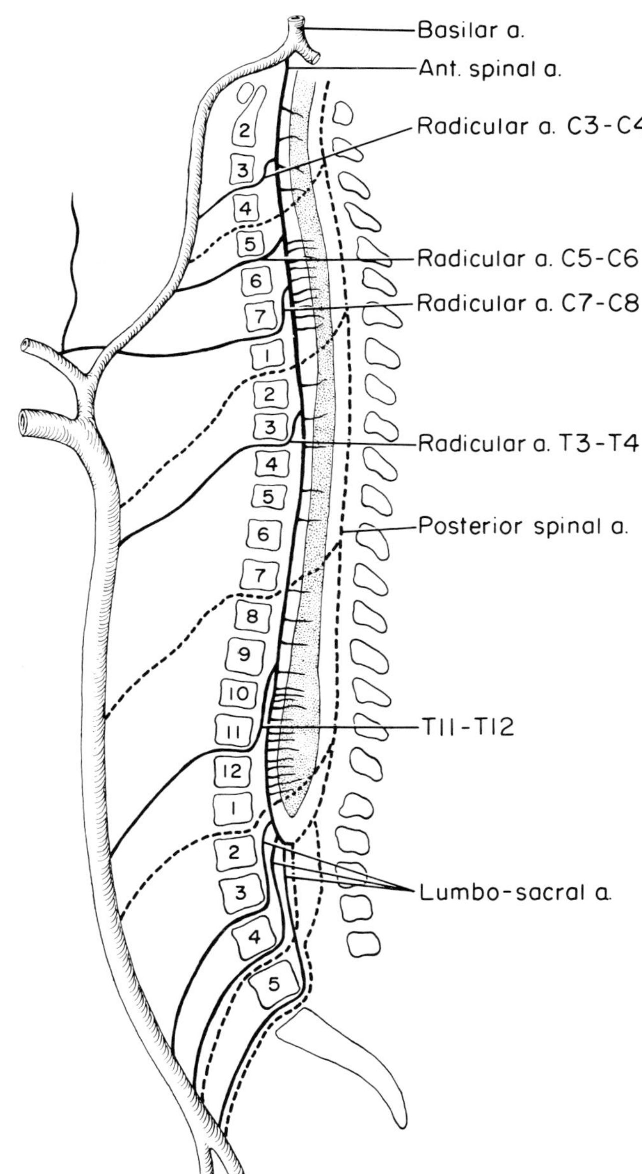

Fig. 106-3. Important arteries via the intervertebral foramina. (After Djindjian R, et al. Courtesy of University Park Press, Baltimore.)

INDICATIONS AND SELECTION OF PATIENTS

The largest series of patients treated by rhizotomy suffered from pain from various causes. When pain is limited to a relatively localized area, use of the extremities as well as bladder and bowel function are not impaired when the nerve roots are cut. Rhizotomy has long been the standard operation for relieving pain from metastatic nodes in the neck, provided the trunk of the brachial plexus is not involved.[15]

Patients are selected for rhizotomy on the basis of a detailed history and a careful physical and neurologic examination. If indicated, myelography should be performed. Routine psychometric testing and psychiatric evaluation are necessary for patients with benign chronic pain before any procedure is undertaken.

DIAGNOSTIC PARAVERTEBRAL BLOCK

As a preliminary procedure, it is generally advisable to inject a local anesthetic into the spinal nerve that is being considered for sensory root section. This procedure should be carried out under fluoroscopic control. Anesthesia equipment should be on hand to treat serious respiratory or cardiac complications, if they occur. This temporary procedure serves a dual purpose: it shows the patient what permanent sensory loss will be like, and it assures the surgeon that the given area of analgesia is likely to relieve the patient's discomfort. It does not guarantee, however, that the pain will not recur.

EXTENT OF POSTERIOR RHIZOTOMY

White and Sweet[6] stated that posterior rhizotomy would be effective when pain was limited to a localized area of the limb, so that an extensive rhizotomy could be avoided. With pain in

Origin or site of pain	Involved nerves	Roots of origin	Extent of rhizotomy	Comment
Occipital scar	Greater or lesser occipital	C2-3	C2-3, C4 if present	Look for possible posterior root of first cervical
Carcinoma of cervical nodes	Superficial and deep cervical plexuses	C2-C4	C2-4, C5, and C4, if present	Eliminate cases of cranial nerve involvement. Include C5 when pain is referred to shoulder or lower neck
Epicondylar fractures and scars along medial side of forearm and hand	Ulnar	C8-T2	C8-T2	Occasional failures will result from C7 overlap
Scarring from chest wounds and thoracotomy operations	Intercostals	Variable	Generally two roots above and below nerves caught in scar	After intercostal drainage for empyema, cut 5 roots. After costectomy, cut 6 roots
Sensitive scar after herniorrhapy	Ilioinguinal and hypogastric	T12-L1	T11-L2	
Retroperitoneal scar and other injuries to nerve in lateral thigh	Lateral femoral Cutaneous	L2-L3	L2-L3	
Coccygodynia	S5 and coccygeal	Same	S4-Cocl	Pain following rectal resection requires additional rhizotomy of S3. This may impair detrusor activity of bladder
Angina pectoris	Thoracic cardiac rami	T1-T4	T1-T4	Bilateral rhizotomy necessary if pain radiates down both arms
Gastric, biliary, and pancreatic	Splanchnic rami	T5-T10	T5-T10	To be recommended only when splanchnicectomy fails because of involvement of somatic nerves in posterior abdominal wall
Renal	Lower splanchnic rami	T10-L1	T10-L1	Preferable to sympathectomy after previous operations on diseased kidney

From White JC, Sweet WH: *Pain and the Neurological Surgeon, A 40-year Experience*. Springfield, Illinois, Charles C Thomas, 1969, p 653

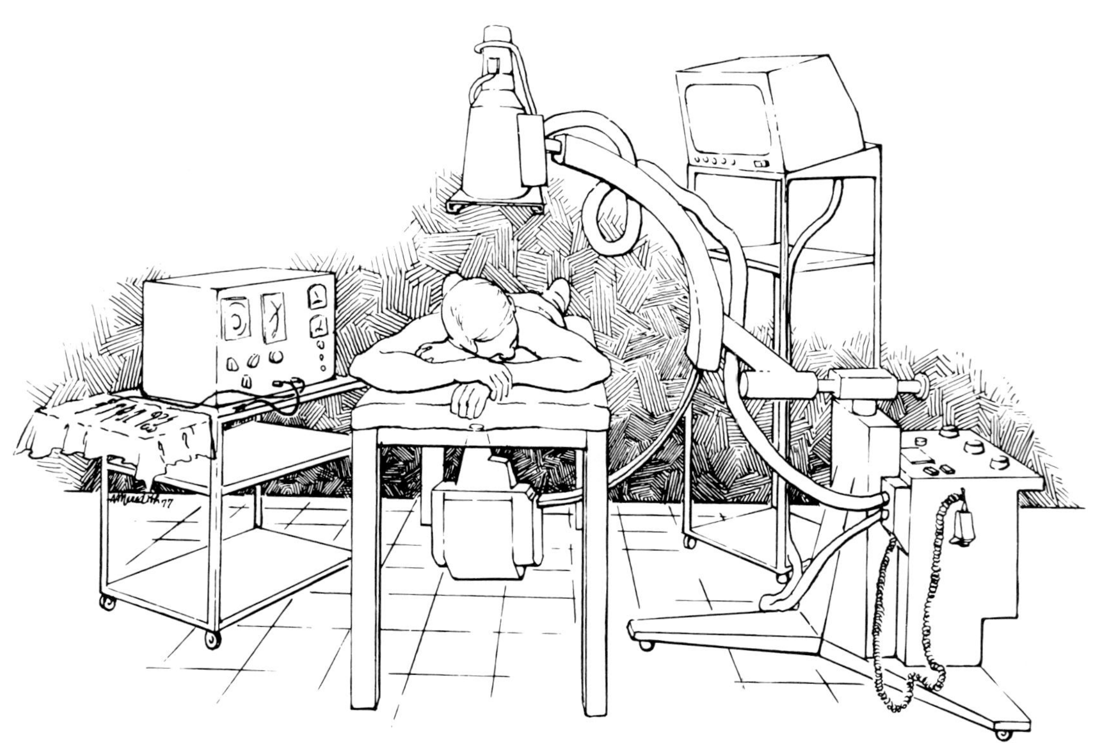

Fig. 106-4. Artist's view of the set-up for the procedure. Note the C-arm fluoroscopic apparatus.

the chest or abdomen, an extensive rhizotomy could be carried out (Table 106-1).

For occipital neuralgia, denervation of C2-3 is indicated. Bilateral denervation of C3-4 should be avoided, however, since it could interfere with diaphragmatic respiration.

Pain in the anterior one third of the tongue and mandibular portion of the neck could be successfully relieved by combined rhizotomy of the fifth cranial nerve and C2-3. Pain of the ear, secondary to infiltrated cancer, could be treated in the same way. Rhizotomy may not be technically feasible, however, when pain is referred to the shoulder or lower neck. These areas are innervated by the lower half of the cervical and upper thoracic nerve (C4-T4). Denervation of C8 to T2 is required to relieve pain of ulnar nerve distribution.

To relieve intercostal neuralgia, two roots above and below the affected area must be interrupted. Denervation from T11 to L2 is recommended for a painful scar after herniorrhaphy. Care should be taken, however, not to injure the Adamkiewicz artery. Pain in the lateral aspect of the thigh requires denervation of L2 to L3. Motor function should be monitored carefully during electrothermocoagulation. Denervation of S4 to the coccygeal nerve is necessary to relieve coccygodynia. Bladder or bowel function is not affected by this procedure; only the dermatome between the posterior portion of the perineum and the coccyx will be denervated. Interruption of S2 and S3, particularly if bilateral, will impair bowel, bladder, and sexual function.

To alleviate pain secondary to malignancy of visceral organs, a combination of sympathectomy and rhizotomy may be required.[6]

TECHNIQUE

PREPARATION AND ANESTHESIA

The patient should have nothing by mouth. Heavy sedation should be avoided: the patient must be alert because patient cooperation is needed to monitor motor and sensory functions during the procedure. A few milliliters of 0.5 or 1 percent lidocaine are injected subcutaneously at the point at which the needle will enter the body. Particular caution should be taken to avoid injecting the anesthetic into the subarachnoid space, especially in the cervical region. During electrothermocoagulation, sodium methohexital (Brevital sodium, Eli Lilly) can be given intravenously by the anesthesiologist for C2 rhizotomy. The patient may experience extreme pain in the area of C2 during treatment. Hence, it is important to explain the procedure in detail, particularly what the patient might experience and the need for his or her cooperation during the procedure. This significantly reduces the amount of premedication and anesthesia required.[16,17]

CERVICAL RHIZOTOMY

The procedure is performed in a room equipped with radiologic image intensification (Figure 106-4). The patient is placed in the supine position, with the neck slightly flexed. The head and neck rest comfortably on a pillow of folded sheets. This position permits fluoroscopic examination of the lateral, oblique, and anteroposterior (AP) views of the cervical spine. The slight flexion, rather than extension, of the cervical spine moves the vertebral artery away from the intervertebral foramina. After the

surgical area is prepared routinely, local anesthesia is injected at the point of needle penetration. The usual puncture site for the C2 foramen is located 1 cm below the mastoid process (Figure 106-5).

A hollow 20-gauge needle with a short bevel and tip, completely insulated except for 5 mm of the tip (Radionics, Inc., Burlington, Massachusetts) is used. The position of the needle is adjusted and the needle advanced under fluoroscopic control in the lateral view. In this view the target posterior ganglion is the midpoint on the rostrocaudal axis and in the dorsal one third of the foramen. On the AP view it is 0 to 2 mm medial to the medial edge of the facet (pedicle) and 2 mm caudal to the caudal margin of the inferior pedicle (Figures 106-6 and 106-7). When the needle is placed in the target, it is gently aspirated. Occasionally, cerebrospinal fluid escapes through the needle, indicating that the tip of the needle is in the subarachnoid space. In this case the needle should be withdrawn about 1 mm and its position rechecked with the image intensifier. The stylet is then replaced with a thermocouple electrode and the nerve root electrically stimulated twice per second by a biphasic square-wave pulse 1 msec in duration at less than 1.0 V. Appropriate sensory or muscle responses should be obtained at less than 0.5 V if the probe is in direct contact with nerve fibers (Table 106-2).

Ground electrodes are placed away from the affected dermatome or myotome. If muscle contraction is observed and the pain response is reproduced, the final position of the electrode is confirmed fluoroscopically. An initial trial at 50° to 70°C is used for a period of 15 seconds, with clinical monitoring. Then a total of 90 to 120 seconds is given. The electrode is then removed and a small pressure dressing applied to the puncture site.

When the electrode tip is in the subarachnoid space it is difficult to generate a temperature sufficient for denervation. Care should be taken not to puncture the vertebral artery when the needle is advanced into the target, as described above, under careful fluoroscopic control. This technique cannot be applied to the atlanto-occipital joint because the vertebral artery takes a redundant course in this area (Figure 106-8) and can be injured. To insert the electrode in the remaining cervical foramen, except for C2, an oblique view of the cervical spine is helpful. Electrothermocoagulation of the level below C6 and the first four thoracic roots should be carried out with extreme caution to avoid injuring the important large radicular arteries. The position of the shoulder muscles and scapula may interfere with the needle puncture and make the procedure more difficult. Open surgical rhizotomy may therefore be a safer approach for this particular region (Figures 106-9, 106-10, and 106-11).

THORACIC RHIZOTOMY

The patient is placed on a fluoroscopic operating table in the prone position with a pillow under the abdomen and the arms hanging over the table. If the upper thoracic nerves are to be blocked, a pillow should be placed under the upper chest and the patient's head should be hanging off the pillow, downward. By palpation and under the image intensifier, the anatomic relationships of the following bony landmarks are studied: the spinous processes, the costotransverse and facet joints on the anteroposterior view, and the intervertebral foramina on the lateral view. The outline of the structure is traced on the skin with methylene blue to determine the entering point, direction, and angulation of the probe to the target foramen. It is helpful to know that in the thoracic region the spinous process of one

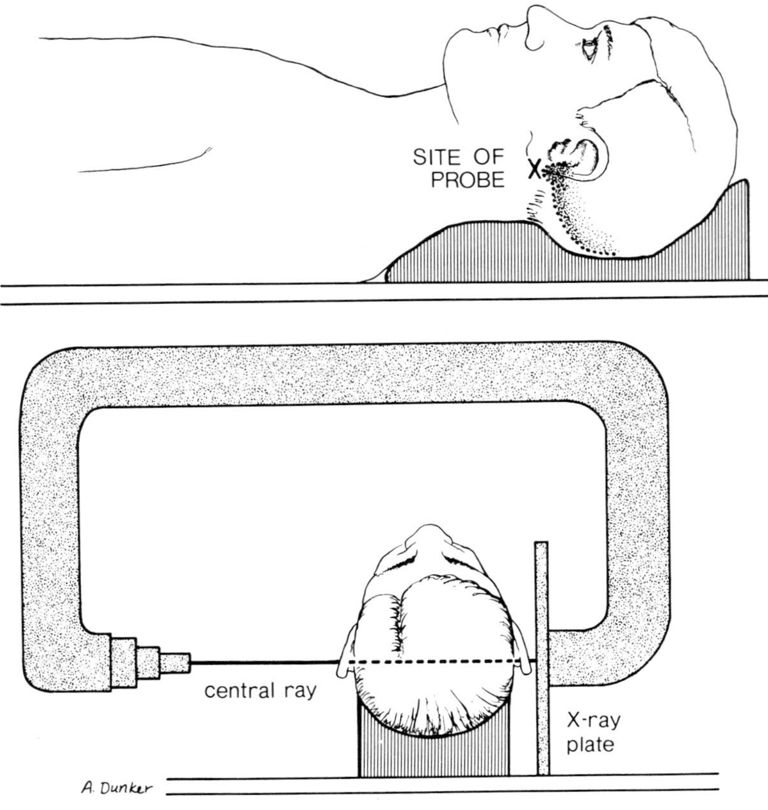

Fig. 106-5. The neck is slightly flexed for C2 rhizotomy. This moves the vertebral artery away from the intervertebral foramina.

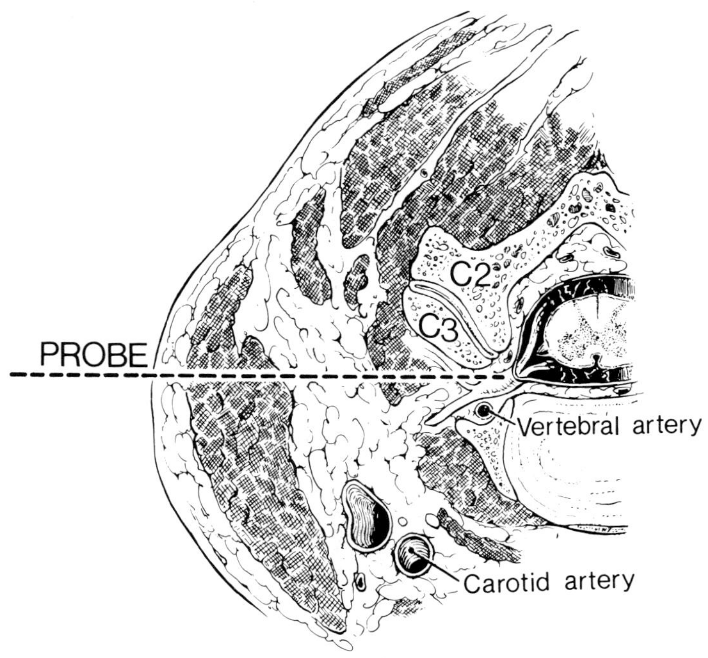

Fig. 106-6. Cross-section at the C2 foramen and the direction of the needle.

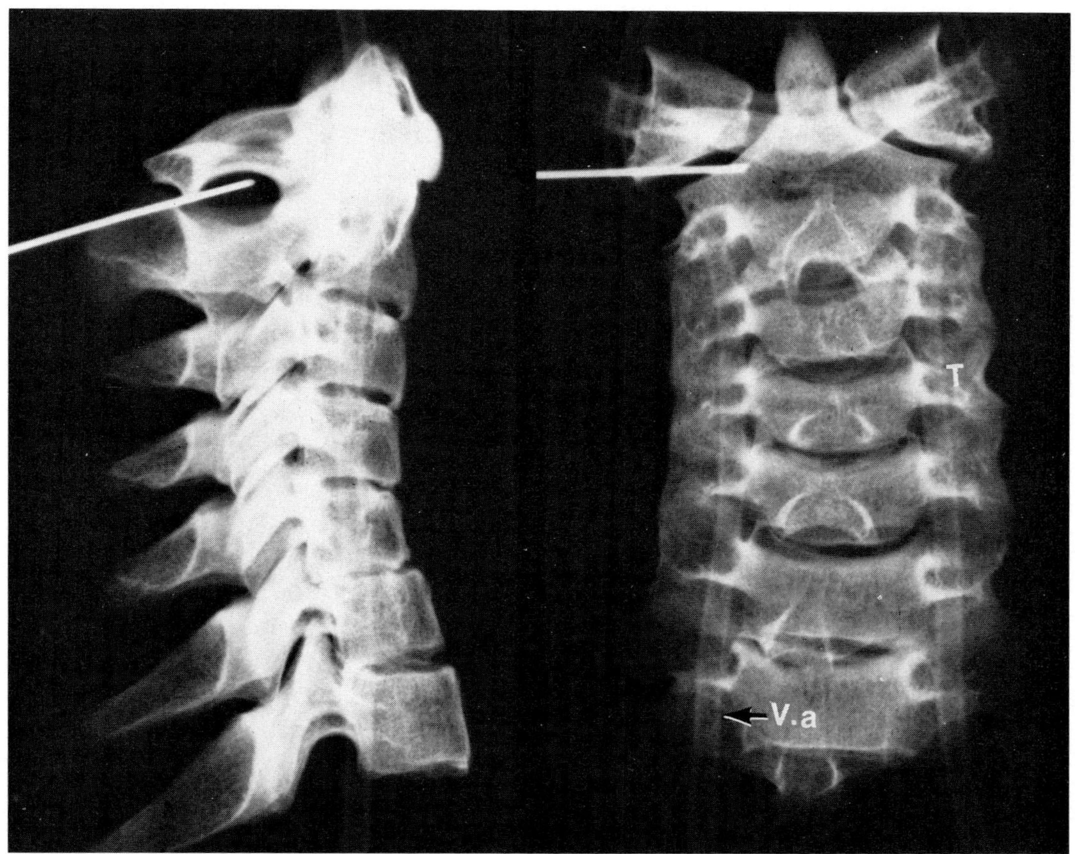

Fig. 106-7. Relationship of the needle to the C2 foramen (x-ray film of a specimen of the cervical spine). V. a = vertebral artery.

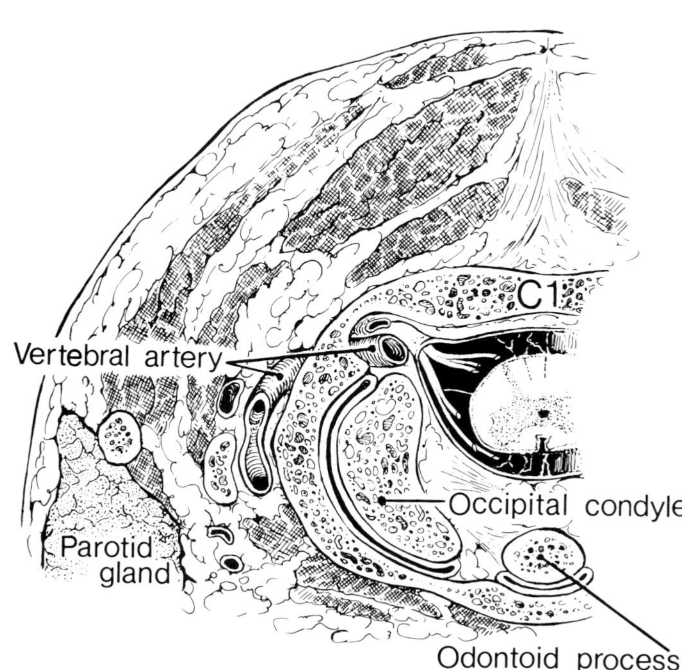

Fig. 106-8. Cross-section at the atlanto-occipital joint. Note the proximity of the vertebral artery and the C1 nerve root.

Table 106-2. Sensory and motor responses at less than 0.5 V with probe in direct contact with nerve fibers

C2	Trapezius
C3	Trapezius
C4	Supraspinatus
C5	Deltoid
C6	Biceps brachii
C7	Triceps
C8	Movement of thumb
T1	Movement of 5th finger
T2 to T5	Sensory response radiating pain to anterior chest wall at appropriate dermatome. Intercostal muscle contraction is often difficult to observe due to subcutaneous adipose tissue
T6 to T12	Abdominal muscle
L1 to L3	Iliopsoas and adductor muscle group of the thigh
L4	Hamstring, quadriceps femoris
L5	Peroneus
S1	Adductor hallucis
S2	Movement of 5th toe
S3 to S5	Sphincter ani

Modified from Raymond CT, Carpenter MB: *Human Neuroanatomy*, ed 6. Baltimore, Williams & Wilkins, 1969, pp 196–198

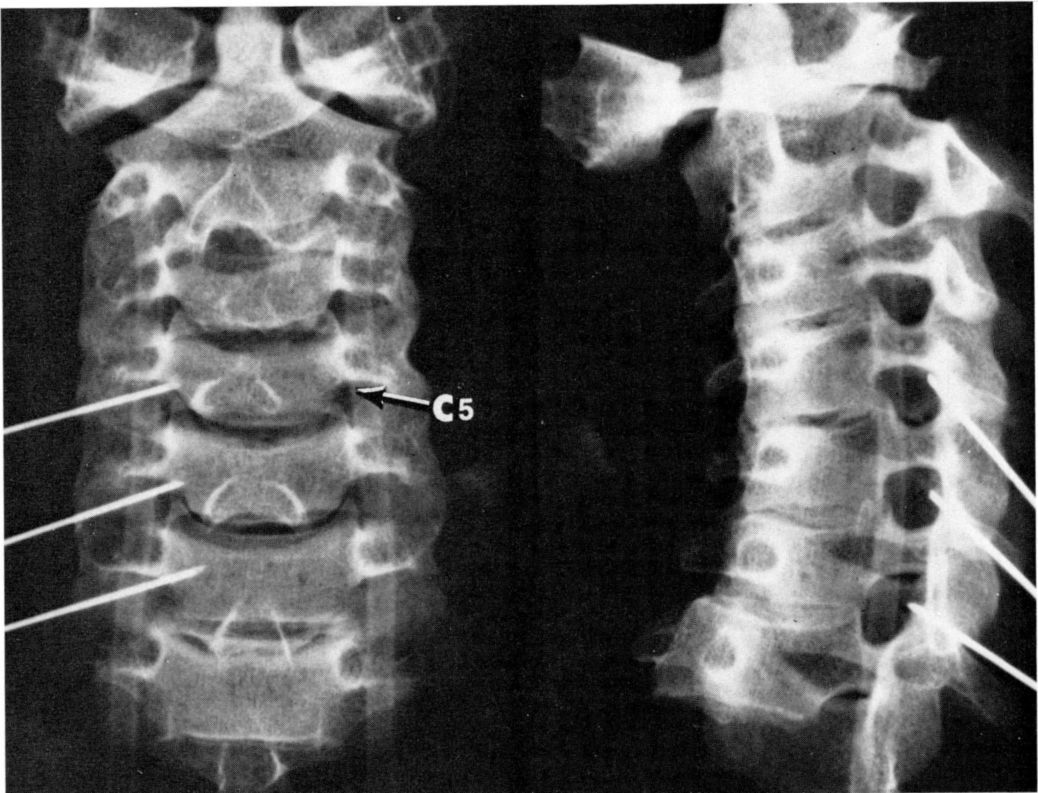

Fig. 106-9.　Relationship of the needles to the lower cervical foramina (oblique x-ray view on the left).

vertebra lies in a line with those of the vertebra immediately below it. For example, the superior edge of the tip of the sixth thoracic vertebra lies in a line with the transverse processes of the seventh thoracic vertebrae (Figures 106-12 and 106-13).

Under fluoroscopic control in the AP view, a line is traced from the head of the transverse process of the vertebra one level below the target foramen to the neck of the transverse process of the target vertebra. For example, using the sixth thoracic vertebra as the target, a line is drawn from the head of the transverse process of the seventh vertebra to the neck of the transverse process of the sixth thoracic vertebra. The needle entry point is approximately 3.5 to 5 cm from the midline of the

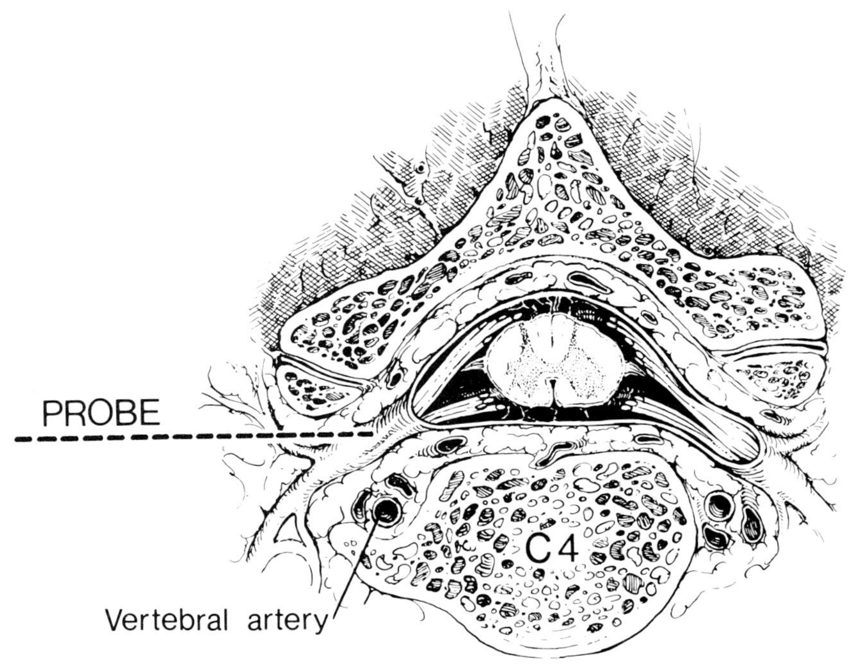

Fig. 106-10.　Cross-section at the C4 foramen and the direction of the needle.

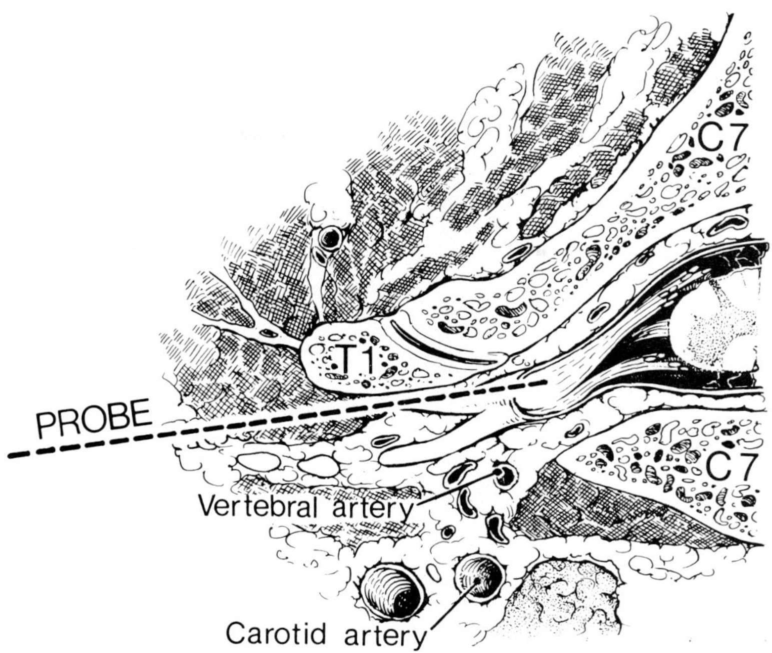

Fig. 106-11. Cross-section at the C7 foramen and the direction of the needle.

vertebral body one level below the target. A local anesthetic is injected and the guiding needle advanced so that it impinges on the head of the transverse process. The needle is then angled toward the neck of the transverse process of the target foramen. Under lateral fluoroscopic control, the target foramen is identified and the needle is then carefully advanced into it. The target, in the AP view, is located 2 to 3 mm caudal to the caudal edge of the facet joint (Figure 106-14).

After the needle is placed in the target, an attempt should always be made to gently aspirate for spinal fluid and blood. If cerebrospinal fluid is observed, the needle is withdrawn 1 to 2 mm. Often the needle tip impinges on the wall of the foramen (pedicle) before it is advanced deeply enough, and multiple attempts to introduce the needle should be avoided. The patient frequently reports radiating pain along the appropriate intercostal nerve to the anterior chest or abdominal wall.

The thermoprobe is introduced after the position of the needle is confirmed. Electrode stimulation is then applied, using the same parameters described for cervical rhizotomy. After the proper location of the needle is confirmed by muscle contraction and by reproducing the pain, trial thermocoagulation is applied at a temperature of 40° to 50°C for 15 seconds, carefully observing flexion and extension movements of all toes, bilaterally, throughout the treatment period. Treatment is given in increments up to a total of 90 to 120 seconds; a maximum temperature of less than 74°C is applied for denervation of pain fibers.

If the needle enters or touches the pleura, the patient may cough while the needle is being advanced or during heating. The needle should not be inserted lateral to the transverse processes nor ventral to the foramen.

As soon as the procedure is completed, chest x-ray films are taken. Two hours after the procedure, follow-up films are taken to be certain that there is no pneumothorax. The patient should be kept under observation in the recovery room for a minimum of 2 hours. Since blood pressure may fall after

multiple roots are denervated, particularly in elderly patients, blood pressure and pulse are closely monitored.

INTERCOSTAL NERVE DENERVATION

Intercostal nerves and vessels lie in the intercostal spaces. The nerves lie a little below the blood vessels. The intercostal

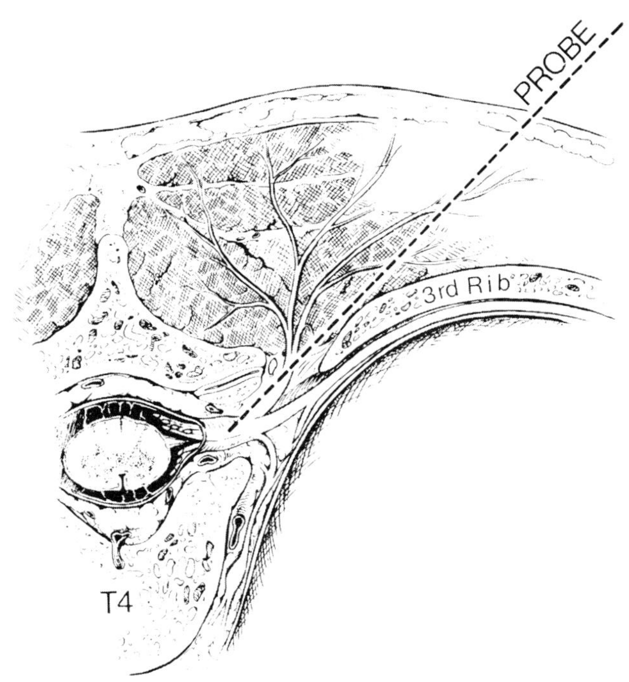

Fig. 106-12. Cross-section at the T4 foramen and the direction of the needle.

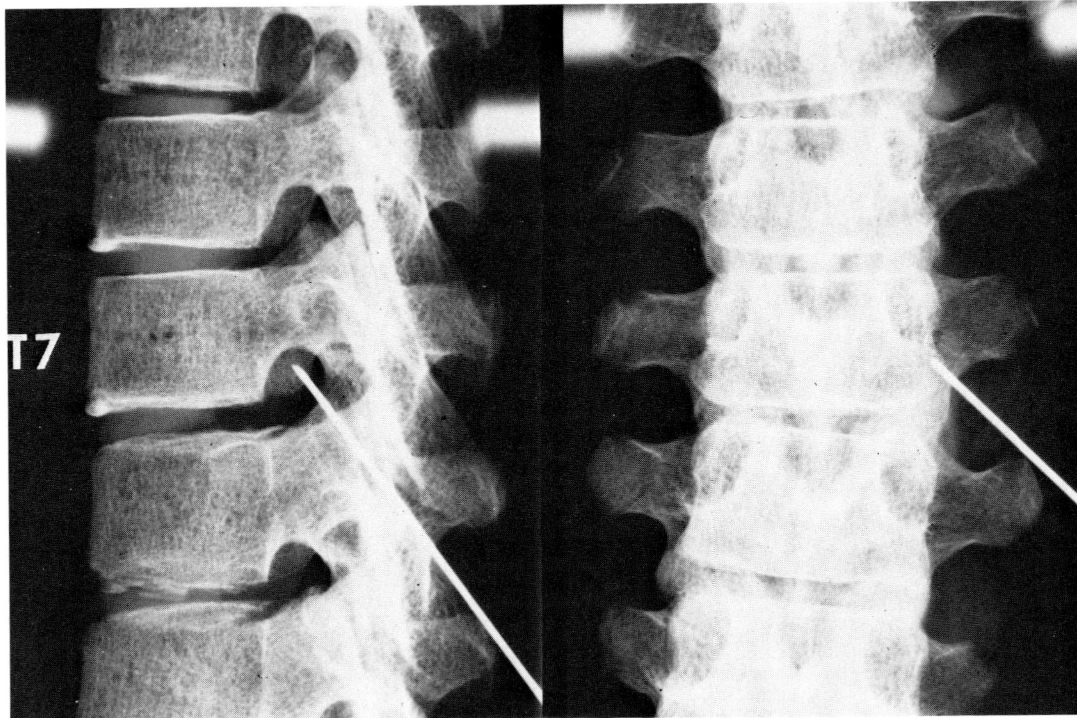

Fig. 106-13. The needle is impinged to the head of the transverse process that is one level below the target foramen and is directed to the target foramen of the thoracic spine.

nerve lies between the pleura and the posterior intercostal membrane, proximal to the angle of the ribs. In the region of the posterior axillary line, the nerves lie between the two muscle layers of the internal and external intercostal muscles. They continue forward in this relationship toward the front of the thorax. The lower six intercostal nerves, at the anterior end of the intercostal space, pass into the abdominal muscles.

The most important branch of each intercostal nerve, from the standpoint of denervation, is the lateral cutaneous. It arises from the intercostal nerve just anterior to the midaxillary line, pierces the external intercostal and anterior serratus muscles, and then divides into anterior and posterior cutaneous branches. Therefore, if the intercostal nerves are not blocked posteriorly or around the posterior axillary line, it is very easy to miss the lateral cutaneous branch and adequate analgesia will not occur. The rib, at this angle, is approximately 0.6 cm thick (Figure 106-15).

Under local anesthesia, at the junction of the posterior axillary line and the inferior edge of the ribs, a 20-gauge needle, as described for cervical rhizotomy, impinges on the ribs at their inferior margin. Then the tip of the needle slides into the visceral aspect of the ribs, only 2 to 3 mm deep from the inner aspect of the rib. At this point, stimulation by 0.2 to 0.5 V, at a rate of 2/sec, is applied to determine the proper location of the needle. After the location is confirmed, incremental heat lesions are made, as described previously. Vital signs should be monitored for 2 hours.[18]

LUMBAR RHIZOTOMY

The patient is placed on the operating table in the lateral recumbent position, with the affected side up. The entry point

of the needle is determined by fluoroscopy in the lateral view. The foramina are easily visualized in this view. The needle entry point is usually 4 cm from the midline and the target point of the intervertebral foramen is located in the slightly rostral portion of the intervertebral disc space. The needle is advanced into the dorsal one third of the foramen. When it is 10 mm away from the target, the x-ray tube is relocated for an anteroposterior examination to advance the needle the remaining depth.

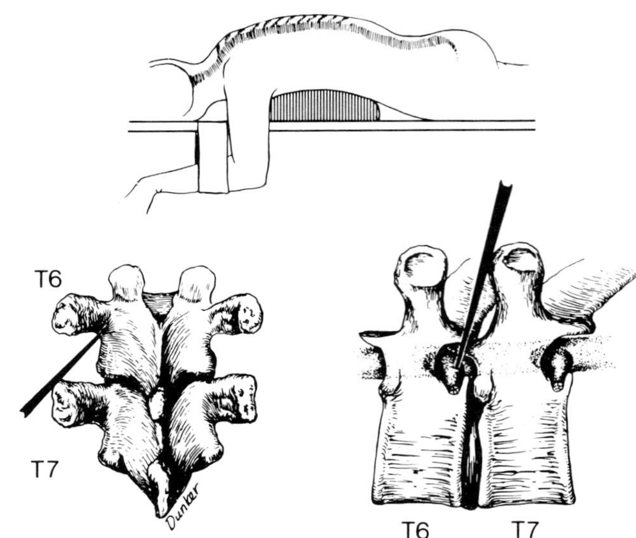

Fig. 106-14. An artist's view of the direction, angulation, and puncture site of the needle for introduction into the thoracic intervertebral foramen.

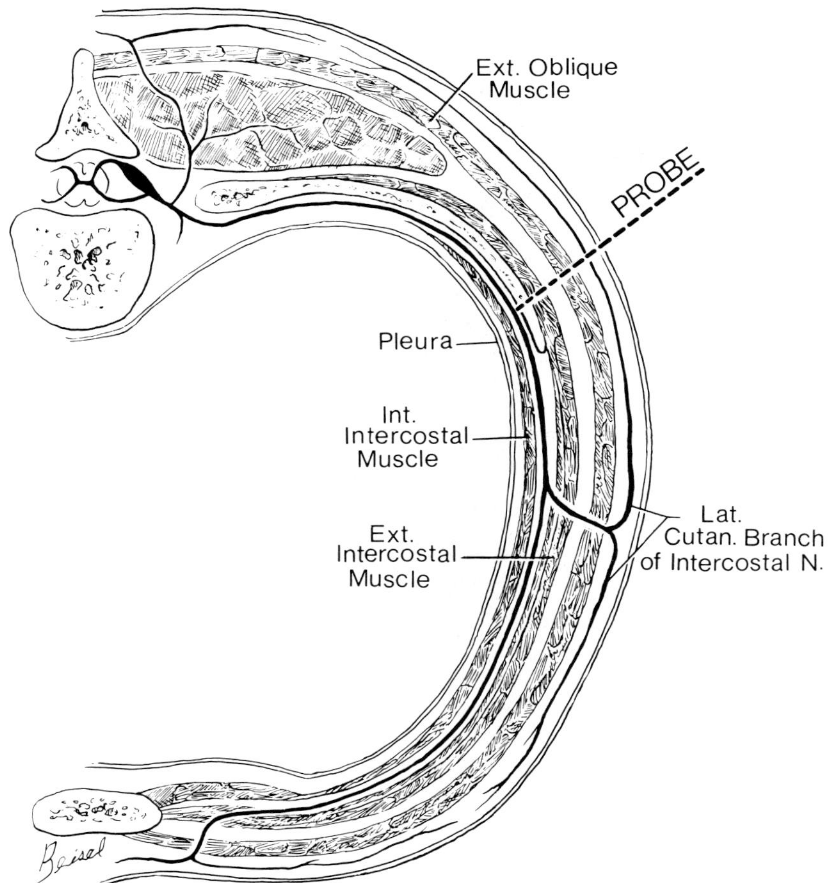

Fig. 106-15. A probe at the posterior axillar line. Note the lateral cutaneous branches.

The target, in the anteroposterior view, is located 0 to 2 mm medial to the medial edge of the facet joint and 2 to 3 mm caudal to the caudal edge of the joint (Figures 106-16 and 106-17).

When the needle is placed in the target, an attempt is always made to gently aspirate for spinal fluid or blood. If cerebrospinal fluid is observed, the needle is withdrawn 1 to 2 mm.

A thermoprobe is introduced after the position of the needle is confirmed. Electrode stimulation is then tried, using the same parameters as described for cervical rhizotomy. After proper muscle contraction and reproduction of pain, trial thermocoagulation is performed with a temperature of 40° to 50°C for 15 seconds. Flexion and extension of the toes, bilaterally, are observed during the entire treatment period. This treatment is then given in increments to a total of 90 to 120 seconds, with a maximum temperature of less than 74°C. It is more important to observe muscle contraction in the lower extremity than in the paravertebral muscles, since the latter could result from direct muscle rather than nerve-root stimulation. Particular care should be taken to avoid injuring the Adamkiewicz artery, which is in the vicinity of T11 to L1. In my opinion, rhizotomy of lumbar or lower cervical nerve roots to alleviate discogenic chronic pain should be used only in patients who already have a sensory or motor impairment, so that the procedure does not increase the degree of disability. It should not be done in patients with chronic pain who have normal sensory and motor functions of the extremity.

THE FIFTH LUMBAR AND SACRAL RHIZOTOMY

The patient is placed in the prone position with a large pillow under the abdomen, at the level of the iliac crest, to

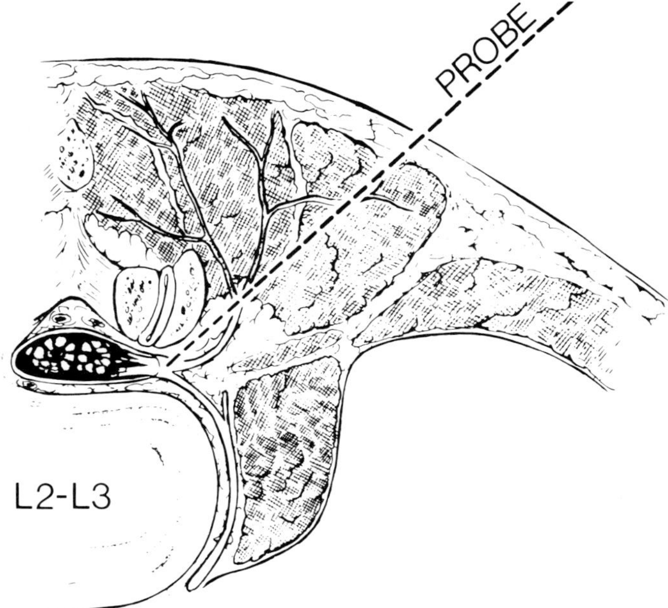

Fig. 106-16. Cross-section of the L2 foramen and the direction of the needle.

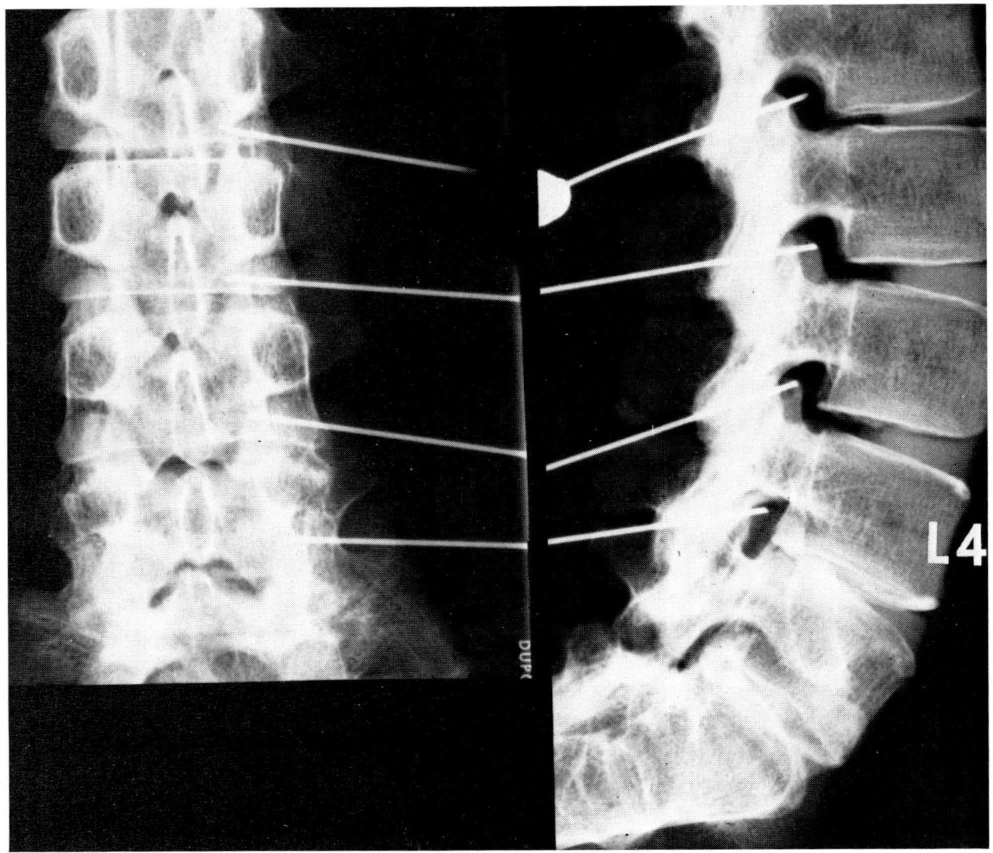

Fig. 106-17. Relationship of the needle to the first, second, third, and fourth lumbar intervertebral foramen as viewed on an x-ray film.

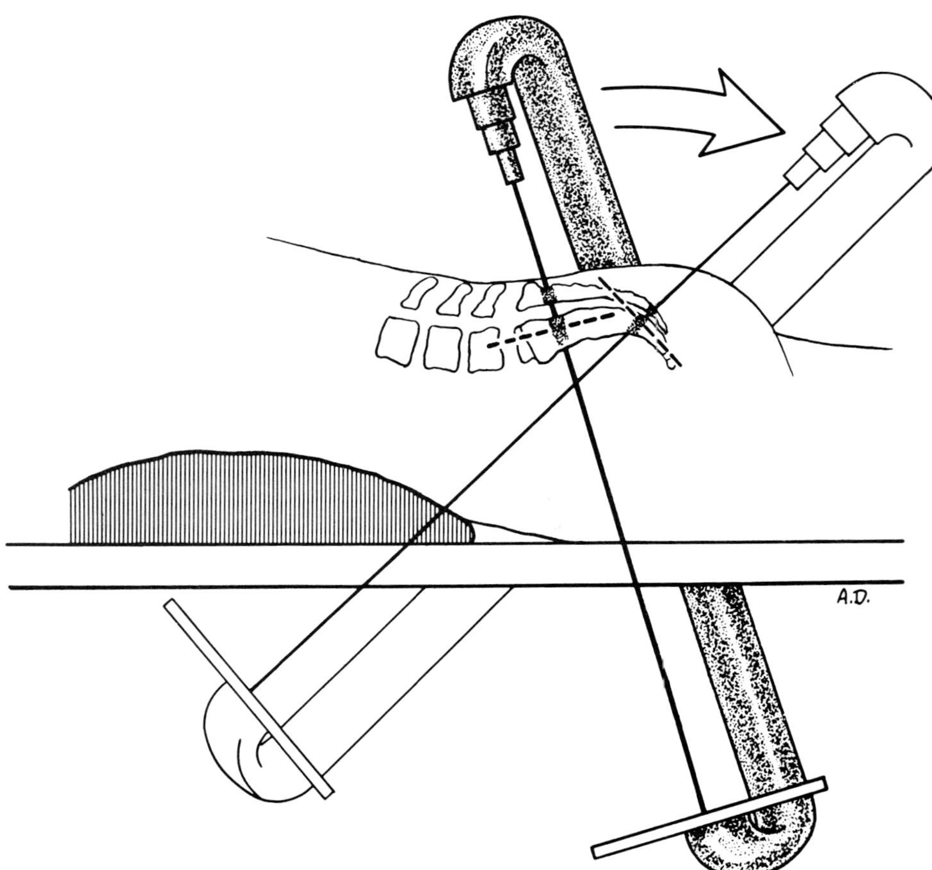

Fig. 106-18. (A) Artist's view of the position of the patient for a sacral rhizctomy. Note the x-ray beam directed at a 90-degree angle toward the longitudinal axis of the sacral spine., This enables fluoroscopic visualization of the sacral foramina.

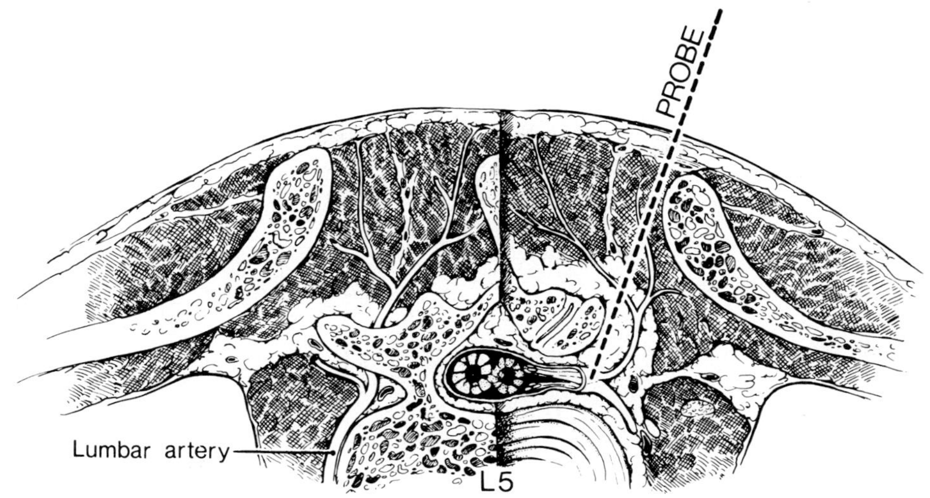

Fig. 106-19. Cross-section at the level of the L5-S1 foramen; the direction of the needle; and the relationship of the needle to the L5 root. Note that the posterior superior iliac spine interferes with the entry of the needle.

create flexion of the lumbosacral joint. This is particularly important for denervation of the fifth lumbar root. An antero-posterior view by fluoroscopic examination locates the fifth lumbar and sacral intervertebral foramina. The x-ray beam must be directed at a 90° angle to the longitudinal axis of the sacral spine (Figure 106-18) to visualize the posterior and anterior sacral foramina. The same type of needle as described previously is introduced through the prepared and anesthetized skin into the posterior surface of the sacrum, just next to the target foramen. This procedure permits the operator to estimate needle depth so that it can be advanced farther through the foramen. The needle then is relocated and aimed at the center of the target foramen, under x-ray control. For fifth-lumbar denervation, the trunk of the nerve is the target. The rootlets and ganglion cannot be reached because the iliac crest and posterior superior spine of the pelvis interfere. The needle enters at the medial edge of the posterior superior iliac spine and is aimed toward the neck of the fifth lumbar transverse process. At times it is difficult to insert the needle because of lumbosacralization or arthritic changes. The depth of the needle is determined by a lateral-view fluoroscopic examination. It is always important to aspirate for blood or spinal fluid before performing local block anesthesia or electrothermocoagulation (Figures 106-19, 106-20, and 106-21). A sponge is placed between the gluteal folds to prevent the antiseptic solution from spilling over the perineum, which would burn the patient.

The patients included in this report had neurologic disorders causing detrusor hyperreflexia. Patients were selected for evaluation if they had one or more of the following conditions: involuntary precipitous micturition, a short interval between catheterization or voiding, and autonomic hyperreflexia. Baseline urodynamic studies included cystometry, anal sphincter electromyography, and a urethral pressure profile. Patients with low-threshold detrusor hyperreflexia were evaluated further with sacral blocks. Various combinations of S2, S3, and S4 nerve roots were anesthetized at the anterior sacral foramen with 1 to 2 ml of bupivacaine hydrochloride injected through the posterior sacral foramen under fluoroscopic control. The initial block included S2, S3, and S4 nerve roots bilaterally to ascertain potential maximum bladder capacity. Patients with fibrotic

bladders not distensible to a capacity of 200 ml were not considered for sacral rhizotomy. Urodynometry was repeated within 1 hour of the sacral block. During the next 8 to 12 hours, the interval between catheterization or voiding, the volume of urine obtained, and each occurrence of involuntary micturition and autonomic hyperreflexia were recorded. Male patients who could obtain a penile erection before the block were asked to determine the effect of the block upon erection. If the bladder

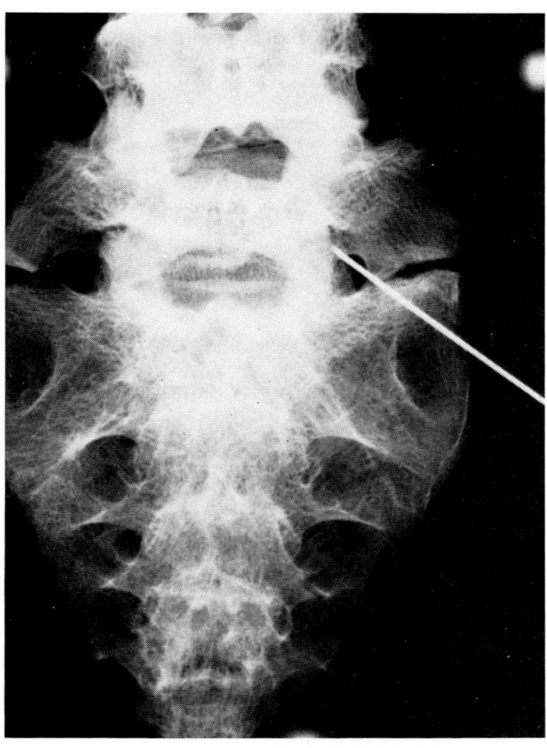

Fig. 106-20. Direction of the needle and its relationship to the fifth lumbar foramen as viewed on an x-ray film.

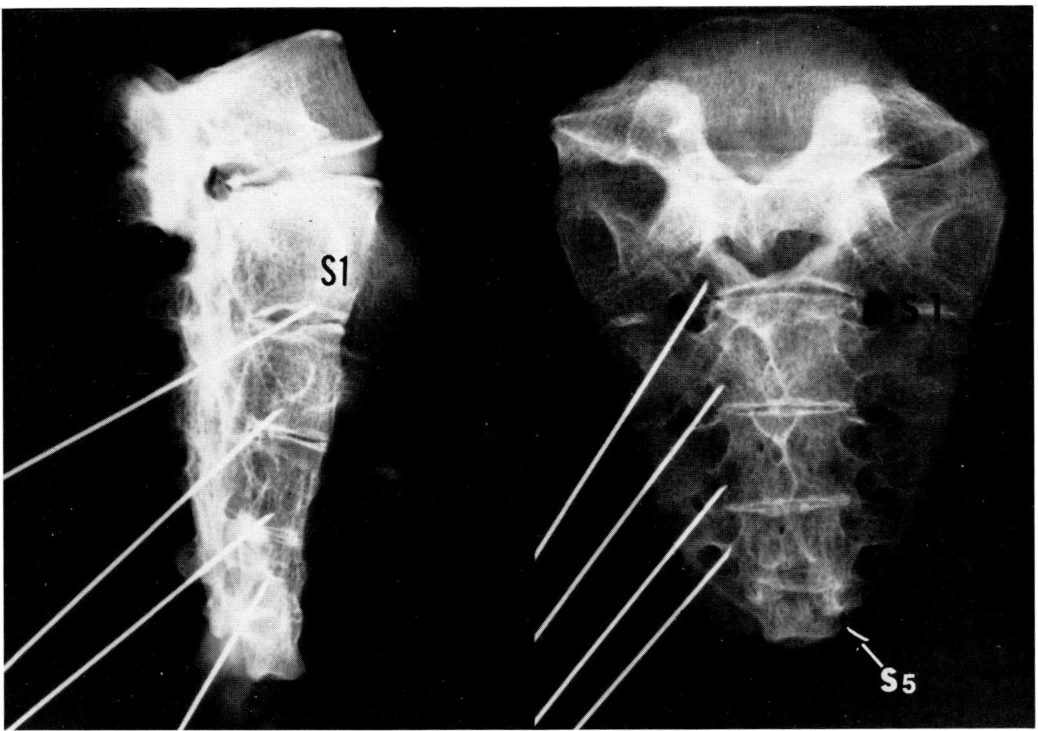

Fig. 106-21.   Relationship of the needle to the first, second, third, and fourth sacral foramina as viewed on an x-ray film.

capacity after the block was increased to at least 200 ml, serial blocks were performed on successive days to determine the predominant roots innervating the detrusor muscle. Percutaneous radiofrequency rhizotomy was performed at the sacral levels providing the predominant bladder nerve supply. When bladder capacity was not increased to at least 200 ml by the rhizotomy, the procedure was repeated or additional roots electrocoagulated.

The procedure was performed by inserting a No. 12 needle with stylet into the selected sacral foramen with the aid of anteroposterior and lateral fluoroscopy. An electrode (1.1 mm in diameter, with a 5-mm tip exposure and a thermistor temperature sensor) was advanced through the No. 12 needle to the anterior foramen. The radiofrequency electrocoagulation lesion was made at a temperature of 70° to 80°C for 3 minutes at each preselected level at the anterior sacral foramen. Stimulation of the nerve root with cystometric monitoring to confirm the accuracy of electrode placement before making the root lesion was later added to the protocol. Frequent fluoroscopic monitoring was done during generation of the lesion to detect any change in the position of the electrode. Particular care was taken to make no lesion anterior to the anterior sacral foramen. Long-term follow-up urodynamic testing was attempted in every case.

Pain secondary to carcinoma of the rectum, with colostomy and loss of bladder control, may be treated by denervation of the second, third, and fourth sacral roots. Bladder function should be monitored cystometrically for denervation of the second, third, and fourth sacral roots when bladder and bowel function are intact.[12] The fifth, fourth, and third roots can be reached through the sacral hiatus. Electrical stimulation and fluoroscopic examination are used to guide the probe toward the target root or ganglion (Figure 106-22).

SUMMARY

A relatively simple technique for interrupting root, ganglion, trunk, and nerve is described as an alternative to open rhizotomy. Clinical observations of trigeminal rhizotomy support the fact that pain can be relieved and proprioception and motor function preserved with this technique. The simple technique of denervation is now available with the use of radiologic image intensification, electrical stimulation, and temperature control. The procedure can be applied to patients who are debilitated as a result of carcinoma, old age, or both, and can be repeated if necessary. Relief of flexor spasms of the hip joint secondary to traumatic paraplegia is a rewarding experience of this author.

ACKNOWLEDGMENTS

Gratitude is due Dr. David Bodian, Department of Anatomy, for his suggestions and for the preparation of the histologic slides used in Figure 106-1.

My thank go to our secretarial and technical staff, Jean Arnett, Erva Baden, Debbie Gilmer, and Richard Kouba, for their careful and conscientious assistance in the completion of the manuscript.

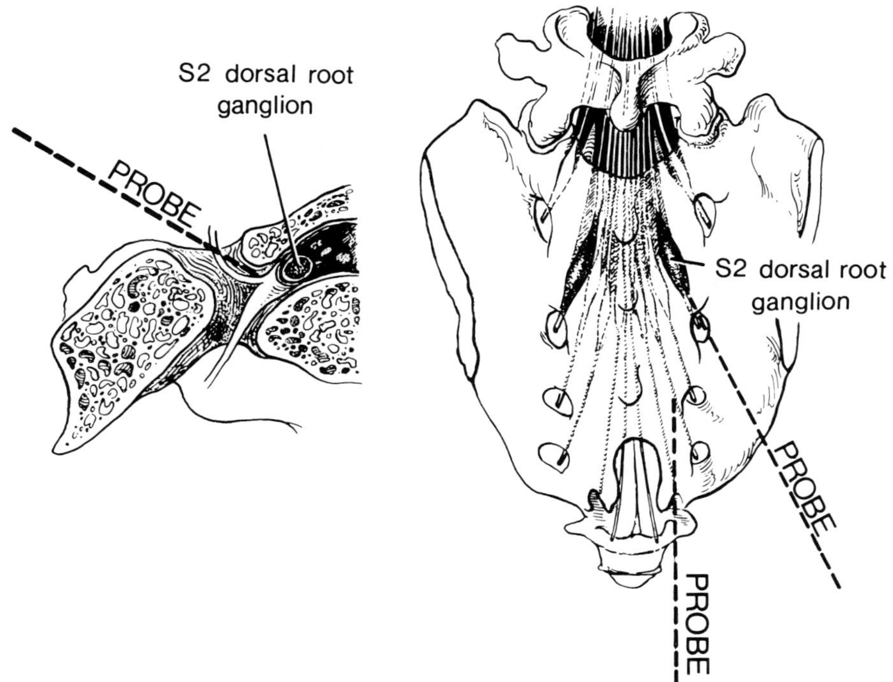

Fig. 106-22. (Left) Cross-section at the level of the second sacral ganglion with a probe inserted through the second sacral foramen. (Right) Superimposed view of the sacral spine with ganglia and roots. Note the probe inserted through the sacral hiatus and its tip in contact with the fifth and fourth root. A second probe is inserted through the second sacral foramen to the second ganglion.

REFERENCES

1. Abbe R: A contribution to the surgery of the spine. Med Rec 35:149, 1889

2. Bennett WH: A case in which antispasmodic pain in the left lower extremity was completely relieved by subdural division of the posterior roots of certain spinal nerves, all other treatment having proved useless. Death from sudden collapse and cerebral hemorrhage on the twelfth day after the operation, at the commencement of apparent convalescence. Med Chir Trans 72:329, 1889

3. Scoville WB: Extradural spinal sensory rhizotomy. J Neurosurg 25:94, 1966

4. Dogliotti AM: Traitement des syndromes douloureux de la peripherie par l'alcholisation subarachnoi dienne des racines posterieures a leur emergence de la moelle epiniere. Presse Med 39:1249, 1931

5. Maher RM: Relief of pain in incurable cancer. Lancet 1:18, 1955

6. White J, Sweet W: Pain and the Neurosurgeon, a 40-Year Experience. Springfield, Ill, Charles C Thomas, 1969, p 662

7. Kirschner M: Die Behandlung der Trigeminus Neuralgie (Nach Erfahrungen an 1113 Kranken). MMW 38:235, 1942

8. Sweet W, Wepsic J: Controlled thermocoagulation of trigeminal ganglion and rootlets for differential destruction of pain fibers. Part 1: Trigeminal neuralgia. J Neurosurg 40:143, 74

9. Uematsu S, Udvarhelyi G, Benson DW, et ai: Percutaneous radiofrequency rhizotomy. Surg Neurol 2:319, 1974

10. Hamby WB, Schiffer: Spasmodic torticollis: Results after cervical rhizotomy in 50 cases. J Neurosurg 31:323, 1969

11. Heimburger R, Slominski O, Griswold P: Cervical posterior rhizotomy for reducing spasticity in cerebral palsy. J Neurosurg 39:30, 1973

12. Rockwold G, Bradley W, Chou S: Differential sacral rhizotomy in the treatment of neurogenic bladder dysfunction. Preliminary report of six cases. J Neurosurg 38:748, 1973

13. Vakili H: The Spinal Cord. New York, Intercontinental Medical Book Corp., p 20

14. Djindjian R, Hurth M, Houdart R, et al: Angiography of the Spinal Cord. Baltimore, University Park Press, 1970, pp 3–10

15. Onofrio BM, Campa HK: Evaluation of rhizotomy. Review of 12 years experience. J Neurosurg 36:751, 1972

16. Pawl P: Percutaneous radiofrequency electrocoagulation in the control of chronic pain. Surg Clin North Am 55:167, 1975

17. Krayenbühl N, et al (ed): Advances and Technical Standard in Neurosurgery, vol 2. New York, Springer Verlag, 1975

18. Moore DC: Regional Block, Handbook for Use in the Clinical Practice of Medicine and Surgery. Springfield, Ill, Charles C Thomas, 1953, pp 113–150

19. White JC: Posterior rhizotomy: A possible substitute for cordotomy in otherwise intractable neuralgias of the trunk and extremities of nonmalignant origin. Clin Neurosurg 13:20, 1966

20. Young B, Mulcahy JJ: Percutaneous sacral rhizotomy. J Neurosurg 53:85, 1980

CHAPTER 107

Surgery of Epilepsy—Current Technique of Cortical Resection

Robert R. Hansebout

DESCRIPTIONS OF THE FALLING SICKNESS are found in the writings of humans since the dawn of recorded history. Fortunately, as a result of the greater understanding of brain physiology that has developed during the past 100 years, attempts at cures for epilepsy have been elevated from those forms with an aura of mysticism and superstition to forms that are more medically oriented.

Although the earliest attempts and successes at reducing seizures appear to have been surgical, the advent of modern drug therapy has allowed many epileptics to become productive. Still, current drugs may be toxic or not tolerated by some,[1] and may fail to control seizures in another 20 percent of epileptics.[2] It is estimated that about 1 in 200 persons today has epilepsy and that 10 percent of the population would be amendable to surgery.[2]

Among the surgical procedures used in the treatment of epilepsy, selective cortical resection has earned its place and has been used at an increasing number of neurosurgical centers during the past few years.[3] The following will illustrate salient features of that procedure.

OVERALL CONCEPTION OF THE TECHNIQUE

In 1870, J. Hughlings Jackson first recognized that epilepsy could be the result of a sudden excessive electrical discharge of a focus in the gray matter in the brain. The experimental demonstration of functional localization in the cortex by Fritsch and associates confirmed Jackson's observations. In his book, published in 1881, William Gowers indicated that cerebral seizures either could be secondary to structural lesions of the brain or idiopathic, in which case there was no visible lesion.[4]

Otfrid Foerster, after World War I, successfully carried out a number of cortical resections in posttraumatic epileptic patients with focal lesions.[5] Wilder Penfield's scholarly elaboration of cortical function based on studies using electrical stimulation during a large series of operations for epilepsy, coupled with Herbert Jasper's neurophysiologic expertise, fully established the usefulness of cortical resection in the neurosurgical armamentarium.[6] Theodore Rasmussen's meticulous surgical technique and analytic observations have broadened the scope and safety of the procedure.[3,7]

Causes of the focal seizure discharge in both adults and children range from tumors and vascular anomalies to scars and atrophic lesions. Such an atrophic cortex was most often found in the medial temporal lobe.[8] This *incisural sclerosis,* as it was termed by the Montreal school, was thought to be due to birth injury, while Falconer associated this *mesial sclerosis* mainly with febrile illness and infantile seizures.[8,9] The seizures could be alleviated by removing the abnormal brain tissue.[10]

In early series discrete cicatricial lesions were surgically removed in nontumoral cases of epilepsy,[5] but subsequently, it became clear that the area of epileptogenic brain tissue usually was larger than the structural abnormality and often was composed of several areas of varying epileptogenicity. When cortex in the region of maximum electrographic abnormality is removed, seizures often cease completely. In other cases seizures then can arise from adjacent cortex, again with lower than normal thresholds for epileptogenicity. It was found that the more complete the removal of epileptogenic brain tissue, the greater the likelihood that the seizure tendency would be abolished.[3] Moreover, initial surgery abolished or reduced seizures, which later recurred or increased in frequency in a few patients. After a second operation and the removal of more epileptogenic cortex, one half of these patients became seizure-free or had a reduced seizure tendency.[3]

Therefore, in patients with drug-refractory focal seizures the current philosophy is to localize the epileptogenic area clinically by electroencephalogram and ancillary methods. Surgery may be considered if this area is deemed to be resectable. The epileptogenic brain tissue is mapped visually, electroencephalographically, and by stimulation during surgery. As much abnormal epileptogenic cortex as possible is removed that is compatible with the least risk of causing or increasing a neurologic deficit.[3]

CRITERIA FOR PATIENT SELECTION

Seizures are a symptom of brain dysfunction, and therefore other entities, such as metabolic disturbances and brain tumor, must be excluded before it is presumed that the patient has a static lesion that requires treatment for the seizure tendency alone. Surgical treatment then is considered according to the following criteria:

1. The patient must have had an adequate trial of maximally tolerable doses of medications without a degree of control adequate to lead a fairly normal life, or must be intolerant to medications. The seizures may interfere with psychologic

OPERATIVE NEUROSURGICAL TECHNIQUES
ISBN 0-8089-1862-1

and intellectual development, preclude employment, or be sufficiently severe to pose a threat of mental deterioration to warrant surgical consideration. Surgery is considered only when all potentially epileptogenic areas have matured, the seizure tendency is stable, and, furthermore, there is no tendency toward spontaneous regression, especially in posttraumatic epilepsy.[11,12] Surgery rarely is advisable until recurrent seizures have been present for 3 to 4 years and the patient is at least 15 to 16 years old. With the newer anesthetic techniques, however, more patients are now being operated upon in late childhood and their early teens.

2. Clinical and electroencephalographic studies should show that attacks are focal in origin and arise from a dispensable portion of brain. The more consistent the attack pattern, the better the chances that surgical extirpation will succeed. The patient must be strongly motivated to cope with an exhaustive diagnostic regimen and a lengthy operative procedure under local anesthesia.[13,14]

INVESTIGATION

CLINICAL

A careful history, especially regarding evidence of birth trauma, seizures early in life, and other potential causes of epilepsy, is necessary. Whether other family members have epilepsy should be known. Handedness should be ascertained. Questioning about what the patient feels at the beginning of attacks and what observers see may indicate the area of lowest seizure threshold. Phenomena such as transient dysphasia or postictal paresis are of considerable lateralizing value.

The neurologic examination, including visual fields, may be normal in temporal lobe epilepsy or show minimal to marked deficits, especially when other lobes are involved.[14]

RADIOLOGIC

Stereoscopic plain x-ray films of the skull may show smallness or asymmetry of one side, indicating brain atrophy from early life. Pneumoencephalography is the most useful method of evaluating subtle atrophic brain changes. Angiography is performed if the previous studies are normal or if a vascular malformation is suspected. A computed tomogram may show a brain tumor or an area of atrophy not demonstrated on previous studies.[14]

ELECTROENCEPHALOGRAPHIC

The electroencephalogram gives the most useful information on the location and size of the epileptogenic area.[13] An interictal epileptiform abnormality repeated on several occasions may be significant. Recordings with pharyngeal or sphenoidal electrodes are useful in temporal lobe epilepsy.[15]

Activation procedures, such as medication withdrawal, hyperventilation, or drug-induced sleep may enhance abnormalities or even provoke a seizure, the recording of which may elucidate the focus if there is not too much muscle artifact. The intravenous injection of methohexital may enhance the epileptiform abnormality in temporal lobe epilepsy, while the intravenous injection of pentylenetetrazol may provoke the patient's habitual seizures.[15]

The intravenous injection of thiopental (the technique of Lombrosa and Erba) may permit the differentiation of primary (corticoreticular) and secondary bilaterally synchronous epileptiform abnormalities that are the result of a unilateral lesion.[16] The intracarotid injection of amobarbital and pentylenetetrazol has been used in the past to lateralize a unilateral lesion. However, because of the magnitude and potential risk of the procedure, it is now rarely used. Instead, in such cases, telemetric EEG recording of seizures during long-term monitoring of the scalp EEG has superceded the intravenous injection procedure.[17] Sometimes, implanted depth electrodes have been used in such cases. In patients with bitemporal foci, stereotactic depth-electrode studies may identify the most active side when conventional recordings have failed.[15]

Telemetric recordings allow the patient freedom of movement while undergoing prolonged recording to increase the likelihood of detecting interictal epileptiform activity or to document an attack. In conjunction with long-term monitoring, video recording of a patient's spontaneous seizures can be very useful.[18] Computer assistance may increase the effectiveness of recording using telemetry or chronic implanted depth electrodes by reducing the recording time of ictal events.[15]

NEUROPSYCHOLOGIC

Neuropsychologic tests help to confirm the location of the focus, since they usually corroborate clinical and electroencephalographic evidence by elaborating deficits, which vary with the lobe involved and the dominance of the hemisphere. Any discrepancy between psychologic and clinical localization may indicate unusual lateralization of speech or bilateral temporal lobe lesions.[19] The intracarotid sodium amobarbital (Amytal) speech test[20] is done preoperatively when lateralization of speech is uncertain, as in left-handers, ambidextrous persons and right-handers who have had left-hemisphere injury in infancy.[13,19] Preoperative lateralization of speech areas adds to the safety of the cortical resection, since electrical stimulation at the time of surgery may give a false-negative response.

Memory testing also is done during the intracarotid sodium amobarbital speech tests. This is especially important in temporal lobe epilepsy when there is independent epileptiform activity or evidence of injury on the side opposite that of the proposed cortical removal. This test identifies the patient in whom surgery carries with it a risk of memory dysfunction, since one hippocampus can be removed only when the other is functional. Thus when the temporal lobe to be operated upon is inactivated by the intracarotid injection and the opposite unactivated temporal lobe cannot provide good memory function, then the temporal lobectomy must carefully spare the hippocampus and hippocampal gyrus to avoid a serious postoperative memory deficit.[13,19,21]

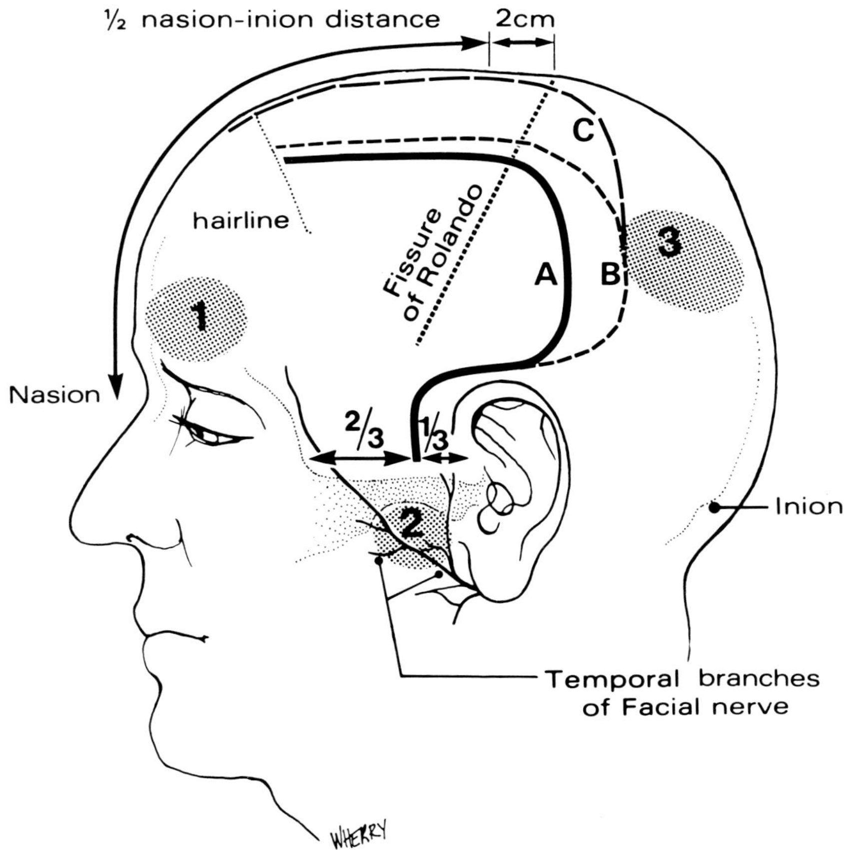

Fig. 107-1. Skin incision for (A) dominant, (B) nondominant, and (C) frontotemporal exposures. 1, 2, and 3 denote points of maximum anesthetic infiltration for major sensory nerves. Note external landmarks for rolandic fissure (central sulcus).

PREOPERATIVE PREPARATION

When surgery is indicated and the patient accepts, it is desirable to have the epileptogenic cortex as active as possible during the operation. Thus, whenever possible, doses of most antiseizure medications are gradually reduced the week before surgery. In patients who have many attacks, an effective but short-lasting anticonvulsant may be continued until the evening before surgery, or until the patient stops all oral intake. Glucocorticoids are begun 24 hours preoperatively. Should an attack occur preoperatively, phenobarbital sodium, 240 mg, can be given by intramuscular injection, or paraldehyde may be given, 10 ml orally or 20 ml rectally.[22]

ANESTHESIA

Whenever possible, local anesthesia, potentiated by analgesic drugs, is used so that motor, speech, and sensory areas can be mapped readily during surgery, a better electrocorticogram can be obtained, and occasionally, auras can be reproduced by stimulation. Under such conditions, motor and speech functions can be tested periodically to assure maximum safety during the removals.[10,23,23]

Atropine (0.4 mg) is given preoperatively. Uncooperative adults and children may require an endotracheal tube and general anesthesia consisting of nitrous oxide, intravenous sodium methohexital (Brevital), fentanyl, and a curariform agent.[24] The nitrous oxide is discontinued before the electrocorticogram, since it obliterates epileptiform activity.[22]

Nupercaine (dibucaine hydrochloride) has proved to be an excellent local anesthesia agent but is no longer available. Lidocaine is suggested as a substitute.[24] Unless there is a medical contraindication, 0.5 ml of 1:1000 epinephrine is added per 125 ml of local anesthetic solution.[20] Lidocaine, 125 ml of a 1 percent solution, is injected into the superficial skin with a 25-gauge needle along the area of the proposed incision, with maximum saturation in the supraorbital, temporal, and occipital regions (Figure 107-1). Then 125 ml of 0.5 percent lidocaine is injected down to the periosteum and in the temporalis fascia and muscle with a 20-gauge needle.[24]

This local anesthesia, fortified by intravenous injections of fentanyl and droperidol, is effective throughout the opening. Other intracranial structures are insensitive to pain, except the dura along the larger meningeal vessels. Here local anesthetic can be injected intradurally with a 27-gauge needle.[10] The patient usually is alert and comfortable throughout the procedure, and is given additional intravenous injections of fentanyl and droperidol as required. If drowsiness ensues, the patient must be roused to check motor and speech functions during cortical resection. Methohexital sodium is given intravenously should a seizure develop at any time.[24] A general anesthetic may become necessary if the patient becomes unruly, espe-

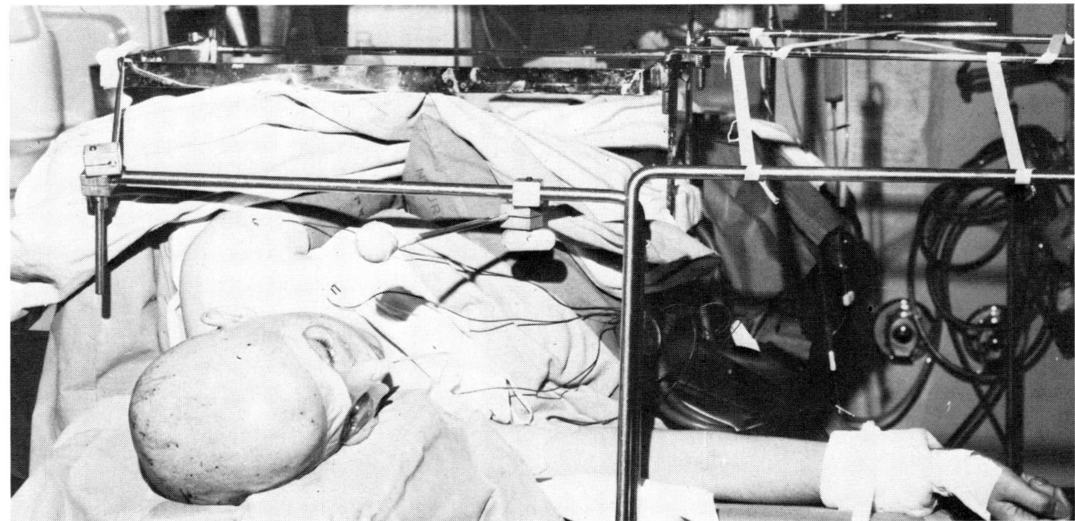

Fig. 107-2. Position for left frontotemporal exposures.

cially after a seizure. A blind transnasal intubation then may be required,[10] and followed by administration of nitrous oxide and intravenous injections of fentanyl and droperidol for balanced anesthesia.[24]

SPECIAL ASPECTS OF THE SURGICAL TECHNIQUE

Surgical techniques for cortical resection are described in detail elsewhere.[7,8,10,22,23,25–27]

POSITIONING

The patient is postured comfortably on the side, with a pillow under the hip and pads protecting other bony prominences. The face is slightly inclined toward the side of the incision. The head of the table is somewhat elevated to reduce venous oozing (Figure 107-2). The skin is sterilized, and a plastic sheet (Pliofilm) is placed around the line of incision. Towels are sutured into place in the anesthetized skin so they do not become dislodged if the patient moves. The anesthetist always has access to the patient's face.

INCISIONS

A generous-sized opening is necessary to afford adequate exposure to map the epileptogenic area and to note its relationship to the central region on either side and the speech areas in the dominant hemisphere. A question-mark incision is the most useful for temporal lobectomy.[9] Adequate incisions for temporal and frontotemporal removals are shown in Figure 107-1. To expose the frontal lobe alone, a C-shaped incision is suggested, with the superior portion at the midline extending up to 2 cm above the frontal sinus and the posterolateral limb extending downward to the level of the zygoma.[22] If the epileptogenic focus is posterior, a C-shaped incision is made with its medial limb in the midline and the lateral limb curved downward to expose the central region.[22]

THE OPENING

A detailed description of the most common cortical resection—partial temporal lobectomy—will follow. The principles are easily modified for cortical resection elsewhere.

The question-mark incision is begun at the superior aspect of the zygoma at the junction of its anterior two thirds and posterior one third (Figure 107-1). If the lowest part of the incision is made too anteroinferior, temporal branches of the facial nerve may be damaged, which causes a frontalis muscle palsy. The superficial temporal artery is coagulated early. The galea is separated from the temporalis fascia for the application of the skin clips. The superior portion of the incision is made down through the periosteum. The temporalis muscle and fascia are divided to the periosteum with electrocautery. Using a periosteal elevator, the skin and muscle are reflected forward over a roll of gauze, and muscle *fishhooks* applied for retraction. Burr holes are made, as in Figure 107-3A. The first two burr holes should be made one above and one below the sphenoid ridge. The intervening bone between these two burr holes is then rongeured away to permit the injection of local anesthetic alongside the middle meningeal vessels. This will permit the placement of the remaining burr holes and elevation of the bone flap with minimum discomfort. Additional sphenoid bone can then be rongeured away to expose the anterior portion of the temporal lobe. Moreover, if a trough is rongeured away inferiorly from each of the two temporal burr holes, access to the inferior temporal region is easier and cosmetic restoration ultimately will be better. A free bone flap provides better exposure and more comfort for the patient than a hinged flap.[22] The edges of the bony opening are waxed. A hole for the electrode post is made along the superior edge of the craniotomy (see Figure 107-7). Dural traction sutures are placed to decrease venous oozing.[7]

The middle meningeal vessels are coagulated and divided. The dura is opened a few millimeters away from the bone edge.

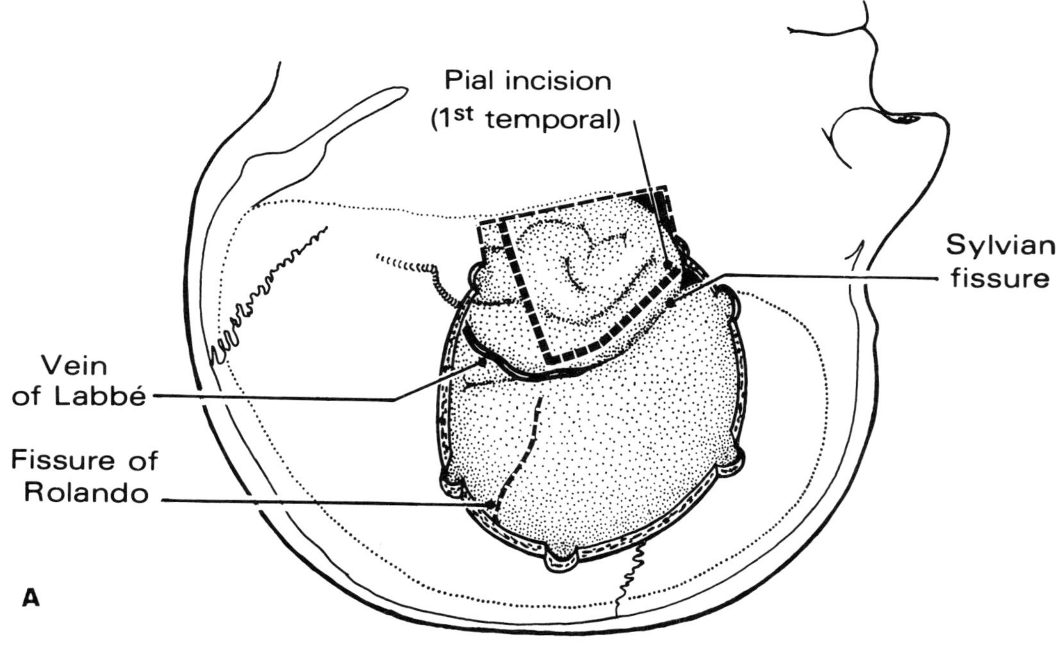

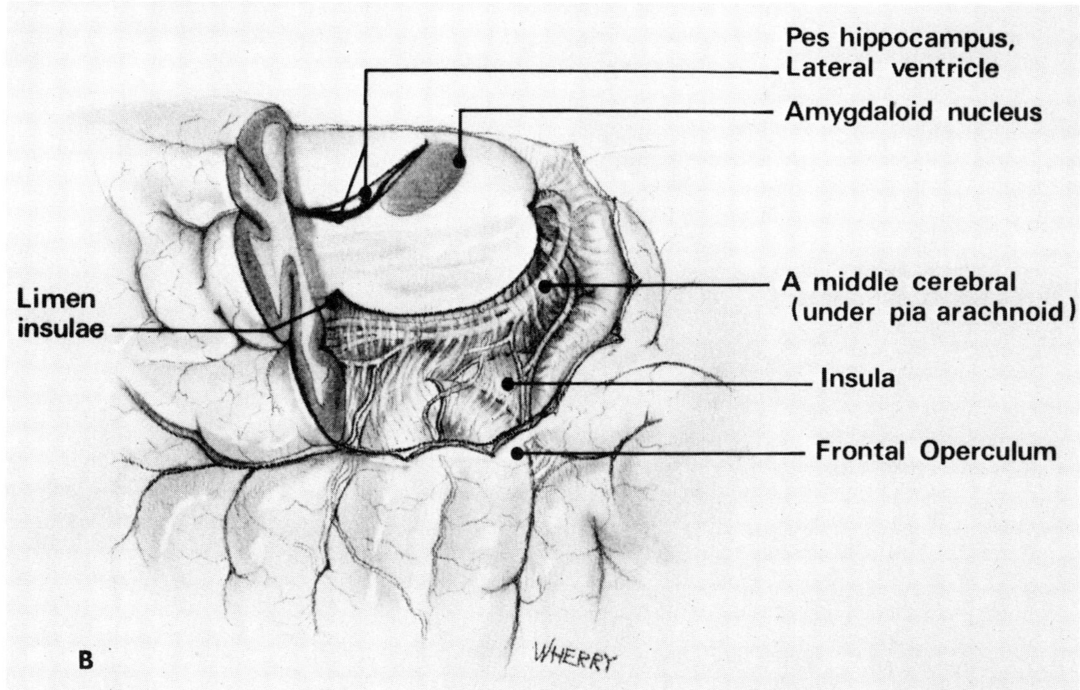

Fig. 107-3

It then is pulled into a small Penrose drain and reflected anteroinferiorly over the temporalis muscle along its remaining 2 cm of attachment. The patient raises the head every 2 hours so the anesthetist can massage the downward side to prevent pressure burns.

THE ELECTROCORTICOGRAM

Electrocorticography and depth electrode recording have proven very useful in mapping epileptogenic regions during surgery.[15,25]

A steel post is screwed into the hole at the superior edge of the craniotomy, and a 16-channel electrode holder is attached. One montage for both monopolar and bipolar recording is shown in Figure 107-4. Wire electrodes can be substituted for the usual contact electrodes for recording on the undersurface of the temporal lobe, the frontal lobe, and medial aspect of the hemisphere. Small lettered tags are placed at any site of electrographic abnormality (see Figure 107-7).

In temporal lobe cases, the inferior eight electrodes are removed and needle depth electrodes with four contacts are inserted perpendicular to the surface of the second temporal convolution to a depth of 3.5 cm at distances of 3 and 5 cm from the tip of the temporal lobe (Figure 107-5A). The deepest

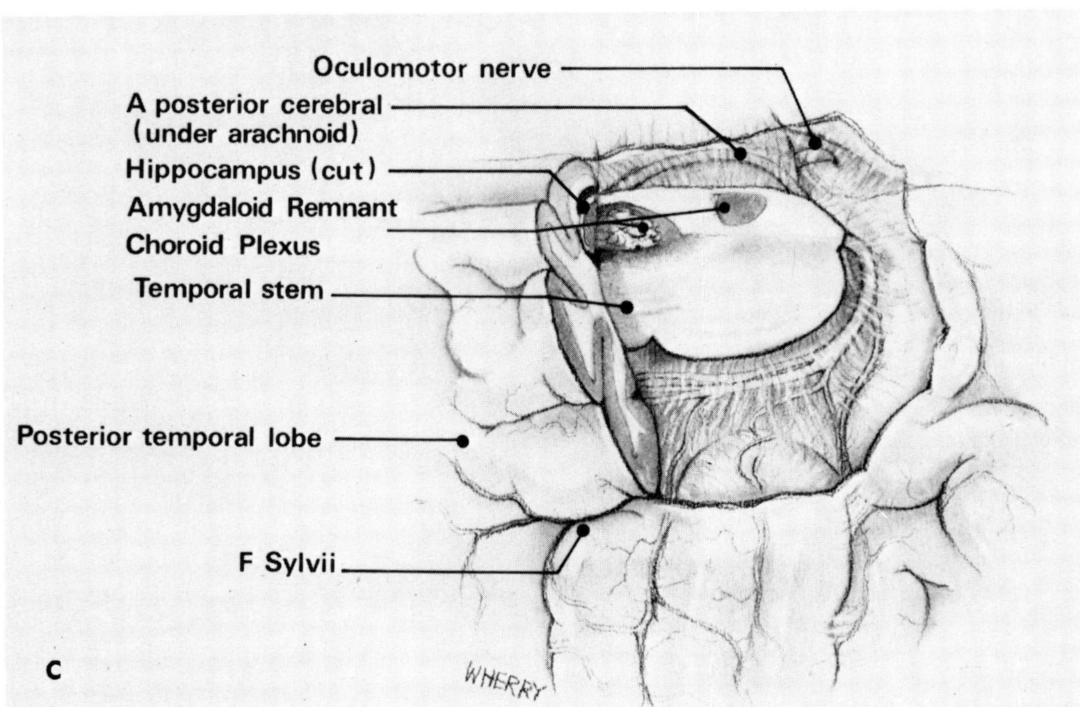

Fig. 107-3. Dominant temporal lobectomy, surgeon's view. (A) Left temporal exposure showing line of proposed cortical resection. (B) Superficial temporal lobe removed, exposing lateral temporal horn and lateral amygdaloid. (C) Following removal of pes hippocampus and most of amygdaloid. Note blood vessels and third nerve protected by pia-arachnoid.

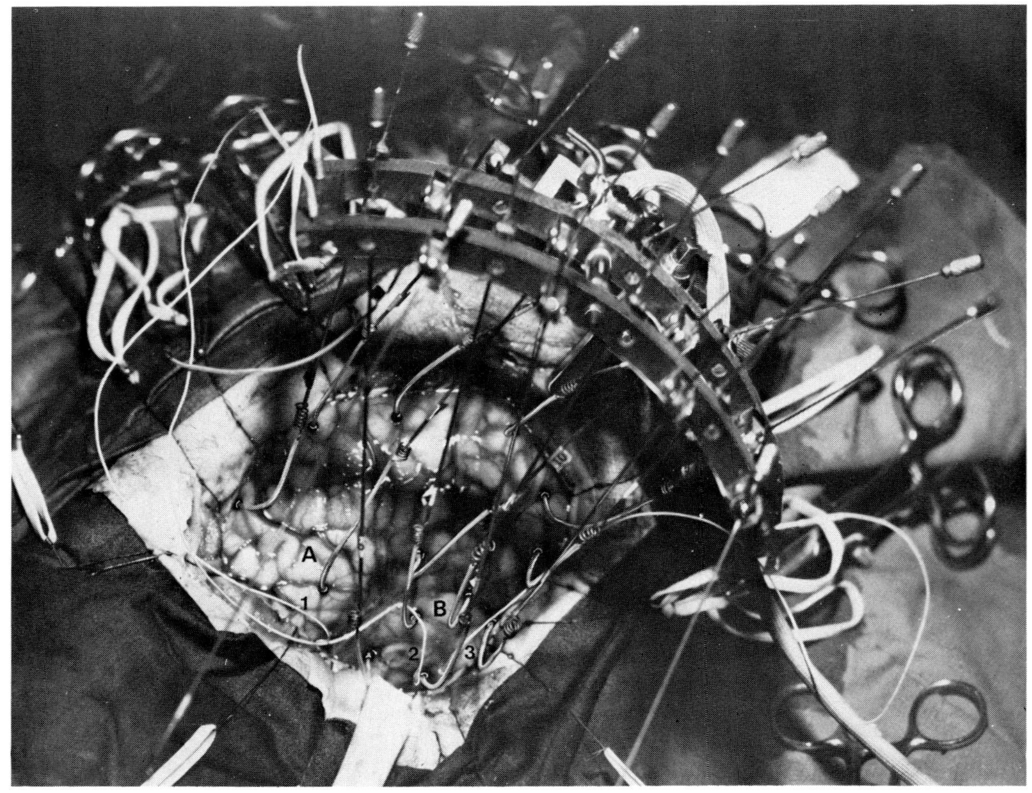

Fig. 107-4. Electrode holder and electrodes over (A) left temporal and (B) temporal and central regions. Wire electrodes for recording from (1) undersurface of frontal and (2,3) temporal lobe.

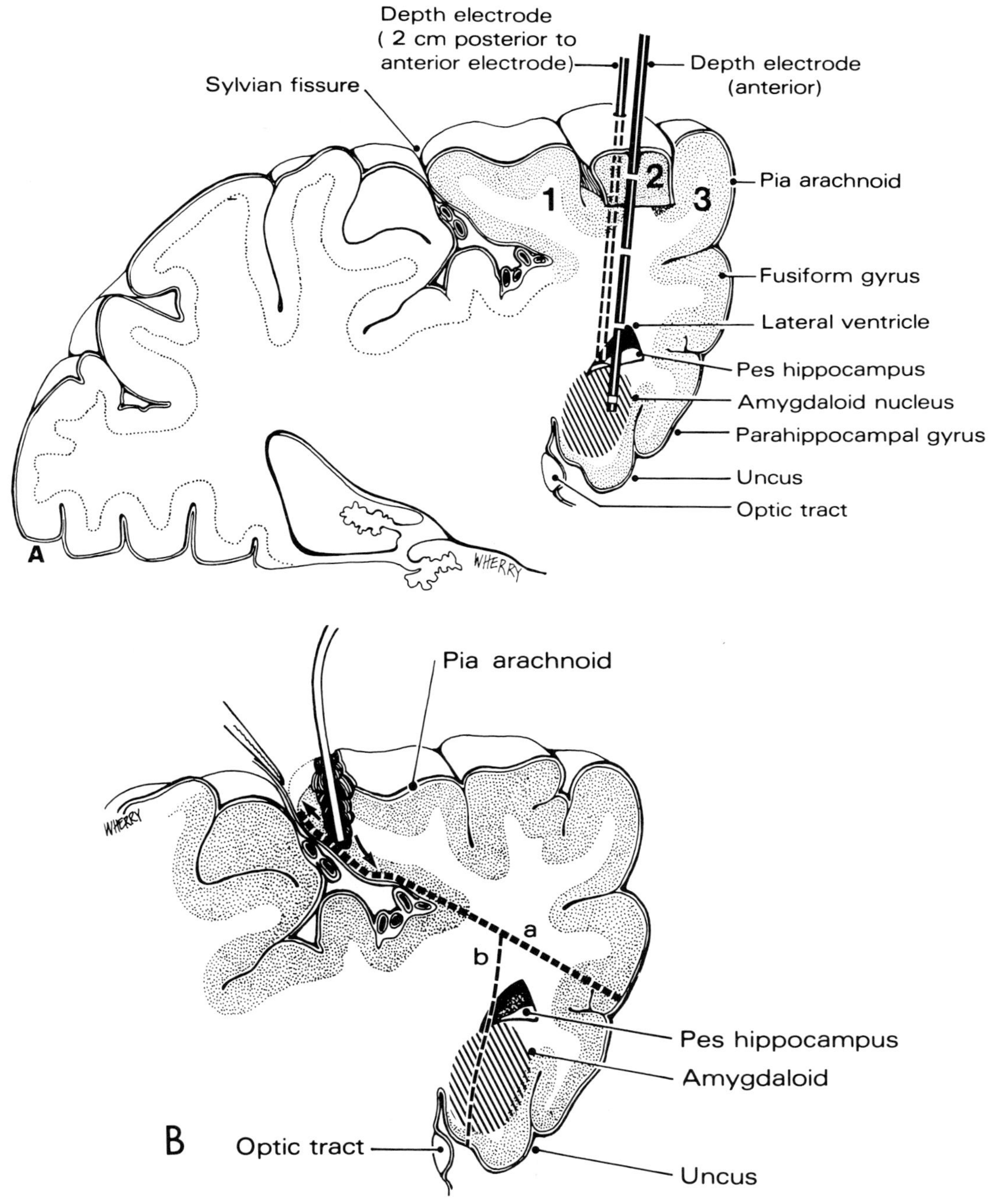

Fig. 107-5. Coronal section of left hemisphere at the tip of the temporal horn. (A) Depth electrodes in place in amygdaloid (anterior) and hippocampus (posterior). (B) Subpial dissection in first temporal convolution while retracting pia-arachnoid. (a) Line of superficial temporal dissection. (b) Line of removal of medial temporal structures.

contact of the anterior depth electrode records from the amygdaloid nucleus, and the posterior electrode from the pes hippocampus. The superficial contacts record from the surface gray matter. The intermediate two contacts of the anterior depth electrode record from circuminsular cortex, and the middle two contacts of the posterior depth electrode from the gray matter in the depths of Heschl's gyri.[25] The superior eight contact electrodes retain their former position. A further electroencephalographic recording is obtained.

ELECTRICAL STIMULATION STUDY

The brain then is electrically stimulated to determine the position of the pre- and postcentral gyri. A 2-msec square-wave pulse at 60 Hz, starting at 1 V and increasing by 0.5-V increments following each negative stimulation is used until a motor response is seen by the anesthetist, oruntil a sensory change is felt by the patient. Positive stimulation points are marked, using numbered tickets (see Figure 107-7). The rolandic fissure (central sulcus) is thus identified. In the dominant hemisphere the speech areas are stimulated while the patient carries out simple verbal tasks.[25] The frontal speech area is indicated by speech arrest, while the posterior temporal area is identified by arrest or a dysphasic reaction during stimulation. A negative stimulation does not always exclude the presence of speech function in the convolution that is stimulated.[23]

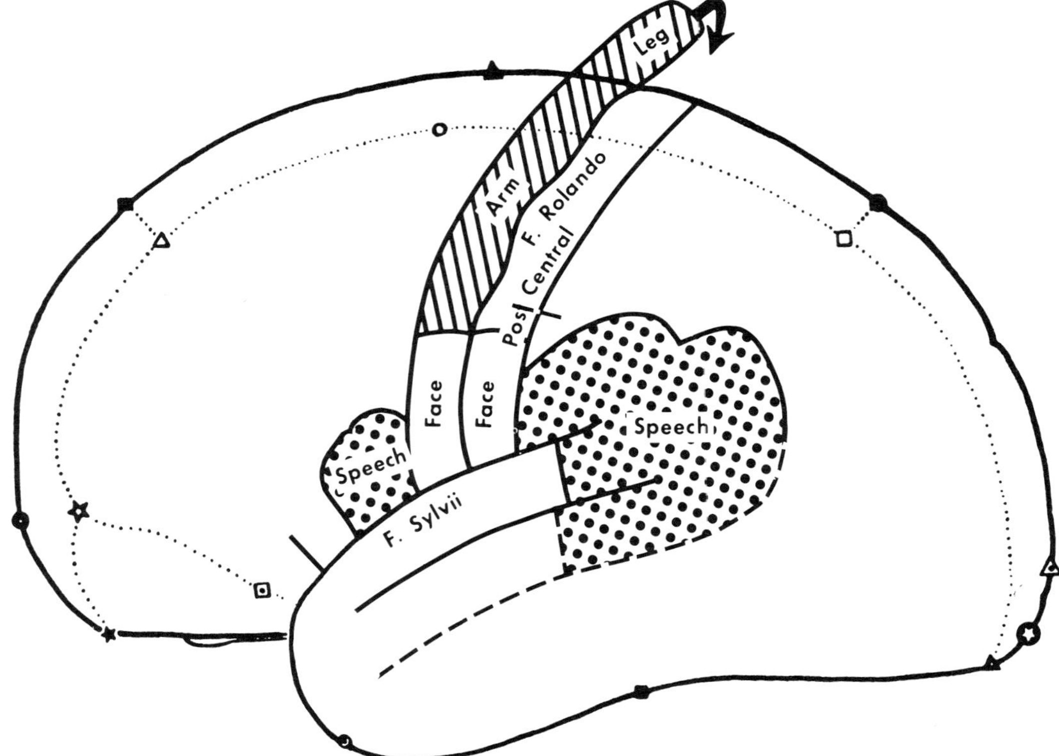

Fig. 107-6.   Most common position of pre- and postcentral gyri and speech areas in dominant hemisphere.

Areas of after-discharge (rhythmic electroencephalographic activity different from the prestimulation activity) may develop at the stimulation site or in adjacent regions. These may indicate areas of hyperirritable cortex,[10] although the clinical significance of this has not yet been documented.[25]

Other areas of the exposed cortex and the depth electrodes then may be stimulated in an endeavor to reproduce the patient's dura. A stimulating voltage more than 3 V higher than that required to elicit motor or sensory responses is dangerous. Above such levels, a nonspecific, full-blown seizure may develop, which precludes the patient's cooperation for some time.[25]

ANATOMIC CONSIDERATIONS— PLAN OF REMOVAL

The frontal (Broca) and posterior speech areas in the dominant hemisphere, as determined by stimulation studies and ablations around these areas, are shown in Figure 107-6.[28] The speech areas are indispensable and their removal is never justified.[10] The pre- and postcentral face area can be removed if pial barriers are respected so the blood supply to the rolandic and speech areas is preserved. This results in contralateral facial paresis, which subsequently improves but may leave some mild facial underaction.[27] Removal of the postcentral arm or leg area causes some persistent astereognosis and rarely is indicated unless markedly epileptogenic cortex in this area is causing a severe seizure tendency.[27] Removal of the precentral arm or leg produces contralateral spastic hemiparesis and is not indicated unless marked preoperative hemiparesis is present.[29]

Originally it was suggested that the anterior 5 to 6 cm of the dominant temporal lobe could be removed,[23] the resection being carried out along the vein of Labbé [8–10] without producing dysphasia. Because of variability in the position of this vein and the size of the temporal lobe, however, the best landmark to use is the junction of the rolandic and sylvian fissures. Removal of the dominant first and second temporal convolutions posterior to this point carries the risk of permanent dysphasia.[28]

The parietal speech zone extends superiorly 1 to 4 cm above the sylvian fissure and from 2 to 4 cm behind the postcentral sulcus. The frontal speech area occupies one or both frontal opercular convolutions anterior to the precentral gyrus.[28]

In the series from the Montreal Neurological Institute a number of epileptic patients without evidence of early damage to the left cerebral hemisphere underwent the carotid amobarbital speech test. In right-handers 96 percent had speech in the left hemisphere and 4 percent in the right hemisphere. In left-handed or ambidextrous individuals 70 percent had speech on the left, 15 percent on the right, and 15 percent had some representation of speech in each hemisphere. Similar studies of speech lateralization in individuals with early left-hemisphere damage show more variability, with larger numbers having speech in the right-hemisphere and those without early damage.[28] In strongly right-handed patients without any clinical evidence of abnormal lateralization of speech functions, the left cerebral hemisphere can be quite accurately considered to be the dominant one, and operation on the right or left hemisphere carried out on that basis without the necessity of doing the carotid amobarbital speech test. Doing the test is necessary in all left-handed and ambidextrous patients. In right-handed patients, the intracarotid amobarbital speech test is necessary when there is some evidence from psychological tests, x-ray films, the electroencephalogram, or the seizure pattern that there may be abnormal localization of the speech functions.

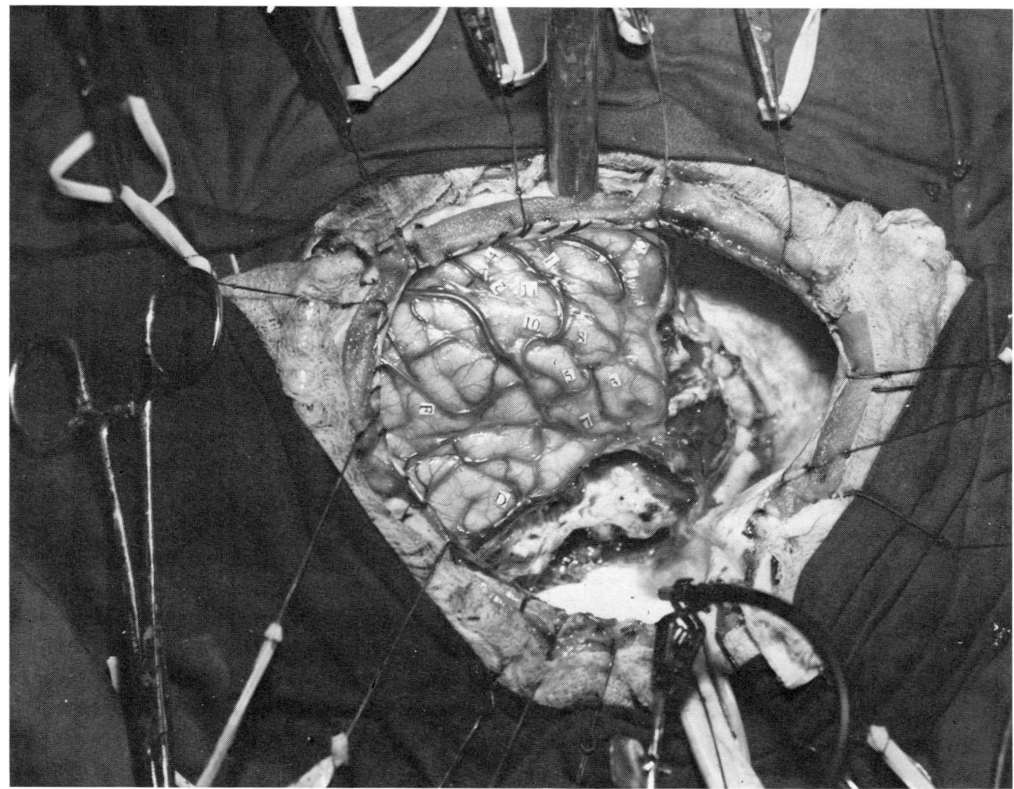

Fig. 107-7. After right frontal and temporal lobectomies with cortical incision following sulci and leaving untraumatized convolutions at removal edge. Note steel post for electrode holder at edge of superior bone margin and fishhooks retracting dura.

When the speech and precentral regions are avoided, *unilateral* removals of frontal, parietal, and temporal cortex are possible without significant additional deficits. When possible, it is best to leave one gyrus between the cortical removal and the indispensable areas of cortex. As much white matter as practicable should be left beneath the cortical removal to reduce any neurologic deficit.

If resection is limited to the anterior 5 cm of a normal-sized temporal lobe,[8] or not posterior to the intersection of the rolandic and sylvian fissures in any temporal lobe a visual field defect is rarely seen following temporal lobectomy.[25] If the temporal horn opening is confined to the anterior 1 cm and the white matter lateral to the ventricle is preserved, geniculo-calcarine tract damage is minimized, and a superior quadrant-anopsia may be avoided even in removals 7 to 8 cm posterior to the temporal tip.[25] Bilateral removal of the temporal lobes is never justified because of the profound memory loss that will result.[30]

CORTICAL RESECTION

Bearing the above principles in mind, the area of proposed cortical resection is outlined, using a piece of thread. The brain is irrigated at intervals and kept moist, especially during recordings. The thin, nonadhesive transparent plastic film is placed over cortical areas to be preserved to prevent drying of the brain and postoperative edema.[10]

In temporal lobectomy, as elsewhere, subpial dissection is stressed. The pia at the summit of the first temporal gyrus is coagulated and incised with a scalpel (Figure 107-3A). With small-bore suction, gray matter is meticulously pulled away from the pia to expose the white matter. The incision line is lengthened anteroposteriorly. The pia-arachnoid is coagulated and divided with scissors, and the incision is deepened by the suction technique. Gradually, sufficient gray matter along this gyrus is removed to expose the pia-arachnoid covering the insula (Figure 107-5B). The superior gray matter of the first temporal convolution is suctioned away from the pia. Deeper gray matter is suctioned away from the intact pia-arachnoid, as illustrated, to expose the insula. Meticulous hemostasis is necessary and movement of the brain must be avoided. Great care must be taken not to traumatize the middle cerebral vessels situated beneath this protective pia-arachnoid in order to prevent postoperative hemiparesis[7] (Figures 107-3B and 107-5B). At the posterior margin of the incision, in the first temporal gyrus, the line of incision is carried inferiorly toward the base of the temporal lobe (Figure 107-3A). Cotton pledgets are placed in the incision, as dissection proceeds distally, and subsequently are removed so that the incision can be deepened using the suction. Only that brain tissue to be removed is retracted away from tissue to be preserved. Larger vessels are coagulated and divided.

When the insular surface is exposed, the incision is carried through the white matter of the temporal stem medially at an angle of about 45 degrees to avoid deep structures in the basal temporal lobe (Figures 107-3B and 107-5B). The posterior end of the incision then is carried forward along the fusiform gyrus and the anterior end of the first temporal gyral incision is carried anteroinferiorly until the two meet on the inferior surface of the temporal lobe. The superficial temporal lobe is lifted out, leaving white matter overlying the lateral ventricle and amygdala (Figure 107-5B). When extremely gliotic brain is encountered, scissors may be used to incise the brain tissue.

The white matter of the anterior temporal lobe inferior to the insula is removed by suction until the ventricle is entered. The pes hippocampus then can be visualized and the amygdala is evident (Figure 107-3B). All but the medial rim of the amygdaloid nucleus and most of the uncus are removed. The remaining portion protects the subjacent optic tract (Figure 107-5B).[25]

If preoperative studies and depth-electrode recordings indicate hippocampal involvement and the opposite hippocampus is functional, the pes hippocampus then is removed together with the anterior parahippocampal gyrus (Figure 107-5B).[25] Great care must be exercised to preserve the pia-arachnoid, separating these structures from the third nerve, posterior cerebral artery, and cerebral peduncle (Figure 107-3C). Heschl's convolution on the dominant side is not removed, unless necessary, since this increases the risk of reducing the blood supply to the posterior speech area.

POSTREMOVAL RECORDING

Wire electrodes are placed on the undersurface of the posterior temporal lobe and orbital surface of the frontal lobe. Cortical electrodes are put on the temporal convexity, insula, amygdaloid, and hippocampal remnants. The remaining cortical electrodes are placed on the dorsolateral convexity of the hemisphere above the sylvian fissure. Persistent spiking from the hippocampus or posterior temporal lobe may require further excision, if no severe neurologic deficit will be produced. In the nondominant hemisphere, excisions are sometimes carried out to 8 cm posterior to the temporal tip. Epileptiform abnormality, recorded from the insular surface, is ignored, since further removal of cortex from that structure does not increase the success rate.[31,32]

The difficult problem of what to do about persistent spiking in the post-excision cortical electroencephalogram, either in the temporal lobe or behind the excision above the sylvian fissure depends on the individual surgeon's judgment. These spikes may not indicate a serious persistent seizure tendency and may abate in the postoperative months. On the other hand, they may indicate a potential persistence of some seizure tendency. More accurate and quantitative methods of assessing the clinical significance of such post-excision spiking are sorely needed.

During any further cortical removal, preservation of the pial barrier protects the adjacent gyri and the sulcal blood vessels supplying those gyri and other portions of the brain.[7] Several such additional excisions may be made before a clear electroencephalographic tracing is obtained or the effort to achieve this is abandoned.[22]

CLOSURE

A subdural drain is left beneath the bone flap. Gelatin is placed over the dural closure. The bone flap is wired intoposition, and burr hole covers are installed. After the galea and skin have been approximated, a wet sulfadiazine-soaked gauze is placed over the incision. A plastic sheet is placed over that and a full head dressing is used that covers the ear on the side of temporal lobectomy. The drain is removed on the first postoperative day.

POSTOPERATIVE CARE

An intravenous solution of glucose and saline containing 250 mg diphenylhydantoin, 240 mg phenobarbital, and 100 mg hydrocortisone per 1000 ml is given until oral intake begins. Fluids are restricted to 1500 ml daily for the first 5 postoperative days to decrease edema. Dexamethasone (6 mg every 6 hours) is given the first 5 days, and the dose then is tapered over the next 7 days. Ambulation begins on the third or fourth day. The sutures are removed on the fifth day.

Unless another medication has proved to be superior, diphenylhydantoin (100 mg, three times daily) and phenobarbital (60 mg, twice daily) are given for the first postoperative year.[22] If the patient then is seizure-free and has a nonepileptiform electroencephalogram, the medications gradually are reduced at 6- to 12-month intervals. Should seizures recur, the original anticonvulsant doses are restarted and reduced only after 2 seizure-free years.[22]

COMPLICATIONS

An aseptic meningitis, accompanied by fever up to 40°C, probably due to breakdown products of blood in the subarachnoid space, may follow large cortical resections.[33] This syndrome clears spontaneously over a 10- to 20-day period.[22]

Long procedures may cause transient cortical dysfunction and seizures during the first 7 to 10 days.[10] Such neighborhood seizures usually originate from cortex adjacent to the removal and have no bearing on the ultimate prognosis.[22] These complications are reduced by the cortisone regime.[34] This temporary postoperative disturbance of neighborhood brain function formerly attributed to cerebral edema and lessened by the use of steroids, has now been shown to be due to temporary dysfunction in glucose utilization in the brain adjacent to the surgical procedure.[35]

An increasing, marked, superior quadrantanopsia occurs when the temporal lobe resection is carried progressively further behind the rolandic-sylvian junction,[13] or if care is not taken to preserve white matter lateral to the temporal horn.[25] When the occipital lobe has been removed, complete contralateral homonymous hemianopsia has resulted.[27] The memory loss that may occur when the remaining functional hippocampus is removed[36] has been avoided since 1958 by preoperative bilateral administration of the amobarbital speech and memory test, when indicated.[25] Of the 250 dominant partial temporal lobectomies done from 1958 to 1975, only 2 patients had mild persistent dysphasia.[25] Mild deficits in verbal fluency may increase after dominant temporal lobectomy,[19,36] but later, verbal fluency often improves compared with preoperative levels, if seizures are reduced.[19] Transient dysphasia may follow cortical removal from the dominant hemisphere.[26,28]

In an earlier series of dominant temporal lobectomies, especially with cortical resections above or medial to the sylvian fissure, a contralateral hemiplegia, homonymous hemianopsia, and dysphasia were sometimes noted. Hemiplegia occurred in 8 (5 percent) of 168 patients with a permanent significant disability in 4 patients (2.5 percent). These complications were felt to be due to manipulation of the middle cerebral arteries over the insula. They can be prevented by preserving the pia-arachnoid over these vessels, avoiding arterial traction, and leaving insular cortex despite electrographic spiking.[7] Such manipulative hemiplegia has been avoided in temporal lobectomy since 1958. Cortical removals above the sylvian fissure have an incidence of hemiparesis or dysphasia of 0.5 percent unless the sensorimotor cortex is involved, in which case the risk becomes greater.[22]

Of the total 1497 operations for nontumoral lesions performed from 1928 through 1974, the operative mortality was 1 percent. From 1957 through 1975, in 820 consecutive operations there were 2 postoperative deaths, i.e., 0.2 percent.[22] In 964 temporal lobe operations carried out from 1950 through 1980, there was one postoperative death (0.1 percent).[37]

RESULTS AND DISCUSSION OF EXPERIENCE

Histopathologic examination of specimens from 506 consecutive patients operated upon at the Montreal Neurological Institute from 1961 through 1970 showed varying etiologies for focal epilepsy. One third had discrete lesions, a further third had essentially normal findings, while the rest had extensive lesions, such as cortical atrophy, hippocampal sclerosis, and chronic encephalitis.[38]

Cortical resection for nontumoral epilepsy was performed in 1267 patients from 1928 through 1971, with a median follow-up of 10 years in 1145 patients (Table 107-1). The seizure tendency was abolished in 36 percent, while in another 28 percent seizures were substantially, although not completely reduced. Variable results were obtained in the remaining 36 percent, with some patients experiencing a 90 percent reduction in seizures and a few essentially unchanged.[22]

In the temporal lobe series (653 patients) seizures were completely or almost completely reduced in 71 percent; in the frontal group (212 patients) in 55 percent; in the parietal group (80 patients) in 59 percent; in the central (sensorimotor) group (63 patients) in 57 percent; in the occipital lobe group (19 patients) in 68 percent; and in the group undergoing total or subtotal hemispherectomy for large destructive lesions (77 patients) in 50 percent.[22,25–27]

Up to 1971 repeat operations were performed on 129 patients who had inadequate seizure reduction, After additional epileptogenic cortex was removed 25 percent became seizure-free and 29 percent had a reduced seizure tendency.[3]

Tumors and arteriovenous malformations, the prime symptom of which was epilepsy rather than increasing neurologic deficit or increased intracranial pressure, were removed in an additional 347 patients. When the causative lesion and the surrounding epileptogenic cortex were removed as completely as possible, the reduction in seizure tendency compared favorably with the nontumor group until neoplasia recurred.[39]

The efficiency of seizure reduction thus correlates with the completeness with which the causative lesion and the epileptogenic cortex are removed rather than with the nature of the lesion or the length of time the patient had seizures.[3] About one fourth of the patients had some postoperative seizures during the first 2 years, but these subsequently ceased. Medications were stopped after 2 years in about one half of the patients. A further one fifth are controlled with medication, whereas this was not possible preoperatively. In addition to the decrease in seizure tendency there may be psychologic improvement in that the patient can often hold a responsible job.[40]

In one center the temporal lobe, including hippocampal and

Table 107-1. Results of cortical excision for focal epilepsy in patients with nontumoral lesions operated on during the years 1928 through 1971

Results	No.	(%)	No.	(%)
Seizure-free since discharge	237	21		
Became seizure-free after some early attacks	179	15	416	36
Free of seizures 3 or more years then rare or occasional attacks	122	11		
Marked reduction in seizure tendency	198	17	320	28
Moderated or less reduction in seizure tendency			409	36
Total patients with follow-up data of 2 to 41 years: median, 10 years			1145	
Inadequate follow-up data	82			
Deaths in 2 years	22			
Postoperative deaths	15			
Total patients	1267			

Data compiled from Rasmussen, TB: Cortical resection in the treatment of focal epilepsy: Neurosurgical management of the epilepsies, in Purpura DP, Penry JK, Walter RD (ed): Advances in Neurology, vol 8. New York, Raven Press, 1975.

amygdaloid regions, is removed en bloc for optimal histologic study, but the removal then is somewhat more complex than in the stages above.[9] Moreover, the contribution of the first temporal convolution to a seizure tendency has been questioned.[1,9] In the present series the best results have been obtained when as much abnormal cortex as possible is removed in addition to the hippocampus and amygdala when feasible.[40]

Stereotactic ablative procedures someday may solve the problem of dealing surgically with generalized, bilateral, or multifocal seizure disorders. To date, targets and methods are not standardized and usually these techniques have been reserved for especially intractable and complicated seizure problems.[41] Corpus callosal section is continuing to undergo evaluation to determine its proper role in the treatment of particularly generalized seizure problems. Cerebral cooling and cerebellar stimulation, formerly of interest[41] are rarely, if ever used at the present time.

Although current medical management with anticonvulsants and controlled drug levels has been extremely effective, such medications may have toxic effects or may fail to control the seizures. In such instances, a place remains for cortical resection in selected epileptic patients, until an ideal medication has been developed.

ACKNOWLEDGMENT

I wish to thank my preceptor and colleague, Dr. Theodore Rasmussen, for his helpful advice and for the use of his detailed records.

REFERENCES

1. Walker AE: Critique and perspective: Neurosurgical management of the epilepsies, in Purpura DP, Penry JK, Walter RD (eds): Advances in Neurology, vol 8. New York, Raven Press, 1975, pp 333–349
2. Robb P: Focal epilepsy: The problem, prevalence, and contributing factors, in Purpura DP, Penry JK, Walter RD (eds): Advances in Neurology, vol 8. New York, Raven Press, 1975, pp 11–12
3. Rasmussen TB: Surgical treatment of epilepsy: The clinical neurosciences, in Tower TB (ed): The Nervous System, vol 2. New York, Raven Press, 1975, pp 277–286
4. Penfield W, Jasper H: Historical introduction, Epilepsy and the Functional Anatomy of the Human Brain. Boston, Little, Brown, 1954, pp 3–20
5. Foerster O, Penfield W: Structural basis of traumatic epilepsy and result of radical operation. Brain 53:99, 1930
6. Penfield W, Japser H: Epilepsy and the Functional Anatomy of the Human Brain. Boston, Little, Brown, 1954, pp 692–815 7. Penfield W, Lende RA, Rasmussen TB: Manipulation hemiplegia, an untoward complication in the surgery of focal epilepsy. J Neurosurg 18:760, 1961
8. Penfield W, Baldwin M: Temporal lobe seizures and technique of subtotal temporal lobectomy. Ann Surg 136:625, 1952
9. Falconer MA, Hill D, Meyer A, et al: Treatment of temporal lobe epilepsy by temporal lobectomy: Survey of findings and results, Lancet 1:827, 1955
10. Penfield W, Jasper H: Surgical Therapy. Epilepsy and the Functional Anatomy of the Human Brain. Boston, Little, Brown, 1954, pp 739–817
11. Caveness WF: Onset and cessation of fits following craniocerebral trauma. J Neurosurg 20:570, 1963
12. Walker AE, Erculei F: Post-traumatic epilepsy 15 years later. Epilepsia 11:17, 1970
13. Rasmussen TB: The role of surgery in the treatment of focal epiiepsy. Clin Neurosurg 16:288, 1969
14. McNaughton FL, Rasmussen TB: Criteria for selection of patients for neurosurgical treatment: Neurosurgical management of the epilepsies, in Purpura DP, Penry JK, Walter RD (eds): Advances in Neurology, vol 8. New York, Raven Press, 1975, pp 37–48
15. Gloor P: Contributions of electroencephalography and electrocorticography to the neurosurgical treatment of the epilepsies, in Purpura DP, Penry JK, Walter RD (eds): Advances in Neurology, vol 8. New York, Raven Press, 1975, pp 59–105
16. Lombroso CT, Erba G: Primary and secondary bilateral synchrony in epilepsy. A clinical and electroencephalographic study. Arch Neurol 22:321, 1970
17. Gloor P, Rasmussen T, Altuzarra A, et al: Role of the intracarotid amobarbital pentylenetetrazol EEG test in the diagnosis and surgical treatment of patients wih complex seizure problems. Epilepsia 17:15, 1976
18. Ives JR, Gloor P: A long term time-lapse video system to document the patient's spontaneous clinical seizure synchronized with the EEG. Electroencephalogr Clin Neurophysiol 45:412, 1978
19. Milner B: Psychological aspects of focal epilepsy and its neurosurgical management: Neurosurgical management of the epilepsies, in Purpura DT, Penry JK, Walter RD (eds): Advances in Neurology, vol 8. New York, Raven Press, 1975, pp 299–321
20. Wada J, Rasmussen TB: Intracarotid injection of sodium amytal for the lateralization of speech dominance. Experimental and clinical observations. J Neurosurg 17:266, 1960
21. Milner B, Branch C, Rasmussen TB: Study of short-term memory after intracarotid injection of Sodium Amytal. Trans Am Neurol Assoc 87:224, 1962
22. Rasmussen TB: Cortical resection in the treatment of focal epilepsy: Neurosurgical management of the epilepsies, in Purpura DP, Penry JK, Walter RD (eds): Advances in Neurology, vol 8. New York, Raven Press, 1975, pp 139–154
23. Rasmussen TB, Jasper H: Temporal lobe epilepsy: Indication for operation and surgical technique, in Baldwin M, Bailey P (eds): Temporal Lobe Epilepsy. Springfield, Ill, Charles C Thomas, 1958, pp 440–460
24. Trop D: Personal communication
25. Rasmussen TB: Surgical treatment of patients with complex partial seizures, in Penry JK, Daly DD (eds): Advances in Neurology. vol 11. New York, Raven Press, 1975, pp 415–449
26. Rasmussen TB: Surgery of frontal lobe epilepsy: Neurosurgical management of the epilepsies, in Purpura DP, Penry JK, Walter RD (eds): Advances in Neurology, vol 8. New York, Raven Press, 1975, pp 197–205
27. Rasmussen TB: Surgery for epilepsy arising in regions other than the temporal and frontal lobes, in Purpura DP, Penry JK, Walter RD (eds): Advances in Neurology, vol 8. New York, Raven Press, 1975, pp 207–226
28. Rasmussen TB, Milner B: Clinical and surgical studies of the cerebral speech areas in man in Zulch KJ, Creutzfeidt O, Galbraith GC (eds): Cerebral Localization. New York, Springer-Verlag, 1975, pp 238–257
29. Penfield W, Rasmussen TB: Excision of cortical regions, The Cerebral Cortex of Man. New York, Macmillan, 1950, pp 183–201
30. Scoville WB, Milner B: Loss of recent memory after bilateral hippocampal lesions. J Neurol Neurosurg Psychiatry 20:11, 1957
31. Ajmone-Marsan C, Baldwin M: Electrocorticography, in Baldwin M, Bailey P (eds): Temporal Lobe Epilepsy. Springfield, Ill, Charles C Thomas, 1958, pp 368–395
32. Silfvenius H, Gloor P, Rasmussen TB: Evaluation of insular ablation in surgical treatment of temporal lobe epilepsy. Epilepsia 5:307, 1964
33. Jackson IJ: Aseptic hemogenic meningitis. Arch Neurol Psychiatr 62:572, 1949
34. Rasmussen TB, Gulati DR: Cortisone in the treatment of a postoperative cerebral edema. J Neurosurg 19:535, 1962
35. Pappius HM: Dexamethasone and local cerebral glucose utilization in freeze traumatized rat brain. Ann Neurol 12:157, 1982
36. Milner B: The memory deficit in bilateral hippocampal lesions. Psychiatr Res Publ 11:43, 1959
37. Rasmussen TB: Personal communication, 1986
38. Mathieson G: Pathologic aspects of epilepsy with special reference to the surgical pathology of focal cerebral seizures: Neurosurgical management of the epilepsies, in Purpura DP, Penry JK, Walter RD (eds): Advances in Neurology, vol 8. New York, Raven Press, 1975, pp 107–138
39. Rasmussen TB: Surgery of epilepsy associated with brain tumors in Purpura DP, Penry JK, Walter RD (eds): Advances in Neurology, vol 8. New York, Raven Press, 1975, pp 227–239
40. Feindel W: Factors contributing to the success, or failure of surgical intervention for epilepsy, in Purpura DP, Penry JK, Walter RD (eds): Advances in Neurology, vol 8. New York, Raven Press, 1975, pp 281–298
41. Ojemann GA, Ward AA, Jr.: Stereotactic and other procedures for epilepsy, in Purpura DP, Penry JK, Walter RD (eds): Advances in Neurology, vol 8. New York, Raven Press, 1975, pp 241–263

CHAPTER 108

Cerebral Hemispherectomy: Indications, Methods, and Results

Theodore Rasmussen

CEREBRAL HEMISPHERECTOMY, more correctly termed hemicorticectomy, was reported independently by Dandy[1] and by L'Hermitte[2] in 1928 as a dramatic effort to cure patients with malignant gliomas of the cerebral hemisphere. Cures were not achieved, however, and neither palliation nor prolongation of life was better than was achieved with more conservative surgical and medical regimes.[3–5] As a result, the operation fell into disfavor in the treatment of tumors and was rarely performed during the late 1930s and the 1940s.

The first reported hemispherectomy for infantile hemiplegia and seizures was carried out by the pioneer Canadian neurosurgeon Kenneth McKenzie[6] at the Toronto General Hospital in 1938, but it was the 1950 report by the South African neurosurgeon R. A. Krynauw[7] of hemispherectomy carried out on 12 patients with infantile type hemiplegia and medically intractable seizures that rejuvenated the procedure. His impressive results in reducing severe, medically refractory seizure tendencies in these young hemiplegic individuals were soon verified by neurosurgical centers in Britain,[8–12] Europe,[13–22] the Middle East,[23,24] Asia,[25,26] North America,[27–32] and South America.[33,34] By 1961 reports on nearly 300 cases had been published.[35] Most centers also reported a significant lessening of the behavioral problems that are frequently present in this patient population and sometimes cause nearly as much difficulty to the patient and his or her family as the seizures themselves.

PATIENT SELECTION

CLINICAL ASPECTS

Hemispherectomy is an operative procedure that is ordinarily considered for patients whose brain lesion has produced a maximal or near maximal hemiplegia and homonymous hemianopsia and has also produced seizures. These seizures arise in the badly damaged cerebral hemisphere and cannot be adequately controlled by tolerable doses of appropriate antiepileptic medications. In most instances the brain injury has occurred in infancy or early childhood, resultant to perinatal trauma or to some inflammatory brain disease such as meningoencephalitis or chronic encephalitis. Postnatal head trauma and severe inoculation reactions are other less common etiologic factors. These patients constitute a relatively small proportion of the overall population of patients with recurring epileptic seizures but often present particularly difficult problems of medical management.

A wide variety of seizure patterns occur in this patient population, with most patients having two or three different seizure types. Focal somatomotor seizures involving the contralateral side of the body are the most common. In some patients these attacks frequently become generalized 1 or 2 seconds after onset. In other patients, secondary generalization is uncommon and most of the somatomotor seizures remain lateralized. In some patients generalized convulsions without lateralizing signs are common, and good evidence of lateralization is seen only in a small percentage of the attacks. Absence and staring attacks occur in some patients and can be distressingly frequent. Minor attacks consisting of head flexion, eye blinking, and limpness or generalized rigidity are also encountered. Regardless of the varied nature of the minor attacks, frequent or occasional generalized convulsions are usually present as well, sometimes with and sometimes without evidence of a lateralized onset. In patients whose hemisphere is being gradually destroyed by chronic encephalitis,[36,37] epilepsia partialis continua of the opposite arm or leg or of the face is common and frequently precipitates the investigation of possible surgical therapy.

ELECTROENCEPHALOGRAPHIC ASPECTS

The EEG usually shows a widespread disturbance of the background activity that is maximal over the damaged hemisphere. Epileptiform abnormalities consisting of high amplitude spikes, sharp waves, and spike-wave complexes are also widespread over the damaged hemisphere as a rule, but sometimes have a focal predominance in the frontotemporal, central, or temporoparietal region. These epileptiform discharges frequently exhibit synchronous spread to the "good" hemisphere, although independent epileptiform discharges are sometimes seen over this hemisphere as well. Occasionally the amplitude of the epileptiform discharges is higher over this hemisphere than over the damaged hemisphere, which is a reflection of the disparity in the number of functioning neurones and neuronal circuits present in the two hemispheres.

Recording the patient's habitual seizures sometimes provides additional assurance that the seizures are arising in the damaged hemisphere, but long-term monitoring to record clinical seizures is less commonly needed than is the case with

OPERATIVE NEUROSURGICAL TECHNIQUES
ISBN 0-8089-1862-1

more restricted epileptic problems such as temporal or frontal lobe epilepsy.

In the presence of radiologic and clinical evidence of widespread damage to the hemisphere, neither the EEG nor the seizure patterns provide as reliable evidence about the extent of the cortical excision necessary to produce a satisfactory reduction in the seizure tendency as is the case in more restricted epileptogenic lesions.

RADIOLOGIC ASPECTS

The skull x-ray films usually shows relative smallness or thickening of the calvarium over the damaged hemisphere. The extent of the brain damage is usually well visualized on both encephalograms and CT scans. There is usually moderate or marked enlargement of the ventricle of the involved hemisphere and often a large porencephalic cyst of the hemisphere as well.

Central angiography is rarely indicated except as part of the carotid amytal speech test[38–40] in the rare instances in which this test is needed to be sure that the speech functions are not present in a damaged left hemisphere.[41]

NEUROLOGIC ASPECTS

When the hemispheral damage has occurred in the perinatal period or during the first year or two of life, the hemiplegic extremities are usually significantly small. A useful grip may be present and the patient may walk with only a moderate limp. If there are no individual finger movements and no voluntary toe or ankle movements, however, hemispherectomy is rarely followed by a significant increase in the motor deficit. When the brain injury has occurred in later childhood or in early adult life, however, a more marked hemiplegia must be present in order for the surgeon to be confident that a hemispherectomy will not produce an unacceptable increase in the motor deficit.

When the homonymous hemianopsia is extensive but not complete, most patients are not significantly handicapped by the complete hemianopsia that follows hemispherectomy. This is particularly the case when the hemispherectomy is carried out in early or middle childhood. When the hemianopsia is minimal or absent, however, a hemispherectomy is rarely advisable, even if maximal hemiplegia is present. In such instances a subtotal hemispherectomy tailored to preserve the posterior third of the cerebral hemisphere is advisable to preserve a useful degree of vision in the contralateral visual field.

Some degree of mental retardation is usually present among these patients. Of the 43 patients in the Montreal Neurological Institute hemispherectomy series as of 1983, the full scale IQ ranged from 36 to 92, with a median level of 65. Intelligence quotient levels in the 40s and 50s do not constitute a contraindication for hemispherectomy. For example, the 21 patients in this series who became and remained seizure free had full scale IQ ratings ranging from 42 to 92, with a median level of 64.

LATE COMPLICATIONS OF TRADITIONAL HEMISPHERECTOMY

In the mid 1960s reports began to appear of increased intracranial pressure associated with progressive neurologic deterioration developing 4 or more years after hemispherec-

tomy in patients who previously had been doing well.[42–45] This late and sometimes fatal complication developed in one quarter to one third of patients in most of the reported series on hemispherectomy in which the patients were followed for 4 years or more. This complication rarely occurs before 3½ years after surgery and has been known to occur as late as 25 years after hemispherectomy. To date, this problem has occurred in 11 of 31 patients with anatomically complete hemispherectomies performed at the Montreal Neurological Institute between 1952 and 1968. Five of these 11 patients died despite shunting; 3 patients had only partial recoveries and were left with significant increases in their previously stable neurologic deficits; the remaining 3 patients, who were diagnosed and treated soon after the onset of the complication, recovered their precomplication neurologic status and subsequently remained neurologically stable.

Numerous reports in the late 1960s of this complication account for a marked reduction of enthusiasm for hemispherectomy in many pediatric neurologic centers and also among many neurosurgeons.[45–48] Few hemispherectomy operations were carried out during the 1970s.

This serious late complication was soon shown to be caused by the gradual accumulation of fluid with a high iron content in the cavity created by removal of the cortex. This ultimately produces the syndrome superficial cerebral hemosiderosis.[49–51] This was initially described by Noetzel in 1940[52] and produced experimentally in dogs by Iwanowski and Olszewski in 1960.[53] The high iron content of this fluid results from the gradual leakage of red blood cells into the hemispherectomy cavity, apparently because of insufficient support of the remaining cerebral hemisphere after the hemispherectomy. This renders the remaining brain vulnerable to minor head trauma and to normal alterations of intracranial pressure produced by coughing or straining. This supposition is supported by the fact that superficial cerebral hemosiderosis has not occurred in a sizeable personal series of patients followed for 4 or more years after subtotal hemispherectomy or hemi-hemispherectomy.[54] It appears that the preservation of a small portion of the damaged hemisphere reduces the vulnerability to the gradual seepage of red blood cells into the large cavity and the development of cerebral hemosiderosis, hydrocephalus, and neurologic deterioration.

Because of this complication, we abandoned the therapeutically effective operation of an anatomically complete hemispherectomy during the decade of the mid 1960s to the mid 1970s and routinely preserved the least epileptogenic one fourth to one third of the hemisphere in those patients who previously would have been candidates for complete hemispherectomy. This tactic effectively eliminated superficial cerebral hemosiderosis as a complication but at the cost of a significant lessening of the effectiveness of the cortical excision in reducing the patient's seizure tendency.[54] In order to achieve the prior effectiveness, the surgical tactic was once again altered. The change consisted of disconnecting the remaining segment or segments of the damaged and epileptogenic hemisphere from the rest of the brain. This procedure produces a functionally complete but anatomically subtotal hemispherectomy. This operation, which we have termed a functional hemispherectomy, provides the therapeutic effectiveness of a standard hemispherectomy with the protection against the late complication of superficial cerebral hemosiderosis of a subtotal or hemi-hemispherectomy.[54]

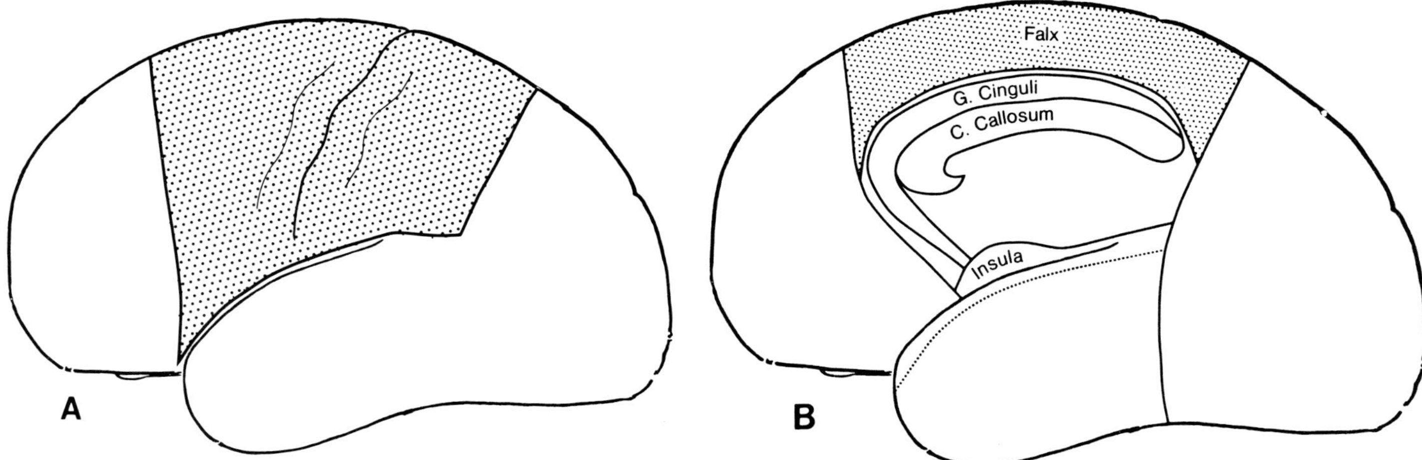

Fig. 108-1. The first stage in functional hemispherectomy. (A) The central suprasylvian cortex (stippled region) is removed to a level just anterior to the rostrum of the corpus callosum and to a level just posterior to the splenium of the corpus callosum. (B) The medial surface of the hemisphere is removed above the gyrus cinguli.

TECHNICAL ASPECTS OF FUNCTIONAL HEMISPHERECTOMY

PREOPERATIVE PREPARATION

The frequency of the seizures in this patient population usually makes it unnecessary to withdraw the patient's antiepileptic medication during the preoperative investigation. Moderate doses of the patient's habitual antiepileptic medication can therefore be continued until the evening before the operation.

The operation is performed with the patient under light general anesthesia. In addition to the usual preanesthetic medications and regime, adult patients are started on oral cortisone acetate (200 mg)[55,56] or a comparable dose of dexamethasone the day before surgery. The steroid dosage is appropriately reduced for children. On the morning of the operation, intravenous hydrocortisone is added to provide a total dosage of 200 mg during the day of the operation.

SURGICAL TECHNIQUE

A large U-shaped skin flap with the medial limb running along the midline is used. A large free bone flap is removed to provide easy access to the frontal lobe at the level in front of the corpus callosum and the parietal lobe at the level just behind the corpus callosum. The bone is removed inferiorly to provide access to the inferior aspect of the temporal lobe. After the dura is reflected a cortical electrogram is obtained for the potential help it might provide in later study of the patient's seizure problem and postoperative course.

The initial cortical incision is made just above the fissure of Sylvius by coagulating the surfaces of the gyri of the frontal, central, and parietal opercular region (Figure 108-1A). The incision is deepened with suction until the insula is exposed. The incision is then extended upward across the frontal and parietal lobes to the midline by suction after the leptomeninx is coagulated and incised. When the ventricle is markedly enlarged, this usually opens into the ventricle. The two limbs of the incision are then extended downward on the medial surface of the hemisphere to the top of the cingulate gyrus (Figure 108-1B). The two limbs of the cortical incisions are then

connected just above the cingulate gyrus. Leaving the cingulate gyrus in situ at this stage protects the anterior cerebral arteries lying on the surface of the corpus callosum against inadvertent injury. The posterior frontal, central, and anterior parietal brain tissue outlined by the cortical incisions is then removed en bloc by sectioning the underlying white matter with the suction tip. The cingulate gyrus is then removed subpially with suction, exposing the anterior cerebral arteries covered by the leptomeninges. The subcallosal gyrus is removed in a similar manner.

The white matter of the frontal lobe is then sectioned with the suction tip just in front of the rostrum of the corpus callosum down to the leptomeningeal layer lying on the falx. The white matter of the parietal lobe is similarly sectioned just behind the splenium of the corpus callosum down to the falx and tentorium. The anterior frontal region and the posterior parietal and occipital regions thus are disconnected from the upper brain stem and also from the corpus callosum (Figure 108-1B).

The temporal lobe is removed completely back to the level of the parietal cortical incision. The cortical incision is initially made just below the fissure of Sylvius and then deepened with suction down to the insula. The incision is carried around the tip of the temporal lobe to the uncus. The incision in the first temporal gyrus is extended posteriorly to the incision across the parietal lobe and then downward to the inferior aspect of the temporal lobe. The incision is then extended anteriorly through the fusiform gyrus to meet the inferior aspect of the incision around the tip of the temporal lobe. This usually opens into the temporal horn of the ventricle when it is markedly enlarged. The circumscribed temporal lobe is then removed en bloc by sectioning any remaining white matter by suction (Figure 108-2).

The bulge of the amygdaloid nucleus is then seen on the medial aspect of the tip of the temporal horn of the ventricle and is removed by suction. The medial rim of the nucleus is preserved to protect against inadvertent damage to the hypothalamus or to the optic tract, which lies just medial and superior to the posterior portion of the nucleus. The pes and the body of the hippocampus are then removed completely from the pial bed, along with any remaining gray matter of the fusiform and hippocampal gyri. The medial leptomeningeal layer is

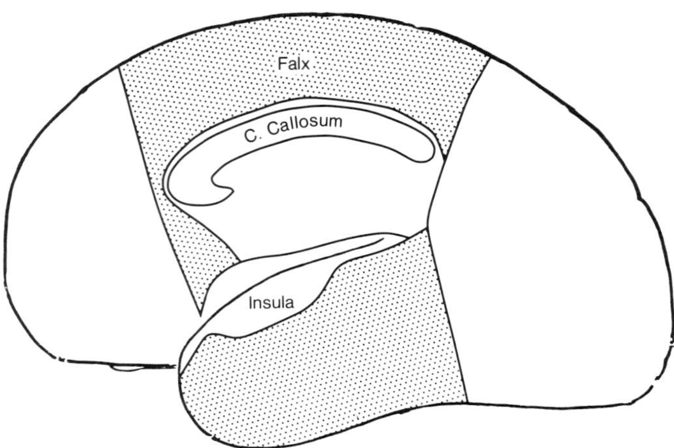

Fig. 108-2. The second stage in functional hemispherectomy. The gyrus cinguli, subcallosal gyrus and temporal lobe are removed and the remaining portions of frontal and parieto-occipital regions are disconnected from the corpus callosum and upper brain stem.

Table 108-1. Early Intracranial Pressure Complications of Large Brain Excisions.

Operations	No. of pts.	Early pressure complication
Anatomical complete hemispherectomy (1 stage................24 pts.) (2,3 or 4 stages......7 pts.)	31	3 pts. (9%)
Functional complete but anatomical subtotal hemispherectomy	14	1 pt. } 8.1 %
Subtotal hemispherectomy 1/5 to 1/3 of hemisphere preserved	6 0	5 pts. }
Hemi-hemispherectomy about 1/2 of hemisphere preserved	78	2 pts. (2.6%)

carefully preserved to protect against injury to the nerves and vessels in the basal cisterns.

Any remaining gray matter of the first temporal gyrus, Heschl's region, and uncus is then removed by suction from the pial surfaces. It is not necessary to remove the insula, which is often so atrophic as to be scarcely identifiable. We have often removed it, however, after clipping and coagulating the sylvian arteries at the anterior margin of the insula as a safeguard against postoperative bleeding.

Depending on the size of the ventricle and the presence and location of a porencephalic cyst, it is sometimes preferable to carry out the temporal lobe excision before the excision above the fissure of Sylvius.

Finally, the choroid plexus is removed as completely as possible to lessen postoperative problems resulting from the extensive removal of the absorbing surface for the CSF. The dura is tacked up at the margins of the bone flap and to the middle of the bone flap through a pair of drill holes. This maneuver, plus the use of an extradural or subgaleal drain for the first 12 hours, protects against postoperative accumulation of fluid beneath the skin flap. The fixation of the bone flap and closure of the skin flap are carried out in the conventional manner.

POSTOPERATIVE CARE

The patient is maintained in a semiprone or semisupine position with the remaining hemisphere down for the first 2 or 3 days to safeguard against complications from brain stem shift. The high dose intravenous steroid regime is maintained until the patient starts oral nourishment, usually on the second or third postoperative day. The steroid medication is then given orally and tapered off over the next 8 to 10 days.

The hemiplegic extremities are usually flaccid and there is an increase in the hemiplegia for the first few days. Strength then returns progressively and is usually back to the preoperative level before the end of the first postoperative month.

A medium dose of the patient's habitual antiepileptic medication is continued during the first year after surgery. If the patient is seizure-free the dose is then reduced 1 dose at a time at 6- to 12-month intervals. If a few attacks occur during the first

postoperative year or if the EEG shows any significant epileptiform activity, it is wise to postpone the gradual reduction of antiepileptic medication until a period of 2 seizure-free years has occurred.

EARLY PRESSURE COMPLICATIONS

Although a low grade increase in intracranial pressure is commonly present for a week or 10 days in nearly all patients who have had large portions of the brain removed, this usually resolves spontaneously during the next few days and without specific treatment. A few patients experience a persistent increase in ICP beyond the usual postoperative period. This finding is the result of inadequate absorption of CSF secondary to the extensive removal of the pia-arachnoidal absorbing surfaces. This is particularly apt to occur in patients in whom the original brain insult has produced chronic fibrosis of the leptomeninges, as happens after head injury with extensive subarachnoid hemorrhage or after meningoencephalitis.

Elevated intracranial pressure as an early complication of hemispherectomy has occurred in 3 (9 percent) of our 31 patients with anatomically complete hemispherectomies (Table 108-1). It also occurred in 1 of the 14 patients with functional hemispherectomies, and in 5 of 60 patients with subtotal hemispherectomies, or in 8.1 percent of these 74 patients. It has occurred in 2 (2.6 percent) of 78 patients following removal of about one half of the cerebral hemisphere.

If the postoperative increased pressure remains even minimally elevated beyond the third or fourth postoperative week, a shunt procedure should be carried out without undue delay, since with prompt shunting, this complication does not have a deleterious long-term effect.

Table 108-2. Late Intracranial Pressure Complications of
Large Brain Excisions

Operations	No. of pts.	Late pressure complication	Interval between operation and complication	Duration of follow-up
Anatomical complete hemispherectomy (1 stage................ 24 pts.) (2,3 or 4 stages......7 pts.)	31	11 pts. (35%)	4 1/2 - 24 yrs. (median 9 yrs.)	7 to 33 yrs. (median 20 yrs.)
Functional complete but anatomical subtotal hemispherectomy	14	1 pt. ⎫ ⎬ 2.6%	3 yrs.	2 to 10 yrs. (median 4½ yrs)
Subtotal hemispherectomy 1/5 to 1/3 of hemisphere preserved	57	1 pt. ⎭	10 yrs.	4 to 34 yrs. (median 29 yrs.)
Hemi-hemispherectomy about 1/2 of hemisphere preserved	71	1 pt. (1.4%)	13 yrs.	4 to 39 yrs. (median 12 yrs.)

RESULTS

SEIZURE STATUS

The current report of the Montreal Neurological Institute experience with hemispherectomy includes 41 patients who survived the first 2 postoperative years following either an anatomically complete or a functional hemispherectomy (Table 108-3). Twenty-one patients (51 percent) became and remained seizure free, 18 since discharge from the hospital and 3 after having a few attacks in the early postoperative months or years. Twelve patients have developed rare or occasional attacks after having been seizure-free for 3 to 28 years, and 1 patient has averaged about 1 major and 1 minor attack per year. We have classified these 13 patients as having had a marked but not quite complete reduction of the seizure tendency. Added to the 21 patients who became and remained seizure free, there are thus 34 patients (83 percent) who have had a complete or nearly complete reduction of the seizure tendency after the hemisphe-rectomy.

Seven patients have had a less satisfactory but still significant reduction in the occurrence of their seizures. In 6, the frequency and severity of the seizures has been reduced to about 1 to 20 percent of the preoperative situation. The seventh patient experienced a reduction in seizures of approximately 50 percent and remains institutionalized but able to perform simple chores.

BEHAVIORAL STATUS

Twenty-four of these 41 patients had significant behavioral abnormalities such as aggressiveness, irritability, and temper tantrums. Each experienced an improvement in behavior that was usually evident within 1 to 2 months after surgery and that continued to improve for months or years before stabilizing.

Seventeen of the 41 patients did not have significant behavioral problems preoperatively, although the range of intelligence in the group was comparable with that of the preceding group. In no instance was there any adverse change in behavior after the hemispherectomy.

INTELLECTUAL STATUS

The full scale IQ rose 5 to 22 points in 19 patients. The rating fell 7 to 12 points in 5 patients, but only early postoperative tests were available for each of these. In the remaining 17 patients the intellectual capacity was unchanged as judged by the full scale IQ rating or by the parents' report for those patients on whom formal testing was not done because of poor cooperation, frequent seizures, or early age.

SOCIOECONOMIC STATUS

Preoperatively the socioeconomic status was determined by three factors: (1) the level of mental retardation, (2) the frequency and severity of the seizures, and (3) the presence or absence of significant behavioral abnormalities. Postoperatively the main determinant of socioeconomic status was the level of intellectual capacity.

Fifteen patients were living at home preoperatively but were unable to go to school because of the severity and frequency of seizures, aggressive behavior, or severe mental retardation. Postoperatively 4 of these patients were able attend a regular school and 10 were able attend either a special school or a special class in a regular school. Four of these patients were ultimately employed on a full-time or part-time basis. All had worthwhile improvement in their social horizons. The remaining patient required custodial care because of marked mental retardation.

Five patients were at a preschool level when their surgery

Table 108-3. Results of Hemispherectomy for Seizures
(operated 1952 through 1983)

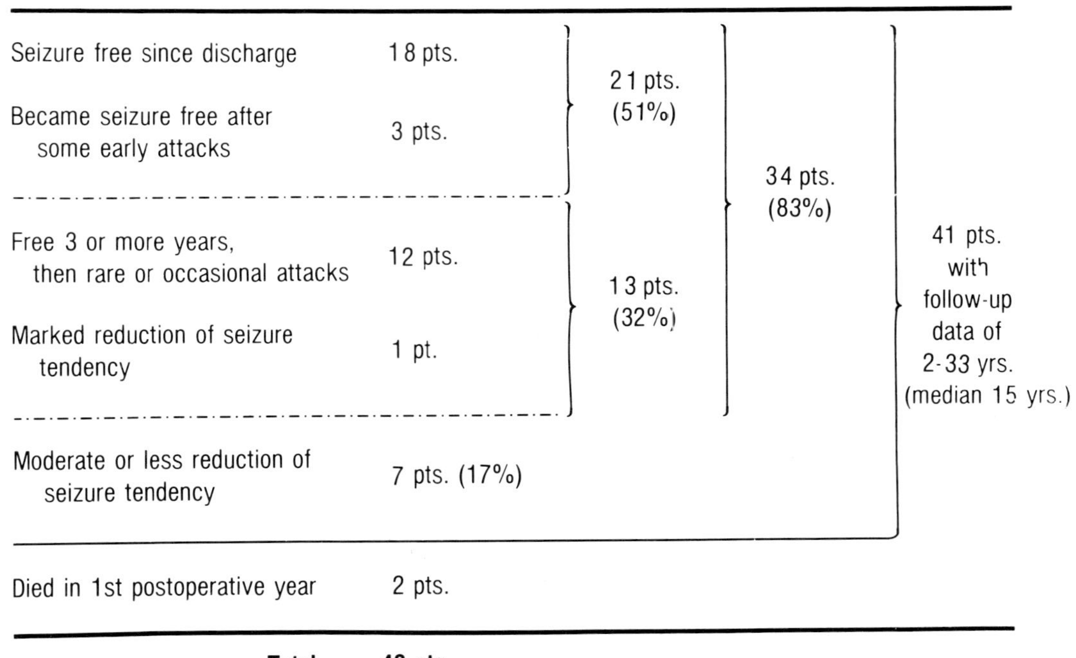

was performed. Postoperatively two attended a regular school, one a special school, and one patient was institutionalized because of severe mental retardation. There was inadequate data on the fifth patient.

Seven other patients were attending a special school or special classes in a regular school preoperatively. All of these patients returned to their schools after surgery and demonstrated a significant improvement in performance. One such patient has subsequently married, has had two 2 children, and manages her home successfully.

Another 7 patients were attending regular school preoperatively. All returned to regular school with improved performance. Five were ultimately employed, married, and managing households or taking vocational training. The other two underwent neurologic deterioration after early improvement as a result of head injuries 9 months and 2 years postoperatively.

Four young adults were employed or working in the home preoperatively. All continued their previous activity with additional responsibilities. Two others were at home preoperatively but not independent. Both became independent at home, but one developed neurologic deterioration after severe jaundice 4 months postoperatively and ultimately required custodial care.

LATE COMPLICATIONS

Among the 31 patients who had anatomically complete hemispherectomies performed between 1952 and 1968, 11 developed superficial cerebral hemosiderosis between 4½ and 25 years after their surgery (Table 108-2). Of these 11 cases, 9 were seizure-free when the complication developed and one had had two major and two minor seizures in 20 postoperative years. The remaining patient, a markedly retarded child operated upon at 3 years of age, had less than 1 percent of his preoperative seizure rate during the 10 postoperative years and then developed superficial cerebral hemosiderosis, from which he died a year later despite a technically satisfactory shunt.

Among the 14 patients in whom a functional hemispherectomy was performed during the decade between 1974 and 1984, 1 patient required a shunt 3 years after surgery. In this patient there was an impairment of absorption of CSF but no evidence of superficial cerebral hemosiderosis or neurologic deterioration. Although the follow-up period is relatively short (2 to 10 years; median 4 1/2 years) in relation to this complication, the long-term results should not be different from the experience with the 57 patients with subtotal hemispherectomy and the 71 patients with hemi-hemispherectomy who have been followed for over 4 years (Table 108-2).

SUMMARY

Hemispherectomy in the treatment of seizures associated with infantile type hemiplegia proved to be a highly successful operation and was widely adopted by neurosurgical centers in many countries during the 1950s and 1960s. Serious late complications developing 4 or more years after anatomically complete hemisphere resection markedly reduced the enthusiasm of the neurosurgical community for the use of the procedure during the late 1960s and 1970s. Subsequently we have used a functionally complete but anatomically subtotal hemispherectomy in which the anterior and posterior portions of the hemisphere are preserved but disconnected from the corpus callosum and from the upper brain stem. This procedure provides the excellent therapeutic results of the classic hemispherectomy while providing the good protection against the late pressure complications that have proved to be the case in long-term follow-up studies of patients who have undergone subtotal or hemi-hemispherectomy.

REFERENCES

1. Dandy W: Removal of right cerebral hemisphere for certain tumors with hemiplegia: Preliminary report. JAMA 90:823, 1928
2. L'Hermitte J: L'ablation complète de l'hémisphère droit dans les

cas de tumeur cérébrale localisée compliquée d'hémiplégie: la décérébration supra-thalamique unilatérale chez l'homme. Encephale 23:314, 1928

3. Gardner WJ: Removal of the right cerebral hemisphere for infiltrating glioma. JAMA 101:823, 1933

4. Gardner WJ, Karnosh LJ, McClure CC, et al: Residual function following hemispherectomy for tumour and for infantile hemiplegia. Brain 78:487, 1955

5. O'Brien JD: Further report on case of removal of right cerebral hemisphere. JAMA 107:657, 1936

6. McKenzie KG: The present status of a patient who had the right cerebral hemisphere removed. Proc Am Med Assoc 11:168, 1938

7. Krynau RA: Infantile hemiplegia treated by removing one cerebral hemisphere. J Neurol Neurosurg Psychiatry 13:243, 1950

8. Cairns H, Davidson MA: Hemispherectomy in the treatment of infantile hemiplegia: With a psychological supplement. Lancet 2:410, 1951

9. Falconer MA, Rushworth RG: Treatment of encephalotrigeminal angiomatosis (Sturge-Weber disease) by hemispherectomy. Arch Dis Child 35:433, 1960

10. McKissock W: Infantile hemiplegia treated by hemispherectomy. Proc R Soc Med 44:335, 1951

11. McKissock W: Infantile hemiplegia. Proc R Soc Med 46:431, 1953

12. Wilson PJE: Cerebral hemispherectomy for infantile hemiplegia. A report of 50 cases. Brain 93:147, 1970

13. Fabisch W, Glees P, MacMillan AL: Hemispherectomy for the treatment of epilepsy in infantile hemiplegia. Monatssch Psychiat Neurol 130:385, 1955

14. Feld M: L'hémisphérectomie totale et subtotale. Considérations de technique opératoire. Rev Neurol 87:525, 1952

15. Frugoni P: L'emisferectomia nel trattamento delle emiplegie spastiche infantili. Minerva Neurochir 5:1, 1961

16. Gros C, Vlahovitch B: L'hémisphérectomie cérébrale. Montpellier, Imprimerie Causse, Graille et Castelnau, 1955

17. Laine E, Gros C: L'hémisphérectomie. Paris, Masson, 1956

18. Obrador SA: Hemisferectomia en el tratamiento de las convulsiones de la hemiplegia infantil por hemiatrofia cerebral. Arq Neuro-psiquiat 9:191, 1951

19. Stepien L, Wocjan J, Wozniak M, et al: Results of hemispherectomy in epileptic patients (Polish). Neurol Neurochir Pol 19:207, 1969

20. Toerma T, Donner M: Hemispherectomy in early hemiplegia and intractable epilepsy. Acta Paediatr Scand 60:545, 1971

21. Wertheimer P, Goutelle A, Fischer G: Les résultats de l'hémisphérectomie. Réflexions sur une statistique. Neuro-Chir 10:554, 1964

22. Zulch KJ: Neurologische Befunde bei Patienten mit Hemispharektomie wegen Frühkindlichen Hirnschaden. Zentralbl Neurochir 14:48, 1954

23. Beller AJ, Streiffler M: Cerebral hemispherectomy in cerebral palsy. Clinical and EEG study. Harefuah Jerusalem 44:221, 1953

24. Haddad FS: Cerebral hemispherectomy in the treatment of epilepsy in patients with infantile hemiplegia (French). Rev Med May Dr 24:240, 1967

25. Fukunaga K, Doi Y, Yamazakit T: Two case reports of hemispherectomy (Japanese). Med J Hiroshima Univ 18:850, 1965

26. Ueki K: Neurological and psychological studies in patients with hemispherectomy. Electroencephalogr Clin Neurophysiol 18:309, 1965

27. Carlson J, Netley C, Hendrick EB, et al: A re-examination of intellectual disabilities in hemispherectomized patients. Trans Am Neurol Assoc 93:198, 1968

28. French LA, Johnson DR, Brown IA, et al: Cerebral hemispherectomy for control of intractable convulsive seizures. J Neurosurg 12:154, 1955

29. Goodall RJ: Cerebral hemispherectomy: Present status and clinical indications. Neurology 7:151, 1957

30. Hendrick EB, Hoffman HJ, Hudson AR: Hemispherectomy in children. Clin Neurosurg 16:315, 1969

31. Ransohoff JC: Hemispherectomy in the treatment of convulsive seizures associated with infantile hemiplegia. Res Publ Assoc Res Nerv Ment Dis 34:176, 1954

32. Verity CM, Strauss EH, Moyes PO, et al: Long term follow-up after cerebral hemispherectomy: Neurophysiologic, radiologic and psychological findings. Neurology 32:629, 1982

33. Christensen JC: Indications for and results of hemispherectomy in infantile hemiplegia. Arch Argent Pediatr 40:67, 1953

34. Matero R, Castro M: Hemisferectomias. Semana Med 123:199, 1963

35. White HH: Cerebral hemispherectomy in the treatment of infantile hemiplegia: Review of the literature and report of 2 cases. Confin Neurol 21:1, 1961

36. Rasmussen T: Further observations on the syndrome of chronic encephalitis and epilepsy. Appl Neurophysiol 41:1, 1978

37. Rasmussen T, Olszewski J, Lloyd-Smith D: Focal seizures due to chronic localized encephalitis. Neurology 8:435, 1958

38. Branch C, Milner B, Rasmussen T: Intracarotid sodium amytal for the lateralization of cerebral speech dominance: Observations on 123 patients. J Neurosurg 21:399, 1964

39. Milner B, Branch C, Rasmussen T: Observations on cerebral dominance, in de Reuck AVS, O'Connor (eds): Ciba Foundation on Disorders of Language. London, Churchill, 1964, pp 220–214

40. Wada J, Rasmussen T: Intracarotid injection of sodium amytal for the lateralization of cerebral speech dominance: Experimental and clinical observations. J Neurosurg 17:266, 1960

41. Basser LS: Hemiplegia of early onset and the faculty of speech with special reference to the effects of hemispherectomy. Brain 85:427, 1962

42. Falconer MA, Wilson PJE: Complications related to delayed hemorrhage after hemispherectomy. J Neurosurg 30:413, 1969

43. Laine E, Pruvet P, Osson D: Résultatséloignes de l'hémisphérectomie dans les cas d'hémiatrophie cérébrale infantile génératrice d'épilepsie. Neuro-Chirurg 10:507, 1964

44. Oppenheimer DR, Griffith HB: Persistent intracranial bleeding as a complication of hemispherectomy. J Neurol Neurosurg Psychiatry 29:229, 1966

45. Till K: Hemispherectomy for infantile hemiplegia. Dev Med Child Neurol 9:773, 1967

46. Brett E: Second thoughts on hemispherectomy in infantile hemiplegia. Dev Med Child Neurol 11:374, 1969

47. Griffith HB: Cerebral hemispherectomy for infantile hemiplegia in the light of late results. Ann R Coll Surg Engl 41:183, 1967

48. Wilson PJE: More second thoughts on hemispherectomy in infantile hemiplegia. Dev Med Child Neurol 12:799, 1970

49. Hughes JT, Oppenheimer DR: Superficial siderosis of the central nervous system. A report of nine cases with autopsy. Acta Neuropathol 13:56, 1969

50. Rasmussen T: Postoperative superficial hemosiderosis of the brain, its diagnosis, treatment and prevention. Am Neur Assoc 98:133, 1973

51. Ulrich J, Isler W, Vassali L: L'effet d'hémorrhagies leptoméningées répétées sur le système nerveux (La sidérose marginale du système nerveux central). Rev Neurol 112:466, 1965

52. Noetzel H: Diffusion von Blutfarbstoff in der innerne Randzone und ausseren Oberflache des Zentralnervensystems bei subarachnoidaler Bluting. Arch Psychiat 111:129, 1940

53. Iwanowski I, Olszewski J: The effects of subarachnoid injections of iron containing substances on the central nervous system. J Neuropathol Exp Neurol 19:433, 1960

54. Rasmussen T: Hemispherectomy for seizures revisited. Can J Neurol Soc 10:71, 1983

55. Galicich JH, French LA: Use of dexamethasone in the treatment of cerebral edema resulting from brain tumors and brain surgery. Am Pract 12:169, 1961

56. Rasmussen T, Gulati DR: Cortisone in the treatment of postoperative cerebral edema. J Neurosurg 19:535, 1962

CHAPTER 109

Section of the Corpus Callosum for Epilepsy

David W. Roberts

SINCE HORSLEY'S first craniotomy for the treatment of a seizure disorder in 1886,[1] the most widely performed surgical procedures for medically intractable epilepsy have shared the fundamental principle of removing the portion of resectable cerebral cortex presumed to represent the primary epileptogenic focus. In those patients in whom such a focus can be identified, the results of operative intervention are generally rewarding. Successful outcome after anterior temporal lobectomy, for example, is achieved in 60 to 80 percent of patients selected for that procedure.[2] There is a large population of patients with poorly controlled seizures, however, in whom a resectable epileptic focus cannot be identified and who therefore are not candidates for resective surgery.

In the 1930s, Van Wagenen, having made the observation that epileptic patients who sustained a stroke involving the corpus callosum often had improvement in their seizure disorders, divided the corpus callosum in a small number of patients.[3] In the early 1960s, Bogen et al. reported on a small series of similarly treated patients with encouraging results,[4–6] and Luessenhop et al. later described comparable success in three of four children.[7,8] In 1971, Wilson[9] chose this procedure as an alternative to hemispherectomy in a 9-year-old boy with infantile hemiplegia and began treating a series of ultimately 20 patients that demonstrated an efficacy to the procedure warranting its wider application.[9–14] The number of centers performing corpus callosotomy has increased dramatically over the past decade, and although numerous questions remain regarding optimal selection criteria and long-term prognosis, most investigators are reporting experiences confirming that of the earlier series.[15–26]

Concurrent with the clinical application of commissurotomy, an extensive body of experimental data has developed. Although the effects of callosotomy had been investigated earlier,[27] Erickson's work[28] remains a landmark for its demonstration of the major role played by the corpus callosum in the propagation of seizures in monkeys. The disruption of seizure generalization by division of the commissure has been demonstrated by numerous investigators,[29–33] and these data have often been cited in support of clinical application. Data suggesting no effect or worsening of seizures after commissurotomy also exist.[34,35] For further discussion of nonclinical investigations, see the excellent collection of papers presented at the 1982 Dartmouth Conference on the Corpus Callosum and Epilepsy[36] and the review papers of Spencer et al.[26] and Blume.[37]

INDICATIONS

Optimal selection criteria derive largely from previous experience and for callosotomy continue to be defined. The intuitive basis for proceeding with such a disconnection procedure has often rested on the presumption that propagation of the spreading seizure discharge could be disrupted and the seizure thus confined to one hemisphere. Many early patients were selected for surgery because of secondarily generalized seizures in the setting of demonstrable, nondiffuse pathologic conditions such as infantile hemiplegia. Early clinical results suggested better outcome in these patients as well as in those with less severe but nonetheless confined disease.[9,10,12–14]

In addition to seizure disorders with secondary generalization, other generalized seizure types have been demonstrated to respond favorably to commissurotomy. Most notable among these are the atonic or akinetic seizures generally characterized by sudden drop attacks. Many series of patients, including those at Dartmouth[13,38] and Minnesota,[19,20] have demonstrated either elimination or attenuation of this seizure type in most patients with such spells. Patients incapacitated by this type of seizure should be seriously considered for callosotomy. Distinguishing between truly primary generalized seizures and rapidly generalizing focal-onset seizures can be exceedingly difficult clinically, and we have not excluded from surgery patients who failed to demonstrate evidence of focal onset. Surgical results in terms of seizure type have been reported[26,38] and will be reviewed below.

In an attempt to improve selection criteria, Williamson[39] reviewed surgical outcomes from various series in terms of clinical diagnoses. Classifying patients into groups of infantile hemiplegia, forme-fruste infantile hemiplegia, Rasmussen's syndrome, Lennox-Gastaut syndrome, frontal lobe epilepsy, and focal/multifocal epilepsy, he found slightly better outcomes in the first two groups but sufficient improvement to justify surgical intervention in all categories.[39]

Electroencephalographic findings have also been correlated with surgical results. Both Geoffroy et al.[21] and Spencer et al.[26] have reported better results in patients with lateralized EEG abnormalities. Bilaterally synchronous epileptiform activity has been present in the majority of patients and does not represent a necessarily bad prognostic sign. The significance of bilaterally independent foci remains undetermined.

Our selection criteria for callosal section include (1) medical intractability of at least 2 and usually 4 years duration with

OPERATIVE NEUROSURGICAL TECHNIQUES
ISBN 0-8089-1862-1

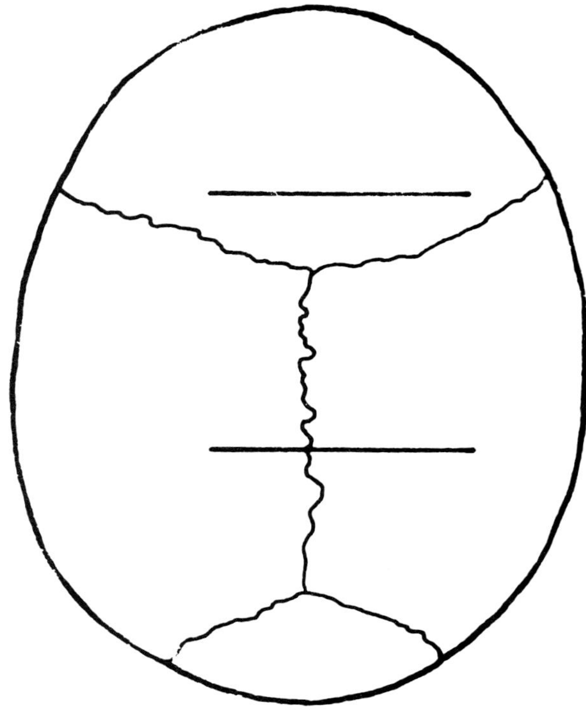

Fig. 109-1. Anterior and posterior callosal section is performed through 9-cm linear incisions and 2-inch trephinations. (Reprinted from Roberts DW: Corpus callostomy: Surgical technique, in Reeves AG (ed): Epilepsy and the Corpus Callosum. New York, Plenum Press, 1985, p 261. With permission.)

exhaustive anticonvulsant regimens and documented adequate serum levels of anticonvulsant medications; (2) generalized seizures, usually but not necessarily major motor or akinetic in type, and (3) potential functional benefit if improvement in the seizure disorder is achieved. Although the likelihood of success may be less in certain instances, we have not automatically excluded patients from surgery because of retardation, age, mixed hemisphere dominance, lack of demonstrable focal seizure onset, or bilaterally independent EEG abnormalities.

OPERATIVE PROCEDURE

A review of the early commissurotomy series shows comparable success rates regardless of whether or not division of the anterior commissure or one fornix was performed at the time of corpus callosotomy. Although there are probably persons in whom these other structures play important roles in seizure propagation, we have restricted our procedure to division of the major commissure and underlying posterior hippocampal commissure only. Whether or not partial callosotomy is preferable to complete division as an initial procedure is less clear. We are currently advocating partial callosotomy in most patients, with division of the anterior one half to two thirds of the corpus callosum unless there is evidence of a predominantly posterior focus. Many of these patients will subsequently require completion of the callosotomy, but it appears preferable to spare those not requiring complete section the effects of greater disconnection.

The surgery is performed under general anesthesia with intraoperative electroencephalographic recording. At least one surgeon has tailored his length of resection based on intraoper-

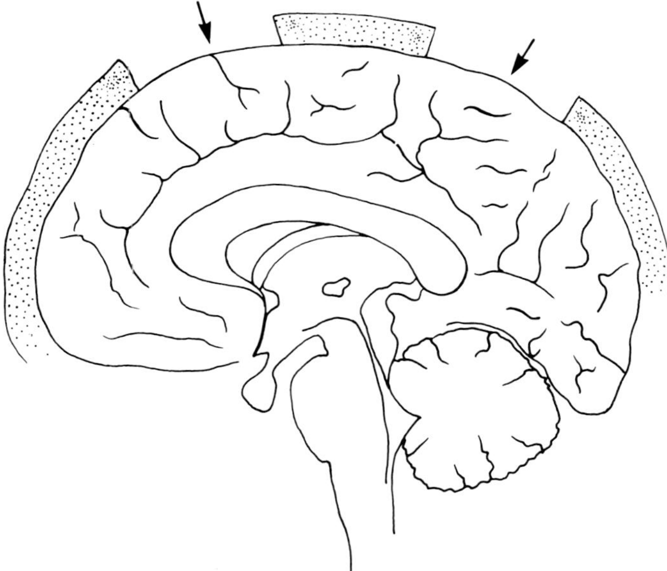

Fig. 109-2. The anterior and posterior approaches provide direct and convenient access to the respective halves of the callosum. (Reprinted from Roberts DW: Corpus callostomy: Surgical technique, in Reeves AG (ed): Epilepsy and the Corpus Callosum. New York, Plenum Press, 1985, p 264. With permission.)

ative EEG information,[22] but having observed subsequent seizure propagation across remaining, adjacent callosal fibers we have not adopted this practice. The patient is placed supine on the operating table and the unturned head is secured in a Gardner head clamp. For the anterior division the neck is left in neutral position; for the posterior division, it is flexed approximately 20 degrees. Decadron (10 mg) is administered the night before surgery and when anesthesia is induced.

We have used linear incisions and 2-inch trephinations

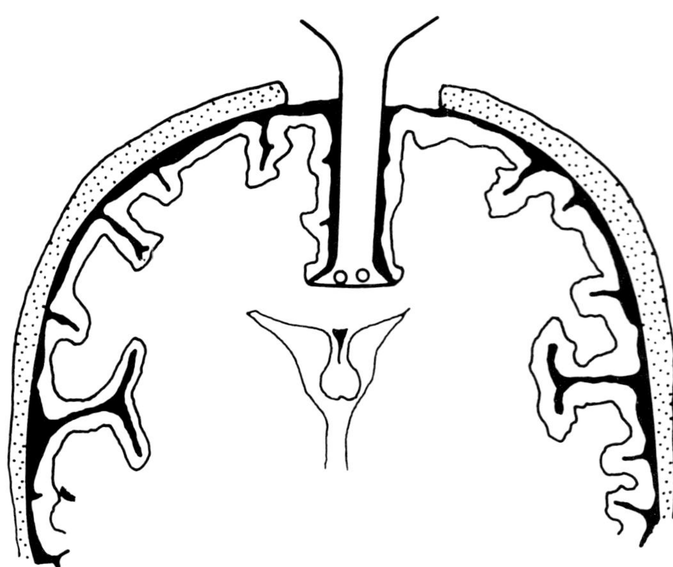

Fig. 109-3. Minimal retraction is required on the nondominant hemisphere. Retraction of the inferior aspect of the falx and contralateral cingulate gyrus is occasionally useful. (Reprinted from Roberts DW: Corpus callostomy: Surgical technique, in Reeves AG (ed): Epilepsy and the Corpus Callosum. New York, Plenum Press, 1985, p 262. With permission.)

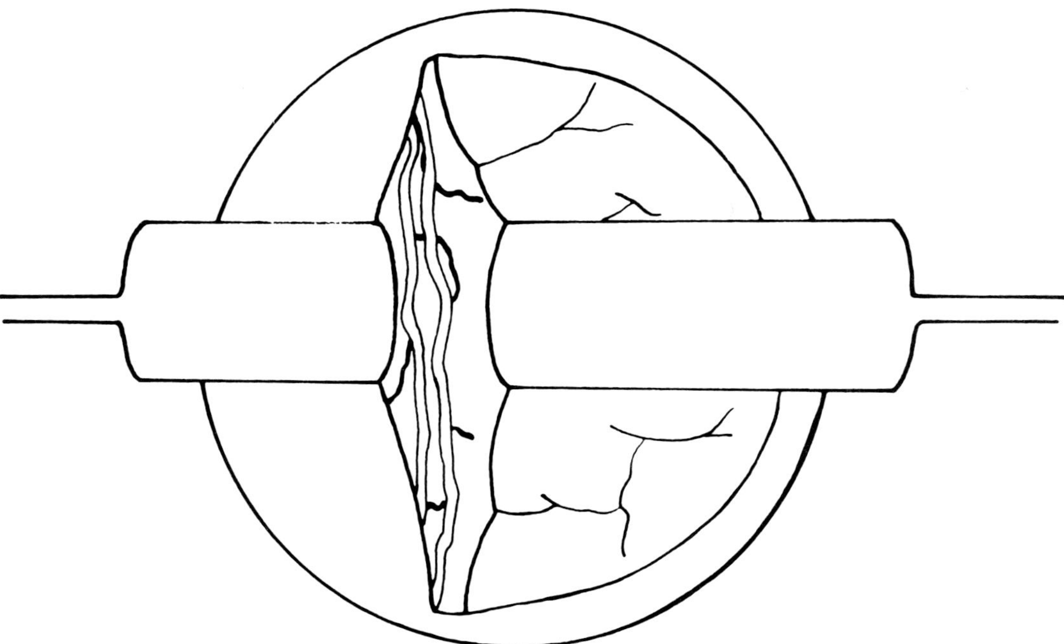

Fig. 109-4. The pericallosal arteries are identified overlying the callosum, and the section is performed wherever most convenient in relation to them. (Reprinted from Roberts DW: Corpus callostomy: Surgical technique, in Reeves AG (ed): Epilepsy and the Corpus Callosum. New York, Plenum Press, 1985, p 262. With permission.)

(Figures 109-1 and 109-2),[12,40] but the type of craniotomy is relatively unimportant. For the anterior procedure, a 9-cm transverse incision with one third of its length across the midline is placed 2 cm in front of the coronal suture. For the posterior procedure a similar incision and trephination is employed at the level of the parietal eminence. The placement of the craniotomy across the sagittal sinus requires increased caution but facilitates later exposure down the interhemispheric fissure. The approach is generally on the side of the nondominant right hemisphere except for those instances in which significant pathology is well lateralized to the other.

Angiography for localization of parasagittal draining veins before transcallosal procedures has been advocated by Apuzzo[41] but has not been a routine study in our series. Using microsurgical technique it has always been possible to work on either or both sides of such a vein without sacrificing it. It is interesting and useful to note nonetheless Apuzzo's observation that in 42 of 100 angiographic studies, significant veins were noted to enter the sagittal sinus within 2 cm of the coronal suture with 70 percent of these posterior to that suture.[41]

The dura is opened in a curvilinear fashion and reflected on the sagittal sinus. Initial dissection down the interhemispheric fissure is performed under loupe magnification, and retraction is aided by the adminstration of mannitol (1 g/kg) during the opening. Pressed Gelfoam (Upjohn, Kalamazoo, Michigan) protects the exposed cortex, and a Greenberg self-retaining retractor (Codman and Shurtleff, Randolph, Massachusetts) is placed before the operating microscope is brought into use. A single retractor blade gently retracts the ipsilateral hemisphere, and, when needed, an additional blade is used on the inferior aspect of the falx or contralateral cingulate gyrus (Figure 109-3).

The glistening white appearance of the corpus callosum distinguishes it from the more superficial cingulate gyrus, and exposure along the length of callosum to be divided is obtained before the commissure is entered. Adhesions between the hemispheres, which are especially common after previous

infection or trauma, can make exposure difficult; approaching the callosum more posteriorly and utilizing the deeper extension of the falx will prove helpful in this situation. The pericallosal arteries are easily identified overlying the callosum, and actual division of callosal fibers is carried out wherever most convenient in relation to these vessels (Figure 109-4).

The magnification and illumination provided by the operating microscope are invaluable during the final exposure and

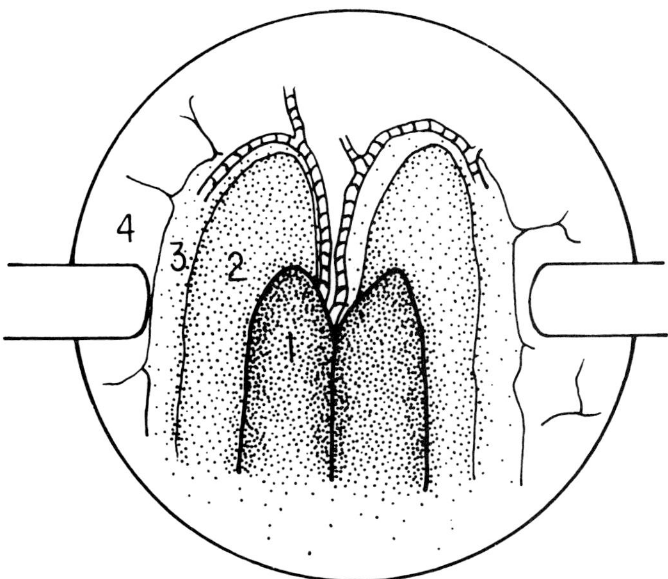

Fig. 109-5. Division of the callosum at the level of the genu. (1) Ependymal surfaces of the frontal horns of the lateral ventricles; (2) the cut surface of the genu; (3) the dorsal aspect of the genu; (4) the cingulate gyrus. The anterior cerebral arteries are visible. (Reprinted from Roberts DW: Corpus callostomy: Surgical technique, in Reeves AG (ed): Epilepsy and the Corpus Callosum. New York, Plenum Press, 1985, p 263. With permission.)

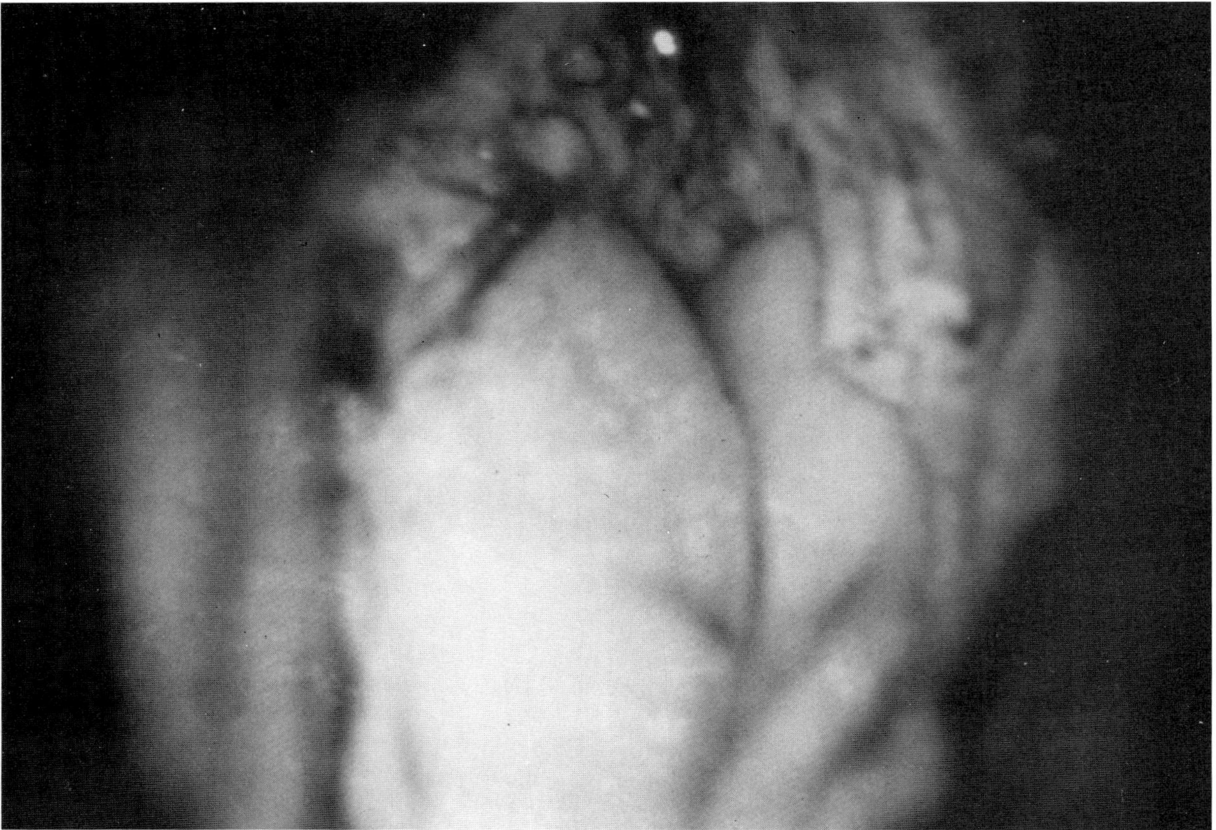

Fig. 109-6. Intraoperative photograph of the divided genu. The ependymal surfaces of the frontal horns, the cut surfaces of the callosum, and the midline cleft are visible (see Figure 109-5).

actual sectioning. We use the Zeiss OPMI 1H microscope on a Contraves stand (both from Carl Zeiss, Inc., Thornwood, New York). The 300-mm objective lens provides a reasonable working distance to the field; 12.5× oculars and settings on the magnification changer of 0.4 to 1.6 (most often 0.6 and 1.0) are used. Small vessels supplying only the callosum itself can be coagulated with bipolar cautery. The actual division of callosal fibers is carried out with the microseptal, Krayenbühl dissector or microsuction tip.

Early descriptions of callosal section describe the bluish appearance of the underlying ventricular ependymal surface and recommend this landmark as the limit of division.[11,12] Over the course of our series of patients, the advantages of identifying the midline during the division have become increasingly evident and include unequivocal assurance of completeness of fiber division, elimination of possible lateral deviation (especially in the frontal region), decreased likelihood of entering the lateral ventricle, and less operative time. A gentle sweeping from side to side of a blunt microinstrument as the callosum is nearly traversed will often expose the midline cleft between the lateral ventricles (Figures 109-5, 109-6, and 109-7). Once this cleft has been identified, the remainder of the sectioning follows easily.

The direction of actual sectioning is not particularly important, but identification of the midline during the anterior division is easiest at the posteriormost portion of the genu or the anterior portion of the body. Subsequent division around the genu and down the rostrum is performed extraventricularly as far as possible. At this point the rostrum is nearly paper-thin and any remaining fibers are insignificant. No attempt is made to divide the anterior commissure blindly.

Attention is now directed to the posterior extent of the division. When plans have already been made to complete the callosotomy regardless of response to an initial procedure, division of approximately one half of the callosum is logical. If an attempt is being made to achieve success with a partial division, it is reasonable to carry the division through the anterior two thirds. When assurance of section and hemostasis is complete, a titanium clip attached to a small piece of Gelfoam is placed at the posterior extent of the divided callosum. At subsequent surgery gliosis can obscure the extent of previous section and such a marker has often been greatly appreciated.

Division of the posterior corpus callosum is similarly performed. As previously mentioned, the more extensive falx cerebri often aids the more posterior exposure. The fibers of the splenium are divided with similar instrumentation, and under magnification the completeness of the section is certain. The underlying arachnoid, beneath which lie the quadrigeminal cistern and the pineal, is preserved. The posterior hippocampal commissure can be indistinguishable from the adjacent callosal fibers, but this is of no practical significance, since it is divided as well. If the posterior section is the initial commissurotomy procedure, a clip is left as a marker at the anteriormost extent of the section. If an anterior section has already been performed, the previously placed clip is retrieved.

After confirmation of hemostasis the dura is closed over Gelfilm (Upjohn, Kalamazoo, Michigan) with 4-0 Vicryl

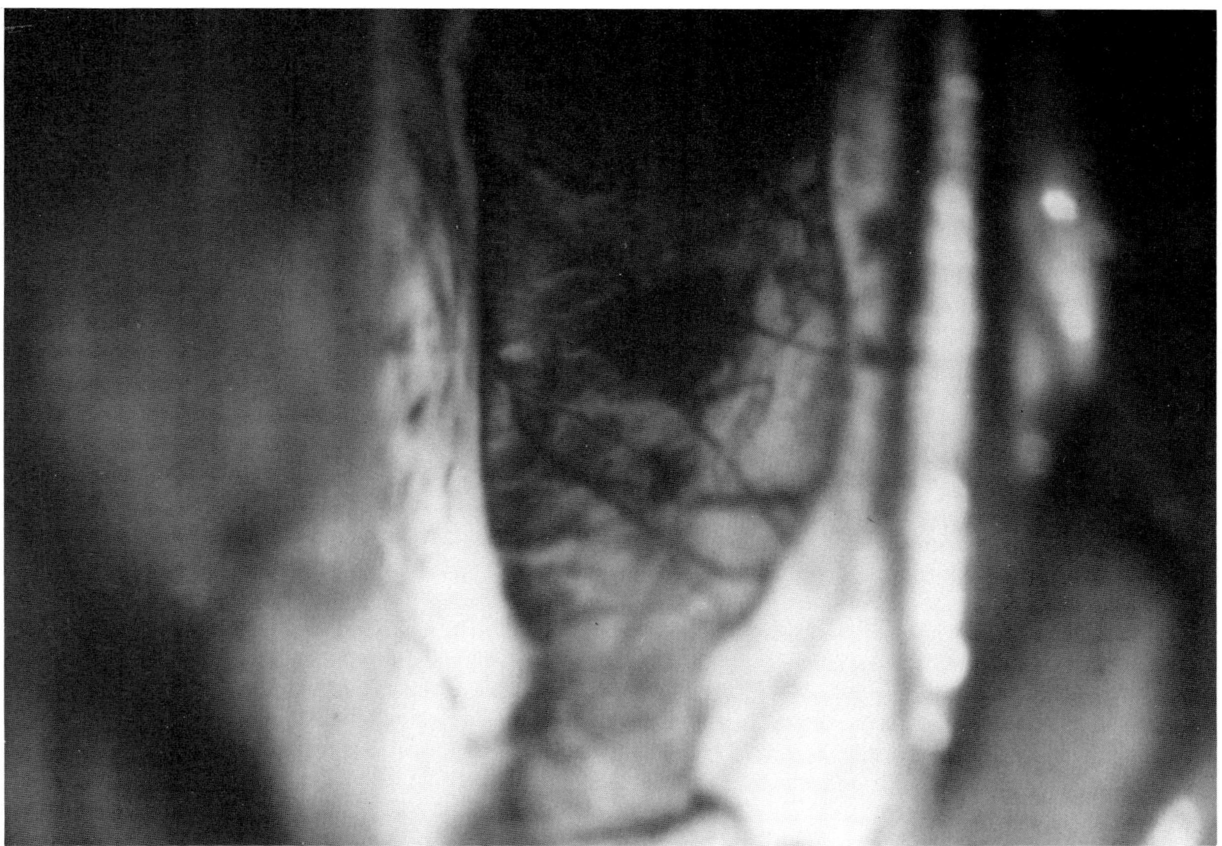

Fig. 109-7. Intraoperative photograph of the divided splenium. The cut surfaces of the callosum and the underlying arachnoid are evident.

(Ethicon). The bone plug is secured through predrilled holes with 2-0 Ethilon; the galea aponeurosis is reapproximated with 2-0 Vicryl; and the skin is closed with either 4-0 Prolene or staples. The patient is observed in the neurosurgical ICU overnight and usually transferred to the neurosurgical ward the next morning. Mobilization begins immediately, and the patient is typically discharged 1 to 1½ weeks later. Anticonvulsant medication is generally left unaltered until at least subsequent follow-up at 1 to 2 months. A decision regarding completion of the callosotomy is made a minimum of 2 months after the first procedure.

RESULTS

Reporting on a total of 20 patients, Wilson et al. noted 16 to have greater than 50 percent reduction in overall seizure frequency.[10,13] Van Wagenen and Herren[3] reported significant improvement in 9 of 10 patients, and Geoffroy et al.[21] had similar success in 6 of 9 patients. Rayport et al.[23] reported 7 of 9 patients significantly improved, Luessenhop et al.[7,8] 3 of 4, Amacher[15] 4 of 4, and Bouvier et al.[17] 6 of 6. An analysis of outcome in 183 patients from 14 centers[18] found 5.5 percent free of seizures, 73.5 percent improved, and 20.7 percent

Table 109-1. Response of major motor seizures to commissurotomy in the 32 of 51 patients who experienced major motor seizures among their seizure types preoperatively

Seizure Response	Number of Patients
No seizures	14
More than 80 percent reduction in frequency	7
50 to 80 percent reduction in frequency	3
Less than 50 percent reduction in frequency	2
No reduction in frequency	6

Table 109-2. Response of focal motor seizures to commissurotomy in the 14 of 51 patients who experienced focal motor seizures among their seizure types preoperatively

Seizure Response	Number of Patients
No seizures	3
More than 80 percent reduction in frequency	2
50 to 80 percent reduction in frequency	1
Less than 50 percent reduction in frequency	0
No reduction in frequency	6
Increased frequency	2

Table 109-3. Response of atonic seizures to commissurotomy in the 21 of 51 patients who experienced atonic seizures among their seizure types preoperatively

Seizure Response	Number of Patients
No seizures	9
More than 80 percent reduction in frequency	7
50 to 80 percent reduction in frequency	2
Less than 50 percent reduction in frequency	0
No reduction in frequency	3

Table 109-5. Response of complex partial seizures to commissurotomy in the 25 of 51 patients who experienced complex partial seizures among their seizure types preoperatively

Seizure Response	Number of Patients
No seizures	10
More than 80 percent reduction in frequency	3
50 to 80 percent reduction in frequency	7
Less than 50 percent reduction in frequency	0
No reduction in frequency	5

unimproved; the range for unimprovement was 10 to 38 percent. Although these figures are not as good as those for temporal lobectomy or extratemporal cortical resection, the patient populations are distinct, with nearly all who underwent division of the corpus callosum having failed to fulfill the selection criteria for other surgery.

The majority of patients undergoing callosal surgery for seizure control have had multiple seizure types, and it is useful to analyze outcome in terms of seizure classification. Tables 109-1 through 109-5 summarize outcome in the Dartmouth series of 51 evaluable patients with a mean follow-up of 53.7 months and a range of 2 to 169 months.

Thirty-two of 51 patients preoperatively had major motor seizures, and of these, 14 have had elimination of those seizures. An additional 7 patients have had greater than 80 percent reduction in their frequency, and 3 a 50 to 80 percent reduction. Two have had less than 50 percent improvement; 6 have had no improvement in frequency, although in 2 the seizures are less severe.

Twenty-one of 51 patients had atonic seizures, generally characterized by sudden falls to the ground. In 9 patients these have been eliminated and in another 7 reduction of greater than 80 percent has been achieved. Although frequency has been less successfully affected in the remaining 5, the actual seizure has been modified in 4 from a fall to head nod or other less injurious manifestation. Absence spells were present in 22 of 51 patients, and although the procedure was not performed for this particular seizure type, 15 patients have had elimination or

Table 109-4. Response of absence seizures to commissurotomy in the 22 patients (of 51 patients) who experienced absence seizures among their seizure types preoperatively

Seizure Response	Number of Patients
No seizures	11
More than 80 percent reduction in frequency	4
50 to 80 percent reduction in frequency	3
Less than 50 percent reduction in frequency	2
No reduction in frequency	2

greater than 80 percent reduction in the frequency of these spells.

The results in focal motor epilepsy, which might be presumed to remain unaffected by a procedure thought to be effective by disruption of propagation, are indeed less successful but nevertheless interesting in this subgroup of 14 patients. Three patients demonstrated no further focal seizure activity and an additional 2 patients had better than 80 percent reduction. Two patients in this group had an increase in frequency for this seizure type, and 12 patients who had not experienced focal motor seizures developed them after surgery. A worsening of this seizure type following callosotomy has been described,[42] and the possibility of the procedure resulting in a loss of an inhibitory influence has been suggested.[26,37,42] Our data confirm the occurrence of increased or new-onset focal seizures, but they have nearly always occurred as the attenuated remnant of previously generalizing seizure activity. In no instance has this represented a deterioration in overall functional outcome.

Corpus callosotomy has not been advocated as a substitute for temporal lobectomy in patients eligible for that procedure, but the results with regard to complex partial seizures in 25 of 51 patients are noteworthy. Ten of 25 have had elimination of this seizure type, and another 3 patients have had greater than 80 percent reduction in their frequency. In 11 patients the seizures have been significantly modified in severity.[43] The role of this procedure in patients with only complex partial seizures but in whom investigations fail to define a resectable focus remains undefined.

Surgical complications early in this series included hydrocephalus in 3 patients; this subsequently has not been encountered. The present surgical technique of remaining extraventricular may be responsible. Wound or bone flap infections occurred in 3 patients. Sterile meningitis was noted in 3 patients; septic meningitis was documented in 1 patient. One patient in whom surgery and the early postoperative course had been unremarkable died of a frontal lobe infarction 12 days after surgery. A second patient died of a cardiopulmonary arrest after readmission to the hospital and development of status epilepticus, pneumonia, thrombophlebitis and possible pulmonary embolus 3 months after surgery.

The behavioral and neuropsychologic effects of commissurotomy have been studied extensively;[44–54] Gazzaniga and colleagues[50–54] are responsible for the most enlightening work. The initial impression following the earliest series had been that callosotomy produced little alteration in cognitive function.[44,45]

Subsequent and more sophisticated investigations have demonstrated numerous effects of disconnection,[50,54] but in general it has been unusual for these to represent significant handicaps.

The majority of patients in the Dartmouth series appear to have improved or remained unchanged in their level of cognitive fuction. This has usually been the result of both diminished seizure activity and decreased anticonvulsant medication. Ferrell et al.[55] reported on formal neuropsychologic testing in eight of the earliest patients and found improvement in six. Of the entire series of 51 patients, 5 patients have decreased cognitive ability according to their families—usually described as poorer memory or concentration—and this has been noted in other series as well.[49,56] Further investigation of this finding has suggested that it may be more of an attentional disorder than actual memory dysfunction.[57] The reason for this disturbance in some patients is unknown.

Speech and motor dysfunction have been frequently noted in the immediate postoperative period, but persistence of these deficits has been rare.[10,58] Antagonism between the right and left hemispheres, usually manifested as opposing actions of the right and left hands, has been similarly reported.[49] In only one patient of our series has this been a chronic difficulty.

CONCLUSIONS

Although the answers to important questions regarding corpus callosotomy for intractable epilepsy continue to evolve, the experience accumulated over nearly 50 years—and especially over the past 15 years—allows a number of important points to be made. Perhaps most important is the recognition that for certain patients who have failed medical management and who are not eligible for other seizure surgery, commissurotomy can successfully reduce seizure frequency and severity. Atonic seizures and secondarily generalized major motor seizures are most likely to be improved, but other seizure types may also respond.

Extraventricular division of the corpus callosum alone achieves the aforementioned success; complete callosotomy may not be required in all patients, and staging of the procedure remains a reasonable approach. Division of the corpus callosum can be safely and confidently performed as a microsurgical procedure.

Behavioral and neuropsychologic sequelae of commissurotomy are well-recognized, but it has been uncommon for these to represent permanent disabilities. In the great majority of patients the benefits resulting from the procedure outweigh any such effects.

REFERENCES

1. Horsley V: Brain surgery. Br Med J 2:670, 1886
2. Spencer SS: Depth electroenecephalography in selection of refractory epilepsy for surgery. Ann Neurol 9:207, 1981
3. Van Wagenen WP, Herren RY: Surgical division of commissural pathways in the corpus callosum: Relation to spread of an epileptic attack. Arch Neurol Psychiatr 44:740, 1940
4. Bogen JE, Vogel PJ: Cerebral commissurotomy in man: Preliminary case report. Bull Los Angeles Neurol Soc 27:169, 1962
5. Bogen JE, Fisher ED, Vogel PJ: Cerebral commissurotomy: A second case report. JAMA 194:1328, 1965
6. Bogen JE, Sperry RW, Vogel PJ: Commissural section and propagation of seizures, in Jasper H, Ward AA, Pope A (eds): Basic Mechansisms of the Epilepsies. Boston, Little, Brown and Co, 1969, p 439
7. Luessenhop AJ: Interhemispheric commissurotomy: (The split brain operation) as an alternate to hemispherectomy for control of intractable seizures. Am Surg 36:265, 1970
8. Luessenhop AJ, dela Cruz TC, Fenichel GM: Surgical disconnection of the cerebral hemispheres for intractable seizures: Results in infancy and childhood. JAMA 213:1630, 1970
9. Wilson DH, Culver C, Waddington M, et al: Disconnection of the cerebral hemispheres: An alternative to hemispherectomy for the control of intractable seizures. Neurology 25:1149, 1975
10. Wilson DH, Reeves AG, Gazzaniga MS, et al: Cerebral commissurotomy for control of intractable seizures. Neurology 27:708, 1977
11. Wilson DH, Reeves A, Gazzaniga M: Division of the corpus callosum for uncontrollable epilepsy. Neurology 28:649, 1978
12. Wilson DH, Reeves A, Gazzaniga M: Corpus callosotomy for control of intractable seizures, in Wada JA, Penry JK (eds): Advances in Epileptology: The Xth Epilepsy International Symposium. New York, Raven Press, 1980, pp 205–213
13. Wilson DH, Reeves AG, Gazzaniga MS: "Central" commissurotomy for intractable generalized epilepsy: Series two. Neurology 32:687, 1982
14. Harbaugh RE, Wilson DH, Reeves AG, et al: Forebrain commissurotomy for epilepsy: Review of 20 consecutive cases. Acta Neurochir 68:263, 1983
15. Amacher AL: Midline commissurotomy for the treatment of some cases of intractable epilepsy. Childs Brain 2:54, 1976
16. Avila JO, Radvany J, Huck FR, et al: Anterior callosotomy as a substitute for hemispherectomy. Acta Neurochir (Suppl) 30:137, 1980
17. Bouvier G, Mercier C, St. Hilaire JM, et al: Anterior callosotomy and chronic depth electrode recording in the surgical management of some intractable seizures. Appl Neurophysiol 46:52, 1983
18. Engel J Jr: Outcome with respect to epileptic seizures, in Engel J Jr (ed): Surgical Treatment of the Epilepsies. New York Raven Press, 1987, pp 553–571
19. Gates JR, Leppik IE, Yap J, et al: Corpus callosotomy: Clinical and electroencephalographic effects. Epilepsia 25:308, 1984
20. Gates JR, Maxwell R, Leppik IE, et al:Electroencephalographic and clinical effects of total corpus callosotomy, in Reeves AG (ed): Epilepsy and the Corpus Callosum. New York, Plenum Press, 1985, pp 315–328
21. Geoffroy G, Lassonde M, Delisle F, et al: Corpus callosotomy for control of intractable epilepsy in children. Neurology 33:891, 1983
22. Marino R Jr, Ragazzo PC: Selective criteria and results of selective partial callosotomy, in Reeves AG (ed): Epilepsy and the Corpus Callosum. New York, Plenum Press, 1985, pp 281–301
23. Rayport M, Ferguson SM, Corrie WS: Outcomes and indications of corpus callosum section for intractable seizure control. Appl Neurophysiol 46:47, 1983
24. Rayport M, Corrie WS, Ferguson SM: Corpus callosum section for control of clinically and electroencephalographically classified intractable seizures, in Reeves AG (ed): Epilepsy and the Corpus Callosum. New York, Plenum Press, 1985, pp 329–337
25. Saint-Hilaire JM, Giard N, Bouvier G, et al: Anterior callosotomy in frontal lobe epilepsies, in Reeves AG (ed): Epilepsy and the Corpus Callosum. New York, Plenum Press, 1985, pp 303–314
26. Spencer SS, Gates JR, Reeves AG, et al: Corpus callosum section, in Engel J Jr (ed): Surgical Treatment of the Epilepsies. New York, Raven Press, 1987, pp 425–444
27. Gozzano M: Biolektrische Erscheinungen bei er Reflexepilepsie. J Psychol Neurol 47:24-39, 1939 [cited by Erickson, 1940]
28. Erickson TE: Spread of the epileptic discharge: An experimental study of the afterdischarge induced by electrical stimulation of the cerebral cortex. Arch Neurol Psychiat 43:429, 1940
29. Marcus EM, Watson CW: Bilateral synchronous spike wave electrographic patterns in the cat. Arch Neurol 14:601, 1966
30. Marcus EM, Watson CW: Symmetrical epileptogenic foci in mon-

key cerebral cortex: Mechanisms of interaction and regional variations in capacity for synchronous discharges. Arch Neurol 19:99, 1968

31. Kopeloff N, Kennard MA, Pacella BL, et al: Section of corpus callosum in experimental epilepsy in the monkey. Arch Neurol Psychiat 63:719, 1950

32. Crowell RM, Ajmone Marsan C: Topographical distribution and patterns of unit activity during electrically induced after-discharge. Electroencephalogr Clin Neurophysiol (Suppl) 31:59, 1972

33. Mutani R, Bergamini L, Fariello R, et al: Bilateral synchrony of epileptic discharge associated with chronic asymmetrical cortical foci. Electroencephalogr Clin Neurophysiol 34:53, 1973

34. Stavraky GW: Supersensitivity Following Lesions of the Nervous System. Toronto, University of Toronto Press, 1961, pp 33–38

35. Kusske JA, Rush JL: Corpus callosum and propagation of afterdischarge to contralateral cortex and thalamus. Neurology 28:905, 1978

36. Reeves AG (ed): Epilepsy and the Corpus Callosum. New York, Plenum Press, 1985

37. Blume WT: Corpus callosum section for seizure control: Rationale and review of experimental and clinical data. Cleve Clin Q 51:319, 1984

38. Reeves AG, O'Leary PM: Total corpus callosotomy for control of medically intractable epilepsy, in Reeves AG (ed): Epilepsy and the Corpus Callosum. New York, Plenum Press, 1985, pp 269–280

39. Williamson PD: Corpus callosum section for intractable epilepsy: Criteria for patient selection, in Reeves AG (ed): Epilepsy and the Corpus Callosum. New York, Plenum Press, 1985, pp 243–257

40. Roberts DW: Corpus callosotomy: Surgical technique, in Reeves AG (ed): Epilepsy and the Corpus Callosum. New York, Plenum Press, 1985, pp 259–267

41. Apuzzo MLJ, Chikovani OK, Gott PS: Transcallosal, interfornicial approaches for lesions affecting the third ventricle: Surgical considerations and consequences. Neurosurgery 10:547, 1982

42. Spencer SS, Spencer DD, Glaser GH, et al: More intense focal seizure types after callosal section: The role of inhibition. Ann Neurol 16:686, 1984

43. Roberts DW, Reeves AG: The effect of commissurotomy on complex partial epilepsy in patients without a resectable seizure focus. Appl Neurophysiol (in press)

44. Akelaitis AJ: Studies on corpus callosum: Higher visual function in each hemisphere's fleld following complete section of the corpus callosum. Arch Neurol Psychiat 45:786, 1941

45. Akelaitis AJ: A study of gnosis, praxis and language following section of the corpus callosum and anterior commissure. J Neurosurg 1:94, 1944

46. Gordon HW, Bogen JE, Sperry RW: Absence of deconnection syndrome in two patients with partial section of the neocommissures. Brain 94:327, 1971

47. Campbell AL Jr, Bogen JE, Smith A: Disorganization and reorganization of cognitive and sensorimotor functions in cerebral commissurotomy: Compensatory roles of the forebrain commissures and cerebral hemispheres in man. Brain 104:493, 1981

48. Oepen G, Schulz-Weiling R, Zimmermann P, et al: Long-term effects of partial callosal lesions: Preliminary report. Acta Neurochir 77:22, 1985

49. Ferguson SM, Rayport M, Corrie WS: Neuropsychiatric observations on behavioral consequences of corpus callosum section for seizure control, in Reeves AG (ed): Epilepsy and the Corpus Callosum. New York, Plenum Press, 1985, pp 501–514

50. Gazzaniga MS, Risse GL, Springer SP, et al: Psychologic and neurologic consequences of partial and complete cerebral commissurotomy. Neurology 25:10, 1975

51. Ledoux JE, Risse GL, Springer SP, et al: Cognition and commissurotomy. Brain 100:87, 1977

52. Volpe BT, Sidtis JJ, Hotzman JD: Cortical mechanisms involved in praxis: Observations following partial and complete section of the corpus callosum in man. Neurology 32:645, 1982

53. Gazzaniga MS, Smylie CS: Dissociation of language and cognition: A psychological proflle of two disconnected right hemispheres. Brain 107:145, 1984

54. Gazzaniga MS: Some contributions of split-brain studies to the study of human cognition, in Reeves AG (ed): Epilepsy and the Corpus Callosum. New York, Plenum Press, 1985, pp 341–348

55. Ferrell RB, Culver CM, Tucker GJ: Psychosocial and cognitive function after commissurotomy for intractable seizures. J Neurosurg 58:374, 1983

56. Zaidel E, Sperry RW: Memory impairment after commissurotomy in man. Brain 97:263, 1974

57. Beniak TE, Gates JR, Risse GL: Comparison of selected neuropsychological test variables pre- and postoperatively on patients subjected to corpus callosotomy. Epilepsia 26:534, 1985

58. Ross MK, Reeves AG, Roberts DW: Post-commissurotomy mutism. Ann Neurol 16:11, 1984

CHAPTER 110

Selective Vestibular Nerve Transection in the Treatment of Meniere's Disease

Richard R. Gacek

THIS CHAPTER reviews the indications, technique, and results of selective vestibular ablation in the treatment of episodic vertigo caused by peripheral ear disease. Although Meniere's disease is the most frequent cause of disabling episodic vertigo, other peripheral disorders such as vestibular neuritis and chronic labyrinthitis are occasionally responsible for disabling dysequilibrium. Accurate diagnosis and evaluation of function are important considerations before the proper surgical approach can be identified for the treatment of vertigo. A review of the pathophysiology responsible for the clinical manifestations of these labyrinthine disorders therefore is essential in the logical choice of the surgical technique of selective vestibular ablation.

PATHOPHYSIOLOGY

MENIERE'S DISEASE

The cardinal symptoms in Meniere's disease are (1) fluctuating sensorineural hearing loss, and (2) episodes of vertigo, which have a usual duration of one to several hours. The pattern of hearing loss usually reflects a greater loss in the low frequencies early in the disease, but eventually all frequency thresholds are elevated as the disease progresses. Tinnitus consistently accompanies the hearing loss and may be a major complaint of the patient. The onset of vertiginous episodes is usually preceded by the sensorineural hearing loss for a period of months to years. The disorder is usually limited to one ear (85 percent), but can be bilateral in approximately 15 to 20 percent of patients. The disease characteristically affects young and middle-aged adults, although occasionally the disorder is seen in the second decade of life. The frequency of the episodic vertigo varies from patient to patient and can even vary within the same patient as the disease progresses.

A variant of the typical clinical presentation of Meniere's disease is a "delayed" form in which the onset of episodic vertigo becomes manifest many years (decades) after the appearance of a (frequently sudden) profound sensorineural hearing loss, often resulting from viral labyrinthitis or head trauma. This form is referred to as delayed Meniere's disease or delayed endolymphatic hydrops.

Although the precise cause of Meniere's disease is unknown, the pathophysiology has received considerable attention. The histopathologic correlate of Meniere's disease is endolymphatic hydrops, which is manifested as distention of the endolymphatic compartment of the pars inferior (cochlea and saccule) (Figure 110-1). Surgical destruction of the endolymphatic sac in the laboratory animal has established that the endolymphatic hydrops occurs as a result of malfunctioning of the endolymphatic sac. The normal resorptive function of the sac is responsible for the proper control of endolymph volume. Specialized structures such as the stria vascularis of the cochlea and secretory (dark) cells of the membranous pars superior which produce endolymph have been described as normal in temporal bones from patients with Meniere's disease.

The prevailing concept explaining the clinical manifestations of Meniere's disease is that a progressive distention of the endolymph compartment occurs after the function of the endolymphatic sac is reduced. Since the endolymph compartment of the pars inferior is contained by more yielding membranes in the labyrinth, (Reissner's membrane, saccular wall) the overdistention of the endolymph compartment initially occurs in the cochlea and saccule. It therefore is not suprising that hearing loss is usually the first manifestation of Meniere's disease. As progressive endolymph accumulation involves the pars superior, distention of the endolymph compartment causes ruptures of the membranous wall (Figure 110-2). Each rupture releases high potassium endolymph into the low potassium perilymphatic space. Theoretical as well as experimental evidence indicates that a change to a high potassium environment surrounding the vestibular and auditory nerve fibers results in significant alterations in their action potentials. Increased hearing loss and episodic vertigo are the clinical manifestations of this potassium intoxication of the neural input of the eighth nerve. Healing of the break in the membranous wall is followed by equilibration of the potassium levels in the perilymph with relief of the vertigo and hearing loss within hours.

The repeated ionic insults to the sensorineural structures of both the auditory and vestibular labyrinth may lead to morphologic changes in the end organs and their nerve supply. Permanent severe hearing loss and reduced vestibular sensitivity (caloric test) reflect these structural changes. The incidence of sensorineural lesions in Meniere's disease varies with individual patients and is unpredictable. Both clinical and experimental trials utilizing diuretics, a reduction in salt, or other fluid regulation methods have failed to demonstrate a significant effect on labyrinthine fluid physiology.

VESTIBULAR NEURITIS

Vestibular neuritis refers to a clinical disorder typified by episodic vertigo in the absence of auditory symptoms or deficits. The vertigo may be a solitary attack lasting one to several

OPERATIVE NEUROSURGICAL TECHNIQUES
ISBN 0-8089-1862-1

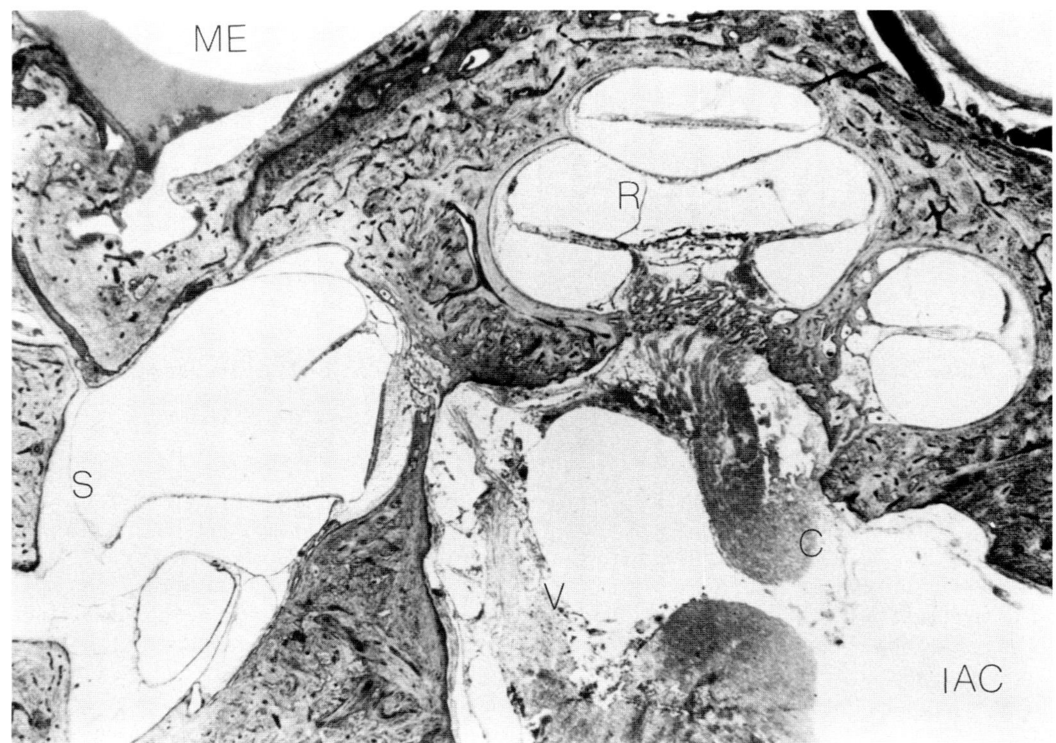

Fig. 110-1. A photomicrograph of the temporal bone demonstrating endolymphatic hydrops in a case of Meniere's disease. S = distended saccular wall; R = displaced Reissner's membrane; IAC = internal auditory canal with the cochlear (C) and vestibular (V) nerves.

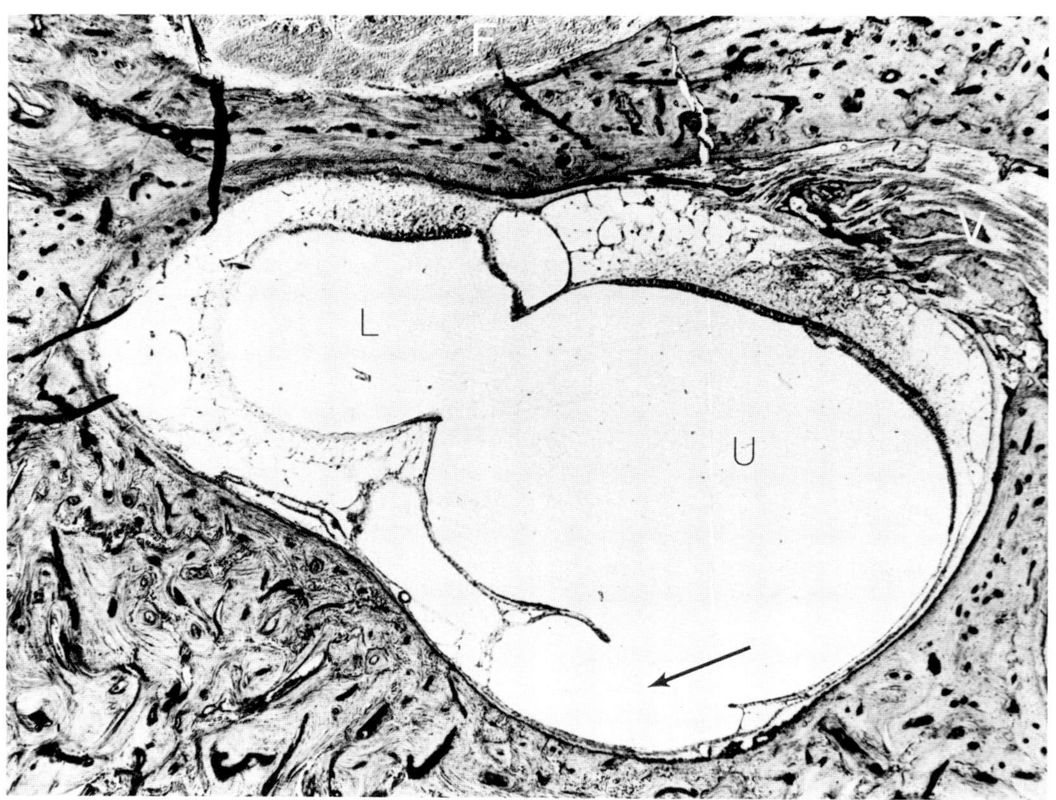

Fig. 110-2. The vestibular labyrinth in Meniere's disease showing a herniation (arrow) in the membranous wall of the utricle (U). L = lateral canal ampulla; V = superior division vestibular nerve; F = facial nerve.

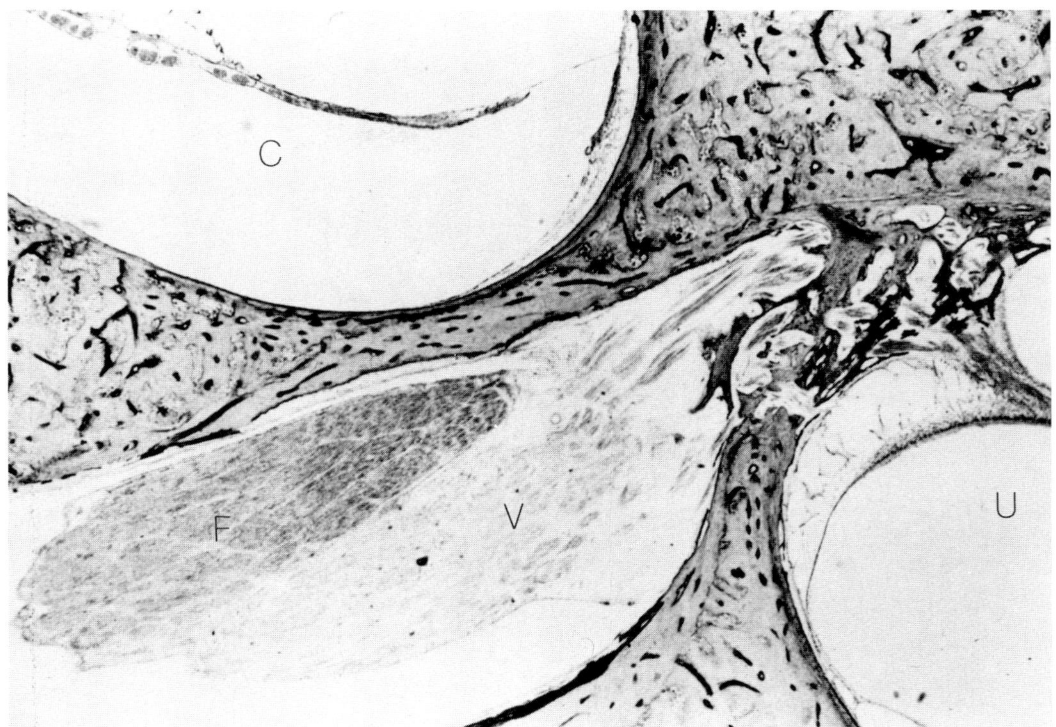

Fig. 110-3. Degenerated superior division of the vestibular nerve (V) in a case of vestibular neuritis. F = facial nerve; C = cochlea; U = utricle.

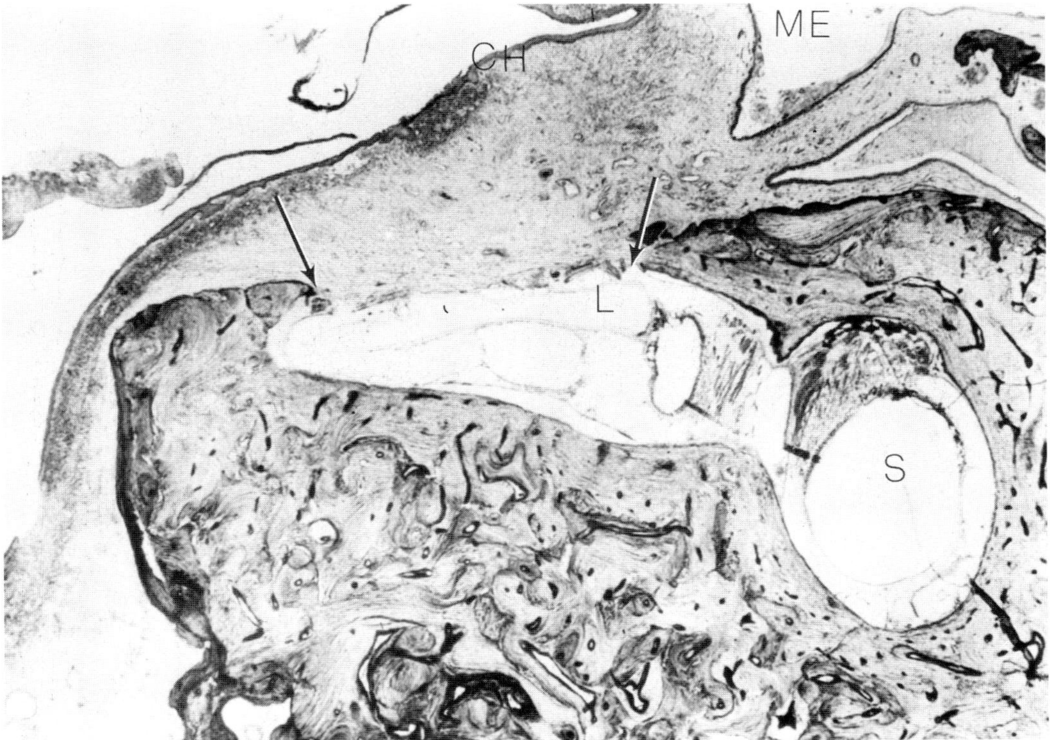

Fig. 110-4. This temporal bone section shows fistulization of the bony lateral semicircular canal (arrows) by cholesteatoma membrane (CH) in chronic otitis media. Note adherence of the inflammatory membrane to the membranous lateral semicircular canal (L). S = superior canal ampulla and sense organ; ME = middle ear space.

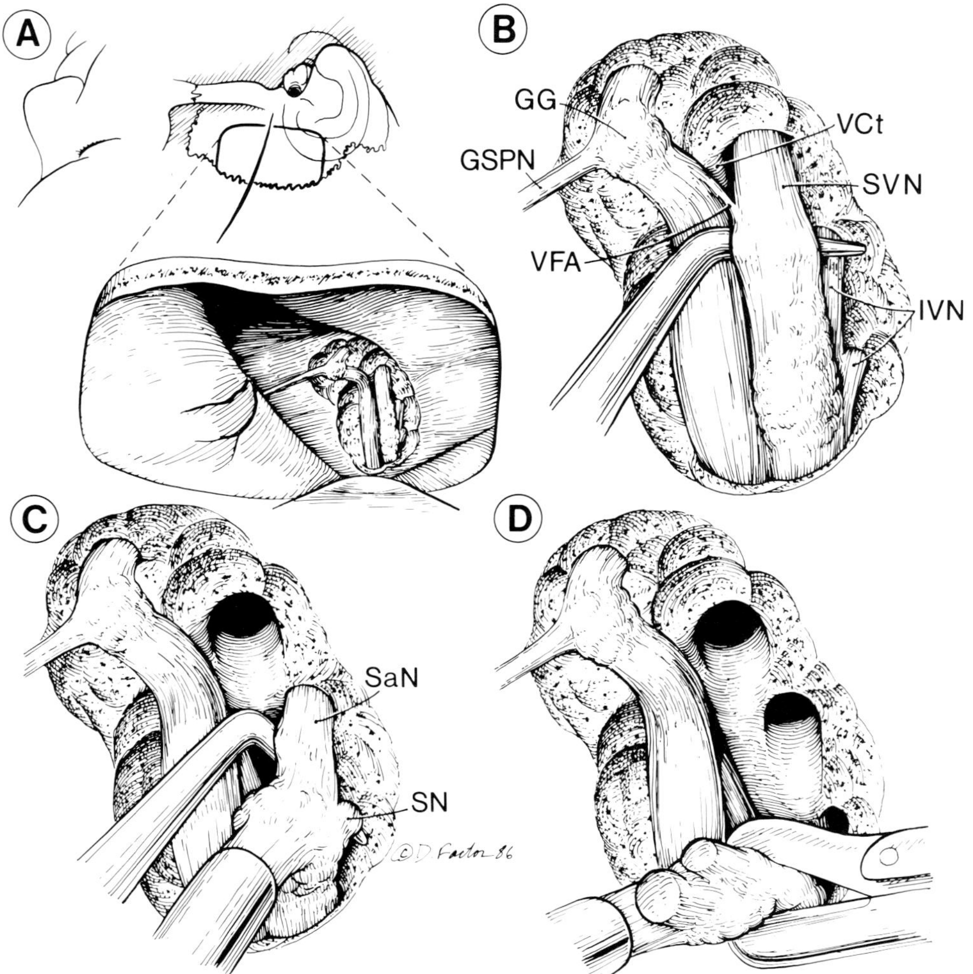

Fig. 110-5. (A through D) The approach and key steps in excision of the vestibular ganglion by the middle cranial fossa approach.

days or may be a recurring vertiginous experience covering a period of months or years. The association of this condition with viral disease has provided support to the concept that it represents viral inflammation of the vestibular ganglion. Histopathologic observations have supported this concept by demonstrating a selective degeneration of the vestibular ganglion and nerve fibers (Figure 110-3). The most common clinical form of vestibular neuritis is the acute form characterized by a solitary episode of vertigo without recurrence. The infrequent recurrent or chronic form of vestibular neuritis rarely reaches a disabling level.

CHRONIC LABYRINTHITIS

Chronic irritation of the labyrinth as a result of inflammatory middle ear disease may be responsible for disabling dysequilibrium. The vertigo is usually relieved after adequate surgical control of the middle ear (mastoid) inflammatory disease. Control may not be achieved if safe removal of inflammatory tissue adjacent to the membranous labyrinth (fistula) is not possible. An example of persistent irritation of the vestibular labyrinth because of incomplete surgical control is a large bony fistula of the semicircular canal where the cholesteatoma membrane cannot be safely removed without disrupting the membranous canal wall (Figure 110-4). Surgical removal of cholesteatoma matrix in this instance carries a high risk of sensorineural hearing loss.[1]

NONSURGICAL TREATMENT

Nonsurgical treatment is initially recommended for peripheral labyrinthine disorders. In the vast majority of patients with Meniere's disease troubled by episodic vertigo, counseling, reassurance, and the judicious use of vestibular suppressants will usually provide sufficient control so that the patient can function adequately. In 20 percent or fewer patients with Meniere's disease, episodic vertigo is refractory to medical therapy and may represent a considerable handicap to daily activities. Surgical relief is then required.

Vestibular neuritis is usually of the self limiting or acute variety and therefore rarely requires surgical treatment. The chronic form of vestibular neuritis usually has a course of decreasingly troublesome vertigo. The clinical course parallels a progressive destruction of the vestibular ganglion. If there is a progressive decrease in vestibular function, surgical ablation may not be necessary. However, occasionally persistent recurring vertigo may be of sufficient magnitude that surgical treatment is warranted.

Successful management of chronic labyrinthitis usually results from surgical control of middle ear inflammatory disease. Vestibular neurectomy is a consideration in the rare case in which vestibular symptoms continue in the presence of controlled middle ear disease and useful hearing function.

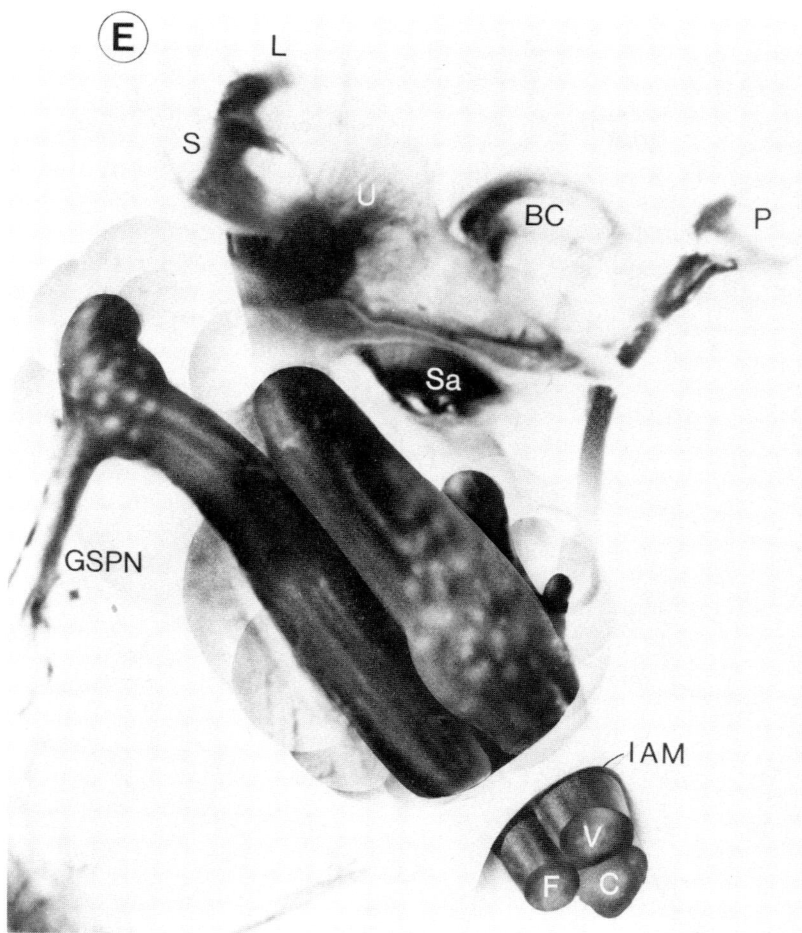

Fig. 110-5   (E) A dissection of the human labyrinth and nerve supply (compare with B). GG = geniculate ganglion; GSPN = greater superficial petrosal nerve; SVN = superior division of vestibular nerve; IVN = inferior division of vestibular nerve: SaN = saccular nerve; SN = singular nerve; VFA = vestibulofacial anastomosis; VCt = vertical crest; L = lateral canal ampulla; S = superior canal ampulla; P = posterior canal ampulla; U = utricle; Sa = Saccule; BC = basal turn of cochlea; IAM = internal auditory meatus; V = vestibular nerve; C = cochlear nerve; F = facial nerve.

SURGICAL TREATMENT

Surgical management is recommended when the degree of disability prevents acceptable social or work life because of the frequency and the severity of vestibular symptoms. The patient should be afforded a final opportunity to live with his or her Meniere's disease. The patient should be aware that ablation surgical treatment will control the vertiginous episodes and that another form of unsteadiness will follow such surgery. The degree of unsteadiness will depend on the patient's ability to adjust to the vestibular deficit.

Factors that determine the type of ablation therapy are (1) the presence of unilateral or bilateral disease; (2) the level of hearing in the involved and the noninvolved ear; and (3) the age and medical status of the patient. This factor determines not only the ability of the patient to undergo general anesthesia but his or her ability to compensate for the loss of vestibular function.

The most reliable treatment principle that is used in the management of intractable episodic vertigo is that of ablation of peripheral vestibular function. The relief of episodic vertigo should approach 100 percent if the ablation procedure has completely eliminated vestibular function in the affected ear.

LABYRINTHECTOMY

Labyrinthectomy is recommended for those patients with unilateral Meniere's disease whose hearing is depressed to a level where it is no longer useful. Generally speaking, when pure tone thresholds exceed 50 dB and speech discrimination scores are less than 50 percent, hearing is not considered useful. Surgical ablation of the vestibular sense organs can be accomplished through either a transcanal or a transmastoid approach. Either approach is effective provided that all five vestibular sense organs are surgically extracted under visual control.[2,3] Achieving this goal requires a familiarity with the location of the vestibular sense organs and technical ability with extra long hooks and other angled instruments that can extract the sense organs from the deep recesses of the vestibule. The sense organ most often overlooked in labyrinthectomy is the posterior canal crista because it resides in a separate inaccessible bony recess posterior to the round window niche. When the transcanal approach to the vestibule is used to accomplish labyrinthectomy, transection of the posterior ampullary nerve in the singular canal (singular neurectomy) ensures complete denervation of the the posterior canal sense organ.[2]

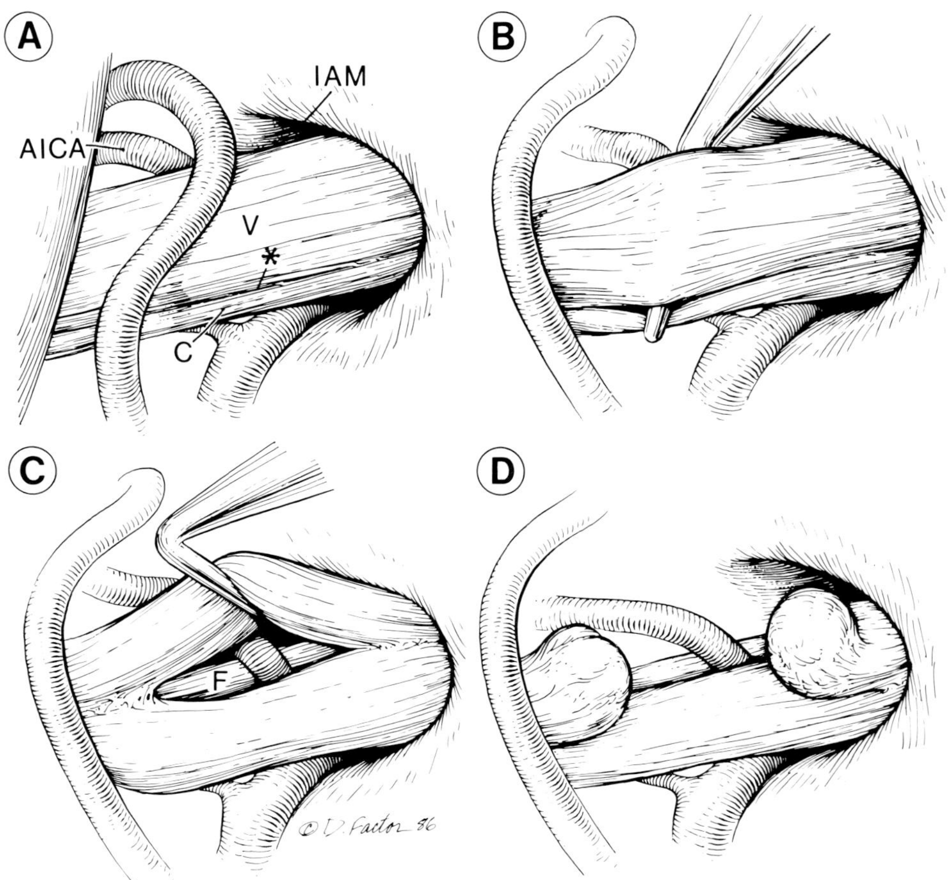

Fig. 110-6. The main steps in selective vestibular nerve transection in the cerebellopontine angle. (A and B) The cleavage plane ( ) between the vestibular (V) and cochlear (C) portions of the eighth nerve is developed with hooks. (C) The facial nerve (F) is identified rostral and ventral to the eighth nerve. (D) The vestibular nerve has been transected. AICA = anterior inferior cerebellar artery; IAM = internal auditory meatus.

VESTIBULAR NERVE TRANSECTION

Selective ablation of vestibular function is indicated in those patients with intractable severe vertigo caused by unilateral pathologic involvement of the labyrinth whose hearing function is at a useful level. Selective transection of the vestibular nerve can be accomplished at two levels: (1) the internal auditory canal (IAC), and (2) the cerebellopontine angle (CPA).

Vestibular nerve transection through a middle cranial fossa approach is used to selectively transect the vestibular nerve with preservation of the cochlear and facial nerves after they are exposed in the IAC.[4] Auditory function is maintained by avoiding surgical exposure of the labyrinth and preserving the cochlear division of the eighth nerve. Since the vestibular and cochlear nerves are separated in the distal end of the IAC, the vestibular nerve branches can be isolated from cochlear nerve fibers. Transection of the distal and proximal ends of the superior and inferior division vestibular neurons within the IAC permits resection of the vestibular ganglion.[5] Excision of this segment reduces the possibility of regeneration of vestibular nerve fiber(s). This exposure of the IAC is accomplished through a middle cranial fossa approach.

The operation should be recommended to those patients with excellent hearing who have intractable vertigo and an excellent hearing level in the affected ear. The hearing level should not exceed a threshhold elevation of 20-30 dB and discrimination scores should not be less than 80 percent. The magnitude and

potential morbidity associated with this procedure suggests that it should be reserved for those patients whose hearing loss is minimal. Furthermore, since progressive endolymphatic hydrops (Meniere's disease) is not halted by the ablation surgery, further deterioration of hearing may occur in subsequent years as a result of progressive hydrops. The selective ablation procedure merely alleviates the disabling vertigo.

Patients with threshhold elevations between 30 and 50 dB and with word discrimination scores between 50 and 80 percent can be considered on a case-by-case basis. For example, if a patient in this group considers his or her hearing to be useful and accepts the possibility of future deterioration of hearing, a middle fossa vestibular nerve section can be recommended provided that the patient is in good health. Patients selected for this procedure should be favorable medical risks for the procedure, e.g., they should be no greater than 60 years of age and in good medical health.

The surgical incision for this procedure is located anterior to the root of the helix and extends superiorly in a curved direction toward the forehead (Figure 110-5A). The incision should stay within the hairline. This incision extends through the temporalis muscle to the squamous portion of the temporal bone until the root of the zygoma is identified. A square or rectangular craniectomy is performed using an electric drill with cutting and diamond burrs. After the bone plate has been elevated from the temporal lobe dura, it is preserved in saline for replacement at the end of the procedure. Satisfactory and

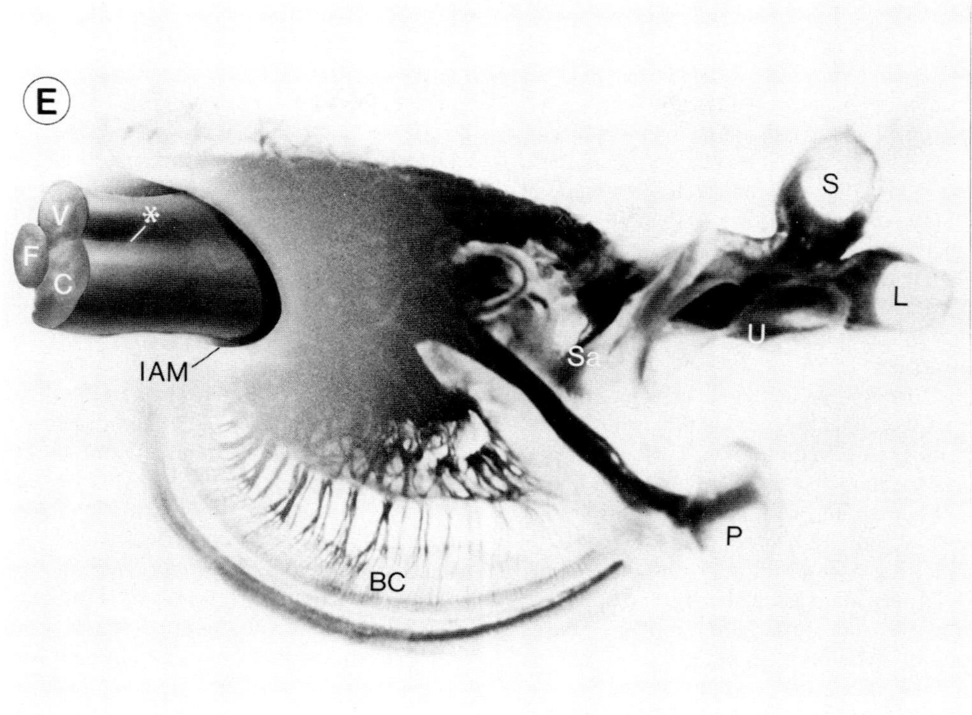

Fig. 110-6.   (E) The relationship of the labyrinth and nerve supply to the cerebellopontine angle.

safe retraction of the temporal lobe is facilitated by the administration of mannitol (1 g/kg of body weight) at the initiation of the procedure. Troublesome bleeding from dural vessels at this stage of the procedure can be controlled with bipolar cautery, absorbable surgical gauze (Surgicel) and either bone wax or a polishing burr if the bleeding vessels are located in bone. The retractor that has been designed by House is useful for retraction of the temporal lobe. Elevation of the temporal lobe dura is carried out with an elevator proceeding from the lateral surface of the temporal bone to the superior aspect of the petrous ridge and anteriorly to a point where the facial hiatus and the greater superficial petrosal nerve can be identified. The blade of the retractor can then be inserted between the dura and the superior aspect of the petrous ridge, thus maintaining retraction of the temporal lobe. If it is not possible to insert the retractor blade over the petrous ridge easily, the blade can be stabilized by fashioning a small groove near the petrous ridge using a small diamond burr. The blade of the retractor is then engaged in this groove in order to maintain satisfactory temporal lobe retraction.

Although the arcuate eminence is a useful classical anatomic landmark for locating the IAC, it is not always a well-formed prominence. A more reliable way of locating the IAC is to trace the facial nerve from the facial hiatus and geniculate ganglion in a retrograde fashion through the labyrinthine segment to the IAC (Figure 110-5). This is accomplished with a small diamond burr assisted by frequent irrigation. The IAC is then exposed in a medial direction to the level of the internal auditory meatus.

After incision of the IAC dura and retraction of the dural flaps, the facial and vestibular nerves can be recognized in the superior compartment of the canal (Figures 110-5A and 110-5E). These nerves can usually be separated at the level of the vertical crest in the IAC. If the vertical crest is not an available landmark, then the cleavage plane between the facial nerve and the superior vestibular nerve can be used as a guide to separate these nerves. The distal end of the superior division of the vestibular nerve should be isolated with a right angled hook and avulsed in a medial direction (Figure 110-5B). The avulsed end of the superior division is then retracted medially using a small gauge (No. 20) suction tip and separated from the facial nerve by blunt dissection until the inferior vestibular division branches come into view. If the vestibulofacial anastomosis is prominent and restricts easy dissection from the facial nerve, it should be transected with microscissors in order to avoid harmful traction on the facial nerve. The inferior vestibular nerve branches (saccular nerve and singular nerve) are then also avulsed with a hooked instrument and retracted in a medial direction (Figure 110-5C). The two divisions of the vestibular nerve are separated with a blunt instrument from the facial nerve to the level of the internal auditory meatus. The proximal end of the vestibular nerve should be cauterized with bipolar cautery and then transected with microscissors (Figure 110-5D). Excision of the vestibular ganglion is accomplished in this way. A small piece of temporalis muscle fascia, obtained at the beginning of the procedure, is then used to obliterate the dural defect in the IAC and is held in place by re-expansion of the temporal lobe dura.

A useful manuever at the termination of this procedure is to secure the temporal lobe dura to the bony edges of the craniectomy defect with fine (7-0) silk sutures. In this way the dura is restricted from any further dissection should an extradural hematoma occur postoperatively. It is extremely important to control not only all epidural bleeders but also the branches of the superficial temporal artery with tightly knotted silk sutures in order to reduce the incidence of postoperative bleeding. The bone plate removed during the craniectomy is then placed on the temporal lobe surface and the temporalis muscle is closed with absorbable sutures. After closure the wound is connected to negative pressure drainage. Steroids are administered intraoperatively and postoperatively.

The results in the control of vertigo, providing the superior and inferior division nerve branches have been transected and excised, is approximately 98 to 100 percent.[6] The incidence of sensorineural hearing loss should be no greater than 10 percent and temporary facial paralysis may occur in approximately 25 percent of patients. The incidence of facial paralysis is probably related to the method used to locate the IAC. This technique is justified by its reliability in locating the IAC and the temporary nature of the facial weakness.

In addition to the 10 percent incidence of sensorineural hearing loss and the 25 percent incidence of temporary facial paralysis, the more serious but infrequent complications are (1) temporal lobe aphasia secondary to edema, (2) epidural hematoma, (3) subdural hematoma, and (4) meningitis.

Selective transection of the vestibular nerve in the CPA can be approached through a transmastoid retrolabyrinthine route or via a suboccipital craniotomy. The retrolabyrinthine approach is used to expose the posterior fossa dura in the mastoid cavity,[7,8] while appropriate incision of the dura and cerebellar retraction exposes the CPA in the suboccipital approach.

The widest exposure of the seventh and eighth nerves is probably best achieved by posterior fossa craniotomy. Retraction on the cerebellum stretches the nerves slightly, bringing them into view across the CPA (Figure 110-6). The advantages of this technique are that the exposure is technically easier to accomplish than the middle fossa approach and the incidence of facial paralysis is less since surgical exposure of the facial nerve is not used to locate the IAC. Advocates of this approach to selective vestibular neurectomy report the same success rate in relieving vertigo. There are five disadvantages to this procedure:

1. The cleavage plane between the cochlear and vestibular divisions of the eighth nerve is often difficult to develop and may not accurately separate the vestibular nerve fibers from cochlear nerve fibers.[9] Therefore, a certain degree of uncertainty is associated with the selective transection of vestibular axons. Either some cochlear fibers may be sacrificed or some vestibular fibers may be spared by surgically developing this cleavage plane.
2. Transection of only the proximal axons leaving the vestibular ganglion intact theoretically allows for the possibility of regeneration neuroma.
3. The traction and manipulation associated with dissection of the nerves raises the possibility of mechanical disruption of cochlear nerve fibers.
4. Since the blood supply to the labyrinth (the labyrinthine artery) is proximal to its peripheral branching at this point, injury to the main vascular supply to the labyrinth is more likely than in the distal IAC where peripheral branches supplying the cochlea are not in the surgical field.
5. If the transmastoid retrolabyrinthine approach is used, retraction of a posterior fossa dural flap containing the endolymphatic sac risks injury to the sac and duct during the exposure of the CPA.

Indications for this procedure are essentially the same as for middle fossa vestibular nerve transection. These are patients with unilateral peripheral labyrinthine disease, usually Meniere's disease or vestibular neuritis with excellent hearing.

Contraindications are poor hearing in the involved ear or intractable vertigo and excellent hearing in an only hearing ear. The former group of patients require labyrinthectomy while the latter are best treated by medical ablation of the vestibular system (streptomycin).

A postauricular incision and a simple mastoidectomy approach is used to expose the posterior fossa dura in the mastoid compartment (retrolabyrinthine approach). A vertical suboccipital incision and craniotomy posterior to the sigmoid sinus can also be used to expose the seventh and eighth nerves in the CPA (suboccipital approach). After the posterior fossa dura has been exposed, it is incised and the CPA visualized by retracting the floccular lobe of the cerebellum. The retraction provides exposure of the seventh and eighth nerve complex in the CPA by applying slight traction to the nerves (Figure 110-6A). A shallow groove on the surface of the eighth nerve is used to identify the separation of the vestibular from the cochlear nerve fibers (Figures 110-6A and 110-6E). This cleavage plane is developed through the eighth nerve complex using knives and hooks (Figure 110-6B) until the caudal and dorsal portion of the eighth nerve containing vestibular nerve fibers is isolated and transected (Figures 110-6C and 110-6D). The blood supply to the labyrinth travels ventral to the seventh and eighth nerve complex and must be avoided during this transection procedure.

Unfortunately this cleavage plane through the eighth nerve is not always easily accomplished (Figure 110-6E). The interface between cochlear and vestibular nerve fibers therefore may not be accurately developed by the surgical cleavage plane.[9] The vestibular nerve transection can result in either an undesirable transection of some cochlear fibers or an incomplete transection of vestibular nerve fibers. The dural defect is closed with a tissue (adipose) graft in the transmastoid approach or repaired with sutures in the occipital approach.

The results are reported to be as good for control of vertigo as the middle fossa vestibular nerve section.[7] The success in preserving hearing is also claimed to be similar to that in the middle fossa procedure. While the short term results for relief of vertigo and hearing preservation are equal by both approaches to selective vestibular nerve transection, significant differences may become apparent over long-term evaluation. The loss of a small portion of auditory neurons (normal = 30,000) would not affect hearing function while a patient is young; however, when the neuronal loss caused by the aging process appears, a significant hearing loss may become more apparent. Furthermore, since the vestibular ganglion cells (normal = 18,000) remain viable in the IAC after transection of axons, the potential for neuroma formation by regenerating axons exists in the CPA. Temporary facial paralysis is less common with the retrolabyrinthine approach compared with the middle fossa approach to the IAC.

Complications that can occur are related to the exposure of the subarachnoid space in the CPA. If an adequate seal of the dural defect is accomplished, neither cerebral spinal fluid leakage or meningitis should result.

MEDICAL ABLATION (STREPTOMYCIN SULFATE)

A description of a medical form of peripheral vestibular ablation is important since it represents the most reliable means of selective vestibular ablation. A large number of histopathologic observations have demonstrated that the degenerative

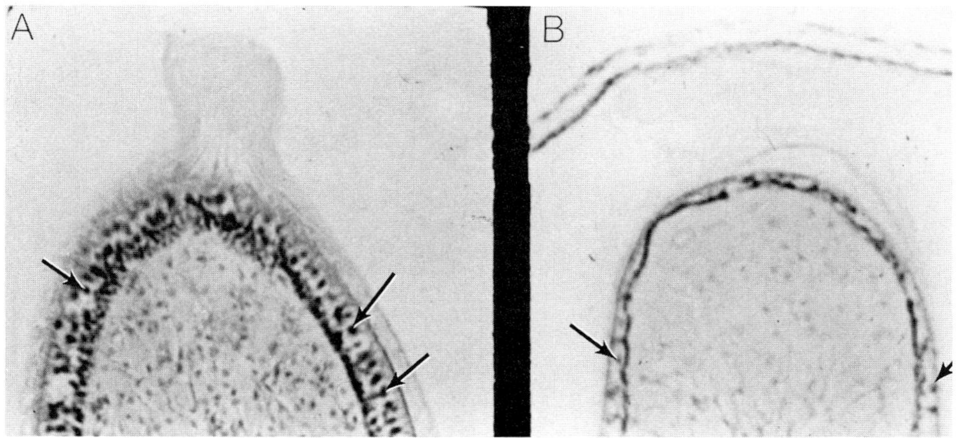

Fig. 110-7. Photomicrographs of the crista ampullaris (A) in a normal animal and (B) in an animal treated with streptomycin sulfate. Note the severe loss of hair cells in (B) compared with the normal complement of hair cells (arrows).

effect of streptomycin sulfate administered parenterally is on the vestibular sensory hair cells.[10] The effect is more pronounced in the vestibular sensory cells of the cristae than on the maculae of the utricle and saccule (Figure 110-7). Streptomycin sulfate administered parenterally is carried through the blood stream into the perilymphatic space of the labyrinth, where it contacts the type I and type II vestibular hair cells of the Zneurosensory epithelium. The effect is selective for the vestibular system if monitored carefully. If the streptomycin sulfate is administered to the point at which the vestibulo-ocular reflex to an ice water stimulus is absent, no cochleotoxic effect will occur. It is only when the end point of vestibular ablation has been surpassed that the danger of cochlear toxicity is significant. This method of ablating the vestibular sensory epithelium has found great therapeutic use in the treatment of bilateral Meniere's disease and in the management of Meniere's disease affecting the only hearing ear. It is the most reliable technique of selective vestibular ablation while preserving hearing. Patients selected for this treatment must be carefully evaluated. The treatment should be restricted to those patients who are severely incapacitated by the episodic vertigo of bilateral Meniere's disease and who have an excellent potential for vestibular adaptation. A reliable general rule limits its use to those patients who are no older than 55 years and in good physical health.

The treatment method basically is to administer streptomycin sulfate intramuscularly in divided doses of approximately 2 to 3 g/day parenterally while the patient is monitored in the hospital. Daily tests of the vestibular ocular reflex (caloric induced nystagmus) and hearing are administered. Streptomycin ablation of vestibular function is considered complete when the nystagmus response to ice water stimulus (5 ml) is absent in both ears (or the only hearing ear). This method has proved to be safe and effective in the treatment of bilateral Meniere's disease and in the management of selective ablation with preservation of hearing when the only hearing ear is affected by endolymphatic hydrops.

CONCLUSION

Selective ablation of vestibular function is a successful treatment of disabling vertigo caused by labyrinthine disorders such as Meniere's disease where preservation of useful hearing is also a goal. Ablation can be achieved by medical (parenteral streptomycin sulfate) or surgical (vestibular nerve transection) methods. Vestibular nerve transection can be accomplished either in the internal auditory canal (middle fossa approach) or in the cerebellopontine angle (posterior fossa approach).

REFERENCES

1. Gacek RR: The surgical management of labyrinthine fistulae in chronic otitis media with cholesteatoma. Ann Otol Rhinol Laryngol 83 (Suppl 10), 1974
2. Gacek RR: "How I do it," Transcanal labyrinthectomy. Laryngoscope 88:1707, 1978
3. Hammerschlag PE, Schuknecht HF: Transcanal labyrinthectomy for intractable vertigo. Arch Otolaryngol 107:152, 1981
4. House WF: Surgical exposure of the internal auditory canal and its contents through middle cranial fossa. Laryngoscope 71:1353, 1961
5. Fisch U: Vestibular neurectomy, in Silverstein H, Norrell H (eds): Neurological Surgery of the Ear. Birmingham, Ala, Aesculapius, 1977, pp 144-149
6. Glassock ME, Kveton JF, Christiansen SG: Middle fossa vestibular neurectomy: An update. Otolaryngol Head Neck Surg 92:216, 1984
7. House JW, Hitselberger WE, McElween J, et al: Retrolabyrinthine section of the vestibular nerve. Otolaryngol Head Neck Surg 92:212, 1984
8. Silverstein H, Norrell H: Retrolabyrinthine Surgery—A direct approach to the cerebellopontine angle. Otolaryngol Head Neck Surg 88:462, 1980
9. Rasmussen AT: Studies of the eighth cranial nerve of man. Laryngoscope 50:67, 1940
10. Schuknecht JF: Ablation therapy in the management of Meniere's disease. Acta Otolaryngol 132:1, 1957

Surgical Management of Spasmodic Torticollis and Adult-Onset Dystonia with Emphasis on Selective Denervation

Claude M. Bertrand

THE UNDERLYING PATHOLOGIC CONDITION of the basal ganglia in spasmodic torticollis and adult-onset dystonia is still undetermined in spite of increasing interest and research.[1-5] However, many aspects of these diseases are now better understood; this has resulted in a gradual improvement in therapy. It is becoming generally accepted that spasmodic torticollis is a limited manifestation of the same disease that causes adult-onset dystonia;[6,7] in fact, it is sometimes difficult to draw the line between severe forms of torticollis and adult-onset dystonia.[8] Although evolution from rotational or laterocollis to dystonia with marked scoliosis of the cervicothoracic spine is unusual,[7] it was present in the history of 5 patients of the 117 surveyed for this chapter, possibly because of the length of time the condition existed and the severity of the cases referred for surgery. In both conditions there may be a personal or familial history of essential tremor[9,10] and, occasionally, involvement of the facial musculature.

It has also been accepted that these manifestations are not psychogenic in the great majority of cases, especially since the rhythmicity and reproducibility of the abnormal movements can be visualized by electromyography.[7,11] Like other extrapyramidal movements they are increased by emotion and they disappear during sleep. Some of these patients may suffer from anxiety and even a reactive depression, which can occasionally delay or preclude surgery. It appears, however, that an emotional shock or trauma can act as a precipitating factor. While in most cases the relationship to trauma is questionable, there have been a few instances in which the onset of symptoms rapidly follow trauma. Definite and persistent remissions are infrequent[12,13] and did not exceed 5 percent in the group of patients surveyed for this chapter.

The unqualified statement that spasmodic torticollis is a bilateral disease, which dates back to the days before electromyography, has been detrimental to the evolution of its surgical management. It has led to the impression that antagonist muscles on either side are usually involved. On the contrary, in a classical case of rotational torticollis without anterocollis or retrocollis, spontaneous abnormal discharges can be found in the sternocleidomastoid on one side and the posterior cervical group, especially the splenius, on the other.[11] The contralateral antagonist muscles do not participate or may even be inhibited. However, when the patient attempts to turn against the abnormal movements, the affected antagonist muscles discharge instead of relaxing. In retrocollis the extensors on either side, which are then synergists, evidently discharge simultaneously, while in laterocollis the muscles that participate are all on the same side, for instance, the posterior cervical group with the ipsilateral sternocleidomastoid and possibly the trapezius. In most instances, however, there is a combination of movements, such as rotation with extension or flexion or inclination, so that the muscles that are implied must be carefully ascertained, since combinations vary from one patient to another. Flexion with inclination of the head to the left and rotation to the right may be caused by involvement of the left sternocleidomastoid and the ipsilateral semispinalis, while rotation to the right with slight inclination and extension of the occiput to the right suggests involvement of the left sternocleidomastoid combined mostly with the right splenius. If the dystonia is more pronounced, there may be simultaneous discharges of the antagonists; sometimes this is an attempt to reduce abnormal discharges, but this is the exception rather than the rule. If there is a component of head tremor, there will also be alternating discharges between one side and the other, but this is another matter. Unfortunately, this false impression of bilaterality has led to the use of indiscriminate bilateral symmetric denervation, such as bilateral rhizotomy, thus suppressing normal uninvolved muscles that are necessary for normal posture and movement.

SPASMODIC TORTICOLLIS

CONSERVATIVE TREATMENT

Medical treatment has been analyzed comprehensively by Fahn,[14] Marsden et al.,[15] and Lee,[16] among others. It is the initial measure in the care of these patients.

Although medication can be of help in treating dystonias,

the great variety of drugs used to alleviate the symptoms of torticollis is an indication of their limited possibilities. Dopaminergics such as levodopa and bromocriptine are still used but with less enthusiasm than initially. The best controlled results seem to have been obtained with anticholinergic drugs, such as trihexyphenidyl (Artane); improvement was noted in a little better than 41 percent of cases in torsion dystonia when the anticholinergic was combined with tetrabenazine and pimozide. Antidepressants such as imipramine combined with alprazolam (Xanax) also seem to be helpful. Anticonvulsants, such as phenytoin, carbamazepine, and clonazepam also have been tried in high doses. Of the patients referred to us for surgery, the majority were receiving diazepam or lorazepam, the neuroleptic haloperidol, trihexyphenidyl, or antidepressants, sometimes in high doses with appreciable side effects. About half of the patients felt that there was some diminution in the severity of the abnormal movements because of the medication, but since these patients were contemplating surgery, few felt that they had obtained an appreciable benefit. Biofeedback[17] and physical therapy, which are aimed at possible relaxation and retraining of the antagonist muscles, can also be useful, but they are infrequently successful over a period of time. Physiotherapy is essential after surgery, particularly to retrain the muscles that were the antagonists to the abnormal movements.

SURGICAL MANAGEMENT

It is impossible to suggest all-inclusive guidelines for at what point and in what instances surgery should be considered, since it varies with the importance and the functional consequences of the procedure. More benign interventions, such as iontophoresis, epidural stimulation, and limited selective denervation may be justifiable if the symptoms have been present for more than 2 years and they are truly bothersome. Others, such as cervical rhizotomy, thalamotomy, or bilateral posterior cervical denervation, should be reserved for severe or incapacitating forms of the disease.

Iontophoresis

Iontophoresis through the eardrum to suppress the vestibular afferents was propounded by Svein and Cody.[18] The primary complication is occasional perforation of the eardrum, especially if the procedure is repeated several times; this can be repaired. Iontophoresis is still being used, but the benefits obtained are usually partial or temporary.

Microvascular Lysis of the Accessory Nerve Roots

Freckmann et al.[19] suggested microvascular lysis of the accessory nerve roots, along the lines of decompression of the facial nerve or the trigeminal nerve. Again, the initial report suggested a certain amount of success, but this was not substantiated afterward. It would be surprising if symptoms that involve so many muscle groups, of which only the sternocleidomastoid and the trapezius are directly innervated by the spinal accessory, could be relieved by a simple decompression of these roots. When the sternocleidomastoid is the main culprit, it seems simpler and more efficient to avulse all the peripheral branches directly in the neck without resorting to a laminectomy.

Epidural Cervical Stimulation

Epidural cervical stimulation has been advocated mostly by Gildenberg[20] and Waltz.[21] In an additional report in 1981,[22] Gildenberg rightly advocated an initial trial period with transcutaneous stimulation. Fourteen patients underwent implantation. Four had excellent results; 7 patients had some relief although there was still appreciable turning of the head. In this text, Gildenberg[23] mentions epidural stimulation using a C1 laminectomy, but only states that one third of patients do not respond. Waltz, reporting on a group of 17 patients with spasmodic torticollis, stated that 6 were markedly improved and 3 were moderately improved. In another group of 9 patients, in whom a four-electrode system was used instead of a two-electrode system, 3 patients were markedly improved and 3 moderately improved.[21]

It is difficult to comment on these results without personal experience in using these three techniques. The patients referred to our clinic are evidently the ones in whom these measures did not succeed. Since epidural stimulation is not a destructive procedure if no laminectomy is used, it might be tried if the patient understands that the benefits could be temporary.

Interruption of the Frontal Capsular Adversive Pathway

Mazars et al.[24] and more recently Stejskal et al.[25] interrupted the corticocapsular head-turning pathway. It is an interesting approach if it is remembered that when the ansa lenticularis is the target for Parkinson's disease, there occasionally is interruption of the frontal adversive pathways and the patient is unable to look to the opposite side or to turn his or her head to the opposite side, sometimes for a period of 2 to 3 days. It is a stereotactic intracerebral procedure, and Stejskal reported good, fair, or excellent results in 71 percent of 17 patients, but very good results in 47 percent.[25]

Thalamotomy or Pallidotomy

Hassler and Hess[26] suggested interrupting the cerebello-dentato-rubro-thalamo-cortical pathways using ventro-oralis internus (VOI) and ventro-oralis posterior (VOP) as the targets, together with the underlying field of Forel. Cooper,[27] Mundinger et al.,[28] and Hassler and Dieckmann[29] reported excellent or satisfactory results in almost two thirds of their patients. After reviewing the cases in which a thalamotomy had been done for spasmodic torticollis in the early 1960s, some with excellent results, we reverted from cervical rhizotomy to this procedure,[30] using the increment obtained during microelectrode recording to ascertain proper positioning, thus increasing our percentage of satisfactory results to 70 percent in a small group of 11 patients. There is, however, the danger of corticobulbar complications in 5 percent.[31] Since this percentage doubles if a lesion is created on the other side, blocking and selective denervation of the still active muscles was done first in an attempt to improve those results and avoid this dreaded complication.[32] For the past 8 years we have used only selective denervation for spasmodic torticollis, thalamotomy combined with pallidotomy usually being reserved for the more severe forms of adult-onset dystonia. Of the group of 117 patients with spasmodic torticollis or dystonia surveyed here, 91 patients were treated exclusively with selective peripheral denervation, while 26 were subjected to a stereotactic procedure. Even in the more diffuse dystonias, when the discharges extend below the cervical musculature, selective denervation is done as the initial procedure, since it may provide the patient enough relief to dispense with stereotactic surgery.

Anterior Cervical Rhizotomy

Anterior cervical rhizotomy has been modified very little since it was described by McKenzie[33] and Dandy.[34] It is probably the one used most frequently for severe torticollis. Essentially, it consists of sectioning the anterior roots of C1, C2, and C3 bilaterally and part or all of the anterior root of C4 on one side with or without section of the ascending roots of the spinal accessory nerve. Since distribution of its fibers to the trapezius and the sternocleidomastoid varies, this can produce an appreciable percentage of shoulder paresis; peripheral denervation is preferable for these muscles, as Tasker suggested.[35] In the reports of Sorensen and Hamby[36] (71 patients), Arseni and Maretsis[37] (52 patients), Hamby and Schiffer[38] (50 patients), Tasker[35] (47 patients), and Fabinyi and Dutton[39] (20 patients), satisfactory results were reported in approximately 70 percent of the patients. There was a 1 to 2 percent incidence of mortality. If an operating microscope is used, fine blood vessels can be spared and possible ischemia of the cord thereby avoided. Cervical subluxation is also rare. In the series of Hamby and Schiffer,[38] in which the follow-up was good, 30 percent of patient used a cervical collar occasionally, 57 percent complained of pain in the neck and shoulders, and 32 percent had dysphagia, which was usually temporary. These complications were probably higher in this series because of the sectioning of the ascending roots of the accessory nerves. Three of the 20 patients who were followed for a long time in Tasker's series had recurrences.[35]

We noted the occurrence of reinnervation of the peripheral portion of C2 after posterior cervical denervation, presumably from cervical anastomoses, in 5 patients who had had a previous cervical rhizotomy, 2 of which were done by me a few years previously. Anterior cervical rhizotomy with peripheral denervation of the sternocleidomastoid muscle, as indicated, was used regularly in our department until 15 years ago. Undoubtedly it helped many patients but it produces certain undesirable side effects. There is marked weakness of the neck postoperatively. Some instability of the neck as well as limitation of movements may persist. At times this occurs without suppression of the abnormal movements, because denervation is limited downward to C4 in order to protect the origin of the phrenic nerve. The posterior rami of C5, C6, and, rarely, C7, contribute definitely to the innervation of the splenius and especially the semispinalis.

Tasker reported that only 1 of 7 patients in whom the procedure was done unilaterally had a satisfactory result.[35] Now that electromyography, nerve blocks, and stimulation are readily available, it would seem that in laterocollis and in most cases of rotational torticollis, when the posterior cervical group is involved only on one side, rhizotomy, if it is still held by the surgeon as the procedure of choice, should be performed unilaterally in order to preserve neck stability and promote rehabilitation.

Bilateral rhizotomy has been abandoned since the advent of selective denervation because it produces too much denervation of useful antagonist muscles as well as incomplete denervation of the ones involved in the abnormal movements. Although there have been some negative reports[12,13] and rare but severe complications have been described (e.g., ischemia of the brainstem or the spinal cord),[40,41] it has produced relief for many patients with severe torticollis.

Muscle Resection

Xinkang[42] advocated selective resection of certain posterior cervical muscles together with section of the spinal accessory nerve when indicated (e.g., the splenius with section of the contralateral spinal accessory nerve for rotational torticollis). The muscles resected varied according to the type of torticollis and the results of electromyography. In 30 patients followed for more than a year, the recovery apparently was permanent in 60 percent. It is contrary to our experience that resection of the splenius only will abolish movements in the synergists and that movements disappear gradually over the months rather than immediately after surgery. Muscle resection undoubtedly is accompanied by a certain amount of denervation, but denervation of the muscles involved must be complete since the least amount of residual denervation will allow the abnormal movements to persist. One must agree with Maccabe that "myotomy . . . is unlikely to be revived".[43]

Selective Peripheral Denervation

Selective peripheral denervation of the muscles involved in abnormal movements while their antagonists are spared has been the procedure used at Hôpital Notre Dame for spasmodic torticollis for the past 8 years.[32,44,45] As mentioned previously, there are many transitional forms of spasmodic torticollis. The movements must be carefully analyzed; repeated review of a videotape is desirable. Palpation during physical examination is helpful in determining which muscles are the main offenders. When surgery is considered, bipolar electromyograms should be obtained in the presence of the surgeon and the clinical neurophysiologist. The needles should be placed in each muscle and proper placement ascertained from voluntary contraction of the muscle concerned. Moreover, when the record is not satisfactory and differs appreciably from the clinical picture, electromyography should be repeated with different needle placements. One also must be wary of discharges originating from the platysma. Besides analyzing the tracings, both observers should compare the sound produced by the discharging muscles. Time relationships should be analyzed and permanent photographic records kept for further comparison. Simultaneous tracings should be done in symmetric muscles, the first ones usually being the two sternocleidomastoid and the two splenius muscles. Both trapezius muscles should also be compared, especially to determine if and how much they are involved, since they must be spared whenever possible. When there is an element of doubt about the origin of the movements, for instance, whether rotation to the right originates from the right splenius or, more rarely, from the left semispinalis, a bipolar depth electrode can be used. A bipolar electrode also is useful for studying the rectus muscles or for the obliques and the longissimus capitis. Not infrequently, a rhythmic tremor is present with alternate discharges in the antagonists. It then is important to tell the patient that, while selective denervation may suppress part or most of the tremor, it cannot be depended on to do so; the procedure is for the abnormal movements and not for the tremor. Electromyographic recordings should be obtained with the patient at rest and during active movement involving different groups of muscles. As mentioned previously, the resistance of the involved muscles to normal movements is particularly revealing.

Stimulation is used mostly to determine the point of

penetration of fairly superficial motor nerves, usually the branches of the spinal accessory to the sternocleidomastoid when it is to be blocked separately from the trapezius. A temporary block with 1-percent lidocaine without epinephrine can be used to determine the relative importance of the involved muscles in the abnormal movements, for instance, the right sternocleidomastoid versus the left posterior cervical group in rotational torticollis or the right sternocleidomastoid and the right posterior cervical group in laterocollis. We block the sternocleidomastoid in most patients. Rarely does the trapezius appear to be involved in abnormal movements, except in marked laterocollis, but whenever there is a doubt, it is also blocked in order to see whether the patient can use the levator scapulae adequately to compensate for the loss of the trapezius, which is possible for some patients. The branch of the trapezius is blocked at its point of penetration into the muscle, where the horizontal and the vertical part join together at the base of the neck, with about 15 ml of 1-percent lidocaine. The sternocleidomastoid block is done fairly deep within the aponeurosis of the muscle and 2 inches below the mastoid to anesthetize the distal branches. The patient should be told that if the lidocaine diffuses further, there may be a temporary block of the recurrent nerve with transitory lowering of the voice and difficulty in swallowing. We now infiltrate directly into the splenius or the semispinalis in the posterior cervical region, as the case may be, rather than infiltrating about the roots of C1 and C2 and the posterior ramus of C3. This is done to avoid penetration of the large venous plexuses, which produced temporary nystagmus and hypotension in 2 patients mentioned in our initial report.[32] Even if the blocks are sometimes incomplete, they indicate what can be expected from denervation. If blocking the sternocleidomastoid produces sufficient although partial relief, denervation may be limited to that muscle and the patient referred for physiotherapy and retraining of the antagonists, knowing that a more extensive procedure may be required later on. In more complex cases, many blocks are done at different times. Rarely is more than 20 ml of 1-percent lidocaine used during one session, so the block is usually limited to one muscle group. Blocking is occasionally dispensed with when the clinical findings and the electromyograms are very definite or if there is any history of allergy to local anesthetics. On the other hand, electromyography is often repeated in doubtful cases to ensure that all the most active muscles have been detected.

Surgical Technique. Except in retrocollis, the surgical procedure commonly involves denervation of a posterior cervical group on one side or the other, together with the ipsilateral or contralateral sternocleidomastoid muscle. This is done under light anesthesia without curare, since stimulation is used throughout the operation to identify all the nervous branches and to ascertain that denervation is complete at the end of the procedure.

Although an incision through the crease of the neck might be preferable from a cosmetic point of view, the spinal accessory is approached through an incision made from the inferior lobe of the ear, along the trajectory of the branch of the trapezius, down to the supraclavicular area;[45] it is desirable to follow the spinal accessory nerve from the level of the styloid process down to its penetration into the trapezius, since there may be recurring branches at or below the posterior border of the sternocleidomastoid muscle coming from the trapezius branch (Figure 111-1). Also, there frequently are anastomotic branches between the spinal accessory nerve and C1 or more

rarely C2, but they are dealt with as the distal branches are severed in this fashion. The latter may come directly from the spinal accessory nerve or may originate from one or two main branches. There are usually four to six fine distal nerves. The large branches are clipped and all the distal nerves are avulsed as completely as possible, since in previous cases we have witnessed reinnervation of the sternocleidomastoid even though the muscle itself was completely sectioned. Only the aponeurosis is closed. Reinnervation, if it occurs, is rarely sufficient to produce abnormal movements in that muscle.

When a contralateral posterior cervical denervation must be performed, the patient is repositioned on the side opposite the one to be denervated. The head is flexed and turned downward,[45] and the shoulder is held down to facilitate the approach. The head and shoulders are slightly above horizontal to minimize oozing from the vertebral venous plexus. The incision extends from the external occipital protuberance to the mastoid and from there downward along the articular facets to the level of C7. It is in the shape of an inverted "L" facing inward. Incidentally, a strong unipolar stimulator must be used (not a disposable battery-operated one), since a certain amount of diffusion is useful to zero in on the nerves. It is best to start with a strong current and gradually reduce it. At the lower end of the incision, subcutaneously, the main branch to the trapezius penetrates this muscle. It must be identified by stimulation and followed upward a few centimeters and then mounted on a Penrose drain, so that it will not be injured. Dissection is then carried through the insertion of the cervical aponeurosis to the occipital bone, cutting through the insertion of the trapezius, the sternocleidomastoid, and then the splenius on the occiput. The greater occipital nerve is sectioned while this is being done or it can be spared temporarily for reference. The branches of the occipital artery are encountered near the mastoid and coagulated. Stimulation is used repeatedly to identify the motor branches, but this is particularly important once the splenius has been sectioned. Afterward, the posterior branches of C2 are pursued and identified by gradually diminishing the intensity of the stimulating voltage, usually from 2 V down to 1/2 V. As dissection proceeds to the posterior lamina of C2, the root of C2 is found to emerge between the laminae of C1 and C2, quite mesial to the articular facets and surrounded by a bothersome vertebral venous plexus, which must be coagulated. It divides immediately into its lateral and posterior branches, both of which must be isolated. It is then mounted on a silk thread. Afterward, stimulation is again used to identify the branches of C1, which lie in the small triangle delimited by the superior oblique, the inferior oblique, and the rectus muscles mesially. Because C1 is the only root to provide a nerve supply to the superior oblique, stimulation along the internal border of the superior oblique is also useful. The inferior oblique, which lies between the laminae of C1 and C2, can then be divided and C1 is pursued toward the posterior arch of the atlas. Surgical loupes and a headlamp usually suffice, but the operating microscope may be used for this portion of the procedure. The C1 nerve is usually spiderlike with multiple branches; the root itself must be carefully identified after some of the branches are severed. It then can be followed to the posterior arch of the atlas, which is partially exposed. It is clipped over the posterior arch and under the vertebral artery to interrupt it before the origin of its lateral branch. Occasionally, it is ruptured during dissection and then the entire area over the posterior arch of the atlas is cauterized. Care should be taken to avoid pulling too intensely on C1, since this may have caused

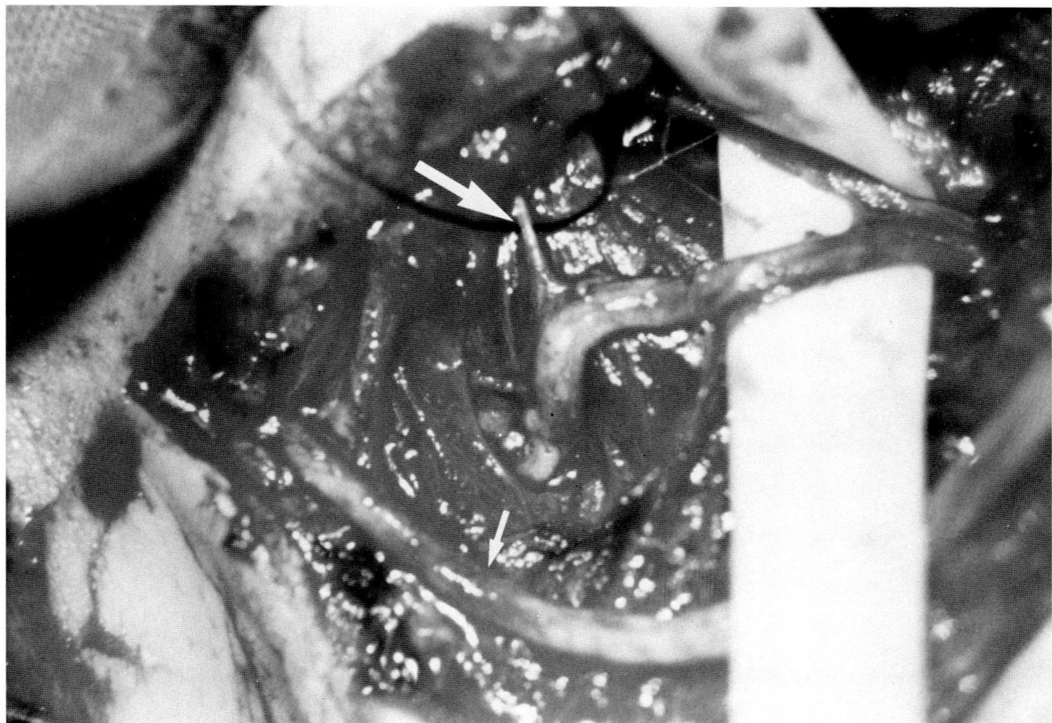

Fig. 111-1.   Photograph showing the two branches of the spinal accessory nerve: one anterior to (above) the sternocleidomastoid muscle, and the other going to (below) the trapezius. The large arrow points to a recurrent nerve from the lower branch to the trapezius, which also innervates the sternocleidomastoid muscle. The small arrow points to a large cutaneous auricular nerve.

edema with temporary difficulty in swallowing in early cases; this has not happened in the past few years. The C1 nerve is interrupted after it is clipped and the distal branches are avulsed. Besides the vertebral venous plexuses, there occasionally is a collateral branch of the vertebral artery close to C1 that can bleed profusely if injured and which must be clipped. Another collateral has also been found along the lateral branch of C2 (Figure 111-2).

The C2 nerve has already been mounted on a silk thread with an aneurysm needle and is kept for orientation, while dissection is pursued along the articular facets, below C2. The posterior primary divisions of C3, C4, C5, and C6 vary somewhat in their position in relation to the articular facets and stimulation is most useful in detecting them initially. The fibers, particularly those from the transversalis muscle that cover the ramus, are gradually dissected and C3 is followed to the point at which the ramus curves around between the articular facets, usually closer to the articulation of C2-3. The posterior rami supply the nerves to the articular facets, as described by Lazorthes.[46] Their removal has no functional consequence. There are usually very definite anastomoses between C1, C2, and C3, and sometimes C3 is large enough and far enough from the articulation that it can be confused with a branch of C2 until it is followed to its origin. A similar process is repeated for the posterior rami of C4, C5, and, if necessary, C6 or C7. These nerves are much smaller but they usually lie close to the notch between the articular facets and can be sought at that point with the stimulator. From the level of C4 one runs into the superolateral portion of the trapezius. The trapezius must be incised mesial to its main nerve supply, which must be protected. These small rami vary in size although C5 is usually larger than the others. Denervation is pursued downward as

long as stimulation produces contractions of the semispinalis or splenius, usually to the level of C6. Occasionally, if the dissection below C5 becomes too difficult, C6 is identified by stimulation and coagulated. In a few instances, the posterior ramus of C7 was also interrupted. After all the rami have been mounted on a silk thread, a clip is placed on the proximal portion at the level of the articular facets, and the distal part of the ramus is avulsed as completely as possible to avoid recurrences.

The root of C2 is interrupted at its point of division into a lateral and posterior branch after a clip is placed on the root. The posterior branch and all its divisions are avulsed completely. To destroy any possible remaining innervation, the semispinalis, the obliques (especially the superior oblique), the recti, and the longissimus capitis may sometimes be sectioned. At the end of the procedure, high voltage stimulation (4 to 5 V) between the articular facets and at the point of emergence of the roots of C1 and C2 should not produce any response in these muscles, and contractions should be seen only in the trapezius. Strong stimulation occasionally reveals that one of the deep branches of the posterior rami was spared inadvertently, particularly at the level of C3 or C4, and an additional avulsion is required; it is possible to carry the dissection from C2 to C4 or to leave a deep branch of C3. After it has been verified that denervation is complete and after careful hemostasis is obtained, the trapezius is sutured. Flexion of the head is reduced and the cervical fascia is sutured tightly; no drainage is used.

In the occasional case of laterocollis in which the trapezius must be denervated together with the ipsilateral sternocleidomastoid, the vertical portion of the incision is carried a little more laterally and the spinal accessory nerve is interrupted before it divides, a clip being placed on the proximal and distal portion, the lower portion being reversed to avoid anastomosis.

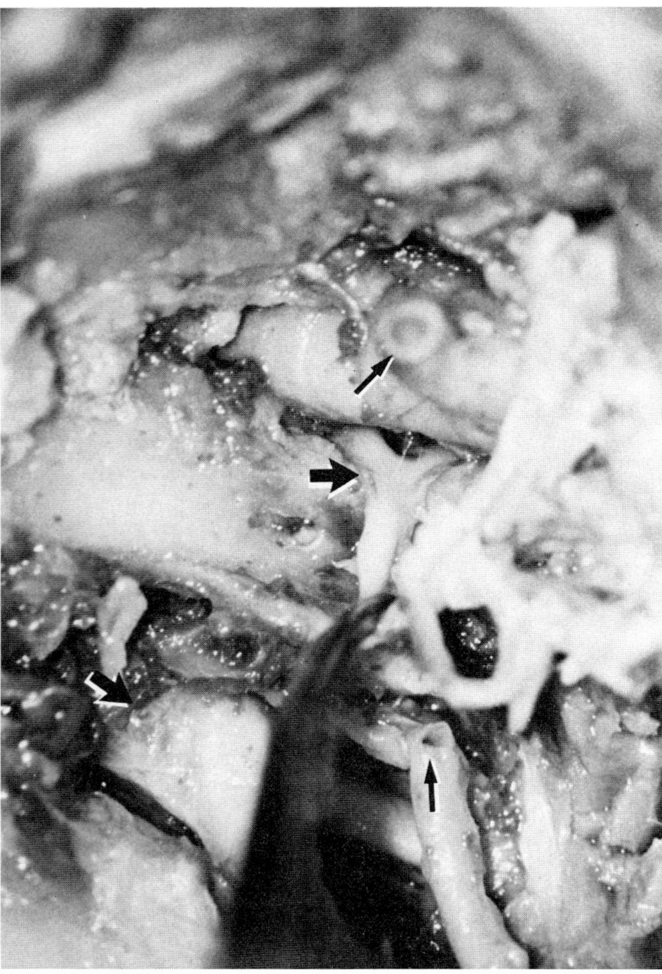

Fig. 111-2.   Microdissection of a cadaver shows the collateral branches of the vertebral artery (small arrows) occasionally found along the roots of C1 and C2 (large arrows).

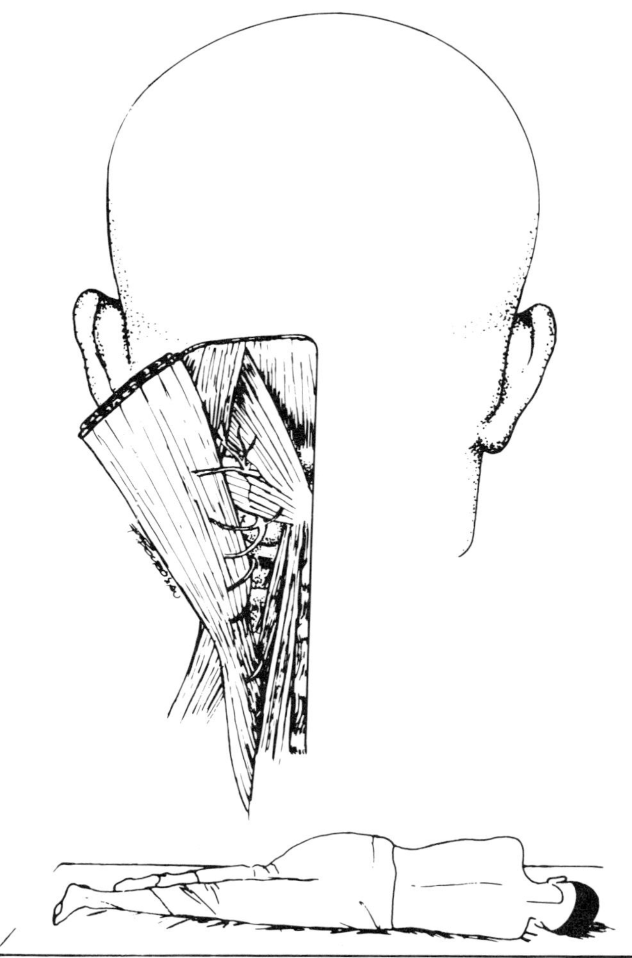

Fig. 111-3.   The approach to C1, C2, and the posterior primary divisions (rami) of C3, C4, C5, and C6 after the semispinalis is sectioned along the occipital bone and reflected laterally.

This is done only if blocks have indicated that the patient can function without the trapezius. Otherwise, an attempt is made to denervate only the vertical part of the muscle and to protect the remaining innervation to the horizontal portion.

From cadaver dissections and recent surgical experience, it seems more simple and expedient to use an incision starting well below the mastoid, coursing over to the external occipital protuberance, and then downward along the midline to C7 after the splenius below the mastoid and the semispinalis along the occipital bone are sectioned. The semispinalis can be everted outward, thus exposing C2 and the posterior rami below it, which can be followed to their point of origin. This also provides an excellent view of C1 (Figure 111-3). This approach was conceived from Bassett's dissection (plate 79) in his *Atlas of Anatomy of the Head and Neck,*[47] where it can best be visualized.

Results.   The following results were tabulated for the International Congress on Neurological Surgery in 1985. It is interesting that, in reviewing the vast majority of these cases at this time, only one patient reported a slight difference in his status a year later. It has been our experience that with avulsion of the peripheral terminations of the nerves the results remain stable over the years.

Between 1976 and 1985, 117 patients with adult-onset dystonia or spasmodic torticollis were treated surgically. Twenty six underwent thalamotomy or pallidotomy or both. At the beginning of this series stereotactic surgery was used frequently for the more severe forms of torticollis as well; at present, selective peripheral denervation is nearly always the first procedure used even when abnormal movements extend beyond the cervical region, since correcting the more severe movements may suffice. In fact, between 1981 and 1985 only six stereotactic interventions were done for adult-onset dystonia and none were done for spasmodic torticollis.

Selective denervation only was performed in 91 patients: 60 received a unilateral ramisectomy (avulsion of C1, C2, and the posterior rami of C3, C4, C5, and usually C6) combined with unilateral peripheral spinal accessory denervation, usually for the sternocleidomastoid muscle; unilateral ramisectomy was done in 11 cases only; in 10, only spinal accessory denervation was done; in 10 others, because of the severity and diffusion of the movements, a multiple approach was used, either a bilateral ramisectomy with or without unilateral spinal accessory denervation, or bilateral spinal accessory denervation with a unilateral ramisectomy (Table 111-1).

In this group of 91 patients, 82 were diagnosed as definitely having spasmodic torticollis, 5 as having adult-onset dystonia, and 4 as having an intermediate form, either because the shoulder was involved, because of a slight scoliosis, or because of discharges below the cervical musculature.

Table 111-1. Procedures used in 91 selective denervations

Procedure	Number of Patients
Combined ramisectomy (R) and spinal accessory denervation (S)	60
Ramisectomy (R)	11
Spinal accessory denervation (S)	10
Multiple approach (SRR-RSS-RR)	10

Table 111-2. Results in 91 consecutive cases treated by selective denervation

Results*	Number of Cases	Percentage
Excellent	28	31
Very good	52	57
Total very good and excellent	80	88
Good	9	10
Poor	2	2

* Excellent = total suppression of symptoms; very good = slight residual rotation or inclination or contraction of no functional significance; good = improvement but with appreciable residual movements.

In 80 patients (88 percent), the result was excellent (28 with total suppression of symptoms) or very good (52 with slight residual rotation or inclination or contraction of no functional significance). Nine patients (10 percent) showed definite improvement but an appreciable amount of residual movement remained. While in some of these, this could be foreseen because of the widespread contractions before surgery, there were a few in which the denervation was not complete; 2 of these patients had severe but purely rotational forms of torticollis. The lateral division of C1 may have escaped, in which case the remaining movement was probably caused by the longissimus capitis. Patients with both retrocollis and laterocollis are more likely to have abnormal residual movements. Extension from the intact contralateral semispinalis or inclination and some degree of extension from the ipsilateral levator scapulae may persist.

The result was poor in 2 patients. In one instance, the patient was sent home before physiotherapy began and some limitation of neck and shoulder movements remained. In another, with long-standing inclination of the head, prolonged elongation of the contralateral musculature was apparently such that the patient could not maintain her head in the vertical position (Table 111-2).

Physiotherapy is an integral part of the treatment. It should be started 3 or 4 days after surgery and continued for a few weeks after the patient returns home. It involves relaxation of the neck musculature, proper posture, and, mostly, retraining of the antagonists and strives toward full movement of the neck. In fact, after the usual ramisectomy with denervation of the sternocleidomastoid, the remaining muscles allow the patient an almost full range of movement since the anterior roots are not touched and posterior cervical denervation is only unilateral in those cases. In patients in whom a multiple approach is required, the patient can recover a surprising range of movements with early and intensive physiotherapy and function adequately. In our series one such patient was a mother and stenographer, another a school teacher, and a third a librarian. Although we still do it with some trepidation, posterior cervical denervation has been performed down to C5 on both sides in five instances, with the patients maintaining good head posture and stability. We prefer to limit it to C4 on one side whenever possible, unless retrocollis is very marked.

There were no complications in our series. Patients rarely complained of anesthesia or paresthesias from the posterior cervical denervation. This was initially reported as bothersome in two instances. When the trapezius has to be incised to pursue the ramisectomy, the patients may complain of pain at the base of the neck, but this is usually of short duration. It is also the reason why denervation of the trapezius is rarely done, since the pain may be more persistent, confirming the experience of Hamby and Schiffer.[30]

COMMENTS

As reported previously, selective peripheral denervation was first used as a complement to thalamotomy;[32] it soon became evident that it was sufficient whenever only the neck musculature was involved. Weir Mitchell apparently suggested a peripheral approach to C1, C2, and C3 to Keen, who reported doing one procedure in 1891.[48] Finney and Hughson wrote a very comprehensive report with excellent historical notes in 1925.[49] They stated that McKenzie's procedure was "an unnecessary dangerous method of resection." However, without the benefit of electromyography, their procedure was no more selective than rhizotomy. It was carried out bilaterally "to make it sufficently comprehensive to include all the offending structures"; it was in fact a bilateral extradural rhizotomy of C1, C2, and C3. Of the 31 patients they followed, they reported that 3 were unimproved, 16 were improved, and 12 were completely cured. One may presume that, in the latter cases, the semispinalis and part of the splenius were not too involved or that the horseshoe incision denervated most of the posterior rami of C4 and C5, since they contribute actively to the innervation of these muscles. This is a fact that is ignored by the proponents of rhizotomy.

As evidenced by the amplitude of movements that can be retained after the atlas and axis are fused, most of the movements of the head occur at the junction between the occiput and the atlas. The anterior cervical group of muscles, which is inserted at the base of the occiput close to the fulcrum, seems to contribute little to abnormal movements, except in the more severe forms of dystonia. Therefore, the muscles of special concern are the rectus muscles, the obliques, the semispinalis, the longissimus capitis, the splenius, and the sternocleidomastoid. The trapezius may be involved in inclination or extension, but seems to have little to do with rotation.

The antagonist muscles are rarely positively involved, but they are frequently inhibited both clinically and on electromyograms. When there are bilateral simultaneous discharges, they occur mostly in the sternocleidomastoids; nerve blocks can be helpful in deciding whether they are the result of resistance to the abnormal movements or an antagonist contraction. It is interesting that the sternocleidomastoid can be denervated bilaterally and the head will still have a fair amount of movement; it can be tilted forward with the anterior cervical group.

It was surprising to find that the area of anesthesia did not extend appreciably beyond the territory of C2 after ramisectomy down to C6, the posterior primary divisions of C3, C4, C5, and C6 having mostly a motor function.

Peripheral avulsion of the nervous branches seems to be important in avoiding recurrences. It was not done in the earlier cases when the sternocleidomastoid was denervated and we noted frequent return of function, although it usually was not sufficient to bring back the abnormal movements. There may be recurring branches from the nerve to the trapezius going to the sternocleidomastoid muscle, which must be sectioned.

The object of selective denervation is to obtain a maximum amount of relief from abnormal movements with minimum impairment of normal movements and with minimum risks and sequelae.

Besides preserving strength and a fuller range of movements than rhizotomy, unilateral peripheral denervation maintains a more normal appearance of the neck.

It is undoubtedly possible to improve on the surgical technique for peripheral denervation, and reflection of the semispinalis appears to be a step in that direction. However, the need for total denervation of the involved muscles must be stressed. As is well known, residual fibers will maintain abnormal movements, so it is worthwhile to use a time-consuming meticulous approach.

Although we do not know as yet precisely which muscles are involved in each of the multiple forms of spasmodic torticollis, it has been established that abnormal movements can be suppressed with selective peripheral denervation while all or almost all of the normal movements of the head are preserved.

ADULT-ONSET DYSTONIA

In its initial stages, adult-onset dystonia may well resemble spasmodic torticollis, which is another reason not to intervene too early or, if the symptoms are bothersome, to use procedures that do not produce important sequelae. Its evolution is quite different from that of spasmodic torticollis, which is usually well established after 2 years. Except in localized dystonias, such as writer's cramp, tardive dystonia of adults involves primarily the axial musculature in contrast to dystonia musculorum deformans of children. During the period from 1976 to 1985, 26 stereotactic procedures were done for adult-onset dystonia or spasmodic torticollis. The five procedures performed for spasmodic torticollis only were done in 1976 and 1977. Also, while there were 20 thalamotomies for these indications until 1981, there have only been 6 since that time, all for adult-onset dystonia. Because of our concern over corticobulbar involvement, only 4 of the 26 were bilateral. Contrary to our statistics from a larger series of a 10 percent occurrence of this complication, 2 of these 4 patients had some dysarthria. This complication is emphasized in the report by Andrew et al.[50] In another patient, with an excellent result from a unilateral lesion and a very severe persistant myoclonic type of dystonia on the other side, a contralateral lesion produced 1 year later was not effective, and after a few weeks the abnormal movements reappeared on the previously operated side for an unexplained reason. We strive to use only unilateral lesions, contralateral to the side where the movements predominate, performing a lesion on the other side later only if absolutely necessary. It was our initial impression that the much higher incidence of corticobulbar complications in these patients was because the lesion was centered on the VOI, further anterior

and closer to the corticobulbar fibers in the internal capsule.[51] Since the degree of hypotonia obtained is essentially the same with a more posterior lesion, we have gradually targeted our lesions 2 or 3 mm further posterior, closer to those used for tremor, in spite of Hassler's theory.[26] The lesion is also limited laterally and anteriorly, but an additional lesion is placed in the globus pallidus internus, the position of which is ascertained by microelectrode recording. While there seems to be little doubt that the clinical improvement depends both on accurate localization on the target and, to avoid compensatory mechanisms, on the size of the lesion, it is better to err on the side of conservatism than to produce dysarthria. Evidently, it is also important to use stimulation and microelectrode recording, especially in these patients, who may be more prone to this complication.

Twenty-four patients were followed. The result was extremely good in 6, very good in 11, fair in 5, and poor in 2, that is, a little better than two thirds of the patients were markedly relieved and it was moderately helpful in the others. Fourteen of these 24 patients also had some form of peripheral denervation, usually a ramisectomy. This has helped considerably when there was marked inclination of the head. Although the degree of improvement is greater, the percentage of patients who have obtained relief has not been increased substantially by ramisectomy. Peripheral denervation is now usually done first, since, at times, it gives the patient adequate relief and it makes a stereotactic procedure easier should one become necessary. Thalamotomy and pallidotomy remain useful procedures in generalized adult-onset dystonia and they may improve functional ability, but, unfortunately, the result remains unpredictable.

SUMMARY AND CONCLUSION

Results in 117 cases of spasmodic torticollis or adult-onset dystonia treated between 1976 and 1985 were reported. Of 91 patients with spasmodic torticollis, selective peripheral denervation produced total or very marked relief in 80 patients, demonstrating that abnormal movements can be suppressed with denervation limited to the muscles involved, with better functional result.

Twenty-four of 26 patients with generalized adult-onset dystonia were submitted to thalamotomy, usually with pallidotomy. In addition, some form of peripheral denervation was performed in 14 of them. The amount of improvement was greater in the latter but marked improvement was obtained only in two thirds of the patients.

REFERENCES

1. Bordeleau J-M (ed): Systèe Extrapyramidal et Neuroleptiques. Montréal, Editions Psychiatriques, 1961
2. Eldridge R, Fahn S (eds): Dystonia. Advances in Neurology, vol 14. New York, Raven Press, 1976
3. Yahr MD (ed): The Basal Ganglia. Research Publications: Association for Research in Nervous and Mental Diseases, vol 55. New York, Raven Press, 1976
4. Marsden CD, Fahn S (eds): Movement Disorders. Neurology II. London, Butterworths, 1981
5. Barbeau A (ed): Disorders of Movements. Current Status of Modern Therapy, vol 8. Lancaster, MTP Press, 1981
6. Fahn S: Torsion dystonia: Clinical spectrum and treatment. Semin Neurol 2:316, 1982

7. Marsden CD: The Problem of Adult-Onset Idiopathic Torsion Dystonia and other Isolated Dyskinesias in Adult Life (including Blepharospasm, Oromandibular Dystonia, Dystonic Writer's Cramp and Torticollis, or Axial Dystonia), in Eldridge R, Fahn S (eds): Dystonia. Advances in Neurology, vol 14. New York, Raven Press, 1976, pp 259–276

8. Fahn S: The Clinical Spectrum of Motor Tics, in Friedhoff AJ, Chase TN (eds): Gilles de la Tourette Syndrome. Advances in Neurology, vol 35. New York, Raven Press, 1982, pp 341–344

9. Couch JR: Dystonia and Tremor in Spasmodic Torticollis, in Eldridge R, Fahn S (eds): Dystonia. Advances in Neurology, vol 14. New York, Raven Press, 1976, pp 245–258

10. Gilbert JG: Familial spasmodic torticollis. Neurology 27:11, 1977

11. Podivinsky F: Torticollis, in Vinken PJ, Bruyn GW (eds): Handbook of Clinical Neurology. Amsterdam, North Holland, 1968, pp 567–596

12. Meares R: Natural history of spasmodic torticollis and effect of surgery. Lancet 2:149, 1971

13. Matthews WB, Beasley P, Parry-Jones W, et al: Spasmodic torticollis: A combined clinical study. J Neurol Neurosurg Psychiatry 41:485, 1978

14. Fahn S: High dosage anticholinergic therapy in dystonia. Neurology 33:1255, 1983

15. Marsden CD, Marion N-H, Quinn N: The treatment of severe dystonia in children and adults. J Neurol Neurosurg Psychiatry 47:1166, 1984

16. Lee MC: Spasmodic torticollis and other idiopathic torsion dystonias. Medical management. Postgrad Med 75:139, 1984

17. Korein J, Brudny J: Integrated EMG Feedback in the Management of Spasmodic Torticollis and Focal Dystonia: A Prospective Study of 80 Patients, in Yahr MD (ed): The Basal Ganglia. Research Publications: Association for Research in Nervous and Mental Diseases, vol 55. New York, Raven Press, 1976, pp 385–424

18. Svein HJ, Cody DTR: Treatment of spasmodic torticollis by suppression of labyrinthine activity: Report of a case. Mayo Clin Proc 44:825, 1969

19. Freckmann N, Hagenah R, Herrmann H-D, et al: Treatment of neurogenic torticollis by microvascular lysis of the accessory nerve roots—Indication, technique, and first results. Acta Neurochir 59:167, 1981

20. Gildenberg PL: Treatment of spasmodic torticollis with dorsal column stimulation. Acta Neurochir (suppl 24):65, 1977

21. Waltz JM: Surgical Approach to Dystonia, in Marsden CD, Fahn S (eds): Movement Disorders. Neurology II. London, Butterworths, 1981, pp 300–307

22. Gildenberg PL: Comprehensive management of spasmodic torticollis. Appl Neurophysiol 44:233, 1981

23. Gildenberg PL: Functional Neurosurgery, in Schmidek HH, Sweet WH (eds): Operative Neurosurgical Techniques. Indications Methods, and Results, vol 2. New York, Grune & Stratton, 1982, pp 993–1043

24. Mazars G, Méienne L, Chodkiewicz JP: La Chirurgie des Dyskinésies d'Orientation Céphalique. Neuro-Chirurgie 14:745, 1968

25. Setjskal L, Vladyka V, Tomanek Z: Surgical possibilities for alleviation for axial dyskinesias—Comparison for forced movements of the head and eyes. Appl Neurophysiol 44:320, 1981

26. Hassler R, Hess WR: Experimentell und Anatomische Befunde über die Drehbewegungen und Ihre Nervosen Apparate. Arch Psychiatr Nervenkr 192:488, 1954

27. Cooper IS: Clinical and physiological publications of thalamic surgery. J Neurol Sci 2:520, 1965

28. Mundinger F, Riechert T, Disselhoff J: Long term results of stereotactic treatment of spasmodic torticollis. Confin Neurol 34:41, 1972

29. Hassler R, Dieckmann G: Stereotactic treatment of different kinds of spasmodic torticollis. Confin Neurol 32:135, 1970

30. Bertrand C: The Treatment of Spasmodic Torticollis with Particular Reference to Thalamotomy, in Morley T (ed): Current Controversies in Neurosurgery. Philadelphia, WB Saunders, 1976, pp 455–459

31. Bertrand C, Molina-Negro P, Martinez SN: Stereotactic Targets for Dystonias and Dyskinesias: Their Relationship to Cortico-Bulbar Fibers and Other Adjoining Structures, in Poirier LJ, Sourkes TK, B é dard PJ (eds): Advances in Neurology, vol 24; The Extra-Pyramidal System and its Disorders. New York, Raven Press, 1979 pp. 395–399

32. Bertrand C, Molina-Negro P, Martinez SN: Combined stereotactic and peripheral surgical approach for spasmodic torticollis. Appl Neurophysiol 41:122, 1978

33. McKenzie KG: Intrameningeal division of the spinal accessory and roots of the upper cervical nerves for the treatment of spasmodic torticollis. Surg Gynecol Obstet 39:5, 1924

34. Dandy WE: Operation for treatment of spasmodic torticollis. Arch Surg 20:10, 1930

35. Tasker RR: The Treatment of Spasmodic Torticollis by Peripheral Denervation: The MacKensie Operation, in Morley T (ed): Current Controversies in Neurosurgery. Philadelphia, WB Saunders, 1976, pp 448–454

36. Sorensen BF, Hamby WB: Spasmodic torticollis: Results in 71 surgically treated patients. JAMA 194:706, 1965

37. Arseni C, Maretsis M: The surgical treatment of spasmodic torticollis. Neurochirurgia 14:177, 1971

38. Hamby WB, Schiffer S: Spasmodic torticollis: Results after cervical rhizotomy in 50 cases. J Neurosurg 31:323, 1969

39. Fabinyi G, Dutton J: The surgical treatment of spasmodic torticollis. Aust NZ J Surg 50:155, 1980

40. Adams CBT: Vascular catastrophy following the Dandy-McKenzie operation for spasmodic torticollis. J Neurol Neurosurg Psychiatry 47:990, 1984

41. Scoville WB, Bettis DB: Motor tics of the head and neck: Surgical approaches and their complications. Acta Neurochir 48:47, 1979

42. Xinkang C: Selective resection and denervation of cervical muscles in the treatment of spasmodic torticollis: Results in 60 cases. Neurosurgery 8:681, 1981

43. Maccabe JJ: Surgical Treatment of Spasmodic Torticollis, in Marsden CD, Fahn S (eds): Movement Disorders. Neurology II. London, Butterworths, 1981, pp 308–314

44. Bertrand C: Stereotactic and Peripheral Surgery for the Control of Movement Disorders, in Barbeau A (ed): Disorders of Movements. Current Status of Modern Therapy, vol 8. Lancaster, MTP Press, 1981, pp 191–208

45. Bertrand C, Molina-Negro P, Martinez SN: Technical aspects of selective peripheral denervation for spasmodic torticollis. Appl Neurophysiol 45:326, 1982

46. Lazorthes G: Les Branches Postérieures des Nerfs Rachidiens et le Plan Articulaire Vertébral Postérieur. Ann Med Phys 15:192, 1972

47. Bassett DL: A Stereoscopic Atlas of Human Anatomy. Section II, Head and Neck. Portland, Oregon, Sawyer's, 1954

48. Keen WW: A new operation for spasmodic wry neck. Namely, division or exsection of the nerves supplying the posterior rotator muscles of the head. Ann Surg 13:44, 1891

49. Finney MT, Hughson W: Spasmodic torticollis. Ann Surg 81:255, 1925

50. Andrew J, Fowler CJ, Harrison MJG: Stereotaxic thalamotomy in 55 cases of dystonia. Brain 106:981, 1983

51. Bertrand C, Martinez SN, Hardy J, et al: Stereotactic Surgery for Parkinsonism: Microelectrode Recording Stimulation and Oriented Sections with a Leucotome, in Krayenb ü hl H, Maspes PE, Sweet WH (eds): Progress in Neurological Surgery, vol 5. Basel, S Karger, 1973, pp 79–112

CHAPTER 112

Surgery of the Sympathetic Nervous System

Russell W. Hardy Jr.   Janet W. Bay

AS DESCRIBED IN GREENWOOD'S ARTICLE, "The Origins of Sympathectomy,"[1] surgeons first employed sympathectomy during the last decade of the 19th century. At that time, Jonnesco performed cervical ganglionectomies for the treatment of epilepsy, exophthalmic goiter, and (somewhat later) for angina pectoris. During these same years, Jaboulay and, later, LeRiche carried out sympathectomies for the relief of trophic ulcers in the lower extremity. Further interest in the operation was stimulated by the work of Royle and Hunter, who believed sympathectomy would relieve spasticity. Although their theory was to prove erroneous, observations made on patients who had undergone sympathectomy led to increased use of the operation for vasospastic disease. Subsequently, this procedure was used to treat a wide variety of conditions, including angina pectoris,[2] hypertension,[3,4] and vascular disease of large and small vessels.[5-7] Currently, many of these conditions are no longer indications for sympathectomy, either because of the advent of more modern methods of treatment (as in the case of angina and hypertension) or because experience has cast doubt on the efficacy of sympathectomy (as in the treatment of claudication of vascular origin).[8]

At present, the use of sympathectomy is limited to a handful of conditions, but it remains an important surgical technique, since it is uniquely effective in treating hyperhidrosis,[9] major causalgia[10-12] and some forms of minor causalgia,[13-18] shoulder-hand syndrome,[10] and certain pain of visceral origin.[19-25] Sympathectomy is also used for the treatment of ischemic ulceration, Raynaud's phenomenon, rest pain, and other sequelae of vascular insufficiency.[6,7]

This chapter will discuss three separate operations. The first is upper thoracic (T2) ganglionectomy as employed to treat hyperhidrosis and causalgia in the upper extremities. The second is splanchnicectomy combined with lower thoracic sympathectomy, which is used in the treatment of pain secondary to pancreatic cancer or (rarely) for the pain of chronic pancreatitis or (even more rarely) for pain of renal origin. The third is lumbar sympathectomy, as used in the treatment of major and minor causalgia in the lower extremities.

UPPER THORACIC GANGLIONECTOMY

ANATOMY

The sympathetic supply to the upper extremity is basically derived from preganglionic fibers leaving the cord from the second through the tenth anterior thoracic roots.[26] These fibers enter the paraspinal sympathetic ganglia via the white rami and synapse in the sympathetic chain. Postganglionic fibers leave the stellate and middle cervical ganglia to join the fifth cervical through the first thoracic roots, although the bulk of these fibers are found in the seventh and eighth cervical and first thoracic roots.[26,27]

According to the above schema, a resection of the second thoracic ganglion should be sufficient to denervate the upper extremity. It has been argued, however, that sympathetic efferents to the arm also are derived from the eighth cervical[28] and, more importantly, the first thoracic,[29,30] roots. In addition, Kuntz has described communications between the third and second thoracic roots, and second and first thoracic roots, which might serve as an extraganglionic sympathetic pathway to the arm.[28-31] Finally, intermediate ganglia have been described in the spinal roots of C8, T1, and T2, which also might supply sympathetic fibers to the arm, independent of traditional pathways.[32]

If these various alternate pathways are viewed as significant, complete sympathetic denervation of the upper extremity would require resection of the middle cervical ganglion, the stellate ganglion, the second and third thoracic ganglia, as well as the intrathoracic nerves of Kuntz. It would also demand section of the anterior roots of T1, T2, and T3, and even then input from anterior cervical roots might persist. In fact, such an extensive procedure has been advocated in the past,[30] and a number of authors recommend at least including the inferior portion of the stellate ganglion, in addition to T2 and T3,[10,31] in order to ensure a complete sympathectomy.

It is relevant to note at this point that the sympathetic outflow to the pupil leaves the cord at T1, but that contributions also may come from T2, T3, T4, and (rarely) C8.[33] These fibers then cross the stellate ganglion and synapse with postganglionic neurons in the superior cervical ganglion. Thus, procedures that require resection of the stellate ganglion will result in a Horner's syndrome, although it has been suggested that resection of the lower half of this ganglion may be performed without risking this complication.[34]

It also should be mentioned that preganglionic sympathectomy (by division of the anterior spinal roots, white rami, and sympathetic chain, but with preservation of the ganglia) was at one time recommended on the grounds that this would avoid "hypersensitivity" of end organs to circulating catecholamines.[35] Many now feel, however, that such hypersensitivity

OPERATIVE NEUROSURGICAL TECHNIQUES
ISBN 0-8089-1862-1

does not occur or is of minimal clinical significance following resection of the ganglia.[10,30]

In our experience, as well as in the experience of others, resection of the T2 (and possibly the T3) ganglia has been sufficient to denervate the upper extremity and serve as adequate treatment for hyperhidrosis and causalgia.[9,36,37] By not resecting the lower portion of the stellate ganglion, the risk of a Horner's syndrome is minimized. We have not observed hypersensitivity following T2 ganglionectomy in the treatment of hyperhidrosis, and it does not occur when postganglionic sympathectomy is performed for the treatment of causalgia.[38,39]

SURGICAL APPROACHES

A variety of approaches to the cervical and upper thoracic chain have been employed. These include posterior thoracic operations via midline,[5] paramedian,[35] or transverse[40] incisions, cervical (unilateral[41] or bilateral[42] incisions), and transthoracic[43] and anterior transthoracic approaches.[44] The operation that we employ is a posterior approach through a midline incision. The anterior and lateral operations have the advantage of providing excellent visualization of the sympathetic chain, but the disadvantage of the exposure being unilateral, which means that a second procedure is required if a bilateral sympathectomy is needed. The posterior paramedian approach can afford a bilateral exposure, albeit through two separate incisions. This approach may carry the disadvantage of providing less adequate visualization of the chain, and in our experience there are occasional difficulties with the upper thoracic paramedian incision. The cervical approach can be done through either a unilateral or midline incision[42] (which affords bilateral exposure), but visualization of the upper thoracic ganglia may be difficult. More recently, upper-thoracic sympathectomy has been carried out via a percutaneous radiofrequency technique.[45] Results were good to excellent in all of 15 patients treated for Raynaud's disease, vascular occlusive disease, and hyperhidrosis. An advantage of this procedure is that it can be performed on an outpatient basis.

Long-term follow-up data on a larger group of patients are necessary in order to assess the permanence of these radiofrequency lesions. The dorsal operation through a midline incision has the advantage of bilateral exposure, and we have felt that this approach afforded adequate visualization of the ganglia to be resected. Moreover, this operation can be performed readily by neurosurgeons, since it is simply an extension of a standard upper thoracic laminectomy exposure.

INDICATIONS

A T2 ganglionectomy is currently used in the treatment of essential hyperhidrosis, and for major causalgia (as described originally by Weir Mitchell),[46] minor causalgia and certain of its variations, and occasionally for shoulder-hand syndrome. A T2 ganglionectomy also may be employed to treat certain conditions of vascular origin.[6]

The use of sympathectomy for the treatment of essential hyperhidrosis was first described by Kotzareff.[9] Hyperhidrosis can be a source of great embarrassment and considerable disability to the patient. It may involve the entire body, including the legs and head, but symptoms are most severe and of the greatest discomfort in the upper extremities. The patients have symptoms that often date from childhood or early adolescence. Such individuals report reluctance to shake hands or touch other people, and often wear gloves to disguise their condition. The diagnosis is readily confirmed by inspection of the extremities.

Experience has confirmed the value of sympathectomy in the treatment of causalgia.[10,12] As originally described, this condition is characterized by severe burning pain, exacerbated by touch, that appears shortly after an injury to a mixed peripheral nerve,[45] most often the median or sciatic nerve. This injury occurs most often during wartime, and is relatively uncommon in civilian practice. It first may be treated by sympathetic blocks, to which a very high proportion of patients will respond. In fact, response to a block is one method of establishing the diagnosis in individuals with typical symptoms. A certain number of patients may be treated without surgery by blocks alone. If the pain recurs, however, sympathectomy may be performed, and relief of pain is obtained in a very high percentage of patients.

Sympathectomy also may be employed in the treatment of a group of ill-defined entities that are characterized by burning pain and trophic changes that may appear following peripheral nerve injury, but also are associated with a variety of other conditions, including fracture, local laceration, infection,[13,18] burns, subcutaneous injection, phlebitis, and arterial embolism. A unifying mechanism has not been postulated for these conditions, other than the suggestion that they may be the result of some form of sympathetic overactivity. Regardless of the etiology, certain of these conditions are said to respond to sympathectomy, although the response to surgery for these conditions may well be less certain than is the response to surgery for major causalgia. Favorable response to sympathetic block will select patients who may do well following surgery, but even this is no guarantee that the operation will be successful.

OPERATIVE TECHNIQUE

The T2 ganglionectomy through a dorsal midline incision is most conveniently done with the patient in the sitting position, although the prone position also may be used (Figures 112-1 through 112-8). The sitting position has the advantage that an intraoperative x-ray film, confirming the level, can be obtained more conveniently than when the patient is prone. We also feel that exposure is somewhat better when the patient is erect. The principal disadvantage of the sitting position, namely air embolus, is minimal or nonexistent when surgery is carried out at this level.

An x-ray film is obtained before the operation, with a marker placed at the spinous process of T2. The spinous process of T2 will be opposite the lamina and medial portion or the rib of T3. These structures are exposed and confirmatory x-ray films are obtained at the T3 level. Following this, the T3 transverse process and underlying rib are removed, either with a Kerrison punch or a rongeur, with care being taken to dissect free the underlying pleura. After resection of the rib and medial transverse process, the lateral border of the vertebral body is exposed by blunt dissection. The lower portion of the second rib also may need to be removed in order to expose the T2 ganglion. At this point, the second intercostal nerve is elevated and the sympathetic chain visualized. The communicating rami and the chain above and below the T2 ganglion are clipped and divided, and the ganglion is removed. If convenient, the T3 ganglion also may be resected. If axillary sweating is a major complaint, both the T2 and the T3 ganglia are removed in entirety.

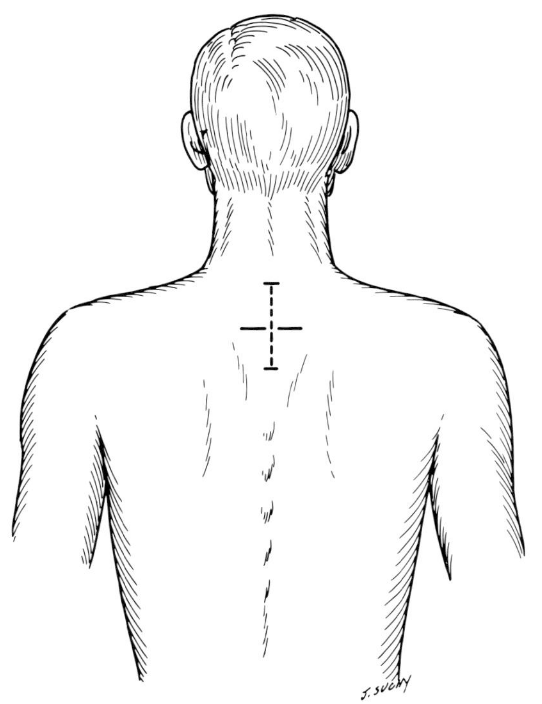

Fig. 112-1.   Location of the skin incision for a T2 ganglionectomy.

Following resection of the ganglion and hemostasis, the incision may be closed in layers, with care being taken to obtain a good closure of the deep fascia over the spinous process of T2 and T3. If a pleural tear has occurred during the course of the dissection, it may be managed by leaving a 12F red rubber catheter in place (within the leaves of the pleura) until a fascial closure is effected. The catheter then is removed with suction as the anesthetist applies positive pressure. This has been adequate to avoid postoperative pneumothorax in most cases.

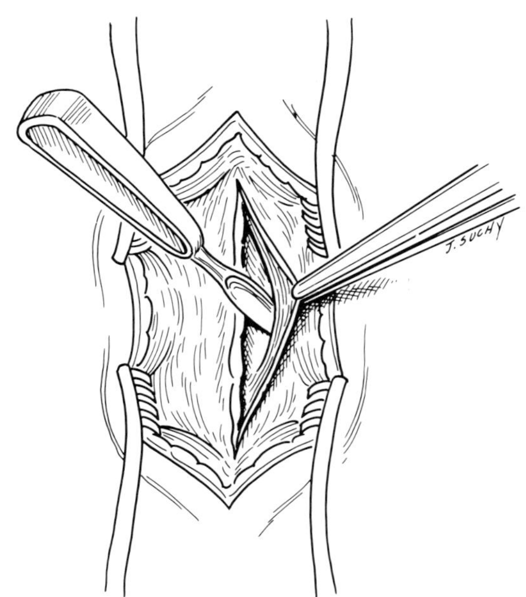

Fig. 112-2.   The beginning of the exposure of the T3 lamina and transverse process.

RESULTS

We have recently reviewed a series of 326 patients undergoing bilateral T2 ganglionectomy for hyperhidrosis at our institution between 1966 and 1983. All patients had immediate relief of palmar sweating. Long-term follow-up data were obtained by questionnaire in 162 patients (49 percent). Eighty-eight percent of these patients remained satisfied with the surgical result for postoperative periods up to 15 years. Causes for dissatisfaction included compensatory sweating, intercostal neuralgia, incisional appearance, and recurrent sweating. The recurrence rate for palmar hyperhidrosis is this series is 1 percent.

COMPLICATIONS

There was no operative mortality in this group of 326 patients. Significant complications were noted in 5 percent of the patients. These included wound infections (9), pneumonia

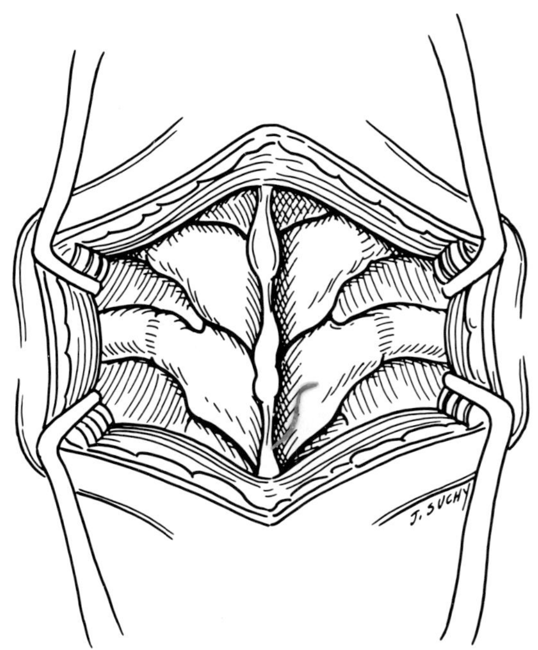

Fig. 112-3.   The completed bilateral exposure of the transverse processes of T3.

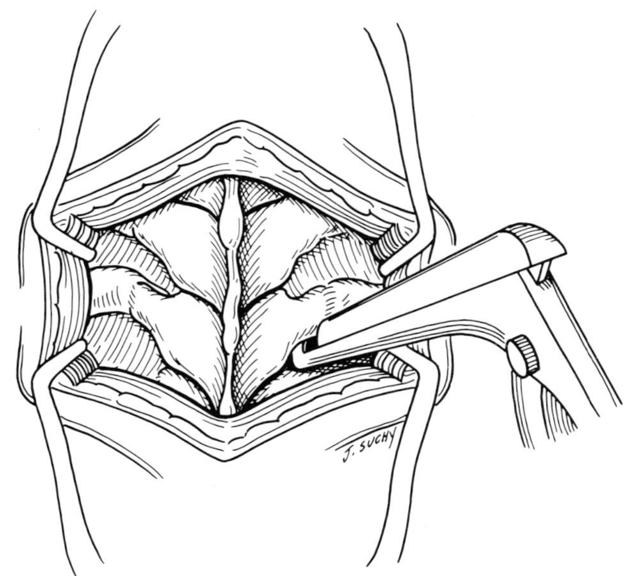

Fig. 112-4.   Resection of the T3 transverse process.

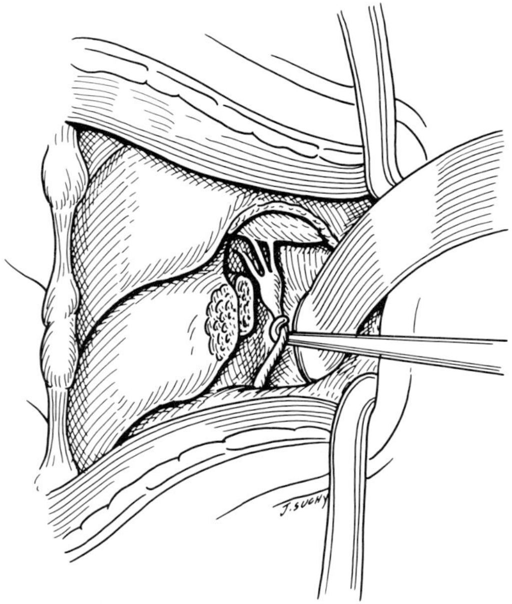

Fig. 112-5. The T3 costotransversectomy has been completed. The nerve hook is under the sympathetic chain.

(2), pneumothorax (2), cerebrospinal fluid (CSF) leak (1), Horner's syndrome (1), spinal cord injury (1), and empyema (1).

SPLANCHNICECTOMY

ANATOMY

Visceral afferents supplying the heart, pancreas, kidneys, gallbladder, and other organs have been described[37,47,48] and serve as a source of pain in various conditions affecting these structures.

Autonomic innervation to the pancreas is derived from the splanchnic nerves and from the vagus. Visceral afferents appear to travel exclusively through the splanchnic chain. These enter the cord via the greater splanchnic nerve after traversing the celiac ganglion. As described by Ray and Neill,[47] the pancreas

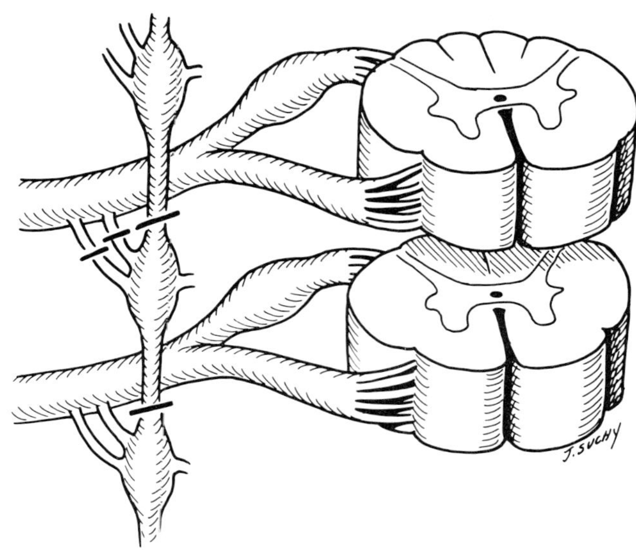

Fig. 112-6. The extent of the sympathetic resection.

receives bilateral innervation not only from the greater splanchnic nerves, which are derived from cord segments T4-T9, but also from the lesser splanchnic nerves and perhaps through the lower portion of the thoracic ganglia and the upper portion of the lumbar chains. Because the pancreas receives bilateral innervation, a bilateral operation will usually be required to effect relief of pain,[22,24] although in certain instances a unilateral operation is said to be sufficient.[21,25] Innervation to the biliary tracts is supplied by the right splanchnic nerves, and the nerve supply to the kidneys is also unilateral (via the lesser and least splanchnic trunks). The minor splanchnic nerves are derived from T10 and T11 and the least splanchnic nerve from T12.

It should be emphasized that while the splanchnic nerves are divided into three separate branches, in actual practice

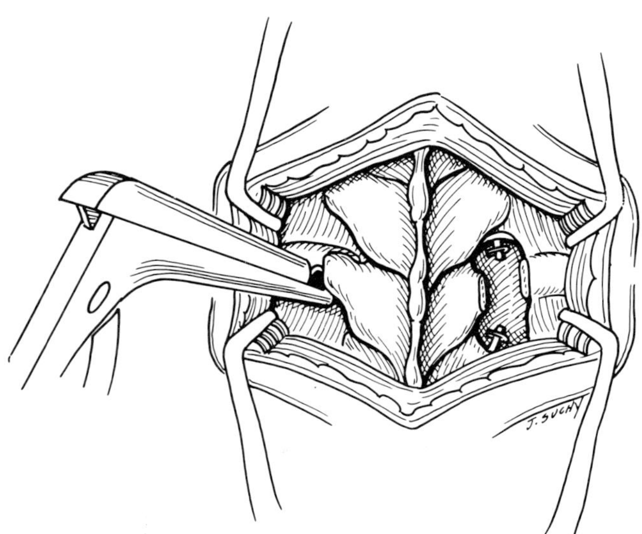

Fig. 112-7. The contralateral T3 costotransversectomy is begun.

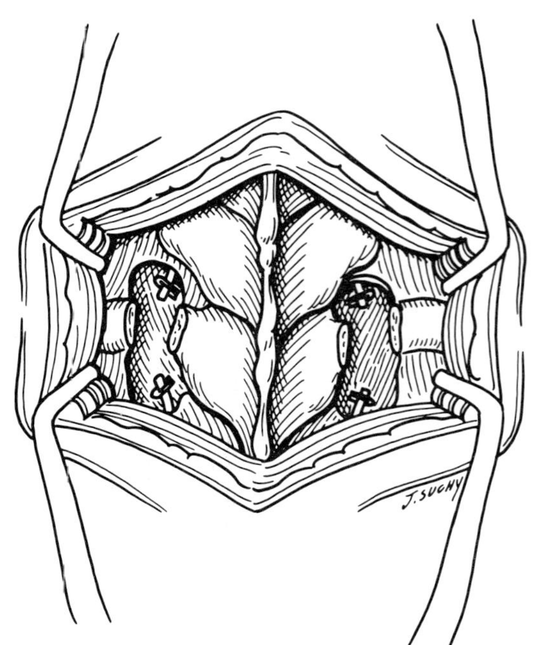

Fig. 112-8. The complete costotransversectomy and bilateral T2 ganglionectomy.

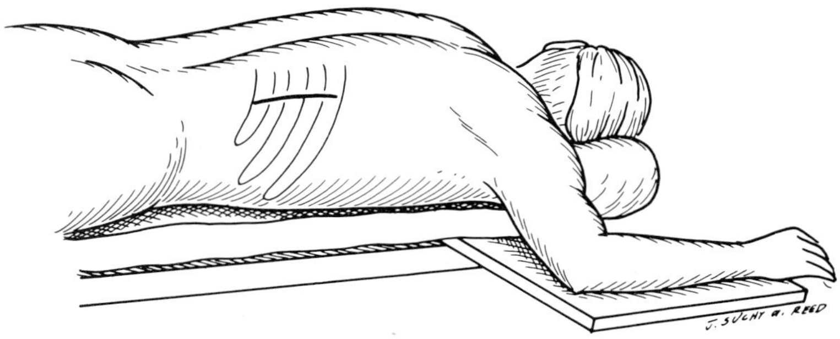

Fig. 112-9. The location of the skin incision for lower thoracic splanchnicectomy-sympathectomy.

identification of these separate trunks may be difficult and there may be considerable variability from patient to patient.

Based on these anatomic considerations, the operation that we employ to denervate the pancreas is resection of the thoracic ganglia from approximately T9 through T12, together with resection of the greater, lesser, and least splanchnic nerves. Other writers have recommended a more extensive operation, including the upper lumbar ganglia, but we have not found such an extensive resection to be necessary, and removal of the upper lumbar ganglia adds technical difficulty and (in the male) the risk of sexual dysfunction.[24,49]

INDICATIONS

Pain from pancreatic carcinoma may result from involvement of visceral afferent fibers or from pain secondary to the involvement of parietal somatic nerves. Any evidence of radicular pain suggests involvement of somatic nerves and is a contraindication to the procedure in the patient with pancreatic carcinoma. If doubt exists, the patient may be evaluated by means of a temporary splanchnic block. Frequently, it is our practice to perform the operation in combination with diagnostic laparotomy. In a patient with upper abdominal and back pain and no evidence of somatic nerve involvement, a bilateral splanchnicectomy can be performed after closure of the abdominal incision and repositioning of the patient. Such a combined operation adds little to the overall morbidity of the laparotomy.

The operation also has been advocated for the pain of chronic pancreatitis,[15,22,25] and such pain may be relieved in certain individuals, but in our experience the operation often fails to help the patient discontinue the use of narcotics (often because the individual will develop new chronic pain at the site of operative incisions or elsewhere). Finally, a rare patient with benign pain of renal or biliary origin may be a candidate for sympathectomy,[37] although operations for these indications are rarely performed at our institution.

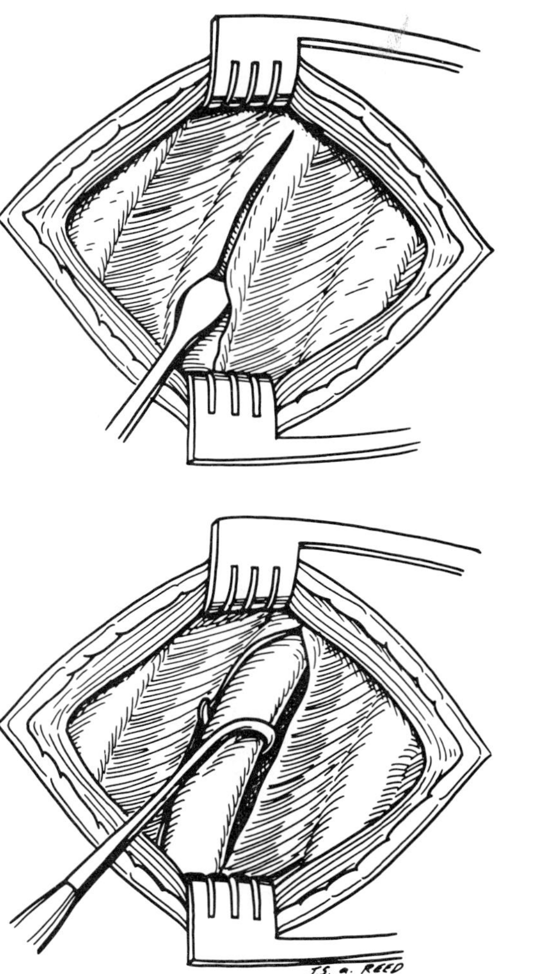

Fig. 112-10. Subperiosteal exposure of the eleventh rib with a periosteal elevator. The underlying periosteum then is stripped with a pigtail periosteal elevator.

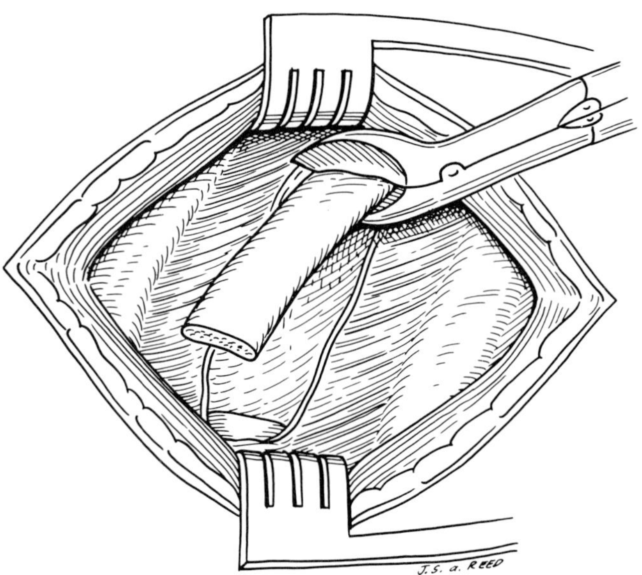

Fig. 112-11. Resection of the eleventh rib. The underlying parietal pleura then is separated from adjacent ribs by blunt dissection.

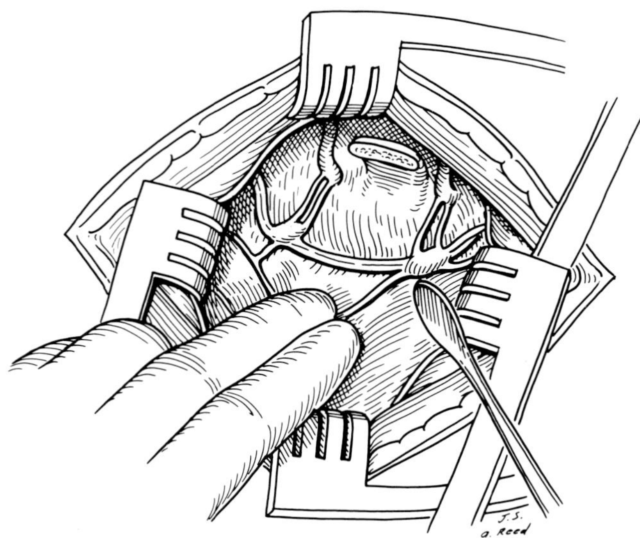

Fig. 112-12.   The exposure of the sympathetic chain and splanchnic nerves.

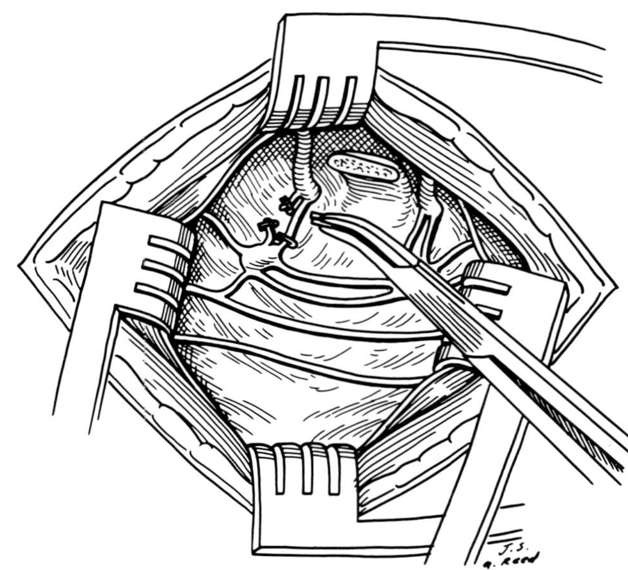

Fig. 112-14.   Resection of the sympathetic chain and splanchnic nerves.

'OPERATIVE TECHNIQUE

The procedure is carried out with the patient in the prone position on a laminectomy frame or with a blanket roll beneath the hips and shoulders (Figures 112-9 through 112-16).[20] An incision is made four fingerbreadths lateral to the spinous process overlying the eleventh rib. Dissection is carried down until the rib is encountered. The periosteum overlying the rib is stripped with an elevator and the pleura then is separated from the underlying rib with a pigtail periosteal dissector. Approximately the lateral 4 to 6 cm of rib are removed with rib cutters and rongeurs. The underlying pleura then is carefully dissected from the medial portion of the rib and also from the undersurface of adjacent ribs. Normally, this is not a particularly difficult maneuver and can be carried out with careful finger dissection. Some large intercostal veins may be encountered as the dissection is carried out medially. These may be easily controlled with either clips or bipolar coagulation. Final

dissection of the pleura from the lateral portion of the spine and the underlying surface of the rib may be carried out with Kittner dissectors. As the pleura is being retracted, it is protected beneath an abdominal sponge.

After the pleura has been swept free of the underlying surface of the rib, the remaining medial portion of the eleventh rib is removed if additional exposure is required. The exposure of the lateral portion of the adjacent vertebrae then is completed. A resection of the sympathetic ganglia and their connections, as well as the greater, lesser, and least splanchnic nerves, then is carried out. As noted above, the splanchnic nerves are not always constant structures, although the greater splanchnic nerve may be identified fairly reliably anterior to the sympathetic chain on the lateral margin of the vertebral bodies. As great a length of splanchnic nerve as possible is resected, together with any other branches of the lesser and least nerves that can be identified. In addition, resection of the ganglia, T9

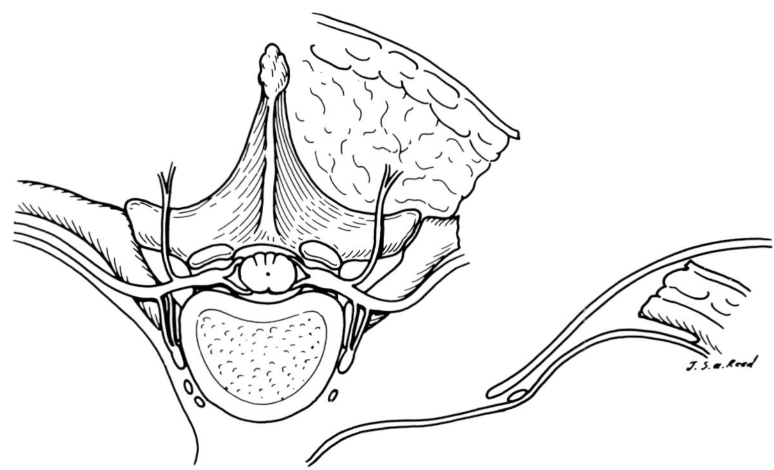

Fig. 112-13.   A cross-sectional view of the exposure. The splanchnic nerves may be inadvertently retracted with the pleura.

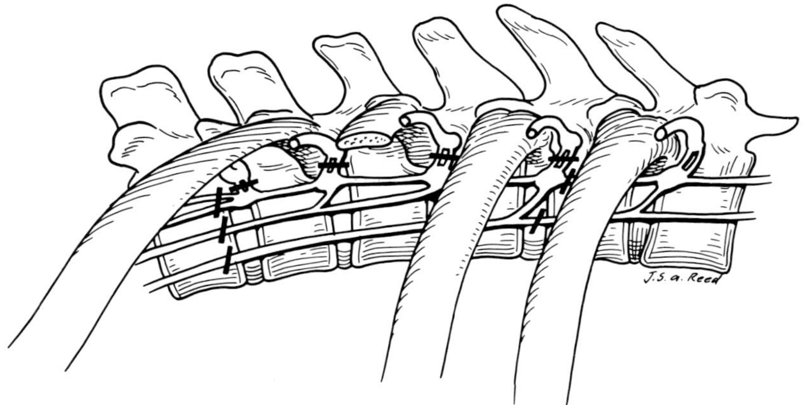

Fig. 112-15. The ideal extent of the resection.

through T12, together with the rami communicantes then is carried out, with the chains being divided between metal clips.

One difficulty that is sometimes encountered is that the splanchnic nerves may be difficult to find. A common cause of this is that the nerve may be swept onto the pleura and is then easily retracted along with the parietal pleura. Careful inspection of the surface of the parietal pleura usually will identify the nerve when it cannot be found adjacent to the vertebral bodies.

If the pleura is torn during the procedure, the situation may be managed by inserting a red rubber catheter through the wound and applying suction and Valsalva's maneuver during closure. If a very large tear has occurred, a chest tube may be

placed at the time of closure, or later if a substantial pneumothorax is seen on postoperative films.

The procedure is carried out bilaterally. As noted, it has not been our custom to divide the diaphragm and remove the L1 ganglia, as has been advocated by some.

RESULTS

In a series of 56 patients undergoing the procedure for pancreatic carcinoma, 70 percent had satisfactory relief of symptoms, 14 percent partial relief, and 16 percent no improvement.[23,24] Recurrence of pain was noted in 23 percent of patients, most often in those who survived for a period of several months; this recurrence of pain was partial and not regarded as a severe problem. The mortality rate in patients with cancer who were undergoing combined laparotomy and splanchnicectomy was 7 percent.

COMPLICATIONS

As noted above, pleural tears occur occasionally and usually can be managed at the time of surgery or with a postoperative chest tube. Superficial wound infections, and 1 case of empyema, have occurred. We have not experienced paraplegia as a complication of this procedure (caused by interference with the blood supply to the cord), but such catastrophes have been reported. In 1 patient it was speculated that the use of electrocautery initiated a vascular thrombosis with a resulting delayed paraplegia.[50]

LUMBAR SYMPATHECTOMY

ANATOMY

The sympathetic supply to the lower extremity is derived from the 5 lumbar ganglia whose efferents leave the spinal canal with the L1 and L2 roots.[26,37] Resection of the second and third lumbar ganglia should be sufficient to denervate the leg, although in a few individuals resection of the L1, L2, and T12 ganglia has been necessary in order to completely abolish the pain of causalgia.[12]

INDICATIONS

The major indication for lumbar sympathectomy by the neurosurgeon is either major or minor causalgia of the lower

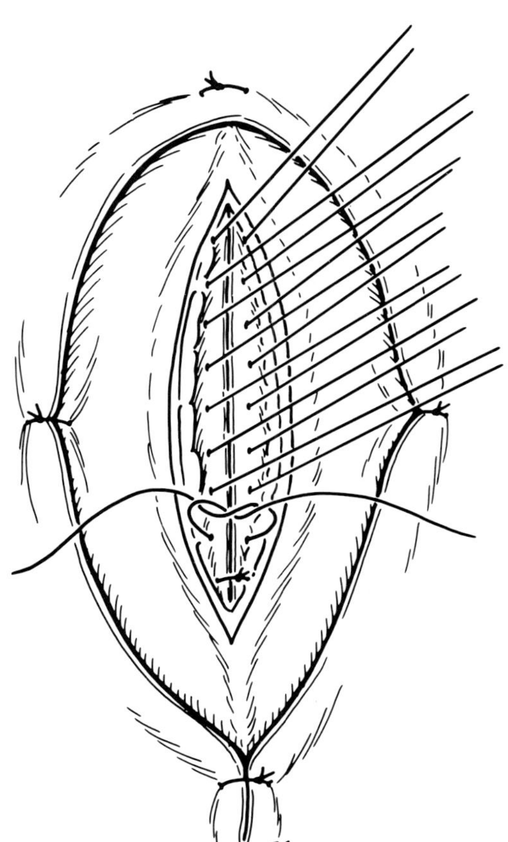

Fig. 112-16. The layered closure of the incision.

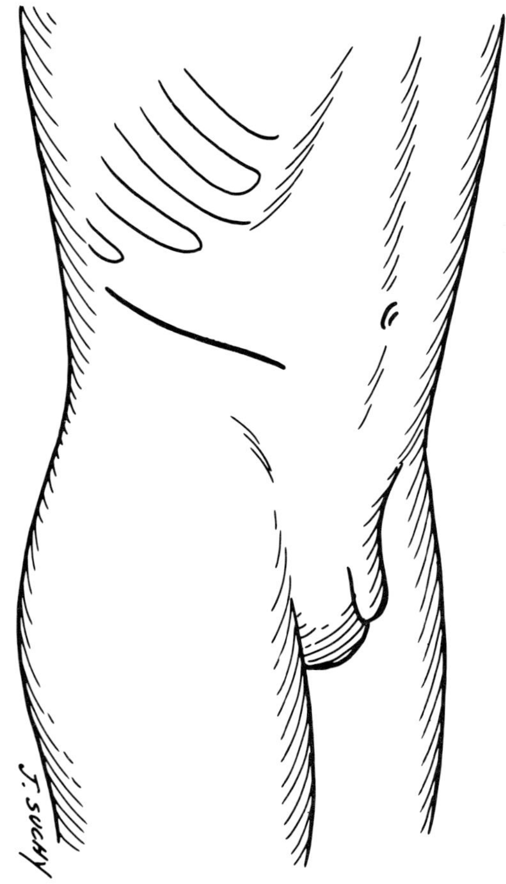

Fig. 112-17.   The incision used for lumbar sympathectomy.

extremity. The procedure also remains useful for the treatment of ischemic rest pain and superficial ulceration secondary to arteriosclerotic vascular disease. We have not employed this operation in the treatment of hyperhidrosis of the lower extremities.

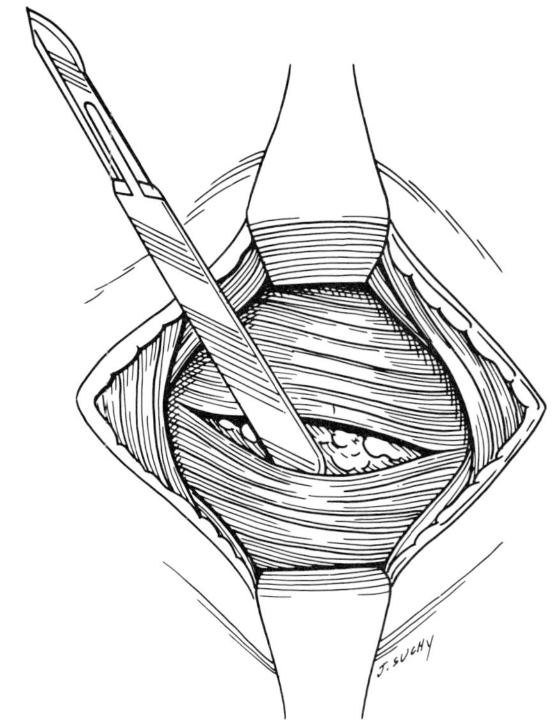

Fig. 112-18.   The abdominal muscles are divided in the direction of their fibers.

SURGICAL TECHNIQUE

The operation may be carried out through a variety of skin incisions. We employ the transverse incision extending obliquely from beneath the costal margin to the right lower quadrant (Figures 112-17 through 112-20). The external oblique, internal oblique, and transversus muscles are divided in the direction of their fibers. The peritoneum and renal fascia then are dissected free of the quadratus lumborum and iliac muscles

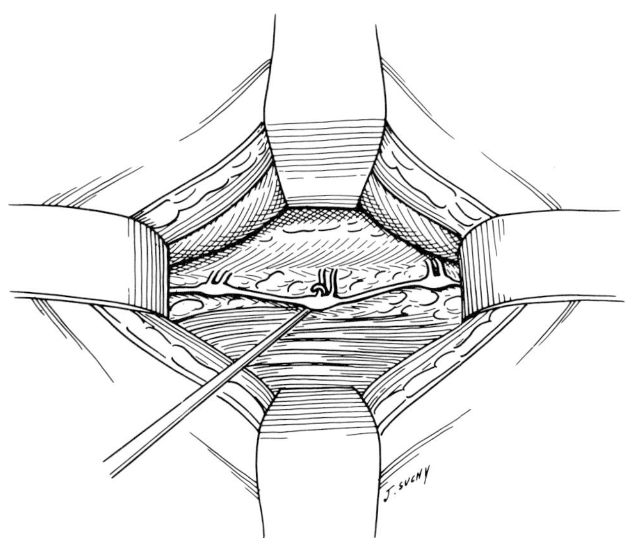

Fig. 112-19.   The sympathetic chain is identified.

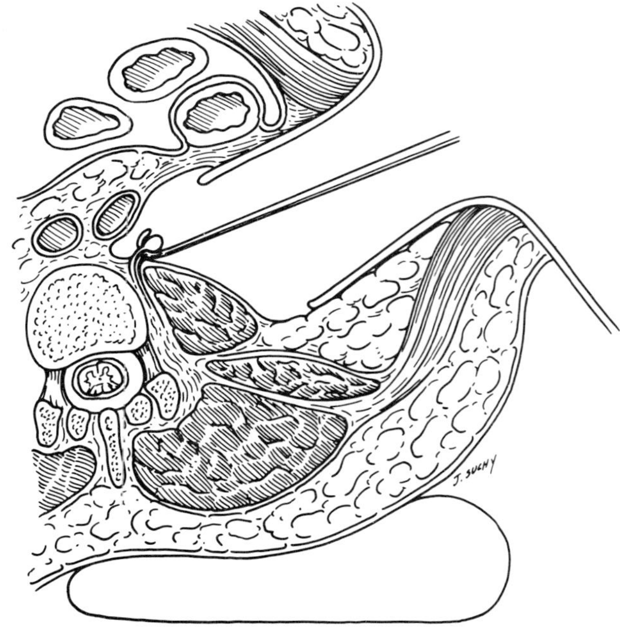

Fig. 112-20.   A cross-sectional view of the exposure following extraperitoneal retraction of the abdominal contents.

with blunt finger dissection. Dissection then is carried medially over the anterior surface of the psoas muscle until the sympathetic chain is encountered between it and the vertebral body.

On the right side, the vena cava will be encountered, and bridging veins may need to be divided and clipped or coagulated. On the left, the aorta may be mobilized and will not overlie the chain.

The chain is identified and at least 2 ganglia are removed. The chain and rami communicantes are divided between metallic clips.

After resection of the ganglia, the muscle layers are closed separately. During this portion of the procedure, the table may be straightened to facilitate closure.

In performing the operation, care should be taken to identify the ureter, which is retracted medially with the kidney, and to avoid injuring somatic nerves passing through the psoas and quadratus lumborum muscles.[41,43]

RESULTS

Peacetime experience in the treatment of causalgia in the lower extremity is limited. Excellent results, similar to those encountered in the upper arm, are generally obtained. As noted by Ulmer and Mayfield,[12] an incomplete result will be obtained in an occasional patient and may require an additional procedure to remove the L1 and T12 ganglia.

COMPLICATIONS

The major neurologic complication is the risk of sexual dysfunction if the procedure is carried out bilaterally in the male. This consideration limits its use in the treatment of hyperhidrosis and other conditions.

REFERENCES

1. Greenwood B: The origins of sympathectomy. Med Hist 11:165, 1967
2. White JC, Bland EF: The surgical relief of severe angina pectoris. Medicine 27:1, 1948
3. Peet MM: Splanchnic resection for hypertension. Univ Hosp Bull, Ann Arbor Mich 1:17, 1935
4. Smithwick RH: A technique for splanchnic resection for hypertension. Surgery 7:1, 1940
5. Adson AW, Brown GE: The treatment of Raynaud's disease by resection of the upper thoracic and lumbar sympathetic ganglia and trunks. Surg Gynecol Obstet 48:577, 1929
6. Dale WA, Lewis MD: Management of ischemia of the hand and fingers. Surgery 67:62, 1970
7. Myers KA, Irvine WT: An objective study of lumbar sympathectomy. II. Skin ischaemia. Br Med J 1:943, 1966
8. Myers KA, Irvine WT: An objective study of lumbar sympathectomy. I. Intermittent claudication. Br Med J 1:879, 1966
9. Dohn DF, Sava GM: Sympathectomy for vascular syndromes and hyperhydrosis of the upper extremities, in Keener EB (ed): Clinical Neurosurgery, vol 25. Baltimore, Williams & Wilkins, 1978, pp 637–650
10. Bergan JJ, Con J: Sympathectomy for pain relief. Med Clin North Am 52:147, 1968
11. Spurling RG: Causalgia of the upper extremity: Treatment by dorsal sympathetic ganglionectomy. Arch Neurol Psychiatry 23:784, 1930
12. Ulmer JL, Mayfield FH: Causalgia: A study of 75 cases. Surg Gynecol Obstet 83:789, 1946
13. Drucker WR, Hubay CA, Holden WD, et al: Pathogenesis of posttraumatic sympathetic dystrophy. Am J Surg 97:454, 1959
14. Echlin F, Owens FM, Wells WL: Observations on "major" and "minor" causalgia. Arch Neurol Psychiatry 62:183, 1949
15. Hardy WG, Posch JL, Webster JE, et al: The problem of major and minor causalgias. Am J Surg 95:545, 1958
16. Homans J: Minor causalgia: A hyperesthetic neurovascular syndrome. N Engl J Med 22:870, 1940
17. McFarlane WV: Causalgic syndromes. Aust NZ J Surg 18:191, 1949
18. Wirth FP, Rutherford RB: A civilian experience with causalgia. Arch Surg 100:633, 1970
19. Connelly JE, Richards V: Bilateral splanchnicectomy and lumbodorsal sympathectomy for chronic relapsing pancreatitis. Ann Surg 131:58, 1960
20. Heisy WG, Dohn DF: Splanchnicectomy for the treatment of intractable abdominal pain. Cleve Clin Q 34:9, 1967
21. Mallet-Guy P, Beaujeu MJ: Treatment of chronic pancreatitis by unilateral splanchnicectomy. Arch Surg 60:233, 1950
22. Ray BS, Console AD: The relief of pain in chronic (calcareous) pancreatitis by sympathectomy. Surg Gynecol Obstet 89:1, 1949
23. Sadar ES, Cooperman AM: Bilateral thoracic sympathectomy—splanchnicectomy in the treatment of intractable pain due to pancreatic carcinoma. Cleve Clin Q 41:185, 1974
24. Sadar ES, Hardy RW: Thoracic splanchnicectomy and sympathectomy for the relief of pancreatic pain, in Cooperman AM (ed): Surgery of the Pancreas. St. Louis, CV Mosby, 1978, pp 141–152
25. de Takats G, Walter LE, Lasner J: Splanchnic nerve section for pancreatic pain. Ann Surg 131:44, 1950
26. Pick J: The Autonomic Nervous System. Philadelphia, JB Lippincott, 1970
27. Sunderland S: The distribution of sympathetic fibres in the brachial plexus in man. Brain 71:88, 1948
28. Kirgis HD, Kuntz A: Inconstant sympathetic neural pathways. Arch Surg 44:95, 1942
29. Kuntz A, Dillon JB: Preganglionic components of the first thoracic nerve. Arch Surg 44:772, 1942
30. Ray BS: Sympathectomy of the upper extremity. J Neurosurg 10:624, 1953
31. Kuntz A: Distribution of the sympathetic rami to the brachial plexus. Arch Surg 15:871, 1927
32. Skoog T: Ganglia in the communicating rami of the cervical sympathetic trunk. Lancet 28:457, 1947
33. Ray BS, Hinsey JC, Geohegan WA: Observations on the distribution of the sympathetic nerves to the pupil and upper extremity as determined by stimulation of the anterior roots in man. Ann Surg 118:647, 1943
34. Palumbo LT: A new concept of the sympathetic pathways to the eye. Surgery 42:,740, 1957
35. Smithwick RH: The rationale and technic of sympathectomy for the relief of vascular spasm of the extremities. N Engl J Med 222:699, 1940
36. Hyndman OR, Wolkin J: Sympathectomy of the upper extremity. Arch Surg 45:145, 1942
37. White JC: Role of sympathectomy in relief of pain, in Krayenbuhl H, Maspes PE, Sweet WH (eds): Progress in Neurological Surgery, vol 7. Basel, S. Karger, 1976, pp 131–152
38. Mayfield FH: Personal communication 39. Nulsen FE: Personal communication
40. Love JG, Juergens JL: Second thoracic sympathetic ganglionectomy for neurologic and vascular disturbance of the upper extremities. West J Surg 72:130, 1964
41. Kempe LG: Operative Neurosurgery, vol 2. Heidelbert, Springer-Verlag, 1970, pp 244–250
42. Lougheed WM: A simple technique for upper thoracic sympathectomy in patients requiring sympathectomy of the upper limb. Can J Surg 8:306, 1965
43. Kleinert HE, Norbert H, McDonough JJ: Surgical sympathectomy—upper and lower extremity, in Omer GE, Spinner M (eds):

Peripheral Nerve Problems. Philadelphia, WB Saunders, 1980, pp 285–302

44. Palumbo LT: Anterior transthoracic approach for upper thoracic sympathectomy. Arch Surg 72:659, 1956

45. Wilkinson HA: Radiofrequency percutaneous upper thoracic sympathectomy. N Engl J Med 311:34, 1984

46. Richards RL: Causalgia: A centennial review. Arch Neurol 16:339, 1967

47. Ray BS, Neill CL: Abdominal visceral sensation in man. Ann Surg 126:709, 1947

48. Richins CA: The innervation of the pancreas. J Comp Neurol 83:,223, 1945

49. Whitelaw GP, Smithwick RH: Some secondary effects of sympathectomy. N Engl J Med 245:,121, 1951

50. Shallat RF, Klump TE: Paraplegia following thoracolumbar sympathectomy. J Neurosurg 34:,569, 1971

CHAPTER 113

Craniovertebral Abnormalities and Their Treatment

John C. VanGilder   Arnold H. Menezes

CRANIOVERTEBRAL JUNCTION ABNORMALITIES can be congenital, inflammatory, developmental, or traumatic in origin.[1-6] To effectively treat these disorders when symptomatic, a knowledge of the embryology and the functional anatomy of the area is necessary. A myriad of abnormal neurologic findings may be present that are secondary to compression or ischemia of neural tissue. The surgical management of these disorders is dependent upon precise identification of the underlying pathophysiologic condition as determined by appropriate radiologic studies. The operative treatment includes anterior and/or posterior approaches to the craniovertebral junction with or without bony fusion. Our experience with 219 patients treated surgically who had neurologic symptoms from craniovertebral abnormalities is the basis for management of these complex disorders (Table 113-1).

HISTORY

Subsequent to the first description of spontaneous atlantoaxial dislocation in 1830 by Bell,[7] lesions of the cervicomedullary junction have emerged from a state of being medical curiosities into an era where they can be effectively managed. Except for acute dislocations, the treatment of occipitoatlantoaxial joint pathologic entities was marked with failure before the era of skeletal traction. Subsequently, it was apparent that the majority of both acute and chronic dislocations could be reduced even years after the initial injury.

The early operative procedures were posterior decompressions of the cervicomedullary junction with and without fusion for stabilization. Posterior decompression in those patients with irreducible decompression of neural tissue at the craniovertebral area often is associated with a high operative risk and a low incidence of improvement. The majority of patients are unchanged or have increased neurologic deficit, especially when the cervicomedullary compromise is ventrally situated.[2,3,8-11]

More recently, transpalatine-transoral[2,3,12-21] and extrapharyngeal[22-24] ventral operations were described for fractures, tumors, congenital abnormalities, infection, and inflammatory conditions at the cervicomedullary junction. Stabilization of the atlantoaxialoccipital joints usually has been done by fusing the spinal column posteriorly. The transpharyngeal route for anterior fusion has met with limited success, and further refinement of the technique may result in its future use.

No single anterior or posterior surgical procedure can be used for all of the patients with craniovertebral abnormalities. It is necessary to select the operation or combination of operations for each patient on an individual basis to correct the pathologic process responsible for the neurologic deficit.[1-6]

EMBRYOLOGY-ANATOMY

By definition, the craniovertebral junction includes the foramen magnum, the atlas, and the axis vertebrae. The occipital bone is formed by fusion of four sclerotomes. The proatlas is the most caudal of these sclerotomes and loses its identity in humans. The neural arch of the primitive proatlas divides into anterior and posterior segments.[25] The former gives rise to the occipital condyles and the latter fuses with the atlas to help form its rostral articular facets. If the posterior segment of the proatlas remains separate, the atlas has bipartite cranial articular facets—a rare anomaly that may result in horizontal instability of this joint. The proatlas also forms the dorsal portion of the C1 lateral masses and gives rise to the distal ossification center of the dens.[26]

The atlas is derived from the first cervical sclerotome as well as the proatlas. The body of the atlas as such disappears and gives origin to the dens. The anterior arch of the atlas has one center of ossification, and at times two centers may be present. The posterior arches of the atlas ossify by the age of 3 to 4 years.

The axis is developed from four primary ossification centers. The dens is formed by the C1 sclerotome, the two neural arches and the body of the axis from the C2 sclerotomes, and the tip of the dens develops from the proatlas. The tip of the dens is fused with the body by the age of 12 years. The remainder of the segments ossify and are fused by the age of 3 years.[27]

Dysgenesis of the odontoid process may encompass a variety of congenital anomalies. Failure of the proatlas and the dens to fuse results in ossiculum terminale. An os odontoideum represents failure of the odontoid process and the axis body to fuse. Hypoplasia and agenesis of the dens is the result of developmental failure of the distal ossification centers. The common pathophysiology that produces neurologic deficit with agenesis or hypoplasia of the dens is instability between the first and second cervical vertebrae because of incompetence of the cruciate ligament.

An occipital vertebra is a bony structure that is separate

OPERATIVE NEUROSURGICAL TECHNIQUES
ISBN 0-8089-1862-1

Table 113-1. Pathologic states in 219 patients with abnormalities of the craniovertebral junction

Pathologic Entity	Number of Patients
Primary Basilar Invagination	
Klippel-Feil	19
Chiari I	10
Hydromyelia	4
Total	32
Traumatic	
Rotational axis location	12
Ligamentous	10
Unfused odontoid fracture with upward migration	4
Total	26
Os Odontoideum	
Dystropic	24
Orthotopic	4
Total	28
Odontoid Dysgenesis	
Spondyloepiphyseal dysplasia	3
Morquio syndrome	2
Hurlers syndrome	1
Unclassified	10
Total	16
Achondroplasia (small foramen magnum paramesial invagination)	4
Down's syndrome	6
Rickets	3
Post infectious	3
Inflammatory	2
Foetal warfarin	1
Rheumatoid	
Cranial settling	53
Atlantoaxial	45
Total	98
Total	219

from the foramen magnum and incorporates the occipital condyles. The anterior arch may be partially or completely fused to the anterior margin of the foramen magnum, and the transverse process, if present, does not have a foramen for the vertebral artery. In contrast, an atlanto-occipital fusion is characterized by ankylosis between the atlas and the skull base, usually with persistence of the normal joints. The transverse process of the atlas has foramina for the vertebral arteries.

The occipitoatlantoaxial joints are complex, both anatomically and kinematically.[28–30] Anatomically, there are two occipitoatlantal articulations. There are four atlantoaxial joints with a common synovial lining between the dens and the anterior arch of the atlas, the dens and the transverse ligament, and between the 4 lateral masses. The second cervical nerve passes through the capsule of each atlantoaxial joint.

The occipitoatlantoaxial joints provide for anti-retroflexion, lateral flexion or tilting and rotation. They therefore function as a ball-and-socket joint. Flexion-extension and lateral bending occurs at the occipitoatlantal joint, flexion-extension and axial rotation occurs at the atlantoaxial joint.

The lateral atlantoaxial joints have convex articular surfaces with a horizontal orientation. Because these convex surfaces are not exactly reciprocal, a telescoping effect occurs during rotation of the head. There is relatively limited movement in the atlantoaxial joint and head-spine motion is basically between the occipital condyles and C2. Because of the intervening C1-C2 convex joint, there is potential decreased stability at the craniovertebral junction with extension, flexion, and rotation. Hypermobility of the occipitoatlantal joint may progressively increase in patients with congenital high cervical fusion. This may be the etiology of basilar invagination associated with the Klippel-Feil abnormality.

The dens is approximated to the anterior arch of the atlas by the transverse ligament, which is anchored to the tubercle on the mesial aspect of each lateral mass of the atlas. This ligament is responsible for the stability of the atlantoaxial joint. The axis is connected to the occiput by the alar ligaments that course obliquely upward from the posterior lateral surface of the dens to the anterior medial aspect of the occipital condyles; the apical dens ligament which continues from the medial aspect of the foramen magnum to the tip of the dens, the tentorial membrane (an extension of the deep layer to the posterior longitudinal ligament) and the cruciate ligament that consists of the transverse ligament plus triangular ascending and descending slips to the anterior rim of the foramen magnum and the axis, respectively (Figure 113-1).

The development of the neck musculature is inadequate to supplement joint stability until the age of 8 years.[1,31] Before this age, laxity of the ligamentous tissue permits excessive movement of the occipitoatlantoaxial articulations.[28,30–32] Forward gliding of the skull in relation to the spine occurs if hypoplastic occipital condyles are present. This is the mechanism for the development of neurologic deficit in children who have spondylo-epiphyseal dysplasia, Conradi's syndrome, and Morquio's syndrome. These syndromes are often associated with ossiculum terminale.[1]

The lymphatic drainage of the occipitoatlantoaxial joints is through retropharyngeal glands to the deep cervical lymphatic chain. In children, since the neck musculature is not fully developed, C1-C2 subluxation may develop secondary to nasopharyngeal infections.[2,33,34]

In the osseoligamentous destruction caused by rheumatoid arthritis, the synovial bursae and associated ligaments that surround the odontoid process are damaged with a resulting loss of stability.[35] Subluxation may occur secondary to the atlas moving anteriorly on the axis (caused by insufficiency of the cruciate ligament or fracture of the odontoid process), the atlas moving posteriorly on the axis (from erosion or fracture of the odontoid process), or by telescoping of the skull on the axis (from destruction of the axis lateral masses and/or apophyseal joints).[3] Chronic subluxation often results in ligamentous hypertrophy and the accumulation of granulation tissue behind the odontoid process from the hypertrophied soft tissue. Even though bone alignment is present on roentgenograms, there may be ventral compression of the cervicomedullary junction by soft tissue.

SIGNS AND SYMPTOMS

Cervicomedullary junction abnormalities produce a myriad of symptoms and signs including myelopathy; brain stem, cranial nerve, and cervical root dysfunction; vascular insufficiency, or any combination of these.[2,3,10,36,37] An abnormal

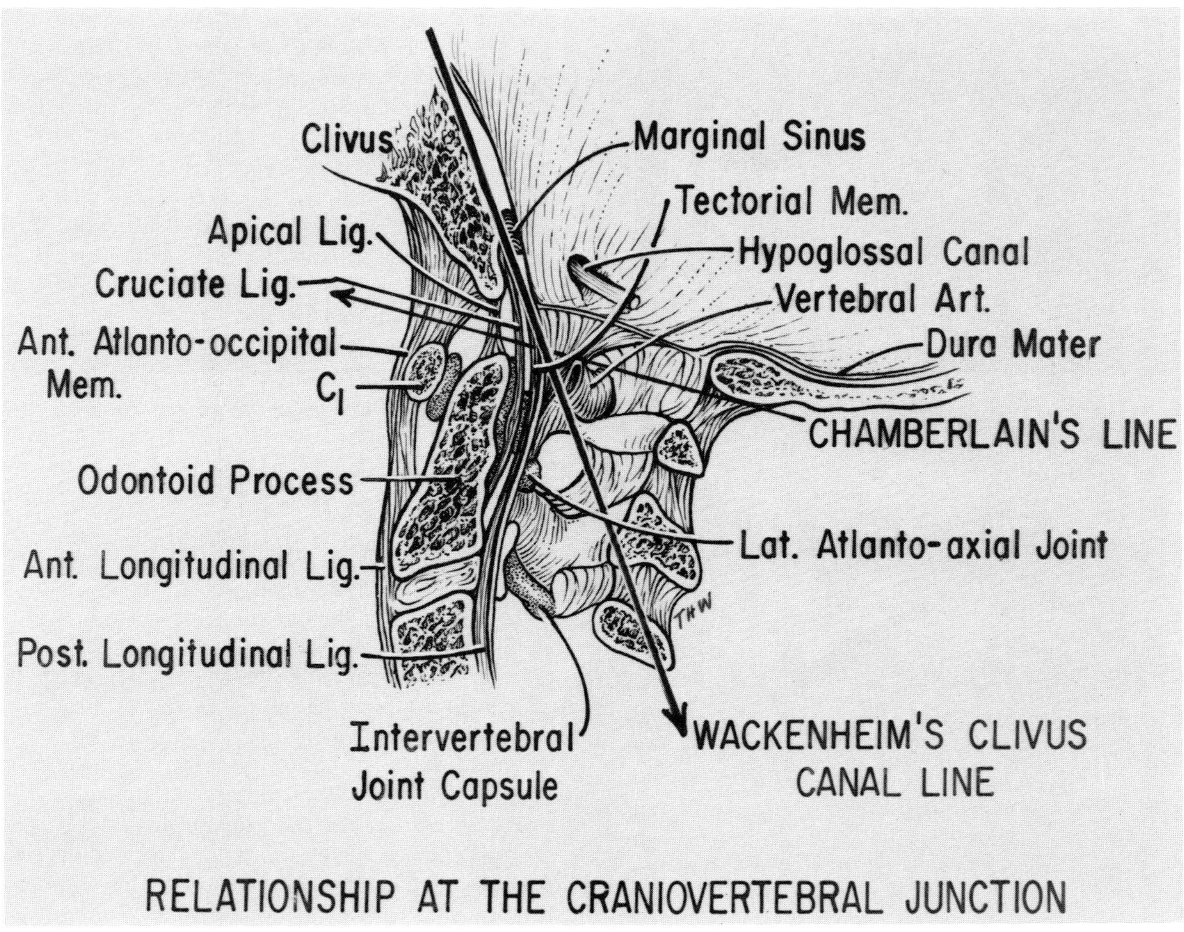

Fig. 113-1. The anatomic relationships of the bone and soft tissue in the midsagittal plane of the craniovertebral junction.

general appearance usually concerning the neck is seen with congenital abnormalities of the craniovertebral junction. The most common congenital anomaly, atlanto-occipital fusion, has a high incidence of associated findings consisting of low hairline, torticollis, short neck, and limitation of neck movement.[38,39] Similarly, the classical triad of shortening of the neck, low posterior hairline, and restriction of neck motion is described in the Klippel-Feil syndrome.[40]

Myelopathy was the most common neurologic deficit in our series, occurring in 202 of 219 patients. The initial symptoms, particularly in younger patients, may be subtle, such as lack of physical endurance. The severity of myelopathy is variable and may present as different degrees of weakness in the upper or lower extremities. False localizing signs were common and motor deficits included monoparesis, hemiparesis, paraparesis, tetraparesis and quadriparesis. A myelopathy mimicking the central cord syndrome often was present in patients having basilar invagination. The pathophysiology of motor myelopathy has been attributed to repetitive trauma to the pyramidal tracts secondary to chronic compression. The false localizing signs have been attributed to stagnant hypoxia of the cervical spinal cord from venous stasis.[41]

Sensory abnormality is usually manifested by neurologic defect relating to posterior column dysfunction, and was present in 112 patients. Hypalgesia, reflecting spinothalamic tract dysfunction was unusual, a finding in only 5 percent of patients and usually associated with severe paralysis. Bladder inconti-

nence was unusual, the most common symptoms being urgency or hesitancy of urination.

Cervical root symptoms usually are manifested by suboccipital headaches in the sensory distribution of the greater occipital nerve. The paresthesias are from irritation of the second cervical nerve as it transverses through the lateral atlantoaxial joint capsule and were present in 181 patients.

Brain stem signs include nystagmus to lateral gaze, and in 9 patients downbeat nystagmus was present. This latter finding has been well documented with cervicomedullary pathologic conditions.[42] Respiratory arrest and sleep apnea were associated with both anterior and posterior compression of the cervicomedullary junction in 8 patients, resolving in each instance after decompression. Dysfunction of the trigeminal, glossopharyngeal, vagus, accessory and hypoglossal cranial nerves have been identified in our patient population in addition to dysmetria, internuclear ophthalmoplegia and facial diplegia. Tinnitus and/or diminished hearing was present in approximately 25 percent of the patients but was an infrequent complaint.

Symptoms attributed to vascular compromise included syncope, vertigo, episodic hemiparesis, altered level of consciousness, and transient loss of visual fields. These symptoms may be secondary to repetitive trauma to spinal cord vessels, intermittent obstruction by angulation, or stretching of the vertebral and/or anterior spinal arteries from excessive mobility of an unstable atlantoaxial joint. Although several patients exhibited vascular symptoms, only 2 patients demonstrated

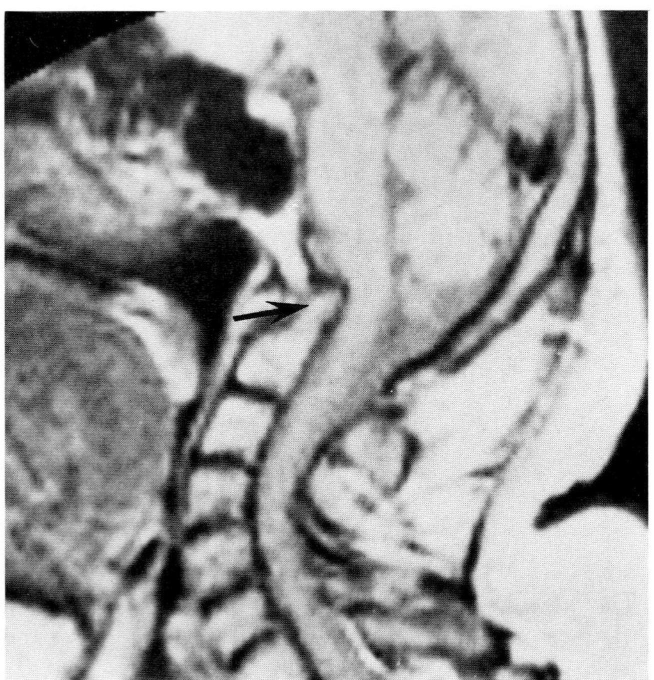

Fig. 113-2. A midline magnetic resonance scan (spin echo T$_2$ weighted image) to illustrate basilar invagination of the odontoid process (arrow) and posterior displacement of the cervicomedullary junction.

magnum from its anterior margin to its posterior margin (average: 35 mm). The Towne's projection is useful for determining the transverse diameter of the foramen magnum (35 mm ± 4 mm). Chamberlain's line is a diagonal from the hard palate to the posterior margin of the foramen magnum (Figure 113-1). The odontoid process should not extend more than one third of its length above this line. Wackenheim's clivus-canal line is drawn along the posterior surface of the clivus (Figure 113-1). Basilar invagination results in intersection of this line by the odontoid process. Fishgold's digastric line is measured on the frontal projections and connects the digastric grooves. The line is normally 11 mm ± 4 mm above the atlanto-occipital junction. The digastric line is the upper limit in position for the odontoid tip. Patients with abnormalities of the craniovertebral junction become symptomatic when the effective diameter of the spinal canal at the foramen magnum (from the posterior surface of the odontoid process to the posterior margin of foramen magnum) is less than 19 mm.[44]

Special radiologic procedures are necessary to clarify the etiology and pathophysiology of the craniovertebral abnormalities.[2–6] These examinations of the cervicomedullary junction include magnetic resonance imaging, computed tomography, and pluridirectional polytomography. These studies provide complimentary information.

The most significant examination of the posterior fossae contents and spinal cord is provided by magnetic resonance imaging. The medullae and cervical spinal cord are demonstrated with great clarity in this examination. Abnormality in size and position of the cervicomedullary junction, cerebellar tonsil position, and the presence or absence of hydromyelia are demonstrated without using ionizing radiation (Figure 113-2). Contrast injection into the subarachnoid space before a computed tomographic study or polytomography is of value to correlate a specific bone abnormality with change in the adjacent arachnoid space. Diagnostic studies of the craniovertebral junction in the flexion-extension positions (with or without

angiographic evidence of vascular compromise at the craniovertebral junction.

DIAGNOSTIC INVESTIGATIONS

To assess the cervicobasilar relationships, there are several reference lines used to evaluate the plain roentgenograms.[43] McRae's line measures the sagittal diameter of the foramen

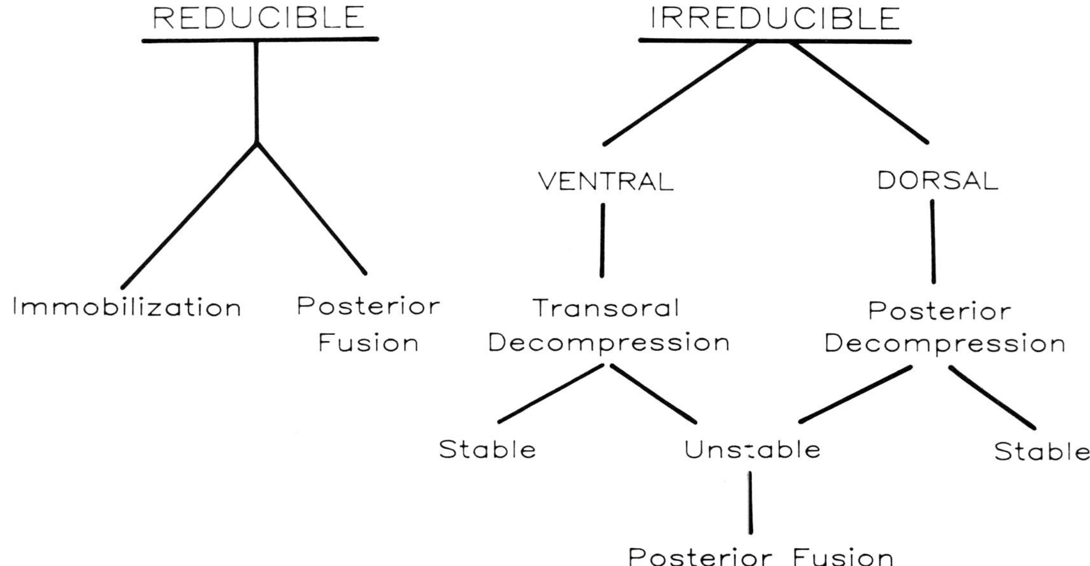

Fig. 113-3. A division for treatment of craniovertebral abnormalities.

contrast material), can only be done with plain x-ray studies or preferably tomographic examination.

OPERATIVE TECHNIQUE

No single anterior or posterior surgical procedure can be used for all the patients with occipitoatlantoaxial abnormalities. It is necessary to select the operation or combination of operations for each patient based on a complete understanding of embryology, functional anatomy, pathophysiology, and investigative radiologic abnormalities as described in the previous sections.

The treatment of craniovertebral junction abnormalities can be divided into those patients whose deformity can be realigned and those whose deformity cannot be realigned (Figure 113-3). Those patients whose deformities are reducible may require immobilization by bracing or posterior fusion. The second group, or patients whose deformities are irreducible, is subdivided into ventral or dorsal compression categories. In the former, the operative procedure is transoral decompression and the latter requires posterior decompression. No further surgery is necessary if following decompression, the craniovertebral junction is stable. If instability is present, both ventral and/or posterior decompression require a posterior fusion for stability. All patients can be classified into these six operative categories for treatment.[2]

REDUCIBLE PATHOLOGIC CONDITION— REQUIRING IMMOBILIZATION ONLY

Fourteen patients had reducible pathologic conditions that required immobilization only as their subsequent treatment. The cause of the deformity was cervicovertebral joint instability following neck infections in 3 patients, posttraumatic atlantoaxial subluxations in 9 patients, and cruciate ligament tears in 2 patients.

We have purposely omitted from this discussion many patients with odontoid as well as atlantoaxial fractures requiring fixation only, since the causes and treatment of these entities are well documented in the literature.[45–47]

Although some patients with reducible pathologic conditions can be realigned by positioning only, the majority will require up to 15 pounds skeletal traction with Crutchfield tongs, Gardner-Wells tongs, or a halo ring. The halo ring with pin fixation has the advantage over other traction devices in that it is not necessary to change the apparatus attached to the skull when the patient is placed in a body brace. An acrylic vest lined with lamb's wool is preferable to the previously utilized plaster of Paris body cast. Light weight metals or alloys have replaced the stainless steel rings, pins, and vertical support bars. Metals such as aluminum, titanium, or graphite alloy do not distort computed tomography or magnetic resonance imaging of patients while immobilized in a brace. The halo brace fixation is preferred for stabilization of the craniovertebral junction because of its superiority over other methods of bracing in the rostral cervical spine.[48]

REDUCIBLE LESIONS— POSTERIOR FUSION

One-hundred-one patients with reducible pathologic conditions were unstable and required posterior fusion for stability. Similar to reducible lesions requiring immobilization only, a few patients could be realigned with positioning only, but the majority required skeletal traction. In this category were 53 patients with rheumatoid arthritis having basilar invagination. Forty-three had an acceptable reduction after cervical traction using either Gardner-Wells tongs or halo ring apparatus. The traction is initiated at 7 pounds followed by graded increases up to 15 pounds maximum. It may be necessary to continue traction 10 to 14 days in order to obtain satisfactory position prior to stabilization. Under certain pathologic conditions, we have not been successful in realigning the craniovertebral junction with cervical traction. These conditions include patients with basilar invagination in which the odontoid process is 20 mm or more above the foramen magnum, those patients with fracture at the base of the dens, or in those patients with complete separation of the atlas posterior-anterior arches.

OPERATIVE TECHNIQUE— POSTERIOR CERVICAL FUSION

Prior to administration of anesthesia, the patient is intubated while awake using regional block and topical anesthesia to the pharynx and larynx. Following intubation, the patient is positioned on the operating table in the prone position. The head is placed in the cerebellar head rest, ensuring that no pressure is placed about the eyes. Skeletal traction is maintained throughout between 5 and 10 pounds, which is sufficient to maintain satisfactory alignment of the cervicomedullary junction.

After positioning the patient on the operating table, a lateral roentgenogram is obtained to confirm that proper occipitocervical alignment has been maintained. The neurologic examination is repeated to ensure no significant change has occurred subsequent to positioning. The patient is then anesthetized. Pin fixation to the head is to be avoided in these patients, since we have observed neurologic deterioration with pin fixation with an unstable spine.

A midline incision is made from the inion to C4 down to the deep cervical fascia. The spinous processes are exposed by incising through the avascular ligamentum nuchae. With precautions to avoid excessive vertebral manipulation, a combination of cutting current and a two periosteal elevator technique (one elevator is used to retract the muscle and the other is used for subperiosteal dissection) is used to dissect the paracervical musculature off the spinous process and lamina in a subperiosteal plane. The suboccipital musculature is dissected from the squamous occipital bone in the subperiosteal plane using both cutting current and sharp-blunt dissection.

In those patients with unstable atlantoaxial articulation, fusion includes only the rostral 2 or 3 cervical vertebrae. In those patients with occipitoatlantoaxial stability, the fusion includes the occiput in addition to the atlantoaxial vertebra. A notch is placed inferiorly and superiorly in each lamina and a hole is drilled through each side of the occipital bone lateral to the foramen magnum. Twisted 25- or 26-gauge stainless steel wire is placed under each lamina and through the occipital bone (Figure 113-4). The twisted wire is prepared by bending the wire into two equal lengths, securing the bent end into a hand drill and grasping the free ends with needle holders. The wire is twisted by turning the drill and keeping equal tension on the free wire ends. This maneuver increases the tensile strength of the wire approximately 16 times.

Bone donor sites are either the rib or ilium. The bone graft is notched adjacent to the lamina and a notch or hole placed in

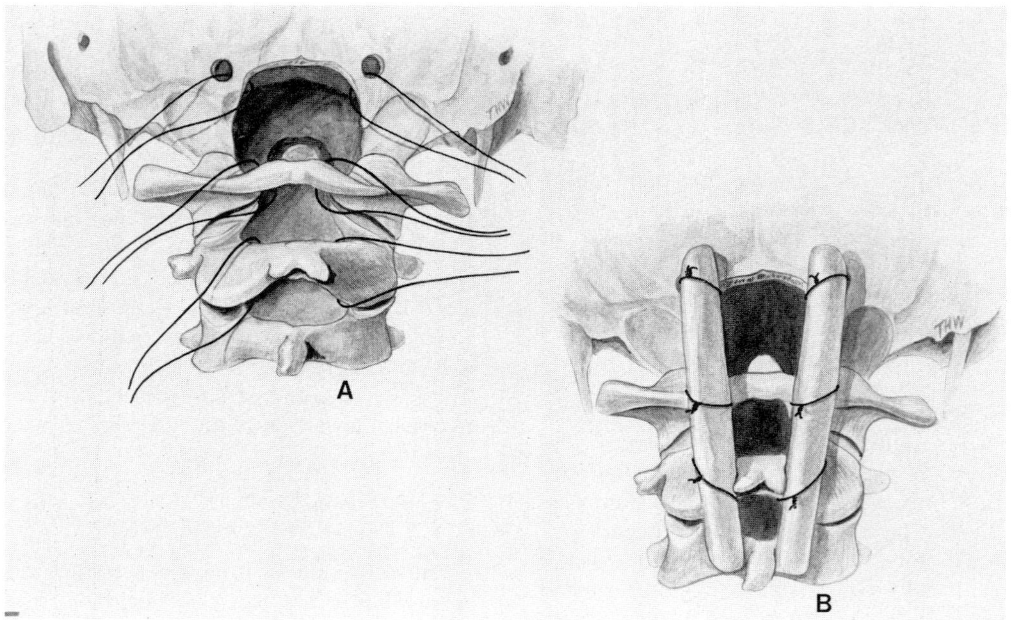

Fig. 113-4. (A) Placement of the wires under the laminae and through the occipital bone. (B) The bone graft is secured to the occiput and the laminae with wire.

the rostral end for the occipital wire. The graft is secured to the opposing laminar surface or suboccipital bone by twisting the end of the wires together (Figure 113-4). Bone chips can be placed along the fusion area for additional strength.

Patients is maintained in skeletal traction for 3 to 7 days after surgery. Prior to ambulation they are immobilized in a halo brace and maintained in the halo until the fusion is solid (Figure 113-5). Immobilization is usually 3 to 4 months for atlantoaxial fusion and 6 to 12 months for occipitoatlantoaxial fusion. For the latter, any less prolonged immobilization may result in nonunion, union in an abnormal position, or in those patients with rheumatoid arthritis, further cranial settling with subsequent increased neurologic deficit.

In severely disabled patients, such as those with rheumatoid arthritis, immediate stabilization can be obtained by supplementing the bone fusion with acrylic and wire fixation.[3,49–54]

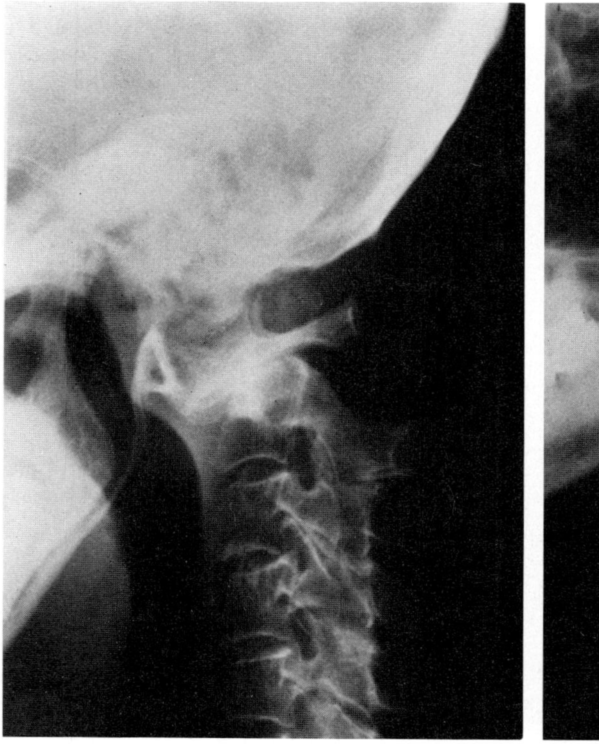
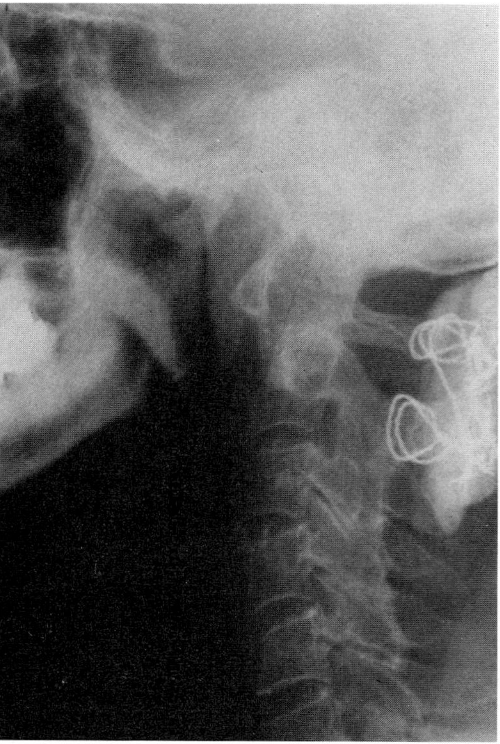

Fig. 113-5. (Left) Preoperative lateral roentgenogram of atlantoaxial subluxation. (Right) Postoperative lateral roentgenogram 12 months after C_1-C_2 posterior fusion (right).

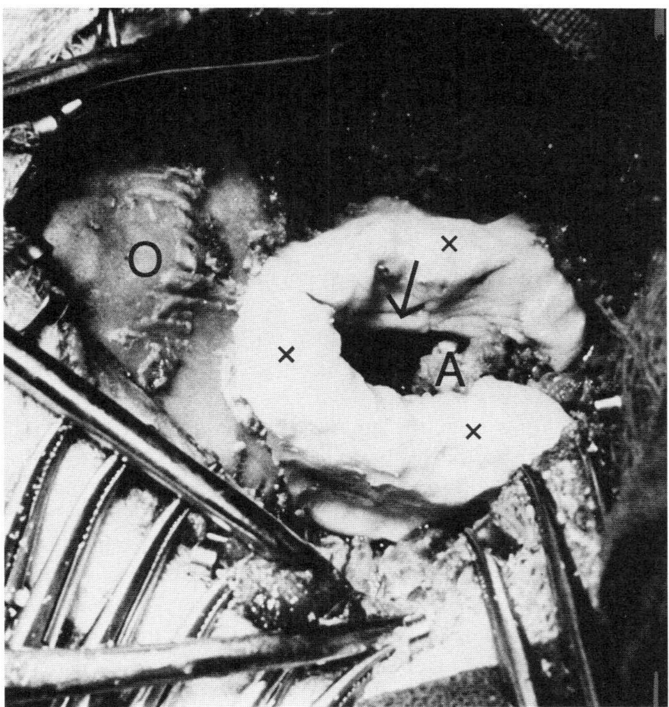

Fig. 113-6. Intraoperative photograph illustrating acrylic overlying the bone fusion. Note the posterior atlas arch has been resected. Occiput (O), arch of C$_2$ (A), bone graft (arrow), acrylic (x).

The technique consists of placing acrylic over the bone fusion incorporating the securing wire for the bone graft into the acrylic (Figure 113-6). With this procedure, there is diminished requirement for external support that allows the use of a SOMI brace or similar fixation apparatus for immobilization. Long-term follow-up results using this fusion technique have demonstrated satisfactory stability.

POSTERIOR DECOMPRESSION— WITH AND WITHOUT FUSION

The patient positioning on the operating table, the anesthesia induction technique, and the operative exposure of the spinous process and the lamina are identical to the description outlined under posterior cervical fusion. A suboccipital craniectomy is done to include the posterior and lateral bone surrounding the foramen magnum. The lamina and spinous processes of C1, C2, and C3 are removed in a rostral caudal direction. The laminectomy should extend laterally to the medial portion of the facets. It is important to excise all compressive soft tissue including the constricting dural band that is frequently present in the Chiari malformation at the level of the foramen magnum.

If stabilization is necessary subsequent to laminectomy, the technique of lateral interfacet fusion is used. The muscles and capsular ligaments from the C1-C2 and/or C3 posterior facets are removed with cutting current, periosteal elevators, and curets. Holes are then drilled through the inferior facet into the interfacet joint of each vertebra. If the suboccipital bone is incorporated into the fusion, a hole is drilled on each side of the occipital bone lateral to the foramen magnum. A 25- or 26-gauge stainless steel twisted wire is prepared as described in the previous section, and is passed through the openings (Figure 113-7). Passing the wire through the interfacet joint is facilitated by spreading the joint with a Freer elevator. Either rib or split thickness iliac bone is placed adjacent to the facets and/or occiput and secured in place by the wires (Figure 113–7).

The postoperative management of the lateral fusion is identical to that described for the posterior fusion without laminectomy. It is necessary to maintain the patient in halo immobilization for a period of 6 to 12 months.

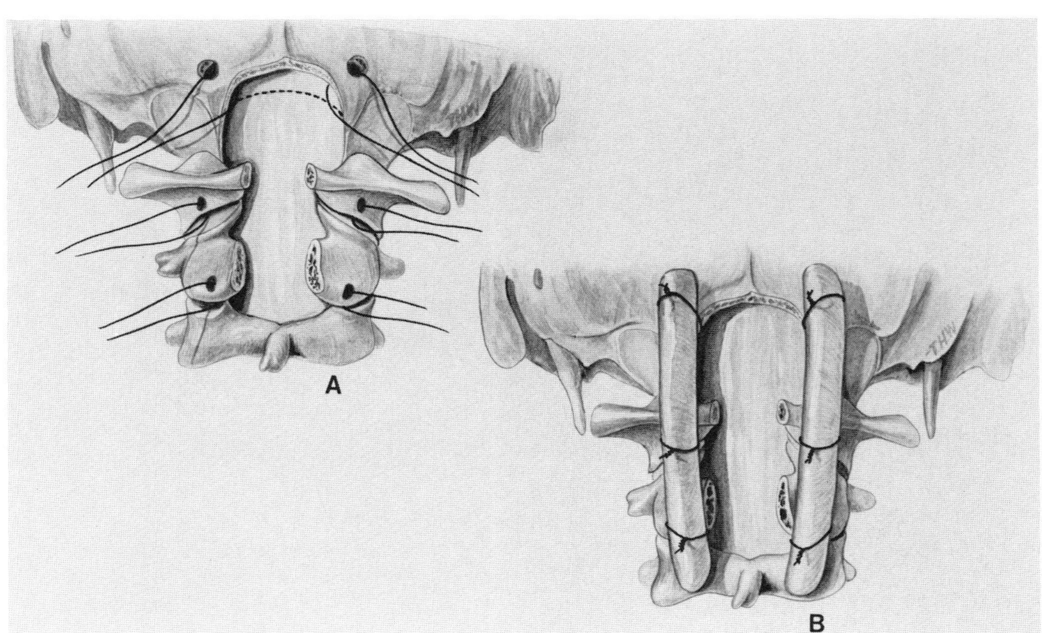

Fig. 113-7. (A) Placement of holes and wire through the occipital bone and the C$_1$-C$_2$ interior facets after laminectomy. (B) The graft is secured to the occiput and facets.

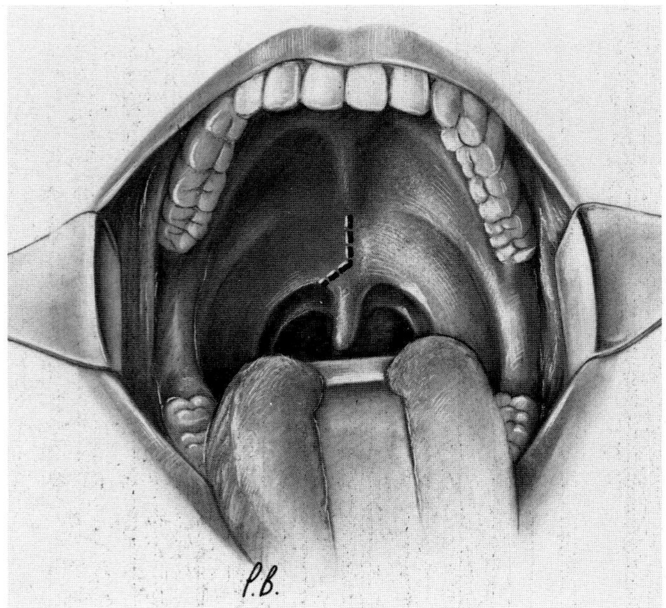

Fig. 113-8. A drawing of the oral cavity illustrating the incision in the soft palate midline (broken line).

ANTERIOR TRANSORAL-TRANSPHARYNGEAL APPROACH

The transoral-transpharyngeal operation is to correct ventral irreducible compression of the cervicomedullary junction. Pharyngeal and nasal cultures are obtained 3 days prior to the proposed surgery in order to treat any pathogenic flora present with antibiotics. If normal flora is present, no antibiotics are

necessary. It is prudent to have the patient's nutritional status in the best condition possible prior to surgery.

The patient is placed supine on the operating table with 5 to 10 pounds skeletal traction to maintain alignment of the craniovertebral junction. The previously outlined techniques of intubation and administration of general anesthesia are adhered to. We perform tracheostomy in each patient to provide for better exposure during the operation and to ensure an adequate airway postoperatively. Following tracheostomy, a gauze packing is used to occlude the laryngopharynx to prevent blood leakage into the stomach.

The mouth is maintained open with a Dingman retractor with placement of a rubber guard over the teeth. Self-retaining retractors are attached to the frame of this instrument to depress the tongue and for lateral retraction of the oral cavity. It is wise to loosen the retraction on the tongue intermittently during the operation to prevent lingual congestion.

The soft palate is infiltrated with 1 percent Xylocaine with 1/200,000 epinephrine or normal saline and a midline incision is made extending from the hard palate diverting from the midline at the base of the uvula (Figure 113-8). This incision ensures a minimum of bleeding and unrestricted healing to the soft palate, because the palatine artery and its accompanying palatine nerve enters the soft palate laterally and terminates in the midline. Stay sutures for retraction are placed on both soft palate flaps to allow for maximum exposure through the pharynx to the caudal portion of the clivus.

The arch of the atlas and caudal extent of the clivus can be palpated by the surgeon through the retropharyngeal musculature. A linear midline incision is made through the posterior pharyngeal wall to the anterior longitudinal ligament and its rostral extension, the atlantooccipital ligament. The retropharyngeal musculature is easily separated from these liga-

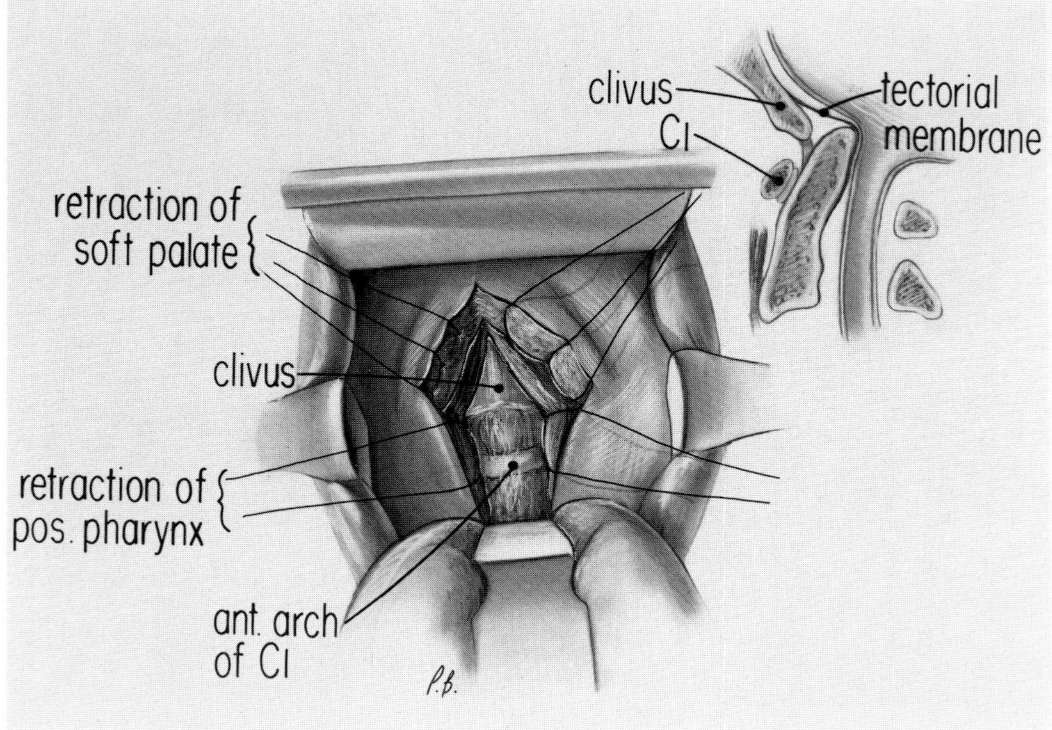

Fig. 113-9. Exposure of the clivus, the anterior arch of the atlas, and the odontoid process with placement of stay sutures in the soft palate and pharynx. The corresponding midline sagittal drawing is in the upper right inset.

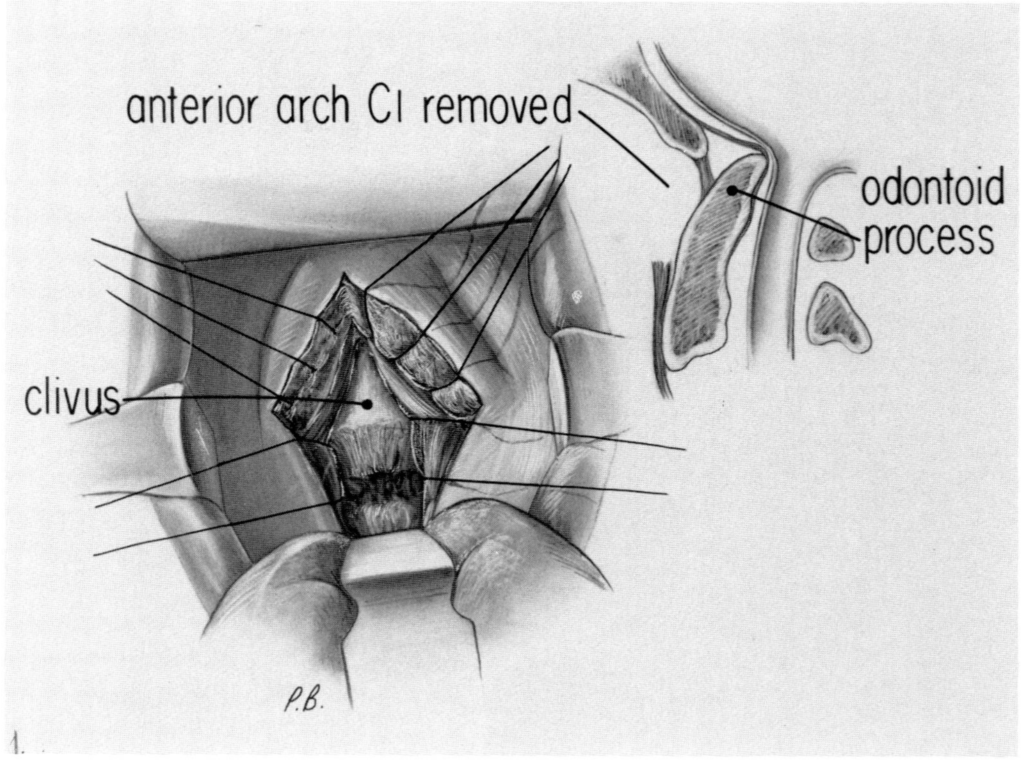

Fig. 113-10.   The operative site after excision of the anterior arch of C$_1$ with the apical ligament still intact. The corresponding midline sagittal drawing is inset upper right.

ments, and stay sutures or a self-retaining retractor is used to maintain lateral retraction of the muscle.

After exposure of the anterior longitudinal ligament, the operating microscope is utilized to provide magnification and a concentrated light source. The ligament is coagulated to reduce bleeding and the anterior body of the axis, anterior arch of the atlas, and caudal anterior clivus are exposed in the subperiosteal plane using a periosteal elevator (Figure 113-9).

The ventral atlantoaxial articulation is separated, and the anterior arch of the atlas is removed using a 1.5 mm foot plate 45-degree angle punch rongeur to expose the caudal odontoid process (Figure 113-10). The apical ligament with its attachment to the caudal clivus is removed, and if the odontoid invagination is severe, it may be necessary to resect a portion of the caudal clivus. If resection of the caudal clivus is required, the tissue posterior to the clivus must be carefully separated from the bone, since the dura can easily be penetrated and troublesome bleeding may occur from the marginal sinus.

The surgeon should next identify the distal tip of the odontoid process by subperiosteal dissection of ligamentous tissue from its osseous ventral surface (Figure 113-11). The bulk of the odontoid process is then removed with a steel cutting burr. A diamond burr is then substituted to remove the tip and thin dorsal bony shell of the dens to avoid tearing of the posterior soft tissue. We prefer a 45-degree angled hand piece attachment to the drill to provide unrestricted visualization of the surgical field. After identifying the posterior tissue plane at the odontoid tip, the odontoid process and body of the axis are removed in a rostral to caudal direction for decompression of the cervicomedullary junction (Figure 113-12).

In those patients with rheumatoid arthritis and other inflammatory disorders, hypertrophy and thickening of the liga-

mentous tissue may be extensive. Adequate ventral decompression is not accomplished until this tissue is removed adjacent to the dura (Figure 113-12). After identification of the dural-ligamentous plane rostrally, the dissection of the granulation tissue is completed in a caudal direction using sharp and blunt instrumentation. The surgeon can be assured that adequate cervicomedullary decompression has been accomplished when the pulsatile dura protrudes ventrally into the decompression site.

If the dura is torn or cerebrospinal fluid is identified, repair of the fistula can be accomplished by placing 2 or 3 layers of fascia over the rent. The fascia is harvested from the external oblique aponeurosis or fascia lata from the anterior lateral thigh. In this situation, a lumbar cerebrospinal fluid drain is inserted and maintained for 7 days after surgery. In our experience, closing the dura with sutures has not been successful, and has resulted in persistent cerebrospinal fluid leak in one case. The leak was successfully repaired using a fascial graft.

The pharyngeal musculature and aponeurosis are closed with interrupted 3-0 polyglycolic acid absorbable sutures in two layers. The soft palate is approximated by closing the nasal mucosa with interrupted polyglycolic acid sutures. Ventral mattress sutures are placed through the oral mucosa to include the muscle and ensure snug approximation. A pre and postoperative roentgenogram of the odontoid resection is illustrated in Figure 113-13.

In children, it is important to preserve the cruciate ligament and tectorial membrane in addition to the periosteum of the dens. This will allow for new bone formation, and spontaneous ventral fusion has occurred in several of our cases. Similarly, it is not uncommon to see spontaneous anterior bone fusion after posterior fusion in children.

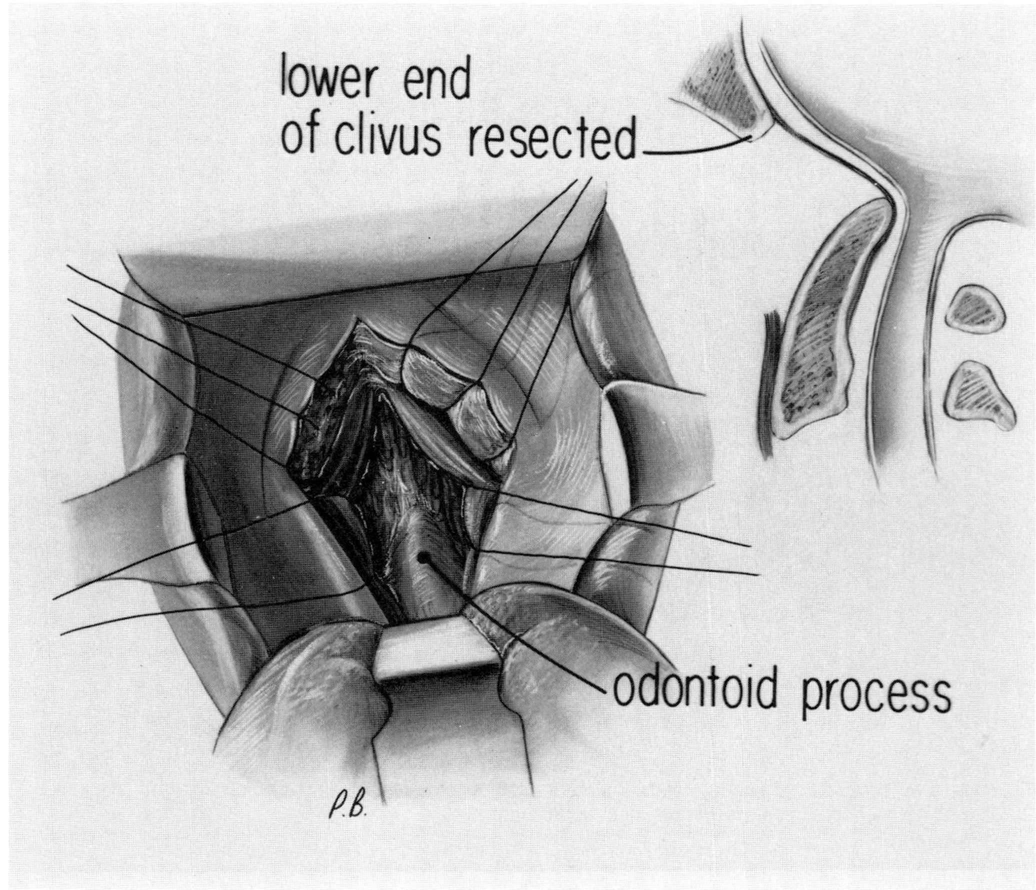

Fig. 113-11.   The operative site after excision of the apical ligament and the caudal clivus to expose the odontoid tip. The corresponding midline sagittal drawing is inset upper right.

Subsequent to surgery, the patient is maintained in 5 pounds of skeletal traction. Intravenous fluids are continued for 5 to 6 days followed by gradual increased feedings to a regular diet by the 10th to 12th day after surgery. Flexion-extension polytomograms are obtained between 5 and 8 days postoperatively to determine craniovertebral stability. If instability is present, a posterior fusion is done as described in the previous section.

If intravenous antibiotics are used, they are discontinued 48 hours after surgery if the dura is intact. If the dura is violated and a fascial graft has been used for repair, intravenous antibiotics

Table 113-2. Summary of surgical treatment (CVJ)

Stability	Compression	Operative Approach	Post Operative Stability	Posterior Fusion
Reducible 115*	—	—	—	101
	Ventral 48	Anterior	Stable 16	—
			Unstable 32	32
Non-reducible				
	Dorsal 52	Posterior	Stable 20	—
			Unstable 32	32

*Immobilization, 14.

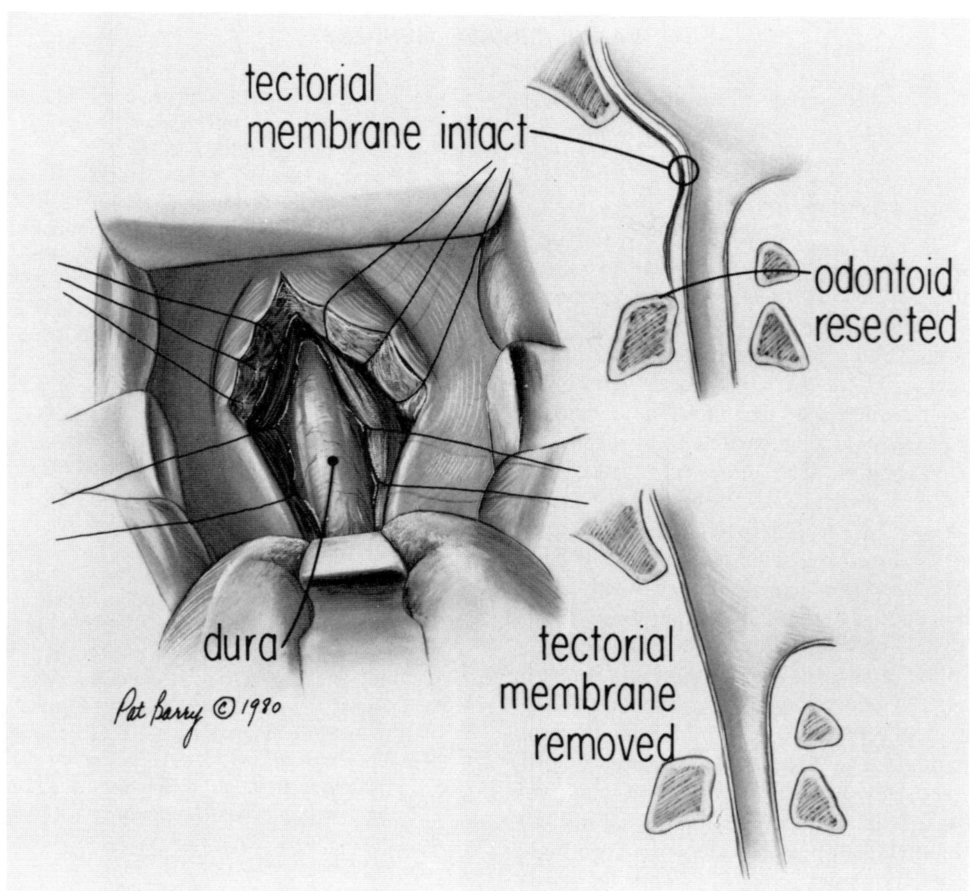

Fig. 113-12. The cervicomedullary junction after removal of the dens. After adequate decompression the dura should protrude into the decompression site. The drawing in the upper right illustrates failure of decompression because of a hypertrophied tectorial membrane. The sagittal reconstruction drawing in the lower right demonstrates adequate ventral decompression following removal of the hypertrophied tissue.

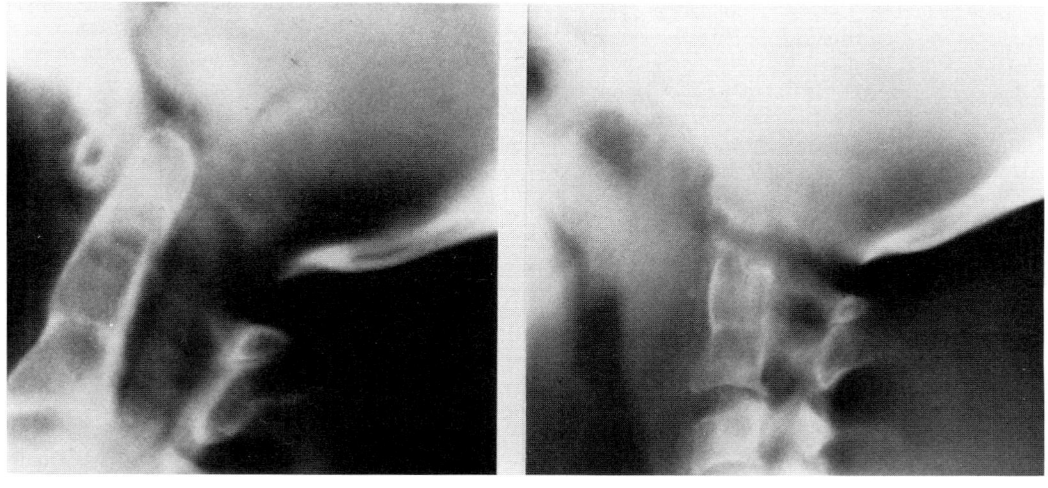

Fig. 113-13. Preoperative lateral polytomogram of basilar invagination with air contrast medium (left). Note congenital C_2-C_3 failure of segmentation. Postoperative polytomogram after odontoid resection (right).

are continued for 14 days after surgery. The tracheostomy is discontinued as soon as the patient's status permits.

RESULTS OF SURGERY

The type and incidence of the operative procedures in our series of 215 consecutive patients with symptomatic craniovertebral junction abnormalities is outlined in Table 113-2.

Two-hundred-thirteen patients recovered or improved neurologically after surgery. There were two deaths following transoral removal of the odontoid. The first, a 66-year-old woman had a rapidly progressive quadriparesis and respiratory arrest from basilar invagination. She underwent anterior removal of the odontoid process and rostral one third of the C2 body followed by posterior fusion. The patient was ambulatory following surgery, but died from sepsis of urinary tract origin 3 weeks after the second operation. A second death occurred in a 79-year-old man with irreducible basilar invagination secondary to rheumatoid arthritis. He was quadriparetic and had been bed ridden for 6 months prior to surgery. Four weeks after anterior odontoidectomy, he died of acute myocardial infarction.

One patient developed cerebrospinal fluid fistula after transoral odontoidectomy. The fistula was repaired with a fascial graft without subsequent complication. One child with spondyloepiphyseal dysplasia and occipitoatlantoaxial instability with ossiculum terminale had posterior decompression with occiput-C1-2 fusion. The bone grafts resolved and the patient required refusion.

REFERENCES

1. Menezes AH, Graf CJ, Hibri N: Abnormalities of the craniovertebral junction with cervico-medullary compression. Childs Brain 7:15, 1980
2. Menezes AH, VanGilder JC, Graf CJ, et al: Craniocervical abnormalities. J Neurosurg 53:444, 1980
3. Menezes, AH, VanGilder JC, Clark CR, et al: Odontoid upward migration in rheumatoid arthritis. An analysis of 45 patients with "cranial settling." J Neurosurg 63:500, 1985
4. VanGilder, JC: Craniovertebral junction abnormalities and their treatment. Neurology and Neurosurgery Update Series, vol 39, 1985
5. VanGilder JC, Menezes AH: Craniovertebral junction abnormalities, in Wilkins, RH and Rengachary SS (eds): Neurosurgery, vol 3. New York, McGraw-Hill, 1985, pp. 2097–2101
6. VanGilder JC, Menezes AH: Craniovertebral abnormalities. Symptoms, etiology and treatment. Contemporary Neurosurgery, vol 3, lesson 7, 1981
7. Bell, C: The Nervous System of the Human Body. London, Longman, Rees, Orme, Brown and Green, 1830
8. Dastur DK, Wadia NH, Desai AD, et al: Medullo-spinal compression due to atlanto-axial dislocation and sudden haematomyelia during decompression. Pathology, pathogenesis and clinical correlations. Brain 88:897, 1965
9. Greenberg AD: Atlanto-axial dislocations. Brain 91:655, 1968
10. List, CF: Neurologic syndromes accompanying developmental anomalies of occipital bone, atlas and axis. Arch Neurol Psychiatry 45:577, 1941
11. Symonds CP, Meadows SP: Compression of the spinal cord in the neighbourhood of the foramen magnum. With a note on the surgical approach, by Julian Taylor. Brain 60:52, 1937
12. Apuzzo MLJ, Weiss MH, Heiden JS: Transoral exposure of the atlanto-axial region. Neurosurgery 3:201, 1978
13. Cannoni M: La voi trans-orale dans l'abord des lesions de la region du clivus. J Fr Otorhinolaryngol 27:81, 1978
14. Delandsheer JM, Caron JP, Jomin M: (The transbucco-pharyngeal approach and malformations of the cervico-occipital joint.) Neurochirurgie 23:276, 1977
15. Estridge MN, Smith RA: Transoral fusion of odontoid fracture. Case report. J Neurosurg 27:462, 1967
16. Fang HSY, Ong GB: Direct anterior approach to the upper cervical spine. J Bone Joint Surg 44:1588, 1962
17. Greenberg AD, Scoville WB, Davey LM: Transoral decompression of the atlantoaxial dislocation due to odontoid hypoplasia. Report of two cases. J Neurosurg 28:266, 1968
18. Mullan S, Naunton R, Hekmatpanah J, et al: The use of an anterior approach to ventrally placed tumors in the foramen magnum and vertebral column. J Neurosurg 24:536, 1966
19. Pech A, Cannoni M, Magnan J, et al: (The trans-oral approach in oto-neurosurgery.) Ann Otolaryngol Chir Cervicofac 91:281, 1974
20. Spetzler, RF, Selman WR, Nash CL Jr, et al: Transoral microsurgical odontoid resection and spinal cord monitoring. Spine 4:506, 1974
21. Sukoff MH, Kadin MM, Moran T: Transoral decompression for myelopathy caused by rheumatoid arthritis of the cervical spine. Case report. J Neurosurg 37:451, 1949
22. Bonney G: Stabilization of the upper cervical spine by the transpharyngeal route. Proc R Soc Med 63:896, 1970
23. DeAndrade JR, MacNab I: Anterior occipito-cervical fusion using an extra-pharyngeal exposure. J Bone Joint Surg 51:1621, 1969
24. Stevenson GC, Stoney RJ, Perkins RK, et al: A transcervical transclival approach to the ventral surface of the brain stem for removal of a clivus chordoma. J Neurosurg 24:544, 1966
25. Ganguly DN, Roy KK: A study on the cranio-vertebral joint in the man. Anat Anz 114:433, 1964
26. Shapiro R, Youngberg AS, Rothman SLG: The differential diagnosis of traumatic lesions of the occipito-atlanto-axial segment. Radiol Clin North Am 11:505, 1973
27. Bailey DK: The normal cervical spine in infants and children. Radiology 59:712, 1952
28. Holmes JC, Hall JE: Fusion for instability and potential instability of the cervical spine in children and adolescents. Orthop Clin North Am 9:923, 1978
29. Werne S: The craniovertebral joints. Acta Orthop Scand 23 (suppl):150, 1957
30. White AA III, Panjabi MM: The clinical biomechanics of the occipitoatlantoaxial complex. Orthop Clin North Am 9:867, 1978
31. Alexander E Jr, Forsyth HF, Davis CH Jr, et al: Dislocation of the atlas on the axis. J Neurosurg 15:353, 1958
32. Gilles RH, Bina M, Sotrel A: Infantile atlantooccipital instability. The potential danger of extreme extension. Am J Dis Child 133:30, 1979
33. Hess JH, Bronstein IP, Abelson SM: Atlanto-axial dislocations. Unassociated with trauma and secondary to inflammatory foci in the neck. Am J Dis Child 49:1137, 1935
34. Sullivan AW: Subluxation of the atlanto-axial joint: Sequel to inflammatory processes in the neck. J Pediatr 35:451, 1949
35. Bland JH: Rheumatoid arthritis of the cervical spine. J Rheumatol 1:319, 1974
36. Michie I, Clark M: Neurological syndromes associated with cervical and craniocervical anomalies. Arch Neurol 18:241, 1968
37. Spillane JD, Pallis C, Jones AM: Developmental abnormalities in the region of the foramen magnum. Brain 80:11, 1957
38. Bharucha EP, Dastur HM: Craniovertebral anomalies. (A report on 40 cases.) Brain 87:469, 1964
39. Spillane JD, Pallis C, Jones AM: Developmental abnormalities in the region of the foramen magnum. Brain 80:11, 1957
40. Klippel M, Feil A: Un cas d'absence des vetebres cervicales avec cage thoracique remmtant jusqu'a la base du craine. Nouv Icon Solpetriere 25:223, 1912
41. Taylor AR, Byrnes DP: Foramen magnum and high cervical cord compression. Brain 97:473, 1974
42. Cogan DG, Barrows LJ: Platybasia and Arnold-Chiari malformation. Arch Ophthalmol 52:13, 1954

43. Dolan KD: Cervicobasilar relationships. Radiol Clin North Am 15: 155, 1977

44. McRae DL: The significance of abnormalities of the cervical spine. Am J Roentgenol Radium Ther 84:3, 1960

45. Apuzzo MLJ, Heiden JS, Weiss MH, et al: Acute fractures of the odontoid process. An analysis of 45 cases. J Neurosurg 48:85, 1978

46. Bohlman HH, Ducker TB, Lucas JT: Spine and spinal cord injuries, in Rothman RH, Simeone FA (eds): The Spine, vol 2. Philadelphia, WB Saunders, 1982, pp 661–757

47. Seljeskog EL, Chou SN: Spectrum of the hangman's fracture. J Neurosurg 45:3, 1976

48. Johnson RM, Hart DL, Simmons EF, et al: Cervical arthrosis. A study comparing their effectiveness in restricting cervical motion in normal subjects. J Bone Joint Surg (Am) 59:332, 1977

49. Duff TA: Surgical stabilization of traumatic cervical spine dislocation using methyl methacrylate. Long term results in 26 patients. J Neurosurg 64:39, 1986

50. Dunn EJ: The role of methyl methacrylate in the stabilization and replacement of tumors of the cervical spine. A Project of the Cervical Spine Research Society. Spine 2:15, 1977

51. Eismont FJ, Bohlman HH: Posterior methyl methacrylate fixation for cervical trauma. Spine 6:347, 1981

52. Kelly DL, Alexander E Jr, Davis CH Jr, et al: Acrylic fixation of atlanto-axial dislocations. Technical note. J Neurosurg 36:366, 1972

53. Panjabi MM, Hopper W, White AA III, et al: Posterior spine stabilization with methyl methacrylate. Biomechanical testing of a surgical specimen. Spine 2:241, 1971

54. Taitsman JP, Saha S: Tensile strength of wire-reinforced bone cement with twisted stainless-steel wire. J Bone Joint Surg (Am) 59:419, 1977

Surgical Treatment of Rheumatoid Arthritis, Ankylosing Spondylitis, and Paget's Disease with Neurologic Deficit

Ghaus M. Malik   James L. Sanders, Jr.

RHEUMATOID ARTHRITIS

RHEUMATOID ARTHRITIS of the spine involves the cervical region more often than any other. Chronic inflammation can lead to erosion of the bone and ligaments with subsequent loss of stability. Involvement of the cervical spine can cause sudden death or symptoms of vertebrobasilar ischemia, tetraparesis, and neck pain.

Both juvenile and adult rheumatoid arthritis carry a high incidence of involvement of the cervical spine. Depending on the particular study and diagnostic criteria, involvement of the cervical spine may be found in 25 to 90 percent of patients with rheumatoid arthritis.[1] Isdale and Conlon, in a long-term follow-up of rheumatoid patients, reported that 80 percent showed radiologic changes in the cervical spine and 50 percent showed atlantoaxial subluxation.[2] In a study by Pellicci et al., 106 patients with rheumatoid arthritis were followed for 5 years. Initially 43 percent of the patients had rheumatoid involvement of the cervical spine. Most common were atlantoaxial subluxation, 61 percent; atlantoaxial subluxation combined with subaxial subluxation, 20 percent; and subaxial subluxation alone in 11 percent. At the completion of the evaluation 36 percent of the patients had progressed neurologically and 80 percent had progressed radiographically.[3]

Rheumatoid arthritis most often affects the upper levels of the cervical spine and produces different clinical features at different ages. In children, the apophyseal joints often fuse and growth is deficient, while subluxation is the predominant feature in adults. In addition to the bony and ligamentous involvement, the presence of rheumatoid nodules, which can lead to destruction and collapse of the vertebral bodies as well as marked thickening and fibrosis of the dura mater, have been reported. The involvement of the spine may be evident in different forms (Table 114-1).

ANTERIOR ATLANTOAXIAL SUBLUXATION

The single most common spinal condition associated with rheumatoid arthritis is anterior atlantoaxial subluxation, which is felt to be caused by destruction or laxity of the transverse ligament or from erosion or fracture of the odontoid process. Davis and Markley have been credited with the first documented case of atlantoaxial subluxation in rheumatoid arthritis causing neurologic deficits.[4]

Atlantoaxial subluxation is considered to be present if the distance between the posterior aspect of the anterior arch of atlas and the anterior aspect of the odontoid is more than 2.5 mm in adults and 4.5 mm in children (measured in flexion). Nakano has reported a 30 to 40 percent incidence of cervical subluxation in patients admitted to the hospital with rheumatoid arthritis.[5] Often these radiologic findings are not associated with neurologic symptoms.

Determination of the exact incidence of neurologic manifestations in atlantoaxial subluxation is difficult, owing to a number of variable factors. Because of the disabling deformities and involvement of major joints causing difficulty in ambulation, some of the symptoms can be disregarded. Sensory symptoms at times are considered to be caused by peripheral neuropathy, which also is associated with rheumatoid arthritis. The neurologic examination is frequently difficult to perform adequately. Conlon et al. found 84 subluxations without any neurologic manifestations in the follow-up of 333 cases of rheumatoid arthritis for 6 years.[6] On the other hand, Stevens et al. had 24 cases with neurologic changes out of 36 patients with subluxations in their study of 100 cases.[7]

CLINICAL PRESENTATION

Rheumatoid subluxation can appear as a neurologic syndrome requiring urgent treatment or even as a cause of sudden death. In addition to direct compression, neurologic symptoms can result from occlusion of the vertebral arteries or intrinsic vascular disease in the spinal cord or the brain stem. Rheumatoid inflammatory tissue also can act as a compressive lesion in the spinal canal. Several factors can be involved in a single patient.

Neck pain is the most frequent symptom. The pain is usually in the upper cervical or suboccipital area with variable radiation to the mastoid, occipital, temporal, or frontal regions. In the review of 106 patients with rheumatoid arthritis by Pellicci et al., neck pain was the most common finding. All the patients with occipital pain were found to have either atlantoaxial subluxation or superior migration of the odontoid process or both.[3] Sometimes this specific information may have

OPERATIVE NEUROSURGICAL TECHNIQUES
ISBN 0-8089-1862-1

Table 114-1. Forms of involvement of the spine in cases of rheumatoid arthritis

Cervical spine
  Craniovertebral region
    1. Anterior atlantoaxial subluxation
    2. Vertical atlantoaxial subluxation
    3. Posterior atlantoaxial subluxation
    4. Transverse or rotatory subluxation
  Subaxial region
    1. Subluxation—single or multiple levels
    2. Vertebral endplate erosion and disc involvement
      (simulating infection)
    3. Apophyseal joint involvement with erosion or
      ankylosis
    4. Intervertebral disc herniation
  Miscellaneous
    1. Pachymeningitis
    2. Rheumatoid granulation tissue
Thoracic and Lumbar Spine
    1. Osteoporosis with compression fractures
    2. Subluxation in lumbar region
    3. Rheumatoid nodules
    4. Vertebral endplate erosion

to be sought by the examining physician. Paresthesias can be caused by head or neck movement, and Lhermitte's sign produced by sudden flexion of the neck may be elicited. Rarely, complaints of vertebrobasilar ischemia (transient visual disturbances, diplopia, vertigo, and sensory or motor phenomena) may be present. Smith et al. reported that in their follow-up of 130 patients with subluxation for an average period of 7 to 8 years, 6 patients developed symptoms consistent with involvement of the vertebral artery.[8]

Compression or ischemia of the spinal cord can produce spastic quadriparesis. As stated earlier, in the majority of the cases, subtle deficits are confused with disability caused by general debilitation and joint involvement. Hyperreflexia and Babinski's sign are probably the most reliable indicators of the involvement of the spinal cord. Paresthesias of the hands and feet are quite common. A significant number of patients have involvement of the first division of the trigeminal nerve as well as sensory disturbance in the distribution of C2.

DIAGNOSTIC STUDIES

Lateral x-ray films of the cervical spine made in neutral, flexion, and extension positions are necessary. In addition to confirming the diagnosis, they serve to demonstrate whether or not subluxation is spontaneously reducible. Lateral tomograms and CT scans of the craniovertebral junction may be needed if visualization of the odontoid process and other structures is not adequate on regular films. It is also important to know the status of the lower cervical spine. Visualization generally is difficult because of shoulder deformities and, again, tomography may be necessary. If neurologic examination points to a lower cervical lesion because of root symptoms or sensory level, this evaluation is even more important. Myelography is indicated whenever involvement of the lower spine is suspected or if the spine films do not show sufficient changes to account for the patient's symptoms. In the latter instance, compression might be due to granulation tissue or pachymeningitis. This was exemplified by

a recent patient of ours who had advanced rheumatoid arthritis and presented with myelopathy. There was a 6 mm anterior atlantoaxial subluxation on flexion, but he complained of Lhermitte's type phenomena with extension of the neck, in contrast to flexion. Myelography showed an almost complete block opposite the C3-4 disc space from hypertrophic changes. The MRI scanner has been found to be particularly helpful in the diagnosis of cervicomedullary compression and will be useful in better delineation of this problem; however, it seems to have limitations in evaluating bony compromise and deformities at the foramen magnum level (Figure 114-1).

In patients with symptoms of vertebrobasilar ischemia, vertebral angiography is indicated. For more detailed aspects, see the monograph by Yves Dirheimer.[9]

TREATMENT

Unless the patient's condition poses definite contraindications to treatment, we feel that patients with neurologic involvement need stabilization of the subluxation. The patient with rheumatoid abnormalities has surgical and anesthetic problems related to a recessed mandible, subluxed cervical spine, rheumatoid lung disease, diminished chest excursion, anemia, and often an increased bleeding time and delicate skin.[10] These patients are also more susceptible to infection, operative fractures, and blood loss.[11] Different types of operative procedures have been described for atlantoaxial subluxation. Most of these utilize a posterior approach. These methods range from a simple internal wire fixation to bony or acrylic fusion. Newman has described an occipitocervical fusion,[12] as has Hamblen,[13] but with different techniques. Others advocate only fusion of C1-C2, since there is less limitation of neck motion and a decreased incidence of nonunion. Alexander and his group have reported that acrylic provides adequate support, and the need for a bone graft is eliminated.[14] With this technique, however, there is long-term reliance on wire, since eventual bony fusion may not occur. Even if minimal displacement persists following the fusion, the stability provided by the fusion prevents further neurologic deterioration by avoiding constant slipping and spinal cord trauma during flexion and extension of the spine.

Ideally, considering the debilitation and disability of these patients, the procedure of choice would be one that provides immediate and long-term stabilization and early ambulation without the necessity of being in heavy orthotic devices. Bryan et al. elaborated on their experience in 11 patients with rheumatoid involvement of the cervical spine who were operated on utilizing methyl methacrylate, wire, and autogenous iliac bone grafts. In brief, they used the wires for internal fixation encased with methyl methacrylate, taking care that the methyl methacrylate did not spill laterally on the lamina. Autogenous iliac bone grafts were then placed over the decorticated lamina. They recommended minimization of the bulk of the methyl methacrylate-metal composite to decrease the potential for wound healing complications.[15] We have been using a modified Gallies fusion, utilizing a bicortical iliac bone H-graft so that two cortical surfaces provide greater immediate strength, and the bony fusion gives long-term stability.[16] The technique of this procedure is described in some detail.

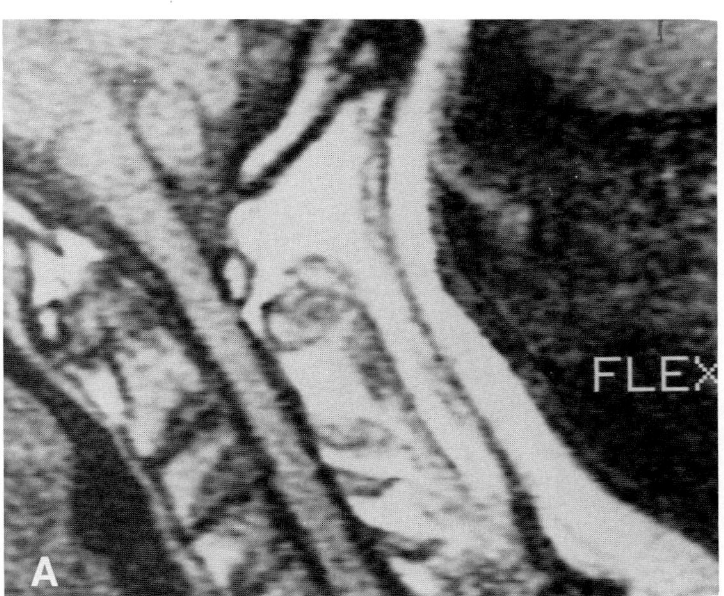
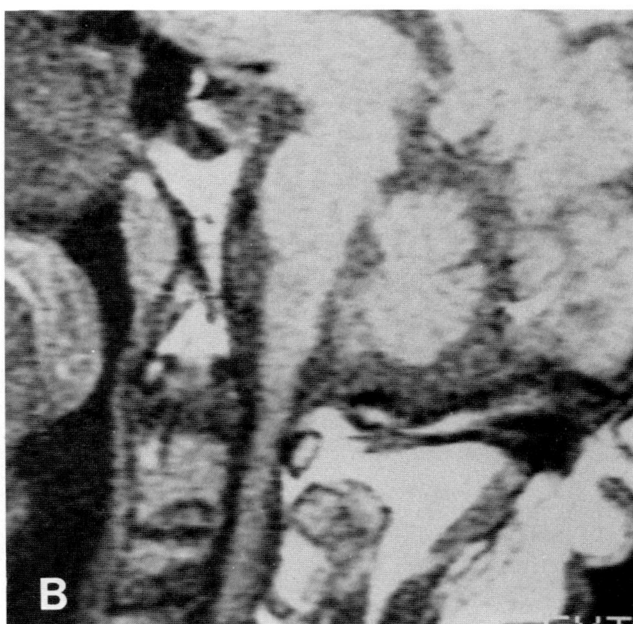

Fig. 114-1. A MRI scan of a patient with rheumatoid involvement of the cervical spine and resultant atlantoaxial subluxation. In flexion (A) there is no compression of the upper cervical cord. On the contrary, in extension (B) there is evidence of compression on the ventral aspect of the upper cervical cord by the odontoid process. Note the excellent visualization of neural elements.

C1-C2 FUSION FOR ATLANTOAXIAL SUBLUXATION

Preparation

The patient is placed in Gardner-Wells tong traction, particularly if the patient has a significant or progressive deficit. Coagulation studies are done, and the patient receives additional steroids, since the majority of these patients have been on long-term steroid therapy. We prefer to use cortisone acetate, 100 mg the night before surgery, and another 100 mg with the preoperative medication on the morning of the operation.

Anesthesia

Since the majority of these patients have joint deformities as well as a limited range of neck motion with subluxation causing neurologic deficit, great care is taken in the induction of anesthesia. We prefer to intubate the patient while he or she is awake, without undue flexion or extension of the neck while the patient is still in traction. The throat is sprayed with Cetacine (Cetylite Industries, Inc. Pennsauken, New Jersey). If the patient is apprehensive, slight sedation with a small dose of Valium is used. We have found that blind nasotracheal intubation while the patient is breathing is well tolerated; however, endotracheal intubation could be done using a fiberoptic laryngoscope.[17]

Positioning

The patient then is turned over to the operating table in the prone position, supported on rolls, while skeletal traction is maintained over an anesthesia screen (Figure 114-2). The head is supported on a horseshoe headrest and held in extension. The pressure points are padded. The table is flexed to avoid hyperextension of the lumbar spine, and a pillow or rolled blanket is used to avoid pressure on the feet. The draw sheet is brought together in such a way that the arms are supported while the upper part of the chest and right flank and buttock areas are left exposed. The right iliac crest is used for the graft, unless other factors dictate differently. A lateral film of the cervical spine is obtained in this position to assess the reduction of the subluxation.

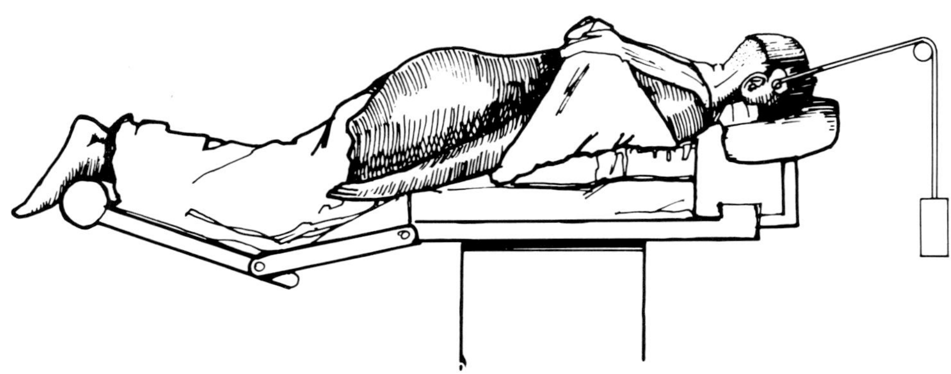

Fig. 114-2. Positioning of the patient.

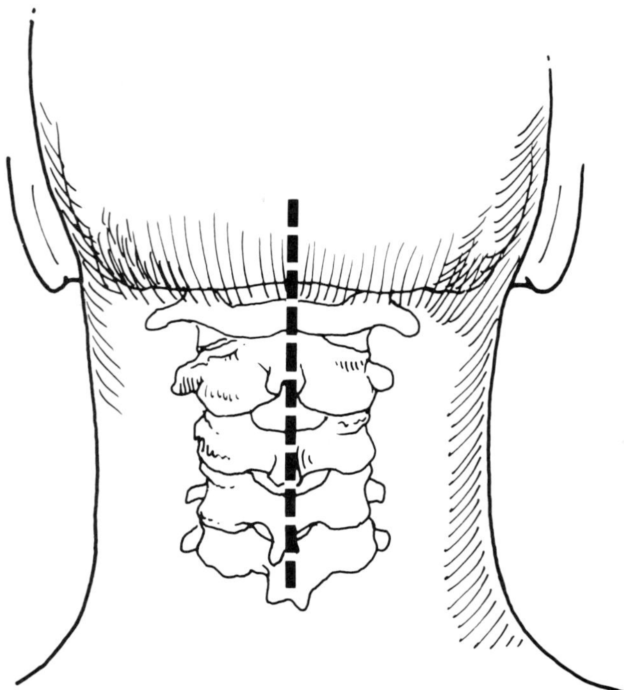

Fig. 114-3.   The line of the incision.

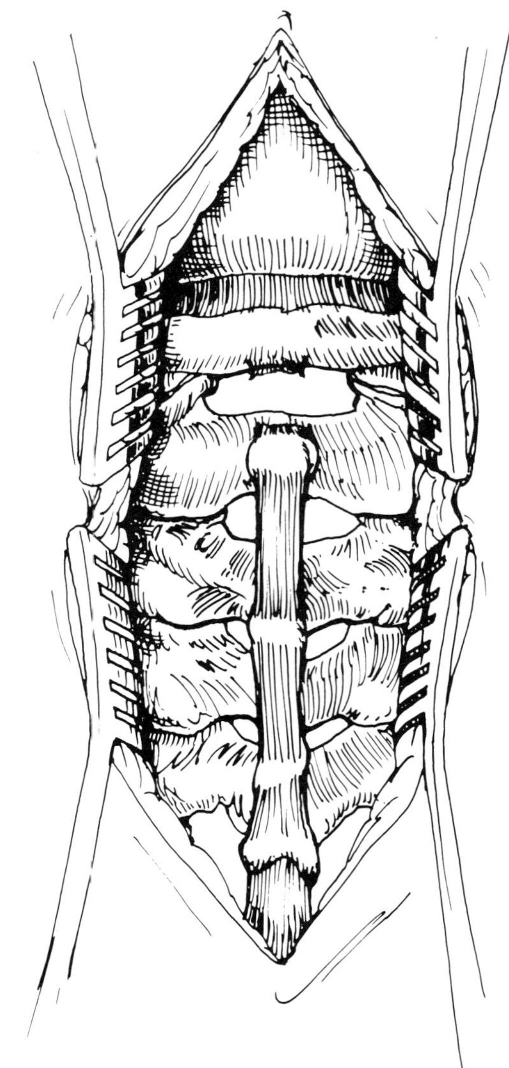

Fig. 114-4.   Exposure of the occipital bone and upper cervical laminae.

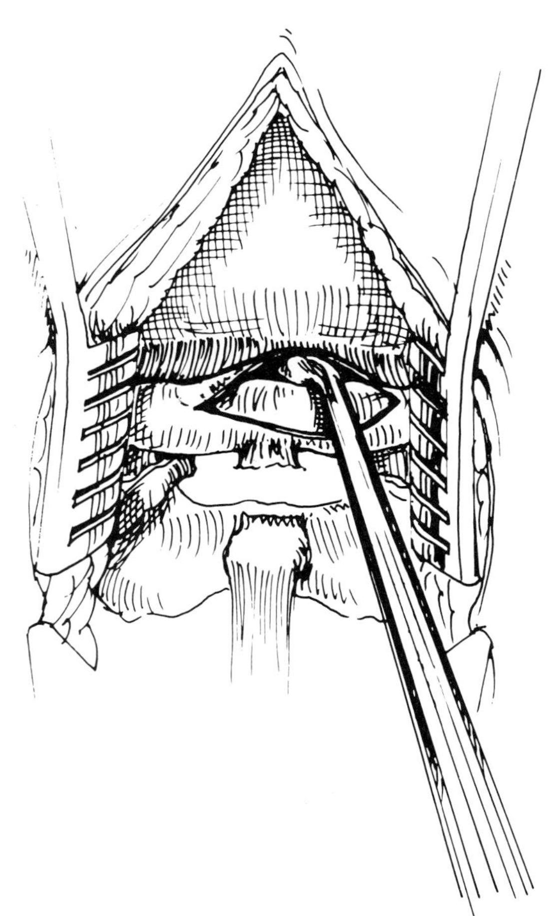

Fig. 114-5.   The periosteum is stipped off the posterior arch of C1 with a small angled curette.

Operation

A midline skin incision is made from the inion to the midcervical region following appropriate preparation and draping (Figure 114-3). The dissection is continued strictly in the midline. The muscles are dissected off the occipital bone and the laminae of C1, C2, and C3. Particular attention is given to the posterior arch of the atlas where, after the muscles in the midline are sharply divided, a periosteal elevator is used gently to dissect the muscles laterally, without disturbing the vertebral arteries or venous plexuses. The exposure is maintained with self-retaining retractors (Figure 114-4). A transverse incision is made over the dorsal aspect of the posterior arch of the atlas with a No. 15 blade, and the periosteum is dissected off the arch, both on the dorsal and ventral surfaces, using a small, angled curette (Figure 114-5). The bony surfaces are roughened with a bone rasp. A notch, about 5 mm in depth, is made at the superior aspect of the base of the C2 spinous process with a narrow-beaked rongeur. Once the arch has been freed, a loop of No. 20 monofilament wire is passed underneath C1 from below, while the arch is gently retracted backward with the curette (Figure 114-6). As the loop becomes slightly visible, it is pulled

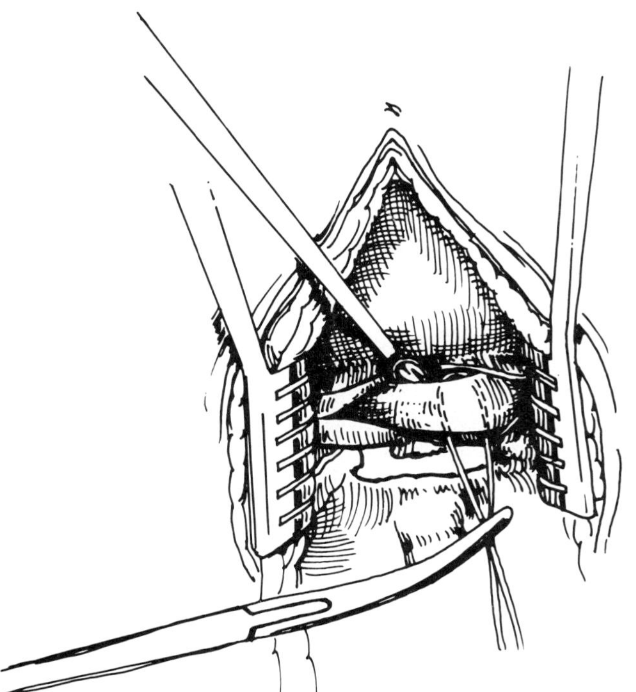

Fig. 114-6. A wire loop is passed beneath the posterior arch of C1 while the arch is gently pulled back with the curette.

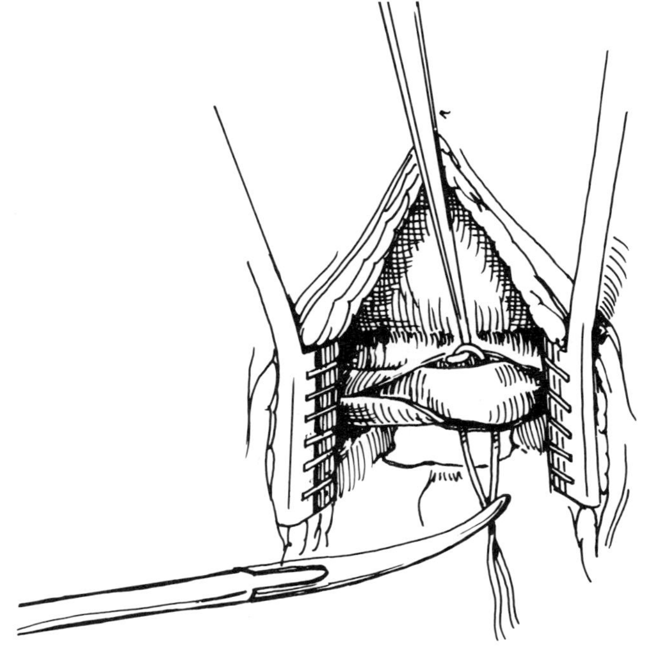

Fig. 114-7. The wire loop is pulled with a nerve hook.

up with a nerve hook (Figure 114-7). At the same time, a bicortical iliac bone graft is removed (Figure 114-8). This requires stripping of abdominal, iliacus, and gluteal muscles from their attachments to the upper, inner, and outer surfaces of the ilium. Four notches are cut on the graft, allowing a close fit between the graft and the posterior elements of C1 and C2. Another wire is then passed under the laminar arch of C2 on each side after stripping the periosteum and ligamentum flavum in the same manner as done under C1. The wire loops are tightened around the graft, pulled downward under tension, and tightly twisted (Figure 114-9). Previously we had passed a wire

through the spinous process of C2 rather than wire loops under the laminar arch of C2. This has been modified to allow for more immediate approximation and stabilization. Cancellous bone chips then are packed into the crevices underneath the iliac graft. Both incisions are closed carefully in layers.

In our experience using this method we have encountered two complications caused by the iliac bone defect resultant in complete fracture through the iliac wing. The fractures, however, healed spontaneously not requiring any specific treatment. This also has the potential for herniation of the bowel through the iliac defect. Recently we started to repair the iliac graft site to prevent a fracture and potential for herniation. Eighteen gauge stainless steel wire is passed through drill holes

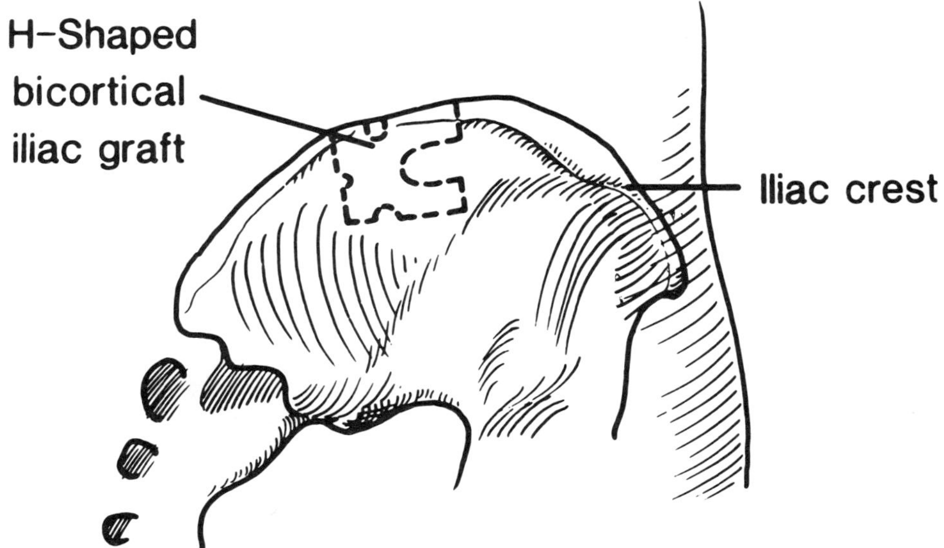

Fig. 114-8. Diagram outlining the donor site for the bicortical iliac bone graft. (Reprinted from Wu KK, Malik GM, Guise ER: Atlanto-axial arthrodesis: A clinical analysis of twenty-two consecutive cases performed at Henry Ford Hospital. Orthopaedics 5:865–871, 1982. With permission.)

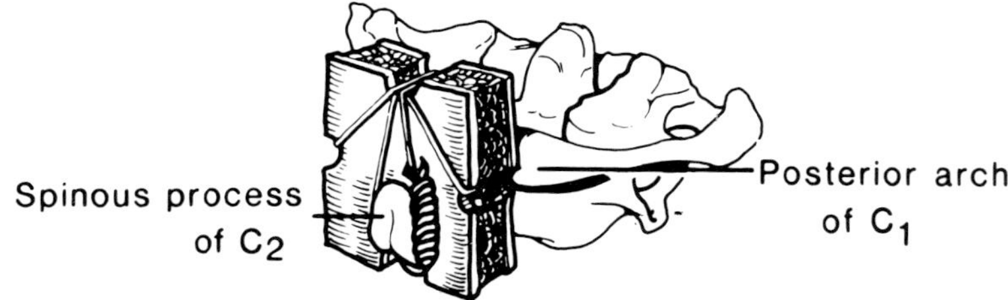

Fig. 114-9. Diagram of the bicortical iliac "H" strut graft in place after it has been intimately wired to the posterior arch of the atlas and the spinous process of the axis. (Reprinted from Wu KK, Malik GM, Guise ER: Atlanto-axial arthrodesis: A clinical analysis of twenty-two consecutive cases performed at Henry Ford Hospital. Orthopaedics 5:865–871, 1982. With permission.)

placed at the perimeter of the iliac bone defect and tightened. The remaining defect is filled with methyl methacrylate encasing the wires. This restores the normal iliac configuration preventing herniation and fracture (Figure 114-10).

Postoperative Care

The patient is placed in a light plastic collar and ambulation is encouraged as tolerated. Roentgenograms of the cervical spine are obtained for 2 to 4 months postoperatively to ensure that adequate reduction and fusion have taken place (Figure 114-11).

VERTICAL ATLANTOAXIAL SUBLUXATION

Greater attention has been given to vertical atlantoaxial subluxation in recent years.[18–20] It has been known by different names such as vertical atlantoaxial dislocation, basilar invagination, upward atlantoaxial dislocation, or upward odontoid dislocation. Vertical subluxation results from: (1) destruction of the ligaments, and (2) erosive changes with bone resorption in the basilar aspect of the skull, the occipital condyles, and the lateral masses of the atlas. The odontoid process projects up into the foramen magnum and generally is associated with some degree of atlantoaxial subluxation, so the odontoid process also is placed posteriorly in the canal. This causes direct compression of the medulla, along with potential ischemia from compression of the vertebral arteries, the anterior spinal arteries, or small perforating vessels of the brain stem and spinal cord.

Several fatal cases, with death caused by sudden-onset medullary ischemia, have been reported.[21,22] In a survey of 476 patients with rheumatoid arthritis admitted to the hospital, Henderson found that 13 cases (3.7 percent) had vertical atlantoaxial subluxation.[18] This form of subluxation was con-

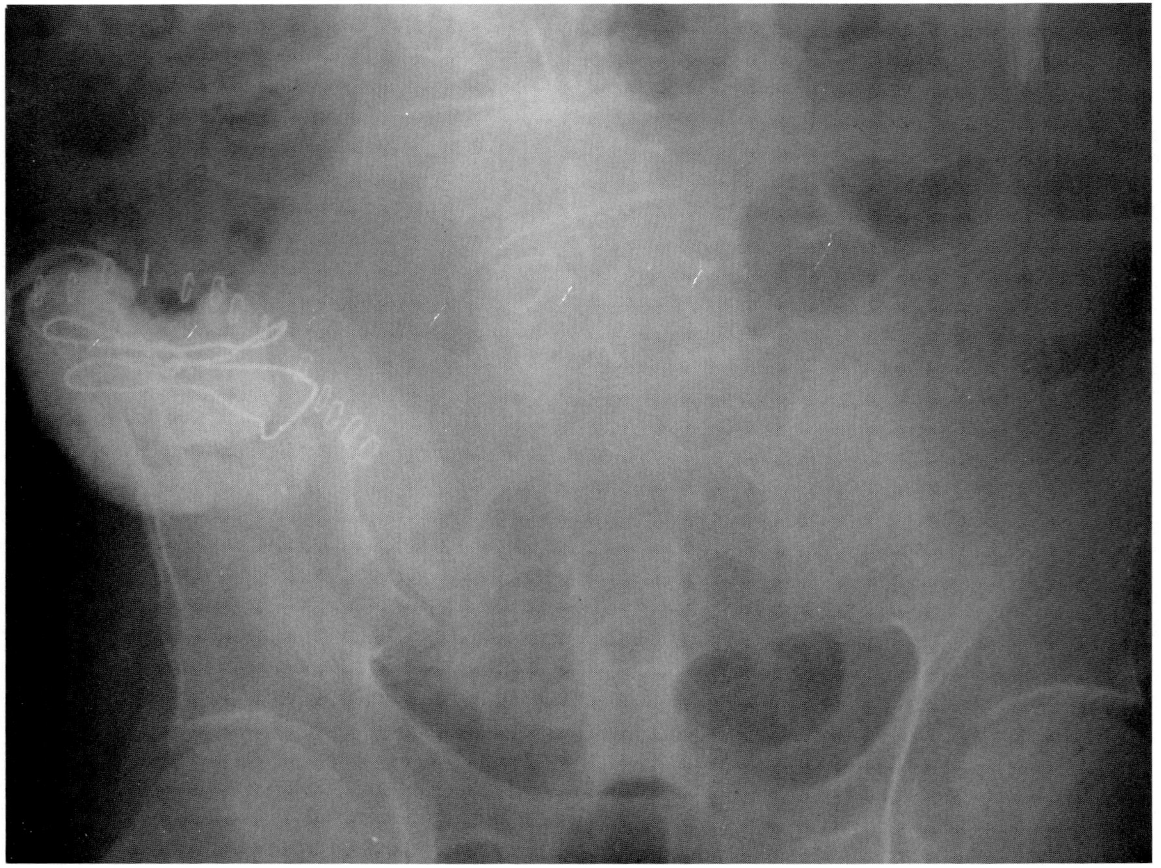

Fig. 114-10. Repair of the iliac bone defect with wire encased in methyl methacrylate.

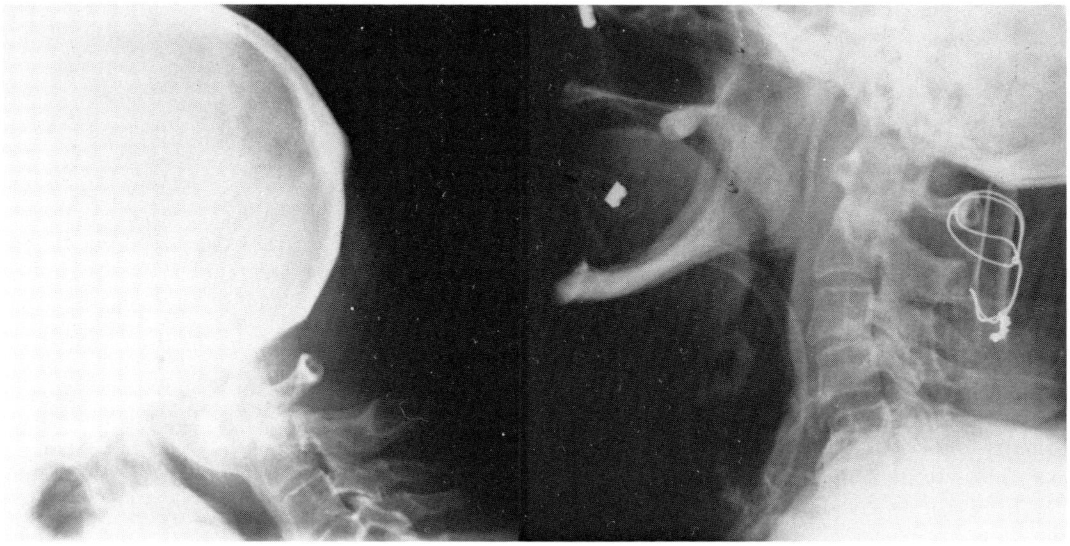

Fig. 114-11. Preoperative and postoperative roentgenograms: (left) a flexion view of the cervical spine showing subluxation; and (right) a lateral film demonstrating reduction of subluxation and position of the graft.

sidered to be present if the tip of the odontoid process lay more than 4.5 mm above McGregor's line. Five of these patients had definite involvement of the brain stem, cervical cord, or upper cervical nerve roots, and two others had pyramidal signs without subaxial subluxation.

The development of brain stem symptoms, especially dysphagia, hoarseness, periods of unconsciousness, and respiratory difficulty, is an ominous sign and requires urgent treatment. The patient should be placed in skeletal traction. Some improvement or stabilization of the neurologic deficit can be obtained with occipitoaxial fusion, with or without removal of the posterior arch of the atlas. When medullary involvement is noted, however, the transoral approach with removal of the odontoid and overlying synovial tissue is recommended.[23,24] This provides the best opportunity to decompress the brain stem. The patient obviously requires a tracheostomy, and transoral decompression has to be followed with occipital-cervical fusion.

In rare cases of atlantoaxial subluxation, as in the one described by Kao et al., reduction is not possible because of the presence of rheumatoid granulation tissue between the anterior arch of the atlas and the odontoid process.[25] Under these circumstances, the transoral approach provides a means of removal of granulation tissue and reduction of the subluxation. This can be followed later with occipitocervical fusion. The alternative method would be resection of the posterior arch of the atlas before fusion of the occiput to C2-3.[26]

SUBAXIAL SUBLUXATION

Spontaneous rheumatoid subluxation below the axis also occurs with some frequency and can cause severe cord damage.[27] Multiple levels may be involved, however, the C4-5 level is most commonly affected. Cervical myelopathy may be caused by intervertebral disc extrusion or rheumatoid granulation tissue in addition to, or at a level different from, that of the subluxation. As pointed out earlier, it also can be associated with atlantoaxial involvement. The difficulty of evaluating lower cervical segments cannot be over emphasized, and therefore tomography may be necessary. Myelography is considered

advisable before surgical treatment unless the clinical level of the involvement of the spinal cord exactly matches the level of subluxation. MRI is a useful adjunct in the diagnostic work up.

Tong traction, followed by anterior cervical fusion by the Cloward method, is the treatment of choice for single-level subluxation.[28] Spinal cord compression from granulation tissue or intervertebral disc herniation also can be treated adequately by this approach. The only problem, encountered occasionally, is the poor quality of graft obtained from the ilium because of severe osteoporosis. One might therefore have to use a strut graft rather than a Cloward plug. A fibular graft could certainly be used, particularly if more than one level is to be treated.

In some patients, however, the only reasonable way to decompress the spinal cord is by cervical laminectomy. If subluxation is already present at this level, this can be treated by anterior fusion. In other cases, one should follow the patient very closely for possible future subluxation. Similarly, if the myelogram reveals compression because of pachymeningitis,[29] decompressive laminectomy and placement of the fascial graft in the dura are necessary.

Obviously, all of these procedures are helpful only if the patient has some neurologic function remaining. Major surgical procedures are fruitless and probably unjustified in a patient who is quadriplegic or on a respirator. It therefore cannot be stressed enough that, despite some reports indicating lack of major neurologic deterioration on long-term follow-up, a thorough initial neurologic evaluation and close follow-up are necessary. If a potentially hazardous situation exists, treatment is necessary before irreversible cord damage occurs.

THORACIC AND LUMBAR SPINE INVOLVEMENT

The neurologic complications from involvement of the thoracic and lumbar spine are rather uncommon.[30] Rheumatoid nodules have been reported to cause nerve root compression.[31] Subluxations are seen in rheumatoid patients, but generally it is difficult to differentiate this from the degenerative disc disease. If the symptoms are referable to the thoracic or lumbar region, myelography is necessary. Occasionally the vertebral end-plate may be destroyed and this may simulate osteomyelitis or discitis. The treatment depends on the pathologic condition.

Obviously a patient suffering from rheumatoid arthritis is not immune to other intraspinal lesion causing myelopathy or radiculopathy that may require appropriate investigations and treatment.

ANKYLOSING SPONDYLITIS

Ankylosing spondylitis is a chronic inflammatory disease that most frequently affects the sacroiliac joints of young men and synovial joints of the whole spine. The incidence of ankylosing spondylitis in the general population is 1–3 per 1000 people with the onset occurring generally in the third decade of life.[32,33] Bony fusion of these joints and ossification along the longitudinal ligaments lead to total immobility of the vertebrae. The condition has been known by different names, such as rheumatoid spondylosis, rheumatoid arthritis of the spine, Marie-Str [umlautu] mpell disease, Bekhterev's disease, pelvospondylitis ossificans, and spondylitis ankylopoietica.

Early symptoms include low back pain or lumbar stiffness or both, which is usually increased in the morning or after periods of inactivity. Interestingly, periods of rest appear to bring on the low back stiffness, and these patients may awaken at night with stiffness of such severity that they must get up and stretch before returning to sleep.[34] In 65 to 70 percent of the patients, the initial symptom is intermittent or persistent low back pain. In rare instances the back pain can be hyperacute and resemble an acute herniated lumbar disc. It is unusual for the pain to have any radicular pattern down the thigh and calf. The possibility of early ankylosing spondylitis must, therefore, be kept in mind while evaluating patients with low back pain and suspected disc disease. Particular attention should be given to sacroiliac joints in patients who do not have neurologic changes of nerve root involvement. The erythrocyte sedimentation rate is elevated in 80 to 90 percent of the patients with obvious active disease. In 1973 Brewerton et al.,[35] and Schlosstein et al.,[36] reported the association between the human histocompatibility antigen, HLA-B27 and ankylosing spondylitis. In population studies it has been found in 90 to 95 percent of patients with ankylosing spondylitis and only 7 to 8 percent of the general white population.[35–37]

The most common neurologic complication in patients with ankylosing spondylitis are caused by: (1) fracture-dislocation of the spine; (2) stress fractures; (3) atlantoaxial subluxation; (4) intraspinal ossifications or pachymeningitis; and (5) cauda equina syndrome.

FRACTURE-DISLOCATION OF THE SPINE

A rigid spine and fragile osteoporotic vertebrae in ankylosing spondylitis make the patient especially susceptible to spinal fracture-dislocation. Unlike an ordinary spinal fracture, the ankylosed spine breaks like a long bone. The fracture line tends to be transverse and may extend to involve more posterior structures. Bergmann stated that the fractures occurred through what had formerly been an interspace.[38] Others have been reported cases, however, in which fracture was primarily through the vertebral body.[39] Hyperextension injuries are most likely to cause a fracture. The spine may be locked in hyperextension, either because of locking of the facts or locking of the neural arches. The more advanced the process of ankylos-

ing spondylitis, the less trauma appears necessary to break the brittle bone and calcified ligaments. At times there may be no definite history of trauma. Woodruss and Dewing reported a case in which the momentary unsupported weight of the head while the patient was being turned on a Stryker frame was enough to result in a fracture of C5-6.[40] The cervical spine is the most commonly involved, although fractures of the thoracic and lumbar spine have been observed. In the cervical region, C5-6 and C6-7 levels are the most frequently affected.

Patients may only complain of pain, but the most dramatic symptom is quadriplegia. Fracture or fracture-dislocation of the vertebral column should be suspected in any patient with severe ankylosing spondylitis who has had trauma, especially if there are complaints of neck or back pain. Approximately 75 percent of ankylosing spondylitis patients who sustain a spine fracture will develop neurologic involvement.[41] Such a patient should be handled as if he had an unstable fracture until thorough clinical and radiologic assessment have ruled out the presence of such a lesion.

Just as in the case of rheumatoid arthritis, certain areas of the spine, particularly the lower cervical and upper thoracic portions, can be difficult to visualize because of the deformities produced by the disease. Tomograms should be obtained if complete visualization is not possible by other means.

A complete transverse fracture converts the spine into two rigid segments. The calcified longitudinal ligaments also can be fractured and are no longer available to assist in maintaining the alignments of the two segments, which move as independent units. Once the diagnosis has been established, every effort should be made to prevent or minimize spinal cord injury.

If there is no neurologic deficit and the subluxation is slight, an efficient immobilization with a Halo or Minerva jacket would be sufficient. The majority of fractures heal within 8 to 10 weeks, although evident nonunion has been reported as late as 6 months.[42] When there is appreciable displacement or instability, however, skeletal traction is needed as initial treatment. The traction should be applied in a neutral position along the axis of the cervical spine. This axis also might be distorted because of flexion deformity of the cervical spine in advanced ankylosing spondylitis. Any hyperextension can cause further compromise of the spinal canal and potential neurologic deterioration. If reduction is achieved, the spine can be stabilized by an anterior approach or simply treated with immobilization.

When reduction is not possible with traction or there is progressive neurologic deficit, immediate operative intervention is necessary. The fracture-dislocation can be associated with epidural hematoma. Open reduction and decompressive laminectomy, followed by a stabilizing procedure, using internal fixation and bone graft at the same time, are essential.[43] The patient then needs to be immobilized in a brace for 2 to 3 months.

If operative intervention becomes necessary, several factors have to be taken into consideration. Endotracheal intubation might risk further neurologic damage because of hyperextension of the neck. Nasotracheal intubation or elective tracheostomy, with the patient awake, may therefore be necessary. Flexible fiberoptic bronchoscopy has several advantages in that it can be utilized in awake patients and with direct visualization and application of topical anesthetics reduces the possibility of larynospasms. With fiberoptic nasotracheal intubation the patient is awake allowing for assessment of the patient neurologically.[17]

Several cardiovascular abnormalities are associated with

ankylosing spondylitis, including aortic insufficiency, persistent conduction disturbances, cardiomegaly, pericarditis, and angina.[44] Complete atrial-ventricular blocks, causing Stokes-Adams attacks, have been reported. Similarly, diffuse rib cage involvement by the ankylosing process leads to the restriction of chest expansion. A peculiar apical or upper lobe fibrosis with occasional cavitation also has been noted. Amyloid is reported to cause up to 6 percent of deaths in ankylosing spondylitis usually because of renal involvement.[45,46] These factors have to be assessed along with the commonly associated problem of severe kyphoscoliosis. These patients generally have been on long-term steroid therapy and require additional steroids at the time of surgery.

The prognosis, in general, is much less favorable in fracture-dislocation of the ankylosed cervical spine than in a similar injury of the normal spine. Hollin et al. reported a 45 percent mortality in their review of 38 cases.[47]

STRESS FRACTURES

The first description of a destructive lesion affecting the rigid spine of ankylosing spondylitis was given by Romanus and Yden in 1955.[48] Infection or a degenerative rheumatoid nodule were initially thought to be the causative factors but more recent studies have identified the etiology as a stress fracture showing nonunion. These fractures present insidiously at all levels of the spine, though most often at the lower thoracic or upper lumbar regions. Patients generally have progressive and disabling pain. The typical site of anterior interbody destruction, the so called Romanus lesion, is probably secondary to a posterior arch fracture.[49] If there is no obvious destructive lesion present on plain roentgenograms and the ankylosing spondylitis patient has severe back pain, the possibility of a stress fracture should be considered. The diagnosis can be confirmed by tomography and radionuclide imaging. Operative treatment by posterior exploration and internal fixation without bone grafting is straight forward and produces immediate pain relief followed by rapid fracture union.

ATLANTOAXIAL SUBLUXATIONS

All types of atlantoaxial subluxation, as described in the section on rheumatoid arthritis, also are seen in ankylosing spondylitis. The frequency, however, is much less and generally is in the range of 2 to 8 percent. When symptomatic, similar treatment is indicated. The problems of a rigid, brittle lower cervical spine and associated cardiovascular and respiratory difficulties need to be taken into consideration when surgical intervention is necessary.

INTRASPINAL OSSIFICATION OR PACHYMENINGITIS

Intraspinal ossification of the posterior longitudinal ligament, as well as the dura, has been reported as a cause of myelopathy in ankylosing spondylitis. Evidently it is more commonly seen in Japanese, and Briedal called this syndrome "the Japanese Disease."[50] Dirheimer, however, reported 2 cases of meningeal ossification evident on radiologic studies. Any patient with ankylosing spondylitis with myelopathy not explained by radiographic changes needs myelography. If a compressive lesion is found, surgical decompression is indicated. If the thickening or ossification of the dura is the source

of compression, placement of a fascial graft in the dura is needed.

CAUDA EQUINA SYNDROME

There are several case reports in the literature of slowly progressive cauda equina syndrome in patients with long-standing ankylosing spondylitis.[51–53] There is loss of function of the lower spinal roots, both motor and sensory. Generally the initial symptom is disturbance of sphincter control. Changes in ankle reflexes and cutaneous sensation, particularly in the sacral dermatomes, are evident. There is variable involvement in the lower nerve roots. Surprisingly, no compressive lesion has been found on myelography in these patients. The spinal canal is said to be quite wide. In some cases, however, posterior diverticula have been noted.[54] In one postmortem evaluation reported by Matthew, the posterior aspect of the lower spinal canal was found to be eroded by numerous large arachnoid cysts, and arachnoid adhesions were present above the level of the diverticula.[55] There also were some degenerative changes in the nerve roots of the cauda equina. No definite cause has been determined, however Matthew suggested the possibility of arachnoiditis occurring at an earlier stage of the disease and possibly being responsible for this syndrome later on. Nothing surgical can be done about it, however, the patient certainly needs investigations, including myelography.

PAGET'S DISEASE

There is some involvement of the spine in almost all patients with Paget's disease. The risk of neurologic involvement is inversely related to the frequency with which the vertebrae are involved, being greatest in the cervical spine where Paget's disease is least common, and least in the lumbar spine where the disease is most common. The thoracic spine is intermediate in both aspects.[56] Although the neurologic complications are relatively uncommon considering the frequency of the disease, they can be treatable and should therefore be recognized. There is a broad spectrum of neurologic sequelae,[57] but only the ones associated with spinal involvement will be discussed here.

Several mechanisms are involved in the etiology of neurologic changes,[57] including.:

1. Pressure exerted by pathologic bone on neural structures.
2. Changes in the ability of the bone to bear weight.
3. Malignant change of the involved bone.
4. Compromise of the vascular supply of neural structures.

Spinal cord compression is a well-known complication of Paget's disease of the vertebral column and was first described by Wyllie in 1923.[58] Sadar et al., in 1973, presented a review of 86 cases, already reported, and 4 of their own with neurologic dysfunction attributable only to Paget's disease of the vertebral column.[59] Eighty-nine percent of the patients were men and 11 percent women. Progressive paraparesis or quadriparesis was the initial feature in most patients. Pain was the only symptom in patients; however, it is a complaint frequently associated with Paget's disease and is secondary to either local bony changes, radicular compression, or flexor spasm at a later stage.

The bony changes in Paget's disease of the spine result from relative effects of the destructive and reparative processes.[57] There is thickening of the pedicles and laminae, and the destructive process causes softening of the bone resulting in the compression of the vertebral bodies. At the same time, reparative changes occur, mainly along the periphery, increasing the width of the vertebral body, which is already increased because of the decreased height secondary to compression. These changes, thus combined, cause narrowing of the spinal canal and the intervertebral foramina, resulting in the compression of the neural elements, i.e., the spinal cord and the nerve roots.

In 101 documented cases of spinal cord and nerve root dysfunction secondary to vertebral Paget's disease without malignant transformation, the most frequent involvement occurred at the thoracic level (76 percent), followed by the lumbar (15 percent) and cervical levels (9 percent).[60]

The upper thoracic spinal cord is most vulnerable to the effects of Paget's disease. Normally the vertebral canal is narrowest in this area and the vascular compromise also is more likely to occur, since this is considered to be the watershed area. Neurologic involvement can follow either a monostotic lesion or diffuse changes affecting a considerable length of the vertebral canal. The radiologic demonstration of a paraspinal mass with neural arch involvement is undoubtedly the most vital clue to the diagnosis.

The patient usually has symptoms of progressive spinal cord involvement. The course is slow with symptoms usually being present for more than 1 year and rarely less than 6 months. Sensory and motor symptoms generally start simultaneously. As noted earlier, the upper thoracic spinal cord is most commonly affected and therefore the patient generally first notices numbness and weakness in the legs. With further progression, spasticity and other upper motor neuron signs appear, and the patient may develop sphincter disturbances. A typical history, however, does not always signify a compressive etiology as explaining the spinal cord dysfunction.[59] Petit-Dutailis et al.[61] described a patient with Paget's disease and progressive paraparesis who had a negative myelogram, but the cerebrospinal fluid protein level was high. Two years later, however, a repeat myelogram showed evidence of spinal cord compression, and decompression resulted in improvement. Similar cases in patients who have had neurologic deficit but no myelographic block have been reported since then. Under these circumstances, vascular insufficiency of the neural elements would have to be considered as the most likely etiologic factor.

Involvement of the atlas and axis with spinal cord compression and subsequent quadriplegia has been reported.[62–64] The involvement of the craniospinal junction results in basilar impression, as described by Wycis.[65] This can be associated with occipital neuralgia, lower cranial nerve signs, medullary compression, cerebellar compression, syringomyelia with ventricular obstruction, hydrocephalus, and vertebrobasilar insufficiency.

Symptoms of compression of the cauda equina result from involvement of the lumbar spine, characteristically of a single vertebra. Paget's disease can be a cause of sciatica through encroachment of the vertebral foramen, through the well-known pelvic outlet (pyriformis) syndrome, or through a lower nerve entrapment between the enlarged ischium and the lesser trochanter.[66]

Malignant degeneration, resulting in osteogenic sarcoma, has been reported.[67] It occurs in approximately 0.15 percent of patients found more commonly with polyostotic disease.[68] The incidence of malignant change in the spine is extremely infrequent in comparison to the humerus and skull. Sadar et al.

found only 7 documented cases.[59] In contrast to slowly progressive neurologic deficit with Paget's disease of the spine, the patient with osteogenic sarcoma has a rapidly deteriorating course over a period of a few weeks. Pain is a prominent symptom, and generally when the patient is first seen, pulmonary metastases are already evident. Operative decompression, in 4 of the 7 patients reported, resulted in minimal and temporary improvement with the longest survival being 5.5 months.

TREATMENT

At the present time, myelography is the only definitive way to determine the extent to which the subarachnoid space is compromised. Myelography, through lumbar puncture, might be difficult if there is involvement of the lumbar spine. In these cases, a lateral C1-2 puncture could be used safely to introduce contrast material.

Computed tomographic scanning of the spine is certainly helpful in delineating the extent of bony involvement. The MRI scanner has added to the existing armamentarium of diagnostic imaging. It allows for an axial evaluation of the extent of Paget's involvement of the spine. Regional angiography is recommended to assess the vascularity of an area before surgery, particularly in the presence of very active or neoplastic disease. It then may be appropriate to consider embolization and occlusion of the major arterial feeders to the involved bone before decompression or excision of tumor.

Several medications are being used in the treatment of Paget's disease of the bone. In the past decade three agents have become available: the calcitonins, disphosphonates, and mithramycin. All three are potent inhibitors of bone resorption but work by different mechanisms.

Calcitonin is a 32-amino-acid polypeptide that inhibits bone resorption via a cyclic-AMP-mediated system.[69] It has proved effective in the relief of pagetic pain in approximately 80 percent of patients.[70] Dramatic therapeutic effects have occurred in patients with paraplegia or paraparesis secondary to myelopathy. Neurologic improvement usually becomes evident after 2 or 3 months and is maximal at 1 year. Up to 70 percent improvement in motor power, sensory levels, and sphincter function have been reported.[70] In a case reported by Melick et al.,[71] it appeared to relieve neurologic dysfunction resulting from spinal compression. This patient showed slow improvement over a period of 8 months. Coincident with therapy, urinary hydroxyproline and serum alkaline phosphatase levels fell. The mechanism of the improvement is unclear, but may be secondary to a reduction in the volume and vascularity of the bone. Histologically there is a reduction in osteoclastic resorption, chaotic bone formation, and marrow fibrosis. A reversion to normal lamellar bone formation occurs along with a decrease in the vascular nature of the bone.[70] Improvement in cranial nerve palsies, ataxia, and myelopathy with spastic paralysis and paraplegia all have been noted during calcitonin therapy, but it must be remembered that only a small number of patients have been documented.[72]

Diphosphonates act as analogues of pyrophosphate and interfere with the growth and dissolution of hydroxyapatite crystals.[73] Pain is relieved in 60 to 70 percent of patients and bone vascularity is reduced. Advantages over calcitonin are that it is taken orally and the remission period is generally at least 1 year.[70]

Mithramycin is a cytotoxic antibiotic that decreases osteoclastic bone resorption by inhibiting RNA synthesis.[74]

Approximately 90 percent of patients show clinical improvement; pain relief is often evident within a few days.[70] Ryan reported having seen considerable return of function in patients with neurologic involvement using mithramycin.[75] The use of mithramycin is generally reserved unless calcitonin and diphosphonates are ineffective and surgery contraindicated. It has significant side effects with toxicity to the liver, kidneys, gastrointestinal tract, and platelets. It is given intravenously, usually over a 12-hour period in doses ranging from 10 to 25 mg/kg.[76]

The medical therapy should be considered in the patient experiencing bone pain without neurologic deficit. Similarly, in the case of a very slow, progressive lesion, drug therapy would be attractive since one is able to monitor the changes on close follow-up. The Metabolic Bone Disease clinic at the Hospital for Special Surgery presented the following medical regimen with two thirds of the patients treated achieving remission without relapse for 5 years. Merkon and Lane recommended serial treatment with calcitonin, 50 units subcutaneously, three times a week for 6 months, followed by diphosphonate, 5 mg/kg/day for 6 months overlapping 1 month.[69]

Douglas, et al. reviewed the English and French literature citing 29 patients reported with spinal dysfunction syndromes treated with calcitonin, diphosphonates, or a combination or sequence of these. Twenty-five patients (86 percent) improved remarkably with twenty-three (79 percent) having complete reversal of paraparesis.[77] None of the patients deteriorated beyond the baseline during treatment.

When the progression of neurologic deficit is more rapid, or other factors dictate early decompression of neural elements in the hope of preserving neurologic function, surgical decompression has to be carried out. The value of surgery in the presence of myelographically documented compression has been repeatedly proven. Sadar et al. reported 55 cases out of 65 treated with decompressive laminectomy showing variable but definite improvement.[59]

The general principles of decompressive laminectomy are the same as they would be for any other similar compressive lesion, such as a metastatic epidural tumor. A few points, however, should be stressed. The bone involved by Paget's disease is extremely vascular and soft. Similarly, the attachments between the paraspinal muscles and laminae are very vascular. The most prominent feature of surgical decompression is difficulty with the hemostasis. The bone bleeds very easily and profusely, making the operation very difficult. Extra attention is therefore necessary in stripping the paraspinal muscles, and judicious use of bone wax helps in reducing blood loss. Excessive blood loss has to be anticipated and appropriate arrangements have to be made for type and cross-match of adequate quantities of blood. It generally is not necessary to open the dura, but one has to make sure that adequate bony decompression has been carried out on both sides of the block.

It has been recommended that patients with very active disease but slow progression receive preoperative treatment, with calcitonin and disphosphonates for 3 to 6 months.[78] It has been cited that this will help decrease intraoperative blood loss and make decompression easier.

Following an initial response to decompression, recurrent neural compression may occur in the course of the disease, secondary to new bone formation, fracture-dislocation, or malignant degeneration. This occurred in 6 out of 65 patients undergoing decompressive laminectomy in the review by Sadar; one patient, however, did not show any improvement

following repeat laminectomy. Plaut also added a representative case in which the patient responded favorably to a second laminectomy.[79]

REFERENCES

1. Bland, JH: Rheumatoid arthritis of the cervical spine. J Rheumatol 3:319, 1974
2. Isdale IC, Conlon PW: Atlanto-axial subluxation. Ann Rheum Dis 30:387, 1971
3. Pellicci PM, Ranawat CS, Tsairis P, et al: A prospective study of the progression of rheumatoid arthritis of the cervical spine. J Bone Joint Surg 63A:342, 1981
4. Davis FW, Markley ME: Rheumatoid arthritis with death from medullary compression. Ann Intern Med 35:451, 1951
5. Nakano KK: Neurological complications of rheumatoid arthritis. Orthop Clin North Am 6:861, 1975
6. Conlon PW, Isdale IC, Rose BS: Rheumatoid arthritis of the cervical spine—an analysis of 333 cases. Ann Rheum Dis 25:120, 1966
7. Stevens JC, Cartlidge NEF, Saunders M, et al: Atlanto-axial subluxation and cervical myelopathy in rheumatoid arthritis. Q J Med 40:394, 1971
8. Smith PH, Benn RT, Sharp J: Natural history of rheumatoid cervical luxations. Ann Rheum Dis 31:431, 1972
9. Dirheimer Y: The Cranio-Vertebral Region in Chronic Inflammatory Disease. Berlin, Springer-Verlag, 1977
10. Stark DC, Miller R: Anesthesia for patients with rheumatoid arthritis. Orthop Rev 7:21, 1978
11. Katz W: Modern management of rheumatoid arthritis. Am J Med 79:24, 1985
12. Newman P, Sweetnam R: Occipito-cervical fusion—an operative technique and its indications. J Bone Joint Surg 51B:423, 1969
13. Hamblen DL: Occipito-cervical fusion: Indications, technique and results. J Bone Joint Surg 49B:33, 1967
14. Kelly DL, Alexander E, Davis C, et al: Acrylic fixation of atlanto-axial dislocation: Technical note. J Neurosurg 36:366, 1972
15. Bryan WJ, Inglis AE, Sculco TP, et al: Methylmethacrylate stabilization for enhancement of posterior cervical arthrodesis in rheumatoid arthritis. J Bone Joint Surg 64A:1045, 1982
16. Wu KK, Malik GM, Guise ER: Atlanto-axial arthrodesis: A clinical analysis of twenty-two consecutive cases performed at Henry Ford Hospital. Orthopedics 5:865, 1982
17. Ovassapian A, Land P, Schafer M, et al: Anesthetic management for surgical corrections of severe flexion deformity of the cervical spine. Anesthesiology 58:370, 1983
18. Henderson DRF: Vertical atlanto-axial subluxation in rheumatoid arthritis. Rheumatol Rehabil 14:31, 1975
19. Rana NA, Hancock DO, Taylor AR, et al: Vertical subluxations of the axis in rheumatoid arthritis. J Bone Joint Surg 55B:471, 1973
20. Swinson DR, Hamilton EBD, Matthews JA, et al: Vertical subluxations of the axis in rheumatoid arthritis. Ann Rheum Dis 31:359, 1972
21. Martel W, Abell M: Fatal atlanto-axial luxation in rheumatoid arthritis. Arthritis Rheum 6:224, 1963
22. Web FWS, Hickman JA, Drew D: Death from vertebral artery thrombosis in rheumatoid arthritis. Br Med J 2:537, 1968
23. Brattstrom H, Elner A, Granholm L: Transoral surgery for myelopathy caused by rheumatoid arthritis of cervical spine. Ann Rheum Dis 32:578, 1973
24. Smith HP, Challa VR, Alexander E: Odontoid compression of the brain stem in a patient with rheumatoid arthritis. J Neurosurg 53:841, 1980
25. Kao CC, Messert B, Winkler SS, et al: Rheumatoid C1-C2 dislocation—pathogenesis and treatment reconsidered. J Neurol Neurosurg Psychiatry 37:1060, 1974
26. Thomas WH: Surgical management of rheumatoid cervical spine. Orthop Clin North Am 6:793, 1975

27. Hopkins JS: Lower cervical rheumatoid subluxation with tetraplegia. J Bone Joint Surg 49B:46, 1967

28. Lidgren L, Ljunggren B, Ratcheson RA: Reposition, anterior exposure and fusion in the treatment of myelopathy caused by rheumatoid arthritis of the cervical spine. Scand J Rheumatol 3:195, 1974

29. Gutmann L, Hable K: Rheumatoid pachymeningitis. Neurology 13:901, 1963

30. Lawrence JS, Sharp J, Ball J, et al: Rheumatoid arthritis of the lumbar spine. Ann Rheum Dis 23:205, 1964

31. Friedman H: Intraspinal rheumatoid nodule causing nerve root compression. J Neurosurg 32:689, 1970

32. West HF: Etiology of ankylosing spondylitis. Ann Rheum Dis 8:143, 1949

33. Lawrence JS: The prevalence of arthritis. Br J Clin Pract 17:699, 1936

34. Smukler N: Arthritis of the spine, in Rothman R, Simeone F (eds): The Spine. Philadelphia, WB Saunders, 1982

35. Brewerton DA, Caffrey M, Hart FD, et al: Ankylosing spondylitis and HL-A27. Lancet 1:904, 1973

36. Schlosstein L, Terasaki PI, Bluesteon R, et al: High association of HLA antigen W27 with ankylosing spondylitis. N Engl J Med 288:704, 1973

37. Neustadt DH: Ankylosing spondylitis. Postgrad Med 61:124, 1977

38. Bergman EW: Fractures of ankylosed spine. J Bone Joint Surg 31A:669, 1949

39. Rand RW, Stern EW: Cervical fractures of ankylosed rheumatoid spine. Neurochirurgia 4:137, 1961

40. Woodruff FP, Dewing SB: Fracture of the cervical spine in patients with ankylosing spondylitis. Radiology 80:17, 1963

41. Hunter T, Dobo H: Spinal fractures complicating ankylosing spondylitis. Ann Intern Med 88:546, 1978

42. Lemmen LJ, Laing PG: Fracture of the cervical spine in patient with rheumatoid arthritis. J Neurosurg 16:542, 1959

43. Grisolia A, Bell RL, Peltier LF: Fractures and dislocations of the spine complicating ankylosing spondylitis. J Bone Joint Surg 49A:339, 1967

44. Calabro JJ: Medical and surgical management of ankylosing spondylitis. Clin Orthop 60:125, 1968

45. Ball J: Symposium on the spondylarthrides. Aspects of Pathology: Rheumatol Rehabil 18:210, 1979

46. Cruickshank B: Pathology of ankylosing spondylitis: Clin Orthop 74:43, 1971

47. Hollin SA, Gross SW, Levin P: Fracture of the cervical spine in patients with rheumatoid spondylitis. Am Surg 31:532, 1965

48. Romanus R, Yden S: Pelvo-spondylitis Ossificans. Chicago, Year Book, 1955

49. Marsh CH: Internal fixation for stress fractures of the ankylosed spine. J R Soc Med 78:377, 1985

50. Briedal P: Ossification of the posterior longitudinal ligament in the cervical spine. "The Japanese Disease" in patients of British descent. Australas Radiol 13:311, 1969

51. Bowie EA, Glasgow GL: Cauda equina lesions associated with ankylosing spondylitis. Br Med J 2:24, 1961

52. Lee MLH, Waters DJ: Neurological complications of ankylosing spondylitis. Br Med J 1:798, 1962

53. Russell ML, Gordon DA, Ogryzlo MA, et al: The cauda equina syndrome of ankylosing spondylitis. Ann Intern Med 78:551, 1973

54. Rosenkranz W: Ankylosing spondylitis-cauda equina syndrome with multiple spinal arachnoid cysts. J Neurosurg 34:241, 1971

55. Matthews WB: The neurologic complications of ankylosing spondylitis. J Neurol Sci 6:561, 1968

56. Parfitt AM, Duncan H: Metabolic bone disease affecting the spine, in Rothman RH, Simeone FA (eds): The Spine. Philadelphia, WB Saunders, 1978, pp 696–702

57. Schmidek HH: Neurologic and neurosurgical sequelae of Paget's disease of bone. Clin Orthop 127:70, 1977

58. Wyllie WG: The occurrence in osteitis deformans of lesions of the central nervous system with a report of four cases. Brain 46:336, 1923

59. Sadar ES, Walton RJ, Gredssman HH: Neurologic dysfunction in Paget's disease of the vertebral column. J Neurosurg 37:661, 1972

60. Reinstein L, Reahl E: Neurologic complications in vertebral Paget's disease. MD State Med J 30:32, 1981

61. Petit-Dutailis D, Marchand J, Garcia Calderon J: Un cas de compression medullaire par maladie osseuse de Paget grandement ameliore par la laminectome. Rev Neurol 66:71, 1936

62. Whalley N: Paget's disease of atlas and axis. J Neurol Neurosurg Psychiatry 9:84, 1946

63. Ramamurthi B, Visvanathan GS: Paget's disease of the axis causing paraplegia. J Neurosurg 14:580, 1957

64. Feldman F, Seaman WB: The neurological complications of Paget's disease in the cervical spine. AJR 105:375, 1969

65. Wycis HT: Basilar impression (platybasia), a case secondary to advanced Paget's disease with severe neurologic manifestations; successful surgical results. J Neurosurg 1:299, 1944

66. Christman OD, Snook GA, Walker HR: Paget's disease a differential diagnosis in sciatica. Clin Orthop 37:154, 1964

67. Finneson BE, Goluboff B, Shenkin HA: Sarcomatous degeneration of osteitis deformans causing compression of cauda equina. Neurology 8:82, 1958

68. Frame B, Mancez GM: Paget's Disease: A review of current knowledge. Radiology 141:21, 1981

69. Merkow R, Lane J: Current concepts of Paget's disease of bone. Orthop Clin North Am 15:747, 1984

70. Wallach S: Treatment of Paget's disease. Adv Intern Med 27:1, 1982

71. Melick RA, Ebeling P, Hjorth RJ: Improvement in paraplegia in vertebral Paget's disease treated with Calcitonin. Br Med J 1:627, 1976

72. MacIntyre I, Evans IMA, Hobitz HHG, et al: Chemistry, physiology and therapeutic applications of Calcitonin. Arthritis Rheum 23:1139, 1980

73. Siris ES, Jacobs TP, Canfield RE: Paget's disease of bone. Bull NY Acad Med 56:285, 1980

74. Dalinka M, Aronchick J, Haddad J: Paget's disease. Orthop Clin North Am 14:3, 1983

75. Ryan WG, Schwartz TB: Mithramycin treatment of Paget's disease of bone. Arthritis Rheum 23:1155, 1980

76. Melick R: Treatment of Paget's disease of bone. Med J Aust 143:394, 1985

77. Douglas DL, et al: Spinal cord dysfunction in Paget's disease of bone and its treatment. Has medical treatment a vascular basis? J Bone Joint Surg 633:495, 1981

78. Merkow R, Pellicci P, Hely D, Salvati E: Total hip replacement for Paget's disease of the hip. J Bone Joint Surg 66A:752, 1984

79. Plaut M: Paget's disease of the vertebrae. J Neurosurg 40:791, 1974

CHAPTER 115
Microsurgery of Syringomyelia and Syringomyelic Cord Syndrome

Albert L. Rhoton, Jr.

THE TERM *SYRINGOMYELIA* has been used to refer to a chronic, relentlessly progressive syndrome that is caused by the destruction of gray and white matter beginning adjacent to the central canal of the spinal cord, and is associated with an enlarging accumulation of fluid within the spinal cord. Its clinical hallmarks are atrophy and dissociated anesthesia beginning in the upper extremities. The first manifestation is often a loss of sensation to pain and temperature in the involved dermatomes (although tactile sensation remains intact) that is caused by destruction of the pain fibers crossing anterior to the central canal of the spinal cord. The area of destruction forms a cavity that then extends into the anterior horn and destroys the motor neurons and causes atrophy and weakness in the involved segments. As the disease progresses, evidence of involvement of the long motor and sensory pathways in the spinal cord often occurs as well. Scoliosis is frequently present, and neurogenic arthropathies develop in the later stages of the disorder. The location of the lesion has led to the constellation of typical neurologic findings being referred to as a central cord syndrome, and the association of these deficits with syringomyelia has led to the name syringomyelic cord syndrome.

The typical spinal syndrome is frequently accompanied by a dysfunction of the lower brain, in which case the syringomyelia is said to be accompanied by "syringobulbia." The common manifestations of this bulbar dysfunction include upper—and lower—motor neuron signs in the bulbar musculature, gait difficulties caused by involvement of cerebellar and corticospinal pathways, and variable nystagmus. Operative experience in 56 patients with syringomyelic syndrome has led the authors to conclude that hydromyelia, a condition in which the central canal of the spinal cord communicates with the fourth ventricle and is distended by cerebrospinal fluid (CSF), is the most common cause of the syringomyelic syndrome, and that the Chiari malformation that invariably accompanies hydromyelia is the cause of the syringobulbic syndrome.

The syringomyelic cord syndrome is a relatively uncommon disorder. In a survey of neurologic disease in an English city, Brewis and his colleagues found a prevalence rate of 8.4 cases for each 100,000 persons.[1]

The pathologic basis of the syringomyelic cord syndrome is frequently misunderstood. Since the initial description of the clinical syndrome in the last century,[2] syringomyelia incorrectly has become synonymous with an untreatable degenerative condition, rather than correctly descriptive of a pressure distension of the spinal cord caused by a developmental anomaly. Authorities as prominent as those writing in *Merritt's Neurology Textbook* classify syringomyelia as a degenerative process for which "there is no satisfactory treatment."[3] This misconception derives from the traditional impression that the syringomyelic type of neurologic deficit is caused by a degenerative cavitation and gliosis beginning adjacent to, but not communicating with, the central canal of the spinal cord; syringobulbia has been assumed to be caused by a rostral extension of the degenerative process into the brain stem.

The inaccuracy of this traditional concept is illustrated by the fact that not one of the more than 50 patients whom we have treated for a spontaneously appearing syringomyelic cord syndrome was found to have degenerative cavitation and gliosis within the spinal cord; approximately three fourths were caused by hydromyelia associated with Chiari malformation (Figure 115-1), and the remainder were caused by an intramedullary tumor.[4,5] These findings correspond with those of other reports on large series[611] in showing that the most frequent cause of the spontaneously appearing slowly progressive central cord deficit that we call the syringomyelic cord syndrome is distension of the spinal cord by a collection of CSF that communicates freely with the central canal of the spinal cord and, at its rostral end, communicates in turn with the fourth ventricle. This syndrome is invariably associated with an Chiari malformation or some other developmental anomaly that occludes the foramen of Magendie.

In response to these findings, Gardner put forward the "hydrodynamic theory of the development of the syringomyelia," by proposing that cystic dilatation of the cord—originating in embryonic life and resulting from overdistension of the neural tube because of a partial or complete obstruction at the foramen of Magendie—results in slowly progressive dilatation of the central canal or a ramifying diverticulum originating in the central canal and in continuity with the spinal fluid pathways through the fourth ventricle.[7]

Earlier authors studying cavitation of the spinal cord suggested that the term syringomyelia be reserved for cavities unconnected with the central canal, and that pathologic dilatation of the central canal as a developmental anomaly be referred to as hydromyelia.[2,12] A review of large series of patients reported in the literature reveals, however, that cavities unconnected with the central canal occur rarely, except in association with intramedullary tumors.[6–11] Barnett and his colleagues agree that a hydromyelic cavity is the most likely cause of a spontaneously appearing central cord syndrome, but they refer

OPERATIVE NEUROSURGICAL TECHNIQUES
ISBN 0-8089-1862-1

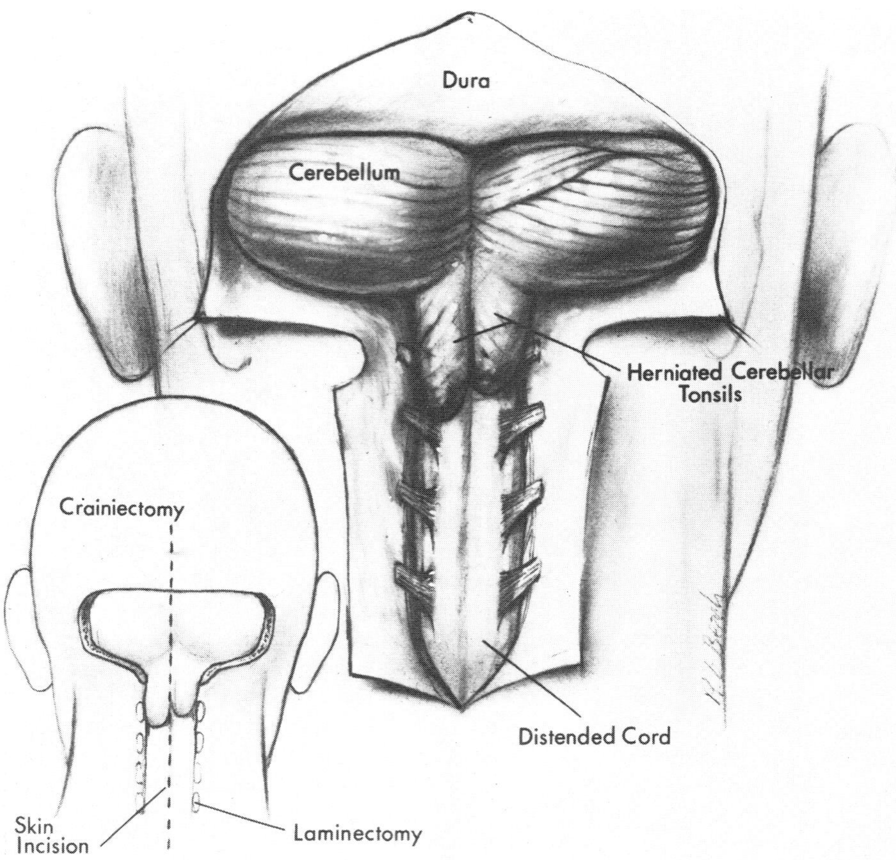

Fig. 115-1. Surgical exposure of an Chiari malformation and hydromyelia. (The operation is performed with the patient in the sitting position). Lower left: A midline incision (dotted line) is used to expose the suboccipital and upper cervical region. Upper right: Surgical exposure of the Chiari malformation showing the caudally displaced cerebellar tonsils, abnormal ascending course of the cervical nerve roots, and the cervical spinal cord distended by the hydromyelic cavity. (Reprinted from Rhoton AL: Syringomyelia, in Wilson CB, Hoff JT (eds): Current Surgical Management of Neurologic Disease. New York, Churchill-Livingston, 1980, pp 29–45. With permission.)

to the condition not as hydromyelia but as communicating syringomyelia.[6] I prefer to refer to the dynamic cord pathology associated with Chiari malformation as hydromyelia because of the traditional association of the term syringomyelia with an untreatable degenerative disease.

Chiari, in 1888, reported that most syringomyelic cavities were, in fact, hydromyelic cavities connected with the central canal of the spinal cord and were associated with the cerebellar deformity that bears his name.[12] The Chiari malformation is characterized by displacement of the cerebellar tonsils, the brain stem, and the fourth ventricle into the upper spinal canal. Because this malformation accompanies hydrocephalus and myelomeningocele in the infant, clinicians who encounter an adult with a spontaneously appearing, slowly progressive central cord syndrome—but no history of hydrocephalus or myelomeningocele—often consider diagnoses other than Chiari malformation and hydromyelia, when in fact that is most frequently the correct diagnosis.

In my series of patients, the second most common cystic spinal lesion producing a syringomyelic-type cord syndrome was an intramedullary tumor associated with a cyst. The cysts did not communicate with the central canal, were not associated with a hindbrain malformation, and contained yellow or brown fluid with an elevated protein content.

Cysts can develop within the spinal cord after traumatic paraplegia, Pott's disease, and arachnoiditis.[6] Posttraumatic

cysts produce a slowly ascending progressive deficit that develops long after the event and causes the acute traumatic paraplegia. Barnett and his colleagues differentiated cystic lesions in the spinal cord into a noncommunicating form and a communicating form, based on whether they communicate with the central canal or with the spinal cord.[6] The noncommunicating form was associated with an intramedullary tumor and posttraumatic paraplegia, and the communicating form resulted from persistent dilatation of the central canal under pressure associated with a developmental anomaly obstructing the foramen of Magendie. The latter is by far the most common cause of a syringomyelic cord syndrome.

The improved understanding of the pathogenesis of syringomyelic cord syndrome that has accrued in recent years has led to a more rational approach to surgical treatment than was previously the case. This chapter focuses on those patients who have the syndrome of hydromyelia associated with an Chiari malformation, because it is the most common cause of a syringomyelic cord syndrome, and because it presents the most difficult problems with respect to diagnosis and treatment.

CLINICAL FACTORS

Most central cervical cord syndromes are caused by hydromyelia associated with an Chiari malformation, which is a surgically treatable condition. For this reason, an active inves-

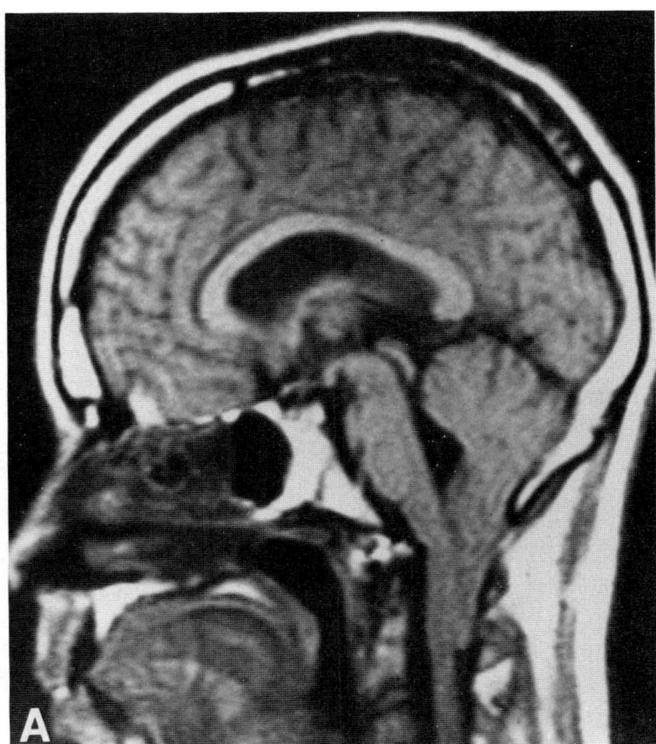

Fig. 115-2A

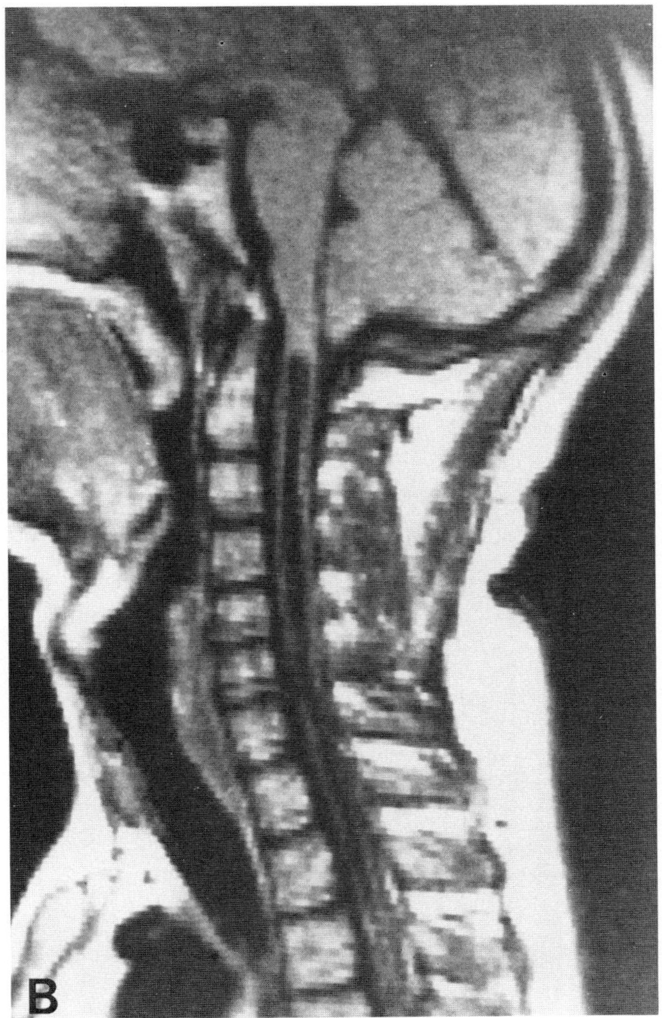

Fig. 115-2B

tigational attitude should be adopted so that the disorder is recognized and treated early, because patients who have progressed beyond a certain stage of disability have little likelihood of achieving a useful recovery.

All of our patients with Chiari malformation and hydromyelia were between the ages of 16 and 72 years. No patient had a prior history of hydrocephalus or myelomeningocele. All patients with hydromyelia had signs and symptoms referable to it, but only one third had signs referable to the Chiari malformation. A number of patients in this series, who were initially diagnosed as having untreatable degenerative disease because the size of the spinal cord (as defined on positive-contrast myelography) was normal, progressed to develop crippling deficits before it was discovered that they had an Chiari malformation with hydromyelia. In approximately one fourth of our patients with a syringomyelic cord syndrome, the cause was a cystic intramedullary tumor. The group of patients with hydromyelia differed from the group with intramedullary tumors, in that patients with hydromyelia commonly had bulbar signs, whereas those with tumors did not.

Sensory loss usually preceded lower motor neuron signs. The deficits produced by the hydromyelia ranged in severity from a minimal motor deficit or subjective sensory loss, or both, to a widespread sensory loss and quadriparesis with marked atrophy of the upper extremities and atrophy or spasticity in the lower extremities. In the early stages, the sensory deficit frequently began and was greater on one side, rather than being bilaterally symmetrical. The weakness and atrophy most commonly began and were greatest in the hands, but in 3 cases, shoulder-girdle involvement was so great that the arms could not be abducted at the shoulders, while strength in the hands was relatively preserved. In the later stages, compression of the corticospinal tracts and long sensory pathways resulted in a spastic gait and sensory loss in the lower extremities. Five patients, who were followed without surgery after the initial

diagnosis because their neurologic deficits were minimal, worsened and were operated upon within 1 year after the initial diagnosis.

The patients with brain stem symptoms caused by the Chiari malformation had a combination of upper and lower motor neuron signs in the bulbar musculature, gait difficulties caused by cerebellar and long tract involvement, and nystagmus. Some patients with Chiari malformation have experienced sudden, severe respiratory stridor caused by bilateral vocal cord paralysis and a rapid onset or progression of other symptoms. Bertrand has described the mechanism for a sudden onset or change of symptoms in cases of the Chiari malformation.[13]

Although defective ventricular drainage is thought to be important in the development of hydromyelia, no patient in this series had either hydrocephalus or evidence of increased intracranial pressure.

DIAGNOSIS

RADIOLOGY

The initial radiologic examination of patients with Chiari malformation and hydromyelia, which consists of plain x-ray films of the skull and cervical spine, frequently shows normal results. In the past, it was assumed that a normal skull and

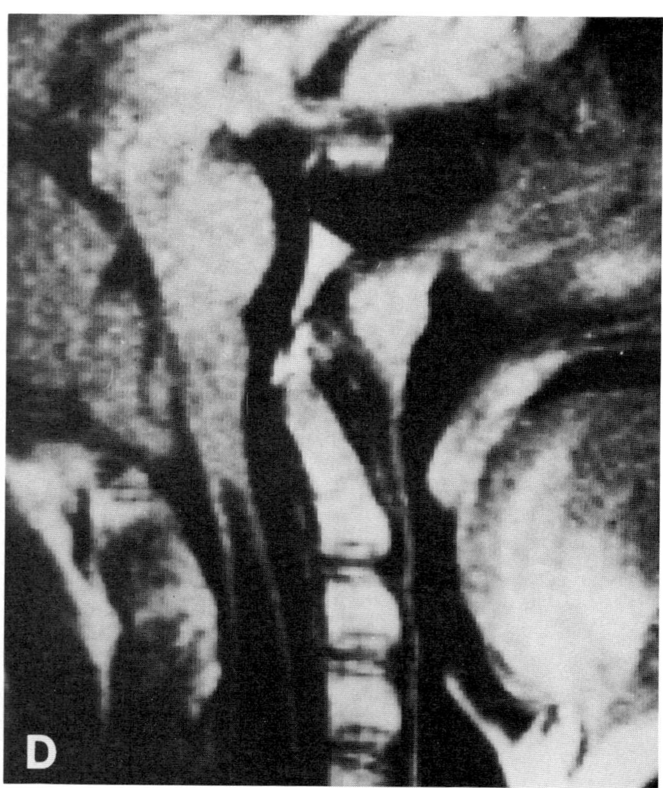

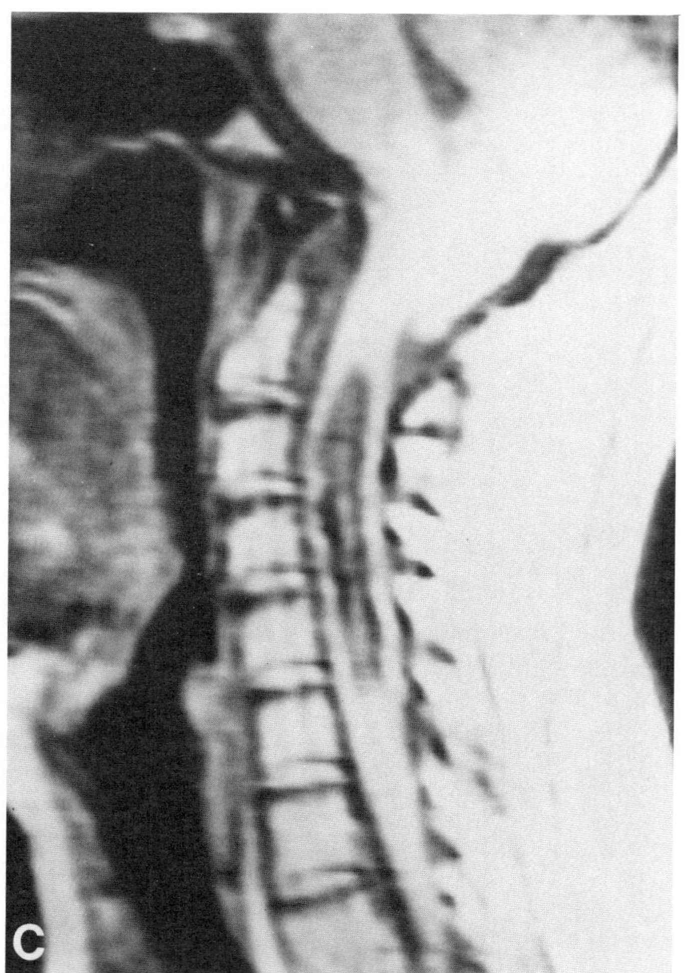

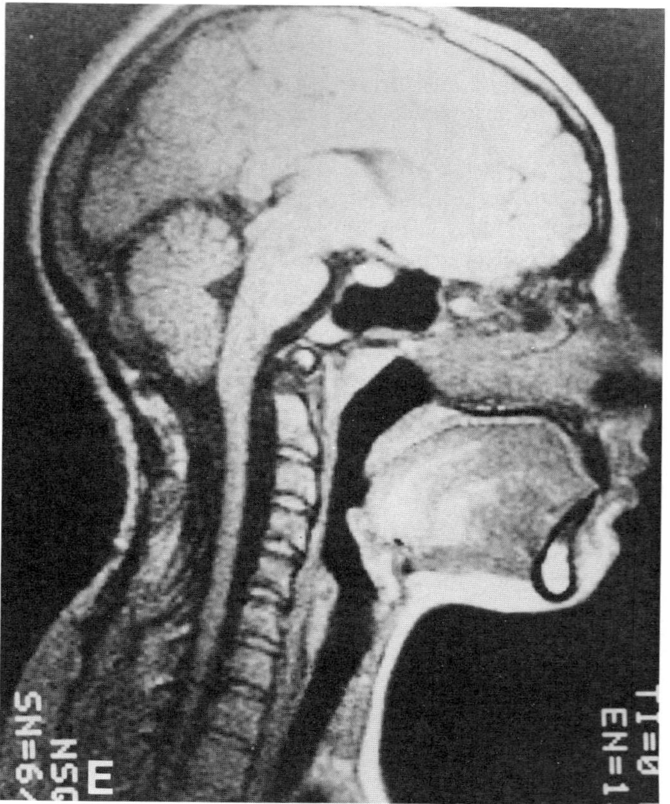

Fig. 115-2. Magnetic resonance images of Chiari malformation and hydromyelia from selected patients. (A) Left lateral view. Chiari malformation without hydromyelia. The cerebellar tonsils are herniated downward to the level of C-2. (B) Left lateral view. This patient with a Chiari malformation also has a hydromyelic cavity. The cavity in the spinal cord extends from the level of the foramen magnum, through the cervical region into the upper thoracic area. (C) Left lateral view. This patient has a hydromyelic cavity with a septum in the central part of the hydromyelic cavity. (D and E) Scan from a patient before (D) and after (E) surgical treatment. (D) MRI before surgical treatment showing the Chiari malformation and the hydromyelic cavity. (E) MRI scan obtained 1 year following suboccipital craniectomy and upper cervical laminectomy and drainage of the cavity through the dorsal root entry zone. Spinal cord size has returned to normal and the cavity within the spinal cord has disappeared.

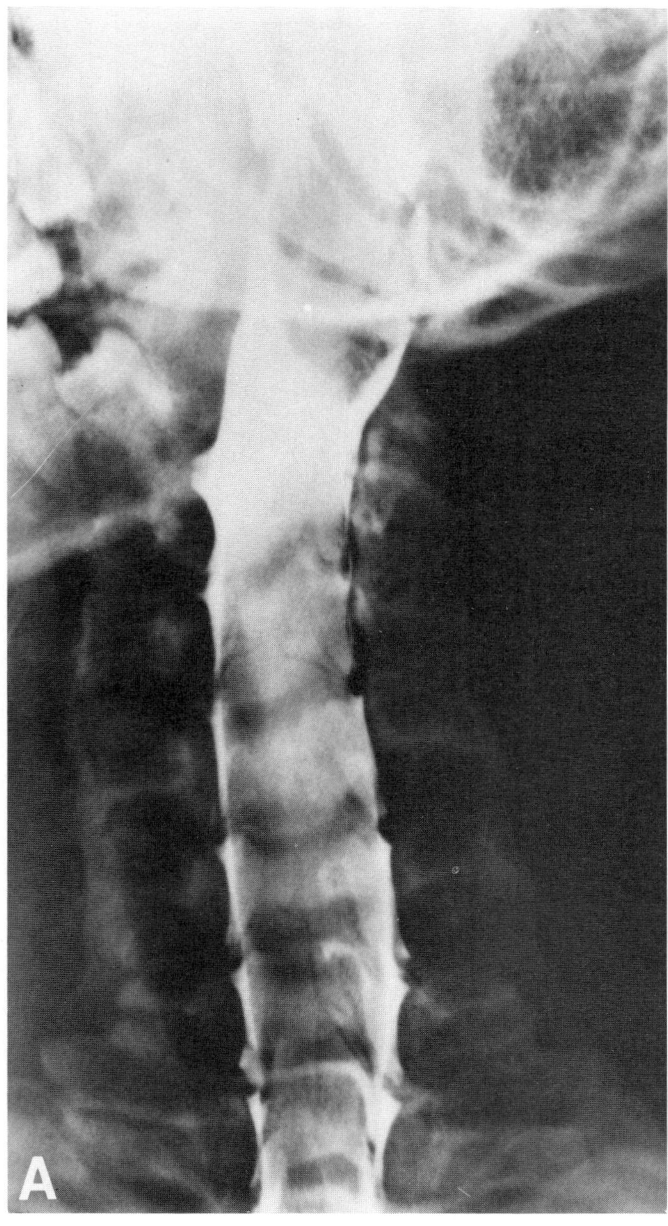

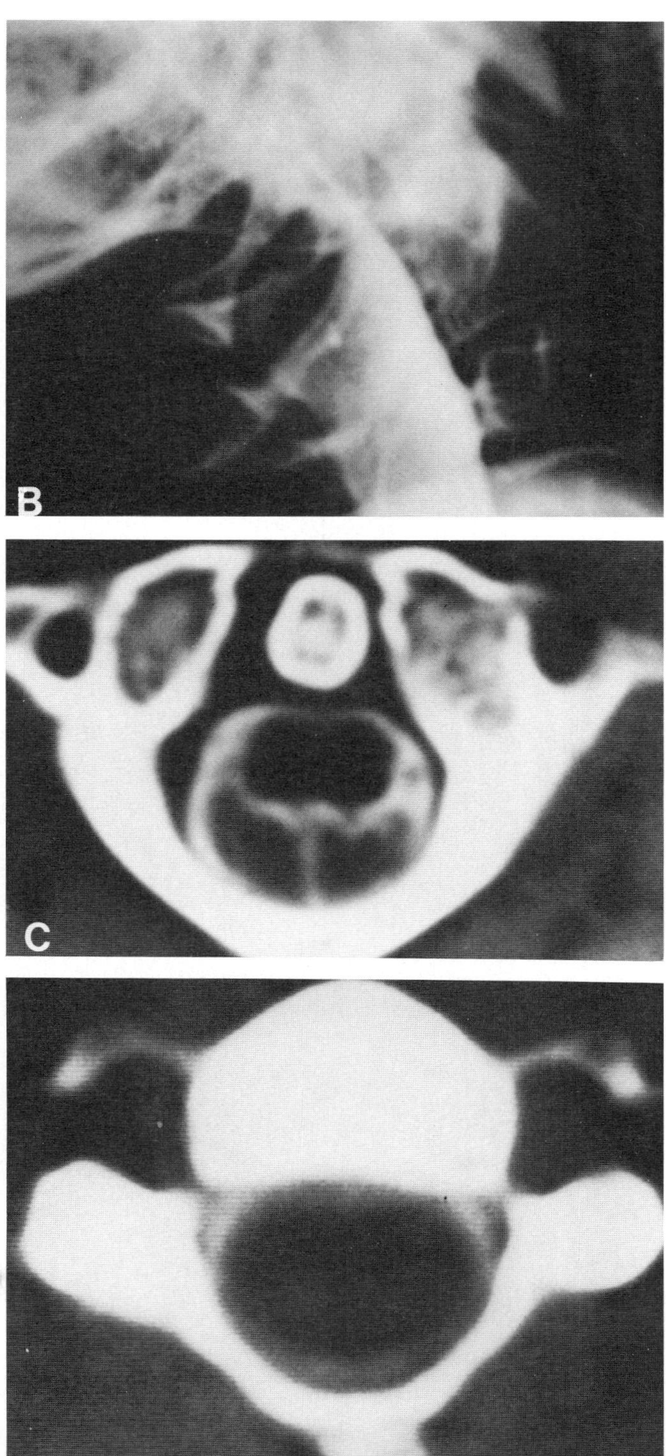

cervical spine excluded the diagnosis of Chiari malformation and hydromyelia; however, our patients infrequently had anomalies of the skull, cervical spine, or craniovertebral junction, such as a basilar impression, Kippel-Feil deformity, atlanto-occipital fusion, or widening of the anteroposterior (AP) diameter of the cervical spinal canal. In patients with an intramedullary tumor, plain x-ray films may reveal focal enlargement of the spinal cord, thinning of the pedicles and laminae, and scalloping of the vertebral bodies. In those with hydromyelia, the AP diameter of the spine may be enlarged, but there are none of the features of focal expansion that are seen with intramedullary tumors.

Magnetic resonance imaging (MRI), if available, is the preferred technique for evaluating patients suspected of having a Chiari malformation and hydromyelia (Figure 115-2). It provides information about the extent of the descent of the cerebellar tonsils and fourth ventricle into the foramen magnum and upper spinal canal, the transverse diameter and rostrocaudal extent of the hydromyelic cavity, and the size of the lateral ventricles. Magnetic resonance imaging will frequently provide all the information needed to plan a surgical approach to these conditions. In addition, it will demonstrate the disappearance of the hydromyelic cavity with successful therapy (Figure 115-2).

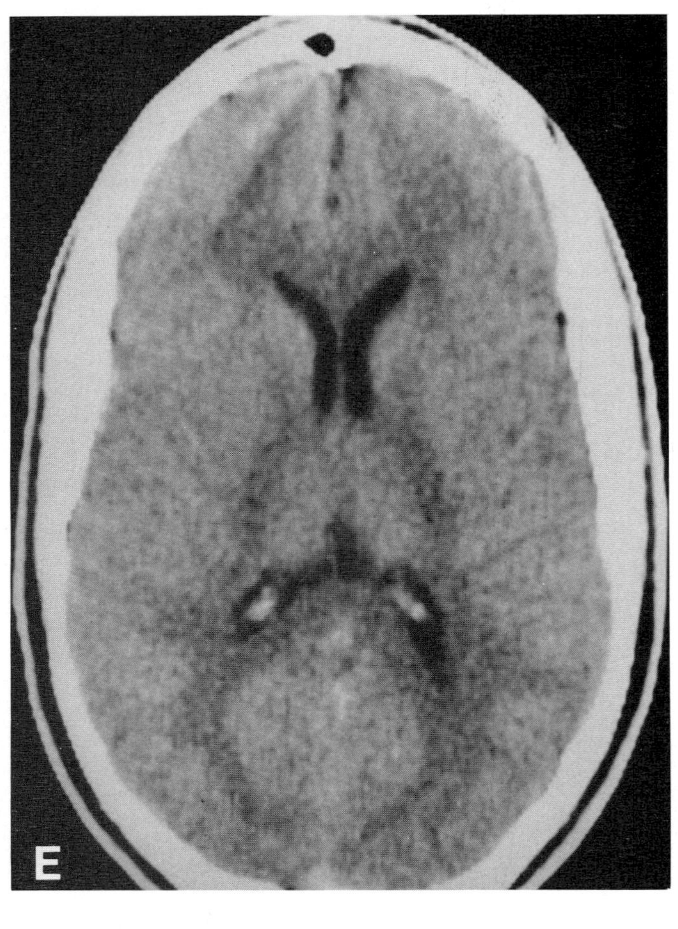

E

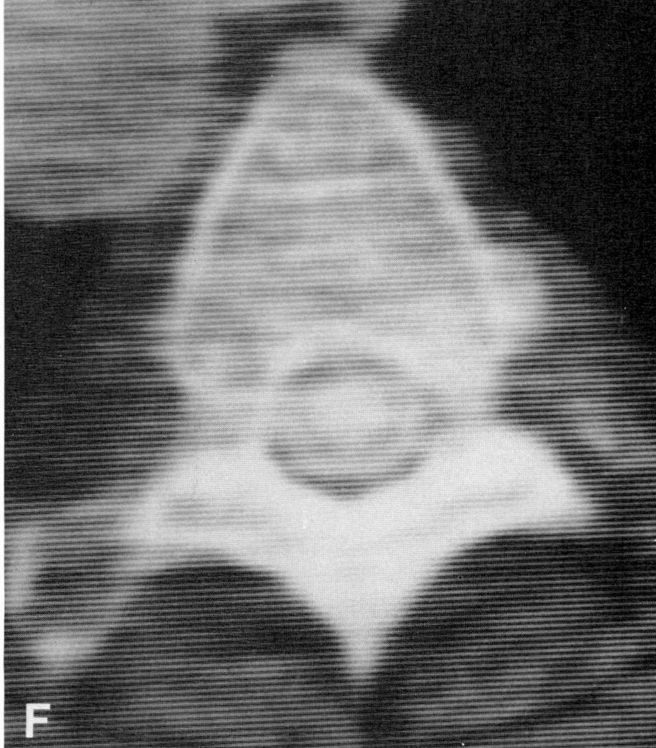

F

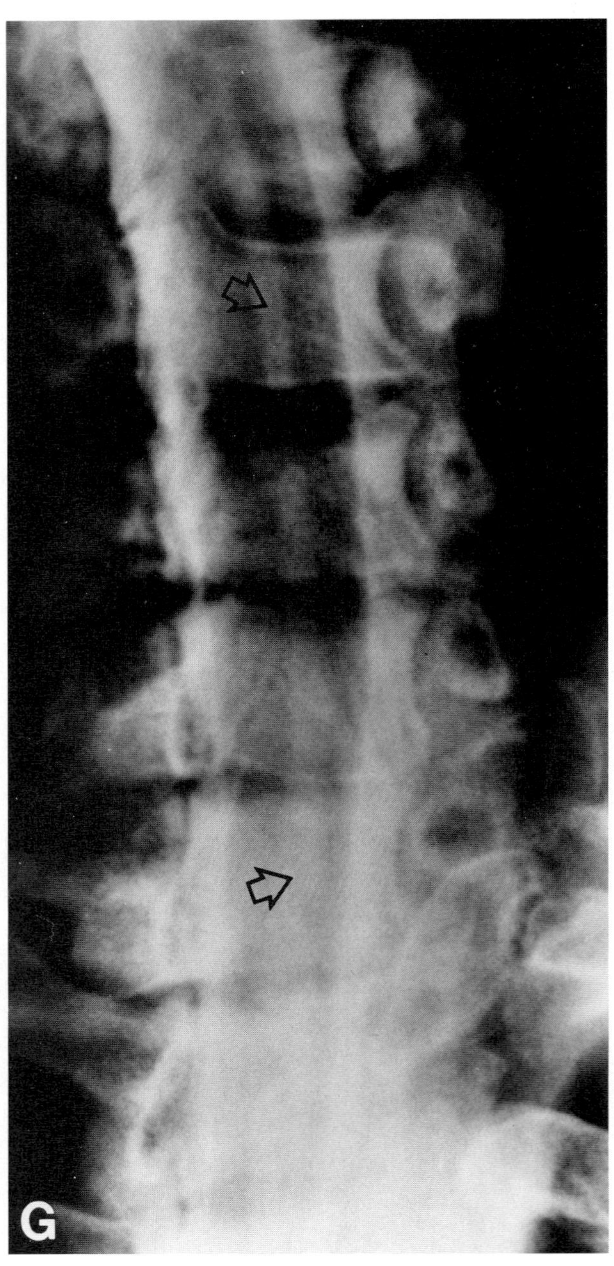

G

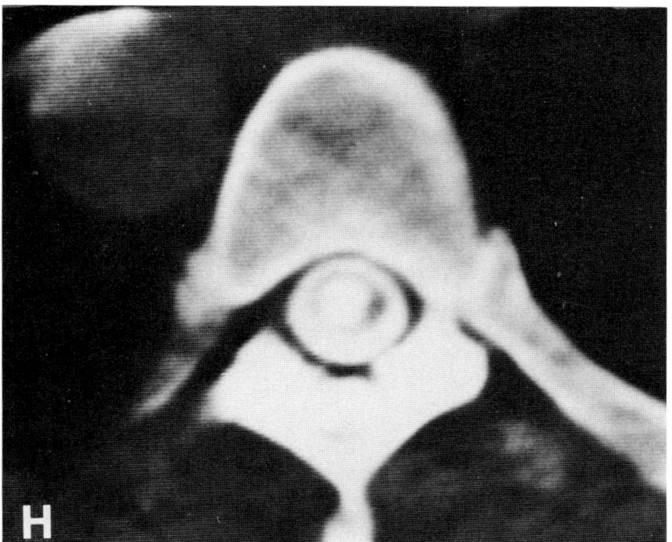

Myelography, using water-soluble contrast medium, when combined with computed tomography (CT), provides another excellent method of evaluating these patients (Figure 115-3). It may also be done if MRI does not provide the information needed for diagnosis and treatment. A CT scan alone will show the caudal displacement of the fourth ventricle and cerebellar tonsils, but has only infrequently shown the enlarged spinal cord and the hydromyelic cavity. A CT scan done after the intrathecal injection of metrizamide will show the tonsillar herniation and the enlargement of the spinal cord (Figure 115-3). A CT scan delayed 8 to 24 hours after infection may show that the contrast medium has entered the cavity in the spinal cord. The hydromyelic cavity may be situated centrally or asymetrically within the cord, and it may vary from level to level in its position (Figure 115-3H and I). Plain x-ray films may rarely show the contrast medium within the hydromyelic cavity (Figure 115-3G).

In the past, the procedure most helpful in defining the cause of syringomyelic cord syndrome was positive-contrast myelography using Pantopaque and obtained with the patient in both the prone and supine positions (Figures 115-4 and 115-5). In patients with hydromyelia, Pantopaque myelography with the patient supine will outline the Chiari malformation; frequently, the prone study will reveal no abnormalities, showing normal cord size even when the patient has a large cavity that produces a marked neurologic deficit (Figure 115-5). A number

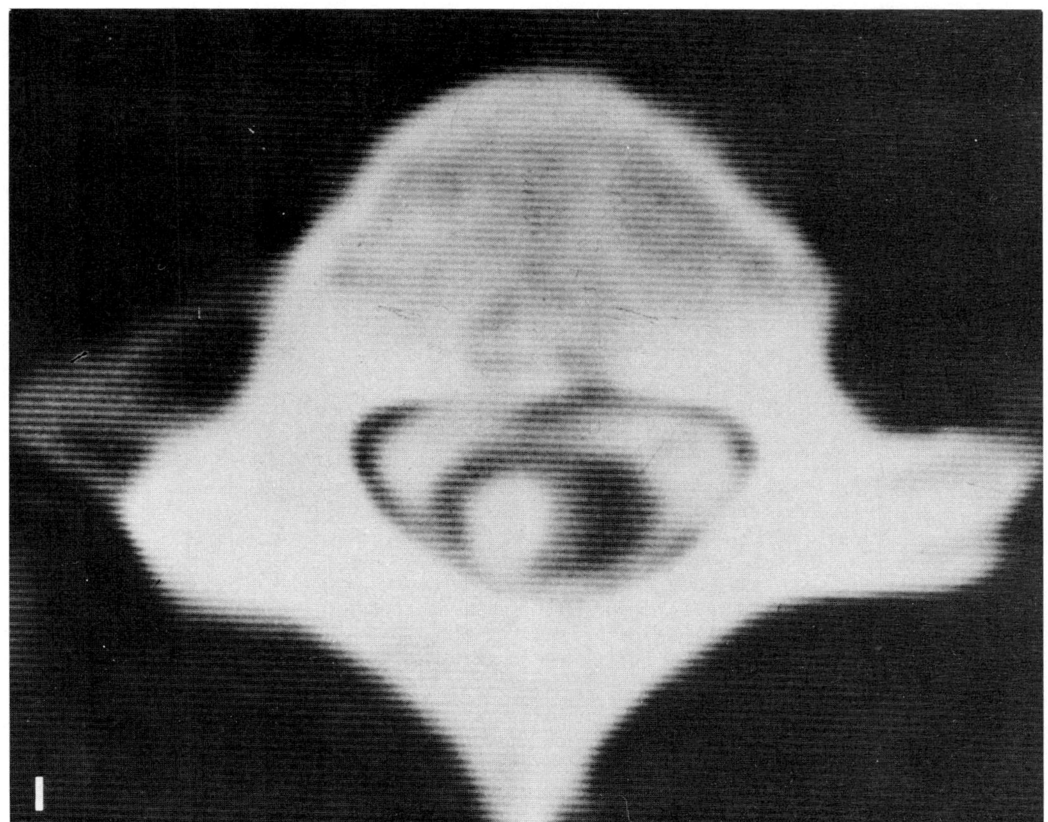

Fig. 115-3.   Myelograms with water-soluble contrast medium and CT scans from selected patients with Chiari malformation and hydromyelia. A-E are from one patient. (A) Myelographic study following the intrathecal administration of metrizamide. Oblique view showing the herniated cerebellar tonsils and the enlarged cervical spinal cord. (B) Right lateral view showing the herniated cerebellar tonsils. (C) Axial CT scan through the level of the odontoid process showing the cerebellar tonsils herniated into the upper spinal canal behind the spinal cord. (D) CT scan showing the enlarged spinal cord. (E) CT scan of head showing the lateral ventricles to be of normal size. (F) CT scan from another patient, 12 hours after intrathecal installation of metrizamide, showing the accumulation of contrast medium within the spinal cord. G-I are from another patient with a Chiari malformation. (G) During the myelogram, the metrizamide entered the hydromyelic cavity (arrows). (H) Axial CT scan showing the metrizamide in the hydromyelic cavity that fills the central part of the spinal cord. (I) Axial CT scan at another level, showing the cavity situated in one half of the cord.

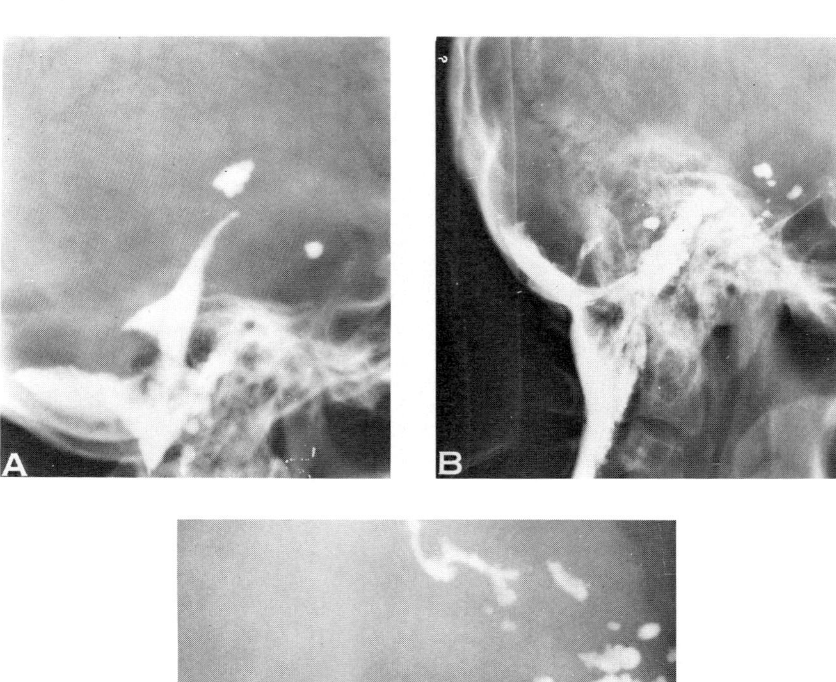

Fig. 115-4. Myelograms, with Pantopaque, of the Chiari malformation from selected patients. (A) Normal lateral view of a Pantopaque study with the patient in the supine position. Pantopaque fills the cisterna magna and the fourth ventricle to the level of the aqueduct. (B) A Pantopaque myelogram done with the patient in the supine position outlines the cerebellar tonsils indicative of the Chiari malformation. (C) A Pantopaque study of the foramen magnum with the patient in the supine position, showing the Chiari malformation. No Pantopaque passes into the cisterna magna above the level of the foramen magnum. At surgery, dense adhesions were found in the area of the cisterna magna that bound the medulla and cerebellum to the dura. (Reprinted from Rhoton AL: Microsurgery of Arnold-Chiari malformation in adults with and without hydromyelia. J Neurosurg 45:473–483, 1976. With permission.)

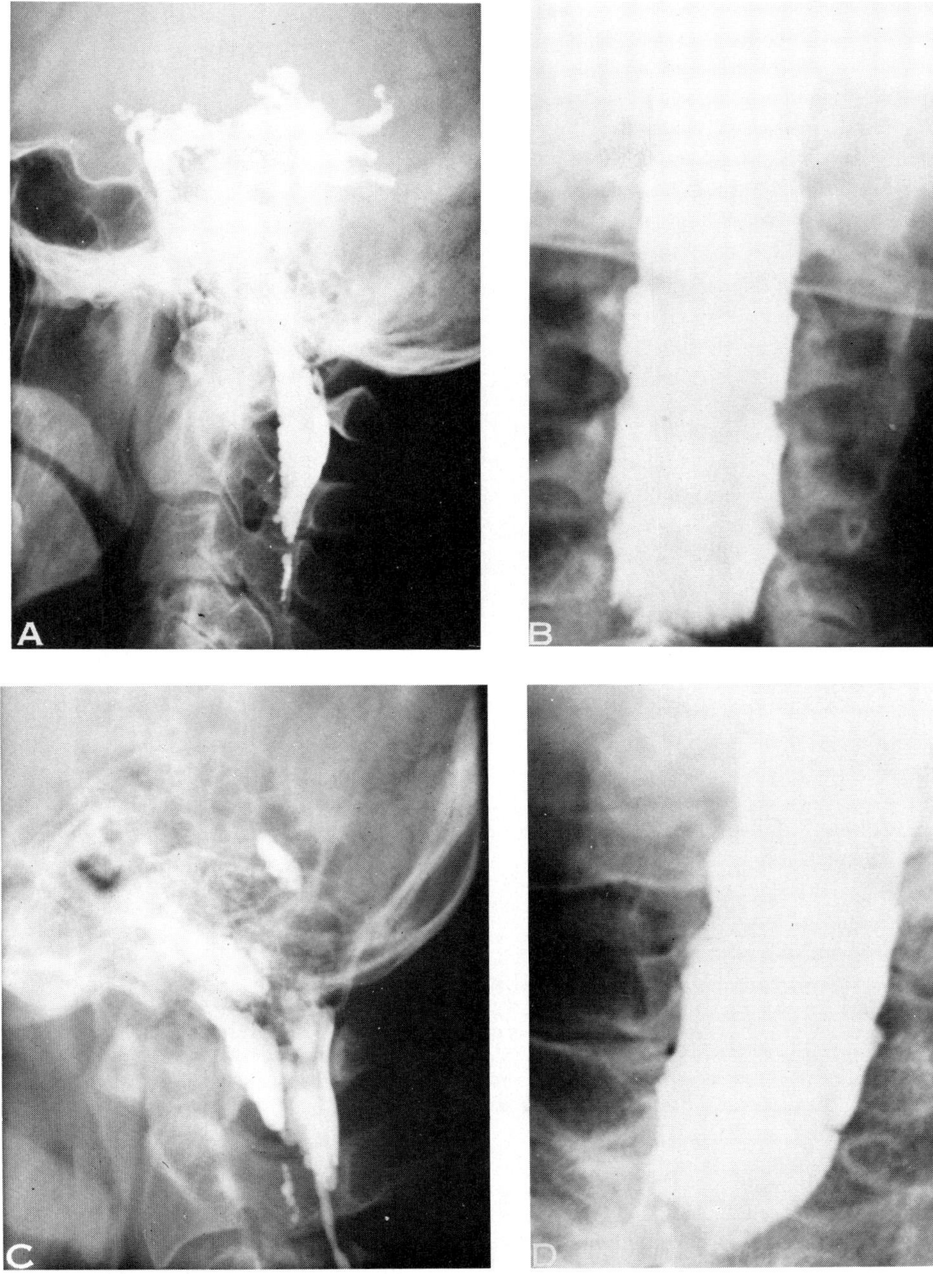

Fig. 115-5. Myelograms with Pantopaque. A and B are from one patient; C and D are from another patient. Both patients had previous myelograms that were reported to be normal. Myelograms B and D show no striking abnormalities in the cervical regions. A diagnosis of degenerative disease had been made because the cord size appeared normal on previous myelograms. Pantopaque studies (lateral view) of the foramen magnum with both patients in the supine position (A and C) show the Chiari malformation causing obstruction to filling of the cisterna magna. The findings from supine Pantopaque myelography led to a diagnosis of Arnold-Chiari malformation with hydromyelia. (Reprinted from Rhoton AL: Microsurgery of Arnold-Chiari malformation in adults with and without hydromyelia. J Neurosurg 45:473–483, 1976. With permission.)

of our patients with hydromyelia were initially diagnosed as having untreatable degenerative disease, because myelography with Pantopaque of the cervical and thoracic regions showed that cord size was normal. In these patients, the disease had progressed, and they developed marked deficits before the correct diagnosis was established. Barnett and his colleagues also noted that myelographic studies of the spinal cord alone may give normal results, even if the patient in fact has hydromyelia.[6]

Spinal cord deficits are assumed to be caused by hydromyelia—even if the cord is of normal size or only minimally enlarged—if the neurologic deficit is typical of syringomyelia and if the myelogram with Pantopaque or metrizamide, or the CT scan, shows the Chiari malformation. We have seen patients in whom deficits caused by a hydromyelic cavity were far advanced, but in whom cord diameter was normal on myelograms, and we would conclude that the pia mater covering the spinal cord apparently restricts the ability of

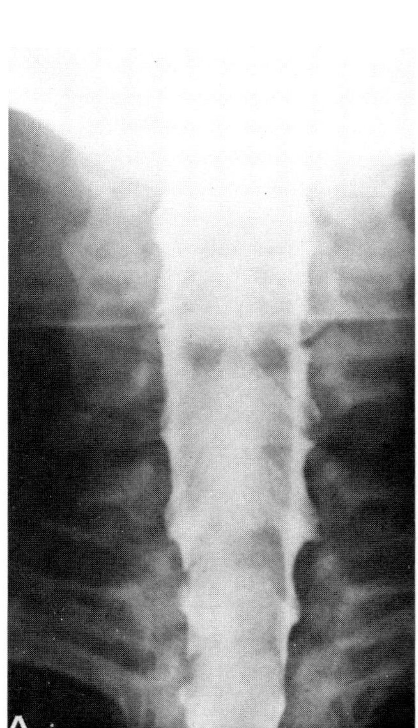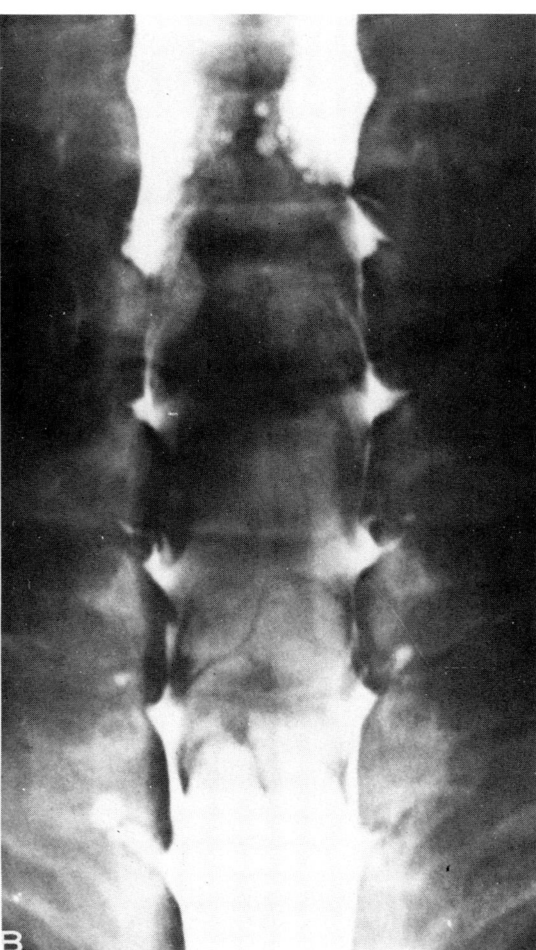

Fig. 115-6. Myelographic studies made using Pantopaque. (A) Pantopaque study of the cervical region, showing dilatation of the cord associated with a hydromyelic deficit that is far advanced. Even in the advanced stages of hydromyelia, the myelographic picture is not as striking as one in which the obstruction is caused by an intramedullary tumor. (B) Pantopaque study showing an intramedullary tumor. The hydromyelia presents a more diffuse enlargement; tumor enlargement is more localized. (Reprinted from Rhoton AL: Microsurgery of Arnold-Chiari malformation in adults with and without hydromyelia. J Neurosurg 45:473–483, 1976. With permission.)

the cord to enlarge with a hydromyelic cavity.

In comparison with hydromyelia, an intramedullary tumor commonly produces a more striking picture of cord enlargement on the myelogram (Figure 115-6). Even when an intramedullary tumor is diagnosed early, it has often caused striking enlargement of the cord, and frequently is associated with an almost complete block. When present, the enlargement produced by hydromyelia is diffuse over many segments, whereas typically the enlargement caused by a tumor is more localized. Exceptions to this rule occur but are uncommon.

The author has limited experience with the use of gas myelography in the investigation of hydromyelia. The hydromyelic cord may appear thin or atrophic on air studies done with the patient upright, because the intramedullary fluid settles to the bottom of the cavity when air surrounds it. The gas delineates the cerebellar tonsils below the foramen magnum and an elongated flaccid cyst of the spinal cord. Ellertsson,[14] by tilting the patient during gas myelography, has demonstrated that the hydromyelic cavity may appear flaccid or distended, fluctuating in size depending on the position of the patient during the study. He also has shown that the enlargement of the spinal cord caused by a tumor is nonfluctuating. Pneumo-

myelography in patients with hydromyelia demonstrates a full cord if the study is done with the patient's head dependent, and demonstrates a thin cord when done with the patient upright.

Angiograms will show the displacement of the cerebellar tonsils associated with the Chiari malformation as defined by the descent of the posterior inferior cerebellar artery, but otherwise angiography is not helpful except to show the size of the lateral ventricles and to diagnostically exclude a tumor in the posterior fossa as the cause of the caudally displaced cerebellar tonsils.

SURGICAL TREATMENT AND RESULTS

CHIARI MALFORMATION WITH HYDROMYELIA

Patients with this condition (Chiari malformation with hydromyelia) should be treated with a suboccipital craniectomy and upper cervical laminectomy to decompress the malformation at the foramen magnum. If the fourth ventricle is blocked, an outlet for it should be established using microsurgical techniques, and the hydromyelic cavity should be drained. The greater accuracy of dissection obtained by the use of surgical magnification techniques facilitates dissection through the scar over the fourth ventricle, the identification of the proper area in which to incise the cord, and the final incision into the spinal cord.

The operation is usually done with the patient sitting, and with the neck in a neutral position. Marked flexion of the neck during the surgery for the Chiari malformation has been reported to increase the neurologic deficit or to cause respiratory problems.[15] A suboccipital craniectomy and a C1-C4 laminectomy are done through a midline skin incision to decompress the Chiari malformation (Figure 115-1). The elongated cerebellar tonsils vary in appearance from those that are normal in color and consistency to those that are white and firm because of scarring and gliosis (Figures 115-7A and 115-8). The caudal loop of the posterior inferior cerebellar artery often descends to the level of C2, marking the lower margin of the cerebellar tonsils (Figures 115-7A and 115-8A).

The degree to which the dura and arachnoid will adhere to the spinal cord and medulla can be predicted from the myelogram. If contrast medium passes freely, although slowly, between the arachnoid and the cerebellar tonsils, the meninges can be separated easily from the tonsils. If the contrast medium passes into the cisterna magna, then the cerebellar tonsils will be found adherent to the arachnoid and the dura. If a plaque of arachnoid and dura is adherent to the dorsal surface of the medulla and the spinal cord, it should be left attached, because an attempt to disconnect it might injure the neural tissue (Figure 115-7B). If the foramen of Magendie is blocked, its lower part should be opened in the midline, and care should be taken to make certain that the dissection is far enough superior to enter the fluid cavity of the fourth ventricle rather than the cord or medulla. After the fourth ventricle is opened, a Silastic wick is attached to the dura and passed up into the new opening in the midline (Figures 115-9 through 115-11). The Silastic wick is used to maintain the patency of the outlet rather than as a conduit for drainage.

The cord should be incised longitudinally in the dorsal root entry zone between the lateral and posterior columns, because inspection with the aid of the surgical microscope has consistently revealed this to be the thinnest area in patients withhydromyelia (Figures 115-9 through 115-11). The natural dissection of the cavity along the dorsal root entry zone also leads to a proprioceptive deficit in the upper extremities; hence, incision here minimizes the possibility of increasing the patient's deficit because the arm fibers course in the lateral part of the posterior columns adjacent to the root entry zone.

The posterolateral myelotomy used in treating cases of hydromyelia is different from the midline myelotomy between the gracile fasciculi (which carry the lower-extremity fibers) that is made to expose and remove an intramedullary tumor (Figures 115-11 through 115-15). The cord usually is thinnest on the side of the greatest neurologic deficit. A needle should be introduced into the cavity at the thinnest area and fluid collected for cell count and protein determinations before the cord is incised. The fluid will be clear CSF with a normal protein level in patients with hydromyelia; an elevated protein value or colored fluid is indicative of an intramedullary tumor. A vertical incision of at least 1 cm in length then is made into the thinnest area along the dorsal root entry zone, and a Silastic wick, anchored to the dura above, is threaded downward into the myelotomy (Figures 115-9 through 115-12). The dura is loosely closed with a dural graft, and care should be taken to make sure the area around the Chiari malformation is not constricted.

There have been no deaths in the author's operative series, and the neurologic deficit was increased in only 2 patients as a result of surgery. One patient developed a mild proprioceptive sensory loss in the right thumb that did not impair the patient in performing work that required moderate dexterity. Another patient, who was quadriparetic and bed-ridden before surgery, experienced a further mild loss of strength in her only functional extremity as a result of surgery. No patient has shown further progression of deficits during follow-up periods ranging from 1 to 14 years.

A careful explanation, preoperatively, about the reasonable potential benefits of the operation are helpful in obtaining an optimal result from surgical therapy. Most patients report that their functional abilities are improved by the operation, although postoperative neurologic examination usually reveals approximately the same deficit as before operation. Because of this, patients are counselled before the operation, regarding the fact that the operation should stop the progression of the deficit, but that it will not restore the patient to normal. The operation commonly arrests the progression of muscle atrophy, prevents the size of areas of numbness from increasing, and may result in some improvement in strength. Most patients with preoperative pain, called anesthesia dolorosa, which is localized to areas of numbness, continue to experience exacerbations of this pain related to emotional stress, hunger, cold weather, and fatigue, after operation. Spasticity will also fluctuate after surgery, under the aforementioned conditions, although, on motor testing, there is no further loss of strength. We have also seen deformities at joints associated with muscle atrophy increase during the years after surgery, even though there has been no further atrophy or loss of strength. Magnetic resonance imaging has provided an excellent way of following these patients. However, even when postoperative MRI shows the hydromyelia to be absent, patients may continue to experience fluctuations in pain and spasticity, even though the size of analgesic areas, extent of muscle atrophy, and loss of strength do not progress.

We have seen 4 patients who were treated previously with a decompressive suboccipital craniectomy and upper cervical laminectomy, plus muscle plugging of the upper end of the central canal at the obex, but who did not have drainage of the hydromyelic cavity. Their neurologic deficits continued to progress. In these cases, we performed a hemilaminectomy in the thoracic region over the lower extent of the hydromyelic cavity, drained the fluid collection through the dorsal root entry zone, and threaded a Silastic wick, anchored to the dura, through the myelotomy (Figure 115-9).

Two patients had myelotomies of the dorsal root entry zone as the initial surgical procedure. If this procedure is to be done as the primary operation, the hemilaminectomy should be performed in the upper thoracic region below the cervical enlargement on the side of the greater deficit. The only patients in this group who were treated by this method were those who had no symptoms caused by their Chiari malformation, but who had a progressive deficit caused by the hydromyelia.

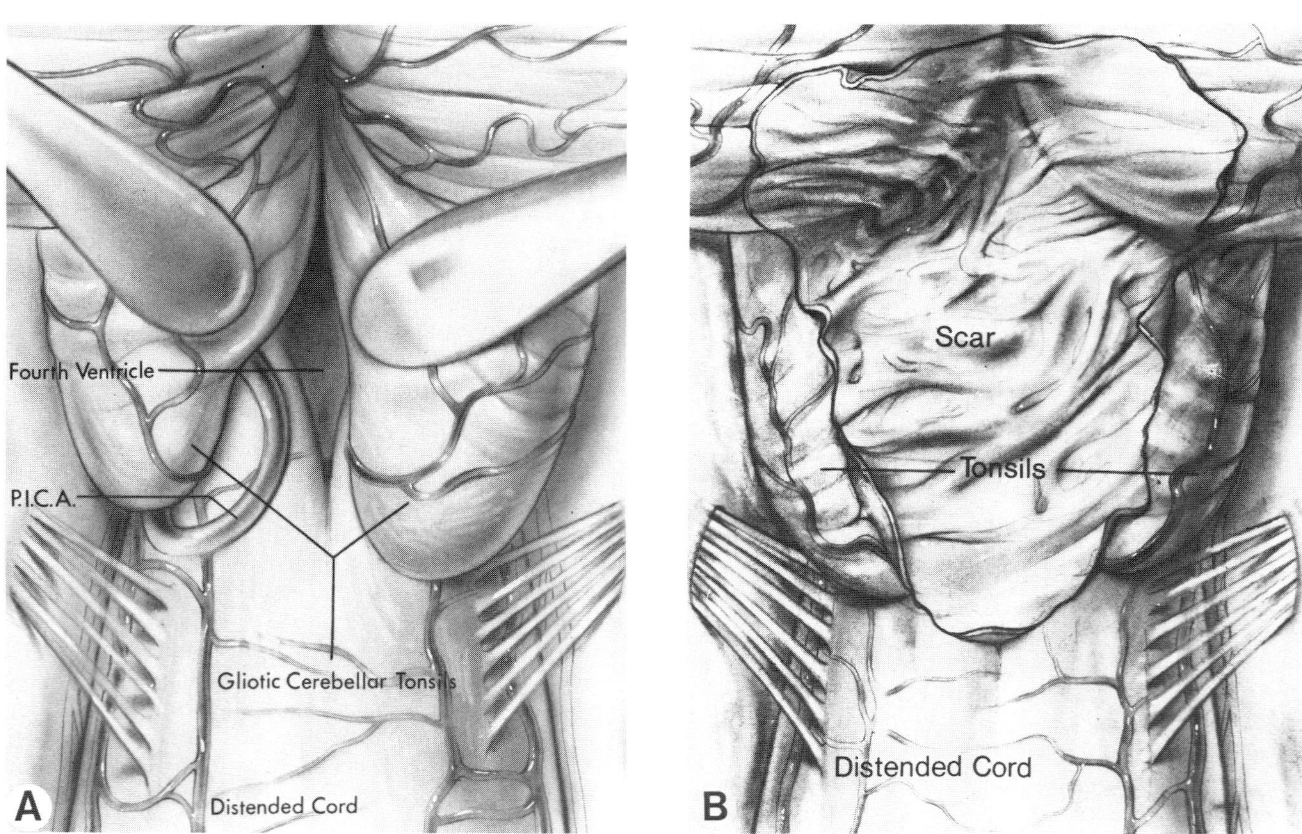

Fig. 115-7. Abnormalities at the outlet of the fourth ventricle with Chiari malformation. The patients are in the sitting position (see Figure 115-1). (A) Less complicated form of Chiari malformation. The herniated gliotic cerebellar tonsils, the ascending course of the cervical nerve roots, the abnormal caudal descent of the posterior inferior cerebellar artery, the loss of normal folial patterns over the tips of the herniated cerebellar tonsils, and the elongated fourth ventricle with the distended spinal cord below are shown. (B) A more complex deformity, with occlusion of the foramen of Magendie by a plaque of scar in which the pia, dura, and arachnoid are adherent to the dorsal medulla and cerebellum, occluding the outlet of the fourth ventricle. Disconnecting this mat of scar from the neural tissue could cause injury to the medulla, the cervical spinal cord, and the structures in the floor of the fourth ventricle; for that reason, the scar is not detached. The dura is opened by incising around the net of scar, which is left attached to the pia over these vital structures. (Reprinted from Rhoton AL: Syringomyelia, in Wilson CB, Hoff JT (eds): Current Surgical Management of Neurologic Disease. New York, Churchill-Livingstone, 1980, pp 29–45. With permission.)

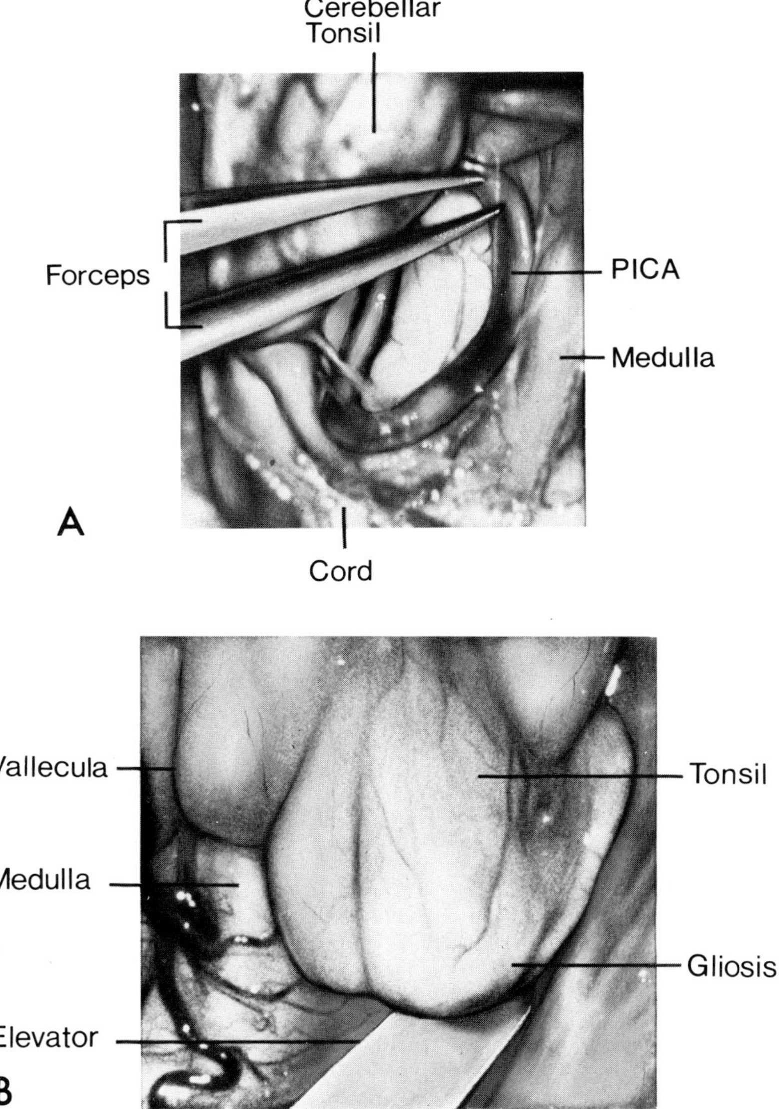

Fig. 115-8. Posterior views of Chiari malformations through suboccipital craniectomies. The photographs were taken through the surgical microscope at 6× magnification and were re-touched and labeled to increase clarity. (A) A caudal loop of the posterior inferior cerebellar artery (PICA) is displaced around the caudal margin of a herniated cerebellar tonsil. The lower margin of the tonsil was at C2. (B) The lower margin of the herniated cerebellar tonsil. Same patient as shown in Figure 115-2B. The pale color at the tip of the left cerebellar tonsil is caused by gliosis in herniated tonsillar tips. (Reprinted from Rhoton AL: Microsurgery of Arnold-Chiari malformation in adults with and without hydromyelia. J Neurosurg 45:473–483, 1976. With permission.)

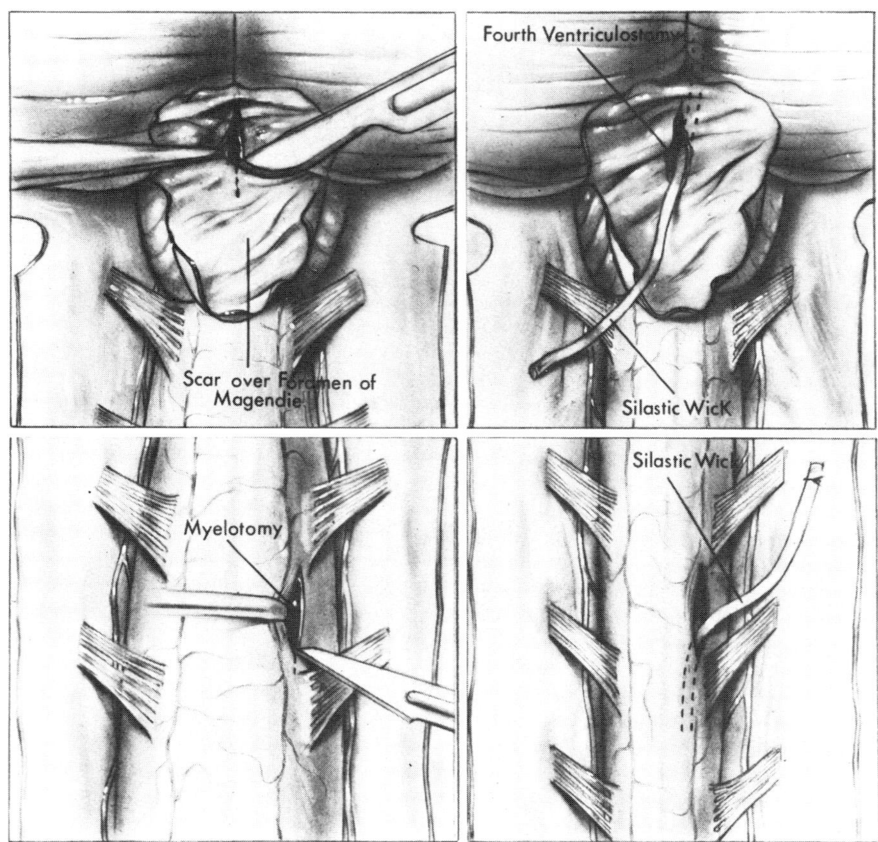

Fig. 115-9. The surgical approach used by the author for treating Chiari malformation with hydromyelia. A suboccipital craniectomy and upper cervical laminectomy has been done to expose and decompress the Chiari malformation (upper right and left) and to expose the hydromyelic spinal cord (lower right and left). The foramen of Magendie is re-established by opening through the upper part of the scar into the fourth ventricle (upper left). A Silastic wick is then anchored to the dura and led through the opening into the fourth ventricle (upper right). The hydromyelic cord is decompressed by opening through the thinnest area, which is consistently through the dorsal root entry zone, using a longitudinal incision placed along the course of the entry of the dorsal roots (lower left). A Silastic wick is then anchored to the dura and led downward into the hydromyelic cavity (lower right). After the incision, the distended cord becomes smaller. (Reprinted from Rhoton AL: Syringomyelia, in Wilson CB, Hoff JT (eds): Current Surgical Management of Neurologic Disease. New York, Churchill-Livingstone, 1980, pp 29–45. With permission.)

Scar over
Foramen of Magendie
cottonoid
Knife
Sharp
Hook
Dorsal
Root
Spinal Cord
Medulla
Scar
A

Scar over Vermis
S
Fourth
Ventricle
Dural
Scar
Dural
Scar
Dorsal
Root
Silastic
Tube
Midline Posterior
Columns
B

Posterior
Columns
Dorsal
Root
Protruding
fluid
collection
Lateral
Column
Midline
Needle
C

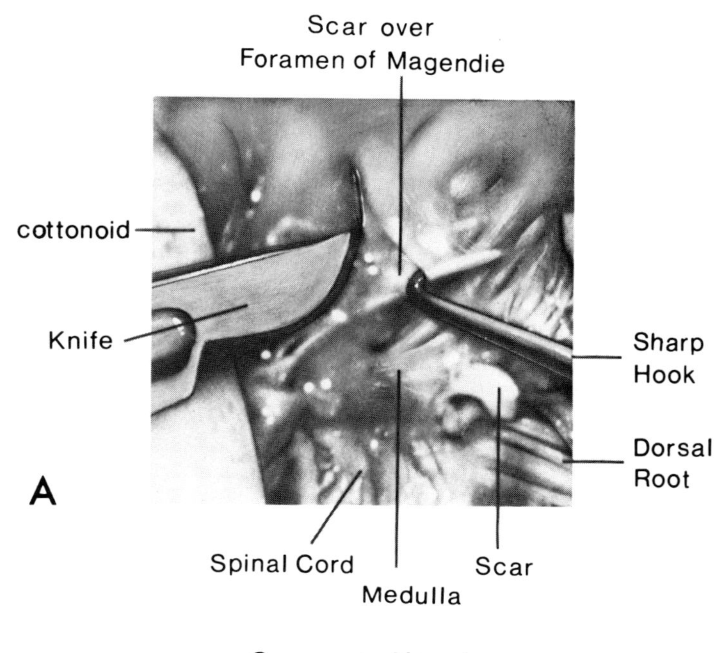

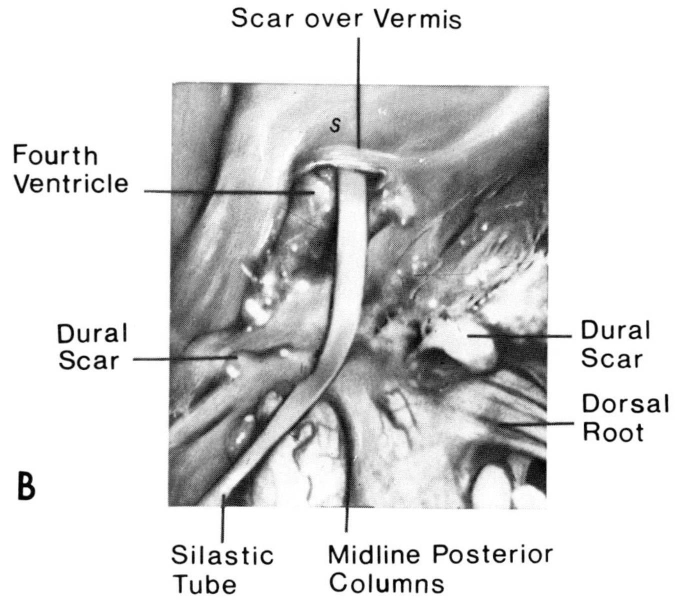

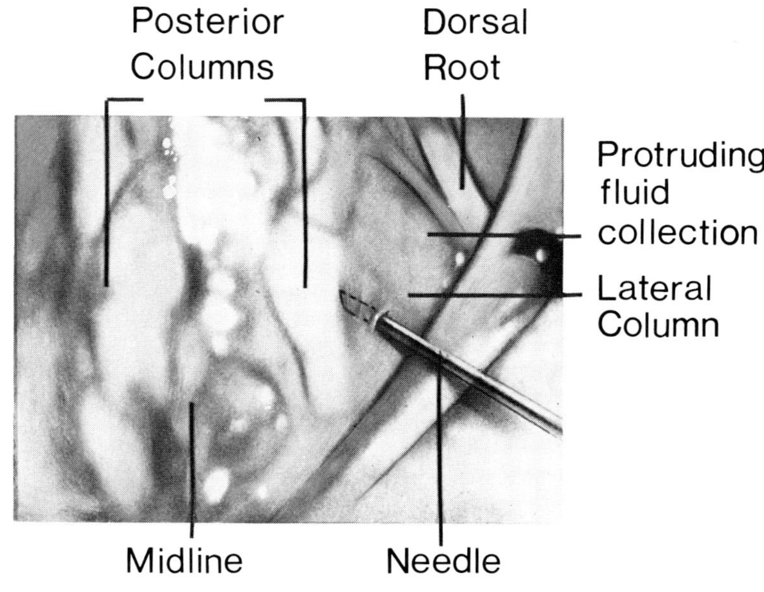

Fig. 115-10

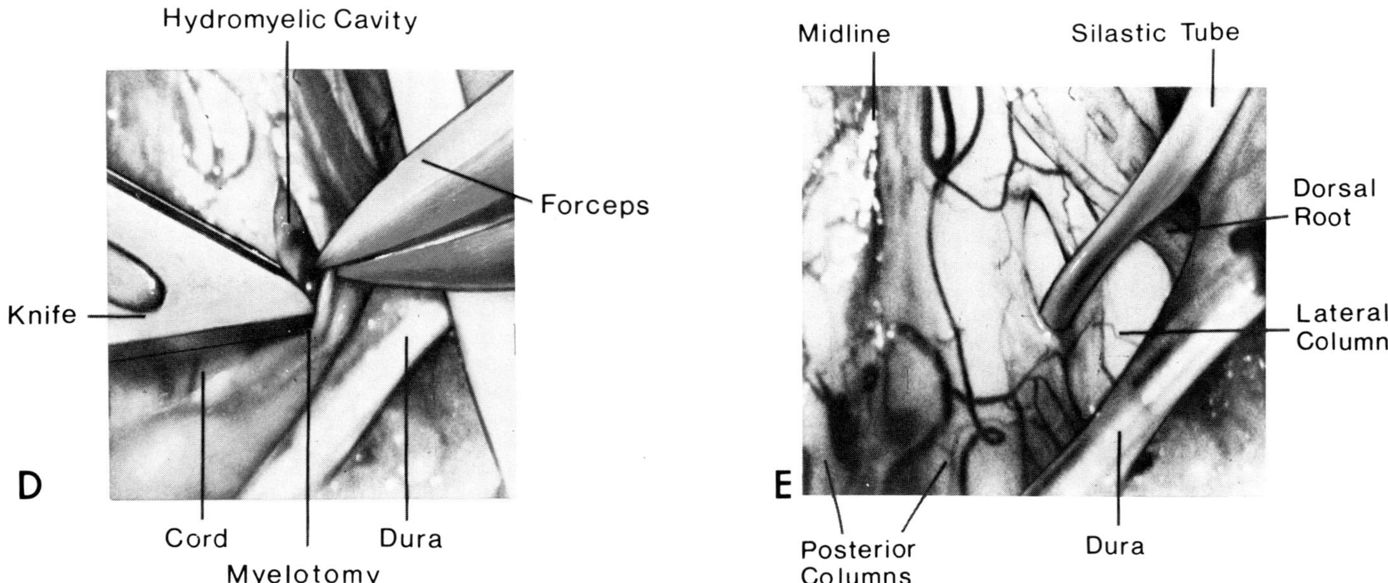

Fig. 115-10. Posterior views of Chiari malformation and hydromyelia through a suboccipital craniectomy and a C1–C3 laminectomy. The photographs were taken at 6× magnification through the surgical microscope and were re-touched for clarity. All photographs are of the same patient. (A) The incision of the dense mat of scar over the foramen of Magendie. (B) The opening into the fourth ventricle is completed and a Silastic tube, anchored to the dura below, is threaded rostrally. (C) A needle is introduced into the right half of the spinal cord lateral to the posterior column near the C3 dorsal root entry zone. Clear fluid was obtained. The cord was so thin in this area that the needle tip could be seen through the bulging surface. (D) An incision 1 cm in length is made in the dorsal root entry zone using a no. 11 knife blade. The cord is thinner than the dura. (E) A Silastic wick is attached to the dura above and led downward into the hydromyelic cavity. (Reprinted from Rhoton AL: Microsurgery of Arnold-Chiari malformation in adults with and without hydromyelia. J Neurosurg 45:473–483, 1976. With permission.)

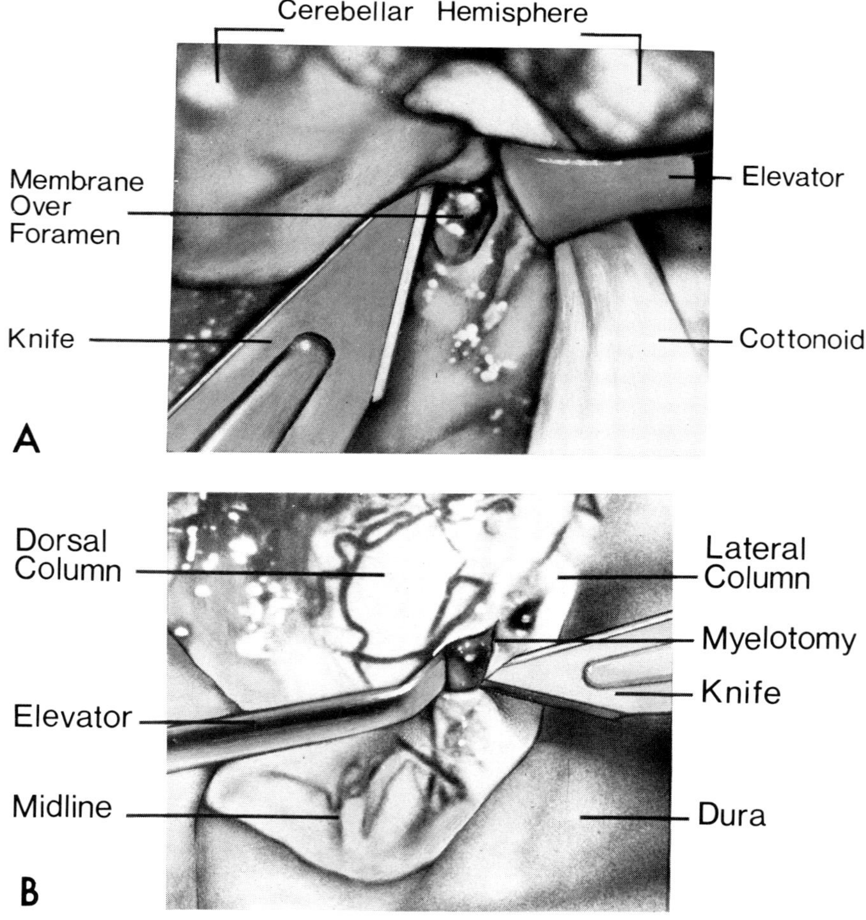

Fig. 115-11. (A) A view through a suboccipital craniectomy of the membrane occluding the foramen of Magendie. A hydromyelia also was present, and is shown in Figure 115–11B. The occluding membrane was incised with a No. 11 blade. (B) The cord was incised at the C3 dorsal root entry zone. The covering over the hydromyelic cavity was only as thick as a layer of dura. A Silastic wick was left in both the fourth ventricle and the cord. (Reprinted from Rhoton AL: Microsurgery of Arnold-Chiari malformation in adults with and without hydromyelia. J Neurosurg 45:473–483, 1976. With permission.)

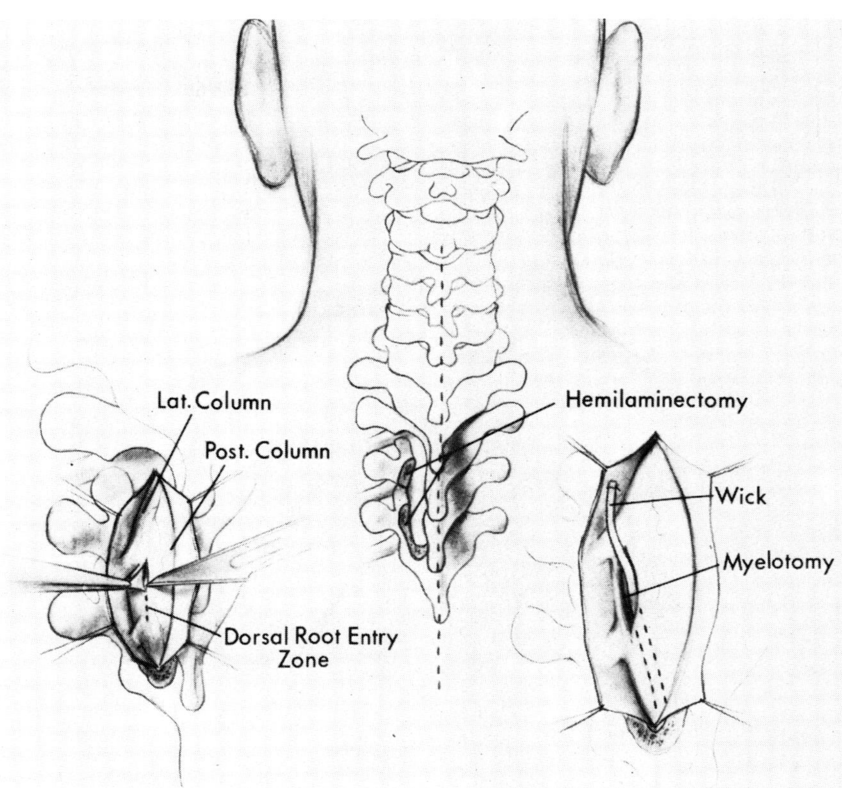

Fig. 115-12.   A myelotomy in the dorsal root entry zone in the upper thoracic region. This approach is used if the patient only has hydromyelic symptoms and no symptoms related to the Chiari malformation, or if a suboccipital craniectomy and decompression of the Chiari malformation has failed to arrest the progression of the spinal cord deficit. Upper center: The site of hemilaminectomy for doing the myelotomy. Lower left: The myelotomy in the dorsal root entry zone being completed. Lower right: The Silastic wick that is anchored to the dura is being threaded into the hydromyelic cavity. (Reprinted from Rhoton AL: Syringomyelia, in Wilson CB, Hoff JT (eds): Current Surgical Management of Neurologic Disease. New York, Churchill-Livingston, 1980, pp 29–45. With permission.)

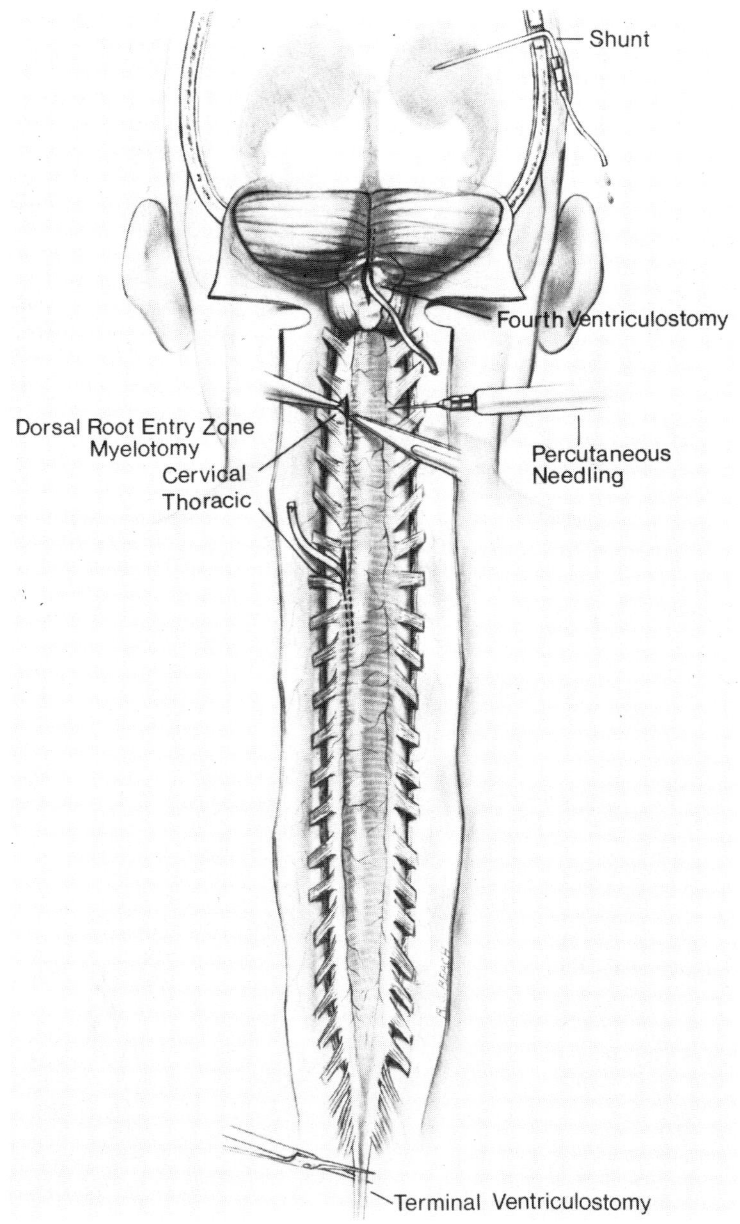

Fig. 115-13.   A summary of the different surgical techniques used to treat Chiari malformation with hydromyelia. A cerebrospinal fluid shunt may be considered if there is significant hydrocephalus. Most adults with Chiari malformation and hydromyelia, however, do not experience hydrocephalus. Decompression of the Chiari malformation may also be achieved by suboccipital craniectomy and upper cervical laminectomy, with insertion of a Silastic wick through a fourth ventriculostomy. Percutaneous needling of the cyst also has been advocated. We combine decompression of the Chiari malformation with a myelotomy in the dorsal root entry zone in the cervical region to drain the hydromyelic cord. If a previous decompression of the Chiari malformation has been done, a myelotomy of the dorsal root entry zone may be done below the cervical enlargement in the thoracic region. If the cavity extends into the filum terminalae, terminal ventriculostomy may be done by dividing the filum terminalae. (Reprinted from Rhoton AL: Syringomyelia, in Wilson CB, Hoff JT (eds): Current Surgical Management of Neurologic Disease. New York, Churchill-Livingstone, 1980, pp 29–45. With permission.)

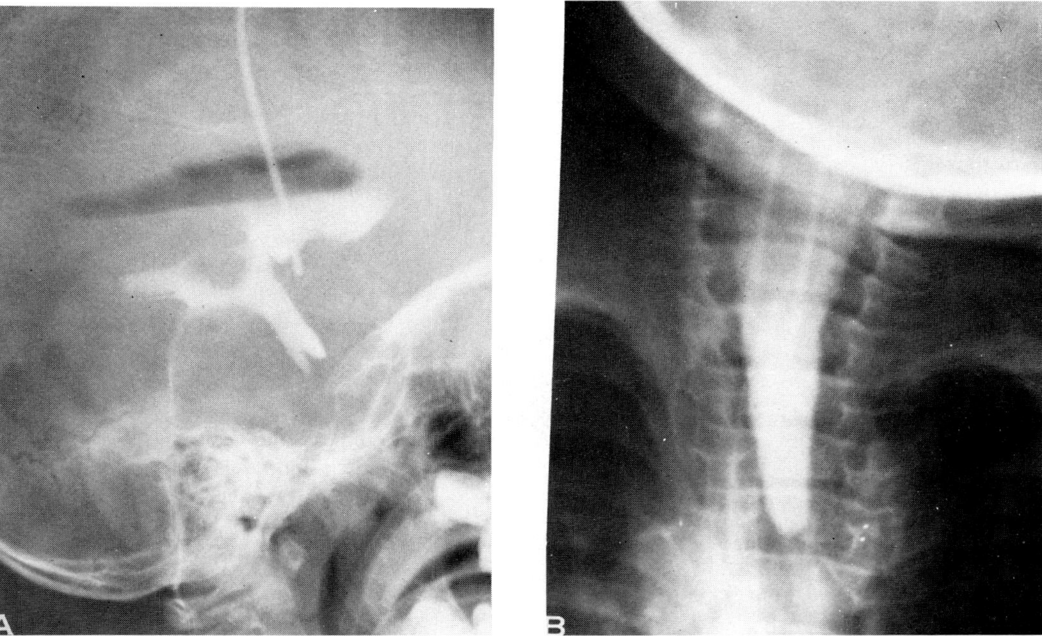

Fig. 115-14.   This infant was previously treated, with a shunt, for hydrocephalus. After the shunt was removed because of infection, the child developed a progressive lower motor neuron deficit in the arms. (A) Positive-contrast ventriculogram showing normal-sized ventricles (lateral view). (B) The contrast medium enters a large cavity in the cervical cord that communicates with the ventricles. (Reprinted from Rhoton AL: Microsurgery of Arnold-Chiari malformation in adults with and without hydromyelia. J Neurosurg 45:473–483, 1976. With permission.)

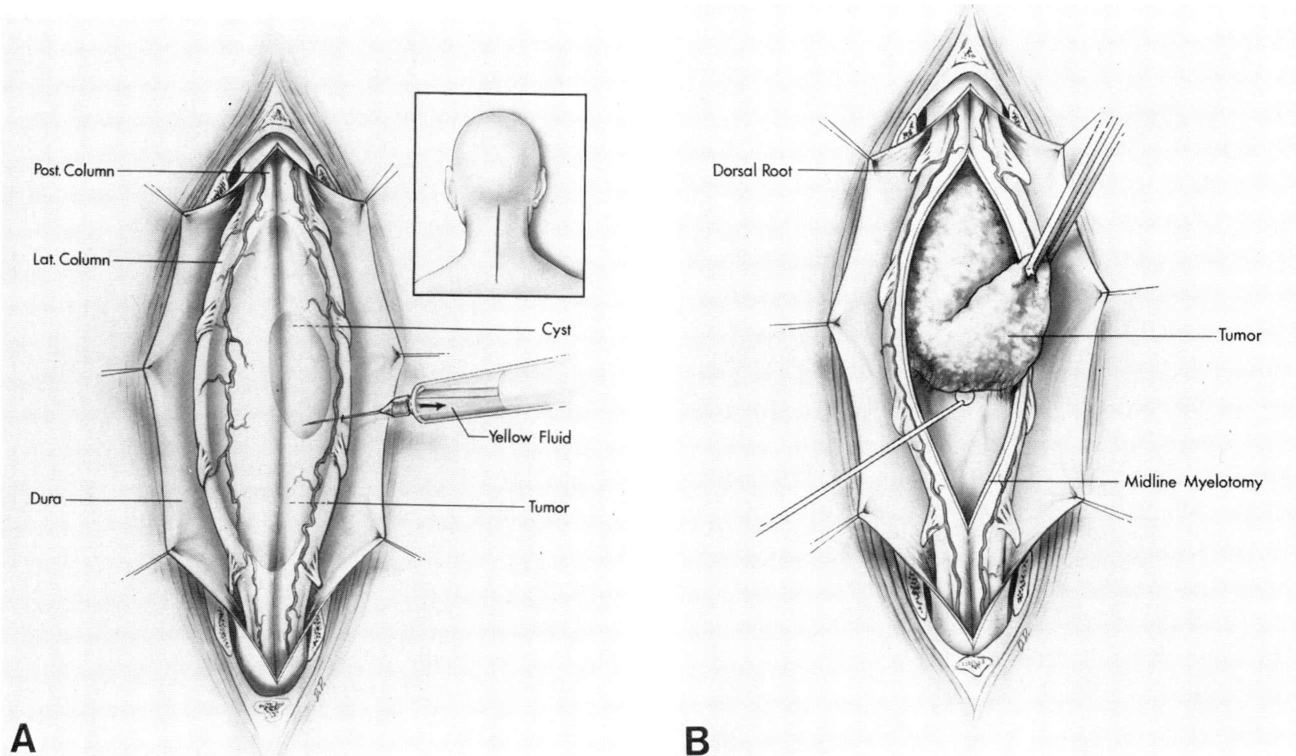

Fig. 115-15.   Exposure and removal of a cystic intramedullary tumor in the cervical region. (A) The insert (upper right) shows the position of the patient for the operation, and the incision (solid line). The illustration shows the tumor in an intramedullary location. The cyst within the tumor is being aspirated with a needle and yields yellow fluid. (B) A midline myelotomy has been performed between the posterior columns, the cleavage plane between the tumor and the spinal cord has been identified, and a small dissector is being used to remove the intramedullary tumor. The myelotomy for removal of the tumor is in the midline, while the incision for drainage of a hydromyelia is usually in the dorsal root entry zone.

INTRAMEDULLARY TUMOR

The surgical treatment of an intramedullary tumor consists of a laminectomy that is as extensive as is required to expose the abnormal cord for decompression. This is followed by a midline myelotomy, biopsy of the tumor, and total removal of the tumor if a cleavage plane can be developed between the tumor and the neural tissue (Figure 115-13). Biopsy only, or incomplete removal, is followed by radiation therapy.

ALTERNATIVE TREATMENTS

Percutaneous needling of the hydromyelic cavity has been advocated as a possible mode of therapy (Figure 115-13);[16] however, aspiration of fluid at surgery is followed by rapid refilling of the hydromyelic cavity from the ventricular system, and it seems unlikely that a needle track would remain patent. In treating hydromyelia, the longitudinal opening into the cord should be long enough to ensure that there is no tendency for spontaneous closure.

Gardner initially recommended surgical treatment consisting of a suboccipital craniectomy and cervical laminectomy to decompress the malformation, and plugging of the upper end of the patent central canal (at the area of the obex) with a small piece of muscle.[7,8] Subsequently, he has reported that most of the patients treated with occlusion of the upper end of the Acentral canal later developed progressive neurologic deficits.[9] I favor making an incision between the posterior and lateral columns of the spinal cord to drain the hydromyelic cavity and have avoided risking damage to the hypoglossal and vagal nuclei, which are located at the obex near the upper end of the central canal.

Gardner and his colleagues have advocated a procedure called terminal ventriculostomy (Figure 115-13).[11] The terminal ventricle is the dilated portion of the central canal that extends below the tip of the conus medullaris into the filum terminalae. A laminectomy is performed over the caudal limit of the fluid sac and the filum is opened. This procedure does not decompress the malformation at the foramen magnum, but may prove satisfactory if the patient has only hydromyelic symptoms. The procedure will not apply in all cases; I have seen numerous cases in which the hydromyelic cavity did not extend into the lumbar portion of the spinal cord or the filum terminalae (Figures 115-9 through 115-12).

Shunting of cerebrospinal fluid from the lateral ventricle to the atrium or peritoneum has been considered as a mode of treatment (Figure 115-13).[17] The patients in our series, however, even those with marked hydromyelic deficits, had no significant ventricular dilatation. Furthermore, the small ventricles would make shunting difficult. In addition, our patients all had normal CSF pressure. Even if shunting were done, a hydrostatic fluid column from the ventricles would remain and act on the cord when the patient was upright. Shunting would be indicated if the ventricles were large or if there was increased intracranial pressure.

The finding of ventricles of normal size in the present series led to the conclusion that intracavity pressure that is too low to dilate the ventricles may cause progressive cord destruction by distension. The following case of an infant supports this concept (Figure 115–14). After birth, this child was found to have hydrocephalus that required shunting; the shunt became infected, was removed, and was not replaced because the head and ventricular size remained normal. The child then developed a progressive, severe, lower motor neuron deficit in the arms. A second series of contrast studies showed ventricles of normal size, but positive-contrast ventriculography showed a hydromyelic cavity in the cervical cord that was hugely dilated. Thus, it appeared that intracavity pressure that was too low to distend the ventricles was distending the hydromyelic cord and causing a neurologic deficit in the arms. The cavity did not extend below the cervicothoracic junction.

REFERENCES

1. Brewis M, Poskanzer DC, Rolland C, et al: Neurological disease in an English city. Acta Neurol Scand (suppl 24) 42:9, 1966
2. Gowers WR: A Manual of Diseases of the Nervous System, vol 1. London, Churchill, 1886
3. Merritt HH: A Textbook of Neurology, ed 5. Philadelphia, Lea & Febiger, 1973
4. Rhoton AL Jr: Microsurgery of Arnold-Chiari malformation in adults with and without hydromyelia. J Neurosurg 45:473, 1976
5. Rhoton AL Jr: Syringomyelia, in Wilson CB, Hoff JT (eds): Current Surgical Management of Neurologic Disease. New York, Churchill-Livingstone, 1980, pp 29–45
6. Barnett HJM, Foster JB, Hudgson P: Syringomyelia. Philadelphia, WB Saunders, 1973, pp 6, 58, 104, 121, 312
7. Gardner WJ: Hydrodynamic mechanism of syringomyelia: Its relationship to myelocele. J Neurol Neurosurg Psychiatry 28:247, 1965
8. Gardner WJ: Myelocele: Rupture of the neural tube? Clin Neurosurg 15:57, 1968
9. Gardner WJ: Personal communication, 1978
10. Gardner WJ, Angel J: The mechanism of syringomyelia and its surgical correction. Clin Neurosurg 6:131, 1959
11. Gardner WJ, Steinberg M, Bell H, et al: Terminal ventriculostomy in the treatment of syringomyelia. Presented at the Annual Meeting of the American Association of Neurological Surgeons, Miami, Florida, April, 1975
12. Chiari H: über die Pathogenese der sogenannten Syringomyelie. Heilkunde 9:307, 1888
13. Bertrand G: Dynamic factors in the evolution of syringomyelia and syringobulbia. Clin Neurosurg 20:322, 1973
14. Ellertsson AB: Syringomyelia and other cystic spinal cord lesions. Acta Neurol Scand 45:403, 1969
15. Mullan S, Raimondi AJ: Respiratory hazards of the surgical treatment of the Arnold-Chiari malformation. J Neurosurg 19:675, 1962
16. Schlesinger ER, Tenner MS, Michelsen WH: Percutaneous spinal cord puncture in the analysis and treatment of hydromyelia. Presented at the Annual Meeting of the American Association of Neurological Surgeons, Houston, Texas, April, 1971
17. Conway LW: Hydrodynamic studies in syringomyelia. J Neurosurg 27:501, 1967

CHAPTER 116
Anterior Cervical Disc Excision in Cervical Spondylosis

Henry H. Schmidek   Donald A. Smith

OVER THE PAST TWO DECADES, operations have been devised in which a direct anterolateral approach has been used to gain access to the spine from the base of the skull to the sacrum. The inventiveness has been particularly apparent with regard to the surgical management of disorders of the cervical spine.[1] In the neck, anterior approaches have undergone constant redevelopment and reassessment so that they could be used to treat cervical disc disease, cervical fractures, tumors, and infections of the bodies of the vertebrae. At the present time at least a half dozen variations of the anterior approach have been fashioned.[2–9] All allow access to the ventral aspect of the dura, the nerve root sheaths, and the vertebral arteries, and all provide for considerable flexibility in the approach available to remove lesions that impinge on these structures or are associated with spinal instability. These approaches allow for the removal of extruded cartilage or bony overgrowth and can also be used with the supine position during surgery and with dissection in avascular planes. Their associated low morbidity has resulted in their widespread acceptance in the treatment of cervical spondylosis and its sequelae.

The anterolateral approaches to the cervical spine originated to explore the tuberculous spine; to reach the site of these lesions, the vertebral bodies had to be approached anteriorly. This approach then was applied to cervical disc disease associated with radiculopathy and myelopathy, beginning with the reports of Robinson[7,10,11] and of Cloward[5,6,12] in the 1960s. Since that time the operation has become a standard part of the neurosurgical armamentarium, since the predominant changes associated with cervical spondylosis are situated ventral to neurovascular structures within the spine and the anterolateral approach allows these structures to be decompressed directly.

SURGICAL INDICATIONS

CERVICAL RADICULOPATHY

Cervical disc disease often involves several levels of the spine, although most often at C4-5, C5-6, and C6-7. These herniations, both of the ''hard'' or ''soft'' type, are situated centrally, laterally, or anterolaterally. The lateral and anterolateral herniations project into the intervertebral foramina, whereas the central disc herniations may be limited to the midline. As the disc degenerates, its nucleus is affected first and begins to bulge transversely. The patient may then experience neck, shoulder, and arm pain, occipital headache, intrascapular

pain, and anterior chest pain. The *painful disc syndrome* produces pain in the neck, shoulders, and arm, often with subjective numbness in a dermatome. In the early stages of the deterioration of the disc, pain may develop when the fibers of the annulus, or anterior and posterior ligaments, become stretched. In these cases, standard radiographic studies remain normal. Further degeneration leads to cracking and fissuring of the disc. These may extend into the joints of Luschka, and nuclear material may be extruded into these joints beneath or through the posterior longitudinal ligament or through the cartilaginous plates into the vertebral bodies. Changes in the cartilage further interfere with nutrition of the disc, contributing to its degeneration. Radiographically there is a loss of the disc space height, and the spine is slightly shortened. Sliding movements between the vertebrae and alterations in the bone adjacent to the disc develop. The end of the vertebral body mushrooms and expands, and bony outgrowths develop with the periosteal activity provoked by the abnormal direction and stresses on lamellar fibers. Osteophytes develop around the lateral margins of the vertebrae. The ''hard'' disc is a degenerative spur mainly associated with outgrowth from the uncovertebral joint, but it may be accompanied by spur formation in the immediate adjacent posterior portion of the disc. The radicular symptoms and signs associated with either ''hard'' or ''soft'' discs are probably due to a combination of neural compression and perineural inflammation.

Surgical decompression is appropriate in cervical radiculopathy with subjective and objective evidence of nerve root compression in which conservative treatment, involving adequate sedation and analgesics, traction, and physical therapy, fails. As mentioned by Scoville,[13] unrelenting symptoms usually should be present for a 3- to 4-week period, although some patients who experience severe pain and neurologic deficit require surgery almost immediately after their symptoms begin. In these patients cervical traction often accentuates their discomfort, and, inevitably, a large disc fragment is found to be responsible for their discomfort (Figure 116-1).

CERVICAL SPONDYLOTIC MYELOPATHY

Cervical spondylotic myelopathy often occurs in patients who have a canal that is narrower than normal (under 14 mm sagittal width) and in whom osteophytes and ligamentous hypertrophy further compromise the size of the canal.[1] The pathogenesis of the disease remains uncertain. Compression of

OPERATIVE NEUROSURGICAL TECHNIQUES
ISBN 0-8089-1862-1

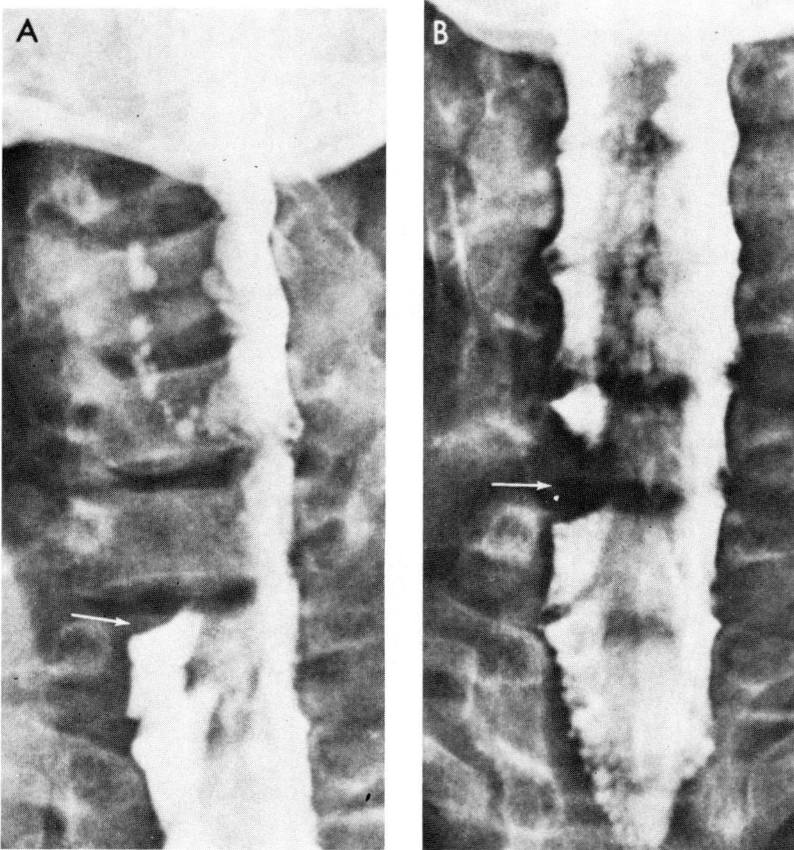

Fig. 116-1. A cervical myelogram showing a laterally situated free disc fragment in a patient with intractable radiculopathy.

the cord by disc material or traction of the cord against osteophytes is etiologically important, particularly in the case of an acute myelopathy; e.g., one associated with traumatic disc protrusion. In chronic myelopathy, however, the factors of disc degeneration, spur formation, foraminal encroachment, and a congenitally narrow canal are probably potentiated by motion and it may be that the motion results in the progression of signs and symptoms. Whether or not compromise of radicular vessel is important in some cases of myelopathy is not known. Acute myelopathy secondary to thrombosis of the anterior spinal artery is very rare and does not explain the progression seen in chronic myelopathy. It may be that, secondary to the spondylotic distortion and flattening of the cord, there is distortion of its intrinsic arterioles and compromise of the feeding and intrinsic vessels of the cord, leading to vascular insufficiency. It has been suggested by Robinson[15] that the stepwise progression of neurologic deficit characteristically seen in certain cases with cervical spondylotic myelopathy actually represents repeated small infarctions within the cord substance.

Cervical spondylotic myelopathy was characterized as a distinct entity by Clarke,[16] who reviewed the case histories of 120 patients with myelopathy and evidence of spinal cord compression, and was further defined by Gregorius[17] as consisting of five distinct syndromes including (1) a transverse lesion syndrome with corticospinal, spinothalamic, and dorsal column involvement; (2) a motor system syndrome with corticospinal tract and anterior horn cell dysfunction; (3) a mixed syndrome with root and cord findings presenting with radicular pain and long tract involvement; (4) a partial Brown-Sequard syndrome; and (5) an anterior cord syndrome with distal arm weakness. They noted that although complete remission was never seen, regression occurred in 2 patients. Of their 120 cases, 75 percent had a series of episodes with progression, 20 percent were steadily and slowly progressing, and 5 percent had a rapid onset of findings, with plateauing before further deterioration at a later date. Of 22 patients managed nonoperatively, 16 were treated with a neck brace alone. In 8 of the 16 patients, walking, the ability to dress, and radicular signs in the arms improved; this improvement was striking in 2. Although the remaining patients did not improve their disease did not progress.

Lees and Turner[18] and Balla[19] also attempted to define the natural history of cervical myelopathy. In Lees' series deterioration often ceased after the first few years; other patients experienced remissions lasting for years and then became worse. Progression and recurrence were particularly evident in patients with a congenitally narrow canal. Balla[19] in a series of 123 patients followed for up to 10 years, found that without treatment 52 percent improved, 35 percent remained unchanged, and 13 percent became worse.

DYSPHAGIA ASSOCIATED WITH CERVICAL SPONDYLOSIS

Compression of the esophagus or hypopharynx by osteophytes had been reported in the literature since 1926. A review, in 1960, reported 36 cases of dysphagia associated with osteo-

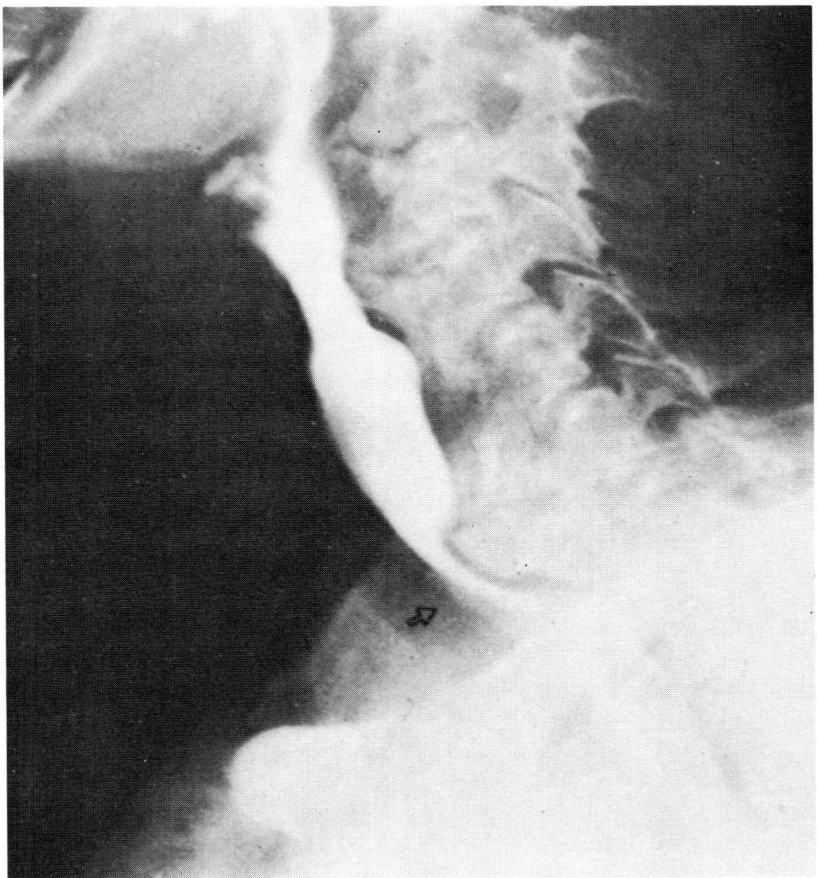

Fig. 116-2.   A cervical osteophyte (arrow) in a patient with dysphagia. (Reprinted from Meeks LW, Renshaw TS: Vertebral osteophytosis and dysphagia. J Bone Joint Surg 55A:197–201, 1973. With permission.)

phytes.[20] In 1971, Maran and Jacobson[21] reported the tenth surgically treated case (Figure 116-2). These authors advocated interbody fusion in addition to excision of the osteophyte to prevent recurrent spur formation at the involved level.[22,23]

Compression of the hypopharynx is experienced as a lump in the throat and is seen with osteophytic compression above C6.

Cervical osteophytes have been reported along the entire cervical spine, with C5-6 being the most common site. In two thirds of the cases, one level is involved, and in the remaining one third, osteophytes at several levels contribute to the symptoms. Surgical removal of the exostosis usually is not indicated, although with persistent dysphagia or lump sensation the lesion can be excised with consideration given at that time to the removal of the involved degenerate disc.

VERTEBRAL ARTERY COMPRESSION ASSOCIATED WITH CERVICAL SPONDYLOSIS

Osteophytes projecting from the uncovertebral joints can intrude into the foramina transversaria and cause vertebral artery compression. To be clinically significant, this compression must impair the flow of blood to the brain stem. Hutchinson and Yates[24] have shown that the effect of vertebral artery compression by osteophytes can be enhanced by rotating the head or extending the neck, which may result in giddiness or drop attacks. These symptoms, however, also may occur in the absence of head movement. Primary or secondary lateral extraspinal extrusions may indent or occlude the vertebral artery in its second portion. In 2 patients with traumatic lateral disc rupture, angiograms showed compression and displacement of the vertebral artery. These patients had radicular pains and motor deficit. Both, however, had normal cervical myelograms, so that this investigation sometimes is useful in delineating ruptured cervical disc.[26]

DIAGNOSTIC EVALUATION

Investigations of cervical spondylosis involve standard roentgenograms and flexion and extension views of the spine to obtain evidence of spinal stability. The musculature of the cervical region, the ligamentous structures, especially the ligamentum nuchae and posterior longitudinal ligament, and the bond between the vertebral bodies because of the discs are major factors responsible for the stability of the cervical spine. White[27] (Figures 116-3 and 116-4), in a biomechanical study of adult cadaver spines, showed that the ligaments normally permit very little motion between vertebrae and that horizontal motions (greater than 3.5 mm) of one vertebral body on another, as seen on plain lateral roentgenograms, indicate instability. If the angulation of one vertebral body with respect to another is 11 percent greater than the angulation of adjacent vertebrae and the vertebral body is not compressed, the spine is relatively unstable. A major number of ligaments must be

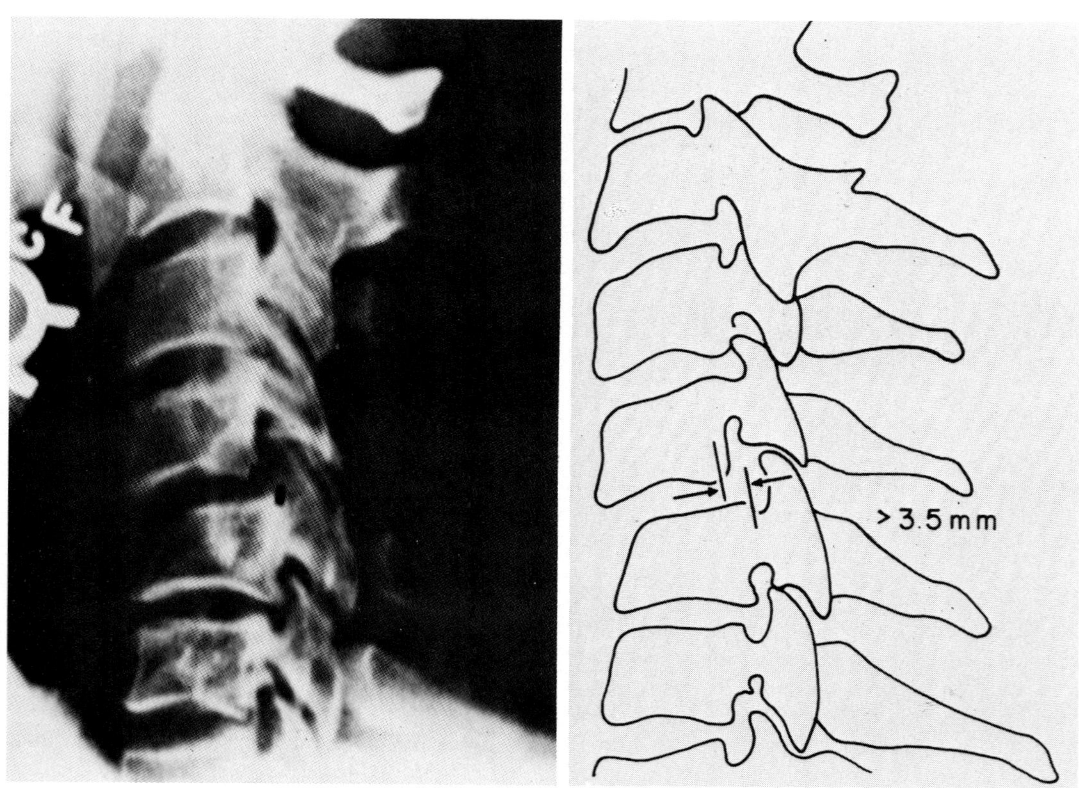

Fig. 116-3. Biomechanical studies have shown that horizontal motion in excess of 3.5 mm as demonstrated on plain roentgenograms indicates instability. (Reprinted from White AA, Johnson RM, Panjabi MM, et al: Biomechanical analysis of clinical stability in the cervical spine. Clin Orthop 109:85–96, 1975. With permission of J.B. Lippincott.)

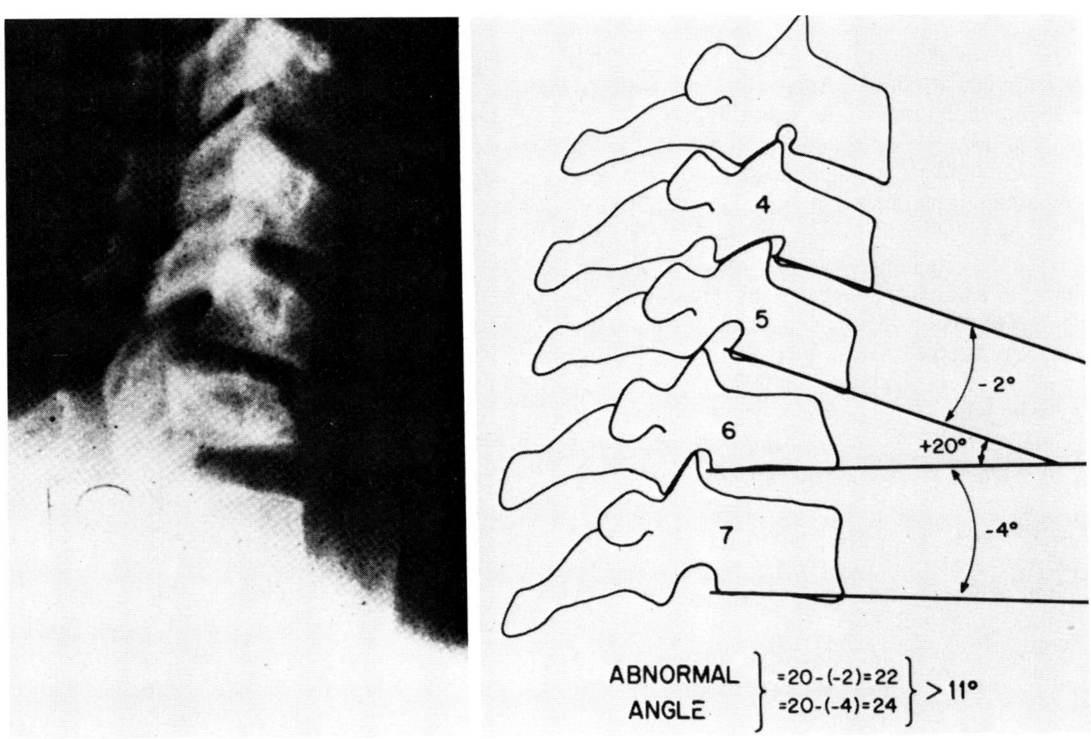

Fig. 116-4. Biomechanical studies have shown that angulation of one vertebral body of more than 11 degrees with respect to another indicates an unstable spine. (Reprinted from White AA, Johnson RM, Panjabi MM, et al: Biomechanical analysis of clinical stability in the cervical spine. Clin Orthop 109:85–96, 1975. With permission of J.B. Lippincott.)

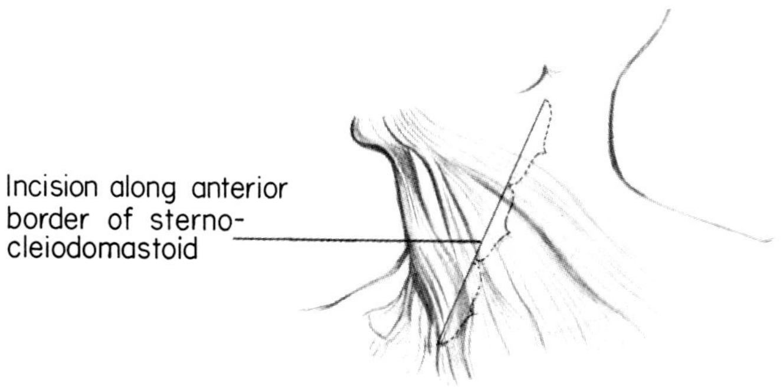

Fig. 116-5. The line of incision for the anterior approach.

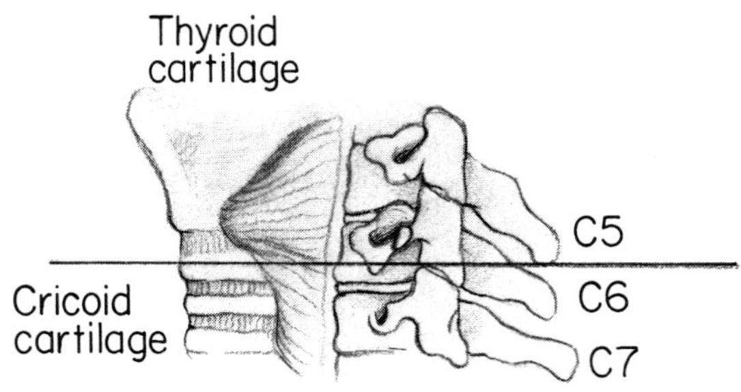

Fig. 116-6. Points for centering the incision opposite C5 and C6.

injured to permit motion exceeding these limits. Instability means that the spine will fail under physiologic loads, causing the spine to lose its ability to move without further deformity, excessive pain, and potential neurologic worsening.

Cervical myelography is performed preoperatively in all cases of cervical myelopathy or radiculopathy. The neurologic examination does not provide all the information required to plan an operation. With severe myelopathy, a lateral C1-2 puncture is preferable to instilling contrast medium by the lumbar route, since the study will not require hyperextension of the cervical spine, which results in maximal impingement on the cord and has been associated with neurologic worsening following myelography. We use metrizamide (Squibb) in conjunction with computed tomography (CT) scanning to outline the cervical cord and establish its relationship to the spinal canal. This agent may be introduced by cervical or lumbar puncture.

Electromyography and nerve conduction studies provide additional objective evidence of root compression in patients with relatively minor neurologic findings. It is also important in differentiating root, plexus, peripheral nerve, and muscle disorders that may mimic cervical radiculopathy, and may help to uncover a second problem that may co-exist with the cervical radiculopathy, such as a carpal tunnel syndrome or ulnar neuropathy.

Computed tomography of the cervical spine with sagittal reconstruction has been found to be extraordinarily helpful in assessing the cervical spine by delineating irregular spurs and the canal topography, and flattening or displacement of the

spinal cord. However, Pantopaque myelography remains the mainstay in the investigation of cases of cervical spondylosis.

Utilizing selective catheterization, digital subtraction or standard angiography to demonstrate cerebral vasculature is occasionally warranted and should include a survey of both intracranial and extracranial vessels for a comprehensive evaluation of cerebral circulation. This is done with head turning to determine whether this further compromises flow in the vertebral artery and reproduces the symptoms.

SURGICAL ANATOMY

The anterior approach is the easiest along the anterior margin of the sternomastoid and medial to the carotid sheath (Figure 116-5). The incision may be centered by noting the hyoid bone at the level of C3, the thyroid cartilage opposite C4, and the cricoid opposite the level of C6 (Figure 116-6).

Dissection is carried out in avascular planes, passing through the pretracheal fascia first and then the prevertebral fascia. The longus colli muscles, covering the lateral parts of the vertebral body, the vertebral canal, and the transverse processes, then can be seen (Figure 116-7). These muscles extend from the atlas to the body of T3. There is no muscle covering the anterior aspect of the vertebrae in the midline (Figure 116-8). The cervical sympathetic chain lies on the longus colli muscles and extends from C2 to T1 (Figure 116-8). Since a Horner's syndrome will result from damage to the spinal cord

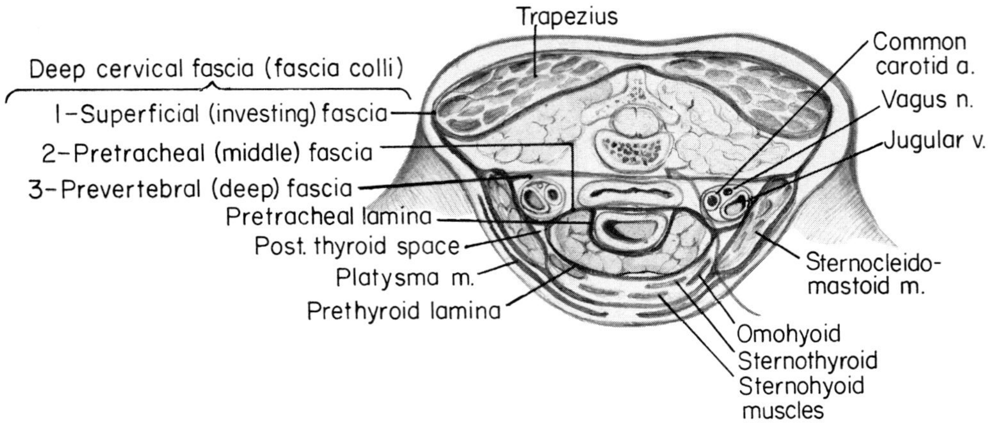

Fig. 116-7. Cross-section representation at the C5 level of the spine indicating the fascial planes and the avascular surgical approach to the anterior spine.

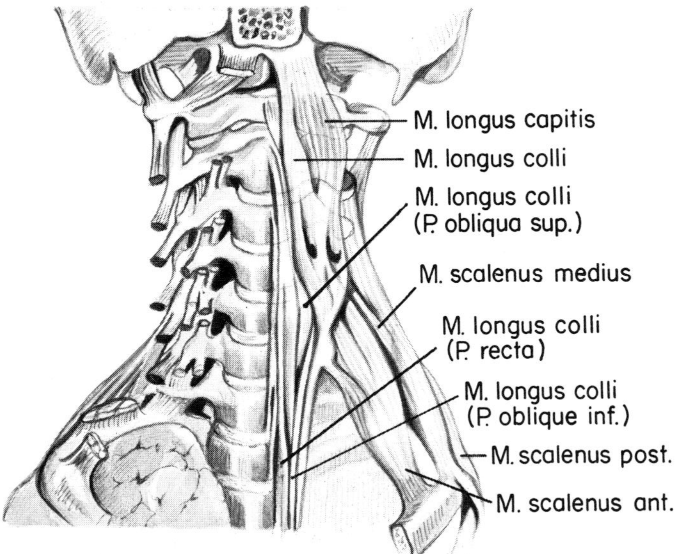

Fig. 116-8. Relationships of the anterior cervical musculature to the cervical spine.

fibers, it is important to retract the longus colli, starting at its medial edge.

The anterior longitudinal ligament is a strong band that extends from the base of the skull to the sacrum (Figure 116-9). It is thickest in its midportion, tapers laterally, and is bound to the anterior annulus, functioning to limit the extension of the spine. The posterior longitudinal ligament also extends as a thick band from the skull to the sacrum, between the posterior annulus and the dura. Since the ligament does not extend laterally over the nerve roots, its normally thick portion, which prevents disc material from extruding into the spinal canal, is absent, permitting disc material to enter the foramen. Functionally, this ligament limits flexion of the spine. Physiologically, the ligamentum flavum does not compress the dura or spinal cord; however, as elasticity is lost the ligamentum buckles and may compress the spinal cord.

The left recurrent laryngeal branch of the vagus nerve arises at the level of the aortic arch, loops beneath the arch, and then passes between the trachea and the esophagus to reach the larynx. On the right side, the recurrent laryngeal nerve has an inconstant course. It usually descends within the carotid sheath, looping beneath the subclavian artery to reach the larynx between the trachea and the esophagus. The nerve may follow one of several aberrant courses, leaving the carotid sheath at a higher level. To avoid injury to an aberrant right recurrent laryngeal nerve, it is preferable to operate on the left side of the neck, irrespective of the side of the radicular symptoms.

SURGICAL PROCEDURE

Prophylactic antibiotics are begun immediately preoperatively. The patient is placed in the supine position on an operating table under general anesthesia. The neck is moderately hyperextended by placing a roll beneath the shoulder blades and a sandbag is placed beneath the opposite hip region. The head is turned about 10 degrees to the right. Dissection is carried out with headlight illumination and magnifying loupes of 3.5–4.5×. The operating microscope may be used instead of the loupes, especially to perform total removal of osteophytes.

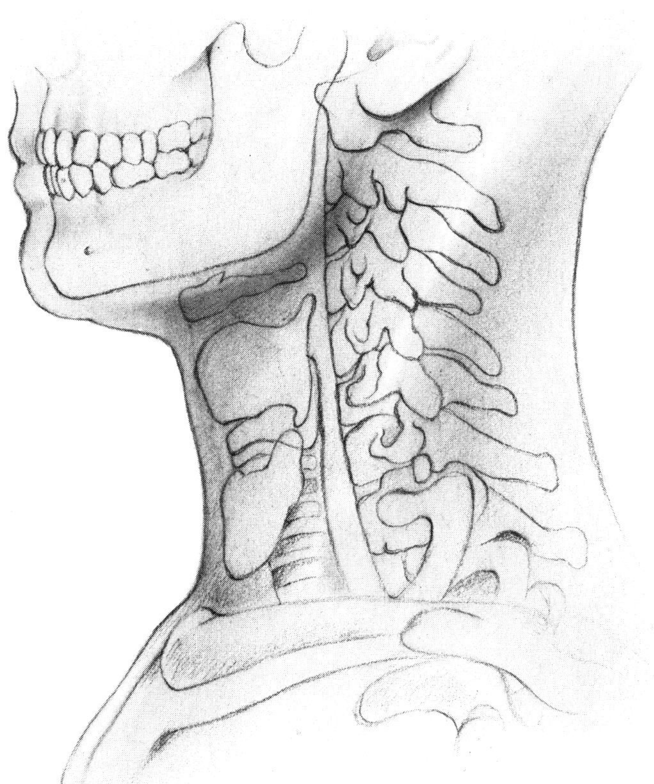

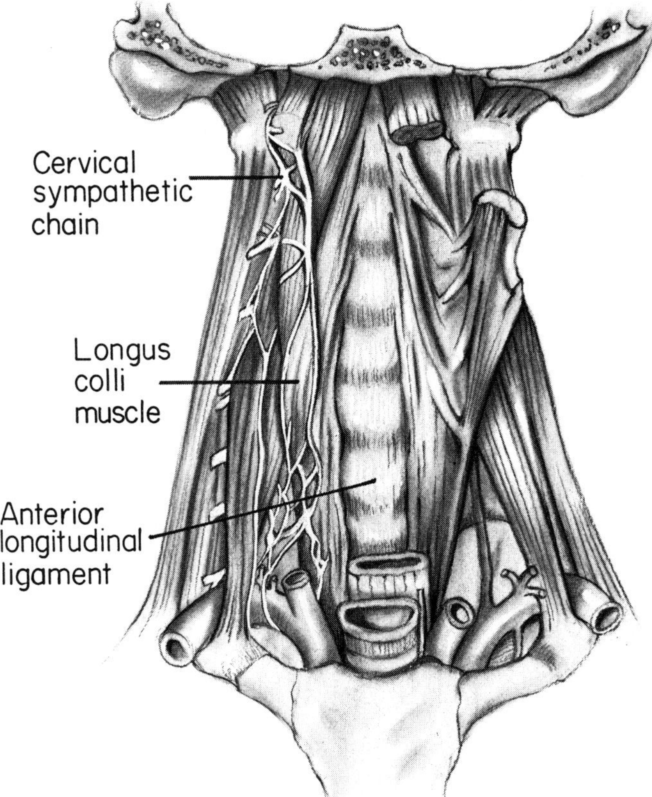

Fig. 116-9. The relationship of the cervical sympathetic chain, anterior spinal musculature, and anterior longitudinal ligament to the spine.

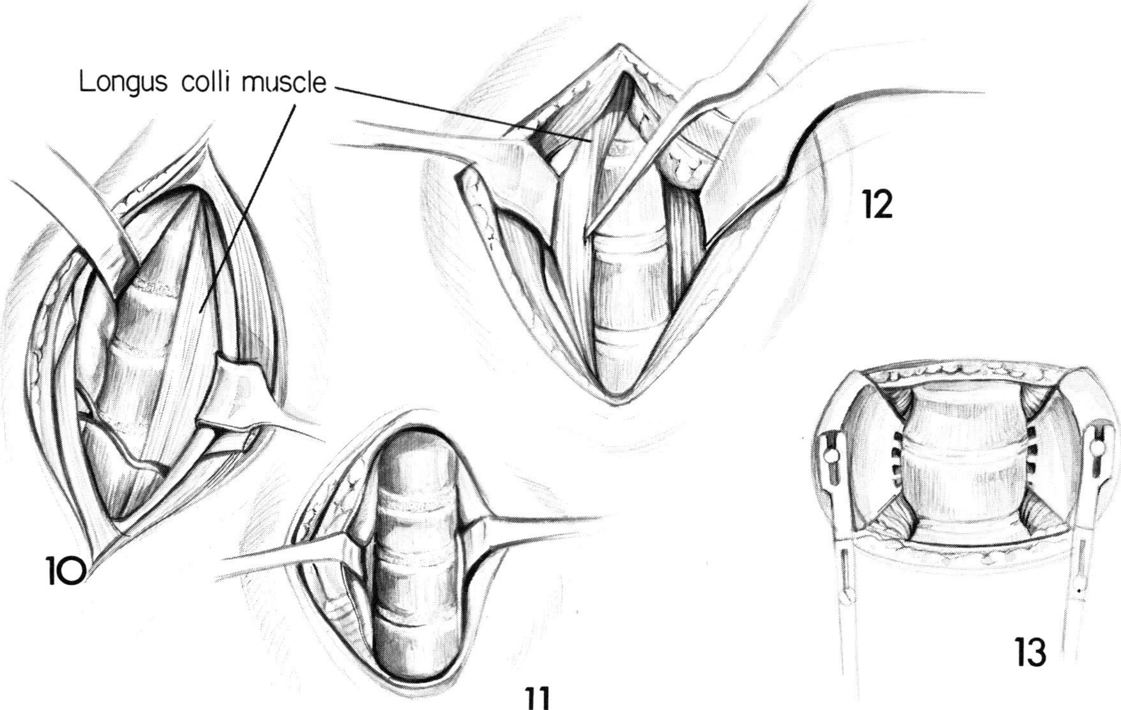

Figs. 116-10 and 116-11.   View of the anterior spine after medial retraction of the trachea and esophagus and lateral retraction of the carotid sheath and its contents.

Routinely a left-sided longitudinal skin incision is used, centered over the anterior border of the sternomastoid muscle and the segment of spine to be exposed (see Figures 116-4 and 116-5). This vertical incision is preferred since different types of anterior and lateral operations on cervical vertebral bodies and intervertebral discs, transverse processes, and vertebral arteries can be carried out without undue traction.

When the platysma has been exposed, it is grasped with forceps and incised with a scalpel parallel to the anterior margin of the sternomastoid. The underlying sternomastoid muscle then is visible (Figure 116-10). The anterior border of the sternomastoid must be clearly identified and mobilized throughout the limits of the exposure so that the medial border of the sternomastoid muscle can be retracted laterally to expose the middle layer of the cervical fascia. The omohyoid muscle crosses the field at C5-6 and may be retracted or transected at

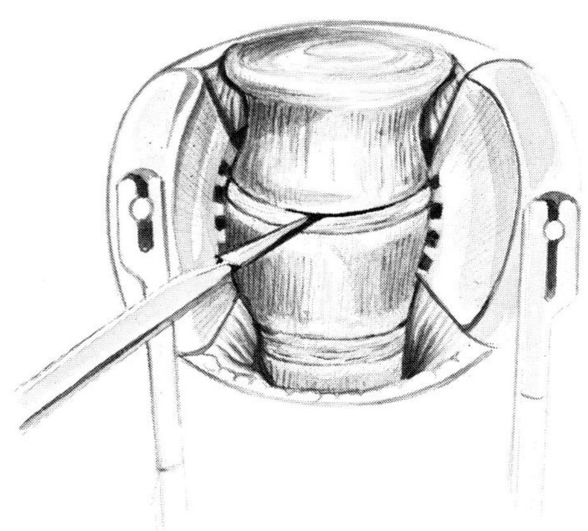

Fig. 116-14.   Incision of the disc space.

its midtendinous segment. The carotid sheath is identified. Using sharp dissection, an avascular plane is developed through the cervical fascia medial and parallel to the carotid sheath. The carotid sheath and the sternomastoid muscle are retracted laterally (Figure 116-11). As this is done, the anterior surface of the cervical spine is seen. The esophagus and trachea are retracted medially. The prevertebral fascia is cauterized with Malis bipolar cautery and incised longitudinally in the midline, exposing the anterior longitudinal ligament. The medial aspect of the longus colli muscles are then cauterized for a length corresponding to the discs to be exposed (Figure 116-12). This helps to keep the wound essentially bloodless. Cloward blades are placed beneath the cauterized medial edges of the longus colli muscles (Figure 116-13). This is probably the most important maneuver in the operation; failure to correctly position the blades is responsible for most of the complications associated with this operation. When the vertical incision is used, a single set of blades placed beneath the muscle edges will suffice to give adequate exposure. A fine needle then is placed in the disc space and a cross-table, cervical-spine roentgenogram is obtained to confirm the disc level. The retractors need not be removed to obtain this study.

The margins of the disc to be entered are cauterized and the disc is incised (Figure 116-14). It is often necessary to remove the bony spurs overhanging the disc space from the upper vertebra before significant amounts of intervertebral disc can be removed. Once the anterior one half to two thirds of the disc and the cartilaginous plates have been removed, the disc-space spreader is introduced laterally in the disc space (Figure 116-15). Dissection up to this point is continued under 3.5-4.5× loupes or the procedure can be completed at 6–15× magnification using the operating microscope. Under magnification the entire disc is excised to the posterior longitudinal ligament, which appears as a structure with glistening white fibers that are

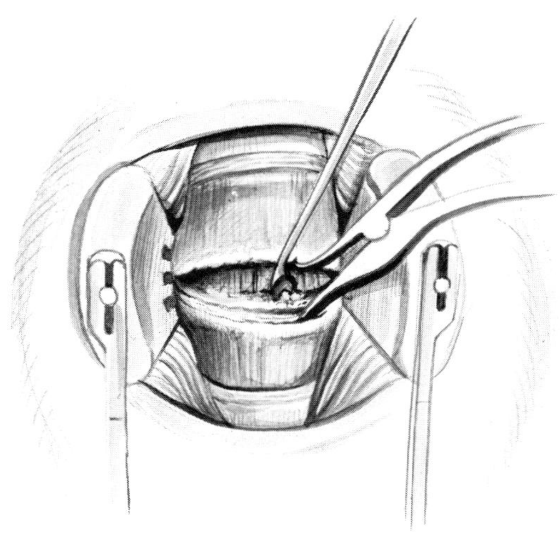

Fig. 116-15. Removal of the contents of the interspace and placement of the intervertebral spreader.

vertically aligned (Figure 116-16A, B, and C). The remaining cartilage and disc are removed with fine curettes. The posterior ligament is incised and removed in order to reach the otherwise inaccessible large fragment beneath it, foraminal spurs, or in the presence of severe cord compression. The defect often can be seen in the posterior ligament through which a fragment of disc is extruding. Lateral dissection will expose the uncovertebral joints and the dura, which is not covered by the posterior longitudinal ligament (Figure 116-17A and B).

Using a 20-degree angled diamond drill the osteophytes above and below the disc space are carefully removed, particularly if one decides to perform an anterior discectomy without fusion, to prevent subsequent nerve root compression.

If a fusion is to be performed, a horseshoe-shaped bone graft with three cortical edges is taken from the ilium using a reciprocating saw. The graft is countersunk in the disc space, and a lateral cervical film is taken to check its alignment (Figure 116-18). The wound is irrigated and a drain is placed above the anterior aspect of the spine, bringing it out through the lower end of the incision. The platysma and skin are closed with fine sutures, and the drain is removed in 12 hours. Improvement following surgery for radiculopathy is apparent to many patients soon after they awaken from anesthesia. Codeine suffices for any pain. The patient is allowed to get out of bed within a day, in a molded plastic cervical collar, and is discharged within 3 to 4 days. The patient remains immobilized in the Philadelphia collar until there is radiologic evidence of bony fusion. Antibiotics are discontinued after a single postoperative dose.

COMPLICATIONS

Tew[25] summarized a combined experience of possible complications of this operation and they appear formidable. Lunsford[29] also quotes a complication rate of 13 percent for discectomy alone and a rate of 23 percent overall in his series; however, the complication rate of the procedure in experienced hands is very modest, and serious neurologic injury is rare.

The exception is the re-operative case in which exploration of the neck can be difficult. In this group of patients serious problems can and do arise.

Retraction-related problems are the most common form of postoperative morbidity, and result in laryngeal edema, hoarseness, dysphagia, or a sensation of a lump in the throat.[30] These problems can be avoided by a vertical incision, preferably on the left side;, meticulous placement of the blades of the Cloward retractor beneath the medial aspect of the longus colli muscles; a gentle degree of retraction; and a drain placed prevertebrally at the end of the operation. Should these retraction-related problems arise, a short course of steroid therapy has been found useful. Occasionally, emergency tracheostomy has been necessary because of upper airway obstruction secondary to extensive retraction.

Profuse bleeding from the disc space is due either to injury to the bone as the cartilaginous plates are removed, injury to the vertebral body with the disc-space spreader, or a small dural tear with a cerebrospinal fluid (CSF) leak, which compresses epidural veins and can result in profuse venous bleeding. In the majority of these cases the bleeding can be controlled with gentle pressure and Avitene in the disc space. Injury to the carotid artery has been reported with resultant cerebral ischemia secondary to excessive compression of the vessel by retraction, and to the vertebral artery by dissection carried into the vertebral canal. The complications that result from excessive bleeding can be reduced by ensuring that if a graft is used there is adequate room to each side of the graft to allow blood to extravasate away from the canal. In addition, a Jackson-Pratt drain is left in place to remove blood and irrigating fluid.

Esophageal and tracheal perforation are retraction-related complications that can be prevented by using the blades properly, but if an esophageal perforation occurs and is recognized this should be repaired immediately. Interrupted nonabsorbable sutures are used to repair the rupture, and the area is drained. Fusion under these circumstances is contraindicated.

Graft extrusion and donor-site problems occur in about 2 to 4 percent of cases and with the interbody technique fusion failed in 10 percent of Tew's cases.[28] The incidence of failures is higher with the Cloward technique. On the other hand, the significant postoperative discomfort that follows discectomy without fusion characterized by a nagging neck, shoulder, and intrascapular pain often lasting several months is a significant consideration when deciding the merit of this modification in the treatment of spondylosis. Although a recent report[29] claims no difference in results following disc excision with or without fusion, it does not address the very real set of complaints seen in patients on our service in whom fusion has not been performed. This same report finds no difference in results between the Cloward and the Smith-Robinson fusion techniques; however, this does not correspond with other reported experiences and we prefer the Robinson technique based on the biomechanical study of Simmons,[31] which demonstrated that the surface area of the rectangular graft is approximately 30 percent more than the surface area of the cylindrical graft of comparable size. Stability studies showed the keystone graft to be more stable than the dowel graft, and that the fusion rate with the keystone graft is 100 percent.

The second consideration is the effect eliminating the graft will have on the stability of the cervical spine. Although interbody fusion is often unnecessary and spontaneous fusion frequently occurs with 6 months after one-, two-, or three-level disc discectomy, the overall results depend on the number of variables responsible for maintaining stability altered by the spondylotic

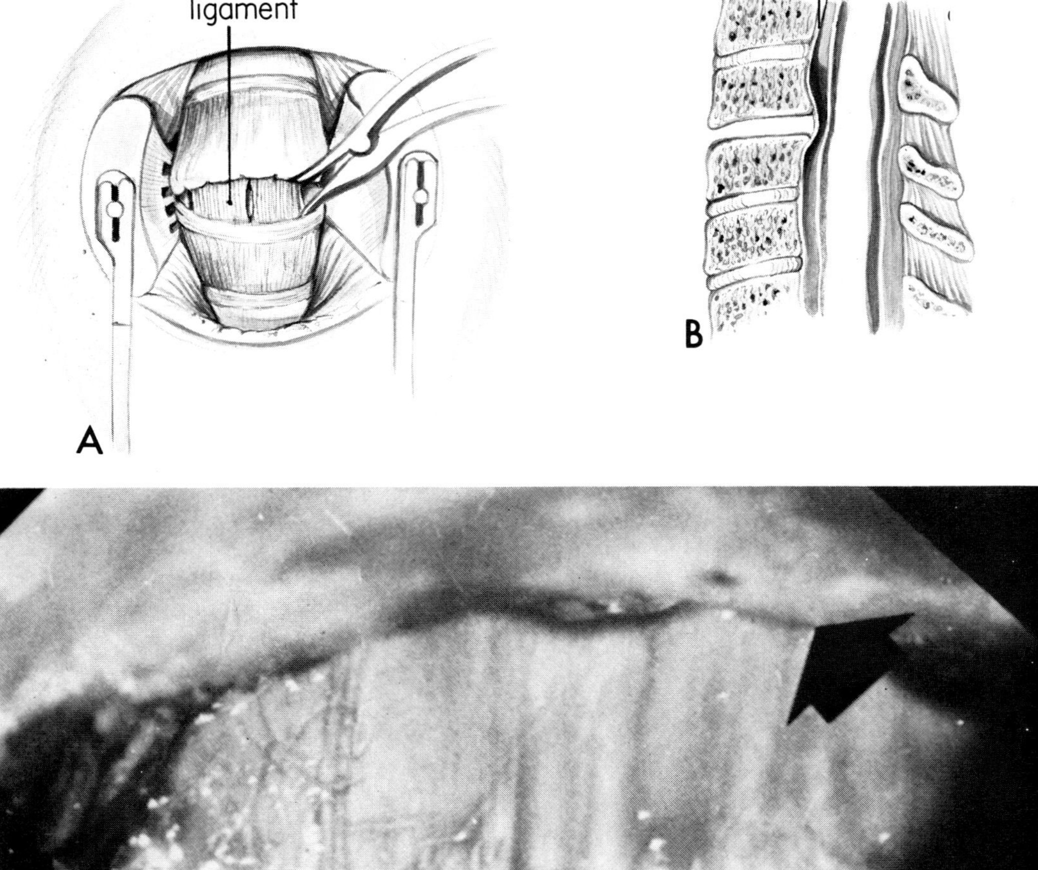

Fig. 116-16. (A) Appearance of the dura following removal of disc material, the cartilaginous plates, and posterior longitudinal ligament. (B) Relationship of the posterior longitudinal ligament to the intervertebral disc and cervical dura. (C) Appearance of the posterior longitudinal ligament under magnification, as seen through the disc space in the cervical region. (Reprinted from Kosary IZ, et al: Microsurgery in anterior approach to cervical discs. Surg Neurol 6:276, 1976. With permission of Paul C. Bucy & Associates.)

processes before surgery. In a patient with degeneration alone, the stability may well be maintained by various muscular and ligamentous structures, and the disc can be removed and fusion occur without a graft. In patients with advanced spondylosis, however, degenerative changes affect the supporting structures of the spine, and subluxation often is seen even before surgery. This latter situation, particularly if it is associated with myelopathy and buckling of the ligamentum flavum, would not favor eliminating the graft. The significant degrees of angulation seen in up to 20 percent of cases in recently reported series according to the criteria discussed earlier represent spinal instability. This instability may eventually escalate into a series of problems significantly worse than the radiculopathy for which the operation was originally performed.

RESULTS OF ANTEROLATERAL DISC EXCISION

CERVICAL RADICULOPATHY

Since the publication of the first edition of this book the results of surgery for cervical radiculopathy have continued to be consistently reported as excellent,[4,6,7,10,13,16,29,32–35] irrespective of whether an anterior or posterior approach was used to decompress the nerve root. Improvement is seen in approximately 85 to 90 percent of the patients, an observation we have reconfirmed with our own series. The advantages of the anterior approach for the treatment of this condition have been enumer-

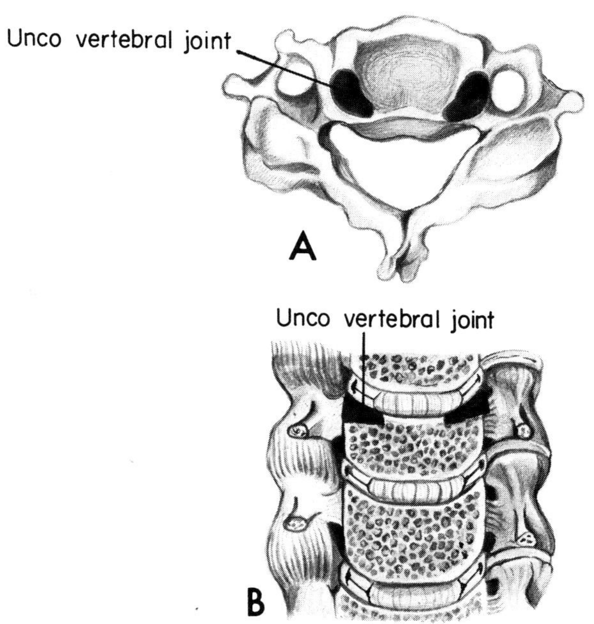

Fig. 116-17. The uncovertebral joints and their local relationships.

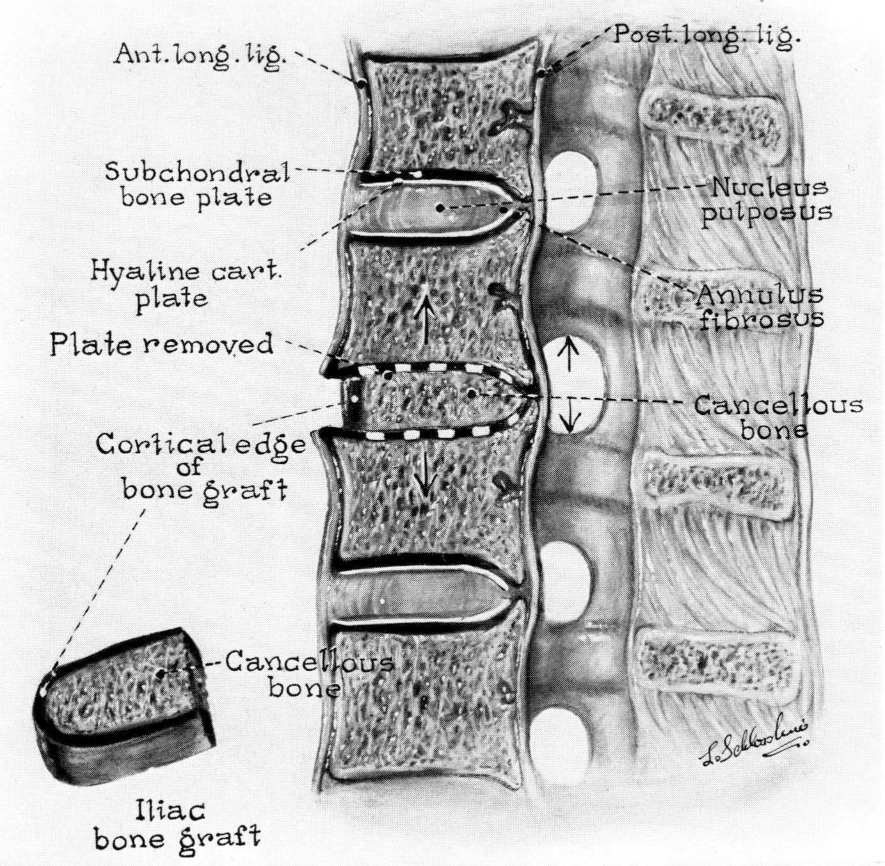

Fig. 116-18. The appearance and positioning of the iliac crest bone graft in a Smith-Robinson-type anterior cervical fusion. (Reprinted from Arthrodesis, in Crenshaw AH (ed): Campbell's Operative Orthopedics, ed 5. St. Louis, C.V. Mosby, 1971, as modified from Robinson RA, Walker AE, Ferlic DC, et al: The results of anterior interbody fusion of the cervical spine. J Bone Joint Surg 44A:1569–1587, 1962. With permission.)

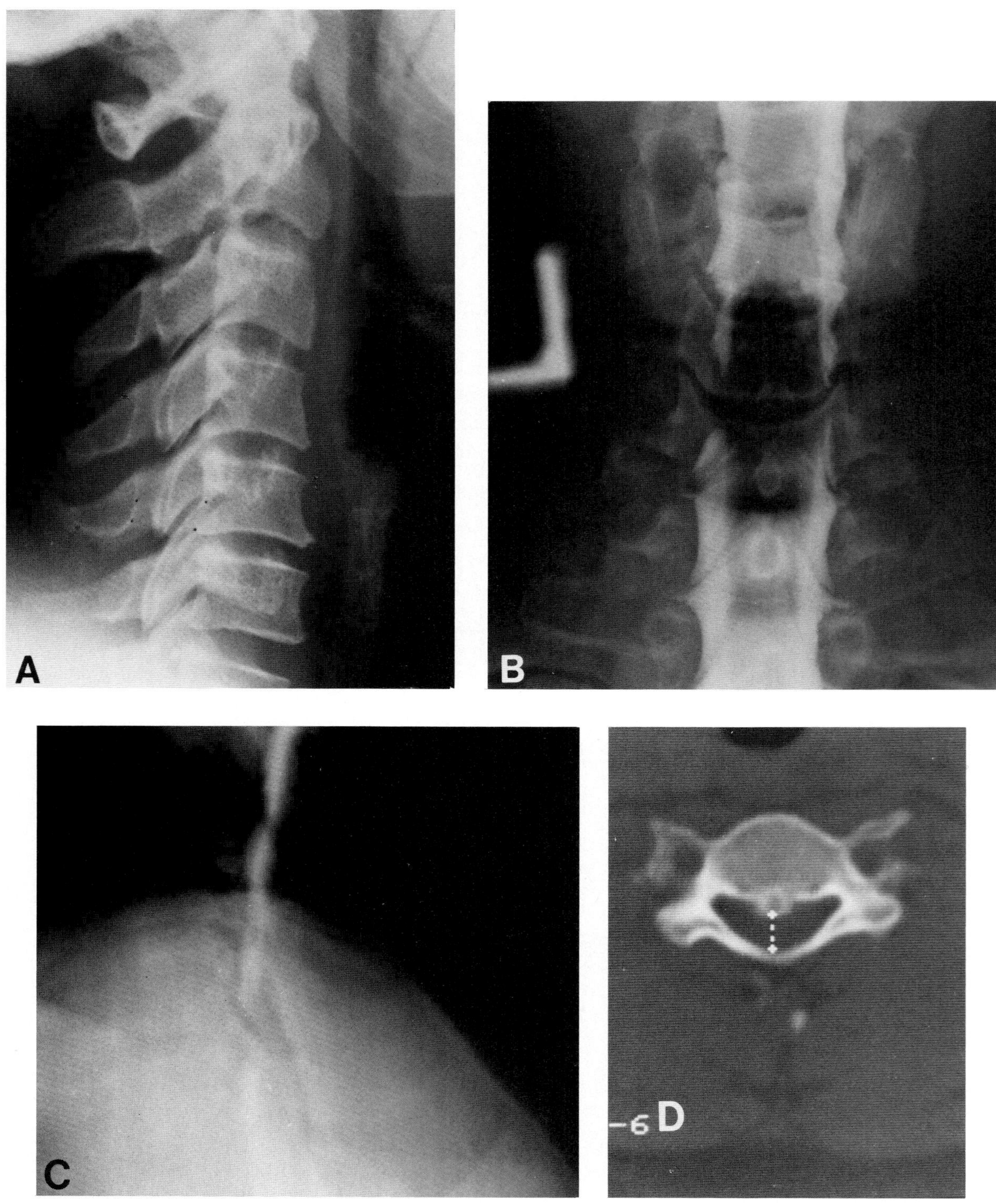

A
B
C
D

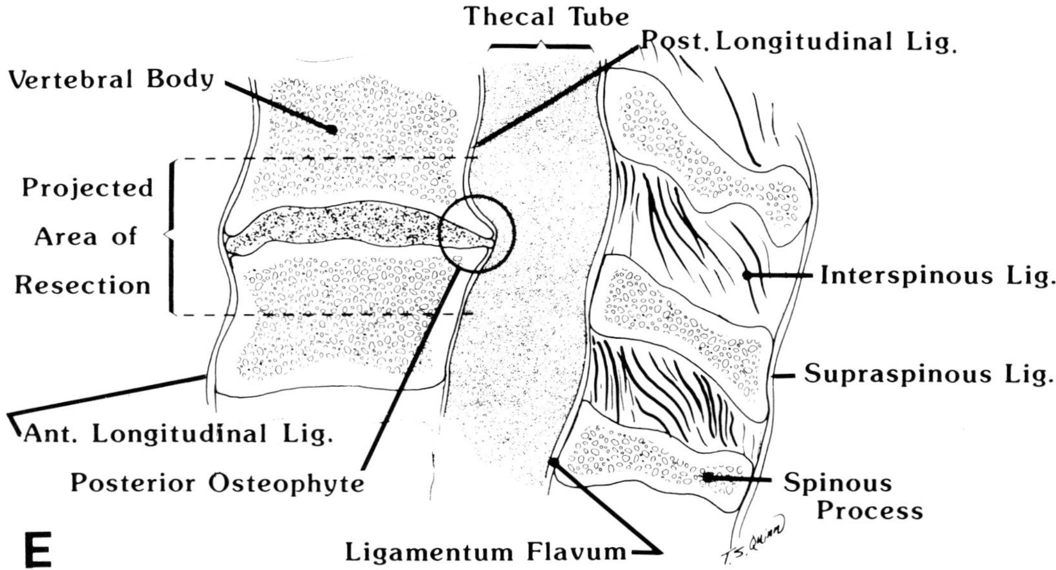

Fig. 116-19 (A) Lateral cervical spine film of a 42-year-old myelopathic man with a congenitally narrow spinal canal and mild superimposed cervical spondylosis. (B) Posteroanterior cervical myelogram of same patient as in A showing high grade obstruction to the passage of contrast at C5-6. (C) Lateral myelographic view of same patient as in A showing obstruction of the dye column by a ventrally situated osteophyte at C5-6. (D) CT image through the C6 body showing marked narrowing of the sagittal diameter of the canal to approximately 8.5 mm by the centrally projecting osteophyte. (E) Projected scope of anterior decompression.

ated, and for these reasons this operation should be standard for the management of cervical radiculopathy due to anterior encroachment at one or two levels at any one time between C3 and T1 levels.

Radiculopathy associated with evidence of disc degeneration at more than one or two levels may be managed without fusion following disc excision. Following discectomy without fusion, intrascapular, neck and shoulder pain are considerably more frequent than with fusion, although the complaints usually subside within 1 to 3 months. Later secondary fusion may be required in some patients with persistent symptoms. If fusion is not performed there is further narrowing of the interspace. One must remove posterior osteophytes to prevent subsequent nerve root compression in these cases.

When radiographic findings are extensive and suggest alterations in the disc, ligamentous, and bony structures, then disc excision with removal of the annulus, anterior longitudinal ligament, and possibly the posterior longitudinal ligament may potentiate the instability of the cervical spine and therefore we prefer fusion and postoperative immobilization of the neck.

CERVICAL MYELOPATHY

When cervical spondylosis was first recognized as a cause of myelopathy, it appeared that favorable results should be produced by removing the mechanical impingement. Allen[36] attempted to remove the protrusions extradurally through a posterior laminectomy with disastrous results. Subsequently, posterior laminectomies and foraminotomies were fashioned to allow the cord to migrate from the spondylotic projections along the anterior aspect of the spine. Collating the various reports, and in our own review of 45 cases, good to excellent results were obtained in approximately 60 percent of patients; another 10 to 15 patients became worse immediately after the surgery. Long-term follow-up revealed that none of the patients ever completely returned to normal. Stoops and King[37] reported 42 patients treated by extensive laminectomy without opening the dura. These patients were followed for up to 6 years. Even though 80 percent were said to show improvement, no prognostic factor could be identified. Crandall,[28] reporting on his long-term study of 55 patients with cervical myelopathy followed from 2 to 25 years, felt that a deficit for less than 1 year was associated with a better prognosis. In contrast, a poor outcome is predictable among patients with sphincteric disturbances shown to be due to the myelopathy. Among these cases, none improved, irrespective of the type of operation.

The debate concerning the appropriate surgical procedure(s) in the management of cervical myelopathy continues. The operative procedure needs to be tailored to the particulars of the case. Posterior cervical laminectomy has a specific indication in patients with prominent dorsal encroachment on the cord due either to bony or ligamentous structures (Figure 116-19A, B, C, and D). Excessive cervical lordosis may be seen in patients with spondylotic myelopathy; overlapping of the lamina, referred to as shingling, may contribute to the myelopathy. Vertebral subluxation may also be seen and may lead to pinching of the cord, from the posterior, by the laminae and infolded ligamentum flavum. Inaccessibility to a disc space; e.g., C2-3 or C3-4 in some cases, is an indication for posterior decompressive cervical laminectomy, as is a secondary procedure in the presence of neurologic progression, particularly with posterior column signs, and in some cases with widespread bony changes and spontaneous fusions anterior to the spinal cord. It has been reported in several series that even in the presence of technically faultless surgery, up to 20 percent of patients treated by laminectomy had an increased deficit after surgery, particularly if the dura is opened and the dentate ligaments are sectioned.

Dereymaeker et al.[50] analyzed two groups of patients with

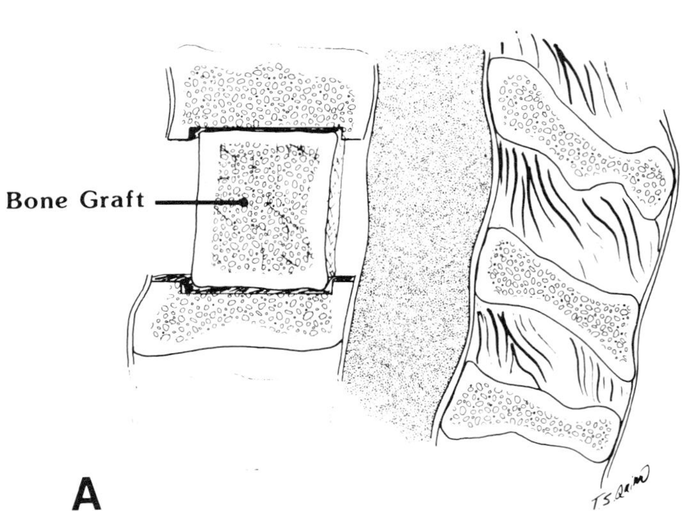

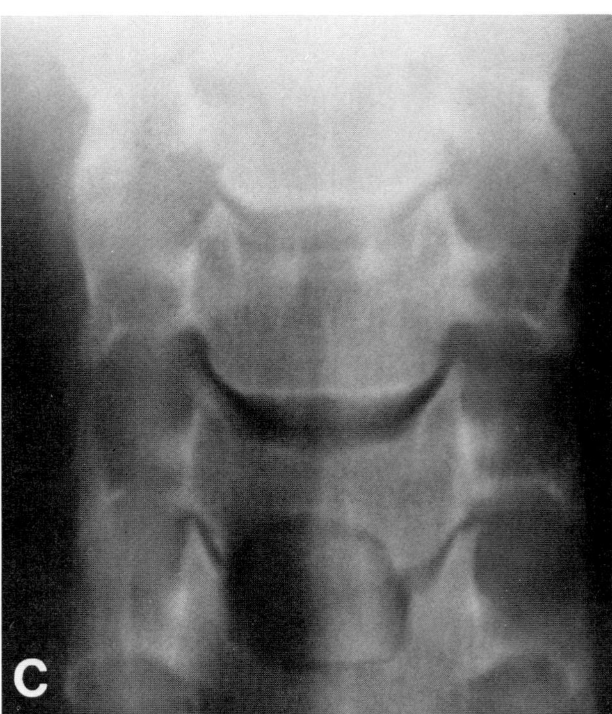

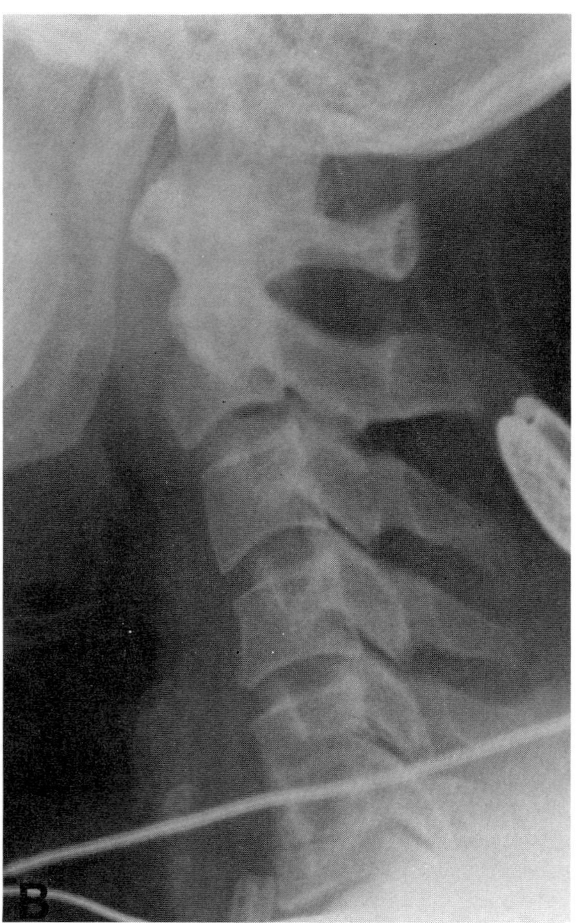

Fig. 116-20 (A) Placement of iliac crest bone graft after radical anterior decompression. (B) Postoperative lateral cervical roentgenogram of same patient as in A following interbody fusion at C5-6. (C) Postoperative AP tomogram of the same patient as in A with an iliac crest bone graft at C5-6.

spondylotic myelopathy operated upon either by the anterior or posterior approach and followed for 2 to 6 years. Clinical and radiographic findings showed that of 31 patients with anterior fusion, 20 were improved; of the 12 who had laminectomy with excision of the disc, 4 were improved. Crandall and Batzdorf[42] reported that of 28 cases of myelopathy treated by anterior discectomy and fusion, 71 percent were improved when posterior projections were removed from the floor of the canal and the involved interspaces were stabilized. No patient was made worse by the operation. This experience was reaffirmed in Crandall's report,[28] showing that none of his patients treated by the Cloward operation was worse postoperatively, but postoperative disability again was increased following decompressive laminectomy. Bohlman[48] has reported his experience with anterior discectomy and interbody arthrodesis in 17 cases of myelopathy. In these cases no attempt was made to remove the posterior longitudinal ligament or osteophytes. Cartilaginous plates and disc material were removed to the posterior longitudinal ligament. Neural function was not lost in any of the 17 patients treated, and of the 17, 14 improved over their preoperative condition. Bone remodeling, but not resorption, occurred at the fused levels and the size of the osteophytes decreased with time.

In Lunsford's series of 32 cases of myelopathy, 92 percent had anterior spondylotic deficits and 13 had a sagittal canal width of under 13 mm at one or more levels. Fifty-nine percent had a myelopathy only, and 41 percent had a myeloradiculopathy. Eight patients had a previous posterior cervical decompressive procedure, and 1 patient a previous anterior operation—so that 24 of the cases address the merits of the anterior approach alone. Surgery involved removal of ventral osteophytes at one or more levels, with 2 patients having four levels operated upon in two stages. One half of the patients improved, and one half of the patients were either unimproved or worse. No predictive indices could be identified, although patients over 60 and symptomatic for more than 2 years tended to have unsatisfactory results. There was no difference in outcome based on the severity of the myelopathy, the number of levels operated upon, or the presence of canal stenosis.

A recent comparative study[51] reviews the experience with 50 cases treated by means of extensive laminectomy, foraminotomy, and excision of osteophytes for cervical myeloradiculopathy. Epstein emphasizes the importance of careful patient selection, adequate laminectomy including two levels above and below areas of significant canal encroachment, and foraminal decompression with removal of only the inner third of the foramen. In this series 85 percent of patients improved and 15 percent were not improved following this operation. In a comparison with other forms of posterior operation, this yielded the best results, and compared to a 73 percent improved category following anterior cervical discectomy.

Based on our assessment of the reported experiences and our own results, we have adopted the following approaches in the management of neurologic sequelae of spondylotic spinal cord with or without root compression, being constantly aware of the very real possibility of increasing the patient's neurologic deficit even when the operation appears to have been technically faultless. In the case of major ventral compression occurring at a single level often reducing the sagittal diameter of the spinal canal under 10 mm and causing a high grade or complete block on cervical myelography, an anterior approach is taken. A Cloward drill is used to remove the bone on either side of the involved disc space for a depth of about 8 to 10 mm. The

remainder of the disc, bone, and osteophyte are then removed with a high speed drill under magnification. The decompression is considered to be complete when the entire ventral aspect of the involved dura is exposed and no further compressive element can be identified rostrocaudally or laterally along the nerve roots. Following this extensive decompression an iliac crest bone graft is fashioned and countersunk into position. In order to prevent the extrusion of the graft, the longus colli muscles are sutured to one another across the midline with 0-0 nonabsorbable suture material. Postoperatively the patient is ambulated within 1 to 2 days depending on the severity of the myelopathy and the neck is kept immobilized in a Philadelphia collar until bony union has been demonstrated radiographically (3 to 4 months).

A similar radical ventral decompression is performed when two contiguous interspaces are involved by severe spondylotic changes resulting in anteriorly situated spinal cord compression. Under these circumstances it is often impossible to attribute the neurologic presentation to one or the other level in spite of the information obtained clinically and radiographically. Under these circumstances the lower of the two levels is decompressed as described above and the decompression is then extended rostrally, This involves removal of a trough of bone constituting the center of the vertebral body between the two interspaces. Decompression is carried superiorly through the disc space and into the body above to ensure radical removal of all ventrally situated disc, osteophytes, and ligament. Examination of the surgical field at this stage shows the dura over a length corresponding to about the height of two vertebral bodies. Following this decompression, carried out with the high speed drill and the operating microscope, an iliac bone graft is fashioned to fill the bony deficit and countersunk into position. Postoperatively the neck is immobilized for 4 to 6 months using an extended Philadelphia collar.

When confronted with a severe degree of cervical spondylotic changes at more than two levels, we generally opt for posterior decompressive laminectomy, usually from C2 to C7 inclusively, using the air drill to cut the laminae at each of these levels and then removing the entire section of laminae plus the spinous processes en bloc. This technique has been adopted to prevent even minimal intraoperative compression of the compromised spinal cord with the Kerrison rongeur or other instruments requiring introduction beneath the lamina prior to their removal. In these cases, unless there is an associated radiculopathy, no specific attempt is made to also decompress the nerve roots. The dura is not opened unless it has been impossible on the basis of the preoperative information to exclude a spinal cord tumor as being responsible for the clinical findings. With the current diagnostic studies including CT, CT with metrizamide, and magnetic resonance imaging this is becoming an increasingly less frequent occurrence. Although much has been written in the orthopedic literature concerning subsequent instability following decompressive cervical laminectomy, we have not seen this complication except in children, in patients with weakness of the cervical musculature due to their underlying neurologic problem, or when there has been a radical removal of the facets bilaterally. Except in these situations the neck does not require external support other than for the patient's comfort.

The anterior approach has evolved into an operative procedure for cervical spondylotic myelopathy provided that the major compressive elements are situated anterior to the spinal cord. Whether the osteophytes require radical removal in this situation is problematic. It is possible with the operating microscope and diamond drills to remove them without substantial risk, and on our service this is done in conjunction with fusion of the involved interspaces in cases of myelopathy.

REFERENCES

1. Adams CBT, Logue V: Studies in cervical spondylotic myelopathy. 3. Some functional effects of operations for cervical spondylotic myelopathy. Brain 94:587, 1971
2. Aronson NI: The management of soft cervical disc protrusions using the Smith-Robinson approach. Clin Neurosurg 20:253, 1973
3. Bailey RW, Badjley CE: Stabilization of the cervical spine by anterior fusion. J Bone Joint Surg 42A:565, 1960
4. Cloward RB: New method of diagnosis and treatment of cervical disc disease. Clin Neurosurg 8:93, 1962
5. Cloward RB: Lesions of the intervertebral disc and their treatment by interbody fusion methods. Clin Orthop 27:51, 1963.
6. Smith GW, Robinson RA: The treatment of certain cervical spine disorders by anterior removal of the intervertebral disc and interbody fusion. J Bone Joint Surg 40A:607, 1958
7. Murphy MB, Bado M: Anterior cervical discectomy without interbody bone graft. J Neurosurg 37:711, 1972
8. Robertson JT: Anterior operations for herniated cervical disc and for myelopathy. Clin Neurosurg 25:245, 1978
9. Robinson RA, Walker AE, Ferlick DE: The results of anterior interbody fusion of the cervical spine. J Bone Joint Surg 44A:1569, 1962
10. Robinson RA: Anterior and posterior cervical fusions. Clin Orthop 35:34, 1964
11. Cloward RB: Treatment of acute fractures and fracture dislocations of the cervical spine by vertebral body fusion. J Neurosurg 18:201, 1961
12. Scoville WB, Dohrmann AM, Corkill AR: Late results of cervical disc surgery. J Neurosurg 45:203, 1976
13. Zulch KJ: Personal communications, 1976
14. Robinson RA: Personal communcation, 1976
15. Clarke, Robinson PK: Cervical myelopathy: Complication of cervical spondylosis. Brain 79:483, 1956
16. Gregorius FK, Estrin T, Crandall PH: Cervical spondylotic radiculopathy and myelopathy: A long-term follow-up study. Arch Neurol 33:618, 1976
17. Lees F, Turner JWA: Natural history and prognosis of cervical spondylosis. Br Med J 2:1607, 1963
18. Roth DA: Cervical analgesic discography: A new test for the definitive diagnosis of the painful disc syndrom. JAMA 235:1713, 1976
19. Hilding DA, Tachdjian MO: Dysphagia and hypertrophic spurring of the cervical spine. N Engl J Med 263:11, 1960
20. Maran A, Jacobson I: Cervical osteophytes presenting with pharyngeal symptoms. Laryngoscope 81:412, 1971
21. Facer JA: Osteophytes of the cervical spine causing dysphagia. Arch Otolaryngol 86:341, 1967
22. Meeks LW, Renshaw TS: Ankylosing vertebral hyperostosis and dysphagia, in Bailey RW (ed): The Cervical Spine. Philadelphia, Lea and Febiger, 1974, pp 242–249
23. Hutchinson EC, Yates PO: The cervical portion of the vertebral artery. A clinicopathological study. Brain 79:319, 1956
24. Verbiest H: From anterior to lateral operations on the cervical spine. Neurosurg Rev 1:47, 1978
25. White AA, Johnson RM, Panjabi MM, et al: Biomechanical analysis of clinical stability in the cervical spine. Clin Orthop 109:5, 1975
26. Tew JM Jr, Mayfield FH: Complications of surgery of the anterior cervical spine. Clin Neurosurg 23:424, 1976
27. Lunsford LD, Bissonette DJ, Jannetta PJ, et al: Anterior surgery for cervical disc disease. J Neurosurg 53:11, 1980
28. Heeneman H: Vocal cord paralysis following approaches to the anterior cervical spine. Laryngoscope 83:17, 1973
29. Simmons EH, Bhalla SK: Anterior cervical discectomy and fusion: A clinical and biomechanical study with eight year follow-up. J Bone Joint Surg 51B:225, 1969
30. Aronson N, Bagan N, Filtzer DL: Results of using the Smith-Robinson approach for herniated and extruded cervical discs. J Neurosurg 32:721, 1970
31. Martins AN: AC discectomy with/without interbody bone graft. J Neurosurg 44:290, 1976
32. Riley LH Jr, Robinson RA, Johnson DA: The results of anterior interbody fusion of the cervical spine. Review of 93 consecutive cases. J Neurosurg 30:127, 1969
33. Bishara SN: The posterior operation in the treatment of cervical spondylosis with myelopathy: A long-term follow-up study. J Neurol Neurosurg Psychiatry 34:393, 1971
34. Brain WR, Northfield DWC, Wilkinson M: Neurological manifestations of cervical spondylosis. Brain 75:187, 1952
35. Brain L, Wilkinson M: Cervical Spondylosis. Philadelphia, WB Saunders, 1967
36. Allen KL: Neuropathies caused by bony spurs in the cervical spine with special reference to surgical treatment. J Neurol Neurosurg Psychiatry 15:20, 1952
37. Stoops WL, King RB: Neural complications of cervical spondylosis: Their response to laminectomy and foraminotomy. J Neurosurg 19:986, 1962
38. Epstein JA, Carras LA, Epstein BS, et al: Myelopathy in cervical spondylosis with vertebral subluxation and hyperlordosis. J Neurosurg 32:421, 1970
39. Cleveland D: Interspace reconstruction and spinal stabilization after disc removal. Lancet 76:326, 1956
40. Epstein JA, Janin Y, Carras R, Lavine LS: A comparative study of the treatment of cervical spondylotic myeloradiculopathy. Acta Neurochir 61:89, 1982
41. Hicks DS, Whitecloud TS, Cracco A, et al: Cervical spondylotic myelopathy: Results of anterior decompression and stabilization. Orthop Trans 4:44, 1980
42. Cervical Spine Research Society: The Cervical Spine. Philadelphia, JB Lippincott Co, 1983

CHAPTER 117

Cervical Discography, Discometry, and Cervical Disc Distension Test

William H. Sweet   Henry H. Schmidek

THE CONTINUING USE in some quarters of diagnostically worthless procedures leads us to include a section on the evolution and devolution of this subject. Injection of radiopaque contrast medium into the intervertebral disc for diagnostic purposes was introduced by Lindblom at Hirsch's suggestion in Sweden in 1948.[1] Later the same year Hirsch, also at the Karolinska Institute in Stockholm, described the injection of normal saline into low lumbar discs with the production of pain "identical with the patient's spontaneous pain."[2] He noted as well that Lindblom's radiography of the disc "is of considerable value"; "it reveals rupture of the annulus." The procedure was extended to the cervical region, Smith and Nichols finding that 0.5 to 1.0 ml of 70 percent Diodrast injected slowly "usually passed readily into the disk space with relatively slight resistance. If the disk space being injected is diseased the patient quickly complains of severe pain . . . or paresthesias . . . simulating his admission complaints. He will complain also of posterior cervical and suboccipital pain, as well as referred interscapular and anterior chest pain, if these have been part of the original syndrome."[3] The procedures of studying the discs with contrast material and of seeking to correlate clinical pain with that induced by injection of specific discs gained many adherents. By 1966 Fox noted that he joined about 100 previous authors publishing on the method.[4] He concluded, "discography in many instances should be the primary diagnostic procedure in preference to myelography." The observation that patients complaints of pain somewhere in the head, neck, upper limb or upper torso might be exacerbated or duplicated by injection of a cervical disc led to the cheerful conclusion that there is a "discogenic syndrome of pain unaccompanied by any sensory, motor, reflex or other objective features implicating the nerve roots or spinal cord."[5,6] We say cheerful because this concept exposes the vista of an almost unlimited number of individuals for whom one might recommend surgical removal of one cervical disc or 2 or 3 or 4 or 5. Thus, Schaerer of St. Louis removed 350 discs from 221 patients between about 1960 and 1968,[7] and Stuck of Denver operated on about 75 percent of the 1200 patients on whom he did cervical discograms.[8] DePalma and Rothman (p. 90) also say that injection of normal saline into various cervical discs will usually yield one that reproduces the patient's symptoms and (p. 100) "This disc distension test will, in practically all instances, locate the disc or discs responsible for the syndrome."[6] To their credit they also state that "the majority of patients with cervical disc disease, either acute or chronic, will respond to a conscientious program of conservative therapy."[9] Aronson and Filtzer add that "cervical myelography and EMGs are usually normal in these individuals"—that "discometry however is markedly positive, and at surgery there is disruption and fissuring of the disc with annular tears . . . the patients are at once relieved of their pain . . . four and even five levels can be done at one sitting with safety."[10]—extremely poor advice in our view.

All of these statements subsequent to the earliest studies ignore dramatic evidence to the contrary. Thus, Smith within 2 years of his original article noted that "since a high percentage of cervical discs shows degeneration, a great number of degenerated intervertebral discs are seen which may not produce spontaneous symptoms and this may give false roentgen-positive information. . . ." "Relatively few normal cervical diskograms are obtained in individuals who have passed the age of 25 or 30 years."[11] This last statement was reinforced by Meyer's observation that "in 32 patients with neck, shoulder or arm pain the cervical diskogram was abnormal in every case" with widespread extravasation of the contrast medium in many directions including the epidural space.[12] Furthermore, "there was no good correlation of pain radiation (during injection) with the patient's clinical symptoms or the roentgenographic findings." In two patients with abnormal discograms "an adequate exploration of the epidural space via the laminectomy approach revealed no abnormality."

The remarkable vulnerability to degenerative change of the intervertebral discs, especially those in the cervical region, has been fully documented as the fact which eliminates the value of radiologic discography. In his earliest edition, the comprehensive studies of Schmorl as well as the later work of Junghanns and the American translation of Besemann all emphasize that early extensive deterioration of disc tissue is "unique in that such changes are hardly encountered in any other organ system of the human body."[13,14] These early aging changes appear to be related to the absence of blood vessels in the discs with the corresponding reliance for nutrition and absorption of wastes on diffusion from and to surrounding tissues. "Beyond age 30 a spine without any undamaged discs is rarely found. Even before age 30 there are a considerable number of disc changes." By 1952 Hirsch and Schajowicz had described early degenerative changes in the lumbar spine.[15] In a monumental study of fresh human autopsy material, these two authors plus Galante studied about 700 discs in 111 cervical spines and over 3000 histologic sections.[16] They found disc fissuration beginning at age 7 and constantly present from age 14 on in the upper disc levels and frequently at the lower discs.'' They found the cervical discs to be avascular tissues from the time of birth, and state, ''The fact that fissures constantly are present early in life, connecting inner parts of the disc with posterolateral regions, allowing leakage of contrast media into foraminal and posterior areas at many disc levels in the same subject eliminates the clinical value of discography as a means of identifying significant disc pathology.'' A recent study confirms for the lumbar spine that ''the major blood supply to the disc for all practical purposes is gone by age 30.''[17]

Probably the most devastating criticisms of both the radiographic and the disc distention tests follow from the studies of Holt on completely asymptomatic men, volunteer criminal prisoners.[8,18,19] His first group of 50 healthy men aged 21 to 50 were selected from 200 volunteers on the basis of no history of cervical injury or of pain in neck or arm. Each man had 3 disc spaces punctured with a 22-gauge needle from C3-4 to C7-T1. Placement in mid-disc was confirmed by biplane x-ray films. Despite premedication with 50 mg meperidine or 90 mg sodium pentobarbital by hypodermic injection, injection of 50 percent sodium diatrizoate (Hypaque) produced great pain in every subject at every space. The pain lasted about 5 minutes, then disappeared. It was referred to the neck, and/or between the shoulder blades or sternum. Despite previous statements in the literature to the contrary, there was no consistent pattern of foci of pain related to disc injected, nor was there any correlation between amount injected with degree of pain. Regardless of the amounts injected—0.5 to 1.0 cc as suggested by Smith[11], or 0.2 to 0.3 cc as suggested by Cloward[5]—there was extravasation of the contrast medium at once beyond the disc in 138 of 148 spaces injected. ''It was a rare space that would not take a full cc if this was desired.'' ''However, if a slow injection was made into the first space, many subjects went into tonic neck spasm, creating intradisc pressures, so that further injection was difficult or impossible.'' ''On the other hand if one cc was injected precipitously, it would be delivered into the space before resistance was met.'' The volume of injectable medium was unreliable as an indication of a pathologic condition since 93 percent of these normal discs allowed rapid extravasation. The amount readily injectable was dependent upon the state of tonus in the neck muscles. ''The claim of reproduction of discogenic pain by injection of the responsible disk space seems likely to be fallacious because injection into any cervical disc causes great pain.''

In 1968, Holt reported similar studies at the lowest 3 lumbar discs in another 30 volunteer prisoners ages 21 to 41 years with an average age of 26.[19] Successful disc injections were made in 69 spaces. Up to 2 cc of Hypaque caused but little discomfort in 45 of those in which the contrast remained central. In 11 discs (15 percent) in which the contrast extended to the annulus, severe pain was usually reported. Actual leakage occurred in 16 discs (22 percent) with pain in the back, the leg, or both sites in each case; this was often severe for several minutes. Holt points out that if there are 37 percent false ±positives in healthy young men there would probably be a higher percentage of these in older age groups. Massie and Stevens also did lumbar discograms on 52 male volunteers aged 20 to 52 years, finding that ''only 60 percent had a normal disc outline in all 3 lower lumbar interspaces.''[20] Gresham and Miller added further evidence as to the infrequency of normal lumbar discograms in normal persons by doing postmortem discography on 63 fresh autopsy specimens of patients aged 14 to 63 years with ''relatively asymptomatic normal backs.'' Even in the group under 35 years of age 10 percent of the discs were '' degenerated''; in the group aged 35 to 60 years 75 percent of the discograms were abnormal with no normal studies at the L5-S1 level in patients 46 to 59 years old. In those over 60 years of age only 5 percent of 60 discs, i.e., 3, yielded normal discograms.[21] Despite the remarkable futility of these procedures as evidenced by such extensive studies, text writers (and we include ourselves) have continued to perpetuate misinformation about them. Thus, Simeone and Rothman (p. 410) erroneously say, ''A normal cervical disc will rarely accept more than 0.1 ml. This seldom induces pain in a normal disc. Pathologic discs will accept a larger quantity of solution, and the injection is usually associated with pain. The location and distribution of this pain is an important additional diagnostic clue . . . . If the induced pain reproduces the patient's symptoms, the disc is implicated.''[22]

However, the control studies in normals have properly led to progressively decreased use of these procedures. Thus the distinguished radiologist Taveras concluded 19 years ago that discography should be limited to the lumbar region, and even there under such rigorous restrictions that he had recommended it in only ''one or 2 dozen cases in 15 years, representing an accumulated experience of some 9000 cases where myelography was required,''[23] which he thought should always precede discography.

Radiographic discography being futile, what is the evidence that reproduction of the clinical pain upon injection of innocuous fluid into a specific disc implicates a lesion of that disc as the cause of the pain? It became clear early that irritation due to the contrast medium was not the cause of the pain. The studies of three papers[2,24,25] of Hirsch all reported the development of pain in some patients upon lumbar intradural injections of 1 to 2 ml of normal saline. If these injections were preceded by injections of 0.5 to 1.0 ml of 1 percent procaine, no pain was caused. The slightly differing finding of Hoen et al. in 12 of 15 patients was that low lumbar intradiscal injections of 3 to 10 ml of either normal saline or 1 percent procaine reproduced or accentuated the patient's pain.[26] Shutkin reports a similar experience of provoking pain in all 6 patients in whom he injected 5 ml of 1 percent procaine into the L5-S1 area.[27] As Fernström pointed out, these observations make it clear that an irritant quality of an injectate is not necessary for the pain to occur.[28] The original proponent of lumbar discography, Lindblom, reported no correlation between intensity of pain and subsequent observations at operation.

Klafta and Collins analyzed 549 disc injections, noting pain in 89 percent of them, and finding a poor correlation between pain responses and discograms.[29] They concluded, ''Pain on injection, similar to the presenting symptom, is of no diagnostic significance.''

In their monograph ''The Spine'' Rothman and Simeone (1975) (p. 468) say regarding lumbar discography ''the amount of dye accepted, the configuration of the opaque media and reproduction of the patient's pain are abnormalities so common that little significance can be placed on the presence of an abnormal discogram in terms of localizing the essence of a patient's pain''[30] By 1985 Simeone had become even more emphatic saying, ''The role of discography has been reduced to insignificance by modern myelography and CT techniques. In particular, lumbar discography, a painful and inaccurate test, can no longer be justified.''[31] Anent cervical discography and the disc distension tests, Hoff in his section on cervical disc disease in the same text has eliminated all mention of these useless procedures.[32]

Our own experiences are that the temporary pain on injection either of saline or contrast medium into the disc may be sufficiently severe and diffuse to make it hard for the patient to compare with the clinical pain. In any event the pain is inconsistently related to the other clinical and radiographic findings. One of us, HHS, had this instructive experience. Under the impression that he had entered the disc space with his needle he injected saline, evoking at once the most convincing statement by the patient of duplication of the main complaint of pain in the neck and upper limb he had encountered. A lateral roentgenogram then showed the needle in the precervical tissues several levels below the clinically indicated disc! The propensity of saline to leave the disc makes it impossible after any intradiscal injection to exclude the possibility that the pain may have arisen from some completely extravertebral site. Further development of both CT and magnetic resonance imaging techniques has eliminated whatever meager justification there may have been for discography and disc distension tests. We have deleted their mention from other chapters for the reasons we have described here in extenso in an attempt to stop the ill advised surgery entailed by reliance on them.

REFERENCES

1. Lindblom K: Diagnostic puncture of intervertebral disks in sciatica. Acta Orthop Scand 17:231, 1948
2. Hirsch C: An attempt to diagnose the level of a disc lesion clinically by disc puncture. Acta Orthop Scand 18:132, 1948
3. Smith GW, Nichols P: The technic of cervical discography. Radiology 68:718, 1957
4. Fox JL: Lumbar discography. A myelographic correlation. Acta Neurol Latinoamer 12:114, 1966
5. Cloward RB: Cervical diskography: Technique, indications and use in diagnosis of ruptured cervical disc. Am J Roentgenol Radiat Therap Nucl Med 79:563, 1958
6. DePalma AF, Rothman RH: Operative treatment of cervical disc disease, in The Intervertebral Disc. Philadelphia, WB Saunders, 1970, pp 97–101
7. Schaerer JP: Anterior cervical disc removal and fusion. Schweiz Arch Neurol Neurochir Psychiat 102:331, 1968
8. Holt EP: Further reflections on cervical discography. JAMA 231:613, 1975.
9. DePalma AF, Rothman RH: Conservative treatment of cervical disc disease, in The Intervertebral Disc. Philadelphia, WB Saunders, 1970, p 90
10. Aronson NI, Filtzer DL: Anterior cervical discectomy and fusion: Smith-Robinson approach. Contemp Neurosurg 4:1, 1982
11. Smith GW: The normal cervical diskogram with clinical observations. Am J Roentgenol Radiat Ther Nucl Med 81:1006, 1959
12. Meyer RR: Cervical diskography. A help or hindrance in evaluating neck, shoulder, arm pain? AJR 90:1208, 1963
13. Schmorl G: The Human Spine in Health and Disease, 5th German Edition H Junghanns, 2nd American translation by EF Besemann. New York, Grune & Stratton, 1971, pp 141–151
14. Junghanns H: Altersveränderungen der menschlichen Wirbelsäule. Die Altersosteoporose. Arch Klin Chir 166:106, 1931
15. Hirsch C, Schajowicz F: Studies on structural changes in the lumbar annulus fibrosus. Acta Orthop Scand 22:184, 1953
16. Hirsch C, Schajowicz F, Galante J: Structural changes in the cervical spine. Acta Orthop Scand Suppl 109:1, 1967
17. Wiesel SW, Bernini, P, Rothman RH: The Aging Lumbar Spine. Philadelphia, WB Saunders, 1982, pp 23–24
18. Holt EP: Fallacy of cervical discography. JAMA 188:799, 1964
19. Holt EP: The question of lumbar discography. J Bone Joint Surg 50A:720, 1968
20. Massie WK, Stevens DB: A critical evaluation of discography. J Bone Joint Surg 49A:1243, 1967
21. Gresham JL, Miller R: Evaluation of the lumbar spine by diskography and its use in selection of proper treatment of the herniated disk syndrome. Clin Orthop 67:29, 1969
22. Simeone FA, Rothman RH: Cervical disc disease, in Rothman RH, Simeone FA (eds): The Spine, vol 1. Philadelphia, WB Saunders, 1975, pp 387–433
23. Taveras J: Is discography a useful diagnostic procedure? J Can Assoc Radiol 19:294, 1967
24. Hirsch C: Studies on the mechanisms of low back pain. 5th International Congress of Orthopedic Surgery and Traumatology, Stockholm, 226, 1951
25. Hirsch C: Studies on the mechanism of low back pain. Acta Orthop Scand 20:261, 1951
26. Hoen T, Druckemiller W, Cook, A: Injection of the lumbar intervertebral disks. US Armed Forces Med J 2:1067, 1951
27. Shutkin NM: Syndrome of the degenerated intervertebral disc. Am J Surg 84:162, 1952
28. Fernström U: A discographical study of ruptured lumbar intervertebral discs. An investigation based on anatomical, pathological, surgical and clinical studies and on experiments in provocation of pain with special reference to simple ruptured lumbar discs and discogenic pain. Acta Chir Scand Suppl 258:560, 1960
29. Klafta LA, Collis JS: The diagnostic inaccuracy of the pain response in cervical discography. Cleve Clin Q 36:35, 1969
30. Rothman RH, Simeone FA: Lumbar disc disease, in Rothman RH, Simeone FA (eds): The Spine, vol 2. Philadelphia, WB Saunders, 1975, pp 443–513
31. Simeone F: Lumbar disc disease, in Wilkins RH, Rengachary S (eds): Neurosurgery, vol 3. New York, McGraw-Hill, 1985, p 2253
32. Hoff JT: Cervical Disc Disease and Cervical Spondylosis. New York, McGraw-Hill, 1985, pp 2230–2239

CHAPTER 118

Posterior Operations for Cervical Disc Herniation and Spondylotic Myelopathy

James C. Collias   Melville P. Roberts

THE TRADITIONAL POSTERIOR APPROACH to decompression of the spinal cord and nerve roots is used less frequently since the development of the anterior approach to the cervical spine.[1,2] Laminectomy and foraminotomy, however, have retained their importance in the surgical treatment of lateral cervical disc herniation and spondylotic myelopathy. In most instances, either the anterior or posterior approach can be used with satisfactory results; the choice is determined by the preference of the surgeon. In some situations, however, the lesion dictates a specific approach. For this reason, expertise in both approaches is necessary. This chapter will describe the techniques used at the Hartford Hospital.

LATERAL CERVICAL DISC HERNIATIONS

Although results with anterior discectomy can be just as gratifying, the posterior approach for lateral disc herniation has certain advantages. It allows immediate mobilization of the neck, the disc structure is preserved, and two or more roots can be explored without additional discectomy. In addition, the morbidity associated with fusions is eliminated, as are the inevitable stresses applied to adjacent interspaces following fusion. Also, the C3-4 and C7-D1 discs are more easily approached by the posterior route. In contrast, centrally located soft disc protrusions are more safely approached anteriorly.

Since Scoville's early contributions to cervical disc surgery,[3-8] laminotomy with foraminotomy has been used to treat most lateral cervical disc protrusions at the Hartford Hospital. We now have an operative experience of more than 2500 cases over a period of 45 years.

INCIDENCE

In a review of 2035 of our surgical cases for ruptured cervical discs (Roberts and Collias, unpublished data), lateral soft disc protrusions occurred in 85 percent, hard disc ruptures in 11 percent, and soft central disc ruptures in 4 percent. The male-to-female ratio was evenly distributed, 49 percent men and 51 percent women. The mean age was 37 years; the oldest patient was 73 years and the youngest 21 years. The most common roots involved were C6 and C7, with 54 percent of disc ruptures occurring at the C6-C7 level, 35 percent at C5-C6, 6 percent at C7-D1, 5 percent at C4-C5, and only two cases at C3-C4.

There was one instance of two extruded fragments found at two adjacent levels on the same side during the same operation. A hard disc protrusion and a soft one at adjacent levels when two discs were explored was more common. Less than 20 percent of the patients had a history of trauma. Recurrent disc rupture on the same side at the same level occurred in only one patient. Nineteen percent of patients developed disc herniations at other locations.[4] Cervical disc protrusion requiring surgery occurred at a ratio of 1:10 compared with lumbar disc protrusion.

CLINICAL MANIFESTATIONS

The classic picture of lateral disc herniation is distinctive and easily recognized. Neck pain occurs, usually without a precipitating event. This pain subsequently extends to the shoulder, the medial scapula, and down the arm to the hand. The pain also can radiate into the anterolateral chest. In acute cases, the head and neck may be held rigidly, flexed and rotated away from the side of the rupture. Extension of the neck to the side of the lesion is resisted (Scoville-Spurling test)[3] and increases the pain. Upward neck traction or elevation of the shoulder and elbow may relieve the pain. Hard disc herniations may cause less acute pain.

Radicular syndromes generally can be recognized easily by dermatomal and myotomal findings. Sensory deficit in overlapping dermatomes without reflex loss or weakness at times may make it difficult to differentiate between the C6 and C7 roots. Weakness of the deltoid, infraspinatus, and supraspinatus with sensory loss over the deltoid occurs in C5 root involvement. Weakness of the biceps and brachioradialis muscles with numbness and paresthesias in the thumb and index finger occurs with C6 root compression in C5-C6 lesions. Weakness of the triceps, wrist, and finger extensors with diminished triceps reflex and numbness in the index and middle fingers occurs with C7 root involvement in C6-C7 ruptures. Weakness of intrinsic hand muscles and ulnar sensory loss occur in C8 root compression with a C7-D1 disc rupture.

OPERATIVE NEUROSURGICAL TECHNIQUES
ISBN 0-8089-1862-1

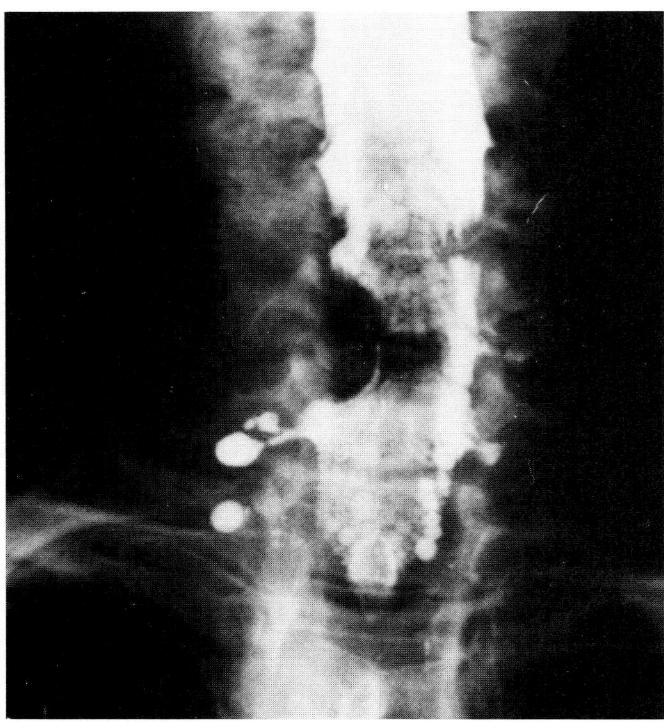

Fig. 118-1. A myelogram showing a large defect on the left at C6-7 caused by a neurofibroma and a smaller defect on the right at C5-6 caused by a ruptured disc.

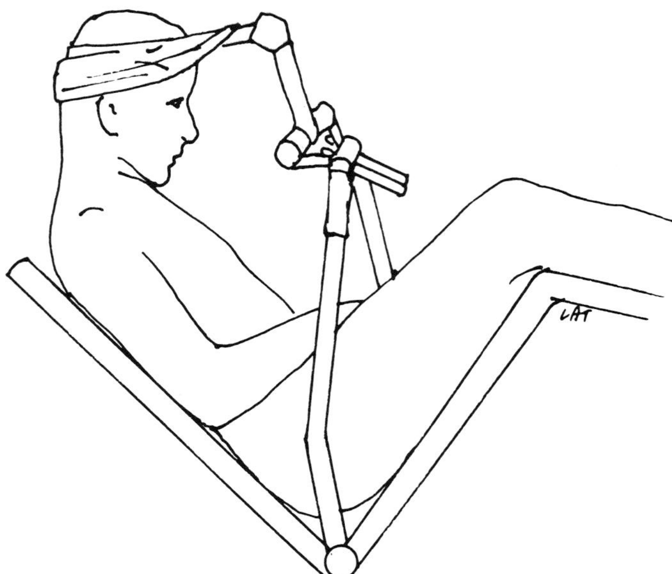

Fig. 118-2. The sitting position used for posterior operations for cervical disc herniation and spondylotic myelopathy.

NONSURGICAL TREATMENT

Initial treatment consists of sedation, analgesics, and traction. Cervical traction with 10 to 15 pounds of weight for 20 to 30 minutes with the neck in the flexed position may help. Traction in extension can exacerbate the pain. Many patients improve without further treatment. It is difficult to set an arbitrary time beyond which nonsurgical treatment should be discontinued and surgery considered. It definitely should be continued as long as the patient is improving.

Severe, unremitting pain and profound neurologic deficit usually require immediate surgical intervention. Decreasing pain with increasing neurologic deficit also warrants concern and merits prompt diagnosis and treatment. The patient's vocation, i.e., surgeon or musician, should be considered, particularly if there is significant dominant arm or hand weakness. Early decompression is frequently indicated so that permanent sensory or motor loss can be avoided. Economic factors may make a long nonsurgical treatment period impractical. Chronic pain that interferes with sleep and work after an initial period of improvement is usually an indication for surgery.

DIAGNOSTIC STUDIES

Flexion, extension, and oblique view roentgenograms of the cervical spine are obtained as initial studies. In our series these studies were normal in 50 percent of patients and showed disc space narrowing and degenerative changes at levels other than that of the disc rupture in 20 percent. Myelography is the definitive study and is carried out on almost all patients considered for surgery to confirm the size, shape, and location of the lesion and also to rule out other unsuspected intradural lesions.

In one case (Figure 118-1) a benign intradural tumor and disc protrusion coexisted and were removed at the same operation.

Multiple minor defects frequently can be seen with associated spondylosis, but the lesion responsible for the patient's symptoms can usually be identified. In our series. myelography was diagnostic in 99 percent of cases. Until recently Pantopaque was used and was usually instilled through the lumbar route. Water-soluble contrast medium such as metrizamide (Amipaque) produced poorer definition and greater toxic reactions. Two patients had seizures after its use. It was useful when diluted for high resolution computed tomographic (CT) scanning. Computed tomographic scanning of the cervical spine without contrast is frequently worthless. We now use a solution of 61 percent iopamidol (Isovue), which produces better contrast and is less toxic than metrizamide. Electromyography is helpful in clarifying confusing root syndromes and in ruling out peripheral nerve lesions. Abnormalities usually cannot be demonstrated by electromyography in acute root lesions before the third week.

PATIENT SELECTION FOR SURGERY

All patients selected for surgery should have unequivocal radicular signs and symptoms. Although nonsurgical treatment is usually initially indicated, there may be exceptions and all of the factors previously noted must be considered. Myelograms should demonstrate a defect that correlates with the patient's signs and symptoms. This frequently is simply a root defect, but larger extradural defects may be seen. Selection of patients for surgery generally is not a problem. Surgery is not performed for neck pain alone or when the myelogram is negative.

SURGICAL PROCEDURE

Keyhole foraminotomy as described by Scoville[8] is used. If further exposure is necessary, additional amounts of the lamina can be removed. Extensive laminectomy is rarely necessary.

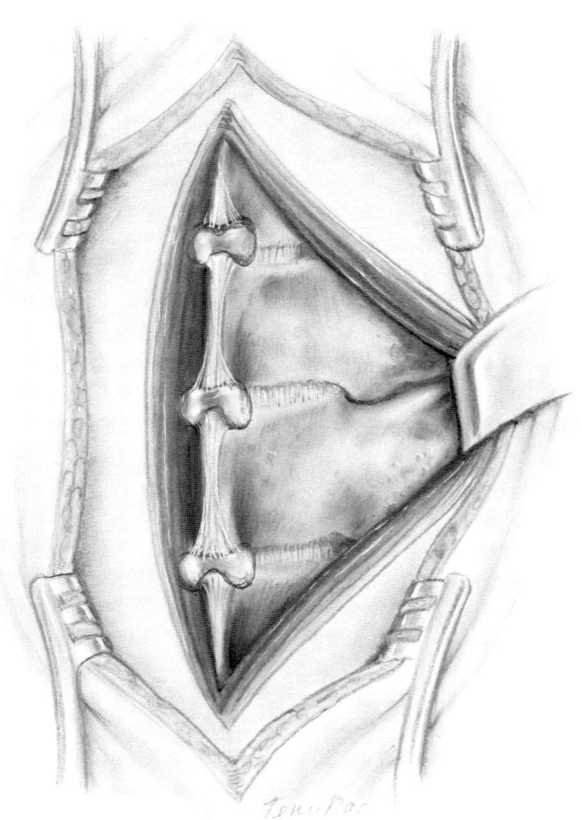

Fig. 118-3.   The initial exposure of laminae and facets.

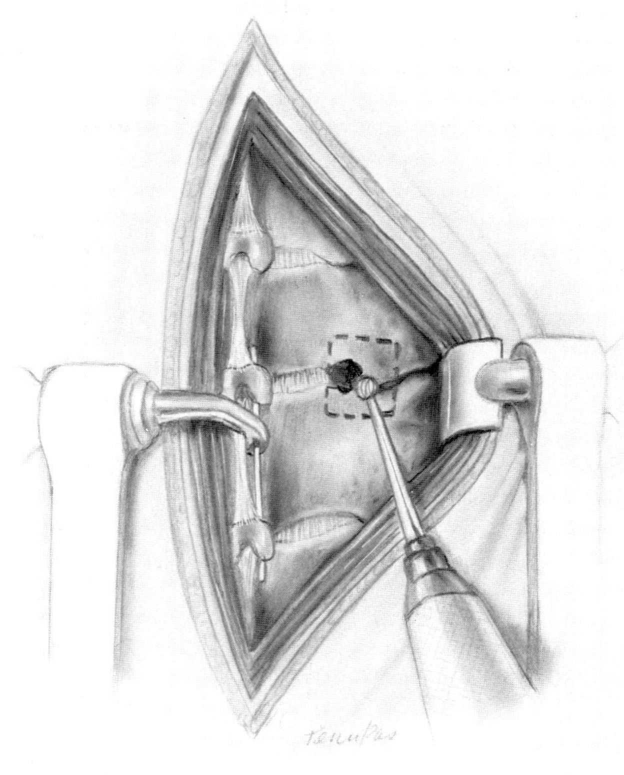

Fig. 118-4.   A diamond burr is used to drill out the medial one third to one half of the facet.

Surgical Technique

The procedure is carried out with the patient under general anesthesia and in the sitting position (Figure 118-2). The patient's legs are wrapped to the mid-thigh with elastic bandages and an abdominal binder is applied. The legs and feet are elevated to the level of the heart. The head is slightly flexed and taped to a Mayfield headrest.

A Doppler monitor is placed on the precordium. A central venous line is passed, generally through the basilic vein, into the superior vena cava. This allows central venous pressure to be monitored and air aspirated if necessary. End tidal CO_2 and arterial pressure are monitored. During induction, dexamethasone (10 mg) and an antibiotic such as Ancef or oxacillin (1 g) are administered intravenously.

A vertical midline incision is made centered over the vertebral level involved and measuring about 3 to 3½ inches in length when a single level is to be explored. To encourage hemostasis, lidocaine with 1:100,000 epinephrine is infiltrated into the subcutaneous tissue and muscle before the skin incision is made. Exposure is carried down to the ligamentum nuchae and an incision made immediately lateral to the spinous process. An Allis clamp is affixed to the spinous process and a lateral roentgenogram is obtained for interspace localization. Following this, the fascial incision is extended. The periosteum and muscles are dissected from the laminae. A hand-held Meyerding retractor facilitates sharply cutting ligamentous and muscle attachments to the laminae and facet. Exposure of a

portion of the lamina above and the lamina below makes lateral retraction easier. A Scoville laminectomy retractor with cross bar adaptation in the hook to prevent slippage through the interspinous ligament is used to maintain muscle retraction and expose the lamina and facet.[8] A small pituitary ronguer is used to peel off any remaining tissue from the lamina, interlaminar space, and facet. The lateral extent of the superior lamina and the most medial extent of the facet are clearly defined (Figure 118-3). The inferior articular process of the superior vertebra generally overhangs the superior articular process of the inferior vertebra. The inferior articular process and then the superior articular process are drilled with an air drill with a small diamond burr and constant irrigation with saline to create a defect in the medial one third or one half of the facet, leaving a thin shell of cortical bone over the foramen and underlying nerve root (Figure 118-4). The cortical bone is then easily lifted off with small, sharp curettes and delicate sella punches to further expose the extension of the ligamentum flavum, which forms a venous-laden membrane over the nerve root.

A small laminotomy of the superior lamina laterally is carried out with punch rongeurs. The bone where the superior articular facet of the inferior vertebra meets the pedicle is removed with punches to gain access to the axilla of the nerve root, where initial exploration should begin (Figure 118-5). Loupe magnification may be helpful at this point. An 0.5-cm vertical incision is then made in the thick ligamentum flavum overlying the dura covering the lateral spinal cord and just medial to the root origin. A thin grooved Woodson (dental) dissector, which is used as a guide, is introduced and manipulated laterally (Figure 118-6); it is pulled backward so that the

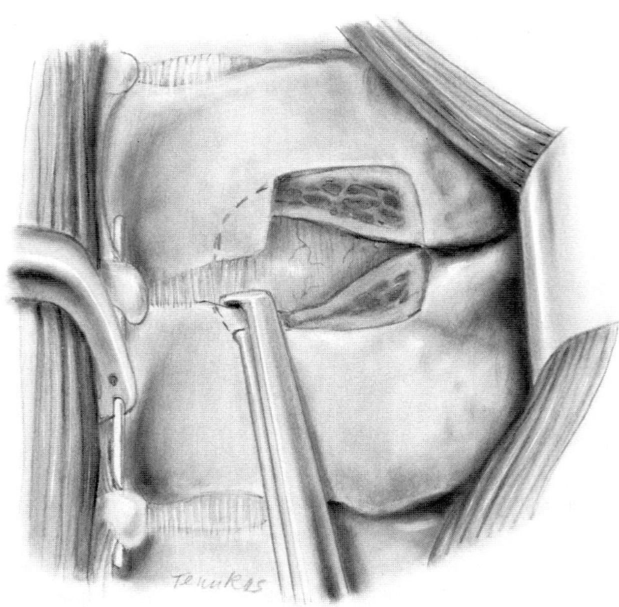

Fig. 118-5. A punch rongeur is used to remove small bits of pedicle and facet to expose the axilla of the root.

underlying compressed root is not compressed any further. The thin extension of ligamentum flavum is incised over the dissector as it is moved laterally, in much the same way as a dural guide is used. A No. 15 Bard-Parker blade is used for cutting. Bleeding in the superior and inferior edges is easily controlled with bipolar coagulation and small cottonoids, which can be inserted epidurally and moved about to provide hemostasis while disc fragments are sought and removed. The root will have a large sensory component superiorly and posteriorly and a smaller motor portion inferiorly and anteriorly.

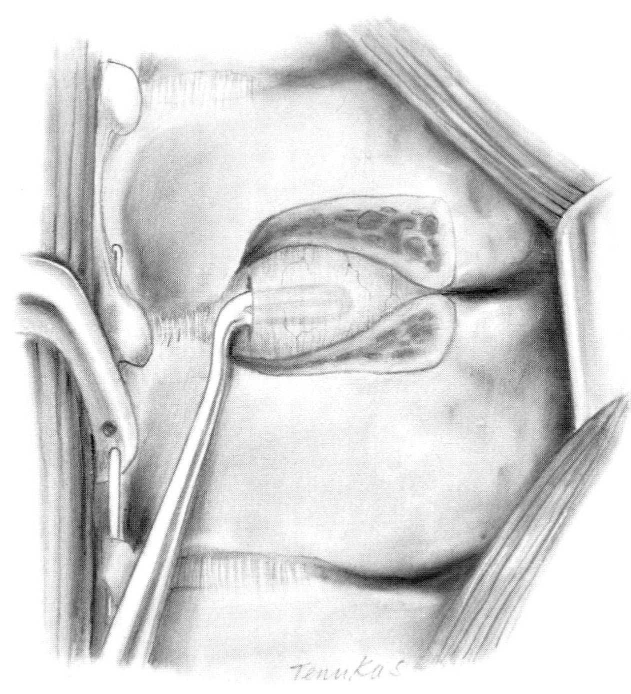

Fig. 118-6. A thin, grooved Woodson dissector is passed laterally beneath the ligamentum flavum and its lateral extension, allowing safe incision.

The root may be tense if an underlying anterior disc fragment or osteophytic spur is present, and care must be taken not to injure the stretched motor division. This should be identified before the root is mobilized and retracted. Exploration is initially carried out in the axilla of the root (Figure 118-7).

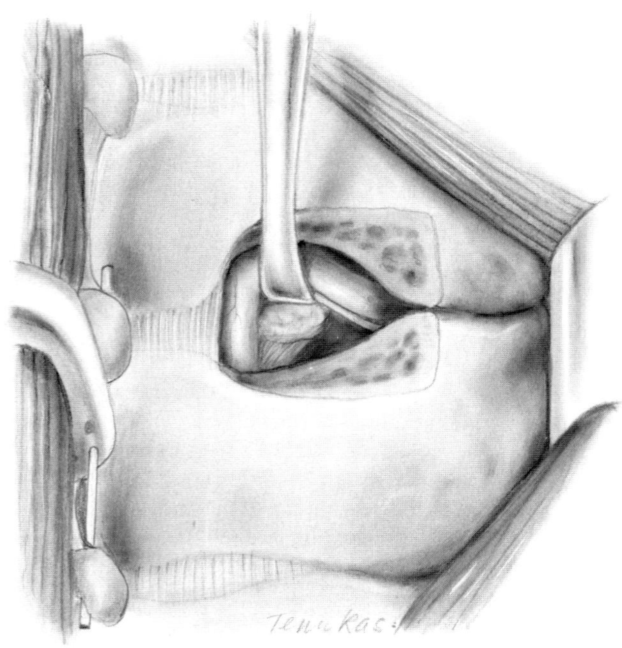

Fig. 118-7. Nerve root being elevated with a root retractor during exploration.

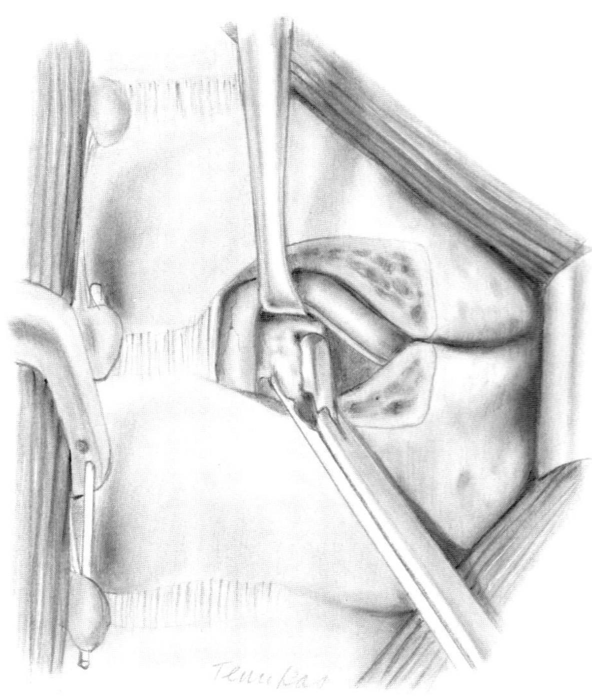

Fig. 118-8. Fragment of disc being removed from beneath the nerve root.

A blunt Stille hook is an excellent instrument for this purpose. Exploration is continued under the dural sac superiorly, medially, and inferiorly with a swirling motion to deliver fragments from beneath the root (Figure 118-8). Not infrequently, the disk is contained within the posterior ligament or annulus and an incision must be made to deliver the fragments. There must be thorough exploration above, below, and medial to the root to be certain that all fragments are removed. They generally are small in comparison with those seen in the lumbar region. Retained fragments are the most common cause of failure of surgery to cure the patient. The dura or cord are not retracted and the interspace is not entered. If an osteophytic spur is encountered, a soft disc fragment should be sought, since these are often asssociated with osteophytic spurs. We have not found it necessary to chisel off the osteophyte; root and foraminal decompression alone have been found adequate. Small pledgets of Gelfoam and bipolar cautery are used to control venous bleeding. After hemostasis is achieved in the muscles, the ligamentum nuchae, subcutaneous fascia, and skin are closed in layers with nonabsorbable sutures. Proper closure leaves an inconspicuous scar. Wound dehiscence has not been a problem. A soft cervical collar is generally applied for the immediate postoperative period, but is removed on the following day, and flexion, extension, and rotation exercises are started. Most patients achieve a full range of neck motion by time of discharge. Dexamethasone is continued at 4 mg every 6 hours postoperatively and tapered over a 3- to 4-day period. We think this contributes to a smoother, less painful postoperative course. Prophylactic antibiotics are not continued postoperatively unless there is a specific reason to do so. Patients can begin ambulation on the evening of surgery. Sutures are removed in 5 days, at the time of discharge from the hospital.

RESULTS AND COMPLICATIONS

The results from this procedure are gratifying. In our series of 2032 patients (Roberts and Collias, unpublished data), 96 percent had a good to excellent result; approximately 4 percent obtained no benefit from the procedure. The radicular pain and root deficits may improve dramatically immediately after the procedure. Recurrences are rare, occurring only in one patient in our series. In a series of 381 cases reported by Scoville[4] and included in our present series, one third of the patients returned to work or former activity within 2 weeks, the average time being 4.2 weeks. Ninety-six percent of the men returned to their previous job. Nineteen percent of patients with lateral disc rupture developed other cervical (8 percent) or lumbar (11 percent) disc herniations that required surgery. Other authors have also reported excellent results with this operation.[9,10,11] Murphy[12] noted 653 cases with 96 percent excellent results and all but 4 percent of the patients returning to their same job.

The morbidity in our series was 0.2 percent. This included transient increased root deficits. This is more apt to occur when more than one root is exposed. Wound dehiscence or infections rarely occurred. Two cases of air emboli with severe brain damage point up the potential risks of the sitting position. Both instances occurred in the early years, when local and block anesthesia were used and before the advent of Doppler monitoring. With Doppler monitoring during the past 12 years, there have been no significant complications from air emboli.

There were 2 patients who developed major postoperative neurologic deficits directly related to the surgery. In one case, a resident plunged a periosteal elevator through the interlaminar space, causing cord injury with a permanent residual Brown-Sequard syndrome. In the other case, the deficit was secondary to cord retraction and injury when a transdural approach was added to an extradural approach for a herniated disc that extended medially. This hazardous approach for central disc herniation is no longer used. Central soft disc herniations are approached anteriorly.

The posterior approach, foraminotomy, provides a reliable, safe, and very effective procedure for the management of lateral cervical disc protrusions. Failures generally occur because of errors in diagnosis or disc fragments that are missed. If severe radiculopathy persists unchanged postoperatively, these errors should be considered and the patient re-examined after a reasonable period of time.

A patient with a lateral cervical disc herniation can be told he or she has a 96 percent chance of being improved or cured by the procedure. There is a 4 percent chance of no benefit and less than 1 percent chance of suffering an adverse effect. Murphy[12] called the results the most gratifying of any neurosurgical procedure except, perhaps, those for trigeminal neuralgia.

SPONDYLOTIC MYELOPATHY

We usually use decompressive laminectomy to treat cervical spondylosis with spinal cord compression. Eighty-four patients operated on during the past 20 years were reviewed (Collias and Roberts, unpublished data). This group does not include 39 cases previously reported by Scoville.[4]

INCIDENCE AND PATHOGENESIS

Cervical spondylotic myelopathy is the most common disease of the spinal cord in middle age and later. Of 84 patients, the mean age was 59 years. There were twice as many women as men. The oldest patient was 84 years and the youngest was 27 years. More than one half of the patients were in the sixth and seventh decades of life.

The cause of the myelopathy is a narrow cervical spinal canal that is further narrowed by a ventral osteophyte, hypertrophic facets, and a thickened, infolding ligamentum flavum. These changes result in compression of the spinal cord, with flattening in its sagittal diameter. The most commonly involved level is C5-6, with one or more of the adjacent levels also affected. Two-level involvement is more common than single-level involvement. Multi-level involvement also occurs, usually between C3 and C7. Congenital blocked vertebrae occurred in 10 percent of patients in one series.[13]

The normal sagittal cervical canal diameter averages 17 mm (at a tube-to-film distance of 6 feet), and the spinal cord diameter averages 10 mm. Any sagittal diameter of the cervical canal less than 12 mm can be associated with cord compression. Cord compression is certain if the cervical canal is less than 10 mm at any level. Spinal canal diameters of 13 mm or greater make spondylosis an unlikely cause of myelopathy.[14]

Although the pathogenesis of myelopathy in cervical spondylosis is imperfectly understood, it is generally accepted that both mechanical and vascular abnormalities are responsible. Flexion and extension movements cause compression and distortion of the spinal cord, creating axial tensions and hemodynamic disturbances producing ischemic lesions. This hypothesis is supported by histologic studies showing ischemic changes in the cord.[15,16] Structural changes of the vessels, however, are not seen. During surgery, Allen[17] noted pallor of the spinal cord associated with spondylosis. The pallor increased with passive flexion of the neck.

Prolonged and repeated episodes of compression can lead to added effects culminating in small areas of cord infarction. The lesions are found most prominently in the lateral columns, the ventral gray matter, and the posterior columns. Early, potentially reversible lesions may in time become fixed. The timing of decompressive surgery must take these facts into consideration. The results of decompression are apt to be better if surgery is done early in the course of the disease.

Degenerative changes resulting in subluxations[18] and kyphotic deformities cause further injury. Kahn[19] suggested that the denticulate ligaments tethered the cord against the ventral osteophytes, preventing dorsal movement and producing increased stresses on the lateral columns. Reid's[20] studies have shown that the denticulate ligaments do not restrict dorsoventral movement of the cord, but do so in a cephalo-caudad direction.

CLINICAL MANIFESTATIONS

Brain[21] aptly described the clinical symptoms and findings in this condition as protean, polymorphic, and without features to distinguish them from other neurologic disorders. The onset is generally insidious, except with acute trauma, and the course intermittent and variably progressive. There can be long periods of remission. Although improvement can occur, function rarely returns to normal.

Spastic weakness of the lower extremities, variable clonus, and pathologic toe signs are the most common manifestations. Ataxia, in part caused by involvement of the spinocerebellar tracts, is also noted. Weakness, atrophy, and clumsiness of the hands with associated stereoanesthesia can occur alone or in combination with spasticity and hyperreflexia in the lower extremities. With upper extremity involvement, it is difficult at times to distinguish myelopathy from associated radiculopathy. Fasciculations are uncommon and limited to the involved myotomes when present.

Neck and arm pain are uncommon except when there is radiculopathy. Lhermitte's sign may be present. Severe sensory loss is not a prominent feature. Hypalgesia may be present as a result of spinothalamic tract involvement. Posterior column dysfunction is less frequent. The bladder and bowel sphincters are usually spared, but may be involved as a late manifestation and generally indicate a poor prognosis.[22] Various syndromes may be seen including transverse cord syndrome (corticospinal, spinothalamic, and posterior column dysfunction), Brown-Sequard syndrome, and central cord syndrome, particularly after trauma.

Cervical spondylotic myelopathy may frequently be confused with other neurologic disorders. These include amyotrophic lateral sclerosis (ALS), multiple sclerosis, combined systems disease, spinal cord tumor, and syringomyelia. With the predominance of motor signs and symptoms, it is not surprising that it is commonly confused with ALS. Widespread fasciculations in ALS (including the tongue) and an increased jaw jerk indicate a lesion above the cervical cord. The absence of sensory findings also provides a strong clue to the diagnosis. Cervical spondylosis should not be accepted as responsible for symptoms attributable to lesions of the spinal cord unless confirmed by a myelogram or CT scan. Errors in diagnosis are common causes of the failure of surgical therapy.

DIAGNOSTIC STUDIES

Flexion, extension, and oblique view x-ray films of the cervical spine are obtained to assess possible abnormalities of movement and kyphotic deformities. Myelography remains the most definitive study and is presently used in conjunction with CT scanning. Pantopaque now has been replaced by water-soluble contrast medium.

A water-soluble medium such as metrizamide (Amipaque) permitted C1-C2 instillation and CT scanning but produced poor contrast. At present we are using iopamidal (Isovue) instilled through the lumbar route, followed by a CT scan in 6 hours with sagittal reconstruction views. This produces excellent visualization of the subarachnoid space and areas of cord compression. It also permits accurate measurement of the sagittal diameter of the spinal canal. Magnetic resonance imaging holds much promise for the future in demonstrating spinal cord lesions but is not as yet generally available. Electromyographic studies are useful in recognizing peripheral nerve lesions, widespread fasciculations (favoring the diagnosis of ALS), and in differentiating radiculopathy from myelopathy in the upper extremities.

NONSURGICAL TREATMENT

Nonsurgical therapy in this disease includes neck immobilization and physical therapy. Continuation of such treatment over a long period is appropriate for elderly patients with longstanding fixed lesions and a poor surgical prognosis. It is also indicated for those patients with severe medical problems in whom a major surgical procedure is contraindicated and for those who decline surgical therapy.

INDICATIONS FOR SURGERY

Decompression is in order when there is progression in the myelopathy and documented compression of the spinal cord. Delay should be avoided, because symptoms of short duration correlate positively with improved results. Age has no such correlation and an older person with a short history of symptoms stands a good chance of significant functional recovery.

SURGICAL CONSIDERATIONS

There are two general approaches in the surgical treatment of cervical myelopathy. The posterior operative procedures commonly employed to decompress the spinal cord consist of laminectomy with or without foraminotomy and section of the denticulate ligaments. Partial removal of anterior bony ridges through a posterolateral approach is used by some surgeons. The anterior procedure consists of discectomy, removal of the protruding ventral osteophyte, and stabilization of the interspace by interbody fusion. Both approaches may give satisfactory results in restoring neurologic function or arresting the progression of the disease. In most instances, statistics do not favor one approach over the other.

Many surgeons use the anterior approach only in patients with one- or two-level involvement when there is no diffuse narrowing of the spinal canal.[13,22–25] Kyphotic angulation or major subluxations require the decompression and stabilization afforded by the anterior approach.

The posterior approach has wide applications and can be used for single-level as well as multilevel involvement. It permits decompression of the extremes of the cervical spine, which are out of reach through an anterior approach. It is the preferred approach if intradural exploration might be necessary or if the diagnosis is in doubt. It is the procedure of choice in congenital spinal narrowing associated with myelopathy.

Combined procedures may be necessary at times. The anterior approach may be required if the result is not satisfactory following posterior decompression and significant anterior compression persists. Instability, kyphosis, and swan neck deformity after a posterior operation with regression in neurologic function may require anterior stabilization.

Posterior Approaches

The aim of decompressive laminectomy is to enlarge the spinal canal by removing posterior compressing elements, which allows the dural tube and spinal cord to migrate posteriorly away from the compressing ventral osteophytes. It also relieves posterior compression caused by infolding and hypertrophy of the ligamentum flavum.

Since the successful case of Horsley,[26] decompressive laminectomy has been used to treat spinal cord compression caused by ventral osteophytes. Limited laminectomies gave results that were no better than those obtained with nonsurgical treatment.[27–30] Total (C1-D1)[31] or extensive laminectomy[32–37] improved results. Some surgeons include intradural section of the denticulate ligaments[32,38,39] to further untether the cord.[19] Reid,[20] however, has shown that contact between the cord and ventral protrusions is not reduced when the denticulate ligaments are sectioned and that these specific structures do not restrict the dorsoventral movement of the cord. Piepgras,[40] in a study of two comparable groups of patients with and without denticulate section, found no difference in surgical results or neurologic recovery. There is, however, an increased risk of damage to the cord and a slightly higher morbidity associated with opening the dura. Some surgeons[33–37,41–43] combine laminectomy with foraminotomy and facetectomy bilaterally at as many as three levels in order to decompress the nerve roots. They are convinced that results are superior and suggest that freeing the roots enables the cord to move posteriorly. There is no substantial evidence to indicate that decompression of the nerve roots involved with epidural fibrosis associated with spondylosis and osteophytic spurs untethers the cord. Reid[20] in his study found no evidence that the roots tethered the cord anteriorly. Epstein[37] has added a ''global decompression'' by curetting the lateral portions of the ventral bar after carrying out foraminotomy at involved levels. Most surgeons are hesitant to remove ventral bars through a posterolateral extradural approach for fear of cord damage.

We have found that laminectomy extending above and below the areas of maximum involvement and carried out widely to expose the posterolateral aspects of the dural sac has been effective. The dura is not opened. Only the medial portion of the facet is removed. Foraminotomies are carried out only if there is associated radiculopathy.

Surgical Procedure

The spinal cord in this disease is highly vulnerable and requires protection. Extreme flexion or extension during intubation for general anesthesia can cause irreparable ischemic cord damage. Determining the limits of neck motion before induction of anesthesia and not exceeding them is most important.

Positioning of the patient should be accomplished with the head and neck supported manually in the neutral position to avoid flexion or extension and cord damage. The surgeon must be present during intubation and positioning. Ischemic cord damage can result if hypotension is not avoided. Experimental work suggests loss of autoregulation and sensitivity to CO_2 in the anesthetized and ischemic cord, and blood flow is dependent on adequate pressure.[44]

Although the procedure is not technically difficult, a careful and unhurried approach is necessary. Rongeurs should have flat heels. Care should be taken not to wedge any instrument into the already crowded epidural space.

The sitting position is optimal. It allows better exposure, improved venous drainage, and easier hemostasis. It unquestionably increases the potential for air embolus. Patients with vascular instability or cardiac disease may do better in the prone position. If the sitting position is used, bone wax should be used on the denuded bone, along with copious irrigation and meticulous hemostasis, to reduce the risk of air embolus. The operating table should be set so that it can be quickly brought to the horizontal position in case of a drop in blood pressure or a significant air emoblus develops.

Surgical Technique

General endotracheal anesthesia and the sitting position are used as described for foraminotomy for cervical disc rupture except that the head and neck are placed in the neutral position. Central venous catheters and monitoring devices are used as previously described.

The incision is made vertically in the midline. A spinous process is isolated, a marker placed, and an x-ray film taken for localization. The spinous processes of the laminae to be removed are exposed. The muscles are sharply dissected from the lamina and facets with a broad periosteal elevator, starting inferiorly and working superiorly, first on one side and then the other. A hand-held Meyerding retractor is helpful in dissection of the muscular and ligamentous attachments to the laminae and facets.

If foraminotomies are to be done, they are carried out at this stage using a Scoville retractor with the spinous processes and laminae intact and by the technique previously described. It is safer to do this before the spinous processes and lamina are removed in order to protect the dura and spinal cord. The spinous processes are then removed (Figure 118-9). Small, sharp curettes are used in separating the ligamentum flavum from the inferior surface of the lamina at each level (Figure 118-10).

The laminectomy can be carried out as an en face or en bloc procedure[32,37] (Figure 118-11). This requires cutting longitudinal channels laterally in each lamina with small punch rongeurs or an air drill and removing the laminae as a single unit. We prefer a piece-meal excision of the laminae with flat heeled rongeurs (Figure 118-12). Leksell rongeurs with a shallow inferior lip or Schlesinger, Kerrison, or Cloward rongeurs with ground down inferior lips are useful for removing laminae in this way.

The laminectomy is extended to the most lateral edge of the dura (Figures 118-13 and 118-14). Portions of the medial facets are removed to barely expose the emerging nerve roots. Complete facetectomy is not required and may result in an unstable cervical spine. The thickened ligamentum flavum is excised, and if the laminectomy is adequate, the dural sac should balloon posteriorly and pulsate normally. It is generally not necessary to include C2 in the laminectomy, because the canal at that level is quite generous unless there is craniocervical junction

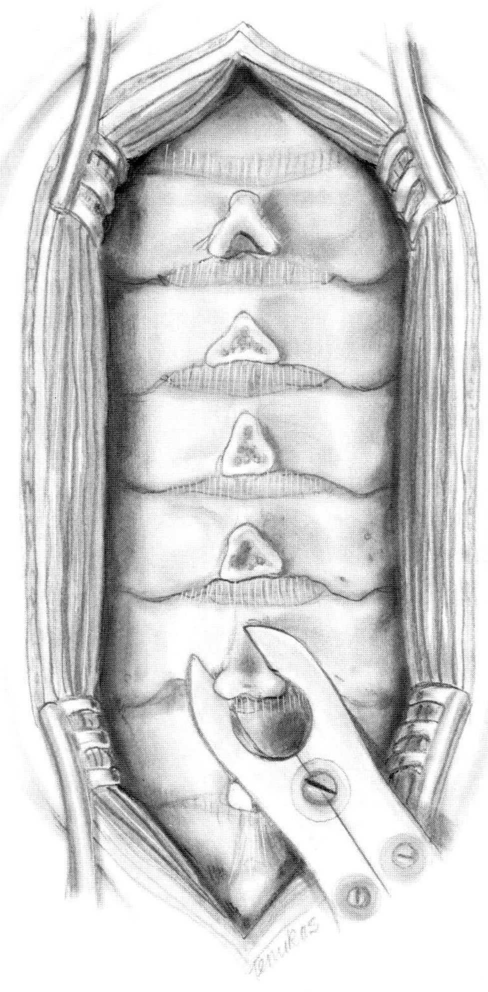

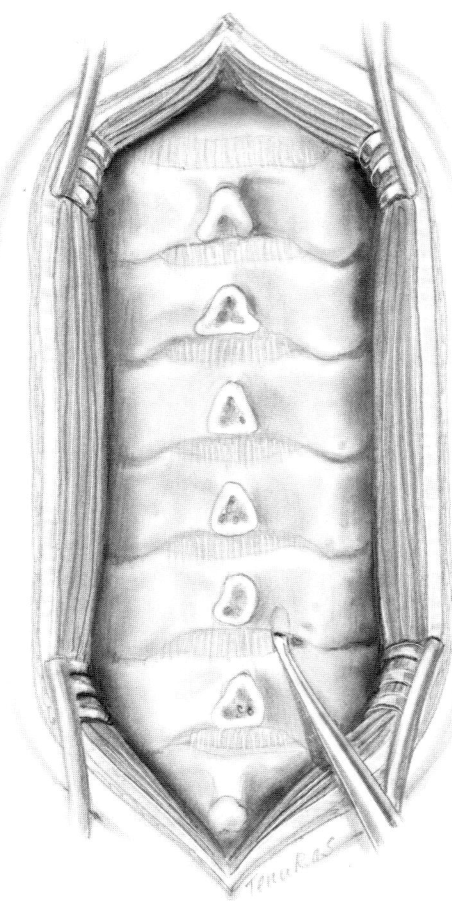

Fig. 118-10. A curette is used to separate the ligamentum flavum from the inferior surface of a lamina.

Fig. 118-9. The initial removal of a spinous process during laminectomy for spondylotic myelopathy.

stenosis. The lamina and spinous process of C2 frequently obscures the upper extent of the C3 lamina, and a portion may have to be removed to ensure complete removal of the C3 lamina.

Bipolar cautery, pledgets of Gelfoam soaked in thrombin, or oxidized cellulose are used to obtain thorough epidural hemostasis. The dura is not opened. A thin layer of Gelfoam strips is placed over the dura. The muscle, fascia, subcutaneous tissue, and skin are closed in layers with nonabsorbable sutures. Prophylactic antibiotic therapy is continued for 24 hours postoperatively. Dexamethasone (4 mg every 6 hours and tapered over 3 to 5 days) reduces postoperative pain.

A soft collar is applied and worn for the first week or two. Lateral flexion and extension x-ray films are obtained to ascertain that there is no postoperative instability. Gentle ''yes and no'' neck exercises are begun during the second week. The patient can get out of bed on the day of surgery. Sutures are removed in 5 to 7 days, and the patient is discharged from the hospital in 7 to 10 days.

Complications

The complications of this procedure are in general less severe than those reported for the anterior procedure.[45–48] There were 10 complications related to surgery in our 84 cases;

none of these was associated with significant neurologic sequelae. There were three mild subluxations, one superficial wound infection, and one extradural hematoma, which was evacuated promptly without significant sequelae. There were no deaths or significant air emboli. There were three errors in diagnosis: one patient had a cerebral thrombosis, one an intramedullary spinal cord tumor, and one had ALS.

Transient worsening occurred in a few patients, but none was permanently worse. In two patients who were considered worse postoperatively there were errors in diagnosis.

In the 39 cases previously reported by Scoville,[4] there were five cases in which minor adverse residuae occurred. There were no infections and no deaths. One patient required further decompression. There was one case of wound dehiscence. There were three incorrect diagnoses: one patient had multiple sclerosis, the second a congenital anomaly of the odontoid, and the third a vascular occlusion.

Air embolus was not a significant problem. There would appear to be few occurrences in series in which the sitting position was used.[4,32,37] In the one instance of postoperative extradural hematoma in our series, the patient awoke from anesthesia with a quadriparesis and was immediately returned to the operating room and the hematoma removed. The quadriparesis cleared immediately and completely. Other causes of quadriparesis such as cord ischemia from positioning or hypotension, intubation injury, or surgical trauma require no

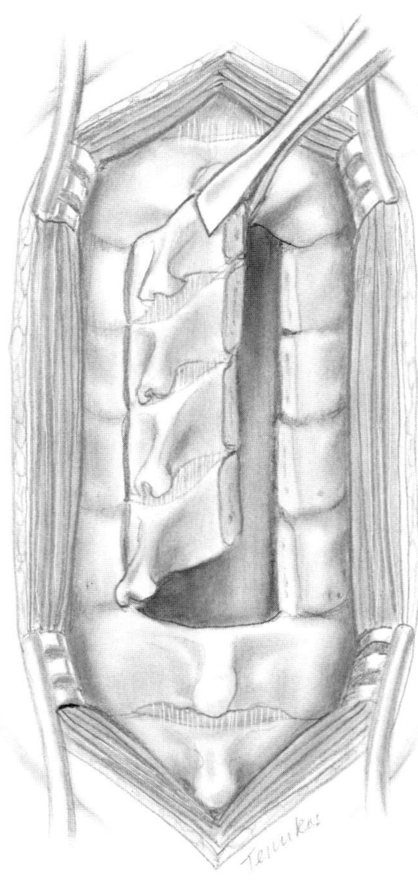

Fig. 118-11. A laminectomy being carried out en bloc.

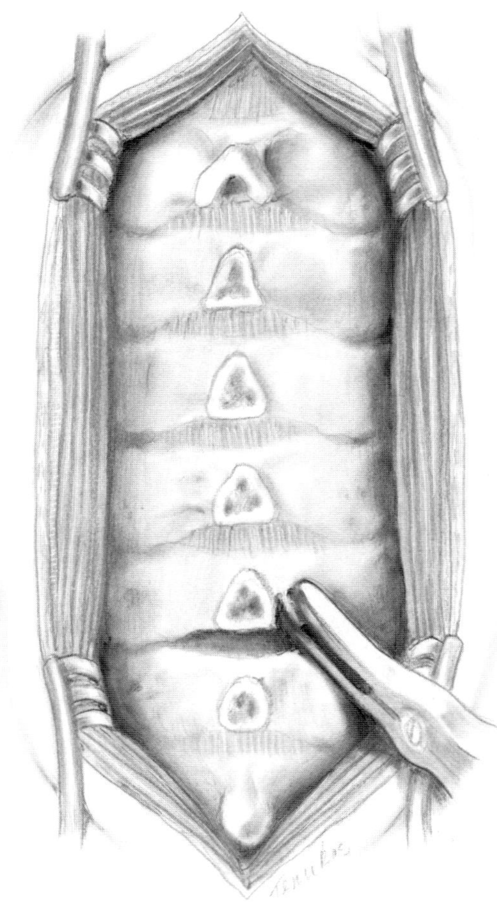

Fig. 118-12. Piece-meal excision of a lamina with a Leksell rongeur with a shallow inferior lip.

further surgical therapy, but if a hematoma is strongly suspected, prompt reopening of the wound is indicated. If the situation appears less urgent, a CT scan may be helpful in diagnosis.

Opening the dura and sectioning the denticulate ligaments is probably accompanied by some increase in morbidity.[32] Piepgras[40] carried out a study of two groups of comparable patients treated with extensive laminectomy, one in which the denticulate ligaments were sectioned and one in which they were not. He found that the complication rates were comparable.

Instability of the spine, which is reported to be one of the drawbacks of the posterior operation,[23,49,50] is, probably, exaggerated.[39] An incidence of 10 percent has been reported.[44] Two kyphotic deformities, one of which required anterior fusion, occurred in our series. Scoville[4] performed bilateral facetectomies in 39 cases with no instability. Epstein[37] noted no postoperative instability after foraminotomies in 50 cases. Stoops and King[33,34] reported on 42 patients with laminectomies and foraminotomies, with as many as six for a single patient, and not one instance of instability.

RESULTS

Our 84 patients were followed from 3 months to 15 years; the average follow-up was more than 2 years. Sixty-nine percent of the patients improved, 28.5 percent remained un-

changed, and 2 patients were worse after the procedure. Seven patients had excellent results. Of the seven, two were over 70 years of age and five had symptoms for a year or less.

There were three errors in diagnosis, and two of these patients were worse after surgery. One had ALS and one had an astrocytoma of the spinal cord. All three had regressed after a previous anterior operation. Fifty-one patients (60 percent) returned to work or equivalent activity.

Scoville,[4] reported on 39 patients from our institution treated by decompressive laminectomy two lamina above and two lamina below the areas of involvement. Bilateral facetectomies of the involved levels were performed in 31 patients and unilateral facetectomies were performed in seven. He noted good to excellent results in 64 percent of cases with clinical cure in three cases and all patients showing an objective arrest of their disease. None was worse after the surgery. The two series from our institution suggest there is no substantial benefit from the addition of facetectomy or foraminotomy to laminectomy.

Stoops and King[34] reported on 42 patients in whom they had carried out extensive laminectomies with bilateral foraminotomies. The dura was not opened. In 83 percent of their patients the condition was improved. Remarkably, five quadriparetic patients returned to normal or near normal. They found no correlation between postoperative improvement and age, sex, duration of symptoms, severity of symptoms,

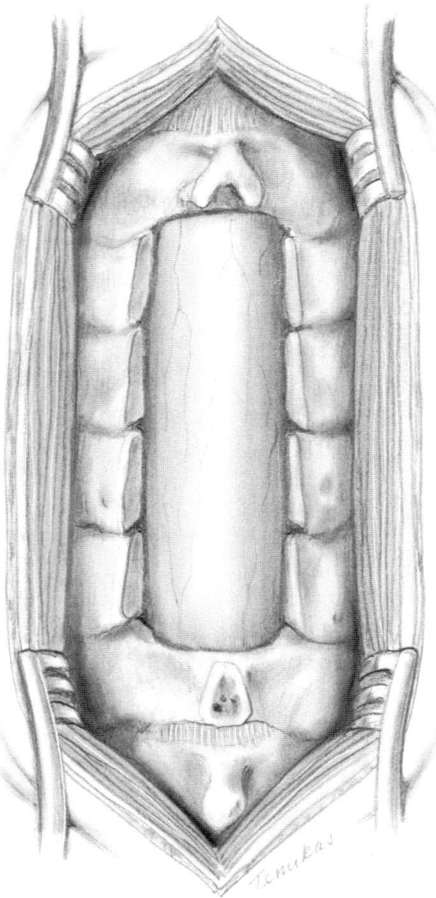

Fig. 118-13. Completed decompression with four-level laminectomy and medial facetectomy.

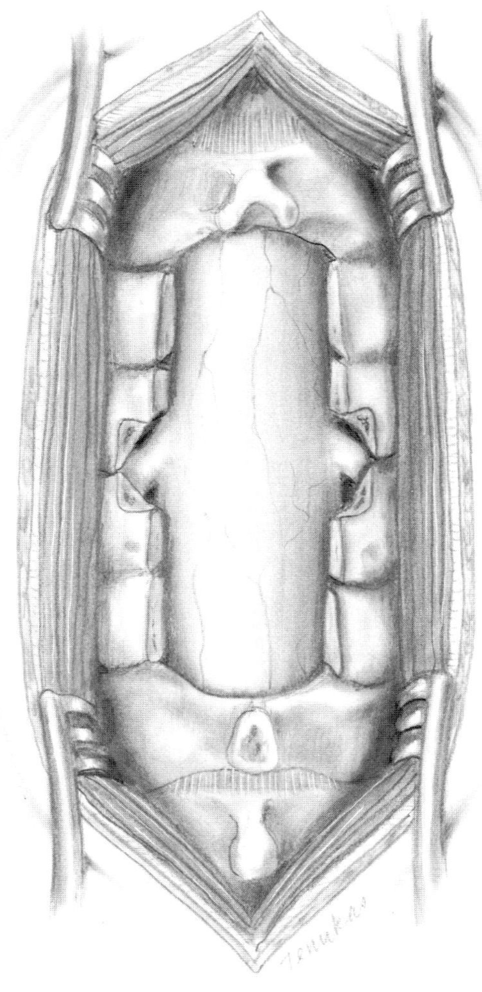

Fig. 118-14. Completed four-level laminectomy with single-level bilateral facetectomy and foraminotomy to relieve root compression.

myelographic findings, or number of osteophytes decompressed.

Epstein[37] studied 1355 patients treated for cervical spondylotic myelopathy. Of 114 patients not treated surgically, 36 percent improved and 64 percent did not improve. Of 353 who underwent an anterior cervical procedure, 73 percent improved and 27 percent did not improve. The remainder had extensive or limited laminectomies with or without foraminotomy, denticulate sectioning, or dural grafting. In these patients, 60 to 85 percent were improved, with the higher figure representing patients with extensive laminectomy, foraminotomies, and excision of osteophytes. He found that age and sex had no specific effect on the results, but none over the age of 70 years had an excellent result. He believed that removal of the ventral osteophyte through a posterolateral approach improved the results significantly, but even if the osteophytes were not removed, a satisfactory result could be obtained in the majority of patients.

Symon and Lavender[51] studied 40 patients who underwent extensive laminectomy without foraminotomy. Seven had the denticulate ligaments sectioned and 70 percent improved. Ten were unchanged and two were worse. They believed that improved results were related to the extent of the laminectomy rather than section of the denticulate ligaments or foraminotomy.

Gorter[52] reviewed a series of patients undergoing an ante-

rior procedure as well as total laminectomies and laminectomies with denticulate ligament section or opening of the dura. Of 345 patients treated with an anterior approach, 73.4 percent were cured or improved and 18.7 percent were unchanged. Of 184 patients who underwent total laminectomy from C2 to D1, 70 percent were cured or improved and 18.2 percent were unchanged. Of 567 patients treated with laminectomy and section of the denticulate ligaments or opening of the dura, 57.4 percent were improved, 22.7 percent unchanged, and 14.8 percent were worse. Surgical results were poorer in procedures in which the dura was opened.

Fager[32] reported on 35 patients who had extensive laminectomies with opening of the dura and section of the denticulate ligament. Sixty-eight percent improved, 26 percent had their disease arrested, and five of the eight most severely afflicted patients improved. None worsened postoperatively during a follow-up period of 1 to 6 years. Piepgras[40] reported on two groups of patients, both with extensive laminectomies. In one group the dura was opened and the denticulate ligaments were sectioned; in the other they were not. He noted there was no significant difference in the results between the two groups.

Gregorius and Crandall[22] reported that some patients with myelopathy had late deterioration after initial improvement.

This could occur 6 to 8 years later. There were six such cases in their series; two were demonstrated to have a pseudomeningocele and three had a retained laminar arch of C3 under an elongated spinous process of C2. One had developed spondylosis above the site of decompression.

In our study of 84 patients, six regressed. Three patients regressed within 1 year, two within 3 years, and one after 14 years. One patient had an anterior surgical fusion at two spaces after regressing, only to have further deterioration 2½ years later.

Hokuda[24] studied 269 patients with cervical spondylotic myelopathy; 191 were followed for 1 to 12 years. One-hundred fifty-six of the patients had a Cloward procedure and 38 had a laminectomy. He noted 15 recurrences in 14 patients for a rate of 5.6 percent. Eleven occurred in the group undergoing an anterior procedure and four in the group undergoing a posterior procedure. He described a constricting membrane as a cause in one patient. Spinal instability after laminectomy occurred in three patients. There was progression of the spondylosis in the anterior group in nine patients. Two patients who had unrecognized stenosis of the canal before their anterior operation required laminectomy. Reports of other series have noted such regressions and point up the need for long-term follow-up for accurate assessment of results.[5,28,31,39,42]

Routine postoperative myelography was not carried out in our patients. Six of the 84 patients who underwent myelography showed improvement in their myelographic picture. There was no significant compressive lesion in five, and one showed persistent anterior compression that required anterior discectomy. Of Scoville's[4] series, 12 patients had complete or nearly complete relief of their block on follow-up myelographic studies.

The most common causes of failure of the surgery are related to patient selection, errors in diagnosis, and inadequate decompression. Laminectomy with adequate decompression in properly selected patients gives satisfactory results in restoring neurologic function or at least in arresting progression of the disease. The duration of symptoms would appear to be the most important prognostic factor and speaks for surgery as soon as it is convenient. Patients with symptoms for less than 6 months do best. Age and severity of symptoms have less prognostic value and do not in themselves mitigate against a beneficial result. An elderly patient with severe myelopathy may have significant recovery, provided the surgery is performed at an early stage.

REFERENCES

1. Cloward RB: New method of diagnosis and treatment of cervical disc disease. Clin Neurosurg 8:93, 1962
2. Robinson RA, Smith GW: Anterolateral cervical disc removal and interbody fusion for cervical disc syndrome. Bull Johns Hopkins Hosp 96:223, 1955
3. Spurling RG, Scoville WB: Lateral rupture of the cervical intervertebral discs. Surg Gynecol Obstet 78:350, 1944
4. Scoville WB, Dohrmann GT, Corkill G: Late results of cervical disc surgery. J Neurosurg 45:203, 1976
5. Scoville WB, Aronson N, Simeone FA: Viewpoint: Soft cervical disc neurosurgery. Neurosurgery 2:89, 1978
6. Scoville WB, Whitcomb BB, McLaurin R: The cervical ruptured disk: Report of 115 operative cases. Transactions of the American Neurology Association 76th Annual Meeting, 1951, pp 222-224
7. Scoville WB, Whitcomb BB: Lateral rupture of the cervical intervertebral disc. Postgrad Med 39:174, 1966
8. Scoville WB: Cervical Disc: Classification, indications and approaches with special reference to posterior keyhole operation, in Dunsker SB (ed): Cervical Spondylosis. New York, Raven Press, 1981
9. Raaf JA: Surgical treatment of patients with cervical disc lesions. J Trauma 9:327, 1969
10. Odom GL et al: Cervical disc lesions. JAMA 166:23, 1958
11. Fager C: Management of cervical disc lesions and spondylosis by posterior approaches. Clin Neurosurg 24:488, 1977
12. Murphey F, Simmons J, Brunson B: Ruptured cervical discs 1939 to 1972. Clin Neurosurg 20:9, 1973
13. Crandall PH, Batdorf U: Cervical spondylotic myelopathy. J Neurosurg 25:57, 1966
14. Wolf BS, Khilnani M, Malis L: Sagittal diameter of bony cervical spinal canal and its significance in cervical spondylosis. J Mt Sinai Hosp 23:283, 1956
15. Mair WGP, Druckman R: The pathology of spinal cord lesions and their relation to the clinical features in protrusion of cervical intervertebral discs. Brain 76:70, 1953
16. Brain R, Wilkinson M: Cervical spondylosis. London, Heineman, 1967
17. Allen KL: Neuropathies caused by bony spurs in the cervical spine with special reference to surgical treatment. J Neurol Neurosurg Psychiatry 15:20, 1952
18. Penning L: Some aspects of plain radiography of the cervical spine in chronic myelopathy. Neurology 12:513, 1962
19. Kahn EA: The role of the dentate ligaments in spinal cord compression and the syndrome of lateral sclerosis. J Neurosurg 4:191, 1947
20. Reid JD: Effects of flexion-extension movements of the head and spine upon the spinal cord and nerve roots. J Neurol Neurosurg Psychiatry 23:214, 1960
21. Brain WR, Northfield DWC, Wilkinson M: The neurological manifestations of cervical spondylosis. Brain 75:187, 1952
22. Gregorius FK, Estrin T, Crandall PH: Cervical spondylotic radiculopathy and myelopathy. Arch Neurol 33:618, 1976
23. Verbeist H: The management of cervical spondylosis. Clin Neurosurg 20:262, 1973
24. Hokuda S, Mochizoki T, Ogata M, et al: Operations for cervical spondylotic myelopathy, a comparison of the results of anterior and posterior procedures. J Bone Joint Surg 67B:000, 1985
25. Koyama T, Handa J: Cervical laminoplasty using apatite beads as implants: Experiences in 31 patients with compressive myelopathy due to developmental canal stenosis. Surg Neurol 24:663, 1985
26. Taylor J, Collier J: The occurrence of optic neuritis in lesions of the spinal cord, injury, tumour, myelitis (an account of twelve cases and one autopsy). Brain 24:17, 1901
27. Haft H, Shenkin HA: Surgical end results of cervical ridge and disk problems. JAMA 186:312, 1963
28. Bradshaw P: Some aspects of cervical spondylosis. Q J Med 26:177, 1957
29. Lees F, Turner JWA: Natural history and prognosis of cervical spondylosis. Br Med J 00:000 1963
30. Nurick S: The natural history and the results of surgical treatment of the spinal disorder associated with cervical spondylosis. Brain 95:101, 1972
31. Aboulker J, Metzger J, David M, et al: Les myelopathies cervicales d'origine rachidienne. Neurochirurgie 11:88, 1965
32. Fager CA: Results of adequate posterior decompression in the relief of spondylotic cervical myelopathy. J Neurosurg 38:684, 1973
33. Stoops WL, King RB: Chronic myelopathy associated with cervical spondylosis: Its response to laminectomy and foramenotomy. JAMA 192:281, 1965
34. Stoops WL, King RB: Neural complications of cervical spondylosis: Their response to laminectomy and foramenotomy. J Neurosurg 19:986, 1962
35. Epstein JA, Carras R, Lavine LS, et al: The importance of removing osteophytes as part of the surgical treatment of

myeloradiculopathy in cervical spondylosis. J Neurosurg 30: 219, 1969

36. Epstein J: Management of cervical spinal stenosis, spondylosis, and myeloradiculopathy. Contemp Neurosurg 7:000, 0000

37. Epstein J, Janin Y: Management of cervical spondylotic myeloradiculopathy by the posterior approach, in xxxxxxxx (ed): The Cervical Spine. Philadellphia, JB Lippincott, 1983

38. Hunt W: Cervical spondylosis: Natural history and rare indications for surgical decompression. Clin Neurosurg 27:466, 1979

39. Bishara SN: The posterior operation in the treatment of cervical spondylosis with myelopathy. J Neurol Neurosurg Psychiatry 34:393, 1971

40. Piepgras D: Posterior decompression for myelopathy due to cervical spondylosis: Laminectomy alone versus laminectomy with dentate ligament section. Clin Neurosurg 24:508, 1977

41. Phillips DG: Surgical treatment of myelopathy with cervical spondylosis. J Neurol Neurosurg Psychiatry 36:879, 1973

42. Northfield DWC: Diagnosis and treatment of myelopathy due to cervical spondylosis. Br Med J 2:1474, 1955

43. Scoville WB: Cervical spondylosis treated by bilateral facetectomy and laminectomy. J Neurosurg 18:423, 1961

44. Hoff JT, Wilson C: The pathophysiology of cervical spondylotic radiculopathy and myelopathy. Clin Neurosurg 24:474, 1977

45. Tew JM Jr, Mayfield FH: Complications of surgery of the anterior cervical spine. Clin Neurosurg 23:424, 1975

46. Mann KS, Khosla V, Gulati DR: Cervical spondylotic myelopathy treated by single stage multilevel anterior decompression. J Neurosurg 60:81, 1984

47. Aronson N: The management of soft cervical disc protrusions using the Smith-Robinson approach. Clin Neurosurg 20:253, 1973

48. Lunsford LD, Bissonette DJ, Zorub D: Anterior surgery for cervical disk disease. Part II: Treatment of cervical spondylotic myelopathy in 32 cases. J Neurosurg 53:12, 1980

49. Mayfield FH: Complications of laminectomy. Clin Neurosurg 23:435, 1975

50. Mayfield FH: Cervical spondylosis: observations based on surgical treatment of 400 cases. Post Grad Med Oct, 1965

51. Symon L, Lavender P: The surgical treatment of cervical spondylotic myelopathy. Neurology 17:117, 1967

52. Gorter K: The influence of laminectomy on the course of cervical myelopathy. Acta Neurochir (Wien) 33:265, 1976

53. Adams CBT, Logue V: Studies in cervical spondylotic myelopathy. 3. Some functional effects of operations for cervical spondylotic myelopathy. Brain 94:587, 1971

The Transthoracic Approach to the Thoracolumbar Spine for Decompression and Spinal Stabilization

Henry H. Schmidek

THE SURGICAL APPROACH to the fractured, unstable thoracolumbar (T1 to L5) spine dates to the early nineteenth century, when Cline[1] resected the injured spinous processes and laminae of a paraplegic patient with a thoracic fracture-dislocation but was unable to reduce the dislocation and the patient subsequently died. In 1827, Tyrrell[2] reported decompressive laminectomy in several cases of spinal dislocation with compression of the spinal cord. Both Cline and Tyrrell removed the spinous processes and laminae through a vertical midline incision centered over the injured portion of the spine. In 1829, Smith[3] operated on a man rendered paraplegic after a fall from a horse. The spinous processes and depressed laminae of three thoracic vertebrae were removed, the dura inspected, and the incision closed. This patient survived and his neurologic condition improved.

Beginning with these operations, posterior laminectomy has evolved into the mainstay procedure for decompression of the spinal cord and nerve roots. In the fractured spine, however, it is now appreciated that the further removal of the posterior elementsmay destabilize the spine and worsen the neurologicand orthopedic condition of the patient. The surgical alternatives to this operation have only recently been used by neurosurgeons except in treating herniated thoracic disc. In this situation, costotransversectomy gained wide acceptance after attempts to remove the disc protrusion via laminectomy were followed by a high incidence of postoperative neurologic deterioration.

Thoracic and thoracolumbar fractures have routinely been treated by decompressive laminectomy and posterior spinal fusion. It is only in the last decade that alternative surgical approaches that allow exploration of the spine by an anterior, anterolateral, posterolateral, or posterior approach, to allow the procedure to be tailored to the particulars of a specific case.[4–8] In the thoracic spine, ventrally situated lesions can be exposed by costotransversectomy, a transthoracic-extrapleural approach, or by a transthoracic-transpleural route. The transthoracic-transpleural approach allows removal, in one stage, of pathologic material ventral to the dura *over several spinal segments* and concurrent stabilization of the spine with bone and fixateurs inserted into the intact vertebral bodies. This operation is useful in some acute thoracic fractures and among those cases treated by decompressive laminectomy in which there is the development of a kyphotic deformity and progressive neurologic deficit (Figure 119-1). These patients have an increasing sharp angular kyphosis over the apex of which the spinal cord is stretched and attenuated (Figure 119-2). Since the posterior elements have been removed, the angulation of the spine makes posterior instrumentation either biomechanically unsound or technically impossible. We have found a one-stage transthoracic-transpleural decompression and stabilization particularly useful in treating this situation. These patients have progressive paraparesis and characteristically after surgery demonstrate marked neurologic improvement and alleviation of all (except their immediate, operatively induced) pain within days even though the problem had been of longstanding duration. The mechanism of this improvement is unclear and may be related to either improved axoplasmic flow within the previously compressed spinal cord or relief of chronic vascular insufficiency. The gratifying experience obtained with these techniques in these cases, in the absence of an increased morbidity associated with their use, has encouraged advocating them to our colleagues.

Fractures of the thoracolumbar region with retropulsed disc and bone arising from a single vertebral body can be adequately decompressed by an extracavitary anterolateral approach and need not be operated on transabdominally or transperitoneally. This operation involves removal of the transverse process, identifying the neural foramen, removal of the ipsilateral pedicle, and then undermining the retropulsed bone rostrocaudally from the body above to that below the level of injury. The entire piece of bone is then removed from the vertebral canal. Following decompression, stabilization is accomplished by (1) bone grafts placed anteriorly between the vertebral bodies, (2) Harrington-rod or other instrumentation posteriorly, and (3) reinforcement by a posterior spinal fusion. Patients who are neurologically intact or who have only partial lesions are not instrumented until their decompression has been accomplished. Both decompression and

OPERATIVE NEUROSURGICAL TECHNIQUES
ISBN 0-8089-1862-1

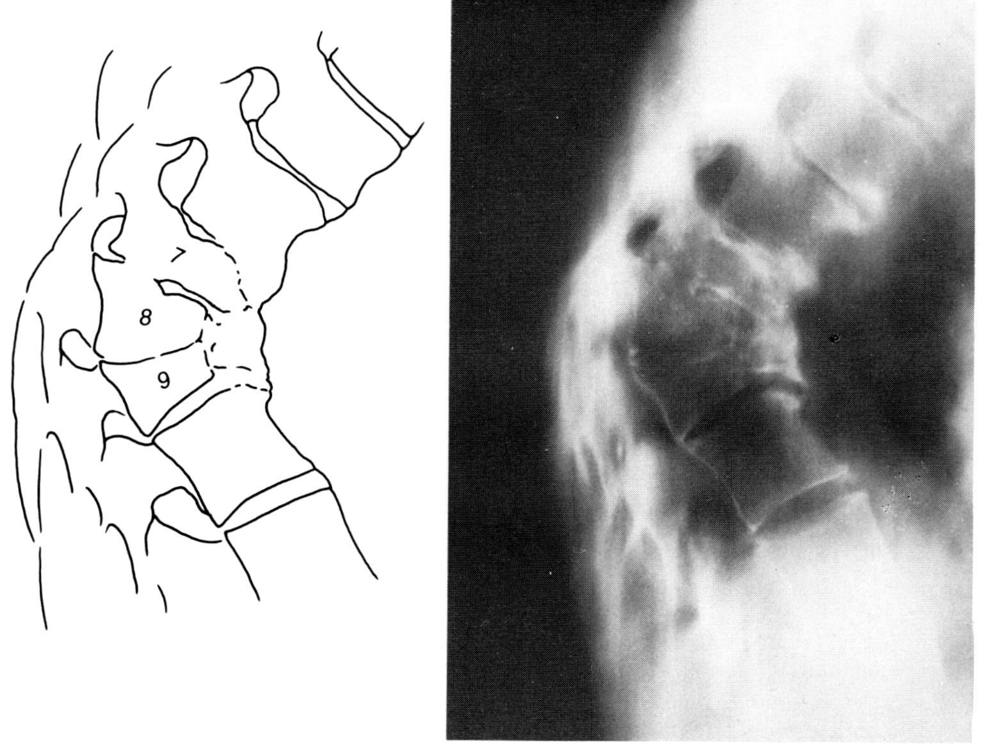

Fig. 119-1. Roentgenographic demonstration of a gibbus deformity at T7, T8, and T9.

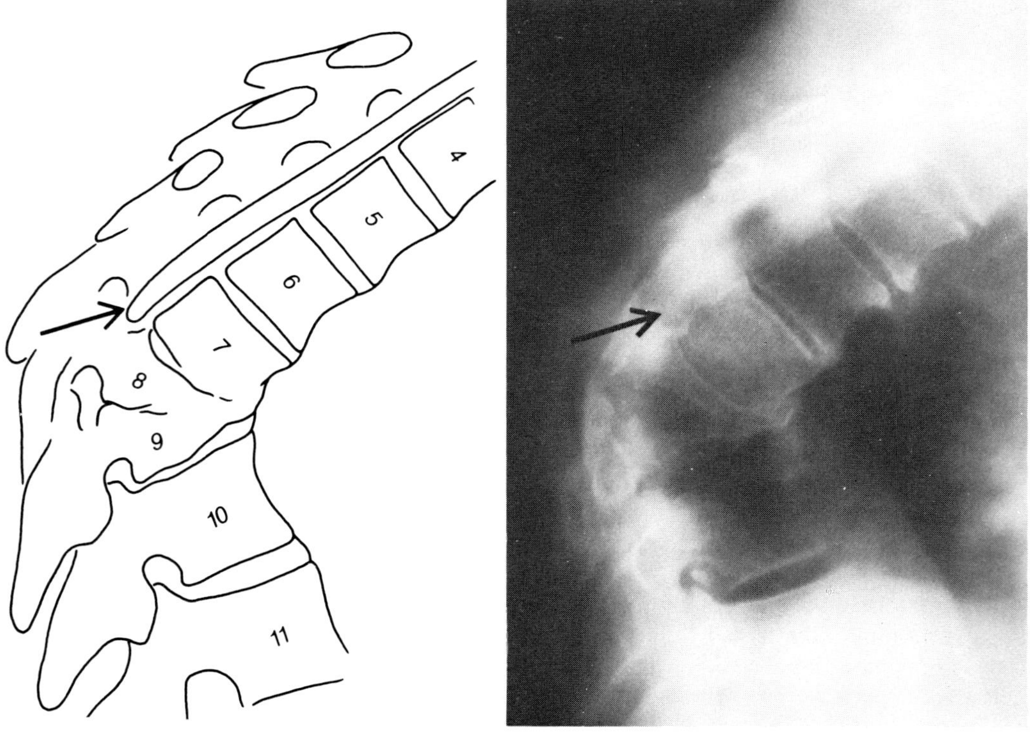

Fig. 11-2. Air myelography and sagittal tomography indicating cord compression over the extent of a gibbus deformity between T7, T8, and T9.

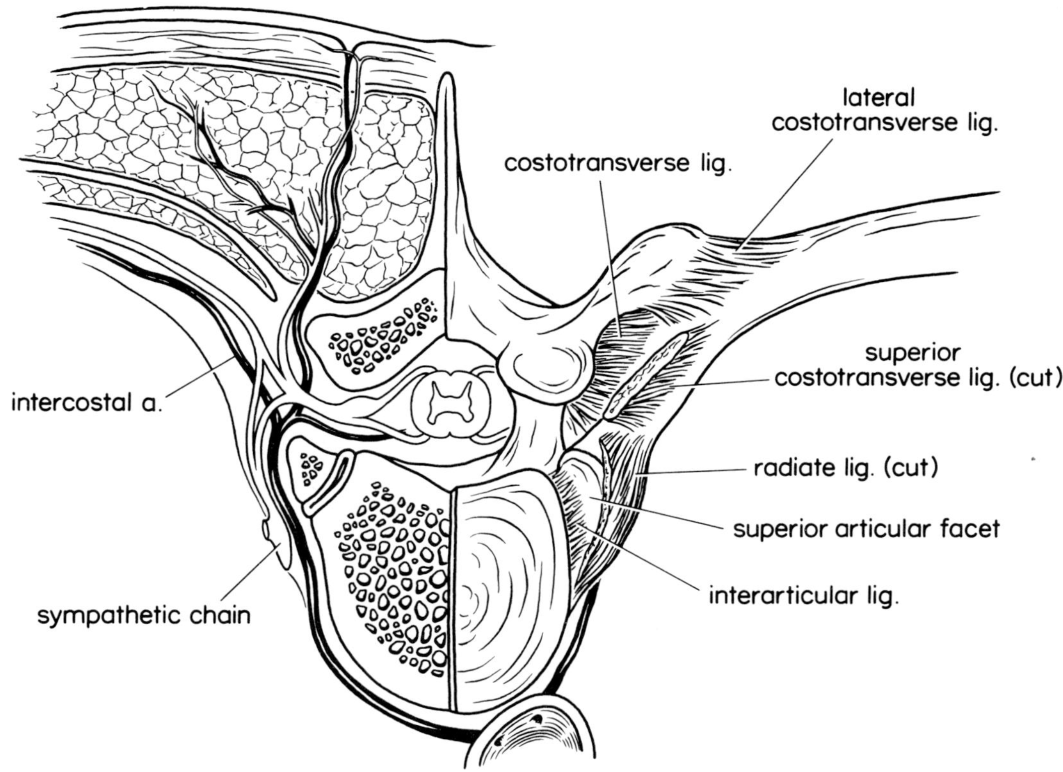

Fig. 119-3. Extent of decompression for one-level anterolateral spinal decompression.

stabilization are carried out as a single operative procedure. Adequate decompression is the exception not the rule is one attempts to accomplish this goal with spinal instrumentation (Figure 119-3).

TRANSTHORACIC APPROACH TO THE THORACIC SPINE FOR DECOMPRESSION AND STABILIZATION

Prior to surgery, the patient undergoing transthoracic or thoracoabdominal exploration, the spine at the level of maximal injury is localized and marked radiographically. Anesthesia is performed with a double-lumen endotracheal tube, and the proper position of the endotracheal tube is confirmed radiographically. An approach to the spine is preferably through a right-sided thoracotomy. The patient is positioned in a three-quarter prone position and draped to allow harvesting iliac crest bone for fusion. To minimize blood loss and to ensure the gentle handling of tissues, the operation is performed with 4.5× loupes and headlight illumination.

The skin incision is carried from the posterior midline overlying the area of deformity to the anterior axillary line (Figure 119-4). The subcutaneous tissues are divided in the line of the incision, and the latissimus dorsi is sectioned. A plane of dissection is developed by running two fingers behind the muscle and dividing the muscle with cutting current. Posteriorly, the trapezius and the rhomboid major muscles are divided in the line of the incision. Some fibers of the sacrospinalis also

may require division. Anteriorly, the serratus anterior is divided over the selected rib.

The ribs may be counted externally anteriorly from the second rib, which is prominent at its junction with the sternum. In the posterolateral position the horizontal border of the first rib may be palpated and used for counting. In lower incisions the ribs may be counted upward from the twelfth rib, which is palpated externally. The intercostal muscles are divided in the same way. The entire rib is resected subperiosteally, and this bone, although not optimal, is reserved for bone graft. The pleural space is entered through the periosteal bed. After placement of a Finochietto rib spreader and collapse of the lung, the sympathetic chain is identified and the intercostal nerve traced into the neural foramen. Depending upon the level chosen for decompression, the azygos vein may require division between ligatures to gain access to the anterior aspect of the vertebral column (Figure 119-5). The overlying pleura, endothoracic fascia, and fibrous tissue is dissected off the vertebral bodies. The thoracic duct lies on the vertebral bodies between the level of the aortic hiatus and T5. If the thoracic duct is known to be injured, it should he ligated with nonabsorbable suture and not clipped. Prior administration of colored cream through a nasogastric tube will help identify this structure.

A thoracoabdominal incision is required to provide exposure of the vertebral bodies of T11-T12, and L1, an incision is planned that extends from the posterior axillary line, in the selected interspace (usually T7-8), and moves forward to the midline of the abdomen. The serratus anterior is split, as are the fibers of the external oblique muscle. The anterior rectus

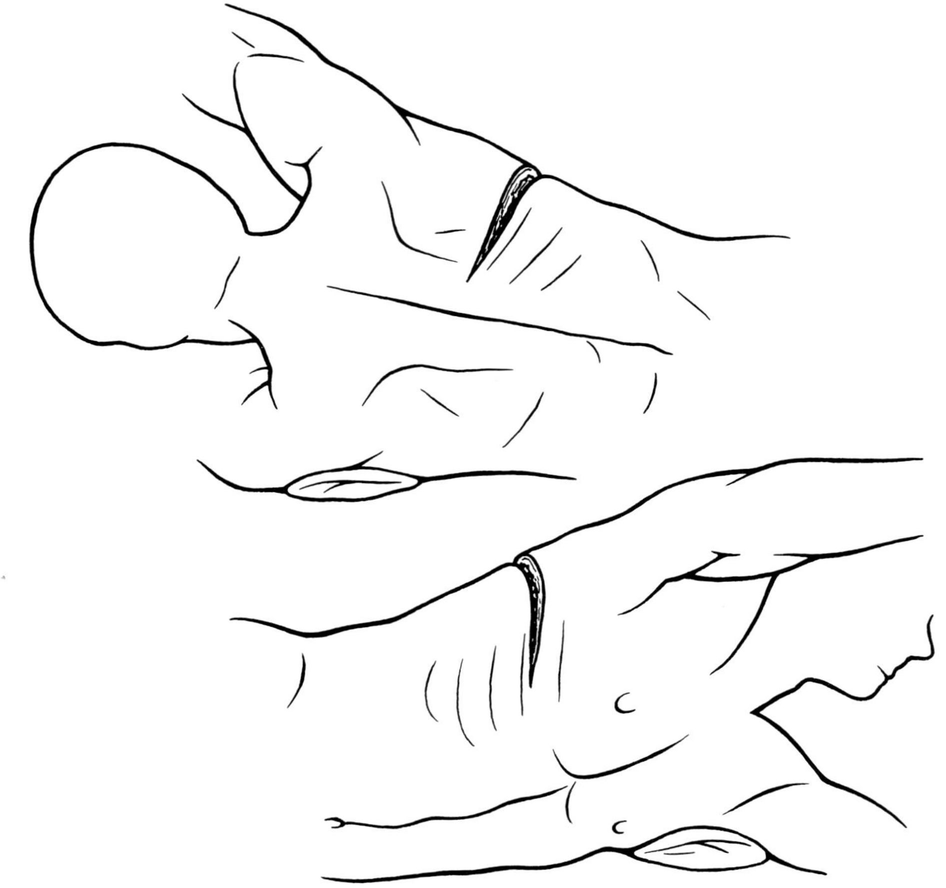

Fig. 119-4. Positioning for transthoracic approach to the thoracic spine.

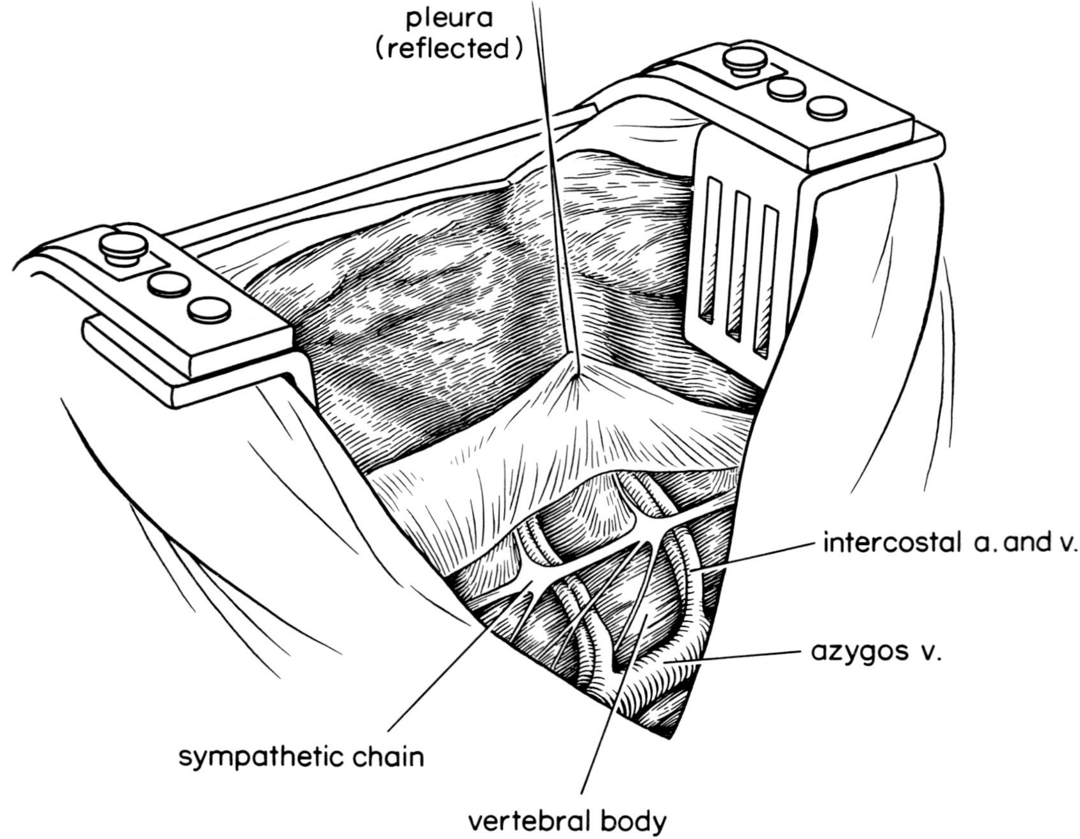

Fig. 119-5. Surgical anatomy: Collapse of the lung, exposing parietal pleura and strictures on the anterolateral aspect of the thoracic spine.

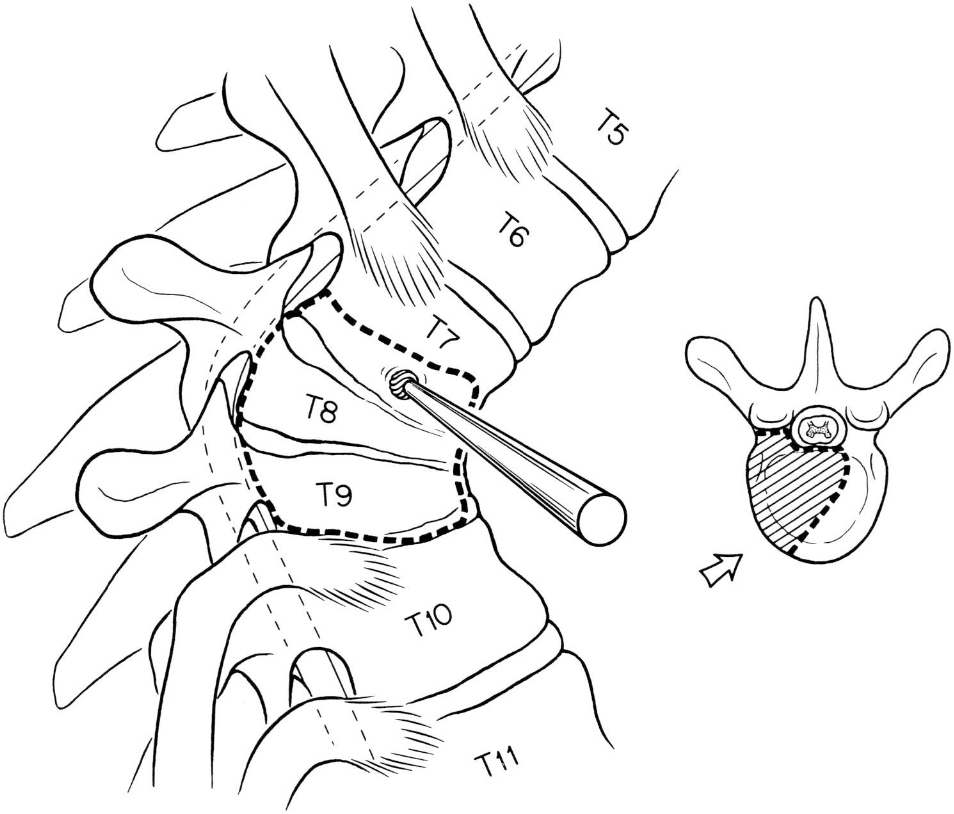

Fig. 119-6. Extent of bone removal, in this case involving three spinal segments, leaving a shell of vertebral body to allow some lateral stability for rib grafts while removing the apex of the gibbus.

sheath, the ipsilateral rectus muscle, the intercostal muscles, and the pleura are cut, thereby entering the chest cavity. In the abdomen, the incision divides the posterior rectus sheath, exposing, but not entering through, the peritoneum. The diaphragm is divided peripherally along its insertion to the spine. This muscle is subsequently repaired with interrupted nonabsorbable sutures. These approaches provide excellent access from approximately T3 to L2 anteriorly. Exposure of T1 to T3 is best accomplished by a posteriorly oriented thoracotomy from midline to the anterior axillary line with lateral displacement of the scapula and its attached musculature. This exposure allows for both neural decompression of these segments and anterior stabilization. Alternatively, a sternal splitting, direct anterior approach to T1-T3 can be used.

After identification of the destroyed or retropulsed bone this is removed under magnification using curettes and a high-speed air drill (Figure 119-6). The intervertebral discs and cartilaginous end plates on the ends of the vertebrae are removed to facilitate subsequent incorporation of the bone placed between the remaining vertebral bodies. Decompression of the spinal cord can be accomplished without removal of the entire vertebral body. Only the bone that is impinging into the spinal canal is removed to reconstitute the cross-sectional diameter of the spinal canal. To accomplish this it is necessary to undermine the bone projecting into the spinal canal with the air drill, which thereby provides adequate space to allow the retropulsed bone fragment to be depressed away from the ventral aspect of the dural sac. This approach is analogous to the technique described for the removal of a herniated thoracic disc; however, the extent of the defect created when dealing with a fracture necessitates removal of one third to one half of

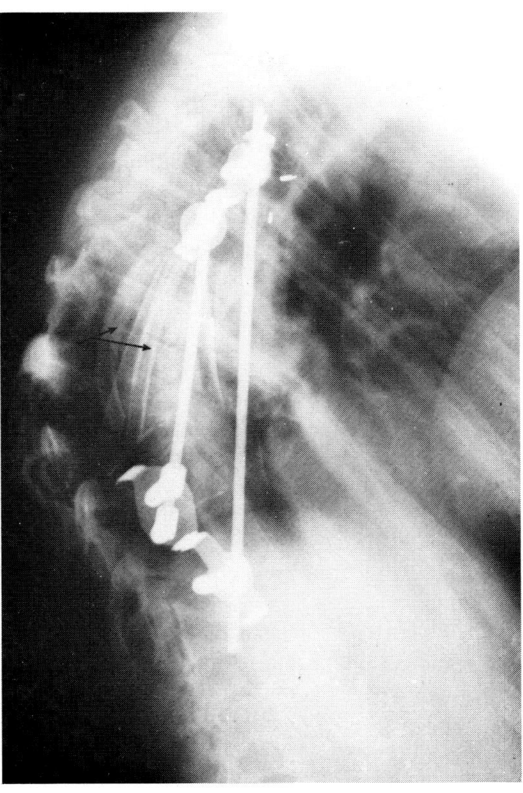

Fig. 119-7. Anterior instrumentation and rib graft stabilization after anterolateral decompression as a one-stage procedure.

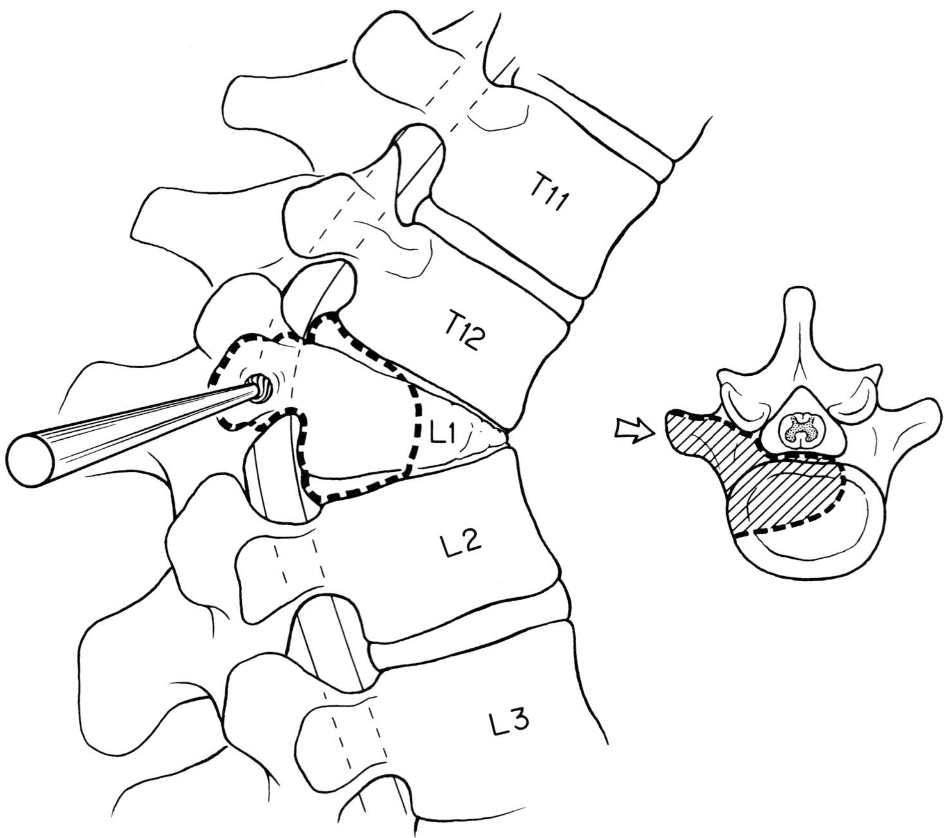

Fig. 119-8.   Extent of decompression for one-level anterolateral spinal decompression.

the vertebral body to achieve an adequate decompression (Figure 119-7 and 119-8).

Following thoracotomy, neurosurgical removal of disc, retropulsed vertebral bone, and hematoma, the levels for a fusion are selected to span the space between the intact vertebral bodies above and below the fracture-dislocation. Screws must be placed in intact vertebral bodies, but the longer the lever arms, the less secure the fixation. The segmental vessels must be suture ligated on the vertebral bodies to be instrumented. The vertebral body is exposed subperiosteally, and it is necessary to be able to feel the surface of the vertebral body from the distal side so that screws can be properly aimed and seated and thoracic injury avoided. Rib struts are used for fusion, although iliac crest bone is preferable. Disc spaces included in the fusion have been previously curetted. Correction of deformity is reserved for those cases without a rigid deficit, and is made by extending the thoracic spine on the operating table. The Santa Casa distractors (DePuy Co.) are useful if marked kyphosis is present over several levels (see Figure 119-3). Slots are cut in the vertebral bodies above and below the site of decompression to receive bone grafts. These grafts are cut and tapped into prepared recesses in the vertebral body with a bone set.

Although a variety of instruments exist, we have used anterior and posterior titanium rods fitted to Dwyer screws for midthoracic stabilization or anterior bone grafts and posterior instrumentation and grafts if the angle of the spine allows this to be carried out. Either single or double staples are used depending upon the configuration present. With a lesser degree of kyphosis and a solid vertebral body, it is possible to seat a double staple into the vertebral body, while with small vertebral

bodies and marked deformity it is safer to use two single staples. Screw and staple size are measured and the proper size selected. Care must be taken that the end of the screw penetrates the distal cortex of the vertebra. Portions of Keith needles inserted in the disc are helpful in guiding the screws so they lie transversely in the vertebral bodies. Staples are measured and set into the disc space, and the screws are turned through the staples so they lie firmly and flush with the vertebral body. Then the titanium rods are cut and guided through the holes in the screws, one anterior and one posterior, to control bending at the level of the fracture. The rods are secured in place in the screws by crimping the screw head. A single chest tube is brought through the anterior axillary line and the collapsed lung is re-expanded with the drainage tube to the posterior paravertebral gutter.

At the time of closure the pleura must be reapproximated with chromic catgut, and a rib approximator is used to appose the ribs above and below the bed from which a rib has been removed. The trapezius, rhomboids, serratus anterior, and latissimus dorsi are reapproximated with nonabsorbable suture material. The subcutaneous tissue is closed with fine, synthetic absorbable suture material and the skin is closed with a running nylon suture.

Postoperatively, the patient is nursed on a rotokinetic frame. The chest tube is removed in 24 to 48 hours if it is adynamic. The patients then gradually are mobilized in a molded plastic orthosis. If the patient is not unstable, ambulation is begun at approximately 1 week.

If posterior instrumentation such as the Harrington system is used in a given case, this is performed to the second intact vertebra above and below the level of injury, and fusion is carried out over approximately 3 segments. In all patients a bone graft is placed in addition to the Harrington instrumentation.

The complication rate attending both the transthoracic-transpleural operation and the anterolateral approach to the thoracolumbar spine has been low. These procedures require 3 to 4 hours to accomplish. When microsurgical techniques are used, blood loss from the neurosurgical portion of the operation is approximately 350 ml. It is during the fusion that 750 to 1000 ml of blood is lost and usually is replaced, since extensive areas of bone are denuded to ensure an adequate fusion. One case of dislodged Harrington rod has occurred to date in the entire series. There has not been an increased incidence of pulmonary complications with these operations. This probably is largely a matter of patient selection; the patients were predominately young, otherwise healthy persons.[16]

REFERENCES

1. Cline HJ Jr, cited by Hayward G: An account of a case of fractures and dislocation of the spine. N Engl J Med Surg 4:1, 1815
2. Tyrrell F: Compression of the spinal marrow from displacement of the vertebrae, consequent upon injury. Operation of removing the arch and spinous processes of the twelfth dorsal vertebra. Lancet 11:658, 1827
3. Smith AG: An account of a case in which portions of three dorsal vertebrae were removed for the relief of paralysis from fracture, with partial success. North Am MESJ 8:94, 1829
4. Cook WA: Transthoracic vertebral surgery. Ann Thorac Surg 12:54, 1971
5. Erickson DL, Leider LL, Browne W: One-stage decompression-stabilization for thoracolumbar fractures. Spine 2:53, 1977
6. Flesch JR, Leider LL, Erickson DL, et al: Harrington instrumentation and spine fusion for unstable fractures and fracture-dislocations of the thoracic and lumbar spine. J Bone Joint Surg 59A:143, 1977
7. Norrell H: The treatment of unstable spinal fractures and dislocations. Clin Neurosurg 25:193, 1978
8. Riseborough EJ: The anterior approach to the spine for the correction of deformities of the axial skeieton. Clin Orthop 9:207, 1973
9. De Oliviera JC: A new type of fracture-dislocation of the thoracolumbar spine. J Bone Joint Surg 60A:481, 1978
10. Dunsker S, Schmidek HH, Frymoyer J, Kahn A (eds): The Unstable Spine: Thoracic, Lumbar, and Sacral Regions. Orlando, Grune & Stratton, 1986
11. Bohlmana HH: Late progressive paralysis and pain following fractures of the thoracolumbar spine. J Bone Joint Surg 58A:728, 1976
12. Dunn HK: Anterior stabilization of thoracolumbar injuries. Clin Orthop 189:116, 1984
13. Hall JE: Dwyer instrumentation in anterior fusion of the spine. Current concepts review. J Bone Joint Surg 63A:1188, 1981
14. Kostiuck JP: Anterior spinal cord decompression for lesions of the thoracic and lumnbar spine: New methods of internal fixation and results. Spine 8:512, 1983
15. Kostiuck JP: Anterior fixation for fractures of the thoracic and lumbar spine with or without neurologic involvement. Clin Orthop 189:103, 1984
16. Gertzbein SD, Offierski C: Complete fracture-dislocation of the thoracic spine without spinal cord injury. A case report. J Bone Joint Surg 61A:449, 1979

CHAPTER 120

Transthoracic Disc Excision

Frederick A. Simeone   Ralph Rashbaum

SYMPTOMATIC HERNIATIONS of thoracic intervertebral discs are the rarest yet most devastating of all disc lesions. They present problems in diagnosis, and, historically, treatment by ordinary laminectomy has been attended with appalling results. Of Mueller's 4 cases, 3 were paraplegic after surgery.[1] Perot and Munro reviewed 91 cases from various sources in 1969.[2] Forty of these patients were not improved by surgery, and 16 were rendered paraplegic as a result of the operation. The results were most unfavorable in cases of central disc herniations, particularly those with advanced preoperative neurologic deficits. As might be expected, patients with lateral disc herniations and minimal neurologic deficit fared better postoperatively. All patients treated by ordinary laminectomy were characterized by the same discouraging conclusions.[3–9]

In 1960, Hulme[10] treated 4 cases through a lateral (costotransversectomy) approach with encouraging results; 3 were cured and 1 showed improvement. Perot and Munro,[2] 9 years later, described the transpleural approach through an ordinary thoracotomy incision in 2 patients, both of whom made a complete recovery. During the same year, Ransohoff and coworkers[9] described a similar procedure. These two approaches will be described in detail below, with additional comments about the use of the operating microscope when dissection near the spinal cord begins. In most of the series of symptomatic disc lesions described, thoracic disc herniations represent 0.25 percent to 0.75 percent of all symptomatic disc lesions. They are seen between the fourth to twelfth thoracic interspaces, with the greatest percentage occurring between T8 and T11. Patients may have pain in a radicular distribution, acute or chronic in nature, with laterally placed lesions. Patients with central herniations develop paraparesis, with or without sensory complaints, and with an acute or chronic onset. There is nothing characteristic about chronic thoracic disc herniations that can lead to a clinical distinction among other causes of thoracic spinal cord compression.

On radiologic examination the offending disc is often calcified, although calcification in thoracic discs is sufficiently common that this finding itself normally just increases the suspicion of thoracic disc protrusion. Accurate myelography, particularly with painstaking efforts to achieve optimum lateral views, is absolutely necessary. No operation for thoracic disc herniation should be undertaken without myelograms that clearly outline the lesion; contrast medium may have to be instilled cisternally. When the offending lesion is identified, great care must be taken to develop criteria for localizing the proper disc intraoperatively. The thoracic spine is approached by the alternative routes described below; it is most difficult to

find the appropriate level during surgery. Consequently, we often will insert a sterile needle into a spinous process on the morning of surgery (with radiologic control) and retain this marker throughout the operation.

SURGICAL TECHNIQUE

COSTOTRANSVERSECTOMY AND DISC EXCISION

Costotransversectomy is carried out with the patient under general anesthesia and intubated with a cuffed endotracheal tube. The anesthesiologist must be able to inflate the patient's lungs should the pleural cavity be entered inadvertently.

The patient lies in a modified lateral decubitus position, elevated 30 degrees from the straight prone, so that the surgeon can stand opposite the abdomen (Figure 120-1). A pad is placed in the axilla and below the shoulders. To avoid increased venous pressure the abdomen must be kept free by carefully placed supports under the chest and iliac crest. The uppermost knee is flexed, and a pillow is placed between the legs. The approach can be made from either side; the choice depends upon the presence of lateralizing features in the clinical presentation. If unilateral root pain is the principal symptom, then the interspace should be approached from the same side. With central disc herniations, or in the absence of lateralizing findings, the right-sided approach has been used because, statistically, the important artery of Adamkiewicz usually originates from the left lower intercostal vessels (roughly T8 to L2).

It is essential to localize the lesion at this point, either with a needle that previously has been inserted into the spinous process, as mentioned earlier, or by marking the rib to be removed by injecting indigo carmine onto it subcutaneously.

The skin incision follows a long semilunar course, extending the length of at least three vertebral bodies above and below the disc space in question (Figure 120-2). The incision extends at least 20 cm laterally from the midline at the apex of the curve. Dissection proceeds through the skin and subcutaneous tissue to the deep fascia, all of which are elevated and retracted medially to the spinous processes (Figure 120-3). The trapezius muscle can be incised in line with the skin incision and retracted medially. This exposes the erector spinae muscle mass (semispinalis longissimus and iliocostalis muscles), which is reflected medially by stripping the muscles from their attachments. Alternatively, the muscle mass can be transected over the rib to be removed and the muscles retracted in a cephalic and caudal direction for easier access to the lamina as well as to

OPERATIVE NEUROSURGICAL TECHNIQUES
ISBN 0-8089-1862-1

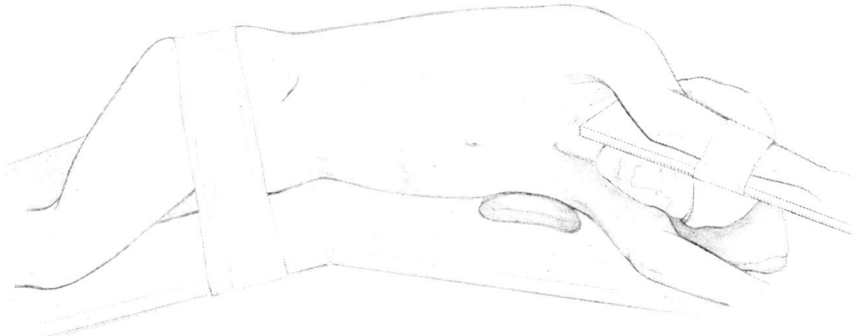

Fig. 120-1.

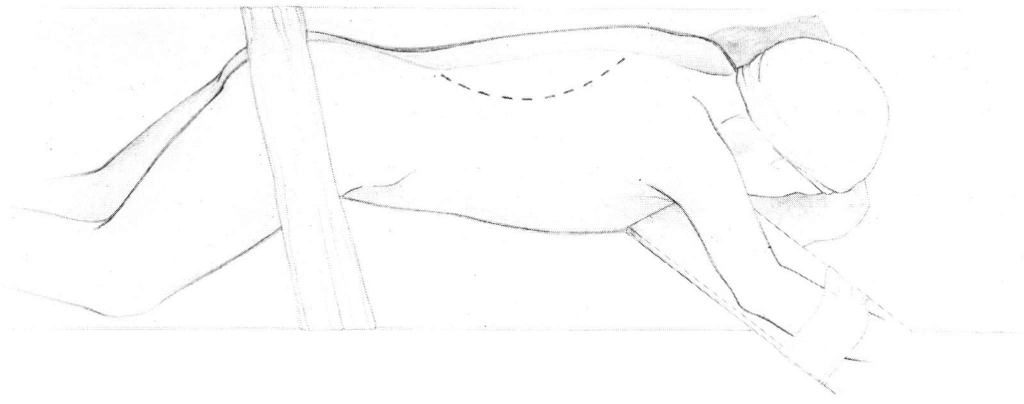

Fig. 120-2.

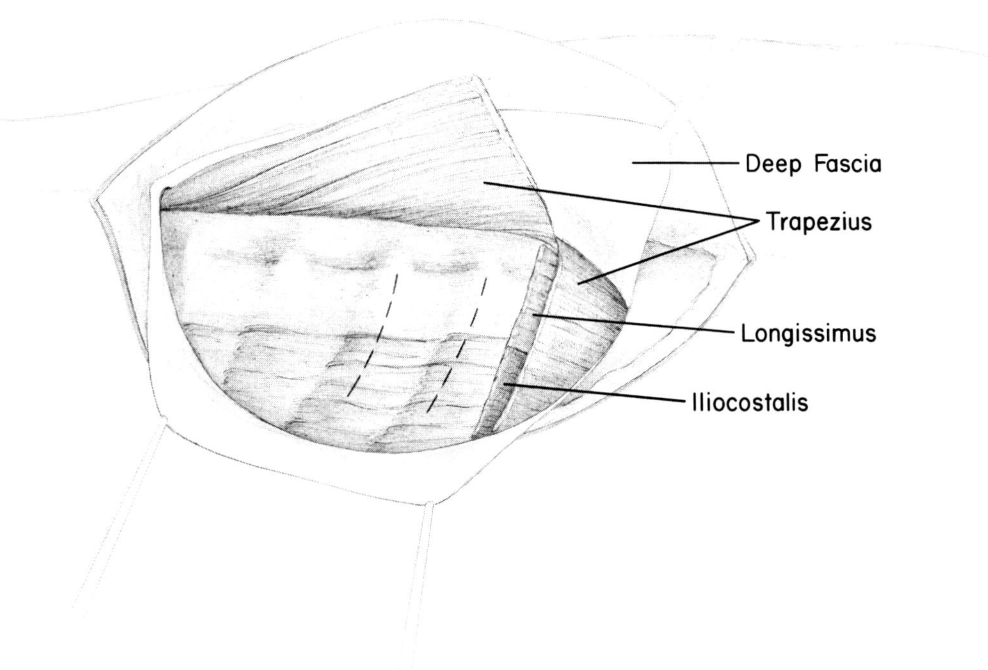

Fig. 120-3.

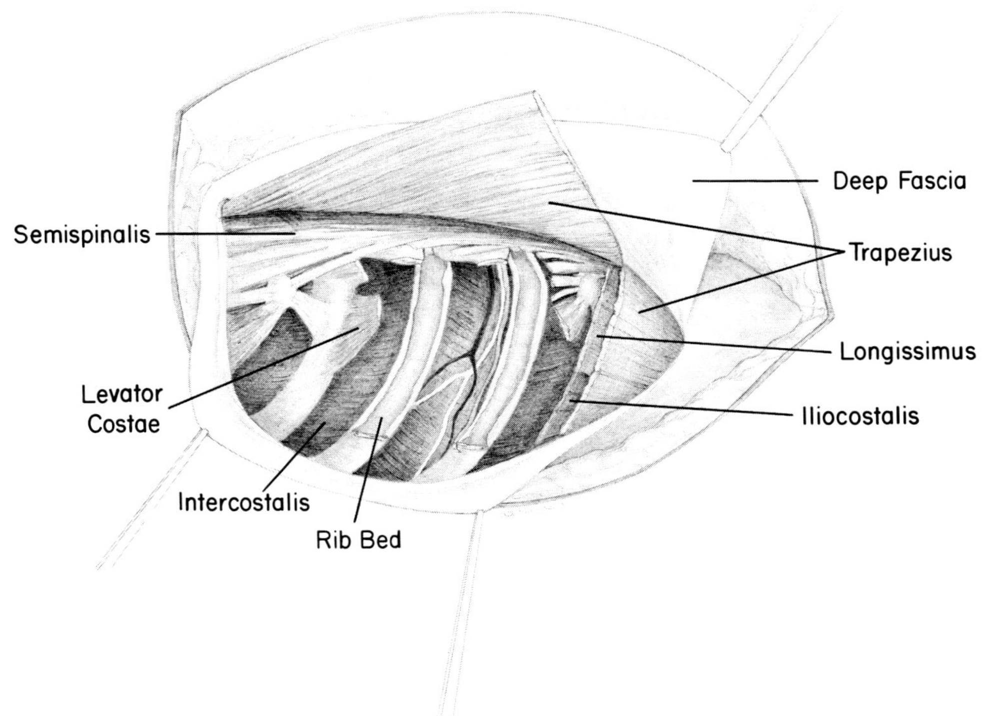

Fig. 120-4.

SIMEONE AND RASHBAUM

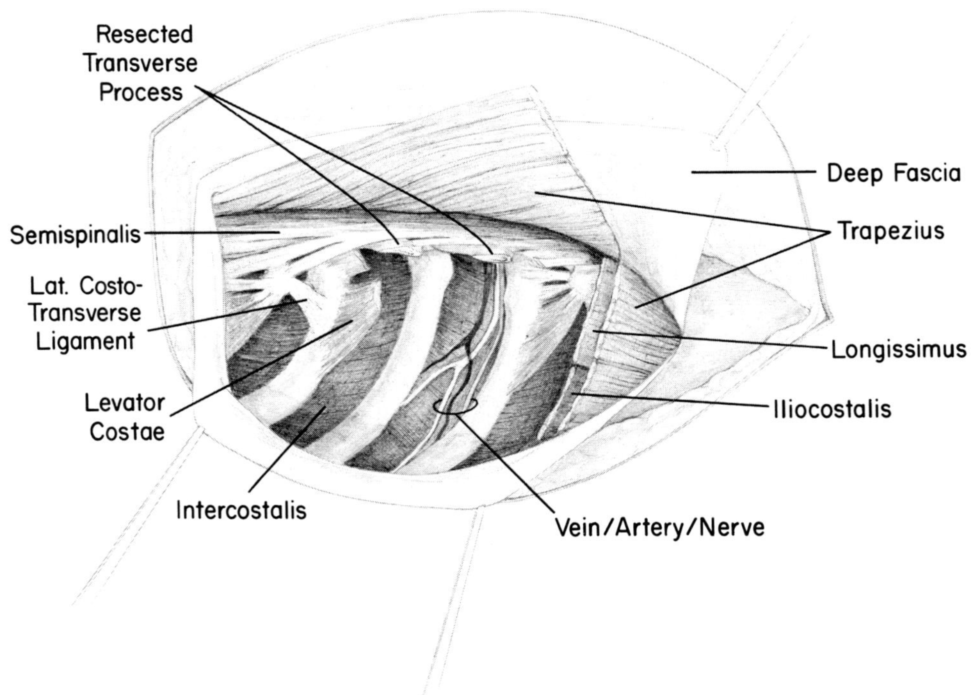

Fig. 120-5.

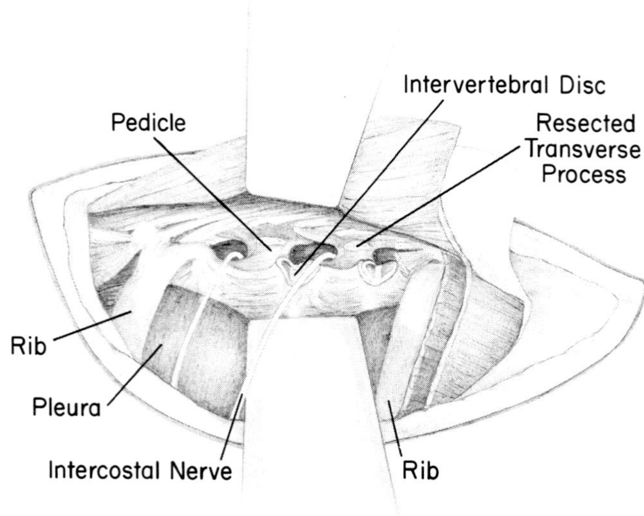

Fig. 120-6.

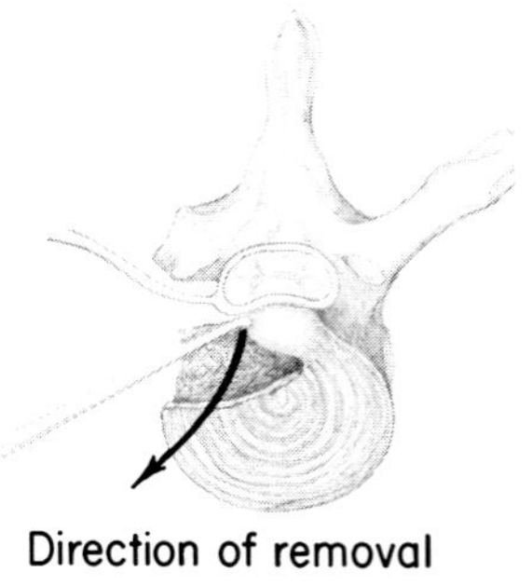

Fig. 120-8.

the rib to be removed. This rib is identified and the intercostal neurovascular complex is separated from its inferior surface. The periosteum is stripped from the rib, about the width of the incision, with a Doyen separator (Figure 120-4).

Attention then is directed to the attachment of the rib with the vertebral bodies. The transverse process is removed with a rongeur so that the articulation of the rib head and its costotransverse and capsular ligaments can be identified and sectioned. The rib is cut at the most lateral portion of the incision (approximately 20 cm of rib is removed), and it is disarticulated from the vertebral body (Figure 120-5).

When the rib is removed, the intercostal vein, artery, and nerve can be followed through their entrance into the spinal canal. It is not necessary to sacrifice any of these structures, although the muscular branches of the intercostal artery can be cauterized as needed (Figure 120-6). The parietal pleura is separated from the ribs, above and below, as well as from the spinal column, and it is depressed with a malleable ribbon or large Deaver retractor. The segmental vessels along the side of the vertebrae are identified. They should not be damaged; if bleeding develops, however, it can be controlled by silver clips or coagulation.

The intervertebral foramen is identified by tracing the intracostal nerve medially. The nerve enters the spinal canal between two pedicles. The latter structures are cleaned with a periosteal elevator and then removed piecemeal with a Kerrison rongeur. A high-speed air drill may facilitate removal of the pedicle. If we use an air drill, we also prefer to use an operating microscope at that time, because it provides excellent illumination and magnification of important neural structures underlying the bone that is to be removed. The microscope is used throughout the rest of the procedure on the vertebra and discs. When the pedicle is removed, the lateral aspect of the dural sac and the intrusion of the disc into the canal can be appreciated (Figure 120-7). An incision is made into the midportion of the disc space, well away from the spinal cord, and the space is emptied by curettage and the use of pituitary rongeurs. A small portion of the opposing margins of the vertebral bodies, nearest the spinal canal, can be curetted away to ease access to the disc space (Figure 120-8). Through this opening, fragments closer to the dural canal may be separated and pushed into the emptied disc space for later removal. A Penfield dissector can be used to palpate the posterior longitudinal ligament for sequestered disc material. This instrument also can depress the annulus fibrosis into the intervertebral disc space to determine if the spinal canal is really fully decompressed.

The interspace is irrigated thoroughly and meticulous hemostasis is achieved. Through positive pressure ventilation, the pleura is checked for leaks. If it has been violated, an extrapleural chest tube may be placed before completing the closure. The wound is closed in layers. A chest x-ray film taken in the

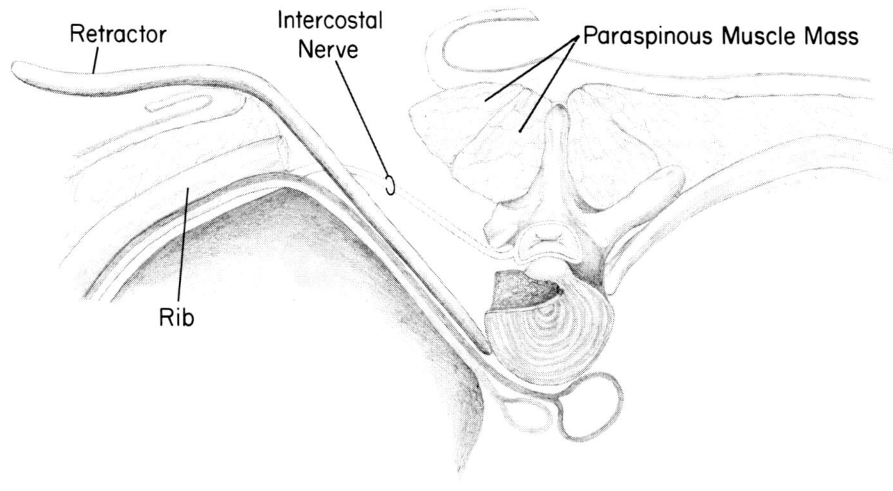

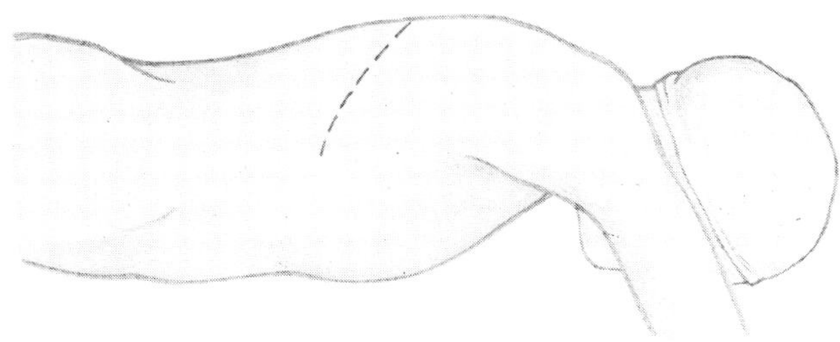

Fig. 120-9.

recovery room will help if there are concerns about a pneumothorax.

TRANSTHORACIC (TRANSPLEURAL) DISC EXCISION

Transthoracic disc excision is considerably more formidable than costotransversectomy, but it provides direct access to the anterior and lateral portions of the disc. A thoracic surgeon is required, at least in the early experiences with this approach. The patient's general medical and pulmonary status must be checked preoperatively. A postoperative unit for the management of thoracotomy patients is required. The degree of postoperative pain is greater, as is the possibility of significant intraoperative bleeding.

The operation is carried out with the patient under general anesthesia and intubated with a cuffed endotracheal tube. A Carlens tube should be used so that each lung may be ventilated separately if the surgical situation requires this.

The chest is entered through a standard right posterior thoracotomy incision (Figure 120-9). The right side is chosen because the artery of Adamkiewicz usually enters on the left side (80 percent of cases) and because the heart and great vessels pose a problem through a left transthoracic incision. The patient is positioned in the straight lateral posture, leaning somewhat toward his or her abdomen so that the chest contents (with the exception of the azygous vein) will gravitate out of the operative field. The surgeon stands on the spinal side of the patient, and a better view is obtained if the patient is tilted slightly toward the surgeon (Figure 120-10). Careful positioning of the patient over the table break or kidney rest will enable the anesthesiologist, at the appropriate time, to flex the thoracic spine laterally, thereby opening the interspace. In younger patients, there will be sufficient elasticity of the rib ligaments so that the rib spreader will provide sufficient exposure. If such is not the case, the rib opposite the offending intervertebral disc can be removed (Figure 120-11). The lateral aspect of the rib is

sectioned first, and the head of the rib can be removed through the endothoracic fascia (Figure 120-12). At least 15 cm of rib, including the rib head, must be removed in order to gain complete exposure to the lateral-most portion of the spinal canal (Figure 120-13). Prior to disarticulation of the rib, identification of the intercostal nerve and vessels is important. The vessels should be preserved and the intercostal nerve may be followed to the appropriate intervertebral foramen. A specifically numbered rib will articulate with a posterior-superior margin of the vertebral body whose number it shares, as well as the posterior-inferior margin of the vertebra above. For example, the T8 rib will articulate with the body of T8 and T7, and it will cross the T7-8 interspace.

Attention now is directed to the lateral aspect of the vertebral body above and below the offending disc. A linear incision is made in the parietal pleura extending from the middle of each vertebral body. The incision is extended at its ends, and the pleura is reflected laterally (Figure 120-14). Careful dissection of the parietal pleura from the vertebral body will expose the intervertebral vessels, as well as the sympathetic chain. It is necessary to ligate the segmental artery and vein above and below the disc lesion to gain adequate exposure. The intercostal nerve is followed to its foramen and gently retracted to expose the pedicles above and below (Figure 120-15). The Kerrison rongeur or high-speed air drill is used to remove the pedicles so that the dural sac above and below the disc lesion is readily demonstrated. With the use of an operating microscope, disc protrusion into the canal is readily seen. The intervertebral disc is incised in its anterior two thirds and its contents are emptied with pituitary rongeurs and curettes. No attempt is made to remove the extruded fragment initially. With flexion of the table or alteration of the kidney rest, the interspace may be opened and a lamina spreader introduced. When the space is emptied, the surgeon may use an air drill to remove a small segment of the vertebral body at the opposing margins (Figure 120-16). A larger window into the spinal canal made in this fashion will enable disc fragments to be picked away from beneath the dural sac with small curettes. The dura is not retracted, but the floor of the spinal canal is palpated repeatedly with flat instruments (Penfield dissectors) to retrieve sequestered fragments and to ascertain the effectiveness of decompression. The annulus fibrosis and its associated ligaments may be forced into the interspace and subsequently retrieved, and the area is irrigated thoroughly when the surgeon is confident that the spinal cord has been decompressed.

The parietal pleura now may be sutured over the vertebral bodies with running sutures of chromic catgut. Following the placement of an apical dependent chest tube through separate stab wounds, the chest is closed in routine fashion. The chest

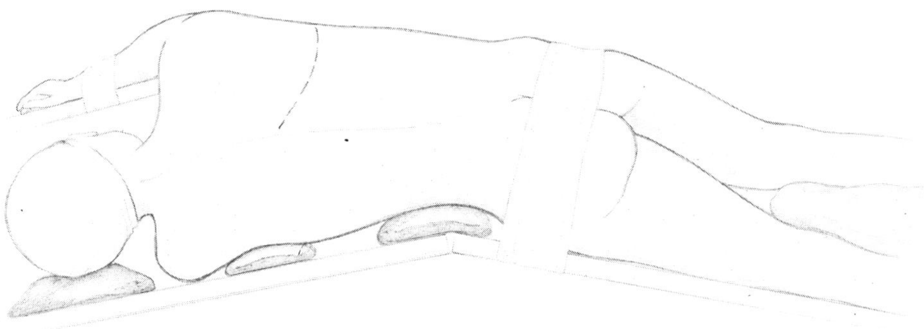

Fig. 120-10.

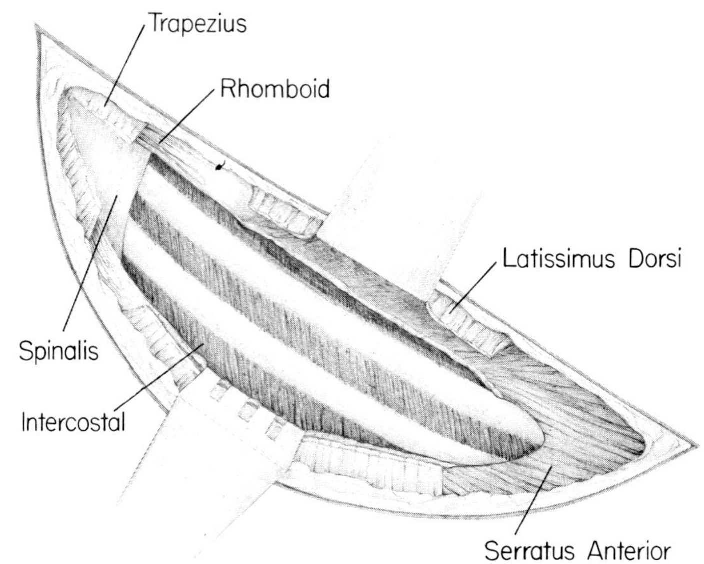

Fig. 120-11.

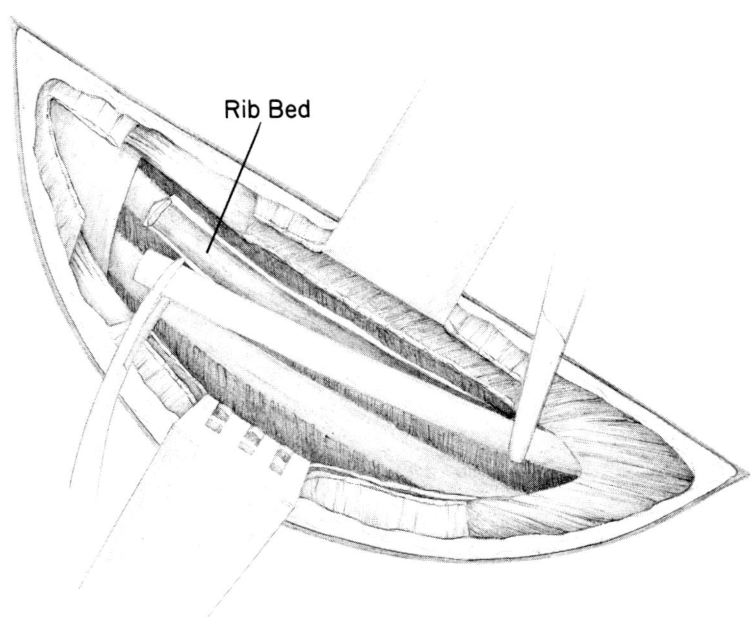

Fig. 120-12.

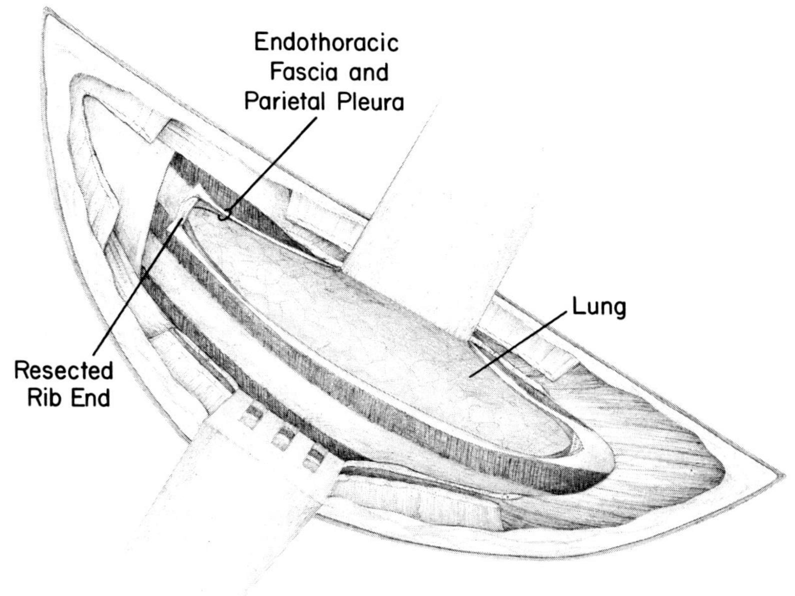

Fig. 120-13.

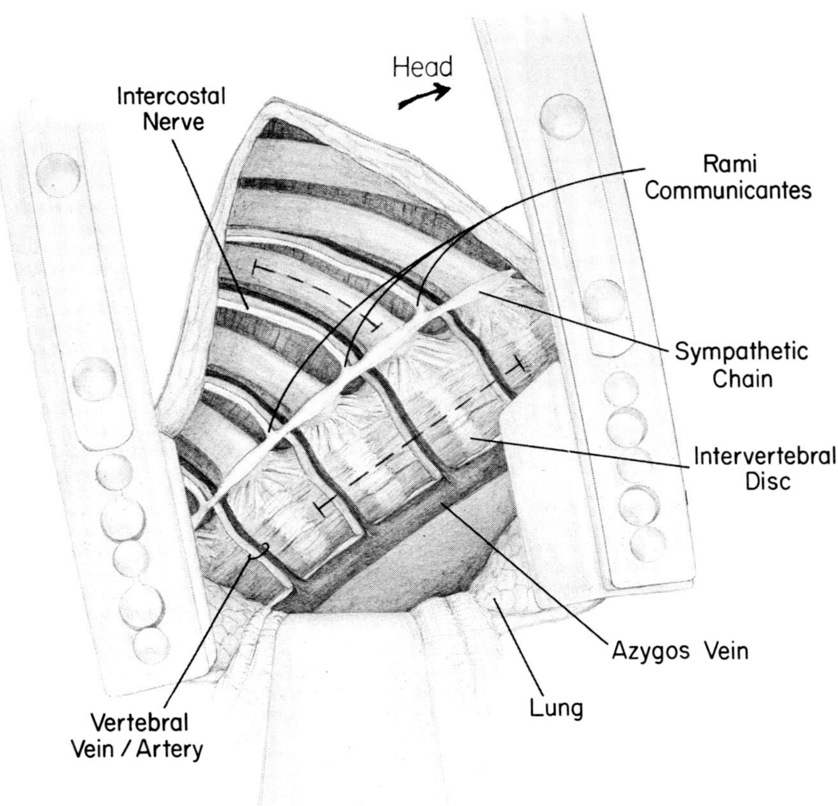

Fig. 120-14.

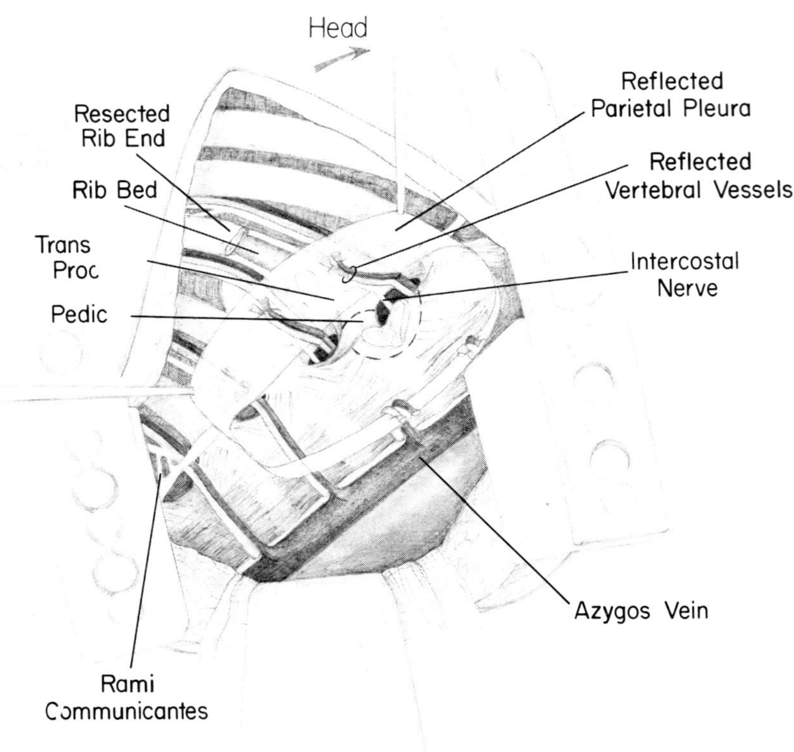

Fig. 120-15.

tubes are subsequently placed to underwater suction drainage, which can be removed when no further air leaks or drainage are present (usually 2 to 4 days). Repeated chest x-ray films are used to follow the size of the pneumothorax if one persists during the immediate postoperative period.

CONCLUSION

Costotransversectomy and the transthoracic approach to thoracic disc herniations have offered patients new hope for cure without great fear of postoperative paraplegia. The costotransversectomy approach is a less formidable operation, and with the operating microscope, provides an adequate exposure to the lateral spinal canal. This approach is probably satisfactory for most symptomatic thoracic disc herniations. Where a more aggressive attack on the anterior surface of the spinal canal is required, transthoracic disc excision provides excellent visualization of the ventral surface of the spinal cord.

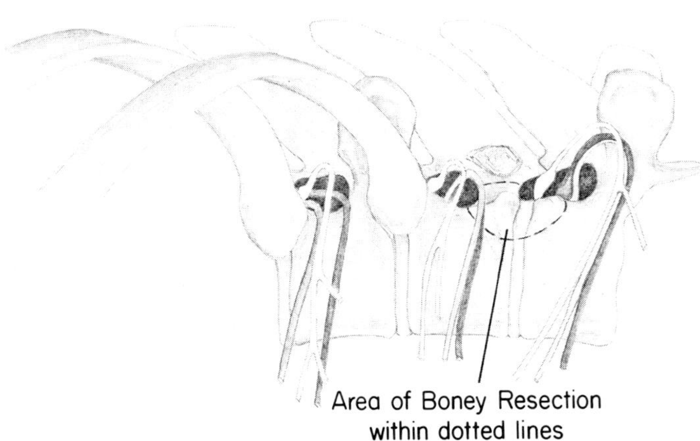

Fig. 120-16.

REFERENCES

1. Mueller R: Prolapse of thoracic intervertebral discs. Acta Med Scand 139:99, 1951
2. Perot PL, Munro OD: Transthoracic removal of midline thoracic disc protrusions causing spinal cord compression. J Neurosurg 31:452, 1969
3. Arseni C, Nash F: Protrusion of thoracic intervertebral discs. Acta Neurochir 11:1, 1963
4. Logue V: Thoracic intervertebral disc prolapse with spinal cord compression. J Neurol Neurosurg Psychiatry 15:227, 1952
5. Love JG, Schorn VG: Thoracic disc protrusions. JAMA 191:627, 1965
6. Reeves DL, Brown, HA: Thoracic intervertebral disc protrusion with cord compression. J Neurosurg 28:24, 1968
7. Svein HJ, Karavitis AL: Multiple protrusions of intervertebral discs in the upper thoracic region: Report of case. Proc Staff Meet Mayo Clin 29:375, 1954
8. Tovi D, Strang RR: Thoracic intervertebral disc protrusions. Acta Chir Scand Suppl 267:1960
9. Ransohoff J, Spencer F, Slew F, et al: Transthoracic removal of thoracic disc. Report of three cases. J Neurosurg 31:459, 1969
10. Hulme A: The surgical approach to thoracic intervertebral disc protrusions. J Neurol Neurosurg Psychiatry 23:133, 1960 J Simeone and Rashbaum

CHAPTER 121

Lumbar Disc Excision

Bernard E. Finneson

CAVEAT DISC SURGEON

THE FIRST DISC OPERATION is relatively easy. The repeat operative procedure, however, presents a problem both in technique and, even more, in satisfactory outcome. The recommended solution to this problem is to avoid the first operation that is apt to lead to a less than satisfactory result, and thus not create a clinical condition that requires repeat disc surgery.

PATIENT SELECTION

The most important consideration affecting the outcome of lumbar disc surgery is patient selection. What factors help predict whether a patient will improve from surgery? The surgeon who can select a patient who will benefit from surgical intervention has won half the battle before the incision is made. It is perhaps even more important for the surgeon to be able to predict those individuals who will not benefit from surgery. The surgeon who operates on this type of patient is handicapped before he starts; a satisfactory clinical result is not likely even with the finest, most meticulous surgical technique. The most that can reasonably be expected is that the patient will not be too discernibly worse after surgery. It should be emphasized that the lack of response to nonsurgical treatment is not, in itself, an indication for surgery. All too often the patient with low back pain who is not readily cured with nonsurgical management is brought to the operating room under the banner of ''we must do something for this poor suffering patient.'' This ''something'' is often a variety of new, and sometimes irreversible, surgically produced signs and symptoms, which are superimposed upon the original complaints. The surgeon should remember that no matter how severe and intractable the pain is, it can always be made worse with surgery.

FALLIBILITY OF THE NEUROLOGIC EXAMINATION

Neurosurgeons, in comparison to their orthopedic colleagues, are perhaps a bit more prone to rely upon the neurologic examination to identify the level of disc protrusion. There are, of course, certain general findings, such as severe paraspinal muscle spasm in the lumbar area or poor mobility of the lumbar spine that are common to most disc syndromes at any level and that are not considered of localizing value. The classic findings of a diminished or absent Achilles reflex and numbness

along the lateral aspect of the foot in the presence of sciatic pain generally would be accepted as representing an L5-S1 disc protrusion. If the lumbar spine films demonstrate a narrow disc space at the level of L5-S1, some disc surgeons might forego the myelogram and proceed with surgery. In most cases they would be right, and a surgically treatable lesion would be found at the L5-S1 level. Three factors can be responsible for neurologic changes, however, that may mislead the surgeon as to the involved interspace.

1. Location of the disc protrusion (Figure 121-1). The disc fragment may extrude laterally into the foramen so that it compresses the exiting root from the interspace above. Such a laterally located fragment at the L5-S1 foramen may produce an L4-5 syndrome.
2. Neuroanatomic changes (Figure 121-2). A partially lumbarized first sacral segment, which may be dismissed as being of no clinical significance, might be associated with a postfixed plexus. In such a situation an L5-S1 disc protrusion may produce weakness of the great toe and numbness over the dorsum of the foot within the L5 dermatome and might be identified as a L4-5 protrusion at the level of L4-5 on the basis of the neurologic examination.
3. Temporal changes. As the patient grows older, degenerative changes within the discs occur in a progressively cephalad direction. This is well documented by discography, which demonstrates that degenerative changes usually occur first at the L5-S1 level; some years later they advance to the L4-5 interspace, and with advancing age, they advance progressively cephalad. For this reason, an individual over the age of 50 who has severe sciatica associated with an Achilles reflex and a narrow L5-S1 disc space could be suffering from an acute lesion at the level of L4-5. The absent Achilles reflex may be a residual finding from a previously protruded lesion at the level of L5-S1 that has long since fibrosed, leaving less mobility at that level, and that is no longer a source of pain. The new painful disc lesion at the level of L4-5 may not have been present long enough to establish hard neurologic findings.

MYELOGRAPHY

Lumbar myelograms should be done on all patients before lumbar disc surgery. These myelograms are used principally to confirm clinical localization and to determine if more than one disc herniation is present. They also help to rule out possible lumbar spinal tumors, which very easily can simulate herniated lumbar discs. Although used mainly as a preoperative test,

OPERATIVE NEUROSURGICAL TECHNIQUES
ISBN 0-8089-1862-1

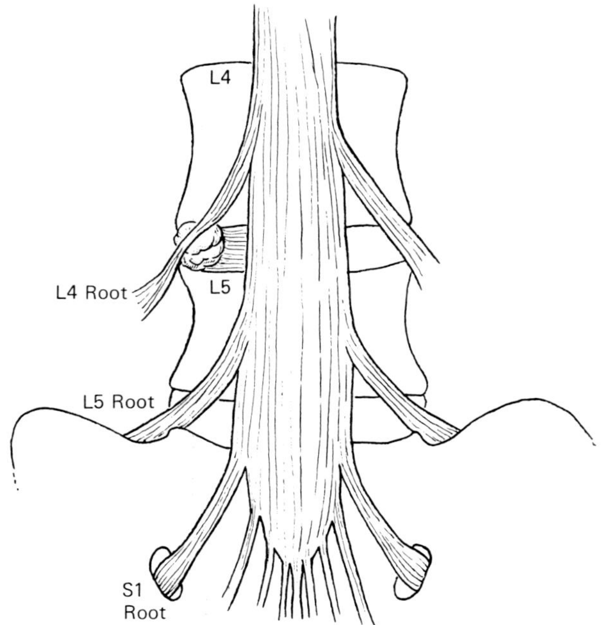

Fig. 121-1. Foraminal root compressive syndrome. The laterally situated L4-5 disc protrusion will extend into the intervertebral foramen impinging upon the L4 root and simulate an L3-4 syndrome. (Reprinted from Finneson BE: Low Back Pain, ed. 2. Philadelphia, JB Lippincott, 1981. With permission.)

myelography is occasionally performed on patients who have not fared well with an adequate course of conservative management and in whom there is significant uncertainty regarding the nature of their complaints. The myelogram is not infallible and is associated with a significant incidence of both false negatives and false positives. Most false negatives are noted at the L5-S1 level, where there is a large space between the anterior dural edge and the posterior bony spine. This space is less wide above the L5-S1 level, so the incidence of false negatives is much less from the level of L4-5 upward. The incidence of false positives is greater in patients over the age of 55 because of the hypertrophic osteoarthritic degenerative changes associated with advancing years.

LUMBAR DISC SURGERY PREDICTIVE SCORE CARD

It must be recognized that any surgical judgment that is based primarily on such a subjective symptom as pain can have as many variables as there are surgeons. All medical judgments relating to therapy are made by assigning positive and negative relative values to various aspects of the clinical picture, with the final decision being made by mentally balancing out these relative values. A numerical value system is not commonly used, but such a system may allow surgeons to communicate more easily about this complex problem.

A review of the various clinical factors that play a role in surgical decision making was carried out in 200 postsurgical patients who had a good result and was compared with 96 postsurgical patients who had a poor result.[1] This clinical review was employed as a base on which to list the major positive and negative factors involved in preoperative selection and to assign these factors positive and negative numerical values. Employment of such a system provides a "predictive

number" indicating the likely outcome of surgery. In an effort to make the system usable by almost all physicians who are involved in lumbar disc surgery, only those criteria that have broad acceptance and that are generally employed were included. Studies that have less widespread use, such as electromyography, discography, lumbar venography, computed tomographic (CT) scanning, and special psychologic studies, were purposely excluded. The result of this study was a Lumbar Disc Surgery Predictive Score Card (Figure 121-3).

POSITIVE SCORE CARD FACTORS

The predictive score card lists 7 positive factors with a total of 115 possible points.

Factor 1. The key word is incapacitating. If pain is not severe enough to hamper activities of daily living, the patient often is likely to be unsatisfied with the results of surgery.

Factor 2. Excision of a herniated lumbar disc usually will relieve nerve root pain. If sciatica is not the major symptom, and surgery provides relief of sciatica but no improvement of the back pain, the unhappy patient may well ignore the disappearance of the minor sciatica and concentrate on the persisting predominant back pain.

Factor 3. Body position should affect a lumbar disc syndrome if it is indeed a mechanical problem. Sciatic syndromes that are unaffected by changes in body position are often nonmechanical in nature and will not be alleviated by the mechanical removal of pressure.

Factor 4. A neurologic examination that demonstrates a single root syndrome indicating a specific interspace obviously increases the possibility of a successful outcome.

Factor 5. It is important that the myelographic defect corroborate the neurologic examination. It must be kept in mind that various reports indicate abnormal lumbar myelographs in (low back) symptom-free patients in percentages varying from 25 percent to 30 percent.

Factor 6. The straight-leg-raising test is a good predictive factor. The crossed-straight-leg-raising test (the nonpainful leg is raised, which produces aggravation of pain radiating into the painful leg) is twice as effective (Figure 121-4).

Factor 7. The patient's realistic appraisal of future life style is an important factor that easily may be ignored by the surgeon. The only way to appreciate the patient's postoperative expectations is to spend some time listening to the patient.

NEGATIVE SCORE CARD FACTORS

The score card lists 6 negative factors with a total of 80 possible points.

Factor 1. Back pain primarily is the reverse of positive factor 2.

Factor 2. Although grossly obese people initially seem to do about the same as those patients with a more normal habitus, after 1 or 2 years the recurrence rate is somewhat higher.

Factor 3. Simultaneous weakness in flexion and extension of the great toe cannot be explained by pressure on a single root, and unless some neurologic explanation can be offered for this finding, it should be considered nonorganic.

Factor 4. Poor psychological background is a "mixed bag," but any of these factors should cause the surgeon to be cautious. The alcoholic, for example, may have demonstrated a very steady work history in the past and may never have been hospitalized previously. It should be recognized, however, that

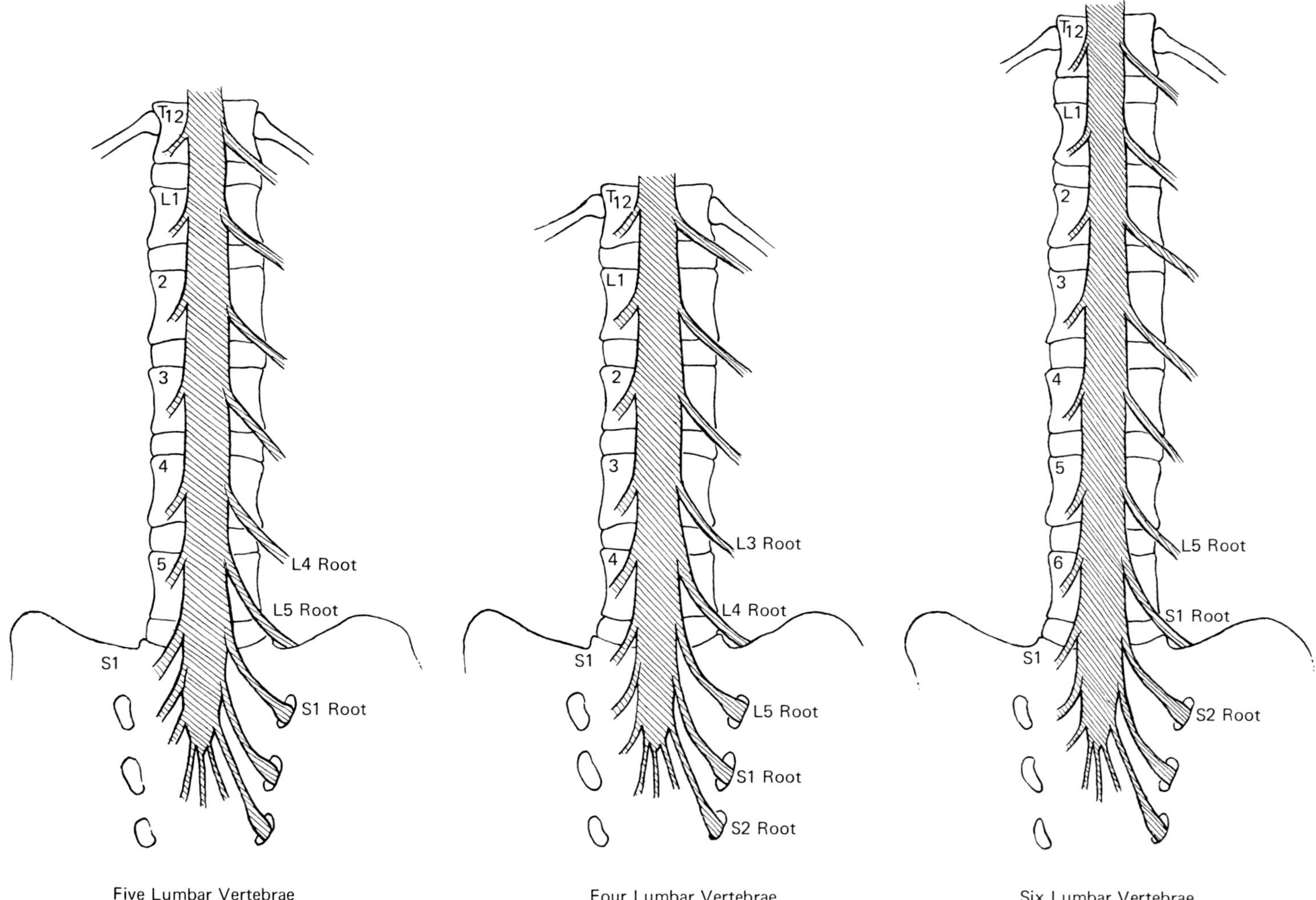

Fig. 121-2. Transitional lumbosacral vertebral and root function. (Reprinted from Finneson BE: Low Back Pain, ed 2. Philadelphia, JB Lippincott, 1981. With permission.)

alcoholics arise every morning and set about their tasks only with great effort and difficulty. Any break in their routine may produce a behavior reversal.

Factor 5, secondary gain, and *Factor 6,* history of lawsuits, are self-explanatory.

By adding the positive scores and adding the negative scores and subtracting the negative total from the positive total, the surgeon can derive a predictive number and compare it against the scoring table (see Figure 121-3) to determine the likely outcome of disc surgery.

PREDICTIVE FACTORS

The four most important factors in determining a satisfactory outcome for surgery are:

1. Sciatic pain more severe than the back pain.
2. An abnormal myelogram that correlates with the clinical picture.
3. Positive Leségue sign.
4. Neurologic deficit.

The crossed Leségue sign is probably the most specific test for lumbar disc herniation. If all four of the above factors are present, technically adequate surgery is likely to produce a satisfactory result. If one of them is absent, the surgeon should be very satisfied with the accuracy of the other three factors before proceeding. Surgery considered when only one or two of these factors is positive is likely to be associated with a high incidence of less than satisfactory results. With these factors in mind, there are four indications for surgery:

1. Intractable pain.
2. Progressively worsening neurologic deficit.
3. Intractable recurrence of pain.
4. Cauda equina syndrome.

With the exception of the cauda equina syndrome, each of these indications is relative and will depend on how well the patient tolerates the symptoms, on the extent of the neurologic deficit, and on the psychologic and sociologic background of the patient.

CONTRAINDICATIONS TO SURGERY

There are five important contraindications to surgery:

1. A first episode of low back and sciatic pain without an adequate trial of conservative management.

LUMBAR DISC SURGERY PREDICTIVE SCORE CARD

This questionnaire is of predictive value when limited to candidates for excision of a herniated lumbar disc who have not previously undergone lumbar spine surgery. It is not designed to encompass candidates for other types of lumbar spine surgery such as decompressive laminectomy or fusion.

Positive Points	POSITIVE FACTORS	NEGATIVE FACTORS	Negative Points
5	1. Low back and sciatic pain severe enough to be incapacitating.	1. **Back pain primarily**	15
15	2. Sciatica is more severe than back pain.	2. **Gross obesity**	10
5	3. Weight bearing (sitting or standing) aggravates the pain; bedrest (in some position) eases the pain.	3. **Nonorganic signs and symptoms** —entire leg numb; simultaneous weakness of flexion and extension of toes; extension of pain into areas not explainable by an organic lesion.	10
25	4. Neurologic examination demonstrates a single root syndrome indicating a specific interspace.	4. **Poor psychologic background**— attempted suicide, unrealistically high expectations from surgery; previous admissions for nonorganic symptoms—hyperventilation—unexplainable chest pains and abdominal pains—intractable incisional pain; alcoholic; not happy with job; physical demands of present occupation excessive; hostility to environment—employer–spouse; much time off from work for medical reasons (man out of work 6 months— woman out of work 16 months).	15
25	5. Myelographic defect corroborating the neurologic examination.		
10	6. Positive straight-leg-raising test.		
20	Crossed-straight-leg-raising test.		
10	7. Patient's realistic self-appraisal of future life style.	5. **Secondary gain**—work-connected accident; vehicular accident; medico-legal adversary situation; near retirement age—eligible for disability pension if symptoms persist.	20
		6. **History of previous lawsuits** for medico-legal problems.	10

<table>
<tr><td>Positive
Total</td><td></td><td>Negative
Total</td></tr>
</table>

Subtract negative total from positive total [ ] **for predictive number.**

```
              SCORING
75 & over ................... good
65—75 ....................... fair
55—65 ................... marginal
below 55 ................... poor
```

Fig. 121-3. A sample Lumbar Disc Surgery Predictive Score Card.

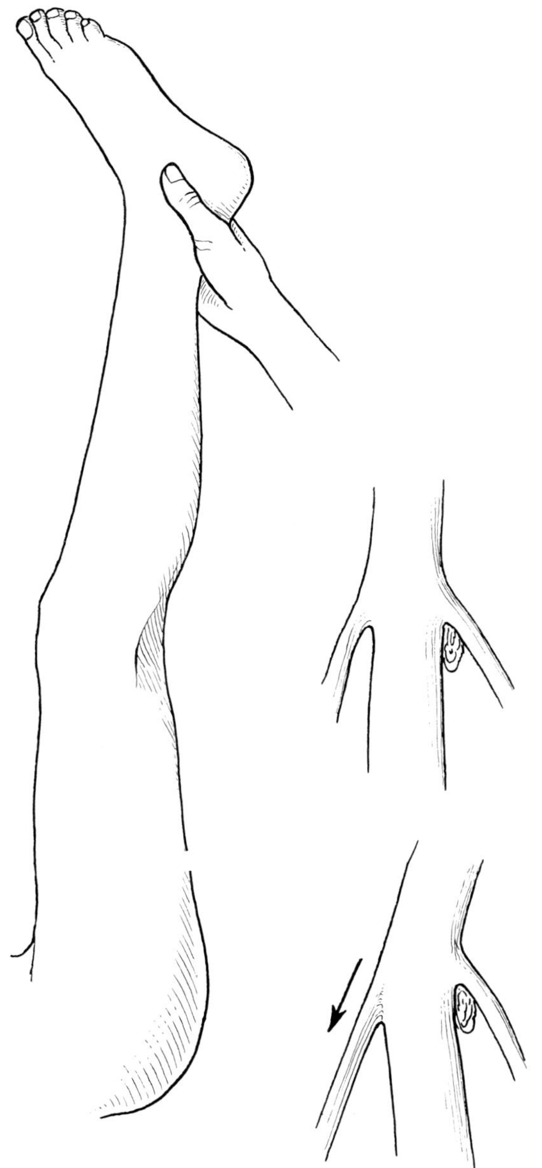

Fig. 121-4. The well leg-raising test of Fajerstajn. (Reprinted from Finneson BE: Low Back Pain, ed 2. Philadelphia, JB Lippincott, 1981. With permission.)

2. Intermittent low back pain associated with occasional pains of an equivocal nature, extending into one or the other lower extremity, and an equivocal myelogram.
3. A prolonged history of intermittent low back pain and an equivocal myelogram.
4. Low back and intermittent sciatic pain with a myelogram demonstrating a lesion on the "wrong" or pain-free side. (I have seen 2 patients on whom disc surgery was performed with "a contralateral myelogram," and the two surgeons who elected to proceed on the basis of this information were divided in choosing the side of surgery upon which to operate. The one who operated upon the painful side used as his justification myelographic evidence of disc dysfunction at a specific interspace; since the pain was on the opposite side, he decided it would be best to decompress the nerve root on the side of the pain rather than on the side of the myelographic defect. The surgeon who elected to operate on the side of the myelographic defect rather than on the side of the pain felt that the disc protrusion might cause a shift of the cauda equina enclosed within its dural sac, which would press the opposite root against the lamina and produce radicular symptoms. Both patients did poorly after surgery.)
5. Improvement of the patient. In the presence of significant motor weakness, if some slight improvement in the pain occurs, it may be justifiable to proceed with surgery. If pain is the primary symptom, however, improvement is an indication to cancel surgery. (I adhere to this principle and have canceled many scheduled cases on the day of surgery upon being told that the patient no longer had pain or that the pain was markedly improved.) Pain surgery performed during an interval of improvement may result in patient dissatisfaction, despite an adequate postoperative result. The patient may be less willing to accept residual symptoms, even of a relatively minor nature, and is more apt to question in retrospect how pressing and indispensable the need was for surgery. If, in the face of improvement, the patient is discharged and subsequently readmitted for surgery with an exacerbation of pain, occasional residual symptoms may be tolerated more kindly. When contemplating lumbar disc surgery, the indications must be clear to the patient as well as to the surgeon.

EXPLORATORY LUMBAR DISC SURGERY

Ten years ago the patient with persisting sciatica and a normal myelogram and who failed to respond to conservative treatment efforts often was considered by many surgeons as a suitable candidate for exploratory lumbar disc surgery. Usually the L5-S1 and L4-5 levels were explored on the symptomatic side. Although some patients possibly benefited by this approach, a significant group either were not improved or were worse after surgery. At this time, with the additional diagnostic help provided by lumbar epidural venography and CT scans of the lumbar spine, surgeons are able to assess those intraspinal areas that previously may have been hidden. Given these new diagnostic tools, a suitable indication for a blind exploration based purely on the persistence of pain is inconceivable. The likelihood of finding a surgically treatable lesion if a myelogram, epidural venogram, and CT scan are all normal is so poor that the era of exploratory lumbar disc surgery is best brought to a close.

SURGERY

HISTORICAL DEVELOPMENT

Fifty years ago an occasional laminectomy was performed for lumbar disc disease and the extruded disc fragments were identified as "chondromata." There was some question regarding the exact nature of these lesions, although many surgeons did recognize them as consisting of displaced intervertebral disc material. The surgical technique used in the removal of such lesions invariably involved an extensive bilateral laminectomy. This usually was followed by opening the dura in the midline, separating the nerve roots to either side, and palpating the anterior spinal canal by means of a narrow probe until the underlying protrusion was identified. The anterior dura then was incised over the most eminent portion of the protrusion, and, through this very limited anterior dural opening, the protruding portion of the disc was exposed and removed.

The entire concept of ruptured intervertebral discs changed after the classic paper of Mixter and Barr.[2] They conclusively and unequivocally demonstrated the origin of these lesions, laid to rest any lingering doubt that they were neoplasms, and documented their etiology as protrusions of the nucleus of an intervertebral disc. They delineated the lumbar disc syndrome and the indications for surgical treatment of this condition. Shortly after the appearance of this paper, the surgical technique for protruding lumbar intervertebral discs underwent an important change, with the dura being left intact and the protruding disc being removed extradurally, although the extensive bilateral laminectomy was continued. Further surgical refinements followed, including the hemilaminectomy, which leaves the spinous process and lamina intact on the pain-free side. Twenty-five or 30 years ago it became common practice to carry out disc surgery in most cases by means of the unilateral interlaminar approach.

In the past 6 or 7 years the combined use of a fiberoptic headlight and 2.5–4.5× operating loupes has been accepted by an increasing number of disc surgeons. The fiberoptic lighting is helpful, not only in providing dependable illumination to the depths of the incision, but in eliminating the technical necessity for the rather long laminectomy incision that extends over three interspaces (although the actual disc surgery was confined to an interlaminar space measuring approximately ½ inch). The lengthy skin and muscle incision was required to allow the standard overhead operating room lighting to illuminate the apex or depth of the operative field. With the brighter beam of light made available with fiberoptic techniques, a much smaller incision is possible. The magnification provided by the operating loupes aids greatly in assuring delicate handling of tissue and helps prevent nerve root damage. Increasing the magnification to 25× with the use of an operating microscope has led to the development of a specific microsurgical discectomy technique involving a distinct departure from prior surgical concepts. A much more limited removal of disc material is performed. This technique avoids laminectomy, curettement of the disc space, and removal of epidural fat, and it avoids incision of the annulus fibrosis with a scalpel; instead, it employs a blunt probe to perforate this surface.

With advances in knowledge and equipment, continued technical changes can be anticipated.

CHOICE OF OPERATIVE PROCEDURE

Once the decision has been made that surgery is indicated, the surgeon must determine which operative procedure is most suitable for the patient's particular low back dysfunction.

Is a disc herniation producing a clear single-root syndrome? If so, interlaminar disc excision is the procedure of choice.

Is it primarily a stenotic lumbar spinal canal syndrome associated with sciatica produced by foraminal impingement and secondary to a bony spur? Attempting to treat this condition with an interlaminar disc excision often is technically difficult and is likely to have a disappointing clinical result. The operation of choice for a stenotic lumbar spinal canal is decompressive laminectomy and foraminotomy at the appropriate level.

If the symptoms are unilateral and the myelographic defect is bilateral, should surgery be confined to the side of the pain or should a bilateral interlaminar disc excision be performed? This is often a gray area and may be open to controversy. As a basic principle, performing the minimal amount of surgery that can adequately relieve the symptoms is preferred rather than attempting prophylactic surgery of symptoms that have not yet developed. Whichever decision is made in this situation can be wrong. Following a bilateral interlaminar operation, the patient may awaken from the anesthesia with postoperative pain in the previously painless leg. Surgery can be confined to the painful side, and in the near or distant future, pain may develop on the nonoperated side.

Should disc excision be followed by a fusion? We do not routinely perform a combined disc excision and spinal fusion, but reserve this combined procedure for the unusual situation.

DOUBLE-CHECKING THE SIDE OF LESION

Performing an operative procedure on the "wrong side" is not a common mishap, but it can occur when surgery is performed on any structure that is paired. Patients who have undergone herniorrhaphies, hip surgery, cataract surgery, or carpal tunnel decompressions occasionally have awakened from anesthesia and have been surprised to find the surgical dressing and the incisional discomfort at an unanticipated site. Because the patient undergoing lumbar disc surgery is in the prone position with his "sides reversed," this error may occur with greater frequency than is likely to happen in the supine position. The best way to preclude this blunder is for the surgeon to remain alert to such a possibility and to establish a preventive behavior pattern.

When reviewing spine x-ray films, the surgeon should make a point of placing the films on the view box as though the patient were in the prone position, with the left marker on the left side. Radiologists, who are trained to visualize films as though the patient is in the anatomic position, may look with mild disfavor at this heresy. It is not the radiologist, however, who will be sued for operating on the wrong side. This practice reinforces a mental image of the spine patient in the prone position.

Another helpful aid to lateralization is the small tatoo that is routinely made at the completion of a myelogram. This permanent mark is radiologically localized at the level of the lesion and is placed laterally on the side of the pain.

Prior to the induction of anesthesia, the patient should always be asked to indicate the painful leg. Of course, the painful side is noted on the chart and the myelograms also are labeled appropriately.

ANESTHESIA

Many surgeons prefer the use of spinal anesthesia, employing a hypobaric solution; epidural anesthesia also has some advocates. Intravenous sodium pentothal supplemented with halothane, nitrous oxide, and oxygen administered through an endotracheal tube is the anesthesia of personal choice and is probably used by the majority of clinics in lumbar disc surgery.

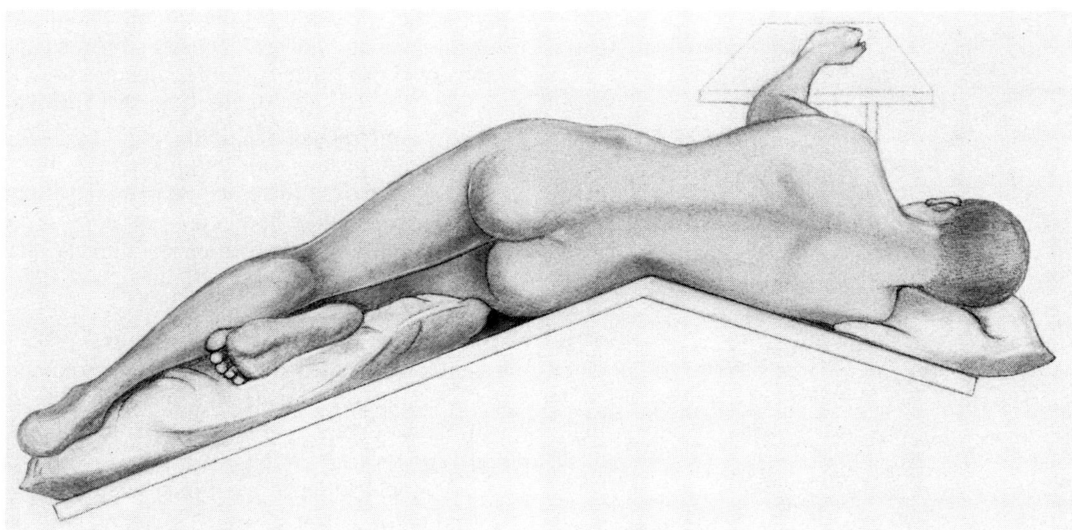

Fig. 121-5. Lateral position for lumbar disc surgery. (Reprinted from Finneson BE: Low Back Pain, ed 2. Philadelphia, JB Lippincott, 1981. With permission.)

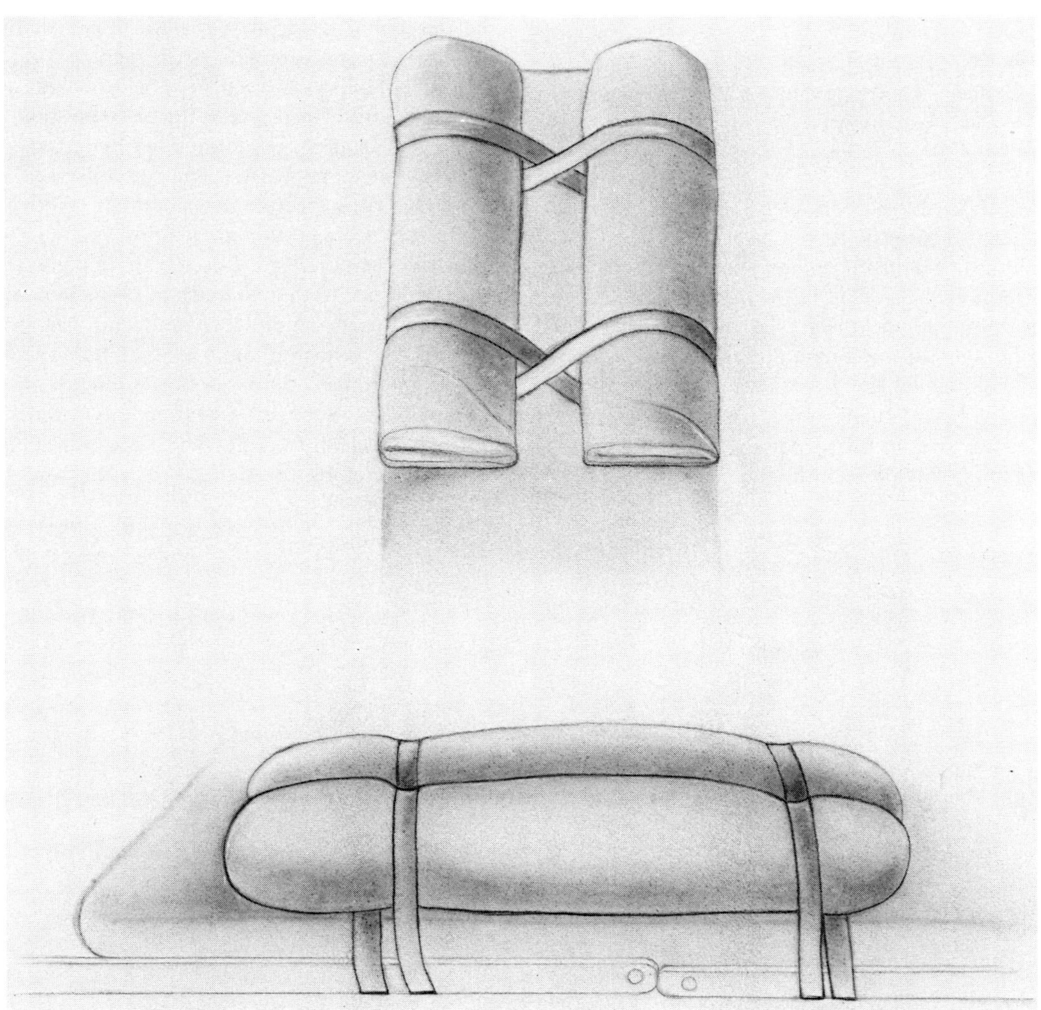

Fig. 121-6. Blanket rolls taped in place. (Reprinted from Finneson BE: Low Back Pain, ed 2. Philadelphia, JB Lippincott, 1981. With permission.)

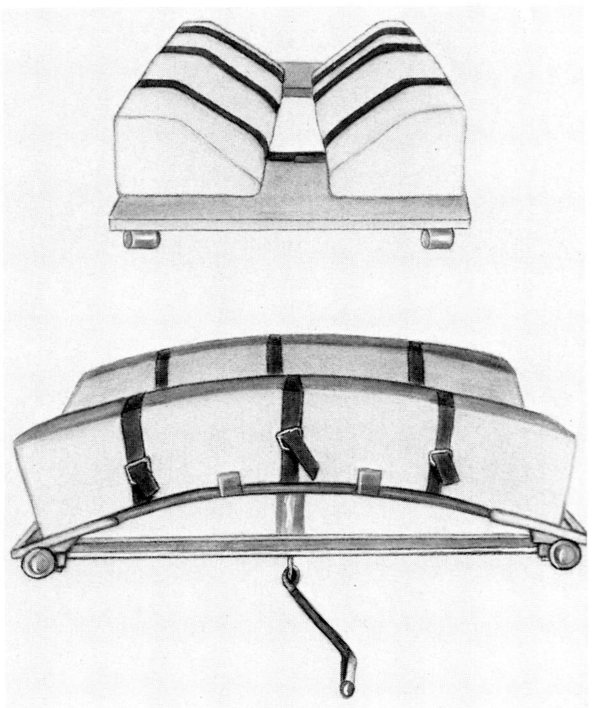

Fig. 121-7. Prone position frame. (Reprinted from Finneson BE: Low Back Pain, ed 2. Philadelphia, JB Lippincott, 1981. With permission.)

POSITION

A variety of positions have been used for operating upon patients with protruded lumbar discs.

For the unilateral disc excision, many surgeons prefer the lateral position (Figure 121-5). This is the position of choice from the point of view of anesthesia, because it does not hamper respiratory excursions as much as the prone position. The principal surgical advantage is that the lateral position allows the abdomen to be relatively free, which reduces pressure on the great veins and, in turn, reduces epidural venous distention and bleeding. This position does not allow blood to pool within the depths of the wound, and it promotes posterior lumbar flexion. Another technical advantage is that the surgeon can spread the uppermost interlaminar space laterally by positioning the patient on the table so that the disc space involved is above the flexion break in the table and then flexing the table.

The disadvantage of this position is more increased difficulty on the part of the assistant in holding the root retractor or in performing other necessary functions. Those who are not experienced with this position may find it technically unsatisfactory.

Most lumbar disc surgeons prefer the prone position, in which the patient is intubated on a litter. After the endotracheal tube has been taped securely in place, the patient is rolled onto the operating table, which has previously been prepared either with blanket rolls or a "prone position frame" (Figures 121-6 and 121-7).

A modification of the prone position can be obtained by flexing the hips and knees 90 degrees, with no effort made to flex the lumbar spine itself. Flexing the hip affords satisfactory flexion of the lumbar spine comparable to the other positions, and it may be associated with somewhat less abdominal pressure. To achieve this position, a minor adjustment of the operating table is accomplished by removing the adjustable headrest and fitting it to the footrest so that it will provide adequate support for the legs (Figure 121-8).

The thin patient with a flat belly will do well either with the prone position frame or with blanket rolls. Such a position, however, is poorly tolerated by the obese individual, since neither the frame nor the blanket rolls will adequately accommodate a large, protuberant abdomen. Abdominal compression is apt to increase lumbar epidural venous distention, and the resulting hemorrhage will be an impediment to satisfactory visualization. In the presence of copious epidural bleeding, the surgeon may have difficulty concentrating on the prime objective of disc excision and adequate nerve root decompression, since the major efforts will be directed at controlling the hemorrhage. Such an irritating environment may lead to a mishap and is not conducive to the calm and deliberate atmosphere so helpful to safe and smooth surgery.

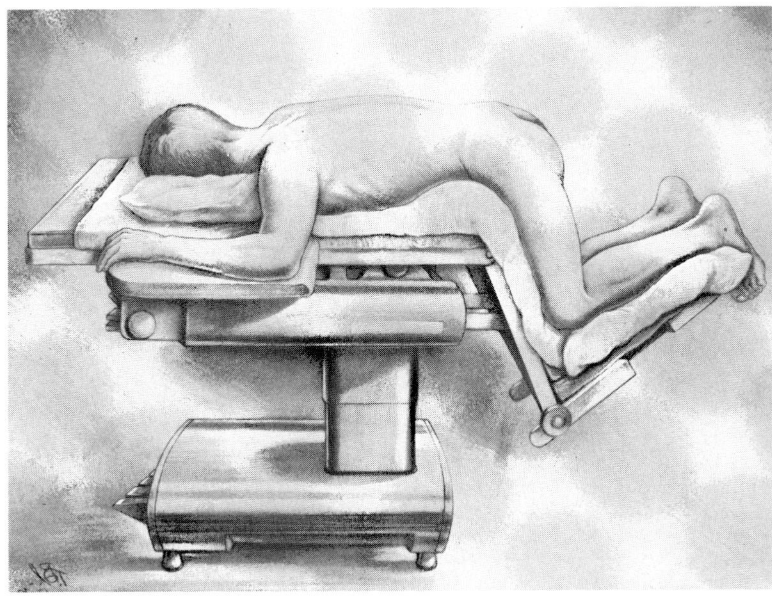

Fig. 121-8. Modified prone position. (Reprinted from Finneson BE: Low Back Pain, ed 2. Philadelphia, JB Lippincott, 1981. With permission.)

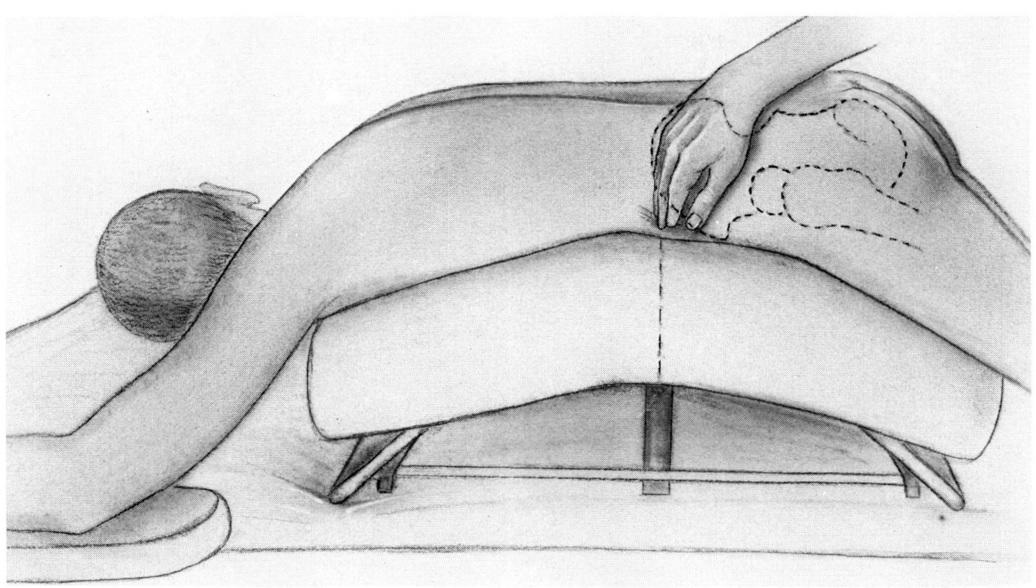

Fig. 121-9. Flexion "break" in table or frame at level of iliac crest. (Reprinted from Finneson BE: Low Back Pain, ed 2. Philadelphia, JB Lippincott, 1981. With permission.)

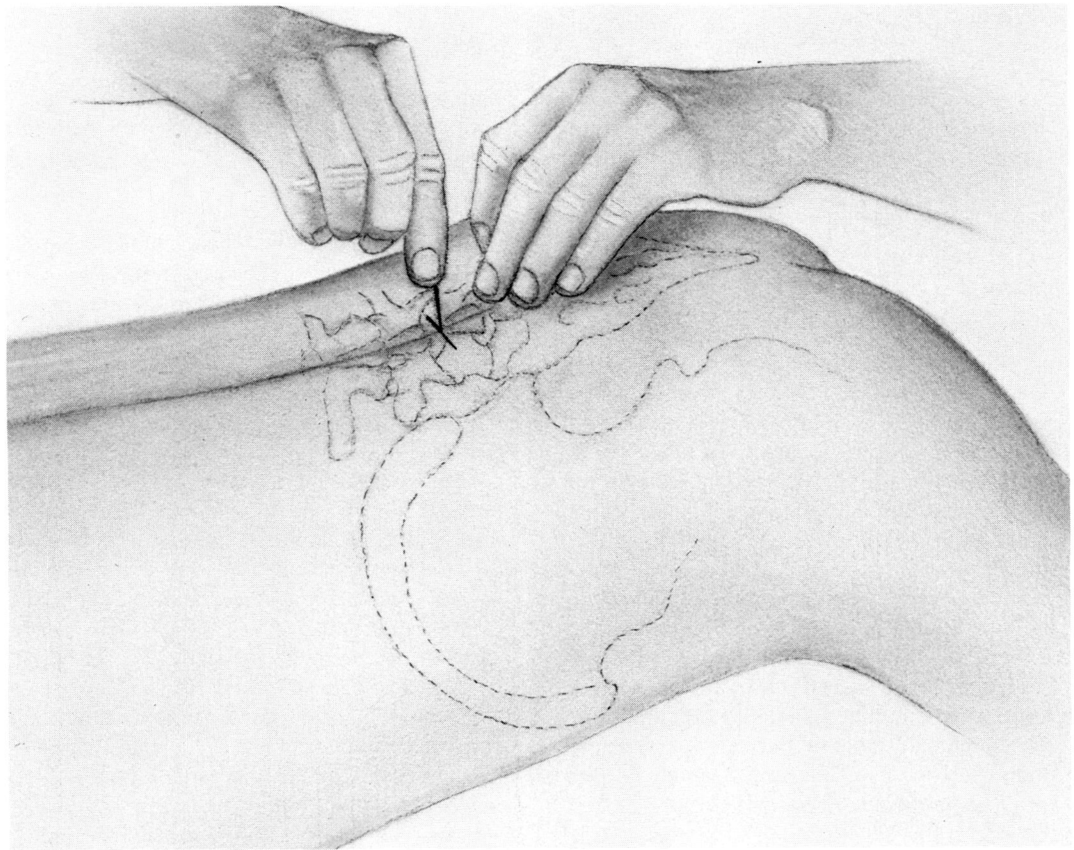

Fig. 121-10. The skin is scratched at the "involved" interspinous space. (Reprinted from Finneson BE: Low Back Pain, ed 2. Philadelphia, JB Lippincott, 1981. With permission.)

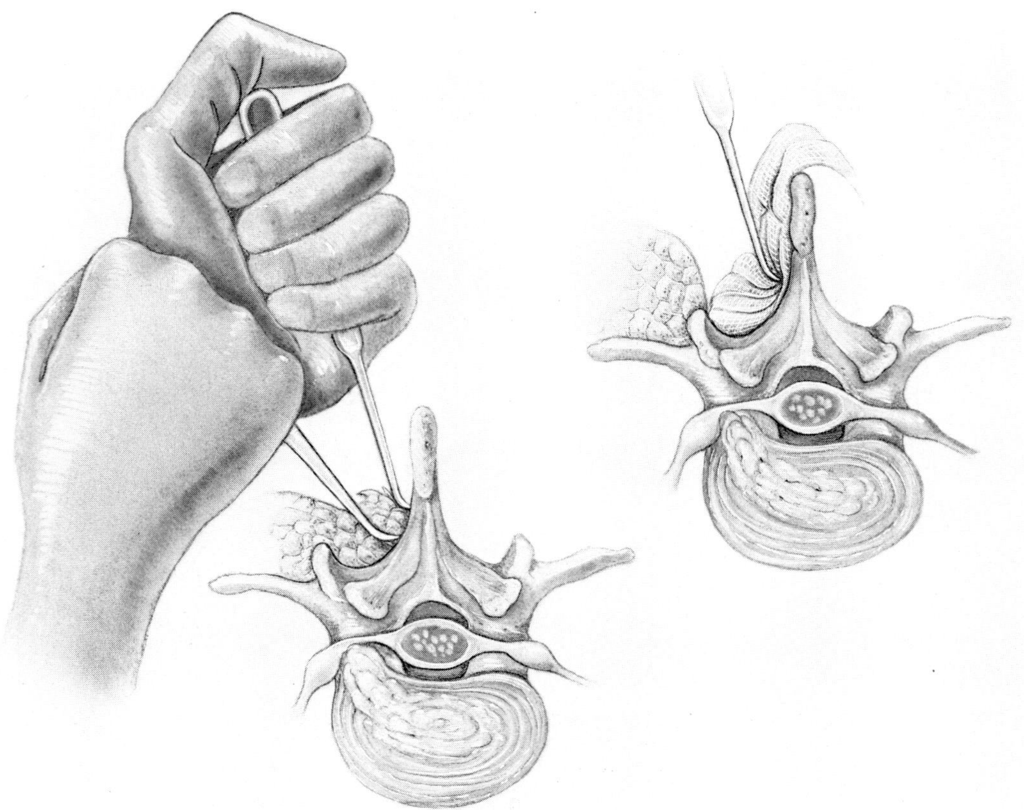

Fig. 121-11.   Subperiosteal dissection technique. (Reprinted from Finneson BE: Low Back Pain, ed 2. Philadelphia, JB Lippincott, 1981. With permission.)

Several positions have evolved in which the abdomen is completely free and unencumbered. Usually some sort of operating table attachment is required to secure and immobilize the hips and thighs. This support is usually assembled by a friendly hospital maintenance machinist or a handy surgeon.

SURFACE LANDMARKS

After the patient is draped, the iliac crests and other bony landmarks that provide approximate relationships to spinal level are obscured. For this reason, it is necessary to prepare a surface guide to interspace identification before draping. Personal preference is the cutaneous tatoo, which is made at the level of the disc protrusion using fluoroscopic guidance after completion of the myelogram. If this is not part of the surgeon's routine, other aids can be employed.

If a myelogram has been done recently, the lumbar puncture mark on the skin can be used as a landmark for the spinal level. For example, if the lumbar puncture needle is seen on the myelogram films to be at the L3-4 interspace, this will serve as an excellent surface guide for identification of the underlying vertebrae. If a myelogram has not been carried out recently, the first interspace at or immediately below the iliac crest can be considered L3-4 (Figure 121-9). Using this as a starting site, one can count down to the involved interspace and scratch a "crosshatch" in the skin at that level with a sterile hypodermic needle subsequent to cleansing the skin with an alcohol sponge (Figure 121-10).

When using surface guides, the elasticity of the skin must be kept in mind, particularly with obese patients. This elasticity may permit a surface marking to shift to the extent of an interspace from the distortion caused by the use of retractors and alterations in the degree of lumbar flexion during surgery.

INCISIONS

For many years my routine incision extended over approximately three spinous processes to allow for interspace localization and for adequate illumination, with the ends of the incision permitting overhead lighting to funnel in. I considered the short incision an ego trip on the part of the surgeon. Further experience has changed my opinion, and I presently believe that the short incision is beneficial to the patient's postoperative recovery.

There is no question that patients feel immeasurably better in the immediate interval after a short-incision operation than after a large or standard-incision operation. Of greater importance is the fact that the long incision, which extends over several spinous processes, produces a band of scar that extends from the skin and attaches to the spinous processes and laminae along the length of the incision. This scar tissue is not as supple as nonscarred muscle and fascia. The lack of elasticity and suppleness is not conducive to a nicely distributed lumbar curvature after the wound has healed. This nonsupple lumbar spine probably makes the patient more vulnerable to recurrent low back dysfunction in the future.

When a small incision is made, the precise location of the involved interspace is crucial, as described under the section "Surface Landmarks."

When the small incision is used, fiberoptic lighting and magnification are a necessity. The fiberoptic lighting and operating loupes or the operating microscope are of great advantage.

These instruments aid greatly in assuring that tissue is handled delicately and they help to prevent nerve root damage. I consider them an integral and essential aid to the surgery.

There are a variety of methods used to control skin bleeding, including Michel clips, Kolodney clamps, and mosquitoes. Weitlaner self-retaining retractors, which place the skin under tension, will stop most of the minor skin bleeding; the several remaining subcutaneous vessels are easily controlled by cautery. Blood vessel cauterization should not be performed with a hemostat, since it invariably results in considerable tissue destruction. When carried out near the surface of the skin, hemostat cauterization may result in a full-thickness skin burn, and the resulting skin slough or necrosis may eventuate into a wound infection. To properly control skin bleeding with cautery, an assistant should use fine-toothed forceps to evert the skin edge, while the surgeon employs suction to locate the bleeding vessel precisely, and then uses a fine-tipped Cushing forceps to cauterize only the vessel, taking care to avoid cautery spread to surrounding tissue.

A second knife ("clean knife") should be used to incise through fat to the fascia. If the patient is extremely obese, the Weitlaner retractors may have to be reset more deeply. Additional bleeding can be controlled with the use of the cautery. When performing the initial incision, the surgeon should not be obsessive about sweeping the fat cleanly away from the fascia. He or she must remember that a surgical procedure is being carried out, not an anatomic exposure. This step can only serve to increase the blood loss and, even more serious, to create a false space that may fill with blood in the postoperative period.

SUBPERIOSTEAL DISSECTION

The subperiosteal muscles can be dissected by a variety of methods (Figure 121-11). I prefer to use a periosteal elevator pressed against the edge of the spinous process and to cut directly against the lateral edge of the spine. In this manner the posterior spinous ligament or supraspinal ligament, which is a strong fibrous cord that extends without interruption along the tips of the spinous processes from C7 to the median sacral crest and which is continuous with the interspinal ligaments, is preserved. It is valuable to preserve this structure and so to avoid unnecessary weakening of the spinal supporting ligaments. To prevent unnecessary tissue destruction and scarring, a scalpel should be used to incise the fascia rather than a cutting cautery. The muscles are best stripped from the spinous processes and lamina with the bimanual two-periosteal-elevator method. One periosteal elevator is used to retract the muscle mass laterally, while the other is used to perform a careful subperiosteal dissection. The periosteum should be peeled as cleanly as possible from the spinous process and lamina without penetrating the muscle which, if torn, may be a source of troublesome bleeding.

After the subperiosteal dissection has been accomplished under direct vision, a sponge extended to its full length is used to strip the bone of any remaining fragments of muscle and fascia. As bone is cleaned with the sponge, it should be allowed to accumulate within the incision to act as a tamponade and prevent muscle bleeding. Any bleeding occurring from the cut edge of the fascia is controlled with cautery. The subperiosteal muscle dissection is carried out laterally to expose the articulation between the superior and inferior articular processes.

After all surface bleeding has been controlled, the sponges are removed and the desired interspace is localized by the time-honored method of palpating the sacrum and then counting up from it. This localization should be checked with the plain x-ray films of the spine to be sure that the patient does not have a lumbarized first sacral segment or sacralized fifth lumbar segment. Skeletal localization then should be correlated with the myelographic defect.

If the sacrum cannot be adequately palpated, or if for some other reason the surgeon is not totally satisfied with the identification of the anatomic level, surgery should be stopped at this point and a definite interspace confirmation obtained with a lateral lumbar spine roentgenogram.

One topic not likely to be discussed at length in the medical literature is the frequency of interspace misidentification at surgery. I occasionally find such an error in a referred patient, and I am aware of two occasions when I myself made such a mistake. Both of my mishaps occurred in the 1950s, when I was less aware of my fallibility and much too decisive to slow up my surgery for an "unnecessary x-ray film." This error is most likely to occur in either grossly obese patients or patients whose partial lumbarization of the first sacral segment dorsal element confuses the surgeon.

When in doubt, it is important to obtain a roentgenogram, not only for the surgeon's peace of mind but also so to be absolutely certain that the interspace being worked on is the proper one. When a pathologic situation is not apparent at first inspection, such knowledge may provide additional incentive for a most thorough and meticulous interspace exploration and decompression, including a generous foraminal decompression.

Once the surgeon is completely satisfied that proper localization has been established, he or she can place the hemilaminectomy retractors in position (Figure 121-12A). A variety of hemilaminectomy retractors is available, the simplest being the Taylor spinal retractor, which consists of a right-angled metal ribbon with a slightly hooked tip that can be inserted laterally and cephalad to the articular facet. The great disadvantage is that it has to be either hand-held by the assistant or tied to the base of the operating table or to the foot of the surgeon. Also, it has the unfortunate propensity to slip out of place occasionally—invariably at the worst possible moment of the procedure.

Most surgeons prefer a self-retaining hemilaminectomy based on the many modifications of the Hoen hemilaminectomy retractor (Figure 121-12B).

When positioning the hemilaminectomy retractors, the shortest blades possible should be used to achieve adequate exposure, so that the flange of the blades will rest flush with the skin surface. If the flange projects above the skin, it increases the depth through which the surgeon must work. The spinous process blade of the retractor should fit between the spinous interspaces, with the hook or hooks embedded into the interspinous ligaments. The muscle blade should rise above the hump of the articular facet (Figure 121-12C). An occasional error is made by impinging the tip of the muscle blade against the facet; this causes the exposure to be needlessly narrow. By placing the paraspinal muscles under tension, the retractors will stop most muscle bleeding. After the retractors are in place and the exposure is deemed satisfactory, any remaining muscle bleeding is controlled with cautery.

It must be emphasized that the remainder of the surgery takes place in that small keyhole of interlaminar space, and any skin, fascia, or muscle bleeding will funnel directly into the work area. If the assistant has to provide suction to remove the blood, either his or her head will be in the way, which will

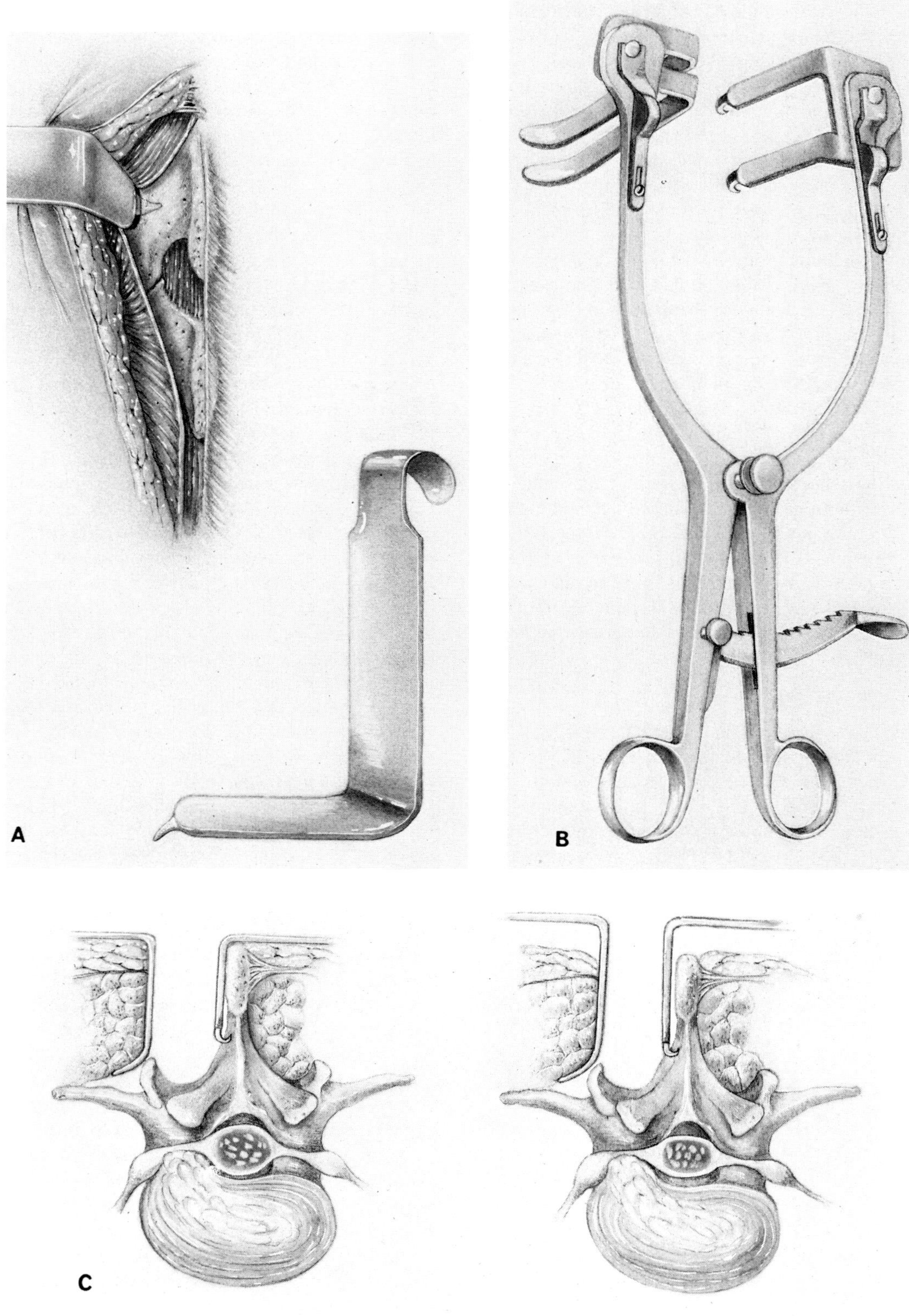

Fig. 121-12. (A) Taylor hemilaminectomy retractor. (B) Hoen hemilaminectomy retractor. (C) If the hemilaminectomy retractor blades are longer than necessary, the depth through which the surgeon must work is increased. (Reprinted from Finneson BE: Low Back Pain, ed 2. Philadelphia, JB Lippincott, 1981. With permission.)

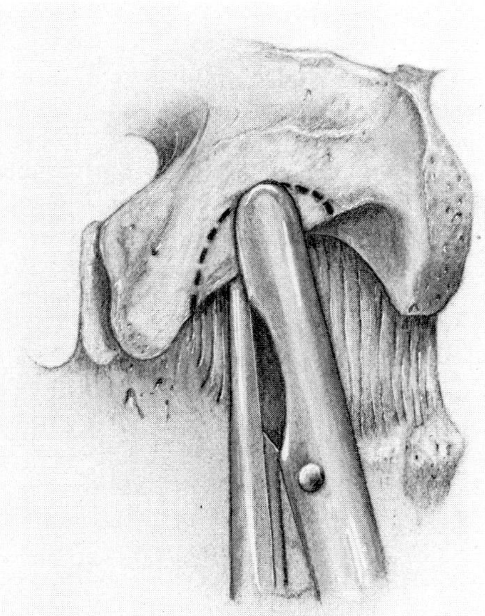

Fig. 121-13.   The overhanging edge of the superior lamina is rongeured. (Reprinted from Finneson BE: Low Back Pain, ed 2. Philadelphia, JB Lippincott, 1981. With permission.)

obstruct the surgeon's vision, or the assistant will be poking the suction tip into the wound blindly, which also has its disadvantages. The other alternative is for the surgeon to hold the suction in one hand and operate with the other; this also is not really satisfactory. Control of bleeding at this stage is therefore a must for smooth, safe surgery.

DEVELOPING THE INTERSPACE

The laminae vary greatly in width, in angulation, and in position relative to each other, so that occasionally the interlaminar space is sufficiently wide to permit exposure and removal of a protruding intervertebral disc without removal of any, or very little, bone. This widened interlaminar space is seen most commonly between the L5-S1 levels and less frequently above the interspace.

The more strenuous bone work of the operation is followed by relatively delicate dissection of the soft tissue interspace involving yellow ligament, nerve root, and dura. This strenuous manual work tends to create a hand tremor that is distressingly obvious when the surgery is being performed with magnification techniques such as loupes or an operating microscope. Air-powered rongeurs can be used for much of the bone work in the hope of reducing a postexertion tremor that may develop while manipulating the nerve root and other soft tissues within the interspace.

When dealing with an interspace of normal dimensions, any rongeur, including duckbilled, Leksell, or Kerrison, can be used to remove the overhanging, inferior edge of the superior vertebrae (Figure 121-13). If working on the L5-S1 interspace, this would be the inferior edge of the L5 lamina. Some surgeons prefer rongeuring away the inferior half of the superior lamina, which exposes the superior border of the yellow ligament. This can be grasped with an Allis tissue forceps and the remainder of the ligament excised by sharp dissection with a scalpel. I prefer to remove only the inferior one third of the superior lamina so

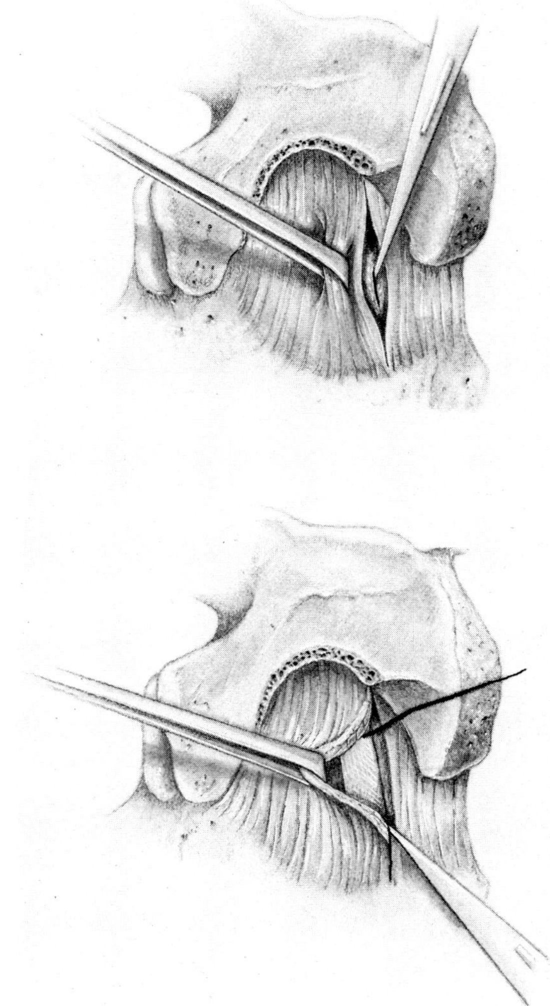

Fig. 121-14.   The yellow ligament is cut. (Reprinted from Finneson BE: Low Back Pain, ed 2. Philadelphia, JB Lippincott, 1981. With permission.)

that the edge of the yellow ligament is not exposed. Bone wax is used to control all bone bleeding from the rongeured edge of the lamina. After the one third overhang of the superior lamina has been removed, an ample area of the ligamentum flavum will be exposed to view. A No. 11 blade on a long handle then is used to make a shallow incision in the ligamentum flavum along the direction of its fibers. The edge of the incision is grasped with an Allis forceps and tugged laterally in order to spread the incision. This allows the No. 11 blade to be used to incise the entire thickness of the yellow ligament down to the epidural fat (Figure 121-14). After a small, moistened cotton patty has been introduced beneath the ligamentum flavum to separate it from the dura, this incision is extended from the superior lamina to the inferior lamina. Care should be taken to insert merely the tip of the blade beneath the ligament to avoid accidentally cutting into the dura. A second Allis forceps is used to get a firmer grasp on the full thickness of yellow ligament. A curette is introduced below the yellow ligament against the inferior surface of the superior vertebra, which permits a flap of yellow ligament to be curetted laterally while the remainder is left attached to the dorsal surface of the inferior lamina. This attachment then can be safely excised with a scalpel or scissors (Figure 121-15).

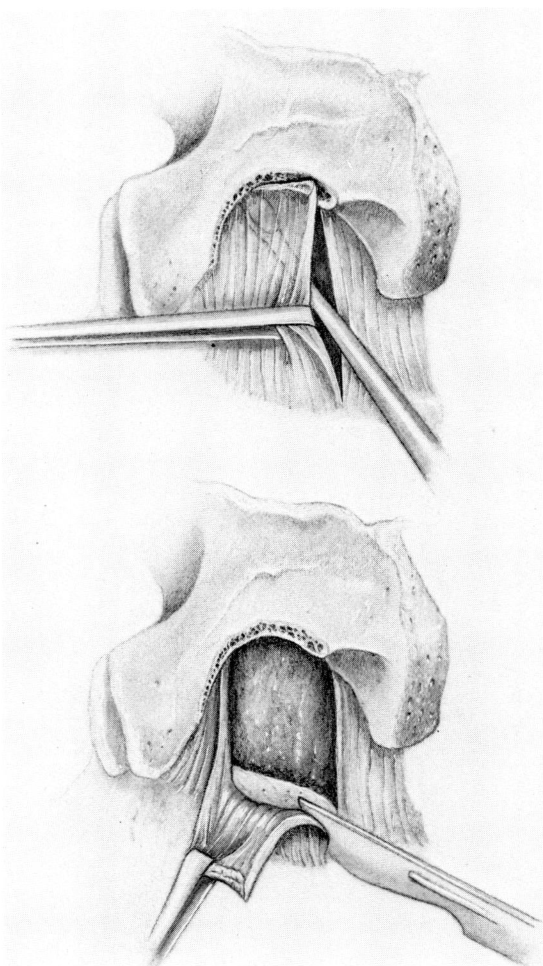

Fig. 121-15. The yellow ligament is curetted. (Reprinted from Finneson BE: Low Back Pain, ed 2. Philadelphia, JB Lippincott, 1981. With permission.)

EPIDURAL FAT AND NERVE ROOT DAMAGE

Once the yellow ligament has been excised, the epidural fat can be clearly visualized. Treatment of the epidural fat recently has developed into a conjectural issue. It is now generally agreed that preservation of a layer of epidural fat, especially around the nerve root, will be helpful in preventing subsequent encasement of the root within the dense epidural scar tissue that forms following an interspace exploration. For this reason, surgeons attempt to carry out disc excision without disturbing the epidural fat. This fatty layer, however, almost always obscures the dura and nerve root. In this laudable effort to prevent future damage of the root by postoperative scar tissue, the surgeon may create immediate and possibly persisting injury to the root during surgery because of his inability to visualize this structure adequately.

Frequently, a flap of epidural fat can be retracted so that good visualization of the root and dura is obtained. After completion of this procedure, the epidural fat can be tucked back into position around the root. If satisfactory root identification and visualization are not possible with preservation of the fat, however, it should be excised. A surgeon is not able to protect a structure that cannot be adequately visualized, and I am aware of two recent postoperative nerve root injuries that two separate surgeons attributed to their desire to preserve the epidural fat. If the epidural fat has been removed, a small stamp of subcutaneous fat can be placed over the dura and nerve root as a free fat graft. Subsequent dissections and explorations have demonstrated a reasonably high rate of "take" of this type of graft.

It is important to remember that the goal of surgery is adequate decompression of the root, while at the same time gently and safely handling the root. At this stage of the surgery, nerve root damage may occur in two ways. One occasional error is to mistake the lateral reflection of the yellow ligament immediately over the root for the root itself. Sometimes after excision of the medial portion of the yellow ligament, the lateral portion rolls up on itself, creating a cylindrical appearance that may be quite deceptive (Figure 121-16). If this cylinder is retracted medially, the underlying root may be mistakenly identified as a bulging disc, which is then attacked with vigor.

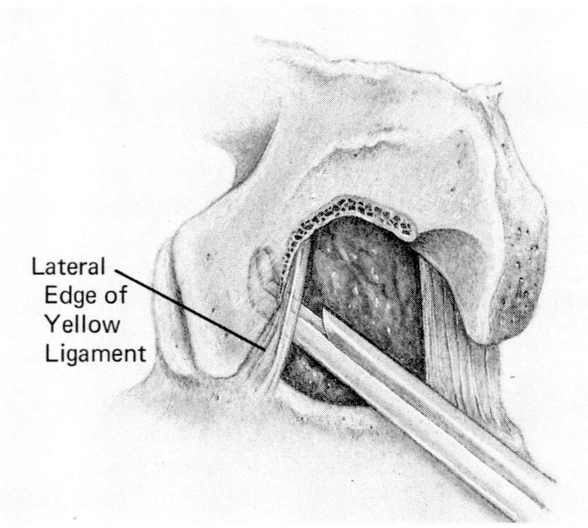

Fig. 121-16. In widening the interspace, do not mistake the rolled-up lateral edge of yellow ligament for the root. (Reprinted from Finneson BE: Low Back Pain, ed 2. Philadelphia, JB Lippincott, 1981. With permission.)

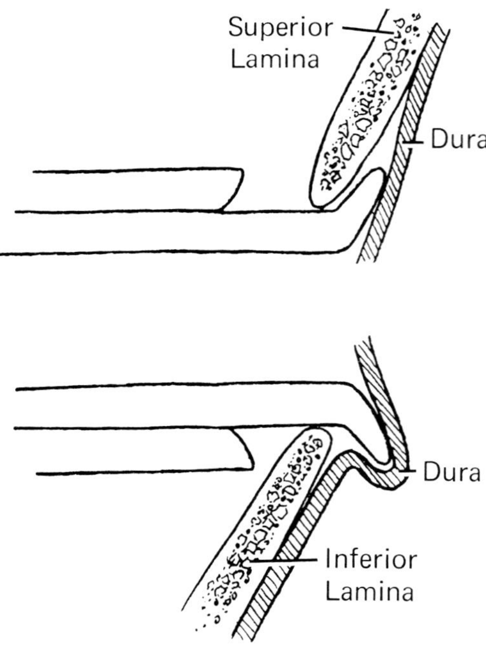

Fig. 121-17. The laminectomy punch with a 40-degree angled jaw is helpful when working on the superior lamina, but is not suited for the slope of the inferior lamina and may produce a dural tear. (Reprinted from Finneson BE: Low Back Pain, ed 2. Philadelphia, JB Lippincott, 1981. With permission.)

Another error may occur when the interlaminar exposure is extended laterally and the lateral reflection of yellow ligament and bone is trimmed. This portion of the exposure must be performed under good visualization, with care being taken to hug the inferior bony and ligamentous surface with the jaws of the Schlesinger punch. If the tip of this rongeur is inserted too deeply, it may grasp a bit of the root along with the edge of the yellow ligament and bone. As the surgeon tugs on the instrument, a fairly long, glistening piece of tissue, resembling spaghetti, comes out, followed by bloody spinal fluid. These errors are classifiable as surgical tragedies and usually can be avoided by proper hemostasis, good visualization, and a cautious pace at this point in the operation.

A thin edge of bone is removed from the superior edge of the inferior lamina using a laminectomy punch that is not angled downward. The 40-degree angled jaw is helpful in working on the superior lamina and laterally, but may produce a dural tear at the inferior lamina (Figure 121-17). A slight fold of dura may bulge and be pinched and torn in the jaws of the bone-biting instrument. Most of the fibers in the dura are longitudinal (running up and down); if the instrument catches a fiber and the surgeon pulls without adequate visualization, to quote that outstanding spinal surgeon George Ehni, "The dura will rip open like a seam." Just a small bit of bone easily can cause a tear an inch long in the dura. If the dura is opened inadvertently, a small hole is usually easier to close than a large one. Dissection should therefore proceed cautiously on the inferior lamina. A bite of bone should not be taken with the rongeur and ripped out. The instrument should be closed carefully and the bone eased out very slowly, so that if the dura is tugged even slightly, the surgeon will be able to visualize the tenting of the dura and can then release the instrument and inspect the area carefully before proceeding further. This type of complication always occurs before an adequate exposure has been obtained. Cerebrospinal fluid may fill the wound suddenly, becoming tinged with blood, so that it is impossible to see the damaged area. There is a tendency to try to close this opening immediately, but this is a mistake. It is also a mistake to try to visualize the damage by putting a sucker directly into the wound, because the roots may float out of the dural tear with the escaping spinal fluid, catch on the tip of the sucker, and sometimes be severely damaged. Instead of direct suction, a cottonoid should be inserted into the opening, and suction should be applied only on the cottonoid until the structures can be seen. Then a square of Gelfoam can be placed over the dural tear and a cottonoid can be placed on top of the Gelfoam square. The table should be tilted head down so that spinal fluid pressure will decrease in the lumbar region. If the table or laminectomy frame is flexed, it should be flattened. The surgeon then can proceed as though the dura had not been opened. After the disc has been excised and the root has been decompressed, full attention can be given to the torn dura. Before closing the dural tear, it is necessary to expose both sides and both ends of the tear. Dural closure must be watertight; 4-0 or 5-0 suture material should be used.

In carrying out a lateral bony exposure, a partial excision of the facet may be necessary for exposure of the lateral margin of the nerve root. This does not cause pain or an unstable spine when performed unilaterally. Bilateral facet excision and disc excision at that level may produce spinal instability and pain.

An adequate intervertebral lateral exposure may be of value for three reasons:

1. It facilitates satisfactory disc excision because there is less

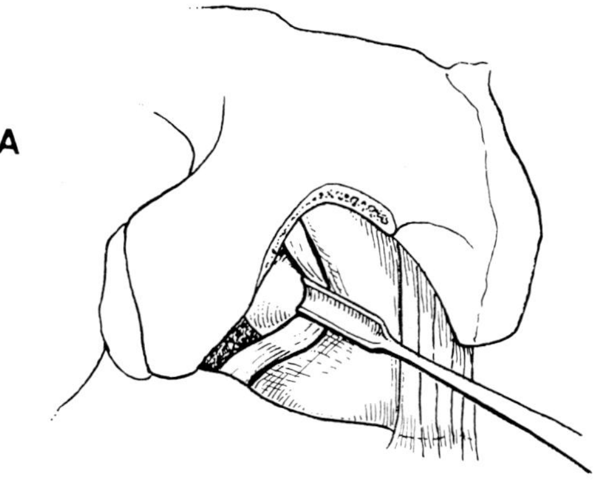

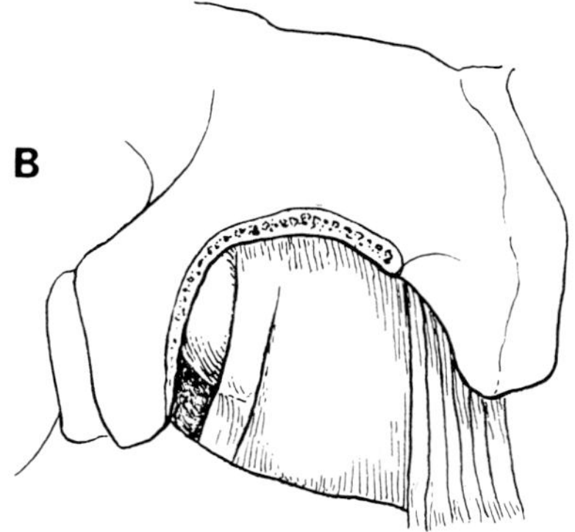

Fig. 121-18. (A) Overstretched root and dural sac with an inadequate lateral bony exposure. (B) Very little root retraction is necessary with adequate lateral bony exposure. (Reprinted from Finneson BE: Low Back Pain, ed 2. Philadelphia, JB Lippincott, 1981. With permission.)

danger of overstretching the nerve root and dural sac as these structures are retracted medially. With an adequate lateral exposure, much less root retraction is necessary to afford good access to the disc (Figures 121-18A and B).

2. A satisfactory lateral exposure is the first step of a foraminotomy that provides bony decompression of the involved root, and almost always manifests some degree of edema and swelling.

3. In the years after surgery, hypertrophic osteoarthritic bony spurring, in association with postoperative epidural and perineural scarring, will be less likely to lead to root compression symptoms in the presence of a generous lateral exposure and foraminotomy.

Following an adequate bony exposure, the epidural fat will be visible. If the nerve root is obscured by the fat, two Cushing forceps can be used to separate the fat from the underlying dura and nerve root. In order to preserve the fat, it should be peeled medially to form a retractable flap that can be tucked back into place around the root after disc excision. Only after exposure of the nerve root can blood vessels within the epidural fat be safely cauterized without danger of damage to the root by cautery current. The Malis bipolar coagulator with bipolar forceps allows current to flow only from one forceps tip to the other. This isolated current, which produces much less heat, reduces the likelihood of inadvertent nerve root irritation or damage.

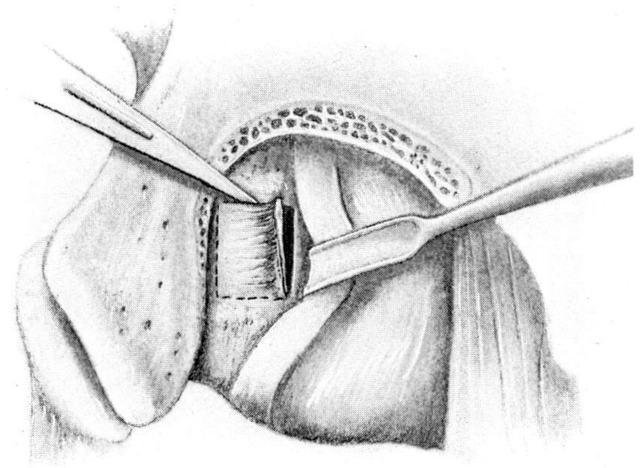

Fig. 121-19. Incision of rectangular window through the annulus fibrosus. (Reprinted from Finneson BE: Low Back Pain, ed 2. Philadelphia, JB Lippincott, 1981. With permission.)

INTERLAMINAR SURGERY

Although the interlaminar space is rather small, the minute anatomy of this area does vary considerably. It is always amazing to see how much can be hidden within this tiny space. An orderly and systematic approach to the area is paramount to successful disc surgery.

INSPECTION

The field should be dry at this stage. If bleeding remains a problem, decreasing lumbar flexion to a flatter position may reduce abdominal pressure and so reduce engorgement of the lumbar epidural veins. If this change in position is effective in controlling epidural venous bleeding, the surgeon should proceed with surgery in the flatter position.

Is the root elevated or is it flat? Does the root appear swollen or hyperemic, or is it the same color as the rest of the dura?

In patients who have had long-standing symptoms, adhesions between the nerve root and the posterior longitudinal ligament are occasionally quite dense. Very careful dissection of the root and the dura may be necessary to allow free retraction and exposure of the protruding disc.

ROOT TENSION

It should be possible to retract medially, without resistance, a root that is under no pressure, using a narrow blunt retractor. As a rule, the typical protruding disc will be quite apparent when the root is retracted medially and manifests itself by slight elevation of the root and by increased pressure on medial retraction. It is at this stage of the procedure that considerable care must be taken to avoid stretching a compromised root. When the disc protrusion is extensive, it is best not to retract the root too vigorously over it in order to avoid excessive stretching of the root. When the root is under too much pressure to be retracted medially with ease, the root should not be retracted but should be decompressed by working laterally to it.

If extruded disc fragments are free within the canal, they usually can be manipulated laterally, grasped with the pituitary forceps, and gently removed. If the disc is not extruded but is bulging so much that the nerve cannot be moved medially easily, the surgeon should work lateral to the disc, introduce the

pituitary forceps into the intervertebral disc space, and remove disc fragments piecemeal until the root can be retracted more easily over the partially decompressed annular shell.

The major error at this point comes under the heading of "grandstanding." There is a temptation to demonstrate the pathology to any and all present in the operating room. The root is retracted medially and maintained in an overstretched position while residents, interns, nurses, and visitors are invited to inspect the protruding disc. This is not the time to "entertain the troops," and a herniated disc is not a very spectacular sight in any event. Retraction of such a swollen, inflamed nerve is best kept to a minimum to avoid adding to the irreversible damage already caused by the disc protrusion.

Sometimes a disc protrusion is a bit more medial, and the nerve root does not appear elevated or under pressure. On attempting to retract the nerve root medially, however, an obstruction is encountered. The surgeon then must be careful to lift the root and dura to determine whether a medially protruding disc is present.

INTERVERTEBRAL DISC EXCISION

Once the disc has been partially excised, there is little difficulty in retracting the root medially. A nerve root retractor then can be used to expose the disc space more completely. A No. 11 blade is used to make a rectangular slab-shaped window through the annulus, and through this opening an adequate subtotal excision of disc contents is performed. This window extends from the most medial exposure of the annulus to the lateral limits of the bony exposure and comprises the entire width of the intervertebral disc, which is bounded by the bodies of the superior and inferior vertebrae (Figure 121-19). Pituitary forceps of various sizes and shapes, as well as a curette, can be used to free up loose fragments of disc material. Excision of a rectangular slab of annulus may prevent the remaining shell of annulus from buckling as the disc space narrows. This buckling is to be prevented because it may fibrose and provide a source of root compression a year or two postoperatively. It is generally accepted that some reduction of the intervertebral space will occur. This seems likely in view of the fact that patients with long-standing disc disease who have not had surgery will often demonstrate interspace narrowing.

In using intervertebral disc rongeur forceps within the intervertebral space, great care is necessary to avoid penetrating the instrument through the anterior annulus fibrosus and the anterior longitudinal ligament. Such penetration is precarious and may result in laceration of one of the great vessels located anterior to the vertebral space (Figure 121-20). Experienced and competent lumbar disc surgeons have suffered this calamity, and when working deep within the intervertebral space, the surgeon must remain alert to the possibility of this mishap. Degenerative changes affecting an intervertebral disc are generalized and may cause softening of the anterior annular fibers and anterior longitudinal ligament. These structures, when reasonably firm, will usually offer resistance to instrument penetration; but when softened, the surgeon may unknowingly poke through the anterior annular fibers with disc rongeur forceps. After such inadvertent penetration, the iliac artery may be grasped and torn by the forceps. Various methods have been advocated to avoid this problem, including marking the instruments 1½ inches from the tip as a visual reminder of depth penetration. Good lighting and magnification aid in depth perception and in visualization of the interior of the disc space.

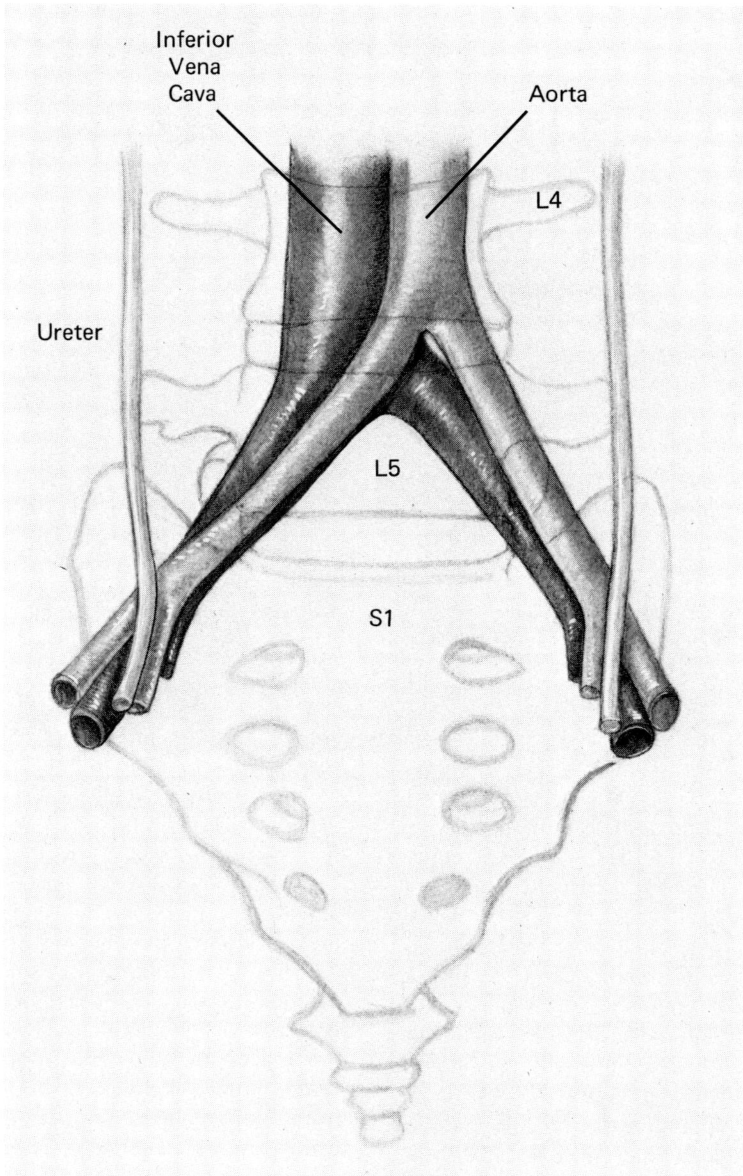

Fig. 121-20.   The major vessels and ureters and their relationship to the anterior lumbar spine. (Reprinted from Finneson BE: Low Back Pain, ed 2. Philadelphia, JB Lippincott, 1981. With permission.)

FREE DISC FRAGMENTS

Occasionally the protruded disc is in the "axilla" between the dural sac and the nerve root. A most meticulous dissection of this extruded fragment is necessary, and care should be taken when this fragment is grasped with an intervertebral disc rongeur forceps to avoid damage to the adjacent laterally displaced nerve root. It is occasionally difficult to recognize a completely free extruded fragment within the axilla. It may resemble epidural fat, and in some cases, only the tip of the extruded fragment presents dorsally, with the bulk of it not being visible and indenting the inferior portion of the dural sac medially. The surgeon, unaware of this large extrusion, may retract the nerve root and dural sac medially together with the free fragment and expose a bulging or protruding annulus. The disc protrusion will be excised and the interspace evacuated as thoroughly as possible by the usual methods, including curettage and the use of the intervertebral disc forceps. The offending free fragment that is causing root pressure, however, will inadvertently be left untouched. The lack of free nerve root mobility may be an indication that such a fragment is present. When the nerve root is not free, further inspection is necessary.

A free disc fragment may extrude beneath the posterior spinal ligament. It occasionally will produce a sizable mass that is capable of producing symptoms that will not be evident to casual inspection. Palpation over the posterior spinal ligament with a thin elevator will disclose this extrusion, and it can be "milked" laterally to expose an amount of disc tissue sufficient enough to be grasped with the intervertebral disc forceps and removed.

SURGICAL JUDGMENT

In those patients in whom there is no gross protrusion of the disc but rather a slightly humped-up annulus, the surgeon must use judgment in deciding whether to excise the high

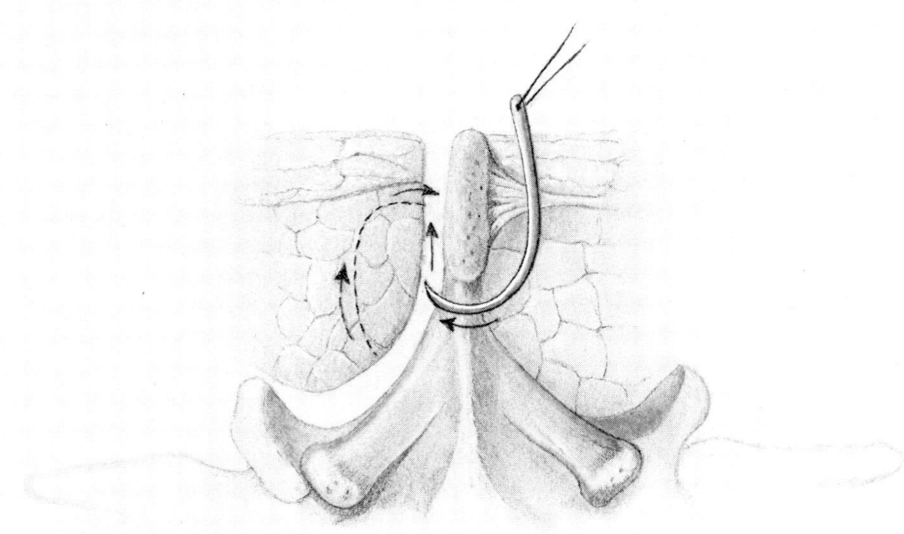

Fig. 121-21.   Muscle closure to eliminate "dead space." (Reprinted from Finneson BE: Low Back Pain, ed 2. Philadelphia, JB Lippincott, 1981. With permission.)

annulus and curette the intervertebral disc space, or to be content with posterior bony decompression of the nerve root by means of a foraminotomy.

A disc should not be violated unless it can be seen to be causing nerve root pressure. Once the disc is violated, however, thorough disc excision is probably advisable. A bulging annulus does not have to be removed, particularly if the nerve root can be adequately decompressed. The root can easily go over a slight hump as long as there is no bony counterpressure above it. Sometimes a generous foraminotomy alone is adequate. In equivocal cases, injection of saline into the disc with a 10 ml syringe may be helpful. If the bulging disc does not take more than 1 or 2 ml of saline without a great deal of pressure, it might be tempting to limit the approach to a decompressive foraminotomy. On the other hand, if the entire 10 ml of the saline can be injected into the intervertebral disc space without a great deal of difficulty, the disc could be considered more pathologic.

NERVE ROOT ANOMALIES

Occasionally the nerve root exiting from the foramen above the surgically exposed interspace will descend medially beneath the facets of the next lower interspace. This minor deviation is not significant unless the surgeon happens to carry out a rather extensive lateral interlaminar exposure. Because the surgeon's attention is focused on the nerve root under direct vision, he may be unaware of an equally vital neural structure that is partially hidden by the lateral reflection of the yellow ligament. Even more rarely, two nerve roots may exit from the same foramen. When the dura and its nerve root is exposed, there is a second root just lateral to the first root. If it is recognized as a nerve root, there is no problem, but occasionally the laterally positioned root is mistaken for a bulging disc, and attempts are made to excise it. In doing so the root may be injured beyond repair. There is no substitute for good lighting and magnification. In addition, the operation should always be done questioningly, since the surgeon is working through a "k

eyhole," and identification of structures is extremely important.

After the protruded intervertebral disc has been adequately excised, the operating room table or spinal rest is flattened, so that the original flexed position is now a relatively straight one. This change in position places the root under less tension, narrows the posterior intervertebral disc space, and increases the depth between the skin surface and the interlaminar space. The interspace then is re-explored, and occasionally several additional fragments of disc material can be removed with the posterior vertebral bodies closer together. At the termination of the procedure, the nerve root should be under no pressure whatsoever, either anteriorly from the intervertebral disc or from bony constriction within the intervertebral foramen, which should have been partially opened during the bony dissection.

Bleeding from epidural veins should be carefully controlled before closure of the wound. Occasionally, a small pledget of Gelfoam is required to control venous bleeding.

WOUND CLOSURE

The suture material of personal preference is 2-0 chromic gut for muscle and fascia, 3-0 plain gut for subcutaneous tissue, and monofilament nylon for skin.

An important, but often overlooked, hemilaminectomy closure technique is the elimination of the dead space, which may fill with clot and contribute to postoperative discomfort (Figure 121-21). This is accomplished with 2-0 chromic suture passed through the interspinous ligament and then into the paraspinal muscles to approximate the paraspinal muscles against the laminae and spinous processes. This hemostatic suture should not be tied so tight that it causes muscle necrosis.

REFERENCES

1. Finneson BE: A lumbar disc surgery predictive score card. Spine 3:186, 1978
2. Barr, JS, Mixter WJ: Posterior protrusion of the lumbar intervertebral discs. J Bone Joint Surg 23:444, 1941

Commentary: Lumbar Disc Excision

Edward Tarlov

Dr. Finneson has emphasized the importance of patient selection. This is another way of saying that a correct diagnosis is important, especially since most patients with low back and leg pain do not require surgery.

Two fundamentally different kinds of pathologic conditions can occur in the lumbar discs as a result of the combination of trauma and aging. Disc degeneration is the most common and is nearly ubiquitous in the population. It is not commonly enough recognized that disc degeneration can cause referred pain in the buttock and down the thigh. All too often it is assumed that if there is leg pain there must be nerve root compression. This is not the case. This important point cannot be over emphasized. True sciatica radiating down the back of the thigh, below the knee, involving the calf may indicate nerve root compression by herniated disc. Less well defined pains and particularly those involving the buttock or thigh predominantly without radiation in a full sciatic distribution, or bilateral buttock or thigh pains, or pains which vary from side to side—all these are most likely to be referred pain from disc degeneration. Obviously, these will not be helped by surgery—almost no matter what their myelograms or scans are felt to demonstrate.

Dr. Finneson discusses the fallibility of the neurologic examination and the relationship of the location of a disc herniation to the lumbar nerve roots and plexus. These are important points. The most common disc herniations, which occur at the L4-5 level, typically affect the L5 nerve root. Although there may be weakness of the extensor halluces longus with involvement of the L5 nerve root, it is quite common even with a very large disc rupture at L4-5 to have no obvious neurologic deficit. This is a fallibility of the neurologic examination that should be added to those listed by Dr. Finneson.

The use of preoperative studies to diagnose or more properly, to confirm the clinical diagnosis of lumbar disc rupture is changing. Lumbar myelography, which can now be carried out on an outpatient basis, with the cautious use of small quantities of the new water soluble contrast media, is still overall probably the most reliable test. Computed tomographic scanning, which can demonstrate disc herniation, requires special attention on the part of the radiologist to get good films and requires an experienced and careful evaluation by the surgeon. The CT changes with disc rupture may not be as obvious as on myelography but there is a great danger that the films will be over interpreted in my experience. Disc protrusion, rupture or herniation is diagnosed too frequently from CT scans. In other words, CT scans are often over read. Once the radiologist, who has less real responsibility for diagnosis than the surgeon, has suggested a pathologic condition, it is all too likely that the phenomenon reported by Hans Christian Anderson in his short story "The Emperor's New Clothes" will prevent subsequent viewers of the scan from recognizing normal anatomy. This problem will be compounded with increasing use of MRI scanning. So far MRI scanning seems to be less accurate and less practical than CT for ordinary garden variety disc problems.

It is important to emphasize the pathology of lumbar disc rupture. The strong posterior longitudinal ligaments in the midline cause most disc herniations to occur laterally, in other words, to one side. Disc herniation rarely affects both legs; the painful syndrome is in the vast majority of instances unilateral, e.g., right or left, not both. Midline bulging of discs occurs so frequently that it should hardly be considered pathologic. Lateral views on myelograms as well as CT and MR scans that demonstrate disc bulging usually do not indicate a need for, or in other words, a likely benefit from surgery.

We have used a system of grading disc ruptures in order to distinguish free fragments, major disc ruptures and normal discs with minimal bulging, from one another. We consider the disc grade 0 or grade I if there is no bulge or little bulging; grade II if there is a marked herniation with a few fibers of the annulus intact; and grade III if there is an extruded free fragment. Grade II and grade III are the pathologic conditions most likely to be helped by surgery.

Dr. Finneson's lumbar disc surgery predictive score card is a graphic way to draw attention to negative risk factors. From the practical viewpoint its value is, to me, somewhat questionable. For example, in the list of positive factors, a neurologic examination demonstrating a single root syndrome indicating a specific interspace is given 25 positive points. As mentioned above, a major disc rupture at L4-5, which is the most common level at which disc rupture occurs, may be unassociated with any identifiable neurologic deficit. Does this mean a major disc rupture at L4-5 carries a less favorable prognosis than one at L5-S1? Obviously not. I would suggest in addition to the positive factors listed that the importance of true sciatica in diagnosis be emphasized and that a number of points be given if the pain is typical, in other words down the back or one leg below the knee. On the other hand, atypical variations which are not true sciatica, namely pain confined to the buttock or back of the thigh, variable pain, and variable nonsciatic pain involving both legs, are negative factors and tend to be correlated with a poor outcome from surgery.

The inclusion of progressively worsening neurologic deficit among indications for surgery is often stated, perhaps most

OPERATIVE NEUROSURGICAL TECHNIQUES
ISBN 0-8089-1862-1

often in orthopedic circles. In fact it is extremely unusual for disc rupture to cause a progressive neurologic deficit. I would suggest that this be removed from the list. Intractable pain is also listed as indication for disc surgery and should also be removed. The pain from typical disc rupture typically fluctuates and motivated patients do not stop work because of it in most instances. In general, injuries that occur in the work place do not cause disc rupture. The severe twisting shearing forces that are necessary to rupture the annulus do not occur after lifting and after falls in the work place. The failure of conservative treatment is definitely not an indication for surgery in the absence of diagnosis of true and typical disc rupture. Dr. Finneson has listed among contraindications to surgery a first episode of sciatic pain without an adequate trial of conservative management. There are instances in which pain is so severe that it may be worse at bed rest. I fully agree that pain on the wrong side means that a correct diagnosis has not been reached and certainly if the patient is significantly improved surgery is not indicated.

It is worth mentioning now with widespread use of CT scanning that the combination of a negative CT scan and a negative myelogram makes it extremely unlikely that a surgically remediable disc rupture will be found. For this reason exploratory lumbar surgery is almost never advisable.

Dr. Finneson mentions epidural venography. In my opinion this and discography are of no value at all.

Regarding the technical aspects of surgery I fully agree with the use of fiberoptic illumination and loupes. The microscope is an option but probably does not add to the efficacy of operation. In fact, at times visualization of the entire disc fragment may be hindered by inexperienced use of the microscope.

A variety of patient positions have been used. Dr. Finneson describes one commonly used. My own preference is for the knee chest position, in which the laminae are spread apart, the depth of the wound is reduced to the absolute minimum, the epidural veins are totally decompressed and the great vessels in the abdomen must hang away from the spine to some extent. It is important to avoid neck extension during any prone operation in order to prevent cervical spinal cord injury.

Regarding surface landmarks, I would add only that the relaxed hand with the thumb and little finger spread apart corresponds to the size of the sacrum in almost all patients and that if the little finger is placed on the tip of the coccyx the thumb with the hand in this relaxed position will lie on the lumbosacral interspace. This has been of greater help to me in localizing the level than any other method.

I would like to make a few points regarding operating on the correct level. It is important to emphasize that if only patients with major disc ruptures are being operated upon, then the correct level is the level with the obvious disc rupture most—often a free fragment or at least a most obvious major prolapse—what we call grade II or grade III if the patients are well selected. Several errors must be made for the surgeon to operate on the wrong level. One possible error is to operate on the wrong patient—in other words to make the wrong diagnosis. If the patient has no disc rupture there is no correct level. This is an error made more often than one might like to think. The

same is true for minimally herniated discs. The taking of x-ray films in such instances can confirm the level being operated upon but there is usually a more fundamental problem—no matter what level is operated the outcome will be poor.

If a large disc rupture is expected and no disc rupture is found then one is at the wrong level. If no disc rupture is expected the operation should probably not have been carried out to begin with.

Regarding the technique of dissection, I prefer to place the muscles on a slight stretch by using a periosteal elevator to retract laterally and then using the cutting cautery at low setting to divide the attachments of the paraspinous muscles to the spines.

Rather than using the rongeur in the manner depicted in Figure 121-13, it seems important to me to emphasize that the Leksell rongeur has a special feature incorporated in the beauty of its design. It can be held to cut in a position nearly vertical. The lower cutting jaw of the instrument should never be inserted beneath the lamina in the manner depicted in this picture because of the likelihood of injury to the underlying nerve root.

The points made about the yellow ligament and avoiding injury to the nerve root at this point are very important and the danger of using the Kerrison punch, which may pick up the edge of the dura, is also of great importance. My own method once the fragment has been removed is to use a curved curette to curette residual loose disc material from the interspace. Nerve root anomalies and wound closure have been well covered.

I feel that it is very important for the patient to know what to expect. Faulty expectation on the part of the patient or surgeon has often led to unnecessary re-operation.

The patient should know on leaving the hospital after lumbar disc excision that no movement, stress or strain is likely to cause a further disc rupture. The interspace is structurally strong from the onset of the recovery period. There will be symptoms that can occur, including pain down the leg but these do not indicate a recurrence of disc rupture in the early postoperative period. Return to work is possible as soon as the patient feels able to do so. Although there may be discomfort no harm will come from this. Recurrent disc ruptures occur in about one out of ten patients who have had bona fide disc rupture. No restriction of activity on the part of the patient will prevent this. Referred pain down the back of the thigh is quite common. An exercise program should be followed, particularly if the patient seems to be helped by it. Obese patients should keep weight down. A sympathetic conveying of these viewpoints will likely reduce the patient's anxiety and help to bring about a confident and speedy recovery and an early return, within a very few weeks, to full activities. Improved awareness on the part of doctors and patients of these viewpoints can reduce the morbidity of appropriately carried out disc surgery in the same way that improved awareness of doctors and patients has reduced the length of hospitalization for obstetrical patients. Well performed disc surgery can and should be the obstetrical part of neurosurgical practice with happy outcomes in most cases.

CHAPTER 122

Microsurgical Lumbar Disc Excision

Robert E. Harbaugh

THE USE of the operating microscope for the excision of herniated lumbar discs has been advocated since 1973.[1] Williams's technique of microlumbar discectomy stresses the use of a small incision, no coagulation in the epidural space, and minimal removal of nucleus pulposus.[2] Microsurgical discectomy as described by Wilson and his colleagues[3–5] also uses a small incision but differs from Williams's procedure in that bipolar cautery is used for coagulation of epidural veins and as much of the nucleus pulposus is removed as is feasible. Wilson also advocated sparing the ligamentum flavum when possible to inhibit epidural scarring.[4] Maroon's technique of microdiscectomy is very similar to Wilson's but no attempt is made at sparing the ligamentum flavum.[6] Similar procedures have been described by others.[7–12]

Although excellent results have been achieved with these procedures, microsurgical lumbar disc excision has been criticized on the grounds of inadequate exposure and gimmickry.[13] Presented here are the rationale of microsurgical lumbar disc excision, the operative technique as performed by the author, published results, personal observations on the advantages and disadvantages of this procedure, and a brief discussion of the criticism of this technique.

RATIONALE OF THE PROCEDURE

The surgical goals of adequate exposure and atraumatic dissection are as important for lumbar disc surgery as for any other neurosurgical procedure. The bright coaxial lighting and magnification provided by the operating microscope allow the surgeon to reach these goals with a somewhat smaller incision than is used for standard discectomy procedures. However, the length of the incision is not an important feature of microsurgical lumbar discectomy; longer skin incisions do not add to the morbidity of discectomy. Far more important is the precise identification of tissue and the meticulous tissue handling that is possible with the operating microscope.

TECHNIQUE

PATIENT SELECTION

Patient selection criteria for microsurgical lumbar discectomy are identical to selection criteria for standard discectomy procedures. Symptoms of radicular pain into one or both lower extremities with or without back pain must be present. In addition, at least one of the following should be present on examination: (1) a positive straight leg raising test, (2) sensory or motor deficits in the lower extremities, or (3) reflex abnormalities in the lower extremities. A computed tomographic scan or myelogram consistent with lumbar disc herniation is also required.

PREOPERATIVE PREPARATION

The night before surgery all patients are instructed to shower with an antiseptic soap. In the operating room the patient is placed under endotracheal anesthesia and positioned in the knee-chest, prone, or lateral position at the surgeon's discretion. I routinely use the knee-chest position to ensure abdominal decompression and minimize epidural bleeding. The back is shaved if necessary and prepared with antiseptic detergent and solution. If there is any question about the location of the correct interspace, a spinal needle is inserted between the appropriate spinous processes and a lateral roentgenogram is obtained. It is helpful to obtain radiographic localization in all cases.

OPERATIVE PROCEDURE

A midline incision is made extending from the upper border of the superior spinous process to the lower border of the inferior spinous process. If the patient is obese or if at any time during the procedure the exposure is inadequate, the incision is elongated. Dissection proceeds through the subcutaneous tissue to the lumbodorsal fascia.

The electrocautery knife is then used to incise the fascia and to develop a plane for subperiosteal dissection. The paraspinous muscles are dissected from the spinous processes and hemilaminae of the appropriate vertebrae laterally to the facet. A Williams self-retaining retractor is placed to expose the superior and inferior hemilaminae, the medial aspect of the facet, and the interlaminar space (Figure 122-1). The operating microscope is then brought into the field.

Kerrison rongeurs are used to remove as much bone from the superior hemilamina, inferior hemilamina, and medial facet as is necessary for adequate exposure. The ligamentum flavum is grasped and sharply incised along its medial border parallel to the spinal axis (Figure 122-2). A small curette is inserted into the opening and used to detach the ligamentum flavum superiorly and inferiorly. Laterally, the ligament and medial facet are removed with a small angled Kerrison rongeur, with care being taken to avoid the nerve root, which may be closely applied to the undersurface of the ligament. Blunt dissection beneath the

OPERATIVE NEUROSURGICAL TECHNIQUES
ISBN 0-8089-1862-1

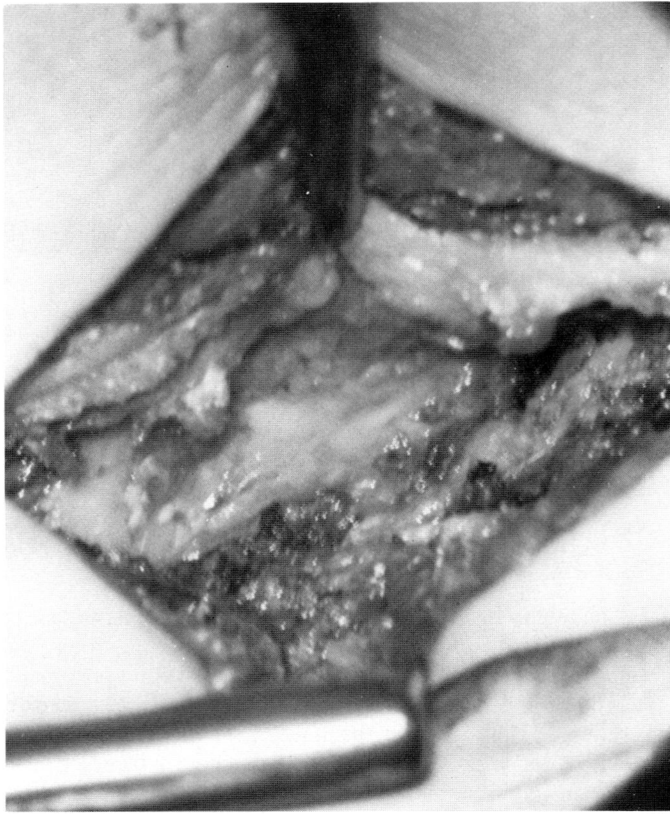

Fig. 122-1. An intraoperative photograph of a microsurgical disc excision at L4-5. The spinous process of L5 is at the extreme left and the spinous process of L4 at the extreme right. A laminotomy has been performed and the interlaminar space is clearly visible.

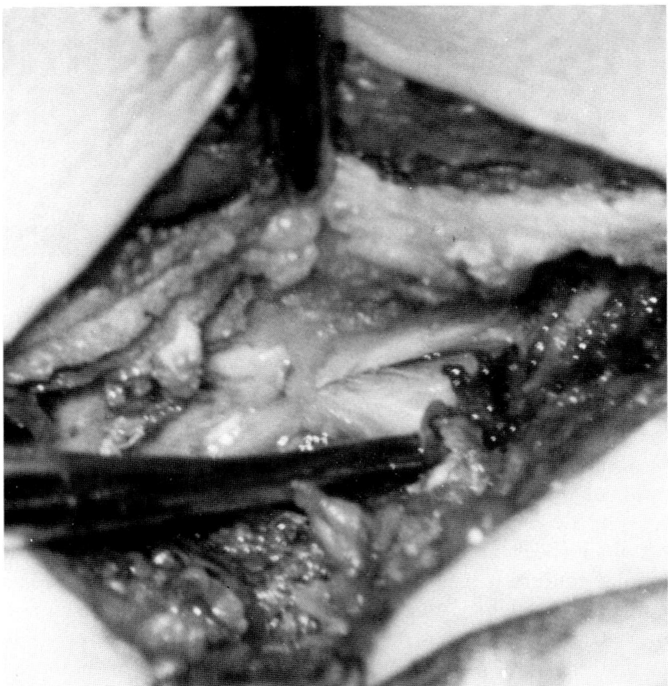

Fig. 122-2. An intraoperative photograph with ligamentum flavum incised.

ligament with a Woodson-Adson dissector before using the rongeur has been helpful in avoiding root injury.

After the ligament is removed, dissection proceeds through the epidural fat. Epidural veins are located, coagulated with bipolar cautery, and sharply divided with microscissors. Epidural fat is separated by sharp dissection and by the use of a No. 4 Penfield dissector.

The nerve root and herniated disc are now clearly identified (Figure 122-3). Free disc fragments are mobilized with a blunt nerve hook and removed with the Williams disc forceps or small pituitary forceps. If the disc fragment is incarcerated under the posterior longitudinal ligament, the ligament is incised in a cruciate fashion and the disc mobilized and removed as described above.

The disc space is entered and various pituitary rongeurs are used to remove as much nucleus pulposus as can be done safely. Curetting of the end plates is not done. Thorough exploration with the blunt hook or Woodson-Adson dissector is carried out to make sure that no retained disc fragment exists. If the nerve root foramen is not capacious, the small angled Kerrison rongeur is used to perform a foraminotomy, and the root is explored in the foramen.

When thorough exploration and decompression have been accomplished, meticulous hemostasis is achieved with bipolar cautery. The operative site is copiously irrigated with saline, and the incision is closed with absorbable sutures in the lumbodorsal fascia and subcutaneous tissues. The skin edges are approximated with nonabsorbable sutures or sterile tapes.

POSTOPERATIVE CARE

Patients are allowed unrestricted ambulation as soon as they are fully alert from the anesthetic. Prolonged sitting, driving, and heavy lifting are discouraged in the initial postoperative period. Patients are routinely discharged from the hospital 3 to 4 days after surgery and are seen for follow-up 4 to 6 weeks after discharge. Following postoperative evaluation in

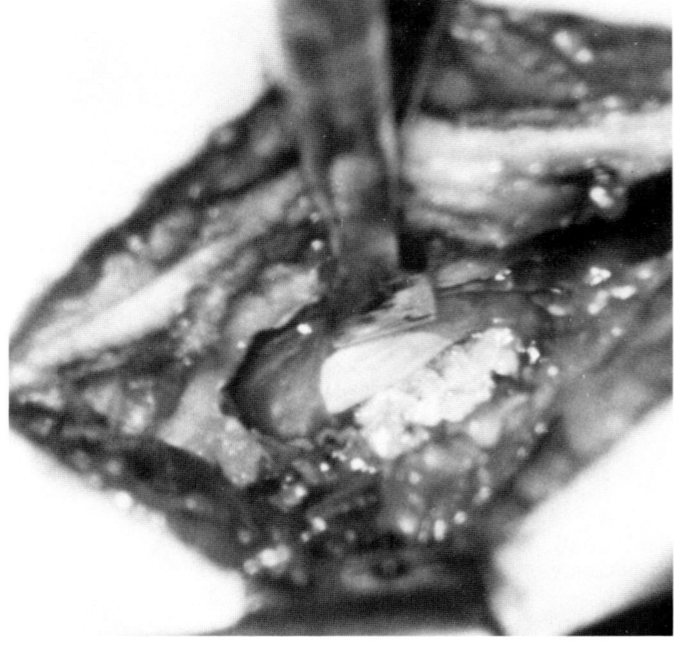

Fig. 122-3. An intraoperative photograph after removal of the ligamentum flavum and division of epidural veins and fat. The L5 nerve root and the underlying disc fragment are clearly visible.

the clinic, patients are encouraged to resume all of their normal activities.

RESULTS

Operative results for patients treated by microsurgical lumbar discectomy have been presented by a number of authors.[1–12] The published results have been excellent, with greater than 90 percent of patients having a good outcome from surgery. In a comparative study of microdiscectomy versus standard discectomy, the microsurgical procedure was somewhat better in regards to speed of recovery.[3] Microdiscectomy also appears to be clearly superior to chemonucleolysis in the initial postoperative period in at least one published study.[6]

Complications are infrequent and qualitatively not different from those of standard discectomy procedures.[1–12] Concern about an unusually high incidence of postoperative discitis[3] has not been borne out in other studies[6,10] nor in patients subsequently treated at Dartmouth-Hitchcock Medical Center.

ADVANTAGES AND DISADVANTAGES

During my residency training I was fortunate to work with four neurosurgeons, all of whom had active discectomy practices. Two of these surgeons performed microsurgical lumbar disc procedures and two performed standard lumbar discectomies. More recently I have had the responsibility of teaching neurosurgical residents to perform lumbar disc surgery. Experience from both perspectives has been valuable in pointing out the advantages and disadvantages of microsurgical lumbar disc excision. I think the advantages are preponderant.

The bright coaxial lighting and magnification of the operating microscope are clearly superior to loupe magnification and overhead lighting. The intraspinal structures are more clearly seen; and precise, meticulous hemostasis is much easier to accomplish. For teaching purposes, the operating microscope allows both the surgeon and assistant an unobstructed view of the operative field throughout the procedure. This is reassuring when one is the student; it is even more reassuring when one is the instructor. In addition, the microsurgical techniques learned in microdiscectomy can be readily applied to other microneurosurgical procedures. Our junior residents are adept in the use of the operating microscope primarily because of experience gained with microsurgical lumbar disc excision.

The disadvantage of microsurgical lumbar disc excision is a tendency to use too small an incision. Microsurgical lumbar disc excision has been criticized, rightly I think, on this point.[13]

The advantages of improved lighting and magnification can be negated by forcing oneself to work with a restricted exposure. Lumbar disc surgery using the operating microscope will allow wholly adequate exposure through a somewhat smaller incision than is used for standard discectomy procedures. However, a small incision should not be the point of the exercise.

SUMMARY

Microsurgical lumbar disc excision is an alternative to other standard discectomy procedures for the treatment of patients with herniated lumbar discs. The use of the operating microscope can result in more precise identification and delicate manipulation of intraspinal tissue. These advantages are negated if an inadequate exposure is obtained by using a needlessly small incision.

REFERENCES

1. Williams RW: The microsurgery of lumbar disc disease. Presented at the meeting of the American Association of Neurological Surgeons, Chicago, 1973
2. Williams RW: Microlumbar discectomy: A conservative surgical approach to the virgin herniated lumbar disc. Spine 3:175, 1978
3. Wilson DH, Harbaugh R: Microsurgical and standard removal of the protruded lumbar disc: A comparative study. Neurosurgery 8:422, 1981
4. Wilson DH, Harbaugh R: Microsurgical lumbar disc excision, in Schmidek HH, Sweet WH (eds): Operative Neurosurgical Techniques, vol 2. New York, Grune & Stratton, 1982, pp 1311–1318
5. Wilson DM, Kenning J: Microsurgical lumbar discectomy: Preliminary report of 83 consecutive cases. Neurosurgery 4:137, 1979
6. Maroon JC, Abla A: Microdiscectomy versus chemonucleolysis. Neurosurgery 16:644, 1985
7. Casper W: A new surgical procedure for lumbar disc herniation causing less tissue damage through microsurgical approach. Adv Neurosurg 4:79, 1977
8. Goald H: Microlumbar discectomy: Followup of 477 patients. J Microsurg 2:95, 1980
9. Goald HJ: Microlumbar discectomy. Spine 3:183, 1978
10. Hudgins RW: The role of micro dissectomy. Orthop Clin North Am 14:589, 1983
11. Roberts D: Microdiscectomy. Presented at the 32nd Annual Meeting of the Congress of Neurological Surgeons, Toronto, Ontario, October 3–8, 1982
12. Yasargil MG: Microsurgical operation for herniated lumbar disc. Adv Neurosurg 4:81, 1977
13. Saunders RL: Microsurgical lumbar discectomy: A dissenting view, in Schmidek HH, Sweet WH (eds): Operative Neurosurgical Techniques, vol 2. New York, Grune & Stratton, 1982, p 1319

Commentary: Microsurgical Lumbar Discectomy

Richard L. Saunders

In 1982, my commentary on the so-called microdisc procedure was one of cautious skepticism, if not condemnation. It seemed at that time the procedure was more contrived to result in a small scar than to affect a fundamental change in surgical outcome. Indeed, Wilson's own data indicated no difference between the ''microdisc'' and the conventional procedure of laminotomy in his hands.[1] The danger seemed not so much the redundancy of the microscope but the deliberate compromise of surgical exposure. The consequent missed pathology was familiar to many neurosurgeons doing the second operation and raised questions as to the wisdom of minimal exposure but greater precision to effect less surgical trauma.

This procedure of removing the lumbar disc protrusion with the benefits of the operative microscope, i.e., brilliant light, avoidance of needless soft tissue trauma, precise definition of venous and root anatomy, and preservation of epidural fat, has now stood the test of many neurosurgeons. Whether from the viewpoint of the enthusiast or the sensible surgeon, the results of using the microscope as a refinement of a properly performed procedure have been certainly no worse, and probably much improved, over conventional laminotomy. Such critical and experienced surgeons as Caspar, Harbaugh, and Hannesson have found that they can do the procedure of lumbar disc excision better with the help of the microscope: whatever one cares to call such a procedure is not critical.[2,3,4]

Unfortunately, it would be difficult to determine without bias whether the use of the operating microscope in disc surgery represents anything more than personal technical preference, an easily supervised method for resident microsurgical experience, or simply a fad. Nevertheless, adhering to traditional surgical fundamentals of adequate exposure of the pathologic condition, incorporating the advantages of microsurgical technique, simply cannot be bad. Through preservation of epidural fat and the maintenance of an absolutely unbloodied epidural space, the consequent epidural scar and arachnoidal reaction following disc surgery are probably minimized. Again, this has not been critically analyzed, but my personal experience and that of Nystrom with subsequent laminotomy following microdiscectomy suggests that improved results may well bedue in part to the minimizing of epidural scar.[5] Although it is not known whether scar indeed does compromise outcome, its amelioration is clearly a logical goal.

As Harbaugh has outlined, the microscope's contribution to the procedure of disc surgery, while obviously making feasible less paraspinal injury, is actually to refine an already perfected operative method.[4] The use of the microscope will not change the poor technique of sloppy hemostasis, excessive root manipulation, and careless exploration. Indeed, a surgeon with such problems will likely suffer even poorer results through prolonged operative time in getting lost, inadequate address of pathologic conditons, and obsession with affecting a tiny bikini-attractive incision. Without doubt, the poor disc surgeon will remain such, the poorly selected case will still be a failed back, and the societal condition of chronic back pain will continue to plague the compensation system regardless of whether or not one chooses to use the microscope. The microscope, like other surgical instruments, can be most important to a given surgeon's method, but it must be seen as such, not the avenue to a new operation, not a gimmick, and most importantly not a means to otherwise nonexistent surgical indications.

REFERENCES

1. Wilson DH, Harbaugh RE: Microsurgical lumbar disc excision, in Schmidek HH, Sweet WH (eds): Operative Neurosurgical Techniques. Indications, Methods and Results. New York, Grune & Stratton, 1982
2. Caspar W: Comparison of conventional and microsurgical lumbar disc surgery techniques. Presentation of Joint Section Spinal Disorders AANS/CNS, San Diego, California, February 19, 1986
3. Hannesson B, Gudmundson K, Gudmondson G: Lumbar disc microsurgery in Iceland from August, 1981–December, 1984—patients self-evaluation. Presentation at Scandinavian Neurosurgical Society, Reykjavik, Iceland, June 13, 1986
4. Harbaugh RE: See preceding chapter.
5. Nystrom B: Experience from microsurgical versus conventional technique in lumbar disc surgery. Presentation at Scandinavian Neurosurgical Society, Reykjavik, Iceland, June 12, 1986

OPERATIVE NEUROSURGICAL TECHNIQUES
ISBN 0-8089-1862-1

CHAPTER 123

Posterior Lumbar Interbody Fusion

Paul M. Lin

INDICATIONS

THE IDEAL OPERATION for lumbar spondylosis should decompress the neural elements, distract the vertebral bodies, and stabilize the motion segment. Although lumbar discectomy decompresses the neural elements, it does not distract and it may increase the settlement of the disc space and it does not stabilize the motion segment. Lumbar laminectomy does decompress, but does not distract and potentially increases the spine's instability. Lateral lumbar spinal fusion, while stabilizing the motion segment, neither decompresses nor distracts the vertebral bodies. Anterior interbody fusion stabilizes the motion segment, but does not decompress and only partially distracts the vertebral bodies.[1,2] Posterior lumbar interbody fusion (PLIF) fulfills all three criteria for the ideal spondylotic surgery, decompressing the neural elements, distracting the vertebral bodies, and stabilizing the motion segment.

Lumbar spondylosis is defined as degenerative changes of the motion segment as a result of settlement of the disc space. There are six different changes of anatomic alignment occurring as a result of the disc space settlement:[3]

1. Posterior bulging of the intervertebral disc and the posterior limiting membrane.
2. ''Shingling'' of the laminae and telescoping of the ligamentum flavum.
3. Structural narrowing of the intervertebral canal or foramen.
4. Overriding of the facet joint.
5. Hypertrophic arthrosis of the facet.
6. Retrolisthesis secondary to instability.

Posterior lumbar interbody fusion rectifies all the six anatomic changes seen in lumbar spondylosis and relieves any combination of neural compression, settlement of the disc space, and segmental instability. It therefore could be useful in the definitive correction of lumbar spondylosis, be it degenerative or postsurgical (Figure 123-1A and B).

The definition of segmental instability should be expanded to include three categories:

1. Anatomic instability. There is a structural loss of the motion segment, such as the facet, pars interarticularis, spinous processes or the supraspinous ligament. Massive disc debulkment, chemical[4,5] or surgical, can produce settlement of the disc space and an instability of the motion segment. Adams and Hutton[6] showed, in an experimental model, that a 0.7 mm settlement of the disc space results in increased stress on the superior facet resulting in altered stability of the motion segment.

2. Dynamic instability. There is a malalignment of forces of the motion segment, as occurring in lumbar spondylolisthesis, retrospondylolisthesis, excessive lumbar lordosis or rotational scoliosis.
3. Functional instability. The motion segment is visibly unstable, as can be seen either on flexion-extension roentgenograms or loose motion segment demonstrated at the time of surgery.

Indications for PLIF in segmental instability are varied. It is very useful in a segmentally unstable spinal stenosis, with or without disc herniation.[7–11] As a single-level fusion above the L5-S1 level, PLIF has a high rate of successful floating fusion.[12] A successful chemonucleolysis debulks the disc space and it should result in a disc-space settlement and acceleration of spondylosis of the injected disc space. In the future, segmental instability and spondylosis after chemonucleolysis may be the most frequent indication for PLIF.[4,5,13] In obese patients with lateral extrusion of disc material, discectomy with PLIF may prevent the rapid postoperative settlement of the disc space and the instant segmental instability brought on by excessive body weight.[12]

Posterior lumbar interbody fusion is indicated for recurrent disc disease especially in association with segmental instability and spondylosis.[9,10]

Posterior lumbar interbody fusion should be considered as the primary procedure for large midline discs requiring radical bilateral disc removal.[14,15] Posterior lumbar interbody fusion is a useful tool in the management of the ''failed back'' syndrome, especially if there is evidence of nerve root compression associated with segmental instability.[15–17]

Even without apparent evidence of segmental instability, PLIF is indicated for unoperated cases if the patient is a laborer or has associated spondylosis and a history of chronic back pain.[12,15,18]

BIOMECHANICAL CONSIDERATION

The current understanding of the biomechanics of the lumbar spine makes it difficult to refute the need for spinal fusion in selected patient.[13,19–21] Wiltse[22,23] called the 1970s the ''decade of decompression'' and believes that the dynamics of fusion might be clarified in the 1980s. He also stated that despite the plethora of techniques for lumbar spinal fusions, none has been ideal. The failure rate of solid lumbar arthrodesis is still distressingly high, especially with posterior fusions.

The greatest advantage of PLIF is that it dynamically decompresses the neural structure by distracting the vertebral

OPERATIVE NEUROSURGICAL TECHNIQUES
ISBN 0-8089-1862-1

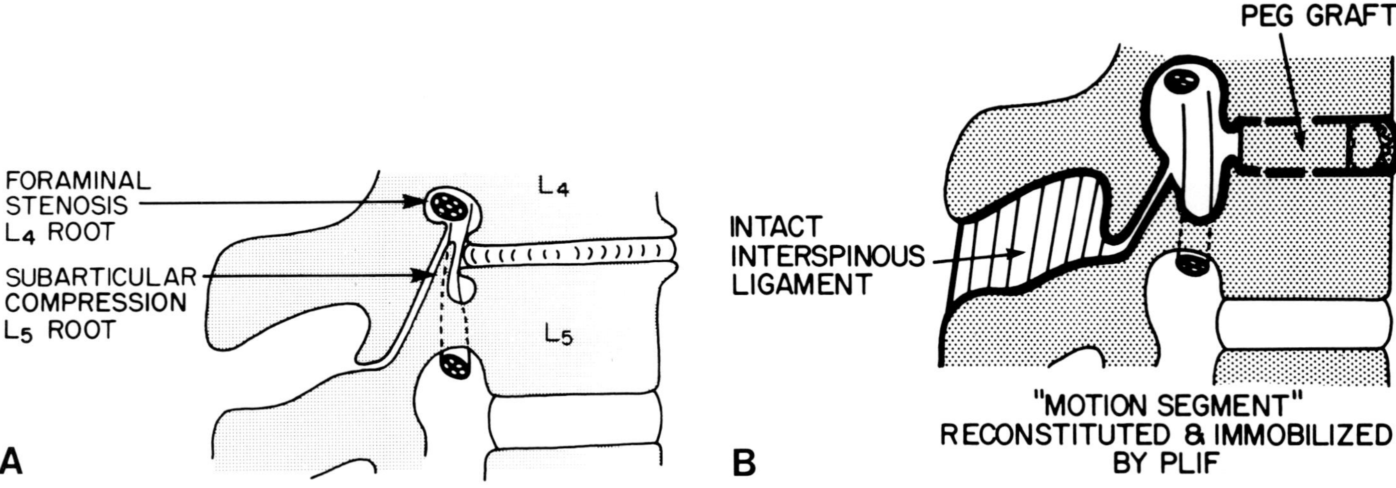

Fig. 123-1. (A) Lumbar spondylosis: changes of anatomical malalignment as a result of disc settlement. (B) PLIF corrected the changes of anatomical malalignment seen with lumbar spondylosis.

bodies apart and fusing it into a single-motion segment.[24,25] Compared with other types of lumbar spinal fusions, PLIF has the following biomechanical advantages:[10,18,26]

1. In spondylosis with a herniated disc, PLIF reconstitutes the normal anatomic relation between the motion segment and

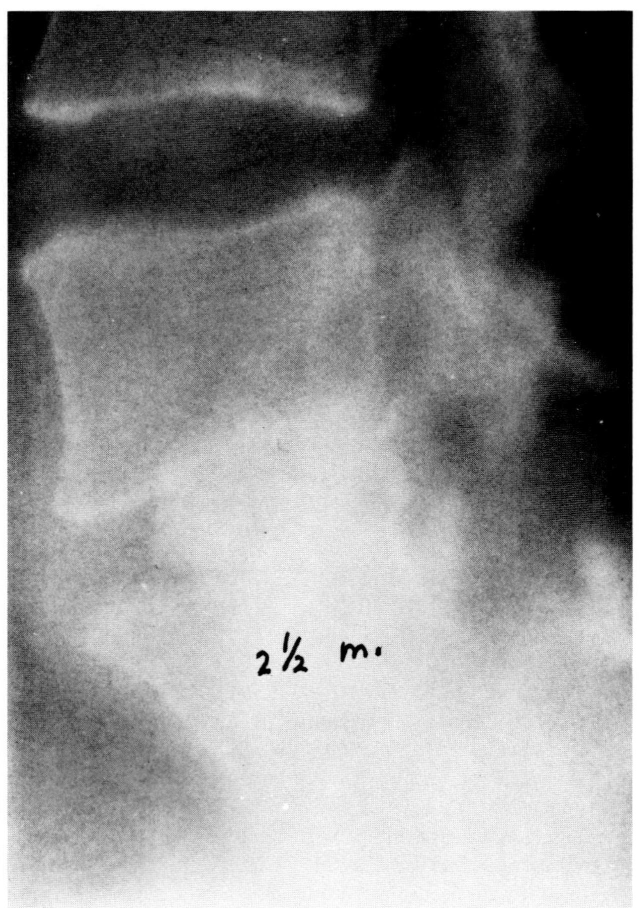

Fig. 123-2. Posterior lumbar interbody fusion using autogenous graft with sandwiched cortical and high density cancellous graft showing evidence of osteosynthesis 2½ months after surgery.

the neural structures. The motion segment is restored to its normal anatomic alignment.

2. A successful PLIF with arrest of motion by fusion prevents disc-space collapse, degenerative changes, or spondylosis seen usually after discectomy.

3. The total discectomy needed for PLIF prevents recurrent lumbar disc herniation at that level.

4. Laminotomy, mesial facetectomy, and foraminotomy integrated with PLIF relieve neural structures of bony compression in segmental spinal stenosis.

5. The fusion achieved in PLIF may prevent painful nerve root irritation by postoperative perineural adhesions. The lack of motion prevents mechanical traction on the nerve root from the surrounding scar tissue.

As proposed by Cautilli,[24] PLIF has definite mechanical advantages compared with other types of lumbar spinal fusion techniques: (1) a wider area of bone surface is involved; (2) adequate blood supply is obtained through the cancellous portion of the vertebral body once the cortical end-plate has been partially or totally removed; (3) the fusion is proximate to the center of motion and compression forces.

Evans[25] proposed additional advantages: (1) posterolateral siting of load-bearing grafts is the optimal location in relation to the load-bearing capacity of the vertebral bodies (cancellous bone strength is greatest in these regions); (2) posterior distraction is enhanced by maintaining the anterior annulus and ligament, which act together as a fulcrum or pivot; (3) when adequate soft-tissue connections are maintained between posterior spinous processes or when they are supplemented (e.g., by wire-ties), the graft is stable and strong enough for early weight bearing.

Schlegel and Pon[27] also advocate preservation of the facet and dorsal structures be accomplished in PLIF. It is their contention that with maximal impaction of grafts, the natural gravitational force would be translated into compression of grafts and enhancement of bony healing, the principle of compact compression grafting.[13,25,27–29]

In PLIF the autogenous bone provides the best graft material with the highest success rate for solid osteosynthesis (Figure 123-2).[30,31] The stroma cells within the marrow of the autogenous cancellous bone are the progenitors of

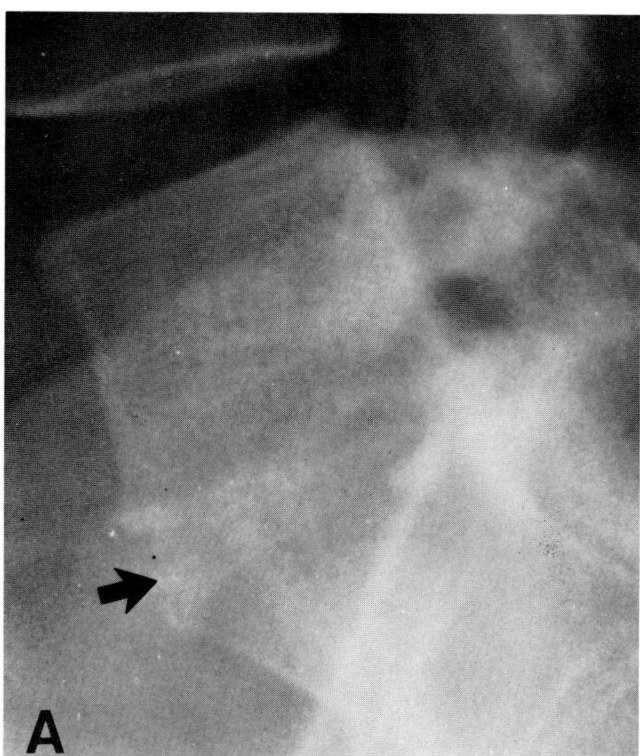

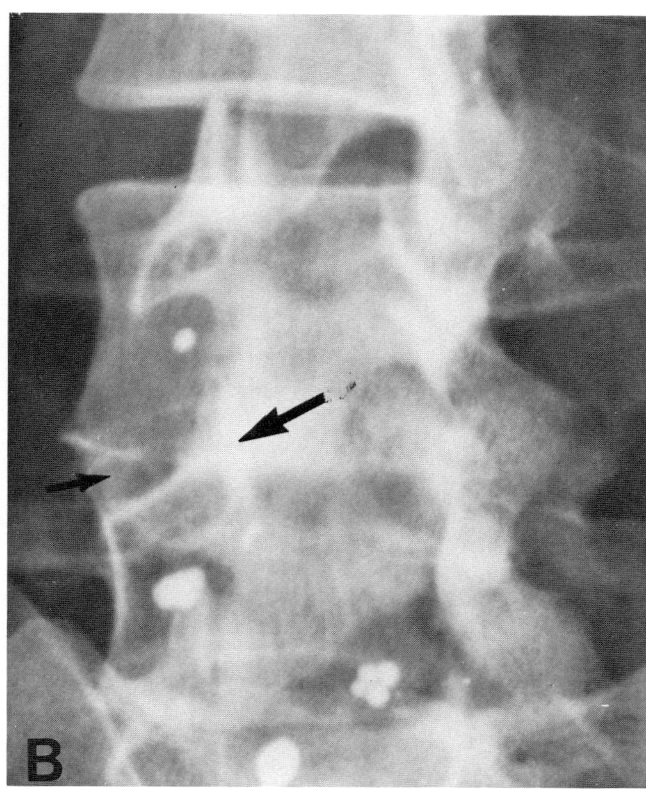

Fig. 123-3. (A) Maturing PLIF graft advancing up to the anterior limiting membrane. (B) Maturing PLIF showing spontaneous fusion of the facet.

osteoblasts.[32] The autogenous cancellous bone further contains high concentration of osteogenetic factor, the bone morphogenetic proteins (BMP).[33] Unlike lateral fusion, in which the grafts are surrounded by vascular muscle tissue, grafts placed within the disc space are relatively avascular. Therefore, if the thick tricortical homologous bone is employed within the disc space, the linear process of osteolysis and osteosynthesis proceeds at a predictably slower rate. The larger the graft, the slower the rate of osteosynthesis.[34] Clinically and experimentally, high density autogenous bone grafting, using the compact compression principle, gives the fastest rate of osteosynthesis.[14,27,30]

The usual criterion for arthrodesis in PLIF is evidence of osteosynthesis in lateral radiographic tomograms. Evidence of trabeculation on a simple roentgenogram is difficult to discern. In matured PLIF one frequently notes filling of the disc space with new bone formation up to the anatomic barrier of the anterior limiting membrane. In AP roentgenograms one also observes increased bone density of the interpedicular line, the line of stress. Elimination of motion by solid fusion in PLIF also absorbs the anterior spurring seen preoperatively. Spontaneous fusion of the facet joint can often be demonstrated in a matured PLIF (Figures 123-3A and B and 123-4A and B).

Early evidence of osteosynthesis as seen on CT scans is an attempt to mix the new cortical and cancellous bone grafts.[35] The matured PLIF graft then assumes the normal osseous architecture of a vertebral body, namely cancellous marrow in the centrum and cortical bone along the margin. This is the most physiologic evidence of fusion in PLIF and it may take 9 to 12 months to be so fully integrated (Figure 123-5A and B).

In anterior cervical interbody fusion, there are four biomechanic principles that ensure the high fusion rate. To achieve an equally high fusion rate in PLIF, these four principles should be followed.[10,12,21,26,36]

PRESERVATION OF THE POSTERIOR PORTION OF THE MOTION SEGMENT

In anterior cervical interbody fusion, the intact cervical supraspinous ligament (the ligamentum nuchae) and the facet joints are important restricting forces that prevent excessive motion of the bone graft within the disc space (Figure 123-1B). With distraction of the disc space and insertion of the grafts, additional tension is produced in the intact posterior portion of the cervical motion segment, further stabilizing the graft within the disc space. Using the same rationale, the posterior portion of the motion segment in PLIF should be maintained.[8,14,37] The spinal canal is entered only through a laminotomy and mesial facetectomy, thereby preserving the integrity of the locking mechanism of the facet joint, especially the strong lateral fibrous capsule (Figure 123-6). The spinous process and the interspinous and supraspinous ligament are not violated, allowing the reattachment of muscles to the lumbar motion segment. The importance of this concept corresponds to observations of Wiltse and Murphy[22] that the fusion rate in PLIF is low when the posterior portion of the motion segment is removed.[9,14]

Preservation of the posterior portion of the motion segment in PLIF would also prevent a slippage of the adjoining vertebral bodies in the event of failure of osteosynthesis.

TOTAL DISCECTOMY

Total excision of the disc material is easily accomplished in anterior cervical interbody fusion. In PLIF, 80 to 90 percent of the disc material should be removed. This creates a larger area

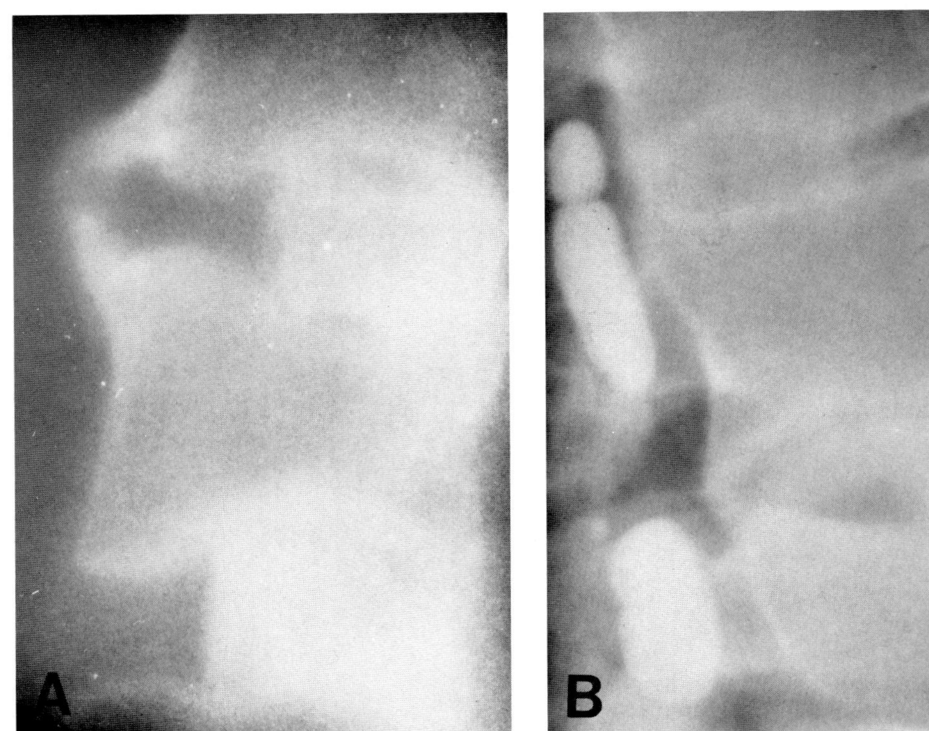

Fig. 123-4.   (A) Lateral tomogram of two levels, L)3 and L)4, four months after PLIF surgery. (B) Note trabeculation and slight settlement of the graft seen 2 years after the surgery. The anterior spurring of L)3 and L)4 interspaces is absorbed and is replaced with a calcification of the anterior limiting membrane.

of bony contact between the grafts with the vertebral bodies and thus heightens the chances of successful interbody fusion.

PARTIAL DECORTICATION

In young people the lumbar cortical end-plates are thin. By curetting down to the layer of oozing cortical bone or by using a cortical perforator, vascularization to the grafts can be achieved in a high percentage of cases. In matured cortical end-plates, it is necessary to establish many islands of decortication down to the cancellous bone. This can be accom-

plished with the sonic curette or the use of a large, sharp curette, and with a rotational force, a thin surface of the cortical end-plate can be sheared off. Jackson[38] has recently advocated the use of the high speed drill in decortication.

THE UNIGRAFT CONCEPT

In anterior cervical interbody fusion, a single piece of tricortical horseshoe iliac crest graft or dowel graft is inserted and fills the entire excavated disc space. Obviously, it is not possible to achieve a single "unigraft" in the lumbar area. The

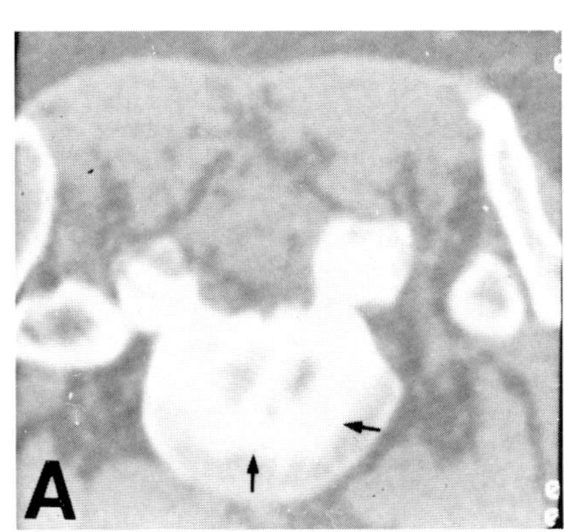
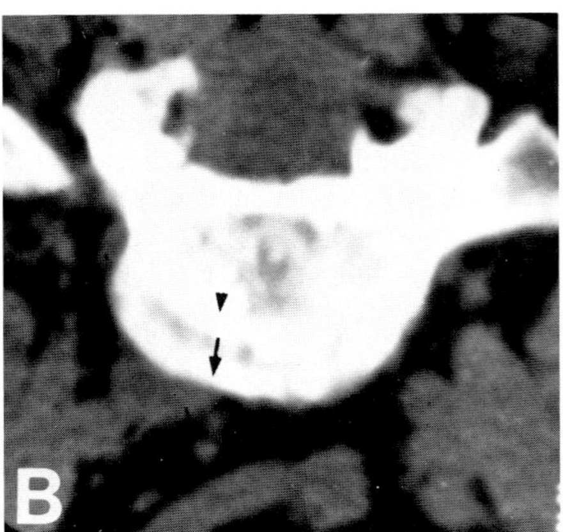

Fig. 123-5.   (A) A CT scan of a matured PLIF showing reorganization of graft to assume normal osseous architecture of a vertebral body, cancellous in the center and cortical ring peripherally. (B) Very matured PLIF shows on the CT scan a double ring phenomenon. Second ring represents further bone growth to the anterior limiting membrane.

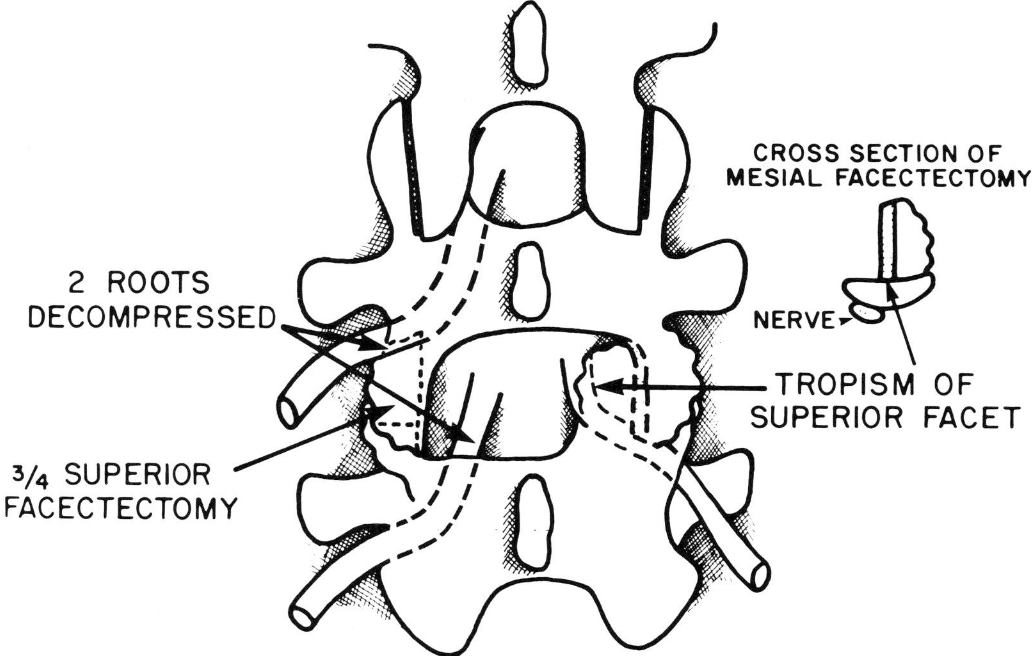

Fig. 123-6. Mesial inferior facetectomy by an osteotome, exposing the underlying superior facet (right). After mesial facetectomy of the superior facet (left) the intervertebral foramen is decompressed by amputation of the remaining tip of the superior facet. Note the extent of the inferior laminotomy.

unigraft concept in PLIF is established by inserting four to six unicortical autogenous peg grafts, keeping the cortical plate of the peg grafts parallel to the longitudinal axis of the body. Every effort is then made to forcefully fill the space between the peg graft and all remaining empty spaces with autogenous cancellous bone strips. The end-product is a tightly packed mixture of unicortical peg grafts and high density cancellous bone filling almost the entire disc space. Functionally and mechanically, it is similar to a one-piece "unigraft." Bunnell,[30] in his experimental anterior lumbar interbody fusion in dogs, indicated that the highest chance of success occurs when the graft consists mainly of cancellous bone packed tightly in the disc space. McNab[39] suggested that if a bone graft is inserted into the disc space, it will be dissolved by the osteolytic properties of the surrounding fibrous tissue. However, if all spaces are filled with osseous materials, preventing fibrous tissue invasion, successful osteosynthesis in PLIF is enhanced.

SURGICAL TECHNIQUE OF PLIF

POSITION

The patient is placed in a prone position. To avoid excessive epidural bleeding during surgery, two firm rolls are used to support the iliac crest, the lateral rib cage, and the clavicle, thereby preventing compression of the anterior abdominal wall and the inferior vena cava. The operating table is not flexed, which helps to decrease intra-abdominal pressure. A Foley catheter is inserted to avoid intra-abdominal pressure during surgery as a result of bladder distension. The incision is horizontal (Figure 123-7A and B). Grafts are removed from the posterior iliac crest through the same incision.

EXPOSURE

When possible, the integrity of the supraspinous ligaments and the spinous processes is preserved. The inferior laminotomy is performed first, after which the mesial portion of the inferior facet is removed by sharp dissection with a thin ¼-inch osteotome. A horizontal cut is made, followed by a vertical cut. The mesial half of the inferior facet is removed, and the underlying superior facet, which often presents as a tropism, is exposed. The mesial half of the superior facet is then removed either with an osteotome or a bone punch. Superior laminotomy can be done first to facilitate mesial facetectomy. With the osteotome a horizontal cut on the superior facet just above the pedicle is made first, followed by a vertical cut up to the lateral limit of the exposure (Figure 123-6). This is followed by a forceful swiveling rotatory action of the osteotome to avulse the remaining tip of the superior facet, which helps to decompress the intervertebral foramen. The intervertebral foramen and its contents are exposed and, if necessary, decompressed, preferably from the opposite side of the table. This can be accomplished with an angled bone punch, angled curette, or a sonic angled curette. The sonic curette consists of a hand tool (Quintron, Inc., Galena, Ohio) and cutting tip, e.g., a curette or gouge. It forms a resonant structure that is driven by a pair of piezoelectric crystals at about 25,000 Hz/sec. The motion of the tip, typically 0.001-0.002 mm, is maintained under a range of load or use conditions by the amount of energy (typically 10 W) supplied to the hand tool. The frequency feedback control circuit ensures that efficient resonance is maintained under all tip and load combinations. The sonic curette is ultrasonic instrumentation, and decreases the resistance between the curette and the bone structure. As with any curetting action on the bone, a perched anchorage on the bone structure should be obtained before forceful rotating action is applied. The sonic curette generates energy mainly at the tip and the degree of heat

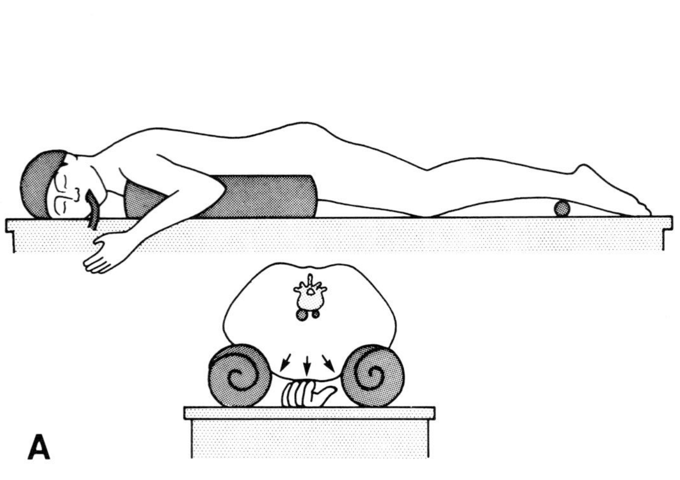

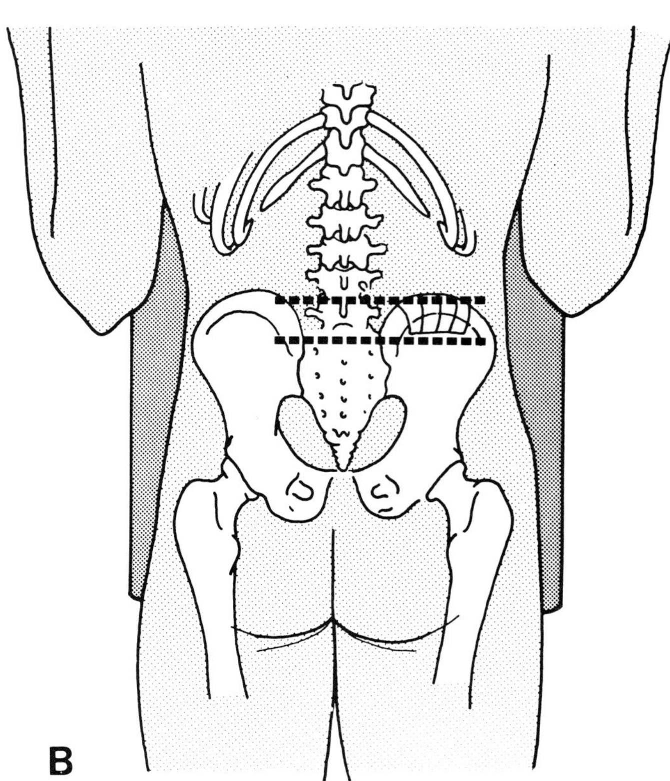

Fig. 123-7. (A) (Top) Positioning for posterior lumbar interbody fusion. Rolls are firm. Flexion of the table is not needed. (Bottom) Testing the tension of the anterior abdominal wall. (B) Incision is horizontal extended laterally so the graft can be removed from the posterior iliac crest.

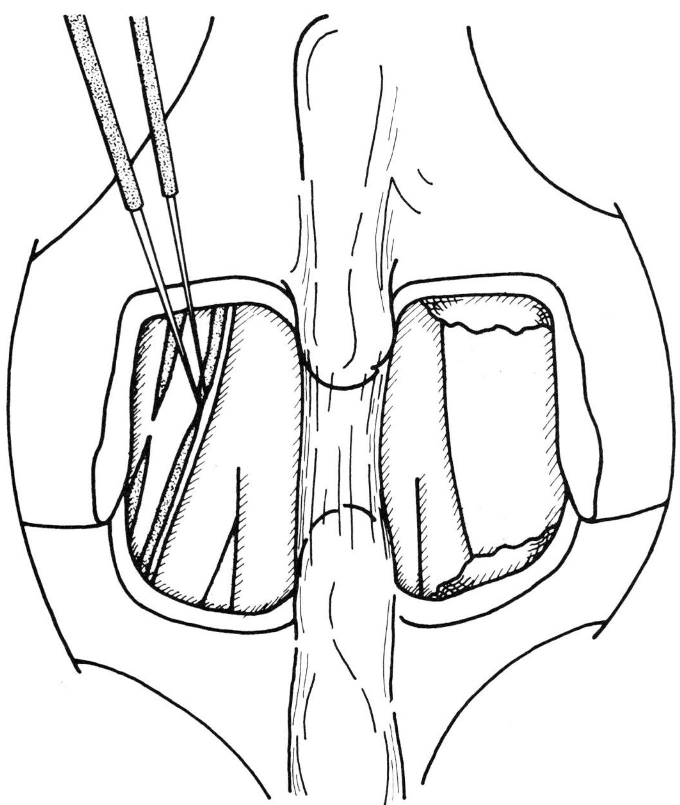

Fig. 123-8. After mesial facetectomy the spinous processes, supraspinous ligaments, and facets are preserved. Control of epidural hemorrhage by bipolar or insulated coagulation forceps is used on the left side. On the right side the epidural hemorrhage is controlled by Surgicel tampons. Impacted Surgicel tampons also push the nerve root medially and expose the disc space without requiring use of a nerve root retractor.

it generates is proportional to elapsed time. Therefore, cutting tips of the sonic instrument must be scrupulously sharpened to avoid dull and slow curetting. The sonic curette in contact with a metal nerve root retractor could reduce the vibration to that of the sonic frequency range, resulting in increased energy per vibration; harmless mechanical stimulation of the nerve root may occur.

EPIDURAL HEMOSTASIS

The epidural veins should be coagulated by bipolar coagulation and then severed. The improved sparkless version of the bipolar coagulation unit is much preferred. Surgicel (Johnson & Johnson, New Brunswick, New Jersey) is used for hemostasis placed above and below the disc space, pushing the veins away from the disc space and lying like a tampon lateral to the dura and nerve root (Figure 123-8). Prior soaking of the Surgicel in a double-strength thrombin solution (Parke-Davis, Morris Plains, New Jersey) enhances hemostasis in problematic epidural bleeding. Occasionally, small arterial bleeding may appear in the epidural space requiring careful hemostasis by bipolar coagulation. By using Surgicel as a tampon above and below the disc space, the dura and nerve root are displaced medially, thus avoiding use of a nerve root retractor.

TOTAL DISCECTOMY

The disc space is entered by cutting a large square plug of annulus, revealing the bony edges of the adjoining vertebral bodies. The adjoining intervertebral rim is removed by first using a ¼-inch thin osteotome for the two vertical parallel cuts on each side of the exposed intervertebral rim. With a ¼-inch or ⅜-inch osteotome, a horizontal cut is then made in the lower rim (Figure 123-9). The horizontal cut is made with slight

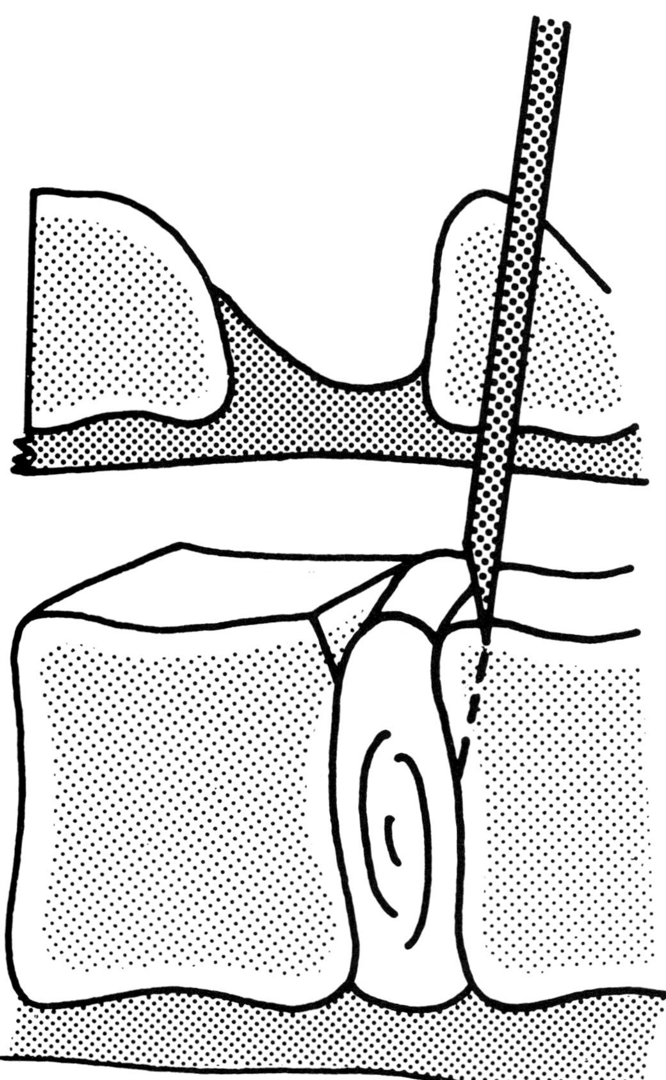

Fig. 123-9. The intervertebral rims are removed by an osteotome. The entrance should be made smaller than the body of the disc space so as to retain the locking mechanism (keystone effect) when grafts are countersunk.

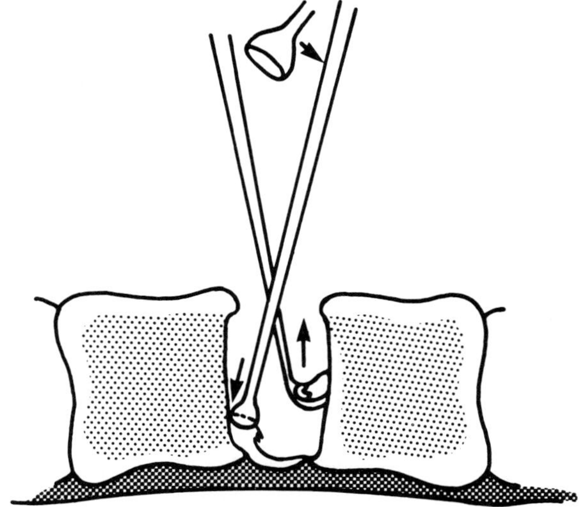

Fig. 123-10. After the intervertebral rims are removed, the cleavage of the disc attachment to the cortical end-plate is identified. A downbite curette is used to detach the disc materials from the cortical end-plate. A curved up-bite curette is used to remove the concave centrum of the lower cartilaginous plate. The detached large chunks of disc material are then removed with a rongeur.

discectomy to the limit of the anterior limiting membrane or approximately 30 mm in depth is attempted with a sharp curette or an ultrasonic curette using only side-to-side motion to avoid anterior vascular injury.

The midline bar, or the disc under the dural space, requires special attention. With a sharp, pointed cervical osteophyte osteotome, the disc material is carefully dissected from the posterior limiting membrane, and with downward pressure the

angulation caudally, in accordance with the alignment of the disc space. The normal concavity of the disc space allows removal of the intervertebral rim and the underlying subchondral bone, before the osteotome enters the disc space. The thickness of the rims to be removed varies from 2 to 8 mm inferiorly and 1 to 3 mm superiorly. Removal of the rims allows wide and straight access to the disc space, and effectively decorticates about 1 cm of the inferior cortical plate. It is not necessary to remove the disc material in a piecemeal fashion as in conventional discectomy. The cleavage between the cortical end-plate and the disc material is easily defined after removal of the intervertebral rim (Figure 123-10). Using a down-bite horizontal cutting edge curette, the disc material is scraped from the cortical end-plate along the cleavage line. An up-biting angle curette is placed as low as possible, and the partially detached disc material is scraped upward and detached. The detached disc materials can then be removed easily with a serrated disc rongeur. A peapod angled rongeur or bone punch is useful for removal of the disc from the lateral recesses. Complete

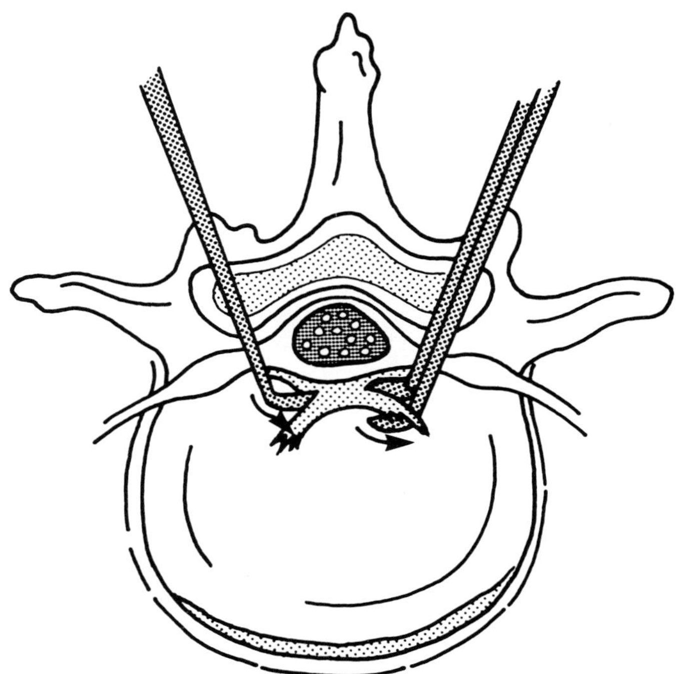

Fig. 123-11. Removal of the midline bar with sharp downward movement of a downbite curette or a pea pod rongeur, separating the disc from the posterior limiting membrane and then preserving the latter.

remaining intervertebral rim can also be removed (Figure 123-11). The midline bar can then be removed by a down-bite curette and an up-bite peapod. At times, the remnants of the midline bar can only be removed after a peg graft is inserted from the contralateral side, pushing and anchoring the disc material laterally, to be removed with a disc rongeur.

DECORTICATION

Decortication of the cortical end-plate is accomplished with a large, sharp, straight curette. The curette is inserted into the disc space, parallel to the cortical end-plates, and a rotational force is applied. The disc space is opened, and at the same time a thin sliver of cortical end-plate is removed. Using the sonic curette for decortication, only slight finger-touch rotational force is needed (Figure 123-12). The lower cortical end-plate often recedes behind the vertical cut of the posterior invertebral rim, requiring use of an up-bite curette for complete disc removal and also for decortication. In a younger person the cortical end-plate is thin and very similar to that in the cervical area. A triangular cortical perforator with a sharp point and a 135-degree angle from the handle is used (Figure 123-13). Using a levering action, multiple perforations are made through the thin cortical end-plate. To prevent possible posterior graft migration, a shallow undercut or "keystone effect," below the vertebral rim can easily be accomplished with a sonic curette.

The decortication need only be superficial, scraping down to the oozing cortical bone layer. Total decortication with an osteotome down to the anterior limiting membrane, as advocated by Cloward,[16,17,40–43] carries with it the inherent danger of anterior vascular injury and has discouraged many surgeons from attempting PLIF. The arterial supply to the cortical end-plate consists of end arteries. The removal of only a very thin layer of cortical end-plate, evidenced by a change in color from white cortical end-plate to brownish subcortical cancellous bone is sufficient to ensure an adequate source of vascularization.[44]

The collateral veins lie horizontally 2 or 3 mm below the surface of the cortical end-plate and frequently are the source of brisk bleeding (Figure 123-14A and B).[44] Because the bony texture is more porous in the central portion of the vertebral body,[25] thin decortication prevents settlement of the graft due to softness of cancellous bone.

GRAFT PREPARATION

The autogenous bone graft is removed through the same horizontal incision from the posterior iliac crest, usually from the right side in a single-level PLIF. With subperiosteal dissection, and avoiding excessive electrocoagulation the lateral portion of the iliac crest and the posterior surface of the iliac bone are exposed. A split-thickness unicortical graft is removed by osteotome. The cortical graft is usually about 8 to 9 cm long along the iliac crest, about 3 cm wide, and 8 to 10 mm thick. The harvesting of peg grafts can be augmented by obtaining a wider 5-cm graft rather than the usual 3-cm graft. A single 5-cm-long peg graft can then be cut into 1½ peg grafts. For a two-level fusion the grafts are preferably removed from the posterior iliac crest of both sides. After the block of cortical graft is removed, 10 to 12 pieces of cancellous bone strips are then removed with a gouge. A sonic gouge facilitates removal of the cancellous graft material. The cortical graft is then cut into four to six peg grafts, with the width determined by the measurement of the

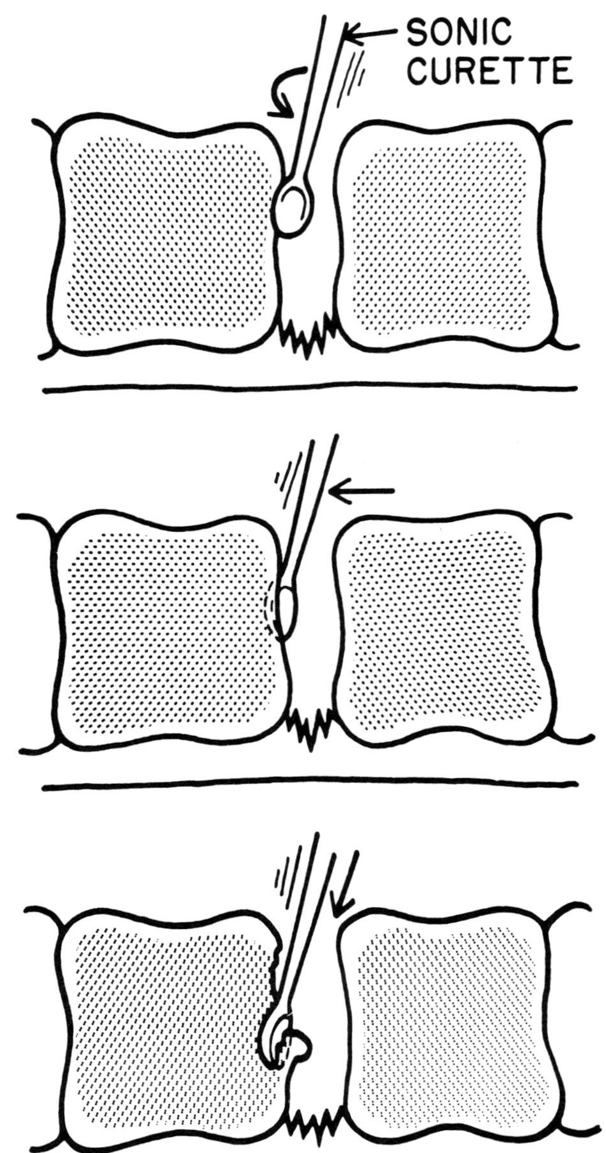

Fig. 123-12. Use of an ultrasonic curette, which can deliver 25,000 cycles per second constant vibration at the tip, helps ease significantly the decortication of the sclerotic cortical end-plates. It also helps sculpturing or undercutting below the intervertebral rim to achieve a keystone type of locking mechanism of the grafts.

height of the disc space when maximally distracted and the length determined by the depth of the decorticated disc space usually 25 to 30 mm in length.

GRAFT INSERTION

The disc space is distracted by a laminal or vertebral body spreader.[16] The laminal spreader tends to open the disc space posteriorly and may actually close the space anteriorly, whereas a vertebral body spreader distracts the disc space more evenly.

The prying action of a blunt end impactor (Cloward's "Puka" stick) within the disc space can also distract the disc space sufficiently to allow placement of one of the two large central peg grafts from the opposite aide. This should be repeated on the other side before the lateral grafts are inserted.

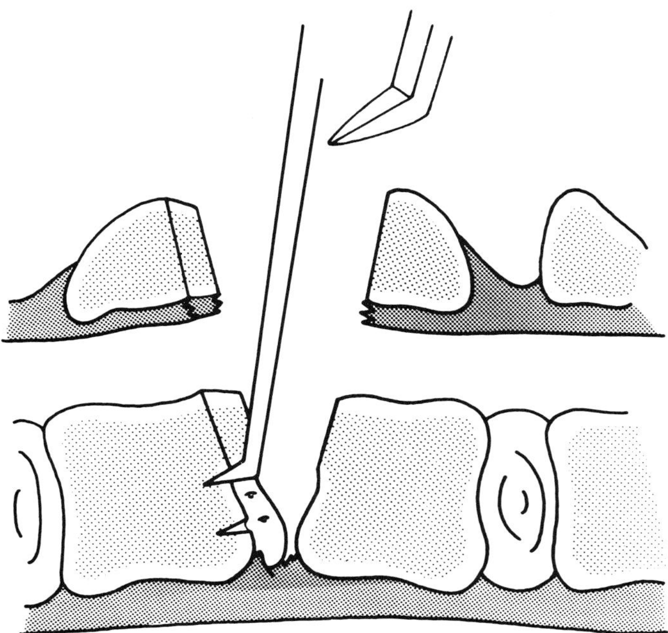

Fig. 123-13. Removal of the intervertebral rim, preservation of the central cortical plate, and fenestration of the cortical plate to enhance revascularization of grafts from cancellous bone. The perforator used had a 135-degree angle and a sharpened tip. A downward tap of the perforator drives the sharp tip into the cancellous bone of the vertebral body.

The first piece of graft is usually a cancellous strip inserted horizontally into the base of the disc space. The larger piece of the peg graft is then placed in the central portion of the disc space. Migration of the graft toward the midline is effected by a swiveling action of the "Puka" stick or by a pushing action from the tip of an up-bite disc rongeur. I avoid placing the largest possible peg graft within the disc space. The hard, pounding action necessary to drive in a large graft can be

traumatic. With excessive distraction and without proper keystone undercutting below the intervertebral rim, a larger graft may slowly induce posterior graft migration. The disc space should be filled with moderately sized peg grafts that are snug but can be packed into the disc space easily. Good keystone preparation under the intervertebral rims may prevent insertion of a graft that is larger than the entrance but adequate for the larger prepared beds within the disc space. Under these circumstances one can place the graft within the disc space with the graft lying horizontally, then with the grasping action of a disc rongeur the graft is firmly rotated to a position where the cortical plate of the graft is parallel to the longitudinal axis of the body (Figure 123-15). The lateral recess is filled with cancellous pieces before the second peg graft is inserted lateral to the first central graft. The lateral graft should be thinner and shorter and it should be placed at a level lower than the central peg graft. Two or three peg grafts are used on each side, depending on the thickness of the graft or the width of the disc space. Every effort is then made to pack cancellous strips tightly between the two peg grafts in a manner described as high density cancellous bone grafting. An osteotome is placed between the two peg grafts; prying action of the "Puka" stick is then used for further separation of the space between the peg grafts. A suction tip is then kept in the separated space and a cancellous strip is packed beside it, thus keeping the peg grafts separated by the high density cancellous bone impaction (Figure 123-16A, B, and C).

It is important that all other crevices between the peg grafts or vertebral bodies be filled with cancellous bone. Before insertion of the second central graft, insertion of two to three cancellous strips to the center of the disc space is recommended. The strips are pushed toward the midline to fill all possible spaces between the two central peg grafts. A laminal retractor may be used on the side already packed to facilitate graft insertion on the opposite side. The only tissue in the disc space should be bone graft. Loose or empty spaces will be invaded by fibrous tissue and thus delay osteosynthesis.[39] The

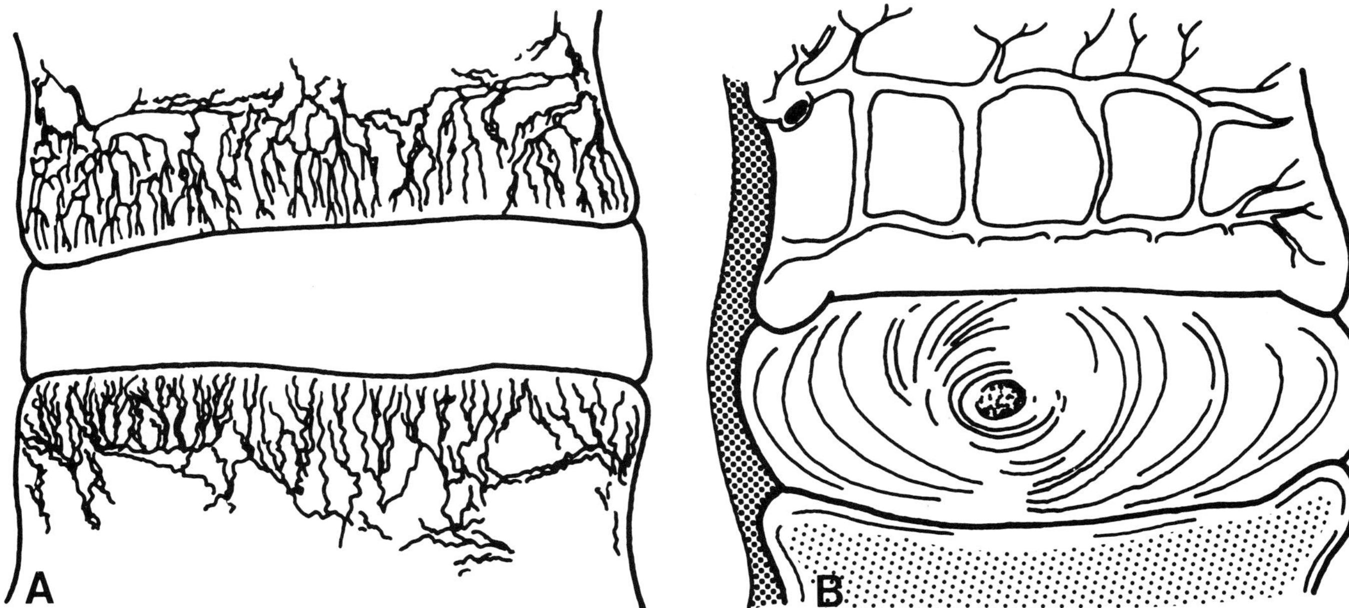

Fig. 123-14. (A) Schematic drawing of the arterial system of the vertebral body.[44] Note the end arteries ending at the cortical end-plates. (B) Schematic drawing of the venous system of the vertebral body.[44] Note the horizontal venous channel situated 2–3 mm below the cortical end-plates. They are the source of brisk bleeding in vigorous decortication.

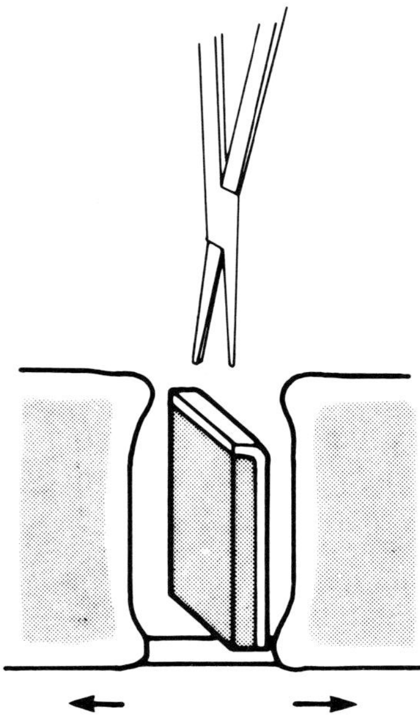

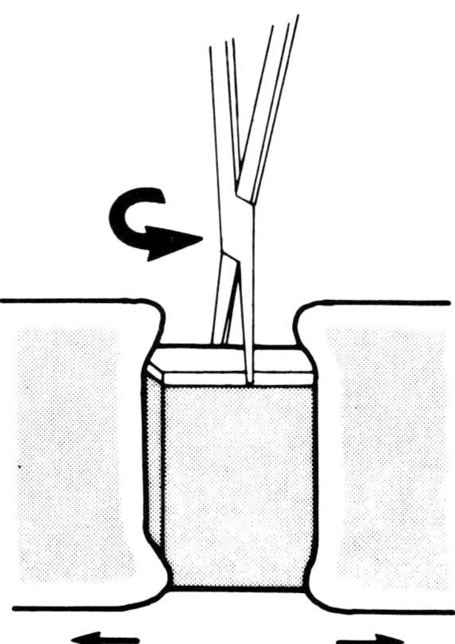

Fig. 123-15. Rotating the graft within the disc space to utilize the keystone locking mechanism. Top. Graft slightly larger than the entrance but smaller than the width of the disc space is in place with cortical plate horizontal to the disc space. Bottom. Graft grasped with disc rongeur is rotated so that the cortical bone is parallel to the longitudinal axis of the body. Graft is now tightly impacted in the disc space underneath the keystoned intervertebral rim.

three most common factors in failure of fusion at this stage are: (1) an inadequate number of grafts; (2) inadequate space within the disc space to accept the grafts; and (3) the presence of spaces between the grafts. The exposed portion of the graft should lie 1 to 2 mm below the surfaces of the adjoining vertebral bodies. When the compression forces are applied in a normal, upright lordotic curvature, the graft is securely locked within the disc space. Locking of the graft may be improved by a slight keystone undercutting below the intervertebral rims (Figure 123-17).

By far the most frequent and serious complication that can arise during graft insertion is breaking off of the cortical end of the lateral graft. The broken pieces are usually pushed laterally

into the intervertebral foramen, where they exert pressure on the intervertebral nerve (Figures 123-18 and 123-19). The intervertebral disc is an oval structure, thus the disc surface is curved; all peg grafts therefore should not lie in a horizontal level. The lateral graft should lie deeper than the central graft. All attempts should be made to avoid compression of the nerve root by a graft that is in place or by a graft that has been displaced from its confinement within the disc space. With adequate foraminal decompression the nerves leaving the intervertebral foramen can be visualized as they pass over the graft and exit freely into the intervertebral foramen.

CLOSURE

After the Surgicel is removed, the epidural space is filled with fat graft or Gelfoam (Upjohn Laboratories, Kalamazoo, Michigan). With the intact midline structures, there is generally no dead space to warrant a drain. However, in a repeat surgical procedure, especially with the absence of the posterior components of the motion segment, the large dead space should be drained by continuous bulb suction. A very strong wound closure can be obtained by suturing the preserved supraspinous ligaments to the adjoining aponeurosis. If the supraspinous ligaments are rudimentary or removed, fixation of the adjoining spinous processes by using a 24-gauge wire through the spinous processes in a double or triple loop figure 8 manner is recommended.

POSTOPERATIVE CARE

1. Antibiotic treatment. I routinely administer antibiotics during operation and for 24 hours after operation. The drug of choice is a cephalosporin.
2. Immobilization. For 4 months the patient should wear a corsetted Knight's lumbar spinal brace with Velcro straps, day and night, except when showering. The patient must be cautioned not to flex the lumbar spine during physical activities. For patients with deficiency or in isthmic spondylolisthesis of the posterior portion of the motion segment, a unilateral hip lock or spica attachment is added to the Knight's brace.
3. Exercise program. Exercise in the form of brisk walking, 6.0 km/hour or faster (4.5 km/hour for females), 6–9 km/day, should be accomplished by the third or fourth month after operation. Half-knee bend exercises are also useful.
4. De-immobilization. Generally, fusion with PLIF occurs about 4 months after surgery. The degree of osteosynthesis is determined routinely from a lateral tomogram. If the fusion is not satisfactory, the bracing is prolonged for 2 to 4 months. The homogeneous mix of the graft with the adjoining vertebral bodies on the tomogram is sufficient evidence of satisfactory osteosynthesis. The patient should then be weaned from the brace. Swimming is a good de-immobilization exercise.
5. Pain control. Methylprednisolone, 40 mg every 12 hours for 2 or 3 days, decreases postoperative discomfort by diminishing tissue edema. Nonsteroidal prostaglandin inhibitors are often used to control postoperative incisional and graft site discomfort during the convalescence period. Intraoperative intrathecal Duromorph (Elkins-Sinn, Inc., Cherry Hill, New Jersey) at a dose of 0.75 mg injected through a 27-gauge needle just before wound closure generally gives

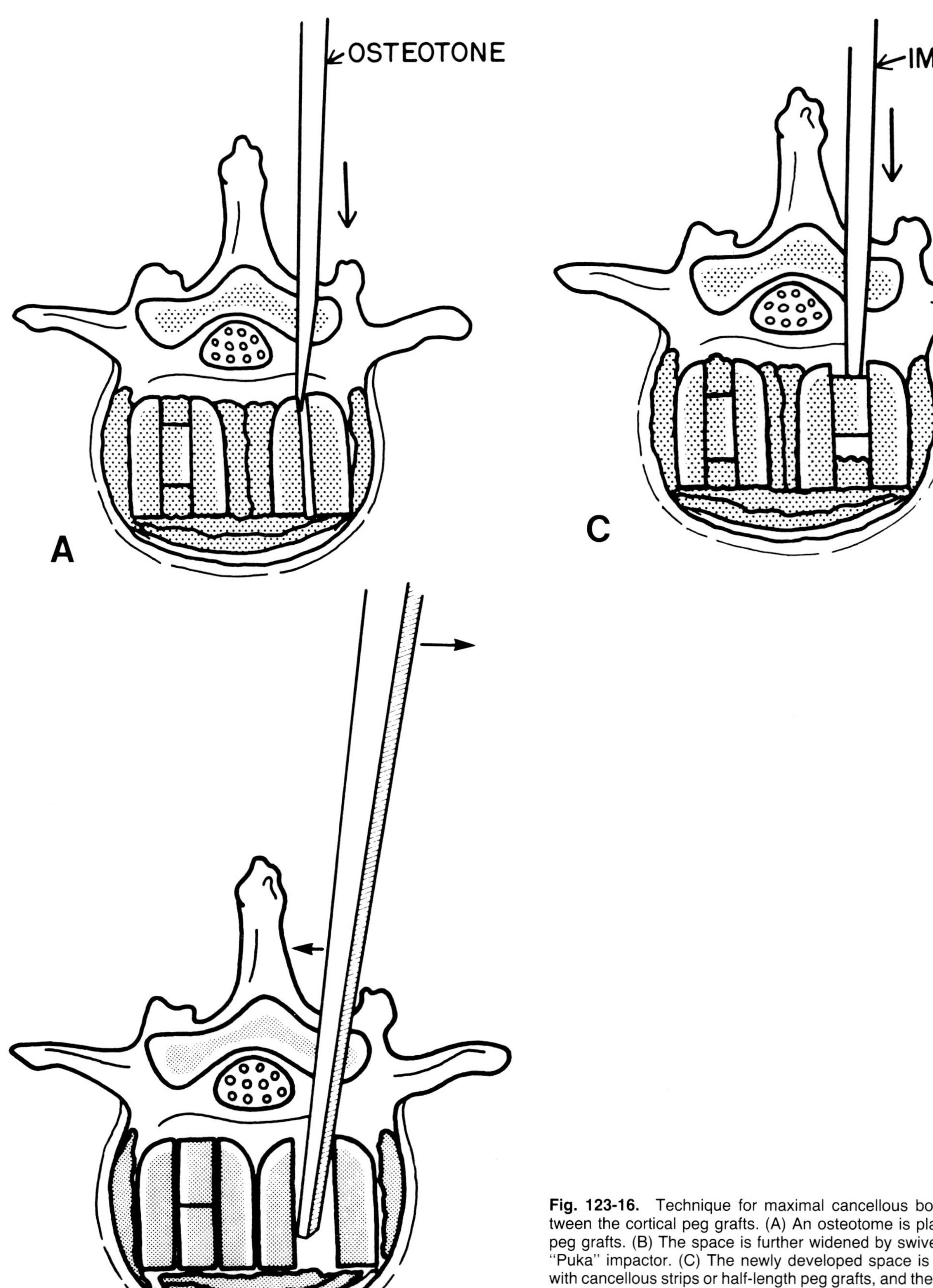

Fig. 123-16. Technique for maximal cancellous bone impaction between the cortical peg grafts. (A) An osteotome is placed between the peg grafts. (B) The space is further widened by swiveling action of the "Puka" impactor. (C) The newly developed space is forcibly impacted with cancellous strips or half-length peg grafts, and they should lie below the surfaces of the adjoining peg grafts. Note that the cancellous bone grafts are already impacted in the lateral recesses at the base of the disc space and the central portion between the two central peg grafts.

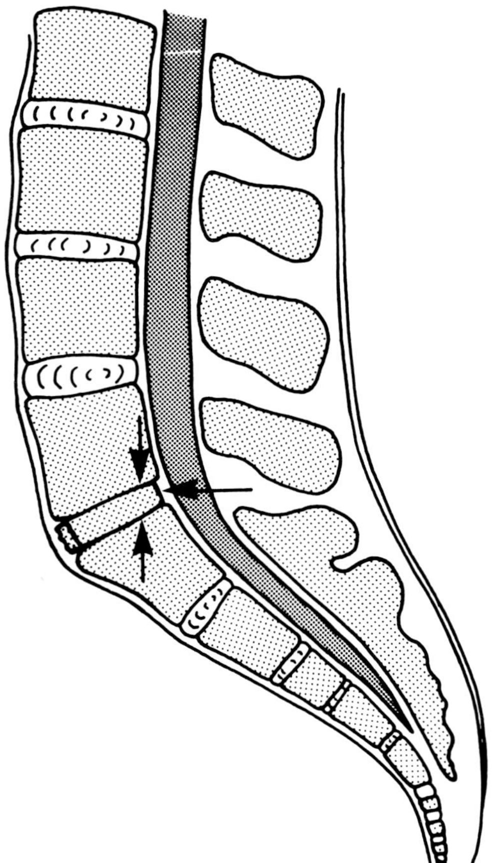

Fig. 123-17. The entrance to the disc space before graft insertion should be smaller than the centrum of the disc space. When the graft is then countersunk below the level of the intervertebral rim, a keystone like locking mechanism develops and it stabilizes the grafts within the disc space.

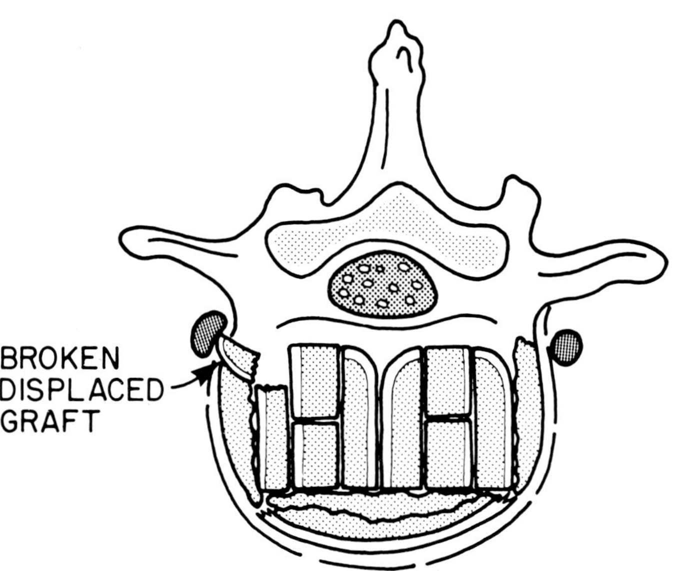

Fig. 123-18. Schematic drawing showing the displaced broken left lateral graft impinging on the nerve within the intervertebral foramen.

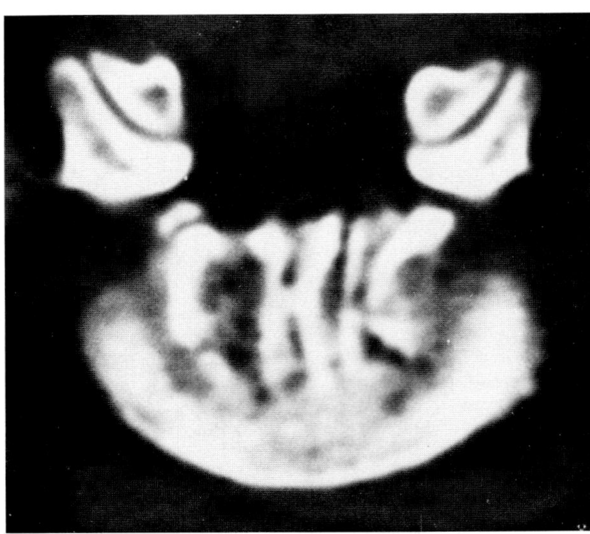

Fig. 123-19. A CT scan of a postoperative PLIF showing the lateral graft impinging into the intervertebral foramen. The lateral grafts should lie lower than the central grafts to conform with the normal oval shape of the intervertebral disc.

the most gratifying pain relief in the first 24 hours. Apnea monitoring has been recommended by the manufacturer.[45]

6. Osteoporosis. Women above the age of 30 begin to develop negative calcium balance. It is therefore imperative that all mature female postoperative patients receive a daily antiosteoporosis regimen such as calcium, 1000–1500 mg, Rocaltrol, 0.25 mg, and sodium fluoride, 10–40 mg.

PITFALLS AND COMPLICATIONS

Pitfalls and complications of PLIF are numerous but mostly avoidable.[14]

INCORRECT LEVEL

When a horizontal incision is used, one must be certain that the sacrum is thoroughly exposed. If a lumbarization or sacralization anomaly is found, the first apparent interlaminal space may not be mobile. In case of doubt, an intraoperative or preoperative verification by roentgenogram is of great help in properly identifying the level. When there is a congenital anomaly of the lumbosacral junction, both anteroposterior and lateral roentgenograms should be obtained.

DISRUPTION OF THE INTEGRITY OF THE POSTERIOR PORTION OF THE MOTION SEGMENT

Only the mesial half of the facet joint is removed by osteotome. However, when the facet joint is rudimentary and mesially located, or when previous surgery was attempted and the integrity of the facet joint would not be preserved, a 24-gauge wire can be used to fix the adjoining spinous processes.

EPIDURAL BLEEDING

Proper positioning of the patient is essential in controlling epidural venous bleeding. Flexion of the lumbar spine can increase the epidural bleeding. We do not flex the patient

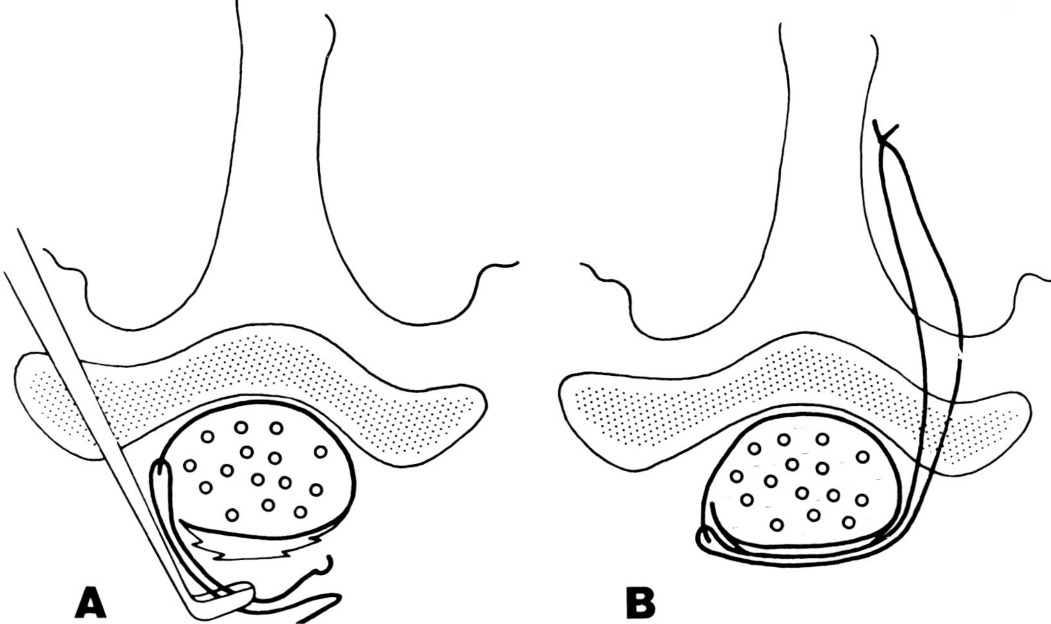

Fig. 123-20. (A) Technique of closing dural defect located on the undersurface of the dural sac. After total discectomy, the silk suture is attached to one end of the dura. (B) The silk is passed below and around the posterior limiting membrane and attached to the muscle or aponeurosis on the opposite side.

because the exposure of the disc space is facilitated by distraction either of the laminae or of the vertebral bodies. Flexion and early distraction of the disc space by a vertebral or laminal spreader will increase the epidural bleeding. The exact cause of this phenomenon is not known. Any support that would decrease the intra-abdominal pressure is helpful in decreasing epidural bleeding.

ADHESION SECONDARY TO PREVIOUS DISC SURGERY

The problem of dissecting the dura and the nerve root free from the surrounding scarred fibrous tissue can be avoided by making the bony exposure lateral to the nerve root through a mesial facetectomy. This would expose the relatively uninvolved lateral recess of the spinal canal. The dissection is continued down to the level of the bony margin of the vertebral body and the disc space. By use of that as a plane of dissection, all the neural tissues are pushed mesially by sharp dissection with a small curved osteotome. Entrance to the disc space can then be achieved through the exposed lateral recess. In most instances, it is advisable to decompress the disc space first before attempting to search for the extruded disc materials. The sonic curette is most useful to free the scar tissue from the bone.

SCLEROTIC CORTICAL END-PLATE

Adequate decortication is most essential in the sclerotic cortical end-plates. There must be adequate vascularization to ensure osteosynthesis. The use of the smaller-sized sonic curette is more effective in decortication of the hard cortical end-plates. Decortication of the deeper portion of the lower cortical end-plate by curetting may be a blind procedure. The surgeon must recognize the changing resistances among the three layers of tissues, i.e., disc, cortical end-plate, and cancellous bone. The latter is usually self-evident when the cancellous

bone chips appear in the curetted material. In order to receive the rectangular shape of peg grafts snugly, the deeper end of the disc space should be sculpted, preferably with a sonic curette or by impacting with a blunt-ended "Puka" stick (Codman and Shurtleff, Inc., Randolph, Massachusetts) to achieve a square-to-square recipient area. Use of Ma's[46] mortised instrumentation heightens the concept of the square-to-square recipient area. Jackson[38] recently advocated the use of a very high speed drill in intradiscoid decortication and sculpturing of a keystone locking mechanism beneath the intervertebral rims.

EXCESSIVE VENOUS BLEEDING FROM CANCELLOUS BONE OF THE VERTEBRAL BODIES

The anatomic location of the large collateral venous channels lying 2 to 3 mm beneath the cortical end-plates dictates that one should avoid deep decortication. Cloward's recommendation of using Gelfoam soaked in double-strength thrombin in contact with the bleeding cancellous bone surface for 1 minute is often effective in controlling venous bleeding in deep cancellous bone.[16]

VASCULAR INJURY

Arterial bleeding in the epidural space should be controlled with bipolar coagulation and hemaclips. I have encountered only one episode of arterial bleeding from the lateral recess of the disc space, presumably arising from a branch of the intervertebral artery in the muscle layer. The arterial bleeding in that case was controlled by Avitene (Alcon Laboratories, Fort Worth, Texas), and the PLIF procedure was safely completed. No major anterior vascular injury has been encountered. The importance of staying behind the anterior limiting membrane and using only side-to-side motion when curetting the deeper area must be stressed. To avoid inadvertent penetration of the anterior limiting membrane, the jaws of the disc

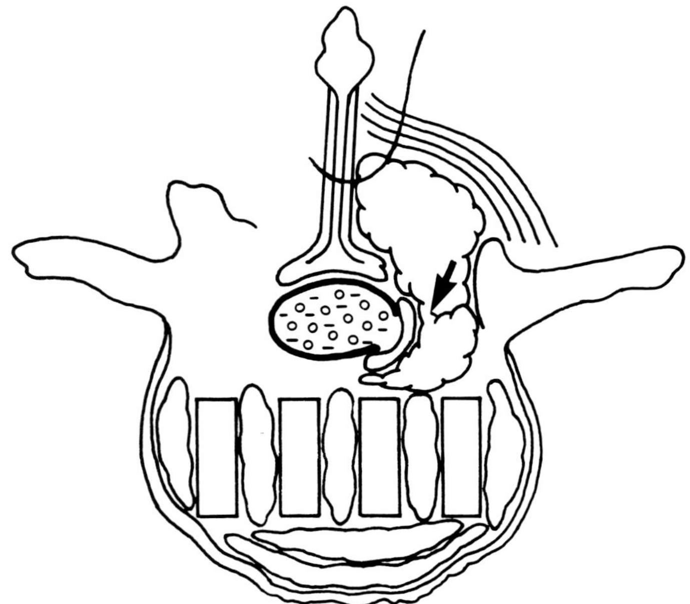

Fig. 123-21. Dural laceration that cannot be repaired by suturing should be covered by Gelfoam or muscle. The epidural space is then packed tightly with a large piece of free fat graft. The fat graft is anchored in place either by a muscle flap or by suturing the overlay muscle to the interspinous ligament.

rongeur must be kept open while approaching the deeper layers of the disc tissue.

CLUNEAL NERVE INJURY AND GRAFT SITE PAIN

The posterior iliac crest should be exposed through a limited exposure; one should undercut beneath the subcutaneous fatty tissue, staying just above the periosteum. This would avoid injury to the cluneal nerve and artery, which lies in a more superficial layer. Strict observation of the subperiosteal dissection technique, and the limited resection of ligaments containing the pain fibers, minimizes the incidence of postoperative graft site discomfort. To obtain the split-thickness posterior iliac bone graft only the lateral half of the ligamentum attachment of the iliac crest need be dissected free.

GRAFT PROTRUSION

All grafts should fit snugly into the recipient area. I favor a peg graft 1 mm smaller than the distracted disc space measurement. The cross-section contour of a disc is an oval one; therefore, the top of the lateral graft must be impacted lower than the central graft. Failure to observe this basic concept is often the cause of postoperative residual root irritation (Figure 123-19). After graft insertion is completed, one must always search very diligently for loose or fragmented bone grafts laterally in the intervertebral foramen. A postoperative CT scan is a learning experience. The PLIF surgeons should appreciate the proper graft site impaction in their early series.

DURAL LACERATION

During the graft insertion, the dura must be protected against the intrusion of the peg graft and the impactor. All dura tears should be repaired with 6-0 silk sutures. The tears along

Table 123-1. Satisfactory results in noncompensation and compensation groups

Pathologic Condition	Noncompensation (%)	Compensation (%)
Narrow disc	79 (65)*	89 (42)
Lateral disc	94 (77)	93 (64)
Midline disc	91 (76)	78 (50)
Recurrent disc	80 (44)	61 (27)
Spinal stenosis	80 (50)	71 (29)
Instability	83 (54)	87 (12)

* Number in parentheses represents number with excellent result.

the nerve root often do not involve the arachnoid layer, and when there is no apparent spinal fluid leakage, suturing is not needed. Dural laceration involving the undersurface of the dural sac can present a technical difficulty. One can repair it, however, by first suturing the visible edge of the dural defect, then passing the suture through the excavated disc space to the opposite side. One should then suture and tie to the muscle, thus effectively obliterating the dural defect (Figure 123-20A and B). If the dura laceration cannot be sutured, then the exposed dura should be covered and packed with Gelfoam or muscle, and the patient should be kept in bed for 2 to 3 weeks.

Obliteration of the epidural space with a large piece of free fat graft secured in place by suturing the overlying muscle tissue to the interspinous ligament is also helpful in controlling the spinal fluid leakage from the dural laceration that cannot be repaired by suturing (Figure 123-21).

PSEUDOARTHRODESIS[12]

If the osteosynthesis is not adequate as demonstrated on the tomogram 4 months after surgery, continuation of immobilization is suggested until satisfactory fusion is seen on repeat roentgenograms. After 9 months, the immobilization therapy can be discontinued in spite of poor radiographic evidence of osteosynthesis. Further treatment, such as a repeat PLIF or lateral intertransverse process fusion, depends on whether the osteofibrous union is symptomatic. Lateral fusion performed for pseudoarthrodesis of PLIF often brings about a solid refusion of the PLIF.

COMPLICATIONS[12]

In the first 500 patients treated with PLIFs the following complications were encountered: A superficial infection developed in one case. There were 24 cases of thrombophlebitis, 21 clinically diagnosed in the hospital (4 verified by venogram) and three clinically diagnosed after discharge from the hospital (1 fatality from pulmonary embolism). Of two cases of myocardial infarction, one was diagnosed 1 week after surgery and the patient recovered, and the other patient died suddenly at home 30 days after surgery.

Neurologic deficits included foot drop in 25 cases, including patients who had preoperative foot drop (12 of these patients needed temporary foot drop braces, and all except 3 improved or recovered in 6 months); urinary incontinence in two cases (1 case was mild and the patient improved, and 1 was moderate and the patient also improved); and anterolateral femoral cutaneous neuritis, generally mild and transient (6 percent of all patients).

Reoperation for immediate graft extrusion was necessary in four cases. Reoperation for the incorrect level of surgery was performed in two cases. Late reoperation for pseudoarthrodesis was performed in 14 cases, re-PLIF in five and lateral fusion in nine (7 of which were in the compensation group).

RESULTS

CLINICAL RESULTS

Four-hundred sixty-five patients who underwent PLIF during a 10-year period from 1972 to 1981 have been evaluated with at least 1 year follow-up[12]; 260 were men and 205 were women. The age distribution peaks were between the third and fourth decades of life for men and during the fourth decade for women.

Clinical results were rated as follows. An excellent result indicated complete recovery, resumption of normal activity, and no medication for pain. Patients who had good results returned to work, took occasional mild analgesics, and enjoyed work and recreation activities. Patients in whom results were rated as fair worked with discomfort, took occasional medication, and improved after surgery. Patients who had poor results required medication in a dependent fashion, were unable to return to work, and denied any improvement.

For purposes of clinical evaluation, excellent and good results are considered satisfactory. Fair and poor results are considered unsatisfactory. Since PLIF was done in a variety of cases, evaluation of results was based on the varying pathologic conditions. Discogenic disorders were classified as: (1) spondylosis with narrow disc space (113 patients), (2) lateral herniated disc (62 patients); (3) midline herniated disc (158 patients); and (4) recurrent disc (143 patients). Also included were spinal stenosis (71 patients) and various types of spinal instability (43 patients), including spondylolisthesis with spondylolysis of the pars interarticularis (12 patients).

The number evaluated by diagnosis (590) is higher than the total number of patients (465) because some patients had two different diagnoses concurrently. Overall, satisfactory results were obtained in 485 cases, 82 percent (excellent, 56 percent). Satisfactory results are distributed as follows: narrow disc, 91 patients, 81 percent (excellent, 61 percent); lateral disc, 58 patients, 94 percent (excellent, 74 percent); midline disc, 139 patients, 88 percent (excellent, 70 percent); recurrent disc, 106 patients, 74 percent (excellent, 35 percent); spinal stenosis, 55 patients, 74 percent (excellent, 48 percent); and instability, 36 patients, 83 percent (excellent, 46 percent).

In the present series of 465 cases there were 111 Workmens' Compensation cases and 30 litigation-pending cases, a total of 141 (31 percent) with secondary gain problems.

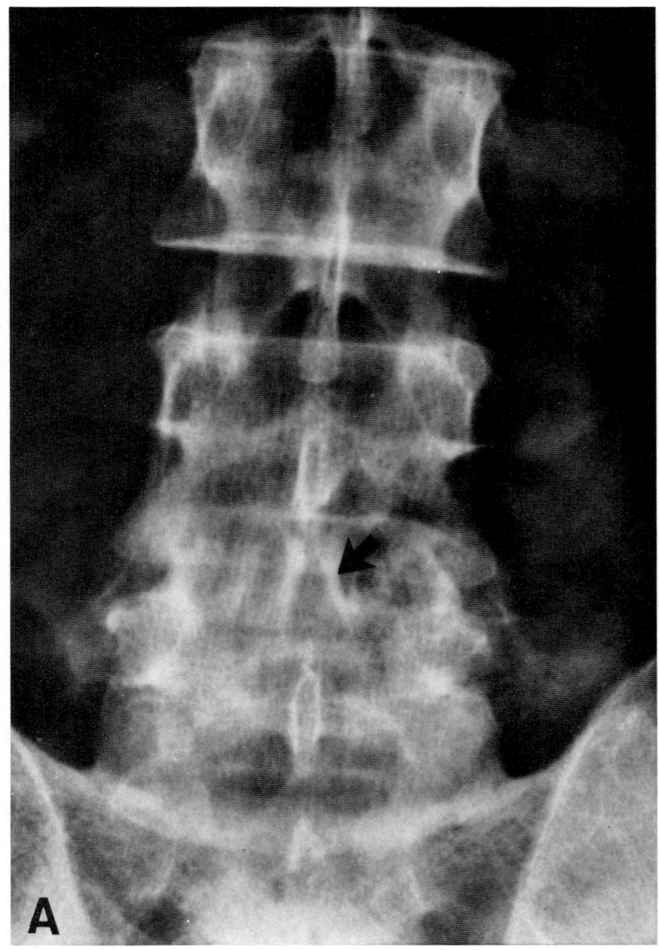
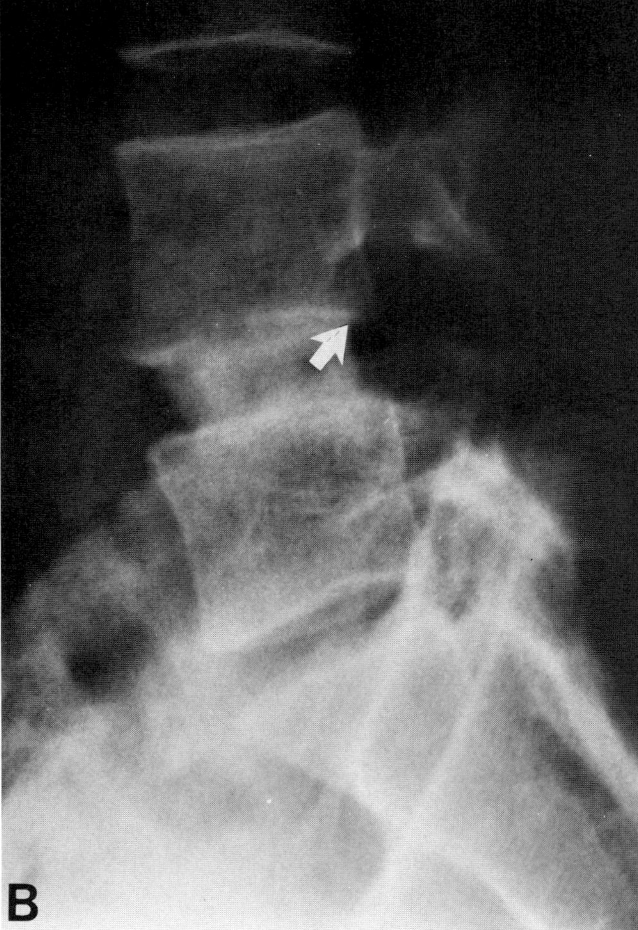

Fig. 123-22.   Satisfactory PLIF at L4-5 interspace, 4 months after surgery. (A) AP and (B) lateral roentgenograms.

Table 123-2. Functional result in the noncompensation and compensation groups (431 patients)

Functional Result	Noncompensation (%)	Compensation (%)
Full duty (262 patients; 61%)	71	39
Light duty (139 patients; 31%)	24	50
Total disability (30 patients; 7%)	5	11

All of these cases were categorized in the compensation group. When excellent results were separated from the statistic of satisfactory results, the compensation group fared less favorably. Satisfactory results for the noncompensation and compensation groups are shown in Table 123-1.

Clinical evaluation was compared with clinical results as assessed by the patients by questionnaire. Of the 465 patients operated on, only 380 were private patients. Of the 380 questionnaires sent to this selected group, 245 were returned, a response rate of 61.5 percent. Two-hundred-twenty-three patients (90.1 percent) reported satisfactory results and 22 (9.9 percent) unsatisfactory results. A fair correlation appears to exist between the clinical evaluation and the patients' evaluation through the questionnaire.

FUNCTIONAL RESULTS

In terms of patients' ability to return to work, there were 431 cases in which the functional result was obtainable. Of these 431, 298 were noncompensation and 133 were compensation cases. Results are shown in Table 123-2.

FUSION RATE

Fusion as evaluated on lateral radiographic tomograms 4 months after surgery was rated on a scale from IV to I: IV = total assimilation between the graft and cortical end-plates; III = 75 percent assimilation of the graft and cortical end-plates; II = 50 percent or less assimilation of the graft or cortical end-plates; and I = disintegration of the graft and settlement of the disc space pseudoarthrodesis.

Ratings of IV and III are considered satisfactory fusion, while II and I are considered unsatisfactory fusion (Figures 123-22A and B and 123-23A and B).

Of 465 patients, 378 had one-level interbody fusion, 84 had two-level fusion, and three had three-level fusion. In eight cases the second level of fusion was done by the lateral fusion technique.

Fusion ratings were obtainable in 440 of 465 cases. Overall, satisfactory results were obtained in 88 percent of patients. Again, the results are divided by pathologic condition. Satisfactory fusion (ratings of IV or III) was distributed as follows: narrow disc, 107 patients (79 percent); lateral disc, 61 patients (98 percent); midline disc, 143 patients (93 percent); recurrent disc, 149 patients (92 percent); spinal stenosis, 69 patients (93 percent), instability, 43 patients (77 percent); and spondylolisthesis with spondylosis, 12 patients (83 percent).

A recent series of 50 consecutive PLIFs done for spondylolysis with spondylolisthesis shows a 73 percent satisfactory result (excellent or good) and if the 47 percent compensation cases are excluded then the percentage increases to 89 percent. A satisfactory fusion rating was obtained in 78 percent of cases, but if the repeated operations are excluded then the satisfactory rating rises to 87 percent. When PLIFs were done with a simultaneous lateral intertransverse process fusion and a

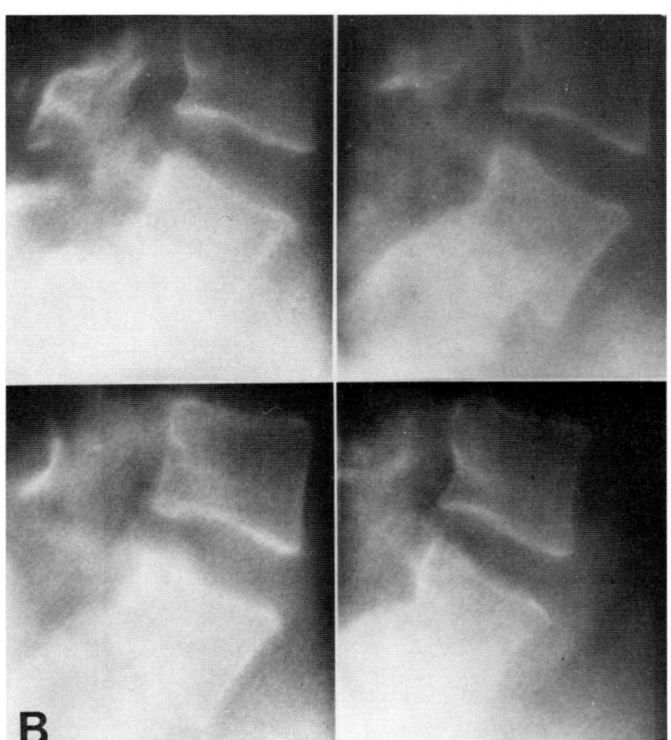

Fig. 123-23. Satisfactory lateral tomogram 4 months after PLIF surgery. (A) L-4 PLIF. Note the keystone locking mechanism at the intervertebral rim. (B) L-5 PLIF for grade I isthmic spondylolisthesis. The smooth line between posterior vertebral bodies and the graft suggests solid fusion.

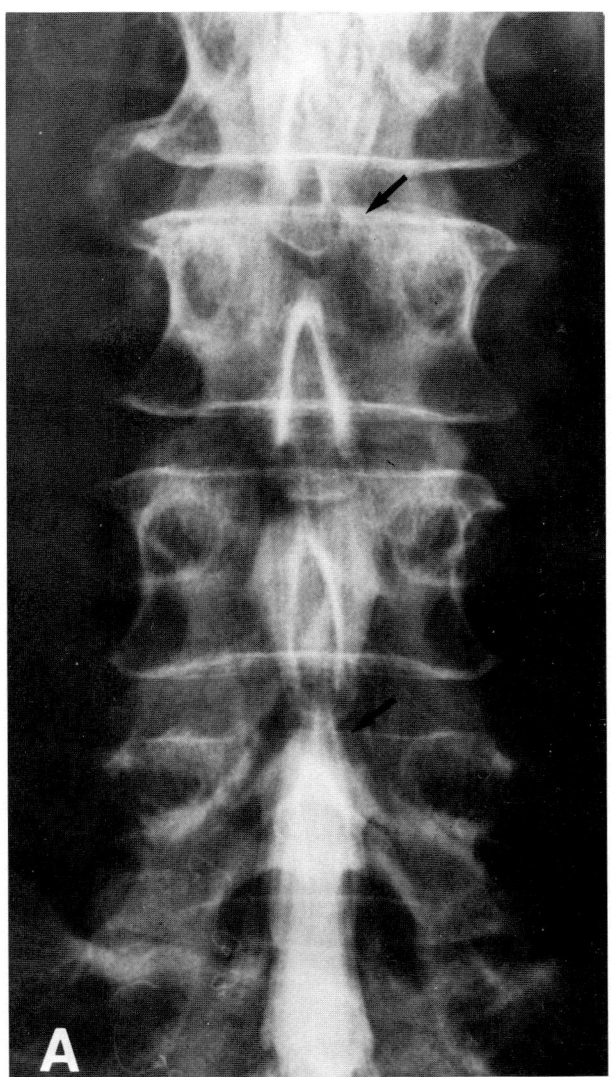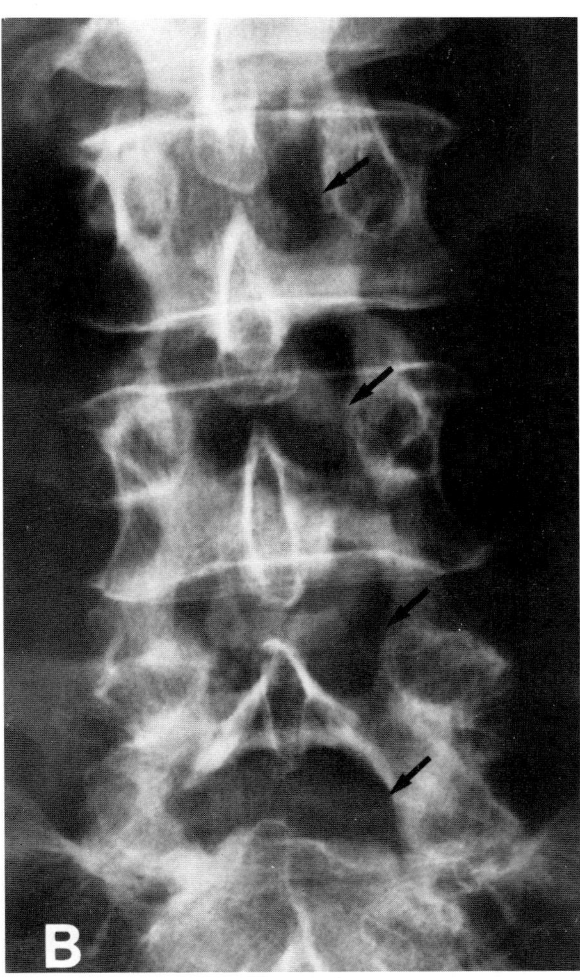

Fig. 123-24. (A) AP myelogram showing multiple levels of lumbar spinal stenosis at L-2, 3, 4, and 5. (B) Postoperative AP roentgenogram showing effect of internal decompression for spinal stenosis (IDSS) at L-2, 3, 4, and 5 (arrows). Note preservation of the spinous processes and the facets' integrity.

unilateral spica process fusion and a unilateral spica brace (19 cases), the clinical results in that smaller series were all satisfactory (excellent and good), and those with a satisfactory fusion rating were 94 percent.

In 7 cases the fusion rating improved with time, and in 10 cases the fusion rating regressed. Thus, the 4-month postoperative tomogram prediction of accuracy for long-term osteosynthesis was better than 96 percent.

Comparison of the fusion rate in 100 cases of L4-L5 PLIF and a similar 100 cases of L5-S1 PLIF revealed no differences. Results were excellent (IV) in 73 percent of patients in both groups. The fusion success rate apparently is not influenced by the anatomic level of the PLIF.

Twenty-five patients in the present study were considered obese (35 kg greater than ideal body weight). Six of these patients were men and 19 were women. In this group the 11 women who had primary discogenic disease all had excellent results.

Previous studies[15] indicated that the fusion rating is not directly related to functional return in the compensation group. However, solid fusion appears to be a prerequisite for excellent results in the noncompensation group. The present study sup-

ports this conclusion. The improved clinical results and fusion rating of the present, larger series are the result of strict adherence during the past 4 years to the four basic biomechanical principles discussed in the introduction to this paper.

DISCUSSION

Posterior lumbar interbody fusion decompresses neural elements, distracts the vertebral bodies and stabilizes the lumbar motion segment. It thus complies with criteria of an ideal surgical procedure for lumbar spondylosis. With the definition of segmental instability expanded to include anatomic loss, dynamic malalignment, and functional instability, the concept of a segmental fusion should be more acceptable to neurosurgeons, at least conceptually.[13,19,27,28,37,38,40-43,46]

Normally, in patients who undergo discectomy, variable degrees of settlement of the motion segment do develop and pave the way to postdiscectomy spondylosis and lateral spinal stenosis.[47,48] In younger patients PLIF would appear to be the procedure of choice as definitive treatment for lateral spinal

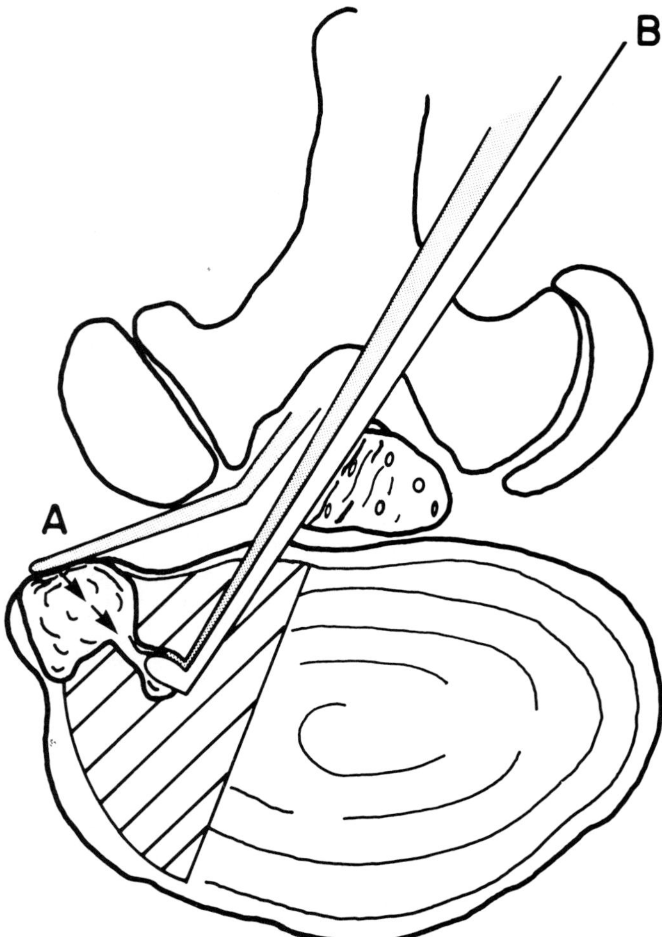

Fig. 123-25. Retrograde extraction of an extreme lateral disc herniation. After radical discectomy of the lateral recess, the surgeon standing on the opposite side of the table can push the disc down (A) and extract the extreme lateral disc herniation in a retrograde manner (B).

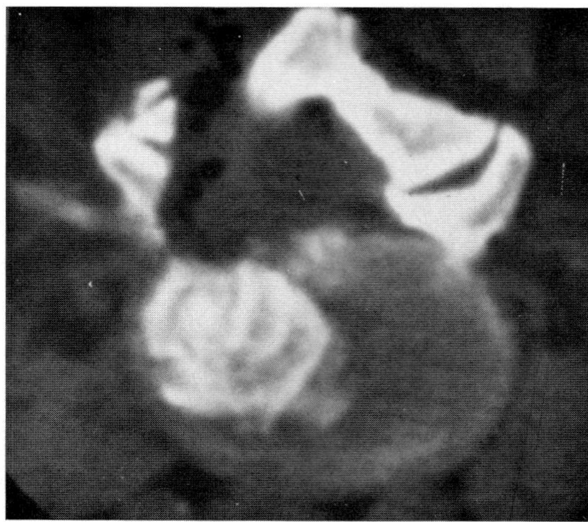

Fig. 123-26. Left unilateral PLIF showing less than 50 percent disc space replacement.

stenosis (subarticular and foraminal stenosis), with or without associated lumbar disc herniation. This is a valuable, logical option, in contrast to the conventional treatment of spondylosis with lateral spinal stenosis by wide decompressive laminectomy or facetectomy, with or without lateral lumbar spinal fusion. The other significant advantage of PLIF is the higher rate of successful single-level fusion in levels above the L5-S1 segments (floating fusion).

The graft in a successful PLIF assumes the physiologic functions of the adjoining osseous structures. The bone graft in the disc space frequently grows anteriorly up to the anterior limiting membrane and fills the entire disc space, conforming to the adjoining bony contour. The growing graft does not protrude beyond either the anterior or posterior limiting membrane. Frequently, AP roentgenograms of mature PLIFs show increased bone density along the interpedicular line, presumably the line of stress. A CT scan of a mature PLIF shows the normal anatomic features of a vertebral body. The grafts reorganize and present cancellous marrow in the centrum surrounded by a dense cortical ring in the periphery. In a very matured graft (3 years or over) a double ring phenomena of two cortical layers can be differentiated (Figures 123-3A and B and 123-5A and B).

Spinal canal stenosis is a frequent late complication of posterolateral lumbar spinal fusion. I have not noted this in

PLIF. However, evidence of foraminal stenosis occurring 6 years after a successful and solid PLIF was noted recently in one case.

In the present series of 465 cases, postoperative lateral tomograms 4 months after the operation were obtained in 107 cases of spondylosis with a narrowed disc space. The satisfactory fusion results in this group were only 79 percent. The lower fusion rating is the result of the earlier technique of inadequate decortication of the sclerotic cortical end-plates. Moreover, the cancellous grafts were not impacted in the high density fashion as advocated by the current A-O system for treatment of nonunion fracture.[27] With the advent of the sonic curette and stricter adherence to the four biomechanical principles needed for successful PLIF, in 1981 a successful fusion rate was obtained in all of the 15 patients with a narrow degenerative disc space.

My technique for obtaining graft involves subperiosteal removal of a split-thickness unicortical graft from the posterior iliac crest along with an equal volume of cancellous bone. Therefore, postoperative graft site discomfort should be no greater than the pain observed after other types of posterolateral fusion.

Lumbar interbody fusion has been found effective in the treatment of back pain with or without radicular symptoms. Forty-six patients in the present series were in this category, and results were excellent in 35 and good in 6, giving 89 percent satisfactory results. This compares favorably with relief of back pain by anterior lumbar interbody fusion, as reported by Chow et al.[1] (89 percent) and Goldnor et al.[49] (78 percent). A patient with single-level spondylosis and chronic intractable back pain should be considered as a reasonable surgical candidate for PLIF.

A secondary gain in the development of PLIF has been better understanding of the treatment of lumbar spinal stenosis. The technique developed for exposing the disc space, i.e., inferior and superior laminotomy, inferior and superior mesial facetectomy, and thorough decompression of the intervertebral foramen with visualization of the nerve root freely leaving the foramen, is quite adequate for relieving segmental spinal stenosis without sacrificing the integrity of the posterior motion segment. This decompressive procedure could be repeated at multiple levels and can be accurately described as an internal decompression for spinal stenosis (IDSS).[50] The postoperative instability observed in wide decompressive laminectomy at one level, and particularly at multiple levels, should be avoided. Fusion is not attempted for pathologic conditions at multiple levels. However, if instability exists, wire fixation of multiple spinous processes is recommended (Figure 123-24).

Another gain from the development of PLIF is the transdiscoid approach to the extreme lateral disc herniation, also known as paralateral or foraminal disc herniation (5 percent incidence in our series). Radical discectomy of the superior lateral recess can afford a space whereby the extruded extreme lateral disc can be pushed into the disc space and be removed in a retrograde manner (Figure 123-25). For better visualization the surgeon must stand on the other side of the table. Transdiscoidal approach for the extreme lateral disc in the foramen affords dissection underneath the facet without the need of disruptive total facetectomy. In a series of 17 cases operated in a 24-month period during 1983–1985, we were able to extract successfully 16 cases of extreme lateral disc by transdiscoidal approach without total facetectomy.

Massive midline disc should be removed in a similar manner, namely an initial radical discectomy bilaterally before the herniated massive disc fragment is extracted downward into the excavated disc space. This would avoid undue pressure from retraction of the neural elements. In these cases of massive disc debulkment we recommend PLIF.

Unilateral PLIFs were performed on 5 patients. Impaction of the bone graft up to 50 percent of the disc area had been attempted (Figure 123-26). We do not have an adequate series to warrant a definitive comment as to whether it can replace the total bilateral PLIFs. The fusion rate for total PLIF even in expert hands is around 90 percent. Blume[51,52] advocated unilateral PLIF with dowel technique, however, unless one can consistently replace more than 50 percent of the total disc space with bone grafts through a unilateral approach, in which case a replacement of more than 50 percent by the bilateral route would be preferred.

As a result of solid fusion at one level the degenerative changes of the adjoining motion segment would be enhanced as a result of increased stress and motion. In the present series only 14 patients required subsequent fusion at an adjoining level, above or below the previous PLIF. One patient required fusion two levels above the previously fused area. It does not appear that PLIF increased degenerative changes of the adjoining motion segment to any significant degree in the present series. However, this observation may be skewed, since we strongly advocate absolute avoidance of flexion of the lumbar spine after the surgery.

The increasing application of chemonucleolysis in the treatment of discogenic disease may lead to the frequent application of PLIF as a salvage procedure.[4,13] Chemonucleolysis, by its nature of disc dissolution or disc debulking, frequently produces persistent postinjection back pain, apparently secondary to settlement of the disc space, and increased segmental instability. Sepulveda indicated that in his series of 56 patients who had undergone chymopapain lumbar disc injections, 10 had persistent back pain and had developed instability. Symptoms in all of these patients were satisfactorily relieved by PLIF.[5]

In female patients with osteoporosis the potential benefits of PLIF may be negated by delayed osteosynthesis in the disc space, which often results in disc space settlement and poor clinical result.[15] Aggressive antiosteoporotic treatments with cyclic hormonal replacement, calcium, Rocaltrol and fluoride appears to be helpful.

Employment of the intraoperative intrathecal morphine therapy (0.75 mg Duromorphine) has consistently produced dramatic pain reduction during the first two postoperative days. Patients' positive attitude from the reduction of suffering during the immediate postoperative period may well affect the eventual clinical result from a procedure designed to reduce chronic low back pain.

Posterior lumbar interbody fusion is not presented as an easy technical procedure. On logical grounds, it must be assumed that fusion by this approach is superior to the more formidable transabdominal anterior interbody fusion. If the interbody fusion is done by the posterior approach the nerve roots can be adequately inspected and decompressed, and the fusion rate is at least as good as that of lateral or posterolateral spinal fusion. The delayed acceptance of this procedure is probably due to technical difficulties and the inability to obtain consistent bony fusion. Jackson recently introduced very high speed drill technology into the PLIF procedure to facilitate the decortication and undercutting of the intervertebral rims.[38] He also utilizes the very osteogenetic bone dusts produced from the drilling and fills them in all crevices after the homologous grafts are in place within the disc space. It is hoped that with increased interest in the PLIF and further refinement in technology similar to Jackson's innovative contribution, PLIF will be established as a standard surgical armamentarium for a spinal surgeon.

It is urged that those who attempt this procedure should not proceed directly without either studying carefully the available video tapes or practicing on a cadaver. Most importantly, the inexperienced surgeon should understudy those who have done this procedure previously.

REFERENCES

1. Chow SP, Leong JCY, Yau AC: Anterior spinal fusion for deranged lumbar intervertebral disc. Spine 5:452, 1980
2. Lunsford LD, Bissanetter DF, Janetta PF, Shiptake PE, Zorub DS: Anterior surgery for spinal disc diseases. J Neurosurg 53:1, 1980
3. Schneck, CD: The anatomy of lumbar spondylosis. Clin Orthop 193:20, 1985
4. Lin PM: Post chemonucleolysis instability treated with PLIF. Alternatives in Spinal Surgery 2:6, 1985
5. Sepulveda, R, Kant AP: Chemonucleolysis failures treated by PLIF. Clin Orthop 193:68, 1985
6. Adams MA, Hutton WC: The relevance of torsion to the mechanical derangement of the lumbar spine. Spine 6:241, 1981
7. Cloward RB: Modifications of PLIF for spinal stenosis, in Lin PM (ed): Posterior Lumbar Interbody Fusion. Springfield, Ill, Charles C Thomas, 1982, p 140
8. Hutter CG: Spinal stenosis and PLIF. Clin Orthop 193:103, 1985
9. Lin PM: Posterior lumbar interbody fusion, in Sweet WH, Schmidek HH (eds): Current Techniques in Operative Neurosurgery, vol 2. New York, Grune & Stratton, 1982, p 1339
10. Lin PM: Introduction of PLIF: Biomechanical principles and indications, in Lin PM (ed): Posterior Lumbar Interbody Fusion. Springfield, Ill, Charles C Thomas, 1981, p 1
11. Lin PM: Applications of PLIF in lateral spinal stenosis, in Lin PM: Posterior Lumbar Interbody Fusion. Springfield, Ill, Charles C Thomas, 1982, p 178
12. Lin PM, Cautilli RA, Joyce MF: Posterior lumbar interbody fusion. Clin Orthop 180:154, 1983

13. Lin PM: PLIF symposium, Editorial comment. Clin Orthop 193:90, 1985

14. Lin PM: PLIF complications and pitfalls. Clin Orthop 193:90, 1985

15. Lin PM, Cautilli RA, Joyce MF: Posterior lumbar interbody fusion. J Neurosurg Orthop Surg 1:1, 1979

16. Cloward RB: Technique of posterior lumbar interbody fusion, in Lin PM (ed): Posterior Lumbar Interbody Fusion. Springfield, Ill, Charles C Thomas, 1982, p 140

17. Cloward RB: Long term result of PLIF, in Lin PM (ed): Posterior Lumbar Interbody Fusion. Springfield, Ill, Charles C Thomas, 1982, p 161

18. Lin PM: Posterior lumbar interbody fusion, in Cauthen J (ed): Lumbar Spine Surgery. Baltimore, Williams & Wilkins, 1982, p 105

19. Keim HA: Indication for spinal fusion and techniques. Clin Neurosurg 25:266, 1977

20. Larson S: Biomechanical principles of lumbar stabilization procedures, in Lin PM (ed): Posterior Lumbar Interbody Fusion. Springfield, Ill, Charles C Thomas, 1982, p 72

21. Lin PM: A technical modification of Cloward's posterior lumbar interbody fusion. J Neurosurg 1:118, 1977

22. Wiltse LL: Spinal fusion in intervertebral joint disease, in Cauthen J (ed): Lumbar Spine Surgery. Baltimore, Williams & Wilkins, 1982, p 128

23. Wiltse LL, Kirkaldy-Willis WH, McIvor GWD: The treatment if spinal stenosis. Clin Orthop 115:83, 1976

24. Cautilli RA: Theoretical superiority of PLIF, in Lin PM (ed): Posterior Lumbar Interbody Fusion. Springfield, Ill, Charles C Thomas, 1982, p 82

25. Evans JH: Biomechanics of lumbar fusion. Clin Orthop 193:38, 1985

26. Lin PM: Technique of posterior lumbar interbody fusion, in Lin PM (ed): Posterior Lumbar Interbody Fusion. Springfield, Ill, Charles C Thomas, 1982, p 94

27. Schlegel KF, Pon A: The biomechanics of PLIF in spondylolisthesis. Clin Orthop 193:115, 1985

28. Rathke FW, Schlegel KF: Operation of the lumbar spine. Atlas of Orthopaedic Operations, vol 1. Philadelphia, WB Saunders, 1977

29. Rathke FW, Walker N: Indications, technique and result of PLIF. Presented at the First International Symposium on PLIF, Philadelphia, 1983

30. Bunnel WP: Anterior spinal fusion: Experimental evaluation of technique. J Pediatr Orthop 1:469, 1982

31. Edmonson AS, Crenshaw AH (eds): Campbell's Operative Orthopedics. St. Louis, CV Mosby, 1980, p 21

32. Burwell RG: The function of bone marrow in the incorporation of a bone graft. Clin Orthop 200:125, 1985

33. Urist MR: Bone transplantation, in Urist MR (ed) Fundamental and Clinical Bone Physiology. Philadelphia, JB Lippincott, 1980 pp 331–368

34. Simmons JW: PLIF with posterior elements as chip grafts. Clin Orthop 193:85, 1985

35. Rothman SLG, Glenn WV: CT evaluation of interbody fusion. Clin Orthop 193:47, 1985

36. Robinson RA, Smith GW: Anterolateral cervical disc removal and interbody fusion for cervical disc syndrome. Bull Johns Hopkins Hosp 96:223, 1955

37. Hutter CG: Posterior lumbar interbody fusion, 500 cases with 25 year followup. Clin Orthop 179:86 1983

38. Jackson J: Alternative technique in PLIF. Presented at Challenge of the Lumbar Spine. December, 1–3, 1984, New Orleans

39. McNab I: Backache. Baltimore, Williams & Wilkins, 1977, p 166

40. Cloward RB: New treatment of ruptured intervertebral disc. Presented at the Annual Meeting of the Hawaii Territorial Medical Association, 1945

41. Cloward RB: The treatment of ruptured lumbar intervertebral discs by vertebral body fusion. Indications, operative technique, aftercare. J Neurosurg 10:154, 1953

42. Cloward RB: Lesions of the intervertebral discs and their treatment by interbody fusion methods. The painful disc. Clin Orthop 27:51, 1963

43. Cloward RB: History of PLIF—Forty years of personal experience, in Lin PM (ed): Posterior Lumbar Interbody Fusion. Springfield, Ill, Charles C Thomas, 1982, p 58

44. Crock HV: Practice of Spinal Surgery. New York, Springer-Verlag, 1983, p 58

45. O'Neill P, Knickenberg C, Bogahalanda S, et al: Use of intrathecal morphine for post operative pain relief following lumbar spine surgery. J Neurosurg 63:413, 1985

46. Ma G: Post lumbar interbody fusion with specialized instruments. Clin Orthop 193:57, 1985

47. Epstein JA: The role of spinal fusion. Spine 6:281, 1981

48. Epstein JA, Epstein BS, Lavine LS, et al: Degenerative spondylolisthesis with an intact neural arch (pseudo-arthrodesis). J Neurosurg 44:139, 1976

49. Goldner JS, Wood KE, Urbaniak JR: Anterior discectomy and interbody fusion, in Sweet WH, Schmidek HH (eds): Current Techniques in Operative Neurosurgery, vol 2. New York, Grune & Stratton, 1982, p 1373

50. Lin PM: Internal decompression for multiple levels of lumbar spinal stenosis—A technical note. Neurosurgery 11:546, 1982

51. Blume HG: Unilateral lumbar interbody fusion (posterior approach) utilizing dowel grafts: Experience in over 200 patients. J Neurosurg Orthop Surg 2: 171, 1981

52. Blume HG: Unilateral lumbar interbody fusion by posterior approach with dowel grafts, in Lin PM (ed): Posterior Lumbar Interbody Fusion. Springfield, Ill, Charles C Thomas, 1982, p 252

CHAPTER 124

Anterior Lumbar Discectomy and Interbody Fusion: Indications and Technique

J. Leonard Goldner
James R. Urbaniak

Kenneth E. Wood

IF SPINAL FUSION is occasionally required for the management of patients with intervertebral disc disease, then anterior lumbar discectomy and fusion have a place in the management of patients with chronic low-back pain. We believe that regardless of the technique used, certain patients are relieved of pain if the spine is stabilized. After one operation has failed to relieve intervertebral disc symptoms, fusion of the spine should be seriously considered as a part of the second operative procedure. This is a generality and exceptions do exist, but that philosophy has been helpful in managing patients with recurrent low-back pain who are candidates for operative treatment.

Those who believe in anterior cervical discectomy and fusion should also recognize the value of the same procedure in the lower lumbar and lumbosacral segments. Removal of an intervertebral disc by the anterior approach in either the cervical or lumbar regions will decompress nerve roots without actually manipulating them. Immobilization is almost complete immediately postoperatively, and relief of nerve-root irritation is, temporarily, prompt.

The anterior procedure is not currently popular. It is reserved for salvage patients and is considered a last resort. Our experience is that it will resolve the problem of failed discectomy at one or two interspaces, and that it might be the procedure of choice in certain patients before posterolateral fusion, and certainly before wide extensive laminectomy is done posteriorly to relieve patients who have nerve-root irritation and who do not have free fragments compressing the roots.

HISTORICAL REVIEW

Anterior lumbosacral fusion was first used in the mid-1930s for spondylolisthesis.[1–5] In 1948[6] the procedure was used for lumbosacral intervertebral disc disease.

Sacks,[7] in 1961, reported 150 patients treated by anterior arthrodesis. He stated that 26 percent of these patients were asymptomatic, 62 percent were improved, and 12 percent were unchanged. In 1970, the same author[4] indicated that the functional results of the anterior lumbar fusion series were ''about the same,'' as those for his posterolateral fusion series. Our experience has been similar. The arthrodesis rate of posterolat-

eral fusions at Duke University Medical Center is only slightly better than the rate of healing of anterior interbody fusion.[8–10]

In 1972, Stauffer and Coventry[11] reported on 77 patients treated by anterior lumbar fusion. They observed a single interspace fusion rate of 68 percent and reported 36 percent ''good clinical results.'' They stated that they reserved the procedure for salvage. They do not indicate why 64 percent were considered failures.

Kotcamp[12,13] has used anterior lumbar fusion in the management of over 500 patients. He stated that he frequently uses this operation as a primary method of managing discectomy, and indicates that he has observed a fusion rate of 90 percent for a single interspace.

Several years ago the results of this procedure and the fusion rate obtained by authors using calf bone[14–16] and by a technique using circular plug grafts were thought to be very high. Harmon[17] has altered his reported technique and more recently has obtained a higher fusion rate by using fibular graft and screw fixation.

INDICATIONS FOR ANTERIOR DISCECTOMY AND LUMBAR FUSION

The nonoperative treatment of intervertebral disc disease has a high priority in our management of patients with chronic low-back pain. We apply all currently available nonoperative techniques in an effort to ''avoid the first operative procedure.'' If this treatment fails, then posterior nerve-root decompression and hemilaminectomy after myelography is the program selected for treating the patient with persistent radiculopathy. If this treatment fails, then reoperation and possibly posterolateral fusion are considered. The latter approach depends on whether or not the nerve roots require re-exploration and further decompression or whether the interspace, proximally or distally, requires exploration. Patients in this first category also have been managed by anterior discectomy and fusion. They have had one or more prior operations, but pain has not been relieved.[8–10]

A second group of patients may have persistent pseudoarthrosis if fusion has been attempted, or instability,

OPERATIVE NEUROSURGICAL TECHNIQUES
ISBN 0-8089-1862-1

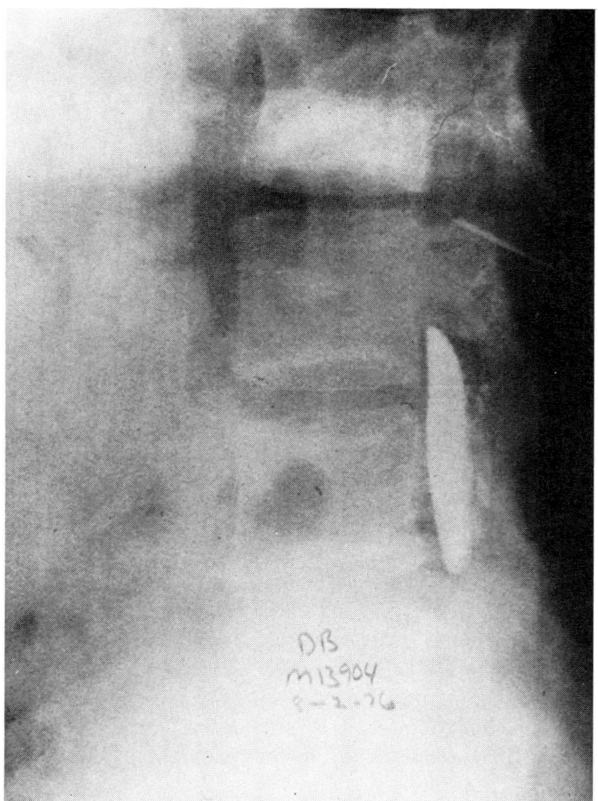

Fig. 124-1. A lateral x-ray film of a 20-year-old man who has had three operative procedures of discectomy and hemilaminectomy for management of pain in the back and lower extremity. This myelogram shows the column of contrast blocked at the L4-5 interspace. Two years have elapsed since the original operation was done. The patient was almost completely incapacitated because of the pain in his back and lower extremity.

incongruity, or nerve-root irritation secondary to specific pathologic conditions.

A third group is the fourth-decade woman with a narrow lumbosacral joint, sclerosis of the interspaces, chronic severe low-back pain, and intermittent radiculopathy. The myelogram usually has been negative, but the patient does have evidence of buttock, thigh, and calf pain. Anterior discectomy and fusion usually relieve the back pain and radiculopathy without interfering with the nerve roots.

A fourth indication is seen in patients who have had posterior operations and developed infection. Persistent back pain and radiculopathy in these patients should be managed by anterior removal of the residual intervertebral disc material and localized arthrodesis. The interspace may or may not have been affected by the prior infection, but tissue usually is sterile after antibiotic therapy has been given.

The fifth group includes patients who have had posterolateral fusion and laminectomy for management of spondylolisthesis and who still have pain and pseudoarthrosis. They usually can be managed successfully by anterior discectomy and fusion. As a primary procedure for management of spondylolisthesis, however, this is not recommended.[16,18]

In the sixth group, patients with proven spinal stenosis and arachnoiditis have been improved by anterior discectomy and fusion, particularly if the myelogram showed anterior indentations rather than posterior compression (Figure 124-1). A sec-

ond-stage posterior laminectomy was done, with less instability resulting if vertebral bodies were fused.

DIAGNOSTIC STUDIES

Information obtained from the patient's history, physical examination, and roentgenograms usually is essential to making the decision concerning which approach to use for spine stabilization. Other studies that can be selected, as indicated, are listed and the particular reasons for each are mentioned briefly.

1. Laboratory studies should include a battery of chemical analyses, including enzymes, uric acid, and blood sugar, to detect any subtle systemic disease and, particularly, to determine any elevation of liver enzymes. This study is described elsewhere. If liver enzymes are elevated, general anesthesia should be avoided until the cause of the elevation is determined. Also, studies related to rheumatoid arthritis or ankylosing spondylitis are important, as, occasionally, the patient with chronic back pain has a primary condition other than intervertebral disc disease.

2. Roentgenograms should be taken in multiple planes and, if the patient has been operated upon previously, a lateral flexion and extension as well as an anterior, posterior right, and left lateral bending-stress exposure should be done. This will give information about motion at the interspaces and aid in determining whether or not pseudoarthrosis exists. Tomography also helps to determine if pseudoarthrosis is present.

3. A differential spinal test will aid in determining whether the patient has total relief of extremity or back pain at certain concentrations of injected anesthetic. If the patient's pain is relieved by saline, then the severity of this complaint is questioned. If pain is not relieved by a total motor and sensory block, the other considerations concerning its origin are reviewed.[18]

4. Psychiatric consultation is important in managing the patient who has had multiple operations and is being considered for another operation. Reactive depression, frank neuroses, or subtle psychoses may exist, and the psychiatrist can recommend appropriate medication and proper timing of an operation, if indicated, in this particular patient. The psychiatrist may be able to give advice to the family through the social worker and information to the employer that is helpful in rehabilitating the patient.

5. Clinical psychologic studies have proved to be valuable in assessing the patient's behavior profile, response to injury and operation, and characteristics as they appear on the scale of conversion hysteria, hypochondriasis, or depression. This information is very important in postoperative management and in deciding whether or not the operative procedure, if not clearly indicated, should be done at all.

6. Discography has proved to be valuable for us in reproducing pain at a space that has not been operated upon, in providing information about the amount of fluid that can be injected into an interspace, and for providing information about a normal intervertebral disc that takes a minimal amount of contrast and does not result in pain at the time of the injection. An intervertebral disc that appears abnormal but does not cause pain at the time of injection usually can be ignored. Abnormalities seen by discography are not an indication for surgery.[19] Renografin (American Critical Care, McGaw Park, Illinois) is the contrast

used for discography. If the injection is painful, it can be followed by an injection of 40 mg of Depomedrol. We believe this diminishes the irritation caused by the iodide contrast (Figure 124-2).

7. Electromyography by a trained observer, if used to sample enough muscles, will provide invaluable information about the condition of the lower extremities. There is a high correlation between positive electromyography and positive myelography and discography. If the electromyogram is positive and the myelogram is negative, that information is particularly helpful. If the electromyogram is negative and the myelogram is positive, the electrical studies should be repeated by an experienced electromyographer and special tests such as H reflex should be done.

8. A metrizamide myelogram is helpful in localizing root-compression lesions and in ruling out a significant posterior block or posterior compression. A large defect, noted at the time of the initial myelogram, usually was a contraindication to anterior discectomy (Figures 124-1 and 124-3). Patients who have had multiple operative procedures, however, and who had perineural fibrosis or arachnoiditis demonstrated that the block was not a contraindication to anterior discectomy and fusion.

9. Nerve-root block has been helpful in localizing the pain and the particular nerve root that required decompression. This test is an adjunct to the differential spinal test in that it provides information about complete or partial relief of pain.

10. Thermography has provided some information about the inflammatory aspect of the patient's complaints. A positive thermogram suggests the process may be inflammatory rather than a primary mechanical deficiency. Occasionally this test has suggested ankylosing spondylitis and has resulted in other studies that aided proper diagnosis.

11. Epidural venography aids in localizing a compression lesion and may provide evidence of nerve-root involvement when the myelogram is negative. False-negative venograms may be a problem, and the data must be interpreted in conjunction with other findings (Figure 124-4A and B).

12. Computed tomography (CT) complements the studies already mentioned (Figure 124-5A and B).

13. Technetium 99 bone scan will aid in determining the presence of nonunion, an inflammatory process, or an infection.

CONTRAINDICATIONS TO ANTERIOR LUMBAR DISCECTOMY AND FUSION

1. If nerve-root exploration is essential, then the posterior approach is desirable. We have not depended on nerve-root decompression from the anterior approach, although we have in the cervical spine.

2. Other contraindications are multiple interspace, advanced intervertebral disc disease (more than three interspaces), particularly in a patient over 60 years of age and in those with severe osteoporosis.

SURGICAL TECHNIQUE

Patients usually have been operated upon under general anesthesia supplemented with muscle relaxants. The Trendelenburg position, with the head down about 10 degrees, is

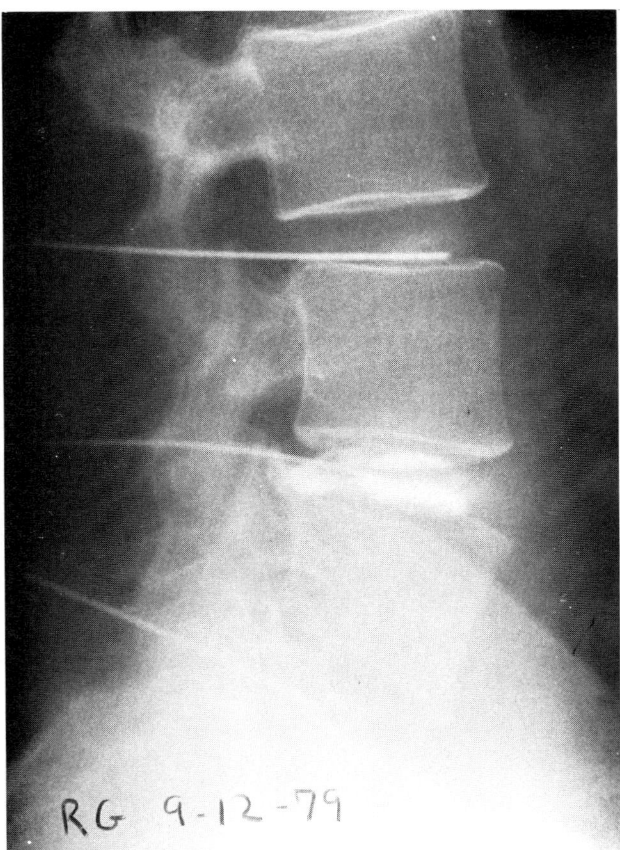

Fig. 124-2. Discography is an adjunct procedure that gives information about the production of pain. Renografin is injected to determine if there is a leak in the annulus and irregularity of the annulus and nucleus. An abnormal test does not require an operative procedure. A normal discogram is helpful in eliminating the diagnosis of intervertebral disc disease and directs attention to the paravertebral structures. The injection shown here between L4-5 is abnormal and shows leakage of the contrast through a defect in the posterior longitudinal ligament. The patient had pain during the injection, as the Renografin irritated sensory receptors outside of the annulus. The needle at L3-4 is not well centered and was readjusted before injection. This interspace showed a "cotton ball" appearance and was considered normal.

desirable as it allows displacement of the abdominal contents proximally and reduces venostasis in the lower extremities. This position is arranged after induction. A thin, folded sheet is placed under the left buttock to elevate the iliac crest. The upper extremities are placed so as to avoid stretch on axillary structures and compression on ulnar nerves at the elbows.

The anesthetist then is asked to locate handles on the table that provide hyperextension of the lumbar spine. This position is not used when the incision is made, but is used while a discectomy is being done.

The abdomen and iliac crest are prepared with soap, water, and Betadine, and the skin is covered with a transparent adhesive dressing. The patient also is tilted to the left side 10 degrees if the surgeon is standing on the left while exposure is being made, or to the right side 10 degrees if the surgeon prefers to stand on the right while the left retroperitoneal exposure is performed.

The left paramedian incision is made through the skin and superficial fascia, the anterior rectus sheath is opened, and the muscle belly is retracted laterally to the lateral gutter (Figure 124-6). If the rectus sheath is incised in the midline, the

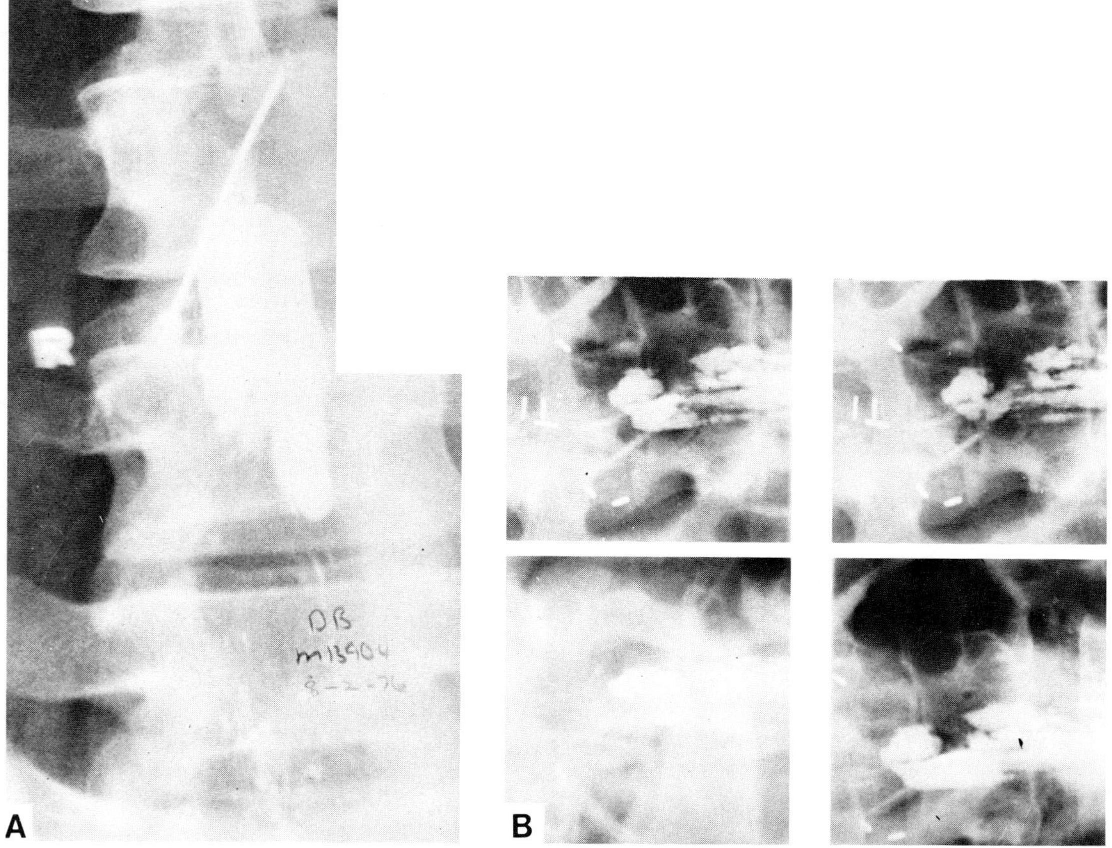

Fig. 124-3. The same patient as in Figure 124-1. (A) This anteroposterior view shows the column of contrast blocked at L4-L5 level. The presumptive diagnosis was arachnoiditis and perineural fibrosis. The appearance of the myelogram was the same after the second and third operations. Note that the spinous processes have been removed and that a segment of the laminal arches has been removed from the fifth lumbar vertebra and the inferior segment of the fourth lumbar vertebra. The facets are intact. (B) A postoperative AP view of the L4-5 interspace with the bone grafts visible between the vertebral bodies and the contrast at the same level as preoperatively.

peritoneum will be entered. The retroperitoneal space is entered, initially, inferiorly at the linea semilunaris, and the peritoneum is carefully and slowly separated by blunt dissection from the undersurface of the rectus sheath. The proximal incision into the posterior sheath should not be made until the peritoneum is separated from the fascia. Small peritoneal tears may occur during this step in the procedure, and they should be repaired with chromic catgut. The rectus sheath is incised from the semilunar notch inferiorly to its superior border proximally. The psoas muscle is identified, and the iliac artery and vein then are palpated or visualized on the left side. The left ureter is located, after which the lumbosacral interspace is palpated. This space is identified between the right and left iliac arteries and veins (Figure 124-7). The sacral promontory is identified by palpation without disturbing the sympathetic nerves crossing over the sacral promontory or the major sympathetic nerves on either side of the lumbar vertebrae. The soft tissue over the interspace of the vertebrae and lower half of the fifth lumbar vertebral body is dissected off with a small dissector, and the venous tributaries from the iliac vein and vena cava are clamped with silver clips. The lumbosacral interspace is exposed by retracting the left iliac artery and vein to the left side and the right iliac artery and vein to the right side with blunt vein retractors (Figure 124-8). Spike retractors, driven into the body of the fifth lumbar vertebra, are helpful in maintaining the

exposure (Figure 124-9A). The vessels are protected from the spike by a small abdominal pack, and the peripheral pulse is palpated distal to the spike, indicating that excessive tension is not placed on the artery or vein. No dissection is done on the first sacral segment. Bleeding and the decussating fibers of the sympathetic chain, which partially control ejaculation, are avoided. Venous bleeding is avoided by frequent use of vascular clips, both large and small, by preclamping of venous tributaries, and by slow and deliberate mobilization of the vena cava. This structure may be adherent and may require partial clipping or suturing to prevent tearing. Angulated vascular clamps in addition to the vascular clips should be readily available. Also, synthetic clotting material should be readily available to stop bleeding from an irregular surface. A fiberoptic headlight provides visibility.

In exposing the fourth lumbar interspace, the left iliac artery and vein and the ureter are displaced to the right side of the spine and are held in place by spike retractors. During exposure of this interspace there is even more likelihood of obliterating the left iliac artery by applying excessive tension on the retractor.

The anterior longitudinal ligament at the L5-S1 interspace is elevated from the annulus as a flap, with the base attached at the left (Figures 124-8 and 124-10). This flap, when tagged with sutures, affords additional retraction and protection for the

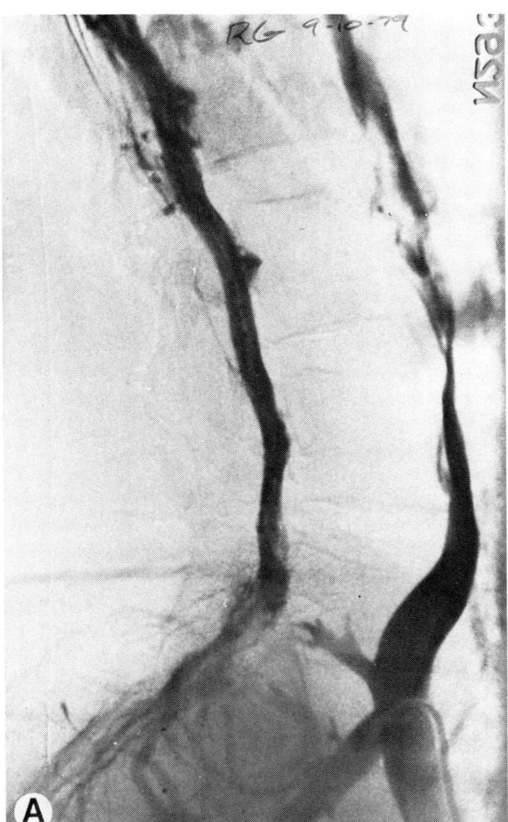
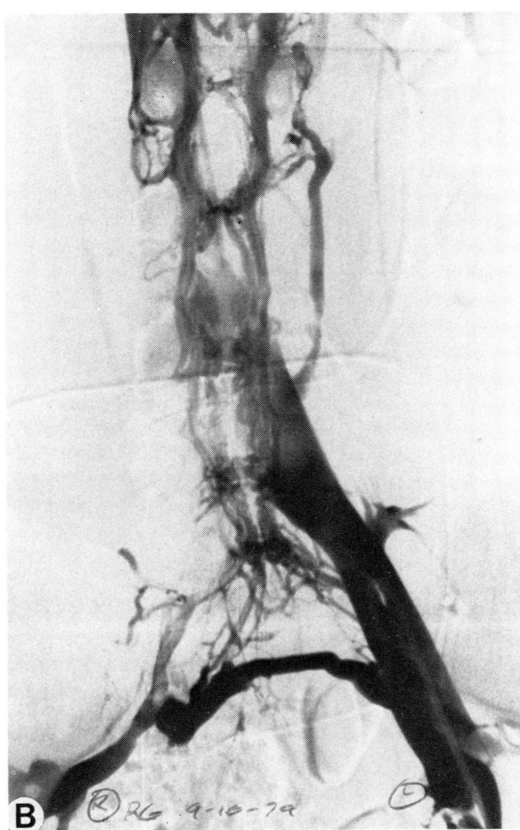

Fig. 124-4. (A) This epidural venogram subtraction film shows the pattern of the vena cava, the iliac arteries, and the anterior and posterior venous pattern over the vertebral bodies and the interspaces. This information is helpful not only in determining an extrusion from the interspace and the extent of fibrosis at the interspace but also in determining any alterations that might be present in the vena cava or the iliac vessels. (B) Epidural venogram subtraction study shows incomplete filling of the radicular veins and the lumbar veins on the right side and cross flow of venous return from right to left through the sacral and iliac veins. This information is helpful in determining the presence of collateral circulation, the size of the venous vessels, and the areas of fibrosis.

vessels. Hyperextension of the operating table brings the spine closer to the surface of the wound and affords better exposure of the interspace (Figure 124-11). The intervertebral disc and the annulus are separated from the cartilaginous plates of the vertebra with a knife or a thin osteotome. Once detached from the vertebral body above and below, the disc complex can be removed easily with a large pituitary rongeur and large curettes (Figure 124-9B). The space is cleaned out thoroughly, back to the posterior longitudinal ligament, before any bone is removed. In this way, bleeding is minimal and dissection can be done under direct vision. The lateral recesses are cleaned thoroughly. Cartilage surfaces are removed from the vertebral bodies with an osteotome until bleeding bone is encountered. Vigorous bleeding may occur from the posterior aspect of the vertebral bodies and can be controlled with small amounts of bone wax or cautery. The undersurface of the L5 vertebra is concave and requires special attention in removing soft tissue.

After the soft tissue and cartilage have been removed from the interspace, the dimensions of the interspace are measured with a caliper and ruler. The grafts then are cut individually from the left ilium, which is prepared by subperiosteal dissection so that full-thickness grafts, with inner and outer cortex of the ilium, can be obtained.[11] The graft is cut slightly larger than the height of the interspace so that firm impaction can be obtained (Figure 124-12A and B). The lateral recesses of the intervertebral space are packed first with short vertical struts,

with the cortices at right angles to the vertebral bodies. The central graft is usually 3.5 cm deep and the width varies from 0.8 to 1.0 cm. After the lateral grafts are placed, the center graft is packed into place so that the anterior edge is countersunk about 2 mm. The second center graft then is inserted and compressed, both to the right and to the left sides. A wedging technique is used by inserting two osteotomes between the center grafts and spreading the osteotomes to the right and to the left, thereby compressing the grafts and allowing space for an additional piece of bone (Figure 124-11C). Small segments of cortical and cancellous bone can be packed between the grafts. The grafts should not be countersunk excessively as they may extend posteriorly through holes in the posterior longitudinal ligament and irritate the nerve roots.

The spine then is straightened by correcting the hyperextended position of the table. This holds the grafts in place by wedging the vertebral bodies.

The L4-5 interspace is exposed by retracting the left iliac artery, vein, and ureter toward the right side and replacing the spike retractors in the L5 vertebral body. The spine then is hyperextended and the L4-5 interspace is cleaned out and prepared for insertion of the iliac bone graft (Figure 124-13). If the L3-4 interspace is to be done, the dissection is completed proximally and the lumbar artery and vein ligated.

After the bone grafts are in place, a small piece of Surgicel is placed over the grafts, and the anterior longitudinal flaps are

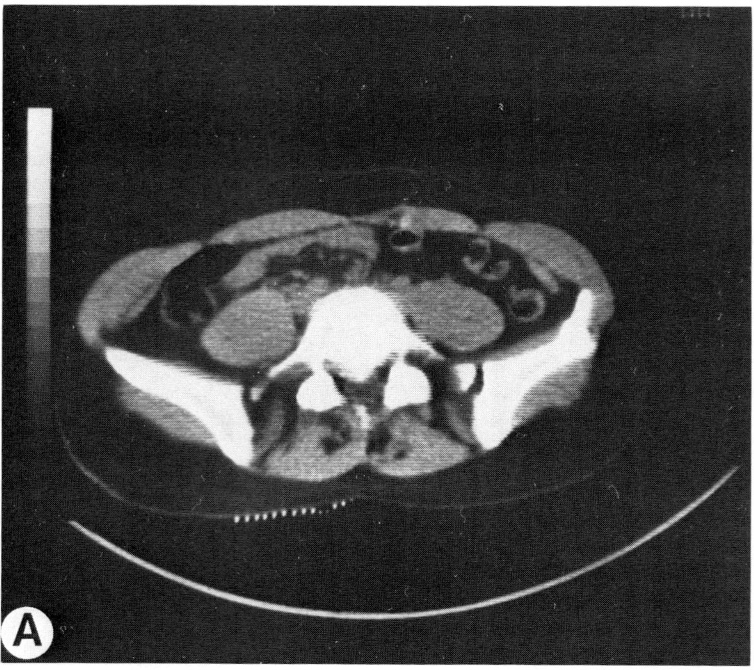

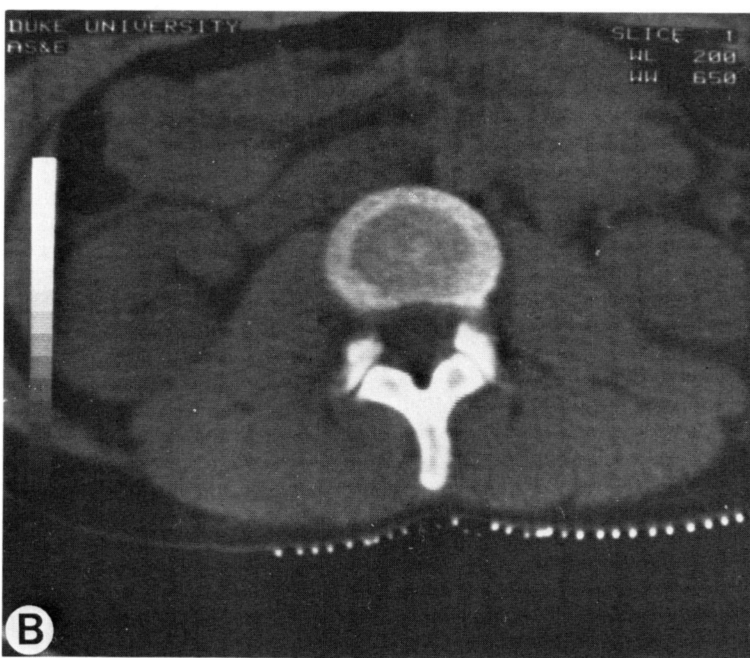

Fig. 124-5. (A) A CT scan shows the absence of the spinous process and part of the laminal arch and impingement in the region of the lateral recess. The bulging in the posterior aspect of the vertebral body is significant only after sections above and below this location are reviewed. (B) This CT exposure through the L3 spinous process and vertebral body shows slight irregularity of the facets but no impingement from the vertebral body. This method of diagnostic study is important in determining "napkin ring" constriction proximal to the site of prior posterior fusion or spontaneous spinal stenosis.

replaced with a single nonabsorbable suture. All deep fascia layers are closed with nonabsorbable sutures and subcutaneous tissues are closed with absorbable sutures. Four tension sutures of nylon are placed through the skin, subcutaneous tissue, and fascia and the dressing is sutured in place in order to absorb hematoma. This is removed after 5 days.

The average blood loss for a one-interspace operation is 500 ml and 1200 ml for a two-interspace operation. Replacement is done during the operative procedure with whole blood or packed cells; selection depends upon the volume of blood and the rapidity of loss. Packed cells may be given postoperatively if necessary.

POSTOPERATIVE MANAGEMENT

Nasogastric intubation is not always necessary but is used in some patients for maximum abdominal comfort, even though the tube itself may be uncomfortable. A low negative pressure

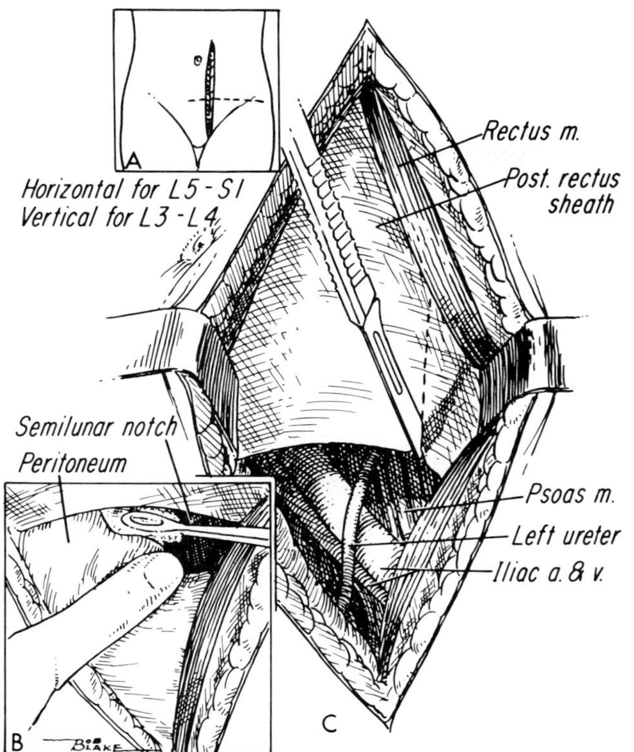

Fig. 124-6. A periumbilical incision has been made, the anterior sheath of the rectus has been incised, and the rectus muscle has been retracted laterally. The posterior rectus sheath is identified anteriorly and far laterally. The semilunar notch is used as a guide for reflecting the peritoneum from the undersurface of the rectus sheath. The peritoneum and abdominal contents are swept medially. The posterior rectus sheath is incised laterally and proximally and these same flaps are sutured with nonabsorbable suture at the time of closure.

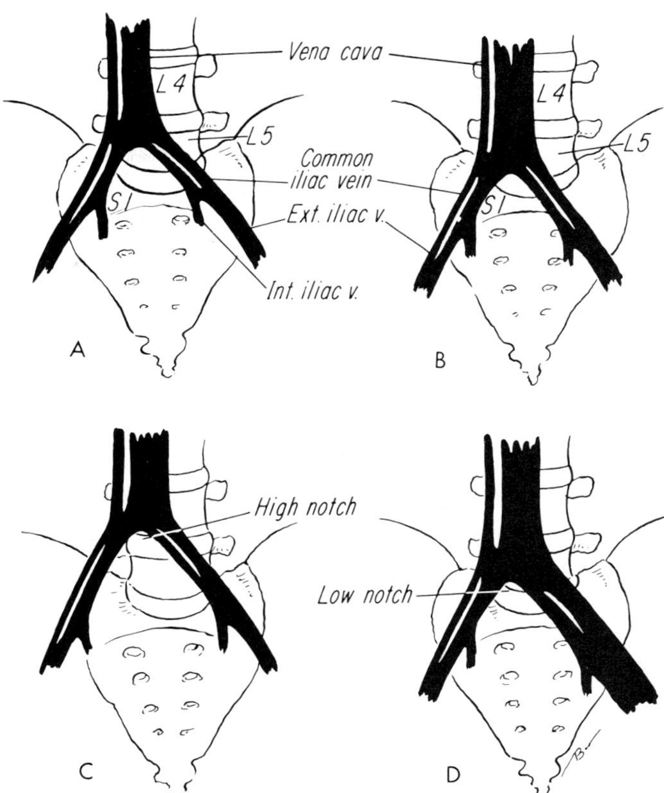

Fig. 124-7. Several patterns of bifurcation of the vena cava into the iliac veins exist. The bifurcation may be opposite the middle of the fifth lumbar vertebra, at the level of the last intervertebral disc space, or even as high as the middle of fourth lumbar vertebral body. The decision to reflect the artery, vein, and ureter to the right, in order to expose L4-5, depends on the height of the notch. Over 90 percent of the time, this reflection is necessary and makes the exposure easier. In each instance, isolation of the L5-S1 interspace has been possible just below the bifurcation.

is connected to the nasogastric tube until active peristalsis occurs, which is usually within 36 to 48 hours. The patient's head and chest are elevated slightly; also, the lower extremities should be higher than heart level. Elastic stockings are used immediately postoperatively, but no elastic wrappings are used during the operation. The patient is encouraged to initiate active motion of the feet immediately upon awakening. The patient should be encouraged to turn frequently, to place a pillow on the abdominal wall in order to decrease pain of coughing, and to breathe deeply several times each hour. A trapeze is placed on the bed and the patient encouraged to use it.

Anticoagulation has been used in all patients who have anterior lumbar fusion. Our current anticoagulation routine is therapeutic low-dose heparin; 5000 units are given subcutaneously on call, and 3000 subcutaneously postoperatively, with the first dose beginning about 6 hours after the operation has been completed. The heparin is monitored daily by activated partial thromboplastin time. High therapeutic levels are not necessary. The level should be prolonged only slightly more than normal. Heparin is continued about 5 days, the platelet count is observed every third day, and the patient is started on Coumadin on the fourth postoperative day. Heparin is continued until the ratio of Coumadin is 1.5:1. Coumadin is monitored for a total of 3 weeks. Prothrombin time is maintained at 1.5 times normal level. The patient may leave the hospital 10 to 14 days after the procedure, and the family physician is asked to monitor the anticoagulant. Certain medications alter the

prothrombin time and the physician should be familiar with these.

Straight-leg raising is started on the third postoperative day and continued for several months. By the fifth postoperative day, the patient is allowed to sit and to walk. A low-back corset has been used to support abdominal muscles and to encourage deep breathing and coughing. The iliac donor site usually is more painful than the abdomen or back.

The pain relief associated with radiculopathy has been consistently noted on the day after surgery. Because of early relief of pain, many patients tend to overexert physically, and they must be warned that total pain relief will not persist and may not be present for several months. Recurrent episodes of discomfort are to be expected.

Patients are asked to avoid driving an automobile for 6 to 8 weeks. Walking should be increased in a graduated way and the patient should attempt to go 2 to 3 miles daily after 4 to 6 weeks have passed. Isometric, abdominal, and gluteal exercises are encouraged. The patient is maintained on a high-protein, low-fat diet with adequate daily vitamin intake and modest doses of anti-inflammatory medication.

Anteroposterior and lateral roentgenograms of the lumbosacral spine are taken just before the patient leaves the hospital. These provide a base line for judging the appearance of the graft, psoas shadows, bone density, and the height of the interspace. Three months after surgery, lateral flexion and

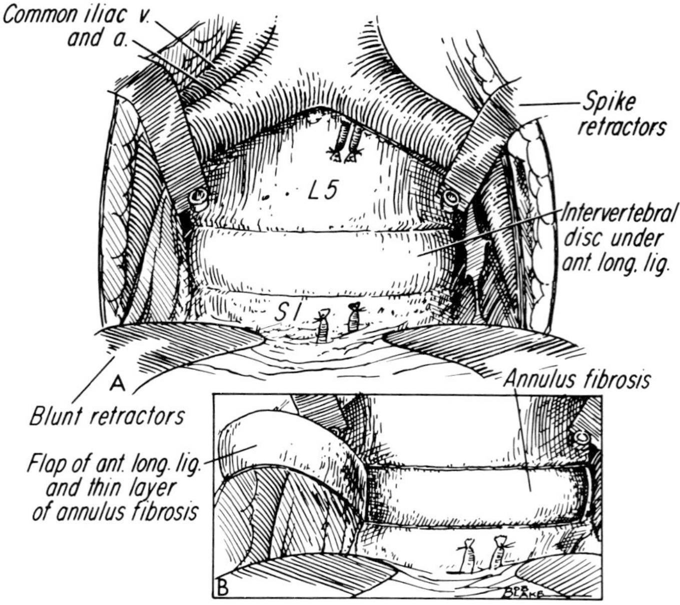

Fig. 124-8. The notch of the vena cava, where it divides into the iliac veins, may be high or low. In this instance the midportion of the fifth lumbar vertebra is clearly visible, the intervertebral disc is exposed widely to the right and left, and no dissection is carried out over the sacral prominence other than to interrupt the veins and arteries with silver clips. Spikes are not inserted into the sacrum, since this may result in additional dissection and cause trauma to the decussating nerve fibers over the first sacral segment. These fibers should be avoided. A long flap of anterior longitudinal ligament, to which is attached a thin layer of the annulus fibrosis, is isolated and reflected either right or left, depending upon which interspace is involved. This flap will protect the artery and vein at the fourth interspace.

extension roentgenograms are taken with the patient in the standing position. Radiographic studies are repeated again at 6 to 12 months. A solid fusion cannot be confirmed until at least a year after the operation, and even at that time trabeculations across both sides of the interspace are not always present. Delayed union can be established at 12 months after surgery, and nonunion can be established at 18 to 24 months if the condition is relatively static.

COMPLICATIONS AND SEQUELAE

Immediate complications have occurred infrequently. These diminished as experience with the procedure increased. Complications have included thromboembolism and pseudoarthrosis.

THROMBOEMBOLISM

Thromboembolism has been avoided by the use of anticoagulation therapy in all of the patients done during the past 6 years. Low-molecular-weight or regular Dextran was used for 3 or 4 years, with a diminished incidence of venous thrombosis. About 1970, therapeutic low-dose heparin was introduced. After 7 to 10 days of receiving heparin, the patient was given Coumadin and maintained on a limited anticoagulation regimen for a total of 4 weeks. Coumadin alone, or Dextran and aspirin, or aspirin alone also are used by certain members of the staff. A recent review of all patients who had major orthopedic operations and received anticoagulation showed that therapeutic low-dose heparin had a predictable protective effect against thromboembolism. Other preventative measures, such as elevation of the extremities during and after the procedure, adequate hydration, and early ambulation (on the third or fourth day), are important measures in diminishing the incidence of thromboembolism. The high-risk patient is defined as one who is known to have had thromboembolic disease or who has a known collagen disease or a family history of hypercholesterolemia. Obesity also is a factor associated with an increased incidence of thromboembolic disease.

PSEUDOARTHROSIS

As the number of spaces operated upon increases in a particular patient, the pseudoarthrosis rate also increases. Studies of successful fusion in the first 100 cases operated upon in our series are listed in Table 124-1. Patients with successful fusion cannot be determined for at least 1 year after the operative procedure has been completed, and, preferably, follow-up should be at least 2 years; nonunion not evident at 1 year may be evident at 2 years. Likewise, what appeared to be an early pseudoarthrosis may progress to a stable spine at about 1 year.

The arthrodesis rate has been reviewed for the second 100 cases, and patients who have had one interspace arthrodesed showed a rate of fusion of about 90 percent; those who had two spaces arthrodesed had a fusion rate of about 80 percent. Individual surgeons, however, demonstrated smaller series in the group with a higher fusion rate, indicating that there is a direct relationship between the technique used, the placement of the bone grafts, the stability of the interspace after the operative procedure has been completed, and the patient's activities during the next several months.

Our analysis of the last 200 patients shows a definite correlation between successful spine arthrodesis, subsequent relief of symptoms, and diminution of pathologic physical findings. A few patients who were relieved of radiculopathy did not have a solid fusion. Their back pain usually persisted. Other patients obtained a solid fusion and were not relieved of all their complaints. Factors known to be related to the persistence of pain, such as perineural fibrosis, intraneural fibrosis, and involvement of areas outside the spine as well as the interspaces proximally, must be considered in the total management of these patients.

When arthrodesis failed in patients who had undergone a two-space fusion, the pseudoarthrosis was usually in the upper interspace. Stress, torque, and abnormal motions persist at that space, whereas the L5-S1 interspace is compressed more readily. Almost all patients who developed anterior pseudoarthrosis were managed subsequently by posterior lateral fusion. A combination of prior anterior and additional posterior fusion provided a high degree of success in obtaining fusion in these patients (98 percent). A prior ununited anterior fusion always showed evidence of union, with trabeculations crossing the vertebral bodies within a year after the posterior lateral fusion was done. Anterior fusion enhanced a failed posterior fusion as well. Reoperation anteriorly was done only if there was a contraindication to posterior exposure, such as prior infection or small transverse processes.

We advise patients who are to have an anterior discectomy and fusion to expect about a 20 percent chance of having to undergo an additional operative procedure in order to obtain a solid fusion. Considering the fact that many of these individuals

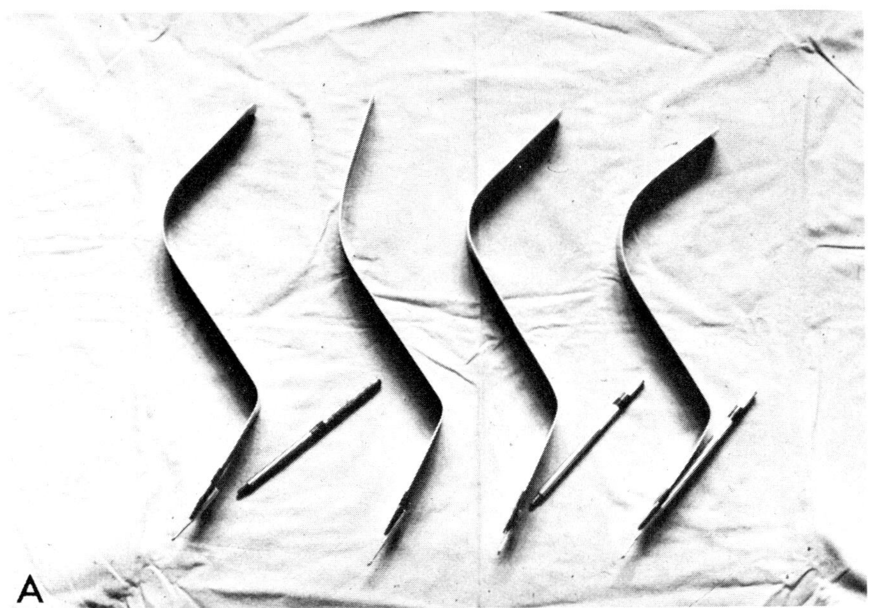

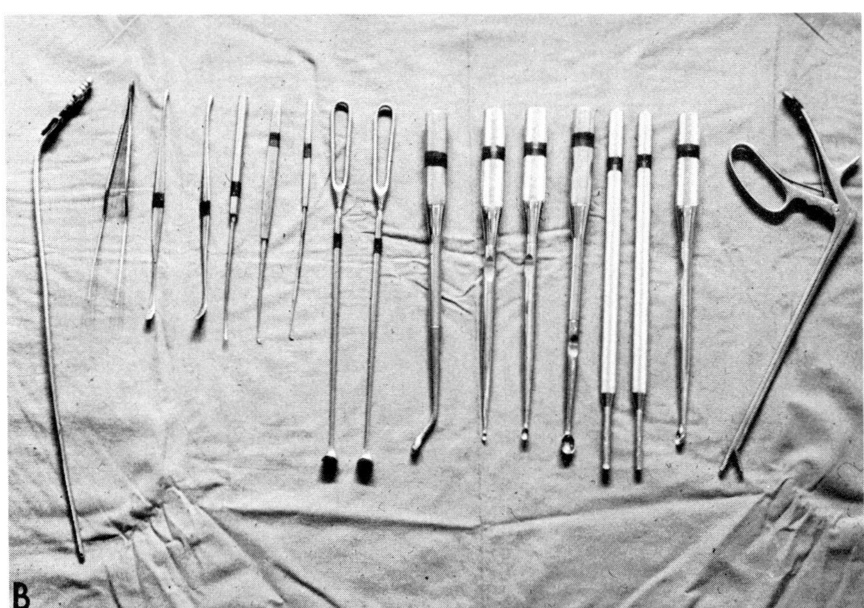

Fig. 124-9. (A) The spiked retractors are very helpful in doing the procedure. The extension screws on and off and is used to impact the spike into the vertebral body. Two retractors usually are used with one being placed on the right and one on the left in order to retract the artery and vein. The spike should be covered with a sponge pack on one side so that pressure from the metal does not irritate the vessels. When the spikes are removed, a small amount of bone wax is used to fill the bone hole in order to diminish bleeding. (B) Special instruments used in doing anterior lumbar discectomy and fusion. The large pituitary rongeur was made by an instrument company at our request. The large curettes and long-handled impactors are helpful in cleaning out the interspace and in placing the bone grafts. The long-handled vein retractors are helpful in displacing the iliac vein and the vena cava, while silver clips are used to clamp the small tributaries.

have anywhere from two to five prior operations, we feel that this is an acceptable method of management.

If prior discectomy without fusion has resulted in persistent signs and symptoms that interfere with the patient's daily activities, then anterior discectomy and fusion are performed. If pain relief has not been acceptable and if evidence of progressive arthrodesis has not occurred within 6 to 12 months, the additional procedure of supplementary posterior lateral fusion or decompression and fusion are included.

DISCUSSION OF OTHER COMPLICATIONS AND SEQUELAE

DONOR SITE DISTURBANCE

Donor site disturbance can be avoided if the anterior superior spine is not removed when the bone graft is taken. The lateral femoral cutaneous nerve should not be subjected to traction or laceration, as this is the most common cause of

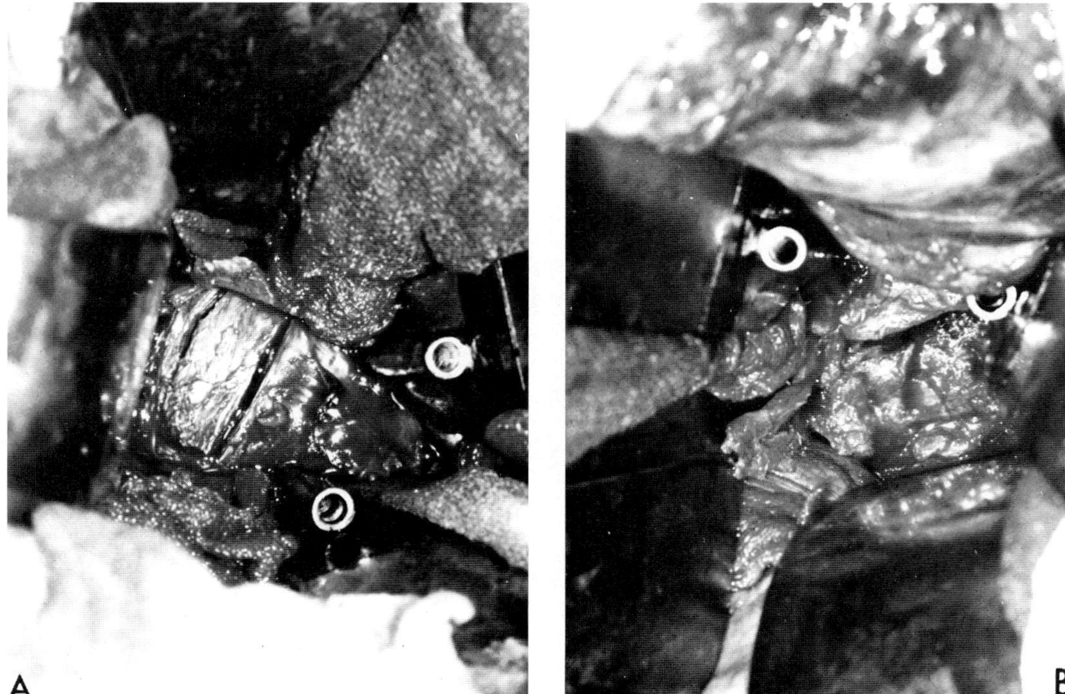

Fig. 124-10.   (A) The anterior ligament has been removed and the annulus incised. The soft tissue remaining in the interspace is made up of residual fragments of annulus, fibrous tissue, cartilaginous fragments, and minimal nucleus. All of this material is removed completely until the cartilage plates are clearly visible. (B) The 2.0 cm spikes of the metallic retractor are driven into the L5 vertebral body. Cuts have been made into the anterior longitudinal ligament superiorly and inferiorly. A flap of anterior longitudinal ligament has been elevated and retracted to the patient's right. Packs are used to protect the vessels, the ureter, the sympathetic chain, and the presacral decussation. (C) The anterior longitudinal ligament flap has been elevated, the anterior, medial, and lateral segments of the annulus have been removed, and the soft tissues remaining superiorly, interiorly, and posteriorly must be removed so that good bone contact can be obtained between the autogenous bone graft and the vertebral bodies.

postoperative discomfort. Pain at the site of the bone graft after operation usually is more noticeable than abdominal pain. Gluteal and abdominal muscles should be removed with a small flake of bone attached to them. An osteotome is used to do this. This allows firm closure of periosteum with a bone attachment. There usually is quicker recovery of muscle tone and less pain if this is done. Suction draining is always used. Bone wax is used to cover the bleeding surfaces. "Hip limp" may persist for 3 months, but there have been no permanent problems from the bone graft site after 6 months. Even after the entire iliac crest is used for full-thickness bone for three interspaces, the reconstitution of stability of the origin of the gluteus muscles and the external oblique muscles has been adequate and allowed unimpeded gait and resumption of ordinary activity.

THROMBOEMBOLISM

Thromboembolism has been avoided by administering anticoagulants as mentioned; elevating the foot of the operating table during the procedure; maintaining the lower extremities higher than the heart level postoperatively; and ensuring that the patient is active in bed postoperatively, using foot exercises and an overhead trapeze, coughing frequently, using blow bottles, and maintaining adequate hydration. Antithromboembolic stockings are used and these must contour above the knee, or below knee stockings are selected. Aspirin is used for several weeks after the primary anticoagulant is stopped.

URINARY TRACT DISTURBANCE

Indwelling catheters are avoided. Preoperative assessment for bacterial infection is done and the patient is not operated upon if there is evidence of a symptomatic bacterial infection. These infections are treated initially. Postoperatively, Urecholine, manual compression, and other methods are used to maintain adequate bladder tone. One patient in 200 received a small puncture wound of the left ureter. This was demonstrable postoperatively by retroperitoneal urinoma. This was treated by an indwelling catheter and healed.

IMPOTENCE (RETROGRADE EJACULATION)

In none of the 200 patients, both males and females, and in no instance in the management of a man was impotence related to neurogenic involvement recognized. Those patients who had difficulty with erection several weeks or months postoperatively had the same problem preoperatively. Three of the 200 patients demonstrated retrograde ejaculation. They were included in the first 30 patients done, and more extensive dissection over the first sacral segment anteriorly had been performed. The decussating fibers of the upper sacral plexus may have been involved in this dissection. No dissection is carried below the anterior edge of the L5-S1 interspace. Hand-held, blunt-nosed retractors are used over the superior body of S1. No cauterization is done over the superior sacral segment and none over the body of L5. Soft tissues are swept aside with blunt dissectors and silver clips are used to manage the venous

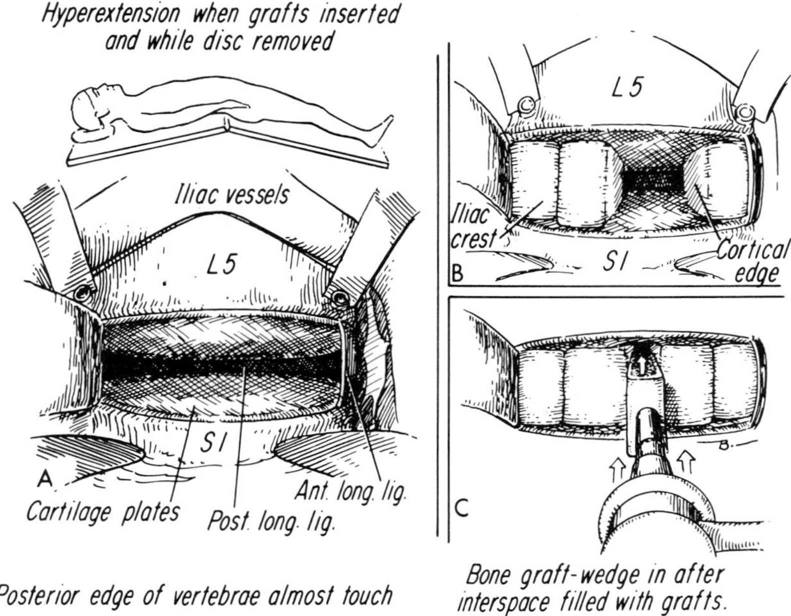

Fig. 124-11. The intervertebral disc, which is relatively avascular, has been removed without breaking through the cartilage plates. After the annulus and nucleus have been excised, the cartilage plates are partially removed, perforated, and roughened, so that bone surfaces that bleed exist. Lateral bone grafts are packed so that the right and left edges of the interspace are filled with a graft. Additional bone grafts then are placed in the center of the interspace and the last bone graft is wedged in between the seemingly tight impacted grafts.

collaterals. We are confident that if this technique is followed, the procedure can be done in male patients of any age without affecting sexual function.

Fear of sexual dysfunction associated with anterior lumbar fusion has been emphasized in the literature. That possibility, of course, does exist because of the anatomic location of the operative procedure. Our experience has shown, however, that this is not an expected or necessary complication of this operative procedure.

INFECTION

Bacterial infection occurred in 2 patients of the initial 100; both of these infections were accounted for by Gram-negative involvement from the urinary tract. Infection was controlled by draining the hematoma and by antibiotics. The fusion rate was not affected. No infections have occurred in the last 100 cases, and the senior author has performed approximately 200 anterior discectomies and fusions during the past 15 years with no deep infections. Ultraviolet light was used during the procedure on each of these patients and one half of the patients received prophylactic antibiotics.

POSTOPERATIVE HEMATOMA

Persistent bleeding from an epigastric vessel resulted in a large progressive retroperitoneal hematoma in 1 patient, which was managed by evacuation and by ligating the vessel on the sixth postoperative day. The patient's progress was satisfactory subsequent to that. If the hematocrit drops and if the patient shows evidence of enlarged abdominal girth, re-exploration is essential in order to locate the bleeding point. This usually will be either on a branch of the iliac artery, a branch of the vena cava, or an abdominal vessel. Re-exploration was required in 2 of 200 patients.

PROLONGED ABDOMINAL ILEUS

Prolonged abdominal ileus is prevented by inserting a nasogastric tube if the patient does not show rapid recovery of bowel sounds after the operative procedure. We do not use the nasogastric tube routinely, although there is much less likelihood of ileus if this is done. The patient is encouraged to assume a side-lying position and to avoid intake by mouth until bowel sounds occur and flatus is passed. A rectal tube is helpful.

INTRAOPERATIVE HEMORRHAGE

Excessive blood loss during the operative procedure has rarely occurred. The surgeon must be prepared, however, to manage a tear in the thin or adherent vena cava, bleeding from a retracted lumbar vein, bleeding from sacral veins that might be punctured from insertion of the spiked retractors into the sacrum (this procedure is not recommended), and arterial bleeding from branches of the iliac artery that might be torn during retraction. Patients who have had prior interspace infection or multiple posterior discectomies show significant reaction around the vena cava and the iliac vessels anteriorly. The surgeon should have available small and large hemoclips, blood vessel sutures, right-angle hemostats, and bipolar cautery. Avitene (American Critical Care, McGaw Park, Michigan), Gelfoam (Upjohn, Kalamazoo, Michigan), and thrombin, and direct compression all aid in stopping venous bleeding. Blood replacement has averaged 3 units per patient but larger quantities must be available if an emergency occurs.

PROBLEM-ORIENTED PATIENTS

Case 1. A 22-year-old nurse gave a history of having had acute back and lower extremity pain, initially treated by bedrest and anti-inflammatory agents. Recurrent radiculopathy was

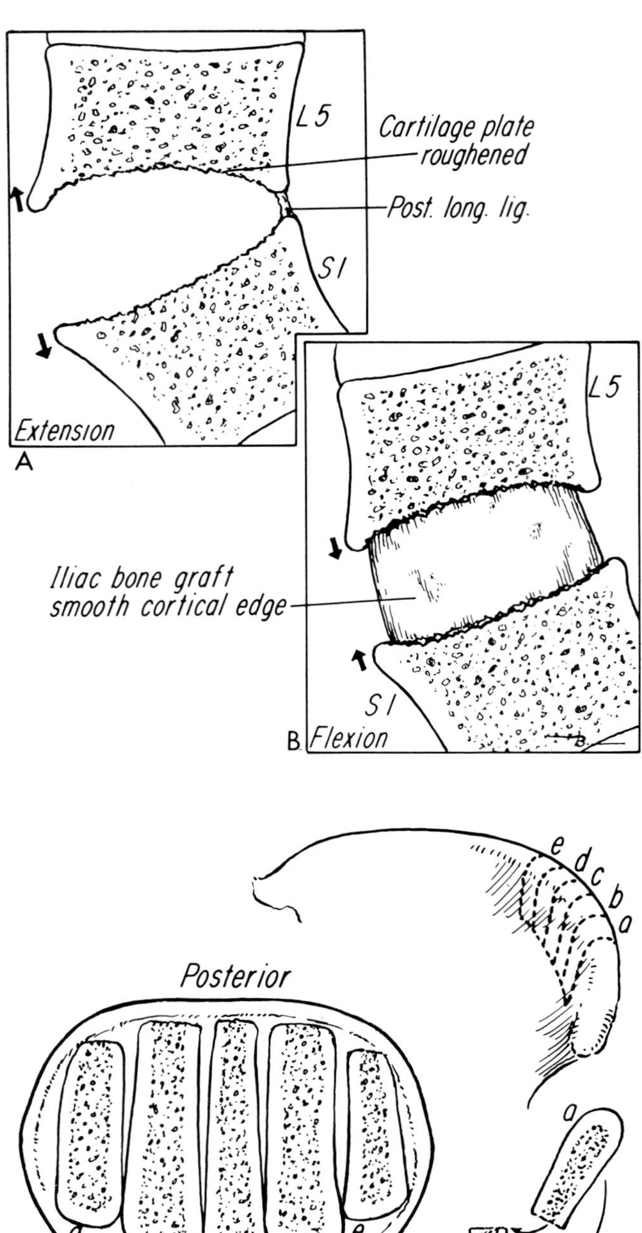

Fig. 124-12. A lateral view of the vertebral bodies in the hyper-extended position showing the posterior longitudinal ligament intact, the roughened edges of the cartilage plates, and perforations into the subchondral bone. After the bone graft is inserted and the convex edge is placed into the inferior surface of the upper vertebra, the trunk is flexed for impaction and compression. The graft is countersunk, with the anterior edge resting just below the edge of the vertebral bodies. The muscle origins attached to the anterior iliac spine are left in place and the anterior-superior iliac spine is not removed. The full-thickness grafts then are rotated before insertion, so that the cortical edges provide vertical support for the vertebral bodies. The bone grafts are contoured so that there is a convex edge superiorly and a straight edge inferiorly. The iliac crest eventually rests in the outer two thirds of the interspace, and the narrower portion of the graft is deep. Wide exposure of the interspace is needed in order to place bone at the periphery of the interspace. The width of the iliac crest and the size of the lumbar interspace determine the number of bone grafts that can be pressed into the interspace.

followed by a myelogram by her attending neurosurgeon, who subsequently performed a hemilaminectomy and removed a soft, bulging intervertebral disc. The patient's symptoms improved during the subsequent 4 months, but back pain and buttock aching persisted, serial x-ray studies showed rapid narrowing of the interspace. Her pain worsened, straight-leg raising tests became strongly positive, and a second myelogram was done. A decompressive laminectomy was performed as the second operation, and spinal fusion was not done at that time. Improvement was slight. Several months elapsed, and she was unable to work at her nursing job. She continued to have evidence of nerve-root irritation and facet joint and interbody pain. One and one-half years after her initial onset of pain and radiculopathy she was still disabled.

Diagnostic studies included electromyography, which showed abnormal polyphasic action potentials in the S1 root distribution. The differential spinal test gave a physiologic response and the clinical psychologic studies showed the patient was not an hysterical type, nor was she somatizing. A discogram was done at the L4-5 level while the patient was awake. There was no pain associated with injection of the contrast and only 0.8 ml could be injected. The retroperitoneal approach was selected for the anterior discectomy and fusion. Only the L5-S1 interspace was included because of the normal discogram. Postoperatively, the straight-leg raising tests were possible to 70 degrees compared with 30 degrees preoperatively. Her relief of extremity pain was almost immediate. The nerve root that is fibrotic or compressed in a small canal can be decompressed by immobilizing the interspace and distracting it minimally with the bone graft. By 3 months her back pain had been eliminated, and by 6 months she was doing limited nursing. Within 1 year there were trabeculations across the interspace, and she was fully active in her occupational and social life.

There are many advantages to directly decompressing a nerve root. Spinal fusion will not cure a nerve root with intraneural fibrosis, but perineural fibrosis may be helped by immobilization. At least the constant trauma of incongruity and instability are removed and the root is protected somewhat.

If anterior discectomy and fusion and posterior discectomy and interbody fusion are compared, greater ease in cleaning out the intervertebral space, placing the bone grafts under compression, and placing the grafts in such a way that they follow the contour of the vertebral bodies will be noted if performed through an anterior approach. If the nerve roots do not require retraction, there is much less chance of involving the dura or the roots during the operative procedure. Anterior stabilization provides a safe way of obtaining stability of the spine and of cleaning out the interspace before posterior decompression if prior posterior operations have been completed.

If there continues to be evidence of anterior-posterior narrowing of the spinal canal or nerve root compression, appropriate decompression is performed posteriorly at a time when the vertebral bodies are relatively stable as a result of the anterior discectomy and fusion. Enhanced computed tomography with metrizamide is helpful in determining the need for posterior decompression.

Case 2. A 19-year-old man developed acute back pain with radiculopathy and had the physical findings and myelographic defect compatible with a ruptured disc at the L4-5 interspace. A hemilaminectomy was done by the attending

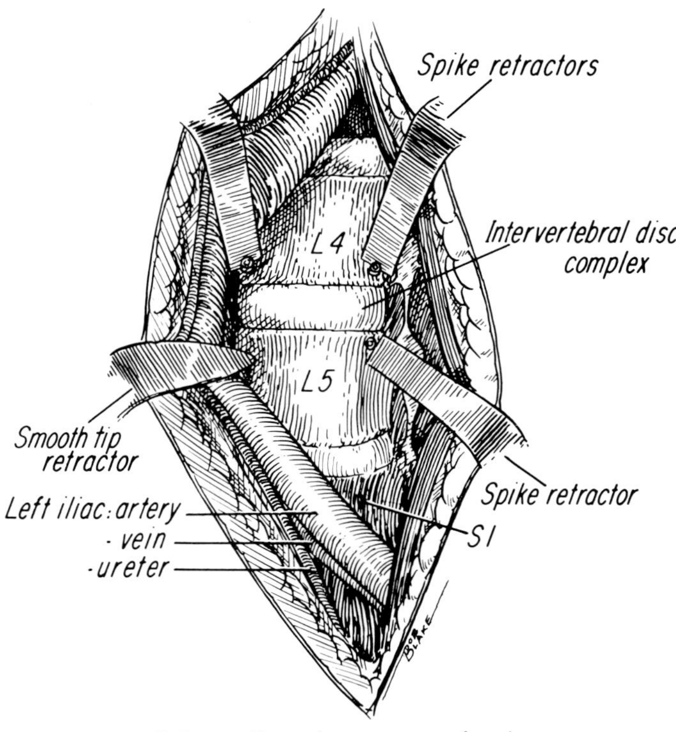

Fig. 124-13. Retroperitoneal exposure of L4, L5, and S1 through a retroperitoneal incision. The iliac artery, vein, and ureter have been displaced medially, the left sympathetic chain is recognized and avoided, and the spike retractors are used to provide exposure of the intervertebral disc complex. Compression of the artery and vein by the retractors must be avoided and the pulsation of the vessels should be felt from time to time. If L3 is to be exposed, the lumbar artery and vein must be ligated and the vessels dissected to the level of the upper edge of the third lumbar vertebra.

neurosurgeon, and a soft, bulging disc was removed. Temporary improvement occurred, but with increased physical activity, pain recurred in approximately 6 months. A second myelogram was done followed by a second decompression, and neurolysis was performed. Temporary improvement occurred while the patient was at bedrest, but within 4 months severe back pain and lower-extremity radiculopathy were present. The x-ray films showed gradual narrowing of the L4-5 interspace and the myelogram showed a partial block and a defect at L4-5 (Figures 124-1A, B, and C). The patient had a physiologic response to the differential spinal test, the electromyogram was positive, involving the L5 root on the left, and a discogram at L3-4 was normal, but resulted in pain at both L4-5 and L5-S1. An anterior discectomy and fusion through a retroperitoneal approach were done at L4-5 and L5-S1. Full-thickness iliac bone grafts were used and both spaces were adequately immobilized by the procedure. immediately postoperatively, straight-leg raising was possible to 70 degrees on the left and was painful on the right at about 60 degrees, which had not been the case preoperatively. After 6 months, straight-leg raising was possible on both sides to 70 degrees and back pain was eliminated about 80 percent. The x-ray study shows fusion is progressing satisfactorily.

The diagnosis was arachnoiditis and perineural fibrosis, and incongruity and instability secondary to removal of the intervertebral disc in the young man.

Spinal fusion is recommended in young people, particularly if the first operation for bulging or soft intervertebral disc fails and definitely if a second procedure fails. Discography is helpful, if performed properly and interpreted correctly. An abnormal discogram means that a pathologic lesion exists, but this does not mean that an operative procedure is necessarily indicated. If the clinical findings are abnormal, however, and if the electromyogram coincides, then operative treatment may be indicated. Furthermore, a normal discogram is much more helpful in many instances than an abnormal one (see Figure 124-2).

Case 3. A 25-year-old female pharmacist with an intervertebral disc syndrome at L4-5 had a 4-year history of back pain with radiculopathy. A bulging disc had been removed initially with temporary relief. Six months later the persistent pain resulted in re-exploration of the lower two interspaces posteriorly. Minimal improvement occurred temporarily and worsened as time passed. Serial x-ray studies showed moderately rapid narrowing of both lower interspaces. Because of her slow response, the question of emotional problems and the influence of possible litigation had been introduced by the attending neurosurgeon.

Our studies included an electromyogram, which was positive for S1 nerve-root irritation. The differential spinal test was physiologic, a selective nerve block gave temporary relief of pain in one extremity, and the discogram was normal at the L3-4 space. We do not usually include spaces operated upon previously in the discogram procedure, although this is done occasionally to determine if pain can be reproduced. A selective nerve block will provide the same information by encouraging the patient to undergo physical activity in order to aggravate the pain and then attempt to relieve it with the nerve block.

A two-space anterior lumbar discectomy and fusion was done. Radiculopathy was diminished, back pain improved gradually, and by 1 year after the procedure, the L5-S1 interspace was solid but a fibrous union was present at L4-5 space. The patient had buttock and thigh pain on the left side after standing and walking for moderately long distances. This root was decompressed by hemilaminectomy and neurolysis with unroofing of the foramen. A posterior lateral fusion was then done from L4 to L5 using iliac bone. The patient's radiculopathy was improved within 2 months and the back pain improved during the next 6 months. Both interspaces were solid at 1 year, and the patient was back at work.

Case 4. A 21-year-old doctor's daughter with back pain and radiculopathy was treated by excision of a bulging intervertebral disc at L5-S1. Pain and limitation of motion persisted and several months later the myelogram showed a bulging intervertebral disc at L4-5. This was excised with

Table 124-1. Anterior discectomy and fusion:
Incidence of successful fusion

	Patients	Successful fusion	% Fusion
Single-space	46	42	91
Two-space	46	33	72
Three-space	8	5	62
Total	100	80	

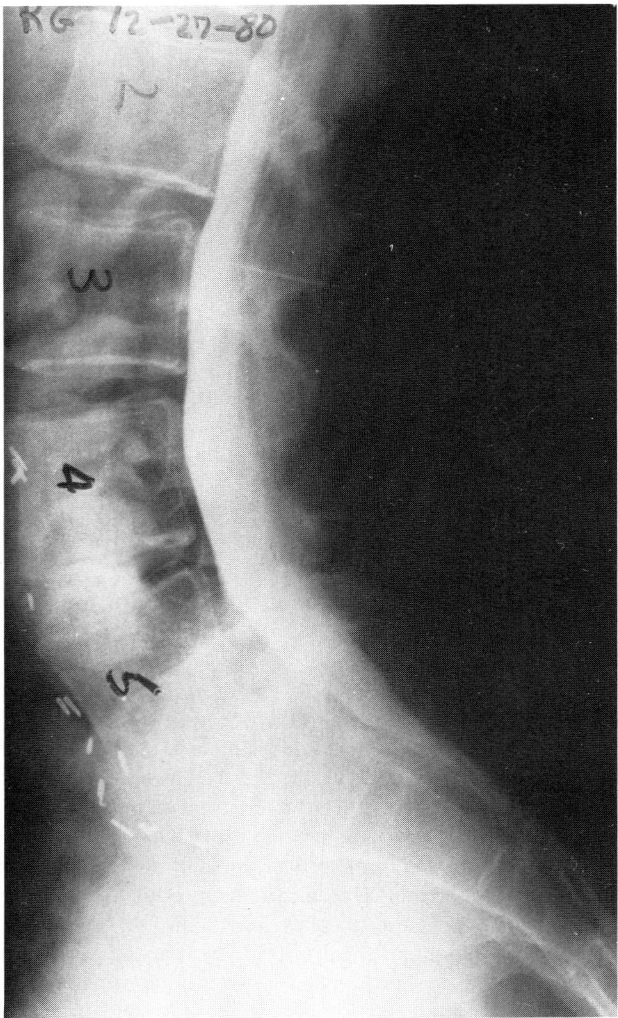

Fig. 124-14. A postoperative anterior discectomy and fusion at L4-5, L5-S1, approximately 8 months after surgery. The hemoclips controlled bleeding from branches of the iliac vessels and the vena cava and small arterioles. The bone graft between L4-5 is definitely fused to L5 and shows early fusion to L4. The interspace has been widened moderately, both anteriorly and posteriorly. The bone graft between L5 and S1 has healed and trabeculae are forming across this interspace. A myelogram was performed because the patient had recurrent lower extremity pain indicative of persistent posterior fibrosis around one root. His back pain had been relieved, and the pain in his opposite extremity had been eliminated. Posterior nerve-root decompression and wide foraminotomy and partial facetectomy diminished the extremity pain. A fusion of the posterior lateral transverse process was performed at the same time and the spine was solid within 1 year after the anterior and posterior procedures. The patient's pain has been eliminated significantly, and he has now returned to work as a truck driver.

temporary relief, but back and buttock pain persisted. A third exploratory operation was done at the lower two spaces, four nerve roots were decompressed, and hemilaminectomies were done bilateral. Subsequent to this procedure, the patient was unable to sit more than 30 minutes without developing severe pain, she walked with the trunk flexed about 30 degrees, and she was comfortable only when lying flat on her back with the hips and knees flexed.

We performed a discogram at the L3-4 level, which was normal. An electromyogram was positive with abnormal action potentials at the L4-5 and L5-S1 roots. X-ray studies showed the interspaces to be narrowed about 70 percent of normal, and

flexion-extension stress x-ray studies showed distinct motion at the interspaces. A two-space anterior discectomy and fusion through a retroperitoneal approach, using iliac bone graft, was done. Recovery was moderately slow, and pain, although improved, persisted for 4 additional months. The patient could sit for longer periods of time, however, could stand erect, and by 4 months after surgery was able to drive her car. X-ray studies showed evidence of a solid fusion by 1 year; the radiculopathy had been eliminated and she returned to school.

Case 5. A 35-year-old female physician had been partially incapacitated because of chronic low back and lower extremity pain for over 5 years. She had been managed by laminectomy, attempted stabilization by posterior lateral fusion with a total of four previous operations. She was using two canes, was required to spend half the day in bed, and was carrying out limited general practice. The physical findings showed positive stretch tests, pain on manipulation of the spine, and weakness of dorsiflexion of the foot.

She was taking urecholine, 25 mg three times a day, for management of her atonic bladder. Cystometrograms showed minimal neurogenic involvement.

A differential spinal test was physiologic, the discogram was negative at L3-4, and the electromyogram was strongly positive, involving the L4-5 and L5-S1 nerve roots bilaterally. There was no evidence of spinal infection. The sedimentation rate was normal, and a thermogram showed no excessive increase in heat.

A psychiatric assessment and clinical psychologic testing showed that the patient did need treatment for reactive depression and anxiety.

Stress x-ray films in the right and left lateral position and forward flexion and extension showed definite motion at both spaces with evidence of pseudoarthrosis and incongruity.

Anterior discectomy and fusion were done through a retroperitoneal approach including the L4-5 and L5-S1 interspaces. A minimal amount of material was found at L5-S1, but a considerable amount of annulus and fibrous tissue was removed from the L4-5 interspace. Full-thickness iliac bone grafts were used to stabilize the two lower intervertebral spaces.

Postoperatively, the straight-leg raising improved, over a period of 2 weeks, to about 60 degrees. Bladder function improved to where urecholine was reduced to 10 mg/day. During the next 3 months, the patient's progress was one of slow but steady improvement, with diminution of pain, increased strength, and increased activity. By 6 months after the operation, she was ready to return to work for half a day. Foot dorsiflexion had improved and bladder control was almost normal. One and one-half years postoperatively this patient was working full time and was relatively free of back and lower extremity pain.

RESULTS

One hundred patients were followed for a minimum of 8 years and a maximum of 15 years after anterior discectomy and fusion as part of their total management. The results were based on the patients' subjective descriptions, the physician's objective findings, and the patients' activity pattern at least 4 years after treatment was completed. The results of this study were based on an assessment of the degree of relief of back or lower

Table 124-2. Overall results of anterior lumbar fusion 100 patients

	Complete relief	Moderate relief	Slight relief	No change	Worse
Lower back pain	47	31	15	7	0
Lower extremity pain	58	27	12	3	0

extremity pain and rated as excellent, good, fair, slight, none, or worse (Figure 124-14).

Table 124-2 can be interpreted as showing that 78 percent of the patients had moderate or complete relief of low-back pain, and 85 percent had complete or moderate relief of lower extremity pain. No patients were worse after treatment. Eighty-five percent of the patients who had one or two interspaces fused were shown to have had complete or moderate relief. Eighteen of the 100 patients continued to have pain and accepted additional back operations after the anterior discectomy and fusion. Fifteen of these had posterior lateral fusions and some had nerve root decompressions. Nine of these patients were improved significantly by the additional surgery. None of these patients were worse; 3 were subjectively the same, but were objectively improved significantly.

Accessory characteristics, such as personality and occupation, of 200 patients were reviewed in 1975. Patients who were considered to have good results were analyzed from an occupational as well as an emotional standpoint. About one half of those with good results were sponsored by workers' compensation. About one half had abnormal clinical psychologic findings, even though the result was satisfactory, and about two thirds of the total patients had a ''normal'' emotional profile. Those patients with abnormal clinical psychologic results required a longer time to reach maximum improvement than did those individuals without personality conflicts and significant secondary gain or other reasons why they did not return to their usual work.

CONCLUSIONS

1. No single method of treatment is sufficient to treat all patients with low-back pain and radiculopathy successfully.
2. There is a direct relationship between patients who obtain a solid fusion and those who show improvement or relief of pain. Patients with persistent pseudoarthrosis have a greater chance of having persistent pain.
3. Detailed preliminary assessment is necessary, using several diagnostic studies as aids in determining the proper method of management and prognosis.
4. Anterior discectomy and arthrodesis with autogenous bone is a safe procedure that allows the diminution of radiculopathy and back pain by removing fragments from the interspace and stabilizing the vertebral bodies.
5. The pseudoarthrosis rate associated with anterior lumbar fusion has been diminished by meticulous removal of the intervertebral soft tissue, by shaping the bone graft, and by the addition of a maximum amount of autogenous bone wedged into the interspace under compression.
6. Bone union as determined by roentgenography may not be accurate with plain films or stress x-ray studies until at least 1 year after the interbody fusion.
7. Spondylolisthesis, in our experience, should be managed by nerve root decompression and posterior lateral fusion at a single interspace if mild (grade 1 or 2) and two spaces if severe (grade 3 or 4). If pseudoarthrosis develops, anterior interbody spinal fusion of the involved interspace can be done provided that the degree of displacement is not excessive. If the spondylolisthesis is graded 3 or 4, the plan is to arthrodese L4 to L5 and remove the disc and insert the iliac bone grafts at that level only. If L4 fuses to L5, the severe forward displacement and movement of L5 on S1 will be diminished. This additional single anterior vertebral body fusion of the superior aspect of the involved vertebra proximal to the defects of the neural arch usually stabilizes the severely displaced spine and avoids extensive dissection about the venous and arterial channels as well as the sympathetic nerve fibers in the region of excessive forward displacement of L5 on S1.
8. Anterior discectomy and fusion have been helpful in diminishing pain and radiculopathy associated with perineural fibrosis and arachnoiditis.
9. Anterior interbody fusion is helpful in treating spinal stenosis and nerve-root stenosis. A stable spine anteriorly allows wide decompression posteriorly without causing incongruity and instability. We have observed several patients who had direct midline posterior fusions who subsequently developed napkin-ring constriction at the upper end of the fusion, encroachment of the fusion on the superior facets, and stenosis of the meninges associated with overgrowth of bone from the laminal arches and facets. A posterior decompression may be performed initially if stenosis is obvious on the CT scan. The surgeon may consider anterior discectomy and fusion if instability is an evident problem after decompression or if it becomes a problem eventually.
10. Sexual dysfunction associated with anterior discectomy and fusion has not been a problem for these patients.
11. A meticulous surgical technique is essential in order to obtain a high rate of fusion of the vertebral bodies.

REFERENCES

1. Burns BH: An operation for spondylolisthesis. Lancet 224:1233, 1933
2. Capener N: Spondylolisthesis. Br J Surg 24:80, 1936
3. Hartman JT, Kendrick JI, Lorman P: Discography as an aid in evaluation for lumbar and lumbosacral fusion, Clin Orthop 81:77, 1971
4. Sacks S: Anterior spinal surgery and ballarat. J Bone Joint Surg 52B:392, 1970
5. Speed K: Spondylolisthesis. Treatment by anterior bone graft. Arch Surg 37:175, 1938
6. McCollum DE, Stephen CR: The use of graduated spinal anesthesia in the differential diagnosis of back and lower extremities. So Med J 57:410, 1964
7. Sacks S: Intervertebral disc excision and lumbar spine fusion by transperitoneal approach. J Bone Joint Surg 43B:401, 1961
8. Goldner JL, McCollum DE, Urbaniak JR: Anterior disc excision and interbody spine fusion for chronic low back pain. American Acad-

emy of Orthopaedic Surgeons, Proceedings-Symposium on the Spine. St. Louis, CV Mosby, 1969

9. Goldner JL, McCollum DE, Urbaniak JR: Anterior intervertebral discectomy and arthrodesis for treatment of low back pain with or without radiculopathy, in Ojemann RJ (ed): Clinical Neurosurgery, vol 15. The Congress of Neurological Surgeons, 1968, pp 352–383

10. Goldner JL, Urbaniak JR, McCollum DE: Anterior disc excision and interbody spinal fusion for chronic low back pain. Orthop Clin North Am 2:543, 1971

11. Stauffer RN, Coventry MB: Anterior interbody spine fusion. J Bone Joint Surg 54A:756, 1972

12. Kotcamp WW: Indications for anterior spine fusion. Clin Orthop 70:235, 1970

13. Hodgson AR, Stock FA: Anterior spine fusion for treatment of tuberculosis of the spine. J Bone Joint Surg 42A:295, 1960

14. Harmon P: Anterior extraperitoneal disc excision and vertebral body fusion. Clin Orthop 18:169, 1961

15. Harmon P: Anterior disc excision and fusion of the lumbar vertebral bodies. J Int Col Surg 40:572, 1963

16. Shanewise RP: Anterior intervertebral lumbar spine fusion. West J Surg 71:212, 1963

17. Harmon P: Personal communication, 1975

18. Freebody D: Motion picture shown at the Vancouver Meeting of the American Orthopaedic Association, 1965

19. Collis JS Jr: Lumbar Discography. Springfield, Ill, Charles C Thomas, 1963

CHAPTER 125

Chemonucleolysis

Walter William Whisler

HISTORY OF CHYMOPAPAIN AND CHEMONUCLEOLYSIS

THE USE OF CHYMOPAPAIN and chemonucleolysis has been surrounded by almost continuous controversy since its introduction by Lyman Smith in 1964.[1] After looking for a material that would dissolve intervertebral discs, Smith, along with a pharmacologist from Baxter Laboratories, in 1963 described the pharmacology of the chondrolytic enzyme in the chymopapain fraction of papaya latex and speculated on its role for dissolution of the nucleus pulposus.[2] He followed this by further animal studies and finally the intradiscal injection of 10 "operative cases" of sciatica.[1] Smith teamed up with J. Brown of Cleveland to publish a study on 75 patients in 1967.[3] One of the cases in this series became paraplegic within 6 hours of injection and the subsequent laminectomy demonstrated severe hemorrhagic arachnoiditis. They believed this to be secondary to blood and Pantopaque from a myelogram 5 days earlier. A second patient in the series developed an anaphylactic reaction, a third developed a disc space infection, while a fourth patient was mistakenly diagnosed and had chymopapain injected into a meningeal endothelioma. Although the results in the other patients in the series were encouraging, it is upon this battleground of safety and efficacy that the resulting controversy has continued. Although reported neurotoxicity studies showed chymopapain to be safe,[4] Shealy claimed it produced a chronic granulatomous inflammation.[5] Ford[6] was unable to duplicate Shealy's work, and Shealy's original slides, when reviewed by McNab, allegedly demonstrated birefringent crystals in the granulations that he felt were consistent with talc granulomas.[7] Further studies by others on the neurotoxicity of chymopapain demonstrated that its only effect was a dose-related rupture of the microvasculature upon contact with the enzyme.[8]

Baxter-Travenol conducted a phase I clinical trial from 1963 to 1969 on a total of 451 patients, with a reported 73 percent good results.[9] Buoyed up by a wave of optimism and excitement, Baxter-Travenol bypassed a phase II study of efficacy and began a phase III study, which continued to 1975 and included over 16,985 patients.[10] In the meantime, because of the loose design and poorly controlled study, serious questions were raised regarding the safety and efficacy of chymopapain, which hardened the skepticism of the medical community.[11] In spite of weaknesses in design and the difficulty of performing a phase II study at such a late date in the investigation, an effort was undertaken in 1974 to perform a phase II controlled double-blind study. The study showed no significant clinical differences between chymopapain and placebo.[12] Baxter-Travenol withdrew its IND for chymopapain

from the Food and Drug Administration in 1975,[13] but continued to market it in Canada, where its use flourished. In the late 1970s, Smith Laboratories was formed in the United States by a nephew of Lyman Smith, who applied for a new IND for their purified form of chymopapain.[14] In 1980, Smith Laboratories undertook a carefully designed double-blind randomized study at seven institutions to compare the efficacy of the intradiscal injection of chymopapain with injections of placebo in patients with a herniated lumbar disc. With a total of 108 patients in the study, using code-brake criterion, it was demonstrated that chymopapain was more effective than placebo for the treatment of patients with herniated lumbar discs ($P = 0.002$).[15] Following these favorable results, a multicenter, open-label trial was conducted entirely within the state of Illinois from September, 1981, to December, 1982. This trial consisted of 1498 patients in which 87 percent of the patients reported excellent to good results. There was an associated anaphylactic rate of 0.9 percent.[16] With the impending approval of Chymodiactin in the early part of 1983, a joint educational effort was undertaken by the American Academy of Orthopedic Surgeons and the American Association of Neurological Surgeons to train approximately 7000 of their members in intradiscal therapy. Chymopapain was approved by the FDA for use on November 10, 1982, with the labeling requirement that its use be restricted to "physicians who are qualified by training and experience to perform laminectomy . . . and who have received specialized training in chemonucleolysis."[17] The controversy of safety still continues.

CHEMISTRY AND PHARMACOLOGY

Chymopapain was isolated and purified from the latex of the fruit of the Carica papaya tree by Jansen and Balls in 1941.[18] Slightly more purified versions of chymopapain are now marketed as Chymodiactin by Smith Laboratories and Discase by Baxter-Travenol. Chymodiactin contains L-cysteinate hydrochloride as a reducing agent. Discase contains cysteine hydrochloride monohydrate as a reducing agent, plus disodium edetate dihydrate and sodium bisulfite as stabilizers.

Chymopapain hydrolyzes the mucopolysaccharide protein "proteoglycan" of the nucleus pulposus. Since 90 percent of the nucleus pulposus is chondromucoprotein, there is an immediate change in the consistency and mass of the herniated disc, which reduces the pressure on the nerve root. The enzyme is almost completely bound on initial contact with the disc substrate so that none of the enzyme escapes into the bloodstream.[8] There is a temporary increase of urinary mucopolysaccharides "glycosaminoglycans" after the injection of chymopapain.[19]

OPERATIVE NEUROSURGICAL TECHNIQUES
ISBN 0-8089-1862-1

Table 125-1. Anaphylaxis in different ethnic groups after intradiscal injection of Chymodiactin

Ethnic Group	Males	Females	Total
White	45/17,129 (0.3%)	71/10,589 (0.7%)*	116/27,718 (0.4%)
Black	3/971 (0.3%)	15/767 (2.0%)*	18/1,738 (1.0%)
Hispanic	2/502 (0.4%)	2/206 (1.0%)	4/708 (0.6%)

* The incidences in white and black females are significantly different ($P = < 0.001$), as are the incidences between males and females.

While the intravenous intradiscal and epidural injection of chymopapain is very well tolerated up to a dosage of 100 times the therapeutic dose, intrathecal injection is highly toxic and can be lethal. The toxic effects appear to be secondary to rupture of the vessels of microcirculation.[4]

INDICATIONS

The use of chymopapain should be restricted to injections at a single level in those patients who have sciatica secondary to a herniated lumbar disc.

Since chymopapain acts only on the nucleus pulposus, it cannot relieve symptoms that are not directly related to pressure caused by the nucleus pulposus. A candidate for injection must have significant radicular pain with a positive straight-leg-raising test, objective evidence of a herniated disc as determined by myelography or computed tomography, appropriate neurologic signs for that level, and would otherwise be considered a candidate for laminectomy. Patients should be excluded if they are pregnant, have had a previous chymopapain injection, a known sensitivity to papaya or papaya derivatives, previous back surgery at the proposed injection level, rapidly progressive neurologic deficits, evidence of an almost complete block on myelograms, spinal cord tumor, spinal stenosis, spondylolisthesis, diabetes, or multilevel disease. Patients should also be excluded if they have bony disease or spondylosis that may be contributing to their symptomatology.

ANAPHYLAXIS

Anaphylaxis occurs in approximately 1 percent of unscreened patients, and in screened patients it is 0.6 percent under general anesthesia and 0.4 percent under local anesthesia. As shown in Table 125-1, it occurs more frequently in females than in males and more frequently in black than white patients.[20]

Anaphylaxis is an acute, severe systemic hypersensitivity reaction resulting from an antigen antibody reaction with the release of histamine and other mediators, which then act on vessels or other target organs. Following the injection of the antigen (chymopapain), a reaction occurs with the IGE antibodies that are attached to the surface membranes of mast cells or basophils, which then release histamine and other mediators.

Any patient who is allergic to papaya or papaya derivatives is not a candidate for chymopapain injection. In the absence of a reliable skin test, the best method of predicting chymopapain sensitivity is the FAST test (fluoroallergeosorbent test), which measures the IGE concentration in a patient's serum. With a negative report, there is a 99.6 percent predictability that anaphylaxis will not occur.[21] Anaphylaxis can occur very quickly and with great severity, so that it is necessary for the surgeon and anesthesiologist to know how to treat an anaphylactic reaction and have epinephrine available. As soon as the reaction begins, the receptors are flooded with histamines. The use of antihistamines, competitive inhibitors, as a pretreatment will lessen the severity of the reaction (Table 125-2). Recent research in immunology has suggested that pretreatment with both H_1) and H_2-histamine receptor antagonists may be more effective than H_1 antagonists alone[22,23,24] (H_1-receptor antagonist: diphenhydramine (Benadryl); H_2-receptor antagonist: cimetidine (Tagamet)).

SURGICAL TECHNIQUE

RADIOLOGIC MONITORING

In order to properly perform chemonucleolysis, it is an absolute requirement to have excellent fluoroscopy with an image intensifier that can visualize the disc space on the lateral view. Unless adequate space to accommodate anesthesia in an environment that permits sterile injection of the disc space can be provided in the radiology suite, the procedure should be done in the operating room using the C-arm image intensifier.

POSITIONING

Irrespective of whether the lateral or prone position is used, it is absolutely necessary that the patient be maintained in position so that there is perfect alignment of the lateral and AP position with the image intensifier. The slightest rotation may interfere with the three-dimensional conceptualization by the

Table 125-2. Anaphylaxis precautionary regime

1. Exclude all patients with a history of sensitivity to papaya or papaya extracts.
2. Prescreen patients using the fluroroallergeosorbent (FAST) test.
3. Pretreat with cimetidine, 300 mg PO every 6 hours, and diphenhydramine, 50 mg PO every 6 hours, for the 24 hours before injection.
4. Since the severity and length of the anaphylactic reaction can be increased with increased amounts of antigen, a test dose of 0.2 to 0.3 ml of chymopapain should be delivered intradiscally. If no adverse reaction is observed within 15 minutes, the remaining therapeutic dose of the enzyme should be administered.
5. Any systemic manifestation of anaphylaxis, no matter how mild, should be considered as part of a potentially lethal process and the patient should be treated immediately and vigorously beginning with 1:10,000 epinephrine.

surgeon, with the result that needle placement will be difficult, if not impossible.[25]

Most surgeons have been trained to operate on patients in the lateral position and under general anesthesia. This allows the anesthesiologist easy access to the endotracheal tube and permits the surgeon to stand close to the patient while the needle is inserted without interfering with the C-arm visualization of the lateral spine. In this position, the knees are flexed, pillows are placed between the knees and the patient secured in position with 3-inch tape. The true AP and lateral alignment with the image intensifier is then verified. Following a soap and water scrub, the surgical site is cleansed with Betadine. A sterile plastic drape is placed over the site of injection and the image intensifier is then draped.

Recently, I have been carrying out this procedure using local anesthesia with increasing frequency. It is much more comfortable for the patient to be in the prone position when awake. Under local anesthesia in the lateral position, it is often difficult for the patient because the slightest amount of pain will cause him or her to move and thus disturb the alignment. This is not as much of a problem with the prone position, which is more natural, and the patient tends to be more relaxed and to resettle back into the original position of alignment. There is some inconvenience to the surgeon since the C-arm fluoroscope tends to get in the way for the lateral fluoroscopy of the spine. I now use this position for both local and general anesthesia. Shields angulates the fluoroscope so that its beam is centered and aligned with the disc space on the AP view. He then guides the needle into the disc space on the AP view and uses the lateral view to confirm his needle position.[26]

ANESTHESIA

An anesthesiologist should be in attendance for all procedures, monitoring the patient, giving supplemental oxygen, and prepared to treat anaphylaxis. If general anesthesia is used, it should be light and the patient not paralyzed so that if the needle touches the nerve root the leg will jump. For local anesthesia it is usually adequate to use 1 percent lidocaine in the skin and deep subcutaneous area with systemic fentanyl and diazepam. If, under local anesthesia, a nerve root is touched by the needle the patient will experience pain and will be able to inform the surgeon of this discomfort.

NEEDLE PLACEMENT

Before the patient is brought to the operating room, plain spine roentgenograms are obtained and reviewed for transitional vertebra and used to verify exactly on the lateral view which disc space is to be injected. If the L5-S1 disc space is narrow, the angle of the intervertebral space too flat, the iliac crest too high, the transverse process too large, or there is a large transitional transverse process, it may be impossible to place the needle at L5-S1.

Using a skin-marking pencil, the iliac crest is outlined and the porous processes are marked. A position 9 cm lateral to the spine is then marked. This distance can be greater or less depending on the size of the patient. With the visualization of the lateral spine on the fluoroscope, a radiopaque rod is held in the x-ray beam and aligned with the angle of the disc space. This plane on the disc space is then marked where it crosses the 9 cm lateral mark, and this point on the skin is injected with local anesthesia. A 6-inch, 18-gauge needle is then inserted in a

series of 2-cm steps and guided toward the center of the disc space along this angle of the plane to the center of the disc space and at a 45 degrees to the sagittal plane of the spine. This angle can vary depending on the size and build of the patient and the distance from the midline. The needle should be checked on the fluoroscope and the angle readjusted after each 2-cm advance. After the needle has been guided to the center of the disc space using the lateral fluoroscopic view, an AP view is taken to verify the position of the needle. If the needle is not in the center of the disc on the two views, the needle should be withdrawn and the angles corrected, and the procedure started again. Once the needle is inserted for more than 2 inches beneath the skin, it is difficult to redirect the needle. It may be best to completely remove the needle and start over. If the needle touches the nerve root, the patient will experience pain in the leg. Pain in the back, hip, or groin indicates that either the facet or the annulus is being touched. As the needle is advanced, rotating the bevel will sometimes help control the direction of the needle, since the bevel can act as a rudder and cause the needle to move in one direction or the other; this will also help the needle slide over the edge of a bony obstruction. It is necessary that the surgeon be certain of the anatomy of the spine and be able to recognize a transverse process or facet on the lateral view so that the cause of obstruction to the needle passage can be recognized and adjustment made.

At the L4-5 disc space, slight changes of the angle of the needle from the sagittal plane may allow passage of the needle past a facet, although it is usually necessary to move the needle caudad or cephalad to get it past the transverse process.

At the L5-S1 interspace, usually the needle can be inserted at or very near the same point in the skin as the L4-5 needle, keeping the same angle from the sagittal plane as was used for the L4-L5 interspace. The needle tip is angled approximately 30 degrees caudad and slowly advanced to the interspace. Since the L4-L5 needle is an excellent guide, it is frequently inserted even though only the L5-S1 interspace is to be injected. As the needle tip enters the L5-S1 interspace, it is often helpful to rotate the needle with the bevel caudad; this enables the needle to bend and slide into the L5-S1 interspace. In some instances where it has been very difficult to insert a needle, it is helpful to use a two-needle technique where the bevel of an 18-gauge needle is inserted to the posterior lateral edge of the disc space and then the stylet is replaced with a 22-gauge, 8-inch needle that has been gently pre-curved over the distal 3 to 4 cm. The 22-gauge needle is then inserted into the L5-S1 disc.[27]

The final position of the needle tip should be as close as possible to the midline. If the needle is in the nucleus pulposus, it should be within the middle one third of the AP and lateral diameter of the vertebral body. There should be little resistance to injection of saline in an abnormal disc, while firm resistance will be met if the needle is in either the annulus or in a normal disc. An abnormal disc will easily accept 2 ml or more of saline. Following fluoroscopic confirmation that the needle is in the nucleus pulposus and a positive saline acceptance of more than 1 ml, the enzyme is reconstituted for injection. A 0.2-ml test dose of the enzyme is then injected and the patient observed for 15 minutes for evidence of an allergic reaction. If no allergic reaction occurs, an additional 1.0–1.5 ml of enzyme (2000–3000 units) is injected. Prior to the test injection, the drapes are removed from the patient so that the patient's skin and extremities can be observed. Following administration of the remaining enzyme, the patient is observed again for 15 minutes before being moved to a stretcher and taken to the recovery area for at least another 30 minutes of further observation.

POST-INJECTION TREATMENT RECOVERY

On return from the operating room, the patient receives pain medication as needed, and is encouraged to get out of bed and walk to the bathroom. The patient is usually discharged from the hospital with prescriptions for pain medication and muscle relaxants within 24 hours of the procedure. He or she is instructed to walk as much as possible, to stand in a hot shower for 10 minutes twice a day, not to return to work, to do no lifting, and to desist from any activity that causes or exacerbates his or her back or leg pain. The patient is routinely seen in follow-up 2 weeks after the procedure and activity increased as tolerated. During the post-injection period, almost every patient will develop some degree of back pain. This may occur immediately or may be delayed in time, and may be mild and last a few days or quite severe and persist for 6 to 8 weeks. The patient should be warned in advance of this possibility and reassured the back pain is temporary. The back pain is probably the result of a chemical discitis or an acute facet syndrome, and is manifested by localized back pain, pain in the buttock, hip or groin. This pain usually responds to nonsteroidal anti-inflammatory agents, hot showers, analgesics, and muscle relaxants, and will occasionally require the use of a back support. Unlike laminectomy, response to chemonucleolysis is quite variable. Some patients will return from the operating room with no further back pain and no sciatica, while other patients will be so handicapped by back pain that they will be essentially immobile for 6 to 8 weeks. Although sciatic pain may persist, it should decrease and if still present in its original intensity 6 weeks after injection, the patient should be evaluated as a possible failure.

PROCEDURAL FAILURES

Chemonucleolysis is a procedure in which the surgeon cannot see the pathologic process under direct vision and therefore cannot be certain the pathologic process has been corrected. Special caution is necessary in identifying a potential failure. The CT scan and myelogram may not revert to normal, even 6 months after a successful injection. This, coupled with the back pain that most patients temporarily develop following injection, may cause both the patient and the physician to make the unwarranted assumption that the injection has failed. The following criteria are indicative of actual failure of the procedure: worsening of objective findings, significant worsening of radicular symptoms, appearance of new and significant findings, and symptoms (excluding back discomfort) or failure of any symptomatic or objective improvement 6 weeks after injection. Approximately 5 percent of chymopapain injections are failures and require subsequent laminectomy.[16] These failures are usually caused by either sequestered disc material that cannot be reached by the enzyme, or a fragment of annulus or bone that is compressing the nerve root and is unaffected by the enzyme. These conditions are remedied by laminectomy. The other causes of failure are incorrect diagnosis, improper technique, unrealistic expectation, denial of success in a compensation patient, acute facet syndrome, precipitation of impending spinal stenosis, or traumatic sensory dysesthesia (more frequent in diabetics). Except in the diabetic patient, the single

puncture of a nerve root usually does not produce any long-lasting symptoms.

COMPLICATIONS

There were 401 complications reported to the manufacturer out of 13,700 patients who had received chymopapain before 1975, when the clinical studies in the United States were stopped.[28] This included 207 sensitivity reactions, 49 neurologic reactions, and 8 deaths. With the resumption of investigations in 1981, there were 1498 patients enrolled in a carefully documented, open-label study that was completed a year later. In this study, there were 13 anaphylactic reactions (including two deaths) and 2 patients with paraplegia.[16] A post-marketing surveillance study of 29,075 patients in 1984 recorded 194 anaphylactic reactions, 22 serious adverse neurologic experiences, 22 cases of discitis, and 11 deaths. In this group of adverse neurologic experiences, 3 patients had seizures, 3 patients had cerebral hemorrhages secondary to vascular lesions (aneurysms, arteriovenous malformations), 4 patients became paraplegic more than 1 week after the enzyme injection (one patient had a Guillain-Barré syndrome), and one had an extruded disc fragment. Of the remaining 11 patients, 3 had hemorrhagic cerebral lesions only; 4 had blood in the CSF as well as spinal and cerebral lesions (hemorrhagic encephalomyelopathy). In almost half the cases, there was either direct or probable evidence of violation of the spinal cord by the needle. It was therefore felt that the cases of paraplegia were "primarily due to needle trauma, or injection of contrast material and enzyme into the subarachnoid space."[29]

These suspicions were strengthened by a study in which either chymopapain, Conray, Amipaque, or Renografin was injected into a series of baboons with no adverse effects, except for two of nine baboons in which Renografin was used. A second series of baboons was injected with contrast material plus chymopapain, and the results were disastrous in almost half of the animals in the groups.[30] This has helped reinforce the warning that care be taken not to inadvertently inject the contrast material into intrathecal space, as well as to caution against the use of Pantopaque contrast material, which in itself may be toxic or enhance the toxicity of chymopapain.[31] As of February, 1985, approximately 95,000 patients have received Chymodiactin and 51 serious adverse neurologic experiences have been reported to the manufacturers. This includes 20 deaths (0.02 percent), 15 cerebral hemorrhages, 1 quadriplegic and 28 paraplegics or paraparesis.[32] Although the inadvertent introduction of chymopapain into the CSF is certainly the mechanism behind some of the neurologic complications, some are coincident processes, and some remain unexplained. One of the patients subsequently studied by myself was found to have a thrombosis of the artery of Adamkiewicz. Another curiosity is the high incidence of ruptured aneurysms and arteriovenous malformations that have occurred following an injection of chymopapain.[33]

REFERENCES

1. Smith L: Enzyme dissolution of the nucleus pulposus in humans. JAMA 187:177, 1964
2. Smith, L, Garvin PJ, Gesler RM, et al: Enzyme dissolution of the nucleus pulposus. Nature 198:1311, 1963
3. Smith L, Brown JE: Treatment of lumbar intervertebral disc lesions

by direct injection of chymopapain. J Bone Joint Surg 49B:502, 1967

4. Gavin PJ, Jennings MD, Smith L, Gesler RM: Chymopapain: A pharmacologic and toxicologic evaluation in experimental animals. Clin Orthop 42:204, 1965

5. Shealy CN: Tissue reactions to chymopapain in cats. J Neurosurg 26:327, 1967

6. Ford LT: Experimental study of chymopapain in cats. Clin Orthop 67:68, 1969

7. Brown MD: Intradiscal Therapy—Chymopapain or Collagenase. Chicago, Year Book, 1983, p 9

8. Gesler RM: Pharmacologic properties of chymopapain. Clin Orthop 67:47, 1969

9. Brown MD: Intradiscal Therapy—Chymopapain or Collagenase. Chicago, Year Book, 1983, p 16

10. Discase Injection (Chymopapain) (Product Information Brochure). Illinois, Omnis Surgical (Affiliate of Baxter-Travenol Laboratories), 1984, p 9

11. Brown JE, Nordby EJ, Smith L: The investigation and approval of chymopapain chemonucleolysis, in: Chemonucleolysis. New Jersey, SLACK, 1985, pp 1–11

12. Schwetschenau PR, Ramirez A, Johnston J, et al: Double-blind evaluation of intradiscal chymopapain for herniated lumbar discs. J Neurosurg 45:622, 1976

13. Chymopapain pulled off IND status. Med World News 16:38, September 8, 1975

14. Brown JE, Nordby EJ, Smith L: Chemonucleolysis. New Jersey, SLACK, 1985 p 7

15. Javid MJ, Nordby EJ, Ford, LT, et al: Safety and efficacy of chymopapain (Chymodiactin) in herniated nucleus pulposus with sciatica: Results of a randomized, double-blind study. JAMA 249:2489, 1983

Commentary—Chymopapain

Charles A. Fager

EFFICACY

The value of chymopapain in the treatment of patients with ruptured intervertebral discs remains open to serious question. In fact, it was predicted that chemonucleolysis as a treatment alternative for a ruptured disc could be more regressive than beneficial.[1-3] Surgeons unwilling to accept the rigid criteria for proper patient selection and appropriate surgical technique perceived intradiscal therapy as a benign substitute. Since chemonucleolysis was proclaimed as the method that could eliminate much lumbar disc surgery, many patients who previously underwent surgery that should not have been performed now undergo chemonucleolysis (often at multiple levels), which also should not be undertaken. Others who may be candidates for surgery endure injection of the enzyme without benefit and then require surgery as well (Figures 125-1 and 125-2).

The intradiscal use of proteolytic agents is faulted by the well-established observation that most disc fragments, which eventually require surgical intervention of some kind, are either extruded or incarcerated outside the disc space. These loosened particles have usually burst in a mushroomlike fashion through a small opening in the annulus and are sometimes contiguous with the disc space but not with intradiscal cartilage (Figures 125-3 and 125-4). Although chymopapain may exert its proteolytic effect on cartilage within the disc space, its influence on such ruptured fragments must be considered dubious, making the procedure useless if not worthless.

Spontaneous recovery from protruded and even ruptured discs is so common that results of successful treatment are delusive (Figure 125-5). Of the numerous studies reported thus far, little evidence exists to conclude that the effect of chymopapain is better than that of a placebo.[4] In the initial study[5] that became the basis for the approval of chymopapain by the Food and Drug Administration in 1982, an overall success rate of 73 percent was claimed. Yet in three of the seven centers chymopapain proved no better than the placebo. Furthermore, treatment was deemed a "success" if the result was excellent, good, or fair. Patients with a fair result were able to perform only very light work and experienced frequent pain that required the use of moderate or strong analgesic agents.

In a recent 9- to 12-year review of 105 patients, Javid[6] reported that among 79 patients who showed marked improvement, results in 67 patients were classified as excellent (pain free) and in 12 as good (50 to 85 percent relief of pain). These findings are hardly comparable with the surgical success rate reported by Scoville and Corkill[7] or with my results,[8] which have been duplicated by a number of other surgeons.

ADVERSE REACTIONS AND MORTALITY

Statements in the literature concerning the dangers of chymopapain have been misleading. Agre et al.[9] compared the mortality rate of chemonucleolysis with that of laminectomy and claimed 11 deaths in 60,000 patients (0.02 percent), but the study, which reported 11 deaths and 11 instances of paraplegia, had data on only 29,075 patients. Recently, 21 deaths have been reported[10] in an "estimated" 98,000 patients who received chemonucleolysis. No data whatsoever on these 98,000 patients were published, and we have no way of knowing whether the latest figures on mortality and adverse reactions are still approximately 50 percent, as they were at the time of the report in 1984.[9]

The same postmarketing surveillance[9] demonstrated some of the abuses of chymopapain, disclosing that approximately 24 percent of the 29,075 patients had received injections at more than one level even though simultaneous symptomatic rupture of more than one disc is extremely rare, if it occurs at all. Inappropriate applications of the procedure are common, and many normal discs, "bulging" discs, degenerative discs, and protruded or ruptured discs have been injected with chymopapain.

The warning to surgeons in June, 1984, from Smith Laboratories and Omnis Surgical (Letters to Physicians, June 19, 1984, Smith Laboratories Inc., Northbrook, Illinois, and Omnis Surgical Inc., Deerfield, Illinois) must raise a serious conflict for surgeons who have relied on contrast radiography to avoid spinal injection or rapid venous absorption of the enzyme. Ray,[11] in commenting on the latter phenomenon, proposed that lateral discography be considered for all patients before injection of chymopapain.

OTHER ADVERSE EFFECTS

Most reports on chemonucleolysis have dealt with the success and failure of the procedure. Few reports have given any indication that some patients are worse as a direct result of the injection. Some of the deleterious sequelae that resemble iatrogenic problems seen after inappropriate surgery are occurring with increased frequency as the agent is administered to larger numbers of patients.

Forty-eight patients were referred to the Lahey Clinic Medical Center because of increased pain and disability after chemonucleolysis. Previous records and all available roentgenograms of these patients were evaluated. Of the 48 patients, 32 (67 percent) were determined to have had nonspecific back pain

OPERATIVE NEUROSURGICAL TECHNIQUES
ISBN 0-8089-1862-1

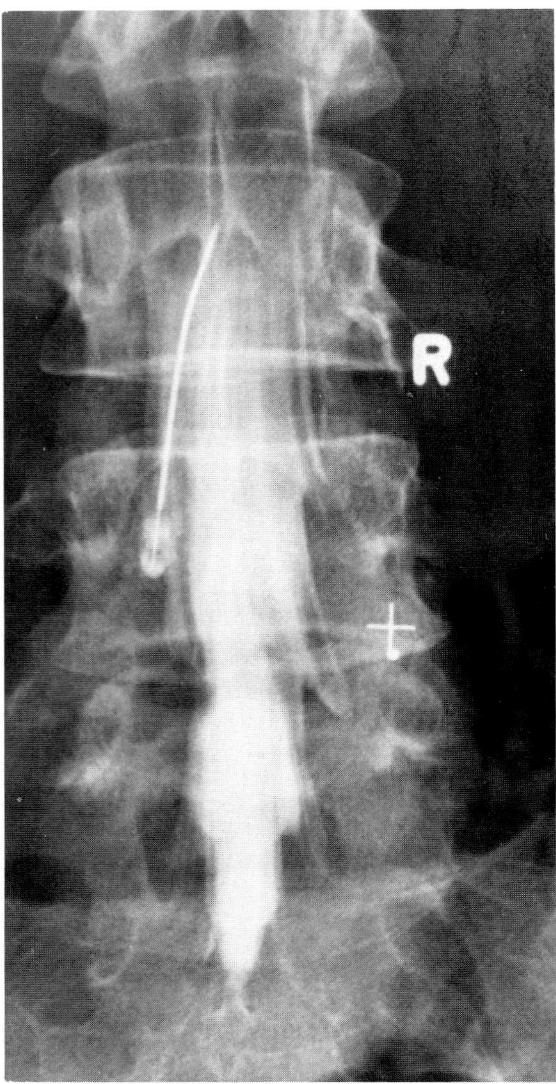

Fig. 125-1.   A myelogram of 33-year-old woman with a disc fragment extruded below the disc space at the left of L4-L5 through a marginal tear. There was persistent severe compression of the left L5 root after injection of enzyme.

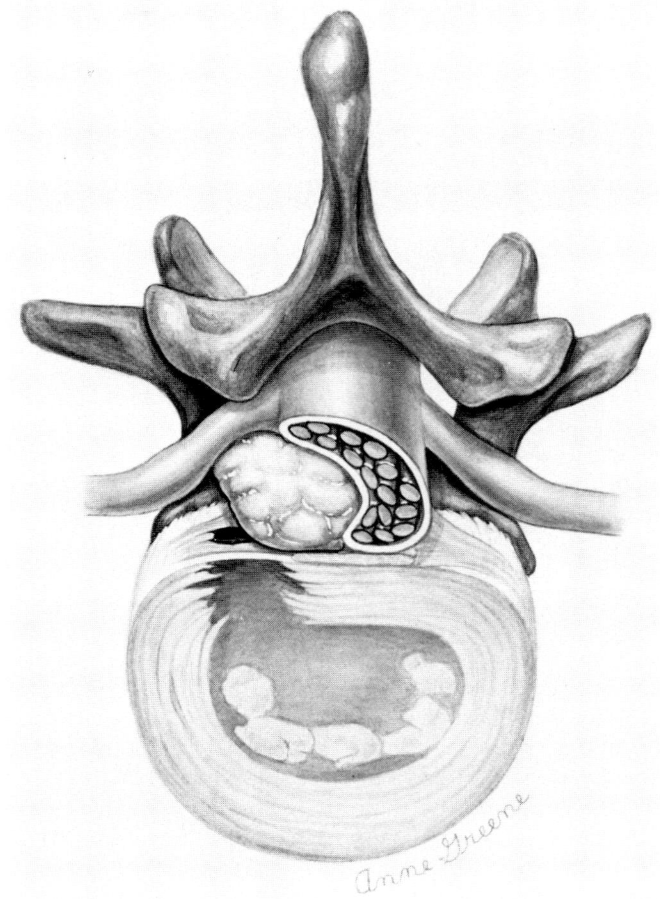

Fig. 125-3.   A typical extruded fragment that ruptured through the annulus and posterior longitudinal ligament. (Reprinted from Fager CA: Lumbar microdiscectomy: A contrary opinion. Clin Neurosurg 33:423, 1986. With permission.)

before chemonucleolysis, 5 had neural compression from spondylosis, and 11 had protruded or ruptured discs (Table 125-3). Of 21 patients (44 percent) who gave a history of trauma, 19 had industrial- or vehicular-related accidents (Table 125-4).

More than half of the patients with nonspecific back pain had some type of pain extending to the lower extremity, usually to the hip or upper thigh, and several had sciatic pain extending below the knee. None of these 32 patients complained of weakness in the lower limb, numbness, or tingling, and no positive neurologic signs were recorded. Positive results in tests of straight leg raising, localized tenderness, and limited movement of the back were common physical findings preceding treatment. Myelograms or CT scans of these patients indicated either a normal or a ''bulging'' disc at one or more levels; 7 patients had degenerative disc disease, facet arthropathy, or both (Table 125-3). In several patients neither myelography nor computed tomography had been performed, and discography was ostensibly the only diagnostic procedure that preceded

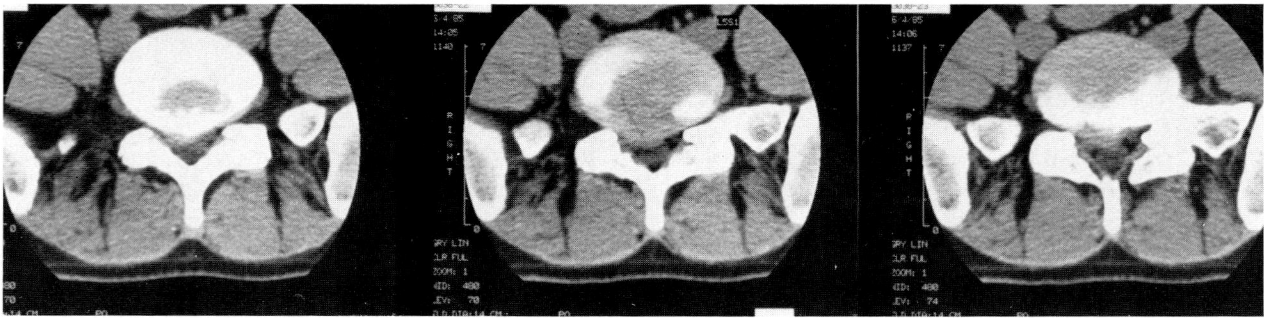

Fig. 125-2.   A CT scan of the lumbar spine of a 28-year-old woman with a subligamentous fragment of disc who failed to obtain relief from injection of chymopapain.

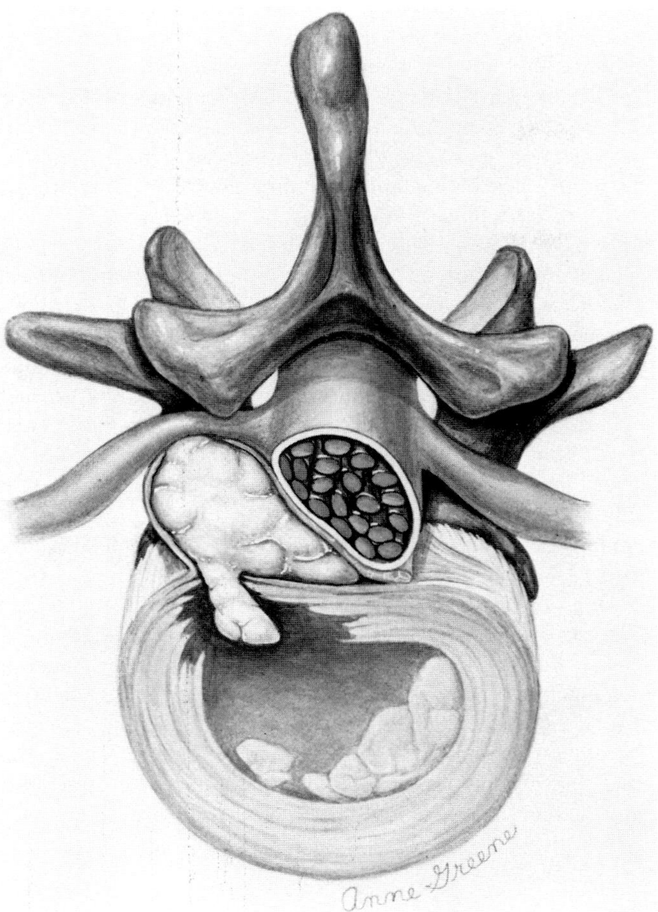

Fig. 125-4. An illustration characteristic of a subligamentous fragment that ruptured through a small opening and is not connected to residual intradiscal cartilage. (Reprinted from Fager CA: Lumbar microdiscectomy: A contrary opinion. Clin Neurosurg 33:422, 1986. With permission.)

Table 125-3. Status of 48 patients before injection of chymopapain

Status	Number of Patients
Nonspecific back pain	32
Spondylosis	
Degenerative disc or facet arthropathy	7
Undetermined or posttraumatic	
''Bulging'' discs	17
Normal roentgenograms or myelograms	8
Disc protrusion or rupture	11
Spondylosis with neural compression	5
Total	48

injection of the enzyme. In some patients no roentgenograms of the spine had been obtained before the operation.

Most of these 32 patients reported severe pain in the back immediately after the injection that at times required hospitalization for 1 or 2 weeks. Others did not have this reaction but within days began to notice a return of the original or similar pain that became increasingly severe, limited movement of the back, and produced progressive disability. The condition of a number of these patients stabilized at a reasonable level, and the patients are no longer worse than they were before injection. Several returned to work, and others are functioning in limited capacity.

The patients with a protruded or ruptured disc and those with neural compression from spondylosis had evidence of involvement of a nerve root on myelograms or CT scans. Of 8 patients who required surgery, 5 had persistent spondylotic nerve root or cauda equina compression, and 3 had ruptured

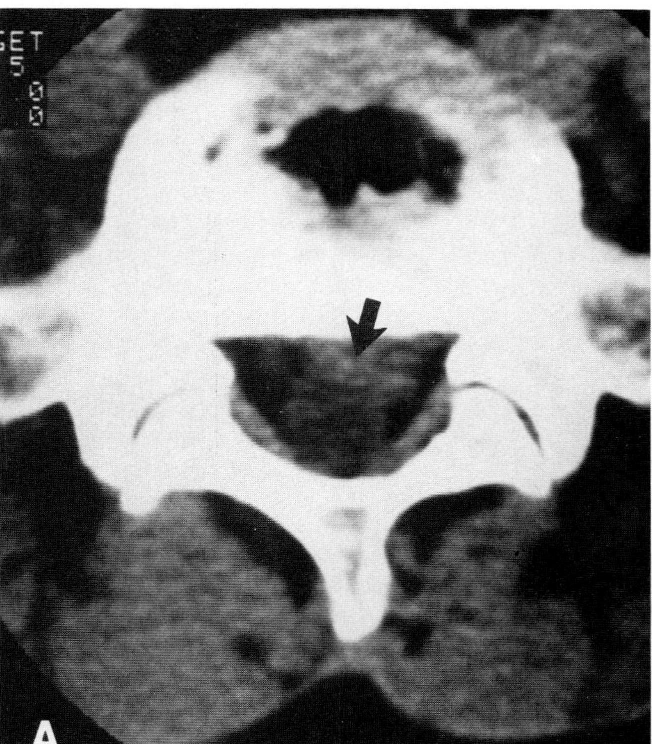

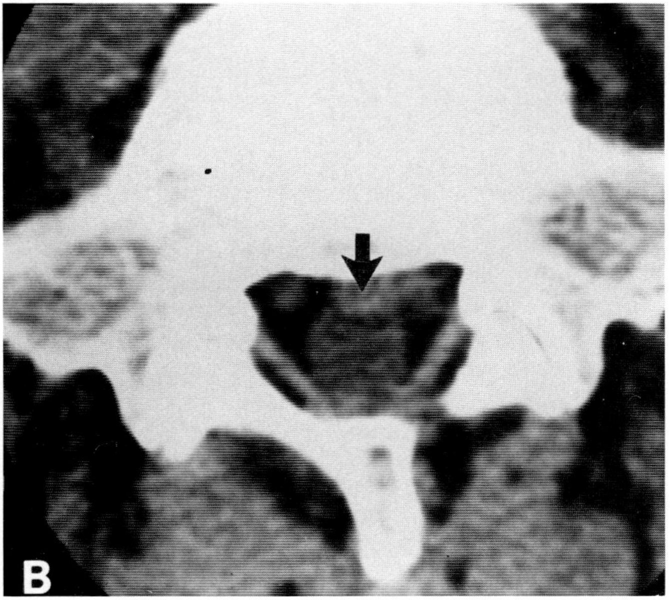

Fig. 125-5. (A) A lumbar CT scan of a 43-year-old man shows left paramedian disc rupture (arrow). The patient had a complete spontaneous recovery in 6 weeks. (B) A CT scan of the same patient 9 months later. The patient remains asymptomatic with partial resolution of the ruptured fragment (arrow).

Table 125-4. Status of 48 patients before injection of chymopapain

Status	Number of Patients
History of trauma	21
Industrial	14
Vehicular	5
Noncompensible	2
No trauma	27
Total	48

Table 125-5. Status of 40 nonsurgical patients after injection of chymopapain

Findings	Number of Patients
Back pain alone	26
Back/leg pain—no deficit	11
Back/leg pain—radiculopathy	3
Disc space narrowed	24
Discitis/osteomyelitis	2

discs. All had a satisfactory recovery and are free of radicular pain, although 3 patients still have serious pain in the back, are limited to light activities, and require analgesics.

Of the other 8 patients believed to have had a protruded or ruptured disc, 2 no longer have pain in the lower extremity since injection of chymopapain and show no signs of compression of the nerve root although they complain of continued activity-related pain in the back of varying severity. Two patients in this group who appeared to have satisfactory criteria for enzyme injection and small myelographic defects continue to have disabling pain in the lower back and lower extremity although the results of myelograms obtained after injection are normal. Three others in the same category had a neurologic deficit from the injection with objective radiculopathy; in each instance the deficit was limited to one lower extremity (Table 125-5). None of these three patients had severe motor or sensory loss before injection. Two patients in the group of 48 required antibiotic therapy for discitis with osteomyelitis and have improved; one of these patients had a metastatic infection at the L1-L2 level after chemonucleolysis at L4-L5.

One conspicuous finding in the 48 patients is a strikingly rapid narrowing of the disc space, which was evident in 20 patients who were seen from 2 to 12 months after injection when compared with roentgenograms of the lumbar spine taken before the procedure (Figures 125-6, 125-7, 125-8, and 125-9). In four other patients similar narrowing of the disc space was found, but no comparison could be made because roentgenograms had not been obtained before the procedure. In an initial

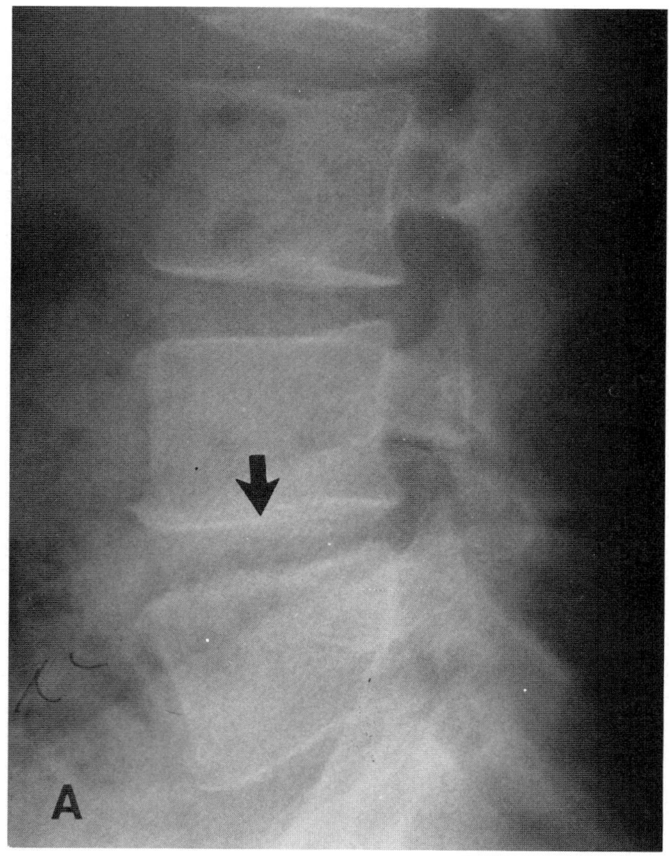
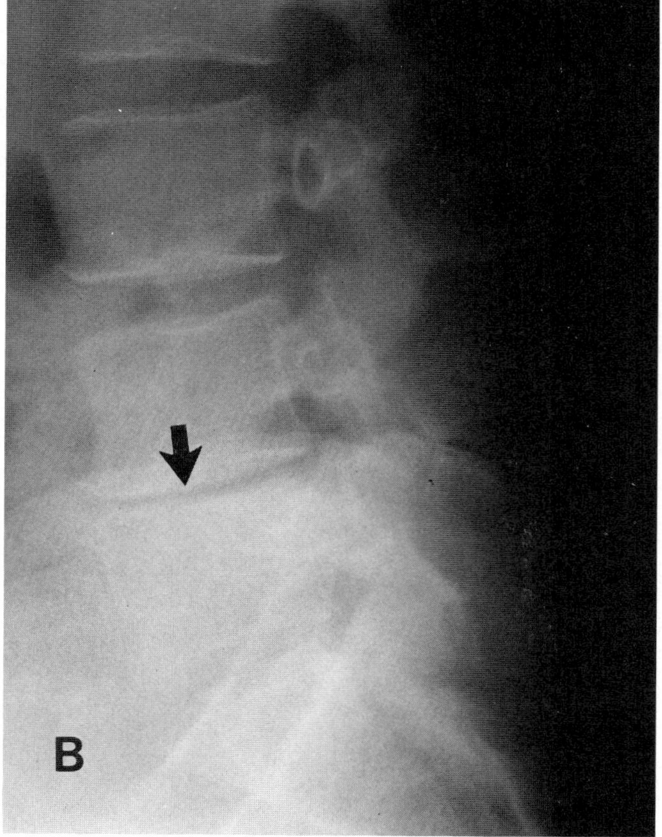

Fig. 125-6. A lateral roentgenogram of the lumbar spine showing the L4-L5 disc space (arrow) (A) before chemonucleolysis and (B) 2 months after injection in a patient with continued severe back pain.

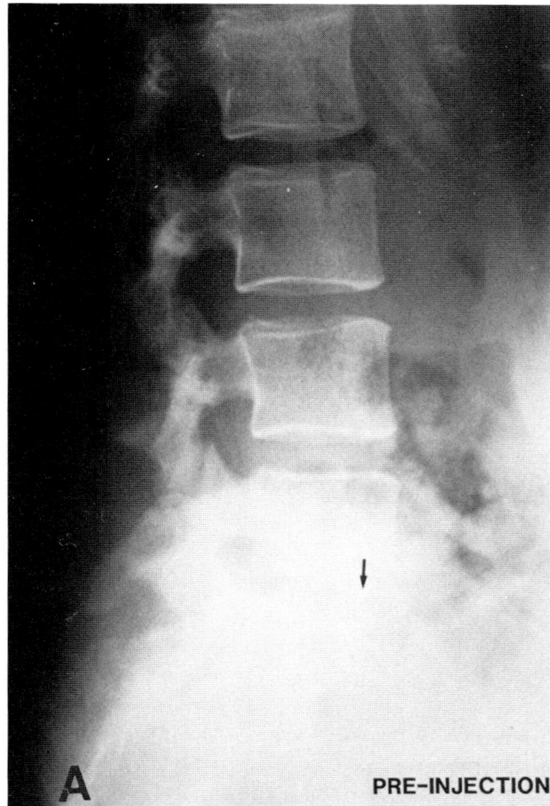

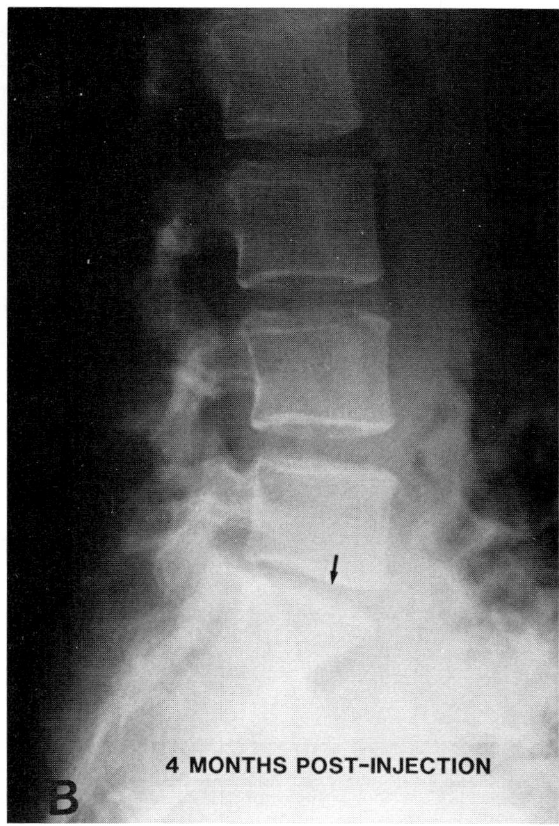

Fig. 125-7. Appearance of the lumbosacral disc space (A) before injection of enzyme and (B) 4 months after injection in a patient with continued severe back pain.

group of 38 patients, this finding was observed in 16 patients who were seen 4 to 10 months after the injection (Fager, unpublished data). Almost all of these patients reported early pain, back spasm, or stiffness immediately after injection. Most have experienced some improvement, with a decrease in the severity of the pain in the back and lessened limitation after several months. Some continue to improve, but most have some degree of residual pain in the back. Several others have

back pain and abnormal results on myelograms but are not considered suitable for surgery (Figure 125-7). The proteolytic effect of the enzyme, which remains in disc tissue when injected, seems well established in these patients. The resultant narrowing, which occurs within months of the injection, must represent a form of subacute degenerative change manifested by pain instead of chronic degenerative disc disease, which can either be painful or asymptomatic.

The symptoms and signs in patients that suggest radiculopathy after injection and in one patient with metastatic infection of the disc space three segments away raise ongoing speculation about the effects of the enzyme employed alone or mixed with a contrast agent that has escaped into the spinal canal (epidural or subarachnoid).

COMMENT

It is difficult to escape the conclusion from this small sampling of unhappy patients that the degree of destruction of cartilage and subsequent narrowing of the disc space may be proportional to the concentration of enzyme within the intervertebral disc space. Some leakage of the agent into the surrounding tissue or absorption into the venous circulation may occur in those patients in whom no postinjection narrowing develops.

These patients obviously represent only those with bad results. While reports of failures of chemonucleolysis have been numerous, the procedure is not innocuous, the adverse effects represent serious complications, and other harmful effects lead to prolonged pain and disability. Considering all the undesirable

Fig. 125-8. (Left) A lateral myelogram of a patient without clear evidence of a ruptured disc and (right) the radiographic appearance of the spine 1 year after injection at L4-L5 and L5-S1. Note the narrowing of both spaces (arrows) associated with persistent disabling pain.

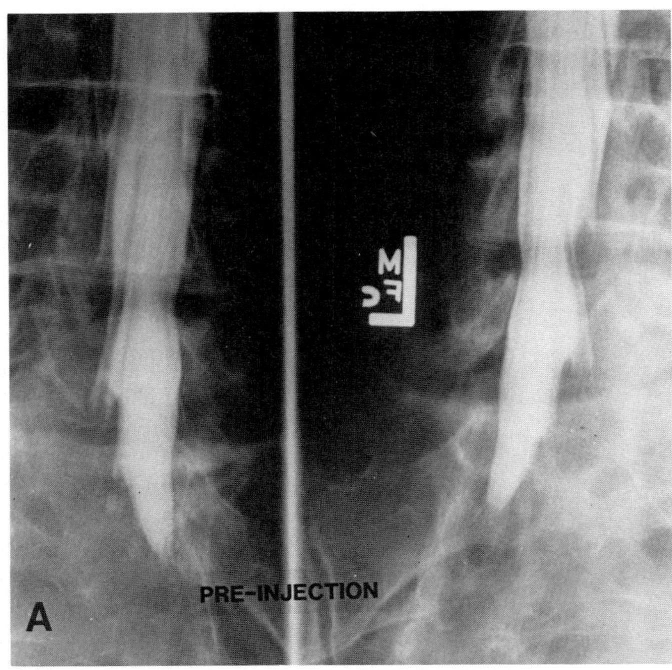

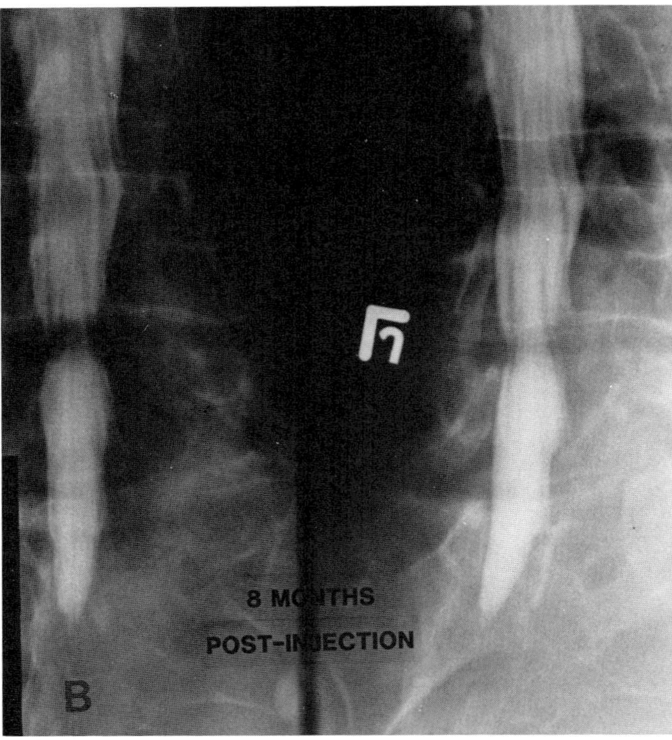

Fig. 125-9.   (A) A preinjection myelogram of 52-year-old woman with symptoms and signs of a protruded disc at L4-L5 on the right. (B) A myelogram 8 months after injection shows additional abnormality related to degenerative narrowing of the disc space and spondylosis. The patient had less pain in the leg but more intense back pain.

side effects, the question must be asked whether the placebo effect of this procedure, which must account for "success" in many patients, justifies its continued use.

REFERENCES

1. Fager CA: Comment and response: Chymopapain for chemonucleolysis for lumbar disk disease in U.S. Orthop Rev 8: 189, 1979
2. Fager CA: The age-old back problem: New fad, same fallacies. Spine 9:326, 1984
3. Fager CA: Chymopapain—a counter comment. Surg Neurol 21: 617, 1984
4. Deyo RA: Chymopapain for herniated intervertebral disc: A methodologic analysis and an agenda for future research. Spine 9: 474, 1984
5. Javid MJ, Nordby EJ, Ford LT, et al: Safety and efficacy of chymopapain (Chymodiactin) in herniated nucleus pulposus with sciatica: Results of a randomized, double-blind study. JAMA 249: 2489, 1983
6. Javid MJ: Efficacy of chymopapain chemonucleolysis: A long-term review of 105 patients. J Neurosurg 62:662, 1985
7. Scoville WB, Corkill G: Lumbar disc surgery: Technique of radical removal and early mobilization. Technical note. J Neurosurg 39: 265, 1973
8. Fager CA: Ruptured median and paramedian lumbar disk: A review of 243 cases. Surg Neurol 23:309, 1985
9. Agre K, Wilson RR, Brim M, et al: Chymodiactin postmarketing surveillance demographic and adverse experience data in 29,075 patients. Spine 9:479, 1984
10. Javid MJ: Response. Neurosurgical forum. J Neurosurg 63:992, 1985
11. Ray CD: Danger of intravenous injection during chemonucleolysis (letter).

CHAPTER 126
Surgical Management of Trauma to the Spine

David Yashon

FRACTURE-DISLOCATION of the vertebral column with or without involvement of the spinal cord or nerve roots continues to present a series of difficult therapeutic problems. Various modes of treatment, including skeletal traction, Halo jacket, neck brace, open fixation, posterior fusion, anterior fusion, or decompressive laminectomy followed by fusion and stabilization, entail immobilizing and hospitalizing the patient for long periods of time. The value of any one form of treatment has been difficult to assess in terms of neurologic recovery, and, indeed, the indications for surgery as well as the virtues of particular operations are controversial. The indications for surgery are not absolute, and this will be discussed when possible. This chapter concerns itself with surgical indications and the types of surgical treatment currently available for injuries to the vertebral column, beginning with the methods of skeletal traction and the anesthetic considerations in the patient with a spinal injury. Computed tomographic scanning has all but supplanted myelography in deciding whether bone fragments or other space-consuming lesions are causing pressure within the spinal canal. Magnetic resonance imaging (MRI) can also be useful in diagnosis.

SKELETAL TRACTION

The use of skull tongs to reduce fracture-dislocation and to maintain alignment of cervical spine fractures is now universal.[1,2] It is also now generally agreed that skeletal traction and reduction offer an important means of protecting and internally decompressing the cervical spinal cord and nerve roots following fracture-dislocation.[3] Halter traction is useful in the treatment of minor neck injuries and as a temporizing maneuver until skeletal traction can be established. Traction for thoracic and lumbar spine injuries is not used because the enormous forces required for distraction and realignment render it impractical.

Halter traction was first employed in 1929 by Taylor,[4] and its use has since become so widespread that most authors do not explore its origin. In acute spinal and vertebral injury, halter traction is not indicated except for temporary immobilization. Many implanted skeletal devices were described in the early 20th century. The tongs primarily used by physicians in the past were described by Crutchfield.[5-8] Many modifications of these tongs have been designed.[9] In 1938, Crutchfield[7] reported 43 patients treated with tongs, with the single complication being

osteomyelitis at the tong site in a patient with pre-existing infection. Gardner[10] described the tongs most utilized at present and Rimel et al.[11] modified them. They are known as University of Virginia tongs. All types involve some manner of fixation of the skull.[12] In 1948, Vinke[13] described a new set of tongs that had interlocking devices between the inner and outer tables of bone. In the past, we preferred Crutchfield tongs, but we have also used Vinke and Barton tongs.[14,15] Now Gardner and University of Virginia tongs (Figure 126-1) are best and can be used in children.

Tongs should be placed as soon as possible after the injury, since, in essence, realignment affects an internal decompression of the spinal contents.[16,17] Delay in treatment following an injury poses a philosophical question much akin to that concerning laminectomy, as to whether tongs should be placed and reduction carried out. We generally place tongs even after 1 week has elapsed, since adequate bone healing diminishes the chance of further neurologic damage, even if that damage is confined to a single nerve root in a tetraplegic patient. Also, adequate bone healing lessens the possibility of pain later. The second indication for placement of tongs is immobilization. We use turning frames and rocking beds exclusively in treatment and advise against circoelectric beds because of excessive loading of the fracture. The University of Virginia tongs have a lower profile, thus allowing easier turning and preventing occipital decubiti.

The length of time that tongs should be left in place is variable. We have left tongs in place for 12 weeks without ill effect. With use of halo traction, this length of time is seldom necessary. The tong sites are treated daily with antibiotic ointment and kept clean with soap and water. Tongs must be gently tightened daily or every other day. With Gardner or Virginia tongs, self-seating occurs and neither tightening nor shaving the hair is required. Skull x-ray films can be valuable in detecting complications. The position can be changed if skull penetration or osteomyelitis becomes a problem. One should watch for perforation of the skull or even brain abscess. At present, in our hospital, tongs are left in place up to 8 weeks, depending on the fracture. They are used during cervical surgery (both fusion and laminectomy) for maintenance of alignment and are left in place until fusion occurs spontaneously or is surgically induced. In all cervical spine fractures, we have used tongs initially until halo traction devices can be applied. On occasion, when doubt exists about the presence of a fracture-dislocation or stability, tongs have been installed only

OPERATIVE NEUROSURGICAL TECHNIQUES
ISBN 0-8089-1862-1

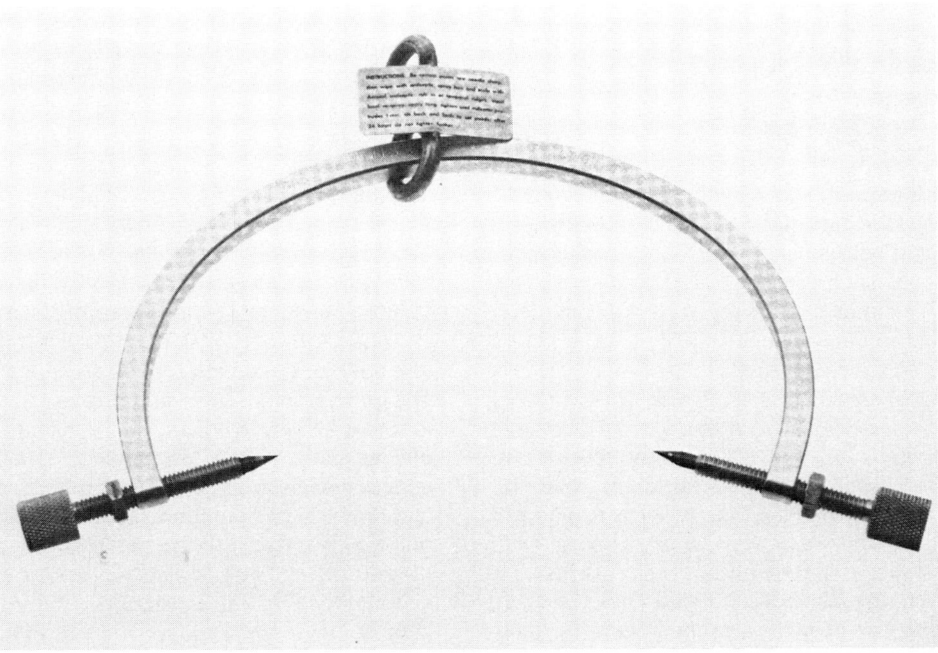

Fig. 126-1. The Gardner-Wells traction tongs. (Courtesy of Codman and Shurtleff, Inc.)

to be removed shortly thereafter when the physician felt that they were unnecessary. When stability is questionable, it is prudent to place tongs until the situation is fully clarified.

In deciding the amount of weight to be utilized, it should be remembered that skeletal traction is employed for alignment and reduction. Traction is begun using 1 to 2 kg per vertebra to the level of injury; for example, 5 kg for a C5-6 dislocation. Additional weights are added under radiographic control until reduction is achieved or about 28 kg of traction has been applied. Once satisfactory alignment has been achieved the applied traction is decreased to a level that maintains the reduction, prevents overdistraction, and is comfortable to the patient. Serial roentgenograms are used to monitor alignment and identify over distraction.

In the four decades since Crutchfield[5] reported tong traction to reduce a fracture-dislocation of the upper cervical spine, most proponents of various tongs, wires, and hooks have used traction weights of no more than 35 pounds to reduce cervical fracture-dislocations over several hours or even days.[5,6,8,18–26] Although greater weights have been used to reduce cervical fracture-dislocations complicated by locked facets,[27–29] Bailey,[30,31] Bovill et al.,[27] and Hollin and Gross[32] have suggested that weights greater than 45 to 50 pounds are excessive, and that operative reduction is indicated when such weights fail to produce satisfactory vertebral alignment in 24 to 48 hours.

Indeed, Crutchfield[5,7] cautioned against using heavy weights to achieve more rapid reduction, believing that force sufficient to speed reduction would add further injury to supporting tissues and endanger the spinal cord. Instead, he advocated a minimal corrective pull of up to 18 pounds[5] followed by gradual completion of reduction with no more than double this weight.

There is at least a theoretical argument in favor of more rapid reduction, and this is our preference.[14,15] Cervical fracture-dislocations often represent emergencies[33] in which the extent and duration of neurologic dysfunction may depend upon the time interval between the injury and spinal cord decompres-

sion.[33,34] A minimum of 60 to 90 minutes commonly elapses before a patient with a cervical fracture-dislocation is brought to the Emergency Service and placed in skull traction. In many cases, there is little useful information concerning improvement or deterioration in the patient's neurologic status during this period. Theoretically, prompt closed internal reduction provides relief of direct bony pressure on the spinal cord, thus diminishing further damage.

In the presence of severe cord injury and radiographic evidence of a cervical fracture-dislocation with or without locked facets, application of a minimal corrective pull to protect neural structures from further injury may represent less than optimal acute treatment. When no neurologic functional loss is apparent such rapidity is not necessarily indicated. In our clinic we attempt to reduce the dislocation as completely as possible, no longer than 2 hours after traction is applied.[14,15] Our goal is to decompress the spinal cord quickly by restoring the anteroposterior diameter of the cervical spinal canal and by achieving satisfactory positioning of bone fragments.

The technique consists of intravenous administration of muscle relaxants to reduce paraspinous muscle spasm, elevation of the head of the bed to exert countertraction through tongs inserted in a coronal plane determined by the cervical transverse processes and the external auditory meati. Traction force thus is exerted along the longitudinal axis of the vertebral bodies with the neck in a neutral position. Five to 10 pounds are added every 10 minutes. The neurologic examination and lateral cervical spine films are repeated after each increment. Once reduction is achieved, traction is maintained with 10 to 15 pounds. It should be emphasized that during reduction attention must be paid to the patient's description of additional neurologic symptoms, such as paraesthesia, pain, and neurologic loss. In patients without neurologic deficit the same technique and precautions may be employed, but haste is not so important.

Among patients in our hospital successfully treated in this manner over past years, the greatest amount of weight used in the first hour was 75 pounds. Operative reduction and decompression is considered in patients with severe neurologic signs in whom we cannot restore the anteroposterior diameter of the cervical spinal canal to within approximately 3 mm of normal[20] with traction over 1 to 2 hours. The inability to establish appropriate alignment by traction usually signifies locked or jumped facets[28] which require operative correction. This remains a controversial issue and the acceptance of imperfect alignment is necessitated occasionally for practical reasons.

Because of variables such as subsequent operative intervention (decompressive laminectomy, fusion, stabilization), it cannot be proved that rapid reduction of cervical fracture ±dislocations by means of skull traction ultimately yields a better neurologic result than gradual reduction. In many patients with significant neurologic deficit whom we have treated with this technique in the past 12 years, however, there have been no cases of neurologic deterioration that could be attributed to traction itself. It is our opinion that the low incidence of neurologic complications reported for reduction of cervical fracture-dislocations with skeletal traction[5,29] is not the result of speed of reduction or the amount of weight used, but rather that neurologic examination is performed carefully and sequentially during the procedure. Our concern for possible harm to supporting soft tissue structures is diminished both by our greater concern for preservation and restoration of neurologic function and by our tendency to ensure stability by subsequent operative fixation and fusion.[14,15]

ANESTHESIA

The risk of damaging the spinal cord by the slightest movement of the neck or head after cervical injury is a prime concern of the surgeon and anesthesiologist.[9,35] Movement after thoracic and lumbar injuries is similarly of concern. Because damage can occur during transport, induction of anesthesia, intubation, or positioning, the anesthesiologist is extremely careful to avoid excessive moving of the patient. In cervical cord injuries, skeletal traction along the spinal axis to stabilize the head and to protect against inadvertent movement is maintained during induction and intubation as well as throughout the operative procedure, and is continued postoperatively.

In patients undergoing emergency operation a full stomach is an added hazard during the induction of anesthesia.[35] Regurgitation is more probable than vomiting, because of paralysis of the abdominal muscles. Factors that predispose to regurgitation include head-down tilt, airway obstruction, intermittent positive pressure breathing before intubation, and the use of depolarizing muscle relaxants. Emptying of the stomach by nasogastric tube before induction of anesthesia not only does not guarantee an empty stomach, but, in fact, may facilitate regurgitation if the tube is left in place during induction. Head-up tilt decreases the likelihood of regurgitation, but may initiate or aggravate hypotension and may add to the technical difficulty of intubation.[36]

Awake intubation is widely advocated because it protects against possible failure to intubate the trachea, with loss of patent airways, and somewhat decreases the risk of inhalation of vomitus.[36] Attempts to visualize the larynx and intubate the trachea by direct oropharyngeal laryngoscopy in an awake patient with severe cervical spasm may be difficult and traumatic. Therefore, blind nasotracheal intubation may be the

procedure of choice; alternatively, the intubating fiberoptic laryngoscope may be the best way in experienced hands. Topical transtracheal and nasal-anesthetic spray is used; however, if the larynx is anesthetized, the risk of aspiration is increased.

Blind nasal intubation does not require a deep level of anesthesia, and in fact can be done without anesthesia. Blind nasal intubation obviates the need for muscle relaxants and traumatic endoscopy; the tube is easier to fix in place than the oral tube and is well tolerated by the conscious patient after operation. Suctioning the trachea is more difficult through a nasotracheal tube. Risk of damage to the mucous membrane of the nose and nasal pharynx is high, but this is balanced against the greater importance of nontraumatic intubation. Lubrication of the tube with a nonanesthetic bland jelly and prespraying of the nose with a 5 percent cocaine solution to shrink nasal mucosa will lessen the likelihood of epistaxis. A tube about 1 to 2 mm smaller than an oral tube with its bevel directed toward the nasal septum is most easily introduced.

Awake intubation can be carried out by nasal passage of the endotracheal tube. Blind oral or nasal intubation while the patient is awake helps to prevent additional injury, since the awake patient can report untoward neurologic symptoms. The patient can be examined during and after intubation. Elective tracheostomy can be performed in unusual cases, but by and large this has been unnecessary.

A patient positioned on the Stryker frame may be anesthetized, intubated, and then turned to the prone position for surgery. We frequently do not anesthetize the patient until he or she is in final (i.e., prone) position. A folded towel or sandbag under the chest causes the head to angulate so that adequate flexion for C1-C2 fusions and laminectomy can be accomplished with the head in the neutral position. The Stryker frame is ideal for such procedures; the circoelectric bed is not recommended because blood pressure may fall while the patient is erect, and loading of the fracture with consequent further damage can occur with change in position. While the patient is prone, prolonged pressure to the eyes must be avoided. Such pressure may exceed the normal retinal artery pressure and result in thrombosis of the retinal artery and blindness. Severe uneven and prolonged pressure on the face may result in necrosis about the zygomatic arch, the supraorbital ridges, and the mandible. Other areas of concern are the feet, the breasts, and the genitalia.

To prevent spinal cord injury during procedures such as the Harrington operation for idiopathic scoliosis, intraoperative evaluation of spinal cord function can be accomplished using evoked response monitoring. The value of this procedure remains in doubt.

CARDIOVASCULAR CONSIDERATIONS

Cardiovascular instability due to the loss of the sympathetic influence on the heart and blood vessels is a serious concern associated with spinal injury since this results in bradycardia, peripheral vasodilation, and hypotension. Circulatory disturbances may be further intensified by anesthetics or narcotics, which result in myocardial depression and vasodilatation. Hypovolemia is poorly tolerated by quadriplegic patients and should be remedied immediately during operation. It is essential to replace blood as it is lost as well as to maintain postoperative fluid balance. Transfusion of blood, however, solely because of hypotension caused by impaired sympathetic activity is not justified.

The central venous pressure level may be misleading in quadriplegic patients, because it may reflect a balance between changes in cardiac output and diminished venous return. Therefore, any tendency of central venous pressure to rise owing to cardiac depression or hypervolemia might be masked by venous pooling resulting from reduction of peripheral venous tone. Severe hypotension in the absence of hypovolemia can be corrected by temporary use of a vasopressive drug having both cardiac and peripheral action. For bradycardia, atropine may be given.

One must be alert to hypertensive crises due to autonomic hyperreflexia during anesthesia in patients with spinal injuries. Hypertension can be controlled with an intravenous drip of Arfonad (trimethaphan) or other medications. Fatal cerebral hemorrhage can occur during such a hypertensive crisis. In addition to paroxysmal hypertension, the symptoms include bradycardia, sweating, severe headache, and pilomotor erection. The syndrome can be initiated by almost any stimulus including distention of the bladder and rectum and pain.

Stone[37] as well as others warned against massive hyperkalemia in patients with musculoskeletal disease such as quadriplegia following relaxation with succinylcholine. A likely explanation for increase in serum potassium is that the denervated muscle cell membrane is altered, resulting in an atypical response to the depolarization produced by succinylcholine. The increased sensitivity to succinylcholine commences on about the sixth day after injury and may continue for over 12 weeks.

Frankel[38] reviewed mechanisms of reflex cardiac arrest in tetraplegic patients. They presented 4 patients not under anesthesia who suffered cardiac arrest within 6 weeks of a complete high cervical spinal cord injury. All required intermittent positive pressure ventilation in the stage of spinal shock; stimuli to the trachea-induced bradycardia, and in two patients, cardiac arrest resulted. Bradycardia occurred when the patients were hypoxic and seemed to be due to vasovagal reflex. This reflex is normally opposed by sympathetic activity, but during hypoxia by increased pulmonary vagal reflex activity due to increased breathing. In spinally injured patients, compensatory sympathetic activity occurs because ventilation is mechanical and does not increase with hypoxia. Treatment of such emergencies includes administration of atropine and adequate oxygenation. Cardiac resuscitation can be performed adequately on the Stryker frame without placing a backboard beneath the patient.

PULMONARY CONSIDERATIONS

A cervical spinal cord injury requires that the patient's ventilatory capability be assessed serially by spirometry and arterial blood gas studies. Pulmonary emboli are a danger during the course of the illness and low-dose heparin may be helpful in preventing this complication. Full dosage is contraindicated because of the dangers of bleeding. An inferior vena caval umbrella may have to be inserted should the patient embolize while under heparin treatment.

Halothane, although a suppressant of sympathetic activity, is potent in low concentration, so that it is preferred for maintenance of an easily controlled level of anesthesia. Halothane also has the advantage of being nonirritating to the respiratory tract, effecting early depression of pharyngeal and laryngeal reflexes, thus facilitating intubation under anesthesia.

Intermittent positive pressure ventilation (IPPV) interferes with venous return by increasing intrathoracic pressure. Nevertheless, it may be necessary. Normally the Valsalva's maneuver in the presence of elevated mean intrathoracic pressure compensates for the decreased venous return by increasing peripheral vascular tone, thus maintaining the pressure gradient between intrathoracic veins and peripheral circulation. This compensatory response is a reflex mechanism mediated through baroreceptors in the aorta and carotid sinuses. These receptors send afferent impulses to the vasomotor center in the medulla, which, in turn, sends down activating impulses for sympathetic outflow. The latter efferent pathways are interrupted in cervical cord injury. Fraser and Edmonds-Seal[39] emphasized that high spinal injury may be accompanied by loss of spontaneous respiration during sleep (Ondine's curse).

In the use of IPPV in paralyzed patients, the inspiratory phase should be reduced to a minimum (1 second) with a longer than normal expiratory pause (3 seconds). The incorporation of a subatmospheric pressure phase during expiration is claimed to help venous return and augment cardiac output. When the operative site lies above the heart level, however, a subatmospheric phase increases the risk of air embolism.

After cervical spinal cord injury, respiratory insufficiency develops late and is due to dysfunction of the thorax rather than to intrinsic pulmonary disease. Paradoxic respiratory movements may be present. Coughing may be inadequate, and frequent suctioning may be necessary. Ventilation in these patients may be worsened by the sitting position but not by the application of braces to support posture.

Pledger[40] discussed disorders of temperature regulation in acute traumatic quadriplegia and suggested that the acute spinal cord injury deprives the patient of essentially all means of compensating for changes in environmental temperatures. He emphasized that fever in these patients may not necessarily be a sign of infection and that presence of the latter should be decided on clinical and bacteriologic grounds.

SURGICAL TECHNIQUE

As a result of an injury to the spine, the bony structures, ligaments, and muscles may be stretched, crushed, fractured, or dislocated, and the spinal cord and nerve roots may be crushed, contused, compressed, or severed. However, secondary circulatory impairment, vasomotor disturbances, venous stasis, hemorrhage, thrombosis, and edema may convert a partial cord injury to a complete one.

The goal of surgical treatment in the acute stage it is to furnish the spinal cord and nerve roots with the best possible conditions for improvement and recovery. There are legitimate differences of opinion among neurosurgeons concerning the optimal approach to any particular problem of spine or spinal cord injury; however, the sparing of even a single nerve root is often crucial to the quadriplegic because it may provide some hand function and may make the difference between total dependence and some ability for self-care. Judicious surgical treatment may prevent future pain resulting from spinal instability and compression of nerve roots that can seriously hinder the patient's rehabilitation either acutely or in months after injury.

Timing of surgical intervention for acute spinal injury remains controversial, although early realignment or decompression or both is my own preference.

It should be stressed that no absolute criteria exist for either operative or nonoperative treatment in the closed, acute spinal cord injury. Various degrees of functional improvement have been reported in patients treated either operatively or nonoperatively. Both points of view have strong advocates, although no statistically valid study can be quoted at present.

ANTERIOR FUSION

Anterior fusion operations have been devised to allow anterior stabilization of the injured spine in any of its regions from the base of the skull to the sacrum.

Upper Cervical Spine

Several authors have described anterior approaches to the C1-C2-C3 region either through the oropharynx[41] or by an extrapharyngeal approach.[42] Murray and Seymour[42] described an anterior extrapharyngeal suprahyoid approach to the first, second, and third cervical vertebrae. Grote et al.[41] described removal of the odontoid process (dens epistropheus) by a transpharyngeal approach. Indications for removal of the dens are very uncommon and include situations in which a persistently dislocated dens continues to impinge on the spinal cord anteriorly following posterior cervical fusion. Stabilization of the upper cervical spine by the transoral transpharyngeal route also has been described by Bonney,[43] Fang and Ong,[44,45] Grote et al.,[41] as well as Estridge and Smith.[46]

In performing a transoral fusion, the palate is elevated, the mouth held open with a McIvor gag, and a 3–4-cm vertical incision is made into the pharynx overlying the involved segment of the spine. Using periosteal elevators, fibrous tissue and soft tissue are removed to expose the fracture site. The bone in the area then is removed under magnification with a high-speed burr, and a bone dowel is positioned for insertion into the defect using the technique of Estridge and Smith.[46] The dowel graft of bone is inserted as manual traction is applied to the head. When the traction is released, the graft is locked in position. Bonney[43] recommended preoperative tracheostomy. Stabilization is secured by inserting two struts of cortical bone into the body of the axis. These are notched into the anterior arch of the atlas with the space between them packed with cancellous bone. Alternatively, Bonney stated that stability could be assured by packing with cancellous chips after partial decortication of the upper vertebra. He then used halo traction. Fang and Ong[44] describe various approaches to the upper cervical spine. The transpharyngeal, transoral route was advocated, and they placed bone from an iliac crest into the lateral masses between the atlas and axis to achieve fusion following removal of the anterior arch of the atlas and odontoid process in certain cases. The anterior extrapharyngeal suprahyoid approach is described by Murray and Seymour[42] as well as Fang, Ong, and Hodgson[45] (Figure 126-2). A collar incision is made along the uppermost crease of the neck at the level between the hyoid bone and the thyroid cartilage, extending as far as the carotid sheaths. The sternohyoid and the sternothyroid muscles are divided, and the thyrohyoid membrane is exposed and detached as close to the hyoid bone as possible to avoid damage to the internal laryngeal nerve and superior laryngeal vessels. The hypopharynx is entered by cutting into the exposed mucous membrane from the side to avoid damaging the epiglottis. Traction on the hyoid bone and epiglottis exposes the posterior pharyngeal wall, and a midline vertical incision is made to bone; the bodies of the second and third or fourth vertebrae can be exposed sufficiently

to remove diseased or abnormal bone or to achieve fusion, although it may be necessary to dislocate the jaw to attain adequate exposure. Fusion is achieved by inserting strut grafts of autogenous bone into a prepared graft with slots made in the opposing vertebral bodies. The insertion of the grafts is made easier by extending the cervical spine during the operative procedure and then permitting resumption of the original somewhat flexed or neutral position. The need for tracheostomy may be avoided by this approach.

Middle and Lower Cervical Spine

The introduction of the anterior approach to the management of fractures and dislocations of the cervical, thoracic, and lumbar spine has added a new dimension to the treatment of spinal injury. The work of Smith and Robinson[47] and Bailey and Badgley[31] first drew attention to the feasibility of the anterior approach in cervical fracture-dislocations. Cloward[48–50] popularized the concept and introduced a set of instruments that has made this operation considerably simpler. That technique generally is satisfactory.

In bursting fractures of an anterior cervical body, at least two levels of fusion followed by prolonged immobilization may be required for adequate healing without subsequent angulation. Anterior cervical fusion between C3 and C7 can be performed through a transverse or longitudinal skin incision. The recommended transverse skin incision is sufficient for exposing three consecutive vertebral bodies and two consecutive intervertebral discs. A longitudinal skin incision should be used in the unusual circumstance that a longer segment of the cervical spine is to be exposed. The landmark for placing either incision is the palpable anterior border of the sternomastoid muscle. A transverse skin incision should be centered over the anterior border of the sternomastoid muscle overlying the segment of the spine to be exposed. Generally the fifth, sixth, and seventh cervical segments should be approached through a transverse skin incision placed two to three finger breadths superior to the clavicle, and the third, fourth, and fifth cervical segments through a transverse incision placed three to four finger breadths superior to the clavicle.

A longitudinal incision should be made in the skin overlying the anterior border of the sternomastoid muscle and may be extended from the tip of the mastoid process to the suprasternal notch. The platysma muscle is grasped between forceps and sharply incised at the lateral limb of the transverse incision or at the caudal limb of the longitudinal incision, bluntly separated from the underlying structures by passing a blunt, curved hemostat or Metzenbaum scissors deep to the muscle, and sharply incised in line with the skin incision. If the platysma muscle is bluntly separated from the deeper structures before it is incised, inadvertent incision of the underlying sternomastoid muscle will be avoided. The anterior border of the sternomastoid muscle must be clearly identified and mobilized throughout the boundaries of the incision. The middle layer of cervical fascia is demonstrated as the sternomastoid muscle is retracted laterally. The omohyoid muscle may be seen crossing the field in the midportion of the neck at this level and may be mobilized and retracted inferiorly or superiorly, or transected to secure adequate exposure. The carotid artery then is palpated. After accurately identifying the artery, the middle layer of cervical fascia is sharply incised just medial to and parallel with the carotid sheath. As the sternomastoid muscle and the carotid sheath are retracted laterally, the anterior surface of the cervical spine may be palpated.

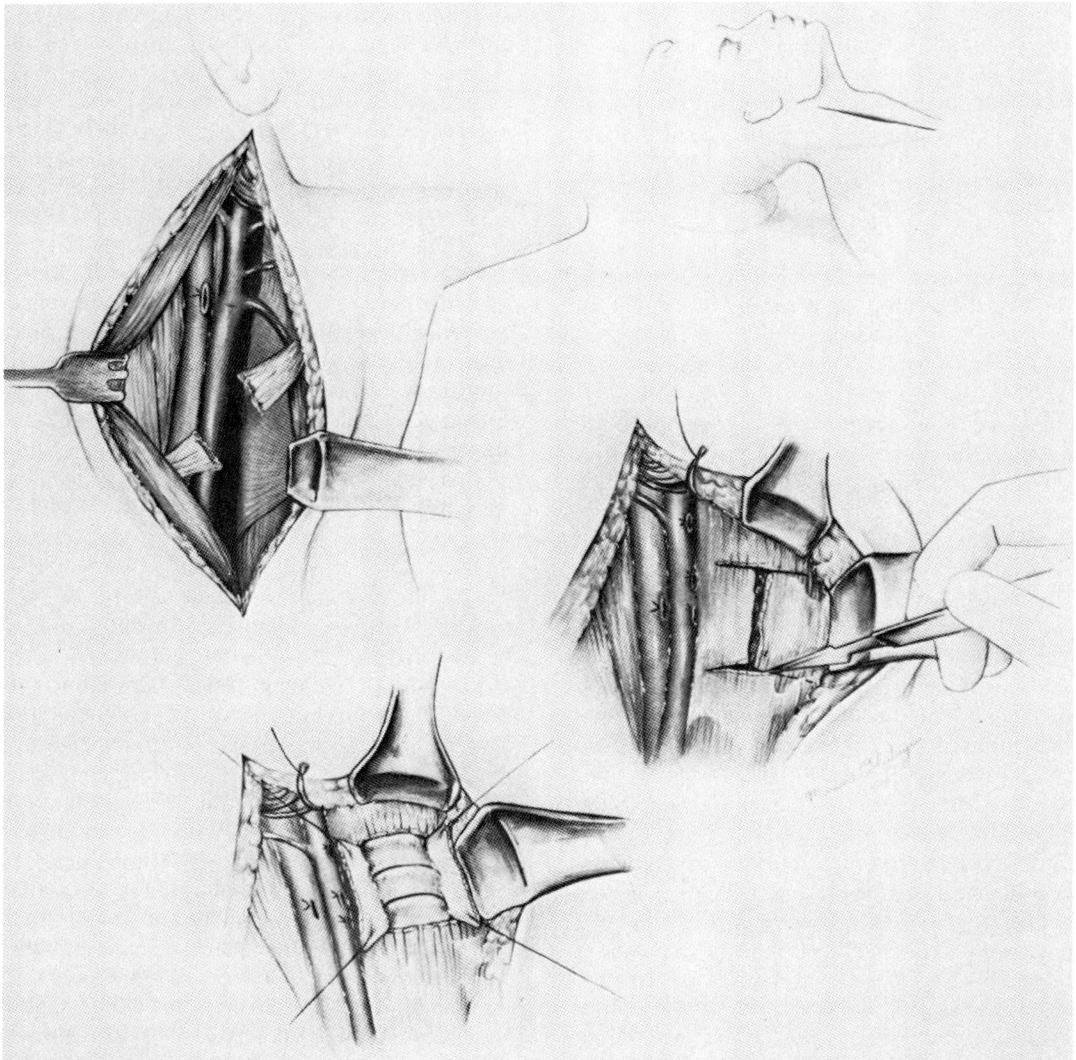

Fig. 126-2. The anterolateral approach to the upper cervical spine (after De Anrade and MacNab).[53] (Reprinted from Yashon D: Spinal Injury. New York. Appleton-Century-Crofts, 1978. With permission.)

The esophagus lies just posterior to the trachea, or more superiorly, posterior to the larynx. After having retracted the esophagus, trachea, and thyroid gland medially, the prevertebral fasciae are incised longitudinally in the midline of the neck and retracted to either side by periosteal elevation. It is important that the palpable anterior tubercles of the transverse processes not be mistaken for the vertebral bodies, or an incision, which should be made through the prevertebral fasciae in the midline, will be made through the longus colli muscle with resulting damage to the cervical sympathetic chain or to the vertebral artery, which lies deep to the longus colli muscle. The longus colli muscle may be sharply elevated from the intervertebral discs and the vertebral bodies in order to allow more complete exposure of the entire segment of the vertebral bodies and the intervertebral discs.

The resulting exposure is sufficient for anterior cervical discectomy and fusion, and anterior decompression of the cervical portion of the spinal cord following comminuted fractures of the vertebral bodies.

Identification of the space usually is done by x-ray study after a needle is inserted into the disc space or by palpation of bony displacement. The dislocation can also be palpated for

identification. At this point the graft can be prepared. The hip has been previously elevated on a sand bag. An incision 8 cm long is made parallel to and 2 to 4 cm below the crest of the ilium. Following skin retraction, the aponeurosis and muscles are cut perpendicular to the iliac crest. Dissection of the muscles from the external side of the crest to allow placement of the Cloward dowel cutter for removal of one or two grafts is sufficient. The dowel cutter is impinged against the bone and always is placed perpendicular to its surface. To ensure this, a cerebellar extension with the Hudson brace is useful. The dowel must be cylindrical in shape with the end surfaces at right angles, otherwise a poorly fitting dowel that is cut at an odd angle may result. This can cause poor fusion and vertebral collapse (Figure 126-3). We have not advised the use of Kiel bone in fracture-dislocations.

Returning to the neck, the selected space then is drilled with Cloward instruments with due consideration for the angle of the intervertebral space. The drilling should be in the plane of the space between the bodies to avoid undesirable angulation and excessive bleeding from venous channels in bone. The offset position of the dowels when two or more spaces are used also is important, as is leaving sufficient bone tissue between

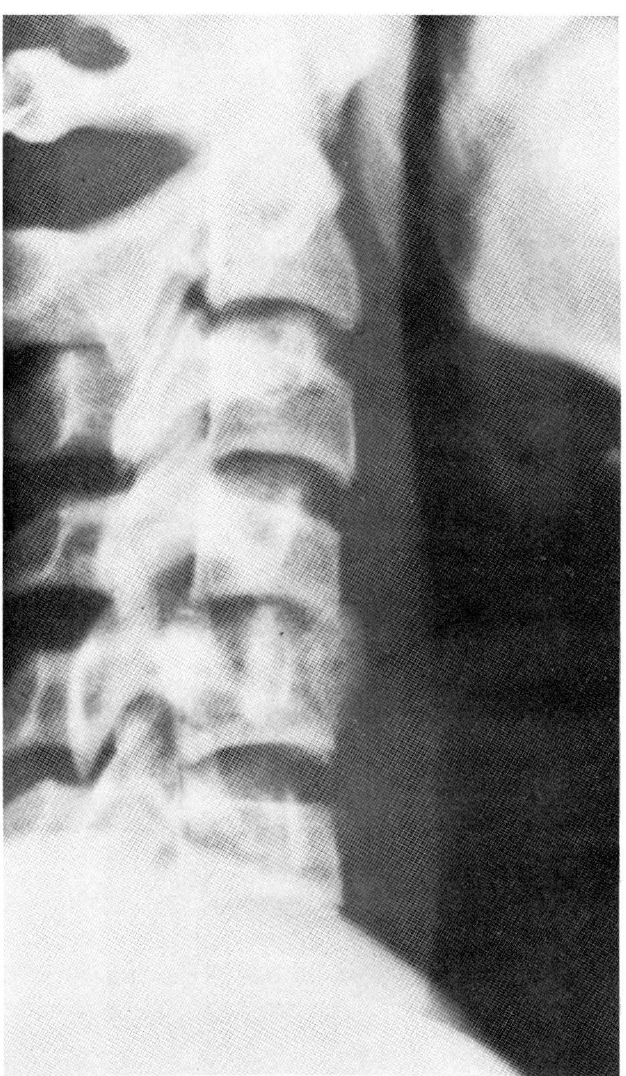

Fig. 126-3. A recent cervical interbody fusion at C4-5. Fusion is adequate but has less purchase than would be ideal. (Reprinted from Yashon D: Spinal Injury. New York. Appleton-Century-Crofts, 1978. With permission.)

the drilling spaces. Initial drilling is carried to a depth of 20 mm in adults. Further drilling is done cautiously in 2-mm steps. The posterior longitudinal ligament may be removed with angular cervical punches. The remaining pieces of disc can be removed with small curettes or rongeurs.

The bone dowel is inserted with either traction or the vertebral spreader. It is desirable that the anterior cortical surface of the dowel be inserted to a depth of at least 1 to 2 mm below the surface of the vertebral bodies. The strength of the fusion rests mostly on the cortical segment and not on the cancellous portion of the dowel (Figures 126-4 and 126-5). Additional fixation for increased stability can be obtained by the use of an H or HH AS IF plate. Closure of the incision is accomplished by approximation of the platysma muscle and skin edges.

The Smith-Robinson type of graft, which is not prefitted as in the Cloward technique, does not seem as efficacious in cervical spine injury. In this technique the iliac bone is fashioned into a plate that is placed between the vertebral bodies after traction, or a vertebral body spreader is used to distract

the vertebral bodies (Figure 126-6). Robinson emphasizes perforation of the subchondral bony end plates for vascular access to the graft.

A vertebral body that has been crushed may be excised and replaced with a bone graft (Figure 126-7). Complete excision of one or more vertebral bodies may be required when a fracture is extensive. A tibial, iliac, or fibular bone graft then can be used to maintain alignment and stability. With exposure of the involved vertebral body by the anterior approach, the involved vertebra is resected with rongeurs and curettes. Care must be exercised to prevent further injury to the spinal cord. Often the posterior longitudinal ligament is torn or frayed. After several days, the natural line of demarcation between the posterior longitudinal ligament and the vertebral body is lost. The vertebra may be vascular, and hemorrhage may be encountered. The upper and lower intact vertebral bodies should be notched so that the graft can be fitted into a trough and lodged tightly. The cervical spine may be extended for insertion of the graft. Cancellous bone chips then can be laid over the graft before replacement of the longitudinal vertebral muscles. The anterior longitudinal ligaments then may be approximated.

Certain pitfalls must be avoided in surgery of the anterior cervical spine. These include paralysis of the recurrent laryngeal nerve, collapse of vertebrae, nonfusion, and infection. Although complications are uncommon, some have occurred and spinal paralysis following such complications has been reported.

Transthoracic surgical decompression of acute spinal cord injuries can be accomplished. The thoracic cord is decompressed by removal of the pedicle (Figures 126-8 and 126-9). The vertebral column is stabilized by fixing a bone graft in place with screws. In the lumbar region, anterior transperitoneal fusion also has been advocated. This operation is uncommonly used for lumbar stabilization following fracture-dislocation.

Acrylic plastics have been used for stabilization of the spine. Kelly et al.[51] as well as Stowsand and Muhtaroglu[52] used acrylic fixation in atlantoaxial dislocation for posterior stabilization. It is our view that in fracture-dislocation use of autologous bone is preferred since it appears to be more stable in the long run and possibly has a lower incidence of infection.

ANTEROLATERAL APPROACH TO THE UPPER CERVICAL SPINE

DeAndrade and MacNab[53] described an approach to the basiocciput and anterior upper cervical spine. Figure 126-2 shows this lateral approach and the anatomic structures involved. Access to the basiocciput anteriorly is limited by the mandible and subglottic structures superficially and by the internal carotid artery, cranial nerves, and pharynx deeper. Access to this area is limited, and the potential hazards are many. Such an approach generally is not useful in spinal injury, but possibly could be employed for fusion using autologous bone. A trough is fashioned and bone is laid into the trough. Some surgeons advocate preliminary tracheostomy, but this is not necessary in all cases. The patient should be immobilized for about a month; some of this time should be spent in skeletal traction. External stabilization is maintained by bracing until fusion is established radiographically in 4 to 6 months. Halo traction may replace a long period of recumbency. This approach can be used for fusing the occiput to C1 and C2, but inclusion of the occiput is not necessary in most cases.

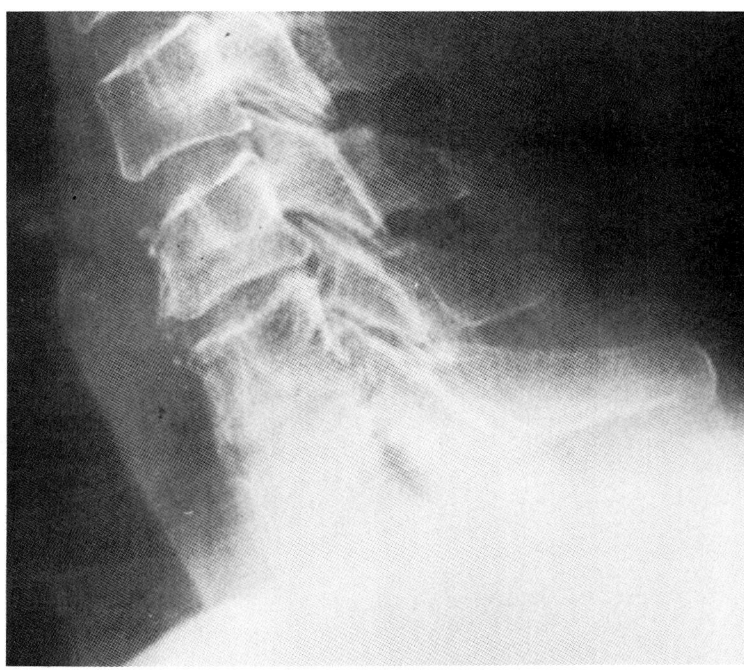

Fig. 126-4.   An interbody fusion, 3 months after it was done. (Reprinted from Yashon D: Spinal Injury. New York. Appleton-Century-Crofts, 1978. With permission.)

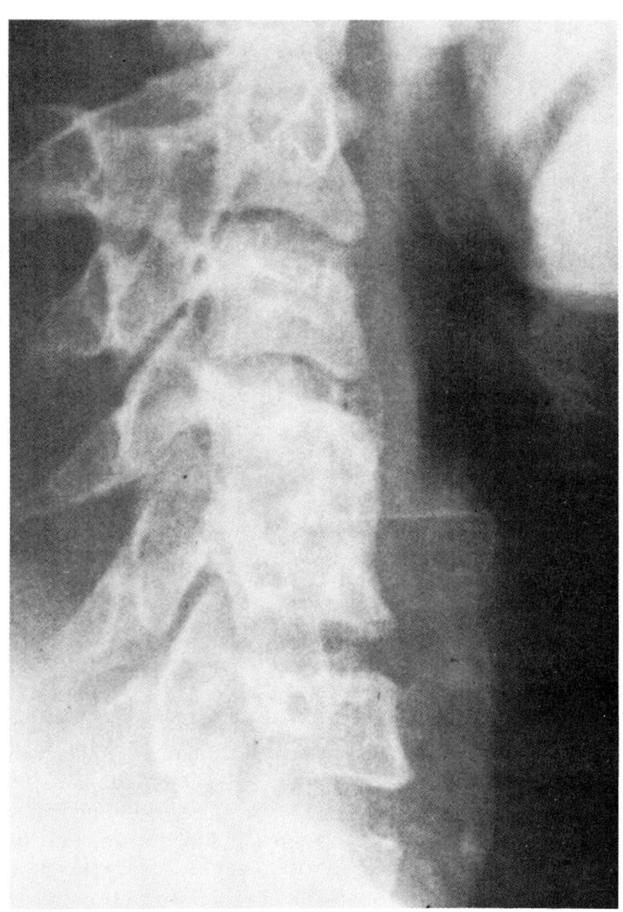

Fig. 126-5.   An ancient interbody fusion at C4-5. (Reprinted from Yashon D: Spinal Injury. New York. Appleton-Century-Crofts, 1978. With permission.)

TRANSORAL ODONTOID RESECTION AND FUSION

Several authors have described anterior approaches either through the oropharynx or via extrapharyngeal routes. Murray and Seymour[42] described an anterior extrapharyngeal suprahyoid approach to the first, second, and third cervical vertebrae. Grote et al.[41] described removal of the odontoid process (dens epistropheus) by a transpharyngeal approach. Indications for removal of the dens are very uncommon and include situations in which, when fusion is carried out posteriorly, a persistently dislocated dens impinges on the spinal cord anteriorly. Masferrer et al.[54] provided, in an excellent description, the technique of transoral microsurgical resection of the odontoid process (Figures 126-10 through 126-14). With proper reduction and fusion, removal is rarely required. Stabilization of the upper cervical spine by the transoral transpharyngeal route has also been described by Bonney,[43] Fang and Ong,[44,45] Grote et al.,[41] and Estridge and Smith.[46] Sakou et al.,[55] Louis,[56] and Spetzler et al.,[57] advocated anterior transoral odontoid removal.

There are different approaches to the transoral fusion. The patient must be intubated and have adequate airway. The palate is elevated and the mouth held open with a McIvor gag. Operative localizing x-ray films can be obtained after a needle is inserted in the operative site if necessary. C-arm fluoroscopy is helpful. A vertical incision 3 to 4 cm in length is made into the pharynx. Using periosteal elevators fibrous tissue and soft tissue are scraped away from the bone. Following the technique of Estridge and Smith[46] a dowel of bone is inserted into the actual fracture line in the odontoid, after a high-speed burr is used to roughen and undercut sclerotic bone margins. The dowel graft of bone is inserted as manual traction is applied to the head. When the traction is released, the graft is locked in position. Bonney[43] recommended preoperative tracheostomy.

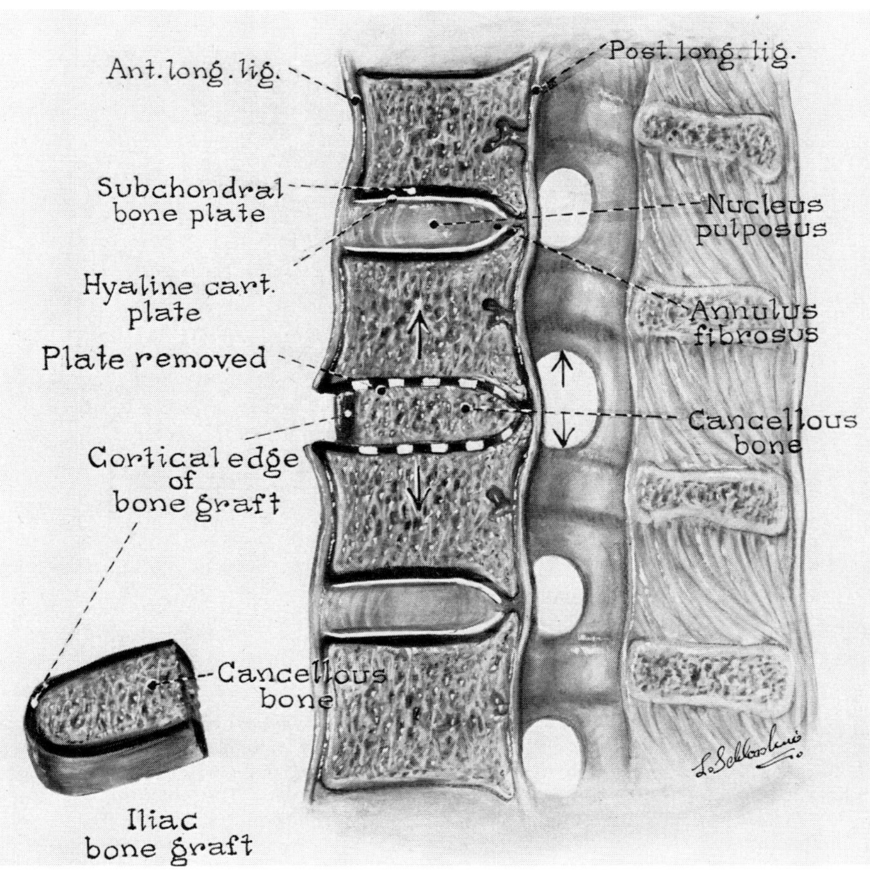

Fig. 126-6. A Smith-Robinson cervical graft. (Reprinted from Robinson RA, Walker AE, Ferlic DC et al: The results of anterior interbody fusion of the cervical spine. J Bone Joint Surg 44A:1569–1587, 1962. With permission.)

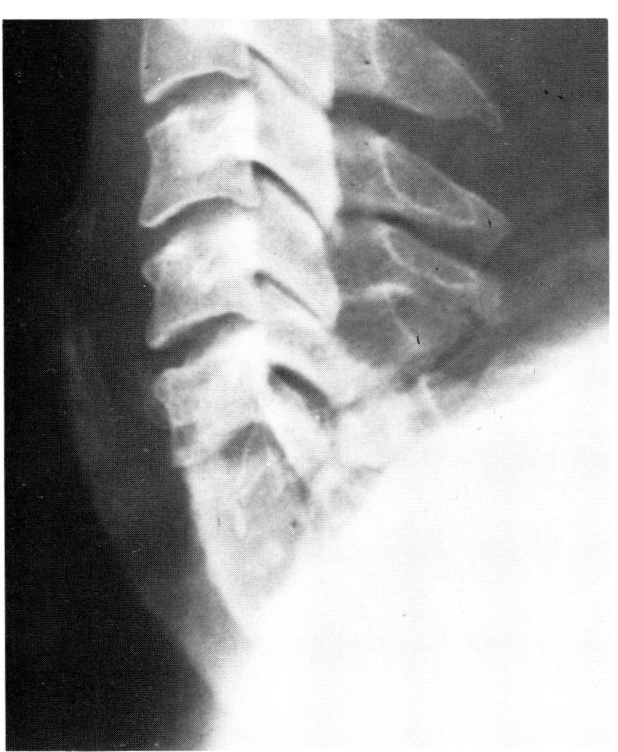

Fig. 126-7. Replacement of a vertebral body after a burst fracture. (Reprinted from Yashon D: Spinal Injury. New York. Appleton-Century-Crofts, 1978. With permission.)

Stabilization was secured by insertion of cortical bone grafts or insertion of cancellous bone. He stated that two struts of cortical bone can be slotted into the body of the axis and notched into the anterior arch of the atlas. The space between them can be filled with cancellous bone. Alternatively he stated that stability could be assured by packing with cancellous chips after partial decortication of the upper vertebrae. He then used halo traction. Fang and Ong[44] and Fang et al.[45] describe several approaches to the upper cervical spine. The transpharyngeal, transoral route was advocated, and the used placement of bone from an iliac crest into the lateral masses between the atlas and axis for achievement of fusion. They removed the anterior arch of the atlas and the odontoid process in certain cases.

The anterior extrapharyngeal suprahyoid approach is used by Murray and Seymour,[42] Kommisar and Tabaddor[58] as well as Fang et al.[45] A collar incision is made along the uppermost crease of the neck at the level between the hyoid bone and the thyroid cartilage extending as far as the carotid sheaths. The sternohyoid and the sternothyroid muscles are divided and the thyrohyoid membrane exposed and detached as near to the hyoid bone as possible to avoid damage to the internal laryngeal nerve and superior laryngeal vessels. The hypopharynx is entered by cutting into the exposed mucous membrane from the side to avoid damaging the epiglottis. Traction on the hyoid bone and epiglottis exposes the posterior pharyngeal wall, and a midline vertical incision is made to bone; the bodies of the second and third or fourth vertebrae can be exposed sufficiently to remove diseased or abnormal bone or to achieve fusion. Fusion is achieved by inserting strut grafts of autogenous bone

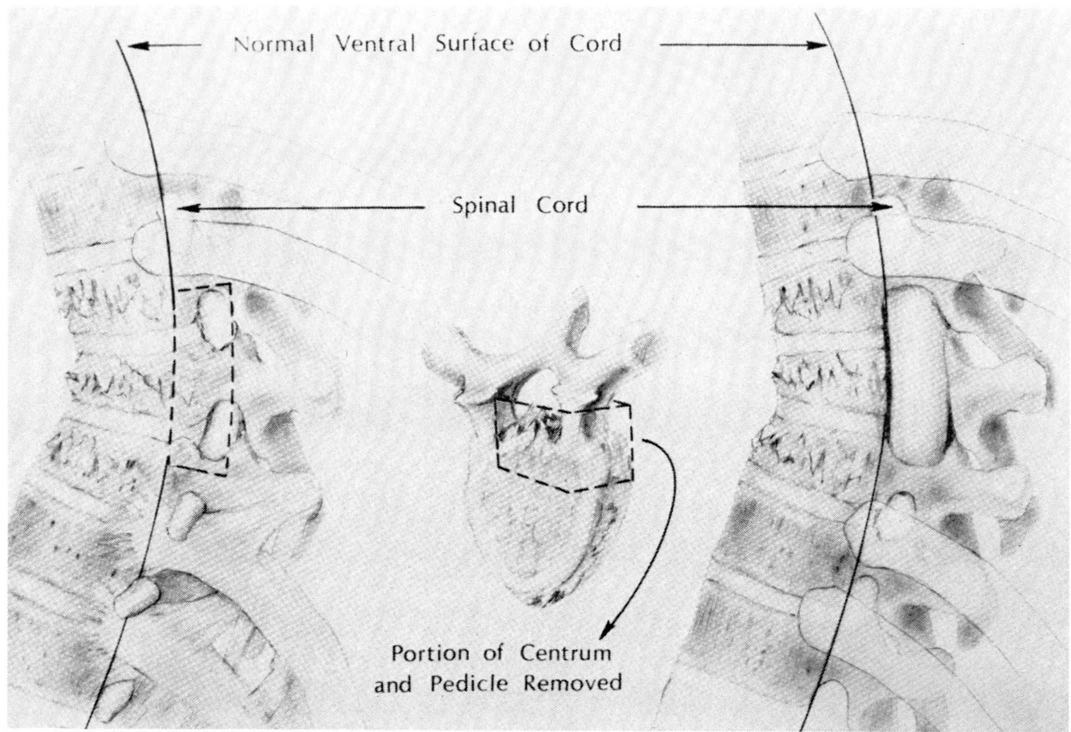

Fig. 126-8. (Left) The heads of the fifth and sixth ribs have been removed to expose the foramina between T5-7. Compression of the ventral spinal cord is in the area outlined by the broken rectangle. The osteotomy begins with resection of the pedicle of T6 (center). The extent of the completed bone resection in the coronal plane is outlined by the broken line. (Right) The completed resection in the longitudinal plane. The facets remain intact. (Reprinted from Paul RL, Michael RL, Dunn JE, et al: Anterior transthoracic surgical decompression of acute spinal cord injuries. J Neurosurg 43:299–307, 1975. With permission.)

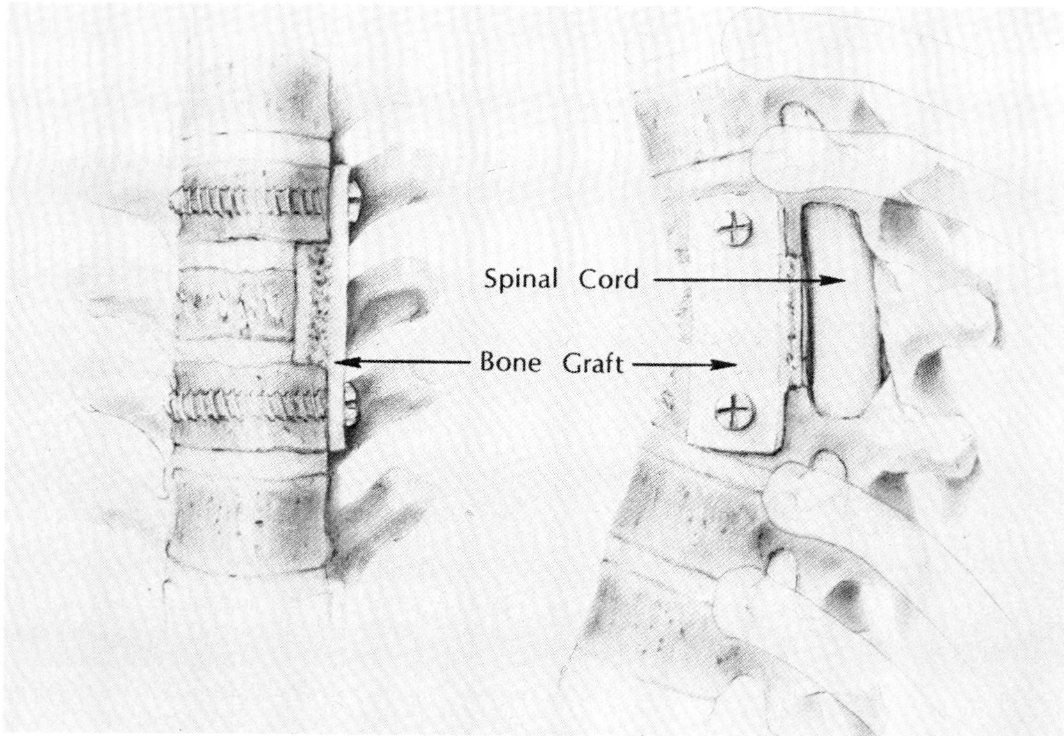

Fig. 126-9. Lateral fusion after the decompression illustrated in Figure 126-8. The template of bone is shown in both anteroposterior and lateral views. The screws should pass from cortex to cortex of the vertebral body. (Right) The relationship of the graft to the decompression. (Reprinted from Paul RL, Michael RL, Dunn JE, et al: Anterior transthoracic surgical decompression of acute spinal cord injuries. J Neurosurg 43:299–307, 1975. With permission.)

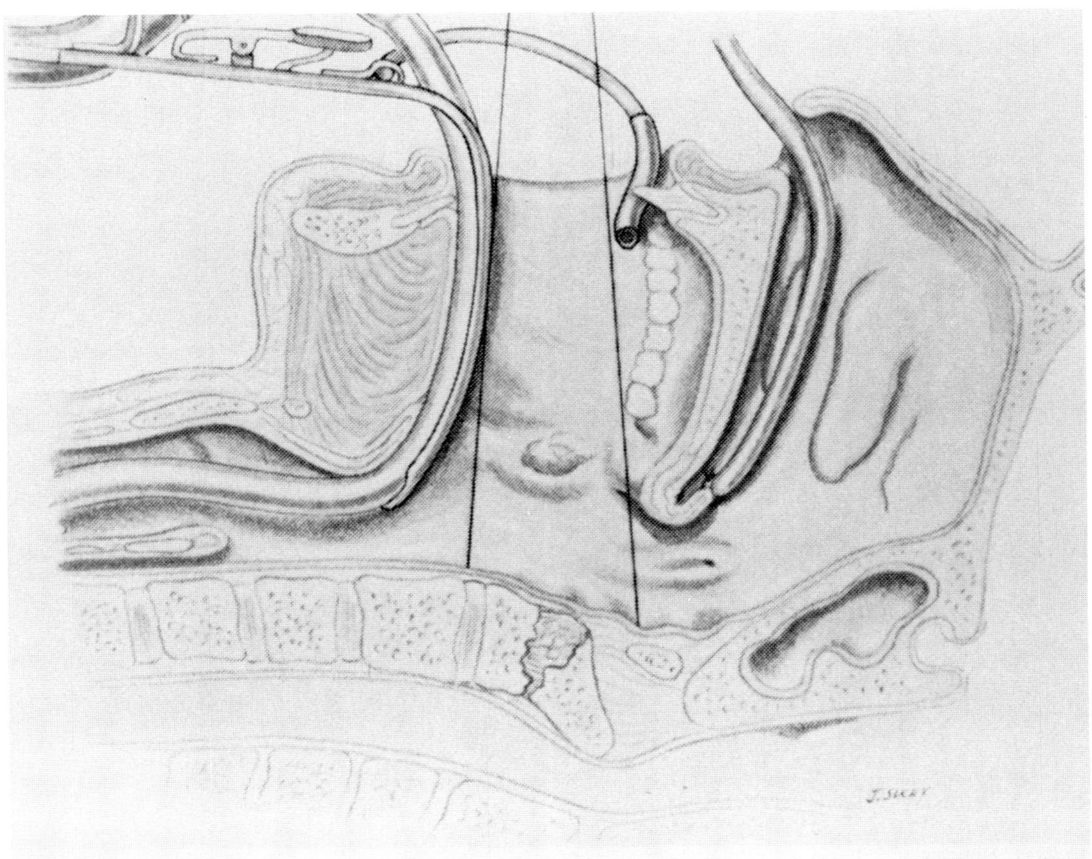

Fig. 126-10. Transoral microsurgical odontoid resection operative exposure. Note retraction of uvula and soft palate cephalad and tongue caudad. Solid lines depict field of view through operating microscope. (Reprinted from Masferrer et al: Transoral microsurgical resection of the odontoid process. BNI Quarterly 1:34–40, 1985.[54])

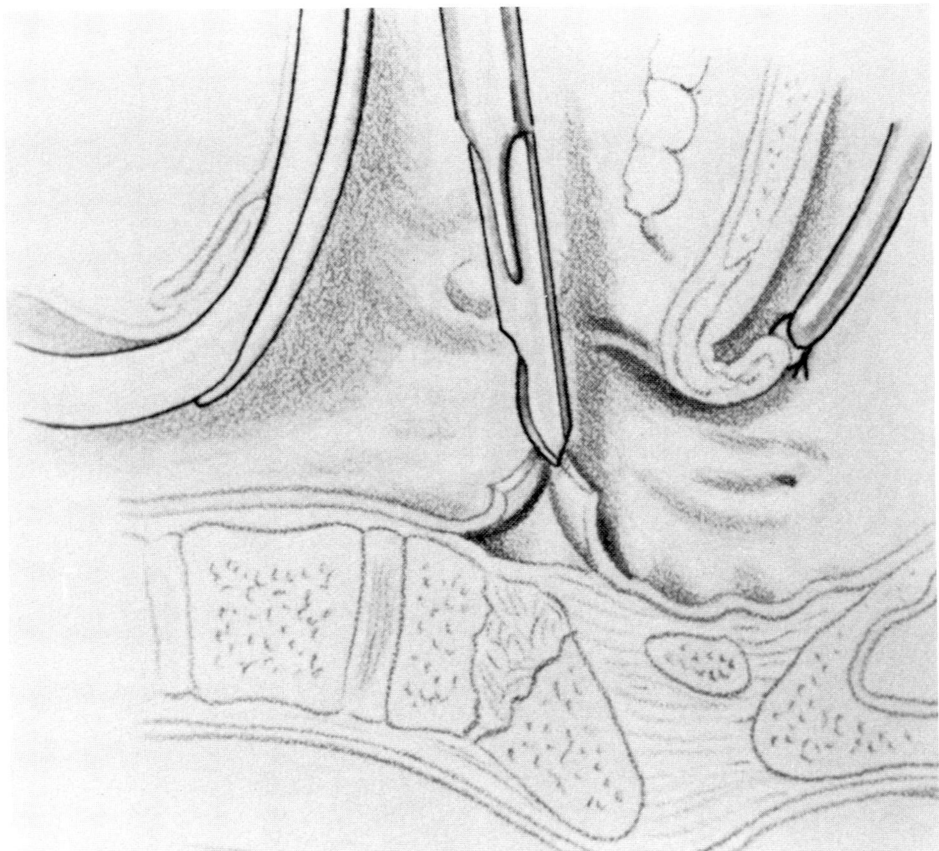

Fig. 126-11. Transoral microsurgical odontoid resection mucosal incision over body of C2.

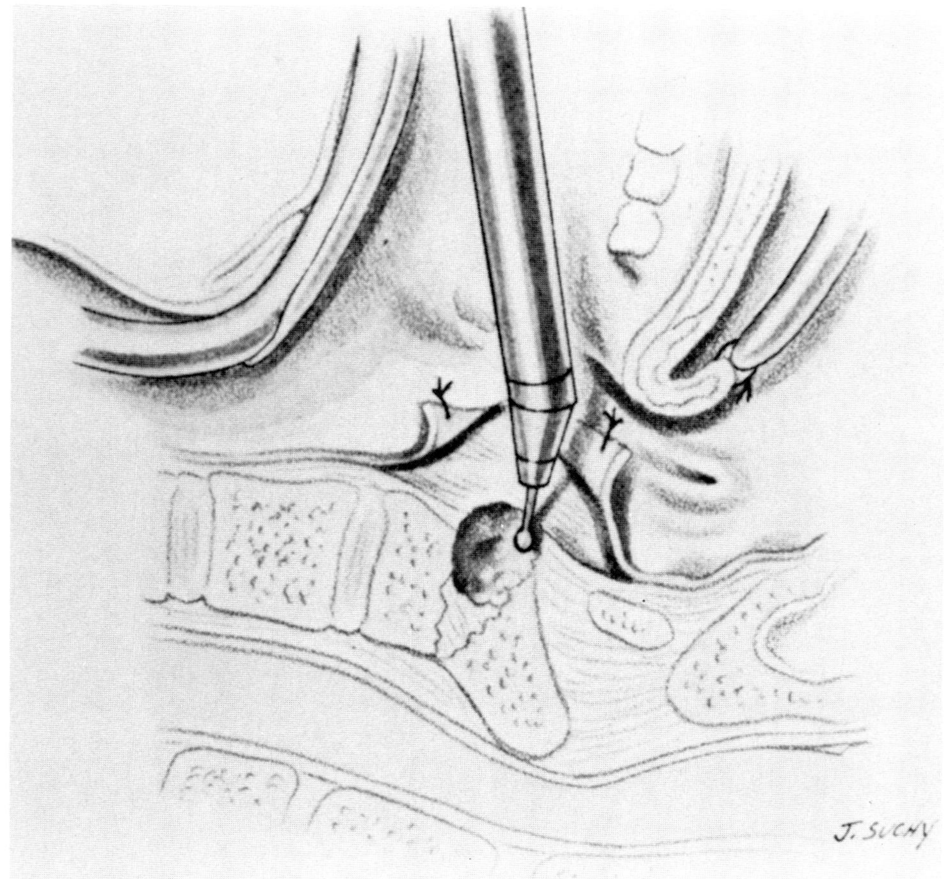

Fig. 126-12. Transoral microsurgical odontoid resection high speed drill dissection of midline portion of body of C2.

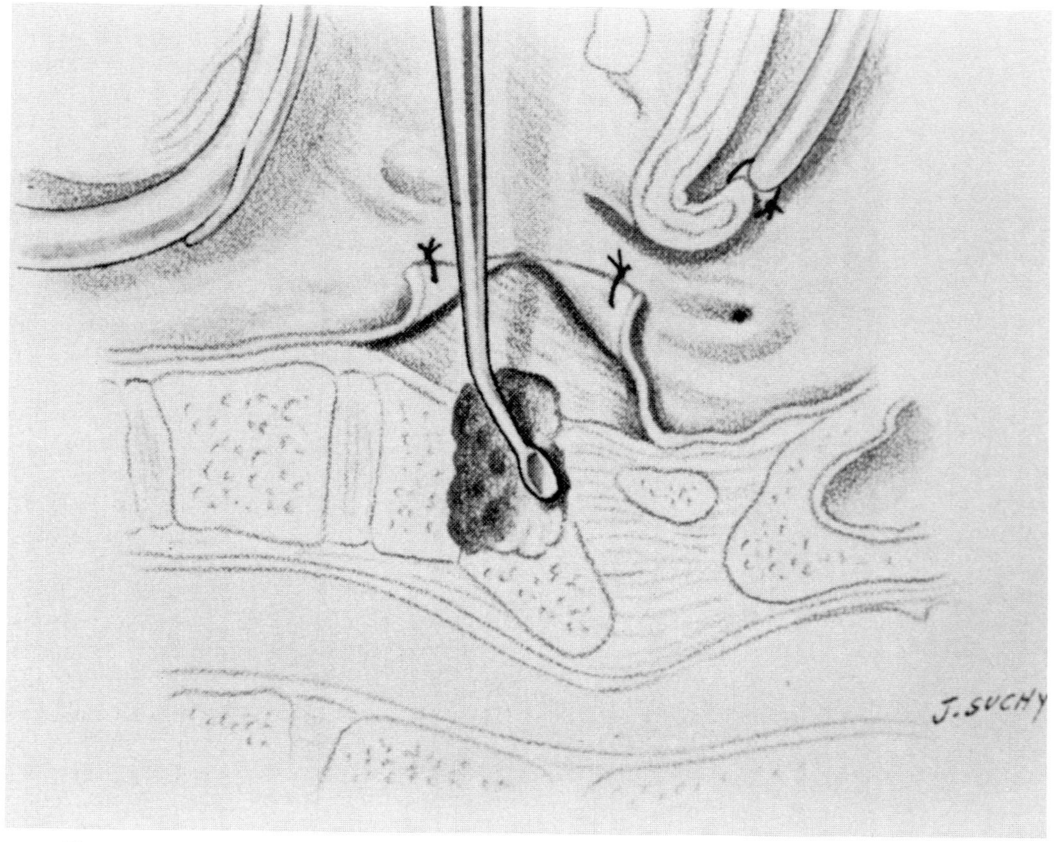

Fig. 126-13. Transoral microsurgical odontoid resection curettage of remaining odontoid process.

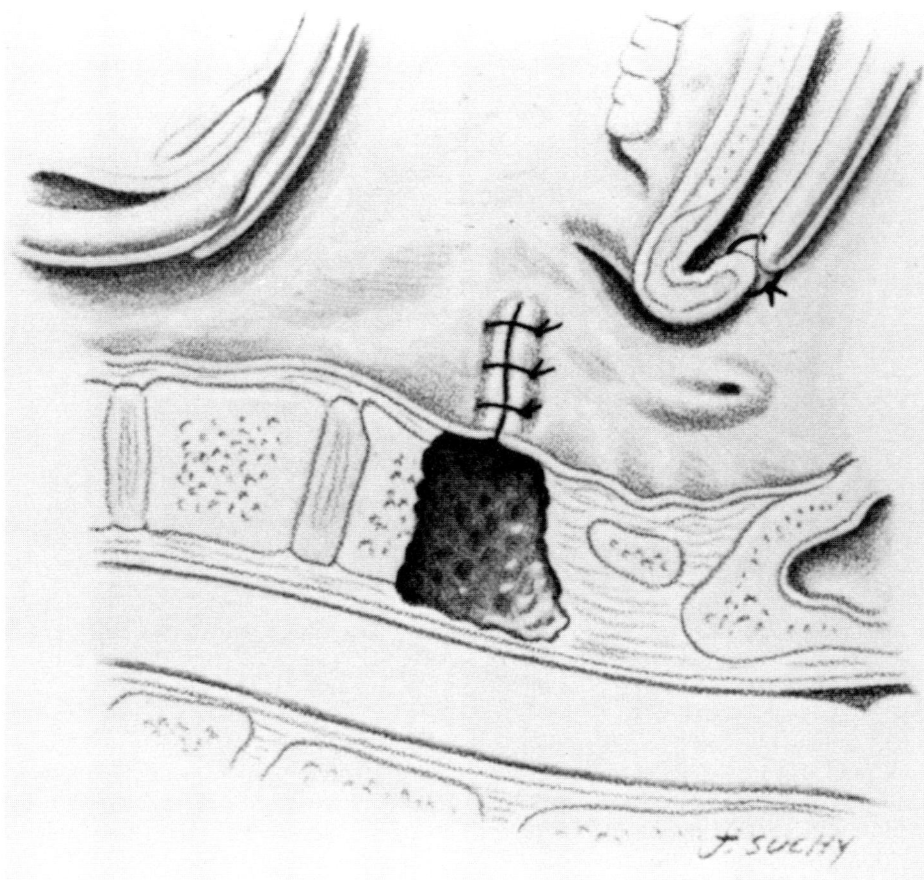

Fig. 126-14. Transoral microsurgical odontoid resection single layer closure of posterior pharyngeal wall.

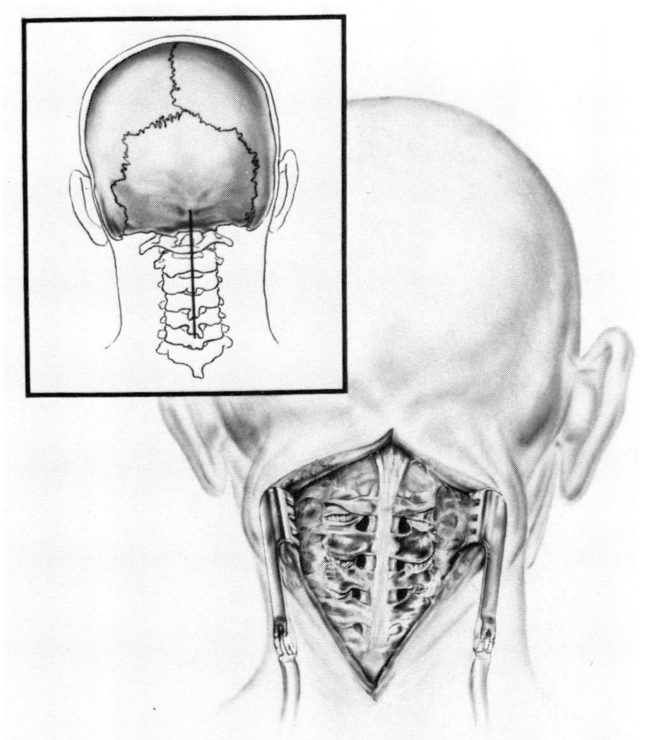

Fig. 126-15. The incision and exposure for a C1-C2 fusion. (Reprinted from Yashon D: Spinal Injury. New York. Appleton-Century-Crofts, 1978. With permission.)

into a prepared graft with slots made in the opposing vertebral bodies. The insertion of the grafts is made easier by extending the cervical spine during the operative procedure, and then permitting resumption of the original somewhat flexed or neutral position. It should be pointed out that the upper vertebral bodies can also be reached by the routine anterior approach.

POSTERIOR SPINAL FUSION

Posterior spinal fusion is a widely accepted technique in the cervical, thoracic, and lumbar spine (Figures 126-15 through 126-25). Indications for this procedure frequently overlap those for anterior fusion, particularly in the cervical spine. We prefer posterior cervical fusion only in burst fractures of the vertebral bodies when multiple levels are involved and in atlantoaxial dislocations. Thus, in the cervical spine it is not used as frequently as anterior fusion. Posterior fusion is most frequently employed in the thoracic and lumbar spine.

Several different operations have been advocated for the treatment of atlantoaxial fracture-dislocations. Posterior fusion of the C1 and C2 vertebrae seems to be the procedure most often chosen (Figures 126-15, 126-16, and 126-17). Mixter and Osgood[59] originated the concept of posterior fixation of C1 and C2. They described a technique that makes use of a strong silk thread wound around the posterior arch of the atlas and tied to the spinous process of the axis. Cone and Turner[19] were pioneers in the use of wires and bone grafts for C1 and C2 fusions. Gallie[21] fused the adjacent articular facets while also wiring C1 to C2. Although they reported good results with early

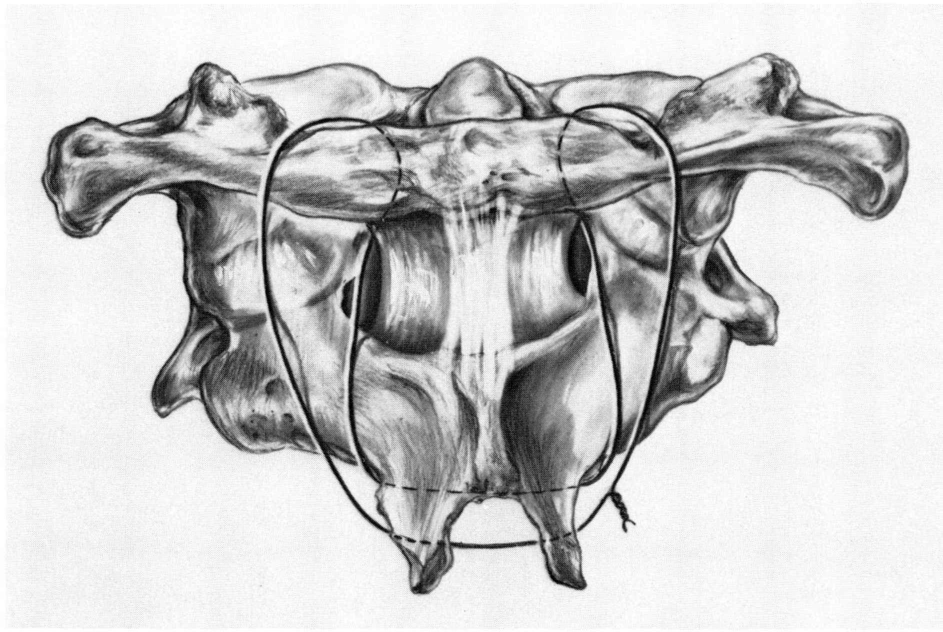

Fig. 126-16.   The wiring configuration for a C1-C2 fusion. (Reprinted from Yashon D: Spinal Injury. New York. Appleton-Century-Crofts, 1978. With permission.)

fusion for the treatment of atlantoaxial fracture-dislocations, neither Gallie[21] nor Cone and Turner[19] published sufficient details for comparison with other methods of treatment. Alexander et al.[60] claimed that fusion of only C1 and C2 gave unsatisfactory results. Fusion from C1 to C3 was advocated.

The general principles of posterior cervical fusion are virtually identical, whether the upper, middle, or lower cervical spine is to be fused. Once the normal relationships between the vertebrae are established, and following exposure of the spinous processes and lamina from behind, wires are passed under the affected laminae bilaterally (Figures 126-18 through 126-25). An alternative approach is to pass wires around only the normal vertebral laminae above and below the fracture site. Passage of the wire is facilitated by removal of small portions of the laminae with a Kerrison punch using No. 20 or 22 wire (Figure 126-19). The dura is separated from the lamina with a small periosteal elevator (Figure 126-20). The cortical bone of the lamina and spinous process is denuded of periosteum and a high-speed drill is used to roughen the bone. Autogenous bone struts, usually obtained from the iliac crest (Figure 126-25) then are wired into place. As an alternative, wires may be passed through bone beneath the spinous processes. A towel clip can provide the passage hole, and the bone struts are wired (Figure 126-20). The periosteum should be denuded from the graft.

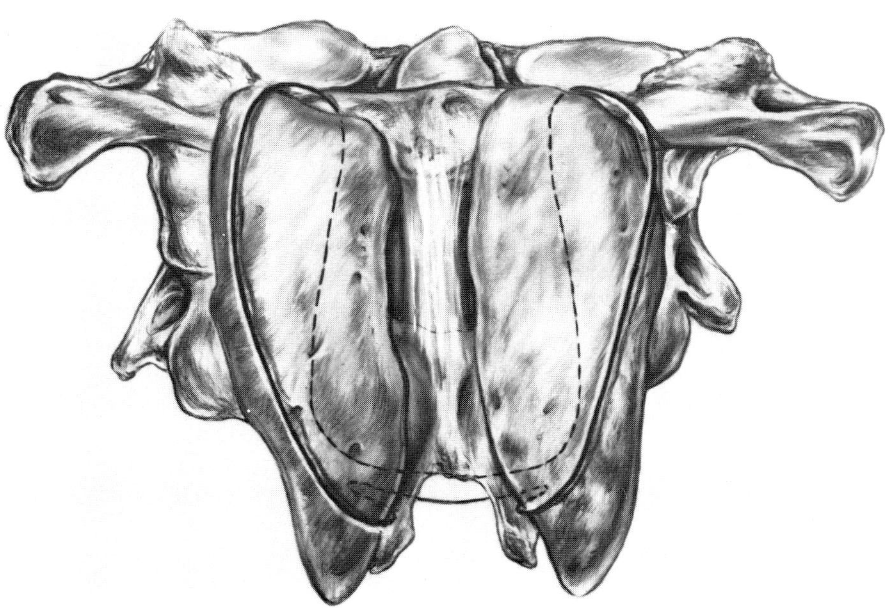

Fig. 126-17.   The bone wired into place—C1-C2 fusion. (Reprinted from Yashon D: Spinal Injury. New York. Appleton-Century-Crofts, 1978. With permission.)

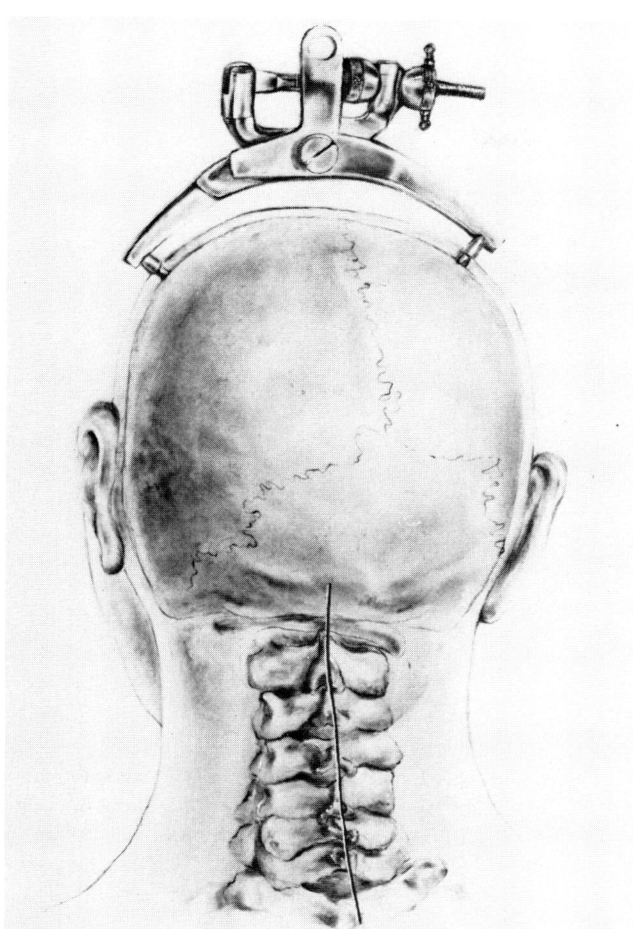

Fig. 126-18. The incision for posterior cervical fusion. (Reprinted from Yashon D: Spinal Injury. New York. Appleton-Century-Crofts, 1978. With permission.)

Small bone chips are packed in the crevices. Fusion of the occiput to the atlantal arch and axis has been advocated but is not used by most surgeons at present because dislocation between the occiput and the atlas is rare. Including the occiput in the fusion for a C1-C2 dislocation does not add to stability, but C3 may be added.

Lewis and McKibben[61] described treatment of unstable fracture-dislocations of the thoracolumbar spine accompanied by paraplegia. They concluded that to preserve long-term spinal function, open reduction and internal fixation are indicated in displaced fractures. Although no differences in the degree of neurologic recovery could be detected between the surgically and nonsurgically treated groups, the surgically treated patients had significantly less residual spinal deformity and significantly less serious pain. In fact, they stated that no serious pain developed in any of their surgically treated patients.

Schmidek et al.[62] employ a one-stage anterolateral decompression of the thoracolumbar spine with Harrington rod alignment and posterior fusion with bone grafting. As adjuncts, they use somatosensory-evoked responses both preoperatively and postoperatively and intraoperative myelography to confirm the adequacy of decompression.

LAMINECTOMY

For many years laminectomy has been carried out to relieve compression on the injured spinal cord. A block to lumbar puncture demonstrated by myelography has been suggested as a prerequisite. We do not subscribe to this, since an opening only the size of the spinal needle need be present for normal cerebrospinal fluid (CSF) dynamics, and have carried out decompressive laminectomy without prior myelography in the presence of severe neurologic deficit and spinal dislocation. Vertebral CT scan has been helpful in delineating candidates for laminectomy as the coronal cuts best show spinal alignment.

Whether the dura should be opened at the time of

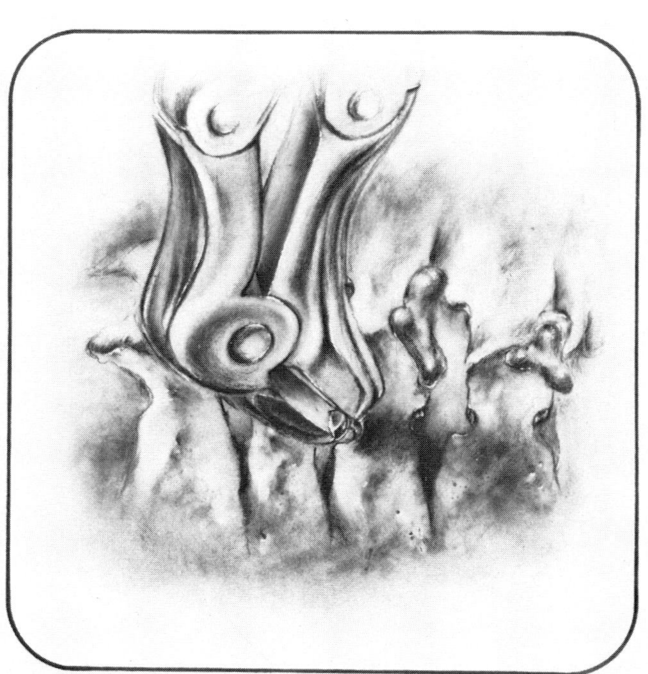

Fig. 126-19. Removal of part of the lamina for passage of the wire. (Reprinted from Yashon D: Spinal Injury. New York. Appleton-Century-Crofts, 1978. With permission.)

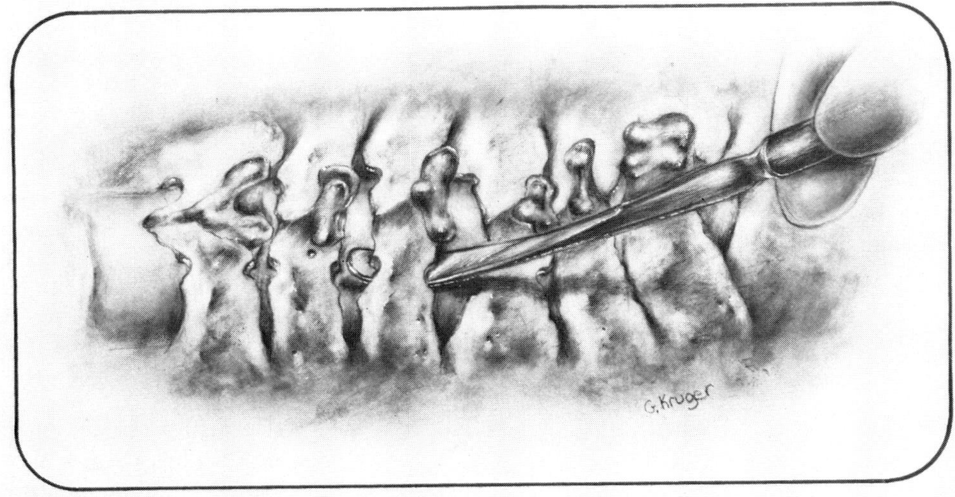

Fig. 126-20.   A periosteal elevator is placed under the lamina in preparation for passing the wire. (Reprinted from Yashon D: Spinal Injury. New York. Appleton-Century-Crofts, 1978. With permission.)

laminectomy is a matter of individual preference. If the dura is not opened, a significant intradural hematomata may be overlooked; however, if the dura is opened, closing it frequently is difficult, so that it either must be left open or a dural substitute must be used for closure. The herniation of a swollen and acutely injured spinal cord may result in neurologic worsening in the patient with a partial lesion or the development of a cerebrospinal fluid leak if the dura is not closed. After laminectomy, posterior fusion is possible and frequently is carried out. The fusion need be only lateral, involving facets and transverse processes.

Luque developed a subliminar 16-gauge wire and segmental rod system in response to the problems occurring with other types of fixation, particularly Harrington rods. The latter rod has a diameter of ³⁄₁₆ inch. Lahde[63] described the procedure as did Bowen.[64] A disadvantage is the necessity of passing the wires under each lamina, which theoretically could cause spinal injury. Thomas[65] has described the nursing care of a patient undergoing surgery with the Luque system. Bernard et al.[66] described their favorable experiences using this system in 11 cases.

POSTERIOR LATERAL FACET FUSION

The technique for posterior lateral facet fusion has been described by Robinson and Southwick.[67] The facet surfaces are fused from one level above the area of laminectomy to one level below, using corticocancellous bone wired to the facets at each level. A small drill hole is made with a ⁷⁄₆₄-inch drill in the

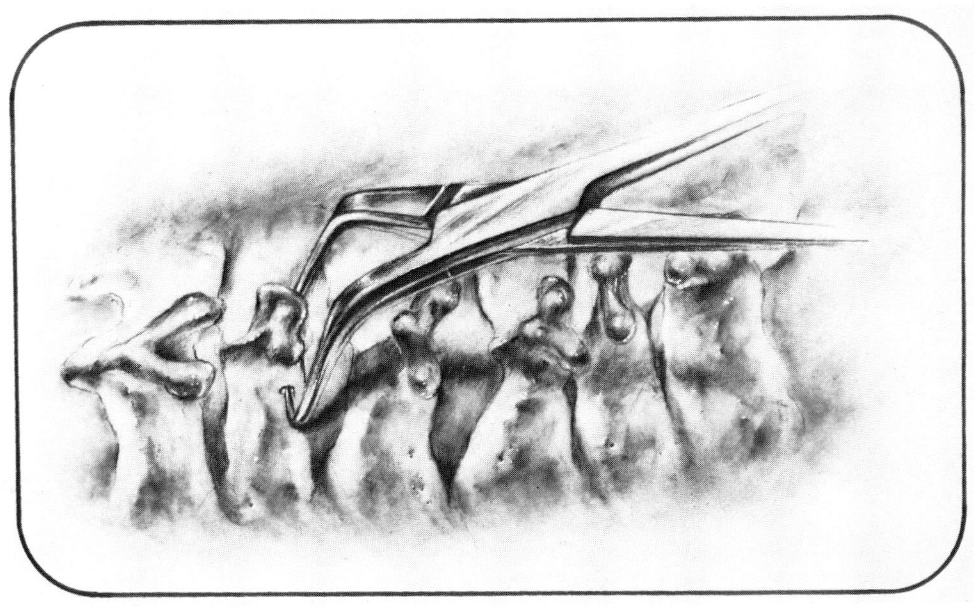

Fig. 126-21.   A towel clip is used for a wire hole at the base of the spinous process. (Reprinted from Yashon D: Spinal Injury. New York. Appleton-Century-Crofts, 1978. With permission.)

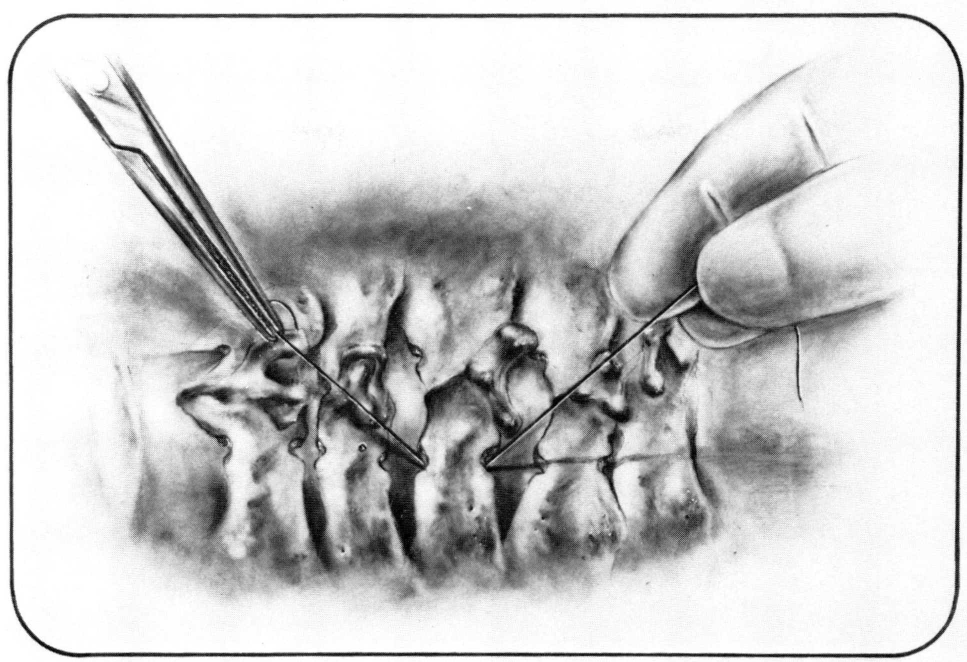

Fig. 126-22. The wires are passed for posterior fusion. (Reprinted from Yashon D: Spinal Injury. New York. Appleton-Century-Crofts, 1978. With permission.)

inferior articulating facet with a periosteal elevator wedged between the inferior and superior articulating facets. The wire then is brought out above the superior articulating facet, and the longitudinal graft from the iliac crest is wired into place at several levels. This technique may be used when a laminectomy has been performed. The procedure is carried out bilaterally.

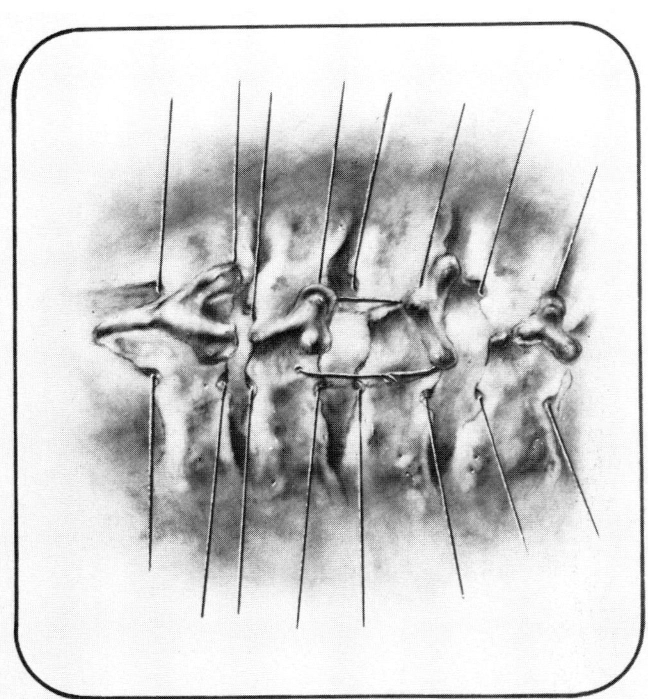

Fig. 126-23. The wires are passed under the laminae and at the base of the spinous processes. Generally the wires need not be passed around each lamina. (Reprinted from Yashon D: Spinal Injury. New York. Appleton-Century-Crofts, 1978. With permission.)

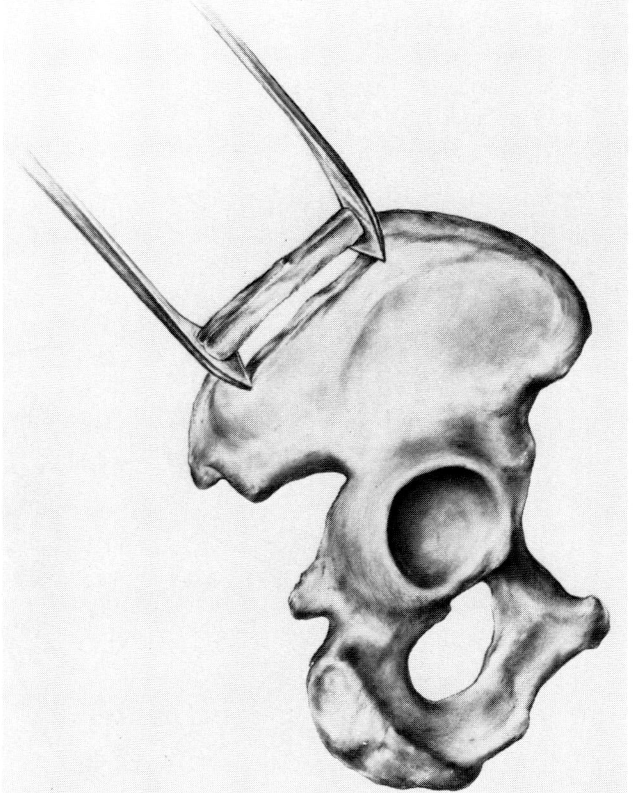

Fig. 126-24. The technique for removing bone from the iliac crest. (Reprinted from Yashon D: Spinal Injury. New York. Appleton-Century-Crofts, 1978. With permission.)

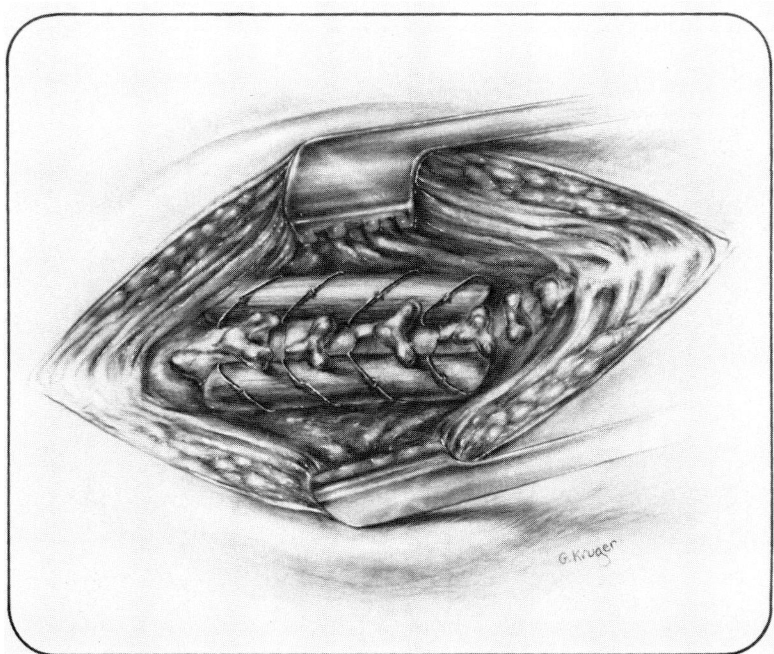

Fig. 126-25.   The bone is wired into place—fusion is completed. (Reprinted from Yashon D: Spinal Injury. New York. Appleton-Century-Crofts, 1978. With permission.)

The facet fusion extends over four levels. A posterior intraspinal fusion is carried out below the fused facets to the second thoracic spinous process. This prevents subsequent development of kyphosis below the fused facets. Support in the form of tong traction or halo traction should be maintained for a considerable period of time.

THORACOABDOMINAL APPROACH TO THE LOWER THORACIC AND UPPER LUMBAR SPINE

It is occasionally necessary to expose the lower thoracic and upper lumbar spine in continuity (see Figures 126-8, and 126-9). This presents a problem in exposure because of the

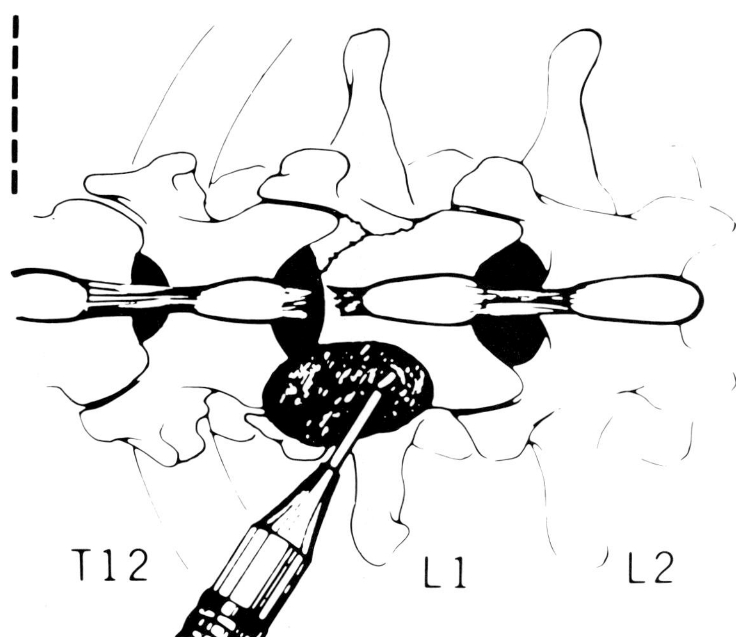

Fig. 126-26.   Initiation of lateral decompression in a one stage decompression-stabilization for a thoracolumbar fracture. Dorsoventral view. Note the use of the air drill for removal of the lateral lamina, facet, and pedicle. (Reprinted from Erikson DL, Leider LL Jr, Brown WE: One stage decompression-stabilization for thoracolumbar fractures. Spine 2:53–56, 1977. With permission.)

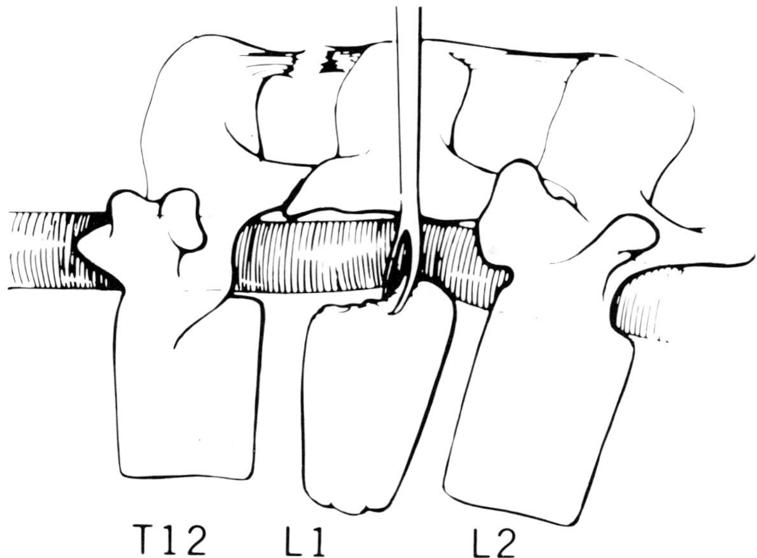

Fig. 126-27. Removal of the retropulsed portion of a comminuted vertebral body in a one-stage decompression-stabilization or a thoracolumbar fracture. Lateral view. (Reprinted from Erikson DL, Leider LL Jr, Brown WE: One stage decompression-stabilization for thoracolumbar fractures. Spine 2:53–56, 1977. With permission.)

diaphragm. A lower thoracotomy incision is made at the level of the seventh to the eleventh rib depending upon the desired level of the section. The incision extends from the plane of the scapula to the anterior margin of the rib cage. The latissimus dorsi muscle is transected across its fibers and the serratus anterior is divided and spread over the intended rib level. Intercostal muscles are divided and the thoracic cavity is opened, using a self-retaining retractor. The lung is deflated and retracted anteriorly and superiorly. A circumferential incision is made in the muscular portion of the diaphragm adjacent to the costal margin. This should be extended posteriorly to the area of the lateral arcuate ligament. The incision then is extended through the peritoneal reflexion of the diaphragm, and the spleen and the contents of the left upper quadrant of the abdomen are exposed. The retroperitoneal space is opened by blunt dissection. Abdominal organs are gently retracted medially with a Deaver retractor. The vertebral bodies and aorta then are exposed. The aorta is mobilized by a combination of sharp and blunt dissection, and segmental vessels are ligated and divided to permit visualization of the involved vertebral bodies. Grafting and even resection of a vertebral body can be carried out. Fusion and inlayed bone grafting in a trough can be accomplished through this exposure. The anterior longitudinal ligament may be closed over the vertebral bodies. Various anatomic structures are reapproximated, and chest tubes attached to water-seal suction should be employed. Erickson et l.[68] advocated internal decompression stabilization for fracture-dislocation (Figures 126-26 through 126-29).

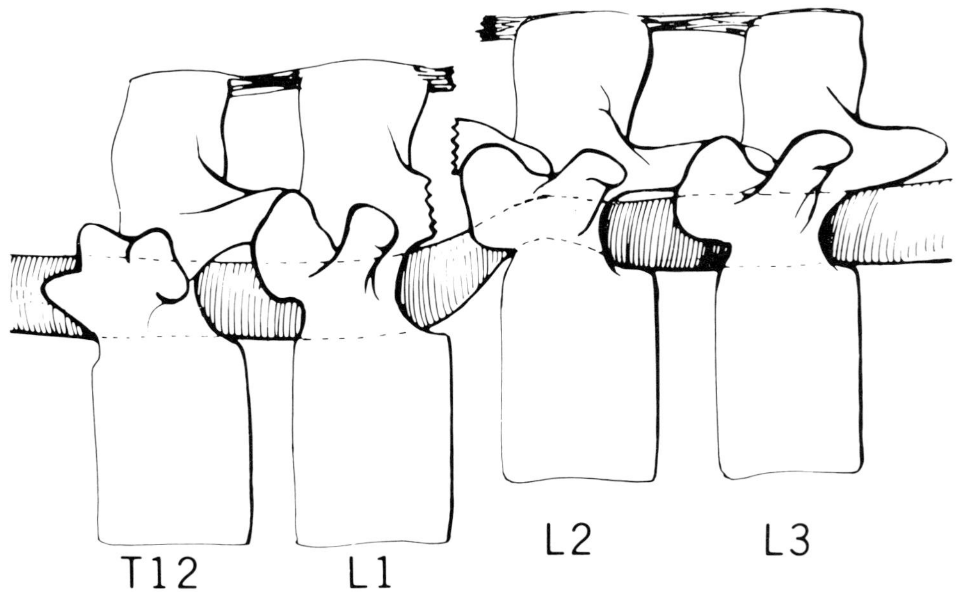

Fig. 126-28. Thoracolumbar dislocation before realignment, relocation, or removal of the retropulsed portion of a vertebral body. Lateral view. (Reprinted from Erikson DL, Leider LL Jr, Brown WE: One stage decompression-stabilization for thoracolumbar fractures. Spine 2:53–56, 1977. With permission.)

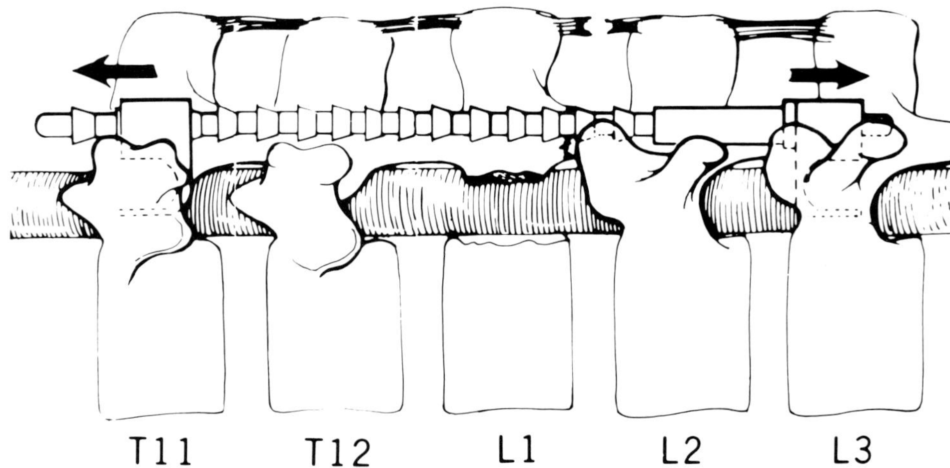

Fig. 126-29.   Restoration of alignment after placement of a Harrington rod. Lateral view. In addition, intervening zygaphophyseal joint fusion and the addition of autologous bone can enhance fusion. (Reprinted from Erikson DL, Leider LL Jr, Brown WE: One stage decompression-stabilization for thoracolumbar fractures. Spine 2:53–56, 1977. With permission.)

ANTERIOR LATERAL APPROACH TO THE LUMBAR VERTEBRAL BODIES

An anterior lateral approach to the lumbar vertebral bodies through a long, oblique flank incision can provide direct access to all lumbar vertebral bodies. In the case of spinal injury, grafting can be carried out for anterior interbody fusion, but abdominal viscera and major vessels must be carefully retracted. In addition, the hypogastric nerve plexus should be protected to avoid postoperative complications of impotence and sterility in males. The anterior lateral approach to the lumbar vertebrae is similar to that used for lumbar sympathectomy.

REFERENCES

1. Harris P, Wu PH: The management of patients with injury of the cervical spine using Blackburn skull calipers and the Stryker turning frame. Paraplegia 2:278, 1965
2. Prather GC, Mayfield FH: Injuries of the Spinal Cord. Springfield Ill, Charles C Thomas, 1953, p 396
3. Gallie WE: Skeletal traction in the treatment of fractures and dislocations of the cervical spine. Ann Surg 106:770, 1937
4. Taylor AS: Fracture dislocation of the cervical spine. Ann Surg 90:321, 1929
5. Crutchfield WG: Skeletal traction for dislocation of cervical spine. Report of a case. Southern Surg 2:156, 1933
6. Crutchfield WG: Further observations on the treatment of fracture dislocations of the cervical spine with skeletal traction. Surg Gynecol Obstet 63:513, 1936
7. Crutchfield WG: Treatment of injuries of the cervical spine. J Bone Joint Surg 20:696, 1938
8. Crutchfield WG: Skeletal traction in treatment of injuries to the cervical spine. JAMA 155:29, 1954
9. Yashon D: Spinal Injury, ed 2. Norwalk, Conn, Appleton-Century-Crofts, 1978
10. Gardner WJ: The principle of spring-loaded points for cervical traction. J Neurosurg 39:543, 1973
11. Rimel RW, Butler AB, Winn HR, et al: Modified skull tongs for cervical traction. J Neurosurg 55:848, 1981
12. Nicholson MW: Treatment of cervical spine dislocation. JAMA 219:1764, 1972
13. Vinke TH: A skull-traction apparatus. J Bone Joint Surg 30A:522, 1948
14. Yashon D, Tyson G, Vise WM: Rapid closed reduction of cervical fracture dislocations. Surg Neurol 4:513, 1975
15. Yashon D, White RJ: Injuries of the vertebral column and spinal cord, in Feiring EG (ed): Brock's Injuries of the Brain and Spinal Cord and Their Coverings. New York, Springer, 1974, pp 688–743
16. Abbott KH, Hale N: Cervical trapeze. J Neurosurg 10:436, 1953
17. Verbiest H: Anterolateral operations for fractures and dislocations in the middle and lower parts of the cervical spine. J Bone Joint Surg 51A:1489, 1969
18. Cave E: Immediate fracture management. Surg Clin North Am 46:771, 1966
19. Cone W, Turner WG: The treatment of fracture-dislocations of the cervical vertebrae by skeletal traction and fusion. J Bone Joint Surg 19:584, 1937
20. Crenshaw AH (ed): Campbell's Operative Orthopedics, vol 1. St Louis, Mosby, 1971, pp 616–630
21. Gallie WE: Fractures and dislocations of the cervical spine. Am J Surg 46:495, 1939
22. Hoen TI: A method of skeletal traction for treatment of fracture dislocation of cervical vertebrae. Arch Neurol Psychiatr 36:158, 1936
23. Loeser JD: History of skeletal traction. J Neurosurg 33:54, 1970
24. McKenzie KG: Fracture, dislocation and fracture-dislocation of the spine. Can Med Assoc J 32:263, 1935
25. Neubeiser BL: A method of skeletal traction for neck extension. J Miss State Med Assoc 30:495, 1983
26. Peyton WT, Hall HB, French LA: Hook traction under zygomatic arch in cervical spine injuries. Surg Gynecol Obstet 791:311, 1944
27. Bovill EG, Eberle CF, Day L, Aufranc OE: Dislocation of the cervical spine without spinal cord injury. JAMA 218:1288, 1971
28. Dowman C: Reduction of cervical fracture dislocation with locked facets. JAMA 219:1212, 1972
29. Rogers WA: Fractures and dislocations of the cervical spine. J Bone Joint Surg 39A:341, 1957
30. Bailey RW: Fractures and dislocations of the cervical spine. Surg Clin North Am 41:1357, 1961
31. Bailey RW, Badgley CE: Stabilization of the cervical spine by anterior fusion. J Bone Joint Surg 42A:565, 1960
32. Hollin SA, Gross SW: Management of cervical spine dislocations with locked facets. Surg Gynecol Obstet 124:521, 1967
33. Ellis VH: Injuries of the cervical vertebrae. Proc R Soc Med (Secton of Orthopaedics) 40:19, 1946

34. Evans DK: Reduction of cervical dislocations. J Bone Joint Surg 43B:552, 1961

35. Daw EF, Svien HJ, Michenfelder JD, Terry HR: The role of the anesthesiologist in the management of acute intracranial and spinal cord emergencies. Surg Clin North Am 45:910, 1965

36. Demian YK, White RJ, Yashon D, Kretchmer HE: Anesthesia for laminectomy and localized cord cooling in acute cervical spine injury. Br J Anaesth 43:973, 1971

37. Stone WA, Beach TP, Hamelberg W: Succinylcholine-induced hyperkalemia in dogs with transected sciatic nerves or spinal cords. Anesthesiology 32:515, 1970

38. Frankel HL, Mathias CJ, Spalding JMK: Mechanisms of reflex cardiac arrest in tetraplegic patients. Lancet 2:1183, 1975

39. Fraser A, Edmonds-Seal J: Spinal cord injuries. Anesthesia 37:1804, 1982

40. Pledger HG: Disorders of temperature regulation in acute traumatic tetraplegia. J Bone Joint Surg 44B:110, 1944

41. Grote W, Romer F, Bettag W: Der ventrale zugang zum dens epistropheus. Langenbecks Arch Chir 331:15, 1972

42. Murray JWG, Seymour RJ: An anterior, extrapharyngeal suprahyoid approach to the first, second and third cervical vertebrae. Acta Orthop Scand 45:43, 1974

43. Bonney G: Stabilization of the upper cervical spine by the transpharyngeal route. Proc R Soc Med 63:40, 1970

44. Fang HSY, Ong GB: Direct anterior approach to the upper cervical spine. J Bone Joint Surg 44A:1588, 1962

45. Fang HSY, Ong GB, Hodgson AR: Anterior spinal fusion. The operative approaches. Clin Orthop 35:16, 1964

46. Estridge MN, Smith RA: Transoral fusion of odontoid fracture. Case report. J Neurosurg 27:462, 1967

47. Smith GW, Robinson RA: The treatment of certain cervical-spine disorders by anterior removal of the intervertebral disc and interbody fusion. J Bone Joint Surg 40A:607, 1958

48. Cloward RB: The anterior approach for removal of ruptured cervical discs. J Neurosurg 15:602, 1958

49. Cloward RB: Treatment of acute fractures of the cervical spine. J Neurosurg 18:201, 1961

50. Cloward RB: Lesions of the intervertebral discs and their treatment by interbody fusion methods. The painful disc. Clin Orthop 27:51, 1963

51. Kelly DT Jr, Alexander E Jr, Davis CH Jr, et al: Acrylic fixation of atlanto-axial dislocations. Technical note. J Neurosurg 36:366, 1972

52. Stowsand D, Muhtaroglu U: Dorsale stabilisierug bei luxationsfrakturen des 1. and 2. halswirbels mit palacos und drahtumschlingung. Neurochirurgia 18:120, 1975

53. DeAndrade JR, MacNab I: Anterior occipito-cervical fusion using an extra-pharyngeal exposure. J Bone Joint Surg 51:1621, 1969

54. Masferrer R, Hadley MN, Bloomfield S, et al: Transoral microsurgical resection of the odontoid process, BNI Quarterly 1:34, 1985

55. Sakou T, Morizono Y, Morimoto N: Transoral atlantoaxial anterior decompression and fusion. Clin Orthop 187:134, 1984

56. Louis R: Atloido-axoid surgery by a transoral approach. Rev Cir Orthop 69:381, 1983

57. Spetzler RF, Selman WR, Nash CL, Brown RH: Transoral microsurgical odontoid resection and spinal cord monitoring. Spine 4:506, 1979

58. Komisar A, Tabaddor K: Extrapharyngeal (anterolateral approach to the cervical spine). Head Neck Surg 6:600, 1983

59. Mixter WT, Osgood RB: Traumatic lesions of the atlas and axis. Am J Orthop Surg 7:348, 1910

60. Alexander E Jr, Davis CH Jr, Forsyth HF: Reduction and fusion of fracture dislocation of the cervical spine. J Neurosurg 27:588, 1967

61. Lewis J, McKibben B: The treatment of fracture dislocation of the thoracolumbar spine. J Bone Joint Surg 56B:391, 1974

62. Schmidek HH, Gomes FB, Seligson D, et al: Management of acute unstable thoracolumbar (T11-L1) fractures with and without neurological deficit. Neurosurgery 7:30, 1980

63. Lahde RE: Luque rod instrumentation. AORN Journal 38:35, 1983

64. Bowen JR: Operative technique: Posterior spinal fusion with luque instrumentation. Orthop Nurse 2:16, 1983

65. Thomas PC: Nursing care of patients undergoing posterior spinal fusion with segmental (Luque) spinal instrumentation. Orthop Nurse 2:13, 60, 1983

66. Bernard TN Jr, Whitecloud TS III, Rodriguez RP, et al: Segmental spinal instrumentation in the management of fractures of the thoracic and lumbar spine. South Med J 76:1232, 1983

67. Robinson RA, Southwick WO: Surgical approaches to the cervical spine. Instructional course lecture. The American Academy of Orthopaedic Surgeons, publ. XVII, St Louis, CV Mosby, 1960, pp 299–330

68. Erickson DL, Leider LL Jr, Brown WE: One-stage decompression-stabilization for thoracolumbar fractures. Spine 2:53, 1977

69. Dunsker S, Schmidek HH, Frymoyer J, Kahn A (eds): The Unstable Spine (Thoracic, Lumbar Sacral Regions). Orlando, Florida, Grune & Stratton, 1986

70. Freyschuss U, Knutsson E: Cardiovascular control in man with transverse cervical cord lesions. Life Sci 8:421, 1969

71. Jacobs RR, Dahners LE, Gertzbein SD, et al: A locking hook spinal rod: Current status of development. Paraplegia 21:197, 1983

72. Thompson CE, Witham AC: Paroxysmal hypertension in spinal cord injuries. N Engl J Med 239:291, 1948

CHAPTER 127

Techniques of Fusion in the Cervical, Thoracic, and Lumbar Spine

Robert C. Cantu

WHILE AN ASSORTMENT of wire, silk, rods, screws, and, more recently, plastics have been employed individually and in combination to stabilize the vertebral column, spinal fusion refers to a surgical procedure performed on adjacent vertebrae that leads to an immobilized bony continuity. Using this definition, Russell A. Hibbs and Fred H. Albee in New York City ushered in the history of spinal fusion in 1911.[1] For Hibbs, intervertebral fusion was the natural end result of his interest in arthrodesing techniques that commenced some 29 years earlier in 1882 with Albert in Vienna. Among the earliest to popularize arthrodesis in the United States, Hibbs carried out the first recorded operation of fusion of the spine at the New York Orthopedic Hospital on January 9, 1911.[2] The fusion was achieved by overlapping osseous elements locally derived. Eventually this included spinous processes, laminae, and intervertebral articulations (facet joints). It was reported on May 28, 1911 in the New York State Medical Journal,[3] and it became known throughout the orthopedic world as the Hibbs fusion operation. With only minor modifications, it has remained the standard for over half a century.

Fred H. Albee, also of New York City, was primarily interested in improving bone graft operations. After exposing the spinous processes and laminae, he split the former in the sagittal plane and inserted a tibial cortical graft into the cleft thus formed. He first performed such a fusion in 1909, and he reported his work before the American Orthopedic Association in 1911.[1] His paper was subsequently published in the *Journal of the American Medical Association.*[4] Albee's fusion had considerable acceptance during his lifetime because of his worldwide travels, but eventually lost popularity to the Hibbs procedure.

Other major contributions to spinal fusion include a report by MacKenzie-Forbs of Montreal in 1920 of denuding the cortical surfaces of the spinous processes and laminae, leaving the cortical slivers overlapping adjacent counterparts.[5] In 1922, Samuel Kleinberg first reported the use of beef-bone grafts and continued to use beef bone until his death in 1957.[6]

Ralph Ghormley of the Mayo Clinic in 1933 recognized the easily accessible abundant supply of autogenous bone from the iliac crest.[7] His report led to a flood of reports regarding the relative merits of cancellous bone versus the stiffer bracing factor offered by the rigid cortical bone. A third minor voice advocated specially prepared beef bone, but cancellous bone from the ilium won the most adherents.

The first two anterior approaches to the lumbar spine both appeared in British journals in 1936. Walter Mercer of Edinburgh described using bone from the iliac crest as an anterior bone graft between the fifth lumbar vertebra and the sacrum.[8] J. A. Jenkins reported in the *British Journal of Surgery* on an abdominal approach for exposing the fifth lumbar vertebra and the sacrum. A bone drill was passed from L5 into S1, and a cortical tibial graft was inserted into the hole.[9] Both of these reports were on cases of spondylolisthesis.

Interfacet screws—metal screws placed across denuded articular facets—were suggested in an effort to improve the efficiency of spinal fusion by James W. Toumey of the Lahey Clinic in Boston in 1943[10] and by Don King of San Francisco in 1944.[11]

Posterior interbody fusion through a laminectomy exposure following disc excision was first reported in *Surgery, Gynecology, and Obstetrics* in 1946 by Irwin A. Jaslow, an orthopedic surgeon in New Bedford, Massachusetts.[12] Ralph B. Cloward of Honolulu in 1952 reported the first large series of his variation of this procedure.[13]

Anterior cervical spine fusion was reported by Robinson and Smith in 1955[14] and by Ralph Cloward in 1958.[15]

Having presented a sketch of the salient milestones in the history of spine fusion, I wish now to be very practical regarding the indications and recommended types of spinal fusion for conditions of the cervical, thoracic, and lumbar regions.

FUSION OF THE CERVICAL SPINE

In his chapter in the first edition of this text, Robert A. Robinson covered the posterior, anterior, anterolateral, and lateral approaches to the cervical spine. He discussed posterior fusions including both the standard wire and bone C1-C2 or C1-C2-C3 fusions for odontoid instability, as well as the anterior approach to fusing C1-C3. Robinson also discussed the role of skull traction and Halo-cast cervical traction and immobilization.

In this edition, Schmidek and Smith (Chapter 116) recount in detail the anterolateral approach to the cervical spine and the use of either the Cloward or Smith-Robinson anterior spinal fusion in cervical spondylosis. With these excellent descriptions of the indications for and various approaches to the cervical spine, my remarks will be confined to posterior cervical spinal fusion below C2 whether for instability secondary to fracture-dislocation, traumatic subluxation, or instability fol-

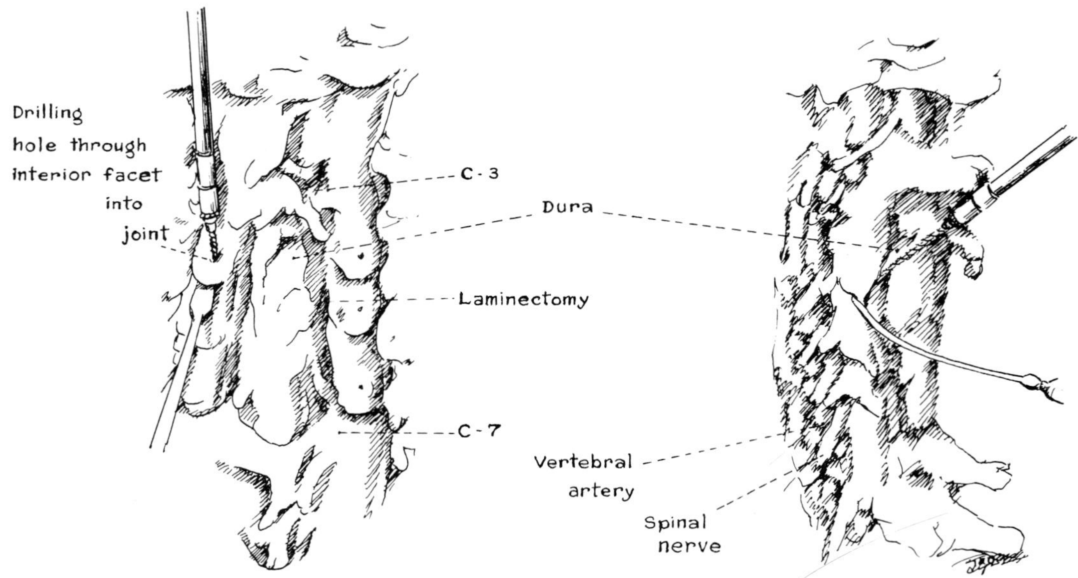

Fig. 127-1. Cervical vertebrae. (A) Posterior view. (B) Left lateral view.

lowing extensive laminectomy. Yashon in Chapter 126 discusses the surgical management of spinal trauma per se. The modified posterior fusion of Robinson and Southwick discussed here is equally applicable to stabilizing iatrogenic extensive instability following decompressive laminectomy as that following fracture-dislocation.

After the laminectomy has been completed, the last exposed facet joint at the cranial end is slightly opened with an osteotome, and either a suction tip or a No. 4 Penfield dissector then is inserted and the osteotome removed. Using a Hall air drill, a hole is drilled through the inferior facet into the joint space (Figure 127-1). A No. 20 wire then is passed through the

hole. Bilaterally, this is carried out from the cranial-most exposed facet to the level below of the first intact spinous process. A corticocancellous graft 2 cm wide by whatever length is required is taken from the outer table of the posterior iliac crest. Cancellous side down, the graft is securely wired to the facets (Figure 127-2). Additional cancellous bone may be tucked laterally. The careful wiring of the graft at each facet ensures the most rapid and secure union.

Comments. I would like to express certain personal biases regarding cervical spinal fusion gleaned from more than 15 years of practice and reflection. The comments of Robinson

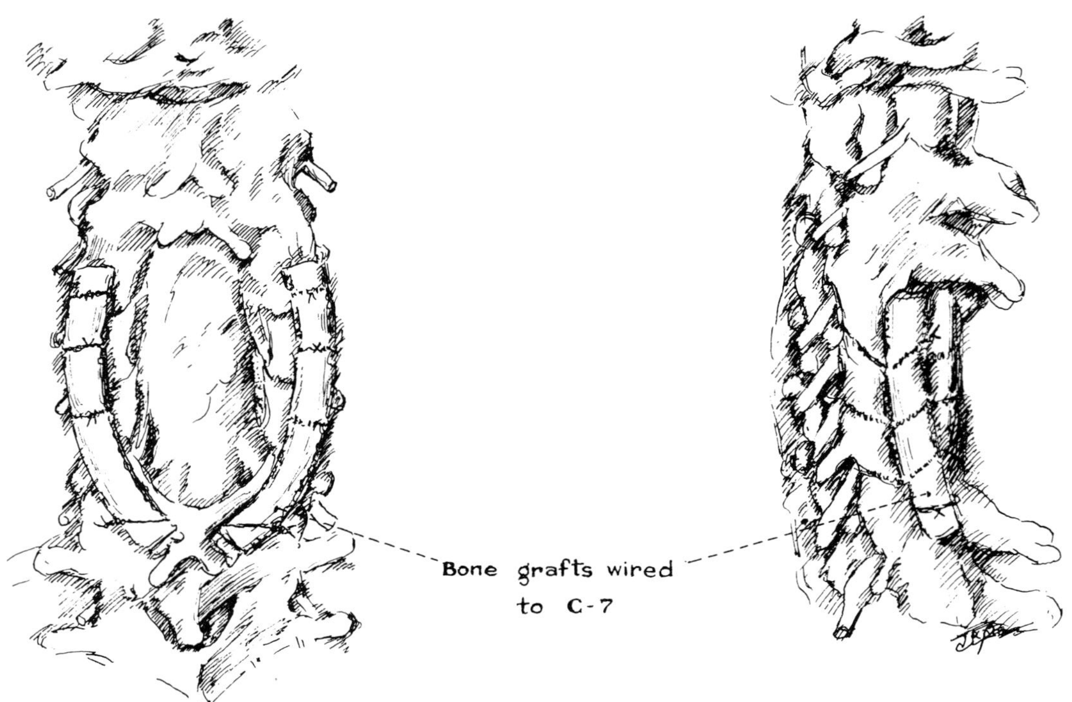

Fig. 127-2. Bone grafts wired to C7.

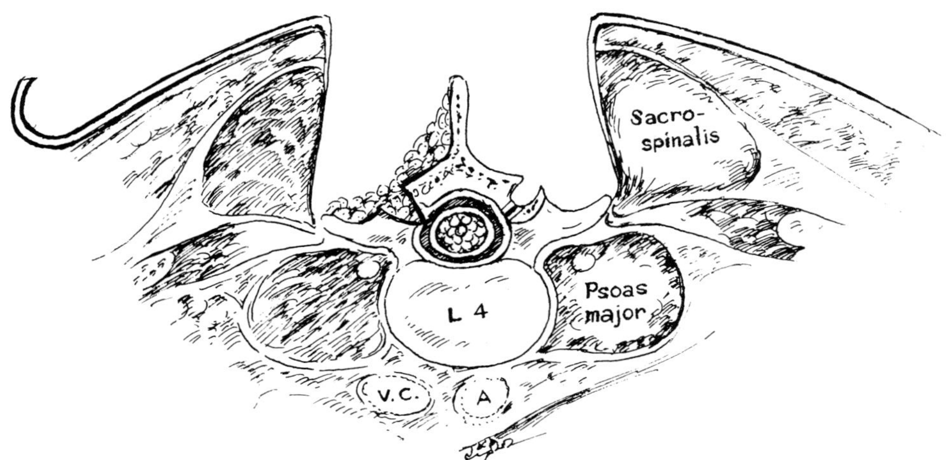

Fig. 127-3. Skin incision is midline and all tissues are stripped from spinous processes, laminae, and transverse processes. Anterior two thirds of facets are excised.

regarding the remodeling of bone are certainly true. Since the central nervous system is unforgiving of transgressions, the major charge to the neurosurgeon must be not to harm or inflict neurologic deficit on the patient. The simplest, safest, successful procedure should be the one employed. It has been my experience with cervical spondylotic disease that if 2 to 3 mm of disc space and resultant neuroforamen distraction can be accomplished, that there is no need to attempt the more risky osteophyte removal in the neuroforamen. With distraction, there will be room for the nerves to exit, and with firm fusion, the osteophytes will be largely absorbed within 18 months.

It has been said that in posterior cervical fusion all that has to be done is clean the lamina and lay on the bone. In my experience, I have found that roughening the bed, i.e., lamina, facets, and spinous processes, with a Hall burr, using wire fixation, employing corticocancellous grafts from the posterior iliac crest with the cancellous side down and using many additional slivers of cancellous bone obtained with gouges maximally ensures the rapidity and solidarity of the fusion.

FUSION OF THE THORACIC AND LUMBAR SPINE

Today, the indication for fusion of the thoracic and lumbar spine is primarily instability resulting from traumatic, congenital, degenerative, or neoplastic disease. Unlike the situation shortly after the turn of the century, tuberculosis is now rarely an indication for spinal fusion. The indications for fusion in the minds of most spine surgeons, be they orthopedists or neurosurgeons, are currently more limited than in the past. Among the common anomalies once considered as indications for spinal fusion that are generally no longer thought to be such are cases of laminectomy with marked disc-space narrowing, transitional vertebrae, tropism, degenerative spondylolisthesis, increased lumbar lordosis, and lumbosacral tilt. Because of the low rate of solid fusion, except when internal fixation is used, such as with the Harrington technique, lumbar three-level fusions now are rarely done.

Paul Lin in Chapter 123 comprehensively covers the technique of posterior lumbar interbody fusion while Goldner, Wood, and Urbaniak accomplish the same for anterior lumbar interbody fusion in Chapter 124. While neither technique is as widely used as the standard posterior and posterolateral fusions

I will discuss, each still has special indications, and the reader is referred to Lin and Goldner's chapters for their discussion.

TECHNIQUES OF THORACIC AND LUMBAR SPINE FUSION—HIBBS FUSION

Initially described in 1911, the most popular technique for posterior spinal fusion remains, with minor variations, the Hibbs fusion. By this technique, bony union is attempted at two points bilaterally—the laminae and the articular processes (facet joints). The skin, subcutaneous tissues, deep fascia, and supraspinous ligaments are incised in the midline. With Cobb or other periosteal elevators, the periosteum is stripped from the sides of the spinous processes and the dorsal surface of the laminae. Bleeding is controlled by electrocautery of frank arterial sources and packing for the ooze. Interspinous ligaments are incised, muscles are elevated from the ligamentum flavum, and the fossa distal to the articular facet joint is exposed. The fat pad in this fossa is removed with a scalpel or curette. The spinous process is removed with rongeurs. The posterior layer (about two thirds) of the ligamentum flavum is freed with a curette from the proximal and distal laminae. The articular cartilage and cortical bone are removed with osteotomes, either straight or curved, from the facet joints. Then additional small cuts into the articular processes are made parallel with the joint line so these thin slivers of bone fill the joint space (Figure 127-3). All cortical bone of the lateral fossa, facet joint, and lamina is cut into chips with a gouge. Additional chips of cortical bone and especially cancellous bone taken from the iliac crest may be added to the lamina slivers. The periosteum, ligaments, and muscles then are snugly sutured over the bone chips with interrupted 0 Dexon sutures. The subcutaneous tissues are closed with 3-0 Dexon and the skin with nylon or subcuticular suture.

While King in 1940 inserted metal screws across the articular facets after removal of the articular cartilage (Figure 127-4), this author agrees with Bosworth, who believes that screw fixation is not of value when evaluated relative to the difficulties encountered by its use. Another popular modification of the Hibbs technique is to use a solid "clothespin" graft between the spinous processes of the fifth lumbar and first sacral vertebra. The cancellous side is placed down against the roughened lamina and the cortical side is dorsal (Figure 127-5).

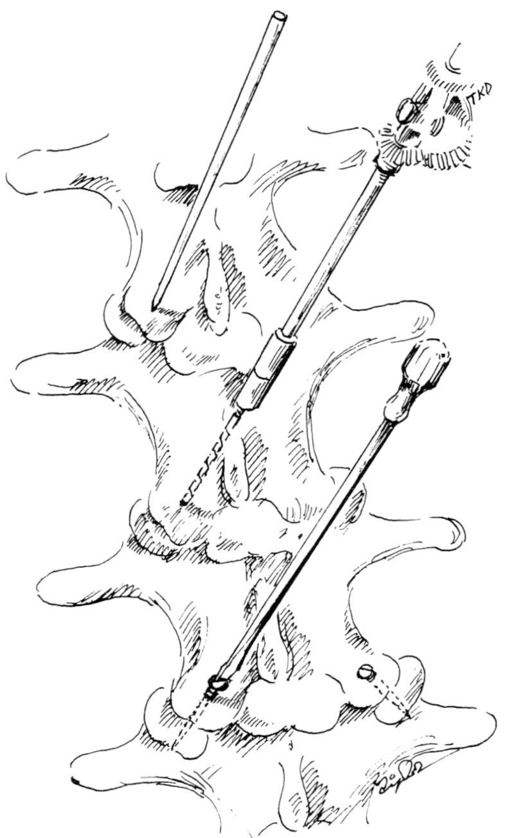

Fig. 127-4. Technique of inserting screws across apophyseal joints.

POSTEROLATERAL OR INTERTRANSVERSE FUSION

Initially described by Cleveland, Bosworth, and F. R. Thompson in 1948[16] as a technique for pseudoarthrosis repair, the lateral fusion was quickly adopted for use in congenital or surgical laminal defects, spondylolisthesis, and postlaminectomy patients with chronic pain that was thought to be due to instability. The operation may be unilateral or bilateral and cover one or more levels.

The skin may be incised either along the lateral border of the paraspinal muscles or in the midline. The distal end curves across the posterior crest of the ilium. The lumbodorsal fascia is incised an inch or more lateral to the midline and the sacrospinalis muscle is split longitudinally. The lamina, articular facets, and transverse processes are exposed, and the cortical surfaces are removed with osteotomes (Figure 127-6). Cartilage is removed from the facets with an osteotome. Bone now is taken from the iliac crest. One long strip with cortical bone on one side and many cancellous slivers are desired for each side to be fused. Half of the cancellous slivers, usually most easily obtained from the iliac crest with a gouge, are fitted against the denuded facets, the pars interarticularis, and the base of the transverse process at each level. The long strip then is firmly packed with its cancellous side down into this bed of cancellous chips. The remaining chips of cancellous bone from the ilium then are packed about the graft.

When there is no laminal defect, others such as Wiltse, Truckly, and Thompson have suggested including the lamina as well as the articular facets and transverse processes in this fusion—the posterolateral fusion.

LATERAL EXTRAPLEURAL AND EXTRAPERITONEAL FUSION

Initially designed for treatment of tuberculous spondylitis by Alexander[17] and Capener,[18] the lateral extrapleural and extraperitoneal approach to the thoracic and lumbar spine is useful in any case in which the pathologic process is extradural and anterior to the thoracic spinal cord or cauda equina. It affords removal of lesions that cannot safely be reached by

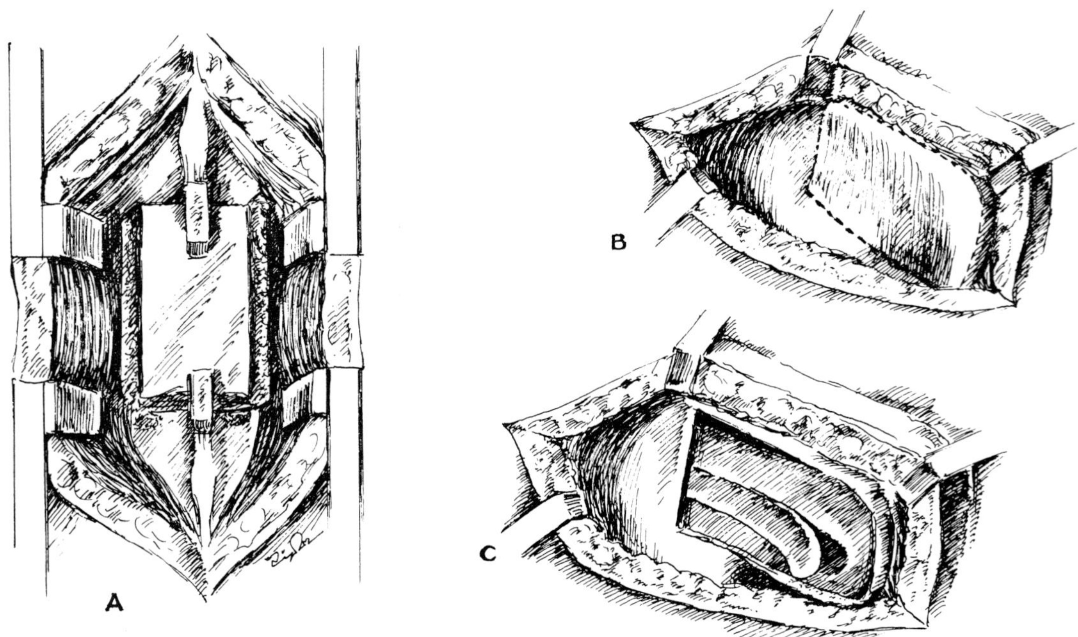

Fig. 127-5. (A) Clothespin graft firmly seated between spinous processes. (B) Graft fashioned from posterior crest of ilium. (C) Reinforcing cancellous iliac grafts.

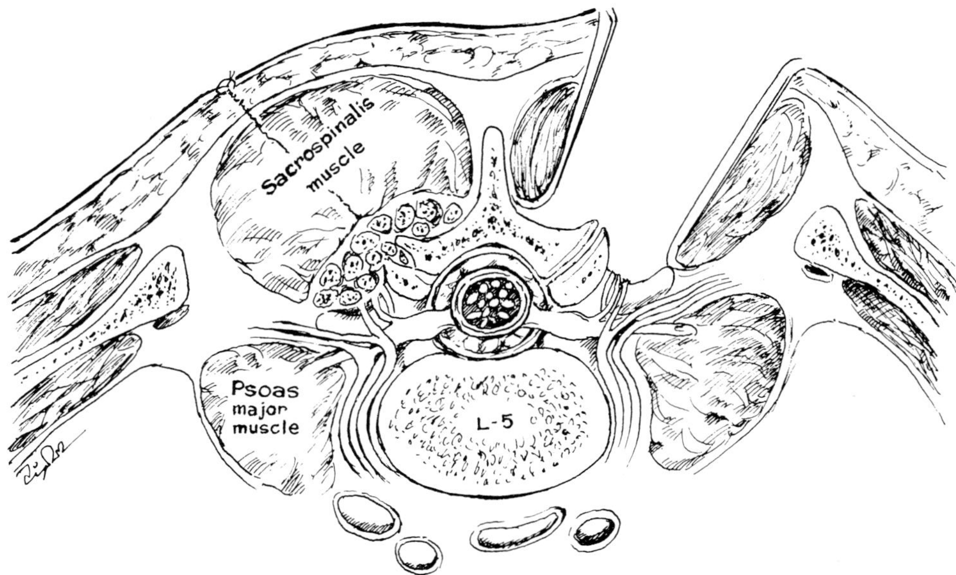

Fig. 127-6.   Posterolateral fusion. The sacrospinalis muscle is split longitudinally and laminae, articular facets, and transverse processes are all included in fusion.

laminectomy or costotransversectomy and has a lower morbidity and complication rate than thoracotomy or laparotomy.

Lateral Thoracic Extrapleural Fusion

The patient is placed in the prone position and a midline incision made from well above to well below the lesion, curving laterally inferiorly for about 10 cm. The back muscles are stripped from the ribs. The number of vertebral levels to be approached determines the number of ribs to be removed, but usually at least two are desirable. The rib is transected 8 cm lateral to the costotransverse joint and is removed with rongeurs (Figure 127-7). The pleura is very carefully stripped from the endothoracic fascia with blunt finger dissection, the neurovascular bundle is located, and the intercostal nerve is separated from the vessels. The costovertebral articulation and transverse processes are removed (Figure 127-7). The intercostal nerve is traced to its foramen and it along with the segmental artery and vein are doubly clipped and divided. The pedicle is removed with a rongeur. When the anatomy is particularly distorted, it is often advantageous to first remove the pedicle above and below the lesion. At this point, turning the operating table on a 30- to 45-degree tilt laterally aids in viewing the spinal canal. The annulus is now incised below the level of the posterior longitudinal ligament and the entire disc and adjacent cartilaginous plates are removed with curettes. The curette stroke is always downward and laterally into the cavity. Epidural bleeding can be controlled with cottonoids. An angled dental mirror may aid in assessing the completeness of the disc excision. I prefer a Smith-Robinson type bone graft from the iliac crest that with the aid of Cloward spreaders is tapped into place with a mallet and tamper. The wound is now closed in layers. If a bronchopleural fistula has occurred, a chest tube connected to a closed drainage system is required.

Lateral Lumbar Extraperitoneal Fusion

A skin incision similar to that used for lateral thoracic extrapleural fusion is employed. The lumbodorsal fascia is incised laterally, and the latissimus and erector spinae muscles are split. At least two transverse processes are identified (an x-ray film may be required), and their superior and inferior surfaces are cleared of erector spinae and quadratus lumborum muscles respectively. Then the transverse processes and associated intertransversarii muscles are removed (Figure 127-8). The lumbar plexus now is identified and the spinal nerve, which has just exited from the level above, is noted. Complete removal of the transverse process affords exposure of the nerve at the level of the lesion. It may be necessary to remove the pedicles above and below to afford good exposure of the spinal canal. Division of connecting rami to the sympathetic chain permits sufficient mobility of the spinal nerves to allow good exposure for removal of the disc and adjacent cartilaginous plates. The technique of disc excision and lateral interbody fusion using a Smith-Robinson bone graft is the same as that described for the thoracic spine (Figure 127-8).

HARRINGTON-ROD THORACOLUMBAR FUSION

David Yashon in Chapter 126 covers the surgical treatment of spinal trauma. I wish, however, to conclude this chapter with a discussion of the Harrington distraction system. Although initially devised to treat scoliosis,[19] it has come to be widely used in the treatment of fracture of the thoracolumbar spine with and without paraplegia.

Controversy still exists regarding the treatment of unstable fractures and fracture-dislocations of the thoracic and lumbar spine. Investigators such as Frankel, Guttman, Lewis, and McKibbin support the nonoperative approach while Dickson, Harrington, Kaufer, Whitesides, Bradford, and others advocate operative management. There also is a wide divergence of opinion regarding the best operative approach. Laminectomy has recently fallen from favor because it frequently fails to relieve spinal compression and furthers instability. In the 1980 edition of *Campbell's Operative Orthopedics*, the statement is made that laminectomy "is to be condemned in these fracture-dislocations."[20]

It is my personal opinion that this is incorrect. I take issue

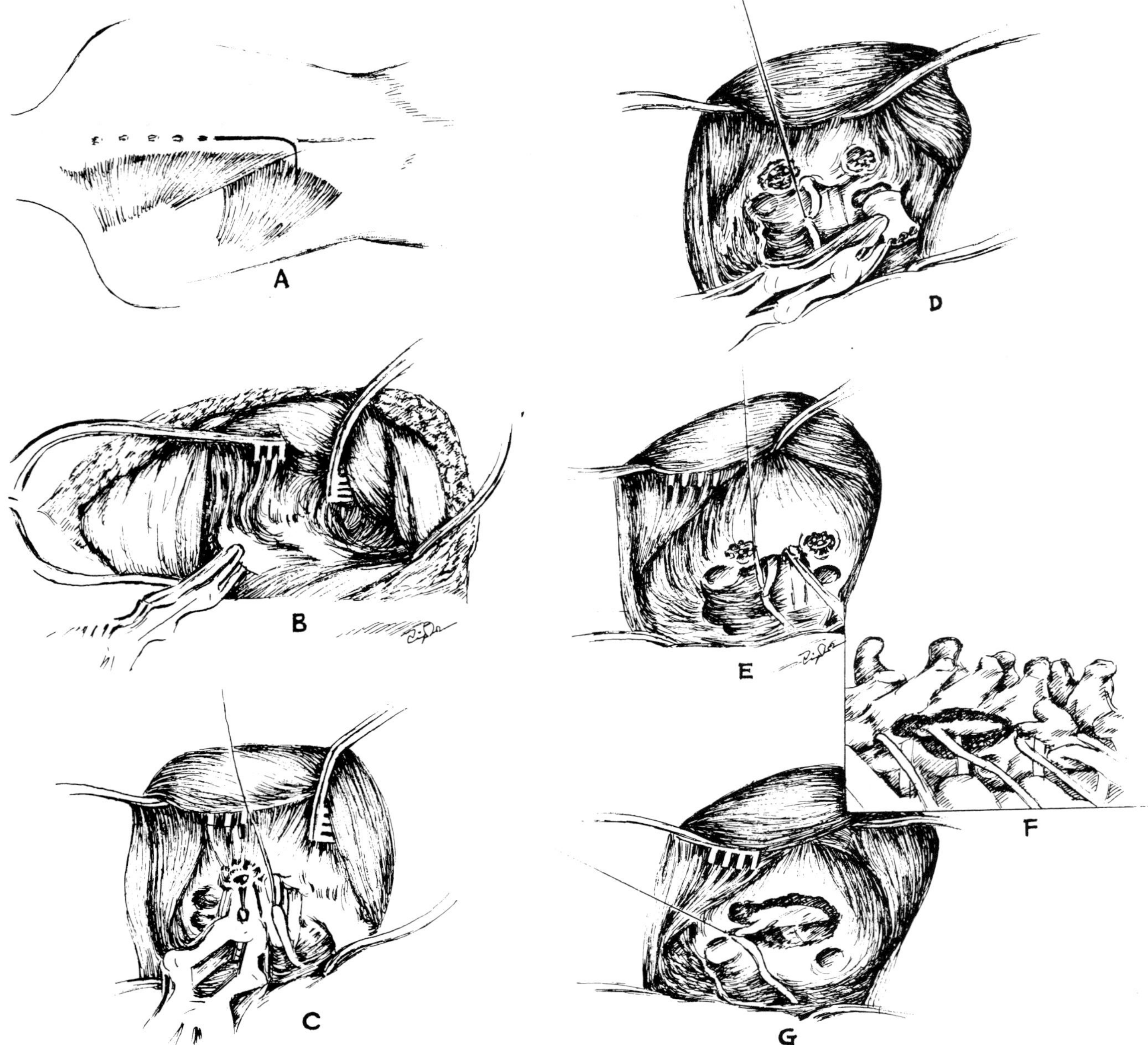

Fig. 127-7.   Lateral retropleural approach: (A) Skin incision in midline and curved laterally; (B) muscles retracted to expose ribs; (C) rib resected; (D) rib, including costovertebral articulation removed; (E) annulus incised and disc removed; (F,G) contiguous portions of bone removed from dorsal portions of vertebral bodies.

with Guttman and Bedbrook that all neural tissue damage occurs at the time of injury.[20] Over my 15-year neurosurgical experience, I have seen incomplete compressive spinal lesions that worsen over a period of hours or several days and then rapidly start to improve with adequate relief of the block by laminectomy and, when unstable, internal fixation. When there is an incomplete lesion of the cord or cauda equina with a high-grade or complete block on myelogram, I favor relief of the block as soon as the patient is stable. I believe a needless delay in some patients will lead to vascular compression and further cord infarction. If the cord lesion is complete, then stabilization may be deferred a week or more, as the indication for stabilization is to lessen local back pain and facilitate a future wheelchair existence, not neurologic recovery.

My own preference for relief of the block with incomplete

lesions is a decompressive laminectomy—especially when there is evidence of neurologic worsening—coupled with Harrington distraction instrumentation and lateral fusion. The laminectomy should be at least a level above and below the fracture and should preserve the articular facets. I favor intraoperative x-ray films to confirm the realignment with the Harrington apparatus, but also direct inspection via the laminectomy to be certain that no disc or bone fragments are left within the spinal canal. If alignment is achieved by x-ray control and inspection shows no intraspinal fragments yet the dura remains tense or "apparently" bulging, then I favor opening the dura to inspect the cord. If the cord is partially pulped, I do not favor a myelotomy, but do favor a fascia lata or sacrospinalis dural fascial graft. I believe that by combining laminectomy and Harrington distraction instrumentation and fusion that maximal cord and root decompression, anatomic align-

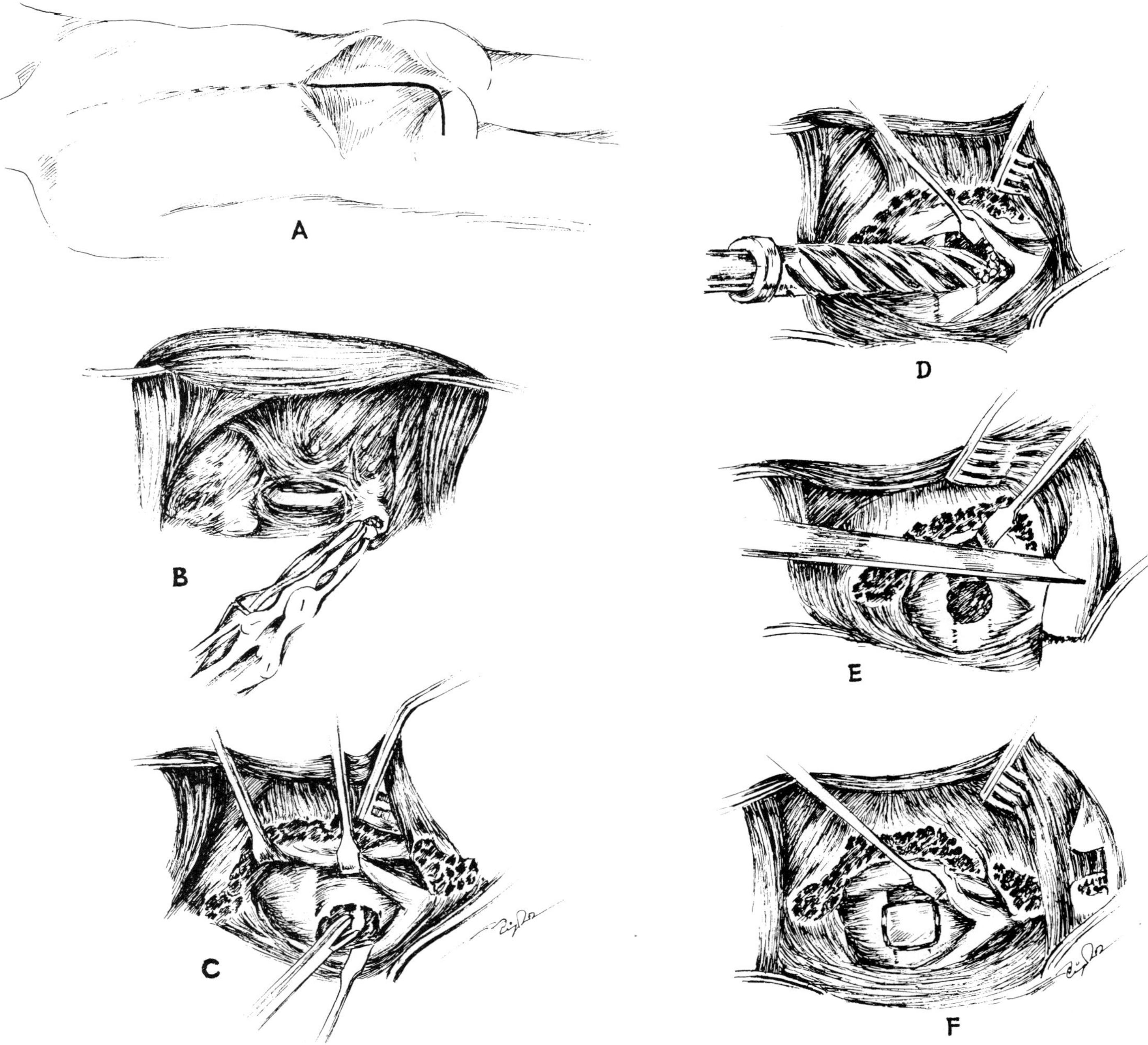

Fig. 127-8. Lateral retroperitoneal approach: (A) Lumbar incision is comparable to that used in thoracic area; (B) lumbar fascia is incised, transverse processes and intertransversarii muscles resected; (C) disc is removed; (D,E,F) bone is removed from vertebral body and fusion achieved with iliac bone graft.

ment, and long-term stabilization are achieved. Depending on one's training, both in residency and subsequently, the above combined procedure may be carried out by a neurosurgeon or orthopedist alone or working together. Following surgery, we prefer to use a Stryker frame for 1 week. Thereafter, a body jacket is used, and the patient is ambulated. External support is continued for 5 to 6 months.

The use of this combined approach is exemplified by the case of a 26-year-old male who sustained a fracture-dislocation of L1 with a resultant incomplete conus lesion. Numbness was present in the perineal and sacral areas. The anal wink, cremasteric, and bulbocavernous reflexes were lost, but knee and ankle reflexes were preserved. The patient was incontinent of urine and stool. Figure 127-9 shows the fracture-dislocation and Figure 127-10 the high-grade but incomplete myelographic bloc. Figure 127-11

shows the Pantopaque trapped above L1. Two No. 1252 Harrington hooks were notched into the facet joints several levels about the fracture and two No. 1254 hooks several levels below the fracture. The outrigger was installed and extended to correct the dislocation and realign the spine (Figure 127-12). With the outrigger in place, twin distraction rods were inserted until snug. X-ray films then were taken to assess alignment. Some surgeons prefer to awaken the patient at this point to test neurologic function. After a final intraspinal inspection, a posterolateral fusion with iliac crest bone was carried out, as described earlier in this chapter, from hook to hook of the instrumentation. Figures 127-13 and 127-14 show the distraction rod and the anatomic alignment attained. Following surgery, perineal and anal sensation rapidly started to improve. Bowel, bladder, and sexual function returned within the first month.

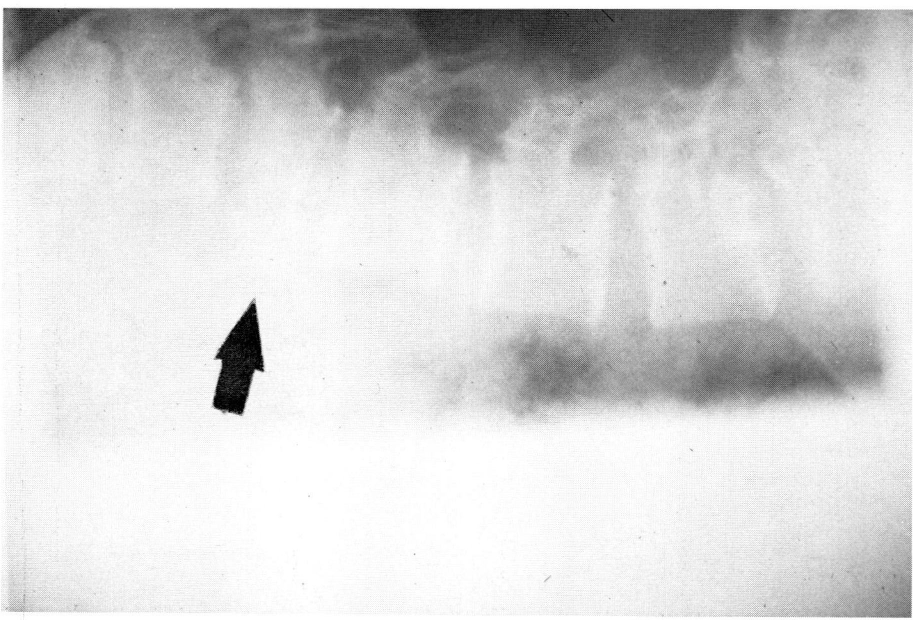

Fig. 127-9

POSTOPERATIVE CARE AND PSEUDOARTHROSIS

No chapter on spinal fusion would be complete without covering the postoperative care including the evaluation of the solidarity of the fusion. My comments here will apply primarily to the posterior and posterolateral fusion, as other authors have covered the anterior approach.

While there is no unanimity of opinion as to the precise day a patient should first be allowed up after surgery, most favor ambulation within a week. There is no concrete evidence that several weeks of bedrest decreases the incidence of pseudoarthrosis, but it does increase the risk of pulmonary embolism. I tend to allow age, condition of the patient, and the degree of postoperative pain to be taken into account, but I like to ambulate most patients by the third or fourth day after surgery. A rigid low-back brace or fiberglass cast is worn for 4 to 6 months until the fusion is solid, as determined by AP and lateral forward, backward, and right and left lateral bending films. Williams low-back exercises are commenced before the brace is discarded and are recommended for the rest of the patient's life.

Pseudoarthrosis will occur in about 10 percent of lumbar

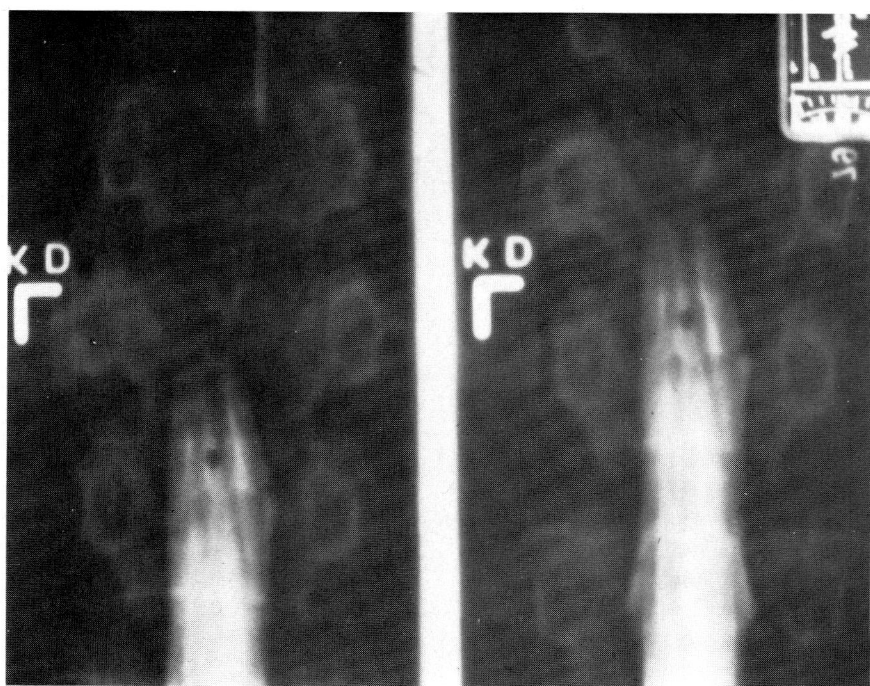

Fig. 127-10

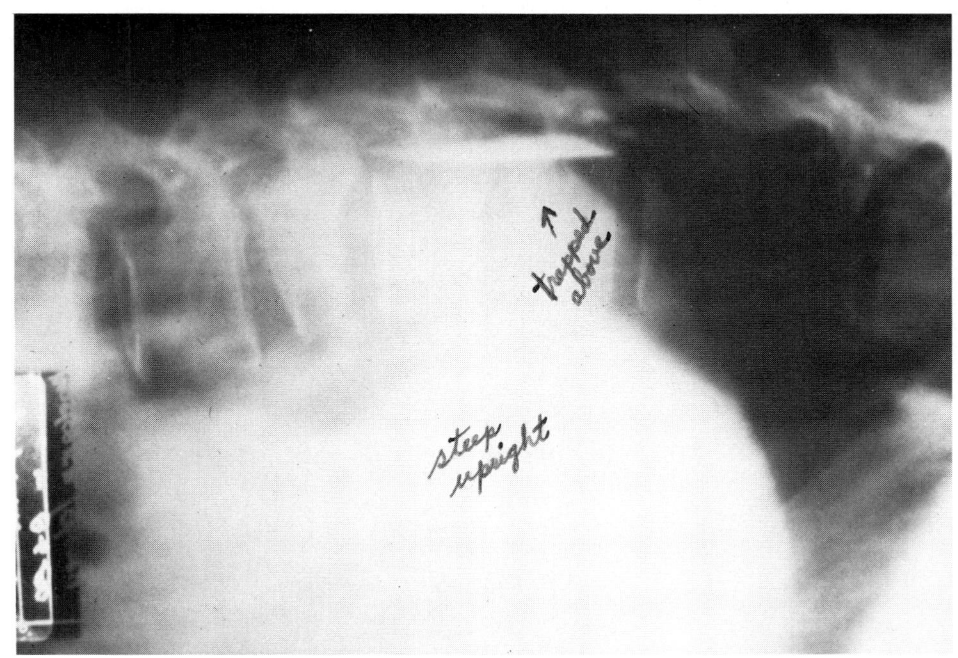

Fig. 127-11

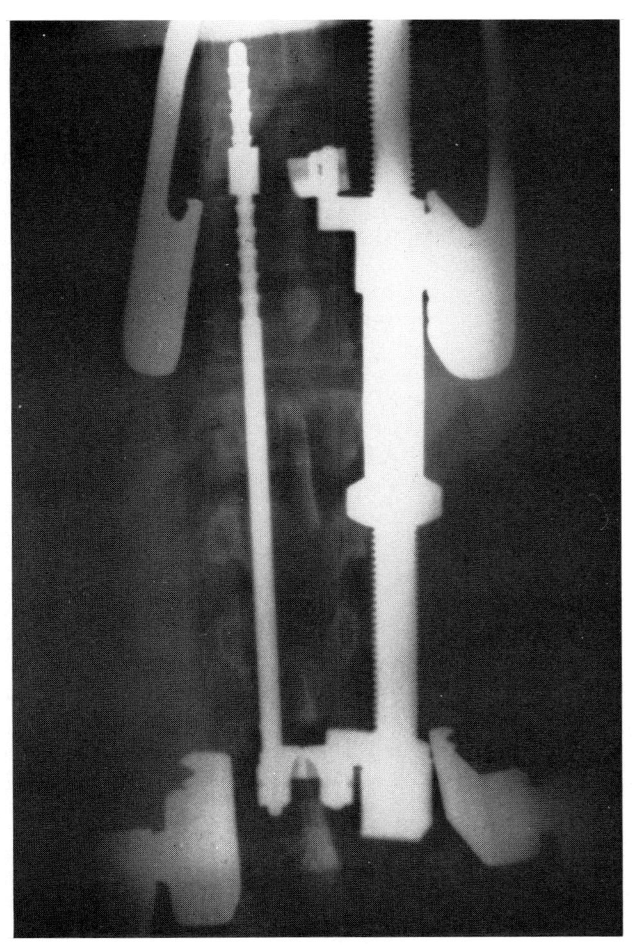

Fig. 127-12

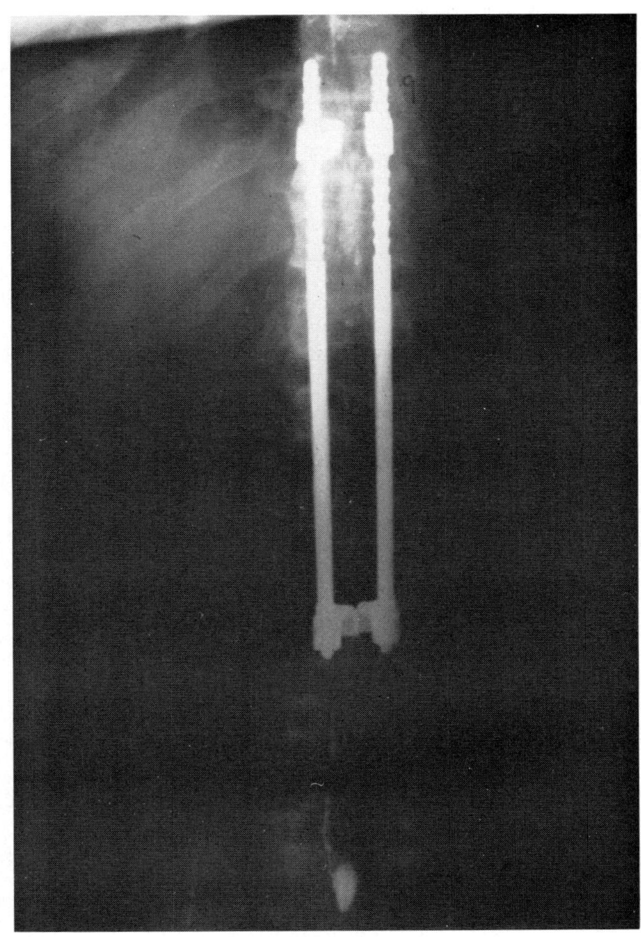

Fig. 127-13

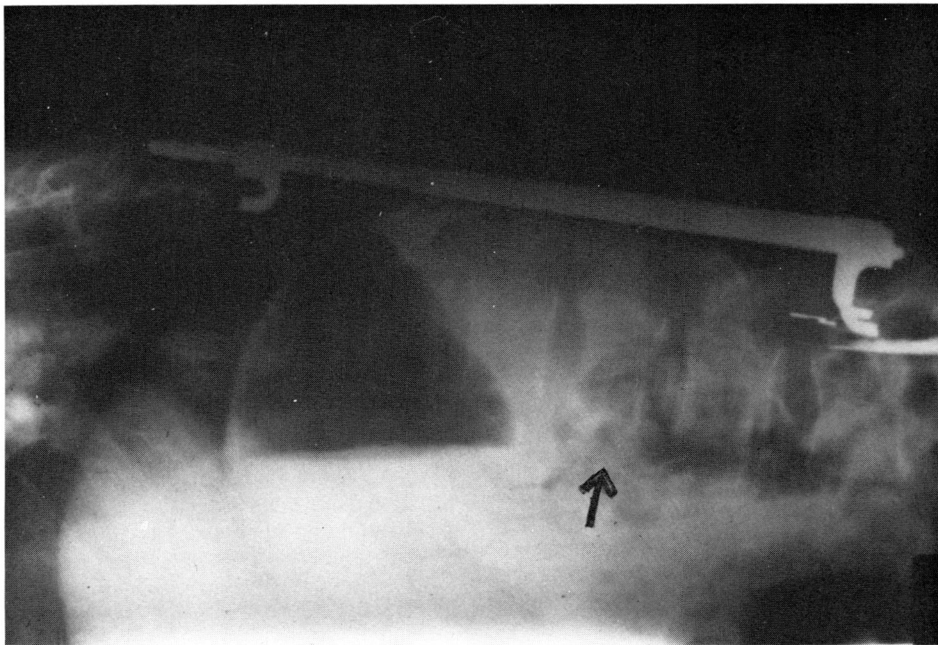

Fig. 127-14

one-level fusions, slightly less in cervical and thoracic fusions. The incidence increases with the number of levels fused; more than two is not recommended in the lumbar area excluding the Harrington procedure. *In this litigious era, it is especially important to frankly discuss the possibility of pseudoarthrosis preoperatively.* It is estimated that up to 50 percent of pseudoarthroses are asymptomatic.[20] In patients in whom severe pain and tenderness are sharply localized over a single level of non-union demonstrated by x-ray studies, and who obtain significant partial relief from a brace, however, pseudoarthrosis repair should be considered. Since there are may reports of successful pseudoarthrosis repair in which pain persists, it is probably wise to insist on favorable preoperative psychometric studies; it certainly is wise to make no promises that the pain will be relieved, and to not operate on cases of pseudoarthroses in which pain is slight or absent unless unacceptable progression of deformity or disease persists.

There is no one favored technique for repair of pseudoarthrosis, as posterior, posterolateral, as well as anterior interbody fusion all can achieve the desired arthrodesis. Rather, operative judgment and technical excellence are of the utmost importance.

REFERENCES

1. Bick EM: An essay on the history of spine fusion operations. Clin Orthop 35:9, 1964
2. Bick EM: Source Book of Orthopedic Surgery, ed 2. Baltimore, Williams & Wilkins, 1948
3. Goodwin GM: Russell A. Hibbs. New York, Columbia University Press, 1935
4. Albee FH: Transplantation of portions of the tibia into the spine for Pott's disease. JAMA 57:885, 1911
5. MacKenzie-Forbes A: Technique of an operation for spinal fusion as practiced in Montreal. J Orthop Surg 2:509, 1920
6. Kleinberg S: Operative treatment for scoliosis. Arch Surg 5:631, 1922
7. Ghormley RK: Low back pain. With special reference to the articular facets with presentation of an operative procedure. JAMA 101:1773, 1933
8. Mercer W: Spondylolisthesis. Edinb Med J 43:545, 1936
9. Jenkins JA: Spondylolisthesis. Br Med J 24:80, 1936
10. Toumey JW: Internal fixation in fusion of the lumbosacral joints. Lahey Clin Bull 3:188, 1943
11. King D: Internal fixation for lumbosacral fusion. Am J Surg 66:357, 1944
12. Jaslow IA: Intercorporal bone graft in spinal fusion after disc removal. Surg Gynecol Obstet 82:215, 1946
13. Cloward RB: Changes in vertebra caused by ruptured intervertebral discs. Observations on their formation and treatment. Am J Surg 84:151, 1952
14. Robinson RA, Smith GW: Anterolateral cervical disc removal and interbody fusion for cervical disc syndrome. Bull Johns Hopkins Hosp 96:223, 1955
15. Cloward RB: The anterior approach for removal of ruptured cervical discs. J Neurosurg 15:602, 1958
16. Cleveland M, Bosworth DM, Thompson RR: Pseudarthrosis in the lumbosacral spine. J Bone Joint Surg 30A:302, 1948
17. Alexander GL: Neurological complications of spinal tuberculosis. Proc Roy Soc Med 39:730, 1946
18. Capener N: The evolution of lateral rhachotomy. J Bone Joint Surg 36:173, 1954
19. Harrington PR: Treatment of scoliosis. J Bone Joint Surg 44:591, 1962
20. Edmonson AS, Crenshaw AH: Campbell's Operative Orthopedics, vol 2. St. Louis, CV Mosby, 1980

CHAPTER 128
Surgical Management of Thoracolumbar Fractures: Indications, Methods, Results

Carrie L. Walters Henry H. Schmidek

THE IMMEDIATE SURGICAL GOALS in the treatment of thoracolumbar fractures are decompression of compromised neural structures and stabilization of the vertebral column. The long-term goals are to prevent delayed onset of spinal deformity, pain, and further neurologic deficit. Early operative intervention also shortens hospitalization time and allows immediate ambulation, thus lessening pulmonary, vascular, urologic, and psychological complications.

The surgical intervention in fractures of the thoracic and lumbar spine has evolved in recent years coincident with the development of spinal instrumentation and better diagnostic techniques. Spinal internal fixation devices that were originally developed to correct scoliotic deformities have subsequently been adopted and modified for fracture stabilization. The second factor facilitating surgical intervention has been improved case selection based on a clear delineation of the characteristics of the bony injury made possible by computed tomography. Our experience indicates that surgical intervention can reduce acute pain, improve spinal stability, shorten hospitalization time, and decrease complications related to spinal injuries. In addition, there is evidence that patients not adequately decompressed during the acute phase of their illness have an increased risk of developing neurologic deficits and pain syndromes months to years after the injury.[1–5]

PREOPERATIVE ASSESSMENT AND TREATMENT

The current classification of thoracolumbar fractures is a combination of Holdsworth's original classification based on mechanisms of injury and the additional information obtained by CT scanning.[6–9]

1. Axial loading injury. Comminuted fracture of the vertebral body with bone retropulsed into the spinal canal, intact posterior ligamentous complex.
2. Flexion injury. Disruption of the posterior ligaments without associated bony injury.
3. Flexion-axial loading injury.
   Type A. Anterior wedge fracture of the vertebral body less than 50 percent of its height, usually with intact posterior spinous elements and ligamentous structures.
   Type B. Anterior wedge fracture of the vertebral body exceeding 50 percent of its height, usually with posterior ligamentous disruption with or without posterior bony element fractures.
   Type C. Burst fracture-dislocation with vertebral body fragments retropulsed into the spinal canal, disruption of the posterior ligamentous complex and frequently with fracture of the posterior bony elements (Figure 128-1).
4. Flexion-rotation injury. Rotational fracture-dislocation with the cephalad vertebral body rotated upon the caudal vertebral body, carrying with it a "slice fragment" of the upper portion of the lower vertebra. The rotational force results in a unilateral facet fracture of the caudal vertebra, while the flexion force often results in a concomitant wedge or burst fracture.
5. Hyperextension injury. Anterior ligamentous disruption with posterior displacement of the cephalad vertebral body in relation to the caudal one.
6. Flexion-distraction injury (seat belt injury, Chance fracture). A transverse disruption of the vertebral body and neural arch through the pedicles with intact posterior ligamentous structures.

To determine whether the spine is unstable requires that two of the following conditions exist: (1) loss of integrity of the vertebral body; (2) loss of integrity of the posterior ligamentous or bony structures; (3) loss of spinal alignment manifested by its angulation or rotation.[12,13] The following fractures are considered to be unstable or potentially unstable: burst fractures, wedge compression fractures if there is a loss of greater than 50 percent of vertebral body height or evidence of posterior ligamentous complex rupture on physical examination or on the x-ray studies, flexion-rotational injuries, hyperextension injuries, and flexion-distraction injuries. Since x-ray films may not reflect the maximal displacement present at the time of injury, a neurologic deficit is considered as evidence of instability until this aspect can be fully clarified.

The treatment of thoracolumbar fractures depends on the assessment of the extent of both the bony and ligamentous injury. The latter is important since ligamentous injury may not heal even with prolonged immobilization. Based on the above classification and our concepts regarding the mechanism or extent of injury, a flexion injury is treated by reduction,

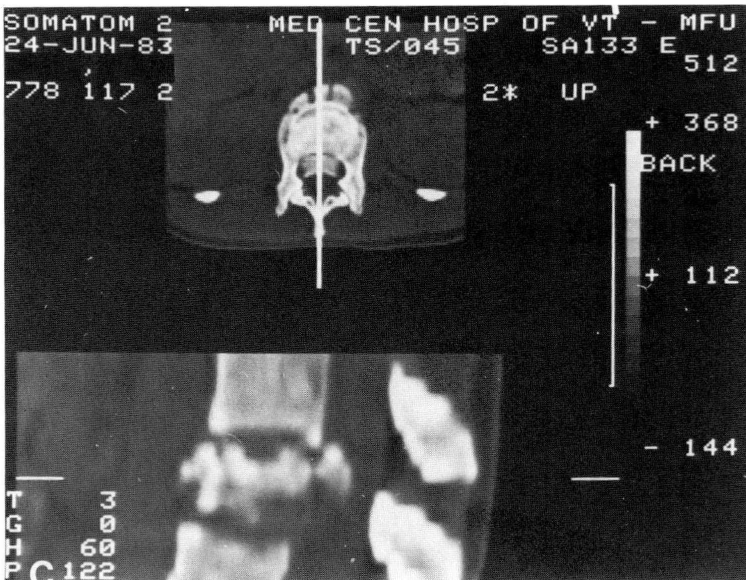

Fig. 128-1. (A) A burst fracture-dislocation in lateral and sagittal views. (B) Lateral x-ray film of a burst fracture-dislocation. The retropulsed body fragment is hidden behind the pedicle. (C) A CT scan of a burst fracture-dislocation with sagittal reconstruction demonstrating the retropulsed fragment at the level of the pedicle.

Harrington compression rods, and a three-segment bone graft. A burst fracture is usually treated by anterolateral decompression of the spinal canal, Harrington distraction rods, and bone grafting. Wedge compression fractures of less than 50 percent do not require operation, whereas fractures of over 50 percent are treated with Harrington distraction rods and bone fusion. Flexion-rotation fractures are treated by reduction, internal fixation, and bone fusion. Since these fractures are frequently very unstable they can often be totally or partially realigned preoperatively by postural reduction. Hyperextension injuries are treated by reduction, Harrington instrumentation and bone grafts. Although flexion-distraction fractures may heal without operative intervention, internal fixation and bone grafting are employed to facilitate early mobilization and rehabilitation.

The merits of spinal realignment; internal fixation and fusion in thoracolumbar dislocations; and of decompression, internal fixation, and fusion in burst fractures with partial neurologic deficits is reasonably well established. However, the optimal treatment of a burst fracture with significant bony encroachment within the spinal canal in the paraplegic patient and the neurologically intact patient remains problematic. In our series of 67 surgically treated patients with thoracolumbar fractures, four patients with burst fractures were paraplegic.[10] One of these cases was treated by open reduction, Harrington rod fixation, and bone grafts; three underwent anterolateral decompressive procedures in addition to the insertion of Harrington rods and bone grafts. The patient who did not undergo a surgical decompression subsequently developed severe bilateral burning pain in the legs. One of the three patients who underwent decompression has back pain radiating around the abdomen; the other two are free of pain. Two patients in the decompression group improved to a grade C postoperatively. The management of the 8 patients with burst fractures who were neurologically intact included Harrington rod stabilization and autogenous bone grafting in 4 patients. One of these patients now has severe back pain and 3 patients are asymptomatic. Of the 4 patients treated by decompression of neural

structures plus insertion of Harrington rods and bone grafts, none subsequently developed a chronic pain syndrome.

Continuous monitoring of somatosensory evoked responses during surgical decompression of thoracolumbar fractures is, in our experience, of questionable value in alerting the surgeon to intraoperative compromise of neural function. Since SSERs are thought to be transmitted primarily in the dorsal columns,[9] it has been the general impression that particularly in the area of the conus it would be unlikely that significant motor damage could occur without detectable change in the SSERs. Our experience, however, has not borne this out. To date 2 patients in our series, both with L1 burst fractures, subjected to decompression and stabilization have exhibited a transient increase in motor deficit postoperatively without an alteration of their intraoperative SSERs. Both of these patients had normal proprioceptive function preoperatively and postoperatively. Presently we restrict the use of intraoperative SSERs to cases requiring spinal alignment alone.

In patients who are neurologically stable and do not have injuries to other systems, surgery is not performed as an emergency but as an elective procedure several days after injury. In patients with thoracolumbar dislocations, realignment is technically easier to accomplish if carried out within the first week after injury. Our experience has been that most patients improve over the first several days, especially in their sensory function; in these patients in particular surgery is delayed until the degree of improvement reaches a plateau. Patients with major life-threatening trauma to other organ systems are operated upon when their overall condition permits. In our series, this consideration has been the primary cause of delay in surgical intervention. Patients who are neurologically deteriorating are emergencies and surgery is performed after adequate neuroradiologic investigation to determine the cause of their deterioration. Epidural hematomas, further dislocation of the spinal vertebrae, further migration of the bone fragment into the canal, infarction of neural tissue secondary to hypotension, and increasing spinal cord or root edema have all been implicated in the worsening of the patient's neurologic condition after thoracolumbar fracture.

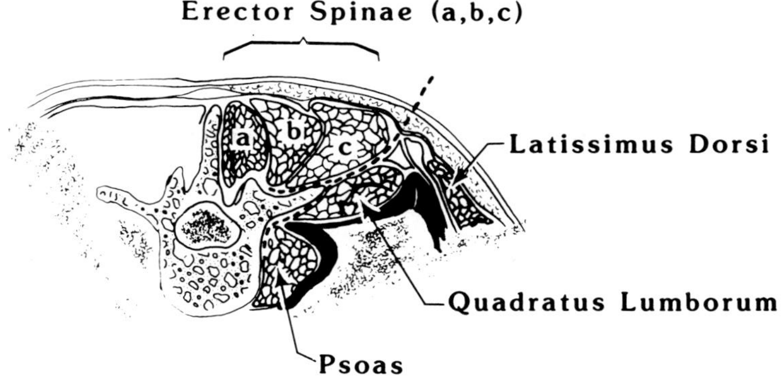

Fig. 128-2.   Cross-sectional view of a lumbar vertebra and its surrounding musculature showing the plane of dissection between the erector spinae and quadratus lumborum muscles.

Patients with thoracolumbar fractures undergo anteroposterior and lateral spine x-ray films to identify the level(s) of injury and computed tomography with sagittal reconstruction of the injured area. Metrizamide-enhanced CT scanning is used to identify the level of the conus in T12-L2 fractures and the relationship of the neural elements to the bony fragments.

Patients are initially immobilized on the rotokinetic bed (Roto-Rest Mark 1, Kinetic Concepts, San Antonio, Texas). This bed gradually rotates from side to side so that the patient need not be turned prone—a feature that is particularly useful when caring for patients with injuries requiring chest tubes, external fixators, and close observation of the abdomen. Patients with neural injury received 4 mg dexamethasone every 6 hours for the first 3 days following injury. Physical therapy is started within the first 3 days of hospitalization.

SURGICAL MANAGEMENT OF THORACOLUMBAR FRACTURES

The basic approach in the management of thoracolumbar fractures with bone in the canal (types 1 and 3c) is to obtain neural decompression before internal fixation and distraction. This is designed to prevent further injury to neural elements by protruded bone fragments or spicules. This tactic is also adopted since spinal instrumentation alone does not routinely or predictably re-establish the normal dimensions of the spinal canal.

The operative approach chosen for decompression is determined by the exact location of the compressing bone fragments. Decompression of anteriorly situated spinal encroachment is accomplished by using either a transthoracic-transpleural approach (applicable only in thoracic fractures), or an anterolateral extracavitary approach. This operation is performed with the patient in a three-quarters lateral position with the side of maximal bone encroachment uppermost. The surgical level to be decompressed is first identified radiographically. One may then use either a vertical incision centered in the midline over approximately five segments or a longitudinal muscle-splitting incision along the lateral margin of the erector spinae muscles 6 to 8 cm from the midline to begin the exploration. The dissection in the latter case is carried to the lumbar dorsal fascia, the anterior leaf of which separates the erector spinae and quadratus lumborum muscles (Figure 128-2). Using this fascial plane the dissection is carried anteromedially. The transverse process of the involved vertebra is identified and removed. When the fracture occurs in the thoracic

spine, 6 to 8 cm of the rib is resected, leaving the neurovascular bundle intact. The pedicle of the damaged vertebra is then removed using a high-speed air drill. Magnification with either surgical loupes or the operating microscope is required for the remainder of the decompression. The nerve root exiting the neural foramen at the level of the fracture is frequently trapped between the pedicle and the retropulsed bony fragment. Care must be taken not to damage it further. In the majority of burst fractures, the retropulsed fragment, located between the pedicles, does not extend below the caudal margin of the pedical (Figure 128-1A and C). Thus, bone removal usually does not need to extend caudally beyond the pedicular level, minimizing the amount of intact bone removed (Figure 128-3). The spinal dura is identified at the junction of the nerve root sleeve and the dural sac. Decompression is begun by removing bone just anterior to the retropulsed bone fragment, thus undermining the retropulsed fragment across the width of the spinal canal. This allows the residual rim of bone compressing the anterior dura to be depressed, using back-angled curettes, into this cavity. The objective is to restore the normal cross-sectional diameter of the spinal canal (Figure 128-4). The intervertebral disc above the fractured vertebra is usually so significantly damaged that it is routinely excised, even though free disc fragments are usually not present. The inferior disc is usually not significantly disrupted and therefore is not surgically disturbed. Dural tears secondary to the original injury are frequently present. These are treated by lining the site with Gelfoam. No attempt is made to formally repair the dural tear.

Following neural decompression spinal stabilization is accomplished by a combination of internal fixation and bone grafts. Since these grafts provide essentially no initial stability, the construct is initially reinforced with spinal instrumentation until the grafts have matured enough to provide structural strength. Harrington rod instrumentation is usually the internal fixation device of choice.

Through a separate midline longitudinal incision, electrocautery is used to develop the dissection down to the surface of the supraspinous ligament. A bilateral subperiosteal dissection is performed exposing the spinous processes and lamina of the fractured vertebrae and the three vertebrae immediately above and below the injured level. The erector spinae muscles are retracted until the lateral tips of the transverse processes of the fractured vertebrae and the one above and below are exposed. Using the technique of Jacobs,[11] dissection is now been carried up and down sufficiently far to allow placement of the superior hooks under the inferior articular processes of the third vertebra above the fractured level and placement of the lower hooks

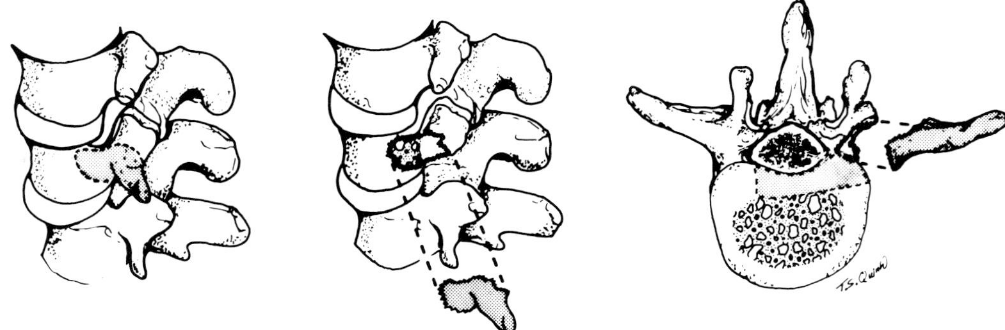

Fig. 128-3.   Lateral and cross-sectional views of lumbar vertebrae demonstrating the degree of bone removal necessary to decompress an axial compression or burst fracture-dislocation injury.

on the superior edge of the lamina of the third vertebra below the fractured level. The facet joint capsules of the superior and inferior articular processes of the fractured vertebra are excised as well as the articular cartilage on both sides of these four facet joints. The exposed bone is decorticated at three levels (the fractured vertebra, one above and one below) out to the tips of the transverse processes. After placement of the hooks, the rods are selected such that the ratchet-rod junction is as close to the upper hook as possible, thereby minimizing the stress at this critical location on the rod.[18] The rods may either be contoured as needed, in which case square-ended Moe rods are used to prevent axial rotation of the rod, or Edwards' sleeves may be used. Bone grafts are harvested from the iliac crest through a separate incision and placed posterior to the transverse process, facet joints, and laminae at the level of the fracture plus one vertebra above and below.

Postoperatively patients are immediately placed into regular hospital beds and fitted with a custom-molded bivalved spinal orthosis within 3 to 7 days. Mobilization either independently or with a wheelchair is begun as soon as the orthosis is fitted. The Harrington rods are removed electively at approximately 6 months and the orthosis is continued for a total of 8 to 9 months postoperatively, after which spinal mobility exercises are started.

COMPLICATIONS

In our 67 most recently treated patients with thoracolumbar fractures, no life-threatening complications attributable to the surgical procedure occurred. One patient died of a massive head injury. Reoperation was required for dislodged or broken Harrington rods in 6 patients and inadequate surgical decompression in 1 case. Because problems with the Harrington rods usually occurred 6 months or more after their insertion, these rods are now removed electively before this time. Thrombophlebitis occurring in the lower extremities has been reduced by earlier mobilization, physical therapy from the time of admission, and the use of the rotokinetic bed. Low-dose heparin has not been used. Three patients developed transient brachial plexus palsies due to improper intraoperative positioning of the dependent arm. Psychological problems, especially depression, have been reduced by early mobilization and transfer to the rehabilitation unit. Psychological evaluation is done shortly after admission and the patient and family are then supported by either a psychiatrist or psychologist throughout and subsequent to hospitalization. Long-term counseling is provided if necessary.

Urinary tract infections remain a problem. Almost every patient unable to void on his or her own had a urinary tract infection at some time during the acute or rehabilitative hospitalization. Intermittent self-catheterization is used. The patients are not routinely placed on prophylactic antibiotics. With earlier ambulation acute hospitalization has been reduced from 57 to 34 days and total hospitalization (acute plus rehabilitation hospital) from 80 to 52 days.

DISCUSSION

The treatment of thoracolumbar fractures has continued to evolve as the characteristics of the various fracture types occurring in this region have come to be appreciated. We can now tailor the surgical approaches to each of these different injuries. The CT scan provides a better delineation of the full extent of vertebral body damage and of canal encroachment than previously available techniques. In addition, certain fractures of the lamina, pedicles, and facets that were often missed on standard x-ray films can now be visualized and their potential impact on the spine's stability assessed. Sagittal reconstruction of the CT scan is helpful in demonstrating the cephalocaudal extent of the bony injury. Metrizamide-enhanced CT scanning is used to demonstrate the relationship of the bone elements of the spine to the dura, the location of the conus, and for evidence of soft tissue encroachment upon neural structures. The latter is particularly important if the bony derangement does not provide an adequate explanation for the neural deficit. Conventional anteroposterior and lateral spinal x-ray films remain useful both for surveying the spine for other injuries, for determining the degree of angulation and rotation at the fracture site, as well as in the postoperative assessment of the instrumentation, bony alignment, and progress of the bony fusion. With the improved delineation of these injuries based on CT scan data, we now appreciate that studies antedating CT did not accurately assess the frequency of the different types of injury. Burst fractures were particularly underdiagnosed. In a 1969 series only 6 of 394 patients were classified as having burst fractures[14]; in 1977 Flesch reported 2 of 40 patients with this type of fracture[2]; whereas 36 of the 67 cases in our recently reported series were represented by burst fractures.[10] This increase most probably is the result of increased recognition of these fractures since the mechanisms and spinal level of injury are essentially the same in all three series. This is important when considering the optimal operative approach. Another observation related to improved fracture delineation and more accurate assignment of the injury to a classification system is that there now

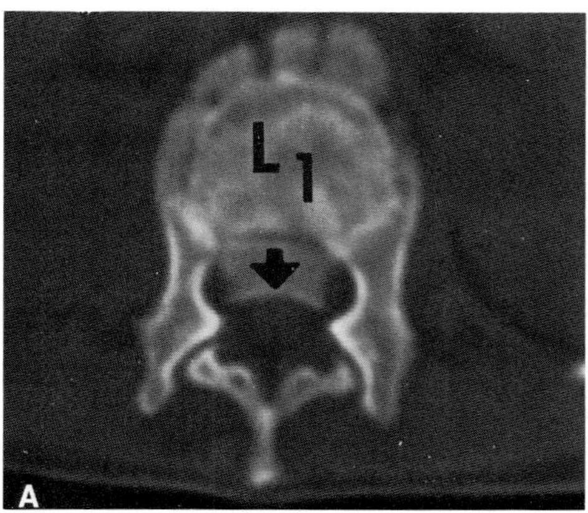

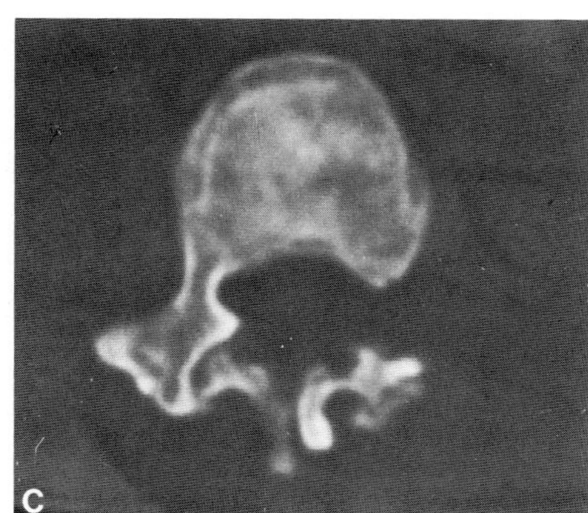

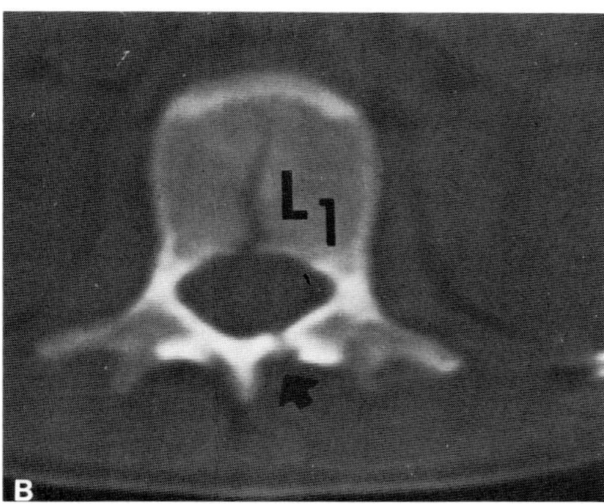

Fig. 128-4.   (A) CT scan of a L1 burst fracture demonstrating the stellate nature of the body fracture and the retropulsed fragment of bone at the pedicular level. (B) CT scan of the same vertebra as shown in Figure 128-3A, but at the caudal level of the pedicle showing only a vertical fracture in the body, no bony fragment in the canal, and a fractured lamina (arrow). (C) Postoperative CT scan of the L1 burst fracture shown in Figure 128-3A demonstrating the decompressed canal and the degree of bone removal necessary (pedicle and transverse process) to achieve it.

appears to be a correlation between fracture type and the patient's initial neural state. This finding is in contradistinction to Frankel's series in which it was not possible for such a correlation to be made.[14] In our experience of 67 cases of thoracolumbar fractures none of the 8 patients with a flexion-rotation injury was initially ambulatory, while over half of the 54 patients with axial loading and flexion-axial loading injuries were ambulatory. There were too few patients in the other categories to allow comment. In this same group of patients, neural recovery occurred in 21 of 67 patients, another 21 patients were initially neurologically normal and could not improve. This is comparable with the results obtained by others in both operative and nonoperative series, suggesting that recovery is determined by the extent of neural damage at the time of injury.[4,14,15,16] Although operative intervention does not increase neurologic recovery, the evidence suggests that realignment and internal fixation decreases spinal deformity and subsequent pain, while decompression of the spinal cord and nerve roots prevents later deterioration in neurologic function.[1–4] Bolhman reported 10 patients, 8 of whom developed increasing pain and 6 of whom developed progressive new paralysis 9 months to 10 years after incompletely treated thoracolumbar fracture.[1] These 10 patients required surgical decompression either by a transthoracic approach (1 patient) or a transpedicular approach with fusion (9 patients). Seven of the 8 were relieved of pain, 4 of the 6 recovered neurologic function, and 2 remained unchanged. McAfee[5] reported gradual neurologic deterioration in 2 nonoperatively treated patients with burst fractures that produced a

reduction in vertebral height of over 50 percent. The patients, originally intact neurologically, developed progressive collapse of the vertebral body, kyphosis, and evidence of neural compression (paresthesias, radicular symptoms, and focal deficits). One patient improved following spinal decompresssion. Nash[17] reported 2 cases of burst fracture in which the patients also developed a progressive kyphosis during conservative treatment. One patient developed a Brown-Sequard syndrome; whereas the second patient's kyphotic deformity increased from 19 to 30 degrees during treatment in an extension body jacket. Ten to 15 years following thoracolumbar fractures, premature degenerative spinal stenosis may occur in the absence of either progressive kyphosis or further protrusion of bony fragments into the spinal canal, especially if the lateral recesses are compromised by fracture fragments.[5] To date we have encountered 4 patients with increasing symptoms 9 months to 8 years after injury as a result of either inadequate primary surgical decompression, increasing kyphosis or spinal adhesive arachnoiditis.

REFERENCES

1.   Bohlman HH: Late progressive paralysis and pain following fractures of the thoracolumbar spine. J Bone Joint Surg 58A:728, 1976
2.   Flesch JR, Leider LL, Erickson DL, et al: Harrington instrumentation and spine fusion for unstable fractures and fracture-dislocations of the thoracic and lumbar spine. J Bone Joint Surg 59A:143, 1977

3. Jacobs RR, Ashen MA, Snider RK: Dorsolumbar spine fractures: Recumbent vs. operative treatment. Paraplegia 18:358, 1980

4. Lewis J, McKibbin B: The treatment of unstable fracture-dislocations of the thoracolumbar spine accompanied by paraplegia. J Bone Joint Surg 56B:603, 1974

5. McAfee PC, Yuan HA, Lasda NA: The unstable burst fracture. Spine 7:365, 1982

6. Holdsworth FW: Fractures, dislocations, and fracture- dislocations of the spine. J Bone Joint Surg 45B:6, 1963

7. Bohlman HH, Ducker TB, Lucas JT: Spine and spinal cord injuries, in Rothman R, Simeone F (eds): The Spine. Philadelphia, WB Saunders, 1982, pp 661–757

8. McAfee PC, Yuan HA, Frederickson B, et al: The value of computed tomography in thoracolumbar fractures. J Bone Joint Surg 65A:461, 1983

9. Dennis F: The three column spine and its significance in the classification of acute thoracolumbar spinal injuries. Spine 8:817, 1983

10. Whitesides TE, Shah SGA: On the management of unstable fractures of the thoracolumbar spine. Spine 1:99, 1976

11. Dickson JH, Harrington PR, Erwin WD: Results of reduction and stabilization of the severely fractured thoracic and lumbar spine. J Bone Joint Surg 60A:799, 1978

12. Walters CL, Schmidek HH, Krag M, Brier, L: The Management of Thoracolumbar Fractures, in Dunsker SB, Schmidek HH, Frymoyer J, Kahn A (eds): The Unstable Spine. New York, Grune & Stratton, 1986

13. Jacobs RR, Nordwall A, Nachemson A: Reduction, stability and strength provided by internal fixation systems for thoracolumbar spinal injuries. Clin Orthop 171:300, 1982

14. Edwards CC, Griffith P, Levine AM, DeSilva JB: Early clinical results using the spinal rod sleeve method for treating thoracic and lumbar injuries. Orthop Trans 6:345, 1982

15. Frankel HL, Hancock DO, Hyslop G, et al: The value of postural reduction in the initial management of closed injuries of the spine with paraplegia and tetraplegia. Paraplegia 7:179, 1969

16. Holdsworth FW, Hardy A: Early treatment of paraplegia from fractures of the thoracolumbar spine. J Bone Joint Surg 35B:540, 1953

17. Jacobs RR, Asher MA, Snider RK: Dorsolumbar spine fractures: Recumbent vs. operative treatment. Paraplegia 18:358, 1980

18. Nash CL, Schatizinger LH, Brown RH, Brodkey J: The unstable stable thoracic compression fracture. Spine 2:261, 1977

CHAPTER 129

Surgical Management of Spinal Cord Tumors and Arteriovenous Malformations

Kalmon D. Post   Bennett M. Stein

INTRAMEDULLARY SPINAL CORD TUMORS

ALTHOUGH VON EISELSBERG totally excised a neurofibrosarcoma from the spinal cord in 1907 and Cushing operated on an 8-year-old child and completely removed an intramedullary ependymoma extending from C1 to T2 in 1924,[1] the first well-documented surgical effort to remove an intramedullary tumor was reported by Elsberg[2] in 1925. Of the 13 tumors he reported on, 3 were totally removed and the remainder were partially removed. He stressed that because some of these tumors were infiltrating, they defied removal; nevertheless, he emphasized that the surgeon must search out those tumors with well-defined cleavage planes that permit total removal of the neoplasm. Considering his lack of magnification techniques and previous surgical experience with such tumors, these results were remarkable. When a definitive plane between the tumor and the spinal cord was not visible, Elsberg proposed a second operation when the tumor might present through the myelotomy, making total removal possible. Later, Matson[3] also advocated this technique. With the exception of these reports, little experience with two-stage removal has been published. Following Elsberg's early reports, others[1,3–9] have described successful removals of intramedullary tumors. Successful surgical removal of these tumors was mounted on a firm foundation when Greenwood presented his experience with 10 intramedullary tumors, primarily ependymomas, which he totally removed with no mortalities.[5] These results, with useful survival, justified his enthusiasm for an aggressive surgical approach to these lesions. He also emphasized the use of magnification techniques and microsurgical instrumentation.

Guidetti[6] published his experience with a large group of intramedullary tumors and noted the difficulty in totally removing astrocytomas. In the presence of intramedullary ependymomas and other tumors, however, he felt that every effort should be made to achieve total removal, although only a line of cleavage between the normal spinal cord and the tumor would make this possible. Once a cleavage was established, gentle dissection separated the tumor from the normal spinal cord on each side; then the tumor could be lifted carefully by one end or the other and slowly removed from its bed. Blood vessels were severed close to the tumor by bipolar cautery with irrigation. Guidetti achieved an overall total removal of 24 of 71 tumors, representing a wide variety of histologic types, with a 10 percent operative mortality.

In the famous case of Horrax and Henderson,[7] an intramedullary ependymoma extending the entire length of the spinal cord was totally enucleated during a series of operations, resulting in recovery and long-term survival.

Our series comprises 40 cases of intramedullary tumor.[4,10] A range of histology is represented, with astrocytoma and ependymoma the most common tumors and teratomatous types less frequent. No lipomas are included in this group.

Some patients had undergone previous treatment, including decompressive laminectomy, tapping of cysts associated with the tumors, and radiotherapy. The effects of treatment other than total removal are difficult to evaluate. It is clear, however, that the degree of neurologic deficit caused by the disease process before surgery often determined the postoperative result.

CLINICAL PRESENTATION

Although intramedullary tumors occur most commonly in adults,[2,4–6,10] a significant incidence has been reported in children.[3,11,12] The symptomatology in both age groups is similar. It is quite amazing at times to see an extensive tumor filling the majority of the intramedullary space yet causing few symptoms. Often, however, an end point is reached when compensatory ability fails, and marked neurologic deterioration occurs rapidly. Persistent pain involving the dorsal root dermatomes in the area of tumor involvement is often the signature of an intramedullary neoplasm. Dysfunction of the posterior column may occur in a progressive fashion, with sensory dysesthesias in the arms, torso, and legs, depending upon the site of the intraspinal neoplasm. Sacral sparing may or may not be present and is not an invariable finding with intramedullary neoplasms. Lower motor neuron symptomatology and signs usually occur at the level of the tumor. Well-defined central cord syndromes, as seen in syringomyelia, with disassociated sensory loss and the classic signs of anterior horn cell involvement may be lacking. Children often have a scoliosis. The symptomatology generally is progressive with few remissions or exacerbations. Symptoms are usually bilateral, but in rare instances neurologic abnormalities are confined to one extremity. The duration of symptoms generally is measured in years, although some neoplasms may have histories of 6 months or less.

OPERATIVE NEUROSURGICAL TECHNIQUES
ISBN 0-8089-1862-1

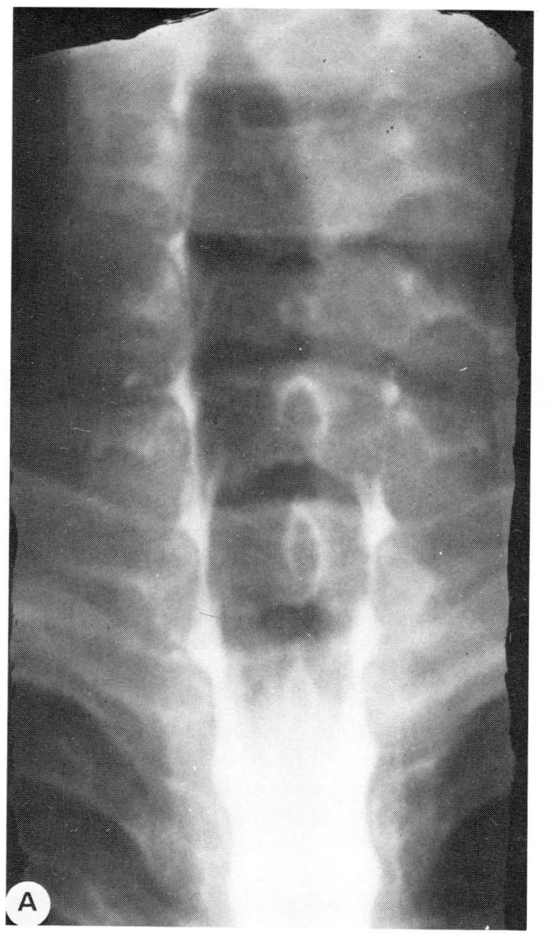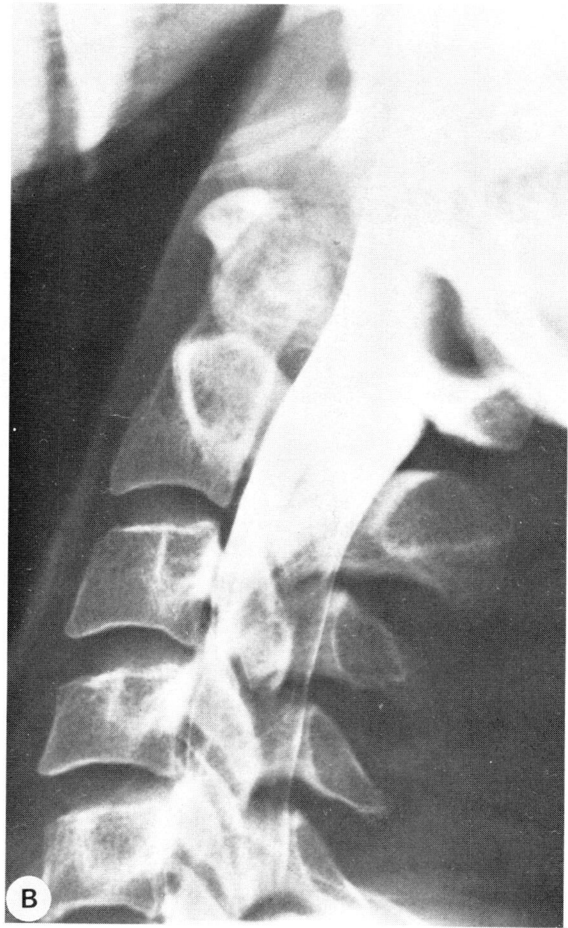

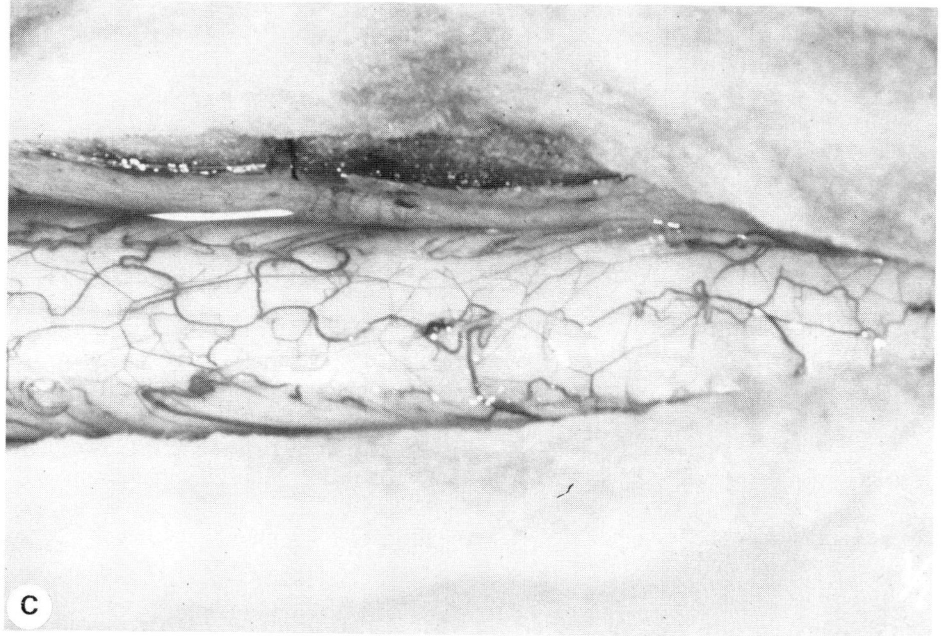

DIAGNOSTIC EVALUATION

The radiologic demonstration of intramedullary tumors was dependent upon myelography with either iohexal, a nonionic water-soluble agent or Pantopaque—iophendylate.[13] A fusiform dilatation of the cord in the region of the tumor usually was seen, while a complete block was not generally present (Figure 129-1). If a block was present, dye was also instilled from the opposite end of the spinal canal to define the complete extent of the tumor. Since the introduction of water-soluble contrast agents, radiologic definition has been significantly improved. Dilated venous channels at the caudal aspect

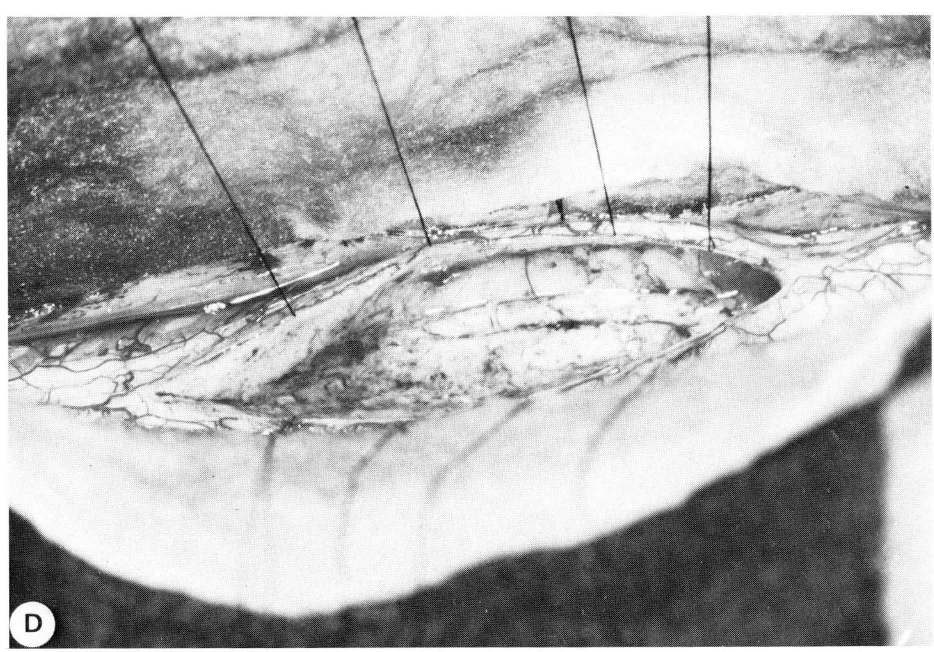

Fig. 129-1. (A) An AP cervical myelogram showing widened spinal cord. (B) Lateral cervical myelogram showing widened spinal cord. (C) Operative view of exposed spinal cord at C2-T2. Note the widened full appearance. (D) Operative view of spinal cord after cystic ependymoma was removed.

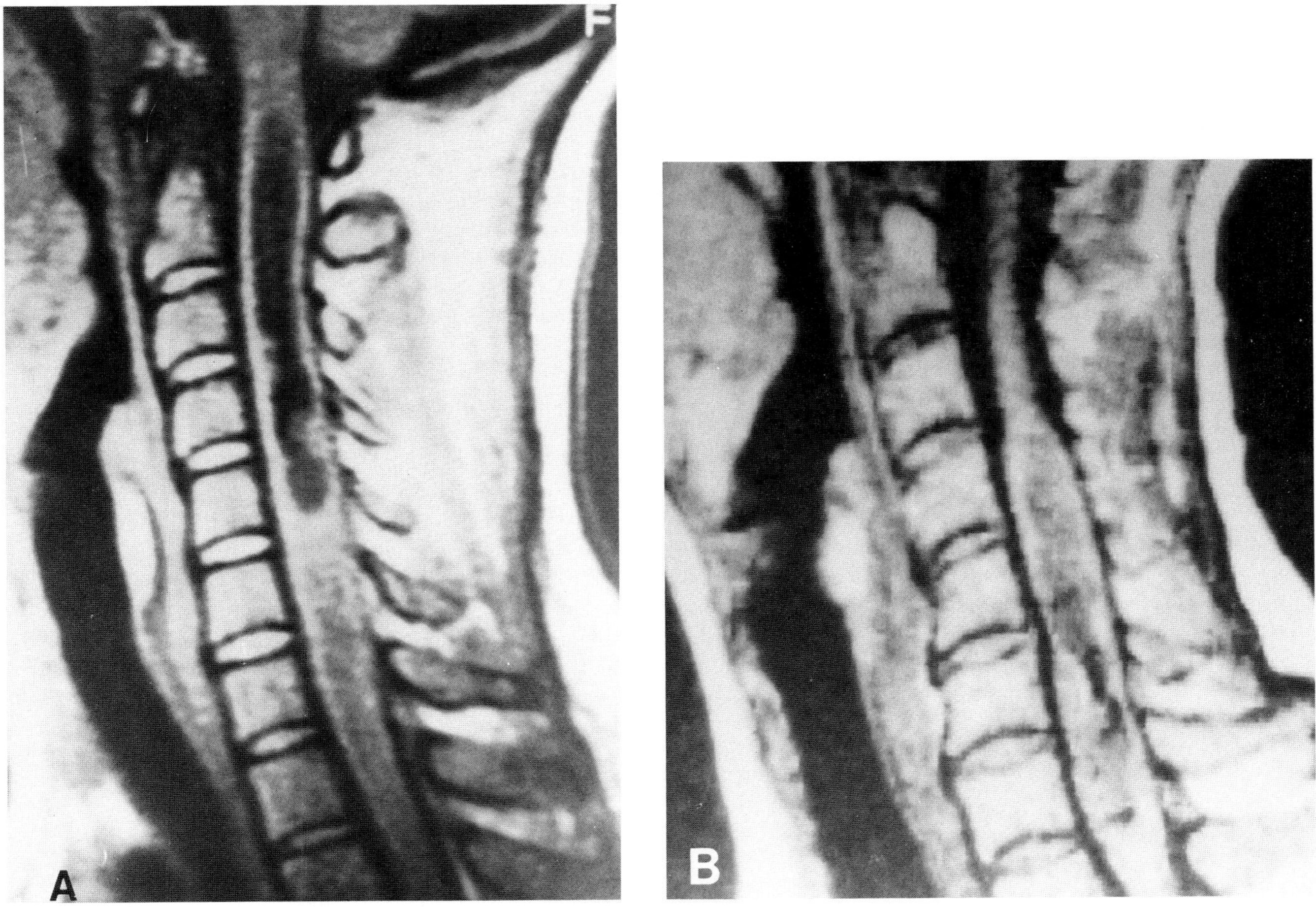

Fig. 129-2. (A) Sagittal MRI scan demonstrating cyst within the cervical spinal cord and a mural hemangioblastoma at the C4-5 level. (B) Sagittal MRI scan demonstrating a wide cervical spinal cord with an intramedullary tumor.

of small intramedullary tumors may suggest the differential diagnosis of a vascular malformation. This differential is rarely a problem, and spinal angiography has not been of diagnostic value except for the identification of an intramedullary hemangioblastoma. The exception is the intramedullary AVM which can mimic a vascular intramedullary tumor.

Routine computed tomographic (CT) scanning of the spinal canal has not been of practical use in the diagnosis of these neoplasms. We have retrospectively scanned a number of patients with large tumors, failing to visualize the tumors. CT scanning with water-soluble contrast agents aids in the diagnosis of a wide spinal canal. It also assists in the definitive diagnosis of syringomyelia. CT scanning has shown metrizamide leaking into the fluid within a syrinx,[14,15] particularly with a 6-hour delayed scan. The use of MRI has facilitated the localization of tumors and the identification of cysts (Figure 129-2). It relies on a quiescent patient and will fail to define these lesions if there is movement. The thoracic region has been particularly difficult. A presurgical histologic diagnosis of the lesion cannot be made from MRI scans other than the fact that it may or may not be associated with a cyst. Manipulation of different pulse sequences and additional surface coils may add to the tumor characterization.

Angiography has been carried out in the presence of dilated vessels and has been helpful in the diagnosis of hemangioblastoma and AVMs.[9] A point should be made here about radiologic changes that appear to be unique to the hemangioblastoma. We have observed in four or five cases of hemangioblastoma extensive widening of the spinal cord in either direction from the primary lesion, which in these cases has been discrete and confined to one or two spinal segments. At operation, we have not been able to define the nature of this widening as seen on myelograms. It does not appear to be due to a cyst extending from the tumor or to multiple hemangioblastomas. We have been perplexed as to the nature of the widening and assume it is due to congestion and edema of adjacent spinal cord secondary to the high vascularity of these lesions. Follow-up myelography done in two of these cases show the spinal cord has returned to normal size following removal of the primary lesion.

Percutaneous cord puncture and myelocystography have been reported,[16] and were performed once in our series. Our patent had a percutaneous puncture to distinguish a cord tumor from a syrinx rather than for relief of symptoms.

SURGICAL PATHOLOGY

Intramedullary spinal cord tumors account for one third of primary intraspinal neoplasms.[2,6,8,10] Astrocytomas and ependymomas constitute the largest group of intramedullary tumors and occur with about equal frequency. They are generally low grade and extend over many segments of the spinal cord. Astrocytomas most commonly appear in the cervical and thoracic regions of the spinal cord, whereas the ependymomas have a higher incidence in the caudal regions because of their prevalence in the conus medullaris and filum terminale.[17]

Tumors that occur less frequently include dermoids, epidermoids, teratomas, oligodendrogliomas, hemangioblastomas, and either primary or metastatic malignant tumors. Lipomas, common in children, have different growth patterns and therapeutic implications and will not be discussed further.

Intramedullary ependymomas often have a distinct plane between the neoplasm and spinal cord tissue. These tumors generally are soft, solid, and have a pseudocapsule. They are not highly vascular and may have necrotic areas. Astrocytomas usually are infiltrative with an ill-defined margin between the neoplasm and the normal spinal cord tissue. Where a well-defined margin between the neoplasm and the normal spinal cord exists, a pseudocapsule is found. This variety is similar to the cerebellar astrocytoma, which has a uniformly soft consistency and minimal vascularity sometimes associated with cysts containing yellow fluid high in protein.

At times, astrocytomas may appear to have a plane between the tumor and the normal cord tissue, yet pathologically they demonstrate infiltration (Figure 129-3). The pathologic grade may also vary in different parts of the tumor, just as it does within brain tumors. Astrocytomas and ependymomas produce a fusiform enlargement of the spinal cord, often without any indication of their presence on the surface of the cord other than an occasional dilated vein at the caudal end of the tumor. In some cases the dorsal surface of the cord will be so thin that it will be transparent. Glioblastomas produce a discoloration of the cord and are associated with a plethora of enlarged arterialized veins and obvious feeding arteries. Ependymomas of the conus or filum terminale region often grow in an exophytic fashion from the intramedullary locus into the cauda equina, displacing and sometimes adhering to the nerve roots. Because of the expanding nature of these neoplasms, structural changes in the osseous spinal canal may be produced.

Teratomas and dermoid tumors have varying amounts of grumous material in their central portions, are frequently variegated, and have a capsule that is adherent to the surrounding spinal cord tissue; often there is a pedicle of fibrous tract involving the dura and overlying bone and soft tissues. Radiographic defects may be present in the overlying bone if a fibrous tract is present.

Intramedullary tumors receive their blood supply from perforating branches of the anterior spinal artery that enter the ventral aspect of the tumor. These vessels are small and are not associated with a high degree of vascularity within the tumor. Small vessels also enter the tumor from the dorsal and lateral positions of the spinal cord. The tumors tend to be eccentric and located in the more dorsal portion of the spinal cord. Invariably there is a thin layer of compressed spinal cord tissue overlying the dorsal surface of these tumors, and they rarely present directly on the surface of the cord.

In our series, 80 percent of the tumors were divided almost equally between astrocytoma and ependymoma.[10] Fortunately, only three of the astrocytomas were glioblastoma. There were five cases of hemangioblastomas, a relatively rare intramedullary tumor. Four of these hemangioblastomas involved the cervical thoracic region while one involved the thoracolumbar region. Teratomas generally occurred in the lumbosacral region. A cavernous malformation occupied the lumbar region and gave rise to a 21-year history. A rare intramedullary pigmented neurofibroma was successfully removed extending from the mid-cervical region to the obex of the medulla in an elderly patient.

SURGICAL TECHNIQUE

Turnbull[1] stated: "A surgeon exploring a spinal cord for a suspected intramedullary tumor must be prepared to face a formidable problem and also have the courage of conviction to make every attempt to remove the tumor. Anything less than this, with a cursory inspection of the spinal cord or aspiration

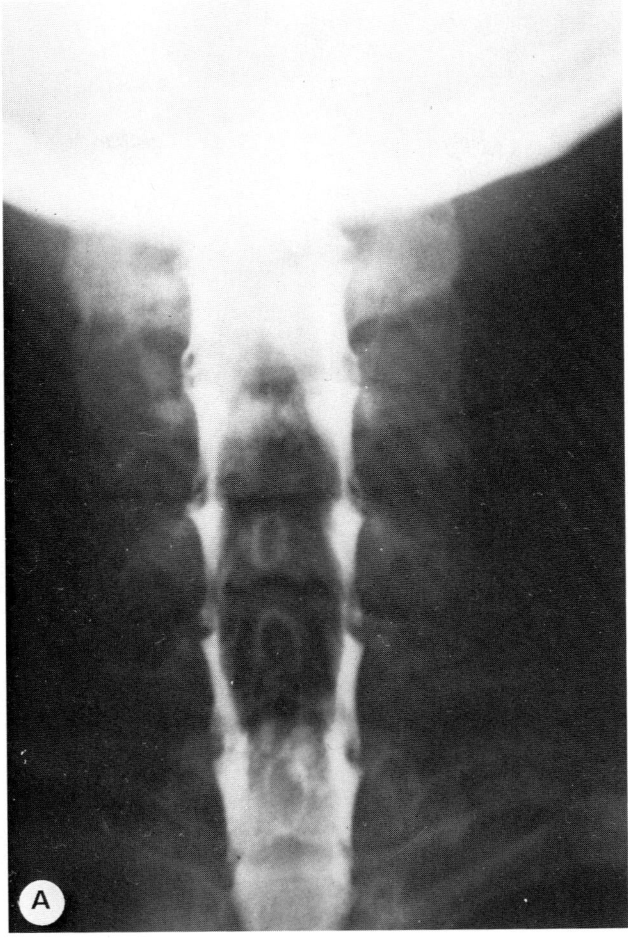

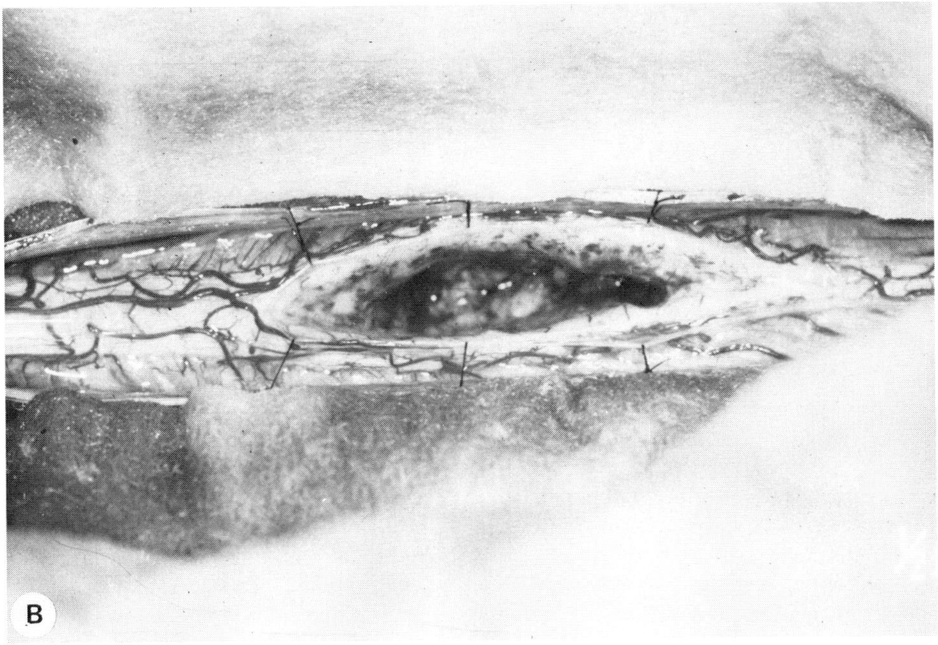

Fig. 129-3

thereof, can only create problems of a more complex nature for the subsequent surgical effort to remove such tumors.''

Surgery is the primary treatment for intramedullary tumors. Radiotherapy has little to offer even for malignant tumors.[10,12,17,18] In timing surgery, the sooner the better in terms of tumor growth. There is nothing to be gained by allowing the tumor growth to devastate the patient while withholding surgery. The surgical results are generally predicated on the preoperative condition of the patient, no matter how large the tumor. If the patient preoperatively has minimal neurologic findings, then the postoperative course should be gratifying, especially if the tumor can be resected in toto. Those patients

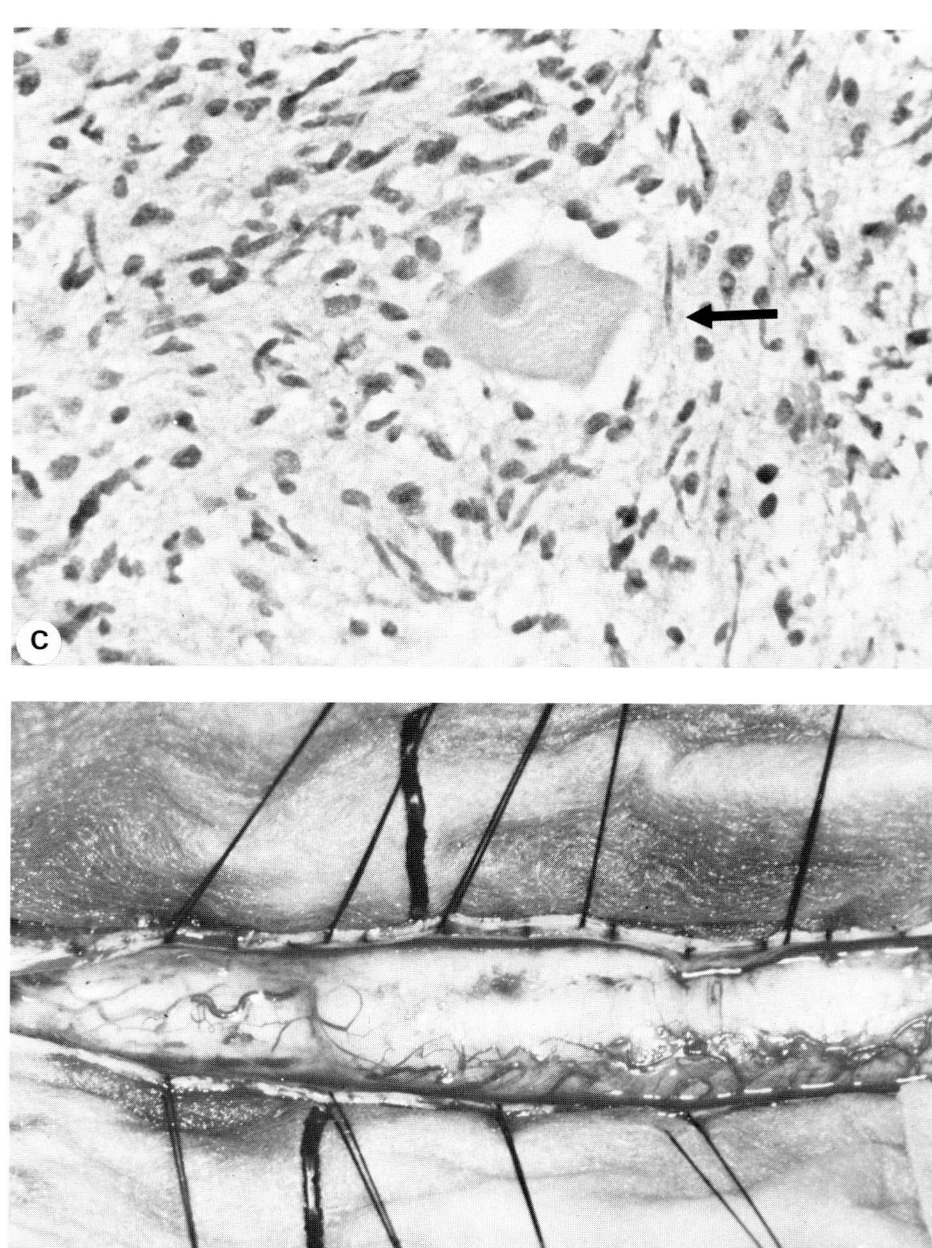

who arrive for surgery in a wheelchair or with severe paralysis, or sensory loss may regain little of this function even after a successful operation.

The prone position is generally used now for all intramedullary cord tumors, although early in our experience the sitting position was used for some cervical cord cases. The prone position is preferred now because it decreases the potential for vasomotor collapse, which can be significant when the autonomic pathways are compromised by the tumor or surgery; it also allows the assistant to take a more active role in the operation, providing traction, irrigation, or assistance with the dissection.

All operations are carried out with evoked potential monitoring of dorsal column function. This has been of some use in guiding the surgery, although we prefer to rely on observations through the operation microscope as to the extent of dissection. In the future, we hope to utilize with greater efficiency recordings from the cortical spinal tract. General anesthesia with endotracheal intubation is always used and the endotracheal tube is frequently left in place for 24 to 48 hours after surgery on more extensive cervical intramedullary tumors.

The full extent of the tumor must be known before the surgery. This usually is demonstrated on a myelogram, often taken from above as well as from below. In the case of a suspected hemangioblastoma, the vasculature should be demonstrated by arteriography to aid in the surgical removal. A wide laminectomy then is performed over the entire extent of the tumor, extending to a level above and below. The dura must

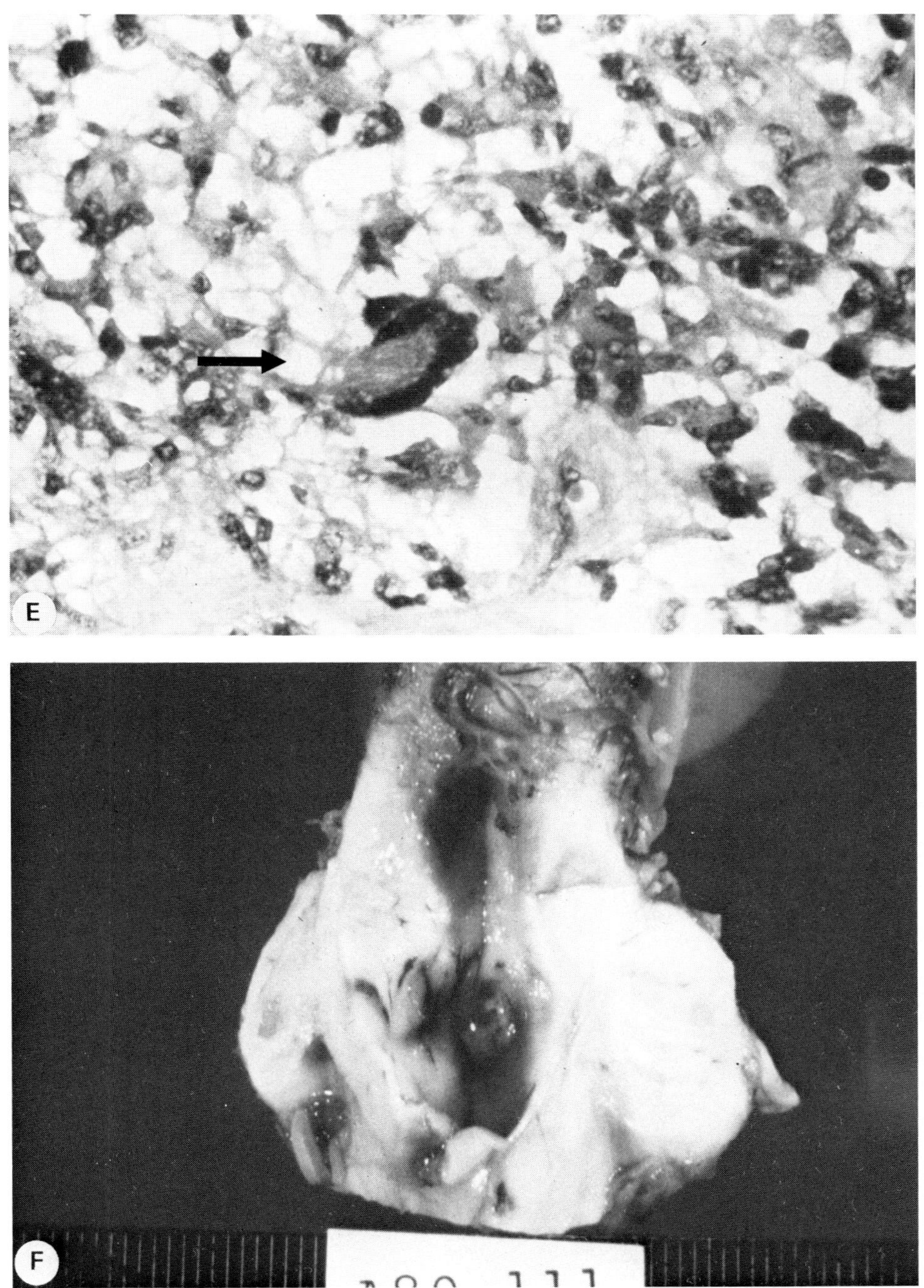

Fig. 129-3.   (A) AP view of cervical myelogram showing widened spinal cord. (B) Operative view of exposed spinal cord during first operation. (C) Microscopic picture of tissue removed during first operation. Pathology was mixed ependymoma-astrocytoma grade II. Note invasion with the tumor surrounding a neuron. (D) Operative view of exposed spinal cord during second operation. Note extreme fullness of spinal cord. (E) Microscopic picture of tissue removed during second operation. Pathology was glioblastoma. Note giant cell. (F) Pathologic specimen, postmortem. Note metastatic nodules along the floor of the fourth ventricle.

be opened carefully since the pia-arachnoid of the enlarged spinal cord often adheres to the underside of the dura. It is important to prevent any injury to the cord vasculature since hemorrhage during this phase of the operation will obscure all landmarks and significantly compromise the surgical effort. In the event of previous surgery, particularly if the dura has been left open, this early dissection is tedious, but care must be taken to reestablish all anatomic landmarks. In those cases, both with and without previous surgery, the initial appearance of the cords generally was similar; the cords appeared widened, often without evidence of tumor on the surface. The widening of the spinal cord and the presence of dilated veins at the caudal end of the tumor site were indications of the underlying pathologic process. When observing a widened spinal cord, the surgeon must not be misled in those rare instances of anterior extramedullary lesion in which the cord is splayed out over the lesion.[19]

The dorsal surface of the cord at the area of greatest enlargement then is inspected for the site of the myelotomy. Generally, myelotomies are performed in the midline with a

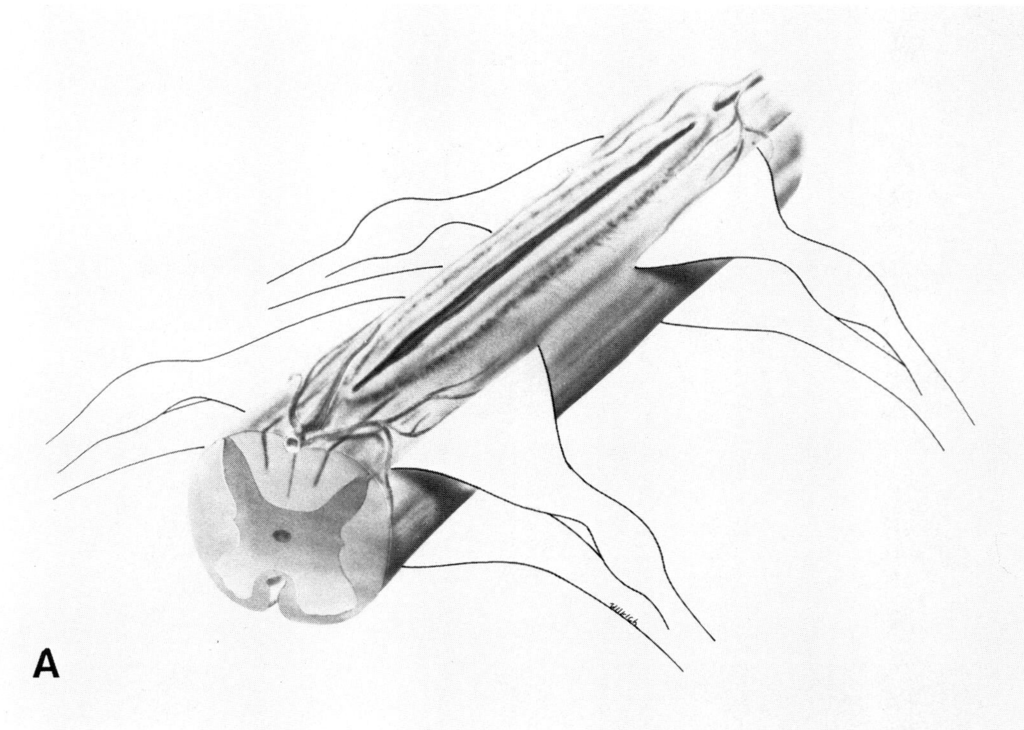

A

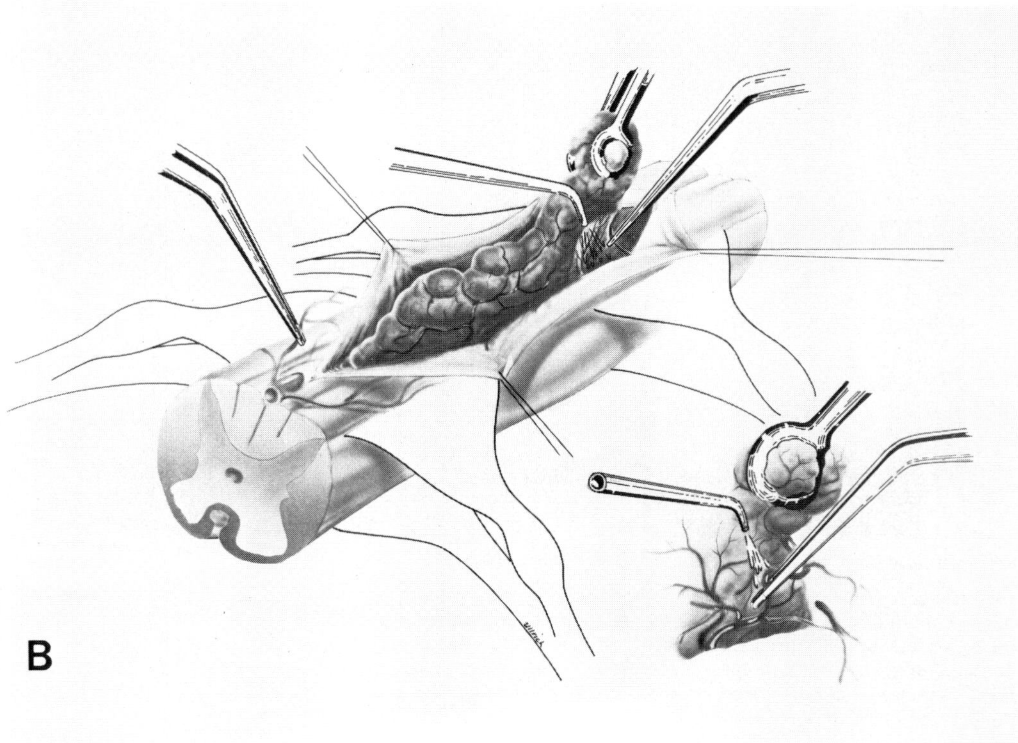

B

preference for the thinnest and most avascular areas; at times, however, it is more expeditious to use a paramedian approach (Figure 129-4).

Some of the vasculature will be sacrificed during this myelotomy. An initial incision of approximately 1 to 2 cm is performed over the greatest enlargement of the spinal cord to evaluate the plane between the tumor and the spinal cord tissue. In some instances the presence of a cyst associated with the tumor may be easily noted; if so, additional room may be gained by aspirating some of the cystic contents through a small-bore needle. To facilitate dissection, however, these cysts should not be completely evacuated. Once it is determined that the neoplasm is cystic or has well-defined planes, the myelotomy is lengthened over the extent of the tumor. With teratomas, a stalk between the cord and the dura should be removed as an integral part of the lesion. With ependymomas extending from the

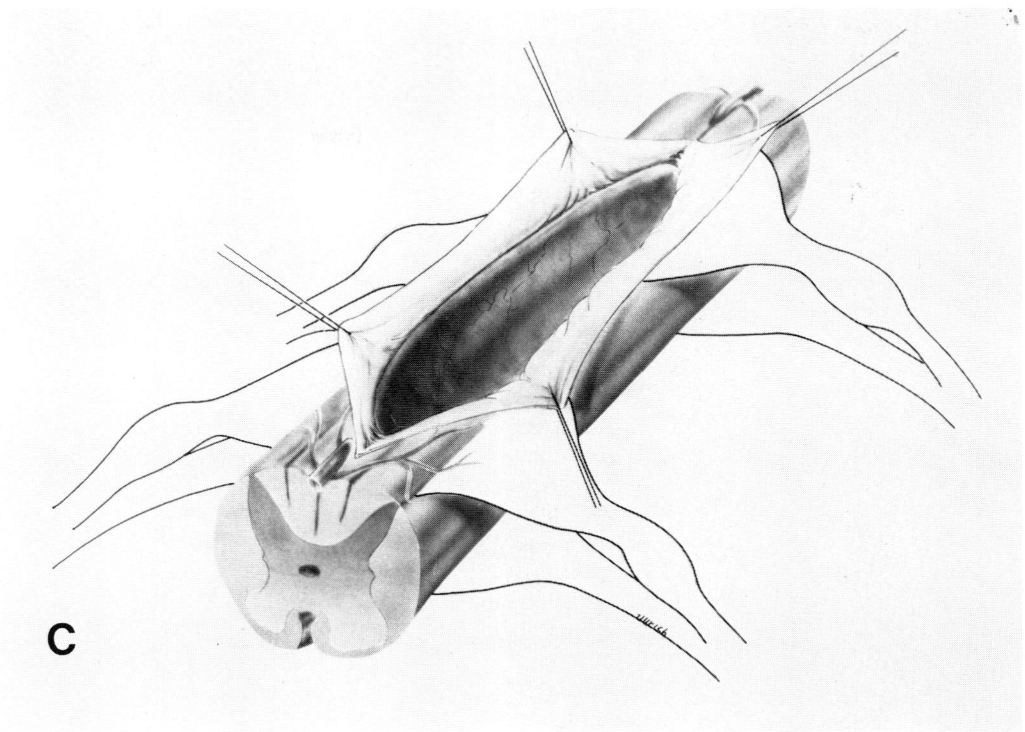

Fig. 129-4. A myelotomy over an intramedullary tumor. (B) Removal of an intramedullary tumor. (C) The open cord after removal of an intramedullary tumor.

conus, the extra-axial portion in the cauda equina may be removed first, providing adequate decompression and visualization of the residual tumor involving the intramedullary portion of the conus. The draining veins of intramedullary hemangioblastomas must be left to the latter part of the surgical resection.

Following the myelotomy, 6-0 or 7-0 traction sutures are placed through the pial margins on either side to expose the interior of the spinal cord (Figure 129-4). Generally, the tumor is visible a few millimeters under the dorsal surface of the spinal cord. There is often a soft gliotic interface between the tumor and the spinal cord proper. With the operating microscope and microsurgical techniques, using bipolar cautery, small suction tubes, and various dissectors, a plane is developed around the margin of the tumor, taking care to retract primarily on the tumor and not on the spinal cord. The surgeon works to one or the other end of the tumor. At the pole where the tumor is the narrowest, it may be possible to grasp the end and gently extract it from the interior of the cord. All the fine vascular adhesions to the spinal cord, especially on the ventral aspect of the tumor, should be cauterized with bipolar cautery and sharply divided. No blunt dissection should be carried out in areas where vascular channels connect the tumor to the spinal cord. Most tumors are amazingly avascular and present no threat of hemorrhage or the loss of control of large blood vessels. It is important to keep the operative field meticulously dry so that the plane between the tumor and the spinal cord may be readily identified (Figure 129-4). If the tumor is too large to remove in toto or necessitates too much retraction on the spinal cord, its interior may be decompressed. We prefer to use the CUSA unit (Cavitron ultrasonic surgical aspirator; Cooper Medical, Stamford, Conn) to debulk the tumor facilitating dissection around its capsule and its removal. This has a minor

disadvantage of spilling the contents of the tumor into the dissection plane or obscuring the dissection plane by bleeding. In most instances, however, the tumors are relatively avascular and bleeding is not a major problem even with the use of the Cavitron. Gradually, the entire tumor may be removed. For those tumors (usually astrocytomas) that are infiltrating, a debulking procedure is valuable, especially in children. The CO_2 and argon lasers have also been utilized for this.[20]

Cystic collections at the margins of the tumor, as in the case of astrocytomas, facilitate the tumor resection. We make no attempt, however, to remove the wall of the cyst, which is thin and nonneoplastic. If there is any doubt about the totality of removal, small biopsies may be obtained from the margin of the resection and evaluated by frozen section during surgery. In most instances, the margins are well defined and there is no question about the removal of the tumor (Figures 129-4 and 129-6). Malignant tumors such as the glioblastoma respond poorly to surgery and do not appear to respond to radiation therapy. These are usually hopeless cases.

In children, the syndrome of holo spinal cord widening is associated with extensive astrocytomas or localized astrocytomas and extensive cysts.[12] Here we must localize the tumor either through clinical or radiologic evaluation and remove it while only draining the cyst. A subtotal radical removal with the Cavitron or laser appears to pay dividends in these children with long-term remission of the disease process. Although these astrocytomas are histologically identical to those in adults, they may have different growth behavior related more to the child's development than to the histologic appearance.

Special attention is given to the removal of hemangioblastomas. These are highly vascular tumors and if they are decompressed or cut into, the bleeding will not only obscure the

Table 129-1. Intramedullary spinal cord tumors

No.	Age	Location	History	Removal	Result	Follow-up
1	26	C	Ependymoma	T	I	3 mos.
2	24	Conus	Ependymoma	T	I	1½ yrs.
3	49	C	Ependymoma	T	I	5 yrs.
4	28	C-D	Ependymoma	T	S	4½ yrs.
5	38	C	Ependymoma	T	S	4½ yrs.
6	45	Conus	Ependymoma	T	S	2 yrs.
7	35	Conus	Ependymoma	T	S	2 yrs.
8	20	Conus	Ependymoma	T	S	2 yrs.
9	35	C	Ependymoma	T	I	1½ yrs.
10	12	C	Astrocytoma	P	S	6 mos.
11	60	C-D	Astrocytoma	90%	S	6 yrs.
12	13	D-L	Astrocytoma	T	S	4 yrs.
13	3	C-D	Astrocytoma	95%	I	4 yrs.
14	48	C	Astrocytoma	T	I	4½ yrs.
15	38	C	Astrocytoma	T	I	5 yrs.
16	7	C	Astrocytoma	T	I	1½ yrs.
17	5	C-D-L-S	Astrocytoma	50%	S	1 yr.
18	14	C	Malignant glioma	P	W	1 yr. (died)
19	20	C	Malignant glioma	P	W	6 mos. (died)
20	13	D	Teratoma	T	I	4½ yrs.
21	12	Conus	Dermoid	T	I	11 yrs.
22	4 mos.	Conus	Epidermoid	T	I	11 yrs.
23	28	D-L	Mixed	P	W	2 yrs.
24	52	D	Metastatic	P	S	1 mo. (died)
25	57	C	Hemangioblastoma	T	I	2 mos.

C = cervical; D = dorsal; L = lumbar; T = total; P = partial; I = improved; S = same; W = worse.

anatomic planes, but may result in catastrophic problems. Therefore, even in large hemangioblastomas, we work around the margin of the tumor interrupting the feeding arteries and finally the primary draining vein as the tumor is rolled out on the last venous pedicle. Often these tumors are associated with a cyst, facilitating their removal. They are identified by their characteristic orange-red appearance and in all instances extrude from the pial surface. Their presence is also identified by large dilated arterialized veins that often surround them. This will mimic an AVM on the myelogram and occasionally on spinal angiography. In some instances hemangioblastomas may be multiple and additional tumors may be removed if they are accessible. In rare instances they will be associated with cranial tumors or the von Hippel-Lindau syndrome.

In cases in which the tumor has been treated with radiation previously, we have noted intense intramedullary gliosis by biopsy, distinctly separate from the margin of the tumor, usually at the caudal or rostral interface. It is assumed that this is an adverse effect of preoperative radiation. Previous surgery with aspiration of a cyst but without definitive removal of the intramedullary tumor has provided transient benefits and reaccumulation of the cyst fluid.

In teratomas, the border of the tumor, although well defined, may be densely adherent to the surrounding spinal cord. Every attempt should be made to remove this capsule, which is a potential source of regrowth. There may be extensive involvement of central areas of the spinal cord and the tumors may extend from the posterior to the anterior surface. Teratomatous tumors also may have a dumbbell configuration within the substance of the spinal cord, and the surgeon must be wary not to miss satellite portions of the primary tumor.

When the margins of the cord are allowed to fall back into position, the remarkable decompressive effect of tumor removal is quite apparent. The dorsal columns are often thin to the point of being transparent. If there has been minimal retraction on the cord, these fiber tracts function in a satisfactory way and will show progressive functional recovery. Rarely has the function of the spinal cord been made permanently worse by this dissection. Gentleness of dissection may be gauged by the vascular pattern on the dorsal surface of the cord at the completion of tumor resection. Distended veins that were present before removal, usually at the caudal end of the tumor on the surface of the spinal cord, will not be less prominent. No attempt has been made to sew the pial surfaces of the spinal cord together. The dura is closed in a watertight fashion; it is rarely necessary to use a fascial graft other than in those cases in which the dura was left open after previous surgery. If total removal of an intramedullary tumor is not feasible, the dura should be reconstructed, preferably with a fascial graft, so that subsequent surgical endeavors may be facilitated.

The most important factor determining the ease of the operation is the presence and nature of previous operations. In patients who have had previous surgery and in whom the dura mater was left open, the initial exposure of the tumor and the dissection of adjacent tissues from the spinal cord has prolonged the operating and made exposure more difficult. In those cases in which radiation was administered previously, gliotic areas in the dorsocentral portion of the spinal cord have been verified by biopsy. There have been no histologic changes in the tumor that were attributed to radiation. Similarly, none of the tumors that were previously irradiated showed malignant changes. Problems with wound healing also were encountered frequently in those cases in which radiotherapy was used previously.

POSTOPERATIVE TREATMENT

Steroids are routinely used pre- and postoperatively in high doses (dexamethasone 10–20 mg IV q4h) with a slow taper dependent upon the neurologic condition. Prophylactic antibiotics are used intraoperatively and for 48 hours postoperatively. If the surgery involved extensive areas of the cervical region, the endotracheal tube is left in place for at least 24 hours, regardless of the patient's condition at the termination of surgery.

Radiation therapy is considered postoperatively for children with astrocytomas, but we generally wait with adults and consider re-operation if recurrence should occur.

Careful orthopedic follow-up and possible bracing are necessary for the pediatric patients.

RESULTS

Removal of large intramedullary tumors can be performed with a fair degree of safety (Table 129-1) and can offer significant neurologic improvement in many situations. Generally, those patients with only mild to moderate neurologic deficit before surgery did extremely well, regardless of the size of the tumor. The total removal of these tumors offers a much improved outlook for patients who have not responded to previous decompressive laminectomy and radiotherapy. Our follow-up in the astrocytoma and ependymoma group has been too short to draw definite conclusions regarding a recurrence rate, although many patients are now 5 years or more postoperative without evidence of recurrence. Experience would indicate that the recurrence rate should be low following total removal.[2,5,7,8,21,22]

Case Report. A 35-year-old woman was asymptomatic until 6 months before admission when she developed sharp pains radiating around the right breast, as well as progressive numbness in a suspended pattern over the right side from the nipple line to the umbilicus level. Subsequently, she developed numbness in the right V2 distribution as well as around the shoulders. Minimal weakness was present in the upper arms.

Examination showed hypalgesia in the right V1 and V2 distribution. Strength was uniformly good except for minimal weakness of the left biceps muscles. Sensory examination showed a marked suspended sensory level loss from T1 to T8 with a lesser loss extending up to C2. Posterior column function was good. Reflexes were decreased in the left biceps, while slightly increased in the lower extremities. Babinski signs were absent.

Myelography was performed, which demonstrated a widened cord extending from T2 to C2 (Figure 129-1). Subsequently, a laminectomy from C2 through T2 was performed with myelotomy and total removal of a cystic ependymoma (Figure 129-1). Follow-up examination at 4½ years postoperatively showed the patient to be functioning extremely well at home. She noted some numbness under the right breast and tingling in her left fingers. Examination showed full muscle power with a decreased left biceps and triceps reflex. Joint position sense and vibratory sensation were decreased in the lower extremities but normal in the uppers.

Radicular pain in the distribution of the nerve roots associated with the tumor has been a distressing postoperative problem. This pain has a burning quality, severely disturbing to the patient and extremely difficult to control. Derangement of the physiologic pathways for pain at the dorsal route entry zone has been postulated as the cause. Unfortunately, we have not had satisfactory results in the treatment of these postoperative dysesthetic or pain syndromes.

Our experience[4,10] and that of others[5,6] indicate that a decompressive laminectomy, whether or not a tumor cyst has been evacuated, with or without radiotherapy, has had little beneficial effect on the course of most intramedullary spinal cord tumors. Some reviews[6,23] of the effects of radiation on these tumors are clouded by incomplete knowledge of the pathology, the natural course of these tumors, and the number of associated variables, including decompression and partial surgical removals.

One report by Schwade et al.[24] retrospectively reviewed 34 patients, 25 of whom had confirmed histology. They recommended conservative surgery to remove as much tumor as safely possible. Postoperative radiation therapy was given to 4500 to 5000 rad in 5 to 6 weeks, through portals that cover the tumor generously. Twelve of 12 patients with ependymomas were alive without recurrence with a minimum follow-up of 3 years. Five of 6 patients with low-grade astrocytomas survived longer than 3 years. Although encouraging, longer follow-up may be needed to evaluate this fully. In most reports there has been little objective follow-up of reduction in tumor size following radiation therapy. A significant number of reports indicate that surgical removal is the treatment of choice.[3–6,8–12] Improvement in the patient's condition or at least an arrest of the neurologic deterioration may be anticipated in most cases following surgery. Postoperative result is determined by the degree of preoperative neurologic involvement. Many surgeons have reported difficulty in totally removing astrocytomas. In our series we were able to totally remove about half the astrocytomas with no more significant problems than those encountered in the removal of ependymomas.

Through the use of microsurgical techniques and strict attention to postoperative pulmonary function, negligible mortality and morbidity rates can be expected, even with removal of extensive tumors in the cervical region.

We have not used postoperative radiation for intramedullary tumors that have been totally removed and do not advocate postoperative radiation for benign intramedullary tumors that have been incompletely removed, except occasionally in children. The patient's course should be monitored closely, facilitated by the use of water-soluble contrast agents and CT and MRI scanning. A second surgical attempt should be made to remove the tumor at the time of recurrence. Following this radiation may be considered.

SPINAL CORD ARTERIOVENOUS MALFORMATIONS (AVMS)

Arteriovenous malformations of the spinal cord are relatively rare, being only one tenth as common as cerebral AVMs and one tenth as common as primary spinal neoplasms. They appear more commonly in males (4:1) and generally occur in an older age group than those of the brain. Eighty percent occur in the thoracolumbar spinal cord, although they may involve the entire cord from cervical to sacral levels.[25,26]

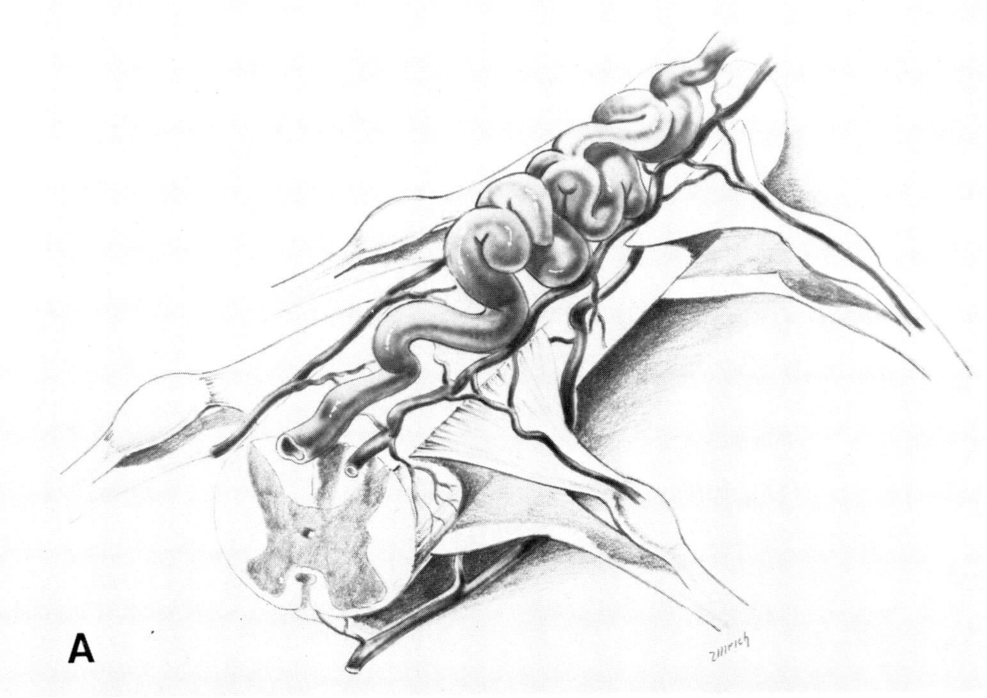

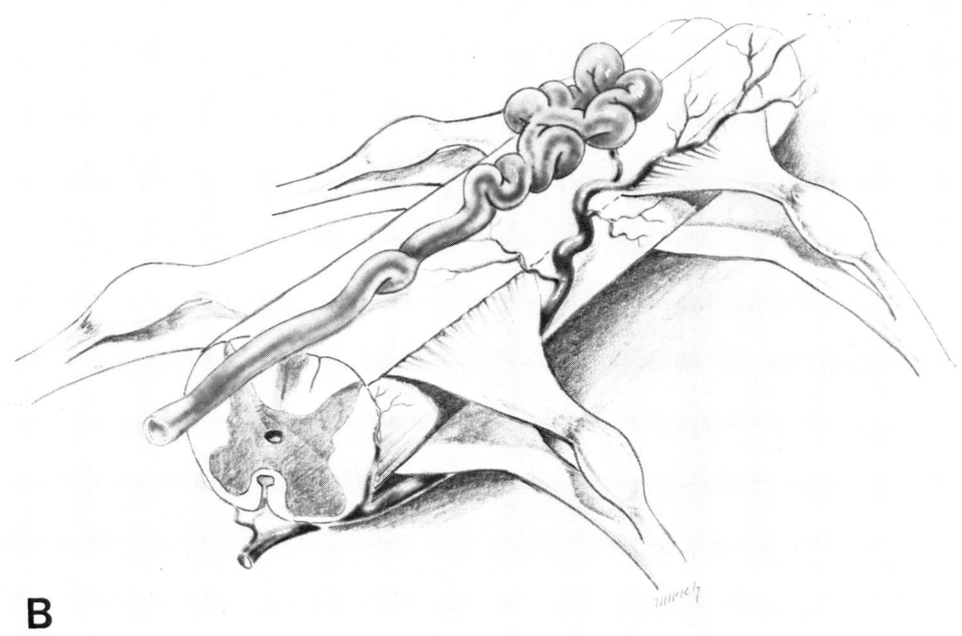

ANATOMY

There are two arterial systems of the spinal cord: an anterior one and a posterior one. These are supplied by the anterior and posterior radiculomedullary arteries, respectively. The anterior spinal artery usually is a well-defined single artery running in the anterior-median fissure and supplying approximately the anterior two thirds of the spinal cord.[27] The posterior arteries while paired on either side of the midline are variable and often are represented by numerous interlacing smaller arteries. They supply the posterior one third of the cord.[27] The largest and most important radicular artery supplying the cord is the artery of Adamkiewiez (great anterior medullary artery), which arises most frequently on the left side between T8 and L4.[28] After entering the spinal canal, it ascends and makes a hairpin turn with its largest branch directed caudally and a smaller branch cephalad. It anastomoses caudally with the artery accompanying the first sacral root. The posterior arteries have rich anastomoses with the anterior ones around the circumference of the cord[27,29,30] Because the dorsal arteries enter at almost every level, forming a very complete collateral network, they are much smaller than the ventral arteries and are normally demonstrated angiographically only with difficulty. The venous system is similar to the arterial in that it is paired

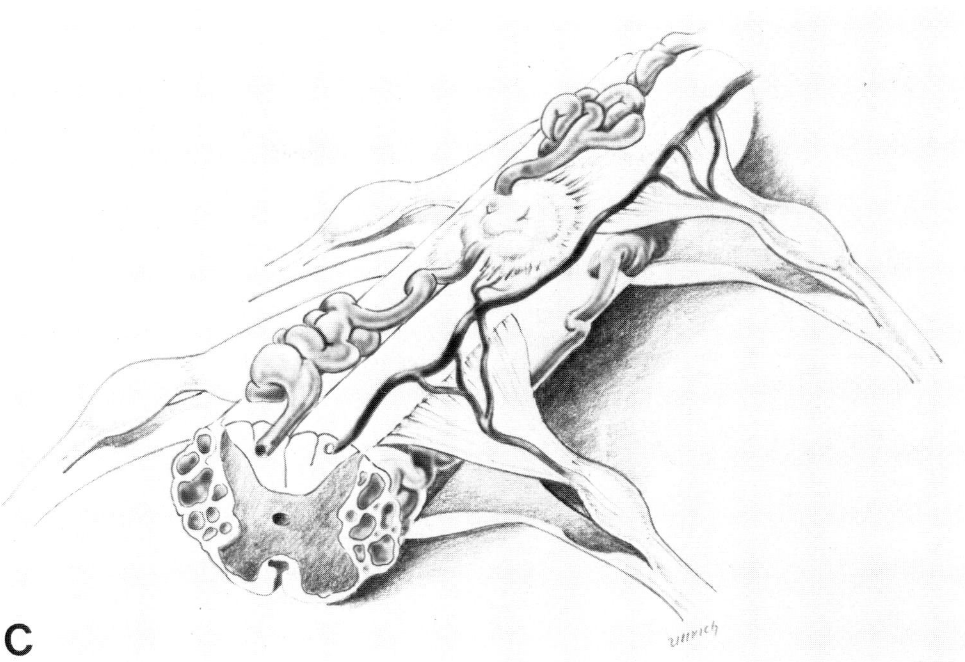

C

Fig. 129-5. AVMs of the spinal cord. (A) Abnormal arterialized tortuous veins cover the dorsal aspect of the cord (lighter and larger vessels). These are fed by numerous arterial branches at multiple levels (smaller and darker vessels). (B) A nidus with a feeding artery (dark vessel) and a localized tangle of abnormal draining veins (lighter and larger vessels.) (C) This AVM lies both within and on the surface of the spinal cord. It consists of large cavernous channels and multiple arteriovenous shunts. (Reprinted with permission of Baker HL Jr, Love JG, Layton DD Jr: Angiographic and surgical aspects of spinal cord vascular anomalies. Radiology 88:1078–1085, 1967.)

and more diffuse over the dorsal aspect than it is on the anterior aspect. Those vascular malformations that are primarily located intramedullary receive the bulk of their arterial supply from median and paramedian penetrating branches of the anterior spinal artery. Their venous drainage is either dorsal or ventral.

The artery of Adamkiewiez often contributes to spinal AVMs, as it supplies the most commonly involved area of the spinal cord. The intercostal arteries, the dorsal segmental arteries, and the lumbosacral radicular arteries also may contribute blood supply to the AVM. In the cervical region, the vertebral arteries and the costocervical or thyrocervical trunks of the subclavian artery may also supply the AVM. The majority of these AVMs are supplied by the dorsal radicular arteries, as the AVMs tend to be dorsal. In some instances, however, the anterior spinal artery sends perforating branches to supply portions of the AVM in the central or dorsal portion of the cord. The feeding arteries often are limited to a few radicular arteries, but on occasion there may be multiple small twigs at numerous levels shunting into an extensive venous draining system. These lesions primarily involve the pial surface of the cord rather than the parenchyma, but at times a portion of the malformation or a venous aneurysm may extend into the center of the spinal cord.[31] Because of the dorsal pial position, their surgical removal is often feasible.

In the past, such terms as "cavernous" and "racemose" angiomas, both arterial and venous, were often used descriptively[32,33]; with the advent of spinal angiography, however, and the operating microscopic exposure, a more practical scheme has been developed.[34–36]

The majority of these lesions represent arteriovenous communications of varying extent and degree. The communication between arteries and veins develops primarily between the

dorsal radicular arteries and the dorsolateral veins of the spinal cord. The classification of Ommaya is useful in the surgical evaluation of these lesions.[35] His type 1, the most common, represents an extensive single-coiled vessel with one or two arterial feeders entering at various levels. (These small arteries are not visualized at arteriography and are difficult to see without the operating microscope.) The flow is slow and the blood supply appears distinct from that of the cord.

The lesion appears at the pial level of the cord, rarely penetrates the cord, may extend laterally but is usually dorsal in location. The ligation of major arterial feeders to these lesions will often significantly decrease the flow in the malformation and lead to stasis, but small arterial contributions at numerous other levels keep the malformation "alive." These latter arteries, however, may be insignificant. The major feature of these malformations is a will identified arterial contribution at the one or two levels.

Type 2 is a glomus or nidus type of malformation. The lesion is angiographically and surgically well visualized and well defined[37] (Figures 129-5 and 129-6). It is generally a discrete coil of arteriovenous vessels supplied by well identified arteries at the margin of the glomus or nidus. A subgroup of this type is the intramedullary vascular malformation.[31] The intramedullary type has been reported in the cervical region by Malis,[38] and has been seen at many other regions of the spinal cord including the conus. These malformations are generally high pressure and can be well demonstrated by arteriography. They can be resected discretely. Venous aneurysms are commonly associated with this type of malformation, especially when intramedullary.

Type 3, the so-called juvenile type, most commonly seen in children, is a more diffuse, comprehensive arteriovenous lesion

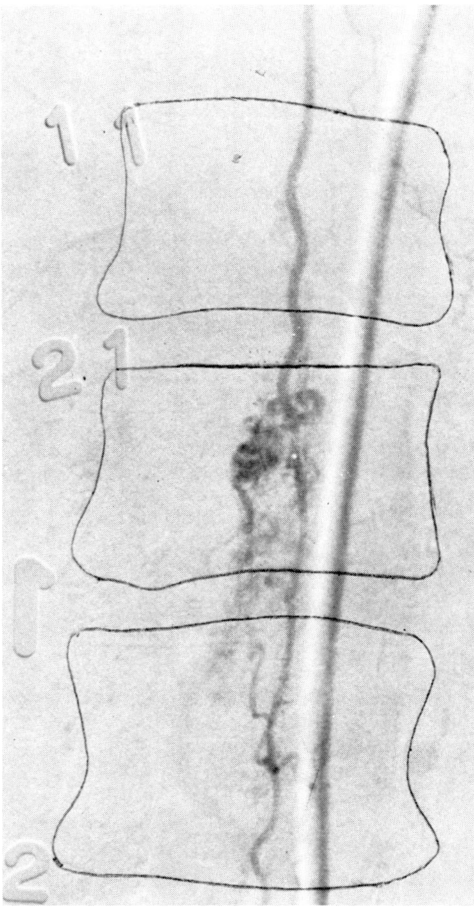

Fig. 129-6. Anteroposterior spinal cord arteriograms with subtraction technique. The nidus of the AVM is seen at the small arrows. The feeding artery is present at the open arrow. (Reprinted with permission of Kasdon DL, Wolpert SM, Stein BM: Surgical and angiographic localization of spinal arteriovenous malformations. Surg Neurol 5:279–283, 1976.)

of the cord, which often encircles it in a cuirass configuration (Figure 129-5). A better term is a diffuse intra and extra medullary AVM since these lesions permeate the spinal cord making their obliteration impossible (Figure 129-5). They have varying degrees of arterial contributions which may or may not be visualized at arteriography. Flow is rapid and the blood supply of the AVM and the cord may be closely related. Doppman[37] emphasizes the "nidus" concept in regard to some of these lesions. In these cases, angiography will demonstrate discrete arteriovenous communications with limited involvement of the rostrocaudal extent of the spinal cord. A detailed picture of the vascular anatomy is therefore essential when one is considering the extent of laminectomy and whether or not a lesion can be totally removed. Ventral lesions are most difficultto treat surgically.

The lesions that do not have arteriovenous communications and that represent pure venous or arterial abnormalities are exceedingly rare and have not been demonstrated by arteriography. The concept that such lesions exist is primarily based on data from autopsy specimens. Whether this concept has any validity in the present-day evaluation of these lesions is open to question.

CLINICAL PRESENTATION AND NATURAL HISTORY

Spinal AVMs tend to occur in males (2–4:1, male:female) in the 30- to 70-year age group, primarily at the thoracolumbar levels.[25] Frequently, AVM is not suspected and a diagnosis of tumor or disc disease is made. In the planning of therapy, which may involve procedures of considerable risk, the natural history of these lesions must be considered. Aminoff and Logue,[39,40] in an extensive review of 60 cases, reported that the vast majority had an insidious onset with progressive deterioration, while 50 percent of the patients were severely disabled within 3 years of the onset of the disorder. Only 20 percent of the cases had an acute onset, and subsequently many of these had progression of symptoms. Subarachnoid hemorrhage occurred at one time or another in 10 percent of the cases, but was an initial symptom in only 5 percent. Herdt et al.[41] found that only 6 percent of the patients had definite proof of subarachnoid hemorrhage. Tobin and Layton,[25] reviewing the Mayo Clinic experience with 71 patients, found a slowly progressive course in 73 percent and an abrupt onset with subarachnoid hemorrhage in 10 percent. The symptom complex of leg weakness, sensory loss, pain, and early sphincteric involvement was the most common presentation. The prognosis once the lesion becomes symptomatic generally is poor and is represented by a progressive and disabling disease. In a small number of cases the threat of instantaneous neurologic disaster is present. In such instances the onset may be devastating with all of the manifestations that go with a ruptured intracranial aneurysm.

Subarachnoid hemorrhage with the sudden onset of neurologic symptomatology is unusual, however, except in patients under 30 years of age.[42] An insidious progressive course is most common; it is accentuated by pain of radicular origin, depending upon the location of the lesion. The location of the pain, however, is often not a reliable indication of the levels of involvement.[25] Progressive upper or lower motor neuron involvement is the rule, with spasticity or absent reflexes, depending upon location. Involvement of the dorsal columns with paresthesias, loss of position, and other sensory modalities is also part of the progressive picture.

These lesions appear to produce symptoms because of ischemic changes in the spinal cord secondary to a vascular steal and the mass effect of the lesion.[36,43,44] On occasion, the arterialized veins that compose these malformations are layered four to five deep on the surface of the spinal cord (Figure 129-7). When the lesions are removed, grooves from the dilated vascular channels can be noted on the surface of the spinal cord. Many of the symptoms associated with spinal AVMs may relate to increased venous pressure altering the dynamics of blood flow within the spinal cord, and leading to venous congestion and infarction within the substances of the spinal cord.

DIAGNOSIS

On examination, two signs are helpful if present. A bruit over the spine is virtually diagnostic[45] and the presence of a cutaneous angioma helps diagnostically and also in localizing the level of the lesions.[46] Plain x-ray films of the spine generally are noncontributory. Cerebrospinal fluid evaluation shows some abnormality in 75 percent with protein elevation and pleocytosis being most common.[25,47]

Spinal myelography with Pantopaque was often diagnostic.[39,40] Since most of these lesions occurred on the dorsal surface of the cord, it was necessary to insert the Pantopaque,

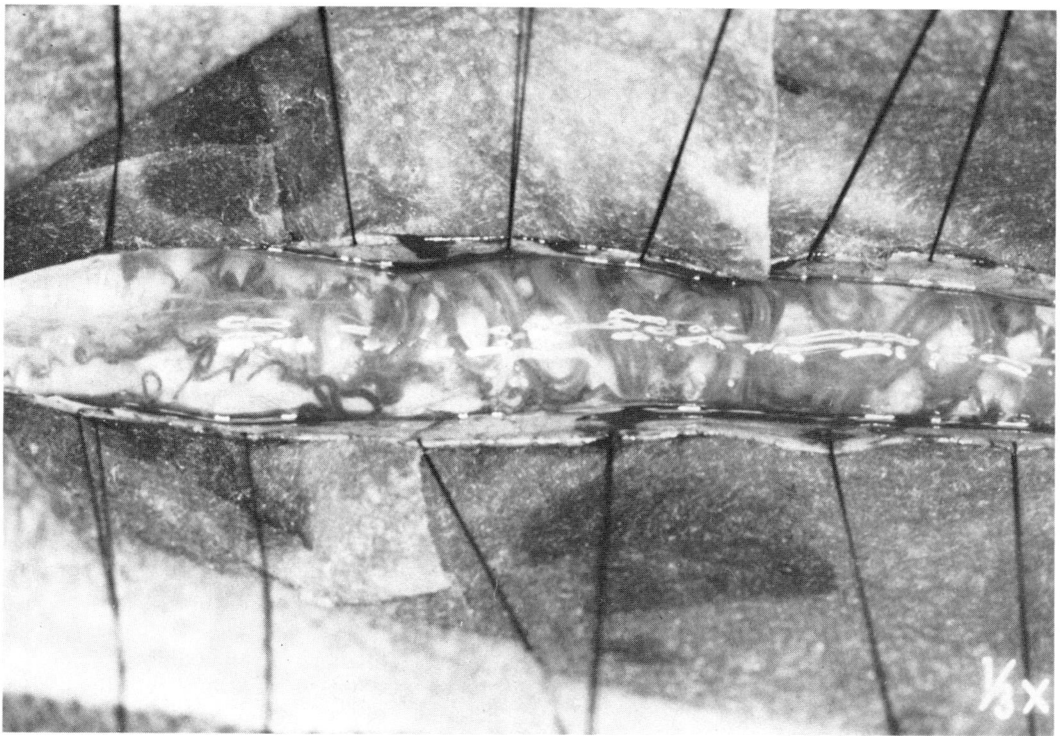

Fig. 129-7. Operative exposure of a large AVM of the spinal cord composed principally of tortuous, distended, arterialized veins.

turn the patient supine, and run the Pantopaque up the dorsal surface of the spinal cord. Often the webbing or trabeculation of the dorsal arachnoid led to the erroneous diagnosis of a vascular malformation, and occasionally tortuous nerve roots, spinal metastases and dilated vessels associated with intramedullary tumors could produce a false-positive diagnosis. (Figure 129-8).

Myelography is now performed with nontoxic contrast agents that are water soluble, nonelectrolyte, and will coat the spinal cord. It is easier to study the dorsal as well as other aspects of the spinal cord and visualize the malformations. The diminished density of these agents and the refined detail also facilitate the diagnosis. A CT scan may also augment these studies.[48] Often, myelography will indicate the longitudinal extent of the malformation and then spinal angiography can be helpful in pinpointing the arterial anatomy.

Spinal angiography with selective injection of the relevant arteries and a serial study with subtraction technique are important. In the cervical region, selective injection of the subclavian branches, including the vertebral, thyrocervical, and costocervical trunks should be done. Spinal angiography must be comprehensive. If there is no myelographic clue to the location of the AVM, the procedure is extremely laborious and tedious.

Unfortunately, a lesion must represent a significant arteriovenous shunt or arteriography may be unsuccessful in the demonstration of all of the ramifications of the lesion. Opacification of the posterior spinal arteries is rare, while the thoracic anterior spinal artery is small and often hard to visualize under normal circumstances.

It should be understood that there is a certain risk in performing spinal angiography since the catheter is frequently wedged into the feeding artery and the cord become temporarily ischemic during the injection. Flexor spasms have occurred during the injection, especially when a pathologic process is present and collateral circulation comprised.

A flush of the aorta may show a flash filling of the lesion but is contraindicated because of spinal cord toxicity. Selective arteriography must be done at individual levels to demonstrate these malformations properly. In some instances, arteriography may fail to define the arterial contribution to an extensive malformation of dilated arterialized veins extending over multiple segments of the spinal cord. In other instances, where a nidus exists, it may be difficult to tell from angiography whether the lesion is intra- or extramedullary in location.[49]

The variability of the position of the spinal cord in the anteroposterior plane within the spinal canal plays a major role in the difficulty of precise localization. Displacement of the spinal cord by thrombosed portions of malformations, which are not visualized with contrast material, is an additional source of error in localization by spinal angiography. A CT scan of the spine with intravenous contrast enhancement may hold some promise for screening and follow-up of patients with spinal AVMs. The axial-transverse view of the lesion may permit a better appraisal of the anatomic relationships of the extrathecal extension of the malformation.[48]

Evoked potentials have been most useful during surgery and radiologic procedures.[50] As a clinical tool prior to operation, these studies have not shown great promise, especially in definitively locating and diagnosing the presence of a spinal AVM. It is unlikely that MRI will lead to as detailed an evaluation as angiography often accomplishes.

TREATMENT

Because the prognosis is poor for patients with spinal arteriovenous malformations that are untreated or simply decompressed, we feel that surgical exploration to assess resect-

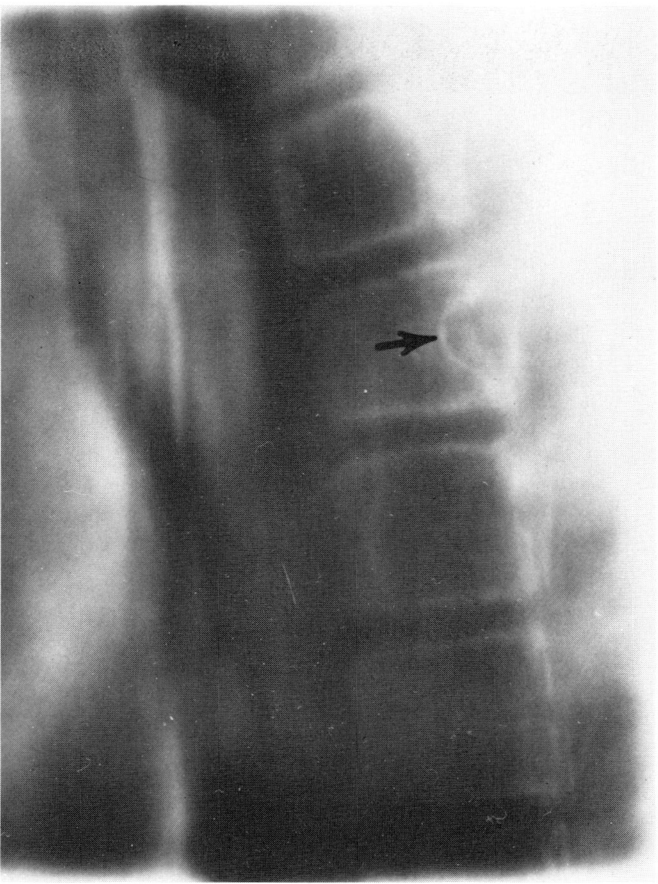

Fig. 129-8. Lumbar thoracic myelogram demonstrating tortuous shadows suggestive of abnormal vascular channels but representing redundant nerve roots (arrows). (Reprinted with permission of Stein BM: Arteriovenous malformations of the brain and spinal cord, in Practice of Surgery, Hagerstown, Md, Harper & Row, 1979.)

ability is important. This should be carried out in spite of an angiographic appearance suggesting a largely intramedullary localization of the malformation.

The only completely satisfactory treatment for spinal AVMs is total obliteration or excision, Thus far, the usefulness of embolization has been limited.

Embolization

Various techniques have been used, including silicone emboli that are placed via catheter into the feeding arteries.[51–53] This technique is limited because of the small size of the feeding arteries and the fact that these arteries, which are proximal to the lesion, may be significant contributors to the normal spinal cord circulation. Furthermore, in lesions with comparatively low blood flow there is an additional hazard of inadvertent embolization of normal vessels.

Surgical Excision

The cornerstone of treatment for spinal AVMs is microsurgical obliteration.[34–36,42,49,54–56] The lesions lend themselves to surgery since the vast majority lie on the dorsal surface of the spinal cord and are thereby accessible (Figures 129-7, 129-9 and 129-10). They also represent low flow and low pressure systems in which there is a limited arterial contribution with a significant venous component that is readily visualized on the surface of the spinal cord. Uncommonly, the lesion

invades portions of the spinal cord. Even in such instances the AVM occasionally may be removed microsurgically with satisfactory results.[31]

The axiom that the preoperative neurologic status is often related to the postoperative outcome is particularly pertinent in these lesions. Surgery should be accomplished early in the disease before major neurologic deficits. Function is unlikely to improve in the face of severe incapacitation.

The patient is prepared with dexamethasone prior to surgery. Malis[38] prefers to use the sitting position for those lesions located in the upper thoracic, cervical, and cervicomedullary region. This creates a certain degree of hypotension which may be useful. It also minimizes respiratory movement artifact. In those lesions located at the lower levels, he prefers an oblique position so as to limit respiratory excursions. Both of these positions preclude the effective use of an assistant during the operation, which we consider a major disadvantage. We prefer to operate on all of these lesions in the prone position with the patient's abdomen and chest free for respiratory excursions. The surgeon and assistant work together across the operating table. The extent of the lesion as identified by myelography and spinal angiography determines the exposure. The laminectomy should be moderately broad and the dura opened widely with preservation of the arachnoid until the extent of the lesion is determined by visualization through the arachnoid. The operating microscope is always used from the point of dural opening. The arachnoid is then opened widely with small scissors or arachnoidal knife. It may be necessary to rotate the cord, cutting the dentate ligament and grasping it to see the lateral supply to the malformation. In many cases of long dorsal AVMs the malformation may extend over different regions of the spinal cord and a few cases have been described where the lesion extends the entire length of the spinal cord. As reported recently,[57] it may not be necessary to remove the entire malformation. Interrupting the fistula between the major arterial supply and the arterialized venous system may suffice.[57] However, there may be minor arterial contributions, and in such cases the malformation may remain turgid with the veins containing arterialized blood under pressure. It may be necessary in one or multiple stages to remove the entire arterialized venous system interrupting even the smallest arterial contribution.

Those lesions of the juvenile variety or those which permeate the spinal cord will be easily identified by visualization of the dorsal, dorsolateral and ventrolateral portion of the spinal cord. Those lesions which are primarily intramedullary may be identified by a local bulge of the spinal cord with draining veins coming out over the dorsal surface of the spinal cord. Occasionally, discoloration due to old hemorrhage or thrombosis within the lesion is seen. These are treated by myelotomy and techniques similar to intramedullary tumor surgery.

Microbipolar cautery is utilized under constant moisture during the occlusion of the AVM vessels. Only the largest vessels are clipped and from a practical point of view this means none, one or two arteries during the removal of the usual spinal AVM. It is extremely difficult to use the standard metallic clips in the removal of an intramedullary lesion which must be accomplished by bipolar cautery. We prefer to approach the lesions from the arterial side first. The venous flow, even though arterialized, is often slow and can be managed easily should rupture occur on the venous side. We see no advantage in attacking the lesion primarily from the venous side, if definitive arterial contributions are easily visualized. The lesion

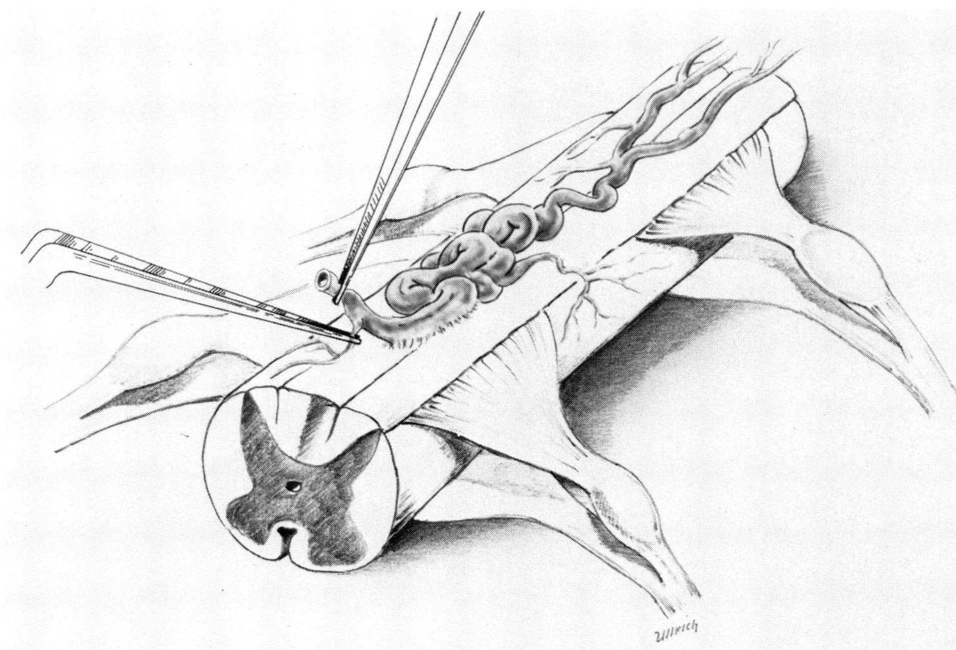

Fig. 129-9.   The surgical resection of an AVM showing meticulous cautery of the feeding arteries and gradual peeling away of the abnormal venous channels from the surface of the spinal cord. (Reprinted with permission of Stein BM: Arteriovenous malformations of the brain and spinal cord, in Practice of Surgery, Hagerstown, Md, Harper & Row, 1979.)

is generally peeled away from the spinal cord while additional arterial contributions are coagulated and divided (Figure 129-9). In general, malformations located within the spinal cord are associated with large venous aneurysms, often partially thrombosed. These are rather dangerous "bombs" and we do not want to threaten the venous drainage or the aneurysm more than necessary to collapse it so that it may be removed safely from within the spinal cord. We have not been using hypotension during the removal, especially if the patient is in the sitting position. In the prone position, hypotension is not necessary because of the low flow in these systems. The dura is always closed, no matter what has been accomplished at the time of the operation.

Lesser surgical procedures such as decompressive laminectomy with or without opening the dura appear to have little or no merit in the treatment of these malformations. In fact, such operative "explorations" may be detrimental in that they make future definitive surgery more difficult. If the lesion is found to be inoperable and all that can be offered is decompression with opening of the dura, then the dura should be closed with a patch graft of fascia to prevent adhesions to the surface of the spinal cord. If there is a possibility that surgery will be performed in the future, it is mandatory to close the dura, since the adhesions that will otherwise form will preclude subsequent, definitive surgical ventures.

SPECIAL CONSIDERATIONS

Long Dorsal AVM

There is no question that these large coiled arterialized veins are fed by one or two primary arteries which are part of the dorsal radiculomedullary arteries. Anyone who has resected the entire coil of veins will also note small arterial contributions at numerous levels. If a segment of the malformation is isolated from its major blood supply, it will still bleed from the contribution of these small arterial feeders. It has been general practice to gradually sweep the entire malformation off the dorsal aspect of the cord, interrupting all arterial feeders to it until the venous system turns blue.

Oldfield et al[7] recently reaffirmed the suggestion of others[35,58,59] that only the major arterial contribution be interrupted. These studies suggest a significant reduction in the flow of the malformation, but not complete obliteration following this maneuver. They also point out that this fistula may occur at the dura where the radicular arteries enter the dural root sleeve. Postoperative arteriographic studies have shown no visualization of the AVM in such cases. However, since the residual arterial feeders are tiny they are not ordinarily shown by arteriography. Clinically, this limited procedure has led to dramatic improvement in many cases. It remains to be seen what will be accomplished over the long term. It is quite possible the malformation will reactivate with time. That has been the case with many cerebral malformations partially treated by obliteration of the major feeders.

At the present time, it is our recommendation that observations at surgery be considered in determining the extent of the surgery and that the major coils of veins that remain arterialized should be obliterated. This may also be accomplished by selective cautery rather than by stripping of the entire dorsal venous system. There is some evidence that this stripping procedure may cause compromise of the normal cord blood supply and ischemic changes beyond the area of the malformation. After the stripping of large coiled veins from the dorsal surface of the cord, it appears significantly devascularized (Figure 129-10). In those cases in which we have interrupted the major arterial fistula and then selectively cauterized portions of the remaining dorsal venous system the circulation

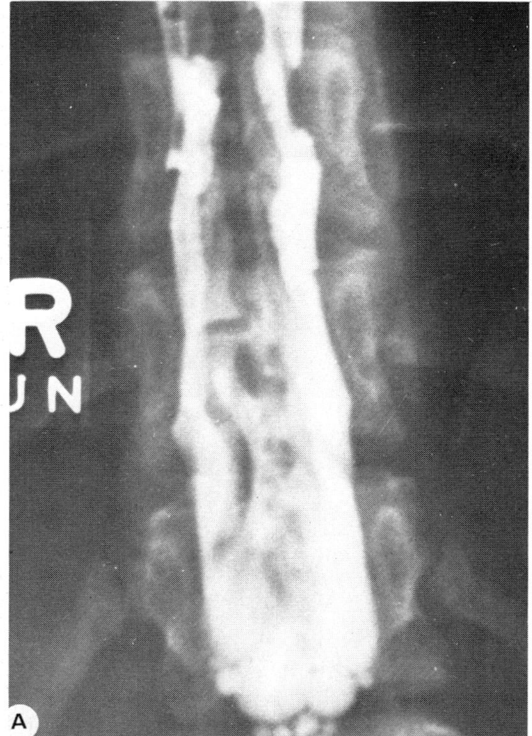
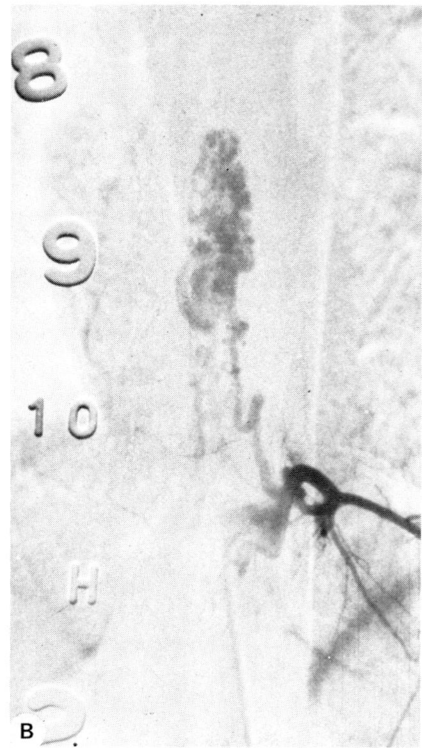

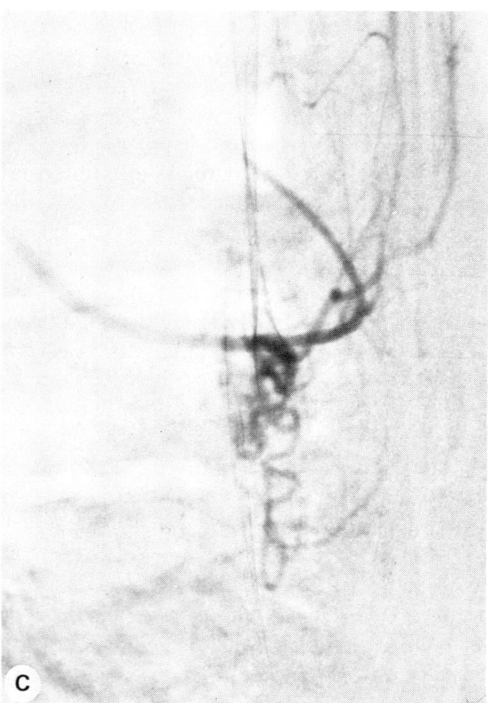

has a more appealing appearance. Long-term follow-up is lacking to determine which is the correct procedure.

Glomus AVM

The malformations in the form of a nidus or glomus are the easiest to comprehend and treat. These lesions produce symptoms of mass hemorrhage or venous thrombosis. They can be circumscribed by interruption of their feeding arteries at the exact margin of the glomus. Interruption of the major venous

drainage first may jeopardize the operation by creating intolerable intraluminal forces within the malformation resulting in hemorrhage.

Malformations that are primarily intramedullary are usually glomus in configuration. A rare one will be associated with a long dorsal type of malformation in conjunction with the primary intramedullary lesion. We have had an unusually high incidence of intramedullary lesions; approximately 20 percent of all spinal cord AVMs[1] They are managed in the fashion of removing a glomus from the dorsal or dorsolateral surface of the cord with the additional considerations akin to removal of an intramedullary tumor. The locus of the lesion is visualized as the cord is exposed. A myelotomy is made in a longitudinal direction from the polar aspects of the lesion, allowing visualization of the rostral and caudal margin of the lesion. Dissection is carried carefully around the appropriate margin depending upon the anatomy of the venous drainage and arterial supply as determined from angiograms and intraoperative observations. These lesions are preferably approached from the arterial side using bipolar cautery for interruption of the arterial feeders while the malformation is rolled toward the venous pedicle. In some occasions, the venous pedicle is in direct relationship to the major supply from the anterior spinal artery. It should be possible to approach the lesion from the arterial side and once this is interrupted the venous pedicle is easy to manage. Clips are rarely used. Sharp dissection is always preferred in the removal as opposed to blunt or a tearing type of dissection technique. These lesions are frequently associated with a large aneurysmal dilatation, often partially thrombosed, but still active and thin-walled, predisposing to intraoperative hemorrhage secondary to excessive manipulation. Careful use of a broad bipolar tip under irrigation may be utilized to shrink venous aneurysms but care must be taken that the wall is not violated. In many cases the venous aneurysm may be gently

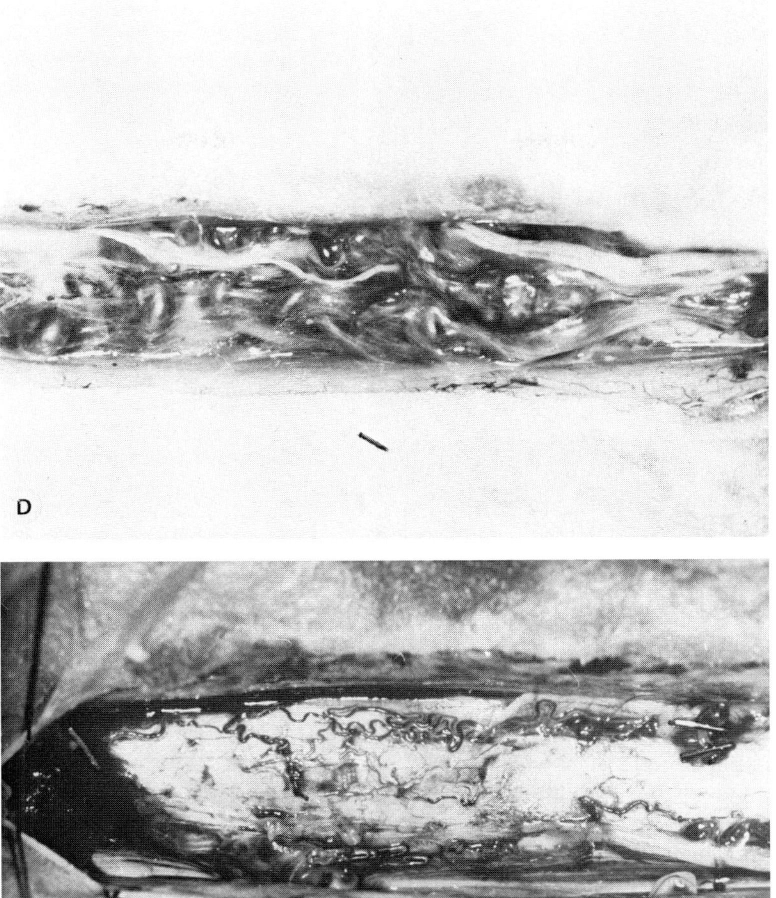

Fig. 129-10. (A) A low thoracic myelogram (AP projection) demonstrating serpiginous filling defect suggestive of an AVM. (B) A selective spinal arteriogram (AP view) demonstrating spinal AVM opposite T8-T10. (C) A selective spinal arteriogram (lateral view) demonstrating spinal AVM with components appearing dorsal, ventral, and possibly within the spinal cord. (D) Operative exposure of spinal cord from T7-T11 with extensive AVM. (E) Operative view after dorsal and lateral portions of the AVM were removed.

teased out of the cord intact. The venous aneurysm is often on the edge of the shunt component of the malformation. The cavity left by removal of these lesions is similar in size and configuration to that left by the total removal of a large intramedullary tumor. It is remarkable how thin the surrounding cord structure can be and still result in a functional neurological state.

Juvenile or Diffuse AVM

These are the most difficult lesions to treat. They permeate the cord and histologic examination indicates functional neural tissue interspersed with vascular channels of the malformation. It is obvious that they do not have well-defined margins permitting resection and that they comprehensively involve both the interior and exterior of the spinal cord over many segments. It is our opinion that confirmation of these lesions must be left to surgical exploration and that definitive knowledge as to their presence, which would preclude intraoperative interventions, cannot be obtained by the usual radiographic studies. Perhaps MRI will answer this question in the future. Although these are nonresectable lesions, in one instance under evoked potential monitoring, we were able to clip a major radicular artery and witness a rather remarkable clinical improvement in an individual who had been plagued by progressive deterioration of spinal cord function. In most cases, these lesions can be treated with little more than a decompressive procedure and perhaps, in exceptional cases, selective ligation of arteries under evoked potential monitoring. These maneuvers are of questionable benefit.

RESULTS

In those patients in whom surgical obliteration or resection of the lesion has been accomplished, good results in terms of an improved or arrested neurologic status are seen in approximately 80 to 90 percent of the patients.[35,36,38–40,42,55] Unfortunately, the results are often predicated on the preoperative condition of the patient, so that those with neurologic devastation or severe advanced disease are less apt to make gratifying recoveries following successful resection of the lesion. On the other hand, individuals who have mild or modest neurologic deficits before surgery will receive the most benefit and often return to normal or near normal status. Resection of these malformations precludes the possibility of devastating neurologic deficit from subsequent hemorrhage.

Luessenhop and Dela Cruz[34] reported, in a broad review of the literature, that decompressive procedures resulted in improvement in 19 percent and deterioration in 81 percent, while ligation of some feeders resulted in improvement in 34 percent and worsening in 66 percent. When these figures are compared with those of surgical resection, it is clear that the latter procedure, if feasible, is preferable. Radiation plays no role in the therapy of these lesions and may be deleterious, producing scar tissue that would make subsequent definitive operative procedures on these lesions difficult or impossible.

A postoperative arteriogram may or may not be obtained to define the completeness of resection. We do not feel postoperative angiography is as important in these cases as in the treatment of cerebral AVMs, since one is better able to gauge the effectiveness of resection while at the same time realizing the limitations of spinal arteriography in fully defining these lesions.

In addition to the AVMs that directly involve the spinal cord, there are similar situations existing in the meninges or parameningeal areas. These are often represented by enormous arteriovenous communications involving the intercostal or cervical arteries and involving not only the dura and sometimes the spinal cord but also often extensively the muscles and surrounding soft tissues. These are associated with bruits and may not manifest themselves with the spinal cord syndrome so familiar to true AVMs of the spinal cord. Unfortunately, these lesions, being extensive with large shunts between arteries and veins, are difficult to treat by embolization, surgery, or both. In many instances, emboli will transverse the fistula and enter into the systemic venous circulation. Because of the extensive nature of these lesions, it is often impossible to remove the entire lesion, even with thoracotomy and massive resection. They are similar to cirsoid aneurysms of the scalp and some of the soft-tissue AVMs that involve the face and tissues at the base of the skull.

REFERENCES

1. Turnbull F: Intramedullary tumors of the spinal cord, in Clinical Neurosurgery, vol 8. Baltimore, Williams & Wilkins, 1962, pp 237–247
2. Elsberg CA: Tumors of the Spinal Cord. New York, Paul B. Hoeber, 1925, pp 206–239
3. Matson DD: Neurosurgery of Infancy and Childhood. Springfield, Ill, Charles C Thomas, 1969, pp 647–688
4. Garrido E, Stein BM: Microsurgical removal of intramedullary spinal cord tumors. Surg Neurol 7:215–229, 1977
5. Greenwood J Jr: Surgical removal of intramedullary tumors. J Neurosurg 26:276, 1967
6. Guidetti B: Intramedullary tumors of the spinal cord. Acta Neurochirugia 17:7, 1967
7. Horrax G, Henderson, DG: Encapsulated intramedullary tumor involving whole spinal cord from medulla to conus: Complete enucleation with recovery. Surg Gynecol Obstet 68:814, 1939
8. Malis LI: Intramedullary spinal cord tumors. Clin Neurosurg 25:512, 1978
9. Yasargil MG, Antic J, Laciga R, et al: The microsurgical removal of intramedullary spinal hemangioblastomas: Report of twelve cases and a review of the literature. Surg Neurol 6:141, 1976
10. Stein BM: Spinal intradural tumors, in Wilkins RH, Rengachary SS: Neurosurgery. New York, McGraw-Hill, 1985, pp 1048–1061
11. Rand RW, Rand CW: Intraspinal Tumors of Childhood. Springfield, Ill, Charles C Thomas, 1960
12. Epstein F, Epstein N: Surgical treatment of spinal cord astrocytomas of childhood: A series of 19 patients. J Neurosurg 57:685, 1982
13. Tievsky AL, Davis DO: Radiology of spinal cord neoplasia, in Wilkins RH, Rengachary SS: Neurosurgery. New York, McGraw-Hill, 1985, pp 1039–1048
14. Vigneud J, Aubin MD, Jardin C: CT in 40 cases of syringomyelia (abstract). AJNR 1:112, 1980
15. Kan S, Fox AJ, Vineula F, Barnett HJM, Peerless SJ: Delayed CT metrizamide enhancement of syringomyelia secondary to tumor. AJNR 4:73, 1983
16. Quencer RM, Tenner MS, Rothman LM: Percutaneous spinal cord puncture and myelocystography. Radiology 118:637, 1976
17. Fischer G, Mansuy L: Total removal of intramedullary ependymomas: Follow-up study of 16 cases. Surg Neurol 14:243, 1980
18. Guidetti B, Mercuri S, Vagnozzi R: Long-term results of the surgical treatment of 129 intramedullary spinal gliomas. J Neurosurg 54:323, 1981
19. Stein BM: Case records of the Massachusetts General Hospital—case 26. N Engl J Med 293:33, 1975
20. Powers SK, Edwards SB, Boggan JE, et al: Use of the Argon surgical laser in neurosurgery. J Neurosurg 60:523, 1984
21. Greenwood J Jr: Intramedullary tumors of the spinal cord. A follow-up study after total surgical removal. J Neurosurg 20:665, 1963
22. Love JG, River MH: Thirty-one year cure following removal of intramedullary glioma of cervical portion of spinal cord. Report of case. J Neurosurg 19:906, 1962
23. Wood EH, Berne AS, Taveras JM: The value of radiation therapy in the management of intrinsic tumors of the spinal cord. Radiology 63:11, 1954
24. Schwade JG, Wara WM, Sheline GE, et al: Management of primary spinal cord tumors. Int J Radiat Oncol Biol Phys 4:389, 1978
25. Tobin WD, Layton DD: The diagnosis and natural history of spinal cord arteriovenous malformations. Mayo Clin Proc 51:637, 1976
26. Krayenbuhl H, Yasargil MG: Die Varicosis spinalis und ihre Behandlung. Schweiz Arch Neurol Psychiatr 92:74, 1963
27. Doppman JL, DiChiro G, Ommaya AK: Selective Arteriography of the Spinal Cord. St. Louis, Warren Green, 1969
28. DiChiro G, Doppman J, Ommaya AK: Selective arteriography of arteriovenous aneurysms of spinal cord. Radiology 88:1065, 1967
29. Djindjian R, Faure C, Houdart R, et al: Exploration angiographique des malformations vasculaires de la moelle epiniere. Acta Radiol (Diagn) 5:145, 1966
30. Djindjian R: Arteriography of the spinal cord. Am J Roentgenol Radium Ther Nucl Med 107:461, 1969
31. Cogen P, Stein BM: Spinal cord arteriovenous malformations with significant intramedullary components. J Neurosurg 59:471, 1983
32. Bergstrand A, Hook O, Lidvall H: Vascular malformations of the spinal cord. Acta Neurol Scand 40:169, 1964
33. Wyburn-Masson R: The Vascular Abnormalities and Tumors of the Spinal Cord and Its Membranes. London, Krimptom, 1943
34. Luessenhop AJ, Dela Cruz T: Surgical excision of spinal intradural vascular malformations. J Neurosurg 30:552, 1969
35. Ommaya AK, DiChiro G, Doppman, JL: Ligation of arterial supply in the treatment of spinal cord arteriovenous malformations. J Neurosurg 30:679, 1969
36. Krayenbuhl H, Yasargil MG, McClintock HG: Treatment of spinal cord vascular malformations by surgical excision. J Neurosurg 30:427, 1969
37. Doppman JL: The nidus concept for spinal cord arteriovenous

malformations. A surgical recommendation based on angiographic observations. Br J Radiol 44:758, 1971

38. Malis LI: Microsurgery for spinal cord arteriovenous malformations. Clin Neurosurg 26:543, 1979

39. Aminoff MJ, Logue V: Clinical features of spinal vascular malformations. Brain 97:197, 1974

40. Aminoff MJ, Logue V: The prognosis of patients with spinal vascular malformations. Brain 97:211, 1974

41. Herdt JR, DiChiro G, Doppman JL: Combined arterial and arteriovenous aneurysms of the spinal cord. Radiology 99:589, 1971

42. Houdart R, Djindjian R, Hurth M: Vascular malformations of the spinal cord; the anatomic and therapeutic significance of arteriography. J Neurosurg 24:583, 1966

43. Kaufman HH, Ommaya AK, DiChiro G, et al: Compression vs. "steal." The pathogenesis of symptoms in arteriovenous malformations of the spinal cord. Arch Neurol 23:173, 1970

44. Djindjian M, Djindjian R, Hurth M, et al: Steal phenomenon in spinal arteriovenous malformations. J Neuroradiol 5:187, 1978

45. Matthews WB: The spinal bruit. Lancet 2:1117, 1959

46. Doppman JL, Wirth FP Jr, DiChiro G, et al: Value of cutaneous angiomas in the arteriographic localization of spinal cord arteriovenous malformations. N Engl J Med 281:1440, 1969

47. Yasargil MG: Diagnosis and treatment of spinal cord arteriovenous malformations. Prog Neurol Surg 4:355, 1971

48. DiChiro G, Doppman J L, Wener L: Computed tomography of spinal arteriovenous malformations. Radiology 123:351, 1977

49. Kasdon DL, Wolpert SM, Stein BM: Surgical and angiographic localization of spinal arteriovenous malformations. Surg Neurol 5:279, 1976

50. Berenstein A, Young W, Ransohoff J, et al: Somatosensory evoked potentials during spinal angiography and therapeutic transvascular embolization. J Neurosurg 60:777, 1984

51. Doppman J L, DiChiro G, Ommaya AK: Percutaneous embolization of spinal cord arteriovenous malformations. J Neurosurg 34:48, 1971

52. Hilal SK, Sane P, Michelson WJ, et al: The embolization of vascular malformations of the spinal cord with low-viscosity silicone rubber. Neuroradiology 16:430, 1978

53. Djindjian R: Embolization of angiomas of the spinal cord. Surg Neurol 4:411, 1975

54. Kunc Z, Bret J: Diagnosis and treatment of vascular malformations of the spinal cord. J Neurosurg 30:436, 1969

55. Yasargil RW, DeLong WB, Guarnaschelli JJ: Complete microsurgical excision of cervical extramedullary and intramedullary vascular malformations. Surg Neurol 4:211, 1975

56. Latchaw TW, Harris RD, Chou Sn, et al: Combined embolization and operation in the treatment of cervical arteriovenous malformations. Neurosurgery 6:131, 1980

57. Oldfield EH, DiChiro G, Quindlen EA, et al: Successful treatment of a group of spinal cord arteriovenous malformations by interruption of dura fistula. J Neurosurg 59:1019, 1983

58. Bailey WL, Sperl MP: Angiomas of the cervical spinal cord. J Neurosurg 30:560, 1969

59. Baker HL Jr, Love JG, Layton DD Jr: Angiographic and surgical aspects of spinal cord vascular anomalies. Radiology 88:1078, 1967

CHAPTER 130
Spinal Deformities Following Neurosurgical Procedures in Children

Edwin G. Fischer   John E. Hall

IATROGENIC INTERFERENCE with the normal development of the spine is an important consideration in pediatric neurosurgery. Deformities can be induced experimentally by surgical, radiation, or metabolic injury to neural, bony, ligamentous or muscular portions of the spine.[1-6] In children, deformities of the spine can be a major problem either before or after surgery for spinal tumors, trauma, malformations, and syringomyelia or following placement of a lumbar shunt. Seventy-five percent of patients with myelomeningocele develop kyphoscoliosis. In some the curvature is the only manifestation of hydromyelia related to untreated hydrocephalus or an obstructed shunt.

RADIOLOGY

Detailed reviews of radiology of the spine of children can be found in the works of Caffey[7] and of Harwood-Nash and Fitz.[8] Posterior arches may appear bifid up until 3 years of age when the ossification centers of the laminae fuse. Lines of delayed or incomplete fusion of ossification centers may be mistaken for fractures. Bony fusion of the lateral masses to the bodies is not completed until a child is 6 or 7 years old. The odontoid does not fuse with the body of C2 until late childhood. There is also greater mobility of the cervical spine in children, compared with adults. Up to 3 mm of movement may be seen normally at C2-C3, and up to 3 or 4 mm between the odontoid and C1.

As in adults, the selection of special imaging procedures will depend on the nature of the specific problem at hand. Magnetic resonance imaging is of increasing value and availability. Myelography is presently performed using nonionic, water-soluble contrast media[9,10] and polytomographic or computed tomographic (CT) scanning. General anesthesia is usually required for children under 10 years of age and prophylactic anticonvulsants are generally give for 24 hours.

INTRASPINAL TUMORS AND RADIATION THERAPY

Tachdjian and Matson were among the first to draw attention to progressive kyphosis and scoliosis following laminectomy for intraspinal tumors in children.[11] Their observations have been confirmed and elaborated upon by others.[12-20] In 117 children spinal deformities were present in 17 patients at initial examination and developed in 26 other following laminectomy. Deformities were more likely in children under 2 years of age or when laminectomy was performed over more than 3 levels. Five patients required fusion. The combination of neurologic deficit, loss of support by posterior elements, and radiation-induced arrest of growth of the vertebral bodies is a triple threat to stability of the spine. If the kyphosis is allowed to progress beyond 50 degrees, combined anterior and posterior stabilization may become necessary.

Fraser did not note an increase in spinal deformity after radiation of spinal tumors in children.[16] Trachdjian and Matson felt it was a significant factor in their patients,[11] however, and it has been well documented that radiation alone and in the absence of neurologic deficit frequently causes changes in vertebral growth that may result in pronounced spinal deformity, especially in children under the age of 2 years.[1,21-26] Spinal fusion may be more problematic after radiation.[27] Bracing is useless in this group of patients and delay in considering surgery leads to the necessity of more complex procedures to correct and stabilize the spine.

INCREASED RISK OF CERVICAL DEFORMITIES

There is a special propensity for spinal deformity following cervical laminectomy (Figures 130-1 and 130-2).[13,16,28,29] Some authors have even considered posterolateral cervical fusion at the time of laminectomy in certain patients,[13,30] rather than waiting for the deformity to occur.[31] Cervical and craniocervical instability are also seen without surgery in conditions such as congenital anomalies of the odontoid, direct and nearby infection, mucopolysaccharidoses, Down's syndrome, rheumatoid arthritis, and trauma.[19,31-40] Both anterior and posterior fusions are employed to manage cervical deformities[13,31,37,41] and in some instances anterior-transoral or posterior decompression are required.[35,38,42-44]

PREVENTION OF DEFORMITY AND POSTOPERATIVE MANAGEMENT

Intraoperative measures that may decrease the risk of subsequent deformity include subperiosteal exposure of the posterior elements, which in the very young will allow considerable reformation of bone; simultaneous fusion during cervical laminectomy, as mentioned above; preservation of facet joints[17]; and en-bloc removal and replacement of laminae.[45,46] The latter involves

OPERATIVE NEUROSURGICAL TECHNIQUES
ISBN 0-8089-1862-1

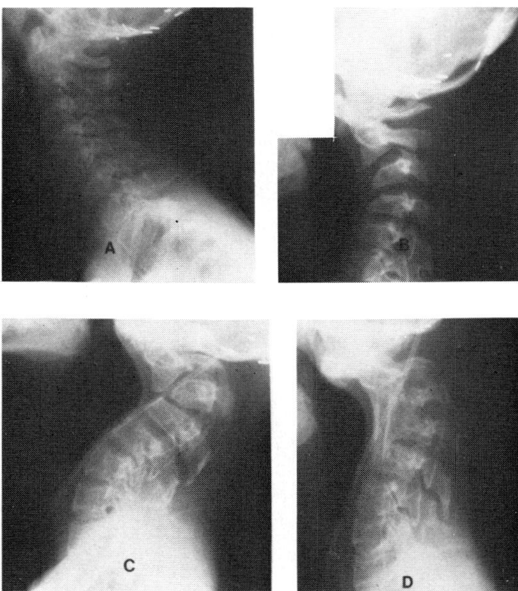

Fig. 130-1.   At 5 months of age this boy was noted to have communicating hydrocephalus. Because the fourth ventricle could not be filled with air at ventriculography, the posterior fossa was explored, leaving C1 intact. A large cisterna magna was found and it was specifically noted that an Arnold-Chiari malformation did not exist. A lumboureteral shunt was inserted and the patient did well until 9 years of age, when he developed bilateral spinal accessory nerve palsies, a spastic quadriparesis and hypalgesia bilaterally in the dermatomes of C2 to C4. Suspecting a tumor, the posterior fossa was re-explored and a laminectomy from C1 to C4 performed. The cerebellar tonsils were found to have descended to the level of C2, and adhesions were present between the spinal cord and dura. Although the upper cervical cord was widened, fluid could not be aspirated from it. It is presumed that the lumbar shunt created a pressure gradient from the intracranial to the spinal compartment, resulting in displacement of the cerebellar tonsils through the foramen magnum, obstruction of the outlets of the fourth ventricle and a syrinx.[24] His neurologic condition stabilized, but repeated episodes of meningitis and shunt malfunction led to a revision, a ventriculoureteral, and eventually to a ventriculoperitoneal shunt. Eight years after the second exploration of the posterior fossa and upper cervical laminectomy, he developed increasing weakness, and a severe cervical kyphosis was noted. This was treated by a transoral anterior decompression of C2 through C4 and anterior fusion using iliac bone. He has remained unchanged neurologically over the subsequent 4 years. The figure shows: (A) a roentgenogram of the cervical spine 1 year before cervical laminectomy; (B) a roentgenogram 1 year after cervical laminectomy; (C) a roentgenogram 7 years after cervical laminectomy; and (D) a roentgenogram 1 year after anterior decompression and fusion.

cutting the chosen laminae on either side medial to the facets. The interspinous ligaments above and below the laminectomy are divided in such a way that they can be reapproximated during closure. The interspinous and yellow ligaments between the segments to be removed are preserved. The entire mass is secured in place at the end of the procedure by sutures in the interspinous ligaments above and below and by sutures from the laminae to the lateral masses laterally. The spine is immobilized until fusion of the "laminotomy" is demonstrated by x-ray study. The extent to which deformities can be prevented or reduced by intraoperative measures remains uncertain and patients should continue to be followed closely for subsequent spine deformity regardless of the operative technique used.

Early recognition of developing deformity will minimize eventual treatment, although nonoperative methods are rarely effective. Bracing generally provides only temporary control of curvature and then often at the expense of pressure scores or distorted mandibular growth. In the neck, bracing is particularly ineffective in supporting paralytic spine or arresting progressive curvature.

SPINAL COMPLICATIONS OF LUMBAR SHUNTS

Spinal deformities and nerve root irritation can occur in as many as 25 percent of patients following lumboureteral or lumboperitoneal shunts, especially when polyethylene tubing is used.[47,48] The extent of the laminectomy does not seem to be related.[48] The use of Silastic tubing may decrease the problem.[47,49] Even with this material, root irritation and spine deformity may occur (Figure 130-3). Root irritation may subside following the removal or replacement of the lumbar tubing.[49] Syringomyelia presenting as scoliosis also can occur many years after lumbar shunting, probably the result of caudal migration of the cerebellar tonsils because of the pressure gradient created by the shunt between the intracranial and the spinal compartments (see Figure 130-1), causing an acquired Chiari I "malformation."[50,51] All children with lumbar shunts should be considered at risk for syringomyelia and spinal curvature.

SPINAL DEFORMITIES AND HYDROMYELIA IN MYELOMENINGOCELE PATIENTS WITH MALFUNCTIONING SHUNTS

Hall, reporting on 11 cases, contended that scoliosis is a common clinical manifestation of hydromyelia in myelomeningocele patients with unshunted hydrocephalus or an otherwise asymptomatic malfunctioning shunt.[52] In 7 patients the curvature improved after shunting. Winston et al. noted the danger of ligating the spinal dura before resecting nonfunctioning spinal cord in the course of kyphosis surgery in meningomyelocele

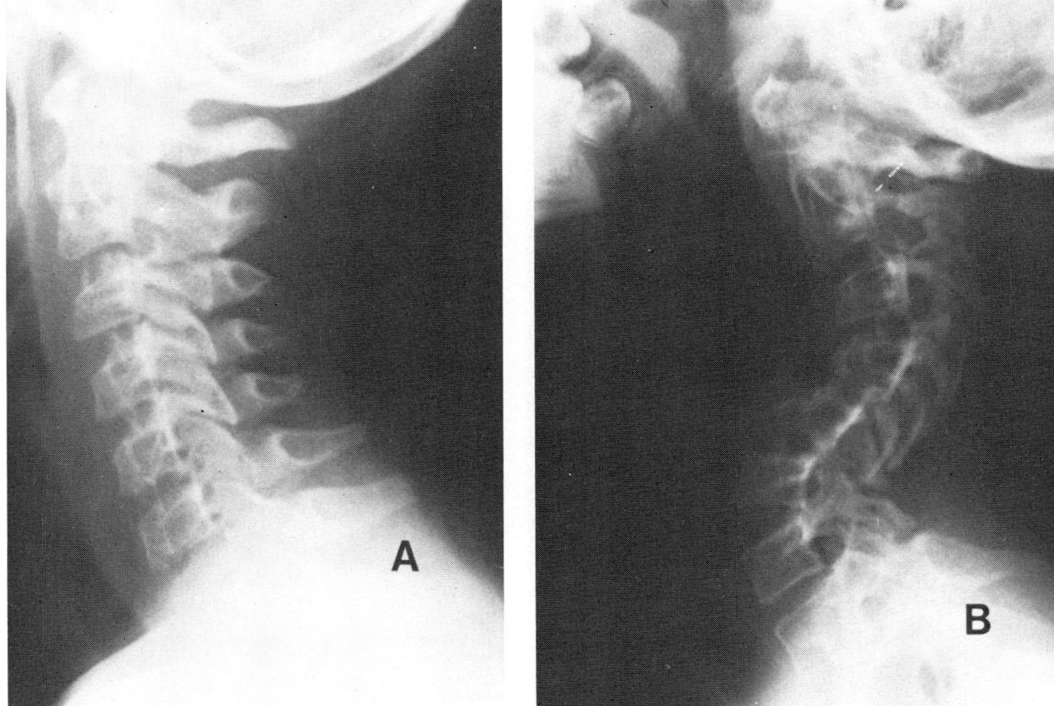

Fig. 130-2. The cervical spine before (A) and 1 year after (B) laminectomy from C1 through C7, biopsy, and radiation (4860 rad) for a grade II astrocytoma of the cervical spinal cord in an 11 year-old-girl. Initially she had a 3-week history of rapidly progressing, severe left arm and leg weakness that were unchanged after treatment. During the 2 months before detection of the deformity she developed weakness of the right arm and an increased sensory deficit. The tumor was re-explored and an intramedullary cyst fenestrated. Her neck is supported by a brace, and if tumor growth appears arrested, a fusion will be considered.

patients.[53] Intracranial pressure may become elevated acutely and a cardiorespiratory arrest may occur if the patient has an asymptomatic malfunctioning shunt and is using the central canal as a conduit for cerebrospinal fluid. It is advisable to divide the cord intradurally and close the dura in a generous pouch over the cut end of the cord.

SURGICAL TREATMENT OF THORACIC AND LUMBAR SPINAL DEFORMITIES

The principles of management of spinal deformities are complex and beyond the scope of this chapter. Reviews of the subject can be found in such monographs as that by Moe and colleagues.[54]

The timing of fusion operations is important. Fusion masses do not grow and deformities may worsen significantly during growth spurts. When a fusion must be performed over many segments, as not infrequently occurs in patients with idiopathic or paralytic scoliosis, it is often desirable to delay surgery until the patient reaches 10 years of age to allow maximum growth. Attempts to "buy time" with bracing must be monitored closely and failure to control progression of the deformity is a signal to abandon bracing and recommend surgery, regardless of age. Early operations often are preferable in progressive congenital kyphosis or lordosis because of the possibility of a better result with a limited early procedure, or in radiation-induced kyphosis where there is a high failure rate because of poor bone substance. In unilateral defects of segmentation (unilateral bars) there is no possibility of longitudinal growth of the affected segment. Growth of the "normal side"

causes only increased deformity, not lengthening of the spine. Serious and progressive spinal deformity and pain frequently follow thoracolumbar fractures that have been subjected to laminectomy without stabilization. Early reduction of deformity and internal fixation by such methods as Harrington instrumentation currently are considered to give the best chance for root recovery, protection of cord function, and permanent spinal stability.[54]

The type of procedure selected depends on many factors, and more than one procedure may be required. When there is an anterior compression of the spinal cord, as in a sharply angulated kyphosis, anterior decompression is necessary. Anterior release by osteotomy and anterior fusion with inlay grafts is the preferred procedure for kyphosis following multiple-level laminectomy, and frequently is used in radiation kyphosis, supplemented by Harrington compression rod stabilization posteriorly. Harrington rod instrumentation may be used to provide corrective distraction and may add internal stabilization to many fusions, thereby permitting ambulation in a brace or cast without loss of correction. Lateral curvatures may be corrected by the Dwyer method, which includes lateral compression of the vertebral bodies by a cable apparatus fixed in place with screws, but it is contraindicated in the presence of a kyphosis. The Dwyer method has its best use in patients with deficiencies of the posterior spinal elements, as in myelodysplasia.

Recent developments in the stabilization of spinal deformities have included the use of sublaminar or spinous process wires[55] associated with either Harrington or Luque rods.[56] The use of these supplemental wires has enabled the operating surgeon to obtain greater stability from the metallic implants, so

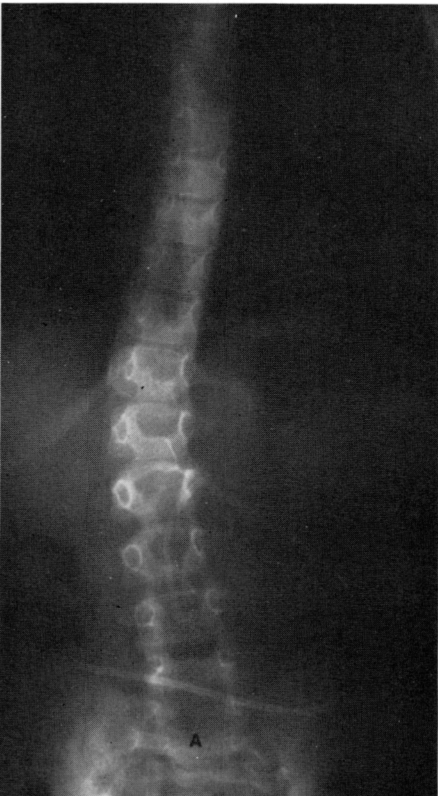
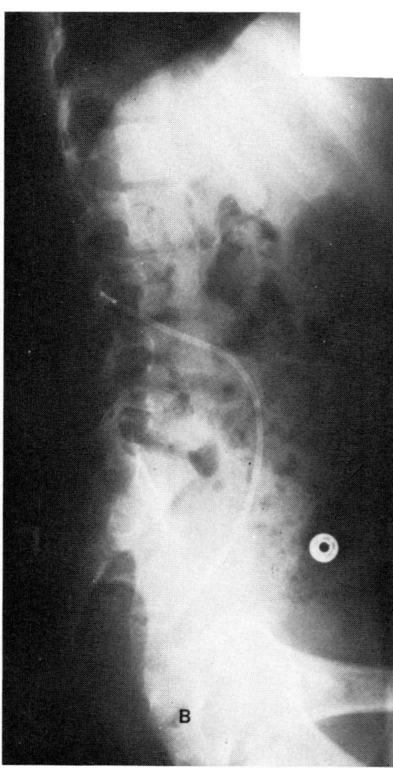

Fig. 130-3. This 10-year-old boy with Apert's syndrome had a lumboperitoneal shunt with Silastic tubing inserted at 2.5 years of age for communicating hydrocephalus. A moderate scoliosis was noted at 10 years of age when he developed distal weakness in his legs and loss of ankle reflexes. The lumbar shunt was removed and a ventricular shunt inserted, but this could not be maintained because of small ventricles. A new lumbar shunt was inserted using tapered Silastic tubing. His strength has returned but the scoliosis remains.

that many patients can be treated in the postoperative period without outside support by either casts or braces.

An even more recent development from France, known as the Cotrel-Dubousset system of spinal instrumentation provides even more intrinsic stability and has several types of implants that are useful in the management of idiopathic scoliosis but also in the management of fractures.[57]

It is extremely important that once the deformity has become established or it is apparent that a deformity is inevitable, the orthopedic surgeon who attempts to repair it is familiar with the use of all current methods of instrumentation, because each of them has its specific merits and only a surgeon familiar with all of them can decide which is best for any individual patient.

Neurologic deficits can result from Harrington rod distraction in patients with unyielding congenital kyphosis or when the cord is tethered, as in myelomeningocele, diastematomyelia, or thickened filum terminale. A tethered cord must be released before an associated spinal curvature is corrected. Neurologic deficits from operative traction on the spine often can recover to a significant degree if they are considered to be true surgical emergencies and the traction apparatus is removed immediately. Spinal cord deficits can be detected intraoperatively by awakening the patient to test lower extremity function[58] or by monitoring posterior column function by cortical or spinal somatosensory evoked potentials.[59–62] During anterior operations, neurologic complications can occur because of direct damage to or subsequent thrombosis of the anterior spinal artery, or more rarely, because of interruption of the segmental vessels to the cord. If these vessels are ligated in the midline, vascular anastomoses provide adequate collateral circulation. Problems may arise if the final common pathway is interrupted within or near the intervertebral foramen.

REFERENCES

1. Arkin AM, Simon N: Radiation scoliosis, an experimental study. J Bone Joint Surg 32A:396, 1950
2. Hass SL: Experimental production of scoliosis. J Bone Joint Surg 21:963, 1939
3. Langenskiold A, Michelsson JE: The pathogenesis of experimental progressive scoliosis. Acta Orthop Scand [[]Supp[]] 59, 1962
4. Liszka O: Spinal cord mechanisms leading to scoliosis in experimental animals. Acta Med Pol 2:45, 1961
5. Ponsetti IV, Shepard RS: Lesions of the skeleton and of other mesodermal tissues in rats fed sweet-pea (Lathyrus odoratus) seeds. J Bone Joint Surg 36A:1031, 1954
6. Schwartzmann JR, Miles M: Experimental production of scoliosis in rats and mice. J Bone Joint Surg 27:59, 1945
7. Caffey J: Pediatric X-Ray Diagnosis, ed 6. Chicago, Yearbook, 1972
8. Harwood-Nash DC, Fitz CR: Neuroradiology in Infants and Children. St. Louis, CV Mosby, 1976
9. Wolf GL: Safer, more expensive iodinated contrast agents: How do we decide? Radiology 159:557, 1986
10. White RI, Halden WJ Jr: Liquid gold: Low-osmolality contrast media. Radiology 159:559, 1986

11. Tachdjian ME, Matson DD: Orthopedic aspects of intraspinal tumors in infants and children. J Bone Joint Surg 47A:225, 1965

12. Audic B, Maury M: Secondary vertebral deformities in childhood and adolescence. Paraplegia 7:11, 1969

13. Cattell HS, Clark GL: Cervical kyphosis and instability following multiple laminectomies in children. J Bone Joint Surg 49A:713, 1967

14. Citron N, Edgar MA, Sheehy J, et al: Intramedullary spinal cord tumors presenting as scoliosis. J Bone Joint Surg 66:513, 1984

15. DeSousa AL, Kalsbeck JE, Mealy J, et al: Intraspinal tumors in children. A review of 81 cases. J Neurosurg 51:437, 1979

16. Fraser RD, Paterson DC, Simpson DA: Orthopedic aspects of spinal tumours in children. J Bone Joint Surg 59B:143, 1977

17. Lonstein J E: Post-laminectomy kyphosis. Clin Orthop 128:93, 1977

18. Reimer R, Onofrio BM: Astrocytomas of the spinal cord in children and adolescents. J Neurosurg 63:669, 1985

19. Sim FH, Svien HJ, Bickel WH, et al: Swan neck deformity following extensive cervical laminectomy. A review of twenty-one cases. J Bone Joint Surg 56A:564, 1974

20. Zajtchuk R, Bowen TE, Seyfer AE, et al: Intrathoracic ganglioneuroblastoma. J Thorac Cardiovasc Surg 80:605, 1980

21. Delinka MK, Mazzeo VR Jr: Complications of radiation therapy. CRC Crit Rev Diagn Imaging 23:235, 1985

22. Katzman H, Wauhg T, Berdon W: Skeletal changes following irradiation of childhood tumors. J Bone Joint Surg 51A:825, 1969

23. Neuhauser EBD, Wittenborg MA, Berman CZ, et al: Irradiation effects of roentgen therapy on the growing spine. Radiology 59:637, 1952

24. Riseborough EJ: Irradiation induced kyphosis. Clin Orthop 128:101, 1977

25. Smith R, Davidson JK, Flatman GE: Skeletal effects of orthovoltage and megavoltage therapy following treatment of nephroblastoma. Clin Radiol 33:601, 1982

26. Thomas PR, Griffith KD, Fineberg BB, et al: Late effects of treatment for Wilms' tumor. Int J Radiat Oncol Biol Phys 9:651, 1983

27. King J, Stowe S: Results of spinal fusion for radiation scoliosis. Spine 7:574, 1982

28. Daussange J, Rigault P, Renier D, et al: Instability and kyphosis following cervical laminectomy in children. Rev Chir Orthop 66:423, 1980

29. Taddonio RF Jr, King AG: Atlantoaxial rotatory fixation after decompressive laminectomy. A case report. Spine 7:540, 1982

30. Callahan RA, Johnson RM, Margolis RN, et al: Cervical facet fusion for control of instability following laminectomy. J Bone Joint Surg 59A:991, 1977

31. Holmes JC, Hall JE: Fusion for instability and potential instability of the cervical spine in children and adolescents. Orthop Clin North Am 9:923, 1978

32. Aung MH: Atlanto-axial dislocation in Down's syndrome. Report of a case with spinal cord compression and review of the literature. Bull Los Angeles Neurol Soc 38:197, 1973

33. Blaw ME, Langer LO: Spinal cord compression in Morquio-Brailsford's disease. J Pediatr 74:593, 1969

34. Brill CB, Rose JS, Godmilow MSW, et al: Spastic quadriparesis due to C1-C2 subluxation in Hurler syndrome. J Pediatr 92:441, 1978

35. Kaplan RJ: Neurological complications of infections of head and neck. Otolaryngol Clin North Am 9:729, 1976

36. Malik GM, Crawford AH, Halter R: Swan-neck deformity secondary to osteomyelitis of the posterior elements of the cervical spine. Case report. J Neurosurg 50:388, 1979

37. McWhorter JM, Alexander E, Davis CH, et al: Posterior cervical fusion in children. J Neurosurg 45:211, 1976

38. Menezes AH, Van Gilder JC, Graf CJ, et al: Craniocervical abnormalities: A comprehensive approach. J Neurosurg 53:444, 1980

39. Nathan FF, Bickel WH: Spontaneous axial subluxation in a child as a first sign of juvenile rheumatoid arthritis. J Bone Joint Surg 50A:1675, 1968

40. Sherk HH, Nicholson JT: Rotatory atlanto-axial dislocation associated with ossiculum terminale and mongolism. A case report. J Bone Joint Surg 51A:957, 1964

41. Roy L, Gibson DA: Cervical spine fusions in children. Clin Orthop 73:146, 1970

42. Gilsbach J, Eggert HR: Transoral operations for craniospinal malformations. Neurosurg Rev 61:199, 1983

43. Hall JE, Dennis F, Murray J: Exposure of the upper cervical spine for spinal decompression by a mandible and tongue splitting approach. J Bone Joint Surg 59A:121, 1977

44. Lesoin F, Jomin M, Pellerin P, Pruvo JP, Carini S, Servato R, Rousseaux M: Transclival transcervical approach to the upper cervical spine and clivus. Acta Neurochir 80:100, 1986

45. Hulme A, Dott NM: Spinal epidural abscess. Br Med J 1:64, 1954

46. Raimondi AJ, Gutierrez FA, DiRocco C: Laminotomy and total reconstruction of the posterior spinal arch for spinal canal surgery in childhood. J Neurosurg 45:555, 1976

47. Hoffman HJ, Hendrick EB, Humphreys RP: New lumboperitoneal shunt for communicating hydrocephalus. Technical note. J Neurosurg 44:258, 1976

48. Kushner J, Alexander E, Davis CH, et al: Kyphoscoliosis following lumbar subarachnoid shunts. J Neurosurg 34:783, 1971

49. Eisenberg HM, Davidson RI, Shillito J: Lumboperitoneal shunts. Review of 34 cases. J Neurosurg 35:427, 1971

50. Fischer EG, Welch K, Shillito J: Syringomyelia following lumboureteral shunting for communicating hydrocephalus. J Neurosurg 47:96, 1977

51. Welch K, Shillito J, Strand R, et al: Chiari I "malformation"—an acquired disorder? J Neurosurg 55:604, 1981

52. Hall P, Lindseth R, Campbell R, et al: Scoliosis and hydrocephalus in myelocele patients. J Neurosurg 50:174, 1979

53. Winston K, Hall J, Johnson D, et al: Acute elevation of intracranial pressure following transection of non-functional spinal cord. Clin Orthop 128:41, 1977

54. Moe J H, Winter RB, Bradford DS, et al: Scoliosis and Other Spinal Deformities. Philadelphia, WB Saunders, 1978

55. Drummond D, Guadagno J, Keene JS, et al: Interspinous process segmental spinal instrumentation. J Ped Orthop 4:397, 1984

56. Luque ER: Segmental spinal instrumentation for correction of scoliosis. Clin Orthop 163:192, 1982

57. Cotrel Y, Dubousset J: Personal communication

58. Hall JE, Levine CR, Sudhir KG: Intraoperative awakening to monitor spinal cord function during Harrington instrumentation and spine fusion. Description of procedure and report of three cases. J Bone Joint Surg 60A:533, 1978

59. Allen AR, Starr A: Sensory evoked potentials in the operating room. Neurology 27:358, 1977

60. Cohen AR, Young W, Ransohoff J: Intraspinal localization of the somatosensory evoked potential. Neurosurgery 9:157, 1981

61. Machida M, Weinstein SL, Yamada T, et al: Spinal cord monitoring. Electrophysiological measures of sensory and motor function during spinal surgery. Spine 10:407, 1985

62. Mostegl A, Bauer R: The application of somatosensory-evoked potentials in orthopedic spine surgery. Arch Orthop Trauma Surg 103:179, 1984

CHAPTER 131

Metastatic Tumors of the Spine

Eugene A. Quindlen

INCREASINGLY, neurosurgeons are asked to evaluate and treat patients with metastatic tumors of the central nervous system. As the average age of the population increases and the prevalence of cancer increases, this trend is likely to continue. The increased use of chemotherapy and other adjuvant therapy for cancer also may increase the numbers of patients who survive to develop metastatic cancer to the spine. Approximately 5 percent of all cancer patients will develop metastatic tumors to the spine.[1] Since most of these patients have an evolving paraparesis or other neurologic syndrome, there is often great anxiety surrounding their care and treatment. The neurosurgeon should know not only what surgical treatment can offer, but also what medical treatment can offer these patients.

RADIATION THERAPY VERSUS SURGERY

Several retrospective studies of patients with spinal metastases[1] and a recent small prospective study[2] have indicated that radiation therapy alone achieves results equal to or superior to either surgery alone or surgery and radiation therapy. These studies, however, combine patients with many different types of tumors and different types of clinical presentation, which makes it difficult to draw clear indications for the type of treatment to be instituted. At the same time it is also clear that the clinical result depends most on the type of tumor and the neurologic condition of the patient before treatment, regardless of the mode of therapy.

Radiation therapy is clearly the treatment of choice for all tumors that are highly sensitive to radiation, such as lymphoma, Ewing's sarcoma, myeloma, and neuroblastoma, even in the presence of spinal block or paraplegia. The treatment should be instituted immediately on an emergency basis. Most other cancers are radiation sensitive to some degree and should be treated with radiation therapy as long as there appears to be any beneficial effect.

Despite the apparent usefulness of radiation therapy, there are several clinical situations in which surgery should be considered as the optimal therapy:

1. To achieve a histologic diagnosis in a patient without a known primary tumor.
2. To decompress a known radioresistant tumor.
3. To decompress the spinal cord of the patient who is deteriorating neurologically during radiation therapy.
4. To decompress the spinal cord compressed by bony encroachment of the canal caused by vertebral body collapse or displacement.
5. To decompress the spinal cord with recurrent tumor in an area with previous maximal irradiation.

If the neurologic condition permits, a metastatic work-up can be instituted in the patient who has a spinal metastasis and unknown primary tumor. The surgeon should determine if the patient has previously received radiation therapy for the primary tumor or other metastatic lesion; if this radiation was not effective in reducing tumor growth, surgery should be performed to decompress a spinal metastasis. Certain tumors are known for their relative radioresistance, such as prostatic carcinoma and renal cell carcinoma. Occasionally these tumors do respond to radiation, however, and this may be tried if the patient's neurologic condition permits. Otherwise, surgical decompression of epidural tumors is warranted if the patient has severe pain or is rapidly developing paraparesis.

It is felt that in some cases of epidural tumor, the tumor swells and increases its bulk during radiation therapy. This would explain why some patients begin to deteriorate rapidly after radiation therapy has been instituted. Surgical decompression may be of benefit in that situation. Although the neurologic decline of most patients is directly related to the presence of an epidural tumor, the surgeon should be alert to the possibility that a few patients have their spinal cords compromised by a collapsed vertebral body that has been displaced posteriorly into the spinal canal. This mechanical compromise of the canal will obviously not be relieved by radiation, and surgical decompression may be required.

CLINICAL PRESENTATION

The clinical presentation of a patient with a spinal tumor metastasis is fairly typical and was well characterized by Wright.[3] The patient first experiences vague back pain or local root pain. This symptom may precede the onset of neurologic deficit by weeks to months and is such a constant finding that cancer patients with this first symptom should be regarded as having a spinal metastasis until it is proven otherwise. Since the results of treatment so heavily depend on the early recognition and treatment of the spinal metastasis, this symptom must be recognized as important by any physician caring for cancer patients. Motor weakness is the next stage in the illness. it is often subtle and not recognized initially in a patient who is already ill and weak. The patient may notice increased difficulty in getting out of a chair or climbing stairs, or may experience unsteadiness while walking. The patient who goes to bed because of back pain may feel that he or she is weaker because of the bed rest.

OPERATIVE NEUROSURGICAL TECHNIQUES
ISBN 0-8089-1862-1

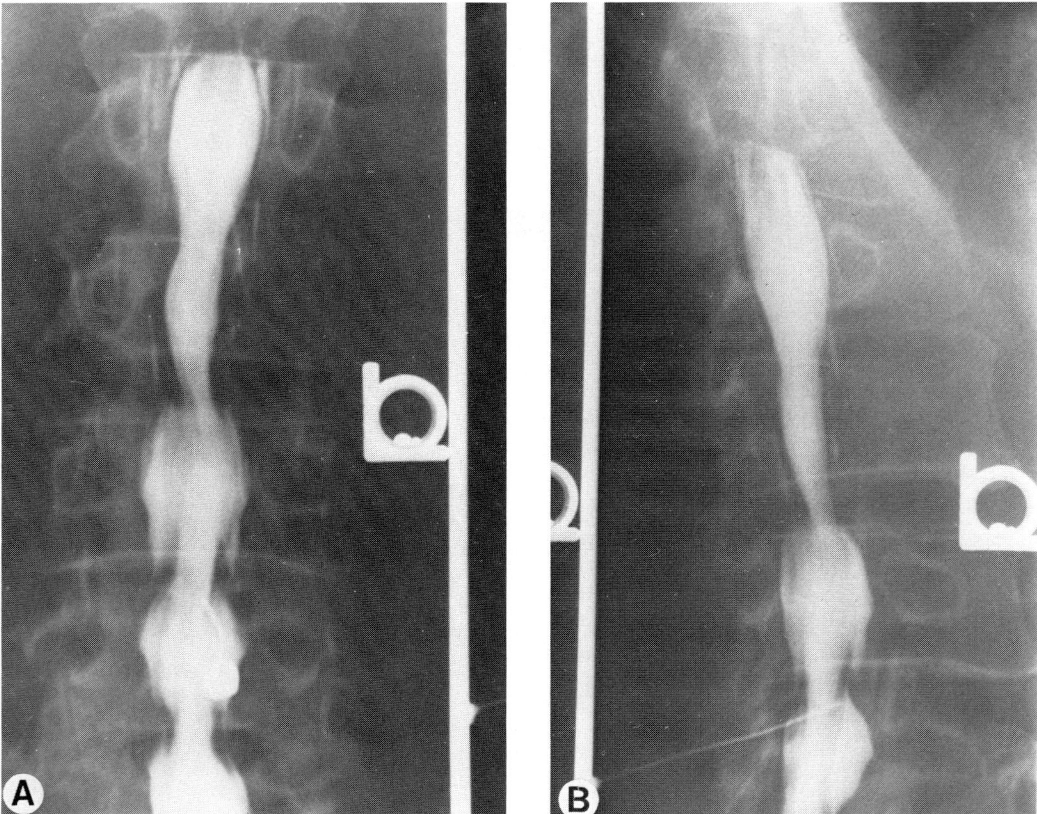

Fig. 131-1. Anteroposterior (A) and oblique (B) lumbar Pantopaque myelograms of a patient with root pain and metastatic breast cancer. Note the hour-glass configuration of the thecal sac caused by lumbar spondylosis. The absent pedicle and the compression of L3, however, are the clues for metastatic involvement of the spine.

Although the initial motor loss may be subtle and gradual, the next stage of the illness tends to evolve over a matter of a few days. The patient notices daily decreases in the strength in the lower extremities, and about the time the patient can no longer walk, he or she begins to develop numbness in the distal extremities. Bladder or bowel incontinence rapidly follows, which heralds complete physiologic transection of the spinal cord.

When the surgeon sees the patient for the first time, it is important to do a careful neurologic examination so that the surgeon can arrive at some impression of the stage the patient's illness has progressed to and what level of the spinal column is affected. In a patient with a single metastasis, local percussion tenderness may locate the affected level of the spine. In testing muscle power, one finds that the hip flexors usually are the most prominently affected group. Careful examination of the skin with a pin may demonstrate a sensory level or a dermatomal sensory loss. The abdomen should be examined for a distended bladder and the anal sphincter checked for tone.

In general, a few tests that are repeated often will give the surgeon a clear idea of the progress of the patient's illness. The majority of patients have myelopathic signs referable to the lower extremities in both cervical and thoracic tumors. Cauda equina compression may be similar in presentation to an early cord compression, and because the latter can progress much more rapidly and with more irreversible potential, early radiologic evaluation should be instituted regardless of the clinical diagnosis. Roughly two thirds of the patients will have metastatic tumors in the thoracic region, while the remainder are divided between the cervical and lumbar areas.

RADIOLOGIC INVESTIGATIONS

Radiologic procedures that are performed properly are crucial in understanding the location and extent of the patient's disease as well as the best approach to treatment. Early in the course of spinal metastasis, radionuclide scanning of the spinal column may be the most sensitive technique available to detect the presence of tumor. If the tumor is confined to the epidural space, however, and has not involved the bony vertebra, bone scan and plain roentgenograms of the spine may be negative. Consequently, even in patients who only have back pain or root pain, myelography should be the next step. Bone scans and roentgenograms of the spine, however, should not be omitted since these studies may alert the surgeon and radiotherapist to other areas of the spine that may require treatment and that may not be seen in myelography.

The plain roentgenograms of the spine may disclose vertebral collapse or, characteristically, the destruction of a pedicle (Figure 131-1). In the case of palpable tumors of the paravertebral soft tissues, the plain x-ray film can nicely demonstrate the extent of local invasion of the bony spinous process (Figure 131-2). If the plain x-ray films show vertebral collapse or instability, polytomography should be performed to assess the diameter of the spinal canal and the extent of bony destruction.

The introduction of ''fourth-generation'' computed tomography (CT) scanners with bone-review options has allowed the physician to scrutinize the spine and its associated soft tissue structures on the same scan. In this mode the section is scanned with the normal window width up to 300 and the high-density window up to 4000; both can be presented on the same scan.

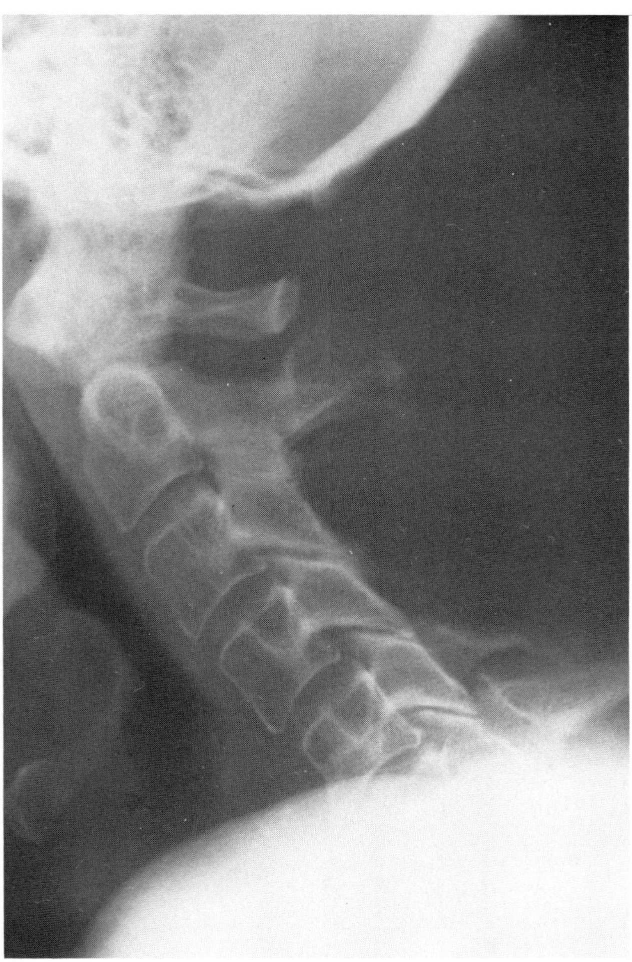

Fig. 131-2. A plain roentgenogram of the lateral cervical spine of a patient with a locally invasive sarcoma of the neck, showing extensive destruction of the spinous processes and lamina.

This allows detailed examination of the bone structure and the soft tissue, as demonstrated in Figure 131-3.

Magnetic resonance imaging (MRI) is a new tool which allows noninvasive imaging of the spine and the contents of the spinal canal. Although the images obtained do not correlate with a tissue's traditional x-ray density, changes in tissue structure can be detected and imaged. The ability to quickly obtain sagittal images of the spine, thecal sac, and spinal cord makes MRi a technique that can rival traditional myelography in the evacuation of patients with spinal cord and epidural lesions. Magnetic resonance imaging is increasingly becoming the initial procedure of choice for evaluating the patient with a suspected spinal lesion and can replace myelography in those situations in which the tumor can be adequately imaged (Figure 131-4).

Myelography is a most important investigation to pursue in patients with spinal metastasis, as it is in patients with primary intraspinal tumors. It should be considered even in patients with back pain or root pain only, since it may disclose disease much more extensive than suspected by clinical examination or routine radionuclide scanning (Figure 131-5).

The most widely used form of myelography is Pantopaque fluorography. When a spinal block is suspected, as in a patient with a progressing myelopathy, 2 to 3 ml of Pantopaque is instilled into the subarachnoid space via a lumbar needle (Figure 131-6). If no block is found, more Pantopaque can be instilled to obtain adequate visualization of the thecal sac. In a patient who has a complete block to the dye column, or is suspected of having a lumbar epidural tumor, a C1-C2 lateral cervical puncture of the subarachnoid space is used to introduce the contrast agent. Instilling the dye in both the cervical and lumbar segments in a case of complete block will nicely define the upper and lower extent of the tumor.

At the time of myelography it is convenient to mark the level of the block on the patient's skin by making a scratch with

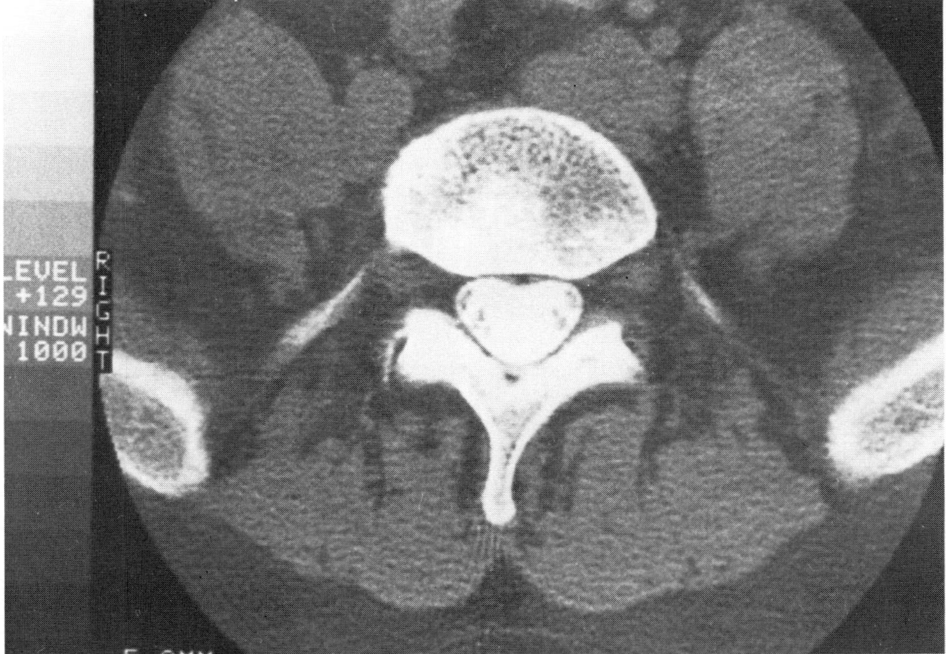

Fig. 131-3. A CT scan of a patient with a painful neuropathy caused by prostate carcinoma involving the pelvic nerves. The scan was performed during metrizamide myelography at the level of L5 on a General Electric 880 scanner with a bone review option. Note the fine detail of the bony structures and soft tissue on the same scan. Review of this scan and the other slices indicated that the patient's disease had not spread into the canal or spine.

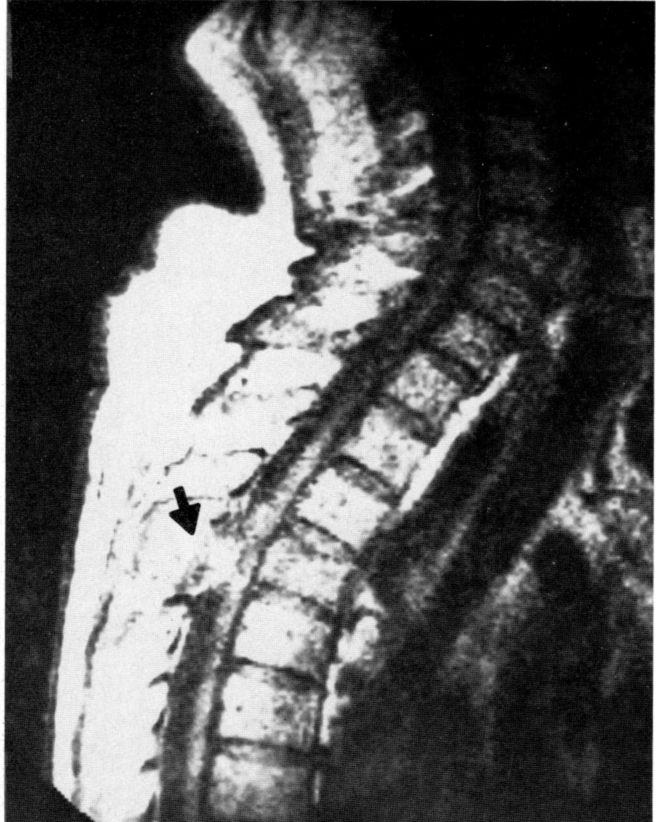

Fig. 131-4. A sagittal MRI scan of the spine demonstrating an epidural metastasis (arrow) compressing the cord at T4.

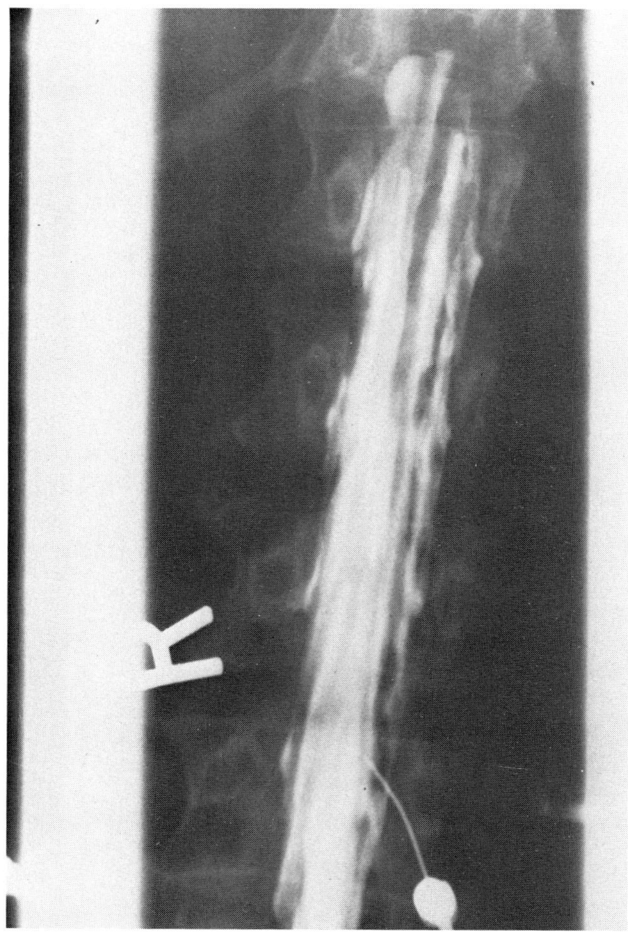

Fig. 131-5. A Pantopaque myelogram of a patient with metastatic adenocarcinoma of the colon. The patient had back and root pain. Plain x-ray films and a bone scan were normal. The myelogram shows the thickened irregular roots characteristic of carcinomatous radiculopathy of the cauda equina.

a sterile needle under fluoroscopic control. Alternatively, a radiopaque marker such as a paper clip can be taped to the skin at the site of the block. This maneuver will greatly aid in planning the incision for subsequent surgery.

Another form of myelography is now being used with increasing frequency with the advent of CT scanning and water-soluble contrast agents. Metrizamide myelography combined with CT scanning can quickly and easily locate the site of an epidural tumor with minimal discomfort to the patient.

This procedure requires much less contrast agent than standard metrizamide myelography. The usual procedure consists of the introduction of 4 to 5 ml metrizamide at a concentration of 170–200 mg/ml of iodine. After allowing 30 to 60 minutes for diffusion of the agent in the subarachnoid space, the patient is scanned at consecutive levels above and below the site of the suspected tumor (Figure 131-7). This type of myelography is extremely useful in demonstrating ventral and ventrolateral lesions in the canal that at times may be difficult to see on standard myelograms (Figure 131-8). The CT machine can produce a scout film of the area examined with a slice location marker on the plain x-ray film.

PREOPERATIVE EVALUATION AND PREPARATION

In addition to a thorough physical examination, adequate laboratory investigations should be performed, including chest x-ray studies, electrocardiogram, complete blood count, platelet count, prothrombin time, partial thromboplastin time, liver function tests, urea nitrogen, creatine level, and urinalysis. Specific tests that may aid in the diagnosis of a particular tumor, such as acid phosphatase in prostate carcinoma, also should be performed. The clotting function test and platelet count are important if one is contemplating surgery:, any deficiencies should be corrected before the operation. In addition, four units of packed red cells or whole blood should be cross-matched for the preoperative patient, and the possibility of more blood for transfusion should be available since some epidural tumors can occasionally be quite vascular and produce bleeding that is difficult to control.

If the patient does not have a rapidly progressing myelopathy and the diagnosis is unknown, then a thorough metastatic work-up can be initiated. This might include a metastatic bone series, lung tomography, and contrast studies of the gastrointestinal and urinary tracts. A bone marrow test may show lymphoma or other metastatic tumor.

If the patient's myelopathy is progressing rapidly and surgery rather than radiation therapy is decided upon as discussed above, then one should proceed with the operation after the basic laboratory studies listed above have been performed.

As soon as the diagnosis of a progressive myelopathy is made, the administration of high-dose steroids such as dexamethasone (4-10 mg PO/IM/IV every 6 hours) has been found to temporarily improve or reduce a progressing neuro-

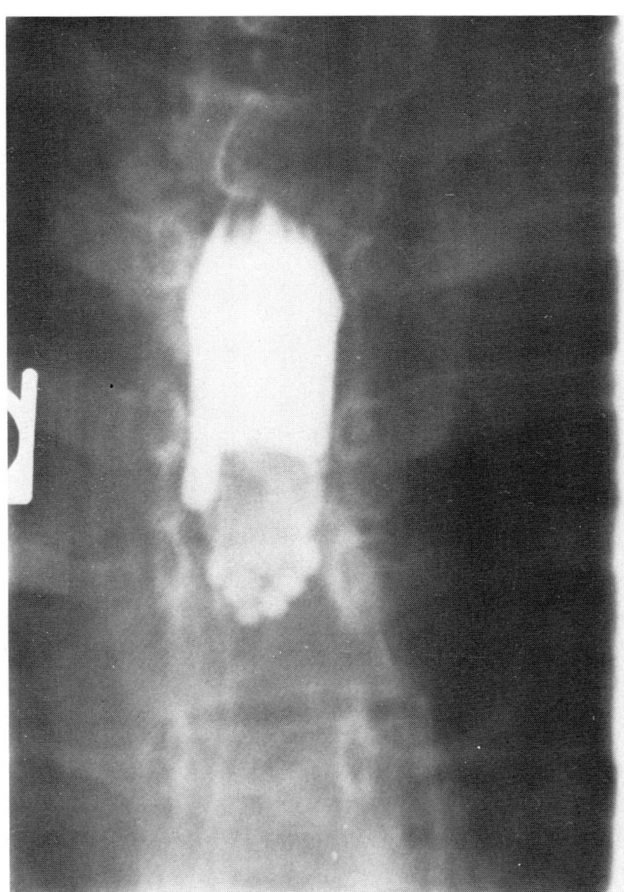

Fig. 131-6. A Pantopaque myelogram of a patient with Ewing's sarcoma who had back pain and mild paraparesis. Three milliliters of Pantopaque was instilled via a lumbar needle. Note the characteristic "paintbrush" appearance of the dye block caused by the epidural tumor.

logic deficit. Most surgeons today are convinced that steroids can reduce spinal cord edema resulting from compression to such an extent that steroids are continued through the operative and postoperative periods. It should be emphasized, however, that improvement in the patient's condition may be minimal or very brief and that steroids are no substitute for a timely decompressive operation.

DECOMPRESSIVE LAMINECTOMY

A decompressive laminectomy is the most common procedure required for alleviating spinal cord compression from a posteriorly situated epidural tumor. If the myelogram shows the tumor mass to be predominantly posterior or posterolateral with little or no ventral body encroachment on the canal, then this is the procedure of choice.

After the patient has been intubated and general anesthesia has been instituted, the patient is carefully rolled into the prone position on the operating table. The body is supported by pillows or blanket rolls extending along the anterolateral chest wall to the anterior iliac crests (Figure 131-9). Alternatively, a padded laminectomy frame may be used. The supports used should be high enough so that the abdomen will not be compressed, thus preventing high pressure and distention in the epidural and paravertebral veins. The operating table is flexed slightly to allow expansion of the interlaminar spaces. The arms can be brought forward and above the head and should be properly padded and supported on arm boards. The surgeon should keep in mind that the emaciated cancer patient is much more susceptible to compression neuropathy than a normal individual, and great care is needed in positioning the patient.

In the case of cervical epidural tumors, the three-point Mayfield or Gardner type of head prongs is a sure way to fix the head and give controlled neck flexion and stability for the

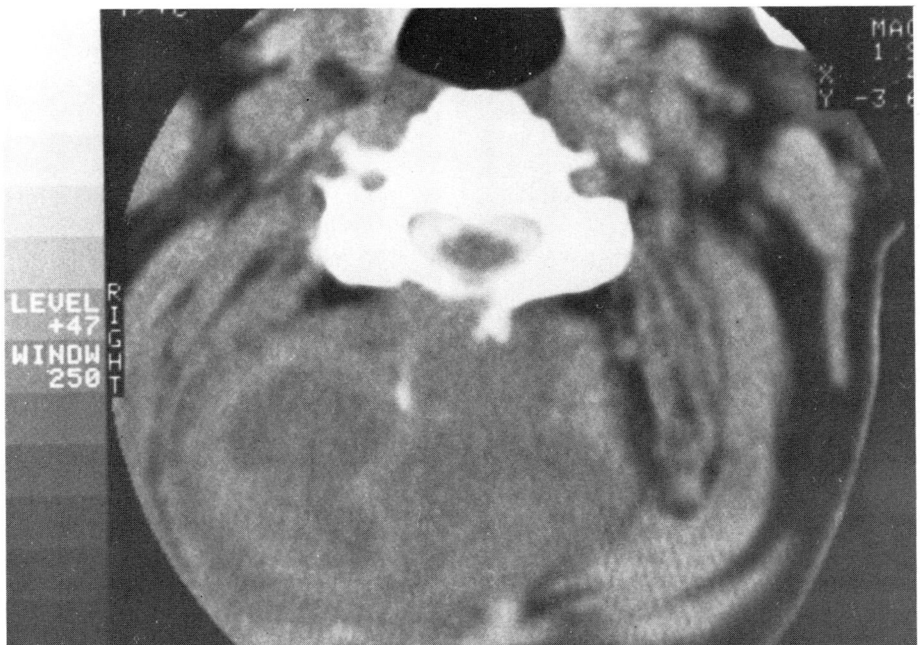

Fig. 131-7. Metrizamide myelogram of the patient in Figure 131-2. The scan demonstrates the extensive tumor of the soft tissue of the neck with involvement of the posterior arch of the spine, but no distortion of the subarachnoid dye column. At operative resection, the tumor extended down to but did not invade the dura.

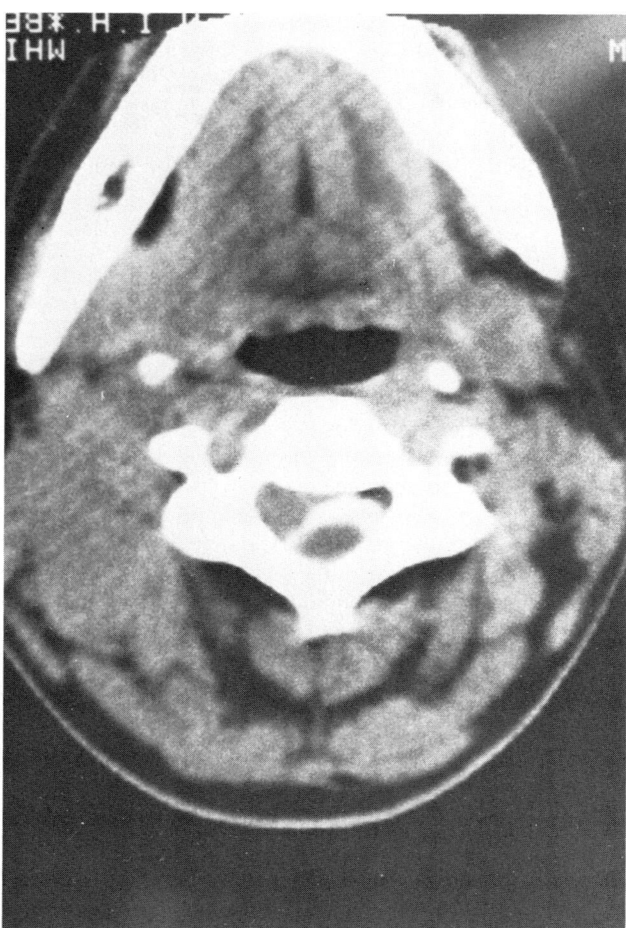

Fig. 131-8. A metrizamide myelogram with CT scan imaging of a patient with a metastatic hemangiopericytoma involving the cervical spine. The patient had neck pain. The ventrolateral tumor mass is easily seen on this scan.

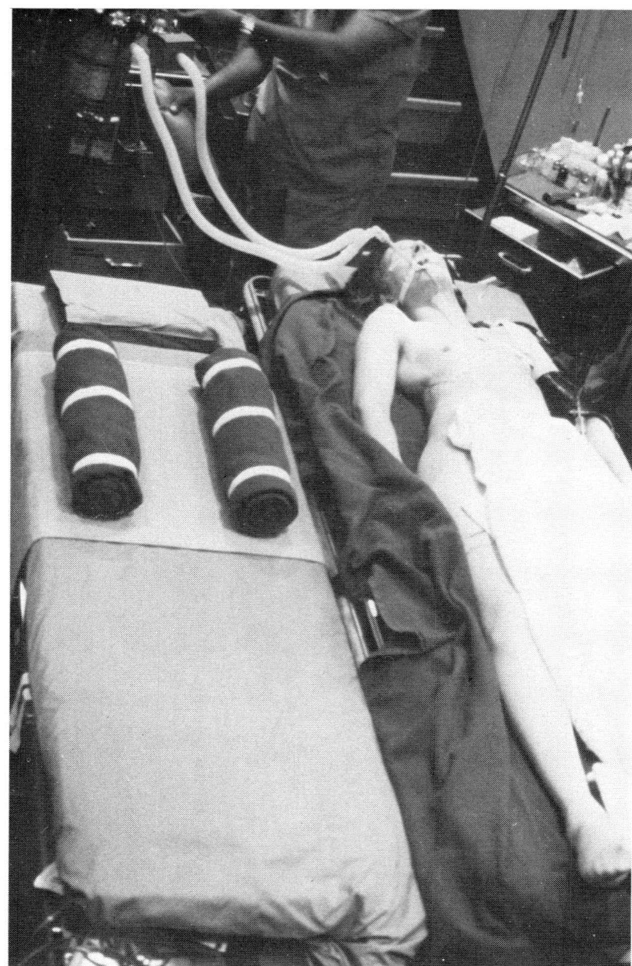

Fig. 131-9. The patient is anesthetized on the mobile stretcher and will be turned prone and lifted onto the blanket rolls on the operating table.

operation. If preoperative x-ray films and tomograms indicate an unstable spine because the tumor has invaded the cervical vertebral bodies, then preoperative stabilization should be instituted before general endotracheal anesthesia. This can be accomplished by placing the patient in a Halo jacket and adjusting the support rods until satisfactory reduction and alignment of the spine is achieved. The patient then is anesthetized and operated upon while in the Halo jacket. Postoperative radiation to the affected vertebrae may bring about healing and subsequent stability.

Another technique is to place the patient in cervical traction with skull tongs on a Stryker frame with 5 to 8 pounds of traction. After definitive decompression of the tumor a lateral fusion with autogenous or homologous bone can be carried out. The patient is then nursed postoperatively in cervical traction and a Halo jacket is applied after 7 to 10 days of initial healing.

After the patient has been positioned properly, a wide area of the trunk or neck is shaved and prepared. The skin is marked with a marking pen or gentian violet for a sagittal midline incision that is bisected by the previously marked level of tumor determined at myelography. The drapes should be placed so that the incision can be extended superiorly or inferiorly if necessary.

The skin is incised with a blade down through the dermis. The electrocautery then is used to divide the subcutaneous

tissue. Small bleeding points can be coagulated using the electrocautery and insulated forceps. The spinous processes are palpated and the paraspinal muscle fascia divided in the midline with the electrocautery. The attachments of the paraspinal muscles to the spinous processes are divided with the electrocautery and the processes palpated to determine if they are loose or destroyed by tumor. Infiltration and softening of the spinous processes and lamina by tumor should be suspected in every case, and as a result the paraspinal muscles are best removed from these structures by sharp dissection. Then gentle blunt dissection of the paraspinal muscles laterally can be achieved. Self-retaining retractors are used to hold the muscles and wound open (Figure 131-10). Attempted movement of the processes may confirm instability or softening of the vertebra, usually at the level of the spinal block. In any case, the spinous processes are removed using bone cutters (Figure 131-11). The remnants of the processes and the lamina are then thinned and nibbled away with bone rongeurs (Figure 131-12).

The actual laminectomy is begun at a location away from the suspected site of the epidural tumor so that normal tissue and structure can be recognized. Ideally this should be at a site above the level of the block, since sudden decompression of the canal below may cause the tumor to shift caudally and further impact against the cord. In the lumbar region this mechanism may not be as important as in areas over the spinal cord proper.

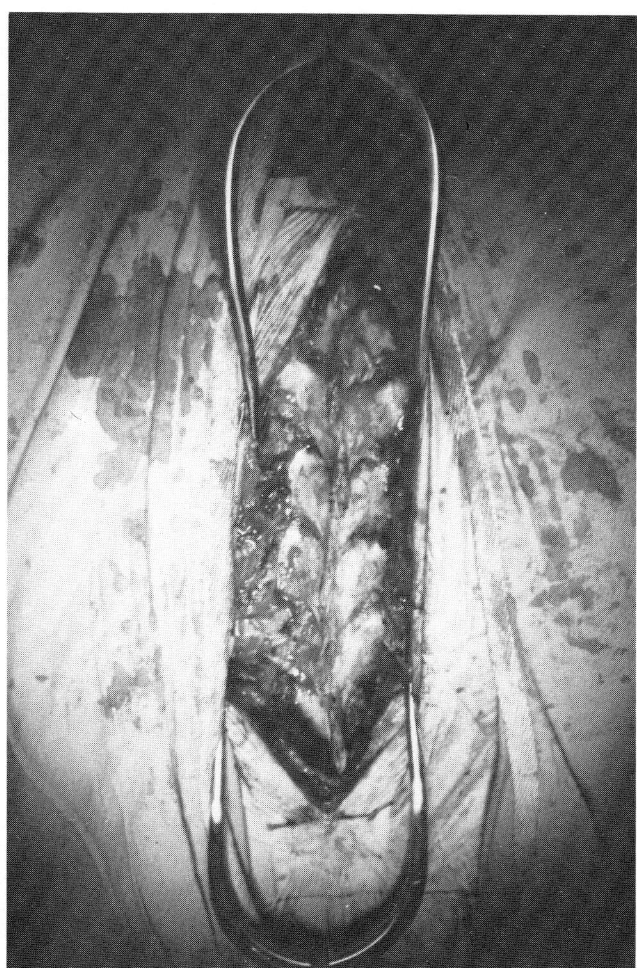

Fig. 131-10. A decompressive thoracic laminectomy. The dissection of the paraspinal muscles from the spinous processes and lamina has been carried out. Self-retaining retractors have been inserted and hemostasis has been achieved.

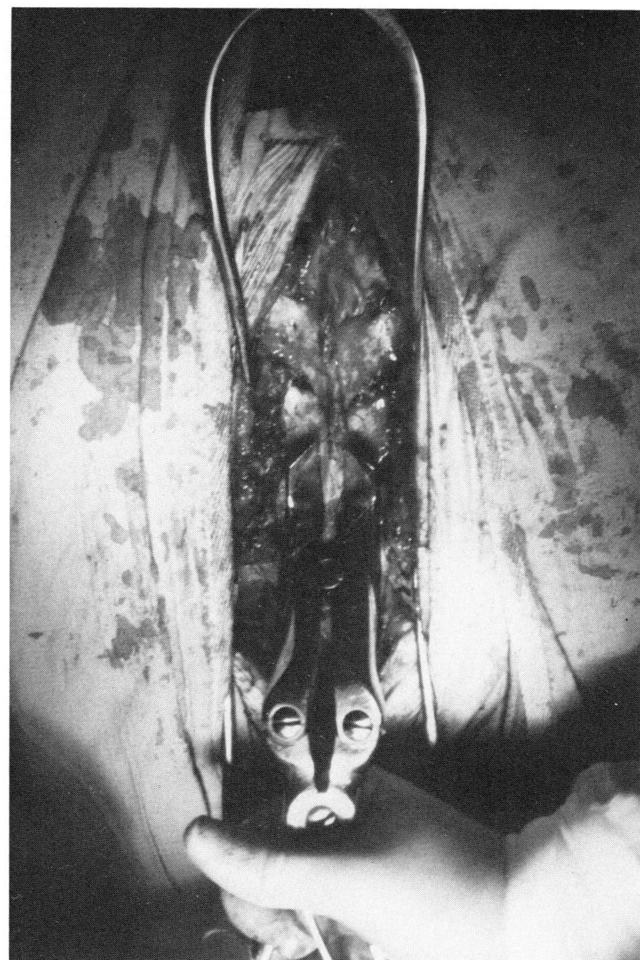

Fig. 131-11. Decompressive thoracic laminectomy. The laminectomy is begun with the sharp removal of the spinous processes with bone cutters and without twisting or tearing.

The removal of the lamina is accomplished with a Kerrison punch inserted beneath the bony inferior edge of the lamina and above the ligamentum flavum (Figure 131-13). Once one lamina is removed, the ligamentum flavum can be removed along with the bone with the Kerrison punch. The punches used should be sharp and the bone removed by a biting action rather than a twisting or tearing action, which could turn a fragment of bone into the spinal cord. The bone may be soft and infiltrated with tumor, and it is a good practice to send all of the bone removed to the pathology laboratory for examination. Occasionally this can aid the pathologist in making a diagnosis.

When the epidural tumor is encountered, normal epidural fat will disappear or will be infiltrated with tumor. The laminectomy is continued right over the surface of the tumor and beyond until normal epidural fat is encountered again. This usually can be accomplished without taking a bite of the tumor, which will result in bleeding. If bleeding is encountered, the bipolar coagulating forceps can be used to gently coagulate the surface of the tumor or surrounding veins. At times, even though the laminectomy is carried out two levels above and below the level of the block, the epidural tumor is found to extend much further in the epidural space than the laminectomy has exposed. If one is sure that the level of the block has been uncovered, then this continuation of tumor, which is usually

diminutive, is left alone. If, however, the tumor still occupies a considerable portion of the canal, extension of the laminectomy should be done until the tumor bulk becomes insignificant. Bleeding from the bone edges is controlled with bone wax.

The tumor generally receives its blood supply from the epidural arteries and veins situated laterally in the canal. After identifying normal dura, the epidural tumor is grasped laterally with the bipolar forceps and coagulated. If this maneuver is repeated on each side for a distance of 1 cm, the coagulated tumor can be cut and the process repeated. In this way the tumor can be rolled up like a rug with minimal bleeding and without tearing the epidural veins (Figure 131-14).

Some tumors have minimal blood supply and can be elevated right off the dura with a No. 3 Penfield dissector and coagulation of a few feeding vessels. Others are tenaciously bound to the dura and cannot be removed by blunt dissection. These tumors often bleed extensively when removal with sharp dissection is attempted. In such a case it is best to remove enough tumor for pathologic examination and to the leave the decompressed tumor attached to the dura. Although any metastatic tumor can be hemorrhagic, melanoma, hypernephroma, and some breast tumors can bleed profusely. This often occurs when the lamina are removed from the tumor. Control of the bleeding may not be possible with the bipolar cautery, in which case oxidized cellulose or gelatin sponge and gentle pressure

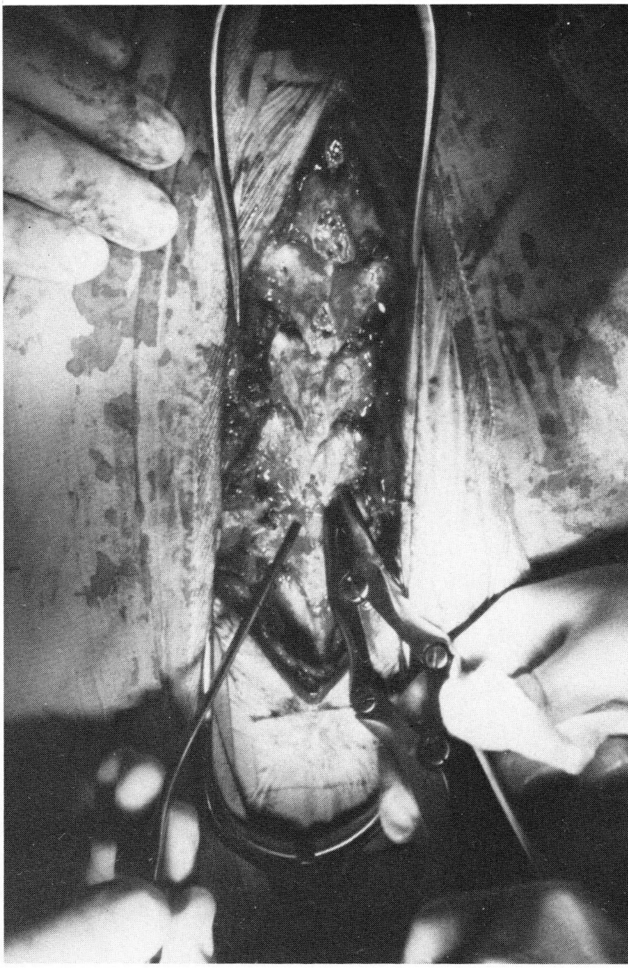

Fig. 131-12. Decompressive thoracic laminectomy. Bone rongeurs are used to nibble away the remaining stumps of the spinous processes and to thin the lamina so that minimal force will be exerted with the Kerrison punch.

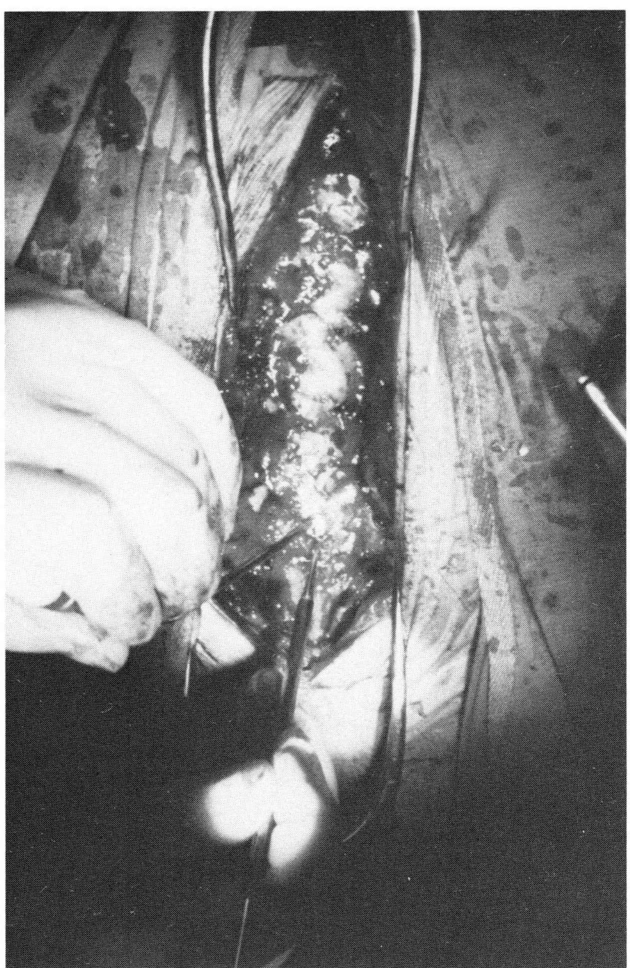

Fig. 131-13. Decompressive thoracic laminectomy. The lamina have been thinned and waxed with bone wax. The dental instrument is used to create a plane beneath the edge of the lamina that will accept the footplate of the Kerrison punch visible on the right.

with a cottonoid will often control the bleeding. After the tumor is removed or at least decompressed, the normal respiratory pulsations of the dural sac will often, but not always, return.

A frozen section of the tumor tissue performed at the time of surgery is useful in helping the surgeon conduct the operation. If the pathologist reports that the tumor is a lymphoma or some other radiation-sensitive tumor, the surgeon can be less aggressive in removing all the tumor that can be seen, knowing that radiation will be effective in controlling any residual tumor.

After the removal of the tumor is completed, hemostasis is achieved by waxing all bone edges and coagulating any epidural veins with the bipolar cautery. Any bleeding points not discrete enough to be coagulated can be controlled with cellulose or gelatin sponge. Despite extensive hemostatic maneuvers, there still may be a slow ooze of blood from the epidural space, in which case the surgeon should consider placing a drain tube in the epidural space and bringing it out to drain through a separate site (Figure 131-15). Drains connected to a closed container system that allows gentle suction on the draining tube are particularly valuable for this purpose. The drain is rarely required for more than 12 to 24 hours after the operation.

The paraspinal muscles and fascia are reapproximated in the midline over the drain tube with interrupted 0 silk or synthetic absorbable sutures. The subcutaneous tissue is closed

with interrupted 3-0 silk or synthetic absorbable sutures. The skin is best closed with interrupted 3-0 nylon sutures. Because of its nonreactive quality, this suture material may be left in the skin for up to 14 days with minimal skin reaction. Some surgeons prefer wire sutures for this purpose. A sterile gauze dressing taped in place completes the operation.

Generally most patients with epidural metastatic tumors have adequate stability of the spine. Since most of the epidural metastases occur in the thoracic region, the surgeon can rely on the ribs and chest wall to stabilize this area, provided extensive destruction of the vertebrae has not taken place. The patient can be simply nursed flat on the bed with appropriate ''log-rolling'' maneuvers. Often, after postoperative radiation therapy, x-ray films will show healing of the affected vertebrae. In the case of extensive destruction of the thoracic and lumbar vertebrae with gross kyphosis, however, the insertion of Harrington rods at the time of decompression should be considered and an orthopedic colleague consulted. The cervical spine is best stabilized with a Halo jacket as described earlier.

In the uncommon situation in which only one vertebra is completely destroyed and presents with angulation, one can perform intraoperative methyl-methacrylate fusion using a technique similar to that described for vertebral fractures of the spine.[4] In order to apply this technique, firm and sound spinous

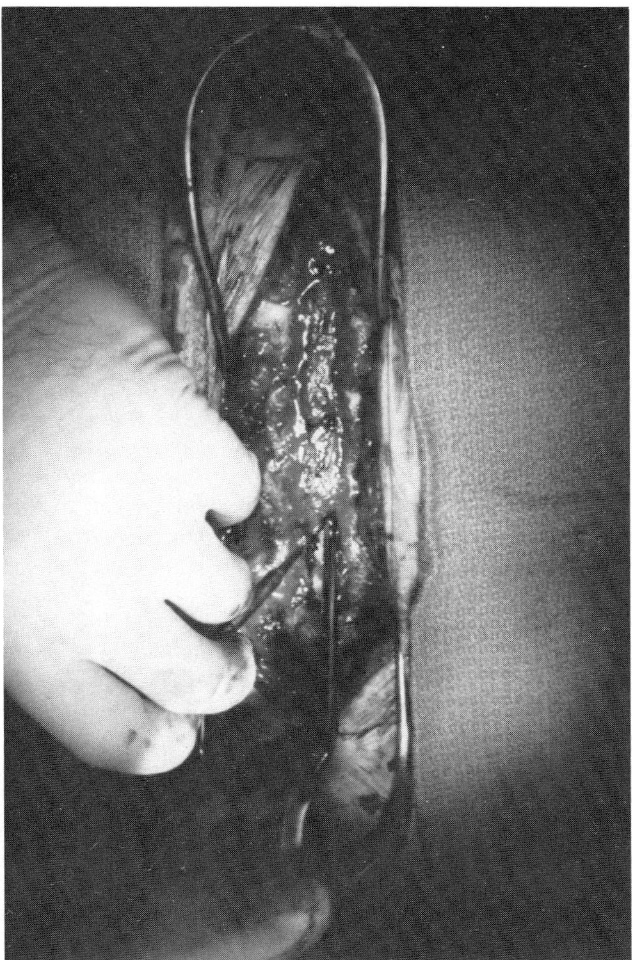

Fig. 131-14. Decompressive thoracic laminectomy. The laminectomy has been completed. A plane between the normal dura and the epidural tissue is developed at the lower edge of the wound. The bipolar forceps then are used to coagulate the lateral epidural veins and tumor tissue as the mass is gently elevated from the dura.

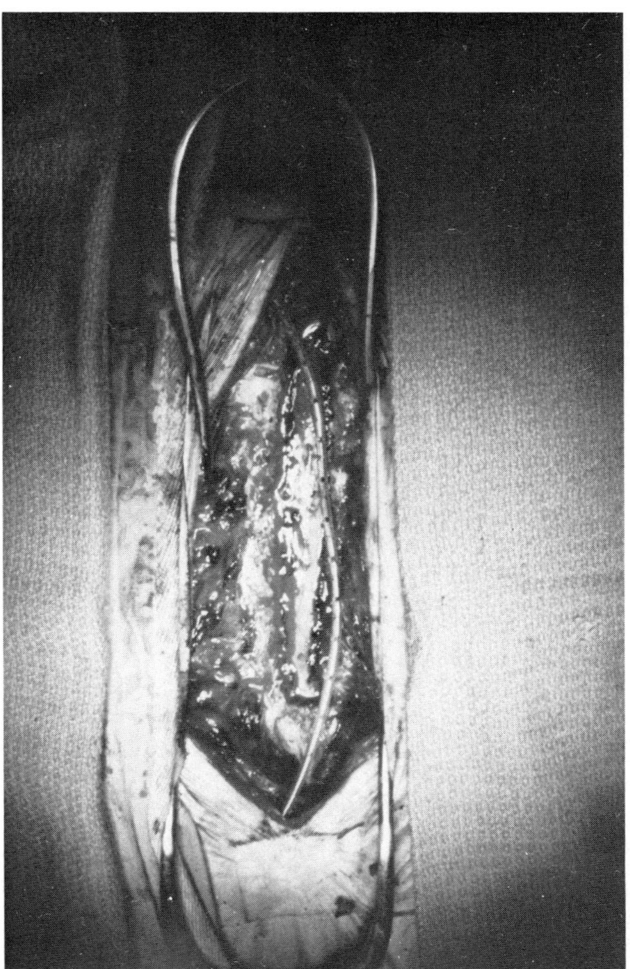

Fig. 131-15. Decompressive thoracic laminectomy. The tumor mass has been successfully removed from the dura and a perforated drain tube has been inserted into the epidural space and is brought out through a separate stab wound before the wound is closed.

processes and lamina should be present above and below the two or three segments that have been decompressed. Instead of making logs of plastic as originally described, I prefer to pass heavy stainless wires through and around the spinous processes above and below the decompression site. Then the methyl-methacrylate plastic is molded on top of and around the wires to form a single large strut of posteriorly situated plastic. The underlying dura is protected with several sheets of gelatin sponge, which can be removed after the plastic hardens. It is important to use the skeletal type of methyl-methacrylate that is designed for orthopedic uses. This plastic sets more slowly than the material used by neurosurgeons for cranioplasty, which allows the plastic to be modeled while it is in its puttylike state. In addition, it is radiopaque and can be visualized by standard x-ray study for continuity and position.

ANTERIOR DECOMPRESSION OF THE SPINAL CANAL

All of the techniques developed for the anterior decompression of the spinal canal in cases of disc herniation and vertebral fracture can be used with modification to remove ventrally placed tumor masses.

Usually the mass consists of a vertebral body that has been replaced by tumor and has impinged on the cord, which results in a myelopathy. The posterior elements—lamina, spinous processes, and facets—may also be invaded by tumor. This fact usually requires that intraoperative stabilization or fusion be performed. Anterior decompression is required in only a minority of patients with metastatic spinal disease, but it is important to recognize those that require it since posterior laminectomy may not achieve a satisfactory result. The description of the general operative technique for approaching the anterior spine is already adequately outlined in the literature and in the chapters dealing with disc disease. It would therefore be best to comment on those modifications and salient features that pertain to metastatic involvement of the spine.

The general operative approach of Cloward can be used to perform a vertebral corpectomy in the cervical region.[5] Instead of using the Cloward drill, however, the softened vertebral body is best removed piecemeal with sharp bone curettes and a high-speed drill with dental burrs. This prevents the displacement of infiltrated and loosened bone fragments into the canal, which can be a problem with the Cloward drill. The disc material is likewise removed with a bone curette until normal vertebral bodies are encountered above and below the lesion. If fragments of the diseased vertebral body remain attached to the underlying dura but are decompressed, they are best left in place. Rarely, more than one vertebral body must be removed. After the decompression has been achieved, a bone graft or plastic vertebral body replacement may or may not be necessary. When a single diseased vertebral body is removed along with the adjacent discs and cartilaginous plates, no fusion is necessary. In fact, the diseased vertebral body usually has already collapsed in height and the small defect left after its removal is easily bridged by the settling of the spine. The patient's neck of course should be immobilized with a Halo jacket, or, if there is no involvement of the posterior elements, a rigid cervical collar.

When two or more vertebral bodies are removed, the resulting defect must be bridged with a bone graft or a methylmethacrylate. The fibula provides a bone graft that is easy to obtain and has the ideal dimensions. The remaining normal superior and inferior vertebral bodies should be hollowed slightly with a drill to accept and secure the correct length of fibula. If a plastic graft is used, short K-wires or screws are driven into the vertebral bodies at either end of the defect.[6] The underlying dura is protected with 2 to 3 layers of gelatin sponge, and the plastic is molded into place when it has a puttylike consistency. In order to dissipate the heat of polymerization, the plastic is irrigated continuously with water while it is curing. After the plastic has set, excess gelatin sponge is removed from beneath the graft. Immobilization of the neck with a rigid collar is maintained for 6 weeks.

The techniques of vertebral body removal in the thoracic region are similar to those described above for the cervical region. There are two major approaches to the thoracic vertebral bodies. One approach is by a thoracotomy at the level of interest, which gives a view of the vertebral bodies that is almost directly anterior. This technique gives the best exposure and is technically quite simple.[7,8] Likewise, a bone graft or plastic graft is used. Recently, the use of stainless steel mesh for reinforcing a thoracic plastic graft has been reported.[9] This technique does expose the patient to the possible pulmonary complications of a thoracotomy. The other approach is a costotransversectomy, which does not require entering the pleural space but gives a more limited and strictly lateral approach to the vertebral bodies. This operative approach has been used for many years, first to treat Potts' disease of the spine and presently for thoracic disc herniations. The actual technique is described in detail elsewhere.[10]

Several points about this technique are worth mentioning, however. The exposure is quite limited and generally affords access to only one vertebral body. The surgeon must therefore be sure to operate at the correct level and use intraoperative x-ray studies if necessary. Although the thoracic cavity is not intentionally opened, the parietal pleura may be violated with a resulting pneumothorax. This may not be noticed at the time of the operation, making an immediate postoperative chest x-ray film mandatory. The surgeon should be prepared to insert a chest tube if necessary. Finally, the operation is easiest in patients with a slender build who already have a dorsal kyphosis caused by vertebral collapse and angulation.

POSTOPERATIVE CARE

Following decompressive laminectomy, patients are nursed flat in bed using log-rolling techniques for the first 3 or 4 days. After this they are mobilized into a chair or are assisted in walking if their condition permits. The same regimen is followed for patients who have had an anteriorly placed bone graft or plastic fusion. Prolonged unnecessary bed rest will invite complications such as pulmonary embolism or pneumonia. Periodic postoperative x-ray films of the spine should be obtained, however, to detect any early subluxation or graft displacement. The dressing is checked daily for any evidence of cerebrospinal fluid (CSF) leakage. If it is found, the wound is immediately oversewn with a running suture of 4-0 or 3-0 nylon and the patient is given meningeal doses of intravenous antibiotics. If the CSF leak continues the patient will require re-exploration to locate the source of leak and to close it.

Preoperative antibiotics are used only in those patients who have a current bacterial infection and require emergency decompressive surgery. Cancer patients are known to be more susceptible to sepsis, however, so that postoperative atelectasis, pneumonia, or urinary tract infection should be diagnosed and treated promptly. Steroids are given to those patients who had a progressing myelopathy preoperatively and are continued for 7 to 10 days or until the neurologic condition stabilizes.

RESULTS AND COMPLICATIONS

In general, the neurologic condition of the patient at the time of surgery can be the expected postoperative condition. A survey of several different operative series showed an overall improvement of only 30 percent.[1] In most cases operative intervention prevented the patient from worsening. This same survey found an average mortality rate of 9 percent, with 12 percent of the patients becoming neurologically worse. Postoperative complications such as wound infection, CSF fistula, epidural hematoma, and spine subluxation occurred in 11 percent of the cases. Complications such as wound infection or hematoma should be treated promptly by a second operation and suitable debridement or closure of the wound. If postoperative x-ray studies show gross displacement of a bone or plastic graft, surgery may be required when the patient's neurologic condition is threatened or when adequate stability cannot be assured.

REFERENCES

1. Black P: Spinal metastasis: Current status and recommended guidelines for management. Neurosurgery 5:726, 1979
2. Young RF, Post EM, King GA: Treatment of spinal epidural metastases. J Neurosurg 53:741, 1980
3. Wright RL: Malignant tumors in the spinal extradural space: Results of surgical treatment. Ann Surg 157:227, 1961
4. Kelly DL, Alexander E, Davis CH, et al: Acrylic fixation of atlantoaxial dislocation. J Neurosurg 36:366, 1972
5. Cloward RB: The anterior approach for removal of ruptured cervical discs. J Neurosurg 15:602, 1958
6. Cross GO, White HL, White LP: Acrylic prosthesis of the fifth cervical vertebra in multiple myeloma. J Neurosurg 35:112, 1971
7. Perot P, Munro DD: Transthoracic removal of midiine disc protrusions causing spinal cord compression. J Neurosurg 31:452, 1969
8. Paul, RL, Michael RH, Dunn JE, et al: Anterior transthoracic surgical decompression of acute spinal cord injuries. J Neurosurg 43:299, 1975
9. Galicich JH: Management of metastatic tumors to the nervous system at the Sloan-Kettering Institute. Presented at the Central Neurosurgical Society Meeting, Chicago, 1980
10. Hulme A: The surgical approach to thoracic intervertebral disc protrusions. J Neurol Neurosurg Psychiatry 23:133, 1960

CHAPTER 132

Surgical Approaches to Primary and Metastatic Tumors of the Spine

Narayan Sundaresan
James E. O. Hughes

George V. DiGiacinto

DURING THE PAST DECADE, improvements in neuroradiologic diagnosis by computed tomography (CT) as well as magnetic resonance imaging (MRI), together with the development of effective multidisciplinary treatment have considerably expanded the role of surgery in the treatment of neoplasms of the spine.[1] The goal of surgery previously was limited largely to providing tissue diagnosis as well as palliation of pain and neurological deficit by decompressive laminectomy. With the radiological demonstration that the majority of metastases and primary tumors are ventral to the cord, it is obvious that tumor resection requires exposures of the anterior spine that are not generally familiar to most neurosurgeons. The development of anterolateral exposures in the thoracic and lumbar region have now provided the impetus for more attempts at ''curative'' rather than palliative surgery. From the standpoint of the surgical oncologist, the goal of surgery is obtaining local tumor control, as is the case at sites elsewhere. The concept of ''cure'' requires in addition a multidisciplinary effort to eradicate overt or silent metastases elsewhere by the use of systemic approaches, i.e., chemotherapy. In addition to tumor resection, a major goal of surgery is the achievement of stability of the spine. Resected segments may be stabilized either by methyl methacrylate and spinal instrumentation or by physiologic bone fusion using autologous bone grafts. With the advent of effective instrumentation, it is technically feasible to remove an entire vertebra (spondylectomy) in either a staged or a single approach.

INCIDENCE

Involvement of the vertebral column is a relatively common feature of many solid tumors. The propensity for some tumors to metastasize selectively to bone has been termed ''osteotropism,'' and a clearer understanding of this phenomenon may one day allow efforts to prevent the development of bone metastases. At present, clinical data suggest that 20 to 70 percent of patients with metastatic disease from the breast, lung, prostate, and hematopoietic system will have involvement of the axial spine.[2] (The vertebral column consists of the true vertebra in the cervical, thoracic, and lumbar regions, as well as the sacrum.) In most series, four primary sites alone account for more than two thirds of all causes of neoplastic cord compression—breast, lung, hematopoietic system, and prostate.[3–5] Clin-

ically, compression of the spinal cord results from extension of a focus to the vertebral body; other possible mechanisms include direct invasion of the spine from a paraspinal tumor, as well as extension through the intervertebral foramina along the perineurium or its lymphatics without bone involvement. Most oncology centers encounter between 40 and 80 patients with this complication every year; in many surgical series of neoplastic cord compression, involvement of the spine may be the initial feature of malignancy in 10 to 40 percent of the patients. In addition to metastases, primary bone tumors and multiple myeloma not infrequently involve the spinal column; many retroperitoneal tumors (sarcomas, neuroblastomas) also involve the spine by direct extension. Approximately 1000 bone tumors and 5000 soft part sarcomas are diagnosed each year in the United States, of which approximately 10 percent involve the spine. Using extrapolated data, we estimate that spinal neoplasms currently outrank trauma as the major cause of paraplegia.

CLINICAL PRESENTATION

The typical clinical syndrome of neural compression is easily recognized—more than 90 percent of patients have back pain, which may be associated with a referred or radicular component. The median duration of pain is about 6 weeks, and it may be followed by the subacute onset of neurologic deficits. If undiagnosed, the deficit may evolve to complete paraplegia or quadriplegia with bladder and bowel involvement. Unfortunately, despite the emphasis on early diagnosis, up to 50 percent of patients have severe deficits at initial examination and 10 percent of patients have acute onset of weakness (less than 24 hours), while 10 to 20 percent deteriorate either before or shortly after undergoing conservative treatment (radiotherapy).

Since spinal involvement may result in an array of clinical manifestations other than the classical presentation above, we believe it is useful to classify the various syndromes into four major categories (Table 132-1). Since most patients are promptly treated with high dose corticosteroid therapy following diagnosis, the deficits represent assessments made after high dose corticosteroid therapy and serve as a guide to the need for ''emergency'' versus ''urgent'' treatment. Asymptomatic patients with spinal involvement are generally detected

OPERATIVE NEUROSURGICAL TECHNIQUES
ISBN 0-8089-1862-1

Table 132-1. Syndromes of spinal metastases

Clinical Manifestations	Myelographic Findings
Asymptomatic	Varying degrees of intraspinal extension
Back pain, no deficit	Intraosseous or epidural disease
Neurologic deficit; stable on steroids	Varying degrees of epidural block
Neurologic deficit; unstable on steroids	Complete block; unstable spine

during myelography performed for the evaluation of posterior mediastinal or retroperitoneal tumors—examples being neurogenic tumors of the posterior mediastinum, superior sulcus tumors, and paraspinal sarcomas. In the patients with solid tumors, radionuclide bone scanning or MRI may identify spine involvement when performed as a routine staging procedure; such spinal involvement may be unifocal or multifocal. Other patients may have back pain alone with minor neurologic deficits, i.e., radiculopathy. The back pain frequently may resolve on high dose corticosteroid therapy. At the time of myelography, the major question is whether epidural extension of the tumor is present; currently, patients with purely intraosseous tumors are treated with systemic therapy whenever possible, while those with epidural extension are often given "emergency RT." Patients with neurologic deficits may be ambulatory or nonambulatory. We propose that neurologic deficits be classified as stable or unstable on steroid therapy; in view of the current emphasis on ambulation as the major end-point of therapy, these deficits may be further subclassified on the basis of ambulatory status (Tables 132-2 and 132-3).

RADIOLOGIC EVALUATION

Accurate radiologic assessment of the spinal segments involved, including bone and soft tissue components, as well as the extent of systemic metastases may require several days. To a large extent, the pace of radiologic evaluation should be based on the urgency for treatment, but every effort should be made to obtain as complete an evaluation as possible. Plain roentgenography, involving spot films, should preferably be the initial study. Classical signs of spinal metastases include (1) vertebral

Table 132-2. Classification of neurologic deficit

Status	
Ambulatory	Normal neurologic examination
	Radiculopathy
	Plexopathy
Nonambulatory	Pain only, compression fracture, unstable spine
	Radiculopathy
	Plexopathy
	Cauda equina compression
	Paraparesis—mild, moderate, severe
	Other causes—Brown-Sequard syndrome, ataxia, etc.

Table 132-3. Classification of anterior spinal approaches

Segment	Levels	Approach
Cervical	C1-C2	Transoral, transmandibular
	C3-C7	Transcervical (Cloward)
Cervicothoracic	C7-T1	Transsternal, transthoracic
Thoracic	T3-T10	Transthoracic, posterolateral thoracotomy
Thoracolumbar	T11-L1	Transthoracic, extrapleural, thoracoabdominal
Lumbar	L2-L4	Retroperitoneal
Lumbosacral	L5-S1	Transabdominal
Sacral	S2-S5	Extra- or intra-abdominal, transperineal

collapse, (2) destruction of the pedicle, (3) lytic destruction or focal osteopenia, and (4) malalignment of the spine. In patients with normal x-ray studies, the decision to perform the next procedure is generally based on the evolving neurologic deficit—patients with paraparesis generally undergo myelography, while those with pain alone may be further evaluated by MRI, CT, or radionuclide bone scans. Radionuclide bone scans are particularly useful in demonstrating multifocal versus unifocal involvement.

Myelography is recommended in most patients with spinal metastases for several reasons: it is currently the most accurate test for distinguishing intraosseous from epidural disease; discontinuous epidural blocks may be seen in 10 percent of patients, especially those with breast cancer, lymphoma, or prostate cancer; other causes of spinal pain and neurologic deficits in the cancer population may be diagnosed; proper identification of epidural extension allows planning of treatment portals for RT; finally, the residual dye can be used for refluoromyelography to assess the effectiveness of therapy. Myelography is not suggested for patients with unstable spines and may be dispensed with for those with adequate demonstration of the subarachnoid space by MRI.[6] If a complete block is identified, the upper limits of the block should be identified by a C1-C2 puncture. It is not uncommon for patients with complete block to show some degree of neurologic deterioration following lumbar puncture; therefore, all patients with epidural extension of tumor should be treated with an intravenous bolus of Decadron (dexamethasone 20–100 mg) after the myelography procedure; this should be followed by 6 hourly dose of intravenous corticosteroid therapy. Based on myelographic extension, spinal metastases can be classified into varying grades depending on the extent of myelographic block: grade I = intraosseous only; grade IIA = minimal epidural extension (0–25 percent); grade IIB = moderate epidural extension (25–75 percent); grade IIC = high grade (75–100 percent); grade IID = paraspinal tumor with varying degrees of epidural extension. These subclassifications are offered for two reasons: patients with grade I lesions have better prospects for control by local RT, whereas patients with grade IIC and IID lesions have a poorer prognosis. In all patients, we believe that spinal CT should follow myelography to determine the actual extent of tumor.

In patients with hypervascular tumors, spinal angiography

may be indicated to diminish tumor vascularity, demonstrate feeding vessels, and determine the location of critical spinal arterial supply such as the artery of Adamkiewicz.[7] A variety of therapeutic agents can be used for presurgical embolization. Temporary materials (such as autologous clot, gelatin foam, and microfibrillar collagen) are easy to handle, associated with minimal risk of permanent damage, and are used for temporary embolization until operative resection is scheduled within several days. Permanent materials include polyvinyl alcohol foam (Ivalon) in particulate form, Silastic spheres, silicone polymers, and absolute alcohol. Particles of Ivalon (150–500 μ in diameter) are mixed with solutions of warmed saline and radiographic contrast in proportions designed to produce a liquid slurry of a concentration and viscosity appropriate to the lesion. In our experience, patients with primary tumors, metastases from the kidneys or thyroid, and sarcomas have been safely embolized, resulting in lowered morbidity from intraoperative blood loss. In addition to Ivalon, absolute alcohol can also be used as a sclerosing agent for permanent tumor necrosis before surgery.

INDICATIONS FOR SURGERY

Attempts to define absolute indications for surgery are hampered by the fact that treatment has to be individualized in many patients. A knowledge of important prognostic factors may be helpful in the decision-making process. In most series, the site of the primary tumor and histologic type, as well as the pretreatment neurologic deficit are considered the most important pretreatment variables.[8,9] For optimum results, surgeons therefore should seek intervention in patients who are ambulatory; there is little purpose in subjecting paraplegic or near-paraplegic patients to extensive surgery. Patients who have rapidly evolving deficits (less than 24 hours) probably are destined to have a poor outcome regardless of therapy, especially if the deficits progress on high dose steroid therapy. Patients with structural abnormalities (instability, retropulsed bone fragments, acute collapse of the vertebral body) do not respond to RT alone, since compression of the neural elements results from bone. The extent of myelographic block (complete versus incomplete) has been noted to be an important factor, but we believe that this is true only if patients with extensive paraspinal masses are excluded. Patients who respond favorably to steroid therapy also are likely to respond to therapy. Finally, the phase in the cancer patient's illness in which treatment is undertaken is important. Patients with advanced widespread disease and those who have failed previous treatments are much less likely to respond to surgery. With these generalizations, we believe that RT and steroid therapy are the treatment of choice in the following conditions: (1) patients with advanced systemic metastases such that survival is measured in weeks; (2) patients with lymphoma and other round cell malignancies such as neuroblastoma, Ewing's sarcoma, etc.; (3) patients with breast and prostate cancer without structural abnormalities of the spine. In all other patients with spinal metastases, neurosurgical evaluation should be sought. Since the goal of therapy in any individual patient may differ, we have classified indications for surgery along five major categories: cancer therapy, stabilization, neurologic salvage, tissue diagnosis, and pain relief.

CANCER THERAPY

In patients with primary osseous neoplasms, localized paraspinal tumors with direct spine involvement, and those with solitary sites of relapse, local treatment has a major bearing on overall survival.[10,11] Other patients with pathologic compression fractures and radioresistant tumors such a kidney cancer with limited systemic disease also fall into this category. In these patients, the extent of epidural extension and the presence or absence of neurologic deficit have little bearing on the timing of surgery; rather the goal of surgery should be maximal reduction of tumor bulk.

STABILIZATION

A second but especially major goal of surgery is the restoration or maintenance of stability of the spine involved by tumor. Patients with fracture-dislocations, localized kyphosis, collapsed vertebrae with retropulsion of a bone fragment may require operative decompression in conjunction with RT.[12–16] In these patients, the radiosensitivity of the primary tumor has little bearing on the indication for therapy. A major subgroup of patients in this category have ''segmental instability'' of the spine. This is clinically manifest by pain aggravated by movement, and is usually seen after radiotherapy. Plain roentgenograms may show progressive collapse of the vertebral bodies, or MRI may show retropulsion of bony elements with a local kyphosis. Surgical reduction of movement across this motion segment will generally result in prompt relief of pain. This can be accomplished by anterior stabilization following vertebral body resection or by posterior stabilization with or without instrumentation.

NEUROLOGIC SALVAGE

For patients who have an acutely evolving deficit, surgery offers the potential of neurologic palliation even though there may be little impact on overall survival. Similarly, patients who deteriorate while undergoing RT or those who cannot receive further RT may be relieved for several months by surgical decompression. In such patients, the goal of therapy is more limited, since it is being performed for salvage. Since these patients have received both RT and prolonged steroid therapy, morbidity from extensive operative procedures may be considerable, and more limited decompression by posterior or posterolateral approaches may be appropriate.[17–19] In our experience, local tumor recurrence is inevitable in almost all patients at a year after resection.

TISSUE DIAGNOSIS

With current radiologic evaluation, the need for a major procedure to document a diagnosis of malignancy should be rare. The primary site frequently is obvious, i.e., on chest x-ray films, abdominal CT scans, or a more accessible site may be seen on radionuclide bone scan. If no site is evident, the diagnosis of malignancy can frequently be established by a CT-guided needle biopsy, especially if a paraspinal soft tissue mass is present. A major indication for operative intervention is to differentiate benign from malignant compression, e.g., disc disease versus metastatic tumor, or in the occasional intradural lesion in which distinction from a primary intraspinal tumor such as meningioma versus metastases must be made. If open biopsy of a tumor is required, the site of laminotomy and extent of bone removal must be minimized to prevent loss of stability as well as to reduce contamination of tissue planes along the biopsy tract.

PAIN RELIEF

In most patients, resection of tumor and restoration of stability frequently results in pain relief; especially in patients with intractable pain either from local plexus or nerve root invasion, the goal of therapy may be pain relief even though motor deficits are permanent and irreversible. The role of local rhizotomies, cordotomy, and resection of lesions compressing the brachial plexus fall into this category.[20,21]

PREOPERATIVE EVALUATION AND ASSESSMENT

Many patients with spinal cord compression are referred for neurosurgical evaluation either with an evolving neurologic deficit or after a myelogram has demonstrated a complete block. This may result in a hasty decision to decompress the cord on an emergency basis in an effort to preserve or improve neurologic function. While such clinical situations cannot always be avoided, we recommend that emergency surgery be considered only in patients who with unstable neurologic deficits on steroid therapy. With an initial bolus dose (Decadron 20–100 mg IV) and continuous high dose corticosteroid therapy, most patients stabilize long enough for more complete radiologic assessment. At a minimum, a spinal CT scan should be obtained to determine the proper operative approach.

In patients with a pathologic compression fracture without a prior history of cancer, two diagnostic possibilities exist: (1) a primary cancer is evident on chest x-ray films or abdominal CT scans, or (2) no primary site is seen. Radiologic evaluation should include a radionuclide bone scan; extensive radiologic studies looking for a primary site are not indicated.

Specific laboratory tests that aid in the diagnosis include serum acid phosphatase, serum and urine immune electrophoresis, and CEA levels. A bone marrow examination should be performed if myeloma is suspected. Since the majority of patients may require thoracotomy, we believe that preoperative pulmonary function tests should be performed whenever feasible; as a minimum, arterial blood gas studies should be obtained. In patients with chronic obstructive pulmonary disease and those with recent respiratory compromise, therapy with Bronchosol or ultrasonic nebulizers a few days before surgery will promote a smoother recovery. In vascular tumors, a complete coagulogram should be performed, and between 4 to 10 units of packed red cells or whole blood should be crossmatched for the patient. In view of the need for blood products such as fresh frozen plasma and platelets, we generally recommend a formal hematologic consultation. A final, most important aspect of preoperative care is to have the patient evaluated for a custom made or prefabricated orthosis.

CHOICE OF OPERATIVE APPROACH

There are three basic approaches to the spine: (1) posterior approaches by laminectomy, (2) lateral approaches by transverse osteotomy, and (3) anterior approaches by vertebral body resection (Figure 132-1). In addition, complete spondylectomy

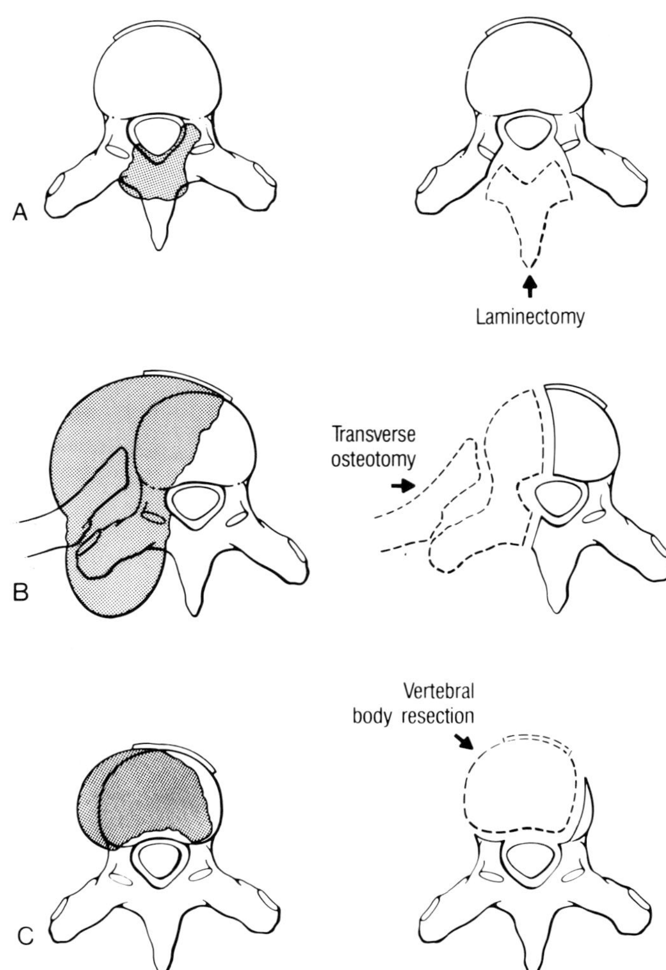

Fig. 132–1.   Line drawing depicting the three basic approaches to tumors (shaded areas) involving the spine.

can be performed by a combination of an anterior or posterior approach. The choice of surgical approach should be based on the radiographic extent of tumor, the ability of the patient to tolerate the proposed operation based on clinical and laboratory criteria, and the desired goal of therapy. If an operation is planned for biopsy of a spinal neoplasm, the incision and execution of the procedure should be such that the tract can be excised later without contamination of tissue planes. Whenever feasible, an anterior approach should be used to obtain biopsy specimens of tumors involving a vertebral body. In addition, we emphasize the usefulness of intraoperative radiography to confirm correct spinal levels and restrict removal of normal bone.

LAMINECTOMY

Laminectomy is indicated for posteriorly placed tumors, for neural decompression and pain relief caused by secondary hypertrophic stenosis, and whenever extensive intradural exploration is indicated. In addition, laminectomy may allow tumor resection within the vertebral body if the pedicles and facet are removed, thus allowing a posterolateral approach to the spine. Our major indications for laminectomy in metastatic cancer are in patients with prostate cancer and lymphoma who relapse after radiation therapy. In patients with primary neoplasms and in those with solitary radioresistant metastases, laminectomy is indicated with posterior instrumentation and bone grafting to complete a staged spondylectomy.

In the thoracic and lumbar region, laminectomies can be performed with the patient in the lateral or prone position; we prefer the lateral position on the Olympic Vac-pac unit because of the ease of patient positioning and because it minimizes intraoperative blood loss. The lateral position also allows extension of the posterior procedure via a lateral osteotomy approach by T-ing the skin incision. In the cervical region, operations are performed in the prone position either with the patient held by the Mayfield skull clamps or the halo apparatus if the head is considered unstable.

A generous midline incision is used after adequate skin preparation and draping with Vi-drapes and skin towels. We prefer the use of skin staples instead of towel clips on the skin to facilitate intraoperative radiography. The skin incision is infiltrated with local anesthetic (Xylocaine ½ percent with epinephrine 1:200,000) to minimize bleeding. If the patient has not undergone RT, we use a midline incision. In previously irradiated patients, an off-midline incision with skin flaps or transverse incisions are suggested. After the dermis is incised, the cautery unit is used to divide the subcutaneous tissue, and the midline located by palpating the spinous processes. The paraspinal muscles are stripped off the spine and lamina, but if the posterior elements are destroyed by tumor, this dissection is best carried out sharply with the Cobb elevators or wide-bladed osteotomes to retract the paraspinous muscles. The spinous processes are removed with bone cutters, and the lamina thinned out with the Adson and Leksell rongeurs. The bone can also be thinned out with a high-speed drill after all ligamentous and soft tissues are stripped away. The final layers of bone are generally removed with curettes and Kerrison punches. The ligamentum flavum should then be removed by sharp dissection. When the epidural space is infiltrated by tumor, normal epidural fat will be absent or will be replaced. Bone removal should be carried out until normal epidural fat is seen, but we emphasize preserving as much normal spine as possible to facilitate either stabilization or instrumentation if required later. Bleeding from the epidural space can be controlled with bipolar current, and tumor resection is facilitated if the Cavitron ultrasonic instrument is used. Profuse bleeding from the epidural space frequently may be encountered. Enough tumor should be removed to minimize postoperative bleeding, and the tumor bed gently packed with hemostatic agents such as Avitene (microfibrillar collagen). Often, repeated gentle packing with cottonoids will be required in between tumor dissection to control bleeding. In some patients the tumor may invade the outer sheath of dura, or the nerve roots. These can be removed by sharp microdissection. Following tumor resection, hemostasis is secured by waxing all bone edges and coagulating bleeding points. In addition, drainage of the epidural space by suction drains isolated from the dura by Gelfoam (gelatin foam) is often required. If instrumentation or bone fusion is required, it is performed at this juncture. The indications and techniques are described elsewhere.[22]

Closure of the paraspinal muscles is carried out with heavy 2-0 Vicryl or 0 Vicryl sutures, and the subcutaneous tissues with 00 Vicryl sutures. The skin is closed with 000 nylon sutures or staples. In the patient who requires a plaster of Paris jacket (after bone fusion), subcuticular stitches and Steri-strips are used. A sterile dressing is then applied.

Patients are nursed flat with "log-rolling" maneuvers, and

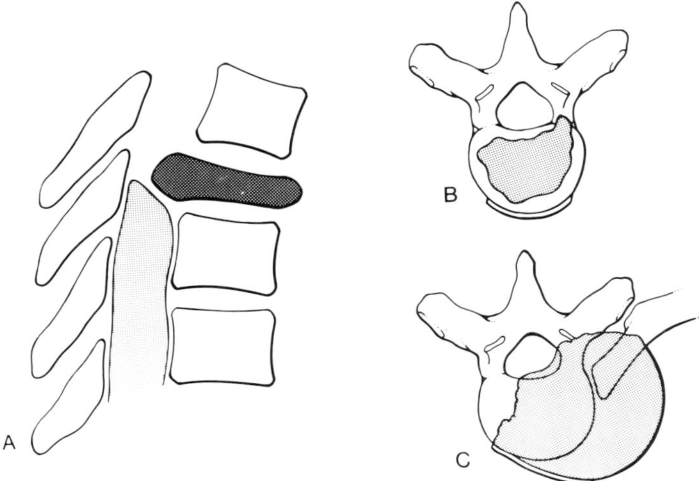

Fig. 132-2. Line drawing indicating radiologic findings that indicate a need for an anterior approach by vertebral body resection: (A) kyphotic deformity secondary to vertebral collapse; (B) anterior osseous destruction by tumor: (C) presence of an anterolateral tumor mass.

care is taken to prevent pulmonary emboli by the use of Venodyne intermittent pressure stockings or low dose heparin therapy.

VERTEBRAL BODY RESECTION

In our experience, the anterior approach by vertebral body resection fulfills the basic principles of tumor surgery: it provides extensive exposure, thus allowing complete resection of all gross tumor, and allows adequate access for anterior stabilization (Figures 132-2 through 132-5). In patients with neoplasms, the importance of immediate stabilization cannot be overemphasized. Stabilization allows immediate ambulation

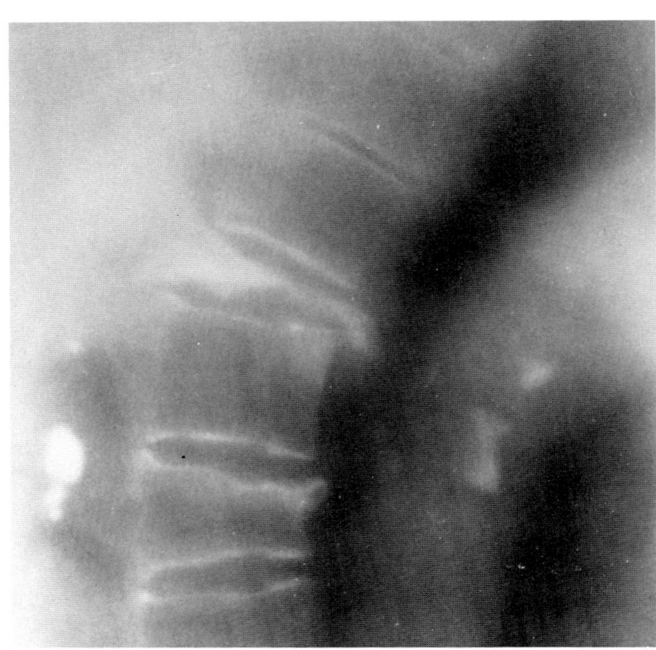

Fig. 132-3. Localized collapse with kyphosis secondary to breast cancer. The presence of collapse exceeding 50 percent of the vertebral body height indicates instability and requires anterior decompression and stabilization.

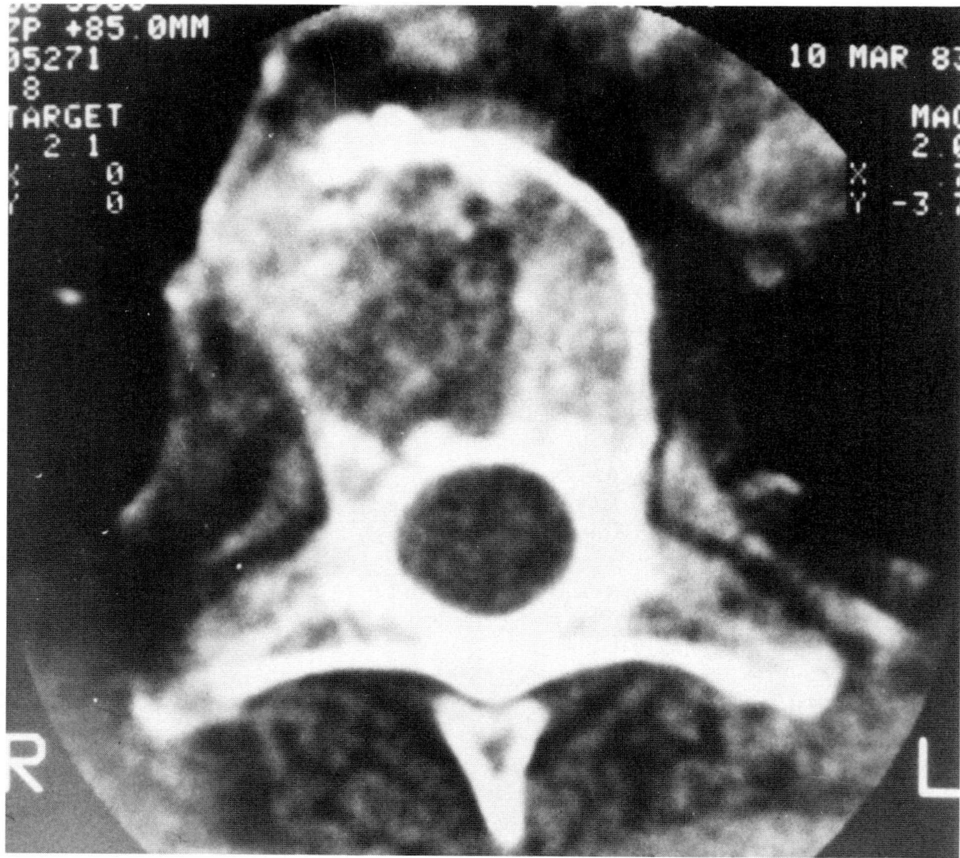

Fig. 132-4. A CT scan of the spine demonstrating destruction of the vertebral body by metastatic kidney cancer. In patients with solitary foci of relapse, surgical resection is indicated regardless of epidural invasion.

and minimizes pulmonary and embolic complications. In view of the limited life expectancy of cancer patients and the need for postoperative radiation therapy, we believe that polymethyl methacrylate (PMMA) as an immediate stabilizing agent allows major advantages over bone grafts. Polymethyl methacrylate is an acrylic polymer belonging to the polyolefin group of synthetic plastics. It is commercially available as a liquid monomer (40 ml) which is mixed with the powdered polymer (20 g). "Curing" or self-polymerization occurs through a self-catalytic process and from the addition of agents. During polymerization, intense heat is generated (80° to 100°C) for periods of 5 minutes. The orthopedic polymethyl methacrylate is impregnated with 10 percent barium sulfate and is available from three major sources: Howmedica, Zimmer, and Richards. There is no bonding at the bone–cement interface, and therefore the brittle acrylic has to be kept in place with additional instrumentation. Although a variety of techniques have been described to achieve this, three methods described in the literature require emphasis.[23–25] All three techniques are relatively simple, easy to master, and should be part of the armamentarium of all spinal surgeons; in this section, we will describe the use of Steinmann pins for anterior fixation of the acrylic.

The anterior spine requires a variety of approaches because of the complex soft part anatomy anterior to the prevertebral space (Table 132-3). In this review, we will focus on the transthoracic approach, which will serve as the model for approaches to the other segments. An initial consideration is the side from which an anterolateral exposure should be performed. In the majority of cases, the side that allows maximal

tumor resection should be chosen. This can usually be ascertained by CT. If a CT scan is not available, then either the side of increased pedicle destruction or collapse or the symptomatic side of radiculopathy or plexopathy probably indicates the site of tumor compression. In equivocal cases, a right-sided approach is chosen for thoracic segments, and a left-sided approach for lumbar segments.

The upper two thoracic segments form the posterior border of the thoracic inlet: this region can be exposed by a direct anterior trans-sternal approach[26] or indirectly by a posterolateral thoracotomy with resection of the upper three ribs for extensive tumors with lateral extension. The trans-sternal anterior operation is performed with the patient in the supine position with the head extended (the range of extension and flexion is tested with the patient awake before surgery). A T-shaped incision is used. The horizontal limb of the T extends 1 cm above the clavicle and extends past the sternomastoid on either side; and the vertical limb is carried down to the body of the sternum. Subplatysmal flaps are elevated and retained by sutures (Figure 132-6). Several veins (anterior jugular veins and the jugular venous arch) and the medial supraclavicular nerves cross the field and must be sectioned. The sternal and clavicular heads of the sternomastoid are detached from their bony origins by cautery and retracted superiorly and posteriorly. The inferior strap muscles (sternohyoid and sternothyroid) are sectioned inferiorly and retracted superiorly and medially (Figure 132-7). The fatty and areolar tissues in the suprasternal space are cleared. The sternal origin of the pectoralis major is cleared from the sternum, and the clavicle stripped subperiosteally. The

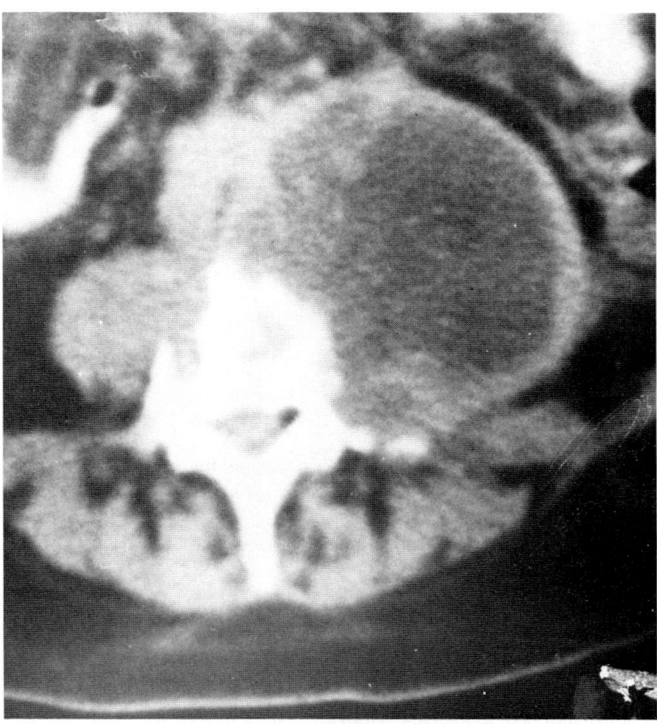

Fig. 132-5. A CT scan demonstrating paraspinal soft part sarcoma with spine destruction and epidural extension. An anterolateral approach is required for tumor resection.

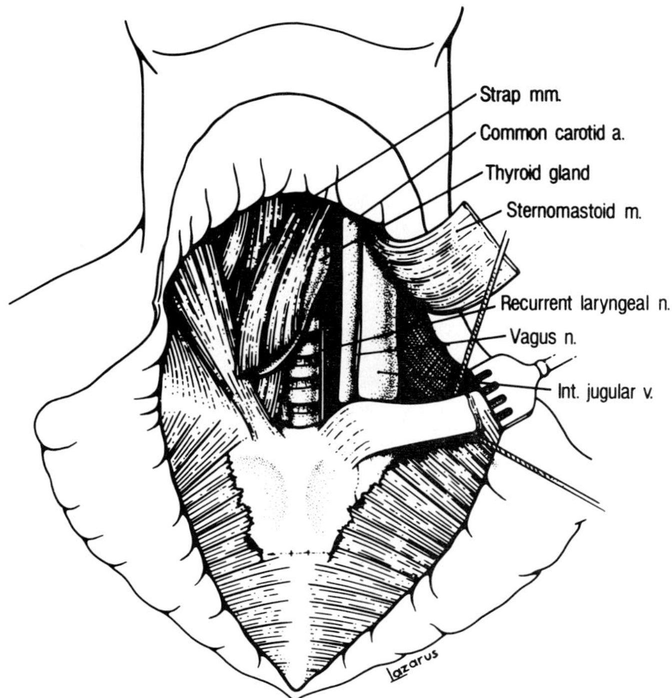

Fig. 132-7. The sternomastoid muscle is sectioned and retracted laterally; the inferior strap muscles are sectioned and retracted medially; the medial third of the clavicle is removed after subperiosteal stripping.

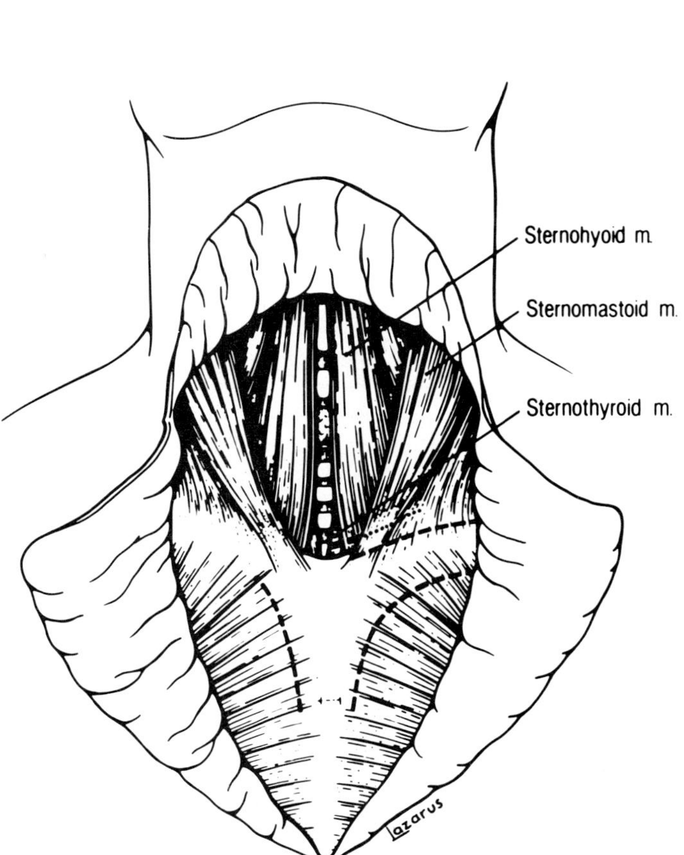

Fig. 132-6. Surgical exposure of the upper two thoracic vertebra. Subplatysmal flaps are elevated, and dotted lines indicate muscles that have to be stripped from the clavicle and manubrium (sternomastoid and pectoralis major).

medial third of the clavicle is sectioned with a Gigli saw, and the medial end disarticulated from the sternum. A power drill is used to thin the edges of a rectangular piece of manubrium, which is then cut off with scissors. Once the periosteum is removed, the vascular structures beneath are exposed. The inferior thyroid veins are ligated but the innominate vein can be retracted out of the field. The thymus and surrounding fat should be dissected and resected. The avascular plane between the trachea and esophagus medially and the vascular sheath laterally is developed (Figure 132-8). The recurrent laryngeal nerve should be identified. The prevertebral space is then opened in the midline, and the longus colli muscles stripped laterally with the periosteum. Intact discs above and below the level of involvement are identified. Self-retaining Cloward retractors or an Oberhill retractor (V. Muller, Chicago, Ill) are placed under the longus colli muscles (Figure 132-9). The involved vertebra is then resected piecemeal with curettes, rongeurs, and osteotomes. If the bone is markedly sclerotic, a high-speed drill can be used. All involved bone and soft tissue tumor and devitalized tissues are removed down to the dura. Meticulous hemostasis is achieved with the bipolar current. After the dura is cleaned of all tumor, a sheet of Gelfoam is used to protect the dura. The resected vertebra is then replaced using the clavicle as a strut graft by impacting it in place under gentle traction. Additional cancellous bone from the sternum is also laid along the strut. Immediate stability can also be achieved by the use of Steinmann pins and methyl methacrylate that is allowed to polymerize in situ. Suction drains are placed, and the wound closed in layers. Postoperatively, a cervicothoracic orthosis is prescribed (generally a Philadelphia collar with thoracic extension). Patients are allowed to ambulate immediately and can begin chemotherapy in a week. If a bone graft is used, RT should be delayed for 6 weeks. In our experience, all

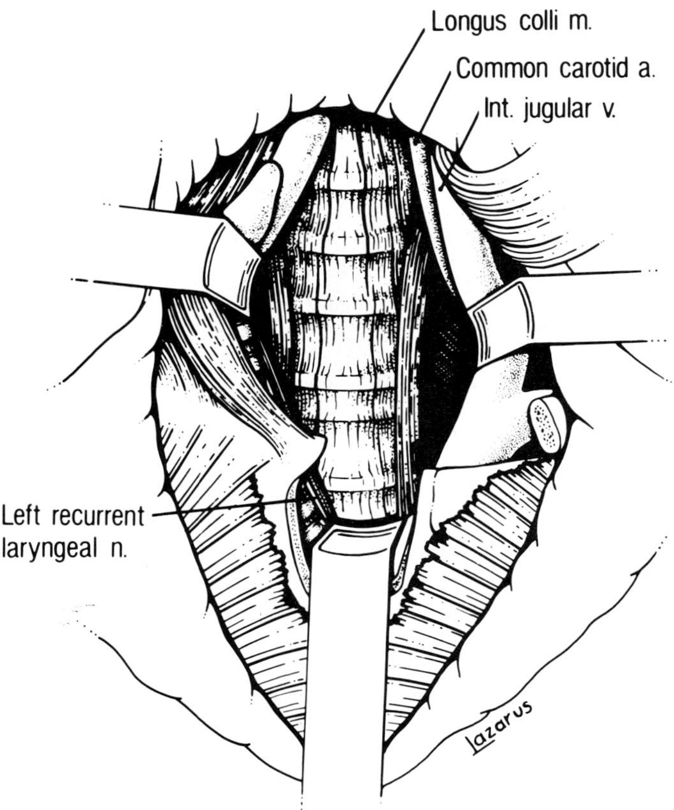

Fig. 132-8. Following removal of a portion of the manubrium sterni, the trachea and esophagus are retracted medially and the carotid sheath retracted laterally.

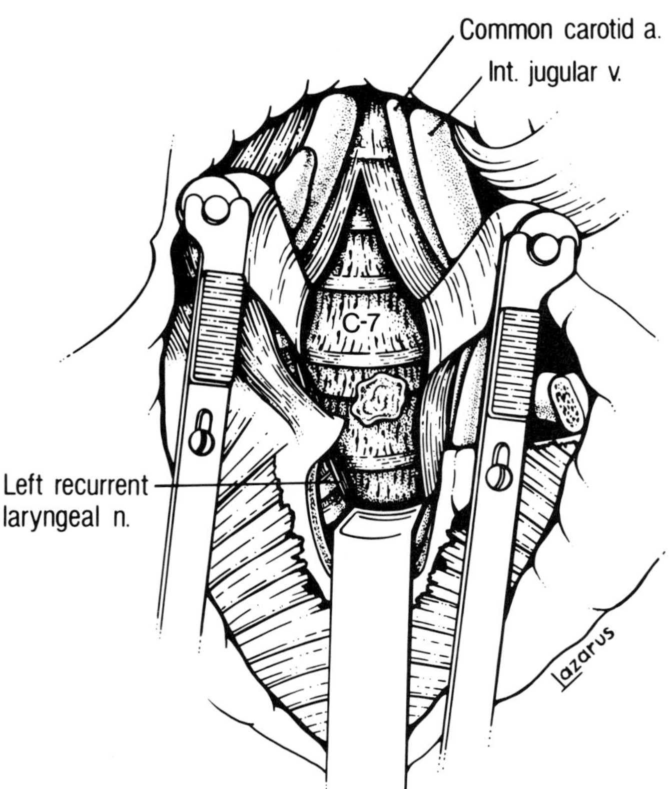

Fig. 132-9. The longus colli muscles are stripped from the anterior aspect of the spine, and self-retaining Cloward retractors are positioned to expose the bony thoracic inlet posteriorly.

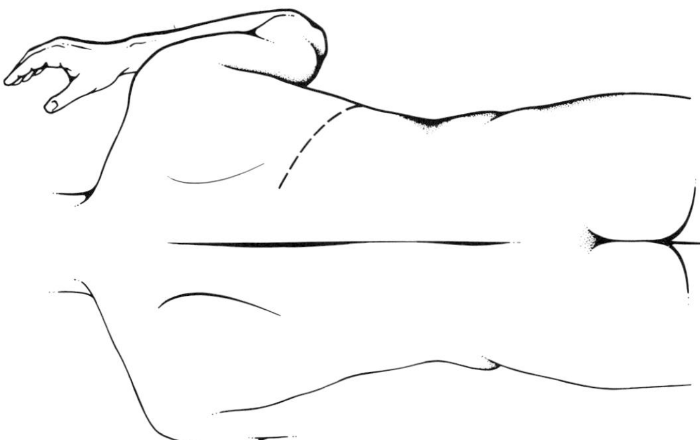

Fig. 132-10. A standard posterolateral thoracotomy incision is used for exposures of the thoracic segments.

patients will probably require a secondary posterior fusion following antitumor therapy.

The transthoracic approach is used for tumors below the third thoracic segment. Patients are positioned in the lateral position on an Olympic Vac-Pac unit, and general endotracheal anesthesia with a double lumen tube is used. A generous skin incision similar to a posterolateral thoracotomy is placed below the scapula (Figure 132-10). The posterior incision should be parallel to the paraspinal muscles but not extend to the midline unless a second-stage spondylectomy is planned. After the skin incision is made, we use the electrocautery to cut through the chest wall muscles (trapezius, serratus, latissimus, and pectoralis major) to reach the rib cage.

When the interspace is entered, it should be above the body that one has to work with since the ribs turn caudally proximal to the angle. In the lower thoracic segments, at least two spaces above the level of involvement are chosen because of the rising dome of the diaphragm. Only the posterior 5-10 cm of rib needs to be removed (Figure 132-11). Rib resection is performed by using the cautery to detach the periosteum of the rib, and using Doyen periosteal elevators to strip the periosteum from the neurovascular bundle. The intercostal bundle should be carefully isolated with right-angle clamps and cleanly ligated or clipped. During the initial phase of tumor resection, the head of the ribs overlies the pedicle and should be kept intact to prevent injury to the cord. A self-retaining thoracic retractor is placed, and the lung held out of the field with a malleable Hurson retractor. The anterior spine is then exposed by retraction of the lung, which can be gradually deflated if required. To expose the spine, the pleura is then reflected in the form of a window. Intercostal vessels (which are direct tributaries of the aorta or vena cava) are carefully identified, and ligated as well as clipped. This maneuver also allows mobilization of the major vessels over the surface of the vertebra. All soft tissues anterior to the vertebra are dissected off (including the sympathetic ganglia). The isolated segments are packed off with lap pads, and if a prevertebral tumor is identified, we can be reasonably sure of the proper location of the segment to be resected. If no tumor is evident on the surface, it is important to establish the correct level, not only by counting the ribs from within the chest, but also by obtaining an intraoperative roentgenogram. Before commencing work on the spine, the anterior surface of the vertebral body is cleared by periosteal elevators. Intact disc structures above and below the

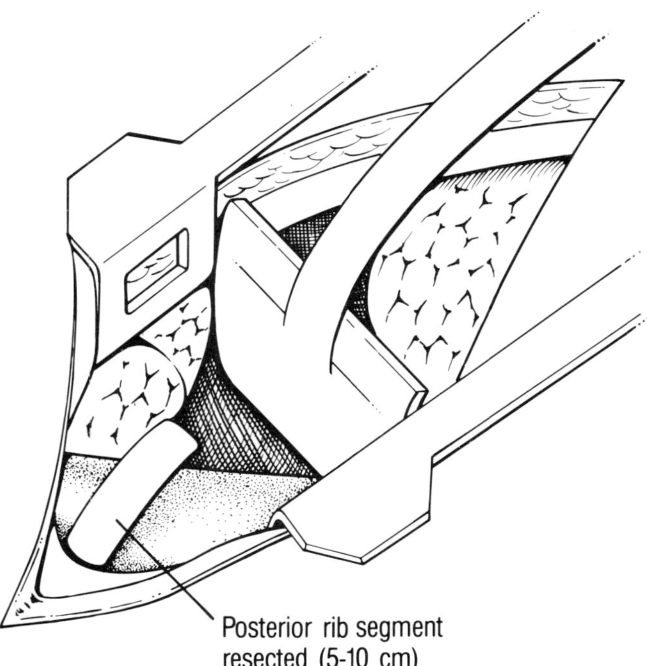

Fig. 132-11. After the thoracic cavity is opened, self-retaining retractors are positioned. Only the posterior 5–10 cm of rib has to be resected as shown.

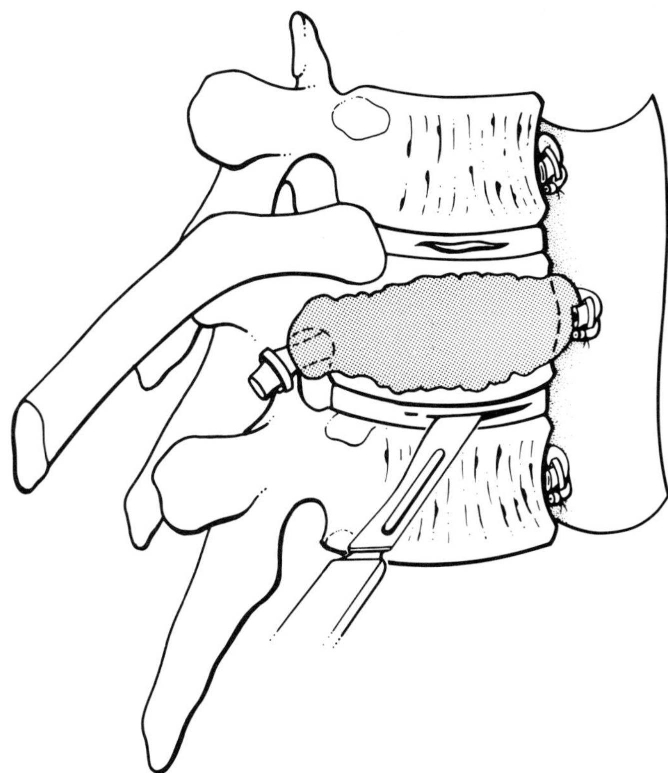

Fig. 132-12. The pleura is reflected off the anterior spine as shown. Vascular bundles are isolated, ligated, and clipped as shown. Dissection of the diseased segments begins by excision of discs above and below the vertebra.

level of involvement are identified (Figure 132-12); the discs are incised with a No. 15 blade, and the vertebral segments removed with rongeurs, curettes, and osteotomes. Tumor resection should be complete, and the posterior longitudinal ligament should be removed. In patients who have not received prior radiation, this resection is relatively easy to accomplish. In radiated patients, the bone and tumor may be fibrotic, and the posterior longitudinal ligament densely adherent to the dura. By tracing the epidural tumor posteriorly, it is possible to decompress the dura laterally and posteriorly by performing a facetectomy and removing the pedicle. To allow additional posterior decompression, a hemilaminectomy can be performed at this time. The anterior longitudinal ligament is left intact if it is not destroyed. A high-speed drill is then used to drill out the opposite half of the body until a thin cortical shell is left. If a curative resection is contemplated, every effort must be made to remove all bone and soft tissue so that the spondylectomy can be completed by a second-stage posterior approach. We emphasize the importance of complete tumor resection even to the extent of using a Cavitron ultrasonic tumor aspirator to remove all gross tumor. Following tumor resection, all soft tissues on the endplates above and below are removed to provide the broadest possible support for the methyl methacrylate reconstruction. Hemostasis is secured by the use of the fine-tipped bipolar current, and the use of hemostatic agents such as Avitene (microfibrillar collagen) or Gelfoam pledgets. Prior to stabilization, the surgeon must be sure that all vertebral segments involved by tumor have been resected, since fixation of the acrylic to a diseased vertebra will result in postoperative displacement. In half the patients, more than one vertebra has to be removed; we have resected up to four vertebrae including the involved chest wall in the thoracic region with little morbidity.

The next phase of the operation is stabilization. Steinmann

pins varying in size from 5/64 to 19/64 inch in diameter are selected and cut to straddle the bony defect (Figures 132-13, 132-14). We prefer to use the smooth pins instead of the threaded variety. The pins are bent at each end in the shape of hockey sticks and introduced with two heavy sternal needle holders. These pins should straddle the resected segments and be securely in place

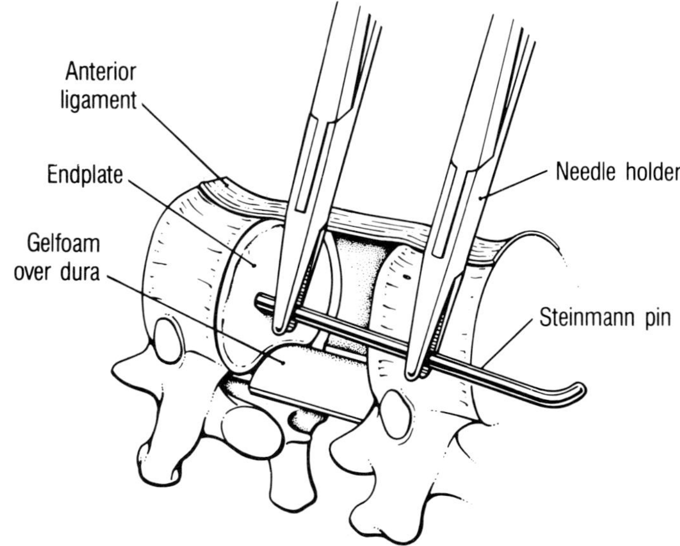

Fig. 132-13. Following tumor resection, the endplates are carefully cleaned with curettes and Steinmann pins bent at each end introduced with heavy needle holders.

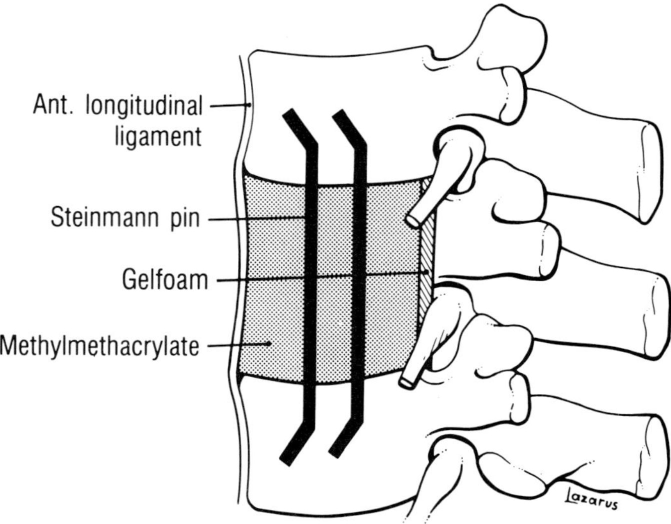

Fig. 132-14. The Steinmann pins should straddle the resected segments and are incorporated within the methyl methacrylate construct; during the heat of polymerization, saline irrigation is used and a sheet of Gelfoam protects the dura.

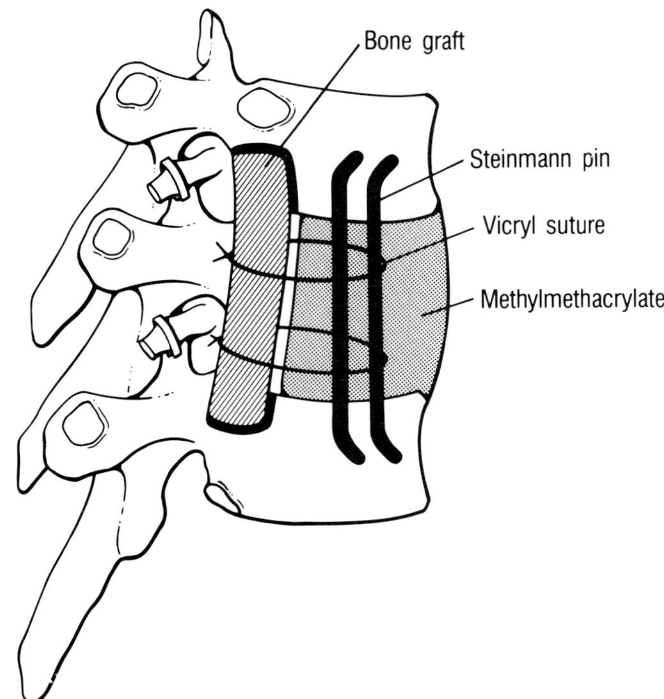

Fig. 132-15. The rib segment may be used as a lateral fusion mass as shown; it is held in place by Vicryl sutures and tied to the Steinmann pins before insertion of the semisolid acrylic cement.

to the vertebrae above and below. Once the pins (generally two) are secured, methyl methacrylate is injected into the space and molded to recreate the resected bodies. At the same time, Penfield dissectors and tongue blades are used to keep the hardening acrylic away from the dura, which is protected by strips of Gelfoam. Copious irrigation with saline is used to dissipate heat during the polymerization process. The epidural space should be kept free of all trapped fluid, and no effort should be made to pack this space tightly. The resected rib can be placed adjacent to the bodies and tied in position with Vicryl sutures as a lateral fusion mass (Figure 132-15). If the angulation of the spine or technical difficulties do not allow safe introduction of Steinmann pins, we use anterior distraction devices such as Knodt or Harrington rods. The anterior distraction devices are then incorporated within the acrylic construct.

The chest cavity is drained by chest tubes, and the closure is that of a standard thoracotomy. Postoperatively, patients are kept in intensive care for a few days, and the chest tube drainage is monitored. When less than 100 ml is drained over 24 hours, it is removed. Extensive chest tube drainage over a week suggests a CSF leak into the pleural cavity. To minimize respiratory complications, we allow early ambulation. A Knight-Taylor brace or a Prenyl jacket is used for patient comfort. Broad spectrum antibiotics are used routinely during the operation and for 48 hours following surgery. A refluoromyelogram is generally performed to check clearing of the block and alignment of the spine (Figure 132-16). If postoperative radiation therapy is decided upon, it is begun after a week.

ANTERIOR APPROACH TO LOWER THORACIC AND UPPER LUMBAR SEGMENTS

A variety of approaches are available for the thoracolumbar region because the diaphragm separates this region into two cavities. The lower thoracic approach can also be performed by a completely extrapleural procedure, but the widest

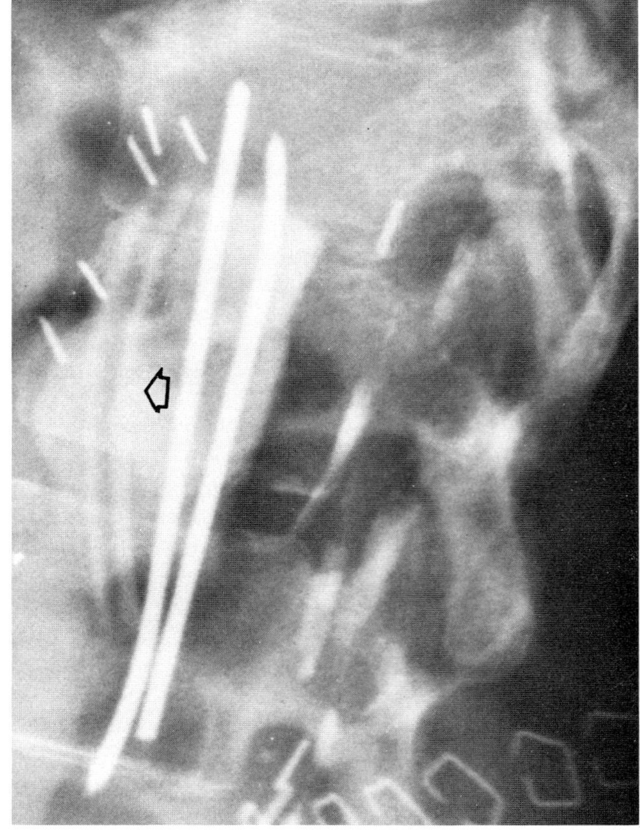

Fig. 132-16. A postoperative lateral roentgenogram demonstrates normal alignment of the spine and clearing of myelographic block. Arrow indicates rib graft.

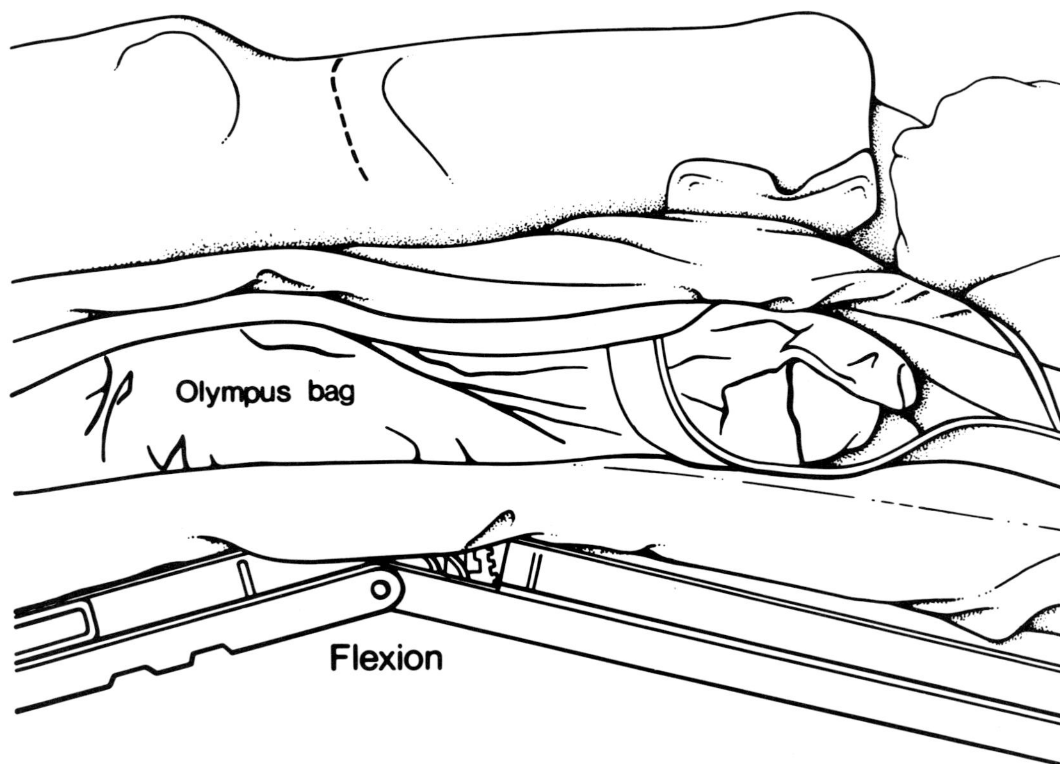

Fig. 132-17. For exposures of the lumbar segments, a retroperitoneal flank approach is used. The patient is positioned on an Olympic Vac-Pac unit, and the table flexed to allow a subcostal exposure.

exposures are obtained by a transthoracic approach with detachment of the diaphragm.

The diaphragm is a dome-shaped muscle that is muscular around its periphery and tendinous centrally. Anteriorly, it arises from the xiphoid and cartilaginous portions of the lower six ribs, posteriorly it originates from the crura that are attached to the anterior longitudinal ligament; superiorly they arise from the medial and lateral arcuate ligaments, which are attached to the transverse processes of the first lumbar and the 12th rib. The widest exposures are obtained by resection of the 10th or 11th ribs, and detaching the muscle from the costal articulations as well as the arcuate ligaments.

For the widest and most direct anterior exposure to the thoracoabdominal spine, a long skin incision centered on the 10th or 11th ribs is required. Posteriorly, the incision should extend to the paraspinous muscles. The latissimus dorsi and serratus anterior muscles are divided, and the ribs to be resected identified. The oblique muscles are detached from the rib with cautery, or cut in the intercostal space. The endothoracic fascia and parietal pleura are opened and the ribs spread. The diaphragm is then put under tension by retraction and circumferentially detached toward the arcuate ligaments. The retroperitoneal space is gradually enlarged by blunt dissection, and the spleen retracted downward. The sympathetic trunk and the areolar tissue around the aorta are cleared. Segmental intercostal vessels are carefully ligated and cut. The anterior surface of the thoracolumbar spine is then exposed and the soft tissues cleared to expose the cortical surface. Tumor resection then proceeds as described earlier in this chapter. Following tumor resection and stabilization, repair proceeds by closure of the diaphragm and insertion of chest tubes. The muscles and skin are then closed in routine fashion.

To approach the lumbar spine from the second to the fourth segments, an oblique retroperitoneal flank approach is used (Figures 132-17, 132-18). The 12th rib is resected subperiosteally, and the retroperitoneal space behind the fascia transversalis developed. The kidney and ureters are displaced anteriorly, and the space kept open by a Balfour retractor. It is important to identify the relatively avascular space behind the peritoneum and Gerota's fascia, and to approach the lumbar spine anterior to the psoas major and quadratus lumborum muscles. A helpful anatomic guide to this region is the crural attachment of the diaphragm, which generally is seen only to the second lumbar segment. The sympathetic chain should be retracted laterally and preserved whenever possible. To remove tumors involving the fifth lumbar vertebra, a retroperitoneal approach is inadequate, and an anterior transabdominal approach should be used. In this segment, Knodt rods are useful because Steinmann pins are difficult to place.

LATERAL OSTEOTOMY APPROACH

The spine can also be approached from the side by the lateral osteotomy approach, which is performed by cutting through the transverse process of the vertebra and fracturing the osteotomized portion of the paraspinal structures anteriorly. The major indications for this procedure are superior sulcus tumors or other lung cancers with chest wall involvement, as well as large paraspinous sarcomas with both anterolateral and posterolateral components. The skin incision can be oblique, as in the thoracic region, or a T with the shorter limbs of the T in the midline. Initially, the paraspinal tumor mass is dissected free from the lateral and anterior attachments including the intra-abdominal and intrathoracic vessels; secondly, it is

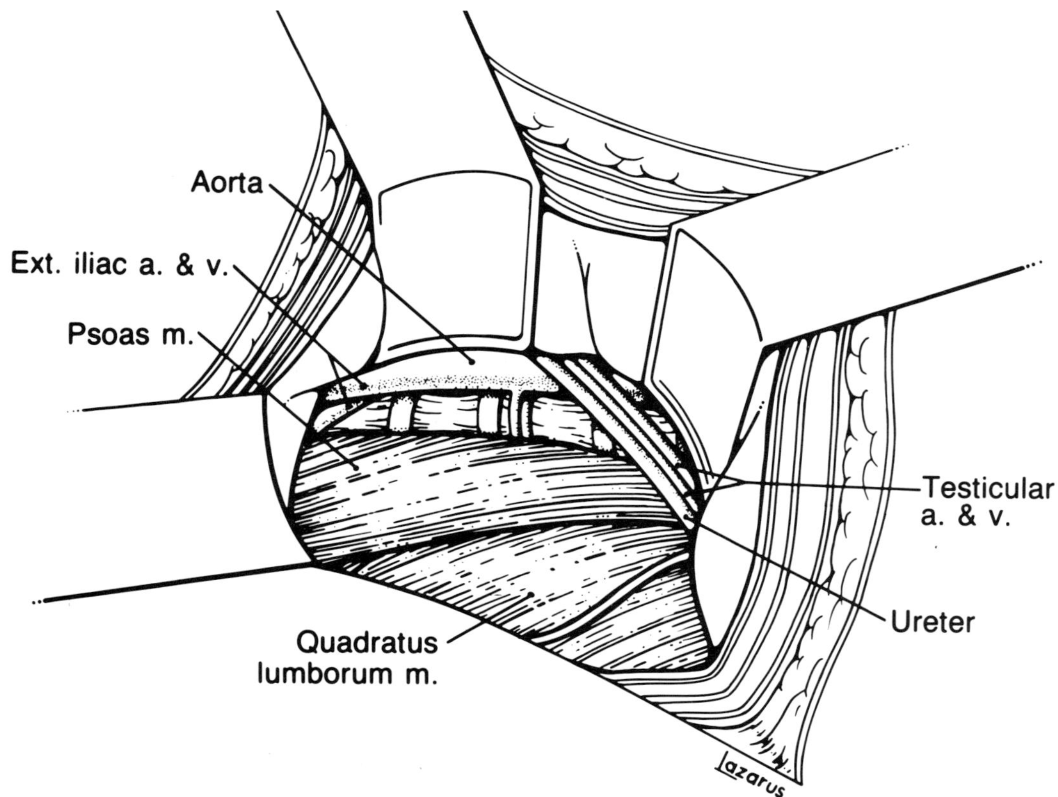

Fig. 132-18.   For exposures of the lumbar segments, the retroperitoneal approach with anterior displacement of the kidney and ureter is used. Note that exposure is anterior to the psoas major muscle.

freed superiorly and inferiorly by resection of the chest wall or the paraspinous muscles. Finally, the paraspinous muscles are cut over the transverse processes and the main mass of the tumor fractured forward. Nerve roots are carefully isolated and clipped. If the intraspinal extensions of tumor are noted, the spinal resection should include a partial hemilaminectomy and facetectomy. No additional reconstruction is required after such lateral osteotomy procedures. Following extensive chest wall resection, extensive skeletal defects may require reconstruction with a Maarlex mesh prosthesis.

POSTOPERATIVE MANAGEMENT AND DISCUSSION

Patients undergoing anterior spinal surgery and stabilization procedures require monitoring in the intensive care unit because of the potential for respiratory complications in addition to the other common postoperative problems such as ileus, venous thrombosis, and infection. Despite their apparent magnitude, these procedures are well tolerated by most cancer patients, and the morbidity is lower than that of decompressive laminectomy. We allow early ambulation and recommend rapid tapering of steroid therapy. In our experience, patients who have received recent radiation therapy as well as high dose steroid therapy for more than a month are particularly likely to develop perioperative complications.

In our experience with the first 160 patients, the 30-day mortality was 6 percent and an additional 15 percent developed surgical complications. The mortality, however, for patients undergoing de novo operation was 4 percent and the morbidity was 10 percent. No serious permanent neurologic defect was

encountered, and all other complications were effectively treated without sequelae. The neurologic improvement rate exceeded 80 percent, and 80 percent of patients with spinal pain experienced pain relief. In long-term survivors, the long-term ambulation rate exceeded 80 percent at 1 year, although repeat anterior or posterior decompressions were necessary in 20 percent of patients. These figures are superior to those reported for external RT and steroid therapy alone. In patients with potentially curable tumors, we believe that this operation is indicated even before cord compression has developed, i.e., in patients with intra-osseous disease. For primary malignant neoplasms of the spine, a two-stage approach is required: vertebral body resection as the initial debulking procedure followed by posterior resection and stabilization. With such aggressive surgery, long-term disease-free survivors and cures may be anticipated with malignant spine tumors. The concept that these patients cannot be cured because the spine has been considered an "inaccessible" site is no longer valid. Our results suggest that the logic of treating malignant bone tumors elsewhere can now be applied equally successfully to lesions involving the spine.

REFERENCES

1. Sundaresan N, DiGiacinto GV, Hughes JEO: Surgical treatment of spinal metastases. Clin Neurosurg 33:503, 1986
2. Boland PJ, Lane JM, Sundaresan N: Metastatic disease of the spine. Clin Orthop 169:95, 1982
3. Constans JP, De Vitiis E, Donzelli, et al: Spinal metastases with neurological manifestations. J Neurosurg 59:111, 1983
4. Gilbert RW, Kim JH, Posner JB: Epidural spinal cord compression

from metastatic tumor: Diagnosis and treatment. Ann Neurol 3:40, 1978

5. Stark RJ, Henson RA, Evans SJW: Spinal metastases: A retrospective survey from a general hospital. Brain 1O5:189, 1982

6. Krol G, Heier L, Becker R, et al: MRI and myelography in the evaluation of epidural extension of primary and metastatic tumors, in Volk J (ed): Neuroradiology 1985–1986. Amsterdam, Elsevier, 1986, pp 91–97

7. Russell EJ, Berenstein A: Neurological applications of interventional radiology. Neurol Clin 2:873, 1984 8. Barcena A, Lobato RD, Rivas JJ, et al: Spinal metastatic disease: Analysis of factors determining functional prognosis and choice of treatment. Neurosurgery 15:820, 1984

9. Tang SG, Byfield JE, Sharp TR: Prognostic factors in the management of metastatic epidural cord compression. J Neuro-oncol 1:21, 1981

10. Sundaresan N, Scher H, Yagoda A, et al: Surgical treatment of spinal metastases in kidney cancer. J Clin Oncol 1986 (in press)

11. Sundaresan N, Hilaris BH, Martini N: The combined neurosurgical-thoracic management of superior sulcus tumors. Arch Surg 1986 (in press)

12. Sundaresan N, Galicich JH, Lane JM: Treatment of odontoid fracture in cancer patients. J Neurosurg 52:187, 1981

13. Sundaresan N, Galicich JH, Lane JM: Harrington rod stabilization for pathological fractures of the spine. J Neurosurg 60:282, 1984

14. Harrington KD: Anterior cord decompression and spinal stabilization for patients with metastastic lesions of the spine. J Neurosurg 61:1O7, 1984 15. Flatley JJ, Anderson MH, Anast GT: Spinal instability due to metastatic disease. J Bone Joint Surg 66(A):47, 1984

16. Clark CR, Keggi KJ, Panjabi MM: Methyl methacrylate stabilization of the cervical spine. J Bone Joint Surg 66(A):40, 1984

17. Martenson JA, Evans RL, Lie MR: Treatment outcome and complications in patients treated for malignant cord compression. J Nenro-Oncol 3:77, 1985

18. Overby MC, Rothman AS: Anterolateral decompression for metastatic epidural spinal cord tumors. J Neurosurg 62:344, 1985

19. Macedo N, Sundaresan N, Galicich JH: Decompressive laminectomy for metastatic cancer: What are the current indications? Proc Am Soc Am Oncol 4:278, 1985

20. Foley KH: The treatment of cancer pain. N Engl J Med 31:84, 1985

21. Sundaresan N, DiGiacinto GV: Antitumor and anti-nociceptive approaches to cancer pain. Med Clin North Am 71:329, 1987

22. Siegel T, Siegal T: The management of malignant epidural tumors compressing the spinal cord, in Schmidek H, Sweet W (eds): Operative Neurosurgical Techniques, ed 2. Orlando, Grune & Stratton, 1987

23. Siegel T, Tikva P, Siegel T: Vertebral body resection for epidural compression by malignant tumors. J Bone Joint Surg 67A:375, 1985

24. Sundaresan N, Krol G, Hughes JEO: Treatment of malignant tumors of the spine, in Youmans J (ed): Neurological Surgery. Philadelphia, WB Saunders, 1987 (in Press)

25. Sundaresan N, Galicich JH, Lane JM, et al: Treatment of neoplastic epidural cord compression by vertebral body resection and stabilization. J Neurosurg 63:676, 1985

26. Sundaresan N, Shah J, Feghali JG: A trans-sternal approach to the upper thoracic vertebra. Am J Surg 148:473, 1986

CHAPTER 133

The Management of Malignant Epidural Tumors Compressing the Spinal Cord

Tzony Siegal   Tali Siegal

THE MANAGEMENT of spinal column metastases that cause neurologic deficits has been the subject of debate for many years. The last two decades have witnessed significant shifts in therapeutic approaches, ranging from urgent laminectomy to a combination of laminectomy and radiotherapy to nonsurgical treatment by radiotherapy alone. More recently, attention has been directed to radiotherapy[1–6] or to anterior surgical decompression[7–10] as preferred treatment modalities. Some attempts have been made to compare various management methods, but the absence of satisfactory controlled trials still leaves no clear consensus on management.[1–6,11,12] A synopsis of the current knowledge and concepts related to various therapeutic measures and prognostic factors will be presented in this chapter.

Metastatic cord and cauda equina compression are often considered together under the name *spinal cord compression,* because in recent series there has been no difference in outcome.[2,3,13,14] Diagnosis of cord compression required evidence of a high degree extradural myelographic block, greater than 80 percent. The management of extradural metastases that partially obliterate the spinal canal (to less than 60 percent) will not be considered in this chapter.

INCIDENCE

Nearly 5 percent of patients with systemic cancer develop spinal extradural metastases,[12,15] and nearly 20 percent of the patients with vertebral column involvement will develop spinal cord compression.[16] In large series, the three most frequent types of primary tumors spreading to the spine and extradural space are bronchogenic carcinoma, breast carcinoma, and lymphoma.[6] The origin of metastases cannot be identified in 9 percent of the cases. Although spinal metastases generally occur in patients with known malignancy, in 8 percent of the patients with spinal cord compression this is the initial symptom of cancer.[2,6]

TUMOR LOCATION

The involvement of any area of the spine by metastatic deposits corresponds roughly to the number of vertebrae contained therein. The thoracic spine thus is involved in about 60 percent of cases.[2,6] A large majority of tumors are localized to one or two vertebral segments, but in 17 percent of patients two or more sites may show evidence of epidural compression at some time during the course of the disease.[2,3,6]

When the metastasis invades the spinal canal, it is usually restricted to the extradural space, with variable involvement of the anterior (ventral) compartment, the lateral gutters, the posterior compartment, or any combination of these sites. However, the majority of epidural tumors (85 percent) arise in a vertebral body, invade the epidural space anteriorly, and remain largely anterior to the spinal cord.[2,15,17,18]

The location of the extradural metastasis has important surgical implications. A metastatic tumor in the posterior extradural compartment is easily accessible by laminectomy, whereas the accessibility of a ventral mass by this approach is largely limited and requires an anterior or anterolateral approach. The location of the tumor within the spinal canal can usually be inferred from the spinal x-ray studies. However, accurate definition of the compressive mass as either posterior, lateral, cuff, or anterior usually requires the combination of metrizamide myelography and computed tomography of the spine (Figure 133-1). Magnetic resonance imaging (MRI) studies, where available, constitute an excellent noninvasive alternative procedure for the pretreatment investigation.

SYMPTOMS AND SIGNS

The onset of symptoms of spinal cord or nerve root compression may be acute or insidious. The duration of symptoms varies widely before diagnosis. Pain is usually the initial symptom (in 96 percent of cases), preceding other symptoms by 5 days to 2 years (median, 7 weeks).[2,3,6] The pain can be localized close to the site of the lesion or can be radicular. Radicular pain results from compression or infiltration of the nerve roots at the affected level[6] (Figure 133-2). By the time of diagnosis, neurologic signs are common[2,6] and include various degrees of muscle weakness in 76 percent of cases, bladder and bowel dysfunction in more than 50 percent, and sensory symptoms in about 50 percent. It is important to note that nearly half of the severely affected patients will develop a complete deficit (no residual cord function) after diagnosis and before undergoing any treatment. Twenty-eight percent of the paraparetic patients become paraplegic in less than 24 hours as a function of time elapsed before treatment.[11] It therefore seems critical to treat patients with cord compression as soon as possible.

OPERATIVE NEUROSURGICAL TECHNIQUES
ISBN 0-8089-1862-1

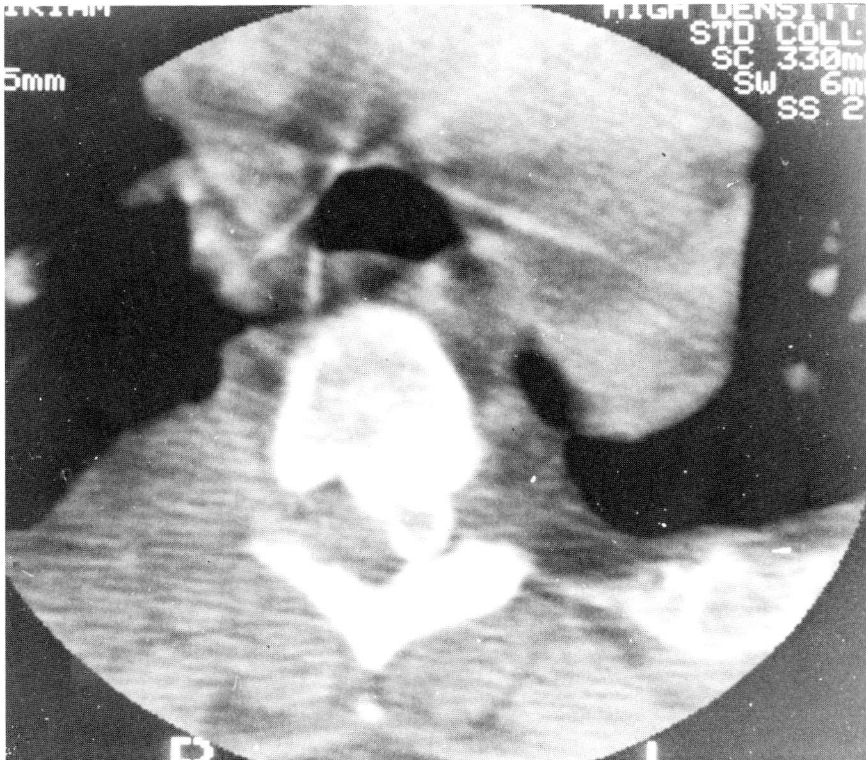

Fig. 133-1. Computed tomographic myelogram of the thoracic spine in a paraparetic patient with metastic breast carcinoma. The epidural tumor lies in a posterolateral position displacing and compressing the spinal cord.

PATHOPHYSIOLOGY

The pathophysiologic mechanisms involved in neoplastic cord compression were investigated in experimental animal tumor models.[19–22] The expanding extradural tumor causes early obstruction of the spinal epidural venous plexus and enhances production of a vasogenic type of edema. The edema involves initially the white matter and eventually the gray matter in the late stage of compression. In the end stage, the spinal cord blood flow decreases rapidly at the site of compression. The ischemia may play the final deleterious role, leading to irreversible loss of function if the compression is not rapidly alleviated. The spinal cord can adjust to gradual compression over a period of weeks or months but is unable to tolerate rapid compression such as that caused by rapidly growing malignant tumors. In such cases it is not uncommon for the spinal cord tolerance to be reached within a matter of hours or days after the onset of the first symptoms. This results in the rapid development of paralysis below the level of compression.

SURVIVAL AND SPINAL CORD COMPRESSION

Malignant spinal cord compression usually occurs in patients with metastatic systemic cancer. In spite of the overall grim prognosis of the basic disease, treatment is warranted in many cases[6] and is aimed at preserving or restoring spinal cord function (ambulation and continence) or at alleviating intractable pain. Spinal cord compression in itself is generally not fatal (except in the upper portion of the cervical spine). Depending upon the natural history of the systemic malignancy, patients may survive for extended periods: 30 percent may be expected to survive beyond a year and rarely as long as 4 to 9 years.[23,24] Patients with widespread metastatic disease have a more limited life expectancy of a few months.[7,25,26]

The overall effect of successful treatment on survival is not clear. Some investigators have suggested that treatment of spinal cord compression is unlikely to prolong survival.[23,27] However, three separate studies[17,24,26] have shown improved survival in patients responding to treatment. It appears that effective treatment is associated with improved survival, but

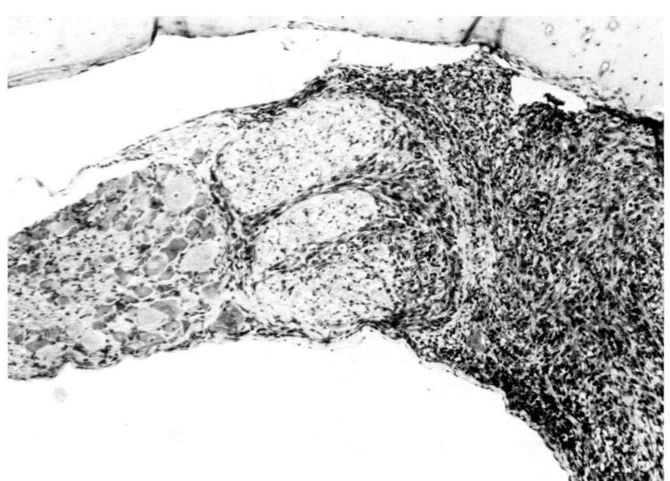

Fig. 133-2. A malignant fibrous histiocytoma infiltrating a thoracolumbar nerve root continuous with the epidural tumor mass.

the precise significance of this association is uncertain, since factors not related to treatment (e.g., tumor histology) can also influence a patient's ability to walk and to survive.

FACTORS INFLUENCING THE RECOVERY OF FUNCTION

Some factors have been considered as important determinants of functional prognosis in patients with spinal metastases: (1) tumor biology; (2) pretreatment neurologic status; (3) progression rate of symptoms; (4) location of tumor within the spinal canal; and (5) therapy employed.[5,6,11,12,23,27,28]

TUMOR BIOLOGY

Cell Type

The biologic activity of the primary neoplasm determines both systemic and local aggressiveness, which are represented, respectively, by posttreatment survival rate and the rate of success of therapy.[11,27] Patients with myeloma, lymphoma, Ewing's sarcoma, neuroblastoma, or carcinoma of the breast have a favorable prognosis for recovery of function.[2,3,6,11] The outlook for patients with metastatic bronchogenic carcinoma is generally poor. However, exceptions to these results make it difficult to prognosticate in individual cases. In general, high tumor radiosensitivity is significantly related to favorable prognosis and the contrary is true for radioresistant tumors. It also appears that the tumor cell type has a greater importance in determining outcome than the type of treatment. This is suggested by a critical review of the results of management obtained by radiotherapy alone and by laminectomy plus radiotherapy.[2,3,6,11]

Response to High-Dose Dexamethasone

The use of steroids in the treatment of spinal cord compression is widely accepted.[2,3,6,7,10,11,29,30] The scientific basis for their use stems from animal models of spinal cord compression, in which reduction of spinal cord edema and delayed onset of paraplegia were observed after treatment with dexamethasone.[19,20,31] Greenberg et al.[3] recommended the use of high-dose steroids based on their experience of rapid relief of symptoms in some patients receiving initial doses of 100 mg dexamethasone. However, they were unable to demonstrate a superior outcome in comparison with their historical group, which had received lower doses of steroids.[2] Several other reports have noted a dramatic reduction in the severity of symptoms following treatment with steroids alone.[29,30,32,33] The response to dexamethasone was considered to have a prognostic value in one series of patients with spinal metastases.[29] Steroid-related improvement, however, was closely related to the type of tumor and probably represented a direct oncolytic effect[30] as in lymphomas and leukemias. The response to dexamethasone therefore has no proven intrinsic prognostic value.[11]

PRETREATMENT NEUROLOGIC STATUS

The results obtained by radiotherapy and by laminectomy plus radiotherapy relate to neurologic status at the time of treatment. There is a positive correlation between the pretreatment motor status and the functional outcome[2,6,11,12]; 70 percent of the patients who can walk at the time of diagnosis retain that ability after treatment; 35 percent of those who are initially paraparetic become ambulatory and only 5 to 7 percent (range 0 to 25 percent) of paraplegic patients regain the ability to walk. These success rates show no significant difference between the two modalities of management when the proportion of tumors with a favorable histologic type is comparable.[11,12] The success rate achieved by all therapies in *paraplegic* patients[11] is different, depending on whether the patient has complete functional cord transection or whether there is preservation of some neurologic function. The fact that only 2 percent of the former patients recovered the ability to walk after treatment, compared with 20 percent of the latter, indicates the strong prognostic significance of residual neurologic function. Complete paraplegia carries a bad functional prognosis regardless of the mode of therapy employed. The results of treatment emphasize the value of early diagnosis and treatment, and it therefore is discouraging that only 25 percent of patients are diagnosed while they are still able to walk.[2,3,6,7,10,12]

PROGRESSION RATE OF SYMPTOMS

It has been claimed that rapid onset and progression of neurologic symptoms are associated with a worse prognosis when compared with gradual onset and slow progression.[2,27,34] It has also been stated that the outlook for recovery is worse if bladder function is also impaired. However, these results should be analyzed in relation to completeness of spinal cord damage. If this is taken into account, it appears that in patients with rapidly developing symptoms (less than 24 hours) the neurologic grade itself has a greater influence on prognosis than has the symptom progression rate.[11] Twenty percent of paraparetic patients whose deficit evolved in less that 24 hours recovered compared with 0 percent of paraplegic patients.[2,11,27]

The rapidity of neurologic deterioration may be related to other prognostic variables, such as tumor cell type or tumor topography within the spinal canal. In one series[34] in which metastases of lung and prostatic carcinoma caused paraparesis, the proportion of patients with a sudden deficit (developing within a few hours) was 15 percent and 14 percent, respectively. These findings indicate that two lesions with significantly different surgical prognoses (22 percent and 49 percent success rate with laminectomy for lung and prostate, respectively) produce a similar symptom progression rate. Unfortunately, the current available information related to tumor topography and the rate of progression of symptoms is rather contradictory[2,11,27,34] and a definite relationship cannot be established. It seems that the rapidity of neurologic deterioration is unrelated to other prognostic variables and that the progression rate of symptoms should not be given intrinsic prognostic value unless further controlled studies indicate the contrary. On the other hand, the residual cord function should be taken into consideration in a rapidly evolving deficit as an important prognostic variable. Once paraplegia has set in, the duration of paralysis does have a prognostic significance, although recovery has been reported even after long periods of time (4 to 8 weeks).[7,8,10,35]

LOCATION OF TUMOR WITHIN THE SPINAL CANAL

It has been claimed that there is a positive correlation between the location of the extradural metastatic deposit and the response to surgical treatment.[27,28,36] A significantly better prognosis for a posterior rather than anterior compression has been demonstrated.[11,12,28] Futhermore, with regard to vertebral collapse, some authors stated that collapse reduced the chances of neurologic recovery.[12,27] It should be emphasized, however, that these statements are based on success rates obtained by laminectomy performed in ventrally located tumors. Following laminectomy only 9 percent to 16 percent of patients with ventral tumor masses retained the ability to walk, and these figures are considerably less than the overall rates of 30 percent to 50 percent ambulation for tumors located posterolaterally.[11,12,28]

When the epidural tumor is situated anterior to the spinal cord, the accessibility of the tumor to surgical removal by laminectomy is limited. Accordingly, an alternative approach to the spine by way of an anterolateral route has recently been developed.[7–10] The anterior approach yielded favorable results; 70 percent to 80 percent of the patients regained or maintained the ability to walk. In only one study was the surgical approach for decompression carefully selected according to tumor topography in the spinal canal.[7] The success rate for the ventrally located tumors was 80 percent when decompressed by an anterior approach, but only 39 percent for the posteriorly located tumors decompressed by laminectomy. Although the figure for posterior compartment tumors seems inferior, the results should not be considered discouraging, since only 8 percent of the patients with posterior compression were ambulatory at initial examination.

We conclude that the currently available information presents no clear evidence that tumor topography within the spinal canal carries an intrinsic prognostic factor. It is important to realize, however, that all the available studies are nonrandomized, and noncomparable variables may affect final outcome. Until randomized studies are carrier out, it is suggested that treatment endeavors be aimed at rapid and efficient decompression if surgery is selected as the preferred modality of treatment.

THERAPY USED

The retrospective analysis of different series of spinal metastases shows that the rate of favorable responses obtained by either radiotherapy or laminectomy plus radiotherapy is overall the same, with posttreatment ambulation rates of 46 percent and 40 percent, respectively.[2,5,6,11,12,37] Because cure is usually beyond expectation, palliation is generally accepted as a reasonable goal in the management of patients with spinal metastases. Preservation or restoration of neurologic function—ambulation and bladder control—are the criteria of successful therapy. Pain relief is also an important but secondary goal. Since treatment of malignant cord compression can rarely be curative in its own right, it emphasizes the importance of considering not only the success rates, but also the treatment effect on the quality of further survival of the entire group.[12] When the limited success rate of laminectomy was critically reviewed, it was balanced by an almost equal rate of adverse neurologic effects. Thus, when combined with other non-neurologic complications and mortality, the role of laminectomy as the first-line therapy for malignant cord compression has been questioned.[2,5,6,7,11,12] There is little doubt that radiotherapy supported by steroids can give comparable results[2,3] and that patients treated by radiotherapy can deteriorate neurologically in the same way as surgical patients. However, they are spared the other adverse effects of surgery. Reviewing patients treated by primary radiotherapy or by laminectomy with radio-

therapy, approximately 25 percent of patients ambulant on initial examination will deteriorate neurologically. Similarly, of those paraparetic before therapy, about 20 percent will get worse.[2,3,5,6,7,12] However, patients who do deteriorate following radiotherapy could still undergo surgery as a treatment option at an early stage in their deterioration.

Based on this data some trends have emerged regarding surgical indication. It has been recommended that surgery be reserved for (1) cases in which the nature of spinal cord compression is unknown; (2) cases in which there is spinal instability or bone collapse into the spinal canal; (3) cases with reactivation of a spinal lesion, in which additional radiotherapy cannot be given; (4) cases in which the tumor is known to be radioresistant; and (5) cases in which there is further clinical deterioration while on radiotherapy. These guidelines for surgery may have to be modified in response to new clinical experience with anterior decompression[7–10] and research data in the future. It should be emphasized here that anterior decompression that was carried on along the recommended guidelines for surgical intervention yielded encouraging results, with 70 to 80 percent ambulation rates. In one series,[7] one third of the patients who underwent anterior decompression received no combination of postsurgical radiotherapy since they faced their second episode of cord compression and had already burnt out any option for further irradiation. It is interesting that the rate of success in this group was similar to that obtained in the rest of the patients. It is not yet clear whether anterior decompression should be recommended as the primary modality of therapy in cord compression; it should be critically examined in a controlled prospective study.

In the case of radiosensitive neoplasms such as lymphomas, Ewing's sarcoma, neuroblastoma, seminoma, and myeloma, radiotherapy is most clearly indicated as the primary modality and therapy for cord compression. The success rate with radiotherapy varies between 44 percent and 83 percent with a pooled improvement rate of 60 percent.[2,7,11,29,35,38–42]

THE CHOICE OF TREATMENT

Recent trends in management of malignant epidural cord compression are outline here (Figure 133-3).

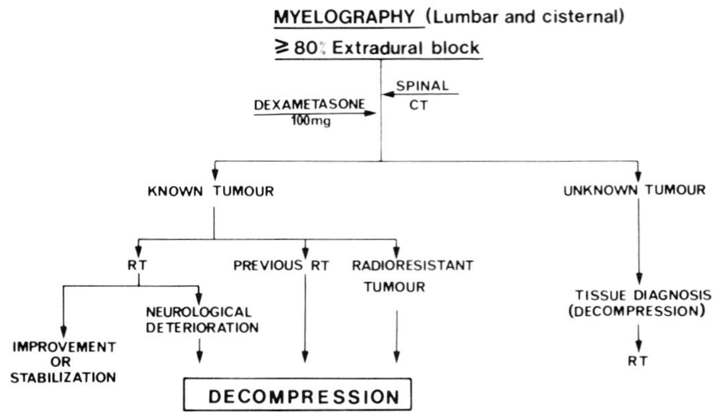

Fig. 133-3. The selection of the appropriate therapeutic modality for neoplastic epidural compression of the spinal cord and cauda equina. When surgical decompression is indicated, the approach (anterior or posterior) is decided upon according to tumor location within the spinal canal.

RADIOTHERAPY AS THE FIRST-LINE THERAPY

Radiotherapy is most clearly indicated for radiosensitive tumors, but it also may well be the primary therapy for moderately radiosensitive tumors, such as breast carcinoma. In the latter group (relatively sensitive tumors), the need for surgical intervention should be critically reviewed for each patient. We have no doubt that in stable patients who are ambulatory or paraparetic on initial examination, radiotherapy should be tried out first. However, in severely paraparetic and paraplegic patients, surgical decompression should be considered. This is based on the knowledge that the use of radiotherapy implies a delay in the reduction of spinal cord damage. In a group of 16 patients harboring lymphomas and other radiosensitive tumors who were extracted from different series,[40–42] improvement as a result of radiotherapy, which occurred in 83 percent of the cases, began 5.6 days (mean) after the initiation of therapy. Thus, when using radiotherapy, one may expect 28 percent of severely paraparetic patients to become paraplegic within 24 hours of treatment.[11] Moreover, the 25 percent favorable response rate obtained in this type of patient with any form of therapy[27,34–36] will decrease to 17 percent when radiotherapy is used.[11] That this group of patients may benefit from surgery is further supported by the high rate of ambulation obtained in the unfavorable prognostic group by *anterior decompression* of the spine.[7,10] If surgery is contraindicated, radiotherapy should be used. This means that patients with a poor general medical status, patients with multiple myelographic blocks, and those with long-standing paraplegia would be offered radiation therapy only.

The indication for radiotherapy is less clear-cut for tumors generally regarded as radioresistant; even here, however, radiotherapy should be tried as a primary modality if the patient's neurologic deficit is not severe and the rate of progression of the deficit is such that there would be time to resort to surgical decompression should radiotherapy fail. In situations in which surgical decompression is used as the primary modality of therapy, postoperative radiation should generally be used in the hope that this may help eradicate or suppress residual tumor, as well as to contribute to pain relief.

INDICATION FOR SURGICAL INTERVENTION

It is usually recommended that surgery be reserved for specific situations.

Diagnosis in Doubt

When the cause of the spinal lesion is in doubt, surgical decompression is advisable to establish a tissue diagnosis and to achieve rapid decompression. The source of the primary tumor cannot be identified in 9 percent of cases of spinal metastases[6] and in an additional 8 percent spinal involvement is the initial sign of cancer.[2] Thus, up to 17 percent of the patients may require surgical intervention by this indication.

Previous Radiation Exposure

When radiotherapy cannot be used, surgical decompression is indicated as the primary modality of therapy. This applies even in highly radiosensitive tumors because of the risk of exceeding spinal cord tolerance by adding further irradiation. Surgery is warranted for relapse occurring months or even years after a successful previous treatment in hope of preserving neurologic function.

Radioresistant Tumors

When dealing with a radioresistant tumor, decompressive surgery might be considered as the primary mode of therapy. Postoperative radiotherapy is administered hopefully to retard tumor regrowth. However, this indication is not generally accepted and sometimes, especially in neurologically stable patients, radiotherapy may be tried out first.

Neurologic Deterioration During Radiotherapy

Neurologic deterioration that occurs during radiotherapy of a relatively radiosensitive tumor should prompt early consideration of surgical decompression. The decline in neurologic function may reflect radioresistance, progressive spinal instability, or bone compression secondary to vertebral collapse. All these may be most effectively treated by spinal decompression and stabilization.

There has been concern that radiation therapy may result in neurologic deterioration, presumably by inducing radiation edema in the tumor or spinal cord.[43] Experimental studies do not support the concept of radiation edema.[44]

It therefore is most likely neurologic deterioration that occurs during the course of radiotherapy suggests its failure, and serious consideration should be given to surgery as an alternative treatment.

Spinal Instability or Bone Compression

When spinal instability endangers spinal cord or nerve root function or when a pathologic fracture produces direct compression on neural structures, surgical decompression and stabilization are essential. Metrizamide myelography combined with CT study is generally recommended in assessing the patient with vertebral column involvement, regardless of the severity of neurologic dysfunction. This study is often of value in determining whether there is bony encroachment on the spinal cord or nerve roots as well as in detecting associated tumor deposits (Figure 133-4).

Spinal instability is present whenever one of the following situations arises: a bone loss of more than 50 percent of the width of the vertebral body, a bone loss extending over two or more vertebrae, or the presence of additional involvement of the posterior elements at the same level (Figure 133-5; Table 133-1). The instability is augmented by any combination of the above. However, not every case of instability requires surgical intervention. If the tumor is radiosensitive, a course of radiotherapy not infrequently results in satisfactory settling and relief of pain over a period of weeks or months. The patient is followed closely and cautioned to report promptly any neurologic dysfunction, in which case surgical intervention may have to be considered.

The vertebral bodies when destroyed by tumor will collapse into a localized kyphosis that is associated with increasing pain and eventual neural deficit. The loss in the height of the vertebrae results in a relative laxity and redundancy in the surrounding soft tissues. This is the essential mechanism in every case of segmental instability in the spine. Whatever stabilization method is used, the kyphosis should not be left alone and every effort should be made to correct it and thus put those soft tissues in optimal tension. The alignment and the stability of the spine then will be restored, the pain will be less, and neural integrity will be maintained. However, not every vertebral fracture requires fixation. In the thoracic spine, stable vertebral

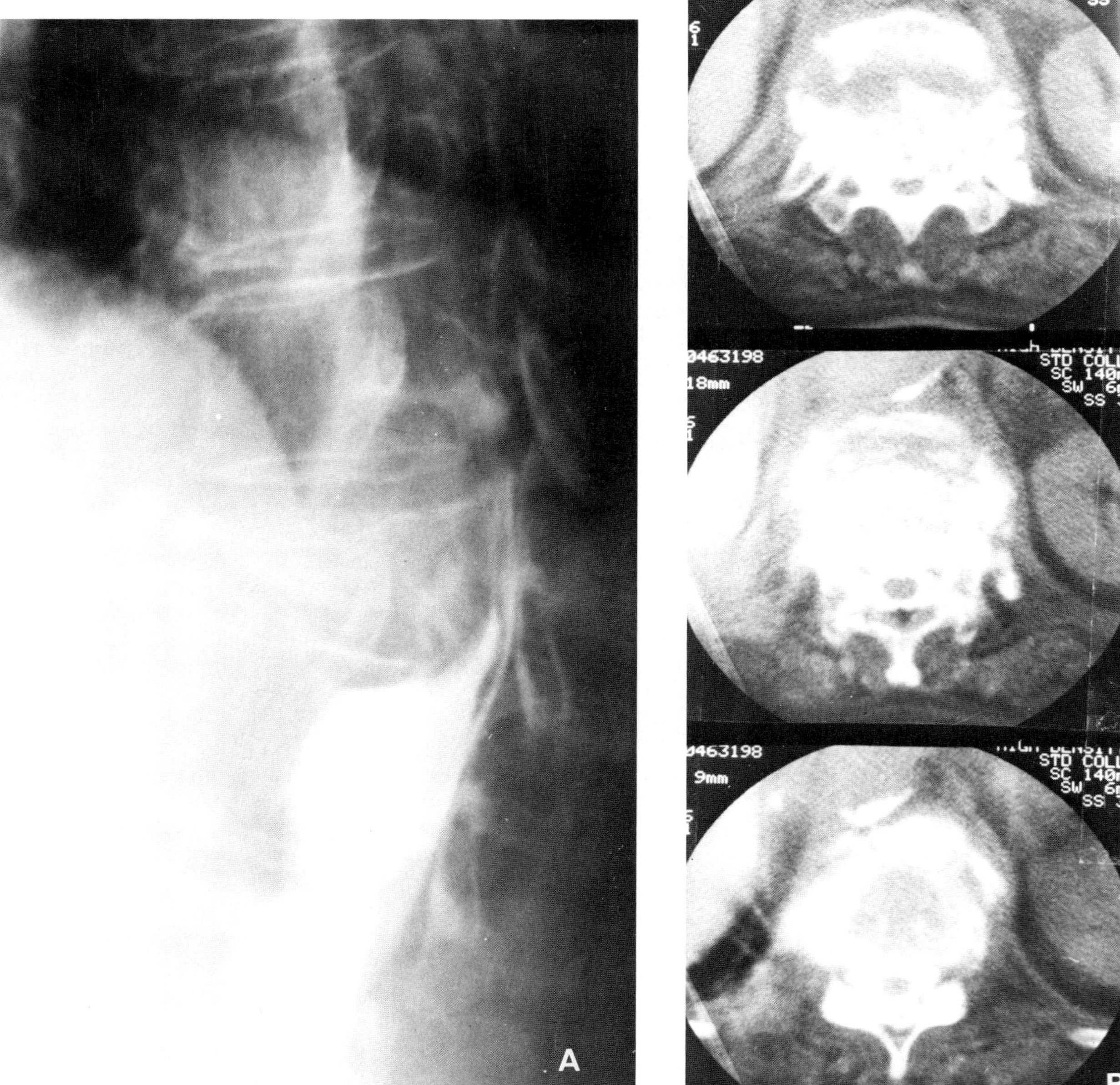

Fig. 133-4. Metrizamide-enhanced myelogram and CT scan of the T11 pathologic fracture in a patient with a single metastasis of lung carcinoma. (A) There is a complete myelographic block caused by the retropulsed diseased vertebral body, which compresses the spinal cord anteriorly. (B) CT-myelogram (at and below the level of the myelographic block) demonstrates intact posterior elements and anterior impingement by the pathologic bone fragments on the spinal cord. Anterior surgical decompression is indicated to alleviate the pressure on the neural tissue by the displaced vertebral bone.

fractures may not require surgical intervention because of the support provided by the rib cage; in the surgical region, it is our experience that the need to operate on patients with metastatic vertebral involvement is not frequent. Most of these are amenable to conservative treatment (external supports and irradiation). Unstable pathologic fractures in the cervical region may require reduction and stabilization[14] by a skull-halo fixation apparatus attached to a plaster body jacket. Subsequently, the patient should be treated with local irradiation of the neck. Only rarely will further internal fixation be needed.

When surgical intervention and stabilization is performed, it is often associated with the removal of the epidural tumor. Therefore, the selection of the anterior, posterior, or combined approach should be determined by the main sight of instability as well as by the location of the tumor inside and outside the spinal canal (Table 133-1).

OPERATIVE TECHNIQUES

The anterior and posterior surgical approaches to the spine at every level have been covered in depth in other chapters of this book. To avoid redundancy, the technical notes will be restricted to issues specific to patients with malignancies in the spinal column.

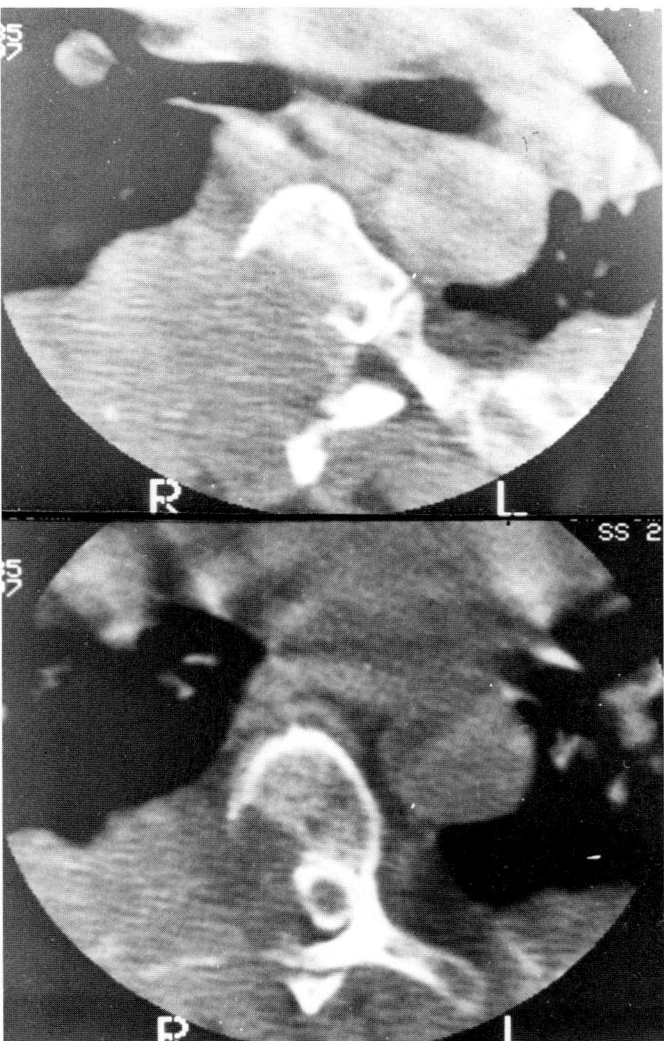

Fig. 133-5. Computed tomographic myelogram of a large paravertebral metastatic tumor involving the posterior chest wall, penetrating the spinal canal, and destroying anterior and posterior spinal elements at the same level. The spinal cord is displaced and compressed laterally.

POSTERIOR DECOMPRESSION AND INSTRUMENTATION

Laminectomy for decompression of the posterior aspect of the spinal canal is indicated when the compressive tumor is in a posterior or posterolateral location. It can also be required as a second stage procedure where a considerable residual tumor is left beyond the equator of the dura at the end of an anterior decompression.

The intubated patient is placed face down on a spinal frame. This will prevent an increase in intra-abdominal pressure and lessen epidural bleeding during surgery. If a frame is not available, the patient is placed with rolls placed laterally under the weight-bearing areas of the chest and pelvis, leaving the abdomen and lower chest free for breathing movements. The head is positioned on a horseshoe headrest, which allows free access to the connections of the anesthesia apparatus. After the field is prepared, space is allotted for large skin flaps and possible lengthening of the incision when the back is dropped.

Skin incisions through radiation portals must be avoided at all costs. Some of these surgical wounds can dehisce and some

Table 133-1. Epidural compression by malignant tumors: Assessment of location and extent of pathologic process for determination of surgical approach

I. Myelography
　　Single or multiple blocks
　　Block related or unrelated to the bone lesion
　　Number of segments involved
　　Position of the compressing mass: Anterior, posterior, or encircling
II. Bone involvement at the site of myelographic block (spinal radiography and computed tomography)
　　Vertebral body and pedicles, posterior elements or a combination of both
　　Number of vertebrae involved
　　Percentage of bone loss of the vertebral cut surface
III. Spinal instability
　　Involvement of two or more adjacent vertebrae
　　Involvement of both anterior and posterior elements at the same level
　　Loss of more than 50 percent of the vertebral width
　　Any combination of the above will increase instability
IV. Paravertebral mass
　　Location
　　Extent
　　Involvement of adjacent structures

will never heal, being further complicated by chronic discharge. Therefore, the area of intended decompression is reached through an incision placed laterally in healthy tissue, circumventing the irradiated area. Thus, a generous skin flap is created to be elevated and retracted. The extent of the lateral placement of the incision is dictated by the width of the radiation portal, which can usually be determined by discoloration of the skin or, in inveterate cases, by the loss of the subcutaneous fat. The incision is usually placed 8 to 10 cm lateral and parallel to the midline, long enough to allow exposure of four to five spinal segments above and below the planned area of decompression, if the use of spinal instrumentation is anticipated. The incision is carried down to reach spinous processes and 5 cm beyond them. Traction on the flap is applied by sutures in the subcutaneous tissue with hemostats on their ends.

The fibrous caps of the spinous processes are split in the midline with diathermy, and subperiosteal dissection of the paravertebral soft tissues is carried out. Tissues even mildly resistant to dissection are released by cautery. Possible involvement of the posterior arch elements with tumor dictates caution; a bone fragment can be pushed or turned into the dura during elevation of the paravertebral muscles. In most cases, involvement of a posterior arch involvement will point to the level in need of decompression. However, it is not unusual to detect tumor deposits at other levels that may have been designated for anchorage of the stabilizing instrumentation. This necessitates the dissection of additional segments to ensure firm placement of rods and wires.

Identification of the spinal levels by an intraoperative x-ray film is mandatory, since it determines the site at which laminectomy is carried out and avoids unnecessary removal of posterior elements. The x-ray film must include an anatomic landmark (such as the cervicothoracic, thoracolumbar, or lumbosacral junction) that is close to the area of the intended decompression. A towel clip is attached to the base of a spinous process close to its superior margin in that area. If so placed, the location of the tongs of the towel clip on the PA x-ray film corresponds to the midportion of the vertebral body at the same level. When the x-ray film has been obtained, the spinous process is nicked for further reference to this vertebra.

Laminectomy is begun one level distal to the lower border of the myelographic block. Decompression is continues cephalad, the posterior elements are carefully removed and instruments are placed between the lamina and the underlying compressing tumor, especially in the presence of neurologic deficit. Only after the tumor borders, both proximal and distal, have been exposed, is its removal considered.

The neoplasm is most conveniently approached from its distal margin. In the area adjacent to the tumor, the epidural fat is split in the midline with a freer to reach the normal dura underneath. The split is advanced until the tumor margin is encountered. A dissection plane is sought, gently elevating the tumor edge from the dura. Some tumors present no problem at removal because they are flexible or friable or easily detachable. Some other tumors are of firm consistency; elevating one end may cause the other to impinge on the dura. Removal is piecemeal with sharp instruments. The tumors that adhere tenaciously to the dura (e.g., osteoblastoma, lung carcinoma) deserve special notice. They are also excised piecemeal, but here one must accept neoplastic residua on the dural surface. Caution must be exercised not to violate the dura when the tumor is scraped off its surface. The malignant remnants are treated by irradiation, if practical.

In many cases the tumor encircles the dura. In these cases the tumor is cut open either by sharp incision or by incision or by bipolar diathermy; it is elevated off the dura and then incised in the midline from its undersurface up. This is continued until the cut margin of the tumor can be grasped. It then can be gently peeled laterally. The segmental nerves are sought and, if possible, the tumor is peeled off them too. In the lateral compartment, the overlying tumor is removed with sharp instruments, preferably sharp curettes of appropriate size. These cut the tumor against the local bone elements and so allow evacuation without pulling on the dura or the tumor itself.

Neurologic deterioration as a direct result of laminectomy in cancer patients is not uncommon,[2,6,7,11,12,28] so that every effort must be made to minimize possible iatrogenic insult. Loupes or an operating microscope may be indicated in some cases. The dura matter is usually an effective barrier to tumor penetration. The segmental nerves are protected by the dural sleeve to their point of exit at the intervertebral foramen. Distally, however, tumor invasion of the nerves may and does occur (see Figure 133-2). This is one of the causes of the intractable pain often encountered in these unfortunate patients. In the thoracic region, a segmental nerve, when involved with tumor, is litigated and severed. In the lumbar or cervical regions, gentle peeling of the tumor off the nerves is attempted to preserve motor function.

Intraoperative bleeding can be very significant. It is controlled by application of either Gelfoam or Surgicel with gentle pressure on the bleeding surface. Vascular feeders of the tumor mass are difficult to control from the posterior aspect of the spine. The walls of the tumor vessels may be devoid of contractile components and thus lack the ability to contract. The continuous gentle pressure is to encourage coagulation. Excess blood should only be removed by suction. Rubbing an oozing tumor surface with gauze removes any clot that has already formed.

When removal of the tumor is complete or optimal for the specific case, the bare dura and roots are routinely covered with free fat grafts harvested from the available subcutaneous tissue at the incision site. The fat grafts are fixed to soft tissues with a few sutures to prevent displacement.

Evaluation of residual spine stability is done at this stage. The spine is considered unstable if tumor excision has necessitated removal of apophyseal joints bilaterally at the same level, if the preoperative studies revealed vertebral body involvement at the same level (see Figure 133-5) or if a pathologic fracture dislocation is present (see Table 133-1). It is a sound policy to aim for a firm, solid, and stable spine. If there is doubt whether decompression has led to an unstable situation, it is best to go ahead with spine stabilization. A stable spine will maximize neurologic function and save the patient the severe intractable pain of instability. We usually use the double Harrington rod distraction system supplemented by segmental sublaminar wiring. At this point in time, it satisfies the two main requirements for re-establishing spinal stability: distraction and fixation. The gradual distraction obtained by the Harrington instrumentation will cause optimal tension in the spinal and paraspinal soft tissues (ligaments, joint capsules, muscles), removing the slack that accompanies vertebral compression. It can also correct local deformity (kyphosis), restore lost vertebral height, and lessen compression at the level of the intervertebral foramina. When coupled with sublaminar wiring, which fixes the spine segmentally to the parallel rods, it results in a firm and solid internal fixation system with instant spinal stability (Figure 133-6). No external appliances (braces, jackets, etc.) are required.

The technique entails placement of two upper Harrington hooks (No. 1251, Zimmer, Warsaw, Indiana) in the apophyseal joints, under the inferior facets of the fourth vertebra above the laminectomy area. The two lower laminar hooks (No. 1256) are placed on the laminae of a vertebra four levels caudal to the distal end of the laminectomy site.

Passing of the sublaminar wires bilaterally is preceded by incision of the ligamenta flava above and below the lamina. If spinous processes are in the way, their overhang is osteotomized. Stainless steel wires, 16 gauge and 30 cm in length, are bent in the middle in a hairpin fashion. This straight double wire is then gently bent so that the hairpin end can be passed under the lamina. It is usually introduced under the caudal edge of the lamina and surfaces cephalad. As it is pulled out, the wire ends are crossed on the lamina to prevent the wire from wandering and from possibly being pushed against the dura during further instrumentation endeavors.

When the sublaminar wires have been passed above and below the laminectomy site, the distance between the upper and lower hooks is measured. Two Harrington rods 3 cm longer than the measured distance are positioned in the hooks. The upper hooks are moved up on the ratchets until optimal tension is reached for both rods. The purpose of the doubled wire is to resist breakage and to distribute the pressure over a larger area of the lamina and so possibly avoid cutout. The wires are tightened by crossing the ends forcefully across the rod. The wires are then fixed by twisting the ends around each other. Excess twisting can cause wire breakage; therefore, no more

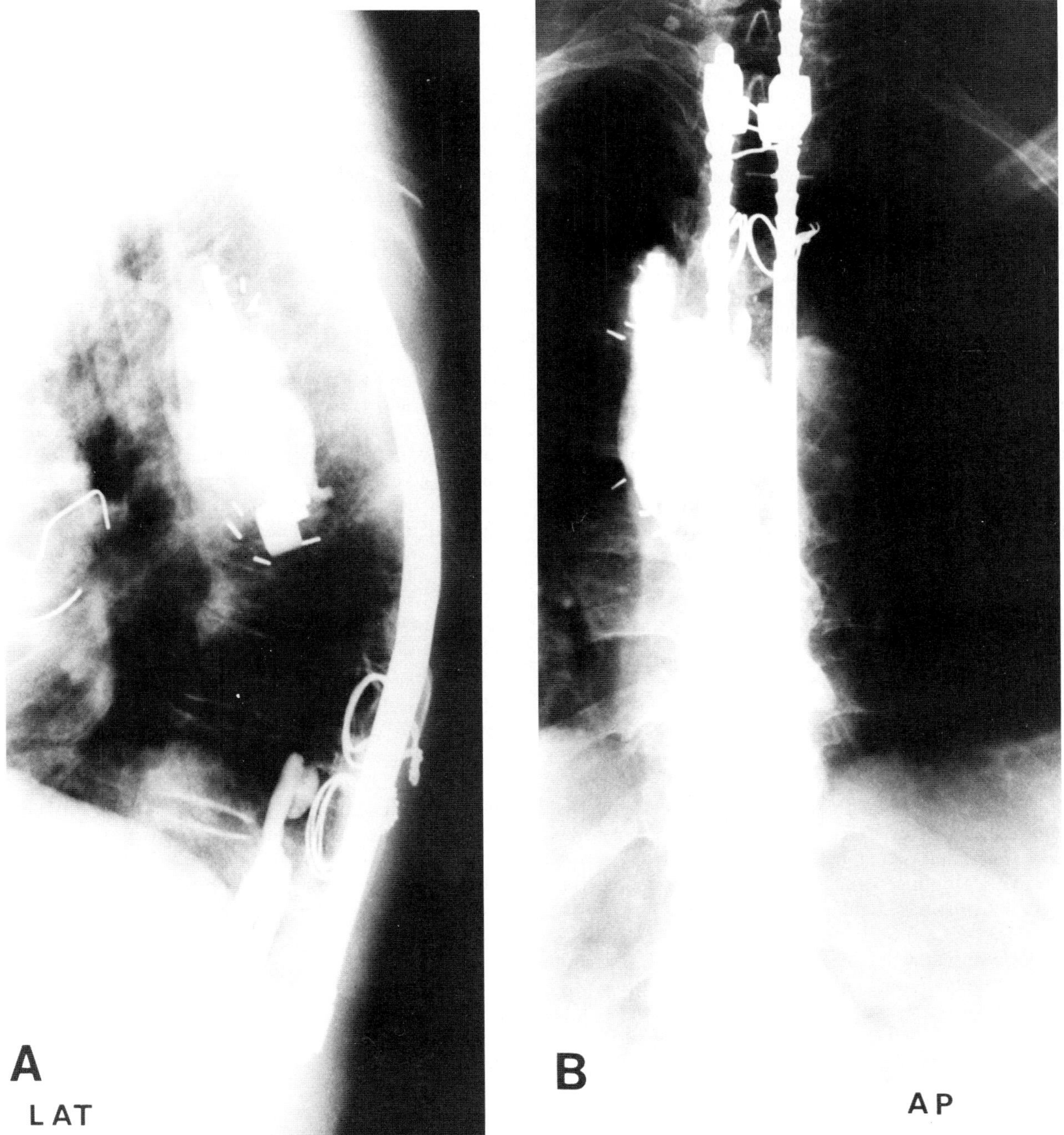

Fig. 133-6. Thoracic vertebral body replacement supplemented by posterior decompression and instrumentation. Lateral (A) and AP (B) views. Immediate stability was obtained following placement of distraction rods with segmental sublaminar wiring. Distal extension of the exposure was indicated to enable placement of the instrumentation on tumor-free posterior elements.

than three full circle twists are allowed. The wire ends are cut and the ''braids'' are bent towards the rod shaft to avoid future discomfort.

The Issue of Bone Grafting

Before wound closure, the advisability of bone grafting to achieve bony arthrodesis must be considered. This is a matter of debate. Orthopedic surgeons have traditionally regarded bone grafting as an integral part of spine fusion with internal fixation. This is because experience has shown that single or even double Harrington rodding can end in rod breakage, especially in young and active people, if solid bone arthrodesis

has not been obtained. However, the great majority of patients with primary or metastatic spinal deposits are not young, and with the advent of segmental instrumentation, rod breakage is a rare occurrence. In many cases, activity is restricted by some neurologic deficit, by pain, or by a less-than-optimal medical status. It is therefore reasonable to assume that in these conditions the internal fixation alone will provide durable spinal stability.

When the addition of bone grafts is considered, the time factor must also be taken into account. If bone autografts are employed, the time required for spinal arthrodesis to occur is about 6 months, and 6 more months are needed for the arthrodesis to mature. When bank bone (allografts) is used, the required time is longer, especially if postoperative irradiation is scheduled. The median survival of patients with spinal cord compression caused by metastatic spread is 12 to 18 months.[7,23–26] Therefore, our main indication for adding iliac cancellous bone grafts is a benign or slow-growing tumor in children and young adults (osteoblastoma, giant cell tumor, aneurysmal bone cysts, etc.).

There are three additional arguments against bone grafting: (1) it requires a separate incision with an increase in operating time and morbidity in patients with active disease; (2) the iliac bone graft can be microscopically involved with tumor; and (3) the bone graft incorporation can be inhibited by postoperative radiotherapy. When a decision has been reached to use bone grafts, either autologous grafts or allografts, decortication is limited to the transverse and spinous processes, since access to the lamina is obstructed by the presence of rods and segmental wiring. An ample quantity of grafts is applied to the decorticated areas in continuity. If internal fixation obtained by instrumentation is adequate, there is no need for external appliances.

We have used posterior spine stabilization with Harrington rods and segmental sublaminar wiring without bone grafting in 36 cancer patients. Stabilization was satisfactory in all of them. The instrumentation did not dislodge, nor was there any mechanical failure. Hook cut-out or dislodgement was encountered before the institution of segmental wiring. Eleven patients were followed for 6 months or more, five of them for more than 1 year. The longest follow-up was 51 months. Three of the earlier cases were complicated by skin breakdown because the skin incision was placed in irradiated areas. However, it was noted that in these three cases the purchase on the upper hooks was reinforced by bone cement (methyl-methacrylate). Before the skin breakdown, the area of the cement fixation was the site of a significant sterile serous accumulation, which had to be evacuated by repeated percutaneous puncture. We have since abandoned the use of bone cement for fixation in the posterior approach to the spine, the only exception being the cervical area.

We conclude that with proper technique the Harrington distraction instrumentation coupled with segmental wiring provides a reliable corrective posterior fixation for cancer patients with unstable spines following posterior decompression.

Postoperative bleeding from the residual tumor or the tumor bed in some cases may account for the neurologic deterioration observed after surgery. It therefore is our routine to cover the dura and segmental nerves with a free fat graft and then place a large bore noncollapsible drain next to one of the Harrington rods near the decompression area. Care is taken that the rod separates the fat graft from the drain, because the free fat graft may dislodge with suction, obstruct the drain, stop the evacuation of the hematoma, and leave the dura bare. Further care is taken to position the drain so that it does not get caught in the wire ends on removal. The drain exit is lateral (posterior axillary line) and certainly not through irradiated tissue.

Meticulous technique is used in closing the wound. The paravertebral muscles are tightly closed over the rods. The skin flap is brought down by sutures in sequential rows to cause the flap to adhere to its bed and eliminate potential spaces. The sutures also release tension on the flap edges, having the skin on both sides of the incision lean toward each other to a touch. No skin overriding is accepted. Sutures are used only for the alignment of the skin flap and so need not be tight. Since sutures

are routinely left in place for at least 20 days, a tight suture will submerge, knot and all, under the skin.

Postoperative Care

The patient is kept flat on his or her back for at least 10 hours. The heels and sacrum are protected from weight-bearing contact with the mattress. Even for paraplegics, turning frames are not used, because patients find them very uncomfortable. Regular beds are used and following the initial 12 postoperative hours, free turning in bed is allowed.

Perioperative antibiotics are discontinued on the third postoperative day, unless otherwise indicated. The patient is allowed to sit up on the second postoperative day and to walk on the fourth, if able to do so. Radiotherapy, when indicated, can be administered on the fourth postoperative week, provided healing of the surgical wound is per primum. Before discharge, standing and supine x-ray films of the spine are obtained to evaluate stability. A fluoroscopic myelogram is also routinely obtained. Since some Pantopaque is usually left in the subarachnoid space from the preoperative myelogram, there is no need for repeated lumbar punctures for periodic assessments of the patency at the site of the previous myelographic block.

ANTERIOR DECOMPRESSION OF THE SPINE AND VERTEBRAL BODY REPLACEMENT

The majority of operations for resection of tumors located anterior to the spinal cord are performed in the thoracic spine. Most of the principles of the anterior surgical approach to the thoracic spine (patient positioning, intraoperative identification of the level for decompression, exposure of the vertebral bodies, tumor removal, vertebral body replacement, etc.), apply as well to other anatomic areas of the spine. Therefore, we present in detail the technical measures for the transthoracic approach and limit the description in the other areas to the variations in the technique dictated by the difference in anatomy.

The Thoracic Spine (T3-T11)

The transthoracic approach to the spine is by thoracotomy, right or left sided, according to the preoperative assessment of tumor location and bone destruction. The induction of general anesthesia is on a stretcher and the patient is intubated with a double lumen endotracheal tube. This will enable the anesthesiology team to deflate the lung at thoracotomy and enhance the exposure. The midsection of the operating table is bent (Figure 133-7) and the anesthetized patient is rolled onto the table and placed in the right or left lateral decubitus position. The mid-thoracic level is positioned over the acute bend in the table. This manuever will stretch the side of the chest facing the surgeon. It is an important technical detail that greatly facilitates exposure; when thoracotomy is in progress, retraction is almost unnecessary.

The level of the thoracotomy is determined before the patient is prepared. We have repeatedly found that skin scratches done by the radiologists to indicate the site of the myelographic block are of little help, because the positioning of the patient and the stretching of one arm causes the skin to be drawn away from the position it was in at the time of myelography. To determine the thoracotomy level, we consult the x-ray films of the chest, of the thoracolumbar junction, and the thoracic spinal segments awaiting decompression. The chest x-ray films reveal the slant of the ribs. Entry into the chest is obtained by a partial rib resection. If the ribs are horizontally aligned, then the rib to be excised is the one that articulates with the diseased vertebral body. If the rib cage is drooped, the downward inclination of the ribs will interfere with visualization. Therefore, the rib selected for removal is one or two levels above the upper level of the vertebral bodies to be exposed. Locating the rib is easy; inspection of AP thoracolumbar x-ray film reveals which is the lowest palpable rib—either a long 12th rib or the 11th rib in case of a hypoplastic 12th rib. By palpating and counting rostrally, the desired rib is reached and the skin overlying it is superficially scratched along the anterior two thirds of its length.

The skin incision over the rib is placed from just lateral to the bulk of the paraspinal muscles ventrally to the costochondral junction. The incision is deepened by cautery down to the rib and carried along it. By subperiosteal dissection the anterior two thirds of the rib is freed of soft tissues. For expediency, an opened gauze is passed under the rib and by successive pulls of the gauze to each side, a fast and thorough soft tissue stripping is obtained. The rib is cut ventrally close to the costochondral junction and dorsally close to the lateral border of the paravertebral muscles. These muscles should not be incised, because bleeding is usually profuse. Cutting through them does not improve the surgical exposure and, when intact, they may contribute to spine stability. The proximal one third or one quarter of the rib is usually not removed unless it is involved with the tumor. If intact, the costovertebral joints contain ligamentous structures that contribute considerably to the stability of that spinal segment. In addition, since the head of the rib is situated astride the intervertebral disc, it firmly binds the two adjacent vertebral bodies. Other stabilizing components worth preserving are the costotransverse, costovertebral, and costocostal ligaments. Entry into the pleural cavity is gained through the rib bed. The lung is inspected for metastatic spread and for tumorous adhesions of the visceral pleura to the chest wall or spinal column. In most cases, the pleural adhesions are good indicators of the location of the metastatic deposit in the spinal column. These adhesions can be separated by blunt dissection, and the associated bleeding is easily controlled. Rarely, separating the adhesions off the spine can be tedious and ligation of feeding vessels should be undertaken before the blunt dissection. When the lung is free and mobilized, warm wet towels are applied to both sides of the incision, an automatic chest retractor is positioned, and gentle retraction of the ribs is obtained. A wet towel is applied to the lung and a malleable retractor is placed on it, the toe of which is located in the angle between the pulsating aorta and the spinal column.

The spine is inspected for a paravertebral mass, a deformation, discoloration, or a change in consistency. Normally, the circumference of the vertebral body is significantly smaller than that of the intervertebral disk, causing it to appear as a decompression between the bordering disks. The segmental arteries and veins usually cross the narrow midportion of the vertebral body. Most tumors will appear as a swelling with a reddish or blue tint (or black in the case of melanoma) localized to one or two vertebral bodies. The swelling may be soft or rubbery and must be palpated for pulsation. A pulsating tumor usually has substantial vascular feeders that must be located and litigated.

The parietal pleura overlying the anterolateral aspect of the vertebrae to be decompressed is cut longitudinally with a No. 15 blade. The pleura is peeled off the disks by gentle blunt

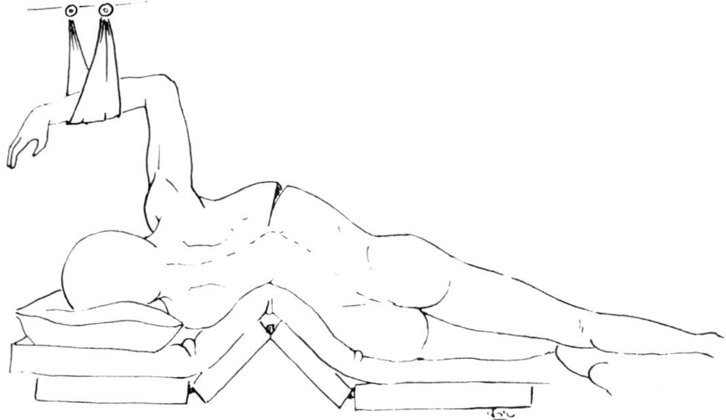

Fig. 133-7. Patient positioning for anterior decompression of the spine. The acute bend of the operating table is placed under the area intended for decompression. It stretches on the side of the trunk facing the surgeon and keeps the surgical wound wide, minimizing the need for retraction and greatly facilitating exposure.

dissection. This usually is a bloodless stage. The longitudinal structures usually encountered are sympathetic nerves, which can be cut or preserved at the discretion of the surgeon.

Bleeding is minimized by ligation of the vascular bundles as they cross the waists of the vertebral bodies. The vertebral waist, covered by areolar tissue, is examined for the segmental bundle, which sometimes may show through. The tip of a long curved hemostat is brought down on the bone close to one disk. It is swept toward the other disk with its tip close to the bone surface. As it emerges near the other disk, the vascular bundle will be elevated on the jaws of the hemostat. Opening the instrument will stretch the vessels across the jaws and so allow clipping or ligating on both sides of the instrument. No effort is made to separate the segmental artery from the vein, since both are contained in the same ligature. The two ligatures are placed as far away from each other as possible. The vascular bundle is then cut midway between the ligatures. The procedure is repeated at each level of interest. With the segmental vessels ligated, a thorough subperiosteal dissection is carried out anteriorly across the midline of the vertebral bodies, displacing the aorta of vena cava and protecting it with a malleable retractor inserted between it and the spine. In some instances, the segmental vessels may have been obliterated by the chronic localized pressure of the tumor. In other cases, the vessel is embedded within the tumor capsule. Every effort is made to localize and ligate these vessels, although a torn segmental artery can be controlled. The dissection is controlled laterally, elevating all soft tissues off the vertebral bodies and disks to the anterior margin of the intervertebral foramina. Dissection is not carried onto the pedicles unless there is need for lateral decompression as well.

At this stage, the tumor-bearing vertebrae are easily identified, but if the tumor is contained within the vertebral body and no localizing deformation can be perceived, then the level to be decompressed is pinpointed according to the preoperative radiologic studies. In the operative field, the vertebra is identified by the rib to which it is connected. This is done by palpating and counting the ribs on the inner aspect of the chest wall, starting either from the almost circular first rib down or from the 12th rib up. One must remember that the head of the rib is located on the superior disc (for example, the 7th rib is situated on the intervertebral disc T6-7).

Because of the possibility of serious bleeding, all partici-

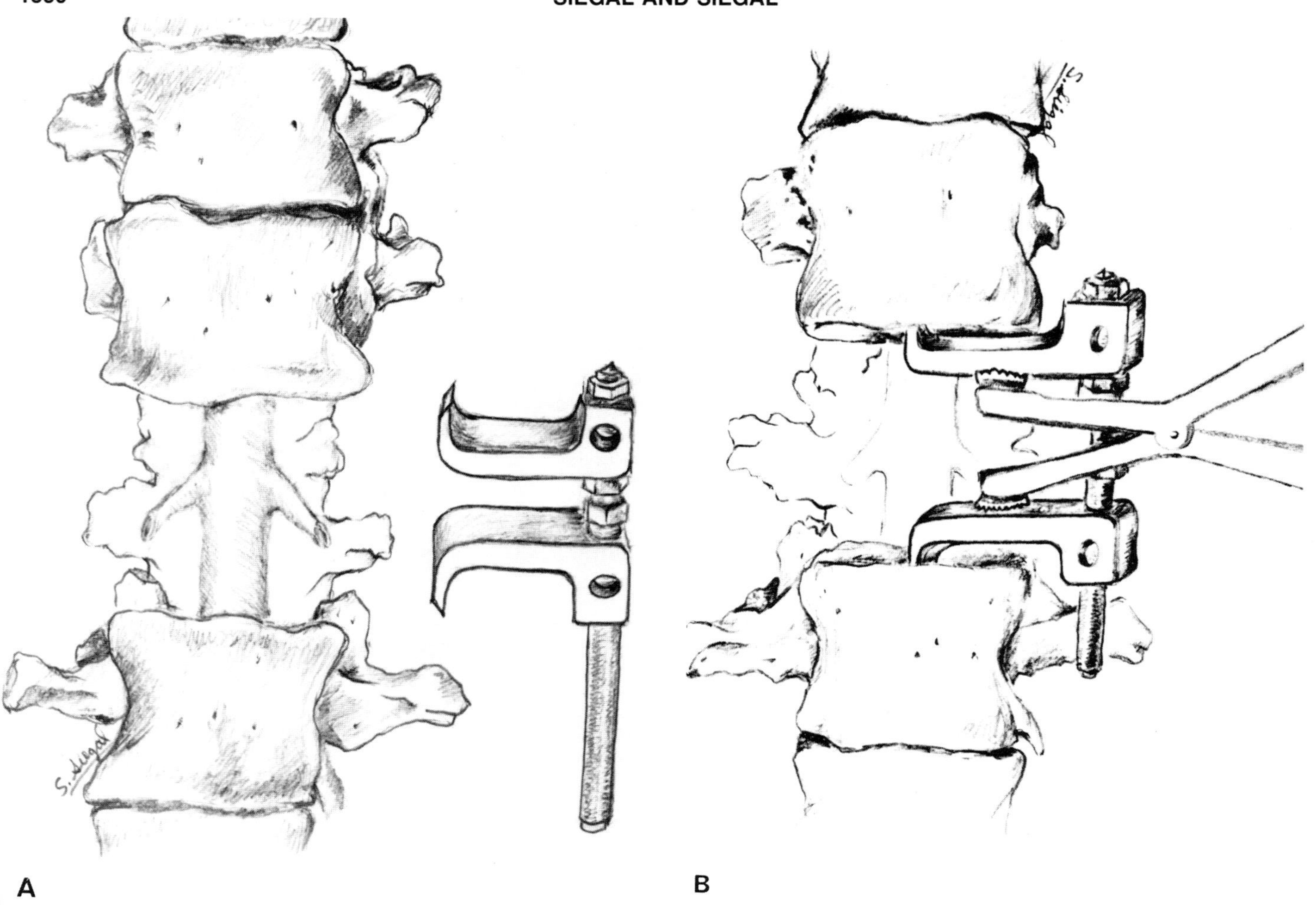

A　　　　**B**

Fig. 133-8. Steps in the vertebral body replacement procedure: (A) The spinal cord is decompressed; a heavy threaded rod is cut 1 1/2 inches longer than the distance to be spanned by the replacement. On one end a Moe sacral hook is fixed by two nuts. A third nut is added and then the second mobile hook, facing the other way. (B) The hooks-and-rod assembly is placed in the gap in a coronal plane. Gradual distraction by a lamina spreader will embed the hook blades into the intact vertebrae above and below. The third nut is moved on the thread to back up the departing mobile hook.

pants, especially the anesthesiology team, must be told when excision of the tumor has begun. In case of a vertebra soft with tumor, large curettes are appropriate for expedient removal of large lumps of tissue; these provide the pathologist with a better, uncrushed specimen for examination. The vertebral body is removed all the way back to the posterior longitudinal ligament. If there is evidence of tumor in the spinal canal, the ligament, if still present, has to be removed to visualize the dura and decompress it. Pulsations of the dura, if present, signify opening of the myelographic block. Reaching the epidural space safely can be achieved by following the segmental nerve exit at the intervertebral foramen, decompressing it there, and, once in epidural space, introducing a curved No. 2 curette into the space with the active edge hugging the posterior wall of the vertebral body. By slow rotation of the curette, the rounded blunt end will gently peel off the soft tissue adhering to the bone. When the surgeon is confident of the dissection, a short controlled pull will dislodge the bone segment forward. Care must be taken not to pull on the segmental nerve.

The segmental roots can be encased in tumor tissue. In the thoracic area these nerves are dispensable. Releasing the nerves may be time consuming and the release incomplete. There is also a possibility of direct penetration of the nerve root by the tumor, which may lead to intractable pain (see Figure

133-2). Therefore, the thoracic nerve root is ligated close to its outlet to avoid CSF leakage and amputated.

When the main bulk of the tumor has been removed, the anatomy is assessed. Bleeding may interfere with the inspection, so it is wise to palpate posteriorly to correctly locate the decompressed dura. Passing a piece of thin rubber tubing above and below the decompressed area is an innocuous method of assessing the patency of the epidural space. When necessary, more vertebral segments are decompressed in the same fashion.

In the case of a tumor that has not violated the anterior cortex of the vertebral body, access to the tumor is gained by opening the cortical bone with a chisel and hammer. The opening is enlarged and the tumor is scooped out with curettes of appropriate size. It is convenient to have a wide initial opening to ensure optimal exposure and complete decompression. In case of bleeding, frequent checking is done with a finger to assess the location of the dura.

The blood loss during anterior decompression of the spine is usually 1500 ml or less, but in some cases (carcinoma of the thyroid, hypernephroma, multiple myeloma) it can be profuse. The bleeding can originate from overlooked major vascular feeders of the tumor, from pathologic vessels within the tumor, which will not contract when severed, from spongy vertebral bone, or from the epidural venous plexus. We have not experienced accidental tears of large vessels. Expeditious removal

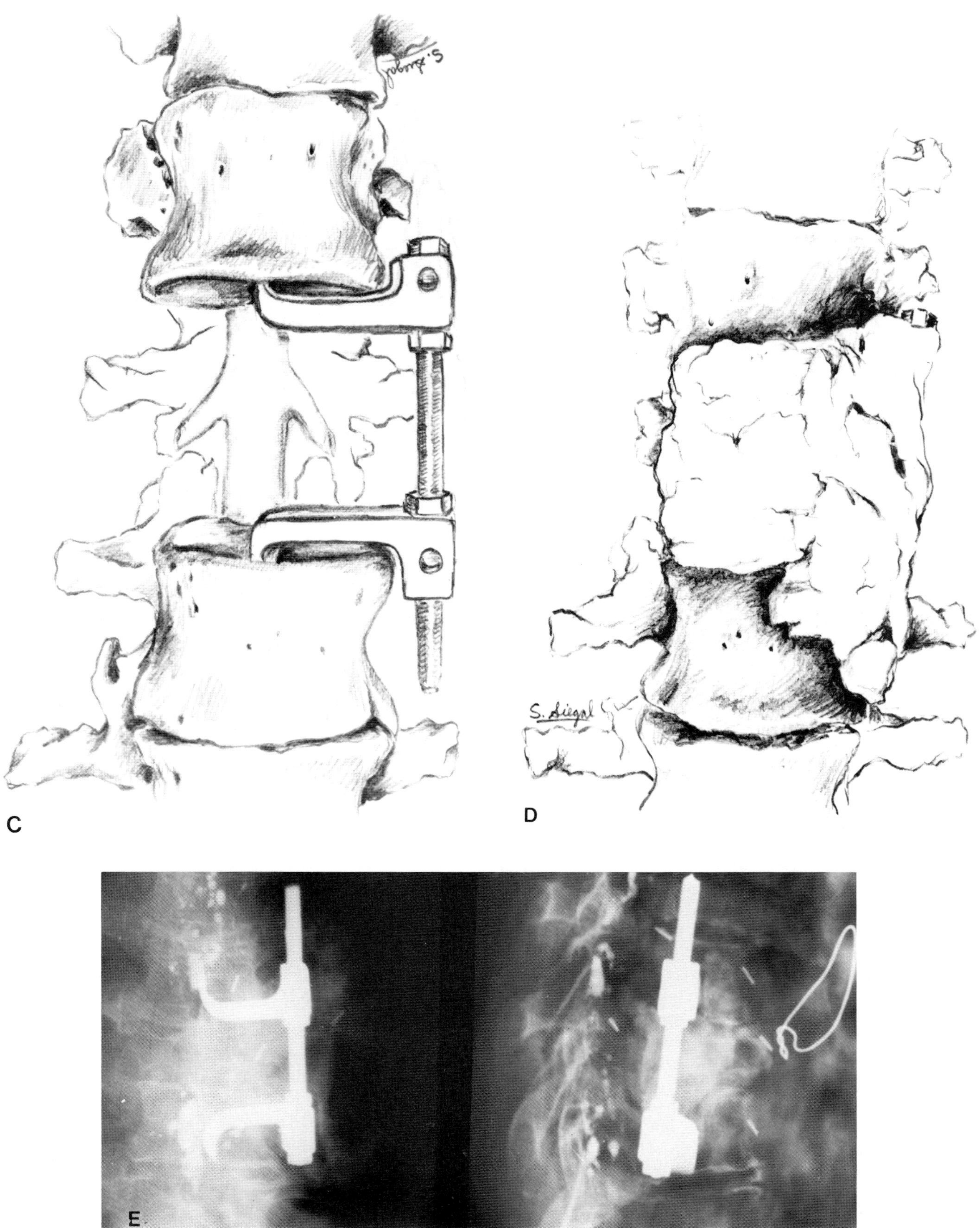

Fig. 133-8 (continued) (C) The assembly firmly placed, with hook blades reaching across the midline. Kyphosis is corrected and vertebral height reconstituted. (D) Methyl-methacrylate bone cement is placed, while still soft, in the spinal gap and around the projecting metal components of the vertebral replacement construct. It is molded to a rounded contour in line with the spinal column. (E) AP and lateral views of a thoracic vertebral body replacement in a patient with follicular thyroid carcinoma. The wire loop is for approximation of the ribs at wound closure.

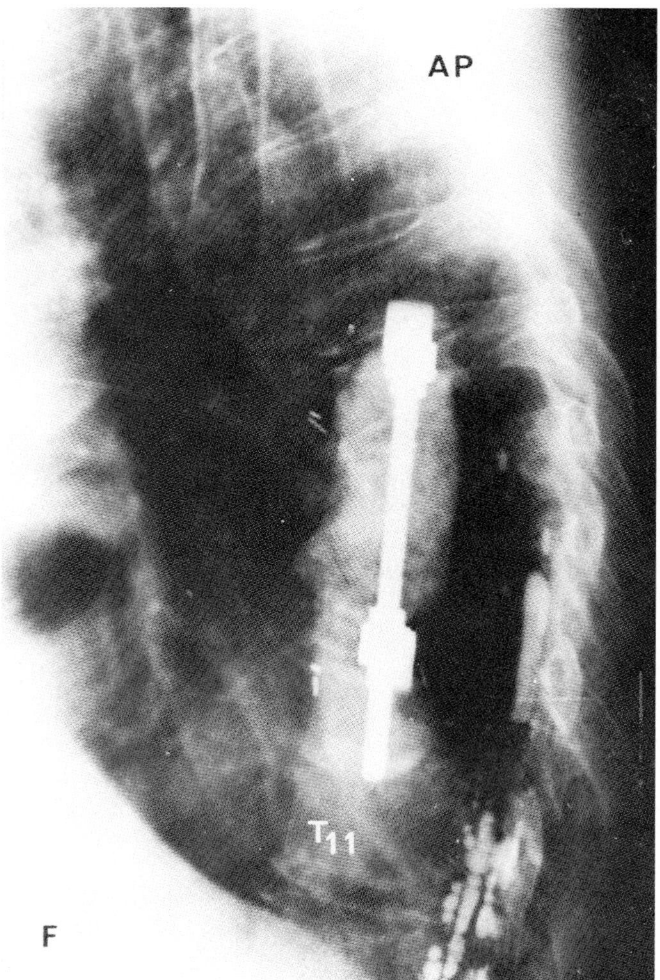

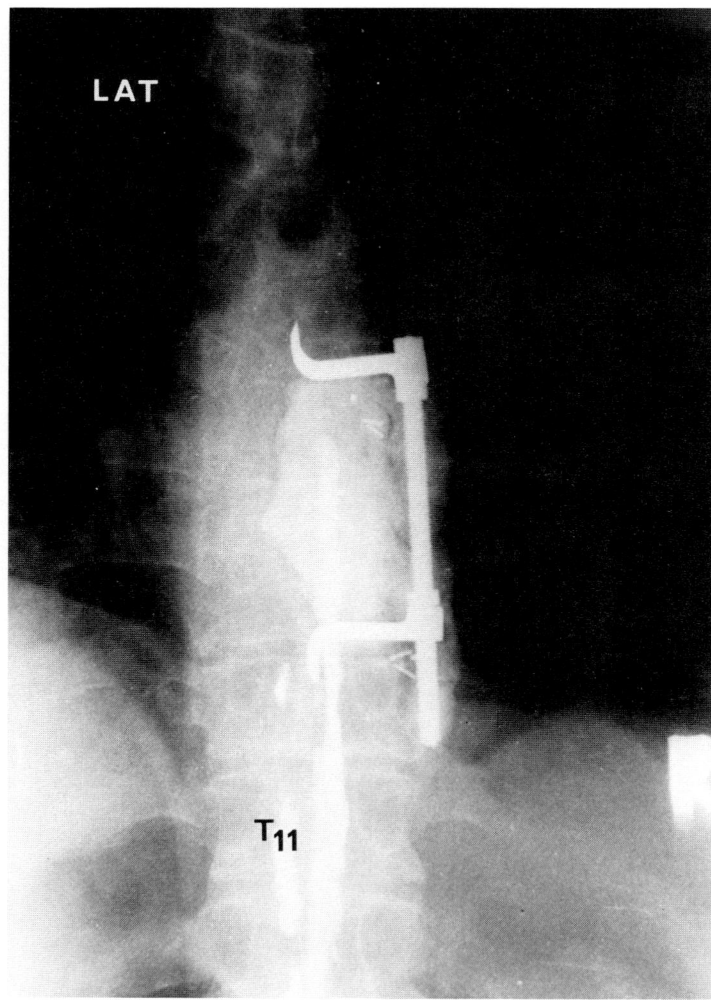

Fig. 133-8 (continued) (F) AP and lateral views of a replacement spanning three thoracic vertebrae in a patient with multiple myeloma. The free flow of the Pantopaque documents opening of the myelographic block.

of the tumor is recommended, since after a major debulking the bleeding is likely to lessen, more so in cases of complete excision. When bleeding continues, we usually apply Gelfoam or Surgicel on a gauze to the bleeding area and wait for the anesthesiology team to catch up with fluid replacement. With bleeding under good or even partial control, decompression is completed and vertebral body replacement is considered.

Vertebral body replacement is a spine stabilizing procedure. The spine is considered unstable if more than 50 percent of the vertebral cut surface is lost because of tumor expansion or as a result of decompression, if the bone loss extends for two vertebras or more, or if there is bone destruction of both anterior and posterior elements at the same level (Table 133-1). Any combination of the above will greatly increase instability. Adequate decompression of the spinal cord, correction of deformity, and stabilization of the spinal column are inherent to the technique and, if obtained, will maximize spinal cord function. The optimal technique for vertebral body replacement has yet to be devised. Several solutions to this problem have been described[8,45–54]; some of them include specially developed instruments and devices. We feel that the vertebral body replacement method should be reliable, simple to use, economical on operating time, and include elements well known and in wide use by most spinal surgeons. We have reported on our experience with vertebral body replacement using components

of the Harrington instrumentation system, namely threaded rods, nuts, and hooks.[7,10] In our hands it has proved efficient and durable, with the additional advantage of not enlarging the surgical armamentarium.

Of all vertebral body replacements, thoracic replacement is the most often done and the easiest to master. Replacements in other areas of the spine are in essence variations of the same technique. Therefore, a detailed account of the steps of the technique is given here.

The Vertebral Body Replacement Technique

A heavy threaded Harrington rod is cut about 1½ inches longer than the distance to be spanned by the vertebral replacement construct. On one end of the rod, a sacral Moe hook is fastened in place with two nuts, one on each side (Figure 133-8). Another nut is added followed by the second hook, facing the other way. Clamps are applied to both hooks to allow insertion of the assembly into the spinal gap in a coronal plane. The assembly is positioned at the widest vertebral diameter with the blades of the hooks reaching across the midline of the intact vertebral bodies, above and below. The hooks are then distracted so that their blades sink into the vertebral bodies. After the initial manual distraction, a large lamina spreader is positioned between and in direct contact with the hooks, rather than the clamps. Opening the spreader will gently drive the hooks into the vertebral bodies. The mobile hook on the rod can be backed up in the advanced position by moving the nut on the thread. The gentle distraction is done in stages as it is ascertained that the distraction forces are correctly directed and do not dislodge the assembly. Special care is taken to avoid impingement on the spinal canal. The spreader and hook clamps are removed when optimal height of the replacement has been obtained and the kyphosis is corrected. A manual testing of the stability of the inserted assembly is carried out by pulling gently on the rod. A thorough rinsing with warm saline is followed by packing of gauze into the decompressed area.

A long-standing kyphosis will resist correction because of ligamentous or bone tethers. To overcome this, the anterior longitudinal ligament is sectioned and the residual vertebral shell on the opposite side of the decompression may have to be removed as well. Radiopaque methyl-methacrylate (bone cement) is used to reconstruct the excised vertebral bodies. It is inserted into the gap while still soft and applied around and over the metal instrumentation (Figure 133-8). The cement is pushed into the spongy bone interstices of the proximal and distal vertebrae to improve the purchase on the bony elements and then the remainder of the cavity is filled. The cement covers the sharp edges of the rod and hooks to prevent direct contact with the large vessels or lungs. Special care is taken not to exert any pressure on the dura mater. While hardening, the cement is kept at a distance from the dura with a Freer elevator, and thus a cleft is formed leading from the epidural space into the pleural cavity, allowing free drainage of postoperative bleeding. Excess bone cement is removed. When the methyl-methacrylate has set, the area is rinsed again. If possible, the construct is covered with parietal pleura, although this is not absolutely necessary. In most of our cases, coverage was not attained. After lavage of the pleural cavity, one or two large bore thoracic drains are inserted in the midaxillary line, preferably distal to the thoracotomy incision. The operating table is straightened and the wound edges are brought together by passing 18-gauge wire around the marginal ribs. The gap is closed by pulling up and crossing the ends of the wires. The wires are then twisted (not more than three full twists to avoid wire breakage) and the wound is closed in layers. The skin is meticulously approximated and sutured without tension. The drains are connected to a suction system. The patient is transferred to the intensive care unit and extubated a few hours later. Extubation is usually delayed when paraplegia is high thoracic or cervical in origin.

Postoperative Care

Turning in bed is not restricted. In case of paraplegia, the patient is turned every 3 hours and such noted on the bed chart. Regular hospital beds are used because turning frames are uncomfortable. Intravenous antibiotics are continued for 48 hours postoperatively. Dexamethasone is tapered by 50 percent every second day, as tolerated, starting on the third day after surgery. Chest x-ray films are obtained daily with the patient in the sitting position to check on the draining efficacy. When draining per 24 hours is less than 100 ml the drain is removed. The wound is covered again and left undisturbed until the 20th postoperative day. Sutures are then alternatively removed. If wound dehiscence is probable or edge necrosis begins to show, suture removal is delayed. The patient is allowed to sit up the first or second postoperative day and ambulation is considered

the day after the chest drain is removed if the neurologic status allows. There is no need for corsets, plaster jackets, or any other external fixation devices. Evaluation of stability at the site of the vertebral body replacement is by spine x-ray films taken with the patient standing and supine. Assessment of patency at the site of the preoperative myelographic block is done by observing the movement of the Pantopaque left in the subarachnoid space on a fluoroscope.

Excision of the Thoracic Wall

Neoplastic involvement of the posterior thoracic wall contiguous with the thoracic spine will require resection of that area. The tumor usually destroys or encases a few adjacent ribs and extends medially into the spinal column and canal (Figures 133-5, 133-9).

The patient is positioned in the lateral decubitus position, as with the transthoracic approach, and the skin incision is planned as in anterior decompression of the spine. The ribs to be excised are identified and the intact overlying muscles are dissected free. The osteotomy of the ribs is placed 5 cm ventral to the tumor margin. The rib ends are elevated, the neurovascular bundles ligated and cut, and the entire segment of the posterior thoracic wall containing the tumor is pulled up. The tumor is detached from the spine by severing all structures, especially the segmented nerves. It is important to make sure the nerves extending into the resected segment are completely resected, to avoid inadvertent pulling on the compressed spinal cord. Once the tumor is removed, the exposure of the spine is wide and very comfortable.

The chest wall is reconstructed with a synthetic fabric. The resulting paradoxical breathing movement of the chest wall lessens with time as a result of scar tissue formation. The postoperative management and follow-up are the same as for transthoracic decompression of the spine.

The High Thoracic Spine (T1-T3)

The approach to a vertebral body in the high thoracic area (T1-T3) is through costotransversectomy.[55] The patient is positioned face down on a spinal frame with the head on a horseshoe cerebellar frame. The upper extremities are brought forward; this pulls the scapulae away from the midline. The skin incision is placed parallel to and 6 to 8 cm lateral to the spine. The incision is deepened to the fascia of the paravertebral muscles. By undermining medially at this level, a flap is created with its base along the spinous processes.

The paravertebral muscles are incised longitudinally with diathermy in a line parallel to the spine and 5 to 6 cm lateral to it. Deepening the incision reveals the transverse processes. The muscles are subperiosteally peeled off the laminae and transverse processes two levels above and two below the level of required decompression. The ribs are denuded in a similar manner 7 to 8 cm lateral to spinous processes. The subperiosteal stripping is extended all around the proximal quarter (or third) of the ribs, with care taken not to violate the pleural space. The entire procedure is extrapleural. When circumferential rib stripping has been completed, a rib cutter is introduced 8 cm lateral to the midline, and the ribs are osteotomized at least one level above and one below the intended level of decompression. The proximal rib segments are elevated at the

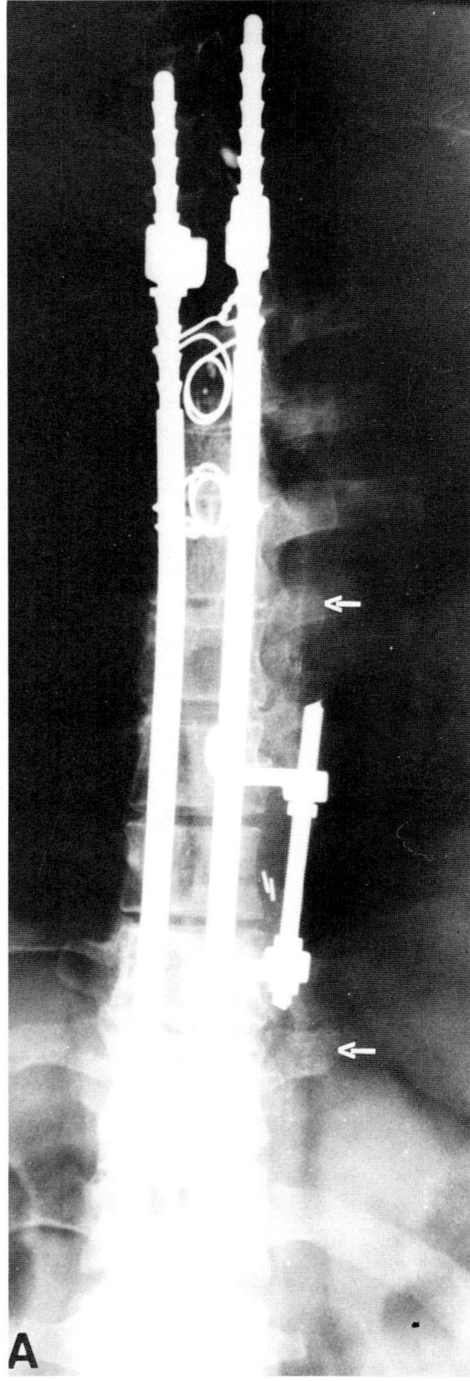

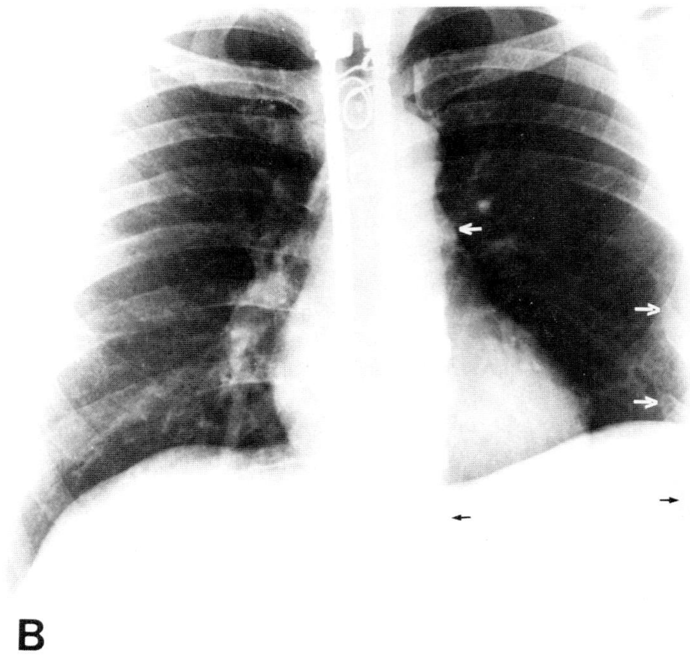

Fig. 133-9. (A) Involvement of the posterior thoracic wall continuous with epidural tumor in local recurrence of chondrosarcoma. Staged survey was indicated for resection of the posterior chest wall, the involved anterior and posterior vertebral elements, and the compressing epidural tumor. Stabilization was achieved by vertebral body replacement and posterior instrumentation with the Harrington distraction system and segmental wiring. (B) Arrows indicate the extent of chest wall resection. Reconstruction was undertaken with a synthetic fabric.

osteotomy end and the soft tissue stripping is completed on their undersurface, including the costovertebral joint and the head of the rib. Cutting the transverse processes leaves the rib connected to the vertebral body by irradiate ligament. Before the proximal rib segment is freed from this joint by simple twisting, one must ensure that the segmental nerves are totally detached from the rib and are not pulled inadvertently. A rib attached to the site of pathologic involvement is easy to detach and constitutes an affirmative indication to the site of prospective decompression. Often the head of the rib is involved with tumor and may break on twisting. The remaining rib fragment can be removed with curettes.

Once the proximal rib segments have been removed, the soft tissues are gently peeled off the anterolateral and anterior aspects of the vertebral bodies, and the field is open for decompression. The tumor is scooped out with curettes. If the segmental root is followed medially, it will safely indicate the position of the intervertebral foramen and lead to the epidural space. If feasible, the T1 and T2 roots are preserved to maintain ulnar functions. Removal of the compressing tumor is done as described in the transthoracic approach.

Once the extrapleural removal of tumor is completed, the dura free and pulsating, and bleeding reduced, reconstruction of the vertebral segments is considered. The upper thoracic ver-

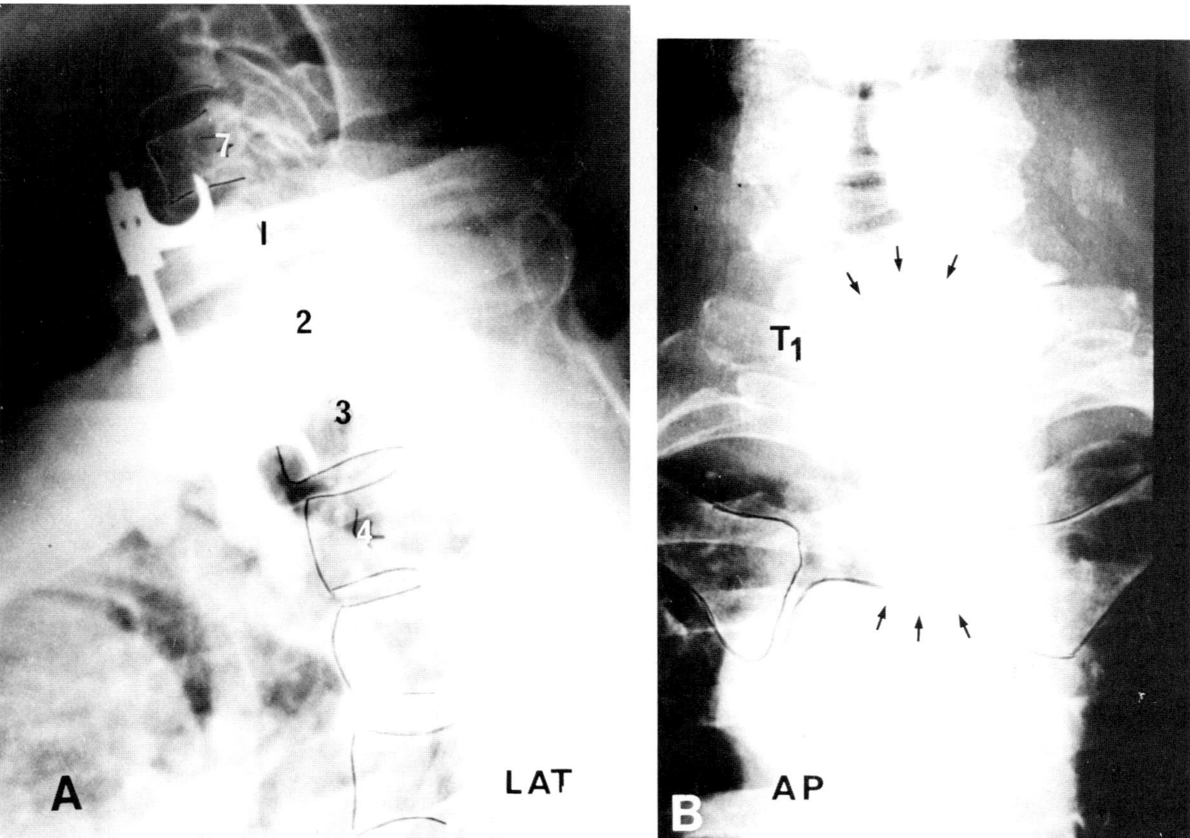

Fig. 133-10. (A,B) Vertebral body replacement at the thoracocervical junction in a 61-year-old patient with carcinoma of the colon. Anterior decompression was feasible since the diminished thoracic kyposis causes the junction to be erect and face the surgeon. The manubrium and clavicles are also set low. Adjustment to the reduced dimensions of the vertebral bodies requires use of the smaller Harrington compression hooks fitting the thin threaded rod. Placement of the construct is sagittal and spans the distance from C7 to T3 (black arrows on the AP view (B). There were no complaints of dysphagia.

tebrae are smaller than the lower thoracic or lumbar vertebrae. Vertebral body replacement may require smaller hooks. Use of Harrington compression hooks (Zimmer, No. 1259) on a thin threaded rod may suffice (Figure 133-10). After a thorough lavage to provide optimal vision for locating the dura, the assembly is inserted, with the fixed hook being manually pushed into the spongy bone of the caudal vertebra in the gap. Caution is taken when positioning the rostral hook, since in the prone patient the spine takes a downward dip following the normal kyphotic pattern. This requires positioning of the vertebral construct on a slope, with its rostral end pointing downward.

Placing the instrumentation is accompanied by repeated visual and palpatory examination to avoid unintentional impingement on the spinal canal. When the direction has been ascertained, the lamina spreader is placed on the hook blades and gradual distraction is applied; the spine is observed constantly to ascertain that the distraction is done in the correct axis. With each acquired length segment, the third nut is advanced on the rod to back up the departing rostral hook. When optimal distraction has been obtained, stability is checked by manual testing of the local fixation.

Once the instrumentation is firmly placed, methyl-methacrylate reconstruction is carried out as described for thoracic vertebral body replacement. After a final lavage, a large bore drain (chest drain) is placed on the cement-covered construct and the wound is closed in layers. The route of drain insertion should not pass through irradiated skin, but rather laterally a distance from the midline. If the pleural space has not been violated, no additional drain is necessary. Postoperative care and follow-up are outlined above in the description of the transthoracic approach.

The Cervicothoracic Junction

The cervicothoracic junction is the area most demanding of the spinal surgeon's skill and ingenuity. Tumors at the C7-T1 junction present a serious surgical and biomechanical challenge. The very flexible cervical spine, which is lordotic, joins the thoracic spine, which is rigid and kyphotic, C7-T1. The junction is therefore on a slope, withstanding compressive forces that become shearing in quality, with increased forward inclination of the transitional segment. Deficiency in either anterior or posterior bony structures evolves into an unstable situation leading to neurologic compromise, which at this site can impair function in the upper extremities as well. We recommend that in this area decompression and stabilization be carried out in two stages. The first state in a posterior approach, at the conclusion of which the cervicothoracic junction is rendered stable. The second stage is anterior, and following removal of tumor one may not include a vertebral body replacement if posterior fixation is adequate. To date, however, there is no available standard instrumentation, either anterior or posterior, to stabilize this segment. The Harrington hook-and-rod distraction system was not engineered to include the cervical vertebrae. The apophyseal joint anatomy does not allow upper hook placement and the restricted cervical epidural space is unable to accommodate sublaminar hooks or even wires without almost certain neurologic compromise. This definitely holds true in elderly patients, in whom the cervical canal is in many cases subclinically stenotic because of inward bulging of the annulus fibrosus and ligamentum flavum. Therefore, segmental wiring is unacceptable and other stabilizing procedures must be sought. The bone stock on which one can hope to obtain purchase for instrumentation is the joint masses and the spinous processes. The laminae are thin and purchase on them is precarious at best.

The solution we have developed is relatively simple. The patient is placed face down on the horseshoe head rest. The head is positioned as high as possible to correct the kyphosis at C7-T1. The skin incision is carried up to C2 and distally down to T7 or T8 about 6 to 8 cm lateral to the spinous processes and down to the fascia. The flap is elevated, and the posterior elements are stripped subperiosteally off the soft tissues and examined for discrete involvement with tumor at sites distant from the cord compression area. This dictates the extension of the exposure; the instrumentation must rest on at least three sound and stable segments above and below the decompressed area, unaffected by metastatic deposits.

A decompressive laminectomy is undertaken at C7 and T1 only if the preoperative studies suggest that there is tumor in the posterior compartment. When the dura and C8 and T1 roots have been released from compression, the exposed neural elements are covered with a free fat graft harvested from the wound edge in the high thoracic area.

Purchase on the cervical spine is obtained by attaching wires to the spinous processes and screws to the articular masses. The wires are 18-gauge stainless steel, and the screws are of the small spongy bone type with wide threads used by hand surgeons. The screws are inserted bilaterally into the articular masses of C4, C5, and C6 if these are not affected by tumor. The heads of the screws are allowed to project posteriorly for about 10 to 12 mm (Figure 133-11). The vertebral arteries lie anterior to the articular masses, the thickness of which is 5 to 7 mm. The screws therefore are positioned at the superior edge of the articular mass and no deeper than 5 mm. Each screw is placed in a somewhat different direction to avoid parallel placement of the screws. This enhances the hold of the instrumentation.

The wires engage the cervical spinous processes (C4-6) by being pulled through holes made by small towel clips. The wires are twisted on each spinous process and cut to leave a 2–3-cm long braid. The wires and screws projecting from the bone surface of the posterior elements constitute the anchorage to which the bone cement (methyl-methacrylate) is attached. Assuming the lower edge of the laminectomy to be at T1 or T2, sublaminar wires are passed bilaterally under T4, T5, and T6. If some posterior elements are damaged by metastatic deposits, a further distal segment is engaged.

Two sharp hooks (Zimmer No. 1256) are placed on the transverse processes of T7 or T8, facing caudally. Two Harrington rods are chosen to span the length from C4 to T8. It is usually necessary to give them a bend to accommodate the existing normal thoracic kyphosis, with the collar end toward the neck and the ratchet end directed caudally. The rachet ends are placed within the hooks already positioned on the T7 or T8 transverse processes. The collar ends of both rods rest on the laminae of C5.

The methyl-methacrylate mix is applied to the screws, wires, cervical spinous processes, and collar ends of the Harrington rods. When the bone cement has hardened, all these

elements are solidly encased together. Controlled distraction of the hooks at the ratchet ends now may be undertaken. If stability is satisfactory, C-washers are clamped on the ratchets close to the hooks and the sublaminar wires are twisted on the rods bilaterally (Figure 133-11). The wound is closed on a large bore drain, preferably a chest drain, connected to a suction system. It is discontinued when discharge is less than 50 ml per 24 hours. Sutures are left in for 20 days. No external supporting device is necessary. X-rays films with the patient standing are obtained within a week.

Timing of the second stage for anterior decompression for excision of C7 and T1 depends on the patient's medical status, the rate of neurologic worsening, and the surgeon's preference. Anterior access to this region is problematic in most cases and depends on there variables: (1) the height of the sternum (and clavicles) in relation to the cervicothoracic junction; (2) the diameter of the thoracic inlet; and (3) the extent of the high thoracic kyphosis. The last variable needs explanation. A high thoracic kyphosis, encountered quite often in elderly patients, increases in the forward inclination of the cervicothoracic junction; in severe cases this segment is almost parallel to the ground. An attempt at vertebral body resection in these cases through an anterior suprasternal approach[57] is futile, since visualization of the cervicothoracic junction is minimal. In these cases a lateral rachotomy may be indicated.[55] In cases with a normal thoracic configuration of hypokyphosis with a low-set manubrium and clavicles, one may resect through the anterior approach the vertebral bodies to T2 and place the lower end of instrumentation on T3. This is feasible because the cervicothoracic junction is erect, faces the surgeon, and is thus approachable.

Anterior instrumentation of the spine at the cervicothoracic junction implies manipulation of vital structures in the thoracic outlet. It also implies placement of the sharp metallic components of the vertebral replacement in close proximity to these structures. Because this is an area in which neurosurgeons or spine surgeons need to operate infrequently, the cooperation of colleagues from the ENT department, who are familiar with the regional anatomy, should be sought.

The patient is placed supine on the operating table and extreme neck extension is avoided. Endotracheal intubation is nasal. The preferable skin incision is transverse.[57] The trachea and esophagus are pulled to one side. The nasogastric tube delineates the position of the esophagus. The sternomastoid muscle and large ascending vessels are retracted laterally. the anterior longitudinal ligament is then visualized as it crosses the somewhat prominent cervical discs. Discoloration, swelling, and softening of the vertebrae at the compression site facilitate identification of the correct level for resection. If the level is in doubt, an intraoperative AP x-ray film is obtained. After ligation of all visible vascular feeders, resection is carried out to the guidelines outlined for transthoracic decompression of the spine. Magnification is helpful although not absolutely necessary.

Removal of the intervertebral disc may not be required. The avascular cartilaginous tissue is known to be rather resistant to tumor invasion and so may act as a barrier to local tumor propagation. The small dimensions of the cervicothoracic vertebrae necessitate use of the smaller compression hooks. These smaller hooks are made to fit the thin threaded compression rods. The instrumentation is carried out in a fashion similar to the thoracic vertebral body replacement. Excess methyl-methacrylate is removed and the surface molded manually to

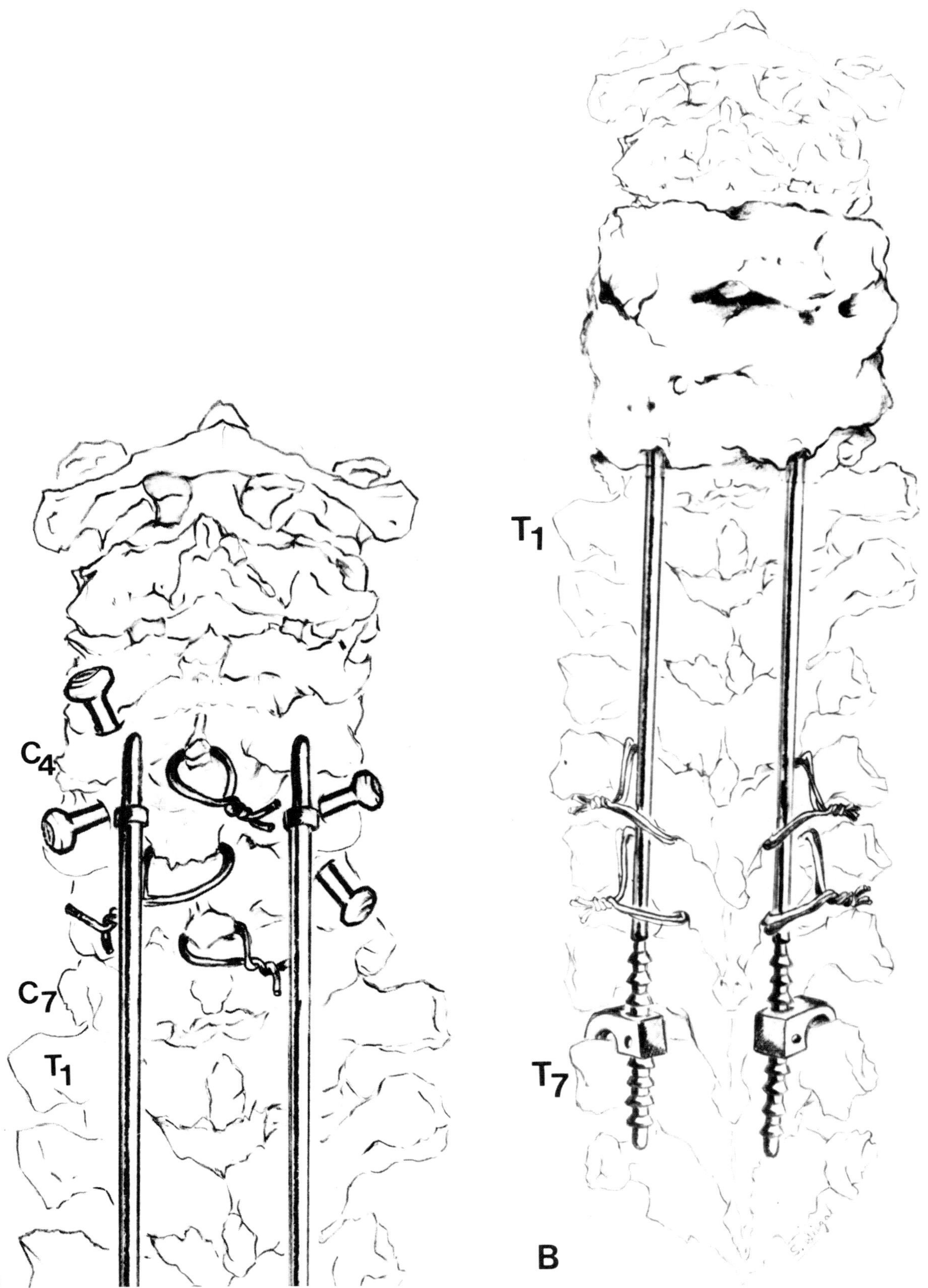

Fig. 133-11. Stabilization of the cervicothoracic junction by posterior instrumentation. (A) Purchase on the spine rostral to the C7-T1 area is obtained by nonparallel screws placed in the cervical articular masses two to three levels rostral to the area to be stabilized. To avoid vertebral artery damage, insertion of the screws should not exceed a depth of 5 mm. The screw heads are left to project 10 to 12 mm posteriorly. For further purchase on the posterior elements, 18-gauge stainless steel wire loops are passed through holes made in the spinous processes with small towel clips. The collar ends of the Harrington distraction rods come to rest on the laminae. (B) Harrington hooks are placed on the transverse processes of T7 and doubled sublaminar wires are passed bilaterally for two to three levels (T4-T5). The distraction rods are placed with the ratchet end in the hooks and the collar end resting on the laminae of the cervical spine. Methyl-methacrylate mix is applied to the screws, wires, cervical spinous processes, and collar ends of the H-rods, encasing all elements in a solid mass. The hooks are then moved distally on the ratchet, obtaining distraction and immediate stabilization of the spine. C-washers are tightened on the ratchet to avoid hook migration (not shown). The sublaminar wires are tightened segmentally over the rods.

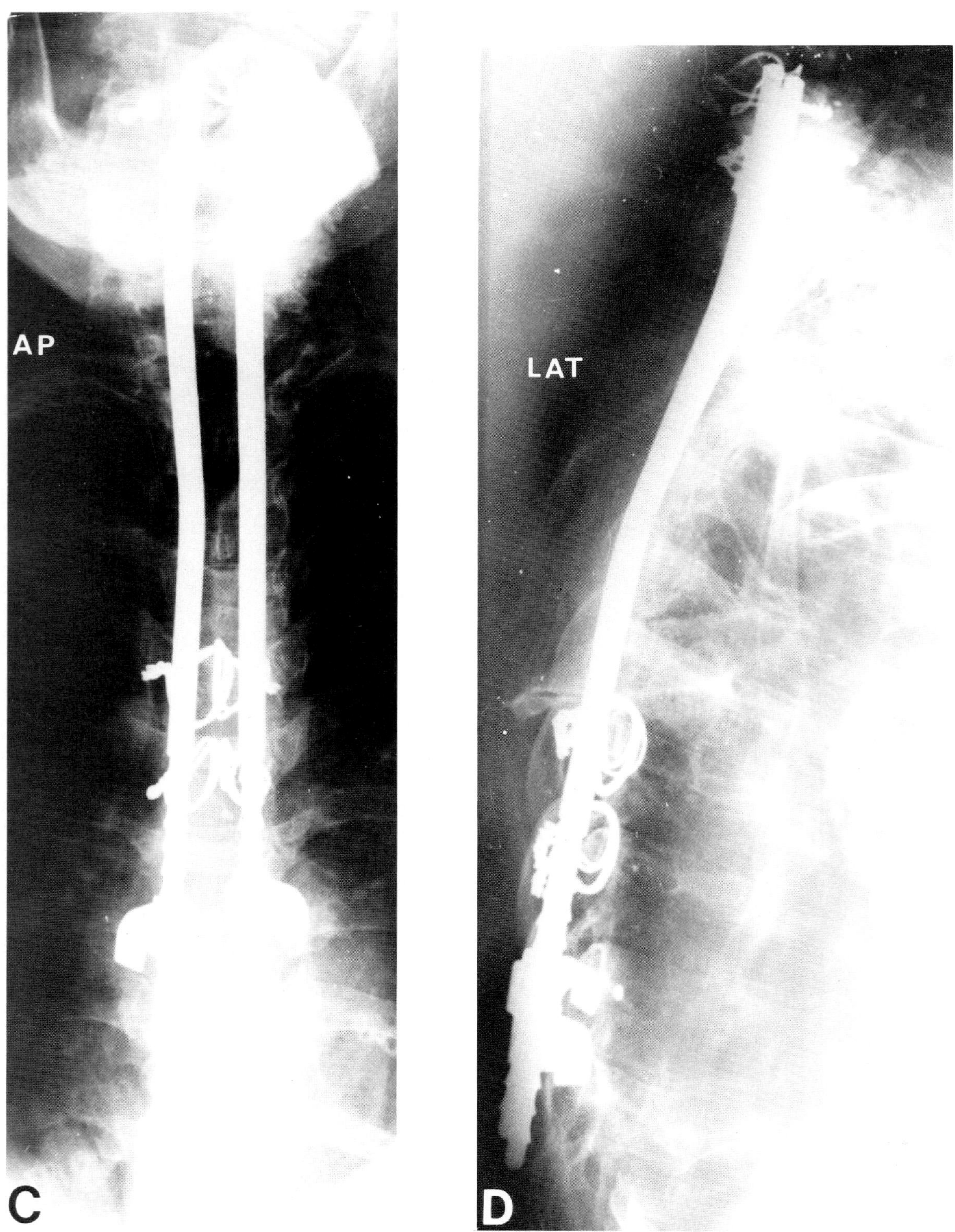

Fig. 133-11 (C,D) The AP (C) and lateral (D) views of the thoracocervical spine stabilization in a 59-year-old patient with breast carcinoma following laminectomy and decompresssion of the C7-T1 levels. Note the bend in the rods to accomodate normal thoracic kyphosis. The segmental wires are doubled to share pressure on the laminae and to avoid a cut out.

form a rounded construct in line with the structure of the spinal column. Sharp edges or protuberances must be eliminated to avoid late vascular or esophageal damage. The wound is closed on a large bore drain placed close to the vertebral construct. Postoperative care is similar in all vertebral body reconstruction procedures.

The Thoracolumbar Spine (T11-L1)

The transition zone at the thoracolumbar junction is somewhat more difficult to expose, but otherwise all other steps of spinal decompression and vertebral body replacement are identical to those in the thoracic or lumbar regions. To approach the T11-L1 area, one must displace not only the lungs and the abdominal contents, but also the diaphragm, separating the two. The insertion of the diaphragm is at L2, but the slope of its dome obstructs the approach to the spine.

The intubated patient is placed in the lateral decubitus position with the low thoracic area positioned over the acute bend in the operating table. The approach is through the bed of the tenth rib. After the skin over the anterior two thirds of this rib is incised the incision is carried obliquely down to the lateral aspect of the rectabdominis on the same side, then down to the bone and continued to the costochondral junction. The distal two thirds of the rib is excised down the junction after the usual subperiosteal stripping of soft tissues. The thoracic cavity is entered with care because it is much narrowed at this level by the ascent of the dome of the diaphragm. Now the chondral end of the tenth rib is longitudinally split, since at this point one can localize the anterior border of the diaphragmatic insertion. Blunt dissection separates the peritoneum from the undersurface of the diaphragm, the lateral and posterior abdominal walls, the iliopsoas muscle, and the upper lumbar spine. With the abdominal contents and the lung retracted forward, the diaphragm is well visualized. From the split end of the tenth rib, the diaphragm is cut along its insertion line, leaving a 2-cm wide strip attached to the chest. Long sutures are placed every 4 or 5 cm on both sides for later precise approximation during wound closure. The crus is detached as well, and vertebral body excision and replacement are carried out as outlined in the transthoracic approach. Before closure, large bore drains are positioned both in the chest cavity and in the retroperitoneum. It is interesting to note that although the diaphragm is sutured back over the synthetic vertebral construct and there is no chance of any biologic adhesion between the two, we have not encountered symptoms of transdiaphragmatic herniation.

The Lumbar Spine (L2-L5)

The intubated patient is placed in the right or left lateral decubitus position according to the tumor location as assessed from the preoperative studies. The lumbar area is positioned over the acute bend of the table (see Figure 133-7). The incision is started at the lateral border of the paravertebral muscle group at the midlumbar level and carried laterally and ventrally to the lateral border of the rectus abdominis. The incision is deepened by cautery to the peritoneum. By blunt dissection with a finger, the peritoneum is peeled off the lateral abdominal wall, extending the dissection to the iliopsoas posteriorly. In the same manner, the peritoneum is detached from the undersurface of the diaphragm. Attention is then directed centrally to the iliopsoas; the peritoneum is peeled off the muscle medially until the lumbar spine is visualized. This is carried out close to the iliopsoas muscle; no intentional dissection is done to reveal the

ureter or kidney. When the peritoneum has been entirely removed from the diaphragm, the posterior abdominal wall, the iliopsoas, and the spine, the abdominal contents will fall forward, opening the way for surgery on the vertebral bodies. If the patient has been conveniently placed over the bend of the operating table, the incised lateral abdominal wall stays widely open, necessitating minimal retraction.

The iliopsoas muscles cover the lateral and anterolateral aspects of the lumbar spine and between them is the anterior longitudinal ligament, which runs as a strong white strip in the midline, segmentally elevated by the bulge of the intervertebral discs.

Intraoperative location of the diseased vertebrae is done in much the same way as in the thoracic spine. The surgeon inspects the iliopsoas muscle for a swelling indicating an underlying or infiltrating paravertebral tumor. In addition, discoloration or bulging of the anterior longitudinal ligament, the presence of frank anterior penetrating tumor, or an abnormally short interdiscal distance are all good localizing signs of the area to be decompressed. If the tumor is contained within the vertebra and its level difficult to identify, it is a sound policy obtain an intraoperative AP film of the lumbar spine with a heavy IV needle hammered lightly into the lateral aspect of a vertebra. To expose the lumbar spine, a round-ended retractor is placed under the medial border of the iliopsoas, kept in close contact with the vertebral bodies, and pulled laterally to the intervertebral foramina.

The vertebral waist, covered by areolar tissue, is now examined to locate the segmental vascular bundle. The tip of a long curved hemostat is positioned on the bone close to one disc and is swept toward the other disc with its tip close to the bone surface. As it emerges near the other disc, the segmental vascular bundle is elevated on the hemostat's jaws. Opening the instrument stretches the vessels to allow clipping or ligating on both sides. (For details of the technique, see transthoracic anterior decompression of the spine above.)

Regardless of the number of vertebrae to be replaced, the steps of anterior instrumentation of the spine (vertebral body replacement) are essentially the same. The lumbar vertebrae are the largest, therefore the large Moe sacral hooks are adequate for a sound purchase across the vertebral bodies (Figure 133-12). The technique of replacement has been described above. However, a few points deserve special notice. The lumbar spine at its lower segments is in close contact with the bifurcations of the aorta and vena cava, and the lateral aspects of L5 are in close relation to the iliac artery and vein. Careful manipulation and retraction therefore are indicated, and the vertebral replacement construct should not be in the way of the pulsating large vessels. We have not yet encountered any vascular complications such as tears of the vena cava or iliac veins or late occurrence of iatrogenic aneurysms. Here, as elsewhere along the spinal column, the rod and hooks are covered by methyl-methacrylate cement, which also fills the gap left after excision of the diseased vertebrae. While hardening, the cement is kept from pressing on the dura. At the same time, a cleft is fashioned between the dura and the cement, leading into the retroperitoneum to allow free drainage of postoperative bleeding. After a thorough lavage with warm saline, a noncollapsible large bore drain is introduced into the retroperitoneum close to the outlet of the cleft. The drain exit is distal to the incision wound and in the posterior axillary line. The acute bend in the operating table is straightened and the wound is meticulously close in layers. The approximation

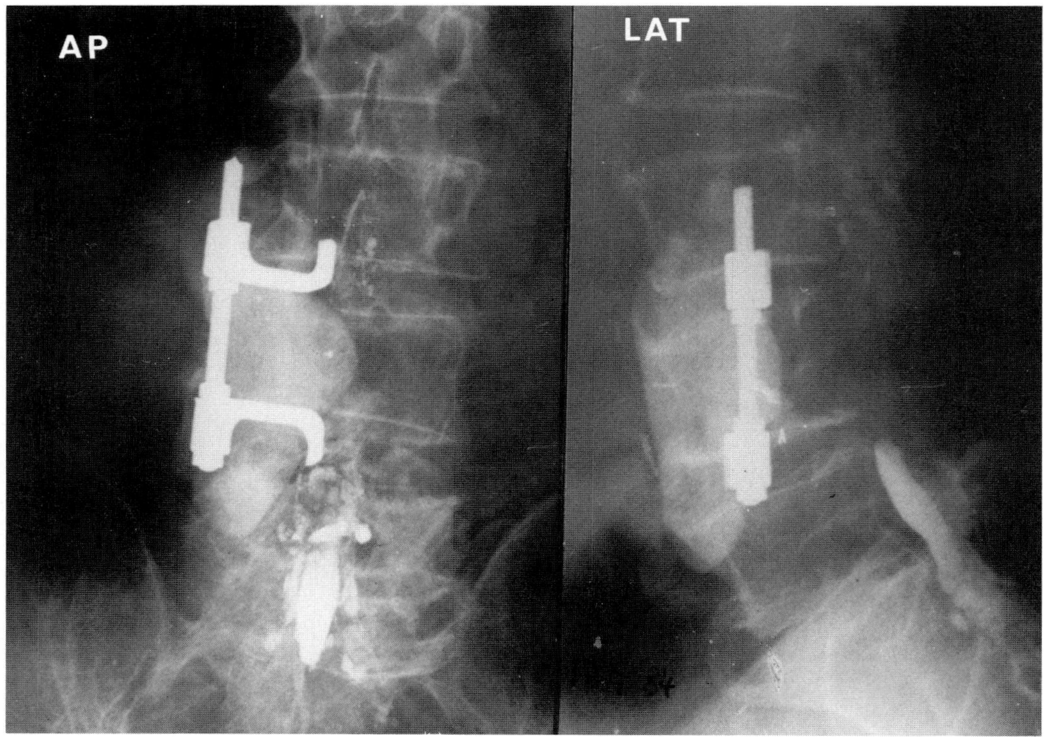

Fig. 133-12.   Vertebral body replacement of L4 in a patient with prostatic carcinoma. Standard sacral Moe hooks are used on a heavy threaded rod. Special attention is given to smooth covering of the metal components by bone cement to avoid direct contact with pulsating large vessels.

forces at the incision wound are carried by the fascial and subcutaneous layers. The skin sutures are intended only to maintain alignment of wound edges and must not be tightened. Postoperative care and follow-up are similar to those outlined for transthoracic decompression.

COMPLICATIONS OF THERAPY

RADIOTHERAPY

Most papers dealing with radiotherapy alone do not comment on complications of therapy or mortality. There has been concern that radiation edema may bring about neurologic deterioration.[43] However, it is still unclear whether such an edema accumulates in the irradiated spinal cord.[44] In any case, most patients are covered with high doses of dexamethasone.[2,3,6,7]

Death in the first month after radiotherapy is likely to be a result of primary disease. In our experience, 70 percent of the patients considered severely ill at the time of diagnosis of spinal cord compression died within 30 days after diagnosis.[7] All these patients were offered radiotherapy because of poor general medical status.

SURGICAL COMPLICATIONS

Mortality

The incidence of death within the first month after decompressive laminectomy ranges from 3 to 14 percent with an average mortality of 9 percent.[2,5,6,7,12] Surgical mortality after vertebral body resection falls within the same range and does not exceed the rate reported for laminectomy.[7-10]

Morbidity

Worsening Neurologic Status.   The risk of neurologic deterioration as a result of surgery is a major concern in patients who are still able to walk or with paraparesis. Worsening of neurologic status occurred to 7 to 26 percent of the patients after unselective decompressive laminectomy, with an overall mean of 12 percent.[6,12] In a group of patients with posterior compartment epidural tumors who underwent laminectomy, neurologic deterioration occurred in 20 percent as a direct result of the operation.[7] Although the vertebral body resection procedure seems to be more formidable, neurologic worsening is a rare complication, in only 2 to 4 percent of the patients.[7-10]

Nonneurologic Complications.   In patients undergoing laminectomy combined with radiotherapy, nonneurologic complications include wound infection, dehiscence, spinal epidural hematoma, CSF leak, and spinal instability. The frequency of these complications ranges from 8 to 43 percent, with a mean of 11 percent.[6,12] Only a few authors specifically mentioned the problem of instability,[2,27] reporting its occurrence in about 9 percent of the cases.

The incidence of nonneurologic complications in vertebral body resection is similar to the reported rate in laminectomies. Dislodgement of the vertebral replacement construct can cause severe pain and neurologic deterioration as a result of spinal instability and subluxation. It occurred in 5 percent of our patients before June 1982, because of faulty anchorage of the construct to adjacent vertebrae.[7] Since the introduction of our improved technique, no dislodgement has occurred in 80 patients who underwent vertebral body replacement procedures. However, the operation and instrumentation techniques require considerable expertise. The anterior approach to the spine may subject the patient to a variety of potentially serious complications, such as severe bleeding, damage to the adjacent vital organs, infection, and poor healing of irradiated tissues. We therefore believe that these procedures should be undertaken by a surgeon familiar with the anterior surgical approach to the spine and the technique of spinal instrumentation with its different options.

Pain and Recompression

Neurologic examination is carried out at 3-month intervals and stability is reassessed. Recurrence of instability is heralded by local or radicular pain, elicited by motion or physical activity. Recurrence of pain in a persistent or radicular pattern may indicate nerve root compression or in infiltration by tumor (see Figure 133-2). Recurrence of neurologic symptoms suggests either severe instability or regrowth of the epidural tumor. In these situations, reassessment and repeat myelography is indicated. If a high degree myelographic block is present or instability is evident, decompression and additional stabilizing instrumentation is considered.

REFERENCES

1. Cobb CA, Leavens ME, Eckles N: Indications for non-operative treatment of spinal cord compression due to breast cancer. J Neurosurg 47:653, 1977
2. Gilbert RW, Kim JH, Posner JB: Epidural spinal cord compression from metastatic tumor: Diagnosis and treatment. Ann Neurol 3:40, 1978
3. Greenberg HS, Kin JH, Posner JB: Epidural spinal cord compression from metastatic tumor: Results with a new treatment protocol. Ann Neurol 8:361, 1980
4. Stark RJ, Henson RA, Evans SJW: Spinal metastases—a retrospective survey from a general hospital. Brain 105:189, 1982
5. Young FR, Post EM, King GA: Treatment of spinal epidural metastases. Randomised prospective comparison of laminectomy and radiotherapy. J Neurosurg 53:741, 1980
6. Black P: Spinal metastases: Current status and recommended guidelines for management. Neurosurgery 5:726, 1979
7. Siegal T, Siegal T: Surgical decompression of anterior and posterior malignant epidural tumors compressing the spinal cord: A prospective study. Neurosurgery 17:424, 1985
8. Harrington KD: Anterior cord decompression and spinal stabilization for patients with metabatic lesions of the spine. J Neurosurg 61:107, 1984
9. Sundaresan N, Galicich JH, Bains MS, et al: Vertebral body resection in the treatment of cancer involving the spine. Cancer 53:1393, 1984
10. Siegal T, Siegal T: Vertebral body resection for eipdural compression by malignant tumors. Results of forty-seven consecutive operative procedures. J Bone Joint Surg 67A:375, 1985
11. Barcena A, Lobato RD, Rivas JJ, et al: Spinal metastatic disease: Analysis of factors determining functional prognosis and the choice of treatment. Neurosurg 15:820, 1984
12. Findlay GFG: Adverse effects of the management of malignant spinal cord compression. J Neurol Neurosurg Psychiatry 47:761, 1984
13. Dunn RC Jr, Kelly WA, Whons RN, et al: Spinal epidural neoplasia: A 15-year review of the results of surgical therapy. J Neurosurg 52:47, 1980
14. Livingston KE, Perrin RG: The neurosurgical management of spinal metastases causing cord and cauda equina compression. J Neurosurg 49:839, 1978
15. Barron KD, Hirano A, Araki S, et al: Experiences with metastatic neoplasms involving the spinal cord. Neurology 9:91, 1959
16. Schabert J, Gainor BJ: A profile of metastatic carcinoma of the spine. Spine 10:19, 1985
17. Torma T: Malignant tumors of the spine and psinal epidural space—a study based on 250 histologically verified cases. Acta Chir Scand 225:1, 1957
18. Arseni CN, Simionescu MD, Horwath L: Tumors of the spine. Acta Psychiatr Neurol Scand 34:398, 1959
19. Ushio Y, Panser R, Posner JB, et al: Experimental spinal cord compression by epidural neoplasms. Neurology 27:422, 1977
20. Ikeda H, Ushio Y, Shimizu K, et al: Experimental spinal cord compression by epidural neoplasms. Neurol Surg 6:891, 1978
21. Ikeda H, Ushio Y, Hayakawa T, et al: Edema and circulatory disturbance in the spinal cord compressed by epidural neoplasms in rabbits. J Neurosurg 52:203, 1980
22. Kato M, Ushio Y, Hayakawa T, et al: Circulatory disturbance of the spinal cord with epidural neoplasm in rats. J Neurosurg 63:260, 1985
23. Vieth R, Olson G; Extradural spinal metastases and their neurosurgical management. J Neurosurg 23:501, 1965
24. Benson H, Scarffe J, Todd ID, et al: Spinal cord compression in myeloma. Br Med J 1:1541, 1979
25. Bernat JL, Greenberg ER, Barrett J: Suspected epidural compression of the spinal cord and cauda equina by metastatic carcinoma. Cancer 51:1953, 1983
26. Martenson JA, Evans RG Jr, Lie MR, et al: Treatment outcome and complications in patients treated for malignant epidural spinal cord compression. J Neuro-Oncol 3:77, 1985
27. Brice J, McKissock W: Surgical treatment of malignant extradural spinal tumors. Br Med J 2:1341, 1965
28. Hall AJ, Mackay NNS: The results of laminectomy for compression of the cord and cauda equina by extradural malignant tumor. J Bone Joint Surg 55B:497, 1973
29. Marshall LF, Langfitt TW: Combined therapy for metastatic extradural tumors of the psine. Cancer 40:2067, 1977
30. Posner JB, Howieson J, Cvitkovic E: "Disappearing" spinal cord compression: Oncolytic effect of glucocorticoids (and other chemotherapeutic agents) on epidural metastases. Ann Neurol 2:409, 1977
31. Ushio Y, Posner R, Kim J, et al: Treatment of experimental spinal cord compression caused by extradural neoplasms. J Neurosurg 47:380, 1977
32. Clarke P, Saunders M: Steroid-induced remission in spinal canal reticulum cell sarcoma. Report of two cases. J Neurosurg 42:346, 1975
33. Canta RC: Corticosteroids for spinal metastases. Lancet 2:912, 1968
34. Smith R: An evaluation of surgical treatment for spinal cord compression due to metastatic carcinoma. J Neurol Neurosurg Psychiatry 28:152, 1965
35. Mullan J, Evans JP: Neoplastic disease of the spinal extradural space: A review of fifty cases. Arch Surg 74:900, 1957
36. Constans JP, de Divitiis E, Donzelli R, et al: Spinal metastases with neurological manifestations: A review of 600 cases. J Neurosurg 59:111, 1983
37. Brady LW, Antonaides J, Prasasvinichai S, et al: The treatment of metastatic disease of the nervous system by radiation therapy, in Seydel HG (ed): Tumors of the Nervous System. New York, John Wiley, 1975, pp 176–189
38. Williams HM, Diamond HD, Craver LF, et al: Neurological Complications of Lymphomas and Leukemias. Springfield, Ill, Charles C Thomas, 1959
39. Friedman M, Kim TH, Panahom AM: Spinal cord compression in malignant lymphoma: Treatment and results. Cancer 37:1485, 1976

40. Mones RJ, Dozier D, Berrett A: Analysis of medical treatment of malignant extradural spinal cord tumors. Cancer 19:1842, 1966

41. Rubin P, Mayer E, Poulter C: Extradural spinal cord compression by tumor; Part II: High daily dose experience without laminectomy. Radiology 93:1248, 1969

42. Silverberg IJ, Jacobs EM: Treatment of spinal cord compression in Hodgkin's disease. Cancer 27:308, 1971

43. Lawes FAE, Ham HJA: A case of Hodgkin's disease with spinal cord involvement treated by nitrogen mustard. Med J Aust 1:104, 1953

44. Rubin P: Extradural spinal cord compression by tumor. Part I: Experimental production and treatment treatment trials. Radiology 93:1243, 1969

45. Dunn EJ: The role of methylmethacrylate in the stabilization and replacement of tumors of the cervical spine: A project of The Cervical Spine Research Society. Spine 2:15, 1977

46. Ono K, Tada K: Metal prosthesis of the cervical vertebra. J Neurosurg 42:562, 1975

47. Scoville WB, Palmer AH, Samra K, et al: The use of acrylic plastic for vertebral replacement or fixation in metastatic disease of the spine: A technical note. J Neurosurg 267:274, 1967

48. White AA III, Panjabi MM: Surgical construct employing methylmethacrylate, in: Clinical Biomechanics of the Spine. Philadelphia, JB Lippincott, 1978, pp 423–431

49. Clark CR, Keggi KJ, Panjabi MM: Methylmethacrylate stabilization of the cervical spine. J Bone Joint Surg 66A:40, 1984

50. Sundaresan N, Bains M, McCormack P: Surgical treatment of spinal cord compression in patients with lung cancer. Neurosurgery 16:350, 1985

51. DeWald RL, Bridwell KH, Prodromas C, et al: Reconstructive spinal surgery as palliation for metastatic malignancies of the spine. Spine 10:21, 1985

52. Fidler MW: Anterior decompression and stabilization of metastatic spinal fractures. J Bone Joint Surg 68B:83, 1986

53. Dunn HK: Anterior stabilization of thoracolumbar injuries. Clin Orthop 189:116, 1984

54. Kostuik JP: Anterior spinal cord decompression for lesions of the thoracic and lumbar spine: Techniques, new methods of internal fixation, results. Spine 8:512, 1983

55. Capener N: The evolution of lateral rachotomy. J Bone Joint Surg 36:173, 1954

56. Harrington PR: Treatment of scoliosis. J Bone Joint Surg 44A:591, 1962

57. Cloward RB: The anterior approach for removal of ruptured cervical discs. J Neurosurg 15:602, 1958

CHAPTER 134

Surgery of the Peripheral Nerves and Brachial Plexus

Robert D. Leffert

I would like to see the day when somebody would be appointed surgeon somewhere who has no hands, for the operative part is the least part of the work.

Harvey Cushing, November, 1911

ACCOMPLISHMENTS IN PERIPHERAL NERVE SURGERY in the 75 years since Dr. Cushing's statement was written are undeniable proof that it cannot be accepted verbatim. It is, however, immediately apparent to anyone with more than trivial clinical experience that re-establishment of the axonal continuity with the end organ, although of major importance to functional recovery, cannot guarantee it. Furthermore, it has been increasingly obvious that despite significant advances in microneurosurgical technique, optics, and suture material, the ultimate ability of the severed peripheral nerve to regenerate depends on biological, not mechanical factors. The control of scar, correct direction of the axon and preservation of the end organ are all critical in neural regeneration. Restoration of function of the paralytic or sense-deficient part depends on a variety of operative and nonoperative techniques involving such nonneural tissue as skin, muscle, bone, and joint. To achieve optimal functional results from the nerve operation, a surgeon must be familiar with these techniques, as well as their indications and timing, so that alternatives can be evaluated and proper decisions made. Above all, these must be relevant to the patient and his or her particular needs.

The focus of this work is on current operative neurosurgical techniques, so these will be described in detail and context. Since a thorough and all-inclusive discourse on the subject is impossible in the space available, see the extensive array of pertinent literature, including several major texts and monographs devoted to the subject.[1,2] The advances since Cushing's day have come largely from the carefully documented clinical experience of two world wars[3–6] (and several lesser ones), as well as laboratory research.

Many of the peripheral nerve techniques are identically applicable to the brachial plexus, but the specialized nature of this area makes certain individual considerations of diagnosis and treatment necessary. These will be described later.

Before proceeding further, a brief comment should be made on some anatomic, physiologic, and pathologic features of the peripheral nervous system that differentiate it from the central nervous system. The unique potential, under optimal circumstances for regeneration in the periphery make successful surgical manipulation possible. This phenomenon, however, primarily depends upon survival of the cell body, without which

new axoplasm cannot be synthesized. If the supporting stroma of the injured nerve is in continuity, or if alignment of the severed distal segment can be restored and scar does not unduly obstruct the juncture, regeneration can then take place. The mechanisms of neurotaxis and the significance of nerve growth factor in this process remain to be determined. The metabolic background within which it occurs is complex and only partially understood. Recent work on the effect of Leupeptin and its effect on the process of Wallerian degeneration and maintenance of the end organs raises some intriguing potential avenues for changing the basic approach to the repair of nerves.[7]

In addition to the interdependence of the cell body and axon, the complex structure of the peripheral nerve itself contributes to the difficulty of repair. Although the axon is the conducting medium for the nerve impulse, the supporting fibrous elements and myelin sheathings are of great importance both under normal and pathologic conditions. Until recently, the various elements of the supporting stroma of the peripheral nerve were simply labeled epineurium, which as its name would imply, is an areolar tissue that allows for gliding of nerves with movement of the joints and for entry of the segmented blood supply to the fascicles it encloses. What has become apparent as nerves were more closely examined is that the epineurium continues into the substance of the nerve between the fascicles. We therefore have further to define external epineurium from internal or epifascicular epineurium to account for this anatomic finding. The perineurium has two major functions—it resists traction elongation of the nerve and also keeps the contents of the fascicles under positive pressure. Endoneurium surrounds the individual fiber and Schwann-myelin sheath complex.

Unfortunately, the simplistic comparison of the peripheral nerve with a telephone cable has led to many illogical and unsuccessful attempts at surgical repair of damaged nerves. The monumental work of Sunderland[2] in demonstrating the intraneural topography of major peripheral nerves has provided an anatomic framework within which the surgeon may work. More recent work by Jabaley[8] has further elucidated the complex nature of the intraneural topography (Figure 134-1).

The constantly changing pattern of groups of fibers within a nerve as it traverses the limb, helps to explain why long gaps caused by injury often lead to poor operative results. Since the pattern does not remain constant along the nerve, this imposes a limit on just how many potential axon-bearing sheaths can be

OPERATIVE NEUROSURGICAL TECHNIQUES
ISBN 0-8089-1862-1

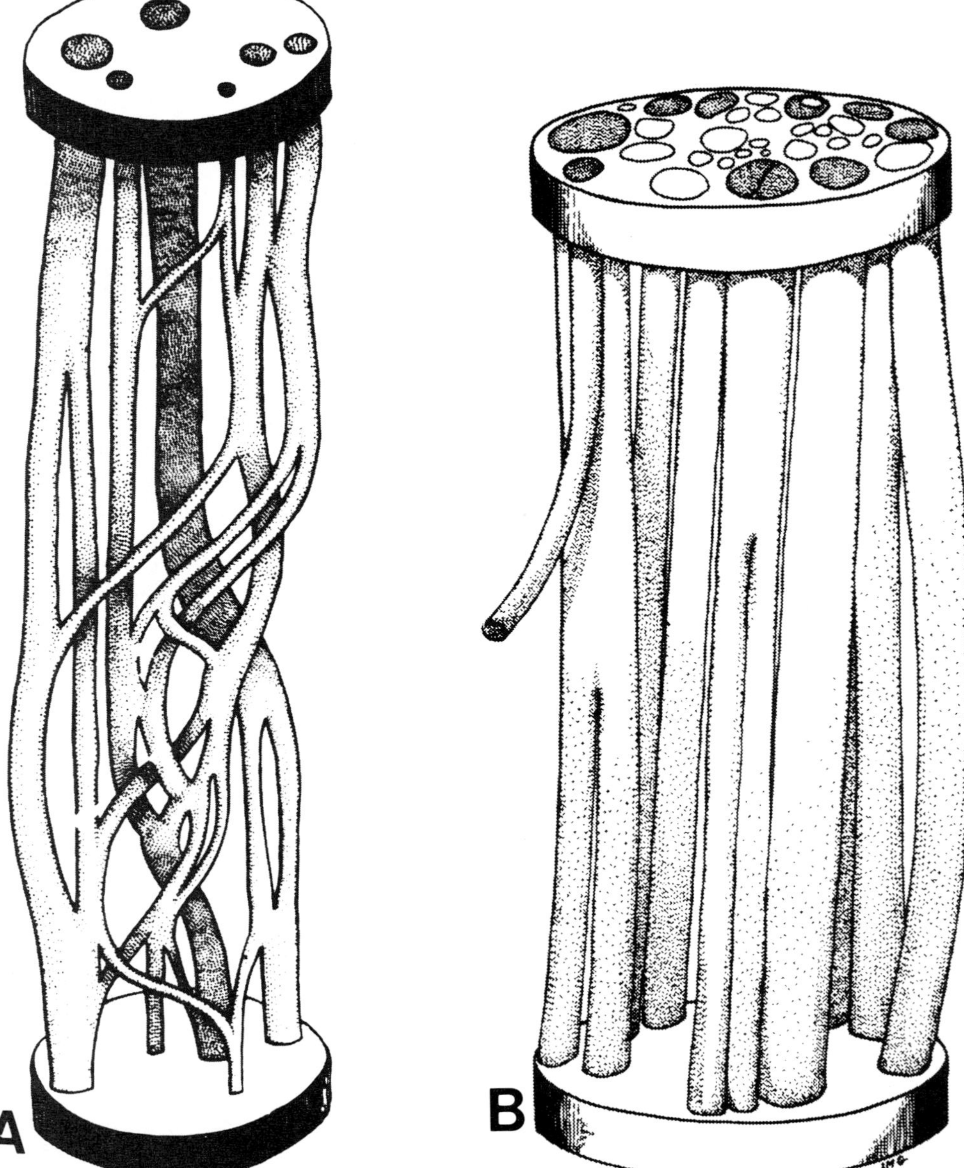

Fig. 134-1. (A) Funicular plexus formations in a 3-cm segment of a specimen of the musculocutaneous nerve of the arm, according to Sunderland. (Reprinted by kind permission of Churchill Livingstone Ltd, Edinburgh, and Sir Sidney Sunderland.) (B) Jabaley's concept of the internal topography of a 3-cm section of the median nerve in the midportion of the forearm. (Reprinted from Jabaley EJ, Wallace WH, Heckler FR: Internal topography of major nerves of the forearm and hand. J Hand Surg 5:1, 1980. With permission.)

reunited following a lengthy resection. Furthermore, even though peripheral nerves are abundantly supplied with blood vessels at all structural levels, and these are arranged both segmentally and longitudinally, it cannot be assumed that extensive mobilization will not have an adverse effect on their nutrition, or that destruction or ligation of adjacent vessels will not prejudice the ultimate result.[9,10] Lundborg's work on the blood supply of nerve and the result of mobilization is a valuable contribution[12–14] (Figure 134-2).

There are two specific situations wherein the presence of an intraneural artery may prove troublesome. Both the sciatic nerve and the median nerve have well-developed and relatively constant arteries. In the sciatic, a laceration of the intraneural artery that leaves the bulk of the nerve intact can cause catastrophic pressure necrosis of the surrounding fascicles, if it is not relieved promptly.

A suture of the median nerve done under tourniquet ischemia may rupture once arterial flow is established if the artery is not microcoagulated and the epineurial closure is tight.

MECHANISM OF INJURY

The peripheral nerves can be injured by a variety of types of trauma, which can act singly or in combination (Table 134-1).

These may not only involve different components of the nerve, but different lengths as well. For example, knife wounds are characteristically discrete and usually involve small seg-

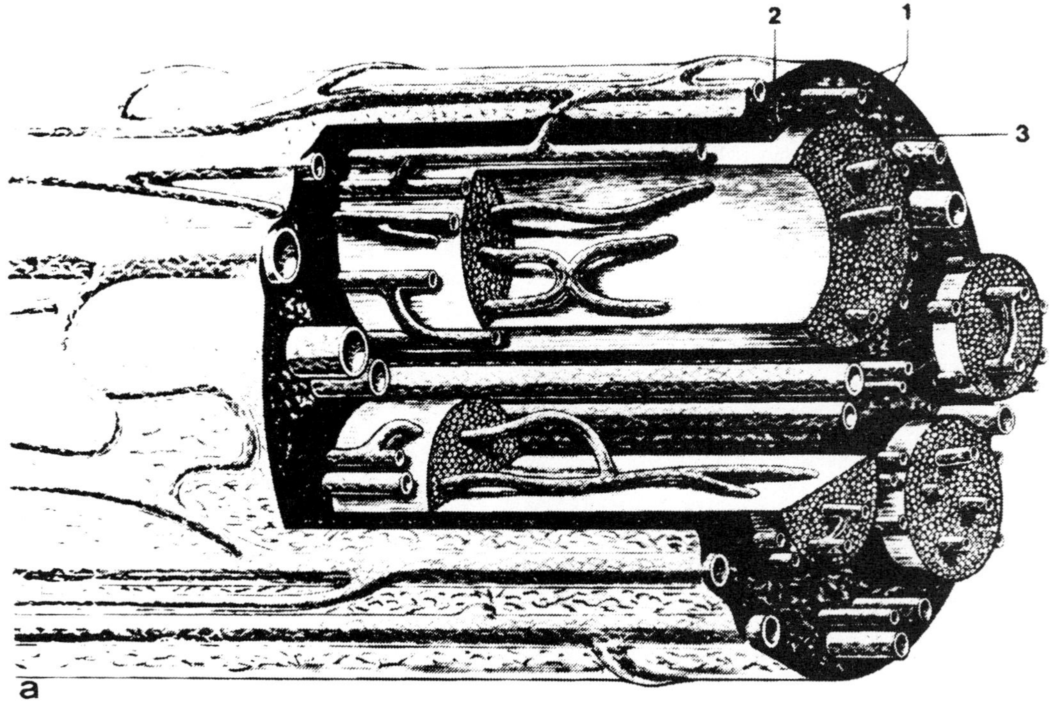

Fig. 134-2. Schematic representation of the intraneural microvascular system. (Reprinted from Lundborg G: Structure and function of the intraneural microvessels. J Bone Jt Surg 57A:7, 1975. With permission.)

ments, while traction injuries usually involve longer lengths and are harder to delineate.

In addition, the injury may be immediate, such as a gunshot wound, or delayed, as in the traction-friction neuropathy presenting as a tardy ulnar palsy years after an elbow fracture. Therefore, an almost infinite variety of clinical presentations of nerve injury is possible, leaving the surgeon with a pathologic condition very difficult to define on which to attempt to formulate rational management. Fortunately, however, traumatized nerves react in a reasonably predictable fashion. There are presently two systems of classification of the pathologic process of nerve injury in common use. Although they have common elements and do overlap, that of Sunderland[2] is more detailed with reference to subdividing the varieties of axonotmesis and neurotmesis as defined by Seddon. Both are presented, since the surgeon should be conversant with them (Table 134-2, Figure 134-3).

DEGENERATION AND REGENERATION

A brief discussion of the sequence of events involved in the process of degeneration of a transected nerve and regeneration following repair will serve as a physiologic background against which to interpret the technical procedures available.

Table 134-1. Mechanism of injury

Compression	Ischemia
Traction	Chemical injury
Laceration	Thermal or cold injury
	Electrical injury

Within 72 hours after the nerve is severed, all conductivity in the distal segment is lost. Axons and myelin sheaths disintegrate and are ingested by macrophages and Schwann cells. This active process is called wallerian degeneration. A proliferation of Schwann cells and endoneurial fibrocytes causes the cut end of the distal stump to swell, with the result that it is initially enlarged. With time, the cellular population diminishes, endoneurial tubes shrink and collagen is laid down around them so that the whole distal part of the nerve is smaller in diameter. The proximal segment undergoes similar changes in its stump over a very short segment, without shrinkage, but significant effects of the injury are also recorded in the cell body. Depending on the severity and proximity of the injury, the neuron may experience minor changes or even undergo complete destruction. More usually, it will begin manufacturing increased amounts of RNA in preparation for regeneration. The axoplasm streams out of the tangle of Schwann cells and collagen to form a randomly arranged and bulbous neuroma. If, however, with a primary suture, the supporting elements of the nerve have been accurately aligned and opposed, vigorous proliferation of Schwann cells and fibroblasts of the distal segment causes them to reach proximally, in an orderly fashion, and align themselves longitudinally. With correct orientation, then, more of the axons may find their way into the proper distal endothelial tubes. Suture within 3 months of injury is called early secondary suture. The cellular hyperplasia is then at its highest level and the epineurium is thickened, so that if epineurial sutures are used, they will hold solidly. The extent of scarring is delineated more easily than immediately after injury, but greater resection usually is necessary. Beyond 3 months, suture will be late secondary, and although Schwann tubes may remain open for longer than 6 months, there is proportional diminution in their available number and size with decreased quality of the end

Table 134-2. Three types of nerve injury

	Neurapraxia	Axonotmesis	Neurotmesis
Common causes	Compression Traction Freezing Ischemia Missiles	Compression Traction Missiles Ischemia Freezing Friction	Lacerations Missiles Traction Injections Ischemia
Pathology (may involve all or part of anatomic nerve circumference)	Local Demyelination no axonal interruption	Axonal interruption supporting stroma (Schwann sheaths intact)	Axonal and sheath interruption
Clinical findings	Complete motor paralysis, incomplete or lesser sensory loss	Complete motor and sensory loss	Complete motor and sensory loss
EMG	Rare fibrillations, no voluntary action potentials	Fibrillations > 3 weeks. No voluntary action potentials	Fibrillations > 3 weeks. No voluntary potentials.
Operative findings	Continuity preserved	Continuity preserved. Occasional neuromatous swelling	Anatomic gap surgically repaired, then 1 mm/day with delays
Spontaneous recovery and timing	Usually by 4–6 weeks in no regular order of innervation	1 mm/day in order of innervation	None unless surgically repaired, then 1 mm/day with delays
Quality of recovery	Normal	Usually normal	Never completely normal even after surgical repair

result. During the period of denervation, both motor and sensory end organs undergo involutional changes that have been well documented. In general, if a muscle has been denervated for 18 months, it is unlikely to make a functional recovery following reinnervation. The outer time limits for sensory recovery are less well-defined, so that, particularly in young patients, it may be worthwhile to attempt nerve repair to regain sensibility as long as 5 years after injury.

DIAGNOSIS OF PERIPHERAL NERVE INJURY

When in doubt, do a history and physical . . ." Anonymous

Although this maxim would seem both inappropriate and unnecessary, many nerve injuries escape initial detection in a massively traumatized patient or a situation wherein a surgeon caring for an injured extremity is introduced to a patient already under anesthesia. The implications of first noting the nerve deficit after treatment are obviously unfortunate. Careful notation of when the neurologic loss occurred is mandatory, both in fresh cases and those seen after a delay. Since many patients are seen late, it is necessary to establish whether motor and sensory loss have changed in the interval. The presence of associated injuries in the limb and their sequelae must be considered, since they can affect what is done to a significant degree. Information about the patient's occupation and previous function, as well as the circumstances and mechanism of injury are pertinent parts of the record, as is the presence or absence of pain.

Physical examination, in addition to discrete neurologic examination, must include an accurate assessment of the posi-

tion of wounds, character of scarring, and tissue quality, as well as the range of motion of joints, the presence of contractures, and vascular status.

For peripheral nerve injuries involving the limbs, it is necessary to determine that there are no nerve lesions proximal to the obvious one under consideration.

The assessment of motor power depends on the ability of the examiner to perform manual muscle tests accurately and with full knowledge of so-called trick and supplementary motions. Although the virtual disappearance of paralytic poliomyelitis has made this technique harder to master, several available manuals are quite helpful.[16]

Records should be detailed, accurate, and standardized. An acceptable scale is that of the British Medical Research Council.[3]

Sensory testing in the presence of nerve injury should include determination of light touch, using a fine brush, wisp of cotton or Semmes-Weinstein filaments, and a pin for pain sensibility. Where applicable, in the fingertips, two point discrimination should be tested with a blunt caliper. There is evidence that testing moving two point discrimination may offer advantages over the static test.[17] This examination is an indication of stereognosis, a higher type of sensory function without which the hand may have protective sensibility, but may still be blind, especially for activities where eye-hand coordination cannot compensate for deficient feedback. The coin test provides additional data on function of the hand. This and other functional evaluations may be far more informative than the standardized neurologic testing of individual modalities, but are not ordinarily used in acute situations.

The value of Tinel's sign, eliciting paresthesias in the distribution of an injured peripheral nerve by percussion over its course, has been much debated and misunderstood.[18,19] If

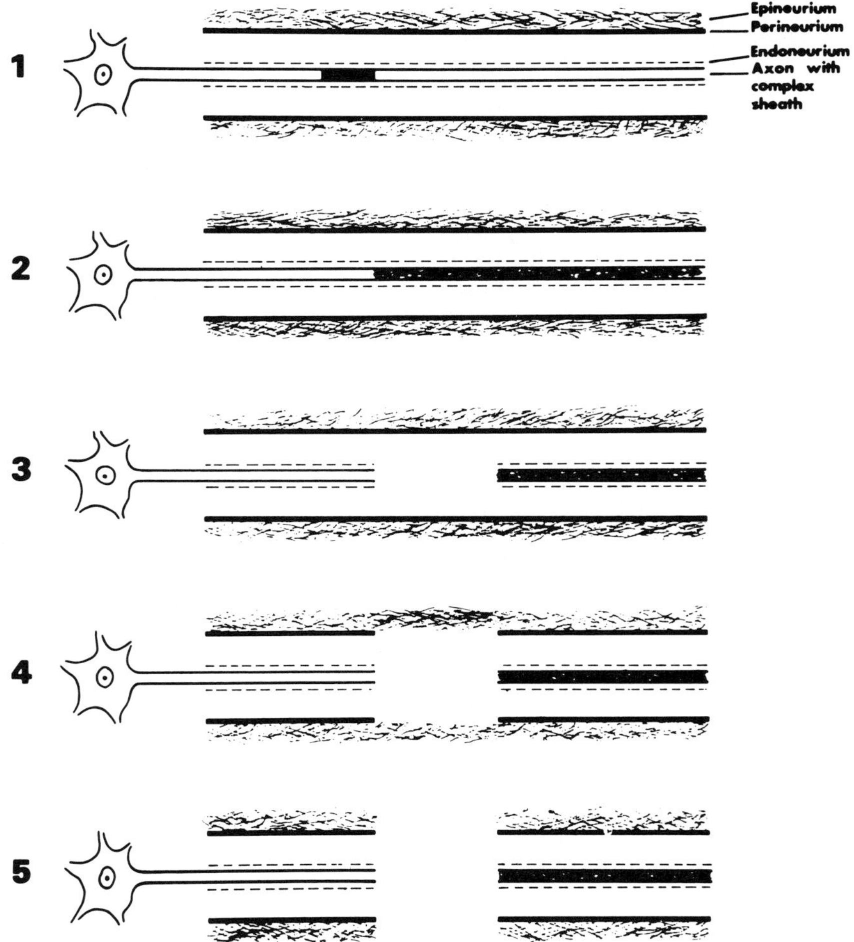

Fig. 134-3. Diagrammatic representation of the five degrees of nerve injury according to Sunderland. (1) Conduction block; (2) transection of the axon with an intact endoneurium; (3) transection of the nerve fiber (axon and Schwann sheath) inside an intact perineurium; (4) transection of funiculi, nerve trunk continuity being maintained by epineurial tissue; (5) transection of the entire nerve trunk. (Reprinted from Sunderland S: Nerves and Nerve Injuries, ed 2. Edinburgh, Churchill Livingstone Ltd, 1978. With permission.)

one taps over the point of injury, assuming the nerve is not deeply buried, a tingling sensation will be felt distally. Since it is a central phenomenon, this would happen even if the limb were amputated at that level. If some time has elapsed during which regeneration could have taken place, however, and tapping over the nerve distal to the injury produced tingling, then one can assume that at least some axons have reached this point. If, with further passage of time, the sign becomes less positive at the point of injury and more distally, this indicates that further down growth of axons has occurred. A persistently positive response at the site of injury and nothing distally bodes ill for recovery, but since only part of the total area of a nerve may have been injured and has been providing this response, an advancing Tinel's sign cannot be taken as assurance that functional recovery will ensue. Furthermore, since smaller and immature axons are responsible for the response, there is no way of determining by this method that more and larger-diameter axons eventually will follow.

Objective electrodiagnostic testing in the form of electromyography and nerve conduction velocity determination has emerged from studies in the neurophysiologic laboratory to provide a most useful adjunct to the management of nerve injuries.[20–23] Although an inexperienced or ill-advised electro-myographer may serve only to obfuscate, when viewed within the perspective of the clinical situation, the test is often of critical value.

By means of small percutaneous needle electrodes, fibrillation potentials may be detected at rest in partially or completely denervated muscle after about three weeks, when Wallerian degeneration has taken place. Since they are entirely outside of the patient's control, they have total objectivity, dependent, of course, on the ability of the observer to correctly interpret them. The pattern, on attempted voluntary contraction, may indicate partial denervation, or sequential observations may document recovery before it can be detected clinically.

Nerve conduction velocity determination, an offshoot of electromyography, may be used to localize the site of a lesion of a peripheral nerve, and is particularly useful in compression lesions. Both motor and sensory components may be measured. Measurement of evoked potentials in the evaluation of neuromas in-continuity at surgery has greatly expanded the use of this modality.[24,25]

Although of historic interest, chronaxie and strength-duration curves have been virtually discarded with the refinement of the preceding techniques.

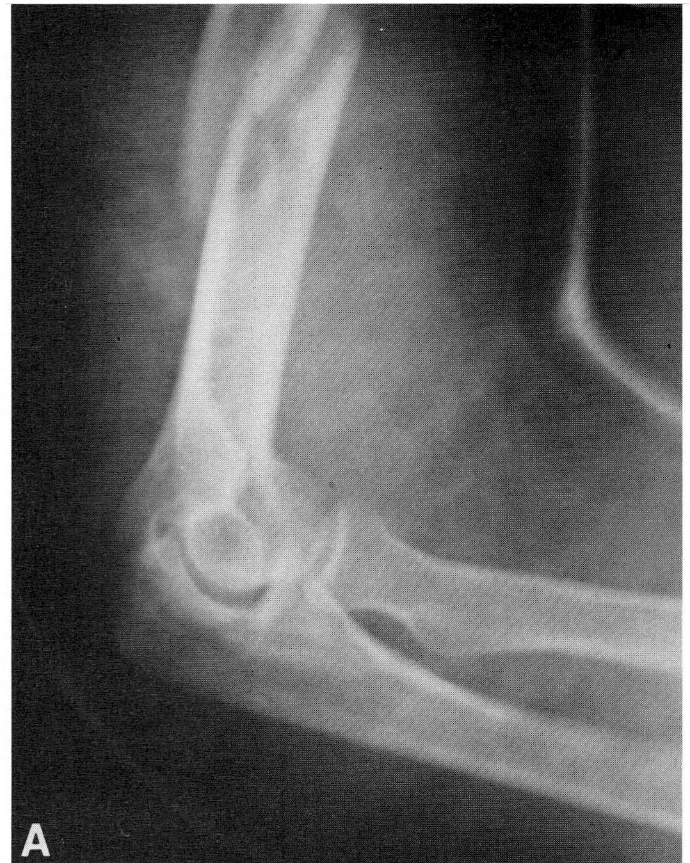

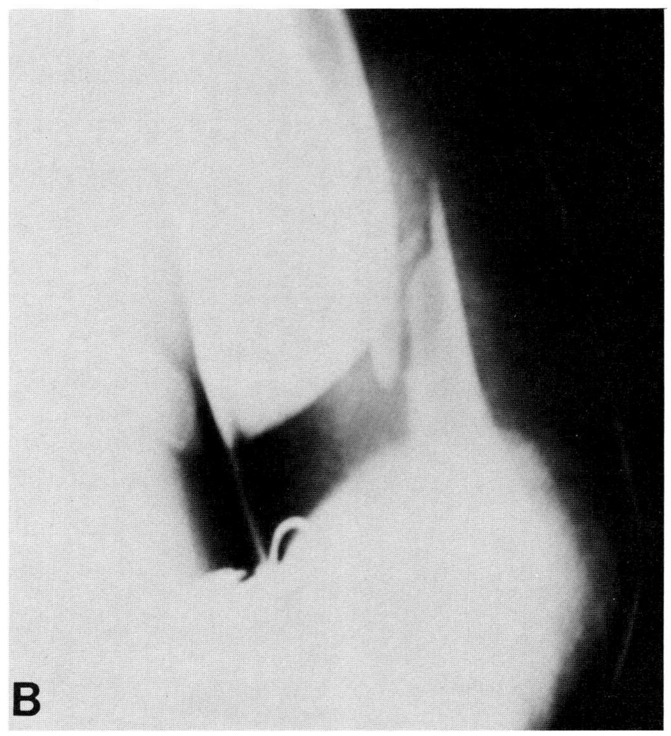

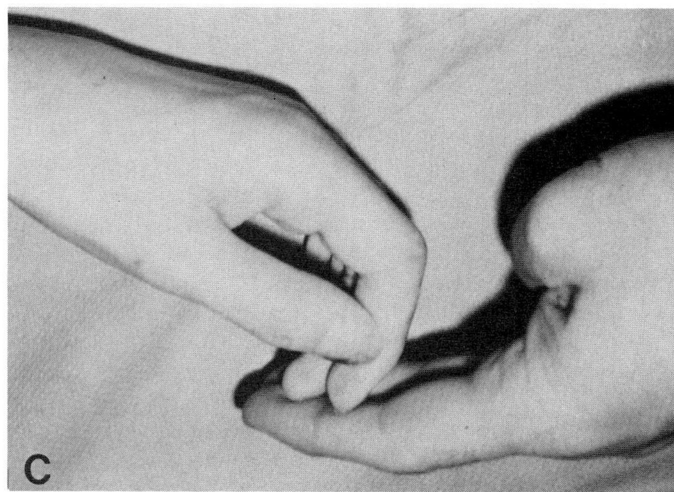

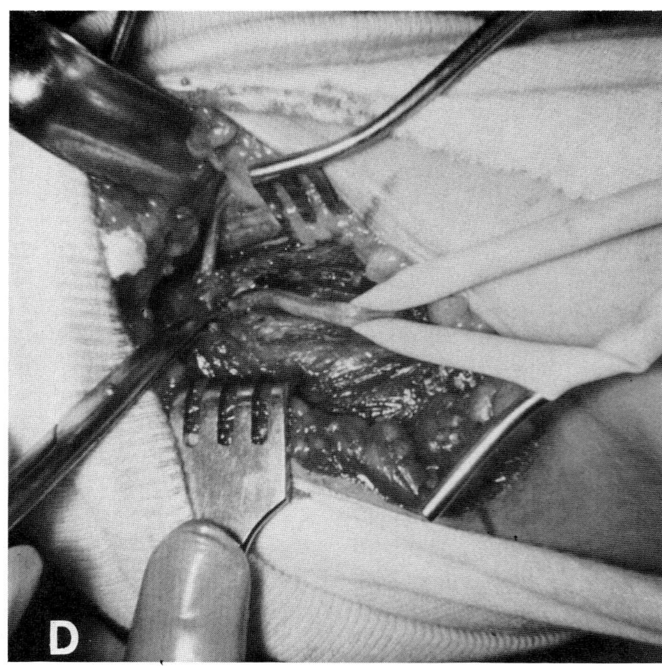

Since the autonomic fibers supplying the skin have the same distribution as sensory fibers, observation of sudomotor function can be a useful adjunct to evaluation. A magnifying glass for visualization, a micro-ohmmeter to measure electrical skin resistance, or Moberg's ninhydrin test all essentially provide the same information.

GENERAL OPERATIVE INDICATIONS

It is most important to know when not to attempt to repair an injured peripheral nerve. Although few dicta can realistically be accepted as absolute, the following can be useful in formulating operative indications in particular cases.

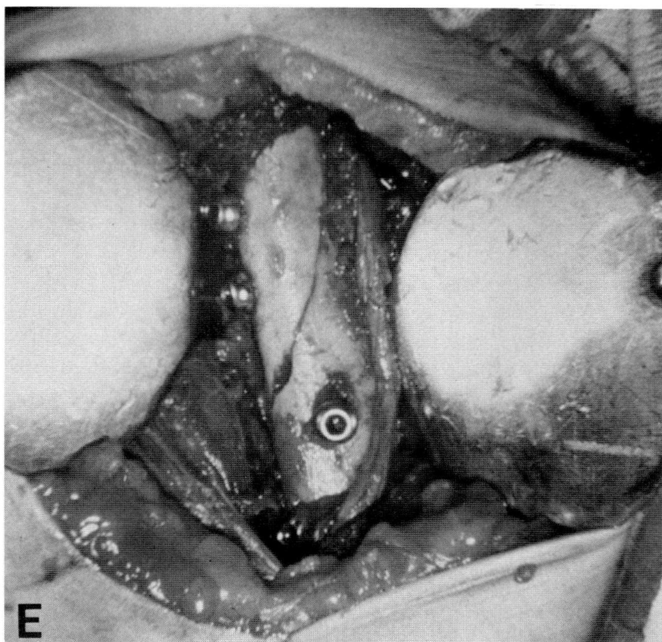

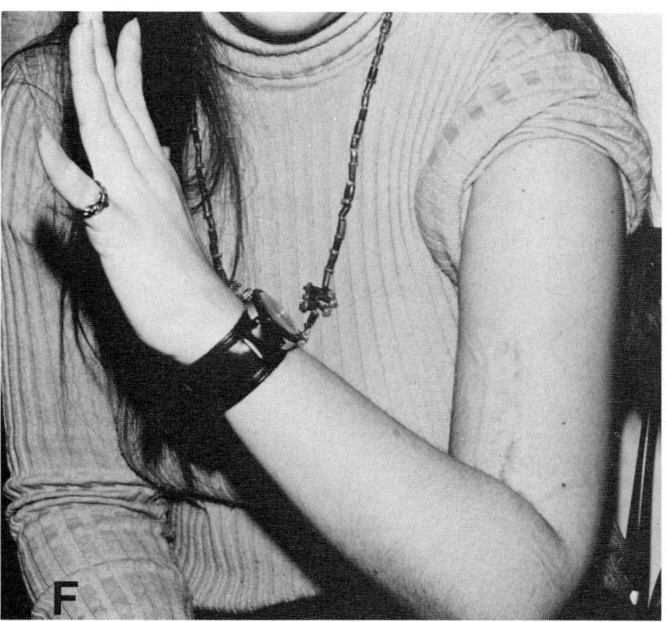

Fig. 134-4. (A) Lateral roentgenogram of a fracture of the humerus at the junction of the upper two thirds and lower one third. (B) Anteroposterior view of the same humerus. Note the long-oblique nature of the fracture. (C) Complete radial nerve palsy at 3 months. (D) Operative view showing the radial nerve (retracted by the Penrose drain) incarcerated in the fracture site. The branch to the brachioradialis is indicated by the point of the scissor. (E) Following internal fixation of the fracture. The nerve, somewhat bruised but intact, is shown to the right of the humerus. (F) Recovery of radial nerve function 3 months following surgery. The hypertrophic scar can be minimized by the use of a zig-zag incision and subcuticular closure.

When the muscles to be reinnervated are severely atrophic, fibrotic, or so distant that years would be required for recovery; if sensibility is present or of much lesser importance; or if the motor lesion is partial, then restoration of deficient motor function by appropriate tendon transfers rather than by nerve repair should be done. This is particularly applicable to intrinsic muscles in the hand, but is valid in other areas as well. Lesions that have a generally poor prognosis, such as severe traction injury of the peroneal nerve accompanying rupture of the lateral knee ligaments in adults often are better not explored secondarily to "see what happens," although individual cases may rarely be benefited. The use of tendon transfers or light plastic braces, or both, may ultimately provide better function. An elderly patient with a high radial nerve lesion caused by a laceration will usually derive considerably more functional benefit immediately and in the long term from tendon transfer to restore wrist and finger extension than from attempts to suture or graft the nerve. A patient seen years after a median nerve injury may not regain motor function after nerve repair, but since median sensibility is so important, an attempt to restore it even partially is reasonable, as long as five years later, particularly in a young person. Recent developments in free tissue transfer have enlarged the possibilities for sensory reconstruction.

Isolated complete lesions of the posterior tibial nerve low in the adult leg may, if repaired, regenerate imperfectly and result in disabling dysesthesia of the skin of the plantar surface of the foot. This lesion must be carefully considered preoperatively, since if the adjacent cutaneous nerves are intact, the sole rarely would be completely anesthetic.

Finally, local conditions in the limbs, such as poor soft tissue cover for the proposed repair, which will predispose to scarring, must be corrected preoperatively. If posturing of joints will be necessary to accomplish coaptation of a nerve following mobilization, then those joints must be mobile to allow for this maneuver.

Gunshot wounds constitute a dilemma because the nerve deficit is often caused by a near-miss and the shock wave that momentarily deforms the nerve. Unless there is a concomitant bone or vascular injury that requires immediate attention, or the path of the bullet could not possibly have missed the nerve, there is little to be gained from immediate exploration, and one should wait out the period of neurapraxia—usually 6 weeks.

Because of the likelihood of nerve division when a sharp object, such as a knife or glass has caused a significant neural deficit, all such wounds should be explored, although a small percentage of them will recover spontaneously. The timing of the procedure, however, seems to be debated between those who favor immediate primary repair and those who will electively postpone definitive surgery. Although numerous clinical theories endorsing each approach exist,[1,2,16] they generally suffer from a lack of precise statistical comparability to account for all pertinent factors. The surgeon should be aware of the advantages and disadvantages to be weighed in each particularly case. In order to allow for primary repair, a nerve wound should be a clean laceration, without significant additional tissue damage or contamination in a patient whose general condition will not be endangered by what could be a lengthy operative procedure. An experienced surgeon and operating team should be available and the wound should be fresh. On the basis of experience gleaned from war time injuries, the general recommendation was that the wound should not be over 18 hours old. However, the judicious use of wound toilet and antibiotics have extended this interval at least for several days.

Children are good candidates for primary repair, since their prognosis for functional recovery is superior to adults. Digital nerves and clean lacerations of median and ulnar nerves at the wrist should be repaired primarily, since in the latter case, fascicles are readily identifiable. Because of the high percentage of fascicular tissues in the nerves at this level and the composition of the bundles themselves, the penalty for mal-rotation is severe in terms of axons that go astray. It is generally agreed that nerve injuries incurred at the time of replantation should be primarily repaired for fear of disruption of reconstructed vascular supply during secondary procedures.[27]

The negative side of primary repair, in addition to the possibly increased risk of infection because of additional surgical manipulation and the time required to accomplish it, is a very real difficulty of being able to accurately assess and delineate the lesion. However, to delay, usually requires greater resection of the nerve ends. The issue has become less of a problem since the operating microscope has been available. At high magnification, a more informed picture of the condition of the fascicles is possible.

The management of nerve injuries accompanying fractures and dislocations should be divided into: (1) closed injuries, where a skeletal injury may be assumed to have caused the nerve injury; (2) open injuries, where the fracture usually is incidental to the wounding agent that also injures the nerve. In the latter case, indications are those of the isolated nerve injury. Closed fractures and dislocations rarely cause neurotmesis, although they may if the fracture fragments are sharp or in a configuration that with displacement might divide the nerve.

In most cases, expectant treatment eventuates in recovery. The best example of this is a closed transverse fracture of the mid-shaft of the humerus with a radial palsy. The anatomic position of the nerve relative to the fracture makes it unlikely that the nerve is caught in fracture fragments. Therefore, knowing the level of the fracture and nerve injury and the distance to the first motor branch, the brachioradialis, calculation at the rate of 1 inch per month should set an outer limit of time allowed for spontaneous recovery. If this interval is exceeded and neither electromyographic nor clinical evidence of recovery is present, then the nerve should be explored. Although this point is quite controversial, I believe that radial palsy accompanying a long oblique fracture of the humerus at the junction of the upper two thirds and lower one third with significant displacement is likely to result in the nerve becoming entrapped at the fracture site.[28] For this reason, I continue to recommend immediate exploration in this situation with internal fixation of the fracture (Figure 134-4).

In general, sciatic nerve injury accompanying hip dislocations recovers spontaneously, while those injuries with acetabular fractures more often require operative intervention. A palsy that arises after manipulation of a fracture or dislocation, where no such lesion pre-existed, in my opinion, usually should be explored.

ANESTHESIA

The prolonged and meticulous nature of peripheral nerve surgery makes general anesthesia preferable in most cases. Since nerve grafts may have to be obtained from the lower extremities in procedures on the upper extremity, this would necessitate a general anesthesia. Since the continued use of muscle relaxants may interfere with intraoperative diagnostic nerve stimulation and electrophysiologic measurement, this

phase of the procedure must be discussed with the anesthetist in advance. The work of Hakstian[29] and Gaul[30] involves electrical stimulation of the freshly transected nerve in an awake patient under local anesthesia so that intraneural topography may be mapped, allowing precise alignment of the fascicles. The patient may then be given general anesthesia for the subsequent neurorrhaphy.

Some operative procedures, such as carpal tunnel release, have been demonstrated by Lichtman[31] and others to be accomplished satisfactorily with the use of local anesthesia, and this has become my preferred method. In general, I believe that regional nerve block is undesirable because of the possibility of inducing further neural damage in an already compromised limb. Intravenous regional anesthesia precludes the essential deflation of the tourniquet so that hemostasis may be assured before neurorrhaphy.

AIDS TO SURGERY

Time is well spent in planning the sequence of maneuvers in an operation on a peripheral nerve, especially if it is done along with tendon, bone, or vascular repair. This precaution usually will avoid embarrassing compromise during or after the procedure. Assuming it will not impose additional hazards to the patient under anesthesia, the position chosen should be selected for ease of surgical approach. The surgeon and operating team are comfortably seated at an absolutely steady table that permits the surgeon to support his forearms to avoid fatigue. A number of hand tables have been designed and are available, but they need not be elaborate, as long as they fulfill the above criteria. In addition, as a result of the technologic explosion accompanying microsurgery, a number of complicated, motorized surgeon's chairs have been marketed. We continue to use conventional operating room stools.

Preparation and draping should be done to allow for extensive exposure and, if necessary, posturing of the limbs. potential graft sites are covered with sterile drapes before the procedure begins so that if the sites are needed, breaks in technique will not be likely. If sural grafts are to be used, the lower extremities should be prepared to the tips of the toes and the limb left mobile and draped free. The aggravation of having to ''stand on one's head'' to harvest the graft may be avoided by positioning the patient prone, securing the grafts and then repositioning the patient for the neurorrhaphy. This carries the potential risk of having to discard the graft if, for some reason, it cannot be used.

Although tourniquet ischemia and a bloodless field are not absolutely essential to peripheral nerve surgery, they can markedly facilitate exposure and identification of vital structures, especially in a scarred or previously explored area. Unless there is an anatomic or physiologic contraindication to the tourniquet, I use it routinely for at least the preliminary exposure and preparation of the nerve. Obviously it is contraindicated in the presence of significant vascular disease. In some situations in which the configuration of the part or position of the wound prevents the use of a standard pneumatic tourniquet, a pediatric-size cuff may be used with benefit. A gas-sterilized or disposable pneumatic cuff may be very useful, but the rubber bandage should be restricted to preliminary exsanguination rather than used as the definitive tourniquet in an awkward situation. If it is used, there is no way of quantifying the amount of compression produced by multiple turns of the rubber bandage at the root of the limb. The risk of tourniquet palsy with this method is significant, but it may be considered acceptable under rare circumstances.

Even with commercially available pneumatic tourniquets, the continued accuracy of a pressure gauge cannot be ensured, so periodic and frequent calibration against a mercury manometer is a good safety measure. Even better is the inclusion of a mercury manometer in the system so that accurate readings may be obtained at any time.[32] The recommended inflation pressures for the adult upper extremity range from 250–375 mm Hg, and for the lower extremity 350–550 mm Hg. These should be adjusted according to the measured systolic blood pressure and the size of the patient's limb. There is no universally accepted time limit for tourniquet ischemia. My own practice is not to exceed 2.5 hours in the upper extremity. By the end of this period, that part of the procedure requiring the tourniquet usually has been accomplished. A double tourniquet cuff may be used in situations in which prolonged ischemia is required, since alternating the portion of the cuff that is inflated will diminish the total time that any particular segment of nerve is subjected to significant compression. It should be remembered that if the electrical stimulation of the nerve is to be part of the procedure, it will have to be accomplished before 20 to 30 minutes of ischemia have passed, since nerve transmission normally ceases under these circumstances.

The management of a neuroma-in-continuity may be considerably improved by the use of intraoperative electrical stimulation and electrophysiologic measurements. Correct decisions regarding the alternatives of neurolysis or resection for part or all of a segment of damaged nerve may simply not be possible on the basis of gross or even microscopic examination. Kline and Nulsen,[24] as well as Terzis[33] and others have described in detail the techniques of evoked potentials and the use of nerve action potentials in the evaluation of lesions in continuity. These are extremely useful, but require sophisticated electromyographic equipment and personnel to provide technical support.

Because the routine use of magnification in nerve repair has made possible the accurate approximation of groups or even individual fascicles, it has become increasingly important to correctly identify and differentiate motor from sensory bundles. The electrophysiologic techniques have already been mentioned. Engle et al.[34] have demonstrated the use of choline acetyl transferase stains within the practical time frame of the operative procedure to differentiate motor from sensory fascicles. The proliferation of specialized instruments for microsurgery has created a large array of available equipment that can be used for nerve suture. In addition to the usual forceps, needle holders and scissors, which are part of the armamentarium of any neurosurgical cabinet, many new instruments, including approximators, have evolved from microvascular surgery. Many of these are suited to peripheral nerve repair and surgeons tend, somewhat arbitrarily, to prefer one instrument type or another. In general, needle holders that do not lock are advantageous, since they do not jar when opened and closed under high magnification. Forceps, too, are varied, but we tend to use simple jeweler's forceps without teeth. They are minimally traumatic, but, as with all such instruments, their tips must be protected against damage, especially during sterilization and storage, when it is wise to keep them and all microinstruments in cases specially designed for the purpose.

If epineurial suture or a cable graft is to be performed, then it will be desirable to cut all fascicles at the same level and at right angles to the length of the nerve. Since normal peripheral nerve fascicles have the consistency and rigidity of wet spaghetti, it is often difficult to achieve the desired neat, sharp cut by simply drawing a scalpel blade across the nerve. The nerve tends to deform as it is cut, with the result that the epineurium may shred or fascicles may be cut on the bias or at different levels. To obviate this problem, a number of ingenious neurotomes and miniature miter boxes have been designed. They may be helpful in achieving the desired result, since even a very experienced surgeon using a very sharp blade can have difficulty steadying a nerve against a wooden tongue depressor. The indelicate practice of pinning the nerve to the tongue depressor proximal to the line of section to steady it so it can be put in tension is to be avoided. A simple, practical, and economical way of aiding the right-angle section of nerves before repair has been proposed by Clark.[35] He enclosed the nerve within a paper sheath and grasped the free leaves of paper with a right angle clamp before sectioning through it. This allows the axons to be held in a cylindric form without being crushed or rolled under the pressure of a razor blade. Rubber dam may be substituted for the paper.

Suture material has been the subject of much discussion. There are many advantages and disadvantages of various materials demonstrated in animal experiments. Although there have been great technical advances in the uniformity, tensile strength and reactivity of suture materials, there is still no ideal material because all of them produce suture reaction and scar. The same sutures that are used for microvascular repairs, 8-0, 9-0 and 10-0 monofilament nylon swaged on needles can be used for most peripheral nerve repairs. The use of plasma clot as a means of joining nerves has been shown to be effective by Tarlov[36] and others. In an attempt to use as few sutures as possible, plasma clot may be employed to reinforce the suture in combination with it or may be used as a substitute.

The successful application of the argon laser to surgery has been demonstrated by Almquist et al.[37] in the repair of peripheral nerves. Although there are advantages to this method, it has not yet reached the status of standard application. There is now no serious doubt that magnification must be employed in the surgery of peripheral nerves. What remains to be seen is just how much magnification is necessary, assuming a constant degree of surgical ability and visual acuity. From a purely practical point of view, most surgeons (and nurses) can barely see 10-0 suture without magnification. The available visual aids are operating loupes and microscopes. Each have their applications, but no absolutely rigid rules are followed. In general, preliminary dissection can be done with 3.5×, and epineurial suture performed with 4.5 or 6× loupes. Unfortunately, as the optics multiply, so does the weight, as well as the need for a focused light source. Therefore, a fiberoptic headlight is of advantage. For repair of nerves at the level of groups of fascicles or smaller units, the operating microscope will be required. In most cases, a 200–300 mm focal length objective will be suitable. This will determine the working distance, which can be varied according to the topography and location of the operative field. Eyepieces ranging from 10 to 20× are available. The addition of zoom optical systems and foot controls for focusing and shifting fields have greatly enhanced the ease of the use of the microscope.

TECHNIQUE

The operative approaches to major peripheral nerves in the limbs have been well-illustrated in standard references.[1,38] Time and space do not permit their recapitulation here. The peripheral nerve surgeon must be prepared to expose the nerve throughout its length with due regard for avoiding the vital structures, hypertrophic scars and contractures, but without apology for the length of the incision, if anatomic considerations so dictate. In the presence of scarring and neuroma formation, the dissection should begin in normal tissue, both proximally and distally if possible, so that all important structures can be identified and preserved. Dissection is then carried centripetally to expose the area of nerve damage.

If one is dealing with a compression lesion, or by reason of the pathogenesis, an incomplete clinical deficit, then simple decompression is indicated, and the prognosis for recovery should be favorable. A common example of this is the carpal tunnel release. Even here, if the nerve shows evidence of epineurial thickening or the surface vascular pattern remains interrupted after the transverse carpal ligament has been divided, then careful partial epineurectomy under magnification is indicated. This should be restricted to the volar half of the epineurium since the blood supply is largely dorsal at this level. Other indications for epineurectomy at the time of carpal tunnel release have been advanced. These include a profound sensory defect, significant atrophy or very prolonged distal latency of conduction of the median nerve, 7 msec and above. I do not use saline injection under the epineurium as a test of the adequacy of decompression or a substitute for manual neurolysis, since without relieving the constriction of tight epineurium, little would appear to be gained. Whether one should perform an additional intraneural neurolysis under magnification is debated, since cross connections between fascicles, the blood supply, or the bundles themselves could conceivably be injured during the dissection. Curtis and Eversman[39] have reported favorably on their extensive experience with intraneural lysis.

Neurolysis, the act of mechanically freeing a nerve from scar, would appear to be a logical and reasonable operation. Yet there are fewer procedures more often done for poorer indications than this one, and quite commonly, either nothing positive is accomplished or the recovery that is observed postoperatively would have occurred spontaneously had the surgeon waited a while longer.

The least controversial and best indication for neurolysis is documented compression, and if it can be relieved without likelihood of supervening scarring, then the chances of recovery are significantly enhanced. If, however, nothing more is done than to simply incise the scar and observe the nerve, the procedure will produce, at best, a temporary improvement. If the basic anatomic surroundings of the nerve or its blood supply can be favorably influenced, however, there may be substantial benefit. A transposition of a nerve into a favorable bed would be a positive example, as for traction-friction neuropathy of the ulnar nerve at the elbow.[40] There is always the risk of intraoperative mechanical injury to the nerve itself, or of stripping it of its remaining blood supply. Neurolysis in situations where recovery has been documented as having ceased or actually regressed is legitimate.

Although for a long time peripheral nerves were felt to be extremely resistant to the effects of radiation, there is now abundant documentation that radiation, even in therapeutic doses, such as is used for the treatment of breast cancer, can produce late fibrosis and scarring with progressive loss of nerve function.[41,42] This will be further discussed in the section on surgery of the brachial plexus.

The treatment of various types of injection injury to nerves remains controversial and specific to the nature of the noxious agent and time elapsed since surgery.[43,44,45] Penicillin is particularly neurotoxic and injection injuries caused by penicillin should be subjected to neurolysis if they are seen within the first day or so. The indications for neurolysis for infections are extremely narrow since peripheral nerves are ordinarily remarkably resistant to infection, with the leprosy bacillus being a significant and invasive exception. The final two conditions often cited as reasons for doing a neurolysis, pain and poor results from suture are, in my opinion, usually poor indications although the occasional case for the former situation may occur.

If the lesion is of long duration, the neurologic deficit is complete, and a neuroma in continuity is encountered at surgery, it still may be possible that the lesion is an axonotmesis rather than a neurotmesis. Obviously, to experience recovery without having to do a formal resection and neurorrhaphy or graft will eventuate in a better result, but the proper identification of the nature of the lesion may be difficult. The appearance of the neuroma may be deceptive, although the extremely attenuated or very large and firm ones usually are not functional and require resection. The intraoperative electrodiagnostic techniques have already been commented upon.

The management of documented complete transections of peripheral nerves is the most difficult and controversial aspect of the subject under discussion. Simply stated, the object of the procedure is to re-establish axonal continuity with the periphery in such a fashion that maximal neurologic function is restored. An ecumenical and complete historical review might prove interesting (or tedious), but a series of straw men erected only to be knocked down is of little comfort to the surgeon faced with the immediate problem of managing a neurotmesis. The question of primary or secondary nerve repair has already been discussed. Having made either choice, the remaining decisions concern how to get the correct fascicles together when that part determined to be damaged has been resected. Inspection of the cut end of the nerve under magnification is an indicator of adequate resection but does not assure the absence of fibrosis or other impediments to regeneration. The variable gap that results may call for more than a single solution and one ought to be prepared to consider alternatives. There is general agreement that excessive tension on the suture line is the most deleterious factor mitigating against success in nerve repair, assuming fascicular orientation is correct.[46,47] In order to avoid tension at the suture line, mobilization of the nerve from its bed (and segmental blood supply), may be carried out. The question remains just how far this can be done before it becomes self-defeating.

The first half of this century saw the establishment of empirically determined critical resection lengths[1] for each nerve, limits within which one could expect regeneration following removal of a segment of the nerve and neurorrhaphy. Of course, the absolute lengths of nerve were really very rough guides, not referable to the height and length of the extremity of the patient under consideration, and based on rather indefinite criteria for success of the procedure. They are, therefore, of historical value only. Assuming the nerve was sufficiently mobilized proximally and distally, then in order to coapt the ends, the adjacent joints would have to be postured accordingly and held with a splint or cast for 3 weeks until healing of the suture line was sufficient to allow gradual stretching. Although it may be possible by total mobilization, transposition, and acute posturing of all joints to actually get the nerve ends together, such maneuvers usually end in failure because when the extreme position is reduced, the result is either a rupture, or more likely, a severe traction lesion of the nerve with failure of the blood supply or axon itself that precludes recovery. In general, for repairs of the median or ulnar nerves, if the elbow must be flexed more than 90 degrees or the wrist 40 degrees to achieve coaptation, then excessive tension will be present when full range is resumed and the prognoy is poor. At the knee, 90 degrees of flexion with the hip in neutral should not be exceeded.

Epineurial suture in which sutures are placed only in the outer layer of epineurium without surgical manipulation of the fascicles themselves has been the accepted and most widely employed method of joining severed nerves until the recent emergence of microsurgical techniques. As surgeons realized that they not only could clearly visualize individual fascicles within a nerve but actually place sutures in them, enthusiasm grew for repairing progressively smaller subunits of peripheral nerves until virtually no fascicle was immune to the needle and thread of the aggressive repairer of nerves. The controversy continues, but I believe that Sir Sidney Sunderland's observations[2,48] as well as recent experimental work[49,50,51] have helped considerably in providing perspective in a field where the "triumph of technology over reason" is a constant threat. In general, I believe that with the exceptions to be described, if suture (rather than a graft) is possible, then it should be epineurial rather than fascicular, since the evidence is not convincing that the additional time, obligatory intraoperative trauma to the nerve elements, and additional suture material that undoubtedly causes scarring will eventuate in a superior result. The exception is in situations where the fascicular pattern can be clearly defined in both ends of the nerves and the ratio of fascicles to epineurium is high. The intraneural topography maps of Sunderland[9] and Jabaley[8] may be very helpful here. Groups of like fascicles can be sutured in order to avoid having their axons misdirected into intraneural epineurium or foreign endoneural tubes.

The technique of epineurial, group fascicular, as well as fascicular repair will be described.

In all nerve repair, the handling of the nerve must be minimized, and then it should be handled only gently, with microinstruments, rubber drain retractors, or fingers. Hemostasis is essential, so the tourniquet should be deflated and all bleeding points stopped using a bipolar coagulator before suture is performed. A suitable background that will allow visualization of the fascicles and fine sutures may be provided by a piece of sterilized light-colored plastic or the backgrounds that are used for microvascular repair. Correct fascicular orientation may be aided by matching the alignment of surface blood vessels, if these are visible. Sometimes the nerve will simply lie in correct rotary position, but it may not, especially if it has been malrotated by a previous attempt at repair. Inspection under magnification of the fascicular pattern at the resection surfaces is the best guide to alignment and although exact correspondence usually is not found, major groups of bundles can be identified and approximated. Once this has been established, the epineurial repair is commenced by means of two traction sutures in the epineurium at a distance from the end, 180 degrees apart and using 7-0 or 8-0 suture to take the tension

off the repair site and allow for use of a minimal number of 9-0 sutures to approximate the epineurium. If the ends of the nerves are impacted by the traction sutures, then the fascicles will be deflected and accurate approximation will not be possible. If there is too much tension, then the fascicles will retract from the epineurium and a fibrous gap will result. Only as many sutures as are required to achieve accurate coaptation are used, varying from two to six in most cases. It should be remembered that the suture material is a foreign body that may, with remodeling, actually become incorporated within the substance of the nerve. Despite claims that wrapping the suture line with foreign material will diminish fibrosis and improve results, there is no conclusive proof that this is so, but the list of materials that have been so employed is long and varied. Most of these have actually proved to be deleterious on long-term evaluation and their use is not recommended. To date, there is no ideal substance for the purpose. The work of Bora[49] and Pleasure[52] in the use of both systemic and local pharmacologic methods of attempting to reduce local scarring at the suture line is of great interest and promise, but it is not in widespread use today.

In situations wherein the intraneural topography is clearly defined and like groups of fascicles can be approximated, group fascicular repair can be employed. Lacerations of the median and ulnar nerves at the wrist are commonly treated in this way. Although this method has been incorrectly called perineurial repair, in fact, sutures are placed in the intraneural epineurium that surrounds the groups of fascicles rather than in the perineurium. The epineurium may either be circumferentially resected or, as has been suggested by Jabaley, a portion of the circumference may be retained and separately sutured so as to serve as an internal splint for the group fascicular repair. Using the operating microscope and $10\times$ magnification, the major groups of fascicles are identified and separated in normal tissue. Once the corresponding bundles in the two sides of the nerve have been identified, they can be coapted by placing 9-0 or 10-0 suture, usually two per group, in the epifascicular epineurium under $15–20\times$ magnification.

The indications for repair of individual fascicles, the smallest subunit of a peripheral nerve are, in my opinion, very restricted. The technique would be applicable, for example, in partial lacerations of the digital nerve where accurate coaptation would otherwise not be feasible. The disadvantage for other situations is that the amount of dissection required, the preservation of local blood supply, and the amount of suture material that will be required all have deleterious effects on the regeneration of the nerve.

For lesions that result in gaps that cannot be overcome, as described with posturing the joints or anatomic maneuvers such as anterior transposition of the ulnar nerve, grafting provides a useful alternative. It is now generally accepted that fresh autogenous grafts are the material of choice. Usually cutaneous nerves are preferred because they can be sacrificed with less significant residual deficit and their smaller diameter makes central necrosis during revascularization less likely. The sural nerve is the most popular donor, and in an average adult, as much as 35 cm may be obtained by multiple transverse incisions in the calf and mobilizations in the intervals. A long incision from the popliteal space to the lateral ankle is easier technically but rarely necessary, and it is less desirable in its ultimate appearance and the scarring it produces. Cutaneous nerves in the upper extremity may be used, but it would be imprudent to sacrifice one that is providing sensibility to an area adjacent to that already denervated. If a mixed nerve has been severed and

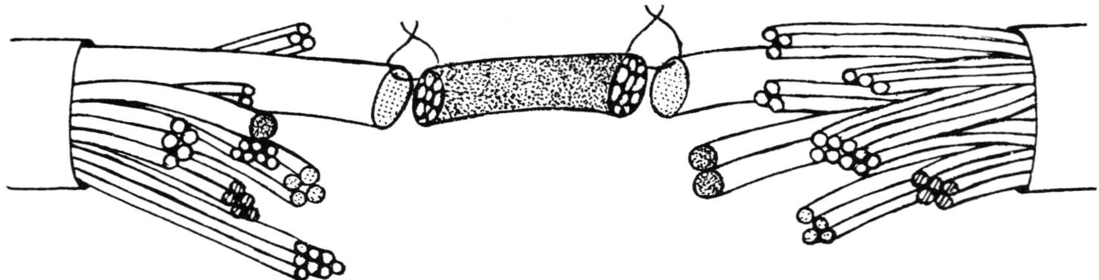

Fig. 134-5.   Schematic drawing of an interfascicular nerve grafting. (Reprinted from Millesi H: Treatment of nerve lesions by fascicular free nerve grafts in traumatic nerve lesion of the upper limb, in Michon J, Moberg E (eds): G.E.M. Monograph 2. Edinburgh, Churchill Livingstone Ltd, 1975. With permission.)

is not to be reconstituted, it may serve as a donor but this situation is becoming progressively less common, and the risk of central necrosis of the thicker graft is a disadvantage in its use.

The manner in which the grafts are to be employed has changed as a result of the work and impetus of Millesi and his colleagues.[46,53,54] Formerly, nerve grafting was available as a technique for salvage of the situation in which a gap could not be overcome after that had been essentially proved by means of an unsuccessful attempt at mobilization. The Millesi concept was designed to avoid the devascularization inherent in extensive mobilization and to achieve better anatomic realignment by placing the grafts between major groups of fascicles to essentially achieve the "graft" equivalent of a group fascicular repair. The technique evolved from the realization of the deleterious effects of tension at the suture line. The criteria for the median and ulnar nerves according to Millesi et al. are as follows. All cases are grafted except:

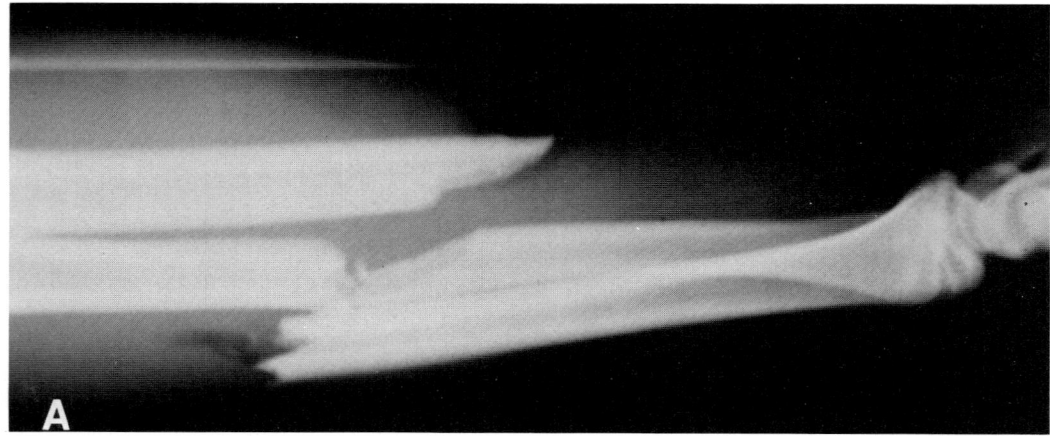

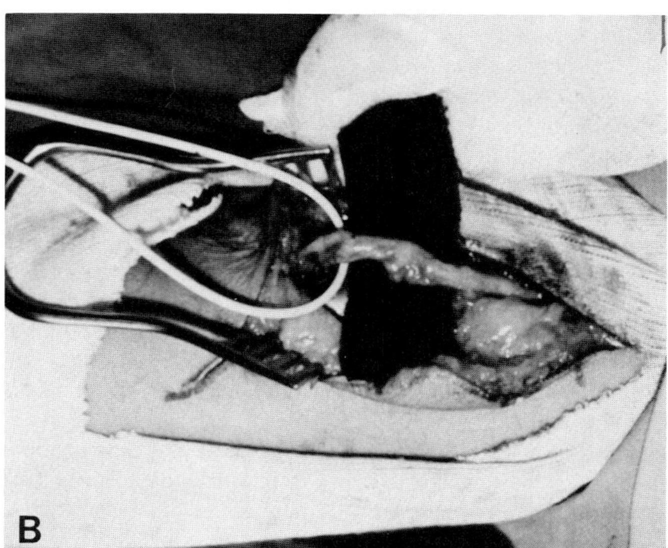

Fig. 134-6.   (A) Roentgenogram of a compound fracture of both bones of the forearm of an 11-year-old boy whose ulna transected the ulnar nerve. A single coaptation suture was placed in the nerve by the initial treating surgeon. (B) The neuroma at surgery 3 months later. (C) Interfascicular sural nerve grafts used to close a 5 cm gap. Note the staggered placement of the grafts.

1. If the gap in the nerve is 2 cm or less and the nerve ends can be approximated without tension when the joints of the extremity are in full extension.
2. For the ulnar nerve at the elbow, gaps of up to 4 cm that can be closed without tension by anterior transposition.
3. A nerve gap accompanying nonunion of a fracture that requires surgery may be closed and sutured following shortening of the bone.

Millesi advocates interfascicular grafting rather than epineurial bridging. Under magnification, the neuroma is approached from both ends, but rather than preserving the epineurium and transecting all fascicles at the same level, he dissects and transects each major fascicle and group of minor ones at the point of injury and then maps them before proceeding to the distal stump, where the same process is repeated. The epineurium is resected from both ends and then corresponding fascicles or groups are united by interposed grafts, usually of sural nerve, with the epineurium of each graft fixed by one fine suture to the epifascicular epineurium surrounding the host fascicles. The suture lines are therefore staggered as the pathologic condition dictates (Figures 134-5 and 134-6).

The exact technique and results have been documented both by Millesi and others who have followed his techniques. Some surgeons have felt that the criteria are too rigid in terms of imposing two suture lines and a graft in situations where a relatively small degree of mobilization and possibly some joint posturing would allow for a group fascicular repair. For secondary nerve repairs done after a month, scarring and nerve retraction generally result in gaps that need to be grafted.

As with situations of primary nerve suture where a distinct fascicular pattern is not readily identifiable, the technique of group fascicular repair by graft will not be possible either. Under these circumstances, the historical technique of cable grafting can be used. In this case, the donor nerves, usually sural nerves, are placed side-by-side in the manner of a cable and sutured to the epineurium of the host proximally and distally, usually with one suture per strand. It is then possible to cover the cross-sectional area of the nerve and preserve longitudinal orientation. Presumably, the fascicles will find their way to the corresponding segment of the distal end of the nerve. Again, it should be stated that this type of repair by graft is indicated in situations where the fascicular pattern is not readily apparent or clearly defined, and the gaps are long, as per the illustration (Figure 134-7). When groups of fascicles are recognized, it is preferable to excise host epineurium and suture the grafts between corresponding groups in order to preserve orientation and apposition that might otherwise be lost. For partial lesions, or lateral neuromas, an inlay graft of this type rather than a loop suture may provide good results, despite the theoretical objections to two suture lines as opposed to one.

A number of unusual methods of handling special situations in peripheral nerve surgery have been developed. Both nerve transfer and pedicle grafts have proved useful in some cases. The pedicle graft as described by Strange[55,56,57] was originally used in situations where both peripheral nerves supplying the hand or foot were extensively damaged over a bad bed. These conditions might well be found in either a localized crush injury or a compartment syndrome, i.e., the disorder in which adverse pressure develops in a circumscribed anatomical area. The retention of the longitudinal blood supply within the nerves allowed this technique to be used under very adverse conditions, although it did involve sacrifice of one nerve to reconstitute the other. Obviously, one would never sacrifice an intact nerve for this purpose, with the median nerve and tibial nerve selected for preservation over the peroneal and ulnar. With the advent of the free vascularized nerve graft and other free tissue transfer techniques, the indications for the use of pedicle nerve graft have all but disappeared. The one circumstance where it is very useful is in the sciatic nerve with a large gap. Such a case is illustrated by a patient I recently treated. The nerve injury was caused by a homemade bomb that exploded prematurely and injured the perpetrator's tibial and peroneal divisions in the popliteal fossa. Because the peroneal division was virtually destroyed at this level, and the gap was 15 cm, it was an ideal indication for the Strange technique, since the total circumference of the tibial nerve could not be matched by even a massive harvest of available cutaneous nerves from the same patient. The result after a year was a grade 4/5 plantar flexor of the ankle and foot, although obviously, no recovery of the peroneal division is expected. At this writing, the patient does have protective sensibility in the sole of his foot.

Whether the addition of vascularized nerve grafts improves the result of nerve repair remains to be determined, although reports by Taylor et al.[58,59] are favorable.

POSTOPERATIVE MANAGEMENT

If a suture repair has been done that involves posturing of joints, immobilization normally is maintained for 3 weeks before the limb is mobilized. Depending on the degree of mobilization, it may well be prudent to gradually allow extension of the joints under controlled conditions of approximately 30 degrees per week. In light of the tendency to avoid such situations, however, and to treat these patients with grafts, we rarely see the necessity for prolonged immobilization. In fact, Millesi recommends immobilization for only 10 days following nerve grafting procedures, since the length of the grafts is usually 15 percent greater than the gaps they are used to close, thus allowing for shrinkage.

If immobilization is used, it is important that during this time adjacent joints must be kept mobile and contractures prevented by splinting and passive exercise. It is indeed unfortunate to regain motor power after many months of waiting for nerve regeneration only to find that it is functionally useless because these joints are stiff. Not all patients require formal physical or occupational therapy, and these treatments must be individualized. When indicated, orthoses (braces) may be used to support or protect limb or to assist in weakened functionally necessary motions (Figure 134-8).

The efficacy of electrical stimulation during the period of regeneration has not been clearly established. Many of the studies that have been done have been on animal models[60] and some have been poorly controlled. I do not believe that sufficient evidence, based on experience with humans, exists either to have my patients come to the hospital for daily stimulation or to urge them to buy or rent home stimulators.

FACTORS INFLUENCING RESULTS OF NERVE REPAIR

A number of technical factors that influence the result of nerve repair have been mentioned. In addition, there is little question that the experience and technical skill of the surgeon are of tremendous importance.

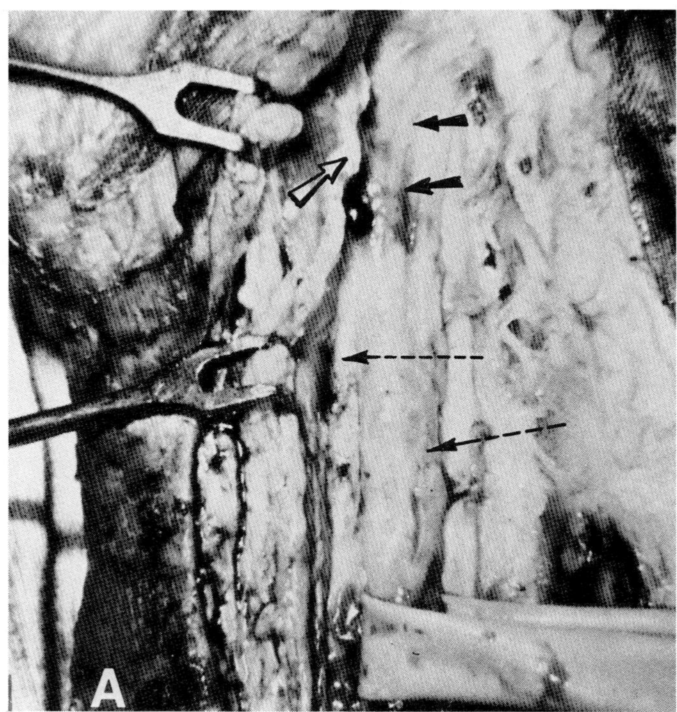

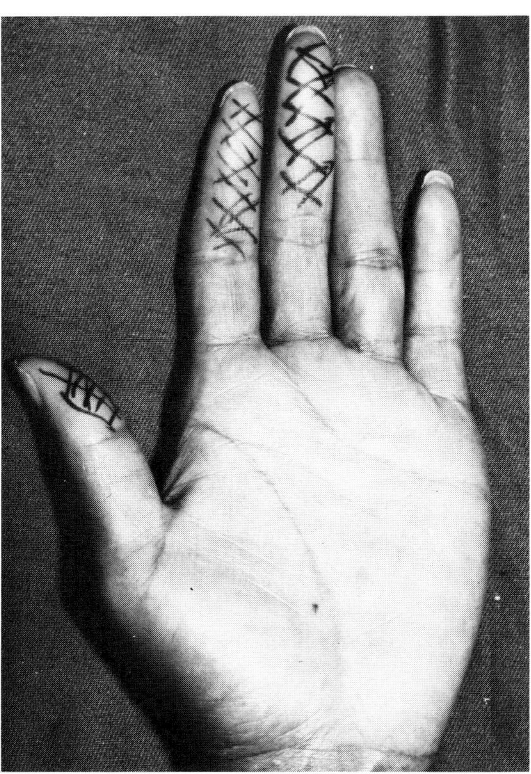

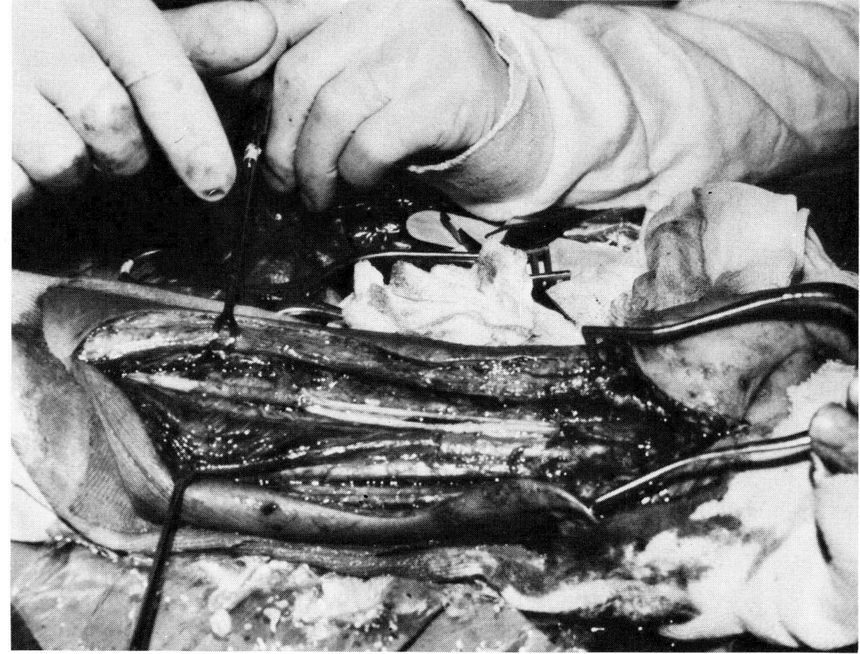

Fig. 134-7. (Upper left) The volar aspect of the distal forearm 5 months following a close range shotgun wound. The median nerve is embedded in the scar in the carpal tunnel. (Upper right) A 10 cm segment of the scarred median nerve has been replaced by four cables of sural nerve graft. (Bottom) Clinical appearance of the hand 10 months after grafting. The thenar muscle bulk had been regained and sensibility had returned proximal to the cross-hatched area. The patient was lost to follow-up thereafter.

Other factors independent of the surgeon or control, however, are significant determinants of the result:

1. Age. The power of regeneration and adaptability of children gives them considerably better results than those obtained in comparable situations in adults. This may be a combination of the fact that their nerves are still growing or the benign plasticity of their central nervous systems.

2. Mechanism of injury. In general, those wounds caused by greater trauma tend to exert a more deleterious effect on the nervous system than those of lesser magnitude, i.e. blast wounds tend to do worse than clean knife wounds.

3. Length of resection. In general, lesions involving greater length require more elaborate maneuvers for repair, have greater dissimilarity of the fascicular pattern and tend not to do as well.

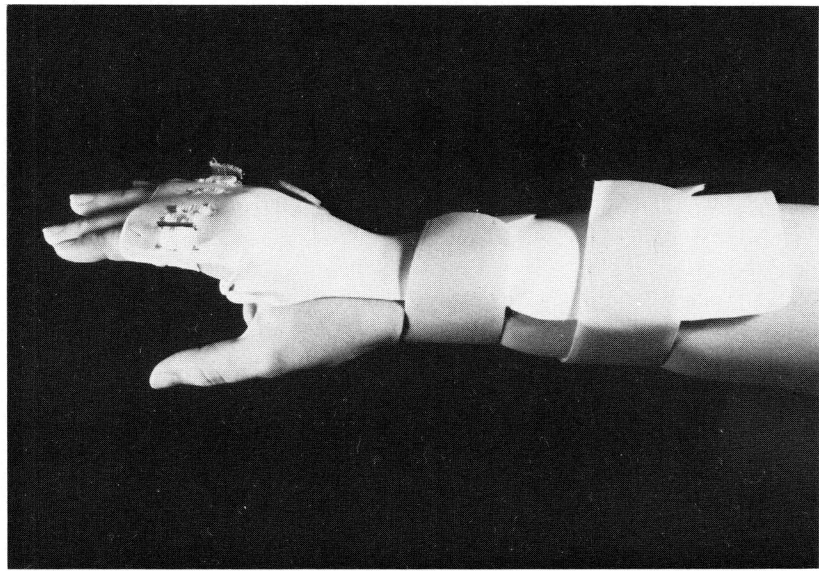

Fig. 134-8. A low profile radial palsy splint made by Occupational Therapy at the Massachusetts General Hospital.

4. Duration between injury and repair. Ordinarily, after three months, the greater the delay in repair, the poorer the result.
5. Location of the lesion. The closer to the spinal cord, or the more proximal the lesion, the poorer the prognosis. This may result from retrograde neurologic change, exhaustion of axoplasmic production, atrophy of the end organ with time, or a combination of all of these factors.

Because of the great number of variables that can be identified with any particular clinical situation, it is not possible simply to consult one of the many series of results of peripheral nerve repair to be able to advance a prognosis for a particular case. Not only are all of the aforementioned factors important, but it should be remembered that civilian injuries[61] are not comparable to wartime injuries,[5] and repairs done under the microscope in contemporary conditions cannot be compared with the traditionally quoted series wherein either the naked eye or low powered magnifying glasses were used along with various types of suture material, many of which were very reactive. A tabulation of all of the possibilities in this chapter would not be possible, and the reader is referred to the references.[1–3,26,43,46,54,62–65]

SURGERY OF THE BRACHIAL PLEXUS

Many of the diagnostic and therapeutic techniques already discussed in detail are directly applicable to surgery of the brachial plexus. Sufficiently specialized differences exist, however, to merit separate consideration[66,67]

The anatomic complexity of the brachial plexus makes both diagnosis and treatment considerably more difficult than the problem posed by single or even multiple peripheral nerve injuries. If compression lesions are excluded, most of the remaining trauma can be considered under the general headings of closed and open injury. The latter will be considered first.

OPEN WOUNDS OF THE BRACHIAL PLEXUS

Open wounds of the brachial plexus often are accompanied by serious vascular or pulmonary complications that may obscure recognition of the nerve injury or even kill the patient.[6] Surgical maneuvers to treat these problems obviously must take preference over the nerve lesion. But what are the indications for surgical exploration of open wounds of the plexus? The answer depends, in addition to the above considerations, on several factors. The nature of the wound is obviously important. A knife or glass cut is unlikely to be anything less than a neurotmesis, so that awaiting recovery calculated at the rate of 1 inch a month is pointless. If the upper or intermediate trunk or their distal outflow is injured, it is worth exploring the lesion, since a discrete injured area may be amenable to suture or graft. The muscles innervated are mainly proximal, often large, and not of great functional complexity (but not invariably). Careful neurorrhaphy, therefore, has at least a chance of improving function. For the lower trunk and its terminal branches, the prognosis for recovery is so poor that in my opinion, it is not worthwhile.

If an open wound of the plexus produces a clinically unimportant deficit, mainly motor, then it may be elected not to explore the plexus at all and to decrease the deficit by means of peripheral tendon transfer.

With the increasing use of chain saws by home owners and others not necessarily skilled in their use, there has been an increase in the number of very serious injuries to the region of the neck and the brachial plexus. These may be fatal, or they may result in very serious injury to the neurovascular supply to the upper limb. Because of the ripping and tearing that such injuries involve, there may be actual avulsion of the spinal nerves from the cord, in addition to whatever damage is done distally in the supraclavicular fossa or axilla. Consequently, as such patients are explored secondarily, it is prudent to obtain electrodiagnostic studies and myelograms, as well as vascular studies.

For patients whose brachial plexus injuries follow

iatrogenic maneuvers such as angiography or the placement of invasive lines, the appearance of a neurologic deficit is, in my opinion, an indication for surgical exploration.

Gunshot wounds, however, constitute a completely different situation and they are much harder to assess. The passage of a bullet through the tissues causes momentary deformation that spreads like a wave through the surrounding area. Hence, the spectrum of injury may be quite broad in an individual case and there is no way of knowing immediately which parts are transected and which are going to recover. Brooks[68] on the basis of World War II experience, demonstrated how difficult it is to assess open wounds of the brachial plexus at surgery. He explored 54 cases, thought 16 to be amenable to surgical repair and achieved a functional result in only one, a lesion of an upper trunk. It should be remembered that this was a wartime series. More contemporary work has clarified the issue somewhat in that gunshot wounds of the brachial plexus rarely result in a complete deficit, and if they do, within a relatively short time, they become partial. The indication for exploration of the gunshot wound, therefore, is far less urgent than that of the sharp transection assuming there is no life-threatening vascular or pulmonary complication. The operating microscope and modern techniques have brightened the outlook for treatment of sharp wounds of the brachial plexus.

CLOSED INJURIES OF THE BRACHIAL PLEXUS

Closed injuries of the brachial plexus can be divided into supraclavicular and infraclavicular injuries, and since they have significantly different prognoses, they will be considered separately. Infraclavicular injuries of the brachial plexus result from skeletal injuries in the region of the shoulder girdle.[69] Often accompanying shoulder dislocations, fractures, or fracture-dislocations, they are of lesser severity than the supraclavicular variety, because the bony lesions are the cause of the nerve injury by direct compression or traction, and root avulsion or infraganglionic neurotmesis usually do not occur. The prognosis for recovery, even of hand function, is generally good, and their treatment differs considerably from the larger group of supraclavicular injuries. Criteria for their identification and management have been advanced by Leffert and Seddon.[69] Rarely, because of sharp bone fragments, neurotmesis of the infraclavicular plexus may occur and require surgical repair, or occasionally, blunt trauma may produce a similar indication.

It should be realized, however, that traction injuries involving the supraclavicular portion of the plexus may extend below the level of the clavicle and will therefore determine both prognosis and method of treatment. If, for example, a patient has a Horner's syndrome, supraclavicular hematoma or swelling, evidence of involvements of branches known to be located above the clavicle, or fractured clavicle, these are indicative of supraclavicular injury and should be handled as detailed below.[70]

The supraclavicular injuries usually are caused by high-velocity vehicular accidents, and most often by falls from motorcycles. The patient often falls so that the head and shoulder are forced apart. With lateral flexion of the cervical spine, great force is brought to bear in producing a traction lesion of the nerve. The damage may vary from frank avulsion of cervical roots from the spinal cord (a supraganglionic lesion) to lesser or greater degrees of damage to the trunks or divisions

or cords (infraganglionic), which can range from neurapraxia to neurotmesis. Differential involvement of motor and sensory components also is possible, so that an almost infinite spectrum of pathologic conditions can be observed. Detailed and accurate anatomic knowledge is essential for diagnosis. In addition to the usual techniques of clinical and electrodiagnostic evaluation, several indirect methods of study are useful at arriving at an accurate picture of the damage before surgery is considered.

Plain films of the cervical spine and shoulder girdle can provide clues to the fate of the unseen plexus. If a transverse process is avulsed, this is good presumptive evidence that the nerve root at that level has suffered a like fate. If the clavicle is fractured, it almost always accompanies a supraclavicular rather than an infraclavicular injury because of the greater excursion that it allows between the head and the shoulder. The prognosis is correspondingly worse.

Cervical myelography can be used to demonstrate rupture of the meninges surrounding the spinal nerves, called traumatic pseudomeningoceles.[71] Usually, we perform this test 1 month following injury to allow the meninges to retract at the site of avulsion and form pockets that will allow the contrast medium to pool and be seen on x-ray films. It should be noted that because of variations in the root innervation, the observed pseudomeningoceles may not correspond exactly to the level of presumed injury arrived at by clinical neurologic deduction. Usually the variation is not greater than a single segment, however. Furthermore, both false-positive and false-negative deductions do occur,[72,73,74] especially if the only criterion is the presence or absence of a pseudomeningocele. The use of water-soluble contrast material and the improved imaging allowed by CT scanning has improved our ability to define the fate of the plexus at the root level. Whether MRI will produce correspondingly greater improvements is not known at this time.

The use of the axon reflex by studying the response to intradermal histamine has been used as an additional indicator of the level of the lesion. The improvement of other means of evaluation, potential problems with adverse reactions to the drug and the relatively lower yield of this test, however, have discouraged me from its use.[70]

Because the erector spinae musculature posterior to the cervical spine is innervated segmentally in its deepest layers by the posterior primary rami of the same spinal nerves that provide the anterior primary rami forming the brachial plexus, electromyographic examination of these muscles, as described by Bufalini and Pescatori[75] provides yet another means of determining whether a particular root is likely to have been avulsed as a supraganglionic lesion. Nerve conduction velocity determinations and somatosensory evoked potentials may contribute similar information.

All of these methods of evaluation, used in conjunction with the clinical and electromyographic studies, make cervical laminectomy unnecessary in determining the presence of root avulsion, which, with the present state of technology, is not amenable to surgical repair. The patient with a flail-anesthetic arm was, until relatively recently, felt not to be a candidate for any attempt at surgical reconstruction of the plexus, especially if there were two or more traumatic pseudomeningoceles seen on myelograms. Seddon, who probably had the greatest accumulated experience in the evaluation and management of traction injuries, thought that exploration in such cases was only for the purpose of clearly establishing a prognosis, since in the presence of a combination of multiple root avulsions and distal

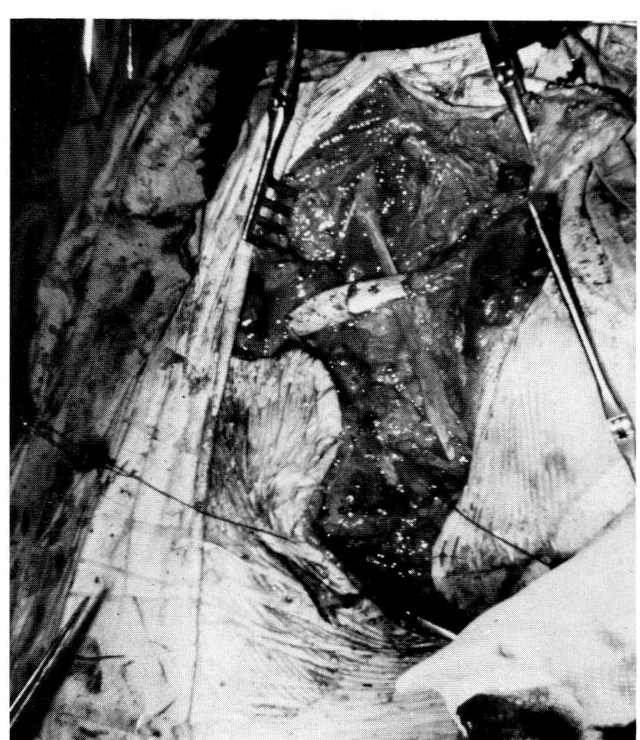

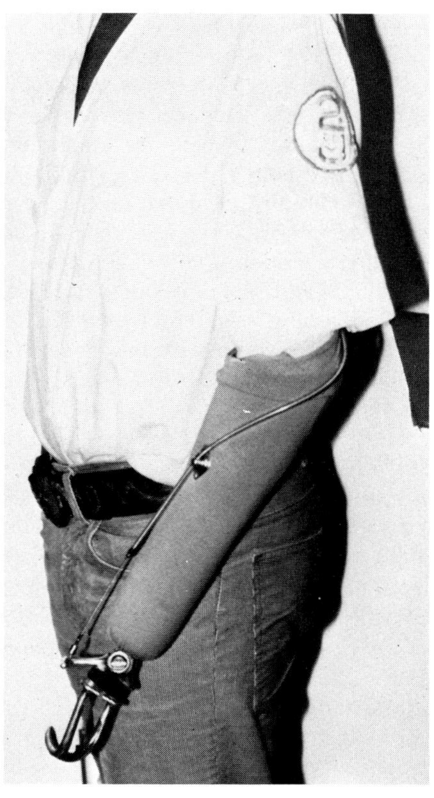

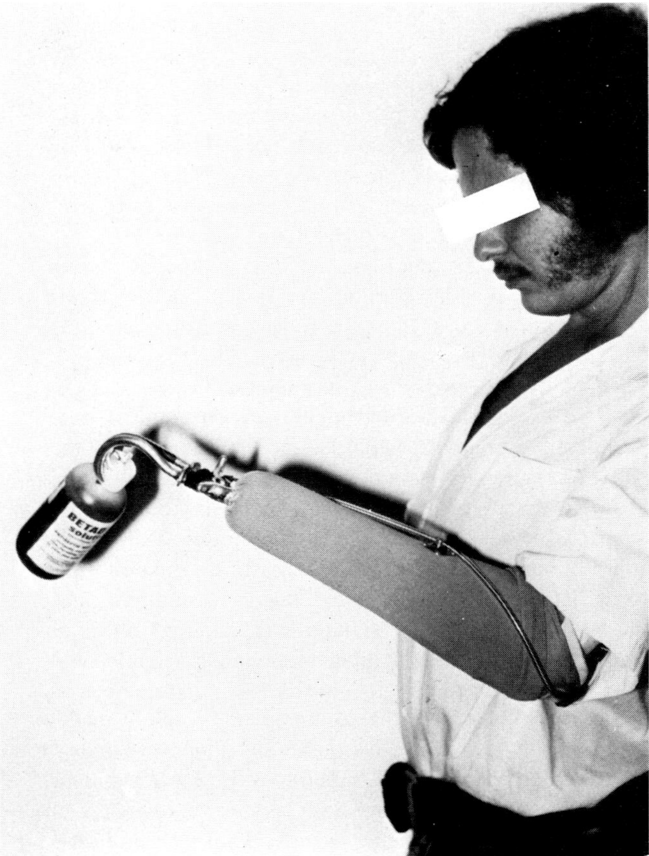

Fig. 134-9. (Upper left) A 16-cm sural nerve graft of four cables from the upper trunk to the lateral cord in a patient whose C7, C8 and T1 have been avulsed. (Right) Eighteen months following nerve grafting with shoulder fusion, forearm amputation, and prosthetic fitting. The active elbow flexion is of significant benefit to the patient's ability to use the prosthesis.

rupture within the plexus, one could then proceed with amputation of the arm and fitting of a prosthesis.[76] In this way, the patient with a flail-anesthetic arm could preserve some semblance of bimanuality. The pioneering work of Millesi et al.[77,78] and Narakas[79,80] as well as Lusskin et al.,[81] Alnot,[82] Allieu,[83] and Sedel[84] in the mid 1960s and 1970s has demonstrated that it is possible to restore the function mediated by parts of the plexus damaged by traction if they are ruptured in the infraganglionic portion. Although the results differ between different centers, it is generally agreed that for the patient with a total plexus lesion, the strong recommendation would be for surgical exploration if any portion is felt to be ruptured distally and therefore is potentially reparable. As a practical matter, this usually is confined to the upper three roots and their outflow. The prognosis for recovery of voluntary elbow flexion has been the best of all the functions sought, but some success has been achieved in restoration of shoulder control, wrist extension and, to a lesser degree, in finger flexion. For details of the results of individual workers, see their publications. In general, such explorations should, after appropriate work-up, be done as early as 2 to 3 months following injury, and are not worthwhile after 18 months. In patients in whom the entire plexus has been irrevocably damaged at the level of the spinal cord, it still may be possible to provide some function by neurotization from innervation either above or below the level of the plexus. The spinal accessory nerve has been used, as have the intercostal nerves.[85] It should be remembered, however, that if a substantial portion of the spinal accessory nerve is taken for this purpose, the trapezius will be denervated, and no longer available to power abduction of the shoulder joint complex in the event that an arthrodesis is required. Patients who have less than complete lesions of the brachial plexus may be benefited by neurologic reconstruction in selected cases. Again, it should be remembered that reconstitution of the outflow of the upper trunk for elbow flexion should not be attempted if the patient has useful sensibility in the thumb and index finger, lest it be lost when the nerve trunk is transected.

Exploration of the plexus requires extensive exposure, long operating time, and a surgical team familiar with the regional anatomy and the specialized techniques specific to this type of procedure. In addition to the sterile field encompassing the neck, hemithorax and arm, both legs must be sterilely prepared, should the harvesting of a sural nerve be required. Ideally, the incision begins in the supraclavicular fossa at the mid-point of the posterior border of the sternomastoid muscle and would drop vertically to 1 inch below the mid-point of the clavicle. However, unless this limb of the incision is directed medially in an oblique direction, a significant skin contracture from hypertrophic scarring will occur. The incision then proceeds laterally beneath the clavicle and then into the deltopectoral groove from which it can be extended into the arm. The platysma muscle is carefully divided and retained for later closure and usually the external jugular vein must be ligated and removed. The transverse cervical and suprascapular vessels, as well as the omohyoid muscle are oriented transversely to the plexus and all must be divided. The pectoralis minor is detached from the coracoid process for exposure of the infraclavicular portion of the plexus. Even though the clavicle would appear to be an impediment if it is not divided for exposure, all efforts should be made to avoid osteotomy, since there is a significant risk of nonunion. If it is necessary, the osteotomy should be oblique and preceded by a fitting of a compression plate, so that

this device may be used for osteosynthesis at the end of the procedure.

Meticulous dissection through dense scar may be required to delineate the nerves and to decide which are potentially reparable. The use of the operating microscope and somatosensory evoked potentials greatly facilitate this stage of the procedure. If grafting can be accomplished, it is more likely to succeed the further it is done from the intervertebral foramen, but grafts may be directed from the proximal intact portions of the plexus distally, as shown in Figure 134-9. The goals of such surgery often are limited, but they may be extremely gratifying, especially if combined with other conventional means of management. For the patient who would otherwise have nothing, a little gained is a lot. The alternative of primary amputation or surgical reconstruction of the flail-anesthetic limb as advocated by Hendry,[86] has, in my opinion, been made largely unnecessary. The now well-documented experience with direct surgical attack on the plexus has meant that more patients who formerly either would have had amputations or no treatment are being considered for neurologic reconstruction or neurolysis. Neurolysis is particularly indicated in patients with documented infraclavicular injuries, whose recovery does not proceed as expected or who actually experience a plateau or a reversal of this process. It may also be applied to supraclavicular injuries, but should not be thought of as an alternative to resection and grafting when indicated. Although surgical approach to obstetrical brachial palsy was practiced at the turn of the century, subsequent experience with it resulted in virtual abandonment of the technique by the 1930s. The well-documented work of Gilbert has shown that in cases of obstetrical palsy without voluntary movement by three months, the degree of function can be significantly enhanced by surgical reconstruction of the plexus.[87,88]

Radiation neuropathy of the brachial plexus is a clinical entity that presents problems in diagnosis and management. It results from therapeutic radiation in the region of the brachial plexus, usually performed because of breast cancer, but it may be associated with other entities, as well. Because the latency between treatment and the onset of symptoms may be as long as 5 or more years, there may be difficulty in differentiating radiation neuropathy from plexopathy caused by recurrent tumor.[89] Both conditions may present similarly with paresthesias and progressive neurologic loss. However, the presence of severe pain in the arm is more often a sign of tumor than radiation injury. CT scanning or MRI may clarify the diagnosis, or one may observe metastasis of breast cancer confined to the brachial plexus. Some patients will require surgical exploration in order to verify a tissue diagnosis.

In patients who have received therapeutic radiation, the dissection of the brachial plexus may be both difficult and hazardous, and the risks of further neurologic deterioration or severe hemorrhage are significant.[41] Whether neurolysis is effective in relieving the pain of radiation neuropathy or alleviating the neurologic symptoms is a subject of continued debate. My personal experience of neurolysis in these circumstances has been confined to three cases, and relief of pain was only temporary. The use of vascularized omentum following neurolysis has been reported with some favorable results.[90,91] This area remains one of continued evolution and will require continued clinical experiments.

It is obvious, then, that the management of patients with brachial plexus injuries has undergone important and continuing changes within the past few years in response to improvements in technology. The surgeon who must advise and treat a patient with a brachial plexus injury must have a well-ordered concept of not only what is available in neurosurgical treatment, but what peripheral reconstruction can offer as well.[67] To attempt to graft the lower trunk of the plexus when chances for restoring the intrinsics by this means are virtually nil, especially when tendon transfer in the hand usually is successful, is to ignore the goal of a functional outcome. The burden imposed on the surgeon is, therefore, one that crosses specialty borders, and must be dealt with. In patients with lesser degrees and distribution of neurologic loss, successful rehabilitation of the upper limb depends on whether a useful hand potentially or actually is present. Many of the peripheral reconstructive procedures may be adapted from their use in poliomyelitis, with the important difference that in the latter disease, sensibility is preserved. The same procedure may be employed in patients with peripheral nerve injuries, where deficits usually are less extensive than in the brachial plexus population. A detailed discussion of these operations is beyond the scope of this chapter.

The problem of pain in patients with brachial plexus injuries is major and has been difficult to treat. Many patients have severe pain, which can be unresponsive even to narcotics. Fortunately, it tends to abate with time, but for some it is intractable. Neurolysis usually is not effective treatment. The dorsal root entry zone radiofrequency lesion as described by Nashold[92] (DREZ) appears to offer significant advantages in terms of the permanence of the pain relief that is obtained. Amputating the arm does not help to cure the pain and actually may be contraindicated when pain is significant; the pain simply continues in the phantom limb and/or the stump.[76,93]

REFERENCES

1. Seddon HJ: Surgical Disorders of the Peripheral Nerves, ed 2. Edinburgh, Churchill Livingstone, 1975
2. Sunderland S: Nerves and Nerve Injuries, ed 2. Edinburgh, Churchill Livingstone, 1978
3. Seddon HJ: Peripheral Nerve Injuries. London, Her Majesty's Stationery Office, 1961
4. Spurling RG, Woodhall B: Surgery in World War II, Neurosurgery, vol 2. Washington, D.C., Office of the Surgeon General, Department of the Army, 1959
5. Nulsen FE and Slade HW: Peripheral nerve regeneration, VA medical myelograph, in Woodhall B, Beebe GW (eds): A Follow-up Study of 3,656 World War II Injuries, Chapter 9, Recovery following injury to the brachial plexus. 1956, p 389
6. Nelson KG, Jolly PC, Thomas PA: Brachial plexus injuries associated with missile wounds of the chest. J Trauma 8:268, 1968
7. Hurst LC, Badalamente MA, Ellstein J, Stracher A: Inhibition of neural and muscle degeneration after epineural neurorrhaphy. J Hand Surg 9A:564, 1984
8. Jabaley ME, Wallace WH, Heckler FR: Intraneural topography of major nerves of the forearm and hand: A current view. J Hand Surg 5:1, 1980
9. Sunderland S: Blood supply of nerves of the upper limb in man. Arch Neurol Psychiatry 54:280, 1945
10. Smith JW: Factors influencing nerve repair. Blood supply of peripheral nerves. Arch Surg 93:335, 1966
11. Smith JW: Factors influencing nerve repair. Collateral circulation of peripheral nerves. Arch Surg 93:433, 1966
12. Lundborg G, Branemark PI: Microvascular structure and function of peripheral nerves. Vital microscopic studies of the tibial nerve in the rabbit. Adv Microcirculation 1:66, 1988
13. Lundborg G: Structure and function of the internal microvessels as related to trauma, edema formation and nerve function. J Bone Joint Surg 57A:938, 1975
14. Lundborg G: The intrinsic vascularization of human peripheral nerves. J Hand Surg 4:35, 1979
15. Seddon HJ: Three types of nerve injury. Brain 66:237, 1947
16. Kendall HO, Kendall FP, Wadsworth GE: Muscles, Testing and Function, ed 2. Baltimore, Williams & Wilkins, 1975
17. Dellon AL: The moving two-point discrimination test: clinical evaluation of the quickly-adapting fibre system. J Hand Surg 3:474, 1978
18. Tinel J: Le signe du fourmillement dans les lesions des nerfe peripheriques. Presse Med 47:388, 1955
19. Henderson WR: Clinical assessment of peripheral nerve injuries. Tinel's test. Lancet 2:801, 1948
20. Leffert RD, Frankel VH: The value of determination of conduction velocity of peripheral nerves in orthopaedic surgery. Bull Hosp Joint Dis 25:32, 1963
21. Kimura J: Electrodiagnosis in Diseases of Nerve and Muscle. Philadelphia, FA Davis, 1983
22. Smorto MP, Basmajian JU: Clinical Electroneurography, ed 2. Baltimore, Williams & Wilkins, 1979
23. Thompson LL: The Electromyographer's Handbook. Boston, Little, Brown, 1981
24. Kline DG, Nulsen FE: The neuroma in continuity. Its preoperative and operative management. Surg Clin North Am 52:1189, 1972
25. Landi A, Copeland SA, Wynn Parry CB, et al: The role of somatosensory evoked potentials and nerve conduction studies in the surgical management of brachial plexus injuries. J Bone Joint Surg 62B:492, 1980
26. Michon J, Moberg E: Traumatic Nerve Lesions of the Upper Limb. Edinburgh, Churchill Livingstone, 1975
27. Urbaniak J: Fascicular nerve suture. Clin Orthop 163, 1982
28. Holstein A, Lewis GB: Fractures of the humerus with radial nerve paralysis. J Bone Joint Surg 45A:1382, 1963
29. Hakstian RW: Funicular orientation by direct stimulation: an aid to peripheral nerve repair. J Bone Joint Surg 50A:1178, 1968
30. Gaul JS Jr: Electrical fascicle identification as an adjunct to nerve repair. J Hand Surg 8:289, 1983
31. Lichtman DM, Florio RL, Mack GR: Carpal tunnel release under local anesthesia: evaluation of the outpatient procedure. J Hand Surg 4:544, 1979
32. Neimkin RJ, Smith RJ: Double tourniquet with linked mercury manometers for hand surgery. J Hand Surg 8:938, 1983
33. Terzis JK, Dykes RW, Hakstian R: Electrophysiological recordings in peripheral nerve surgery. J Hand Surg 1:52, 1976
34. Engel J, Ganel A, Melamed R, et al: Choline acetyl transferase for differentiation between human motor and sensory nerve fibres. Ann Plast Surg 4:376, 1979
35. Clark GL: Method of preparation of nerve ends for suturing. Plast Reconstr Surg 34:233, 1964
36. Tarlov IM: Plasma Clot Suture of Peripheral Nerves and Nerve Roots. Springfield, Ill, Charles C Thomas, 1950
37. Almquist EE, Nachemson A, Aurth D, et al: Evaluation of use of argon laser in repairing rat and primate nerves. J Hand Surg 9A;792, 1984
38. Henry AK: Extensile Exposure, ed 2. Baltimore, Williams & Wilkins, 1957
39. Curtis RM, Eversmann WW: Internal neurolysis as an adjunct to the treatment of the carpal tunnel syndrome. J Bone Joint Surg 56A:733, 1973
40. Leffert RD: Anterior transposition of the ulnar nerve by the Learmonth technique. J Hand Surg 7:197, 1982
41. Match RM: Radiation induced brachial plexus paralysis. Arch Surg 110:384, 1975
42. Stoll BA, Andrews JT: Radiation-induced peripheral neuropathy. Br Med J 1:834, 1956
43. Gentile F, Hudson AR, Kline D, et al: peripheral nerve injection injury. Neurosurgery 4:244, 1979
44. Gentile F, Hudson AR, Hunter D, et al: Nerve injection injury with

local anesthetic agents. A light and electron microscope, fluorescent microscopic and horseradish peroxidase study. Neurosurg 6:263, 1980

45. Hudson AR, Kline DG, et al: Injection injury of nerve, in Omer GE Jr, Spinner M (eds): Management of Peripheral Nerve Problems. Philadelphia, WB Saunders, 1980

46. Millesi H: Microsurgery of peripheral nerves. Hand 5:157, 1977

47. Terzis JK, Faibisoff R, Williams HB: The nerve gap: Suture under tension vs. graft. Plast Reconstr Surg 56:166, 1975

48. Sunderland S: The pros and cons of fascicular nerve repair. J Hand Surg 4:201, 1979

49. Bora FW, Lane JM, Prockop DJ: Inhibitors of collagen biosynthesis as a means of controlling scar formation in tendon injury. J Bone Joint Surg 54A:1501, 1972

50. Bora FW, Pleasure DE, Didizian NA: A study of nerve regeneration and neuroma formation after nerve suture by various techniques. J Hand Surg 1:138, 1976

51. Cabaus HE, Rodkey WG, McCarroll HR, et al: Epineural and perineurial fascicular nerve repairs: a critical comparison. J Hand Surg 1:131, 1976

52. Pleasure D, Bora FW, Lane J, et al: Regeneration after transection: effect of inhibition of collagen synthesis. Exp Neurol 45:72, 1974

53. Millesi H, Meissl G, Berger A: The interfascicular nerve grafting of the median and ulnar nerves. J Bone Joint Surg 54A:727, 1972

54. Millesi H, Meissl G, Berger A: Further experience with interfascicular grafting of the median, ulnar and radial nerves. J Bone Joint Surg 58A:209, 1976

55. Strange FGStC: An operation for nerve pedicle grafting, preliminary communication. Br J Surg 34:423, 1947

56. Strange FCStC: Case report on pedicle nerve graft. Br J Surg 37:331, 1950

57. Alpar EK, Brooks DM: Long-term results of ulnar to median pedicle grafts. Hand 10:61, 1978

58. Taylor IG, Horn FJ: The free vascularized nerve graft. Plast Reconstr Surg 57:412, 1976

59. Taylor IG: Nerve grafting with simultaneous microvascular reconstruction. Clin Orthop 133:56, 1978

60. Gutmann E, Gutmann L: Effect of galvanic exercise on denervated reinnervated muscles in rabbit. J Neurol Neurosurg Psychiatry 7:7, 1944

61. Nicholson OR, Seddon HJ: Nerve repair in civil practice: Results of median and ulnar nerve lesions. Br Med J 2:1065, 1957

62. Brooks DM: The place of nerve grafting in orthopedic surgery. J Bone Joint Surg 37A:299, 1955

63. Omer GE: The evaluation of clinical results following peripheral nerve suture, in Omer GE Jr, Spinner M (eds): Management of Peripheral Nerve Problems. Philadelphia, WB Saunders, 1980

64. Omer GE: Injuries to nerves of the upper extremity. J Bone Joint Surg 56A:1615, 1974

65. Seddon HJ: Nerve grafting. J Bone Joint Surg 45B:447, 1963

66. Leffert RD: Lesions of the brachial plexus, including thoracic outlet syndrome. Instructional Course Lectures, vol 31, American Academy of Orthopedic Surgeons. St Louis, CV Mosby, 1977

67. Leffert RD: Brachial Plexus Injuries. New York, Churchill Livingstone, 1985

68. Brooks DM: Open wounds of the brachial plexus. J Bone Joint Surg 31B:17, 1949

69. Leffert RD, Seddon HJ: Infraclavicular brachial plexus injuries. J Bone Joint Surg 47B:9, 1965

70. Bonney G: The value of axon responses in determining the site of

the lesion in traction injuries of the brachial plexus. Brain 77:588, 1954

71. Murphy F, Hartung W, Kirklin JW: Myelographic demonstration of avulsing injury of the brachial plexus. AJR 58:102, 1947

72. Heon M: Myelogram: A questionable aid in diagnosis and prognosis in avulsion of brachial plexus components by traction injuries. Conn Med 29:260, 1965

73. Jelasic F, Piepgres U: Functional restitution after cervical avulsion injury with "typical myelographic findings". Eur Neurol 11:158, 1974

74. Yeoman PM: Cervical myelography in traction injuries of the brachial plexus. J Bone Joint Surg 50B:2, 1968

75. Bufalini C, Pescatori G: posterior cervical electromyography in the diagnosis and prognosis of brachial plexus injuries. J Bone Joint Surg 51B:627, 1969

76. Yeoman PM, Seddon HJ: Brachial plexus injuries: Treatment of the flail arm. J Bone Joint Surg 43B:3, 1961

77. Millesi H, Meissl G, Katzer H: Therapy of brachial plexus injuries: Proposal for an integrated therapy (German). Bruns Beitr Klin Chir 220:429, 1973

78. Millesi H: Surgical management of brachial plexus injuries. J Hand Surg 2:367, 1977

79. Narakas A: plexo braquial terapeutica quirrigica directa. Rev Orthop Traumatol 16:855, 1972

80. Narakas A: Surgical treatment of traction injuries of the brachial plexus. Clin Orthop 133:71, 1976

81. Lusskin R, Campbell JB, Thompson WAL: Post-traumatic lesions of the brachial plexus: Treatment by transclavicular exploration and neurolysis or autograft reconstruction. J Bone Joint Surg 55:1159, 1973

82. Alnot JY: Technique chirgicale dans les paralysies du plexus brachial. Rev Chir Orthop 63:75, 1977

83. Allieu Y: Exploration et traitement direct des lesions nerveuses dans les paralysies traumatiques par elongation du plexus brachial chez l'adults. Rev Chir Orthop 83:107, 1977

84. Sedel L: Results of surgical repair in brachial plexus injuries. J Bone Joint Surg 64B:54, 1982

85. Tsuyama N, Hara T: Intercostal nerve crossing in the treatment of brachial plexus injury of root avulsion type. Proceedings of the 12th Congress of the International Society of Orthopaedic Surgery and Traumatology. Tel Aviv, 1972. Amsterdam, Excerpta Medica, 1972, p. 351

86. Hendry AM: The treatment of residual paralysis of brachial plexus injuries. J Bone Joint Surg 31:42, 1949

87. Gilbert A, Khouri N, Carlioz H: Exploration chirurgicale du plexus brachial dans la paralysie obstetricale. Rev Chir Orthop 68:33, 1980

88. Tassin JL: paralysies obstetricales du plexus brachial evolution spontance, resultats des interventions reparatrices precoces. Thesis, University of Paris, VII, 1983

89. Thomas JE, Colby MY: Radiation induced or metastatic brachial plexopathy? JAMA 222, 1972

90. Brunelli G: Neurolysis and free microvascular omentum transfer in the treatment of post-actinic palsy of the brachial plexus. Int Surg 65:6, 1980

91. Clodius L, Uhlschmid G, Hess K: Irradiation plexitis of the brachial plexus, in Terzis J (ed): Clinics in Plastic Surgery, Peripheral Nerve Microsurgery. Philadelphia, WB Saunders, 1984

92. Nashold BS Jr: Current status of the Drez operation, 1984. Neurosurgery 15:942, 1984

93. Fletcher I: Traction injuries of the brachial plexus. Hand 1:129, 1969

CHAPTER 135

Surgical Management of Peripheral Entrapment Neuropathy

Henry A. Young

EXPERIMENTAL AND CLINICAL OBSERVATIONS on the etiology and pathogenesis of peripheral entrapment neuropathy suggest that the two predominant causative agents are ischemia and compression. The precise role of each factor is not established, although the more recent studies emphasize the importance of direct mechanical compression of the nerve.

Local compression results in damage to peripheral nerves. Severe compression may crush fibers and lead to wallerian degeneration with a loss of distal excitability that requires months to resolve. Very mild compression produces physiologic block, which is reversed as soon as the pressure is released. Based on studies with pneumatic cuffs or clamps in humans, Lewis et al.[1] concluded that this physiologic block was caused by local asphyxia. Compression of an intermediate degree produces local conduction block with preservation of distal excitability that may take several weeks to recover.[2] Denny-Brown and Brenner[3,4] found the anatomic basis for this to be demyelination with preservation of axonal continuity, and concluded that this lesion was caused by local asphyxia of the nerve rather than by mechanical deformation. In support of this concept were the experimental observations of Grundfest,[5] who showed that very high pressures were necessary to abolish conduction in the excised nerves of frogs enclosed in an oxygenated pressure chamber.

More recent clinical and experimental work has emphasized the importance of direct mechanical compression. Gilliatt et al.,[6] using a cuff inflated to 1000 mm Hg for 1 to 2 hours around the legs of baboons, found that the anatomic lesions were concentrated under the edges of the cuff, with sparing in the center, where the lesions might have been expected to be maximal if ischemia had played an important role. The characteristic lesion produced in this experiment was damage to large myelinated fibers with displacement of the node of Ranvier from its usual position under the Schwann cell junction, accompanied by stretching of the paranodal myelin on one side of the node and invagination of the paranodal myelin on the other. This nodal lesion is followed by a breakdown of the paranodal myelin. Repetition of the experiment with nylon cords attached to peripheral nerves in animals with attached weights designed to simulate human pressure palsies produced the same characteristic anatomic lesions. Thus, displacement of the node of Ranvier accompanied by stretching of paranodal myelin on one side of the node and invagination of myelin on the other side, followed in time by paranodal or segmental demyelination, may

be regarded as the characteristic anatomic lesion caused by an acutely evolving compression neuropathy.

Neary et al.,[7] by careful microscopic examination of segments of ulnar and median nerves in cadaver specimens without clinical evidence of entrapment neuropathy, found a characteristic set of microscopic lesions in ulnar nerve segments in the area of the cubital tunnel and in median nerve segments at the flexor retinaculum, both clinically common sites of entrapment. In a high percentage of nerve segments, they found that the appearance of internodes was altered as a result of bulbous swelling at one end and thinning and retraction of myelin at the other; in some nerves intercalated segments indicative of previous demyelination also were present. Previous studies[8] indicated that the distortion of internodes resulted from slippage of myelin lamellae away from the site of the pressure, the bulbous ends of the internodes consisting of redundant folds of myelin. This process is thought to represent the earliest change to occur in nerve fibers subject to chronic recurrent compression and thus is the anatomic substrate of chronic compressive neuropathy.

Both the early lesion of acutely evolving compression neuropathy (displacement of the node of Ranvier with stretching of paranodal myelin on one side and invagination of myelin on the other side) and the early lesion of chronic compressive neuropathy (bulbous swelling at one end of the internode and retraction at the other end) are followed by segmental demyelination, which has been shown to be the characteristic lesion in chronic compression neuropathy in experimental animals.[9] Given time and continued compression, the neurapractic lesion of segmental demyelination may evolve into axonotmetic and neurotmetic lesions, culminating in complete fibrosis of a segment of nerve.

The predominant role of mechanical compression in producing entrapment is not universally accepted. Sunderland[10] emphasized the importance of vascular factors in the production of a carpal tunnel syndrome. He visualized the carpal tunnel syndrome as an entity passing through three stages. In stage 1, chronic mechanical compression leads to increased intrafunicular pressure, eventually resulting in slowing of intrafunicular capillary circulation. The nerve fibers are afflicted by vascular insufficiency and become hyperexcitable, resulting often in pain and paresthesias. The pain and paresthesias are aggravated by venous stasis. Relief is obtained by vigorously exercising the hand or arm, which promotes venous return. In stage 2, capillary circulation slows to the point that the capillary

OPERATIVE NEUROSURGICAL TECHNIQUES
ISBN 0-8089-1862-1

endothelium is damaged, with intrafunicular edema and leakage of proteinaceous exudate into funiculi. Enlargement of the nerve may be observed grossly at the level of the flexor retinaculum. In stage 3, fibroblasts proliferate in the protein exudate, leading to intrafunicular fibrosis associated with destruction of increasing numbers of nerve fibers. Eventually, nutrient vessels are completely obliterated with conversion of the affected segment of nerve into a fibrous cord. Sunderland pointed out that this hypothesis applies only to the carpal tunnel syndrome. It appears, however, that both direct mechanical deformation of myelin and vascular factors may play a role in the production of entrapment neuropathy, although the precise role of each variable has not been precisely defined.

GENERAL MANAGEMENT OF COMPRESSIVE NERVE LESIONS

Two systems of classification of peripheral nerve lesions are in use. Seddon used the terms neurapraxia, axonotmesis, and neurotmesis, while Sunderland classified nerve injury into five degrees of severity. The fifth-degree nerve lesion is not applicable to neural compression lesions. It occurs when a nerve is completely severed and the ends retract. A first-degree Sunderland lesion is equivalent to neurapraxia, while a second-degree lesion is equivalent to axonotmesis. The fourth-degree lesion is neurotmetic and implies a neuroma in continuity. In third-degree lesions, intrafunicular fibrosis is present. These lesions may be reversible or axonotmetic, but they also may be neurotmetic with irreversible intrafunicular fibrosis.

In neurapraxia the nerve fiber is physiologically transected at the point of compression. Wallerian degeneration does not occur, however, and the axonal basement membrane is intact. Neurapraxia may be due to the following anatomic and physiologic causes: (1) electrolyte imbalance, including disturbances of sodium, potassium, and adenosine triphosphatase function,[11] occur at the site of compression and can result in neurapraxia; (2) displacement of the node of Ranvier with stretching and invagination of internodal myelin, discussed above as the earliest anatomic change of acutely evolving compression neuropathy, results in neurapraxia; (3) bulbous swelling of myelin at one end of the internode with thinning and retraction at the other, the earliest change in chronic compression neuropathy, may produce neurapraxia; (4) processes (2) and (3) above result in segmental demyelination over time, which produces neurapraxia; (5) intrafunicular anoxia, thought by Sunderland to be the cause of the carpal tunnel syndrome, also may play a role in the production of neurapraxia. If neural compression continues over time, neurapractic lesions may evolve into axonotmetic and neurotmetic lesions.

Axonotmesis is characterized by complete interruption of the axons and their myelin sheaths, but the stroma of the nerve remains in continuity-Schwann tubes, endoneurium, and epineurium. Electron microscopy has shown that even the Schwann basement membranes persist. Axonal damage and loss of function are as complete as that occurring after nerve transection. Distal to the level of axonotmetic compression, complete wallerian degeneration occurs; however, regeneration can occur spontaneously and is often of good quality because intact endoneurial tubes guide outgoing streams of axoplasm toward appropriate peripheral connections. Classically, regeneration occurs at the rate of 1 mm per day, or roughly 1 inch per month, and this is the expected rate of clinical recovery, which

exhibits a sequential pattern depending upon the distance from the point of compression to the point of reinnervation of muscle fiber or sensory end-organ.

Neurotmesis describes a nerve that either has been completely severed or is disorganized by scar tissue to the point that spontaneous regeneration is impossible. Neurotmetic compression lesions require resection and suture, with or without the interposition of nerve grafts.

A neural compression lesion persisting for 60 days with no improvement requires surgical therapy. If neurologic deficit is not rapidly progressive, a neural compression lesion may be followed for 60 days after the diagnosis and conservative measures adopted, such as splinting in the case of the carpal tunnel syndrome. Neurapractic lesions that will resolve without surgery will exhibit evidence of recovery during this period, while axonotmetic lesions that will not require surgery exhibit reinnervation proceeding distally at the rate of 2.5 cm or 1 inch per month. During this period of observation, evidence for return of function may be sought by serial physical examination and electrical testing. An advancing Tinel's sign provides evidence of reinnervation often before motor and sensory recovery, but many patients with the advancing Tinel's sign will nonetheless exhibit poor spontaneous functional recovery.[12] It is important to test the autonomous sensory zone of the damaged nerve so that sensory overlap from other peripheral nerves is not mistakenly interpreted as regeneration in the injured nerve. In performing serial motor and sensory examination, one should have a clear idea of the expected schedule of functional recovery. In neurapractic lesions, distal functions return simultaneously after resolution of conduction block in the area of compression. Neurapractic lesions caused by local nodal electrolyte imbalance may be corrected within several days, with sudden reappearance of all motor and sensory functions distal to the compressed area. Neurapractic lesions caused by local myelin damage in the area of compression-whether myelin paranodal intussusception or segmental demyelination-require a 60-day period for local remyelinization and resolution of conduction block to occur. Therefore, within a 60-day period of observation and conservative therapy, the bulk of neurapractic lesions responding to conservative therapy should exhibit evidence of recovery. Axonotmetic lesions exhibit a proximal-to-distal march of sensory and motor recovery that occurs at the rate of 1 mm per day or 1 inch per month, which roughly corresponds to the rate of axonal regeneration.

Serial electrical testing also may be used to confirm that reinnervation is proceeding at the desired rate. When regeneration is occurring, serial EMGs show a decrease in the number of fibrillations and denervation potentials, which are replaced by nascent motor action potentials. These findings, however, cannot predict the quality or completeness of regeneration. Serial conduction velocities across affected segments may be obtained, to test for resolution of conduction block. Simple percutaneous nerve stimulation also is a valuable test. Muscle contraction distal to the point of compression indicates that useful clinical function in that muscle will occur in several weeks. If, after a 60-day period of observation of a neural compression lesion, physical and electrical examination shows that the expected rate of recovery is not occurring, surgical exploration is necessary.

Preoperatively, careful clinical examination and electrical testing are necessary to localize the area of entrapment and to be certain that the nerve is not compressed in more than one place, i.e., the "double crush" syndrome.[13] For example, the ulnar nerve may be compressed both at Guyon's tunnel in the wrist and at the cubital tunnel in the elbow. Decompression at only one level in such a situation is of minimal value.

Surgical exposure must be generous because several centimeters of normal nerve should be identified proximal and distal to the area of entrapment. Dissection proceeds from the proximal and distal sides to separate the epineurium from surrounding scar, thickened fascia, and fibrous bands. Many times this external neurolysis alone provides adequate treatment and decompression.

Indications for internal neurolysis, with dissection of individual funiculi, are less well established. Extensive internal neurolysis may provoke fibrosis in all layers of the nerve.[14] Spinner[15] pointed out that internal neurolysis should be limited to those fasciculi that are clinically involved. In cases of carpal tunnel syndrome where pain and dysesthesias are most severe in the long finger, he obtained excellent results by selective internal neurolysis of the medial two or three funiculi of the median nerve. He cautioned against internal neurolysis of all fasciculi of the median nerve in this condition. Curtis and Eversmann,[16] reporting 96 cases of carpal tunnel syndrome treated with both external and internal neurolysis, found that internal neurolysis increased the success of surgery in a subgroup of patients with constant sensory loss or thenar atrophy or both. Brown[17] emphasized the value of internal neurolysis for a wide variety of lesions in continuity, including those resulting from chronic entrapment. He pointed out that many lesions in continuity are accompanied by intraneural scarring, which can only be treated definitively by internal as well as external neurolysis. No patient in his series was made worse by internal neurolysis.

An intraoperative finding that is frequently encountered, particularly in neural compression lesions of long standing, is a neuroma in continuity, the management of which has been well outlined by Kline and Nulsen.[18] Direct nerve stimulation proximal to the neuroma may be attempted first. If distal muscle contraction is elicited, the lesion may be treated by external and, if indicated, internal neurolysis. If no motor response is elicited, an attempt is made to record nerve action potentials. This procedure is done by placing bipolar stainless electrodes proximal to the neuroma in continuity and then attempting to evoke a nerve action potential distal to the neuroma after stimulating proximal to the neuroma. Evoked responses are obtained by means of bipolar electrodes placed distal to the neuroma and recorded by an amplifier and an oscilloscope. The presence of a nerve action potential distal to the lesion after proximal stimulation means that neurolysis is indicated. Inability to evoke a nerve-action potential through the neuroma after a 60-day period of conservative management of a neural compression lesion indicates that satisfactory regeneration is not occurring and that resection of the neuroma, with or without intrafascicular nerve grafting, is indicated.

All peripheral nerve entrapment surgery is performed with headlight illumination under $3.5–4.5\times$ magnification. The microscope is reserved for internal neurolysis, intrafascicular nerve grafting, and suturing of individual fascicles after resection of neuromas in continuity.

A variety of anesthetic options is available: (1) General endotracheal intubation with or without tourniquet on the extremity. This type of anesthesia should be used whenever a procedure lasting more than several hours is anticipated, particularly if the microscope will be required. (2) General anesthesia without intubation with or without tourniquet. This is of value in apprehensive patients when the procedure is of short duration. (3) Local anesthesia alone. This limits the scope of the procedure, particularly if unexpected intraoperative findings are encountered. It is seldom adequate for anything more complicated than simple carpal tunnel release. (4) Intravenous regional anesthesia is an excellent technique, which can be used in both the upper and the lower extremities. It provides adequate analgesia and, in addition, tourniquet effect. The maximal duration of a procedure with such anesthesia is approximately 2 hours. In general, we prefer systematic meticulous hemostasis to the use of tourniquet. Bleeding after tourniquet release must be thoroughly controlled to prevent postoperative wound hematoma, which can predispose to neural scarring and thus give a poor surgical result. A tourniquet must be used carefully in elderly patients and in those with a history of peripheral vascular insufficiency. We usually prefer general anesthesia to local and intravenous regional anesthesia because it is often difficult to tell preoperatively if a prolonged procedure with intrafascicular dissection and nerve grafting under the microscope will be necessary.

INDIVIDUAL NERVE COMPRESSION LESIONS

MEDIAN NERVE ENTRAPMENT

Median nerve entrapment occurs distally in the carpal tunnel, or, less commonly, in the proximal forearm.

Entrapment of the median nerve at the wrist results in the carpal tunnel syndrome. The disease occurs more frequently in females, with the peak incidence between the ages of 40 and 60 years. The syndrome most often is caused by narrowing of the carpal tunnel. A history of repeated occupational trauma to the hand and wrist often may be elicited. Carpal tunnel syndrome also may be associated with a wide variety of systemic diseases. Amyloid infiltration of the transverse carpal ligament due to either primary or secondary amyloidosis (as in multiple myeloma) may produce a carpal tunnel syndrome. Diseases such as rheumatoid arthritis, acromegaly, and hypothyroidism, which result in thickening of connective tissue, may thicken the transverse carpal ligament sufficiently to result in median nerve compression.

The most common clinical finding of the syndrome is pain and paresthesias in the radial 3½ fingers, often more severe at night and relieved by shaking of the hand. Diagnosis is easily arrived at when a complete set of signs and symptoms of the fully evolved syndrome is present—positive Tinel's and Phalen's signs, hypesthesia in the radial 3½ digits, thenar atrophy, and EMG abnormalities in the distal median nerve. The disease, however, may present atypically as pain in the proximal upper extremity and shoulder.[19] Unexplained shoulder or proximal upper extremity pain is a clear indication for a detailed physical and electromyographic examination of the median nerve at the wrist. At times the diagnosis must be made purely on clinical grounds because EMG and nerve conduction time at the wrist are normal in up to 25 percent of cases.[15]

Conservative therapy consists of splinting the wrist in a neutral position. Local injections of Xylocaine or steroid have not been useful in our experience. Indications for surgery include motor weakness, persistent arm and hand discomfort or paresthesias, and lack of response to conservative therapy.

The procedure of carpal tunnel release, including the skin

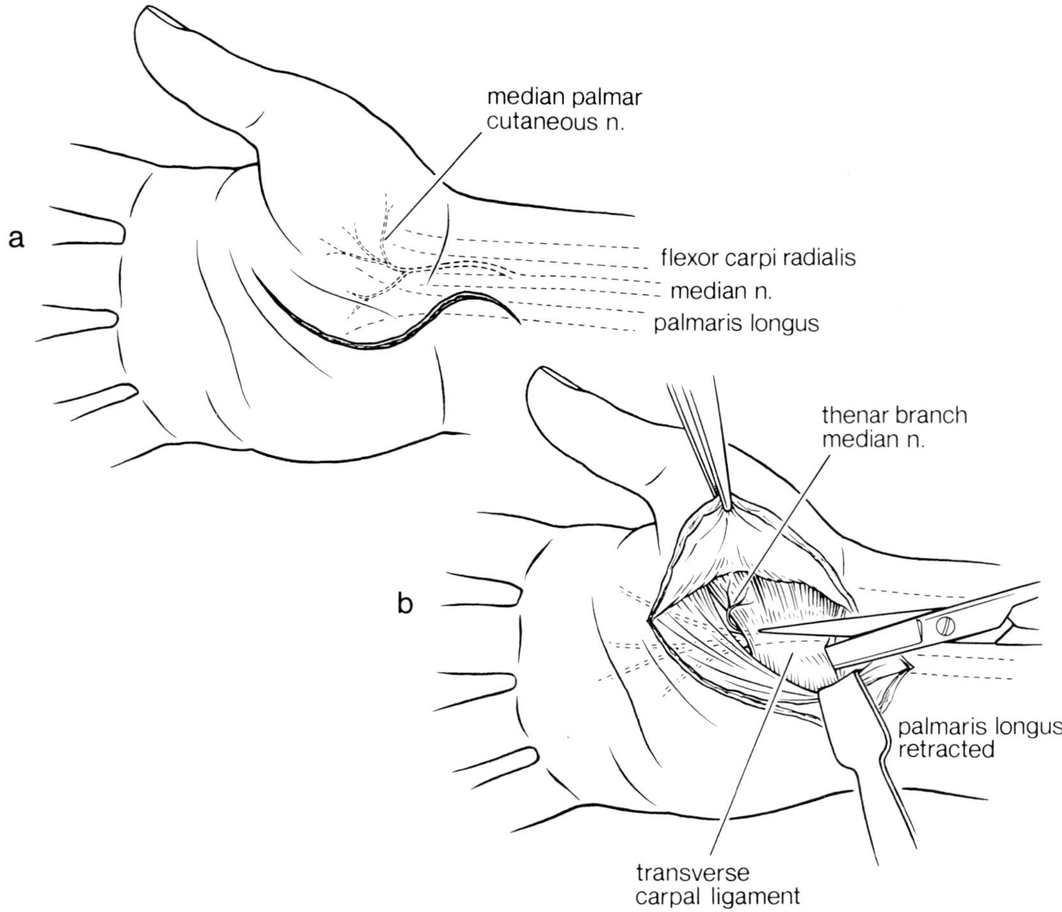

Fig. 135-1. Surgical exposure of the median nerve at the wrist. A curvilinear incision avoiding the branches of the medial palmar cutaneous nerve is utilized.

incision preferred by the author, taking into account the position of the motor branch of the median nerve, is illustrated in Figure 135-1. After the incision is made, dissection is continued through the antebrachial fascia. The palmaris longus tendon is retracted, and the underlying median nerve is identified as it enters the carpal tunnel between the flexor digitorum superficialis and the flexor carpi radialis tendons. The transverse carpal ligament is divided along its entire length parallel to the median nerve, and the nerve is freed of all ligamentous structures as far as the proximal crease of the hand. Incomplete division of the transverse carpal ligament is a major cause of failure of this procedure to relieve symptoms.

Several special points regarding carpal tunnel surgery must be noted. Injury to the medial palmar cutaneous nerve recently has been emphasized as a cause of postoperative pain. This nerve arises 5.5 cm proximal to the radial styloid from the radial aspect of the median nerve. It then crosses the space between the median nerve and the flexor carpi radialis tendon and attaches to the undersurface of the antebrachial fascia under the ulnar margin of the flexor carpi radialis tendon. From this point it continues ulnarward to enter the transverse carpal ligament and passes via a tunnel of its own through the ligament 9 to 16 mm within the ligament.[20] Transverse incisions for carpal tunnel release should be avoided because of the possibility of injuring the main trunk of the medial palmar cutaneous nerve. At the level of the heel of the hand, the incision is best placed ulnar to the longitudinal axis of the fourth metacarpal to avoid injury to the distal branches of the nerve. At the wrist the skin

incision may be curved either radially or ulnarward in an S configuration, which is helpful in avoiding contracture.

The presence of significant thenar atrophy is an indication for operative exposure and examination of the thenar branch of the median nerve. This recurrent branch usually arises distal to the transverse carpal ligament from the radial portion of the median nerve trunk. Frequently, however, the thenar branch may pass through a foramen of its own in the distal portion of the transverse carpal ligament,[15] which may constitute an area of neural compression and require release.

A less common but significant area of median nerve entrapment is the proximal forearm. In its course down the arm, the median nerve initially lies lateral to the brachial artery, but it gradually crosses the ventral surface of the artery in the lower part of the arm and lies medial to it at the bend of the elbow, where it is deep to the lacertus fibrosus and superficial to the brachialis. In the forearm it passes between the two heads of the pronator teres and continues distally between the flexor digitorum sublimis and profundus. The median nerve branches innervating the flexorpronator group originating from the medial epicondyle arise from the medial aspect of the nerve. The anterior interosseous nerve arises from the lateral aspect of the nerve as it passes between the heads of the pronator teres. The anterior interosseous nerve innervates the flexor pollicis longus, the radial half of the flexor digitorum profundus, and the pronator quadratus. It is important to preserve all of these branches.

The surgical approach to the median nerve in the proximal

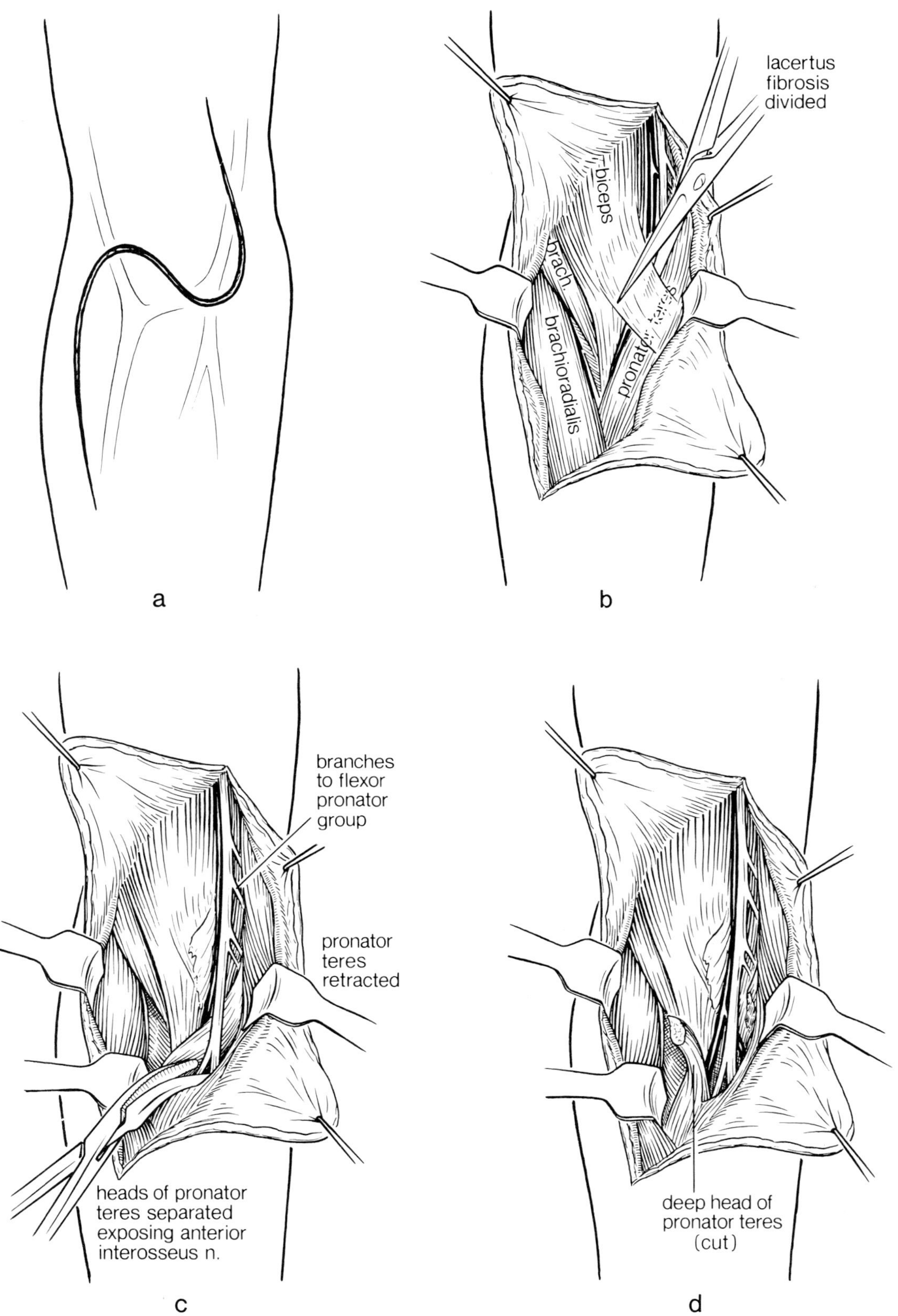

Fig. 135-2. Steps in the operative exposure of the median nerve and its anterior interosseous branch at the elbow.

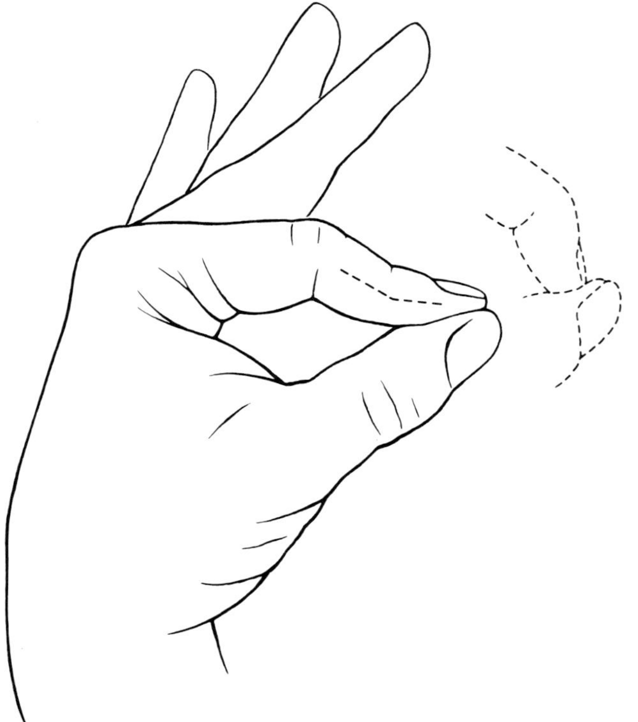

Fig. 135-3. The patient with anterior interosseous palsy is unable to pinch the distal phalanges of the first and second fingers together because of paralysis of the flexor pollicis longus and of the flexor digitorum profundus of the index finger.

forearm is illustrated in Figure 135-2. A Z-shaped incision overlying the pronator teres is used. The incision begins 5 cm above the medial epicondyle, continues transversely following a flexion crease across the antecubital fossa, and then is carried distally along the medial margin of the brachioradialis muscle. The median nerve is identified as it lies on the brachialis muscle proximal to the lacertus fibrosus and then is traced distally. The lacertus fibrosus is divided and the nerve traced distally as it passes medial to the bicipital tendon into the antecubital fossa. The nerve then is traced distally as it passes between the two heads of the pronator teres. The tendinous origin of the deep head is divided when exploring the anterior interosseous nerve.

Two different types of median nerve compression syndrome prevail in the proximal forearm: (1) the pronator syndrome, and (2) the anterior interosseous syndrome. The pronator syndrome consists of a pain in the proximal volar aspect of the forearm, exacerbated on pronation of the forearm, weakness of intrinsic muscles innervated by the median nerve, paresthesias in the radial 3½ digits, and normal function of the flexor pollicis longus, pronator quadratus, and flexor digitorum profundus of the second and third fingers—all of which are innervated by the anterior interosseous nerve. The most important cause of pronator syndrome is median nerve compression by a hypertrophic pronator teres and adhesions within the pronator teres. Less frequent causes include compression by the lacertus fibrosus or by a thickened flexor superficialis arch as well as passage of the median nerve posterior to both heads of the pronator teres. The anterior interosseous syndrome results in selective paralysis of the flexor digitorum profundus of the second and third fingers, the pronator quadratus, and the flexor pollicis longus. There are no sensory changes. The patient is unable to pinch the distal phalanges of the thumb and

index finger together (Figure 135-3). The most common cause of selective anterior interosseous compression neuropathy is compression by the tendinous origin of the deep head of the pronator teres. Treatment is by release of the tendinous origin of the deep head.

ULNAR NERVE COMPRESSION

Ulnar nerve compression occurs most commonly at the elbow, and, less often, at the wrist. The ulnar nerve in the arm runs medial to the axillary artery within the medial intermuscular septum. In the middle of the arm it angles dorsally, pierces the medial intermuscular septum, and follows the medial head of the triceps through the groove between the olecranon and medial epicondyle. In passing from the extensor surface behind the humerus to the forearm flexor surface, the nerve passes through the elliptical cubital tunnel bounded laterally by the elbow joint and its transverse ligament, and medially by the aponeurosis between the two heads of the flexor carpi ulnaris. It enters the forearm between the two heads of the flexor carpi ulnaris and continues distally between this muscle and the flexor digitorum profundus. A significant anatomic variation is the arcade of Struthers, a thickening of muscle and connective tissue passing medial to the nerve between the medial intermuscular septum and the medial head of the triceps. It is present in 70 percent of cadaver specimens.[21]

Ulnar nerve compression in the vicinity of the elbow has many causes. The nerve can be compressed at the cubital tunnel where it enters the forearm between the heads of the flexor carpi ulnaris because there is a fascial connection between the two muscle heads that can act as a compressing force, particularly during flexion. Within the ulnar groove repetitive frictional forces may damage the nerve, since the nerve may elongate as much as 0.5 cm during flexion.[22] Local elbow pathology such as ganglion cysts, rheumatoid synovitis, osteoarthritis, and old medial epicondyle fractures may injure the nerve by direct local compression.

Medial epicondylectomy has been advocated for ulnar compression at the elbow,[23] and recent publications also claim success for simple division of the fibrous arch between the heads of the flexor carpi ulnaris.[24] Our surgical approach to the ulnar nerve at the elbow (Figure 135-4) combines anterior translocation with division of the arcade of Struthers and the medial intermuscular septum proximally, and division of the aponeurosis between the heads of the flexor carpi ulnaris distally. This approach provides complete decompression above and below the elbow, and anterior translocation effectively removes the nerve from frictional forces in the ulnar groove. After translocation, the nerve lies subcutaneously at the elbow crease. Major causes of recurrent symptoms after anterior transposition include kinking caused by incomplete division of the medial intermuscular septum, compression at the entrance to the cubital tunnel by scar or incomplete division of the heads of the flexor carpi ulnaris, dense scarring of the nerve bed, and constriction where the fascial sling is created to hold the nerve in its anterior position. Submuscular transposition of the ulnar nerve[25] requires division of the flexor-pronator group of muscles close to their origin from the medial epicondyle, rerouting of the nerve deep to them, and resuturing of the muscles over the nerve. This technique is useful for reoperation,[26] especially when dense scarring has occurred after anterior subcutaneous transposition, because the nerve can be

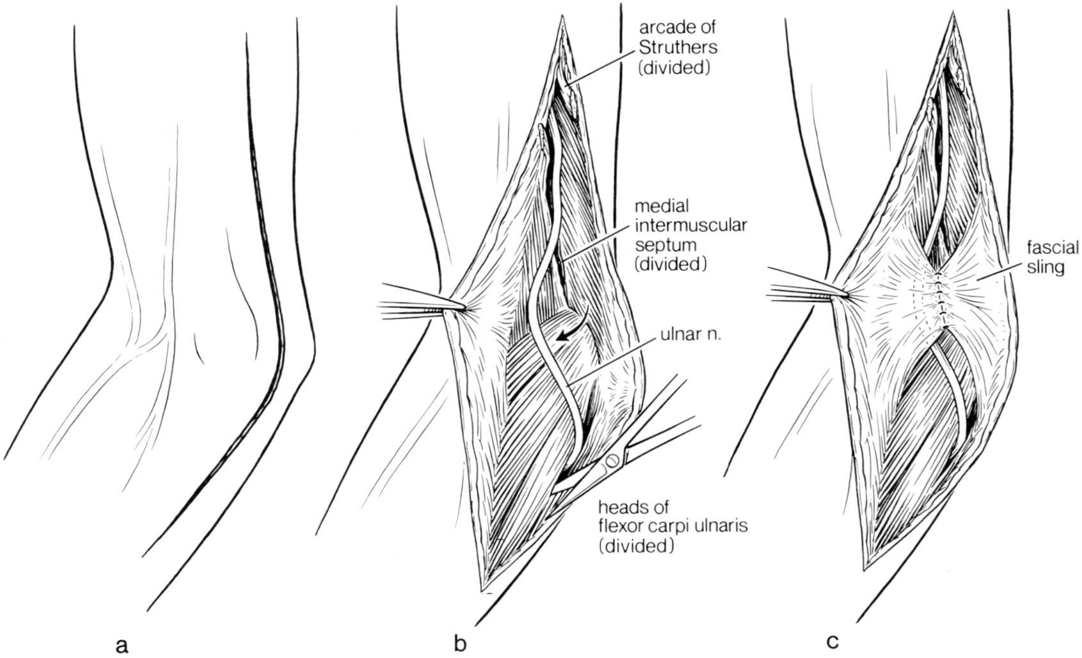

Fig. 135-4.　Steps in the anterior transposition of the ulnar nerve at the elbow.

redirected deep to the flexor-pronator group into an unscarred bed.

At the wrist the ulnar artery and nerve pass superficial to the flexor retinaculum and under a thickened aponeurosis, which is an extension of the flexor carpi ulnaris. The area of passage under this aponeurosis is called Guyon's tunnel. Ulnar nerve entrapment in this area occurs at Guyon,s tunnel, or at the pisiform or hook of the hamate. Ulnar nerve entrapment at the wrist may result from anomalous muscles, ganglia, osteoarthritic bony spurs, or ligamentous thickening. Treatment consists of division of the aponeurosis forming the roof of the tunnel (Figure 135-5). The underlying ulnar nerve then can be identified and neurolysis carried out. A diligent search also should be made for compression by bony spurs and anomalous muscles.

RADIAL NERVE ENTRAPMENT

The radial nerve is most susceptible to acute injury when fracture of the midshaft of the humerus occurs, injuring the nerve within the musculospiral groove. Chronic spontaneous entrapment is more likely to occur below the level of the elbow, where the nerve divides into superficial and deep (posterior interosseous) branches. After piercing the lateral intermuscular septum in the lower arm, the radial nerve runs between the brachialis and brachioradialis to the front of the lateral epicondyle and divides into superficial and deep portions. The superficial branch runs along the lateral border of the forearm under the brachioradialis and supplies sensation to the dorsal portions of the radial 3½ fingers. The deep posterior interosseous branch passes between the two heads of the supinator and continues dorsolaterally around the neck of the radius.

Posterior interosseous entrapment occurs most commonly as the nerve passes between the heads of the supinator. The nerve enters the supinator through an inverted arch—the ''arcade of Frohse''—formed by the edge of the proximal border of the superficial head of the supinator. The arcade may compress the nerve just as the carpal ligament compresses the median nerve at the wrist.

Complete posterior interosseous palsy has the following features: (1) inability to extend the fingers at the metacarpophalangeal joints; (2) dorsiflexion of the wrist in a radial direction because of paralysis of the extensor carpi ulnaris; (3) inability to

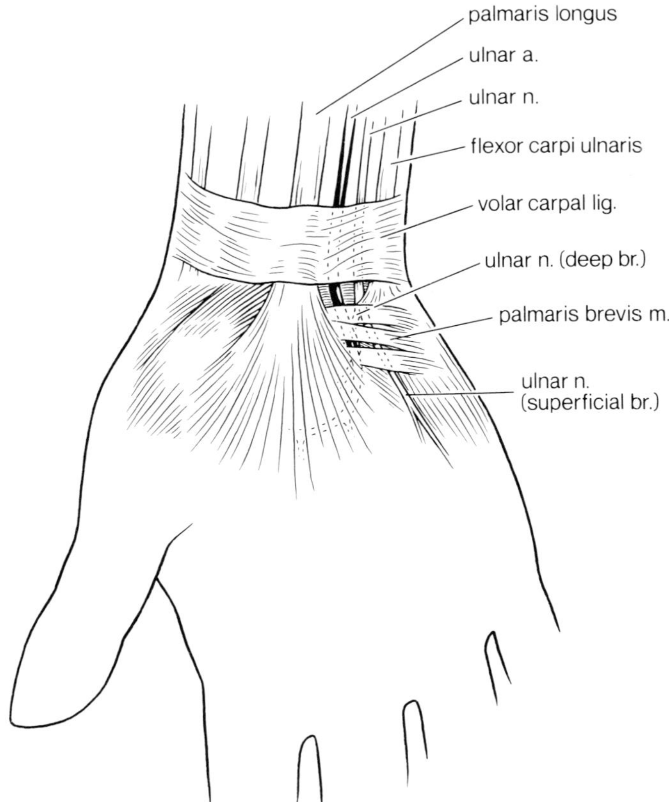

Fig. 135-5.　In decompressing the ulnar nerve at the wrist, it is necessary to divide the volar carpal ligament and the palmaris brevis.

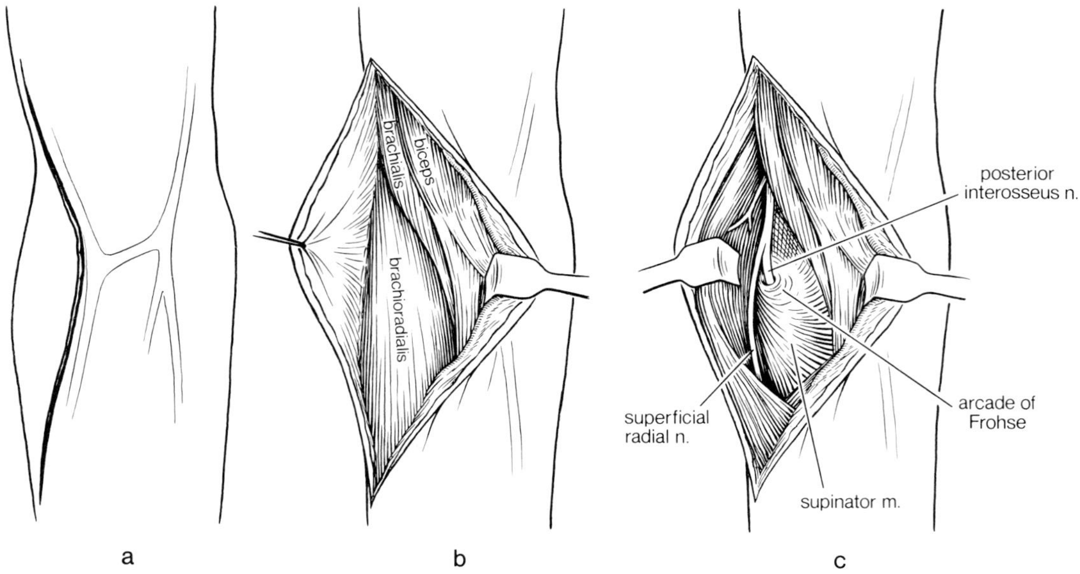

Fig. 135-6. Operative exposure of the posterior interosseous nerve. The arcade of Frohse, which runs between the heads of the supinator, may compress the posterior interosseous nerve just as the transverse carpal ligament compresses the median nerve at the wrist.

extend the thumb in a metacarpal plane; and (4) no sensory abnormalities.

The operative approach to the posterior interosseous nerve involves a curvilinear incision that avoids the cubital flexion crease (Figure 135-6). The nerve is identified as it runs between the brachialis and brachioradialis and is followed along its course beneath the brachioradialis to its point of division into superficial and deep branches. The posterior interosseous branch then is traced through the arcade of Frohse between the two heads of the supinator. Surgical treatment consists of division of the arcade of the Frohse. If clear evidence of compression by the arcade is absent intraoperatively, the nerve should be traced within the supinator muscle itself because adhesions within the supinator muscle may rarely cause posterior interosseous entrapment.

SUPRASCAPULAR NERVE ENTRAPMENT

Suprascapular nerve entrapment may occur as the nerve passes under the transverse scapular ligament through the suprascapular foramen[27] (Figure 135-7). Arising from the upper trunk of the brachial plexus, the suprascapular nerve runs laterally, deep to the trapezius and omohyoid muscles, and,

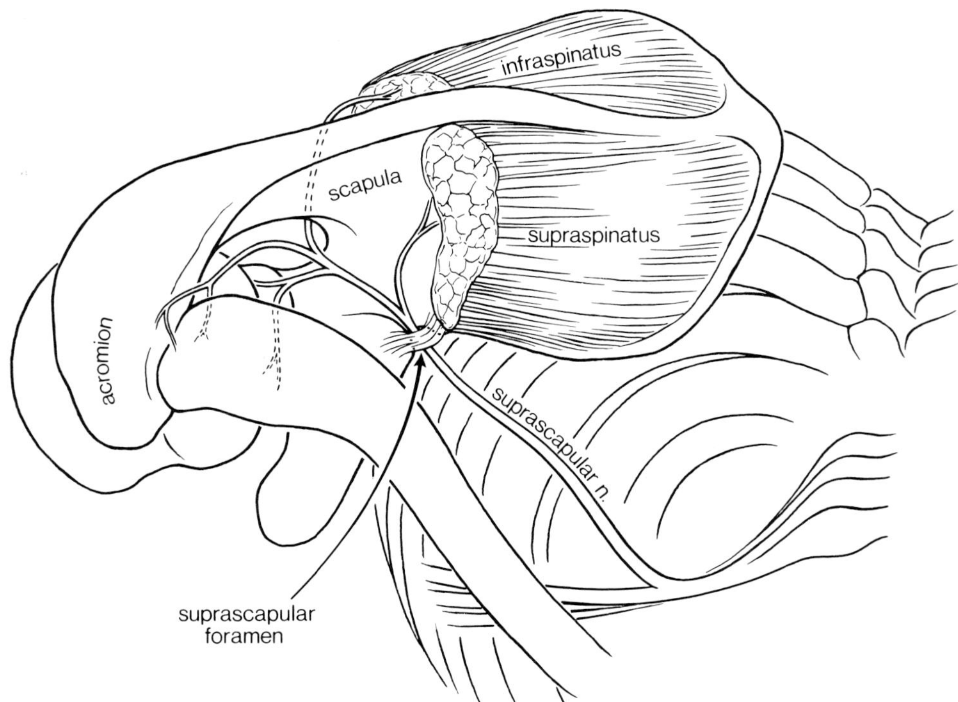

Fig. 135-7. Schematic diagram of the course of the suprascapular nerve.

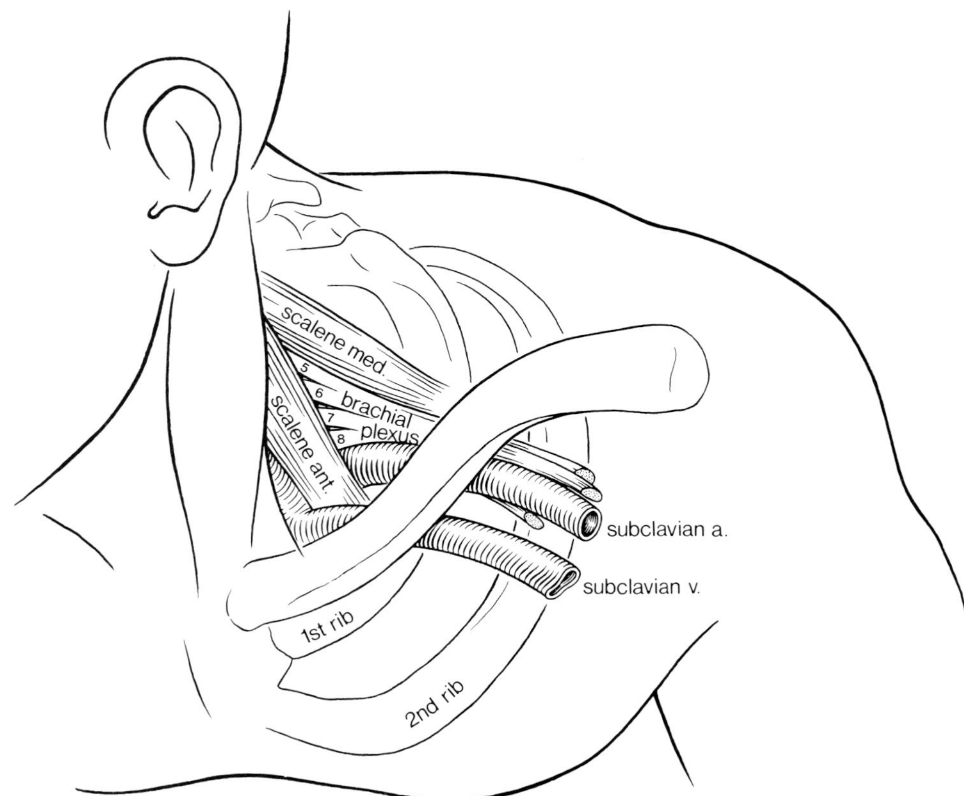

Fig. 135-8.   Anatomy of the thoracic outlet.

passing under the transverse scapular ligament through the suprascapular foramen, enters the supraspinous fossa. In the supraspinous fossa, the nerve gives branches to the supraspinatus muscle and then curves around the lateral border of the spine of the scapula to enter the infraspinous fossa, where it gives branches to the infraspinatus muscle. The nerve is relatively fixed at the level of the suprascapular foramen beneath the transverse scapular ligament, but the foramen constantly moves because of motion of the scapular during arm movement. Inflammatory reaction and swelling of the nerve beneath the ligament within the foramen may result.

Patients usually give a history of trauma to the shoulder area, either direct trauma, repetitive shoulder movements, or exaggerated shoulder movements. Pain is dull and aching and may radiate into the neck, medially into the interscapular area, or laterally down the arm. Wasting of the spinati muscles, pain on shoulder movement, and marked weakness on external rotation of the arm are prominent features. There are no sensory changes. The most accurate diagnostic test is EMG, showing denervation of the spinati muscles.

Surgical therapy consists of division of the transverse scapular ligament. The surgical procedure is as follows. With the patient in lateral position, a transverse incision is made parallel to and 1 inch above the spine of the scapula. The trapezius muscle is identified and divided along the length of its fibers. After identification of the underlying supraspinatus muscle, the upper border of the scapula is identified just medial to the origin of the omohyoid muscle. The transverse scapular ligament then is identified, and a flat dissector is inserted between the ligament and the underlying nerve. The ligament then is divided by cutting down on the dissector. When neural compression has been severe and of long standing, the nerve

bulges into the defect. Relief of pain is prompt following surgery, while recovery of motor function proceeds more slowly.

THORACIC OUTLET SYNDROME

Compression of the neurovascular bundle in the area of the thoracic outlet is the neuroanatomic common denominator for a variety of conditions described in the literature as hyperabduction syndrome,[28] scalenus anticus syndrome,[29] costoclavicular syndrome,[30] and Paget-Schroetter syndrome (subclavian-axillary vein thrombosis of effort).[31] All of these conditions are in reality merely special cases of thoracic outlet syndrome. The condition is best viewed as a special variety of peripheral entrapment neuropathy. Symptoms are more complex because they may be neural, vascular, or both. The same compressive force may affect the brachial plexus, the subclavian artery, and the subclavian vein. Successful surgical treatment requires adherence to several major principles: (1) The anatomic basis of neurovascular compression at the thoracic outlet must be thoroughly understood. (2) Diagnostic work-up must rule out a wide variety of other conditions often confused with thoracic outlet syndrome. Detailed inquiry must be made for vascular symptoms, since the vascular complications of the disease are potentially disastrous. (3) Successful surgical treatment involves complete decompression and a search for multiple areas of compression.

The anatomy of the thoracic outlet is illustrated in Figure 135-8. Neurovascular compression may have multiple causes: (1) The brachial plexus may be compressed at the interscalenic hiatus by the scalene muscles. Common insertion of the scalenus anticus and medius, posterior displacement of the normal scalenus anterior insertion, and unusually broad costal insertions of the scalenus minor and minimus all are anatomic variations that narrow the scalenic hiatus and may contribute to brachial plexopathy.[32] The upper cords of the brachial plexus may pass directly through the fibers of the scalene muscle.[33] The C7, C8, and T1 nerve roots may pass through the belly of the middle scalene muscle.[34] Gage and Parnell[33] postulated that trauma of the scalene muscle was a major cause of symptoms of thoracic outlet syndrome and reported microscopic changes in the scalene muscles including hypertrophy, inflammation, and degeneration. Sanders et al.,[34] however, detected microscopic changes in only 18 percent of cases in a large series of scalenectomies. Scalenus muscle spasm alone, in the absence of other predisposing anatomic causes, is now thought incapable of producing compressive symptoms.[35] (2) A wide variety of ligamentous structures and adhesions may cause neurovascular compression. Costocostal bands may originate from the anterolateral surface of the first rib and pass directly across the thoracic outlet to insert behind the scalene tubercle of the first rib. Fibrous bands are frequently associated with cervical ribs or elongated cervical transverse processes and extend from the tip of the first rib or elongated transverse process behind the brachial plexus to insert on the first rib. Scalenopleural bands[32] have been reported to cause compression of the lower roots of the brachial plexus. (3) A cervical rib may readily compress the overlying neurovascular bundle, both because of direct compression and because of the frequent presence of ligamentous bands between cervical ribs and the first rib. (4) The first rib is an extremely important structure because it forms part of the superior thoracic outlet, the scalenic hiatus, and the costoclavicular passage. Any abnormality of the first rib-thickening, unusual angulation, or bony exostoses-may compress the neurovascular bundle at any of these levels. Cadaveric dissection of asymptomatic patients[36] has demonstrated that the lower trunk of the brachial plexus composed of C8 and T1 makes contact with the first rib in all cases. Frequently the seventh cervical nerve makes contact with the first rib as well. (5) The costoclavicular hiatus is a potential site of neurovascular compression because of the repetitive scissoring action of the clavicle against the neurovascular bundle. The costoclavicular syndrome, pain and paresthesias in the upper extremity first described in soldiers carrying knapsacks in the military position, is due to this mechanism. Subclavian vein thrombosis at the costoclavicular passage, often occurring after extreme exercise or heavy labor, also is thought to be caused by shearing of the vein at the costoclavicular passage between the first rib and the subclavian muscle and costoclavicular ligament.[37] (6) Hyperabduction syndrome consists of pain and paresthesias and fatigability of the upper extremities produced upon hyperabduction of the arms. It often occurs in patients whose occupation entails prolonged abduction of the arms. The point of neurovascular compression is thought to be where the pectoralis minor tendon inserts on the coracoid process. Treatment is conservative, often by change of occupation.

The most common symptoms of thoracic outlet syndrome are supraclavicular pain, arm pain, and paresthesias, often in the fourth and fifth digits or in the entire hand, and, less often, in the first three fingers. Only 10 percent of patients have vascular symptomatology such as obliteration of the brachial or radial pulses, edema, peripheral cyanosis, and claudication. Physical examination often reveals supraclavicular tenderness, a fullness to palpation in the supraclavicular area, and tenderness over the brachial plexus, where evidence of a Tinel's sign

may be sought. Placing the upper extremity in provocative positions is of value. When the arm is abducted and externally rotated, it often is possible to reproduce the patient's symptoms. The shoulder also may be placed in the military position and the arms pulled forcefully downward, with production of paresthesias and pain. Adson's maneuver is no longer used because it is often positive in normal subjects. Evidence of Tinel's signs at the wrist and elbow should be sought to exclude a carpal tunnel or cubital tunnel syndrome, and local orthopedic pathology such as bicipital tendonitis and shoulder bursitis excluded.

Detailed electromyelography of the upper extremities is performed to rule out associated carpal tunnel syndrome, cubital tunnel syndrome, or cervical radiculopathy—any of which may mimic thoracic outlet syndrome. Ulnar nerve conduction studies across the thoracic outlet may be slowed in up to 61 percent of cases,[38] but are often only minimally depressed. Normal ulnar conduction across the outlet in no way excludes the diagnosis of thoracic outlet syndrome. Where necessary, cervical myelography is performed to exclude a herniated cervical disc when this diagnosis remains a possibility. Apical lordotic views of the chest are done to exclude a tumor of the pulmonary apex infiltrating the brachial plexus. Cervical spine films and plain x-ray films of the upper ribs are useful to exclude osseous abnormalities such as cervical rib and elongated transverse processes. Doppler ultrasonography[39] will detect significant arterial obstruction with the arm in provocative positions. The presence of vascular symptomatology is a definite indication for subclavian angiography and venography. Vascular complications of thoracic outlet syndrome occur in less than 10 percent of cases but are extremely serious. Poststenotic dilatation, aneurysm, mural thrombus with distal embolization, and total occlusion of the subclavian artery have been reported.[40] Retrograde thrombosis of the subclavian artery may result in a stroke.[41] These arterial complications may endanger the life of the patient and the viability of the extremity. Although these arterial complications may be due to compression by fibrous bands or adhesions, they are more often associated with osseous abnormalities[42] such as cervical rib, hypoplastic first ribs joining the second rib at the insertion of the anterior scalene muscle, osseous exostoses of the first rib, or elongated seventh cervical transverse processes with associated fibrous bands. The presence of arterial symptomatology demands a detailed radiographic search for bony abnormalities. Positional angiography[43] has to be interpreted cautiously, since normal subjects may obliterate their pulses in provocative positions.

Indications for surgery include significant vascular pathology, and, among patients with primarily neural symptoms, lack of response to conservative therapy such as heat, massage, and exercises to strengthen the musculature of the shoulder girdle. Scalenectomy alone is often but not invariably an inadequate procedure, carrying up to a 50 percent recurrence rate.[44] This procedure ignores the important restraining influence of the first rib at the superior thoracic outlet, scalene hiatus, and costoclavicular passage. The infraclavicular and posterior thoracoplasty approaches to the thoracic outlet are now rarely used. Two major approaches to the thoracic outlet are used in most centers: (1) transaxillary resection of the first rib combined with scalenectomy,[45] and (2) a supraclavicular approach. Advantages of the transaxillary procedure are that the first rib may be more completely removed posteriorly than through the supraclavicular approach. Also, the second rib may act to compress the neurovascular bundle even after the first rib is removed; the second rib may be inspected after removal of the first rib to see if it is compressing the brachial plexus, and, if necessary, resected—all of which is not possible through the supraclavicular approach. We prefer the supraclavicular approach, however, because the pathologic anatomy is better displayed, the phrenic nerve can be identified fully and protected, the brachial plexus can be thoroughly inspected for the presence of fibrous bands, and the plexus and axillary vessels can be viewed directly as the first rib is removed. When causalgic symptoms accompany thoracic outlet syndrome, sympathectomy of the lower stellate ganglion and the first three thoracic sympathetic ganglia can be performed through either approach.

Our own surgical approach emphasizes complete decompression (Figure 135-9). Scalenectomy and resection of the first rib are performed, cervical ribs are resected if they are compressing the brachial plexus, and the plexus is explored in detail for evidence of fibrous bands. We use a supraclavicular incision over the lateral aspect of the sternocleidomastoid. After the deep cervical fascia is incised, the phrenic nerve and the anterior scalene muscles are identified. The phrenic nerve and accessory phrenic nerves are dissected free from the fascia investing the anterior scalene muscle. On the left side the thoracic duct and associated lymphatic channels pass in a loop toward the angle formed by the subclavian and internal jugular veins. These should be treated gently, and the thoracic duct should be protected with wet cottonoids. The scalene muscles then may be divided close to the first rib. The anterior and middle scalene muscles are sectioned and allowed to retract so that the scalene hiatus is completely free. The undersurface of the brachial plexus then is explored for the presence of aberrant muscle fibers and restricting bands inserting on the first rib. The first rib then is removed with Kerrison rongeurs from the costochondral junction to the transverse process posteriorly. Cervical ribs are resected if they are adjudged to be causing neurovascular compression. Any fascial tissue extending from transverse processes of cervical vertebrae or from cervical ribs over the cupola of the lung is divided. By this procedure, the neurovascular bundle is freed of fibrous bands and osseous restraints, and, in addition, a patulous passage for the neurovascular bundle from the cervical to the axillary regions is created by removal of the first rib. Thrombectomy and vascular reconstruction, if indicated, are performed by vascular surgeons. If necessary, the supraclavicular incision may be extended below the clavicle and claviculectomy performed if it is necessary to trace the axillary vessels into the axilla for major vascular reconstruction.

LATERAL FEMORAL CUTANEOUS NERVE ENTRAPMENT

The lateral femoral cutaneous nerve, which supplies sensation to the lateral aspect of the thigh, arises from the roots of L2 and L3 and, after running under the iliac fascia, passes through an opening in the lateral attachment of the inguinal ligament at the anterior superior pubic spine into the subcutaneous tissue of the thigh (Figure 135-10). Entrapment neuropathy occurs where the nerve pierces the inguinal ligament and results in burning dysesthesias in the anterolateral aspect of the thigh—"meralgia paresthetica."

The condition most often appears without antecedent history of trauma. The mechanism of nerve injury is probably a pulling of the nerve by fascial attachments in the thigh against the opening for the nerve at the lateral edge of the inguinal ligament. Conservative therapy consists of weight reduction and anti-inflammatory medication. If these fail, surgical neurolysis, involving decompression of the nerve as it passes through its canal within the inguinal ligament, is indicated. The nerve is approached through an incision beginning 2 to 3 cm above the anterior superior iliac spine, passing along the edge of the ilium, and extending around and medial to the anterior superior iliac spine down toward the thigh, overlying the interspace between the sartorius and tensor fascia lata muscles. The nerve is identified distally as it passes beneath the tensor fascia lata and penetrates the fascia lata; it then can be traced to the area of entrapment within the inguinal ligament. Neurolysis is carried out several centimeters proximal to the point where the nerve penetrates the inguinal ligament, in order to free the nerve proximally from its fascial investments.

POSTERIOR TIBIAL NERVE ENTRAPMENT

Entrapment neuropathy of the posterior tibial nerve may occur immediately below and behind the medial malleolus. The neurovascular bundle, accompanied by the tendons of the tibialis posterior, flexor digitorum longus, and flexor hallucis longus, occupies a groove behind the medial malleolus. The lancinate ligament provides a roof under which these structures pass through a tunnel known as the tarsal tunnel (Figure 135-11). Entrapment neuropathy at this point is called the tarsal tunnel syndrome and is analogous to the carpal tunnel syndrome at the wrist. Beyond the edge of the lancinate ligament the nerve branches into medial plantar, lateral plantar, and calcaneal branches. They supply the sole of the foot, the plantar surface of the toes, and the plantar intrinsic musculature.

Compression at the level of the lancinate ligament results in pain and dysesthesias in the toes and sole of the foot, progressing to sensory and motor loss. Pain may be referred retrograde along the sciatic axis to the buttock. When motor disturbance occurs, the foot assumes a pes cavus position and clawing of the toes occurs. Pressure over the retromalleolar region often results in pain radiating into the sole of the foot. Putting the ankle in the valgus position aggravates the pain, while the varus position lessens the pain because it slackens the lancinate ligament. Electromyographic and nerve conduction studies are useful in diagnosis, but muscle sampling in the foot is extremely painful.

The condition may occur as a sequela of fracture, posttraumatic edema with resultant fibrosis, tenosynovitis, or venous engorgement of the posterior tibial veins due to peripheral vascular insufficiency. It also may be caused by thickening of the lancinate ligament secondary to systemic connective tissue diseases.

Conservative therapy consists of anti-inflammatory agents and correction of abnormal foot mechanics by use of a support, when necessary. Potential causative factors such as tenosynovitis or venous insufficiency should be corrected by medial or surgical means if they are present. Neurosurgical intervention becomes necessary when persistent pain or motor deficit occurs, or when conservative measures fail. Satisfactory relief is obtained by section of the lancinate ligament and external neurolysis of the nerve. It is advisable to trace the nerve distally to its trifurcation and to visualize the entrance of each of the plantar nerves into the foot so that compressive lesions of these branches distal to the lancinate ligament are not overlooked.

scalene med.
brachial plexus
ext.
jugular v.
phrenic n.
clavicle
scalene ant.
subclavian a.
thoracic duct
A
B

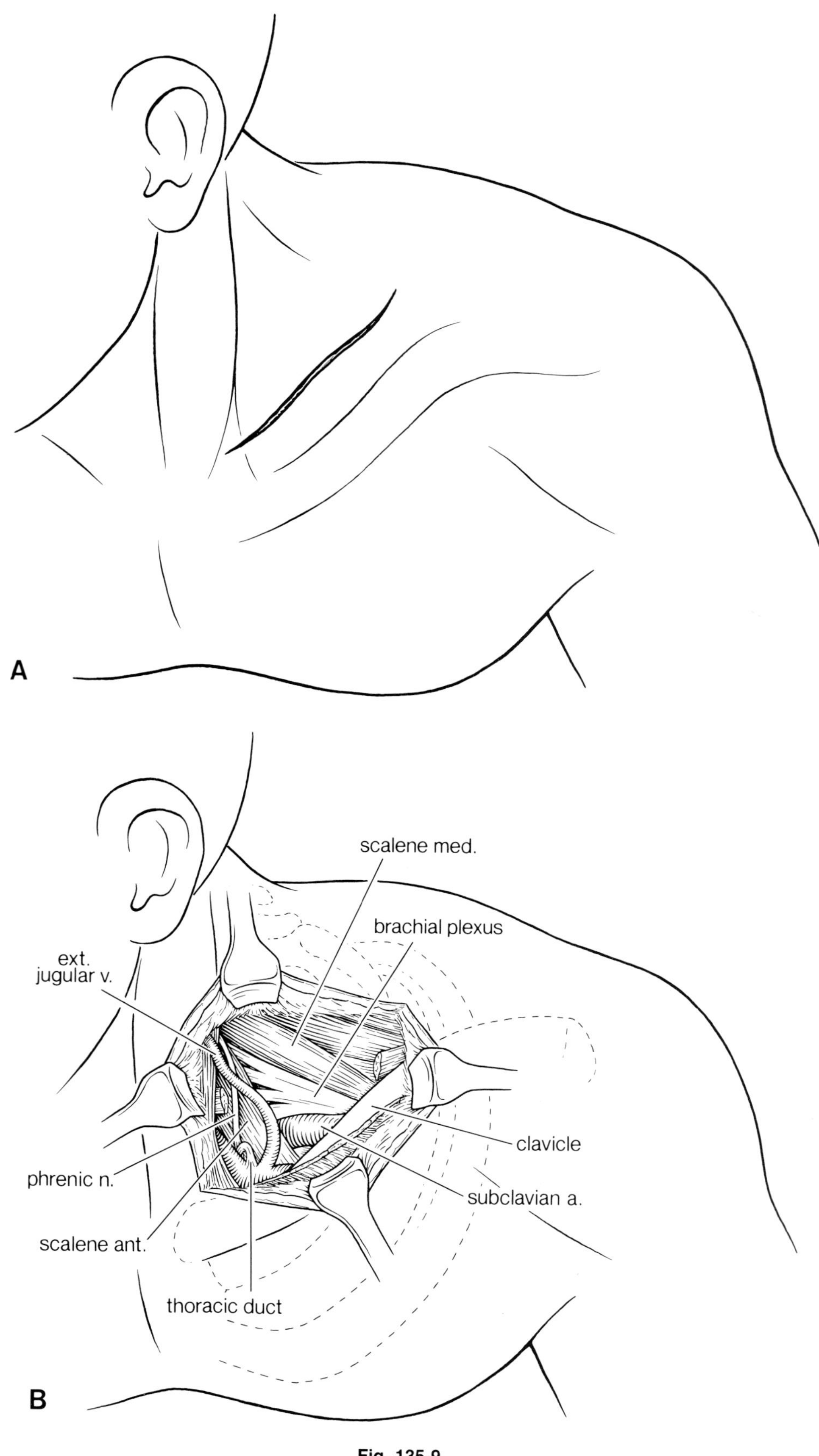

Fig. 135-9

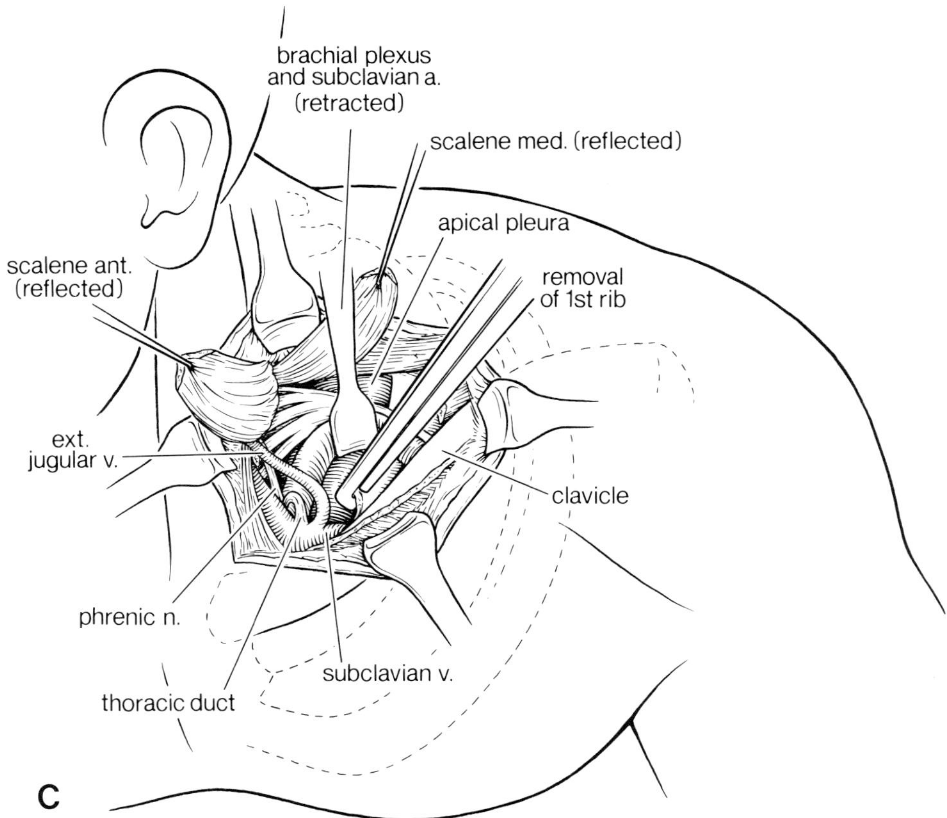

Fig. 135-9. (A through C) Steps in the supraclavicular approach to thoracic outlet decompression.

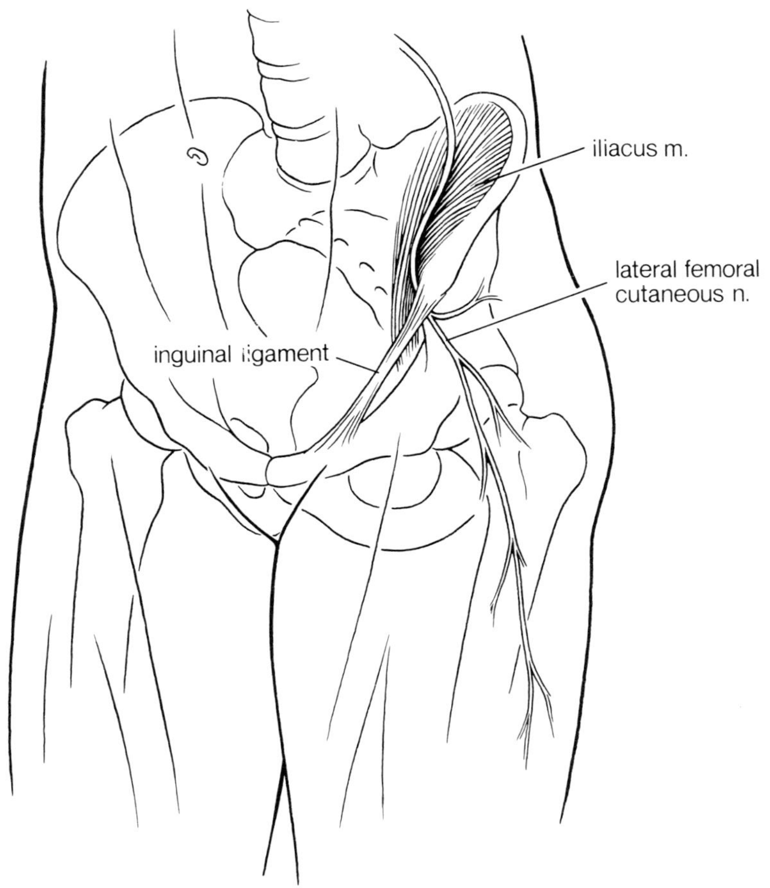

Fig. 135-10. Schematic diagram of the course of the lateral femoral cutaneous nerve.

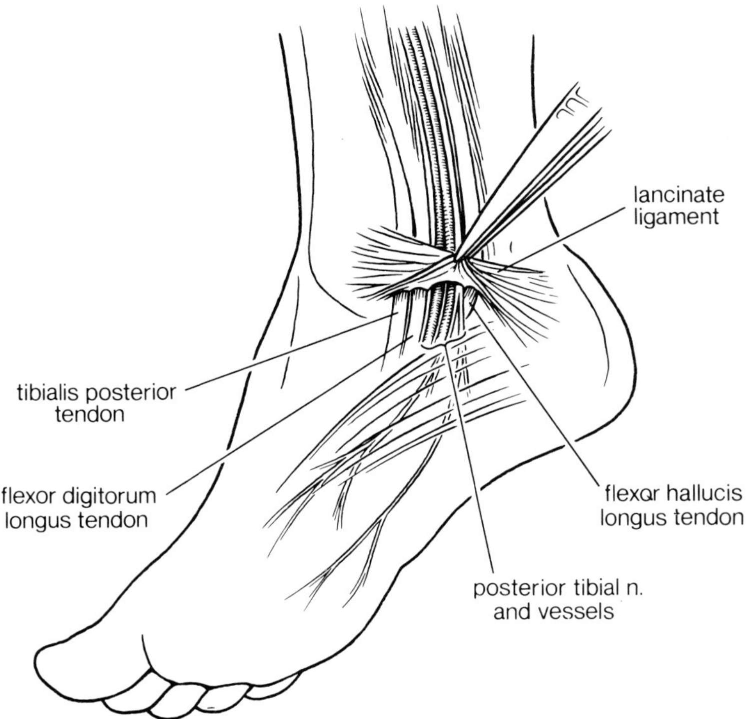

Fig. 135-11. Schematic diagram of the tarsal tunnel.

COMMON PERONEAL NERVE COMPRESSION

The common peroneal nerve is vulnerable to compression neuropathy in the area of the fibular neck. The common peroneal nerve is derived from the bifurcation of the sciatic nerve in the lower thigh. It runs down the lateral aspect of the popliteal fossa and passes between the biceps femoris tendon and the lateral head of the gastrocnemius. It then pierces the deep fascia and passes around the neck of the fibula through an opening in the origin of the peroneus longus muscle. This opening is essentially a gap between the sites of attachment of the peroneus longus to the head and to the body of the fibula. At or immediately beyond the opening in the origin of the peroneus

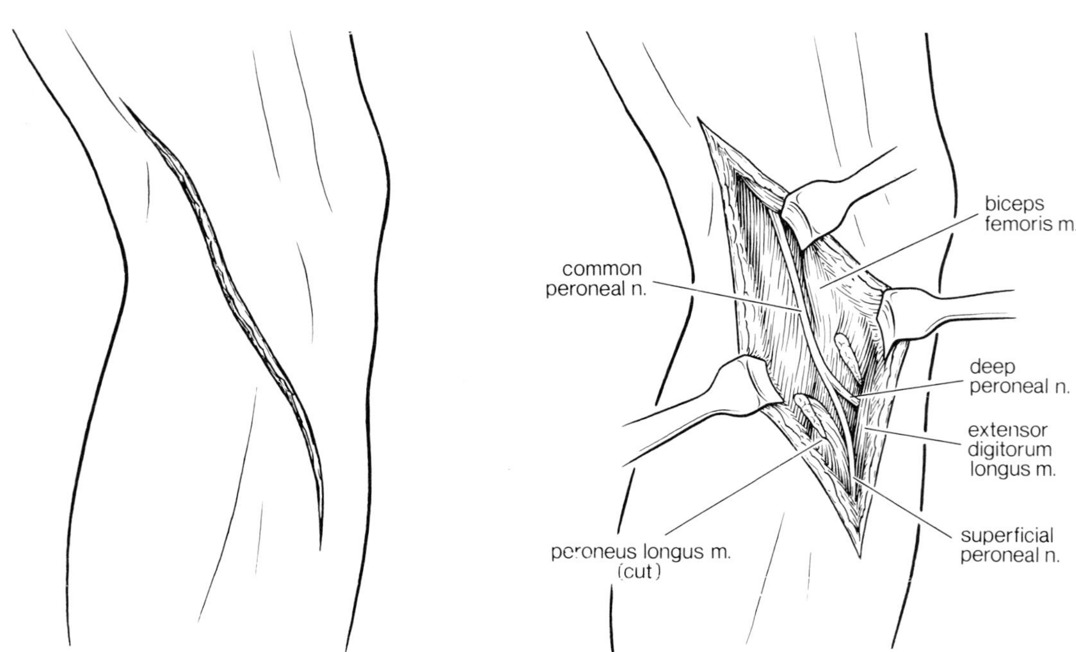

Fig. 135-12. Operative exposure of the common peroneal nerve at the fibular head. Surgical decompression is achieved by division of the superficial portion of the peroneus longus.

longus, the nerve divides into its superficial and deep components.

The nerve is extremely vulnerable to injury as it crosses the fibula through the opening in the peroneus. Usually a history of trauma is elicited. Direct blunt trauma may injure the nerve at this level by impacting it against the fibula. Fibular fracture places the nerve at risk because of the possibility of both laceration by bony fragments and fibrosis secondary to local soft tissue edema. Trauma producing sudden, strong inversion at the ankle may produce a traction injury of the nerve as it passes over the fibular head through the origin of the peroneus longus. Pressure palsy is quite common at the fibular neck and may occur when patients lie on their side. Structural lesions in the popliteal fossa—such as laterally located popliteal cysts—may produce the lesion.

Pain in the lateral aspect of the leg and foot is a common presenting symptom. Pain may radiate up the sciatic axis to the buttock. Sensory loss in the dorsum of the foot and weakness of dorsiflexion and eversion of the foot may result.

So vulnerable is the common peroneal nerve as it curves around the fibular head that exposure of the nerve in this area is the most common neural decompression procedure in the lower extremity. The surgical procedure is illustrated in Figure 135-12. The incision extends from proximal to distal along the medial border of the biceps femoris, to the level of the fibular neck, and over the peroneal compartment distally. After opening the fascia lata, the biceps femoris is identified, and medial and deep to it the common peroneal nerve is found. It is then traced distally as it passes between the tendinous insertion of the biceps femoris and the lateral portion of the gastrocnemius. The lateral sural cutaneous nerve, arising high from the medial portion of the common peroneal nerve, should be identified and protected. The nerve is traced as it passes behind the biceps femoris toward the fibular neck. After the nerve has been identified as it passes through the peroneus longus, the more superficial portion of the peroneus longus may be divided and detached and the superficial and deep peroneal branches identified. The division of the small superficial portion of the peroneus and resultant close approximation of the nerve to the subcutaneous tissues carry no significant complication.

REFERENCES

1. Lewis T, Pickering GW, Rothschild P: Centripetal paralysis arising out of arrested blood flow to the limb, including notes on a form of tingling. Heart 16:1, 1931
2. Seddon HJ: Three types of nerve injury. Brain 66:237, 1943
3. Denny-Brown D, Brenner C: Paralysis of nerve induced by direct pressure and by tourniquet. Arch Neurol Psychol 51:1, 1944
4. Denny-Brown D, Brenner C: Lesions in peripheral nerve resulting from compression by spring clip. Arch Neurol Psychol 52:1, 1944
5. Grundfest H: Effects of hydrostatic pressures upon the excitability, the recovery, and the potential sequence of frog nerve. Cold Spring Harbor Symp Quant Biol 4:179, 1936
6. Gilliatt RW, Ochoa J, Rudge P, et al: The cause of nerve damage in acute compression. Trans Am Neurol Assoc 99:71, 1974
7. Neary D, Ochoa J, Gilliatt RW: Subclinical entrapment neuropathy in man. J Neurol Sci 24:283, 1976
8. Ochoa J, Marotte L: The nature of the nerve lesion caused by chronic entrapment in the guinea pig. J Neurol Sci 19:491, 1973
9. Fullerton PM, Gilliatt RW: Median and ulnar neuropathy in the guinea pig. J Neurol Neurosurg Psychiatry 30:393, 1967
10. Sunderland S: The nerve lesion in the carpal tunnel syndrome. J Neurol Neurosurg Psychiatry 39:615, 1976
11. Kuczynski K: Functional micro-anatomy of the peripheral nerve trunks. Hand 6:1, 1974
12. Woodhall B, Nulsen F, White J, et al: Neurosurgical Implications in Peripheral Nerve Regeneration. Washington, D.C., Veterans Administration Monograph, 1957, pp 569–638
13. Upton ARM, McComas AJ: The double-crush in nerve entrapment syndromes. Lancet 2:359, 1973
14. Rydevik B, Lundborg G, Nordborg C: Intraneural tissue reactions induced by internal neurolysis. Scand J Plast Reconstr Surg 10:3, 1976
15. Spinner MS: Injuries to the Major Branches of Peripheral Nerves of the Forearm. Philadelphia, WB Saunders, 1978, p 37
16. Curtis RM, Eversmann WW: Internal neurolysis as an adjunct to the treatment of the carpal tunnel syndrome. J Bone Joint Surg 55A:733, 1973
17. Brown BA: Internal neurolysis in traumatic peripheral nerve lesions in continuity. Surg Clin North Am 52:1167, 1972
18. Kline DG, Nulsen FE: The neuroma in continuity. Its preoperative and operative management. Surg Clin North Am 52:1189, 1972
19. Kummel BM, Zazanis GA: Shoulder pain as the presenting complaint in carpal tunnel syndrome. Clin Orthop 92:227, 1973
20. Taleisnik J: The palmar cutaneous branch of the median nerve and the approach to the carpal tunnel. J Bone Joint Surg 55A:1212, 1973
21. Kane E, Kaplam EB, Spinner M: Observations on the course of the ulnar nerve in the arm. Ann Chir 27:487, 1973
22. Apfelberg DB, Larson SJ: Dynamic anatomy of the ulnar nerve at the elbow. Plast Reconstr Surg 51:76, 1973
23. Neblett C, Ehni G: Medial epicondylectomy for ulnar palsy. J Neurosurg 32:55, 1970
24. Osborne G: Compression neuritis of the ulnar nerve at the elbow. Hand 2:10, 1970
25. Learmonth JR: Technique for transplanting the ulnar nerve. Surg Gynecol Obstet 75:792, 1942
26. Broudy AS, Leffert RD, Smith RJ: Technical problems with ulnar nerve transposition at the elbow: findings and results of operation. J Hand Surg 3:85, 1977
27. Rengachary SS, Burr D, Lucas S, et al: Suprascapular entrapment neuropathy: a clinical, anatomical, and comparative study. Part 2: Anatomical study. Neurosurgery 5:447, 1979
28. Wright IS: The neurovascular syndrome produced by hyperabduction of the arms; immediate changes produced in 150 normal controls, and effects on some persons of prolonged hyperabduction of arms as in sleeping, and in certain occupations. Am Heart J 29:1, 1945
29. Adson AW, Coffey JR: Cervical rib, method of anterior approach for relief of symptoms by division of the scalenus anticus. Ann Surg 83:839, 1927
30. Falconer MA, Weddel G: Costoclavicular compression of the subclavian artery and vein; relation to the scalenus anticus syndrome. Lancet 2:539, 1943
31. Hughes ESR: Collective review, venous obstruction in the upper extremity (Paget-Schroetter's syndrome), review of 320 cases. Surg Gynecol Obstet (Suppl):88, 1949
32. Pollak EW: Surgical anatomy of the thoracic outlet syndrome. Surg Gynecol Obstet 150:97, 1980
33. Gage M, Parnell H: Scalenus anticus syndrome. Am J Surg 73:252, 1947
34. Sanders RJ, Monsour JW, Gerber WF, et al: Scalenectomy versus first rib resection for treatment of the thoracic outlet syndrome. Surgery 85:109, 1979
35. Clagett OT: Presidential address: Research and prosearch. J Thorac Cardiovasc Surg 44:153, 1962
36. Williams HT, Carpenter NH: Surgical treatment of the thoracic outlet compression syndrome. Arch Surg 113:850, 1978
37. Etheredge S, Wilbur B, Stoney RJ: Am J Surg 138:175, 1979
38. McGough EC, Pearce MB, Byrne JP: J Thorac Cardiovasc Surg 77:169, 1979
39. Pisko-Dubienski ZA, Hollingsworth J: Can J Surg 21:145, 1978

40. Judy KL, Heymann RI: Vascular complications of thoracic outlet syndrome. Am J Surg 123:521, 1972
41. Samiy E: Thrombosis of the internal carotid artery caused by a cervical rib. J Neurosurg 12:181, 1955
42. Dorazio RA, Ezzet F: Arterial complications of the thoracic outlet syndrome. Am J Surg 138:246, 1979
43. Winsor T, Borw R: Costoclavicular syndrome, diagnosis and treatment. JAMA 196:697, 1966
44. Raaf J: Surgery for cervical rib and scalenus anticus syndrome. JAMA 157:219, 1955
45. Roos DB: Experience with first rib resection for thoracic outlet syndrome. Ann Surg 173:429, 1971

CHAPTER 136

Peripheral Nerve Tumors

Alan R. Hudson   Fred Gentili   David Kline

THE SURGEON who undertakes the management of patients harboring peripheral nerve tumors should have absolute mastery of the gross anatomy of the region, a complete appreciation of the internal structure of nerves, and a thorough understanding of the normal histology of peripheral nerves and aberrations of cell growth which result in peripheral nerve neoplasm.[1] While the range and complexity of cellular pathology in the entire spectrum of peripheral nerve tumors is extensive, fortunately the commonly encountered neoplasms have characteristic macroscopic and microscopic features that are easily recognizable.[2] The writings of Harkin on this topic are lucid and are required reading for any neurosurgeon undertaking peripheral nerve tumor surgery.[3] The peripheral nerve surgeon must work in close conjunction with a truly expert neuropathologist. Few neurosurgeons or neuropathologists gain the necessary experience and, in most instances, it is far preferable to refer a patient to a center specializing in this type of work. This arena is not one for the occasional operator or the occasional neuropathologist.[4] The risk of significant neurologic deficit, nonneurologic morbidity, and even death is significant, and inadequate technical surgery or histologic diagnosis can result in catastrophic disability.

CLASSIFICATION OF PERIPHERAL NERVE TUMORS

The sophisticated classification of peripheral nerve tumors based on histologic characteristics is a matter of interest and fascination.[5] Because there is considerable debate surrounding the relationship of Schwann cells, perineurial cells, and endoneurial fibroblasts, it is scarcely surprising that there is considerable debate over the exact nomenclature that should be employed in the classification of neoplasms derived from these cells.[6] The practicing surgeon, however, while appreciating just how complex a matter this is, is best served by adopting a simple, practical classification that will guide him or her in the judgments required for patient management (Table 136-1).

CLINICAL DIAGNOSIS

The clinical diagnosis of nerve tumor may present significant difficulty insofar as a nerve tumor is frequently not considered in the differential diagnosis of a mass or of a pain. The classical clinical feature is that the mass can be displaced at right angles to the course of the peripheral nerve but not in a longitudinal manner. While the surgeon is palpating the mass, the patient may complain of induced paresthesia in a distribution appropriate to that particular peripheral nerve. Tapping the mass may likewise give rise to appropriate sensory phenomena. If a peripheral nerve tumor is suspected, evidence of other nerve tumors and Von Recklinghausen's disease is sought. Computed tomographic and MRI scanning may be useful in delineating the true extent of a tumor and, on occasion, angiography and myelography are required (Figure 136-1). Any suspected nerve tumor situated close to the spine should have the medial extent of the tumor carefully defined (Figure 136-2). Dumbell neurofibromas require prior spinal surgery in the majority of cases. If the diagnosis of a peripheral nerve tumor is made on clinical grounds, the surgeon must appreciate that he or she cannot ascertain, at that stage, whether or not he or she is dealing with a schwannoma or neurofibroma or malignant nerve tumor, so it is best to refer such a patient to an appropriate center so that the definitive diagnosis and definitive surgery can be undertaken.

INTRAOPERATIVE DIAGNOSIS

Because peripheral nerve tumors are infrequently regarded during the differential diagnosis of a mass, it is not unusual for such a mass to be discovered during an exploratory operation. The expertise of the surgeon making such a discovery is usually related to his or her own specialty and not to the management of peripheral nerve tumors. Hopefully, the anatomic relationship of the mass to the peripheral nerve structure is appreciated either as a result of inspection of the structures or as a result of muscle contraction following cautery of blood vessels close to the mass, before significant neurologic damage is created. If a surgeon is not an expert peripheral nerve surgeon and if expert neuropathologic help is not available, the appropriate maneuver is then to close the skin without a biopsy. Injudicious biopsy by itself can create significant neurologic disability (Figure 136-3).

INTRINSIC PERIPHERAL NERVE TUMORS

SCHWANNOMA

The outstanding principle guiding the peripheral nerve surgeon is that the schwannoma is a benign tumor and that it is possible to resect the tumor with no or minimal neurologic loss as a result of the surgical maneuver.

OPERATIVE NEUROSURGICAL TECHNIQUES
ISBN 0-8089-1862-1

Table 136-1. Classification of peripheral
nerve tumors

Intrinsic Peripheral Nerve Tumors
    Schwannoma
    Neurofibroma
    Malignant peripheral nerve tumor
    Miscellaneous
Extrinsic Peripheral Nerve Tumors
    Compressive
    Invasive

Anaesthesia

The operation is conducted under general anaesthetic but the anesthetist must be warned that the surgeon may wish to stimulate the nerve during the operation. The effect of short acting agents used for intubation will have worn off by the time the mass is exposed.

Position

The patient is positioned so as to allow easy access to the mass. The draping should be appropriately arranged to allow observation of distal musculature during nerve stimulation. A single leg is prepared in case a sural nerve graft is required. At this time it is appropriate to decide the future positioning of the microscope so that the operator and his or her assistants will be able to sit comfortably during the microsurgical phase of the operation. As in any neurosurgical procedure, a few extra

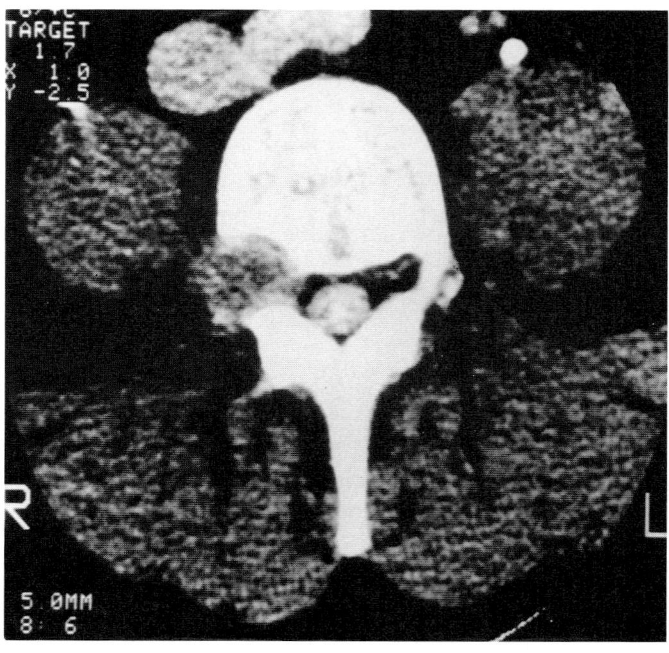

Fig. 136-2. This patient presented with pain and neurologic disability. The myelogram was normal. The scan clearly delineates the position of the schwannoma within the intervertebral foramen (right).

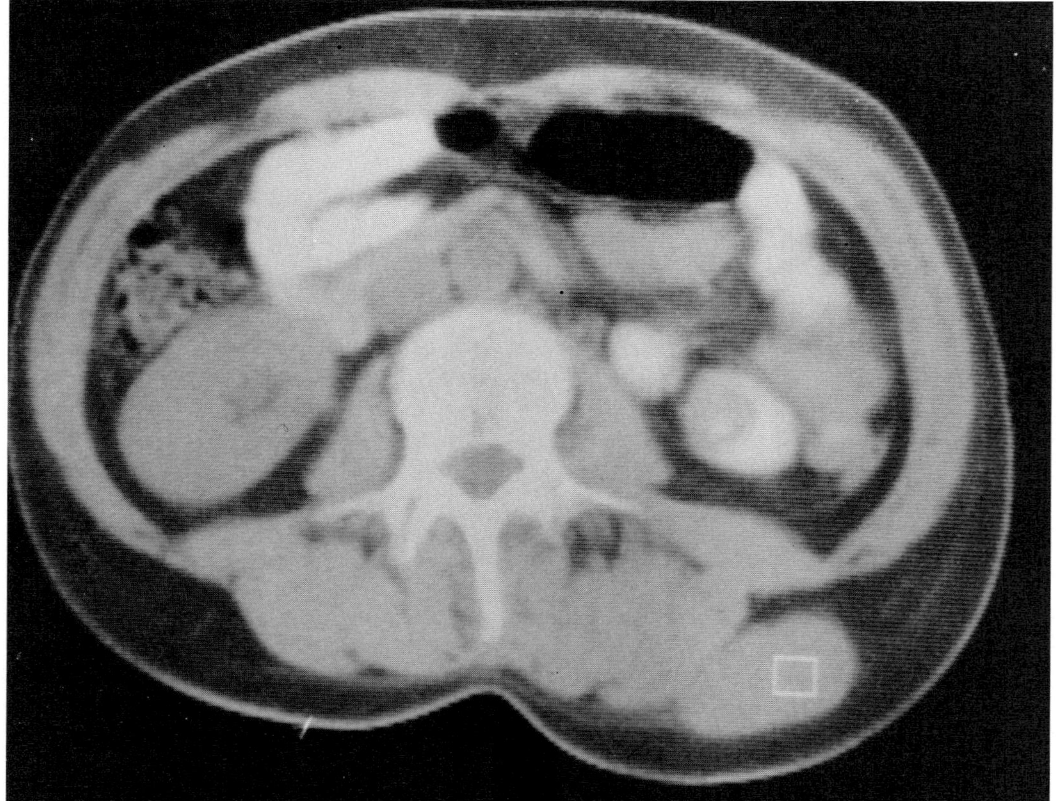

Fig. 136-1. The patient presented with a mass. The CT scan clearly outlines the extent of this malignant peripheral nerve tumor. (Cursor is superimposed over the neoplasm.)

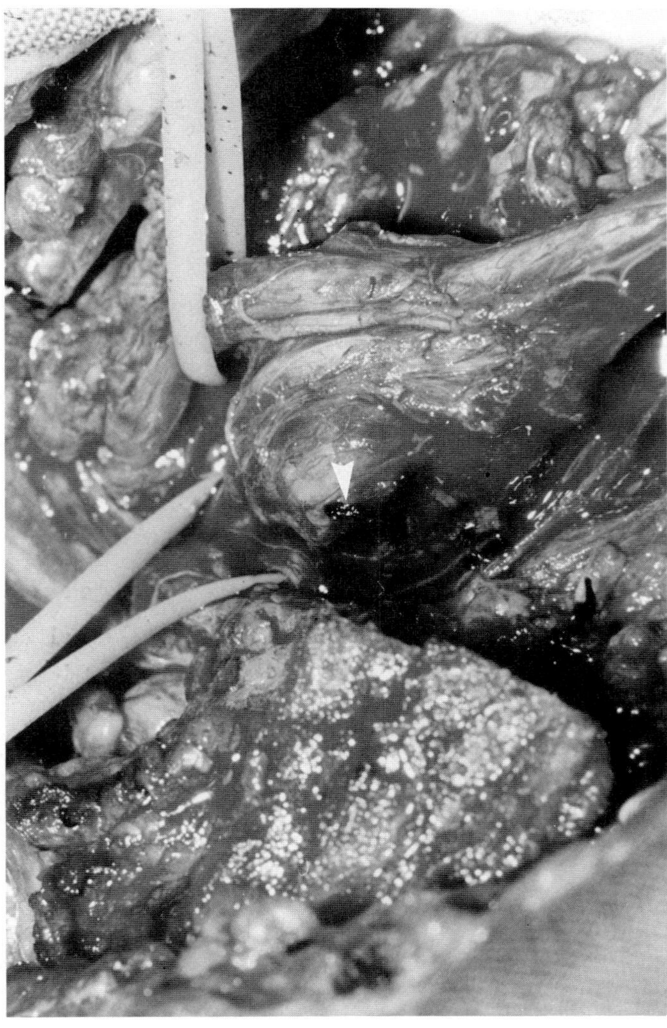

Fig. 136-3. Brachial plexus tumor. Previous biopsy and suturing (arrow) of this schwannoma resulted in significant neurologic loss.

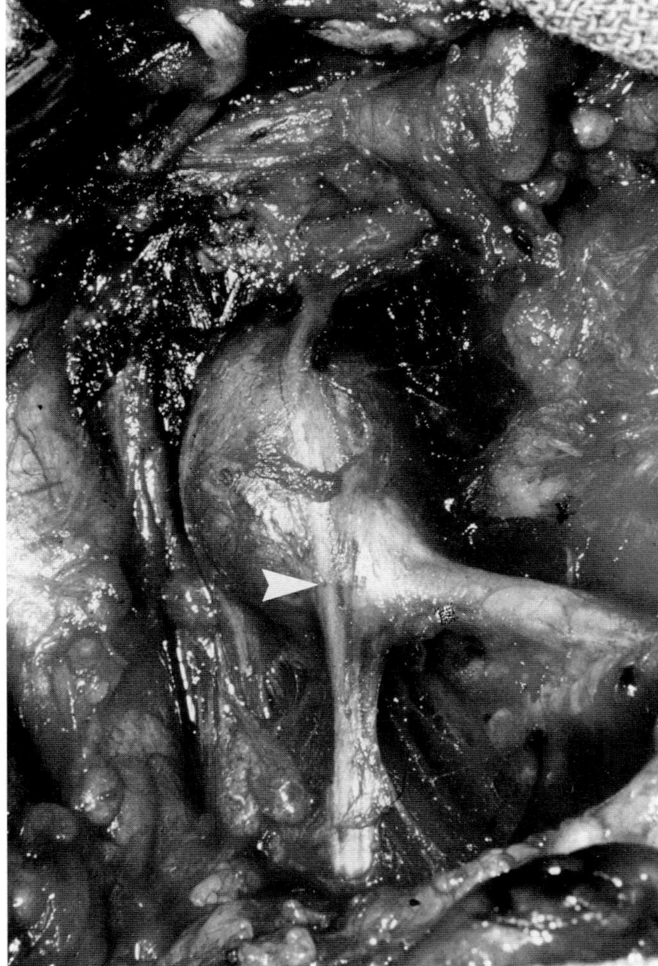

Fig. 136-4. Brachial plexus tumor (left). The initial dissection outlines the phrenic nerve, which is adherent to the anterior aspect of this proximally placed schwannoma. (Arrow: phrenic nerve.)

minutes invested at this phase of the operation will pay dividends at a later stage of the surgery.

Instrumentation

Two sets of instruments are required. The first is a standard set to allow dissection of the appropriate region and the second is a standard microsurgical set. A variable voltage nerve stimulator with its sterilized electrodes should be available if required.

Operation

The exposure of the nerve bearing the mass is usually a matter of standard surgical technique. The incision should be generous to allow a clear view of normal nerve on either side of the mass (Figure 136-4). If the operation is being performed close to an entrapment area, e.g., the carpal tunnel, such entrapment sites should be divided at this stage.[7] A dissection of the nerve trunk is facilitated by passing Silastic slings around the nerve proximal and distal to the mass. All adjacent structures should be dissected free and the surgeon should be certain that self retaining retractors are not compromising important structures (Figure 136-5). Finally, an appropriate plastic sheet is

passed behind the mass, providing a background for microsurgical dissection.

The microscope is then brought into position and the arrangement of the fascicles relative to the tumor mass is studied. In the case of smaller tumors, e.g., less than 0.5 cm, the mass may be situated within the center of the nerve, with fascicles and groups of fascicles equidistant from one another as they flow around the spindle shaped mass. As the tumor grows larger, the tendency is for the mass to expand between certain fascicular groups and the surgeon is likely to observe that the majority of fascicles are grouped together on one side of the tumor (Figure 136-6). Just as dissection in a plane parallel to the main nerve trunk is least likely to result in injury during the macroscopic phase of the operation, so should incision of the epineurial tissues superficial to the capsule be made in a longitudinal direction to avoid damaging fascicular groups. The plane around the capsule of the tumor is usually quite obvious and once the surrounding tissues have been incised from the proximal to the distal pole in a longitudinal fashion, the mobilized fascicles or fascicular groups can be slid around the mass as if one was raising or lowering a bucket handle (Figure 136-7). It is essential to dissect in the correct plane, which is immediately superficial to the tumor capsule. It is usually unnecessary

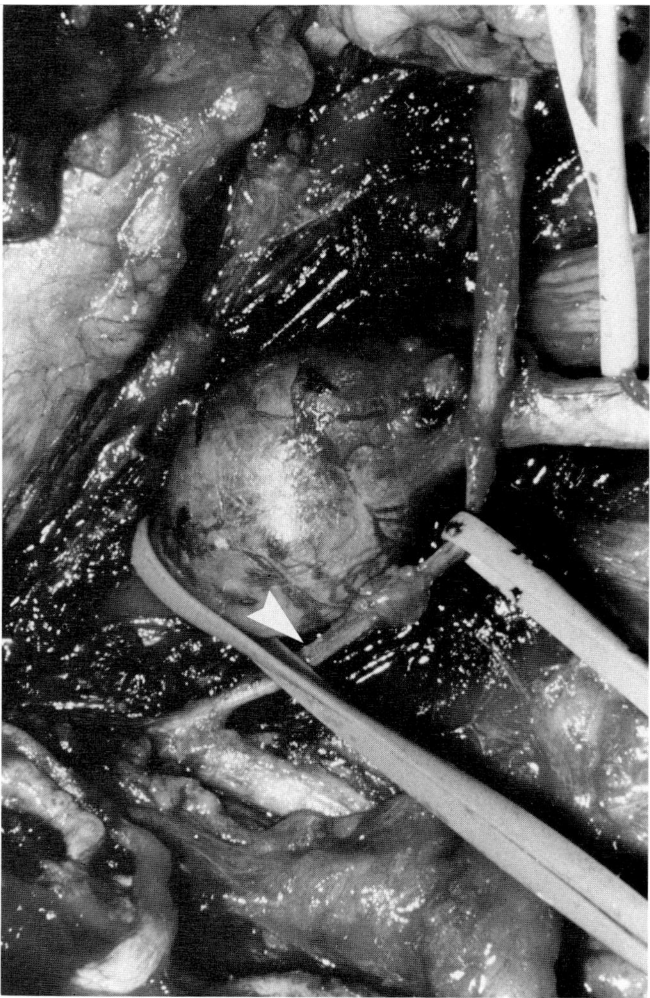

Fig. 136-5.   Brachial plexus tumor (left). The macroscopic dissection of the region clearly defines the adjacent structures and these are identified and maneuvered with the aid of Silastic slings. (Arrow: phrenic nerve.)

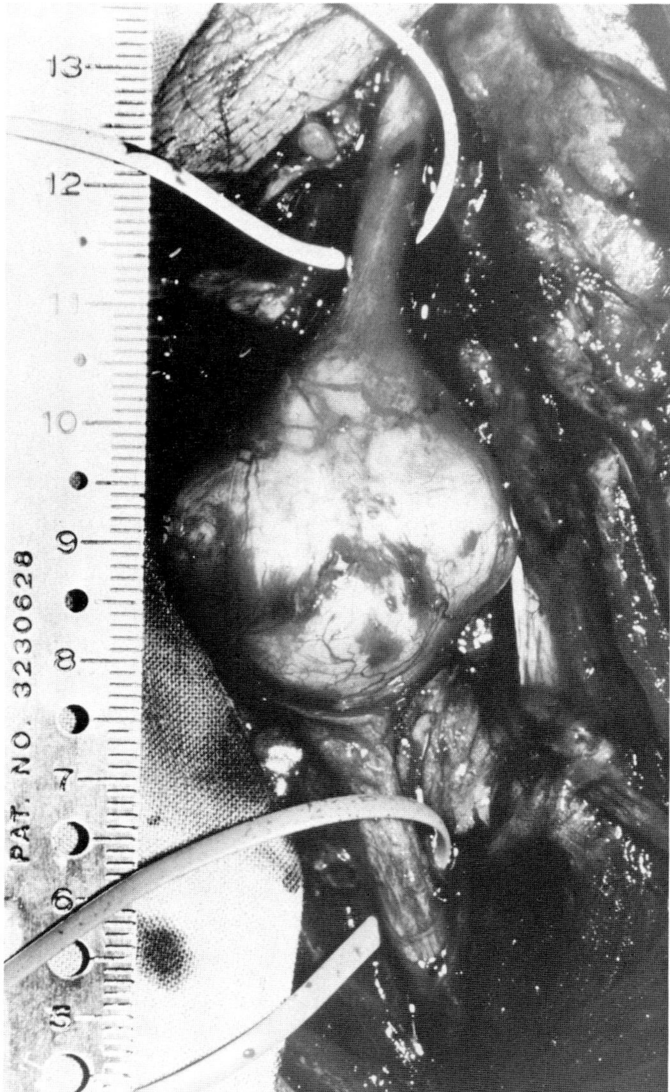

Fig. 136-6.   Schwannoma. The proximal and distal nerve trunks are clearly defined and surrounded with Silastic slings. This slightly irregular tumor has grown out between the majority of the fascicular bundles, which lie on the deep aspect of the tumor.

to debulk the tumor (although this is easily accomplished, if necessary) and, although care must be exercised, the dissection is not particularly difficult. The tumor may be cystic. Finally, a stage is reached in which all fascicles and fascicular groups have been freed up with exception of a small fascicle from which the mass itself is arising (Figure 136-8). Usually this small fascicle has to be sacrificed. This decision must not be made too early, since careful dissection at this stage frequently reveals that the final groups of fascicles can also be mobilized from the tumor capsule so that at the end of the dissection only a small component of the nerve trunk is sacrificed in removing the tumor. It is usually a matter of no difficulty to determine that the dissection is made between normal nerve fascicle at either pole, thus, totally removing the mass, leaving the bulk of the peripheral nerve trunk intact (Figure 136-9). Nerve stimulation should confirm the fact that the nerve trunk is conducting an impulse.

On rare occasions it is impossible to spare significant fascicles as they blend into the tumor mass itself at either pole. In this situation a sural nerve graft should be employed to restore continuity of those particular fascicles.[8] Histology of

these troublesome tumors may reveal features of both schwannoma and neurofibroma.

If the schwannoma arises from a small and insignificant cutaneous nerve, the detailed microscopic dissection is not required and the mass and parent nerve are simply excised.

An inflatable tourniquet may be used in appropriate circumstances. The tourniquet must be deflated prior to closure so that all blood vessels can be secured and the field be made completely dry. Standard and micro bipolar forceps are an essential part of the armamentarium and bleeding epineural vessels must be coagulated with accuracy, under a saline pool, so as not to damage immediately adjacent fascicles.

While the wound is being closed, a quick section should be reviewed by an expert pathologist. In most cases there is no difficulty in making the diagnosis after reviewing the classical histology.[3] Occasionally, cellular features may give rise to concern, e.g., an excessive number of mitoses in an "ancient" schwannoma, and in this circumstance particular care must be

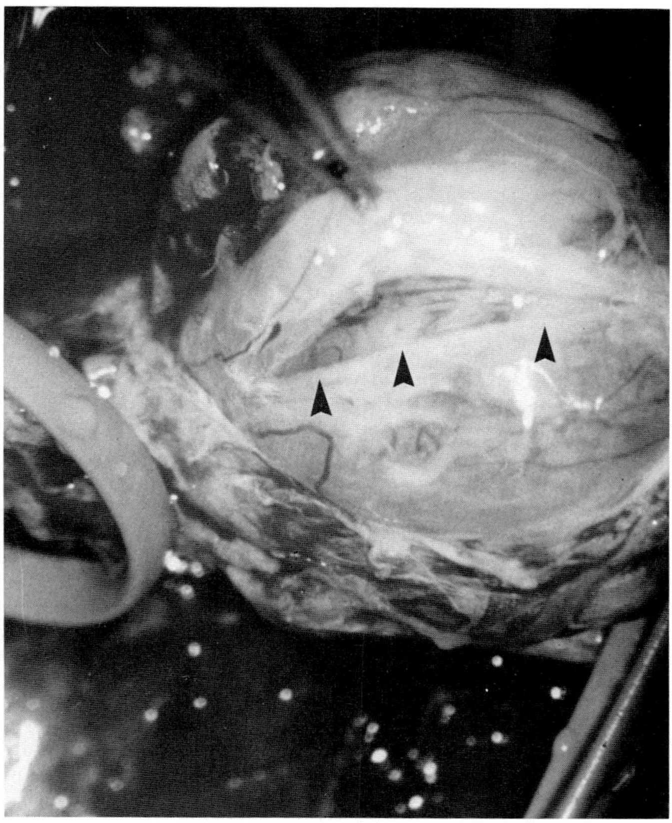

Fig. 136-7. Schwannoma. A fascicular group is being mobilized (arrow). A few individual fascicles will subsequently be dissected and slid around the periphery of the underlying schwannoma (double arrow).

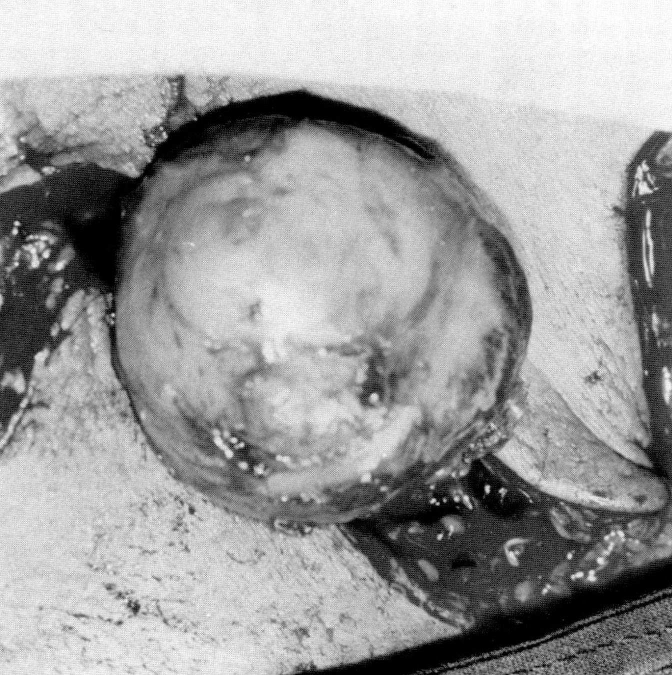

Fig. 136-9. Brachial plexus schwannoma. The size of this large schwannoma necessitated division of the clavicle. The mass was totally excised without creating any neurologic deficit.

given to the preparation and interpretation of routine histologic material. The consequences of diagnosing an unexpected malignancy are significant and may include massive nerve resection or amputation so that such decisions should be made after very careful study of the sections and usually not following the initial review of a frozen quick section alone.

The surgeon should be confident of cure once a schwannoma has been totally resected.

NEUROFIBROMA

The outstanding principle relating to neurofibroma surgery is that, in the majority of cases, resection of a neurofibroma will result in loss of function of that nerve element harboring the neoplasm. Usually, a discrete mass is not found but, instead, a swollen nerve trunk is present, with indistinct upper and lower polar margins (Figure 136-10). Solitary neurofibromas are encountered with far less frequency than solitary schwannomas. When such a tumor is identified, a careful appraisal of evidence of Von Recklinghausen's disease must be made in that patient.

Axial incision of encasing epineural tissues reveals that fascicles are grossly enlarged with significant irregularity of caliber. The appearance is quite characteristic and totally unlike a classical schwannoma. Fascicular biopsy is essential and 5 mm of a plump, glarey, translucent fascicle should be sent for quick section and routine section. If the mass has previously been biopsied at another institution, it is essential that the neuropathologist review those slides prior to the operation. The pathologist must assure the surgeon that the biopsy accurately reflects the pathology of neurofibroma and not scarring resulting from a previous biopsy at that site. This distinction may, on occasion, be a difficult one.

On rare occasions, it becomes apparent that the bulk of the mass is, indeed, composed of neurofibroma in only some of the

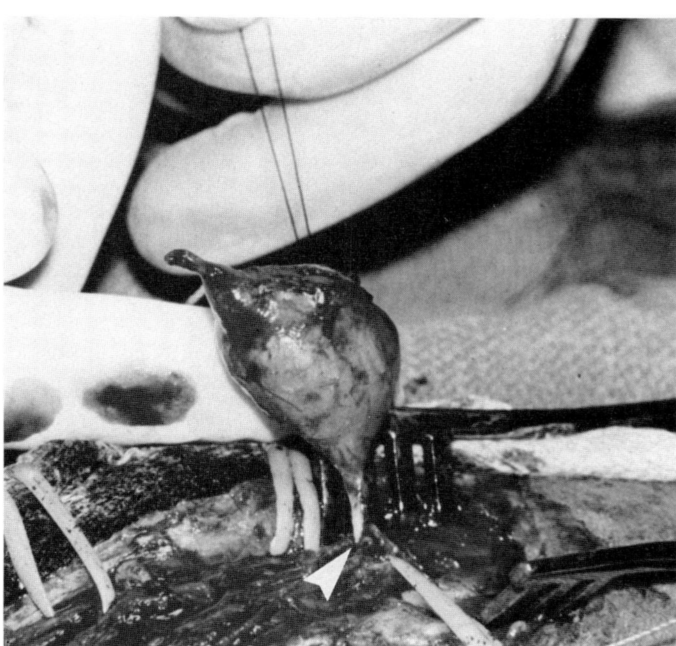

Fig. 136-8. Schwannoma of peroneal nerve. The schwannoma is being removed. A single fascicle has been transected proximally and a single fascicle, continuous with the distal pole of the tumor, is about to be divided (arrow).

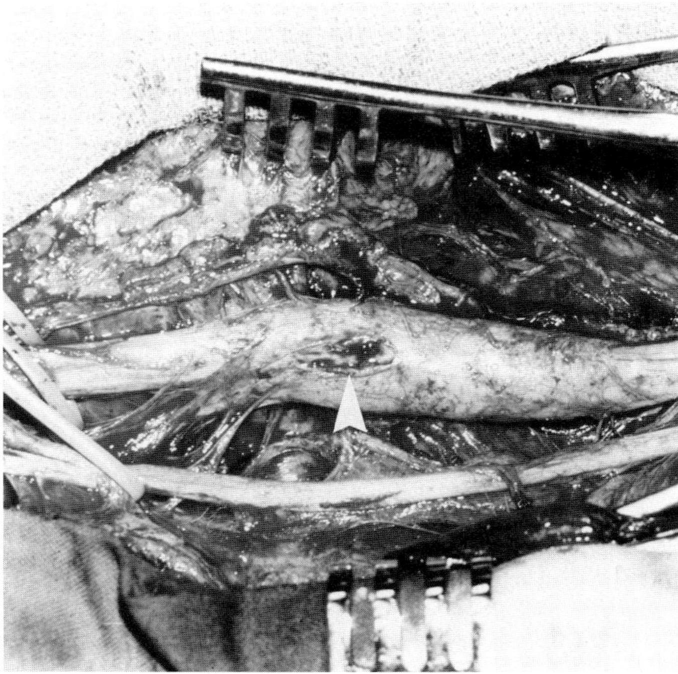

Fig. 136-10. Neurofibroma. A typical rather diffuse swelling of the nerve trunk is seen. A fascicular biopsy specimen confirmed the diagnosis of neurofibroma (arrow).

fascicles. In this circumstance, the bulk of the mass can then be resected, leaving normal or near-normal appearing fascicles intact (Figures 136-11 and 136-12). Continuity of the divided fascicles may be restored by the use of sural nerve grafts, if appropriate. Thus, it is incorrect to state that neurofibromas can never be resected without loss of function but, unfortunately,

the opportunity of selective resection presents itself rarely and it is frequently difficult in those circumstances to be certain that one has cleared the pathologic process in a proximal and distal direction, since there is no well-formed capsule to delineate the conclusion of the dissection.

The question of whether or not to resect a neurofibroma mass is based on a number of factors and the options available to the surgeon are :

1. Establishment of the diagnosis by fascicular biopsy and closure. This option should be considered in the presence of good neurologic function and in the absence of any evidence of malignancy. Some neurofibromas grow extremely slowly and, indeed, appear to be more akin to hamartomas than neoplasms. These patients can be followed at 6-month intervals and in the absence of significant increase in bulk or progressive neurologic disability, nothing further need be done. The results of significant resection of nerve trunk and subsequent nerve grafting are likely to be disappointing.
2. Resection of the bulk of the neurofibroma, leaving the majority of the nerve intact. As already stated, this is a rare opportunity but the surgeon will find that the greater his or her microsurgical peripheral nerve tumor experience, the more frequently he or she is able to accomplish this feat.
3. Resection of the mass and grafting. The resections are likely to be significant in length so that the surgeon can be certain that he or she is proximal and distal to the pathologic process. Total resection therefore is rarely indicated in tumors involving major nerves but can be accomplished in examples in which minor nerves are involved. If previous partial resection has been performed, the pathologist must be certain to distinguish between postoperative

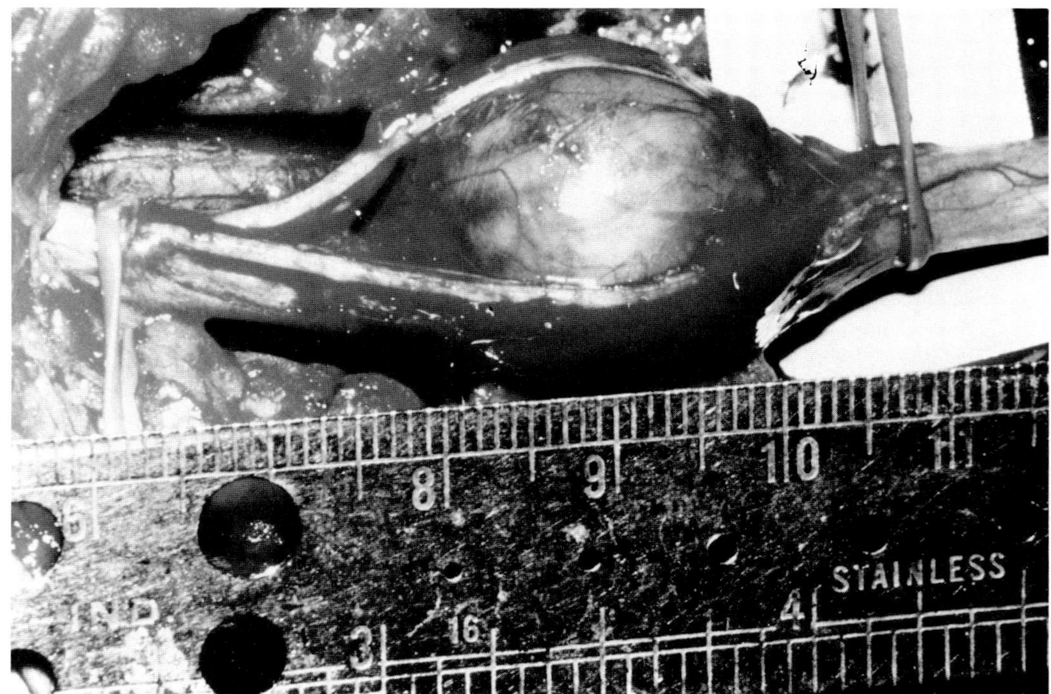

Fig. 136-11. Neurofibroma. At operation this tumor was initially thought to be a schwannoma. It was possible to isolate surface fascicular bundles. The bulk of the mass, however, proved to be a neurofibroma and this was resected.

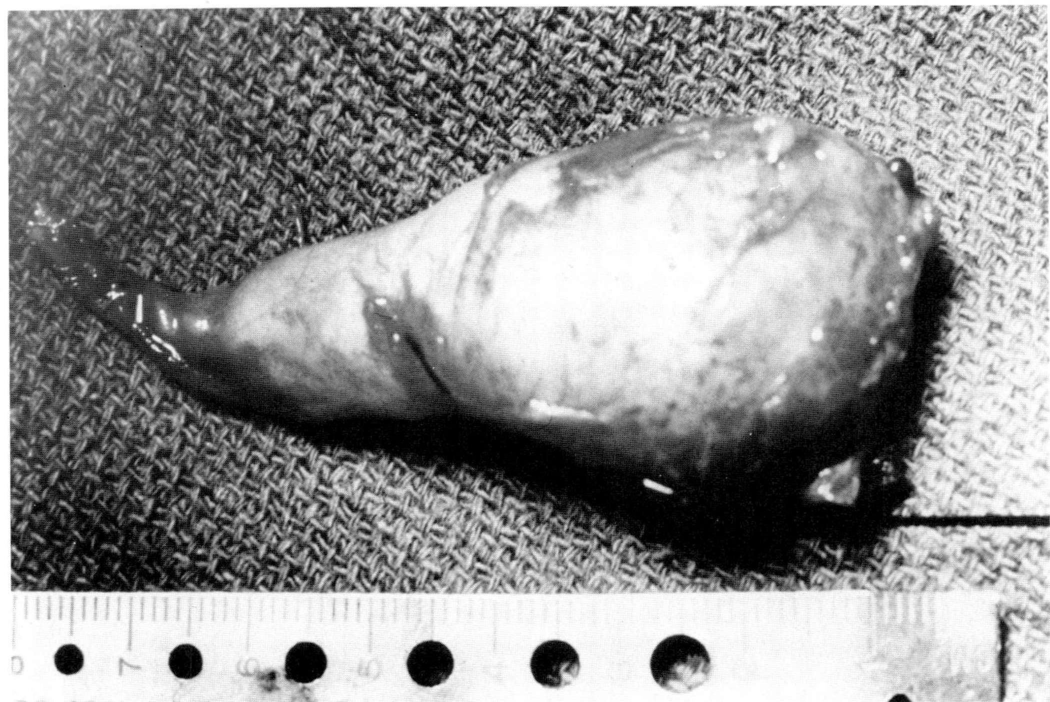

Fig. 136-12. Neurofibroma. This operative specimen is an example of what can occasionally be achieved. Only minor neurologic deficit followed resection of this mass from the parent trunk.

scarring and neurofibroma formation in assessing proximal and distal stumps (Figure 136-13).

VON RECKLINGHAUSEN'S DISEASE

In the patient with multiple tumors, the surgeon must be completely satisfied that the patient's initial symptomatology is related to a specific peripheral nerve tumor and not to some other pathologic entity harbored by the patient (e.g., syringomyelia or intracranial glioma) (Figure 136-14). Having satisfied himself or herself on clinical grounds that the problem is related to a specific mass, it is appropriate to explore the mass, define whether or not a schwannoma, neurofibroma, or malignant nerve tumor is present, and then manage the situation appropriate to the particular pathologic entity. These patients may harbor extensive, complex, interweaving masses. These are plexiform neurofibromas and are quite different in appearance at surgery compared with the swollen nerve trunk of the discrete neurofibroma.[9] Radical excision of these irregular clumps of abnormal tissue is required if recurrence is to be avoided, and if surgery is indicated because of mass size, pain, or neurologic deficit.

MALIGNANT PERIPHERAL NERVE TUMORS

The outstanding principle relating to the management of patients harboring malignant nerve tumors is that these malignancies are extremely dangerous tumors and that 5-year survival rates are low. Nomenclature problems are avoided by the surgeon's adoption of the general term "malignant peripheral nerve tumor" (Figure 136-15 and Table 136-2). Malignant nerve tumors arise from within the substance of the peripheral nerve. A characteristic feature is the axial spread of the malignancy within the substance of the parent nerve trunk. Blood-borne tumor emboli result in metastatic deposits in the lungs and liver. Radiation and chemotherapy have little to offer so that the

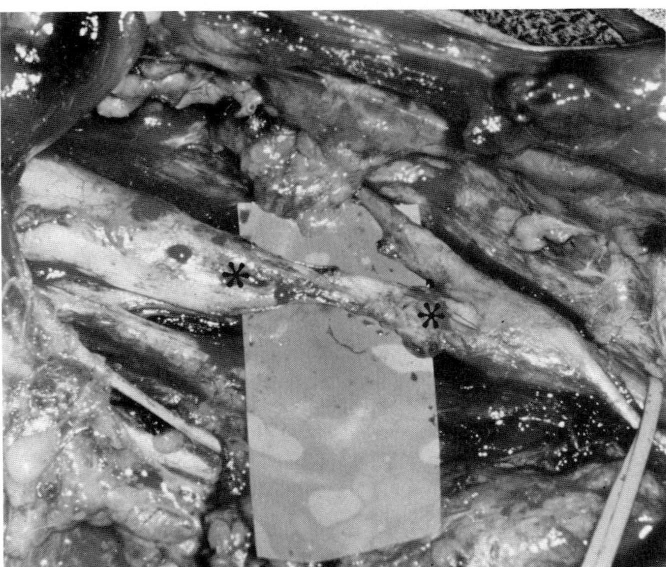

Fig. 136-13. Brachial plexus upper trunk. Resection of an unidentified mass resulted in almost complete destruction of the upper trunk of the plexus. Expert neuropathologic quick section advice is required to distinguish between scarring of the proximal and distal stumps (stars) and tumor prior to reconstructive grafting.

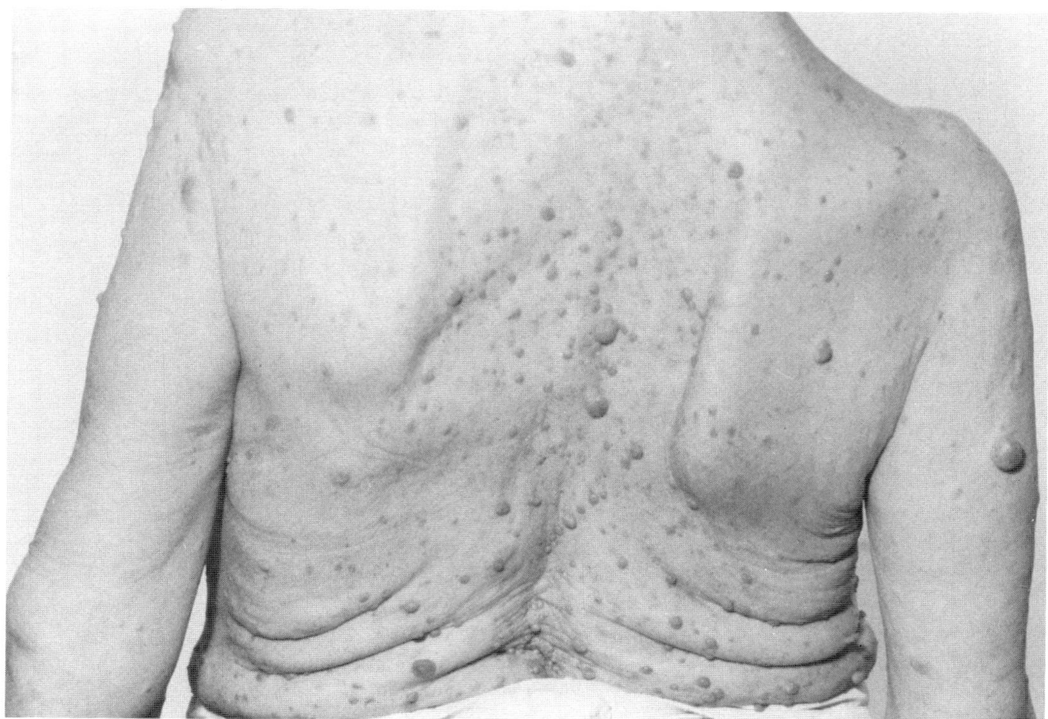

Fig. 136-14. Von Recklinghausen's disease. The patient was referred for management of a brachial plexus tumor. In fact, the initial symptoms and signs were related to cervical syringomyelia.

tendency is to advise aggressive and radical surgery. Few centers have acquired sufficient experience to state unequivocally that major ablative surgery of the limb improves the cure rate but it can be stated with certainty that lesser forms of surgery are certain to lead to disaster. Gentili and Rewcastle have analyzed the pathology register of malignant intrinsic nerve tumors at the University of Toronto and the data presented here are based, in part, on their researches.[10]

Presentation

The surgeon may suspect that he or she is dealing with a malignant nerve tumor because of rapid increase in size of a nerve tumor (Figures 136-16 and 136-17; Table 136-3). It is generally agreed that benign schwannomas undergo malignant transformation extremely rarely, if at all. In a patient suffering from Von Recklinghausen's disease the risk of malignant presentation appears to be approximately 12 percent. Clinical or radiologic demonstration of metastases makes a preoperative

Table 136-2. Terms that neuropathologists have applied to peripheral nerve tumors

Malignant schwannoma
Malignant neurilemoma
Neurogenic sarcoma
Neurofibrosarcoma
Sarcoma of peripheral nerve
Nerve sheath fibrosarcoma
Malignant neurofibroma
Neuroepithelioma of peripheral nerve

diagnosis more certain and guides the surgeon to palliative rather than curative surgery.

Biopsy

It has previously been emphasized that the parent nerve trunk should be cleanly exposed and the mass isolated during operations for schwannoma and neurofibroma. This is not the initial tactic if malignancy is suspected. At this stage, the

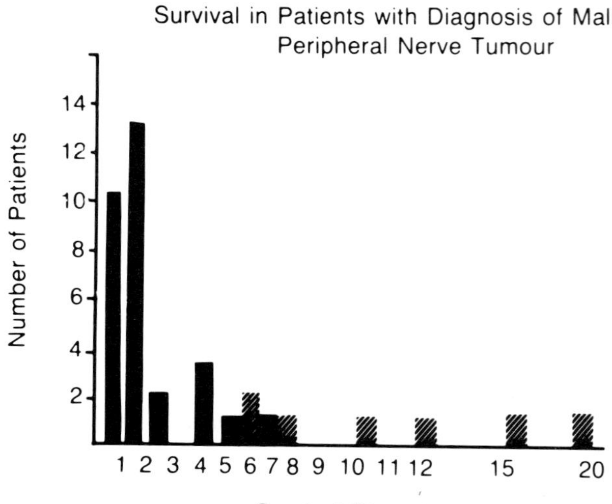

Fig. 136-15. Survival rates of patients in the University of Toronto malignant peripheral nerve tumor pathology registry. Patients surviving longer intervals (cross hatches) may display specific histologic characteristics on biopsy, but this issue is not yet settled.

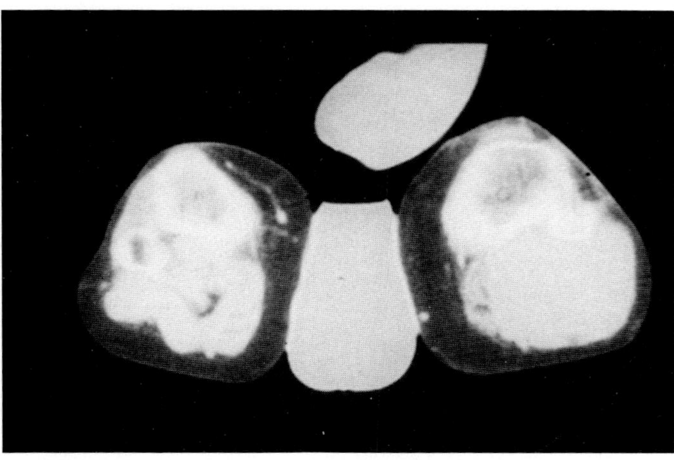

Fig. 136-16. A CT scan of a malignant peripheral nerve tumor. Rapid increase in size of this mass in the left popliteal fossa suggested the preoperative diagnosis of malignancy.

Table 136-3. Clinical presentation of patients harboring malignant peripheral nerve tumors in the University of Toronto pathology registry

Clinical Presentation	Number of Patients	Percentage
Painless mass	24	55
Painful mass	12	28
Nerve dysfunction	12	28
History of previous lump excision	12	28
Association with neurofibromatosis	12	28

surgeon does not know whether he or she is dealing with a soft tissue sarcoma invading nerve or with a malignant nerve tumor invading the surrounding tissues or with a malignant nerve tumor which is, as yet, well encapsulated. One of the options that will be available to the surgeon is that of a radical block resection of the mass and its surrounding tissues in a classical en block cancer operation. Therefore, the surgeon should make a more limited approach to a confined area of the tumor and an appropriate biopsy specimen is then taken. The procedure should then be terminated. The sections are then prepared and studied with great care using all appropriate tinctorial stains, electron microscopy, cell culture, and immunofluorescent techniques.

If there is no evidence of metastatic disease and if the diagnosis of an intrinsic malignant nerve tumor is made with certainty, there appear to be very few options available to the patient (Table 136-4).

1. A radical block resection of the mass and its surrounding tissues and of 3 or 4 cm of nerve trunk on either side of the mass with quick section control to be certain that the nerve resection line is through clean tissue.
2. Limb amputation. Malignancies presenting proximally in the limb present even greater difficulties (Figure 136-18). Spread to the subarachnoid space renders the patient incurable. If cure is attempted, the forequarter amputation must be performed with care. The brachial plexus is divided at the tips of the transverse processes and the thoracic duct carefully exposed and divided if this maneuver is required to resect the mass and its surrounding tissues.[11]

These shocking facts may present great difficulties to the patient who has a lump in his or her limb. The situation is aggravated by the fact that no guarantee can be given that major ablative surgery will cure the patient. Radiation and chemotherapy have little to offer, however, and local minor surgery has nothing to offer.

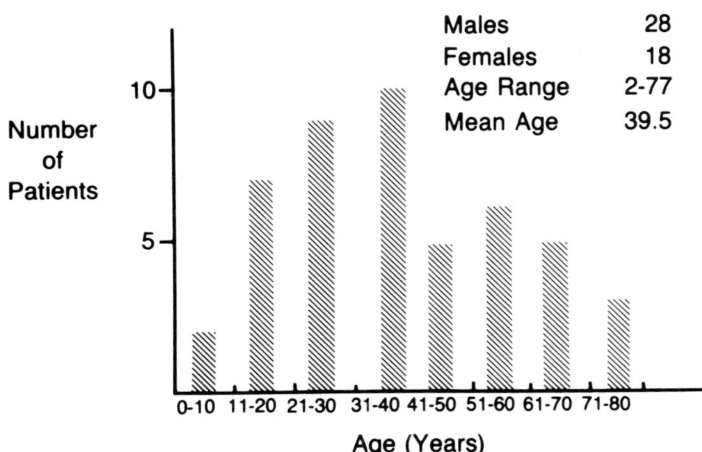

Fig. 136-17. Clinical presentation of patients harboring malignant peripheral nerve tumors in the University of Toronto pathology registry.

Table 136-4. Recurrence following minor surgery of malignant peripheral nerve tumors (University of Toronto)

Primary Treatment	Total Number of Patients	Number of Recurrences	Percentage
Biopsy	8	8	100
Subtotal resection	11	11	100
Radical local excision	24	19	80
Major amputation	1	1	100

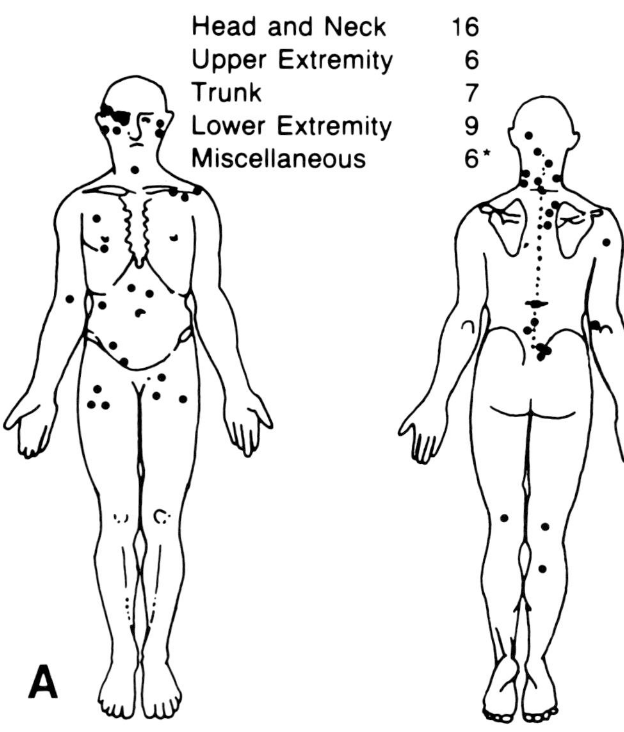

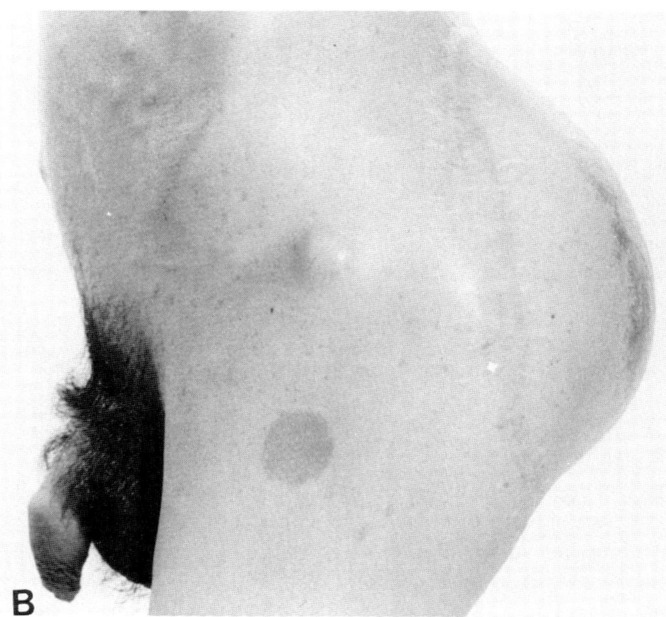

Fig. 136-18. (A) Disposition of malignant peripheral nerve tumors in the University of Toronto series. (B) Malignant peripheral nerve tumor in the buttock of a patient with Von Recklinghausen's disease. Initial operative biopsy specimens had suggested neurofibroma but subsequent clinical behavior and biopsy revealed frank malignancy.

MISCELLANEOUS INTRINSIC TUMORS

The surgeon and his or her neuropathology colleagues should be aware of the wide range of miscellaneous intrinsic tumors that may rarely be encountered. Few surgeons or pathologists gain any great experience in these areas. On occasion the distinction between a hypertrophic neuritis and a true neoplasm (perineuroma) may be difficult.[12] Compression of a peripheral nerve by a ganglion in the canal of Guyon is a well recognized entity but the finding of a ganglion within the substance of a nerve is a rare occurrence.[13,14] Unusual neoplasms or hamartomas may occasionally be encountered and should be managed in as conservative a fashion as is consistent with prolongation of normal neurologic function. Thus, intraneural lipomas should be excised but lipofibromatous hamartomas should not (Figure 136-19).

EXTRINSIC PERIPHERAL NERVE TUMORS

COMPRESSIVE TUMORS

Peripheral nerves may be compressed by neoplasms arising from adjacent structures (Figure 136-20). Nerves may also be injured in the course of operations on neoplasms that lie in the vicinity of the peripheral nerve (Figure 136-20). Such unfortunate accidents are rarely defensible in a medical-legal setting. Any surgeon approaching a neoplasm should, of course, be a master of the regional anatomy and any appropriate nerves should be clearly identified proximal and distal to the mass before the mass is excised.

INVASIVE TUMORS

Invasion of peripheral nerve by surrounding carcinomas or sarcomas will give rise to motor-sensory disability and regional pain. Local recurrence of dermoid tumors may give rise to painful neuropathy and require repeated local surgery in an attempt to prevent direct peripheral nerve invasion. Not infrequently the distinction between radiation neuritis and direct tumor invasion may be a difficult diagnostic point. While the problem of peripheral nerve invasion by malignancy may occur at any site in the body, brachial plexus involvement by Pancoast's tumor or carcinoma of the breast constitutes a particularly difficult management entity (Figure 136-21). In our experience there is no easy way of distinguishing direct plexus invasion from postradiation plexitus. Specifically, the temporal sequence of the onset of neurologic disability and pain has been an unreliable indicator of the true pathologic process and the identification of the particular element of the plexus involved has also proved to be unreliable in distinguishing tumor invasion from fibrosis. In our experience, decompression of the neural elements has given reasonably good pain relief, but we have never achieved satisfactory restoration of neurologic dysfunction once it has occurred.

POSTOPERATIVE CARE

Wound care following peripheral nerve tumor surgery is conventional and no specific comment is required. Areas of reduced sensation should be guarded for injury and paralyzed joints should be splinted and exercised appropriately. The overall management of patients postoperatively is related to basic surgical principles and there are few specific requirements related to the fact that the patient had previously harbored a nerve neoplasm.[15] In patients who have undergone relatively conservative surgery and who continue to harbor an unresected neurofibroma, serial clinical and CT scanning follow-up is required. Patients harboring malignant nerve tumors require close follow-up looking for evidence of either local or distant recurrence.

SUMMARY

The management problems confronting a peripheral nerve neoplasm surgeon range from relatively simple issues, e.g., the resection of a well-defined peripherally situated schwannoma, through areas that require a keen sense of appropriate judgment, e.g., whether or not to resect a neurofibroma, to arenas in which extremely difficult management and technical problems may have to be faced, e.g., intrinsic malignant tumor of the brachial plexus. The patient is best served by a team consisting of an expert peripheral nerve microsurgeon and an expert peripheral nerve neuropathologist.

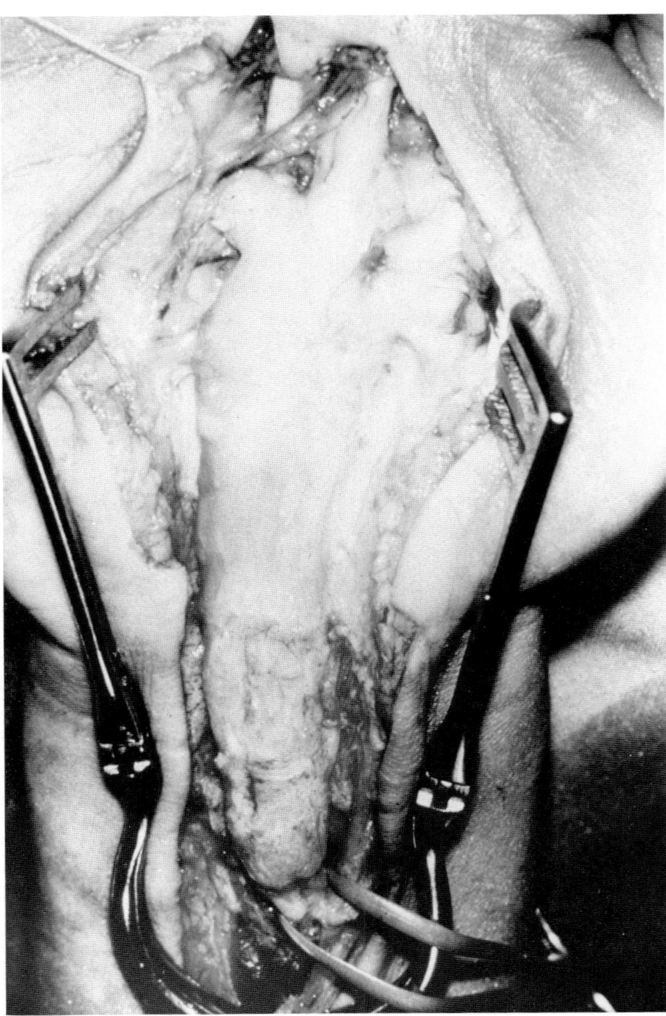

Fig. 136-19. Median nerve. The patient had carpal tunnel syndrome. Operation revealed diffuse fatty infiltration of the median nerve. The symptoms were relieved by the division of the transverse carpal ligament (lipofibromatous hamartoma).

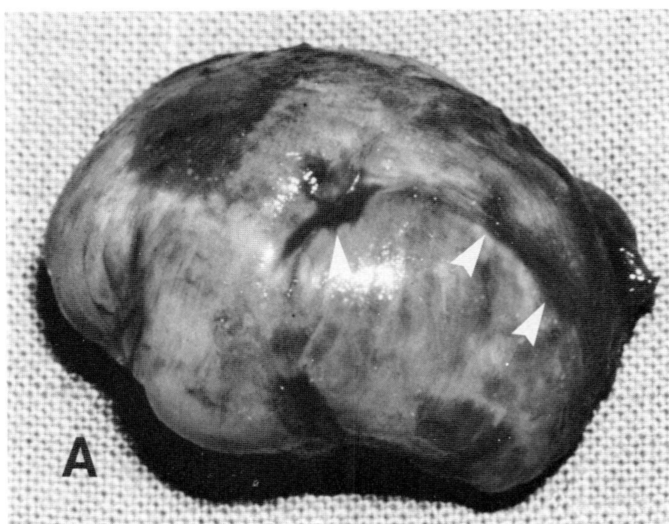

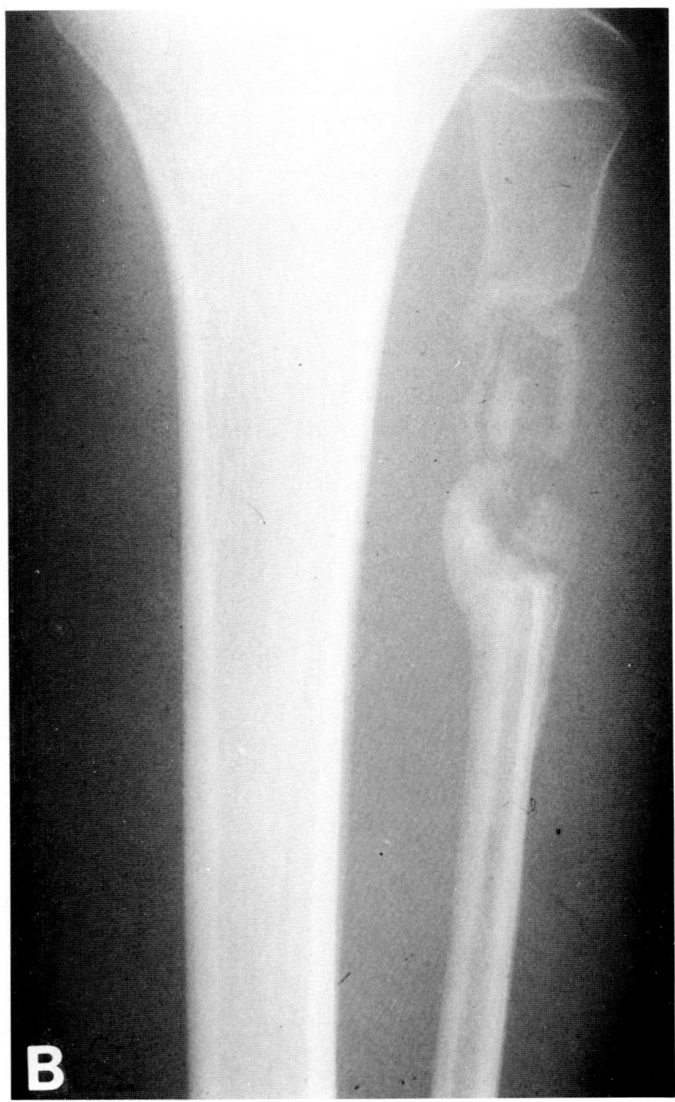

Fig. 136-20. (A) Osteoma of the neck of the radius. The patient had a posterior interosseous nerve syndrome and at surgery the nerve was found to occupy a groove on the surface of this benign bone tumor (arrow). (B) Benign tumor of the proximal fibula. Normal preoperative neurologic examination. Postoperative foot drop was found to be resultant on a total division of the peroneal nerve, which occurred during the bony surgery.

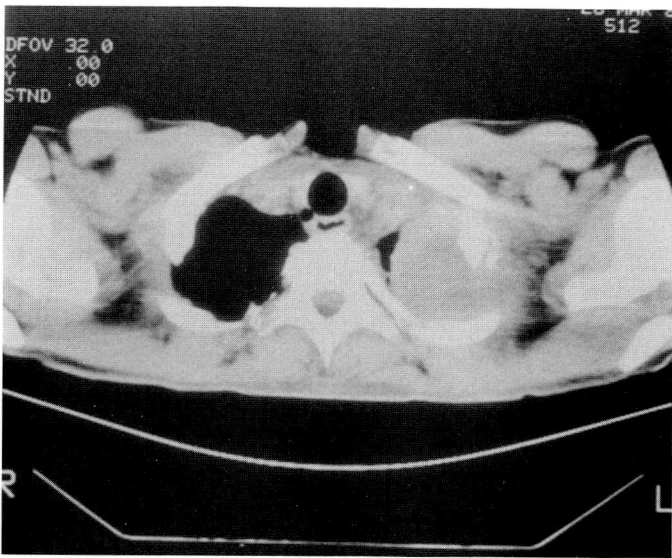

Fig. 136-21. A CT scan of the brachial plexus demonstrating invasion by an apical thoracic tumor. This left-sided mass resulted in a severe pain syndrome with associated loss of small muscle function and anesthesia of the left hand.

REFERENCES

1. Morris J, Hudson AR, Weddell G: A study of degeneration and regeneration in the divided rat sciatic nerve based on electron microscopy. Z Zellforsch 124:76, 1972
2. Seddon Sir H, Livingstone, C: Nerve Tumours in Surgical Disorders of the Peripheral Nerves. 1972, pp 153–170
3. Harkin JC, Reed, RJ: Tumours of the Peripheral Nervous System. Fascicle 3, Atlas of Tumour Pathology, Armed Forces Institute of Pathology, 1969
4. Weller R, Cervos-Navarro J: Tumours of the peripheral nervous system, in Pathology of Peripheral Nerves. London, Butterworths, 1977, pp 144–207
5. Asbury, Johnson: Tumours of the peripheral nerve, in Pathology of Peripheral Nerves. Philadelphia, WB Saunders, 1978, pp 206–249
6. Das Gupta T: Tumours of the peripheral nerves. Clin Neurosurg 25:574, 1977
7. Hudson AR, Berry H, Mayfield F: Chronic injuries of peripheral nerves by entrapment, in Youmans JR (ed): Neurological Surgery, ed 2. Philadelphia, WB Saunders, 1982, pp 2430–2474
8. Kline DG, Hudson AR, Bratton BR: Use of grafts to repair nerves with serious gaps, in Gorio A, Millesi H, Minigrin S (eds): Posttraumatic Peripheral Nerve Regeneration: Experimental Basis and Clinical Implications. New York, Raven Press, 1981, pp 339–342
9. Brooks D: Clinical presentation and treatment of peripheral nerve tumours, in Bunge R, Dyck P, Lambert E, Thomas P (eds): Peripheral Neuropathy. Philadelphia, WB Saunders, 1984, pp 2236–2251
10. Gentili F, Rewcastle B: Malignant peripheral nerve tumours. Presented at the Eighth International Congress of Neurological Surgery, Toronto, 1985
11. Hudson AR, Tranmer B: Brachial plexus injuries, in Wilkins RH, Rengachary SS (eds): Neurosurgery. New York, McGraw-Hill, 1985, pp 1817–1832
12. Bilbao JM, Briggs SJ, Hudson AR, et al: Perineurioma (localized hypertrophic neuropathy). Arch Pathol Lab Med 108:557, 1984
13. Scherman BM, Bilbao JM, Hudson AR: Intraneural ganglion: A case report with electron-microscopic observations. Neurosurgery 8:487, 1981
14. Tindall SC: Ganglion cysts of peripheral nerves, in Wilkins RH, Rengachary SS (eds): Neurosurgery. New York, McGraw-Hill, 1985, p 1900
15. Hudson AR: Peripheral nerve surgery, in Bunge R, Dyck P, Lambert E, Thomas P (eds): Peripheral Neuropathy, vol 2. Philadelphia, WB Saunders, 1984, pp 420–438

Index

Abscess. *See specific sites and diagnoses*
Accident, emergency care, 19
Acoustic neuroma, 705–708
  anatomy, 687–689
  anesthesia for, 689–690
  cerebellopontine angle, 673–674
  cerebrospinal fluid rhinorrhea with, 702–703
  closure, 701–702
  differential diagnosis, 572
  four quadrants dissection, 699–701
  gutting procedure, 699
  hematoma with, 702
  hemostasis, 701
  patient positioning, 690
  postoperative complications, 702–703
  postoperative management, 702
  postradiosurgery complications, 521
  removal, 696–699
  results, 703
  stereotactic radiosurgery, 520–521
  surgical management, 690–692
  translabyrinthine dissection, 692–696
  translabyrinthine operation, 685–704
Acoustic tumor (bilateral), 681
Acquired immune deficiency syndrome, 419, 422
Acromegaly, 299
  stereotactic radiosurgery, 518
ACTH assay, in pituitary adenoma, 300
Adult respiratory distress syndrome, with acute head injury, 27–28
Affective disorders
  surgery for, 1057–1060
  surgical anatomy, 1058
  surgical controversies, 1059–1060
  surgical indications, 1060
Air embolism, in tentorium tumor, 648
Alloplastic grafting materials, for skull defects, 11, 14–16
Alpha fetoprotein, in intracranial germ cell tumor, 398
Amnesia, after transcallosal interfornicial approach to third ventricle, 389–390
Amphotericin B, in fungus infection, 90
Amyotrophic lateral sclerosis, 1352, 1354, 1355
Analgesia, implanted electrode brain stimulation for, 1089–1095
Anaphylaxis, from chymopapain chemonucleolysis, 1437, 1438, 1440
Anesthesia. *See also specific diagnoses and procedures*
  anatomophysiologic factors in children, 103–116
  for head injury, 113–114
  for neuroradiographic procedures, 112–113
Anesthetic agents
  for children, 104
  epidural infusion for intractable pain, 1145

Aneurysm, 1003–1007. *See also specific sites*
  age factor, 1003, 1005
  arteriography in, 1004, 1006
  asymptomatic, 1006
  bleeding potential, 1004
  clinical parameters, 1004, 1006
  computed tomography in, 1004, 1006
  diagnosis, 1003–1004
  electroencephalography in, 1004, 1006
  hypertension and, 1003, 1006
  incidence, 1003, 1006
  intraoperative ultrasonography visualization, 217
  laser occlusion, 226
  multiple, 1003, 1006
  nonsurgical management, 1006
  risk of rupture, 1005
  ruptured, 1004, 1005
  sex factor, 1003
  site, 1003
  subarachnoid hemorrhage with, 1004, 1005
  surgical criteria, 1005
  surgical morbidity, 1005
  surgical treatment, 1005, 1006
  unruptured, 1005–1006
Aneurysm (giant)
  internal carotid artery at anterior communicating region, 1026
  at middle cerebral artery, 1026
  of vertebrobasilar circulation, 1026
Aneurysm (intracerebral)
  balloon catheter management, 831–832
  traumatic, 991–995
Aneurysm (unclippable), 1023–1034
  aneurysmorrhaphy in, 1032–1033
  angiography, 1029–1030
  balloon occlusion, 1024, 1033
  computed tomography, 1029–1030
  configuration factor, 1029–1030
  deep hypotension in, 1030, 1032
  evaluation at surgery, 1030–1033
  indirect procedures, 1033
  ingenious clip techniques, 1033
  intra-aneurysmal thrombosis, 1033
  preoperative evaluation, 1023–1030
  Sendai cocktail, 1032
  site factor, 1023
  size factor, 1025–1029
  temporary proximal occlusion or trapping, 1030–1032
  wrapping of, 1032
Aneurysmorrhaphy, 1032–1033
Angiography
  in arterial aneurysm, 1011, 1013
  in anterior communicating artery aneurysm, 940, 949, 951, 953
  in anterior skull base tumor, 612
  in arteriovenous malformation, 523–525, 900, 902, 1011, 1017

  in anteroinferior dural venous fistula, 849–854
  in bacterial intracranial aneurysm, 997, 998–999
  in carotid artery lesion, 753, 754, 757
  in carotid cavernous fistula, 846
  in carotid ophthalmic aneurysm, 918, 925, 927
  in cerebellar hemangioma, 660
  in cervical spondylosis, 1332
  in Chiari malformation with hydromelia, 1316
  in clivus and basioccipital region tumor, 638
  in craniopharyngioma, 356
  in dural fistula, 828
  in dural sinus malformation, 861
  in gunshot wounds of head, 38–39
  in internal carotid artery aneurysm, 837, 930
  in intracerebral hemorrhage, 885
  in intramedullary spinal cord tumor, 1490, 1492
  in medial sphenoid wing meningioma, 538
  in meningioma, 550–551, 564–566, 572
  in middle cerebral artery aneurysm, 957, 970
  in moyamoya disease, 798–801, 803
  in olfactory groove meningioma, 540
  in optic nerve decompression, 270
  in spine tumor, 1526–1527
  in STA-MCA bypass, 783, 791
  in suprasellar germinoma, 398
  in suprasellar meningioma, 531
  in tentorium tumor, 647
  in traumatic aneurysm, 991, 992
  in traumatic carotid cavernous fistula, 822, 825
  in unclippable aneurysm, 1029–1030
  for vertebrobasilar insufficiency, 808, 810, 812
Angiography (digital), with stereotactic intra-axial tumor resection, 481, 483
Ankle clonus, stimulation management, 1056–1057
Ankylosing spondylitis, 1300–1303
  atlantoaxial subluxation, 1303
  cauda equina syndrome, 1303
  intraspinal ossification, 1303
  pachymeningitis, 1303
  spinal fracture/dislocation, 1302–1303
  stress fracture, 1303
Annulus of Zinn, 235, 236
Anterior communicating artery aneurysm, 939–955, 1032
  anesthesia, 940
  aneurysm neck dissection, 945–946
  aneurysm obliterating, 946–948
  aneurysm rupture management, 946
  angiography, 940, 949, 951, 953

Anterior communicating
  artery aneurysm *(continued)*
  bipolar neck cauterization, 948
  brain tension reduction, 941
  carotid balloon occlusion, 951
  case reports, 949–952
  cerebral blood flow studies, 939, 949, 950,
    951, 954
  clipping alternatives, 946–948
  closure, 948
  complications, 954
  computed tomography in, 939, 949, 952
  controlled hypotension in, 941
  deterioration with, 939, 940
  dome aspiration, 948
  exposure, 942–943
  incision, 941–942
  indirect surgical attack, 948–949, 954
  ligature placement, 948
  magnetic resonance imaging in, 939
  medical management, 939–940
  microsurgical dissection, 944–945
  patient positioning, 941
  periarterial hematoma removal, 950–951
  postoperative management, 949
  preoperative management, 939
  reinforcement with muslin, 948
  results, 952–953
  surgical technique, 941–949
  temporary clipping and cerebral
    protection, 945, 954
  vasospasm with, 941, 954
Anterior lumbar discectomy/interbody
    fusion, 1421–1436
  abdominal ileus with, 1431
  anticoagulation therapy after, 1427
  case reports, 1431–1434
  complications, 1428–1431
  computed tomography, 1423
  contraindications, 1423
  donor site disturbance, 1429–1430
  electromyography, 1423
  impotence with, 1430–1431
  indications for, 1421–1422
  infection with, 1431
  intraoperative hemorrhage, 1431
  metrizamide myelography for, 1423
  postoperative hematoma, 1431
  postoperative management, 1426–1428
  pseudoarthrosis with, 1428–1429
  radiography, 1422, 1427–1428
  results, 1434–1435
  technetium 99 bone scan, 1423
  technique, 1423–1426
  thermography, 1423
  thromboembolism with, 1428, 1430
  urinary tract disturbance with, 1430
  venography for, 1423
Anterior skull base tumor
  angiography, 612
  computed tomography, 611
  craniofacial resection, 609–618
  radiography, 611
Antibiotic prophylaxis
  in cerebrospinal fluid leakage, 61, 62
  with missile injury, 52
Anticholinergic agents, in torticollis, 1262
Anticoagulation therapy
  after anterior lumbar discectomy, 1427

in carotid artery lesion, 753, 756, 760
Anticonvulsants
  in cerebral glioma, 435–436
  in missile injury, 52
  in torticollis, 1262
  in tuberculoma, 82
Antidepressants, in torticollis, 1262
Antituberculosis agents
  in tuberculoma, 81–82
  in tuberculous meningitis, 84
Arachnoid cyst
  extra-axial, 658–659
  reconstruction technique, 331
Argon laser, 223–224, 226
Arnold-Chiari malformation, posterior fossa
    decompression, 111
Arterial aneurysm (cerebral)
  angiography, 1011, 1013
  case reports, 1013–1017
  preoperative stereotactic calculations,
    1011–1012
  stereotactic clipping, 1009–1022
    indications/contraindications, 1012–1013
    instrumentation, 1010–1011
    results, 1013–1017
    technique, 1012
Arteriography
  in aneurysm, 1004, 1006
  in arteriovenous malformation, 905, 908
  in glomus jugulare tumor, 742, 744
  in pineal tumor, 403
  after proton beam therapy, 911–912
  in scalp/skull tumor, 604
  in spinal cord arteriovenous malformation,
    1501, 1502, 1506
  in vertebrobasilar insufficiency, 771–775
Arteriosclerotic vascular disease, lumbar
    sympathectomy for pain and
    ulceration, 1278
Arteriovenous malformation
  angiography, 523–525
  case reports, 525–526
  cerebellar, 908
  cerebellopontine angle-brain stem, 908
  in children, 109
  computed tomography, 523, 526
  dural, 908
  embolization in, 905, 906, 908, 909
  intraoperative ultrasonography
    visualization, 217
  intraventricular, 908
  magnetic resonance imaging, 523, 905
  postoperative evaluation, 908–909
  preoperative evaluation, 905–906
  radiation therapy, 906
  radiosurgery results, 526–528
  recurrent hemorrhage after radiosurgery,
    528
  stereotactic radiosurgery, 521–528
  stereotactic resection, 489
  surgical management, 906–908
  with tumor, 909
Arteriovenous malformation (cerebral), 899,
    905–910
  angiography, 1011, 1017, 1018
  arteriography, 905, 908
  block resection, 901
  with bucrylate and calibrated leak balloon,
    829–830

case reports, 1019–1021
computed tomography, 905
direct coagulation and obliteration, 900
embolization management, 828–831, 903,
    911
fistula with, 827
headache with, 914
hemorrhage with, 905, 913–914
intraoperative embolization, 830–831
liquid agent embolization, 829
marginal resection, 900–901
natural history, 899
neurologic deficit with, 914
operative staging, 902
postoperative management, 902
preoperative evaluation, 900
preoperative stereotactic calculations,
    1011–1012, 1018
proton beam therapy, 911–915
regional cerebral blood flow in, 1018
results, 831, 903, 911–912
steal effect, 829
stereotactic clipping, 1009–1022
  indications/contraindications, 1012–
    1013
  instrumentation, 1010–1011
  results, 1017–1021
  technique, 1012
surgical access difficulty, 902–903
surgical complications, 901
surgical risk, 899–900
surgical technique, 900–901
Arteriovenous malformation (spinal cord),
    832–835, 1497–1506
  anatomy, 1498–1500
  anterior vs. posterior, 832–833
  arteriography, 1501, 1502, 1506
  balloon catheter management, 832–833
  clinical presentation, 1500
  computed tomography, 1501
  diagnosis, 1500–1501
  embolization, 1502
  glomus, 1504–1505
  juvenile (diffuse), 1505
  long dorsal, 1503–1504
  myelography, 1500–1501
  natural history, 1500
  radiography, 1500–1501
  results, 1505–1506
  with small dural fistula, 833, 835
  somatosensory evoked potentials, 1501
  surgical excision, 1502–1503
  types, 1499–1500
Aspirator, ultrasonic surgical, 226–227
Astrocytoma
  cystic pilocytic of cerebral hemispheres,
    431–432
  grades 3 and 4, 431
  intramedullary spinal cord, 175–185, 1490,
    1495
  intraoperative ultrasonography
    visualization, 216
  malignant, 182, 184, 185
  optic nerve, 239
  stereotactic resection, 487–488
  supratentorial grade, 1–2, 431
Atherosclerosis, carotid artery bifurcation
    lesions, 753, 757
Axonotmesis, 1584

Back pain (low), anterior lumbar discectomy and interbody fusion for, 1421–1436
Backlund biopsy instrument, 467–468
Bacterial endocarditis, aneurysm with, 997–1001
Bacterial intracranial aneurysm, 997–1001
  angiography, 997, 998–999
  clinical manifestations, 997–998
  computed tomography, 998
  culture in, 997–998
  diagnosis, 998–999
  incidence, 997
  medical treatment, 999
  multiple, 999–1000
  sites, 998
  surgical treatment, 999–1000
Ballism, stereotactic surgery for, 1053
Ballistics
  of gunshot wounds, 37
  missile injury relation, 49–50
Balloon catheter
  calibrated-leak balloon, 820
  catheter and guide wires available, 821–822
  detachable balloon, 819
  embolic agents with, 820–821
  instrumentation, 819–822
  in intracerebral vascular lesion management, 819–836
  latex balloon, 819, 820
  silastic balloon, 819, 820, 824
Balloon embolization, 873
Balloon occlusion, of unclippable aneurysm, 1024, 1033
Basilar-anterior inferior cerebellar artery aneurysm, 984–986
Basilar artery aneurysm, 973–989
  anesthesia, 973–974
  monitoring techniques, 973–974
  patient positioning, 974
  subtemporal approach, 975
  surgical technique, 975–979
  unclippable, 1026–1029, 1031
Basilar artery occlusive disease, interposition vein graft to posterior cerebral artery, 793
Basilar bifurcation aneurysm, 979–982
  giant/bulbous, 983
Basioccipital region. See Clivus and basioccipital region
Biliary tract, splanchnicectomy for pain, 1276
Biologic markers, in pineal tumor, 403
Biopsy. See also Stereotactic biopsy; specific diagnoses
  Backlund instrument, 467–468
  with Brown-Roberts-Wells stereotactic frame, 475–480
  computed tomography in, 463–474
  free-hand computed tomography techniques, 463
  magnetic resonance imaging in, 463–474
Bischof's myelotomy, 1177–1184
  circular griseotomy, 1181, 1183
  complications, 1182–1183
  exploration, 1178–1179
  indications for, 1178
  lateral longitudinal, 1179–1180
  lesion production, 1179–1181

in lower limb spasticity, 1177–1184
  posterior longitudinal, 1180
  postoperative care, 1182
  preoperative management, 1178
  results, 1182–1183
  technical factors, 1177
Bladder function, with spinal dysraphism, 166
Blast injury, 51
Body temperature regulation, in children, 106, 108
Bone chips, with missile injury, 50
Bone grafts, for skull defects, 11
Boston Brace, 193
Brachial plexus avulsion, dorsal root entry zone thermocoagulation for pain, 1170–1171, 1173–1174
Brachial plexus injury
  closed, 1578–1581
  computed tomography, 1578
  infraclavicular, 1578
  myelography, 1578
  open wounds, 1577–1578
  pain management, 1581
  radiation neuropathy, 1580
  radiography, 1578
  supraclavicular, 1578
  surgical technique, 1580
Brachycurietherapy, 491, 499–502
  indications for, 507–512
  results, 507
Bracing, in scoliosis, 191–194
Brain abscess, 72–74
  computed tomography in, 73
  intraoperative ultrasonography visualization, 217
Brain biopsy, 419–422
  complications, 421–422
  indications for, 419
  intraoperative ultrasonography in, 219
  legal/moral/ethical considerations, 419
  operative techniques, 419–421
  preferred sites, 420
  results, 420
Brain lesion
  computed tomography, 215–217
  intracranial ultrasonography, 215
  normal vs. pathologic ultrasonography visualization, 215–216
  preoperative localization, 215
Brain metastasis, intraoperative ultrasonography visualization, 217
Brain revascularization (direct), 783–795
Brain stem auditory evoked potentials, in brain stem tumor, 716
Brain stem glioma, 709–737
  anatomic categories, 710–714
  computed tomography in, 716–718
  diagnosis, 714–716
  growth types, 713–714
  histology, 710
  magnetic resonance imaging in, 716–718
  postoperative neurological signs, 722
  postoperative radiotherapy, 724, 735
  removal, 719–722
  results, 722–724
  sites, 710
  surgical approach, 719–722
  symptomatology, 714–716

Brain stem tumor, 709–737
  case reports, 724–733
  caudal, 711
  computed tomography in, 716–718
  evoked potentials in, 716
  hyperkinesis with, 722, 724
  magnetic resonance imaging in, 716–718
  midbrain, 711–712
  thalamic, 712
  treatment, 719
Brain stimulation
  for cancer pain, 1047
  for denervation pain, 1049
  electrode implantation for, 1039, 1041–1043
  with implanted electrodes for analgesia, 1089–1095
  periventricular/periaqueductal area, 1041–1042
  sites for, 1041–1043
  somatosensory system, 1042–1043
Brain tumor, stereotactic biopsy with radionuclide implantation, 491–514
Brown-Roberts-Wells stereotactic frame, 475–480, 1037
  biopsy with, 476–477
  cases, 477–478
  complications, 478
  computed tomography with, 477
  instrumentation, 477
  postoperative care, 478
  potential applications, 478
  results, 477–478
  target localization, 475–476
  target selection, 475–476
Brown-Roberts-Wells stereotactic system, 466–467
Bucrylate, as embolic agent, 821
Burr holes, exploratory, 22
Bypass grafts. See specific procedures

Campotomy, for movement disorder, 1051
Cancer pain. See also Pain (intractable)
  ablative procedures for, 1043
  of cervical and craniofacial region, 1079–1088
  commissural myelotomy for, 1185–1190
  intraventricular morphine for, 1077–1088
  management of, 1043
  narcotics for, 1043
  neurosurgical management, 1043–1047
  percutaneous cordotomy for, 1191–1205
  percutaneous electrode implantation for, 1047
  percutaneous rhizotomy in, 1125–1127
  spinal sensory rhizotomy for, 1209, 1211
Canthotomy, lateral, 254
Carbon dioxide laser, 223, 224, 225
  in meningioma surgery, 559
  wet-field, 226
Carotid artery
  in dural venous sinus lesions, 872–873
  trapping procedure, 872–873
Carotid artery (extracranial), 753–764
  aneurysms, 763
  angiography, 753, 754, 757
  anticoagulation, 753, 756, 760
  asymptomatic lesions, 754

Carotid artery (extracranial) *(continued)*
　atherosclerosis, 753, 757
　computed tomography, 753
　embolization, 753
　fibromuscular dysplasia, 763
　kinking, 762–763
　lesion diagnosis, 753–755
　lesion symptomatotology, 753–755
　traumatic injury, 762
Carotid artery aneurysm, subarachnoid
　　hemorrhage with, 917, 918, 927
Carotid cavernous fistula
　angiography in, 846
　anterior approach, 846
　balloon catheter management, 822–827
　balloon embolization, 873
　with basilar skull fracture, 21–22
　classification, 845
　embolization, 873
　lateral approach, 846–847
　percutaneous jugular approach, 847
　posterior approach, 847
　preoperative planning, 846
　results, 847
　superficial temporal artery catheterization,
　　846
　thrombosis technique, 845–847
　thrombosis via positive current, 873
Carotid cavernous fistula (spontaneous), 827
　dural subtypes, 827
　embolization management, 827
Carotid cavernous fistula (traumatic), 822–
　　827
　angiography, 822, 825
　arterial approach, 825
　clinical presentation, 822
　diagnosis, 822–825
　direct surgical approach, 825
　results, 825, 827
　steal effect, 823–824
　venous approach, 825
Carotid endarterectomy, 765–769
　anesthesia, 755
　bilateral, 760
　closure, 757–760
　complications, 760–761
　indications for, 753–754
　intraoperative shunt, 757
　patient positioning, 755
　postoperative care, 760
　preoperative preparation, 754–755
　restenosis management, 760
　results, 762
　risk factors, 753
　technique, 755–760
Carotid fistula (external), balloon catheter
　　management, 827
Carotid ligation, for internal carotid artery
　　aneurysm, 1025
Carotid occlusion, for internal carotid artery
　　aneurysm, 1023
Carotid ophthalmic aneurysm, 917–928
　anatomy, 917
　anesthesia, 918
　angiography, 918, 925, 927
　brain tension reduction, 918
　case report, 927
　cerebral blood flow studies, 918, 927
　cervical carotid occlusion for, 925

　clinoid process removal, 921–922
　computed tomography, 917–918
　contralateral aneurysm clipping, 924–925
　controlled hypotension in, 918–919
　dissection, 922
　extubation, 919
　incision, 919
　magnetic resonance imaging, 917
　medical management, 917–918
　microsurgical dissection, 921
　obliteration, 923–924
　patient positioning, 919
　postoperative management, 925, 927
　pterional (frontotemporal) craniotomy
　　exposure, 920
　results, 927
　STA-MCA bypass in, 927
　superior hypophyseal, 925
　surgical technique, 919–925
　symptomatology, 917
　vasospasm management, 919
　wound closure, 925
Carpal tunnel syndrome, 1583–1584
　medial palmar cutaneous nerve and, 1586
　surgical management, 1585–1588
Catecholamines, in glomus jugulare tumor,
　　744
Caudal brain stem tumor, 711
　symptomatology, 714–716
Cauda equina syndrome, 1303
Causalgia, 1271, 1272
　lower extremity, 1277–1278
　sympathectomy for, 1049
Cavitron ultrasonic surgical aspirator, 178,
　　184, 650
　in craniofacial resection, 613
Central nervous system cyst, toxin-leaking,
　　373–374
Central nervous system infection, 79–91
Central retinal artery occlusion, with
　　radiofrequency rhizotomy, 1141–1142
Cerebellar artery (anterior inferior)
　　aneurysm, 984–986
Cerebellar artery (superior) aneurysm, 983–
　　984
Cerebellar astrocytoma
　computed tomography, 660
　magnetic resonance imaging, 660
　surgical management, 659–660
Cerebellar hemangioblastoma
　angiography, 660
　computed tomography, 660
　radiation therapy, 660
　surgical management, 660
Cerebellar metastasis, surgical management,
　　660
Cerebellopontine angle
　anatomy, 674
　middle fossa approach, 675
　posterior cranial fossa transmeatal
　　approach, 676–680
　surgical approaches, 675–680
　translabyrinthine approach, 676
Cerebellopontine angle tumor, 673–683
　clinical features, 673–674
　surgical approaches, 675–680
　surgical complications, 680–681
Cerebral angiography, anesthesia for, 112
Cerebral artery (posterior) aneurysm, 984

Cerebral blood flow (regional)
　in arteriovenous malformation, 1018
　in moyamoya disease, 798–799, 803
　in vertebrobasilar insufficiency, 807–808
Cerebral contusion, with acute head injury,
　　24
Cerebral palsy, stereotactic surgery for, 1054
Cerebritis, with fungus infection, 89
Cerebrospinal fluid
　with intraventricular hemorrhage, 119
　in suprasellar germinoma, 398
　morphine injections, 1078–1088
Cerebrospinal fluid drainage
　catheter management, 62–63
　complications, 62
　infection prevention, 62
　technique, 62
Cerebrospinal fluid fistula, 57–69
　with basilar skull fracture, 21
　diagnosis, 58–60
　external drainage, 62
　extralabyrinthine, 61
　with glomus jugulare tumor, 750
　high-pressure vs. low-pressure, 61
　intralabyrinthine, 61
　with missile injury, 53
Cerebrospinal fluid leakage, 57–69
　anatomic considerations, 60–61
　anterior fossa craniotomy, 63–64
　antibiotic prophylaxis, 61, 62
　cerebrospinal fluid shunt in, 66
　contrast studies, 60
　craniotomy for, 63
　dural repair for, 110
　epidemiology, 58
　etiology, 58
　extracranial surgical approach, 65–66
　facial fracture reduction with craniotomy,
　　65
　glucose concentration, 59
　in gunshot wound of head, 45
　headache with, 59
　immunofixation technique in, 60
　intensive care for, 61
　lumbar drainage in, 66
　management with sella turcica
　　reconstruction, 324–325
　meningitis with, 58, 61, 63
　methylmethacrylate repair, 66
　middle fossa craniotomy, 64–65
　patient position, 61
　in pituitary adenoma, 306
　pneumocephalus with, 58
　posterior fossa craniotomy, 65
　postoperative, 58
　radiography in, 59
　radioisotope scan in, 59–60
　reservoir sign, 59
　in sella turcica surgery, 304–305, 306
　site delineation, 58, 59, 60–61
　spinal, 66–67
　surgical indications, 63
　surgical management, 63
　target sign, 59
　tissue adhesives in, 66
　traumatic vs. spontaneous (nontraumatic),
　　57–58, 60–61
Cerebrospinal fluid rhinorrhea
　with acoustic nerve tumor, 702–703

posthypophysectomy, 348
  as postoperative complication, 331, 333
Cerebrospinal fluid shunt, in cerebrospinal
    fluid leakage, 66
Cervical deformity, after laminectomy in
    children, 1509
Cervical disc excision (anterior)
  in cervical myelopathy, 1339–1341
  in cervical radiculopathy, 1337–1339
  in cervical spondylosis, 1327–1342
  complications, 1335–1337
  fusion with, 1335, 1337
  procedure, 1333–1335
  surgical anatomy, 1332–1333
  surgical indications, 1327–1329
Cervical disc herniation, 1347–1358
Cervical disc herniation (lateral), 1347–1351
  clinical manifestations, 1347
  complications, 1351
  diagnosis, 1348
  incidence, 1347
  nonsurgical treatment, 1348
  patient selection for surgery, 1348
  radiography, 1348
  results, 1351
  surgical treatment, 1348–1351
Cervical fracture-dislocation, skeletal
    traction in, 1449–1451
Cervical laminectomy, postoperative spinal
    deformity in children, 1509
Cervical meningocele, 158
Cervical radiculopathy
  anterior cervical disc excision in, 1327
  anterolateral disc excision results, 1337–
    1339
Cervical rhizotomy, percutaneous
    electrothermo-coagulation technique,
    1211–1216
Cervical rhizotomy (anterior), in torticollis,
    1263
Cervical spinal cord injury
  anesthesia, 1451, 1452
  anterior fusion, 1453–1461
  anterolateral approach to upper spine,
    1461–1462
  posterior fusion, 1464–1466
  pulmonary considerations, 1452
  transoral odontoid resection and fusion,
    1462–1464
  in children, 175
Cervical spine fusion
  anterolateral approach to upper spine,
    1461–1462
  transoral odontoid resection with fusion,
    1462–1464
Cervical spine fusion (anterior)
  in middle/lower spine injury, 1454–1461
  in upper spine injury, 1453–1454
Cervical spine fusion (posterior), 1471–1480
  in atlantoaxial fracture-dislocation, 1464
  lateral facet, 1467–1468
Cervical spondylosis
  angiography, 1332
  anterior cervical disc excision in, 1327–
    1342
  computed tomography, 1332
  diagnosis, 1329–1332
  dysphagia with, 1328–1329
  myelography, 1332

radiography, 1329–1332
  surgical anatomy, 1332–1333
  surgical complications, 1335–1337
  surgical management, 1333–1335
  vertebral artery compression with, 1329
Cervical spondylotic myelopathy, 1351–1357
  anterior cervical disc excision in, 1327–
    1328
  anterolateral disc excision results, 1339–
    1341
  clinical manifestations, 1352
  complications, 1354–1355
  diagnosis, 1352
  incidence, 1351–1352
  nonsurgical treatment, 1352
  pathogenesis, 1351–1352
  radiography, 1352
  surgical approaches, 1352–1353
  surgical indications, 1352
  surgical results, 1355–1357
  surgical technique, 1353–1354
Cervicothoracic junction epidural tumor
    (metastatic), 1555–1557
Chemonucleolysis, 1419, 1437–1441
  anaphylaxis with chymopapain, 1437,
    1438, 1440
  anesthesia, 1439
  with chymopapain, 1437–1441
  complications, 1440
  failures, 1440
  indications for, 1438
  in intervertebral disc disease, 1443–1448
  needle placement, 1439–1440
  patient positioning, 1438–1439
  postoperative course, 1440
  radiography, 1438, 1439
  technique, 1438–1440
Chemotherapy
  with balloon catheter management of
      intracerebral vascular lesion, 835
  in cerebral glioma, 448
  in intracranial metastasis, 455, 456, 460,
    461
  in pineal region tumor, 399
  for pineal tumor, 404–405
Chiari malformation with hydromelia
  angiography, 1316
  diagnosis, 1309–1316
  cerebrospinal fluid shunting in, 1326
  clinical factors, 1308–1309
  computed tomography, 1313
  magnetic resonance imaging, 1311
  microsurgical technique, 1316–1317
  myelography, 1313–1316
  percutaneous cyst needling, 1326
  radiography in, 1309–1316
  surgical management, 1316–1317
  surgical results, 1317
  terminal ventriculostomy for, 1326
  treatment alternatives, 1326
Chiari II malformation, 123
Children. *See also* Neonate, *specific
    childhood condition*s
  anesthesia management, 103–116
  computed tomography in, 1509
  head injury in, 113–114
  holo spinal cord widening, 1495
  intracranial pressure in, 103, 106
  magnetic resonance imaging in, 1509

myelography in, 1509
  neuroradiographic procedures for, 112–
    113
  postoperative care, 107
  preoperative assessment, 106
  spinal cord injury, 114–115
  spinal deformity after neurosurgery, 1509–
    1513
Chordoma
  of clivus, 651
  of clivus and basioccipital region, 635–
    636, 637, 645
Choreoathetosis, stereotactic surgery for,
    1055
Chymopapain, 1437–1441
  anaphylaxis, 1437, 1438
  chemistry, 1437
  pharmacology, 1437
  toxicity, 1437, 1440
Chymopapain chemonucleolysis, 1419
  adverse reactions, 1443–1444
  in intervertebral disc disease, 1443–1448
  mortality, 1443
Cingulate gyrus
  anatomy, 1069–1070
  physiologic factors, 1069–1070
Cingulotomy, for cancer pain, 1047
Cingulotomy (stereotactic)
  for chronic pain, 1069–1075
  equipment, 1071
  patient selection, 1070–1071
  postoperative management, 1073
  for psychiatric disorder, 1069–1075
  results, 1072–1075
  technique, 1071–1072
Circle of Willis, moyamoya disease of, 797–
    806
Cisternography
  metrizamide, 60
  radioisotope, 60
Clivus
  anatomy, 635
  embryology, 635
Clivus and basioccipital region tumor, 635–
    646
  angiography in, 638
  chordoma, 635–636, 637, 645
  clinical presentation, 637
  computed tomography in, 639
  extradural anterior approaches, 642–643
  extradural posterolateral approaches, 644
  intradural approaches, 640–642
  magnetic resonance imaging in, 639–640
  meningioma, 637, 645
  radiography, 637–640
  surgical approach, 640–644
  surgical approach selection, 645
  transbasal approach, 644
  transoral median labiomandibular
      approaches, 643–644
  transsphenoidal approach, 643
Clivus tumor, 650
  chordoma, 651
  classification, 650–651
  computed tomography, 650
  radiography, 650
  surgical approaches, 650–651
Clonogenic assay, in intracranial metastasis,
    456

Cluster headache (chronic migrainous
    neuralgia)
  glycerol injection for, 1136
  radiofrequency heating for, 1136
Coagulation disorders, with acute head
    injury, 30
Cobalt 60 Gamma Unit, 515–529
Commissural myelotomy, 1185–1190
  for cancer pain, 1044
  postoperative care, 1187
  results, 1187, 1189
  technique, 1185–1187
Common peroneal nerve compression, 1596
Computed tomography
  in acute head injury, 19
  in aneurysm, 1004, 1006
  in anterior communicating artery
      aneurysm, 939, 949, 952
  for anterior lumbar discectomy, 1423
  in anterior skull base tumor, 611
  in arteriovenous malformation, 523, 526,
      905
  in bacterial intracranial aneurysm, 998
  in brachial plexus injury, 1578
  in brain abscess, 73
  in brain lesion localization, 215, 216, 217
  in brain stem tumor, 716–718
  in carotid artery lesion, 753
  in carotid ophthalmic aneurysm, 917–918
  in cerebellar astrocytoma, 660
  in cerebellar hemangioblastoma, 660
  in cerebral glioma, 432–433, 436, 444, 445
  in cerebrospinal fluid leakage, 59
  in cervical spondylosis, 1332
  in cervical spondylotic myelopathy, 1352
  in children, 113, 1509
  in clivus and basioccipital region tumor,
      639, 650
  in craniofacial abnormality, 135
  in craniopharyngioma, 355–356, 357
  in cysticercosis, 86, 94, 98
  data transposition to stereotactic films,
      463–464
  in dural fistula, 827
  in dural sinus malformation, 861
  in exophthalmos, 229
  free-hand techniques, 463
  in fungus infection, 89
  in glomus jugulare tumor, 742, 743
  in gunshot wounds of head, 38
  in internal carotid artery aneurysm, 837,
      930
  in intracerebral hematoma, 890–891
  in intracerebral hemorrhage, 881, 884–886
  in intracranial metastasis, 457–458, 459
  in intramedullary spinal cord tumor, 1490
  in intraorbital tumor, 238
  for intraventricular morphine injection,
      1079
  in lateral ventricle tumor, 583
  in lesion localization and biopsy, 463–474
  of lumbar intervertebral disc, 1393, 1394
  in medial sphenoid wing meningioma, 537–
      538
  in meduloblastoma, 658
  in meningioma, 549–550, 564, 571–572
  in metastatic spine tumor, 1516, 1520
  in middle cerebral artery aneurysm, 957,
      958, 968
  in missile injury, 49, 54

  in moyamoya disease, 798
  in olfactory groove meningioma, 540
  in optic glioma, 279
  in optic nerve decompression, 270
  in orbit pathology, 249, 250, 251
  in Paget's disease, 1304
  in pineal tumor, 403
  in posterior fossa tumor, 653–654
  in Rathke's cleft cyst, 373, 374
  in rheumatoid arthritis, 1296
  in scalp/skull tumor, 604
  of sella turcica, 300–301, 356
  in spinal cord arteriovenous malformation,
      1501
  in spinal cord astrocytoma, 176, 177, 184
  in spinal dysraphism, 168
  in spine trauma, 1449
  in spine tumor, 1525, 1526, 1527, 1528,
      1530
  with stereotactic biopsy, 495–498, 502
  stereotactic frame modification for, 464–
      466
  with stereotactic intra-axial tumor
      resection, 481–490
  in stereotactic surgery, 463, 1061–1062
  in subdural hematoma, 33–35
  in suprasellar cyst, 375
  in suprasellar germinoma, 398
  in suprasellar meningioma, 531
  in synostosis, 126–127, 130, 132, 133
  in tentorium tumor, 647, 648
  in thoracolumbar fracture, 1481, 1483,
      1484–1485
  in traumatic aneurysm, 991, 993
  in trigonal meningioma, 597
  in tuberculoma, 80–81
  in tuberculosis meningitis, 84
  in unclippable aneurysm, 1029–1030
  in vertebrobasilar insufficiency, 807
Computer analysis, for stereotactic
    resection, 483–484, 485, 486
Contusion, with missile injury, 51
Cordis Brain State Analyzer, 177
Cordotomy
  for cancer pain, 1043–1044
  percutaneous, 1191–1205
Cordotomy (open)
  anesthesia, 1158
  anterolateral, spinal cord anatomy and,
      1156
  bilateral, 1155–1156, 1163
  bladder dysfunction after, 1163
  corticospinal tract anatomy and, 1156–
      1157
  dentate insertion variations and, 1157
  dysesthesias after, 1165
  electrophysiologic monitoring, 1158
  failures, 1164
  indications for, 1155–1156
  instrumentation, 1157–1158
  for intractable pain, 1155–1168
  mortality, 1164
  patient positioning, 1159
  postoperative complications, 1163
  postoperative hypotension, 1163, 1165
  postoperative sleep apnea, 1163
  postoperative weakness, 1163, 1165
  preoperative preparation, 1157–1158
  respiratory complications, 1164
  results, 1163–1164

  sexual dysfunction after, 1165
  spinal cord width variations and, 1157
  spinothalamic tract anatomy and, 1156
  unilateral, 1155, 1159–1163
Coronal synostosis
  complications, 131
  diagnosis, 130
  lateral canthal advancement, 131
  results, 131
  surgical technique, 131
Corpus callostomy
  commissurotomy results, 1247–1249
  commissurotomy technique, 1244–1247
  complications, 1248
  for epilepsy, 1243–1250
  neuropsychological effects, 1248–1249
Cortical resection
  anesthesia for, 1225
  complications, 1232–1233
  for epilepsy, 1223–1234
  incision, 1226
  partial temporal lobectomy, 1223–1234
  patient positioning, 1226
  postoperative care, 1232
  results, 1233–1234
Corticosteroids
  in cerebral glioma, 435
  in intracranial metastasis, 453, 461
  in missile injury, 51
  in orbit pathology, 251
  in spinal cord compression, 1541
  in subdural hematoma, 33
  in tuberculoma, 82
Costotransversectomy, in thoracic disc
    herniation, 1367–1371
Cotrel-Dubousset fixation, in scoliosis, 201–
    202
Cranial nerve(s), nociceptive afferents, 1165–
    1166
Cranial nerve disorders, 1097–1109, See also
    specific diagnoses
Cranial nerve injury
  with basilar skull fracture, 21
  after stereotactic radiosurgery, 521
Cranial nociceptive tract (descending),
    medullary tractotomy of, 1165–1166
Cranial suture, histology, 125
Craniofacial abnormality, 134–137
  classification, 135
  complications, 137
  computed tomography in, 135
  diagnosis, 135
  genetic factor, 135
  hypertelorism with, 137
  LeFort III midface advancement, 137
  radiography in, 135
  results, 137
  treatment, 135
Craniofacial repair, anesthesia for, 111–112
Craniofacial resection
  for anterior skull base tumor, 609–618
  Cavitron ultrasonic tumor aspirator in, 613
  complications, 616–617
  for epidermoid cancer, 609
  for nasal tumor, 611
  for paranasal sinus tumor, 609
  patient selection, 612
  postoperative management, 615–616
  preoperative evaluation, 612
  results, 617

for salivary gland tumor, 609
skull base reconstruction in, 615
technique, 612–615
Craniopharyngioma, 349–379
angiography, 356–357
calcification removal, 363
in children, 109
clinical presentation, 355
computed tomography, 355–356, 357
desmopressin acetate in, 365
endocrine management, 364–365
extracerebral removal, 359–360
growth characteristics, 349–355
growth direction, 349–352
growth rate, 349
histology, 352–354
lateroposterior transpetrosal-transtentorial
approach, 362
magnetic resonance imaging, 355–356
metabolic management, 364–365
microscopic features, 352–355
pituitary stalk sacrifice in, 363
pterional approach, 362
radiation therapy, 368–372
radical surgery, 357–368
radiography, 355–357
reconstruction technique, 331
removal of bone anterior to sella, 360
reservoir drainage system for, 364
results, 365–367, 369
retrochiasmal removal, 360–362
sequelae, 365
shunting procedures, 364
site, 349–352
size/cystic content relation to operation
type, 362–363
small tumor management, 367–368
stereotactic radiosurgery, 515–516
suboccipital approach, 364
subtemporal approach, 362
transcallosal approach, 364
transcorticoventricular approach, 364
transfrontal approach, 358–359
transsphenoidal approach, 317–318, 363–
364
visual deficit, 355
Cranioplasty
brain protection factor, 12
complications, 14
cosmetic considerations, 12
indications for, 12, 14
infection with, 14
methyl methacrylate for, 11, 14–16
technique, 14–16
Craniosynostosis, 125–134. *See also specific
deformities*
anatomy, 125–126
anesthesia for, 111
associated abnormalities, 125
pathophysiology, 125–126
preoperative evaluation, 125–126
Craniotomy
basic trauma, 22–23
for cerebrospinal fluid leakage, 63
exploratory burr holes, 22
for neonate, 117–119
Craniovertebral junction abnormality, 1281–
1293
anatomy, 1281–1282
anterior transoral-transpharyngeal

approach, 1288–1292
diagnosis, 1284
embryology, 1281–1282
immobilization management, 1285
posterior decompression for, 1287
posterior fusion for, 1285–1287
radiography, 1284
surgical procedures for, 1281
surgical results, 1292
surgical technique, 1285–1292
symptoms, 1282–1284
Curietherapy, 491, 499–503
indications for, 507–512
Currarino triad, 160
Cushing's disease, 299–300
stereotactic radiosurgery, 516–518
Cyanoacrylate tissue adhesive, in
cerebrospinal fluid leakage, 66
Cysticercosis, 85–88, 93–102
cerebrospinal fluid blockage with, 98, 99
in chiasmatic region, 98
clinical features, 86, 93–94
computed tomography in, 86, 94, 98
cysts (*Cysticercus cellulosae*), 93
diagnosis, 86, 94–95
diagnosis, 94–95
drug therapy, 87
epidemiology, 93
incidence, 85
increased intracranial pressure with, 98
management, 87
medical management, 95
pathology, 85–86, 93
prognosis, 95
racemose lesions, 96
seizures with, 95, 96
serology, 94–95
spinal, 98
surgical approaches, 98–99
surgical indications, 95–96
surgical management, 87–88, 95–99
Taenia solium transmission, 93
of ventricular pathways, 96
Cysticercus cellulosae, 93

Dandy-Foerster operation, 1054
Dandy-Walker malformation, 121, 123, 658–
659
Decompression, in cerebral glioma, 436,
442–443
Decompression laminectomy, in metastatic
spine tumor, 1519–1523
Denervation pain, 1042
stimulation therapy for, 1049
Dermal sinus pore, 166
Dermoid cyst, posterior fossa, 658–659
Descending cranial nociceptive tract. *See*
Medullary tractotomy
Desmopressin acetate, in
craniopharyngioma, 365
Dexamethasone suppression test, 300
Diabetes insipidus, 300, 398
with pituitary adenoma, 307
posthypophysectomy, 348
Diabetic retinopathy, stereotactic thermal
hypophysectomy for, 345–348
Diastematomyelia, 164–165
surgery for, 169–170

Dinorphin, 1078
Diplomyelia, 165
Disc distention test, 1343–1345
Discography, 1343–1345
for anterior lumbar discectomy, 1422–1423
Discometry, 1343
Disseminated intravascular coagulation, with
acute head injury, 27
Distal vertebral endarterectomy
results, 811–812
technique, 810–811
for vertebrobasilar insufficiency, 810–812
Dopaminergic agents, in torticollis, 1262
Dorsal column stimulation, for denervation
pain, 1049
Dorsal root entry zone, anatomy, 1169
Dorsal root entry zone thermocoagulation,
1169–1175
at conus, 1173
electrophysiologic control, 1173
indications for, 1170–1172
patient selection, 1170–1172
physiologic basis, 1169–1170
results, 1173–1174
technique, 1172–1174
Dorsal spinal cord stimulation, electrode
implantation for, 1039
Dura tear repair, 110
Dural arteriovenous malformation (lateral/
sigmoid sinuses), 855–862
craniotomy, 856
embolization, 855
patient positioning, 855
preoperative embolization, 855
scalp flap, 855
sinus ligation, 856–857
soft-tissue dissection, 855
surgical technique, 855–859
Dural fistula
angiography, 828
anteroinferior dural, 849–854
balloon catheter management, 827–828
computed tomography, 827
Dural sinus laceration, 875–879
anatomy, 876–877
diagnosis, 875
exposure, 875
patient positioning, 875
surgical preparation, 875
surgical technique, 877–879
Dural sinus malformation
angiography, 861
arterial supply, 861
bridging veins, 861
closure, 859
computed tomography, 861
diagnosis, 861
magnetic resonance imaging, 861
pathogenesis, 860
pathophysiology, 860
results, 859
symptomatology, 859–860
technical considerations, 861
venous drainage, 861
Dural sinus repair, with penetrating missile
injury, 53
Dural venous fistula (anteroinferior)
case reports, 850–854
obliteration, 849–854
transvenous approach, 849–854

Dural venous sinuses
  abnormal vascular channel elimination, 872–873
  abnormal vascular communication management, 872–873
  compressive obstruction control, 863, 868
  dural tunnel construction, 865
  embolization for abnormal vascular communication, 873
  hemorrhage control, 863
  intima-lined stent placement, 868, 871
  normal flow reinstitution, 868–876
  replacement graft, 868
  surgical management, 863–874
  trapping for abnormal vascular communication, 872–873
Dwyer instrumentation, in scoliosis, 203–204
Dysphagia, with cervical spondylosis, 1328–1329
Dystonia (adult-onset), 1261, 1269
  medical treatment, 1261
  peripheral denervation in, 1268
  surgical management, 1268
Dystonia musculorum deformans, stereotactic surgery for, 1053

Electric current thrombosis, 873
Electrical stimulation
  in scoliosis, 191–194
  with temporal lobectomy, 1229–1230
Electrocorticography, in temporal lobectomy, 1227
Electrode brain stimulation
  for analgesia, 1089–1095
  electrode internalization, 1094–1095
  implantation procedure, 1090–1094
  patient selection, 1089
  postimplantation care, 1094
  postoperative constant point screening, 1094
  results, 1095
Electroencephalography
  in aneurysm, 1004, 1006
  in epilepsy, 1224
  in infantile hemiplegia, 1235–1236
  in meningioma, 551
  in moyamoya disease, 799, 801, 804
  with stereotactic surgery, 1038
Electrolyte balance, with acute head injury, 29–30, 114
Electromyelography
  in compressive nerve lesions, 1584, 1585
  in thoracic outlet syndrome, 1592
Electromyography
  for anterior lumbar discectomy, 1432
  in cervical disc herniation, 1348
  in cervical spondylotic myelopathy, 1352
  in peripheral nerve injury, 1567, 1571
  in torticollis, 1263–1264
Electroneuroprosthesis, 1062–1064
Electronic stimulators (implantable), 1039
  implantation technique, 1039–1040
Electrophysiologic monitoring, for open cordotomy, 1158
Electrothermocoagulation (percutaneous), of spinal nerve trunk/ganglion/rootlets, 1207–1221
Embolic agents
  for intracerebral vascular lesion

management, 820–821
  liquid substances that solidify, 820–821
  solid particles, 820
Embolization
  in arteriovenous aneurysm, 905, 906, 908, 909
  in arteriovenous malformation, 828–831, 903, 911
  in atherosclerotic carotid artery lesion, 753
  in carotid cavernous fistula, 873
  in dural arteriovenous malformation, 855
  of glomus jugulare tumor, 744
  for meningioma, 551–553
  for spinal cord arteriovenous malformation, 1502
  in spine tumor, 1526
Encephalocele
  frontal nasal, 121
  intraorbital, 239
  occipital, 120–121
Encephaloduroarteriosynangiosis, in moyamoya disease, 802, 804
Encephalomyosynangiosis, in moyamoya disease, 802, 804
Endocrine factor
  in craniopharyngioma, 364–365
  in pituitary adenoma, 299–300, 305
  in sella turcica lesion, 299–300
  in third ventricle tumor, 398
Endorphins, 1078
Endoscopy (neurologic), 423–430
  operative procedures, 426
  optical system, 425–428
  preoperative procedures, 425
  prospectus, 424–425
  stereotactic protocol, 428–430
Endotracheal intubation, in children, 104
Enkephalins, 1078
Ependymoma, intramedullary spinal cord, 1490
Epidermoid cancer, craniofacial resection for, 609
Epidural cervical stimulation, in torticollis, 1262
Epidural hematoma, with acute head injury, 23
Epidural implantation systems
  availability, 1147–1148
  complications, 1149–1152
  for intractable pain, 1147–1148
Epidural tumor (metastatic)
  anterior decompression and vertebral body replacement, 1548–1559
  bone compression factor, 1543–1544
  bone grafting in, 1547–1548
  cell type factor, 1541
  of cervicothoracic junction, 1555–1557
  complications, 1560
  corticosteroids response factor, 1541
  functional prognosis, 1541
  incidence, 1539
  location, 1539, 1541–1542
  of lumbar spine, 1559
  morbidity, 1560–1561
  mortality, 1560
  neurologic deterioration with, 1541
  pathophysiology, 1540
  posterior decompression and instrumentation, 1545–1548
  postoperative care, 1548, 1553

pretreatment neurologic status, 1541
  radiation therapy, 1542, 1543, 1560
  radioresistance, 1543
  with spinal cord compression, 1539–1562
  spinal instability factor, 1543–1544
  surgical indications, 1543–1544
  surgical management, 1543–1559
  surgical techniques, 1544–1559
  survival, 1540–1541
  symptomatology, 1539
  therapy alternatives, 1542
  therapy selection, 1542
  of thoracic spine, 1553–1555
  thoracic wall excision, 1553
  of thoracolumbar spine, 1557–1559
  vertebral body replacement technique, 1552–1553
Epilepsy
  in children, 110
  clinical investigation, 1224
  corpus callosum section for, 1243–1250
  cortical resection for, 1223–1234
  electroencephalography in, 1224
  neuropsychologic examination in, 1224
  operative procedure for corpus callostomy, 1244–1247
  patient positioning, 1226
  postoperative care, 1232
  preoperative preparation, 1225
  radiography in, 1224
  stereotactic surgery for, 1060–1061
  surgical complications, 1232–1233
  surgical criteria, 1223–1224
  surgical indications, 1243–1244
  surgical results, 1233–1234, 1247–1249
Epsilon-aminocaproic acid, 931
Esthesioneuroblastoma, 611
Ethambutal, 81
Ethanol, as embolic agent, 821
Ethmoidectomy (external), in optic nerve decompression, 270
Exophthalmos
  in adults, 229
  bilateral, 229–233
  in children, 229
  computed tomography in, 229
  differential diagnosis, 229–233
  unilateral, 229–233
Extralemniscal myelotomy, for cancer pain, 1044
Extraocular muscles, 236
Extrapyramidal system, in movement disorders, 1050–1051
Extrathoracic common carotid-subclavian bypass, 781

Facial fracture, with cerebrospinal fluid leakage, 65
Facial neuralgia (atypical), glycerol injection for, 1136
Facial neuralgia (post-traumatic), glycerol injection for, 1136
Facial pain, percutaneous rhizotomy/ microvascular decompression complications, 1139–1143
Facial pain (atypical), trigeminal rhizotomy for, 1120–1121
Facial pain (intractable), percutaneous rhizotomy for, 1111–1123

Facial palsy
  cross-facial nerve graft, 705
  dynamic muscle reconstruction, 707
  local/distant muscle transfer in, 707
  nerve transfer in, 705
  neurectomy/myomectomy for, 707
  peripheral nerve surgery, 705
  static procedures for, 707
  surgical correction, 705–708
Facial paralysis, surgical management, 681–683
Fawn's tail, 166
Fiberoptic endoscopy, 423–430
Fibrillation potentials, in peripheral nerve injury, 1567
Fibrin clot adhesives, in cerebrospinal fluid leakage, 66
Firearms, ballistic data, 37
Fistula. See specific sites
Flucytosine, in fungus infection, 90
Fluid balance
  with acute head injury, 29–30, 114
  in children, 105–106
Fluorescein scan, in cerebrospinal fluid leakage, 59
Fourth ventricle ependymoma
  radiation therapy, 658
  surgical management, 658
Frontal lobectomy
  in cerebral glioma, 436–439
  exposure, 437–438
  patient positioning, 437
  postoperative deficits, 439
Frontal nasal encephalocele, 121
Frontotemporal approach, to clivus, 640
Functional neurosurgery, 1035–1068. See also specific disorders
  chronic stimulation techniques, 1039–1040
  indications for, 1040–1057
  stereotactic techniques, 1035–1039
Fungus infection, 79, 88–90
  cerebritis with, 89
  computed tomography, 89
  diagnosis, 89
  drug therapy, 90
  granuloma with, 89
  management, 90
  pathology, 89
  surgical management, 90

Gadolinium-diethylenetriamine pentaacetic acid, 280, 550
Gelfoam, as embolic agent, 820
Germ cell tumor
  alpha fetoprotein in, 398
  human chorionic gonadotropin in, 398
Germinoma. See also specific sites
  chemotherapy, 399
  suprasellar, 397
Genetic factor
  in craniofacial abnormality, 135
  in moyamoya disease, 797
  in myelomeningocele, 151
  in synostosis, 126
Gigantism, 299
Glasco Coma Scale, in subdural hematoma, 33
Glioblastoma multiforme, 431

Glioma. See also specific diagnoses
  intraoperative ultrasonography visualization, 217
  preoperative assessment, 432
Glioma (intracranial), 431–450
  anticonvulsants in, 435–436
  biopsy in, 436
  chemotherapy, 448
  computed tomography, 432–433, 436, 444, 445
  corticosteroids in, 435
  decompression in, 436, 442–443
  frontal lobectomy in, 436–439
  immunotherapy, 448
  intraoperative management, 436
  Karnofsky rating in, 444–445
  magnetic resonance imaging, 433
  neuropsychologic testing, 434–435
  occipital lobectomy in, 441–442
  postoperative care, 443–444
  preoperative management, 435–436
  radiation therapy, 448
  radiography, 432–433
  reoperation for, 444–446
  surgical alternatives, 436
  survival rates, 436
  temporal lobectomy in, 439–441
  visual fields in, 433–434
Glomus jugulare tumor, 739–752
  anatomy, 741
  anesthesia in, 745
  arteriography, 742, 744
  biochemistry, 742
  bleeding with, 750
  case, 747
  cerebrospinal fluid fistula with, 750
  classification, 741
  clinical material, 742
  complications, 749
  computed tomography, 742, 743
  cranial nerve dysfunction, 742, 750
  dental evaluation, 745
  diagnosis, 742–743
  differential diagnosis, 742
  embolization, 744
  epidemiology, 741
  pathology, 741
  postoperative management, 746, 747
  preoperative medical management, 744
  preoperative procedures, 745
  radiation therapy, 739, 743–744, 749
  results, 748–749
  sigmoid-jugular control, 746
  skull base approach, 745–746
  skull base exposure, 745–746
  small tumor management, 747
  surgical approach, 749
  surgical approach review, 739–741
  surgical technique, 749–750
  symptoms, 742
  temporal bone exposure, 746
  treatment selection, 743
  tumor removal, 746
  very large tumor management, 747
  wound closure, 746
Glossopharyngeal neuralgia, 1108–1109
  percutaneous rhizotomy for, 1121–1122, 1125–1127
Glucose (CSF), in cerebrospinal fluid leakage, 59

Glycerol chemoneurolysis, in trigeminal neuralgia, 1098
Glycerol injection (retrogasserian)
  for atypical facial neuralgia, 1136
  biological effects, 1134–1136
  for cluster headache, 1136
  complications, 1131
  hemorrhagic diasthesis with, 1133
  mechanism of action, 1134–1136
  for multiple sclerosis, 1134
  results, 1129–1133
  for post-traumatic facial neuralgia, 1136
  technique, 1133–1134
  in trigeminal neuralgia, 1129–1137
Grafts. See specific reconstruction techniques
Granuloma, with fungus infection, 89
Griseotomy, radiofrequency, 1181
Growth hormone, in pituitary adenoma, 299
Gunshot wounds
  ballistic data, 37
  of brachial plexus, 1578
Gunshot wounds (head), 37–48
  angiography, 38–39
  bacterial contamination, 38, 43
  bone fragment removal, 39
  case reports, 41–44
  cerebrospinal fluid leakage with, 45
  computed tomography, 38
  debridement, 39, 40, 43
  diuretics preoperatively, 39
  exit wound, 39
  hemostasis, 39, 40
  laceration and crushing, 37–38
  neurologic deficit, 38
  postoperative care, 47–48
  preoperative evaluation, 38
  prognosis-wound type relation, 45
  radiography, 38–39
  retained bone management, 45, 47
  shock waves, 38
  with spent bullet, 44–45
  surgical pathology, 37–38
  surgical technique, 39–41
  temporary cavitation, 38
  watertight closure, 39–40

Håkanson procedure, 1129
  results, 1129–1133
Harrington rod instrumentation, 198
Harrington-rod thoracolumbar spine fusion, 1475–1478
Head injury
  anesthesia for, 113–114
  in children, 113–114
  gunshot wound management, 37–48
  nonoperative management, 114
  optic nerve lesion with, 269
Head injury (acute). See also specific lesions
  blood pressure management, 25
  coagulopathy with, 30
  complications, 25–30
  computed tomography in, 19
  emergency room care, 19
  fluid and electrolyte management, 29–30
  gastrointestinal complications, 30
  infection with, 26–27
  intracranial pressure monitoring with, 25–26, 27

Head injury (acute) *(continued)*
  postoperative management, 24–25
  preoperative care, 19
  respiratory complications, 27–29
  seizures with, 30
  specific injury management, 20–24
  surgical management, 19–31
  traumatic mass lesion, 22–24
  triage for, 19, 20
  ventilatory assistance with, 27–29
Headache
  with arteriovenous malformation, 914
  with cerebrospinal fluid leakage, 59
Hearing, electroneuroprosthesis, 1063
Hearing loss
  in Meniere's disease, 1251
  after stereotactic radiosurgery, 521
Hemangioblastoma, intramedullary spinal
    cord, 1492, 1495–1496
Hemangioma (cavernous) stereotactic
    resection, 489
Hematoma. *See also specific lesions*
  with acoustic nerve tumor, 702
  with missile injury, 51
Hematoma (intracerebral)
  case reports, 893–897
  computed tomography, 890–891
  preoperative calculations, 890–891
  results, 892
  stereotactic evacuation, 889–898
  stereotactic instrumentation, 889–890
  surgical technique, 891
  with traumatic aneurysm, 991
Hemiballism, stereotactic surgery for, 1053
Hemifacial spasm, 1105–1108
  Jannetta microvascular decompression,
    1106–1108
  results, 1108
  surgical complications, 1108
Hemiplegia (infantile)
  electroencephalography, 1235–1236
  etiology, 1235
  hemispherectomy for, 1235–1241
  homonymous hemianopsia with, 1235,
    1236
  mental retardation with, 1236
  neurologic aspects, 1236
  radiography in, 1236
  seizures with, 1235
Hemispherectomy (cerebral), 1235–1241
  behavior modification, 1239
  clinical aspects, 1235
  hemianopsia and, 1235, 1236
  hemosiderosis with, 1236
  intellectual status results, 1239
  intracranial pressure complications, 1238
  late complications, 1236, 1240
  patient selection, 1235–1236
  postoperative care, 1238
  preoperative preparation, 1237
  results, 1239–1240
  socioeconomic status postoperative, 1239–
    1240
  technique, 1237–1238
Hemorrhage. *See specific sites*
  with artervenous malformation, 913–914
Hemosiderosis, with cerebral
    hemispherectomy, 1236
Hemostatis
  with laser, 226

in meningioma surgery, 558, 560
Herpes simplex encephalitis, 419
Herpes zoster
  dorsal root entry zone thermocoagulation
    for pain, 1171–1172, 1174
  medical management, 1172
  postherpetic neuralgia, 1049
Hibbs spine fusion, 1473
Holo spinal cord widening, 1495
Homonymous hemianopsia, 1235, 1236
Horsley-Clark stereotactic apparatus, 491,
    492, 494, 1035, 1037
House-Urban rotary dissector, 650
Human chorionic gonadotropin, in
    intracranial germ cell tumor, 398
Huntington's chorea, stereotactic surgery
    for, 1052–1053
Hydrocephalus, 141–150. *See also* Shunting
    procedure
  in children, 110
  clinical findings, 141–142
  endoscopy in, 423
  in intracranial metastasis, 459
  with missile injury, 53
  with myelomeningocele, 119
  in neonate, 119
  pathophysiology, 141
  with spinal cord astrocytoma, 182
  after stereotactic radiosurgery, 521
  surgical shunting indications, 141
  surgical treatment, 142–150
  with tuberculous meningitis, 83–85
  ventricular drainage, 573
Hydromyelia, with Chiari malformation,
    1307–1326
Hyperhidrosis, 1271, 1272
Hyperkinesis, with brain stem tumor, 722,
    724
Hypertelorism, 137
Hypertension, aneurysm and, 1003, 1006
Hypertensive hematoma, stereotactic
    evacuation, 889–898
Hypoglossal-facial nerve anastomosis, 682–
    683
Hypoglossal nerve, transfer in facial palsy,
    705
Hyponatremia, with acute head injury, 30
Hypophysectomy. *See also* Stereotactic
    thermal hypophysectomy
  reconstruction technique, 331
  replacement therapy, 347–348
  transsphenoidal approach, 315–316
Hypotension (controlled)
  in anterior communicating artery
    aneurysm, 941
  in carotid ophthalmic aneurysm, 918–919
  in children, 107
  in unclippable aneurysm, 1030, 1032
Hypothermia (induced)
  in children, 108
  in neonate, 117
  in saccular aneurysm, 839, 841

Immunofixation technique, in cerebrospinal
    fluid leakage, 60
Immunotherapy
  in cerebral glioma, 448
  in intracranial metastasis, 460

Impedance monitoring, in percutaneous
    cordotomy, 1195, 1198
Implantable electronic stimulators, 1039
Implantable systems, for intractable pain,
    1145–1153
Indigo carmine scan, in cerebrospinal fluid
    leakage, 59–60
Infection. *See also specific diagnoses*
  with acute head injury, 26–27
  with skull fracture, 14
Infratemporal fossa approach
  to clivus, 644
  to posterior cranial fossa, 668, 671
Infratentorial approach, to posterior fossa
    tumor, 660–662
Intercostal nerve denervation, percutaneous
    electrothermocoagulation technique,
    1215–1216
Interfornicial approach, to third ventricle,
    382, 389
Internal carotid artery
  complications of distal exposure, 769
  distal exposure, 765–769
  distal exposure alternatives, 765
  dissection, 767
  lesions requiring distal exposure, 765
  reconstruction, 769
Internal carotid artery aneurysm,
  angiography in, 930
  at anterior choroidal artery, 929, 930, 932
  at carotid bifurcation, 929, 930, 931, 932,
    1025
  carotid ligation, 1025
  carotid occlusion for, 1023
  clipping procedure, 934–935
  computed tomography, 930
  diagnosis, 930–931
  paraclinoid, 1032
  at posterior communicating artery
    junction, 929, 930, 931–932, 1025
  preoperative management, 931
  results, 935–936
  subarachnoid hemorrhage with, 929, 930,
    931, 936
  supraclinoid, 930
  surgical anatomy, 931
  surgical management, 929–955
  surgical procedure, 932–935
  symptoms, 929–930
Internal carotid artery aneurysm
    (intracavernous), 837–844
  angiography, 837
  computed tomography, 837
  developmental vs. traumatic, 837
  diagnosis, 837
  direct surgical repair, 839–842
  epistaxis with, 837, 838
  hemorrhage control, 838–839
  hypothermia in, 839, 841
  radiography, 837
  treatment, 837–842
Intervertebral disc (cervical)
  disc distention test, 1343–1345
  discography, 1343–1345
  discometry, 1343
Intervertebral disc (lumbar)
  anesthesia selection, 1380
  computed tomography, 1393, 1394
  degeneration, 1393
  epidural fat management, 1388–1389

excision, 1390
exploratory surgery, 1379
free disc fragments, 1391
herniation pathology, 1393
interlaminar surgery, 1390
interspace dissection, 1387
lesion site confirmation, 1380
microsurgical discectomy, 1399
myelography, 1375–1376, 1393, 1394
nerve root anomalies, 1392
nerve root damage, 1388–1389, 1394
neurological changes evaluation, 1375, 1393
procedure selection, 1380
prognostic factors, 1377
root tension management, 1390
sciatica and, 1393
subperiosteal dissection, 1385–1387
surface landmarks, 1384
surgery—historical development, 1379–1380
surgery—predictive score card, 1376–1378, 1393
surgical contraindications, 1377, 1379
surgical criteria, 1375
surgical field inspection, 1390
surgical incision, 1384–1385
surgical positioning, 1382–1384, 1394
wound closure, 1392
Intervertebral disc (thoracic)
costotransversectomy, 1367–1371
excision technique, 1367–1374
transthoracic (transpleural) approach, 1371–1374
Intervertebral disc disease
anterior lumbar discectomy and interbody fusion for, 1421–1436
chymopapain chemonucleolysis in, 1443–1448
diagnosis, 1422–1423
Intervertebral disc herniation, intraoperative ultrasonography visualization, 221
Intra-axial tumor
approach alternatives, 484–485
stereotactic definition of approach, 485
stereotactic resection, 481–490
volume interpolation, 483–484
Intracerebral hematoma, with acute head injury, 24
Intracerebral hemorrhage, 881–888
angiography, 885
classification, 881
clinical presentation, 881–882
computed tomography, 881, 884–886
diagnosis, 884–885
etiology, 881
general management, 885
postoperative care, 887
primary, 881
prognosis, 884–885
subependymal/intraventricular in infants, 884
surgical management, 885–887
surgical technique, 887
symptomatic, 882–884
Intracranial infection, 71–77
Intracranial extradural abscess, 71
Intracranial lesion, stereotactic biopsy, 495–498
Intracranial pressure

with acute head injury, 25–26, 27
anesthesia management and, 103, 106
in children, 103, 106
with head injury, 114
with hemispherectomy, 1238
with intraventricular hemorrhage, 119
with missile injury, 51, 52
in subdural hematoma, 34
with synostosis, 125–126
Intracranial subdural abscess, 71–72
Intracranial tumor
approach, 239
stereotactic radiosurgery, 515–529
Intracranial tumor (deep-seated), stereotactic resection, 481–490
Intramedullary spinal cord astrocytoma
anterior subarachnoid spinal fluid loculation, 182
in children, 175–185
clinical presentation, 175
computed tomography in, 176, 177, 184
congenital, 184
focal, 177
holocord, 176, 184, 185
hydrocephalus with, 182
magnetic resonance imaging in, 177, 184
malignant, 182
neurodiagnostic evaluation, 176, 184
postoperative morbidity relation to segmental location, 184
radiation therapy for, 180, 185
results, 184
rostral or caudal tumor fragment, 181–182
surgical complications, 181–184
surgical procedure for, 177–180
transcutaneous ultrasonography in, 177, 184
Intramedullary tumor, with syringomyelia, 1307, 1326
Intraneural artery, in peripheral nerve repair, 1564
Intraorbital tumor, 235–244
anatomy, 235–238
anesthesia, 239
case selection, 238–239
closure, 243
complications, 244
computed tomography in, 238
diagnosis, 238
instrumentation, 239
lateral orbital approach, 243
magnetic resonance imaging in, 238
medial orbit approach, 241
operative procedure, 240–244
polytomography in, 238
postoperative care, 244
preoperative management, 239
tarsorrhaphy in, 244
Intraspinal infection, 71–77
Intraspinal tumor, postoperative kyphosis/scoliosis in children, 1509–1513
Intraventricular hemorrhage, in premature infant, 119
Iontophoresis, in torticollis, 1262
Isoflurane, in children, 108
Isobutyl-2-cyanoacrylate, 744
Isoniazid, 81–82

Jannetta microvascular decompression
anesthesia for, 1099

complications, 1104–1105
for glossopharyngeal neuralgia, 1108–1109
for hemifacial spasm, 1106–1108
instrumentation, 1101–1102
positioning for, 1099
postoperative considerations, 1103–1104
preoperative evaluation, 1099
results, 1104–1105
surgical procedure, 1099–1103
for trigeminal neuralgia, 1097–1098
Jugular foramen syndrome, 743

Karnofsky rating, 444–445
Kidney disease, with myelomeningocele, 151
Krönlein procedure, 270
Kyphosis, 187–211. *See also* Scoliosis
classification, 187
after intraspinal tumor surgery in children, 1509–1513
natural history, 190–191
after radiation therapy in children, 1509

Labbé's vein, 857, 861
Labyrinthectomy, in Meniere's disease, 1255
Labyrinthine disorders. *See also specific diagnoses*
nonsurgical treatment, 1254
Labyrinthitis (chronic)
nonsurgical treatment, 1254
pathophysiology, 1254
Lacrimal gland tumor, 264–265
Lambdoid synostosis, 132–133
complications, 133
diagnosis, 132
lambdoid synostectomy, 132–133
results, 133
surgical technique, 132–133
Laminectomy, in spinal cord injury, 1466–1467
Laminectomy (decompressive), in Paget's disease, 1305
Laryngoscopy, in children, 104
Laser technology, 223
aneurysm occlusion, 226
argon, 223–224, 226
biologic effects, 223–225
carbon dioxide, 223, 224, 225
clinical applications, 225–226
with computer-assisted stereotactic resection, 485–486
evaluation, 223
hemostasis, 226
in meningioma surgery, 559
Nd:YGA, 223, 226
neoplasm excision, 223–228
pain surgery, 226
perspectus, 226
physics, 223
stereotactic laser microsurgery, 226, 1062
systems, 225
techniques, 225
tissue bonding, 226
wet-field carbon dioxide, 226
Later particle agglutination test, in tuberculous meningitis, 84
Lateral femoral cutaneous nerve entrapment, 1593
Lateral osteotomy approach, to spine tumor, 1535–1536

Lateral sinus, dural arteriovenous malformation, 855–862
Lateral ventricle meningioma (trigonal)
  computed tomography in, 597
  surgical approaches, 597–599
Lateral ventricle tumor, 583–596
  approaches, 583
  case report, 592–595
  computed tomography in, 583
  postoperative care, 592
  preoperative studies, 583
  surgical complications, 591–592
Lateral ventricle tumor (frontal horn), 589–591
  anatomy, 589–590
  surgical approach, 590–591
  transcallosal approach, 590–591
Lateral ventricle tumor (midbody), 588–589
  anatomy, 588
  surgical approach, 588–589
  transcallosal approach, 588–589
Lateral ventricle tumor (temporal horn), 591
  anatomy, 591
  surgical approach, 591
Lateral ventricle tumor (trigonal), 583–588
  anatomy, 584
  approaches, 584–588
  lateral temporal parietal lobe incision, 584
  middle temporal gyrus incision, 584
  occipital lobectomy, 585
  superior parietal occipital incision, 585
  transcallosal approach, 585–586
  transtemporal horn occipital temporal gyrus incision, 586–587
Lateroposterior transpetrosal-transtentorial approach, to craniopharyngioma, 362
LeFort III midface advancement, 137
Leksell stereotactic system, 464–465, 492, 1037
Limbic system surgery, 1069–1070
Lipoma, transpinal, 163, 170–172
Lipomyelomeningocele, 163
Lobectomy. See specific approaches
Localization technique
  computed tomography in, 463–474
  magnetic resonance imaging in, 463–474
Low back pain, stimulation management, 1049
Lower extremity causalgia, lumbar sympathectomy for, 1277–1278
Lumbar disc excision (microsurgical)
  advantages/disadvantages, 1397
  patient selection, 1395
  postoperative care, 1396–1397
  results, 1397
  preoperative preparation, 1395
  procedure rationale, 1395
  technique, 1395–1397
Lumbar disc herniation
  chymopapain chemonucleolysis, 1437–1441
  microsurgical disc excision, 1395–1397
Lumbar drainage, in cerebrospinal fluid leakage, 66
Lumbar epidural tumor (metastatic), 1559
Lumbar interbody fusion (posterior)
  biochemical considerations, 1401–1405
  closure, 1410
  complications, 1414–1415

decortication with, 1404, 1408
  epidural hemostasis with, 1406
  exposure, 1405–1406
  grafting, 1402–1403, 1404–1405, 1408–1410, 1418
  indications for, 1401
  for lumbar spondylosis, 1401–1420
  patient positioning, 1405
  posterior motion segment preservation, 1403
  postoperative care, 1410, 1412
  pseudoarthrosis with, 1414
  results, 1415–1417
  surgical pitfalls, 1412–1414
  technique, 1405–1410
  total discectomy with, 1403–1404, 1406–1408
  unigraft concept, 1404–1405
Lumbar meningocele, 158–159
Lumbar rhizotomy
  fifth lumbar denervation, 1217–1220
  percutaneous electrothermocoagulation technique, 1216–1220
Lumbar shunt, spinal complications after, 1510
Lumbar spinal deformity, surgical treatment, 1511–1512
Lumbar spine fusion, 1473
  extraperitoneal, 1474–1475
Lumbar spine injury, anterior lateral approach, 1468
Lumbar spondylosis
  anatomic alignment changes with, 1401
  instability categories, 1401
  posterior lumbar interbody fusion in, 1401–1420
  postoperative care, 1410, 1412
  radiography, 1403
  surgical results, 1415–1417
Lumbar sympathectomy, 1277–1279
  anatomy, 1277
  complications, 1279
  indications for, 1277–1278
  results, 1279
  surgical technique, 1277–1279
Lumbosacral spine fusion, 1474

Magnetic resonance imaging
  anesthesia for, 113
  in anterior communicating artery aneurysm, 939
  in arteriovenous malformation, 523, 905
  in brain stem tumor, 716–718
  in carotid ophthalmic aneurysm, 917
  in cerebellar astrocytoma, 660
  in cerebral glioma, 433
  in cerebrospinal fluid leakage, 59
  in cervical spondylotic myelopathy, 1352
  in Chiari malformation with hydromyelia, 1311
  in children, 1509
  in clivus and basiocciptial region tumor, 639–640
  in craniopharyngioma, 355–356
  in dural sinus malformation, 861
  in intraoribital tumor, 238
  in lesion localization and biopsy, 463–474
  in meningioma, 550, 566–567, 572

in metastatic spine tumor, 1517
  in optic glioma, 279–280
  in pineal tumor, 403
  in posterior fossa tumor, 654
  in rheumatoid arthritis, 1296, 1301
  in sella turcica lesion, 301
  in spinal cord astrocytoma, 177, 184
  in spinal dysraphism, 168
  in spine trauma, 1449
  in spine tumor, 1525, 1526
  with stereotactic biopsy, 495–498, 502
  stereotactic frame modification for, 464–466
  with stereotactic intra-axial tumor resection, 481–490
  in stereotactic surgery, 463
  in tentorium tumor, 647
Mandibular subluxation, with distal internal carotid artery exposure, 765–767, 769
Marcus-Gunn pupil, 269, 270
Mauer's triad, 837
Mebendazole, in cysticercosis, 87
Medial nerve, intraneural artery, 1564
Medial palmar cutaneous nerve, in carpal tunnel syndrome, 1586
Medial sphenoid wing meningioma, 537–539
  angiography, 538
  computed tomography, 537–538
  presentation, 537–538
  radiography, 537–538
  results, 539
  surgical technique, 538–539
Median nerve entrapment, 1585–1588
  anterior interosseous syndrome, 1588
  conservative management, 1585
  diagnosis, 1585
  pronator syndrome, 1588
  proximal forearm, 1586–1587
  surgical management, 1586
Mediolongitudinal myelotomy. See Commissural myelotomy
Medullary tractotomy
  anatomic basis, 1165–1166
  anesthesia, 1166–1167
  for cancer pain, 1045
  complications, 1167–1168
  indications for, 1166
  instrumentation, 1166
  for intractable pain, 1165–1168
  patient positioning, 1167
  results, 1167–1168
  technique, 1167
Medulloblastoma
  computed tomography, 658
  postoperative radiation therapy, 658
  recurrence, 658
  surgical management, 658
Meniere's disease, 1251–1259
  labyrinthectomy in, 1255
  nonsurgical treatment, 1254
  pathophysiology, 1251
  streptomycin sulfate ablation of vestibular nerve, 1259
  surgical treatment, 1255–1258
  vestibular nerve transection in, 1251–1259
Meningeal carcinomatosis, 460
Meningioma
  angiography, 550–551, 564–566, 572
  bone flap elevation, 557–558

carbon dioxide laser surgery, 559
cerebellopontine angle, 673–674
of clivus and basioccipital region, 637, 645
computed tomography, 549–550, 564, 571–572
differential diagnosis, 572
dural opening, 558
encephalography in, 551
excision, 559
exposure, 558–559
hemostasis, 558, 560
histology, 547–548
intraoperative ultrasonography visualization, 217
magnetic resonance imaging, 550, 566–567, 572
myelography, 572–573
NdYAG laser surgery, 559
optic nerve, 235, 236, 239, 241
patient positioning, 556
postoperative care, 561
preoperative embolization, 551–553
preoperative evaluation, 547–553
preoperative preparation, 553
prognosis, 547–548
radiation therapy, 551
radiography, 548–551, 564–567, 571–573
recurrence, 547
scalp incision, 556–557
sites, 547
of skull base, 627, 629
stereotactic radiosurgery, 519
surgical principles, 556–561, 567–570, 575–581
surgical treatment, 551
ultrasonic aspiration, 559
ventriculography, 573
wound closure, 560
Meningioma (cerebellopontine angle), 572
computed tomography, 572
magnetic resonance imaging, 572
surgical technique, 578–579
Meningioma (convexity), 555–562
classification, 555
coronal, 555
occipital, 556
pararolandic, 555
parietal, 555
postcoronal, 555
precoronal, 555
symptomatology, 555–556
temporal, 555–556
Meningioma (falx), 563–570
angiography, 564–566
excision, 569
exposure, 569
radiography, 564–567
surgical principles, 567–570
Meningioma (foramen magnum), surgical technique, 578–579
Meningioma (parasagittal), 563–570
angiography, 564–566
bone flap, 567, 569
computed tomography, 544
dural opening, 569
excision, 569
exposure, 569
magnetic resonance imaging, 566–567
patient positioning, 567

radiography, 564–567
sagittal sinography, 566
scalp incision, 567
site, 563
surgical principles, 567–570
symptomatology, 563–564
Meningioma (posterior fossa), 571–582
anesthesia, 574
angiography, 572
classification, 571
computed tomography, 571–572
magnetic resonance imaging, 572
myelography, 572–573
obstructive hydrocephalus control, 573
patient positioning, 574–575
radiography, 571–573
site-symptoms relationship, 571
surgical approach, 575–581
surgical technique, 575–581
ventriculography, 573
Meningioma (posterior petrous ridge), surgical technique, 575–578
Meningioma (tentorium cerebelli), surgical technique, 575–578
Meningitis. *See also* Tuberculous meningitis
with cerebrospinal fluid leakage, 58, 61, 63
Meningitis (chemical), with Rathke's cleft cyst, 373–374
Meningocele
anterior sacral, 159–161
anterolateral spinal, 158–161
cervical, 158
intrasacral, 159–161
lumbar, 158–159
posterior spinal, 157–158
thoracic, 158–159
Meningocele manqué, 164
surgery for, 169
Mental retardation, with infantile hemiplegia, 1236
Mesencephalotomy, for cancer pain, 1045–1046
Metastasis (intracranial), 451–462
biopsy in, 454, 457, 459
chemotherapy, 455, 456, 460, 461
clonogenic assay, 456
combined surgical and radiation therapy, 454
computed tomography in, 457–458, 459
corticosteroids in, 453, 461
differential diagnosis, 459
distribution, 451
immunotherapy, 460
incidence, 451
latency of, 451–452
leptomeningeal, 451, 460
lesion characteristics, 451
mortality and morbidity, 456
origin, 451
postoperative complications, 456
primary tumor factor, 459
radiation therapy, 453–454, 460, 461
results, 455, 456
shunt for hydrocephalus, 459
solitary and accessible, 458–459
solitary vs. multiple, 451
stereotactic biopsy in, 457
surgical indications, 458–459
surgical management, 454–458

terminal illness, 461
treatment modalities evaluation, 452–453
Metastatic tumor (intra-axial), stereotactic resection, 488–489
Methylmethacrylate
in cerebrospinal fluid leakage repair, 66
for skull implant, 11, 14–16
spine fusion, 1522–1523
Metopic synostosis, 133–134
complications, 134
diagnosis, 133
"floating forehead," 134
metopic syntectomy, 134
results, 134
surgical treatment, 133–134
Metrizamine, computed tomography enhancement, 176, 184, 1332
Metrizamine cisternography, 60
Metrizamide instillation, in posterior fossa tumor, 654
Metrizamide myelography, 1518
for anterior lumbar discectomy, 1423
Microslad, for stereotactic resection, 486
Microvascular decompression
for facial pain, complications, 1139–1143
for glossopharyngeal neuralgia, 1108–1109
for hemifacial spasm, 1107
Microvascular replantation
in scalp avulsion, 6–9
for trigeminal neuralgia, 1097–1098
Midbrain, stereotactic surgery, 472
Midbrain tumor, 711–712
symptomology, 714–716
Middle cerebral artery aneurysm, 957–971, 1026, 1032
angiography, 957, 970
at bifurcation, 959
computed tomography, 957, 958, 968
giant aneurysm, 963–967
patient positioning, 959–960
postoperative care, 968, 970
preoperative medication, 957–958
proximal, 959
results, 970
sites, 959
somatosensory evoked response monitoring, 967–968
subarachnoid hemorrhage with, 957, 958, 970
surgery timing, 958–959
surgical approach, 959
surgical procedure, 960–963
temporary vascular occlusion in, 967–968
at trifurcation, 962–963
Middle cranial fossa approach
to cerebellopontine angle, 675
to posterior cranial fossa, 665–666, 671
Middle fossa-infratemporal fossa approach, to posterior cranial fossa, 669, 671
Milwaukee Brace, 193
Missile injury (penetrating), 49–55
antibiotic prophylaxis with, 52
anticonvulsants in, 52
ballistics factor, 49–50
blast injury with, 51
bone chips, 50
bone fragment management, 52
bone fragment replacement, 53–54
bullet track factor, 50

Missile injury (penetrating) *(continued)*
  cerebrospinal fluid fistula with, 53
  computed tomography in, 49, 54
  contusions, 51
  corticosteroids in, 51
  debridement, 52
  dural sinus repair, 53
  explosive bullets management, 53
  hematoma with, 51
  hydrocephalus with, 53
  intracranial pressure with, 51, 52
  issues, 49
  migrating metallic fragments, 52–53
  nutrition with, 51–52
  pathophysiology, 50
  skull fracture with, 51
  strategic considerations, 54
  surgical principles, 51
  tangential injury, 51
  velocity factor, 50
Morphine test, 1089–1090
Morphine therapy, opioid system and, 1077–1078
Morphine therapy (intraventricular)
  for cancer pain, 1077–1088
  case reports, 1079–1085
  cerebrospinal fluid injection, 1078–1088
  computed tomography, 1079
  instrumentation, 1079, 1086
  patient selection, 1079
  results, 1079, 1086
  surgical technique, 1079
Movement disorders
  extrapyramidal system in, 1050–1051
  neurosurgical management, 1050–1057
  stereotactic surgery for, 1051
Moyamoya disease, 797–806
  angiography, 798–801, 803
  computed tomography, 798
  electroencephalography, 799, 801, 804
  encephaloduroarteriosynangiosis in, 802, 804
  encephalomyosynangiosis in, 802, 804
  epidemiology, 797–798
  etiology, 797–798
  genetic factor, 797
  medical management, 801
  omentum transplantation in, 801
  regional cerebral blood flow in, 798–799, 803
  results, 804
  pathology, 798–801
  STA-MCA anastomosis in, 802, 804
  surgical management, 801–804
  sympathectomy in, 801, 804
  transient ischemic attacks with, 797, 801, 804
  types, 797
Multiple sclerosis
  retrogasserian glycerol injection for, 1134
  stimulation management, 1055–1056
  trigeminal neuralgia with, 1105
  trigeminal rhizotomy in, 1120
Muscle reconstruction, in facial palsy, 707
Mycobacterium tuberculosis, 79–85
Myelocystocele, 166
  terminal, 158
Myelography
  anesthesia for, 112

  in brachial plexus injury, 1578
  in cervical disc herniation, 1348
  in cervical spondylosis, 1332
  in cervical spondylotic myelopathy, 1352
  in Chiari malformation with hydromyelia, 1313–1316
  in children, 1509
  in intramedullary spinal cord tumor, 1492
  of lumbar intervertebral disc, 1375–1376, 1393, 1394
  in meningioma, 572–573
  in metastatic spine tumor, 1517–1518
  in Paget's disease, 1304, 1305
  in rheumatoid arthritis, 1296
  in spinal cord arteriovenous malformation, 1500–1501
  in spine tumor, 1526
  in third ventricle tumor, 398
Myelomeningocele, 151–162
  anesthesia for, 111
  closure-site reconstruction, 156–157
  concurrent care considerations, 151
  demographic factor, 151
  genetic factor, 151
  with hydrocephalus, 119
  kidney disease with, 151
  postnatal care, 152–154
  postoperative care, 156
  spinal deformity with hydromyelia and malfunction shunt, 1510–1511
  surgical closure technique, 154–157
  survivals, 151–152
  treatment criteria, 152
Myelotomy (longitudinal-Bischof's), 1177–1184
  for cancer pain, 1044
  commissural, 1185–1190
Myofascial syndrome, trigger point blocks for, 1049

Nasal cavity tumor
  craniofacial resection for, 611
  patient selection, 612
  preoperative evaluation, 612
Nasal structures, reconstruction techniques, 331–337
Nasopharyngeal cancer, percutaneous rhizotomy for pain, 1125–1127
Needlescope, 424
Nelson's syndrome, stereotactic radiosurgery, 518
Neodymium:ytterium argon garnet laser, 223, 226
  in mengioma surgery, 559
Neonate
  Chiari II malformation, 123
  Dandy-Walker malformation, 121, 123
  frontal nasal encephalocele, 121
  head trauma, 119–120
  hydrocephalus in, 119
    with myelomeningocele, 119
  intraoperative considerations, 117–119
  intraventricular hemorrhage in, 117
  neurosurgical management in, 117–123
  occipital encephalocele, 120–121
  positioning precautions, 117
  temperature regulation in, 117
  vein of Galen malformation, 120

  venipuncture in, 117
Neoplasm
  laser excision, 223–228
  ultrasonic surgical fragmentation, 227
Nerve conduction velocity, in peripheral nerve injury, 1567
Nerve graft, in facial palsy, 705
Nerve root microvascular lysis, in torticollis, 1262
Nerve transfer, in facial palsy, 705
Neural decompression, in thoracolumbar fracture, 1481, 1482, 1483
Neuralgia, spinal sensory rhizotomy for, 1211
Neurapraxia, 1584
Neurocysticercosis, 79, 93–102
Neurofibroma, 1603–1605
  optic nerve, 239, 243
  surgical indications, 1604
Neurofibromatosis. *See* Von Recklinghausen's disease
Neurologic deficit, with arteriovenous malformation, 914
Neurolysis, in peripheral nerve injury, 1572
Neuroma, with peripheral entrapment neuropathy, 1585
Neuromuscular blockade, in children, 104–105
Neuromuscular disease, scoliosis and, 191
Neuropsychologic testing, in cerebral glioma, 434–435
Neurotmesis, 1584
Neurotransmitters, 1070
Niclosamide, 87
Nitroprusside (sodium), in children, 107–108
Nucleus pulposus, chemonucleolysis with chymopapain, 1437–1441
Nutrition, in penetrating missile injury, 51–52

Occipital artery–anterior inferior cerebellar artery bypass
  in vertebrobasilar insufficiency, 814–815
  results, 814–815
  technique, 814
Occipital artery–middle cerebral artery bypass, 792–793
Occipital artery–posterior inferior cerebellar artery bypass, 793
  results, 813
  technique, 812–813
  in vertebrobasilar insufficiency, 810, 812–814
Occipital encephalocele
  anesthesia for, 110–113
  in neonate, 120–121
Occipital lobectomy
  in cerebral glioma, 441–442
  exposure, 441–442
  patient positioning, 441–442
Occipital transtentorial approach, to pineal region, 411–418
Occlusive cerebrovascular disease
  direct brain revascularization, 783–795
  interposition vein graft to posterior cerebral artery, 793
  long vein grafts, 792

occipital artery–middle cerebral artery bypass, 792–793
occipital artery–posterior inferior cerebellar artery bypass, 793
short vein graft, 791
STA-MCA bypass for, 783–791
vertebrobasilar revascularization, 793–794
Odontoidectomy, transoral, 1289
Olfactory groove meningioma
  angiography, 540
  computed tomography, 540
  presentation, 539–540
  radiography, 540
  results, 545
  surgical technique, 541–545
Oligodendroglioma, 432
  stereotactic resection, 488
Omentum transplantation, in moyamoya disease, 802

Ommaya reservoir, 219
Ophthalmic artery, 236–237
Opthalmic artery aneurysm. *See* Carotid ophthalmic aneurysm
Opthalmic vein, 237
Ophthalmologic testing, in cerebral glioma, 433–434
Opiates
  epidural infusion for intractable pain, 1145–1147
  epidural system availability, 1147–1148
  epidural therapy complications, 1149–1152
  epidural therapy results, 1148–1149
  indications for epidural implantation systems, 1147
  preparation for epidural administration, 1147
Opioid system, morphine therapy and, 1077–1078
Optic glioma, 235, 239, 241, 279–298
  calcification, 279
  case reports, 280–282, 290–293
  chiasma/optic nerve/brain involvement, 279, 287–295
  computed tomography in, 279
  cystic component, 289
  diagnosis, 279–286, 287–288
  diagnostic controversies, 280–286
  with edema/without neoplastic invasion, 288–289
  exophytic tumor growth, 289–290
  hemorrhagic component, 289
  hypothalamic invasion, 293–294
  magnetic resonance imaging, 279–280
  of one optic nerve, 285–286
  partial vs. complete resection, 288–290
  radiation therapy, 295
  spontaneous regression, 284–285
  surgery for, 286–295
  visual evoked potentials in, 280
Optic nerve, 235
  sphenoethmoid approach, 269–277
  visual deficit after head trauma, 269
Optic nerve decompression
  angiography, 270
  case reports, 272–276
  computed tomography, 270
  external ethmoidectomy approach, 270

indications for, 271–272
  Krönlein procedure, 270
  sphenoethmoid approach, 270–271
  surgical requirements, 269
  transantralethmoidal approach, 270
  transantrosphenoidal approach, 270
  transfrontal craniotomy approach, 269–270
  transsphenoidal approach, 270, 275
Optic nerve lesions, with radiofrequency rhizotomy, 1140–1141
Optic nerve tumor, 235
  approach, 238, 239, 241–243
  radiation therapy, 239
Orbit
  anatomy, 235
  arterial supply, 236–237
  nerve supply, 237–238
  venous drainage, 236–237
Orbit pathology
  anterior approach, 248, 251–252, 261–264
  computed tomography, 249, 250, 251
  contrast media in diagnosis, 249–250
  contrast orbitography, 250–251
  corticosteroids in, 251
  instrumentation, 252
  lacrimal gland tumor, 264–265
  lateral approach, 247–248, 249, 252–253
  lateral canthotomy, 254
  lateral orbitotomy, 254–261
  microsurgical approaches, 245–267
  noninvasive vs. invasive diagnostic procedures, 249
  postoperative complications, 266
  radiography, 250
  superior approach, 251
  surgical anatomy, 245–249
  surgical approaches, 251–265
  surgical complications, 265–266
  surgical indications, 252
  venography, 250
Orbital surgery, 235–244
Orbitography (contrast), in orbit pathology, 250–251
Orbitotomy, lateral, 254–261
Osteoma, intraorbital, 239
Osteomyelitis
  of skull, 71
  of spine, 76–77
Owl percutaneous cordotomy electrode, 1194–1195

Pachymeningitis, 1303
Packing substances
  for pituitary fossa, 321
  for sphenoidal sinus, 322
Paget's disease, 1303–1305
  computed tomography in, 1304
  decompressive laminectomy in, 1305
  medical management, 1304–1305
  myelography in, 1304, 1305
  spinal cord compression, 1303–1304
Pain
  anatomy of, 1040–1041
  deep-brain stimulation for, 1041–1043
  denervation, 1042
  functional neurosurgery for, 1040–1050
  laser surgery for, 226
  lower body segments/thoracic region,

commissural myelotomy for, 1185–1190
  nociceptive vs. deafferentation, 1191, 1199
  pathways of, 1041
  perception of, 1041
Pain (chronic). *See also specific syndromes*
  indications for surgery, 1047
  management, 1047–1050
  medication addiction and, 1048
  multiple management factors, 1048
  patient classification, 1047–1048
  patient selection for stereotactic cingulotomy, 1071
  postcingulotomy management, 1074
  psychopathology with, 1048–1049
  sympathectomy for, 1049
  stereotactic cingulotomy for, 1069–1075
  trigger point blocks for, 1049
Pain (intractable)
  dorsal root entry zone thermocoagulation for, 1169–1175
  epidural anesthetic infusion for, 1145
  epidural morphine therapy complications, 1149–1152
  epidural morphine therapy results, 1148–1149
  epidural opiate infusion for, 1145–1147
  implantable systems for management of, 1145–1153
  implanted electrode brain stimulation for, 1089–1095
  medullary tractotomy for, 1165–1168
  morphine test for, 1089–1090
  open cordotomy for, 1155–1168
  paramedian, midline, bilateral: bilateral cordotomy for, 1156
  types of, 1040–1050
  unilateral somatic cancer: unilater cordotomy for, 1155
  unilateral visceral: bilateral cordotomy for, 1155–1156
Painful disc syndrome, 1327
Pallidotomy
  in dystonia, 1268
  in torticollis, 1262–1263
Pan synostosis, 134
Pancreas cancer, splanchnicectomy for pain, 1275
Pancreatitis, splanchnicectomy for, 1275
Pan-hypopituitarism, 300
Papaya latex, 1437
Papilledema, 235
Para-aminosalicylic acid, 81
Paranasal sinus tumor
  craniofacial approach, 609
  patient selection, 612
  preoperative evaluation, 612
Paranasal structures, reconstruction techniques, 331–337
Paraplegia, scoliosis and, 191
Paraplegia (traumatic), dorsal root entry zone thermocoagulation for pain, 1172, 1174
Parasite infection, 93–102. *See also specific diagnoses*
Parkinson's disease
  campotomy for, 1052
  stereotactic procedures for, 1051, 1052
  thalamotomy for, 1052

Pattern visual evoked potentials, 280
Percutaneous cordotomy, 1191–1205
  analgesia maintenance, 1200
  anesthesia for, 1194, 1195, 1199
  bilateral, 1192, 1199, 1202
  complications, 1202–1203
  cord structure identification, 1198
  dermatome level factor, 1192
  impedance monitoring, 1195, 1198
  instrumentation, 1194–1195
  lateral high cervical, 1191
  lateral spinothalamic tract identification,
    1196–1198, 1200
  lesion making, 1198
  lesion tailoring, 1199
  local pathology factor, 1192–1193
  for midline pain, 1192
  nociceptive vs. deafferentation pain factor,
    1191, 1199
  in nonmalignant disease, 1201
  vs. open procedure, 1193
  pain location factor, 1192
  pain persistence after, 1200–1201
  pain recurrence, 1201–1202
  pain relief results, 1199, 1202
  patient positioning, 1194
  patient selection, 1191
  physiologic localization, 1195–1198
  postcordotomy dysesthesia, 1200–1201
  postoperative care, 1199
  preoperative preparation, 1194
  radiographic localization in, 1195, 1198
  respiratory function factor, 1192
  results, 1199–1203
  surgical technique, 1193–1199
  technique selection, 1193
Percutaneous electrode implantation, 1040
  for cancer pain, 1047
Percutaneous electrothermocoagulation, of
    spinal nerve trunk/ganglion/rootlets,
    1207–1221
Percutaneous rhizotomy
  for cancer pain, 1125–1127
  commentary, 1125–1127
  for facial pain, complications, 1139–1143
  in trigeminal neuralgia, 1125–1127
Percutaneous trigeminal neurolysis, 1097–
    1098
Periaqueductal gray matter, stimulation site
    in pain control, 1089, 1091, 1094
Periorbita, 235–236
Peripheral denervation
  in dystonia, 1268
  results, 1266–1267
  surgical technique, 1264–1266
  in torticollis, 1263–1268
Peripheral entrapment neuropathy, 1583–
    1597
  classification, 1584
  common peroneal nerve compression,
    1596
  compression and, 1583
  compressive lesions, 1584–1596
  electromyelography, 1584, 1585
  ischemia and, 1583
  lateral femoral cutaneous nerve, 1593
  median nerve, 1585–1588
  neurolysis, 1585
  neuroma with, 1585

  posterior tibial nerve, 1593
  radial nerve entrapment, 1589–1590
  suprascapular nerve, 1590–1591
  surgical management, 1585
  thoracic outlet syndrome, 1591–1593
  ulnar nerve compression, 1588–1589
Peripheral nerve(s)
  anatomy, 1563–1564
  blood supply, 1564
  degeneration/regeneration, 1565–1566
  injury mechanism, 1564–1565
Peripheral nerve injury
  anesthesia, 1570
  complete transection, 1572
  compression lesion, 1572
  diagnosis, 1566–1568
  electromyography in, 1567, 1571
  epineurial suture, 1573
  fascicular/group fascicular repair, 1573–
    1574, 1575
  fibrillation potentials, 1567
  with fracture/dislocation, 1570
  grafting in, 1574, 1575
  injection, 1572
  magnification requirements, 1571
  microsurgical instrumentation, 1571
  nerve conduction velocity, 1567
  neurolysis in, 1572
  patient positioning, 1570
  postoperative management, 1575
  radiation injury and, 1572
  resection length criteria, 1572–1573
  results variables, 1575–1577
  sensory testing, 1566
  sudomotor function, 1568
  surgical indications, 1568–1570
  surgical technique, 1572
  suture material, 1571
  sympathectomy for sequela, 1272
  Tinel's sign, 1566–1567
  tourniquet management, 1570–1571
Peripheral nerve lesions, classification, 1584
Peripheral nerve surgery, in facial palsy, 705
Peripheral nerve tumor, 1599–1610
  biopsy, 1606–1607
  classification, 1599
  clinical diagnosis, 1599
  extrinsic compressive, 1608
  extrinsic invasive, 1608
  intraoperative diagnosis, 1599
  malignant, 1605–1607
  neurofibroma, 1603–1605
  postoperative care, 1608–1609
  schwannoma, 1599–1603
  Von Recklinghausen's disease, 1605
Phantom limb pain, stimulation
    management, 1049
Photoradiation therapy, 226
Phrenic–facial nerve anastomosis, 683
Physiotherapy, in torticollis, 1267
Pig tape worm, 79
Pineal region, occipital transtentorial
    approach, 411–418
Pineal region tumor, 397–399
  associated syndromes, 397
  benign vs. malignant, 397
  chemotherapy, 399
  neuro-ophthalmologic examination, 398
  radiation therapy, 399

  sterotactic radiosurgery, 518–519
  suprasellar germinoma, 397
  surgical management, 398–399
  symptomatology, 397
  third ventricle lesion, 398
  tumor markers in, 398
Pineal tumor
  arteriography in, 403
  biologic markers in, 403
  chemotherapy, 404–405
  classification, 404–405
  clinical features, 402
  computed tomography, 403
  diagnosis, 402–404
  incidence, 401
  magnetic resonance imaging in, 403
  occipital transtentorial approach, 411–418
  posterior fossa approach, 405–407
  radiation therapy, 404–405
  radiography in, 403
  site distribution, 401
  supracerebellar approach, 401–409
  surgical alternatives, 401–402
  surgical complications, 407–408
  surgical criteria, 403–404
  surgical indications, 401
  surgical results, 408
  surgical technique, 405–407
  therapeutic alternatives, 404
  ventriculography in, 403
Pituitary adenoma, 299–307
  ACTH assay in, 300
  cerebrospinal fluid leak, 306
  dexamethasone suppression test, 300
  diabetes insipidus with, 307
  endocrine function in, 299–300
  endocrine results, 305
  empty sella complication, 330
  ghost sella complication, 330–331
  growth hormone level, 299
  intrasella, 325–326
  pan-hypopituitarism with, 300
  postoperative considerations, 305
  radiofrequency electrode application,
    302
  sella turcica reconstruction, 325–326
  serum prolactin, 299
  sinusitis with, 306
  suprasellar extension with, 326–329
  surgical complications, 306–307
  surgical identification, 305
  surgical results, 305–306
  transsphenoidal approach, 299–307, 309–
    319
  visual results, 306
Pituitary fossa
  anchored intradural packing, 323–324
  cerebrospinal fluid leakage management,
    324–325
  combined extradural-intradural packing,
    324
  extradural packing, 324
  packing substances, 321
  reconstruction complications, 333–334
  reconstruction techniques, 321–337
  simple intradural packing, 323
  transsphenoidal approach, 321–337
Pituitary gland, transethmoidal
    sphenoidotomy approach, 339–343

Pituitary microadenoma
  sella turcica reconstruction, 325
  transsphenoidal approach, 314
Pituitary stalk, sacrifice in
    craniopharyngioma, 363
Pituitary tumor (hypersecreting), stereotactic
    radiosurgery, 516–518
Pneumocephalus, with cerebrospinal fluid
    leakage, 58
Pneumography, of sella turcica, 356
Polymethyl methacrylate, 1530
Polytomography, in intraorbital tumor, 238
Polyvinyl alcohol foam, for embolization,
    552, 820
Pons, stereotactic surgery, 472
Positioning. *See also specific diagnoses and
    procedures*
  of children, 105, 106
Positive-end-expiratory pressure, in acute
    head injury, 27–28
Positron emission tomography, 433
Posterior cerebral aneurysm, 973–989. *See
    also* Basilar artery aneurysm
  anesthesia, 973–974
  anterior-projecting, 983
  monitoring techniques, 973–974
  patient positioning, 974
  posterior-projecting, 982–983
Posterior cranial fossa
  case reports, 669–670
  infratemporal fossa approach, 668, 671
  middle fossa approach, 665–666, 671
  middle fossa–infratemporal fossa
      approach, 669, 671
  retrolabyrinthine approach, 667
  skull base approach, 667–668, 671
  suboccipital approach, 665, 670
  suboccipital–translabyrinthine approach,
      668, 671
  transcanal approach, 667, 671
  transcochlear approach, 668, 671
  translabyrinthine approach, 665, 670–671
  transmeatal approach to cerebellopontine
      angle, 676–680
  transtemporal approaches, 665–672
Posterior fossa approach, to pineal tumor,
    405–407
Posterior fossa craniectomy
  midline, 655–658
  unilateral, 659
Posterior fossa cyst, surgical management,
    658–659
Posterior fossa revascularization, 807–818
  indications for, 807–808
Posterior fossa tumor, 653–664
  cerebrospinal fluid diversion, 654
  in children, 109
  combined supratentorial and infratentorial
      approach, 660–662
  computed tomography, 653–654
  diagnosis, 653–654
  magnetic resonance imaging, 654
  metrizamide instillation, 654
  midline posterior fossa craniectomy, 655–
      658
  neurologic consequences, 653
  pathology, 656
  patient positioning, 655
  surgical management, 654–659

symptomatology, 653
Posterior tibial nerve entrapment, 1593
Postherpetic neuralgia
  stimulation management, 1049
  surgical management, 1049
Praziquantel, 87
Prefrontal lobotomy, 1057, 1069
Prematurity, intraventricular hemorrhage
    with, 119
Premedication, for children, 106
Prolactin (serum), in pituitary adenoma, 299
Prolactinoma, 299
Proptosis, 235, 238
Proton beam therapy
  arteriography after, 911–912
  for arteriovenous malformation, 911–915
  complications, 912, 914
  hemorrhage with, 913–914
  incubation period with, 913
  ionizing event with, 913
  lesion tissue changes from, 912
  response variation, 914
  risk, 914
  tissue histology, 912–913
Pseudoarthrosis, with spine fusion, 1478,
    1480
Psychiatric disorder
  patient selection for stereotactic
      cingulotomy, 1070–1071
  postcingulotomy management, 1073–1074
  prefrontal lobotomy, 1069
  stereotactic cingulotomy for, 1069–1075
Psychosurgery, 1057–1060
Psychotrophic drugs, 1070
Pterional approach
  in craniopharyngioma, 362
  to sella turcica, 303–304
Pyrazinamide, 81

Quadriplegia, electroneuroprosthesis for,
    1062–1063

Radial nerve entrapment, 1589–1590
Radiation therapy. *See also specific
    modalities*
  in arteriovenous malformation, 906
  brachial plexus neuropathy and, 1580
  in brain stem glioma, 724, 735
  in cerebellar hemangioblastoma, 660
  in cerebral glioma, 448
  contact radiation devices, 504–507
  in craniopharyngioma, 368–372
  for fourth ventricle ependymoma, 658
  for glomus jugulare tumor, 739, 743–744,
      749
  in intracranial metastasis, 453–454, 460,
      461
  in intramedullary spinal cord tumor, 1496
  in medulloblastoma, 658
  in meningioma, 551
  in metastatic epidural tumor, 1542, 1543
  in metastatic spine tumor, 1515, 1522,
      1560
  for optic glioma, 295
  in optic nerve tumor, 239
  in pineal region tumor, 399
  for pineal tumor, 404–405

postradiation kyphosis/scoliosis in
    children, 1509
  peripheral nerve injury and, 1572
  for spinal cord astrocytoma, 180, 186
  in spine tumor, 1526, 1527, 1530, 1531
Radiofrequency electrode, in pituitary
    adenoma resection, 302
Radiofrequency griseotomy, in lower limb
    spasticity, 1181
Radiofrequency heating
  for cluster headache, 1136
  for trigeminal neuralgia, 1134
Radiofrequency rhizotomy
  central retinal artery occlusion with, 1141–
      1142
  optic nerve lesions with, 1140–1141
Radiofrequency thermocoagulation, in
    trigeminal neuralgia, 1098
Radiography. *See also specific procedures*
  in anterior lumbar discectomy, 1422, 1427–
      1428
  in anterior skull base tumor, 611
  in brachial plexus injury, 1578
  in cerebral glioma, 432–433
  in cerebrospinal fluid leakage, 59
  in cervical disc herniation, 1348
  in cervical spondylosis, 1329–1332
  in cervical spondylotic myelopathy, 1352
  in Chiari malformation with hydromyelia,
      1309–1316
  in chymopapain chemonucleolysis, 1438,
      1439
  in clivus and basioccipital region tumor,
      637–640
  in clivus tumor, 650
  in craniofacial abnormality, 135
  in craniopharyngioma, 355–357
  in craniovertebral junction abnormality,
      1284
  in epilepsy, 1224
  in gunshot wounds of head, 38–39
  in infantile hemiplegia, 1236
  in internal carotid artery aneurysm, 837
  in intramedullary spinal cord tumor, 1488–
      1490
  in lumbar spondylosis, 1403
  in medial sphenoid wing meningioma, 537–
      538
  in meningioma, 548–551, 564–567, 571–573
  in metastatic spine tumor, 1516–1518,
      1520, 1522
  in olfactory groove meningioma, 540
  in orbit pathology, 250
  in percutaneous cordotomy, 1195, 1198
  in pineal tumor, 403
  in rheumatoid arthritis, 1296
  in scalp/skull tumor, 604
  in scoliosis, 191
  in sella turcica lesion, 299, 300–301
  in spinal cord arteriovenous malformation,
      1500–1501
  in spinal dysraphism, 167–168
  in spinal sensory rhizotomy, 1211, 1215,
      1216, 1220
  of spine in children, 1509
  in spine tumor, 1526–1527, 1528
  with stereotactic surgery, 1037–1038
  in suprasellar germinoma, 398
  in suprasellar meningioma, 531

Radiography *(continued)*
in synostosis, 125, 126, 130, 132, 133
in tentorium tumor, 647
for third ventricle lesion, 382, 391–392
in thoracolumbar fracture, 1483
in tuberculoma, 80–81
in vertebrobasilar insufficiency, 771–775
Radioisotope scan
in cerebrospinal fluid leakage, 59–60
in spine tumor, 1526, 1528
Radionuclide implantation
indications for, 507–512
nuclides for, 500
permanent (curietherapy) technique, 491,
499–503
results, 507
stereotactic biopsy with, 491–514
temporary (brachycurietherapy) technique,
491, 499–502, 503–504
Radiosurgery, stereotactic, 515–529
Rathke's cleft (epithelial) cyst, 349, 372–374
chemical meningitis with, 373–374
computed tomography, 373, 374
Renal pain, splanchnicectomy for, 1275
Retrolabyrinthine approach, to posterior
cranial fossa, 667
Revascularization. *See specific sites and
procedures*
Reye-Johnson syndrome, anesthesia
management, 115
Rheumatoid arthritis, 1295–1306
anterior atlantoaxial subluxation, 1295–
1301
C1-C2 fusion for subluxation, 1296–1300
computed tomography in, 1296
diagnostic studies, 1296
lumbar spine involvement, 1300
magnetic resonance imaging in, 1296, 1301
myelography in, 1296
radiography in, 1296
subaxial subluxation, 1299–1300
subluxation presentation, 1295–1296
subluxation stabilization in, 1296
thoracic spine involvement, 1300
vertical atlantoaxial subluxation, 1300–
1301
Rhizotomy. *See specific procedures*
Rhinopharyngeal tumor, of skull base, 630,
633
Rhodes-Glenn stereotactic system, 467
Riechert-Mundinger stereotactic system,
464–465, 495
Rifampicin, 81–82
Rigidity, stereotactic surgery for, 1051

Sacral meningocele
anterior, 159–161
intrasacral, 159–161
Sacral rhizotomy, percutaneous
electrothermocoagulation technique,
1217–1220
Sagittal sinography, 566
Sagittal sinus, dural laceration, 875–879
Sagittal synostosis, 126–130
complications, 130
diagnosis, 126–128
midline sagittal crainectomy, 128–129
pi procedure, 129

results, 130
surgical management, 128–130
surgical technique, 129–130
vault remodeling, 129–130
Salivary gland tumor, craniofacial resection
for, 609
Saphenous vein graft, to posterior cerebral
artery, 793–794
Scalp
anatomy, 1
circulation, 1, 3
congenital aplasia, 5
innervation, 1
vasculature, 1
Scalp avulsion
anatomy, 7
microvascular replantation, 6–9
vascular/coagulation status after
replantation, 9
Scalp burn
electrical, 6
thermal, 6
Scalp defect. *See also specific defects*
assessment, 1
back cutting, 4
flaps available, 3
free skin grafts, 2–3
local attached flaps, 3
management principles, 1–2
reconstructions available, 2
repair technique, 4
rotation flaps, 3
tissue expansion in reconstruction, 4–5
Scalp laceration, 5, 20
Scalp tumor, 601–607
arteriography, 604
case report, 602–603
computed tomography, 604
postoperative management, 606
preoperative management, 603–604
radiography, 604
surgical management, 604–606
Schwannoma, 1599–1603
anesthesia, 1600
instrumentation, 1601
patient positioning, 1600–1601
surgical management, 1601–1603
Sciatic nerve, intraneural artery, 1564
Sciatica, 1393
chymopapain chemonucleolysis, 1437–
1441
Scoliosis, 187–211
anterior surgical approach, 195–196, 202–
204
bone graft in, 197–198
bracing in, 191–194
classification, 187
complications of therapy, 205–206
congenital, 187
Cotrel-Dubousset fixation, 201–202
diagnostic evaluation, 191–192
Dwyer instrumentation, 203–204
electrical stimulation in, 191–194
etiology, 187
fusion procedures, 194–195, 197–198
Harrington rod instrumentation, 198
with hydromyelia with shunt malfunction
in myelomeningocele, 1510–1511
idiopathic, 187, 190–191, 195

incidence, 190
after intraspinal tumor surgery in children,
1509–1513
mechanical complications, 206
natural history, 190–191
neurologic complications, 206
neuromuscular development and, 191
nonoperative treatment, 191–194
paraplegia and, 191
posterior surgical approach, 196–198
postoperative management, 204–205
after radiation therapy in children, 1509
radiography, 191
segmental instrumentation, 200
spinal cord monitoring, 207
spinal fracture and, 191
surgical approaches, 195–196
surgical indications, 194–195
surgical treatment, 194–204
transpedicle fixateurs, 202
tumor and, 191
Wisconsin system, 201
Seizures. *See also* Epilepsy
with acute head injury, 30
with cysticercosis, 95, 96
with infantile hemiplegia, 1235, 1237, 1238,
1239, 1240
Sella turcica
computed tomography, 356
empty sella complication, 330
floor closure, 321–322
ghost sella complication, 330–331
pneumography, 356
reconstruction techniques, 321–337
transsphenoidal approach, 309–319
Sella turcica lesion, 299–307
cerebrospinal fluid leak with, 304–305, 306
classification, 299
computed tomography in, 300–301, 356
endocrine factor, 299–300
intraoperative bleeding, 304
magnetic resonance imaging in, 301
postoperative considerations, 305
preoperative evaluation, 299
radiography, 299, 300–301
subfrontal approach, 303
subtemporal approach, 304
surgical complications, 304
surgical results, 305–306
transcranial approach, 302–303
transethmoid approach, 302
transsphenoidal approach, 301–304
visual examination, 299, 301
Sendai cocktail, 1032
Sex factor, in aneurysm, 1003
Sheldon-Jacques tumorscope, 430
Sheldon tumorscope, 427
Shunting procedure
for craniopharyngioma, 364
for hydrocephalus, 142–152
intraoperative ultrasonography with, 219
postoperative care, 148
preoperative preparation, 143
shunts available, 143
technique, 143
with transcallosal approach, 386
Sigmoid sinus, dural arteriovenous
malformation, 855–862
Silicone oil, as embolic agent, 821

Sinusitus, with pituitary adenoma, 306
Sleep apnea, after open cordotomy, 1163
Somatomedin C, 299
Somatosensory evoked potentials
 in middle cerebral artery aneurysm, 967–
  968
 in spinal cord arteriovenous malformation,
  1501
 in spinal cord astrocytoma, 177
 in thoracolumbar fracture, 1482
Skeletal traction, in cervical fracture-
  dislocation, 1449–1451
Skin abnormality, with spinal dysraphism,
  166
Skull osteomyelitis, 71
Skull base approach
 to glomus jugulare tumor, 745–746
 to posterior cranial fossa, 667–668, 671
Skull base tumor. *See also* specific lesions
 clivus removal, 625, 626
 closure, 625–626
 combined approaches, 626
 exposure, 622–623
 meningeal repair, 623–624
 meningioma, 627, 629
 mucosal plane preservation, 621–622
 preoperative management, 619, 621
 removal, 624–625
 of rhinopharyngeal origin, 630, 633
 skull base repair, 625
 surgical indications, 627–633
 transbasal approach, 619–633
 true bone tumor, 630
Skull defect, 11–17. See also Cranioplasty
 in children, 11–12
 complications, 14
 cosmetic considerations, 11
 grafting materials, 11
 infection with, 14
 preoperative evaluation, 11–14
 repair principles, 11–14
 from trephine, 14
 ventricular migration with, 12
Skull fracture
 basilar, 21–22
 depressed, 20–21
 with missile injury, 51
 parasellar saccular aneurysm with, 837
Skull traction, in cervical fracture
  dislocation, 1449
Skull tumor, 601–607
 case reports, 601–602
 computed tomography, 604
 postoperative management, 606
 preoperative management, 603–604
 radiography, 604
 surgical management, 604–606
Spasticity
 stereotactic surgery for, 1054–1055
 stimulation management, 1055–1056
Spasticity (lower limb)
 Bischof's myelotomy for, 1177–1184
 radiofrequency griseotomy, 1181
Sphenoethmoid approach
 disadvantages, 275
 to optic nerve, 269–277
 in optic nerve decompression, 270–271
Sphenoidal sinus, packing and closure,
  322

Sphenoidotomy, approach to pituitary, 339–
  343
Spiegel-Wycis apparatus, 1037
Spina bifida, 163–173
Spina bifida occulta
 dermal sinus with, 165, 166
 with spinal dysraphism, 166
Spine
 anterior atlantoaxial subluxation, 1295–
  1301
 degenerative changes, 1343–1344
 atlantoaxial subluxation, 1295–1299
 growth and development, 189–190
 osteomyelitis, 76–77
 in Paget's disease, 1303–1305
 radiography in children, 1509
 subaxial subluxation, 1299–1300
 vertical atlantoaxial subluxation, 1300–
  1301
Spine anomaly, cerebrospinal fluid leakage
  with, 66–67
Spine fracture, scoliosis and, 191
Spine fracture (thoracolumbar), 1359–1365
 decompression and stabilization, 1361–
  1365
 transthoracic approach, 1361–1365
Spine fusion
 Cotrel-Dubousset fixation, 201–202
 extraperitoneal, 1474–1475
 Harrington rod instrumentation, 198
 Harrington-rod thoracolumbar, 1475–1478
 Hibbs technique, 1473
 intertransverse, 1474
 in intervertebral disc disease, 1421–1436
 after laminectomy, 198
 lateral extrapleural, 1474–1475
 lumbar spine, 1473
 methyl-methacrylate, 1522–1523
 posterior cervical spine, 1471–1480
 posterolateral, 1474
 postoperative care, 1478
 pseudoarthrosis with, 1478, 1480
 in scoliosis, 194–195, 197–198
 segmental instrumentation, 200
 thoracic spine, 1473
 transpedicle fixateurs, 202
 Wisconsin system, 201
Spine trauma, 1449–1469
 anesthesia in, 1451, 1452
 anterior cervical approach, 1453–1461
 anterolateral cervical approach, 1461–1462
 anterolateral lumbar approach, 1468
 cardiovascular considerations, 1451–1452
 computed tomography in, 1449
 laminectomy in, 1466–1467
 magnetic resonance imaging, 1449
 posterior approach, 1464–1466
 posterior lateral approach, 1467–1468
 pulmonary consideratons, 1452
 surgical management, 1452–1468
 thoracoabdominal approach, 1468
 transoral odontoid approach, 1462–1464
 ventilatory assistance in, 1452
Spine tumor, 1525–1537
 angiography, 1526–1527
 biopsy, 1527–1528
 clinical presentation, 1525–1526
 computed tomography, 1525, 1526, 1527,
  1528, 1530

corticosteroid therapy, 1525, 1526, 1527,
  1528
 incidence, 1525
 laminectomy in, 1528–1529
 lateral osteotomy approach, 1535–1536
 magnetic resonance imaging in, 1525, 1526
 myelography, 1526
 neurological deficits with, 1526
 neurological salvage, 1527, 1528
 pain relief, 1528
 postoperative care, 1534, 1536
 preoperative assessment, 1528
 presurgical embolization in, 1527
 radiation vs. surgical treatment, 1515, 1522
 radiation therapy, 1526, 1527, 1530, 1531
 radiography, 1526–1527, 1528
 radionuclide scan in, 1526, 1528
 stabilization in, 1527, 1529, 1533
 surgical approach, 1528–1536
 surgical goals, 1525, 1527
 surgical indications, 1527
 surgical results, 1536
 thoracolumbar region approach, 1534–1535
 tissue diagnosis, 1527–1528
 transabdominal approach, 1535
 transthoracic approach, 1530, 1532, 1535
 vertebral body resection, 1529–1534
Spine tumor (metastatic), 1515–1524
 anterior spinal canal decompression, 1523–
  1524
 clinical presentation, 1515–1516
 complications, 1524
 computed tomography, 1516, 1520
 decompression laminectomy in, 1519–1523
 magnetic resonance imaging, 1517
 methyl-methacrylate fusion in, 1522–1523
 myelography, 1517–1518
 postoperative care, 1524
 preoperative evaluation, 1518–1519
 preoperative preparation, 1518–1519
 radiography, 1516–1518, 1520, 1522
 results, 1524
Spinal accessory–facial nerve anastomosis,
  683
Spinal cord biopsy, intraoperative
  ultrasonography in, 222
Spinal cord compression
 corticosteroids in, 1541
 from epidural metastasis, 1539–1562
Spinal cord decompression, in epidural
  metastatic tumor, 1545–1548
Spinal cord injury, anesthesia for, 114–115
Spinal cord lesion
 intraoperative ultrasonography, 219–222
 normal vs. pathologic ultrasonography
  visualization, 219–222
Spinal cord stimulation
 for cancer pain, 1047
 electrode implantation for, 1039–1040
Spinal cord tethering, 163, 166
Spinal cord tumor, 1487–1507
 astrocytoma, 175–185
 in children, 175–185
 scoliosis and, 191
Spinal cord tumor (extramedullary),
  intraoperative ultrasonography
  visualization, 220–221
Spinal cord tumor (intramedullary), 1487–
  1497

Spinal cord tumor *(continued)*
  angiography, 1490, 1492
  clinical presentation, 1487
  computed tomography, 1490
  diagnosis, 1488–1490
  intraoperative ultrasonography
      visualization, 221–222
  myelography, 1492
  postoperative care, 1497
  radiation therapy, 1496
  radiography, 1488–1490
  results, 1497
  surgical management, 1490–1497
  surgical pathology, 1490
Spinal deformity, 187–211. *See also specific
      diagnoses*
  classification, 187
  with hydromyelia with shunt malfunction
      in myelomeningocele, 1510–1511
  fusion operation for, 1511
  after lumbar shunt, 1510
  after neurosurgery in children, 1509–1513
  prevention after neurosurgery in children,
      1509–1510
  stabilization procedures, 1511–1512
Spinal dysraphism (occult), 163–173
  bladder function with, 166
  clinical presentation, 166–167
  computed tomography, 168
  diagnosis, 167–168
  follow-up, 172
  magnetic resonance imaging, 168
  pathology, 163–166
  radiography in, 167–168
  results, 172
  skin abnormalities with, 166
  with spina bifida occulta, 166
  spine abnormalities with, 166
  surgical indications, 167–168
  surgical technique, 168–172
Spinal extradural abscess, 74–75
Spinal intramedullary abscess, 75–76
Spinal meningocele
  anterolateral, 158–161
  posterior, 157–158
Spinal nerves, rootlets, ganglion, trunk
      anatomy, 1207–1208
Spinal sensory rhizotomy
  anatomy, 1207–1209
  anesthesia, 1211, 1215
  cervical procedure, 1211
  diagnostic paravertebral block, 1209
  indications for, 1209
  intercostal nerve denervation, 1215–1216
  patient preparation, 1211
  patient selection, 1209
  physiology, 1207–1209
  posterior rhizotomy extent, 1209–1211
  radicular arteries in, 1208–1209
  radiography, 1211, 1215, 1216, 1220
  thoracic procedure, 1211–1215
Spinal subdural abscess, 75
Splanchnicectomy,
  anatomy, 1274–1275
  for biliary tract pain, 1275
  for cancer pain, 1044–1045
  complications, 1277
  indications for, 1275
  for pancreas cancer pain, 1275
  for renal pain, 1276

results, 1277
surgical technique, 1276–1277
Spondylotic myelopathy, 1351–1357
Stereotactic atlas, 1036–1037
Stereotactic biopsy, 463–474
  in cerebral glioma, 436
  computed tomography with, 495–498, 502
  consecutive procedures after, 498–499
  of intracranial lesion, 495–498
  in intracranial metastasis, 457
  with magnetic resonance imaging, 495–
      498, 502
  with radionuclide implantation, 491–514
  results, 498
Stereotactic Bragg peak proton beam
      therapy, in arteriovenous
      malformation, 911–915
Stereotactic head holder, 481–482
Stereotactic instrumentation, 491–495, 1035,
      1037
  Brown-Roberts-Wells apparatus, 1037
  Leksell's apparatus, 492, 1037
  Horsley-Clarke apparatus, 491, 492, 494,
      1035, 1037
  Riechert-Mundinger apparatus, 495
  Spiegel-Wycis apparatus, 1037
  Talairach apparatus, 491–492
  Todd-Wells apparatus, 1037
  types, 1037
Stereotactic laser microsurgery, 226
Stereotactic radiosurgery, 515–529
Stereotactic resection, 481–490
  accessory instruments, 486
  clinical experience, 487–488
  computer analysis, 483–484, 485, 486
  data acquisition, 481
  instrumentation, 485–486
  for large deep-seated tumor, 489–490
  for metastacic tumor, 488–489
  microslad for, 486
  patient rotation for, 485
  stereotactic frame for, 485–486
  surgical approach definition, 485
  surgical planning, 484–485
  surgical procedure, 486–487
  for vascular malformation, 489
Stereotactic retractors, 486
Stereotactic surgery. *See also* Cingulotomy
      (stereotactic); *specific diagnoses*
  arterial aneurysm clipping, 1009–1022
  arteriovenous malformation clipping,
      1009–1022
  with Brown-Robert-Wells frame, 475–480
  clipping indications/contraindications,
      1012–1013
  clipping instrumentation, 1010–1011
  clipping operation results, 1013–1021
  clipping technique, 1009–1010, 1012
  computed tomography in, 463, 1061–1062
  computed tomography data transposition
      to film, 463–464
  development of, 1057–1058
  electrode insertion, 1038
  electroencephalography with, 1038
  electroneuroprosthesis, 1062–1064
  as functional neurosurgery modality,
      1035–1039
  hematoma evacuation results, 892
  indications for, 467–468
  instrumentation, 889–890

in intracerebral hematoma, 889–898
  with laser, 1062
  lesion production, 1038–1039
  lesion site, 470–471
  magnetic resonance imaging in, 463
  of midbrain and pons, 472
  for motor disorders, 1051
  preoperative calculations, 1011–1012
  Presbyterian-University Hospital
      (Pittsburgh) technique, 468–472
  radiography with, 1037–1038
  results, 470–472
  stereotactic atlas, 1036–1037
  technique, 891
  ventrolateral nucleus lesion, 1051
Stereotactic system
  Brown-Roberts-Wells, 466–467, 1037
  CT-compatible, 467
  device alternatives, 464
  frame modification for CT and MRI, 464–
      466
  Rhodes-Glenn, 467
  Leksell, 464–465, 492, 1037
  Todd-Wells, 464, 466, 1037
Stereotactic thermal hypophysectomy, 345–
      348
  anesthesia, 345
  complications, 348
  indications for, 345
  patient preparation, 345
  postoperative management, 347–348
  procedure, 345–347
  replacement therapy, 347–348
Stimulation techniques (chronic), 1039–1040.
      See also specific diagnoses
Storz pediatric-type Hopkins endoscope, 426
Streptomycin
  in tuberculoma, 81
  in tuberculous meningitis, 84
  in vestibular nerve ablation, 1258–1259
Stroke, 881–888. *See also* Intracerebral
      hemorrhage
  direct brain revascularization, 783
  posterior fossa revascularization, 807
Subarachnoid hemorrhage
  with aneurysm, 929, 930, 931, 936, 1004,
      1005
  with anterior communicating artery
      aneurysm, 939, 954
  with carotid ophthalmic artery aneurysm,
      917, 918, 927
  with middle cerebral artery aneurysm,
      957, 958, 970
Subclavian-carotid stenosis, 781
Subcutaneous electrode implantation, 1039,
      1040
Subdural hematoma, 33–35
  acute, chronic, subacute, 33
  with acute head injury, 24
  anesthesia management, 34
  computed tomography in, 33–35
  corticosteroids in, 33
  diagnosis, 33
  intracranial pressure monitoring, 34
  postoperative complications, 35
  preoperative management, 33
  surgery for acute condition, 33–35
  surgery for chronic condition, 35
Subfornicial approach, to third ventricle,
      381–382

Subfrontal approach, to sella turcica, 303
Suboccipital approach
    to clivus, 642
    to craniopharyngioma, 364
    to posterior cranial fossa, 665, 670
    to vertebral junction aneurysm, 986
Suboccipital craniectomy, with upper
        cervical laminectomy for Chiari
        malformation, 1317
Suboccipital-translabyrinthine approach, to
        posterior cranial fossa, 668, 671
Subtemporal approach
    to AICA aneurysm, 984
    to basilar artery aneurysm, 975
    to clivus, 640–642
    to craniopharyngioma, 362
    to sella turcica, 304
    to superior cerebellar artery aneurysm,
        984
Sudomotor function, in peripheral nerve
        injury, 1568
Superficial temporal artery–middle cerebral
        artery bypass, 783–791
    anastomosis, 789
    anesthesia, 784
    angiography, 783, 791
    in carotid ophthalmic aneurysm, 927
    closure, 789, 791
    complications, 791
    exposure, 787
    instrumentations, 784, 787
    long vein grafts, 792
    MCA preparation, 789
    in moyamoya disease, 801–804
    patient positioning, 784
    postoperative management, 791
    preoperative evaluation, 783–784
    results, 791
    short vein graft in, 791
    STA preparation, 789
    technique, 784–791
Superficial temporal artery–superior
        cerebellar artery bypass
    results, 816
    technique, 815–816
    in vertebrobasilar insufficiency, 808, 813
Supracerebellar approach, to pineal region
        neoplasms, 401–409
Suprascapular nerve entrapment, 1590–1591
Suprasellar cyst, 349, 375
    computed tomography, 375
Suprasellar germinoma, 397
    angiography, 398
    cerebrospinal fluid cytology, 398
    chemotherapy, 399
    computed tomography, 398
    radiography, 398
    symptoms, 397
Suprasellar meningioma
    angiography, 531
    approach, 532
    computed tomography, 531
    presentation, 531
    radiography, 531
    results, 536–537
    surgical technique, 532–535
Supratentorial approach, to posterior fossa
        tumor, 660–662
Sympathetic nervous system, 1271–1280
Sympathectomy, 1271–1280

for causalgia, 1049
    lumbar, 1277–1279
    in moyamoya disease, 801, 804
    preganglionic, 1271–1272
    splanchnicectomy, 1274–1277
    upper thoracic ganglionectomy, 1271–1274
Synostosis, 125. *See also specific
        deformities*
    computed tomography, 126–127, 130, 132,
        133
    etiology, 126
    genetic factor, 126
    intracranial pressure with, 125–126
    radiography, 125, 126, 130, 132, 133
    surgical indications, 126
    syndromes with, 126
Syringobulbia, 1307
Syringomyelia, 1307–1326. *See also* Chiari
        malformation with hydromelia
    hydrodynamic theory for, 1307
    intramedullary tumor with, 1307, 1326
Syringomyelic cord syndrome, 1307–1326
    cyst formation with, 1308
    pathology, 1308

Taenia solium, 79, 93
Talairach stereotactic apparatus, 491–492
Tarsorrhaphy, in intraorbital tumor, 244
Technetium 99 bone scan, for anterior
        lumbar discectomy, 1423
Temperature regulation, in neonate, 117
Temporal lobectomy
    in cerebral glioma, 439–441
    cortical resection in, 1231–1232
Temporal lobectomy (partial)
    anatomic considerations, 1230–1231
    closure, 1232
    complications, 1232–1233
    electrical stimulation study in, 1229–1230
    electrocorticography in, 1227
    for epilepsy, 1223–1234
    postexcision recording, 1232
    postoperative care, 1232
    results, 1233–1234
Temporary vascular occlusion in middle
        cerebral artery aneurysm, 967–968
Tentorium tumor, 647–651
    air embolism in, 648
    anesthesia, 647
    angiography, 647
    computed tomography, 647, 648
    diagnosis, 647
    instrumentation, 650
    magnetic resonance imaging, 647
    microsurgery, 650
    radiography, 647
    retraction technique, 650
    surgical approaches, 648
    surgical positioning, 647–648
Teratoma, intramedullary spinal cord tumor,
        1496
Terminal ventriculostomy, for Chiari
        malformation with hydromelia, 1326
Thalamic glioma, 710
Thalamic pain syndrome, 715–716
Thalamic tumor, 712
    symptomatology, 714–716
Thalamotomy
    for cancer pain, 1046–1047

    in dystonia, 1268
    for Parkinson's disease, 1052
    in torticollis, 1262–1263
Thalamus, stimulation site in pain control,
        1089, 1092, 1094
Thermocoagulation, of dorsal root entry
        zone, 1169–1175
Thermography, for anterior lumbar
        discectomy, 1423
Thoracic epidural tumor (metastatic), 1557–
        1559
    anterior decompression and vertebral
        body replacement, 1548–1559
    high thoracic spine approach, 1553
Thoracic lateral extrapleural spine fusion,
        1474–1475
Thoracic meningocele, 158–159
Thoracic outlet syndrome, 1591–1593
    electromyelography, 1592
    etiology, 1591–1592
    surgical management, 1591–1593
    symptoms, 1592
Thoracic rhizotomy, percutaneous
        electrothermocoagulation technique,
        1211–1215
Thoracic spinal cord tumor, in children,
        175–176
Thoracic spinal deformity, surgical
        treatment, 1511–1512
Thoracic spine fusion, 1473
    lateral facet, 1467–1468
Thoracolumbar fracture, 1481–1486
    approach, 1483
    burst fracture, 1481, 1482, 1485
    classification, 1481
    complications, 1484
    computed tomography, 1481, 1483, 1484–
        1485
    grafting in, 1483, 1484
    immobilization management, 1483
    neural decompression in, 1481, 1482, 1483
    postoperative management, 1484
    preoperative management, 1481–1483
    radiography, 1483
    somatosensory evoked responses in,
        1482
    spine stabilization in, 1483–1484
    surgical management, 1483–1484
    unstable vs. stable, 1481
Thoracolumbar Harrington-rod spine fusion,
        1475–1478
Thoracolumbar spine fusion, 1464–1466
Thoracolumbar spine injury
    posterior spine fusion in, 1464–1466
    thoracoabdominal approach, 1468
Third ventricle
    lesions encountered, 381
    surgical approaches, 381–382, 389
    transcallosal approach, 381–387
    transcallosal interfornicial approach, 389–
        395
    preoperative evaluation of lesion, 382
Third ventricle colloid cyst, intraoperative
        ultrasonography visualization, 218
Third ventricle lesion, stereotactic resection,
        489
Third ventricle tumor (posterior)
    endocrine function in, 398
    myelography in, 398
    surgical management, 398–399

Thrombosis technique, for carotid cavernous fistula, 845–847
Tic convulsif, 1108
Tinel's sign, 1566–1567
Tissue adhesives, in cerebrospinal fluid leakage, 66
Tissue aspiration, ultrasonic, 226–227
Tissue bonding, with laser, 226
Tissue expander, in scalp reconstruction, 4–5
Todd-Wells stereotactic system, 464, 466, 1037
Torticollis
  anterior cervical rhizotomy in, 1263
  iontophoresis, 1262
  muscle resection in, 1263
  physiotherapy in, 1267
  selective peripheral denervation in, 1263–1268
  surgical management, 1262
Torticollis (spasmodic), 1261–1268
  conservative treatment, 1261–1262
  Dandy-Foerster operation for, 1054
  electromyography in, 1263–1264
  epidural crevical stimulation in, 1262
  frontal capsular adversive pathway interruption, 1262
  medical treatment, 1262
  nerve root microvascular lysis, 1262
  pallidotomy in, 1262–1263
  stereotactic surgery for, 1053–1054
  thalamotomy in, 1262–1263
Transantralethmoidal approach, in optic nerve decompression, 270
Transantrosphenoidal approach, in optic nerve decompression, 270
Transbasal approach
  to clivus, 644
  closure, 625–626
  goals, 619
  hazards, 619
  indications for, 627–633
  limits, 626
  meningeal repair, 623–624
  mucosal plane preservation, 621–622
  skull base exposure, 622–623
  to skull base tumor, 619–633
Transcallosal approach
  cingulate gyrus exposure, 383
  closure with, 386
  corpus callosum exposure, 383
  to craniopharyngioma, 364
  foramen of Monro in, 382–386
  to frontal horn lateral ventricle tumor, 590–591
  intraventricular exposure, 384
  to midbody lateral ventricle tumor, 588–589
  patient positioning, 382
  shunt with, 386
  surgical procedure, 382
  to third ventricle tumor, 381–387
  to trigonal lateral ventricle tumor, 585–586
Transcallosal interfornicial approach
  advantages, 391
  anatomy, 390–391
  bone flap with, 392–393
  choroid plexus in, 395
  cingulate gyri in, 393
  complications, 389–390

corpus callosum in, 393
  dural incision, 393
  lateral ventricle entry, 394
  patient positioning, 392
  physiology, 390–391
  preoperative planning, 391–392
  results, 389
  risk factors, 390–391
  septum pellucidum in, 395
  surgical technique, 392–395
  to third ventricle, 389–395
  transcalvarial entry, 392–393
Transcanal approach, to posterior cranial fossa, 667, 671
Transcervical approach, to clivus, 642
Transcochlear approach, to posterior cranial fossa, 668, 671
Transcorticoventricular approach, to craniopharyngioma, 364
Transcranial approach, to sella turcica, 302–303
Transethmoid approach, to sella turcica, 302
Transethmoidal sphenoidotomy
  advantages, 339
  approach to pituitary, 339–343
  complications, 339
  contraindications, 339
  disadvantages, 339
  indications, 339
  preoperative evaluation, 339–340
  procedure, 342–343
  technique, 340–342
Transforaminal approach, to third ventricle, 389
Transfrontal approach
  to craniopharyngioma, 358–359
  to third ventricle, 381
Transfrontal craniotomy approach, for optic nerve decompression, 269–270
Transient ischemic attacks
  direct brain revascularization, 783, 791, 794
  with moyamoya disease, 797, 801, 804
  posterior fossa revascularization in, 807
Translabyrinthine operation
  for acoustic nerve tumor, 685–704
  acoustic nerve tumor removal, 696–698
  advantages/disadvantages, 685–686
  anatomy, 687–689
  anesthesia for, 689–690
  at cerebellopontine angle, 676
  cerebrospinal fluid rhinorrhea with, 702–703
  dissection, 692–696
  four quadrants dissection, 699–701
  gutting procedure, 699
  hematoma with, 702
  hemostasis, 701
  closure, 701–702
  patient positioning, 690
  at posterior cranial fossa, 665, 670–671
  postoperative complications, 702–703
  postoperative management, 702
  procedure, 690–692
  results, 703
Transoral approach, to clivus, 642–643
Transoral median labiomandibular approach, to clivus, 643–644
Transoral odontoid resection and fusion, in cervical spinal cord injury, 1462–1464

Transoral-transpharyngeal approach, to craniovertebral junction abnormality, 1288–1292
Transpedicle fixateurs, in scoliosis, 202
Transsphenoidal approach, 299–307
  to clivus, 643
  complications, 319
  to craniopharyngioma, 363–364
  hemitransfixion incision, 309
  indications for, 309
  operative procedure, 309–318
  in optic nerve decompression, 270, 275
  patient positioning, 309
  risk factors, 334–335
  to sella turcica, 301–304, 309–319, 321–337
  sublabial incision, 309
Transtemporal approaches
  case reports, 669–670
  infratemporal fossa, 668, 671
  middle fossa, 665–666, 671
  middle fossa-infratemporal fossa, 669, 671
  to posterior cranial fossa, 665–672
  retrolabyrinthine, 667
  skull base, 667–668, 671
  suboccipital, 665, 670
  suboccipital-translabyrinthine, 668, 671
  transcanal, 667, 671
  transcochlear, 668, 671
  translabyrinthine, 665, 670–671
Transtemporal horn occipital temporal gyrus incision, to trigonal lateral ventricle tumor, 586–587
Transthoracic approach
  to spine tumor, 1530, 1532, 1535
  to thoracic spine, 1361–1365
Transthoracic (transpleural) approach, to thoracic intervertebral disc, 1371–1374
Transvenous approach, to anteroinferior dural venous fistula, 849–854
Transverse sinus, dural laceration, 875–879
Traumatic aneurysm, 991–995
  angiography, 991, 992
  computed tomography, 991, 993
  intracerebral hematoma with, 991
  surgical management, 991–994
  symptomatology, 991
Traumatic mass lesions, 22–24
Tremor, stereotactic surgery for, 1051–1052
Trephine defects, 14
Triage, for acute head injury, 19, 20
Trigeminal nerve injury, after stereotactic radiosurgery, 521
Trigeminal neuralgia, 1097–1105
  herpes simplex with, 1119
  Jannetta microvascular decompression procedure, 1097–1098
  medical management, 1097, 1111, 1117
  microvascular decompression for, 1111
  motor paresis with, 1119
  with multiple sclerosis, 1105
  ocular complications, 1117, 1119
  patient evaluation, 1111
  percutaneous rhizotomy for, 1111–1120, 1125–1127
  percutaneous rhizotomy/microvascular decompression complications, 1139–1143
  percutaneous trigeminal neurolysis, 1097–1098
  radiofrequency heating for, 1134

recurrence, 1119
retrogasserian glycerol injection, 1129–1137
sensory complications, 1117, 1119
surgical management, 1097–1105
surgical procedures comparison, 1119–1120
surgical results, 1116–1117
Trigeminal rhizotomy
for atypical facial pain, 1120–1121
electrode locatization for, 1115–1116
hemorrhage with, 1139–1140
lesion production, 1116
for multiple sclerosis, 1120
percutaneous technique, 1112–1116
for trigeminal neuralgia, 1111–1120
Tuberculoma
age factor, 80
anticonvulsants in, 82
antituberculosis agents, 81–82
clinical features, 80
computed tomography, 80–81
corticosteroids in, 82
incidence, 79
location, 79
pathology, 80
radiography, 80–81
results, 83
sex factor, 80
surgical management, 82–83
treatment, 81
Tuberculosis, 79–85
Tuberculous meningitis, 83–85
antituberculosis agents, 84
computed tomography, 84
diagnosis, 84
hydrocephalus with, 83–85
later particle agglutination test in, 84
results, 85
surgical management, 84–85
ventriculoatrial/ventriculoperitoneal shunts in, 84
Tumor. *See specific diagnoses and sites*
Tumor markers, in pineal region tumor, 398
Tumorscope, 424, 427

Ulnar nerve compression, 1588–1589
Ultrasonic surgical aspirator, 226–227
applications, 227
biologic effects, 227
in meningioma surgery, 559
neoplasm fragmentation, 227
system, 227
Ultrasonography (intraoperative), 213–222
biopsy guide for, 215
in biopsy procedures, 219, 222
in brain lesion localization, 215
equipment, 214
equipment sterilization, 214
history, 213–214
intracranial, 215
intraspinal, 219–222
7.5-MHz crystal for, 213–214
normal brain tissue visualization, 215–216
normal spinal cord tissue visualization, 219–220
pathologic brain tissue visualization, 215–216

pathologic spinal cord tissue visualization, 220–222
techniques, 214–215
Ultrasonography (transcutaneous), in spinal cord astrocytoma, 177, 184
Upper extremity, sympathetic denervation, 1271
Upper thoracic ganglionectomy, 1271–1274
anatomy, 1271–1272
for causalgia, 1271, 1272
complications, 1273–1274
for hyperhidrosis, 1271, 1272
indications for, 1272
results, 1273
surgical approach, 1272
surgical technique, 1272–1273

Vascular disorders, in children, 109
Vascular lesions (intracerebral)
balloon catheter management, 819–836
chemotherapy infusion, 835
embolic agents for, 820–821
Vascular malformations, stereotactic resection, 489
Vasoglossopharyngeal neuralgia, percutaneous rhizotomy in, 1121–1122, 1125–1127
Vein of Galen aneurysm
balloon catheter management, 828
in children, 109
Vein of Galen lesion, occipital transtentorial approach, 411–418
Vein of Galen malformation, 120
Venipuncture, in neonate, 117
Venography
for anterior lumbar discectomy, 1423
in orbit pathology, 250
Venous fistula, anteroinferior dural, 849–854
Venous hypertension, with anteroinferior dural fistula, 849
Ventilation management
in children, 104
with head injury, 27–29, 114
in spine trauma, 1452
Ventricular drainage, for obstructive hydrocephalus, 573
Ventricular migration, with skull defect, 12
Ventriculography
anesthesia for, 113
in meningioma, 573
in pineal tumor, 403
Ventriculoperitoneal shunt, in tuberculous meningitis, 84–85
Ventrolateral nucleus, stimulation lesion production, 1051
Vertebral artery (extracranial), 771–782
Vertebral artery compression, with cervical spondylosis, 1329
Vertebral artery endarterectomy, 771–782
technique, 775–781
Vertebral body replacement, in epidural metastatic tumor, 1552–1553
Vertebral to carotid transposition
results, 810
technique, 808–810
for vertebrobasilar insufficiency, 808–810
Vertebral column
embryology, 189
fracture-dislocation, 1449–1469

Vertebral fistula, balloon catheter management, 827
Vertebral junction aneurysm, 986
Vertebrobasilar insufficiency, 771–782
arteriography, 771–775, 808, 810, 812
cerebral blood flow (regional) measurement in, 807–808
clinical evaluation, 771–775
computed tomography, 807
distal vertebral endarterectomy for, 810–812
OA-AICA bypass in, 814–815
OA-PICA bypass for, 810, 812–814
pathology, 771–772, 774
posterior fossa revascularization in, 807–818
postoperative management, 817
preoperative preparation, 808
radiography, 771–775
results, 818
STA-SCA bypass for, 808, 813, 815–817
surgical indications, 772
symptoms, 771, 772
vertebral to carotid transposition for, 808–810
Vertebrobasilar revascularization, 793–794
Vertebrobasilar system aneurysm, 973–989
Vertigo
in chronic labyrinthitis, 1254
medical ablation of vestibular nerve in, 1258–1259
in Meniere's disease, 1251
nonsurgical treatment, 1254
surgical treatment, 1255–1258
in vestibular neuritis, 1251, 1254
Vestibular nerve ablation, with streptomycin sulfate, 1258–1259
Vestibular nerve transection
cerebellopontine angle (posterior fossa approach), 1258
complications, 1258
internal auditory canal (middle fossa) approach, 1256–1258
in Meniere's disease, 1251–1259
procedure, 1256–1258
results, 1258
Vestibular neuritis
nonsurgical treatment, 1254
pathophysiology, 1251, 1254
Vietnam Head Injury Study, 49
Vision, electroneuroprosthesis, 1063
Visual deficit
in craniopharyngioma, 355
after head trauma, 269
Visual evoked potentials, 280
with head trauma, 269, 270
Visual examination, in sella turcica lesion, 299, 301
Visual fields, in cerebral glioma, 433–434
Volume interpolation, for intra-axial tumor, 483–484
Von Hippel-Lindau disease, 660
Von Recklinghausen's disease, 158, 1605

Wada intra-arterial sodium amytal test, 433
Wallenberg syndrome, 772
Weapons, ballistic design-injury relation, 50
Wisconsin system, of spine fusion, 201
Wounds. *See* Gunshot wounds; *specific sites*